Merritt's Neurology

THIRTEENTH EDITION

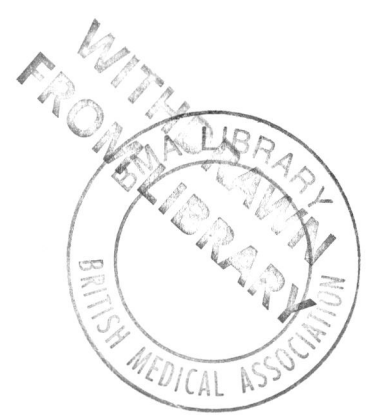

Merritt's Neurology

THIRTEENTH EDITION

Edited by

Elan D. Louis, MD, MS
Professor of Neurology and Epidemiology
Chief, Division of Movement Disorders
Departments of Neurology and Chronic Disease Epidemiology
Yale School of Medicine and Yale School of Public Health
Yale University
New Haven, Connecticut

Stephan A. Mayer, MD, FCCM
Professor of Neurology and Neurosurgery
Icahn School of Medicine at Mount Sinai
Director, Neurocritical Care
Mount Sinai Health System
New York, New York

Lewis P. Rowland, MD
Professor of Neurology
Chairman of Neurology, Emeritus
Director of the Neurology Service, Emeritus
The Neurological Institute of New York
Columbia University Medical Center
New York, New York

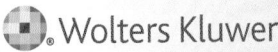

Philadelphia • Baltimore • New York • London
Buenos Aires • Hong Kong • Sydney • Tokyo

Acquisitions Editor: Jamie Elfrank
Product Development Editor: Andrea Vosburgh
Editorial Assistant: Brian Convery
Marketing Manager: Stephanie Kindlick
Production Project Manager: Marian Bellus
Design Coordinator: Joan Wendt
Manufacturing Coordinator: Beth Welsh
Prepress Vendor: Absolute Service, Inc.

Thirteenth Edition

9 8 7 6 5 4 3 2 1

Printed in China

Library of Congress Cataloging-in-Publication Data

Merritt's neurology / edited by Elan D. Louis, Stephan A. Mayer, Lewis P. Rowland. — Thirteenth edition.
    p. ; cm.
  Neurology
  Includes bibliographical references and index.
  ISBN 978-1-4511-9336-7
  I. Louis, Elan D., editor. II. Mayer, Stephan A., editor. III. Rowland, Lewis P., editor. IV. Title: Neurology.
  [DNLM: 1. Nervous System Diseases. WL 140]
  RC346
  616.8—dc23
                    2015021976

LWW.com

Preface

When H. Houston Merritt first published this *Textbook of Neurology* in 1955, he was the sole author. The book became popular, and he revised it himself through the fourth edition. The body of neurologic knowledge increased and, in the fifth edition, he finally accepted contributions from colleagues. Even then, he wrote most of the book himself, and he continued to do so for the sixth edition despite serious physical disability. He died in 1979, just as the sixth edition was released for distribution.

The seventh edition, published and edited in 1984 by Lewis P. Rowland, was prepared by 70 of Merritt's former students. Thirty of them headed neurology departments and others had become distinguished clinicians, teachers, and investigators. That edition documented the human legacy of a singular leader whose career had set models for clinical investigation (when it was just beginning), clinical practice, teaching, editing books and journals, administering departments and medical schools, and commitment to national professional and voluntary health organizations.

With the passage of 60 years, Merritt's has become one of the time-honored textbooks in the field of clinical neurology. We now provide the 13th edition, with Elan D. Louis, Stephan A. Mayer, and Lewis P. Rowland as coeditors.

As with any dynamic book, the list of authors has changed progressively. The editors have substantially broadened the authorship. With more than 180 authors, the editors have tapped into the best expertise across the country. Yet the ties to Merritt persist. Many of his personal students are still authors, as are their students as Merritt's intellectual grandchildren. Along the same lines, we have tried to maintain Merritt's literary style: direct, clear, and succinct writing; emphasis on facts rather than unsupported opinion; and ample use of illustrations and tables.

While maintaining ties with its tradition, this edition of Merritt's has undergone considerable reorganization. In short, our goal was to extensively revamp the book, with substantial consolidation and reduction in the number of chapters. While retaining its best elements and traditions, we aimed to create the essential modern neurology textbook with a global worldview. The main change in content is that the 13th edition emphasizes evidence-based medicine practice guidelines, diagnostic and treatment algorithms, management checklists, and practical pearls. Authors were encouraged to include more tables and figures as well as videos, when applicable. The book is designed for access from tablet, phone, and computer screens. The chief idea for our readers is to provide useful information at the bedside when they need it. The Internet is full of information, but it is difficult to sort through. Merritt's provides trusted and cohesive information from an expert.

The book has changed in other ways. The number of tables has expanded from 298 to 545 and the number of figures from 343 to 400. The figures themselves have been substantially updated and replaced. The book includes moving images for the first time, with more than 40 instructive videos, showing a broad range of involuntary movement disorders. Finally, the black and white text and photos of the 12th edition have now bloomed into full color text and illustrations.

We have also reordered the sections of the book, as the face of clinical neurology has changed. A new opening chapter reviews the global burden of neurologic disease, and the sections that follow cover neurologic diseases in order of their impact on international public health, starting with cerebrovascular disease, trauma, and dementia.

This edition of Merritt's also includes a new section in the front of the book, *Common Problems in Neurology*. These syndrome-based chapters are designed to provide immediate expert access to clinicians on the front lines who confront common neurologic problems such as headache, dizziness, seizures, and stroke. These chapters provide a practical structured approach to managing undifferentiated neurologic syndromes in the office, emergency department, or hospital. They focus on history, examination, localization, diagnosis, and initial management. This is where the classic neuroanatomy and description of clinical signs may be found. These chapters share a common structure that naturally flows with the course of evaluation and management.

For the first time, Merritt's specifically cites all level 1 standards for prevention, diagnosis, or treatment. The specific citation to back up a level 1 recommendation provides the single most authoritative trial, guideline, or meta-analysis.

A book of this clinical breadth and detail cannot be written by one or even a handful of authors. Moreover, the evolving complexity of subspecialty areas within neurology demands additional oversight of chapter content. With this edition of Merritt's, we have enlisted the careful assistance of 20 section editors. The content of each chapter has been reviewed both by a section editor and one of the three coeditors.

This edition includes comprehensive revisions demanded by the progress of research in every chapter listed in the table of contents. In addition, many new chapters have been added to reflect the evolution of clinical neurology, including neurocritical care monitoring, interventional neuroradiology, brain death, concussion, hypoxic–ischemic encephalopathy, autoimmune meningitis and encephalitis, vascular dementia, restless legs syndrome, and autonomic storming.

In the years since the last edition was published, the electronic world has expanded rapidly. To meet demands for easily accessible content, the 13th edition includes an interactive e-book, which offers tablet, smartphone, and online access to the complete content with enhanced navigation, search tools, and videos.

We thank all the authors for their devoted and skillful work. We also thank the many section editors for their thoughtful guidance and painstaking efforts.

This project would never have moved forward without the help of many people at Wolters Kluwer. Indeed, a full roster of people has been involved in the project, from its conception to completion. There are Julie Goolsby and Jamie Elfrank (acquisitions editors), Kristina Oberle and Andrea Vosburgh (product development editors), Brian Convery (editorial assistant), Joan Wendt (design coordinator), Marian Bellus (production project manager), and Stephanie Kindlick (marketing manager). Special thanks should go to Andrea Vosburgh, whose tireless efforts guided this book to completion.

We formally rededicate the book to H. Houston Merritt. Dr. Louis also dedicates this book to his late father, Dr. Sydney Louis, an academic neurologist who inspired his career in neurology—a role model as a humanist, an educator, a perceptive clinician with a keen eye for nuance and detail, and a patient-centered physician. Countless friends and colleagues with whom we have worked at The Neurological Institute of New York at Columbia University over the years deserve credit for inspiring us, most notably John Brust, E. Sander Connolly, Stanley Fahn, Matthew E. Fink, Laura Lennihan, Linda Lewis, Karen Marder, Richard Mayeux, J. P. Mohr, Timothy Pedley, and Robert A. Solomon. Finally, we would like to personally dedicate this book to the spouses and children of all the contributors and especially to our own families. The Louis family includes Elan Louis and Dr. Vinita Sehgal and children, Devin, Ravi, and Kiran. The Mayer family includes Dr. Elissa Fory and children, Philip, Catherine, and Chloe. The Rowland family comprises Esther E. Rowland; children, Andrew, Steven, and Joy; their spouses, Darryl and Kathleen; and grandchildren, Mikaela, Liam, Cameron Henry, Mariel, and Zuri.

Neeraj Badjatia, MD
Medical Director, Neurocritical Care
University of Maryland Medical Center
Baltimore, Maryland

Carl W. Bazil, MD, PhD
Caitlin Tynan Doyle Professor of Clinical Neurology
Director, Division of Comprehensive Epilepsy Center and
    Sleep Center
Columbia University
New York, New York

John C. M. Brust, MD
Professor of Neurology
Columbia University College of Physicians and Surgeons
New York, New York

Denise E. Chou, MD
Assistant Professor
Department of Neurology
Columbia University Medical Center
Assistant Attending Neurologist
Department of Neurology
New York-Presbyterian Hospital
New York, New York

Andrew B. Lassman, MD
John Harris Associate Professor and Chief
Neuro-Oncology Division, Department of Neurology
Medical Director, Clinical Protocol & Data Management Office
Herbert Irving Comprehensive Cancer Center
Columbia University Medical Center
New York, New York

Kiwon Lee, MD, FACP, FAHA
Vice-chairman of Neurosurgery and Neurology for Critical Care
Associate Professor of Neurosurgery and Neurology
Chief, Division of Critical Care
Departments of Neurology and Neurosurgery
The University of Texas Health Science Center at Houston
Mischer Neuroscience Institute
Memorial Hermann-Texas Medical Center
Houston, Texas

Laura Lennihan, MD
Professor of Neurology
Vice-chair, Department of Neurology
Chief, Division of Critical Care and Hospitalist Neurology
Columbia University Medical Center
New York, New York

Elan D. Louis, MD, MS
Professor of Neurology and Epidemiology
Chief, Division of Movement Disorders
Departments of Neurology and Chronic Disease Epidemiology
Yale School of Medicine and Yale School of Public Health
Yale University
New Haven, Connecticut

Karen S. Marder, MD, MPH
Sally Kerlin Professor of Neurology
Gertrude H. Sergievsky Center
Department of Neurology
Columbia University Medical Center
New York, New York

Stephan A. Mayer, MD, FCCM
Professor of Neurology and Neurosurgery
Icahn School of Medicine at Mount Sinai
Director, Neurocritical Care
Mount Sinai Health System
New York, New York

Paul C. McCormick, MD, MPH
Herbert and Linda Gallen Professor of Neurological Surgery
Columbia University College of Physicians and Surgeons
New York, New York

James M. Noble, MD, MS, CPH
Assistant Professor of Neurology
Taub Institute for Research on Alzheimer's Disease and the Aging
    Brain
Department of Neurology
Columbia University Medical Center
New York, New York

Claire S. Riley, MD
Assistant Professor of Neurology
Department of Neurology
Columbia University College of Physicians and Surgeons
Assistant Attending Neurologist
New York-Presbyterian Hospital
Columbia University Medical Center
New York, New York

Fred Rincon, MD, MSc, MBE, FACP, FCCP, FCCM
Assistant Professor of Neurology and Neurosurgery
Thomas Jefferson University
Philadelphia, Pennsylvania

James J. Riviello Jr, MD
Sergievsky Family Professor of Neurology and Pediatrics
Department of Neurology
Columbia University
New York, New York

J. Kirk Roberts, MD
Associate Professor of Neurology
College of Physicians and Surgeons
Columbia University Medical Center
New York-Presbyterian Hospital
New York, New York

Karen L. Roos, MD
John and Nancy Nelson Professor of Neurology
Department of Neurology
Indiana University School of Medicine
Indianapolis, Indiana

Lewis P. Rowland, MD
Professor of Neurology
Chairman of Neurology, Emeritus
Director of the Neurology Service, Emeritus
The Neurological Institute of New York
Columbia University Medical Center
New York, New York

David H. Strauss, MD
Associate Professor and Vice-chair
Research Administrator, Ethics and Policy
Director, Psychiatric Research
Department of Psychiatry
Columbia University
New York State Psychiatric Institute
New York, New York

Louis H. Weimer, MD, FAAN, FANA
Professor of Neurology
Director, EMG Laboratory
Department of Neurology
Columbia University Medical Center
New York, New York

Contributors

Gary M. Abrams, MD
Professor of Neurology
University of California, San Francisco
San Francisco, California

Sachin Agarwal, MD, MPH
Assistant Professor of Neurology
Neurocritical Care
Columbia University College of Physicians and Surgeons
New York-Presbyterian Hospital/Columbia Medical Center
New York, New York

Teresa A. Allison, PharmD, BCPS
Clinical Pharmacist Specialist
Program Director, PGY2 Critical Care Residency
Department of Pharmacy
Memorial Hermann-Texas Medical Center
Houston, Texas

Tareq Saad H. Almaghrabi, MD
Fellow, Division of Neurocritical Care
Department of Neurosurgery
The University of Texas Health Science Center at Houston
Houston, Texas

Fawaz Al-Mufti, MD
Neurocritical Care Fellow and Assistant Attending Neurologist
Division of Neurocritical Care
The Neurological Institute of New York
Columbia University Medical Center
New York, New York

Peter D. Angevine, MD, MPH
Assistant Professor
Department of Neurological Surgery
Columbia University College of Physicians and Surgeons
New York, New York

John Ausiello, MD
Assistant Professor of Medicine
Columbia University
New York-Presbyterian Hospital
New York, New York

Neeraj Badjatia, MD
Medical Director, Neurocritical Care
University of Maryland Medical Center
Baltimore, Maryland

Kelly J. Baldwin, MD
Department of Neurology
Geisinger Medical Center
Danville, Pennsylvania
Clinical Assistant Professor
Temple University School of Medicine
Philadelphia, Pennsylvania

Jacob S. Ballon, MD, MPH
Clinical Assistant Professor
Director, INSPIRE Clinic
Department of Psychiatry
Stanford University
Stanford, California

Tracy T. Batchelor, MD, MPH
Giovanni Armenise Harvard Professor of Neurology
Harvard Medical School
Executive Director, Stephen E. and Catherine Pappas Center for Neuro-Oncology
Massachusetts General Hospital
Coleader, Brain Cancer Program
Dana-Farber/Harvard Cancer Center
Boston, Massachusetts

Carl W. Bazil, MD, PhD
Caitlin Tynan Doyle Professor of Clinical Neurology
Director, Division of Comprehensive Epilepsy Center and Sleep Center
Columbia University
New York, New York

Michelle Wilson Bell, MD
Fellow in Clinical Neurophysiology (Epilepsy)
Department of Neurology
Columbia University
New York, New York

Gary L. Bernardini, MD, PhD, FANA
Professor of Neurology
Chair, Department of Neurology
New York Hospital Queens
Vice-Chair, Department of Neurology
Weill-Cornell Medical Center
New York, New York

Thomas H. Brannagan III, MD
Professor of Neurology
Director, Peripheral Neuropathy Center
Columbia University College of Physicians and Surgeons
New York, New York

Susan B. Bressman, MD
Chair and Professor
The Mirken Family Clinical Neuroscience Institute
Department of Neurology
Icahn School of Medicine at Mount Sinai
New York, New York

Carolyn Barley Britton, MD, MS
Associate Professor of Clinical Neurology
Department of Neurology
Columbia University College of Physicians and Surgeons
New York, New York

Jeffrey N. Bruce, MD
Edgar M. Housepian Professor and Vice-chairman
Department of Neurological Surgery
Columbia University College of Physicians and Surgeons
New York, New York

Charles A. Bruno Jr, DO
Clinical Fellow, Interventional Neuroradiology
Department of Radiology
New York-Presbyterian Hospital
Columbia University Medical Center
New York, New York

John C. M. Brust, MD
Professor of Neurology
Columbia University College of Physicians and Surgeons
New York, New York

Robert E. Burke, MD
Departments of Neurology and Pathology and Cell Biology
Columbia University Medical Center
New York, New York

David Cachia, MD
Neurooncology Fellow
Department of Neuro-Oncology
The University of Texas MD Anderson Cancer Center
Houston, Texas

Joshua Cappell, MD, PhD
Assistant Professor of Pediatrics and Neurology
Columbia University Medical Center
Morgan Stanley Children's Hospital of New York-Presbyterian
New York, New York

Alejandro S. Cazzulino, BA
Research Assistant
Integrative Neuroscience
Columbia University
New York, New York

Tiffany R. Chang, MD
Assistant Professor
Departments of Neurosurgery and Neurology
The University of Texas Medical School at Houston
Houston, Texas

Claudia A. Chiriboga, MD, MPH
Associate Professor of Neurology
Division of Pediatric Neurology
Department of Neurology
Columbia University Medical Center
New York, New York

Enid Choi, MD, PhD
Radiation Oncology
University of Maryland
Baltimore, Maryland

Huimahn Alex Choi, MD, MS
Assistant Professor of Neurology and Neurosurgery
The University of Texas Health Science Center at Houston
Houston, Texas

Denise E. Chou, MD
Assistant Professor
Department of Neurology
Columbia University Medical Center
Assistant Attending Neurologist
Department of Neurology
New York-Presbyterian Hospital
New York, New York

Daniel S. Chow, MD
Department of Radiology
Columbia University Medical Center
New York, New York

Comana M. Cioroiu, MD
Assistant Professor of Neurology
Columbia University College of Physicians and Surgeons
New York-Presbyterian Hospital
Columbia University Medical Center
New York, New York

Jan Claassen, MD, PhD, FNCS
Associate Professor of Neurology
Head of Neurocritical Care and Medical Director of the
    Neurological Intensive Care Unit
Columbia University College of Physicians and Surgeons
New York, New York

Gary D. Clark, MD
The Blue Bird Circle Endowed Chair for the Chief of
    Child Neurology
Section Chief, Section of Neurology and Developmental Neuroscience
Professor of Pediatrics, Neurology, and Neuroscience
Baylor College of Medicine
Chief, Neurology Service
Texas Children's Hospital
Houston, Texas

Stephanie Cosentino, PhD
Assistant Professor of Neuropsychology
Department of Neurology
Columbia University Medical Center
New York, New York

John F. Crary, MD, PhD
Department of Pathology, Fishberg Department of Neuroscience,
    Friedman Brain Institute
Ronald M. Loeb Center for Alzheimer's Disease
Icahn School of Medicine at Mount Sinai
New York, New York

Barry M. Czeisler, MD, MS
Assistant Professor of Neurology
Division of Neurocritical Care
NYU Langone Medical Center
New York, New York

Randy S. D'Amico, MD
Department of Neurological Surgery
Columbia University Medical Center
New York, New York

Jahannaz Dastgir, DO
Assistant Professor of Neurology
Columbia University Medical Center
New York, New York

Darryl C. De Vivo, MD
Sidney Carter Professor of Neurology
Professor of Pediatrics
Associate Chairman (Neurology) for Pediatric Neurosciences
Director, Pediatric Neurology, Emeritus
Director, Colleen Giblin Research Laboratories
Director, Pediatric Neuromuscular Disease Center
Codirector, Center for Motor Neuron Biology and Disease
Columbia University College of Physicians and Surgeons
New York, New York

Anna Lopatin Dickerman, MD
Assistant Professor of Psychiatry
Weill Cornell Medical College
Assistant Attending Psychiatrist
Consultation-Liaison Service
New York-Presbyterian Hospital/Weill Cornell Medical Center
New York, New York

Salvatore DiMauro, MD
Lucy G. Moses Professor of Neurology
Department of Neurology
Columbia University Medical Center
New York, New York

Nancy J. Edwards, MD
Assistant Professor of Neurology and Neurosurgery
The University of Texas Health Science Center at Houston
Mischer Neuroscience Institute
Memorial Hermann-Texas Medical Center
Houston, Texas

Mitchell S. V. Elkind, MD, MS, FAAN, FAHA
Professor of Neurology and Epidemiology
Department of Neurology
College of Physicians and Surgeons
Department of Epidemiology
Mailman School of Public Health
Columbia University
New York, New York

Charles C. Esenwa, MD
Chief Resident and Clinical Instructor
Department of Neurology
Columbia University Medical Center
New York, New York

Stanley Fahn, MD
Movement Disorders Founding and Emeritus Director
H. Houston Merritt Professor of Neurology
Division of Movement Disorders
Department of Neurology
Columbia University Medical Center
New York, New York

Charles L. Francoeur, MD, FRCPC
Postdoctoral Clinical Fellow
Institute for Critical Care Medicine
Icahn School of Medicine at Mount Sinai
New York, New York

Pamela U. Freda, MD
Professor of Medicine
Department of Medicine
Columbia University College of Physicians and Surgeons
New York, New York

Jennifer A. Frontera, MD, FNCS
Associate Professor of Neurology
Cerebrovascular Center, Neurologic Institute
Cleveland Clinic
Cleveland, Ohio

Steven J. Frucht, MD
Professor of Neurology
Mount Sinai Medical Center
New York, New York

Licínia Gananca, MD
Division of Molecular Imaging and Neuropathology
New York State Psychiatric Institute
Columbia University
New York, New York

James H. Garvin Jr, MD, PhD
Professor of Pediatrics
Columbia University Medical Center
Attending Pediatrician
Morgan Stanley Children's Hospital of New York-Presbyterian
New York, New York

Nicolas Gaspard, MD, PhD
Associate Professor
Department of Neurology
Université Libre de Bruxelles-Hôpital Erasme
Brussels, Belgium
Assistant Professor (Adjunct)
Department of Neurology
Yale University
New Haven, Connecticut

Michelle L. Ghobrial, MD
Assistant Professor
Department of Neurology
Division of Cerebrovascular and Neurocritical Care
Thomas Jefferson University Hospital
Philadelphia, Pennsylvania

Mark R. Gilbert, MD
Professor
Department of Neuro-Oncology
Division of Cancer Medicine
The University of Texas MD Anderson Cancer Center
Houston, Texas

Emily J. Gilmore, MD
Assistant Professor of Neurology
Staff Neurointensivist, Neuroscience Intensive Care Unit
Yale University School of Medicine
New Haven, Connecticut

Peter J. Goadsby, MD, PhD, DSc, FRACP, FRCP
Professor of Neurology
King's College London
Professor of Neurology
University of California
San Francisco, California

Jill S. Goldman, MS, MPhil, CGC
Taub Institute for Research on Alzheimer's Disease and the
   Aging Brain
Columbia University Medical Center
New York, New York

Clifton L. Gooch, MD
Professor and Chair
Department of Neurology
University of South Florida
Tampa, Florida

Paul Greene, MD
Department of Neurology
Icahn School of Medicine at Mount Sinai
New York, New York

Noam Y. Harel, MD, PhD
Assistant Professor
Departments of Neurology and Rehabilitation Medicine
Icahn School of Medicine at Mount Sinai
James J. Peters Veterans Affairs Medical Center
New York, New York

Michio Hirano, MD
Professor of Neurology
Department of Neurology
Columbia University Medical Center
New York, New York

Lawrence S. Honig, MD, PhD, FAAN
Professor of Neurology
Columbia University Medical Center
New York, New York

Edward D. Huey, MD
Herbert Irving Assistant Professor of Psychiatry and Neurology
Taub Institute for Research on Alzheimer's Disease and
   the Aging Brain
Gertrude H. Sergievsky Center
Columbia University
New York, New York

Christopher G. Hughes, MD
Assistant Professor
Department of Anesthesiology and Critical Care Medicine
Vanderbilt University School of Medicine
Nashville, Tennessee

Emitseilu K. Iluonakhamhe, MD
Vivian L. Smith Department of Neurosurgery
The University of Texas Health Science Center at Houston
Houston, Texas

Fabio M. Iwamoto, MD
Deputy Director, Division of Neuro-Oncology
Department of Neurology
Columbia University
New York, New York

Sarah C. Janicki, MD, MPH
Assistant Professor in Neurology
Gertrude H. Sergievsky Center
Department of Neurology
Columbia University Medical Center
New York, New York

Joseph Jankovic, MD
Professor of Neurology
Distinguished Chair in Movement Disorders
Director, Parkinson's Disease Center and Movement
   Disorders Clinic
Department of Neurology
Baylor College of Medicine
Houston, Texas

Jasmin Jo, MD
Neurooncology Fellow
Department of Neurology
Dana Farber Cancer Institute
Massachusetts General Hospital
Boston, Massachusetts

Burk Jubelt, MD, FAAN
Professor
Departments of Neurology, Microbiology/Immunology, and
   Neuroscience
State University of New York Upstate Medical University
Syracuse, New York

Michael G. Kaiser, MD
Associate Professor of Clinical Neurological Surgery
Associate Director, Spine Center
Department of Neurosurgery
Columbia University Medical Center
New York, New York

Thomas J. Kaley, MD
Assistant Attending Neurologist
Department of Neurology
Memorial Sloan Kettering Cancer Center
Assistant Professor of Neurology
Department of Neurology
Weill Cornell Medical College
New York, New York

Un Jung Kang, MD
H. Houston Merritt Professor of Neurology
Chief, Division of Movement Disorders
Department of Neurology
Columbia University Medical Center
New York, New York

Petra Kaufmann, MD, MSc
Director, Division of Clinical Innovation
National Center for Advancing Translational Sciences
National Institutes of Health
Bethesda, Maryland
Adjunct Associate Professor of Neurology
Columbia University
New York, New York

Steven G. Kernie, MD
Associate Professor of Pediatrics, Pathology, and Cell Biology
Columbia University College of Physicians and Surgeons
New York, New York

Alexander G. Khandji, MD, FACR
Professor of Radiology
Departments of Neurological Surgery and Neurology
Columbia Presbyterian Medical Center
New York, New York

Adam B. King, MD
Assistant Professor
Department of Anesthesiology and Critical Care Medicine
Vanderbilt University Medical Center
Nashville, Tennessee

Barbara S. Koppel, MD
Professor of Clinical Neurology
New York Medical College
Valhalla, New York
Chief, Neurology Service
Metropolitan Hospital
New York, New York

Andreas H. Kramer, MD, MSc, FRCPC
Clinical Associate Professor
Departments of Critical Care Medicine and Clinical Neurosciences
Hotchkiss Brain Institute
University of Calgary
Calgary, Alberta, Canada

William Charles Kreisl, MD
Assistant Professor of Neurology
Taub Institute for Research on Alzheimer's Disease and the Aging Brain
Division of Aging and Dementia, Department of Neurology
Columbia University Medical Center
Assistant Attending Neurologist
New York-Presbyterian Hospital
New York, New York

Shouri Lahiri, MD
Fellow, Neurocritical Care
New York-Presbyterian Hospital
Columbia University Medical Center
Weill Cornell Medical Center
New York, New York

Andrew B. Lassman, MD
John Harris Associate Professor and Chief
Neuro-Oncology Division, Department of Neurology
Medical Director, Clinical Protocol & Data Management Office
Herbert Irving Comprehensive Cancer Center
Columbia University Medical Center
New York, New York

Kiwon Lee, MD, FACP, FAHA
Vice-chairman of Neurosurgery and Neurology for Critical Care
Associate Professor of Neurosurgery and Neurology
Chief, Division of Critical Care
Departments of Neurology and Neurosurgery
The University of Texas Health Science Center at Houston
Mischer Neuroscience Institute
Memorial Hermann-Texas Medical Center
Houston, Texas

Laura Lennihan, MD
Professor of Neurology
Vice-chair, Department of Neurology
Chief, Division of Critical Care and Hospitalist Neurology
Columbia University Medical Center
New York, New York

Angela Lignelli, MD
Department of Radiology
Columbia University Medical Center
New York, New York

Elan D. Louis, MD, MS
Professor of Neurology and Epidemiology
Chief, Division of Movement Disorders
Departments of Neurology and Chronic Disease Epidemiology
Yale School of Medicine and Yale School of Public Health
Yale University
New Haven, Connecticut

Jennifer L. Lyons, MD
Director, Division of Neurological Infections
Brigham and Women's Hospital
Instructor of Neurology
Department of Neurology
Harvard Medical School
Boston, Massachusetts

Julia Mallory, BA, MS4
Ophthalmology Research Fellow
Columbia University College of Physicians and Surgeons
New York, New York

Hani R. Malone, MD
Department of Neurological Surgery
Columbia University Medical Center
New York, New York

Elliott L. Mancall, MD
Emeritus Professor of Neurology
Jefferson Medical College
Thomas Jefferson University
Philadelphia, Pennsylvania

Arthur M. Mandel, MD, PhD
Assistant Professor of Clinical Neurology and Pediatrics
Department of Neurology
Columbia University
New York, New York

Christopher E. Mandigo, MD
Assistant Professor of Clinical Neurosurgery
Department of Neurosurgery
Columbia University Medical Center
New York, New York

Karen S. Marder, MD, MPH
Sally Kerlin Professor of Neurology
Gertrude H. Sergievsky Center
Department of Neurology
Columbia University Medical Center
New York, New York

Randolph S. Marshall, MD, MS
Elizabeth K. Harris Professor of Neurology
Columbia University College of Physicians and Surgeons
Director, Stroke Center
Attending Neurologist
New York-Presbyterian Hospital
Columbia University Medical Center
New York, New York

Stephan A. Mayer, MD, FCCM
Professor of Neurology and Neurosurgery
Icahn School of Medicine at Mount Sinai
Director, Neurocritical Care
Mount Sinai Health System
New York, New York

Richard Mayeux, MD
Sergievsky Professor and Chair
Department of Neurology
Director, Gertrude H. Sergievsky Center
Columbia University
New York, New York

Paul C. McCormick, MD, MPH
Herbert and Linda Gallen Professor of Neurological Surgery
Columbia University College of Physicians and Surgeons
New York, New York

Minesh P. Mehta, MD, FASTRO
Professor, Radiation Oncology
Medical Director, Maryland Proton Treatment Center
University of Maryland
Baltimore, Maryland

Charles B. Mikell, MD
Resident
Department of Neurological Surgery
Columbia University Medical Center
New York, New York

Vesselin Zdravkov Miloushev, MD, PhD
Postdoctoral Clinical Fellow
Department of Diagnostic Radiology
Columbia University
New York-Presbyterian Hospital
New York, New York

Hiroshi Mitsumoto, MD, DSc
Professor of Neurology
Department of Neurology
Columbia University
New York, New York

J. P. Mohr, MD, MS
Daniel Sciarra Professor of Neurology
Doris and Stanley Tananbaum Stroke Center
Department of Neurology
The Neurological Institute of New York
Columbia University Medical Center
New York, New York

Shibani S. Mukerji, MD, PhD
Department of Neurology
Massachusetts General Hospital
Brigham and Women's Hospital
Boston, Massachusetts

Philip R. Muskin, MD
Professor of Psychiatry
Columbia University Medical Center
Chief, Consultation-Liaison Psychiatry
New York-Presbyterian Hospital/Columbia Campus
Faculty
Columbia University Center for Psychoanalytic Training
    and Research
Research Psychiatrist II
New York State Psychiatric Institute
New York, New York

Barnett R. Nathan, MD
Associate Professor
Department of Neurology
University of Virginia School of Medicine
Charlottesville, Virginia

James M. Noble, MD, MS, CPH
Assistant Professor of Neurology
Taub Institute for Research on Alzheimer's Disease and the
    Aging Brain
Department of Neurology
Columbia University Medical Center
New York, New York

Douglas R. Nordli Jr, MD
Epilepsy Center
Ann & Robert H. Lurie Children's Hospital of Chicago
Northwestern University
Chicago, Illinois

Jeffrey G. Odel, MD
Professor of Ophthalmology
Columbia University Medical Center
Edward S. Harkness Eye Institute
New York, New York

William G. Ondo, MD
Professor of Neurology
The University of Texas Health Science Center at Houston
Houston, Texas

Maria A. Oquendo, MD
Professor and Vice-chair for Education
Department of Psychiatry
Columbia University and New York State Psychiatric Institute
New York, New York

Natalie Organek, MD
Neurology Resident
Department of Neurology
Cleveland Clinic
Cleveland, Ohio

Edward (Mel) J. Otten, MD, FACMT, FAWM
Professor of Emergency Medicine and Pediatrics
Director, Division of Toxicology
Department of Emergency Medicine
University of Cincinnati College of Medicine
Cincinnati, Ohio

Alison M. Pack, MD, MPH
Associate Professor of Neurology
Department of Neurology
Columbia University Medical Center
New York, New York

Gunjan Y. Parikh, MD
Assistant Professor
Division of Neurocritical Care
Department of Neurology
Program in Trauma
R Adams Cowley Shock Trauma Center
University of Maryland School of Medicine
Baltimore, Maryland

Marc C. Patterson, MD, FRACP
Chair, Division of Child and Adolescent Neurology
Professor of Neurology, Pediatrics, and Medical Genetics
Departments of Neurology, Pediatrics, and Medical Genetics
Mayo Clinic
Rochester, Minnesota

Toni S. Pearson, MBBS
Assistant Professor of Neurology
Icahn School of Medicine at Mount Sinai
New York, New York

Timothy A. Pedley, MD
Henry and Lucy Moses Professor of Neurology
Chairman, Department of Neurology
Columbia University College of Physicians and Surgeons
Neurologist-in-Chief
The Neurological Institute of New York
The New York-Presbyterian Hospital Columbia University
   Medical Center
New York, New York

Jonathan Perk, MD, PhD
Assistant Professor of Neurology
Neurology Residency Program Director
SUNY Downstate Medical Center
Brooklyn, New York

John Pile-Spellman, MD
Neuroradiologist
Department of Neurosurgery and Radiology
Winthrop University Hospital
Mineola, New York

Chiara Pisciotta, MD, PhD
Department of Neurology
University of Iowa Carver College of Medicine
Iowa City, Iowa

Leon D. Prockop, MD
Professor of Neurology
College of Medicine
University of South Florida
Tampa, Florida

Seth L. Pullman, MD
Professor
The Neurological Institute of New York
Columbia University Medical School
Director
Clinical Motor Physiology Laboratory
New York, New York

Ashwini K. Rao, EdD, OTR, FAOTA
Associate Professor of Rehabilitation & Regenerative Medicine
   (Physical Therapy)
Gertrude H. Sergievsky Center
Columbia University Medical Center
New York, New York

Alexandra S. Reynolds, MD
Resident
Department of Neurology
New York-Presbyterian Hospital
Columbia University Medical Center
New York, New York

Claire S. Riley, MD
Assistant Professor of Neurology
Department of Neurology
Columbia University College of Physicians and Surgeons
Assistant Attending Neurologist
New York-Presbyterian Hospital
Columbia University Medical Center
New York, New York

Alden Doerner Rinaldi, MD
Resident
Department of Neurology
Columbia University Medical Center
New York-Presbyterian Hospital
New York, New York

Fred Rincon, MD, MSc, MBE, FACP, FCCP, FCCM
Assistant Professor of Neurology and Neurosurgery
Thomas Jefferson University
Philadelphia, Pennsylvania

Mikael L. Rinne, MD, PhD
Instructor in Neurology
Dana-Farber Cancer Institute, Center for Neuro-Oncology
Department of Neurology
Brigham and Women's Hospital
Harvard Medical School
Boston, Massachusetts

James J. Riviello Jr, MD
Sergievsky Family Professor of Neurology and Pediatrics
Department of Neurology
Columbia University
New York, New York

Daphne Robakis, MD
Movement Disorders Clinical Fellow
Department of Neurology
Columbia University Medical Center
New York, New York

J. Kirk Roberts, MD
Associate Professor of Neurology
College of Physicians and Surgeons
Columbia University Medical Center
New York-Presbyterian Hospital
New York, New York

David Roh, MD
Neurocritical Care Fellow
Department of Neurocritical Care
Columbia University College of Physicians and Surgeons
New York, New York

Gustavo C. Román, MD, DrHC
Jack S. Blanton Distinguished Endowed Chair
Houston Methodist Neurological Institute
Professor of Neurology
Weill Cornell Medical College
Houston, Texas

Roger N. Rosenberg, MD
Zale Distinguished Chair and Professor of Neurology
Director, Alzheimer's Disease Center
University of Texas Southwestern Medical Center at Dallas
Dallas, Texas

Sara K. Rostanski, MD
Department of Neurology
The Neurological Institute of New York
Columbia University Medical Center
New York, New York

Lewis P. Rowland, MD
Professor of Neurology
Chairman of Neurology, Emeritus
Director of the Neurology Service, Emeritus
The Neurological Institute of New York
Columbia University Medical Center
New York, New York

Tatjana Rundek, MD, PhD
Professor of Neurology and Public Health Sciences
Department of Neurology
University of Miami Miller School of Medicine
Miami, Florida

Jennifer F. Russo, BA
Department of Neurological Surgery
Columbia University Medical Center
New York, New York

Ned Sacktor, MD
Professor of Neurology
Johns Hopkins University School of Medicine
Johns Hopkins Bayview Medical Center
Baltimore, Maryland

Daniel H. Sahlein, MD
Departments of Radiology, Neurosurgery, and Neurology
Columbia University Medical Center
New York, New York

Jacinda B. Sampson, MD, PhD
Assistant Professor of Neurology
Gertrude H. Sergievsky Center
Columbia University Medical Center
New York, New York

Sophie Samuel, PharmD, BCPS
Department of Pharmacy
Memorial Hermann-Texas Medical Center
Houston, Texas

Rachel Saunders-Pullman, MD, MPH
Associate Professor of Neurology
Icahn School of Medicine at Mount Sinai
Mount Sinai Beth Israel
New York, New York

Nikolaos Scarmeas, MD, MS, PhD
Associate Professor of Neurology
Columbia University
New York, New York
National and Kapodistrian University of Athens
Athens, Greece

Lauren R. Schaff, MD
Resident Physician
Department of Neurology
New York-Presbyterian Hospital
Columbia University Medical Center
New York, New York

Heidi Schambra, MD
Assistant Professor of Neurology
Department of Rehabilitation and Regenerative Medicine
Columbia University
New York, New York

David Schiff, MD
Harrison Distinguished Teaching Professor of Neurology, Neurological Surgery, and Medicine
Division of Neuro-Oncology, Department of Neurology
University of Virginia
Charlottesville, Virginia

Hyman M. Schipper, MD, PhD, FRCP©
Professor
Department of Neurology and Neurosurgery
Department of Medicine (Geriatrics)
McGill University Faculty of Medicine
Montreal, Quebec, Canada

Franklin R. Schneier, MD
Special Lecturer
Department of Psychiatry
Columbia University Medical Center
Research Psychiatrist
Anxiety Disorders Clinic
New York State Psychiatric Institute
New York, New York

David B. Seder, MD, FCCP, FCCM
Director of Neurocritical Care
Maine Medical Center
Portland, Maine
Assistant Professor of Medicine
Tufts University School of Medicine
Boston, Massachusetts

Jennifer Sevush-Garcy, MD
Neurology Resident
College of Physicians and Surgeons
Columbia University
New York, New York

Tina Shih, MD
Associate Clinical Professor of Neurology
Department of Neurology
University of California at San Francisco
San Francisco, California

Michael E. Shy, MD
Professor of Neurology, Pediatrics, and Physiology/Biophysics
University of Iowa Carver College of Medicine
Iowa City, Iowa

Reet K. Sidhu, MD
Assistant Professor of Neurology
Department of Neurology, Division of Child Neurology
Columbia University Medical Center
New York, New York

Michael B. Sisti, MD, FACS
James G. McMurtry III, MD, Associate Professor in Clinical
    Neurological Surgery, Radiation Oncology, and Otolaryngology
Codirector, Center for Radiosurgery
Department of Neurosurgery
Columbia University Medical Center
The Neurological Institute of New York
New York-Presbyterian Hospital
New York, New York

Scott A. Small, MD, PhD
Boris and Rose Katz Professor of Neurology
Director, Alzheimer's Disease Research Center
Departments of Neurology, Radiology, and Psychiatry
Columbia University
New York, New York

Robert A. Solomon, MD
Byron Stookey Professor and Chairman
Department of Neurological Surgery
Columbia University College of Physicians and Surgeons
New York-Presbyterian Hospital
New York, New York

Shraddha Srinivasan, MD
Assistant Professor of Neurology
Columbia Comprehensive Epilepsy Center
The Neurological Institute of New York
New York, New York

Yaakov Stern, PhD
Professor of Neuropsychology
Departments of Neurology and Psychiatry
Taub Institute for Research on Alzheimer's Disease and the
    Aging Brain
Columbia University College of Physicians and Surgeons
New York, New York

Ian S. Storper, MD
Director, Otology Program
New York Head and Neck Institute
Lenox Hill Hospital
New York, New York

T. Scott Stroup, MD, MPH
Professor of Psychiatry
Columbia University Medical Center
New York State Psychiatric Institute
New York, New York

Sally M. Sultan, MD, MS
Instructor in Pediatric Neurology/Pediatric Neurovascular
Department of Neurology
Columbia University Medical Center
New York, New York

Kurenai Tanji, MD, PhD
Professor of Pathology and Cell Biology (in Neurology)
Departments of Pathology and Cell Biology and Neurology
Columbia University Medical Center
New York, New York

Claudio E. Tatsui, MD
Assistant Professor
Department of Neurosurgery
The University of Texas MD Anderson Cancer Center
Houston, Texas

Pichet Termsarasab, MD
Neurology Fellow
Department of Neurology
Icahn School of Medicine at Mount Sinai
New York, New York

Kiran Thakur, MD
Postdoctoral Fellow
Division of Neuroinfectious Diseases and Neuroimmunology
Department of Neurology
Johns Hopkins Hospital
Baltimore, Maryland

Mathula Thangarajh, MD, PhD
Director of Neuromuscle Program
Department of Neurology
Children's National Medical Center
Washington, District of Columbia

Rebecca Traub, MD
Assistant Professor
Department of Neurology
Columbia University
New York, New York

Christina M. Ulane, MD, PhD
Assistant Professor of Neurology
Department of Neurology
Columbia University Medical Center
Division of Neuromuscular Diseases and EMG Laboratory
Medical Director, Adult Neurology Resident Clinic
Associate Director, Adult Neurology Residency Program
The Neurological Institute of New York
New York, New York

Julio R. Vieira, MD, MS
Neurology Resident
Department of Neurology
The Neurological Institute of New York
New York-Presbyterian Hospital
Columbia University Medical Center
New York, New York

Natalie R. Weathered, MD
Postdoctoral Clinical Fellow
Assistant Attending Neurologist
New York-Presbyterian Hospital
Columbia University Medical Center
New York, New York

Louis H. Weimer, MD, FAAN, FANA
Professor of Neurology
Director, EMG Laboratory
Department of Neurology
Columbia University Medical Center
New York, New York

Michael L. Weinberger, MD
Associate Clinical Professor of Anesthesiology
Columbia University College of Physicians and Surgeons
New York-Presbyterian Hospital
New York, New York

Patrick Y. Wen, MD
Professor of Neurology
Harvard Medical School
Director, Center for Neuro-Oncology
Dana-Farber Cancer Institute
Director, Division of Neuro-Oncology
Department of Neurology
Brigham and Women's Hospital
Boston, Massachusetts

Andrew J. Westwood, MD, MRCP(UK)
Assistant Attending Neurologist
Columbia University College of Physicians and Surgeons
New York-Presbyterian Hospital
Columbia University Medical Center
New York, New York

Eelco F. M. Wijdicks, MD, PhD, FACP, FNCS, FANA
Professor of Neurology
Mayo Clinic
Rochester, Minnesota

Joshua Z. Willey, MD, MS
Assistant Professor
Department of Neurology
Columbia University
New York, New York

Christopher J. Winfree, MD, FACS
Assistant Professor
Department of Neurological Surgery
Columbia University Medical Center
New York, New York

Graeme F. Woodworth, MD
Assistant Professor
Department of Neurosurgery
University of Maryland School of Medicine
Baltimore, Maryland

Marianna Shnayderman Yugrakh, MD
Assistant Professor of Neurology
Columbia University Headache Center
Department of Neurology
Columbia University
New York, New York

Christopher Zammit, MD
Assistant Professor of Emergency Medicine and Neurology
Department of Emergency Medicine
University of Cincinnati
Cincinnati, Ohio

Joseph R. Zunt, MD, MPH
Professor, Departments of Neurology and Global Health
Adjunct Professor, Departments of Medicine (Infectious Diseases)
    and Epidemiology
University of Washington
Seattle, Washington

Contents

SECTION XX

PSYCHIATRY AND NEUROLOGY 1305
Section Editor: *David H. Strauss*

SECTION XXI

RECOVERY AND END-OF-LIFE CARE 1335
Section Editor: *Laura Lennihan*

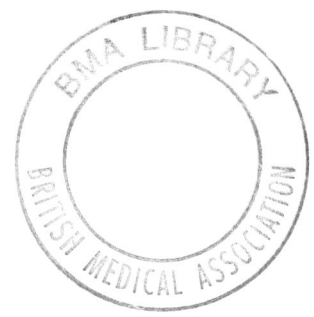

Videos

Hereford cattle. There were generalized myoclonic jerks with somesthetic stimuli.

Video 78.5. Propriospinal myoclonus. This video demonstrates reflex myoclonus, axial jerks shown as truncal flexion after being tapped with a reflex hammer. Note the relatively long latency between the taps and truncal flexion due to slow conduction via propriospinal pathways, in contrast to the short latency in cortical myoclonus due to conduction through corticospinal pathways.

Video 78.6. Hemifacial spasm. The first patient demonstrated clonic twitching of the left orbicularis oculi, especially in the lower portion, greater than left zygomaticus. There was synkinesis: When she puffed her cheek, there was also contraction of the left orbicularis oculi seen as left eye closure. The second patient demonstrated clonic and tonic twitching of the left facial muscles including orbicularis oculi and zygomaticus as well as left platysma. There was also synkinesis, similar to the first patient.

Chapter 79

Video 79.1. A 29-year-old woman with SCA2 exhibits a wide-based, ataxic gait. (Courtesy of Sheng-Han Kuo, MD, Department of Neurology, Columbia University.)

Chapter 80

Video 80.1. Classic orobuccolingual dyskinesia and limb dyskinesia. The patient has typical orobuccal movements resembling chewing and swallowing as well as tongue popping and lip puckering. Oral movements cease when she talks and do not significantly interfere with speech. She also shows repetitive finger extension and flexion. The right thumb is in extended position, suggesting a dystonic component. She has similar flexion and extension movement of toes and wrist when standing up.

Video 80.2. Tardive dystonia. The patient shows excessive eye blinking and closure (blepharospasm) as well as lower facial grimacing movement. Her eyes open better when talking than listening to examiner.

Video 80.3. Tardive akathisia. The patent sits with crossing and uncrossing of his legs and arms, repeatedly touching his hat, and rocking his trunk back and forth. He jumps out of chair and paces around.

Chapter 81

Video 81.1. Sydenham disease. A 13-year-old boy with a 2-month history of left hemichorea and prior history of sore throat; serum antistreptolysin O (ASO) titer is greater than 600. The chorea completely resolved in 6 months.

Video 81.2. Kernicterus. An 11-year-old boy with a history of marked and prolonged neonatal jaundice, delayed developmental milestones, generalized choreoathetosis, vertical ophthalmoparesis, and deafness, typical of kernicterus.

Chapter 82

Video 82.1. Motor signs of Huntington disease.

Chapter 83

Video 83.1. Tremor. The patient has arm tremor at rest. The right arm tremor subsides for a second while he is moving his arm from the resting to outstretched position. Once his arm is in an outstretched position, the tremor reemerges. On the left, the tremor continues from rest to kinetic and to posture-holding positions. He has no kinetic tremor with finger-to-nose maneuvers on the right and slight intention tremor on the left. He also has jaw tremor at rest. The patient's rest tremor continues in both arms while walking.

Video 83.2. Bradykinesia and gait difficulty. The patient has mildly slurred speech. She has decreased facial expression with decreased blinking and partially open mouth. She has mild oral dyskinesia. Her rapid alternating movements are more impaired on the left side than the right side. Her finger tapping is slow, small in amplitude, and irregular, more severely affected in the left side. She stands up by pushing against the arm rest. Her posture is mildly stooped forward. She takes good strides, normal base, but without heel strike and with decreased arm swing on both sides. She takes five steps to turn 180 degrees. On pull test, she takes four steps of retropulsion before her fall was stopped by the examiner.

Video 83.3. Levodopa-induced dyskinesia. The patient has truncal, oral, and arm dyskinesia, with some dystonic posture of the left arm activated by voluntary movement of the right arm. She has excessive swinging of the left arm and oral dyskinesia while walking. She fails to regain her balance on pull test. With a few minutes, she turns "off" and shows left-sided rest tremor and akinesia. She continues to have oral dyskinesia, however.

Video 83.4. Freezing of gait. The patient freezes after reaching a destination and turning. He develops tremulous movements in the legs while attempting to take steps. After a few seconds, he is able to resume walking again.

Chapter 84

Video 84.1. Patient with mild signs and symptoms of progressive supranuclear palsy (PSP) for 2 years. Continuous, tiny square wave jerks are visible when he fixates. He has extremely limited upgaze and downgaze. He does not generate saccades when asked to look left or right. He is able to open his eyes after lid closure but there is a delay on the left. Tongue movements are mildly slow. He has marked axial bradykinesia (slowed shoulder shrug on the right) with mild slowing of rapid succession movements of the hands of feet. His blink rate is markedly reduced and he has a stare. He is able to rise from a chair with arms crossed, although slowly. He has a mildly broad based, slow gait with right > left arm abduction ("gunslinger's walk") and decreased arm swing.

Video 84.2. Patient with more severe PSP. She has the characteristic facial dystonia of PSP producing a troubled or angry look. She has poor balance, cannot rise from a chair safely with arms crossed, and falls in all directions. She also has a mildly broad-based stance and gait. When instructed to step backwards when pulled from behind, she falls backwards.

Video 84.3. Patient seen initially with mild signs and symptoms of cortical–basal ganglionic degeneration (CBGD). She has dystonic posturing of the right hand with twisting, slightly jerky movements of the right forearm, wrist, and fingers. Rapid succession movements of the upper extremities are mildly slowed on the left and markedly slowed on the right. She can rise slowly from a chair using her left hand. Her gait is slow, with mildly broad base, short stride on the left, dystonic posturing of both arm and leg on the right with even shorter stride, and no heel strike on either side. She turns en bloc, barely lifting the right foot. Two years later, she spends almost all her time in a wheelchair. She has severe dystonic posturing of the right arm and hand. She has overflow elevation of the right arm and left leg when she lifts the left. She has almost no function of the right hand or arm, requiring the left for simple actions like raising or lowering the arm. The left side is slow but significantly more functional than the right. She needs assistance to rise from a chair, and when she does, her right leg elevates and she can barely lower it to the ground and cannot support her weight with her legs alone.

Chapter 103

Video 103.1. Gross total resection of the thoracic meningioma seen in Figure 103.6. After standard posterior thoracic laminectomy and midline opening of the dura mater is completed, microsurgical technique is used to dissect the arachnoid plane and separate the tumor from the spinal cord, nerve roots, and radiculomedullary artery and veins. Subsequently, the tumor capsule is incised, and a debulking followed by piecemeal resection is performed. After gross total resection is achieved, the dural insertion is cauterized to reduce risk of recurrence. We opted not to remove the dura given the anterior location and potential morbidity of a CSF leak.

Video 103.2. Gross total resection of an intramedullary ependymoma. After standard posterior thoracic laminectomy and midline opening of the dura mater is completed, microsurgical technique is used to perform a midline posterior myelotomy at the level of the posterior midline sulcus. The myelotomy is extended to allow complete exposure of the tumor. A plane of cleavage is developed and the dorsal and lateral border of the mass are gently separated from the surrounding spinal cord. Subsequently, the tumor is mobilized away from the ventral columns and all feeders from the anterior spinal artery are cauterized and cut allowing en bloc resection of the ependymoma.

Chapter 115

Video 115.1. Typical Takotsubo.
Video 115.2. Atypical Takotsubo.

Global Burden of Neurologic Disease 1

Jennifer Sevush-Garcy and Mitchell S. V. Elkind

INTRODUCTION

Neurologic disorders are globally among the most important causes of human illness and mortality. Quantifying the burden of neurologic disease and its impact on populations throughout the world is challenging for several reasons, however. First, neurologic disease includes disorders that primarily affect the brain as well as diseases that affect other body systems but have prominent neurologic manifestations. Second, neurologic diseases are notable for more frequently causing disability than death. Commonly used measures of disease impact, such as hospitalization or mortality rates, may not capture the impact of nonfatal neurologic problems such as migraine or epilepsy. Third, there are often disparities in neurologic disorders caused by socioeconomic and geographic factors. Assessment and diagnosis of neurologic disease may also depend on resources available for their measurement that are not available in all environments. Despite these limitations, present estimates of the burden of neurologic disorders suggest that they have an enormous impact on human health.

THE CLASSIFICATION OF DISEASE: WHAT IS A NEUROLOGIC DISORDER?

The classification of neurologic disorders can be broken down into two general categories: primary neurologic disorders affecting the nervous system only and secondary neurologic disorders, in which injury or dysfunction of the nervous system occurs as a result of a disease that primarily affects another organ system or in which dysfunction of the nervous system occurs along with dysfunction of several other organ systems. Examples of primary neurologic disorders include Alzheimer disease, migraine, and multiple sclerosis. Examples of secondary neurologic disorders include seizures secondary to infection with malaria, paraneoplastic syndromes associated with primary systemic cancer, and peripheral neuropathy occurring in the setting of nutritional deficiencies.

The distinction between primary and secondary neurologic disorders complicates the task of estimating global disease burden. For instance, do we classify diabetic neuropathy as a neurologic disorder or as a complication of an endocrinologic disorder? Should stroke be considered a neurologic disorder or a cardiovascular disease? Should head injury in the context of a motor vehicle accident be counted toward the burden of disease of neurologic disorders or of accidents? Various approaches have been taken to answer these questions, and in some instances, the definitions may shift depending on the purpose of the analysis. Although these distinctions may seem academic at first glance, they could have implications for public health campaigns and approaches to measuring, reporting, and acting on the relative burden of illness caused by different diseases.

ESTIMATING DISEASE BURDEN

There are several measures used to evaluate disease burden, including incidence, prevalence, morbidity, case fatality, mortality, disability, quality of life, pain, and cost. Incidence and prevalence are used to determine how common a disease is. The number of first cases of a disease over a defined time interval in a defined population determines its incidence. Prevalence measures the total number of cases, new and old, at a particular time in a defined population. Both indices depend on the accurate and complete enumeration of cases and adequate knowledge of the underlying population at risk. Case fatality refers to the proportion of patients with a disease who die from it. Mortality refers to the overall number of deaths due to the disease in a given time period.

Traditional approaches to estimating the impact of illness have focused on mortality because it is relatively easy to measure. The impact of some neurologic disorders may be reasonably captured by reference to their case fatality or mortality. For example, malignant brain tumors, strokes, and head injuries are often severe and may lead to death. A metric focused exclusively on mortality, however, will fail to capture the impact of many neurologic disorders that are chronic and slowly progressive, or intermittent and disabling, but that do not cause their sufferers to die. For example, multiple sclerosis is a disease process that has low mortality but inflicts a rather high level of disability on its patients; however, it is relatively rare. Alternatively, migraine is a neurologic disorder that also has low mortality but has moderate disability and is extremely common. Clearly, attempts to measure this type of disease burden require a more versatile metric than mortality alone.

More recent attempts to measure disease burden have therefore aimed at capturing not only mortality but also morbidity, which captures the disability, handicap, and other physical costs associated with the disease. One common approach to measuring burden of disease is to consider a time-based metric that incorporates premature mortality (the number of years of life lost due to premature death, based on an expected life span) and disability (years of healthy life lost as a result of disability weighted by the severity of the disability). The combination of both of these measures yields disability-adjusted life years (DALYs). DALYs are a well-established metric of disease burden that measure the number of healthy years of life lost as a result of both death and disability caused by a particular disease. One DALY constitutes 1 year of healthy life lost in an ideal world in which everyone lives into old age free of any disease or disability. One advantage to using the DALY to measure disease burden is that it allows comparisons of impact across very different disease states, in effect serving as a common measure for acute severe illness (stroke, head injury, myocardial infarction) and less severe chronic illnesses (epilepsy, migraine). The DALY metric thus reflects the impact of disease on both early mortality and on

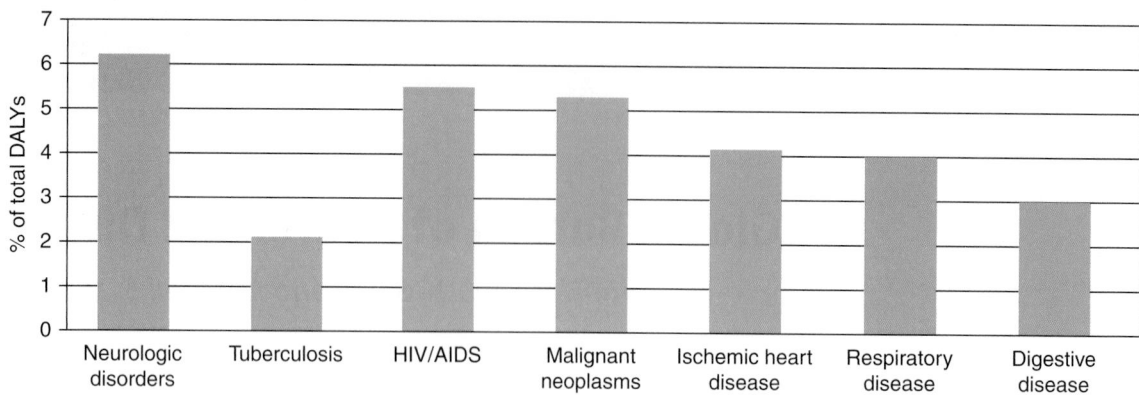

FIGURE 1.1. Percentage of total DALYs for selected diseases and neurologic disorders.

disability, both of which are particularly important for assessing the overall impact of neurologic disease.

Neurologic disorders account for the largest proportion of DALYs of any category of disease, more so than cancer, heart disease, or pulmonary disease (Fig. 1.1). Within the category of neurologic disorders, the greatest proportion of DALYs is due to cerebrovascular disease, which represents just over half of the DALYs due to all neurologic disorders. Alzheimer disease and other dementias, together with epilepsy and tetanus, comprise another quarter of the DALYs seen with neurologic disease. Perhaps surprisingly, migraine encompasses 8.3% of DALYs among neurologic disorders, which is double that encompassed by Parkinson disease and multiple sclerosis combined, although it contributes little to the occurrence of deaths. Likewise, although epilepsy contributes to almost 8% of DALYs, it is responsible for less than 2% of deaths. Stroke, on the other hand, which is also frequently fatal, is responsible for 85% of deaths when compared to other neurologic disorders (Figs. 1.2 and 1.3).

Among neurologic disorders, stroke carries the largest burden of disease. Estimates from the Global Burden of Diseases,

Injuries, and Risk Factors Study, sponsored by the World Health Organization (WHO), ranked stroke as the second most common cause of death and the third most common cause of DALYs worldwide in 2010. These numbers may still underestimate the burden of disease, however, because they are limited to the clinical stroke syndromes that lead patients to seek medical attention. They generally do not include the subclinical disease burden from cerebrovascular disease, such as subclinical infarcts and white matter injury from ischemia, which may lead to cognitive impairment and functional decline.

THE SHIFTING CHARACTER OF NEUROLOGIC DISEASE OVER TIME

The relative importance of different neurologic disorders over time has changed not only as a consequence of changes in population demographics and risk factors but also as a consequence of world events and scientific knowledge. For example, tremendous advances in our understanding of peripheral nerve injuries, including phantom limb pain, occurred during the civil war, through the examination of amputees and injured soldiers by Silas Weir Mitchell and colleagues. Further advances in our understanding of head injuries occurred during the First World War. Early in the 20th century, neurologists also frequently

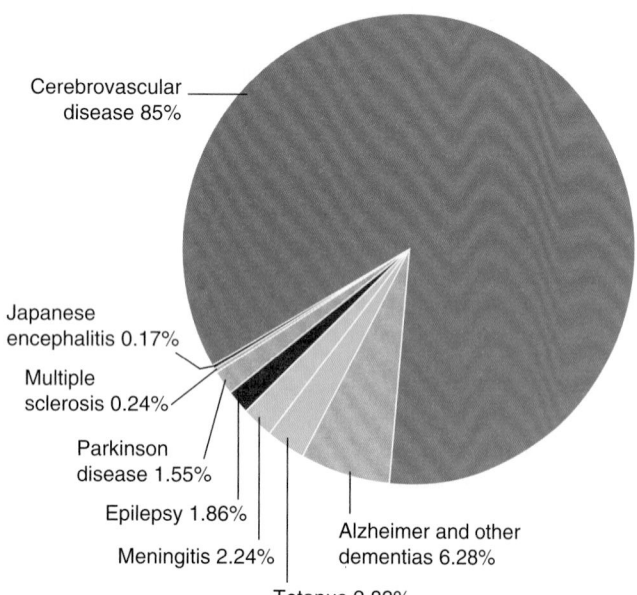

FIGURE 1.2. Deaths from selected neurologic disorders as percentage of total neurologic disorders. (From World Health Organization. *Neurological Disorders: Public Health Challenges.* Geneva, Switzerland: World Health Organization; 2006.)

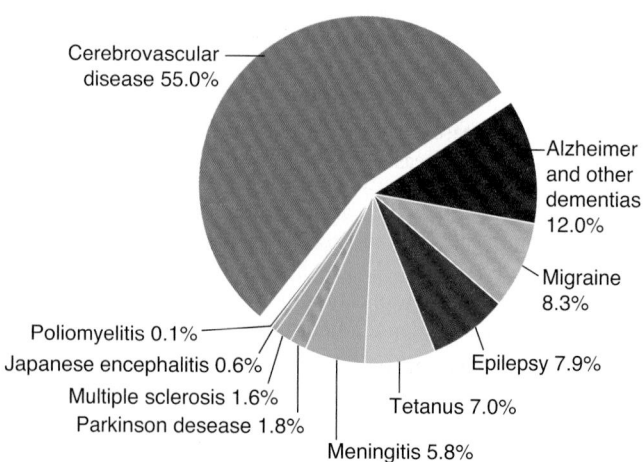

FIGURE 1.3. DALYs for individual neurologic disorders as percentage of total neurologic disorders. (From World Health Organization. *Neurological Disorders: Public Health Challenges.* Geneva, Switzerland: World Health Organization; 2006.)

encountered brain injury as a direct or indirect consequence of infections, including syphilis, tuberculosis, and viral encephalitis. For example, the Spanish flu pandemic of 1918 to 1919 gave rise to many cases of postencephalitic parkinsonism, a disorder made familiar to many through Oliver Sacks' *Awakenings*. Later in the century, as life expectancy in developed countries increased, disorders of the elderly, including stroke and neurodegenerative disorders such as Parkinson disease and Alzheimer disease, were commonly encountered. Infectious neurologic disorders resurfaced again, however, in the 1980s in the form of the HIV/AIDS epidemic, with its well-known complications of toxoplasmosis and cerebral lymphoma. Rare and initially mystifying neurologic diseases have also captured the popular imagination and generated interest beyond what would be expected from the numbers of patients affected; the spongiform encephalopathies caused by prions, such as new variant Creutzfeldt–Jakob disease (or mad cow disease) had a tremendous impact in terms of teaching us about how diseases can jump from one species to another.

THE EPIDEMIOLOGIC TRANSITION AND THE DOUBLE BURDEN OF DISEASE

The concept of the "epidemiologic transition" has been used to explain the shift in the types of diseases that often occur in countries as they pass through different stages of development. As nations industrialize and develop, the major causes of death and disability shift from a predominance of nutritional deficiencies and infectious diseases toward degenerative and chronic diseases, such as diabetes and cardiovascular disease. Investigators have described at least five stages of transition. The first stage (pestilence and famine) includes nutritional deficiencies and infection and characterizes regions such as sub-Saharan Africa and rural South Asia. In the second stage (receding pandemics), during which the pandemics of infectious disease and malnutrition recede, diseases related to hypertension, such as hemorrhagic stroke, become more common. China is an example of a region in this stage. During the third stage (degenerative and man-made diseases), life expectancy improves but high-fat diets, sedentary lifestyles, and cigarette smoking are introduced, allowing chronic, degenerative, and "man-made" diseases, including cardiovascular disease and ischemic stroke, to become more prominent. Urban India serves as an example of a country in this stage. As countries become more industrialized, populations are also exposed to new environmental hazards. In a study conducted in Taipei, Taiwan, urban air pollution was associated with increased numbers of emergency admissions for cerebrovascular diseases. In the fourth stage (delayed degenerative disorders), there are increased efforts to prevent, diagnose, and treat these lifestyle-related diseases, which allows for a delay in their age of onset as well as the increase in degenerative diseases affecting the elderly. Western Europe and North America are considered to be in this fourth stage of the epidemiologic transition. Finally, a fifth stage may exist (social upheaval and social regression) in which social upheaval and war break down the existing health structures, leading to a resurgence of conditions seen in the first two stages as well as to the effects of violence and accidents. Post-Soviet Russia has been suggested as an example of this fifth stage.

As countries develop, they may also fall prey to the adverse consequences of a Western lifestyle (high-fat diet, sedentary lifestyle) before they fully emerge from the problems of underdevelopment. This phenomenon has been referred to as the *double burden* of disease and explains why countries in the middle levels of development have the highest rates of many illnesses. Developing and middle-income regions such as Latin America and urban India, for example, are experiencing an increased incidence of cardiovascular disease while simultaneously facing the lingering effects of infection and malnutrition.

Neurologic disorders are also subject to this epidemiologic staging. At any given time, different regions throughout the world may be in different stages of this transition. In particular, empirical evidence of the epidemiologic transition of stroke was nicely described in the Sino-MONICA-Beijing project. In this community-based surveillance study, investigators examined temporal trends in stroke incidence in Beijing over two decades from 1984 to 2004, a particularly rapid period of economic development in China. Four characteristics of the epidemiologic transition were observed: declining incidence of hemorrhagic stroke due to improved treatment of hypertension, reduced case fatality due to improved treatment after stroke, increased age of stroke onset, and an expanded proportion of ischemic heart disease deaths with a decreased proportion of stroke deaths in the study population. Additionally, an increase in the incidence of ischemic stroke was found, which was felt to be secondary to increased atherosclerotic risk factors.

DISPARITIES

Populations can be stratified by geography and income, and there are often disparities in neurologic disorders based on these factors. The WHO recognizes 6 geographic regions (Africa, Americas, Southeast Asia, Europe, Eastern Mediterranean, and Western Pacific) and 14 subregions, stratified according to child and adult mortality in those regions. The World Bank categorizes countries into four groups on the basis of gross national income per capita: low, lower middle, upper middle, and high-income. Varying types of neurologic disorders and degrees of disease burden occur in the different regions and income groups (Figs. 1.4 and 1.5). Low-income countries have a higher proportion of deaths from HIV, tuberculosis, and malaria infection, which can lead to infection within the nervous system, compared with high and middle-income countries. In the Southeast Asia region, tuberculosis, HIV, AIDS, and meningitis are four of the major causes of death in the region. WHO estimates that this region contributes 27% of the global burden of infectious and parasitic diseases and 35% of nutritional deficiencies. This is just one example of how countries in the WHO high mortality stratum or low-income category face major challenges from diseases associated with poverty, underdevelopment, and ineffective health care systems.

Worldwide, stroke accounts for approximately 10% of all deaths. The highest numbers of stroke deaths occur in Northern Asia, Eastern Europe, Central Africa, and the South Pacific. Systematic reviews of population-based studies from 28 countries showed that stroke incidence has increased in low-income and middle-income countries, whereas high-income countries have experienced a 42% decrease in incidence over the past four decades. According to a recent global analysis contained in the estimates from the Global Burden of Diseases, Injuries, and Risk Factors Study, stroke mortality has decreased in the past two decades, whereas global stroke burden, rated in terms of yearly stroke survivorship, related deaths, and DALYs lost, has increased with the brunt of the burden in low-income and middle-income countries. Within high-income countries, improved health services and preventative stroke care may explain the reduction in stroke incidence, mortality, and DALYs lost and the converse for low-income and middle-income regions. In areas such as sub-Saharan Africa, there are high stroke mortality rates and low rates of reduction in DALYs lost.

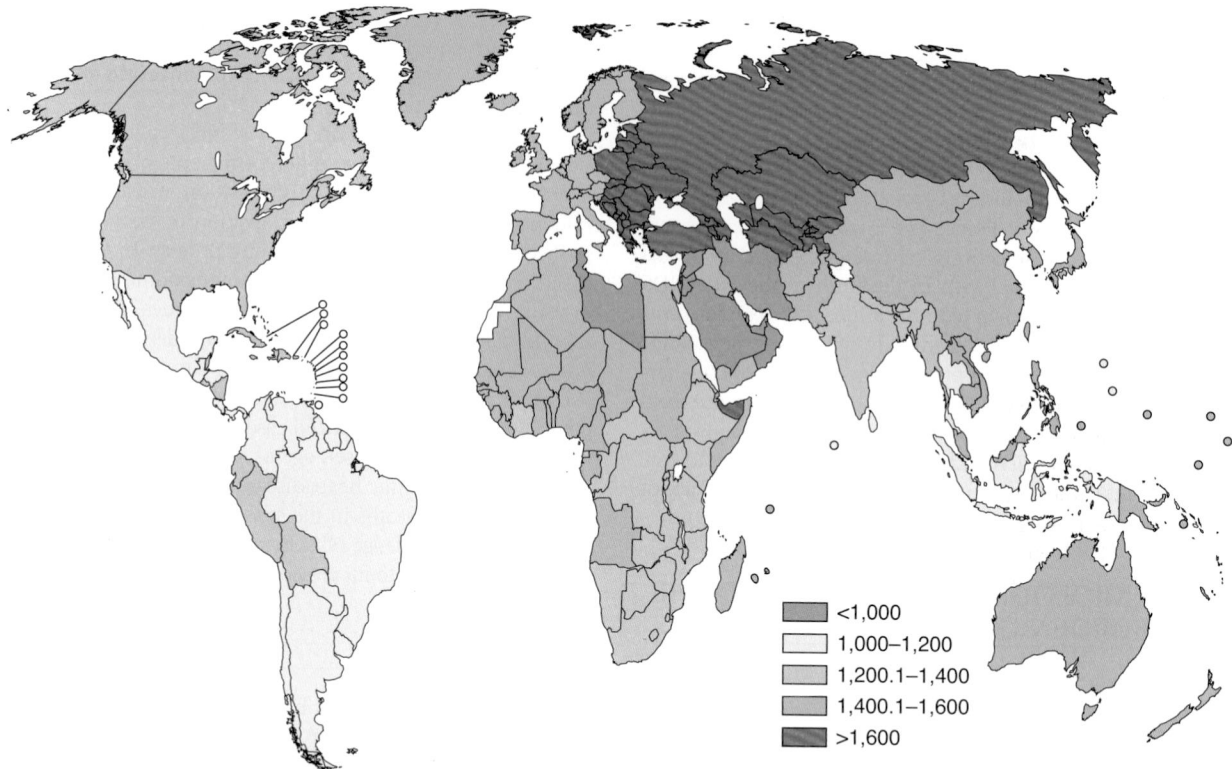

	<1,000
	1,000–1,200
	1,200.1–1,400
	1,400.1–1,600
	>1,600

FIGURE 1.4. DALYs per 100,000 population associated with neurologic disorders by WHO region and mortality stratum. (From World Health Organization. *Neurological Disorders: Public Health Challenges.* Geneva, Switzerland: World Health Organization; 2006.)

Stroke disparities are not limited to the developing world; in fact, global disparities are reflected within nations. In the United States, racial minorities suffer increased stroke mortality and disability rates compared to non-Hispanic whites. African-Americans have the highest mortality rates due to stroke and Hispanics have a higher stroke incidence than whites. Within the United States, a geographic distribution in stroke incidence and mortality can be discerned. In the southeastern United States, within a region referred to as the *Stroke Belt*, stroke mortality and incidence rates are increased. The highest rates are found along the coast, in Georgia and the Carolinas, in a region nicknamed the *Stroke Buckle*. Variations in the race or ethnicity of people comprising the popu-

lation do not appear to explain the disparities in stroke mortality and incidence that exist in the southeastern United States because African-Americans in that region seem to have increased stroke risks compared to African-Americans in other parts of the country. The difference may be attributable to socioeconomic factors limiting access to care, producing an increase in the prevalence of stroke risk factors. It has been noted that, at the age that Medicare becomes available to elderly Americans, African-Americans have no higher in-hospital mortality than do whites and no higher incidence in stroke rates or hypertension than do Hispanics. This provides indirect evidence that it is the lack of access to care that may be responsible for some of the racial and regional disparities.

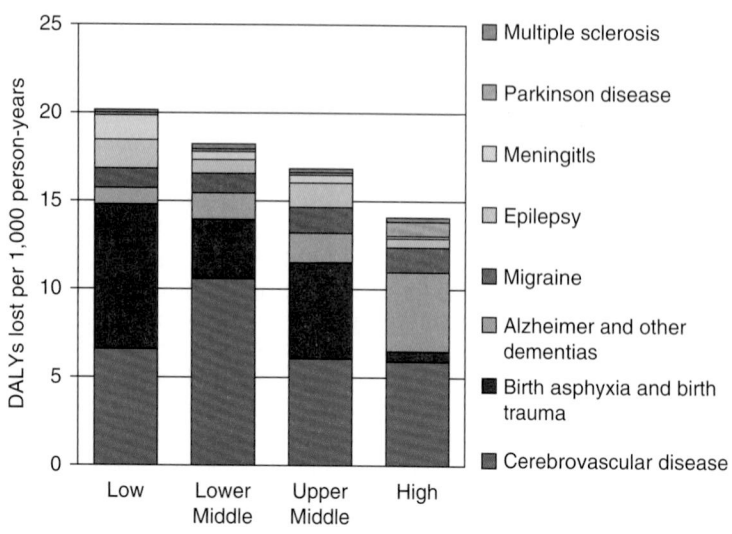

FIGURE 1.5. Burden of neurologic diseases in lost DALYs per 1,000 person-years by World Bank national income level. (From Johnston SC, Hauser SL. Neurological disease on the global agenda. *Ann Neurol.* 2008;64:11–12.)

Global disparities in neurologic disease are not limited to stroke. In a population-based survey of residents older than age 65 years in seven countries with low and middle incomes (China, India, Cuba, Dominican Republic, Venezuela, Mexico, and Peru), dementia was overwhelmingly found to be the most important independent contributor to disability for elderly people in these countries. Chronic disease disability in countries with low and middle incomes is expected to increase by 224% in the least developed regions over the next four decades. Similarly, in a cross-sectional study of elderly Chinese people living in Hong Kong, dementia, stroke, and Parkinson disease were the chronic conditions most strongly associated with severe debility.

Limitations in neurologic resources and variability in resource allocation to neurologic problems contribute to the disparities in the global burden of neurologic disease. In a WHO/World Federation of Neurology survey of neurologic services, conducted from 2001 to 2003, there were marked disparities in availability of neurologists, neurosurgeons, subspecialized neurologic services, and methods of financing neurologic care across regions and income strata. The Americas and Southeast Asia had the highest regional availability of neurologic facilities at the primary health care level, whereas countries in the Western Pacific and Africa had limited emergency care or follow-up care for patients. Worldwide, the median number of neurologists per 100,000 people was 0.91. There was great variability, however: In Europe, the number of neurologists was four times higher, and in regions of Africa and Southeast Asia, the number of neurologists was substantially lower (Fig. 1.6). A similar regional pattern was identified regarding the availability of neurosurgeons and neurologic nurses around the world. Additionally, in 83% of countries from Africa, out-of-pocket payments represented the primary method of financing neurologic care, compared with 25.6% worldwide. Similarly, out-of-pocket

payments represented the primary method of financing neurologic care in 84.2% of low-income countries. This survey illustrates the existence of inadequate resources for neurologic disorders in most countries and highlights the inequalities in access to neurologic care particularly present in low-income countries.

Variation in allocation of attention and research resources may contribute to the disparities seen in neurologic care worldwide. For example, of the 685 manuscripts published in the *Annals of Neurology* from 2005 through 2008, 91% had a corresponding author in either North America or Europe. Thus, 97% of manuscripts were produced in high-income countries where only 15% of the global population resides. Furthermore, the vast majority of clinical studies of neurologic disease describe people in high-income countries. A paradox has been observed within the pharmaceutical research realm where 90% of medical research funds are spent on 10% of the world's population. Apparently, research and development expenditures for diseases of poverty, including malaria, tropical diseases, and tuberculosis, are considered more likely to provide low returns and thus are considered high risk for failure and are not pursued.

SOCIOCULTURAL DIFFERENCES IN INTERPRETATION OF DISEASE

Cultural differences in disease screening, reporting, and management may contribute to the variation in identified global neurologic disease burden. A skew in the number of neurologic diagnoses identified in developing countries, as compared to high-income countries, might be a result of neurologically afflicted patients in developing countries not coming to medical attention. In one analysis of health systems constraints in Timor-Leste, one of the

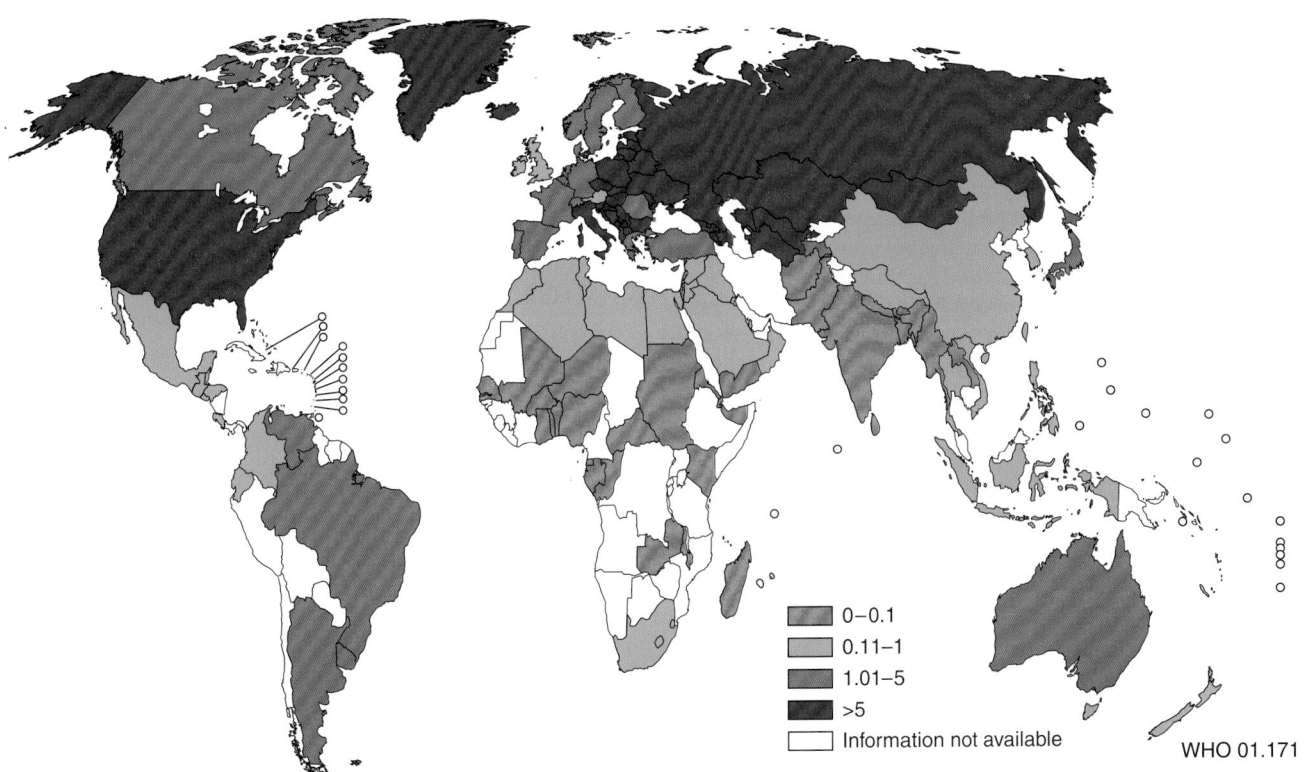

FIGURE 1.6. Global number of neurologists per 100,000 population. (From Janca A, Aarli JA, Prilipko L, et al. WHO/WFN survey of neurological services: a worldwide perspective. *J Neurol Sciences.* 2006;247:29–34.)

poorest countries in Asia, it was found that poverty, strong beliefs in traditional medicine and healers, and low levels of education were barriers to people seeking care. Diagnostic equipment that is crucial for neurologic care, such as electroencephalography, electromyography, computed tomography, and magnetic resonance imaging, were absent. There were no manufacturers of medicine in the country, requiring importation of all necessary medicines.

In a study examining the reportable neurologic diseases in refugee camps in 19 countries within Africa, the Eastern Mediterranean, and Southeast Asia, a variety of diagnoses were revealed. Epilepsy represented more than 9 out of every 10 visits for neurologic disease in these refugee camps. The underlying causes of epilepsy in refugee camps, although unknown, were presumably similar to those for other inhabitants in the region, including perinatal injury, head trauma, cerebral malaria, and previous stroke. Within refugee camps throughout sub-Saharan Africa, the monitoring of meningitis and newer initiatives for vaccination were found to be crucial for preventing epidemic outbreaks, particularly those due to *Neisseria meningitidis*. However, there were limitations in accurate reporting in these regions, with many of the diagnoses not being verified by physicians and conditions such as meningitis being unlikely to have received cerebrospinal fluid confirmation. Regional and cultural differences in diagnosis and disease reporting can have an impact on the accurate assessment of the total global burden of neurologic disease.

Regional differences in the management of neurologic disease are also seen worldwide. Infectious disease, including meningitis, encephalitis, and cerebral malaria, is a major cause of critical neurologic illness in developing countries. Ischemic and hemorrhagic stroke, severe head injury, and epilepsy are major unaddressed causes of morbidity and mortality in many developing countries. In addition, neurologic manifestations of rabies, tetanus, eclampsia, and tuberculosis contribute to the burden of disease in these regions. The largest share of tuberculosis infection is seen in Africa and Asia where resource constraints hamper efforts to control new infections and prevent drug resistance. Infections of the nervous system by *Mycobacterium tuberculosis*, including meningitis, tuberculoma, tuberculous abscess, and nonosseous spinal tuberculoma, affect more than 10% of patients in the region. Tuberculosis is the leading cause of death in HIV-infected individuals in this population. Many low- and middle-income countries with high tuberculosis burdens have limited laboratory capacity to perform smear microscopy or run cultures for drug susceptibility testing. Unfortunately, in low-resource settings, patients often present late for medical care and are sometimes misdiagnosed and treated inappropriately, which can lead to a more severe clinical course. In some of even the least developed countries, governments fund hospitals that include intensive care unit–level care and, in addition, humanitarian efforts and military hospitals also contribute to offer some form of neurologic disease management, showing that neurocritical care can sometimes be practiced even in extremely resource-poor locations. There are, however, limitations in available resources. Many medications are not universally available. For example, although tissue plasminogen activator is a standard of care in high-income settings, developing countries still struggle with poor availability of this drug. Alternatives such as snake venom or urokinase may be employed instead. Finally, there remains a need for attention to neurologic recovery after the illness to allow for a seamless continuum between prevention, intervention, and rehabilitation from neurologic illness.

Cultural differences worldwide are an additional contributor to the differences seen in neurologic care around the world. For example, in many countries, patients with recurrent seizure may be considered to be possessed rather than as having epilepsy. In a cross-sectional study performed in Dar es Salaam, Tanzania, it was shown that of 100 traditional healers interviewed, 30% believed that epilepsy was caused by witchcraft, whereas 19% thought epilepsy had a genetic origin that could be inherited. The traditional healers treated epilepsy with up to 60 different plants, and some of these plants have demonstrated anticonvulsant activity. Among the Maasai population living throughout East Africa, who hold fast to their traditional and nomadic lifestyle, patients presenting with HIV/AIDS, epilepsy, and cerebral palsy are treated in remote sites using "bush medicine" within tents and working by sunlight with no electricity. In Maasai traditional medicine, herbs, roots, and bark are commonly boiled down into a soup. These examples serve as reminders that cultural differences in disease management and medication usage may vary greatly throughout the world.

There are a number of international organizations dedicated to neurologic care globally. Several member organizations within the United Nations, including the WHO, the World Bank, and the United Nations Children's Fund have played roles in policy matters related to neurologic disease. Nongovernmental organizations provide care for people with neurologic disease in some of the least developed regions globally. Similarly, the World Federation of Neurology is an international organization of country-level neurologic societies composed of community-based and academic neurologists, who have successfully come together in the past to tackle international issues within neurologic disease.

SUMMARY

Neurologic disease has a tremendous impact on human illness and mortality globally. Despite the challenges in quantifying the burden of neurologic disease and assessing its impact on populations throughout the world, several points are clear. Neurologic diseases, whether they are primary or secondary, more frequently cause disability than death. This has been an obstacle to research employing common measures of disease impact. Additionally, disparities in incidence, diagnosis, disease management, and outcomes for patients in different geographic and socioeconomic sectors proffer a unique signature on the global burden of neurologic disease.

SUGGESTED READINGS

Chan CC, Chuang KJ, Chien LC, et al. Urban air pollution and emergency admissions for cerebrovascular diseases in Taipei, Taiwan. *Euro Heart J.* 2006;27:1238–1244.

Chin J, Mateen F. Central nervous system tuberculosis: challenges and advances in diagnosis and treatment. *Curr Infect Dis Rep.* 2013;15:631–635.

Cruz-Flores S, Rabinstein A, Biller J, et al. Race-ethnic disparities in stroke care: the American experience: a statement for healthcare professionals from the American Heart Association/American Stroke Association Council on Stroke. *Stroke.* 2011;42:2091–2116.

Cushman M, Cantrell RA, McClure LA, et al. Estimated 10-year stroke risk by region and race in the United States: geographic and racial differences in stroke risk. *Ann Neurol.* 2008;64(5):507–513.

Elkind MS. Epidemiology and risk factors. *Continuum.* 2011;17:2013–2032.

Feigin VL, Forouzanfar MH, Krishnamurthi R, et al. Global and regional burden of stroke during 1990-2010: findings from the Global Burden of Disease Study 2010. *Lancet.* 2014;383:245–255.

Feigin VL, Lawes CM, Bennett DA, et al. Worldwide stroke incidence and early case fatality reported in 56 population-based studies: a systematic review. *Lancet.* 2009;8(4):355–369.

Gupta I, Guin P. Communicable diseases in the South-East Asia Region of the World Health Organization: towards a more effective response. *Bull World Health Organ.* 2010;88(3):199–205.

Horton R. GBD 2010: understanding disease, injury, and risk. *Lancet.* 2012;380:2053–2054.

Janca A, Aarli JA, Prilipko L, et al. WHO/WFN Survey of neurological services: a worldwide perspective. *J Neurol Sci.* 2006;247:29–34.

Johnston SC, Hauser SL. Neurological disease on the global agenda. *Ann Neurol.* 2008;64:A11–A12.

Johnston SC, Mendis S, Mathers CD. Global variation in stroke burden and mortality: estimates from monitoring, surveillance, and modelling. *Lancet Neurol.* 2009;8(4):345–354.

Lloyd-Jones D, Adams RJ, Brown TM, et al. Heart disease and stroke statistics—2010 update: a report from the American Heart Association. *Circulation.* 2010;121(7):e46–e215.

Mateen F. Neurocritical care in developing countries. *Neurocrit Care.* 2011;15:593–598.

Mateen F. Neurology and international organizations. *Neurology.* 2013;81: 392–394.

Mateen F, Carone M, Haskew C, et al. Reportable neurologic diseases in refugee camps in 19 countries. *Neurology.* 2012;79:937–940.

Mateen F, Martins N. A health systems constraints analysis for neurologic diseases: the example of Timor-Leste. *Neurology.* 2014;82:1274–1276.

McWilliams JM, Meara E, Zaslavsky AM, et al. Differences in control of cardiovascular disease and diabetes by race, ethnicity, and education: U.S. trends from 1999 to 2006 and effects of medicare coverage. *Ann Intern Med.* 2009;150(8):505–515.

Moshi MJ, Kagashe GA, Mbwambo ZH. Plants used to treat epilepsy by Tanzanian traditional healers. *J Ethnopharmacol.* 2005;97(2):327–336.

Pruss-Ustun A, Corvalan C. *Preventing Disease Through Healthy Environments. Towards an Estimate of the Environmental Burden of Disease.* Geneva, Switzerland: World Health Organization; 2006.

Sheikh AL. Pharmaceutical research: paradox, challenge, or dilemma. *East Mediterr Health J.* 2006;12:42–49.

Sousa RM, Ferris CP, Acosta D, et al. Contribution of chronic diseases to disability in elderly people in countries with low and middle incomes: a 10/66 Dementia Research Group population-based survey. *Lancet.* 2009;374:1821–1830.

Strong K, Mathers C, Leeder S, et al. Preventing chronic diseases: how many lives can we save? *Lancet.* 2005;366:1578–1582.

Trimble B, Morgenstern LB. Stroke in minorities. *Neurol Clin.* 2008;26(4): 1177–1190.

Woo J, Ho SC, Lau S, et al. Prevalence of cognitive impairment and associated factors among elderly in Hong Kong Chinese aged 70 years and older. *Neuroepidemiology.* 1994;13:50–58.

World Health Organization. *Neurological Disorders: Public Health Challenges.* Geneva, Switzerland: World Health Organization; 2006.

Yusuf S, Reddy S, Ounpuu S, et al. Global burden of cardiovascular diseases. *Circulation.* 2001;104:2746–2753.

Zhao D, Liu J, Wang W, et al. Epidemiological transition of stroke in China: twenty-one-year observational study from the Sino-MONICA-Beijing Project. *Stroke.* 2008;39:1668–1674.

Zumla A, Raviglione M, Hafner R, et al. Current concepts: tuberculosis. *N Engl J Med.* 2013;368:745–755.

Signs and Symptoms in Neurologic Diagnosis: Approach to the Patient 2

Lewis P. Rowland and Timothy A. Pedley

INTRODUCTION

Accurate diagnosis is essential to making rational decisions about management and, increasingly in neurology, instituting effective treatment. Making a neurologic diagnosis requires a systematic approach to the patient. The history and physical examination provide essential but complementary data that form the cornerstone of diagnosis. Of course, laboratory tests are often necessary and are sometimes pathognomonic. They should, however, be ordered selectively, and students have to learn which tests are appropriate and when to order them. It is therefore necessary to know which diagnostic possibilities are reasonable considerations for a particular patient. Overreliance on laboratory tests and technology and analysis that is uninformed by clinical reasoning and appropriate differential diagnosis can lead to errors and delay suitable therapy.

The clinical data obtained by a careful history and physical examination are used to address three questions:

1. **What anatomic structures of the nervous system are affected?** Progressive weakness in the legs, for example, could be due to a myopathy, peripheral neuropathy, or myelopathy, but each of these possibilities can usually be distinguished by the presence or absence of characteristic symptoms and signs. It is usually not possible to make a specific etiologic diagnosis without knowing what parts of the nervous system are affected. In addition, knowing the probable anatomic substrate restricts the etiologic possibilities. Thus, making an accurate *anatomic diagnosis* should be the first step in analyzing a neurologic disorder. Clues to identifying the anatomic sites of neurologic disorders are discussed in the following section and later in this chapter.
2. **What is the nature of the neurologic disorder?** An individual patient's symptoms and signs usually cluster into broad syndromes or categories of disease: developmental disorder, peripheral neuropathy, acute encephalopathy, progressive dementia, parkinsonian syndrome, cerebrovascular syndrome, and so on. A syndromic diagnosis assists in clarifying the nature of the disease and further focuses on possible specific causes.
3. **What are the most likely etiologies for the patient's illness?** These derive from consideration of the anatomic and syndromic diagnoses in light of the tempo (rapid or slow) and course (fixed from onset, steadily progressive or stepwise) of the illness, relevant past history and family history, and whether there is evidence of systemic involvement. The possible etiologies listed in order of probability constitute the differential diagnosis, and this in turn determines which laboratory tests need to be ordered and the urgency with which the evaluation should proceed.

An experienced clinician is likely to deal with these three questions simultaneously or even reverse the order. To take an obvious example, if a patient suddenly becomes speechless or awakens with a hemiplegia, the diagnosis of stroke is presumed. The location is then deduced from findings made upon examination, and both site and pathophysiologic process are ascertained by computed tomography (CT) or magnetic resonance imaging (MRI). If there are no surprises in the imaging study (e.g., demonstration of a tumor or vascular malformation), further laboratory tests might be considered to determine the precise cause of an ischemic infarct.

NEUROLOGIC HISTORY

A reliable and accurate history is essential. This should be obtained directly from the patient if at all possible, but it is often necessary to verify the patient's account or obtain additional information by speaking with relatives or close friends. This is particularly true if the illness has compromised the patient's mental function or use of language. Particular attention should be paid to the onset of symptoms, the circumstances in which they occurred, and their subsequent evolution. Have any of the symptoms resolved? Have similar or different neurologic symptoms occurred previously? To avoid errors, it is important that the physician avoids leading questions and clarifies what the patient means by ambiguous terms, such as *dizziness* or *weakness*. Discrepancies and inconsistencies in details obtained by different examiners are often the source of diagnostic confusion and must be resolved.

NEUROLOGIC EXAMINATION

Performing an accurate neurologic examination (Chapter 3) requires practice and skill. It begins with observations made as the patient enters the room and continues while his or her history is being obtained. Abnormalities of gait and balance may be readily apparent. The manner in which the patient tells the history may reveal confusion, aphasia, or memory loss. It is preferable to record exact observations (what the patient actually did or did not do) rather than interpretations that may introduce ambiguity. It is best to perform the examination in a standard sequence to avoid omissions, although it may be necessary to modify this based on the patient's condition and ability to cooperate. The usual order is mental status, cranial nerves, strength and coordination, sensation, and reflexes.

The specific nature of different symptoms and findings obtained from examination are reviewed in the following chapters. Other considerations that influence diagnosis are briefly described here.

IDENTIFYING THE SITE OF DISORDER

Aspects of the patient's history may suggest the nature of the disorder; specific symptoms and signs suggest the site of the disorder.

Cerebral disease is implied by seizures or by focal signs that may be attributed to a particular area of the brain; hemiplegia, aphasia, or hemianopia are examples. Generalized manifestations of cerebral disease are seizures, delirium, and dementia.

Brain stem disease is suggested by cranial nerve palsies, cerebellar signs of ataxia of gait or limbs, tremor, or dysarthria. Dysarthria may be the result of incoordination in disorders of the cerebellum itself or its brain stem connections. Cranial nerve palsies or the neuromuscular disorder of myasthenia gravis may also impair speech. Ocular signs have special localizing value. Involuntary movements suggest *basal ganglia disease*.

Spinal cord disease is suggested by spastic gait disorder and bilateral corticospinal signs, with or without bladder symptoms. If there is neck or back pain, a compressive lesion should be suspected; if there is no pain, multiple sclerosis is likely. The level of a spinal compressive lesion is more likely to be indicated by cutaneous sensory loss than by motor signs. The lesion that causes spastic paraparesis may be anywhere above the lumbar segments.

Peripheral nerve disease usually causes both motor and sensory symptoms (e.g., weakness and loss of sensation). The weakness is likely to be more severe distally, and the sensory loss may affect only position or vibration sense. A more specific indication of peripheral neuropathy is loss of cutaneous sensation in a glove-and-stocking distribution.

Neuromuscular disorders and *diseases of muscle* cause limb or cranial muscle weakness without sensory symptoms. If limb weakness and loss of tendon jerks are the only signs (with no sensory loss), electromyography and muscle biopsy are needed to determine whether the disorder is one of motor neurons, peripheral nerve, or muscle. The diseases that cause these symptoms and signs are described in later sections of this book.

AGE OF THE PATIENT

The symptoms and signs of a stroke may be virtually identical in a 10-year-old, a 25-year-old, and a 70-year-old patient, but the diagnostic implications are vastly different for each patient. Some brain tumors are more common in children, and others are more common in adults. Progressive paraparesis is more likely to be due to spinal cord tumor in a child, whereas in an adult, it is more likely to be due to multiple sclerosis. Focal seizures are less likely to be fixed in pattern and are less likely to indicate a specific structural brain lesion in a child than in an adult. Myopathic weakness of the legs in childhood is more likely to be caused by muscular dystrophy than polymyositis; the reverse is true in patients older than 25 years. Muscular dystrophy rarely begins after age 35 years. Multiple sclerosis rarely starts after age 55 years. Hysteria is not a likely diagnosis when neurologic symptoms start after age 50 years. These ages are somewhat arbitrary, but the point is that age is a consideration in some diagnoses.

GENDER SPECIFICITY

Only a few diseases are gender-specific. X-linked diseases (e.g., Duchenne muscular dystrophy) occur only in boys or, rarely, in girls with chromosome disorders. Among young adults, autoimmune diseases are more likely to affect women, especially systemic lupus erythematosus and myasthenia gravis, although young men are also affected in some cases. Women are exposed to the neurologic complications of pregnancy and may be at increased risk of stroke because of oral contraceptives. Men are more often exposed to the possibility of head injury.

ETHNICITY

Stating the race of the patient in every case history is an anachronism of modern medical education. In neurology, race is important only when sickle cell disease is considered. Malignant hypertension and sarcoidosis may be more prevalent in blacks, but whites are also susceptible. Other diseases are, however, more common in certain ethnic groups: Examples include Tay–Sachs disease, familial dysautonomia, and Gaucher disease in Ashkenazi Jews; familial inclusion body myopathy in Iranian Jews; familial Creutzfeldt–Jakob disease in Libyan Jews; thyrotoxic periodic paralysis in Japanese and perhaps other Asians; nasopharyngeal carcinoma in Chinese; sickle cell disease in people of African descent; Marchiafava–Bignami disease in Italian wine drinkers; and hemophilia in descendants of the Romanovs. Ethnicity is rarely important in diagnosis.

SOCIOECONOMIC CONSIDERATIONS

In general, social deprivation leads to increased mortality, and the reasons are not always clear. Ghetto dwellers, whatever their race, are prone to the ravages of alcoholism, drug addiction, and trauma. Impoverishment is also accompanied by malnutrition, infections, and the consequences of medical neglect. For most other neurologic disorders, however, race, ethnicity, sex, sexual orientation, and socioeconomic status do not affect the incidence.

Inequities of access affect prevention, early diagnosis, and treatment of neurologic conditions in the United States. Globally, poor countries suffer from tragedies of malnutrition, parasitic diseases, and AIDS. Embargos have become popular political weapons but impose punishment on innocent civilian adults and children. It is not just poverty that impedes access; rural areas in any continent may have limited access to imaging or advanced therapeutic technology (a problem that has generated helicopter transfer and telemedicine). The many millions of U.S. citizens without health insurance have limited access.

TEMPO OF DISEASE

Seizures, strokes, and syncope are all abrupt in onset but differ in manifestation and duration. Syncope is the briefest. There are usually sensations that warn of the impending loss of consciousness. After fainting, the patient begins to recover consciousness in a minute or so. A seizure may or may not be preceded by warning symptoms. It may be brief or protracted and is manifested by alteration of consciousness or by repetitive movements, stereotypical behavior, or abnormal sensations. A stroke due to cerebral ischemia or hemorrhage strikes "out of the blue" and manifests as hemiparesis or other focal brain signs. The neurologic disorder that follows brain infarction may be permanent, or the patient may recover partially, or completely, in days or weeks. If the signs last less than 24 hours, the episode has traditionally been called a *transient ischemic attack* (TIA). Sometimes, it is difficult to differentiate a TIA from the postictal hemiparesis of a focal motor seizure, especially if imaging shows no lesion and the seizure was not witnessed. Another syndrome of abrupt onset is subarachnoid hemorrhage, in which the patient is struck by a headache that is instantaneously severe and sometimes followed by loss of consciousness.

Symptoms of less than apoplectic onset may progress for hours (intoxication, infection, or subdural hematoma), days (Guillain–Barré syndrome), or longer (most tumors of the brain or spinal cord). The acute symptoms of increased intracranial pressure (ICP) or brain herniation are sometimes superimposed on the slower progression of a brain tumor. Progressive symptoms of brain tumor may be punctuated by seizures. Heritable or degenerative diseases tend to progress slowly, becoming most severe only after years of increasing disability (e.g., Parkinson disease, Alzheimer disease, essential tremor).

Remissions and exacerbations are characteristic of myasthenia gravis, multiple sclerosis, and some forms of peripheral neuropathy. Bouts of myasthenia tend to last for weeks at a time; episodes in multiple sclerosis may last only days in the first attacks and then tend to increase in duration and leave more permanent residual neurologic disability. These diseases sometimes become progressively worse without remissions.

The symptoms of myasthenia gravis vary in a way that differs from any other disease. The severity of myasthenic symptoms may vary from minute to minute. More often, however, there are differences in the course of a day (usually worse in the evening than in the morning but sometimes vice versa) or from day to day.

Some disorders characteristically occur in bouts that usually last minutes or hours but rarely longer. Periodic paralysis, migraine headache, cluster headaches, and narcolepsy are in this category. To recognize the significance of these differences in tempo, it is necessary to have some knowledge of the clinical features of the several disorders.

DURATION OF SYMPTOMS

It may be of diagnostic importance to ask patients how long they have been having similar symptoms. Long-standing headache is more apt to be a migraine, tension, or vascular headache, but headache of recent onset is likely to imply intracranial structural disease and should never be underestimated. Similarly, a seizure or drastic personality change for days or months implies the need for CT, MRI, and other studies to evaluate possible brain tumor or encephalopathy. If no such lesion is found or if seizures are uncontrolled for a long time, perhaps video-electroencephalographic monitoring

should be carried out to determine the best drug therapy or surgical approach.

MEDICAL HISTORY

It is always important to know whether there is any systemic disease in the patient's background. Common disorders, such as hypertensive vascular disease or diabetes mellitus, may be discovered for the first time when the patient is examined for neurologic symptoms. Because they are common, these two disorders may be merely coincidental, but, depending on the neurologic syndrome, either diabetes or hypertension may actually be involved in the pathogenesis of the neural signs. If the patient is known to have a carcinoma, metastatic disease is assumed to be the basis of neurologic symptoms until proven otherwise. If the patient is taking medication for any reason, the possibility of intoxication must be considered. Cutaneous signs may point to neurologic complications of von Recklinghausen disease or other phakomatoses or may suggest lupus erythematosus or some other systemic disease.

SUGGESTED READINGS

Amarenco P. "Telethrombolysis": stroke consultation by telemedicine. *Lancet Neurol.* 2008;7(9):763–765.

Blumenfeld H. *Neuroanatomy Through Clinical Cases.* Sunderland, MA: Sinauer Associates; 2002.

Brust J. *Current Diagnosis and Therapy in Neurology.* New York: Lange Books, McGraw-Hill; 2007.

Campbell WW. *DeJong's The Neurological Examination.* Philadelphia: Lippincott Williams & Wilkins; 2005.

DeMyer WE. *Technique of the Neurologic Examination.* 5th ed. New York: McGraw-Hill; 2004.

Epstein AM. Health care in America—still too separate, not yet equal. *N Engl J Med.* 2004;351(6):603–605.

Fuller G. *Neurological Examination Made Easier.* 4th ed. New York: Elsevier; 2008.

Marshall RS, Mayer S. *On Call Neurology.* New York: Elsevier; 2007.

Navarro V. Race or class versus race and class: mortality differences in the United States. *Lancet.* 1990;336:1238–1240.

Vastag B. Health disparities report [abstract]. *JAMA.* 2004;291(6):684.

Wang DZ. Telemedicine: the solution to provide rural stroke coverage and the answer to the shortage of stroke neurologists and radiologists [editorial]. *Stroke.* 2003;34:2957.

Woolf SH, Johnson RE, Fryer GE Jr, et al. The health impact of resolving racial disparities: an analysis of US mortality data. *Am J Public Health.* 2008;98(9) (suppl):S26–S28.

The Neurologic Examination 3

James M. Noble

INTRODUCTION

Of all the chapters presented in this book, the one most likely to remain nearly 100% relevant, if not also accurate, decades from now is that of the neurologic examination. Clearly new handheld and bedside examination tools continue to and will make implementation and interpretation of the exam different over time, but the general principles and approach have not substantially changed for decades and are unlikely to substantially differ over a trainee's career. This chapter should be used in close conjunction with the guidelines for developing the neurologic history that are presented in Chapter 2.

One must recognize that an exhaustively comprehensive neurologic examination cannot be defined within the scope of this chapter. Instead, this chapter provides a set of guiding principles on which the neurologic examination can be built to support, augment, or refute findings suggested by the neurologic history.

A thorough neurologic history and examination are designed to accurately localize neurologic dysfunction and develop a differential diagnosis of the most likely disease processes. The history and physical should be used in a complementary manner rather than as stand-alone devices. With the patient or family members as informants and physician as historian, the neurologic history should be a logical, linear story told such that the history leads sensibly into the examination, without many surprises to the examiner or another physician hearing about the encounter.

SETTING GOALS OF EXAMINATION VERSUS NEUROLOGIC TESTS

As is the case in many professions, there are likely as many ways to accomplish an examination as there are examiners performing the examination itself. However, some approaches may be far more efficient, understandable, and sensible than others. There are numerous neurologic examination techniques known, sufficient to comprise a substantial book, let alone a single chapter.

The approach presented here is intended to demystify the reasons and the methods by which a comprehensive neurologic examination is accomplished. It is well recognized that most trainees in neurology will not go on to become professionals or practitioners in advanced neurology. However, it must be the case that every graduate of any medical training program has a sufficient confidence, skill level, and knowledge base to begin to develop a proficient neurologic examination for each context it requires.

This chapter attempts to strike a balance between the comprehensive examination that neurologist can accomplish, with the base expectation of all practitioners being able to approach a neurologic patient without trepidation, concern, misdiagnosis, or more importantly, a missed urgent neurologic diagnosis. A comprehensive neurologic examination is one typically done in the context of a focused neurologic assessment. All physicians should be familiar with how to accomplish each of these tests in the appropriate context. However, it is likely good practice to perform a screening neurologic examination in any patient encounter seen in a general medical inpatient or outpatient assessment, as major neurologic diseases can likely be identified through such an approach or alternatively provide a good point of reference should the patient subsequently develop neurologic problems. Elements suggested to be included in comprehensive and screening neurologic examinations are provided in Table 3.1. An in-depth review of the coma examination is provided in Chapter 18.

A TOP-DOWN APPROACH

The manner in which the neurologic examination should be presented follows a structured approach that facilitates a complete and comprehensive neurologic examination. Anatomically and generally speaking, this follows a "top-down" approach, which begins with the mental status examination and cranial nerve examination at the top with the head, followed by the body including motor and deep tendon reflex examinations, followed by sensory and coordination exams, and finally gait. The neurologic examination can be temptingly approached in an excitedly, symptom-focused manner, but this method introduces the risk of unintentionally forgoing an essential element of the neurologic examination. This approach is also designed to improve efficiency during the first pass assessment, to be followed by more focused and detailed examination based on relevant initial findings.

HELPING YOUR PATIENT THROUGH THE NEUROLOGIC EXAMINATION

There is a good chance that a neurologic examination performed on a patient may be perceived the most comprehensive medical examination the patient has experienced, with many elements even seemingly strange during the exam. Accordingly, some patients may unintentionally embellish the examination or even provide nonsensical physical exam responses, in an effort to impress their physician during demonstration of their neurologic system. In some cases, it may be helpful to tell the patient very specifically what is going to be done, as well as the expected outcome or finding, particularly when a normal examination is expected based on a benign relevant history. On the other hand, it may be more worthwhile to provide no instructions to patients with psychogenic disorders who are also prone to purposeful embellishment or feigned signs. It is certainly allowable for an unexpected neurologic examination finding to be repeated on a patient after coaching for expected findings has been given.

SOFT VERSUS HARD NEUROLOGIC EXAMINATION FINDINGS

In some cases, the examiner may be inclined to search unnecessarily for an abnormality on neurologic examination based on history provided or alternatively identify a subtle unexpected finding referred to as a "soft" neurologic sign. Commonly, faces may be asymmetric, strabismus persists into adulthood, memory may be imperfect, or

TABLE 3.1   The Neurologic Exam

Comprehensive	Screening
Mental Status	
Level of alertness	Level of alertness
Language function (fluency, comprehension, repetition, and naming)	Appropriateness of responses
Memory (short-term and long-term)	Orientation to date and place
Calculation	—
Visuospatial processing	—
Abstract reasoning	—
Cranial Nerves	
Vision (visual fields, visual acuity, and funduscopic examination)	Visual acuity
Pupillary light reflex	Pupillary light reflex
Eye movements	Eye movements
Facial sensation	—
Facial strength (muscles of facial expression and muscles of facial expression)	Facial strength (smile, eye closure)
Hearing	Hearing
Palatal movement	—
Speech	—
Neck movements (head rotation, shoulder elevation)	—
Tongue movement	—
Motor Function	
Gait (casual, on toes, on heels, and tandem gait)	Gait (casual, tandem)
Coordination (fine finger movements, rapid alternating movements, finger-to-nose, and heel-to-shin)	Coordination (fine finger movements, finger-to-nose)
Involuntary movements	—
Pronator drift	—
Tone (resistance to passive manipulation)	—
Bulk	—
Strength (shoulder abduction, elbow flexion/extension, wrist flexion/extension, finger flexion/extension/abduction, hip flexion/extension, knee flexion/extension, ankle dorsiflexion/plantar flexion)	Strength (shoulder abduction, elbow extension, wrist extension, finger abduction, hip flexion, knee flexion, ankle dorsiflexion)
Reflexes	
Deep tendon reflexes (biceps, triceps, brachioradialis, patellar, Achilles)	Deep tendon reflexes (biceps, patellar, Achilles)
Plantar responses	Plantar responses
Sensation	
Light touch	One modality at toes—can be light touch, pain/temperature, or proprioception
Pain or temperature	—
Proprioception	—
Vibration	—

From Gelb DJ, Gunderson CH, Henry KA, et al. The neurology clerkship core curriculum. *Neurology.* 2002;58(6):849–852.

balance may be less than pristine especially with advancing age. Slight asymmetries, particularly in the face, are commonly found during neurologic examination in normal individuals and likely do not hold much clinical relevance. Some reviews have suggested that soft neurologic signs including poor motor coordination, sensory perception, and motor sequencing may occur in as much as half of all healthy individuals. Understanding when to strongly consider finding, simply record it, or to discard it altogether often takes a very skilled examiner cautiously interpreting each finding. However, this need not take a fully refined neurologist to make such decisions, particularly if one approaches the neurologic examination with a clear sense of the likely localization as suggested by a fully developed history. When findings are found in isolation, particularly without a clear connection to the history that has just been developed, it may be justifiable to recognize and record the finding but not necessarily dwell on it. A neurologist typically will take these findings into consideration and tailor, repeat, or perform additional elements of the neurologic examination to assure that the finding is simply an isolated finding (and perhaps even a normal variation) or a relevant new finding. In addition, it is certainly acceptable upon discovery of a subtle neurologic finding to reask a newly relevant history, which may not have otherwise been apparent despite a seemingly comprehensive initial history.

DESCRIPTIONS VERSUS IMPRESSIONS

Whenever possible, a description of neurologic findings should be included in the examination rather than the synthesis of the findings themselves. Changes in the neurologic examination day to day can be remarkably subtle and only a descriptive neurologic examination may reveal such changes and sometimes only in retrospect. For example, a patient may be described on a series of examinations by different examiners to be lethargic, yet substantially different levels of stimulus are required to result in the same response from the patient, ranging from light tactile to verbal stimuli to other more rigorous stimuli applied yet inadequately described. Such a failure to accurately describe patient, particularly in an era increasingly reliant on effective care transitions, can jeopardize true understanding of neurologic disease progression in both inpatient and outpatient practices.

POSITIONING THE PATIENT (AND EXAMINER)

Appropriately positioning the patient and examiner is an important first step in many aspects of the neurologic examination and is described in each of the relevant sections. Positioning of the patient and examiner is important throughout the patient encounter, including initial moments of a patient encounter when developing patient trust and rapport. At the bedside, correct position with each component of the neurologic examination is essential in both effective and efficient performance and interpretation of the neurologic examination. Positioning is most relevant not only to assessment of visual fields, funduscopy, strength, and deep tendon reflexes but also during times of potential injury during provocative or potentially risky elements of the exam, such as pull testing for assessing postural stability, or even when standing a patient affected by frailty or imbalance suggested in the history or during gross inspection.

REPEATED EXAMINATIONS ARE THE KEY TO IMPROVE SKILL

Skill and ability in any medical field, or in any field involving adult learners, likely relates to the prior volume of experience had in that field. A well-described cognitive heuristic suggests that adult learners transition from a hypothetical deductive approach in learning to a more automated approach through progressive experience.

A set of rich and deeply understood normative values can be determined for simple yet essential components of the neurologic examination, including determining the relatively normalcy of interpersonal interactions, conversations, or even walking. With this set of normal findings, an examiner can begin to dissect a subtly abnormal neurologic examination into its principal components. By the same measure, one cannot know how an abnormal funduscopic examination or tandem gait may appear until having seen normal findings in many patients. Although a specific diagnosis, particularly among patients with complicated history, may remain elusive even in the hands of an accomplished neurologist, an accomplished dissection of abnormal findings on the neurologic examination, used in conjunction with the history, can facilitate localization and diagnostic approach.

THE PATIENT EXAMINATION

GENERAL MEDICAL EXAMINATION

All neurologists participate in substantial training in internal medicine, whether in the adult or pediatric setting. Thus, it is expected that any patient with a neurologic disease should have a comprehensive general medical examination performed on them at least once in the course of their initial neurologic assessment. However, it is typically the case that a relatively brief overview of the general medical examination will be included in any neurologic case presentation with only the elements most germane to the neurologic diagnosis presented. For example, description of cardiac and carotid auscultation should be described for a patient presenting with stroke, and a rash should be described in a patient presenting with proximal myopathy.

However, each patient should have a complete and accurate description of the general impression—the essence of the strong first impression each patient may have provided to the examiner. Specific points to mention may include general appearing of wellness, nourishment, habitus, manner of dress, or other related elements. Some of these elements may be reinforced in the mental status examination.

MENTAL STATUS EXAMINATION

In contrast to other elements of the neurologic examination, the mental status examination is composed of a potentially variable set of tasks tailored to each patient. Rather than beginning with the prespecified set of neurologic examination tasks, a far preferable approach is one that aims to develop a description of the function of the cognitive domains based on a set of often interdependent tests. It is difficult, if not impossible, to find any single test that can comprise and completely describe an entire neuropsychological cognitive domain. Instead, many tests map to several cognitive domains and vice versa. In graphical or mathematical terms, the brain expresses its cognitive functions in a series of overlapping domains, conceptually representable as Venn diagrams (Fig. 3.1), which can broadly be broken down into domains of language, memory, attention and executive function, visuospatial function, and processing speed. Predicated on each of these is that the patient has a sufficient level of consciousness in order to participate in the examination.

The neurologic examination should include a standardized assessment of mental status for several reasons. First, any

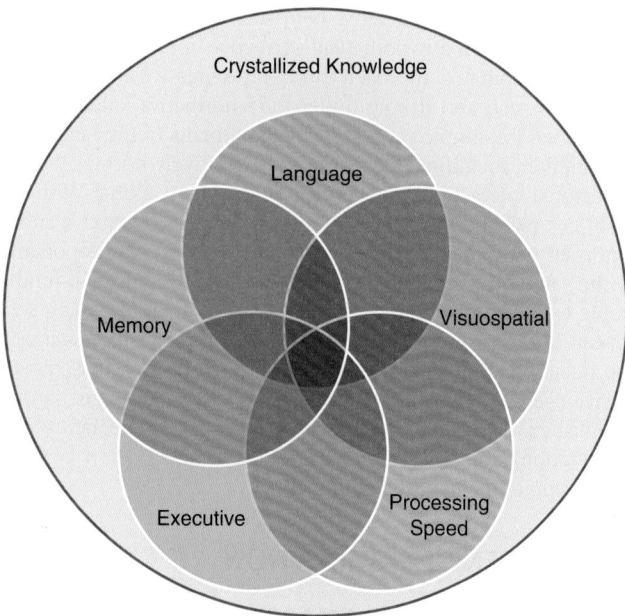

FIGURE 3.1 Conceptual framework for the mental status examination and interpretation. Each of the five principal cognitive domains (language, memory, visuospatial, processing speed, and executive function) are drawn from a series of tests comprising the mental status examination. Relative strengths and weaknesses in each domain may be inferred based on a series of related tests which map potentially to several domains but relatively consistently identify a domain of impairment. The interpretation of each abnormality must be considered within the context of each test, including normative information if known. The relative function of each domain is likely influenced by and superimposed on crystallized knowledge, which conceptually summarizes education, life experiences, and cognitive reserve.

standardized cognitive screening examination will often have been developed in the context of hundreds, if not thousands, of applications and multiple social economic and cultural contexts, making its interpretation more generalizable. Second, at the level of the examiner, use of the same examination repeatedly may give the examiner greater confidence in examination skill and interpretation based on a learned experience of typical or expected responses developed over the course of giving the same test in multiple clinical contexts. Third, most standardized mental status examinations allow for a hierarchical approach to understanding someone's cognitive abilities. For instance, for a task of delayed recall, it is important to understand not only what a patient can freely recall but also what the patient may recognize either through the contextual or categorical clue given for recognition tasks or subsequently through list of forced choices. Using a sequential, hierarchical approach to assessing memory abilities allows for determination of free word retrieval (presumably a harder response) versus recognition (by choices), which are thought to be independent of registration tasks. Finally, serial assessments of an individual patient may require adjustment of exam techniques to avoid the potential effects of learning or practice.

Many caveats apply to interpreting the mental status examination and thus require understanding and how it is devised for each patient, particularly how it is tailored to each cultural context. For instance, education and lifetime cognitive abilities play a strong role in one's ability to interpret both normal and abnormal mental status examination findings. Prior to each mental status examination, developed within social history must be a clear sense of someone's educational history, literacy, and thus likely expected performance on mental status testing. As a point of comparison, more formal neuropsychological testing will take into consideration two norms: the person's premorbid intellectual capacity as determined by intelligence quotient as well as comparison to normative values based on peer performance matched to age, education, and potentially primary language.

It is important during the mental status examination not only to record whether or not the patient correctly answers the question but also the actual response itself. Much can be learned through some elements of the mental status examination which can, to some degree, be influenced by complex factors including mood. For instance, a patient may be considered to be disoriented to time and place through simple scoring, but when review of the actual answers suggest an exactly wrong response to every single question (including nonsensical dates, often in the future), it might suggest an element of feigned or embellished neurologic examination.

Determining Alertness

The entirety of the formal mental status testing is predicated on a patient being fully awake, alert, and able to engage the examiner. Presuming this is the case, neurologic examination as described in the following section is relevant in such patient. Determining a depressed level of alertness is described in Chapter 18 as relates to the examination of coma and brain stem examination.

Tasks of Attention and Concentration

Typical tasks of attention and concentration relate to the ability of a patient to attend and focus any specific, often narrow set of tasks in real time. Typical bedside techniques in assessing concentration include serial subtraction, spelling a five-letter common word backward, or more simply involving stating the months of the year in reverse, days of the week in reverse, or counting from 20 down to 1, always beginning with the most difficult task first. Elements of these examinations are often appropriately interpreted in the context of related domains such as executive function. For instance, the ability of a patient to count down from 20 may reflect the ability to attend to the task, whereas subtracting a series of changing answers may suggest intact or impaired executive or calculation abilities. Other more practical tasks may involve simple addition and subtraction, presuming appropriate levels of literacy and numeracy. Tasks such as making monetary change may not only give one a sense of the patient's calculation abilities but also any degree of functional impairment should a clear impairment emerge. For a patient residing in a major metropolitan area, the ability to appropriately make change at a hypothetical street-side food vendor can be such an example.

Additional tasks of attention and concentration may be more conventionally thought of in conjunction with other cognitive tests, such having a patient register several words to be later recalled, following a three-step command, or drawing a complex figure. As detailed earlier, it is not the performance on a single test that draws concern but rather an overall pattern that may emerge across the sequence of several tests.

Memory Testing

Differing definitions of working, short-, and long-term memory exist, are often used inappropriately in colloquial examination and presentations, and may have differing meanings depending on the person reviewing the examination described by others. A formal description of various forms of memory is provided in summary in Table 30.2. Working memory is generally considered to be the online or in-the-moment memory, such as what may be used when repeating a series of unrelated words or number sequence. Short-term memory involves testing a set of ideas registered with the patient and specifically queried by the examiner after a delay of several minutes. Items not freely recalled but instead recognized from a list (recognition) can be additionally informative. Long-term memory can either represent a more prolonged delay in testing responses to the task of recollection, or in some other tasks may instead represent long-term general or autobiographical knowledge. It is important to document the content asked to be remembered and the duration of time until asking for retrieval of information. Recall is entirely predicated on the patient's ability to register several items to be recalled, and this begins with preparing patient for this task in a minimally distracting environment.

In its simplest form, memory testing involves having a patient remember several items in the context of an examination to be recalled several minutes later. Certainly, this is an important element of memory testing but is just one method of assessing memory among many. This manner of testing memory, in conjunction with several other tests, such as time and place orientation, may be highly specific in screening out major cognitive disorders, which may adversely affect health care such as medication compliance. However, it largely serves to only test verbal memory of three unrelated words, and does not take into account nondominant hippocampal function such as visuospatial memory or implicit memory associated with programmed motor tasks.

Ideally, a test of three to five unrelated words, or a brief contextually related phrase (name and address of a fictional person), should be given to a patient to register and subsequently recall. It is most important for the examiner to use a series of words that have been rigorously studied to understand their cultural and socioeconomic norms, can be understandably and simply chosen from categorical clues, which may be given to help with recognition after-the-fact (e.g., "the first word was a color"), can be recognizable from a list of similar words, and is also easily memorable to the examiner who may be giving such an examination many times over the course today.

Verbal memory can also be tested through repetition and recall of a simple story. This can be particularly effective in identifying the patient with a confabulatory amnestic syndrome (i.e., Korsakoff syndrome) rather than anterograde amnesia (i.e., Alzheimer disease). For example, a patient may be given a brief story to recall such as "Johnny had a red tricycle. Billy liked Johnny's red tricycle and stole it one day. Billy broke Johnny's red tricycle after he took it. When Johnny found out Billy had stolen the tricycle, he got very upset." A patient with a typical amnestic disorder may respond to this task by providing a few or a restricted set of elements germane to the story with the remainder unrecalled. In contrast, a patient with a confabulatory amnestic disorder may provide the initial basic elements of the story correctly but then provide an idiosyncratic thread far beyond the initial details provided in the story. Moreover, such a patient may begin with the same thread when testing the story on a follow-up examination, only to give a remarkably different yet linear story thereafter.

Nonverbal short-term memory is thought to be localizable to the nondominant hippocampus or most typically the right side in right-handed individuals. Testing visuospatial memory in the office can be somewhat difficult but can be accomplished. For instance, one can hide three objects within a room telling the examinee each time where each object is placed, to be registered and recounted several minutes later. A hospital corridor can be used as a visuospatial memory task by having a patient and examiner pass through a specific path, to be led by the patient immediately to demonstrate registration, and again several minutes later to demonstrate recollection.

Long-term memory likely engages separate circuits, widespread across the cerebrum, and is better categorized as public or autobiographical memory rather than a true function of working or recent memory. This memory type can also be easily conflated and is dependent on knowledge of worldly events and life experiences. Testing long-term memory can be approached by using a standardized set of questions which should be well known to the individual, such as sequential ordering of recent presidents. However, this can be easily tailored to a patient who may lack such conventional knowledge. For example, an elderly sports enthusiast can be tested for his knowledge of recent sports events important to him and hierarchically working back to biographical events which must be corroborated by an informant. A test of recent worldly events likely more reflects function of the same recent memory circuits being tested by recollecting three unrelated words, given the need to both register and recall worldly information gathered through the news.

Language

Language is composed of seven principal components: (1) fluency, (2) prosody, (3) repetition, (4) naming, (5) comprehension, (6) reading, and (7) writing. A language examination is not complete without each of the seven elements. The pattern of dysfunction related to these seven components allows the neurologist to diagnose and classify all types of aphasia (Table 3.2).

Fluency and prosody can often be determined through development of the neurologic history before turning to formal examination. Prosody is the musical component of language, the sing-song nature, and cadence that allows one to understand the nature of a stated expression. For example, prosody allows one to discern when a declarative sentence is stated versus a question. In contrast to normal prosody, aprosodic patients may be identified among those with major neuropsychiatric disorders including schizophrenia or in patients with advanced or untreated Parkinson disease. Fluency is a quality of speech pertaining to the ability of a patient to express him- or herself without hesitation or disruption spontaneously as well as during formal testing. Dysfluent speech may have hallmarks of patient frustration or an unexpected halting pattern, such as that seen in a suddenly acquired Broca area stroke, or progressively developed in a patient with progressive nonfluent aphasia form of frontotemporal dementia. Dysfluent speech is distinct from thought blocking, which is described within the elements of psychiatric examination.

Repetition may be assessed by asking a patient to repeat a simple, understandable phrase and further tested by a longer more complex sentence if the history and examination warrant further exploration. When such a phrase cannot be repeated, repetition of single words should be attempted.

Naming also should be approached in a hierarchical manner when testing knowledge of names of presented objects and virtual pictures. Standard images/figures comprise most neurologic screening examinations but differ among each exam. Objects to be named should be ubiquitous, well-known to the patient, and have elements that offer an opportunity to test parts and not just the sum of the object. This approach may reveal difficulty in describ-

TABLE 3.2   Types of Aphasia

Aphasia Subtype	Fluency	Comprehension	Repetition	Localization
Expressive (motor, Broca)	Effortful speech with paraphasic errors[a] and agrammatism[b]; mutism in severe cases	Normal	Impaired[c]	Frontal opercular region of inferior frontal gyrus (Broca area) in the dominant hemisphere
Receptive (sensory, Wernicke)	Fluent speech, mostly nonsensical in content; frequent paraphasic errors	Impaired	Impaired[c]	Posterior-superior temporal region (Wernicke area) in the dominant hemisphere
Global aphasia (combination of expressive and receptive)	Effortful speech with paraphasic errors[a] and agrammatism[b]; mutism in severe cases	Impaired	Impaired[c]	Both inferior frontal gyrus and posterior-superior temporal region in the dominant hemisphere
Conduction aphasia	Normal	Normal	Impaired	Due to lesions of the arcuate fasciculus connecting Broca and Wernicke areas in the dominant hemisphere

[a]*Literal (phonemic) paraphasic error*: an error made by substituting a similar-sounding word for another (i.e., "pat" substituted for "cat"). *Verbal (semantic) paraphasic error*: an error made by substituting words with similar meaning (i.e., "cup" for "bottle").

[b]*Agrammatism* or *telegraphic speech*: Language content of spontaneously uttered sentences is condensed, missing many filler words, such as definite articles and sometimes verbs.

[c]Normal repetition in the setting of expressive, receptive, or global aphasia denotes transcortical expressive, transcortical receptive, and transcortical mixed aphasia subtypes.

ing low-frequency relative to high-frequency words, as is often seen in disorders like Alzheimer disease. In addition, the naming examination may be tailored to the patient for objects well-known in the context of their life experience or profession, such as images of a set of carpenter's tools. A number of forms of specific categorical dysnomic aphasias are known to exist, such as color dysnomia, and should be tested in the appropriate clinical context.

Comprehension is often tested as a three-step command. As with a memory task, the patient should be prompted to expect the task rather than occurring as a surprise. Numerous three-step commands have been published but should be easily understandable, contextually appropriate, and whenever possible use commonly available objects so that the same task can be repeated by a single examiner in multiple clinical contexts.

Reading testing begins with a patient reading a simple sentence aloud and offers an opportunity to test for comprehension by having the patient act on the sentence provided. Should a patient have difficulty reading a sentence (e.g., "Close your eyes."), then the examiner should move on to simple phrase or a single word if the phrase cannot be read. In a similar approach, writing should begin with an instruction for the patient to write a complete sentence. If this cannot be accomplished, the patient should be asked to write a simple dictated sentence. If this is further not possible, the patient should be asked to write or sign his or her name, although this principally tests for praxis or dysgraphia. Such highly learned written tasks, and even a signature, likely localize to the nondominant frontal lobe as a programmed motor task, or "n-gram," rather than a function of spontaneous written language.

Executive Function

Executive function can be demonstrated through several types of tasks highlighting the abilities or limitations of the frontal lobe or its principal subcortical circuits. Broadly speaking, these can be thought of as tasks which demonstrate the ability of a patient to both maintain and shift between specific tasks or concepts, as demonstrated by examinations of either language or physical/motor abilities.

Common tests of executive function involve repetition of a number series in the reverse order in which it was given, complex tasks of addition or subtraction, or sequential tasks performed by the patient in a specific order and manner. Examples of executive tasks involving the hands may be in a standard set of hand movements such as knocking ("fist"), chopping ("edge"), and slapping ("palm") the hand on a table in sequence after being instructed to register the series, also known as the *Luria sequence*.

Tests of praxis may be considered to some degree to be tests of executive function, as a demonstration of ability or limitation in fine movement of the hands or limbs based on frontal lobe function. In contrast to weakness, praxis is the ability of a patient to coordinate and perform a simple or complex set of tasks based on instruction, independent of simple motor abilities. Simple, or ideomotor, tests of praxis involve single motions with contextually independent movements such as the ability of a patient to open and close their hand either to simple instruction or to demonstration. In contrast, ideational tests of praxis instead involve a complex task often with multiple steps of a well-known or overlearned task used in daily life. Examples include demonstration of brushing one's hair, brushing teeth, or blowing out a match. More specific examples for common daily tasks include putting on a coat known as *dressing praxis*.

Visuospatial Function

Visuospatial function is often tested through tasks which require ability to perceive, plan, orient, and synthesize visual images. As is the case for other cognitive tests one might typically think of as specifically testing one domain, visuospatial abilities inevitably may have a basis in other domains including frontal executive function, but are also reliant on memory (how one may be familiar with an object in daily life such as a clock or cube) or language (understanding the contextual basis for an image). The simplest of drawing tasks may limit the influence of frontal executive function on the ability of a patient to draw but must be taken in consideration relative to other nonvisuospatial tasks in order to fully interpret visuospatial test findings. Visuospatial tasks often involve drawing intersecting pentagons, a circle with a tangentially touching square, or cubes, among other figures. More complex figures used in common practice, such as a clock drawing, can be very helpful in demonstrating visuospatial function but may be also prone to a number of cognitive difficulties including planning, memory, as well as visual field deficits. As is the case with language, visuospatial function may be significantly impacted by a patient educational history, in particular simple literacy. Individuals who may not have held a writing implement for significant period of time in their life may have difficulty with relatively simple drawing tasks.

Higher Order Cognition

Higher order cognitive functions are often placed alongside executive functions but likely represent a separate set of cognitive abilities which are more often predicated on experiential knowledge and social norms. Tests of higher order function include interpretation of proverbs or common sayings and judgment as demonstrated by patient's response to simple hypothetical situations.

The neurologist should select a few proverbs for such tasks, which are culturally sensitive, relatively ubiquitously known, and interpretable by both the patients and the examiner in the response. Using a relatively narrow set of appropriate phrases will also give the examiner better experience in anticipating a typical response from patients. Examples for proverb interpretation include "two heads are better than one," "people in glass houses should not throw stones," and "don't count your chickens before they hatch," or one of many similar phrases. Examples of hypothetical situations to be provided for testing judgment may include asking for patient's response to discovering an unmailed fully addressed letter, or steps taken when facing a simple public emergency. As with any test, these must be interpreted with consideration of education and culturally based normative responses.

Key Psychiatric Examination Elements

The key elements of a conventional psychiatric examination will also be germane to many patients with neurologic disease, particularly those with an acquired cognitive disorder. The patient's reported symptoms of mood are recorded as mood, whereas the examiner's interpretation of the patient's mood is better characterized as affect. These can both be matched or unmatched in the context of examination and both are important distinctions to make for later interpretation.

Thought process is an important component of the psychiatric examination and is often discovered either during or in retrospect when the examiner reflects on a simple or challenging interview. Thought processes can be characterized using the following descriptors, which also have graphical corollaries to better conceptualize how conversation transpires (Fig. 3.2). These thought processes are linear, tangential, thought insertions, thought blocking, circumstantial (too many details, meandering but with spontaneous return), circumlocutions (talking around the subject with eventual arrival), and circumferential (talking around the subject without arrival). Thought content is considered the components and characteristics which make up thought processes and include psychotic and nonpsychotic phenomenology. Important psychotic

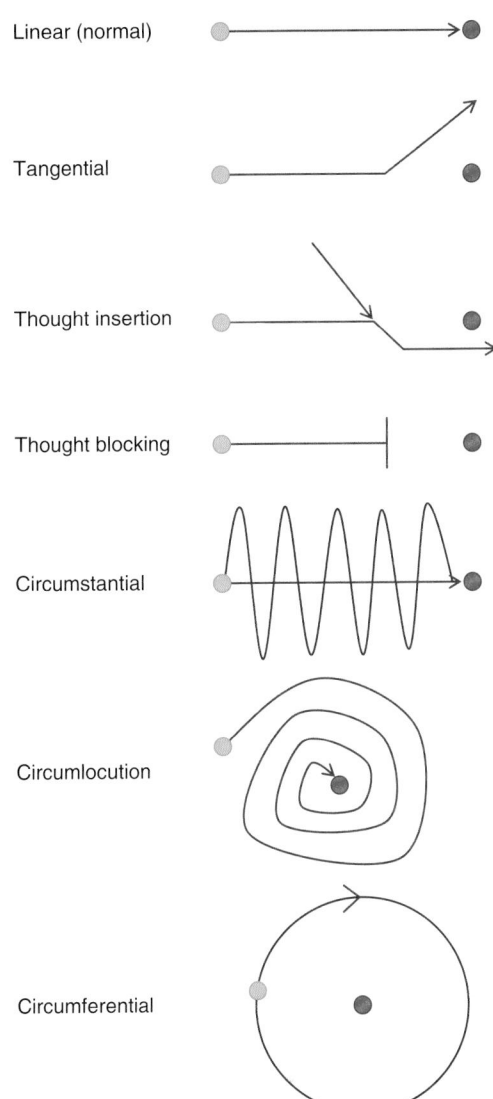

FIGURE 3.2 Graphical representations of thought processes. Starting points are indicated with a *green dot*, final points with a *red dot*. *Lines* represent direction of conversation. (Adapted with permission from Edward R. Norris, MD [personal communication].)

phenomenology either identified during examination or history includes delusions (fixed false beliefs), hallucinations (idiosyncratic, spontaneously perceived visual, olfactory, gustatory, or auditory stimuli), or illusions (misperceived complex visual or auditory perceptions based on normal and present environmental cues). Other types of abnormal thought content include ideas of reference, sense of presence, or other thought idiosyncrasies.

CRANIAL NERVE EXAMINATION

The cranial nerve examination is an essential component of the neurologic examination that requires skilled training and expertise to interpret appropriately. However, when approaching the examination methodically, based on its principal components, rapid interpretation of the individual and localizing findings can be accomplished.

As is the case with the remainder of the general medical and neurologic examinations, the cranial nerve examination should be described in such a manner that only the elements of examination that were performed are those recorded. For instance, one may not assess olfaction in every neurologic examination, and it is unnecessary to state when it was not done. The examiner should demonstrate the findings again in a top-down approach beginning with findings identified in an ordinal manner, presenting the cranial nerves from lowest to highest number (begin with cranial nerve [CN] I and end with CN XII). CN function should be described in the context of the test performed rather than the nerves themselves (e.g., "eye movements fully intact" rather than "CNs III, IV, and VI intact").

Cranial Nerve I (Olfactory Nerve)

Assessment of olfaction is important in certain neurologic diseases including frontal lobe tumor, head trauma, and degenerative disease, among others. Testing is comprised of commonly recognizable smells which are not caustic, toxic, or excessively potent in strength. Examples of commonly used, recognizable, and available smells include coffee, vanilla, and mint. These can be stored within a neurologist's equipment bag using plastic film canisters (although these are increasingly more difficult to find) or opaque contact lenses cases (so that the patient may not see the item to be smelled in advance). To test for smell, with the patient's eyes closed, have a patient fully close one of his or her nares and ask to take a deep breath with the item to be smelled placed immediately below the nares.

Cranial Nerve II (Optic Nerve)

Assessment of CN II includes tests of visual acuity, visual fields, funduscopy, and pupillary light reaction.

VISUAL ACUITY

Most standard physician examination kits include a Snellen card for testing visual acuity. One of the most important steps prior to doing a visual acuity examination is to know the exact distance at which the vision is to be tested. This is typically printed on the card and varies from 14 inches for near vision to 6 ft for far vision (as a surrogate for a standard 20-foot distance examination). Begin by instructing the patient to put the hypothenar eminence of his or her hand against the bridge of the nose such that the eyes completely obstructed by the palm of the hand. If the patient is simply instructed to cover his or her eye with hand, there is a tendency of using the fingers to cover the eye and therefore the possibility of peeking through these fingers in order to improve or embellish the examination findings. Related to this issue, the examiner should always hold a visual acuity card to avoid a patient's temptation to bring the card closer to the face and conflate the exam.

VISUAL FIELDS

This examination should begin with the examiner standing at an arm's distance from the patient. Testing visual fields at a farther distance may only test central vision rather than demonstrate any frank field deficits as is desired by this test. Using the instructions previously described for covering the eye, the examiner should close their ipsilateral eye when facing the patient (the examiner should close his or her own left eye while examining the patient's left eye). With arms held aloft, the examiner should attempt to assess monocular visual fields at the left and right of meridian as well as above and below the equator of each tested eye. Generally speaking, the bedside visual examination test should be used to

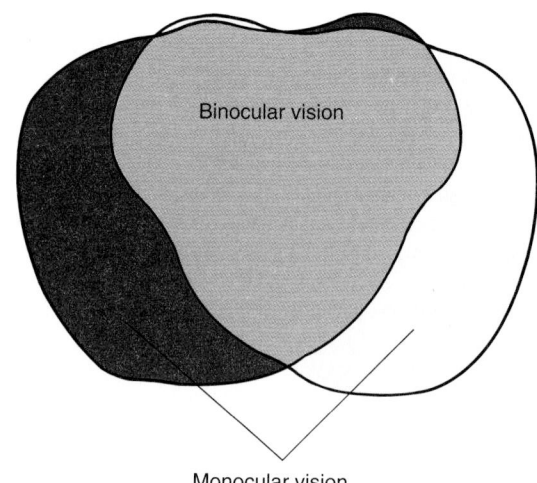

FIGURE 3.3 Visual fields. (From Bickley L. *Bates' Guide to Physical Examination and History-Taking*. 11th ed. Philadelphia: Wolters Kluwer Health/Lippincott Williams & Wilkins; 2013.)

discover quadrantanopsias, binocular visual field loss, or homonymous hemianopsias. Any smaller field deficits would be far more difficult to identify on bedside examination and may require formalized visual field testing as is done in an ophthalmologist office (Fig. 3.3).

Methods of testing visual field include counting fingers within each of these quadrants, identifying a statically held hand with a wiggling finger, or moving a hand into the field being tested. Despite their routine inclusion on examination, most bedside techniques are poorly sensitive but highly specific to identifying visual field deficits.

FUNDUSCOPY (VIA DIRECT OPHTHALMOSCOPY)

An essential element of the neurologic exam, and one which is marvelously distinguished as being the only visualized aspect of the neuraxis and can demonstrate both elements of chronic systemic disease and acute neurologic emergency, yet one which is far too frequently neglected out of examiner discomfort, lassitude, or disinterest, is funduscopy. The quality of the remainder of the exam and history as performed by a referring physician, in the eyes of a consulting neurologist, may be predicated on inclusion or at least attempt of this aspect of the exam for this reason, particularly when called for by the diagnosis. Two main barriers may persist and limit the interest of a physician on performing this exam: perceived difficulty of use of the equipment and simple availability. Two forms of direct ophthalmoscopes exist for the bedside exam: conventional and panoptic. The conventional heads have the benefit of bright light for magnification, portability, and relatively ubiquitous presence of these heads in many clinics, but are limited by perceived difficulty of use perhaps related to partial views of the optic disc even in optimal patients. The conventional heads are available in a normal size, as well as a smaller "micro" version, which offers even greater portability but faces the same limitations. The panoptic head offers the benefit of a wide field of view, but is limited by expense and lower light intensity.

The essential aspects to be identified in funduscopy include characteristics of the optic nerve head including the cup, margins, and vessels as well as the immediately visualizable

FIGURE 3.4 Funduscopic view (right eye). (From Bickley L. *Bates' Guide to Physical Examination and History-Taking*. 11th ed. Philadelphia: Wolters Kluwer Health/Lippincott Williams & Wilkins; 2013.)

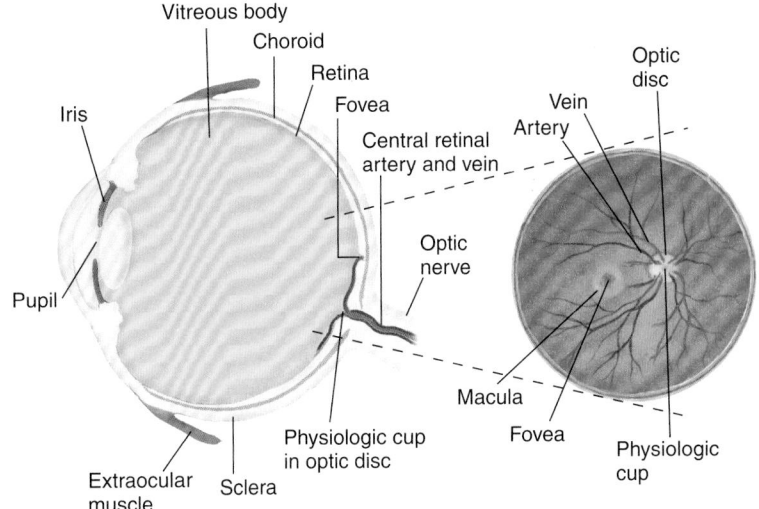

and relevant retinal components including the macula/fovea (Fig. 3.4). Visualizing the retina beyond the width of 2 or 3 optic disc diameters of most patients is particularly difficult by direct ophthalmoscopy.

Care should be taken to describe the color and shape of the disc as well as the cup-to-disc ratio if perceptible. A relative description of vessels can include the quantity and quality including relative diameter, or a suggestion of hypertensive change often described as "copper wiring," or "AV nicking" when the vein appears compressed by a superimposed arteriole. Description of retinopathic changes including color variegations, vascularity, and plaques should be described. Having such an approach will leave more emergent and obvious abnormalities to the end of the focused examination and description.

PUPILLARY LIGHT RESPONSE

Two components of the pupillary response should be considered within each patient. These include the response of the ipsilateral and contralateral eyes to both direct and consensual light responses. While asking a patient to fixate on the examiner's face or another suitable target several feet away, using a light of sufficiently bright intensity, a narrowly focused beam is shown into a single eye with the examiner assessing for the ipsilateral and contralateral responses.

The swinging flashlight (Fig. 3.5) is another component of this test in which the initially examined eye is provided direct light followed by a rapid movement of light to be shown into the contralateral eye followed by a movement back to the initially tested eye. The object of this examination is to identify either a lack of direct response (in the case of severe optic neuropathy) or paradoxical dilatation to direct response (in less apparent cases, termed the relative afferent pupillary defect) as the swinging flashlight is shone back into an eye affected by an optic neuropathy.

In addition, pupillary asymmetries should be described and assessed in both a lit and a darkened environment with the use of tangential light (to assess pupillary size with minimal afferent stimulus).

Extraocular Movements (Cranial Nerves III [Oculomotor Nerve], IV [Trochlear Nerve], and VI [Abducens Nerve])

The elements of testing extraocular movements include demonstration of limitations of excursion of either individual or consensual gaze, rapidity of saccades, preservation of smooth pursuits, and the control of multiple types extraocular movements, both large and small excursions, as well as slow and fast movements.

Prior to any testing of eye movements, the patient should be carefully examined for any spontaneous eye movements when

FIGURE 3.5 Swinging flashlight test. (From Bickley L. *Bates' Guide to Physical Examination and History-Taking*. 11th ed. Philadelphia: Wolters Kluwer Health/Lippincott Williams & Wilkins; 2013.)

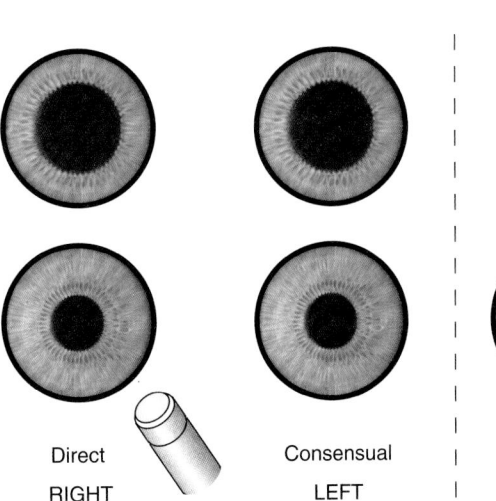
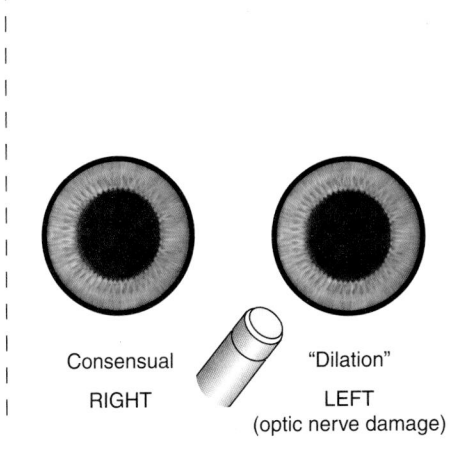

Direct
RIGHT

Consensual
LEFT

Consensual
RIGHT

"Dilation"
LEFT
(optic nerve damage)

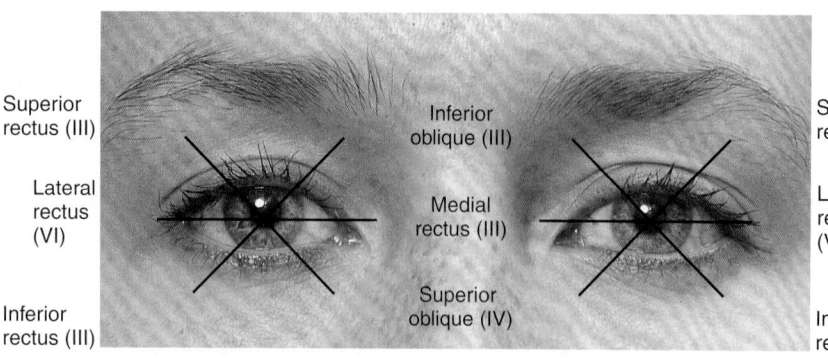

Superior rectus (III)

Inferior oblique (III)

Superior rectus (III)

Lateral rectus (VI)

Medial rectus (III)

Lateral rectus (VI)

Inferior rectus (III)

Superior oblique (IV)

Inferior rectus (III)

FIGURE 3.6 Extraocular movements. (From Bickley L. *Bates' Guide to Physical Examination and History-Taking.* 11th ed. Philadelphia: Wolters Kluwer Health/Lippincott Williams & Wilkins; 2013.)

focusing on a fixed near target placed several feet before the patient. Although this technique may demonstrate spontaneous eye movement abnormalities including so-called square wave jerks, finer perception of such movements may be identified during funduscopic examination which magnifies subtle spontaneous eye movements otherwise missed during casual visual inspection.

To test for restriction of gaze, the patient (Fig. 3.6) should be asked to follow the finger or a similar near target at approximately an arm's length distance from the patient moving through a typical H pattern. Care should be taken not to move through these movements too quickly; otherwise, saccadization of pursuits may occur and potentially mislead the development of the oculomotor examination.

To test for rapidity of saccadic eye movements at a similarly near distance, the patient should be asked to fixate on the examiner's nose while both hands are placed in mid-position between the patient and examiner at about a shoulder width apart. With one hand wiggling (to indicate a target) and the patient staring at the examiner, the patient is instructed to look at the wiggling stimulus, followed by instructions to return to gaze back to the nose. After a series of repeated assessments, the rapidity of saccadizations as well as the ability to accurately fixate on the lateral and midline targets can be assessed using this technique. An alternating bright and dark cloth tape to stimulate optokinetic nystagmus can be an additionally helpful tool in potentially identifying lateralized saccadic eye movement deficit.

To further test for the accuracy of fixation and the ability to maintain fine, fixed, and accurate extraocular movements, the patient can be asked to additionally follow a moving target through an unpredictable series of movements in either the horizontal or vertical planes. A consistent need to provide a corrective saccade in all, or a single direction, provides a localizable deficit.

Cranial Nerve V (Trigeminal Nerve)

Principally, the trigeminal nerve serves to provide facial sensations including touch, temperature, and pinprick of the face and anterior elements of the mouth. Vibratory sensations applied to the face likely reflect neck vibratory sensory function, which is seldom if ever absent on examination and thus cannot be discerned from facial sensation. Joint position sense may only be evident in the jaw and rarely if ever demonstrably found.

As is the case for sensory testing within the torso and limbs, the goal of the sensory examination is to identify the modality of sensory deficit and thus the potential tracts and nerve fiber types involved against the pattern of sensory deficits identified on examination (Fig. 3.7). Patterns include laterality and segmentation in the face. Palpating the face (as well as within the mouth) can be useful in trying to identify trigger points in patients with suspected trigeminal neuralgia.

The fifth nerve also controls the muscles of mastication including the masseter and temporalis. Demonstrating weakness of these muscles may be identified through gross testing of the jaw opening and closure but rarely identified on exam outside of severe muscular weakness. Palpation of a tender temporomandibular joint or identifying crepitus may be useful in assessing a patient with headaches; this may be done by palpating the joint while the patient opens and closes the jaw.

Cranial Nerve VII (Facial Nerve)

The goal of testing the seventh nerve is to identify specific patterns of weakness which may be evident at rest, volitional action, or through unintentional means such as laughter. Although many examiners tend to jump to specific movements to demonstrate either segmental or unilateral weakness of the face, one of the most effective means of identifying facial weakness is through simple inspection, including critical appraisal during the interview. Flattened nasolabial folds will be extinguished by forced movements but may reveal low tone as a presenting sign in acute ischemic stroke or even Bell palsy. Specific facial movements that should be tested include brow raising, forced eye closure including assessment of "burying the eyelashes," smiling, pursing the lips, and puffing the cheeks. Although patients may be able to demonstrate these functions on their own, assessment of force can be made by

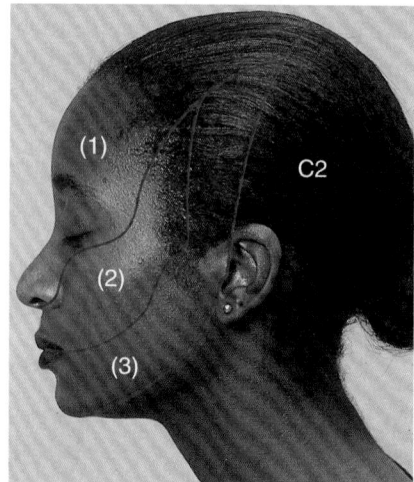

FIGURE 3.7 Dermatomes of the face and head. *(1)*, *(2)*, and *(3)* correspond to divisions of the trigeminal nerve. (From Bickley L. *Bates' Guide to Physical Examination and History-Taking.* 11th ed. Philadelphia: Wolters Kluwer Health Lippincott Williams & Wilkins; 2013.)

the examiner by pulling on any of the muscles being tested one side against the other.

Testing for unilateral loss of taste perception may be helpful in assessing the localization of a Bell palsy. To test for taste, take a commonly perceived recognizable flavor, such as salt or sugar, which are also conveniently typically on hand in most physician office practices or hospital-based settings. Place a small amount of this into a small cup with water and stir with a cotton-tipped applicator. With the patient's eyes closed and tongue protruded, attempt to paint the salty or sweet solution on the side of suspected facial paresis. The patient should be instructed not to draw his or her tongue into the mouth until asked whether or not he or she can taste the applied mixture. Upon demonstration or confirmation that no taste is perceived, the patient is then allowed to draw the tongue into the mouth and swirl around the fluid, and presumably, the taste will be perceived by the normal, contralateral side of the tongue unaffected by the facial paresis.

Cranial Nerve VIII (Vestibulocochlear Nerve)

The bedside examination of the CN VIII typically focuses on hearing but may include additional testing for the patient complaining of dizziness. Testing for hearing includes relatively crude screening measures to be done at the bedside beginning with perceptions of hearing grossly as simply assessed through the interview by the examiner's vocal volume required. Additional tests include using the 512 Hz (or similarly high tone) tuning fork for the Weber test for lateralized hearing loss (Fig. 3.8) and the Rinne test to identify the typical perception of air conduction being longer than bone conduction of sound (Fig. 3.9).

Additional tests include whispering a number into the patient's ear to be then repeated by the patient, or audible hand movements including lightly rubbing the fingertips, escalating to flicking the fingernail, and then snapping. Clearly, such testing cannot supplant more formal audiography. For the severely hearing impaired, history development and examination may be aided by placing the stethoscope earbuds into the patient's ears, with the examiner speaking into the diaphragm.

Vestibular testing in the dizzy patient should focus on attempting to identify central versus peripheral localizations of vertigo. Specific tests to apply to any such patient include the Dix–Hallpike maneuver, head impulse nystagmus test, and the Fukuda marching test, all of which will help to distinguish localization.

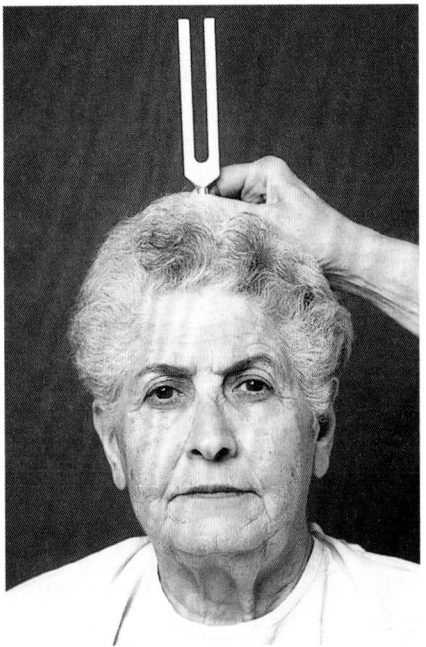

FIGURE 3.8 Weber hearing testing for lateralization of hearing. (From Bickley L. *Bates' Guide to Physical Examination and History-Taking*. 11th ed. Philadelphia: Wolters Kluwer Health/Lippincott Williams & Wilkins; 2013.)

The Lower Cranial Nerves Involved in Speech (IX [Glossopharyngeal Nerve], X [Vagus Nerve], and XII [Hypoglossal Nerve])

Speech, or the articulation of language, can be very helpful in localizing a neurologic disorder. Table 3.3 reviews phonemes of speech and typical neurologic localization. The patient should be asked to speak each of these phonemes with particular attention paid to whether a singular or grossly abnormal speech pattern evident.

Additional testing includes asking the patient to open his or her mouth to assess symmetry in raising the palate (Fig. 3.10), assessment of phonation for vagal nerve abnormalities, and protrusion of the tongue in one direction or another to suggest hypoglossal dysfunction.

FIGURE 3.9 Rinne hearing testing for air > bone conduction. **A:** Bone conduction; once sound extinguishes. **B:** Air conduction is tested. (From Bickley L. *Bates' Guide to Physical Examination and History-Taking*. 11th ed. Philadelphia: Wolters Kluwer Health/Lippincott Williams & Wilkins; 2013.)

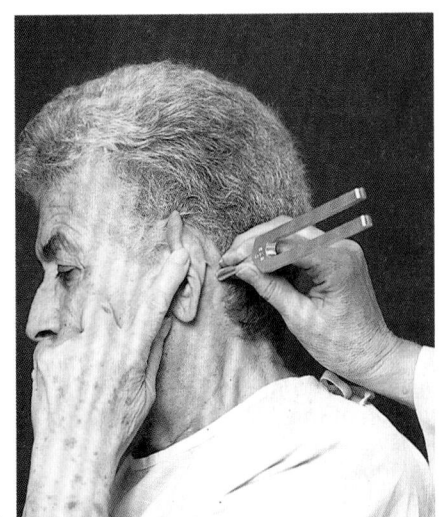

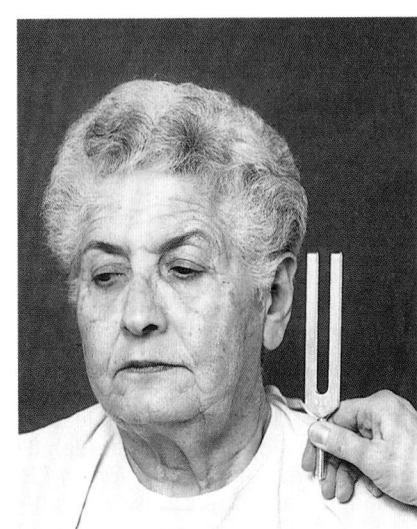

A

B

TABLE 3.3	Phonemes Tested for Patterns of Dysarthria
Phoneme	**Neurologic Localization**
Labial sounds: "ma," "pa"	CN VII
Pharyngeal/guttural sounds: "ga" and "ka"	CN IX, X
Lingual sounds: "la," "ta"	CN XII
Bland dysarthria (all sounds similarly involved)	Corticobulbar tracts to subcortical
Additional Speech Patterns	
Scanning or "metronomic" speech	Cerebellar
Dysphonic (hoarse) voice	CN X

CN, cranial nerve.

Of note, a patient with a seventh nerve paresis may give the false impression of having an ipsilateral hypoglossal dysfunction simply because of the formation of the shape of the mouth. Thus, in patients with facial nerve weakness having tongue protrusion tested, the examiner should begin by forcibly opening the mouth in a symmetric fashion such that the tongue is allowed to exit the mouth in an unobstructed manner.

Cranial Nerve XI (Accessory Nerve)

The spinal accessory nerve has two principal functions including shoulder shrug by the trapezius muscle and head turning by the sternocleidomastoid muscles. Forcibly testing each of these movements may be of lower yield than simply observing shoulder shrug, which may demonstrate either low tone or slow or clumsy movement in a patient presenting with hemiparesis. Although frequently tested and included in neurologic examinations, head turning and shoulder shrug may only rarely be focally affected and thus infrequently provides additional information to the examination above and beyond the history and other findings on examination.

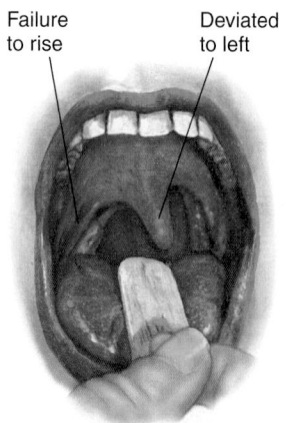

Failure to rise   Deviated to left

FIGURE 3.10 Examination of palate/uvula elevation to command. Weakness on the right leads to a deviation of the uvula to the left (unaffected side). (From Bickley L. *Bates' Guide to Physical Examination and History-Taking.* 11th ed. Philadelphia: Wolters Kluwer Health Lippincott Williams & Wilkins; 2013.)

MOTOR EXAMINATION

The motor examination has several principal components, including inspection, palpation, tone, power, and drift testing and other tests for identifying subtle lateralized motor deficit.

Inspection is an essential element of the neurologic examination particularly for a patient being assessed for the first time. Relatively straightforward diagnoses are often missed by failing to place the patient into a gown. Inspection may identify focal or global patterns of atrophy, fasciculations, or rashes which may be germane to muscular disorders. In determining the presence of fasciculations, it is often necessary to use a tangential light or observe subtle movements in the muscles affecting the overlying hair. Palpation of the muscles is indicated in a patient presenting with weakness or chronic pain, seeking to identify trigger points, but may be additionally helpful in other conditions, such as chronic low back pain in discerning musculoskeletal from neurogenic pain.

Tremor may also be identified to casual inspection or more formally during strength, tone, and coordination testing. Tremor should be described in each limb using the following features: its relative frequency (fast vs. slow), context in which it appears (with action [including specific actions if relevant], rest, posture, or multiple contexts), the consistency with which it appears during the examination (how frequently it is present), the severity of the movements (ranging from mild to disabling), and the quality of the movements themselves (ranging from sinusoidal and monotonous to irregular and chaotic or myoclonic).

Of all the components of the neurologic examination, muscle tone testing is one that requires particular attention to nuance and is learned principally through practice when working alongside a skilled examiner. Tone of the neck, arms, and legs should be assessed in all patients. Tone testing begins by moving a limb through several planes of motion simultaneously to prevent the patient from either contributing or diminishing tone in a volitional manner. To facilitate tone, the patient should be instructed to perform distracting tasks, such as contralateral movements, or even a complex arithmetic question, simply to further diminish the influence of volitional control of tone. Tone abnormalities may be static (rigidity), velocity-dependent with a sudden release at high speeds and extremes of joint flexion/extension (spasticity), or velocity-dependent without sudden changes (paratonia or *gegenhalten*— "holding against").

Drift testing is an essential component of the motor examination because through its subtle nature, it may be one of the few highly reliable and easily identifiable findings in the early presentation of hemiparesis such as may be seen with stroke. Drift testing is accomplished by having a patient either sitting or lying in bed, with hands outstretched before the patient, palms facing upward. With eyes closed for approximately 10 seconds, the patient's hand position should remain static. Pronation may be demonstrable but so may be an altitudinal drift such that the hand does not pronate but moves in either an upward or downward or even a variable vertical direction. Drift testing in the foot involves bringing the leg off the bed and an approximate 30 degrees angle and with the patient's eyes closed instructing them to maintain that position for approximately 10 seconds. Any drift including a drop of the leg backed onto the bed suggests a positive finding. Other tests that can be used to detect or confirm the presence of a subtle lateralized motor deficit include the arm roll test (in which the unaffected arm tends to "orbit" the affected, less mobile arm), and the finger tap test (with velocity and amplitude of the finger or toe taps reduced on the affected side).

TABLE 3.4	Medical Research Council Strength Assessment Scale
Strength Rating	**Description**
5	Full power to confrontational testing by the examiner (normal)
4	The examiner is able to overcome the strength of the patient but near full strength remains
3	Sufficient strength to overcome gravity only
2	Flexion possible when out of the plane of gravity
1	Demonstration of muscle contraction but without any demonstrable joint movement
0	No appreciable movement

Motor strength examination, or power testing, is often focally pursued by trainees while dropping other essential elements of the motor examination. In each patient, power testing must be considered in the context of other principal motor components. The score to evaluate all motor examination findings (0 to 5) has been modified over time and may be idiosyncratically applied by differing examiners. The scale often leaves the neurologist to adjust findings using subtleties in the scale such as +/− symbols rather than just relying on numbers as the scale suggests. The definitions of each strength value are listed in Table 3.4.

Several essential elements of the motor examination include testing a single muscle side to side rather than testing an entire side of the patient compared with the other. A direct comparison of each muscle or joint side to side allows for a far more instructive examination and allows subtle asymmetries to be revealed. Correct positioning of the patient and examiner is essential in order to accurately interpret strength. Whenever possible, the examiner's body position should mimic the patient. Muscles being tested for strength should always be at mid position (Fig. 3.11), as at extremes of the joint position may convey inaccurate perception of superb strength or frank weakness. Other references are suggested as an additional guideline for testing each muscle

group in a comprehensive manner, which is beyond the scope of this review.

Additional components of the strength examination may also include an assessment of fatigability as may be seen with myasthenia gravis, or facilitation as may be seen with the Lambert–Eaton myasthenic syndrome. Fatigability may be assessed by having a patient hold up his or her arms aloft for approximately 30 seconds and assess for fatigability when myasthenia is suspected. In contrast, facilitation may be elicited by having a patient's strength tested before and after sustained contraction (e.g. sustained biceps contraction).

Coordination

The coordination examination is used to principally identify abnormalities grossly associated with ataxia and cerebellar dysfunction. Cerebellar examination techniques include assessments of appendicular and axial functions. Appendicular coordination may be demonstrated by asking the patient to extend a pointed index finger to a target provided as far away from the patient as possible, followed by touching a near target such as the nose or chin (preferable for an obviously ataxic patient given the risk for eye injury). Axial coordination may be assessed using a heel-to-shin test, in which the patient places the heel of one foot against the shin of the opposite leg, with it moved vertically several times. Tests of coordination additionally include rapid movements such as finger taps (or more finely demonstrated as an index finger tapping on the thumb interphalangeal joint), rapid alternating movements (flipping the hand over, opening/closing the hand), and heel/toe tapping. These tasks are also essential in patients with suspected movement disorders. Additional coordination testing is comprised within the gait examination listed in the following section.

Gait, Station, and Body Movements

Observation of a patient's gait and station may be the first and importantly impressionistic examination done in the course of a visit as the patient enters from the waiting room, but also the last done as part of a formal examination. The assessment begins with watching casual gait, assessing for stride length and speed, and lateralizing findings such as a shoulder droop, asymmetric arm swing, or leg circumduction, followed by tandem gait, as well as assessments of balance on individual feet if indicated by the clinical context. Special attention should also be given to ability to stand, quality of turns (en bloc or with appropriate, distinct steps), and passage through

FIGURE 3.11 Testing strength. The example of biceps brachialis strength testing is provided to demonstrate the importance of (1) isolation of the muscle being tested, (2) testing force at mid position, and (3) the examiner's own arm similarly positioned to the patient. (From Bickley L. *Bates' Guide to Physical Examination and History-Taking.* 11th ed. Philadelphia: Wolters Kluwer Health/ Lippincott Williams & Wilkins; 2013.)

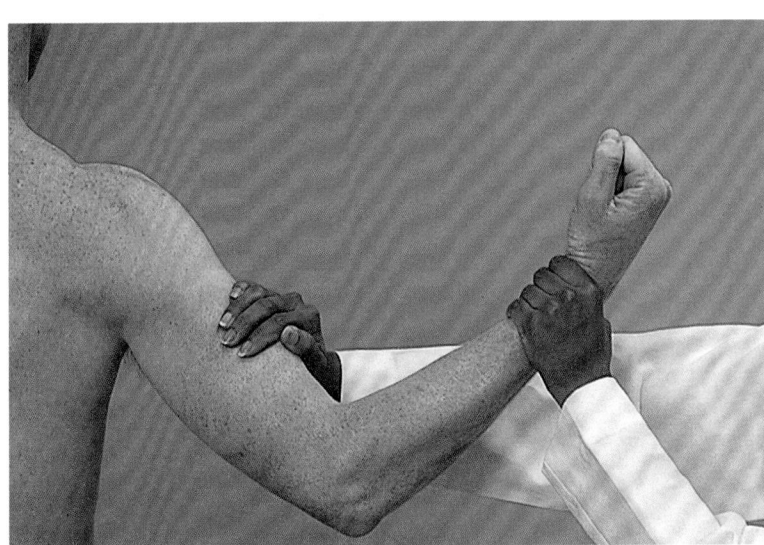

thresholds (doorways). Romberg testing and assessment of postural stability (pull testing) are additional essential exam elements. The Romberg test is performed by having the patient stand feet together, arms outstretched, followed by eye closure once the examiner is able to determine no postural sway, which could be due to other causes such as cerebellar disease. Once eyes are closed, a tendency to sway or fall is indicative of either a defect in vestibular or proprioceptive function. The pull test, which evaluates postural stability, is performed by having the examiner stand behind the patient pulling suddenly backward on the shoulders. In a normal response, the patient makes a quick corrective step to maintain balance. An abnormal response is characteristic of parkinsonism and other diseases that affect postural stability. Toe walking assesses gastrocnemius strength as much as it does test balance, although this may be distinguished when the examiner offers a steadying hand.

Deep Tendon and Other Motor Reflexes

As is the case for motor examination, several essential elements allow for accurate interpretation of the deep tendon reflexes. These include correct positioning of the patient and assessing reflexes for subtle asymmetry. Histories have been written about the various neurologic reflex hammers, and most neurologists have their favorite type. Trainees should identify and use a hammer of heavy mass which allows for consistent low-velocity strike to consistently test the deep tendon reflex, as opposed to a low-mass, high-velocity strike which may be more likely to injure the examiner than elicit the actual response intended.

As is the case for muscle testing, other resources are suggested to identify the optimal locations in which to strike the tendon of each respective deep tendon reflex, but several principal ones are provided in Table 3.5.

TABLE 3.5   Deep Tendon and Other Motor Reflexes

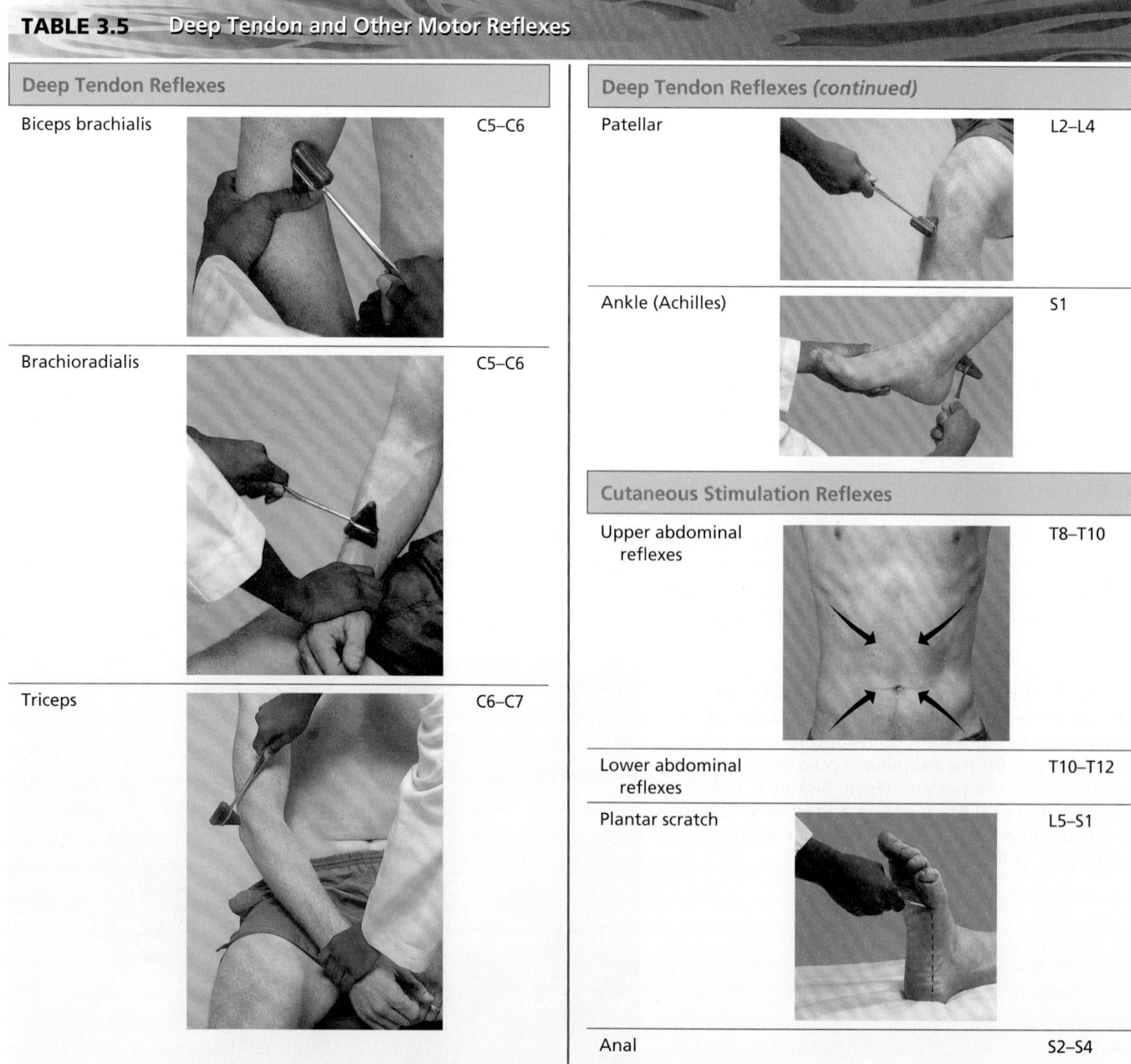

Deep Tendon Reflexes		Deep Tendon Reflexes *(continued)*	
Biceps brachialis	C5–C6	Patellar	L2–L4
Brachioradialis	C5–C6	Ankle (Achilles)	S1
Triceps	C6–C7	**Cutaneous Stimulation Reflexes**	
		Upper abdominal reflexes	T8–T10
		Lower abdominal reflexes	T10–T12
		Plantar scratch	L5–S1
		Anal	S2–S4

Images from Bickley L. *Bates' Guide to Physical Examination and History-Taking*. 11th ed. Philadelphia: Wolters Kluwer Health/Lippincott Williams & Wilkins; 2013.

TABLE 3.6	Deep Tendon Reflex Assessment Scale
4	Pathologic; with sustained clonus elicited and typically light percussion to elicit brisk reflexes
3	Usually pathologic; several beats of clonus or spread to adjacent ipsilateral muscle group or same group tested contralaterally are evident
2	Normal reflex; may have a brisk upstroke but without pathologic features
1	Hyporeflexic; contraction of the muscle as expected but insufficient force to move the joint
0	Hyporeflexic; no movement of the muscle or joint

Trainees are encouraged to test for biceps brachialis, brachioradialis, triceps, patellar, crossed adduction in the legs, and ankle jerks on all newly assessed patients. Finger flexion (Hoffman sign) and plantar scratch response ("Babinski sign" when positive) should be routinely assessed. Additional tests of the tendon reflex including jaw, shoulder, abdominal scratch, and deep abdominal reflexes may be relevant and pursued in the appropriate context (Table 3.6).

Frontal release signs, including snout, glabellar (Meyerson sign), and palmomental signs, are commonly included in neurologic examinations but are of questionable sensitivity and specificity. These are not true reflexes but are instead thought to represent loss of normal cortical circuitry which ordinarily inhibits these "primitive" adaptive responses and can be seen in a host of neurologic disorders including stroke, trauma, and degenerative disease.

SENSORY EXAMINATION

Similar to guidelines suggested in trigeminal nerve assessment, the approach of these sensory examination is intended to identify the nerve fiber type and tract involved, as based on the tested modality. Additionally, patterns of deficit are a principal goal of sensory examination, including laterality, dermatomal distribution (both radicular and peripheral dermatomal patterns), possible spinal level, and determination of a distal or proximal pattern of abnormality (Fig. 3.12). Each domain should be assessed with these in mind.

Essential components of the sensory examination include assessment of light touch (using a cotton-tipped applicator or fine gauze), pinprick (using disposable implement such as a safety pin or a broken wood handle of a cotton-tipped applicator), temperature (actually heat conduction of a metal damper on a low-frequency tuning fork), vibratory sensation, and joint position sense.

One of the great challenges of the sensory examination is determining objective measures within a largely subjective examination. Of all of the modalities included, only joint position sense is truly objective nature. Patients either do not perceive (totally anesthetic), occasionally misperceive (partially anesthetic patient), or exactly misperceive (somatoform presentation) the stimulus.

Light touch, pinprick, and temperature sensations are all assessed in a relatively similar manner by asking the patient whether or not they perceive the intended stimulus. An appropriate reference point may be to provide the stimulus to the cheek (for light touch, temperature, and pin prick sensation) or finger (for vibration) followed by the area being tested and asking the patient to assess whether they are equivalent. Although percentages of difference may be appropriate to determine the nature deficit, other

analogies proportions may be more understandable such as considerations of money ($1.00 v 10c in lieu of percentages).

Vibration sense is crudely assessed by using a 128-Hz tuning fork struck and then with its base applied to the distal most boney prominence available on a patient's limb, such as the interphalangeal joint of the great toe or the tip of the finger (Fig. 3.13). The patient is then asked to assess the presence and persistence of the vibratory stimulus until it is no longer perceived, at which time it may then be applied to the more proximal limb, such as moving from the toes to the finger and asking if the stimulus is still perceived. Two control conditions are established—one within the patient as well as the examiner presuming vibratory sensory function is normal in the examiner.

Joint position sense is performed by having the examiner touch the lateral aspects of the distal interphalangeal joint and asking the patient to close his or her eyes (Fig. 3.14). Using the smallest excursion possible, the patient is asked to perceive the movement (either up or down). The examiner should be careful to record the responses in a patient incorrectly identifying the position change, as consistently wrong answers may suggest a feigned response.

As is the case with vibratory sensory testing, assessment of the patient's sensation should begin with the most distal position and then moved proximally.

Higher order cognitive sensory testing should be included in patients with suspected cognitive impairment but can only be fully interpreted when performed in limbs/hand unaffected by primary sensory loss. These tests are myriad but commonly include assessment of graphesthesia (by drawing a number or letter on a patient's palm while eyes are closed; several training trials may be required), stereognosis (placing a single or similar objects within the palm of the patient such as paperclip/key or various familiar coins), and assessment of perception of simultaneously applied bilateral stimuli (by touching both hands after assessment of primary sensory function).

ADDITIONAL NEUROLOGIC TESTS FOR SPECIAL CONDITIONS

Dix–Hallpike Maneuver

The Dix–Hallpike maneuver is useful to apply to a patient with suspected benign paroxysmal positional vertigo (or a similar vertiginous syndrome) who is actively or very recently affected. Patients in a quiescent period will most likely be asymptomatic and have no demonstrable signs on examination. As demonstrated in the Figure 3.15, the patient begins seated with the head turned about 45 degrees in a single direction. The patient is then positioned supine with the head slightly extended (either hanging off the exam table or supported by the examiner's arm beneath the shoulder). With the patient's eyes open, looking at the examiner's face, the expected positive test will reveal a 5- to 10-second delay in onset of rotatory nystagmus and recapitulation of symptoms. These should resolve after 10 to 30 seconds. A brief vertical nystagmus phase may occur upon sitting. In most cases, the finding should be unilateral and serves as the first step of the Epley maneuver.

The Head Impulse Test

One of the newest bedside diagnostic tests may be better at identifying some brain stem strokes than diffusion-weighted imaging. One component of the head impulse–nystagmus test of skew (HINTS) is the head impulse test. The test can only be applied and appropriately interpreted in a patient acutely symptomatic with

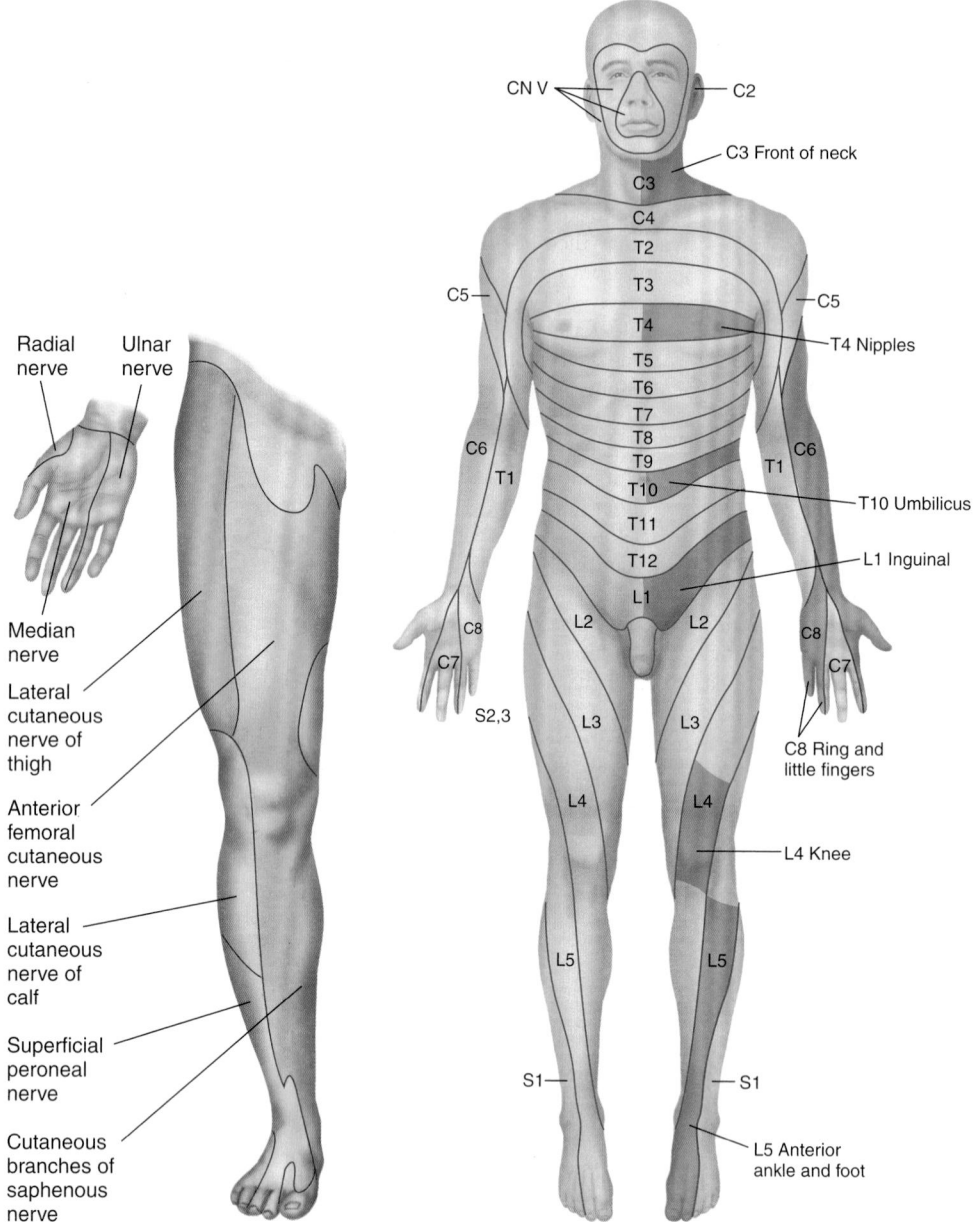

FIGURE 3.12 Dermatome maps. (From Bickley L. *Bates' Guide to Physical Examination and History-Taking*. 11th ed. Philadelphia: Wolters Kluwer Health/Lippincott Williams & Wilkins; 2013.)

vertigo or a suspected related disorder (i.e., cerebellar dysfunction). As demonstrated in the Figure 3.16, the examiner rotates the patient's head about 30 degrees off mid position. With the patient's gaze fixated on the examiner's face, the head is rapidly rotated to midposition. If a catch-up saccade is repeatedly identified, particularly unilaterally, a peripheral vestibular etiology is suggested but must be interpreted in the context of other neurologic examination findings, as ischemic vestibular mimics do occur.

Phalen and Tinel Signs

When considering the diagnosis of carpal tunnel syndrome, in addition to inspection of the hand and assessment of weakness of the opponens, two additional tests can be helpful. The Tinel sign (Fig. 3.17A) involves percussing the course of the median nerve across the wrist, whereas the Phalen sign (Fig. 3.17B) involves keeping a sustained position of flexed wrists. Both the Phalen and Tinel signs seek to recapitulate the patient's specific neurologic syndrome and not simply discomfort. A Tinel sign

can also be identified anywhere a suspected focal neural compression may have occurred, such as across the olecranon or the fibular head.

Straight Leg Raise

The straight leg raise test is used in the context of diagnosing sciatica. As demonstrated in the Figure 3.18 with the patient lying down, the heel of the ipsilateral (affected) leg is raised straight off the bed by the examiner to about 30 to 45 degrees; at its conclusion, the toe may be passively dorsiflexed.

A contralateral (crossed) straight leg raise test may be applied to the opposite leg, only if the affected leg has a positive finding; the contralateral test seeks to recapitulate the affected leg symptoms, still on the affected side. To be considered a positive sign, the patient should report the specific pain (typically lancinating) syndrome which led to the patient to seek attention. The ipsilateral test is highly sensitive but weakly specific, whereas the contralateral test is highly specific but weakly sensitive.

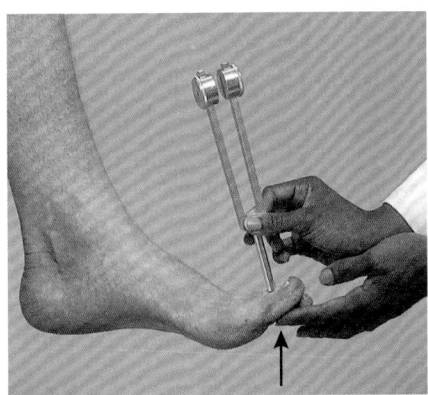

FIGURE 3.13 Vibration sensation testing. (From Bickley L. *Bates' Guide to Physical Examination and History-Taking*. 11th ed. Philadelphia: Wolters Kluwer Health/Lippincott Williams & Wilkins; 2013.)

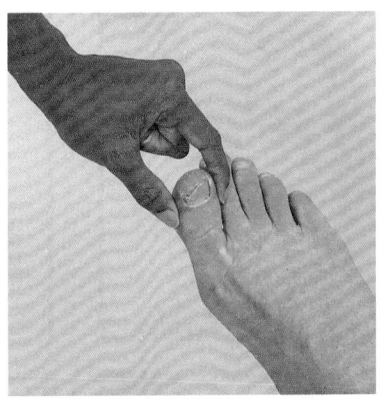

FIGURE 3.14 Joint position sense testing. (From Bickley L. *Bates' Guide to Physical Examination and History-Taking*. 11th ed. Philadelphia: Wolters Kluwer Health/Lippincott Williams & Wilkins; 2013.)

Additional Spinal Reflexes (Male Patients Only)

THE CREMASTERIC REFLEX

The cremasteric reflex tests for the L1–L2 reflex arc and may be considered as a localizing test finding when considering a patient with a lower spinal cord neurologic disorder or as confirmatory reflex examination in patients exhibiting evidence of reflex abnormalities in ipsilateral limb muscle groups. The response will be absent in both central and peripheral neurologic disorders. It is performed by lightly stroking a slightly noxious tactile stimulus proximally along the inner aspect of the thigh (suggest a disposable item such as tongue depressor or hard end of a wooden swab stick). The testicle will normally rise ipsilaterally in conjunction with the applied scratch.

BULBOCAVERNOSUS REFLEX

The bulbocavernosus should be applied specifically to individuals suspected of experiencing acute spinal cord injury. The test involves two potential stimuli: (1) squeezing on the glans penis or clitoris or (2) gently tugging on a Foley catheter while monitoring for anal sphincter contraction; this can be done electrophysiologically or manually. The response will be lost in acute spinal shock.

As is the case with any potentially sensitive element of physical examination, but particularly with these tests, given their involvement of examination of genitalia, inclusion of an examination chaperone, particularly one of the same gender as the patient, should be included in all such examinations.

Tests of Malingering

Myriad tests have been proposed to potentially identify patients with embellished, feigned, or malingered signs. Of those which have been studied to identify their sensitivity and specificity, most are imperfect. However, as detailed earlier, when findings are identified in the context of others on the neurologic examination, some of these additional tests can be useful in the appropriate context. Whenever considering applying these tests, it is most important to do so tactfully, as both the act of applying and interpreting the findings takes a very skilled and advanced examiner to both appropriately perform and inform the patient about their findings with appropriate sensitivity and respect for the patient. Although some may consider these examination components potentially deceitful of the patient, they can be highly instructive, potentially avoid substantial evaluative cost and even morbidity (particularly when they may obviate invasive, unnecessary, or misleading diagnostic measures), and when appropriately disclosed, potentially highly therapeutic. The following are several techniques that can be particularly useful on examination.

FIGURE 3.15 Dix–Hallpike maneuver. *1* and *2* correspond to the first and second positions of the maneuver. (From Fife TD, Iverson DJ, Lempert T, et al. Practice parameter: therapies for benign paroxysmal positional vertigo [an evidence-based review]: report of the Quality Standards Subcommittee of the American Academy of Neurology. *Neurology*. 2008;70:2067–2074.)

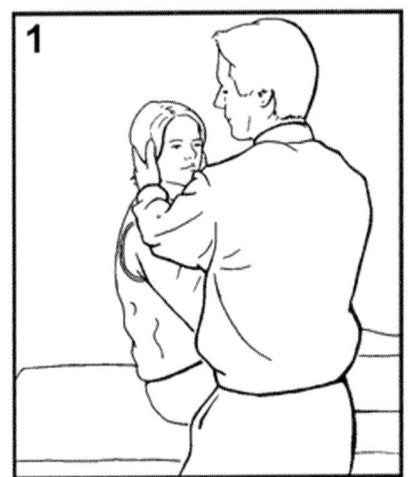

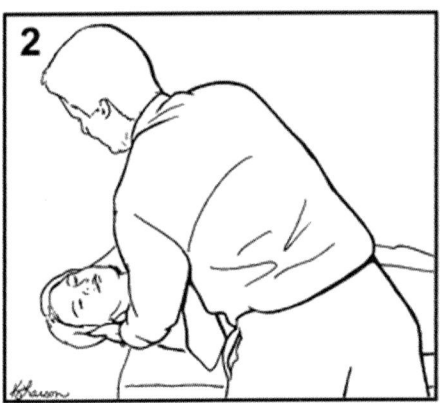

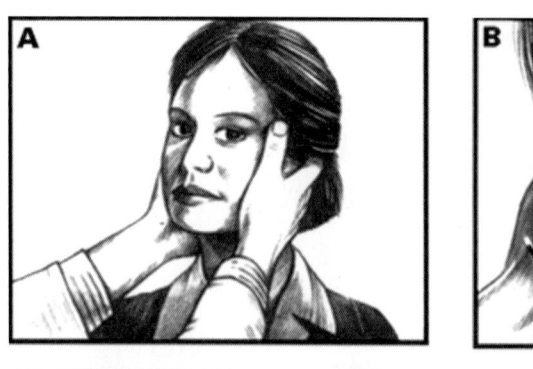
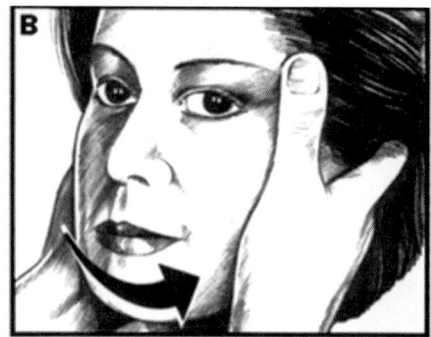
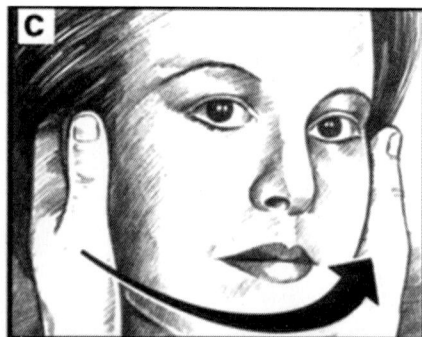
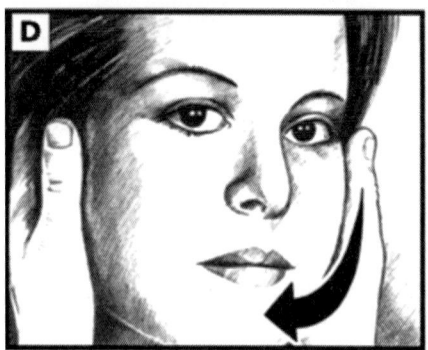
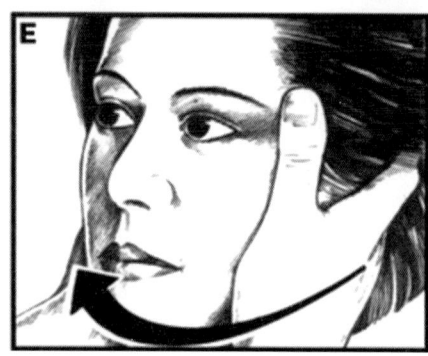
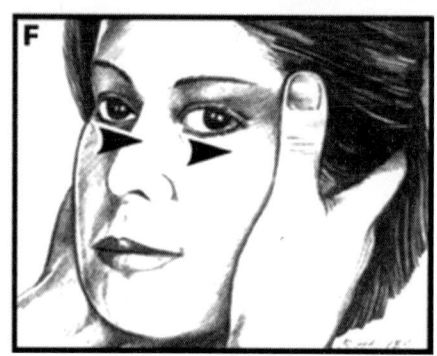

FIGURE 3.16 Head impulse test. With the patient fixated on a distant target, the examiner rapidly turns the head from 15 degrees to the right to 15 degrees to the left **(A–C)**, with normally maintained fixation demonstrated. Testing in the opposite direction, **D–F** illustrate a right peripheral vestibular lesion with a severe loss of right lateral semicircular canal function and no vestibulo-ocular reflex as demonstrated by loss of fixation **(E)** followed by a voluntary corrective saccade **(F)**. (From Halmagyi GM, Cremer PD. Assessment and treatment of dizziness. *J Neurol Neurosurg Psychiatry*. 2000;68:129–134.)

HOOVER SIGN

This test is used to identify feigned unilateral leg weakness. Following assessment of the normal leg, with the patient lying down supine, the examiner places their hand beneath the heel of the normal leg and asks the patient to raise the left leg. Normally, a patient attempting to raise the affected leg should depress the normal leg toward the examination surface, with the force felt by the examiner. Caution in its interpretation should be raised in the patient with evidence of dyspraxia or delayed responses.

HEAD VIBRATORY HEMIANESTHESIA

Patients with psychogenic examinations may have hemianesthesia affecting the entire body including the face, often to all modalities

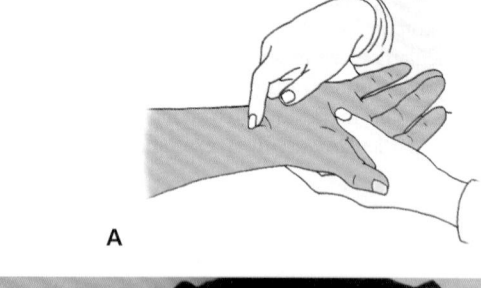

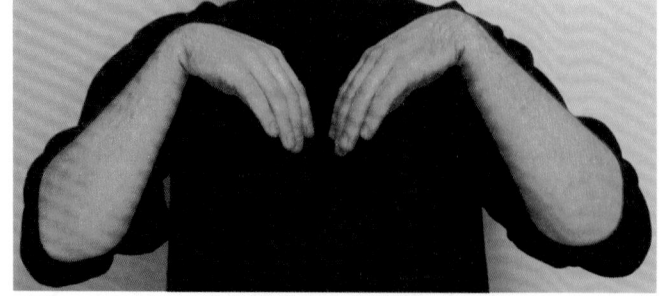

FIGURE 3.17 A: Tinel sign. (From Bickley L. *Bates' Guide to Physical Examination and History-Taking*. 11th ed. Philadelphia: Wolters Kluwer Health/Lippincott Williams & Wilkins; 2013.) **B:** Phalen sign. (Courtesy of James M. Noble, MD.)

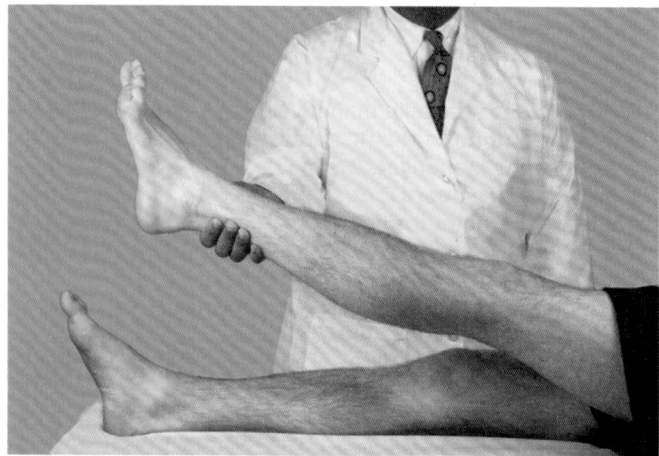

FIGURE 3.18 Straight leg raise test. (From Bickley L. *Bates' Guide to Physical Examination and History-Taking*. 11th ed. Philadelphia: Wolters Kluwer Health/Lippincott Williams & Wilkins; 2013.)

FIGURE 3.19 Bowlus and Currier test. Sequence of the Bowlus and Currier test, followed **A, B, C,** then **D**. Pinprick sensory testing is performed using a normal approach, comparing the left and right hand at baseline. When a nonphysiologic sensory examination is suspected, instruct the patient to position the hands in to that shown in **D**. Sensory testing is repeated quickly to identify discrepancies in examination. (Photos by James M. Noble, MD.)

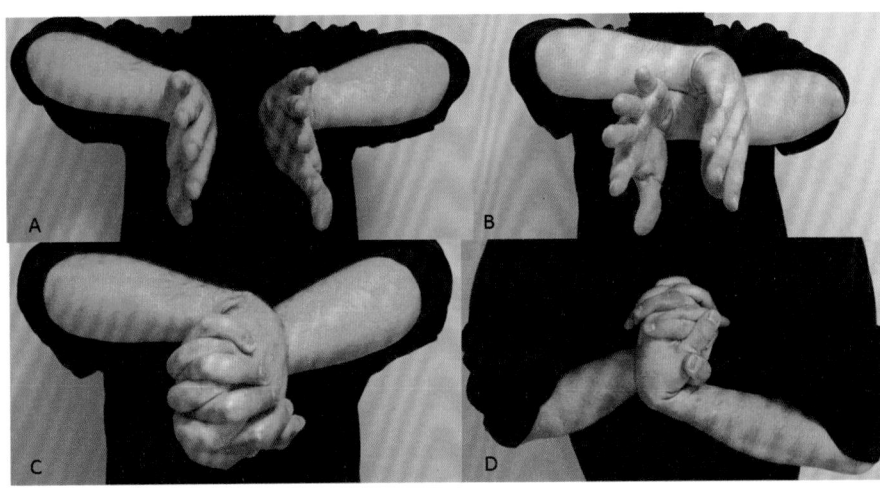

tested. Vibratory sensation in the head is likely principally or at least partially perceived by transmitted signal to the neck and to a lesser extent the head. Several methods to identify feigned from true facial hemianesthesia using vibratory sensation have been proposed. One approach involves, with the patient's eyes open, placing a 128-Hz tuning fork centrally above the brow, visible to the patient. While keeping the base position of the fork static, tilt the fork toward the affected (anesthetic) side followed by a tilt to the normal side. Record the patient's responses. Repeat the measure, out of sequence, with the eyes closed to discern an exam discrepancy.

BODY HEMIANESTHESIA

The Bowlus and Currier test (Fig. 3.19) can be a useful approach in distinguishing the patient with psychogenic hemianesthesia. As shown in the figures, the patient begins by pointing the thumbs down with the arms outstretched before them. Then the right wrist is crossed over the left and fingers are then interdigitated and flexed. Keeping the fingers locked together, the elbows are flexed, and the forearms supinated such that the hands are nearly at the patient's chin, thumbs pointing upward. Quickly thereafter, the examiner tests pinprick sensation on the knuckles of either hand, seeking not only for consistency but also for the rapidity with which the patient provides the answer. Substantial hesitation or inconsistency with primary sensory examination supports a feigned neurologic examination.

ACKNOWLEDGMENT

Dr. Noble would like to acknowledge the contributions of Drs. John Brust and Blair Ford in developing this approach to the neurologic examination.

SUGGESTED READINGS

Bowlus WE, Currier RD. A test for hysterical hemianalgesia. *N Engl J Med*. 1963;269:1253–1254.

Brain. *Aids to the Examination of the Peripheral Nervous System*. London: W. B. Saunders; 2000.

Burgess N, Maguire EA, O'Keefe J. The human hippocampus and spatial and episodic memory. *Neuron*. 2002;35(4):625–641.

Clements SD, Peters JE. Minimal brain dysfunctions in the school-age child. Diagnosis and treatment. *Arch Gen Psychiatry*. 1962;6:185–197.

Croskerry P. A universal model of diagnostic reasoning. *Acad Med*. 2009;84(8):1022–1028.

Dazzan P, Morgan KD, Chitnis X, et al. The structural brain correlates of neurological soft signs in healthy individuals. *Cereb Cortex*. 2006;16(8): 1225–1231.

Deville WL, van der Windt DA, Dzaferagic A, et al. The test of Lasègue: systematic review of the accuracy in diagnosing herniated discs. *Spine (Phila Pa 1976)*. 2000;25(9):1140–1147.

Dyck PJ, Boes CJ, Mulder D, et al. History of standard scoring, notation, and summation of neuromuscular signs. A current survey and recommendation. *J Peripher Nerv Syst*. 2005;10(2):158–173.

Ercan I, Ozdemir ST, Etoz A, et al. Facial asymmetry in young healthy subjects evaluated by statistical shape analysis. *J Anat*. 2008;213(6):663–669.

Fife TD, Iverson DJ, Lempert T, et al. Practice parameter: therapies for benign paroxysmal positional vertigo (an evidence-based review): report of the Quality Standards Subcommittee of the American Academy of Neurology. *Neurology*. 2008;70(22):2067–2074.

Gelb DJ, Gunderson CH, Henry KA, et al. The neurology clerkship core curriculum. *Neurology*. 2002;58(6):849–852.

Greer S, Chambliss L, Mackler L, et al. Clinical inquiries. What physical exam techniques are useful to detect malingering? *J Fam Pract*. 2005;54(8): 719–722.

Halmagyi GM, Cremer PD. Assessment and treatment of dizziness. *J Neurol Neurosurg Psychiatry*. 2000;68(2):129–134.

Jarvik JG, Deyo RA. Diagnostic evaluation of low back pain with emphasis on imaging. *Ann Intern Med*. 2002;137(7):586–597.

Kattah JC, Talkad AV, Wang DZ, et al. HINTS to diagnose stroke in the acute vestibular syndrome: three-step bedside oculomotor examination more sensitive than early MRI diffusion-weighted imaging. *Stroke*. 2009;40(11):3504–3510.

Kerr NM, Chew SS, Eady EK, et al. Diagnostic accuracy of confrontation visual field tests. *Neurology*. 2010;74(15):1184–1190.

Moore FG, Chalk C. The essential neurologic examination: what should medical students be taught? *Neurology*. 2009;72(23):2020–2023.

Phalen GS. The carpal-tunnel syndrome. Seventeen years' experience in diagnosis and treatment of six hundred fifty-four hands. *J Bone Joint Surg Am*. 1966;48(2):211–228.

Tinel J. The sign of "tingling" in lesions of the peripheral nerves. *Arch Neurol*. 1971;24:574–575. Originally published, in French, in: *La Presse Médicale*. 1915;23:388–389.

Dizziness, Vertigo, and Hearing Loss 4

J. Kirk Roberts

INTRODUCTION

Dizziness is an imprecise term used to describe a variety of symptoms including but not limited to vertigo, light-headedness, faintness, giddiness, disequilibrium, confusion, etc. It affects nearly one quarter of the general population and is a common complaint in the emergency room and in the office of the neurologist, otolaryngologist, and internist. The causes of dizziness are varied, span across medical subspecialties, and range from the relatively benign to life threatening. The evaluation of dizziness is made more difficult by the fact that the symptom is difficult for the patient to describe. A first step is an attempt to categorize dizziness into vertigo, presyncope, disequilibrium, and other or nonspecific dizziness as noted in Table 4.1.

Vertigo is an illusion of motion, either the environment or the self, most commonly rotatory but may be translational or tilting. *Presyncope* is the sensation encountered before loss of consciousness and is discussed in Chapter 5. *Dysequilibrium* is not a sensation of motion but a feeling of imbalance or unsteadiness and is discussed in Chapter 14. Other or nonspecific dizziness include those whose symptoms do not easily fit into one of the aforementioned categories or fall into more than one category. Rather than using the qualitative description of dizziness to categorize the subtype, it is often more helpful to use characteristics such as onset, duration, triggers, history of prior episodes, and associated symptoms in evaluating these patients.

VERTIGO

NEUROANATOMY

Vertigo primarily results from disorders of the vestibular system, which includes the vestibular labyrinth, vestibular nerve, vestibular nuclei in the brain stem, vestibular portions of the cerebellum, connections between these structures, and only rarely higher in the cerebrum. The vestibular labyrinth, located in the temporal bones, is composed of the three orthogonally oriented semicircular canals (anterior, posterior, and lateral) and the vestibule, which contains the otolith organs, the utricle and saccule, which are also angled at approximately 90 degrees to each other. The former responds to angular acceleration and the latter to linear acceleration including translation or tilt. When the head is rotated, endolymphatic fluid in the semicircular canals lags behind, leading to a deflection of the gelatinous cupula within the canal, which activates or inhibits the firing of hair cells. Activation on one side is paired with inhibition in the complementary canal on the other. The otolith organs, the utricle and saccule, contain hair cells on which calcium carbonate crystals, the otoconia, rest. Translational motion or tilt (via gravity) will activate or inhibit these cells. From the vestibular labyrinth, neurons travel centrally through the vestibular portion of the eighth cranial nerve into the brain stem to the vestibular nuclei and then project on to the cerebellum, ocular motor nuclei, spinal cord, and, via some less well understood pathways, to the

TABLE 4.1	**Dizziness Subtypes**			
	Vertigo	Presyncope	Disequilibrium	Nonspecific Dizziness
Symptom description	Illusion of motion, imbalance	Going to pass out, faint	Imbalance, unsteady, symptoms not in the head	Light-headed, foggy, floating
Onset	Usually sudden	Usually sudden	Sudden to slow	Poorly defined
Duration	Seconds to hours	Seconds to minutes	Acute to chronic	Subacute to chronic
Triggers	Head motion, position change	Orthostatic maneuvers, urination, cough, dehydration	Standing or walking, not when sitting or lying	Stress, situational, nonspecific
History	None or episodes	None or episodes	Chronic	Chronic
Associated symptoms	Nausea, ear symptoms (hearing loss, tinnitus), brain stem symptoms (diplopia, slurring, numbness, weakness, incoordination, ataxia)	Graying vision, warmth, diaphoresis, nausea, palpitations, chest pain	Slurring, incoordination	Many

TABLE 4.2	Peripheral versus Central Vertigo	
	Peripheral	Central
Nausea/vomiting	Severe	Mild/moderate
Imbalance	Mild/moderate	Severe
Ear symptoms (hearing loss, tinnitus, pain)	Common	Rare
Other neurologic symptoms	Rare	Common

TABLE 4.3	Peripheral versus Central Nystagmus	
	Peripheral	Central
Appearance	Combined torsional, horizontal, and vertical Nystagmus beats away from the affected side.	Often pure vertical, horizontal, or torsional; any trajectory
Fixation	Inhibits	No effect
Gaze	Obeys Alexander law (nystagmus increase when looking toward the side of the fast phase)	May change direction, does not obey Alexander law

cerebrum. Integration of the combinations of activations and inhibitions of the various components of the vestibular system of both ears, along with visual input and proprioceptive input, detects motion, rotation, translation, and tilt and affects eye movements and posture.

Vertigo can result from disorders of the peripheral vestibular system (labyrinth or nerve) or central vestibular system (brain stem, cerebellum, connections, and rarely, cerebrum) and this localization is the natural next step in the evaluation of vertigo. Table 4.2 lists some differentiating features.

MANAGEMENT STRATEGY

In the patient with the acute first presentation of vertigo, the most significant concern is evaluating for stroke (ischemic or hemorrhagic) and differentiating from vestibular neuritis. A history of vascular risk factors and other neurologic symptoms, headache, and complaints related to the brain stem is particularly important. However, the lack of those symptoms does not exclude an ischemic etiology. Patients presenting with isolated vertigo have a threefold increased risk of stroke compared to the general population that increases with the presence of multiple vascular risk factors. In the patient presenting with recurrent attacks of vertigo, the major differential includes benign positional paroxysmal vertigo (BPPV), Ménière syndrome, and migraines. Vertebral artery compression from neck rotation is a very rare case of episodic dizziness or vertigo.

FOCUSED HISTORY

Loss of vestibular function affects eye movements and image stabilization, balance, and spatial orientation. In addition to vertigo, patients may feel tilted, the world jiggling while walking (oscillopsia), spatially disoriented, imbalanced, and rarely, suffer from drop attacks, where they may feel pulled or pushed to the ground. These drop attacks, known as *Tumarkin crises*, are most commonly seen in Ménière syndrome but also may occur in other vestibular conditions.

FOCUSED EXAMINATION

The examination of the patient with vertigo includes all components of the neurologic examination with special attention to certain aspects. The ear must be examined and hearing must be tested. Examination of the eyes is particularly important. Start by observing for nystagmus in primary gaze and with eye movements in all directions. Reobserve after removing the ability to fixate by the use of Frenzel lenses, goggles with magnifying lenses that allow you to see eye movements but does not allow the patient to fixate. If Frenzel lenses are unavailable, fixation can be eliminated during ophthalmoscopic examination of one eye by covering the eye not

being examined with your free hand and observing for nystagmus of the optic disc. Remember that this movement is in the opposite direction of the movement of the front of the eye. Pay attention to the type of motion (horizontal, vertical, torsional, mixed), the effect of fixation, and the effect of gaze. Pendular nystagmus is sinusoidal, whereas jerk nystagmus, the more commonly observed nystagmus, is composed of slow drift in one direction and a rapid correction back. It is caused by an imbalance in vestibular input, either peripheral or central. Characteristics of peripheral versus central jerk nystagmus are listed in Table 4.3. Jerk nystagmus is named for the direction of the fast phase and can be further categorized by its trajectory and the conditions under which it is seen. Some particular forms of nystagmus and their relevance are listed in Table 4.4.

In addition to nystagmus, unilateral peripheral vestibular dysfunction leads to a subtle skew deviation of vertical eye position with the ipsilateral eye lower in the orbit relative to the contralateral eye and conjugate torsion of the eyes to the ipsilateral side. In addition to the ocular motor findings, the patient usually has a small head roll or tilt to the affected side and a tendency to fall toward the same side. They may perceive vertical to be slightly tilted. Testing for past pointing will reveal deviation to the ipsilateral side. Tandem gait and Romberg will be impaired but are not specific. The Fukuda step test, marching in place with the eyes closed, will show deviation toward the side of the vestibular lesion.

Head Impulse Test

The head thrust or head impulse test evaluates for loss of vestibular input from either the vestibular labyrinth or vestibular nerve to the vestibulo–ocular reflex. It is performed (Fig. 4.1) by asking the patient to focus on a target in front of him or her. The head is then rapidly rotated a small amount (approximately 15 degrees). In normal circumstances, the eyes remain focused on the target. A vestibular lesion on the side to which the patient is being rotated will lead to a loss of fixation and the eyes will turn with the head and require a saccade to refixate. The input from the horizontal canal is most commonly tested by rotating the head in the horizontal plane. The other canals may also be tested by rotating the head along the plane of the canal in question. The head impulse test is generally normal in those with central causes of vertigo. In patients presenting with an acute vestibular syndrome, the use of the head impulse test along with the evaluation of nystagmus and the presence of skew can be used to distinguish an acute peripheral vestibular lesion from an acute central lesion such as cerebral infarct with more accuracy than magnetic resonance imaging (MRI). Dynamic visual acuity also

TABLE 4.4 Subtypes of Nystagmus

Jerk Nystagmus

Gaze-evoked: nystagmus at the extremes of gaze beating in the direction of gaze

Physiologic: fine nystagmus, usually fatigues

Drug/medication: often seen with sedatives and anticonvulsants

Brain stem/cerebellar lesions: may be sustained

Rebound nystagmus: After looking eccentrically for approximately 1 min on return to primary gaze, there is nystagmus beating in the other direction associated with brain stem or cerebellar lesions.

Bruns nystagmus: Slow, large-amplitude nystagmus in one direction and rapid, small-amplitude nystagmus in the other direction suggest a cerebellopontine angle lesion on the side of the slow, large-amplitude nystagmus.

Horizontal Nystagmus

Peripheral nystagmus: Nystagmus only beats in one direction, away from the affected side, obeys Alexander law, usually mixed with torsion, and inhibited by fixation.

Central nystagmus: Nystagmus may change directions, may be purely horizontal, does not obey Alexander law, and fixation does not inhibit.

Periodic alternating nystagmus: nystagmus alternating directions every 1–2 min associated with lesions at the cervicomedullary junction or in the cerebellum

Dissociated nystagmus: nystagmus differing between the eyes seen with internuclear ophthalmoplegia or mimicked by myasthenia gravis

Downbeat nystagmus: Nystagmus usually increases on down and lateral gaze seen with involvement of the dorsal medulla or the cerebellar flocculus or projections associated with lesions at the cervicomedullary junction, medications (lithium, carbamazepine, phenytoin), alcohol, hypomagnesemia, thiamine deficiency, paraneoplastic syndromes, cerebellar degenerations, and other.

Upbeat nystagmus: associated with brain stem and cerebellar lesions, most commonly the medulla

Congenital nystagmus: often a mixture of jerk and pendular nystagmus

Convergence–retraction nystagmus: part of Parinaud dorsal midbrain syndrome, convergence and retraction of the eyes

Positional nystagmus: seen with specific head motions and will be discussed more in the following text

Pendular Nystagmus

Acquired: seen with brain stem and cerebellar lesions

Congenital: often a mixture of jerk and pendular nystagmus

Spasmus nutans: infant onset; nystagmus is asymmetric and rapid, often associated with head nodding and head turning; usually resolves

Associated with visual loss

Seesaw nystagmus: opposite conjugate vertical and torsional movements associated with mesencephalic or parasellar lesions

Oculopalatal myoclonus: rhythmic 2–3-Hz movements seen late after lesion of Mollaret triangle

Oculomasticatory myorhythmia: rhythmic movements of eye convergence and contraction of masticatory or other muscles seen in 20% of patients with Whipple disease

evaluates this reflex. It is performed by testing vision while stationary and then while shaking the head at approximately 2 Hz. Most can read no more than two to four lines worse on the eye chart with normal function of at least one labyrinth.

Dix–Hallpike Maneuver

Positional maneuvers must also be performed to look for BPPV and this is discussed in more detail in Chapter 59. In this condition, vertigo is precipitated by characteristic head motions due to otolith debris loose in the semicircular canals, most commonly the posterior canal. To evaluate, the Dix–Hallpike maneuver (see Fig. 3.15) is performed by having the patient sit with the head turned 45 degrees to one side. The patient is then laid back into a supine position with the head extended 30 degrees and is observed for nystagmus for at least 30 seconds. A positive test will result in symptoms of vertigo after a few seconds, lasting up to a minute and the observer will see upbeating and rotatory nystagmus of the upper pole of the eye toward the ground. This response will fatigue with repeated maneuvers.

Less common horizontal canal BPPV might be revealed with horizontal nystagmus on Dix–Hallpike and is more reliably investigated with lateral head and body turns while supine. Anterior canal BPPV is quite rare. If the nystagmus is not characteristic for BPPV in terms of type, latency, and fatigability nystagmus, then a

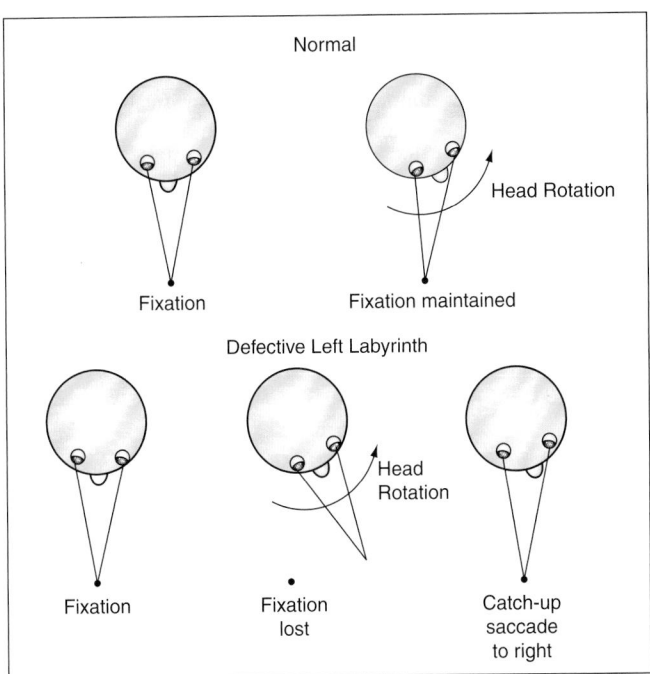

FIGURE 4.1 The head thrust test. (Modified from Barraclough K, Bronstein A. Vertigo. *BMJ*. 2009;339:b3493.)

TABLE 4.5   Causes of Peripheral Vertigo

Cause	Characteristics
BPPV	Brief, recurrent, positional nystagmus only in provoking position
Vestibular neuritis	Acute, single episode, viral prodrome
Ramsay Hunt syndrome (herpes zoster oticus)	Acute, single episode, vesicles in/near the ear, facial nerve palsy, deafness
Ménière syndrome	Recurrent, last minutes to hours, unilateral ear symptoms of fullness, hearing loss, tinnitus
Trauma	History of trauma
Perilymphatic fistula	Episodic, associated with Valsalva, loud sounds (Tullio phenomenon), history of trauma
Superior canal dehiscence	Episodic, associated with Valsalva, loud sounds
Cogan syndrome	Ménière-like syndrome with interstitial keratitis
Acoustic neuroma	Rare vertigo, more imbalance, unilateral hearing loss or tinnitus
Medications	Aminoglycoside exposure
Otitis	Evidence of otitis
Labyrinth ischemia	Presence of vascular risk factors, sudden vertigo, and hearing loss
Recurrent vestibulopathy	Recurrent attacks but without the ear symptoms to suggest Ménière

BPPV, benign positional paroxysmal vertigo.

central lesion must be considered. BPPV is best treated with repositioning maneuvers designed to "roll" the otolith debris out of the affected canal.

Various causes along with characteristics of some of the causes of vertigo are listed in Tables 4.5 (peripheral) and 4.6 (central). More details may be found in other chapters.

DIAGNOSIS

Diagnostic testing that is most useful in patients with vertigo includes comprehensive auditory examination to determine ear involvement especially with any complaints of hearing loss or tinnitus. Imaging is indicated when a central cause is under consideration and in other select cases. Computed tomography (CT) does not image the posterior fossa well and MRI is the imaging modality of choice. In the evaluation of superior canal dehiscence, CT better images the bony dehiscence that is the cause. Videonystagmography (VNG) or electronystagmography (ENG) is helpful if BBPV is considered, but nystagmus is not evident on clinical exam or if a unilateral vestibular lesion is suspected but not confirmed on clinical exam (see also Chapter 28). Rotational chair testing is also helpful in this circumstance and if bilateral vestibular dysfunction is suspected.

TREATMENT

The treatment of vertigo is primarily directed at the causes and is discussed in the appropriate chapters. Nonspecific treatments include antihistamines (meclizine, diphenhydramine, dimenhydrinate), anticholinergics (scopolamine, glycopyrrolate), and benzodiazepines (diazepam, lorazepam, alprazolam, clonazepam). Nausea and vomiting may also be treated with antiemetics. Vestibular rehabilitation is thought to benefit by promoting compensation, facilitating strategic substitution, limiting inactivity, and in the case of BPPV, repositioning otolith debris. There are some concerns that medications may interfere with rehabilitation.

TABLE 4.6   Causes of Central Vertigo

Cause	Characteristics
Migraine-associated vertigo	Migraine history
Cerebral ischemia/hemorrhage	Vascular risk factors, other neurologic symptoms and signs, more prominent dysmetria or ataxia
Multiple sclerosis	History or presence of other neurologic symptoms or signs
Tumor	Presence of other neurologic symptoms or signs
Craniocervical junction abnormalities (Arnold–Chiari, basilar impression, etc.)	Associated with headaches, neck pain, other lower cranial nerve involvement
Episodic ataxia type 2	Episodic vertigo and ataxia lasting hours to days
Cerebellar or spinocerebellar degenerations	More commonly ataxia and not vertigo
Mal de débarquement	After boat travel (or other), sensation of motion persists.

TABLE 4.7 Causes of Tinnitus

Pulsatile Tinnitus
Arteriovenous malformations/arteriovenous fistulas
Vascular stenosis/turbulence
Paragangliomas
Increased intracranial pressure
Jugular dehiscence
Tensor tympani or stapedius muscle spasm or myoclonus
Palatal spasm or myoclonus
Eustachian tube dysfunction
Nonpulsatile Tinnitus
Sensorineural hearing loss (age, toxicity, noise exposure, etc.)
Otosclerosis
Middle or inner ear trauma
Acoustic neuroma/cerebellopontine angle lesions
Temporomandibular joint dysfunction
Craniocervical junction and cervical spine disorders
Medications

TINNITUS

Tinnitus is the perception of sound in the head when there is no external sound present. Disability may range from none to severe. Subjective tinnitus is heard only by the patient, whereas objective tinnitus is also heard by the examiner. Tinnitus can be classified into pulsatile and nonpulsatile tinnitus, with pulsatile tinnitus usually indicating a vascular etiology. Table 4.7 lists various causes of tinnitus.

NEUROANATOMY

Most tinnitus is related to sensorineural hearing loss at the cochlear or cochlear nerve level and the tinnitus is thought to be generated in the central nervous system. Less commonly, tinnitus originates from structures in proximity to the ear, most commonly vascular structures.

FOCUSED HISTORY

One should inquire about the quality of the sound, whether it is episodic or constant, whether it is pulsatile or nonpulsatile, and precipitating and alleviating factors. Pay particular attention to a history of ear disease or trauma, hearing loss, noise exposure, headaches, and conditions that predispose to atherosclerosis such as hypertension, hypercholesterolemia, diabetes mellitus, and smoking. Tinnitus that is pulsatile or humming and changes with exercise or head motion raises more concern for a vascular etiology.

DIAGNOSIS

The ear and surrounding structures must be inspected; hearing must be tested; and one should listen for bruits in the neck, over the skull, and over the eye. If a vascular etiology is suspected, further evaluation might include duplex Doppler, MRI without and with contrast, MR angiography, CT angiography, and in some cases, conventional angiography.

TREATMENT

The treatment of tinnitus from vascular abnormalities or from other nonaudiologic abnormalities are usually treated by treating the underlying condition. Patients with tinnitus thought to be related to disorders of the auditory systems should be referred for complete audiologic evaluation (CAE) and otolaryngology consultation. Unfortunately, the success of treatment of this type of tinnitus is marginal. Hearing aids may benefit patients with presbycusis. Behavioral therapies may help. The success of masking devices producing low-level sounds and electrical stimulation are unproven. Medication trials have largely been disappointing.

HEARING LOSS

Hearing loss is common. It is typically categorized as conductive, usually from a problem in the outer or middle ear, sensorineural, usually from a problem in the inner ear or the along the eighth cranial nerve, or mixed. It can be unilateral or bilateral.

FOCUSED HISTORY

The history should focus on the degree of hearing loss, time course, laterality, types of sounds affected, and precipitating factors, along with associated features such as tinnitus, vertigo, other cranial nerve abnormalities, headache, or other neurologic symptoms. Family history is important especially in those with onset at a younger age.

Outer and middle ear problems causing conductive hearing loss are listed in Table 4.8, whereas inner ear and problems along the eighth cranial nerve causing sensorineural hearing loss are listed in Table 4.9. Central nervous system causes of hearing loss are rare.

SUDDEN HEARING LOSS

The patient with sudden sensorineural hearing loss, usually unilateral, over 1 to 3 days is a particular subcategory of hearing loss.

TABLE 4.8 Causes of Conductive Hearing Loss

Outer Ear
Congenital
Cerumen
Infection
Trauma
Tumor (squamous cell carcinoma, basal cell carcinoma, melanoma, exostoses, osteoma, etc.)
Foreign objects
Middle Ear
Congenital
Infection
Eustachian tube dysfunction
Tympanic membrane perforation
Otosclerosis
Trauma
Tumors (cholesteatoma, paraganglioma)

TABLE 4.9   Causes of Sensorineural Hearing Loss

Congenital

Presbycusis

Infection

Ménière syndrome

Noise exposure

Trauma

Autoimmune/inflammatory

Ischemic

Metabolic

Ototoxic

Structural

The incidence is 5 to 20 per 100,000 people per year and is most common in the middle aged. The etiology in most cases is never identified. Autoimmune, inflammatory, infectious, and ischemic etiologies are postulated. Many report tinnitus and some report vertigo. Urgent evaluation is warranted. A repeated history suggests Ménière or a chronic autoimmune condition. Neck pain might suggest vertebral artery dissection. The internal auditory artery is a branch of the anterior inferior cerebellar artery (AICA). CAE and MRI should both usually be performed. The use of oral glucocorticoids is controversial but many treat with prednisone 60 mg daily for 2 weeks as long as given early. Intratympanic steroids have also been given, particularly to those who might not tolerate oral steroids or those who have not responded to oral steroids, again with a similar lack of evidence. Some, but not most, recommend antiviral therapy, similar to those who recommend it for Bell palsy. Prognosis is related to the severity of hearing loss at onset.

FOCUSED EXAMINATION

Examination must include visual inspection of the ear along with tests of hearing. Patients should be able to hear a finger rub or a whisper a few inches away from the ear. The Weber and Rinne tests provide additional information. The Weber test is performed by placing a 256-Hz tuning fork in the center of the forehead equidistant from both ears. A normal response is hearing the tuning fork similarly in both ears. A patient with a conductive hearing loss will hear the tuning fork louder in the affected ear and a patient with sensorineural hearing loss will hear the tuning fork louder in the unaffected ear. The Rinne test is performed by placing a 512-Hz tuning fork on the mastoid bone behind the ear and asking when the sound is no longer heard. It is then moved to 1 to 2 inches from the external auditory canal. In a patient with normal hearing or sensorineural hearing loss, the sound will still be heard, as air conduction is better than bone conduction. In a patient with conductive hearing loss, bone conduction is better than air conduction. Further hearing testing includes a CAE with pure tone audiometry, speech reception thresholds and discrimination, impedance testing, and acoustic reflexes. Imaging with MRI and/or CT will depend on the clinical situation.

TREATMENT

The treatment of hearing loss is directed at the cause along with hearing amplification and cochlear implantation.

SUGGESTED READINGS

Halmagyi GM, Cremer PD. Assessment and treatment of dizziness. *J Neurol Neurosurg Psychiatry.* 2000;68:129–134.

Halmagyi GM, Curthoys IS. A clinical sign of canal paresis. *Arch Neurol.* 1988;45(7):737–739.

Hillier SL, Hollohan V. Vestibular rehabilitation for unilateral peripheral vestibular dysfunction. *Cochrane Database Syst Rev.* 2007;(4):CD005397.

Kattah JC, Talkad AV, Wang DZ, et al. HINTS to diagnose stroke in the acute vestibular syndrome: three-step bedside oculomotor examination more sensitive than early MRI diffusion-weighted imaging. *Stroke.* 2009;40(11):3504–3510.

Kim JS, Zee DS. Benign paroxysmal positional vertigo. *New Engl J Med.* 2014;370:1138–1147.

Lee CC, Su YC, Ho HC, et al. Risk of stroke in patients hospitalized for isolated vertigo: a four-year follow-up study. *Stroke.* 2011;42:48–52.

Lee H, Yi HA, Lee SR, et al. Drop attacks in elderly patients secondary to otologic causes with Meniere's syndrome or non-Meniere peripheral vestibulopathy. *J Neurol Sci.* 2005;232:71–76.

Neuhauser HK, Radtke A, von Brevern, et al. Burden of dizziness and vertigo in the community. *Arch Int Med.* 2008;168(19):2118–2124.

Newman-Toker DE, Cannon LM, Stofferahn ME, et al. Imprecision in patient reports of dizziness symptom quality: a cross-section study conducted in an acute care setting. *Mayo Clin Proc.* 2007;82(11):1329–1340.

Newman-Toker DE, Hsieh YH, Camargo CA, et al. Spectrum of dizziness visits to US emergency departments: cross-sectional analysis from a nationally representative sample. *Mayo Clin Proc.* 2008;83(7):765–775.

Newman-Toker DE, Kattah JC, Alvernia JE, et al. Normal head impulse test differentiates acute cerebellar strokes for vestibular neuritis. *Neurology.* 2008;70(24, pt 2):2378–2385.

Stachler RJ, Chandrasekhar SS, Archer SM, et al. Clinical practice guideline: sudden hearing loss. *Otolaryngol Head Neck Surg.* 2012;146(3)(suppl): S1–S35.

Waldvogel D, Mattle HP, Sturzenegger M, et al. Pulsatile tinnitus—a review of 84 patients. *J Neurol.* 1998;245(3):137–142.

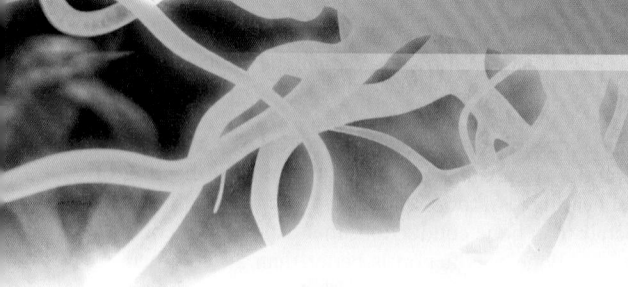

INTRODUCTION

Sudden alteration of consciousness is a common presenting symptom in a variety of clinical contexts, from the emergency room to the outpatient clinic. The vast majority of events can be categorized as either seizure or syncope or the proverbial "fit" versus "faint." This chapter aims to provide a practical framework to help the clinician distinguish between these two diagnoses. When evaluating a patient with a history of transient loss of consciousness, clinicians should spend the majority of their efforts on interviewing the patient and eyewitnesses, eliciting the symptoms and signs in a step-by-step fashion in order to understand the order and tempo of the events as they unfolded.

DIFFERENTIATING SYNCOPE FROM SEIZURE

Syncope is defined as a transient loss of consciousness due to insufficient blood flow to the brain. Epileptic *seizures* are defined as transient alteration in brain function due to abnormal electrocerebral activity. The most important clinical features distinguishing these two conditions are the following: (1) precipitating stimuli or situations, (2) prodromal symptoms before losing awareness, and (3) the postevent recovery (Table 5.1).

Although many patients and witnesses will use terms such as "passing out" or "fainting" to describe either condition, it is important to delve further and elicit a first-person narrative of the patient's actual experience, carefully parsing out what the patient means when using these words.

SYNCOPE

Syncope typically occurs when patients are upright (standing or sitting) and can be triggered by exercise, coughing, bearing down (Valsalva maneuver), venipuncture, prolonged standing, or pain. Presyncope begins with a sense of unwellness accompanied by light-headedness and nausea. Patients may feel weak and unsteady on their feet, followed by a decreased awareness or detachment from their environment. Immediately before losing consciousness, patients experience a "graying of the vision" and/or "muffling" of ambient sounds. Eyewitnesses will often note that the patients appear pale or ashen, diaphoretic, and tachypneic. Sometimes an attack can be aborted if the patients lie down quickly or lower the head below the level of the heart. Once patients lose consciousness, they will lose tone in the muscles of their trunk and legs and they will limply collapse to the floor. On the ground, the limbs are flaccid and patients continue to appear pale and sweaty. The period of unconsciousness is generally brief, lasting only seconds up to 1 to 2 minutes. If the degree of decreased cerebral perfusion is profound enough, patients may display a few jerking movements of the limbs ("convulsive syncope") but this is also typically very brief (lasting only a few seconds). Generally, the pulse and blood pressure quickly return to normal with the patients in the recumbent position; and they rapidly regain consciousness and quickly become oriented and aware of their surroundings. Patients will often realize that they have fainted and remember details of the event up until the moment of losing consciousness. They might experience mild fatigue or brief disorientation after the event, but this should not last more than a few minutes.

SEIZURES

The clinical manifestations of seizures vary widely, depending on brain volume and neuroanatomic location of activation. Seizures can occur day or night, regardless of whether the patient is awake or asleep, and usually are not triggered by a precipitating stimuli or environment. Sometimes, a seizure may begin with the patients reporting an "aura" or warning. These subjective experiences might be described as a sense of déjà vu (a sense of reliving a familiar experience), a noxious smell, sudden anxiety, or tingling over one side of the body. Eyewitnesses might find the patients unresponsive to their direct questions, staring into space, or stopping what they were previously doing (behavioral arrest). Some patients exhibit oral or manual automatisms (lip smacking, chewing, rubbing of their hands, picking at their clothes). If a focal seizure then secondarily generalizes (electrical activity starting off in one area of the brain but then spreading to both hemispheres of the brain), the patients' head and eyes may suddenly and forcibly turn to one side, with stiffening of the limbs, frothing at the mouth, cyanosis of the lips, followed by rhythmic jerking of the limbs. Most secondarily generalized seizures last between 1 and 2 minutes in duration and rarely over 5 minutes in duration, but afterwards, the patients may be confused and disoriented for minutes to hours. Patients may report lateral tongue biting and urinary incontinence after some seizures.

CAUSES OF SYNCOPE

NEURALLY MEDIATED REFLEX SYNCOPE

The most common type of syncope, accounting for over half of cases, is reflex syncope, also known as *neurocardiogenic syncope*. In this form of syncope, an external factor or set of circumstances (apprehension of pain, cough, head turning etc. . . .) leads to bradycardia, hypotension, or a mixture of both phenomena. Reflex syncope is divided into two main categories: vasovagal syncope and carotid sinus syncope (Table 5.2).

Vasovagal Syncope

Vasovagal syncope, the most common type of reflex syncope, is caused by a brief loss of neurally mediated circulatory control and is generally associated with a benign prognosis. Vasovagal syncope can be subdivided into three major categories: postural, central, and situational. In the postural form of vasovagal syncope, a common patient narrative might describe a young person attending a hot and crowded school assembly or concert, standing for a long period of time and having skipped a recent meal and ingested

TABLE 5.1   Clinical Features Distinguishing Syncope from Seizure

Feature	Syncope	Seizure
Before a Spell		
Trigger (change in position, prolonged standing, emotion, Valsalva, exercise)	Common	Rare
Sweating, light-headedness, graying of vision, and/or nausea	Common	Rare
Occurring out of sleep	Rare	Occasional
Aura (déjà vu olfactory hallucination, unilateral symptoms)	Rare	Common
During a Spell		
Pallor	Common	Rare
Cyanosis	Rare	Common (generalized tonic–clonic seizures)
Duration of loss of consciousness	<20 s	>60 s
Movements	A few rhythmic jerking movements of the limbs, lasting <15 s	Prolonged stiffening of the limbs (tonic), transitioning to rhythmic jerking of the limbs (clonic), lasting ~1–2 min
Automatic behavior (lip smacking, picking, patting)	Occasional	Common (focal dyscognitive seizures)
Tongue biting (lateral)	Rare	Occasional
Frothing/hypersalivation/vomiting	Rare	Common
After a Spell		
Confusion/disorientation	Rare, <30 s	Common, several minutes or longer
Diffuse muscle pain	Rare, brief	Common, hours to days
Creatinine kinase (CK) elevation	Rare	Common (especially after 12–24 h)
Focal neurologic signs	Rare	Occasional
Incontinence	Rare	Occasional
Headache	Rare	Common
Amnesia for the event	Less common (sometimes seen in elderly)	Common

some alcohol. In cases of centrally mediated vasovagal syncope, the trigger may involve sudden pain (commonly in the setting of venipuncture), apprehension of pain, or emotional shock immediately preceding the fainting episode. Less commonly, syncope occurs in specific situations or appears to be temporally related to specific triggers. Older men may report symptoms soon after arising from bed and emptying a distended bladder. Some young people describe recurrent syncope after exercise. Others describe syncope after coughing, laughing, or sneezing. It is not unusual for a history of vasovagal syncope to run in families. Surprisingly, despite the prevalence of this condition, the underlying pathophysiology of vasovagal syncope remains a mystery. Physiologists have yet to identify why an emotional state or coughing or prolonged standing can lead to a sudden decrease in blood pressure or why vasovagal syncope can recur frequently in some individuals, rarely in others.

Carotid Sinus Syndrome

A more unusual type of reflex syncope is carotid sinus syndrome, which occurs when normal stimulation of an unusually sensitive carotid sinus leads to hypotension and/or bradycardia. This diagnosis should be suspected in older individuals who report

unexplained falls or syncope with almost no prodromal symptoms; occasionally, a history of head turning, wearing a tight-collared shirt, or shaving preceding syncope is elicited, but in general, this diagnosis is often difficult to make and is considered after extensive diagnostic testing has been inconclusive or negative.

CARDIAC SYNCOPE

The most dangerous type of syncope is cardiac syncope, when a transient loss of consciousness is caused by either cardiac arrhythmia or structural heart disease. In a large population-based study of syncope, cardiac syncope was associated with a twofold increased risk of dying, regardless of etiology, as compared to individuals without a history of syncope.

Arrhythmias are the most common cause of cardiac syncope and both tachyarrhythmias and bradyarrhythmias have been implicated. The most common arrhythmia associated with syncope is sinus node dysfunction. Other arrhythmias include atrioventricular conduction system disease, supraventricular tachyarrhythmias, and ventricular tachyarrhythmias.

Mechanical or structural causes of cardiac syncope include prior myocardial infarction, cardiomyopathy, aortic stenosis,

TABLE 5.2 Causes of Syncope

Neurally Mediated Reflex Syncope

- Vasovagal syncope

  Central (emotional stimuli)

  Postural (prolonged upright position)

- Situational (specific triggers)

  Micturition, defecation, coughing, sneezing, laughing, weight lifting, post exercising, trumpet playing

- Carotid sinus syndrome

Cardiac Syncope (Cardiovascular)

- Arrhythmias
- Structural heart disease/mechanical

Syncope due to Orthostatic Hypotension

- Autonomic failure

  Multiple system atrophy, diabetes, amyloidosis, hereditary polyneuropathy

- Drug-induced

  Antihypertensives, diuretics, antianginal, tricyclic antidepressants, levodopa, lithium, alcohol

- Hypovolemia

  Anemia, failure to thrive, malnutrition

- Postural orthostatic hypotension syndrome (POTS)

mitral stenosis, pericardial tamponade, myxoma, aortic dissection, and pulmonary emboli.

Because of the high morbidity associated with cardiac syncope, it is imperative to consider this diagnosis when evaluating an individual with syncope. The clinical features most predictive of cardiac syncope include age older than 60 years, male gender, known structural heart disease, fewer events (less than three events by history), syncope while supine, and syncope during effort/exercise.

SYNCOPE DUE TO ORTHOSTATIC HYPOTENSION

Unlike individuals with vasovagal syncope (who have an intact autonomic nervous system at baseline), individuals with syncope due to orthostatic hypotension are believed to have underlying autonomic dysfunction involving sympathetic efferent pathways, preventing appropriate vasoconstriction upon standing. Therefore, when an individual with this condition rises from a supine position, he or she experiences an abnormal drop in systolic blood pressure. Patients who present with this form of syncope are usually elderly, and this condition rarely occurs in individuals younger than 40 years of age. The clinical history may reveal other symptoms upon standing, which include light-headedness/dizziness or presyncope, weakness/fatigue/lethargy, diaphoresis, vision disturbances (graying of vision, enhanced brightness, tunnel vision), muffled hearing, and/or pain in the shoulders ("coat hanger" distribution), invariably associated with an upright position.

Causes of orthostatic hypotension include neurodegenerative disorders such as multiple system atrophy, hereditary, toxic or paraneoplastic peripheral neuropathies, secondary neuropathies due to systemic diseases such as diabetes and amyloidosis,

hypovolemia, and medications. A rare form of orthostatic hypotension with dizziness and near syncope is postural orthostatic hypotension syndrome (POTS), a poorly understood syndrome typically seen in young women with chronic fatigue syndrome. The syndrome consists of an increase in heart rate and unstable blood pressure upon standing.

SPELLS POTENTIALLY MISTAKEN FOR SYNCOPE

VERTEBROBASILAR TRANSIENT ISCHEMIC ATTACK

Transient ischemic attack (TIA) of the vertebrobasilar system is a rare cause of brief loss of consciousness. The underlying pathophysiology is believed to be due to temporary ischemia of the brain stem reticular activating system. Almost invariably, TIAs of the vertebrobasilar system are associated with focal neurologic symptoms due to ischemia of the brain stem, cerebellum, and/or occipital lobe. Therefore, patients and family members will typically describe associated dysarthria, diplopia, dysphagia, hemianopsia, ataxia, unilateral weakness, or numbness.

HYPOGLYCEMIA

Hypoglycemia may cause feelings of light-headedness or dizziness and rarely results in a brief loss of consciousness. A more typical presentation of hypoglycemia is a slow and insidious onset of delirium that may last minutes to hours and be associated with diaphoresis, hunger, tremulousness, anxiety, and palpitations. If severe enough, hypoglycemia can progress to coma and/or generalized tonic–clonic seizures.

BASILAR MIGRAINE

Basilar migraine may cause confusion but rarely leads to loss of consciousness. It is associated with headache, ataxia, and positive visual phenomenon developing over minutes to hours and therefore is unlikely to be confused with syncope.

SUBCLAVIAN STEAL SYNDROME

Subclavian steal syndrome is characterized by a reversal of blood flow in the vertebral artery, away from the brain, in order to supply blood flow to an ischemic arm. In this syndrome, exercising the affected arm leads to dizziness, vertigo, dysarthria, dysphagia, ataxia, unilateral weakness, and sometimes loss of consciousness.

FOCUSED EXAMINATION

If the clinician remains uncertain whether the diagnosis is syncope or seizure after taking the history, the physical examination is unlikely to be helpful. In cases of likely syncope, orthostatic blood pressure and auscultation of the neck and heart should be included as part of the routine physical examination and patients should have a routine 12-lead electrocardiogram (ECG).

Carotid sinus massage has been recommended in the evaluation of unexplained syncope in individuals older than age 45 years, but the procedure is generally not performed by neurologists. The generally accepted protocol for carotid sinus massage involves longitudinal massage at the region where the common carotid bifurcates, but the duration of massage should not last longer than 5 seconds and the force applied should not occlude the carotid artery. The procedure should be performed in upright and supine positions with continuous ECG and noninvasive blood pressure monitoring. The procedure should not be performed in individuals with known carotid disease, history of TIA or stroke within the last 3 months, or carotid bruit.

The *active standing test* (having the patient move from lying position to standing position) with simultaneous intermittent manual blood pressure monitoring (sphygmomanometer) may be helpful in diagnosing orthostatic hypotension. A classic finding of orthostatic hypotension is defined as a greater than 20 mm Hg decrease in systolic blood pressure and greater than 10 mm Hg decrease in diastolic blood pressure with 3 minutes of standing. Initial orthostatic hypotension is defined as a blood pressure decrease immediately on standing of greater than 40 mm Hg, whereas delayed orthostatic hypotension is described as a slow, progressive decline in SBP while standing.

DIAGNOSIS

Once the syndrome of syncope has been established but the cause remains uncertain (unlikely reflex syncope or orthostatic hypotension), further laboratory studies to consider might include hemoglobin/hematocrit to look for anemia, chemistry panel to look for electrolyte disturbances, tilt table testing to try to reproduce neurally mediated reflex syncope, echocardiography to evaluate cardiac structure and function, and/or continuous electrocardiographic monitoring to investigate the possibility of a cardiac arrhythmia. The decision to pursue further cardiac testing (continuous ECG or echocardiography) should be strongly considered if there is any suspicion of a potential cardiac cause (Table 5.3). More systematic, protocol-based approaches attempting to stratify high-risk patients have failed to perform consistently when tested in varying patient populations, but expert consensus recommends prompt hospitalization and immediate evaluation for patients with abnormal 12-lead ECG findings, known severe cardiac disease, severe anemia, electrolyte disturbances, and/or clinical features concerning for cardiac syncope (Table 5.4).

TREATMENT

For patients with vasovagal syncope and orthostatic intolerance, nonpharmacologic management strategies are most effective.

TABLE 5.3 "Red Flags": When to Consider a Diagnosis of Cardiac Syncope

Clinical features	• Lack of clear trigger causing syncope
	• Absence of sweating/nausea before syncope
	• Syncope while supine
	• Palpitations at the time of syncope
	• Syncope with exercise/effort
Demographic features	• Older age
	• Family history of sudden death
	• Personal history of structural heart disease
	• Fewer events (less than three syncopal events)

TABLE 5.4 "Red Flags": When to Consider Prompt Hospitalization or Intensive Evaluation

Clinical features	• Severe cardiac structural dysfunction or coronary artery disease
	• Family history of sudden cardiac death
	• Syncope during exercise or while supine
	• Palpitations at the time of syncope
Comorbidities	• Severe anemia
	• Electrolyte disturbance
Abnormal ECG findings	• Bifascicular block or other intraventricular conduction block (QRS duration >120 ms)
	• Inadequate sinus bradycardia (<50 bpm) in absence of negative chronotropic medication or physical training
	• Prolonged or short QT interval
	• Right bundle branch block with ST elevation in leads V1–V3 (Brugada pattern)
	• ECG pattern suggestive of arrhythmogenic right ventricular cardiomyopathy

ECG, electrocardiogram.

Patients benefit greatly from education about the condition, identification and then avoidance of potential triggers, and learning how to perform maneuvers to abort an episode (supine posture; physical counterpressure maneuvers consist of leg crossing, arm-tensing, or hand grip).

If the events are recurrent and clear triggers have not been identified, patients should be counseled about high-risk activities such as driving, operating heavy machinery, and working at unrestricted heights, and in some states, mandatory reporting is required.

SUGGESTED READINGS

Benbadis SR, Wolgamuth BR, Goren H, et al. Value of tongue biting in the diagnosis of seizures. *Arch Intern Med.* 1995;155(21):2346–2349.

Benditt DG, Adkisson WO. Approach to the patient with syncope. *Cardiol Clin.* 2013;31(1):9–25.

Berecki-Gisolf J, Sheldon A, Wieling W, et al. Identifying cardiac syncope based on clinical history: a literature-based model tested in four independent datasets. *PLoS One.* 2013;8(9):e75255.

Birnbaum A, Esses D, Bijur P, et al. Failure to validate the San Francisco Syncope Rule in an independent emergency department population. *Ann Emerg Med.* 2008;52:151–159.

Cornes SB, Shih T. Evaluation of the patient with spells. *Continuum (Minneap Minn)* 2011;17(5 Neurologic Consultation in the Hospital):984–1009.

Hatoum T, Sheldon R. A practical approach to investigation of syncope. *Can J Cardiol.* 201;30(6):671–674.

Hoefnagels WA, Padberg GW, Overweg J, et al. Transient loss of consciousness: the value of the history for distinguishing seizure from syncope. *J Neurol.* 1991;238(1):39–43.

Jardine D. Vasovagal syncope. *Cardiology Clinics.* 2013;31(1):75–87.

Jobst BC, Williamson PD. Anatomical-clinical localization of ictal behavior. In: Kaplan PW, Fisher RS, eds. *Imitators of Epilepsy.* 2nd ed. New York: Demos; 2005:29–44.

Khoo C, Chakrabarti S, Arbour L, et al. Recognizing life-threatening causes of syncope. *Cardiology Clinics.* 2013;31(1):51–66.

Krediet CT, van Dijk N, Linzer M, et al. Management of vasovagal syncope: controlling or aborting faints by leg crossing and muscle tensing. *Circulation*. 2002;106:1684–1689.

Lempert T, Bauer M, Schmidt D. Syncope: a videometric analysis of 56 episodes of transient cerebral hypoxia. *Ann Neurol*. 1994;36(2):233–237.

McKeon A, Vaughan C, Delanty N. Seizure versus syncope. *Lancet*. 2006;5(2): 171–180.

Moya A, Sutton R, Ammirati F, et al. Guidelines for the diagnosis and management of syncope (version 2009). *Eur Heart J*. 2009;30(21): 2631–2371.

Quinn J, McDermott D, Stiell I, et al. Prospective validation of the San Francisco Syncope Rule to predict patients with serious outcomes. *Ann Emerg Med*. 2006;47:448–454.

Seifer C. Carotid sinus syndrome. *Cardiology Clinics*. 2013;31(1):111–121.

Sheldon R, Rose S, Ritchie D, et al. Historical criteria that distinguish syncope from seizures. *J Am Coll Cardiol*. 2002;40(1):142–148.

Soteriades ES, Evans JC, Larson MG, et al. Incidence and prognosis of syncope. *N Engl J Med*. 2002;347(12):878–885.

Sun BC, Costantino G, Barbic F, et al. Priorities for emergency department syncope research. *Ann Emerg Med*. 2014;64(6):649–655.

Tea SH, Mansourati J, L'Heveder G, et al. New insights into the pathophysiology of carotid sinus syndrome. *Circulation*. 1996;93(7):1411–1416.

van Dijk N, Quartieri F, Blanc JJ, et al. Effectiveness of physical counterpressure maneuvers in preventing vasovagal syncope: the Physical Counterpressure Manoeuvres Trial (PC-Trial). *J Am Coll Cardiol*. 2006;48(8): 1652–1657.

Seizures and Status Epilepticus 6

David Roh and Jan Claassen

INTRODUCTION

Seizures are frequently encountered in both the community and hospital setting. Epidemiologic studies in the United States have shown that 11% of the general population will have a seizure at some point in their life. Of these seizure patients, there is an estimated 1 million hospital visits due to seizures per year. The International League Against Epilepsy (ILAE) defines seizures as transient clinical events due to abnormally excessive or synchronous neuronal activity in the brain. These can manifest in a wide array of symptoms ranging from obvious convulsive activity to more subtle signs of twitching or altered mental status.

STATUS EPILEPTICUS

A failure to stop isolated seizures may lead to status epilepticus (SE). Its incidence has seen an increase in recent years with 5 to 30 cases per 100,000. SE is defined as convulsions lasting more than 5 minutes or two or more convulsions in a 5-minute interval without a return to preconvulsive neurologic baseline. Historically, SE had been defined as continuous convulsive seizure activity lasting greater than 30 minutes without complete recovery. However, the minimum time elapsed to qualify for SE was drastically shortened to 5 minutes based on the observation that convulsive seizures rarely last for more than a few minutes. Furthermore, seizures that are of longer duration typically do not stop spontaneously. Animal studies and human data have demonstrated irreversible brain injury can occur as early as 5 minutes of ongoing seizure activity. Delaying effective recognition and treatment of SE dramatically increases the patient's morbidity and mortality. Thus, SE constitutes a neurologic emergency requiring prompt and decisive intervention.

CAUSES OF SEIZURES

It is important to identify any underlying cause for seizures, as management will be tailored to reverse these factors if possible (Table 6.1). In adults without a history of prior seizures, stroke is the most frequent underlying etiology of seizures. The most common cause of SE is a history of epilepsy. Frequent precipitating factors in these patients include medication noncompliance, low antiepileptic drug (AED) levels, and recent changes in AEDs. Other seizures due to underlying metabolic derangements (hypoglycemia, hyponatremia) can be commonly seen but will be difficult to control with AED agents alone. Subsequently, timely investigation into the underlying cause of the seizure will need to be implemented in the management of acute seizures. Many of these provoking factors may be elicited from the patient's history or exam as discussed previously; however, laboratory and imaging workup can further elucidate these factors. See "Initial Workup" section for recommended testing.

TABLE 6.1	Etiology of Seizures
Acute
Stroke: ischemic or hemorrhagic
Metabolic derangement: hypoglycemia, electrolyte abnormalities, renal failure
Infection: CNS infection, sepsis
Head trauma
Drugs: AED noncompliance, withdrawal from alcohol, opiates, benzodiazepines, drug toxicity
Hypoxia/cardiac arrest
Hypertensive encephalopathy (PRES)
Chronic
Epilepsy with breakthrough seizures
Mass lesion: tumor, vascular malformations
Prior cortical CNS lesion: stroke, abscess, dysplasia

CNS, central nervous system; AED, antiepileptic drug; PRES, posterior reversible encephalopathy syndrome.

Adapted from Brophy GM, Bell R, Claassen J, et al. Guidelines for the evaluation and management of status epilepticus. *Neurocrit Care.* 2012;17(1):3–23.

DIAGNOSIS

The diagnosis of acute seizures can be made on clinical grounds depending on the patient's history and symptoms. Symptoms can range from obvious positive signs of rhythmic jerking and posturing to more subtle positive symptoms of twitching, nystagmus, automatisms, and eye deviation. Negative symptoms of seizures include staring, coma, lethargy, confusion, and aphasia. These negative symptoms may raise the suspicion of seizures in the appropriate context; however, the definite diagnosis requires an electroencephalogram (EEG). The differential diagnosis of seizures includes a wide variety of seizure mimics that produce sudden unexplained movements or alteration in level of consciousness (Table 6.2). If the patient is not exhibiting symptoms at the time of assessment, a focused history must be obtained from whoever witnessed the event.

FOCUSED HISTORY

Initial questions should be focused on what symptoms were seen, laterality of symptoms (hemibody or generalized), time of onset, length of activity, if the patient returned to baseline, seizure history, recent illness/fever, trauma, and relevant medications (Table 6.3). Medication history should include antiepileptics or agents that would lower seizure threshold (Table 6.4). These questions may allow the examiner to rapidly differentiate seizure versus SE, direct an initial diagnosis for the underlying etiology, and guide the diagnostic workup.

TABLE 6.2	Common Seizure Mimics
Movement disorders	
Limb-shaking transient ischemic attacks	
Convulsive syncope	
Motor posturing (in coma)	
Sleep disorders	
Transient global amnesia	
Complicated migraine	
Psychiatric nonelectrographic seizure activity	

FOCUSED EXAM

A focused general physical exam should rapidly screen the patient's stability and identify life-threatening etiologies of seizures. These may include meningitis, hemorrhage, ischemic stroke, or mass effect (Table 6.5). Vital signs should be monitored with particular attention to hemodynamic stability and respiratory status. Focus should be paid to the presence of fever, nuchal rigidity, and rash. These findings, if present, should raise suspicion for central nervous system (CNS) infection, prompting further laboratory investigation and empiric treatment.

Observation and neurologic examination may detect obvious positive symptoms of seizures supporting the diagnosis. However, absence of obvious symptoms should not preclude the possibility of seizures. Nearly half of patients with generalized tonic–clonic SE will continue to have electrographic seizures after clinical symptoms disappear. This can result in continued subtle signs such as eye deviation, nystagmus, and facial twitching. Some of these subtle positive findings may have localizing value (Table 6.6). *Comatose patients who have subtle lateralized facial or extremity twitching, nystagmus, or eye deviation should be considered to be in nonconvulsive SE until proven otherwise by EEG.*

TREATMENT STRATEGY

Emergency EEG is indicated for patients who present with SE who fail to awaken after cessation of convulsive seizures. Nonconvulsive seizures occur in up to 40% of patients who fail to awaken after convulsive seizures. This can cause further depression of level of consciousness and increase resistance to antiepileptic therapy if not controlled.

TABLE 6.3	Focused History: Questions to Ask in the Patient with Seizure
What symptoms were seen?	
Hemibody versus generalized activity	
What time was patient last seen normal?	
How long did the activity last?	
Did the patient return to baseline at any point?	
Medication use	
Recent illness or fever	
Preceding trauma	
Prior medical history (e.g., stroke, brain tumor, brain infection)	

TABLE 6.4	Drugs that Lower the Seizure Threshold
Analgesics: narcotics (tramadol, fentanyl, meperidine)	
Antibiotics: penicillins, imipenem, cephalosporins, isoniazid, metronidazole	
Anticholinesterases	
Antidepressants: bupropion, tricyclics	
Antihistamines: diphenhydramine	
Antipsychotics: clozapine, phenothiazine	
Chemotherapy: etoposide, cisplatinum	

Affected patients will not exhibit obvious physical signs of seizures, but electrographic seizure activity will be detected on EEG. As a result, the clinician must be wary of the possibility of nonconvulsive status epilepticus (NCSE) if the patient does not awaken after cessation of seizure activity or displays subtle symptoms of continuing seizures. Please see Chapter 58 for further details on seizure semiology, localizing signs, and seizure syndromes.

EMERGENT TREATMENT OF STATUS EPILEPTICUS

PREHOSPITAL TREATMENT

The most important factor in the treatment of acute seizures is the amount of time it takes to administer the initial treatment. This requires a timely recognition of seizures by bystanders and notification of emergency medical services (EMS). Prehospital EMS care with patient stabilization and medication administration is vital in early treatment of acute seizures and has been associated with improved patient outcomes. Stabilization includes initial assessment of secure airway, stable breathing, and circulation. Once stabilized, prehospital care also involves attempts at obtaining intravenous (IV) access and assessing for reversible causes of seizures such as hypoglycemia.

Following initial assessment, treatment for convulsive seizures can be given by EMS. Benzodiazepines have been the AED of choice in the field (Table 6.7). IV agents have traditionally been used with lorazepam (4 mg) or diazepam (10 mg). In appropriate, targeted dosing, seizure patients that receive IV benzodiazepines have lower instances of respiratory depression/intubation than patients that have prolonged seizures without treatment. Subsequently, the efficacy and safety of IV benzodiazepine use, particularly IV

TABLE 6.5	Red Flags for Life-Threatening Causes of Seizures	
Findings	**Etiology**	
Nuchal rigidity	Meningitis	
Fever		
Rash		
Anisocoria	Transtentorial herniation	
Gaze deviation	Hemispheric mass lesion	
Hemibody weakness	Contralateral stroke	
Periorbital ecchymosis	Trauma	

TABLE 6.6 Localizing Symptoms of Seizures

Signs	Localization
Positive Symptoms	
Hemibody convulsion	Contralateral hemisphere
Generalized convulsion	Generalized cerebral activity
Lateralized facial twitching	Contralateral hemisphere
Eye deviation	Contralateral frontal eye field
Directional nystagmus	Contralateral hemisphere
Echolalia	Temporal or frontal lobe
Automatism	Nonlocalizable
Negative Symptoms	
Aphasia	Dominant hemisphere
Coma	Bilateral hemispheres

lorazepam, has been an important finding in the early prehospital treatment of convulsive seizures [Level 1].[1]

The ability of EMS to establish venous access to appropriately provide IV benzodiazepines along with the storage of IV lorazepam in ambulances have provided limitations to its use. As a result, intramuscular (IM) midazolam (10 mg) has been used increasingly in the prehospital setting. Its study has revealed efficacy and efficiency as an alternative treatment to IV lorazepam [Level 1].[2]

HOSPITAL TREATMENT

Once the patient arrives to the hospital, they should once again be assessed for stable airway, breathing, and circulation (Table 6.8). Supplemental oxygen can be provided. Hemodynamic monitoring should be implemented with particular attention to blood pressure, cardiac monitoring, and oxygenation. IV access, if not already established, should be obtained along with fluid

TABLE 6.7 Emergent First-line Therapy Benzodiazepine Agents and Dosing

Benzodiazepine	Route	Dosing
Lorazepam	IV	0.1 mg/kg IV (max 4 mg per dose) and can repeat at 5–10 min
Diazepam	IV	0.15 mg/kg IV (max 10 mg per dose) and can repeat in 5 min
	PR	0.2 mg/kg PR for >12 yr
		0.3 mg/kg PR for 6–11 yr
		0.5 mg/kg PR for 2–5 yr
Midazolam	IM	0.2 mg/kg IM (max 10 mg)
	Intranasal	0.2 mg/kg intranasal
	Buccal	0.5 mg/kg buccal

IV, intravenous; PR, per rectum; IM, intramuscular.

Adapted from Brophy GM, Bell R, Claassen J, et al. Guidelines for the evaluation and management of status epilepticus. *Neurocrit Care.* 2012;17(1):3–23.

TABLE 6.8 Status Epilepticus Algorithm

Emergent Management

- Recognition and diagnosis of prolonged seizures
- Stabilize patient: ABCs (airway, breathing, circulation). Place IV, supplemental O$_2$, and hemodynamic monitoring.
- Thiamine 100 mg and D50W 50 mL IV (if hypoglycemia)
- Lorazepam 4 mg over 2 min IV; can repeat after 5 min if still seizing; diazepam 10 mg IM or 20 mg per rectum if no IV route available
- Monitor BP and respiratory status during treatment. If no return to baseline:

Second-Line Therapy/Urgent Control Therapy

- Fosphenytoin 20 mg/kg IV at 150 mg/min or valproic acid 40 mg/kg IV over 10 min
- Can consider levetiracetam 1–3 g IV over 2–5 mg/kg/min
- Start maintenance dose of loaded AEDs and order AED levels post loading.
- Order cEEG unless patient is clearly back to baseline.
- Can consider giving additional fosphenytoin 5–10 mg/kg IV ×1 vs. valproic acid 20 mg/kg IV ×1 if no improvement or continued seizure activity. However, do not perform this at the expense of delaying more aggressive RSE treatment measures.
- Monitor BP and respiratory status during treatment. Consider intubation if sedation or seizure compromises airway. If no improvement:

Refractory Status Epilepticus

- Intubate patient and admit to the ICU.
- cEEG should be in place.
- RSE cIV anesthetic agents to goal of burst suppression: See table for RSE medications.
- Monitor hemodynamic stability and add vasopressors if needed.
- Monitor cEEG for 24–48 h for seizure suppression and optimize maintenance AED.

IV, intravenous; O$_2$, oxygen; IM, intramuscular; BP, blood pressure; AED, antiepileptic drug; cEEG, continuous electroencephalography; RSE, refractory status epilepticus; ICU, intensive care unit; cIV, continuous intravenous.

resuscitation to maintain euvolemia. Physicians should reassess glycemic status, and if there is evidence of hypoglycemia, it is important to promptly treat with D50W 50 mL IV with concurrent thiamine 100 mg IV. Handoff between EMS and physicians should establish what treatments were given in the field, including benzodiazepine doses.

Benzodiazepine initial therapy is frequently underdosed due to the seizure treatment dosing being higher than most indications seen by EMS or the emergency department (ED). Attention should be made to provide full appropriate benzodiazepine treatment via additional doses if not given initially. Lorazepam IV has been shown to be the preferred initial agent. A recommended total dose of 0.1 mg/kg (4 mg per dose) can be given [Level 1].[3] A repeat dose of 4 mg can be given after 5 to 10 minutes if needed (for a maximum total of 8 mg). Lorazepam should be administered at a rate up to 2 mg/min. Close attention should be taken to cardiopulmonary status during benzodiazepine administration to avoid uncontrolled hypotension or respiratory depression. Similar to the prehospital management, if there is no IV access readily available, benzodiazepines can be administered via IM, rectal, nasal, or buccal routes. Midazolam is the preferred agent for IM administration. This can be administered at 0.2 mg/kg IM for a total dose of 10 mg (see Table 6.4).

INITIAL WORKUP

Although emergent management is underway, concurrent workup needs to be carried out to establish the underlying cause of seizures as discussed earlier (Table 6.9). All patients should receive basic serum lab evaluation including complete blood count, basic metabolic panel, liver function tests, AED levels, and drug toxicology to evaluate for any metabolic etiologies for seizures. A noncontrast computed tomography (CT) of the brain should be performed for most patients on admission to screen for any obvious structural etiologies of seizures.

The extended workup to be chosen on a case-by-case basis includes a lumbar puncture, magnetic resonance imaging (MRI), and further miscellaneous laboratory tests. If the patient has clear inciting factors (i.e., epilepsy with AED noncompliance or hypoglycemia), a lumbar puncture (LP) may not be necessary. Conversely, in febrile patients, those with an elevated white blood cell count and nuchal rigidity, suspicion should be raised for a CNS infection and an LP is warranted. In addition, if basic metabolic serum workup and CT neuroimaging fail to reveal an obvious etiology of seizures,

TABLE 6.9   Diagnostic Seizure Evaluation

Perform immediately if possible and concurrently with emergent management and treatment.

All Patients
• Glucose fingerstick
• Hemodynamic monitoring and vital signs (blood pressure, cardiac monitoring, O$_2$ saturation, heart rate)
• Neuro checks
• IV access
• O$_2$ administration (if needed)
• Head CT scan
• Serum lab tests: complete blood count, basic metabolic panel, blood glucose, liver function tests, calcium (total and ionized), magnesium, troponin, antiepileptic drug levels, toxicology screen (cocaine and urine), pregnancy test (if female)
• EEG

Consider Depending on Presentation
• Brain MRI
• Lumbar puncture
• Comprehensive toxicology panel: toxins that can cause seizures (isoniazid, tricyclic antidepressants, theophylline, sympathomimetics, organophosphates, cyclosporine)
• Serum blood work: type and hold, coagulation studies, arterial blood gas, inborn errors of metabolism

O$_2$, oxygen; IV, intravenous; CT, computed tomography; EEG, electroencephalography; MRI, magnetic resonance imaging.
Adapted from Brophy GM, Bell R, Claassen J, et al. Guidelines for the evaluation and management of status epilepticus. *Neurocrit Care.* 2012;17(1):3–23.

an MRI of the brain should be performed along with an LP. If infection is suspected, these tests should be pursued without delaying empiric antibiotic treatment. Aggressive measures should be taken to treat life-threatening causes of seizures or SE.

INDICATIONS FOR HOSPITAL ADMISSION

ED policy states that patients with a normal neurologic examination following a seizure can be discharged from the ED with outpatient follow-up. However, if the patient fails to return to baseline in 10 minutes, SE should be suspected and admission is warranted. Failure to control convulsive seizures or persistent unexplained altered mental status requires further evaluation with a continuous EEG (cEEG). These patients with suspected SE require admission to an intensive care unit for further EEG directed treatment and hemodynamic monitoring. cEEG monitoring should be established within 1 hour of SE and should be placed for at least 48 hours in comatose patients to detect nonconvulsive seizures.

TREATMENT ALGORITHM FOR STATUS EPILEPTICUS

In patients with SE, the timely administration of second-line therapy is vital. Second-line therapy administration should ideally occur concomitantly with first-line benzodiazepine therapy. Benzodiazepine therapy alone has a short duration of treatment effect and will not be effective in preventing prolonged seizures or SE. There is no need to delay the administration of second-line therapy to assess if the patient responds to first-line benzodiazepine therapy. The goal of second-line/urgent control therapy is to establish rapid therapeutic levels.

Frequently used second-line agents include phenytoin/fosphenytoin, valproic acid, phenobarbital, and levetiracetam. Prospective studies have not revealed a superior second-line AED agent. However, fosphenytoin/phenytoin is commonly used as the second-line therapy of choice. A 20-mg/kg IV can be given with either formulation. Fosphenytoin can be given at rate of 150 mg/min and phenytoin at 50 mg/min. Care must be taken to avoid rapid infusion, as this may cause hypotension or arrhythmias. Despite preference for phenytoin use, IV valproic acid may be of equal efficacy without the caveats of phenytoin's side effects. A 20- to 40-mg/kg IV can be given over 10 minutes with an option of giving an additional 20 mg/kg over 5 minutes if seizure activity continues. Levetiracetam IV has also been used for second-line therapy for SE. Doses of 1,000 to 3,000 mg IV can be given with administration rate of 2 to 5 mg/kg/min IV.

After second-line or urgent control therapy is administered, AED maintenance therapy is required even if SE is controlled. This requires giving maintenance doses of the AED that was administered IV. Many experts advocate for more aggressive treatment of SE. Rather than treating with second-line AEDs, waiting for a clinical response, and reloading with these agents, the idea of proceeding directly to continuous IV agents while concomitantly using second-line AEDs have been proposed. Studies have shown suboptimal cessation of seizure activity with the sole use of classic second-line agents such as phenytoin. Consequently, when possible, the aggressive escalation of treatment straight to continuous IV AEDs such as midazolam can be considered.

REFRACTORY STATUS EPILEPTICUS

If there is failure to control SE after the use of a benzodiazepine and second-line AED, the patient is considered to be in refractory SE (RSE). RSE occurs in approximately 30% of patients with SE and is

TABLE 6.10   Continuous Intravenous Anesthetic Agents for Refractory Status Epilepticus

Drug	Bolus Dose	Maintenance Dose	Side Effects
Pentobarbital	5–15 mg/kg (up to 50 mg/min) Repeat bolus of 5 mg/kg until seizures stop.	1–10 mg/kg/h	• Hypotension • Ileus • Respiratory/cardiac depression
Propofol	1–2 mg/kg over 3–5 min Repeat bolus every 3–5 min until seizures stop (maximum 10 mg/kg).	30–100 µg/kg/min	• Hypotension • Propofol infusion syndrome (particularly at >80 µg/kg/min for >48 h)
Midazolam	0.2 mg/kg (rate of 2 mg/min) Repeat bolus of 0.2–0.4 mg/kg every 5 min until seizures stop (maximum of 2 mg/kg).	0.05–2.9 mg/kg/h	• Respiratory depression • Hypotension (less than propofol and pentobarbital) • Tachyphylaxis

associated with increased morbidity and mortality compared to SE counterparts. The pathophysiology of propagation to RSE involves the internalization of γ-aminobutyric acid receptors and upregulation of excitatory N-methyl-D-aspartate receptors. Consequently, management of RSE requires rapid and aggressive escalation of care with intubation (if not already performed) and induction of coma with continuous IV (cIV) anesthetic agents with therapeutic targets at these two receptors. It is unclear of the treatment target endpoints as some evidence suggests that RSE outcome is based on the underlying cause of RSE rather than the aggressiveness of treatment. Despite this, many experts agree that aggressive treatment tailored to EEG suppression rather than clinical seizure activity is ideal in the escalation of care. Consequently, cEEG is vital at this point in both evaluating for seizure activity and response to therapy. Attempts to advance therapy should not be delayed with repeat treatments with second-line agents.

Although there is no uniform consensus on optimal RSE therapy, frequently used agents include midazolam, propofol, and pentobarbital (Table 6.10). When intubation is not possible, valproic acid can be used as a viable alternative. There remains a paucity of prospective comparative studies for these agents. However, retrospective analysis and limited prospective studies have given some guidance for future studies and selection of preferred RSE treatments.

Pentobarbital has been seen to have higher treatment efficacy compared to propofol and midazolam. However, longer rates of mechanical ventilation have been seen with barbiturate use due to its long half-life along with increased risk of cardiac side effects. Pentobarbital infusion is preceded by a loading dose of 5 to 15 mg/kg (up to 50 mg/min) with repeated boluses of 5 mg/kg until seizures stop. Maintenance infusion can be started at 1 mg/kg/h with titration up to 10 mg/kg/h for goal of EEG burst suppression.

Propofol is also an effective agent but it requires careful hemodynamic monitoring. It has the caveat of hypotension along with propofol infusion syndrome (circulatory collapse, lactic acidosis, hypertriglyceridemia, rhabdomyolysis). Propofol requires a 1- to 2-mg/kg loading dose over 3 to 5 minutes. Repeat boluses can be given every 3 to 5 minutes until seizures stop (maximum loading dose of 10 mg/kg). Maintenance propofol dosing should be titrated to EEG burst suppression at 30 to 100 µg/kg/min. Doses of greater than 80 µg/kg/min for extended periods of time (>48 hours) may place the patient at risk for propofol infusion syndrome.

Midazolam appears to have less of an effect on blood pressure in comparison to propofol or pentobarbital. However, its use is particularly prone to tachyphylaxis and its mechanism of action is hindered by not having any effect on NMDA receptor sites. Midazolam requires a loading dose of 0.2 mg/kg at a rate of 2 mg/min. Repeat boluses of 0.2 to 0.4 mg/kg boluses every 5 minutes can be given until seizures stop with a maximum loading dose of 2 mg/kg. Maintenance infusion can be titrated for goal of EEG burst suppression at 0.05 to 2 mg/kg/h. However, maintenance infusion rates of as high as 2.9 mg/kg/h can be used safely with lower rates of withdrawal seizures and lower discharge mortality rates.

There is no clear support for the length of treatment and seizure suppression with cIV anesthetic agents before weaning attempts are made. However, general consensus states that patients should remain seizure free for 24 to 48 hours on cEEG monitoring. While waiting for this to occur, the patient's maintenance AED agents should be optimized from a therapeutic level standpoint. Levels can be allowed to be supratherapeutic and should be dictated based on seizure control and side effect profile. Gradual attempts can then be made to wean off of these agents.

KEY POINTS

- Distinguishing between isolated seizures and SE is paramount for effective treatment.
- Focused history/exam should characterize seizure activity, presumed duration of seizures, and pertinent history (i.e., seizures in the past).
- Treatment begins with assessment of airway, breathing, and circulation.
- Prehospital treatment with benzodiazepines should be initiated as soon as possible and may be given by a number or routes (i.e., IV, IM, buccal, rectal).
- Concurrent workup and tests should occur while the patient is being stabilized and treated.
- Treat early with initial line of therapy with benzodiazepines; agent of choice is lorazepam IV.
- Continue therapy with second-line urgent control therapy with phenytoin/fosphenytoin or valproic acid; alternatives include levetiracetam or phenobarbital.
- Start maintenance AED therapy after second-line urgent control therapy.

- If the patient does not return to baseline within 20 minutes after convulsions stop, suspect nonconvulsive seizures or SE.
- cEEG must be ordered to further drive therapeutic management if concerns for SE.
- If evidence of prolonged seizures, intubate and escalate to cIV anesthetic AED agents.
- Do not delay treatment.

LEVEL 1 EVIDENCE

1. Alldredge BK, Gelb AM, Isaacs SM, et al. A comparison of lorazepam, diazepam, and placebo for the treatment of out-of-hospital status epilepticus. *N Engl J Med.* 2001;345(9):631–637.
2. Silbergleit R, Durkalski V, Lowenstein D, et al. Intramuscular versus intravenous therapy for prehospital status epilepticus. *N Engl J Med.* 2012;366(7):591–600.
3. Treiman DM, Meyers PD, Walton NY, et al. A comparison of four treatments for generalized convulsive status epilepticus. *N Engl J Med.* 1998;339(12):792–798.

SUGGESTED READINGS

Berning S, Boesebeck F, van Baalen A, et al. Intravenous levetiracetam as treatment for status epilepticus. *J Neurol.* 2009;256(10):1634–1642.

Brophy GM, Bell R, Claassen J, et al. Guidelines for the evaluation and management of status epilepticus. *Neurocrit Care.* 2012;17(1):3–23.

Claassen J, Hirsch LJ, Emerson RG, et al. Treatment of refractory status epilepticus with pentobarbital, propofol, or midazolam: a systematic review. *Epilepsia.* 2002;43(2):146–153.

Claassen J, Mayer SA, Kowalski RG, et al. Detection of electrographic seizures with continuous EEG monitoring in critically ill patients. *Neurology.* 2004;62(10):1743–1748.

Claassen J, Silbergleit R, Weingart SD, et al. Emergency neurological life support: status epilepticus. *Neurocrit Care.* 2012;17(suppl 1):S73–S78.

DeLorenzo RJ, Waterhouse EJ, Towne AR, et al. Persistent nonconvulsive status epilepticus after the control of convulsive status epilepticus. *Epilepsia.* 1998;39(8):833–840.

Fernandez A, Lantigua H, Lesch C, et al. High-dose midazolam infusion for refractory status epilepticus. *Neurology.* 2014;82(4):359–365.

Fisher RS, van Emde Boas W, Blume W, et al. Epileptic seizures and epilepsy: definitions proposed by the international league against epilepsy (ILAE) and the international bureau for epilepsy (IBE). *Epilepsia.* 2005;46(4):470–472.

Jenssen S, Gracely EJ, Sperling MR. How long do most seizures last? A systematic comparison of seizures recorded in the epilepsy monitoring unit. *Epilepsia.* 2006;47(9):1499–1503.

Jirsch J, Hirsch LJ. Nonconvulsive seizures: developing a rational approach to the diagnosis and management in the critically ill population. *Clin Neurophysiol.* 2007;118(8):1660–1670.

Logroscino G, Hesdorffer DC, Cascino G, et al. Short-term mortality after a first episode of status epilepticus. *Epilepsia.* 1997;38(12):1344–1349.

Lowenstein DH, Alldredge BK. Status epilepticus. *N Engl J Med.* 1998;338(14):970–976.

Mayer SA, Claassen J, Lokin J, et al. Refractory status epilepticus: frequency, risk factors, and impact on outcome. *Arch Neurol.* 2002;59(2):205–210.

Misra UK, Kalita J, Patel R. Sodium valproate vs phenytoin in status epilepticus: a pilot study. *Neurology.* 2006;67(2):340–342.

Pallin DJ, Goldstein JN, Moussally JS, et al. Seizure visits in US emergency departments: epidemiology and potential disparities in care. *Int J Emerg Med.* 2008;1(2):97–105.

Rossetti AO. Which anesthetic should be used in the treatment of refractory status epilepticus? *Epilepsia.* 2007;48:52–55.

Rossetti AO, Logroscino G, Bromfield EB. Refractory status epilepticus: effect of treatment aggressiveness on prognosis. *Arch Neurol.* 2005;62(11):1698–1702.

Rossetti AO, Milligan TA, Vulliémoz S, et al. A randomized trial for the treatment of refractory status epilepticus. *Neurocrit Care.* 2011;14(1):4–10.

Walker M. Status epilepticus: an evidence based guide. *BMJ.* 2005;331(7518):673–677.

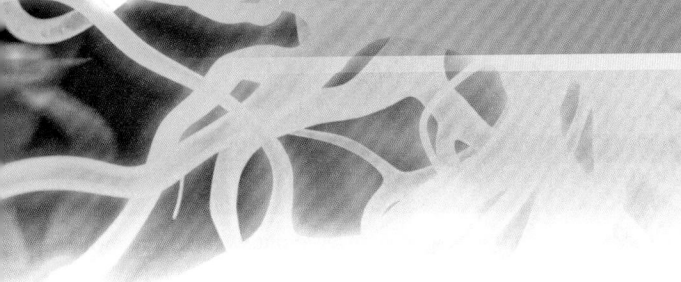

Headache and Facial Pain

Julio R. Vieira and Denise E. Chou

INTRODUCTION

Headache is one of the most frequent reasons for which patients seek medical attention and accounts for more disability on a global scale than any other neurologic problem when including direct and indirect costs. The appropriate management of headache disorders relies on a careful diagnostic approach that is based on an understanding of the physiologic mechanisms of head pain and different characteristics of both primary and secondary headache syndromes.

GENERAL PRINCIPLES

A classification system for headache disorders has been established by the International Headache Society (IHS). The most recent version, *International Classification of Headache Disorders*, 3rd edition, beta version (*ICHD-3* beta) divides headache disorders into *primary syndromes* (in which the headache and associated features constitute the disorder itself) and *secondary disorders* (in which the headache results from exogenous causes).

The most common primary headache syndrome is tension headache comprising 69% of all primary headaches; however, such headaches are rarely debilitating and are generally self-treated with over-the-counter medications. The second most common primary headache disorder is migraine, with a 1-year prevalence of 12% (17% among women and 6% among men peaking around the fourth decade of life). Recurrent and disabling headaches in a primary care setting are most often migraines. Life-threatening headache is infrequent; however, caution and adequate surveillance are needed to properly diagnose and manage these cases.

DIAGNOSIS

The key to the proper diagnosis of headache is obtaining a comprehensive and precise history. Important components of the headache history include the following:

- **Onset:** abrupt versus insidious; context in which headache began (e.g., recent head trauma, including head/neck surgeries, viral illness, pregnancy/postpartum)
- **Timing:** chronicity, duration, and frequency of headache attacks; time to maximal intensity; diurnal versus nocturnal
- **Quality:** for example, sharp, dull, pressure, throbbing, stabbing, lancinating, burning
- **Laterality:** unilateral versus bilateral; side-locked versus alternating
- **Location:** for example, retroorbital, frontal, temporal, occipital
- **Severity:** including disability and interference with work/normal activities

- **Change:** different pattern from prior headaches
- **Associated symptoms:** sensory hypersensitivity (e.g., to light, noise, sound, smell, movement); nausea/vomiting; visual changes; numbness/tingling of the face or extremities; focal motor weakness; impairment of speech; light-headedness/vertigo; cognitive dysfunction
- **Cranial autonomic features:** lacrimation, conjunctival injection, periorbital or facial edema, ptosis, pupillary changes; nasal congestion or rhinorrhea; aural fullness or tinnitus
- **Premonitory features:** symptoms that are experienced days to hours prior to headache attacks (such as yawning, sleepiness, increased thirst, changes in bowel/bladder pattern, neck stiffness)
- **Triggers:** for example, menstrual cycle; skipping meals; lack of sleep or oversleeping; stress or relaxation from stress; altitude or barometric changes; position (lying down vs. standing up); Valsalva maneuvers or physical exertion; bright lights, noise, or smells; alcohol; caffeine; and certain foods (such as those containing nitrates or monosodium glutamate)
- **Family history** of headache disorders

Past medical history, review of systems, social history, concomitant medications, prior imaging, and labwork should also be reviewed in detail, as these may reveal an underlying cause for the headache.

The physical examination should include a comprehensive systemic and neurologic examination with particular attention to the following: bruits of the head or neck, temporal artery tenderness and pulsations, occipital nerve tenderness, pupillary size and symmetry, funduscopic examination (for evaluation of papilledema and retinal venous pulsations), visual field testing and extraocular movements, facial sensation (including corneal responses), and motor function.

The first goal of diagnosis is to differentiate between a benign headache disorder (usually a primary syndrome) and a serious underlying condition (secondary headache). There are a few tools available to help identify a potential life-threatening headache (using so-called red flags); conversely, the presence of "white or green flags" can suggest a more benign scenario.

RED FLAGS

Symptoms that may point to a serious underlying disorder can be evaluated by the mnemonic "SNOOP" (Table 7.1). Despite the use of SNOOP, the neurologic examination remains the best predictor of structural intracranial pathology. The evaluation of a patient with headache in the emergency room is shown in Figure 7.1.

Alarming causes of secondary headaches that require urgent evaluation include meningitis, intracranial hemorrhage, acute ischemic event, tumor or obstructive lesion, glaucoma, purulent sinusitis, cortical vein/cranial sinus thrombosis, carotid/vertebral artery dissection, pituitary apoplexy, posterior reversible encephalopathy

TABLE 7.1	"Red Flags" When Evaluating Headache Symptoms
Systemic	Systemic signs/symptoms: stiff neck, vomiting preceding the headache, fever, night sweats, rash, myalgia, weight loss; also headache during pregnancy or postpartum and comorbid systemic disease (e.g., HIV, malignancy)
Neurologic symptoms	Change in mental status or level of consciousness; papilledema, diplopia; loss of sensation; weakness; ataxia; local tenderness (region of temporal artery); headache induced by Valsalva maneuvers (bending, lifting, cough, sneezing); pain that disturbs sleep or presents immediately upon awakening; history of seizure/collapse/loss of consciousness
Older	Onset after age 50 years
Onset	Onset sudden and/or first ever; severe or "worst" headache of life; "thunderclap" headache (pain reaches maximal intensity in an instant)
Pattern change	Change in frequency, severity, or clinical features of the attack; subacute worsening over days/weeks or accelerating pattern, continuous or persistent headache; pain triggered by sexual activity, Valsalva maneuver, or sleep; worsening with change in position

Adapted from Silberstein SD, Lipton RB, Dodick D, et al. *Wolff's Headache and Other Head Pain*. 8th ed. New York: Oxford University Press; 2008.

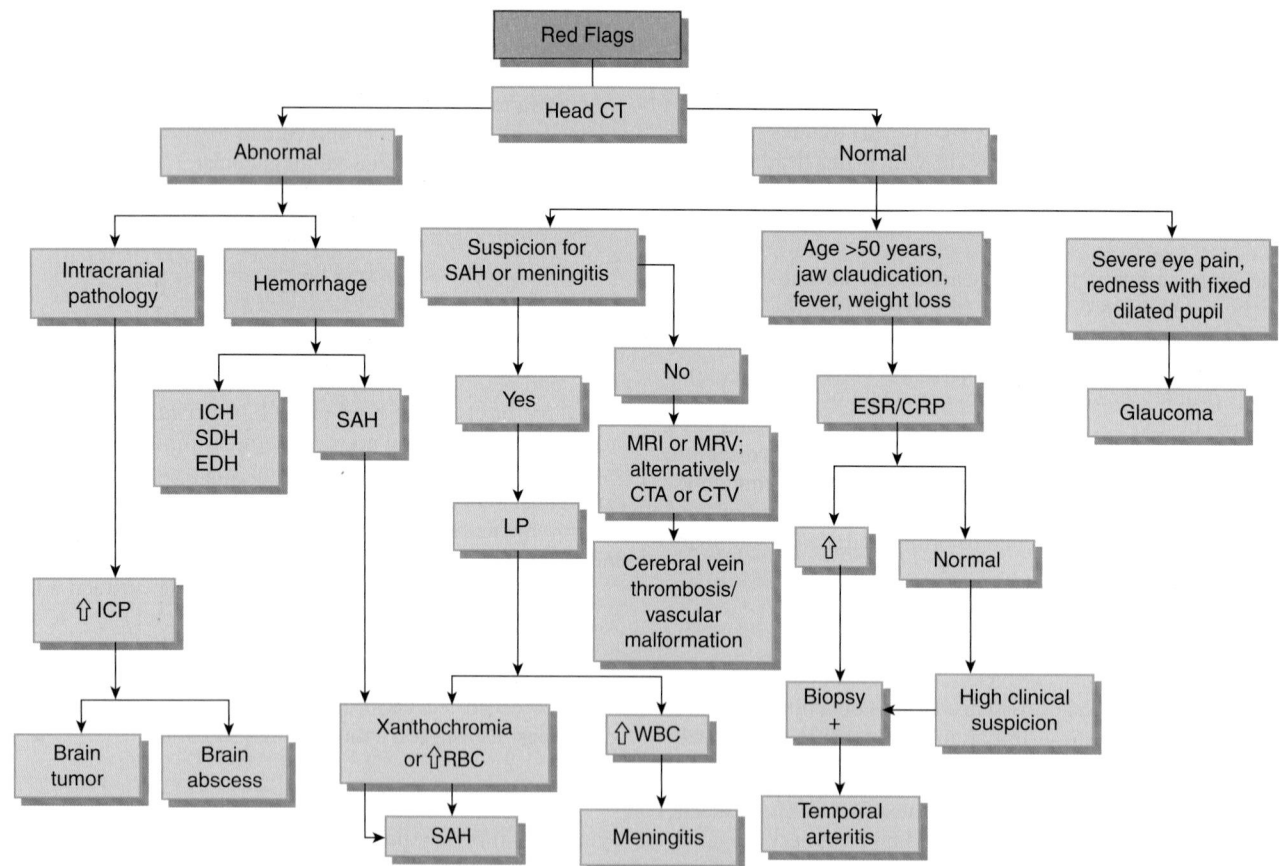

FIGURE 7.1 Evaluation of a patient with headache in the emergency room. CT, computed tomography; SAH, subarachnoid hemorrhage; ICH, intracerebral hemorrhage; SDH, subdural hemorrhage; EDH, extradural hemorrhage; LP, lumbar puncture; MRI, magnetic resonance imaging; MRV, magnetic resonance venography; CTA, computed tomography angiography; CTV, computed tomography venography; ESR, erythrocyte sedimentation rate; CRP, C-reactive protein; ICP, intracranial pressure; RBC, red blood cell; WBC, white blood cell. (Adapted from Gordon DL. Approach to the patient with acute headache. In: Biller J, ed. *Practical Neurology*. 4th ed. Philadelphia: Lippincott Williams & Wilkins; 2012:194–206.)

TABLE 7.2	POUND Mnemonic for Identifying Migraine Headache
Pulsatile quality of headache	
One-day duration (4–72 h)	
Unilateral location	
Nausea or vomiting	
Disabling intensity	

syndrome (PRES), and reversible cerebral vasoconstriction syndrome (RCVS). Patients who had a recent ischemic infarct and develop new-onset headache should also undergo immediate head computed tomography (CT) to rule out hemorrhage, particularly those patients who received thrombolysis. Thyroid disorders (most commonly hypothyroidism) are also frequently associated with headache.

GREEN FLAGS

Certain clinical features support a benign primary headache disorder. Simple tools that can help identify migraine include *ID Migraine*, a set of three questions regarding photophobia, nausea, and disability simplified as "PIN" (photophobia, inability to function, and nausea). If two out of the three features are present, a diagnosis of migraine is likely (with sensitivity of 81% and specificity of 75%). If all three are present, there is a 93% probability of meeting IHS diagnostic criteria for migraine. Another tool is the *POUND mnemonic* (Table 7.2), in which the presence of four out of five features can accurately predict a diagnosis of migraine.

Despite present guideline recommendations, many clinicians overorder imaging in benign scenarios. The American Headache Society (AHS) created the "Choosing Wisely" recommendations to address the need for neuroimaging as follows:

- No need for imaging in patients with stable headache that meet migraine criteria
- No CT for headache when magnetic resonance imaging (MRI) is available except in emergency settings.

SECONDARY CAUSES OF HEADACHE

MENINGITIS

Presence of fever, stiff neck, and Kernig and Brudzinski signs (poor sensitivity but good specificity) warrant further workup with imaging (CT/MRI) followed by lumbar puncture for cerebrospinal fluid (CSF) analysis to rule out an infectious or inflammatory meningitis. If suspecting meningitis, cover with empiric antibiotics while awaiting CSF results.

SUBARACHNOID HEMORRHAGE

History of a "thunderclap headache" or "worst headache of life" can be suggestive of subarachnoid hemorrhage. In addition, focal neurologic deficits can be present on examination. A third nerve palsy suggests a possible posterior communicating (PComm) artery aneurysm, whereas a sixth nerve palsy can suggest a posterior fossa lesion or increased intracranial pressure, as can nystagmus or ataxia. Bilateral leg weakness or abulia may signify an anterior communicating (AComm) artery aneurysm; aphasia, hemiparesis, or neglect can suggest a middle cerebral artery (MCA) aneurysm. Patients with these presenting symptoms should undergo immediate noncontrast head CT imaging; if this is negative and subarachnoid hemorrhage is still suspected, lumbar puncture should be performed (checking for the presence of red blood cells or xanthochromia). Note that patients presenting with headache for more than 2 weeks with a negative CT and clear CSF may still have subarachnoid hemorrhage requiring further workup with MRI and vessel imaging with computed tomography angiogram (CTA), magnetic resonance angiogram (MRA), or conventional angiogram.

BRAIN TUMOR

Approximately 30% of patients diagnosed with a brain tumor report headache at presentation; however, only 1% present with headache as the *only* clinical symptom. Apart from focal neurologic deficits, clues that may suggest an intracranial lesion include sudden change in pattern of a preexisting headache disorder, worsening of headache with Valsalva maneuvers and exertion, or headache that awakens one up from sleep. However, these characteristics are also commonly seen in primary headache disorders, such as migraine and cluster headache.

SUBDURAL HEMATOMA

Headache is reported in 80% of cases and is more insidious in onset than subarachnoid hemorrhage. Otherwise, headache characteristics may resemble those of a brain tumor (due to mass effect). Mental status changes and gait instability are common in the elderly who are prone to acute-on-chronic subdural bleeding (often from nonwitnessed or nonreported falls).

CERVICAL ARTERY DISSECTION

Headache with carotid artery dissection is typically unilateral and may be associated with ipsilateral neck pain or Horner syndrome. Headache from vertebral artery dissection is posterolateral and may be accompanied by meningismus when subarachnoid hemorrhage has resulted from dissection of blood through the vessel wall of the intracranial segment.

CEREBRAL VENOUS THROMBOSIS

Approximately 90% of cases present with headache (most common feature but not specific); other signs include seizures, altered mental status, papilledema, and focal neurologic deficits. This condition is most common among young adult women.

REVERSIBLE CEREBRAL VASOCONSTRICTION SYNDROME

This condition often presents with thunderclap headache resembling subarachnoid hemorrhage. The diagnosis is established by demonstrating the absence of blood in the CSF, the presence of diffuse cerebral arterial vasospasm, and a relatively benign clinical course with resolution of the syndrome over a period of weeks.

GIANT CELL ARTERITIS

New-onset headache at age 50 years or older, with associated temporal artery tenderness or decreased temporal artery pulse, should raise suspicion for giant cell arteritis (temporal arteritis). Other associated symptoms include jaw claudication, unanticipated weight loss, fatigue, and/or myalgias. An elevated erythrocyte sedimentation rate (ESR) and/or C-reactive protein (CRP) should be checked in such cases; if these are normal but clinical suspicion remains high, a temporal artery biopsy should be pursued. Headache typically resolves or greatly improves within 3 days of starting high-dose corticosteroids.

SPONTANEOUS INTRACRANIAL HYPOTENSION

Headache is exquisitely orthostatic in nature, occurring in the upright position and resolving or notably improving upon lying supine. Pain may also be worsened by Valsalva maneuvers and especially in the Trendelenburg position. Stiff neck and nausea are prevalent. If intracranial hypotension is suspected, an MRI brain with and without contrast should be performed, which may reveal subdural fluid collections, pachymeningeal enhancement, engorgement of venous structures, pituitary hyperemia, and/or sagging of the brain with cerebellar tonsil displacement. If there is no clear precipitating event (such as a recent lumbar puncture), spinal MRI with T2 weighting and CT/magnetic resonance (MR) myelography should be considered to identify potential sites of CSF leakage. Treatment options include bedrest, intravenous fluids and caffeine, and blood patch (if the site of leak is identified). In patients with intractable pain, oral theophylline is a useful alternative.

IDIOPATHIC INTRACRANIAL HYPERTENSION

Idiopathic intracranial hypertension (IIH), formerly called *pseudotumor cerebri*, is a syndrome of elevated intracranial pressure associated with normal brain imaging and CSF findings that occurs primarily in young women. Headache may share features as seen with brain tumors, such as worsening with Valsalva maneuvers, wakening from sleep, and/or intractable nausea or vomiting. Other symptoms include transient visual obscuration, photopsia, and pulsatile tinnitus. Persistently raised intracranial pressure can also trigger migraine symptoms such as photophobia or phonophobia. Abnormal findings on examination include papilledema or cessation of venous pulsations (suggesting elevated intracranial pressure) or diplopia from sixth nerve palsy. IIH is most commonly associated with obesity and women of childbearing age; however, the disorder can also manifest at any age, in men, and in patients who are not overweight. Certain medications may increase the risk for developing IIH, such as estrogen-containing oral contraceptives, excessive intake of vitamin A or retinoic acid derivatives, and lithium. Brain MRI and magnetic resonance venogram (MRV) should be obtained if there is concern; imaging may reveal an empty sella, flattening of the posterior globes, protruding of optic nerve heads, and vertical tortuosity of optic nerves. An elevated opening pressure on lumbar puncture and improvement in headache following removal of CSF is diagnostic. Initial treatment is with acetazolamide 250 to 500 mg twice a day (b.i.d.); topiramate is the next treatment of choice. Severely disabled patients who do not respond to medical treatment require intracranial pressure monitoring and may require ventriculoperitoneal shunting.

EMERGENCY EVALUATION OF HEADACHE

Upon presentation to the emergency department (ED), it is necessary to evaluate for the presence of red flags—if any are present, the algorithm in Figure 7.1 should be followed for further workup. Useful lab work for the evaluation of headache in the emergency room include the following:

- Comprehensive metabolic panel
- Complete blood count
- Coagulation panel, β-human chorionic gonadotropin (β-HCG) (pregnancy test)
- Thyroid studies
- ESR and CRP (if concern for temporal arteritis)

If there is concern for intracranial hemorrhage or space-occupying lesion, a noncontrast head CT should be obtained first; a follow-up MRI brain may be later obtained for further characterization. Vascular imaging (such as with MRA/CTA, MRV/computed tomography venography [CTV], or conventional angiography) may be considered in the circumstances described earlier. In other conditions, lumbar puncture may be required, unless a benign etiology can be otherwise established.

The exclusion of underlying secondary causes suggests a non–life-threatening headache disorder; likewise, the presence of white or green flags provides reassurance of a primary headache syndrome, most commonly migraine. The primary headache syndromes are further covered in Chapter 54.

FACIAL PAIN AND CRANIAL NEURALGIAS

The analysis of facial pain requires a different approach. *Neuralgias* are characterized by paroxysmal, fleeting, and often electric shock–like episodes in the distribution of a particular nerve usually without a background of chronic pain. Such disorders are generally caused by ectatic vascular loops compressing the associated nerve (e.g., trigeminal or glossopharyngeal) at the nerve root entry zone, activating a pain-generating mechanism in the brain stem. Other causes, including demyelinating lesions at the central portions of the nerve root entry zones, are more commonly seen in younger patients who are less likely to have ectatic vascular loops. However, the most common cause of facial pain is dental pathology or irritation; provocation by hot or cold foods is typical. Application of a cold stimulus repeatedly induces dental pain, whereas in neuralgic disorders, a refractory period usually occurs after the initial response, so that pain cannot be induced repeatedly. The presence of refractory periods nearly always may be elicited in the history, thereby saving the patient from a painful testing experience.

Trigger maneuvers characteristically provoke paroxysms of pain. Activation of the pain by chewing points to trigeminal neuralgia, temporomandibular joint dysfunction (TMD), giant cell arteritis, or occasionally angina (jaw claudication), whereas the combination of swallowing *and* taste provocation points to glossopharyngeal neuralgia. Pain on swallowing is common among patients with *carotidynia* (facial migraine) because the inflamed, tender carotid artery abuts the esophagus during deglutition.

As with other painful conditions, many patients with facial pain do not describe stereotypic syndromes and are frequently given a diagnosis of "atypical facial pain." Vague, poorly localized, continuous facial pain can be seen in conditions such as nasopharyngeal carcinoma and other somatic diseases; a burning, painful element often supervenes as deafferentation occurs and evidence of cranial neuropathy appears. Occasionally, the underlying cause may not be promptly uncovered, thus necessitating periodic follow-up examinations until further clues appear. Facial pain syndromes and the cranial neuralgias are further covered in Chapter 55.

TREATMENT

The core principles of effective headache treatment are reassurance, adequate hydration, and the appropriate control of pain and associated symptoms (such as nausea). Treatment goals include accurate diagnosis of the headache syndrome, reduction of disability, and rapid return to normal functioning, as well as avoidance of medication overuse and prevention of recurrent emergency room visits.

Despite evidence against the use of opioids for headache treatment in the emergency setting, administration of such medications has been increasing over recent years. Indeed, opioids are the most commonly prescribed medications for migraine in the emergency room, whereas migraine-specific therapies (such as triptans and dihydroergotamine) are scarcely used in the ED setting.

The Choosing Wisely campaign from the American Board of Internal Medicine (ABIM) recommends avoiding opioids and butalbital-containing medications as first-line treatment for recurrent headache. Butalbital is associated with a high frequency of medication overuse ("rebound") headache and has been banned in some countries. Opioids are not as effective for acute migraine treatment as phenothiazines (e.g., chlorpromazine, prochlorperazine, and promethazine), dihydroergotamine, ketorolac, and butyrophenones and have more side effects. In addition, opioids may decrease the effectiveness of migraine-specific abortive therapies (such as triptans and ketorolac), increase relapse with recurrent ED visits and medication overuse, and accelerate progression to chronic migraine due to a "pain memory state."

HEADACHE TREATMENT IN THE EMERGENCY DEPARTMENT

As previously mentioned, the majority of headache cases presenting to the ED are migraine. For mild headache without nausea, oral nonsteroidal anti-inflammatory drugs (NSAIDs) and/or triptans are recommended as first-line treatments (see Table 54.3 for detailed dosage information). More severe headache with or without nausea can be treated with intravenous fluids along with a single dose of a dopamine receptor antagonist such as chlorpromazine 25 to 50 mg, prochlorperazine 10 to 25 mg, promethazine 25 to 50 mg, or metoclopramide 5 to 10 mg, which have both antiemetic and antinociceptive properties. Patients should be monitored for the development

of akathisia or other extrapyramidal side effects (particularly with use of prochlorperazine and metoclopramide), which can be treated or prevented with concomitant administration of intravenous diphenhydramine.

Intravenous valproic acid 10–15 mg/kg can also be considered for treatment of severe migraine; however, one study showed lower efficacy than metoclopramide or ketorolac alone. Use of valproic acid should be avoided in pregnant women and cautiously used in women of childbearing age, as well as those with liver disease or urea cycle disorders.

The addition of intravenous dexamethasone 4 to 10 mg has been shown to decrease headache recurrence with a number needed to treat (NNT) of 10 when used prior to ED discharge.

For refractory pain, dihydroergotamine (DHE) 1 mg intravenous/intramuscular (IM)/subcutaneous (SC) can be useful; repetitive dosing over a 3- to 5-day course is generally more effective than a single infusion. Contraindications include pregnancy, uncontrolled hypertension, history of coronary artery disease, cerebrovascular disease or severe peripheral vascular disease, acute porphyria, Raynaud disease, and use of any triptan or ergot in the preceding 24 hours. Alternatively, a continuous infusion of intravenous lidocaine (1 to 4 mg/min) over a 7- to 10-day course under cardiac monitoring can be considered in patients with refractory headache who are unable to receive DHE for these reasons.

Headache recurrence after ED discharge is remarkably frequent, occurring in approximately 75% of patients within 48 hours of discharge; thus, close outpatient follow-up is necessary. Oral naproxen (Naprosyn) 500 mg and/or sumatriptan 100 mg at headache onset as abortive therapy are useful options upon discharge to avoid recurrent migraine.

Special conditions include the trigeminal autonomic cephalalgias (TACs), which are further covered in Chapter 54. The acute treatment of cluster headache includes 100% oxygen inhaled via a nonrebreather mask at a rate of 10 to 12 L/min for 15 to 20 minutes and/or sumatriptan 6 mg SC. Alternative options include intranasal sumatriptan 20 mg or zolmitriptan 5 mg or DHE 1 mg administered IM or intravenously. Paroxysmal hemicrania (PH) and hemicrania continua (HC) respond exquisitely to oral indomethacin, which can be started at a dose of 25 mg three times a day (t.i.d.) for 5 to 7 days, if no response then increased to 50 mg t.i.d. for an additional 5 to 7 days and further if needed to 75 mg t.i.d. A single intramuscular dose of indomethacin 100 mg ("Indotest") can be useful to confirm a diagnosis of PH or HC; however, this formulation is currently not available in the United States. SUNCT (**s**hort-lasting **u**nilateral **n**euralgiform headache with **c**onjunctival **t**earing and injection) or SUNA (**s**hort-lasting **u**nilateral **n**euralgiform headache with cranial **a**utonomic symptoms) that is not responsive to oral therapies (such as lamotrigine) may require a short course of intravenous lidocaine 1 to 4 mg/min under cardiac monitoring.

One of the challenges in standardizing headache treatment in the ED is that about half of such cases do not fit IHS criteria, which raises concerns about the external validity of ED studies. The schematic in Figure 7.2 is a suggested general approach to the management of the migraine patient presenting to the ED. However, treatment ultimately should be tailored to the patient's individual headache characteristics, associated features, and medical comorbidities.

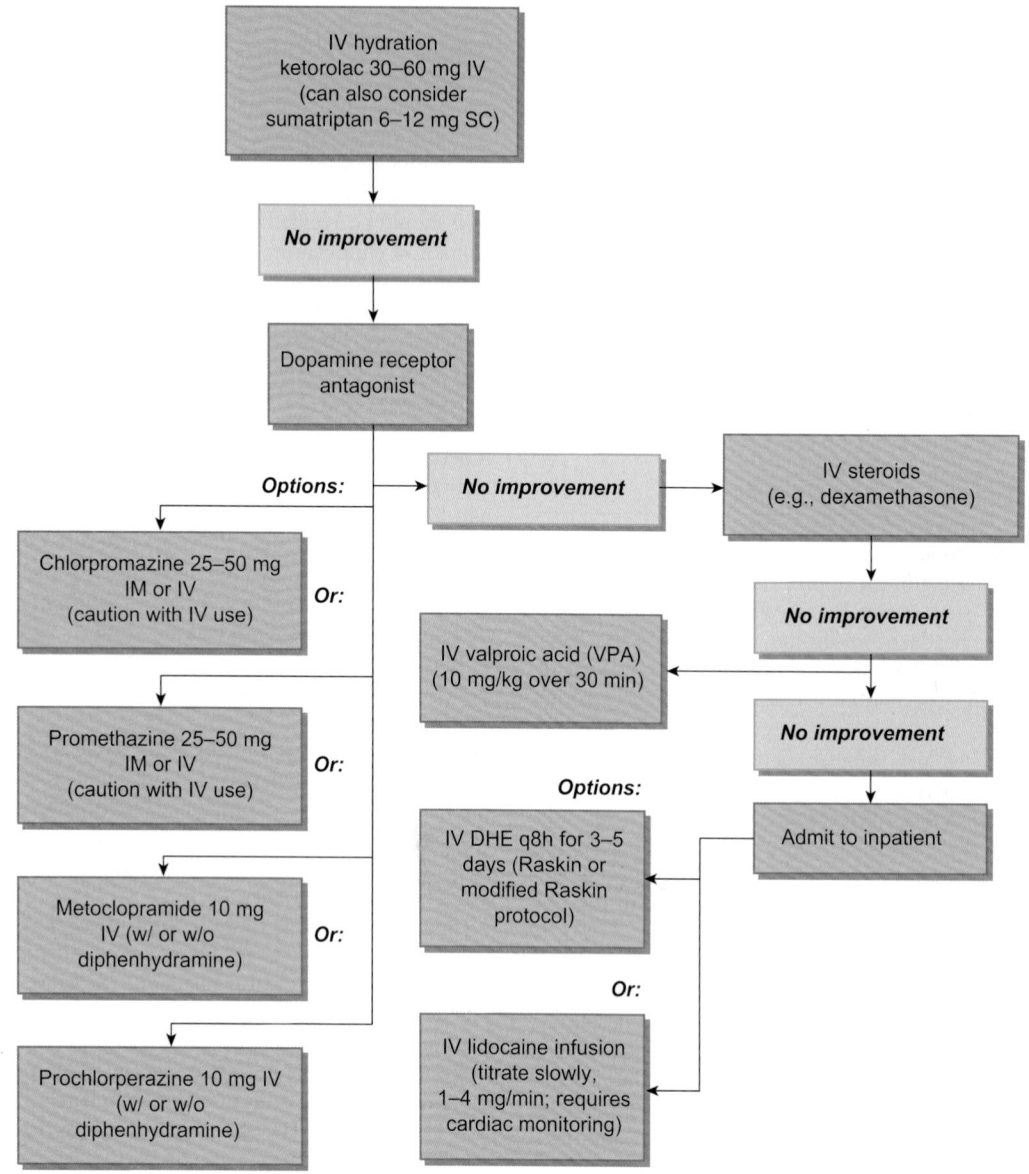

FIGURE 7.2 Treatment algorithm for the migraine patient in the emergency room. IV, intravenous; SC, subcutaneous; IM, intramuscular; DHE, dihydroergotamine.

SUGGESTED READINGS

Ball AK, Clarke CE. Idiopathic intracranial hypertension. *Lancet Neurol.* 2006;5(5): 433–442.

Bigal ME, Lipton RB. Excessive acute migraine medication use and migraine progression. *Neurology.* 2008;71(22):1821–1828.

Burstein R, Collins B, Jakubowski M. Defeating migraine pain with triptans: a race against the development of cutaneous allodynia. *Ann Neurol.* 2004;55(1): 19–26.

Carolei A, Sacco S. Headache attributed to stroke, TIA, intracerebral haemorrhage, or vascular malformation. *Handb Clin Neurol.* 2010;97(chapter 47): 517–528.

Colman I, Rothney A, Wright SC, et al. Use of narcotic analgesics in the emergency department treatment of migraine headache. *Neurology.* 2004;62(10): 1695–1700.

De Luca GC, Bartleson JD. When and how to investigate the patient with headache. *Semin Neurol.* 2010;30(2):131–144.

Detsky ME, McDonald DR, Baerlocher MO, et al. Does this patient with headache have a migraine or need neuroimaging? *JAMA.* 2006;296(10): 1274–1283.

Dilli E. Thunderclap headache. *Curr Neurol Neurosci Rep.* 2014;14(4):437–412.

Dodick DW. Diagnosing headache: clinical clues and clinical rules. *Adv Stud Med.* 2003;3(2):87–92.

Donohoe CD. The role of the physical examination in the evaluation of headache. *Med Clin North Am.* 2013;97(2):197–216.

Edlow JA, Caplan LR. Avoiding pitfalls in the diagnosis of subarachnoid hemorrhage. *N Engl J Med.* 2000;342(1):29–36.

Fiesseler FW, Kec R, Mandell M, et al. Do ED patients with migraine headaches meet internationally accepted criteria? *Am J Emerg Med.* 2002;20(7):618–623.

Friedman BW, Garber L, Yoon A, et al. Randomized trial of IV valproate vs metoclopramide vs ketorolac for acute migraine. *Neurology.* 2014;82(11): 976–983.

Friedman BW, Solorzano C, Esses D, et al. Treating headache recurrence after emergency department discharge: a randomized controlled trial of naproxen versus sumatriptan. *Ann Emerg Med.* 2010;56(1):7–17.

Friedman BW, West J, Vinson DR, et al. Current management of migraine in US emergency departments: an analysis of the National Hospital Ambulatory Medical Care Survey. *Cephalalgia.* 2015;35(4):301–309.

Gelfand AA, Goadsby PJ. A neurologist's guide to acute migraine therapy in the emergency room. *Neurohospitalist.* 2012;2(2):51–59.

Gordon DL. Approach to the patient with acute headache. In: Biller J, ed. *Practical Neurology*. 4th ed. Philadelphia: Lippincott Williams & Wilkins; 2012:194–206.

Grosberg BM, Friedman BW, Solomon S. Approach to the patient with headache. *Headache*. 2013;(chapter 2):28–38.

Kelley NE, Tepper DE. Rescue therapy for acute migraine, part 1: triptans, dihydroergotamine, and magnesium. *Headache*. 2012;52(1):114–128.

Kelley NE, Tepper DE. Rescue therapy for acute migraine, part 2: neuroleptics, antihistamines, and others. *Headache*. 2012;52(2):292–306.

Kelley NE, Tepper DE. Rescue therapy for acute migraine, part 3: opioids, NSAIDs, steroids, and post-discharge medications. *Headache*. 2012;52(3):467–482.

Krymchantowski AV. Naproxen sodium decreases migraine recurrence when administered with sumatriptan. *Arq Neuropsiquiatr*. 2000;58(2B):428–430.

Law S, Derry S, Moore RA. Sumatriptan plus naproxen for acute migraine attacks in adults. *Cochrane Database Syst Rev*. 2013;(10):CD008541.

Leonardi M, Steiner TJ, Scher AT, et al. The global burden of migraine: measuring disability in headache disorders with WHO's Classification of Functioning, Disability and Health (ICF). *J Headache Pain*. 2005;6(6):429–440.

Lipton RB, Bigal ME, Diamond M, et al. Migraine prevalence, disease burden, and the need for preventive therapy. *Neurology*. 2007;68(5):343–349.

Lipton RB, Dodick D, Sadovsky R, et al. A self-administered screener for migraine in primary care: the ID Migraine validation study. *Neurology*. 2003;61(3):375–382.

Loder E, Weizenbaum E, Frishberg B, et al. Choosing wisely in headache medicine: the American Headache Society's list of five things physicians and patients should question. *Headache*. 2013;53(10):1651–1659.

Lynch KM, Brett F. Headaches that kill: a retrospective study of incidence, etiology and clinical features in cases of sudden death. *Cephalalgia*. 2012;32(13):972–978.

Sobri M, Lamont AC, Alias NA, et al. Red flags in patients presenting with headache: clinical indications for neuroimaging. *Br J Radiol*. 2003;76(908):532–535.

McCormack RF, Hutson A. Can computed tomography angiography of the brain replace lumbar puncture in the evaluation of acute-onset headache after a negative noncontrast cranial computed tomography scan? *Acad Emerg Med*. 2010;17(4):444–451.

Mehndiratta M, Nayak R, Garg H, et al. Appraisal of Kernig's and Brudzinski's sign in meningitis. *Ann Indian Acad Neurol*. 2012;15(4):287–288.

Minen MT, Tanev K, Friedman BW. Evaluation and treatment of migraine in the emergency department: a review. *Headache*. 2014;54(7):1131–1145.

Miner JR, Smith SW, Moore J, et al. Sumatriptan for the treatment of undifferentiated primary headaches in the ED. *Am J Emerg Med*. 2007;25(1):60–64.

Mokri B. Spontaneous low pressure, low CSF volume headaches: spontaneous CSF leaks. *Headache*. 2013;53(7):1034–1053.

Murray CJL, Vos T, Lozano R, et al. Disability-adjusted life years (DALYs) for 291 diseases and injuries in 21 regions, 1990–2010: a systematic analysis for the Global Burden of Disease Study 2010. *Lancet*. 2012;380(9859):2197–2223.

Nelson S, Taylor LP. Headaches in brain tumor patients: primary or secondary? *Headache*. 2014;54(4):776–785.

Pareja JA, Álvarez M. The usual treatment of trigeminal autonomic cephalalgias. *Headache*. 2013;53(9):1401–1414.

Purdy RA, Kirby S. Headaches and brain tumors. *Neurol Clin*. 2004;22(1):39–53.

Ramirez-Lassepas M, Espinosa CE, Cicero JJ, et al. Predictors of intracranial pathologic findings in patients who seek emergency care because of headache. *Arch Neurol*. 1997;54(12):1506–1509.

Robertson CE, Black DF, Swanson JW. Management of migraine headache in the emergency department. *Semin Neurol*. 2010;30(2):201–211.

Schievink WI. Spontaneous spinal cerebrospinal fluid leaks and intracranial hypotension. *JAMA*. 2006;295(19):2286–2296.

Silberstein SD, Lipton RB, Dodick D, et al. *Wolff's Headache and Other Head Pain*. 8th ed. New York: Oxford University Press; 2008.

Taylor LP. Mechanism of brain tumor headache. *Headache*. 2014;54(4):772–775.

Vinson DR. Treatment patterns of isolated benign headache in US emergency departments. *Ann Emerg Med*. 2002;39(3):215–222.

Waldman SD. Targeted headache history. *Med Clin North Am*. 2013;97(2):185–195.

Wang S-J, Fuh J-L. The "other" headaches: primary cough, exertion, sex, and primary stabbing headaches. *Curr Pain Headache Rep*. 2010;14(1):41–46.

Pain, Numbness, and Paresthesias 8

Comana M. Cioroiu

INTRODUCTION

For the general neurologist, the evaluation of a patient with complaints of numbness can be a daunting one. Being the most subjective of neurologic complaints, numbness is often a difficult sensation for the patient to explain and often all the more difficult for the clinician to appreciate on examination.

MANAGEMENT STRATEGY

As with all complaints in medicine, the first step is to obtain a detailed history. The first question should be one aimed at best characterizing the sensation (or lack thereof) described by the patient. It is important to differentiate between numbness as a *loss of sensation* as opposed to the *presence of an abnormal sensation*. At times, patients may also use the term *numbness* to describe muscle weakness, and this is important to keep in mind during one's examination.

TYPES OF SENSORY SYMPTOMS

Numbness can occur as a result of pathology at several different parts of the neuraxis, including the cortex, brain stem, spinal cord, and peripheral nerves. *Paresthesias*, spontaneous and abnormal sensations often described as "tingling" or "pins and needles," may imply a different neurologic localization than a complete lack of sensation alone. They also may occur following a period of absent sensation as nerves begin to slowly regenerate.

NEUROPATHIC PAIN

Neuropathic pain (see Chapter 57) is a category of pain specific to that caused by nerve injury and is often described as painful paresthesias, associated with a sensation of burning or radiating pain as can be seen in cases of peripheral neuropathy or radiculopathy (Fig. 8.1). In such cases, patients may exhibit altered sensation or abnormally increased sensations—*hyperesthesia* refers to increased sensation, whereas *dysesthesia* refers to an evoked unpleasant or painful sensation.

An exaggerated response to stimuli that normally evoke pain is known as *hyperalgesia*, whereas an exaggerated response to stimuli that should not normally invoke pain is referred to as *allodynia*. These abnormal sensations can be seen with various nerve injuries, both at the central and peripheral level. Conversely, *hypoesthesia* refers to the diminished perception of pain, *anesthesia* to the inability to perceive pain, and *analgesia* to the inability to feel pain.

Neuropathic pain must be differentiated from somatic pain caused by pathology in bones, ligaments, muscles, and other soft tissues.

Complex regional pain syndrome (CRPS; also known as *reflex sympathetic dystrophy*) is a chronic disease characterized by severe neuropathic pain, skin changes, and swelling in one limb. It may occur in the absence of a known nerve injury (type 1) or in the

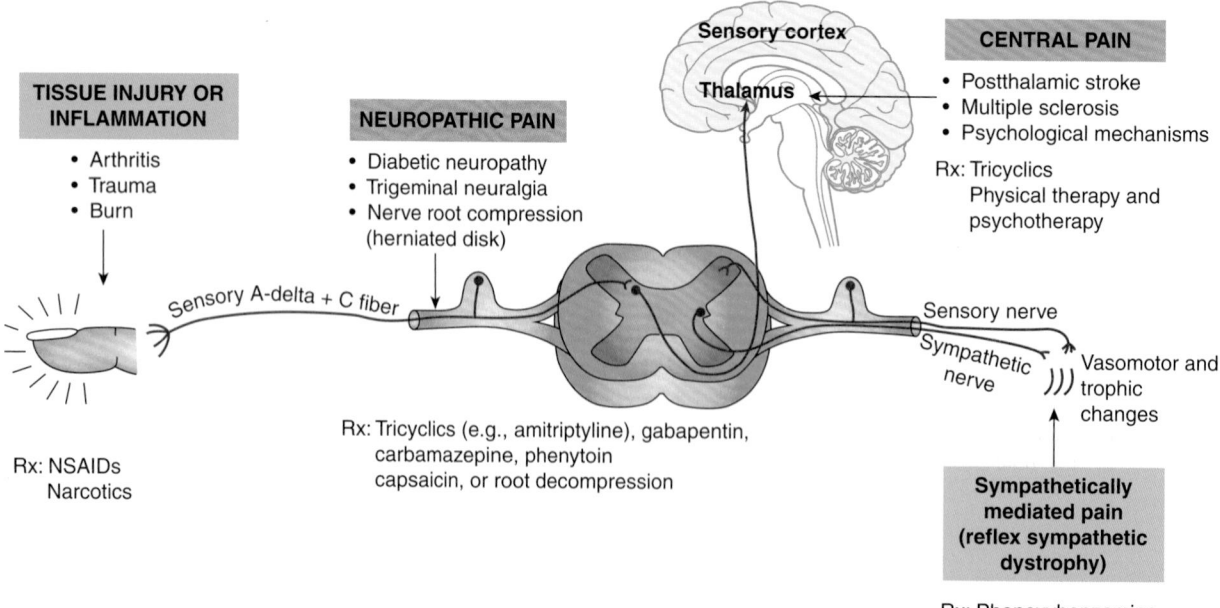

FIGURE 8.1 Sites of origin of pain within the nociceptive pathway. NSAIDs, nonsteroidal anti-inflammatory drugs. (Adapted from Marshall R, Mayer S. *On Call Neurology*. 3rd ed. Philadelphia: Saunders; 2007.)

TABLE 8.1 Patterns of Sensory Loss

Localization	Sensory Pattern	Associated Findings
Cortical	• Contralateral sensory loss	• Cortical sensory loss (i.e., neglect, astereognosis, agraphesthesia) • Visuospatial deficits
Brain stem	• Contralateral sensory loss of arm and leg with ipsilateral loss in face	• Cranial neuropathies (i.e., ophthalmoparesis, facial weakness) • Ataxia • Contralateral weakness • Hyperreflexia
Spinal cord	• Complete transverse lesion: loss of all sensory modalities below the level of the lesion • Central cord lesion (i.e., syrinx): loss of pain and temperature below the level of the lesion • Anterior cord lesion: contralateral loss of pain and temperature sensation below level of the lesion • Cord hemisection (Brown-Séquard syndrome): ipsilateral loss of vibration and joint position below the level of the lesion and contralateral loss of pain and temperature two or three segments below the level of the lesion • Cauda equina syndrome or conus medullaris syndrome: saddle anesthesia	• Contralateral or complete paralysis below the level of the lesion • Change in bladder or bowel control • Areflexia/hyporeflexia at the level of the lesion with hyperreflexia below the lesion • Dissociation between sensory modalities
Brachial plexus	• Ipsilateral sensory loss in the distribution of more than one peripheral nerve or nerve root	• Weakness in the distribution of the involved peripheral nerves or nerve roots • Areflexia • Neuropathic pain
Dorsal root ganglion	• Complete loss of sensation of all modalities in the affected dermatome	• Neuropathic pain • No weakness
Nerve root	• Loss or diminution of all sensory modalities in the affected dermatome	• Radicular pain • Weakness in the corresponding myotome • Areflexia or hyporeflexia
Peripheral nerve (also see Fig. 8.1)	• Mononeuropathy: loss or diminution of all sensory modalities in the distribution of the nerve • Polyneuropathy: distal and symmetric loss of sensation (vibration and joint position in cases of large-fiber neuropathy and pain and temperature in cases of small-fiber neuropathy) • Mononeuritis multiplex: loss of sensation in various peripheral nerves in an asymmetric fashion	• Weakness involving muscles of the corresponding peripheral nerve • Distal and symmetric weakness in cases of large fiber polyneuropathy • Autonomic findings • Neuropathic pain • Areflexia or hyporeflexia

setting of known nerve injury (type 2). Diagnosis and treatment of CRPS is further discussed in Chapter 56.

NEUROANATOMY AND LOCALIZATION

The pattern and distribution of sensory complaints provides important clues regarding the localization of the pathology (Table 8.1). Sensory syndromes that relate to injury at different levels of the neuraxis are discussed in the following section.

CENTRAL SENSORY SYNDROMES

Cortex

Numbness and paresthesias can result from both lesions in the central or peripheral nervous system. Higher cortical sensory functions are localized to the parietal cortex, with the primary sensory cortex being the postcentral gyrus of the parietal lobe. Lesions of the parietal lobe such as tumors or vascular insults (i.e., stroke, vascular malformation, hemorrhage) may cause sensory loss and numbness and are often associated with other impaired parietal lobe functions clinically manifested by poor visuospatial skills and hemineglect. Subcortical lesions in the parietal lobe may also manifest with loss of sensation as can be seen with demyelinating plaques of multiple sclerosis.

Brain Stem

Brain stem lesions involving the trigeminal nucleus, medial lemniscus, or spinothalamic tract may also present with facial or limb numbness but are frequently associated with other brain stem findings such as ophthalmoparesis, weakness, or ataxia. Numbness resulting from spinal cord injury may correspond to a particular dermatome but may also lead to a sensory level, in which the entire body below the lesion is affected (see Chapter 13). Examples of this include cases of transverse myelitis, in which patients may present with a sensory level with complaints of numbness extending down from a particular dermatomal level.

Spinal Cord

The two main central sensory pathways in the spinal cord are the *dorsal columns* also known as the *medial lemniscus* and the *spinothalamic tract* (see Fig. 16.1). Neurons carrying information related to vibration sense and proprioception travel up the cuneate and gracile fasciculus (which form the dorsal columns) in the spinal cord and synapse in their respective nuclei in the medulla, after which they decussate and form the medial lemniscus which carries these fibers to the ventral posterolateral (VPL) nucleus of the thalamus.

Fibers carrying pain and temperature sensation form the lateral spinothalamic tract in the spinal cord and typically ascend two spinal levels in Lissauer tract in the ipsilateral cord before synapsing with a second-order sensory neuron. From there, they decussate (cross over) in the anterior white commissure to the contralateral cord, and the tract then travels up the remainder of the spinal cord and brain stem and synapses again in the thalamus. Pathology of the posterior limb of the internal capsule or VPL nucleus of the thalamus may also cause numbness, and sudden-onset isolated numbness of a limb in a patient with vascular risk factors should raise concern for a possible vascular event in these regions. Similarly, sudden-onset numbness of the face may result from a lesion in the ventral posteromedial (VPM) nucleus of the thalamus.

Numbness resulting from spinal cord injury may also be accompanied by weakness and changes in bowel or bladder function. Depending on which segment of the cord is injured, patients may have preferential involvement of one tract or another and may have only certain sensory modalities affected; one classic example of this is the *Brown-Séquard syndrome*, where a spinal cord hemisection leads to ipsilateral weakness and loss of vibration and joint position sense below the level of the lesion and contralateral loss of cold and temperature sensation two or three segments below the level of the lesion.

PERIPHERAL SENSORY SYNDROMES

Dorsal Root Ganglia

The dorsal root ganglion is a group of nerve cell bodies distal to the spinal cord carrying somatic afferents to the cord. A *sensory ganglionopathy* refers to the selective destruction or involvement of the dorsal root ganglion and clinically typically manifests as a sensory ataxia with profound deficits in proprioception, at times also with marked neuropathic pain and paresthesias. A ganglionopathy of this type may be autoimmune, paraneoplastic (specifically related to anti-Hu antibodies), toxic, or associated with a paraproteinemia or with Sjögren syndrome. Injury to the nerve root just distal to the spinal cord may cause numbness and pain in the setting of a radiculopathy—patient may complain of radiating pain of an electric quality, at times associated with muscle soreness.

Nerve Roots and Plexuses

Sensory loss in a specific dermatomal distribution may be seen on exam (see Fig. 3.12). Processes affecting the brachial or lumbosacral plexus often present with pain as well as numbness and weakness in one limb in the distribution of more than one peripheral nerve or nerve root. *Brachial plexopathy* is the most common of these and can result from trauma, tumor infiltration, a postinfectious autoimmune process, or can often be idiopathic.

Peripheral Nerves

Neuropathic pain and numbness is a classic complaint in diseases of the peripheral nerves, such as in *polyneuropathy* (see Chapter 87). These patients will often complain of numbness and neuropathic pain that is distal and symmetric, typically starting in the feet. Neuropathy may preferentially affect large myelinated nerve fibers (group A fibers) carrying information related to vibration and joint position sense or small unmyelinated nerve fibers (group C fibers) transmitting pain and temperature sensation (see Fig. 8.1). Polyneuropathy can be either primarily axonal (with a predominant loss of axonal integrity) or demyelinating (due to destruction of the myelin sheath and often autoimmune in origin). Diseases of the neuromuscular junction and muscle do not present with sensory complaints, although some patients may complain of proximal muscle pain (as with the inflammatory myopathies).

FOCUSED HISTORY

A detailed history is the best tool a clinician has in the initial evaluation of a patient with sensory complaints. First, one must try to characterize the nature of the complaint. It is helpful to determine the nature of the pain or numbness and whether the patient is referring to a complete lack of sensation or the presence of an abnormal sensation (i.e., paresthesias). One must inquire as to the nature of symptom onset, as an acute or sudden onset of numbness may point more toward a vascular lesion (i.e., stroke) than towards a progressive process, and requires more urgent evaluation. *Red flags suggesting a more serious structural problem in a patient with primary sensory complaints include the presence of fever, weakness, and bowel or bladder changes.*

NUMBNESS AND PARESTHESIAS

When evaluating complaints of numbness or paresthesias, the anatomic distribution is important to determine, as this will help with localization and differential diagnosis: For instance, numbness or paresthesias localized to a specific dermatome will have different implications than numbness involving an entire limb. One must ask about symmetry, duration of symptoms, and any alleviating or exacerbating factors. For instance, neuropathic pain often worsens at night while patients are in bed, and radicular pain/paresthesias may be elicited with specific movements of the neck or back. In order to help formulate a differential diagnosis, it is crucial to ask about various associated symptoms. Numbness associated with changes in bowel or bladder habits may point towards a spinal cord lesion. A recent history of viral infection associated with ascending numbness should alert one to the possibility of Guillain–Barré syndrome. Asking about any recent trauma or injury may also help differentiate between an acute as opposed to a chronic nerve injury. Questions regarding gait are pertinent, as patients with polyneuropathy may complain of imbalance early in the disease course.

PAIN

Acute pain is often managed very different from chronic pain, as the former may respond well to a brief course of a particular kind of analgesic, whereas the latter may require a complex regimen of medications. *Back pain* (see Chapter 109) is one of the most common complaints in neurology, and one must differentiate between benign causes of low back pain and other causes of pain, which may be indicative of a more serious diagnosis. An acute disk herniation is characterized by an abrupt onset often incited by lifting, Valsalva maneuver, or a sudden positional change. Lying down typically relieves this pain, whereas it is exacerbated by movement. It may be associated with radicular pain down the distribution of a particular dermatome. Chronic back pain is often challenging to treat and may require a complex therapeutic approach including medications, physical therapy, pain management, and sometimes surgical intervention.

PAST MEDICAL HISTORY

The patient's past medical history is important as well, as certain systemic illnesses may point toward an underlying etiology of the patient's symptoms. For instance, there are several conditions that may be associated with peripheral neuropathy, such as diabetes mellitus, rheumatologic diseases, or a history of cancer. A prior history of stroke of the thalamus or lateral medulla may contribute to a chronic pain syndrome (*Dejerine–Roussy syndrome*). A comprehensive list of current medications is also important to gather, as paresthesias can at times be a known side effect of certain medications (i.e., paresthesias of the hands with use of topiramate). When obtaining the family history, one must be careful to inquire as to any possible neurologic diseases or any family members with a history of known neuropathy or foot deformities that may, for instance, point toward Charcot–Marie–Tooth disease. Exposure to certain substances such as heavy metals, pesticides, or chemotherapeutic agents may be implicated in those with neuropathy (some of which can be quite painful), and thus, one should ask about these possibilities when no other clear etiology can be found.

FOCUSED EXAM

The examination of a patient complaining of numbness is often challenging, as the sensory exam is the most subjective part of the neurologic exam. See Chapter 3 for a complete description of the neurologic exam.

GENERAL MEDICAL EXAMINATION

As with all other patients, one should begin with a thorough general medical examination to look for any hints of a possible systemic disease or other findings that may be associated with the patient's complaints. For a patient with numbness or neuropathic pain, this should include an examination of the skin, assessing for rashes, hair loss, or trophic skin changes as can be seen in patients with neuropathy. Although often difficult, looking directly at the skin of the affected region may be very telling—for instance, in a patient with neuropathic pain confined to a particular dermatome, patchy erythema with grouped vesicles may be diagnostic of herpes zoster (although zoster may present without a rash, as in zoster sine herpete, or the rash may present after the onset of pain). Any patient with acute onset of numbness in which a vascular event is suspected should have a thorough cardiac evaluation including examination of the carotid arteries.

Examination of the extremities should also involve an assessment of both active and passive range of motion of affected limbs, including a *straight leg raise test* (when indicated) which may be positive in cases of lumbosacral radiculopathy (see Fig. 3.16). A straight leg raise is performed while having the patient lie supine as the examiner raises each leg up vertically. If the test is positive, the patient's radicular symptoms are reproduced with passive lifting of the leg (particularly the contralateral leg), as the nerve roots are stretched. *Lhermitte sign* can at times be elicited with passive flexion of the neck and is positive when the patient reports a feeling of paresthesias radiating down the arms or legs. This is caused by pressure over the posterior columns and suggests a lesion in the posterior cervical cord as can be seen in patients with multiple sclerosis. *Tinel* and *Phalen* signs can elicit signs of median nerve compression from carpal tunnel syndrome in patients with unilateral or bilateral hand numbness (see Fig. 3.15).

NEUROLOGIC EXAMINATION

Mental Status

The majority of patients with complaints of paresthesias or neuropathic pain should have an entirely normal mental status. An abnormal finding in the patient's mental status examination points toward a cortical lesion. Higher cortical sensory function can be assessed by testing for *graphesthesia* (the ability to identify a number or letter written on the skin) and *stereognosis* (the ability to recognize an object placed in one's hand without visual or auditory stimuli). Testing for hemispatial neglect or extinction may also help identify a parietal lobe lesion.

Cranial Nerves

Similarly, a comprehensive examination of the cranial nerves can help to further localize a brain stem problem. A cranial neuropathy of any kind also suggests a central lesion as can be seen with a brain stem process or an intracranial lesion. Facial pain and neuropathies of the trigeminal nerve are discussed in detail in Chapters 55 and 86.

Motor Examination

A thorough motor examination is crucial to the evaluation of a patient with numbness and pain. In cases of chronic peripheral nerve injury, one may see atrophy of muscles in the distribution of the affected nerve. When pain is severe, a reliable determination of strength is often difficult to make. Similarly, when numbness is profound (particularly when proprioception is markedly affected), one may mistake joint position impairment for weakness. Weakness in the same distribution as numbness may point to a central lesion in the brain or spinal cord or a peripheral process in the nerve root or peripheral nerve. Distal and symmetric weakness is often most suggestive of a large-fiber polyneuropathy. Ataxia noted on finger-to-nose tests or heel–knee–shin tests may help localize a lesion to the brain stem; however, one may also find a marked sensory ataxia on coordination testing if joint position is markedly impaired.

Sensory Examination

The sensory examination is the most subjective part of the neurologic examination and often the most challenging. Several modalities can be tested and which ones are tested and how is dictated by the clinical presentation. Paresthesias that are transient and sporadic are infrequently associated with a clear loss of sensation on exam.

TABLE 8.2 **Basic Principles of Sensory Examination**

- Is the sensory loss symmetric?
- Does it follow a distal pattern?
- Does it correspond to a particular territory (i.e., of one dermatome or one peripheral nerve)?

When examining sensation, it is helpful to keep in mind *three basic principles* (Table 8.2). Taking the time to map out a specific distribution of numbness is often diagnostic and of localizing value. For instance, in suspected spinal cord lesions, one should assess for a sensory level, which may suggest the location of the cord pathology. One can begin with an assessment of light touch sensation, for example, using the tip of a cotton swab. Pinprick sensation and temperature sensation evaluate the integrity of the spinothalamic tract and small unmyelinated nerve fibers, whereas a selective loss of vibration or joint position implies injury to the posterior columns or to the large myelinated nerve fibers as seen in polyneuropathy.

Vibration sense is determined using a 128-Hz tuning fork placed over a bony prominence, most commonly the big toe and medial malleolus of the ankle (see Fig. 3.11). Interpretation of the vibratory exam must take into account the patient's age, as vibration sense diminishes with age over time, and can be absent in those older than 80 years old. Joint position is tested by moving the most distal joint passively up or down and asking the patient the direction of movement. Typically, the most subtle of movements should be detected, and if a problem is found in the most distal joint, one should move more proximally to determine the full extent of impairment. In those with severe joint position sense abnormalities, involuntary movements of the fingers may be observed with arms outstretched (*pseudoathetosis*).

Reflexes

Deep tendon reflexes are important to elicit, as they may be pathologically brisk or hyperreflexic in cases of central lesions—for instance, in spinal cord injury, reflexes may be diminished or absent at the level of the lesion but increased below the level of the lesion. In cases of peripheral neuropathies, reflexes are typically diminished or absent.

Gait and Station

A careful assessment of gait, including stance, toe walking, heel walking, and tandem gait are also of importance, for example, as loss balance is often a key complaint in cases of polyneuropathy. A positive Romberg test suggests impaired proprioception as can be seen with disorders of the posterior columns or with advanced large-fiber polyneuropathy.

DIAGNOSTIC EVALUATION

Following a comprehensive history and exam, one should consider appropriate diagnostic studies based on the differential diagnosis and most likely localization.

SEROLOGIC TESTS

Various tests are available to us in working up patients with neuropathic pain and numbness. Serum studies are routinely done early on in the workup and in cases of sensory loss should include electrolyte and vitamin levels (particularly B_{12}, B_6, B_1) as well as a hemoglobin A1c level, as vitamin deficiencies and diabetes are common systemic illness that often contribute to nerve damage. Depending on the clinical scenario and index of suspicion, serum testing can be expanded to include testing for HIV, thyroid function, hematologic malignancies, rheumatologic diseases, and various other illnesses. In those patients with a history of specific environmental exposures, testing can be done to evaluate for the presence of specific toxic agents such as heavy metals. Genetic causes of numbness and paresthesias exist (i.e., Charcot–Marie–Tooth disease, hereditary neuropathy with liability to pressure palsies), and genetic testing should be pursued in those with a family history and the appropriate clinical phenotype.

NEUROIMAGING

If a central lesion is suspected, imaging studies are typically done early to evaluate for a structural lesion. Magnetic resonance imaging (MRI) (see Chapter 21) has the highest sensitivity and is the preferred imaging modality; however, a computed tomography (CT) scan can be done in patients unable to tolerate or undergo MRI testing. Spine imaging in particular can be instructive when considering a lesion at the level of the cord or the nerve root. In those patients in whom MRI is not feasible, CT myelography can be used to assess for structural lesions of the spine and nerve roots. More distally, imaging of the brachial plexus is at times instructive in providing a more clear etiology in cases of plexopathy and can be used to evaluate for hemorrhage, inflammation, or infiltrative lesions.

LUMBAR PUNCTURE

Lumbar puncture (LP) (see Chapter 31) should be performed in cases of suspected inflammatory, infectious, or neoplastic processes. It is particularly helpful in cases of suspected autoimmune demyelinating neuropathies, which will show a characteristic albuminocytologic dissociation with elevated protein in the setting of a normal cell count.

ELECTRODIAGNOSTIC AND QUANTITATIVE SENSORY TESTING

Nerve conduction studies and electromyography (EMG) are important in helping to diagnose conditions of the peripheral nervous system and can help localize a complaint of numbness or neuropathic pain to the nerve root, plexus, or peripheral nerve (see Chapter 25). These tests have long been the standard practice in the diagnosis of neuropathy involving large nerve fibers and can characterize the severity of injury as well as distinguish between generalized and focal forms of either purely axonal or demyelinating forms of neuropathy (such as acute or chronic inflammatory demyelinating neuropathy). Nerve conduction study techniques are not sensitive in the assessment of small nerve fibers and are normal in cases of small-fiber neuropathy. More extensive quantitative sensory testing (QST) can be done in certain patients to more sensitively assess sensory dysfunction. QST uses noninvasive methods to determine the sensory threshold to various modalities including vibration, temperature, and pain and compare it to standardized normal values.

SKIN AND NERVE BIOPSY

Given the inability of routine electrodiagnostic tests to assess for involvement of small unmyelinated cutaneous nerve fibers, a diagnosis of small-fiber neuropathy is typically made via skin biopsy. *Nerve biopsy*, a more invasive test, is typically best reserved for cases in which the diagnosis is in question and there is no known etiology (see Chapter 32). The diagnostic yield and use of nerve biopsy is best seen in cases of inflammatory, demyelinating, or infiltrative etiologies of neuropathy, with the most informative being those done on a nerve with abnormalities demonstrated on nerve conduction studies.

INITIAL MANAGEMENT

IDENTIFY POTENTIALLY SERIOUS CONDITIONS

Most patients with complaints of pain or paresthesias can be safely evaluated on an outpatient basis; however, exceptions certainly do exist. *Acute conditions that may lead to rapid deterioration must be identified promptly and treated as such.* For instance, a patient presenting with acute-onset lateralized numbness with vascular risk factors should be directed to the emergency room for stroke evaluation. Similarly, a patient with suspected Guillain–Barré syndrome or transverse myelitis should be evaluated rapidly and admitted to the hospital, as a delay in treatment could result in rapid deterioration and possible respiratory compromise. Inpatient hospitalization for treatment with steroids, intravenous immunoglobulin (IVIG), plasmapheresis, or other immunomodulatory agents is at times necessary for these patients depending on the clinical situation.

SYMPTOMATIC TREATMENT

Once all diagnostic tests are completed, treatment of pain and paresthesias is twofold. The first approach is to treat the underlying etiology of the symptoms—for instance, if a structural lesion is found, surgical intervention may be appropriate, or if an autoimmune condition is diagnosed, treatment with immunomodulatory therapy is indicated. Patient with diabetes should be counseled regarding glycemic control and diet modification, those with vitamin deficiencies should be repleted, and so forth. Second, symptomatic therapy should be initiated to help with bothersome symptoms. *The treatment of neuropathic pain and paresthesia is vast and is discussed in detail in Chapter 57.* Symptomatic treatment should be multidisciplinary and include a combination of pharmacologic measures, physical therapy, and behavioral modifications. Chronic pain is often markedly challenging to treat and can be frustrating to both patients and practitioners alike.

KEY POINTS

- Characterize the nature of the complaint—what does the patient mean by "numbness"? How can you characterize the pain?
- Obtain a detailed history and examination to help localize the patient's complaints of numbness/paresthesias to a location in either the central or peripheral nervous system.
- When examining a patient with sensory loss, look for asymmetry, a distal versus proximal gradient, and try to identify a pattern of sensory loss to guide your diagnostic impression.
- Look out for red flags that suggest an urgent problem that needs to be addressed and treated rapidly.
- Let your differential diagnosis guide your diagnostic testing.
- Treatment of chronic pain and paresthesias can be complex and often requires a multidisciplinary approach.

INTRODUCTION

No symptom may be as disturbing or dramatic to a patient as acute visual loss. Although acute ocular diseases such as glaucoma, uveitis, and retinal detachment may require urgent evaluation by an ophthalmologist, a high percentage of visual disturbances fall within the province of the neurologist. Neurologic visual symptoms may be reported as blurriness, focal obscurations, or positive visual phenomena. Because the visual pathway from the retina to the calcarine cortex is constant from individual to individual, anatomic localization can be made with a high degree of accuracy on physical examination. The progression, associated symptoms and signs, and clinical setting will help you make the correct diagnosis and suggest the proper acute management.

NEUROANATOMY

The optical system of the eyes focuses images onto the outer retina where the light energy is converted into nervous impulses by rods and cones. These impulses are then conveyed by the axons of the retinal ganglion cells on a path centripetally through the inner retina, converging on the optic nerve head. The impulses then travel along the optic nerve and through the optic chiasm where fibers from the nasal retina (temporal visual field) decussate to join temporal retinal fibers (nasal visual field) from the other eye in the contralateral optic tract. The retinal ganglion cell axons pass from the optic tract into the geniculate body where they synapse. The nervous impulse is conveyed by the geniculocalcarine pathway, composed of the axons from the geniculate body cells that pass through the temporal and parietal lobes, to synapse in the calcarine cortex in the occipital lobe which relays the impulses for higher cortical analyses such as reading and recognition.

COMMON PROBLEMS

Visual loss may be due to abnormalities of the ocular media, the retina, the anterior visual pathway (the optic nerves, chiasm, and optic tracts), or the geniculocalcarine pathway (Fig. 9.1 and Table 9.1).

FIGURE 9.1 Visual field cuts produced by lesions at different points along the visual pathway. (a) Monocular segment anopia produced by a retinal artery branch occlusion in the left eye. (b) Monocular blindness produced by a lesion in the left optic nerve. (c) Bitemporal hemianopia produced by a mass lesion at the optic chiasm. (d) Right segment anopia produced by a lesion in the lateral geniculate body of the left thalamus. (e) Right upper quadrantanopia produced by a lesion in the left temporal optic radiation (Meyer loop). (f) Right lower quadrantanopia produced by a lesion in the left parietal optic radiation. (g) Left homonymous hemianopia produced by a lesion in the calcarine cortex of the right occipital lobe. Note that macular vision is sometimes spared because of middle cerebral artery collateral blood flow to the occipital pole. OS, oculus sinister; OD, oculus dexter. (Adapted from Marshall R, Mayer S. *On Call Neurology*. 3rd ed. Philadelphia: Saunders; 2007.)

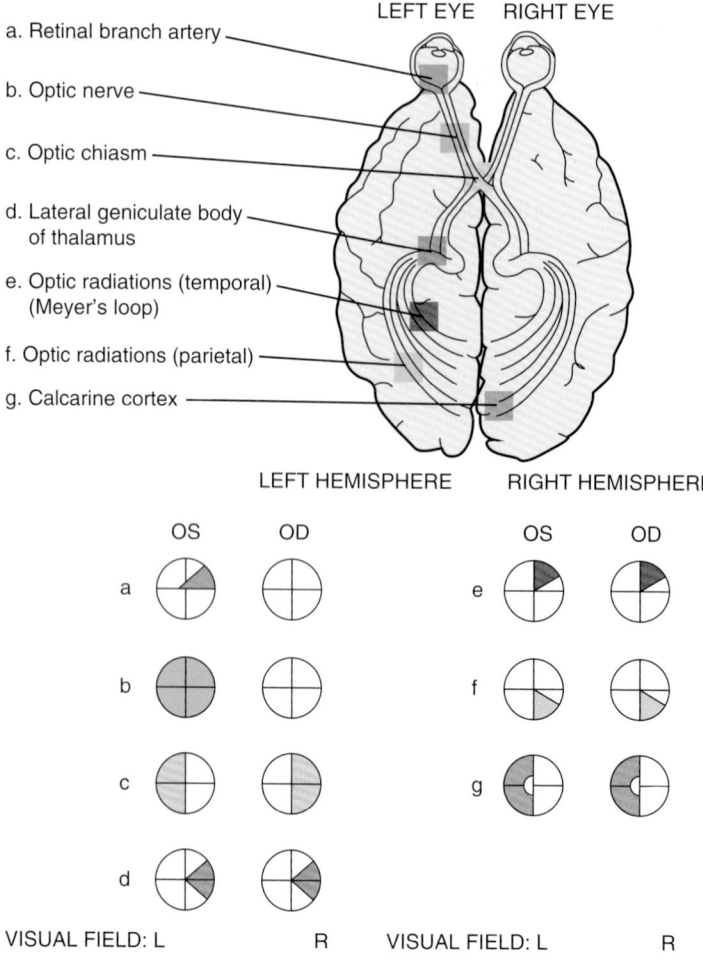

LEFT EYE   RIGHT EYE

a. Retinal branch artery
b. Optic nerve
c. Optic chiasm
d. Lateral geniculate body of thalamus
e. Optic radiations (temporal) (Meyer's loop)
f. Optic radiations (parietal)
g. Calcarine cortex

LEFT HEMISPHERE   RIGHT HEMISPHERE

OS   OD   OS   OD

a   e

b   f

c   g

d

VISUAL FIELD: L   R   VISUAL FIELD: L   R

TABLE 9.1 Signs and Symptoms that Suggest Location in the Visual Pathway

Location of Lesion along Visual Pathway	Signs and Symptoms	Location of Lesion along Visual Pathway	Signs and Symptoms
Anterior segment of the eye	• Blurred vision • Glare or halos • Foreign body sense in eye • Correction with squinting, pinhole, or ophthalmoscope • Response to blinking • Visible opacities on exam	Chiasm	• Bitemporal hemianopia • Band atrophy of optic disc • Postfixation blindness • Hemifield slide phenomena
		Optic tract	• Homonymous hemianopia with optic atrophy and relative afferent pupillary defect in contralateral eye
Retina	• Metamorphopsia • Macropsia or micropsia • Positive scotoma • Geographic scotoma • Central scotoma unconnected to blind spot • Prolonged photostress recovery time • Flashes or floaters • Nyctalopia or hemeralopia • Purple, yellow, or green vision	Geniculate body	• Congruent horizontal homonymous sectoranopsia • Congruent upper and lower sectoranopsias • Incongruent homonymous hemianopia • Optic atrophy
Optic nerve	• Negative scotoma • Decreased brightness and/or color sense • Cecocentral, arcuate, or altitudinal visual field defect or horizontal step in visual field • Relative afferent pupillary defect • Optic disc swelling or atrophy • Nerve fiber layer dropout • Optic nerve head cupping	Geniculocalcarine pathway	• Homonymous hemianopia • "Pie-in-the-sky" hemianopia, temporal lobe • "Pie-on-the-floor" hemianopia, parietal lobe • Optokinetic defect ipsilateral to parietal lobe lesion • Scotomatous hemianopia—occipital lobe • Preserved temporal crescent of field—occipital lobe • Hemiparesis, aphasia, alexia, agnosia, somatosensory disturbance
		Oculomotor/vestibular system	• Oscillopsia • Diplopia

It may also result from a lesion in the oculomotor or vestibular systems from diplopia or oscillopsia. Patients with alexia or agnosia may also complain of visual loss, although their acuity may test normally.

BLURRED VISION

Refractive errors, as in myopia, hyperopia, and astigmatism, cause blurred vision. This blurring may be corrected by having the patient focus through an ophthalmoscope by turning the lens wheel either at distance or with a reading card held at 14 inches. If the ophthalmoscope fails or is not available, having the patient view through a pinhole (with an optimum diameter of 2 mm) corrects most refractive errors. Cataract and corneal edema or opacity may cause glare, halos, or light beams from lights. Tear film disturbance, or dry eye, responds to blinking or artificial tears. Opacities of the ocular media, as in cataract, corneal scar, or aqueous or vitreous hemorrhage, may be visualized during examination using an ophthalmoscope while focusing on the red reflex in the pupil. Opacities anterior to the center of the eye in the cornea, anterior chamber, and lens rise when the patient looks up slightly, whereas those in the posterior half of eye (vitreous) descend.

VISUAL DISTORTIONS

Retinal pathology that distorts the retina may cause straight lines to appear bent, broken, or curved (*metamorphopsia*) or objects to appear small (*micropsia*) or large (*macropsia*). This is caused by distortion of the outer retina by detachment, edema, fibrosis, neovascularization, or hemorrhage. Vitreous traction on the retina will cause photopsias if the vitreous detaches from the retina or vitreous traction tears or pulls a hole in the retina; *floaters* may be seen.

Retinal detachment will occur if fluid accumulates under the retina because of a hole or tear and would be appreciated as a shadow or curtain over the eye. With disease of the rods, as in retinitis pigmentosa or vitamin A deficiency, the patient experiences night blindness (*nyctalopia*) and prolonged dark adaptation. Impaired vision in daylight (*hemeralopia*) suggests cone dysfunction as in cone dystrophy but may be seen with central visual field defects of optic nerve origin. Central scotomas (areas of depressed visual sensitivity surrounded by areas of higher sensitivity) so small as to be unconnected to the blind spot are almost only seen in retinal conditions (Fig. 9.2A). Central ring scotomas are also a strong indicator of a retinal process (Fig. 9.2B).

Impaired visual recovery following bright light exposure suggests a retinal process. Purple vision suggests poor oxygenation to the outer retina from ipsilateral high-grade carotid stenosis or poor choroidal perfusion from giant cell arteritis; this can also be seen in central serous chorioretinopathy. Yellow, green, or snowy vision suggests retinal toxicity from digitalis toxicity. A dark blotch, positive scotoma, suggests a retinal process particularly if associated with photopsia. With visual loss of ocular origin, there may be associated local symptoms or signs, such as pain, photophobia, redness, or soft-tissue swelling.

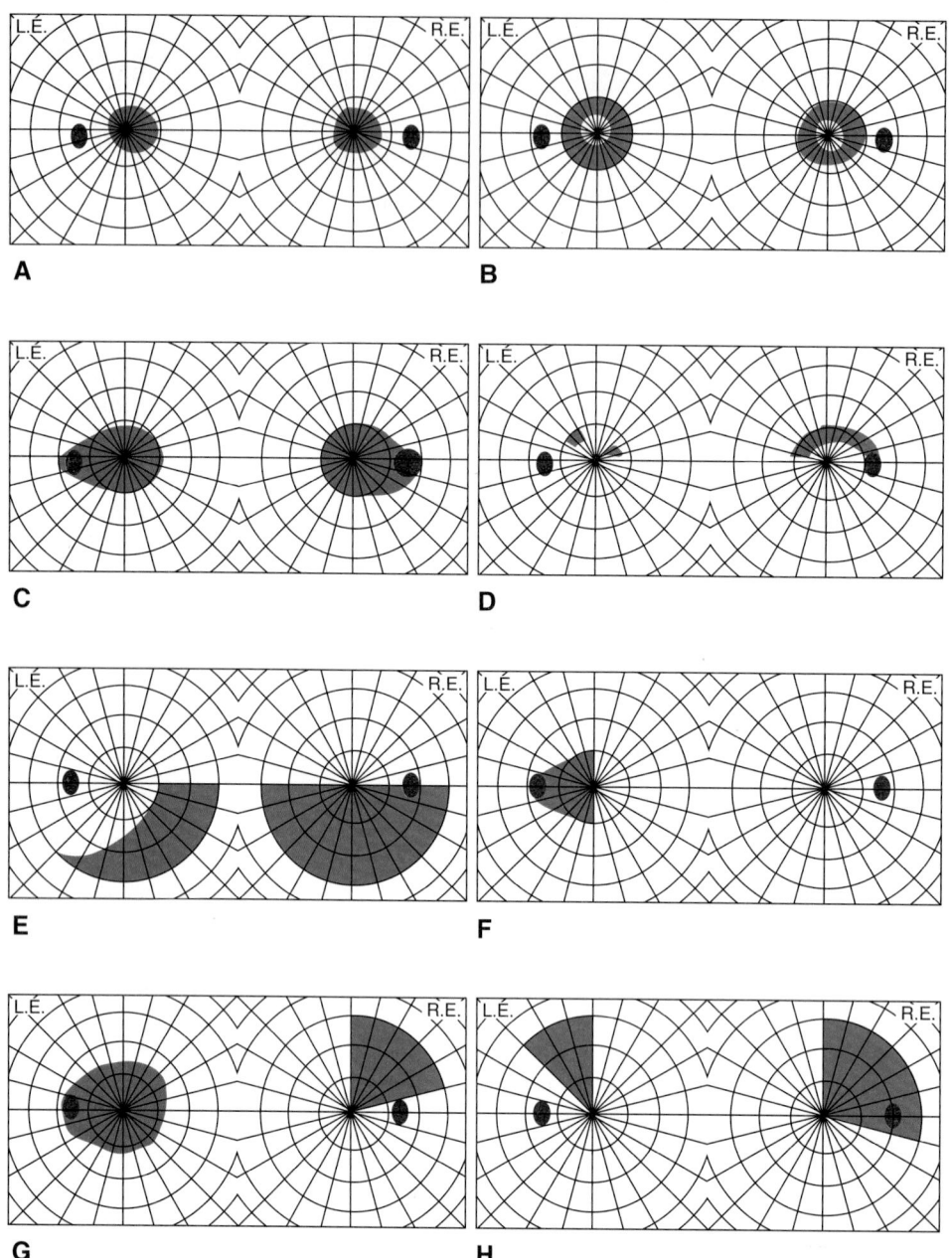

FIGURE 9.2 Examples of visual field loss. Areas in *red* denote the physiologic blind spot created by the optic disc. Areas in *blue* denote pathologic visual loss. **A:** Bilateral small central scotomas at the fovea indicating a retinal condition. **B:** Bilateral central ring scotoma also strongly indicative of a retinal condition. **C:** Bilateral cecocentral scotomas, as in optic neuropathy. **D:** Left eye: paracentral defect. Right eye: paracentral defects that have coalesced to an arcuate defect. **E:** Left eye: nasal horizontal step field defect. **F:** Left eye: junctional scotoma of Traquair. **G:** Left eye: cecocentral defect ipsilateral to the affected left optic nerve. Right eye: junctional temporal defect in the contralateral (*right*) eye. **H:** Variation of BTH as in pituitary adenoma or meningioma attacking the chiasm from above.

VISUAL FIELD DEFECTS

Retinal Nerve Fiber Bundle Defects

The retinal nerve fiber bundle path is determined by the fovea, which is the center of the macula; the optic disc, which is centered about 15 degrees nasal to the fovea slightly above the horizontal; and the horizontal retinal raphe. Fibers coming from the retina temporal and superior to the foveal center arc above the macula, entering the superior optic disc; those temporal and inferior to the

center of the fovea arc below the macula and enter the optic disc inferiorly (Fig. 9.3).

This divergent pathway of the superior and inferior axons in the temporal retina around the macula creates the horizontal retinal raphe in the temporal retina and is the anatomic correlate of the nasal horizontal step field defect (Fig. 9.2E). These defects are more marked in the nasal visual field typically closer to fixation nasally and show respect for the horizontal meridian. Axonal damage may occur in the retina, disc, or retrobulbar optic nerve, as the nerve bundles stay together anterior to the chiasm. The axons from

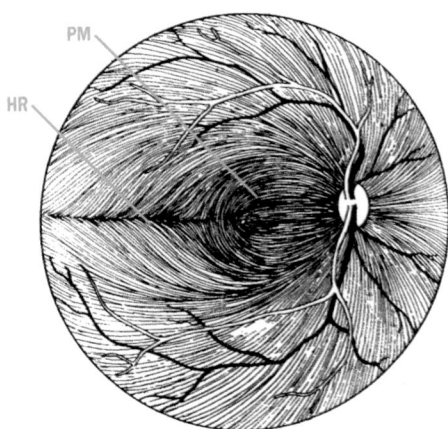

FIGURE 9.3 Retinal nerve fiber anatomy of a right eye as seen on opthalmoscopy, with the optic disc nasal to the fovea, which is the center of the macula. PM is the papillomacular bundle of fibers that carry visual impulses nasally directly from the macula to the optic disc. HR is the horizontal retinal raphe. Nerve fibers arising from the retina temporal to the fovea arch above and below the macula and PM, and insert into the superior and inferior poles of the optic disc respectively. These arcuate paths of fibers from the temporal retina (nasal visual field) are responsible for the characteristic visual field defects of optic nerve disease, including peripheral horizontal nasal steps, arcuate defects, and cecocentral scotomas.

the nasal fovea and axons originating between the fovea and the disc course directly into the temporal disc, and damage to these axons results in a cecocentral scotoma (Fig. 9.2C). This bundle then occupies the center of the optic nerve anterior to the chiasm. Damage to fibers coming from the retina nasal to the disc leads to temporal sectoral defect with an apex at the blind spot.

Symptoms and Signs of Optic Nerve Defects

The hallmarks of optic nerve dysfunction are visual field defects, loss of brightness and color sense, decreased pupillary reaction to light, optic nerve head swelling or optic atrophy, and nerve fiber layer dropout. Optic neuropathy causes cecocentral visual field defects (see Fig. 9.2C), paracentral defects (see Fig. 9.2D left eye), arcuate visual field defects (see Fig. 9.2D right eye), nasal step defects (see Fig. 9.2E left eye), and altitudinal defects (see Fig. 9.2E right eye). In optic neuropathy, the shape of visual field defects corresponds to the path of the arcuate and macular–papillary nerve fiber bundles. Paracentral defects, the smallest defects in the arcuate region may coalesce to form arcuate defects (Fig. 9.2D) as in glaucoma.

Injury of nasal optic nerve fibers anywhere from the back of the eye to just anterior to the chiasm will produce an ipsilateral relative temporal visual field defect that does not respect the vertical meridian. A small lesion right at the nasal junction of the optic nerve and chiasm may result in an ipsilateral central temporal defect that respects the vertical meridian, the monocular junctional scotoma of Traquair (Fig. 9.2F). Injury of temporal fibers of the optic nerve between the optic canal and the chiasm will produce a relative ipsilateral nasal defect that does not respect the vertical. More marked junctional involvement of the optic nerve and chiasm may produce a cecocentral defect ipsilateral to the involved optic nerve and an upper temporal defect in the contralateral eye (Fig. 9.2G). *Thus with loss of vision in one eye, it is critical to check the other eye to look for an unsuspected temporal visual field defect, as this is frequently caused by a mass lesion such as a pituitary adenoma or meningioma.*

Chiasmal Defects

Chiasmal involvement leads to variations of bitemporal hemianopsia (BTH) due to damage to crossing fibers from the nasal retinas, which carry information from the temporal visual fields. Tumors that compress the chiasm from below produce BTH that is greatest superiorly (Fig. 9.2H). Lesions attacking the chiasm from above, such as craniopharyngiomas, produce BTH that starts inferiorly (Fig. 9.4A) The visual field defect of lateral chiasmal compression (typically due to an aneurysm) spares the ipsilateral superior temporal visual field, causing visual loss in the other three ipsilateral quadrants and in the contralateral superior temporal quadrant (Fig. 9.4B).

Optic Tract Defects

Lesions of the optic tract (the continuation of the optic nerve relaying signals from the optic chiasm to the ipsilateral lateral geniculate nucleus) produce *contralateral incongruent homonymous hemianopsias*. These may have elements of chiasmal involvement and are accompanied by optic atrophy. The eye with more visual field loss, typically the contralateral eye, may exhibit a relative afferent pupillary defect. The pattern of optic atrophy is band or bow tie shaped in the eye with the temporal field defect; it is more generalized in the eye with the nasal defect. Some examiners have found congruous homonymous hemianopias in tract lesions.

Geniculate Body Defects

Geniculate body lesions may cause incongruous or congruous visual field defects. Tumors of the geniculate body produce incongruous homonymous hemianopias. There are two syndromes of geniculate infarction that result in striking congruous defects. Lateral posterior choroidal artery infarction results in a *congruous horizontal homonymous sectoranopia*, (Fig. 9.4C), a wedge-shaped hemianopia along the horizontal with the apex pointing to fixation and the wedge spreading out to the contralateral periphery. Anterior choroidal artery occlusion results *in upper and lower homonymous sectoranopias* that spare the horizontal and are complementary in shape to the horizontal homonymous sectoranopia (Fig. 9.4D). Because the optic tract synapses in the geniculate body, optic atrophy may be observed several weeks after a geniculate lesion.

Hemispheric Defects

Homonymous hemianopias are caused by lesions of the geniculocalcarine pathway in the temporal, parietal, or occipital lobes. Traditionally, the more posterior the site of a lesion, the more congruous it was thought to be, with occipital lesions being highly congruous. Recently, however, the rule of congruity has been questioned due to radiographic verification that shows congruous hemianopias at all retrochiasmal locations, even in the optic tract. "Pie-in-the-sky" upper quadranopias that do not respect the horizontal suggest a temporal lobe location (Fig. 9.4E), whereas hemianopias that are greatest inferiorly suggest a parietal localization (Fig. 9.4F). This is especially true when accompanied by a defect in optokinetic nystagmus with targets following to the side of the lesion. The *extinction phenomenon* is an apparent hemianopsia in a seeing area of the visual field that occurs during simultaneous stimulation to right and left hemifields. Extinction can be confirmed by finding a similar defect to tactile simultaneous stimulation that is not present on single-sided stimulation.

Homonymous hemianopic scotomas suggest occipital lesions but are not specific for that location (Fig. 9.4G). Involvement of the calcarine cortex (or primary visual cortex, V1, Brodmann area 17),

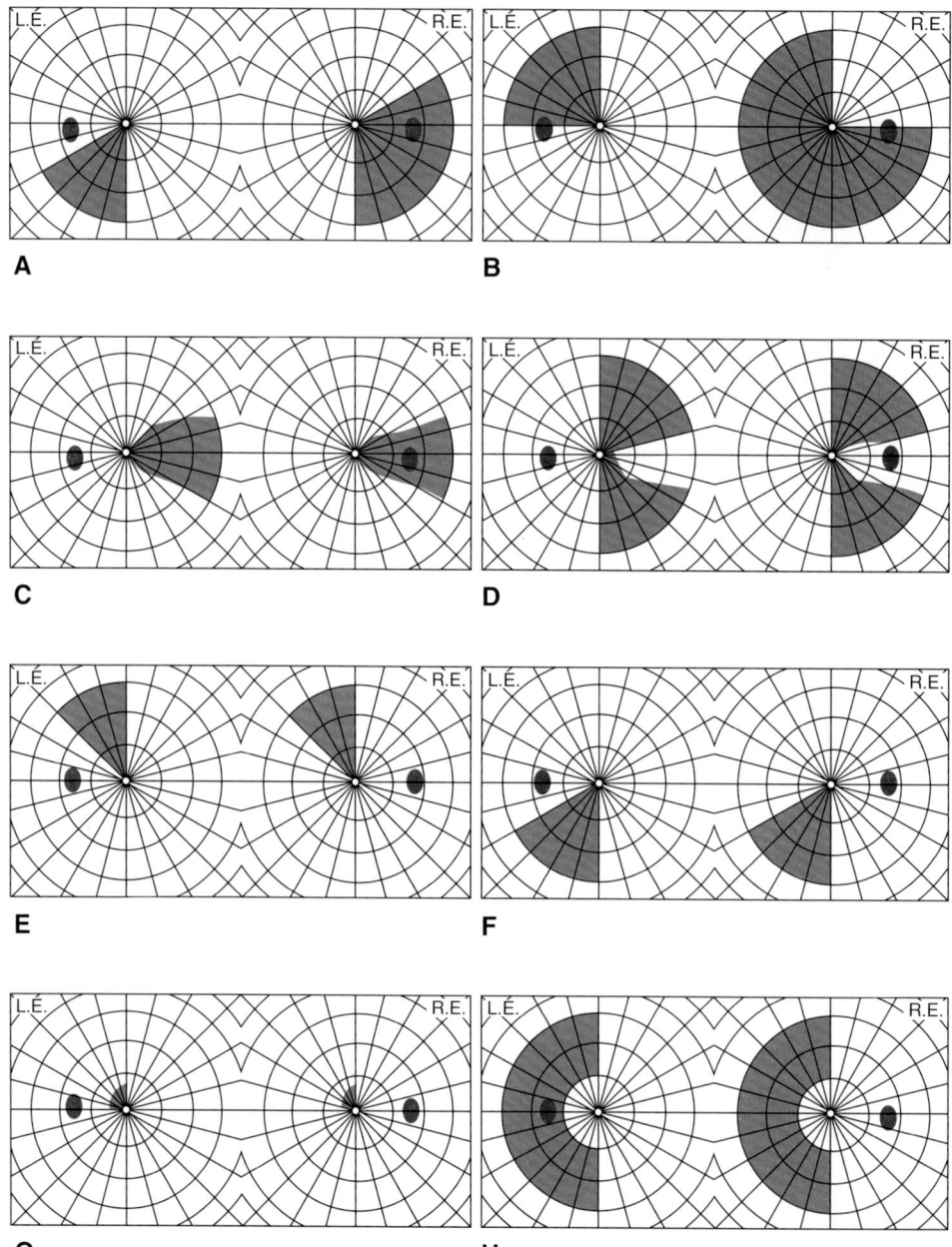

FIGURE 9.4 Examples of visual field loss. Areas in *red* denote the physiologic blind spot created by the optic disc. Areas in *blue* denote pathologic visual loss. **A:** Variable bitemporal inferior quadrantanopsia attacking the chiasm from below. **B:** Variable bilateral visual field defects from a right lateral chiasmal compression from an aneurysm. **C:** Bilateral congruous horizontal homonymous sectoranopia resulting from lateral posterior choroidal artery infarction. **D:** Upper and lower homonymous sectoranopsias that spare the horizontal as in anterior choroidal artery occlusion. **E:** Bilateral pie-in-the-sky upper quadranopsias from a temporal lobe lesion. **F:** Hemianopia greater inferiorly from a parietal lesion. **G:** Homonymous hemianopic scotoma suggesting but not specific for occipital lesion. **H:** Macular-sparing hemianopsia suggesting but not specific for occipital lesion.

anterior in the occipital lobe, where peripheral vision is represented, results in a *monocular temporal crescent visual field defect*. After a retinal detachment has been ruled out, this is specific for an occipital lobe lesion contralateral to the field defect and is usually caused by a tumor. Sparing of the anterior calcarine cortex is common in infarcts of the posterior cerebral artery and results in a preservation of the temporal crescent contralateral to the lesion. It is highly suggestive of occipital localization. A homonymous

hemianopia with sparing of the central visual field is referred to as *macular-sparing hemianopsia* (Fig. 9.4H) and is suggestive of occipital involvement but macular sparing has been reported as anterior as the optic tract. Preservation of motion vision in a hemianopic defect, termed the *Riddoch phenomenon*, is also suggestive of occipital involvement, although it has also been seen as far anteriorly as the optic tract as well. *Anton syndrome*, denial of blindness in the setting of bilateral hemianopsias, represents bilateral calcarine involvement plus an association area infarction. Quadrantic visual field defects precisely respecting the horizontal meridian in each eye have been reported in extrastriatal occipital cortex lesions involving areas V2/V3.

DIPLOPIA

Disturbances of eye movement and ocular alignment result in diplopia. This can result from ocular muscle problems, neuromuscular transmission defects, cranial neuropathies, and ocular motor nuclear and internuclear ophthalmoplegias and cause double vision, which the patient may report as blurry vision. Damage to the central vertical and horizontal gaze pathways and vestibular systems may result in gaze palsies or nystagmus that the patient may report as visual difficulty.

CAUSES OF VISUAL LOSS

Visual loss may be fleeting (unilaterally or bilaterally), acute and slowly remitting, slowly progressive, acute and nonremitting, or acute with ophthalmoplegia. The tempo of visual loss provides important clues regarding etiology.

TRANSIENT MONOCULAR BLINDNESS

Also known as *Amaurosis fugax* (AF), transient monocular blindness (TMB) may be complete or partial and lasts from seconds to 20 minutes with recovery. The most frequent cause is thromboembolism of the retinal artery, but many other conditions can cause the syndrome as well (Table 9.2).

Embolic Transient Monocular Blindness

TMB from *embolism* is frequently described as a descending curtain that covers all or half of the field of vision or may start with quadrant involvement. Less frequently, it is reported as an ascending curtain and rarely, as a sideways moving blind. It may appear as a ground glass, a gray-out, a cloud, or complete blackness. Swirling sparks of light, signifying emboli that are entopically stimulating the retina as they course through the retinal vessels, may occur. TMB may clear like a clearing fog or regress like a curtain that goes

TABLE 9.2	Causes of Transient Unilateral Visual Loss

- Embolism
- Hypotension
- Arterial spasm
- Recurrent erosions of the cornea or corneal basement membrane dystrophy
- Angle-closure glaucoma
- Hyphema
- Vitreous hemorrhage
- Optic nerve head drusen
- Congenital optic nerve anomalies (coloboma, morning glory disc)
- Orbital masses (causes gaze-evoked monocular visual loss)
- Uhthoff phenomenon
- Asymmetric light adaptation

up or down, altitudinally or quadranopically. This pattern of AF suggests embolic origin most frequently from an ulcerative plaque of the carotid bifurcation or originating from the ascending aorta or heart. These cases require emergent evaluation.

Hypotensive Transient Monocular Blindness

Hypotensive TMB usually occurs in the setting of extensive arterial occlusive disease. Hypotensive AF may range from being very brief to lasting longer than embolic AF. The episodes may present with monocular concentric constriction, or blotchy vision, or bright objects appearing brighter, loss of contrast, or photographic negative vision. Bright light may provoke hypotensive TMB, and there may be prolonged photostress recovery of vision. It may be associated with ocular ache and mild signs of cerebral ischemia such as poor concentration, sudden fatigue, or feeling faint. Hypotensive TMB may be precipitated by arterial hypotension, arrhythmias, or venous hypertension. Bending over, standing up, exercising, bright light, and overheating may also precipitate attacks. Giant cell arteritis, Takayasu disease, and other occlusive disorders of the aortic arch or carotid arteries may also be present.

During an attack of hypotensive TMB, the retinal vessels on ophthalmoscopy may be narrow and the disc blanched; just following an attack, the vessels dilate with irregularity of the veins and hyperemia of the disc. Between attacks, the retina may have midperipheral and peripheral retina dot and blot hemorrhage at the end of vessels, venous tortuosity, and microaneurysms. This is referred to as *venous stasis retinopathy* and can be differentiated from vein occlusion by the presence of arterial pulsations spontaneously or with light pressure on the globe.

Arterial Spasm

Arterial spasm in the ophthalmic, retinal, or choroidal circulation may result in TMB in the adolescent or young adult who is otherwise healthy. The description of the visual loss is varied but does not involve a curtain falling over the vision. It more closely mimics the description of hypotensive TMB with blotchy visual loss of several minutes' duration. Previously, it was referred to as *retinal migraine*; however, its relation to migraine is now less certain.

Ocular Erosions

Other ocular abnormalities may cause transient visual blurring. For instance, recurrent erosions of the superficial corneal epithelium, usually seen in the setting of corneal epithelial basement membrane dystrophy, may present with foreign body sensation and generalized hazy vision that may be unilateral or bilateral. These symptoms start upon opening the eyes after sleep, last from minutes to hours, and respond to blinking.

Angle-closure Glaucoma

Angle-closure glaucoma can cause transient visual loss. The episodes of visual loss are unilateral, recurrent, and can be painful or painless. Patients may report seeing halos around lights. During an attack, the eye may exhibit perilimbal injection, a vertically oval pupil, a cloudy cornea, and high intraocular pressure that may normalize if the attack breaks. Angle closure occurs in patients who are middle aged or older and can be precipitated by watching a movie in darkness, exercise, sexual activity, and drugs that dilate the pupil, for example, atropinic drugs used during anesthesia or sulfur drugs that enlarge the ciliary body, for example, topiramate. The neurologist should arrange for slit lamp examination, intraocular pressure check, gonioscopy of the angle, and fundus examination with an ophthalmologist. Release of pigment from the posterior leaf of the iris may cause acute elevations of intraocular pressure called *pigmentary glaucoma*. This form of glaucoma causes transient monocular visual loss after vigorous exercise or in situations that dilate the pupil and again requires ophthalmic consultation.

Ocular Hemorrhage

Hyphema is blood in the anterior chamber of the eye between the cornea and iris. It may trigger hazy vision if it is dispersed as when the patient bends over. *Vitreous hemorrhage* may do the same. *Uveitis–glaucoma–hyphema* (UGH) *syndrome*, as the name suggests, is characterized by uveitis, glaucoma, and hyphema and caused by repeated anterior chamber hemorrhages following intraocular lens surgery. It too may be responsible for repeated bouts of hazy vision.

Drusen

Hyaline bodies in the anterior optic nerve, called *optic nerve head drusen* (ONHD), can cause monocular or binocular transient obscurations of several seconds' duration. ONHD buried within the disc in childhood grow, calcify, and extrude through to the disc surface with age. They are sometimes mistaken for papilledema, particularly before they extrude, but ultrasound and CT scan reveal their calcification. Optic discs with ONHD are small, have no cup, and display early bifurcation of the retinal blood vessels. Visible drusen are usually multiple and may resemble mulberries. Blood vessels can be followed coursing from the disc to the retina unlike those in real disc edema, which are obscured by axoplasmic transport backup in the nerve fiber layer. The adjacent peripapillary retina may have small areas of retinal pigment hypertrophy and scarring from old subretinal hemorrhage. When seen acutely, this appears as a flat, crescent-shaped area adjacent to the disc.

Congenital Optic Disc Anomalies

Congenital optic disc anomalies such as *coloboma* and *morning glory disc* may be associated with transient visual obscurations. Acquired disc elevations, particularly *papilledema* and *central retinal vein occlusion*, may also be associated with transient visual obscurations. These are described as gray or blackouts associated with postural change, can be unilateral or bilateral, and last for seconds.

Others

Acquired disc edema from compression or infiltration of the optic nerve by tumors, for example, meningioma or hemangioma, can be associated with transient visual obscurations. *Gaze-evoked monocular visual loss* occurring on eccentric gaze suggests an orbital tumor with vascular compromise. *Uhthoff phenomenon* of crescendo–decrescendo visual loss over 20 to 30 minutes with exercise, overheating, hot baths, or showers suggests demyelination of the optic nerve; it can also be seen in nerve compression.

Finally, asymmetric light adaptation occurs situationally when one eye is dark adapted compared to the other. This presents when a patient is reading next to a bedside lamp. When the light is turned off, the eye further from the lamp is relatively dark adapted, whereas the eye closer to the light is unable to see in the darkness for several minutes.

FLEETING BILATERAL VISUAL LOSS

Migraine

Migraine is the most frequent cause of bilateral simultaneous transient visual loss (Table 9.3). The migrainous aura typically precedes

TABLE 9.3	Causes of Fleeting Bilateral Visual Loss
• Migraine	
• Vertebrobasilar insufficiency	
• Papilledema	
• Blepharospasm	
• Dry eye	

the headache beginning as a tiny paracentral scintillating scotoma or negative scotoma. The scotoma is experienced homonomously and congruently usually in the shape of a C in the left hemifield or a backward C in the right hemifield. Over 20 minutes, it expands and migrates centrifugally, leaving in its wake an area of transiently depressed field disappearing into the periphery of the involved field. It is variously described as zigzagged, saw-toothed, or lightning-like or if viewing a face imparting a *Picasso effect*. A headache contralateral to the involved field typically begins within minutes of the scotoma's disappearance. Rarely, a structural lesion of the occipital lobe can trigger a migrainous march in which case the aura never switches sides. Occipital epilepsy does not have the characteristic 20-minute expansion and migration and may persist for hours or days.

Vertebrobasilar Insufficiency and Others

Patients with *vertebrobasilar insufficiency* (VBI) may experience bilateral blurry vision as if looking through water. It may be hemianopic or bihemianopic and typically lasts minutes, typically without photopsia, migration, or expansion. It may be accompanied by other symptoms of VBI. A patient with papilledema has transient obscurations of vision that can be bilateral or unilateral. They are typically brief, exacerbated by postural change, and accompanied by optic disc swelling. Clearly, blepharospasm, with its random intermittent closures of the eyelid, leads to interruptions in vision. This cause, however, may not be apparent to the patient who merely complains of unclear vision. Finally, dry eye may cause generalized visual blurring of either or both eyes, which is made worse by wind and relieved by blinking and artificial tears.

ACUTE, SLOWLY REMITTING VISUAL LOSS

Optic Neuritis

Optic neuritis (ON) is the most common cause of acute optic neuropathy in patients younger than age 50 years (see also Chapter 69). ON is characterized by painful, monocular visual loss that typically does not worsen beyond 2 weeks and recovers dramatically in the ensuing months (although persistent pain beyond this timeline may occur). It is usually a manifestation of multiple sclerosis (MS). In 95% of cases, patients experience either pain on motion of the globe, ocular tenderness, or ocular ache. Patients with painless ON typically show magnetic resonance imaging (MRI) involvement limited to the optic canal or intracranial optic nerve. Color vision, as measured by color plates or subjective comparison with the other eye, is more markedly impaired than acuity. The visual field defect is typically a cecocentral scotoma (see Fig. 9.2C) that has sloping borders. Nerve fiber bundle (arcuate) defects may also be seen (see Fig. 9.2D).

Acutely, the majority of adult patients have normal-appearing optic discs indicating retrobulbar ON. Papillitis, or optic disc swelling, however, is present in 40% of adults at the time of presentation. In childhood, papillitis is present in the majority as is simultaneous or sequential bilaterality. Occasionally, one may have demyelination of the chiasm or of the optic tract. Peripapillary hemorrhage is a rarity in demyelinating papillitis. If a patient with papillitis develops macular exudates in the form of a star or hemistar 2 weeks after onset, it is referred to as *neuroretinitis*, which is not related to MS. Neuroretinitis is caused by catscratch fever, syphilis, Lyme disease, tuberculosis, viral and nematode infections, sarcoidosis, and Behçet disease.

The vast majority of cases of typical monocular painful ON in the 20- to 50-year age group will be found to be from MS or to be isolated ON, probably monosymptomatic MS. However, other processes can cause ON such as neuromyelitis optica, leukodystrophies, syphilis, viral infections, postviral reactions, reactions to vaccines, fungal infections, sinusitis, Lyme disease, nematodes, and sarcoidosis. Several poorly characterized variants of ON exist such as relapsing ON, autoimmune ON, and chronic relapsing inflammatory optic neuropathy (CRION). Relapsing ON is a form of isolated ON that occurs and recovers spontaneously multiple times. Autoimmune ON may be of several forms that are identified by the presence of antibodies such as antinuclear antibody (ANA) or aquaporin-4 antibodies. These disorders and CRION may be identified by their steroid dependence or their tendency toward progressive worsening.

Central Serous Chorioretinopathy

Central serous chorioretinopathy occurs in patients 25 to 55 years of age, mostly male, who have "type A" personalities, or take corticosteroids. It presents as painless visual loss with metamorphopsia, prolonged ipsilateral photostress recovery time, and no or a minimal relative afferent pupillary defect. With careful ophthalmoscopy, a yellow oval elevation can be seen in the macula representing a serous detachment of the retina. Most resolve spontaneously within 3 to 4 months but some may require laser or vascular endothelial growth factor inhibitor injections.

SLOWLY PROGRESSIVE VISUAL LOSS

Primary Open-angle Glaucoma

The most common optic neuropathy is *glaucoma* (Table 9.4). The most common form is *primary open-angle glaucoma*. It is painless and causes bilateral, asymmetric, slowly progressive visual field constriction, typically nasally, while sparing central acuity until its late stage. Visual field loss in glaucoma is characterized by steps along the horizontal meridian in the nasal visual field as well as paracentral defects in the arcuate region closer to fixation in the nasal visual field. Glaucoma may be suspected on ophthalmoscopy over time by an increasing diameter of the optic disc cup (and thereby an increase in the cup-to-disc ratio).

Glaucoma may be suspected when the cup-to-disc ratio exceeds 30% or when one eye's ratio is 20% larger than that in the fellow eye. The rim around the cup represents healthy nerve fibers. Typically, the inferior (I) rim is widest, followed by the superior (S) rim, then the nasal (N) rim, and lastly, the temporal (T) rim. This progression has been called the *ISN'T rule*. If the *ISN'T rule* is broken, glaucoma should be suspected. Optical coherence tomography is used to measure the thickness of the nerve fiber layer and the ganglion cell layer complex (ganglion cells plus the inner plexiform layer) in the diagnosis and management of glaucoma and other optic neuropathies. In glaucoma, the intraocular pressure is typically elevated above 22 mm Hg; however, a single intraocular

TABLE 9.4	Causes of Slowly Progressive Visual Loss
• Primary open-angle glaucoma	
• Dominant optic atrophy	
• Compression	
• Pituitary adenoma	
• Meningioma	
• Craniopharyngioma	
• Gyrus rectus syndrome	
• Aneurysm	
• Optic glioma	
• Optic neuropathy degenerations	
• Hereditary	
• Toxic	
• Nutritional	

pressure measurement is not sensitive for detecting glaucoma and in fact, many glaucoma patients do not have elevated intraocular pressure (low-tension glaucoma).

Dominant Optic Atrophy

Several recessive neurologic disorders with associated optic neuropathies frequently present with blindness in infancy. For example, *Wolfram syndrome*, also known as *DIDMOAD* (diabetes insipidus, diabetes mellitus, optic atrophy, and deafness), presents in childhood and is recessively inherited.

Dominant optic atrophy (DOA), the most common hereditary optic neuropathy, presents in adolescence with symmetric mild to moderately decreased acuity (20/25 to 20/200), tritanopic axis (blue-yellow) color vision loss, cecocentral scotomas, and temporal optic disc pallor. It is a progressive neuropathy, but visual loss rarely continues past the third decade of life. DOA has variable penetrance. Some families with DOA have an associated mutation (OPA1). Some patients present with large cups and have "dominant pseudoglaucoma."

Compression

Expansile or proliferative lesions can damage the anterior visual pathway (optic nerves, chiasm, and tract) by compression, infiltration, a combination of infiltration with exophytic compression, leaking of toxic cystic content, apoplectic hemorrhage or infarction, interference with blood supply, meningeal spread, or provocation of a paraneoplastic reaction. The location (intracranial, intracanalicular, orbital, or disc), relation to adjacent structures (meninges, skull and orbital bone, gland, cavernous sinus, nasal sinuses, and blood supply), and nature of the lesion (cyst, solid tumor, aneurysmal, inflammatory, infectious, hemopoietic, lymphoproliferative, or paraneoplastic) determine the presentation.

Pituitary tumors are the most frequent cause of chiasmal compression and BTH. Meningiomas may also present with gradually PPLOV. The pattern of visual field loss and additional signs reflect the location of the mass. Intracranial meningiomas of the medial sphenoid may cause hyperostosis with proptosis and orbital dystopia and orbital venous congestion with upper lid edema after recumbency. They may compress the optic nerves, chiasm, or tract.

With extension into the cavernous sinus, cranial nerve palsies ensue. Meningiomas of the optic canal are often silent, other than their visual loss, and may be bilateral. An optic nerve sheath meningioma (ONSM) produces axial proptosis and optic disc swelling with pallor. If it blocks retinal venous outflow, optociliary shunt vessels develop on the disc. With pressure on the back of the globe, chorioretinal folds and a hyperopic shift occur. With PPLOV, optociliary shunt vessels, and blurred disc pallor in adult, an ONSM is likely. Meningiomas may spread from the orbit to the intracranial space or vice versa along the optic nerve.

Craniopharyngiomas are cystic suprasellar tumors that attack the anterior visual pathway from above, tending to produce inferior visual field defects. Cystic tumors may produce conduction block along the anterior visual pathways prior to axonal death. As a result, acuity and field loss present prior to optic atrophy and may mislead the examiner to suspect functional visual loss, especially in children.

The *gyrus rectus syndrome* occurs when hemorrhage or swelling in the frontal lobe herniates the gyrus rectus downward onto the ipsilateral optic nerve causing an acute compressive optic neuropathy. *Aneurysms* of the ophthalmic, anterior communicating or carotid arteries can produce optic neuropathy by compression of the optic nerves or chiasm.

Optic gliomas are most frequently pilocytic astrocytomas that appear in the first decade of life and are often associated with neurofibromatosis type 1. They may originate in the orbital or intracranial optic nerve, chiasm, or tract. Orbital gliomas present with visual loss, strabismus, proptosis, and optic disc edema that gives way to optic atrophy. The glioma infiltrates the normal structure resulting in fusiform enlargement of the nerve. Infiltration of the anterior visual pathway causes enlargement, and an exophytic component may even cause compression of the adjacent visual pathway. Chiasmal gliomas are more common than optic nerve gliomas and present with bilateral visual loss, strabismus, nystagmus, optic atrophy, papilledema, hydrocephalus, and endocrine problems. Optic gliomas of childhood have limited growth potential, but because of their location, even limited growth may cause serious disability. *Malignant optic gliomas of adulthood* are rare, high-grade gliomas of middle age. They present with painful loss of vision, which progresses to total bilateral blindness over 3 to 4 months and to death in a year. The tumor infiltrates the anterior pathway rapidly, causing vascular occlusions from compression of the central retinal vessels, papilledema, and marked retinal hemorrhages. Proptosis may occur and the patient ultimately develops signs of a hemispheric glioma.

Hereditary, Nutritional, and Toxic Optic Neuropathies

These neuropathies present with bilateral color and acuity loss, cecocentral scotomas, and temporal pallor of the optic discs (see also Chapter 123). Some toxins, such as methanol, cause disc edema when acutely ingested (see also Chapter 128).

Nutritional amblyopia, formally called *tobacco–alcohol amblyopia*, is frequently seen in middle-aged men who avoid vegetables and get their caloric intake through ethanol, although it can also be seen in nonalcoholics and children with poor nutrition. It can be accompanied by hearing loss and peripheral neuropathy and has been seen epidemically in prisoners of war and in Cuba during a food shortage at the time of the collapse of the former Union of Soviet Socialist Republics (USSR). Isolated optic neuropathy from ethanol is not seen in the setting of good nutrition, and iso-

lated tobacco amblyopia is excessively rare. B_{12} deficiency can present with decreased vision prior to the recognition of combined degeneration of the spinal cord. Complex vitamin B deficiencies and deficiencies of folate and copper are also reported to cause visual loss.

The administration of ethambutol, isoniazid, chloramphenicol, linezolid, and disulfiram can result in a bilateral toxic optic neuropathy. If not recognized, this will progress to optic atrophy, but stopping the drug usually results in slow recovery. Exposure to heavy metals, methanol, and toluene can also result in optic atrophy. A newly recognized syndrome caused by cobalt and chromium metallosis results in optic neuropathy, retinopathy, hearing loss, cardiomyopathy, hypothyroidism, and pseudotumors. It occurs following total hip replacement with a cobalt–chromium metal-on-metal (MoM) implant that follow a failed ceramic total hip replacement where ceramic debris remains in the joint at the time of the MoM hip placement. In these cases, the ceramic debris grinds against the metal ball over time, sending dangerous amounts of cobalt and chromium into the bloodstream. The toxicity is treated by surgical removal of the metal implant and washing out the metal debris.

ACUTE, NONREMITTING VISUAL LOSS

Nonarteritic Anterior Ischemic Optic Neuropathy

Nonarteritic anterior ischemic optic neuropathy (NAION) is the most common acute optic neuropathy in the population older than age 50 years (Table 9.5). It is typically painless, although some ache is present in 10% to 15% of cases. Pain on motion of the globe, present in less than 1% of NAION patients, should make one suspect ON. NAION is usually noted upon awakening as an inferior altitudinal clouding with decreased acuity. Superior and cecocentral loss may also occur. The visual loss is typically stable, although it may progress while the disc is swollen. Some improvement in acuity is noted in a minority of NAION patients, but in contrast to ON, there is little improvement in the visual field. Color vision, as measured by color plate testing, is lost in proportion to acuity loss, which helps differentiate it from ON, where dyschromatopsia is marked. A relative afferent pupillary defect will be present if the process is unilateral and the other eye is normal. The optic disc is swollen, either segmentally or diffusely, and funduscopic exam shows arterial narrowing and splinter hemorrhages at the disc margin. Early in the course, the swelling is hyperemic and later, it becomes pallid. Usually, in 1.5 to 3 months, the disc becomes atrophic and the hemorrhages resorb.

NAION occurs in optic nerves with small cup-to-disc ratios, the so-called disc at risk. Risk factors associated with NAION include hypertension, diabetes, smoking, hyperlipidemia, anemia, obstructive sleep apnea, and nocturnal hypotension. NAION occurs

TABLE 9.5	Causes of Acute, Nonremitting Visual Loss
• Nonarteritic anterior ischemic optic neuropathy (NAION)	
• Arteritic anterior ischemic optic neuropathy	
• Retinal artery occlusion	
• Leber optic neuropathy	
• Subacute loss of vision	
• Pituitary apoplexy	

in patients with ONHD, following cataract extraction, following an attack of migraine, and following hypotensive anesthesia of long duration with blood loss and crystalloid replacement. Amiodarone, PDE-5 inhibitors, and interferon-α may be related to the attacks of NAION. No treatment has proven effective in NAION.

Diabetic papillopathy, a variant of ischemic optic neuropathy, occurs in long-standing insulin-dependent and non–insulin-dependent diabetics. It may be unilateral, sequential, or bilateral with disc swelling and a proliferation of radially oriented telangiectatic capillaries on the disc surface. There is often mild arcuate or altitudinal visual field loss and mild acuity loss. Typically, the patients have no or minimal diabetic retinopathy. The swelling and vessel changes resolve over months, leaving mild visual impairment. Diabetic papillopathy occurs in patients with small cups as does NAION. Interestingly, it often follows when patients achieve rapid glycemic control.

Arteritic Anterior Ischemic Optic Neuropathy

NAION must be distinguished from arteritic anterior ischemic optic neuropathy (AAION) that is caused by giant cell arteritis and rarely by other causes of vasculitis (see also Chapter 42). Giant cell arteritis occurs over age 50 years and may be accompanied by polymyalgia rheumatica, jaw claudication, temporal tenderness, loss of appetite, weight loss, and fever. Acutely, the optic nerve appears pale, even chalk white, and swollen. If suspected, the patient should have an erythrocyte sedimentation rate (ESR), a C-reactive protein (CRP), and a complete blood count performed stat and started on at least 80 mg prednisone by mouth daily until the blood tests return. If blood testing is supportive with elevated ESR, CRP, and platelets, temporal artery biopsy should be performed immediately to secure the diagnosis.

Retinal Artery Occlusion

Retinal artery occlusions are acute and painless causes of visual loss. On early examination, the inner retina is cloudy representing ganglion cell layer and nerve fiber layer ischemic damage and the retinal arteries may exhibit interrupted circulation. In a branch retinal artery occlusion (BRAO), there is edema in the wedge-shaped area of distribution of the vessel. BRAO are nearly always embolic, although they may rarely be angiopathic as in *Susac syndrome*, a microangiopathy characterized by BRAOs, deafness, and encephalopathy (see also Chapter 43). In central retinal artery occlusion (CRAO), cloudy swelling of the inner retina is again seen. However, because there are no ganglion cells or nerve fiber layer in the fovea, the cloudy swelling of the ganglion cells does not extend there. This results in a cherry-red spot (CRS) in the fovea. The CRS represents the normal choroid unobstructed by edema. After 4 to 6 weeks, the CRS and edema dissipate. CRAO does not result in complete blindness, as small vessels coming from the optic disc usually result in a small area of nasal retinal perfusion and thus some remaining temporal vision. Like BRAO, CRAO is frequently embolic (50% of the time; however, CRAO may also be caused by giant cell arteritis). A cilioretinal artery is present in about 17% of the population. It is supplied directly by the choroidal circulation and frequently supplies the macula; occlusion therefore may lead to central vision loss. Conversely, in CRAO, a cilioretinal artery if present may preserve central vision.

In retinal artery occlusions, an embolism may be made up of calcium, cholesterol (Hollenhorst plaque), or a mix of platelets and fibrin. Calcific emboli tend to lodge on or near the disc and are white globs appearing larger than the occluded vessel; they never dissolve. They typically originate from the aortic or mitral valves. Hollenhorst plaques lodge at retinal arterial bifurcations, are reflective yellow shards, and can be made to move slightly with light ocular pressure. They ultimately break up and disappear. They originate from ulcerative plaques at the carotid bifurcation or in the proximal aorta. Finally, platelet fibrin emboli are cream-colored, non-shiny and break up quickly; they may be seen snaking through the vessels and again, originate from ulcerative plaques.

Patients with retinal artery occlusions require emergent ophthalmologic referral for possible paracentesis, ocular digital massage, acetazolamide, carbogen breathing, and consideration of tissue plasminogen activator (TPA) to reestablish circulation. If the retinal circulation has already been reestablished when the patient is examined, these treatments are unnecessary. In general, once cloudy swelling of the ganglion cells is present, visual prognosis is guarded. Both embolic and thrombotic risk factors should be assessed in all retinal artery occlusions.

Ophthalmic artery occlusion results in complete, ipsilateral, painless blindness and marked retinal cloudy swelling frequently without a CRS, as the choroid is ischemic as well. In the elderly, giant cell arteritis should be suspected.

Leber Hereditary Optic Atrophy

Leber hereditary optic atrophy, a disorder of mitochondrial DNA substitution mutations, typically presents in young males but may present in females and patients of all ages. It typically presents with acute to subacute painless monocular loss of vision. If examined acutely, the peripapillary nerve fiber layer may appear swollen, and the small arterioles coming off the major retinal arteries near the disc may appear telangiectatic (microangiopathy). On fluorescein angiography, no staining is seen of the disc or vessels. The nerve fiber swelling and telangiectasias may be seen in the presymptomatic phase and also just after the visual loss. Over several weeks, the nerve fiber layer swelling and telangiectasias are replaced by optic atrophy. Simultaneous eye involvement occurs in 25% of cases. Bilateral involvement may be present without relative afferent papillary defect (RAPD) and be less obvious especially if the nerve fiber layer swelling and the microangiopathy are not seen; these patients may be dismissed as having functional vision loss. There are three common substitutions at the 3460, 14484, and 11778 positions in the mitochondrial DNA genome that account for 95% of cases. Late spontaneous improvement in vision may occur in a minority of patients, most commonly in those with the 14484 mutations and least commonly in those with the 11778 mutation. Some patients have an associated cardiac preexcitation disorder, whereas others have an MS-like presentation.

Finally, there is a rare malignant type of optic glioma occurring in adulthood, which follows an acute, nonremitting course.

ACUTE VISUAL LOSS WITH PAINFUL OPHTHALMOPLEGIA

Pituitary apoplexy may be acute or subacute. It is due to either a hemorrhage or infarction with swelling of a sella or suprasellar tumor into the chiasm, one or both cavernous sinuses, the brain stem, or the subarachnoid space. It may cause a combination of visual loss, severe headache referred to the forehead, meningitis, seizures, adrenal failure, cerebrospinal fluid (CSF) rhinorrhea, and loss of consciousness depending on the direction the hemorrhage or swelling takes. The third nerve is the most medially placed and is therefore closest to the pituitary body and most prone to compression. Pituitary apoplexy should be suspected if band or bow tie atrophy of the optic discs is found in a patient with a history of headache followed by loss of consciousness. Recovery from the ophthalmoplegia of pituitary apoplexy is better than the recovery of the visual loss, although aberrant regeneration may occur.

PAINFUL OPHTHALMOPLEGIA WITHOUT VISUAL LOSS

Cerebral Aneurysms

Several life-threatening syndromes can present with painful ophthalmoplegia; these must be distinguished from self-limited conditions. *Aneurysms* of the junction between the posterior communicating artery and internal carotid artery commonly cause acute, isolated, painful third nerve palsies in adults due to enlargement or bleeding. This presents with a pupil involving third nerve palsy. Patients may complain of a generalized headache, ipsilateral orbital pain, forehead pain, or even signs of meningismus. Any acute third nerve palsy in an adult must be evaluated to rule out posterior communicating artery aneurysms unless the palsy is complete and the pupil is entirely spared (i.e., equal in size and reactivity to the other eye). Partial external third nerve palsies with complete pupillary sparing and complete external third nerve palsies with relative pupil sparing require aneurysm rule out. An isolated, dilated, or nonreactive pupil with or without headache is not from an aneurysm and is instead the result of *Adie tonic pupil*, atropinic exposure, or an intrinsic iris anomaly.

After several months, recovery from aneurysmal ophthalmoplegia may occur and the patient typically develops *aberrant regeneration of the third nerve*. Aberrant regeneration is caused by misdirection of the recovering third nerve axons to all third nerve innervated ocular muscles following traumatic or compressive lesions in the peripheral third nerve. For instance, the levator muscle receives regenerated fibers that were originally innervating the inferior and medial recti. As a result, when the inferior or medial recti receive stimulation for downgaze or adduction, the levator simultaneously fires, and the eyelid retracts. Similarly, on downgaze and adduction, the levator and pupillary sphincter are innervated causing lid retraction and miosis.

Diabetic Ophthalmoplegia

Isolated, acute, painful third, fourth, and sixth nerve palsies, and rarely, combinations of the three may be caused by diabetic ophthalmoplegia (DO). In fact, DO is occasionally the presenting symptom of diabetes mellitus. The pain may be severe and may precede, accompany, or follow the ophthalmoplegia. Pain is not helpful in distinguishing from aneurysm and may last from days to 3 weeks. Recovery from DO occurs within 3 to 4 months. A thorough workup is necessary in adults if recovery does not take place in 3 to 4 months. Rarely, DO presents in children; when it does, a full workup is necessary. Patients can have several bouts of DO involving any combination of cranial nerves III, IV, and VI. When DO involves the third nerve, it must be distinguished from an aneurysmal cause. Although DO tends to spare the pupil, the only sparing that is of diagnostic importance is complete pupillary sparing in the setting of complete third nerve palsy. Aberrant regeneration of the third nerve never follows DO.

Internal Carotid Artery Dissection

Dissection of the internal carotid artery may be accompanied by neck, throat, ear, eye, and forehead pain, bruit, dysgeusia, postganglionic oculosympathetic palsy, retinal artery occlusion; and stroke. If the dissection extends into the cavernous sinus, ophthalmoplegia may result from compression of cranial nerves.

Cavernous Sinus Abnormalities

Aneurysms of the cavernous sinus may present with acute, chronic or episodic pain in the trigeminal distribution. They may also present with sixth or third nerve palsies or postganglionic oculosympathetic paresis. *Carotid–cavernous fistulas* that drain posteriorly, white-eyed shunts, can present with painful third, fourth, or sixth nerve palsies and will not exhibit the scleral, dilated blood vessels typical of other carotid–cavernous fistulae. In white-eyed shunts, the pain may precede the palsy by months.

The cavernous sinus and orbit may also be invaded by nasopharyngeal carcinomas, other sinus and skull-based malignancies, lymphomas, leukemia, Langerhans cell disorders, and inflammatory disease.

Cavernous sinus compressive lesions of the third nerve may spare the fibers to the pupillary sphincter resulting in a pupil-sparing third nerve palsy.

Temporal Arteritis

Temporal arteritis can cause diplopia from cranial nerve or extraocular muscle ischemia, brain stem transient ischemic attack (TIA), or stroke. Pain can come from tenderness of the temporal artery, scalp ischemia, jaw claudication, or ocular ischemia. In any patient older than the age of 50 years presenting with headache, loss of vision, or double vision, temporal arteritis must be excluded. Other vasculitides, namely Granulomatosis with polyangiitis (formerly known as *Wegener granulomatosis*) and polyarteritis nodosa, may present with painful ophthalmoplegia as well.

Infection

Rhinocerebral mucormycosis, seen in diabetics with ketoacidosis and in the immunosuppressed, is a fungal infection that spreads from the nasal sinuses into the orbit, cavernous sinus, and brain. It can spread via blood vessels and results in necrosis of the orbital contents and lids, causing blindness, pain, proptosis, and ophthalmoplegia. A black, necrotic patch may be seen inside the nose. Additionally, syphilis, Lyme disease, tuberculosis, and chronic fungal meningitis can cause painful ophthalmoplegia.

Following or with an attack of trigeminal herpes zoster, patients may present with a painful third, fourth, or sixth nerve palsy. This may be accompanied by postherpetic neuralgia and if the third nerve is involved, aberrant regeneration.

Transneural Tumor Growth

These tumors form along the sensory nerves of the face and results in chronic, unrelenting facial pain; formication; and dysesthesias. This may occur following excision of squamous cell carcinomas and occasionally, basal cell carcinomas and melanomas. With spread to the cavernous sinus, motor cranial nerve palsies and ophthalmoplegia ensue.

Tolosa–Hunt Syndrome

The painful ophthalmologic syndrome known as *Tolosa–Hunt syndrome* (THS) is an idiopathic, presumed granulomatous inflammation of the cavernous sinus, and is a diagnosis of exclusion. It presents with a boring pain, numbness, and paresthesias in the trigeminal distribution with ipsilateral paresis of one or more of the ocular motor nerves. It has a relapsing and remitting course that, together with its dramatic remission in response to high-dose oral steroids, was felt to be diagnostic. Subsequently, however, both masses and infiltrations were found to have the exact same presentation. On MRI, the cavernous sinus in THS is enlarged in about half the cases. Extensive systemic workup to exclude

TABLE 9.6	Key Questions When Evaluating Visual Disturbances

- Is the visual loss unilateral or bilateral?
- What is the time course?
- Is it painful or painless? If so, where and when?
- What's the tempo of any recovery of symptoms?
- Are the symptoms situational?
- Is there any metamorphopsia?
- Is there any red eye or foreign body sensation?
- Was the episode preceded by floaters or flashing lights?
- Are there any symptoms of polymyalgia rheumatica or giant cell arteritis?
- Are there any endocrine symptoms?
- What is the patient's nutritional status?
- Is there any family history of eye disease?
- Are the symptoms more pronounced during the day or night?
- What medications is the patient taking?

TABLE 9.7	Components of Neuroophthalmologic Examination
Visual acuity	• Snellen visual acuity chart • Amsler grid to detect metamorphopsia (distortion of straight lines), which suggests retinal disease
Color	• AO/HRR plates • Color comparison • Look for asymmetry in color perception or color desaturation (red). • Desaturation suggests optic nerve cause.
Confrontation visual fields	• Perform for each eye separately
Pupils	• Record size in dark and in light. • Record response to light. • Perform swinging flashlight test to look for relative afferent pupillary defect (RAPD).
External exam	• Look for ptosis and proptosis. • Look for injection of conjunctiva. • Examine for bruits. • Examine for temporal artery tenderness.
Motility	• Look for restrictions in extraocular movement, presence of phorias or tropias, abnormal saccades, abnormal pursuit, nystagmus, optokinetic nystagmus (OKN).
Funduscopic exam (ophthalmoscopy)	• Examine the fundus for optic nerve and retinal pathology.

lymphomas, primary and secondary tumors of cavernous sinus, IgG4-related disease, syphilis, tuberculosis, and infiltrations, such as sarcoid, should be performed.

FOCUSED HISTORY

Visual disturbances loss can occur due to problems anywhere along the visual system. To determine the cause of the vision loss, break the history down to determine whether it is transient or progressive. The key questions to ask are shown in Table 9.6. Then use physical exam to localize the pathology and further narrow the diagnosis.

EXAMINATION

Table 9.7 shows the essential components of a complete neuro-ophthalmologic examination.

VISUAL ACUITY

If vision is not improved with refraction or pinhole during visual acuity assessment with a Snellen chart or card, an *Amsler grid* should be used to assess for maculopathy. In this test, the patient uses near correction to look at a piece of graph paper for the straightness of its lines while focusing on the paper's central fixation dot. Each Amsler grid graph box represents one degree when viewing at 14 inches. If the lines appear bent, curved, or broken (metamorphopsia), the patient has maculopathy. Rotate the grid 180 degrees around the fixation point and the grid is now a map of where to look at the macula relative to the foveal center for pathology; for scale, the horizontal diameter of the disc is about 5 degrees. Missing areas of the grid suggest neural damage. Maculopathy is suggested by prolonged photostress recovery measured by the time it takes to read one line less than best acuity following a minute of staring into a light; a difference of 30 seconds between eyes is significant.

COLOR

Relative color saturation and brightness sense are useful in unilateral visual loss to distinguish optic neuropathy from maculopathy; they are preserved in retinal disorders and decreased in optic neuropathy. The common forms of hereditary color blindness spare color saturation. Compressive and inflammatory optic neuropathies decrease overall brightness and color sense. Color desaturation can be explained to patients by asking, "What happens to the color of blue jeans after several washings?" Brightness and color saturation may appear equal between eyes in unilateral ischemic optic neuropathy, as it tends to affect the optic nerve focally as in an inferior altitudinal visual field defect; however, the color sense and brightness will be depressed in the area of the visual field defect. In hemianopsias, color and brightness sense will be depressed in the affected hemifield, as it will be inside a cecocentral scotoma from ON. Color vision as measured by color plates as in the American Optical Hardy–Rand–Rittler (AO-HRR) plates is helpful in separating optic neuropathy from maculopathies. Maculopathies spare color vision except for the rare cone dystrophies and hereditary color vision defects, whereas optic neuropathies lose color vision in advance of visual acuity.

VISUAL FIELDS

Visual fields can be performed by confrontation. With one eye covered, the patient fixes on the examiner's nose at a distance of 1 to 2 m and is asked to describe what is seen or missing (Fig. 9.5). The examiners can wink an eye, protrude their tongue, raise their brow, smile, or frown; in this way, subtle central defects may be explored. With the patient fixed on the examiner's nose, the examiner then checks finger counting in the quadrants by placing fingers diagonally in the quadrants about 12 to 18 inches from

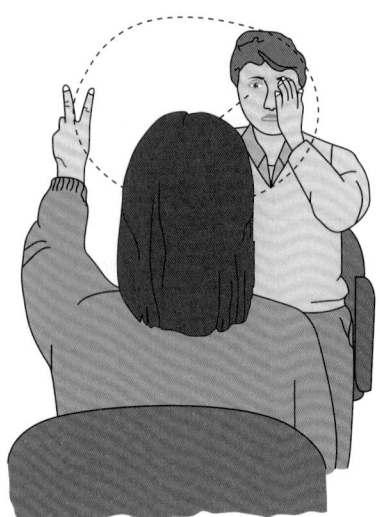

FIGURE 9.5 Visual field technique: Sit 1 to 2 m from the patient and have the patient cover one eye completely while looking at the examiner's nose. In quick succession, flash one, two, or five fingers in all four quadrants. Then switch eyes. (Adapted from Marshall R, Mayer S. *On Call Neurology.* 3rd ed. Philadelphia: Saunders; 2007.)

fixation. If the fingers are not seen, the examiner brings the finger toward the vertical midline checking for a vertical step as seen in hemianopsia. After checking for vertical steps, horizontal steps can be sought. Colored objects can be compared across the horizontal and vertical. Double simultaneous presentation can be used to pick up subtle defects. A laser pointer and a fixation dot on a piece of tape can be used to do an improvised tangent screen visual field exam that can be used on the ceiling in bed-bound patients. In children or adults who have trouble fixating, the head is held and the fingers placed in the temporal field to check for hemianopias.

PUPILS

The size and shape of the pupils are noted while the patient is fixing at distance in a dark room and in the light. The briskness of the pupillary reactions to light and near is recorded and the swinging flashlight test is performed. If the pupil is distorted, an inspection with a slit lamp or magnifier may reveal iris adhesions to the lens, damage to the iris sphincter, or iris stromal damage. A penlight applied to the lid inferotemporally while the eye is open in a dark room transilluminates the globe and reveals a pupillary red reflex. In traumatic, surgical, or inflammatory damage, the iris itself may transilluminate revealing sites of damage.

The RAPD results from an optic nerve lesion in one eye or asymmetric bilateral optic neuropathy; the sign is best shown by the swinging flashlight test. This pupillary sign is not seen if the problem is media opacity, a moderate retinopathy, or a nonorganic visual loss. It may be present to a mild degree in simple amblyopia. In the test, a bright flashlight is swung from one eye to the other, just below the visual axis, while the subject stares at a distant object in a dark room. Constriction of the pupils should be the same when either eye is illuminated. However, if an eye with optic nerve dysfunction is illuminated, the pupil constricts less briskly, less completely, and less persistently in response to the light than when the normal fellow eye is illuminated. If the pupil dilates or if the initial constriction is less brisk than that of the fellow eye, the test is positive. The RAPD may be quantified by placing increasing

amounts of neutral density filter before the good eye until the reaction of the pupils is equal. Both pupils are equal in size at all times in purely afferent defects because there is hemidecussation of all afferent light input to the midbrain with equal efferent stimulation through both third cranial nerves. Therefore, if one pupil is fixed to light because of an efferent defect, the other one may be observed throughout the performance of this test.

EXTERNAL EXAM

A clear understanding of visual disturbances is aided by an examination of the palpebral fissures, lids, and brows. In the normal adult, the upper lid covers 1 to 2 mm of the corneal limbus and the lower lid just kisses the lower limbus. The brows sit symmetrically at the supraorbital ridge. With unilateral or asymmetric facial weakness, the side of the weaker orbicularis oculi will have a wider palpebral fissure. When a patient's brow is below the supraorbital ridge along with an ipsilateral, narrow fissure, there is a blepharospastic disorder. This indicates either diplopia avoidance, aberrant regeneration of the facial nerve, hemifacial spasm, or facial myokymia. If the brow is raised on the side of the narrower fissure, the brow is purposefully being raised to compensate for ptosis.

The height of the palpebral fissure is recorded with a millimeter rule. With the patient looking at a light, the distance from the upper lid to the corneal light reflex is recorded which is the *marginal reflex distance* 1 (MRD 1); normal is about 4.5 mm. The distance from the light reflex to the lower lid is the MRD 2 and normal is about 5.5 mm. The MRD 1 and MRD 2 are equal to the palpebral fissure height that in normals is about 10 mm. The MRD measurements were introduced to clarify the effects of congenital and acquired lower lid anomalies on palpebral fissure height and focus in on levator dysfunction. In levator weakness, if the upper lid covers the corneal light reflex, the MRD 1 is recorded in negative numbers. In lid retraction and proptosis as in Graves disease or orbital tumors, the MRDs are increased; with enophthalmos, the MRDs are decreased. In oculosympathetic palsy with Mueller muscle weakness, the MRD 1 and 2 are both smaller, as there is Mueller muscle in both upper and lower lids. To measure levator function, press the eyebrow to the supraorbital ridge with your thumb and measure the excursion of the upper lid from down-to upgaze. Normal levator function is 15 mm. Decreased levator function implies levator weakness as seen in third nerve palsy, myasthenia gravis, mitochondrial myopathies, and congenital ptosis. Levator aponeurosis dehiscence is the most common cause of acquired ptosis in adults and has normal levator function.

Relative prominence of the globes can be observed by having the patient recline in a chair as the examiner looks directly down over the patient's nose for relative proptosis or enophthalmos. Using a ruler placed horizontally through the corneal light reflex of one eye as the patient stares straight ahead will detect anomalies of vertical globe alignment as seen in blowout fracture of the orbital floor or the silent sinus syndrome where the roof of the maxillary sinus descends.

OCULAR MOTILITY

The examination of eye movements starts with ocular alignment as measured by the cover test. While the patient is comfortably seated and fixing on a distance target straight ahead, the examiner covers one of the patient's eyes with an occluder and watches the other eye for a *refixation movement*. If a refixation movement is seen, a manifest deviation of the eyes is present called a *tropia*. If the eye being watched moves toward the nose, it means that it was deviated out relative to fixation and the term *exotropia* (wall-eyed) applies.

If the watched eye moves away from the nose, it was deviated in and it is termed *esotropia* (cross-eyed). If the eye moves down, it was hypertropic and if it moves up, hypotropic. If the watched eye does not move, it means it was aligned and fixating on the distance target. The next step is to switch and now cover the previously watched eye and observe the other eye for a tropia. The test can be performed in right gaze, left gaze, up gaze, down gaze as well as up and right, up and left, down and right, and down and left to reveal deficits of movement. For instance, a patient who complains of new-onset diplopia and has an esotropia in primary position that increases in right gaze and decreases or is gone in left gaze has a right lateral rectus weakness and may have a right sixth nerve palsy.

The second step is to look for latent disorders of ocular alignment, called *phorias*, with the alternate cover test. With the patient fixating at distance, the examiner covers one eye and then alternates the cover back and forth several times rapidly from one eye to the other eye, looking for movements of the uncovered eye. If the uncovered eye moves toward the nose, the patient has an exophoria and the other eye will act the same. If the eyes move away from the nose, esophoria is present. Phorias can be overcome by the patient's fusion mechanism but may break down into tropias with fatigue, alcohol, medication, or age. The normal patient may have a small exophoria at distance and near. An esophoria for distance or near, however, is always a sign of either congenital tendency to strabismus or neural or muscular dysfunction. Phorias and tropias that are about the same in the different positions of gaze and with either eye fixing are called *comitant deviations*. Comitant horizontal tropias usually occur in patients who had childhood strabismus. Deviations that vary in different directions are deemed incomitant and are a sign of muscular or neural dysfunction. Incomitant phorias may precede tropias as a pathologic process evolves. For example, an early right sixth nerve palsy may have an esophoria in right gaze before a manifest tropia with diplopia develops. A consequence of Herring law of equal innervation of agonist extraocular muscles is that the deviation is greatest with the paretic eye fixing, so in a paretic deviation, the refixation movement will be biggest when the paretic eye fixes.

Next in the eye movement exam is to have the patient follow into the eight different gaze positions looking for lag of movement. Movements with both eyes open are versions; if one eye is checked at a time, they are called *ductions*. Ductions produce larger movements than versions. Notation of the extent of the movements can be recorded using a millimeter ruler or the lag of ductions can be estimated on a scale of 1 to 4, with 4 being no movement at all. The pattern of lag of ductions can be inspected for a neurogenic pattern as in sixth or third nerve palsy; internuclear ophthalmoplegia; or a myogenic pattern with relatively symmetric, bilateral, and reduced movements in all directions with ptosis and pupil sparing as in mitochondrial myopathy or autosomal dominant French–Canadian muscular dystrophy. In isolation, an inability to look up in abduction, mimicking weakness of the superior rectus muscle, is likely Graves disease that has caused fibrosis of the ipsilateral inferior rectus muscle restricting the superior rectus. In isolated inferior rectus weakness, myasthenia gravis is the most likely diagnosis. In inferior rectus weakness seen in the setting of other neurologic signs or acute neurologic dysfunction, a stroke or mass of the midbrain involving the rostral portion of the third nerve nucleus in the inferior rectus subnucleus must be suspected. An eye that cannot elevate in adduction due to an apparent deficit of the inferior oblique muscle is seen in Brown tendon sheath syndrome. This is a congenital malformation of the superior oblique sheath that prevents free movement of the superior oblique tendon through the trochlea and is unaccompanied by diplopia. An acquired version of Brown syndrome occurs in rheumatoid arthritis and is accompanied by diplopia. Duane retraction syndrome is a congenital anomaly more common in women that is unaccompanied by diplopia. It demonstrates decreased abduction, typically on the left, with globe retraction on adduction, which is recognized by narrowing of the palpebral fissure.

Eye movements should next be examined for fast eye movements or saccades. If eye movements are incomplete, saccades should be inspected for slowing. Saccadic slowing suggests neural involvement anywhere from the peripheral cranial nerve, brain stem nuclei, internuclear connections, and supranuclear pathways. Saccadic slowing can be checked for with repetitive, voluntary saccades into the area of interest, or the saccades can be generated using an optokinetic nystagmus flag or drum. Restrictive problems, as in Graves disease, orbital myositis, and orbital blowout fractures, do not slow saccades enough to be recognized by the unaided eye. Slowing of saccades of horizontal and vertical versions may be a result of the lesions of the frontal pontine pathways for gaze, the paramedian pontine reticular formation, the rostral interstitial nucleus of the medial longitudinal fasciculus, or their connections. Saccades should also be checked for dysmetria by having the patient refixate from 30 degrees to the right of center, then from 30 degrees to the left of center.

Finally, examination of the fundus in each eye is critical to a complete assessment with observations of the disc for swelling or atrophy, the nerve fiber layer for dropout, the vessels for diameter, emboli, or occlusion, and the macula for hemorrhages, exudates, or detachments.

SUGGESTED READINGS

Bernstein EF, ed. *Amaurosis Fugax.* New York: Springer-Verlag; 1988.

Fisher CM. Observations of the fundus oculi in transient monocular blindness. *Neurology.* 1959;9:333–347.

Frisen L. Quadruple sectoranopia and sectorial optic atrophy: a syndrome of the distal anterior choroidal artery. *J Neurol Neurosurg Psychiatry.* 1979;42:590–594.

Frisen L, Holmegard L, Rosencrantz M. Sectorial optic atrophy and homonymous, horizontal sectoranopia: a lateral choroidal artery syndrome. *J Neurol Neurosurg Psychiatry.* 1978;41:374–380.

Gerling J, Meyer JH, Kommerell G. Visual field defects in optic neuritis and anterior ischemic optic neuropathy: distinctive features. *Graefes Arch Clin Exp Ophthalmol.* 1998;236:188–192.

Glaser JS. Topical diagnosis: prechiasmal pathways. In: Glaser JS. *Neuro-Ophthalmology.* Philadelphia: Lippincott Williams & Wilkins; 1999:95–198.

Glaser JS, Hoyt WF, Corbett J. Visual morbidity with chiasmal glioma. Long term studies of visual fields in untreated and irradiated cases. *Arch Ophthalmol.* 1971;85:3–12.

Harrington DO. The character of visual field defects in temporal and occipital lobe lesions, localizing value of congruity and incongruity in complete homonymous hemianopia. *Trans Am Ophthalmol Soc.* 1961;59:333–369.

Horton JC. Wilbrand's knee of the primate optic chiasm is an artefact of monocular enucleation. *Trans Am Ophthalmol Soc.* 1997;95:579–609.

Horton JC, Hoyt WF. The representation of the visual field in the human striate cortex: a revision of the classic Holmes map. *Arch Ophthalmol.* 1991;109:816–824.

Horton JC, Hoyt WF. Quadrantic visual defects: a hallmark of lesions of the extrastriate (V2/V3) cortex. *Brain.* 1991;114:1703–1718.

Hoyt WF. Ocular symptoms and signs. In: Wylie EJ, Ehrenfeld WK, eds. *Extracranial Occlusive Cerebrovascular Disease: Diagnosis and Management.* Philadelphia: WB Saunders; 1970:64–95.

Hoyt WF, Beeston D. *The Ocular Fundus in Neurologic Disease: A Diagnostic Manual and Stereo Atlas.* St. Louis, MO: CV Mosby; 1966.

Hoyt WF, Meschel LG, Lessell S et al. Malignant optic glioma of adulthood. *Brain*. 1973;96:121–132.

Imes RK, Hoyt WF. Childhood chiasmal gliomas: update on the fate of patients in the 1969 San Francisco study. *Br J Ophthalmol*. 1986;70:179–182.

Kedar S, Zhang X, Lynn MJ, et al. Congruency in homonymous hemianopia. *Am J Ophthalmol*. 2007;143:772–780.

Kline LB, Hoyt WF. The Tolosa-Hunt syndrome. *J Neurol Neurosurg Psychiatry*. 2001;71:577–582.

Leigh RJ, Zee DS. *The Neurology of Eye Movements*. New York: Oxford University Press; 2015.

Lepore FE. The preserved temporal crescent: the clinical implication of an "endangered clinical finding." *Neurology*. 2001;57:1918–1921.

Miller NR, Newman NJ, eds. *Walsh & Hoyt's Clinical Neuro-Ophthalmology*. Philadelphia: Lippincott Williams & Wilkins; 2005.

Nevalainen J, Krapp E, Paetzold J, et al. Visual field defects in acute optic neuritis—distribution of different types of defect pattern, assessed with threshold-related supraliminal perimetry, ensuring high spatial resolution. *Graefe's Arch Clin Exp Ophthalmol*. 2008;246:599–607.

Petzold A, Wattjes MP, Costello F, et al. The investigation of acute optic neuritis: a review and proposed protocol. *Nat Rev Neurol*. 2014;10:447–458.

Plant GT, Perry VH. The anatomical basis of the caecocentral scotoma: new observations and a review. *Brain*. 1990;113:1441–1457.

Purvin V, Sundaram S, Kawasaki A. Neuroretinitis: review of the literature and new observations. *J Neuroophthalmol*. 2011;31:58–68.

Scott GI. *Traquair's Clinical Perimetry*. London, United Kingdom: Henry Kimpton; 1957.

Skarf B, Glaser JS, Trick GL, et al. Neuro-ophthalmologic examination: the visual sensory system. In Glaser JS. *Neuro-Ophthalmology*. Philadelphia: Lippincott Williams & Wilkins; 1999:7–50.

Smith JL. Homonymous hemianopia. A review of one hundred cases. *Am J Ophthalmol*. 1962;54:616–623.

Thompson HS, Corbett JJ, Cox TA. How to measure the relative afferent pupillary defect. *Survey Ophthalmol*. 1981;23:39–42.

Zhang X, Kedar S, Lynn MJ, et al. Homonymous hemianopias: clinical-anatomic correlations in 904 cases. *Neurology*. 2006;66:906–910.

Delirium 10

Adam B. King and Christopher G. Hughes

INTRODUCTION

Delirium is a clinical syndrome characterized by fluctuations in mental status caused by acute cerebral dysfunction. Patients may present with inattention, disorganized thinking, disorientation, and/or altered levels of consciousness. Other symptoms associated with delirium include sleep disturbances, abnormal psychomotor activity, hallucinations, and emotional disturbances such as fear, depression, or anxiety. Patients may experience symptomatology that is hyperactive or hypoactive or fluctuate between both (mixed delirium). Although hyperactive delirium is more dramatic, hypoactive delirium is more common and much more underdiagnosed.

Development of delirium while in the intensive care unit (ICU) has been associated with increased cost, ICU length of stay, hospital length of stay, and long-term cognitive dysfunction. This risk is independent of preexisting comorbid conditions, severity of concurrent illness, and age. Additionally, duration of delirium has been shown to increase the relative risk of death by 10% per day of delirium.

Delirium is common among hospitalized patients. Upon admission, approximately 11% to 25% of elderly patients are delirious, and an additional 30% or so will go on to develop delirium. Delirium is even more frequent among critically ill patients; it is estimated that up to 80% of patients in the ICU experience an episode of delirium. Given the implications of an episode of delirium on patient outcomes, prevention and treatment is of utmost importance.

MANAGEMENT STRATEGY

- Rule out life-threatening causes of mental status change such as hypoxia, hypercarbia, drug ingestion/withdrawal, or seizures.
- Perform focused history and physical exam including assessment of arousal level and delirium with tools such as the confusion assessment method (CAM) or confusion assessment method for the intensive care unit (CAM-ICU).
- Focus on appropriate and early removal of catheters/restraints, promote sleep, perform early mobilization, provide glasses and hearing aids, and eliminate unnecessary alarms and auditory stimuli (e.g., television).
- Establish a calm, reassuring environment, and promote human contact, especially with loved ones.
- Ensure patient and staff safety. Pharmacologic management may be required in patients whose agitation puts them at risk for harming themselves or others.

CAUSES OF DELIRIUM

The underlying mechanism of delirium or acute brain dysfunction has many proposed mechanisms. Systemic inflammation, cholinergic deficiency, and disturbances in other neurotransmitters such as serotonin and norepinephrine have been implicated in the development of delirium.

Risk factors for delirium can be characterized into patient factors, current illness factors, and iatrogenic causes, as outlined in Table 10.1. Baseline patient factors that have been associated with development of delirium include preexisting dementia, history of hypertension, alcoholism, and a high severity of illness upon admission. Additionally, age has been shown to be an independent risk factor for development of delirium outside of the ICU; however, within the ICU, there is discordance about it as a risk factor.

Clinicians are able to modify several risk factors for delirium by improving sleep hygiene and sedative regimens and avoiding medications that might trigger delirium. For instance, lorazepam administration is an independent risk factor for development of delirium in ICU patients undergoing mechanical ventilation. In addition, midazolam administration has been associated with worse delirium outcomes in mixed ICU patients.

Analgesic regimens, specifically opiates, do not have a clearly defined relationship with development of delirium. In fact, inadequate pain control is a risk factor for development of delirium. In a prospective study that enrolled patients with hip fractures without preexisting delirium, patients who received less than 10 mg of morphine equivalents per day were at increased risk of development of delirium. However, other studies have associated morphine and meperidine administration with the development of delirium. It appears that adequate pain control might be beneficial in protection against delirium, but use of opiates for sedation might place patients at risk for development of delirium.

NEUROANATOMY

Neuroanatomic changes that include brain atrophy and white matter changes have been witnessed in patients with delirium. White matter changes continue to persist even after hospital discharge and may be the cause of long-term cognitive impairment in these patients. In addition, patients have dysregulation of acetylcholine, dopamine, and γ-aminobutyric acid.

TABLE 10.1 Clinical Risk Factors for Delirium

Patient Factors	Acute Illness	Iatrogenic Causes
Baseline cognitive impairment	Electrolyte disturbances	Sedative medications
Age	Hypoxemia	Sleep disturbances
Baseline comorbidity	Global severity of disease	Anticholinergic medications
Frailty	Sepsis	Analgesic medications

FOCUSED HISTORY

Evaluation of the patient with suspected delirium should start with a history and physical exam. Causes of delirium such as drug ingestion, alcohol or drug withdrawal, metabolic derangements, and infection should be sought. Because features of delirium such as confusion or inattention may be present, history may be difficult to obtain from the patient. Assistance from staff or family members may be necessary. In addition, baseline functional status of the patient should be obtained, as this can help differentiate between dementia and delirium.

FOCUSED EXAM

Physical exam should look for possible sources of infection (e.g., pneumonia or urinary tract infection) as the cause of the patient's acute change in mental status. In addition, physical exam findings suggestive of drug exposure may be useful. For example, anticholinergic exposure would reveal increased temperature, flushed dry skin, tachycardia, and pupillary dilation on exam. Focal neurologic findings that could point to seizure activity or stroke should also be sought.

The development of validated instruments now allows for assessment of patient's level of arousal and content of consciousness even when a patient is mechanically ventilated. The Richmond Agitation-Sedation Scale (RASS) (Table 10.2) and the Riker Sedation-Agitation Scale (SAS) are commonly used tools that can be used to assess level of arousal. Assessment for delirium cannot occur if the patient is deemed unresponsive by the sedation scales (RASS −4 to −5 or SAS of 1 to 2). If the patient is responsive to verbal stimuli, then delirium can be assessed using tools such as the CAM, the CAM-ICU, or the Intensive Care Delirium Screening Checklist (ICDSC). Further information about these tools used for diagnosis of delirium can be found in the "Diagnosis" section.

Delirium is a syndrome of brain dysfunction and rarely presents as a single clinical entity. Pure hyperactive delirium is less common despite being the foremost perception of delirium to most clinicians. Patients with hyperactive delirium display prominent agitated motor behaviors such as pulling at lines/catheters and physically or verbally assaulting staff. In contrast, most patients are either hypoactive or have a mixed subtype. Hypoactive delirium is characterized by slow patient movements, decreased speed of cognition, and decreased alertness. It might be associated with worse outcomes; however, patients are often overlooked because they are not displaying disruptive behavior.

DIAGNOSIS

In addition to a history and physical exam, other causes of changes in mental status should be sought. An electrolyte panel, blood count, and liver and thyroid function tests should be obtained. Additionally, infectious causes should be ruled out with appropriate testing such as chest radiograph, urinalysis, and culture data. Hypoxemia and hypercarbia should also be excluded as causes of confusion, which may require arterial blood gas analysis.

After a thorough history and physical exam, the next step is determining the patient's level of arousal through the use of a sedation scale such as the RASS, as described in the physical exam section. If the patient is determined to be unresponsive, RASS −4 or −5, then they are in a coma and cannot be assessed for delirium. There are several validated tools through which delirium diagnosis and screening can be performed.

TOOLS FOR SCREENING AND DIAGNOSIS

Diagnosis of delirium relies on determination from the history and physical that the condition is an acute change in the patients' status. In patients who are not mechanically ventilated, the CAM (Table 10.3) can be used for diagnosis. The CAM assesses the patient for the key features of delirium such as an acute onset, fluctuating course, and inattention. It then assesses the patient for other symptomatology of delirium such as disorganized thinking or altered level of consciousness.

In critically ill or mechanically ventilated patients, the CAM–ICU (Table 10.4) and ICDSC (Table 10.5) have been validated. The CAM-ICU assesses the same four features as the CAM in an abbreviated manner more applicable to patients with critical illness: acute change or fluctuation in mental status, inattention, disorganized thinking, and an altered level of consciousness. The ICDSC uses eight diagnostic features; the diagnosis of delirium requires four or more features to be present.

DIAGNOSIS OF DELIRIUM AFTER STROKE

The incidence of poststroke delirium varies from 10% to 48%. Diagnosis of delirium in this patient population requires the ability to dif-

TABLE 10.2	Richmond Agitation-Sedation Scale	
Score	Term	Description
+4	Combative	Overly combative, violent, immediate danger to staff
+3	Very agitated	Pulls or removes tube(s) or catheter(s); aggressive
+2	Agitated	Frequent or nonpurposeful movements, fights ventilator
+1	Restless	Anxious but movements not aggressive/vigorous
0	Alert and calm	
−1	Drowsy	Not fully alert but has sustained awakening (eye opening/eye contact) to voice >10 s
−2	Light sedation	Briefly awakens with eye contact to voice (<10 s)
−3	Moderate sedation	Movement or eye opening to voice (but no eye contact)
−4	Deep sedation	No response to voice but movement or eye opening to physical stimulation
−5	Unarousable	No response to voice or physical stimulation

TABLE 10.3 Confusion Assessment Method

Diagnosis of delirium requires the presence of BOTH features A and B and the presence of EITHER feature C or D.

A. Acute onset or fluctuating course	Is there evidence of an acute change in mental status from baseline?
	Does the abnormal behavior:
	• Fluctuate over time?
	• Come and go?
	• Increase/decrease in severity?
B. Inattention	Does the patient:
	• Have difficulty focusing?
	• Become easily distracted?
	• Have difficulty keeping track of what is said?
C. Disorganized thinking	Is the patient's thinking:
	• Disorganized?
	• Incoherent?
D. Altered level of consciousness	Is the patient:
	• Alert (normal)?
	• Vigilant (hyperalert)?
	• Lethargic (drowsy but arousable)?
	• Stuporous (difficult to arouse)?
	• Comatose (unarousable)?

ferentiate delirium from mental status changes from the underlying disease process. The CAM-ICU has been validated in stroke patients by comparing it to the *Diagnostic and Statistical Manual of Mental Disorders*, 4th edition (*DSM-IV*), criteria for delirium. The CAM-ICU proved to be 76% sensitive and 98% specific for the diagnosis of delirium after stroke. The positive predictive value was 91%.

DELIRIUM VERSUS DEMENTIA: A DIAGNOSTIC CHALLENGE

It is estimated that 4.5 million elderly Americans have Alzheimer disease (AD). As the population continues to age, this number will continue to increase. The prevalence of delirium in hospitalized patients with coexisting AD is estimated at 60% to 89% of patients, and delirium in patients with preexisting dementia has been associated with long-term cognitive decline that persists for at least 5 years after discharge from the hospital. Diagnosis of delirium in patients with underlying dementia can be difficult; symptoms of delirium can be attributed to the underlying cognitive dysfunction and overlooked as new symptomatology. Trials for validating delirium assessment tools have either excluded or included few patients with underlying dementia; however, based on the available evidence, the CAM and CAM–ICU are currently considered the best available tools.

ELECTROENCEPHALOGRAM FINDINGS IN DELIRIUM

The fluctuating state of awareness in delirium is accompanied by changes in the electroencephalogram (EEG). Changes in level of attention parallel the slowing of background EEG rhythms. There may be deceleration or complete loss of posterior background

TABLE 10.4 Confusion Assessment Method for the Intensive Care Unit

Feature A plus B and either C or D present = CAM-ICU positive

A. Acute onset or fluctuating course	• Is the patient different than his or her baseline?
	OR
	• Has the patient had any fluctuation in mental status in the past 24 h?
B. Inattention	• Letters attention test:
	Say to the patient, "I am going to read to you a series of 10 letters. Whenever you hear the letter 'A,' indicate by squeezing my hand."
	SAVEAHAART or CASABLANCA or ABADABADAAY
	Errors are counted when patient fails to squeeze on the letter "A" and when patient squeezes on any letter other than "A."
	If greater than two errors, patient has inattention.
C. Altered level of consciousness	• Present if the RASS score is anything other than alert and calm or RASS 0.
D. Disorganized thinking	• Ask patient yes/no questions:
	1. Will a stone float on water?
	2. Are there fish in the sea?
	3. Does 1 lb weigh more than 2 lb?
	Errors are counted when the patient incorrectly answers a question.
	• Have the patient follow commands:
	Say to patient "Hold this many fingers up" (show two fingers to patient). Have him or her repeat with the other hand using a different number of fingers.
	An error is counted if patient is unable to complete the entire command.
	If patient makes greater than one error, then he or she is positive for this feature.

CAM-ICU, confusion assessment method for the intensive care unit; RASS, Richmond Agitation-Sedation Scale.

TABLE 10.5 Intensive Care Delirium Screening Checklist

1. Altered level of consciousness

A.	Exaggerated response to normal stimulation	RASS +1 to +4
B.	Normal wakefulness	RASS 0
C.	Response to mild/moderate stimulation	RASS −1 to −3
D.	Response only to intense stimulation	RASS −4
E.	No response	RASS −5

Assessment is terminated if patient is a RASS −4 or RASS −5.

2. Inattention

A. Difficulty in following commands

B. Easily distracted by external stimuli

C. Difficulty in shifting focus

One point if any are present

3. Disorientation

Patient not oriented to person, place, or time

One point if any are present

4. Hallucinations or delusions

A. Equivocal evidence of hallucinations or behavior due to hallucinations

B. Delusions

One point if any are present

5. Psychomotor agitation or retardation

A. Hyperactivity requiring the use of addition sedatives or restraints

B. Hypoactivity or psychomotor slowing

One point if any are present

6. Inappropriate speech or mood

A. Inappropriate, disorganized, or incoherent speech

B. Inappropriate mood

One point if any are present

7. Sleep/wake cycle disturbance

A. Sleeping <4 h per night

B. Waking frequently at night

C. Sleeping >4 h during the day

One point if any are present

8. Symptom fluctuation

Fluctuation of any of the above items over the previous 24 h

Total score is based on adding items up from 1 to 8. A score >4 is concerning for delirium.

RASS, Richmond Agitation-Sedation Scale.

rhythm, global slowing, and intermittent rhythmic delta activity especially in the frontal regions. Triphasic waves may be present when metabolic encephalopathy is a contributing factor.

MANAGEMENT

Delirium is an urgent medical condition and prompt review of possible causes or inciting factors should be performed. Underlying causes such as pain, metabolic derangements, infection, and hypoxemia should be sought and treated.

Treatment consists of two broad categories: *pharmacologic symptom management* and *environmental optimization*. The initial step in management is to ensure patient and staff safety. If the patient is exhibiting signs of hyperactive delirium and is trying to remove medically necessary devices, pharmacologic management is likely needed. If pain is an inciting cause, analgesic therapy with opioids or NSAIDS should be used as the first line of therapy. Symptomatic treatment is usually with dexmedetomidine or an antipsychotic medication such as haloperidol, olanzapine, or quetiapine (Table 10.6). Benzodiazepines can often exacerbate delirium symptoms and should be avoided unless the cause is alcohol withdrawal or if there is a component of severe anxiety. Despite common use among clinicians, there is a lack of large randomized controlled trials of medications for the treatment of delirium, and current evidence is limited to small cohort studies.

PHARMACOLOGIC THERAPY

First-line pharmacologic therapy for delirium prevention and treatment after pain control consists of dexmedetomidine and antipsychotic medications. The Maximizing Efficacy of Targeted Sedation and Reducing Neurological Dysfunction (MENDS) trial compared lorazepam and dexmedetomidine for sedation in critically ill patients, and patients who received dexmedetomidine for sedation had more days free of delirium [**Level 1**].[1] The Safety and Efficacy of Dexmedetomidine Compared with Midazolam (SEDCOM) trial showed that patients sedated with dexmedetomidine achieved adequate levels of sedation while experiencing less episodes of delirium and shorter time to extubation [**Level 1**].[2] A small, open-label trial comparing haloperidol versus dexmedetomidine in delirious, agitated, mechanically ventilated patients showed earlier time to extubation and shorter ICU length of stay in the dexmedetomidine group. Together, these studies support the use of dexmedetomidine as a first-line therapy to prevent and treat delirium in mechanically ventilated ICU patients.

There are several small randomized controlled trials examining the efficacy of antipsychotics for treatment or prevention of delirium. The Modifying the Incidence of Delirium (MIND) study compared ziprasidone (an atypical antipsychotic) with haloperidol (a typical antipsychotic) versus placebo and found no difference in outcomes between groups. Quetiapine was compared to placebo in a small trial of critically ill patients with delirium. Patients in both groups received haloperidol as rescue medication. Quetiapine was shown to decrease the number of hours until resolution of delirium symptoms and reduce rescue medication but was not effective in preventing recurrence of symptoms. Another randomized

TABLE 10.6 Medications Used to Control Delirium Symptoms

Drug	Dose
Dexmedetomidine (Precedex)	0.7–1.4 μg/kg/min IV infusion
Haloperidol (Haldol)	1–10 mg q4–6h
Lorazepam (Ativan)	0.5–4 mg IV q4h
Olanzapine (Zyprexa)	5–10 mg PO q8h
Quetiapine (Seroquel)	25–50 mg q8–12h

IV, intravenous; PO, by mouth.

TABLE 10.7 Key Points for Managing Delirium

- Delirium is common among hospitalized patients; occurring in up to 80% of patients with critical illness.

- Development of delirium increases the patients' hospital length of stay and is associated with long-term cognitive impairment and mortality.

- Treatment is focused on correcting any possible underlying causes of delirium and improving environmental factors. Pharmacologic therapy may be undertaken for symptom management.

- Medications should be used judiciously due to uncertainty about their efficacy and their potential effect on patient's sensorium.

- Improvement in the patient's sleep/wake cycle, early mobility, removal of unnecessary lines/catheters, and frequent stimulating activities may provide some delirium prevention.

controlled trial showed that single dose of risperidone given sublingually after cardiac surgery was more effective than placebo in prevention of delirium. A pre/post trial in the Netherlands found haloperidol prophylaxis decrease the incidence of delirium from 75% to 65% in this group of patients who were at high risk for development of delirium. The HOPE-ICU trial, however, found that intravenous haloperidol given to patients with delirium or coma did not improve outcomes versus placebo. At the present time, there is insufficient data to recommend routine prophylactic therapy with antipsychotic agents to prevent delirium in high-risk patients.

ENVIRONMENTAL OPTIMIZATION

Nonpharmacologic interventions have been shown to be beneficial in patients with delirium, and improving the environmental factors remains the first-line intervention for delirium prevention and treatment. These treatments include sleep hygiene and patient reorientation. A study in medical patients reduced the incidence of delirium by 40% by focusing on regulation of environmental factors [**Level 1**].[3] These factors included appropriate and early removal of catheters/restraints, nonpharmacologic sleep protocols, early mobilization, providing regular stimulating activities, and attention to hydration. In a randomized trial of early physical and occupational therapy in critically ill patients, patients in the early mobilization group had greater return to functional status at hospital discharge and shorter duration of delirium [**Level 1**].[4] In addition to early physical therapy, sedation protocols have also been shown to reduce delirium. The Awakening and Breathing Coordination, Delirium Monitoring/Management, and Early Exercise/Mobility trial (ABCDE) showed that sedation protocols combined with early mobilization can reduce the incidence of delirium and length of mechanical ventilation in critically ill patients.

CONCLUSION

Delirium commonly occurs in hospitalized patients and is independently associated with worse outcomes (Table 10.7). Early recognition of delirium may be achieved through active use of screening tools such as the CAM or CAM-ICU. Treatment should focus on nonpharmalogic therapy such as improvement in the patient's sleep/wake cycle, early mobility, removal of unnecessary lines/catheters, and frequent stimulating activities. Pharmacologic therapy should be used when patient behavior places themselves or staff at risk. These therapies should be used judiciously, as they have unproven efficacy and alter patient sensorium.

LEVEL 1 EVIDENCE

1. Pandharipande PP, Pun BT, Herr DL, et al. Effect of sedation with dexmedetomidine vs lorazepam on acute brain dysfunction in mechanically ventilated patients: the MENDS randomized controlled trial. *JAMA*. 2007;298(22):2644–2653.

2. Riker RR, Shehabi Y, Bokesch PM, et al. Dexmedetomidine vs midazolam for sedation of critically ill patients: a randomized trial. *JAMA*. 2009;301(5):489–499.

3. Inouye SK, Bogardus ST Jr, Charpentier PA, et al. A multicomponent intervention to prevent delirium in hospitalized older patients. *N Engl J Med*. 1999;340(9):669–676.

4. Schweickert WD, Pohlman MC, Pohlman AS, et al. Early physical and occupational therapy in mechanically ventilated, critically ill patients: a randomised controlled trial. *Lancet*. 2009;373(9678):1874–1882.

SUGGESTED READINGS

Balas MC, Burke WJ, Gannon D, et al. Implementing the awakening and breathing coordination, delirium monitoring/management, and early exercise/mobility bundle into everyday care: opportunities, challenges, and lessons learned for implementing the ICU Pain, Agitation, and Delirium Guidelines. *Crit Care Med*. 2013;41(9)(suppl 1):S116–S127.

Barr J, Fraser GL, Puntillo K, et al. Clinical practice guidelines for the management of pain, agitation, and delirium in adult patients in the intensive care unit. *Crit Care Med*. 2013;41(1):263–306.

Bergeron N, Dubois MJ, Dumont M, et al. Intensive Care Delirium Screening Checklist: evaluation of a new screening tool. *Intensive Care Med*. 2001;27(5):859–864.

Dahl MH, Rønning OM, Thommessen B. Delirium in acute stroke—prevalence and risk factors. *Acta Neurol Scand Suppl*. 2010;(190):39–43.

Devlin JW, Roberts RJ, Fong JJ, et al. Efficacy and safety of quetiapine in critically ill patients with delirium: a prospective, multicenter, randomized, double-blind, placebo-controlled pilot study. *Crit Care Med*. 2010;38(2):419–427.

Dubois MJ, Bergeron N, Dumont M, et al. Delirium in an intensive care unit: a study of risk factors. *Intensive Care Med*. 2001;27(8):1297–1304.

Ely EW, Gautam S, Margolin R, et al. The impact of delirium in the intensive care unit on hospital length of stay. *Intensive Care Med*. 2001;27(12):1892–1900.

Ely EW, Inouye SK, Bernard GR, et al. Delirium in mechanically ventilated patients: validity and reliability of the confusion assessment method for the intensive care unit (CAM-ICU). *JAMA*. 2001;286(21):2703–2710.

Ely EW, Shintani A, Truman B, et al. Delirium as a predictor of mortality in mechanically ventilated patients in the intensive care unit. *JAMA*. 2004;291(14):1753–1762.

Fick DM, Agostini JV, Inouye SK. Delirium superimposed on dementia: a systemic reivew. *J Am Geriatr Soc*. 2002;50(10):1723–1732.

Girard TD, Pandharipande PP, Carson SS, et al. Feasibility, efficacy, and safety of antipsychotics for intensive care unit delirium: the MIND randomized, placebo-controlled trial. *Crit Care Med*. 2010;38(2):428–437.

Gross AL, Jones RN, Habtemariam DA, et al. Delirium and long-term cognitive trajectory among persons with dementia. *Arch Intern Med*. 2012;172(17):1324–1331.

Gunther ML, Morandi A, Krauskopf E, et al. The association between brain volumes, delirium duration, and cognitive outcomes in intensive care unit survivors: the VISIONS cohort magnetic resonance imaging study. *Crit Care Med*. 2012;40(7):2022–2032.

Gustafson Y, Olsson T, Erikkson S, et al. Acute confusional states (delirium) in stroke patients. *Cerebrovasc Dis*. 1991;1:257–264.

Inouye SK, van Dyck CH, Alessi CA, et al. Clarifying confusion: the confusion assessment method. A new method for detection of delirium. *Ann Intern Med*. 1990;113(12):941–948.

Jacobson S, Jerrier H. EEG in delirium. *Semin Clin Neuropsychiatry*. 2000;5: 86–92.

Lin SM, Liu CY, Wang CH, et al. The impact of delirium on the survival of mechanically ventilated patients. *Crit Care Med*. 2004;32(11): 2254–2259.

McNicoll L, Pisani MA, Zhang Y, et al. Delirium in the intensive care unit: occurrence and clinical course in older patients. *J Am Geriatr Soc*. 2003;51(5): 591–598.

Mitasova A, Kostalova M, Bednarik J, et al. Poststroke delirium incidence and outcomes: validation of the Confusion Assessment Method for the Intensive Care Unit (CAM-ICU). *Crit Care Med*. 2012;40(2):484–490.

Morandi A, McCurley J, Vasilevskis E, et al. Tools to detect delirium superimposed on dementia: a systematic review. *J Am Geriatr Soc*. 2012;60(11): 2005–2013.

Morandi A, Rogers BP, Gunther ML, et al. The relationship between delirium duration, white matter integrity, and cognitive impairment in intensive care unit survivors as determined by diffusion tensor imaging: the VISIONS prospective cohort magnetic resonance imaging study. *Crit Care Med*. 2012;40(7):2182–2189.

Morrison RS, Magaziner J, Gilbert M, et al. Relationship between pain and opioid analgesics on the development of delirium following hip fracture. *J Gerontol A Biol Sci Med Sci*. 2003;58(1):76–81.

Page VJ, Ely EW, Gates S, et al. Effect of intravenous haloperidol on the duration of delirium and coma in critically ill patients (Hope-ICU): a randomised, double-blind, placebo-controlled trial. *Lancet Respir Med*. 2013;1(7): 515–523.

Pandharipande P, Cotton BA, Shintani A, et al. Motoric subtypes of delirium in mechanically ventilated surgical and trauma intensive care unit patients. *Intensive Care Med*. 2007;33(10):1726–1731.

Pandharipande P, Cotton BA, Shintani A, et al. Prevalence and risk factors for development of delirium in surgical and trauma intensive care unit patients. *J Trauma*. 2008;65(1):34–41.

Pandharipande PP, Girard TD, Jackson JC, et al. Long-term cognitive impairment after critical illness. *N Engl J Med*. 2013;369(14):1306–1316.

Pandharipande P, Shintani A, Peterson J, et al. Lorazepam is an independent risk factor for transitioning to delirium in intensive care unit patients. *Anesthesiology*. 2006;104(1):21–26.

Pisani MA, Kong SY, Kasl SV, et al. Days of delirium are associated with 1-year mortality in an older intensive care unit population. *Am J Respir Crit Care Med*. 2009;180(11):1092–1097.

Prakanrattana U, Prapaitrakool S. Efficacy of risperidone for prevention of postoperative delirium in cardiac surgery. *Anaesth Intensive Care*. 2007;35(5): 714–719.

Reade MC, O'Sullivan K, Bates S, et al. Dexmedetomidine vs. haloperidol in delirious, agitated intubated patients: a randomized open-label trial. *Crit Care*. 2009;13(3):R75.

Robinson TN, Raeburn CD, Tran ZV, et al. Motor subtypes of postoperative delirium in older adults. *Arch Surg*. 2011;146:295–300.

Sampson EL, Raven PR, Ndhlovu PN, et al. A randomized, double-blind, placebo-controlled trial of donepezil hydrochloride (Aricept) for reducing the incidence of postoperative delirium after elective total hip replacement. *Int J Geriatr Psychiatry*. 2007;22(4):343–349.

Shehabi Y, Riker RR, Bokesch PM, et al. Delirium duration and mortality in lightly sedated, mechanically ventilated intensive care patients. *Crit Care Med*. 2010;38(12):2311–2318.

van den Boogaard M, Schoonhoven L, van Achterberg T, et al. Haloperidol prophylaxis in critically ill patients with a high risk for delirium. *Crit Care*. 2013;17(1):R9.

Dementia and Memory Loss 11

Lawrence S. Honig

INTRODUCTION

Dementia is characterized by intellectual deterioration, with concomitant decline in independence and daily social or occupational functions.

With different dementia disorders, various cognitive domains may be dominantly affected including memory, orientation, abstraction, learning ability, visuospatial perception, language functions, constructional praxis, and higher executive functions such as planning, organizing, and sequencing activities. By past convention, now loosened, dementia was not typically diagnosed in the presence of impairment of only a single domain, requiring significant involvement of at least two domains.

In the *Diagnostic and Statistical Manual of Mental Disorders (DSM)* versions I through IV-TR, there was a requirement that at least one of the affected cognitive domains be memory. This requirement, designed originally for Alzheimer disease (see Chapter 50), has been dropped in the most recent *DSM-5* with recognition of various dementias that do not initially or primarily involve memory, for example, frontotemporal dementia (see Chapter 51).

Dementia is diagnosed only when there is some significant decline in ability to function at home or at work. Dementia may be distinguished from mild cognitive impairment (MCI; see Chapter 49) in the requirement of significant impairment of independence in everyday activities such as occupational, social, or self-maintenance activities. The patient with MCI may have cognitive impairment in one or more domains, but this dysfunction is insufficient to cause functional impairment. For this reason, detailed analysis of the patient's need for help from others for simple activities of daily living (e.g., toileting, food preparation, shopping, housework) is crucial.

TERMINOLOGY AND CLASSIFICATION

In the most recent *DSM-5*, the American Psychiatric Association has eliminated the term *dementia* in favor of Major Neurocognitive Disorder. However, the distinction between dementia and MCI remains, as it pertains to functional status. The DSM-5 formulation is of "major" and "minor" neurocognitive disorders, depending on the degree of functional impairment. The major neurocognitive disorders are what were termed dementias, and the minor neurocognitive disorders represent types of MCI that may be precursors to dementias (see Chapter 49). The new *DSM-5* criteria permit both major and minor neurocognitive disorders to involve impairment with even a single domain but keep the distinction as to presence or absence of functional impairment. Despite the revised terminology of the *DSM-5*, the use of the terms dementia and MCI are likely to persist in both neurologic and lay parlances.

Dementia can be classified in various ways. The oldest system was to classify dementias as presenile (i.e., young at onset) or senile (i.e., old at onset). This is not of any present use because each of the dementing disorders can have first symptoms arise over a wide range of age at onset. Older texts also referred to treatable versus untreatable dementias, with the treatable group including conditions such as hypothyroidism or B_{12} deficiency and the untreatable group including Alzheimer disease and other degenerative conditions. Such a classification is not presently useful because treatment is being developed for dementing disorders previously deemed untreatable. For example, as of 2015, five different drugs are approved in the United States, per U.S. Food and Drug Administration labeling, specifically for treatment of Alzheimer disease (see Chapter 50). Another dichotomous categorization of dementia proposed separating disorders into those of genetic origin and others of "sporadic" nature. However, this also has proven to be of minimal use because most dementia disorders may occur in either inherited (familial) forms or sporadic varieties. Dividing dementias into those with principally cortical or subcortical features, or into those with or without motor signs, has not proven useful for diagnosis, prognosis, or treatment and management. Thus, the most useful categorization of dementias is now based on the pathoetiologic basis of disease (Table 11.1). With clinicopathologic correlation, it is now usually possible to provide a specific diagnosis during life with 75% to 85% accuracy. It is important to recognize that even with an excellent clinical history and examination and auxiliary testing, clinical diagnosis of the dementia pathoetiology will not have perfect sensitivity or specificity.

Some patients have subjective complaints of cognitive disturbance, which is objectively verifiable but insufficient in either severity or functional disturbance or activities of daily life to meet criteria for dementia. In these cases, a diagnosis of MCI may be made, with specification of the involved cognitive domains (memory, language, visuospatial, executive, or attention). A large proportion of persons with MCI will develop some form of dementia within 5 to 7 years, with an annual rate of conversion of MCI to dementia as high as 10% to 15%.

CAUSES OF DEMENTIA

Dementing disorders are best etiologically classified as endocrine, metabolic, cerebrovascular, inflammatory, infectious, structural, or neurodegenerative (see Table 11.1). The last category is characterized by absence of the prior-listed etiologies.

NEURODEGENERATIVE DEMENTIAS

In the United States, the most common causes of dementia of the elderly are neurodegenerative. These include Alzheimer disease, Lewy body dementia, frontotemporal dementia, and Creutzfeldt–Jakob disease (CJD).

Alzheimer Disease

Alzheimer disease (see Chapter 50), with prominent memory and language impairment, is the most frequent form of dementia, accounting in the elderly for about 80% of the total number of patients in autopsy, clinical, or population-based series (Table 11.2). Structurally, it is marked by temporal and parietal degeneration.

TABLE 11.1	Dementias Categorized by Pathoetiologic Basis
Primary Neurodegenerative Disorders	
Alzheimer disease (AD)	
Lewy body disorders	
Dementia with Lewy bodies (DLB)	
Parkinson disease dementia (PDD)	
Frontotemporal dementias (FTD)	
Behavioral variant frontotemporal dementia (bvFTD)	
Progressive nonfluent aphasia (PNFA)	
Frontotemporal dementia with motor neuron disease (FTD-ALS, FTD-MND)	
Progressive supranuclear palsy (PSP)	
Corticobasal degeneration (CBD)	
Huntington disease (HD)	
Wilson disease (WD)	
Creutzfeldt–Jakob disease (CJD) and other prion diseases	
Hippocampal sclerosis	
Others: British familial dementia, HDLS, others	
Vascular dementias: multi-infarct dementia, Binswanger disease, CADASIL	
Immune-mediated encephalitides: NMDARAE, VGKCAE, others	
Demyelinating dementias: multiple sclerosis, adreno- and metachromatic leukodystrophies	
Inflammatory dementias: CNS vasculitides, Behçet syndrome, systemic lupus	
Infectious dementias: neurosyphilis, neuroborreliosis, HIV dementia, others	
Neoplastic dementias: tumors, carcinomatous meningitis, paraneoplastic syndromes	
Metabolic or endocrine dementias: B_{12} or rarer vitamin deficiencies, hypothyroidism	
Structural dementias: hydrocephalus, brain trauma	

FTD-ALS, frontotemporal dementia with amyotrophic lateral sclerosis; HDLS, hereditary diffuse leukoencephalopathy with spheroids; CADASIL, cerebral autosomal dominant arteriopathy with subcortical infarcts and leukoencephalopathy; NMDARAE, *N*-methyl-D-aspartate receptor antibody encephalitis; VGKCAE, voltage-gated potassium channel antibody encephalitis; CNS, central nervous system.

TABLE 11.2	Prevalence of Dementing Disorders in the Elderly	
Alzheimer disease[*]	65%–85%	
Lewy body disorders[†]	15%–30%	
Frontotemporal dementias	5%–10%	
Vascular dementias[¶]	2%–10%	
Other dementias	5%–10%	

*Note that Lewy bodies may also be present in 20%–40% of cases.
†Note that concomitant Alzheimer disease is present in 65%–90% of cases.
¶Note that infarcts are noted in ~35% of cases of dementia.

Molecularly, it is characterized as an "amyloidopathy" because the most specific hallmark is abnormal deposits of β-amyloid in plaques, in addition to the less specific hyperphosphorylated tau protein evident in neurofibrillary tangles.

Lewy Body Dementia

Lewy body dementia is the second most frequent cause of dementia in the elderly (see Chapter 52), characterized clinically by parkinsonism, hallucinations, and fluctuations in level of consciousness. Pathologically, the presence of Lewy bodies with molecular composition principally alpha-synuclein has led to the term *synucleinopathy*.

Frontotemporal Dementias

Frontotemporal dementias represent a molecularly heterogeneous group of degenerative disorders marked by frontal and temporal degeneration (see Chapter 51). Frontotemporal degeneration often presents with onset of symptoms at younger ages, in the 50s, and accounts for 5% to 10% of cases. Manifestations typically consist of either frontal-type behavioral disturbances (e.g., disinhibition, apathy, social impropriety, obsessions) or language disturbances. The molecular pathologies of this group of disorders can be broadly divided into those involving tau and those involving TDP-43 protein (TAR DNA-binding protein 43), with less common involvement of FUS, CHMP3, or VCP proteins. Pathologic entities including Pick disease, progressive supranuclear palsy, corticobasal degeneration, tangle dominant dementia, and argyrophilic grain disease are marked by prominent tau abnormalities and all now termed *tauopathies*. Motor neuron disease with dementia (amyotrophic lateral sclerosis dementia), some progressive aphasic disorders, and some behavioral variant frontotemporal dementias are TDP-43 proteinopathies.

Less Common Neurodegenerative Dementias

Other degenerative dementias include Wilson disease (see Chapter 134), a genetic disorder marked by copper deposition in the basal ganglia, dementia, and tremor, and Huntington disease (see Chapter 82), a genetic disorder marked by bicaudate atrophy, clinical dementia, chorea, and gait disorder. Even less frequent neurodegenerative dementing disorders include CJD (see Chapter 68), British familial dementia, neuroaxonal dystrophy, certain spinocerebellar ataxias, fragile X tremor ataxia syndrome, and others.

VASCULAR DEMENTIA

Cerebrovascular disease was once considered to be a major cause of dementia of the elderly but is now recognized to be the principle cause of dementia in less than 5% of cases in the United States. Syndromes of strategic infarct dementia, multiple infarct dementia, severe ischemic white matter disease (Binswanger disease or subcortical arteriosclerotic dementia), and hemorrhagic brain disease may all cause dementia (see Chapter 53). Acute stroke is a common cause of cognitive impairment but does not present as a gradually progressive dementing illness; instead, cognitive deficits follow in the aftermath of acute focal neurologic deficits or may take a stepwise course with discrete episodes of impairment and disability.

STRUCTURAL CAUSES OF DEMENTIA

The most common structural causes of dementia are chronic subdural hematoma (see Chapter 46) and hydrocephalus (see Chapter 106). Both diagnoses are established, in part, by neuroimaging, such as computerized tomography or magnetic resonance imaging, although imaging itself is not sufficient to determine the role of hydrocephalus in dementia. Subdural hematoma typically presents as progressive deterioration in cognition and gait over days to weeks. Headache and lateralized focal deficits may or may not be present. Hydrocephalus represents a relative increase in cerebrospinal fluid in the cranial vault, causing compressive dysfunction of descending cortical pathways and cortex itself. The symptoms classically involve gait disorder, urinary incontinence, and dementia. Risk factors for hydrocephalus include prior history of intracranial hemorrhage, head injury, or meningitis, although these may not be known. Radiologically, distinguishing ventricular enlargement due to hydrocephalus from ventricular enlargement due to brain atrophy can be challenging.

METABOLIC CAUSES OF DEMENTIA

Metabolic causes of dementia include cobalamin (vitamin B12) deficiency, hypothyroidism, hypercalcemic disorders, and rarer vitamin or endocrine deficiencies. Toxic disorders can include inhalant, mercury, or manganese poisoning. Inherited metabolic disorders that may lead to dementia in adults include Wilson disease, the adult form of ceroid lipofuscinosis (Kufs disease), cerebrotendinous xanthomatosis, metachromatic leukodystrophy, adrenoleukodystrophy, mitochondrial disorders such as MELAS (mitochondrial encephalomyopathy, lactic acidosis, and stroke-like episodes). Transient reversible memory loss may occur from acute medical illness, drug intoxications (most notably benzodiazepines), or from the poorly understood syndrome of *transient global amnesia* (Chapter 60). This disorder typically occurs in older persons and consists of an acute circumscribed period of time in which no new memories are acquired, with complete anterograde amnesia. Patients typically repetitively ask questions about their current situation.

INFECTIOUS CAUSES OF DEMENTIA

Infectious causes of dementia are less common in the developed world and mostly more frequent in the younger population. CJD, which results from prion protein infiltration of the brain resulting in a spongiform encephalopathy (see Chapter 68), is the most notorious potentially infectious cause of dementia, although it can only be transmitted by direct exposure to diseased nervous system tissue. Viral disorders include HIV-associated dementia or herpesvirus family disorders (herpes simplex virus, varicella-zoster virus, cytomegalovirus, Epstein-Barr virus, human herpesvirus 6). Bacterial disorders include spirochetal disorders neurosyphilis and neuroborreliosis (Lyme disease) and atypical bacterial infections (tuberculosis). Fungal infections include meningitides owing to infection with *Cryptococcus*, *Coccidioides*, histoplasmosis, or others.

DEMENTIA FROM ENDOCRINE DYSFUNCTION

Undiagnosed hypothyroidism is the most common endocrine abnormality that can present as dementia. Other endocrine disturbances that can cause dementia include Addison or Cushing disease, repeated episodes of hypoglycemia in diabetics, hyperparathyroidism associated with hypercalcemia, and hyperthyroidism (see Chapter 117). Hashimoto encephalopathy is a rare autoimmune encephalitis that occurs in conjunction with autoantibodies to thyroid proteins (see Chapter 71).

INFLAMMATORY CAUSES OF DEMENTIA

Rapidly progressive dementia can be caused by the immune-mediated encephalitides (see Chapter 71), some of which are paraneoplastic disorders.

EPIDEMIOLOGY

Dementia increases in prevalence with age. Although uncommon in younger persons, with a prevalence of 1% by age 60 years, dementia becomes dramatically more common thereafter, with a prevalence of 50% or greater at age 90 years and older. In autopsy studies of individuals with dementia, about 70% to 80% of brains show pathologically definite Alzheimer disease (see Table 11.2). About half of these have concomitant pathology, with evidence of Lewy body involvement or cerebrovascular infarctions. Thus, only one-third of autopsy brains have "pure" Alzheimer disease.

FOCUSED HISTORY AND DIFFERENTIAL DIAGNOSIS

The first symptoms of dementia often include occasional forgetfulness, misplacing objects, and word-finding difficulties (Table 11.3). With aging, a decline in memory may be observed, and thus sometimes the distinction between cognitive decline in old age and early dementia may be difficult. By definition, dementia is associated with progressive decline in functioning and thus is distinguished from a static encephalopathy such as mental retardation or congenital syndromes. Important exclusionary criteria for dementia include syndromes that are better explained by delirium (see Chapter 10) or by a primary psychiatric disorder such as major affective disorder or schizophrenia.

QUESTIONS TO ASK

Evaluation of complaints of cognitive dysfunction, whether self-tendered or enunciated by a family member or caregiver, are first elicited by obtaining a thorough history. Particular attention should be paid as to which symptoms predominated at onset. Symptoms of loss of memory (whether short term or long term), language usage (word-finding problems or decreased fluency, comprehension, or naming), praxis (dressing, use of utensils, or use of mechanical devices such as telephone or remote electronic controls), executive function (disorganization), insight (such as failure to recognize symptoms), dyscalculia, or behavioral dysfunction (agitation, disinhibition, depression, obsessions, delusions, or hallucinations) should be elicited. Symptoms of motor or gait impairment, adventitious movements, autonomic involvement (hypotension, urinary or bowel dysfunction), or sleep disturbance should also be elicited.

TABLE 11.3	**Ten Warning Signs of Alzheimer Disease**
1.	Memory loss that affects job skills
2.	Difficulty performing familiar tasks
3.	Problems with language
4.	Disorientation to time and place
5.	Poor or decreased judgment
6.	Problems with abstract thinking
7.	Misplacing things
8.	Changes in mood or personality
9.	Problems with directions or spatial relations
10.	Loss of initiative

Adapted from the Alzheimer's Association. Retrieved from http://www.alz.org/alzheimers_disease_10_signs_of_alzheimers.asp#signs

DEMENTIA VERSUS MILD COGNITIVE IMPAIRMENT

Attempts have been made to better define cognitive changes associated with aging, and varying sets of criteria have produced multiple terms, including such terms as age-associated memory impairment (AAMI), age-related cognitive change (ARCD), and questionable dementia (QD), among others. The most widely used term for cognitive change insufficient to meet criteria for dementia is *mild cognitive impairment* or, in the most recent psychiatric lexicon (*DSM-5*), *minor neurocognitive disorder* (Chapter 49). Criteria for MCI include subjective cognitive complaints and objective cognitive dysfunction but preserved general cognitive function and activities of daily living, with pursuant absence of dementia diagnosis. Follow-up examinations of individuals with MCI indicate that some, but not all, develop dementia over time.

DEMENTIA VERSUS DELIRIUM

Delirium presents acutely or subacutely and is a state of mental confusion that, unlike dementia, is primarily characterized by inattention to the immediate environment. Dementia is insidious in onset, evolves over months to years with normal consciousness and progressively worsens, whereas delirium is acute in onset, evolving in days to weeks, with fluctuations in consciousness. Both dementia and delirium may involve anxiety, hallucinations, illusions, delusions, and dysautonomia. Delirium is often a consequence of diffuse systemic or cerebral insults, including pain, infections, intoxications, or withdrawal from medications or drugs of abuse, metabolic disorders including hepatic or renal dysfunction, hypoxemia, or other medical or neurologic diseases. It is not possible to diagnose dementia with certainty in the presence of delirium. Delirium in elderly hospitalized patients very often has an underlying substrate of a baseline dementing illness that becomes apparent once the delirium has resolved.

Several features help differentiate dementia from delirium. Attention is not usually impaired in patients with dementia, although it is almost always altered in delirium. Increased or decreased motor activity is inherent in delirium but absent usually in dementia. If the cause is identified, delirium itself can be reversed (although not necessarily an underlying dementia process), although most forms of dementia progressively worsen.

DEMENTIA VERSUS DEPRESSION

Differentiating dementia from depression can sometimes be difficult. Depression (see Chapter 149) may be an early manifestation of Alzheimer disease. In depression, memory loss typically declines as the mood worsens. The onset of memory problems may be more abrupt than usually occurs in dementia and is mild, fluctuating, and nonprogressive. Neuropsychological test results may reflect variability in performance and greater difficulties with learning, concentration, and attention, rather than true memory deficits such as seen with Alzheimer disease.

FOCUSED EXAMINATION

MENTAL STATUS EXAMINATION

The mental status evaluation is an essential part of every neurologic examination but particularly so in the evaluation of patients with cognitive symptoms. Much of the evaluation is predicated upon an attentive and communicative patient. Thus, the evaluation starts with determination of level of consciousness, alertness, and attention and proceeds to basic ascertainment of expressive and receptive language. If these are not intact, the evaluation is necessarily difficult and limited. General assessments include the following:

- Awareness and consciousness
- Verbal behavior including appropriateness
- Motor behavior including agitation or picking movements
- Mood and emotional state

More specific cognitive assessments include the following:

- Orientation to time (hour, day, date, month, year, season) and place (institution, address, floor, city, state)
- Concentration (e.g., spelling a five-letter word in reverse, counting backwards by serial 7s, reciting the months of the year in reverse)
- Detailed language testing (expressive speech, aural and reading comprehension of one-, two, or three-step commands, naming of solid objects or drawings, repetition of easy or difficult [prepositional] phrases, reading comprehension, ability to write a sentence)
- Registration or immediate recall (of three or five objects or words)
- Short-term memory or delayed recall after 3 to 10 minutes of three or five objects or words
- Long-term memory or fund of knowledge (names of current and prior elected officials, birthdates of family members, items of history)
- Visuospatial constructive abilities (copying simple shapes)
- Arithmetic calculations (mentally summing the values of coins, simple one- or two-digit additions or subtractions)
- Abstract reasoning (defining similarities, interpreting proverbs)
- Motor sequencing and praxis (sequential movements and motor commands)

BEDSIDE STANDARDIZED COGNITIVE TESTING

Two widely used brief standardized cognitive assessments are the Mini-Mental State Examination (MMSE) and the Montreal Cognitive Assessment (MoCA). These tests were introduced as standard measures of cognitive function for both research and clinical purposes. They are short, requiring less than 10 minutes, relatively easy to administer, and result in scores of 0 point (failing all items) to 30 points (perfect score).

It is important to emphasize that the MMSE and MoCA, like all brief mental status exams, are not perfectly sensitive or specific for dementia. These tests are sensitive to cultural and language factors and level of education. Well-educated patients may suffer from dementia and nonetheless score a "perfect" 30 points on these 30-point scales, whereas poorly educated patients may score much lower and yet be nondemented. Therefore, the MMSE or MoCA should be used as screening instruments, but they do not replace a detailed history and examination or full neuropsychological testing (see Chapter 30).

GENERAL NEUROLOGIC EXAMINATION

The general neurologic examination is useful in the evaluation of the patient with dementia because certain signs (Table 11.4) may make a diagnosis of Alzheimer unlikely and may point to another causative etiology. For example, focal findings of hemiparesis may suggest a vascular component or, in cases of hemineglect, the degenerative disorder corticobasal degeneration. Prominent visual dysfunction may suggest posterior cortical atrophy, usually a variant of Alzheimer disease, or cerebral amyloid angiopathy. Paralysis of supranuclear gaze with preserved brain stem reflexes may suggest progressive supranuclear palsy or corticobasal degeneration.

TABLE 11.4 Neurologic Signs and Symptoms Atypical for Alzheimer Disease

Sign or Symptom	Possible Significance
Dominant nonmemory Sx (e.g., language, praxis, visuospatial dysfunction)	Frontotemporal degenerations, posterior cortical atrophy
Prominent behavioral, personality, psychotic symptoms	Frontotemporal degenerations, Lewy body dementia
Early parkinsonism (e.g., resting tremor, bradykinesia, cogwheeling)	Lewy body dementia, progressive supranuclear palsy (no rest tremor), corticobasal degeneration, hydrocephalus
Urinary incontinence	Hydrocephalus
REM sleep behavior disorder	Parkinson disease dementia, Lewy body dementia
Seizures	Immune-mediated or infectious encephalitides
Myoclonus	Creutzfeldt–Jakob disease
Frequent falls	Progressive supranuclear palsy
Early unexplained gait abnormalities	Lewy body dementia, progressive supranuclear palsy, corticobasal degeneration, hydrocephalus
Early prominence of bulbar/ brain stem signs	Progressive supranuclear palsy
Unexplained motor or reflex asymmetries	Vascular dementia, corticobasal degeneration
Unexplained (early) UMN signs (e.g., Babinski sign)	Frontotemporal degeneration with motor neuron disease
Unexplained LMN signs (e.g., fasciculations)	Frontotemporal degeneration with motor neuron disease

Sx, symptoms; REM, rapid eye movement; UMN, upper motor neuron; LMN, lower motor neuron.

Lower motor neuron signs, such as fasciculations and atrophy, may suggest frontotemporal dementia with motor neuron disease.

DIAGNOSTIC TESTING

The American Academy of Neurology in 2001 developed the evidence-based practice parameters for evaluation of the diagnosis and cause of dementia. These parameters have been entirely revolutionized by the development of modern neuroimaging, biomarkers, and genetic tests. A workgroup formed by the National Institute on Aging in conjunction with the Alzheimer's Association published in 2011, revised recommendations on diagnostic criteria, which are included in Table 11.5.

NEUROPSYCHOLOGICAL TESTING

Detailed neuropsychological testing (see Chapter 30) may be performed to augment the clinical mental status examination by assessing severity and regional pattern of cognitive impairment through use of standardized tests with normative values. This can be very helpful not only in differential diagnosis but also in monitoring disease progression.

TABLE 11.5 Practice Parameters for Diagnosis of Dementia

Clinical Evaluation
History from patient and an informant
Cognitive assessment – mental status examination
Neuropsychological testing (when above is insufficient for confident diagnosis)

Routine Testing
Complete blood cell count
Serum chemistry – electrolytes, glucose
Serum BUN, creatinine, liver function tests
Serum thyroid function tests (TSH) and B12 level
Serologic tests for syphilis and HIV (optional – depending on risk)

Biomarkers
Measures of cerebrovascular disease
Brain MRI
Measures of neuronal injury
CSF tau measurement
FDG-PET
MRI hippocampal volume
Measures of beta-amyloid
CSF beta-amyloid measurement
PET amyloid imaging
Measure of dopaminergic dysfunction
Ioflupane SPECT scan
Genetic tests (depending on age, family history and clinical presentation)
AD mutations: PS1, PS2, APP
FTD mutations: tau, C9orf, progranulin
Prion protein mutations
Other mutations

BUN, blood urea nitrogen; MRI, magnetic resonance imaging; AD, Alzheimer disease; PET, positron emission tomography; SPECT, single photon computed tomography; CSF, cerebrospinal fluid; FTD, frontotemporal dementia.

This table is based on first practice guidelines published by American Academy of Neurology (2001), more recent National Institute on Aging-Alzheimer's Association Workgroup recommendations (2011), and other practice guidelines.

Memory impairment can be parsed into immediate or working memory, short-term memory, and remote memory. Working memory is typically unaffected in early Alzheimer disease but often significantly affected in depression and subcortical dementias such as Parkinson disease dementia. In contradistinction, short-term recall is severely and early affected in Alzheimer disease and its precursor, amnestic MCI. Remote or long-term memory is affected later in the disease course of Alzheimer disease but may be relatively preserved even late in the course of some of the other dementias.

Language impairments can be assessed. Naming difficulties, common in Alzheimer disease, are less common in subcortical dementias. Verbal fluency for categories (semantic verbal fluency) is much more severely affected in disorders of the temporal lobes, such as Alzheimer disease, compared to verbal fluency for letters (phonemic verbal fluency) which is more affected in disorders of the frontal lobes, such as frontotemporal dementia.

Visuospatial impairments can be assessed. Typically, visuoperceptive impairment is marked in Alzheimer disease, whereas disorganization is more prominent in frontotemporal dementias. Micropraxia (drawing very small shapes) is common in the Lewy body disorders.

LABORATORY BLOOD TESTING

Recommendations for auxiliary testing generally include basic laboratory tests (blood chemistry and cell counts) and, more specifically, laboratory testing for vitamin B_{12} deficiency (with homocysteine and methylmalonate ordered if B_{12} is borderline or low) and thyroid deficiency (thyroid-stimulating hormone [TSH], with free T4 ordered if TSH is out of normal range). The American Academy of Neurology guidelines specify B_{12}, TSH, and structural imaging (generally magnetic resonance imaging [MRI]) to exclude contributory disorders to cognitive symptoms, which might be otherwise unrecognized [**Level 1**].[1] Serologic tests for exposure to syphilis (Venereal Disease Research Laboratory and fluorescent treponemal antibody-absorption test), Lyme disease (screening enzyme immunoassay, with confirmatory Western blots), or HIV (HIV-1/2 antibody and antigen) may be of value.

LABORATORY CEREBROSPINAL FLUID TESTING

Analysis of cerebrospinal fluid (CSF) obtained through lumbar puncture (see Chapter 31) is increasingly used in diagnosis of cognitive dysfunction. CSF provides information in two broad categories: (1) In an exclusionary fashion, it may be used to be certain that various infectious or inflammatory etiologies of dementia discussed earlier are not present, and (2) in an inclusionary fashion, it may provide information with regard to neurodegenerative diseases, such as Alzheimer disease or CJD, through use of protein biomarkers (see Chapter 31). Presence of abnormal numbers of leukocytes, taking into account any blood contamination, is typically indicative of an inflammatory or infectious process. Biomarkers including β-amyloid-42, total tau, phosphotau, and 14-3-3 protein are established as of use in the diagnosis of Alzheimer disease and CJD. In Alzheimer disease, typically β-amyloid-42 is lower than normal, total tau is higher than normal, and phosphotau is higher than normal. These changes are often the earliest biomarker of Alzheimer disease and may be evident prior to clinical symptoms and prior to structural and functional neuroimaging changes seen by MRI or positron emission tomography (PET) scans. Currently, these biomarkers are being increasingly utilized not only for their diagnostic value, but also to potentially provide surrogate indices of dementia severity and progress. For CJD, typically both total tau and 14-3-3 are highly elevated. CSF biomarkers not only may yield improvements in the differential diagnostic process but also allow better assessment of change during investigational therapies designed to affect disease symptoms or modify the disease process (Table 11.6).

NEUROPHYSIOLOGIC TESTING

Electroencephalogram (EEG) testing can be useful in two fashions: (1) It may assist in the assessment of the possibility of subclinical paroxysmal disorders being responsible for abnormal mental status and (2) it may be of use in cases where it is less clear whether a primary psychiatric or neurologic diagnosis is operative. Epileptiform

TABLE 11.6	Dementias Categorized by Protein Pathologies
β-Amyloidopathy	Alzheimer disease
α-Synucleinopathy	Lewy body disorders (DLB), PDD
Tauopathy	Frontotemporal dementia: Pick disease, PSP, CBD (Note that AD has secondary tau pathology.)
TDP-43 proteinopathy	Frontotemporal dementia (FTD-U), ALS with dementia
Prionopathy	Creutzfeldt–Jakob disease, sporadic/familial fatal insomnia, GSS, vCJD

DLB, dementia with Lewy bodies; PDD, Parkinson disease dementia; PSP, progressive supranuclear palsy; CBD, corticobasal degeneration; AD, Alzheimer disease; ALS, amyotrophic lateral sclerosis; GSS, Gerstmann–Sträussler–Scheinker disease; vCJD, variant Creutzfeldt–Jakob disease.

activity may be particularly prominent in the immune-mediated encephalitides or other rapidly progressive dementias such as rabies or herpes simplex encephalitis. In disorders that are purely psychiatric, frequently background EEG rhythm may be normal, whereas conversely neurologic disorders may be accompanied by focal or generalized background slowing.

Electromyography provides an assessment of the lower motor neurons which can be helpful in ascertaining the presence of frontotemporal dementia with motor neuron disease. Sensory nerve studies may be helpful in rarer disorders such as metachromatic leukodystrophy.

NEUROIMAGING

Conventional Computed Tomography and Magnetic Resonance

Structural neuroimaging can be useful in both exclusionary and inclusionary fashions with respect to neurodegenerative dementias. Discovery of significant vascular injury, inflammatory lesions, contrast-enhancing processes, or tumors may be decisive in ruling out degenerative processes and indicating some infectious, inflammatory, or neoplastic process. However, even in cases of "radiologically normal" scans, structural features such as parietal atrophy or temporal atrophy may be indicative of an Alzheimer process. Specialized imaging such as gradient echo sequences can reveal microhemorrhages, which when multiple may be suggestive of amyloid angiopathy, cerebral autosomal dominant arteriopathy with subcortical infarcts and leukoencephalopathy, or less frequently hypertensive cerebrovascular injury. Other specialized sequences such as diffusion-weighted imaging may show strong evidence of prion disease. CJD typically results in diffusion-weighted hyperintensities in cortical regions confined to the gray matter cortical ribbon and also to the deep gray nuclei, including thalami, caudate, and lenticular nuclei.

Biomarker Imaging

Nuclear medicine imaging provides useful information in cases of suspected dementia. Single-photon emission computed tomography (SPECT) imaging (see Chapter 22) using ^{99m}Tc-hexamethyl propylene amine oxime (HMPAO) or ^{99m}Tc-ethyl cysteine dimer (ECD) allows imaging of brain perfusion. These tests, as well as 18O-PET which also images brain blood perfusion, and more frequently used ^{18}F-fluorodeoxyglucose (FDG) PET imaging (see Chapter 22) which images the closely linked feature of brain glucose metabolism, can be of value in displaying topographic patterns of brain dysfunction. These patterns can be relatively disease specific. Typically, Alzheimer disease shows a pattern of biparietal and bitemporal hypoperfusion, or hypometabolism, that may be more or less asymmetric. There is sparing of the primary cortices including sensory, motor, and visual regions, as well as the deep gray nuclei. Lewy body disease shows a similar pattern but often with less prominent temporal involvement and much more parietal and occipital involvement, often involving the visual cortices. Frontotemporal dementias typically involve frontal and/or anterior temporal regions, sometimes quite asymmetrically, with preservation of parietal and other posterior regions. Most recently, the expanding field of molecular imaging has provided more specific imaging biomarker tools for neurodegenerative disorders. Assistance with diagnosis of Lewy body disorders may be provided, albeit with less than excellent sensitivity or specificity, through dopamine transporter imaging, such as ^{123}I- ioflupane SPECT. Most recently, use of amyloid imaging, including ^{18}F-florbetapir, ^{18}F-florbetaben, and ^{18}F-flutemetamol, has allowed in vivo assessment in humans of fibrillar β-amyloid, indicating an Alzheimer process. Currently, this testing has high sensitivity but low specificity because many clinically unaffected individuals older than age 65 years may show evidence of amyloid deposition as determined by binding of these radiopharmaceutical tracers imaged using PET. However, additional investigational molecular imaging tools such as tracers believed to be specific for the tau protein aggregated in neurofibrillary tangles may also prove to be of diagnostic assistance.

LEVEL 1 EVIDENCE

1. Knopman DS, Dekosky ST, Cummings JL, et al. Practice parameter: diagnosis of dementia (an evidence-based review). Report of the Quality Standards Subcommittee of the American Academy of Neurology. *Neurology*. 2001;56(9):1143–1153.

SUGGESTED READINGS

Attems J, Jellinger K. Neuropathological correlates of cerebral multimorbidity. *Curr Alzheimer Res*. 2013;10:569–77.

Downing LJ, Caprio TV, Lyness JM. Geriatric psychiatry review: differential diagnosis and treatment of the 3 D's—delirium, dementia, and depression. *Curr Psychiatry Rep*. 2013;15:365.

Farlow JL, Foroud T. The genetics of dementia. *Semin Neurol*. 2013;33: 417–422.

Folstein MF, Folstein SE, McHugh PR. "Mini-mental state": a practical method for grading the cognitive state of patients for the clinician. *J Psychiatr Res*. 1975;12:189–198.

Fong TG, Tulebaev SR, Inouye SK. Delirium in elderly adults: diagnosis, prevention and treatment. *Nat Rev Neurol*. 2009;5:210–220.

Frisoni GB, Bocchetta M, Chételat G, et al. Imaging markers for Alzheimer disease: which vs how. *Neurology*. 2013;81:487–500.

Hyman BT, Phelps CH, Beach TG, et al. National Institute on Aging-Alzheimer's Association guidelines for the neuropathologic assessment of Alzheimer's disease. *Alzheimers Dement*. 2012;8:1–13.

Jack CR Jr, Barrio JR, Kepe V. Cerebral amyloid PET imaging in Alzheimer's disease. *Acta Neuropathol*. 2013;126:643–657.

Maldonado JR. Neuropathogenesis of delirium: review of current etiologic theories and common pathways. *Am J Geriatr Psychiatry*. 2013;21: 1190–1222.

McKhann GM, Knopman DS, Chertkow H, et al. The diagnosis of dementia due to Alzheimer's disease: recommendations from the National Institute on Aging-Alzheimer's Association workgroups on diagnostic guidelines for Alzheimer's disease. *Alzheimers Dement*. 2011;7:263–269.

Nasreddine ZS, Phillips NA, Bédirian V, et al. The Montreal Cognitive Assessment, MoCA: a brief screening tool for mild cognitive impairment. *J Am Geriatr Soc*. 2005;53:695–699.

Petersen RC. Clinical practice. Mild cognitive impairment. *N Engl J Med*. 2011;364:2227–2234.

Riedl L, Mackenzie IR, Förstl H, et al. Frontotemporal lobar degeneration: current perspectives. *Neuropsychiatr Dis Treat*. 2014;10:297–310.

Sonnen JA, Postupna N, Larson EB, et al. Pathologic correlates of dementia in individuals with Lewy body disease. *Brain Pathol*. 2010;20:654–659.

Warren JD, Rohrer JD, Rossor MN. Clinical review. Frontotemporal dementia. *BMJ*. 2013;347:f4827.

Involuntary Movements 12

Elan D. Louis

INTRODUCTION

Abnormal involuntary movements, often called *dyskinesias*, are uncontrollable movements that are usually evident when a patient is at rest and, with rare exceptions (e.g., palatal myoclonus), these movements disappear during sleep. These movements are continual or easily evoked, although some are intermittent or paroxysmal, such as the *tics*, *paroxysmal dyskinesias*, or *episodic ataxias*. Although convulsions, fasciculations, and reflex clonus are involuntary movements, they are not classified with the types of abnormal involuntary movements that are described in this chapter.

The various dyskinesias are distinguished from one another based primarily on the visual inspection of the patient. Hence, the neurologic examination is of central importance when assigning a diagnosis.

The visual opposite of the hyperkinesias are the hypokinesias. Hypokinesia refers to reduced amplitude of movement or a paucity of movement that is not due to weakness or paralysis, but the term is commonly used synonymously with bradykinesia (slow movement), and the two features typically occur together in the parkinsonian states. Furthermore, hesitation and freezing phenomena (i.e., delays and interruptions of movement) are frequent features of parkinsonian states.

TYPES OF DYSKINESIAS

There are a large number of dyskinesias (Table 12.1), and each of these will be described further in the following text.

CHOREA

Chorea refers to brief, irregular contractions that, although rapid, are not as lightning-like as myoclonic jerks. In classic choreic disorders, such as Huntington disease (see Chapter 82) and Sydenham chorea (see Chapter 81), the movements affect individual muscles as random events that seem to flow from one muscle or muscle group to another (Video 12.1). The movements are neither repetitive nor rhythmic. *Ballism* is a form of chorea in which the movements are more jerk-like and are of large amplitude, producing flinging movements of the affected limbs.

DYSTONIA

Dystonia (see Chapter 76) is a syndrome of sustained muscle contraction that frequently causes twisting and repetitive movements or abnormal postures. The spasms may affect the neck muscles (*torticollis*) (Video 12.2), periocular muscles (*blepharospasm*), facial muscles (*Meige syndrome*), or limb muscles (e.g., *writer's cramp*). Dystonia is represented by the following phenomena: (1) sustained contractions of both agonist and antagonist muscles simultaneously (cocontraction) and persisting in the same muscle groups repeatedly ("patterning"), in contrast to the flowing of choreic movements; (2) an increase of these involuntary contractions when voluntary movement in other body parts is attempted ("overflow");

TABLE 12.1	List of Involuntary Movements
Hyperkinesias	
Akathitic movements	
Asynergia	
Athetosis	
Ballism	
Chorea	
Dysmetria	
Dystonia	
Episodic ataxia	
Hemifacial spasm	
Hyperekplexia and jumping disorders	
Hypnogenic dyskinesias	
Jumpy stumps	
Myoclonus	
Myorhythmia	
Painful legs–moving toes	
Paroxysmal movement disorders (paroxysmal dyskinesias, episodic ataxias, paroxysmal hypnogenic dyskinesias, transient dyskinesias of infants)	
Restless legs syndrome	
Stereotypy	
Tics	
Tremor	
Hypokinesias	
Akinesia/bradykinesia (parkinsonism)	
Hesitation and freezing phenomenon	

(3) rhythmic interruptions of these involuntary, sustained contractions (*dystonic tremor*); (4) inappropriate or opposing contractions during specific voluntary motor actions (*action dystonia*); and (5) torsion spasms that may be as rapid as chorea but differ because the movements are continual, patterned, and of a twisting nature, in contrast to the random and seemingly flowing movements of chorea. The speed of dystonic movements varies considerably from slow (athetotic dystonia) to shock-like (myoclonic dystonia). One of the characteristic features of dystonic movements is that they can often be diminished by tactile or proprioceptive "sensory tricks" (geste antagoniste). Thus, touching the involved body part or an adjacent body part can often reduce the muscle contractions (e.g., patients with torticollis may touch their chin to lessen the spasms).

Inexperienced clinicians might assume that this sign indicates that the abnormal movements are psychogenic; however, the presence of sensory tricks strongly suggests an organic etiology.

MYOCLONUS

Myoclonus (see Chapter 78) refers to an ultrabrief, shock-like movement that may arise from sudden muscle contractions (Video 12.3) or sudden interruption of ongoing muscle contractions with resultant postural lapses (i.e., negative myoclonus). The most common form of negative myoclonus is asterixis, which frequently accompanies various metabolic encephalopathies. In asterixis, the brief flapping of the outstretched limbs is due to transient inhibition of the muscles that maintain posture of those extremities.

Myoclonus can appear when the affected body part is at rest but it may also occur when it is performing a voluntary motor act (i.e., "action myoclonus"). Myoclonic jerks are usually irregular (arrhythmic) but can also be rhythmical (such as in *palatal myoclonus, ocular myoclonus,* or *limb myorhythmia*, with a rate of approximately 2 Hz).

TICS

Tics may be simple jerks or complex sequences of coordinated movements that appear suddenly and intermittently (Video 12.4). When simple, the movements may resemble a myoclonic jerk. Complex tics often include head shaking, eye blinking, sniffing, shoulder shrugging, facial distortions, arm waving, touching parts of the body, jumping movements, or making obscene gestures (*copropraxia*). Tics are usually rapid and brief, but occasionally, they may involve sustained muscle contractions (i.e., dystonic). In addition to motor tics, phonic tics involve sounds through the nose (e.g., sniffing) or throat (throat clearing) as well as other vocalizations. These range from sounds, such as barking or squealing, to verbalizations, including the utterance of obscenities (*coprolalia*) and the repetitions of sounds, words, or phrases (*palilalia* and *echolalia*). Motor and phonic tics are the essential features of the Tourette syndrome (see Chapter 74). One feature of tics is the compelling urge felt by the patient to make the motor or phonic tic, with the result that the tic movement brings relief from unpleasant sensations that develop in the involved body part. Tics may be voluntarily controlled for brief intervals, but such a conscious effort at suppression is usually followed by more intense and frequent contractions. The spectrum of severity and persistence of tics is wide; the milder the tic disorder is, the more control the patient may exert over the tics.

STEREOTYPIES

Stereotypic movements (*stereotypies*) occur as repetitive, sometimes rhythmic movements (e.g., hand flapping, head nodding, body rocking), and they may resemble tics; these are encountered in persons with mental retardation, autism, or schizophrenia, although they also occur in normal developing children. Stereotypic movements are also encountered in the syndrome of drug-induced tardive dyskinesia (see Chapter 80) and refer to repetitive movements that most often affect the mouth; in *orobuccolingual dyskinesia*, there are constant chewing movements of the jaw, writhing and protrusion movements of the tongue, and puckering movements of the lips.

TREMOR

Tremors are rhythmic oscillatory movements. They result either from alternating contractions of opposing muscle groups or from simultaneous contractions of agonist and antagonist muscles. A useful way to differentiate various tremors clinically is to determine whether the tremor is present during different conditions: when the affected body part is at rest, as in parkinsonian disorders; when posture is maintained (e.g., with arms outstretched in front of the body or with elbows flexed with arms in a winged position), as in Wilson disease and essential tremor (see Chapter 73); when action is undertaken (e.g., writing or pouring water from a cup) (Video 12.5), as in essential tremor; or when intention is present (e.g., during finger-to-nose maneuver), as in diseases involving the cerebellum such as ataxias and essential tremor (see Chapters 73 and 79).

ATHETOSIS

Athetosis is a slow, continuous, writhing movement of the limbs, trunk, head, face, or tongue. When these movements are brief, they merge with chorea (*choreoathetosis*). When the movements are sustained at the peak of the contractions, they merge with dystonia, and the term *athetotic dystonia* may be applied.

AKATHISIA

Akathitic movements commonly accompany the subjective symptom of *akathisia*, an inner feeling of motor restlessness or the need to move (Video 12.6). Today, akathisia is most commonly seen as a side effect of antipsychotic drug therapy, either as acute akathisia or tardive akathisia, which often accompanies tardive dyskinesia. In addition to that induced by antipsychotic drugs, pathologic akathisia may be seen in the encephalopathies of confusional states, in some dementias, and in Parkinson disease. Picking at the bedclothes (i.e., carphology) is a manifestation of akathitic movements in patients who are bedridden. Akathitic movements (e.g., crossing and uncrossing the legs, squirming and/or attempting to rise from a chair, pacing the floor) may also be a reaction to stress, anxiety, boredom, or impatience; these may then be termed *physiologic* akathisia.

RESTLESS LEGS SYNDROME

One other neurologic condition in which there are subjective feelings of the need to move is *restless legs syndrome*. This is characterized by formication in the legs, particularly in the evening when the patient is relaxing and sitting or lying down and attempting to fall asleep. These sensations of ants crawling under the skin disappear when the patient gets up and walks around.

PAROXYSMAL MOVEMENT DISORDERS

Paroxysmal movement disorders are syndromes in which the abnormal involuntary movements appear for brief periods out of a background of normal movement patterns. They may be divided into four distinct groups: (1) the *paroxysmal dyskinesias* (either induced by movement or not), (2) *episodic ataxias*, (3) *paroxysmal hypnogenic dyskinesias* (intermittent dystonia and chorea that begins during sleep), and (4) *transient dyskinesias of infants* (e.g., torticollis, body tilt).

HYPEREKPLEXIA

Hyperekplexia (startle disease) consists of dramatic, complex motor responses to sudden tactile or auditory stimuli. It may be hereditary or sporadic. The reaction can consist of a blink; facial contortion; abduction of the arms; and flexion of the neck, trunk, and arm. Sometimes instead of movements, the body becomes stiff and immobile. When it is severe, the patient's movements must be curtailed because a sudden attack may lead to injury from falling. Hyperekplexia, however, is probably distinct from jumping disorders, which are often described with local names, such as jumping Frenchmen of Maine, myriachit (in Siberia), latah (in Malaysia), and ragin' Cajun (in Louisiana); these jumpers may react to a sudden visual threat and may also respond to sudden verbal commands, such as "jump" or "throw." They may incorporate echolalia and echopraxia (repletion or imitation of another person's actions).

OTHER DYSKINESIAS AND MOVEMENT DISORDERS

Continued muscle stiffness due to continuous muscle firing may be seen in patients with neuromyotonia, encephalomyelitis with rigidity, the stiff limb syndrome, and the stiff person syndrome, which tends to involve axial and proximal limb muscles (see Chapter 94).

Cerebellar diseases (see Chapter 79) or lesions involving the pathways to or from the cerebellum result in a variety of abnormalities of movement. *Asynergia* or *dyssynergia* refers to the decomposition of movement due to breakdown of normal coordinated execution of a voluntary movement. Instead of a smooth, continuous movement, the limb moves off its trajectory in attempting to reach a target, with corrective maneuvers that resemble oscillations of the limb. The limb often misses the target (*dysmetria*); the asynergia worsens when the limb approaches the target. Common tests for asynergia and dysmetria are the finger–nose–finger and the heel–knee–shin maneuvers. Limb asynergia is also manifested by *dysdiadochokinesia*, which refers to the breakup and irregularity that occurs when the limb is attempting to carry out rapid alternating movements. The dysmetria in cerebellar disease is due to overshooting (*hypermetria*) and undershooting (*hypometria*) the target. There may be an associated *intention* (or terminal) *tremor*. Asynergia is usually associated with hypotonia, loss of check (when a fast voluntary movement is unable to stop precisely on target as the limb reaches its destination), and rebound (when sudden displacement of a limb results in excessive overcorrection to return to the baseline position). *Ataxia* of gait is typified by unsteadiness on walking with a wide base, the body swaying, and a difficulty with tandem walking (heel-to-toe walking).

Although most of the involuntary movements described are the result of lesions in the central nervous system, some dyskinesias are attributed to peripheral disorders, and these include hemifacial spasm (Video 12.7) (see Chapter 77), painful legs–moving toes, jumpy stumps, and the sustained muscle contractions seen in reflex sympathetic dystrophy (complex regional pain syndrome) (see Chapter 56).

Psychogenic movement disorders may manifest with a variety of movements but particularly shaking, fixed postures, bizarre gaits, or paroxysmal disorders (Table 12.2). Careful evaluation of the phenomenology for inconsistency, incongruity, prolonged fixed postures, deliberate slowness, suggestibility, distractibility, entrainment, false (give-way) weakness, nonanatomic sensory impairment, and marked fatigue and exhaustion from the "involuntary" movements suggest the diagnosis.

NEUROANATOMY

Most of the involuntary movements are the result of central nervous system disorders and more specifically, lesions involving the basal ganglia and cerebellum. For example, the motor features of Parkinson disease are related to a lesion in the substantia nigra pars compacta, chorea is related to disorders of the caudate nucleus but sometimes involving other structures, and ballism is more often related to lesions of the subthalamic nucleus. Ataxia and intention tremor are related to lesions of the cerebellum.

The neural site of origin of myoclonus is more widespread, including the cerebral cortex (cortical myoclonus), brain stem (reticular reflex myoclonus), and spinal cord (propriospinal myoclonus). Rhythmic myoclonias are typically due to structural lesions of the brain stem or spinal cord (therefore also called *segmental myoclonus*).

Dyskinesias attributed to peripheral disorders are hemifacial spasm, painful legs–moving toes, jumpy stumps, and the sustained muscle contractions seen in reflex sympathetic dystrophy.

TABLE 12.2	Red Flags for Psychogenic Movements
Finding	**Explanation**
Inconsistency	Movements that change quality (e.g., change in direction or frequency)
Combination of several hyperkinesias that do not ordinarily occur together	Unusual combinations of movements that do not typically co-occur in organic disease
Fixed postures	Postures that are sustained for prolonged periods of time
Deliberate slowness	Practiced slowness that resolves when the patient is unaware that they are still being observed
Suggestibility	The movement is reproduced when the examiner performs a maneuver that he or she suggests will acutely bring on the movement.
Distractibility	The movement stops when the examiner draws the patient's attention away from the affected body part to perform a task that requires considerable effort and concentration.
Entrainment (in tremor disorders)	Tremor frequency changes to match the frequency of tapping with the opposite limb.
Give-way weakness	During strength testing, the patient initially provides resistance against the examiner's force but then suddenly "gives way" and provides no further muscular resistance.
Nonanatomic sensory impairment	Sensory deficits that do not follow anatomic patterns/boundaries
Marked fatigue and exhaustion	By history, the amount of fatigue is out of proportion to the severity of the movements.

FOCUSED EXAMINATION

The neurologic examination is the most important tool for the diagnosis of involuntary movements. To begin with, it is important to spend time observing the patient and visualizing the movements. Tell the patient that you are going to watch their movements, and then sit in front of them and observe. Patients may sometimes be self-conscious and may try to inhibit their involuntary movements, particularly if these movements are embarrassing. If this is the case, then ask the patient to just let their body "do what it wants to do . . . don't try to stop it." After the observation, it is important to ask the patient to perform certain maneuvers designed to bring out the movement (e.g., writing may bring out a tremor, heel–knee–shin maneuver may bring out asynergia, and walking may bring out a dystonic foot movement). Some movements may be quite elaborate, and the examiner may need to observe for quite some time before being able to detect a consistent pattern or before being able to fully encapsulate and describe the phenomenology.

FOCUSED HISTORY

The neurologic history is also an important step in arriving at the correct diagnosis (Table 12.3). It is important to ask the patient about the location of the movements. Some patients with tremor may feel the movements in body parts that are not visibly shaking. Other features, including the periodicity of the movements and the items that exacerbate and/or relieve the movements, are important to assess. The conditions during which the movements occur (e.g., at rest or which movement) is also of importance in tremor classification, and accompanying feelings of restlessness, urges to move, and relief after the movement are important historical features to consider when diagnosing tics, akathisia, and restless legs syndrome. Family history information is also important, and it may be instructive to examine additional family members. It is important to obtain a list of current medications (as these may be producing, exacerbating, or partially suppressing movements) as well as medication exposures in the past (especially neuroleptics).

DIAGNOSIS

The first step in diagnosing a movement disorder is to recognize the movement phenomenology itself, and this is based primarily on keen and unhurried observation. Once the specific movement or movement types are identified, one may consider the various etiologies that can result in that/those type(s) of movements. In some instances, electromyogram may be helpful by determining the rate, rhythmicity, and synchrony of involuntary movements, as well as the duration of individual contractions. The duration of an individual contraction may distinguish specific types of dyskinesias; for instance, differentiating an organic myoclonic jerk from a psychogenic one. Motor control physiology laboratories typically perform this service. Additional blood work as well as brain imaging may aid in the diagnosis, although these should not be used as a substitute for clinical observation. Psychogenic movements due to somatoform disorders (conversion, hysteria) are subconscious and thus involuntary, in contrast to malingering. A common mistake is to label an abnormal movement not previously encountered by the physician as psychogenic. Experience of seeing a large number of movement disorders brings knowledge that helps in distinguishing psychogenic versus organic movements. It is important to look for positive signs such as give-way weakness, nonanatomic sensory impairment, and a combination of several hyperkinesias that do not ordinarily occur together; distraction; and entrainment (in tremor disorders) to help establish the diagnosis of a psychogenic movement disorder.

TREATMENT

The initial management of involuntary movements is the triaging into those that require acute treatment versus those that do not. There are a small number of movement disorders that must be dealt with acutely, including acute dystonic reactions and the paralytic form of Sydenham chorea. A number of emergent situations may arise in the treatment of patients with involuntary movements, including acute psychosis in patients with Parkinson

---

TABLE 12.3 Questions to Ask the Patient Who Presents with Involuntary Movements

Question	Relevant Involuntary Movement
Where (i.e., in what body regions) are the movements?	All
Do movements occur at rest or with action?	All
Does anything (e.g., movement, startle) trigger the movements?	Paroxysmal movement disorders, hyperekplexia
Are there accompanying vocalizations?	Tics, Tourette syndrome
Does the movement produce a feeling of relief?	Tics
Is there an urge to move?	Akathisia, tics, restless legs syndrome
Is the patient feeling restless?	Akathisia, restless legs syndrome
Is the patient able to suppress the movements?	Tics, chorea (briefly)
Is there pain/discomfort in the region where the movements are occurring?	Dystonia (esp. torticollis)
Is there a pulling feeling in the muscles?	Dystonia (esp. torticollis)
Is there a sensory trick (a place they can touch to lessen the movement)?	Dystonia
What are the current medications?	Tremor, parkinsonism, chorea
What were the past medications (e.g., neuroleptics)?	Tardive movements

TABLE 12.4 Emergent Situations in the Treatment of Patients with Involuntary Movements

Entity	Comments	Acute Management
Dystonic storm	Continuous dystonic spasms	• Admission to ICU • Monitor fluids and electrolytes. • Treat rhabdomyolysis. • Treat with anticholinergic agents (diphenhydramine), baclofen, and benzodiazepines (lorazepam). • Sedation, airway protection, and paralysis may be necessary.
Hemiballismus	Continuous violent flailing, lateralized arm and leg movements seen with injury to the subthalamic nucleus	• May require intubation, sedation, and paralysis in the most severe cases
Acute psychosis in patients with Parkinson disease	Generally due to medication effects	• Acute hospitalization may be necessary. • Reduce and/or withdraw medication. • Treat with antipsychotic agents.
Parkinsonian hyperpyrexia	May occur in a variety of settings	• Admission to ICU • Monitor fluids and electrolytes. • Carbidopa/levodopa, dantrolene, or steroids may be beneficial.
Stridor in patients with multiple system atrophy	More often at night and may result in respiratory arrest	• Nasal continuous positive airway pressure mask • Botulinum toxin injections to the thyroarytenoid muscles • Tracheostomy
Neuroleptic malignant syndrome	Due to drugs with dopamine-blocking activity	• Admission to ICU • Withdrawal of offending medication • Treat with bromocriptine, amantadine, dantrolene, or lorazepam.
Acute dystonic reaction	Due to drugs with dopamine-blocking activity	• Withdraw offending drug. • Treat with IV diphenhydramine.
Oculogyric crisis	Due to drugs with dopamine-blocking activity	• Withdraw or lower dose of offending drug. • Treat with IV diphenhydramine.
Paralytic form of Sydenham chorea	A severe hypotonic state with paralysis	• Treatment with IV steroids

ICU, intensive care unit; IV, intravenous.

disease, neuroleptic malignant syndrome, dystonic storm, and oculogyric crisis (Table 12.4). The initial management of the remaining patients depends very much on the stage and severity of the disease; in many instances, a realistic goal of therapy is to lessen the frequency, severity, and functional impact of movements rather than to aim for complete cessation. Dosages of drugs used in movement disorder emergencies are shown in Table 12.5.

Videos can be found in the companion e-book edition. For a full list of video legends, please see the front matter.

TABLE 12.5 Medications Used in Movement Disorder Emergencies

Amantadine (Symmetrel)	100 mg PO t.i.d.
Baclofen (Lioresal)	10–20 mg PO t.i.d.
Bromocriptine (Parlodel)	5–10 mg PO q8h
Carbidopa–levodopa	25/100 mg PO
Dantrolene sodium (Dantrium)	2.5 mg/kg IV loading dose, 0.25 mg/kg/h IV infusion
Diphenhydramine (Benadryl)	25–50 mg IV q4–8h
Lorazepam (Ativan)	2–4 mg IV q4–6h

PO, by mouth; IV, intravenous.

SUGGESTED READINGS

Albanese A, Bhatia K, Bressman SB, et al. Phenomenology and classification of dystonia: a consensus update. *Mov Disord*. 2013;28(7):863–873.

Bakker MJ, van Dijk JG, van den Maagdenberg AM, et al. Startle syndromes. *Lancet Neurol*. 2006;5(6):513–524.

Barker RA, Revesz T, Thom M, et al. Review of 23 patients affected by the stiff man syndrome: clinical subdivision into stiff trunk (man) syndrome, stiff limb syndrome, and progressive encephalomyelitis with rigidity. *J Neurol Neurosurg Psychiatry*. 1998;65(5):633–640.

Bogan RK, Cheray JA. Restless legs syndrome: a review of diagnosis and management in primary care. *Postgrad Med*. 2013;125(3):99–111.

Deuschl G, Toro C, Hallett M. Symptomatic and essential palatal tremor. 2. Differences of palatal movements. *Mov Disord.* 1994;9(6):676–678.

Dreissen YE, Tijssen MA. The startle syndromes: physiology and treatment. *Epilepsia.* 2012;53(suppl 7):3–11.

Dressler D, Thompson PD, Gledhill RF, et al. The syndrome of painful legs and moving toes. *Mov Disord.* 1994;9(1):13–21.

Elias WJ, Shah BB. Tremor. *JAMA.* 2014;311(9):948–954.

Espay AJ, Chen R. Myoclonus. *Continuum (Minneap Minn).* 2013;19(5)(Movement Disorders):1264–1286.

Fahn S, Jankovic J. *Principles and Practice of Movement Disorders.* Philadelphia: Churchill Livingstone Elsevier; 2007.

Frucht SJ. Treatment of movement disorder emergencies. *Neurotherapeutics.* 2014;11(1):208–212.

Ghosh D, Rajan PV, Erenberg G. A comparative study of primary and secondary stereotypies. *J Child Neurol.* 2013;28(12):1562–1568.

Hallett M. Electrodiagnosis in movement disorders. In: Levin KH, Lüders HO, eds. *Comprehensive Clinical Neurophysiology.* Philadelphia: WB Saunders Company; 2000:281–294.

Jankovic J, Kurlan R. Tourette syndrome: evolving concepts. *Mov Disord.* 2011;26(6):1149–1156.

Kerr S, McKinon W, Bentley A. Descriptors of restless legs syndrome sensations. *Sleep Med.* 2012;13(4):409–413.

Klockgether T. The clinical diagnosis of autosomal dominant spinocerebellar ataxias. *Cerebellum.* 2008;7(2):101–105.

Kulisevsky J, Martí-Fàbregas J, Grau JM. Spasms of amputation stumps. *J Neurol Neurosurg Psychiatry.* 1992;55(7):626–627.

Morgante F, Edwards MJ, Espay AJ. Psychogenic movement disorders. *Continuum (Minneap Minn).* 2013;19(5)(Movement Disorders):1383–1396.

Ondo WG. Restless legs syndrome. *Neurol Clin.* 2009;27(3):779–799.

Reich SG. Painful legs and moving toes. *Handb Clin Neurol.* 2011;100:375–383.

Roper LS, Saifee TA, Parees I, et al. How to use the entrainment test in the diagnosis of functional tremor. *Pract Neurol.* 2013;13(6):396–398.

Singer HS. Motor stereotypies. *Semin Pediatr Neurol.* 2009;16(2):77–81.

Sternberg EJ, Alcalay RN, Levy OA, et al. Postural and intention tremors: a detailed clinical study of essential tremor vs. Parkinson's disease. *Front Neurol.* 2013;4:51.

Tan A, Salgado M, Fahn S. The characterization and outcome of stereotypic movements in nonautistic children. *Mov Disord.* 1997;12(1):47–52.

Walker RH. Differential diagnosis of chorea. *Curr Neurol Neurosci Rep.* 2011;11(4):385–395.

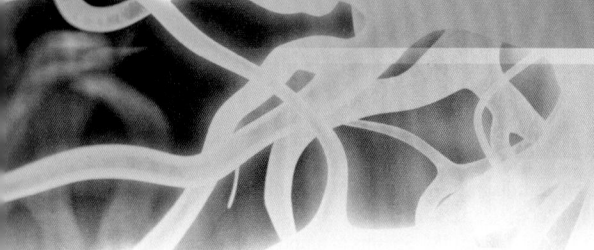

Muscle Weakness, Cramps, and Stiffness 13

Comana M. Cioroiu and Lewis P. Rowland

INTRODUCTION

Weakness is one of the most common complaints in all of neurology; hence, both the scope of the term and its differential diagnosis is broad. A patient may have weakness due to a lesion anywhere in the central or peripheral nervous system from the motor cortex to the muscle itself. Often, patients will use the term *weakness* to describe various functionally limiting symptoms unrelated to loss of strength as with the bradykinesia seen in parkinsonism or the clumsiness experienced with cerebellar ataxia. The concept of weakness is particularly challenging to differentiate from an overall sense of fatigue or asthenia, which is a common complaint in patients with psychiatric (i.e., depression) or systemic diseases such as cancer.

It is not at all uncommon for patients to present to the neurologist with a feeling of poorly described generalized weakness, which can be attributed to various nonneurologic or a specific neurologic cause. The charge of the neurologist in this situation is to focus on the backbone of our specialty: Obtain a comprehensive history and perform a detailed neurologic examination to determine if the patient's complaints are caused by a problem within the nervous system.

MANAGEMENT STRATEGY

Asking the patient about the specific functional consequences of his or her weakness (i.e., trouble climbing stairs, buttoning buttons, opening jars) may help distinguish generalized weakness due to fatigue from weakness with an underlying localizable neurologic cause. Both the history and examination should help the clinician localize the problem to a specific region of the central or peripheral nervous system and give clues to possible etiologies. Symptoms concurrent and associated with the weakness are helpful in formulating a diagnostic impression. Complaints of muscle pain, cramping, or stiffness may invoke a myopathy, whereas numbness or tingling suggests a peripheral neuropathy or central nervous system lesion.

Specific "red flags" in the history or examination may provide important clues and prompt one to institute more acute treatment (Table 13.1). Once a comprehensive differential diagnosis is made, testing is done to confirm or exclude a specific disorder and may include but not be limited to serum studies, imaging, and electrodiagnostic testing. Many weak patients are encountered in the office setting; however, acute weakness may present in the hospital as well and often warrants a more prompt evaluation and rapid institution of therapy (Table 13.2).

NEUROANATOMY AND LOCALIZATION OF WEAKNESS

Weakness can be localized to various regions within the neuraxis, from the cortex to the muscle itself, and can be thought of as originating within either the central or peripheral nervous system.

The central, or pyramidal, motor system is composed of the motor cortex, corticospinal tract, and the various other tracts that modify and interact with it (i.e., the rubrospinal and tectospinal tracts). Weakness related to a central process affecting the corticospinal tract or pyramidal system is typically thought to produce a clinical syndrome of upper motor neuron weakness manifested by spastic tone, hyperreflexia, and pathologic reflexes (i.e., Babinski response).

Weakness due to pathology in the peripheral nervous system characteristically produces a pattern of peripheral lower motor neuron weakness consisting of hyporeflexia, muscle atrophy and wasting, reduced tone, and in some cases, spontaneous muscle activity such as fasciculations. The peripheral motor system is typically considered to include the motor neuron within the anterior horn of the spinal cord (or brain stem for cranial nerves), the peripheral nerve, neuromuscular junction, and muscle distal to it. Both the history and neurologic exam will help localize the problem to a particular part of the neuraxis and thus guide one's differential diagnosis and treatment plan.

TABLE 13.1	Red Flags in the Evaluation of Weakness

- Weakness that becomes severe over a few days or less
- Dyspnea
- Inability to raise the head against gravity
- Bulbar symptoms (e.g., difficulty chewing, talking, and swallowing)
- Loss of ambulation
- Changes in bowel or bladder function

TABLE 13.2	Key Steps in the Diagnosis and Management of Weakness

- Characterize the weakness in terms of tempo, variability, distribution, and associated symptoms.
- Perform a detailed neurologic examination to help localize the weakness within the neuraxis.
- Determine if there are predominantly upper or lower motor neuron findings.
- Look out for red flags (see Table 13.1).
- Order appropriate tests depending on most likely localization and differential diagnosis.
- Beware of diagnoses or signs prompting acute intervention (i.e., Guillain–Barré syndrome, mononeuritis multiplex, or myasthenia gravis).

CENTRAL (UPPER MOTOR NEURON) WEAKNESS

The corticospinal tract or pyramidal system can be damaged anywhere along its tract from the cortex through the corona radiata to the posterior limb of the internal capsule and down to the brain stem via the cerebral peduncles of the midbrain to the medulla and spinal cord. The highest possible lesion is in the primary motor cortex of the brain, where the largest of the pyramidal cells (Betz cells) lie in layer 5 of the cortex. Responsibility for planning and preparation of movement lies within the supplementary and premotor cortices, which regulate the motor action. The actions of the corticospinal tract are further modulated by the cerebellum as well as the basal ganglia and its tracts, which is also known as the *extrapyramidal system*. Pathology within this system can lead to either a paucity or exaggeration of movement, and the functional impairment experienced by the patient can be frequently described as weakness.

The neurologic examination and history can point toward a diagnosis localized within either the cerebellar or extrapyramidal system (such as Parkinson disease) and can include such findings as ataxia, bradykinesia (paucity and slowness of movement), tremor, and postural instability. In many cases, the key to localization is "pattern-matching"—actively looking for a pattern or constellation of findings that point to a specific cause of weakness (Table 13.3).

Cortical Lesions

A variety of diseases can affect the corticospinal tract from large strokes or hemorrhages to tumors and infections. Cortical lesions cause a characteristic pattern of weakness, where one limb is typically preferentially affected due to the distribution of motor representation in the homunculus of the primary motor cortex. For instance, infarcts affecting the middle cerebral artery territory will preferentially affect the arm and face more so than the leg. Often, there are other associated cortical signs such as aphasia or neglect, and patients may also present with headaches or seizures. Cortical weakness can also result from etiologies such as atypical migraine or postictal Todd paralysis; these diagnoses should be considered in the appropriate clinical setting.

Subcortical Lesions

Subcortical lesions, such as those in the internal capsule, will present with more complete unilateral weakness that may or may not spare the face. Demyelinating diseases such as multiple sclerosis (MS) are often implicated in subcortical weakness, although various other etiologies such as infarct or tumor are possible as well. Weakness attributed to a brain stem lesion can present with unilateral weakness of an arm and leg, and the face may be involved as well. There are usually associated symptoms attributable to cranial nerve dysfunction such as diplopia and facial numbness or hemiataxia due to involvement of cerebellar tracts within the brain stem.

Spinal Cord Lesions

After decussating in the pyramids of the medulla, the lateral corticospinal tract is formed within the spinal cord where it travels ipsilateral to the innervated side of the body, lying anterior to the posterior columns and medial to the posterior spinocerebellar tract. Of note, about 10% of fibers in the corticospinal tract do not decussate and travel down into the cord to form the anterior or ventral corticospinal tract. Patients with weakness related to spinal cord pathology will typically present with both motor and sensory complaints, which can be bilateral or localized to one limb. Pain may be present or absent, and its description will vary depending on the cause of weakness. For instance, it may be described as stiffness related to myelopathy, Lhermitte sign (shock-like sensations with back flexion), or diffuse back pain. There may be disturbances in bowel or bladder function requiring prompt evaluation for cord compression.

PERIPHERAL (LOWER MOTOR NEURON) WEAKNESS

Upper motor neurons that form the corticospinal tracts synapse with both interneurons and lower motor neurons within the anterior horn of the spinal cord. The motor unit is defined as one alpha motor neuron within the anterior horn (or brain stem when related to cranial nerves) and all of the muscle fibers it innervates. Pathology within the anterior horn itself may present with a combination of both upper and lower motor neuron signs as seen in amyotrophic lateral sclerosis (ALS) and often includes concomitant bulbar weakness. Patients with weakness localized to the anterior horn will often present with asymmetric weakness, which begins in the bulbar region or within one limb and then progresses segmentally over time. Pain related to muscle cramps and stiffness is a common complaint.

TABLE 13.3 Common Etiologies of Weakness Depending on Time Course

Acute (Seconds to Minutes)	Subacute (Minutes to Hours)	Chronic (Months to Years)
• Infarction	• Demyelinating CNS disease (i.e., MS)	• Neoplasm
• Hemorrhage	• Toxic ingestion	• Neuromuscular junction disorder
• Periodic paralysis	• Plexopathy	• Axonal polyneuropathy
• Complicated migraine	• Acute demyelinating neuropathy (Guillain–Barré syndrome)	• Structural lesion (i.e., herniated disk)
• Trauma	• Metabolic disturbances	• Motor neuron disease
• Postictal Todd paralysis	• Neuromuscular junction disease	• Myopathy
• Conversion disorder	• Infection	
	• Mononeuritis multiplex	

CNS, central nervous system; MS, multiple sclerosis.

The lower motor neuron exits the spinal cord to form the ventral motor portion of the spinal nerve root, after which it meets the dorsal sensory nerve root past the dorsal root ganglion to form the peripheral nerve. At this location, the dorsal nerve root is commonly susceptible to compression by vertebral disk herniation, and patients may present with radiating pain or sensory loss corresponding to a particular *dermatome*. A *myotome* is defined as the group of muscles innervated by one single nerve root. Most muscles are supplied by two or more nerve roots and thus, a single root lesion rarely causes marked weakness due to this overlap within myotomes.

Brachial Plexus

Prior to separating into specific peripheral nerves, the motor and sensory fibers together form a network called a *plexus*, of which there are two (brachial and lumbosacral). The brachial plexus consists of nerve roots from C5 to T1, whereas the lumbosacral plexus consists of those from L1 to S3. The brachial plexus is composed of three trunks (upper, middle, lower) dividing into two divisions (anterior and posterior), which then form three cords (medial, lateral, posterior) ultimately subdividing and ending in terminal peripheral nerves (Fig. 13.1). Different peripheral nerves come off the brachial plexus at different levels; some, such as the phrenic nerve, exit immediately off the nerve roots, whereas others form the terminal branches of the plexus. These terminal nerves may be pure motor, pure sensory, or mixed.

Lumbosacral Plexus

The lumbosacral plexus is arranged somewhat differently, with various nerve roots coming together to form large nerves that then continue to differentiate into terminal branches or peripheral nerves. For instance, nerve roots from L4 to S3 come together to form the sciatic nerve, which later then subdivides into the fibular and tibial nerves. Weakness localized to the plexus typically presents with acute or subacute pain in one limb and is most commonly traumatic but can also result from other various etiologies such as infectious, structural, and inflammatory causes. Weakness is localized to one limb, often in the distribution of various nerves. There may be associated sensory complaints but the sensory examination is frequently normal.

Peripheral Nerves

Terminal or peripheral nerves may be affected in isolation (mononeuropathy) or together in a uniform or multifocal pattern. Mononeuropathies are most commonly due to compression, and symptoms and exam findings are restricted to the distribution of one nerve distal to the injury. Polyneuropathies have a broad differential and can be subdivided into those caused by demyelination and those with predominant axonal involvement.

Demyelinating neuropathies typically also involve the nerve roots and can be referred to as *radiculoneuropathies*. They tend to have a motor greater than sensory predominance, present with more generalized or multifocal rather than length-dependent weakness, and areflexia is typical on examination. Cranial nerves may be affected as well.

Axonal polyneuropathies are usually length-dependent, affect sensory greater than motor function, and spare cranial nerves. The differential for such a polyneuropathy is vast and includes metabolic, infectious, and systemic causes among others. Diabetic neuropathy is by far the most common etiology of length-dependent axonal polyneuropathy.

At times, different peripheral nerves can be affected in an asymmetric and patchy fashion (Fig. 13.2). Such a syndrome of multiple mononeuropathies (also frequently referred to as *mononeuritis multiplex*) is often the result of ischemic injury to different peripheral nerves and present with acute and painful weakness and sensory loss. In these instances, it is crucial to rule out an underlying vasculitis, as management must be prompt to avoid further irreversible injury.

Neuromuscular Junction

Each peripheral nerve ultimately terminates at the motor endplate of the muscle it supplies, where it forms the neuromuscular

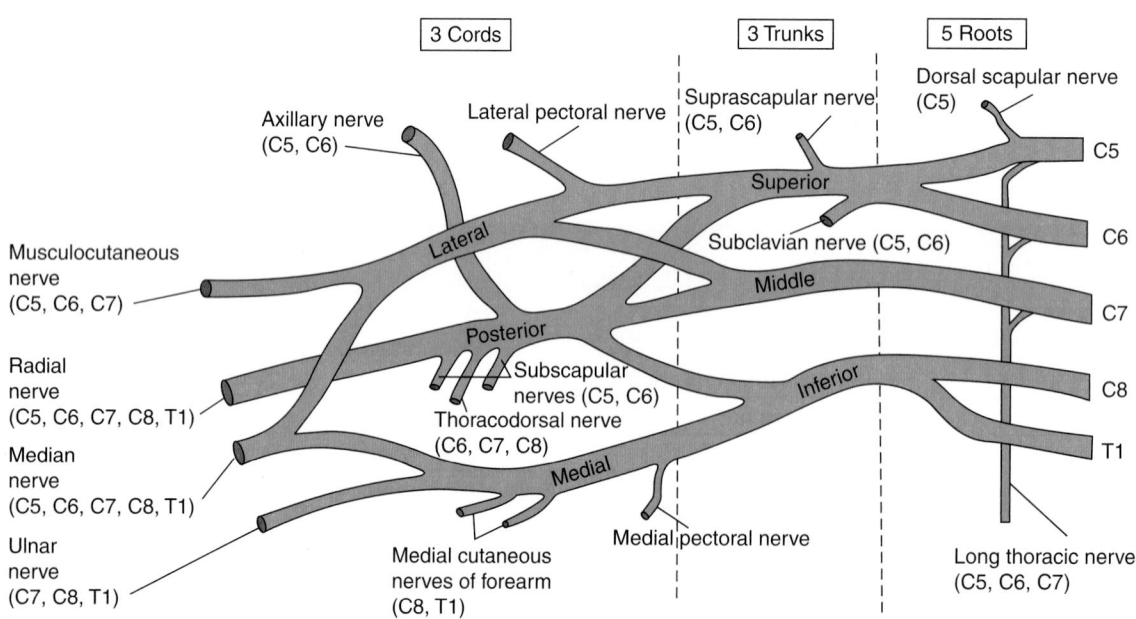

FIGURE 13.1 Brachial plexus. (Adapted from Marshall R, Mayer S. *On Call Neurology*. 3rd ed. Philadelphia: Saunders; 2007.)

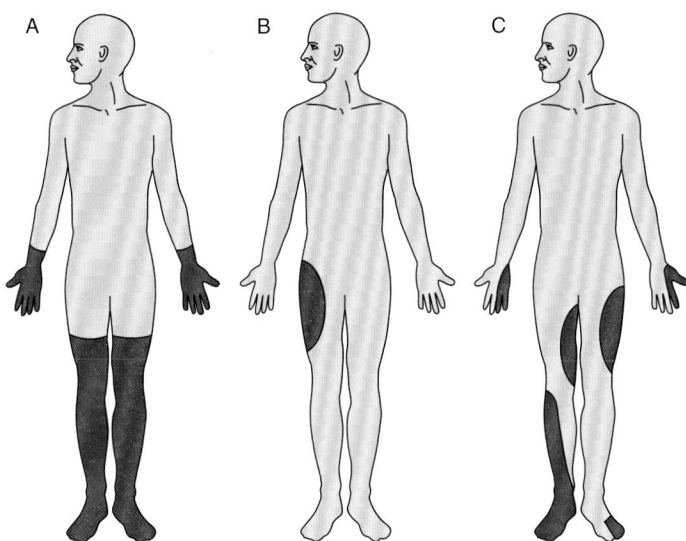

FIGURE 13.2 Patterns of sensory loss in patients with neuropathy. **A:** Polyneuropathy: diffuse stocking-glove pattern. **B:** Mononeuropathy: focal involvement corresponding to a single peripheral nerve. **C:** Mononeuritis multiplex: pattern of multiple, asymmetric regions of sensory loss corresponding to multiple peripheral nerves. (Adapted from Marshall R, Mayer S. *On Call Neurology.* 3rd ed. Philadelphia: Saunders; 2007.)

junction. At this point, calcium influx into the terminal portion of the neuron leads to binding of acetylcholine-containing vesicles to the neuronal membrane and release of Ach into the postsynaptic space. The Ach-release site is known as the *active zone* and is the location of both calcium influx via voltage-gated calcium channels and acetylcholine release. Binding of acetylcholine to its corresponding postsynaptic receptors at the motor endplate leads to opening of sodium channels and consequent depolarization of the muscle membrane and an endplate potential (EPP). The summation of several EPPs is ultimately what leads to a discrete muscle fiber potential and subsequent muscle contraction.

Weakness localized to the neuromuscular junction (see Chapter 89) often presents with proximal and bulbar weakness, which fluctuates with activity and time of day. Autoantibodies may be directed toward components of the presynaptic membrane (i.e., toward the voltage-gated calcium channel in Lambert–Eaton myasthenic syndrome) or the postsynaptic membrane (i.e., myasthenia gravis, where antibodies are formed against acetylcholine receptors). The muscle fiber action potential causes depolarization of the internal portion of the muscle fiber and leads to activation of calcium channels in the sarcoplasmic reticulum of the myocyte leading to calcium release. Calcium then binds to troponin C on the actin filaments of the myofibril, thereby unbinding tropomyosin from the filament, allowing the binding of myosin. The binding of adenosine triphosphate (ATP) to myosin then allows unbinding and release of actin, thereby leading to muscle relaxation.

Myopathy

Muscle weakness due to pathology within the muscle itself is frequently proximal, symmetric, and progressive. There can be associated facial weakness and weakness of eye movements (such as in mitochondrial myopathies). Myalgias are common, and the sensory examination should be normal. Etiologies are variable and can include inflammatory, congenital, and metabolic causes.

FOCUSED HISTORY

DEMOGRAPHICS AND PAST MEDICAL HISTORY

Knowledge of the patient's age and prior medical history is crucial, as various etiologies are more or less likely depending on the age of the patient. A left hemiparesis presenting in a young woman is more likely to be attributable to an MS flare than a stroke, and the opposite is true in an 87-year-old man with hypertension.

One must be careful to obtain a complete list of medications the patient is taking, as certain exposures may provide diagnostic clues (i.e., statin myopathy). The social history is important to obtain, particularly with respect to toxic exposures and travel, as both toxic ingestion (i.e., alcohol, lead) and various infectious agents may lead to weakness of either central or peripheral origin. A detailed family history is required in cases of suspected hereditary disorders and a pedigree is often helpful. Thus, the age and complete medical, social, and family history of a patient will help formulate an appropriate differential diagnosis based on likelihood and help dictate management.

TEMPO OF WEAKNESS

One of the key questions one must ask is the time of onset and whether the weakness is acute, subacute, or chronically progressive (see Table 13.3). Focal weakness that begins abruptly (i.e., over seconds to minutes) is most concerning for a vascular event such as a hemorrhage or infarct and these patients must be emergently assessed and evaluated. Subacute onset of weakness has a broader differential and may be due to demyelinating disease such as MS, a mass lesion, or an acute demyelinating neuropathy, among others. Weakness that evolves chronically over months to years is suggestive of a neurodegenerative disease such as motor neuron disease, peripheral neuropathy, myopathy, or a slowly progressive structural lesion. *The tempo of the course of symptoms dictates the urgency with which the patient should be evaluated and managed.*

VARIABILITY OF WEAKNESS

Another crucial component of a detailed neurologic history includes asking about the nature of the weakness and whether it is transient, fluctuating, or permanent. Transient weakness that fluctuates with the time of day or with exertion may point toward a neuromuscular junction disorder, MS flare, or a channelopathy (i.e., periodic paralysis).

DISTRIBUTION OF WEAKNESS

The distribution and symmetry of weakness is equally important to characterize when formulating a plan for localization and likely etiology. Weakness affecting one arm and leg on the same side is referred to as *hemiparesis*. If the arm and leg are affected on opposite sides, this is known as *crossed hemiparesis*. If the weakness involves only one limb, this is called *monoparesis*, whereas weakness of both legs is known as *paraparesis*. The term *plegia* in the same context refers to complete paralysis.

Certain patterns of weakness give clues regarding localization. Predominantly upper motor neuron weakness of one limb, with or without facial involvement, suggests a cortical lesion in the central nervous system such as a stroke or MS. Given the distribution of the motor homunculus, incomplete upper motor neuron weakness in one limb suggests a lesion in the cortex, whereas complete hemiplegia involving the face is more likely to be localized to subcortical structures or the brain stem. If certain muscles within one limb (corresponding to a particular myotome or peripheral nerve) are preferentially affected, this may indicate a problem in the peripheral nervous system such as a radiculopathy or mononeuropathy. Generalized weakness can involve all four limbs and be related to a process within the spinal cord (i.e., cervical myelopathy), peripheral nerve (i.e., polyneuropathy), neuromuscular junction, or muscle.

Further characterizing the pattern as being *distal* or *proximal* is also helpful. For instance, generalized weakness that is symmetric and distal is commonly related to a polyneuropathy, whereas proximal weakness is more likely referable to a problem in the neuromuscular junction or muscle.

SENSORY SYMPTOMS

Asking about associated symptoms is crucial to determining not only proper localization but also in assisting with thinking of possible etiologies (Table 13.4). One must ask about associated sensory symptoms, as this could point toward a neuropathy, plexopathy, or spinal cord lesion. Sensory disturbances can have a positive quality (tingling, paresthesias, pain), or a negative quality (numbness or loss of sensation). A specific sensory level is indicative of pathology within the spinal cord and should be looked for in the appropriate setting.

Cognitive complaints or language symptoms will always be most suspicious of a cortical process, and weakness in this instance may involve the face and typically affect one limb more than another.

PAIN

Pain can be encountered in the setting of neuromuscular weakness but must be differentiated from the diffuse myalgias that can be related to an underlying systemic medical illness or psychiatric disease. Often, this distinction is difficult to make, as complaints can be nearly identical. Patients with neuropathy often present with burning pain, which is distal and symmetric, and those with radiculopathy or plexopathy may complain of radiating neck, arm, or shoulder pain. Hand pain is a common manifestation of carpal tunnel syndrome, which may eventually progress to hand weakness and clumsiness. Mononeuritis multiplex due to nerve infarcts in the setting of vasculitis can present with acute pain in a variable distribution. Plexopathy is often heralded by acute to subacute pain in the affected limb prior to weakness or sensory complaints. Weakness in the setting of a slowly progressive brain or spinal cord mass may present associated with headaches or back pain.

STIFFNESS AND CRAMPS

Muscle stiffness is commonly encountered in upper motor neuron lesions causing spasticity and can be seen in both weakness due to cortical, subcortical, and brain stem lesions as well as with myelopathy in spinal cord syndromes. *Cramps* (a localized muscle spasm or persistent contraction) are more of a lower motor neuron/muscle phenomenon and are encountered frequently in various peripheral syndromes. It is seen as a frequent manifestation of motor neuron disease, where patients may complain of frequent cramps and intermittent debilitating muscle spasms. Those with polyneuropathy may often also have cramping or stiffness that is more constant and less paroxysmal.

Various primary muscle diseases include cramps as a primary symptom, and often, the distinction must be made between cramps and more diffuse myalgias. Myopathies characterized by *myotonia* (prolonged muscle contraction after voluntary contraction or percussion) such as myotonic dystrophy and certain channelopathies commonly present with cramps as an initial symptom. Metabolic and certain mitochondrial myopathies often also may present with intermittent cramps. *Stiff person syndrome* (see Chapter 94) is an autoimmune disorder characterized by painful muscle spasms caused by diffuse or localized body stiffness usually in the absence of weakness.

VISUAL AND SPEECH DISTURBANCES

If visual complaints are present, it is necessary to characterize them well. A visual field cut or gaze preference may point to a cortical problem, whereas ptosis or diplopia could be a manifestation of a neuromuscular junction disorder or a myopathy.

Trouble with speech in the form of dysarthria must first be differentiated from a language disturbance. The presence of dysarthria may point toward bulbar weakness of various etiologies. A cortical, subcortical, or brain stem lesion may affect tongue fibers; motor neuron disease may present with or lead to bulbar involvement; and similarly, a neuromuscular junction or muscle disorder may involve trouble with speech and swallowing. A complaint of dysarthria should always prompt one to inquire about swallowing difficulties, as this may have important management and prognostic implications.

RESPIRATORY SYMPTOMS

Asking about respiratory involvement is also essential in patients presenting with weakness whether localized or general. Large cortical and brain stem lesions may rapidly lead to respiratory failure when acute. Disorders of the motor neuron, neuromuscular junction, and muscle may often be complicated by respiratory insufficiency, which may present as shortness of breath, early morning headaches, or daytime fatigue. Acute demyelinating inflammatory polyneuropathy at times may lead to diaphragmatic weakness and subsequent respiratory failure, and thus, respiratory function must be carefully monitored in these patients.

AUTONOMIC DISTURBANCES

Urinary complaints (most often incontinence or frequency) are most commonly seen with upper motor neuron lesions, such as those involving the paracentral frontal lobe or spinal cord. A complaint of dark-colored urine may indicate the presence of myoglobinuria indicative of muscle breakdown suggesting a primary muscle disease such as McArdle disease. One should ask about autonomic involvement as well (i.e., symptoms of orthostasis, dry mouth or eyes), as this may play an important role in certain neuropathies. Finally, symptoms suggesting cardiac involvement such as syncope, chest pain, and shortness of breath with activity may be worrisome for a concurrent cardiomyopathy as can be seen with certain myopathies (i.e., Duchenne or Becker muscular dystrophy).

FOCUSED EXAM

A focused and goal-directed neurologic exam is critical to the evaluation of a patient with weakness. Ideally, this should be done with the patient undressed and in a gown. Acquisition of both sitting and standing heart rate and blood pressure, when appropriate, is useful to assess for orthostatic changes suggestive of autonomic nervous system involvement.

MENTAL STATUS

Testing of mental status is important, particularly in cases of weakness due to cortical and subcortical processes (i.e., stroke, neoplasm), as this may further assist in localization. Weakness due to a peripheral nervous system disorder should preserve cognitive and language function.

TABLE 13.4 Symptoms Associated with Various Weakness Syndromes

	Cortex	Brain Stem	Spinal Cord	Motor Neuron	Nerve Root or Plexus	Peripheral Nerve	Neuromuscular Junction	Muscle
Sensory loss	May be in the same distribution of weakness (i.e., stroke, MS plaque)	May be in the same distribution of weakness	Corresponds to level of weakness, usually with sensory level	Absent	Can be in a dermatomal or peripheral nerve distribution	May be in the distribution of one nerve or many nerves (i.e., distal stocking-glove distribution)	Absent	Absent
Cognitive or language deficits	Present	Absent	Absent	Absent (advanced ALS can be associated with cognitive deficits)	Absent	Absent	Absent	Absent
Pain	Headache may be present.	Headache may be present.	Localized or diffuse back pain	Absent	Radicular pain or diffuse pain with plexopathy in the affected limb	Burning or paresthesias (i.e., polyneuropathy), acute pain (i.e., mononeuritis multiplex)	Absent	Myalgias, proximal greater than distal
Cramps or stiffness	Spasticity	Spasticity	Spasticity	Both cramps and stiffness are common.	Absent	Both cramps and stiffness with both polyneuropathy and certain mononeuropathies	Absent	Cramps common in • Myotonic dystrophy • Channelopathies • Metabolic myopathies • Mitochondrial myopathies • Stiff person syndrome
Visual changes	Involvement of frontal eye fields or hemianopsia	Diplopia or nystagmus	Absent	Absent	Absent	Ophthalmoparesis or diplopia can be seen in GBS or Miller–Fisher syndrome	Diplopia or ptosis occurs with myasthenia gravis.	Diplopia as can be seen in mitochondrial myopathies, among others

(table continues on page 100)

TABLE 13.4 Symptoms Associated with Various Weakness Syndromes (continued)

	Cortex	Brain Stem	Spinal Cord	Motor Neuron	Nerve Root or Plexus	Peripheral Nerve	Neuromuscular Junction	Muscle
Speech or swallowing difficulties	Due to tongue/facial weakness	Due to tongue/facial weakness	Absent	Bulbar involvement in motor neuron disease	Absent	Can be seen in demyelinating neuropathies with cranial nerve involvement	Nasal speech, dysphagia in myasthenia gravis	Due to both pharyngeal and tongue weakness
Respiratory compromise	Occurs with large infarcts or hemorrhages	Occurs with infarcts or hemorrhages	Can be present with high cervical lesions	Bulbar involvement in motor neuron disease	Phrenic involvement in plexopathies	Can be seen in demyelinating neuropathies with bulbar and phrenic nerve involvement	Bulbar involvement in both pre- and postsynaptic neuromuscular junction disorders	Can be present in certain myopathies (i.e., amyloid, distal myopathy with early respiratory failure)
Cardiac symptoms	Absent	Absent	Absent	Absent	Absent	Absent	Absent	Cardiomyopathy can be associated with various myopathies (i.e., myotonic dystrophy, Duchenne or Becker myopathy).
Urinary disturbances	Incontinence with paracentral frontal lesions	Absent	Urinary incontinence with cord compression	Absent	Absent	Absent	Absent	Myoglobinuria with certain myopathies (i.e., McArdle disease)

MS, multiple sclerosis; ALS, amyotrophic lateral sclerosis; GBS, Guillain–Barré syndrome.

CRANIAL NERVES

In testing cranial nerves, particular attention should be paid to examination of the eyes starting with their appearance at rest. One should make note of the presence or absence of ptosis, skew, or other asymmetry at rest. Both central and peripheral processes may lead to pupillary involvement with or without ophthalmoparesis.

A careful assessment of extraocular movements is essential, as they can be abnormal in states affecting supranuclear, nuclear, and peripheral cranial nerve function (i.e., brain stem processes) as well as in diseases of the neuromuscular junction (i.e., myasthenia gravis) and muscle (i.e., mitochondrial myopathies).

Facial strength is examined both by assessment of asymmetry at rest (i.e., a flattened nasolabial fold), as well as by having the patient activate various muscles. Ask the patient to forcefully close his or her eyes and subsequently try to pry them open to assess strength of eye closure. Patients with facial weakness are typically unable to bury their eyelashes with forced eye closure, and eyes are easily pried open. To assess strength in the lower face, ask the patient to purse his or her lips together or whistle. Asymmetric facial weakness sparing the forehead implicates an upper motor neuron facial nerve lesion, whereas facial weakness involving the entire half of the face suggests a peripheral seventh cranial nerve lesion. Symmetric weakness of the facial muscles most typically implies a lesion of the neuromuscular junction or muscle but can rarely also be seen in certain demyelinating neuropathies and in motor neuron disease with bulbar involvement.

Tongue weakness can be evaluated by looking for deviation with tongue protrusion and by having the patient push the tongue against the inner cheek with the examiner's resistance. The tongue should also be carefully inspected for the presence of atrophy and fasciculations as can be seen with motor neuron disease. Pharyngeal weakness should also be assessed by having the patient make guttural sounds and checking for the presence of an intact gag reflex.

MOTOR EXAMINATION

Inspection

The motor examination should always begin with inspection and observation. It is in this part of the examination that one makes the distinction between weakness due to upper motor neuron dysfunction (most commonly related to a process localized to the corticospinal tract) versus lower motor neuron disease localized to the peripheral nervous system. One should look for muscle atrophy and wasting, both in large proximal muscles as well as in the smaller distal muscles such as the intrinsic hand muscles (i.e., first dorsal interosseus) in which subtle atrophy can often be more frequently appreciated.

Adventitious Movements

Abnormal movements such as *fasciculations*, *myokymia*, and *tremor* should be sought in various muscles. The presence of atrophy and fasciculations are indicative of lower motor neuron dysfunction as can be seen with motor neuron disease or chronic mono- or polyneuropathies. Myokymia can be seen in limb muscles but also in the face, where it typically is suggestive of a brain stem lesion such as an MS plaque. The back should also be inspected for both atrophy (i.e., scapular winging) as well as fasciculations. Assessment of tone is also helpful in distinguishing an upper motor neuron from a lower motor neuron problem.

Tone

Increased tone in the arms can manifest as either rigidity (resistance that is consistent and present throughout the full range of motion) related to basal ganglia dysfunction or spasticity (resistance that is velocity dependent) related to corticospinal tract disease and upper motor neuron dysfunction. When testing tone in the arms, it is often helpful to have the patient open and close the opposite hand, which may accentuate mildly increased tone. Examining tone in the legs is often best done in the supine position where the knees are grasped and quickly pulled up. An unintentional lifting of the heels off the bed is indicative of increased tone in the legs, whereas the heels will naturally slide up the bed in the setting of normal tone.

The motor exam is also an appropriate time to check for the presence or absence of *myotonia* when clinically suspected. One approach is to test for grip myotonia by having the patient squeeze the examiner's hand for 10 seconds, then asking the patient to quickly let go. In the presence of myotonia, the patient will be unable to relax the grip. Similarly, one can check for percussion myotonia by tapping on a muscle—those with myotonia will demonstrate subsequent prolonged muscle contraction (typically, the abductor pollicis brevis is used, but the tongue can be checked as well).

Power

Assessment of strength can be done both by objectively examining different muscle groups and by observation. The first step in examination of strength is often testing of *pronator drift* where the arms are outstretched with the palms up and the patient's eyes closed. Those with subtle or overt hemiparesis due to an upper motor neuron lesion will exhibit pronation and a downward drift. Testing of *rapid finger taps* and *arm rolling* may also demonstrate subtle weakness in the setting of a mild hemiparesis. Particularly in cases of suspected peripheral causes of weakness, a detailed examination of various muscle groups is necessary. One must remember to test strength of neck flexion and extension, as this may have important implications particularly in motor neuron disease, neuromuscular junction disorders, and myopathies. Strength of neck flexion is often correlated with respiratory insufficiency due to respiratory muscle weakness and is important to check in all cases of motor neuron disease, neuromuscular junction disease, myopathy, and acute inflammatory demyelinating polyneuropathy.

Objective testing of muscle power is traditionally based on the Medical Research Council (MRC) scale from 0 to 5, with 5 representing full strength and 0 being complete absence of muscle movement. A score of 1 implies a discernable muscle twitch without movement of a full muscle. A score of 2 indicates movement in the same plane of gravity, whereas movement against gravity but not resistance is a score of 3. A score of 4 represents active movement against resistance and can be further assigned a "+" or a "−" when appropriate to make a more subtle distinction between variations in resistance.

When testing power, each muscle should be tested in a position in which it is at its maximal mechanical advantage—for instance, finger abduction should be tested with the wrist in the neutral position and not flexed. At times, weakness may be too subtle to detect with formal testing of power. It is helpful at times to ask the patient to perform certain functional movements, which may be impaired in cases of subtle weakness. For instance, someone with full strength on testing of power may have trouble standing up from a squatted position or hopping on one foot. A recognition and identification of a specific pattern of weakness is important, as different diseases will manifest with different patterns of weakness. For instance, weakness in one limb following a specific myotome may point toward a root or plexus problem, whereas symmetric proximal weakness may suggest either a neuromuscular junction or muscle disorder. Knowledge of the innervation and action of various muscle groups is essential in localization of weakness due to a peripheral cause, as the pattern of muscle involvement may point one toward a particular localization and diagnosis (Table 13.5).

SENSORY EXAMINATION

Evaluation of sensory loss is often challenging, as it is the most subjective and thus least reliable portion of the neurologic exam. The best approach is to use the sensory exam to confirm what is clinically suspected. Look for particular patterns of sensory loss to complement the clinical picture, such as sensory loss in a dermatomal pattern consistent with a mononeuropathy or in a distal and symmetric pattern consistent with a polyneuropathy. Testing of different modalities is often helpful in discerning specific spinal cord syndromes (i.e., Brown-Séquard) and in distinguishing a large- from a small-fiber neuropathy.

REFLEXES

The absence of reflexes or hypoactive reflexes point toward a lower motor neuron lesion in the peripheral nervous system, whereas pathologically hyperactive reflexes, particularly when in the presence of a Babinski sign or Hoffmann sign, are indicative of an upper motor neuron lesion and corticospinal tract localization. Examination of reflexes may be an important diagnostic clue; for instance, complete loss of reflexes in the setting of subacute weakness should prompt one to quickly consider a diagnosis of acute inflammatory demyelinating neuropathy.

COORDINATION

Tests of coordination such as finger-to-nose testing are often impaired in the setting of weakness, and the distinction should be made accordingly to avoid confusing subtle weakness for cerebellar or sensory ataxia.

GAIT

Examination of gait is often critical, as the scissoring, spastic gait of myelopathy will look appreciably different from the waddling gait of myopathy with proximal leg weakness. When assessing gait, one can also notice subtle steppage related to a footdrop or circumduction in the setting of a hemiparesis. It is important to differentiate gait disturbance due to weakness from that related to basal ganglia dysfunction as seen with a shuffling, stooped parkinsonian gait or cerebellar disease where a wide-based ataxic gait is the predominant manifestation. More subtle gait testing involving heel, toe, and tandem gait is often sometimes necessary to further complement the rest of the examination and help elucidate the problem.

DIAGNOSIS AND INITIAL TREATMENT

Once one has formed a differential diagnosis based on likelihood of a particular diagnosis (Table 13.6), various tests can be ordered to further confirm or refute one's diagnostic impression. The urgency of certain tests will depend on the clinical context and circumstances. Patients seen in an emergency room or inpatient setting with acute complaints will often require a more prompt evaluation, and tests can be performed on a more urgent basis. Most patients in the office can be managed with tests ordered on an outpatient basis. However, at times, patients can be seen in the outpatient setting that need urgent evaluation, and it is crucial for the clinician to make this distinction following a detailed history and examination.

RECOGNITION OF EMERGENT SITUATIONS

A patient presenting to the office with subacute ascending weakness and areflexia should be promptly admitted to the hospital for evaluation and treatment of probable Guillain–Barré syndrome. Similarly, those with chronic weakness and known diagnoses may present with progressive symptoms requiring hospitalization and more urgent management. For instance, a myasthenic presenting with new-onset shortness of breath and dysphagia needs hospitalization for respiratory monitoring and treatment for likely crisis. It is important to identify patients in need of prompt evaluation where the most important tests to be ordered often include pulmonary function tests and a formal swallowing evaluation.

LABORATORY TESTING

Various tests are available in the evaluation of muscle weakness. Serum studies are important to exclude various metabolic, infectious, inflammatory, or autoimmune conditions. The extent of testing depends on the differential diagnosis. For instance, the workup for causes of axonal polyneuropathy is very broad and can include tests from vitamin levels to heavy metal testing. In cases of suspected neuromuscular junction disease, appropriate antibody testing is necessary, and a creatine kinase should be checked in patients with suspected myopathy.

Genetic tests are now available for those with a family history or other evidence to suggest a congenital or genetic etiology. Imaging is often first line for patients with central causes of weakness.

IMAGING STUDIES

For patients with predominantly upper motor neuron signs and cortical involvement, a computed tomography (CT) scan (see Chapter 20) or magnetic resonance imaging (MRI) (see Chapter 21) of the brain is indicated. Brain imaging is indicated for anyone with a history and exam that localizes to the cortex, subcortex, or brain stem.

In cases of suspected spinal cord pathology, an MRI of the spinal cord is indicated. The exam will guide which particular part of the cord to image, as it can be either cervical, thoracic, or lumbosacral. In some instances, all three may be necessary. Imaging can also be done of the brachial or lumbosacral plexus, and this is often instructive in cases of plexopathy where trauma, structural lesions, or neoplastic infiltration are suspected. A contrast MRI of the plexus can at times be abnormal in cases of idiopathic brachial neuritis. In patients who cannot tolerate MRI, a CT scan can be helpful to exclude structural and neoplastic processes. CT myelography is still performed at times in those who cannot undergo MRI and can provide more detailed imaging of the nerve roots than a CT scan alone.

LUMBAR PUNCTURE

A lumbar puncture (see Chapter 31) is important to consider in various cases of both central and peripheral weakness. For instance, a patient with a suspected inflammatory, autoimmune, infectious, or neoplastic etiology will typically warrant examination of the cerebrospinal fluid looking for cells, abnormal protein, and the presence of various other antibodies and cells which may be diagnostic. It is particularly useful in the diagnosis of Guillain–Barré syndrome where one typically sees a cytoalbuminologic dissociation with elevated protein in the absence of cells.

TABLE 13.5 Common Muscle Groups, Actions, and Innervation

Muscle	Peripheral Nerve	Nerve Root	Action
A. Muscles of the Back, Shoulder, and Neck			
Sternocleidomastoid	Spinal accessory	CN XI, C2, C3	Contralateral rotation of the head
Trapezius	Spinal accessory	CN XI, C3, C4	Shoulder elevation
Diaphragm	Phrenic	C3, C4, C5	Inspiration
Serratus anterior	Long thoracic	C5, C6, C7	Protraction and stabilization of scapula
Rhomboid	Dorsal scapular	C4, C5	Abduction and elevation of scapula
Levator scapulae	Dorsal scapular	C4, C5	Elevation of scapula
Supraspinatus	Suprascapular	C5, C6	Abduction of arm to 90 degrees
Infraspinatus	Suprascapular	C5, C6	Lateral arm rotation
Deltoid	Axillary	C5, C6	Abduction of arm past 30 degrees
Teres minor	Axillary	C4, C5	Medial arm rotation
Teres major	Subscapular	C5, C6, C7	Medical rotation and adduction of arm
Latissimus dorsi	Thoracodorsal	C6, C7, C8	Adduction of arm
B. Muscles of the Arm and Hand			
Biceps brachii	Musculocutaneous	**C5**, C6	Forearm flexion with arm supinated
Brachialis	Musculocutaneous	C5, C6	Forearm flexion with arm pronated
Triceps brachii	Radial	C6, **C7**, C8	Forearm extension
Brachioradialis	Radial	**C6**, C7	Forearm flexion with arm supinated to 90 degrees
Extensor carpi radialis	Radial	**C6**, C7	Hand extension
Supinator	Radial	**C6**, C7	Forearm supination
Extensor digitorum	Radial (posterior interosseus nerve [PIN])	**C7**, C8	Extension of hand and digits two to five
Extensor carpi ulnaris	Radial (PIN)	**C7**, C8	Hand extension toward ulna
Abductor pollicis longus	Radial (PIN)	**C7**, C8	Thumb abduction
Extensor pollicis longus and brevis	Radial (PIN)	**C7**, C8	Thumb extension
Extensor indicis	Radial (PIN)	C7, **C8**	Index finger extension
Flexor carpi ulnaris	Ulnar	C7, **C8**, T1	Ulnar hand flexion
Flexor digitorum profundus	Ulnar	**C8**, T1	Flexion of distal phalanx of digits four and five
Adductor pollicis	Ulnar	C8, T1	Thumb adduction
Abductor digiti minimi	Ulnar	C8, T1	Abduction of fifth digit
Interossei	Ulnar	**C8**, T1	Finger abduction or adduction
Lumbricals three and four	Ulnar	C8	Flexion of proximal phalanx and extension of distal phalanx of digits four and five
Flexor carpi radialis	Median	C6, **C7**	Radial hand flexion
Pronator teres	Median	C6, C7	Forearm pronation

(table continues on page 104)

TABLE 13.5   Common Muscle Groups, Actions, and Innervation *(continued)*

Muscle	Peripheral Nerve	Nerve Root	Action
B. Muscles of the Arm and Hand			
Flexor digitorum superficialis	Median	C7, C8, T1	Flexion of the middle phalanx of digits two to five
Abductor pollicis brevis	Median	C8, **T1**	Abduction of thumb at the metacarpal joint
Flexor pollicis brevis	Median	C8, **T1**	Flexion of thumb at the metacarpal joint
Opponens pollicis	Median	C8, **T1**	Thumb opposition
Lumbricals one and two	Median	C8, **T1**	Flexion of proximal phalanx and extension of distal phalanx of digits two and three
Flexor digitorum profundus	Median (anterior interosseous nerve [AIN])	C7, **C8**	Flexion of distal phalanx of digits two and three
Flexor pollicis longus	Median (AIN)	C7, **C8**	Flexion of distal phalanx of the thumb
Pronator quadratus	Median (AIN)	C8, **T1**	Forearm pronation
C. Muscles of the Hip, Leg, and Foot			
Iliopsoas	Femoral and nerve roots	L1, **L2, L3**	Hip flexion
Sartorius	Femoral	L2, L3	Hip flexion and lateral thigh rotation
Quadriceps femoris	Femoral	L2, **L3, L4**	Knee extension
Adductor longus, brevis, magnus	Obturator	L2, **L3,** L4	Thigh adduction
Gracilis	Obturator	L2, L3, L4	Thigh adduction
Obturator externus	Obturator	L3, L4	Thigh adduction and lateral rotation
Gluteus medius and minimus	Superior gluteal	**L4, L5,** S1	Thigh abduction and medial rotation
Tensor fasciae latae	Superior gluteal	L4, L5	Thigh abduction
Gluteus maximus	Inferior gluteal	**L5, S1,** S2	Hip extension
Biceps femoris (long head)	Sciatic	L5, S1, S2	Knee flexion
Biceps femoris (short head)	Sciatic (fibular)	L5, S1, S2	Knee flexion
Semitendinosus	Sciatic	L5, S1, S2	Knee flexion
Semimembranosus	Sciatic	L5, S1, S2	Knee flexion
Tibialis anterior	Fibular	L4, **L5**	Foot dorsiflexion
Extensor digitorum longus	Fibular	**L5,** S1	Extension of toes two to five
Extensor hallucis longus	Fibular	**L5,** S1	Great toe extension
Extensor digitorum brevis	Fibular	**L5,** S1	Toe extension
Fibularis longus and brevis	Fibular	**L5,** S1	Foot eversion
Tibialis posterior	Tibial	**L5,** S1	Foot inversion and plantarflexion
Flexor digitorum longus	Tibial	S2, S3	Flexion of toes two to four
Flexor hallucis longus	Tibial	S1, S2	Flexion of great toe
Gastrocnemius	Tibial	**S1,** S2	Foot plantarflexion
Soleus	Tibial	**S1**	Foot plantarflexion
Muscles of perineum	Pudendal	S2, S3, S4	Contraction of pelvic floor muscles

The nerve roots in boldface are the dominant roots involved in that particular muscle's innervation.

TABLE 13.6   Common Causes of Weakness

Cortical, Subcortical, or Brain Stem

- Infarct
- Hemorrhage
- Trauma
- Tumor
- Infection (e.g., abscess)
- Vascular malformation
- Complicated migraine
- Postical Todd paralysis
- Demyelinating disease
  - MS
  - ADEM
  - PML

Spinal Cord

- Structural (e.g., disk herniation, syringomyelia)
- Tumor
- Demyelinating disease (e.g., transverse myelitis or NMO)
- Infection (e.g., zoster, HIV, HTLV-1)
- Vascular malformation
- Nutritional (e.g., B_{12} deficiency)
- Spinal cord infarction
- Inflammatory (e.g., lupus, sarcoid)
- Toxic (e.g., nitrous oxide)

Motor Neuron/Anterior Horn

- Amyotrophic lateral sclerosis
- Primary lateral sclerosis
- Progressive muscular atrophy
- Monomelic amyotrophy
- Spinal muscular atrophy
- Poliomyelitis
- Kennedy disease

Nerve Root

- Structural
  - Herniated disk
  - Spondylosis
- Infection
  - CMV polyradiculopathy
  - Lyme

Nerve Root (continued)

- Malignancy
  - Tumor invasion
  - Leptomeningeal metastasis
- Infarction
- Inflammatory
  - Sarcoidosis

Plexus

- Trauma
- Structural
  - Thoracic outlet syndrome
- Idiopathic brachial neuritis (Parsonage–Turner syndrome)
- Radiation plexopathy
- Tumor infiltration
- Diabetic amyotrophy

Peripheral Nerve

- Mononeuropathy
  - Entrapment
    - Carpal tunnel syndrome
    - Ulnar nerve entrapment at the elbow
    - Fibular nerve entrapment at the fibular head
- Mononeuritis multiplex
  - Vasculitis
- Polyneuropathy
  - Demyelinating
    - Acquired
      - AIDP (Guillain–Barré syndrome)
      - CIDP
    - Congenital
      - CMT
- Axonal
  - Associated with systemic disease (diabetes, monoclonal gammopathy, amyloid)
  - Infectious (HIV, Lyme)
  - Nutritious (vitamin deficiency such as B_{12}, B_6, B_1)
  - Toxic (chemotherapy, alcohol, nitrous oxide, arsenic)
  - Autoimmune (anti-MAG, anti-sulfatide)
  - Hereditary (CMT2)

(table continues on page 106)

TABLE 13.6 *Common Causes of Weakness (continued)*

Neuromuscular Junction	Muscle *(continued)*
• Myasthenia gravis	• Endocrine myopathies
• Lambert–Eaton myasthenic syndrome	• Hyper- or hypothyroidism
• Botulism	• Diabetes
• Congenital myasthenia	• Mitochondrial myopathies
Muscle	• MELAS
• Electrolyte imbalance	• Leigh disease
• Hyper-/hypokalemia	• Progressive external ophthalmoplegia
• Hypophosphatemia	• Toxic myopathies
• Hypercalcemia	• Statin
• Metabolic myopathies	• Steroid
• Glycogen storage diseases	• Inflammatory myopathies
• Disorders of lipid metabolism	• Dermatomyositis
• Muscular dystrophies	• Polymyositis
• Dystrophinopathy (e.g., Duchenne/Becker)	• Inclusion body myositis
• Limb girdle muscular dystrophy	• Infectious myositis (e.g., trichinosis)
• Myotonic dystrophy	• Periodic paralysis
• Myotonic dystrophy	• Amyloid myopathy
• Congenital myopathies	• Critical illness myopathy

MS, multiple sclerosis; ADEM, acute disseminated encephalomyelitis; PML, progressive multifocal leukoencephalopathy; NMO, neuromyelitis optica; HTLV-1, human T-lymphotropic virus 1; CMV, cytomegalovirus; AIDP, acute inflammatory demyelinating polyneuropathy; CIDP, chronic inflammatory demyelinating polyneuropathy; CMT, Charcot–Marie–Tooth; MAG, myelin-associated glycoprotein; MELAS, mitochondrial encephalomyopathy, lactic acidosis, and stroke-like episodes.

ELECTRODIAGNOSTIC TESTING

Electrodiagnostic testing (see Chapter 26) is important in the evaluation of weakness due to a peripheral cause. Classically, electrodiagnostic testing consisting of nerve conduction studies and electromyography (EMG) have been the standard practice in the diagnosis of several diseases of the peripheral nervous system. These studies are useful for several reasons. First, they can help to localize the problem to the peripheral nerve and exclude other etiologies such as a primary muscle disease, a plexopathy, or a mononeuropathy. Second, it is of crucial importance in helping to distinguish between generalized and focal forms of either purely axonal or demyelinating forms of neuropathy (such as acute or chronic inflammatory demyelinating neuropathy), which may show evidence of markedly slowed conduction velocity or conduction block. Nerve conduction studies and EMG also help assess the severity of the nerve injury partially in demonstrating whether there is resultant denervation of muscle.

Repetitive stimulation testing can be done to evaluate for neuromuscular junction diseases, which may show evidence of electrodecrement or increment. Single-fiber EMG can be done in certain instances, as it is the most sensitive (although not specific) test for neuromuscular junction disorders. In cases of motor neuron disease, EMG is necessary to demonstrate diffuse active and chronic denervation of several muscles in various distributions. EMG is often abnormal in primary muscle diseases and may show evidence of myopathic changes with or without muscle inflammation.

MUSCLE OR NERVE BIOPSY

In situations where testing is inconclusive, biopsies can be performed on most tissues in an attempt to make a definitive diagnosis (see Chapter 32). This may include biopsy of brain tissue, the meninges, muscle, or nerve. Given the invasive nature of biopsy, this is typically not performed unless there is a clear need and the benefits of the procedure outweigh the risks.

Gait Disorders 14

Ashwini K. Rao

INTRODUCTION

The evolution of locomotion has been very important for humans, as it enabled us to travel greater distances and interact with novel and complex environments. Bipedal locomotion also facilitated the evolution of complex manipulation skills. The capacity for independent gait is crucial for function: For instance, the loss of independent ambulation is a predictor of the need for long-term care in a number of age-related neurologic disorders. In addition to independent gait, achieving a requisite speed is also important for independent mobility in the community. For example, in people who have suffered a stroke, speed of 0.85 m/s is predictive of the ability to independently ambulate in the community.

Gait impairments are very common sequelae of aging and neurologic disorders. At the age of 60 years, about 15% people have gait impairments. Among people older than the age of 85 years, approximately 80% report gait impairments. Even among middle-aged individuals, approximately 40% report mild difficulties with mobility functions. Gait impairments can have devastating consequences, such as falls and injury. Approximately one-third of community-dwelling individuals older than the age of 65 years fall and fall-related injuries increase with age. An unfortunate consequence of gait impairments is that individuals often reduce their mobility in order to prevent falls and related incidents. However, reduced mobility further increases risk for falls by reducing muscle strength and worsening balance.

The purpose of this chapter is to briefly describe the gait cycle, the neural pathways underlying gait, the most commonly seen disorders of gait, and methods for clinical assessment of gait. Finally, we present the risk factors and assessment of falls in the elderly.

INTRODUCTION TO THE GAIT CYCLE

The gait cycle consists of repetitive sequential movements of the limbs that help propel the body forward along a predetermined line of progression. The gait cycle is defined by foot contact with the ground and extends from the heel strike of one lower limb to the subsequent heel strike of the same limb (Fig. 14.1). We define two phases within each gait cycle: a stance phase, which consists of approximately 60% of the gait cycle and a swing phase, which consists of approximately 40% of the gait cycle. Stance phase begins with heel strike and ends with toe off and consists of three events—foot flat, midstance, and heel off. The function of the stance phase is to accept the weight of the body on to the supporting (stance) limb. At the beginning of stance (from heel strike to foot flat on the right side) and at the end of stance (from heel off to toe off on the right), both feet are on the ground simultaneously. The period of double support comprises approximately 20% of the gait cycle. During midstance, body weight is supported by one limb (single limb support). During a typical gait cycle, the lower limbs move in a symmetric alternating movement with a phase lag of 0.5 (indicating that when one limb initiates swing, the opposite limb is in the middle of stance phase).

The swing phase of a limb begins with toe off and ends with heel strike. The events within the swing phase (foot clearance and midswing) serve to allow the foot to clear the floor as it propels the body forward in preparation for the subsequent step. The events within the gait cycle described earlier pertain to walking at a comfortable preferred speed. As speed of gait increases, the percentage of time spent in double support decreases. During running, there is no double support phase. Gait can be described quantitatively

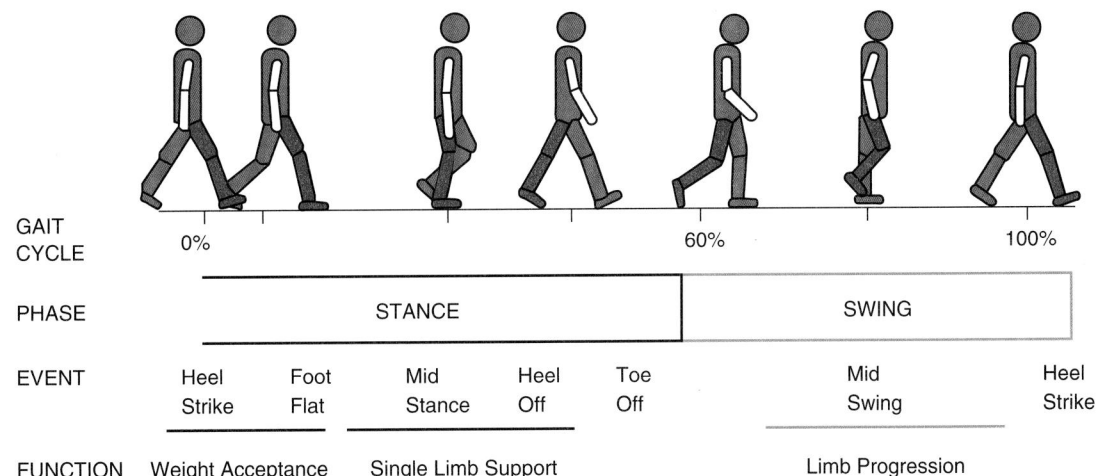

FIGURE 14.1 The gait cycle. The position of the right leg (*shaded red*) shows major events within the gait cycle during stance and swing phases.

TABLE 14.1   Definition of Clinical Gait Measures

Gait Variable	Definition
Speed	Distance covered in unit time (e.g., meters per second)
Cadence	Step frequency—number of steps in a given time (steps per minute)
Step length	Distance (measured in meters along the line of progression) between successive heel strikes of the lower limbs
Stride length	Distance (measured in meters along the line of progression) between successive heel strikes of the same limb
Step width	Distance (measured in meters perpendicular to the line of progression) between successive heel strikes of the lower limbs
Step height	Vertical clearance of the foot from the floor during swing
Step symmetry	Ratio of step length on the right and left sides
Step continuity	Ratio of step time on the right and left sides
Foot angle	Angle formed by the long axis of the foot with the line of progression
Walking path	Direction of the line of progression

with respect to its spatial and temporal features. Gait measures that can be assessed in the clinical setting are described in Table 14.1 and Figure 14.2.

NEURAL CONTROL OF GAIT

Gait is a complex task that requires the coordinated activity of several brain circuits. Even walking in an uncluttered environment at a preferred speed (considered an easy task) elicits activity in higher cortical regions. The following description briefly discusses the role of different circuits in controlling gait. Readers interested in additional details are referred to excellent recent reviews in the suggested readings list. In order to successfully initiate and control gait, the nervous system needs to perform the following tasks:

- Maintain balance against the force of gravity under static (e.g., during stance) and dynamic conditions (e.g., during walking). Maintenance of balance under dynamic conditions includes predictive and reactive control of destabilizing forces that are either generated internally (e.g., destabilizing forces generated by movement of the arms) or externally (e.g., destabilizing forces generated by bumping into another person).

- Coordinate movements of the lower limbs to propel the body forward.
- Help navigate complex environments, which may include stationary obstacles (e.g., furniture) and moving obstacles (e.g., people walking).
- Perform concurrent tasks with walking, such as talking, listening, or manipulating objects (e.g., mobile phone).

Most of the experimental work in understanding the neural control of gait has come from experiments with quadruped and biped animals. These experiments suggest that distinct neural circuits perform specific functions. Cortical circuits (including premotor and motor areas, parietal and occipital areas) are involved with *activation* and *guidance*. Reciprocal circuits between the cortex–basal ganglia and cortex–cerebellum are involved with *regulation* of gait (including postural tone, balance, and coordination of limb movement). Finally, brain stem and spinal cord circuits are involved with the *execution* of gait (including gait initiation, step frequency, reciprocal movements of the lower limbs). A simplified diagram of the neural structures involved in control of gait is presented in Figure 14.3 and functions of brain structures are summarized in Table 14.2.

ACTIVATION AND VISUAL GUIDANCE OF GAIT

Gait can be activated either by a volitional process under the control of cerebral cortical circuits or by emotional cues (fight or flight reaction) under the control of limbic circuits. Volitional guidance of gait requires precise visual information about the environment, which is processed in the visual areas of the occipital cortex. The posterior parietal cortex (PPC) receives information from the visual cortex and project to the motor areas in the frontal cortex. An important function of the PPC is to construct maps of space, which are very important for visual guidance of locomotion. The premotor areas, in particular the supplementary motor area (SMA), are important for postural control during gait. The motor cortex projects to interneurons and motor neurons in the spinal cord and is important in the control of limb movements during gait.

REGULATION OF GAIT

The basal ganglia and cerebellum have a major influence on motor output even though they do not directly project to the spinal cord. The basal ganglia input nuclei, in particular the putamen, receive inputs from the premotor and motor cortex. The output nuclei of the basal ganglia (*globus pallidus internal segment and substantia nigra pars reticulata*) project back to the premotor and motor cortex via the thalamus. These projections are thought to be important for regulating movement amplitude and speed. In addition, the basal ganglia send inhibitory projections to the midbrain locomotor region (MLR) and the pedunculopontine nucleus (PPN). The projection from the basal ganglia to the MLR is responsible for

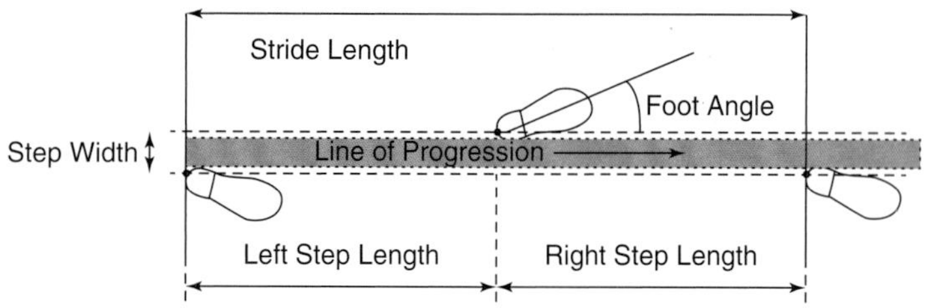

FIGURE 14.2 Spatial characteristics of gait. Spatial gait variables defined by foot placement along the line of progression.

FIGURE 14.3 Neural control of gait. Schematic illustration of neural structures involved in the control of gait. Efferent connections are shown in *blue arrows* and afferent connections in *red arrows*. PPC, posterior parietal cortex; MLR, midbrain locomotor region; PPN, pedunculopontine nucleus; CPG, central pattern generator.

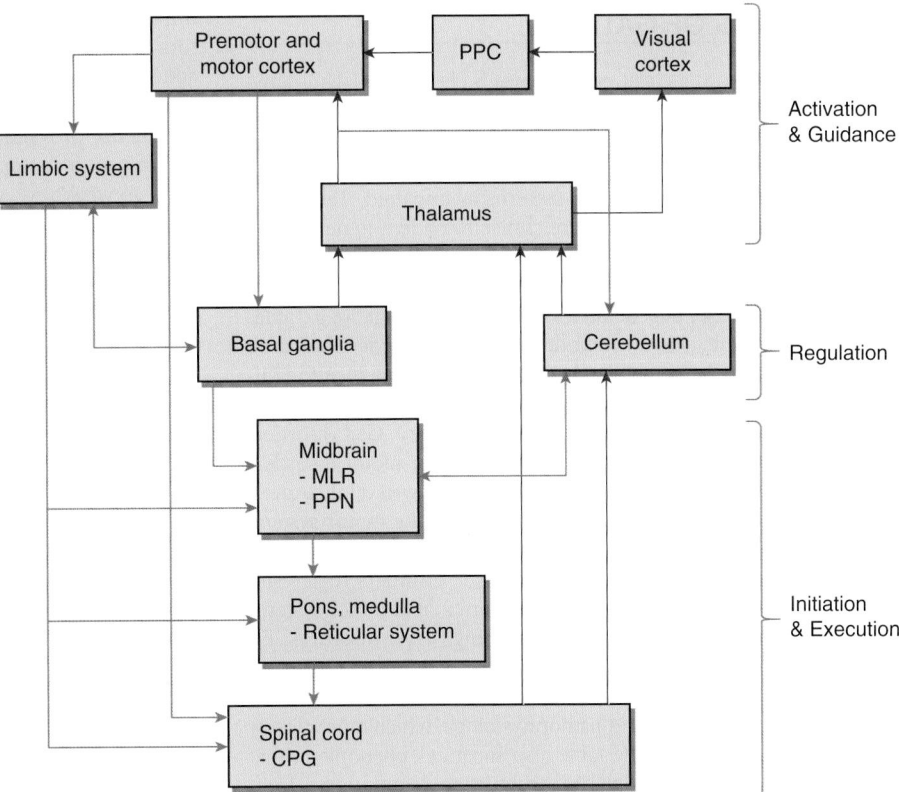

regulating the rhythmic aspects of gait. When there is damage to these projections, as seen in Parkinson disease and Huntington disease, rhythmic control of gait is impaired. The projection from the basal ganglia to the PPN is responsible for regulating muscle tone. Damage to these projections lead to disorders of postural muscle tone, as seen in Parkinson disease.

The cerebellum receives a tremendous amount of afferent information from the limbs and vestibular apparatus. In addition, projections from the cerebral cortex to the cerebellum provide information regarding the upcoming movement. The output of the cerebellum is directed to the motor areas of the cerebral cortex,

midbrain (MLR and PPN), and brain stem (vestibular and reticular nuclei). A major function of the cerebellum is to evaluate disparities between intended movement and actual movement (based on feedback). The cerebellum is important for regulating balance and limb coordination during gait and for providing adaptability to novel conditions based on trial and error learning.

EXECUTION OF GAIT

Two areas in the brain stem are important for initiating and executing locomotion—the MLR and the PPN. The MLR receives inputs from the cerebral cortex, limbic system, basal ganglia, and cerebellum. A primary function of the MLR is activation of spinal cord circuitry to initiate gait. Inputs from the motor areas and the limbic system to MLR provide the neural substrate for activation of gait based on volitional (motor areas) and emotional (limbic system) cues. The PPN also receives inputs from the motor areas of the cerebral cortex, limbic system, basal ganglia, and cerebellum. The PPN inhibits spinal interneurons and motor neurons. A major function of the PPN is to modulate muscle tone during stance and gait. The spinal cord circuitry includes networks of interneurons (central pattern generators) and motor neurons that innervate skeletal muscles. There are two sets of interneurons, termed *half centers*, that project to flexor and extensor motor neurons. The half centers mutually inhibit each other and are responsible for producing the basic locomotor pattern. Although the half centers do not require sensory input to generate the basic locomotor pattern, their activity can be modulated by sensory input from the limbs. For example, signals from proprioceptors of the hip flexors may be used to signal the end of stance phase. In addition, skin afferents from the limbs are important for adjusting stepping movements in the presence of obstacles. Thus, the function of the spinal cord is to execute the rhythmic movement pattern of gait.

TABLE 14.2	**Neural Control of Gait**	
Region	**Area**	**Function**
Cortex	Motor areas	Volitional activation
		Visual guidance
	Limbic system	Emotional activation
Subcortical	Basal ganglia	Inhibition of postural tone
		Regulate rhythmic aspects of gait
	Cerebellum	Balance
		Limb coordination
		Adaptation
Brain stem	MLR	Initiation of locomotor pattern
	PPN	Postural muscle tone
Spinal cord	Interneurons	Control locomotor pattern

MLR, midbrain locomotor region; PPN, pedunculopontine nucleus.

DISORDERS OF GAIT

In neurologic disorders, gait performance is classified as disordered based on comparison with healthy subjects, for whom normative values through the course of aging are available. However, given the large variability of what is considered "normal" gait, caution must be used in order to describe gait patterns as impaired. Table 14.3 highlights gait impairments that are clinically evident in neurologic disorders. Several classifications have been proposed for gait disorders including anatomic, hierarchical (e.g., low, mid, and high level), etiologic (e.g., degenerative) or phenomenologic (e.g., antalgic gait). Anatomic classification describes gait disorders based on brain pathology (e.g., cerebellar gait). Hierarchical classification differentiates gait disorders into three categories based on the level of pathology (e.g., low level, midlevel, and high level). Gait disorders due to peripheral sensory (e.g., sensory ataxic) or motor disorders (e.g., spinal muscular atrophy) are classified as low-level disorders. Disorders that occur as a result of pathology in the motor system, including motor cortical areas, basal ganglia, and cerebellum, are classified as midlevel disorders. Finally, gait disorders that result from the interaction of cognitive (frontal cortex) and motor systems (e.g., Alzheimer disease) are classified as high-level disorders. Finally, classification of gait disorders by phenomenology takes into account etiology and clinical features. In this chapter, gait disorders are classified by hierarchy and pathophysiology, which more closely reflects clinical practice. The table also separates phenomena that may be observed throughout gait observation (continuous) from those that are unpredictable (episodic). According to this classification, continuous phenomena reflect the underlying pathology and compensatory mechanisms, whereas episodic phenomena are those that the patient cannot adapt to because of their unpredictability.

FALLS IN THE ELDERLY

Falls are defined as "unexpected events in which a person comes to rest on the floor, ground, or supporting surface." Falls are considered an inevitable consequence of aging and may result in serious adverse events in older adults. Approximately one-third of community-dwelling people older than the age of 65 years fall each year. The number of falls is much higher for older people living in nursing homes: approximately 1.5 falls per bed per year. The high incidence of falls coupled with the susceptibility to injury (because of comorbidities and age-related physiologic changes) leads to adverse events in the elderly. Falls may result in injuries such as abrasions, bruising, lacerations, and sprains. It is important to note that falls resulting in minor injuries may be underreported by patients. A careful ascertainment of history of falls is very important in clinical practice. About 10% of falls result in fractures, the type of fracture depending on the nature of the fall. Forward or backward falls on outstretched hands result in wrist fractures, falls to the side result in hip fractures, and falls resulting in impact to the head may result in head injury and loss of consciousness. Backward falls on the buttocks result in lower rates of fractures, although fractures of the vertebrae can occur.

Falls account for two-thirds of accidental deaths. The other negative consequences of falls include increased fear of falls and reduced mobility. This results in a negative spiral: Reduced mobility leads to reduction in muscle strength, flexibility and postural stability, and gait impairments, all of which, in turn, increase the risk for additional falls. Falls have a significant negative impact on the quality of life of elders.

Risk factors for falls can be classified as intrinsic or extrinsic. Intrinsic factors include age, muscle strength, gait and balance impairments, and neurologic or cognitive disorder. Extrinsic factors include medications, environmental hazards, and type of activity (based on hazard). The greatest risk factors for falls are previous history of falls, muscle weakness, gait and balance impairments, use of walking aids, vertigo, Parkinson disease, and medication use. It is important to note that a number of these factors, such as weakness, gait and balance impairments, use of walking aids, and medications are modifiable factors. Often, patients report near falls, defined as a "loss of balance that would have resulted in a fall if sufficient recovery mechanisms (movement of the trunk or arms, change in stride length or velocity) were not activated." Near falls often precede falls and are more frequent than falls. Clinical assessment of falls should include information on near fall events. More information on fall assessment appears in the following section. Physical exercise (under the supervision of a physical or occupational therapist) is effective in reducing the frequency of falls and preventing future falls. In addition, home hazard assessment and reduction (under the supervision of occupational therapists) reduces the frequency of fallers and the number of falls. Clinicians should consult physical and occupational therapists, as needed.

CLINICAL ASSESSMENT OF STANCE, GAIT, AND FALLS

Assessment should include a detailed medical history and clinical exam, which consists of two parts: clinical observation and standardized assessment. A summary of the clinical assessment procedures is provided in Table 14.4.

HISTORY

It is important to document the history of acute and chronic medical problems, history of near falls and falls, history of problems with balance and gait, and level of physical activity. Ask the patient about the most recent fall and ascertain the circumstances around the fall, including what the patient was doing, what caused the fall, where the fall occurred, environmental hazards that may have caused the fall, and the consequence of the fall.

MEDICATIONS

Note the list of prescribed medications and if any medications and/ or dosages have been recently modified.

FOCUSED EXAMINATION

Physical examination should include an assessment of musculoskeletal function and footwear. Neurologic examination should include tests of cognitive function (using an assessment such as the Montreal Cognitive Assessment), muscle strength, reflexes, sensation, coordination, and presence of involuntary movements.

BALANCE AND GAIT ASSESSMENT

The examination begins with observation of a patient in a quiet stance. Clinicians should observe the patient from the front, back, and side. Determine if head is flexed, translated forward or backward, or tilted to one side. It is important to note if the shoulders are level or positioned asymmetrically. Examine if shoulders are hunched (rotated) forward. Note the position of the trunk to determine if it is kyphotic (rounded) as seen in disorders of aging or lordotic (hyperextended). Examine if trunk is tilted to one side, as this may be an indication of pain, diminished sensory feedback, or impaired vestibular system.

TABLE 14.3   Disorders of Gait

Disorder	Continuous Phenomena (Speed, Support Base, Arm Swing, Symmetry, Path)	Episodic Phenomena (Freezing of Gait, Gait Initiation, Falls)
High-Level Gait Disorders		
Alzheimer disease Gait disorder occurs late in the disease.	Slow gait speed Short step length Lower cadence Increased percentage of time in double support Increased variability, particularly when performing cognitive dual task	Increased risk for falls
Mild cognitive impairment (MCI)	Slow gait speed Short step or stride length Increased percentage of time in double support Gait variability is higher in amnestic MCI but not in nonamnestic MCI Poor limb coordination (foot tapping) compared with controls	Increased risk for falls and fear of falls
Vascular dementia Gait disorder occurs early in the disease.	Slow gait speed Short step length Wide support base Rigidity	Freezing of gait Imbalance and falls seen
Normal pressure hydrocephalus Gait disorder seen early in the disease in conjunction with cognitive impairment and urinary incontinence.	Slow gait speed Short step length Wide support base and outward rotation of foot (may be compensation for poor balance) Asymmetric steps Low step height (shuffling steps)	Increased risk for falls
Dementia with Lewy bodies Gait impairments seen in conjunction with visual hallucinations.	Slow gait speed Reduced arm swing Flexed trunk posture Rigidity	Increased risk for falls
Frontotemporal dementia Gait impairments seen in the presence of behavioral disturbances (impulsivity, disinhibition).	Slow gait speed Involuntary trunk movements Postural instability	Increased risk for falls
Psychogenic gait disorder Gait impairments seen in the presence of psychiatric disorders such as anxiety, depression, or personality disorder.	Gait impairments are not consistent from one session to the next, may have sudden onset, very severe impairments at onset, and spontaneous remissions. Astasia-abasia Knee buckling during stance Wide support base and short step length (waddling) Excessive retropulsion	Tremor and dystonia seen although may not be observed when the patient is distracted

(table continues on page 112)

TABLE 14.3   Disorders of Gait *(continued)*

Disorder	Continuous Phenomena (Speed, Support Base, Arm Swing, Symmetry, Path)	Episodic Phenomena (Freezing of Gait, Gait Initiation, Falls)
Midlevel Gait Disorders		
Hemiparesis	Slow gait speed	Increased risk for falls
	Asymmetric stepping	
	During swing	
	Impaired lower limb moves in circumduction; hip hiking seen (Trendelenburg sign)	
	Ankle may be maintained in plantar flexion and inversion leading to loss of heel strike at the beginning of stance.	
	During stance, knee joint may hyperextend.	
	Reduced arm swing on impaired side and reduced trunk rotation	
	During dual-task gait, impairments worsen.	
Paraparesis	Slow gait speed	Increased risk for falls due to weakness and imbalance
	Low cadence	
	Low step height	
	Circumduction may be seen.	
	Decreased support base (scissoring gait) seen in patients with spasticity	
Parkinson disease	Slow gait speed	Freezing of gait
Gait impairments seen in the presence of tremor, rigidity, and postural instability.	Very short step length	Difficulty initiating gait
	Poor foot clearance during swing (which leads to shuffling gait)	Increased fear of falls and increased risk for falls as disease progresses
	Increased temporal variability	
	Postural instability and impaired balance seen (missteps during tandem gait)	
	During dual-task gait, Parkinson disease patients pay greater attention to secondary cognitive task as opposed to gait leading to greater gait impairments (posture second strategy).	
Multiple system atrophy	May present like Parkinson disease (slow speed, short step length)	Increased risk for falls as disease progresses
Gait impairments seen in the presence of autonomic dysfunction and urinary incontinence.	May present like cerebellar ataxia (gait ataxia—increased support base, path deviation, postural instability, impaired balance—missteps during tandem gait)	
Progressive supranuclear palsy	Postural instability	High risk for falls, increased fear of falls
	Wide support base	
	Rigid support base	
	Slow gait speed	
	Difficulty turning (turn en bloc)	
Huntington disease	Slow gait speed	Increased fear of falls and greater number of falls as disease progresses
	Decreased step/stride length	
	Decreased cadence	
	Increased time in double support	
	Asymmetric step length	
	Inconsistent step time	
	Increased temporal variability	
	Gait impairments worsen during secondary dual task	
	Chorea of limbs or trunk may increase instability.	

TABLE 14.3 Disorders of Gait (continued)

Disorder	Continuous Phenomena (Speed, Support Base, Arm Swing, Symmetry, Path)	Episodic Phenomena (Freezing of Gait, Gait Initiation, Falls)
Essential tremor	Slow gait speed Decreased cadence Increased time in double support Asymmetric step length Wide support base Increased temporal variability Prominent balance impairment (missteps during tandem gait)	Increased fear of falls and greater number of falls
Cerebellar ataxia	Inconsistent step time Asymmetric step length Short step length and low step height Wide support base Increased temporal variability Increased postural sway Greater missteps during tandem gait	High risk for falls, increased fear of falls

Low-Level Gait Disorders

1. Peripheral sensory disorders (peripheral neuropathy, posterior *column* disorder, vestibular and visual deficit)

Sensory ataxic gait	Wide support base Postural instability increased when standing with eyes closed Increased step height (steppage gait) Short step length Foot slap evident at the beginning of stance phase Patients tend to look at their feet while walking.	Increased risk for falls when not using vision

2. Peripheral *motor* disorders

Antalgic gait	Decreased weight bearing on painful limb leading to shorter stance phase Short stride length Reduced range of motion in affected joint(s) Trendelenburg sign may be seen due to pain at the hip joint.	
Spinal muscular atrophy	Slow gait speed Decreased step/stride length Decreased cadence Wide support base Trendelenburg sign Impairments (particularly speed and cadence) worsen with fatigue during continuous walking.	Increased risk for falls
Duchenne muscular dystrophy	Lordotic posture and anterior pelvic tilt Waddling gait (short step length, wide support base) Knee hyperextension during stance Ankle plantar flexion during swing Gait pattern does not change with continuous walking.	Increased risk for falls

TABLE 14.4   Clinical Assessment

History	Falls and near falls
	Level of physical activity
	Complaints of gait and balance
Medications	Prescribed medications
	Change in medication or dosage
Most recent fall incident	1. What was the patient doing?
	(Standing, walking, turning, bending, reaching for objects, transfers, climbing on step-stool or ladder, recreational activity)
	2. What caused the fall?
	(Dizziness, loss of balance, weakness, dual-task performance, slip/trip, fatigue, bumped into object)
	3. Where did the fall occur?
	(Indoor level surface, indoor uneven surface, outdoor level surface, outdoor uneven surface)
	4. Did environmental hazard cause fall?
	(Icy or wet surface, clutter, rugs/carpet, darkness, moving objects)
	5. What was the result of the fall?
	(Minor injury, major injury)
Physical examination	Cognitive function
	(e.g., Montreal Cognitive Assessment [MoCA])
	Musculoskeletal examination
	(Range of motion, joint pain, swelling)
	Footwear
	(Sandals, flip-flops, sneakers)
Neurologic examination	Muscle strength
	Reflexes
	Sensation
	Presence of involuntary movements
	Coordination
Balance and gait assessment	Clinical observation and standardized assessments. Please see Table 14.5.
Environmental assessment	Presence of safety grab bars
	Clutter and presence of area rugs or carpets
	Adequacy of lighting
	Height of chairs
	Surfaces (uneven, incline, stairs)
	Use of walking aids (cane, walker)

Upper Extremities

Healthy people tend to maintain their arms next to the trunk with slight internal rotation at the shoulder and extension at the elbows. Observe if the arm is maintained in a flexed and internally rotated posture (as is often the case in people with stroke) and if involuntary movements are present (such as writhing choreic movements in Huntington disease or resting hand tremor seen in Parkinson disease). Also note if the hand is maintained in a fixed posture, as this may be a sign of dystonia.

Lower Extremities

Healthy people stand with the pelvis in a neutral position and lower limbs extended with the feet pointing straight ahead. Note if the hip and knee joints are maintained in flexion, as is sometimes seen in people with muscle tightness or weakness.

Ensure that there is adequate space (length of 7 to 10 m) to conduct a comprehensive gait assessment. Observe the patient from the front, back, and sides. Note the position of the head and trunk during gait, presence or absence of arm swing, and instability during walking and turning.

- *Standard walk*: Ask the patient to walk at their comfortable pace. Observe position of the head and trunk, walking path, and length and symmetry of steps. Note presence of instability during gait.
- *Turns*: Ask the patient to turn and observe the number of steps taken to turn. Note presence of instability during turns.

TABLE 14.5   Standardized Assessments of Mobility, Balance, and Fall Risk

Assessment	Details	Clinical Indication
Timed up and go	Time taken to get up from a seated position, walk 3 m, turn around, walk back, and take a seat	Increased fall risk in the following: a) Community-dwelling elderly: >13.5 s b) Parkinson disease: >11.5 s c) Stroke: >14 s
Tinetti performance–oriented mobility assessment	Balance scale consists of nine items that assess balance in sitting, standing, transitions, and turning.	Total score is 28. Score >25 indicates low fall risk, score between 19 and 24 indicates medium fall risk, and scores <19 indicate high fall risk.
Berg Balance Scale	Measures performance on 14 functional tests of sitting and standing balance, transfers, turning, etc.	Total score is 56. Scores <45 indicative of increased fall risk.
Dynamic Gait Index	Measures ability to walk a distance of 6.1 m (20 ft) under external demands (such as head turns)	Total score is 24. Score <19 indicative of fall risk.
Walking while talking	Examines whether patients are able to walk while reciting the alphabet (simple) or every alternate alphabet (complex)	Community-dwelling elderly: >20 s for simple task; >30 s for complex task indicative of falls.
10-m walk	Patient is asked to walk a distance of 10 m at either a self-selected comfortable speed or fast speed. Time taken to cover middle 6-m distance is measured to eliminate the effect of acceleration and deceleration.	Household ambulator = speed <0.4 m/s; Limited community ambulator = speed between 0.4 and 0.8 m/s; Community ambulator = speed >0.8 m/s
Tandem walk	Measures ability to walk 10 steps tandem (heel to toe) walk	<2 completed steps indicative of fall risk
6-min walk test	Measures the distance walked in a period of 6 min along a 30-m long walkway	Distance <400 m indicates lack of aerobic capacity.

- *Narrow doorway*: Ask the patient to walk through a narrow doorway. This test is provocative for freezing of gait. Note presence of freezing.
- *Tandem walk*: Ask the patient to walk heel to toe for 10 steps. Note whether the patient can perform the task without support and the number of steps taken away from a straight line.
- *Dual-task walk*: Ask the patient to walk at his or her comfortable speed while performing a secondary motor or cognitive task. Typical secondary motor tasks include carrying a cup of water or carrying a tray with a cup on it. Several secondary cognitive tasks have been employed and include the following:
  - Count backwards: Give the patient a number and ask him or her to count backwards by 3 (serial 3) or by 7 (serial 7). Note that performance on the serial 7 task is dependent on level of education and may be too difficult for several patients.
  - Verbal fluency: Ask the patient to generate words that begin with a certain letter (such as "d") or words that belong to a category (e.g., animals).
  - Walking while talking: Ask the patient a question (such as "What did you have for breakfast today?")

In addition to clinical observation, several standardized assessments of mobility, balance, and fall risk are available, summarized in Table 14.5.

SUGGESTED READINGS

Aarsland D, Ballard C, McKeith I, et al. Comparison of extrapyramidal signs in dementia with Lewy bodies and Parkinson's disease. *J Neuropsychiatry Clin Neurosci.* 2001;13:374–379.

Aarsland D, Larsen JP, Tandberg E, et al. Predictors of nursing home placement in Parkinson's disease: a population-based, prospective study. *J Am Geriatr Soc.* 2000;48:938–942.

Alexander NB, Goldberg A. Gait disorders: search for multiple causes. *Cleve Clin J Med.* 2005;72:586, 589–590, 592–584 passim.

Al-Yahya E, Dawes H, Smith L, et al. Cognitive motor interference while walking: a systematic review and meta-analysis. *Neurosci Biobehav Rev.* 2011;35:715–728.

Al-Zahrani KS, Bakheit AM. A study of the gait characteristics of patients with chronic osteoarthritis of the knee. *Disabil Rehabil.* 2002;24:275–280.

Arkadir D, Louis ED. The balance and gait disorder of essential tremor: what does this mean for patients? *Ther Adv Neurol Disord.* 2013;6:229–236.

Beauchet O, Allali G, Berrut G, et al. Gait analysis in demented subjects: interests and perspectives. *Neuropsychiatr Dis Treat.* 2008;4:155–160.

Behrman AL, Bowden MG, Nair PM. Neuroplasticity after spinal cord injury and training: an emerging paradigm shift in rehabilitation and walking recovery. *Phys Ther.* 2006;86:1406–1425.

Berg KO, Wood-Dauphinee SL, Williams JI, et al. Measuring balance in the elderly: validation of an instrument. *Can J Public Health.* 1992;83(suppl 2):S7–S11.

Bilney B, Morris ME, Churchyard A, et al. Evidence for a disorder of locomotor timing in Huntington's disease. *Mov Disord.* 2005;20:51–57.

Bloem BR, Haan J, Lagaay AM, et al. Investigation of gait in elderly subjects over 88 years of age. *J Geriatr Psychiatry Neurol.* 1992;5:78–84.

Bohannon RW. Comfortable and maximum walking speed of adults aged 20–79 years: reference values and determinants. *Age Ageing.* 1997;26:15–19.

Bowden MG, Balasubramanian CK, Behrman AL, et al. Validation of a speed-based classification system using quantitative measures of walking performance poststroke. *Neurorehabil Neural Repair.* 2008;22:672–675.

Bugalho P, Alves L, Miguel R. Gait dysfunction in Parkinson's disease and normal pressure hydrocephalus: a comparative study. *J Neural Transm.* 2013;120:1201–1207.

Cameron ID, Gillespie LD, Robertson MC, et al. Interventions for preventing falls in older people in care facilities and hospitals. *Cochrane Database Syst Rev.* 2012;12:CD005465.

Cooper KH. A means of assessing maximal oxygen intake. Correlation between field and treadmill testing. *JAMA.* 1968;203:201–204.

D'Angelo MG, Berti M, Piccinini L, et al. Gait pattern in Duchenne muscular dystrophy. Gait Posture. 2009;29:36–41.

Deandrea S, Lucenteforte E, Bravi F, et al. Risk factors for falls in community-dwelling older people: a systematic review and meta-analysis. Epidemiology. 2010;21:658–668.

DeLong MR, Wichmann T. Circuits and circuit disorders of the basal ganglia. *Arch Neurol.* 2007;64:20–24.

Delval A, Krystkowiak P, Delliaux M, et al. Role of attentional resources on gait performance in Huntington's disease. Mov Disord. 2008;23:684–689.

Drew T, Andujar JE, Lajoie K, et al. Cortical mechanisms involved in visuo-motor coordination during precision walking. *Brain Res Rev.* 2008;57: 199–211.

Drew T, Prentice S, Schepens B. Cortical and brainstem control of locomotion. *Prog Brain Res.* 2004;143:251–261.

Fasano A, Bloem BR. Gait disorders. *Continuum (Minneap Minn).* 2013;19: 1344–1382.

Fogel JF, Hyman RB, Rock B, et al. Predictors of hospital length of stay and nursing home placement in an elderly medical population. *J Am Med Dir Assoc.* 2000;1:202–210.

Franssen EH, Souren LE, Torossian CL, et al. Equilibrium and limb coordination in mild cognitive impairment and mild Alzheimer's disease. *J Am Geriatr Soc.* 1999;47:463–469.

Giladi N, Horak FB, Hausdorff JM. Classification of gait disturbances: distinguishing between continuous and episodic changes. *Mov Disord.* 2013;28: 1469–1473.

Gillespie LD, Robertson MC, Gillespie WJ, et al. Interventions for preventing falls in older people living in the community. *Cochrane Database Syst Rev.* 2012;9:CD007146.

Grillner S, Wallen P, Saitoh K, et al. Neural bases of goal-directed locomotion in vertebrates—an overview. *Brain Res Rev.* 2008;57:2–12.

Gurevich T, Giladi N. Freezing of gait in multiple system atrophy (MSA). *Parkinsonism Relat Disord.* 2003;9:169–174.

Hallett M, Weiner WJ, Kompoliti K. Psychogenic movement disorders. *Parkinsonism Relat Disord.* 2012;18(suppl 1):S155–S157.

Hausdorff JM, Cudkowicz ME, Firtion R, et al. Gait variability and basal ganglia disorders: stride-to-stride variations of gait cycle timing in Parkinson's disease and Huntington's disease. *Mov Disord.* 1998;13:428–437.

Hollman JH, McDade EM, Petersen RC. Normative spatiotemporal gait parameters in older adults. *Gait Posture.* 2011;34:111–118.

Karlsson MK, Vonschewelov T, Karlsson C, et al. Prevention of falls in the elderly: a review. *Scand J Public Health.* 2013;41:442–454.

Koenraadt KL, Roelofsen EG, Duysens J, et al. Cortical control of normal gait and precision stepping: an fNIRS study. *Neuroimage.* 2014;85(pt 1): 415–422.

Lamb SE, Jorstad-Stein EC, Hauer K, et al. Development of a common outcome data set for fall injury prevention trials: the Prevention of Falls Network Europe consensus. *J Am Geriatr Soc.* 2005;53:1618–1622.

Lim MR, Huang RC, Wu A, et al. Evaluation of the elderly patient with an abnormal gait. *J Am Acad Orthop Surg.* 2007;15:107–117.

Litvan I. Progressive supranuclear palsy and corticobasal degeneration. *Baillieres Clin Neurol.* 1997;6:167–185.

Litvan I, Campbell G, Mangone CA, et al. Which clinical features differentiate progressive supranuclear palsy (Steele-Richardson-Olszewski syndrome) from related disorders? A clinicopathological study. *Brain.* 1997;120(pt 1):65–74.

Maidan I, Freedman T, Tzemah R, et al. Introducing a new definition of a near fall: intra-rater and inter-rater reliability. *Gait Posture.* 2014;39: 645–647.

Martin LG, Freedman VA, Schoeni RF, et al. Trends in disability and related chronic conditions among people ages fifty to sixty-four. *Health Aff (Millwood).* 2010;29:725–731.

Montes J, Blumenschine M, Dunaway S, et al. Weakness and fatigue in diverse neuromuscular diseases. *J Child Neurol.* 2013;28:1277–1283.

Montes J, Dunaway S, Montgomery MJ, et al. Fatigue leads to gait changes in spinal muscular atrophy. *Muscle Nerve.* 2011;43:485–488.

Moretti R, Torre P, Antonello RM, et al. Gait and equilibrium in subcortical vascular dementia. *Curr Gerontol Geriatr Res.* 2011;2011:263507.

Morris ME, Huxham F, McGinley J, et al. The biomechanics and motor control of gait in Parkinson disease. *Clin Biomech (Bristol, Avon).* 2001;16:459–470.

Morton SM, Bastian AJ. Mechanisms of cerebellar gait ataxia. *Cerebellum.* 2007;6:79–86.

Nevitt MC, Cummings SR. Type of fall and risk of hip and wrist fractures: the study of osteoporotic fractures. The Study of Osteoporotic Fractures Research Group. *J Am Geriatr Soc.* 1993;41:1226–1234.

Olney SJ, Griffin MP, McBride ID. Multivariate examination of data from gait analysis of persons with stroke. *Phys Ther.* 1998;78:814–828.

Peel NM, Kassulke DJ, McClure RJ. Population based study of hospitalised fall related injuries in older people. *Inj Prev.* 2002;8:280–283.

Perry J, Garrett M, Gronley JK, et al. Classification of walking handicap in the stroke population. *Stroke.* 1995;26:982–989.

Pijnenburg YA, Gillissen F, Jonker C, et al. Initial complaints in frontotemporal lobar degeneration. *Dement Geriatr Cogn Disord.* 2004;17:302–306.

Plummer-D'Amato P, Altmann LJ, Saracino D, et al. Interactions between cognitive tasks and gait after stroke: a dual task study. *Gait Posture.* 2008;27: 683–688.

Podsiadlo D, Richardson S. The timed "Up & Go": a test of basic functional mobility for frail elderly persons. *J Am Geriatr Soc.* 1991;39:142–148.

Pugh KG, Lipsitz LA. The microvascular frontal-subcortical syndrome of aging. *Neurobiol Aging.* 2002;23:421–431.

Rao AK, Gillman A, Louis ED. Quantitative gait analysis in essential tremor reveals impairments that are maintained into advanced age. *Gait Posture.* 2011;34:65–70.

Rao AK, Muratori L, Louis ED, et al. Spectrum of gait impairments in presymptomatic and symptomatic Huntington's disease. *Mov Disord.* 2008;23: 1100–1107.

Rao AK, Uddin J, Gillman A, et al. Cognitive motor interference during dual-task gait in essential tremor. *Gait Posture.* 2013;38:403–409.

Rochester L, Galna B, Lord S, et al. The nature of dual-task interference during gait in incident Parkinson's disease. *Neuroscience.* 2014;265:83–94.

Rubenstein LZ. Falls in older people: epidemiology, risk factors and strategies for prevention. *Age Ageing.* 2006;35(suppl 2):ii37–ii41.

Rubenstein LZ, Josephson KR, Robbins AS. Falls in the nursing home. *Ann Intern Med.* 1994;121:442–451.

Sheridan PL, Hausdorff JM. The role of higher-level cognitive function in gait: executive dysfunction contributes to fall risk in Alzheimer's disease. *Dement Geriatr Cogn Disord.* 2007;24:125–137.

Shimada H, Suzukawa M, Tiedemann A, et al. Which neuromuscular or cognitive test is the optimal screening tool to predict falls in frail community-dwelling older people? *Gerontology.* 2009;55:532–538.

Shumway-Cook A, Baldwin M, Polissar NL, et al. Predicting the probability for falls in community-dwelling older adults. *Phys Ther.* 1997;77:812–819.

Sjogren M, Andersen C. Frontotemporal dementia—a brief review. *Mech Ageing Dev.* 2006;127:180–187.

Snijders AH, van de Warrenburg BP, Giladi N, et al. Neurological gait disorders in elderly people: clinical approach and classification. *Lancet Neurol.* 2007;6:63–74.

Sofuwa O, Nieuwboer A, Desloovere K, et al. Quantitative gait analysis in Parkinson's disease: comparison with a healthy control group. *Arch Phys Med Rehabil.* 2005;86:1007–1013.

Steffen TM, Hacker TA, Mollinger L. Age- and gender-related test performance in community-dwelling elderly people: six-minute walk test, berg balance scale, timed up & go test, and gait speeds. *Phys Ther.* 2002;82:128–137.

Stolze H, Klebe S, Petersen G, et al. Typical features of cerebellar ataxic gait. *J Neurol Neurosurg Psychiatry.* 2002;73:310–312.

Stolze H, Kuhtz-Buschbeck JP, Drucke H, et al. Comparative analysis of the gait disorder of normal pressure hydrocephalus and Parkinson's disease. *J Neurol Neurosurg Psychiatry.* 2001;70:289–297.

Takakusaki K. Neurophysiology of gait: from the spinal cord to the frontal lobe. *Mov Disord.* 2013;28:1483–1491.

Takakusaki K, Tomita N, Yano M. Substrates for normal gait and pathophysiology of gait disturbances with respect to the basal ganglia dysfunction. *J Neurol.* 2008;255(suppl 4):19–29.

Talley KM, Wyman JF, Gross CR, et al. Change in balance confidence and its associations with increasing disability in older community-dwelling women at risk for falling. *J Aging Health.* 2014;26:616–636.

Thach WT, Bastian AJ. Role of the cerebellum in the control and adaptation of gait in health and disease. *Prog Brain Res.* 2004;143:353–366.

Tinetti ME. Performance-oriented assessment of mobility problems in elderly patients. *J Am Geriatr Soc.* 1986;34:119–126.

Tinetti ME, Speechley M, Ginter SF. Risk factors for falls among elderly persons living in the community. *N Engl J Med.* 1988;319:1701–1707.

van Iersel MB, Hoefsloot W, Munneke M, et al. Systematic review of quantitative clinical gait analysis in patients with dementia. *Z Gerontol Geriatr.* 2004;37:27–32.

Verghese J, Buschke H, Viola L, et al. Validity of divided attention tasks in predicting falls in older individuals: a preliminary study. *J Am Geriatr Soc.* 2002;50:1572–1576.

Verghese J, Robbins M, Holtzer R, et al. Gait dysfunction in mild cognitive impairment syndromes. *J Am Geriatr Soc.* 2008;56:1244–1251.

Waite LM, Broe GA, Grayson DA, et al. Motor function and disability in the dementias. *Int J Geriatr Psychiatry.* 2000;15:897–903.

Wenning GK, Ben Shlomo Y, Magalhaes M, et al. Clinical features and natural history of multiple system atrophy. An analysis of 100 cases. *Brain.* 1994;117(pt 4):835–845.

Wheelock VL, Tempkin T, Marder K, et al. Predictors of nursing home placement in Huntington disease. *Neurology.* 2003;60:998–1001.

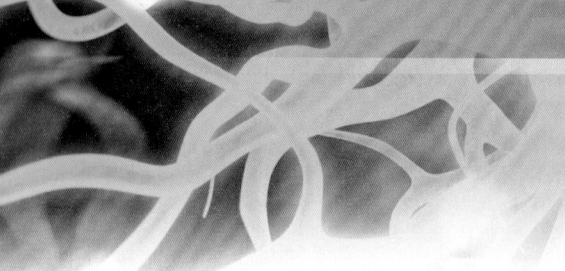

Acute Stroke: The First Hour 15

Barry M. Czeisler and Stephan A. Mayer

INTRODUCTION

Sudden focal neurologic deficits can result from a variety of causes, the most frequent and concerning of which is acute stroke. The two most common forms of stroke that cause sudden onset of focal neurologic deficits without antecedent symptoms are acute ischemic stroke (AIS) and intracerebral hemorrhage (ICH). Both conditions are neurologic emergencies. The symptoms of AIS and ICH (Table 15.1) have significant overlap necessitating imaging studies to distinguish the two conditions.

The greatest opportunity to positively impact on the ultimate outcome of the patient with stroke occurs within the first hour of diagnosis and within 4 hours of the onset of symptoms. Emergency management of AIS is focused on attaining vascular reperfusion as soon as possible, most commonly with the administration of intravenous tissue plasminogen activator (IV tPA) for thrombolysis. In most cases, the outer limit of the time window for effective intervention is 4.5 hours after symptom onset. It has been estimated that every 15-minute reduction in onset-to-treatment time translates into a meaningful reduction in the risk of long-term disability at 3 months. In the case of ICH, emergency care is focused on blood pressure control, reversal of anticoagulation, and management of intracranial pressure (ICP).

This chapter focuses on the emergency management of the patient presenting with an acute focal neurologic deficit. Subsequent management after the first hour is discussed in Chapter 35 for AIS and in Chapter 38 for ICH.

PHASE 1: INITIAL MANAGEMENT AND IMAGING

Due to the importance of early intervention in stroke, the emphasis of emergency department (ED) management should not be on identifying subtle, unusual, or interesting neurologic signs but on the following five simple priorities. These tasks are ideally performed in parallel by four different personnel immediately upon

TABLE 15.1   Symptoms of Acute Stroke

Facial asymmetry
Lateralized limb weakness or clumsiness
Lateralized numbness or paresthesias
Slurred or confused speech
Visual disturbances (diplopia or difficulty seeing)
Dizziness or vertigo
Gait instability
Headache
Alterations in level of consciousness

patient arrival (e.g., the ED attending, resident, nurse, and stroke neurologist):

1. Assess level of consciousness and ensure adequate airway, breathing, and circulation.
2. Obtain the history with precise attention to the specific time of onset (or discovery) of symptoms along with a list of current medications.
3. Establish large-bore (preferably 18 gauge) intravenous access, and obtain admission labs.
4. Perform a National Institutes of Health (NIH) Stroke Scale examination.
5. Obtain head computed tomography (CT) imaging as soon as possible.

Modern emergency stroke management is evolving toward a paradigm that resembles trauma resuscitation. The initial goal is to minimize door-to-CT time because subsequent management is entirely dependent on the results of the scan. For AIS, the conventional goal is to obtain CT within 20 minutes and to start tPA infusion within 60 minutes of arrival to the ED (Figure 15.1). Currently, most hospitals struggle to have half of their AIS patients meet these targets.

New acute stroke care delivery models emphasizing parallel processing and lean management principles that exclude unnecessary steps have been shown to significantly reduce door-to-needle time for AIS. In the Helsinki model, physicians have proven the feasibility of safely administering IV tPA within 20 minutes of hospital arrival. In this paradigm, prehospital notification by ambulance triggers the stroke code, which then leads to the following:

1. Notification of the stroke team and ED staff, which assembles to meet the patient at the CT scanner
2. Transmitting the mobile phone number of any first responders or eyewitnesses to the stroke team to facilitate obtaining the history
3. Establishing a medical record number and hospital chart prior to arrival
4. Preordering the CT scan
5. Notification of pharmacy so that tPA or an anticoagulation reversing agent can be provided as soon as possible after CT

Given the complexity of coordinated personnel, resources, preparation, and teamwork that is required, most municipalities triage acute stroke patients directly to hospitals that are designated as primary stroke centers. After the initial resuscitation is completed, if the patient is unusually complex or critically ill, consideration should be given to transferring the patient to the nearest comprehensive stroke center.

INITIAL SURVEY AND VITAL SIGNS PRIOR TO COMPUTED TOMOGRAPHY

Level of Consciousness

ICH with mass effect as well as ischemic strokes of the brain stem, thalami, or large cortical regions can cause impairment in

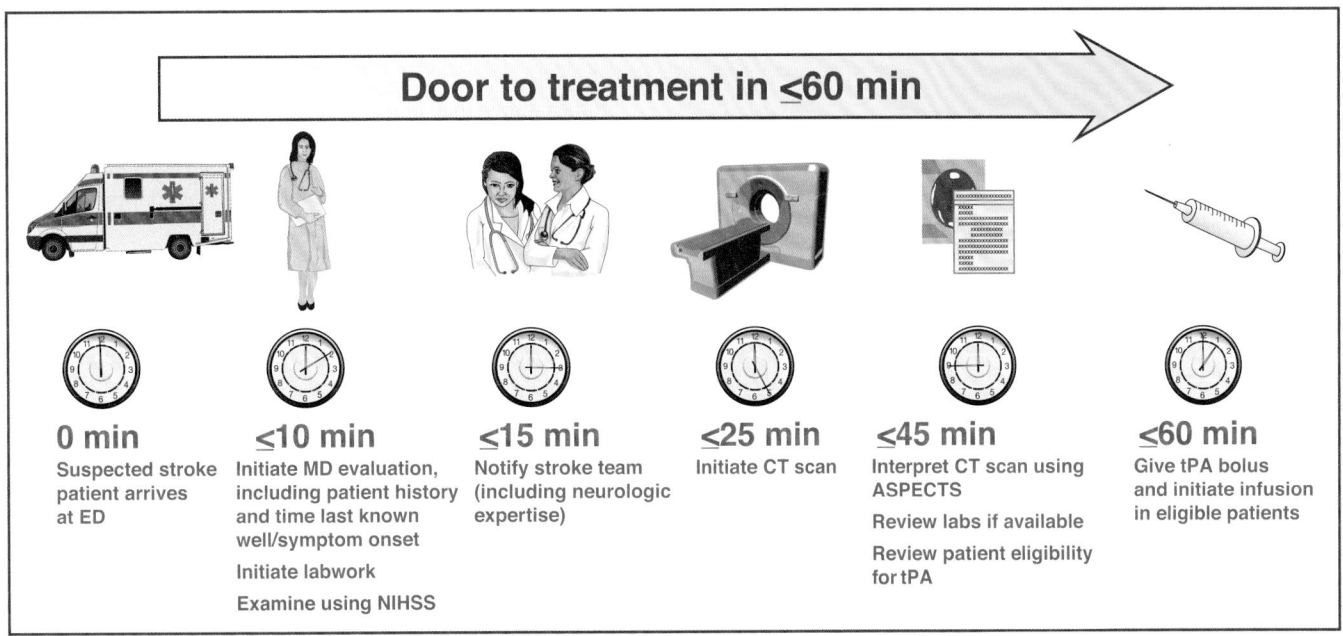

FIGURE 15.1 NINDS timeline targets for attaining an IV tPA door-to-needle time of 60 minutes or less. ED, emergency department; MD, doctor of medicine; NIHSS, National Institutes of Health Stroke Scale; CT, computed tomography; ASPECTS, Alberta Stroke Program Early CT Score; tPA, tissue plasminogen activator.

mental status. Depressed level of consciousness may in turn lead to aspiration of oropharyngeal contents or ineffective respirations due to upper airway obstruction, either of which may necessitate endotracheal intubation prior to further evaluation and management.

Blood Pressure

Hypertension occurs commonly as a nonspecific response to cerebral injury and can be present in both AIS and ICH. Elevated blood pressure (BP) is a strong indicator that the patient is actually having a stroke as opposed to a stroke mimic. Early BP elevation may be advantageous in AIS, allowing for increased cerebral perfusion to the *ischemic penumbra*, areas of marginally perfused brain. Aggressive BP reduction within the first few hours of AIS onset can lead to worsening of the neurologic deficit and therefore should be avoided.

BP should only be lowered prior to noncontrast CT if the systolic BP is higher than 220 mm Hg, diastolic BP is higher than 120 mm Hg [**Level 1**],[1] or it is suspected that hypertension is leading to acute end-organ damage (e.g., acute myocardial infarction, aortic dissection, or cardiogenic pulmonary edema). If BP is lowered, a systolic BP of 180 mm Hg is the preferred target. The preferred agents and their dosages for emergency BP control in acute stroke are shown in Table 38.3. BP goals are reevaluated after CT imaging has established the etiology of the symptoms and, for AIS, once decisions are made regarding reperfusion therapy.

Heart Rate

Atrial fibrillation (AF) with rapid ventricular response (RVR) or other tachyarrhythmias can occur on presentation and may necessitate stabilization prior to obtaining CT. Diltiazem 10 mg IV or metoprolol 5 mg IV are commonly used initial therapies for AF with RVR in this setting. A cardiac monitor should be placed if there is any concern about heart rate or if the patient reports chest pain or palpitations. Routine electrocardiography should be obtained in acute stroke patients but is only required prior to CT if there is significant dysrhythmia or if an acute coronary syndrome is suspected.

Respirations and Breathing

Obvious respiratory distress should trigger placement of an oxygen saturation monitor and oxygen via nasal cannula. A decision whether to proceed directly to CT or to defer until adequate airway and ventilation can be assured then needs to be made. Patients with severe dyspnea or significantly impaired level of consciousness (stupor or coma) should be intubated prior to CT scan, as failure to control the airway can lead to respiratory arrest or severe aspiration.

Temperature

In general, it is not necessary to measure body temperature prior to CT in a patient with acute stroke unless meningitis is suspected.

INITIAL HISTORY

If eyewitnesses are available, obtain a collateral history from them to corroborate the patient's account. Whenever possible, confirm the patient's history with emergency medical system (EMS) personnel, and ask prehospital providers to provide mobile phone numbers of eyewitnesses who might not be immediately present in the ED. Be sure to inquire about the following points.

1. *Exactly when did the stroke symptoms first begin?*

If the onset of symptoms cannot be reported by the patient and were not witnessed, ask when the patient was last known well. For those who present on waking from sleep, the physician must determine whether the symptoms were present immediately upon awakening or shortly thereafter after a brief period of normalcy. If they truly awoke with the symptoms, the last known well time may be the time when they went to sleep the prior evening but often will be a time that they awoke transiently in the middle of the night.

2. *What were the initial symptoms?*

A maximal deficit at onset in a fully alert patient supports cerebral infarction and suggests embolism in particular. Ask specifically if the patient's deficits have worsened or fluctuated since onset. Early headache, vomiting, or change in level of consciousness supports

ICH. Inquire specifically about lateralized weakness, numbness, or other classic symptoms of acute stroke (see Table 15.1).

3. Was any seizure activity observed?
Postictal deficits from seizures can mimic stroke. Seizures manifesting as focal motor convulsions or generalized tonic–clonic activity can also occur at the onset of ICH or AIS, but this is unusual.

4. What is the patient's medical history and neurologic baseline?
Assess for stroke risk factors such as hypertension, diabetes mellitus, dyslipidemia, cigarette smoking, AF, carotid stenosis, and prior transient ischemic attacks (TIAs) or strokes. A patient presenting with worsening of an existing or previously resolved neurologic deficit may have the "peeling-the-onion" syndrome (Table 15.2), with their symptoms resulting from unmasking of their prior deficit due to systemic derangements such as fever, hypoglycemia, or hypoxia.

5. What medications is the patient taking?
Ask particularly about anticoagulants or antiplatelet agents. Use of these agents not only predisposes to ICH but can also limit therapeutic options in the setting of ischemic stroke.

ESTABLISH INTRAVENOUS ACCESS AND DRAW ADMISSION LABS

Ideally, two peripheral IVs should be placed, at least one of which ideally should be 18 gauge to facilitate advanced imaging studies (i.e., CT angiography) if necessary. Labs should be drawn for complete blood count, serum chemistries, prothrombin time (PT)/partial thromboplastin time (PTT)/international normalized ratio (INR), troponin I, and other tests as indicated (e.g., liver function tests, toxicology screen, etc.). Point-of-care finger stick blood glucose level should also be obtained.

NATIONAL INSTITUTES OF HEALTH STROKE SCALE EXAMINATION

The National Institutes of Health Stroke Scale (NIHSS, Table 15.3) is a simple algorithm for quantifying the severity of neurologic deficits in patients with acute hemispheric or cerebellar syndromes. Eleven items are tested, and a score is generated on a scale ranging from 0 (no deficit) to 42 (comatose and quadriplegic). In expert hands, the test takes only several minutes to administer. When obtained within 6 hours of symptom onset, an NIHSS score greater than or equal to 7 indicates a nearly 85% chance of detecting a large-vessel intracranial occlusion by CT angiography. In hospitals that offer intra-arterial (IA) endovascular intervention for AIS, this cut point can be used to select patients for immediate CT angiography after the noncontrast CT has excluded blood in order to expedite endovascular therapies. Scores higher than 20 in patients with AIS imply a high risk of large territory infarction and a very poor prognosis if reperfusion is not attained. Once the history and examination are completed, the lesion should be able to be localized clinically.

PERFORM NONCONTRAST COMPUTED TOMOGRAPHY IMAGING

Noncontrast CT is by far the most readily available test for differentiation of AIS and ICH and the only one that must absolutely be obtained prior to administering thrombolytic therapy for AIS. The ability to obtain timely CT scans is greatly improved by having the CT scanner located within the ED. To minimize any delays in treatment, the patient should ideally be taken directly from the ambulance to the CT scanner with coordinated evaluation and intervention performed just outside the CT suite or on the CT table.

Studies show that obtaining CT imaging is the rate-limiting step in acute stroke management, so optimization of door-to-CT times should be of high priority. *The main differential diagnosis in acute stroke is infarction versus hemorrhage. All further management decisions will depend on making this distinction.*

Analysis for Hemorrhage

Blood is hyperdense (bright) and easily identifiable on noncontrast helical computed tomography (NCHCT) (Fig. 15.2A). ICH appears as a discrete focus of blood that displaces the surrounding brain parenchyma. ICH volume, a strong predictor of 30-day mortality and functional outcome, can be quickly measured using the ABC/2 method (see Fig. 38.3). Two diameters (A + B), measured at right angles on the slice that corresponds to the epicenter of the hemorrhage, are measured in centimeters. The third diameter perpendicular to that plane (C) is measured by multiplying the number of slices on which the bleed is apparent by each slice thickness (usually 5 mm, expressed 0.5 cm). The product of these three diameters is divided by two as a simplification of the equation for the volume of an ellipsoid. Patients with ICH volumes of less than 30 mL have potential for a good prognosis and have a small risk of early deterioration, whereas those with ICH volumes between 30 and 70 mL are at higher risk for early deterioration due to mass effect. Patients with hemorrhages greater than 70 mL were traditionally considered to be uniformly lethal, although survival with reasonable recovery can be attained in this group with emergency surgery, most often hemicraniectomy.

Whenever ICH is present, be sure to check for the following radiographic findings:

- *Subarachnoid hemorrhage* (Fig. 15.2B) in association with intraparenchymal hemorrhage suggests a ruptured aneurysm and requires angiography.
- *Intraventricular hemorrhage* (Fig. 15.2C) in association with ventricular enlargement requires neurosurgical evaluation for possible emergent ventriculostomy.
- *Fluid/fluid levels* within a hematoma (Fig. 15.2D) result from separation of red blood cells and plasma and are indicative of a coagulopathy.
- *Edema, mass effect, and midline shift* usually lead to delayed neurologic deterioration when associated with a large hemorrhage (>30 mL). Perihematomal edema takes several hours to develop after ICH and is therefore not usually seen on initial head CT. An abnormally large or an irregular amount of edema associated with hemorrhage on initial presentation suggests (1) hemorrhagic conversion of infarcted tissue, (2) bleeding associated with neoplasm, or (3) venous infarction from dural sinus thrombosis.

Analysis for Ischemic Stroke

Infarction does not cause consistent changes on CT within 6 hours of stroke onset. *Infarction is suspected when a patient presenting with sudden onset of neurologic deficits has a normal CT scan.* Over a period of approximately 6 hours, regions of ischemia will gradually develop into an area of hypodensity as the tissue infarcts. The presence of a large hypodensity on NCHCT in an AIS patient should prompt reevaluation and careful scrutiny of the reported time of onset.

TABLE 15.2   Differential Diagnosis of Acute Neurologic Deficits

Diagnosis	Clinical Characteristics	Diagnosis	Clinical Characteristics
Stroke		**Stroke Mimics (continued)**	
Ischemic stroke	• Deficits that are maximal at onset suggest embolism • Sometimes preceded by transient ischemic attacks • Headache is uncommon • BP often elevated	Subdural hematoma	• May not have a clear history of recent trauma in elderly patients with acute-on-chronic bleeding • Typically presents with focal deficits or subacute confusion and gait disturbance in an elderly patient • Headache is common but not universal
Intracerebral hemorrhage	• Often presents with headache and/or nausea and vomiting • Deficit commonly worsens over minutes to hours as hemorrhage expands • Loss of consciousness at onset is rare • BP often extremely elevated	Brain tumor or abscess	• Usually has a subacute to chronic presentation but can suddenly worsen due to associated seizure or bleeding into the tumor • Often with symptoms of headache, especially when recumbent
Subarachnoid hemorrhage	• Typically presents with sudden "thunderclap headache" • Often associated with transient loss of consciousness • Focal symptoms are unusual	Multiple sclerosis or other demyelinating disease	• Usually has a more subacute presentation but can mimic acute stroke at times • Often has history of prior deficits in varying locations • Can be differentiated from ischemic stroke with DWI MRI • Affects younger patients with no stroke risk factors
Stroke Mimics			
Seizure with postictal deficit	• Occurs in aftermath of focal motor activity or an unwitnessed seizure • Deficits gradually improve and resolve over minutes to hours after onset • Can be differentiated from ischemic stroke with diffusion-weighted (DWI) MRI • EEG may show corresponding epileptiform activity	Peripheral (labyrinthine) vertigo	• Can mimic an infarct in the brain stem or cerebellum causing acute vertigo • Can be differentiated from ischemic stroke with careful examination (horizontal head impulse test, characterization of nystagmus, and cover–uncover test[a]) in most but not all cases • Definitive exclusion of ischemic stroke requires DWI MRI, although DWI can also miss small brain stem infarcts
Migraine with aura	• Typical patient has a history of migraine and prior similar events • Can present with weakness, aphasia, neglect, visual changes, and/or sensory loss • Symptoms may precede, be concurrent with, or follow a typical migraine headache • Typically occurs in younger women with no stroke risk factors	Hypertensive encephalopathy (posterior reversible encephalopathy syndrome)	• Most commonly presents with altered mental status, headache, vision changes, or seizures • Usually does not cause unilateral symptoms • BP usually elevated • Can occur in younger patients with no stroke risk factors
Unmasking of a prior focal deficit (i.e., "peeling-the-onion" phenomenon)	• Sudden worsening of old stroke symptoms (does not cause new symptoms) • Triggered by fever, hypoxia, hypoglycemia, hyponatremia, or other metabolic disturbances • Focal deficits are typically accompanied by features of encephalopathy	Conversion disorder	• A diagnosis of exclusion • Detailed neurologic exam sometimes reveals inconsistencies suggesting a nonphysiologic cause of symptoms • Positive signs of misdirected effort may be elicited (e.g., Hoover sign)

BP, blood pressure; MRI, magnetic resonance imaging; EEG, electroencephalogram.

[a]See Chapter 4 for details of the Head Impulse Nystagmus Test of Skew (HINTS) examination for differentiating central from peripheral vertigo.

TABLE 15.3 The National Institutes of Health Stroke Scale

1a. Level of consciousness (LOC):

0 = Alert; keenly responsive

1 = Not alert but arousable by minor stimulation to obey, answer, or respond

2 = Not alert; requires repeated stimulation to attend or is obtunded and requires strong or painful stimulation to make movements (not stereotyped)

3 = Responds only with reflex motor or autonomic effects or totally unresponsive, flaccid, and areflexic

1b. LOC questions: The patient is asked the month and his or her age.

0 = Answers both questions correctly

1 = Answers one question correctly

2 = Answers neither question correctly

1c. LOC commands: The patient is asked to open and close the eyes and then to grip and release the nonparetic hand.

0 = Performs both tasks correctly

1 = Performs one task correctly

2 = Performs neither task correctly

2. Best gaze: horizontal eye movements

0 = Normal

1 = Partial gaze palsy; gaze is abnormal in one or both eyes.

2 = Forced deviation or total gaze paresis not overcome by the oculocephalic maneuver

3. Visual loss:

0 = No visual loss

1 = Partial hemianopia

2 = Complete hemianopia

3 = Bilateral hemianopia (blind including cortical blindness)

4. Facial palsy:

0 = Normal symmetric movements

1 = Minor paralysis (flattened nasolabial fold, asymmetry on smiling)

2 = Partial paralysis (total or near-total paralysis of lower face)

3 = Complete paralysis of one or both sides (absence of facial movement in the upper and lower face)

5. Motor arm: The limb is elevated for 10 s, scored separately for left and right.

0 = No drift; limb holds 90 (or 45) degrees for full 10 s.

1 = Drift; limb holds 90 (or 45) degrees but drifts down before full 10 s; does not hit bed or other support

2 = Some effort against gravity; limb cannot get to or maintain (if cued) 90 (or 45) degrees, drifts down to bed, but has some effort against gravity.

3 = No effort against gravity; limb falls.

4 = No movement

6. Motor leg: The limb is elevated for 5 s, scored separately for left and right.

0 = No drift; leg holds 30-degree position for full 5 s.

1 = Drift; leg falls by the end of the 5-s period but does not hit bed.

2 = Some effort against gravity; leg falls to bed by 5 s but has some effort against gravity.

3 = No effort against gravity; leg falls to bed immediately.

4 = No movement

7. Limb ataxia:

0 = Absent

1 = Present in one limb

2 = Present in two limbs

8. Sensory:

0 = Normal; no sensory loss

1 = Mild to moderate sensory loss; patient feels pinprick is less sharp or is dull on the affected side; or there is a loss of superficial pain with pinprick, but patient is aware of being touched.

2 = Severe to total sensory loss; patient is not aware of being touched in the face, arm, and leg.

9. Best language:

0 = No aphasia; normal

1 = Mild to moderate aphasia

2 = Severe aphasia; all communication is through fragmentary expression.

3 = Mute, global aphasia; no usable speech or auditory comprehension

10. Dysarthria:

0 = Normal

1 = Mild to moderate dysarthria; patient slurs at least some words and, at worst, can be understood with some difficulty.

2 = Severe dysarthria; patient's speech is so slurred as to be unintelligible in the absence of or out of proportion to aphasia.

11. Extinction and inattention:

0 = No abnormality

1 = Visual, tactile, auditory, spatial, or personal inattention or extinction to bilateral simultaneous stimulation in one of the sensory modalities

2 = Profound hemi-inattention or extinction to more than one modality; does not recognize own hand or orients to only one side of space

Total score ranges from 0 (normal) to 42 (comatose and quadriplegic). For informational purpose only. Accurate and reliable scoring of the NIHSS requires strict adherence to a standardized testing protocol. Refer to www.ninds.nih.gov/doctors/NIH_Stroke_Scale.pdf for complete instructions on how to conduct and score the test and for smartphone applications than can assist in performance and scoring.

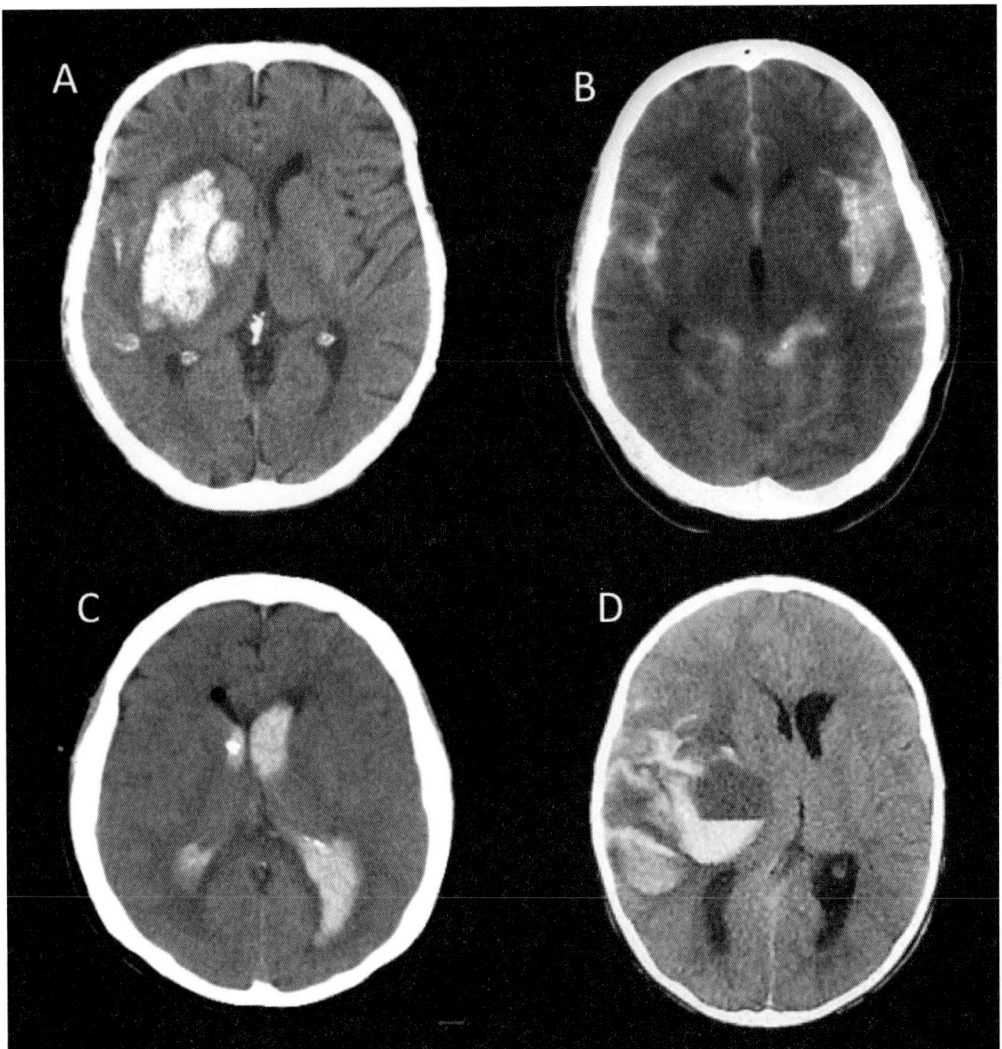

FIGURE 15.2 CT scans of brain hemorrhage. **A:** Intracerebral hemorrhage. **B:** Subarachnoid hemorrhage. **C:** Intraventricular hemorrhage. **D:** Acute hemorrhage with fluid/fluid level indicative of a coagulopathy.

The Alberta Stroke Programme Early CT Score (ASPECTS) was developed to quantify the extent of infarction on initial CT imaging (Fig. 15.3). Loss of differentiation between gray and white in the cortex and deep structures such as the caudate, putamen, or globus pallidus results from early ischemic injury and portends eventual progression to irreversible infarction (Fig. 15.4). The score is composed of seven cortical regions and three subcortical regions of the middle cerebral artery (MCA) territory totaling 10 points for a normal study from which 1 point is subtracted for each area of visualized infarct. This score has high interrater reliability and serves to quantify infarction, predict outcome, and stratify patients regarding the use of reperfusion therapies. The risk of hemorrhagic conversion after thrombolysis is increased in patients with ASPECTS lower than 7.

Acute thrombus in a proximal vessel such as the MCA ("dense MCA sign") or basilar artery can create a hyperdense appearance to the vessel on NCHCT. The presence of a hyperdense vessel may have clinical use in the acute setting, as it helps to confirm the diagnosis of large-vessel occlusion (LVO) and may lead clinicians to mobilize neurointerventional teams for clot extraction.

PHASE 2: POST–COMPUTED TOMOGRAPHY EMERGENCY MANAGEMENT

INTRACEREBRAL HEMORRHAGE

The following management guidelines apply specifically to spontaneous intraparenchymal ICH. Refer to Chapter 39 for management of *subarachnoid hemorrhage* and Chapter 46 for management of *traumatic brain injury*.

Diagnose and Reverse Coagulopathy and Platelet Dysfunction

The presence of blood on CT mandates that a PT/INR, PTT, and platelet count are send as STAT tests to confirm normal values as soon as possible. Next, confirm whether or not the patient is taking any anticoagulants that do not significantly affect these values (e.g., dabigatran, rivaroxaban, apixaban, low molecular weight heparins). Also inquire about antiplatelet agents (e.g., aspirin, clopidogrel, dipyridamole, prasugrel). A basic metabolic panel is also useful to show evidence of uremia, which can cause a qualitative platelet defect.

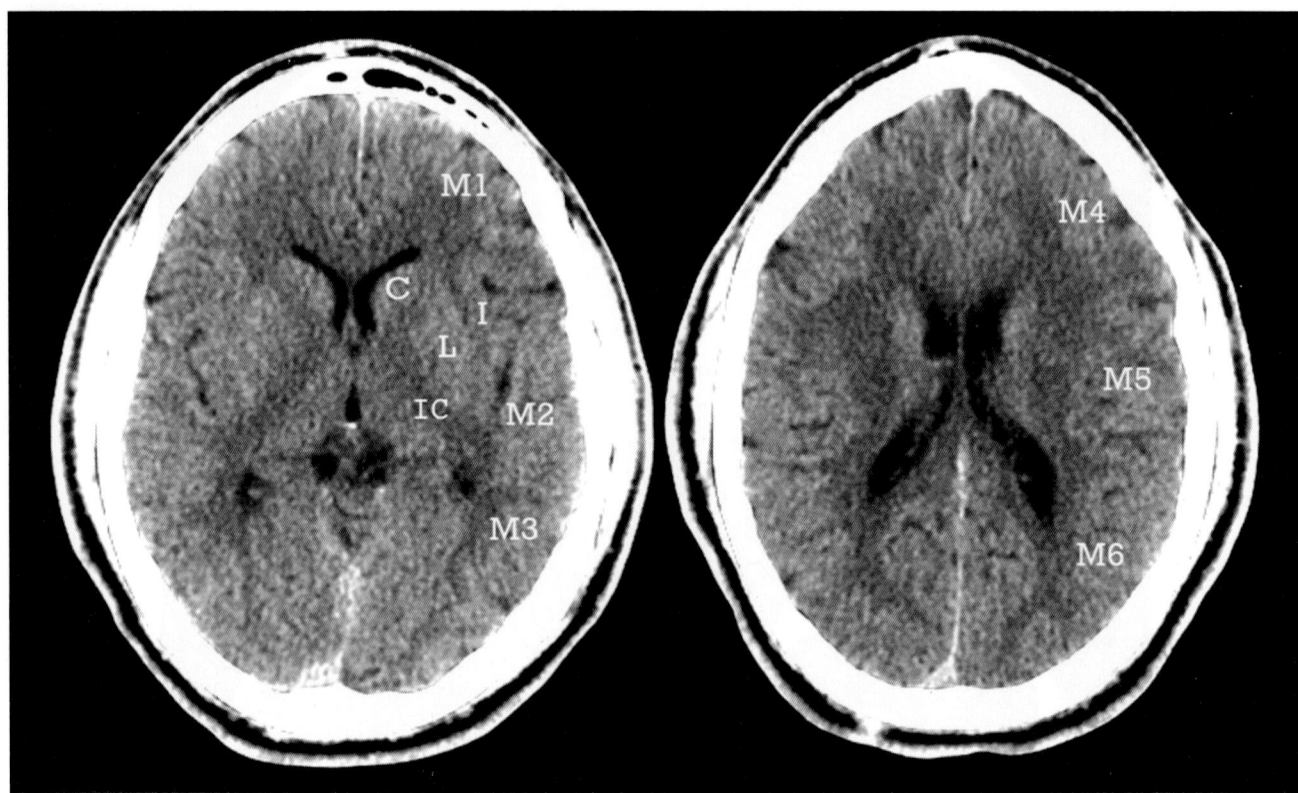

FIGURE 15.3 Anatomic regions evaluated in the ASPECTS. A score of 10 indicates no evidence of early ischemic change from which 1 point is subtracted for each region of infarction. Patients with scores below 7 are at high risk for hemorrhagic transformation if given IV tPA. C, caudate; I, insula; L, lentiform nucleus; IC, internal capsule; M, middle cerebral artery territories 1 through 6.

Suggested protocols for the reversal of different forms of anticoagulation or platelet dysfunction are shown in Table 15.4. *If there is a clear history of current use, steps to reverse anticoagulation or restore platelet function should not be delayed by waiting for coagulation testing or a platelet count* [**Level 1**].[2] In patients with oral anticoagulant-associated ICH, successful reversal of the INR to <1.3 and reduction of systolic BP to <160 mm Hg is associated with a reduced risk of hematoma enlargement.

Control Severe Hypertension

In contrast to the AIS patient, continued hypertension can harm the ICH patient by causing expansion of the hemorrhage and worsened perihematomal edema. Older guidelines suggest lowering the systolic BP to lower than 180 mm Hg, whereas a more recent randomized trial (Intensive Blood Pressure Reduction in Acute Cerebral Hemorrhage Trial [INTERACT]) showed that lowering to systolic BP lower than 140 mm Hg is safe and may be of clinical benefit [**Level 1**].[3] Nicardipine or clevidipine infusion is preferable because of their reliable dose-response characteristics and quick onset and offset times. If these short-acting agents are unavailable, labetalol can be administered initially as IV pushes followed by an infusion (see Table 38.3). Nitrates such as sodium nitroprusside should be avoided due to their potential to cause cerebral vasodilation and elevated ICP.

Treat Suspected Elevated Intracranial Pressure or Symptomatic Mass Effect

If the NCHCT shows significant mass effect (midline shift, effacement of the basal cisterns, or both) and the patient has depressed level of consciousness, empiric treatment of ICP should be initiated. Hyperventilation causes vasoconstriction that will lower cerebral blood volume and thus lower ICP. It should be used transiently as a bridge to further intervention in intubated patients who show signs of transtentorial herniation (i.e., dilated pupil). In general, a partial pressure of carbon dioxide (PCO_2) level of 30 is targeted. If the patient is intubated and agitated or coughing, sedation should be considered. Bolus osmotherapy with mannitol 1 to 1.5 g/kg IV can be easily administered through a peripheral IV. Alternatively, 30 mL of 23.4% hypertonic saline can be given, but this requires central venous access. Steroids should not be administered, as they have been shown to be ineffective for management of cerebral edema after ICH [**Level 1**][4] and may increase the risk of infectious complications (see also Chapter 107).

Consider External Ventricular Drain Placement or Placement of an Intracranial Pressure Monitor

Obstructive hydrocephalus typically develops in ICH patients who also have a significant amount of intraventricular hemorrhage in the third or fourth ventricles. Any new enlargement of the temporal horns of the lateral ventricles on NCHCT in a patient with altered level of consciousness should prompt consideration of external ventricular drain placement for management of hydrocephalus and control of ICP. Without diversion of cerebrospinal fluid, patients with hydrocephalus can deteriorate rapidly. If significant mass effect is present in a patient who is ineligible for surgical evacuation, a parenchymal ICP monitor may be considered to allow for optimization of ICP management (see Chapter 33).

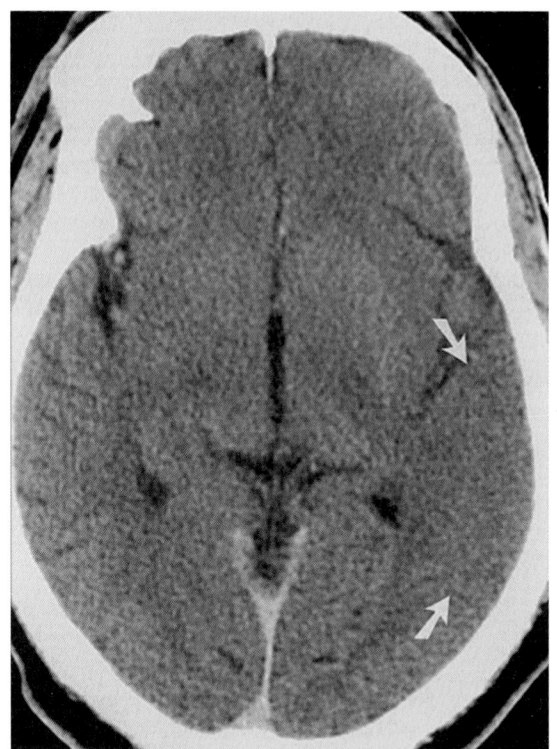

FIGURE 15.4 Early cerebral infarction with loss of gray–white definition and sulcal effacement. (*Arrows* indicate anterior and posterior borders of the involved territory of the MCA.)

Consider Emergent Surgical Hematoma Evacuation

For cerebellar hemorrhage greater than 3 cm in diameter, suboccipital surgical decompression with or without hematoma evacuation is recommended if the patient shows decreased level of consciousness and CT shows evidence of mass effect [**Level 1**].[2] For supratentorial hemorrhage, however, there is far less consensus. The Surgical Trial in Intracerebral Hemorrhage (STICH) was unable to show definitive benefit for craniotomy with evacuation of supratentorial ICH within 72 hours of onset compared with best medical therapy [**Level 1**].[5,6] Most likely, the incision in cerebral cortex required to surgically evacuate deeper hemorrhage leads to further neurologic injury that negates any benefit. Despite these results, there is some suggestion that younger patients with active deterioration due to mass effect may still benefit from surgical evacuation, as these patients were not randomized into the trials.

Consider Anticonvulsant Therapy

Hemorrhage can cause cortical irritation and the development of seizure activity. If seizures occur, patients should be given an IV antiepileptic medication (commonly used agents are levetiracetam 1 to 2 g IV, fosphenytoin 20 mg/kg IV, or phenytoin 20 mg/kg IV) [**Level 1**].[2] Prophylactic treatment with anticonvulsants for 7 days after onset can be considered in unstable patients with cortical hemorrhage, as these patients are at higher risk for seizures.

Consider Advanced Imaging

ICH is most commonly due to hypertension when it occurs in the putamen, globus pallidus, caudate, thalamus, pons, or cerebellum.

Cortical ICH occurs more frequently in the elderly and usually results from *amyloid angiopathy*, the deposition of amyloid into the arterial wall. However, ICH may also be caused by aneurysms (if adjacent to the subarachnoid space), arteriovenous malformations (AVMs), cavernous malformations, tumors, or other less common etiologies. Young patients, those with atypical CT findings, and those without a history of hypertension or anticoagulant use should undergo further imaging studies to evaluate for an underlying lesion. Imaging options include CT angiography, magnetic resonance imaging/magnetic resonance angiography (MRI/MRA), or catheter angiography. CT angiography can be performed on the CT table immediately after NCHCT identifies ICH, provided the patient remains stable and does not urgently require any additional treatments.

Disposition

Due to high risks of neurologic deterioration and development of medical complications, all patients with acute ICH should ideally be admitted to an intensive care unit for further evaluation and management.

ACUTE ISCHEMIC STROKE

For patients presenting with an acute neurologic deficit who show no signs of hemorrhage on noncontrast CT, the presumptive diagnosis is ischemic stroke and the primary goal is to provide eligible patients with reperfusion therapy as soon as possible. Thrombolysis with IV tPA loses its efficacy rapidly as acute ischemia progresses to infarction. Optimization of each step of acute stroke management is required to ensure timely therapies. When done successfully, thrombolysis with IV tPA can be administered within 20 minutes after ED arrival.

Indications for Intravenous Tissue Plasminogen Activator

With the completion of the National Institute of Neurological Disorders and Stroke (NINDS) trial in 1995, administration of IV tPA has become the standard of care for acute reperfusion therapy in AIS within 3 hours of symptom onset [**Level 1**].[7] Thrombolysis with tPA increases the chances of a good recovery at 3 months after infarction from approximately 26% to 39% corresponding to a number needed to treat of 8 with no effect on mortality. Unfortunately, tPA also carries a 6% risk of symptomatic hemorrhagic conversion, most commonly in patients given tPA at later time points relative to symptom onset or in those with extensive signs of early ischemic change as evidenced by an ASPECTS lower than 7.

More recently, the European Cooperative Acute Stroke Study III (ECASS III) trial confirmed the safety and efficacy of IV tPA up to 4.5 hours after symptom onset in a subgroup of patients who were younger than 80 years of age. The benefit of tPA in this subset is less than those treated within 3 hours. Patients given tPA within the 3.0- to 4.5-hour window also have increased rates of hemorrhagic conversion and worsened mortality compared with patients given tPA within 3 hours of onset [**Level 1**].[8]

Speed of attaining reperfusion is by far the most important determinant of the efficacy of tPA. The number needed to treat to achieve one functionally independent patient after ischemic stroke increases from as little as 5 for patients treated within 90 minutes of onset to 15 when tPA is given within the 3.0- to 4.5-hour window. For patients who present beyond 4.5 hours from onset, IV tPA is not of proven benefit and may cause harm, as the risk of hemorrhagic conversion increases significantly [**Level 1**].[9]

TABLE 15.4	Strategies for Reversal of Anticoagulation or Platelet Dysfunction in Acute Intracerebral Hemorrhage	
Agent	**Treatment Strategy**	**Comments**
Warfarin (vitamin K antagonist that results in reduced synthesis of factors II, VII, IX, and X)	Administer vitamin K 10 mg IV over 30 min. *and* Four-factor prothrombin complex concentrate (PCC) 25–50 U/kg IV *or* Fresh frozen plasma (FFP) 2–4 200 mL units IV	If available, PCC is preferable, as it results in a substantially quicker time to INR reversal than FFP using a much smaller volume of infusion. The goal should be to lower the INR to <1.5.
Dabigatran (direct thrombin inhibitor)	Give activated charcoal if the medication was ingested within the past 2 h. *and* Consider emergency hemodialysis.	There is limited data to support other therapies, but four-factor PCC or factor VIIa can be considered.
Rivaroxaban, apixaban, edoxaban (Xa inhibitors)	Consider a four-factor PCC 25–50 U/kg IV.	In one study, PCC was shown to be superior to FFP for normalizing the INR in normal subjects treated with rivaroxaban. These drugs are heavily bound to plasma protein, so plasma exchange can be considered, but there is limited experience with its use.
Unfractionated heparin (UFH)	For IV bolus UFH given <1 h ago, administer 1 mg of protamine sulfate for every 100 units of UFH. If UFH was given 1–2 h ago, give 1 mg of protamine sulfate for every 200 units of UFH. If UFH was given >2 h ago, give 1 mg of protamine sulfate for every 400 units of UFH.	For patients receiving an IV infusion of UFH, administer protamine sulfate 1 mg for every 100 units given in the past 2 h.
Enoxaparin, dalteparin (low molecular weight heparin [LMWH])	If LMWH was given <8 h ago, give 1 mg of protamine sulfate per 100 anti-Xa units of LMWH. If LMWH was given 8–24 h ago, give 1 mg of protamine sulfate per 200 anti-Xa units of LMWH. If bleeding continues, an additional dose of 0.5 mg per 100 anti-Xa units can be administered.	Enoxaparin has 100 anti-Xa U/mg, whereas dalteparin has 156 anti-Xa U/mg.
Antiplatelet agents, platelet abnormalities (i.e., uremia), or thrombocytopenia	Give DDAVP 0.3 μg/kg IV over 30 min *and/or* 1 unit of single-donor platelets (or 6 units of pooled platelets)	Limited data is available to support these interventions. For thrombocytopenia, transfuse platelets to goal of >50,000/cm^3.

INR, international normalized ratio; IV, intravenous; DDAVP, desmopressin acetate.

Contraindications to Tissue Plasminogen Activator Administration

The 1995 NINDS trial used strict exclusion criteria derived from expert opinion at the time, which were subsequently translated into contraindications for tPA administration. However, these rigorous contraindications may not necessarily define the full population of patients who might benefit from tPA. Table 15.5 shows the relative strength of various contraindications to tPA therapy. These updated recommendations largely reflect case series, cohort studies, and 20 years of clinical experience since the original approval of tPA. It is crucial to use sound clinical judgment when giving tPA in the setting of a relative contraindication and to fully explain how this may alter the risks of therapy relative to the expected benefit. The most commonly encountered exclusions are discussed in the following sections.

EARLY INFARCT SIGNS

Early ischemic changes on imaging are clearly associated with higher rates of hemorrhagic conversion. Early ischemic changes should not exclude patients from thrombolysis if the extent of these changes is small (ASPECTS of 7 to 9).

IMPROVING OR MILD SYMPTOMS

Although as many as 30% of AIS patients are not administered tPA due to rapidly improving or minor stroke syndromes, 25% of these patients still have poor functional outcomes or death after stroke. AIS patients with minor or resolving deficits may still benefit from thrombolysis and should be considered on a case-by-case basis.

BLOOD PRESSURE HIGHER THAN OR EQUAL TO 185/110 MM HG

Severe hypertension is thought to increase the risk of hemorrhagic transformation after thrombolysis, although good evidence of cause and effect is scant. It is reasonable to rapidly control BP to lower than 185/110 mm Hg and start tPA while continued efforts are made to attain target BP with a continuous infusion agent such as nicardipine or clevidipine (Table 38.3).

TABLE 15.5	Strength of Evidence for Contraindications to Tissue Plasminogen Activator Therapy	
Clinical Scenario	Strength of Contraindication	
CT evidence of hemorrhage	Absolute	
Early infarct signs involving >1/3 of the MCA territory	Absolute	
Time of symptom onset unknown	Absolute	
History of coagulopathy or anticoagulant use or documented elevation of INR (>1.7) or aPTT (>1.5 × control)	Relative, strong	
Thrombocytopenia (platelet count <100,000)	Relative, strong	
SBP >185 mm Hg or DBP >110 mm Hg[a]	Relative, moderate	
Major surgery or serious trauma within preceding 14 days	Relative, moderate	
Glucose <50 or >400 mg/dL[a]	Relative, moderate	
Pregnancy	Relative, moderate	
Stroke or serious head trauma within preceding 3 mo	Relative, weak	
Seizure at onset of stroke	Relative, weak	
Rapidly improving or minor symptoms (e.g., pure sensory, minimal weakness)	Relative, weak	
Gastrointestinal, urinary tract, or other significant bleeding within preceding 21 days	Relative, weak	
Significant MI within past 4 wk or symptoms of post-MI pericarditis	Relative, weak	
Arterial puncture at a noncompressible site within preceding 7 days	Relative, weak	
Lumbar puncture within preceding 7 days	Relative, weak	

This information is intended to serve only as a guideline. Successful and safe use of IV tPA has been reported despite the presence of one or more of these complications. Decisions regarding the risks and benefits of tPA should be individualized.

[a]Blood pressure and glucose can be urgently corrected and then tPA can be administered.

CT, computed tomography; MCA, middle cerebral artery; INR, international normalized ratio; aPTT, activated partial thromboplastin time; SBP, systolic blood pressure; DBP, diastolic blood pressure; MI, myocardial infarction.

SEIZURE AT ONSET

Seizures at onset are unusual in AIS and raise the strong possibility that the patient may have a postictal rather than ischemic deficit. Nevertheless, tPA is safe in patients with seizures at onset, and it is reasonable to give tPA if the index of suspicion for AIS is very high, especially in the setting of an LVO seen on imaging.

WARFARIN WITH INTERNATIONAL NORMALIZED RATIO GREATER THAN 1.7

A history of warfarin use in patients with AIS mandates a STAT INR. Otherwise, there is no need to check coagulation routinely prior to giving tPA. There is conflicting evidence as to whether tPA is associated with an increased risk of hemorrhagic transformation when the INR is either below or mildly above 1.7 among patients taking warfarin.

ABNORMAL BLOOD GLUCOSE

Elevated blood glucose has been associated with a decreased likelihood of neurologic improvement, decreased rates of recanalization, and a higher risk of hemorrhagic conversion after thrombolysis for AIS. Treatment of hyperglycemia has not yet been shown to modify outcome, but it nevertheless is prudent to control blood glucose within a tight normal range when administering tPA. Both hyper- and hypoglycemia raises the possibility of a stroke mimic due to "unmasking" of a prior focal deficit.

OLD AGE

Although those older than age 80 years do not benefit as much from thrombolysis, patients given tPA still show improved outcomes compared with those in whom tPA is withheld. Thrombolysis with IV tPA should not be withheld from elderly patients without other contraindications.

Tissue Plasminogen Activator and Stroke Mimics

The prevalence of potential AIS that prove to be stroke mimics is as high as 20% to 25% in some regions, most of which represent seizure, complicated migraine, or conversion disorder. MRI, which can more definitively differentiate stroke from mimics, leads to delays that reduce the efficacy of tPA in improving neurologic outcomes. Fortunately, several studies show that tPA administration to stroke mimics is not associated with ICH or other complications. A rate of treating stroke mimics with thrombolysis of up to 15% is considered acceptable in most active stroke centers.

Dosage of Intravenous Tissue Plasminogen Activator

tPA is supplied in powder form and must be reconstituted with sterile water prior to administration. For eligible patients, 0.9 mg/kg of IV tPA is administered up to a maximum dose of 90 mg with the initial 10% given as an IV push and the remainder infused over 1 hour.

Post–Tissue Plasminogen Activator Blood Pressure Management

BP should be strictly maintained at lower than 180/105 mm Hg for at least 24 hours after tPA is administered to minimize the risk of hemorrhagic conversion. Because the half-life of tPA is extremely short, a radial arterial line can be safely placed for BP monitoring 1 hour after discontinuation of the infusion, as direct pressure can be effectively applied if bleeding occurs at this location. Intravenous short-acting drip antihypertensive agents that can be easily titrated are optimal to definitively achieve this goal and to avoid large swings in BP.

Aspirin

Patients who do not receive IV tPA should be given aspirin 81 to 325 mg as soon as possible. For those who receive IV tPA, aspirin administration should be delayed for 24 hours after tPA infusion to prevent hemorrhagic conversion and then started thereafter. Early aspirin administration after AIS has been shown to decrease the risk of early recurrent stroke, death, and dependency [**Level 1**].[10,11]

Role of Interventional Therapy

An important limitation of tPA is that it fails to recanalize the occluded vessel in 40% of cases. When larger clots occlude the major large intracranial vessels—the proximal MCA, internal carotid artery (ICA) terminus, or basilar artery—recanalization rates are even worse and outcomes remain poor despite IV tPA administration. Interventional bridging therapy is the strategy of proceeding immediately to endovascular intervention while tPA is infusing. If a persistent LVO is detected, endovascular intervention to extract the clot from the vessel using a suction, corkscrew, or retrievable stent device can then be attempted (see Chapter 35 for details).

In 2013, the Interventional Management of Stroke III trial (IMS III), Systemic Thrombolysis for Acute Ischemic Stroke (SYNTHESIS) trial, and Mechanical Retrieval and Recanalization of Stroke Clots Using Embolectomy (MR RESCUE) trials all failed to show benefit of endovascular intervention in the setting of AIS. These trials used less effective devices than are available today and most patients were recanalized many hours after the onset of symptoms. More recent clinical trials reported in 2015, including Multicentre Randomised Clinical Trial of Endovascular Treatment for Acute Ischemic Stroke in the Netherlands (MR CLEAN) [**Level 1**],[12] Endovascular Treatment for Small Core and Anterior Circulation Proximal Occlusion with Emphasis on Minimizing CT to Recanalization Times (ESCAPE) [**Level 1**],[13] and five additional trials (Table 35.5), used modern retrievable stent technology, achieved better recanalization rates, and showed that urgent intra-arterial intervention combined with IV tPA can improve outcome. Interventional therapy can also be considered in patients with certain contraindications to IV tPA, such as patients already on anticoagulation or those with recent major surgery.

In the absence of widely accepted practice guidelines, clinical practice at this level varies widely. Many primary stroke centers in the United States do not offer endovascular intervention, although most comprehensive stroke centers do. To be successful, rapid evaluation and mobilization of the interventional team requires preparation and interdisciplinary teamwork.

Emergency Computed Tomography Angiography for Detecting Large-Vessel Occlusion

Increasingly, major stroke centers are incorporating CT angiography into their acute stroke algorithms with the goal of detecting a treatable LVO (Fig. 15.5) during tPA therapy or in patients who present acutely but have a contraindication to its use. A high NIHSS score very early in the course of stroke implies a high probability of a LVO. One study showed that among AIS patients who present within 6 hours with a baseline NIHSS higher than or equal to 7, CT angiography demonstrates a potentially treatable LVO in nearly 85% of patients. By contrast, in the MR CLEAN Trial mechanical thrombectomy within 6 hours of onset improved outcome in AIS patients with documented LVO and NIHSS scores as low as 2. Many stroke centers have established protocols in which tPA therapy is initiated in the CT scanner immediately after the noncontrast CT is obtained. This allows the team to proceed directly with a CT angiogram without delaying tPA administration. In these protocols routine documentation of a normal serum creatinine level is waived owing to the urgency of the situation and the low risk of serious contrast-induced nephropathy (<1%). Demonstration of LVO then triggers an interventional "secondary page" that mobilizes the interventional team with the goal of beating a 60-minute "picture-to-puncture" time interval.

Even if mechanical thrombectomy is not being pursued, vessel and perfusion imaging may clarify or confirm sites of cervical vessel occlusion, guide BP management, affect disposition, and establish prognosis. For patients with severe or fluctuating stroke syndromes presenting beyond 4.5 hours who are therefore not

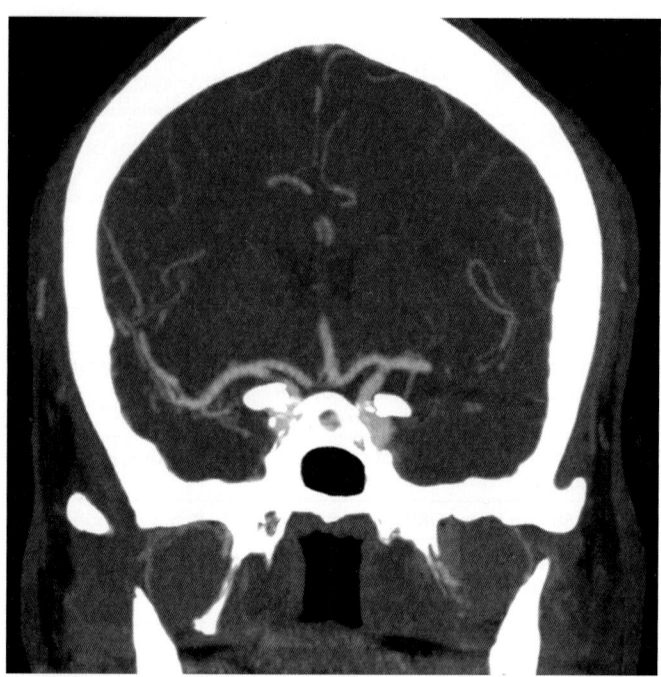

FIGURE 15.5 CT angiogram maximum intensity projection (MIP) image (coronal view) demonstrating total occlusion of the left M1 segment of the middle cerebral artery.

eligible for IV tPA, CT angiography/CT perfusion or MRA/MR perfusion can be considered at the time of initial imaging to allow for the possibility of pursuing endovascular intervention.

Disposition

Ischemic stroke patients should be transferred to a stroke unit or a neuro-ICU whenever possible depending on the clinical scenario, including active comorbidities and the immediate risk of neurologic deterioration.

LEVEL 1 EVIDENCE

1. Jauch EC, Saver JL, Adams HP, et al. Guidelines for the early management of patients with acute ischemic stroke: a guideline for healthcare professionals from the American Heart Association/American Stroke Association. *Stroke.* 2013;44(3): 870–947.

2. Morgenstern LB, Hemphill JC, Anderson C, et al. Guidelines for the management of spontaneous intracerebral hemorrhage: a guideline for healthcare professionals from the American Heart Association/American Stroke Association. *Stroke.* 2010; 41:2108–2129.

3. Anderson CS, Heeley E, Huang Y, et al. Rapid blood-pressure lowering in patients with acute intracerebral hemorrhage. *N Engl J Med.* 2013;368(25):2355–2365.

4. Poungvarin N, Bhoopat W, Viriyavejakul A, et al. Effects of dexamethasone in primary supratentorial intracerebral hemorrhage. *N Engl J Med.* 1987;316(20):1229–1233.

5. Mendelow AD, Gregson BA, Fernandes HM, et al. Early surgery versus initial conservative treatment in patients with spontaneous supratentorial intracerebral haematomas in the International Surgical Trial in Intracerebral Haemorrhage (STICH): a randomised trial. *Lancet.* 2005;365(9457):387–397.

6. Mendelow AD, Gregson BA, Rowan EN, et al. Early surgery versus initial conservative treatment in patients with spontaneous supratentorial lobar intracerebral haematomas (STICH II): a randomised trial. *Lancet.* 2013;382(9890):397–408.

7. The National Institute of Neurological Disorders and Stroke rt-PA Stroke Study Group. Tissue plasminogen activator for acute ischemic stroke. The National Institute of Neurological Disorders and Stroke rt-PA Stroke Study Group. *N Engl J Med.* 1995;333(24):1581–1587.

8. Hacke W, Kaste M, Bluhmki E, et al. Thrombolysis with alteplase 3 to 4.5 hours after acute ischemic stroke. *N Engl J Med.* 2008;359(13):1317–1329.

9. The IST-3 Collaborative Group. The benefits and harms of intravenous thrombolysis with recombinant tissue plasminogen activator within 6 h of acute ischaemic stroke (the third international stroke trial [IST-3]): a randomised controlled trial. *Lancet.* 2012;379(9834):2352–2363.

10. International Stroke Trial Collaborative Group. The International Stroke Trial (IST): a randomised trial of aspirin, subcutaneous heparin, both, or neither among 19435 patients with acute ischaemic stroke. *Lancet.* 1997;349(9065):1569–1581.

11. Cast Collaborative Group. CAST: randomised placebo-controlled trial of early aspirin use in 20,000 patients with acute ischaemic stroke. CAST (Chinese Acute Stroke Trial) Collaborative Group. *Lancet.* 1997;349(9066):1641–1649.

12. Berkhemer OA, Fransen PSS, Beumer D, et al. A randomized trial of intraarterial treatment for acute ischemic stroke. *N Engl J Med.* 2015;372(1):11–20.

13. Goyal M, Demchuk AM, Menon BK, et al. Randomized assessment of rapid endovascular treatment of ischemic stroke. *N Engl J Med.* 2015;372(11):1019–1030.

SUGGESTED READINGS

Balucani C, Grotta JC. Selecting stroke patients for intra-arterial therapy. *Neurology.* 2012;78(10):755–761.

Barber PA, Demchuk AM, Zhang J, et al. Validity and reliability of a quantitative computed tomography score in predicting outcome of hyperacute stroke before thrombolytic therapy. ASPECTS Study Group. Alberta Stroke Programme Early CT Score. *Lancet.* 2000;355(9216):1670–1674.

Barber PA, Zhang J, Demchuk AM, et al. Why are stroke patients excluded from TPA therapy? An analysis of patient eligibility. *Neurology.* 2001;56(8):1015–1020.

Broderick JP, Palesch YY, Demchuk AM, et al. Endovascular therapy after intravenous t-PA versus t-PA alone for stroke. *N Engl J Med.* 2013;368(10):893–903.

Chernyshev OY, Martin-Schild S, Albright KC, et al. Safety of tPA in stroke mimics and neuroimaging-negative cerebral ischemia. *Neurology.* 2010;74(17):1340–1345.

Ciccone A, Valvassori L, Nichelatti M, et al. Endovascular treatment for acute ischemic stroke. *N Engl J Med.* 2013;368(10):904–913.

Cocho D, Belvis R, Marti-Fabregas J, et al. Reasons for exclusion from thrombolytic therapy following acute ischemic stroke. *Neurology.* 2005;64(4):719–720.

De Herdt V, Dumont F, Hénon H, et al. Early seizures in intracerebral hemorrhage: incidence, associated factors, and outcome. *Neurology.* 2011;77(20):1794–1800.

Ford AL, Williams JA, Spencer M, et al. Reducing door-to-needle times using Toyota's lean manufacturing principles and value stream analysis. *Stroke.* 2012;43(12):3395–3398.

Ford GA, Ahmed N, Azevedo E, et al. Intravenous alteplase for stroke in those older than 80 years old. *Stroke.* 2010;41(11):2568–2574.

Frontera JA, Gordon E, Zach V, et al. Reversal of coagulopathy using prothrombin complex concentrates is associated with improved outcome compared to fresh frozen plasma in warfarin-associated intracranial hemorrhage. *Neurocrit Care.* 2014;21:397–406.

Furlan A, Higashida R, Wechsler L, et al. Intra-arterial prourokinase for acute ischemic stroke. The PROACT II study: a randomized controlled trial. Prolyse in Acute Cerebral Thromboembolism. *JAMA.* 1999;282(21):2003–2011.

Heldner MR, Zubler C, Mattle HP, et al. National Institutes of Health stroke scale score and vessel occlusion in 2152 patients with acute ischemic stroke. *Stroke.* 2013;44(4):1153–1157.

Hemphill JC, Bonovich DC, Besmertis L, et al. The ICH score: a simple, reliable grading scale for intracerebral hemorrhage. *Stroke.* 2001;32(4):891–897.

Hopyan JJ, Gladstone DJ, Mallia G, et al. Renal safety of CT angiography and perfusion imaging in the emergency evaluation of acute stroke. *Am J Neuroradiol.* 2008;29:1826–1830.

Kidwell CS, Jahan R, Gornbein J, et al. A trial of imaging selection and endovascular treatment for ischemic stroke. *N Engl J Med.* 2013;368(10):914–923.

Kuramatsu JB, Gerner ST, Schellinger PD, et al. Anticoagulant reversal, blood pressure levels, and anticoagulant resumption in patients with anticoagulation-related intracerebral hemorrhage. *JAMA.* 2015;313:824–836.

Lees KR, Bluhmki E, von Kummer R, et al. Time to treatment with intravenous alteplase and outcome in stroke: an updated pooled analysis of ECASS, ATLANTIS, NINDS, and EPITHET trials. *Lancet.* 2010;375(9727):1695–1703.

Lindsberg PJ, Häppölä O, Kallela M, et al. Door to thrombolysis: ER reorganization and reduced delays to acute stroke treatment. *Neurology.* 2006;67(2):334–336.

Meretoja A, Strbian D, Mustanoja S, et al. Reducing in-hospital delay to 20 minutes in stroke thrombolysis. *Neurology.* 2012;79(4):306–313.

Meretoja A, Weir L, Ugalde M, et al. Helsinki model cut stroke thrombolysis delays to 25 minutes in Melbourne in only 4 months. *Neurology.* 2013;81(12):1071–1076.

Morgenstern LB, Hemphill JC, Anderson C, et al. Guidelines for the management of spontaneous intracerebral hemorrhage: a guideline for healthcare professionals from the American Heart Association/American Stroke Association. *Stroke.* 2010;41:2108–29.

Newman GC. Clarification of abc/2 rule for ICH volume. *Stroke.* 2007;38(3):862.

Nogueira RG, Lutsep HL, Gupta R, et al. Trevo versus Merci retrievers for thrombectomy revascularisation of large vessel occlusions in acute ischaemic stroke (TREVO 2): a randomised trial. *Lancet.* 2012;380(9849):1231–1240.

Prabhakaran S, Naidech AM. Ischemic brain injury after intracerebral hemorrhage: a critical review. *Stroke.* 2012;43(8):2258–2263.

Riedel CH, Zimmermann P, Jensen-Kondering U, et al. The importance of size: successful recanalization by intravenous thrombolysis in acute anterior stroke depends on thrombus length. *Stroke.* 2011;42(6):1775–1777.

Rost NS, Masrur S, Pervez MA, et al. Unsuspected coagulopathy rarely prevents IV thrombolysis in acute ischemic stroke. *Neurology.* 2009;73(23):1957–1962.

Smith EE, Fonarow GC, Reeves MJ, et al. Outcomes in mild or rapidly improving stroke not treated with intravenous recombinant tissue-type plasminogen activator: findings from Get With The Guidelines-Stroke. *Stroke.* 2011;42(11):3110–3115.

Tsivgoulis G, Alexandrov AV, Chang J, et al. Safety and outcomes of intravenous thrombolysis in stroke mimics: a 6-year, single-care center study and a pooled analysis of reported series. *Stroke.* 2011;42(6):1771–1774.

Tsivgoulis G, Katsanos AH, Butcher KS, et al. Intensive blood pressure reduction in acute intracerebral hemorrhage: a meta-analysis. *Neurology.* 2014;83(17):1523–1529.

Vespa PM, Martin N, Zuccarello M, et al. Surgical trials in intracerebral hemorrhage. *Stroke.* 2013;44(6)(suppl 1):S79–S82.

INTRODUCTION

Patients presenting with acute spinal cord syndromes represent true neurologic emergencies. Pathologic damage to the cord is usually incomplete. Therefore, there is opportunity to salvage (and peril of losing) vital cord tissue and function over the ensuing minutes and hours after presentation. As with other neurologic presentations, clinicians must first localize and then differentiate the type of damage in order to initiate the most effective interventions.

DIFFERENTIAL DIAGNOSIS

The differential diagnosis for an acute cord syndrome ranges from mechanical to vascular, infectious, inflammatory, neoplastic, and toxic etiologies (Tables 16.1 and 16.2). A careful history regarding remote or recent trauma, other systemic symptoms, or toxic habits may help narrow your differential. Determining the rate of symptom progression proves critical, as patients whose symptoms reach maximal involvement within minutes are more likely to have a mechanical or vascular cause rather than an infectious, inflammatory, or neoplastic cause.

SPINAL CORD ANATOMY

To aid with localization, recall that the caudal spinal cord segments do not align with the vertebrae bearing the same names. The spinal cord ends around L1, with the roots of the cauda equina below that vertebral level. Additionally, within the cervical cord, the spinal roots exit the spinal canal above the associated vertebral level except for root C8, which exits between C7 and T1. Thereafter, each spinal root exits below the corresponding vertebral body.

MOTOR SYSTEM

The majority of the corticospinal tract, mediating a large proportion of our volitional limb movements, decussates in the medulla before descending in the contralateral lateral corticospinal tract. The minority of motor axons that do not decussate within the medulla form the anterior corticospinal tract. The lower motor neurons, receiving input from corticospinal fibers as well as segmental interneurons, reside within the ventral horn (Fig. 16.1).

SENSORY SYSTEM

Afferent sensory fibers from the dorsal root ganglia enter the spinal cord at the dorsal horn. From there, their course depends on the type of modality being transmitted.

Pain and Temperature

These fibers travel rostrally within Lissauer tract for one or two spinal segments before synapsing within the dorsal horn and crossing to the contralateral anterolateral system. The anterolateral system is composed of the anterior spinothalamic tract, which carries crude touch sensory fibers, and the lateral spinothalamic tract, which carries pain and temperature fibers.

TABLE 16.1	Differential Diagnosis for Acute Spinal Syndromes	
Compressive/mechanical	**Infectious**
Trauma	Viral gray matter/acute flaccid paralysis
Disk herniation	
Epidural abscess	Poliovirus
Epidural hematoma	Enterovirus
Epidural neoplasm/ metastasis	Coxsackieviruses A & B
	West Nile virus (WNV)
Vertebral compression fracture	Japanese encephalitis (JE)
Vascular	Tick-borne encephalitis
Ischemic stroke	Viral white matter/ longitudinal myelitis
Dural arteriovenous fistula	
Arteriovenous malformation	Herpes simplex virus (HSV)
Cavernous malformation	Varicella-zoster virus (VZV)
Inflammatory	Cytomegalovirus (CMV)
Multiple sclerosis	Epstein–Barr virus (EBV)
Neuromyelitis optica	Influenza
Transverse myelitis	**Bacterial**
Acute disseminated encephalomyelitis (ADEM)	*Mycoplasma pneumoniae*
	Syphilis
Sarcoidosis	Tuberculosis
Paraneoplastic	Lyme
Systemic lupus erythematosus (SLE)	**Fungal**
	Cryptococcus neoformans
Antiphospholipid antibody syndrome (APS)	*Coccidioides immitis*
Sjögren syndrome	*Blastomycetes dermatitides*
Mixed connective tissue disease (MCTD)	*Histoplasma capsulatum*
	Candida species
Behçet disease	*Aspergillus* species
Toxic/metabolic	Zygomycetes
Heroin	**Parasitic**
Konzo	*Schistosoma* species
Arachnoiditis after angiographic/myelographic contrast agents	*Toxoplasma gondii*
	Taenia solium (cysticercosis)
Methotrexate toxicity	
Cytarabine toxicity	
Amphotericin B toxicity	
Neoplasm	

TABLE 16.2 Classic Spinal Cord Syndromes

Syndrome	Typical Causes	Clinical Characteristics
Central cord syndrome (syringomyelia)	Underlying cervical spondylosis with hyperextension injury; damage relatively greater to gray than white matter	Weakness in upper extremities > in lower extremities; may have neurogenic bladder dysfunction and varying degrees of sensory loss at or below the lesion (often in a "cape-like" distribution).
Brown-Séquard syndrome	Penetrating trauma (many nonpenetrating injuries show partial asymmetric syndromes)	Ipsilateral motor and vibration/proprioception loss below the lesion, contralateral pain/temperature loss two levels below the lesion
Anterior cord syndrome	Hypotensive event leading to infarct within the midthoracic region, or hyperflexion injury leading to compression of the anterior spinal artery	Bilateral loss of motor, pain/temperature sensation below the lesion with preservation of vibration/proprioception/two-point discrimination
Posterior cord syndrome	B_{12} deficiency, MS, vascular malformations, atlantoaxial subluxation	Bilateral loss of vibration/proprioception/two-point discrimination with preservation of motor, pain/temperature sensation below the lesion
Cauda equina syndrome	Disk herniation, tumor	Asymmetric lower extremity weakness, patchy impaired sensation to all modalities, loss of deep tendon reflexes as well as bulbocavernosus reflex and anal wink, often with low back and radicular pain
Conus medullaris syndrome	Disk herniation, trauma, tumor	Symmetric sacral > lumbar weakness (may have normal leg strength), saddle anesthesia, bowel/bladder dysfunction

MS, multiple sclerosis.

Vibration, Proprioception, and Two-Point Discrimination

These fibers travel within the ipsilateral dorsal columns to the gracilis and cuneatus nuclei of the lower medulla. Axons from the legs (fasciculus gracilis) are pushed medially by entering axons from the arms (fasciculus cuneatus) (see Fig. 16.1).

AUTONOMIC SYSTEM

Sympathetic

Sympathetic preganglionic neurons are located within the intermediolateral nucleus of the thoracic and upper lumbar (L1–L2) spinal cord. Their axons exit via the ventral roots and synapse on the postganglionic sympathetic neurons in the paravertebral ganglia (the "sympathetic chain ganglia") or the prevertebral ganglia.

Parasympathetic

Parasympathetic preganglionic neurons are found within four brain stem nuclei (cranial nerve [CN] III, VII, IX, X) of which only the vagus nerve contributes to autonomic control below the head. Additionally, parasympathetic preganglionic axons originating in cord segments S2–S4 exit via the sacral ventral roots. The vagus innervates the heart, bronchi, pancreas, kidney, and

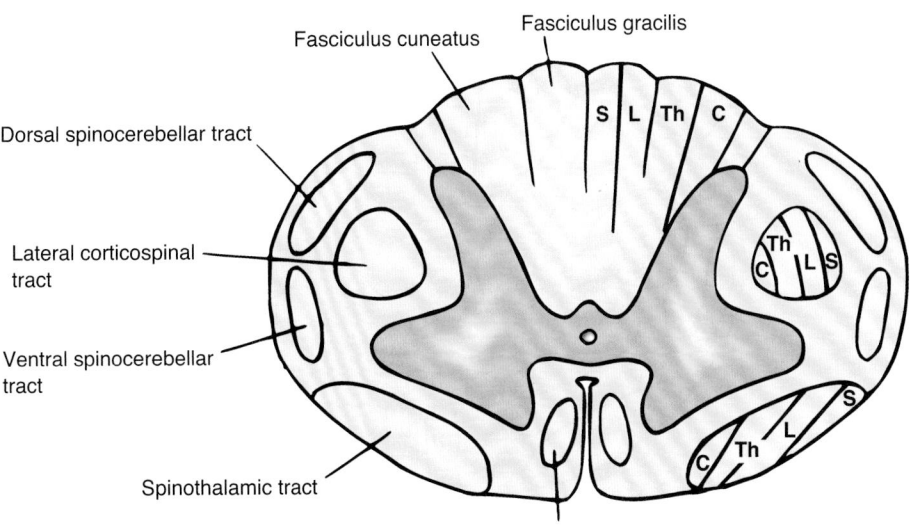

FIGURE 16.1 Anatomy of the spinal cord (cross-section). Tract lamination: S, sacral segments; L, lumbar segments; Th, thoracic segments; C, cervical segments. (From Brazis PW, Masdeu JC, Biller J. *Localization in Clinical Neurology.* 5th ed. Philadelphia: Lippincott Williams and Wilkins; 2007.)

Fasciculus cuneatus

Fasciculus gracilis

Dorsal spinocerebellar tract

Lateral corticospinal tract

Ventral spinocerebellar tract

Spinothalamic tract

Anterior corticospinal tract

the upper portion of the gastrointestinal tract, whereas sacral parasympathetics innervate the sexual organs, bladder, descending colon, and rectum.

Cardiovascular Innervation

The vagus nerve tonically reduces heart rate through effects on the sinoatrial node. Sympathetics arising from the upper thoracic levels (T1–T5) increase heart rate and contractility, whereas sympathetics from T5 to T12 increase vasoconstriction in the splanchnic bed and lower extremities. Splanchnic vasoconstriction can increase systemic blood pressure to dangerous, even lethal levels, in the phenomenon of autonomic dysreflexia, which is seen in some individuals with severe injuries at or above the T6 level.

Pulmonary Innervation

The phrenic nerve, which innervates the diaphragm, arises from C3 to C5. Although preservation of the phrenic nerve allows independent respiration, more subtle impairment of respiratory function may still be seen in those with lower injuries as a result of weakness in the intercostal or abdominal musculature.

VASCULAR ANATOMY OF THE SPINAL CORD

Three primary arteries run longitudinally along the spinal cord: the anterior spinal artery and two posterior spinal arteries. Branches of the single anterior spinal artery are responsible for two-thirds of the cord's cross-sectional area, whereas branches of the two posterior arteries serve a combined one-third of the cord's area. Therefore, the anterior portion of the cord is more susceptible to ischemia (Fig. 16.2).

The spinal arteries are fed by segmental radicular arteries, which are notoriously variable between individuals. The artery of Adamkiewicz is one of the largest radicular arteries that most commonly arises from the 9th to 12th intercostal arteries on the left. The artery of Adamkiewicz serves a critical role in supplying the anterior spinal artery's distribution over the lower third of the spinal cord including the conus medullaris. This artery is vulnerable to occlusion by aortic aneurysms and aortic repair procedures, resulting in a high rate of catastrophic cord ischemia and paraplegia. Rostral to the artery of Adamkiewicz, there is a relative paucity of collateral blood flow, making the midthoracic region particularly susceptible to ischemia from systemic hypotension.

FOCUSED HISTORY: KEY QUESTIONS

Depending on the level of injury, patients with spinal cord lesions are at risk for catastrophic acute cardiac and respiratory complications. Therefore, before taking the history, one must quickly assess airway, breathing, and circulation.

LOCALIZATION

- Does the patient have any *weakness*, and if so, what is its distribution? Does it involve only the lower extremities or the upper extremities or both?
- Does the patient have any *numbness* or *paresthesias*, and if so, what is its distribution?
- Is there any *pain* present? Is it local to the back or does it follow a radicular distribution?
- Is there any evidence of *bowel* or *bladder dysfunction*? In acute presentations without prior symptoms, the bladder may be prone to retention and overflow incontinence. In cases presenting with acute exacerbation of subacutely or chronically progressing lesions, the bladder may be spastic, with a history of increasing frequency, nocturia, and urge incontinence over the preceding weeks to months. Conversely, lesions affecting the lumbosacral cord segments may cause bladder hypotonia, leading to retention and frequent urinary tract infection.

DIFFERENTIAL DIAGNOSIS

- Is there a history of *trauma* or falls?
- Did the patient recently have *surgery* that may have led to hypotension or local cord ischemia?
- Does the patient have a known history of *cancer* or recent unexplained weight loss?
- Has the patient had any recent *infectious symptoms* such as fevers, chills, or cough?
- Has the patient had a *rash*?

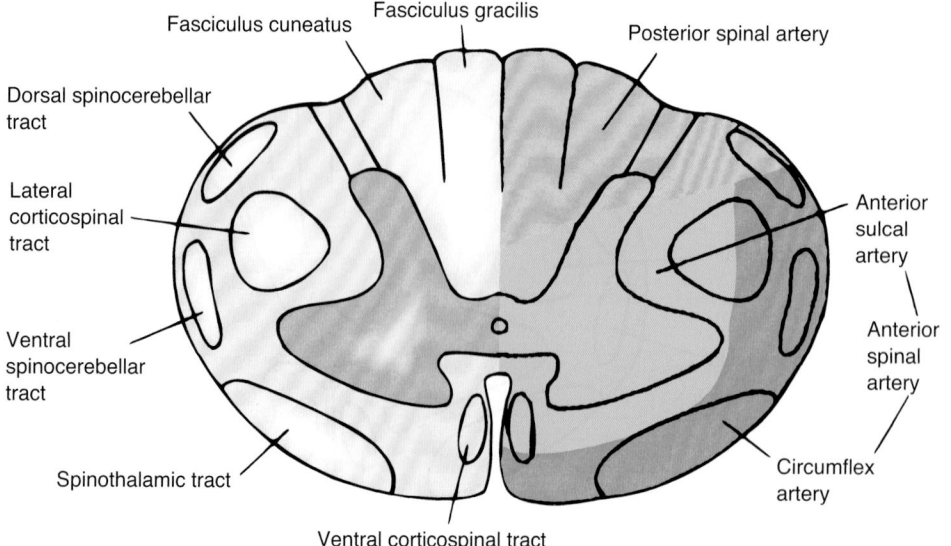

FIGURE 16.2 The vascular supply of the spinal cord. (From Brazis PW, Masdeu JC, Biller J. *Localization in Clinical Neurology*. 5th ed. Philadelphia: Lippincott Williams and Wilkins; 2007.)

Fasciculus gracilis

Fasciculus cuneatus

Posterior spinal artery

Dorsal spinocerebellar tract

Lateral corticospinal tract

Ventral spinocerebellar tract

Spinothalamic tract

Ventral corticospinal tract

Anterior sulcal artery

Anterior spinal artery

Circumflex artery

- Is the patient *immunocompromised* due to medications, cancer, or HIV? This may predispose to infection or medication-induced myelopathy.
- Is there a history of *vision loss* in either eye that later resolved partially or completely?
- Is there a history of *substance abuse* or workplace/*environmental exposures*?

FOCUSED EXAM

GENERAL EXAM

Recall that with cervical lesions, the *respiratory* and *cardiovascular* systems may be compromised (Table 16.3).

Respiratory

Shortness of breath or frank respiratory failure may occur. Careful observation must be paid to assess not only for hypoxia but also for hypercapnic respiratory failure and increased work of breathing using accessory muscles.

Cardiovascular

Lesions at or above T6 place the patient at risk of unbalanced sympathetic–parasympathetic drive. These patients may present with neurogenic shock: hypotension (resting and orthostatic), bradycardia, or other cardiac arrhythmias including asystole. At later time points, affected patients are also at risk for autonomic dysreflexia: episodes of extreme hypertension (due to excessive sympathetic vasoconstriction of the splanchnic vessel bed) with corresponding autonomic signs or symptoms such as diaphoresis, piloerection, facial flushing, and bradycardia (due to parasympathetic-mediated vasodilation above the lesion), and headache. These episodes most often have an identifiable trigger such as bladder or bowel irritation.

Autonomic

Effects on bowel and bladder function are not as straightforward as often perceived. During acute spinal shock, tone is decreased, leading to urinary retention, decreased rectal tone, and loss of bulbocavernosus reflex. Therefore, the rectal exam and checking the postvoid residual are required.

TABLE 16.3	Summary of Exam Findings
System	**Exam Signs/Symptoms**
Respiratory	Tachypnea, shallow breathing, complaints of shortness of breath
Cardiovascular	Hypotension, bradycardia, arrhythmia
Dermatologic	Presence of a rash may aid in narrowing the differential
Motor	Weakness below lesion; decreased tone initially, transitioning to increased tone/spasticity
Sensory	Sensory level at lesion
Reflexes	May be depressed initially then below lesion then transition to hyperreflexia
Autonomic	Evaluate for decreased rectal tone (heart rate, etc.)

Dermatologic

A cutaneous rash, if present, helps narrow the differential diagnosis to a stronger consideration of infectious or autoimmune mechanism.

NEUROLOGIC EXAM

Strength and Reflexes

Involvement of the lateral corticospinal tract results in upper motor neuron weakness: Below the lesion, one observes increased tone in velocity-dependent fashion (spasticity), as well as hyperreflexia (often but not always including an extensor response to noxious plantar stimulation). Ventral horn involvement results in lower motor neuron weakness *at* the lesion levels with decreased or flaccid tone as well as hyporeflexia. Atrophy takes weeks or longer to develop. Note that cervical injuries often demonstrate *both* types of weakness—lower motor neuron weakness at the cervical level (due to damage of the ventral horn) and upper motor neuron weakness below the lesion (due to damage of the passing corticospinal tracts).

A period of *spinal shock* lasting up to several days may result in the patient presenting with flaccid tone and diffuse hyporeflexia regardless of upper or lower motor neuron involvement. On examining any patient with an injury not involving the sacrum, spinal shock is confirmed by absence of the bulbocavernosus reflex. Key muscle groups useful for localizing spinal levels include elbow flexors (C5), wrist extensors (C6), elbow extensors (C7), intrinsic hand muscles (C8–T1), hip flexors (L2), knee extensors (L3), ankle dorsiflexors (L4), and ankle plantarflexors (S1).

Sensory

A sensory "level," with sharply demarcated decreased or absent sensation below the level of the lesion, may be seen. Depending on the distribution of the lesion in the anteroposterior and mediolateral axes, different combinations of bilateral, ipsilateral, and contralateral sensory loss may be observed, such as loss of vibration and proprioception (dorsal columns) and/or loss of pain and temperature (anterolateral system). Useful dermatomal landmarks include the nipple line (T4) and navel line (T10).

DIAGNOSTIC TESTING

IMAGING

To visualize the cord parenchyma, intervertebral disks, and surrounding soft tissues, magnetic resonance imaging (MRI) with T2-weighted imaging is the gold standard (see also Chapter 21). If an infectious, inflammatory, or neoplastic process is suspected, post-intravenous gadolinium contrast sequences should be performed as well, unless the patient's renal function is compromised. If an ischemic process is suspected, then diffusion-weighted and apparent diffusion coefficient sequences warrant special attention, with consideration of magnetic resonance angiography. In general, MRI should focus on the cord region suspected to harbor the lesion. For example, the clinician should avoid the common mistake of imaging the lumbosacral cord in a patient presenting with bilateral leg weakness, leg hypertonia, and hyperreflexia. This upper motor neuron presentation strongly argues for a thoracic, not a lumbosacral lesion. It should be noted that a total spinal cord survey may be warranted in many situations, such as to assess for multiple lesions or diffuse meningeal involvement.

TABLE 16.4   Laboratory Evaluation for Acute Spinal Cord Syndromes

Source	Laboratory Test
Lumbar puncture	Cell count with differential
	Glucose
	Total protein
	Gram stain and culture
	HSV 1 and 2 PCR
	VZV PCR
	VZV IgG/IgM
	EBV PCR
	Enterovirus PCR
	VDRL
	Oligoclonal band profile (needs matching serum sample)
	IgG index
	Angiotensin-converting enzyme (ACE)
	Aquaporin-4 antibody
Serum	ACE
	ANA
	dsDNA antibodies
	Anti-Smith antibodies
	Anti-Ro/SSA antibodies
	Anti-La/SSB antibodies
	Anti-RNP antibodies
	Anti-slc-70 antibodies
	RPR
	Paraneoplastic

HSV, herpes simplex virus; PCR, polymerase chain reaction; VZV, varicella-zoster virus; IgG, immunoglobulin G; IgM, immunoglobulin M; EBV, Epstein–Barr virus; VDRL, Venereal Disease Research Laboratory; ANA, antinuclear antibodies; RPR, rapid plasma reagin.

LABORATORY TESTING

A lumbar puncture should be performed as part of the diagnostic evaluation in patients with suspected infectious, inflammatory, or image-negative etiology. A list of tests to consider are listed in Table 16.4.

INITIAL MANAGEMENT

SPINAL STABILIZATION

As part of the "ABCs" (airway, breathing, circulation) of emergency medicine, any acute traumatic spinal cord presentation should be immediately stabilized with a rigid cervical collar in the emergency department (ED) if not already applied in the field (Table 16.5). Please see Chapter 47 for more on the management of acute spinal trauma.

INTENSIVE CARE UNIT ADMISSION

Intensive care, within a neurologic intensive care unit (ICU) if available, is preferred in any patient who has cardiovascular or

TABLE 16.5   Acute Spinal Cord Management Checklist

1. Stabilize cervical spine in all patients with traumatic or suspected traumatic etiology.
2. Assess need for ICU admission.
3. Consider neurosurgical consultation.
4. Pulmonary management: pulse oximetry, ABG, bedside pulmonary function tests
5. Cardiovascular management: telemetry, frequent or continuous blood pressure monitoring
6. Bowel care: neurogenic bowel protocol
7. Bladder care: frequent bladder scans with catheterization as appropriate
8. Skin care: aggressive monitoring and early treatment to prevent pressure ulcers
9. DVT prophylaxis: early initiation of chemoprophylaxis and mechanical devices

ICU, intensive care unit; ABG, arterial blood gas; DVT, deep vein thrombosis.

pulmonary symptoms associated with the lesion or who has rapid progression of neurologic symptoms. The ICU setting allows for the frequent neurologic examination and urgent pulmonary and cardiovascular care that is often necessary to prevent further deterioration in the setting of acute cord pathology.

NEUROSURGICAL CONSULTATION

If the etiology of the patient's presentation is compressive, neurosurgical consultation is emergently required.

PULMONARY MANAGEMENT

Patients with high cervical or elongated multilevel cervical or thoracic lesions should be monitored for respiratory compromise even if intubation is not immediately needed. Not all patients will decompensate immediately. Hypercarbia often precedes hypoxia, so abnormalities are often present on arterial blood gas (ABG) before they become evident on pulse oximetry.

Regardless of lesion location, all patients with spinal cord compromise are at high risk of developing pulmonary complications such as atelectasis, pneumonia, and embolism. Incentive spirometry, chest physiotherapy, and early mobilization can mitigate these risks.

CARDIOVASCULAR MANAGEMENT

During the acute period, spinal shock may result in decreased sympathetic outflow leading to neurogenic hypotension, bradycardia, and arrhythmia. Therefore, patients should be closely followed using telemetry and frequent or continuous blood pressure monitoring. To prevent exacerbation of cord dysfunction from systemic hypoperfusion, a mean arterial pressure of at least 85 mm Hg for the first 7 days is recommended using fluid resuscitation and vasopressors as necessary.

BLADDER CARE

Urinary retention during the acute period places the patient at increased risk for urinary tract infection and renal complications. If the patient is still able to void, bladder scanning or catheterization for postvoid residuals is required every 6 hours. If the patient is unable to void acutely, a Foley catheter should be placed initially, with the goal of transitioning to intermittent catheterization as soon as feasible to avoid complications in the postacute period.

BOWEL CARE

Clinicians often assume that spinal cord injury simply causes bowel incontinence. However, the far more common bowel sequela is severe constipation or even an utter inability to defecate. Bowel retention can trigger episodes of life-threatening autonomic dysreflexia. In addition to an aggressive bowel protocol consisting of stool softeners, fiber, hyperosmotic agents, and intermittent colonic irritants, digital stimulation is often needed to trigger the rectocolic reflex. Patients with hand function should be trained by nurses experienced in spinal cord injury bowel care to self-perform digital stimulation on a fixed daily or every-other-day schedule.

SKIN CARE

Patients with cord dysfunction may lack the sensorimotor feedback required to make subtle adjustments in body position to relieve pressure on bony prominences. Hence, pressure ulcers are a critical concern during both the acute and chronic periods. Vigilant monitoring and aggressive treatment at the first sign of skin breakdown (erythema) are required. Frequent rotation by nursing or a rotating bed will aid in ulcer prevention.

DEEP VEIN THROMBOSIS PROPHYLAXIS

Patients with spinal cord lesions are at highly increased risk of developing deep vein thromboses (DVTs) and pulmonary emboli. Consequentially, multimodal DVT prophylaxis with both medication and sequential compression devices is warranted. Routine placement of prophylactic vena cava filters is not recommended.

STEROIDS

The extremely high-dose methylprednisolone protocol previously recommended during the first 24 to 48 hours after acute traumatic injury has fallen out of favor (see Chapter 47). However, the role of lower or moderate-dose glucocorticoids (decadron 4-10 mg IV q6H) in reducing inflammation and vasogenic edema from tumor or epidural abscess still warrants their use in many situations.

NEXT-GENERATION SPINAL CORD TREATMENTS

Clinicians caring for patients with acute spinal cord syndromes would be well served to treat their patients with the same mindset as they do for patients with acute brain injury—viable tissue can be saved through quick intervention and development of "next-generation" treatments. In the following section are some promising avenues for improving care and outcomes in acute spinal cord syndromes. Although these treatments are not evidence-based, the poor prognosis for recovery associated with acute spinal cord injury encourages many practitioners and teams to offer these interventions.

LIMITING SECONDARY DAMAGE

Therapeutic Hypothermia

In parallel to its use in ischemic cardiac and brain settings, the goal of mild to moderate hypothermia is to reduce cellular metabolic demand during the acute stages of spinal cord compression and ischemia. To date, only nonrandomized, noncontrolled cohorts have been reported using this modality in patients with spinal injury.

Antiexcitotoxic Agents

Many putative neuroprotective drugs have been trialed for efficacy in the setting of stroke and neurodegenerative disease. To date, all have failed. However, several neuroprotectants that have shown early promise in spinal cord injury are currently undergoing efficacy trials: riluzole (sodium channel and glutamate antagonist), magnesium (N-methyl-D-aspartate [NMDA] antagonist), and minocycline (anti-inflammatory and antiapoptosis).

Perfusion Pressure Support

Maintenance of a mean arterial perfusion pressure above 85 mm Hg with the use of fluid resuscitation and vasopressors has been cited as a method for reducing secondary ischemic injury after acute spinal cord injury.

Intrathecal Pressure Relief

Decompression of vertebral or neoplastic tissue is a basic approach in situations involving trauma or metastatic encroachment. Necrosis, edema, and inflammation may cause ongoing increased intradural pressure and resultant hypoperfusion of the cord parenchyma. For this reason, work in animals as well as preliminarily in humans has begun to focus on the potential of performing durotomy or even myelotomy in the acute setting to improve local perfusion.

IMPROVING NEURAL PLASTICITY AND RECOVERY

Spared neural tissue persists even after clinically severe spinal cord syndromes. Therapies that increase activity and sprouting of residual neural circuitry show great promise in animal models. Multiple human trials on agents listed below are either underway or in planning stages. Importantly, these approaches are not mutually exclusive—optimal treatment will require combinations of drugs, electrical, and cellular approaches with intense physical rehabilitation.

Intrinsic Neural Reactivators

These drugs stimulate intrinsic neuronal second-messenger pathways: rolipram (cyclic adenosine monophosphate [AMP] agonist), SUN13837 (basic fibroblast growth factor agonist), dalfampridine (potassium channel antagonist), and lithium (glycogen synthase kinase 3 inhibitor).

Extrinsic Inhibitor Antagonists

These drugs block the inhibitory role played by myelin proteins and chondroitin sulfate proteoglycans in limiting neural regeneration: ATI 355 (anti-Nogo-A antibodies), chondroitinase ABC, and BA-210 (Rho antagonist).

Neural Reactivating Devices

Exoskeletal robotic devices for improving arm and leg function are rapidly evolving. But implanted epidural stimulation represents the most promising device-based approach to truly reactivating spared neural circuits. Early human results show that when implanted over the lower cord, these devices, already U.S. Food and

Drug Association (FDA) approved as spine stimulators for patients with chronic pain, can amplify endogenous signals from residual circuitry to result in voluntary leg movement in patients that previously had complete motor paraplegia.

Stem Cells

Long heralded as the cure for most ills, stem cells continue to make slow progress toward practical clinical application. In spinal injury, implantation of predifferentiated stem cells may improve recovery through release of neurotrophic growth factors as well as through improved remyelination of residual axons.

SUGGESTED READINGS

Alexander M, Biering-Sorensen F, Bodner D, et al. Internation standards to document remaining autonomic function after spinal cord injury. *Spinal Cord.* 2009;47:36–43.

Angeli CA, Edgerton VR, Gerasimenko YP, et al. Altering spinal cord excitability enables voluntary movements after chronic complete paralysis in humans. *Brain.* 2014;137:1394–409.

Becker D, McDonald JW. Approaches to repairing the damaged spinal cord: overview. *Handb Clin Neurol.* 2012;109:445–461.

Casha S, Christie S. A systematic review of intensive cardiopulmonary management after spinal cord injury. *J Neurotrauma.* 2011;28:1479–1495.

Consortium for Spinal Cord Medicine. Early acute management in adults with spinal cord injury: a clinical practice guideline for health-care professionals. *J Spinal Cord Med.* 2008;31:403–479.

Cree B. Acute inflammatory myelopathies. *Handb Clin Neurol.* 2014;122: 613–667.

Dhall SS, Hadley MN, Aarabi B, et al. Deep venous thrombosis and thromboembolism in patients with cervical spinal cord injuries. *Neurosurgery.* 2013;72:244–254.

Dhall SS, Hadley MN, Aarabi B, et al. Nutritional support after spinal cord injury. *Neurosurgery.* 2013;72:255–259.

Dididze M, Green B, Dietrich W, et al. Systemic hypothermia in acute cervical spinal cord injury: a case-controlled study. *Spinal Cord.* 2013;51:395–400.

Fink JK. Hereditary myelopathies. *Continuum (N Y).* 2008;14:58–73.

Flanagan E, McKeon A, Lennon V, et al. Paraneoplastic isolated myelopathy: clinical course and neuroimaging clues. *Neurology.* 2011;76:2089–2095.

Francis K. Physiology and management of bladder and bowel continence following spinal cord injury. *Ostomy Wound Manage.* 2007;53:18–27.

Furlan JC, Fehlings MG. Cardiovascular complications after acute spinal cord injury: pathophysiology, diagnosis and management. *Neurosurg Focus.* 2008; 25:E13.

Gorman PH, Qadri SFA, Rao-Patel A. Prophylactic inferior vena cava (IVC) filter placement may increase the relative risk of deep venous thrombosis after acute spinal cord. *J Trauma.* 2009;66:707–712.

Hadley MN, Walters BC, Aarabi B, et al. Clinical assessment following acute cervical spinal cord injury. *Neurosurgery.* 2013;72:40–53.

Hansebout RR, Hansebout CR. Local cooling for traumatic spinal cord injury: outcomes in 20 patients and review of the literature. *J Neurosurg Spine.* 2014;20:550–561.

Ho EL. Infectious etiologies of myelopathy. *Semin Neurol.* 2012;32:154–160.

Hurlbert RJ, Hadley MN, Walters BC, et al. Pharmacological therapy for acute spinal cord injury. *Neurosurgery.* 2013;72:93–105.

James W, Mass J. Inherited myelopathies. *Semin Neurol.* 2012;32:114–122.

Kakulas B. The clinical neuropathology of spinal cord injury: a guide to the future. *Paraplegia.* 1987;25:212–216.

Ko HY, Ditunno JF Jr, Graziani V, et al. The pattern of reflex recovery during spinal shock. *Spinal Cord.* 1999;37:402–409.

Kumar N. Metabolic and toxic myelopathies. *Semin Neurol.* 2012;32:123–136.

Kwon B, Sekhon L, Fehlings M. Emerging repair, regeneration, and translational research advances for spinal cord injury. *Spine.* 2010;35:S263–S270.

Lemons VR, Wagner FC. Respiratory complications after cervical spinal cord injury. *Spine.* 1994;20:2315–2320.

McKinley W, Santos K, Meade M, et al. Incidence and outcomes of spinal cord injury clinical syndromes. *J Spinal Cord Med.* 2007;30:215–224.

Mihai C, Jubelt B. Infectious myelitis. *Curr Neurol Neurosci Rep.* 2012;12: 633–641.

Moftakhar P, Hetts SW, Ko NU. Vascular myelopathies. *Semin Neurol.* 2012;32:146–153.

Nagpal S, Clarke JL. Neoplastic myelopathy. *Semin Neurol.* 2012;32:137–145.

Ramer L, Ramer M, Bradbury E. Rescue, reactivate, rewire: restoring function after spinal cord injury. *Lancet Neurol.* 2014;13(12):1241–1256.

Ryken TC, Hurlbert RJ, Hadley MN, et al. The acute cardiopulmonary management of patients with cervical spinal cord injuries. *Neurosurgery.* 2013;72:84–92.

Theodore N, Hadley MN, Aarabi B, et al. Prehospital cervical spinal immobilization after trauma. *Neurosurgery.* 2013;72:22–34.

West TW, Hess C, Cree BA. Acute transverse myelitis: demyelinating, inflammatory and infectious myelopathies. *Semin Neurol.* 2012;32:97–113.

Winslow C, Rozovsky J. Effect of spinal cord injury on the respiratory system. *Am J Phys Med Rehab.* 2003;82:803–814.

Yoshioka K, Niinuma H, Ehara S, et al. MR angiography and CT angiography of the artery of Adamkiewicz: state of the art. *Radiographics.* 2006;26:S63–S73.

Focal Mass Lesions 17

Michelle Wilson Bell, Alexander G. Khandji, and Fabio M. Iwamoto

INTRODUCTION

The differential diagnosis of an undifferentiated focal brain mass lesion is broad and the clinical presentation quite variable. This chapter will discuss the major etiologic categories of focal brain mass lesions—namely tumors, abscesses, and other inflammatory lesions—and present an algorithm for implementing empiric management in stable patients while a definitive diagnosis is pursued.

EMERGENT MANAGEMENT OF SYMPTOMATIC INTRACRANIAL MASS EFFECT

The first step in management of a focal mass lesion is to assess for increased intracranial pressure (ICP) and signs of herniation in patients with radiographic signs of mass effect and midline shift.

Common symptoms and signs of increased ICP include headache, vomiting, depressed level of consciousness, papilledema, abducens nerve palsies, and hypertension with or without bradycardia (Cushing reflex). As mass effect worsens, in addition to the expected contralateral hemiparesis, patients develop motor signs *ipsilateral* to the lesion as a result of lateral and rotation displacement of both corticospinal tracts. Common signs include

stiffening, hyperreflexia, and extensor plantar responses. With further brain tissue displacement, transtentorial herniation leads to ipsilateral third nerve palsy ("blown pupil").

If the clinical assessment is concerning for elevated ICP, it is imperative to take immediate measures to reduce it. First-line interventions include head elevation to 30 degrees and bolus osmotherapy with either 20% mannitol 1 g/kg intravenously (IV) or 30 mL of 23.4% hypertonic saline if there is central venous access. If level of consciousness is depressed with inability to maintain and protect the airway, the patient should be intubated and hyperventilated to PaCO$_2$ of 30 mm Hg while awaiting definitive treatment (see Chapter 107 for further details).

If there is no evidence of increased ICP, further management should be determined by the clinician's assessment of the most likely underlying cause of the mass lesion. This chapter will discuss the diagnostic evaluation of undifferentiated mass lesions and the initial steps in management depending on the suspected diagnosis.

CAUSES OF FOCAL BRAIN LESIONS

Figure 17.1 shows common causes of focal lesions of the brain not consistent with stroke or trauma based on location.

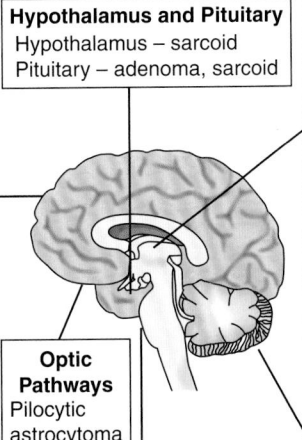

Hemispheres
Metastases: 80% of metastases go to the cerebral hemispheres, mainly at the gray–white junction
Adult Primary Brain Tumors: GBM (23% are in the frontal lobe, 24% parietal, 31% temporal, occipital lobes usually spared); lymphoma (40% go periventricular white matter, 38% coating of ventricles)
Bacterial: Bacterial abscess from otitis media or mastoiditis (streptococci, *Bacteroides*, *Pseudomonas*, *Haemophilus*) often go to inferior temporal lobe; bacterial abscess from ethmoid/frontal infection (streptococci, staphylococci); usually go to frontal lobe
Viral: HSV, usually in medial temporal lobe
Inflammatory: Tumefactive multiple sclerosis

Hypothalamus and Pituitary
Hypothalamus – sarcoid
Pituitary – adenoma, sarcoid

Optic Pathways
Pilocytic astrocytoma

Basal Ganglia and Deep Midline Structures
Metastases: 3% of metastasis go to the basal ganglia
Adult Primary Brain Tumors: GBM (can involve the deep gray and white matter more than other gliomas)
Lymphoma: Located in deep gray matter nuclei/subcortical 27% of the time
Pediatric Primary Brain Tumors: Diffuse fibrillary astrocytoma (occurs supratentorially in the deep midline structures)
Bacterial: Whipple (lesions in hypothalamus, thalamus, basal parts of telencephalon)
Viral: Eastern Equine Virus (EEV), Japanese encephalitis, rabies, measles virus, St. Louis encephalitis virus
Fungal: *Cryptococcus* tends to affect basal ganglia

Cerebellum
Metastases: 15% of mets go to cerebellum. Colorectal metastasis affect the cerebellum disproportionately
Pediatric Primary Brain Tumors: Pilocytic, astrocytoma, medulloblastoma (usually arise from the vermis then grow into the inferior or superior velum of the fourth ventricle and can distort the fourth ventricle)
Bacterial: Bacterial abscess from otitis media/mastoiditis
Viral: EBV
Fungal: Coccidioidomycoses

Brain Stem
Pediatric Primary Brain Tumors: Pilocytic astrocytoma, diffuse fibrillary astrocytoma (can occur at the cervicomedullary junction), ependymoma (most often localized to the floor of the fourth ventricle)
Viral: EBV, EEV, Japanese encephalitis, rabies
Fungal: Cryptococcus can occur in the midbrain
Inflammatory: Behçet, sarcoid

FIGURE 17.1 Common causes of focal lesions in the brain based on location. GBM, glioblastoma; HSV, herpes simplex virus; EBV, Epstein–Barr virus.

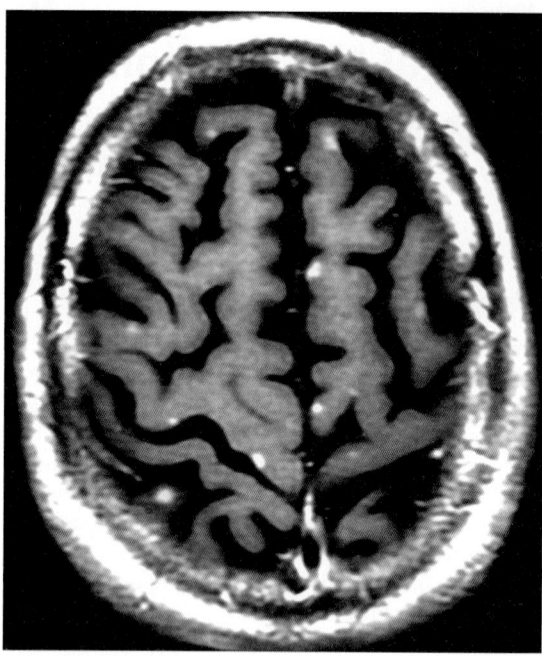

FIGURE 17.2 Metastatic small cell lung cancer. T1 MRI of the brain shows multiple small enhancing metastatic nodules.

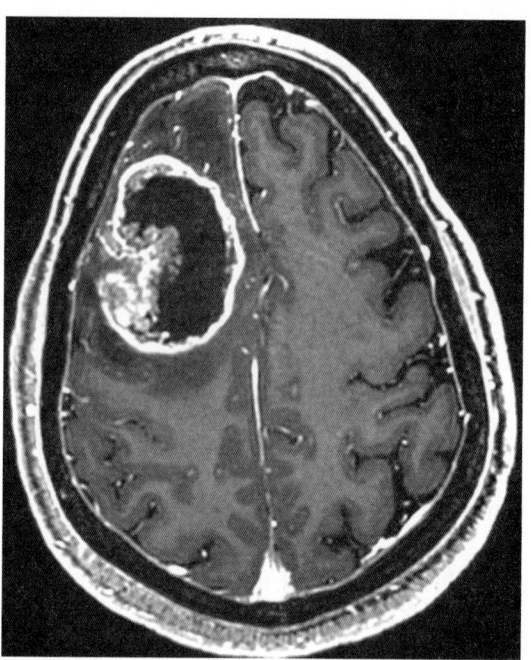

FIGURE 17.4 Glioblastoma multiforme. T1 MRI shows central necrosis and ring enhancement with a nodular component extending into the center of the lesion.

BRAIN TUMORS

Tumors account for the majority of focal brain mass lesions. In adults, *metastatic tumors* account for approximately 50% of symptomatic brain tumors (Fig. 17.2). The most common primary tumor to metastasize to the brain is lung cancer. Approximately 50% to 60% of brain metastasis originate from lung cancer, with 25% to 40% being of non–small cell lung cancer (NSCLC) origin and 5% to 15% being of small cell lung cancer (SCLC) origin. About 20% of lung cancer brain metastases are found at the time of initial diagnosis. The next most common sources of brain metastases are breast cancers (15% to 30%), melanoma (10%), renal cancer (5%), and gastrointestinal cancers (5%) (see Chapter 97).

Approximately 70,000 primary brain tumors are diagnosed each year. The most common form of primary brain tumor found in adults are *meningiomas* (35%). These dural-based masses enhance densely with gadolinium on magnetic resonance imaging (MRI) (Fig. 17.3) and are easy to identify prior to surgery due to their highly characteristic appearance (see Chapter 98). *Gliomas* are the second most common form of primary tumor accounting for 30% of all brain tumors (see Chapter 97). Glioblastoma multiforme is the most common form of glioma and account for 80% of all malignant brain tumors (Fig. 17.4). Anaplastic astrocytoma and oligodendrogliomas (Fig. 17.5) are lower grade tumors that show less prominent enhancement and no necrosis. Less common

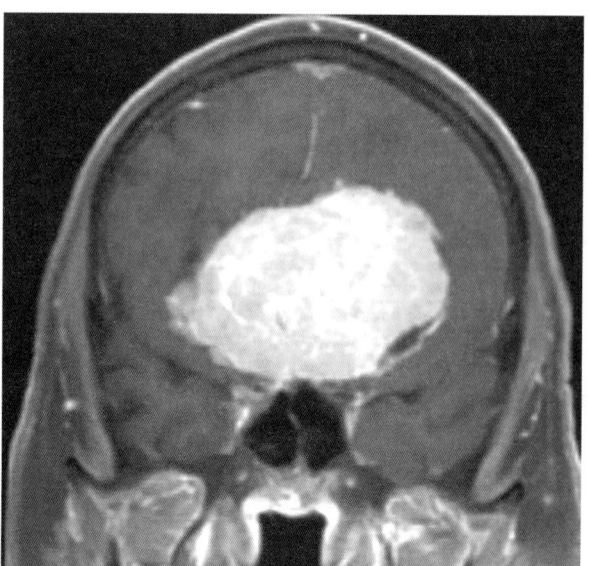

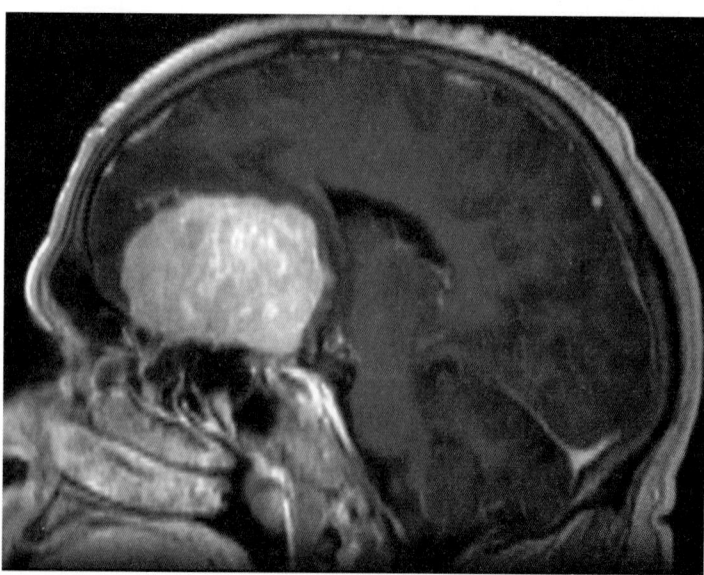

A   B

FIGURE 17.3 Large parasagittal olfactory groove meningioma strongly enhancing after contrast. Note the small cleft of CSF noted along the left margin of the lesion (coronal image, panel A).

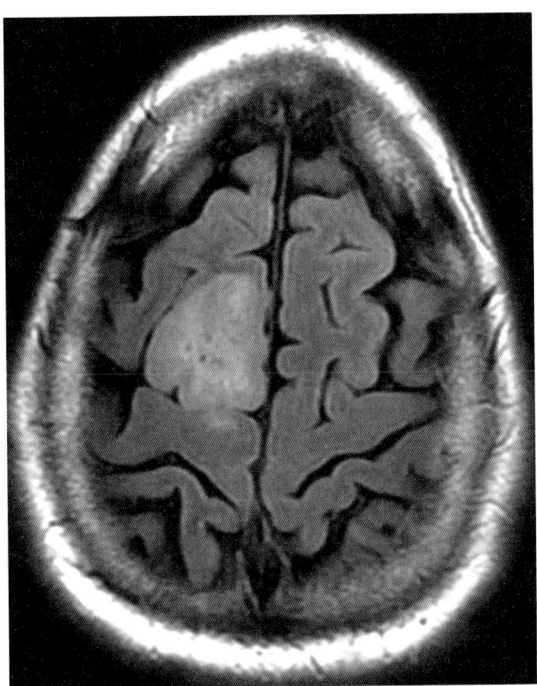 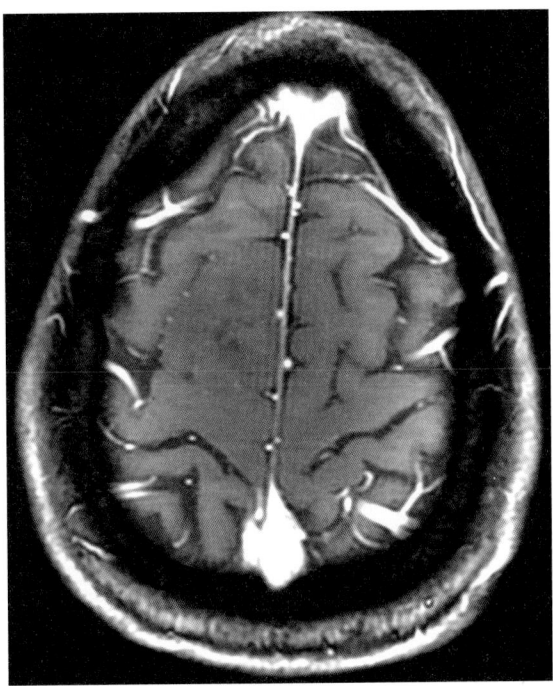

A

B

FIGURE 17.5 FLAIR **(A)** and T1 gadolinium enhanced **(B)** MR of a right frontal oligodendroglioma showing very little contrast enhancement and very little surrounding edema.

adult primary brain tumors, in order of frequency, are pituitary adenomas (Fig. 17.6 and Chapter 100), nerve sheath tumors such as acoustic neuromas (see Chapter 102), and primary central nervous system (CNS) lymphomas (Fig. 17.7 and Chapter 99). Table 17.1 outlines typical clinical features, imaging findings, and suggested ancillary testing in adult patients with suspected brain neoplasm.

In children, the most common primary brain tumors are gliomas (40%) including pilocytic astrocytoma (Fig. 17.8), embryonal tumors (15%) including medulloblastoma (Fig. 17.9), and ependymoma (~5%). Table 17.2 outlines typical clinical features, imaging findings, and suggested ancillary testing in children with suspected brain neoplasm (see also Chapter 145).

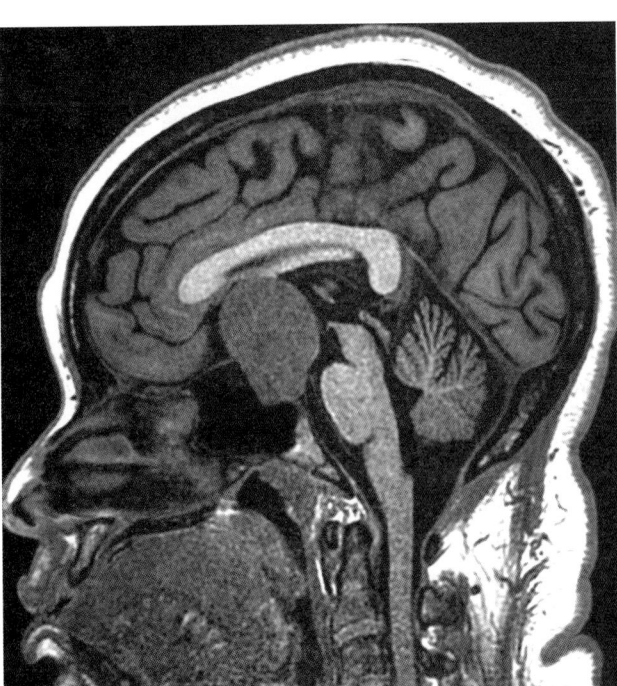 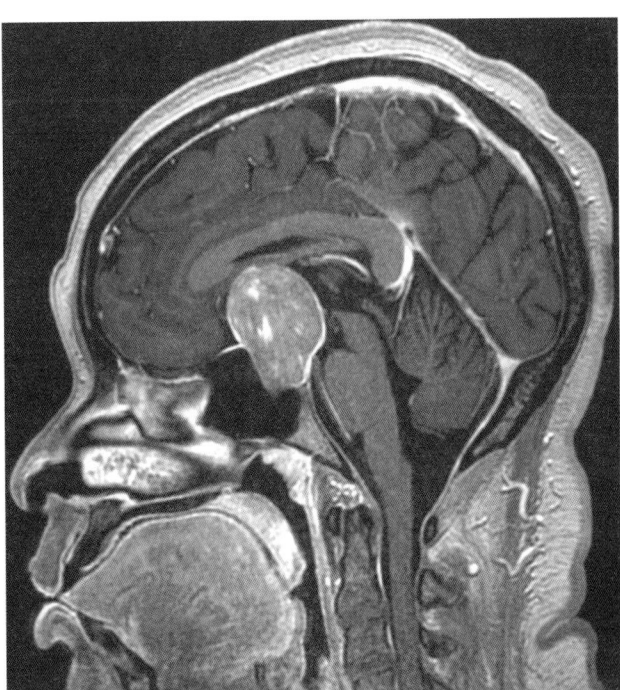

A

B

FIGURE 17.6 Pituitary macroadenoma. **A:** Hypointense on T1. **B:** Enhancing postcontrast.

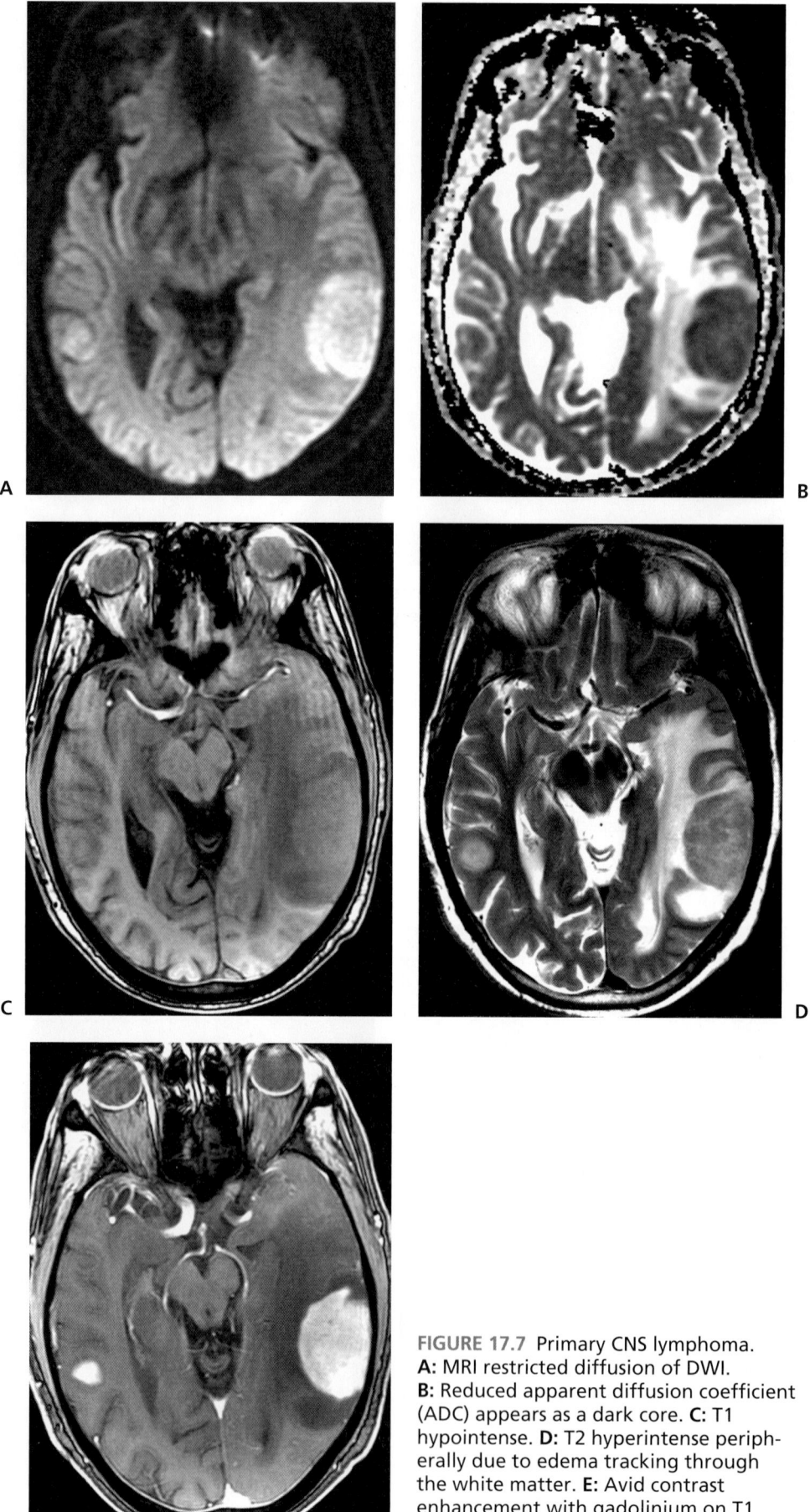

FIGURE 17.7 Primary CNS lymphoma.
A: MRI restricted diffusion of DWI.
B: Reduced apparent diffusion coefficient (ADC) appears as a dark core. **C:** T1 hypointense. **D:** T2 hyperintense peripherally due to edema tracking through the white matter. **E:** Avid contrast enhancement with gadolinium on T1 imaging.

TABLE 17.1 Common Adult Brain Tumors

	Clinical Pearls	Imaging Features	CSF Studies and Systemic Workup
Metastatic tumors (in order of decreasing frequency)	Lung • Small cell lung cancer eventually metastasized to the brain in up to 50% of cases. Breast • HER2+/ER− receptor status portends a higher likelihood of metastasis to the brain. Melanoma • Head, neck, and primary oral lesions have a higher rate of metastasis. Renal • In up to 10% of patients, a new metastasis later develops in patients who were thought to have been cured of their primary tumor. Colorectal • Left-sided cancers are more likely to metastasize to the lung and brain, whereas right-sided tumors usually go to liver.	• 80% of brain metastases occur in the cerebral hemispheres, 15% in the cerebellum, and 5% in the basal ganglia. • Metastases tend to localize to the gray–white junction location and the border zone between two major arterial distributions. • Brain metastases are multiple, approximately 50% of cases. • FLAIR imaging tends to reveal a large amount of associated vasogenic edema. • MR spectroscopy shows low *N*-acetylaspartate (NAA) and creatine levels and elevated choline levels reflecting cell membrane and myelin turnover. • Gradient echo or SWI may demonstrate hemosiderin deposits in cancers that tend to hemorrhage (e.g., melanoma, choriocarcinoma, renal cell, and thyroid cancer). Melanoma tends to be hyperdense on CT scan even in the absence of hemorrhage. On MRI, melanoma is hyperintense on T1 and hypointense on T2. • Colorectal metastases involve the cerebellum disproportionately.	More than 60% of patients with brain metastases will have a mass demonstrated on chest imaging that is either due to a primary lung cancer or lung metastases from a primary tumor elsewhere. Tests to consider when brain metastases are suspected: • Mammogram • Skin exam • Whole-body CT • Whole-body FDG-PET
Meningoma	• 35% of all primary brain tumors • 67% of cases occur in women • Peak incidence, age 40–60 yr	Dural based with dense, homogeneous enhancement • Isointense to hypointense on T1 • Isointense to hyperintense on T2 Anatomic predilection in order of frequency • Parasagittal • Convexity • Sphenoid ridge • Cerebellopontine angle • Olfactory groove Can elicit a bony reaction leading to hyperostosis of the overlying calvarium Calcification occurs in approximately 20% of cases.	None

Gliomas	• 30% of all primary brain tumors
	• Average age of diagnosis:
	  • Glioblastoma: 65 yr
	  • Anaplastic astrocytoma: 50 yr
	  • Oligodendroglioma: 40 yr
	  • Anaplastic astrocytoma usually evolves from a lower grade astrocytoma.
		Glioblastoma (GBM)
		• Causes extensive edema in the deep white matter
		• Enhances with gadolinium
		• Central areas of necrosis restrict on DWI (bright)
		• May have satellite lesions
		• Tumor often crosses the corpus callosum and anterior commissure.
		• MR spectroscopy: Cho/NAA ratio >2.2 is thought to be high grade.
		
		Anaplastic astrocytoma
		• Some contrast enhancement but no necrosis
			Order lower extremity Doppler in patients with GBM. Ultimately, up to 25% of these patients suffer from venous thromboembolism during the first year of diagnosis.

(table continues on page 142)

TABLE 17.1 *Common Adult Brain Tumors (continued)*

	Clinical Pearls	Imaging Features	CSF Studies and Systemic Workup
		Oligodendroglioma • 40%–80% rate of calcification • Enhances in 50%–70% • Hemorrhage or cyst formation occurs in 20%. • Usually, there is little edema.	

Pituitary adenoma	10% of all primary brain tumors
	
	Classified as secretory (75%) and nonsecretory (25%)
	
	Prolactinoma
	• Amenorrhea
	• Galactorrhea
	• Gynecomastia
	• Erectile dysfunction or impotence
	• Infertility
	• Decrease in body hair
	
	Growth-hormone–producing tumor:
	• Gigantism
	• Acromegaly
	
	Adrenocorticotropic hormone (ACTH)–producing tumors
	• Cushing syndrome
	
	Thyroid-stimulating hormone (TSH)–producing tumors:
	• Primary hyperthyroidism
		• Tends to be hypodense on CT
		• Microadenomas are generally hypointense on T1 and variable intensity on T2.
		• Adenomas do not enhance as much, and enhance later, than normal pituitary tissue. Dynamic contrast-enhanced MRI scans are best of delineate adenomas.
		• Macroadenoma are adenomas >10 mm. They have a propensity for hemorrhage and infarction (pituitary apoplexy).
		• Differential diagnosis:
		  • Rathke cyst: hyperintense on T1 and does not enhance
		  • Craniopharyngioma: has cystic lesions and calcifications
			Pituitary hormone panel
			• Prolactin
			• FSH
			• LH
			
			Serum and 24-h urine cortisol levels
			
			TSH and T3/T4 levels
			
			Growth hormone
			
			Formal visual field testing and ophthalmologic evaluation are critical.
			
			Serum prolactin >200 μg/L with an adenoma >10 mm in size is diagnostic of a prolactinoma.

Primary central nervous system lymphoma (PCNSL)	• Causes <5% of all primary brain tumors • Immunocompromised state (e.g., HIV, transplant) is a major risk factor. • Among immunocompetent patients, the mean age of onset is 60 yr and there is a slight male predominance.	Tends to be hypodense on CT MRI features • T1 hypointense and T2 hyperintense • DWI shows diffusion restriction (bright) Anatomic predilection • Periventricular white matter in 40% • Coating of ventricles in 40% • Deep gray matter nuclei/subcortical in 30% • Unusual multifocal distribution of tumor can occur. Diffusely enhancing in the immunocompetent patients; necrotic center can occur in immunocompromised patients. Spread across corpus callosum is suggestive of PCNSL. Masses tend to be <2 cm in patients with AIDS and >2 cm in non-AIDS patients.	Slit lamp examination reveals intraocular involvement in 15% of patients.

CSF, cerebrospinal fluid; FLAIR, fluid-attenuated inversion recovery; MR, magnetic resonance; SWI, susceptibility-weighted imaging; CT, computed tomography; MRI, magnetic resonance imaging; FDG-PET, ^{18}F-fluorodeoxyglucose positron emission tomography; DWI, diffusion-weighted imaging; FSH, follicle-stimulating hormone; LH, luteinizing hormone.

FIGURE 17.8 Pilocytic astrocytoma with high signal intensity on FLAIR imaging invading the midbrain.

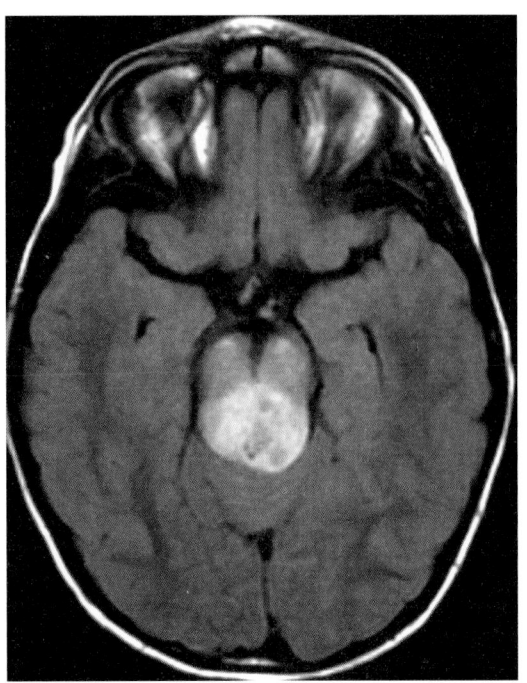

FIGURE 17.9 Medulloblastoma with distortion of the fourth ventricle and secondary hydrocephalus. **A and B:** Hypointense on T1. **C:** Moderate partial gadolinium enhancement.

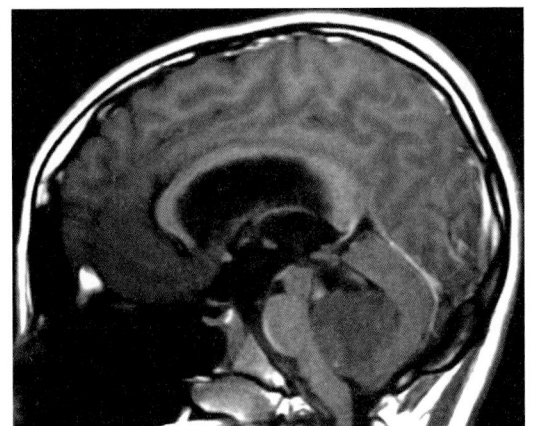

A

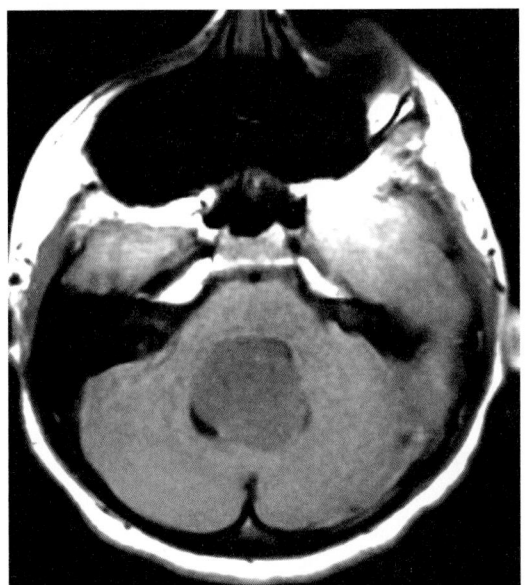

B

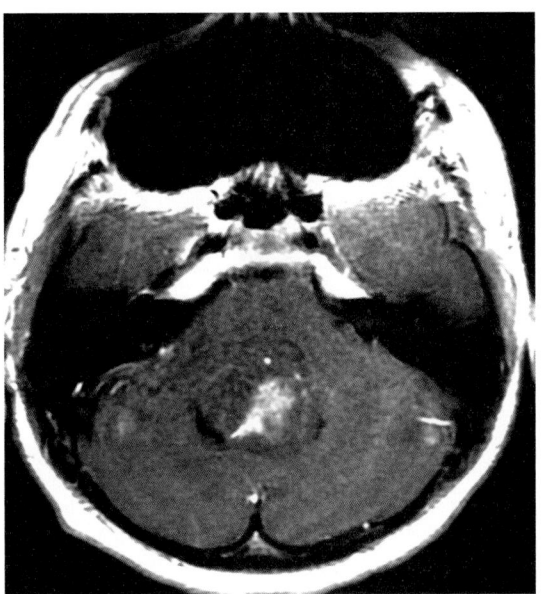

C

TABLE 17.2   Common Pediatric Brain Tumors

	Clinical Pearls	Imaging Features	CSF Studies and Systemic Workup
Gliomas • Grade 1: pilocytic astrocytoma (see Fig. 17.7) • Grade 2: diffuse fibrillary astrocytoma	Two main types in children: • Pilocytic astrocytoma • Diffuse fibrillary astrocytoma	• Pilocytic astrocytoma is predominately located in the cerebellum, optic pathways, and the dorsal brain stem. • Well circumscribed with a cystic component and an enhancing mural nodule • Diffuse fibrillary astrocytoma occurs more often supratentorially in deep midline structures and at the cervicomedullary junction. • Hypointense on T1 and hyperintense on T2 with varying degrees of enhancement	None
Medulloblastoma	Peak incidence is approximately between 5 and 10 yr of age Occurs in boys twice as often as girls	• Accounts for 50% of cerebellar tumors in children • Usually arise from the vermis then grow into the inferior or superior velum of the fourth ventricle • As opposed to ependymoma, medulloblastoma distorts the fourth ventricle. • Well circumscribed and hyperdense on CT. Up to 20% have calcification or cystic changes. • MRI often has diffusion restriction on DWI. Medulloblastoma tends to enhance to a moderate degree.	None
Ependymoma	Among pediatric patients, peak incidence among infants, toddlers, and preschoolers Another peak of incidence occurs in adults.	• Intracranial in 90% of pediatric patients (more often spinal in adults); most often localized to the floor of the fourth ventricle • Hypodense to isodense on CT • Calcification in up to 50%, cystic changes in 15%. Mild enhancement is the rule.	Spinal MRI is mandatory if cranial ependymoma is suspected. Spinal drop metastasis occurs in 5% of cases.

CSF, cerebrospinal fluid; CT, computed tomography; MRI, magnetic resonance imaging; DWI, diffusion-weighted imaging.

CEREBRITIS AND ABSCESSES

Approximately 1,500 cases of brain abscess occur annually in the United States with an incidence of 0.3 to 1.3 cases per 100,000 of the population annually. Brain abscess (see Chapter 62) is most commonly caused by bacterial infection (Fig. 17.10), most commonly streptococci and staphylococci. Focal brain infection resulting in cerebritis or abscess can also be caused by *fungi* (Table 17.3). Among fungal infections, aspergillosis (Fig. 17.11), cryptococcosis (Fig. 17.12), candida, mucormycosis, and nocardia are most common in immunosuppressed patients. *Blastomyces*, *Histoplasmosis*, and

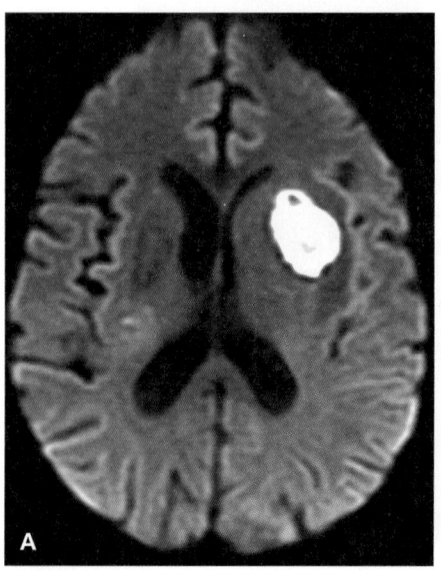
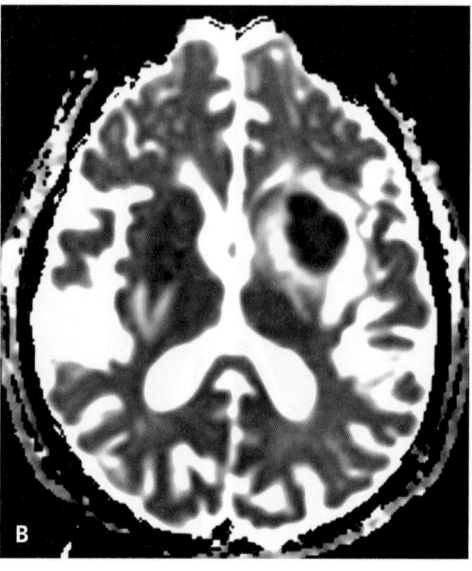

FIGURE 17.10 Left basal ganglia abscess. **A and B:** Bright on DWI **(A)** with restricted ADC. *(continued)*

FIGURE 17.10 *(continued)* Left basal ganglia abscess. **C and D:** T2 images show hyperintense core and a hypointense ring **(C)** and postcontrast T1 image shows sharply demarcated thin rim enhancement post contrast.

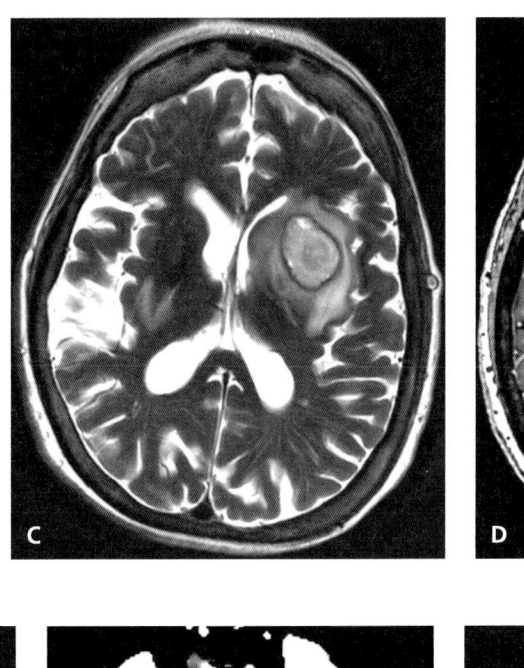
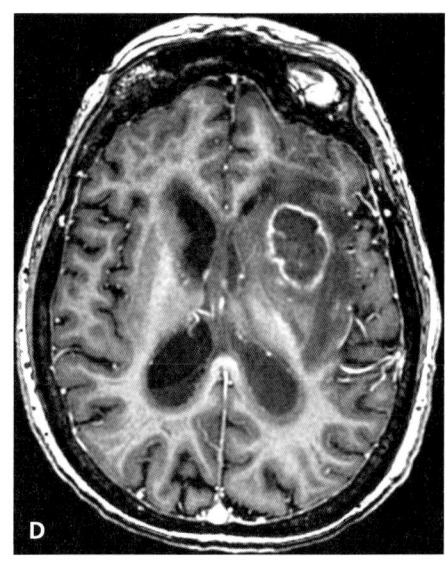

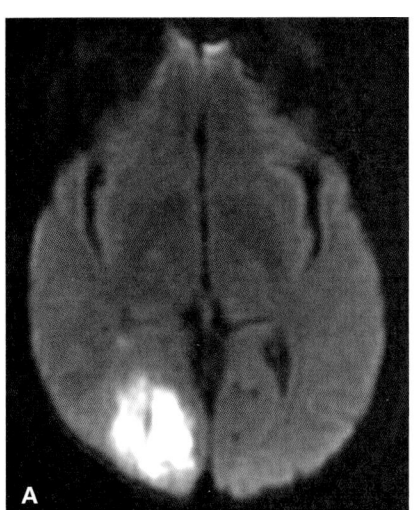
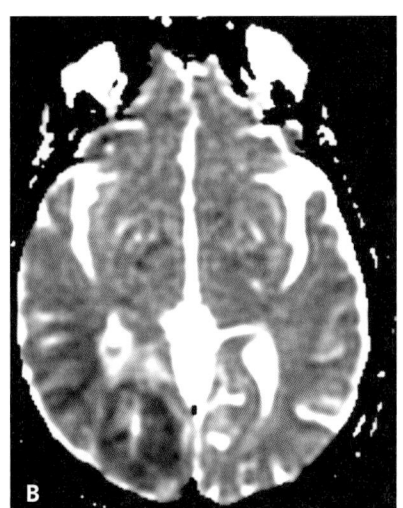
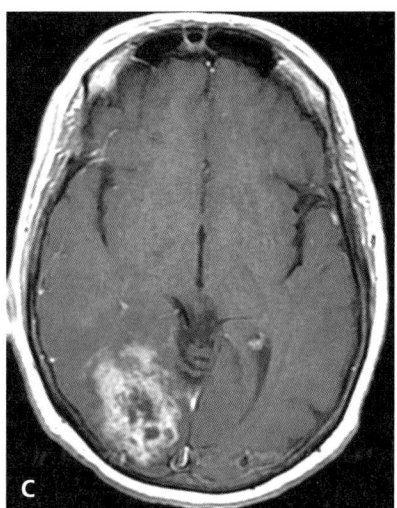

FIGURE 17.11 Focal *Aspergillus* infection with little edema or mass effect. **A:** Bright on DWI with restriction. **B:** Dark on ADC suggesting necrosis. **C:** Heterogeneous coarse irregular enhancement on T1 with gadolinium.

FIGURE 17.12 Cryptococcal meningitis with hydrocephalus and small punctate areas of enhancement in the midbrain **(A)** and basal ganglia **(B)** on T1-enhanced imaging.

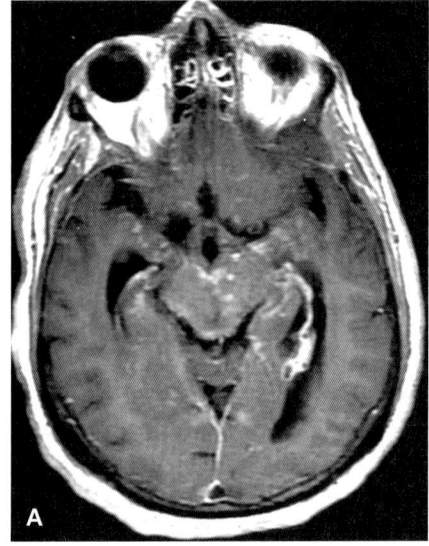
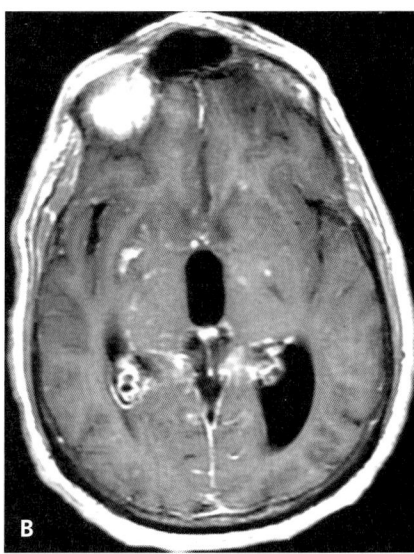

TABLE 17.3 Common Infectious Etiologies of Mass Lesions

	Clinical Pearls	Imaging Features	CSF Studies and Systemic Workup

Bacterial abscess	Most abscesses in immunocompetent individuals are bacterial.
	
	Only 50% of patients have fever on initial presentation.
		• Characterized on T2 imaging as hyperintense core and hypointense ring, both of which restrict on DWI.
		• Ring enhancement with contrast imaging
		• MRS features:
		  • Pyogenic aerobic abscess: Amino acids, lactate, and lipid are elevated.
		  • Pyogenic anaerobic abscess: Succinate and acetate are elevated.
		  • Tuberculosis (TB): Only lipid is elevated.
			• Blood cultures
			• Transesophageal echocardiography to detect a valvular vegetation
			• LP may reveal concurrent meningitis.

Tuberculoma	When the caseous core of the tuberculoma liquefies, a tuberculous abscess results.	CT appearance • Solid-enhancing, ring-enhancing, or mixed lesions • Occasionally, there is the "target sign," which is pathognomonic of TB: central calcification surrounded by a hypodense area with peripheral ring enhancement. MRI appearance • DWI: no abnormalities or can be bright with restriction like a bacterial abscess • T1: isointense in gray matter with a hyperintense ring • T2: noncaseating: hyperintense with nodular enhancement; caseating: iso-/hypointense with ring enhancement	Tuberculin skin test is positive in up to 85% of patients. Chest CT suggests pulmonary TB in 50%–80% of patients.
Gummatous neurosyphilis	Histology reveals that the central portion of the mass is necrotic material, and the peripheral region is infiltrated with plasma cells.	• CNS gummas can arise from the meningeal surfaces and extend directly into the brain or may arise directly from the parenchyma. • Presents as a ring-enhancing mass lesion	Serum RPR and FTA-ABS CSF VDRL
Viral encephalitis	HSV-1 only rarely causes a typical vesicular skin eruption in the setting of meningitis.	• DWI sequences on MRI are most sensitive for detecting tissue injury from encephalitis. • Herpes encephalitis can cause significant swelling and mass effect of the temporal lobes, mimicking tumor.	CSF shows lymphocytic pleocytosis with normal or decreased glucose but can be normal.
Fungal	Immunocompromised • Aspergillosis • Cryptococcosis • Candida • Mucormycosis • Nocardia Immunocompetent • *Blastomyces* • *Histoplasma* • *Coccidioides*	• DWI shows restricted diffusion in the wall of a fungal abscess. Typically, the core does not show restriction (unlike in a bacterial abscess). • MRS can show increased trehalose, amino acids, and lactate. • Anatomic predilations • *Cryptococcus*: predominately in midbrain and basal ganglia • Coccidioidomycosis: predilection for the cerebellum • Mucormycosis: rim of soft-tissue thickness along the walls of the paranasal sinus. In some cases, bony destruction is present. • Nocardial: enhancing capsule containing multiple loculations • Aspergillosis: Aggressive forms manifest as meningoencephalitis; less aggressive forms manifest as solitary abscess or isolated granulomas.	CSF shows lymphocytic predominance, although neutrophils may predominate early in the course. *Histoplasmosis* causes CSF mononuclear pleocytosis. *Coccidioides* may cause CSF eosinophilia.

TABLE 17.3   Common Infectious Etiologies of Mass Lesions (continued)

	Clinical Pearls	Imaging Features	CSF Studies and Systemic Workup
Helminthic infection	Travel history • Coenurosis cerebralis: sheep-raising areas North America/Europe/South America/Africa • Cysticercosis: endemic in Latin America, sub-Saharan Africa, and some regions of Asia • *Echinococcus granulosus*: reported in the Americas as well as Mediterranean countries • *Ascaris*: endemic in North America. Host are raccoons. • *Paragonimus*: Asia and South Pacific Islands • *Schistosoma japonicum*: Southeast Asia • *Spirometra*: Southeast Asia and the Americas • *Toxocara*: worldwide • *Trichinella*: worldwide • *Strongyloides*: Latin America, Caribbean, Africa, Asia	Cyst-forming • Coenurosis • Cysticercosis • *Echinococcus granulosus* Granuloma-forming • *Ascaris* • *Paragonimus* • *Schistosoma japonicum* • *Spirometra* • *Toxocara* • *Trichinella* Abscess • *Strongyloides*	CSF shows lymphocytic predominance except: *Trichinella*, which demonstrates eosinophilic pleocytosis. *Strongyloides*, which demonstrates a neutrophilic pleocytosis.
Protozoal infections	Immunosuppressed • *Acanthamoeba*: transmitted via swimming in freshwater pools • Toxoplasmosis: transmitted via food or congenitally • *Entamoeba histolytica* is associated with liver abscess.	Granulomatous encephalitis • *Acanthamoeba* • Toxoplasmosis Brain abscess • *Entamoeba histolytica*	• *Acanthamoeba* • CSF protein and glucose usually normal • Toxoplasmosis • The presence of IgG antibodies indicates prior exposure to the parasites and potential for reactivation

CSF, cerebrospinal fluid; DWI, diffusion-weighted imaging; MRS, magnetic resonance spectroscopy; LP, lumbar puncture; MRI, magnetic resonance imaging; CT, computed tomography; CNS, central nervous system; RPR, rapid plasma reagin; FTA-ABS, fluorescent treponemal antibody absorption; VDRL, Venereal Disease Research Laboratory; HSV-1, herpes simplex virus 1; IgG, immunoglobulin G.

Coccidioides are most common in immunocompetent patients. The most common *parasitic* organisms that causes brain abscess are by far toxoplasmosis (Fig. 17.13) and cysticercosis (Fig. 17.14), although *Strongyloides* and *Entamoeba histolytica* are also common causes (see Chapter 65). *Tuberculosis* forms solid tuberculomas; after the caseous core liquefies, the tuberculoma becomes a tuberculous abscess (see Chapter 64). *Syphilis* can form gummas, cysticercosis can cause an inflammatory mass lesion when the cyst degenerates and dies, and viruses such as *herpes simplex 1* (see Chapter 66) can cause encephalitis complicated by acute swelling and inflammation of the affected temporal lobes (Fig. 17.15).

OTHER INFLAMMATORY LESIONS

Occasionally, noninfectious inflammatory processes can also cause mass lesions (Table 17.4). Most notoriously, *multiple sclerosis* (see Chapter 69) can form a large demyelinating mass lesion known as *Marburg variant* or *tumefactive multiple sclerosis* (Fig. 17.16). *Sarcoidosis* (see Chapter 72) can also present as an inflammatory intraparenchymal mass lesion. *Radiation necrosis* can present as a space-occupying mass lesion months to decades after prior radiation treatment (see Chapter 105).

FOCUSED HISTORY

DEMOGRAPHICS

Age is an important factor for narrowing the differential diagnosis particularly for brain tumors. Children develop a very different set of brain tumors than do adults. Ependymoma affects the youngest children (high incidence among infants, toddlers, and preschoolers), followed by medulloblastoma and pilocytic astrocytoma (peak incidence between 5 and 10 years of age), oligodendroglioma (incidence peak at 40 years of age), anaplastic astrocytoma (incidence peak at 50 years of age), and glioblastoma (incidence peak at 65 years of age). The average age at diagnosis for pituitary adenomas and meningiomas straddle several decades, with pituitary adenomas primarily being diagnosed between age 20 and 50 years and meningiomas between age 40 and 60 years. Pituitary adenoma and meningiomas occur more commonly in women.

TIME COURSE

Symptoms associated with abscesses tend to develop acutely to subacutely (with bacterial infections presenting more acutely and

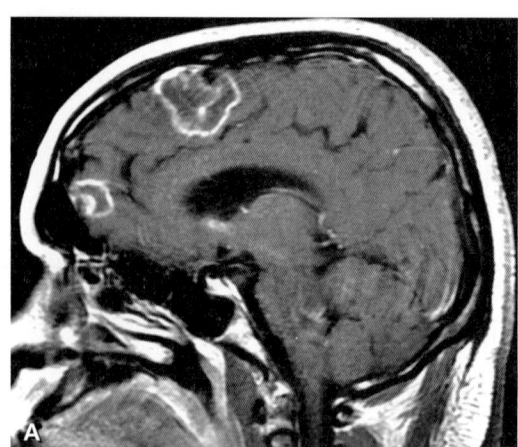

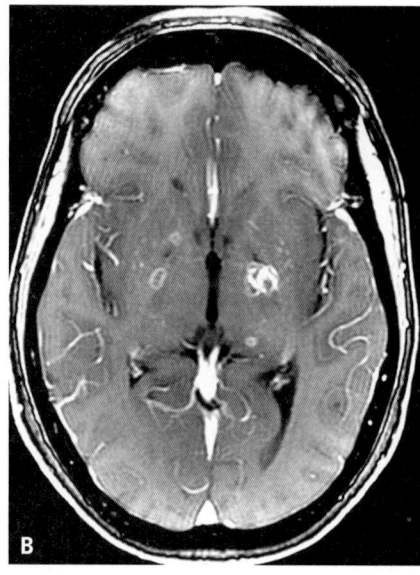

FIGURE 17.13 Toxoplasmosis. Multiple ring-enhancing lesions in the cortex **(A)** and basal ganglia **(B)** on T1 imaging with gadolinium.

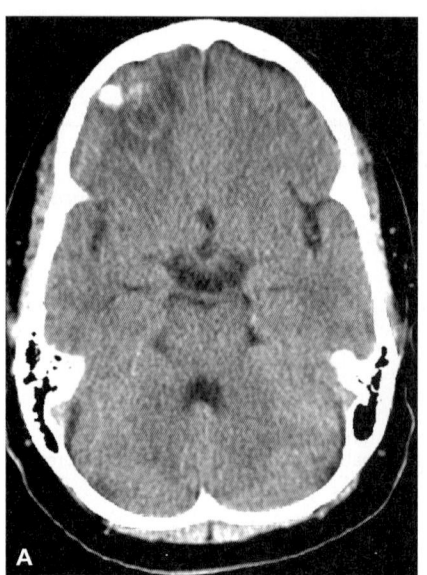

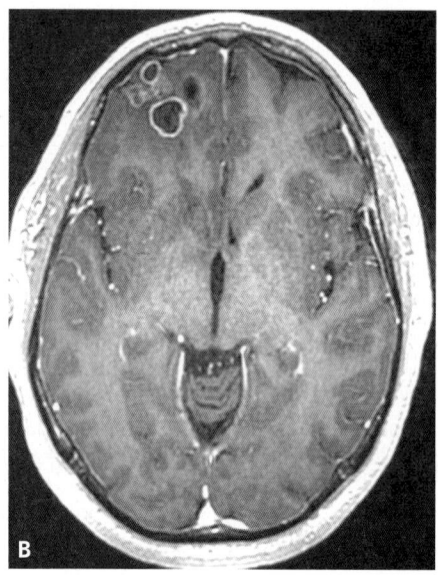

FIGURE 17.14 Cysticercosis. **A:** Partially calcified right frontal lesion with a 1-cm ringlike lesion on noncontrast CT. **B:** Multiple cortical ring-enhancing cystic lesions in T1 gadolinium-enhanced imaging.

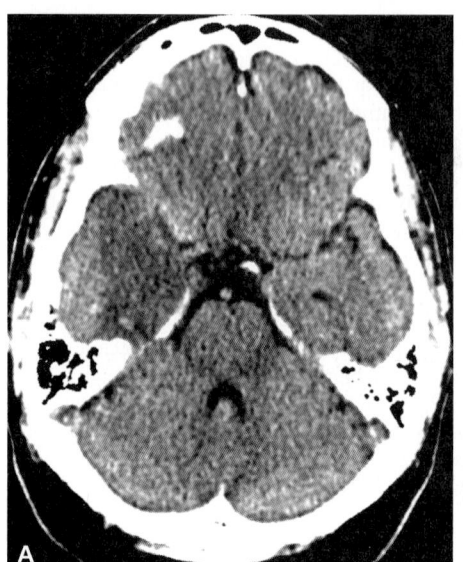

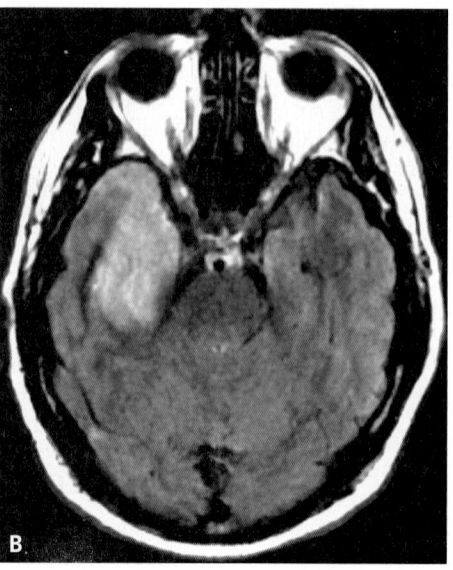

FIGURE 17.15 HSV1 encephalitis. **A:** CT scan showing early punctate hemorrhage. **B:** MRI with abnormal FLAIR signal with swelling of the medial temporal lobe.

TABLE 17.4   Select Inflammatory Causes of Focal Brain Lesions

	Clinical Pearls	Imaging Features	CSF Studies and Systemic Workup
Sarcoidosis	• Sarcoidosis primarily occurs in the third and fourth decade. • Five percent of cases of systemic sarcoid have neurologic involvement.	• Intraparenchymal sarcoid masses may or may not enhance. • Nodules may be calcified, have an increased density, or be isodense and can occur throughout the brain parenchyma. • Nodular meningeal enhancement is common. • The nodules are not usually associated with edema. • Sarcoid nodules do not cavitate as frequently as tuberculosis.	• Chest CT • Gallium scan • Lacrimal gland biopsy • CSF and serum ACE activity
Whipple disease	• Mean age of onset is around 50 yr. • Men are more commonly affected (80%). • In about 5% of the cases, the presentation is solely neurologic. In other cases. the small bowel is involved. • Granuloma formation is a delayed hypersensitivity to Whipple disease.	• The lesions are in the gray matter, in the basal part of the telencephalon, the hypothalamus, and the thalamus.	• *Tropheryma whippelii* PCR • Small bowel biopsy
Behçet disease	• Most common in the countries around the eastern shores of the Mediterranean, the Middle East, and Eastern Asia • Mean age of onset of neurologic symptoms is about 30 yr of age. • Triad of recurrent genital ulcerations, skin or eye lesions, and meningitis	• Predilection for brain stem • Enhancement may occur as a ring or nodule.	• May also present as cortical vein thrombosis or isolated increased intracranial pressure
Tumefactive multiple sclerosis	• Mean age of onset is approximately 35 yr of age. • The female-to-male prevalence is 1.2:1. • May have had previous neurologic symptoms isolated in space and time supportive of multiple sclerosis as a diagnosis	• Demyelinating lesion ≥2 cm in size • Incomplete ring enhancement open on the gray matter side of the lesion • Does not restrict on DWI • MR perfusion normal	• C-spine MRI

CSF, cerebrospinal fluid; CT, computed tomography; ACE, angiotensin-converting enzyme; PCR, polymerase chain reaction; DWI, diffusion-weighted imaging; MR, magnetic resonance; MRI, magnetic resonance imaging.

fungal infections more subacutely), whereas tumors present more subacutely to chronically based on their grade (for instance, glioblastoma tends to have a more subacute presentation as compared to meningiomas which tend to have a more chronic presentations).

PAST MEDICAL HISTORY

It is essential to learn whether there was a past history of cancer and/or a history of immunosuppression. In patients with a history of systemic cancer, certain details are helpful in determining the likelihood that brain mass is a metastatic tumor. SCLC metastasizes to the brain in about 50% of instances as opposed to 7% in cases of NSCLC. In patients with prior breast cancer, HER2+/ER− status portends a higher likelihood of metastasis to the brain. The same applies for melanoma patients with head/neck/oral lesions and colorectal cancer patients with left-sided cancers. Regarding immunosuppression,

a history of HIV is a major risk factor for primary central nervous system lymphoma (PCNSL) and toxoplasma infection (see Chapter 67), whereas neutropenia and steroid use is a major risk factor for aspergillosis, candida, mucormycosis, and nocardia infections.

Other important history elements include the following:

• A prior distant (usually 5 to 30 years prior) history of irradiation, which increases the long-term risk of meningiomas and malignant glioma
• A recent history of radiation treatment, which can lead to radiation necrosis
• A history of systemic sarcoidosis, which increases the likelihood that a brain mass is due to neurosarcoidosis
• Prior diagnoses of amenorrhea, galactorrhea, erectile dysfunction, infertility, or hyperthyroidism, which can be seen in pituitary adenomas

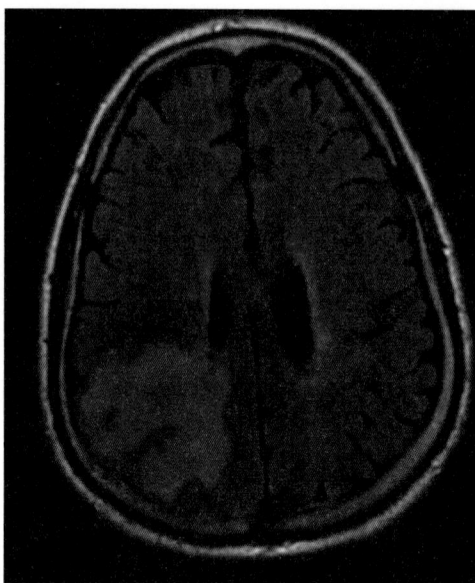

FIGURE 17.16 Tumefactive multiple sclerosis with a large high-intensity focal mass lesion in the right parietal lobe on FLAIR imaging. Note the periventricular lesions.

SOCIAL HISTORY

The social history portion of the interview may reveal HIV risk factors and/or risk factors for systemic cancers such as smoking history. Additionally, the patient's travel history may be helpful, particularly for identifying potential fungal and helminthic infections (see Table 17.1).

REVIEW OF SYSTEMS

In the neurologic review of systems, a history of episodic changes in neurologic status may indicate either an epileptic seizure or an ICP plateau wave. Plateau waves are thought to be the result of a sudden increase in cerebral blood volume because of a sudden decrease in cerebral vascular resistance. Patients who have diminished blood flow absorption, either from an intracranial mass or leptomeningeal disease, are more likely to develop plateau waves than patients with normal cerebrospinal fluid (CSF) absorption.

Another important point of query should focus on prior episodes of focal neurologic deficits lasting days in distributions characteristic of multiple sclerosis attacks, such as unilateral vision loss, bilateral leg paresthesias, unilateral arm weakness/paresthesia, or double vision. This can point to tumefactive multiple sclerosis as the causative etiology.

Symptoms of subacute to chronic weight loss can point to an occult malignancy and when combined with fever and night sweats may indicate either a CNS lymphoma or tuberculosis, given the clinical context. History of galactorrhea or gynecomastia can raise concern for pituitary adenoma (see Chapter 100).

FOCUSED EXAM

In patients with focal mass lesions of the brain, the most important role of the exam is to assess for increased ICP and herniation. A pale optic disc, red desaturation, partial internuclear ophthalmoplegia, and increased leg reflexes with normal arm reflexes can all be indications of prior multiple sclerosis demyelinating episodes.

The next most important elements of the exam are found in the general exam. Patients with undetermined focal mass lesions require a careful lung, breast, skin, and gastrointestinal exam to assess for lumps or masses suggestive of malignancy.

The breast exam is also helpful to assess for gynecomastia, which can occur with pituitary adenoma. Skin examination may also be helpful to look for herpes simplex rashes, melanoma, Kaposi sarcoma, or peripheral manifestations of bacterial endocarditis such as Janeway lesions (nontender, small erythematous macular lesions on the palms or soles only a few millimeters in diameter that are indicative of infective endocarditis).

DIAGNOSIS

The diagnostic cornerstones for brain masses are imaging, lumbar puncture, and biopsy.

IMAGING

Usually, a computed tomography (CT) scan (see Chapter 20) is the first radiographic study performed when a patient presents with a new neurologic symptom. Most focal brain lesions from tumor or abscess tend to be hypodense on CT. Admixture of heterogenous hyperdense signal usually represents hemorrhage into a tumor (typically glioblastoma multiforme) or less commonly an abscess. A homogenous hyperdense pattern can result from melanoma, medulloblastoma, or meningioma. Calcification, usually punctate, occurs in 40% of ependymomas, 20% of meningiomas, and 10% of medulloblastomas. Tuberculomas have a pathognomic "target sign" resulting from central calcification surrounded by a hypodense area with peripheral ring enhancement with IV contrast.

Although the CT scan can sometimes be helpful, an MRI (see Chapter 21) is always recommended unless there is a contraindication (e.g., pacemaker). The important MRI sequences are diffusion-weighted imaging (DWI), fluid-attenuated inversion recovery (FLAIR), susceptibility-weighted imaging (SWI), T1 precontrast, and T1 postcontrast. Important imaging features are reviewed in Table 17.1.

Magnetic resonance (MR) spectroscopy is sometimes pursued, although its use is limited. Primary brain tumors are classically thought of as having an increased choline/N-acetylaspartate (NAA) ratio (with ratio >2 suggestive of a high-grade tumor). In high-grade brain tumors, the surrounding FLAIR hyperintensity is thought to represent infiltrative tumor and also has an elevated choline/NAA ratio, whereas in metastatic tumor, this surrounding FLAIR hyperintensity is thought to represent vasogenic edema and therefore has a low choline level. Additionally, lactate is thought to be very elevated in infections, although it can also be elevated in necrotic tumors, making the distinction somewhat difficult.

Brain positron emission tomography (PET) scans (see Chapter 22) can be helpful in distinguishing between radiation necrosis and recurrent tumor in that radiation necrosis is hypometabolic and recurrent tumor is hypermetabolic. The PET scan would also demonstrate increased metabolism in a high-grade tumor as opposed to a low-grade tumor. PET scans, however, have poor spatial resolution and are not useful for lesions smaller than 1 cm.

Whole-body CT scanning should be pursued whenever metastatic disease is being entertained.

LUMBAR PUNCTURE AND BIOPSY

Lumbar puncture (see Chapter 31) is an essential part of the neurologic examination in patients with intracranial mass lesions. CSF examination can reveal an infectious organism or the presence

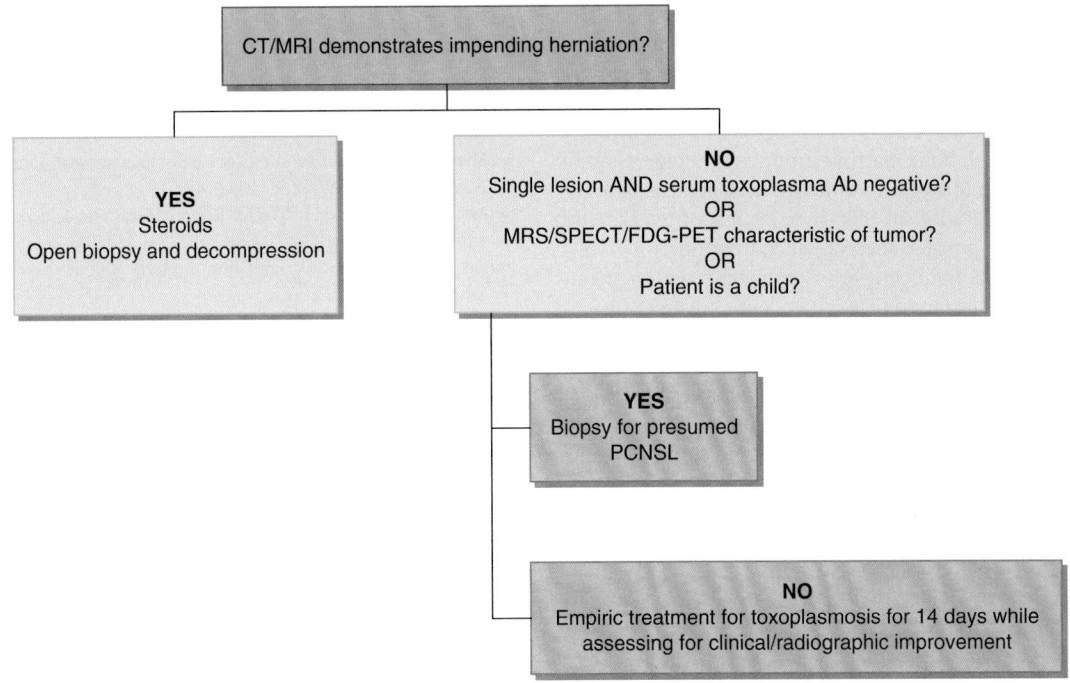

FIGURE 17.17 Algorithm for diagnosis and management of enhancing mass lesions in an AIDS patient. CT, computed tomography; MRI, magnetic resonance imaging; MRS, magnetic resonance spectroscopy; SPECT, single-photon emission computed tomography; FDG-PET, 18F-fluorodeoxyglucose positron emission tomography; PCNSL, primary central nervous system lymphoma.

of malignant cells by cytology when CNS lymphoma, germ cell tumors, or carcinomatous meningitis is suspected.

For most primary brain tumors, however, lumbar puncture is not diagnostic and when there is evidence of impending herniation, it is also not safe. CSF in the setting of cerebral abscess formation is often nondiagnostic. An important exception is in patients with HIV/AIDS who often can be infected with multiple opportunistic infections. In the case of encephalitis, whether viral, parasitic, or fungal, lumbar puncture is essential for establishing the diagnosis. Lumbar puncture is also routinely performed for the diagnosis of inflammatory masses resulting from sarcoidosis or multiple sclerosis.

The diagnostic method of choice for suspected malignancy or abscess is tissue biopsy or CT-guided drainage and culture, respectively (see Chapter 32). Eventually, the majority of patients with suspected brain tumor are diagnosed by pathologic examination of surgically resected tissue as the result of a diagnostic biopsy or as part of a partial debulking or gross total resection of the lesion.

INITIAL MANAGEMENT

If imaging reveals significant vasogenic edema, corticosteroids can be used to prevent further neurologic injury in the case of impending herniation or for symptomatic relief if the cause is felt to be tumor or abscess. Most often, the corticosteroid regimen is dexamethasone 10 mg IV as an initial dose followed by 4 to 6 mg every 6 hours. Use of steroids should be avoided when PCNSL is a main consideration, as steroids can significantly lead to loss of the main histologic findings if the lesion is biopsied.

One situation in which lymphoma should be seriously considered is the case of the AIDS patient (CD4 <100/μL). In this case, the two most common etiologies of enhancing focal mass lesions are toxoplasmosis and PCNSL. Figure 17.17 outlines an algorithm for managing to diagnosis, and Table 17.5 outlines the imaging

differences between lymphoma and toxoplasmosis. The standard approach is to withhold steroids unless absolutely necessary and proceed directly to biopsy in patients at high risk for PCNSL and otherwise to proceed with empiric therapy for toxoplasmosis. Therapy for toxoplasma encephalitis is oral pyrimethamine (adults: an initial loading dose of 50 to 200 mg followed by 25 to 50 mg/day; children: 2 mg/kg/day administered in divided doses every 12 hours for 1 to 3 days, then 1 mg/kg daily or as divided doses every 12 hours to a maximum of 25 mg/day) and sulfadiazine (adults: 6 to 8 g/day divided into four equal doses; children: 120 mg/kg/day in divided doses every 6 hours in doses not to ex-

TABLE 17.5	Imaging Differences between Lymphoma and Toxoplasmosis	
Lymphoma	**Toxoplasmosis**
Periventricular propensity	Basal ganglia propensity
Hypodense on T2/FLAIR	Hyperdense on T2/FLAIR
Single or multiple lesions	Lesions more numerous and smaller than lymphoma lesions
Does not tend to bleed except after steroids	May bleed pretreatment
Thallium spectroscopy and MR perfusion demonstrate increased uptake.	Thallium spectroscopy and MR perfusion demonstrate decreased uptake.
MR spectroscopy shows moderately elevated lactate and lipid and markedly elevated choline.	MR spectroscopy shows markedly elevated lactate and lipid.

FLAIR, fluid-attenuated inversion recovery; MR, magnetic resonance.

ceed the adult dose). Individuals allergic to sulfadiazine may be desensitized to sulfadiazine or alternatively treated with clindamycin 2,400 mg/day in three equal doses. Other treatment alternatives include atovaquone or azithromycin. In conjunction with the anti-toxoplasmosis agents, folinic acid (5 to 10 mg/day) is concurrently administered to diminish bone marrow suppression. Regression of the lesion on follow-up MR or CT confirms the diagnosis of toxoplasmosis. The total duration of therapy is at least 6 weeks and longer if the clinical response is incomplete at that time.

Another question that frequently arises in patients with new-onset mass lesions is whether to initiate antiepileptic treatment. Generally, unless the patient has had a seizure, antiepileptic treatment is not recommended. If the patient has significant increase in ICP with impending herniation, it is reasonable to initiate antiepileptic treatment even without a clinical history of a seizure. The thought in this circumstance is that by causing an increased cerebral metabolic demand, a seizure can lead to further increase in ICP and herniation.

SUGGESTED READINGS

American Academy of Neurology. Evaluation and management of intracranial mass lesions in AIDS: report of the Quality Standards Subcommittee of the American Academy of Neurology. *Neurology*. 1998;50(1):21–26.

Beckham J, Tyler K. Neuro-intensive care of patients with acute CNS infections. *Neurotherapeutics*. 2012;9(1):124–138.

Kennecke H, Yerushalmi R, Woods R, et al. Metastatic behavior of breast cancer subtypes. *J Clin Oncol*. 2010;28(20):3271–3277.

Prasad G, Haas-Kogan D. Radiation-induced glioma. *Expert Rev Neurother*. 2009;9(10):1511–1517.

Roser F, Rosahl SK, Samii M. Single cerebral metastasis 3 and 19 years after primary renal cell carcinoma: case report and review of the literature. *J Neurol Neurosurg Psychiatry*. 2002;72(2):257–258.

Schuette W. Treatment of brain metastases from lung cancer: chemotherapy. *Lung Cancer*. 2004;45:S253–S257.

Tan WS, Ho KS, Eu KW. Brain metastases in colorectal cancers. *World J Surg*. 2009;33(4):817–821.

Stupor and Coma 18

Jan Claassen, Stephan A. Mayer, and John C. M. Brust

INTRODUCTION

"Normal human consciousness consists of a serially, time-ordered, organized, restricted, and reflective awareness of self and the environment. Moreover, it is an experience of graded complexity and quantity." Schiff and Plum, J Clin Neurophys, 2000.

Philosophical and religious frameworks may influence definitions of consciousness. Consciousness is classically defined as awareness of self and the environment and requires both arousal (i.e., wakefulness) and cognitive content (i.e., thoughts and perceptions).

Coma is a state of unconsciousness that differs from sleep in that it represents a neurologic deficit and is not readily reversed. Cerebral oxygen uptake (cerebral metabolic rate of oxygen [$CMRO_2$]) is normal in sleep, and brain electrical activity progresses thorough organized stages of synchronized activity on electroencephalography (EEG). In coma, $CMRO_2$ is abnormally reduced and EEG activity progressively slows and becomes attenuated, with loss of normal reactivity to sensory stimuli.

DEFINITIONS

Coma is clinically defined by the neurologic examination, especially responses to external stimuli. Terms such as *lethargy, obtundation, stupor,* and *coma* usually depend on the patient's response to normal verbal stimuli, shouting, shaking, or pain. These terms are not rigidly defined, and it is useful to record both the response and the stimulus that elicited it. Occasionally, the true level of consciousness may be difficult or impossible to determine due to coexisting behavioral disturbances (i.e., catatonia in severe depression) or neurologic deficits (i.e., akinesia plus aphasia) that blunt responses to stimuli.

The chronicity of the impaired mental status differentiates acute disorders of consciousness such as stupor and coma from their long-term correlates: the chronic disorders of consciousness known as unresponsive wakefulness (UW) or persistent vegetative state (PVS) and minimally conscious state (MCS). UW/PVS is characterized by eyes-open unresponsiveness, purely reflexive behavior, and lack of the ability to follow verbal commands. MCS differs from PVS in that the patient is able to follow simple commands, albeit sometimes inconsistently, consistent with partial preservation of conscious awareness.

Induced states of altered consciousness such as those seen during general anesthesia or with sedation in the intensive care unit (ICU) share some similarities with coma induced by brain injury and may confound the assessment of comatose patients. Sedatives are frequently required in critically ill patients to facilitate ventilator management or to manage pain or agitation. *Accurate neurologic assessment of level of consciousness in the ICU can only be performed when sedatives have been stopped or interrupted.* For this reason, short-acting continuous infusion agents such as propofol, midazolam, or fentanyl are preferred in the setting of acute brain injury.

NEUROANATOMY

Confusional state and *delirium* are terms that refer to a state of inattentiveness, altered cognitive content, and sometimes hyperactivity, rather than to a decreased level of arousal; these conditions may presage or alternate with obtundation, stupor, or coma.

The anatomic substrate of consciousness lies within the reticular activating system, thalamus, and cerebral cortex. Location for classic structural brain lesions associated with stupor and coma have been derived from lesion studies and more recently confirmed and expanded based on structural and functional brain imaging studies such as diffusion tensor and resting state magnetic resonance imaging (MRI) (Fig. 18.1).

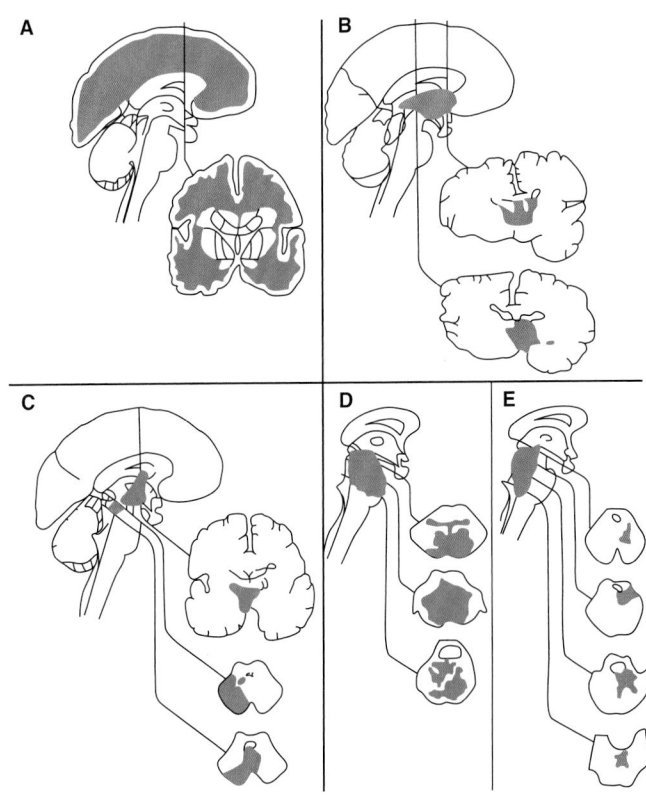

FIGURE 18.1 Anatomy of coma. Classic brain lesions that cause coma include those located diffuse bihemispheric **(A)**, diencephalic **(B)**, paramedian caudal midbrain and caudal diencephalic **(C)**, high pontine and lower midbrain paramedian tegmental regions **(D)**, and pontine **(E)**. (From Posner JB, Saper CB, Schiff ND, et al. *Plum and Posner's Diagnosis of Stupor and Coma.* 4th ed. New York: Oxford University Press; 2007 by permission of Oxford University Press, USA.)

MANAGEMENT STRATEGY

A suggested algorithm for the initial management of new-onset coma is shown in Figure 18.2.

INITIAL RESUSCITATION

Initial management of the comatose patient should always focus on the ABCs: airway, breathing, and circulation. Assuring a patent airway, securing adequate ventilation, and restoring or maintaining circulation should take precedence, as it does with any critically ill patient. Vascular access needs to be obtained as soon as possible and may include central venous access and large bore peripheral access. Detection and treatment of immediately life-threatening systemic conditions may include stopping a hemorrhage; supporting the circulation by administration of fluids, blood products, or pressors; intubation when necessary (e.g., to prevent aspiration in a patient who is vomiting); and obtaining an electrocardiogram to detect dangerous arrhythmias. Fingerstick glucose should be obtained immediately and if in doubt, 50% dextrose should be given intravenously with parenteral thiamine. (Administering glucose alone to a thiamine-deficient patient can precipitate Wernicke–Korsakoff syndrome.) When opiate overdose is a possibility, naloxone hydrochloride (Narcan) 0.4 mg IV is given. If trauma is suspected, damage to internal organs and cervical fracture should be assumed until radiographs determine otherwise and emergency ultrasound scanning (i.e., focused assessment with sonography for trauma [FAST]) or other imaging has ruled out major internal bleeding or organ injury.

HISTORY AND GENERAL PHYSICAL EXAMINATION

The next step is to localize and identify the underlying cause of coma. A history is obtained from whoever accompanies the patient,

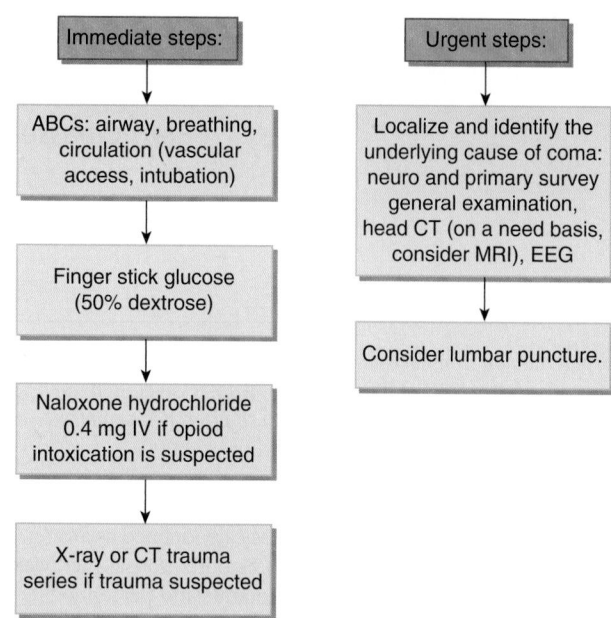

FIGURE 18.2 Management algorithm for new-onset coma. IV, intravenous; CT, computed tomography; MRI, magnetic resonance imaging; EEG, electroencephalography.

including emergency medical service providers. Table 18.2 lists a number of practical pearls to look for that can aid in the diagnosis of nontraumatic coma. Order an emergent EEG to evaluate for nonconvulsive seizures or status epilepticus if even minor involuntary facial or extremity twitching is observed.

FOCUSED NEUROLOGIC EXAMINATION

In their classic monograph, Plum and Posner divided the causes of coma into supra- and infratentorial structural lesions and diffuse or metabolic diseases. By concentrating on motor responses to stimuli, respiratory patterns, pupils, and eye movements, the clinician can usually localize the cause and identify the category of coma. However, immediate computed tomography (CT) imaging should not be delayed after stabilization of the vital signs.

Motor Responses

The patient is observed to assess respiration, limb position, and spontaneous movements. Myoclonus or seizures may be subtle (e.g., twitching of one or two fingers or the corner of the mouth). More florid movements, such as facial grimacing, jaw gyrations, tongue protrusion, or complex repetitive limb movements, may defy ready interpretation. Asymmetric movements or postures may signify either focal seizures or hemiparesis.

Assessment of motor tone is crucial in the examination of coma. Asymmetry of muscle tone suggests a structural lesion, but it is not always clear which side is abnormal. *Gegenhalten*, or *paratonia*, is variable resistance to passive movement that often increases with the velocity of the movement; it is attributed to diffuse forebrain dysfunction and is often accompanied by a grasp reflex. *Rigidity* is present throughout the entire range of movement, is often seen in combination with cogwheeling, and usually indicates basal ganglia dysfunction (e.g., parkinsonism) or symptomatic hydrocephalus. *Spasticity* has a characteristic "catch" midway through passive movement and indicates corticospinal pathway dysfunction. Acute transtentorial herniation often produces exaggerated lower extremity spasticity and clonus.

TABLE 18.1	Glasgow Coma Scale	
Eye opening	Spontaneous	4
	To voice	3
	To pain	2
	None	1
Best motor response	Obeys commands	6
	Localizes to pain	5
	Withdraws to pain	4
	Flexor posturing	3
	Extensor posturing	2
	None	1
Best verbal response	Conversant and oriented	5
	Conversant and disoriented	4
	Inappropriate words	3
	Incomprehensible sounds	2
	None	1
Total score		3–15

Although a total score can be calculated, proper notation of the Glasgow Coma Scale involves delimitation of the three subscores. For instance, e3 m5 v3 applies to a patient who opens eyes to voice, localizes to pain, and is capable of uttering words but not sentences.

From Teasdale G, Jennett B. Assessment of coma and impaired consciousness. A practical scale. *Lancet.* 1974;2(7872):81–84.

TABLE 18.2   Practical Pearls in the Physical Examination of the Comatose Patient

System	Positive Finding
Body temperature	• Fever (implies infection or heatstroke) • Hypothermia (cold exposure, sepsis, cardiac arrest, hypothyroidism, hypoglycemia)
Peripheral pulses	• Asymmetry of pulses suggests dissecting aortic aneurysm.
Head and scalp	• External signs of trauma (e.g., mastoid ecchymoses consistent with Battle sign) • Ears and nose are examined for blood or CSF.
Skin, nails, and mucous membranes	• Pallor • Cherry redness (carbon monoxide poisoning) • Cyanosis • Jaundice • Sweating • Uremic frost • Myxedema (dry, flaky, cool skin) • Petechiae • Dehydration • Decubiti • Signs of trauma
Breath	• Acetone • Alcohol • Fetor hepaticus
Optic fundi	• Papilledema (suggests elevated ICP), hypertensive or diabetic retinopathy, retinal ischemia • Roth spots (suggests endocarditis) • Subhyaloid hemorrhages (suggests subarachnoid hemorrhage)
Neck	• Resistance to passive neck flexion but not to turning suggests meningitis, subarachnoid hemorrhage, or foramen magnum herniation. • Resistance to manipulation in all directions suggests bone or joint disease, including fracture.
Urinary or fecal incontinence	• May signify an unwitnessed seizure, especially in patients who subsequently awaken

CSF, cerebrospinal fluid; ICP, increased cranial pressure.

Motor responses to stimuli may be appropriate, inappropriate, or absent. Even when patients are not fully awake, they may be roused to follow simple commands. Some patients who respond only to noxious stimuli (e.g., pressure on the sternum or supraorbital bone; pinching the neck or limbs; or squeezing muscle, tendon, or nail beds) may make voluntary avoidance responses. The terms *decorticate* and *decerebrate* posturing are physiologic misnomers but refer to stereotyped hypertonic flexion or extension in response to noxious stimuli (Fig. 18.3). In *decorticate rigidity*, the arms are flexed, adducted, and internally rotated, and the legs are extended; in *decerebrate rigidity*, the arms and legs are all extended. These postures are most often associated with cerebral hemisphere disease, including hypoxic–ischemic or metabolic encephalopathy, but may follow upper brain stem lesions or

FIGURE 18.3 Decerebrate or extensor posturing **(A)** and decorticate or flexor posting **(B)**.

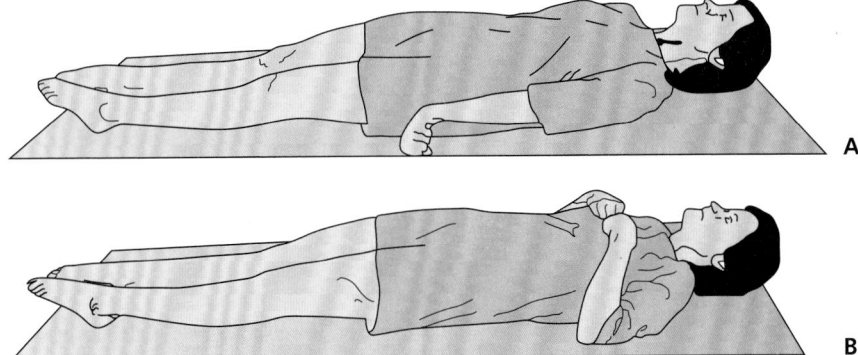

transtentorial herniation as well (see later section for a discussion of herniation syndromes). Flexor posturing generally implies a more rostral lesion and has a better prognosis than extensor posturing, but the pattern of response may vary with different stimuli, or there may be flexion of one arm and extension of the other. When these postures seem to occur spontaneously, there may be an unrecognized stimulus (e.g., airway obstruction or bladder distention). With continuing rostrocaudal deterioration, there may be extension of the arms and flexion of the legs until, with lower brain stem destruction, there is flaccid unresponsiveness. However, lack of motor response to any stimulus should always raise the possibility of limb paralysis caused by cervical trauma, Guillain–Barré neuropathy, or the locked-in state.

Respiration

In Cheyne–Stokes respiration (CSR), periods of hyperventilation and apnea alternate in a crescendo–decrescendo fashion. The hyperpneic phase is usually longer than the apneic, so arterial gases tend to show respiratory alkalosis. CSR occurs with bilateral cerebral disease or metabolic encephalopathy. It usually signifies that the patient is not in imminent danger. Long-cycle CSR, with brief periods of apnea occurring every 1 to 2 minutes, is a stable breathing pattern and does not imply impending respiratory arrest. Conversely, "short-cycle CSR" (*cluster breathing*) with less smooth waxing and waning is often an ominous sign of a posterior fossa lesion or dangerously elevated ICP.

Sustained hyperventilation is usually due to metabolic acidosis, pulmonary congestion, hepatic encephalopathy, or during acute herniation (see Fig. 18.3). Rarely, it is the result of a lesion in the rostral brain stem. *Apneustic breathing*, consisting of long inspiratory pauses, is seen with pontine lesions, especially infarction; it occurs infrequently with metabolic coma or transtentorial herniation.

Respiration having a variably irregular rate and amplitude (*ataxic breathing*) indicates medullary damage and may progress to apnea, which also occurs abruptly in acute posterior fossa lesions. Loss of automatic respiration with preserved voluntary breathing (*Ondine curse*) occurs with medullary lesions; as the patient becomes less alert, apnea may be fatal. Other ominous respiratory signs are end-expiratory pushing (e.g., coughing) and "fish-mouthing" (i.e., lower jaw depression with inspiration). Stertorous breathing (i.e., inspiratory noise) is a sign of airway obstruction.

Pupils

Pupillary abnormalities in coma may reflect an imbalance between input from the parasympathetic and sympathetic nervous systems or lesions of both. Although many people have slight pupillary inequality, anisocoria should be considered pathologic in a comatose patient. Retinal or optic nerve damage does not cause anisocoria, even though there is an afferent pupillary defect. Parasympathetic lesions (e.g., oculomotor nerve compression in uncal herniation or after rupture of an internal carotid artery aneurysm) cause pupillary enlargement and, ultimately, full dilation with loss of reactivity to light. Sympathetic lesions, either intraparenchymal (e.g., hypothalamic injury or lateral medullary infarction) or extraparenchymal (e.g., invasion of the superior cervical ganglion by lung cancer), cause Horner syndrome with miosis. With involvement of both systems (e.g., midbrain destruction), one or both pupils are in mid position and are unreactive. Small but reactive pupils following pontine hemorrhage are the result of damage to descending intra-axial sympathetic pathways.

With few exceptions, metabolic disease does not cause unequal or unreactive pupils. Fixed, dilated pupils after diffuse anoxia–ischemia denote a bad prognosis. Anticholinergic drugs, including glutethimide, amitriptyline, and antiparkinsonian agents, abolish pupillary reactivity. Hypothermia and severe barbiturate intoxication may cause not only fixed pupils but also a reversible picture that mimics brain death. Bilateral or unilateral pupillary dilation and nonreactivity may accompany (or briefly follow) a seizure. In opiate overdose, miosis may be so severe that a very bright light and a magnifying glass are necessary to detect reactivity. Some pupillary abnormalities are local in origin (e.g., trauma or synechiae).

Eyelids and Eye Movements

Spontaneous blinking may occur with or without purposeful limb movements. Eyes that are conjugately deviated away from hemiparetic limbs indicate a destructive cerebral lesion on the side toward which the eyes are directed. Eyes turned toward paretic limbs may indicate a pontine lesion, an adversive seizure, or the wrong-way gaze paresis of thalamic hemorrhage. Eyes that are dysconjugate while at rest may indicate paresis of individual muscles, internuclear ophthalmoplegia, or preexisting tropia or phoria.

When the brain stem is intact, the eyes may rove irregularly from side to side with a slow, smooth velocity; jerky movements suggest saccades and relative wakefulness. Repetitive smooth excursions of the eyes first to one side and then to the other, with 2- to 3-second pauses in each direction (*periodic alternating* or

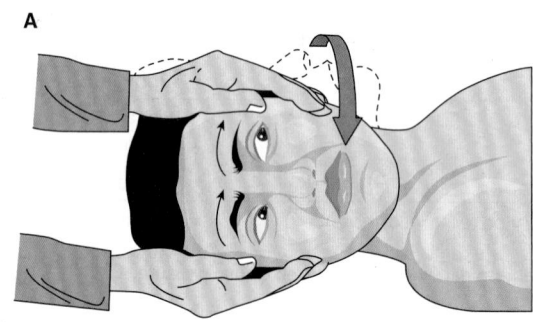

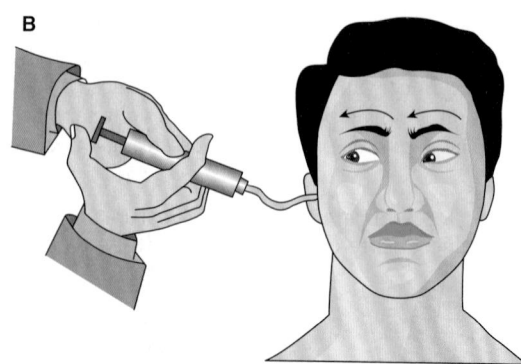

FIGURE 18.4 A: Doll's eye maneuver (oculocephalic reflex): With intact brain stem (cranial nerves III through VIII), the eyes remain relatively stationary and move opposite to the direction of head turning. **B:** Cold caloric test (oculovestibular reflex): With intact brain stem, cold water in the auditory canal results in tonic conjugate eye deviation toward the cold ear.

ping-pong gaze), may follow bilateral cerebral infarction or cerebellar hemorrhage with an intact brain stem.

If cervical injury has been ruled out, oculocephalic testing (the *doll's eyes maneuver*) is performed by passively turning the head from side to side; with an intact reflex arc (vestibular system → brain stem → eye muscles), the eyes move conjugately in the opposite direction (Fig. 18.4). A more vigorous stimulus is produced by irrigating each ear with 30 to 60 mL of ice water. A normal, awake person with head elevated at 30 degrees has nystagmus with the fast component in the direction opposite the ear stimulated, but a comatose patient with an intact reflex arc has deviation of the eyes toward the stimulus, usually for several minutes. Simultaneous bilateral irrigation causes vertical deviation, upward after warm water and downward after cold water.

Oculocephalic or caloric testing may reveal intact eye movements, gaze palsy, individual muscle paresis, internuclear ophthalmoplegia, or no response. Cerebral gaze paresis may often be overcome by these maneuvers, but brain stem gaze palsies are usually fixed. Complete ophthalmoplegia may follow either extensive brain stem damage or metabolic coma, but except for barbiturate or phenytoin poisoning, eye movements are preserved early in metabolic encephalopathy. Unexplained disconjugate eyes indicate a brain stem or cranial nerve lesion (including abducens palsy due to increased ICP).

Downward deviation of the eyes occurs with lesions in the thalamus or midbrain pretectum and may be accompanied by pupils that do not react to light (*Parinaud syndrome*). Downward eye deviation also occurs in metabolic coma, especially in barbiturate poisoning and after a seizure. Skew deviation, or vertical divergence, follows lesions of the cerebellum or brain stem, especially the pontine tegmentum.

Retraction and convergence nystagmus may be seen with midbrain lesions, but spontaneous nystagmus is rare in coma. *Ocular bobbing* (i.e., conjugate brisk downward movements from the primary position) usually follows destructive lesions of the pontine tegmentum (when lateral eye movements are lost). Preservation of voluntary vertical eye movements with loss of lateral eye movements and quadriplegia is consistent with *locked-in syndrome*. Unilateral bobbing (i.e., nystagmoid jerking) signifies pontine disease.

DIAGNOSTIC TESTS

CT or MRI should be promptly performed whenever coma is unexplained. Unless meningitis is suspected, imaging should precede lumbar puncture. If imaging is not readily available, a spinal tap is cautiously performed with a 20- or 22-gauge needle. If imaging reveals frank, transtentorial, or foramen magnum herniation, the comparative risks of performing a lumbar puncture or of treating for meningitis without CSF confirmation must be weighed individually for each patient.

Other emergency laboratory studies include serum levels of glucose, sodium, calcium, and BUN or creatinine; determination of arterial pH and partial pressures of oxygen (PO_2) and carbon dioxide (PCO_2); and blood or urine toxicology testing (including testing serum levels of sedative drugs and ethanol). Blood and CSF should be cultured and liver function studies and other serum electrolyte levels determined. The use of coagulation studies and other metabolic tests is based on the index of suspicion.

The EEG may distinguish coma from psychic unresponsiveness or locked-in state, although alpha-like activity in coma after brain stem infarction or cardiopulmonary arrest may make the distinction difficult. In metabolic coma, the EEG is always abnormal, and early in the course, it may be a more sensitive indicator of abnormality than the clinical state of the patient. The EEG may also reveal asymmetries or evidence of clinically unsuspected seizure activity. Infrequently, patients without clinical seizures demonstrate repetitive electrographic seizures or continuous spike-and-wave activity; conversely, patients with subtle motor manifestations of seizures sometimes display only diffuse electrographic slowing. Distinguishing true status epilepticus from myoclonus (common after anoxic–ischemic brain damage) is often difficult, both clinically and electrographically; if any doubt exists, anticonvulsant therapy should be instituted.

COMA PRESENTATIONS AND TREATMENT

Many structural and nonstructural pathologies can result in impaired consciousness, necessitating a structured diagnostic approach with a broad differential. For rapid efficient communication between providers, generalizable scales such as the Full Outline of UnResponsiveness (FOUR) score may be helpful (Fig. 18.5). A more commonly used alternative is the Glasgow Coma Scale (see Table 18.1).

COMA FROM SUPRATENTORIAL HERNIATION SYNDROMES

Coma may result from bilateral cerebral damage or from sudden large unilateral lesions that functionally disrupt the contralateral hemisphere (*diaschisis*). Herniation syndromes result from mass lesions that shift the brain out of its normal position. CT studies indicate that with acute hemisphere masses, early depression of consciousness correlates more with lateral brain displacement than with downward transtentorial herniation. The different types of herniation syndromes are described in (Table 18.3). It is important to keep in mind that different herniation syndromes can occur in a sequence or combination. For instance, an expanding hemispheric mass lesion resulting in lateral brain displacement may initially produce subfalcine herniation, followed by uncal herniation as a combination of downward and lateral displacement ensues.

Subfalcine herniation results from lateral displacement of the brain from mass lesions that are positioned rostrally in the cranial vault, at the level of the lateral ventricles or above (Fig. 18.6). *Transtentorial herniation* can result from lateralized (uncal) or bilateral (central) downward displacement. In *uncal herniation*, brain stem signs are initially lateralized. Typically, there is early compression of the oculomotor nerve by the inferomedial temporal lobe with ipsilateral pupillary enlargement. Alertness may not be altered until the pupil is dilated, at which point there may be an acceleration of signs, with unilaterally and then bilaterally fixed pupils and oculomotor palsy, hyperventilation or ataxic breathing, and progressive unresponsiveness. Typically, a lateralized motor deficit progresses to symmetric and bilateral flexor and then extensor posturing, as the caudal most level of injury progresses to the upper brain stem. During the downward course of transtentorial herniation, there may be hemiparesis ipsilateral or oculomotor nerve compression contralateral to the cerebral lesion, which can be attributed to compression of the contralateral midbrain peduncle against the tentorial edge (*Kernohan notch*). Aqueduct obstruction and posterior cerebral artery compression may further raise supratentorial pressure. If the process is not halted, there is progression to deep coma, apnea, bilaterally unreactive pupils, ophthalmoplegia, and eventually, circulatory collapse and brain death.

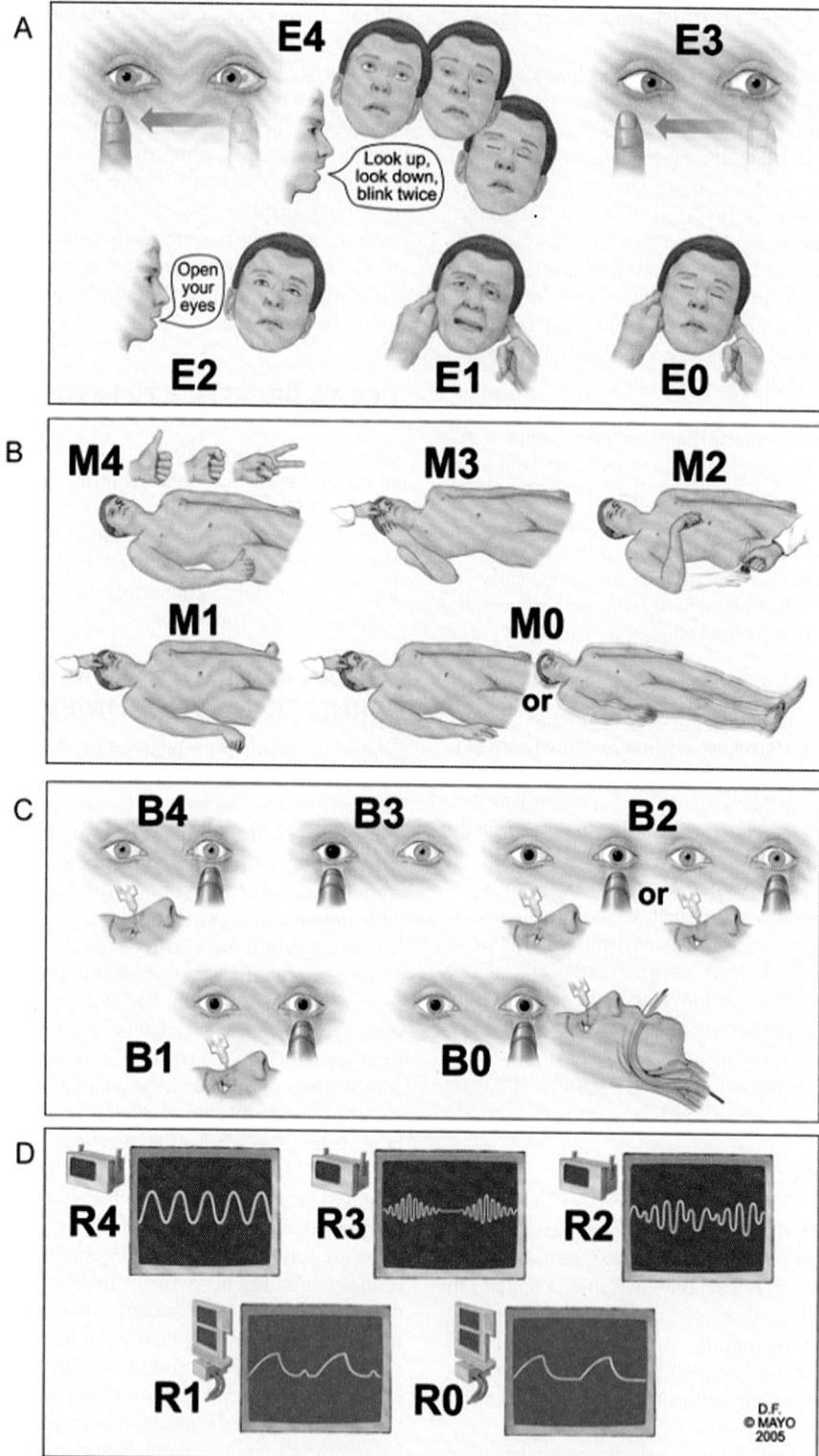

FIGURE 18.5 Eye response: *E4*, eyelids open or opened, tracking, or blinking to command; *E3*, eyelids open but not tracking; *E2*, eyelids closed but open to loud voice; *E1*, eyelids closed but open to pain; *E0*, eyelids remain closed with pain. Motor response: *M4*, thumbs-up, fist, or peace sign; *M3*, localizing to pain; *M2*, flexion response to pain; *M1*, extension response to pain; *M0*, no response to pain or generalized myoclonus status. Brain stem reflexes: *B4*, pupil and corneal reflexes present; *B3*, one pupil wide and fixed; *B2*, pupil or corneal reflexes absent; *B1*, pupil and corneal reflexes absent; *B0*, absent pupil, corneal, and cough reflex. Respiration pattern: *R4*, not intubated, regular breathing pattern; *R3*, not intubated, Cheyne-Stokes breathing pattern; *R2*, not intubated, irregular breathing; *R1*, breathes above ventilatory rate; *R0*, breathes at ventilator rate or apnea. (From Wijdicks EFM, Bamlet WR, Maramattom BV, et al. Validation of a new coma scale: the FOUR score. *Ann Neurol.* 2005;58[4]:585–593.)

TABLE 18.3   Herniation Syndromes

Types	Mechanism of Herniation/Complications
Subfalcine	• Mechanism: lateral shifting displacement of the brain by a compartmentalized hemispheric mass lesion at the level of the ventricles or above • Classic causes: malignant MCA infarction, acute subdural or epidural hematoma • Imaging: midline shift with ipsilateral widening of the perimesencephalic cisterns • Clinical: contralateral hemiparesis progressing to bilateral motor posturing and coma, with late ipsilateral CN III palsy due to stretching of the oculomotor nerve • Complications: delayed ipsilateral ACA pericallosal infarction due to compression against the falx
Central transtentorial	• Mechanism: downward displacement of the brain by a bilateral supratentorial mass lesion, with craniocaudal pressure on diencephalon with downward displacement • Classic causes: massive bilateral intraventricular hemorrhage leading to acute obstructive hydrocephalus, massive global cerebral edema • Imaging: bilateral loss of the perimesencephalic cisterns and downward displacement of the midbrain tectum into the posterior fossa • Clinical: early Parinaud syndrome (loss of upgaze and convergence, retraction nystagmus) followed by rostrocaudal loss of brain stem reflexes associated with progression from decorticate to decerebrate posturing • Complications: stretching of small penetrating vessels leading to diencephalic and brainstem infarction, sometimes pituitary damage • Less common dorsal pressure leading to Parinaud syndrome (limitation of upward eye movements, usually with impairment of pupillary light reflex and difficulty with convergence)
Uncal transtentorial	• Mechanism: displacement of medial temporal lobe over free tentorial edge by a temporal lobe mass lesion or during the late stages of lateral and downward herniation • Classic causes: intracerebral mass lesions for example intracerebral hematoma, subdural hematoma, brain tumor • Imaging: prominent medial displacement of the uncus into the tentorial notch • Clinical: early ipsilateral dilated pupil due to CN III compression and ipsilateral or contralateral hemiparesis/posturing • Complications: trapping of the contralateral lateral ventricle due to compression of the third ventricle and aqueduct; compression of posterior cerebral arteries with resultant infarction
Tonsillar	• Mechanisms: displacement of cerebellar tonsils into the foramen magnum → compression of medulla and fourth ventricle • Classic cause: acute cerebellar ICH or rapidly expanding tumor • Imaging: herniation of cerebellar tonsils into the foramen magnum at level of the medulla • Clinical: impaired respiratory and cardiac function, neck stiffness, flaccid paralysis, and coma • Complications: secondary obstructive hydrocephalus due to obstruction of the fourth ventricle
Upward herniation	• Mechanisms: displacement of superior cerebellar vermis upward leading to compression of dorsal mesencephalon, blood vessels, and aqueduct • Classic cause: acute cerebellar ICH or rapidly expanding tumor • Imaging: cerebellar mass lesion with effacement of quadrigeminal cistern and upward displacement of midbrain tectum • Clinical: impaired consciousness, loss of pupillary and oculocephalic reflexes • Complications: secondary obstructive hydrocephalus due to obstruction of the cerebral aqueduct

MCA, middle cerebral artery; CN, cranial nerve; ACA, anterior cerebral artery; ICH, intracranial hemorrhage.

In *central transtentorial herniation* (as in thalamic hemorrhage), consciousness is rapidly impaired, and abnormalities of brain stem reflexes progress in rostrocaudal fashion. Pupils initially are of normal or small diameter and react to light, lateral eye movements and corneal reflexes are preserved, and bilateral spasticity progresses to flexor posturing. This stage is referred to as *diencephalic syndrome* because the level of injury is localized to the level of the thalamus. As herniation progresses, the pupils become fixed in mid position (midbrain pupils); this is followed by loss of pontine level brain stem reflexes (cornmeal and oculocephalic) and sometimes by pinpoint unreactive pupils (pontine pupils). Eventually, only medullary function remains (gag and cough), and after this, abolished brain death ensues.

The major lesions causing transtentorial herniation are traumatic (e.g., epidural, subdural, or intraparenchymal hemorrhage), vascular (e.g., ischemic or hemorrhagic), infectious (e.g., abscess or granuloma, including lesions associated with AIDS), and neoplastic (primary or metastatic). CT or MRI locates and often defines the lesion.

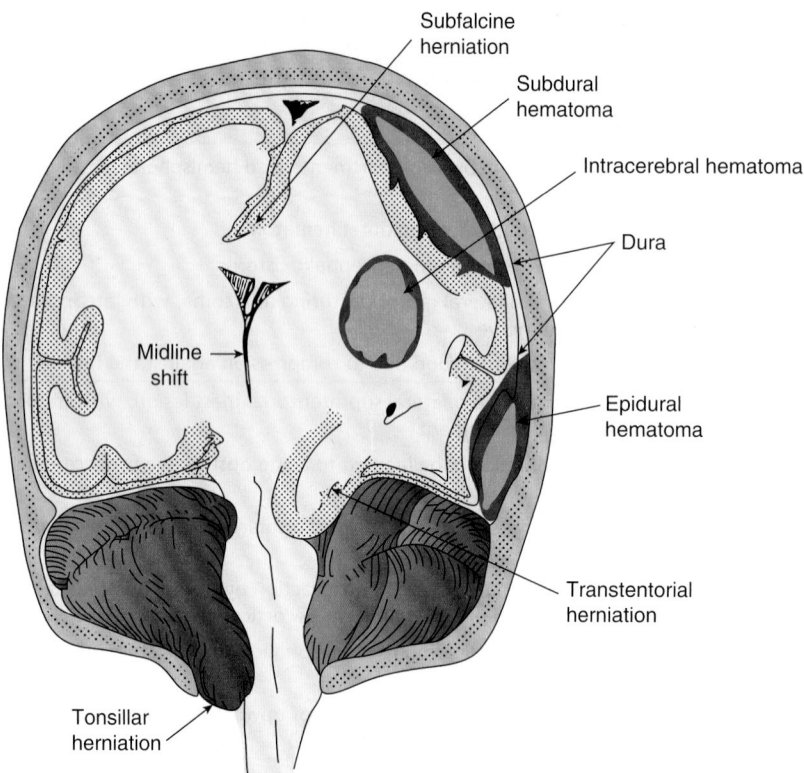

FIGURE 18.6 Herniation syndromes.

COMA FROM INFRATENTORIAL STRUCTURAL LESIONS

Infratentorial structural lesions may compress or directly destroy the brain stem. Such lesions may also cause brain herniation either transtentorially upward (with midbrain compression) or downward through the foramen magnum, with distortion of the medulla by the cerebellar tonsils. Abrupt tonsillar herniation causes apnea and circulatory collapse; coma is then secondary, for the medullary reticular formation has little direct role in arousal. In coma, *primary infratentorial structural lesions* are suggested by bilateral weakness or sensory loss, crossed cranial nerve and long-tract signs, miosis, loss of lateral gaze with preserved vertical eye movements, dysconjugate gaze, ophthalmoplegia, short-cycle CSR, and apneustic or ataxic breathing. The clinical picture of pontine hemorrhage (i.e., sudden coma, pinpoint but reactive pupils, and no eye movement) is characteristic, but if the sequence of signs in a comatose patient is unknown, it may not be possible to tell whether the process began supratentorially or infratentorially without the use of imaging. Infrequent brain stem causes of coma include multiple sclerosis and central pontine myelinolysis.

COMA FROM METABOLIC OR DIFFUSE BRAIN DISEASE

In metabolic, diffuse, or multifocal encephalopathy, cognitive and respiratory abnormalities occur early; there is often tremor, asterixis, or multifocal myoclonus. Gegenhalten, frontal release signs (e.g., snout, suck, or grasp), and flexor or extensor posturing may occur. Except in anoxia–ischemia and anticholinergic intoxication, the pupils remain reactive. The eyes may be deviated downward, but the presence of sustained lateral deviation or disconjugate eyes argues against the diagnosis of a metabolic disturbance. Metabolic disease, however, may cause both focal seizures and lateralizing neurologic signs, often shifting but sometimes persisting (as in hypoglycemia and hyperglycemia).

Arterial blood gas determinations are especially useful in diagnosing metabolic coma. Of the diseases listed in Table 18.4, psychogenic hyperventilation is more likely to cause delirium than stupor but may coexist with hysterical coma. Cognitive change associated with metabolic alkalosis is usually mild. Metabolic and diffuse brain diseases causing coma are numerous, but the diversity is not overwhelming. Most entities listed in Table 18.5 are described in other chapters.

HYSTERIA AND CATATONIA

Hysterical (conversion) unresponsiveness is rare. Clinically indistinguishable from malingering, it is usually associated with closed eyes, eupnea or tachypnea, and normal pupils. The eyelids may resist passive opening and, when released, may close abruptly rather than with smooth descent; lightly stroking the eyelashes causes lid fluttering. The eyes do not slowly rove but move with saccadic jerks, and ice water caloric testing causes nystagmus rather than sustained deviation. The limbs usually offer no resistance to passive movement, yet demonstrate normal tone. Unless organic disease or drug effect is also present, the EEG pattern is one of normal wakefulness.

Catatonia is a behavioral disturbance characterized by wakeful unresponsiveness with minimal or no spontaneous purposeful behavior or speech. It is most commonly associated with depression, schizophrenia, toxic psychosis, or other brain diseases. There may be akinetic mutism, grimacing, rigidity, posturing, catalepsy, or excitement. Respirations are normal or rapid, pupils are large but reactive, and eye movements are normal. The EEG is usually normal.

LOCKED-IN SYNDROME

Infarction, hemorrhage, or rarely, central pontine myelinolysis may destroy the basis pontis, producing total paralysis of the

TABLE 18.4 Causes of Abnormal Ventilation in Unresponsive Patients

Hyperventilation

Metabolic acidosis

Anion gap

Diabetic ketoacidosis[a]

Diabetic hyperosmolar coma[a]

Lactic acidosis

Uremia[a]

Alcoholic ketoacidosis

Acidic poisons (ethylene glycol, methyl alcohol, paraldehyde)[a]

No anion gap

Diarrhea

Pancreatic drainage

Carbonic anhydrase inhibitors

NH_4Cl ingestion

Renal tubular acidosis

Ureteroenterostomy

Respiratory alkalosis

Hepatic failure[a]

Sepsis[a]

Pneumonia

Anxiety (hyperventilation syndrome)

Mixed acid–base disorders (metabolic acidosis and respiratory alkalosis)

Salicylism

Sepsis[a]

Hepatic failure[a]

Hypoventilation

Respiratory acidosis

Acute (uncompensated)

Sedative drugs[a]

Brain stem injury

Neuromuscular disorders

Chest injury

Acute pulmonary disease

Chronic pulmonary disease

Metabolic alkalosis

Vomiting or gastric drainage

Diuretic therapy

Adrenal steroid excess (Cushing syndrome)

Primary aldosteronism

Bartter syndrome

[a]Common causes of stupor or coma.

From Posner JB, Saper CB, Schiff ND, et al. *Plum and Posner's Diagnosis of Stupor and Coma.* 4th ed. New York: Oxford University Press; 2007.

lower cranial nerve and limb muscles, with preserved alertness and respiration. At first glance, the patient appears unresponsive, but examination reveals voluntary vertical eye movements, including blinking. (Even with facial paralysis, inhibition of the levator palpebrae may produce partial eye closure). Communication is possible with the use of purposeful blinking or eye movements to indicate "yes," "no," or in response to letters.

VEGETATIVE STATE AND MINIMALLY CONSCIOUS STATE

Persistent impairment of consciousness in the postacute hospitalization phase is categorized into MCS and UWS, formerly known as vegetative state. Patients with UWS have sleep–wake cycles, intact cardiorespiratory function, and primitive responses to stimuli but without evidence of inner or outer awareness present for at least 1 month (Table 18.6). In contrast, patients with MCS intermittently show signs of self or environmental awareness, which may include those verbal command, visual tracking, and context-specific emotional responses. Identifying this state is important, as it may represent a transitory state on the road to recovery.

Patients who survive coma usually show varying degrees of recovery within 2 to 4 weeks; those who enter UWS may recover further, even fully. Emerging data indicate that much of our formerly pessimistic assumptions regarding outcome of comatose patients are likely based on self-fulfilling prophecies. Recent studies indicate that one-third of UWS patients die in the ICU, whereas one-fifth remain in the UWS state and half recover consciousness by the time they are discharged from the ICU. In the Multi-Society Task Force study, patients remaining in the UWS 3 months after traumatic brain injury were associated with a 35% rate of recovery of consciousness at 1 year and 16% of these patients recovered independent function by 1 year after injury. The majority (>80%) of patients remaining in MCS at 3 to 6 months after injury will improve, some eventually demonstrating no disability. Patients with traumatic brain injury tend to have better recovery compared to those with anoxic–ischemic injury. Much research is currently directed toward identifying predictors of who will recover to which state at what time. Amantadine hydrochloride 100 mg t.i.d. has been shown to accelerate the pace of functional recovery among patients with UWS and MCS after severe traumatic brain injury [**Level 1**].[1] Also under study are the use of the pharmacologic interventions (e.g., zolpidem) and thalamic stimulation.

BRAIN DEATH

Unlike the UWS in which the brain stem is intact, the term *brain death* means that the cerebrum and the brain stem are both permanently destroyed. The only spontaneous activity is cardiovascular; apnea persists in the presence of hypercarbia sufficient for respiratory drive, and the only reflexes present are those mediated by the spinal cord. In adults, brain death rarely lasts more than a few days and is always followed by circulatory collapse despite persistence on a ventilator. In the United States, brain death is equated with legal death. When criteria are met, artificial ventilation and BP support are appropriately discontinued, regardless of whether or not organ harvesting is intended. Detailed information on how to diagnose and manage brain death in the ICU is provided in Chapter 19.

TABLE 18.5 Diffuse Brain Diseases or Metabolic Disorders that Cause Coma

Deprivation of oxygen, substrate, or metabolic cofactor

Hypoxia

Diffuse ischemia (cardiac disease, decreased peripheral circulatory resistance, increased cerebrovascular resistance, widespread small-vessel occlusion)

Hypoglycemia

Thiamine deficiency (Wernicke–Korsakoff syndrome)

Disease of organs other than brain

Liver (hepatic coma)

Kidney (uremia)

Lung (carbon dioxide narcosis)

Pancreas (diabetes, hypoglycemia, exocrine pancreatic encephalopathy)

Pituitary (apoplexy, sedative hypersensitivity)

Thyroid (myxedema, thyrotoxicosis)

Parathyroid (hypo- and hyperparathyroidism)

Adrenal (Addison or Cushing disease, pheochromocytoma)

Other systemic disease (cancer, porphyria, sepsis)

Exogenous poisons

Sedatives and narcotics

Psychotropic drugs

Acid poisons (e.g., methyl alcohol, ethylene glycol)

Others (e.g., anticonvulsants, heavy metals, cyanide)

Abnormalities of ionic or acid–base environment of CNS

Water and sodium (hypo- and hypernatremia)

Abnormalities of ionic or acid–base environment of CNS (continued)

Acidosis

Alkalosis

Magnesium (hyper- and hypomagnesemia)

Calcium (hyper- and hypocalcemia)

Phosphorus (hypophosphatemia)

Disordered temperature regulation

Hypothermia

Heat stroke

CNS inflammation or infiltration

Leptomeningitis

Encephalitis

Acute toxic encephalopathy (e.g., Reye syndrome)

Parainfectious encephalomyelitis

Cerebral vasculitis

Subarachnoid hemorrhage

Carcinomatous meningitis

Primary neuronal or glial disorders

Creutzfeldt–Jakob disease

Marchiafava–Bignami disease

Adrenoleukodystrophy

Gliomatosis cerebri

Progressive multifocal leukoencephalopathy

Seizure and postictal states

CNS, central nervous system.

Modified from Posner JB, Saper CB, Schiff ND, et al. *Plum and Posner's Diagnosis of Stupor and Coma*. 4th ed. New York: Oxford University Press; 2007.

TABLE 18.6 Criteria for Determination of Unresponsive Wakefulness State (Formerly Known as Vegetative State)

1. No evidence of awareness of self or surroundings. Reflex or spontaneous eye opening may occur.

2. No meaningful and consistent communication between examiner and patient, auditory or written. Target stimuli not usually followed visually, but sometimes, visual tracking present. No emotional response to verbal stimuli.

3. No comprehensible speech or mouthing of words

4. Smiling, frowning, or crying inconsistently related to any apparent stimulus

5. Sleep–wake cycles present

6. Brain stem and spinal reflexes variable, e.g., preservation of sucking, rooting, chewing, swallowing, pupillary reactivity to light, oculo-cephalic responses, and grasp or tendon reflexes

7. No voluntary movements or behavior, no matter how rudimentary; no motor activity suggesting learned behavior; no mimicry. Withdrawal or posturing can occur with noxious stimuli.

8. Usually intact BP control and cardiorespiratory function. Incontinence of bladder and bowel.

BP, blood pressure.

FUTURE DIRECTIONS

Functional imaging and EEG studies applying task-based or resting state paradigms may offer more objective means to study patients with impaired consciousness. These studies have indicated that some patients who appear comatose may have preserved higher cognitive processing suggesting intact consciousness. These imaging and electrophysiologic techniques may offer more quantifiable and objective endpoints to study impairment of consciousness in natural history studies and clinical trials.

LEVEL 1 EVIDENCE

1. Giacino JT, Whyte J, Bagiella E, et al. Placebo-controlled trial of amantadine for severe traumatic brain injury. *N Engl J Med.* 2012;366(9):819–826.

SUGGESTED READINGS

Childs NL, Mercer WN. Late improvement in consciousness after post-traumatic vegetative state. *N Engl J Med.* 1996;334:24–25.

Claassen J, Mayer SA. Continuous electroencephalographic monitoring in neurocritical care. *Curr Neurol Neurosci Rep.* 2002;2:534–540.

Fisher CM. The neurological examination of the comatose patient. *Acta Neurol Scand.* 1969;45(suppl 36):1–56.

Giacino JT, Kalmar K. Diagnostic and prognostic guidelines for the vegetative and minimally conscious states. *Neuropsychol Rehabil.* 2005;15:166–174.

Goudreau JL, Wijdicks EFM, Emery SF. Complications during apnea testing in the determination of brain death: predisposing factors. *Neurology.* 2000;55:1045–1048.

Michelson DJ, Ashwal S. Evaluation of coma and brain death. *Semin Pediatr Neurol.* 2004;11(2):105–118.

Owen AM, Coleman MR, Boly M, et al. Detecting awareness in the vegetative state. *Science.* 2006;313:1402.

Parvizi J, Van Hoesen GW, Buckwalter J, et al. Neural connections of the postero-medial cortex in the macaque. *Proc Natl Acad Sci U S A.* 2006;103:1563–1568.

Posner JB, Saper CB, Schiff ND, et al. *Plum and Posner's Diagnosis of Stupor and Coma.* 4th ed. New York: Oxford University Press; 2007.

Robinson LR, Mickleson PJ, Tirschwell DL, et al. Predictive value of somatosensory evoked potentials for awakening from coma. *Crit Care Med.* 2003;31:960–967.

Saper CB, Scammell TE, Lu J. Hypothalamic regulation of sleep and circadian rhythms. *Nature.* 2005;437(7063):1257–1263.

Saposnik G, Bueri JA, Maurino J, et al. Spontaneous and reflex movements in brain death. *Neurology.* 2000;54:221.

Schiff ND. Recovery of consciousness after brain injury: a mesocircuit hypothesis. *Trends Neurosci.* 2010;33(1):1–9.

Schiff ND, Giacino JT, Kalmar K, et al. Behavioural improvements with thalamic stimulation after severe traumatic brain injury. *Nature.* 2007;448(7153):600–603.

Schiff ND, Ribary U, Rodriguez Moreno D, et al. Residual cerebral activity and behavioural fragments can remain in the persistently vegetative brain. *Brain.* 2003;125:1210–1234.

Schiff ND, Rodriguez-Moreno D, Kamal A, et al. fMRI reveals large-scale network activation in minimally conscious patients. *Neurology.* 2005;64:514–523.

Sitt JD, King JR, El Karoui I, et al. Large scale screening of neural signatures of consciousness in patients in a vegetative or minimally conscious state. *Brain.* 2014;137(pt 8):2258–2270.

Wijdicks EF, Bamlet WR, Maramattom BV, et al. Validation of a new coma scale: the FOUR score. *Ann Neurol.* 2005;58(4):585–593.

Wijdicks EFM, Pfeifer EA. Neuropathology of brain death in the modern transplant era. *Neurology.* 2008;70:1234–1237.

Wijdicks EFM, Varelas PN, Gronseth GS, et al. Evidence-based guideline update: determining brain death in adults *Neurology.* 2010;74:1911–1918.

Eelco F. M. Wijdicks

INTRODUCTION

Brain death is the preferred term to summarize an apneic patient with not only irreversible coma from a massive brain injury but loss of all brain stem reflexes and uncontrolled diuresis and hypotension from loss of vascular tone. Nothing else should explain this condition and characteristically, it is due to an acute catastrophic bihemispheric and diencephalic injury. Brain death remains uncommon because such progression would require not only involvement of both hemispheres of the brain but also loss of brain stem function. Typically, this clinical situation would be an acute massive hemispheric lesion (e.g., cerebral hemorrhage) compressing and sequentially damaging the mesencephalon, pons, and medulla oblongata (Fig. 19.1). The brain stem is very resilient to injury and it would take a substantial shift (from mass effect) or poor perfusion (from basilar artery occlusion or massively increased intracranial pressure) for it to get permanently damaged. This core neurologic principle—the brain stem to be the last brain structure to go out of function—is the most important attribute to our understanding of brain death. Once brain stem function is lost, breathing stops first and the heart soon thereafter. If in the acute phase the patient can be intubated, placed on a mechanical ventilator, sufficiently oxygenated, fluid resuscitated, and vasopressors and vasopressin added, this agonal sequence can potentially be prevented.

Once an untreatable catastrophic neurologic structural injury has been proven and the brain stem reflexes have disappeared, recovery does not occur, and there is no known effective medical or surgical intervention. Irreversibility is determined by this diagnosis and involves testing of absent motor responses, loss of all brain stem reflexes, and observation of apnea after a CO_2 challenge in a patient temporarily detached from the ventilator.

The determination of brain death is a fundamental skill for the neurologist but experience could be waning. In many regions, the incidence of brain death has declined over the last decade. It is possible that family members may decide to withdraw when the situation is already hopeless and do not want to wait any further. Improved neurosurgical care, in particular early decompressive craniotomy, may also have contributed.

Brain death determination is relatively straightforward. Physicians should work through a set of criteria and not be swayed by supposedly quicker options. This chapter provides ways on how to proceed with this evaluation and how to prevent common pitfalls.

THE CLINICAL DIAGNOSIS OF BRAIN DEATH

Declaring a patient brain dead can be considered in a comatose patient with a major destructive brain injury, loss of at least three brain stem reflexes, and no evidence of a breathing effort. A more formal assessment, however, may only proceed when the patient worsens even more, when all medical or neurosurgical interventions are futile, and when there are no confounding factors or alternative explanations. The clinical examination starts when

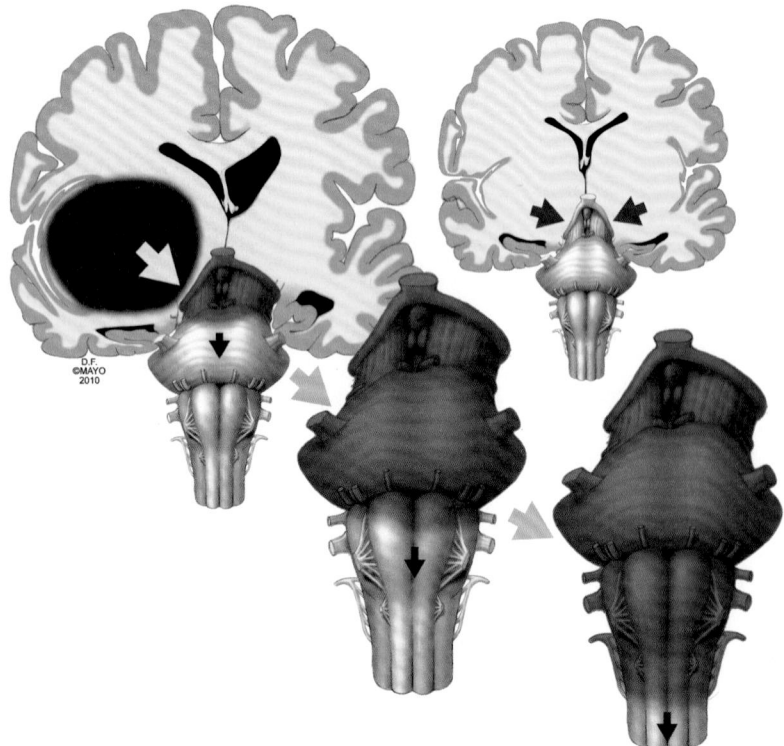

FIGURE 19.1 Supratentorial lesions (mass, cerebral edema) leading to rostrocaudal damage of the brain stem and eventually to brain death. *Arrows* point at direction of tissue compression and loss of function. (Courtesy of the Mayo Foundation for Medical Education and Research.)

a patient with a massive acute brain injury has no motor response to pain, fails to grimace to pain, has absent brain stem reflexes, and does not trigger the ventilator. Commonly, the patient has become hypotensive and polyuric from diabetes insipidus and has been placed on vasopressors. Using this starting point, many patients will fulfill the criteria of brain death after detailed neurologic examination. With any other (earlier) starting point, there is a greater chance that there will be retained brain stem function and even spontaneous breathing when the patient is briefly disconnected.

DETERMINE THE CAUSE OF BRAIN DEATH

Brain death evaluation involves several sequential steps. First, there is nothing more important than to be very certain that all possible confounding factors have been excluded. This implies there can be no lingering effects of prior sedation, other confounding medications, or prior use of illegal drugs or alcohol. A reasonable guideline is to calculate five to seven times the drug's elimination half-life in hours and allow that time to pass before clinical examination is performed. Examples of long elimination half-life drugs are phenobarbital (100 hours), diazepam (40 hours), amitriptyline (24 hours), primidone (20 hours), and lorazepam (15 hours). A commonly used short-acting benzodiazepine is midazolam, but the elimination may still take 3 hours. Prior use of therapeutic hypothermia may substantially slow down the metabolism of medications such as lorazepam and fentanyl used to support the procedure. Substantial alcohol levels should be excluded, but alcohol content below the legal alcohol limit for driving (blood alcohol content 0.08%) is acceptable to determine brain death. Absence of neuromuscular blockade (defined by the presence of four twitches with a train of four with maximal ulnar nerve stimulation) should be demonstrated but is likely if the patient has tendon reflexes (or breathes). Furthermore, absence of severe electrolyte, acid–base, or endocrine disturbances (defined by marked acidosis or any substantial deviation from the normal values) should be documented. A core temperature greater than 32°C must be present, but preferably, there should be near normothermia (36°C to 37°C), which can be achieved with a warming blanket—assuming the patient is not a victim of environmental severe hypothermia. Systolic blood pressure should be greater than 90 mm Hg because pupil size and light reflex can fully disappear with lower values. Only after these confounders have been addressed should a more formal examination proceed.

IMAGING CONFIRMATION OF BRAIN DEATH

Next, the computed tomography (CT) scan should be carefully reviewed and expectedly demonstrate massive brain destruction. Abnormalities may include a large mass with brain tissue shift, multiple hemorrhagic lesions, or diffuse cerebral edema with obliteration of basal cisterns. CT scan can be initially normal if the patient has been imaged very early after cardiopulmonary arrest. However, in the patients with anoxic–ischemic encephalopathy who eventually fulfill these criteria, brain edema or marked hypodensities in thalami, caudate nuclei, and basal ganglia are typically seen on a repeat CT scan. A normal CT should under no circumstances be acceptable. In some cases of cardiac arrest, a magnetic resonance imaging can be helpful to demonstrate the full extent of ischemic tissue damage compatible with brain death.

CLINICAL EXAMINATION

The main components of neurologic examination and technique of the apnea test in a patient suspected of brain death are summarized in Table 19.1.

Cranial Nerves

Clinical examination can proceed after these aforementioned hurdles have been cleared. The examination begins with evaluation of pupillary responses. Pupils should be midposition (4 to 6 mm) and unresponsive to light. A magnifying glass or handheld pupillometer can be helpful, in particular, when there is an uncertainty about the reactivity of pupils. One should be aware that atropine used during cardiopulmonary resuscitation may cause pupillary dilation, but intravenous (IV) drugs do not change reactivity. The corneal reflex is tested with squirting water on the cornea or by touching with a tissue and no blink response should be seen. (Subtle blink responses may be only a movement of eyelashes.) Oculocephalic reflexes ("doll's eyes") should be absent bilaterally (fast turning of the head to both sides should not produce any ocular movement). The oculovestibular response ("cold calorics") should be absent. The head should be elevated 30 degrees. Approximately 50 mL of ice water is then infused in the external auditory canal. No eye movement should be observed for 2 minutes. The examination then proceeds with evaluation of gag and cough reflexes, both of which should be absent. Gag reflex could be tested by a movement of the endotracheal tube but is far more reliable with sticking a gloved finger of the examiner deep in the back of the throat moving the uvula. Cough reflex should be tested by deep bronchial suctioning and with at least two passes.

Motor Responses to Pain

The comatose patient should be unresponsive to verbal or painful stimuli. Standard noxious stimuli include compression of the supraorbital nerves, forceful nail bed pressure, and bilateral temporomandibular joint compression. Eye opening to noxious stimuli should be absent. No motor response should be observed. Some motor responses may be preserved and the challenge is to label them as "spinal responses." They may occur with neck flexion and nail bed compression but are absent with supraorbital nerve compression. These responses are not classifiable as decorticate or extensor responses because that would imply an intact subcortical circuitry. These responses are uncommon—and far less common than claimed in the literature—but include triple flexion responses, finger flexion or extension, head turning, and slow arm lifting. These movements do, on occasion, cause concern for the family members (and later even transplant surgeons) and have to be properly explained and documented in the medical record.

Apnea Testing

Finally, absent breathing is proven with a formal apnea test. The apnea test is best performed under controlled circumstances and with disconnection of the mechanical ventilator. The ventilator may spuriously indicate a breathing drive of the patient and this phenomenon—caused by minimal pressure or volume changes in the breathing circuit—is quite commonly not recognized. There is a real concern that some patients with "retained breathing drive" may have been excluded from formal testing, or worse, a prolonged waiting time for the respiratory drive to "disappear" may have led to premature cardiac arrest in a potential organ donor.

The apnea test is a complex testing procedure. The patient is prepared (preoxygenation, reducing positive end-expiratory pressure to 5 cm of H_2O and drawing a baseline blood gas), then disconnected from the ventilator, while an oxygen source is provided with an oxygen flow catheter placed at the level of the carina. The oxygenation diffusion method is very safe method with few aborted tests. Demonstration of apnea with a rise in PCO_2 to

TABLE 19.1 Twenty-five Clinical Assessments to Diagnose Brain Death

Prerequisites (all must be checked)	Apnea testing (all must be checked)
1. Coma, irreversible and cause known	17. Patient is hemodynamically stable (systolic blood pressure ≥100 mm Hg).
2. Neuroimaging explains coma.	18. Ventilator adjusted to normocapnia (PaCO$_2$ 35–45 mm Hg)
3. Sedative drug effect absent (if indicated, order a toxicology screen)	19. Patient preoxygenated with 100% FiO$_2$ for 10 min (PaO$_2$ ≥200 mm Hg)
4. No residual effect of paralytic drug (if indicated, use peripheral nerve stimulator)	20. Patient maintains oxygenation with a PEEP of 5 cm H$_2$O.
5. Absence of severe acid–base, electrolyte, or endocrine abnormality	21. Disconnect ventilator.
6. Normal or near-normal temperature (core temperature ≥36°C)	22. Provide oxygen via an insufflation catheter to the level of the carina at 6 L/min or attach T-piece with CPAP valve at 10 cm H$_2$O.
7. Systolic blood pressure >100 mm Hg	23. Spontaneous respirations absent
8. No spontaneous respirations	24. Arterial blood gas drawn at 8–10 min, patient reconnected to ventilator
Examination (all must be checked)	25. PaCO$_2$ ≥60 mm Hg or 20 mm Hg rise from normal baseline value or
9. Pupils nonreactive to bright light	Apnea test aborted and ancillary test (EEG or cerebral blood flow study) confirmatory
10. Corneal reflexes absent	**Documentation**
11. Eyes immobile, oculocephalic reflexes absent (tested only if C-spine integrity ensured)	• Time of death (use time of blood gas result or time of ancillary test)
12. Oculovestibular reflexes absent	**Brain death guideline recommendations**
13. No facial movement to noxious stimuli at supraorbital nerve or temporomandibular joint or absent snout and rooting reflexes (neonates)	• Newborn (≥37 wk gestational age) to 30 days: two examinations, two separate physicians, 24 h apart
14. Gag reflex absent	• 30 days to 18 yr: two examinations, two separate physicians, 24 h apart
15. Cough reflex absent to tracheal suctioning	• 18 yr or older: one examination (A second examination is needed in six U.S. states: CA, CT, FL, IA, KY, LA.)
16. No motor response to noxious stimuli in all four limbs (Spinally mediated reflexes are permissible and triple flexion response is most common.)	

C-spine, cervical spine; PEEP, positive end-expiratory pressure; CPAP, continuous positive airway pressure; EEG, electroencephalogram; CA, California; CT, Connecticut; FL, Florida; IA, Iowa; KY, Kentucky; LA, Louisiana.
Courtesy of the Mayo Foundation for Medical Education and Research.

60 mm Hg or 20 mm Hg about a normal baseline value after completion of the brain stem reflexes defines brain death and death of the patient (the time of the second blood gas is best used as the official time of death).

ANCILLARY TESTS TO CONFIRM THE DIAGNOSIS OF BRAIN DEATH

Technical tests to support the clinical diagnosis of brain death have been developed and may demonstrate absent blood flow to the brain or absent electrical activity of the cortex (Table 19.2). These tests have considerable inaccuracy and should not replace, in any way, a clinical assessment. Interpretation of these tests, when results are not obvious, remains difficult and results of multiple tests may not be matching. Elevating an ancillary test to a diagnostic test may lead to errors in brain death determination. Ancillary tests are used in less than 5% of patients diagnosed with brain death and are better generally avoided. These tests have mostly been used when there is an inability to perform an apnea test (due to poor oxygenation of the patient, hemodynamic instability, or evidence of prior chronic CO$_2$ retention). Some countries in the world legally require performing these tests, but in the United States, there is no such requirement. Once the patient is declared brain dead and time of death is documented in the medical record, decisions can be made without further hesitation

TABLE 19.2 Tests Commonly Used for the Confirmation of Brain Death

1. **Electroencephalography (EEG):** Confirmation of neocortical death can be documented by at least 30 min of electrocerebral silence, using a 16-channel instrument with increased gain settings, according to guidelines developed by the American Electroencephalographic Society. If any brain wave is present, the diagnosis of brain death cannot be made. EEG confirmation of brain death is also not valid in patients exposed to sedatives or toxins because they can directly suppress the brain electrical activity.

2. **Digital subtraction or CT angiography:** Complete absence of intracranial blood flow above the level of the proximal internal carotid and vertebral arteries confirms the diagnosis of brain death.

3. **Radioisotope cerebral imaging:** The complete absence of cerebral perfusion can also be established using radionuclide angiography or single-photon emission computed tomography (SPECT).

4. **Transcranial Doppler ultrasonography:** A velocity profile showing systolic spikes with absent or reversed diastolic flow is consistent with the cessation of cerebral blood flow and brain death.

CT, computed tomography.

and should first involve notification of organ donation agencies. Refusal of organ donation (in estimated 30% of cases) will lead to withdrawal of support.

BRAIN DEATH IN CHILDREN

Brain death in children was recently revisited by a multidisciplinary task force. Most concerns regarding interpretation of neurologic examination are in neonates several months old, and the advanced skills of a neonatologist are needed to obtain reliable findings. Examination of a child in an incubator remains limited, and neurologists should be aware of incompletely developed brain function and motor response. The new pediatric guideline suggests a 24-hour interval between examinations by two physicians in neonates and children from 37-week gestation to the end of the first month. However, in children aged 1 month or older, the pediatric guidelines still impose two examinations 12 hours apart by two different attending physicians. Two examinations in children are different from adults but the need for such a distinction is highly questionable. The guideline also recommends that physicians be competent to perform examinations in infants and neonates but speculatively suggest that these examinations be performed by pediatric intensivists and neonatologists, pediatric neurologists and neurosurgeons, pediatric trauma surgeons, and pediatric anesthesiologists with critical care training.

COMMON DIAGNOSTIC CHALLENGES AND PITFALLS

The examination and later communication with distraught family members requires experience. There are situations that can easily create unease and uncertainty. Some common mistakes are shown in Table 19.3. Most pitfalls relate to premature assessment of the patient and suggesting the patient might be brain dead when there has not been a formal evaluation.

Therapeutic hypothermia has become a common treatment of comatose patients following cardiopulmonary resuscitation. However, the category of patients who fulfill brain death after cardiopulmonary resuscitation more often are hemodynamically unstable, and many of them die from irreversible cardiac shock before brain death can be determined. The clinical examination of brain death may be difficult to complete due to persistent hypotension and use of multiple vasopressors. The apnea test may also be compromised due to the presence of significant pulmonary edema from cardiac failure. How to assess these patients after prior use of therapeutic hypothermia and use of sedative drugs remains unclear, and it may be prudent not to proceed with a brain death examination at all.

TABLE 19.3 Common Misjudgments in the Diagnosis of Brain Death

- Incomplete testing
- Examination in a patient with confounders (mostly recently administered medication, drug, and alcohol use)
- Use of cerebral blood flow study as a diagnostic test
- Misinterpretation of ancillary test
- Misinterpretation of "spinal reflexes"
- Premature discussion with family about brain death and organ donation

The most important challenge for physicians is to perform a complete examination in patients with primary lesion in the brain stem. More often than not, physicians will find patients with a primary brain stem lesion or a compressed brain stem from a cerebellar lesion that do not fulfill all criteria of brain death and may even benefit from aggressive intervention (ventriculostomy or suboccipital craniotomy). A destructive primary brain stem lesion is as irreversible lesion as the one that involves the hemispheres and brain stem, and it is therefore unnecessary to perform an ancillary test. These tests often will show preserved blood flow when the intracranial pressure has not increased to extreme values, and early electroencephalography may show nonreactive alpha or spindle coma patterns.

Ancillary testing demonstrating complete intracranial circulatory arrest by catheter or CT angiography or a radionuclide brain perfusion study remains very problematic if used to confirm brain death in the setting of confounding medications, hypothermia, or metabolic disarray.

INTENSIVE CARE UNIT MANAGEMENT OF THE POTENTIAL ORGAN DONOR

Brain death eventually leads to severe homeostatic derangements and cardiac arrest, despite mechanical ventilation and aggressive life support measures. This inexorable progression toward multisystem organ failure creates a challenge in managing the potential organ donor, in whom the goal is to maintain and optimize organ viability for transplantation.

A suggested algorithm for critical care management of the potential organ donor is shown in Table 19.4. Most patients become hypotensive due to sudden loss of resting sympathetic tone and require IV pressors at the time brain death occurs, and soon thereafter, they develop diabetes insipidus (because antidiuretic hormone secretion ceases). *Arginine vasopressin* is the first-line therapy for hypotension in brain death because it works effectively and also because it guards against central diabetes insipidus, which also occurs in the majority of brain dead patients. Adrenergic vasopressors such as norepinephrine or dopamine can also be added, but their usefulness can be limited by tachyarrhythmias, severe peripheral vasoconstriction, or aggravation of sympathetically mediated myocardial injury. In some cases, continued hypotension will respond to thyroid and glucocorticoid hormone replacement, indicating a relative deficiency of these hormones.

To maintain adequate systemic organ perfusion, large volumes of isotonic fluid resuscitation in the form of normal saline, plasmalyte, or lactated Ringer solution should be given in the range of 100 to 250 mL/h. The goal of euvolemia can be assessed targeting mean arterial pressure of greater than 65 mm Hg, central venous pressure of greater than 5 mm Hg, and a cardiac index of greater than 3.0 L/min/m^2 and be documenting lack of respiratory variation of the inferior vena cava diameter with ultrasound. Reversal of hypernatremia due to untreated diabetes insipidus is best accomplished by calculating the free water deficit and replacing it over 24 to 48 hours with a concomitant infusion of 5% dextrose solution.

The situation usually deteriorates when brain dead patients are maintained on a ventilator for a prolonged period of time. Hypothermia, metabolic acidosis, renal failure, and adult respiratory distress syndrome may all occur. The key to management is to be ready for these complications. Even with meticulous attention to cardiovascular, acid–base, and electrolyte homeostasis, organ viability in most adult patients with brain death can be maintained for only 72 to 96 hours.

TABLE 19.4 Protocol for Management of the Potential Organ Donor in the Intensive Care Unit

1. **Insert a central venous catheter or two large-bore peripheral IV lines.**

2. **Insert an arterial line for continuous BP monitoring. Maintain mean arterial pressure >65 mm Hg with stepwise intervention:**

    A. 1,000 mL 0.9% saline fluid bolus (two times at 10-min intervals)

    B. Arginine vasopressin (Pitressin) 2.4–4.0 U/h

    C. Norepinephrine starting at 5 µg/kg/min, titrated up to a maximal dose of 30 µg/kg/min

    D. If hypotension is refractory to dopamine and/or IV vasopressin, perform a thyroxine (T_4) replacement protocol:

        i. Administer as sequential IV boluses:

            a. Dextrose 50% (1 amp)

            b. Methylprednisolone 1 g

            c. Regular insulin 4–10 units

            d. Levothyroxine 20 µg

        ii. If the BP responds to the above boluses, start levothyroxine 5 µg/h as a continuous infusion and titrate to maintain the MAP >65 mm Hg. Note that thyroxine can precipitate cardiac arrhythmias, particularly in younger, hypokalemic patients.

3. **Start baseline maintenance IV flow: 0.9% saline at 100–250 mL/h.**

    A. Adjust the maintenance IV flow to target a euvolemic state with CVP >5 mm Hg.

4. **Correct any existing free water deficits due to untreated diabetes insipidus.**

    A. Check serum sodium levels every 6 h.

    B. If sodium level is >150 mmol/L, calculate the free water deficit and replace it with an infusion of D5W over 24–48 h.

5. **Adjust fraction of inspired oxygen and positive end-expiratory pressure to maintain oxygen saturation >94%.**

6. **Transfuse blood for a hemoglobin level <7.0 g/dL.**

7. **Insert a Foley catheter. Measure fluid input and urine output and monitor urine specific gravity every 2 h. If the urine output over 2 h is >500 mL with specific gravity of 1.005 or lower, begin treatment for DI:**

    A. If the patient is in frank DI with negative fluid balance, administer arginine vasopressin 6–10 units IVP.

    B. Start IV pitressin 2.4–4.0 U/h titrated to maintain UO <200 mL/h.

8. **Check the fingerstick glucose level every 4 h. If fingerstick glucose level is >180 mg/dL, begin an insulin drip (100 units regular insulin in 1,000 mL 0.9% saline) starting at 20 mL/h (2 U/h), titrated to maintain blood glucose between 120 and 180 mg/dL.**

IV, intravenous; BP, blood pressure; MAP, mean arterial pressure; CVP, central venous pressure; D5W, 5% dextrose in water; DI, diabetes insipidus; IVP, intravenous push; UO, urine output.

CONCLUSIONS

Brain death examination requires expertise and follows a stepwise protocol. It is an obvious enough fact that the diagnosis of brain death is complex due to its clinical testing, in determination of confounding factors, and in the interpretation of ancillary tests. The responsibilities of neurologists are substantial also because it eventually involves organ transplantation.

SUGGESTED READINGS

Ashwal S, Schneider S. Brain death in children: part I. *Pediatr Neurol.* 1987; 3(1):5–11.

Ashwal S, Schneider S. Brain death in children: part II. *Pediatr Neurol.* 1987; 3(2):69–77.

Bueri JA, Saposnik G, Mauriño J, et al. Lazarus' sign in brain death. *Mov Disord.* 2000;15:583–586.

Datar S, Fugate J, Rabinstein A, et al. Completing the apnea test: decline in complications. *Neurocrit Care.* 2014;21(3):392–396.

Martí-Fàbregas J, López-Navidad A, Caballero F, et al. Decerebrate-like posturing with mechanical ventilation in brain death. *Neurology.* 2000;54(1): 224–227.

Nakagawa TA, Ashwal S, Mathur M, et al. Guidelines for the determination of brain death in infants and children: an update of the 1987 Task Force recommendations. *Crit Care Med.* 2011;39(9):2139–2155.

Saposnik G, Bueri JA, Mauriño J, et al. Spontaneous and reflex movements in brain death. *Neurology.* 2000;54(1):221–223.

Shemie SD, Pollack MM, Morioka M, et al. Diagnosis of brain death in children. *Lancet Neurol.* 2007;6(1):87–92.

Webb AC, Samuels OB. Reversible brain death after cardiopulmonary arrest and induced hypothermia. *Crit Care Med.* 2011;39(6):1538–1542.

Wijdicks EFM. *Brain Death.* 2nd ed. New York: Oxford University Press; 2011.

Wijdicks EFM. The case against confirmatory tests for determining brain death in adults. *Neurology.* 2010;75(1):77–83.

Wijdicks EFM, Rabinstein AA, Manno EM, et al. Pronouncing brain death: contemporary practice and safety of the apnea test. *Neurology.* 2008;71(16): 1240–1244.

Wijdicks EFM, Varelas PN, Gronseth GS, et al. There is no reversible brain death. *Crit Care Med.* 2011;39(9):2204–2205; author reply 2206.

Yee AH, Mandrekar J, Rabinstein AA, et al. Predictors of apnea test failure during brain death determination. *Neurocrit Care.* 2010;12(3):352–355.

Computed Tomography 20

Daniel S. Chow and Angela Lignelli

INTRODUCTION

This chapter provides a framework for understanding the basic principles of x-ray (roentgenogram) production and computed tomography (CT) image formation along with appropriate window and level parameters for evaluation of intracranial pathologies. In addition, the common indications for CT are discussed along with precautions and recommendations related to CT usage and iodinated contrast. Advanced CT modalities including CT perfusion and CT angiogram are given special consideration.

DESCRIPTION

CT is based on image reconstruction from sets of quantitative x-ray measurements through the head. A beam of x-rays serves as the source of photon energy, which is received by a detector. Although the exact physics of x-ray production is beyond the scope of this chapter, this section will try to simplify the basic principles of x-ray production important for image formation. Briefly, x-ray beams are generated when electrons, produced in the cathode of the tube unit, strike the anode target. The potential difference across the tube is measured as peak kilovoltage (kVp). Thus, increasing the kVp increases the energy of x-rays produced, which will increase penetration of the beam during image production but decrease contrast (and vice versa). Imaging intravenous (IV) or oral contrast in CT imaging is based on the differential attenuation of the x-ray beam through various tissues. As the electron density of the tissue increases, the attenuation increases (giving a "whiter" image). Therefore, the bony calvarium appears "white" compared to soft tissue and air because of its greater attenuation.

Modern CT scanners use highly collimated x-ray beams, which are rotated over many different angles to obtain a differential absorption pattern across various rays through a slice of a patient's body. A circular scanner gantry houses the x-ray source and detectors; the plane of the circle can be tilted to perform scans at a range of angles from axial to coronal, depending on head position and scanner specifications. The x-ray source rotates around the patient's head, and the x-ray attenuation through the section plane is measured in compartments called *voxels*. A voxel is a volume element similar to a picture element, or pixel, with the added dimension of section thickness to create an image volume component. Through projection reconstruction, the computer creates or builds the image from more than 800,000 measurements per image plane and assigns a number to each voxel according to its x-ray attenuation (which is proportional to tissue electron density averaged over the volume of the voxel). These values are termed *Hounsfield units* (HU) (Table 20.1) in honor of Nobel Prize winner Sir Godfrey Hounsfield who first developed CT technology in 1973.

CT of the head differentiates cerebrospinal fluid (CSF) and brain as well as white matter and cortical gray matter, delineates the deep gray nuclei from the internal capsule, and images the skull and skull base in detail. Noncontrast computed tomography (NCCT) of the brain is especially useful for identifying acute hemorrhage, which is easily and reliably visualized as higher density than normal brain or CSF. Typically, intracranial arteries are not well delineated on standard NCCT. Iodinated water-soluble contrast agents, which have high x-ray density, when administered intravenously enhance differences in tissue density, demonstrate vasculature and vascular pathology, and detect areas of blood–brain barrier breakdown.

A major limitation of CT has been imaging the posterior fossa, where linear artifacts appear because bone selectively attenuates the low-energy components of the x-ray beam; the resulting "beam hardening" creates dense or lucent streaks that project across the brain stem and may obscure underlying lesions in the brain stem and cerebellum. However, new detector technology and image-processing algorithms have reduced this artifact in the latest CT scanners, improved spatial resolution, and reduced the radiation dose. Current CT technology allows scan time per section ("slice") to be shortened to less than 1 second to minimize motion artifact. Multisection helical CT can acquire contiguous thin sections to produce three-dimensional (3D) data sets of an entire body part, such as the neck or head. Rapidly, repeated acquisitions can be used to acquire dynamic computed tomography angiography (CTA) and computed tomography perfusion (CTP) studies, which will be discussed later in this chapter.

TABLE 20.1	Hounsfield Units for Common Structures
Structure	**HU**
Air (blackest)	−1,000
Fat	−100 to −50
Water	0
Cerebrospinal fluid	0–15
White matter	20–30
Gray matter	35–45
Acute hemorrhage[a]	45–65
Bone (whitest)	>500

[a]In patients with anemia or iron deficiency, Hounsfield unit values for hemorrhage may be lower.

HU, Hounsfield unit.

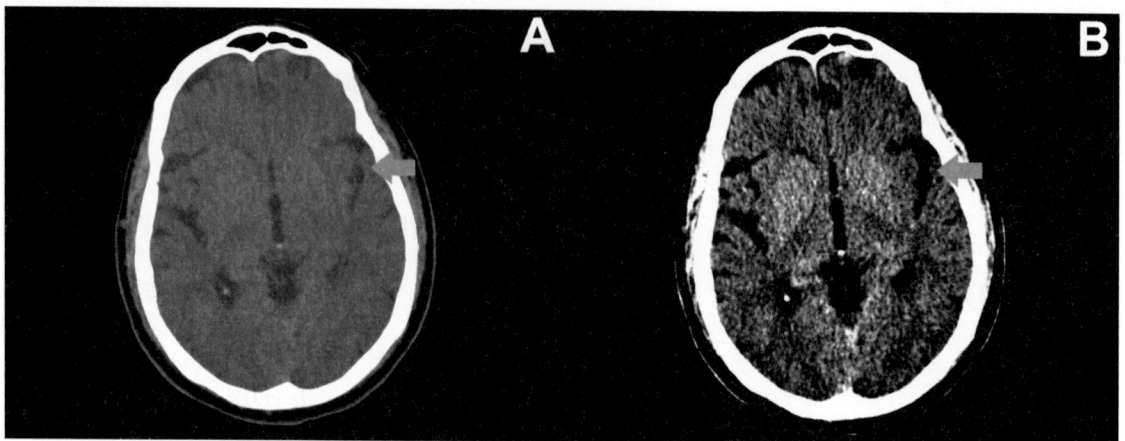

FIGURE 20.1 NCCT of the head with standard brain **(A)** and narrow stroke **(B)** windows in a patient with acute right-sided weakness. Stroke windows reveal loss at the left insular ribbon (*arrow*), which was not clearly visualized on conventional windows.

WINDOWS AND LEVELS

Although CT imaging can display 4,096 shades of gray, the human eye can only visualize between 16 and 32 shades of gray, which is well beyond human perception. "Windowing" allows users to narrow the range of shades of gray, which in turn adjusts the contrast scale. Two factors that can be adjusted by the user are the window width (W) and the window level (L). The W determines the range of shades of gray that can be displayed. Therefore, "narrowing the window" would increase the contrast of the image. The L determines the center of the W. By convention, users can decrease the W by dragging the mouse from right to left, increasing the contrast. The L can be decreased by dragging the mouse from top to down on monitors.

Although the default "brain window" (80 W 40 L) is suitable for assessing a wide range of pathologies, there are several other important windows for neuroimaging to assess for subtle abnormalities. For example, evaluation of parenchymal hypodensity as a marker for early infarct in stroke patients may be improved by using narrow windows (35 W 35 L) (Fig. 20.1). Additionally, subdural hemorrhages are often located at the convexities adjacent to bone and may be difficult to identify due to beam hardening and volume averaging. Using wider windows may assist in countering these limitations (Fig. 20.2). Lastly, bone windows (2,000 W 200 L) are formed with wide ranges and centered above soft tissues and are best for evaluating for subtle nondisplaced calvarial fractures (Fig. 20.3).

ROLE OF COMPUTED TOMOGRAPHY

For reasons of cost, speed, and availability, CT remains widely used for screening in the acute evaluation of trauma, stroke, and infections (Table 20.2). CT is widely accepted as the more reliable method for detection of acute brain parenchymal or extra-axial hemorrhage, especially subarachnoid hemorrhage. It is particularly useful for patients who are neurologically or medically unstable, uncooperative, or claustrophobic, as well as for patients with pacemakers or other metallic implants that may be contraindications for magnetic resonance imaging (MRI). The principle drawback of CT is its use of ionizing radiation, which will be discussed at the end of this chapter. Although there are numerous indications for obtaining a CT examination of the central nervous system, this section will briefly focus on the appropriate use of CT in common clinical scenarios.

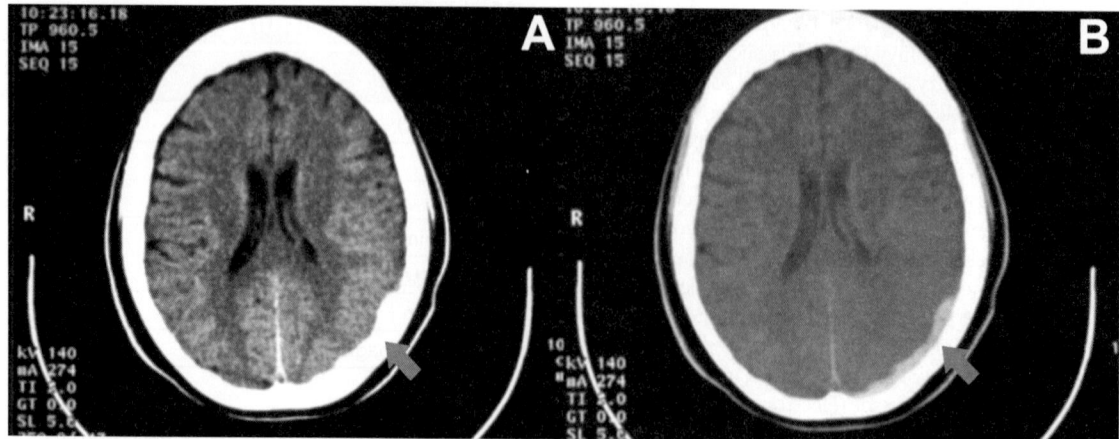

FIGURE 20.2 NCCT of the head with standard brain **(A)** and wider subdural windows **(B)** in a patient after fall. Subdural windows reveal a subdural hematoma at the left parietal convexity (*arrow*), which is not clearly visualized on conventional windows.

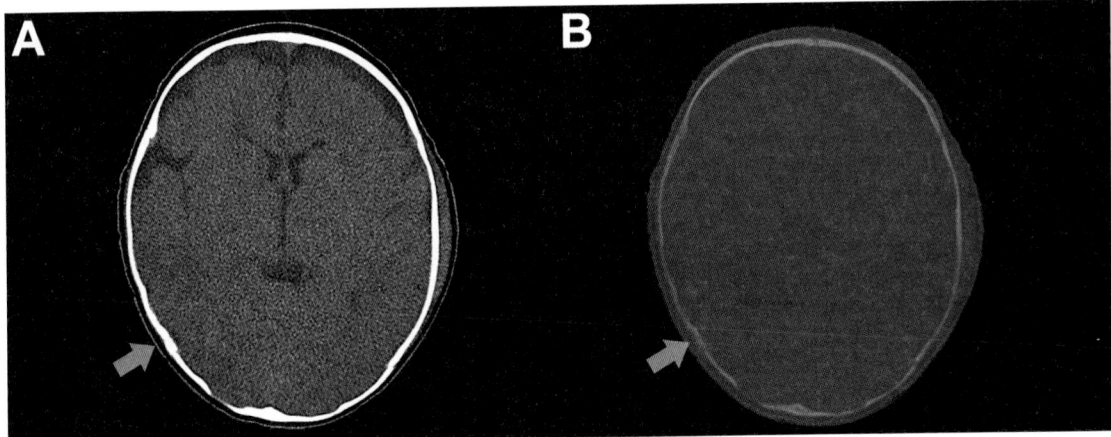

FIGURE 20.3 NCCT of the head with standard brain **(A)** and bone **(B)** windows in a pediatric patient after fall. Bone windows (*right, at arrow*) reveal a nondisplaced hairline fracture at the right temporal bone, which is not visualized on conventional windows.

HEAD TRAUMA

An NCCT is the most appropriate first study for evaluation of acute head trauma. In patients with moderate or high risk for intracranial injury, there is consensus that postinjury NCCT is useful in excluding intracerebral hematoma, midline shift, or increased intracranial pressure. Additionally, NCCT is also very sensitive for identification of acute trauma in patients with minor head injury with the following risk factors: headache, vomiting, drug/alcohol intoxication, age older than 60 years, short-term memory deficit, physical findings of supraclavicular trauma, and/or seizure. CT's advantage for evaluation of traumatic injury includes its sensitivity for acute hemorrhage, fractures, and mass effect. CT is limited by its relative insensitivity to lesions adjacent to bony surfaces (i.e., at the greater sphenoid wing) due to streak artifact. Additionally, diffuse axonal injury (DAI) may go undetected.

HEADACHE

Routine screening head CT is generally not warranted in patients with chronic headaches in the absence of focal neurologic symptoms, change in headache pattern, or history of seizure activity. Several studies have confirmed the low yield of neuroimaging in individuals with isolated headaches and have reported a 0.4% yield for treatable lesions. However, neuroimaging is likely to be of greater yield for particular patient populations. For example, patients with cancer, immunocompromised status, or other systemic illness are more likely to have a "positive" scan. Imaging may also offer greater yield in headaches associated with trauma, abrupt or worsening headache, headache radiating to the neck or suspected meningitis, positional headache, or temporal headaches in older patients. Regarding suspected meningitis, CT imaging is often performed prior to lumbar puncture to assess for elevated intracranial pressure.

SUBARACHNOID HEMORRHAGE

NCCT imaging remains the most appropriate choice of imaging for patients with suspected subarachnoid hemorrhage (SAH), and failure of obtaining a head CT accounts for 73% of misdiagnosis. Patients diagnosed with SAH require imaging of the cerebral vasculature, which may include CTA, magnetic resonance angiography (MRA), or direct catheter angiography. CTA has gained popularity and is frequently used for its noninvasiveness and sensitivity and specificity comparable to that of cerebral angiography.

STROKE

Initial workup for patients with suspected acute stroke is an NCCT in patients who are candidates for IV tissue plasminogen activator (TPA) in order to differentiate between hemorrhagic and ischemic infarcts. NCCT remains the standard of care imaging modality for exclusion of intracranial hemorrhage. In considering patients for endovascular therapies, the American Society of Neuroradiology, American College of Radiology, and Society of NeuroInterventional Surgery have recommended that appropriate imaging options include NCCT followed by digital subtraction angiography, or NCCT with CTA and perfusion CT, or MRI (with perfusion) and MRA. Although NCCT has relatively low sensitivity to early ischemic injury compared to magnetic resonance diffusion imaging, it is not recommended that these findings be used to withhold IV TPA treatment. With regard to CTP and CTA, its use has gained increased popularity in acute stroke evaluation and will be discussed in the subsequent section.

COMPUTED TOMOGRAPHY PERFUSION AND ANGIOGRAPHY

Spiral CT increases scanning speed and image acquisition to less than 1 second per section and allows large-volume acquisitions that can be used for 3D presentation of anatomic information. Advances in CT technology have widened the extent of coverage per scan rotation from 2 cm (32 slices) to 4 cm (64 slices) and most recently, to 16 cm (320 slices), which allows a set of images of the entire head to be obtained in a few rotations as the patient moves through

TABLE 20.2	Common Indications for Emergency Computed Tomography Examination
Acute or chronic focal neurologic deficit	
Head or facial trauma	
Headache	
Change in mental status	
New-onset seizure	

the scanner or in as little as a single subsecond scan rotation in a stationary patient using the widest detector array. Rapidly repeating the scan acquisitions at two or three times per second during a bolus of IV contrast produces a set of "dynamic" images through a volume of tissue as wide as the detector array. This approach, with the widest detector array on a cone beam computed tomography (CBCT), can be used to produce whole-brain "real-time" 4D images of blood flow through the intracranial vessels (CTA) combined with "functional" images of brain parenchymal blood flow (CTP) in a total time of 1 minute, with a single IV contrast bolus injection.

CTA allows vascular imaging with IV contrast agents. Without contrast, intracranial vessels are not well seen on CT, unless abnormally large or dense—as with a thrombus. As previously described, modern CT scanners allow for rapid imaging, which permits noninvasive arterial phase imaging. Advantages of CTA over catheter angiography include more widely available technology; less specialized skill requirements; and no risk of dissection, stroke, or pseudoaneurysm at groin site. A limitation of CTA is the time-consuming processing required to edit out bone and calcium and to generate 3D surface renderings, although this has improved with the availability of specialized software that partially automates this process. *Maximum intensity projection* (MIP) reformations or 3D renderings with surface shading can be used to display vascular anatomy and abnormalities such as stenosis or aneurysm with either of these approaches.

CT perfusion allows quantitative measures of cerebral blood volume (CBV), cerebral mean transit time (MTT), time-to-peak (TTP), and cerebral blood flow (CBF). These parametric maps can be easily generated at a work station, following the IV bolus administration of contrast. Perfusion imaging measurements can be used as a quick screening method in assessment of acute cerebral ischemia in major vascular territories and for differentiating between infarct and penumbra, with results comparable to MRI perfusion. Specifically, the infarct core, that is, region of irreversible injury, has been described as prolonged MTT, decreased CBV, and decreased CBF. The ischemic penumbra, potentially salvageable tissue, is described as prolonged MTT and TTP with normal or increased CBV and resultant mildly reduced CBF, thought to reflect compensatory vasodilatation. The combination of NCCT, CTA, and CTP allows CT imaging to provide a complete evaluation of acute stroke.

IODINATED CONTRAST ADMINISTRATION

Contrast-enhanced computed tomography (CECT) is used to detect lesions that involve breakdown of the blood–brain barrier, such as brain or spinal tumors, infections, and inflammatory conditions. CECT is often used to rule out cerebral metastases. However, it is less sensitive than gadolinium-enhanced MRI (Gd-MRI), which is also better for detection of primary intracranial tumors and infections. IV CT contrast agents are based on iodine, and the older agents are classified as high-osmolar contrast media (HOCM). Newer, nonionic agents, classified as low-osmolar contrast media (LOCM), are less allergenic, and they cause less morbidity than do HOCM. The majority of patients receiving IV iodinated contrast media will have suffer no ill effects. With use of LOCM, the overall incidence of reactions is between 0.2% and 0.7% with severe and life-threatening reactions occurring between 0.01% and 0.02%.

With regard to the risk factors, history of prior contrast reaction is associated with a five times greater likelihood of a subsequent contrast reaction. Other risk factors include history of anaphylaxis, atopy, asthma, and significant cardiac disease. Of note, history of shellfish allergy is no longer considered a risk factor for

TABLE 20.3	Premedication Strategies for Patients with Known Risk Factors to Intravenous Iodinated Contrast Agents
Elective	Prednisone: 50 mg PO at 13 h, 7 h, and 1 h before contrast injection
	or
	Methylprednisolone: 32 mg PO 12 h and 2 h before contrast injection
	plus
	Diphenhydramine: 50 mg IV, IM, or PO 1 h before contrast
Emergent	In decreasing order of desirability:
	Methylprednisolone sodium succinate: 40 mg
	or
	Hydrocortisone sodium succinate: 200 mg IV q4h until contrast injection
	plus
	Diphenhydramine: 50 mg IV 1 h prior to contrast injection

PO, by mouth; IV, intravenous; IM, intramuscular.
Data from the American College of Radiology. *ACR Manual on Contrast Media, Version 9.* Reston, VA: American College of Radiology, ACT Committee on Drugs and Contrast Media; 2013.

contrast administration. In patients at increased risk for allergic reaction, several premedication strategies have been proposed by the American College of Radiology (Table 20.3).

Another important consideration for iodine-based IV contrast agents is contrast-induced nephrotoxicity (CIN), which is defined as an acute deterioration in renal function following IV iodinated contrast administration in the absence of other nephrotoxic event. However, the majority of the prior literature studying the incidence of CIN has failed to include a control group. In one study with a control group by Newhouse et al. involving 30,000 patients at a single institution, half of the control group (patients who did not receive contrast medium) displayed a change in serum creatinine of at least 25% and a change of 0.4 mg/dL in 40%. This study concluded that had some of these patients received IV iodinated contrast, a creatinine rise would have been attributed to it, rather than to physiologic variation. Nonetheless, it is important to recognize risk factors described for CIN, which includes preexisting renal insufficiency.

There is no universally agreed upon threshold of serum creatinine elevation (or degree of renal dysfunction) to contraindicate intravascular iodinated contrast administration. With regard to prevention against CIN in patients receiving contrast, studies suggest that adequate hydration is beneficial. Although an accepted ideal infusion rate has yet to be established, isotonic fluids are

TABLE 20.4	Premedication Strategies for Patients at Risk for Contrast-Induced Nephropathy

1. A 3 mL/kg bolus 1 h prior to procedure followed by 1 mL/kg/h for 6 h postprocedure

2. N-acetylcysteine 600 mg PO/IV 12 h preprocedure, followed by 600 mg q12h PO/IV postprocedure × three doses

PO, by mouth; IV, intravenous.

preferred (i.e., lactated Ringer or 0.9% normal saline). Protocols using sodium bicarbonate solution infusion or N-acetylcysteine exist for reducing the risk of CIN (Table 20.4). These are safe and reasonable therapeutic options when IV contrast is required for patients with chronic renal insufficiency, although their efficacy is not established.

SUGGESTED READINGS

Adams HP Jr, del Zoppo G, Alberts MJ, et al. Guidelines for the early management of adults with ischemic stroke: a guideline from the American Heart Association/American Stroke Association Stroke Council, Clinical Cardiology Council, Cardiovascular Radiology and Intervention Council, and the Atherosclerotic Peripheral Vascular Disease and Quality of Care Outcomes in Research Interdisciplinary Working Groups: the American Academy of Neurology affirms the value of this guideline as an educational tool for neurologists. *Stroke.* 2007;38:1655–1711. doi:10.1161/STROKEAHA.107.181486.

Campbell BC, Christensen S, Levi CR, et al. Cerebral blood flow is the optimal CT perfusion parameter for assessing infarct core. *Stroke.* 2011;42:3435–3440. doi:10.1161/STROKEAHA.111.618355.

Gilbert JW, Johnson KM, Larkin GL, et al. Atraumatic headache in US emergency departments: recent trends in CT/MRI utilisation and factors associated with severe intracranial pathology. *Emerg Med.* 2012;29:576–581. doi:10.1136/emermed-2011-200088.

Haydel MJ, Preston CA, Mills TJ, et al. Indications for computed tomography in patients with minor head injury. *N Engl J Med.* 2000;343:100–105. doi:10.1056/NEJM200007133430204.

Jayaraman MV, Mayo-Smith WW, Tung GA, et al. Detection of intracranial aneurysms: multi-detector row CT angiography compared with DSA. *Radiology.* 2004;230:510–518. doi:10.1148/radiol.2302021465.

Kowalski RG, Claassen J, Kreiter KT, et al. Initial misdiagnosis and outcome after subarachnoid hemorrhage. *JAMA.* 2004;291:866–869. doi:10.1001/jama.291.7.866.

Lee B, Newberg A. Neuroimaging in traumatic brain imaging. *NeuroRx.* 2005;2:372–383. doi:10.1602/neurorx.2.2.372.

Newhouse JH, Kho D, Rao QA, et al. Frequency of serum creatinine changes in the absence of iodinated contrast material: implications for studies of contrast nephrotoxicity. *AJR Am J Roentgenol.* 2008;191:376–382. doi:10.2214/AJR.07.3280.

Reinus WR, Erickson KK, Wippold FJ II. Unenhanced emergency cranial CT: optimizing patient selection with univariate and multivariate analyses. *Radiology.* 1993;186:763–768. doi:10.1148/radiology.186.3.8430185.

Sandrini G, Friberg L, Coppola G, et al. Neurophysiological tests and neuroimaging procedures in non-acute headache (2nd edition). *Eur J Neurol.* 2011;18:373–381. doi:10.1111/j.1468-1331.2010.03212.x.

Sempere AP, Porta-Etessam J, Medrano V, et al. Neuroimaging in the evaluation of patients with non-acute headache. *Cephalalgia.* 2005;25:30–35. doi:10.1111/j.1468-2982.2004.00798.x.

Stiell IG, Wells GA, Vandemheen K, et al. The Canadian CT Head Rule for patients with minor head injury. *Lancet.* 2001;357:1391–1396.

Suarez JI, Tarr RW, Selman WR. Aneurysmal subarachnoid hemorrhage. *N Engl J Med.* 2006;354:387–396. doi:10.1056/NEJMra052732.

Wardlaw JM, Mielke O. Early signs of brain infarction at CT: observer reliability and outcome after thrombolytic treatment—systematic review. *Radiology.* 2005;235:444–453. doi:10.1148/radiol.2352040262.

Wintermark M, Flanders AE, Velthuis B, et al. Perfusion-CT assessment of infarct core and penumbra: receiver operating characteristic curve analysis in 130 patients suspected of acute hemispheric stroke. *Stroke.* 2006;37:979–985. doi:10.1161/01.STR.0000209238.61459.39.

Wintermark M, Sanelli PC, Albers GW, et al. Imaging recommendations for acute stroke and transient ischemic attack patients: a joint statement by the American Society of Neuroradiology, the American College of Radiology, and the Society of NeuroInterventional Surgery. *AJNR Am J Neuroradiol.* 2013;34:E117–E127. doi:10.3174/ajnr.A3690.

Magnetic Resonance Imaging 21

Vesselin Zdravkov Miloushev and Angela Lignelli

INTRODUCTION

Magnetic resonance imaging (MRI) is a noninvasive medical imaging technique. The images created by MRI often appear similar to gross-anatomic specimens. The major strength of MRI is the ability to distinguish different soft tissues and identify pathologic abnormalities. It is indispensable to modern neurologic practice for diagnosis, confirmation, and characterization of neurologic conditions, as well as for monitoring response to therapy. Although MRI signal abnormalities can be very sensitive to pathologic processes, in isolation, the findings may lack specificity, requiring thorough integration of clinical information. The main weaknesses of MRI are cost, inherent low signal to noise necessitating high magnetic fields as well as lengthy exam times, and distortion of images by artifacts. The MRI scanner consists of a bore that is generally small and constricting, creating anxiety or claustrophobia in many patients. In addition, implanted devices can be ferromagnetic and therefore contraindicated for MRI imaging, for example, most pacemakers. As in all radiologic procedures, contrast agents should be administered when the benefit of improved diagnostic accuracy outweighs their generally low risk. In the following paragraphs, the physics of MRI and technical considerations will be discussed. In addition, the application of basic imaging sequences and advanced imaging methods will be reviewed.

PHYSICS OF MAGNETIC RESONANCE IMAGING

MRI is based on Fourier transform nuclear spin spectroscopy of water protons. Clinical imaging is performed on the nuclear spin of water protons because water is abundant in biologic tissues and protons have relatively greater sensitivity in a magnetic resonance than other nuclei.

In the classical description relevant for clinical imaging, MRI can be understood by considering the spin properties of protons to be equivalent to small magnetic dipoles that align in a magnetic field. In the quantum mechanical description of proton magnetic resonance, individual proton spins exist as a combination (superposition) of two quantized energy states, transitions between which can be manipulated using radiofrequency pulses and delays. The very large number of water protons leads to behavior of biologic tissues in the magnetic field that can be thought of as net magnetization. This longitudinal magnetization can be *tipped* from the aligned state by a radiofrequency excitation pulse. The change in angle from the original aligned state is called the *flip angle*. Once in the transverse plane, the magnetization begins to rotate (precess) around the magnetic field at a specific resonant frequency called the *Larmor frequency* (~43 MHz per tesla for protons). This precessional motion in turn generates a time-varying voltage in a receiver coil. The specific resonance frequency depends on the nucleus being imaged, its local environment, and the magnetic field strength.

Relaxation of the signal back to equilibrium is described by the T1 and T2 exponential time constants. Relaxation of magnetization is not a spontaneous process but rather a phenomenon that is due to underlying molecular motion and molecular interactions. The BPP theory of relaxation named after Bloembergen, Purcell, and Pound has proven accurate and permits calculation of relaxation times from first principles. The two principal relaxation mechanisms are termed *T1* and *T2 processes*, which are relevant to clinical imaging and approximately depend on the molecular tumbling rate or rather the rotational diffusion of individual molecules. The T1 time constant describes the recovery of longitudinal magnetization back to the equilibrium aligned state (after a time T1 ~63% of the magnetization has realigned). The T2 time constant describes the decay of magnetization in the transverse plane (after a time T2 ~63% of the magnetization has decayed).

IMAGE CREATION

MRI creates images by applying linear spatial magnetic field gradients so that different parts of the human body resonate at different frequencies. One dimension can be sampled directly (called the *frequency dimension*), whereas other dimensions can be sampled indirectly (called *phase dimensions*). By combining multiple gradient directions, two-dimensional or three-dimensional images can be constructed.

The MRI signal is composed of time-dependent damped sinusoids and requires Fourier transformation to convert it to a power spectrum that is the image. The term *k-space* is used to refer to the time-dependent data. This is sometimes a source of confusion because the Fourier transform is very similar to its own inverse and acquisition of time-dependent MRI data in k-space is essentially equivalent to acquisition of different frequency components of the image. For this reason, it is often noted that the center of the k-space image determines image contrast (low-frequency components), whereas the edges of the k-space image determine detail in the image (high-frequency components).

Since the first live human images were obtained in the late 1970s, the field has drastically expanded to include a wide variety of clinical applications. The sequence of radiofrequency pulses, gradient pulses, and intervening time delays used to prepare magnetization and the methods of sampling k-space are referred to as the *pulse sequence*. Different pulse sequences are also tailored for specific applications. The two basic sequences are gradient echo and spin echo techniques, upon which additional sequences can be derived. Gradient echo sequences refocus magnetization following a radiofrequency pulse using a field gradient, whereas spin echo sequences refocus magnetization using a radiofrequency inversion (180-degree) pulse. Spin echo sequences are generally less susceptible to artifacts because artifacts are also inverted by the refocusing pulse and subsequently cancel out.

CLINICAL MAGNETIC RESONANCE IMAGING SYSTEMS

Clinical imaging systems are rated by the strength of the main magnetic field, referred to the as the B_0 field, measured in tesla (1 T = 10,000 gauss ~15,000–40,000 the earth's magnetic field). The majority of clinical imaging systems use field strengths of 1.5 or 3 T. The term *high field* in the context of clinical imaging refers to magnet systems operating at 7 to 9 T. High-field systems have clear benefits in terms of improved anatomic resolution and increased signal to noise but are more prone to artifacts and require more radiofrequency power (higher specific absorption rate). Higher field magnets are typically closed-bore, meaning that they are shaped like long tube or cylinder. A variety of open-bore magnets is also commercially available. These magnets are more accommodating to variations in patient body habitus and typically create a less claustrophobic environment. Completely open-bore magnets operate at lower field strengths than closed-bore systems, with resultant lower resolution that may compromise clinical diagnosis.

Multiple components of the magnetic imaging system influence the ultimate sensitivity in detecting the magnetic resonance signal and generating a distortion-free image. One important physical factor that is changed between different applications is the radiofrequency coil. A variety of receive and transmit/receive coils are available for specific applications to the brain, head, neck, and spine. These include including bird cage–type coils for imaging the brain, surface coils, multichannel, and parallel imaging coils, all of which have different trade-offs in terms of size of allowed imaging volume, as well as sensitivity and speed of imaging.

MAGNETIC RESONANCE IMAGING SAFETY

The main safety considerations in MRI include the powerful main magnetic field, rapidly changing magnetic field gradients, deposition of radiofrequency power, sound pressure levels, and safety concerns related to contrast agents. The powerful magnetic field produced by an MRI scanner is a major safety consideration because objects can become dangerous projectiles when placed in the field. Moreover, non-MRI–compatible implanted devices or metallic foreign bodies pose a danger because of local tissue-heating effects and movement of the object in respect to critical structures. Commonly encountered devices in clinical practice include implanted cardiac devices (e.g., cardiac pacemakers) as well as others such as infusion pumps, cochlear implants, and a variety of surgical implants such as some aneurysm clips. Recently, MRI-compatible cardiac devices have been devised and new MRI-compatible implanted surgical devices are being developed. However, precaution needs to be taken with every implanted device to ensure MRI compatibility and patient safety. Before the patient is even brought near the magnetic field, which is never turned off, a thorough safety check by appropriately trained medical personnel must be performed.

Once inside the MRI scanner, some patients may experience a variety of physical effects in addition to the possibility of claustrophobia. Federal limits on the main magnetic field strength imposed by the U.S. Food and Drug Administration are 8 T for adults and 4 T for neonates. Fields greater than these limits may pose a risk. Limits are also placed on the speed of the rapidly switching magnetic field gradients in MRI due to the possibility of neural or cardiac depolarization resulting in pain, auras, or possibly cardiac arrhythmias. Regulatory limits are also placed on the rate of energy deposition by radiofrequency pulses (similar to limits placed on cell phones for example). This limit is referred to as the *specific absorption rate* and meant to prevent heating damage of body tissues.

Gadolinium chelates are commonly used contrast agents in MRI because of the local relaxivity effects that lead to T1 shortening and resultant bright signal on T1-weighted images. Other contrast agents including manganese-based contrast agents and superparamagnetic iron oxides are currently less common in clinical practice. The risk of contrast administration in the context of MRI includes contrast reactions that may be life threatening. The deposition of gadolinium in tissues and resulting fibrosis, commonly known as *nephrogenic systemic fibrosis* (NSF), has been reported in patients with significantly reduced renal function necessitating appropriate screening.

BASIC SEQUENCES

For the purpose of clinical imaging, there are many sources of image contrast. Dynamic processes on the molecular level such as flow-related and diffusion effects and a variety of relaxation mechanisms are responsible for the power of MRI to generate contrast between different biologic tissues.

The basic sequences that are weighted for specific sources of image contrast are as follows:

- T1-weighted
- T2-weighted
- Fluid-attenuated inversion recovery T2-weighted
- Diffusion-weighted
- Susceptibility-weighted
- Post–contrast-enhanced images

T1-WEIGHTED AND T2-WEIGHTED IMAGING

The two core sequences in magnetic resonance are T1-weighted and T2-weighted sequences, which individually emphasize either the T1 or the T2 relaxation time of tissues. *T1-weighted* imaging emphasizes *short T1* relaxation times as bright signal; tissues composed of spins with long T1 relaxation times will appear relatively lower signal intensity (dark) on T1-weighted images. The main clinical use of T1 imaging is to display brain and spinal cord anatomy. However, T1-weighted images are also useful to evaluate for subacute hemorrhage, lipids, paramagnetic metals, or proteinaceous composition of lesions, which all shorten the T1 relaxation time and appear bright on T1-weighted images. T1-weighted images also serve as the baseline comparison to contrast-enhanced images. T1-weighting can be accomplished by either decreasing the *repetition time* (TR) between successive excitations thus preventing magnetization from fully relaxing to equilibrium or by changing phase of successive radiofrequency pulses thus causing destructive inference (referred to as *spoiled gradient echo* or SPGR).

The main clinical use of T2 imaging is to display brain and spinal cord pathology, as evidenced by increased tissue water content. *T2-weighted* images emphasize *long T2* relaxation times as a bright signal. Tissues composed of spins with short T2 relaxation times will appear dark on T2-weighted images. However, susceptibility effects resulting in local field inhomogeneities also decrease the T2 time (this type of effect is sometimes referred to as *T2**). T2 weighting can be accomplished by increasing the time the magnetization spends in the transverse plane, or *time to echo* (TE), prior to acquisition. Different from both T1-weighted and T2-weighted images, proton-density (PD) weighted images are obtained with a short TE to minimize relaxation losses and long TR to allow more magnetization to recover between successive excitations.

Fluid-attenuated inversion recovery (FLAIR) is the preferred sequence for demonstrating subtle brain pathology. FLAIR images are obtained by preparing magnetization with a radiofrequency inversion pulse, which inverts the equilibrium alignment. As the magnetization relaxes back to the aligned state with the T1 time constant, it temporarily becomes negligible as it crosses zero and timing detection at this time can essentially null signal from spins with a specific T1. Although FLAIR sequences can be T1-weighted or T2-weighted, in common clinical parlance, the FLAIR method refers to FLAIR T2-weighted images. The main advantage of FLAIR images is sensitivity to detect a broad array of pathologic processes and is specifically useful for the evaluation of white matter diseases in the brain. The archetypal example is multiple sclerosis, which is characterized by periventricular white matter lesions, radially oriented to the bodies of the lateral ventricles (requiring both axial and sagittal FLAIR sequences for complete assessment) (Fig. 21.1; see Fig. 21.6).

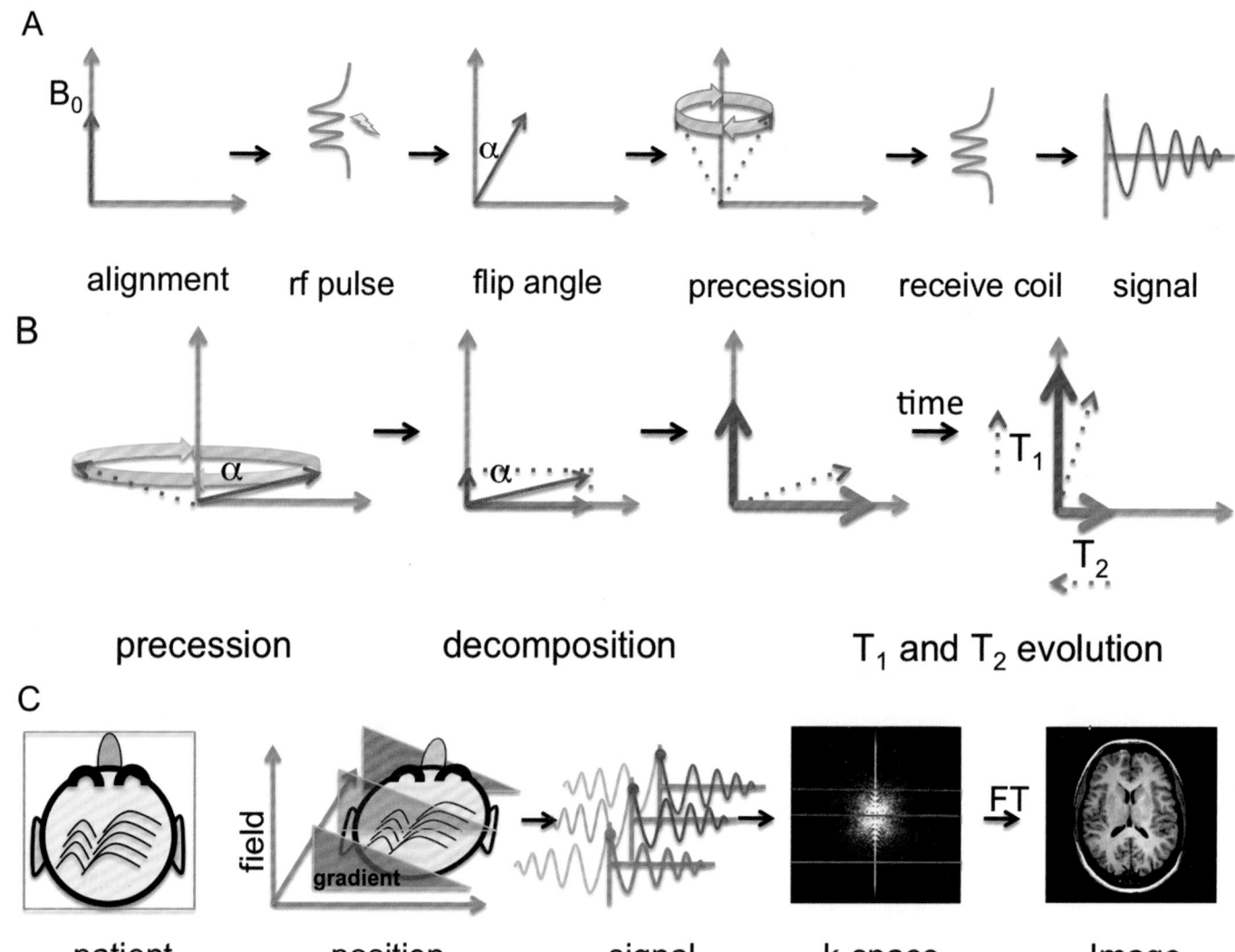

FIGURE 21.1 Schematic representation of magnetic resonance. **A:** Magnetization (*red arrow*) aligns along the main magnetic field (B_0). A radiofrequency pulse generated by a transmit coil tips the magnetization from the aligned state by a flip angle (α). The magnetization precesses around the main magnetic field. The precessional motion results in a time-varying voltage in a radiofrequency receive coil, which is recorded as the magnetic resonance signal. **B:** While the magnetization precesses around the magnetic field, the decay of magnetization can be described by two separate exponential time constants. The magnetization vector can be decomposed into a longitudinal component parallel to the main magnetic field and a transverse component orthogonal to the main magnetic field. The T1 time describes the relaxation of magnetization back to the equilibrium-aligned state. The T2 time constant describes the decay of transverse magnetization. **C:** Images are created in magnetic resonance by applying multiple field gradients, which positionally encode the magnetic resonance signal. In this schematic of a patient's head, directly acquiring signal from each gradient direction allows encoding of the frequency dimension. Applying an additional increasing orthogonal gradient with every frequency encoding gradient allows encoding of the phase dimension. The signal from one gradient direction thus corresponds to one line of k-space. Once all of the lines of k-space are filled, a Fourier transform (FT) is used to make an image representation.

Individual tissues have characteristic appearance on T1-weighted, T2-weighted, and FLAIR images. For example, cerebrospinal fluid (CSF) has a relatively long T1 and long T2 relaxation time and thus appears dark on T1-weighted images and bright on T2-weighted images (Fig. 21.2A and B). CSF appears dark on FLAIR images because these images are specifically calibrated to suppress CSF or "free" water (Fig. 21.2C). White matter in the adult is fully myelinated and appears slightly bright on T1-weighted images and dark on T2-weighted images (see Fig. 21.2A and B). Gray matter is brighter than white matter on T2-weighted images, whereas the reverse is true for T1-weighted images. Parenchymal hemorrhage can have a variety of appearances on T1- and T2-weighted images based on its components. In the brain, hemorrhage evolves predictably and its appearance can be used to infer its age. T2 prolongation (bright on T2-weighted images) correlates with hyperacute hemorrhage and late subacute hemorrhage, whereas T1 shortening (bright on T1-weighted images) correlates with early and late subacute hemorrhage. These characteristic appearances are summarized in Table 21.1.

QUANTIFICATION OF T1 AND T2 TIMES

T1 and T2 relaxation time constants can be quantified to provide information of dynamic properties on a molecular level. Relaxation can also be measured during the application of a continuous radiofrequency pulse; in this case, the relaxation time constants are referred to as *T1-rho* and *T2-rho* (rho referring to a rotating reference frame used in the theoretical description). Magnetization transfer imaging, as well as chemical exchange saturation transfer (CEST) imaging are additional methods that rely on using a radiofrequency pulse to attenuate magnetization. These emerging methods are currently confined to the research setting but hold promise for future clinical applications.

DIFFUSION-WEIGHTED IMAGING

Diffusion-weighted imaging (DWI) is invaluable for the detection of early ischemic brain injury (Fig. 21.3). Like T1 and T2 processes, DWI creates image contrast by exploiting dynamic molecular properties, specifically translational diffusion, by applying multidirection

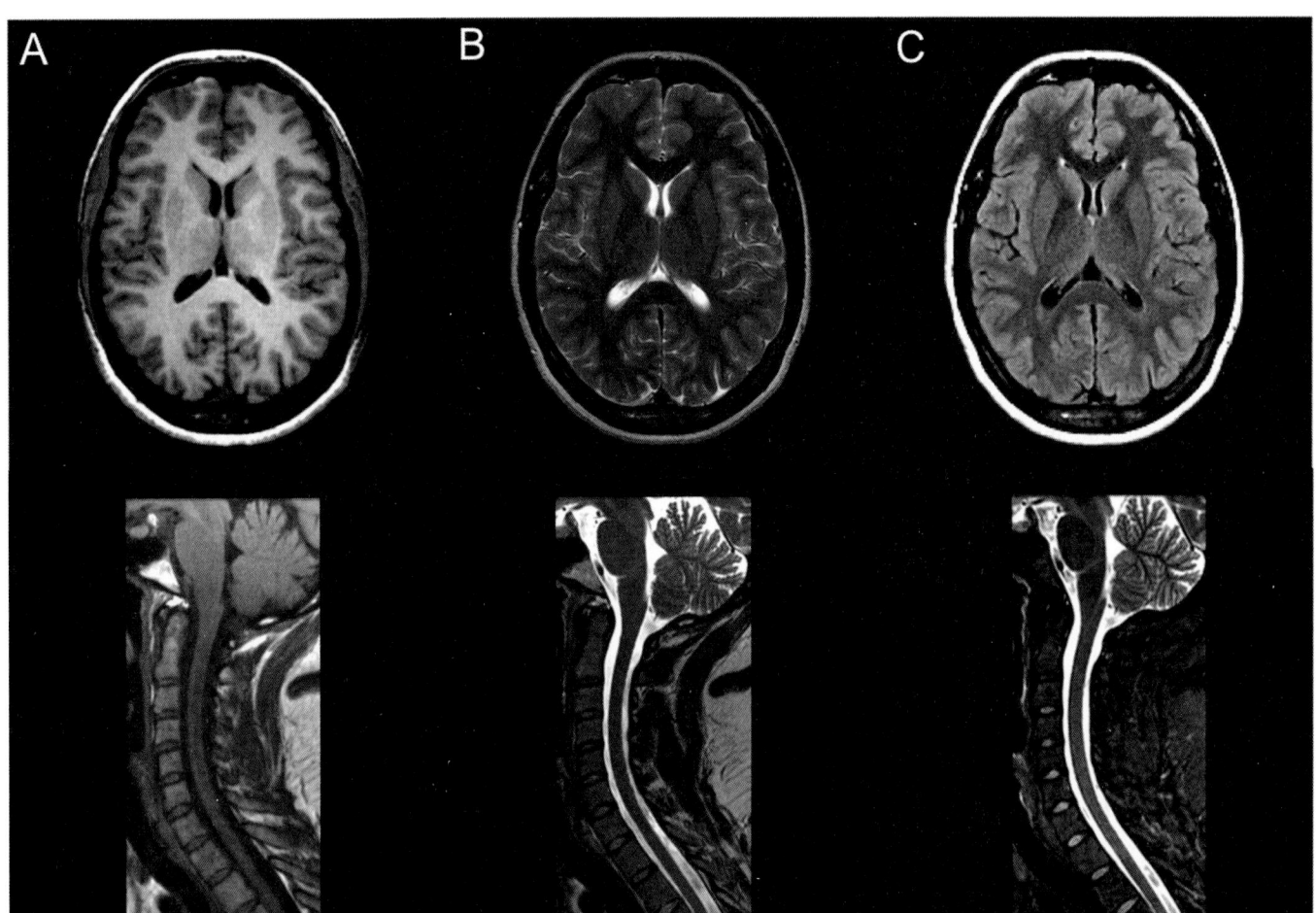

FIGURE 21.2 Normal T1-weighted, T2-weighted, FLAIR, and inversion recovery (IR) images. **A:** Normal T1-weighted images of the brain and cervical spine. White matter is bright and gray matter is dark. CSF signal is dark. **B:** Normal T2-weighted images of the brain and cervical spine. Gray matter is bright and white matter is dark. CSF signal is bright. **C:** Normal FLAIR image of the brain and IR image of the cervical spine. On the FLAIR image, CSF signal is suppressed and appears dark; white matter is dark and gray matter is bright similar to a T2-weighted image. On the IR image of the cervical spine, fat is suppressed and there is increased contrast in the spinal cord.

TABLE 21.1   Usual Appearance of Normal Structures on T1-Weighted, T2-Weighted, FLAIR, DWI/ADC, and GRE or SWI Images

	T1-Weighted	T2-Weighted	FLAIR	DWI/ADC	GRE or SWI
CSF	Dark	Bright	Dark	Dark/bright	Bright
White matter or gray matter brighter	White matter brighter	Gray matter brighter	Gray matter brighter	Gray matter brighter/white matter brighter	Variable
Acute infarct	Dark	Bright	Bright	Bright/dark	Variable
Hemorrhage	Bright if early or late subacute	Bright if hyperacute or late subacute	Variable	Variable	Dark
Edema	Dark	Bright	Bright	Variable/bright	Isointense

FLAIR, fluid-attenuated inversion recovery; DWI, diffusion-weighted imaging; ADC, apparent diffusion coefficient; GRE, gradient-recalled echo; SWI, susceptibility-weighted imaging; CSF, cerebrospinal fluid.

diffusion sensitizing field gradients. In clinical practice, DWI is typically performed for water although applications to other molecules have been reported. The "effect" of the diffusion gradient sequence is often quantified using a b-value. For adults, a b-value = 1,000 s/mm^2 is typically used, whereas b- value = 1,500 s/mm^2 is sometimes preferred in pediatric cases. In routine clinical practice, DWI is typically detected using an echo planar imaging (EPI) technique due to the speed of imaging. EPI is a gradient echo technique that can acquire the entirety of k-space within one excitation by interweaving frequency and phase dimensions.

Diffusion imaging is considered a quantitative technique, permitting the calculation of an apparent diffusion coefficient (ADC), which measures the extent to which the diffusivity of water is restricted from free diffusion, presumably due to structural barriers such as cell membranes or association of water with larger molecules that have lower diffusion coefficients. The most useful application of DWI is in acute stroke imaging (see Fig. 21.3A). This occurs most frequently in the setting of cellular bioenergetic failure and cytotoxic brain edema due to cerebral hypoxia/ischemia. Acute and early subacute infarcts display restricted diffusion and are easily detected as bright regions on DWI. Differentiation of acute infarcts from late subacute infarcts, both of which can appear bright on DWI (known colloquially as *T2 shine through*), can

be accomplished by examination concurrent ADC image. Acute to early subacute infarcts truly demonstrate restricted diffusion and appear dark on the ADC image (see Fig. 21.3B). Subacute to chronic infarcts are bright on DWI due to T2 shine through and appear isointense to bright on the ADC image.

Other conditions including uncontrolled status epilepticus and prion diseases (e.g., Creutzfeldt–Jakob disease) may demonstrate increased cortical DWI signal. Restricted diffusion can also be observed in hemorrhage and for tissues/neoplasms with high cellular density in the case of active inflammation and within the center of abscesses. DWI is specifically useful in the evaluation of brain tumors, where foci of restricted diffusion raise suspicion for an aggressive hypercellular tumor component, which may predate contrast enhancement.

GRADIENT-RECALLED ECHO AND SUSCEPTIBILITY-WEIGHTED IMAGING

The primary clinical use of gradient-recalled echo (GRE) or susceptibility-weighted imaging (SWI) is sensitivity to the presence of small amounts of hemorrhage. SWI or GRE images generate image contrast from differences in underlying magnetic susceptibility. Differences in susceptibility are interpreted to represent

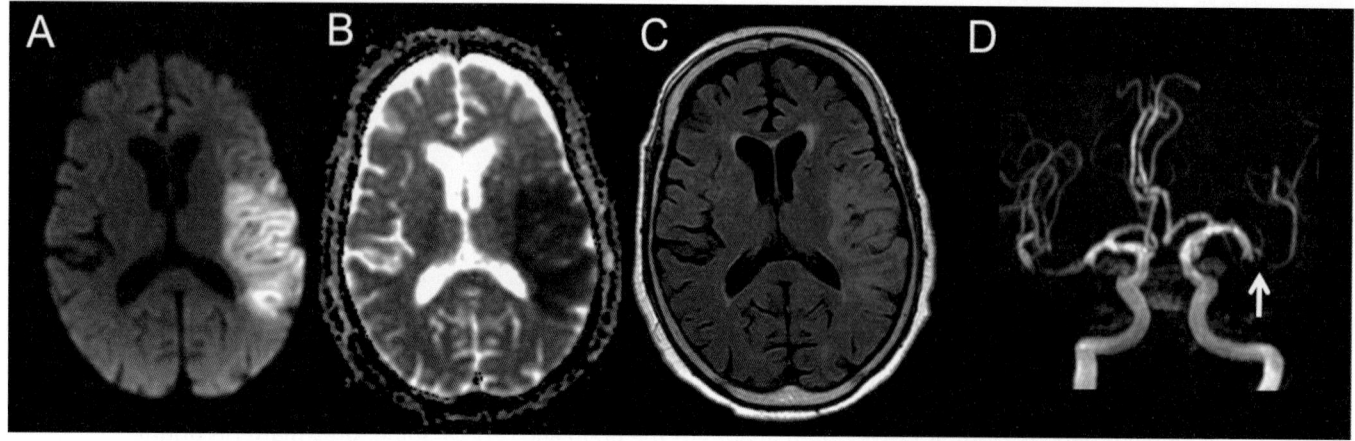

FIGURE 21.3 Acute left middle cerebral artery (MCA) infarct. **A:** The DWI image shows bright signal in the left MCA territory. **B:** The corresponding ADC image shows dark signal confirming an acute or early subacute infarct. **C:** The corresponding FLAIR image shows mild associated increased signal compatible with edema. **D:** MRA of the circle of Willis shows absent flow-related enhancement of the left distal M1 MCA segment (*arrow*) compatible with occlusion. Irregularity is also noted of the contralateral right M1 segment.

underlying paramagnetic or diamagnetic species and have important implications for characterizing tissue components such as calcification or iron content. SWI are slightly different from GRE images in that they depict intracranial vessels and are considered more sensitive than conventional GRE. Methods to quantify susceptibility are called *quantitative susceptibility mapping* (QSM). In the research setting, quantitative methods have applications in more accurate dating of hemorrhage, quantifying contrast agent enhancement, and in the evaluation for neurodegenerative disease associated with heavy metal deposition.

GADOLINIUM CONTRAST ENHANCEMENT

The use of intravenous paramagnetic contrast agents, typically gadolinium chelates, is invaluable in MRI. Enhancement is defined as increased T1 shortening following administration of contrast, and the concept is further developed in the context of magnetic resonance perfusion imaging. The presence of contrast enhancement in the brain parenchyma signifies a breakdown of the blood–brain barrier and has important implications for characterizing lesions from brain tumors and metastases to infectious and inflammatory etiologies (see Fig. 21.3D).

Several structures in the brain lack a blood–brain barrier such as the pineal gland and pituitary gland and normally enhance. Vascular enhancement is variable. Vessels are typically bright on SPGR type T1 postcontrast images but have a variable appearance on spin echo T1-type images, depending on flow rate and other imaging parameters. In the spine, enhancement can be observed in the epidural veins as well as the soft tissues. Dedicated magnetic resonance angiographic images may be necessary to characterize some vascular malformations, and conventional catheter angiography may be necessary to evaluate subtle vascular malformations.

In some situations, contrast-enhanced imaging may not be appropriate. Examples include contraindications to contrast such as prior severe allergic reactions or renal failure. In the setting of possible or prior allergic reaction, premedication with a standard steroid algorithm is necessary if the benefit of contrast to make a diagnosis outweighs the risks. Many imaging protocols such as for the evaluation of infarct, hypertensive hemorrhage, or acute spinal cord compression do not typically require postcontrast imaging. In the setting of an evolving infarct or parenchymal hemorrhage, contrast enhancement is sometimes seen and may in fact present a diagnostic dilemma in the absence of adequate clinical history.

MAGNETIC RESONANCE ANGIOGRAPHY AND MAGNETIC RESONANCE VENOGRAPHY

Vascular structures in the head and neck can be imaged noninvasively using MRI without the use of intravenous contrast agents as well as with contrast. Primary clinical applications include evaluating for stenosis, thrombosis, dissection, and aneurysm in the vascular structures of the head or neck. The *time-of-flight* (TOF) method relies on vascular flow to bring *fresh* unrelaxed spins into the imaging volume. As a result, vessels that contain flowing spins appear bright and are easily delineated. The *phase contrast* (PC) or *velocity encoding* (VENC) method detects phase changes of spins moving through a gradient. *Contrast-enhanced magnetic resonance angiography* (MRA) methods rely on the T1 shortening effects of gadolinium chelates, which are directly injected intravenously. Appropriate timing of a bolus of contrast and imaging can provide individual arterial and venous phases.

In the neck, MRA is commonly used to assess the patency of the carotid and vertebral systems, although ultrasound (US) and neck computed tomography angiography (CTA) may be used as well. Specific protocols used at individual imaging facilities depend on the resources available and the pretest probability for abnormalities in the specific patient population. The American College of Radiology (ACR) Appropriateness Criteria give equally high recommendations for carotid US, CTA, and MRA for screening in the setting of a physical exam finding, such as a carotid bruit. However, in the setting of focal neurologic deficit, MRA and CTA are preferred over US.

Noncontrast MRA of neck, using two-dimensional (2D) and three-dimensional (3D) TOF methods may be sufficient to exclude hemodynamically significant carotid stenosis. One limitation of noninvasive TOF techniques, however, is turbulent or slow flow, which can lead to loss of signal and overestimate the degree of stenosis, leading to false-positive results. This is specifically true in the carotid bulb or the V3 vertebral artery segments, which are sensitive to flow artifacts (Fig. 21.4A and B). Contrast-enhanced MRA is considered the most sensitive noninvasive imaging method for the diagnosis of 70% to 99% internal carotid artery stenosis with meta-analytic estimates of sensitivity equal to 85% (95% CI, 69% to 93%) and specificity equal to 85% (76% to 92%). Furthermore, in cases of carotid or vertebral arterial dissection, subtle luminal changes may be better evaluated with additional T1-weighted or proton-density weighted fat-saturated images in addition to contrast-enhanced methods.

In the intracranial circulation, TOF MRA methods are well suited to evaluate for vessel patency and aneurysm formation (Fig. 21.4C and D). In the setting of screening for aneurysm, for example, when there is a positive family history, the ACR Appropriateness Criteria gives slightly higher recommendations to the use of CTA over MRA given the higher resolution of CTA and absence of flow artifacts.

The use of contrast-enhanced MRA methods is preferred when evaluating aneurysms following intervention, such as coiling or stenting or when evaluating cerebrovascular malformations. Time-resolved contrast-enhanced methods (in which successive acquisitions can provide multiple arterial and venous phases) in the head and neck are typically applied when the temporal profile of enhancement is important. Examples include differentiating low- from high-flow vascular malformations or slow flow from complete occlusion.

Magnetic resonance venography is used clinically to evaluate for patency of the dural venous sinuses in the setting of venous sinus stenosis or thrombosis. 2D TOF (Fig. 21.4E) and velocity encoding (VENC) techniques (Fig. 21.4F) are typically employed. Time-resolved postcontrast methods are useful, however, when an abnormality is identified to differentiate flow artifacts or partial stenosis/occlusion from complete occlusion.

Outside of the head and neck, MRA can be applied to the spine to evaluate for vascular malformations. Lastly, although magnetic resonance angiography and venography are useful techniques, some subtle vascular malformations may only be identified on conventional catheter angiography, and this must be considered if there is the need to completely exclude an underlying vascular malformation.

MAGNETIC RESONANCE IMAGING ARTIFACTS

MRI is subject to a multitude of artifacts, which in general refers to image representations that are distortions of the true underlying anatomy. Artifacts can both introduce nonexistent structures or obscure anatomy. Artifacts can originate from any of the multiple

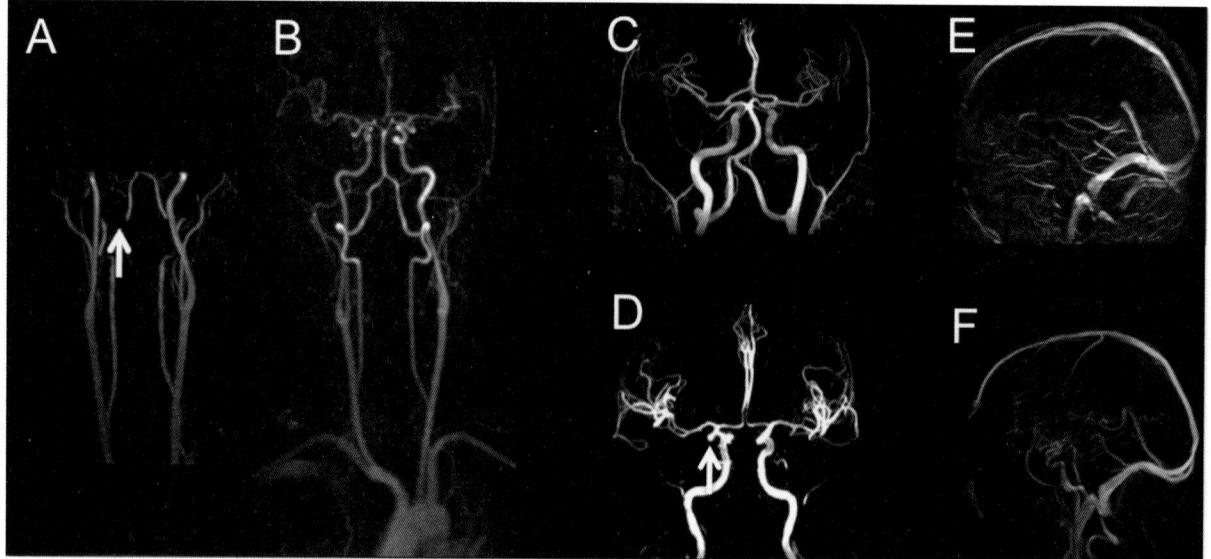

FIGURE 21.4 MRA and magnetic resonance venography. **A:** MRA of the neck delineates the carotid and vertebral arteries. Note the in-plane flow artifact (*arrow*) in the V3 segments of the vertebral artery. **B:** Contrast-enhanced MRA arterial phase shows resolution of flow artifacts. **C:** Normal MRA of intracranial vessels. **D:** MRA depicts a right supraclinoid carotid artery aneurysm (*arrow*). **E:** 3D TOF magnetic resonance venography depicts the dural venous sinuses. **F:** Velocity encoded magnetic resonance venography of the dural venous sinuses.

steps in signal generation, acquisition, and processing in addition to the underlying properties of biologic tissues and patient cooperation.

Some of the most commonly encountered artifacts arise from motion, either due to voluntary or involuntary patient motion (Fig. 21.5A) or biologic flow phenomena such as in vascular structures or pulsation of CSF (Fig. 21.5B). Flow phenomena lead to either increased or decreased signal within vascular structures, similar to effects exploited in noncontrast *TOF* MRA. Patient motion or pulsating structures such as vessels result in ghosting-type artifacts in clinical images (Fig. 21.5C). Ghosting artifacts also arise in EPI (called *N/2 ghosts*) due to distortions between successive echoes.

Susceptibility artifacts arise when there are distortions of the local magnetic field. This can be due to air–tissue interfaces or implanted metallic material. These artifacts are commonly encountered in the setting of dental hardware (such as fillings or braces), aneurysm clips, or spine fusion hardware. Usually, these artifacts lead to loss of signal in adjacent structures, but they may also result in increased signal, for example in FLAIR imaging (Fig. 21.5D and E).

Aliasing artifacts are common when the field of view in the phase encoding dimension is too small; structures outside the field wrap within the image. It is important to note that these artifacts can arise from any phase encode direction.

Stray radiofrequency interference leads to so-called zipper artifacts (Fig. 21.5F). For this reason, MRI rooms are electrically shielded and must be operated with the door closed. Many additional artifacts are described in MRI, related to chemical shift effects, coil, and radiofrequency inhomogeneity.

CLINICAL MAGNETIC RESONANCE IMAGING

MRI attains significantly higher contrast between different biologic tissues compared to other cross-sectional imaging techniques such as CT or US. For this reason, MRI is considered the most precise and sensitive imaging modality for detecting CNS tissue pathology.

Appropriateness criteria comparing MRI and CT in the select neurologic scenarios are provided in Table 21.2. The approach to three major paradigms, infarction, white matter disease, and tumors is discussed in the following sections.

CEREBROVASCULAR DISEASE

MRI has revolutionized stoke imaging. Acute infarcts are bright on DWI and display restricted diffusion on ADC images (see Fig. 21.3). Mass effect and vasogenic or cytotoxic edema can be evaluated on associated T2-weighted or FLAIR images. The presence of hemorrhage can be identified on SWI or GRE images. The size of the infarct can be quantified and the specific vascular territories involved can be delineated. Various scoring scales may be used to determine prognosis or indicate treatment based on imaging. Concurrently, performed vascular imaging can show causative vascular disease, such as stenosis, thrombosis, or dissection.

The approach to stroke imaging begins with close inspection of the DWI for increased diffusion-weighted signal relative to the background of normal structures. Once a lesion is identified, evaluation of the ADC image can confirm an acute or early subacute infarct, which is dark relative to background. Evaluation of the SWI or GRE images is used to look for evidence of hemorrhage or hemorrhagic conversion. It is important not to confuse hemorrhage with an acute infarct, both of which may show restricted diffusion. Additional sequences including T2 and FLAIR images are used to evaluate for mass effect, cytotoxic and vasogenic edema. Some authors suggest that inspection of the concurrent FLAIR images may differentiate between acute and subacute infarcts when clinical information is incomplete or unavailable.

The specific structures involved in stroke and multiplicity of infarcts help to differentiate individual vascular territories from embolic-type infarcts and diffuse ischemia/hypoxia. Stroke imaging typically is performed in conjunction with vascular imaging such as MRA or CTA of the head and neck with attention specifically focused on determining if vascular occlusion is responsible for the

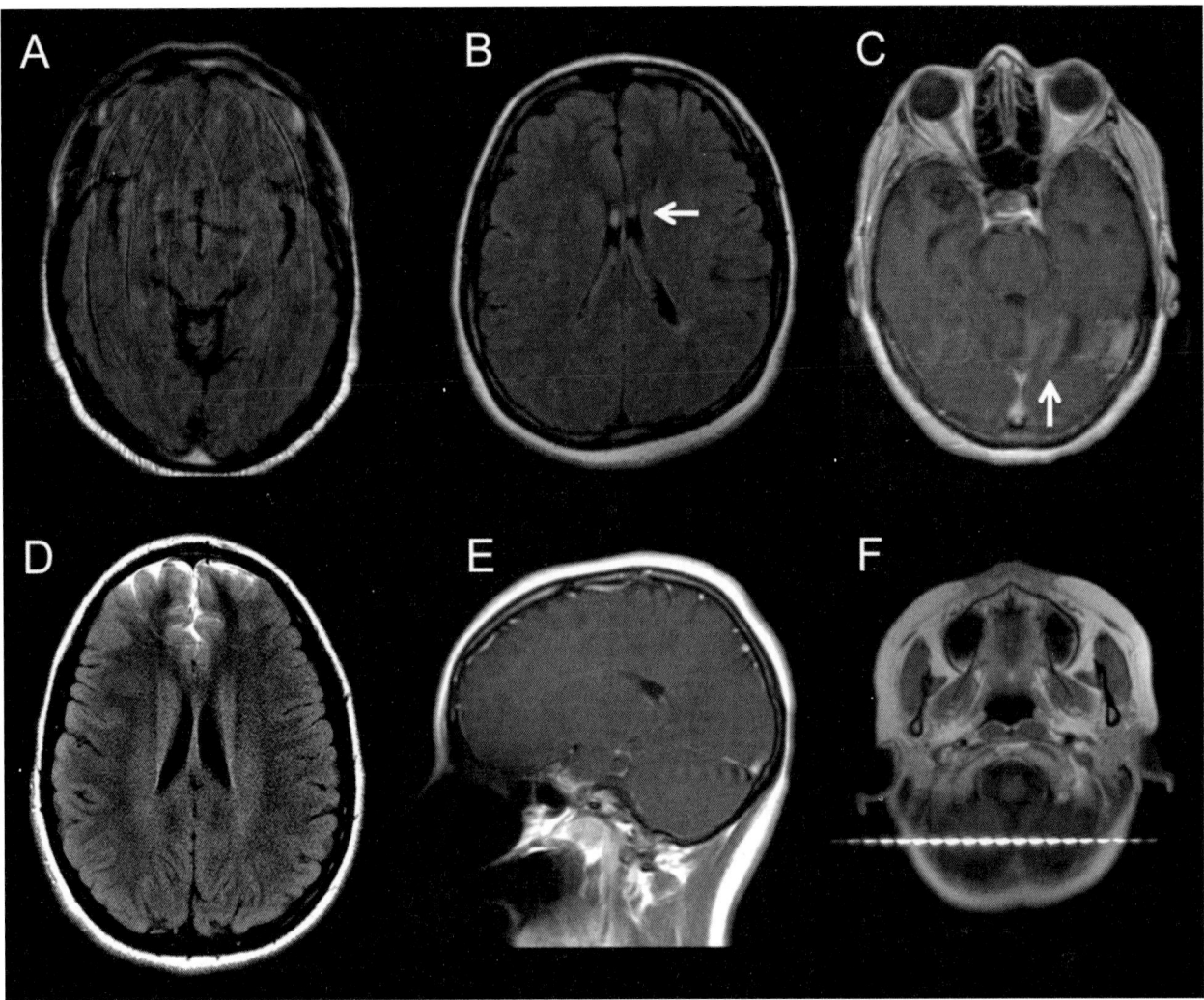

FIGURE 21.5 MRI artifacts. **A:** Motion artifact results in ghosting on a FLAIR image. **B:** Flow artifact due to CSF pulsations in the lateral ventricles (*arrow*). **C:** Ghosting artifact due to pulsatile flow in the transverse sinuses (*arrow*). **D:** Susceptibility artifact leads to increased signal in the frontal region due to failure of CSF suppression. **E:** Corresponding susceptibility artifact due to dental hardware is shown on a T1-weighted image. **F:** Zipper artifact due to stray radiofrequency interference.

TABLE 21.2   American College of Radiology Appropriateness Criteria

	MRI Brain without Contrast	MRI Brain without and with Contrast	CT Head without Contrast	CT Head without and with Contrast
New focal neurologic deficit <3 h (e.g., acute stroke)	8	8	9	3
Transient ischemic attack	8	8	8	3
Suspected parenchymal hemorrhage	6	6	9	7
Ataxia, slowly progressive	7	8	5	6
Possible Alzheimer disease	8	7	5	6

Appropriateness ratings for brain MRI versus head CT without and with contrast (non-MRA/CTA) are provided for selected neurologic conditions. The ratings range from 1 to 9, with "usually appropriate" studies rated 7 to 9, "may be" appropriate rated 4 to 6, and "usually not appropriate" rated 1 to 3. Level of evidence is generally based on expert opinion. A complete list and background evidence may be obtained at www.acr.org/Quality-Safety/Appropriateness-Criteria.

MRI, magnetic resonance imaging; CT, computed tomography.

infarct (see Fig. 21.3D). Perfusion imaging in stroke is sometimes performed to determine the size of the territory at risk and guide intervention.

WHITE MATTER DISEASE

Abnormalities in the white matter are best identified on FLAIR images. The differential diagnosis of white matter disease includes demyelinating and dysmyelinating etiologies, vasculitic and vasospastic processes, infection and inflammatory processes, toxic/metabolic etiologies, edema, trauma, seizures, as well as neoplasm and hypoxic/ischemic processes including arterial and venous infarcts. Characterizing these processes and narrowing the differential diagnosis require concurrent integration of clinical information and a complete set of MRI sequences.

As an example, we discuss an approach to multiple sclerosis (MS), an archetypal disease process with imaging abnormalities on brain and spine MRI (Fig. 21.6). The approach to MS begins with thorough inspection of the FLAIR images for abnormal signal specifically involving the white matter. Supratentorially, lesions are typically identified in the periventricular, deep, and subcortical/juxtacortical white matter and corpus callosum, as well sometimes the basal ganglia, although cortical disease burden in MS is not well delineated on FLAIR imaging. Sagittal FLAIR images are invaluable for confirming subtle lesions on axially acquired sequences and for evaluating the corpus callosum. T2-weighted images are preferred for the evaluation of white matter lesions in the brain stem and cerebellar white matter due to artifacts in the posterior fossa on FLAIR images. After lesions are identified, their acuity is estimated based on associated diffusion abnormality and contrast enhancement, both of which would suggest acute demyelinating lesions. Finally, because MS patients undergoing treatment may be immunosuppressed, it is important to evaluate for superimposed infection such as progressive multifocal encephalopathy (PML).

In the spine, the approach to MS concentrates on using T2-weighted images and IR T2-weighted images. IR T2-weighted images are similar to FLAIR images in that they also employ an inversion pulse; however, they are timed not to suppress CSF signal but rather to increase the conspicuity of lesions and suppress signal from fat. As in the brain, the presence of contrast enhancement is used to identify acute lesions. It is important to remember that patient symptoms may not be due to demyelinating lesions in the spinal cord but rather to degenerative changes, such as disk herniations.

BRAIN AND SPINAL CORD TUMORS

Tumors are defined by the presence of mass effect, where normal structures are displaced or infiltrated and display abnormal signal characteristics including postcontrast enhancement. Despite common belief, contrast enhancement does not always correlate with World Health Organization (WHO) tumor grade. For example, both grade I pilocytic astrocytoma and grade IV glioblastoma typically display postcontrast enhancement. On the other hand, grade III anaplastic astrocytoma may not display contrast enhancement. FLAIR imaging is indispensable in brain tumor imaging because FLAIR imaging demonstrates nonenhancing tumor components but also associated mass effect and edema (Fig. 21.7). One of the main problems in evaluating brain tumors is distinguishing tumor recurrence (progression) from posttreatment changes (pseudoprogression). For this reason, tumor imaging typically entails advanced MRI methods such as magnetic resonance perfusion imaging and magnetic resonance spectroscopy, in addition to correlation with other modalities such as nuclear medicine ^{18}F-fluorodeoxyglucose positron emission tomography (FDG-PET) or thallium single-photon emission computed tomography (SPECT).

The approach to assessment of brain tumors begins with localization of the lesion in the intra-axial or extra-axial space. Subsequent evaluation of mass effect and definition of the mass on T1-weighted, T2-weighted, FLAIR, or postcontrast images is performed. The adjacent parenchyma is evaluated for associated edema or infiltration. Diffusion-weighted images are used to evaluate associated ischemic changes or hypercellular components of the tumor. SWI or GRE images are used to evaluate for associated hemorrhage or calcifications. Given the heterogeneity of brain tumors, the location, appearance, signal characteristics, enhancement, or comparison to prior studies are all integrated to arrive at a differential diagnosis.

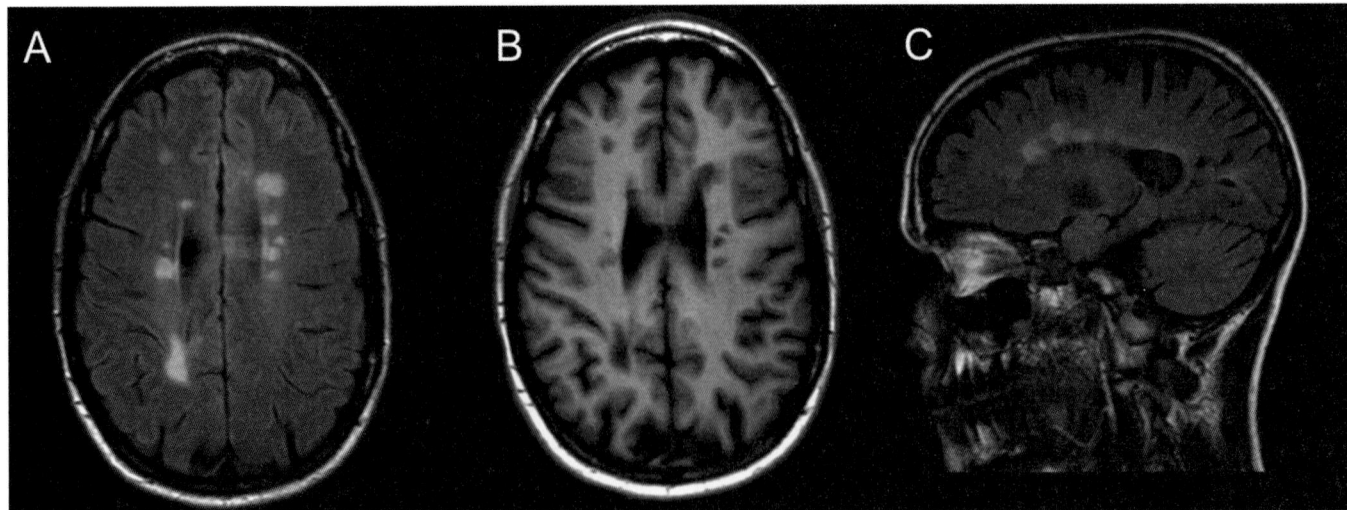

FIGURE 21.6 Multiple sclerosis. A: Characteristic white matter lesions of multiple sclerosis depicted on an axial FLAIR image. **B:** Low signal intensity of the lesions on T1-weighted images suggests chronic lesions. **C:** Sagittal FLAIR image depicts the radial orientation of white matter lesions characteristic of multiple sclerosis.

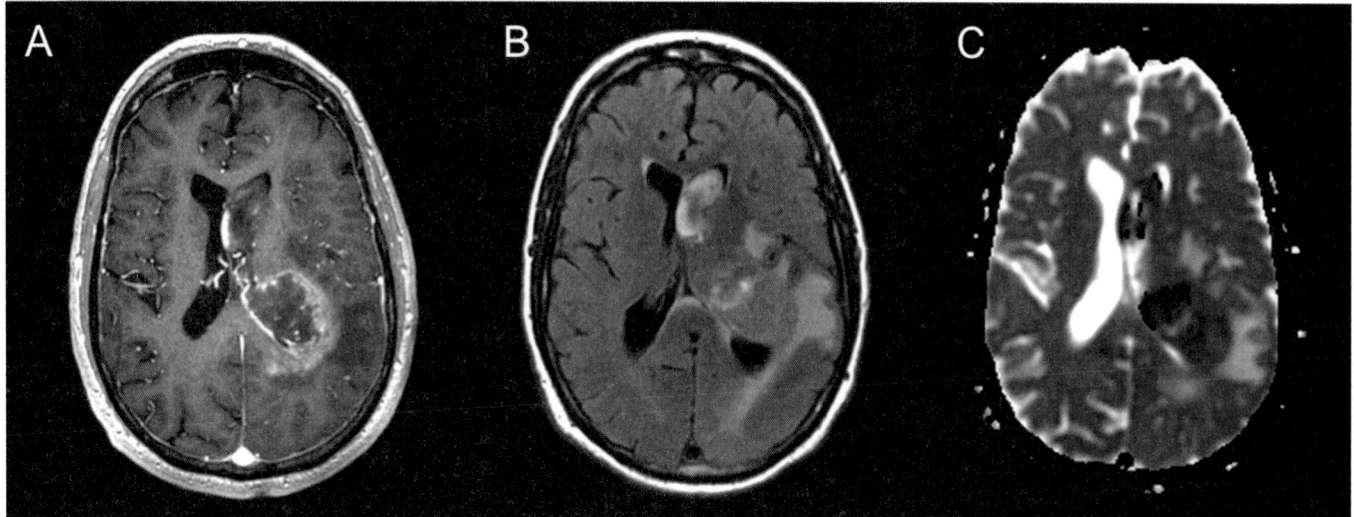

FIGURE 21.7 Glioblastoma. **A:** Post–contrast-enhanced image shows a large enhancing mass with central necrosis. **B:** FLAIR image depicts the associated white matter abnormality compatible with a combination of edema and nonenhancing tumor. **C:** ADC image shows restricted diffusion in components of the tumor suggestive of increased cellular density.

ADVANCED MAGNETIC RESONANCE IMAGING METHODS

FUNCTIONAL MAGNETIC RESONANCE IMAGING

Functional magnetic resonance imaging (fMRI) refers to the use of magnetic resonance for the localization of cerebral activation. The most commonly employed technique takes advantage of hemodynamic coupling of cerebral activation to indirectly infer cerebral activation. The blood oxygen level–dependent (BOLD) contrast mechanism results from a relative increase in the concentration of oxyhemoglobin (a paramagnetic species) compared to deoxyhemoglobin (a diamagnetic species) in response to cerebral activation. This change can be detected using rapid MRI sequences typically employing gradient echo sequences sensitive to T2* contrast, allowing cerebral activation to be imaged in the brain. Some authors have proposed using DWI to map cerebral activation but this is not common.

fMRI can be performed in conjunction with specific task paradigms (Fig. 21.8A and B). This type of fMRI has current clinical applications for mapping the cortical location of known cognitive and motor functional units and has specific use in presurgical and pretherapeutic planning. Examples include mapping the primary motor and visual cortices or localizing language activation areas.

In the research setting, the technique has been applied to monitor a variety of psychiatric disorders. When acquired without a specific task paradigm, the technique is referred to as *resting state fMRI*, which maps connectivity features of the so-called default-mode neural networks (DMN).

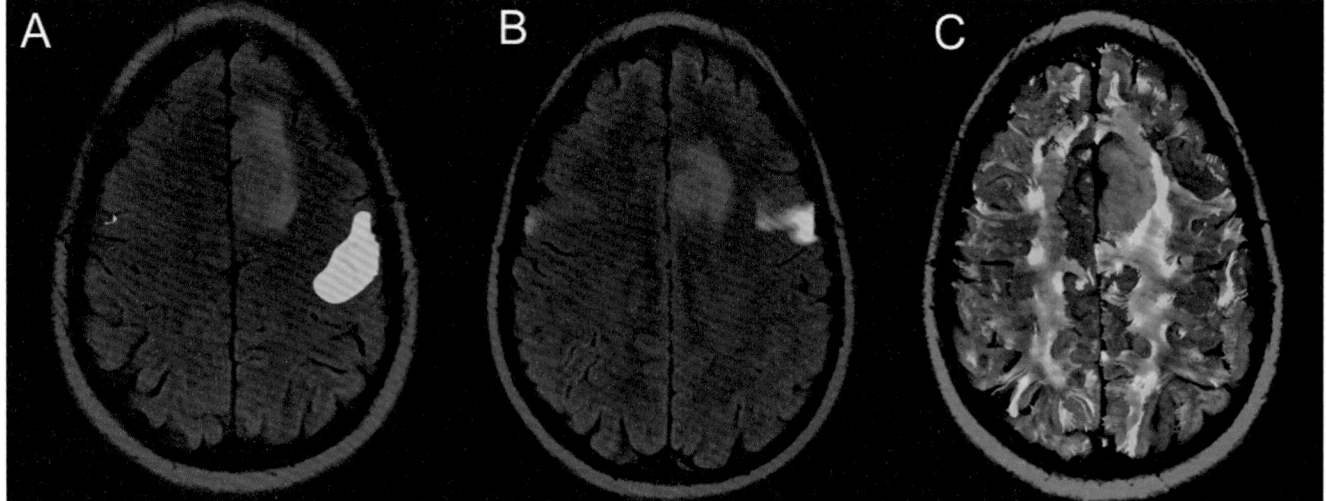

FIGURE 21.8 fMRI and diffusion tensor imaging. **A:** Preoperative fMRI showing activation of primary motor cortex during a motor task in a patient with a left frontal neoplasm. **B:** Preoperative fMRI showing activation of left frontal language processing area during a verb generation task. **C:** Fiber tracking performed based on diffusion tensor data showing displacement of the left frontal tracts by the left frontal mass.

DIFFUSION TENSOR IMAGING

Diffusion tensor imaging (DTI) is a technique that can quantify the directional dependence of diffusion of water. Clinically, DTI is most commonly applied to assess the integrity of white matter tracts (Fig. 21.8C). Normal white matter tracts are densely packed, which creates an anisotropic environment. Diffusion perpendicular to white matter tracts is relatively hindered compared to diffusion parallel to white matter tracts. Therefore, measuring the direction of greatest diffusion will estimate the dominant orientation of white matter tracts. Measuring multiple directions of diffusion can subsequently be used to define a diffusion tensor. The diffusion tensor information can then be postprocessed to generate images with white matter tracts. More advanced approaches, such as Q-ball and diffusion spectrum imaging, provide a more general description of diffusion and have improved performance in resolving crossing white matter fibers. The current clinical application of DTI is definition of white matter tracts in presurgical and pretherapeutic planning. A multitude of applications of DTI to variety of neurologic conditions including stroke, MS, dementia, and traumatic brain injury primarily reside in the research setting. In part, this is due to lack of standardization of acquisition and postprocessing techniques as well data lacking on clinical use and effect on patient outcomes.

MAGNETIC RESONANCE SPECTROSCOPY

Magnetic resonance spectroscopy (MRS) is considered an advanced imaging technique within MRI, although it is an integral part in the formation of anatomic magnetic resonance images. In the absence of an applied field gradient, different nuclei can be resolved by their chemical shift. MRS in clinical practice typically refers to spatially selective acquisition (single or multiple voxel) of proton spectra, where care has been taken to suppress the dominant water resonance, thus increasing sensitivity for the resonances of small molecules. In the brain, the most commonly observed resonances belong to N-acetylaspartate (NAA) (2.0 ppm—interpreted to signify normal neuronal tissue), creatine (3.0 ppm—interpreted to signify energy stores), choline (3.2 ppm—interpreted to signify components of the cell membrane and myelin), and lactate (doublet at 1.3 ppm—interpreted to signify anaerobic metabolism) (Fig. 21.9). The lactate doublet resonance corresponding to the lactate methyl protons is inverted at an echo time of 144 milliseconds compared to 288 milliseconds due to J-coupling effects with the lactate methine proton.

Additional metabolites such inositol/myoinositol (interpreted as a marker of astrocytes and astrogliosis seen in MS lesions), glutamate/glutamine, and several amino acids such as alanine (described in meningiomas) and glycine can also be observed. The relative amplitude of the resonance peaks reflects the relative concentrations of metabolites; however, it should be noted that in general, relaxation effects may alter resonance amplitudes, highlighting attention to the time-to-echo (TE). In general, more metabolites are seen with a shorter TE. In routine clinical practice, spectroscopy is often used as a problem-solving technique, for example, in an attempt to differentiate tumor recurrence from posttreatment effects (higher choline-to-creatine ratios tend to be observed with recurrent brain tumors than radiation necrosis; see Fig. 21.10C) or to evaluate for inborn errors of metabolism such as mitochondrial disorders and leukodystrophies (the presence of a lactate peak may signify a mitochondrial disorder such as mitochondrial encephalomyelopathy, lactic acidosis, and stroke [MELAS]). MRS has also been used to directly observe 2-hydroxyglutarate, a metabolite that accumulates in isocitrate dehydrogenase (IDH) mutant glioblastoma tumors, and thus constitutes a biomarker for IDH status in glioma.

MAGNETIC RESONANCE PERFUSION IMAGING

Magnetic resonance perfusion is a method of quantifying blood flow through biologic tissues. The method is usually applied to the brain but has been extended to other parts of the body including the spine. The relevant measures include measurement of cerebral blood volume, cerebral blood flow, and mean transit time.

This is achieved in MRI using a *first-pass* or *bolus-tracking* method that records the signal reduction that occurs when rapidly repeated images are acquired during the first passage of an intravascular bolus of paramagnetic contrast, usually a gadolinium chelate. The images produced are called *perfusion-weighted images* (PWI) or *dynamic susceptibility contrast* (DSC) *images*. Gradient echo images with EPI type detection are usually used because they provide the ability to image very rapidly to track the contrast bolus.

The time course of the signal change during the passage of the bolus can be used to obtain the cerebral blood volume (CBV), mean transit time (MTT), and their ratio, the cerebral blood flow (CBF = CBV/MTT). Because of the technical difficulty in measuring the arterial input function of the contrast bolus, perfusion maps are semiquantitative and are best interpreted as relative rather than absolute perfusion values (rCBV, rMTT, and rCBF). If the arterial

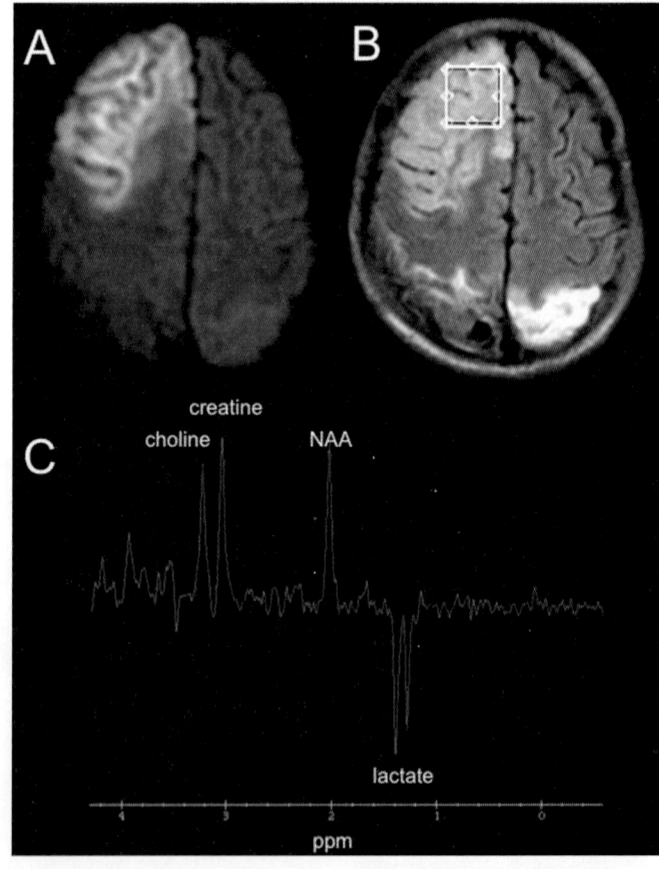

FIGURE 21.9 MRI spectroscopy. **A:** DWI shows an acute infarct in the right superior frontal lobe. **B:** Voxel (*square*) is placed in the right superior frontal image on the corresponding FLAIR image. **C:** MRS performed at an echo time of 144 milliseconds shows choline, creatine, and NAA resonances with relative decrease of the NAA resonance. An inverted lactate doublet is present compatible with anaerobic metabolism in the setting of an infarct.

input function is known, then a measure of permeability of the extravascular–extracellular space known as *k-trans* can be calculated. Algorithms exist in clinical practice for quantifying the permeability of tissues to contrast (called *leakage*) from modeling of the perfusion time course without knowledge of the exact arterial input function.

Magnetic resonance perfusion can be performed without contrast with the arterial spin labeling (ASL) method. Similar to TOF MRA, the ASL method depends on inflow of spins through vessels. ASL may provide more quantitative information without the need for arterial input functions but is less widely available than contrast bolus tracking methods.

Clinical applications of magnetic resonance perfusion include cerebrovascular disease. In cases of stroke or vasospasm, measures of perfusion delay, such as MTT, are sensitive indicators of small reductions in cerebral perfusion that can delineate relatively hypoperfused vascular territories. In this way, magnetic resonance perfusion is similar to CT perfusion methods, but can be performed without ionizing radiation, and permits direct correlation with other magnetic resonance images. Outside of cerebrovascular disease imaging, clinical applications of magnetic resonance perfusion include brain tumors and metastases. These applications focus on assessment of CBV, which correlates with histologic tumor grade and characterizes response to treatment of the tumor (Fig. 21.10A and B).

EMERGING MAGNETIC RESONANCE IMAGING METHODS

Recent advances in MRI aim to drastically improve the resolution of images and speed of imaging as well as to significantly extend clinical applications. The emergence of high field (>7 T) imaging systems promises improvements in signal to noise and image resolution as well as functional imaging. Similarly, improvements in imaging speed have been a constant focus since the inception of MRI. Recent advances rely on undersampling and subsequent reconstruction using nonlinear methods. One of the most popular of such methods called *compressed-sensing* holds promise for implementing near real-time imaging, especially when combined with methods to improve signal to noise.

Although magnetic resonance is a very powerful technique to study structure and dynamic processes on a molecular level, its application to biologic systems is primarily limited by its inherent low signal to noise. As a result, low-concentration molecules involved in metabolism and other cellular functions are essentially inaccessible by conventional techniques. This limitation is primarily evident in MRS, where multidimensional experiments could in theory characterize a multitude of metabolites, provided there was sufficient signal to noise. The goal of emerging methods called *hyperpolarization* (HP) is to increase nuclear spin polarization and

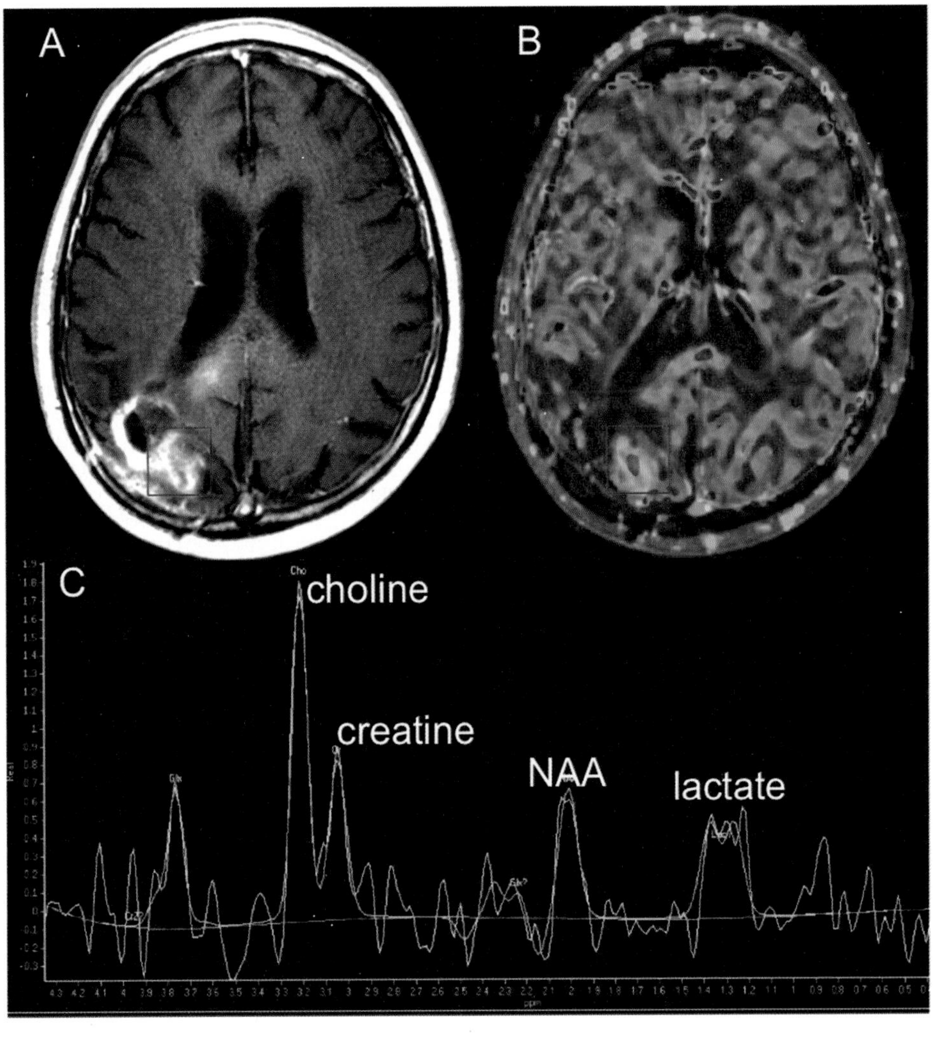

FIGURE 21.10 Magnetic resonance perfusion imaging and MRS in recurrent high-grade glioma. **A:** Post–contrast-enhanced image showing abnormal enhancement (*red square*) in the posterior right parietal region. **B:** Magnetic resonance perfusion image shows a focus of increased relative cerebral blood volume (*red square*) suggestive of recurrent tumor. **C:** MRS at a TE of 288 milliseconds shows elevated choline and decreased NAA resonances suggestive of recurrent tumor. A lactate doublet is present.

thus drastically increase signal to noise. A primary application of HP-MRI is the study of in vivo transient interactions through HP of small metabolites suited to probing varied processes such as metabolism and oxidative stress or as agents of perfusion. HP-MRI is a promising technique for combining the intrinsic biologic tissue contrast, temporal and chemical shift resolution, as well as sensitivity to dynamic processes of magnetic resonance with molecular imaging.

Perhaps the most important advancement in clinical imaging comes from contemporary advances in information technology and quantitative image-processing methods. The availability of electronic medical records and digitally archived images has permitted the correlation of imaging features with molecular pathology and development of a new field of *radiogenomics*. This field is predicated on correlation of quantitative image analysis features with molecular markers and information pertaining to patient diagnosis, prognosis, and treatment response available within the electronic medical record. This revolution in medicine embraces the heterogeneity of pathologic processes and individual responses in the patient population and seeks to tailor therapeutics for maximal efficacy.

SUGGESTED READINGS

Acosta-Cabronero J, Williams GB, Cardenas-Blanco A, et al. In vivo quantitative susceptibility mapping (QSM) in Alzheimer's disease. *PLoS One.* 2013;8(11):e81093.

American College of Radiology. ACR Appropriateness Criteria®. American College of Radiology Web site. http://www.acr.org/Quality-Safety/Appropriateness -Criteria. Accessed January 1, 2015.

Andronesi OC, Kim GS, Gerstner E, et al. Detection of 2-hydroxyglutarate in IDH-mutated glioma patients by in vivo spectral-editing and 2D correlation magnetic resonance spectroscopy. *Sci Transl Med.* 2012;4(116):116ra4.

Chappell FM, Wardlaw JM, Young GR, et al. Carotid artery stenosis: accuracy of noninvasive test—individual patient data meta-analysis. *Radiology.* 2009;251(2):493–502.

De Coene B, Hajnal JV, Gatehouse P, et al. MR of the brain using fluid-attenuated inversion recovery (FLAIR) pulse sequences. *AJNR Am J Neuroradiol.* 1992;13(6):1555–1564.

de Rochefort L, Brown R, Prince MR, et al. Quantitative MR susceptibility mapping using piece-wise constant regularized inversion of the magnetic field. *Magn Reson Med.* 2008;60(4):1003–1009.

Deoni SC. Quantitative relaxometry of the brain. *Top Magn Reson Imaging.* 2010;21(2):101–13.

Duong TQ, Yacoub E, Adriany G, et al. Microvascular BOLD contribution at 4 and 7 T in the human brain: gradient-echo and spin-echo fMRI with suppression of blood effects. *Magn Reson Med.* 2003;49(6):1019–1027.

Fox MD, Snyder AZ, Vincent JL, et al. The human brain is intrinsically organized into dynamic, anticorrelated functional networks. *Proc Natl Acad Sci U S A.* 2005;102(27):9673–9678.

Geurts JJ, Bö L, Pouwels PJ, et al. Cortical lesions in multiple sclerosis: combined postmortem MR imaging and histopathology. *AJNR Am J Neuroradiol.* 2005;26(3):572–577.

Goldman M. *Quantum Description of High-Resolution NMR in Liquids.* Oxford, United Kingdom: Clarendon Press; 1988.

Gupta A, Young RJ, Karimi S, et al. Isolated diffusion restriction precedes the development of enhancing tumor in a subset of patients with glioblastoma. *AJNR Am J Neuroradiol.* 2011;32(7):1301–1306.

Haacke EM, Cheng NY, House MJ, et al. Imaging iron stores in the brain using magnetic resonance imaging. *Magn Reson Imaging.* 2005;23(1):1–25.

Hajnal JV, Bryant DJ, Kasuboski L, et al. Use of fluid attenuated inversion recovery (FLAIR) pulse sequences in MRI of the brain. *J Comput Assist Tomogr.* 1992;16(6):841–844.

Keshari KR, Wilson DM. Chemistry and biochemistry of 13C hyperpolarized magnetic resonance using dynamic nuclear polarization. *Chem Soc Rev.* 2014;43(5):1627–1659.

Krings T, Reinges MH, Erberich S, et al. Functional MRI for presurgical planning: problems, artefacts, and solution strategies. *J Neurol Neurosurg Psychiatry.* 2001;70(6):749–760.

Kuo PH, Kanal E, Abu-Alfa AK, et al. Gadolinium-based MR contrast agents and nephrogenic systemic fibrosis. *Radiology.* 2007;242(3):647–649.

Lansberg MG, Thijs VN, O'Brien MW, et al. Evolution of apparent diffusion coefficient, diffusion-weighted, and T2-weighted signal intensity of acute stroke. *AJNR Am J Neuroradiol.* 2001;22(4):637–644.

Le Bihan D, Urayama S, Aso T, et al. Direct and fast detection of neuronal activation in the human brain with diffusion MRI. *Proc Natl Acad Sci U S A.* 2006;103(21):8263–8268.

Levitt MH. *Spin Dynamics: Basis of Nuclear Magnetic Resonance.* 2nd ed. Chichester, United Kingdom: John Wiley & Sons; 2008.

Linfante I, Linas RH, Caplan LR, et al. MRI features of intracerebral hemorrhage within 2 hours from symptom onset. *Stroke.* 1999;30(11):2263–2267.

Lustig M, Dohono D, Pauly JM. Sparse MRI: the application of compressed sensing for rapid MR imaging. *Magn Reson Med.* 2007;58(6):1182–1195.

Mader I, Rauer S, Gall P, et al. (1)H MR spectroscopy of inflammation, infection and ischemia of the brain. *Eur J Radiol.* 2008;67(2):250–257.

McRobbie DW, Moore EA, Graves MJ, et al. *MRI from Picture to Proton.* 2nd ed. Cambridge, United Kingdom: Cambridge University Press; 2006.

Mitterschiffthaler MT, Ettinger U, Mehta MA, et al. Applications of functional magnetic resonance imaging in psychiatry. *J Magn Reson Imaging.* 2006;23(6):851–861.

Ogawa S, Tank DW, Menon R et al. Intrinsic signal changes accompanying sensory stimulation: functional brain mapping with magnetic resonance imaging. *Proc Natl Acad Sci U S A.* 1992;89(13):5951–5955.

Parizel P, Makkat S, Van Miert E, et al. Intracranial hemorrhage: principles of CT and MRI interpretation. *Eur Radiol.* 2001;11(9):1770–1783.

Prince MR, Grist TM, Debatin JF. 3D contrast MR angiography. Berlin, Germany: Springer-Verlag; 2002.

Prince MR, Zhange HL, Roditi GH, et al. Risk factors for NSF: a literature review. *J Magn Reson Imaging.* 2009;30(6):1298–1308.

Sorensen AG, Buonanno FS, Gonzalez RG, et al. Hyperacute stroke: evaluation with combined multisection diffusion-weighted and hemodynamically weighted echo-planar MR imaging. *Radiology.* 1996;199(2):391–401.

Thomalla G, Cheng B, Ebinger M, et al. DWI-FLAIR mismatch for the identification of patients with acute ischaemic stroke within 4-5 h of symptom onset (PRE-FLAIR): a multicentre observational study. *Lancet Neurol.* 2011;10(11):978–986.

Warach S, Chien D, Li W, et al. Fast magnetic resonance diffusion weighted imaging of acute human stroke. *Neurology.* 1992;42(9):1717–1723.

Watts R, Andrews T, Hipko S, et al. In vivo whole-brain T1-rho mapping across adulthood: normative values and age dependence. *J Magn Reson Imaging.* 2014;40(2):376–382.

Zhuo J, Gullapalli RP. AAPM/RSNA physics tutorial for residents: MR artifacts, safety, and quality control. *Radiographics.* 2006;26(1):275–297.

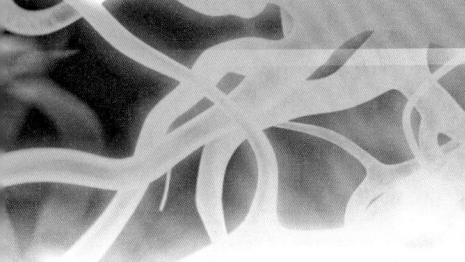

Positron Emission Tomography and Single-Photon Emission Computed Tomography

22

William Charles Kreisl

INTRODUCTION

Molecular imaging is used in the clinical practice of nuclear medicine and in medical research to better understand the biochemical processes that underlie human disease. Two examples of molecular imaging are positron emission tomography (PET) and single-photon emission computed tomography (SPECT). In both PET and SPECT, patients are administered a radioactive compound with a pharmacokinetic behavior that targets a molecular pathway related to the pathology of a certain disease.

PET and SPECT allow highly sensitive and selective measurement of specific biologic changes in the human body. Agents are administered in amounts too small to cause pharmacologic effects ("trace" doses) so as to avoid perturbation of the biochemical pathway being studied. Many radioactive compounds used in PET and SPECT reversibly bind to a target protein via ligand-receptor kinetics. In these cases, the radioactive ligand is referred to as a radioligand. However, some radioactive compounds used for PET or SPECT do not bind a target protein. For example, $[^{15}O]H_2O$ is used to measure perfusion, as the uptake of this compound reflects the flow of blood into a given tissue. A $[^{15}O]H_2O$ PET scan therefore does not measure the binding of water to any receptor, but rather it traces the flow of blood to different tissues (Fig. 22.1). In this case, the term radiotracer is more appropriate. A broader term that applies to all compounds used with PET or SPECT is radiopharmaceutical, reflecting that the radioactive compounds used in molecular imaging are given the same regulatory considerations as drugs.

BASIC PRINCIPLES

Both PET and SPECT employ the physical phenomenon of radioactive decay, which occurs in radionuclides that are unstable due to incompatible number of protons and neutrons or excess energy.

In PET imaging, radionuclides are proton rich and as a result undergo decay and emission of a positron. An example of a radionuclide is carbon-11 (^{11}C), which has six protons and five neutrons. Unstable due to the greater number of protons than neutrons, ^{11}C undergoes a decay event in which a proton is converted to a neutron and the nucleus emits a positron and a neutrino. The positron will then zigzag around the vicinity of the decay event, losing energy as it collides with electrons of neighboring atoms, until it comes almost to rest and combines with an electron. Because a positron and electron are of equal mass but opposite charge, this event results in an annihilation encounter, with two 511 keV gamma rays (photons) emitted at about 180 degrees from each other. Other examples of positron-emitting radionuclides used for PET are ^{18}F, ^{15}O, and ^{13}N.

In SPECT imaging, radionuclides exist in a metastable state and decay from their excited state to ground state, resulting in emission of a single photon. The gamma-emitting radionuclides ^{99m}Tc and ^{123}I are commonly used for SPECT.

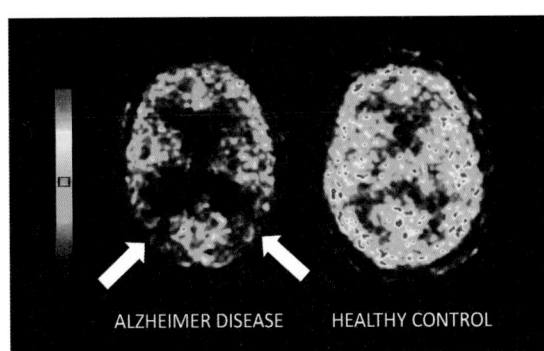

FIGURE 22.1 Example of $[^{15}O]H_2O$ perfusion scan. The patient with Alzheimer disease has lower cerebral perfusion in the parietal cortex bilaterally (*arrows*) than the age-matched cognitively normal control subject. (Image courtesy of Robert Innis and William Charles Kreisl, Molecular Imaging Branch, National Institute of Mental Health.)

RADIOPHARMACEUTICALS AND SELECTION OF RADIONUCLIDES

Radionuclides are combined with a pharmaceutical through a series of synthetic steps to create a radiopharmaceutical. Radiopharmaceuticals are administered either intravenously or orally and once in the biologic system, they interact with different molecules based on the kinetic properties of the pharmaceutical to which the radionuclide is attached. The radionuclide will then undergo nuclear decay as described earlier, ultimately resulting in the emission of two photons in the case of PET and a single photon in the case of SPECT. The radiation exposure to the patient is a function of the radionuclide used and the amount of radiopharmaceutical administered. Radionuclides with longer half-lives (e.g., ^{18}F, $t_{1/2} = 110$ minutes) result in larger exposure than those with shorter half-lives (e.g., ^{11}C, $t_{1/2} = 20.5$ minutes). However, the advantage of radiopharmaceuticals with long half-lives is that they may be synthesized offsite and delivered to medical facilities, providing greater availability for clinical use. Use of radiopharmaceuticals with short half-lives is limited to facilities capable of onsite synthesis.

DETECTION, ACQUISITION, AND DISPLAY OF SIGNAL

When radiopharmaceutical decay events occur inside a PET or SPECT scanner, crystals in a scintillation detector absorb the photons and then emit pulses of light that are then amplified, sorted, and registered as a count. The sum of these counts creates a tomographic map of all the decay events that occur within the view of the scanner. The result is an image that represents the different densities of radioactivity throughout the tissues captured by the scanner. The basis of PET and SPECT imaging is that the majority of decay events occur in proximity to where the radiopharmaceutical is acting on the molecular target of interest. The sensitivity of PET and SPECT is a function of the fraction of emitted photons that contribute to the total image. In PET, coincidence detection of the pair of photons that are emitted per decay event allows greater efficiency than in SPECT, which captures only the single photons that approach the detector at certain angles. Therefore, PET is generally more sensitive than SPECT and is more frequently used for quantitative imaging, although absolute quantitation has been reliably attained with SPECT.

PET and SPECT images reflect only the amount of radioactivity detected by the scanner. The scanner cannot distinguish between sources of radioactivity (which radionuclide or which radiopharmaceutical was administered). Therefore, sufficient time (at least six half-lives of the radionuclide) must pass between consecutive scans on the same subject; otherwise, the second scan will be contaminated from residual signal from the first. In addition, once injected, radiopharmaceuticals are broken down by enzymes in the liver and other tissues (including brain in some instances) leading to the generation of radiolabeled metabolites. If these metabolites are generated in the brain or cross from the blood into the brain, they will contribute to the total signal in the resulting images, potentially confounding accurate quantification. For this reason, using radiopharmaceuticals that do not generate radiometabolites that cross the blood–brain barrier is beneficial. Another problem is cross-selectivity and nonspecific binding. If a radiopharmaceutical binds more than one receptor in the brain, the resulting image will overestimate the density of the intended target. As radiopharmaceuticals must be lipophilic to cross the blood–brain barrier, they often bind nonspecifically to lipids throughout the brain. Both specific binding to the target protein and nonspecific binding contribute to the signal seen on the resulting image. However, only the specific binding component represents the density of the target protein. Therefore, a high ratio of specific to nonspecific binding is favorable for reliable PET and SPECT measurements.

CLINICAL APPLICATIONS

The sensitivity of PET and SPECT are ideal for measuring specific biochemical changes in the brain. However, the expense of molecular imaging limits its cost-effectiveness in clinical practice. This is particularly true when diagnoses can be made with reasonable confidence using other techniques or when the results of molecular imaging are unlikely to alter management of the patient. Therefore, PET and SPECT imaging have a limited role in clinical neurology. However, as new disease-modifying therapies for neurologic disorders become available, molecular imaging may provide a critical role in predicting and monitoring treatment response.

The following radiopharmaceuticals are currently approved by the U.S. Food and Drug Administration (FDA) for indications in clinical neurology.

GLUCOSE IMAGING

The 2-deoxy-2-[^{18}F]fluoro-D-glucose (FDG) is structurally identical to D-glucose except for the substitution of ^{18}F for a hydroxyl group at the 2' position. Like glucose, FDG is taken up by cells using the glucose transporter and phosphorylated by hexokinase in the first step of glycolysis. Once phosphorylated, FDG becomes charged and therefore trapped in the cell. Lacking a 2' hydroxyl group, [^{18}F]FDG-6-phosphate cannot undergo further metabo-

lism. The concentration of FDG in cells therefore reflects the metabolic activity, both in taking up FDG via active transport and its phosphorylation during glycolysis.

Positron Emission Tomography Using ^{18}F-fluorodeoxyglucose in Epilepsy

Although the most widely used PET radiopharmaceutical for clinical applications, FDG is only approved by the FDA for cancer staging and evaluation, measuring myocardial viability in patients with coronary artery disease, and detecting seizure foci in epilepsy patients. In the case of epilepsy, during a seizure, the cells at the focus of epileptic activity will have greater metabolic demand and take up more FDG than surrounding cells. Therefore, focal increase in FDG-PET signal can identify epileptic foci if the scan is performed during a seizure. Between seizures, the epileptic focus often has lower metabolic demand than normal brain tissue, as repeated seizures are associated with decrement in baseline function. Therefore, interictal FDG-PET may show an area of hypometabolism (reduced FDG uptake) in the seizure foci. These findings may aid the neurosurgeon in planning surgical excision for treatment of refractory epilepsy.

Positron Emission Tomography Using ^{18}F-fluorodeoxyglucose in Dementia

FDG-PET is often used off-label to assist in diagnosis of dementia, particularly when attempting to distinguish Alzheimer disease from frontotemporal dementia (Fig. 22.2). Patients with Alzheimer disease typically show a signature pattern of FDG hypometabolism in the temporal and parietal cortices bilaterally. Patients with frontotemporal dementia, in contrast, show early hypometabolism in the prefrontal cortex, particularly in behavioral variant frontotemporal dementia. These differing patterns of hypometabolism may aid the clinician in making the correct diagnosis, particularly when both behavioral and memory symptoms are present in the same patient. Although not FDA approved for this purpose, the Centers for Medicare & Medicaid Services (CMS) provides reimbursement for FDG-PET when used for this indication.

DOPAMINE IMAGING

Ioflupane I^{123} (DaTscan) is a SPECT radiopharmaceutical that binds to presynaptic dopamine transporters (Fig. 22.3). Ioflupane I^{123} is approved to aid clinicians in distinguishing tremor caused

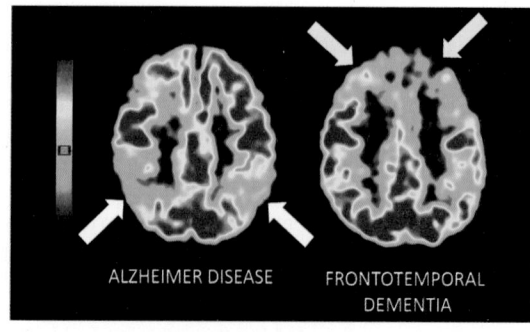

FIGURE 22.2 Using FDG-PET to distinguish Alzheimer disease from frontotemporal dementia. The Alzheimer disease patient on the left shows biparietal hypometabolism (*white arrows*), whereas the frontotemporal dementia patient on the right shows bifrontal hypometabolism (*yellow arrows*). (Image courtesy of Robert Innis and William Charles Kreisl, Molecular Imaging Branch, National Institute of Mental Health.)

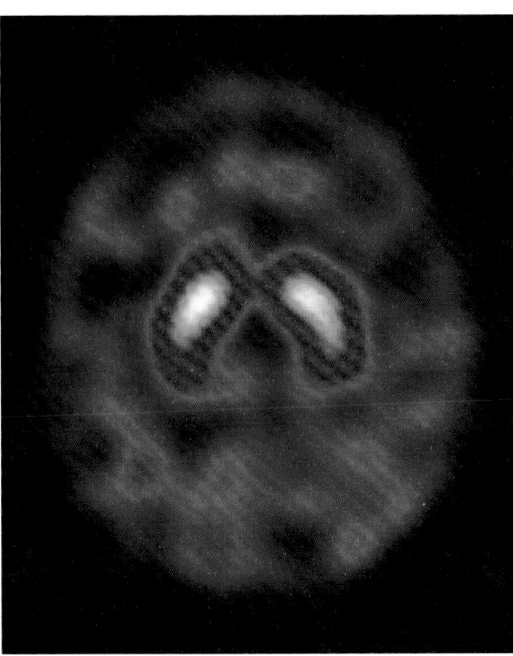

FIGURE 22.3 A normal Ioflupane I¹²³ (DaTscan) SPECT scan. The SPECT signal is concentrated in the striatum bilaterally, reflecting normal density of presynaptic dopamine transporters and intact nigrostriatal dopaminergic innervation.

by neurodegenerative parkinsonian syndromes from that caused by essential tremor. In the former, loss of dopaminergic neurons that originate in the substantia nigra will result in fewer presynaptic dopamine transporters in the striatum. Patients with neurodegenerative parkinsonian syndrome will have reduced striatal signal on DaTscan, whereas a patient with essential tremor will have normal signal.

PERFUSION IMAGING

[⁹⁹ᵐTc]-hexamethyl-propylene amine oxime (HMPAO) (*Neurolite*) and [⁹⁹ᵐTc] ethylcysteinate dimer (ECD) (*Ceretec*) are SPECT radiopharmaceuticals approved as adjunct in detecting areas of abnormal cerebral perfusion in patients who have had a stroke. These SPECT scans are often performed after vasodilatory challenge with acetazolamide to measure cerebrovascular reserve. SPECT perfusion imaging can also be used to identify ictal foci in patients with seizures or status epilepticus. Because reduced blood flow typically localizes to neurodegeneration, perfusion SPECT may also be used to distinguish different types of dementia.

AMYLOID IMAGING

Several PET radiopharmaceuticals that label the β-amyloid plaques found in Alzheimer disease have been developed (Fig. 22.4). These compounds bind to amyloid in neuritic plaques more strongly than diffuse plaques and do not label soluble amyloid at all. As studies suggest that amyloid plaque deposition occurs years prior to symptom onset, amyloid PET may be of particular use in early diagnosis of Alzheimer disease to distinguish mild cognitive impairment caused by Alzheimer disease versus that caused by other entities. Because non-Alzheimer diagnoses such as cerebral amyloid angiopathy and dementia with Lewy bodies may be associated with amyloid deposition in brain, and up to one-third of older cognitively normal adults have incidental amyloid positivity

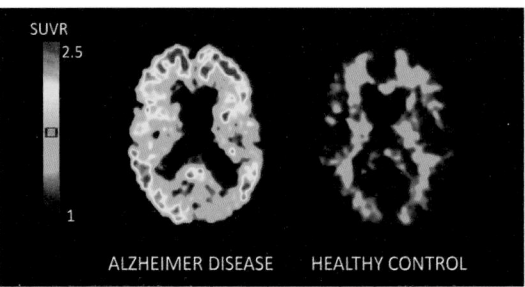

FIGURE 22.4 Example of amyloid PET imaging. [¹¹C] Pittsburgh compound B PET shows binding in amyloid plaque–rich cortical areas in the patient with Alzheimer disease but not the age-matched cognitively normal control subject. Binding in the control subject is limited to nonspecific binding in white matter. (Image courtesy of Robert Innis and William Charles Kreisl, Molecular Imaging Branch, National Institute of Mental Health.)

on PET, a positive amyloid scan should not be taken as proof positive of an Alzheimer disease diagnosis. However, a negative scan is considered inconsistent with the known neuropathology of Alzheimer disease. The amyloid-detecting radiopharmaceutical [¹¹C] Pittsburgh compound B has been widely used in Alzheimer disease research; however, the short half-life of ¹¹C makes its clinical use impractical. [¹⁸F] Florbetapir (*Amyvid*), [¹⁸F]flutemetamol (*Vizamyl*), and [¹⁸F]florbetaben (*Neuraceq*) have longer half-lives and have been approved by the FDA to assist clinicians in the diagnosis of Alzheimer disease. In 2013, the CMS decided not to provide coverage for amyloid PET imaging for diagnosis of Alzheimer disease, except for patients participating in certain studies under a Coverage with Evidence Development program. As the cost of amyloid imaging remains prohibitive to most patients, the most practical advantage may be in enriching clinical trials so as to avoid accidental inclusion of patients with non-Alzheimer diagnoses.

SUGGESTED READINGS

Abi-Dargham A, Gandelman M, Zoghbi SS, et al. Reproducibility of SPECT measurement of benzodiazepine receptors in human brain with iodine-123-iomazenil. *J Nucl Med*. 1995;36(2):167–175.

Accorsi R. Brain single-photon emission CT physics principles. *AJNR Am J Neuroradiol*. 2008;29(7):1247–1256.

Benamer TS, Patterson J, Grosset DG, et al. Accurate differentiation of parkinsonism and essential tremor using visual assessment of [123I]-FP-CIT SPECT imaging: the [123I]-FP-CIT study group. *Mov Disord*. 2000;15(3):503–510.

Blennow K, Hampel H, Zetterberg H. Biomarkers in amyloid-beta immunotherapy trials in Alzheimer's disease. *Neuropsychopharmacology*. 2014;39(1):189–201.

Fox PT, Mintun MA, Raichle ME, et al. A noninvasive approach to quantitative functional brain mapping with H2 (15)O and positron emission tomography. *J Cereb Blood Flow Metab*. 1984;4(3):329–333.

Friedland RP, Budinger TF, Ganz E, et al. Regional cerebral metabolic alterations in dementia of the Alzheimer type: positron emission tomography with [18F]fluorodeoxyglucose. *J Comput Assist Tomogr*. 1983;7(4):590–598.

Gomperts SN, Locascio JJ, Marquie M, et al. Brain amyloid and cognition in Lewy body diseases. *Mov Disord*. 2012;27(8):965–973.

Grimmer T, Diehl J, Drzezga A, et al. Region-specific decline of cerebral glucose metabolism in patients with frontotemporal dementia: a prospective 18F-FDG-PET study. *Dement Geriatr Cogn Disord*. 2004;18(1):32–36.

Innis RB, Cunningham VJ, Delforge J, et al. Consensus nomenclature for in vivo imaging of reversibly binding radioligands. *J Cereb Blood Flow Metab.* 2007;27(9):1533–1539.

Jack CR Jr, Knopman DS, Jagust WJ, et al. Tracking pathophysiological processes in Alzheimer's disease: an updated hypothetical model of dynamic biomarkers. *Lancet Neurol.* 2013;12(2):207–216.

Juni JE, Waxman AD, Devous MD Sr, et al. Procedure guideline for brain perfusion SPECT using (99m)Tc radiopharmaceuticals 3.0. *J Nucl Med Technol.* 2009;37(3):191–195.

Ly JV, Donnan GA, Villemagne VL, et al. 11C-PIB binding is increased in patients with cerebral amyloid angiopathy-related hemorrhage. *Neurology.* 2010;74(6):487–493.

Mazziotta JC, Engel J Jr. The use and impact of positron computed tomography scanning in epilepsy. *Epilepsia.* 1984;(25)(suppl 2):S86–S104.

Owen DR, Matthews PM. Imaging brain microglial activation using positron emission tomography and translocator protein-specific radioligands. *Int Rev Neurobiol.* 2011;101:19–39.

Pike KE, Ellis KA, Villemagne VL, et al. Cognition and beta-amyloid in preclinical Alzheimer's disease: data from the AIBL study. *Neuropsychologia.* 2011;49(9):2384–2390.

Rowe CC, Villemagne VL. Amyloid imaging with PET in early Alzheimer disease diagnosis. *Med Clin North Am.* 2013;97(3):377–398.

Saha GB. *Basics of PET Imaging Physics, Chemistry, and Regulations.* 2nd ed. New York: Springer; 2010:1–67.

Sokoloff L, Reivich M, Kennedy C, et al. The [14C]deoxyglucose method for the measurement of local cerebral glucose utilization: theory, procedure, and normal values in the conscious and anesthetized albino rat. *J Neurochem.* 1977;28(5):897–916.

Zanotti-Fregonara P, Lammertsma AA, Innis RB. Suggested pathway to assess radiation safety of (1)(8)F-labeled PET tracers for first-in-human studies. *Eur J Nucl Med Mol Imaging.* 2013;40(11):1781–1783.

Zoghbi SS, Liow JS, Yasuno F, et al. 11C-loperamide and its N-desmethyl radiometabolite are avid substrates for brain permeability-glycoprotein efflux. *J Nucl Med.* 2008;49(4):649–656.

Tatjana Rundek

INTRODUCTION

Neurovascular ultrasound includes two major ultrasound imaging technologies: extracranial ultrasound (duplex ultrasound or Color Doppler) and transcranial ultrasound (transcranial Doppler). Together, these techniques provide a real-time, noninvasive, comprehensive, and affordable evaluation of the major brain-supplying arteries. Besides, these imaging technologies are repeatable and portable and therefore can be performed at bedside, emergency rooms, or at any other patient care settings. Extracranial Doppler and transcranial Doppler have become an integral part of the evaluation of patients with cerebrovascular disease or in asymptomatic individuals at an increased risk of vascular disease. These technologies are also an integral part of primary and comprehensive stroke centers. The most established clinical situations for the use of neurovascular ultrasound include the early detection and characterization of extracranial and intracranial atherosclerosis and occlusive disease; the evaluation of cerebral hemodynamic consequences of proximal arterial occlusive disease; monitoring of response to treatment of acute or chronic occlusive atherosclerotic disease; the time course and reversibility of cerebral vasospasm after subarachnoid hemorrhage; the detection of cerebral emboli in patients with cardiac, aortic, and carotid disease; and selection of sickle cell patients for blood transfusion as an effective imaging technology in primary stroke prevention. Neurovascular ultrasound is often used to complement other neuroimaging technologies such as magnetic resonance angiography (MRA) and computed tomography angiography (CTA). All of these neuroimaging techniques provide concordant results when performed in accredited laboratories. If discrepancies arise, conventional two-dimensional angiography may be indicated, mainly if an immediate interventional revascularization procedure is considered.

EXTRACRANIAL ULTRASOUND (DUPLEX ULTRASOUND OR COLOR DOPPLER)

Extracranial ultrasound is the noninvasive method of screening the extracranial carotid and vertebral arteries for an atherosclerotic disease with the lowest risk and cost. It provides real-time imaging of anatomy, physiology (hemodynamics), and pathophysiology of the extracranial circulation. Extracranial ultrasound is used in the risk stratification of patients with symptomatic or latent cerebrovascular disease as well as in asymptomatic patients to detect the presence of carotid stenosis and to evaluate other carotid artery phenotypes, including carotid plaque size, plaque echomorphology, intima-media thickness (IMT), and carotid stiffness.

Imaging modes of extracranial ultrasound include the *brightness* or *B mode*, where ultrasound echoes are displayed in various levels of gray; *color* or *C mode*, where the Doppler signal of blood flow velocities is displayed in color; *Doppler* or *D mode*, where shift in echoes is obtained from the moving blood particles and displayed as a Doppler spectrum of blood flow velocities; *power mode*, where the Doppler signal of blood flow is displayed independent of the angle of insonation and is therefore magnified; and *motion* or *M mode*, where motion of interfaces is recorded along the depth axis. An ultrasound system that combines the B and D modes is called *duplex ultrasound*, and if B, C, and D modes are combined, it is called "triplex" or *Color Doppler*. All modern ultrasound systems are now equipped with all of these imaging modes.

CAROTID ULTRASOUND CRITERIA FOR DETECTION OF CAROTID STENOSIS

Traditionally, carotid stenosis is usually defined as stenosis greater than 50% by carotid ultrasound criteria. The most important ultrasound measures in assessing carotid stenosis are peak systolic (PS) velocity, end-diastolic (ED) velocity, and velocity ratios. These are applied in prestenotic, stenotic, and poststenotic regions. The degree of stenosis is also assessed visually from gray-scale ultrasound images and crosschecked with Color Doppler imaging, which can guide Doppler velocity determination in order to select the most critical part of stenosis for Doppler velocity examination. The examples of carotid ultrasound criteria for the degree of carotid stenosis are widely available. The Society of Radiologists in Ultrasound has published multidisciplinary consensus on diagnostic criteria to grade the internal carotid artery (ICA) stenosis using Duplex ultrasound [**Level 1**][1] (Table 23.1). These criteria can be used as a template for new vascular laboratories as well as to validate individual laboratory criteria for the estimation of carotid stenosis (Fig. 23.1). Because of Doppler velocity measurement variability and specific patient populations, there are discrepant criteria for Doppler parameters of carotid stenosis. Each carotid ultrasound laboratory must, therefore, develop and validate its own criteria to grade carotid stenosis. These parameters must be validated with other imaging modalities and/or surgical findings and an ongoing quality control program must be implemented.

ASSESSMENT OF CAROTID ARTERY AFTER CAROTID ENDARTERECTOMY AND STENTING

Carotid imaging shows changes in the carotid artery wall after successful carotid surgery or stenting. Special attention needs to be paid to the evaluation of the arterial wall changes at the edges of carotid reconstruction where incomplete plaque removal and residual stenosis can be detected. In addition, Doppler velocities may show values above normal through the reconstructed part of the artery likely due to flow remodeling or increased stiffness in the stented segments. If PS velocities at maximal narrowing in the reconstructed artery is greater than 150 cm/s and the PS ratio between stenotic and prestenotic (or prestented) segment is greater than 2, then significant restenosis likely occurred (Fig. 23.2).

TABLE 23.1	The Society of Radiologists in Ultrasound Multidisciplinary Consensus Criteria for Carotid Stenosis			
Degree of Stenosis	ICA PSV (cm/s)	Plaque	ICA/CCA PSV ratio	ICA EDV (cm/s)
Normal	<125	None	<2	<40
<50%	<125	<50% diameter reduction	<2	<40
50%–69%	125–230	≥50% diameter reduction	2.0–4.0	40–100
70% to near occlusion	>230	≥50% diameter reduction	>4	>100
Near occlusion	High, low, or undetectable	Visible, detectable lumen	Variable	Variable
Occlusion	Undetectable	Visible, no detectable lumen	Not applicable	Not applicable

ICA, internal carotid artery; PSV, peak systolic velocity; CCA, common carotid artery; EDV, end-diastolic velocity.

Data from Grant EG, Benson CB, Moneta GL, et al. Carotid artery stenosis: gray-scale and Doppler US diagnosis—Society of Radiologists in Ultrasound Consensus Conference. *Radiology.* 2003;229(2):340–346.

SENSITIVITY AND SPECIFICITY OF DUPLEX ULTRASOUND IN DETECTING CAROTID STENOSIS

Extracranial ultrasound is accurate and reliable in detecting carotid stenosis. The positive predictive value (PPV) of carotid ultrasound as compared to conventional angiography is 82% to 97%. In a large meta-analysis of 17 studies comparing carotid ultrasound with carotid angiography, carotid ultrasound had a pooled sensitivity of 86% (95% CI, 84% to 89%) and a pooled specificity of 87% (95% CI, 84% to 90%) for carotid stenosis [Level 1].[2] For diagnosis of occlusion, carotid ultrasound had a sensitivity of

96% (95% CI, 94% to 100%). Although there can be considerable variation in the accuracy of duplex scanning among laboratories, accreditation programs such as Intersocietal Accreditation Commission (IAC) set standards for performance and accuracy of vascular testing.

CAROTID ULTRASOUND OF CAROTID PLAQUE SIZE, MORPHOLOGY, AND CAROTID INTIMA-MEDIA THICKNESS

Carotid ultrasound provides information on plaque size (regardless of the degree of stenosis) and plaque echomorphology.

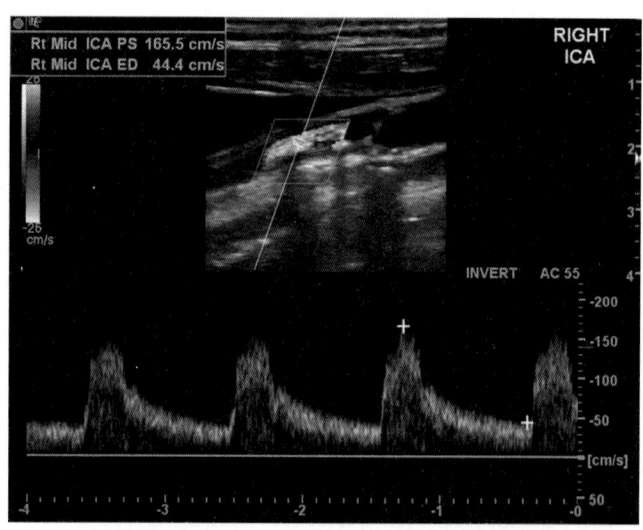
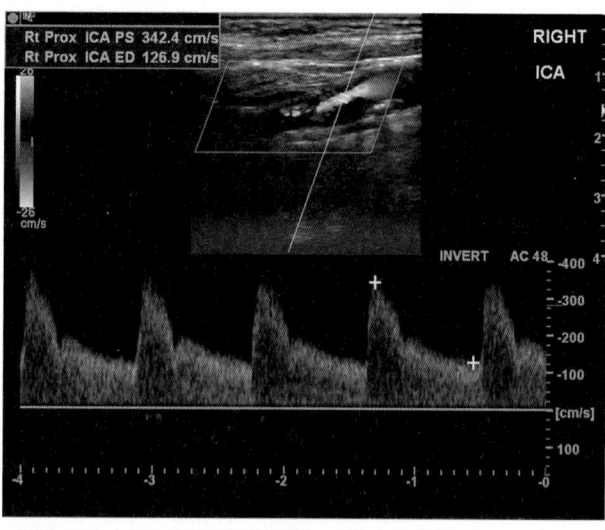

FIGURE 23.1 Two Color Doppler carotid artery studies, each showing different degree of the extracranial internal carotid stenosis. The studies show B mode (brightness mode) ultrasound image (gray scale) of the internal carotid artery (*ICA*) with corresponding atherosclerotic plaque, C mode (color mode) with color-coded blood flow velocity in the chosen volume sample (*the selected box in the image*), and D mode (Doppler mode) with the blood flow waveforms representing the velocity profile calculated from the Doppler shift (waveforms shown with velocity in cm/s in each picture from the chosen volume sample (represented by the *diagonal line* within the color-selected box). The peak systolic (*PS*) and end-diastolic (*ED*) velocities are marked with the yellow calipers in both pictures and used for the assessment of the degree of carotid stenosis. Two examples of varying degrees of ICA stenosis are presented: **(A)** ICA stenosis of 40% to 60%, with PS velocity of 165.5 cm/s and ED velocity of 44.4 cm/s (or 50% to 70% stenosis using the Society of Radiologists in Ultrasound Multidisciplinary Consensus Criteria[1]); and **(B)** with ICA stenosis of 60% to 80% (or >70% using the Society of Radiologists in Ultrasound consensus), with PS velocity of 342.4 cm/s and ED velocity of 126.9 cm/s and moderate turbulent blood flow.

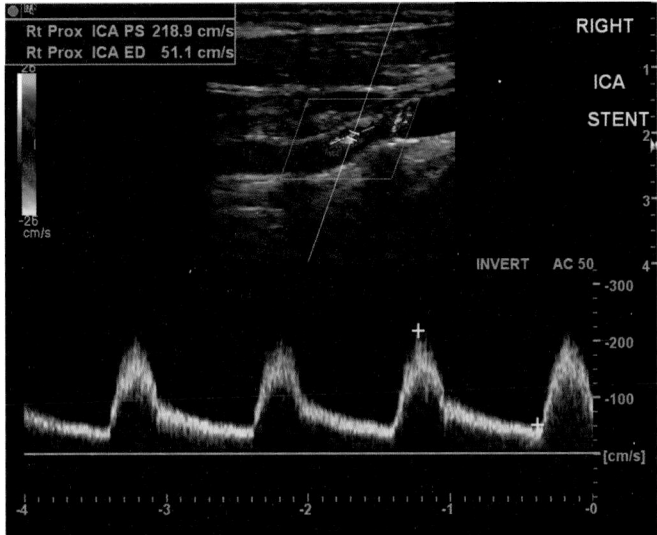

FIGURE 23.2 Carotid in-stent stenosis. Color Doppler of the common carotid artery and the internal carotid artery shows stent placed in both arteries. The lumen in the proximal internal carotid artery is reduced. The peak systolic (*PS*) and end-diastolic (*ED*) velocities are marked with the *yellow calipers* in spectral image and used for the assessment of in-stent stenosis. In the narrowing segment, PS velocity was 218.9 cm/s and ED velocity 51.1 cm/s, which indicates in-stent stenosis greater than 50%.

The *presence of small nonstenotic carotid plaque* on ultrasound is an independent predictor of future stroke and other cardiovascular disease independent of the degree of stenosis, although it is related to the degree of carotid stenosis. Detection of *plaque ulceration* by ultrasound imaging is limited. However, *plaque surface irregularity* is easy to detect on ultrasound and was shown to be associated with an increased risk of stroke. Ultrasound may help characterize plaque using a qualitative scoring system (echolucent or echodense; homogenous or heterogeneous plaque) as well as by the quantitative, computer-assisted echodensity parameters, such as the *gray-scale median* (GSM) *index*, recently shown to be clinically relevant in the prediction of stroke. *Echolucent carotid plaque* (soft) has been associated with an increased risk of first-ever stroke or myocardial infarction in asymptomatic individuals. *Echodense carotid plaque* (calcified) is in general considered to be of a good prognostic feature based on the lower rates of stroke, but recent studies have shown opposite results with an increased risk of stroke. Similar observation was reported for coronary calcium score. This presumably paradoxical effect of plaque calcification may be explained by the fact that echodense plaque is not a cause of stroke but rather a marker of presence of an "active" plaque in other vascular beds, which then can explain its association with increased vascular risk.

Carotid IMT is a measure of subclinical atherosclerosis shown to be associated with an increased risk of stroke and other cardiovascular disease. It has been used extensively as an outcome measure in numerous clinical trials testing the effect of lipid, blood pressure, and glucose-lowering medications. It has been associated with traditional vascular risk factors across different age groups, including in children and young adults. The American Society of Echocardiography and Society for Vascular Medicine have supported the use of carotid IMT in vascular risk stratification in moderate-risk individuals and outlined the recommendations for the IMT protocols [**Level 1**].[3]

DUPLEX ULTRASOUND OF THE VERTEBRAL ARTERIES

The ultrasound evaluation of the vertebral arteries (VAs) is similar to that of the carotid arteries. Examination of the VA is, however, limited by its anatomy because VA, unlike the carotid, cannot be traced continuously when it passes within the transverse processes of cervical vertebrae. Therefore, ultrasound examination of the extracranial VA is reliable only at the origin, intervertebral segments, and at the atlas-loop portion. Color Doppler and Power Doppler are particularly useful in assessing the caliber of VAs. Use of other diagnostic technologies (MRA, CTA, and even conventional angiography) is often recommended in symptomatic patients with suspected VA stenosis on Duplex ultrasound.

CONTRAST-ENHANCED ULTRASOUND

Contrast-enhanced ultrasound vascular imaging has been recently introduced as a novel extracranial ultrasound imaging. Intravenous ultrasound contrast agents are gas-filled microbubbles, which serve as intravascular reflectors of ultrasound waves. The potential clinical use of contrast-enhanced ultrasound has been proposed in different vascular beds including the carotid arteries. It is particularly useful in the situations of poor visualization of high-grade carotid stenosis or suspected occlusion, complex carotid plaques, and evaluation of plaques with suspected ulcerations. It also provides a novel, noninvasive method for the assessment of the vasa vasorum and the vascularization of the atherosclerotic plaque neovascularization, possibly helping in the risk stratification of patients with high risk of plaque rupture. In the future, the use of targeted microbubbles may further enhance the diagnostic capabilities of vascular ultrasound by detecting specific molecular processes important in the pathophysiology of atherosclerosis.

INDICATIONS FOR EXTRACRANIAL ULTRASOUND EXAMINATION

The guidelines for noninvasive vascular testing and indications for vascular ultrasound has been proposed by the American Society of Echocardiography and the Society for Vascular Medicine and Biology and adopted by other professional organizations, Centers for Medicare and Medicaid Services (CMS), and private insurers [**Level 1**].[4] *Indications for carotid artery ultrasound* include the following:

- Evaluation of patients with cerebral ischemia, stroke, or TIA
- Evaluation of patients with a cervical bruit
- Evaluation of pulsatile mass in the neck
- Evaluation of blunt neck trauma
- Preoperative evaluation of patients undergoing major cardiovascular or other major surgical procedures, including cardiac, liver, and kidney transplant
- Drop attacks or syncope (rare indications primarily seen in vertebrobasilar insufficiency or bilateral carotid artery disease)
- Vasculitis involving extracranial arteries
- Follow-up of patients with known carotid artery disease
- Evaluation of postoperative patients following carotid endarterectomy or carotid stenting
- Evaluation of suspected subclavian steal syndrome
- Evaluation of suspected carotid or VA dissection

INTRACRANIAL ULTRASOUND (TRANSCRANIAL DOPPLER)

Transcranial Doppler (TCD) is a noninvasive ultrasound technology that monitors blood flow velocity and blood flow direction in large intracranial arteries. Using a probe with great tissue-penetration properties, it is possible to insonate the major vessels of the circle of Willis, the distal intracranial segments of the VAs, and much of the length of the basilar artery (BA). Current TCD devices have a color-coded B mode and Power Doppler display. TCD provides only spectrum analysis of blood flow velocities, whereas transcranial Color Duplex Imaging (TCDI) provides spectrum analysis as well as color-coded imaging of the intracranial vessels and visualization in Power Doppler. Recently, transcranial Power Motion Doppler (PMD) has been introduced. PMD continuously displays flow intensity and direction of blood flow over 6 cm of intracranial space. Its advantage is in easier insonation, which allows inexperienced individuals to learn technique faster. Any of these TCD technologies produce the spectral signal that allows estimation of the degree of arterial stenosis.

Arteries of the circle of Willis are insonated through temporal, orbital, suboccipital (foramen magnum), and submandibular acoustic "windows." The measures used include distance from the probe, direction of flow (toward or away from the probe), flow velocities, and waveform characteristics.

INDICATIONS FOR TRANSCRANIAL DOPPLER ULTRASOUND

The American Institute of Ultrasound in Medicine (AIUM) has published practice guidelines [Level 1][5] for the performance of TCD for adults and children. *TCD indications in adults* include the following:

- Detection and follow-up of stenosis or occlusion in a major intracranial artery in the circle of Willis and vertebrobasilar system and monitoring of thrombolytic therapy in acute stroke

- Detection of cerebral vasculopathy
- Detection and monitoring of vasospasm in patients with sub-arachnoid hemorrhage
- Evaluation of collateral pathways of intracranial blood flow, including after intervention
- Detection of circulating cerebral microemboli
- Detection of right-to-left shunts
- Assessment of cerebral vasomotor reactivity
- As an adjunct in the confirmation of the clinical diagnosis of brain death
- Intraoperative and periprocedural monitoring to detect cerebral embolization, thrombosis, hypoperfusion, and hyperperfusion
- Evaluation of sickle cell disease to determine the stroke risk
- Assessment of arteriovenous malformations
- Detection and follow-up of intracranial aneurysms
- Evaluation of positional vertigo or syncope

Additional *TCD applications in children* include the following:

- Assessment of intracranial pressure and hydrocephalus
- Assessment of hypoxic ischemic encephalopathy
- Assessment of dural venous sinus patency

In the American Academy of Neurology report [Level 1],[6] the highest level of evidence was given to the use of TCD for the screening of children aged 2 to 16 years with sickle cell disease for stroke risk (Type A, Class I) and the detection and monitoring of angiographic vasospasm after spontaneous subarachnoid hemorrhage (Type A, Class I to II) (Table 23.2).

Sickle Cell Disease

TCD is an important tool for the selection of children with sickle cell disease in need of blood transfusion and who should stay on blood transfusion to sustain the benefit for prevention of stroke. In the STOP (Stroke Prevention Trial in Sickle Cell Anemia) trials, TCD detection of time-averaged maximum mean flow velocity

TABLE 23.2	Recommendations and Level of Evidence for the Use of Transcranial Doppler by the American Academy of Neurology Therapeutics and Technology Assessment Subcommittee
Setting/Disease/Condition	Rating of Recommendation/Level of Evidence
Sickle cell disease	Type A, Class I
Detection and monitoring of angiographic vasospasm	Type A, Class I–II
Detection of cerebral circulatory arrest/brain death	Type A, Class II
Intracranial steno-occlusive disease	Type B, Class II–III
Vasomotor reactivity testing	Type B, Class II–III
Monitoring carotid endarterectomy	Type B, Class II–III
Cerebral microembolism detection	Type B, Class II–IV
Monitoring cerebral thrombolysis	Type B, Class II–III
Monitoring coronary artery bypass graft surgeries	Type B–C, Class II–III
Right-to-left cardiac shunts	Type A, Class II
Intracranial occlusive disease	Type B, Class II–IV

Type A, established as useful/predictive recommendation; Type B, probably useful/predictive; Type C, possibly useful/predictive; Class I, evidence provided by prospective study in broad spectrum of persons with suspected condition, using a "gold standard" to define cases, where test is applied in blinded evaluation, and enabling assessment of appropriate tests of diagnostic accuracy; Class II, evidence provided by prospective study in narrow spectrum of persons with suspected condition or well-designed retrospective study of broad spectrum of persons with suspected condition (by gold standard) compared with broad spectrum of controls where test is applied in blinded evaluation and enabling assessment of appropriate tests of diagnostic accuracy; Class III, evidence provided by retrospective study where either persons with established condition or controls are of narrow spectrum and where test is applied in blinded evaluation; Class IV, any design where test is not applied in blinded fashion or evidence provided by expert opinion or descriptive case series.

From Sloan MA, Alexandrov AV, Tegeler CH, et al; Therapeutics and Technology Assessment Subcommittee of the American Academy of Neurology. Assessment: transcranial Doppler ultrasonography: report of the Therapeutics and Technology Assessment Subcommittee of the American Academy of Neurology. *Neurology.* 2004;62(9):1468–1481.

(MFV) of 200 cm/s (not mean velocity) on two separate examinations in middle cerebral artery (MCA) or TICA (terminal ICA) was used to determine the need for blood transfusion that resulted in 90% relative risk reduction of first-ever stroke. Moreover, long-term follow-up results from the STOP trials indicated that persistent elevation in TCD velocities in these patients is indicative of ongoing increased risk of stroke.

Intracranial Stenosis and Occlusion

Stenosis of greater than 50% lumen narrowing can reliably be detected in arterial segments with anatomically favorable insonation angles, particularly in the M1 segment of the MCA. Significant narrowing of intracranial arteries results in focal increases in flow velocities, turbulent flow, and increased waveform pulsatility at the level of stenosis. Compensatory collateral flow from uncompromised vessels to deprived areas may result in flow reversal and augmentation of flow. Because some patients have suboptimal temporal windows, failure to obtain a waveform reading does not imply vessel occlusion unless a prior study had demonstrated vessel patency. An intracranial stenosis of the major intracranial arteries should be suspected when the normal hierarchy of the flow velocities is disrupted. The flow in the MCA should be greater than in the anterior cerebral artery (ACA), where blood flow velocities should be greater than in the posterior cerebral artery (PCA) or BA and VA. The difference in these disrupted MFV should be greater than 20%. According to the SONIA (Stroke Outcomes and Neuroimaging of Intracranial Atherosclerosis) criteria [Level 1],[7] the TCD MFV cutoff for more than 50% stenosis for MCA is greater than 100 cm/s and for VA and BA is greater than 80 cm/s (Fig. 23.3).

Sensitivity and Specificity of Transcranial Doppler in Detecting Intracranial Stenosis

TCD can reliably detect stenosis in M1 segment of MCA, ICA syphon and terminal ICA, terminal VA, proximal BA, and P1 segment of PCA. The sensitivity of TCD for stenosis in these segments is 85% to 90% and specificity is 90% to 95%. PPV is 85% and negative predictive value (NPV) is 98%, with lower accuracy values for posterior circulation. In the SONIA trial [Level 1],[7] the accuracy of TCD in detection of intracranial steno-occlusive disease was superior to CTA or digital subtraction angiography (DSA) for ruling out than ruling in stenosis (having a higher NPV than PPV) for all intracranial arterial segments.

Detection of Arteriovenous Malformations

Arteriovenous malformations (AVMs) are direct communications between the arterial and venous systems, without an intervening capillary bed. No resistance vessels exist to impede or regulate flow, and flow measurements from feeding vessels typically demonstrate elevated velocities and low-resistance waveforms. Because of the large volume of flow that traverses an AVM, flow patterns may also be altered in vessels not directly connected to the AVM, resulting in altered waveform recordings. TCD is sensitive for the detection of medium- to large-sized AVMs. TCDI may provide more information about anatomic characteristics of AVMs than regular TCD.

Vasospasm in Subarachnoid Hemorrhage

TCD has become a standard procedure for the detection, quantification, and monitoring of arterial vasospasm after subarachnoid hemorrhage or head trauma. Most clinically important spasm occurs in the proximal cerebral vessels, which are accessible to TCD insonation. TCD monitoring, however, is limited in identifying vasospasm in distal cerebral arteries. TCD flow velocity criteria appear to be most reliable for detecting angiographic MCA and BA vasospasm. Mean MCA velocities greater than 120 cm/s are indicative of moderate vasospasm, whereas velocities greater than 200 cm/s show severe vasospasm. A Lindegaard ratio (MFV MCA/ICA) greater than 3 is suggestive of vasospasm, whereas a ratio of 6 or greater

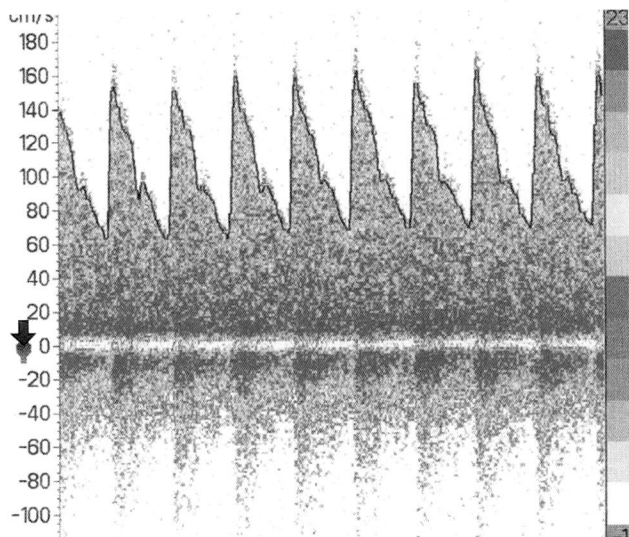
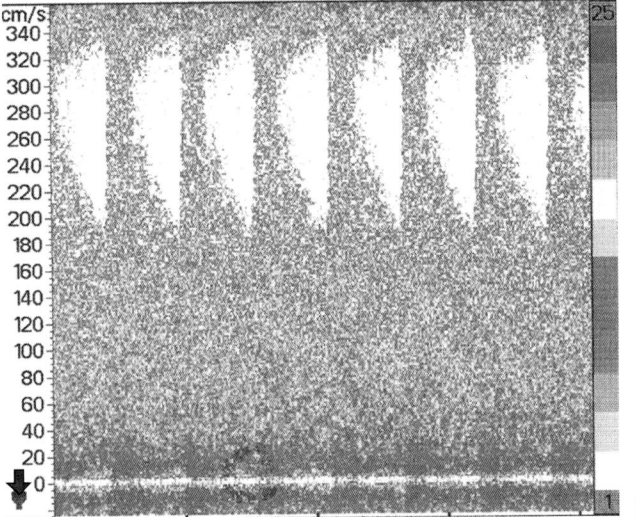

FIGURE 23.3 Example of TCD study of the both MCA (**A, left and B, right**) in patients with the right MCA stenosis. The spectral velocities are obtained at the depth of 50 cm from both sides of the head overlying the temporal bone. The blood flow velocity profile of the Doppler shift is calculated from the blood in the MCA flowing toward the probe (*the blue arrow on the left side of both images directed toward the probe*). The image on the left (**A**) represents the normal spectral flow with PS velocities of about 160 cm/s and ED velocities of about 60 cm/s. The image on the right (**B**) represents the high-grade MCA stenosis with systolic blood flow velocities over 320 cm/s and ED blood flow velocities of 200 cm/s and marked turbulent flow.

reliably predict the presence of clinically significant angiographic vasospasm. In addition, a sudden rise in MCA MFV by greater than 65 cm/s or by 20% increase is suggestive of vasospasm. TCD is most useful in monitoring the temporal course of vasospasm to help guide the timing of diagnostic and therapeutic angiographic interventions.

Cerebral Microemboli Detection

TCD can detect microemboli or high-intensity transient signal (HITS), which account for up to 70% of all ischemic strokes. Most of these emboli originate not only from carotid atherosclerosis but also from cardiac diseases including atrial fibrillation, prosthetic heart valves, right-to-left cardiac shunt (patent foramen ovale [PFO]), aortic arch atheroma, vertebral disease, and stenosis in other intracranial arteries. Criteria for microemboli are established by the consensus committee at the Ninth International Cerebral Hemodynamic Symposium [**Level 1**],[8] which defines microembolus as a TCD signal with (1) random occurrence during the cardiac cycle; (2) brief duration (embolic signals should be transient lasting <300 ms); (3) high intensity (at least 3 dB higher than the background blood flow signal); (4) primarily unidirectional signal within the Doppler spectrum; and is (5) accompanied by an audible component ("snap," "chirp," or "pop").

Cerebral Vasomotor Reactivity Testing

TCD can be used to assess cerebral hemodynamic reserve. When arterial perfusion in compromised, distal regulating arterioles dilate to allow more flow and to prevent cerebral ischemia. However, when perfusion is severely impaired, the arterioles are maximally dilated and cerebral vasomotor reactivity (CVR) decreases or disappears, indicating a state of exhausted cerebrovascular reserve or "misery" perfusion. Impaired CVR may predict impending ischemia in patients with extracranial or intracranial artery stenosis or occlusion. CVR tests include the breath-holding index, blood pressure changes, or the carbon dioxide (CO_2) inhalation test. Impaired CVR has been found in various conditions, including severe carotid artery stenosis, stroke, sleep apnea, and congestive heart failure. CVR is not a direct measure of cerebral autoregulation, but new methods that include correlations between flow velocities and spontaneous fluctuations in blood pressure have been developing to assess cerebral autoregulation.

Sonothrombolysis

TCD may be effective as an adjunct therapy to intravenous thrombolysis after acute MCA occlusion. Application of *intravascular low-intensity ultrasound* at the site of occlusion may enhance the outcome after ischemic stroke without the administration of tissue plasminogen activator (tPA). Also, augmentation of tPA-associated thrombolysis with standard diagnostic TCD monitoring has been safe and associated with a higher arterial recanalization rate. The CLOTBUST trial showed that patients with acute stroke treated with sonothrombolysis (tPA + 2 MHz TCD) had more dramatic clinical recovery and arterial recanalization (25% vs. 8%) without an increased risk of symptomatic hemorrhage. This resulted in a trend toward better outcome, with more patients having modified Rankin score of 0 to 1 at 3 months after stroke (42% vs. 29%). In addition, gaseous microspheres, initially developed as ultrasound contrast agents, can further increase the effectiveness of tPA. A microsphere dose-escalation study showed sustained complete recanalization rates of 67% in patients receiving TCD monitoring with perflutren lipid microspheres compared to controls receiving tPA alone with no increase in hemorrhage rate. TCD with the administration of microspheres is an emerging application in acute stroke management. Currently, a novel operator-independent TCD device for delivery of ultrasound energy has been tested in phase III efficacy trial of sonothrombolysis (named CLOTBUSTER).

LIMITATIONS OF TRANSCRANIAL DOPPLER

TCD is highly operator dependent. It requires technical skills, detailed three-dimensional knowledge of cerebrovascular anatomy and its variations, and global understanding of brain hemodynamics. The use of TCD is also limited by the 10% to 15% rate of inability to perform TCD due to inadequate acoustic windows, which is prevalent in blacks, Asians, and elderly women. This is related to thickness and porosity of the bone, which causes attenuation of the ultrasound energy transmission. TCD examination is also limited to the large cerebral basal arteries, and it cannot directly examine a status of local cerebral blood flow. These limitations of TCD are the main reason for its underutilization, and most of them can be overcome by vascular laboratory accreditation and proper training and certification of sonographers and interpreting physicians.

LEVEL 1 EVIDENCE

1. Grant EG, Benson CB, Moneta GL, et al. Carotid artery stenosis: gray-scale and Doppler US diagnosis—Society of Radiologists in Ultrasound Consensus Conference. *Radiology.* 2003;229(2):340–346.

2. Wardlav JM, Chappell FM, Best JJ, et al; NHS Research and Development Health Technology Assessment Carotid Stenosis Imaging Group. Non-invasive imaging compared with intra-arterial angiography in the diagnosis of symptomatic carotid stenosis: a meta-analysis. *Lancet.* 2006;367(9521):1503–1512.

3. Stein JH, Korcarz CE, Hurst RT, et al; American Society of Echocardiography Carotid Intima-Media Thickness Task Force. Use of carotid ultrasound to identify subclinical vascular disease and evaluate cardiovascular disease risk: a consensus statement from the American Society of Echocardiography Carotid Intima-Media Thickness Task Force. Endorsed by the Society for Vascular Medicine. *J Am Soc Echocardiogr.* 2008;21(2):93–111.

4. Gerhard-Herman M, Gardin JM, Jaff M, et al; American Society of Echocardiography, Society for Vascular Medicine and Biology. Guidelines for noninvasive vascular laboratory testing: a report from the American Society of Echocardiography and the Society for Vascular Medicine and Biology. *Vasc Med.* 2006;11(3):183–200.

5. American College of Radiology, Society for Pediatric Radiology, Society of Radiologists in Ultrasound. AIUM practice guideline for the performance of a transcranial Doppler ultrasound examination for adults and children. *J Ultrasound Med.* 2012;31(9):1489–1500.

6. Sloan MA, Alexandrov AV, Tegeler CH, et al; Therapeutics and Technology Assessment Subcommittee of the American Academy of Neurology. Assessment: transcranial Doppler ultrasonography: report of the Therapeutics and Technology Assessment Subcommittee of the American Academy of Neurology. *Neurology.* 2004;62(9):1468–1481.

7. Feldmann E, Wilterdink JL, Kosinski A, et al. The Stroke Outcomes and Neuroimaging of Intracranial Atherosclerosis (SONIA) trial. *Neurology.* 2007;68:2099–2106.

8. Consensus Committee of the Ninth International Cerebral Hemodynamic Symposium. Basic identification criteria of Doppler microembolic signals. *Stroke.* 1995;26:1123.

SUGGESTED READINGS

Aaslid R, Lindegaard KF. Cerebral hemodynamics. In: Aaslid R, ed. *Transcranial Doppler Sonography*. New York: Springer-Verlag; 1986.

Alexandrov AV. Ultrasound enhanced thrombolysis for stroke. *Int J Stroke*. 2006;1(1):26–29.

Alexandrov AV, Sloan MA, Tegeler CH, et al; American Society of Neuroimaging Practice Guidelines Committee. Practice standards for transcranial Doppler (TCD) ultrasound. Part II. Clinical indications and expected outcomes. *J Neuroimaging*. 2012;22(3):215–224.

Alsulaimani S, Gardener H, Elkind MS, et al. Elevated homocysteine and carotid plaque area and densitometry in the Northern Manhattan Study. *Stroke*. 2013;44(2):457–561.

Brant-Zawadzki M, Heiserman JE. The roles of MR angiography, CT angiography, and sonography in vascular imaging of the head and neck. *Am J Neuroradiol*. 1997;10:1820–1825.

Brown OW, Bendick PJ, Bove PG, et al. Reliability of extracranial carotid artery duplex ultrasound scanning: value of vascular laboratory accreditation. *J Vasc Surg*. 2004;39(2):366–371.

De Bray JM, Baud JM, Dauzat M. Consensus concerning the morphology and the risk of carotid plaques. *Cerebrovasc Dis*. 1996;7:289–296.

Frontera JA, Rundek T, Schmidt JM, et al. Cerebrovascular reactivity and vasospasm after subarachnoid hemorrhage: a pilot study. *Neurology*. 2006;66(5):727–729.

Garami Z, Alexandrov AV. Neurosonology. *Neurol Clin*. 2009;27(1):89–108.

Garami ZF, Bismuth J, Charlton-Ouw KM, et al. Feasibility of simultaneous pre- and postfilter transcranial Doppler monitoring during carotid artery stenting. *J Vasc Surg*. 2009;49(2):340–344.

Hartmann A, Mast H, Thompson JL, et al. Transcranial Doppler waveform blunting in severe extracranial carotid artery stenosis. *Cerebrovasc Dis*. 2000;10(1):33–38.

Helton KJ, Adams RJ, Kesler KL, et al. Magnetic resonance imaging/angiography and transcranial Doppler velocities in sickle cell anemia: results from the SWiTCH trial. *Blood*. 2014;124(6):891–898.

Johnsen SH, Mathiesen EB, Joakimsen O, et al. Carotid atherosclerosis is a stronger predictor of myocardial infarction in women than in men: a 6-year follow-up study of 6226 persons: the Tromsø Study. *Stroke*. 2007;38(11):2873–2880.

Kolkert JL, Meerwaldt R, Loonstra J, et al. Relation between B-mode gray-scale median and clinical features of carotid stenosis vulnerability. *Ann Vasc Surg*. 2014;28(2):404–410.

Komotar RJ, Zacharia BE, Valhora R, et al. Advances in vasospasm treatment and prevention. *J Neurol Sci*. 2007;261(1–2):134–142.

Lennihan L, Petty GW, Fink ME, et al. Transcranial Doppler detection of anterior cerebral artery vasospasm. *J Neurol Neurosurg Psychiatry*. 1993;56(8):906–909.

Marshall RS, Rundek T, Sproule D, et al. Monitoring of cerebral vasodilatory capacity with transcranial Doppler carbon dioxide inhalation in patients with severe carotid disease. *Stroke*. 2003;34:945–949.

Mast H, Mohr JP, Thompson JL, et al. Transcranial Doppler ultrasonography in cerebral arteriovenous malformations. Diagnostic sensitivity and association of flow velocity with spontaneous hemorrhage and focal neurological deficit. *Stroke*. 1995;26:1024–1027.

Molina CA, Barreto AD, Tsivgoulis G, et al. Transcranial ultrasound in clinical sonothrombolysis (TUCSON) trial. *Ann Neurol*. 2009;66(1):28–38.

Moussa I, Rundek T, Mohr JP, eds. *Risk Stratification and Management of Patients with Asymptomatic Carotid Artery Disease*. New York: Taylor & Francis Group of London; 2007:95–105.

Moussouttas M, Trocio S, Rundek T. Vascular ultrasound: carotid and transcranial Doppler imaging. In: Orloff L, ed. *Head and Neck Ultrasound*. San Diego, CA: Plural Publishing; 2008:257–290.

Nederkoorn PJ, Brown MM. Optimal cut-off criteria for duplex ultrasound for the diagnosis of restenosis in stented carotid arteries: review and protocol for a diagnostic study. *BMC Neurol*. 2009;9:36.

Nussel F, Wegmuller H, Huber P. Comparison of magnetic resonance angiography, magnetic resonance imaging and conventional angiography in cerebral arteriovenous malformation. *Neuroradiology*. 1991;33:56–61.

Ortega-Gutierrez S, Petersen N, Masurkar A, et al. Reliability, asymmetry, and age influence on dynamic cerebral autoregulation measured by spontaneous fluctuations of blood pressure and cerebral blood flow velocities in healthy individuals. *J Neuroimaging*. 2014;24(4):379–386.

Prabhakaran S, Rundek T, Ramas R, et al. Carotid plaque surface irregularity predicts ischemic stroke: the Northern Manhattan Study. *Stroke*. 2006;37(11):2696–2701.

Prabhakaran S, Singh R, Zhou X, et al. Presence of calcified carotid plaque predicts vascular events: the Northern Manhattan Study. *Atherosclerosis*. 2007;195(1):e197–e201.

Rundek T. Beyond percent stenosis: carotid plaque surface irregularity and risk of stroke. *Int J Stroke*. 2007;2(3):169–171.

Rundek T, Arif H, Boden-Albala B, et al. Carotid plaque, a subclinical precursor of vascular events: the Northern Manhattan Study. *Neurology*. 2008;70(14):1200–1207.

Rundek T, Spence JD. Ultrasonographic measure of carotid plaque burden. *JACC Cardiovasc Imaging*. 2013;6(1):129–130.

Saqqur M, Tsivgoulis G, Molina CA, et al; CLOTBUST Investigators. Symptomatic intracerebral hemorrhage and recanalization after IV rt-PA: a multicenter study. *Neurology*. 2008;71(17):1304–1312.

Staub D, Partovi S, Imfeld S, et al. Novel applications of contrast-enhanced ultrasound imaging in vascular medicine. *Vasa*. 2013;42(1):17–31.

Touboul PJ, Hennerici MG, Meairs S, et al. Mannheim carotid intima-media thickness and plaque consensus (2004-2006-2011). An update on behalf of the advisory board of the 3rd, 4th and 5th watching the risk symposia, at the 13th, 15th and 20th European Stroke Conferences, Mannheim, Germany, 2004, Brussels, Belgium, 2006, and Hamburg, Germany, 2011. *Cerebrovasc Dis*. 2012;34(4):290–296.

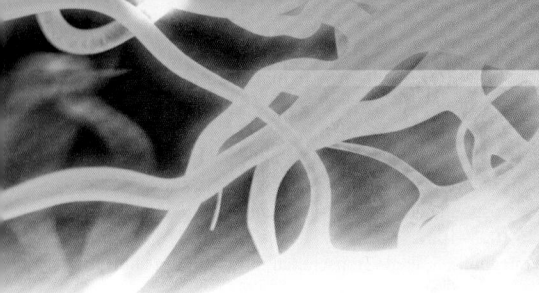

Angiography and Endovascular Neuroradiology 24

Charles A. Bruno Jr and Daniel H. Sahlein

INTRODUCTION

Interventional neuroradiology (INR) or endovascular surgical neuroradiology (ESNR) encompasses all invasive diagnostic and therapeutic interventions for diseases, often neurovascular, of the central nervous system and often the skull base, neck, spinal cord, and paraspinal soft tissues. INR is a continually evolving field that has made tremendous strides over the last several decades based largely on technologic advances leading to more therapeutic options and improvements in procedure safety and efficacy, leading to increasing acceptance of endovascular therapies by the biomedical neuroscience community.

TECHNIQUE

Cerebral angiography provides high-resolution images of the extracranial and intracranial cerebral vasculature (Fig. 24.1). The procedure is performed by accessing the femoral artery and threading a small catheter into the precerebral vessels.

The first cerebral angiogram in a living patient was performed by Egas Moniz in the early 1920s. During its infancy, cerebral angiography was performed via direct percutaneous puncture of the cervical carotid and vertebral arteries. This remained the principle technique for cerebral angiography until the late 1960s when the transfemoral approach was introduced. Transfemoral catheterization offered several advantages, not the least of which

included access to all four cerebral vessels with one puncture, improved patient comfort, less need for general anesthesia, the ability to perform cerebral angiography on an outpatient basis, and diminished stroke risk because of limited trauma to the precerebral arterial circulation. In the modern medical era, cerebral angiography is overwhelmingly performed via the transfemoral approach.

Although advances in noninvasive imaging of the cerebral vasculature have markedly improved over the last two decades, catheter angiography remains the gold standard for imaging cerebral blood vessels. Catheter angiography has two significant advantages over noninvasive vascular imaging; improved temporal resolution, meaning images can be acquired at a rate of 10 per second versus approximately 1 per second for computed tomography (CT) and magnetic resonance imaging (MRI); and spatial resolution—the voxel size (smallest unit for which there is only one signal, akin to a pixel on a cathode ray television) for fluoroscopy on the latest equipment is 0.1×0.1 mm versus an average of $0.4 \times 0.4 \times 3$ mm for CT and $1.0 \times 1.0 \times 0.9$ mm for an average clinical MRI. Figure 24.2 demonstrates both the differences in spatial and temporal resolution between postcontrast MRI and digital subtraction catheter angiography.

Mastery of both its acquisition and interpretation serves as the foundation for all interventional procedures. Modern catheter angiography is a relatively safe procedure associated with a low complication rate when performed by neurointerventionalists even in a highly complex patient population.

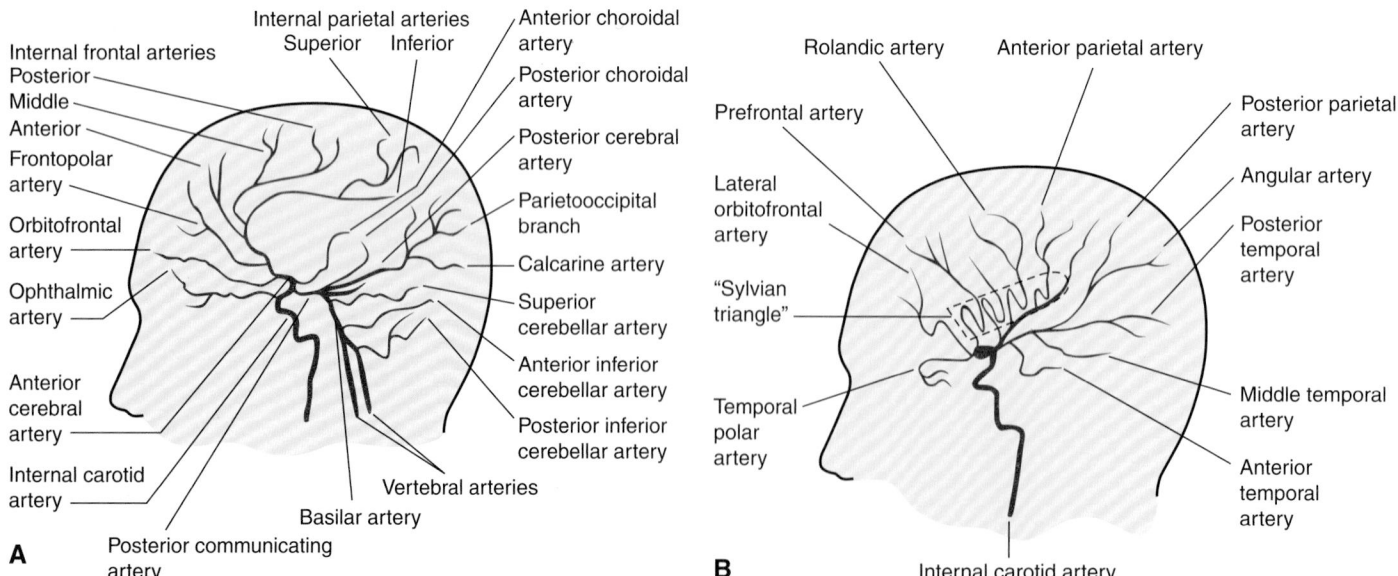

FIGURE 24.1 Major arterial vessels that supply the brain as viewed on a lateral angiogram. **A:** Anterior and posterior cerebral arteries. **B:** Biddle cerebral artery. (Adapted from Marshall R, Mayer S. *On Call Neurology.* 3rd ed. Philadelphia: Saunders; 2007.)

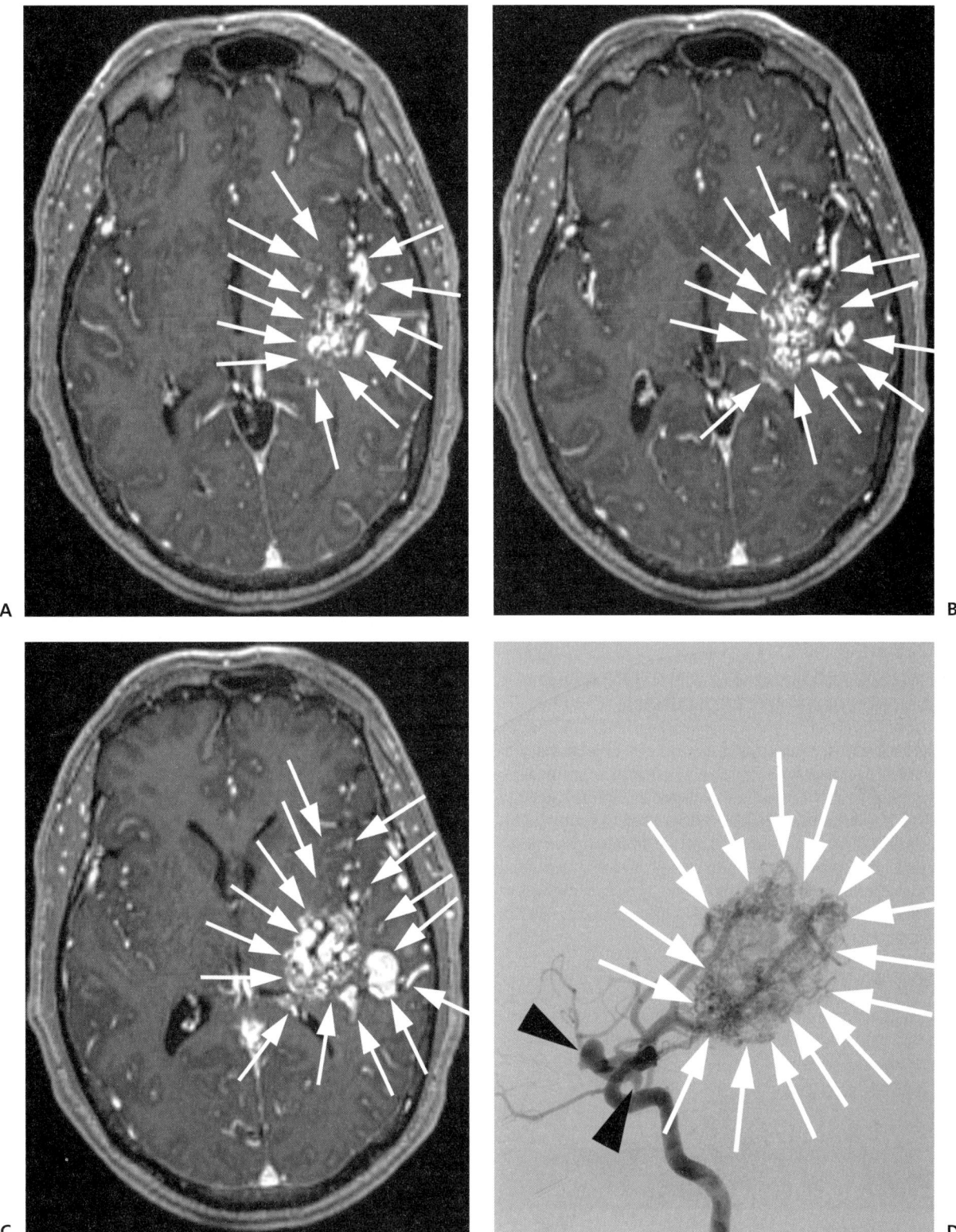

FIGURE 24.2 A–C: Three sequential transaxial T1-weighted postcontrast images from a 64-year-old male who presented with seizure. The images demonstrate a left frontotemporal brain arteriovenous malformation (AVM) (*white arrows*). On the MRI, it is difficult to distinguish nidus from draining vein. Nidal measurements are important for surgical and radiotherapy risk assessment. **D–F:** Lateral images from a catheter cerebral angiogram from the same patient. **D:** Early arterial phase. Note the very clear identification of nidus on an image with no draining veins (*white arrows*). Also note two proximal arterial aneurysms (*black arrowheads*). *(continued)*

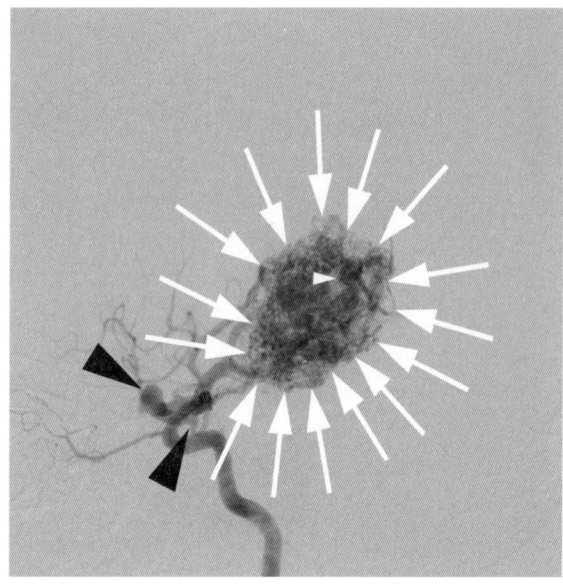
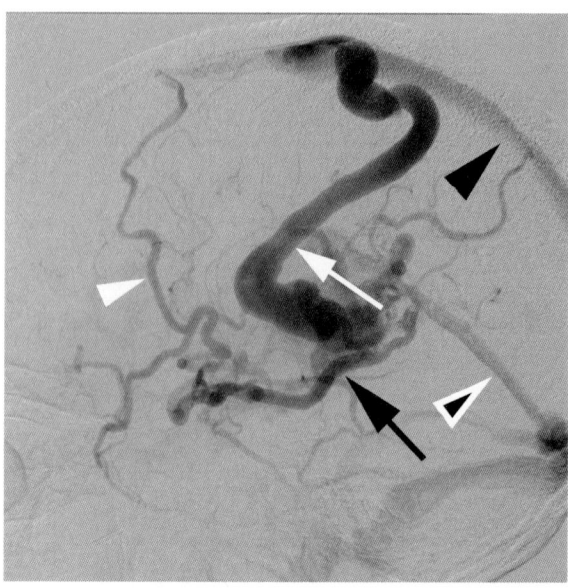

E   F

FIGURE 24.2 *(continued)* **E:** Slightly later in the arterial phase. The nidus has now completely opacified (*white arrows*) and there is the suggestion of very early venous opacification (*white arrowhead*). **F:** Venous phase: an excellent demonstration exclusively of veins draining the nidus. The nidus is drained by the vein of Trolard (*white arrow*), which drains secondarily into the anterior frontal veins (*white arrowhead*). There is deep venous drainage into the basal vein of Rosenthal (*black arrow*), which drains out via the Vein of Galen and straight sinus (*white and black arrowhead*).

CONDITIONS DIAGNOSED AND TREATED WITH ANGIOGRAPHIC TECHNIQUES

Angiography is useful for diagnosing a variety of conditions that affect the brain and spinal cord (Table 24.1). Because of its invasive nature, angiography functions as both a diagnostic and therapeutic modality. Major conditions that can be diagnosed or treated with angiographic techniques are discussed in the following sections. The most common complications of diagnostic and interventional angiographic procedures include stroke due to vessel occlusion or thrombosis and hemorrhage due to vessel perforation, dissection, and groin hematoma.

CEREBRAL ANEURYSMS

Cerebral aneurysms constitute a relatively common cerebrovascular abnormality with a prevalence of approximately 4%. Subarachnoid hemorrhage (SAH) is the most feared and common clinical presentation (see Chapter 39). Endovascular treatment of cerebral aneurysms has evolved dramatically over the past two decades and can now be offered as a viable alternative to craniotomy and microsurgical clipping in most cases.

Early endovascular endeavors to treat intracranial aneurysms used detachable balloons, pushable microcoils, and liquid embolic agents with varying degrees of procedural efficacy and safety. In 1991, Guido Guglielmi revolutionized endovascular treatment of cerebral aneurysms with the Guglielmi detachable coil (GDC). The GDC is designed with a thrombogenic platinum coil attached to a stainless steel delivery guide wire or mandrel. Once the coil is correctly positioned within the aneurysm, an electric current is applied to the guide wire, thereby electrolytically dissolving the soldered connection between the coil and delivery mandrel. The guide wire is subsequently removed and another coil can be advanced into the aneurysm until the aneurysm is completely excluded from the arterial circulation (i.e., no longer fills with contrast). A wide range of aneurysm morphologies can be treated because of the intrinsic compliance of the coil helix.

Treatment with GDC offers durable, long-term protection from aneurysm rebleeding. The rate of rebleeding following coil embolization is directly proportional to the percentage of the aneurysm that remains patent. Not surprisingly, the percentage of residual aneurysm patency following coil embolization is dependent on aneurysm neck size—the size of the opening connecting the aneurysm to the flowing blood. Small aneurysms with wide necks and large aneurysms (which typically have large necks as well) are most likely to be incompletely treated following coil embolization. To aid in the endovascular coil embolization of wide-necked aneurysms, balloon remodeling was introduced.

The *balloon remodeling technique* involves temporary inflation of a nondetachable balloon within the parent artery over the aneurysm neck during coil placement. The inflated balloon provides a resistive barrier to keep the coil within the aneurysm during and after deployment, preventing migration into the parent artery. The balloon

TABLE 24.1	Conditions Diagnosed by Angiography
1. Occluded or stenotic vessels	
2. Arterial dissections	
3. Aneurysms	
4. Arteriovenous malformations and other vascular malformations	
5. Vasculitic narrowing ("beading")	
6. Dural venous sinus thrombosis ("venous phase")	

remodeling technique is particularly useful in treating ruptured aneurysms with challenging neck anatomy because of the necessity of double antiplatelet therapy (usually aspirin and clopidogrel) when a permanent intravascular stent is used. Disadvantages of the technique include potential ischemia secondary to blood flow arrest, migration of the coil mass after the balloon is deflated, and intimal damage and thrombosis related to repeated inflation of the balloon.

A more recent iteration in the evolution of endovascular aneurysm treatment involves moving the matrix of reconstruction from the aneurysm sac (endosaccular) to the parent artery lumen (endoluminal) via the use of a stent. The procedure involves placement of a permanent cylindrical cage or stent (current available devices include the Neuroform stent, Enterprise stent, LVIS Device, and LVIS Jr. Device) across the neck of an aneurysm to act as a resistive barrier, preventing the deployed coils from herniating into the parent artery. There are three traditional techniques for coiling with stent assistance. One technique involves placing a stent within the parent artery across the neck of an aneurysm and subsequently accessing the aneurysm with a microcatheter through the wall of the stent. An alternative approach involves using two catheters in which a coil catheter tip is advanced into the aneurysm after which a stent is deployed across the aneurysm neck, effectively "jailing" the first catheter between the stent and the arterial wall. The final technique involves coiling the aneurysm with balloon assistance and subsequently placing a stent across the neck of the aneurysm. *Stent-assisted coiling* offers several advantages over coiling alone or balloon remodeling including creating a permanent buttress for the coil mass, decreasing blood flow across the neck of the aneurysm (potentially facilitating hemostasis within the aneurysm), and providing a scaffold for endothelialization.

The newest technology in aneurysm treatment namely *flow-diverting stents* are designed as endoluminal-only aneurysm treatment constructs. The first of these devices, the *Pipeline embolization device* (PED), represents a major paradigm shift in the endovascular treatment of intracranial aneurysms (Fig. 24.3). The PED is a braided stent with approximately 30% total metallic coverage versus less than 10% for the Neuroform and Enterprise stents. The PED is ideal for the treatment of large or giant, wide-necked, and fusiform aneurysms, as the stent construct can be deployed across the diseased segment of artery, rapidly resulting in hemostasis and slowly endothelializing over the course of months. In a cohort of anterior circulation aneurysms with a mean aneurysm size of 18 mm and a mean neck size of 9 mm treated with the PED, 74% of aneurysms were completely cured at 6 months and 87% at 1 year, with a 6% incidence of major ipsilateral stroke or neurologic death. Although flow diversion is a promising technique, careful analysis and follow-up of treated patients is required to determine its safety and efficacy. Stent placement requires the long-term use of dual antiplatelet agents to prevent thrombosis, potentially problematic in the setting of acute SAH.

Choosing between endovascular and open surgical treatment of intracranial aneurysms is a complex decision, often dependent on local preferences and physician skill and experience. Nevertheless, two randomized trials have compared the two options in the setting of SAH. The International Subarachnoid Aneurysm Trial (ISAT) was a prospective, randomized, multicenter trial designed to compare the safety and efficacy of endovascular coiling with microsurgical clipping [**Level 1**].[1,2] The study enrolled 2,143 patients between 1994 and 2003 with ruptured cerebral aneurysms and randomly assigned them to microsurgical clipping ($n = 1,070$) or endovascular coiling ($n = 1,073$). The primary outcome was death or dependence for activities of daily living at 1 year. This study showed that in this population of patients with small to moderate size anterior circulation aneurysms, endovascular coiling was safer

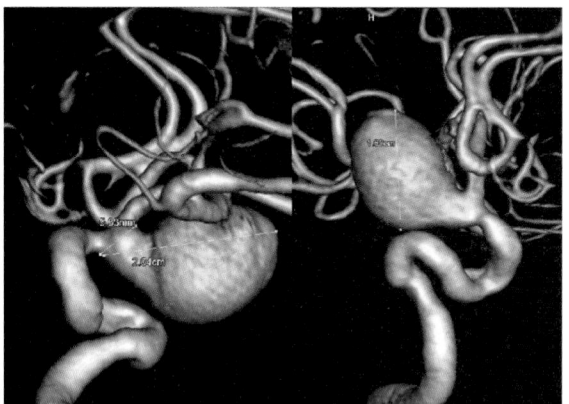

A

FIGURE 24.3 **A:** Two volumetric reconstructions from a catheter cerebral angiogram demonstrating a wide neck, giant aneurysm in a 72-year-old patient with worsening headaches. **B:** Three lateral catheter cerebral angiograms (left internal carotid artery injection). On the *left* is the pretreatment angiogram that demonstrates the aneurysm (*white arrows*). In the *center* is the angiogram immediately following placement of three pipeline embolization devices. Note that the angiogram is in the venous phase and yet contrast is still opacifying the aneurysm (*white arrows*), a function of the hemostatic feature of the flow-diverting stent. On the *right* is the 6-month follow-up angiogram demonstrating complete aneurysm cure.

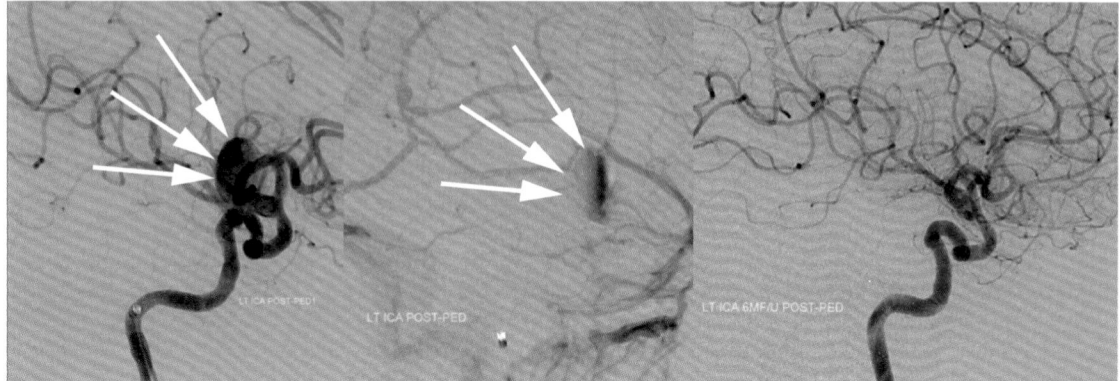

B

than surgical clipping: 24% of patients in the coiling arm were dead or dependent versus 31% in the clipping arm, a 23% relative risk reduction. At 5 years, there was a small but statistically significant increased risk of recurrent bleeding in the coil arm, but the risk of death was slightly albeit statistically significantly lower in the coiled group than in the clipped patients [**Level 1**].[3] The Barrow Ruptured Aneurysm Trial (BRAT) reported remarkably similar results. BRAT prospectively treated 471 aneurysm patients, alternating between coiling and clipping. Overall, 34% of patients in the clipping arm were dead or dependent at 1 year compared to 23% in the coil arm, a statistically significant difference [**Level 1**].[4] Nevertheless, 33% of those originally assigned to coiling crossed over to the clipping arm, reinforcing the need for open surgical treatment of difficult-to-coil aneurysms for the foreseeable future.

ARTERIOVENOUS MALFORMATIONS

Brain arteriovenous malformations (AVMs; see also Chapter 41) are subpial connections between arteries and veins that lack a normal capillary bed and articulate via a tangled network of dysplastic vessels known as a *nidus*, resulting in a direct connection between the arterial and venous systems. As is the case with aneurysms, rupture is the most feared complication of an AVM, with a risk of 1% to 4% per year.

Current therapeutic options for brain AVMs include microsurgical resection, radiosurgery, and endovascular embolization. Endovascular embolization tends to play an adjunct role in the treatment plan, typically in devascularizing the nidus prior to microsurgical resection, although it has been used increasingly as the sole treatment option. Embolization can also be used prior to or following radiosurgery and has also been used successfully to alleviate clinical symptoms and preserve or improve neurologic function in inoperable lesions. The liquid embolic agents n-butyl-cyanoacrylate (NBCA) and Onyx, a copolymer of ethylene vinyl, are the primary agents used for the endovascular treatment of cerebral AVMs.

Treatment of unruptured brain AVMs remains controversial. The Randomized trial of Unruptured Brain Arteriovenous malformations (ARUBA) compared outcomes in patients with unruptured brain AVMs who were treated with medical management with those treated with surgical or interventional therapy [**Level 1**].[5] A total of 223 patients were enrolled in the study: 114 were assigned to interventional therapy, whereas 109 patients received medical management alone. The study was prematurely halted because the risk of death or stroke was significantly lower in the medical management group than in the interventional therapy group.

DURAL ARTERIOVENOUS FISTULAS

Cranial or spinal dural arteriovenous fistulas (DAVFs; see also Chapter 41) are acquired pathologic shunts between dural arteries and dural venous sinuses. DAVFs are located within the leaflets of the dura matter and lack a distinctive vascular nidus. The pathogenesis of DAVFs is unknown, although multiple associations have been described including head trauma, infection, hypercoagulable states, and sinus thrombosis. Signs and symptoms include pulse-synchronous tinnitus and exophthalmos, cranial nerve deficits, cognitive impairment, venous infarction, intracranial hemorrhage, and even death, depending on fistula location, duration of disease, and venous drainage pattern. DAVFs most commonly occur in the transverse/sigmoid and cavernous sinuses.

DAVFs are dynamic lesions that may either spontaneously regress or progress. For this reason, close clinical and radiologic monitoring is critical. Treatment should be pursued for all lesions with cortical venous drainage or intolerable symptoms. First-line management of DAVFs is endovascular embolization via the transarterial route, transvenous route, or a combination of both. Transarterial embolization is typically performed with a liquid embolic agent such as NBCA or Onyx. Although cures are sometimes difficult to achieve through the transarterial route, it may be the only viable option in certain circumstances where transvenous embolization is not possible because of limited venous access to the fistula site due to stenosis or thrombosis.

Transvenous embolization is performed by retrograde catheterization of the involved dural sinus or cortical vein followed by deposition of coils and/or liquid embolic material at the site of inflow of the arteriovenous shunt. Transvenous embolization has been shown to have a high likelihood of cure and is often used to treat transverse/sigmoid sinus and cavernous sinus DAVFs. Detachable coils are deployed to form a scaffolding, after which pushable fibered coils, which are more thrombogenic and much less expensive, can then be added to achieve complete occlusion of the venous segment.

ACUTE ISCHEMIC STROKE

Globally, stroke remains the leading cause of disability and the second leading cause of death worldwide. Over the last two decades, the management of acute ischemic stroke (AIS) has dramatically changed with the introduction of novel pharmacologic and endovascular therapies aimed at arterial recanalization and reperfusion of ischemic brain tissue (see Chapter 35). Although the mainstay of emergency treatment for AIS is tissue plasminogen activator (TPA), endovascular therapy is increasingly being used in conjunction with thrombolytic therapy for patients with large-vessel occlusion (LVO) (see also Chapter 15).

Initial efforts at endovascular stroke therapy focused on intra-arterial (IA) administration of thrombolytics. The Prolyse in Acute Cerebral Thromboembolism II (PROACT II) study demonstrated that prourokinase, when given to patients with proximal middle cerebral artery (MCA) occlusion within 6 hours of onset of AIS, significantly improved clinical outcome at 90 days as compared to a control group given only intravenous heparin [**Level 1**].[6] Patients who received IA prourokinase demonstrated a 66% recanalization rate, with 40% having good clinical neurologic outcomes at 90 days as compared to 25% in the control arm. PROACT-II remains the only randomized trial supporting IA thrombolysis, which is not U.S. Food and Drug Administration (FDA) approved for the treatment of AIS. Many neurointerventionalists use IA thrombolytics off-label as adjunct to mechanical thrombectomy for distal small branch occlusions that may be difficult to access with larger mechanical devices.

The Mechanical Embolus Removal in Cerebral Ischemia (MERCI) retriever system was approved by the FDA in 2004 as the first mechanical thrombectomy device for removing clot in AIS patients. The MERCI retriever is a nitinol corkscrew-shaped microcatheter-deployed device that is advanced through occlusive thrombus and then pulled back to ensnare clot and allow it to be removed. The mechanical embolectomy is done through an 8- or 9-French balloon guide catheter that arrests antegrade flow and allows for aspiration during the clot retrieval process. The MERCI retriever system has undergone numerous redesigns since its introduction.

In 2008, the FDA approved a second endovascular device, the Penumbra aspiration system. This device is composed of two main components, a reperfusion catheter used for clot aspiration and a

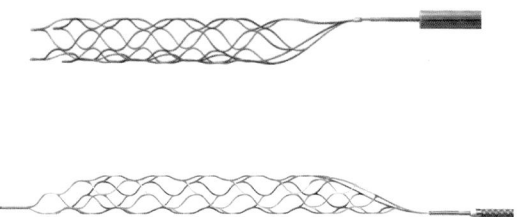

FIGURE 24.4 The "stentriever" stroke devices. The Solitaire device is depicted above the Trevo device.

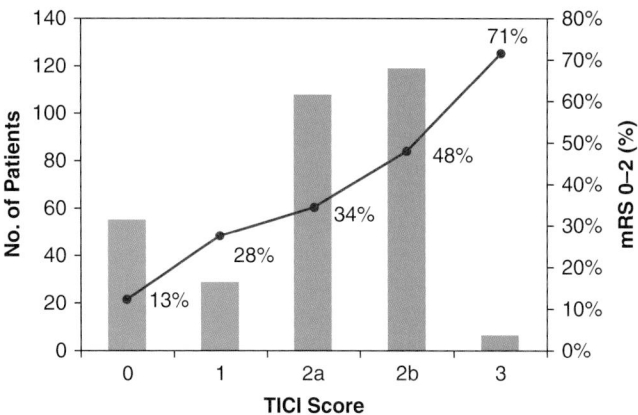

FIGURE 24.5 Ninety-day rates of good functional outcome stratified by degree of arterial recanalization. Note that in patients with good and complete recanalization (thrombolysis in cerebral infarction [TICI] grades 2b and 3), met the prespecified end point of 10% greater good functional outcome. (From Manning NW, Campbell BC, Oxley TJ, et al. Acute ischemic stroke: time, penumbra, and reperfusion. *Stroke.* 2014;45:640–644.)

separator or wire with a short segment of thickness near the tip used for mechanical breakdown of the thrombus. In the Penumbra Pivotal Stroke trial, a single-arm study of AIS patients presenting within 8 hours of onset, recanalization was achieved in 82% of the treated occluded arteries. More recently, Penumbra has introduced a larger aspiration catheter, the 5 Max Ace, which is designed for clot aspiration without the separator. ADAPT, a direct aspiration first-pass technique using this device, has been shown to be safe and effective for arterial thrombectomy.

Stent retrievers (or *stentrievers*) are the latest devices available for acute stroke treatment. These soft, self-expanding stents are adherent to and deployed at the end of a guide wire. Two devices are commercially available in the United States at present, the Solitaire (Medtronic) and Trevo (Stryker) devices (Fig. 24.4). Stentrievers are temporary self-expanding stents that when deployed capture thrombus and simultaneously restore blood flow by displacing clot peripherally against the artery wall. This positioning often temporarily restores blood flow, giving the brain a few minutes of restored perfusion. After a waiting period of several minutes, the stent is retrieved with the hope that the thrombus is removed as well, typically adherent to the stent. Several "passes" may be required to achieve satisfactory results and there is a possibility of breaking up the clot and creating distal emboli. Nevertheless, the stentrievers are a safe and effective tool for thrombectomy in AIS, with recanalization rates approaching 80% [Level 1].[7,8]

Uncontrolled cohort studies of patients with LVO treated with endovascular therapy have consistently shown that outcome is improved when vessel recanalization is achieved. Despite these observations, three large studies published in 2013 comparing endovascular therapy (alone or in combination with TPA) with TPA alone failed to show clinical benefit, raising serious questions about the efficacy of this approach [Level 1].[9–11] These trials were characterized by low recanalization rates in the endovascular treatment arms related to use of the older clot removal systems, long treatment windows, and variable patient selection criteria. In an unplanned post hoc analysis of these trials, LVO patients who were successfully recanalized again were shown to have better outcome than those who were not (Fig. 24.5). In 2014, the Multicenter Randomized Clinical Trial of Endovascular Treatment for Acute Ischemic Stroke in the Netherlands (MR CLEAN) reported significant improvement in 3-month outcome with no effect on mortality when TPA followed by endovascular therapy was compared to endovascular therapy alone (33% vs. 19% with good outcome) [Level 1].[12] Unlike these prior studies, MR CLEAN enrolled only patients with LVO documented by CT angiography, attained shorter intervention times, and relied exclusively on stent retriever technology, resulting in a near complete or complete recanalization rate of 75% compared to 33% in the patient treated with TPA alone (see Chapter 35 for details) [Level 1].[12]

EXTRACRANIAL AND INTRACRANIAL ARTERIAL OCCLUSIVE DISEASE

Endovascular treatment of carotid atherosclerotic disease is now considered to be a viable alternative to the gold standard treatment, carotid endarterectomy (CEA), in appropriately selected patients [Level 1].[13,14] Using current devices and techniques, carotid artery balloon angioplasty and stent placement (CAS) and CEA have nearly equivocal rates of complications, making the choice of therapy based more on medical comorbidities, carotid artery anatomy, and local clinical practice and expertise. A multidisciplinary team approach should be used to determine the most appropriate treatment for an individual patient. The risks and benefits of best medical management versus CEA versus CAS must be weighed before any intervention is considered.

CAS can be performed under conscious sedation or general oroendotracheal anesthesia. Prior to the procedure, patients are placed on dual antiplatelet agents, typically aspirin 81 mg and clopidogrel 75 mg for 7 to 10 days. Aspirin function and P2Y12 inhibition studies (platelet aggregometry) are performed before the procedure to ensure adequate platelet inhibition. Once femoral access is obtained, anticoagulation in the form of heparin is given to achieve an activated clotting time (ACT) of greater than 250. The ACT is checked every 30 to 60 minutes throughout the case and heparin is redosed as needed. A guide catheter is advanced just proximal to the stenosis, which is then crossed with a distal embolic protection device, a semipermeable membranous filter on a wire, which is placed within the distal cervical internal carotid artery. Alternatively, a proximal flow reversal system can be used in which a balloon tip catheter in the common carotid artery is used to establish antegrade flow arrest and a second balloon in positioned in the external carotid artery. Blood therefore flows retrograde down the internal carotid artery into the catheter. A venous shunt can be temporarily established via external tubing connecting to a femoral venous sheath to promote retrograde arterial flow during the period of arterial occlusion. After angioplasty with a balloon, stent deployment is performed. In general, the stent should be longer than the lesion and have a diameter corresponding to the largest diameter of the artery where stent placement is anticipated.

The use of intracranial balloon angioplasty for treatment of intracranial atherosclerotic disease has become increasingly controversial. The Stent Placement versus Aggressive Medical Management for the Prevention of Recurrent Stroke in Intracranial Stenosis (SAMMPRIS) was a randomized, multicenter trial comparing revascularization using stent angioplasty of the cerebral arteries versus medical therapy alone for symptomatic intracranial atherosclerotic disease. The study was stopped by the data safety monitoring board after 451 patients were enrolled because of significantly higher 30-day stroke or death rate in the stenting group than the medical management group (14.7% vs. 5.8%) [**Level 1**].[15] The study made no effort to distinguish between patients with thromboembolic versus perfusion failure–related infarcts, a critical physiologic difference in patients being assessed for reperfusion [**Level 1**].[15] Nevertheless, the selection criteria for use of intracranial stents has become more stringent, and use has declined.

LEVEL 1 EVIDENCE

1. Molyneux A, Kerr R; International Subarachnoid Aneurysm Trial Collaborative Group, et al. International Subarachnoid Aneurysm Trial (ISAT) of neurosurgical clipping versus endovascular coiling in 2143 patients with ruptured intracranial aneurysms: a randomized trial. *J Stroke Cerebrovasc Dis.* 2002;11:304–314.
2. Molyneux A, Kerr R, Stratton I, et al. International Subarachnoid Aneurysm Trial (ISAT) of neurosurgical clipping versus endovascular coiling in 2143 patients with ruptured intracranial aneurysms: a randomised trial. *Lancet.* 2002;360:1267–1274.
3. Molyneux AJ, Kerr RS, Birks J, et al. Risk of recurrent subarachnoid haemorrhage, death, or dependence and standardised mortality ratios after clipping or coiling of an intracranial aneurysm in the International Subarachnoid Aneurysm Trial (ISAT): long-term follow-up. *Lancet Neurol.* 2009;8:427–433.
4. McDougall CG, Spetzler RF, Zabramski JM, et al. The Barrow ruptured aneurysm trial. *J Neurosurg.* 2012;116:135–144.
5. Mohr JP, Parides MK, Stapf C, et al. Medical management with or without interventional therapy for unruptured brain arteriovenous malformations (ARUBA): a multicentre, non-blinded, randomised trial. *Lancet.* 2014;383:614–621.
6. Furlan A, Higashida R, Wechsler L, et al. Intra-arterial prourokinase for acute ischemic stroke. The PROACT II study: a randomized controlled trial. Prolyse in acute cerebral thromboembolism. *JAMA.* 1999;282:2003–2011.
7. Saver JL, Jahan R, Levy EI, et al. Solitaire flow restoration device versus the Merci Retriever in patients with acute ischaemic stroke (SWIFT): a randomised, parallel-group, non-inferiority trial. *Lancet.* 2012;380:1241–1249.
8. Nogueira RG, Lutsep HL, Gupta R, et al. Trevo versus Merci retrievers for thrombectomy revascularisation of large vessel occlusions in acute ischaemic stroke (TREVO 2): a randomised trial. *Lancet.* 2012;380:1231–1240.
9. Broderick JP, Palesch YY, Demchuk AM, et al. Endovascular therapy after intravenous t-PA versus t-PA alone for stroke. *N Engl J Med.* 2013;368:893–903.
10. Ciccone A, Valvassori L; SYNTHESIS Expansion Investigators. Endovascular treatment for acute ischemic stroke. *N Engl J Med.* 2013;368:2433–2434.
11. Kidwell CS, Jahan R, Gornbein J, et al. A trial of imaging selection and endovascular treatment for ischemic stroke. *N Engl J Med.* 2013;368:914–923.
12. Berkhemer OA, Fransen PS, Beumer D, et al. A randomized trial of intraarterial treatment for acute ischemic stroke. *New Engl J Med.* 2015;372(1):11–20.
13. Brott TG, Hobson RW II, Howard G, et al. Stenting versus endarterectomy for treatment of carotid-artery stenosis. *N Engl J Med.* 2010;363:11–23.
14. Yadav JS, Wholey MH, Kuntz RE, et al. Protected carotid-artery stenting versus endarterectomy in high-risk patients. *N Engl J Med.* 2004;351:1493–1501.
15. Chimowitz MI, Lynn MJ, Derdeyn CP, et al. Stenting versus aggressive medical therapy for intracranial arterial stenosis. *N Engl J Med.* 2011;365:993–1003.

SUGGESTED READINGS

Becske T, Kallmes DF, Saatci I, et al. Pipeline for uncoilable or failed aneurysms: results from a multicenter clinical trial. *Radiology.* 2013;267:858–868.

Brinjikji W, Murad MH, Lanzino G, et al. Endovascular treatment of intracranial aneurysms with flow diverters: a meta-analysis. *Stroke.* 2013;44:442–447.

Chalouhi N, Zanaty M, Whiting A, et al. Safety and efficacy of the pipeline embolization device in 100 small intracranial aneurysms. *J Neurointerv Surg.* 2014;6(suppl 1):A46–A47.

Cognard C, Januel AC, Silva NA Jr, et al. Endovascular treatment of intracranial dural arteriovenous fistulas with cortical venous drainage: new management using onyx. *AJNR Am J Neuroradiol.* 2008;29:235–241.

de Paula Lucas C, Piotin M, Spelle L, et al. Stent-jack technique in stent-assisted coiling of wide-neck aneurysms. *Neurosurgery.* 2008;62:ONS414–ONS416; discussion ONS416–ONS417.

De Vries J, Boogaarts J, Van Norden A, et al. New generation of flow diverter (surpass) for unruptured intracranial aneurysms: a prospective single-center study in 37 patients. *Stroke.* 2013;44:1567–1577.

DeMeritt JS, Pile-Spellman J, Mast H, et al. Outcome analysis of preoperative embolization with n-butyl cyanoacrylate in cerebral arteriovenous malformations. *AJNR Am J Neuroradiol.* 1995;16:1801–1807.

D'Urso PI, Lanzino G, Cloft HJ, et al. Flow diversion for intracranial aneurysms: a review. *Stroke.* 2011;42:2363–2368.

Fifi JT, Meyers PM, Lavine SD, et al. Complications of modern diagnostic cerebral angiography in an academic medical center. *J Vasc Interv Radiol.* 2009;20:442–447.

Gobin YP, Starkman S, Duckwiler GR, et al. Merci 1: a phase 1 study of mechanical embolus removal in cerebral ischemia. *Stroke.* 2004;35:2848–2854.

Guglielmi G, Vinuela F, Dion J, et al. Electrothrombosis of saccular aneurysms via endovascular approach. Part 2: preliminary clinical experience. *J Neurosurg.* 1991;75:8–14.

Halbach VV, Higashida RT, Dowd CF, et al. The efficacy of endosaccular aneurysm occlusion in alleviating neurological deficits produced by mass effect. *J Neurosurg.* 1994;80:659–666.

Higashida RT, Halbach VV, Dowd CF, et al. Initial clinical experience with a new self-expanding nitinol stent for the treatment of intracranial cerebral aneurysms: the cordis enterprise stent. *AJNR Am J Neuroradiol.* 2005;26:1751–1756.

Hinck VC, Judkins MP, Paxton HD. Simplified selective femorocerebral angiography. *Radiology.* 1967;89:1048–1052.

Hong B, Patel NV, Gounis MJ, et al. Semi-jailing technique for coil embolization of complex, wide-necked intracranial aneurysms. *Neurosurgery.* 2009;65:1131–1138; discussion 1138–1139.

Hu YC, Newman CB, Dashti SR, et al. Cranial dural arteriovenous fistula: transarterial onyx embolization experience and technical nuances. *J Neurointerv Surg.* 2011;3:5–13.

Jafar JJ, Davis AJ, Berenstein A, et al. The effect of embolization with n-butyl cyanoacrylate prior to surgical resection of cerebral arteriovenous malformations. *J Neurosurg.* 1993;78:60–69.

Kallmes DF, Ding YH, Dai D, et al. A new endoluminal, flow-disrupting device for treatment of saccular aneurysms. *Stroke.* 2007;38:2346–2352.

Kole MK, Pelz DM, Kalapos P, et al. Endovascular coil embolization of intracranial aneurysms: important factors related to rates and outcomes of incomplete occlusion. *J Neurosurg*. 2005;102:607–615.

Luessenhop AJ, Velasquez AC. Observations on the tolerance of the intracranial arteries to catheterization. *J Neurosurg*. 1964;21:85–91.

Mokin M, Snyder KV, Levy EI, et al. Direct carotid artery puncture access for endovascular treatment of acute ischemic stroke: technical aspects, advantages, and limitations. *J Neurointerv Surg*. 2015;7(2):108–113.

Moret J, Cognard C, Weill A, et al. The "remodelling technique" in the treatment of wide neck intracranial aneurysms. Angiographic results and clinical follow-up in 56 cases. *Interv Neuroradiol*. 1997;3:21–35.

Murayama Y, Nien YL, Duckwiler G, et al. Guglielmi detachable coil embolization of cerebral aneurysms: 11 years' experience. *J Neurosurg*. 2003;98:959–966.

Pasqualin A, Scienza R, Cioffi F, et al. Treatment of cerebral arteriovenous malformations with a combination of preoperative embolization and surgery. *Neurosurgery*. 1991;29:358–368.

Penumbra Pivotal Stroke Trial Investigators. The penumbra pivotal stroke trial: safety and effectiveness of a new generation of mechanical devices for clot removal in intracranial large vessel occlusive disease. *Stroke*. 2009; 40:2761–2768.

Raymond J, Guilbert F, Weill A, et al. Long-term angiographic recurrences after selective endovascular treatment of aneurysms with detachable coils. *Stroke*. 2003;34:1398–1403.

Saatci I, Geyik S, Yavuz K, et al. Endovascular treatment of brain arteriovenous malformations with prolonged intranidal onyx injection technique: long-term results in 350 consecutive patients with completed endovascular treatment course. *J Neurosurg*. 2011;115:78–88.

Sahlein DH, Mora P, Becske T, et al. Nidal embolization of brain arteriovenous malformations: rates of cure, partial embolization, and clinical outcome. *J Neurosurg*. 2012;117:65–77.

Sanders WP, Burke TH, Mehta BA. Embolization of intracranial aneurysms with guglielmi detachable coils augmented by microballoons. *AJNR Am J Neuroradiol*. 1998;19:917–920.

Sedat J, Chau Y, Mondot L, et al. Endovascular occlusion of intracranial widenecked aneurysms with stenting (neuroform) and coiling: mid-term and long-term results. *Neuroradiology*. 2009;51:401–409.

Shapiro M, Becske T, Sahlein D, et al. Stent-supported aneurysm coiling: a literature survey of treatment and follow-up. *AJNR Am J Neuroradiol*. 2012;33:159–163.

Siddiqui AH, Abla AA, Kan P, et al. Panacea or problem: flow diverters in the treatment of symptomatic large or giant fusiform vertebrobasilar aneurysms. *J Neurosurg*. 2012;116:1258–1266.

Sluzewski M, van Rooij WJ, Beute GN, et al. Balloon-assisted coil embolization of intracranial aneurysms: incidence, complications, and angiography results. *J Neurosurg*. 2006;105:396–399.

Smith WS, Sung G, Starkman S, et al. Safety and efficacy of mechanical embolectomy in acute ischemic stroke: results of the merci trial. *Stroke*. 2005;36:1432–1438.

Stiefel MF, Albuquerque FC, Park MS, et al. Endovascular treatment of intracranial dural arteriovenous fistulae using onyx: a case series. *Neurosurgery*. 2009;65:132–139; discussion 139–140.

Turk AS, Frei D, Fiorella D, et al. Adapt fast study: a direct aspiration first pass technique for acute stroke thrombectomy. *J Neurointerv Surg*. 2014; 6:260–264.

van Rooij WJ, Jacobs S, Sluzewski M, et al. Curative embolization of brain arteriovenous malformations with onyx: patient selection, embolization technique, and results. *AJNR Am J Neuroradiol*. 2012;33:1299–1304.

Vinuela F, Dion JE, Duckwiler G, et al. Combined endovascular embolization and surgery in the management of cerebral arteriovenous malformations: experience with 101 cases. *J Neurosurg*. 1991;75:856–864.

Vinuela F, Duckwiler G, Mawad M. Guglielmi detachable coil embolization of acute intracranial aneurysm: perioperative anatomical and clinical outcome in 403 patients. *J Neurosurg*. 1997;86:475–482.

Yadav JS, Wholey MH, Kuntz RE, et al. Protected carotid-artery stenting versus endarterectomy in high-risk patients. *N Engl J Med*. 2004;351: 1493–1501.

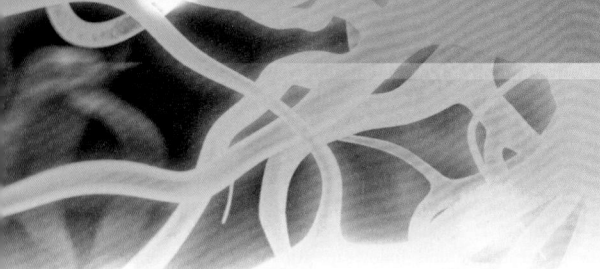

Electroencephalography and Evoked Potentials 25

Nicolas Gaspard and Emily J. Gilmore

ELECTROENCEPHALOGRAPHY

INTRODUCTION

Electroencephalography (EEG) and evoked potentials (EPs) measure the electrical activity generated by neural structures. They allow for the functional assessment of the central nervous system and are often complimentary to imaging studies. Electrophysiologic studies are especially important to the differential diagnosis when neurologic disorders are unaccompanied by detectable alterations in brain morphology. This chapter is an overview of the current capabilities and limitations of these techniques in clinical practice.

NORMAL ELECTROENCEPHALOGRAPHY

The EEG measures electrical potentials resulting from the summation of the postsynaptic activity of cortical neurons. Although generated by cortical cells, these potentials are influenced by ascending projections from subcortical structures such in the thalamus and upper brain stem. Most commonly, the EEG is recorded with electrodes placed on the scalp. The scalp EEG presents a very low resolution view of electrical activity of the brain that favors contributions from the lateral convexities due to attenuation and blurring from overlying tissue layers.

The EEG varies greatly with the state of arousal. The main feature of the normal EEG during wakefulness in adults is the posterior dominant rhythm (PDR), also called *alpha rhythm*. This rhythm consists in an 8- to 13-cycle-per-second (cps) sinusoidal activity that is best observed over the parietal and occipital regions

bilaterally (Fig. 25.1). In a relaxed individual, the alpha rhythm manifests with eye closure and attenuates with alerting or eye opening.

Sleep is divided in four stages on the basis of EEG, eye movements, and muscle activity. Stage N1, or drowsiness, is characterized by the disappearance of the posterior dominant rhythm, which is replaced by low-voltage slower activity. Sharp waves maximal at the vertex, called *vertex sharp waves*, also occur. Stage N2 is defined by the presence of sleep spindles (12 to 14 cps sinusoidal activity that is maximal over the central regions) but also features vertex sharp waves, K complexes (large amplitude diphasic slow waves usually brought up by auditory stimulation and often occurring in close temporal proximity to a spindle [Fig. 25-2]), and positive occipital sharp transients of sleep (POSTS; surface-positive check mark–like waveforms occurring singly or in trains in the occipital regions). Slow waves of sleep (0.5–1 cps) progressively occupy most of the recording during stage N3. During REM sleep, the EEG resembles the EEG of drowsiness, but rapid eye movements and general atonia are present. In adults, REM occurs about 90 minutes after sleep onset and thus is not usually seen on routine studies.

EEG activity undergoes major changes with age. In neonates, these changes occur on a nearly daily basis and knowledge of the conceptional age is required for proper interpretation. Sleep–wake cycles can be identified on the basis of characteristic EEG patterns that are beyond the scope of this chapter. A PDR that is reactive to eye opening becomes visible in most children by 4 months of age. With increasing age, the frequency of the PDR progressively increases, reaching 6 cps in most children at 1 year and 8 cps in

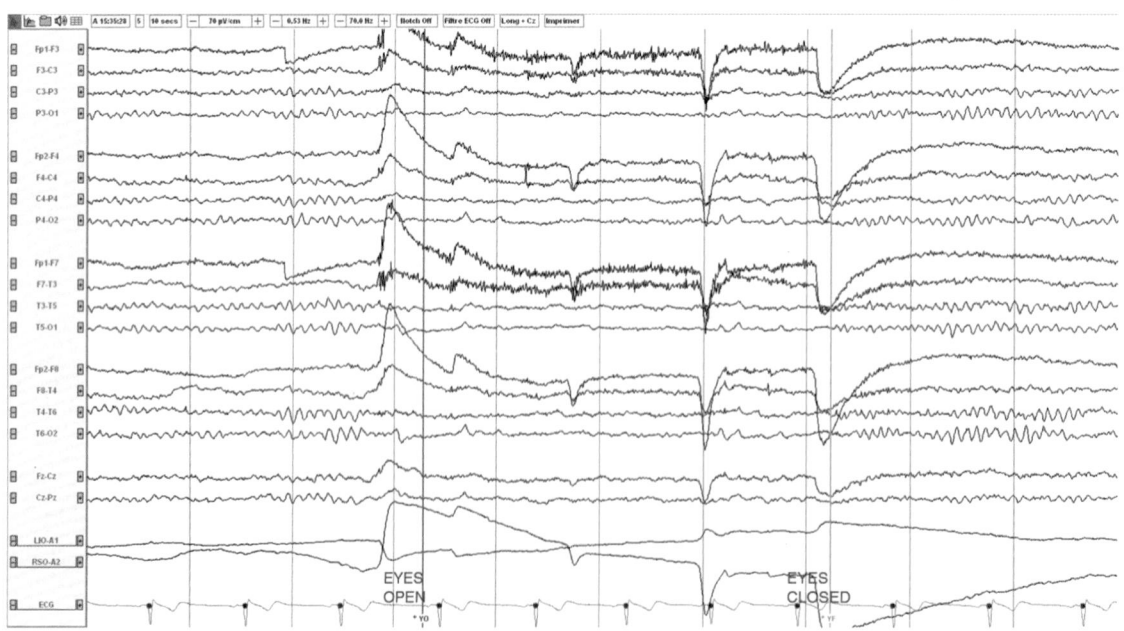

FIGURE 25.1 Normal EEG in an awake 37-year-old man. The posterior dominant rhythm attenuates with eye opening.

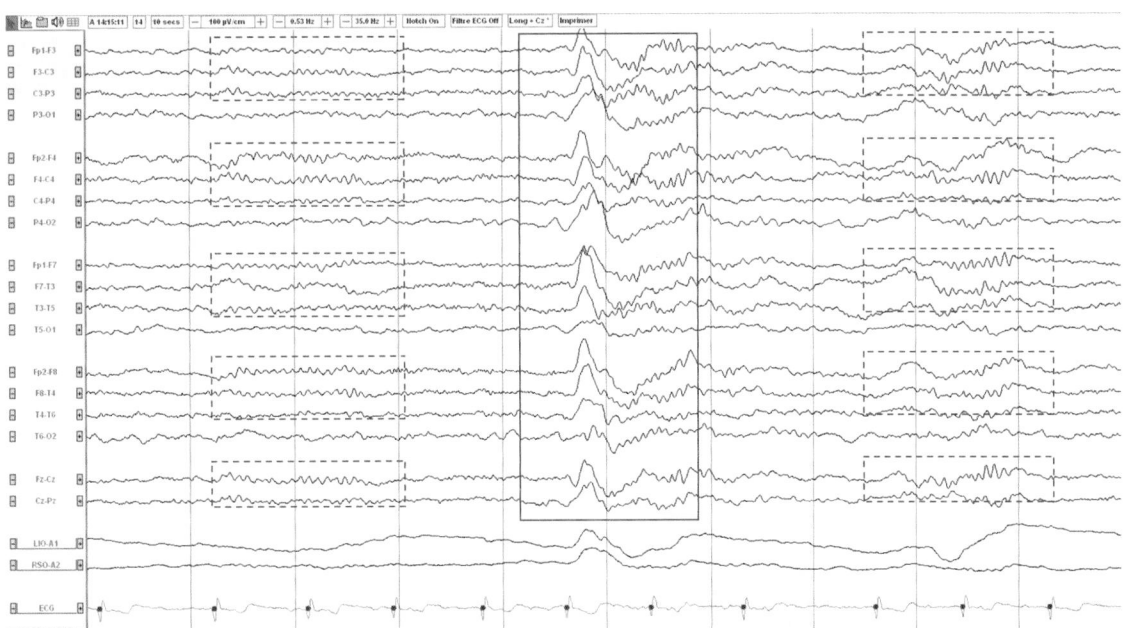

FIGURE 25.2 Normal EEG in a 25-year-old man during stage N2 sleep. Sleep spindles (*dashed boxes*) and K complex (*solid box*).

most children at 4 years. Sleep spindles appear at 2 months but do not become synchronous in most children until the age of 2 years. Normal delta activity persists during wakefulness through childhood, adolescence, and early adulthood but becomes progressively less prominent and more intermittent and restricted to the posterior regions (*posterior slow wave of youth*).

ABNORMAL ELECTROENCEPHALOGRAPHY

Epilepsy

The EEG is the most single important ancillary test for the diagnosis of epilepsy. Epileptiform discharges include spikes (<70 ms), polyspikes, sharp waves (70–200 ms), spike-and-slow-wave complexes, sharp-and-slow-wave complexes. Other nonspecific findings in epilepsy include focal polymorphic slowing and intermittent rhythmic delta activity.

Not only can the presence of epileptiform discharges (EDs) confirm a clinical suspicion of epilepsy, but the localization and type of discharge also helps to identify the diagnosis of a specific syndrome (Table 25.1). A proper syndromic classification is paramount to ensure adequate management, as different syndromes may call for different treatments. It should be noted that EDs may occasionally be absent in a minority of patients who have epilepsy. The first routine EEG obtained after an inaugural seizure demonstrates EDs in approximately 30% to 50% of cases. This proportion increases to a maximum of 80% to 90% after the third routine EEG and subsequent EEGs do not raise this proportion further. Longer recordings, sleep recordings, and so-called activation procedures, such as hyperventilation, intermittent photic stimulation, and sleep deprivation can be performed to increase the sensitivity of the EEG.

Conversely, EDs are seen in 1% to 2% of EEGs of individuals without a history of epilepsy. This proportion is higher in children and in siblings of patients with epilepsy.

In addition to diagnosis, EEG results also help with the management of epilepsy. A finding of interictal EDs after a single seizure increase the likelihood of seizure recurrence and therefore influences the decision about whether to treat with antiepileptic drugs. Similarly, the presence of interictal EDs increases the likelihood of seizure recurrence when consideration is being given to discontinuing antiepileptic drugs after a period of seizure control. Finally, in the setting of convulsive status epilepticus, EEG can be extremely helpful in determining whether individuals with prolonged postictal cognitive impairment (usually >30 minutes) are experiencing electrographic seizures (up to 50%) or nonconvulsive status epilepticus (up to 14%).

Finally, so-called benign epileptiform variants should not be confused for *bona fide* EDs. These variants are physiologic activity with a somewhat sharp morphology that may resemble spikes or sharp waves but can be readily dismissed after careful inspection. This distinction is important, as it is not uncommon to encounter patients who carry a diagnosis of medically refractory epilepsy but turn out to have nonepileptic spells and in whom a normal variant has been mislabeled as an ED.

Focal Brain Lesion or Dysfunction

With the advances of brain imaging, the usefulness of EEG for the diagnosis of focal brain injury has significantly decreased. However, EEG remains the only way to assess the epileptogenic potential of a cerebral lesion. The hallmark of focal brain injury is the presence of localized nonrhythmic delta (1 to 4 cps) or theta (5 to 7 cps) activity, referred to as *focal polymorphic slowing* (Fig. 25.3). As a rule of thumb, delta activity is associated with more destructive lesions than theta activity. *Focal attenuation of fast activity*, the absence of normal alpha or beta (14 to 30 cps) activity over a region of the scalp indicates focal cortical injury. Both focal slowing and attenuation can be seen in the absence of a focal lesion (Fig. 25.4). In this case, they represent the presence of focal cerebral dysfunction as a result of a postictal state or, rarely, migraine. *Lateralized periodic discharges* (LPDs; also referred to as *periodic lateralized epileptiform discharges* or PLEDs) usually indicate the presence of an acute destructive lesion with a high epileptogenic potential, usually stroke, neoplasm, or encephalitis, as up to 85% of patients will experience seizures during the acute phase of their illness (Fig. 25.5). They

TABLE 25.1   Electroencephalography Features of Major Epileptic Syndromes

Syndrome	EEG Features
Ohtahara syndrome	Suppression-burst pattern during sleep and wakefulness
Early myoclonic encephalopathy	Suppression-burst pattern during sleep
West syndrome	Hypsarrhythmia (highly disorganized background with arrhythmic and asynchronous high-amplitude slow waves and multifocal spikes)
Lennox–Gastaut syndrome	Slow (≤2.5 cps) generalized spike-and-wave complexes
	Generalized paroxysmal fast activity
	Slowed background
Benign idiopathic focal epilepsy of childhood	Focal (often bilateral independent or multifocal) sharp waves or spikes
	Normal background
Childhood absence epilepsy	≥3 cps generalized spike-and-wave complexes
	Normal background
Juvenile myoclonic epilepsy	≥3 cps (often up to 6 cps) generalized spike-and-wave and polyspike-and-wave complexes
	Normal background
Localization-related epilepsy	Focal spikes, sharp waves, or spike-and-wave complexes
	Sometimes focal polymorphic or rhythmic slow activity

EEG, electroencephalography.

can occasionally be seen in the aftermath of a seizure in patients with chronic epilepsy or with a remote brain injury. Rarely, LPDs are associated with clinical manifestations (time-locked contralateral myoclonus, visual hallucinations, etc.).

Diffuse Brain Dysfunction or Injury

Toxic, metabolic, diffuse hypoxic–ischemic, and other global insults to the brain result in generalized nonspecific EEG changes. Mild encephalopathy is characterized by slowing of the posterior dominant rhythm and a generalized excess of polymorphic theta activity. With more pronounced brain dysfunction, the posterior dominant rhythm is lost and replaced by a mixture of theta and delta activity. These changes are described as *generalized polymorphic slowing*. In more severe cases, cerebral activity consists mostly of delta activity, which may become monotonous. At this point, *reactivity to external stimulation* (noise, noxious stimuli) may be lost. In the most severe forms of encephalopathy, there is attenuation (<20 μV) or even suppression (<2 μV) of all cerebral activity.

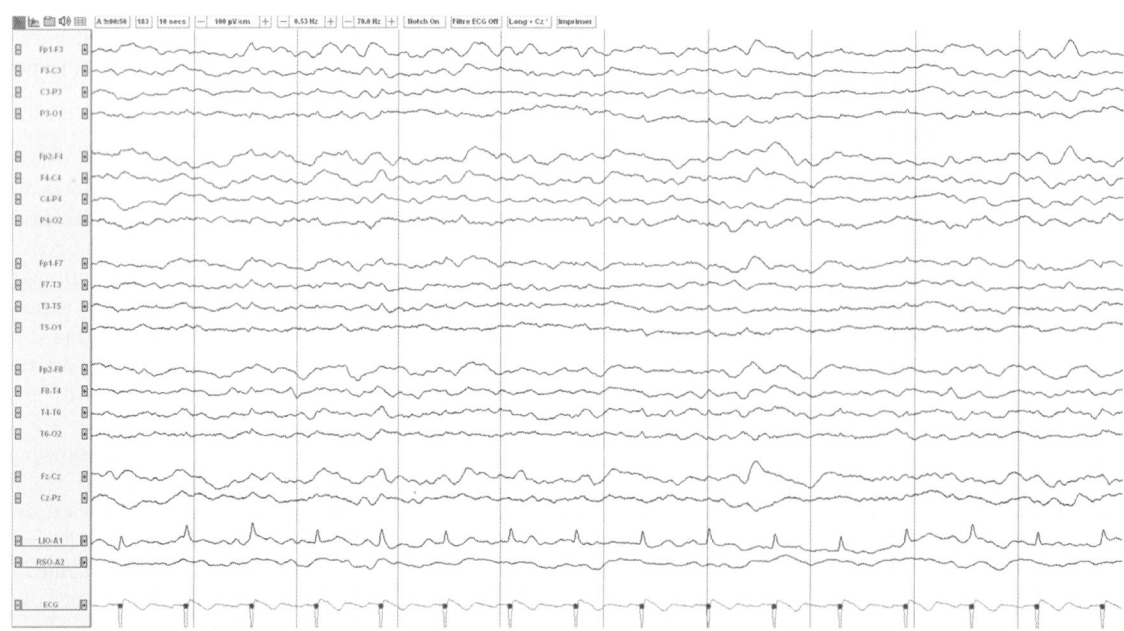

FIGURE 25.3 Diffuse slowing in a 72-year-old woman with sepsis. The posterior dominant rhythm is not visible. The background consists of admixed theta and delta activity.

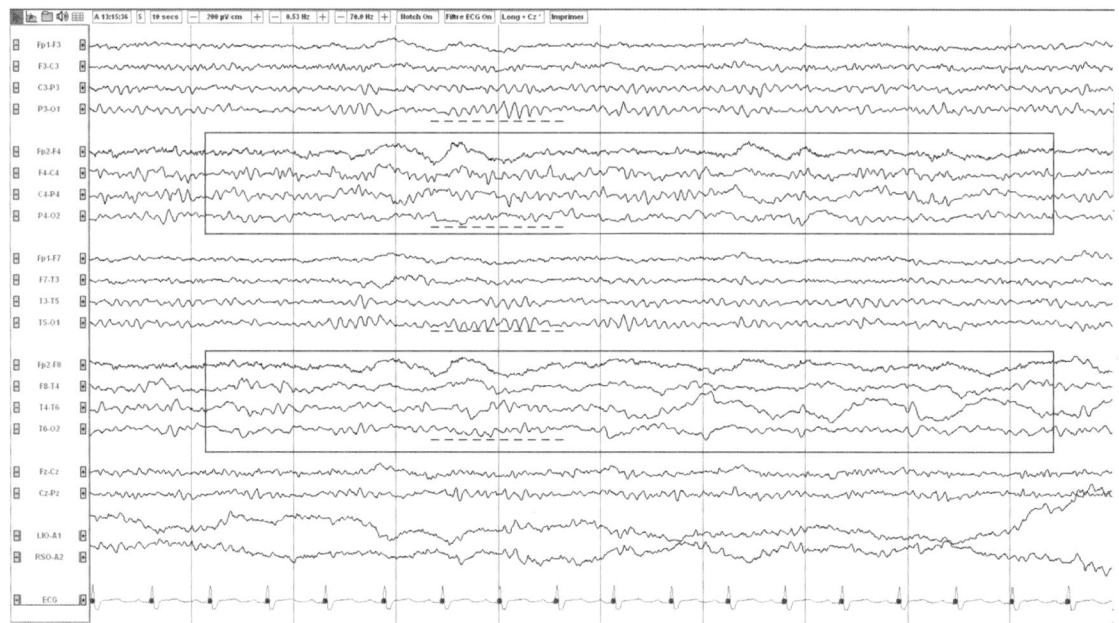

FIGURE 25.4 Focal slow activity (*boxes*) with attenuation of the posterior dominant rhythm (*dashed lines*) over the right hemisphere in a 64-year-old woman with a glioblastoma multiforme.

A *suppression-burst pattern* in which periods of suppression alternate with bursts of high amplitude activity, can also be seen in severe cases (Fig. 25.6). *Generalized rhythmic delta activity* (GRDA; often frontal and intermittent; FIRDA) is another nonspecific finding of encephalopathy, although it can be seen with lesions in the frontal lobes. *Generalized periodic discharges* (GPDs) are repetitive waveforms that occur either at periodic or quasiperiodic intervals of 0.5 to 3 cps. They can be encountered in any type of encephalopathy, at a moderate to severe stage, and are associated with an increased risk of seizures. *Triphasic waves* are a subtype of GPDs with a typical morphology (Fig. 25.7). They were initially thought

to be specific of hepatic encephalopathy. They can in fact be seen in most metabolic or toxic encephalopathies and even during or after status epilepticus. A major role of the EEG in patients with acute confusion and obtundation is to identify those who suffer from nonconvulsive status epilepticus.

Neurodegenerative disorders affecting the cortex and subcortical structures can be associated with similar nonspecific findings, albeit most often mild (i.e., slowing of the posterior dominant rhythm, diffuse excess of theta activity, and FIRDA).

Occasionally, the EEG discloses patterns that point toward a specific diagnosis. In Creutzfeldt–Jakob disease, severe

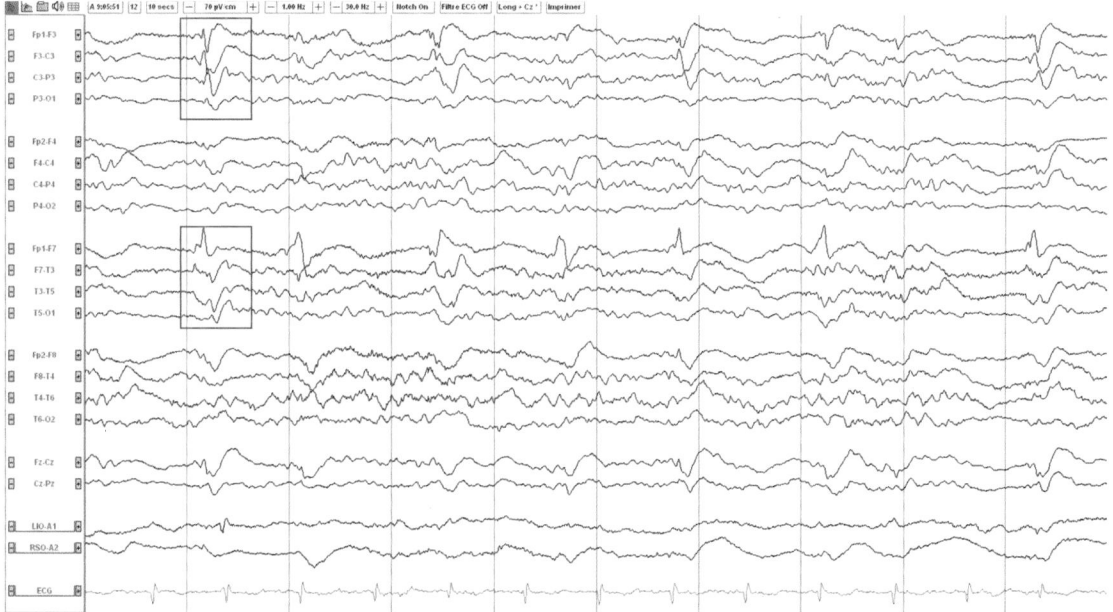

FIGURE 25.5 Left hemispheric lateralized periodic discharges (LPDs; *boxes*) at approximately one per second in a 52-year-old man with herpes encephalitis.

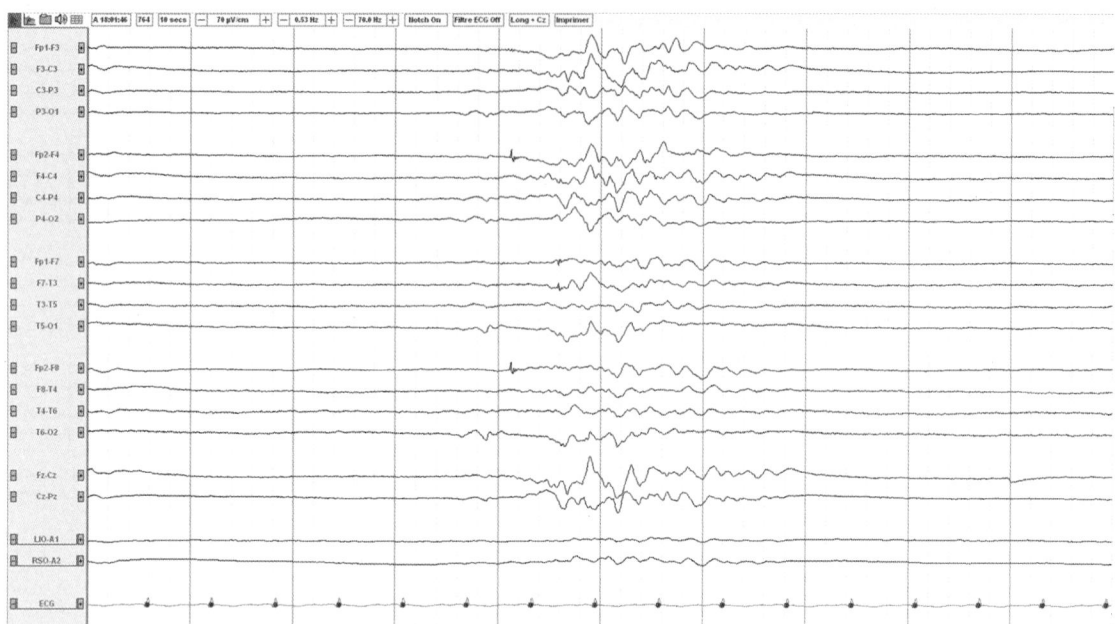

FIGURE 25.6 Suppression-burst pattern following cardiac arrest in a 54-year-old man. Periods of suppression are interrupted by bursts of sharply contoured delta and theta activity.

disruption of the background and periodic discharges (LPDs or more commonly GPDs) occur, always within 3 months after the onset. Huntington disease is associated with a progressive attenuation of cerebral activity. At least 50% of patients with anti–N-methyl-D-aspartate (NMDA) receptor encephalitis show a typical pattern of rhythmic delta activity overridden by beta activity, which has been termed *extreme delta brush* due to its resemblance to normal delta brushes of neonates.

LONG-TERM MONITORING

Epilepsy Monitoring Unit

Long-term EEG monitoring, simultaneously with audio and video recording, can be performed in dedicated epilepsy monitoring units (EMU) to not only capture interictal epileptiform activity but also characterize patients' typical spells. These recordings are useful to clarify the nature of spells of uncertain etiology and assist in the

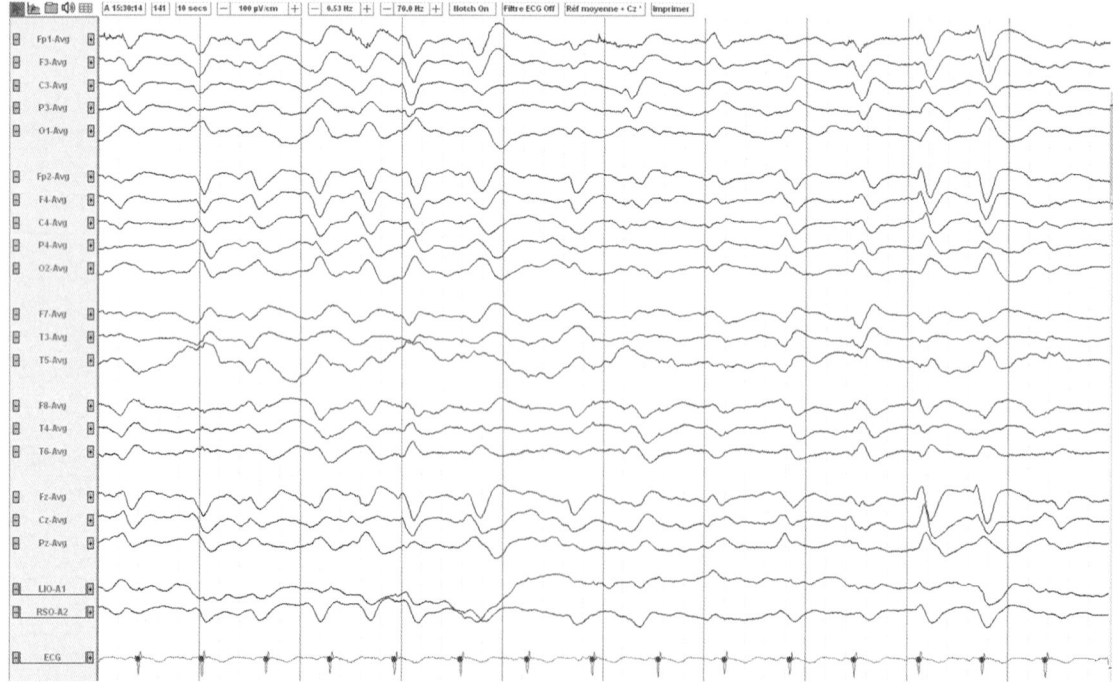

FIGURE 25.7 Generalized periodic discharges with triphasic morphology (triphasic waves) at 1.5 per second in a 35-year-old man with acute liver failure. Each discharge consists of three phases: (1) a small-amplitude negative sharp wave followed by (2) prominent positive sharp wave and (3) a negative slow wave.

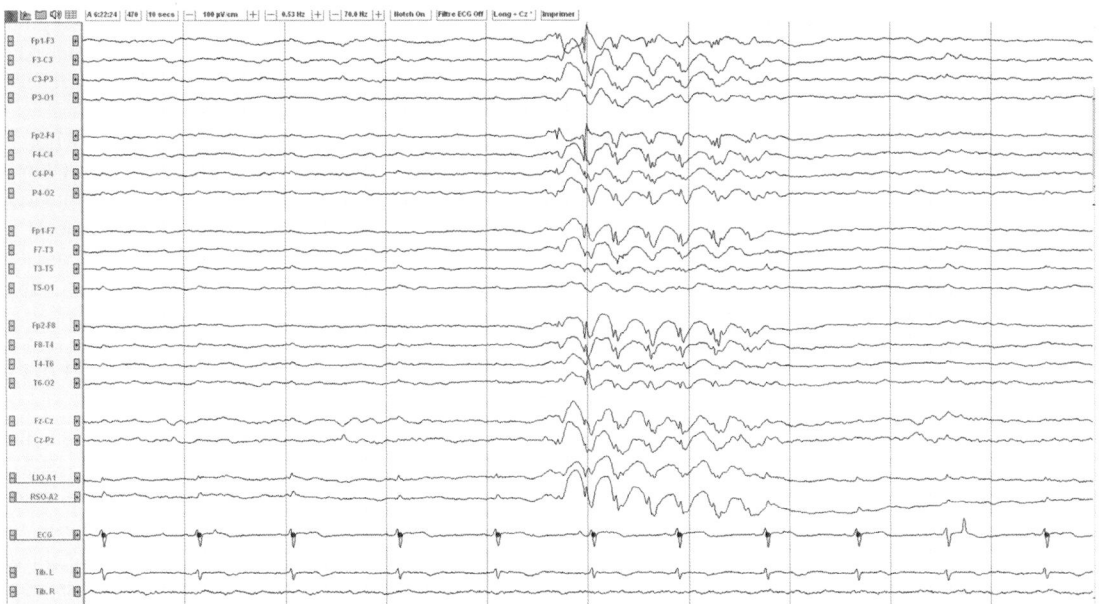

FIGURE 25.8 Three-cycle-per-second generalized spike-and-wave complexes in a 6-year-old girl with childhood absence epilepsy.

determination of seizure type and epilepsy syndrome (Figs. 25.8 and 25.9). The EEG shows typical changes in all patients during generalized or complex partial seizures but can remain normal during simple partial seizures. In patients with medically refractory epilepsy, long-term monitoring provides invaluable electroclinical correlations that will contribute to the assessment of potential candidates for resective surgery. If the results of monitoring with scalp EEG and other ancillary tests (magnetic resonance imaging [MRI], positron emission tomography [PET] scan with 18F-fluorodeoxyglucose [FDG], etc.) are inconclusive, patients may benefit from invasive EEG, either with cortical electrodes (electrocorticography, ECoG) or with depth electrodes implanted stereotactically (stereo-EEG).

These invasive studies offer better spatial resolution and can identify a seizure focus that was not detected or well-circumscribed with scalp EEG. They also permit the delineation of functional cortical areas through electrical cortical stimulation mapping.

Intraoperative Neuromonitoring

Given the exquisite sensitivity of cortical neurons to ischemia, the EEG can detect reduction in cortical perfusion at an early and reversible stage. This can be advantageously used to monitor for cerebral ischemia secondary to carotid clamping during carotid endarterectomy. EEG monitoring may identify those patients who would benefit from the use of a vascular shunt during

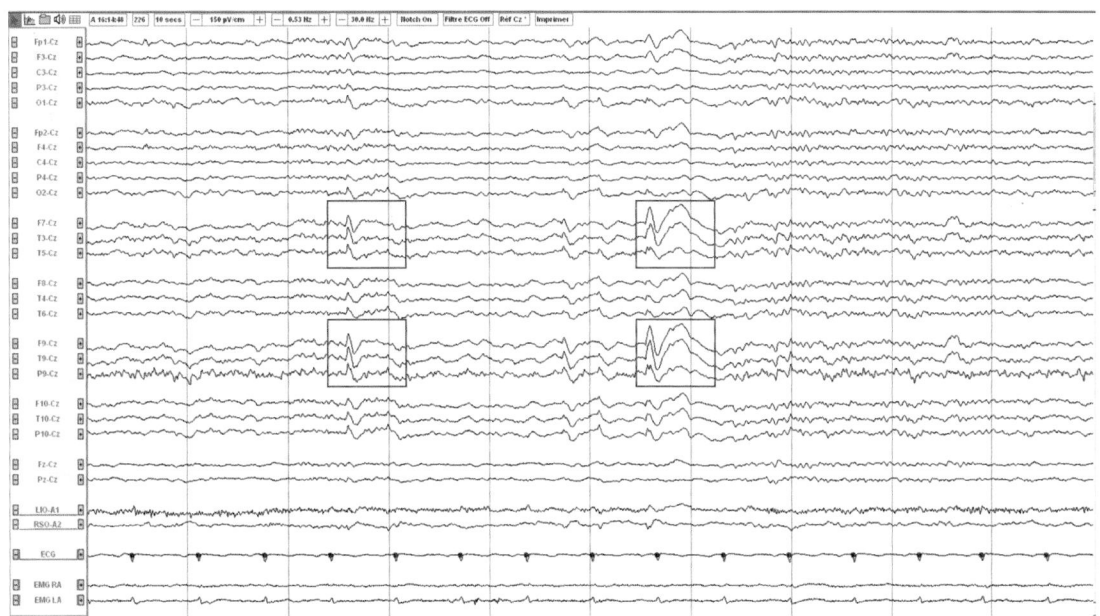

FIGURE 25.9 Left temporal spike-and-wave discharges in a 32-year-old man with mesial temporal lobe sclerosis and epilepsy. The discharges (*boxes*) are maximal over the left anterior inferior temporal region (F7, T3, F9, and T9).

the procedure in order to restore adequate perfusion. Conversely, shunts, which have an associated risk of complications, can be avoided in those patients in whom the EEG remains normal. EEG monitoring has also been advocated during cardiac and aortic surgery, but its use in this indication has been limited to selected academic centers.

ECoG can be used during awake neurosurgery to map functional cortical areas and to delineate the critical limits of a resection. Intraoperative ECoG recordings can also be used to identify epileptogenic regions for resection.

Critical Care Electroencephalography Monitoring

Continuous EEG monitoring is increasingly used in the critical care setting. These prolonged recordings are currently indicated to detect and monitor treatment of nonconvulsive seizures, clarify the nature of abnormal motor activity, and to monitor brain function during drug-induced coma.

Between 15% and 20% of critically ill patients develop seizures during their acute illness. Half of them will develop status epilepticus. Risk factors include acute brain injury, a chronic seizure disorder, younger age, sepsis, and severe alteration of consciousness (i.e., stupor and coma). Up to 90% of these seizures are nonconvulsive and will be missed if EEG monitoring is not performed. There is mounting evidence that nonconvulsive seizures have detrimental metabolic and hemodynamic effect and contribute to secondary brain injury and poorer outcome. A monitoring period of 24 hours is required to detect 90% of these seizures. A longer period is required in comatose patients and in patients with LPDs. A 60-minute EEG will miss half of the patients who have seizures. Episodes of abnormal spontaneous motor activity do not always correspond to seizures. Nonepileptic myoclonus, tremor, clonus, and rigors are frequent among acutely ill patients. Continuous EEG monitoring will help clarify the nonepileptic nature of these episodes and avoid the unnecessary and potentially harmful prescription of antiepileptic drugs. Deep sedation with high-dose barbiturates is sometimes performed to control refractory intracranial hypertension. In this indication, the EEG is used to monitor sedation, with the aim of maintaining a suppression-burst pattern.

EEG abnormalities have prognostic values after traumatic and anoxic brain injury. Malignant patterns of suppression-burst, suppression, and low-voltage unreactive widespread delta activity are almost invariably associated with poor outcome. Other possible applications of EEG monitoring include early detection of delayed cerebral ischemia after aneurysmal subarachnoid hemorrhage.

EVOKED POTENTIALS

INTRODUCTION

EPs are potentials generated by the nervous system in response to stimuli.

Somatosensory, auditory, and visual pathways can be investigated using simple sensorial stimulation and recording from neural structures, whereas motor pathways are explored by transcranial magnetic stimulation of the motor cortex and recording of muscle response. EPs have a low signal-to-noise ratio, being of much lower amplitude than spontaneous activity, and require the averaging of a large number of responses to be identified.

Clinically, EPs are functional tests, which can be viewed as an extension of the neurologic examination. They can provide objective confirmation of the existence of a lesion that may have been suggested by ambiguous or subtle signs or symptoms. Additionally, they can also reveal dysfunction of sensory pathways that is not clinically apparent. Finally, they have the capacity to localize a suspected lesion.

EPs are composed of a stereotyped sequence of waveforms that are labelled by their polarity (negative [N] or positive [P]) and their peak latency from the time of stimulation (expressed in milliseconds). Dysfunction of sensory or motor pathways due to disease or injury leads to increased waveform latency, whereas complete interruption of conduction or destruction of the neural generators results in the absence of waveforms.

SOMATOSENSORY-EVOKED POTENTIALS

Somatosensory-evoked potentials (SSEPs) are elicited by light electrical stimulation of peripheral nerves and reflect sequential activation of structures along the afferent sensory pathways, principally the dorsal column lemniscal system. Upon stimulation of the median nerve, the following responses are clinically useful: first the N9 (Erb's point potential), representing the afferent volley entering the brachial plexus; the N13, generated by postsynaptic activity in the gray matter of the spinal cord; the P14, generated by the caudal medial lemniscus in the lower brain stem; the N18, generated by the rostral brain stem; and finally the N20, reflecting the activation of the somatosensory cortex (Fig. 25.10). Similar responses can be recorded upon stimulation of the posterior tibial nerves.

SSEPs are altered by most conditions affecting the somatosensory pathways, including stroke, tumors, traumatic injury, and demyelinating disorders. They are abnormal in 50% to 60% of patients with multiple sclerosis (MS), even in the absence of clinical signs or symptoms.

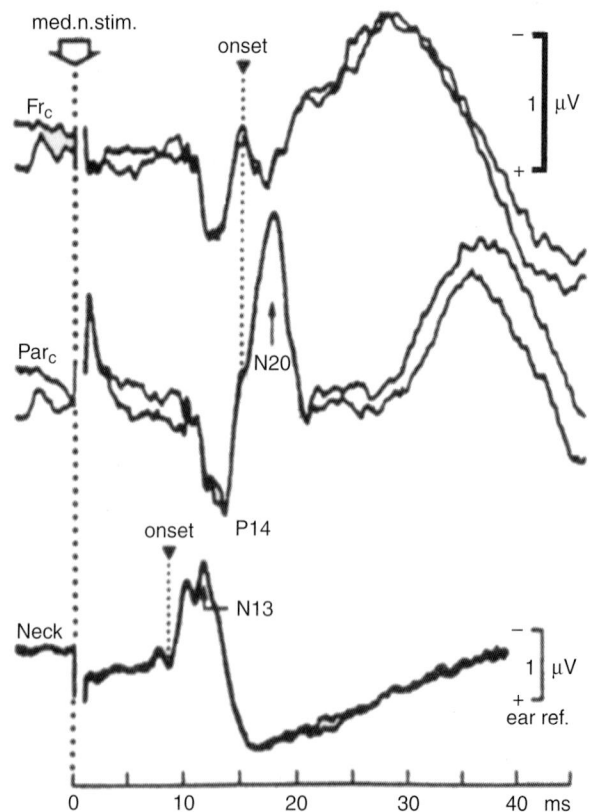

FIGURE 25.10 Normal SSEPs obtained by stimulation of the median nerve at the wrist. (Courtesy of Nicolas Mavroudakis, MD, PhD.)

FIGURE 25.11 SSEP obtained by stimulation of the median nerves at the wrist in a patient with postanoxic brain injury. N13 and P14 potentials, generated in the brain stem, are identified. N20 potentials, generated in the cortex, are not identified, indicating a poor prognosis. (Courtesy of Nicolas Mavroudakis, MD, PhD.)

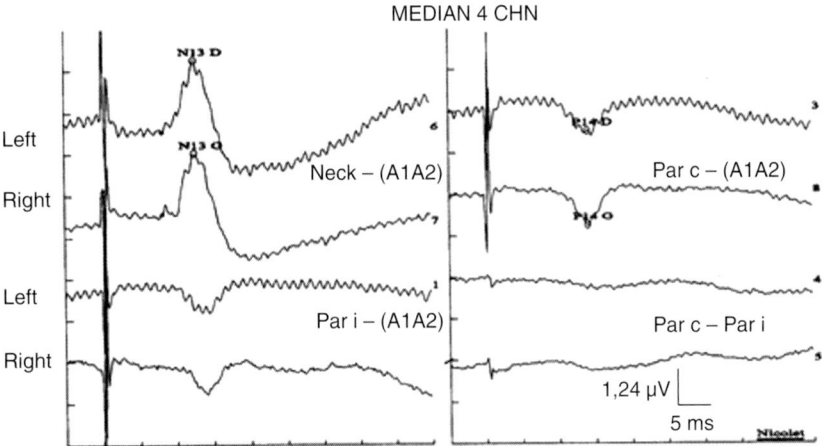

SSEPs are increasingly used for prognostication in comatose patients after anoxic or traumatic brain injury. The absence of N20 after the rewarming period is almost invariably associated with a poor outcome (Fig. 25.11).

SSEPs are also commonly used to monitor the integrity of the spinal cord during high-risk neurosurgical, orthopedic, and vascular interventions. They are also increasingly used to monitor the integrity of the brain function during high-risk cardiovascular surgery, as loss of the N20 indicates early ischemia at a reversible stage.

VISUAL-EVOKED POTENTIALS

Visual-evoked potentials (VEPs) are obtained by stimulation with an alternating checkerboard pattern of black and white squares (i.e., white squares change to black and vice versa at a regular frequency). This stimulation with pattern reversal produces an occipital positive response with a mean latency of 100 milliseconds (P100). VEPs are performed for each eye individually. Because fibers from the temporal side of the retina decussate at the optic chiasm, an abnormal P100 after stimulation of one eye implies the presence of a prechiasmatic lesion, affecting the retina or the optic nerve on the side of the stimulation. An abnormal P100 upon stimulation of both eyes may be caused either by bilateral prechiasmatic and/or retrochiasmatic lesions. Unilateral retrochiasmatic lesions usually do not significantly alter the P100. Acute optic neuritis is initially accompanied by an attenuation of the P100 (Fig. 25.12). In the postacute phase, although the P100 may return to almost normal amplitude, it is significantly delayed. Abnormal VEPs are found in up to 70% of patients with MS, even in the absence of a history of optic neuritis. These findings are nonspecific and can also be seen in other conditions, including demyelinating disorders (acute disseminated encephalomyelitis [ADEM], anti–neuromyelitis optica [NMO] spectrum), ischemic optic neuropathy, compression of the optic nerve, cataracts, glaucoma, toxic and metabolic optic neuropathy, degenerative disorders, and retinal disease. In the setting where a patient reports visual loss, a normal VEP strongly favors a psychogenic disorder (i.e., hysteria or malingering).

BRAIN STEM AUDITORY–EVOKED RESPONSES

Brain stem auditory–evoked potentials (BAEPs) consist of five waveforms, labelled I to V, of which waves I, III, and V are the most important from a clinical point of view. The nature of the generators of the responses is largely unclear but it is believed that wave I is generated by the peripheral portion of the acoustic nerve, whereas

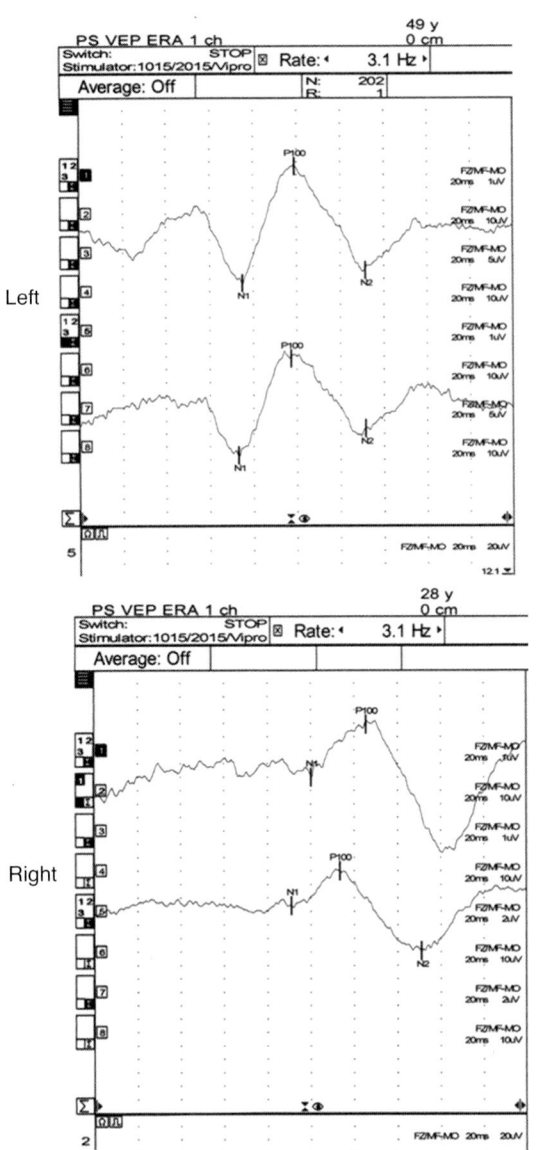

FIGURE 25.12 Visual-evoked potentials in patient with probable multiple sclerosis. The P100 after stimulation of the **left** eye is normal, whereas there is a significant delay after stimulation of the **right** eye. (Courtesy of Nicolas Mavroudakis, MD, PhD.)

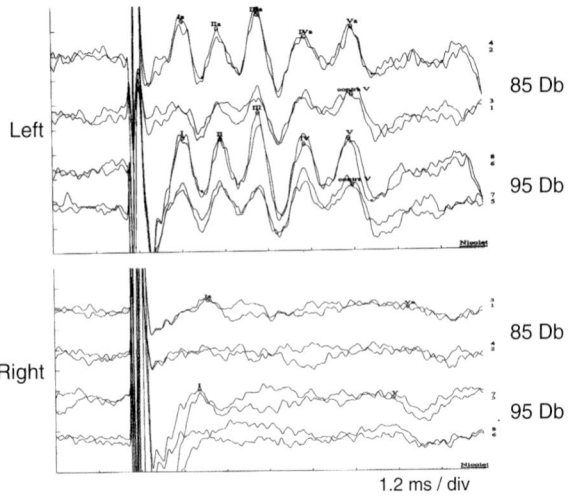

1.2 ms / div

FIGURE 25.13 Auditory-evoked potentials (AEPs) in a patient with a meningioma in the right pontocerebellar angle. With left stimulation, waves I to V are identified and have a normal latency. With right stimulation, only wave I (generated in the peripheral acoustic nerve) is identified; subsequent waves generated in the brain stem are not visible, indicating impairment of auditory pathways in the right pons and/or midbrain. (Courtesy of Nicolas Mavroudakis, MD, PhD.)

wave III and V are probably generated in the brain stem by the superior olivary complex and the inferior colliculus, respectively.

BAEPs are abnormal in most cases of tumors of the cerebellopontine angle, such as acoustic neuroma. Abnormalities include delay or absence of all waves after wave I and absence of all waves (Fig. 25.13).

BAEPs are also sensitive to lesions affecting the auditory pathways in the brain stem. They are almost always abnormal in the case of intrinsic tumors of the brain stem. They are preserved when the auditory pathways are spared, as may occur in vascular lesions of the pontine tegmentum causing a locked-in syndrome. BAEPs abnormalities are frequent in patients with multiple sclerosis and in other demyelinating conditions.

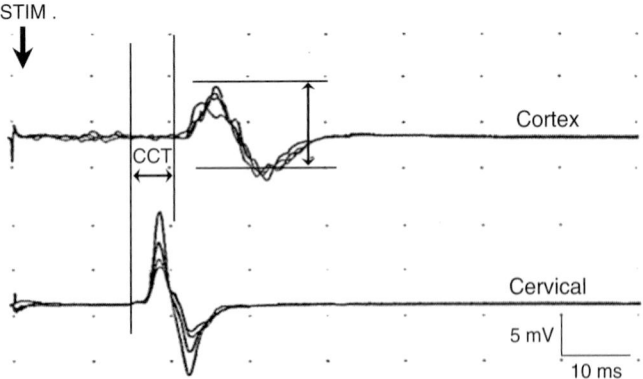

FIGURE 25.14 Motor-evoked potentials by transcranial magnetic stimulation of the motor cortex and by stimulation of the cervical spinal cord. The response is recorded with surface electromyogram (EMG) electrodes over the first dorsal interosseous. The delay between the two responses is the central conduction time in the corticospinal tract. (Courtesy of Nicolas Mavroudakis, MD, PhD.)

In comatose patients, BAEPs are normal when the cause is metabolic or toxic. They are abnormal when the brain stem is directly affected between the midbrain and the lower pons by a primary infratentorial lesion or by herniation due to a supratentorial mass. The absence of all waves subsequent to wave I carries a poor prognosis, whereas the presence of wave V is associated with good outcome. BAEPS are relatively insensitive to sedative drugs, including anesthetic doses of barbiturates. They can be used as a confirmatory test of brain death, even in the presence of doses of barbiturates that induce an isoelectric EEG. Absence of all waves or the sole persistence of wave I indicates brain death.

MOTOR-EVOKED POTENTIALS

Motor-evoked potentials (MEPs) assess the integrity of motor pathways. They are elicited by transcranial magnetic stimulation of the primary motor cortex. Muscle compound potentials are recorded and the latency of response can be measured. Stimulation can also be delivered at the spinal cord level allowing for calculation of central conduction time by subtracting the latency after spinal cord stimulation from the latency after cortical stimulation (Fig. 25.14). MEPs are increasingly used in association with SSEPs to monitor spinal cord integrity during surgery.

SUGGESTED READINGS

Ajmone-Marsan C. Electroencephalographic studies in seizure disorders: additional considerations. *J Clin Neurophysiol.* 1984;1:143–157.

American Clinical Neurophysiology Society. Guidelines in electroencephalography and evoked potentials. *J Clin Neurophysiol.* 2006;23:125–179.

Buzsaki G, Draguhn A. Neuronal oscillations in cortical networks. *Science.* 2004;30:1926–1929.

Chiappa KH. *Evoked Potentials in Clinical Medicine.* 3rd ed. Philadelphia: Lippincott-Raven Publishers; 1997.

Chong DJ, Hirsch LJ. Which EEG patterns warrant treatment in the critically ill? Reviewing the evidence for treatment of periodic epileptiform discharges and related patterns. *J Clin Neurophysiol.* 2005;22:79–91.

Claassen J, Jetté N, Chum F, et al. Electrographic seizures and periodic discharges after intracerebral hemorrhage. *Neurology.* 2007;69:1356–1365.

Claassen J, Mayer SA, Kowalski RG, et al. Detection of electrographic seizures with continuous EEG monitoring in critically ill patients. *Neurology.* 2004;62(10):1743–1748.

Claassen J, Taccone FS, Horn P, et al. Recommendations on the use of EEG monitoring in critically ill patients: consensus statement from the neurointensive care section of the ESICM. *Intensive Care Med.* 2013;39(8):1337–1351.

Claassen J, Vespa P, The Participants in the International Multi-disciplinary Consensus Conference on Multimodality Monitoring. Electrophysiologic monitoring in acute brain injury [published online ahead of print September 11, 2014]. *Neurocrit Care.*

Cruccu G, Aminoff MJ, Curio G, et al. Recommendations for the clinical use of somatosensory-evoked potentials. *Clin Neurophysiol.* 2008;119(8):1705–1719.

DeLorenzo RJ, Waterhouse EJ, Towne AR, et al. Persistent nonconvulsive status epilepticus after the control of convulsive status epilepticus. *Epilepsia.* 1998;39:833–840.

Emerson RG, Pedley TA. Intraoperative monitoring. In: Ebersole JS, Pedley TA, eds. *Current Practice of Clinical Electroencephalography.* 3rd ed. New York: Lippincott Williams and Williams; 2003:936–954.

Epstein Charles E. Visual evoked potentials. In: Levin KH, Lueders HO, eds. *Comprehensive Clinical Neurophysiology.* Philadelphia: WB Saunders; 2000:507–524.

Fisch BJ, Klass DW. The diagnostic specificity of triphasic wave patterns. *Electroencephalogr Clin Neurophysiol.* 1988;70:1–8.

Foreman B, Claassen J, Abou Khaled K, et al. Generalized periodic discharges in the critically ill: a case-control study of 200 patients. *Neurology.* 2012;79(19):1951–1960.

Friedman D, Claassen J, Hirsch LJ. Continuous electroencephalogram monitoring in the intensive care unit. *Anesth Analg.* 2009;109(2):506–523.

Gaspard N, Hirsch LJ. Pitfalls in ictal EEG interpretation: critical care and intracranial recordings. *Neurology.* 2013;80(1)(suppl 1):S26–S42.

Gaspard N, Manganas L, Rampal N, et al. Similarity of lateralized rhythmic delta activity to periodic lateralized epileptiform discharges in critically ill patients. *JAMA Neurol.* 2013;70(10):1288–1295.

Guérit JM, Amantini A, Amodio P, et al. Consensus on the use of neurophysiological tests in the intensive care unit (ICU): electroencephalogram (EEG), evoked potentials (EP), and electroneuromyography (ENMG). *Neurophysiol Clin.* 2009;39(2):71–83.

Hallett M. Transcranial magnetic stimulation and the human brain. *Nature.* 2000;406:147–150.

Hirsch LJ. Classification of EEG patterns in patients with impaired consciousness. *Epilepsia.* 2011;52(suppl 8):21–24.

Hirsch LJ, Claassen J, Mayer SA, et al. Stimulus-induced rhythmic, periodic, or ictal discharges (SIRPIDS): a common EEG phenomenon in the critically ill. *Epilepsia.* 2004;45(2):109–123.

Hirsch LJ, LaRoche SM, Gaspard N, et al. American Clinical Neurophysiology Society's Standardized Critical Care EEG Terminology: 2012 version. *J Clin Neurophysiol.* 2013;30(1):1–27.

Kellaway P. Orderly approach to visual analysis: characteristics of the normal EEG of adults and children. In: Ebersole JS, Pedley TA, eds. *Current Practice of Clinical Electroencephalography.* 3rd ed. New York: Lippincott Williams & Wilkins; 2003:100–159.

Lai CW, Gragasin ME. Electroencephalography in herpes simplex encephalitis. *J Clin Neurophysiol.* 1988;5:87–103.

Lerman P. Benign partial epilepsy with centro-temporal spikes. In: Roger J, Bureau M, Dravet C, et al, eds. *Epilepsy Syndromes in Infancy, Childhood, and Adolescence.* 2nd ed. London: John Libbey; 1992:189–200.

Levy SR, Chiappa KH, Burke CJ, et al. Early evolution and incidence of electroencephalographic abnormalities in Creutzfeldt-Jakob disease. *J Clin Neurophysiol.* 1986;3:1–21.

Lueders HO, Terada K. Auditory evoked potentials. In: Levin KH, Lueders HO, eds. *Comprehensive Clinical Neurophysiology.* Philadelphia: WB Saunders; 2000:525–541.

Mendiratta A, Emerson RG. Transcranial electrical MEP with muscle recording. In: Nuwer MR, ed. *Handbook of Clinical Neurophysiology.* Amsterdam, The Netherlands: Elsevier B.V.; 2008:8:275–288.

Noachtar S, Binnie C, Ebersole J, et al. A glossary of terms most commonly used by clinical electroencephalographers and proposal for the report form for the EEG findings. The International Federation of Clinical Neurophysiology. *Electroencephalogr Clin Neurophysiol Suppl.* 1999;52:21–41.

Noachtar S, Rémi J. The role of EEG in epilepsy: a critical review. *Epilepsy Behav.* 2009;15(1):22–33.

Novotny EJ Jr. The role of clinical neurophysiology in the management of epilepsy. *J Clin Neurophysiol.* 1998;15:96–108.

Nuwer MR, Emerson RG, Galloway G, et al. Evidence-based guideline update: intraoperative spinal monitoring with somatosensory and transcranial electrical motor evoked potentials: report of the Therapeutics and Technology Assessment Subcommittee of the American Academy of Neurology and the American Clinical Neurophysiology Society. *Neurology.* 2012;78(8):585–589.

Oddo M, Carrera E, Claassen J, et al. Continuous electroencephalography in the medical intensive care unit. *Crit Care Med.* 2009;37(6):2051–2056.

Pedley TA, Mendiratta A, Walczak TS. Seizures and epilepsy. In: Ebersole JS, Pedley TA, eds. *Current Practice of Clinical Electroencephalography.* 3rd ed. New York: Lippincott Williams & Wilkins; 2003:506–587.

Pohlmann-Eden B, Hoch DB, Chiappa KH. Periodic lateralized epileptiform discharges: a critical review. *J Clin Neurophysiol.* 1996;13:519–530.

Reeves AL, Westmoreland BE, Klass DW. Clinical accompaniments of the burst suppression EEG pattern. *J Clin Neurophysiol.* 1997;14:150–153.

Salinsky M, Kanter R, Dasheiff RM. Effectiveness of multiple EEGs in supporting the diagnosis of epilepsy: an operational curve. *Epilepsia.* 1987;28:331–334.

Scheuer ML. Continuous EEG monitoring in the intensive care unit. *Epilepsia.* 2002;43:114–127.

Sutter R, Kaplan PW. Clinical and electroencephalographic correlates of acute encephalopathy. *J Clin Neurophysiol.* 2013;30(5):443–453.

Tatum WO IV, Husain AM, Benbadis SR, et al. Normal adult EEG and patterns of uncertain significance. *J Clin Neurophysiol.* 2006;23(3):194–207.

Zifkin BG, Cracco RQ. An orderly approach to the abnormal EEG. In: Ebersole JS, Pedley TA, eds. *Current Practice of Clinical Electroencephalography.* 3rd ed. New York: Lippincott Williams & Wilkins; 2003:288–302.

Electromyography, Nerve Conduction Studies, and Magnetic Stimulation 26

Louis H. Weimer, Clifton L. Gooch,
Thomas H. Brannagan III, and Seth L. Pullman

INTRODUCTION

Advances in electronics enabled clinical assessment of peripheral nerve and muscle physiology in the mid-20th century, spawning the neurologic specialty of clinical neurophysiology. Electrodiagnostic techniques have become increasingly computerized and are indispensable for the proper diagnosis and management of patients with neuromuscular disease. Despite technologic improvements, a basic understanding of the principles, potential errors, and disease-specific effects are essential for meaningful interpretation and conclusions. This chapter provides a brief overview of nerve conduction studies (NCS), needle electromyography (EMG), special neuromuscular junction, and central motor function techniques.

NERVE CONDUCTION STUDIES

SENSORY AND MOTOR NERVE CONDUCTION STUDIES

NCS measure the speed and strength of an electrical impulse conducted along a peripheral nerve. Typically, the impulse is generated using a bipolar stimulator placed on the skin surface over the anatomic course of the tested nerve. The intensity and duration of this transcutaneous stimulus is gradually increased until all available axons within that nerve are depolarized, sparking an action potential that travels down the nerve to the recording site. For *sensory NCS*, the recording electrodes are placed on the skin surface overlying the nerve (usually over a pure sensory branch) at some distance from the stimulation site (Fig. 26.1).

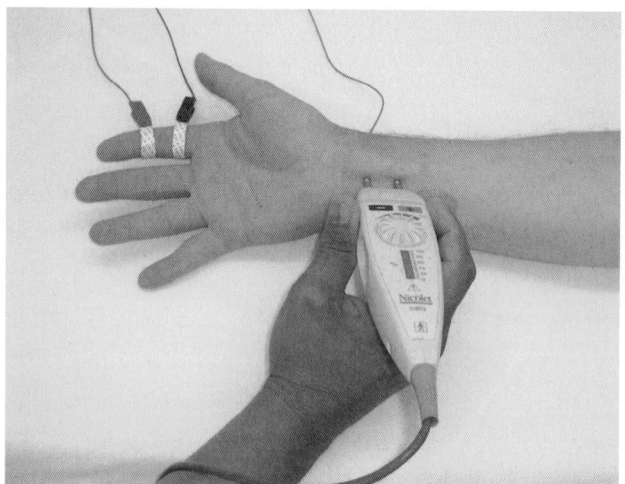

FIGURE 26.1 Setup for sensory NCS. A bipolar stimulator is placed over the median nerve at the wrist, and self-adhesive recording electrodes are placed over the median sensory branches over the index finger, ensuring that only sensory nerve responses are recorded. A self-adhesive ground electrode is placed over the dorsum of the hand.

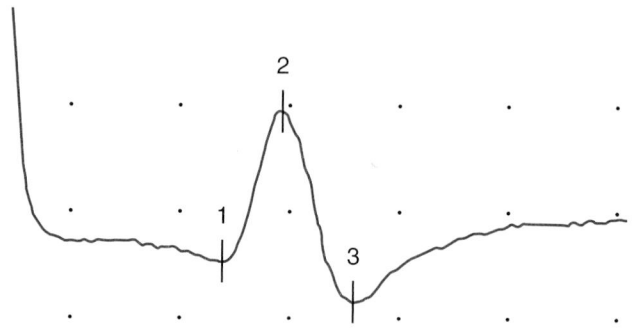

FIGURE 26.2 SNAP, recorded using the setup depicted in Fig. 16.1. The horizontal space between two dots, or graticules (one division), is assigned a specific value (the time base shown is 1 millisecond per division) to enable time measurements. Vertical divisions are also assigned a specific value to enable measurement of stimulus strength (the gain or sensitivity; 10 μV per division as shown). The time between the stimulus artifact and the waveform peak (the sensory peak latency) is 2.75 milliseconds, and the peak-to-peak waveform amplitude is 13.2 μV, within the normal range. Onset latency is needed to calculate a conduction velocity.

When an action potential passes under these bipolar recording electrodes, a *sensory nerve action potential* (SNAP) waveform is recorded and displayed (Fig. 26.2). The SNAP is produced by large Ia sensory axons and not small-diameter A or C fibers.

Motor NCS are performed similarly, except that the recording electrodes are placed over the motor endplate region of an innervated muscle, rather than over the nerve itself (Fig. 26.3).

For motor NCS, the action potential passes down the nerve, triggers acetylcholine release at the neuromuscular junction, and produces muscle membrane depolarization. The recording electrodes capture the electrical potential generated by depolarization of the innervated muscle, subsequently generating a waveform known as the *compound motor action potential* (CMAP) (Fig. 26.4). Care must be taken to maximally but not excessively stimulate nerve axons at each stimulation site. Multiple other technical considerations can impede quality NCS and must be controlled as much as feasible, including standardized procedures, temperature maintenance, accurate electrode placement and measurement, interference avoidance, detection of anatomic anomalies, and stimulation of unintended nerves.

Although modern equipment is computerized with digital processing and storage to capture and analyze the data, the waveform display owes its origins to the cathode ray oscilloscope. By convention, the x-axis of the tracing is the time base (or sweep speed) in milliseconds, whereas the y-axis measures the impulse strength.

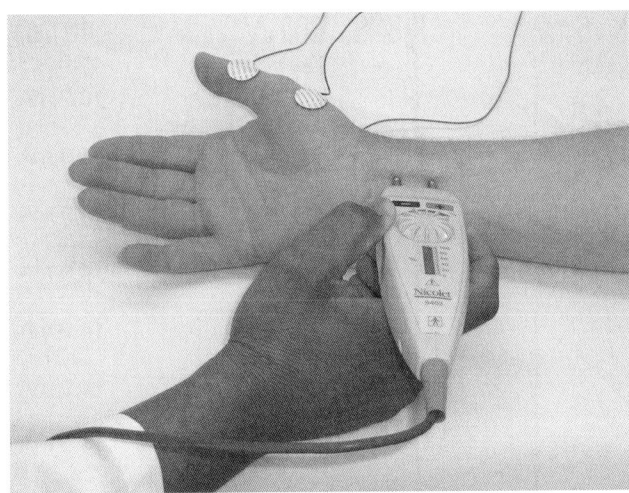

FIGURE 26.3 Setup for motor NCS. The bipolar stimulator is placed over the median nerve at the wrist and recording electrodes are placed over the median-innervated abductor pollicis brevis. The resultant muscle depolarization produces the recorded waveform. Note that sensitivities are in the millivolt, rather than microvolt, range.

The waveform *amplitude*, measured either in microvolts (sensory waveforms) or millivolts (motor waveforms), reflects the summated number of responsive nerve axons. The time difference between the stimulus and the waveform onset, one of several measures of nerve speed, is the *distal latency*. Using this value and the measured distance between the stimulating and recording points, a *nerve conduction velocity* may be calculated for sensory nerves (m/s). Some prefer to measure the latency to the sensory waveform peak instead of the onset and to compare this value to controls. Similarly, the *distal motor latency* is measured from the stimulation point to the waveform onset and compared to control values; some laboratories use a standard distance from the stimulation point and the muscle to improve reliability. Because of the non–nerve-related components of the motor system including the neuromuscular junction and muscle membrane depolarization, motor NCS require additional stimulation sites to calculate conduction velocity. A waveform from a second, typically more proximal, stimulation site is captured and the time difference between the two waveforms is measured. This step subtracts out the time for the nonnerve factors and assesses only the motor nerve components. The distance between the two sites (mm) divided by the time difference (ms) provides the *conduction velocity* of that segment (m/s). Additional segments may be added by stimulating further sites along the nerve course. Accuracy is reduced, however, if the stimulation points are too close together. A difference of 10 cm is typical except for special circumstance, such as short-segment studies across the elbow in the assessment of ulnar neuropathy. Another consideration is the accessibility of the nerve to surface stimulation.

It is important to measure and control limb temperature; cold limbs influence many electrodiagnostic measures. The most significant effect is on conduction velocity, with a conduction velocity fall on average of 2 m/s/°C and latency increase of approximately 0.2 ms/°C below ideal.

Because muscle tissue is much more electrically potent than nerve fibers, the CMAP is approximately 3 orders of magnitude larger than the SNAP, and its amplitude is measured in millivolts rather than microvolts. Otherwise, latency and amplitude measures are similar to the SNAP.

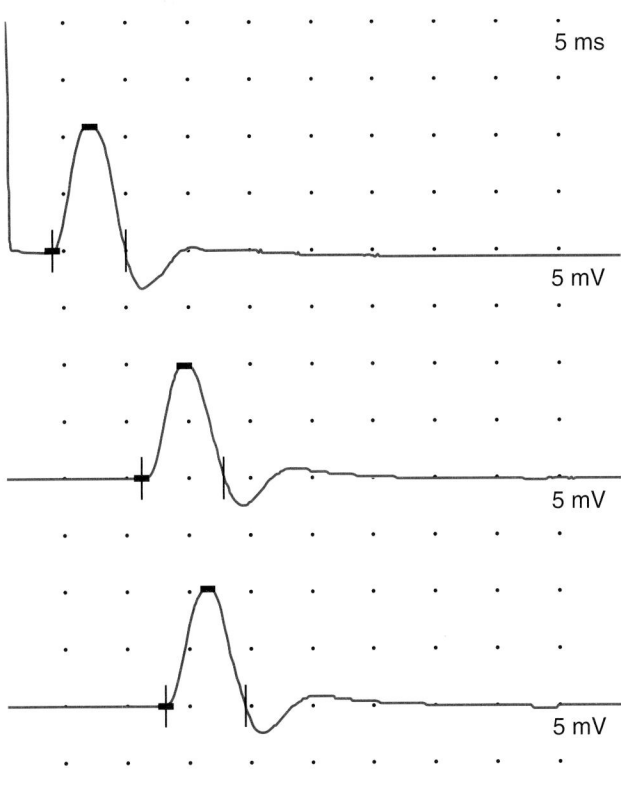

FIGURE 26.4 A CMAP. These three responses were recorded from the extensor digitorum brevis muscle of the foot following stimulation of the peroneal nerve at three different sites: the ankle (*top waveform*), just below the fibular head (*middle waveform*), and above the knee (*bottom waveform*). The recording sensitivity was 5 mV per division, and the sweep speed was 5 milliseconds per division. Onset latencies are 4.0, 11.1, and 13 milliseconds, respectively, predictably increasing as the distance between the stimulating and recording electrodes increases. Subtracting one onset latency from another yields the time for the impulse to travel from one stimulation point to the other. The measured distance is divided by this value to produce the segmental conduction velocity in meters per second. The amplitude is measured from baseline to peak.

Both latency and conduction velocity depend on an intact, myelinated nerve; myelin and the saltatory conduction it fosters are essential for rapid action potential propagation. In contrast, the waveform amplitude depends primarily on the number of functioning axons within the nerve. Significant slowing of conduction velocity or prolongation of latency usually implies demyelinating injury, whereas loss of amplitude usually correlates with axonal loss or dysfunction. However, axonal loss also may mildly slow conduction velocity by eliminating the fastest conducting axons. When demyelination is severe enough, a complete block of transmission in most axons can occur; demyelination results in a loss of local current and an insufficient charge to activate the next node of Ranvier. NCS may be used to demonstrate the conduction block. In this situation, recordings made from nerve stimulation above the site of injury produce waveforms with a much lower amplitude and area than recordings made from stimulation below the site of demyelination of the same nerve. When severe enough, this loss of waveform amplitude due to block of impulse transmission in a

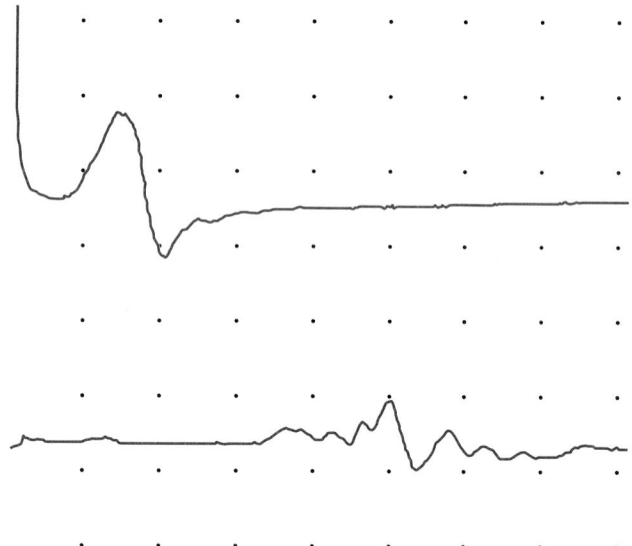

FIGURE 26.5 Conduction block with temporal dispersion. Two CMAPs recorded from the abductor hallucis muscle of the foot following stimulation of the tibial nerve at the ankle and the knee (*top and bottom*, respectively) in a patient with demyelinating neuropathy. The sensitivity was 1 μV per division, and the sweep speed was 5 milliseconds per division. When stimulation is moved from the ankle to the knee, the recorded waveform decreases in amplitude (from 1.1 to 0.5 mV, a 54% decline); its duration lengthens; and its morphology becomes irregular and complex. These findings suggest significant demyelination of the nerve segment between the stimulation sites, with partial conduction block. An increased range of axonal conduction times between different axons, caused by differential involvement, produces increased waveform duration as the distance between stimulation and recording sites increases (*temporal dispersion*). A 30% increase is considered to be significant in motor axons.

group of axons at a single site is known as a *conduction block* and is an important diagnostic feature of acquired demyelinating neuropathies (Fig. 26.5). If some but not all fibers show reduced conduction velocity without a conduction block, the increased range of velocities may produce *temporal dispersion*, a broadened waveform that demonstrates increased waveform duration but a lesser reduction in waveform area. Despite the fact that certain accessible nerves dominate most NCS, techniques are described for most recognized peripheral nerves; studies for uncommon procedures are performed on the basis of clinical necessity.

LATE RESPONSES

Routine NCS are limited to accessible segments in the proximal and distal arms and legs. Nerve roots are not easily stimulated and *long-latency reflex* tests are typically used to assess these most proximal segments. When a stimulus is delivered to the distal nerve, action potentials are propagated both proximally and distally. The impulse traveling up the motor axons (in a direction opposite to the normal flow or *antidromic*) eventually reaches the anterior horn cells. The anterior horn cells then generate a second nonsynaptic action potential that travels back down the axon into the muscle (in the direction paralleling the normal flow or *orthodromic*), where it is recorded as a much smaller waveform known as the *F wave*, named because it was originally recorded foot muscles (Fig. 26.6).

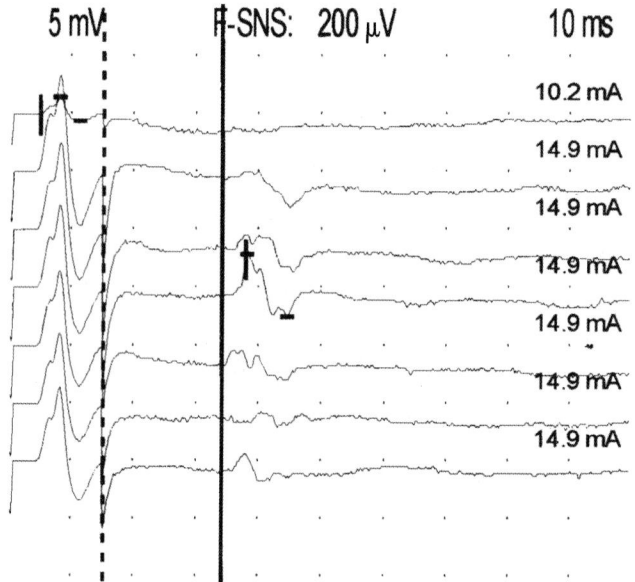

FIGURE 26.6 A series of F waves recorded from the thenar eminence following repeated median nerve stimulations in a patient with cervical radiculopathy. The screen is split with lower sensitivity (5 mV per division) to the left of the dotted line to show the full CMAPs generated by distal stimulation and higher sensitivity (200 μV per division) to the right to allow visualization of the much smaller F-wave responses. The sweep speed is 10 milliseconds per division. The dark vertical line marks the latency of the earliest F-wave potential in the group (minimal F latency).

The time required for this round trip up and down the motor nerve is measured as *the F-wave minimal latency*. Although pathology at any point along the nerve may prolong the F-wave latency, if normal function of the distal nerve is documented by motor NCS in the more distal nerve sites, F-wave prolongation must be the result of slowing in the proximal segment.

A different long-latency response, *the H reflex* (named after Hoffmann, who first described it in 1918), may be elicited in the legs by electrical stimulation of the Ia sensory nerve afferents in the tibial nerve at the knee while recording over the soleus muscle. (The type Ia sensory fiber [also called the *primary afferent fiber*] is a component of the muscle spindle that monitors stretch velocity.) The contraction resulting from soleus activation is analogous to the monosynaptic stretch reflex pathway elicited by testing the tendon reflex. Thus, the H reflex is the electrical equivalent of the ankle jerk reflex and aids primarily in the assessment of S1 nerve root disease and involvement of sensory fibers. In adults, the H reflex is not normally found in other muscles except for the flexor carpi radialis. F waves are present in nearly all nerves. By analyzing motor and sensory nerve conductions and long-latency responses in multiple nerves, the nature of a given neuronal injury (axonal, demyelinating, or both) and its geographic distribution may be identified, aiding in the diagnosis of neuronopathy, radiculopathy, plexopathy, mononeuropathy, and polyneuropathy.

OTHER SPECIALIZED REFLEX TESTS

Numerous other reflex tests are described and uncommonly performed. The *blink reflex* is one exception. This relatively simple to perform test assesses both trigeminal and facial nerve pathways. Recording electrodes are placed on the orbicularis oculi bilaterally and the supraorbital nerve is stimulated. An ipsilateral R1 response is seen on the stimulated side only. A later R2 complex response is seen bilaterally. Differing patterns are evident in trigeminal or facial neuropathy and central pontine or medullary disease.

NEEDLE ELECTROMYOGRAPHY

BASIC CONCEPTS

Complementary to NCS is assessment of clinically relevant muscles using needle EMG. A sterile, disposable, needle recording electrode is placed directly into the selected muscle, which is then activated by voluntary contraction at differing levels of effort. Anterior horn cell action potentials propagate impulses to the end of multiple axonal branches and initiate neuromuscular junction transmission, thereby activating individual muscle fibers; normally every muscle fiber innervated by a motor neuron fires following a nerve action potential. A single motor axon with all of its multiple branches and innervated muscle fibers is known as a *motor unit*. The strength of a muscle contraction is determined primarily by the number of activated motor units and motor unit firing rates. The recording characteristics of the EMG needle enable live recording and analysis of individual and aggregate motor unit waveforms. Two types of electrode are most commonly used. *Monopolar electrodes* are flexible solid stainless steel needles coated with inert material so that only the bare tip can record activity. The reference point is typically a surface electrode on the skin. *Concentric electrodes* are a rigid stainless steel cannula that includes a specialized central wire. The activity is recorded from the wire and referenced to the cannula. Monopolar needles record from a larger territory, which is slightly better for spontaneous activity discussed later. Concentric electrodes record from a smaller area and are better for motor unit analysis also discussed later. Some consider monopolar electrodes to be less painful but the difference is minimal when ultrasharp disposable electrodes are used. Either electrode is acceptable for use.

INSERTIONAL AND SPONTANEOUS ACTIVITY

During the needle EMG examination, three major categories are assessed: *spontaneous activity*, *motor unit configuration*, and *motor unit recruitment*, including the *interference pattern*. Different areas of the muscle are explored to ensure a representative sample and to detect focal changes. Insertional activity is the brief burst of electrical activity provoked by the EMG needle as it moves through the muscle, generating a cluster of transient high-frequency spikes lasting from 50 milliseconds to a few hundred milliseconds. In some disorders, the insertional activity is consistently prolonged or reduced with each movement of the needle, but the distinction is often subjective and not considered by most to be diagnostic. Once needle movement has ceased, no other electrical activity should normally appear as long as the muscle remains at rest. Reduced insertional activity is present in muscle replaced by nonexcitable tissue, such as fat or connective tissue.

Muscle fibers that have lost innervation through motor axon injury or muscle degeneration or necrosis may undergo spontaneous depolarization, generating brief spikes (*fibrillations*) and *positive sharp waves* in the resting muscle; sharp waves usually fire in a regular pattern with a frequency of 0.5 to 15 Hz (Fig. 26.7). This activity is generated by individual myocytes. Waveforms similar to fibrillations normally occur at the muscle endplate region and must be distinguished; the *endplate spikes* also fire at faster semirhythmic rates. Also recorded at the endplate region is

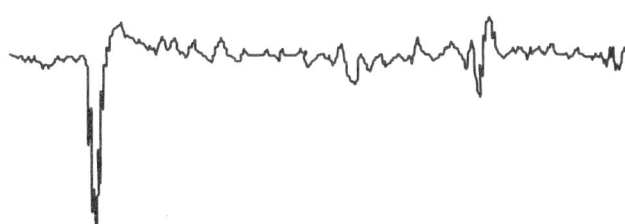

FIGURE 26.7 Spontaneous activity in a resting muscle. This tracing was recorded from the triceps muscle of a patient with cervical radiculopathy. A positive sharp wave, named for its sharp initial positive (downward) deflection, is seen on the *left*. On the *right*, a smaller triphasic fibrillation is seen. These potentials are markers of active denervation and result from the random, spontaneous depolarization of denervated single muscle fibers.

endplate noise, a disturbance of the baseline that correlates with miniature endplate potentials.

Abnormal spontaneous activity is the hallmark of denervating axonal injury at any point from the anterior horn cell to the nerve terminal (e.g., radiculopathy, plexopathy, axonal polyneuropathy, mononeuropathy) but is also prominent in inflammatory myopathies, such as polymyositis or dermatomyositis because of isolation of section of muscle from the endplate region producing functional denervation. Lesser degrees of spontaneous activity may be observed in other myopathies with muscle fiber necrosis (e.g., myotonic dystrophy, Duchenne or limb girdle muscular dystrophy) and in some toxic, metabolic, and infectious myopathies (e.g., myoglobinuria [rhabdomyolysis] or viral myositis). Spontaneous activity typically begins to initially occur at 10 to 14 days after denervation but is more evident 3 to 4 weeks after onset and may persist for a protracted time unless that muscle fiber is reinnervated.

Other aberrant involuntary discharges may appear with certain neurogenic or myopathic disorders. *Fasciculations* are isolated spontaneous discharges of whole or partial motor units and are prominent in motor neuron disease, benign fasciculation syndrome, and disorders of nerve excitability. Fasciculations may be visible as a muscle twitch, EMG needle sudden movement, or recordable discharge. *Complex repetitive discharges* are relatively nonspecific machine-like phenomena more common in chronic neurogenic conditions. These discharges are very regular and start and stop abruptly. The origin is considered to a stable circuit created between several adjacent muscle fibers. *Myotonic discharges* are distinctive revving motor-like discharges with more limited associations, including myotonic dystrophy and myotonia congenita; however, acquired conditions can also demonstrate these finding. Waxing and waning frequency and amplitude are characteristic. *Myokymic discharges* are repetitive, grouped, nerve-generated discharges (doublets or multiplets) and occur commonly in the facial muscles from diverse cause but are uncommon in the limbs. Limb myokymic discharges suggest radiation injury, timber rattlesnake venom, or certain channelopathies. The origin is nerve components. Most rare are the very rapid *neuromyotonic discharges*, characteristic of Isaac syndrome or other forms of motor unit hyperactivity.

MOTOR UNIT CONFIGURATION

Assessment of the waveform generated by motor unit activation (*the motor unit potential* or MUP) yields important information

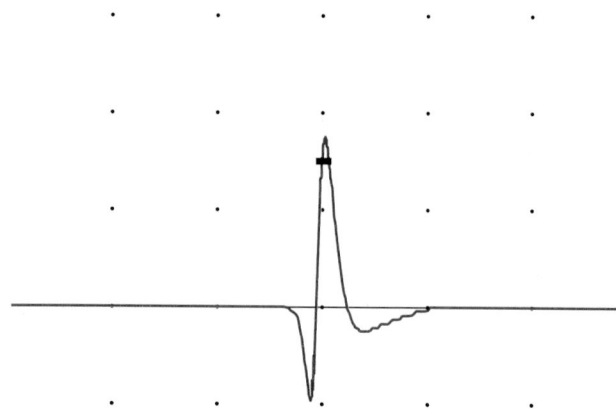

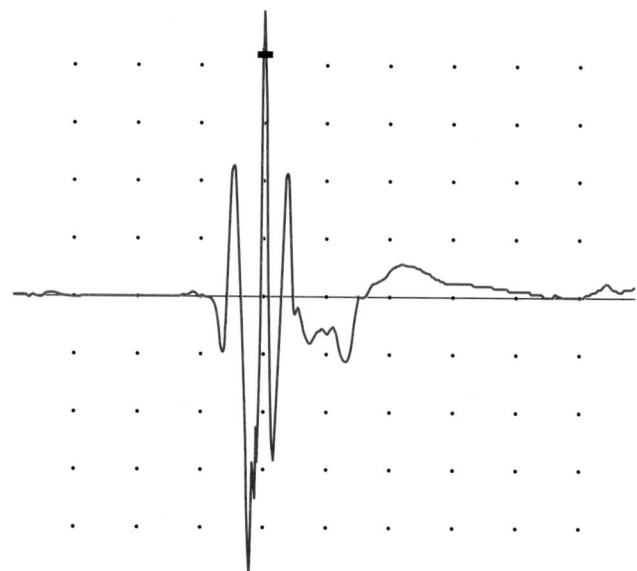

FIGURE 26.8 A normal MUP. This waveform was recorded from the biceps muscle with a concentric needle electrode as the first potential recruited during minimal voluntary contraction in a normal subject. Sweep speed was 10 milliseconds per division and sensitivity was 500 μV per division. This waveform has an amplitude of 1.4 mV, a duration of 12.5 milliseconds, and a simple morphology with three turns.

FIGURE 26.9 A neurogenic MUP. This waveform was recorded during voluntary activation of the gastrocnemius muscle with a concentric needle electrode in a patient with a distal diabetic neuropathy. Sweep speed was 5 milliseconds per division and sensitivity was 1 mV per division. This waveform has a high amplitude of 10 mV and a significantly increased duration of 29 milliseconds, and is highly complex, with more than 10 turns. This motor unit likely innervated a number of muscle fibers denervated from loss of other motor axons, producing the characteristic MUAP changes in neurogenic conditions.

(Fig. 26.8). MUP parameters include waveform duration, amplitude, and morphology (number of turns or baseline crossings). Motor unit characteristics are best assessed by capturing MUPs with the aid of a trigger and delay line, so that the waveform can be frozen and assessed. The duration is measured from the point where the waveform deviates from the baseline to the point where a stable baseline returns following the waveform. The amplitude is typically measured from the largest waveform-positive and waveform-negative peaks. *Polyphasic* waveforms have five or more phases, determined by the number of times the waveform crosses the baseline plus one. Waveform turns or phase reversals are considered as well. MUPs that contain more than seven or more turns are considered by some to be *complex MUPs*. Both polyphasic and complex MUPs are indicators of desynchronization seen in all forms of chronic neuromuscular disease that affects neurogenic or myogenic components. Small percentages of these potentials are evident in normal muscle as well, typically less than 12%. Some MUPs include a small additional time-locked component following a return to baseline—a *satellite potential*. Because a muscle may contain hundreds of motor units, the EMG examination must include a representative sample of motor units collected at varying levels of voluntary contraction.

Diseases of the motor nerve and muscle alter these motor unit parameters in characteristic ways. When motor axons fail, the associated muscle fibers lose their innervation. However, branches from surviving motor axons in the same nerve may reinnervate these denervated muscle fibers in a process called *collateral reinnervation*. Over the course of several months, this compensatory repair process gradually expands both the total number of muscle fibers innervated by surviving motor units, as well as the geographic territory spanned within the muscle. Reinnervated motor units produce abnormally enlarged MUPs of long duration, high amplitude, and increased complexity, which are markers of chronic neurogenic injury (Fig. 26.9).

In contrast, myopathies destroy or inactivate some muscle fibers in most or all of the motor units within a muscle, thereby reducing both the number and distribution of fibers within each unit, producing abnormally small MUPs of short duration, low amplitude, and increased complexity (Fig. 26.10).

In normal individuals as well as patients with neuropathic or myopathic disorders, there is a wide range of sizes of individual MUPs. The size of the motor neuron, motor axon, and corresponding motor unit specifies the available strength, maximal firing rate, and fatigue resistance of that unit. In addition, different muscles may have divergent average motor unit size depending on the muscular function. For example, an extraocular muscle may have relatively few muscle fibers per motor unit to deliver small precise movements in contrast to a proximal hip girdle muscle where high fatigue resistance predominates. Thus, the characteristics of a small number of MUPs are insufficient for a definitive diagnosis. Determining the mean duration of 20 MUPs is one reliable way to separate neuropathic from myopathic disorders. Normal values, generated in Copenhagen, for the mean durations of most muscles in each decade of life were published in 1975 and are widely used. However, qualitative MUP assessment invokes the same process by assessing a number of different MUPs without quantitative measurement. This assessment requires experience with the process and specific muscle undergoing testing.

Disorders of the neuromuscular junction, as in myasthenia gravis, may also prevent activation of enough fibers, owing to cumulative neuromuscular junction blockade, to produce myopathic-appearing MUPs. Following severe nerve injury, the earliest phases of reinnervation and the latest phases of denervation during neurogenic atrophy may also produce short-duration motor units (*nascent units*) when the initial few muscle fibers are reinnervated.

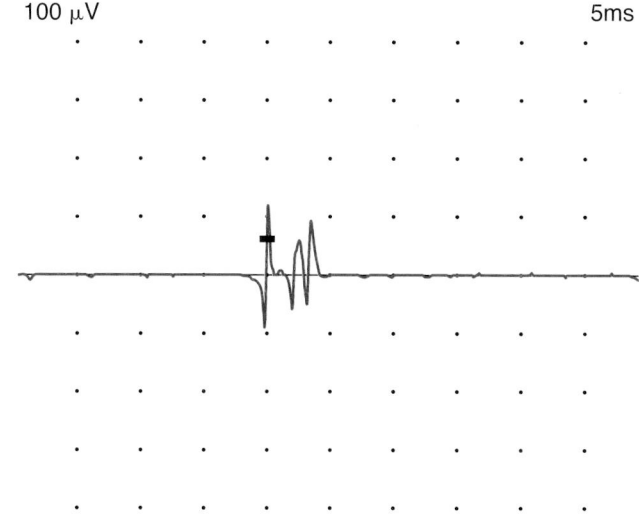

100 μV   5ms

FIGURE 26.10 A myopathic MUP. This waveform was recorded during voluntary activation of the vastus lateralis muscle with a concentric needle electrode in a patient with polymyositis. Sweep speed was 5 milliseconds per division and sensitivity was 100 μV per division. This waveform has a low amplitude of 210 μV and a short duration of 7 milliseconds and is complex with eight turns. As individual muscle fibers within a motor unit drop out during myopathic injury, the electric potential generated shrinks proportionately, resulting in decreased MUAP amplitude and duration and increasingly complex morphology from reduced synchronization.

RECRUITMENT AND INTERFERENCE PATTERNS

Needle EMG also enables assessment of motor unit recruitment patterns. As a muscle begins to contract at the lowest force levels, the first recruited motor unit begins to fire repeatedly at a specific frequency, usually at a minimum of 4 to 5 Hz. As demand for more strength increases, the firing frequency of the motor unit increases until a second motor unit is recruited. The specific firing frequency of the first recruited motor unit at the moment the second motor unit appears is *the recruitment frequency*. Abnormally high recruitment frequencies appear as motor units are lost, forcing surviving units to fire at faster and faster rates before additional units appear because of reduced numbers of motor units available for recruitment. In contrast, because most motor units are smaller and weaker, owing to loss of muscle fibers, lower recruitment frequencies are seen in myopathies (*early recruitment*). Consequently, multiple motor units must be activated earlier than in normal subjects to generate the same levels of force. Following damage to upper motor neuron pathways, recruitment is disordered, and motor units may fire at a slower than needed rate despite true maximal voluntary effort, as disrupted descending impulses improperly modulate firing frequency. The *firing ratio* is calculated by dividing the firing frequency (firing rate of the fastest firing MUP) over the number of different MUPs activated. This ratio is typically around five. In other words, if the fastest MUP fires at 15 Hz, one expects to see three total firing MUPs. Neurogenic processes increase this ratio.

The *interference pattern* is the overlapping pattern generated by the simultaneous activation of large numbers of MUPs during maximal contraction; the spike density and the amplitude of the summated response (*envelope amplitude*) are assessed. This response typically appears as a dense band of competing waveform activity at slow sweep speeds, which normally obscures the baseline tracing (Fig. 26.11).

Normal recruitment from low to intermediate to full contraction should produce a full interference pattern with a conical onset, as amplitudes increase progressively with the recruitment of larger and larger motor units to generate increasing force. *Incomplete or reduced interference patterns* (despite maximal contraction) are seen in advanced denervating disorders as more and more motor units drop out, ultimately leaving a *picket-fence* pattern, termed *discrete recruitment* (Fig. 26.12).

Maximal voluntary effort must be elicited before interference patterns are accurately assessed because poor volitional effort also produces an incomplete pattern; weakness due to central motor neuron injury may also result in reduced recruitment. In contrast, full *interference patterns*, *despite weakness*, occur with myopathic disorders. A full pattern appears almost immediately with minimal effort, owing to the large numbers of weakened motor units that are required to generate low levels of force. This pattern also has low envelope amplitude because the size of the constituent MUPs is reduced. Advanced methods that attempt to minimize the effects of voluntary effort (cloud analysis) are available on most machines but are not routinely applied, partly from limited normative data.

FIGURE 26.11 A normal interference pattern. This dense, overlapping group of MUP waveforms was recorded with a concentric needle electrode from the biceps muscle during maximal voluntary contraction in a normal subject. The pattern represents the simultaneous activation of all the functional motor units within that muscle. The sweep speed was 100 milliseconds per division and the sensitivity was 1 mV per division.

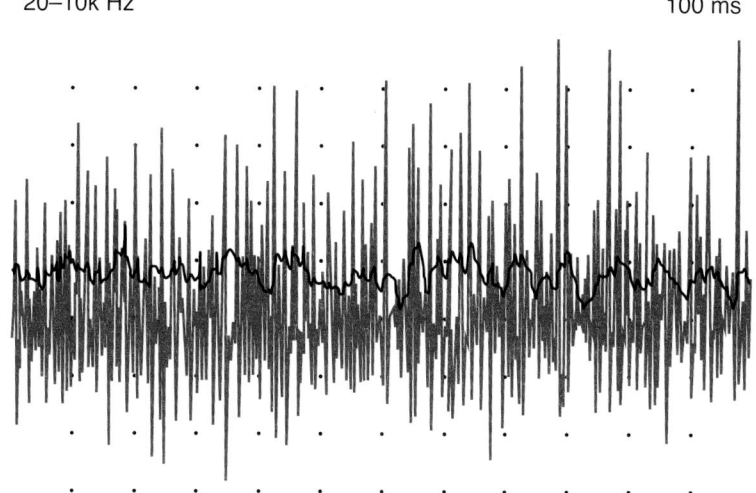

20–10k Hz   100 ms

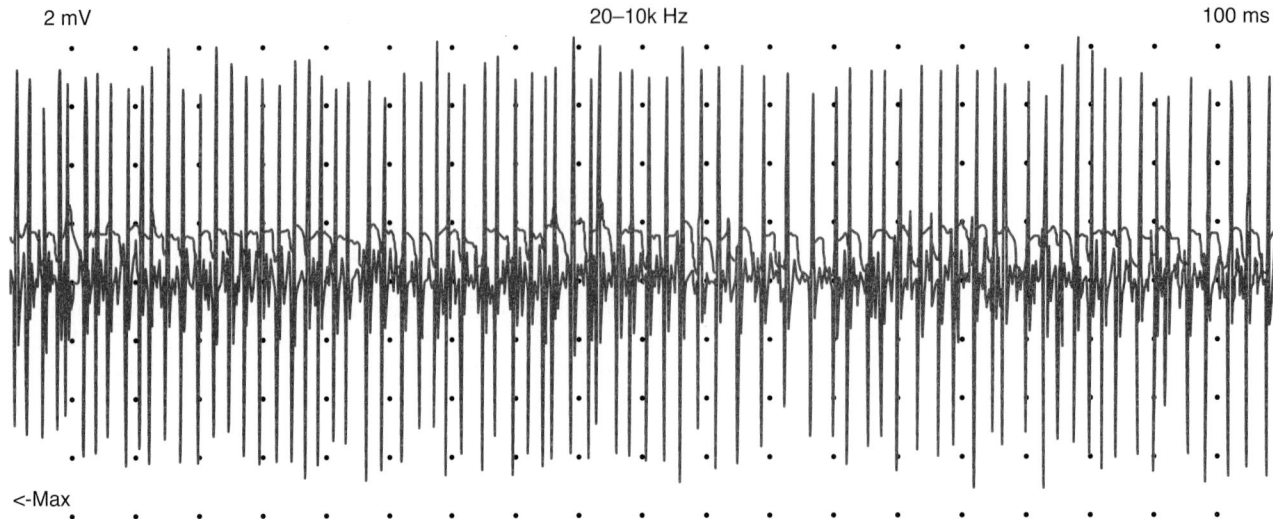

2 mV   20–10k Hz   100 ms

<-Max

FIGURE 26.12 A reduced interference pattern. This pattern of MUP waveforms was recorded with a concentric needle electrode from the biceps muscle of a patient with amyotrophic lateral sclerosis during maximal voluntary contraction. The sweep speed was 100 milliseconds per division and the sensitivity was 2 mV per division. Instead of the normal, dense band of overlapping MUAPs observed in the normal subject (see Fig. 16.11), a "picket-fence" pattern (*discrete recruitment*) representing the activation of only one rapid firing motor unit emerges because so many motor units have been lost. The MUAP amplitude of the most prominent surviving unit is increased (8 to 10 mV), consistent with collateral reinnervation.

NERVE CONDUCTION STUDIES AND ELECTROMYOGRAPHY APPLICATIONS

A wide range of neuromuscular and central disorders may benefit from electrodiagnosis. Many specific applications are discussed in other sections dedicated to specific conditions. Some common examples include focal mononeuropathy, multifocal neuropathy, axonal and demyelinating polyneuropathy, motor neuronopathy, myopathy, myositis, and radiculopathy. A proper electrodiagnostic medicine consultation relies on a targeted clinical assessment so that the study design is focused on the clinical problem at hand and includes assessment of sufficient but not excessive numbers of clinically relevant nerves and muscles. Small-diameter fibers may be assessed by other means, most commonly skin biopsy for determination of epidermal nerve fiber density. Nerves are amenable to ultrasonography; however, this technology is currently considered to be a supplemental adjunct to electrodiagnostic methods described. A guideline found level B evidence for use of ultrasound in the diagnosis of suspected carpal tunnel syndrome. Magnetic resonance imaging (MRI) of nerve is increasing sophisticated with higher power magnetic fields and improved protocols. However, imaging of nerve and muscle is also adjunct information that typically identifies potential sites of nerve swelling and muscle signal changes that do not provide information on the disease type or process. MRI can identify atrophic muscles. Practice parameters and diagnostic criteria exist for some common conditions, including but not limited to carpal tunnel syndrome, ulnar neuropathy, amyotrophic lateral sclerosis, chronic inflammatory demyelinating polyneuropathy, polyneuropathy, and others. In nearly all cases, both sensory and motor NCS and needle EMG are performed. Timely reporting of results is required that includes numeric data described earlier and written assessment of the normality of obtained values. A diagnostic conclusion based on the data acquired

is expected. In some cases, guidance on disease severity, time course, and prognosis is possible.

TESTS OF NEUROMUSCULAR TRANSMISSION

REPETITIVE NERVE STIMULATION

Repetitive nerve stimulation (RNS) studies assess neuromuscular transmission using a standard motor nerve conduction setup (see section "Nerve Conduction Studies") to deliver a series of supramaximal stimulations to a motor nerve at a specific frequency while recording each generated CMAP. CMAP trains of 4 to 10 waveforms are usually recorded at rates from 2 to 3 Hz (low-frequency stimulation). By convention, the waveforms within each train are displayed horizontally on the same baseline from left to right (Fig. 26.13).

Trains are then evaluated either for decreases in consecutive CMAP size (as assessed by area and amplitude, from the first to a later potential, typically the fourth or fifth, and expressed as percentage decrement) or for increases in size (usually expressed in percentage increments). Most protocols include one baseline train, followed by a brief period of voluntary exercise without stimulation, and then followed by one immediate, postexercise train and several more trains at intervals over the next 1 to 5 minutes. The role of exercise is explained in the following text. For high-frequency stimulation studies, either transcutaneous stimulation at rates of 20 to 50 Hz or maximal voluntary contraction itself, which provides painless activation of the nerve at similar rates, is used. However, high-frequency RNS studies are quite painful and very infrequently used in clinical practice; scenarios almost exclusively are for presynaptic disorders such as Lambert–Eaton myasthenic syndrome (LEMS), organophosphate poisoning, or botulism (as described

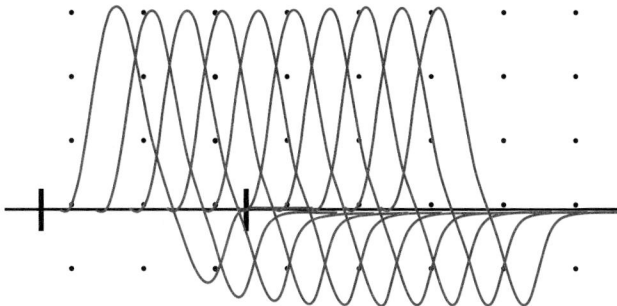

FIGURE 26.13 RNS. A train of 10 CMAPs recorded from the thenar eminence following RNS of the median nerve at a frequency of 3 Hz, arrayed in the order of stimulation (*left to right*). Each individual CMAP is normal, and no significant change in CMAP amplitude or area is observed during repetitive stimulation.

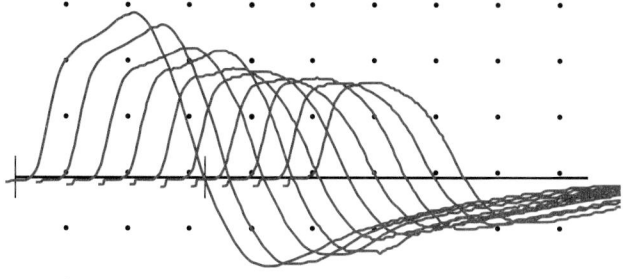

FIGURE 26.14 Decrement during RNS. Progressive decreases in the size of CMAPs were recorded from the thenar eminence during a train of RNS at 3 Hz in a patient with myasthenia gravis. Losses in both amplitude and area of 40% to 50% appeared during RNS, owing to transmission failure at increasing numbers of neuromuscular junctions.

later in the chapter and in Chapter 137) when the patient is unable to provide voluntary muscle activation.

POSTSYNAPTIC NEUROMUSCULAR JUNCTION DYSFUNCTION

Patients with postsynaptic neuromuscular junction dysfunction, most commonly caused by myasthenia gravis, may demonstrate decremental responses following low-frequency stimulation. During normal neuromuscular junction transmission, depolarization of the motor axon induces acetylcholine release from the nerve terminal; the transmitter diffuses across the synaptic cleft to activate a group of acetylcholine receptors on the muscle fiber, each of which generates a local depolarization. These summated depolarizations ultimately reach threshold and generate a muscle action potential, which then initiates muscle fiber contraction. Declining release of acetylcholine normally occurs with stimulation at low frequencies; however, because postsynaptic acetylcholine receptors are abundant, these declines do not affect neuromuscular transmission, ensuring adequate muscle fiber depolarization despite the lower levels of acetylcholine released (*safety margin*). However, in myasthenia and some rare genetic postsynaptic disorders, the decline in acetylcholine release becomes critical because there are fewer functional acetylcholine receptors. The result is failure of neuromuscular transmission at multiple neuromuscular junctions with continued stimulation. As increasing numbers of muscle fibers drop out with successive stimulation, the size of the overall summated CMAP also decreases (Fig. 26.14). Rare hereditary disorders of neuromuscular junction physiology (congenital myasthenia) cause differing effects on this test depending on the affected component.

Additionally, the size (amplitude or area) of a single CMAP immediately after brief exercise, in myasthenia, may increase by 10% to 50% or more compared to the baseline (preexercise) CMAP. This phenomenon, known as *postexercise facilitation* or *posttetanic potentiation*, is attributed to a temporary increase in acetylcholine release after a brief maximal contraction because of transiently heightened presynaptic calcium influx. Postexercise facilitation is assessed by comparing the first CMAP in the first train acquired immediately after exercise to the amplitude of the first CMAP in the preexercise train. In addition to postexercise facilitation of CMAP amplitude, any decrement in the baseline train may transiently improve immediately after exercise (*decrement repair*). However, after this transient repair, decrement typically worsens in trains recorded over the next 3 to 4 minutes, often dipping below baseline (*postactiva-*

tion exhaustion) as reserve acetylcholine levels are exhausted. Decrement ultimately returns to preexercise levels within 10 minutes. The decrement is typically greater in proximal and bulbar muscles but is simpler and more reliably performed in distal muscles.

PRESYNAPTIC NEUROMUSCULAR JUNCTION DYSFUNCTION

In the presynaptic LEMS and some cases of botulism, the CMAP amplitude may be reduced on routine NCS, and low-frequency RNS produces decrement similar to that seen in postsynaptic dysfunction. Both the low baseline CMAP and the decrement seen on low-frequency stimulation are the result of the combination of normal decline in acetylcholine release at low rates of stimulation superimposed on the diminished release of acetylcholine resulting from antibody blockade of the presynaptic voltage-gated calcium channel (LEMS) or disruption of the mechanisms of acetylcholine release (botulism). High-frequency RNS, in contrast, characteristically leads to CMAP increment (facilitation) over 1 to 2 seconds, usually exceeding 100%. The pain of high-frequency stimulation may be avoided by having the patient voluntarily contract the muscle with maximum force for 10 to 20 seconds, after which a second single CMAP is immediately obtained; this "exercise test" shows postexercise facilitation comparable in magnitude to the increment observed after high-frequency stimulation.

SINGLE-FIBER ELECTROMYOGRAPHY

Another test of the neuromuscular junction is single-fiber electromyography (SFEMG). A specialized reusable electrode or small concentric disposable electrode is used that records single muscle fiber potentials. When an axon is selectively stimulated and a single muscle fiber action potential is measured (*stimulated SFEMG*), the interval between stimulus and response varies with each stimulus. This normal variation results from the fluctuating time required for electrochemical transmission across the junction and is quantitated as *jitter*. *Volitional SFEMG* recordings are more commonly performed and measure jitter by assessing the differences between two voluntarily activated muscle fibers from the same motor unit. With neuromuscular dysfunction, jitter increases, and in severe cases, complete block of neuromuscular transmission may be documented. SFEMG is the single most sensitive assay of neuromuscular dysfunction in myasthenia gravis, having a sensitivity of greater than 95% when applied to a clinically affected muscle (Fig. 26.15A and B).

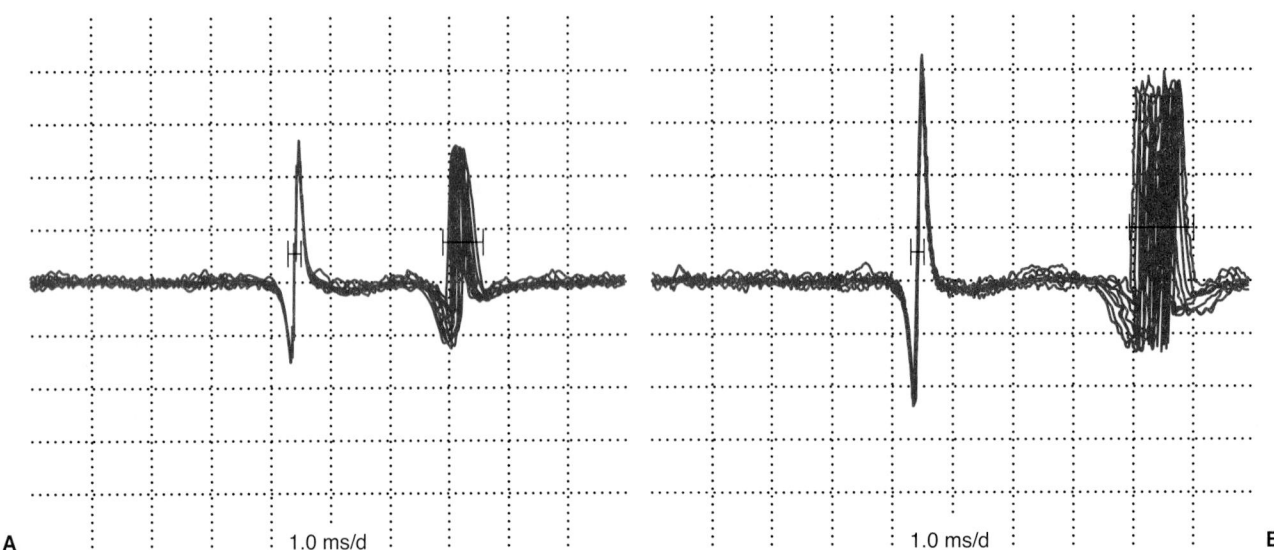

A   1.0 ms/d   1.0 ms/d   B

FIGURE 26.15 **A:** Single-fiber EMG in a normal subject. In this tracing, 50 to 100 consecutive discharges generated by two single muscle fibers from the same motor unit during voluntary activation of the frontalis muscle are superimposed. The tracings are arrayed so that the first (*left*) potential is fixed with each discharge. Consequently, the variability in the time between the firing of the first (*left*) and second (*right*) potential with each discharge (the interpotential interval) is illustrated solely as varia- tion of the second waveform. This effect, quantitated as *jitter*, is due to the variable time required for neuromuscular transmission to produce an action potential from discharge to discharge. **B:** Single-fiber EMG in a patient with myasthenia gravis during volitional activation of the frontalis muscle using the same recording methods described in **A**. This tracing illustrates increased variability in neuromuscular transmission and clearly differs from that of the normal subject above. The jitter in this fiber pair was 160 microseconds, well above the upper limits of the normal range.

Although SFEMG is highly sensitive, it is not specific and may be abnormal in any condition causing damage to nerve or muscle that produces reinnervation. Consequently, it is essential to perform other electrodiagnostic methods and a careful clinical assessment before considering SFEMG. SFEMG is most useful for confirming neuromuscular junction dysfunction in suspected myasthenia gra- vis when other tests are equivocal or negative and other conditions that produce muscle weakness are assessed (see Fig. 26.11).

TRANSCRANIAL MAGNETIC STIMULATION

Transcranial magnetic stimulation (TMS) evokes compound motor potentials through noninvasive stimulation of the cortex. TMS has become an important method for studying the conductivity and excitability of the corticospinal system, abnormal cortical circuitry in neurologic diseases, and the reorganization of sensorimotor and visual systems after peripheral and central lesions. Electromag- netic induction may stimulate neural tissue. TMS is accomplished through the generation of high-intensity current (5 to 10 kiloam- pere) and discharged as a quick pulse through wire coils placed on the surface of the head. The coils induce a magnetic flux of short duration (100 to 200 microseconds) and high intensity (1 to 2 T). The magnetic fields, in turn, induce electrical current in the underlying cerebral cortex. TMS delivery devices are embedded in a nonconductive plastic or rubber material and typically fashioned into figure eight, butterfly, or flat or concave circular shapes and applied near the part of the brain under study. The various shapes and sizes are designed to distribute or focus the induced magnetic fields. Round coils generate more diffuse magnetic fields and figure eight coils produce a narrower region of neural activation.

Stimulus intensity is expressed as a function of either the motor threshold or the percentage of machine output. TMS is less painful than transcranial electrical stimulation (TES), which causes uncom- fortable shocks in the underlying skin and muscle. Unlike TES, which directly excites cortical long tracts, the induced electrical fields of TMS preferentially stimulate neural elements oriented par- allel to the surface of the brain (i.e., primarily interneurons). TMS pulses are associated with benign acoustic clicks and mild scalp or facial muscle activation. A momentary sense of disorientation at maximal stimulation may be felt. However, there are virtually no clinical cognitive or sensory effects at low intensities of TMS stimu- lation. Waveform recordings are usually obtained from a contralat- eral distal limb muscle, the motor-evoked potential (MEP).

TMS may be delivered as a single pulse, in paired pulses, or as repetitive trains of stimulation (rTMS). Paired pulse and rTMS are powerful in studying human brain function, transiently stimulating or inhibiting different brain areas in awake and behaving subjects. Effects of rTMS on cortical excitability and inhibition outlast (for minutes to hours) the stimulation itself, a characteristic that could lead to therapeutic applications. Clinical trials have been con- ducted primarily not only in depression but also in Parkinson dis- ease, epilepsy, obsessive–compulsive disorders, and schizophrenia.

SINGLE-PULSE TRANSCRANIAL MAGNETIC STIMULATION

Following a single TMS, the MEP latency and amplitude measure the integrity of pathways and membrane excitability characteris- tics of the upper motor neuron. Central motor conduction time is calculated by subtracting the peripheral MEP latency (i.e., cervical or lumbosacral proximal roots to distal limb muscles) from the total conduction latency (i.e., TMS to MEP onset of the same muscle) and is obtained with a single, maximal TMS over the primary motor cortex (Fig. 26.16).

Prolongation of the central motor conduction time may originate with the loss of large myelinated motor axons subsequent to degeneration, and the test assesses upper motor neuron (UMN) dysfunction. Central motor conduction time, as well as other TMS measures, is helpful in diagnosing and following progression in patients with upper motor neuron diseases, such as amyotrophic lateral sclerosis (ALS). However, central motor conduction time may be of limited value when large-diameter axons remain normal or in diseases where long-tract integrity is known to be normal, such as Parkinson disease.

As a measure of UMN functional integrity, TMS may detect abnormalities when there are no clinical UMN signs. TMS may reveal subtle subclinical UMN dysfunction and help clarify the diagnosis of ALS, as well as the relationship between ALS and its variants (100), including progressive muscular atrophy where there may be subclinical UMN changes.

MEP amplitudes and latencies are influenced by multiple factors, including configuration and placement of the TMS coil, stimulus intensity, presence of conditioning pulses, muscle facilitation, and degree of phase cancellation. Suprasegmental modulation of MEPs may be inferred in several ways, including demonstration of relatively unchanged F-wave properties under the same stimulus conditions. Motor threshold is defined as the lowest stimulus intensity that evokes MEPs of 50 μV in amplitude in 5 of 10 trials. Stimulus intensity is expressed as a percentage of the TMS device's maximum output. MEP amplitude is usually measured peak to peak, increases with stimulus intensity, and plateaus at 80% of the amplitude of the wave produced by peripheral stimulation.

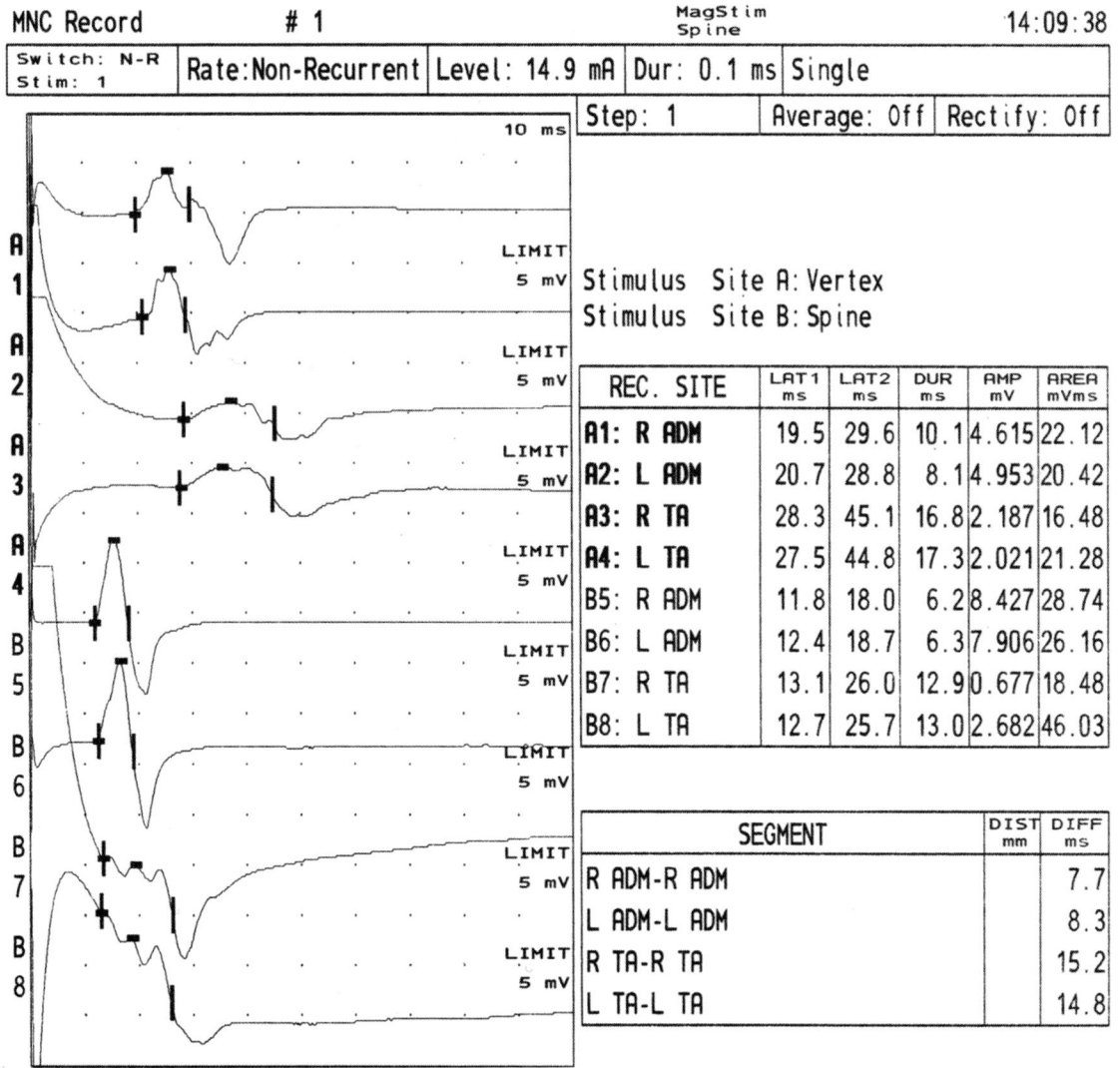

FIGURE 26.16 Transcranial magnetic stimulation (TMS) in a normal subject. These tracings show the motor-evoked responses recorded from the right and left abductor digiti minimi (ADM) muscle of the hand and the right and left tibialis anterior (TA) muscles, following stimulation of the cerebral cortex with the stimulator placed over the vertex of the skull (traces *A1* to *A4*) and following stimulation of the spine; cervical stimulation for the ADM and lumbosacral stimulation for the TA is shown in traces *B5* to *B8*. Latencies, in milliseconds, from stimulation to the onset of the waveform recorded from the muscle are shown in the *first column* (*LAT1*). Central-conduction latency (i.e., time from cortex to spinal segment) is calculated by subtracting the peripheral-conduction latency (i.e., time from spine to muscle) from the total conduction latency (i.e., time from cortex to muscle) and is shown in *SEGMENT table, final column* (*DIFF*).

Voluntary muscle activation during TMS lowers the motor threshold and increases the MEP amplitude and is associated with shorter latency. This facilitation may result from an increased number and synchronization of descending impulses from the motor cortex or from reafferent facilitation at the spinal level. Recruitment is measured by plotting a stimulus–response curve of stimulus intensity versus MEP amplitude. The slope of this curve is normally increased by facilitation, as well as by maneuvers that enlarge cortical representation of muscles, such as highly skilled, fine motor actions. Temporal summation may also follow repeated delivery of stimuli. In the first minutes following rTMS trains at low frequency (1 Hz), the amplitude of single-pulse MEP decreases. Conversely, high-frequency (>10 Hz) stimulation increases the response; these patterns resemble long-term depression and facilitation.

SILENT PERIOD

The cortical or central silent period is measured from an actively contracting muscle, representing suppression of voluntary EMG activity for up to 300 milliseconds after a single TMS. The cortical silent period is an important method of assessing inhibitory mechanisms in neurologic disease. The silent period typically follows an MEP but may be induced by subthreshold stimuli that do not produce an MEP. This *negative effect* is mechanistically distinct from the positive effect seen in MEP induction. Although the origin of the initial segments of the cortical silent period are controversial, the latter part of the silent period is modulated by central mechanisms.

REPETITIVE TRANSCRANIAL MAGNETIC STIMULATION

The first TMS capacitors could recharge only after several seconds and thus allow only single TMS pulses. With technical advances, rTMS output increased from just under 1 Hz to pulse trains up to 50 Hz. rTMS at frequencies greater than 20 Hz increases cerebral blood flow and neuronal excitability, whereas low-frequency rTMS (1 to 2 Hz) has the opposite effect. The therapeutic potential of TMS is of interest as a painless and relatively safe alternative to electroshock therapy, which has lasting motor benefit in severe parkinsonism. Enhanced cortical excitability is suggested by increased MEP amplitude after rTMS and by persistent focal metabolic enhancement as demonstrated by positron emission tomography (PET). However, rTMS may have negative effects on the motor system, so the underlying mechanisms must be more fully understood before widespread use may be expected.

The authors acknowledge significant contributions from authors of earlier editions of this section, especially Dale J. Lange, MD.

SUGGESTED READINGS

Nerve Conduction Studies and Electromyography

American Association of Electrodiagnostic Medicine. Glossary of terms in electrodiagnostic medicine. *Muscle Nerve Suppl.* 2001;10:S1–S50.

Buchthal F. Electromyography in the evaluation of muscle diseases. *Neurol Clin.* 1985;3:573–598.

Cornblath DR, Sumner AJ, Daube J, et al. Conduction block in clinical practice. *Muscle Nerve.* 1991;14:869–871.

Daube JR. Needle examination in clinical electromyography. *Muscle Nerve.* 1991;14(8):685–700.

Falck B, Stalberg E. Motor nerve conduction studies: measurement principles and interpretation of findings. *J Clin Neurophysiol.* 1995;12:254–279.

Gooch CL, Weimer LH. The electrodiagnosis of neuropathy: basic principles and common pitfalls. *Neurol Clin.* 2007;25:1–28.

Gutmann L. Pearls and pitfalls in the use of electromyography and nerve conduction studies. *Semin Neurol.* 2003;23:77–82.

Jones LK Jr. Nerve conduction studies: basic concepts and patterns of abnormalities. *Neurol Clin.* 2012;30(2):405–427.

Kimura J. *Electrodiagnosis in Diseases of Nerve and Muscle, Principles and Practice.* 4th ed. New York: Oxford University Press; 2013.

Oh J. *Clinical Electromyography, Nerve Conduction Studies.* 3rd ed. Philadelphia: Lippincott Williams & Wilkins; 2003.

Olney RK, Lewis RA, Putnam TD, et al; American Association of Electrodiagnostic Medicine. Consensus criteria for the diagnosis of multifocal motor neuropathy. *Muscle Nerve.* 2003;27(1):117–121.

Preston DC, Shapiro BE. *Electromyography and Neuromuscular Disorders: Clinical–Electrophysiologic Correlations.* 3rd ed. London: Elsevier Saunders; 2013.

Ross MA. Electrodiagnosis of peripheral neuropathy. *Neurol Clin.* 2012;30(2):529–549.

Wilbourn AJ. Sensory nerve conduction studies. *J Clin Neurophysiol.* 1994;11(6):584–601.

Tests of Neuromuscular Transmission

AAEM Quality Assurance Committee; American Association of Electrodiagnostic Medicine. Literature review of the usefulness of repetitive nerve stimulation and single fiber EMG in the electrodiagnostic evaluation of patients with suspected myasthenia gravis or Lambert–Eaton myasthenic syndrome. *Muscle Nerve.* 2001;24(9):1239–1247.

Drachman DB. Myasthenia gravis. *N Engl J Med.* 1994;330:1797–1810.

Howard JF Jr. Electrodiagnosis of disorders of neuromuscular transmission. *Phys Med Rehabil Clin N Am.* 2013;24(1):169–192.

Oh SJ. *Electromyography: Neuromuscular Transmission Studies.* Baltimore: Lippincott Williams & Wilkins; 1988.

Sanders DB. Clinical neurophysiology of disorders of the neuromuscular junction. *J Clin Neurophysiol.* 1993;12:167–180.

Sanders DB, Stalberg EV. Single fiber electromyography. *Muscle Nerve.* 1996;19:1069–1083.

Tim RW, Sanders DB. Repetitive nerve stimulation studies in the Lambert–Eaton myasthenic syndrome. *Muscle Nerve.* 1994;17:995–1001.

Transcortical Magnetic Stimulation

Barker AT, Jalinous R, Freeston IL. Non-invasive magnetic stimulation of human cortex. *Lancet.* 1985;1:1106–1107.

Eisen AA, Shtybel W. Clinical experience with transcranial magnetic stimulation. *Muscle Nerve.* 1990;13:995–1011.

Hallett M. Transcranial magnetic stimulation: a tool for mapping the central nervous system. *Electroencephalogr Clin Neurophysiol Suppl.* 1996;46:43–51.

Kobayashi M, Pascual-Leone A. Transcranial magnetic stimulation in neurology. *Lancet Neurol.* 2003;2:145–156.

Mitsumoto H, Ulug AM, Pullman SL, et al. Quantitative objective markers for upper and lower motor neuron dysfunction in ALS. *Neurology.* 2007;68:1402–1410.

Rossini PM, Rossi S. Transcranial magnetic stimulation: diagnostic, therapeutic, and research potential. *Neurology.* 2007;68:484–488.

Turner R, Bowser R, Bruijn L, et al. Mechanisms, models and biomarkers in amyotrophic lateral sclerosis. *Amyotroph Lateral Scler Frontotemporal Degener.* 2013;14(1):19–32.

Wassermann EM, Lisanby SH. Therapeutic application of repetitive transcranial magnetic stimulation: a review. *Clin Neurophysiol.* 2001;112:1367–1377.

Autonomic Testing 27

Louis H. Weimer

INTRODUCTION

Recognition of disorders producing autonomic dysfunction continues to increase the demand for noninvasive clinical testing in order to validate clinical diagnoses. Because autonomic systems affect virtually all organ systems, symptoms produced are multiple and varied, often affecting functions not considered by neurologists. Because many autonomic complaints can appear to be nonspecific, objective assessment is desirable in many instances. Laboratories testing autonomic function are increasingly available in part due to reliable noninvasive techniques. However, formal training opportunities in this neurologic specialty remain limited.

Unlike other systems, autonomic function is not directly assessed. Instead, responses of complex overlapping reflex loops are measured after controlled perturbations, most commonly heart rate (HR), blood pressure (BP), and sweating. Techniques to evaluate autonomic function are numerous and continue to be devised, but only a limited number are considered to be suitable for routine clinical application (Table 27.1). Tests of cardiovagal, adrenergic, and sudomotor function are most commonly performed and are recognized, standard clinical measures. Consensus recommends use of a standardized testing battery in a controlled setting. Bedside screening tests complement a clinical evaluation; some techniques can be performed with limited equipment such as an electrocardiography (ECG) or electromyography (EMG) machine.

TABLE 27.1   Selected Tests of Autonomic Function

Cardiovagal	Microneurography
Well established	Mental stress tests
HR variability to cyclic deep breathing	Cold pressor test
HR response to the VM (VR)	Spectral and transfer function BP analysis
HR response to standing (30:15 ratio)	**Sudomotor**
Other	*Well established*
Diving reflex/cold face test	Sympathetic skin response (SSR)
HR variability at rest	Quantitative sudomotor axon reflex test (QSART)
HR response to cough	Thermoregulatory sweat test (TST)
Spectral analysis of HR signals (frequency domain)	Silastic sweat imprint testing
Transfer function analysis (nonlinear dynamics)	Skin biopsy for sweat gland innervation
Adrenergic	**Additional or Investigational Methods**
Well established	Pharmacologic challenges
BP response to the VM (phase IV and late phase II)	Vasomotor testing
BP response to orthostatic stress	Pupillary testing (pharmacologic)
– Head-up tilt	Pupillometry, pupillography
– Standing	Urodynamics/cystometrogram with bethanechol
Other	GI motility studies
Sustained handgrip test	GI manometry
Squat test	Salivary testing/Schirmer test
BP response to alternate stressors	Penile plethysmography, papaverine injection
– Lower body negative pressure	Neuroendocrine tests
– Neck suction	Neurogenic flare test
– Lying down	Quantitative direct and indirect test of sudomotor function (Q-DIRT)
– Liquid meal	Cardiac PET scanning
Plasma catecholamine levels (supine/standing)	

HR, heart rate; VM, Valsalva maneuver; VR, Valsalva ratio; BP, blood pressure; GI, gastrointestinal; PET, positron emission tomography.

The primary testing goal is to identify autonomic failure and to assess and quantify disease severity. In some cases, determining the systems involved, such as parasympathetic, sympathetic, or pan-autonomic, can refine diagnostic possibilities. In most instances, localization to central, preganglionic, or postganglionic dysfunction is not possible. The effects of medications, environmental conditions, dehydration, and acute illness should be minimized during testing. Selected commonly performed tests are briefly discussed in this chapter.

SELECTED TESTS

HEART RATE VARIABILITY

Measures of HR variability are simple to record and are sensitive indicators of parasympathetic function. Cyclic deep breathing at 6 breaths per minute is the best validated stimulus; both afferent and efferent pathways are vagally mediated and blunted by anticholinergic agents. Most commonly, beat-to-beat HR is recorded, and R-R intervals or sequential HR data are measured, and the resultant enhanced sinus arrhythmia is analyzed with one of numerous methods; the test is currently the best cardiovagal measure available. Age-segregated normative ranges are well described. Other parasympathetic cardiovagal tests include measures of HR variability during rest, coughing, diving reflex, standing, squatting, and active lying down. The HR response to Valsalva maneuver (VM) is discussed later. Spectral and frequency HR analysis is an important research tool that has not been adequately validated for routine clinical application, although commercial automated testing devices using these methods are employed typically by non-neurologists and cardiologists.

SYMPATHETIC MEASURES

The VM is a reliable and reproducible method that provides information for both parasympathetic and sympathetic function if beat-to-beat HR and BP data are recorded. Devices that noninvasively record continuous BP are typically used; multiple machines are commercially available. The subject blows into a closed tube at 40 mm Hg for 15 seconds while HR and BP are recorded. Isolated Valsalva ratio (VR) HR recording requires minimal equipment but more information is gathered with less chance of misinterpretation if continual BP is recorded. The VM BP waveform is divided into four distinct phases (I to IV). Phases I and III signify nonspecific transmitted pressure and release from the maneuver, which initially causes cardiac output and BP to drop, providing the test stimulus. Normally, peripheral vasoconstriction and increased HR produce partial or full reversal of the BP decline, marking early (BP drop) and late (BP recovery) phase II. After Valsalva ends, the BP slowly overshoots and later returns to baseline (phase IV overshoot). Adrenergic insufficiency causes phase II to progressively deepen or fail to correct. Phase IV may fail to overshoot. Phase II recovery is likely mediated by α-adrenergic stimulation and phase IV by β-adrenergic supported by pharmacologic studies. HR normally increases during the Valsalva period and then overshoots below baseline values.

The VR is calculated by dividing the R-R interval of the HR nadir over the HR peak. Normative values are well established and decline with age. The baroreflex index is also measurable and correlates well with traditional invasive methods. The HR response is affected by both atropine and β-blockade. The isolated HR response can be measured on most current EMG devices. Abnormalities are evident in a high percentage of patients with autonomic failure and

significant autonomic neuropathy; the BP findings are more sensitive than tilt studies, which are described later. Abnormalities also correlate with the severity of diabetic autonomic neuropathy and diabetes disease duration. Patients with orthostatic intolerance or the *postural orthostatic tachycardia syndrome* (POTS) may show excessive phase II decline and insufficient recovery but additionally markedly enhanced phase IV overshoot and a high VR.

STANDING AND THE 30:15 RATIO

Standing initiates a coordinated sequence of reflexes to maintain BP and therefore cerebral perfusion. Simple HR and BP responses to standing are important bedside markers of autonomic integrity, but further information is gained by laboratory testing. Most labs, however, use passive tilting. Responses are best measured after a supine rest period of 15 to 30 minutes, but shorter periods suffice. Baseline values are recorded and readings are taken at least every minute for 2 to 5 minutes. Leg muscle contraction necessary for active standing triggers an exercise reflex that transiently reduces BP that can mimic orthostatic hypotension. Pressure normally returns to baseline levels within 1 to 2 minutes but can be delayed for 3 to 15 minutes in patients with mild orthostatic intolerance. This phenomenon is why standing BP measures must be delayed. The 30:15 ratio, the R-R interval ratio of the HR nadir around beat 30 after standing divided by the HR peak near beat 15, is reduced by inadequate parasympathetic function. A BP decrease of 20 mm Hg systolic or 10 mm Hg diastolic within 3 minutes is considered significant; triggered symptoms are also noted. The recognition of delayed or slowly declining BP has been noted that can be missed by shorter measurement periods. Fifteen percent of cases in one series had BP declines between 3 and 10 minutes after head-up tilt, and nearly 40% occurred after 10 minutes suggesting milder adrenergic insufficiency than patients with more acute declines.

TILT TABLE STUDIES

Orthostatic challenge with passive upright tilting is the standard method used in most laboratories. Tilting employs slightly different physiologic mechanisms to active standing; however, testing is more easily controllable, enables reproducible tilting angles, simplifies BP monitoring at heart level, and is easier for patients with neurologic impairment. Neurogenic orthostatic hypotension from autonomic failure or HR changes characteristic of primary orthostatic intolerance are generally evident within the first 5 to 15 minutes of tilting. In contrast, prolonged studies are often needed to trigger reflex or vasovagal syncope, which are further delayed or require pharmacologic challenge. Tilt angles range from 60 to 90 degrees depending on the laboratory (Fig. 27.1). ECG recordings are continuously monitored, and serial BP measurements are recorded with a manual cuff with an automated sphygmomanometer or ideally with continuous BP monitoring. Additional systems can be simultaneously monitored in special circumstances such as electroencephalography (EEG), transcranial Doppler, or noninvasive cardiac impedance plethysmography. The BP measurement point is maintained at heart level. Orthostatic hypotension, however, is a sign and not a disease; diagnosis of central autonomic disorders or autonomic neuropathy also depends on clinical assessment and other autonomic tests (see Chapter 112). Similar to active standing, a systolic BP decline of 20 mm Hg is considered to be abnormal, but most centers require at least a 30 mm Hg drop. Although drops of this magnitude may be asymptomatic, ideally, the patient's typical symptoms are reproduced during testing. Diastolic BP declines of 10 mm Hg are significant.

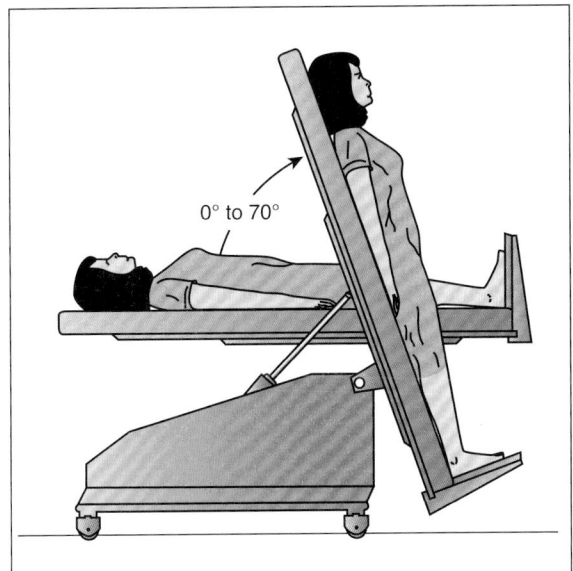

0° to 70°

FIGURE 27.1 Tilt table.

Patients with autonomic failure often have impaired HR response despite orthostatic hypotension. In contrast, orthostatic intolerance (POTS) patients have excessive HR increases commonly defined as a 30-beats-per-minute (bpm) increase usually with a rate exceeding 120 bpm and induced symptoms. Asymptomatic orthostatic hypotension is prevalent, especially in elderly patients. Confirmation of benign, recurrent vasovagal syncope, which comprises the majority of unexplained recurrent syncopal cases, is the most frequent use of cardiologic tilt table testing. Unexplained noncardiac syncope is increasingly recognized in older patients, including reflex or situational triggers, carotid sinus hypersensitivity, and acute events with subclinical autonomic failure.

Multiple other techniques that test adrenergic responses have been devised. Orthostatic stress can be enhanced by lower body negative-pressure chambers but primarily only in research applications. The *sustained handgrip test* is performed by continual handgrip at 30% of maximal strength, which normally elevates diastolic BP by at least 10 to 15 mm Hg within 3 to 5 minutes; some normal controls, however, have minimal BP elevation. *Mental stress* is an older method to elevate BP that has unclear use. The *cold pressor test* is another long-standing means to elevate BP that is surprisingly still performed. The subject immerses a hand into ice water for 3 to 5 minutes and BP increases similar to the handgrip test are produced. Measurement of supine and standing *plasma norepinephrine* and other catecholamine levels is a somewhat useful but relatively insensitive marker of adrenergic function. In this circumstance, supine pressure levels characteristically are low and fail to increase adequately with upright tilting. Levels increase poorly with both central and peripheral causes of autonomic failure and rise excessively in pheochromocytoma and some forms of orthostatic intolerance. Nearly unrecordable norepinephrine and epinephrine and increased dopamine levels are characteristic of dopamine β-hydroxylase deficiency. *Microneurography* directly records sympathetic nerve traffic; insertion of a tungsten microelectrode directly into a nerve fascicle enables recording bursts of muscle or skin sympathetic impulses. This powerful technique has important research applications but has limited clinical use and requires considerable expertise and specialized equipment.

TESTS OF SUDOMOTOR FUNCTION

Heat and cold intolerance are prevalent symptoms. Thermal homeostasis is a complex process that relies on both sweating and vasomotor control for heat elimination and shivering and non-shivering mechanisms for heat production and conservation. Disorders producing excessive sweating, with or without neurologic dysfunction, are generally treated by other specialties, usually dermatologists. Vasomotor assessment is possible using laser Doppler techniques but is not highly reliable; however, measurement of sweat gland activity and assessment of sweat gland innervation are commonly performed methods. Reproducible and generally accepted tests are discussed in this chapter.

The *quantitative sudomotor axon reflex test* (QSART) records chemically induced dynamic sweat output. The test basis is an axon reflex induced by chemically stimulating muscarinic eccrine sweat gland receptors with iontophoresed acetylcholine. This activation induces an antidromic response up a cholinergic axon and induces an orthodromic signal down to a different and isolated group of sweat glands. The sweat produced in this isolated chamber is measured over time. Denervated sweat glands fail to function. Testing requires specialized but commercially available equipment, is reproducible, and correlates variably with epidermal nerve fiber density skin biopsy analysis as a measure of small-diameter nerve integrity. Many, but not most, centers have the necessary equipment. The *thermoregulatory sweat test* (TST) assesses sweat output over the anterior body surface in response to a thermal stimulus. This approach uses a physiologic stimulus (core temperature increase) and simultaneously assesses wide areas of skin. An indicator dye, usually alizarin red and not iodine, is applied. The subject is heated to a predetermined degree in a temperature-controlled chamber and the color change is recorded. Abnormal patterns are readily apparent, but normal variant patterns can complicate interpretation. The test has limited availability, but a simpler more localized testing form is evolving. *Sweat imprint techniques* are additional sudomotor testing methods that rely on inducing sweat using heat or cholinergic agents and recording the resultant output on a recording medium; a special quick-hardening silastic media is typical. Droplet numbers and density are later counted usually by automated and computerized methods using a confocal microscope. Sensitivity and specificity are similar to other methods.

The *sympathetic skin response* (SSR) is a simple to record, popular, and widely available technique well known for over a hundred years. The response, however, is a highly complex multisynaptic reflex with sudomotor activity as the final efferent arm. Both sweat glands and surrounding skin tissue provide the response generators. Interest stems primarily from the simplicity of recording and lack of need for specialized equipment. Multiple protocols are used with various methods. Electrical shock is the most common stimulus; other triggers include startle, cough, deep inspiration, and magnetic stimulation. Responses are best recorded over the palm and sole, ideally all four limbs simultaneously. The evoked amplitude is the most sensitive indicator but is variable and habituates with repeated trials. The range of reported normal values is correspondingly wide; no uniform methods or consensus normative values are accepted. Numerous pitfalls hamper meaningful SSR interpretation, so the test is not recommended in isolation. Anticholinergic medications dampen responses. Sensory deficits such as sensory neuropathy may blunt the noxious effect of electrical, but not respiratory, stimuli. Anxiety and distractions can produce unprovoked responses. Patients with hereditary hyperhidrosis syndromes often have recurrent spontaneous discharges that can blunt measured responses. Responses from the palms are severely reduced or eliminated from sympathectomy but usually eventually return. In addition to epidermal nerve fiber density determination, some skin biopsy samples include sweat glands. The innervating nerves can be stained with PGP9.5 identically to small sensory nerve fibers. However, the simple consensus rules used to count fibers are not applicable with these complex structures. Methods to estimate the density of innervation were devised and are commercially employed and available. Measures reliably distinguish patients with diabetic neuropathy from controls. Reduced sweat gland innervation also correlated with TST measures in one cohort of 10 patients. Other techniques to measure or image small nerve fibers are evolving.

OTHER ORGAN/SYSTEM-SPECIFIC TESTS

Multiple other systems are testable. Some measures are less reliable, difficult to perform, require special expertise, or need further evaluation. Some are performed by specialists in other fields, such as pupillography, gastrointestinal motility and manometry studies, cystometry and urodynamic studies, and sexual dysfunction testing.

USE IN CLINICAL PRACTICE

Current autonomic testing batteries have multiple well-validated, sensitive, and noninvasive tests available that can help confirm, quantify, and characterize clinical autonomic disorders. A multispecialty consensus panel in 2009 recommended that there is level B evidence of autonomic testing to be considered as part of a neuropathy evaluation, especially in the setting of suspected autonomic involvement and there is level C evidence for testing patients with purely sensory neuropathy. Autonomic testing is also potentially useful in the assessment of parkinsonian syndromes, multiple system atrophy, acute and chronic autonomic neuropathy, atypical syncope, and other disorders with suspected autonomic insufficiency or autonomic dysregulation. Multiple clinical syndromes can benefit from testing to guide symptomatic and disease-specific therapy and to aid with diagnosis and management.

SUGGESTED READINGS

Assessment: clinical autonomic testing report of the Therapeutics and Technology Assessment Subcommittee of the American Academy of Neurology. *Neurology.* 1996;46:873–880.

Consensus Committee of the American Autonomic Society and the American Academy of Neurology: consensus statement on the definition of orthostatic hypotension, pure autonomic failure and multiple system atrophy. *Neurology.* 1996;46:1470.

England JD, Gronseth GS, Franklin G, et al. Practice parameter: evaluation of distal symmetric polyneuropathy: role of autonomic testing, nerve biopsy, and skin biopsy (an evidence-based review). Report of the American Academy of Neurology, American Association of Neuromuscular and Electrodiagnostic Medicine, and American Academy of Physical Medicine and Rehabilitation. *Neurology.* 2009;72(2):177–184.

Ewing DJ. Which battery of cardiovascular autonomic function tests? *Diabetologia.* 1990;33:180–181.

Gibbons CH, Freeman R. Delayed orthostatic hypotension: a frequent cause of orthostatic intolerance. *Neurology.* 2006;67:28–32.

Gibbons CH, Illigens BM, Wang N, et al. Quantification of sweat gland innervation: a clinical-pathologic correlation. *Neurology.* 2009;72(17):1479–1486.

Jones PK, Gibbons CH. The role of autonomic testing in syncope. *Auton Neurosci.* 2014;184:40–45.

Kimpinski K, Iodice V, Burton DD, et al. The role of autonomic testing in the differentiation of Parkinson's disease from multiple system atrophy. *J Neurol Sci.* 2012;317(1–2):92–96.

Loavenbruck A, Wendelschaefer-Crabbe G, Sandroni P, et al. Quantification of sweat gland volume and innervation in neuropathy: correlation with thermoregulatory sweat testing. *Muscle Nerve.* 2014;50(4):528–534.

Low PA, Caskey PE, Tuck RR, et al. Quantitative sudomotor axon reflex test in normal and neuropathic subjects. *Ann Neurol.* 1983;14:573–580.

Low PA, Denq JC, Opfer-Gehrking TL, et al. Effect of age and gender on sudomotor and cardiovagal function and blood pressure response to tilt in normal subjects. *Muscle Nerve.* 1997;20:1561–1568.

Low VA, Sandroni P, Fealey RD, et al. Detection of small-fiber neuropathy by sudomotor testing. *Muscle Nerve.* 2006;34(1):57–61.

Report and Recommendations of the San Antonio Conference on Diabetic Neuropathy. Consensus statement. *Diabetes.* 1988;37:1000–1005.

Stewart JD, Low PA, Fealey RD. Distal small fiber neuropathy: results of tests of sweating and autonomic cardiovascular reflexes. *Muscle Nerve.* 1992;15:661–665.

Vogel ER, Sandroni P, Low PA. Blood pressure recovery from Valsalva maneuver in patients with autonomic failure. *Neurology.* 2005;65(10):1533–1537.

Weimer LH. Autonomic testing: common techniques and clinical applications. *Neurologist.* 2010;16(4):215–222.

Vision, Hearing, and Balance Testing 28

J. Kirk Roberts

INTRODUCTION

As with all neurologic complaints, diagnosis begins with a proper history and physical examination.

Appropriate testing supplements the examination and provides more refined measures of neurologic function and impairment. The neurologist may order or request testing that is performed by another physician or a technician in another specialty, or the neurologist may supervise, interpret, or perform the test. In either circumstance, the neurologist should understand the test and its appropriate use. This section will review some commonly performed vision, hearing, and balance tests.

VISION TESTING

VISUAL ACUITY

Visual acuity measures central or foveal vision. Testing usually involves reading letters of different sizes but may involve identifying other symbols. The Snellen chart, which uses letters, and the E chart, which uses the letter E in various orientations, are commonly used tests (Fig. 28.1). Testing is typically done at a distance, to approximate infinity, often 20 ft, and the smallest row read accurately is the visual acuity. If distance vision cannot be performed, then near vision may be tested at a distance of 15.7 inches. For those with such poor vision that the largest letter on the eye chart cannot be read, acuity can be recorded, in order of worsening vision by counting fingers, hand motion, and finally light perception or no light perception. So-called normal vision using the foot as the unit of measurement is defined as 20/20 and means the person can see detail at 20 ft that a person with normal eyesight would see at 20 ft Thus, a person with 20/40 vision can see at 20 ft what a person with normal vision would see at 40 ft In the metric system, normal visual acuity is reported as 6/6 (meters), and in the decimal system, normal eyesight is reported as 1.00. However, many have vision that is better than 20/20. Moreover, distance vision and near vision acuity may differ because of hyperopia, myopia, or presbyopia. Specialized testing has been developed to evaluate visual acuity in infants, preverbal children, and others who cannot identify the letters or symbols.

COLOR VISION

Color vision testing is most commonly evaluated with Ishihara plates. This test consists of a series of plates with colored dots with a pattern of different colored dots forming a number or a shape. This test was originally designed to test for congenital disease, which is most commonly red–green color deficiency. There are other tests of color vision that include blue–yellow testing. Congenital color vision deficiency is not rare and is more common in men than women. Acquired color vision deficiencies typically, although not strictly, divide into loss of red–green vision in optic nerve disorders and blue–yellow vision in retinal or macular disorders.

VISUAL-EVOKED POTENTIALS

Visual-evoked potentials (VEPs), also known as *visual-evoked responses* (VERs), are recorded by measuring brain electrical activity over the occipital lobe in response to repetitive visual stimulation (see Chapter 25). Typically, the P100 wave is the most useful response, and its latency and amplitude are measured. Responses, including latency and amplitude, are measured for each eye, with latency prolongation having the most clinical significance. Ocular, retinal, and visual pathway dysfunction may affect the VEP responses. For the neurologist, the VEP is most commonly used in the evaluation of optic neuritis, where there is a prolonged latency from one eye and/or an elevated interocular latency, as long as ocular and retinal pathology has been excluded.

ELECTRORETINOGRAM

The flash electroretinogram (fERG) tests retinal function and is not affected by damage more central, such as in the optic nerve.

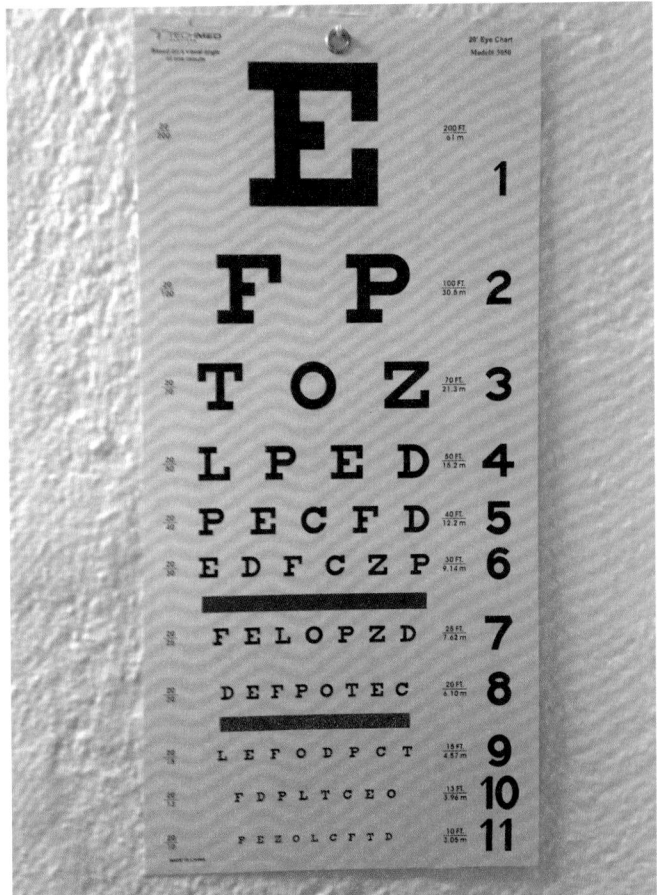

FIGURE 28.1 Snellen chart.

VISUAL FIELDS

Visual field testing is commonly performed in the neurologist office using finger motion and finger counting (see Chapter 3). More formal testing such as Goldman kinetic perimetry uses a test light of various sizes and intensities which is moved from the periphery to the center of the of vision and thus establishes a boundary of visual detection for each level of stimulus. Most visual field testing is now automated (e.g., Humphrey) with lights of varying intensities and sizes appearing in different areas of the visual field while the patient's eye is focused on a specific spot (Fig. 28.2). Although the ophthalmologist uses visual fields to monitor a variety of eye conditions, the neurologist is generally monitoring them in patients with occipital lesions or pituitary lesions with pressure on the optic nerve or chiasm.

OPTICAL COHERENCE TOMOGRAPHY

Optical coherence tomography (OCT) is a relatively recent test that uses light scattering to produce cross-sectional images of the retina with a resolution that allows evaluation of the different layers. It has been used in neurologic applications to measure the retinal nerve fiber layer which reflects the state of the optic nerve. It is reduced, for example, in patients with multiple sclerosis with optic neuritis.

HEARING TESTING

AUDIOGRAM

The audiogram or pure tone testing plots the threshold of hearing in decibels (dB) with standardized frequencies, typically from 125 Hz to 8 kHz. Normal hearing is typically better than 15 dB. Each ear is tested, and both air and bone conduction hearing may be tested. Speech audiometry evaluates how softly someone is able

hear words and to understand them. Impedance audiometry includes tympanometry, which measures the changes in acoustic impedance with changes in air pressure and basically measures the compliance of the eardrum.

BRAIN STEM AUDITORY–EVOKED POTENTIALS

Brain stem auditory–evoked potentials (BAEPs), also known as *brain stem auditory–evoked responses* (BAERs) or *auditory brain stem responses* (ABRs), are the auditory equivalent of the VEP (see Chapter 25). In this test, the patient listens to auditory clicks, and electrical responses are generated at specific anatomic points along the auditory pathway: wave I at the cochlear nerve, wave III at the superior olivary nucleus, and wave V at the inferior colliculi. BAEPs were typically used in the diagnosis of multiple sclerosis and in the evaluation for an acoustic neuroma, but magnetic resonance imaging (MRI) has largely supplanted this testing. Electrocochleography (ECOG) is another evoked potential measuring the electrical response of the cochlea to sound. It is used to aid in the diagnosis of Ménière syndrome and in perilymph fistula, although its use is controversial. Otoacoustic emissions (OAEs) measure sounds produced by the ear and are useful in that, if present, indicate a relatively normal functioning cochlea with at least near-normal hearing. However, they are not that helpful in determining the cause of hearing loss.

BALANCE TESTING

ELECTRONYSTAGMOGRAPHY/ VIDEONYSTAGMOGRAPHY

Electronystagmography (ENG), which uses electrodes to record eye movements, has largely been supplanted in clinical practice by videonystagmography, in which goggles with infrared cameras

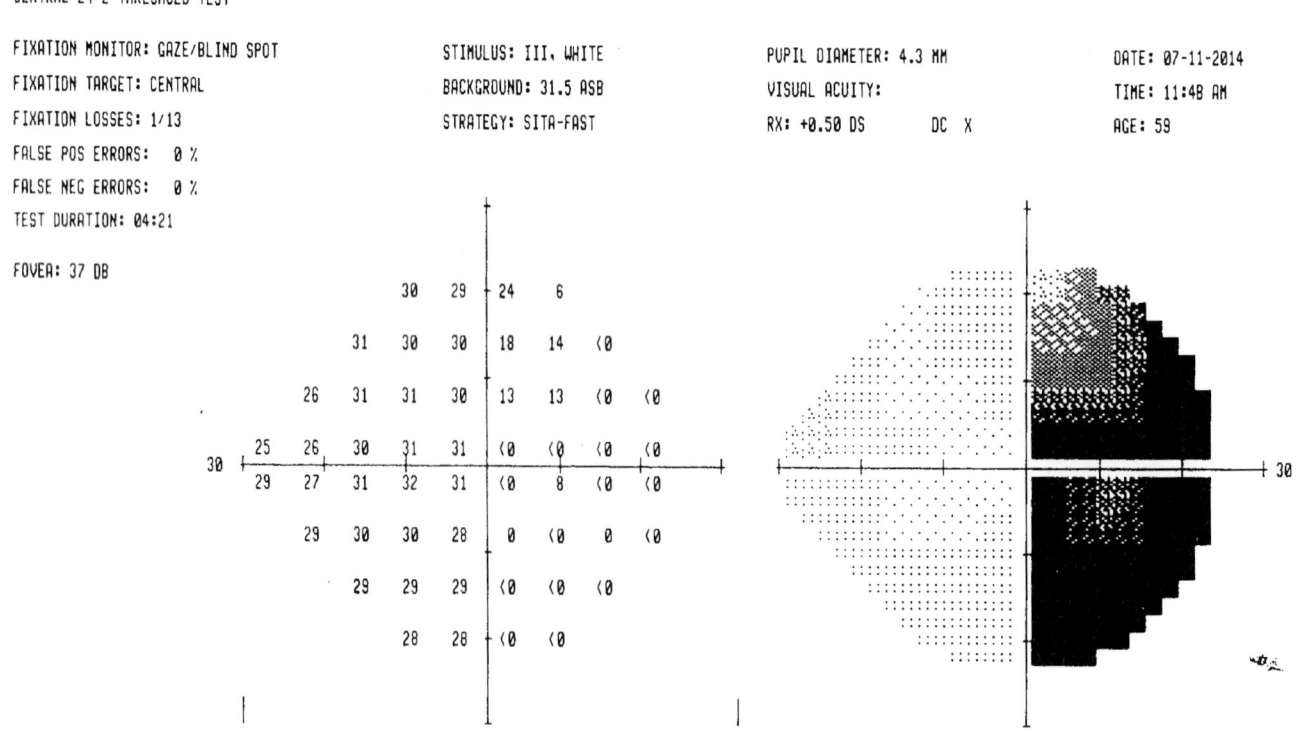

FIGURE 28.2 Computerized automated visual field report showing a right homonymous hemianopia.

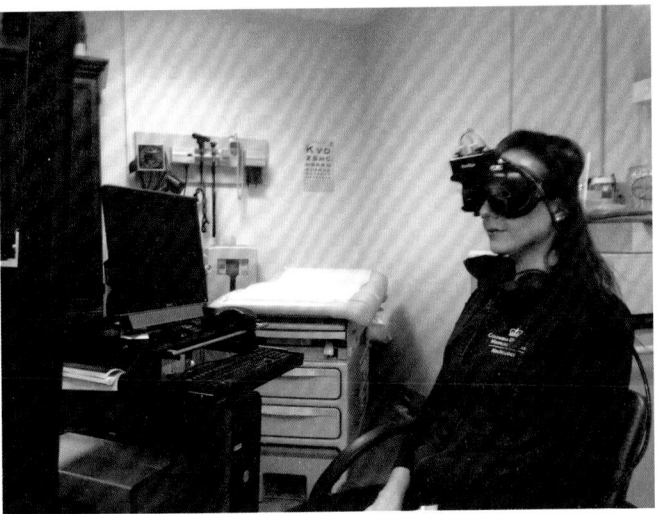

FIGURE 28.3 Videonystagmography.

are used to track eye motion (Fig. 28.3). The test can be divided into three components: ocular motor testing, tests for spontaneous and positional nystagmus, and caloric testing. Ocular motor testing measures saccade velocity, accuracy, and latency along with gain for smooth pursuit and optokinetic nystagmus. The second part includes an evaluation for spontaneous nystagmus with and without fixation. Positional testing includes the Dix–Hallpike maneuver and lateral head and body turn looking for nystagmus associated with canalolithiasis or cupulolithiasis in the posterior, lateral, or anterior canal. Lastly, bithermal caloric testing is completed to evaluate the response of the vestibular system. Conventionally, water irrigation is used, but more and more are using air because of the ease of performing. The vestibular system generates the slow phase, and the velocity of the slow phase is measured in degrees per second, and the responses between the two ears are compared. More specifically, Jongkees formula is used to calculate a relative vestibular reduction by subtracting the sum of the left cool and left warm response from the sum of the right cool and right warm response and then dividing by the sum of all four responses. More than 20% to 25% asymmetry is considered abnormal. Bilateral dysfunction can be suggested by markedly reduced responses (sum total responses <20 degrees per second), but this might also be due to anatomic or technical issues. The use of air, which is potentially less stimulating than water, is of particular concern in this setting.

ROTARY CHAIR

Rotary chair testing adds additional certainty to vestibular testing particularly if the ENG is inconclusive and most importantly if bilateral vestibular dysfunction might be present. The rotary chair may also be useful if mechanical obstruction of the ear canal impedes ENG bithermal caloric testing. As it sounds, in this test, a patient is rotated while eye movements are recorded. The chair is moved either sinusoidally or with step changes in velocity, and eye movements are recorded for gain, phase, and symmetry. Responses to optokinetic stimulation and a test of visual fixation suppression are also measured. In a patient with bilateral vestibular dysfunction, for example, gain is reduced, and there is a phase lead. Although patients with unilateral vestibular dysfunction may also show abnormalities of gain and phase, rotary chair testing is not sensitive to the side of the dysfunction.

VESTIBULAR-EVOKED MYOGENIC POTENTIALS

Vestibular-evoked myogenic potentials (VEMPs) are a relatively less commonly used test meant to evaluate the saccule and the inferior vestibular nerve. In this test, the response of the sternocleidomastoid to auditory stimuli is recorded. Of note, hearing does not seem necessary for VEMPs. In general, VEMPs are considered abnormal if there is a significant asymmetry or they are low or absent. In addition, thresholds to generate VEMPs may be abnormally low in patients with perilymphatic fistula or superior canal dehiscence. Some have reported that VEMPs are low or have a higher threshold in Ménière syndrome, but their use in diagnosing this disorder is questionable. Similar responses may also be seen in muscles other than the sternocleidomastoid, such as the eye muscles.

COMPUTERIZED DYNAMIC POSTUROGRAPHY

Computerized dynamic posturography (CDP) attempts to quantify balance disorders. In this test, the patient stands on a horizontal platform, which can translate or incline, along with measuring the forces exerted by the patient's feet, and can also alter the visual surround. Testing systems that do not include all of the mentioned are less useful. A common testing protocol includes the sensory organization test, which includes six subtests. The subtests grow progressively more difficult by altering the conditions including eyes open or closed, flat or tilted floor, and vertical or tilted visual surround. CDP is not necessarily abnormal in those with vestibular disorders and is therefore complementary to vestibular testing.

SUGGESTED READINGS

Baloh RW, Jacobson KM, Enrietto JA, et al. Balance disorders in older persons: quantification with posturography. *Otolaryngol Head Neck Surg.* 1998;119(1):89–92.

Desmond AL. *Vestibular Function: Evaluation and Treatment.* New York: Thieme; 2004.

Fife TD, Tusa RJ, Furman JM, et al. Assessment: vestibular testing techniques in adults and children: report of the Therapeutics and Technology Assessment Subcommittee of the American Academy of Neurology. *Neurology.* 2000;55:1431–1441.

Handelsman JA, Shepard NT. Electronystagmography and videonystagmography. In: Goebel JA, ed. *Practical Management of the Dizzy Patient.* 2nd ed. Philadelphia: Lippincott Williams & Wilkins; 2008:117–135.

Handelsman JA, Shepard NT. Rotational chair testing. In: Goebel JA, ed. *Practical Management of the Dizzy Patient.* 2nd ed. Philadelphia: Lippincott Williams & Wilkins; 2008:137–152.

Leigh RJ, Zee DS. *The Neurology of Eye Movements.* 4th ed. Oxford, England: Oxford University Press; 2006.

Nashner LM. Computerized dynamic posturography. In: Goebel JA, ed. *Practical Management of the Dizzy Patient.* 2nd ed. Philadelphia: Lippincott Williams & Wilkins; 2008:153–182.

Skarf B, Glaser JS, Trick GL, et al. Neuro-ophthalmologic examination: the visual sensory system. In: Glaser JS, ed. *Neuro-ophthalmology.* 3rd ed. Philadelphia: Lippincott Williams & Wilkins; 1999:7–49.

Sweetow RW, Sabes J. Audiologic testing. In: Lalwani AK, ed. *Current Diagnosis & Treatment in Otolaryngology—Head & Neck Surgery.* 3rd ed. New York: McGraw-Hill; 2012:596.

Valente M. Audiometric tests. In: Goebel JA, ed. *Practical Management of the Dizzy Patient.* 2nd ed. Philadelphia: Lippincott Williams & Wilkins; 2008:183–201.

Welgampola MS, Colebatch JG. Characteristics and clinical applications of vestibular-evoked myogenic potentials. *Neurology.* 2005;64(10):1682–1688.

Andrew J. Westwood and Carl W. Bazil

INTRODUCTION

The National Institutes of Health estimate that 50 to 70 million Americans are affected by sleep problems (see Chapter 114). Sleep deprivation and disorders have been linked to chronic medical diseases such as stroke and diabetes but also to mental health issues and to an increased risk of accidents, particularly motor vehicle accidents. Lack of sleep is not a trivial concern as many patients (and physicians) perceive; it is a very real public health problem.

Evaluation of sleep is complex and is a multidisciplinary analysis. Given the vast spectrum of sleep problems such as sleep-disordered breathing, parasomnias, insomnia, narcolepsy, bruxism, nightmare disorder, circadian rhythm disorders, and nocturnal enuresis, several medical specialties, dentists, and psychologists take an interest in sleep disorders. For physicians, sub-specialty certification in sleep medicine can be obtained following primary certification in anaesthesia, internal medicine, pediatrics, neurology, psychiatry, or otolaryngology. Although detailed medical history and examination are critical in the diagnostic evaluation, subjective reports of sleep concerns are marred by recall bias because the primary problem often occurs during sleep such that the patient may be partly or completely unaware of the problem, and observations by bed partners or housemates will also be limited. Validated questionnaires and sleep logs (including those now available as smartphone applications) provide somewhat more detailed, albeit still subjective, information about sleep and can be helpful. For many disorders, however, testing is required for more objective evaluation of physiologic parameters in sleep and to direct correct treatment.

INDICATIONS FOR DIAGNOSTIC SLEEP TESTING

The need for diagnostic testing, and the specific test required, depends on the clinical suspicion and the question at hand. In general, sleep tests evaluate the quality and quantity of sleep along with other physiologic parameters. The major tests used include polysomnography, a measure of overnight sleep and associated phenomena; multiple sleep latency testing, a measure of the ability to fall asleep during the day; and maintenance of wakefulness test, a measure of the ability to stay awake during the day. Additionally, actigraphy uses movement as a surrogate for sleep and can give useful information about sleep patterns over days to weeks. Each of these will be discussed in detail in the following text.

Polysomnography is not usually indicated for suspected insomnia (delayed or interrupted sleep) or circadian rhythm disturbances, as these are generally diagnosed by history. However, if the condition remains refractory to treatment, polysomnography may be indicated to look for other causes. Obstructive sleep apnea is probably the most common reason for overnight polysomnography, as testing is required for diagnosis no matter how high the suspicion. Signs of sleep apnea include excessive daytime somnolence, snoring, morning headache, frequent nocturia, obesity, and a narrow airway; however, all are rarely present in a given individual. Restless legs syndrome is a clinical diagnosis wherein the patient is aware of uncomfortable sensations in the limbs (usually legs but sometimes arms or trunk) that keep him or her awake at night. This may be treated without testing; however, many of these patients will also have periodic limb movements—repetitive movements during sleep that are typically unrecognized by the patient or bed partner and can result in unrefreshing sleep. Periodic limb movements can also occur in the absence of restless legs syndrome. Suspected narcolepsy requires polysomnography to ensure the absence of other causes of sleepiness. This is followed by multiple sleep latency testing; very short sleep latency and presence of rapid eye movement (REM) in more than one nap are highly suggestive of narcolepsy. Parasomnias may sometimes be diagnosed without testing, but due to the possible confusion between them, association with other sleep disorders such as obstructive sleep apnea, and differential diagnosis that sometimes includes nocturnal seizures, polysomnography is often advisable. Parasomnias include night terrors, rhythmic movement disorder, and sleepwalking (especially in adults) and REM behavior disorder. When nocturnal seizures are in the differential, polysomnography should be performed with simultaneous video electroencephalography (EEG).

POLYSOMNOGRAPHY

The in-laboratory polysomnogram is the gold standard diagnostic test of most sleep disorders (Table 29.1). Clinical polysomnography consists of the simultaneous recording of multiple physiologic variables, allowing objective documentation of sleep state and for evaluation of common sleep disorders. Practitioners will routinely use a minimum of four EEG channels, covering the occipital and central regions required for scoring of sleep, but most will use more. Electro-oculography (EOG); mentalis electromyography (EMG); surface EMG of the anterior tibial muscles for detection of leg movements in sleep; electrocardiography (ECG); and measurement of nasal and oral airflow, respiratory effort, and oxygen saturation as well as audio and video recording are also standard. Additional variables analyzed may include CO_2 monitoring and esophageal manometry.

The recordings are analyzed at 30-second intervals or epochs. Each epoch is evaluated based on muscle tone, EOG, and EEG to determine sleep stage or wakefulness. Each epoch is also evaluated for abnormalities in respiratory flow/pressure, oxygen saturation, heart rate, and any movements (Fig. 29.1). The American Academy of Sleep Medicine provides guidance on recommended scoring for sleep stage, respiratory disturbances (apneas, hypopneas, respiratory-related arousals), as well as limb movements. Once each epoch has been analyzed, a convenient way to display this significant amount of data is the hypnogram. This can show the macroarchitecture over the course of the entire night and can

TABLE 29.1 Indications for Polysomnography

- Diagnosis of sleep-related breathing disorders
- PAP titrations for sleep-related breathing disorders
- Preoperative evaluation prior to upper airway surgery for snoring or obstructive sleep apnea
- Follow-up after good clinical response to oral appliance treatment
- Follow-up after surgical treatment
- Recurrence of symptoms despite initial response to surgical or dental treatments
- Follow-up in patients with substantial weight loss after PAP initiation
- Follow-up in patients with substantial weight gain after PAP initiation
- Insufficient response to PAP therapy despite a good initial response
- Patients with systolic or diastolic heart failure with sleep complaints despite optimal cardiac treatments
- Patients with neuromuscular disorders and sleep complaints despite optimal sleep hygiene
- Narcolepsy (followed by MSLT)
- Periodic limb movement disorder
- Uncertainty of restless legs syndrome

PAP, positive airway pressure; MSLT, multiple sleep latency test.
Based on Kushida CA, Littner MR, Morgenthaler T, et al. Practice parameters for the indications for polysomnography and related procedures: an update for 2005. *Sleep*. 2005;28(4):499–521.

be modified to provide additional information such as timings of respiratory disturbances and body position.

Polysomnography must always be interpreted in the context of potentially relatable history. Therefore, patients should ideally fill out sleep logs for at least 1 week prior to the test. Medications and napping on the day of the study should be noted, and it is often helpful to have the patient's impression of his or her sleep during the study. A patient with 6 hours of documented sleep on polysomnography who believes only 1 to 2 hours of sleep occurred likely has a diagnosis of paradoxical insomnia.

EVOKING PARASOMNIAS

Parasomnias such as sleepwalking and sleep terrors typically arise from slow-wave sleep (stage N3). They may not occur on a nightly basis. In order to increase the yield of recording such events, a patient may sometimes be asked to restrict his or her sleep the night prior in order to provoke a rebound of slow-wave sleep. There is some data that deliberate external stimuli, such as sound, during slow-wave sleep may also cause provocation of the events.

EVALUATING RAPID EYE MOVEMENT BEHAVIOR DISORDER

Recording of dream enactment behavior during REM sleep (Fig. 29.2) is helpful, however not required to support a diagnosis of REM behavior disorder. One of the cardinal features of this disorder is the lack of atonia during REM sleep. Atonia is usually identified in the chin lead; however, it may be present in one or more limb leads. Some practitioners may apply additional leads to all four extremities

in cases where REM behavior disorder is a concern. It is important to note that melatonin can suppress the atonia and should be stopped prior to the study.

PORTABLE POLYSOMNOGRAPHY MONITORING

Obstructive sleep apnea is a prevalent condition within the general population. In those with no significant comorbidities such as neuromuscular weakness, heart failure, seizure disorder, or morbid obesity, a simplified version of the in-laboratory polysomnogram may be warranted. There are many devices for the ambulatory polysomnogram, or home sleep test, and can range from detecting three variables (typically oxygen saturation, pulse, and flow) to a thorough evaluation including ECG and EEG. The benefits of the test are typically in cost-saving as well as being beneficial for individuals who may not sleep well in unknown environment. As portable testing typically does not allow reliable sleep scoring and does not include video or limb EMG, it is not indicated for evaluation of suspected parasomnias, REM behavior disorder, or periodic limb movement disorder.

This home version can be a useful screening tool for obstructive sleep apnea but can lack sensitivity, as it yields limited data in many cases because it relies on the individual to comment if they were asleep and readjust the equipment themselves. In-laboratory polysomnography may be required if the study remains unrevealing or if the apnea-hypopnea index is borderline, yet suspicion for obstructive sleep apnea remains high. Subsequent in-laboratory testing is also needed if portable testing is negative for obstructive sleep apnea and evaluation is then required for other sleep disorders.

OTHER DIAGNOSTIC SLEEP TESTS

MULTIPLE SLEEP LATENCY TEST

Patients with excessive daytime sleepiness may be evaluated by the multiple sleep latency test (MSLT), a series of five nap opportunities (sometimes four or six) with sleep recordings at 2-hour intervals throughout the day. "Normal" sleep for that individual is recommended for 7 days prior to the test and any medications that can disrupt sleep architecture, particularly antidepressants, should ideally be discontinued 2 weeks prior to the study. Polysomnography should be performed the night prior to testing so that prior sleep is documented. If significant obstructive sleep apnea is noted on polysomnography, the MSLT is typically not performed. A minimum of 6 hours of sleep should occur during polysomnography to reliably proceed with an MSLT.

Sleep onset is defined as the first epoch of nonwakefulness. The nap is terminated 15 minutes after sleep onset. If no sleep occurs, each recording session is terminated after 20 minutes. The sleep latency (the time it takes to fall asleep) is determined for each nap and provides an objective measure of daytime sleepiness. If no REM sleep occurs in four naps, the test may be terminated. Similarly, if REM occurs in at least two of four naps, testing is considered complete. If, however, REM has occurred in only one of four naps, the patient is generally given the fifth nap in order to determine whether narcolepsy is likely.

Sleep latency over the course of the naps is averaged (20 minutes is used as time onset if the patient does not fall asleep). Additionally, any REM periods are counted; REM within 15 minutes is considered abnormal. These are described as sleep-onset rapid eye movement periods (SOREMPs). If an SOREMP is obtained in the prior night polysomnography, this can also be taken into consideration.

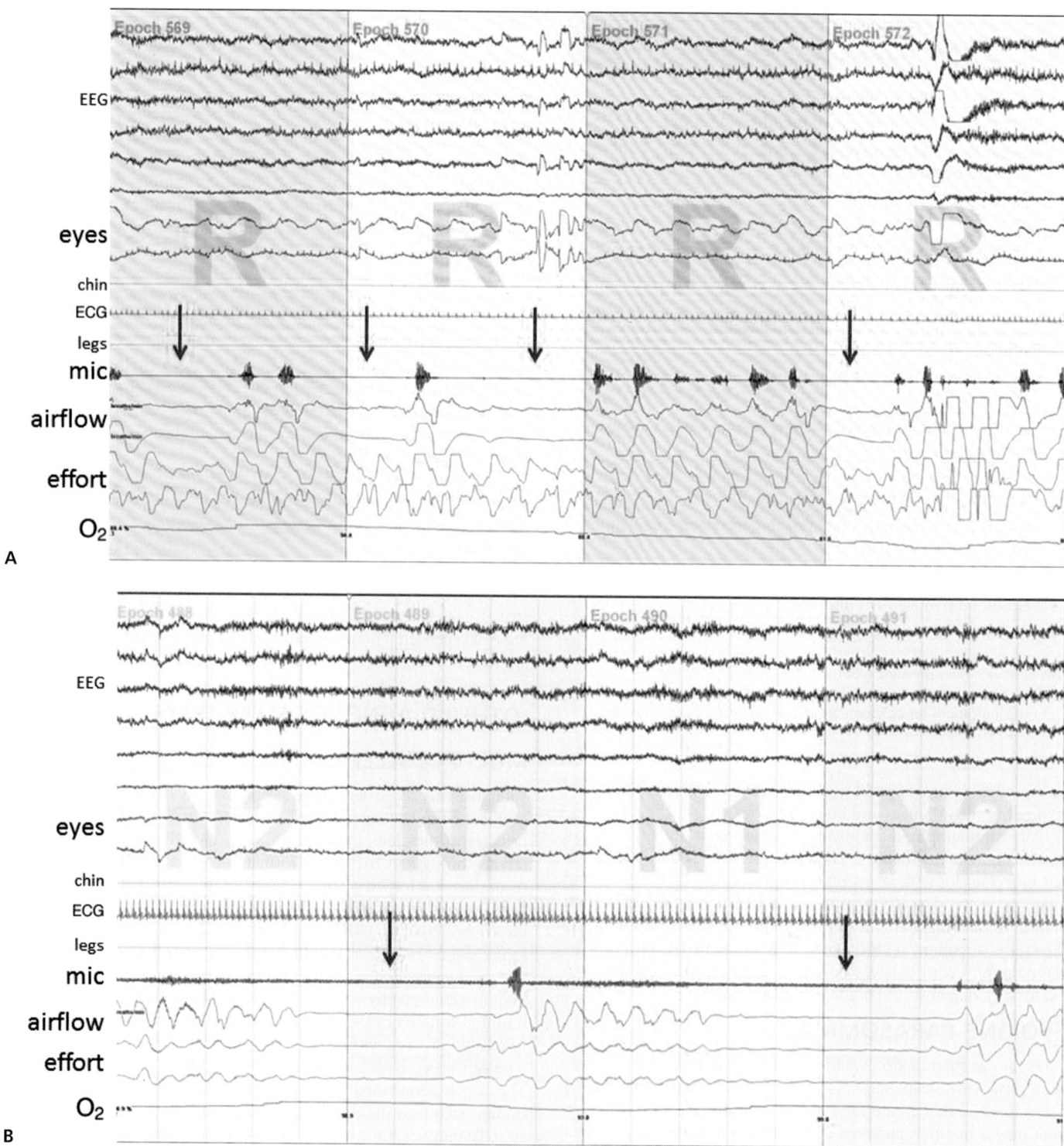

FIGURE 29.1 A: A 4-minute recording of stage R (REM sleep) showing cessation of airflow with continued abdominal and chest movements during apneic pauses illustrated by the *red arrows*. Note the snoring ceases with airflow and oxygen saturation declines. This is consistent with obstructive sleep apnea. **B:** A 4-minute recording of N1 and N2 (non-REM sleep) showing cessation of airflow and abdominal and chest movements illustrated by the *red arrows*. This is consistent with central sleep apnea. EEG, electroencephalography; ECG, echocardiopgraphy; O₂, oxygen.

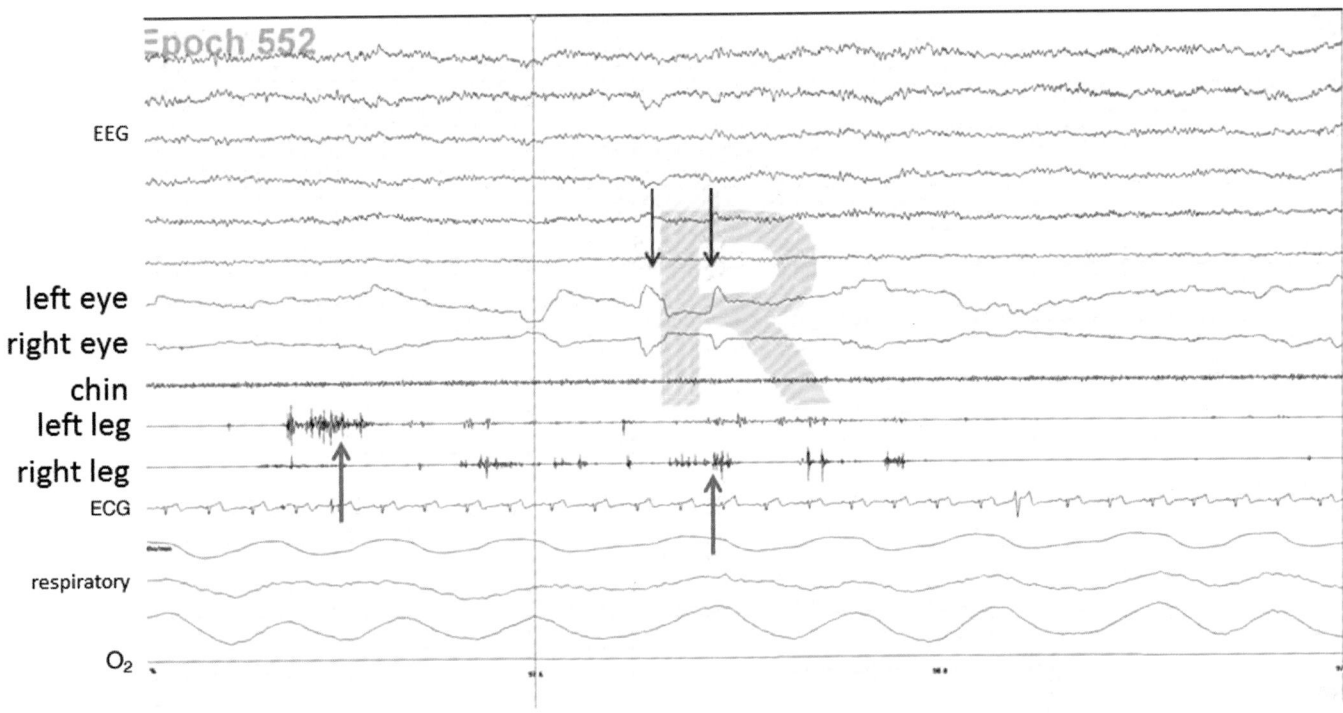

FIGURE 29.2 Single epoch of phasic R sleep (*red arrows* indicate rapid eye movements) with movements of both the left and right legs (*blue arrows*). EEG, electroencephalography; ECG, echocardiopgraphy; O₂, oxygen.

The main indication of this study is to support the diagnosis of narcolepsy. Individuals with narcolepsy tend to have mean sleep latencies of 3 ± 3 minutes. However, 16% of normal individuals will have a sleep latency of less than 5 minutes. Patients with narcolepsy typically have a mean sleep latency of less than 8 minutes and demonstrate at least two naps with sleep-onset REM. Although there is significant overlap of the mean sleep latencies of normal individuals and those who complain of excessive sleepiness, normal is considered to be a mean sleep latency of greater than 10 minutes.

SOREMPs can also be seen as a result of obstructive sleep apnea, sleep deprivation, drugs/drug withdrawal, or narcolepsy; in these cases, only one is typically seen in an MSLT. Two SOREMPs have 78% sensitivity and 93% specificity for narcolepsy. Notably, no large systematically collected repository of normative MSLT data is known to exist, and normal values for individuals younger than 6 years of age have not been established.

MAINTENANCE OF WAKEFULNESS TEST

The maintenance of wakefulness test (MWT) measures the time a patient is able to remain awake in a low-light environment during four 40-minute (sometimes 20-minute) attempts. The patient is instructed to remain awake in a semirecumbent position, without any stimulating behaviors. The test may provide more information about the patient's ability to sustain wakefulness, but the validity of test results to real-life experience is unclear. It is sometimes used to evaluate driving performance in individuals who may be at high risk of daytime sleepiness.

Sleep onset is defined as three epochs (90 seconds) of continuous stage 1 sleep or one epoch of any other stage of sleep. A total of 97.5% of normal sleepers stay awake for an average of 8 minutes or more during the MWT. Falling asleep in an average of less than 8 minutes during the test would be considered abnormal.

Results show that from 40% to 59% of people with normal sleep stay awake for the entire 40 minutes of all four trials.

EVALUATION OF CIRCADIAN RHYTHM DISTURBANCES

As well as the intrinsic characteristic of a person's sleep, extrinsic factors placed on the timing of the sleep–wake cycle may disrupt the ability of an individual to sleep when necessary. Several variants have been described including the delayed and advanced sleep phase syndromes, shift work disorder, and jet lag disorder. Diagnosis may be made simply through history taking; however, patient recall of sleep patterns over time may be limited and there are instruments that may be useful to support the diagnosis.

ACTIGRAPHY

The essence of actigraphy is based on the concept that movement is limited during sleep. A device typically worn on the nondominant wrist monitors movement over a specific duration of time, typically up to 2 weeks, and is typically correlated to a diary of activity (Fig. 29.3). The parameters on some devices can be used to assess specifics such as the frequency of limb movements that occur during sleep. Studies that compare actigraphy to sleep with polysomnography show that it is a reasonable, although not perfect, surrogate measurement for sleep. It is clearly not practical (or necessary) to do formal polysomnography for weeks at a time to determine sleep patterns.

Many commercially available applications now use the principle of actigraphy to allow patients to track their sleep. Actigraphy applications using smartphone accelerometers have limited use, as most require movement of the bed rather than the person, and are

DAY

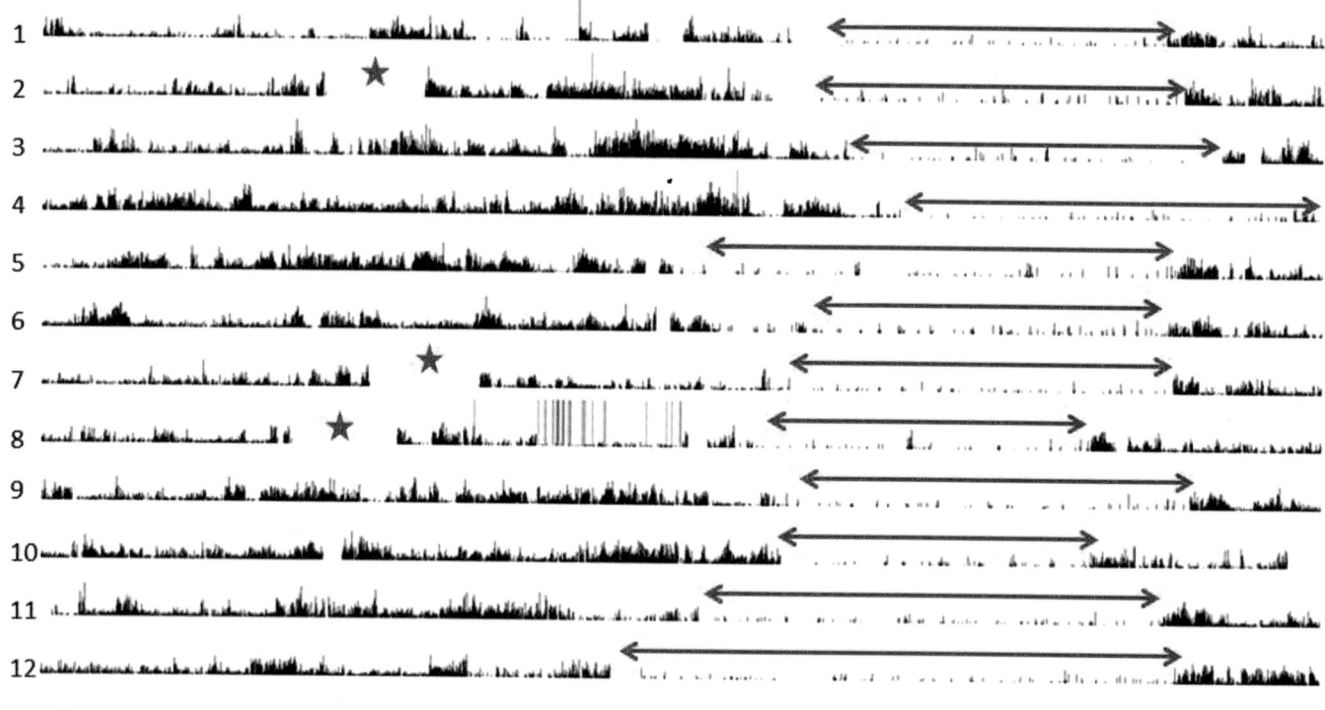

6 AM

6 AM

FIGURE 29.3 Actogram of activity for 12 days. Each day is plotted on a row and quantity of movement is indicated by *black*. This is typically correlated with a log by the individual. Periods with limited movement likely correlate with sleep (*red arrows*). Periods of absolute lack of movement (*red stars*) suggest removal of the watch.

not well correlated with actual sleep. In contrast, other linked accelerometry devices may be worn on the body (typically the arm); these are likely reasonably similar to actigraphy and have potential to be viewed by the clinician to help with diagnosis and to monitor treatment progress.

BIOMARKERS OF CIRCADIAN RHYTHM

Several variables are used to evaluate the sleep–wake rhythm, principally for research purposes and to a lesser extent in clinical practice. Melatonin or its metabolites can be measured in the urine, blood, or saliva. Melatonin secretion begins in the evening hours and peak overnight. During the daytime hours, levels are barely detectable. Dim light melatonin onset (DLMO) is the point at which melatonin levels reach 2 pg/mL in plasma or 4 pg/mL in the saliva. It can also be measured as the mean of three daytime samples plus two twice the standard deviation of these three daytime samples. It typically occurs 2 hours before bedtime provided that lighting is dim. DLMO is considered the standard measure of circadian pattern. For example, a patient with delayed sleep phase phenomenon would have very late DLMO (3 to 5 AM). A patient with shift work sleep disorder would continue to show DLMO during the typical work shift.

Core body temperature usually peaks in the late afternoon. Sleep typically occurs on the downward slope and ends about 2 hours following the nadir. Loss of normal core body temperature rhythm can be diagnosed with continuous temperature monitoring, but this is not a convenient method for determining circadian pattern clinically.

SUBJECTIVE REPORTING OF SLEEP

In addition to reports of sleep complaints, a patient can keep a log of their sleep–wake cycle over time (Fig. 29.4). This can be used in combination with actigraphy, particularly when evaluating for paradoxical insomnia. It can also be used to visually evaluate potential sleep–wake disorders as well as help to ensure the patient is getting sufficient sleep prior to polysomnography, which may otherwise alter sleep architecture.

Many questionnaires related to sleep exist, with most particularly focusing on obstructive sleep apnea or snoring, whereas others may evaluate the quality of sleep, degree of sleepiness, or the inability to sleep. A frequently used questionnaire in many practices is the Epworth Sleepiness Scale. Rating eight situations on a scale of 0 to 3 for severity of sleepiness results in a possible total of 24. A level of 10 or more typically indicates excessive sleepiness. Persons with narcolepsy may have scores around 16, although this is varied between individuals. Not only is it used for diagnostic purposes but can also be quickly and easily used to monitor efficacy of treatment. It is important to know that the Epworth shows very limited correlation with the objective sleepiness seen on MSLT. Patients with severe sleepiness due to obstructive sleep apnea, for example, may be observed to fall asleep in the waiting room but score normally on the Epworth. This supports that patients are often unaware or in denial of their own sleepiness; nevertheless, the Epworth can be useful in documenting a patient's perception of his or her drowsiness.

Other questionnaires are typically used as a screening tool for potential sleep disorders. There are over 14 questionnaires that

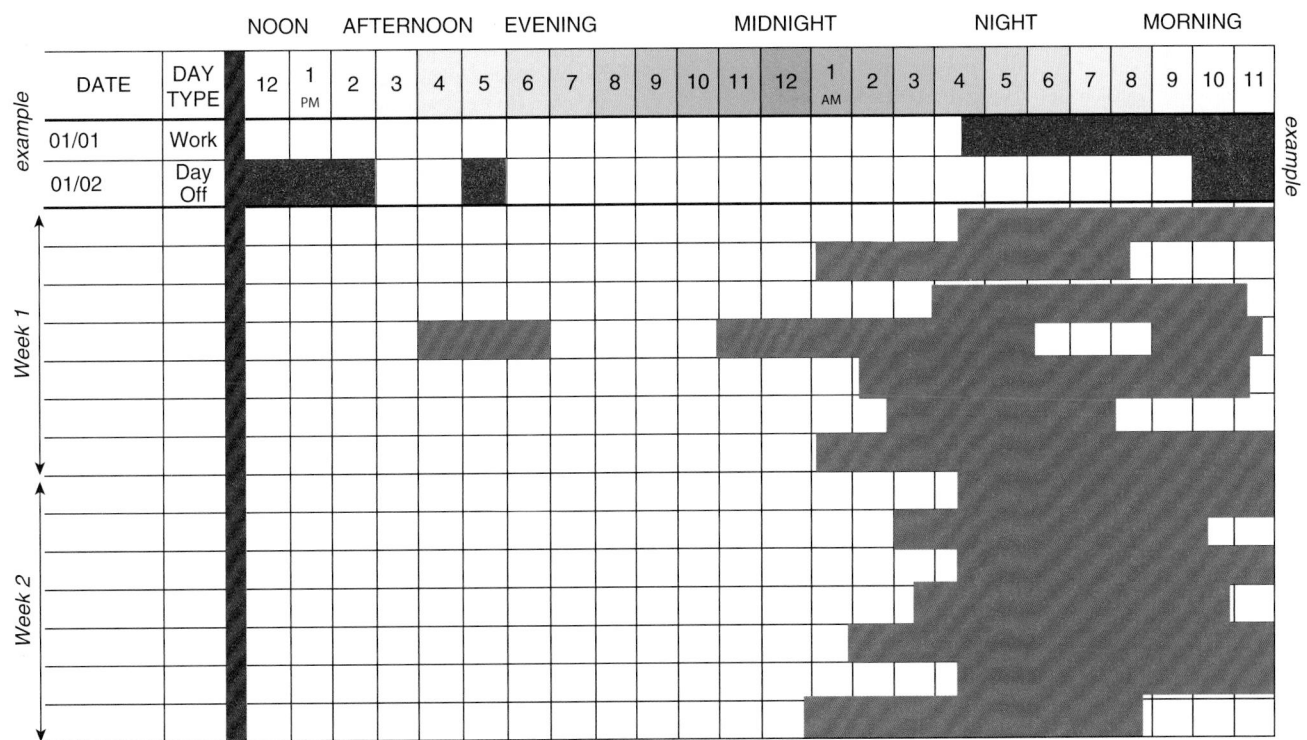

FIGURE 29.4 Sleep diary. The individual is asked to shade the boxes indicating their estimated sleep. Here, the individual has a delayed sleep phase syndrome typically not sleeping until 2 AM or later. Note that on the day of a nap in the afternoon, the individual remains awake during the typical hours of sleep. Further information could be added such as time of medication, times of caffeine intake or exercise, and time getting into and out of bed.

exist for the evaluation of sleep-disordered breathing. Although many can help increase the sensitivity for sleep apnea, the diagnosis can only be made through the use of polysomnography. There are also at least five available questionnaires to evaluate for REM sleep behavior disorder but ultimately, a polysomnogram determines the diagnosis and excluded mimickers such as periodic limb movement disorder or obstructive sleep apnea.

OTHER LABORATORY TESTING

NARCOLEPSY

In rare circumstances or for research purposes, laboratory tests may be useful to confirm a suspicion of narcolepsy. In individuals who have narcolepsy type 1 (associated with cataplexy), a lumbar puncture can be performed. Cerebrospinal fluid (CSF) levels of hypocretin-1 of less than 110 ng/mL are diagnostic with 87% sensitivity and 99% specificity for narcolepsy type 1. The majority of patients with idiopathic hypersomnia and narcolepsy type 2 have normal CSF hypocretin-1 levels. Genetic testing can also be helpful in some circumstances. The allele HLA-DQB1*0602 is present in over 90% of individuals with narcolepsy type 1, 56% of type 2 narcolepsy, and 52% of individuals with idiopathic hypersomnia. However, it is found in between 12% and 35% of healthy individuals.

RESTLESS LEGS SYNDROME

Restless legs syndrome (RLS) is a clinical diagnosis based on an urge to move limbs (not necessarily legs or a leg) that is typically worse in the evening or inactivity that is temporarily relieved by movement and not due to position, cramps, or pain (see Chapter 75). Secondary causes may include anemia, uremia, thyroid dysfunction, or venous disease. Of particular note is that a ferritin level of less than 50 μg/L, sometimes 75 μg/L despite being considered to be within the normal range, is treated with exogenous iron supplementation. Single nucleotide polymorphisms in some genes have been associated with an increased risk of RLS; however, these are not diagnostic. For example, variants in the gene BTBD9 can be seen in 75% of individuals with RLS but also in 65% of those who have never had the syndrome.

IMAGING

Imaging is not routinely performed as part of a workup for sleep disturbances. However, rare presentations of narcolepsy have resulted from strokes or demyelinating lesions in the brain stem. Hypoperfusion in the thalami of individuals with Kleine–Levin syndrome during symptomatic periods can be seen on single-photon emission computed tomography (SPECT) or positron emission tomography (PET) imaging. Brain imaging should be considered in any individual with respiratory arrests not typical of obstructive sleep apnea or that occur during wakefulness. In a subset of individuals with congenital central hypoventilation syndrome—respiratory arrests during sleep, typically seen in childhood as a result of inborn failure of autonomic control of breathing—there is a higher incidence of neural crest tumors such as neuroblastomas.

SUGGESTED READINGS

Berry RB, Brooks R, Gamaldo CE, et al; for the American Academy of Sleep Medicine. *The AASM Manual for the Scoring of Sleep and Associated Events: Rules, Terminology and Technical Specifications*. Version 2.1. Westchester, IL: American Academy of Sleep Medicine; 2014.

Bjorvatn B, Pallesen S. A practical approach to circadian rhythm sleep disorders. *Sleep Med Rev*. 2009;13:47–60.

Brown EN, Czeisler CA. The statistical analysis of circadian phase and amplitude in constant-routine core-temperature data. *J Biol Rhythms*. 1992;7:177–202.

Buysse DJ, Reynolds CF III, Monk TH, et al. The Pittsburgh Sleep Quality Index: a new instrument for psychiatric practice and research. *Psychiatry Res*.1989; 28:193–213.

Carskadon MA, Dement WC, Mitler MM, et al. Guidelines for the multiple sleep latency test (MSLT): a standard measure of sleepiness. *Sleep*. 1986;9: 519–524.

Collop NA, Anderson WM, Boehlecke B, et al. Clinical guidelines for the use of unattended portable monitors in the diagnosis of obstructive sleep apnea in adult patients. Portable Monitoring Task Force of the American Academy of Sleep Medicine. *J Clin Sleep Med*. 2007;3:737–747.

Doghramji K, Mitler MM, Sangal RB, et al. A normative study of the maintenance of wakefulness test (MWT). *Electroencephalogr Clin Neurophysiol*. 1997;103:554–562.

Fedson AC, Pack AI, Gislason T. Frequently used sleep questionnaires in epidemiological and genetic research for obstructive sleep apnea: a review. *Sleep Med Rev*. 2012;16:529–537.

Huang YS, Guilleminault C, Kao PF, et al. SPECT findings in the Kleine-Levin syndrome. *Sleep*. 2005;28:955–960.

Johns MW. A new method for measuring daytime sleepiness: the Epworth sleepiness scale. *Sleep*. 1991;14:540–545.

Johns MW. Sensitivity and specificity of the multiple sleep latency test (MSLT), the maintenance of wakefulness test and the epworth sleepiness scale: failure of the MSLT as a gold standard. *J Sleep Res*. 2000;9:5–11.

Kushida CA, Littner MR, Morgenthaler T, et al. Practice parameters for the indications for polysomnography and related procedures: an update for 2005. *Sleep*. 2005;28:499–521.

Lewy AJ, Bauer VK, Ahmed S, et al. The human phase response curve (PRC) to melatonin is about 12 hours out of phase with the PRC to light. *Chronobiol Int*. 1998;15:71–83.

Littner MR, Kushida C, Wise M, et al. Practice parameters for clinical use of the multiple sleep latency test and the maintenance of wakefulness test. *Sleep*. 2005;28:113–121.

Mignot E, Lammers GJ, Ripley B, et al. The role of cerebrospinal fluid hypocretin measurement in the diagnosis of narcolepsy and other hypersomnias. *Arch Neurol*. 2002;59:1553–1562.

Morgenthaler T, Alessi C, Friedman L, et al. Practice parameters for the use of actigraphy in the assessment of sleep and sleep disorders: an update for 2007. *Sleep*. 2007;30:519–529.

Morgenthaler TI, Lee-Chiong T, Alessi C, et al. Practice parameters for the clinical evaluation and treatment of circadian rhythm sleep disorders. An American Academy of Sleep Medicine report. *Sleep*. 2007;30:1445–1459.

Pilon M, Montplaisir J, Zadra A. Precipitating factors of somnambulism: impact of sleep deprivation and forced arousals. *Neurology*. 2008;70:2284–2290.

Roehrs T, Roth T. Multiple sleep latency test: technical aspects and normal values. *J Clin Neurophysiol*. 1992;9:63–67.

Stiasny-Kolster K, Mayer G, Schäfer S, et al. The REM sleep behavior disorder screening questionnaire—a new diagnostic instrument. *Mov Disord*. 2007;22:2386–2393.

Neuropsychological Evaluation 30

Yaakov Stern

INTRODUCTION

Before the availability of high-resolution imaging, neuropsychological evaluation played a role in lesion localization. Currently, neuropsychological testing remains a valuable adjunct to neurologic evaluation, assisting in the diagnosis of dementia and in evaluating or quantifying cognition and behavior in development, brain diseases, and clinical treatment, as well as in research.

STRATEGY OF NEUROPSYCHOLOGICAL TESTING

Conditions that affect the brain often cause cognitive, motor, or behavioral impairment that can be detected by appropriately designed tests. Defective performance on a test and certain patterns of test performance may suggest specific pathology. Alternatively, patients with known brain changes may be assessed to determine how the damaged brain areas affect specific cognitive functions. Before relating test performance to brain dysfunction, however, other factors that affect test performance must be considered.

Typically, test performance is compared with normal values derived from populations similar to the patient in age, education, socioeconomic background, and other variables. Scores significantly below the mean expected values imply impaired performance. Performance sometimes can be evaluated by assumptions about what might be expected from the average person (e.g., repeating simple sentences or simple learning and remembering).

Unfortunately, comparable data may not exist for the patient being tested. This problem is common in the elderly and those with language and cultural differences. This situation may be addressed by collecting local, normal characteristics that are more descriptive of the local clinical population or by evaluating the cognitive areas that remain intact. In this way, the patient guides the clinician in terms of the level of performance that should be expected in possibly affected domains. Other factors that also influence test performance include the patient's current mood, anxiety, depression or other psychiatric disorders, medication, and the patient's motivation to participate fully.

Patterns of performance, such as strengths in some cognitive domains and weaknesses in others, have been associated with specific conditions based on empiric observation and knowledge of the brain pathology associated with those conditions. Observation of these patterns may aid in diagnosis.

TEST SELECTION

Neuropsychological tests in an assessment battery come from many sources. Some were developed for academic purposes (e.g., intelligence tests) and others for experimental psychology. The typical clinical battery consists of a series of standard tests that have been proved useful and are selected for the referral issue.

These tests should have established reliability and validity. A trade-off exists between the breadth of application and ease of interpretation, available from standard batteries, and the ability to pinpoint specific or subtle deficits offered by more experimental tasks that are useful in research but have not yet been standardized.

Most tests are intended to measure performance in specific cognitive or motor domains, such as memory, spatial ability, language function, or motor agility. These domains may be subdivided (e.g., memory may be considered verbal or nonverbal; immediate, short term, long term, or remote; semantic or episodic; public or autobiographic; or implicit or explicit). However, no matter how focused a test is, multiple cognitive processes are likely to be invoked. An ostensibly simple task, such as the Wechsler Adult Intelligence Scale (WAIS) Coding subtest (previously called *Digit Symbol Coding*), which uses a table of nine digit–symbol pairs to fill in the proper symbols for a series of numbers, assesses learning and memory, visuospatial abilities, motor abilities, attention, and speeded performance. In addition, tests may be failed for more than one reason: Patients may draw poorly because they may not appreciate spatial relationships, because they plan the construction process poorly, or because they are distractible or lack motivation. Relying solely on test scores may lead to spurious conclusions.

TESTS USED IN A NEUROPSYCHOLOGICAL EVALUATION

INTELLECTUAL ABILITY

Typically, a test such as the WAIS-IV or the Wechsler Intelligence Scale for Children-IV is used to assess the present level of intellectual function for adults and children respectively. These tests yield a global IQ score and index scores that are standardized, so that 100 is the mean expected value at any age (with a standard deviation of 15).

The WAIS-IV consists of 10 core and 5 supplemental subtests (Table 30.1). The 10 core subtests comprise the full scale IQ. In previous WAIS versions, verbal and performance IQ estimates were calculated. In contrast, the WAIS IV emphasizes a set of index scores based on groups of subtests, each assessing a broad, separate class of cognitive abilities. These include Verbal Comprehension, Perceptual Reasoning, Working Memory, and Processing Speed. The WAIS-IV also adds a General Ability Index, which consists of selected subtests from the Verbal Comprehension and the Perceptual Reasoning subtests. The intention of this index score is to assess cognitive abilities that are not as susceptible to changes in processing speed and working memory. For the individual subtests, scaled scores range from 1 to 19, with a mean of 10 and a standard deviation of 3; the average range for subtest scaled scores is from 7 to 13.

The overall IQ and index scores supply summary information about the level of general intelligence and broad ability categories. The neuropsychologist is often more interested in the "scatter" of subtest scores, which indicates strengths and weaknesses.

TABLE 30.1	Subtests of the Wechsler Adult Intelligence Scale-IV Arranged by the Four Index Groups	
Verbal Comprehension	**Verbal Concept Formation, Verbal Reasoning, Knowledge Acquired from Environment**
Similarities	Derive relevant superordinate category or similarity for word pairs; abstract verbal reasoning
Vocabulary	Name pictures and define words; often used to assess "premorbid" level of ability
Information	Answer questions that address a broad range of general knowledge topics; ability to acquire, retain, and retrieve general factual knowledge
(Comprehension)	Answer questions based on understanding of general principles and social situations
Perceptual Reasoning	**Perceptual and Fluid Reasoning, Spatial Processing, Visual-Motor Integration**
Block design	Arrange blocks with red, white, and half-red and half-white sides to form 14 designs; spatial perception, visual abstract processing, and problem solving
Matrix reasoning	Identify the picture that completes a pattern using pattern completion, classification, analogy, or serial reasoning; classic measure of fluid intelligence
Visual puzzles	View a completed puzzle and select three response options that, when combined, reconstruct the puzzle; visual perception and organization, nonverbal reasoning
(Picture completion)	Determine the missing feature in pictures; visual perception
(Figure weights)	View a scale with missing weight(s) and select the response option that keeps the scale balanced; quantitative and analogical reasoning
Working Memory	**Attention, Concentration, Mental Control, Reasoning**
Digit span	Standardized assessment of digits forward and backward. In addition, hear a sequence of numbers and recall those numbers in ascending order; attention, concentration, mental control
Arithmetic	Verbal arithmetic problems; mental manipulation, concentration, attention, short- and long-term memory, numeric reasoning ability
(Letter–number sequencing)	Listen to a combination of numbers and letters and recall first the numbers in ascending order and then the letters in alphabetical order. Sequential processing, mental manipulation, attention, concentration, memory span, short-term auditory memory.
Processing Speed	**Ability to Quickly and Correctly Scan, Sequence, and Discriminate Simple Visual Information, Short-Term Visual Memory, Attention, Visual-Motor Coordination**
Symbol search	Scan a search group and indicate whether one of the symbols in the target group matches; processing speed, visual discrimination
Coding	Using a key, copy symbols that are paired with numbers; processing speed, short-term visual memory
(Cancellation)	Scan a structured arrangement of shapes and mark target shapes; processing speed, visual selective attention

Supplementary subtests are indicated by parentheses. Comments describe the subtests and identify some select cognitive features that they tap.

The subtests are often better considered as separate tests, each assessing specific areas of cognitive function. There are many other tests of general intelligence, including some that are nonverbal.

MEMORY

The subclassifications of memory have evolved from clinical observation and experimentation; most are important to the assessment (Table 30.2).

For example, preservation of remote memories, despite the inability to store and recall new information, is the hallmark of specific amnestic disorders. Other subclassifications are used to evaluate different clinical syndromes.

PROCESSING SPEED

Processing speed is defined as either the amount of time it takes to process a set amount of information or the amount of information that can be processed within a certain amount of time.

In the WAIS IV, it is assessed with the Coding and Symbol Search subtests. Another commonly used test is pattern comparison, where two patterns are presented and the test taker must decide as quickly as possible if they are the same or different.

PERCEPTUAL

Neuropsychologists may provide a standardized version of neurologists' perceptual tasks: double (simultaneous) stimulation in touch, hearing, or sight; stereognosis; graphesthesia; spatial perception; or auditory discrimination.

VISUAL PERCEPTUAL AND CONSTRUCTION

Some tasks tap basic perceptual abilities. For example, the Benton Judgment of Line Orientation test assesses a person's ability to match the angle and orientation of lines.

Construction, typically assessed by drawing or assembly tasks, requires both accurate spatial perception and an organized

TABLE 30.2 Typical Subclassifications of Memory Addressed by Neuropsychological Tests

Verbal and nonverbal	Memory for material that is or is not verbally encoded
Immediate, short term	Length of time between exposure to material and recall. The length of time has implications for how long term and remote the memory may be stored and retrieved.
Semantic and episodic	Memory for encodable knowledge, such as vocabulary or facts about the world, as opposed to memory for events
Public and autobiographic	Memory for public, commonly known events vs. events that occurred in one's own life
Implicit and explicit	Memory tested on tasks that do not require conscious, explicit recollection of recent exposures (such as motor skills, procedural skills, classical conditioning, or priming) vs. tasks that demand explicit recall of prior information (such as recall or recognition tasks)
Working	Similar to what in the past has been called short-term memory, working memory provides a buffer for briefly holding on to information, such as a telephone number or the name of a newly met person. It is also important for tasks that require mental manipulation of information, such as multistep arithmetic problems. For many theorists, working memory also has a more important role at the work space where recalled information is actually used, manipulated, and related to other information, allowing complex cognitive processes such as comprehension, learning, and reasoning to take place.

motor response. The Block Design subtest of the WAIS-IV is example of an assembly task. In the Rey–Osterrieth Complex Figure, the patient is asked to copy a figure that contains many details embedded within an organizing framework. In addition to the scores these tests yield, the clinician attends to the patient's construction performance to determine factors that may underlie poor performance (e.g., a disorganized impulsive strategy may be more related to anterior brain lesions, whereas difficulty aligning angles may arise from parietal lobe injury).

LANGUAGE

"Mapping" of different aphasic disorders to specific brain structures was one of the early accomplishments of behavioral neurology. In neuropsychological assessment, this model is often followed. Comprehension, fluency, repetition, and naming are assessed in spoken or written language. Language deficits typically indicate dominant hemisphere pathology, although naming deficits and other verbal difficulties are evident in various forms of dementia as well.

EXECUTIVE

The ability to plan, sequence, and monitor behavior has been called "executive function." These functions, often linked to the prefrontal cortex, rely on and organize other intact cognitive functions that are required components for performance. Several schemes for classifying executive functions: For example, Miyake et al. (2000) identified three separable functions in a meta-analytic study: mental set shifting, information updating and monitoring, and inhibition of prepotent responses. Here we summarize several task classifications typically included under the umbrella of executive function. Others, not described here, include planning, insight, and social cognition and behavior.

Working memory describes the ability to hold several pieces of information in the mind for a short period of time and manipulate them. For example, the Letter–Number Sequencing subtest of the WAIS-IV require patients to listen to a series of randomly ordered letters and numbers and then state first the numbers in numeric order and letters in alphabetical order.

One test of *inhibition* is the Stroop Color–Word Test. The patient is given a series of color names printed in contrasting ink colors (e.g., the word "blue" printed in red ink) and is asked to name the color of the ink. The response set must be maintained while the subject suppresses the alternate (and more standard) inclination to read words without regard to the color of the print.

Set shifting tasks require the patient to shift attention between one task and another or to alternate strategies. One commonly used task is the Wisconsin Card Sort, which uses symbols that may be sorted by color, number, or shape. Based only on feedback about whether each card was or was not correctly placed, the subject must infer an initial sort rule. At intervals, the sort rule is changed without the subject's knowledge; subjects must switch based only on their own observation that the current rule is no longer effective. Other set shifting tasks use explicit cues to indicate which rule should be used.

Fluency refers to the ability to use one or more strategies that maximize the production of responses while avoiding response repetition (Ruff, Allen et al., 1994). Word fluency tests are typically considered measures of executive function because they tap organizational strategies required for retrieval and recall, as well as self-monitoring, self-initiation, and inhibition. Two often-used verbal fluency tasks are letter fluency, where the patient is given a fixed period of time to name as many words as possible that begin with a specific letter and semantic fluency where the task is to name as many words as possible in a specific category.

MOTOR AND PRAXIS

Tests of motor strength, such as grip strength, and of motor speed and agility, such as assessing speed and peg placement, establish lateral dominance and focal point of impairment. In some diseases, such as the dementia of AIDS, reduced motor agility is part of the diagnosis. Tasks such as the grooved pegboard assess manual dexterity and sensorimotor integration. They can identify lateralized brain damage because both hands are tested. The grooved pegboard task contains 25 holes with randomly positioned slots and pegs which have a key along one side. Pegs must be rotated to match the hole before they can be inserted. The patient is asked to insert the pegs into the holes as rapidly as possible.

Higher order motor tasks, such as double-alternating movements or triple sequences, are used to assess motor sequencing or programming, as opposed to pure strength or speed.

ATTENTION

The ability to sustain attention is often tested by cancellation tasks, in which the patient must detect and mark targets embedded in distractors, or by computerized continuous performance tests (CPTs), which measure accuracy, response time, and variability in response time as a function of time on task. CPTs assess sustained attention over relatively long time intervals (10 to 20 minutes) and are frequently used in the assessment of attention deficit disorder. Mental tracking tasks such as Digit Span Forward may also be included in this category.

CONCEPT FORMATION AND REASONING

Brain damage is often associated with concrete reasoning. Tests of concept formation include verbal tasks, such as proverb interpretation, and nonverbal tasks, where underlying concepts must be extracted from visual displays. Tests of abstract reasoning include the Similarities subtest of the WAIS-IV, where the subject must explain how two words are alike. The quality of the response is judged. A general classification response that is pertinent to both words receives a higher score than a specific property or function that is relevant to both.

Perceptual reasoning can be assessed with tasks such as matrix reasoning. This task usually involves a series of figures in which there is a discernible pattern, with one figure in the series left blank. The patient is asked to choose, from an array of possibilities, what figure would complete the series or pattern.

PERSONALITY AND EMOTIONAL STATUS

Mood may affect test performance. At minimum, the neuropsychologist notes the psychiatric history and probes for current psychiatric symptoms. Standardized mood rating scales are also available. Many neurophysiologists use standardized personality scales to aid in diagnosis and test interpretation.

CLINICAL OBSERVATION

Along with the formal scores, the intake interview and testing period afford an extensive period to observe the patient under controlled conditions. These clinical observations are valuable for diagnosis. Formal test scores capture only certain aspects of performance. The patient's problem-solving approach or the nature of the errors made may be telling. Also important in timed tasks is determining whether the patient may complete them with additional time or is actually incapable of solving them. Another important dimension of assessment is the patient's ability to learn and follow directions for the many tests.

More subtle aspects of behavior include responses or coping abilities when confronted with difficult tasks, the ability to remain socially appropriate as the session progresses, and the subjects' appreciation of their own capacities.

REFERRAL ISSUES

Neuropsychological testing is useful for the diagnosis of some conditions and is a tool for evaluating or quantifying the effects of disease on cognition and behavior. The tests may assess the beneficial or adverse effects of drug therapy, radiation, or surgery. Serial evaluations give quantitative results that may change with time. In temporal lobectomy for intractable epilepsy, tests that help identify the location of dysfunction are required in presurgical evaluation to minimize the possibility of adverse effects. Specific referral issues are summarized in the following paragraphs.

DEMENTIA

Testing may detect early dementing changes and discriminate them from "normal" performance. It also helps to obtain information contributing to differential diagnosis, either between dementia and nondementing illness, such as depression versus dementia, or between alternate forms of dementia (e.g., Alzheimer disease, dementia with Lewy bodies, or vascular dementia). Test results may also confirm or quantify disease progression and measure efficacy of clinical interventions.

OTHER BRAIN DISEASE

The effects on cognitive function of stroke, cancer, head trauma, Parkinson disease, Huntington disease, multiple sclerosis, brain infection, or other conditions may be investigated. Testing may be prompted by the patient's complaints. The evaluation helps to clarify the cause or extent of the condition.

EPILEPSY

Testing is part of the presurgical evaluation to determine whether cognitive deficits are consistent with electroencephalography and possibly magnetic resonance imaging (MRI) evidence of focal dysfunction. Additionally, test results, together with knowledge of the proposed surgery, can be used to predict risk of postoperative cognitive decline or the probability of postoperative improvement. Nonsurgical patients are frequently assessed to address memory, attention, and mood issues associated with epilepsy and antiepileptic medications.

TOXIC EXPOSURE

Testing may evaluate the consequences of toxic or potentially toxic exposures, either on an individual basis or for particular exposed groups (e.g., factory workers). Exposures may include metals, solvents, pesticides, alcohol and drugs, or any other compounds that may affect the brain.

MEDICATION

The potential effect of medications on the central nervous system may be evaluated in therapeutic trials or clinical practice. For example, in trials of agents used to treat Alzheimer disease, neuropsychological tests are typically primary measures of drug efficacy. In clinical practice, adverse or therapeutic effects of newly introduced medications may be evaluated.

PSYCHIATRIC DISORDERS

Testing may help in the differential diagnosis of psychiatric and neurologic disorders, especially affective disorders and schizophrenia. It may also assess cognition and areas of competence in patients with these conditions.

LEARNING DISABILITY

Testing may evaluate learning disabilities and the residuals of these disabilities in later life. Behavioral disorders, ADD, autism, dyslexia, and learning problems are common referral issues.

EXPECTATIONS FROM A NEUROPSYCHOLOGICAL EVALUATION

The minimum that a neuropsychological evaluation yields is an extensive investigation of the abilities of the patient. In these cases, although the studies do not lead to a definite diagnosis, they help determine the patient's capacities, establish a baseline from which to track the future, and advise the patient and family.

Sometimes, the evaluation suggests that additional diagnostic tests would be useful. For example, if a patient's pattern of performance deviates substantially from that typically expected at the current stage of dementia, a vascular contribution may be considered. Similarly, evaluation may suggest the value of psychiatric consultation or more intensive electroencephalographic recordings.

Many times the neuropsychologist may offer a tentative diagnosis or discuss the possible diagnoses compatible with the test findings. Neuropsychological evaluation may not yield a diagnosis without appropriate clinical and historical information. In the context of multidisciplinary testing, however, it may provide evidence to confirm or refute a specific diagnosis. In this case, testing might best be considered an additional source of information to be used by the clinician for diagnosis in conjunction with the neurologic examination and laboratory tests.

HOW TO REFER

The more information the examiner has at the start, the more directly the issues may be addressed. For example, if MRI has revealed a particular lesion, tests may be tailored specifically to better understand the lesion. The examination is not an exploration of the ability to detect a lesion but is rather a contribution to understanding the implications of the lesion. Similarly, the more explicit the referral question, the more likely the evaluation may yield use-ful information. Besides providing the relevant history, a useful referral describes the problem to be assessed. This is often a statement of the differential diagnosis being entertained. Alternately, the neurologist or the family may simply want to document the current condition or explore some specific aspect of performance, such as language.

SUGGESTED READINGS

Lezak MD, Howieson DB, Bigler E, et al. *Neuropsychological Assessment*. 5th ed. New York: Oxford University Press; 2012.

Miyake A, Friedman NP, Emerson MJ, et al. The unity and diversity of executive functions and their contributions to complex "frontal lobe" tasks: a latent variable analysis. *Cognit Psychol*. 2000;41(1):49–100.

Ruff RM, Allen CC, Farrow CE, et al. Figural fluency: differential impairment in patients with left vs. right frontal lobe lesions. *Arch Clin Neuropsychol*. 1994;9:41–45.

Salmon DP, Bondi MW. Neuropsychological assessment of dementia. *Annu Rev Psychol*. 2009;60:257–282.

Vliet EC, Manly J, Tang MX, et al. The neuropsychological profiles of mild Alzheimer's disease and questionable dementia as compared to age-related cognitive decline. *J Int Neuropsychol Soc*. 2003;9:720–732.

Wechsler D. *Wechsler Adult Intelligence Scale*. 4th ed. San Antonio, TX: The Psychological Corporation; 2008.

Wechsler D. *Wechsler Intelligence Scale for Children*. 3rd ed. London: Pearson Assessment; 1991.

Wechsler D. *Wechsler Intelligence Scale for Children*. 4th ed. London: Pearson Assessment; 2003.

Nancy J. Edwards, Tareq Saad H. Almaghrabi, and Kiwon Lee

INTRODUCTION

Accessing the cerebrospinal fluid (CSF) compartment—typically via lumbar puncture (LP)—is one of the key skills every neurologist should have. Proper analysis of CSF findings may result in a diagnosis (even if the neurologic examination and neuroimaging have not); furthermore, LP and the removal of CSF may be therapeutic in certain cases. This chapter will review step by step the technique of the LP, including advances in the procedure (e.g., ultrasound guidance); in addition, we outline here a guide for the interpretation of CSF findings in various neurologic disorders ranging from infectious to demyelinating to neoplastic.

LUMBAR PUNCTURE

TECHNIQUES

Careful positioning of the patient is often the key to performing a successful LP. Patients may be placed in either a lateral recumbent position with the spine flexed—head bowed, knees bent, and drawn up into the torso, for example, the "fetal position" (Fig. 31.1). Alternatively, patients may sit upright with the neck and back flexed forward (typically resting on a table). The lateral recumbent position should be used if an opening pressure is needed. As the conus medullaris ends at the level of the L1 and L2 interspace in 94% of adults, this level should be avoided during LP. Instead, the L3–L4, L4–L5, and L5–S1 interspaces are appropriate for needle puncture. These interspaces can be identified via palpation of bony landmarks. The line joining the superior aspect of the iliac crests posteriorly (the intercristal line) identifies the L4 spinous process or L3 and L4 interspace.

The interspace for needle insertion should be marked and the skin overlying the LP site should be sterilized and draped using standard aseptic technique. Local anesthetic—usually 1% lidocaine—is

then applied; the 25-gauge needle should be used to raise a skin wheal at the LP site and the longer, 20-gauge needle should then be used to infiltrate the deeper layers. The spinal needle (with stylet in) is then inserted through the skin wheal into the interspinous space. Ideally, needle insertion should be midline, orthogonal to the plane of the back. To reduce the risk of post-LP headache, the bevel should be parallel to the longitudinal fibers of the dura; if the patient is in the lateral recumbent position, the bevel should face up and if the patient is sitting upright, the bevel should face to one side. Theoretically, this allows dural fibers to be separated rather than cut. The spinal needle is then advanced slowly at a slightly cephalad angle (directed toward the umbilicus) in order to follow the contour of the spinous processes. The needle will pass through the supraspinous ligament and the ligamentum flavum, perhaps resulting in a "pop" when the dura is pierced and the subarachnoid space is entered. The stylet should then be removed and CSF should readily appear at the needle hub if in the subarachnoid space. If instead CSF does not flow, the stylet should be replaced and the needle advanced or withdrawn incrementally, with frequent removal of the stylet, until CSF is obtained or bone encountered.

ULTRASOUND GUIDANCE

Ultrasound visualization of landmarks may significantly improve the rate of LP success. This is particularly true in certain patient populations where palpation of landmarks may be challenging—neonates, pregnant women, obese patients, and patients with generalized edema, for example. One large meta-analysis of 14 studies and 1,334 patients revealed a significant reduction in the risk of failed or traumatic LPs and epidural catheterizations with the use of ultrasound guidance. The absolute risk reduction was 0.63, resulting in a number needed to diagnose of 16 to avoid one failed tap.

To perform an ultrasound-guided LP, the linear probe (higher resolution of superficial structures) should be used. The first view that should be obtained is the transverse view—the goal of this view is to determine an accurate anatomic midline by identification of the spinous process (Fig. 31.2A). To obtain this view, the probe is placed perpendicularly to the long axis of the spine. The spinous process will appear as a hyperechoic white convex rim with an anechoic shadow (or the anechoic shadow itself can simply be used if the rim is not identified). The midline should be marked and the longitudinal view should then be obtained (using the midline as a reference). The goal of the longitudinal view is to determine the spinal interspace—where the spinal needle will be inserted. To obtain this view, the transducer should be rotated into the sagittal/longitudinal plane with the probe marker pointing cephalad. Identify the hyperechoic spinous process again and then adjust the probe cephalad and caudad in order to center the probe/image between two contiguous, crescentic-shaped spinous processes; the interspace will be the hypoechoic gray gap in between (see Fig. 31.2B). This interspace should also be marked. Remove the probe and extend the transverse/longitudinal markings until they intersect; this intersection represents the ideal position for the spinal needle to be inserted.

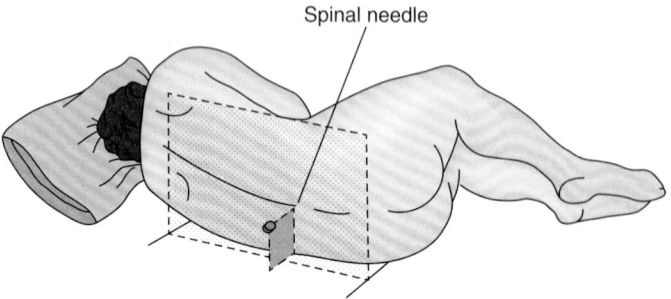

Spinal needle

FIGURE 31.1 Proper positioning for lumbar puncture. Position the patient's back at the edge of the bed with the head flexed and the legs curled up in the fetal position. Place a pillow under the head. Hips are parallel to each other and perpendicular to the bed. The spinal needle should be parallel to the bed. (Adapted from Marshall R, Mayer S. *On Call Neurology*. 3rd ed. Philadelphia: Saunders; 2007.)

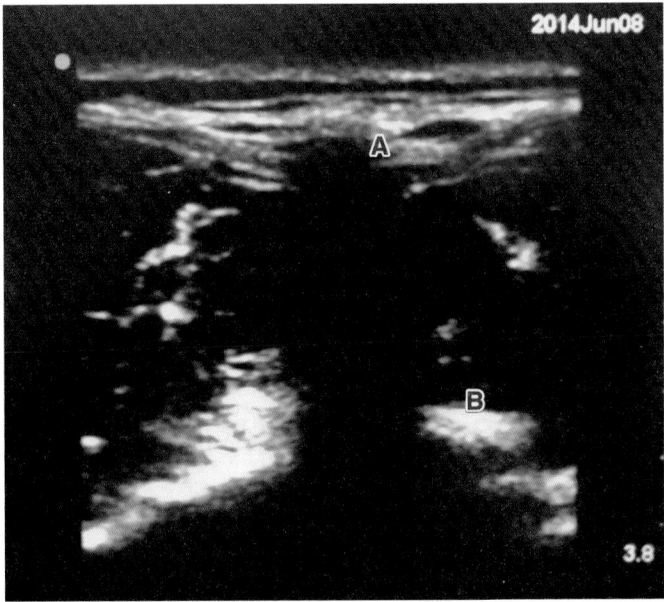
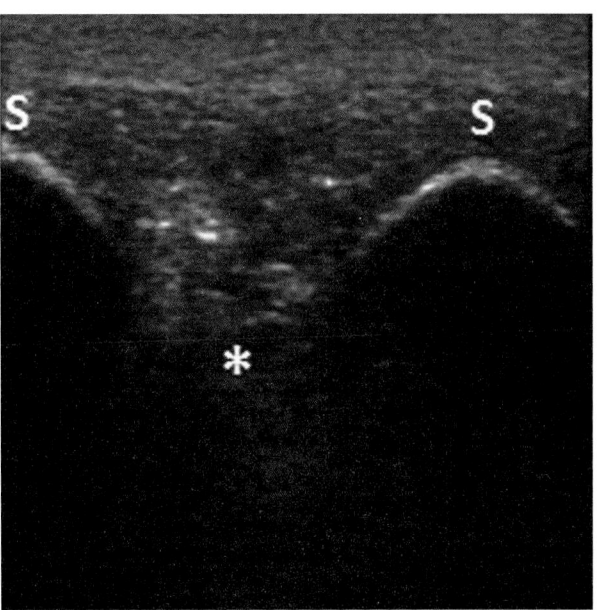

FIGURE 31.2 Ultrasound-guided LP. **A:** Transverse view. The anechoic shadow below *A* represents the spinous process—the midline; *B* localizes the transverse process. **B:** Longitudinal view. The interspace (*asterisk*) is located between the two crescentic-shaped, hyperechoic spinous processes (*S*).

CEREBROSPINAL FLUID ANALYSIS

CEREBROSPINAL FLUID PLEOCYTOSIS

Basic analysis of the CSF begins with red blood cell (RBC) and white blood cell (WBC) analysis and measurements of protein and glucose, although an extensive variety of additional tests can also be ordered (Table 31.1). The normal WBC count of CSF ranges from 0 to 5 lymphocytes or monocytes per cubic millimeter. Rarely, a single polymorphonuclear (PMN) cell may be identified from a large volume tap; the presence of two or greater PMNs, though, should be considered abnormal. A myriad of neurologic disorders can result in a CSF pleocytosis, ranging from acutely life-threatening (bacterial meningitis) to entirely chronic (as can be seen in patients with HIV).

Assessing the magnitude of pleocytosis along with the relative predominance of neutrophils to lymphocytes is often key, as is the clinical history—specifically whether the neurologic symptoms are acute or chronic in nature. For instance, a patient presenting with acute encephalopathy and a neutrophil-predominant CSF pleocytosis should be presumed to have bacterial meningitis (and promptly treated as such). In general, patients with acute bacterial meningitis have a CSF WBC count of several thousand (although the range may be from hundreds to >60,000). Furthermore, a CSF sample with greater than 33% neutrophils, a protein concentration of greater than 100 mg/dL, and a glucose level of less than 50% of the serum glucose level is strongly suggestive of bacterial meningitis. Exceptions include bacterial meningitis due to *Listeria* (often with a lymphocytic rather than neutrophilic pleocytosis), early viral or atypical (fungal/mycobacterial) infections that may initially recruit neutrophils into the CSF, neuroinvasive disease due to West Nile virus, and neuroinflammatory disorders (neuro-Behcet, Sweet syndrome).

In an acutely ill patient with a lymphocytic CSF pleocytosis, viral meningoencephalitis is often the cause. The WBC count generally ranges from 10 to 1,000 cells/mm³ and is composed primarily of

TABLE 31.1 Common Cerebrospinal Fluid Tests

- Cell count
- Protein and glucose levels
- Gram stain and culture
- VDRL test
- India ink test (for *Cryptococcus neoformans*)
- Wet smear (for fungi and amebae)
- Stain and culture for AFB (for tuberculosis)
- Cryptococcal antigen titers
- pH and lactate levels (abnormal in MELAS)
- Oligoclonal bands (abnormal in multiple sclerosis)
- IgG index (intrathecal IgG production)
- IgG and IgM antibody titers (for viral infections, compare to serum)
- Lyme disease antibody titers (compare with serum titers) and Western blot
- Latex agglutination bacterial antigen tests (for pneumococcus, meningococcus, and *Haemophilus influenzae*)
- Viral isolation studies
- Cytology (requires fixation in formalin)
- Polymerase chain reaction for Lyme disease, tuberculosis, and causes of viral encephalitis
- CSF ACE activity (abnormal with tuberculosis or sarcoidosis)
- 13-9-9 protein (elevated in Creutzfeldt–Jacob disease)

VDRL, Venereal Disease Research Laboratory; AFB, acid-fast bacilli; MELAS, mitochondrial encephalomyopathy, lactic acidosis, and stroke; IgG, immunoglobulin G; IgM, immunoglobulin M; CSF, cerebrospinal fluid; ACE, angiotensin-converting enzyme.

mononuclear cells. The cornerstone of etiologic diagnosis is the detection of viral nucleic acid sequences in the CSF via polymerase chain reaction (PCR). In cases of suspected viral meningoencephalitis, CSF PCRs for the enteroviruses along with the herpesviruses (herpes simplex virus 1 and 2, cytomegalovirus, varicella-zoster virus, Epstein–Barr virus (EBV), and in immunocompromised patients, human herpesvirus-6) should be sent, along with serologic testing for HIV. Serologic testing for several additional viruses can be considered (West Nile virus, St. Louis encephalitis virus, Eastern equine encephalitis virus, Venezuelan equine encephalitis virus, and La Crosse virus).

In patients with chronic neurologic symptoms and a lymphocytic CSF pleocytosis, an atypical infection such as fungal, tuberculous, or spirochetal should be considered. Etiologic diagnosis can be made via these CSF studies: India ink staining, fungal cultures, assays for cryptococcal antigen or histoplasma antigen, and *Coccidioides* complement fixation antibodies; acid-fast bacilli smear and culture, PCR for *Mycobacterium tuberculosis*; Venereal Disease Research Laboratory (VDRL) in conjunction with serum testing for syphilis; and antibodies against *Borrelia burgdorferi*. That being said, a chronic lymphocytic CSF pleocytosis may also be caused by various noninfectious disorders, including neoplasm (central nervous system [CNS] lymphoma, leptomeningeal carcinomatosis), paraneoplastic encephalitides, autoimmune/demyelinating disorders (CNS vasculitis, neurosarcoidosis, neuromyelitis optica [NMO], multiple sclerosis [MS]), and even medications or toxins (nonsteroidal anti-inflammatory drugs [NSAIDs], sulfa drugs, intravenous immunoglobulin, carbamazepine). Therefore, the clinical history along with neuroimaging is often vital for the diagnostic interpretation of a chronic lymphocytic CSF pleocytosis.

The CSF findings in the various meningitides are summarized here in Table 31.2.

There are two frequently encountered caveats to the interpretation of a CSF pleocytosis—the first being CSF obtained from a traumatic LP and the second being CSF obtained from an external ventricular drain (EVD). Inadvertent needle trauma to a capillary or venule during LP will introduce additional WBCs from the peripheral blood into the CSF, increasing the total number of WBCs.

A useful rule of thumb if a traumatic LP is suspected is to subtract 1 WBC for every 500 to 1,000 RBCs present in the CSF. Alternatively, the following formula can be used, especially in patients with an abnormal peripheral WBC count:

$$WBC\ (CSF) = \frac{WBC\ (blood) \times RBC\ (CSF)}{RBC\ (blood)}$$

In the neurocritical care unit, patients may have an EVD inserted into the lateral ventricle to aid in CSF diversion or to monitor intracranial pressure. CSF can be easily sampled through this drain and is often sampled to exclude nosocomial meningitis/ventriculitis associated with the drain itself. Whether a truly pathologic pleocytosis (e.g., one due to meningitis/ventriculitis) is present in EVD-sampled CSF can be challenging to ascertain; patients who have EVDs inserted for CSF diversion may have high RBC counts in the ventricular system (for instance, those with subarachnoid hemorrhage or intracerebral hemorrhage) and the aforementioned corrections for RBCs are not entirely valid for EVD CSF samples. Furthermore, patients with large volumes of blood in the subarachnoid or ventricular compartments often develop an inflammatory response with an elevation in the WBC count in ventricular CSF. To aid with the diagnosis of meningitis/ventriculitis in patients with EVDs, the cell index, in conjunction with CSF Gram stain and culture, can be used. The cell index is calculated as follows:

$$Cell\ index = \frac{WBC\ (CSF) \div RBC\ (CSF)}{WBC\ (blood) \div RBC\ (blood)}$$

A cell index of 1 is (by definition) normal. And although there is no explicit cutoff for an "abnormal" cell index, a significant rise in the cell index from one day to the next may signal the presence of infection.

HYPOGLYCORRHACHIA

A reduced CSF glucose level may be caused by impaired glucose transport into the CSF (for instance, due to severe disruption of the blood–brain barrier and its glucose transporter, GLUT1) or as a result of increased glucose use within the CNS. There are a

---

TABLE 31.2 Cerebrospinal Fluid Findings in Various Meningitides

Type	Leukocytes (mm³)	Protein (mg/dL)	Glucose (mg/dL)
Acute bacterial	>1,000 although ranges from several hundred to >60,000; PMNs predominate	100–500, occasionally >1,000	5–40; typically a CSF-to-serum glucose ratio of <0.33
Viral	5–1,000; lymphocytes predominate (although early in the disease course, PMNs may predominate)	Frequently normal or slightly elevated; generally <100	Normal (although rarely reduced in cases of LCMV, CMV, paramyxoviruses, HSV)
Tuberculous	25–100; rarely >500; lymphocytes predominate (although early in the disease course, PMNs may predominate)	Elevated, 100–200	Low; <45 in 75% of cases
Cryptococcal	0–800; lymphocytes predominate	20–500	Often reduced; average 30
Syphilitic	Average 500; primarily lymphocytes	100	Generally normal although may be mildly reduced
Sarcoid	0 to <100	Slight to moderate elevation	May be reduced in 18%–50% of patients
Leptomeningeal carcinomatosis	0 to several hundred; cytology may reveal malignant cells	Elevated	Low in 40%–75% of cases

PMNs, polymorphonuclear cells; CSF, cerebrospinal fluid; LCMV, lymphocytic choriomeningitis virus; CMV, cytomegalovirus; HSV, herpes simplex virus.

TABLE 31.3 Causes of Hypoglycorrhachia
Bacterial meningitis
Fungal meningitis
Tuberculous meningitis
Meningitis due to spirochetes (syphilis, Lyme)
CNS lymphoma
Leptomeningeal carcinomatosis
Neurosarcoidosis

CNS, central nervous system.

handful of pathologies that typically result in an abnormally low CSF glucose and as such, hypoglycorrhachia can be a very helpful diagnostic clue. In general, a CSF glucose of 45 mg/dL to 80 mg/dL is considered normal, although this is dependent on a fairly normal range of serum glucose (70 to 120 mg/dL). Of greater usefulness is the CSF-to-serum glucose ratio, as this is relatively constant through a wide range of serum glucose levels. The normal CSF-to-serum glucose ratio is 0.6 to 0.8; a ratio less than 0.5 is abnormal and should prompt urgent evaluation.

The principal causes of a reduced CSF-to-serum glucose ratio are listed in Table 31.3. Several infectious meningitides—bacterial, fungal, tuberculous, and spirochetal—are often heralded by hypoglycorrhachia. For instance, in one study of adults with bacterial meningitis, 70% had CSF glucose concentrations of less than 50 mg/dL. The CSF-to-serum glucose ratio in patients with bacterial meningitis is generally less than 0.33; a ratio of less than 0.23 in patients with acute meningitis had a positive predictive value of 99% for a bacterial etiology.

Fungal meningitis is also associated with low CSF glucose—generally 20 to 40 mg/dL in one-half to two-thirds of patients. *Mycobacterium tuberculosis* meningitis characteristically depresses the CSF glucose; in one study of CSF culture-positive patients, the mean admission CSF glucose level was 23 mg/dL. Hypoglycorrhachia has also been reported in patients with Lyme disease and syphilitic meningitis, although the reduction in CSF glucose is often modest compared to cases of bacterial meningitis. The CSF glucose level in patients with viral meningitis is classically normal; that being said, rare cases of viral meningitis due to cytomegalovirus (CMV), paramyxoviruses, and lymphocytic choriomeningitis virus have been associated with low CSF glucose.

Other causes of hypoglycorrhachia include CNS lymphoma (approximately 10% of patients), leptomeningeal carcinomatosis (40% of patients), neurosarcoidosis (18% of patients), and lupus cerebritis/vasculitis (8% of patients). Patients with aneurysmal subarachnoid hemorrhage may have transient reductions in their CSF glucose (usually 4 to 8 days postictus). And finally, hypoglycorrhachia has been reported in patients who have received intrathecal injections of corticosteroids.

CEREBROSPINAL FLUID FINDINGS IN INFLAMMATORY AND DEMYELINATING DISORDERS

Although a detailed description of the CSF findings across the gamut of autoimmune and demyelinating neurologic disorders is beyond the scope of this chapter, there are certain CSF generalizations we can refer to. For instance, a mild lympho-cytic pleocytosis and modest elevation in protein is frequently encountered in these patients. Approximately, one-third of patients with MS, optic neuritis, transverse myelitis, and even acute disseminated encephalomyelitis will have a mild lymphocytic pleocytosis. A greater proportion of patients with neurosarcoidosis and NMO will have a lymphocytic pleocytosis, and in the proper clinical context, a CSF pleocytosis of greater than 50 WBC/mm^3 or greater than 5 PMNs/mm^3 is strongly supportive of a diagnosis of NMO.

Even if the CSF cell count and protein are normal, evidence of an active intrathecal humoral immune response is often fundamental to the diagnosis of a neuroinflammatory disorder. During CNS inflammation, CSF immunoglobulin G (IgG) content may preferentially increase above serum levels, reflecting intrathecal synthesis. A routinely used estimate of intrathecal IgG synthesis is the IgG index, calculated as follows:

$$IgG\ index = \frac{IgG\ (CSF) \div IgG\ (serum)}{albumin\ (CSF) \div albumin\ (serum)}$$

An IgG index greater than 0.70 to 0.75 is often considered elevated (although parameters range depending on the clinical laboratory processing the sample). As an adjunct to the IgG index, the detection of unique oligoclonal bands (OCBs) within the CSF—distinct from those found in the serum—provides qualitative evidence of intrathecal Ig production. If 2 or more distinct CSF bands (bands absent from a corresponding serum sample) are detected, OCBs are considered to be positive. In MS patients, for instance, approximately 90% will have either an elevated IgG index or two or greater OCBs in the CSF, and these CSF findings may even precede a diagnosis of MS based on clinical history (or radiology) alone.

CEREBROSPINAL FLUID CYTOLOGY

Diagnosis of a CNS malignancy via CSF cytology is highly specific and relatively noninvasive (compared to biopsy, for instance)—unfortunately, the sensitivity of CSF cytology ranges from low to moderate. Several factors may alter the yield of CSF cytology, including the site sampled (lumbar vs. cisterna magna), the volume of CSF collected, the number of specimens examined, tumor location/grade, and the extent of leptomeningeal disease. The sensitivity of CSF cytology across CNS malignancies is outlined in Table 31.4. In general, repeated sampling will increase the yield of CSF cytology; for instance, in patients with leptomeningeal carcinomatosis, 41% to 71% will have a positive cytopathology on the first CSF sample, whereas 79% to 92% will have a positive cytology with repeated sampling. These findings form the basis for the recommendation that three large-volume (ideally >20 mL; >10 mL at the very least) LPs should be analyzed for malignant cells in patients with presumed leptomeningeal disease. Furthermore, CSF samples should be promptly delivered to the cytopathology laboratory for processing as autolysis begins within 1 to 2 hours of sample collection. In cases where primary CNS lymphoma is suspected, several additional CSF studies may aid in diagnosis. Immunophenotyping the CSF via flow cytometry can considerably increase the diagnostic yield by differentiating monoclonal B lymphocyte populations from reactive polyclonal lymphocytes even if the sample is relatively hypocellular. And in patients with HIV, CNS lymphoma is strongly associated with transformation of malignant cells by EBV; as such, EBV PCR in CSF has a high sensitivity and specificity for the diagnosis of CNS lymphoma in this particular patient population.

TABLE 31.4   Cerebrospinal Fluid Cytology Yield

Type of CNS Malignancy	Percentage of Patients with Positive Cytology	Notes
Malignant glioma	7–66 (more than one sample)	
Parenchymal metastatic lesions	2–10	
Primary CNS lymphoma	16–26 (single sample)	Flow cytometry = higher yields EBV PCR as an adjunct in HIV +
Leptomeningeal carcinomatosis	47–92	41–71 with one sample; increasing yields with repeat sampling

CNS, central nervous system; EBV, Epstein–Barr virus; PCR, polymerase chain reaction.

SUGGESTED READINGS

Boon JM, Abrahams PH, Meiring JH, et al. Lumbar puncture: anatomical review of a clinical skill. *Clin Anat.* 2004;17:544–553.

Cascella C, Nausheen S, Cunha BA. A differential diagnosis of drug-induced aseptic meningitis. *Infect Med.* 2008;25:331–334.

Chakraverty R, Pynsent P, Isaacs K. Which spinal levels are identified by palpation of the iliac crests and posterior superior iliac spines? *J Anat.* 2007;210(2):232–236.

Cinque P, Brytting M, Vago L, et al. Epstein-Barr virus DNA in cerebrospinal fluid from patients with AIDS-related primary lymphoma of the central nervous system. *Lancet.* 1993;342:398–401.

Conly JM, Ronald AR. Cerebrospinal fluid as a diagnostic body fluid. *Am J Med.* 1983;75:102–108.

Dougherty JM, Roth RM. Cerebral spinal fluid. *Emerg Med Clin North Am.* 1986;4:281–297.

Fishman RA. *Cerebrospinal Fluid in Diseases of the Nervous System.* 2nd ed. Philadelphia: WB Saunders; 1992.

Hegde U, Filie A, Little RF, et al. High incidence of occult leptomeningeal disease detected by flow cytometry in newly diagnosed aggressive B-cell lymphomas at risk for central nervous system involvement: the role of flow cytometry versus cytology. *Blood.* 2005;105:496–502.

Hussein AS, Shafran SD. Acute bacterial meningitis in adults: a 12-year review. *Medicine.* 2000;79:360–368.

Irani DN. *Cerebrospinal Fluid in Clinical Practice.* Philadelphia: Saunders Elsevier; 2009.

Kaplan JG, DeSouza TG, Farkash A, et al. Leptomeningeal metastases: comparison of clinical features and laboratory data of solid tumors, lymphomas and leukemias. *J Neurooncol.* 1990;92:225–229.

Kilpatrick ME, Girgis NI, Yassin MW, et al. Tuberculous meningitis—clinical and laboratory review of 100 patients. *J Hyg (Lond).* 1986;96:231–238.

McLean BN, Luxton RW, Thompson EJ. A study of immunoglobulin G in the cerebrospinal fluid of 1007 patients with suspected neurological disease using isoelectric focusing and the log IgG-index. *Brain.* 1990;113:1269–1289.

Noble VE, Bret NA, Sutingco N. Ultrasound for procedural guidance: lumbar puncture. In: Noble VE, Nelson BP, Sutingco AN, eds. *Manual of Emergency and Critical Care Ultrasound.* New York: Cambridge University Press; 2007.

Pfausler B, Beer R, Engelhardt K, et al. Cell index—a new parameter for the early diagnosis of ventriculostomy (external ventricular drain)-related ventriculitis in patients with intraventricular hemorrhage? *Acta Neurochir.* 2004;146:477–481.

Roos KL. Lumbar puncture. *Semin Neurol.* 2003;23:105–114.

Shaikh F, Brzezinski J, Alexander S, et al. Ultrasound imaging for lumbar punctures and epidural catheterisations: systematic review and meta-analysis. *BMJ.* 2013;346:f1720.

Spanos A, Harrell FE, Durack DT. Differential diagnosis of acute meningitis. An analysis of the predictive value of initial observations. *JAMA.* 1989;262:2700–2707.

Thompson RB Jr, Bertram H. Laboratory diagnosis of central nervous system infections. *Infect Dis Clin North Am.* 2001;15:1047–1071.

Tunkel AR, Glaser CA, Bloch KC, et al. The management of encephalitis: clinical practice guidelines by the Infectious Diseases Society of America. *Clin Infect Dis.* 2008;47:303–327.

Wingerchuk DM, Lennon VA, Pittock SJ, et al. Revised diagnostic criteria for neuromyelitis optica. *Neurology.* 2006;66:1485–1489.

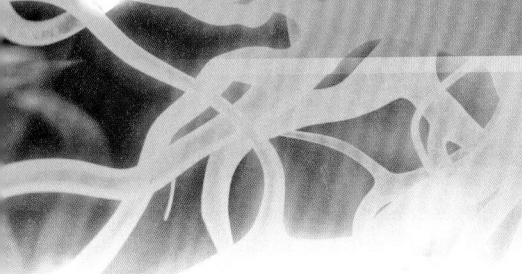

Brain, Nerve, and Muscle Biopsy 32

John F. Crary, Thomas H. Brannagan III, and Kurenai Tanji

INTRODUCTION

Biopsy of nervous and muscle tissue remains a critical tool. Any potential benefits associated with having a tissue-based diagnosis must be carefully weighed against the risks associated with the procedure. Brain, muscle, and nerve biopsies are always performed in the context of an interdisciplinary team, which can include neurologists, internists, neuroradiologists, neurosurgeons, and neuropathologists. To ensure appropriate assessment of the biopsy, a high level of communication between providers is of the utmost importance. In most cases, brain biopsy should be a last resort, reserved for clinical settings where all other diagnostic modalities have been exhausted. However, modern surgical techniques have helped to minimize complications and the risk of obtaining a nondiagnostic biopsy in some disorders, the benefit in establishing a diagnosis and thus treatment plan may outweigh the risks of the procedure. In addition, modern molecular techniques are increasingly being applied, greatly increasing the use of biopsy specimens. Although the widespread deployment of next-generation sequencing technology has obviated the need for biopsy in some settings, these modern ancillary studies have not supplanted classical histomorphologic analysis. In this chapter, we will provide an overview of the critical issues associated with the brain, muscle, and nerve biopsy. We will also discuss the use of skin biopsies for epidermal nerve fiber density analysis.

BRAIN BIOPSY

INDICATIONS

Certain general considerations must be weighed before referring a patient for a brain biopsy. General risks associated with brain biopsy are similar to those associated with any surgical procedure, including deep vein thrombosis, postoperative hemorrhage, infection, etc. Patients on anticoagulant treatment might need to make adjustments given the risk of postoperative intracranial hemorrhage in the brain. Other complications include stroke, seizures, and cerebrospinal fluid (CSF) leak (fistula). Given the risks, it is generally accepted that all other diagnostic modalities must be exhausted before proceeding to brain biopsy.

An essential consideration prior to biopsy is determining the likelihood that the answer will lead to a change in patient management. Should, for example, the expected diagnoses have similar or no disease-modifying treatments, then the decision to proceed to a biopsy should be questioned. Furthermore, there is often a window of opportunity for the biopsy to be useful clinically. If the patient has deteriorated beyond the point to which a reasonable recovery in function can be anticipated, the biopsy might also be of limited value. Further, the ability of the neuropathologist to recognize diagnostic features in the tissue is highest during the active phase of a disease. Once the pathology has run its course, secondary changes in the tissue can predominate and increase the

likelihood of a nondiagnostic biopsy. Treatment effects, such as brain irradiation or steroids, may also mask diagnostic changes. For example, in a patient with a possible diagnosis of central nervous system (CNS) lymphoma, the use of systemic steroids should be deferred unless essential in the context of clinical care (i.e., as a component of treating brain herniation), as treatment can make the biopsy nondiagnostic. Thus, it is essential that empiric treatments be used judiciously should a patient be a candidate for brain biopsy.

Brain biopsies have a prominent place in the treatment and management of CNS neoplasms. For mass lesions, partial brain resection and/or biopsy may be performed, depending on the functional importance of the region that contains the lesion. For malignant brain tumors, resections have the additional advantage of being both diagnostic and therapeutic in the form of debulking. Watchful waiting might be considered for benign brain tumors. Certain brain tumors in vital regions of the brain, such as brain stem gliomas, or eloquent cortical regions might not be amenable to a full resection, but guided stereotactic biopsy might be performed in some cases.

Brain biopsies are generally not required for most CNS infections, as other forms of diagnosis are often definitive. Viral, bacterial, and fungal organisms can be identified with other diagnostic modalities, including with CSF sampling. In ambiguous contexts, a brain biopsy might be performed. Such biopsies are often of highest clinical use when two pathogenic processes with contradictory treatments are under consideration, for example, infectious versus autoimmune. Immunocompromised patients also provide a special setting where a broad differential diagnosis might trigger consideration of a brain biopsy.

In the case of age-related neurodegenerative disorders, brain biopsy is rarely performed. However, a biopsy may be considered in the setting of a rapidly progressive dementia, when there is a reasonable chance that a treatable cause might be uncovered, which cannot be diagnosed by other means. Recent advances have led to the ability to diagnose specific autoimmune encephalitides using antisera. Moreover, CSF biomarkers have shown increasing use in diagnosing Alzheimer disease and prion disease. These advances have altered referral patterns, perhaps decreasing the total number of subjects undergoing brain biopsy for rapidly progressive dementia but increasing the diagnostic yield.

Brain biopsy is not indicated for ischemic stroke, but brain tissue may be sampled in the setting of hemorrhagic stroke to assess the vasculature for cerebral amyloid angiopathy. Vascular abnormalities may be resected surgically, and histopathologic analysis of such lesions is generally of only modest use.

BRAIN BIOPSY REQUIRES AN INTERDISCIPLINARY APPROACH

Brain biopsies are always performed in the context of an interdisciplinary team. The neurologist plays a critical role in the clinical workup and referring patients to biopsy only when all other diagnostic modalities have been exhausted. Next, the neurologist will work closely with both the neuroradiologist and neurosurgeon to identify a radiographically evident lesion that is amenable to biopsy. Although "blind" biopsies of the nondominant (usually right) frontal cortex are often performed, targeting a specific lesion is thought to provide the most informative results. If a biopsy is indicated, an open biopsy consisting of 1 cm³ full-thickness biopsy that contains gray matter, leptomeninges, and subcortical white matter is considered optimal by most neuropathologists. However, if the lesion is located within a vital or eloquent brain region, stereotactic core biopsies, sometimes measuring just a few millimeters, can provide diagnostic material.

During surgery, neurosurgeons often call on the neuropathologist to perform a *frozen section*. These intraoperative consultations are a means to rapidly obtain some diagnostic information and involve rapidly freezing tissue and cutting followed by hematoxylin and eosin (H&E) staining. Although these tissue sections are of only limited diagnostic value, given the severe tissue artifacts that develop, the information provided may be helpful to guide surgical decision making. Another use of the frozen section is confirming the presence of lesional tissue within the biopsy, which also decreases the likelihood of a nondiagnostic biopsy. Critically, the preliminary diagnostic impression obtained through a frozen section must be interpreted with caution, as it is not uncommon for revision following additional sampling and ancillary studies.

NEUROPATHOLOGIC INTERPRETATION OF THE BRAIN BIOPSY

Classical histopathologic examination by a neuropathologist remains the foundation of brain biopsy interpretation. Tissue sections from formalin-fixed brain are mounted on glass slides, stained with the H&E, and examined microscopically. The H&E stain allows for visualization of the cytoarchitecture and all the cellular types in the brain, including neurons and glia. Other stains are in routine use, including variations of the Bielschowsky silver stain, which is excellent for visualizing neuronal processes. Connective tissue stains such as trichrome, reticulin, or van Gieson are particularly useful for vascular pathology. Congo red and thioflavin are useful for visualizing amyloid. Gram, Gömöri methenamine silver (GMS), and the Ziehl–Neelsen (acid-fast bacilli) stains are routinely used for microorganisms.

Various ancillary studies are routinely used in neuropathology. Immunohistochemical stains are commonly employed in various contexts, particularly in the setting of neoplasms, where molecular alterations can be detected with both diagnostic and prognostic relevance. Many molecular tests require fresh (nonfixed) frozen tissue, and a portion of the specimen must be set aside for this purpose prior to processing. Should an infectious etiology be a consideration, tissue cultures are ideally performed using swabs of the surgical site, but fragments of fresh tissue can be submitted after surgery provided that it has not been fixed or contaminated. If lymphoma is a consideration, brain tissue can be used for flow cytometry to characterize the neoplastic population, but CNS lymphoma is most often of the diffuse large B-cell type, and these fragile cells generally do not perform well for this test. Alternatively, cultures of the tissue may be grown for cytogenetic analysis. Electron microscopy is generally of only very limited use in the setting of brain biopsies. Next-generation DNA and RNA sequencing is increasingly being applied to brain tumors for subclassification and targeted treatments. Also, next-generation sequencing can detect very low levels of pathogen DNA/RNA and may become more widely deployed in the future for this use.

MUSCLE BIOPSY

A muscle biopsy may be warranted when neurologic examination, laboratory tests, and electrophysiologic studies suggest a neuromuscular disease. Microscopic examination can help to distinguish between neurogenic and myogenic disorders and can also provide assistance in subclassifying myopathies and in rendering a specific diagnosis. With the advent of new genetic techniques including standard candidate gene sequencing, high-throughput sequencing of specialized gene panels, whole exome, and even whole genome sequencing, several genetic myopathies are diagnosed without invasive muscle biopsy. However, prior to embarking on exhaustive and often costly genetic investigations, a muscle biopsy chosen by thorough history taking and careful neurologic examination may provide an important aid in identifying the most likely cause of the disease that could be treatable. For example, the presence of widespread inflammation suggests an acquired inflammatory myopathy as distinguished from other acquired or hereditary myopathies such as muscular dystrophy. Vasculitis and amyloidosis are often associated with a neuropathy but both disorders may also be identified in muscle. The decision to perform a muscle biopsy should also include noninvasive tools including blood test (e.g., electrolytes, glucose, thyroid-stimulating hormone, vitamin D, creatine kinase [CK], and autoimmune screen), electrodiagnostic studies, and other laboratory tests. Imaging studies, such as magnetic resonance imaging (MRI), have been increasingly incorporated into the evaluation of muscle diseases. When combined with a biopsy, MRI can provide preoperative information about the muscle and adjacent structures (e.g., fascia and subcutaneous tissue). In some cases, the MRI may disclose a characteristic pathologic involvement of muscle groups, which may lead directly to a genetic test and obviate the need for a biopsy.

The best muscles for biopsy are those moderately affected by the disease. MRI may be helpful in selecting a muscle that is most likely to provide diagnostic findings histologically. Severely atrophic muscles, prior injection or electromyography examination sites, or previously traumatized muscles must be avoided. Patients with myoglobinuria or rhabdomyolysis should have the biopsy performed 6 to 8 weeks following the episode to allow muscle to recover from myonecrosis, because extensive and active myonecrosis/regeneration on biopsy may obscure the underlying pathology. The most commonly investigated muscles are the deltoid, biceps, and vastus lateralis, when proximal weakness predominates. In patients with distal weakness, the anterior tibialis or gastrocnemius can be chosen depending on anterior or posterior predominance in weakness or atrophy. The clinical history should be available to the pathologist who examines the biopsy, to apply optimal histologic, histochemical, immunohistochemical, or electron microscopic techniques, to detect the important pathology in the tissue.

Technically, an accurate *morphologic diagnosis* requires formalin-fixed tissue to be processed for routine histology, rapidly and properly frozen tissue for histochemical and immunohistochemical preparations, and glutaraldehyde-fixed tissue for possible electron microscopic examination. Preserving a separate piece of snap frozen muscle is helpful for potential biochemical enzymatic assay(s) of glycogenolytic and glycolytic pathways; lipid metabolism; or mitochondrial respiration, electrophoresis for the protein expression study of muscle proteins, or genetic study.

When the routine histology of muscle demonstrates large or small groups of atrophic fibers, it is most suggestive of a *neurogenic disorder*. In contrast, *myopathic features* include a significantly increased fiber size, an increased number of internally nucleated fibers, necrotic and/or regenerating fibers, and abnormal intracytoplasmic storage material or inclusions. In chronic myopathies, notable endomysial fibrosis is often present. Inflammatory myopathies tend to display widespread, often multifocal, inflammatory infiltrates in the endomysium and/or perimysium. The diagnosis of vasculitis, infectious or noninfectious granulomatous diseases, and amyloidosis can be established by routine histologic evaluation.

Histochemical staining techniques applied on cryosections help classify the fiber types (e.g., myosin adenosine triphosphatase [ATPase]) and delineate cytologic abnormalities. A neurogenic disease can demonstrate fiber-type grouping and/or target/targetoid fibers, best demonstrated by myosin ATPase and nicotinamide adenine dinucleotide tetrazolium reductase, respectively. In certain myopathies, fiber-type predominance (e.g., congenital myopathy) or selective fiber atrophy (e.g., steroid myopathy, critical illness myopathy, and collagen vascular disease) may occur. A variety of cytologic abnormality associated with myopathies, such as cores, nemaline rods, tubular aggregates, caps, hyaline bodies, reduced bodies, cytoplasmic bodies, cytoplasmic mass, significantly increased mitochondria (ragged red fibers), excessive intracytoplasmic glycogen or lipid, and increased lysosomal reactivity with or without fiber vacuolation, are best characterized by proper histochemical preparations. Certain enzymatic deficiencies in metabolic myopathy can be histochemically demonstrated. These include myophosphorylase deficiency (glycogenosis type V), phosphofructokinase deficiency (type VII), myoadenylate deaminase deficiency, and cytochrome c oxidase (respiratory chain complex IV) deficiency (mitochondrial myopathy).

In the new molecular era, immunohistochemical staining using the antibodies against certain proteins, immunoexpressions of which are affected directly or indirectly by DNA mutation, can offer an excellent guide to select candidate gene(s) to be molecularly investigated. Genetic defects of dystrophin, sarcoglycan proteins, dysferlin, caveolin 3, emerin, merosin (α2-laminin), collagen VI, carbohydrate side chain of α-dystroglycan, and others can be reliably tested in the tissue. When a muscular dystrophy demonstrates on biopsy morphologically indistinguishable abnormalities from those of other acquired myopathies, immunohistologic staining may help establish the cause of the disease. Further, immunohistochemical detection of a specific protein deficiency may find the cause of otherwise nonspecific clinical symptoms in patients without typical dystrophic muscle weakness, such as persistent CK elevation (so-called benign hyperCKemia), myoglobulinuria/rhabdomyolysis, myalgia, or cramp. The other advantage of immunohistochemical staining is found in the analysis of inflammatory myopathies. The immunohistochemical detection of inflammatory markers (e.g., major histocompatibility complex [MHC] class I antigens) and immunocytologic typing of lymphocytic infiltrates may aid subclassification of immune-mediated inflammatory myopathies such as dermatomyositis, polymyositis, and inclusion body myositis.

In summary, to promptly establish an accurate and clinically meaningful diagnosis for patients with muscle disorders posing diagnostic challenges, it is essential to wisely minimize the number of investigations that could be extremely costly, especially under the increasing availability of commercial testing. Although new-generation sequencing methods face their own challenges including consent and interpretation of the sequenced data, traditional diagnostic methods such as muscle biopsy remain important tools in narrowing the differential diagnosis.

NERVE BIOPSY

Nerve biopsy is indicated in patients with peripheral neuropathy when additional information about the etiology and severity of the disorder is needed. Although the indications have generally decreased in the last 20 years, mostly due to increasing availability of molecular diagnostic testing for hereditary peripheral neuropathies, certain specific disorders require tissue diagnosis or characterization. These include vasculitis, sarcoid neuropathy, amyloidosis, leprous neuropathy, chronic inflammatory demyelinating polyneuropathy (CIDP), especially cases with clinically and/or electrophysiologically atypical and/or asymmetric presentation, neuropathy associated with monoclonal gammopathy, toxic neuropathy, storage disorders, and other systemic disorders with peripheral nervous system involvement. Several central nervous system diseases, for instance, metachromatic leukodystrophy, adrenoleukodystrophy, Krabbe disease, Lafora disease, neuronal lipofuscinosis, and other lysosomal storage diseases, may clinically involve the peripheral nerve. Nerve biopsy may also be helpful in identifying sporadic cases of genetically defined neuropathy or be required in the follow-up of patients with genetically diagnosed neuropathy with unusual clinical presentations. In children, the pathologically characteristic features in nerve may establish the diagnosis of giant axonal neuropathy and neuroaxonal dystrophy.

The human sural nerve is the most widely studied nerve in health and disease and is generally recommended for biopsy. If mononeuritis multiplex clinically spares the sural nerve, another cutaneous nerve can be selected. For example, in most patients with suspected vasculitic neuropathy, a combined superficial fibular (peroneal) nerve/fibularis (peroneus) brevis muscle biopsy through a single incision on the lateral aspect of the leg is the most efficient and cost-effective procedure. For a comprehensive morphologic diagnosis, the removed nerve specimen is conventionally divided into three parts: buffered formalin-fixed for paraffin-embedded sections; buffered glutaraldehyde-fixed for epoxy resin sections, teasing fiber analysis, and electron microscopic assessment; and frozen for potential immunofluorescent study.

The routine histology of nerves demonstrate diagnostic features of vasculopathy (vasculitis, arteriolosclerosis, embolus, intravascular malignancy, etc.), amyloid deposition, sarcoidosis, inflammation, infiltration of nerve by hematologic neoplasia, leprosy, giant axon neuropathy, and polyglucosan body disease. The hematologic neoplasia invading the nerve may be distinguished from reactive processes using immunocytologic lymphocytic markers. Immunoglobulin light-chain deposition secondary to plasma cell dyscrasia can be identifiable by in situ hybridization or by immunofluorescence study for kappa and lambda light chains. If a sizable amyloid deposit is histologically detected, the tissue may be useful for amyloid typing by mass spectroscopy. In general, however, most neuropathies do not show distinctive or specific morphologic findings in paraffin sections, and usually require examination of semithin epoxy resin sections that are significantly thinner than paraffin sections, offering a better resolution of histology. Combined with observation of the teased myelinated fibers, axonopathy can be distinguished from demyelinating neuropathy. *Axonopathy* is recognized by marked depletion of nerve fibers associated with endoneurial fibrosis, with or without myelin debris or axonal regeneration. Teased fibers may exhibit prominent wallerian degeneration of myelinated fibers in an active phase of the disease. These axonopathic features can be seen in vasculitic neuropathy, toxic (iatrogenic) neuropathies, alcoholic neuropathy, amyloid neuropathy, and various neuropathies associated with metabolic disease, nutritional defect, and infectious disease. Segmental demyelination and remyelination, recognized in section as thinly myelinated fibers or onion bulb (concentric layers of Schwann cell processes) formation, are often the result of *primary demyelinating disorders* (e.g., immune-mediated and inherited). The teasing fiber analysis may further illustrate myelin changes such as excessive myelin wrinkling and folding and tomacula formation (irregular thickening of myelin within internodes), and the semiquantitative analysis of those myelin alterations may be informative in identifying the presence of pathologic demyelinating condition, as a low degree of myelin irregularity can be physiologically associated with aging.

Electron microscopic examination is useful to further delineate the pathology of axons, myelin, Schwann cells, or interstitial tissue (e.g., accumulation of neurofilaments, organelles, or protein aggregation in axon; widened, uncompacted, or irregularly folded myelin lamellae; various intracellular inclusions or deposits) and is essential for the assessment of unmyelinated fibers.

For various autoimmune polyneuropathies, many serum autoantibodies directed against peripheral nerve glycoconjugate antigens have been identified as putative targets to date, and the direct *immunofluorescent study* using nerve frozen sections could be used to demonstrate possible immunoglobulin and compliment deposits within the myelin sheath. For example, intense and widespread deposits of the C3 component of complement and immunoglobulin M (IgM) along the myelin sheath could help distinguish neuropathy associated with IgM paraproteinemia from a morphologically or clinically resembling CIDP.

In summary, in the new genetic era, conventional nerve biopsy can still offer clinically useful information, when it is wisely chosen. However, it is noted that in various neuropathies with a multifocal nature, findings in the nerve biopsy may not be representative of primary pathology taking place at other sites of the nerve, particularly at a nerve root level, and that the diagnostic usefulness of nerve biopsy must be assessed on a case-by-case basis.

SKIN BIOPSY

Skin biopsy is primarily used to evaluate cutaneous sensory and autonomic nerves, and clinically, it has been widely used as a useful diagnostic tool for acquired and hereditary small-fiber neuropathy by the quantification of *intraepidermal nerve fiber density* (IENFD). The clinical course of certain systemic autoimmune diseases including celiac disease and Sjögren syndrome may be complicated by small-fiber symptoms. Skin biopsy has also been used in detection of other neuropathies such as small-fiber–predominant polyneuropathy and distal symmetric neuropathy. Given the minimally invasive nature, it enables multiple sampling from different biopsy sites (e.g., proximal and distal sites in a same limb of the patient) for comparison or monitoring patients over the clinical course. For IENFD analysis, epidermal axons are immunohistochemically visualized in the tissue sections, commonly using the antibody against a panaxonal marker, PGP9.5 (a ubiquitin hydrolase: a major protein of nerve cells including axons and dendrites), and are counted in a given length of the epidermis. The quantitative analysis of nerve fibers requires normative values, and in patients with small-fiber neuropathy, the IENFD tends to be significantly low. Morphologic abnormalities in the epidermal axons (e.g., short length, small diameters, and complicated branching patterns) may precede the actual dropout of the epidermal axons. The *current limitation* of skin biopsy include the following: (1) Skin biopsy does not provide the specific differentiation of pathogenic mechanism/cause of the disease and (2) except in a clinical trial setting, the observation of skin biopsy rarely changes clinical management especially in diseases where the cause of neuropathy is already known.

Recent expansion of skin biopsy use includes evaluation of patients with autonomic disorders such as diabetes, chemotherapy-induced autonomic neuropathy, and autonomic dysfunctions in neurodegenerative disorders by semiquantification of the autonomic innervation to sweat glands or arrector pili muscle. However, reliability and correlation with neuropathy scores have been debatable in the published methods, and availability of normative values is limited. In research, however, skin biopsy has been used to date in a wide range of studies, including detection of changed voltage-gated sodium channel expressions in small-fiber neuropathy and assessment of dermal myelinated fibers in demyelinating disease.

In summary, skin biopsy is a unique minimally invasive biopsy technique, and the quantification of IENFD remains a reliable diagnostic tool for small-fiber neuropathy, with high diagnostic specificity and relatively good sensitivity which cannot be readily detected by nerve conduction study. Indications of skin biopsy may be increased in the future, with potential development of biomarkers to gain further insight into the functional abnormality of small fibers.

SUGGESTED READINGS

Brain Biopsy

Greenfield JG, Love S, Louis DN, et al. *Greenfield's Neuropathology*. London: Hodder Arnold; 2008.

Perry A, Brat DJ. *Practical Surgical Neuropathology: A Diagnostic Approach*. Philadelphia: Churchill Livingstone/Elsevier; 2010.

Muscle Biopsy

Banwell BL, Gomez MR, Daube JR, et al. General approaches to neuromuscular diseases. In: Engel AG, Franzini-Armstrong C, ed. *Myology*. 3rd ed. New York: McGraw-Hill; 2004:599–958.

Dubowits V, Sewry CA. The procedure of muscle biopsy. In: Dubowits V, Sewry CA, ed. *Muscle Biopy*. 3rd ed. London: Elsevier Saunders; 2007:3–20.

Ghaoui R, Clarke N, Hollingworth P, et al. Muscle disorders: the latest investigations. *Intern Med J*. 2013;43:970–978.

Tanji K, Hays AP. Muscle biopsy. In: Aminoff MJ, Daroff RB, ed. *Encyclopedia of the Neurological Sciences*. Vol 3. 2nd ed. Oxford: Academic Press; 2014:174–178.

Nerve Biopsy

Dyck PL, Dyck PJB, Engelstad J. Role of pathology study of peripheral nerve. In: Dyck PL, Thomas PK, ed. *Peripheral Neuropathy*. 4th ed. Philadelphia: Elsevier Saunders; 2005:733–754.

Mendell JR, Erdem S, Agamanolis DP. The role of peripheral nerve and skin biopsies. In: Mendell JR, ed. *Diagnosis and Management of Peripheral Nerve Disorders*. Oxford: Oxford University Press; 2001:90–125.

Vallet JM, Vital A, Magy L, et al. An update on nerve biopsy. *J Neuropathol Exp Neurol*. 2009;68(8):833–844.

Skin Biopsy

Devigili G, Tugnoli V, Penza P, et al. The diagnostic criteria for small fiber neuropathy: from symptoms to neuropathology. *Brain*. 2008;131:1912–1925.

England JD, Gronseth GS, Franklin G, et al. Evaluation of distal symmetric polyneuropathy: the role of autonomic testing, nerve biopsy, and skin biopsy. *Muscle Nerve*. 2009;39:106–115.

McArthur JC, Stocks EA, Hauer P, et al. Epidermal nerve fiber density: normative reference range and diagnostic efficiency. *Arch Neurol*. 1998;55:1513–1520.

Myers MI, Peltier AC. Use of skin biopsy for sensory and autonomic nerve assessment. *Curr Neurol Neurosci Rep*. 2013;13:323–330.

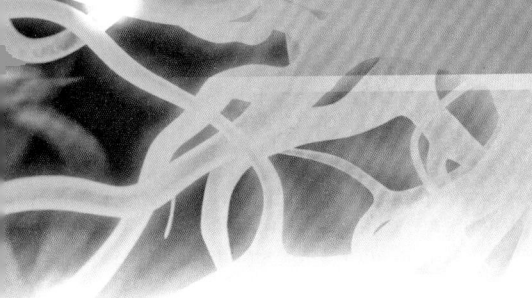

Intracranial Pressure and Neurocritical Care Monitoring 33

Charles L. Francoeur and Stephan A. Mayer

INTRODUCTION

Monitoring plays a fundamental role in the daily practice of neurocritical care. Bedside neuromonitoring supplements clinical evaluation and imaging with the underlying goal of detecting physiologic derangements before neurologic deterioration and irreversible damage occurs. This chapter introduces continuous bedside neuromonitoring modalities that are in use in the most advanced neurocritical care units around the world. Although no study has tested whether "multimodality" monitoring improves outcome, these advanced systems allow for recognition of real-time pathologic events that we were unable to identify just a few years ago and provide new insights into the complex pathophysiology of severe brain injury.

INTRACRANIAL PRESSURE MONITORING

PHYSIOLOGIC PRINCIPLES

Monro–Kellie Doctrine and Intracranial Pressure

The rigid skull is filled with incompressible content, namely brain (1,400 mL), cerebrospinal fluid (CSF) (150 mL), and blood (75 mL). In normal state, with blood outflow being equal to blood inflow, CSF absorption equals CSF production (~20 mL/h) and intracranial pressure (ICP) lies between 5 and 15 mm Hg in the supine position (8 to 20 cm H_2O).

If any one of those compartments increases in volume, as in the case of obstructive hydrocephalus, or a new mass lesion is added (a subdural hematoma for example), buffering mechanisms are called upon. The first adaptive process is egress of CSF in the spinal canal, provided there is no obstruction to flow. The second step is shifting of blood from the capacitance vessels (veins) out of the intracranial compartment. Once these buffering mechanisms are exhausted, intracranial compliance is reduced and ICP quickly rises (Fig. 33.1).

Secondary neurologic injury occurs with ICP over 20 mm Hg, and elevated ICP above this threshold after traumatic brain injury (TBI) or subarachnoid hemorrhage (SAH) correlates with increased mortality. The magnitude of ICP elevation (especially >40 mm Hg), the duration of intracranial hypertension, as well as its refractoriness to treatment are all associated with higher mortality.

Cerebral Perfusion Pressure

Arterial blood carries oxygen and glucose, which are necessary for neuronal function and survival. Cerebral perfusion pressure (CPP), defined as the difference between mean arterial pressure and ICP, is the main determinant of cerebral blood flow (CBF):

$$CPP = MAP - ICP$$

CPP values below 50 to 60 mm Hg can begin to cause cerebral ischemia, and systemic hypotension strongly correlates with mortality in TBI patients.

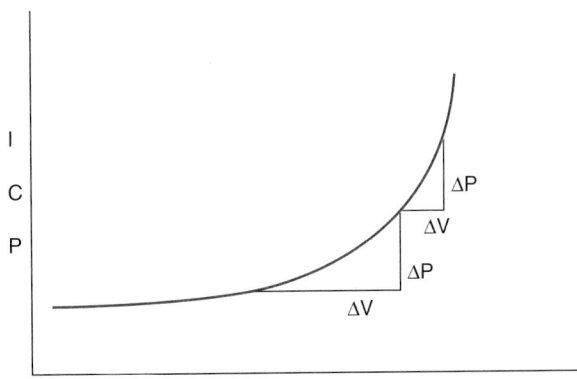

FIGURE 33.1 Compliance is the change in pressure per change in unit of volume ($\Delta P/\Delta V$). Once compensatory mechanisms are overwhelmed, compliance dramatically decreases, meaning that with a smaller increment in intracranial volume, a much more dramatic increase in pressure develops.

Intracranial Pressure Waveform

ICP is pulsatile with pressure deflections that correspond to transient increases in cerebral blood volume with systole. Bedside displays will show an ICP waveform with three components (Fig. 33.2): an initial percussion wave which occurs at the start of systole and under normal conditions in greatest amplitude (called *P1*), a secondary tidal wave then occurs which reflects brain recoil or elastance (*P2*), followed by a third tidal wave created by closure of the aortic valve at the start of diastole (*P3*). In states of reduced intracranial compliance, the ICP pulse pressure typically increases, and the amplitude of P2 exceeds that of P1 in the ICP waveform, as the "shock" of systolic inflow becomes less absorbable.

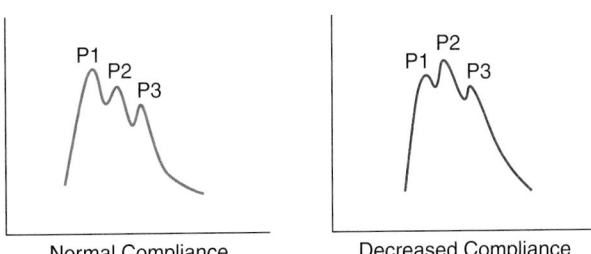

FIGURE 33.2 ICP waveform. *P1*, the percussive wave, comes from arterial transmission through the choroid plexus. *P2*, the tidal wave, reflects brain tissue elastance. As it rises, so does *P2*. When *P2* exceeds *P1*, it has an excellent sensitivity to predict incoming increase in ICP. The third and final wave (*P3*) is secondary to aortic valve closure, a corollary of the arterial dicrotic notch.

Pathologic Intracranial Pressure Elevations

In patients with raised ICP, pathologic ICP waveforms may occur. Lundberg A waves (or plateau waves) represent prolonged periods (>10 minutes) of high ICP (>20 mm Hg) (Fig. 33.3). They are caused by sustained vasodilation and abruptly occur when either CPP or intracranial compliance are low (see also Figure 107.4). Severe plateau waves preceding the onset of brain death can last for hours and reach levels as high as 50 to 100 mm Hg. Lundberg B waves are shorter duration (<10 minutes), low-amplitude elevations (<20 mm Hg) that indicate that intracranial compliance is compromised.

EXTERNAL VENTRICULAR DRAINAGE

Since the landmark study published by Lundberg in 1960, external ventricular drainage (EVD) has been the gold standard for ICP monitoring. It consists of a catheter blindly inserted into the lateral ventricle and connected via fluid-filled tubing to an external pressure transducer. Insertion is usually on the right side just anterior to the coronal suture roughly in the midpupillary line approximately 6 cm deep, although other approaches are described. The fluid-filled system relays the pulsatile waveform to a transducer, which is then converted to a digital signal. The ICP number displayed at the bedside represents the mean pressure. The hydrostatic reference point is the Foramen of Monro, which is estimated using the external acoustic meatus or the tragus.

EVD placement has the advantage of allowing therapeutic CSF drainage, making it the monitoring of choice in case of elevated ICP secondary to hydrocephalus. Depending on the indication, height of the EVD drip chamber is kept from 0 to 20 cm above the tragus, with lower levels causing a higher hourly CSF drainage rate. With

a conventional EVD system, either ICP can be monitored with the system clamped or CSF can be drained but not both at the same time. Some EVD systems are equipped with a fiberoptic pressure transducer at the tip, which allows for simultaneous pressure monitoring and CSF drainage.

The main complications of EVD placement are insertional bleeding and infection. Clinically significant (requiring intervention) bleeding rates are 1% or less, but the risk of infection (ventriculitis) ranges from 5% to 15%. As for any other invasive devices, aseptic insertion technique, limited manipulations, and quick removal are the best ways to keep infectious complications to a minimum.

Safe discontinuation of an EVD is accomplished by performing a 24-hour clamp trial. If the ICP remains below 20 mm Hg, the patient remains stable, and a follow-up CT shows no interval ventricular enlargement, the EVD can be safely removed.

INTRAPARENCHYMAL INTRACRANIAL PRESSURE MONITORS

Intraparenchymal devices are now the most commonly used method of ICP monitoring, and they are as reliable and accurate as EVD. In most systems, a fiberoptic or strain gauge pressure transducer is located at the catheter tip, which is inserted 0.5 to 1 cm into the cerebral parenchyma. Although often placed on the nondominant side, insertion should be ipsilateral to the lesion aiming for the brain parenchyma most at risk of secondary injury. The risk of insertional bleeding with a parenchymal ICP monitor is lower than that of an EVD, and the risk of infection is negligible.

INDICATIONS FOR INTRACRANIAL PRESSURE MONITORING

As a general rule, there are here indications for placement of an EVD or ICP monitor:

1. The patient is comatose (generally Glasgow Coma Scale [GCS] score ≤8).
2. Brain imaging indicates that the patient is at risk for elevated ICP due to the presence of significant intracranial mass effect.
3. Aggressive intensive care unit (ICU) care is warranted.

The Brain Trauma Foundation issued updated recommendations in 2015 regarding indications for ICP monitoring of severe TBI patients (Table 33.1). Other considerations include when clinical exam is likely to be lost for a moderate to long period of

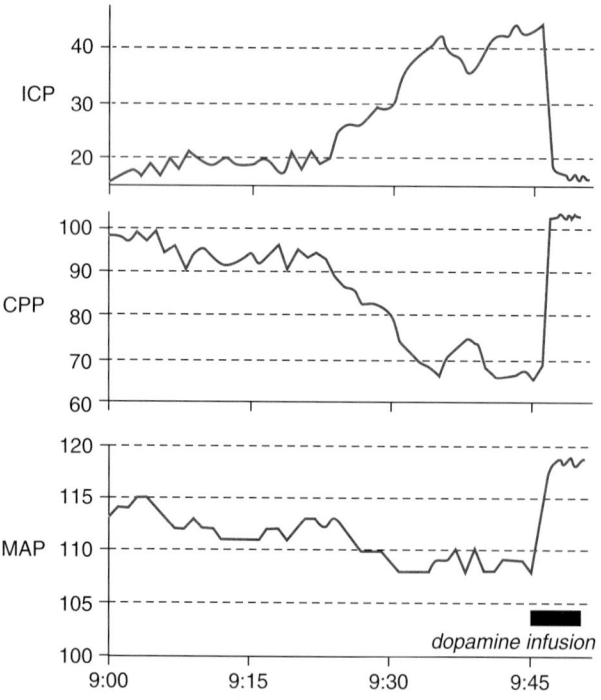

FIGURE 33.3 Lundberg A (plateau) wave, with characteristic "mirror" reduction in CPP. The plateau wave is terminated by an infusion of dopamine, which leads to an elevation in mean arterial pressure and reversal of the brain's vasodilated state. ICP, intracranial pressure; CPP, cerebral perfusion pressure; MAP, mean arterial pressure.

TABLE 33.1	Indications for Intracranial Pressure Monitoring in Traumatic Brain Injury Patients
Level of Evidence	**Indication**
Level I and II A	There is insufficient evidence to support a level I or II A recommendation for this topic.
Level II B	Management of severe TBI patients using information from ICP monitoring is recommended to reduce in-hospital and two-week post-injury mortality.

GCS, Glasgow Coma Scale; CT, computed tomography; TBI, traumatic brain injury.

From Guidelines for the Management of Severe Traumatic Brain Injury, 4th Edition; Brain Trauma Foundation, 2015.

time, especially if associated with physiologic derangement, for example, during major surgery or a difficult to ventilate acute respiratory distress syndrome (ARDS) patient. Obstructive hydrocephalus is also a clear indication for EVD insertion. Recent guidelines from the International Multidisciplinary Consensus Conference on Multimodality issued recommendations for ICP monitoring in non-TBI patients (Table 33.2). Examples given in the consensus include massive ischemic stroke, meningitis, hypoxic–ischemic injury, and hepatic fulminant failure. Any pathology complicated by elevated ICP might benefit of such monitoring when clinical exam is not trustworthy, as it allows optimization of cerebral hemodynamics through CPP manipulation, aggressive ICP treatment, as well as detection of new catastrophic events.

EFFECT OF INTRACRANIAL PRESSURE–DIRECTED THERAPY ON OUTCOME

There is a strong association between elevated ICP, especially if refractory to treatment, and poor outcome. Retrospectives studies, databases analysis, and a meta-analysis show that 20 mm Hg is a powerful threshold for identifying patients at risk for death or poor outcome after TBI and also suggest a mortality benefit with ICP monitor–based management.

Of course, a monitoring device alone cannot improve the outcome of a disease. Only a treatment protocol based on the results of monitoring can impact on survival and recovery.

In 2012, the Benchmark Evidence from South American Trials: Treatment of Intracranial Pressure (BEST TRIP) trial compared two ICP treatment protocols, one triggered by ICP values exceeding 20 mm Hg and the other triggered by clinical examination and serial imaging results alone [**Level 1**].[1] Outcome was similar with a tendency toward more efficiency in the ICP monitor arm (less hypertonic saline, less hyperventilation, less barbiturates). The external validity was problematic with poor prehospital care and even worse postdischarge management with few to no patients receiving rehabilitation. The medical community still believes ICP monitoring is an essential component of severe TBI management, although the possibility has been raised that perhaps more sophisticated triggers of therapy that take into account the state of autoregulation and intracranial compliance need to be explored. Current management algorithms for treatment of ICP are presented in Chapter 107.

TABLE 33.2	Indications for Intracranial Pressure Monitoring in Nontraumatic Brain Injury Patients	
Level of Evidence	**Indication**
Moderate	Patients at high risk or those with clinical or radiologic evidence of acute symptomatic hydrocephalus
Low	SAH, ICH, and other non-TBI conditions in patients at risk for elevated ICP based on clinical and/or imaging features
Low	All poor-grade SAH patients with consideration for multimodality monitoring
Low	Patients who undergo hemicraniectomy in the setting of cerebral edema

SAH, subarachnoid hemorrhage; ICH, intracerebral hemorrhage; TBI, traumatic brain injury; ICP, intracranial pressure.

BRAIN OXYGENATION MONITORING

PHYSIOLOGIC PRINCIPLES

The human brain, although only 2% of the total body weight, consumes 20% of total body oxygen. Approximately 90% of the energy is used by neurons mainly for synaptic activity and to preserve ionic gradients. The energy substrate is high-energy adenosine triphosphate (ATP) produced from glucose through aerobic metabolism. In the absence of continuous oxygen delivery, ATP production ceases within seconds. Osmotic gradients are lost, edema sets in, intracellular calcium rises, and early apoptotic mechanisms are triggered. With new technology, early detection and reversal of brain hypoxia is feasible in the neuro-ICU. Two invasive bedside techniques allow for brain oxygenation monitoring: *brain tissue oxygen partial pressure* ($PbtO_2$) and *jugular venous oxygen saturation* ($SjvO_2$) monitoring.

Both $SjvO_2$ and $PbtO_2$ are dependent on CBF, arterial O_2 content, and cerebral O_2 consumption ($CMRO_2$). $AVDO_2$, the arteriovenous difference in O_2 content, can be simplified as $SaO_2 - SjvO_2$ because other parameters, such as hemoglobin, remain constant during cerebral transit.

$$CMRO_2 = CBF \times AVDO_2, \text{ where } AVDO_2 \approx SaO_2 - SjvO_2$$

$PbtO_2$ is also influenced by arterial oxygen pressure (PaO_2). With other factors being constant, a PaO_2 of less than 65 mm Hg results in impaired ability to perform complex tasks, and with a PaO_2 less than 30 mm Hg, loss of consciousness ensues.

Low $PbtO_2$ values are often seen in severe neurologic injuries sometimes despite normal ICP and CPP values. Imaging cannot reliably predict brain tissue hypoxia because some episodes result from cellular distress and increased oxygen demand related to seizures, shivering, or other hypermetabolic states.

Available data strongly suggest an independent association of the burden of brain tissue hypoxia with poor outcome both in TBI and SAH patients. Taken together, these findings underlie the rationale for incorporating invasive brain oxygenation monitoring as a management option for life-threatening brain injury. Use of either $SjvO_2$ or $PbtO_2$ monitoring is recommended for patients at risk of cerebral ischemia according to the latest International Multidisciplinary Consensus Conference on Multimodality Monitoring.

JUGULAR VENOUS OXYGEN SATURATION MONITORING

This technique employs continuous oximetry in the jugular bulb to analyze oxygen content of cerebral venous drainage. The six major cranial sinuses, running between the dura mater and the cranial periosteum, end up forming the left and right internal jugular veins (IJVs). The IJV starts with the jugular bulb, a small dilation at the jugular foramen, into which the cerebral hemispheres, the cerebellum, and the brain stem drain. Venous blood from extracranial sources make up less than 5% of net blood flow in the jugular bulb. Sampling necessitates retrograde placement of a catheter in the IJV up to the bulb. The tip of the catheter, verified with a lateral or anteroposterior x-ray, should lie at the level of the mastoid bone above the lower border of C1.

Normal $SjvO_2$ values range between 55% and 75%. Low values suggest insufficient O_2 delivery to the brain to meet metabolic needs, which may reflect either high $CMRO_2$, low CBF, or both. Values under 45% are associated with cellular dysfunction. One limitation of $SjvO_2$ is that it reflects global oxygenation; regional ischemia can be missed. It has been estimated that 13% of the brain volume must be ischemic to impact on $SjvO_2$. Another technical point is that improper catheter placement will mean a greater contamination by extracranial blood reducing sensitivity to detect brain hypoxia.

$SjvO_2$ values above 75% suggest hyperemia from loss of autoregulation resulting in excessive cerebral vasodilation, which can occur after TBI or in states of diffuse inflammation or low oxygen consumption, which can occur with hypothermia, barbiturate anesthesia or extensive cerebral infarction.

BRAIN TISSUE OXYGEN PRESSURE MONITORING

The most commonly used technologies for $PbtO_2$ measurement today are based on use of a Clark electrode (Licox) and oxygen quenching methods using a microchip at the catheter tip (Raumedic). The Clark electrode has two metallic electrodes surrounded by electrolytes and a membrane. Oxygen from the interstitial space diffuses through the membrane and is reduced at the cathode, which changes the voltage difference between the two electrodes. The more oxygen, the more the voltage change measured. The oxygen quenching method uses a lanthanide polymeric matrix that luminesces at different wavelengths based on regional oxygen tension. A fiberoptic cable detects these wavelengths and transmits a continuous output signal.

The tip of the probe should be located in the white matter, where normal $PbtO_2$ levels range from 25 to 50 mm Hg (Table 33.3). A postinsertion CT scan is mandatory to confirm positioning and interpret readings because placement in hemorrhagic or infarcted tissue results in uninterpretable readings near zero. An equilibration period of 60 minutes is expected, and an oxygen challenge (5 minutes 100% fraction of inspired oxygen [FiO_2]) is performed daily to make sure of the proper monitor functioning: It should lead to a threefold $PbtO_2$ increase, provided CBF is adequate.

The volume of brain tissue sampled with this focal form of monitoring ranges from 15 to 20 mm^3. As with ICP monitoring, the area of probe insertion should be carefully considered; areas most at risk of secondary injury are the best target. An example would be in the vascular territory of the ruptured aneurysm, which is at highest risk for developing delayed cerebral ischemia.

$PbtO_2$ measured with different technologies are not interchangeable, and the most cited values come from data obtained with Clark electrode technology (see Table 33.3). Values with the oxygen quenching systems tend to run higher.

CLINICAL USE

$PbtO_2$ monitoring is an adjunct to ICP monitoring in comatose patients. A low $PbtO_2$ can help detect a new critical event, such as vasospasm after SAH or seizure. A reassuring value, on the contrary,

TABLE 33.3	Brain Tissue Oxygen Partial Pressure Thresholds (Clark Electrode Technology)
$PbtO_2$ Value (mm Hg)	**Interpretation**
>50	Hyperemia or inability to extract O_2
25–50	Normal
<20	Hypoxia
<10	Severe hypoxia

$PbtO_2$, brain tissue oxygen partial pressure.

may be an argument for permissive ICP. $PbtO_2$ change is a way to evaluate the patient's response to delayed cerebral ischemia (DCI) treatment with hemodynamic augmentation therapy. It can also be used to carefully titrate hyperventilation therapy or to detect a detrimental ventilation strategy. Some observational studies suggest that combining ICP/CPP and $PbtO_2$-based management leads to better outcomes in TBI or SAH patients.

CEREBRAL BLOOD FLOW MONITORING

PHYSIOLOGIC PRINCIPLES

Adequate CBF is critical to proper function and survival of neurons. Avoidance of hypoperfusion is essential to limit secondary injuries (Fig. 33.4). *Autoregulation* is the intrinsic capacity of the cerebral vasculature to adapt to changing pressure and maintain constant CBF by varying the caliber of its resistance vessels at the precapillary level. In healthy individuals, autoregulation allows for a stable level of brain perfusion across a wide range of blood pressures. In pathologic states such as TBI, SAH, ICH, or ischemic stroke, however, autoregulation often fails, putting the brain at high risk for ischemia or hyperemia.

The partial pressure of carbon dioxide also has a potent effect on cerebral resistance vessels. The change is not mediated directly by CO_2 but rather by hydrogen ions that determine the pH level. The effect of respiratory acidosis or alkalosis on CBF is fast (within minutes) but short-lived (<24 hours), as homeostatic mechanisms lead to a reequilibration of pH. Iatrogenic hyperventilation produced with mechanical ventilation (low PCO_2, high pH) can theoretically aggravate ischemia in the acute phase of TBI or ischemic stroke, which is why current guidelines caution against aggressive hyperventilation for ICP control in these conditions.

The partial pressure of oxygen does not affect CBF as long as it is within normal range; however, a PaO_2 below 50 mm Hg will increase CBF significantly as occurs with hypoxia-associated cerebral edema (see Chapter 107).

CONTINUOUS CEREBRAL BLOOD FLOW MONITORING TECHNIQUES

CBF monitoring is meant to detect hypoperfusion before it leads to irreversible ischemia and while it is still amenable to treatment. Two available continuous bedsides modalities are available.

Thermal Diffusion Flowmetry

Thermal diffusion flowmetry (TDF) is an invasive technique that allows quantitative continuous measurement of regional cerebral blood flow (rCBF) measured in mL/100g/min. The probe is inserted 25 mm into the brain and comprises a thermistor at the tip and a temperature sensor a few millimeters proximal. Tiny temperature fluctuations are produced by transiently heating the thermistor tip; according to the Fick principle, the resulting change in temperature at the proximal sensor is inversely related to CBF.

Real-time dynamic rCBF data have been correlated with xenon computed tomography (Xe-CT) perfusion studies and $PbtO_2$ monitoring. Studies relating rCBF to outcome are limited. Because the probe is located in the subcortical white matter, 15 mL/100g/min is a reasonable threshold for defining critical hypoperfusion. Low CBF values alone, however, do not necessarily imply active ischemia because low CBF can also be coupled to a low rate of cerebral metabolism. Concurrent $PbtO_2$ or $SjvO_2$ monitoring is helpful in differentiating low CBF states.

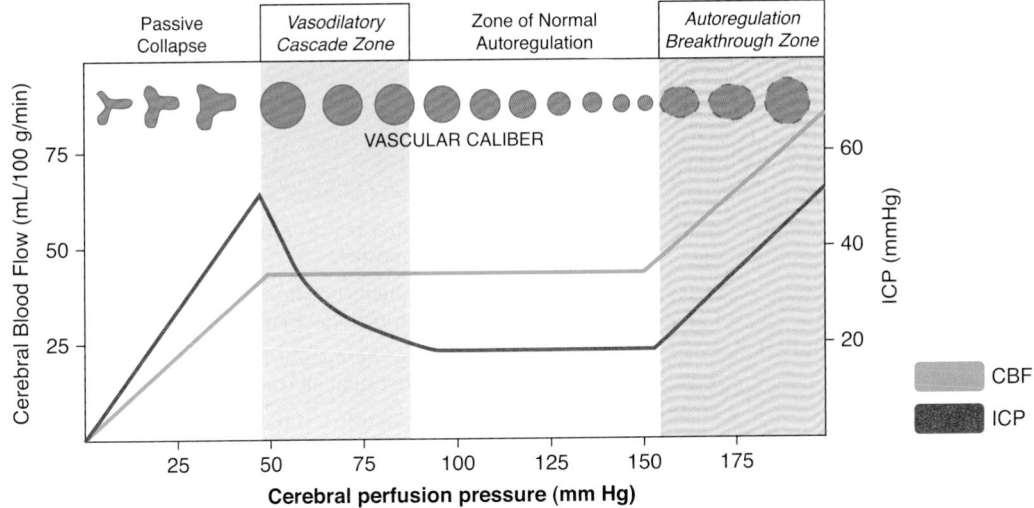

FIGURE 33.4 Autoregulation allows for a constant CBF in the face of changing CPP by varying the vessels caliber (*red line*). Over the limit of around 150 mm Hg of CPP in a healthy brain, there is endothelial injury and blood–brain barrier disruption with luxury perfusion and edema formation. Under 50 mm Hg of CPP, vasodilatation is maximal and CBF becomes directly proportional to CPP with great risks of hypoperfusion. Both hyperemia and reactive vasodilation can increase ICP when intracranial compliance is reduced (*green line*). With vasodilatory cascade physiology (*shaded blue*), vasodilation in response to low CPP drives up cerebral blood volume (CBV) ICP. With perfusion pressure breakthrough physiology (*shaded orange*), vasodilation from hydrostatic forces increases CBV and ICP. CBF, cerebral blood flow; ICP, intracranial pressure.

One of the main limitations of TDF is its focal nature; the data is highly dependent on the probe's location. Other technical limitation is the 5-minute recalibrations that occur every 30 minutes during which monitoring is unavailable. Infectious and bleeding complications are well under 1%.

Laser Doppler Flowmetry

Laser Doppler flowmetry (LDF) is an invasive technique that provides continuous qualitative assessment of local microvascular perfusion. The fiberoptic laser probe emits laser light, illuminating approximately 1 mm^3 of brain tissue, and the photoreceptor detects a portion of the light that is scattered back. The frequency shift of the light, based on the Doppler-effect paradigm, allows for evaluation of red blood cell velocities. Mathematical algorithm correlate the Doppler shift to CBF expressed as arbitrary units. Although correlation with gold standard measurements of CBF is high, LDF does not provide absolute CBF value and can only be used as a trend monitor. It is prone to many artifacts and has limited use in neurocritical care units.

CEREBRAL MICRODIALYSIS

PHYSIOLOGIC PRINCIPLES

Brain energetic function is dependent on ATP production. One molecule of glucose is metabolized to pyruvate and, in the presence of oxygen, will enter the Krebs cycle and produce a total of 38 moles of ATP. In the absence of oxygen, pyruvate will be metabolized into lactate, a much less efficient energy-producing pathway with a yield of only 2 moles of ATP. Lactate can be used as a source of energy production by neurons when glucose is unavailable. If the whole glycolysis process is accelerated, for example, in the

presence of catecholamines or fever, both pyruvate and lactate will be elevated. If hypoxemia is present, only lactate will increase, as pyruvate is anaerobically consumed with lactate as an end product. This is the logic behind the use of lactate-to-pyruvate ratio (LPR) to detect anaerobic metabolism, an important physiologic marker of ischemia (Fig. 33.5).

Another important mechanism of neuronal injury is excitotoxicity. Glutamate is the main excitatory amino acid, and levels are kept low by astrocytes responsible for converting glutamate back to glutamine. This is an energy-dependent process and metabolic failure will lead to elevated glutamate levels. This will mediate excessive intracellular calcium influx and neuronal damage.

When cellular metabolism fails, one of the final common pathways is loss of cellular integrity and membrane degradation. Release of phospholipids ensues, which are converted to free fatty acids and glycerol. This makes glycerol a marker of advanced cellular damage.

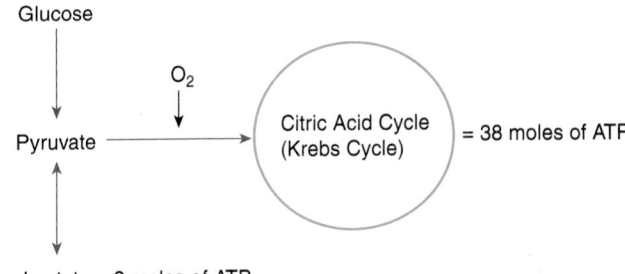

FIGURE 33.5 Efficient ATP production from glucose necessitates oxygen. Without O_2 or if the cells are unable to use it, the pathway shifts to lactate production.

MICRODIALYSIS MONITORING

Microdialysis allows for bedside monitoring of brain tissue biochemistry. The probe is a 0.6-mm double-lumen catheter with a semipermeable membrane that allows free diffusion of water and solutes down a concentration gradient. Isotonic fluid is perfused at a constant rate of 0.3 μL/min and the perfusate is collected and analyzed hourly. The probe is usually 2 cm deep, close to white matter.

Almost any molecule present in the interstitial fluid can be measured in a laboratory setting; the commercially available biomarkers for clinical use are lactate, pyruvate, glucose, glycerol, and glutamate (Table 33.4). One of the most clinically useful indices is the LPR. Values over 20 to 25 correlates with worse outcome in TBI and SAH patients, and a ratio over 40 is used to define "metabolic distress." LPR elevation can be further defined as type I or type II depending on trends in pyruvate levels. Type I LPR elevation is present when pyruvate is decreased with a marked increase in lactate; it is attributed to a lack of oxygen. In type II, pyruvate is normal or elevated indicating mitochondrial failure and a normal supply of metabolic substrates.

Low brain glucose levels (normally 1 to 2 mmol/L) are also related to outcome in SAH and TBI patients, especially when less than 0.50 mmol/L. An LPR ratio greater than 40 combined with a brain interstitial glucose level less than 0.5 mmol/L is termed *metabolic crisis* and is associated with poor outcome and a high risk of death among comatose patients. Active glucose transport across the blood–brain barrier into the central nervous system (CNS) is impaired after severe brain injury, which may further compromise brain energetic function. Low levels of brain glucose associated with metabolic crisis despite normal CBF has been reported with blood glucose levels in the normal range. For this reason, microdialysis is useful for helping to minimize the risk of critical brain tissue hypoglycemia when continuous insulin infusion is used to control stress hyperglycemia.

CLINICAL USE

A useful aspect of microdialysis monitoring is that derangements can precede impending deterioration, including elevated ICP in TBI patients or delayed neurologic injury in SAH patients. Severe derangements can be used to trigger emergent decompressive neurosurgical intervention, induction of hypothermia, or angiography to reverse ongoing ischemia.

CONTINUOUS ELECTROENCEPHALOGRAPHY

Technical advances and the era of digitization have made continuous electroencephalography (cEEG) monitoring an essential tool

TABLE 33.4 Threshold Values in Brain Interstitial Tissue of Selected Biomarkers Associated with Worse Outcome

Biomarker	Threshold Values
Glucose (mmol/L)	<0.7 or >2.6
Lactate (mmol/L)	>4
Pyruvate (μmol/L)	<70
LPR	>40
Glutamate (mmol/L)	>20

LPR, lactate-to-pyruvate ratio.

TABLE 33.5 Indications for Continuous Electroencephalography in the Intensive Care Unit according to the Neurocritical Care Society and the European Society of Intensive Care Medicine

- All patients with ABI and unexplained and persistent altered consciousness
- All patients having suffered a seizure that are not back to their functional baseline 60 min after receiving AED
- During therapeutic hypothermia and within 24 h of rewarming in all comatose patients after cardiac arrest
- All comatose ICU patients without ABI but with unexplained impairment of mental status or unexplained neurologic deficits, particularly in those with severe sepsis or renal/hepatic failure
- In comatose SAH patients, in whom neurologic examination is unreliable, to detect DCI

ABI, acute brain injury; AED, antiepileptic drug; SAH, subarachnoid hemorrhage; DCI, delayed cerebral ischemia.

in neurocritical care. Specific uses include detection of seizures, titration of therapy for status epilepticus, monitoring for DCI in SAH patients, and coma prognostication. Refer to Chapter 25 for a detailed discussion of basic electroencephalography (EEG) physiology and interpretation. Listed in the following sections are some of the recommended indications for EEG monitoring in the ICU setting (Table 33.5).

SEIZURE DETECTION

One of the main goals of cEEG is seizure detection. Ten percent to 50% of comatose patients have nonconvulsive seizures or nonconvulsive status epilepticus (NCSE) when monitored with cEEG depending on the primary diagnosis, and the vast majority are clinically undetectable (Table 33.6). Nonconvulsive seizures can directly produce depressed level of consciousness and are associated with poor outcome after all forms of acute severe brain injury.

TABLE 33.6 Yield of Continuous Electroencephalography for Detecting Nonconvulsive Seizures or Status Epilepticus in Selected Conditions

Condition	Yield
After termination of convulsive status epilepticus	48%
Lobar intracerebral hemorrhage	36%
Encephalitis or meningitis	36%
Cardiac arrest	22%
Traumatic brain injury	22%
Poor grade SAH	18%
Septic encephalopathy	16%

SAH, subarachnoid hemorrhage.

In TBI patients, nonconvulsive seizures are associated with elevated ICP, metabolic crisis, and long-term hippocampal atrophy.

Duration of monitoring is an important factor in the ability to detect seizures: A 30-minute spot EEG has approximately one-third the sensitivity of a 24-hour cEEG study. A minimum of 48 hours of cEEG monitoring is required to attain greater than 90% sensitivity for detecting nonconvulsive seizures or NCSE.

Surface cEEG in comatose patients often detects periodic or rhythmic patterns that appear to be highly epileptiform but fail to meet conventional diagnostic criteria for electrographic seizures. The term *ictal–interictal continuum* has been used to describe these patterns, which typically create vexing diagnostic and treatment dilemmas. Intracortical (or depth) EEG monitoring is an invasive form of focal electrical brain monitoring that can been used in addition to multimodality monitoring of CBF and $PbtO_2$ to determine whether these ictal–interictal patterns are truly ictal or not. Intracortical EEG has two to three times the sensitivity of surface EEG for detecting electrographic seizures in comatose patients.

TITRATION OF THERAPY FOR STATUS EPILEPTICUS

cEEG is essential for guiding therapy for refractory status epilepticus (see also Chapter 6). Delays in efficient treatment of status epilepticus leads to less therapeutic success and higher mortality. Almost 50% of patients who present with convulsive status epilepticus who fail to recover consciousness after initial therapy continue to have evidence of nonconvulsive seizures or NCSE. Failure to urgently detect and treat these seizures leads to prolonged coma and increasing refractoriness to therapy. The EEG target of continuous infusion treatments for NCSE (i.e., midazolam, propofol, ketamine, or pentobarbital) can range from simple elimination of ictal discharges to induction of burst suppression depending on the clinical scenario.

MONITORING FOR DELAYED CEREBRAL ISCHEMIA AFTER SUBARACHNOID HEMORRHAGE

EEG is very sensitive to brain physiology, and changes in the EEG pattern are a promising way to detect DCI after SAH. Reduction in alpha variability and the alpha-to-delta ratio has been found to signal the imminent onset of DCI. Most interestingly, those changes can precede the onset of clinical symptoms by 1 to 2 days.

COMA OUTCOME

Trends in the background EEG over several days of monitoring has prognostic value in coma. After cardiac arrest, improvement of the background from near isoelectric attenuation to burst suppression to a continuous pattern of diffuse slowing implies improving brain function and a more hopeful prognosis. Absence of a posterior dominant (i.e., alpha) rhythm or reactivity of the background EEG to painful stimuli are poor prognostic signs; recovery of these findings implies a better chance of recovery. Comatose patients with electrographic seizures or generalized periodic epileptiform discharges (PEDs) have a worse prognosis than those with lateralized PEDs, who in turn have a worse prognosis than those with no epileptiform activity. The presence normal sleep architecture implies an extremely good likelihood of eventual recovery of consciousness.

LIMITATIONS OF CONTINUOUS ELECTROENCEPHALOGRAPHY

The main limitations of cEEG monitoring are technical and logistic. The recordings are subject to multiple artifacts from eye movement to electrostatic artifacts. The continuous recordings constitute an incredible amount of data to be interpreted, and conclusions can vary from one reader to another. Automated systems are being developed, but cEEG remains for now a cost and labor-intensive modality requiring expert technical and medical staff.

MULTIMODALITY MONITORING DATA ACQUISITION AND ANALYSIS

Since the advent of ICP monitoring, the number of monitored physiologic parameters in neurocritical care has grown faster than our ability to integrate it to a meaningful clinical management plan without special tools that allow us to store, review, and analyze the data. In addition to the brain-specific measurements discussed in this chapter, clinicians must take into account systemic physiologic variables such as heart rate, blood pressure, temperature, and end-tidal CO_2. The amount of data to integrate can be overwhelming.

The primary goal of ICU multimodality monitoring is to act as an alarm system to detect harmful physiologic processes before they lead to irreversible damage. A secondary goal is to allow neurointensivists to optimize the physiologic environment to prevent secondary injury from occurring altogether. In order to do so, modern ICUs will be increasingly grounded within an informatics infrastructure that allows for real-time synchronized data acquisition, storage, and analysis. Raw data must be processed to differentiate signal from noise and to eliminate artifacts. Complex analysis systems are being developed to allow for automated event detection and to minimize unnecessary alarms. Information displays must be optimized to avoid information overload and assist in clinical decision making. All of this implies a greater role for informatics and artificial intelligence in neurocritical care units in the future. A stand-alone data acquisition system is commercially available at present (Moberg Research Inc., Ambler, PA), and two systems exist for data display and analysis (ICU Pilot, Mdialysis, Stockholm, Sweden; ICM+, University of Cambridge, England).

LEVEL 1 EVIDENCE

1. Chesnut RM, Temkin N, Carney N, et al. A trial of intracranial-pressure monitoring in traumatic brain injury. *N Engl J Med.* 2012;367:2471–2481.

SUGGESTED READINGS

Brain Trauma Foundation; American Association of Neurological Surgeons; Congress of Neurological Surgeons. Guidelines for the management of severe traumatic brain injury. *J Neurotrauma.* 2007;24:S1–S106.

Brain Trauma Foundation; American Association of Neurological Surgeons; Congress of Neurological Surgeons; Joint Section on Neurotrauma and Critical Care; et al. Guidelines for the management of severe traumatic brain injury. VI. Indications for intracranial pressure monitoring. *J Neurotrauma.* 2007;24:S37–S44.

Claassen J, Taccone FS, Horn P, et al. Recommendations on the use of EEG monitoring in critically ill patients: consensus statement from the neurointensive care section of the ESICM. *Intensive Care Med.* 2013;39(8):1337–1351.

de Lima Oliveira M, Kairalla AC, Fonoff ET, et al. Cerebral microdialysis in traumatic brain injury and subarachnoid hemorrhage: state of the art. *Neurocrit Care.* 2014;21(1):152–162.

Helbok R, Olson DM, Le Roux PD, et al; Participants in the International Multidisciplinary Consensus Conference on Multimodality Monitoring. Intracranial pressure and cerebral perfusion pressure monitoring in non-TBI patients: special considerations. *Neurocrit Care.* 2014;21:1–10.

Le Roux P, Levine J, Kofke A. *Monitoring in Neurocritical Care.* Philadelphia: Saunders; 2013.

Le Roux P, Menon DK, Citerio G, et al. Consensus summary statement of the international multidisciplinary consensus conference on multimodality monitoring in neurocritical care. *Neurocrit Care.* 2014;21:1–26.

Perez-Barcena J, Llompart-Pou JA, O'Phelan KH. Intracranial pressure monitoring and management of intracranial hypertension. *Crit Care Clin.* 2014; 30(4):735–750.

Sivaganesan A, Manley GT, Huang MC.. Informatics for neurocritical care: challenges and opportunities. *Neurocrit Care.* 2014;20(1):132–141.

Sutter R, Stevens RD, Kaplan PW. Continuous electroencephalographic monitoring in critically ill patients: indications, limitations, and strategies. *Crit Care Med.* 2013;41(4):1124–1132.

Genetic Testing and DNA Diagnosis 34

Jill S. Goldman and Jacinda B. Sampson

INTRODUCTION

Enormous advances in genetic technology are changing what we know about the molecular mechanisms and causes of neurologic disease. As a result, genetic testing is becoming more common and, at the same time, more complicated. The need for both clinicians and patients to understand the various types of genetic tests and the implication of genetic results is greater than ever. This chapter will review the process of genetic counseling, the genetic mechanisms that influence the appropriate choice of different types of genetic tests, and interpretation of genetic results.

THE PROCESS OF GENETIC COUNSELING

OBTAINING THE FAMILY HISTORY

A review of family history and drawing of a pedigree are the essential first steps for determining the likelihood of a neurogenetic disease. A carefully constructed pedigree can guide the differential diagnosis by indicating whether any family history exists and, if it does, the possible mode of inheritance. At least a three-generation family history should be obtained, which includes ethnicity, age of onset of symptoms, age and cause of death, diagnoses determined by genetic testing, and known history of consanguinity. Specific family history questions can help to narrow the differential diagnosis. As an example, consider the patient with ataxia: a family history that includes mental retardation or premature ovarian failure would suggest a diagnosis of fragile X–associated tremor ataxia syndrome. Similarly, for a patient with amyotrophic lateral sclerosis (ALS) and a family history of dementia, a likely cause is a hexanucleotide expansion in *C9orf72*. An Ashkenazi Jewish background in the presence of Parkinson disease could indicate a *LRRK2* or *GBA* mutation and, in the presence of dystonia, a *Tor1A* deletion (Table 34.1).

A lack of family history, however, does not rule out a genetic diagnosis. A negative family history may be due to lack of information, early death, autosomal recessive inheritance, undisclosed adoption, false paternity, or de novo mutations (mutations that first appeared in the patient).

THE GENETIC COUNSELING DISCUSSION

The process of genetic counseling and testing differs, depending on whether the patient is being seen prior to diagnostic testing of a symptomatic patient or for predictive testing of an at-risk family member. Regardless, enough time should be given to genetic counseling to provide the patient/family with the understanding of the implications of testing. Clinicians may refer to the National Society of Genetic Counselors (http://www.nsgc.org) if they wish to locate a genetic counselor in their area. In general, patients should be encouraged to attend all counseling sessions with a support person who can help them interpret the information and support them through the process.

Even when testing is being performed to assist in diagnosis, the nature and genetics of the disorder; the implications of a positive result for other family members; the benefits, risks, and limitations of testing; and an emotional impact of testing should be discussed (Table 34.2).

Pretest counseling for predictive genetic testing is an opportunity for anticipatory guidance. Patients should be asked how they would feel both over the short term and long term upon receiving a positive or negative result. They should consider how a positive or negative result would impact their life decisions including relationships, school or work choices, financial decisions, and reproductive choices. Many patients may need referrals for psychological counseling to help them work through the decision to test. In fact, the Huntington disease genetic testing protocol, which is used by many centers for predictive testing for fatal, untreatable neurogenetic conditions, advocates for a psychiatric assessment of all patients prior to predictive testing (Table 34.3).

As with counseling for diagnostic genetic testing, the benefits, risks, and limitations of testing should be covered. In general, predictive testing should not be performed without confirmation of a genetic diagnosis (and known mutation) in another family member. Without a known mutation in the family, a negative result may falsely reassure the individual, or a discovery of a variant of unknown significance will be inconclusive without other informative cases in the family.

Genetic results should be given in person, especially when they are predictive. While delivering the results, the clinician should review the meaning of the test result for the patient and family members, assess the psychological state of the patient and refer for psychological counseling as necessary, determine a plan of action, and give information about appropriate disease associations and support groups. When a positive result has been given, the clinician should check in with the patient/family following the posttest session.

GENETIC PHENOMENOLOGY

The genetics of neurologic disease is complicated by an array of genetic mechanisms. When considering a genetic etiology, all of these phenomena warrant attention and discussion with patients.

INCOMPLETE AND AGE-DEPENDENT PENETRANCE

Penetrance is the likelihood that an individual carrying a pathogenic mutation will develop the disorder caused by that gene. Incomplete penetrance can be found in many autosomal dominant conditions. Examples of incomplete penetrance include *DYT1* early-onset dystonia (about 30% of carriers develop symptoms) and *LRRK2*-related Parkinson disease (age-dependent penetrance increasing during the life span with 35% to 80% by age 75 years). Penetrance sometimes correlates with certain mutations within the

TABLE 34.1	Family History Questions for Differential Diagnosis of Neurogenetic Disorders		
Disorder	**Specific Questions:** "Has any family member ever had . . ."	**Disorder**	**Specific Questions:** "Has any family member ever had . . ."
Dementia	Dementia	**Movement disorders**	Infertility
	Memory problems or other cognitive problems		Tremor
	Language or speech problems		Seizures
	Personality or behavioral change		Writer's cramp or cramps in other muscles
	Mental illness including depression		Abnormal posture
	Any other neurologic disease such as Parkinson disease, ALS		Tics or other abnormal movements
	Movement or gait disorder		Alcoholism
	Strokes		Clumsiness
	Migraines		Immune deficiency
	Seizures		Cancer
Neuromuscular disease	Gait or walking problems		Heart problems
	Weakness		Hearing loss
	Heart problems	**Neuropathies**	Walking problems
	Developmental delay		Numbness, tingling, or pain in limbs
	Learning disabilities		Clumsiness
	Dementia or cognitive impairment		Difficulty fitting shoes
	Language or speech problems	**Neurocutaneous disorders**	Birthmarks or spots on skin
	Personality or behavioral change		Seizures
	Psychiatric illness including depression		Hearing problems
	Vision problems, including early-onset cataracts		Vision problems
	Infertility		Tumors or growths that were removed
	Diabetes		Bumps on skin
Movement disorders	Dementia or cognitive impairment		Scoliosis
	Learning disabilities or mental retardation		Mental retardation or learning disabilities
	Language or speech problems		Heart problems, arrhythmias
	Personality or behavioral change		Kidney problems
	Mental illness including depression		Stroke
	Gait or walking problems	**Epilepsy**	Seizures, spasms
	Weakness		Periods of staring or seeming vacant
	Vision problems		Headaches
			Vision problems
			Learning disabilities, autism, or autism spectrum disorders

ALS, amyotrophic lateral sclerosis.

gene but may also be influenced by other largely unknown genetic or environmental factors. In some disorders such as myoclonus-dystonia (ε-sarcoglycan or *SGCE*), the sex of the transmitting parent determines penetrance (most symptomatic individuals have inherited the mutation from their father).

PHENOTYPIC VARIABILITY

Neurogenetic disorders can have remarkable inter- and intrafamilial variability in severity of symptoms, type of symptoms, age of onset, and disease course. Consider spinal muscular atrophy (SMA), which can occur in infancy as a severe and rapidly fatal condition (SMA type 1) to onset in childhood (SMA type 2) to onset in adolescence or adulthood (SMA type 3) due to the influence of the modifier gene, *SMN2*. Hexanucleotide repeat expansions in the gene *C9orf72* can cause frontotemporal degeneration, ALS, or both. Additional phenotypes that have been reported with this gene include ataxia, parkinsonism, Alzheimer-like dementia, and psychosis. *DYT1* can cause severe childhood dystonia with contractures, adult-onset writer's cramp, or no symptoms at all.

Some genotype/phenotype correlations exist, as with the D178N mutation in *PRNP*, which, when present on the same

TABLE 34.2	Genetic Counseling Discussion Points

Disorder symptoms and course

Genetics of the disease

- Gene/genes
- Modes of inheritance
- Penetrance
- Degree of variability in symptom expression

Implication of genetic testing for family members

- Recurrence risk for children
- Risk for siblings
- Carrier status of parents

Benefits of genetic testing

- Diagnosis
- Clinical trial candidacy
- Management, if applicable
- Ability to make reproductive choices, including preimplantation genetic diagnosis
- More information for life planning
- End of uncertainty

Risks of genetic testing

- Possible insurance discrimination (life, long-term care, and disability insurances), particularly for presymptomatic individuals
- Emotional impact
  - For diagnostic testing—confirmation of risk to children
  - For predictive testing—knowledge that one will (may) develop disorder

Limitations of genetic testing

- May not discover the genetic cause
- Variants of unknown significance
- For predictive testing: inability to predict age of onset, severity, or exact symptomology, incomplete penetrance (if applicable)
- The need to identify a mutation in an affected family member prior to predictive testing

Communication of test result

- Will the genetic result be shared with family or others? If so, how and when?
- Right of relative not to know—encourage family discussion before results are in.

TABLE 34.3	Huntington Disease Protocol for Predictive Genetic Testing

1. Telephone screen: demographics, family history, motivation for testing, review of protocol, anticipatory guidance
2. Pretest counseling session with support person
3. Psychiatric assessment
4. Neurologic evaluation
5. Informed consent and blood draw
6. In person posttest result and counseling session with support person
7. Follow-up phone call

From International Huntington Association; World Federation of Neurology Research Group on Huntington's Chorea. Guidelines for the molecular genetics predictive test in Huntington's disease. *Neurology.* 1994;44(8):1533–1536.

POLYNUCLEOTIDE REPEAT EXPANSION AND ANTICIPATION

Many examples of polynucleotide repeat disorders are found in neurogenetic disease. These include Huntington disease (HD), many of the spinocerebellar ataxias (SCAs), fragile X–associated tremor ataxia syndrome (FXTAS), and the myotonic dystrophies. Age of onset for these diseases roughly correlates with the number of repeats; however, repeat size is not an accurate clinical predictor of age of onset. Expansion of the allele size occurs during gamete formation so that the repeat number can increase, and therefore, age of onset can decrease with successive generations. This phenomenon is called *anticipation*. Contractions occasionally occur. Depending on the disorder, expansion is more common when being inherited from one parent over the other. For HD, SCAs, and FXTAS, expansion usually occurs in the father. In myotonic dystrophy type 1, large expansions more often occur in the mother and can result in a congenital form of the disease. Additionally, these conditions have ranges of repeats whereby the carrier is asymptomatic or will have a very late onset but can transmit an expansion to their children. Thus, a negative family history for these disorders is not uncommon.

GENETIC HETEROGENEITY

Many neurogenetic diseases are multigenic. Presently, over 25 loci for dystonia and over 50 loci for hereditary spastic paraparesis have been reported. Testing for such conditions can be expensive and problematic. Although certain types of gene panels may be appropriate, the ordering clinician has to evaluate which genes are being tested and how. For some of the genes, such as *PARK2*, when sequencing does not reveal a mutation, duplication/deletion testing should be ordered.

PLEIOTROPY

Many genes causing neurologic conditions can cause problems in other systems as well. Examples of pleiotropy include hearing loss in fascioscapulohumeral muscular dystrophy and cataracts in myotonic dystrophy. For this reason, pointed questions about associated symptoms can help to clarify an otherwise negative family history.

PHENOCOPIES

Neurologic conditions such as Alzheimer and Parkinson diseases represent some of the most common conditions in the population.

chromosome with the polymorphism codon 129M, causes fatal familial insomnia but, when with 129V, causes Creutzfeldt–Jakob disease. Another example is dystrophinopathy, where in-frame deletions are more likely to result in the milder Becker muscular dystrophy phenotype, and out-of-frame deletions result the more severe Duchenne muscular dystrophy phenotype, but there are frequent exceptions to the reading frame rule. At other times, unknown factors seem to influence gene expression.

Finding a genetic etiology for one of these diseases in one family member does not necessitate that another family member has the mutation, especially with an older onset.

TYPES OF GENETIC TESTS

Many options now exist for genetic testing of neurologic disease. Determining the most appropriate test is essential because they do not all analyze the same types of mutations. The ordering physician may want to consult with a geneticist, genetic counselor, or laboratory director before testing to ensure that they are ordering the correct test and that the test has clinical use. The cost of testing, and whether it will be covered by insurance, is another factor to consider. The types of genetic tests and their appropriate use are described in the following section.

MICROARRAY

Microarray detects large deletions and duplications by detecting the relative signal of markers (single nucleotide polymorphisms or SNPs) spaced through the genome; loss of a copy by a deletion results in a decreased signal; a duplication results in increased signal at that point. Microarray does not detect single nucleotide point mutations nor does it define the exact breakpoints of a deletion or duplication, only that it is present between the normal and changed copy number SNP. Microarray cannot pick up balanced translocations that can be seen on karyotypes but can pick up unbalanced ones. Insertions or deletions smaller than the spacing between microarray markers can be detected using a multiple ligation polymerase assay with polymerase chain reaction (PCR) primers designed to bind to an exon in question; if both primers can bind, they are ligated and amplified by PCR. If one primer is not able to bind its target sequence due to a deletion, no signal will be detected for the primer pair for that exon.

TESTING FOR POLYNUCLEOTIDE REPEAT DISORDERS

Small repeat sizes can be directly sequenced after PCR. Larger ones may require southern blot testing, where genomic DNA is cut with restriction enzymes around the repeat motif and separated on a gel. At larger sizes, polynucleotide repeat disorders may appear to be a smear rather than a single band—this reflects a range of repeat sizes called *somatic mosaicism*.

SANGER SEQUENCING

Primers are designed bracketing the sequence of interest, allowing PCR amplification followed by sequencing, an excellent way of detecting missense mutations or small deletions or duplications falling within the bracketing primers.

NEXT-GENERATION SEQUENCING

Genomic DNA is fragmented into small pieces which are then sequenced and aligned by comparison to the reference human genome. This technique is excellent at detecting point mutations and small insertions/deletions but cannot detect larger insertions, deletions, or polynucleotide repeats and can have difficulty aligning highly homologous sequences or detecting areas with high guanine-cytosine content. It can be used for designing panels of genes using a reagent to capture those sequences of interest. It can also be used for the whole exome or the whole genome.

TESTING STRATEGY

More than one type of test may be available for a disorder, and more than one gene may cause a disorder. A panel may be useful by including other genetic disorders on the differential, avoiding serial testing. A single gene or panel may be less expensive, with a faster turnaround time, than exome or genome sequencing.

Pretest counseling is vitally important for genetic testing, as most laboratories require informed consent. Patients and families should be counseled about the cost of testing, time until results, probability of finding a mutation, and limitations of a selected test. Counseling should also include information on whether insurance will cover the costs and their financial responsibility, whether the chosen test is the end of the diagnostic odyssey or if there may be more testing in their future and how a confirmation of genetic diagnosis may affect their prognosis, their medical care, and their family. It is important to allow sufficient time for these discussions and questions.

SUGGESTED READINGS

Bennett RL. The family medical history. *Prim Care*. 2004;31(3):479–495, vii–viii.

Foo JN, Liu J, Tan EK. Next-generation sequencing diagnostics for neurological diseases/disorders: from clinical perspective. *Hum Genet*. 2013;132(7): 721–734.

International Huntington Association; World Federation of Neurology Research Group on Huntington's Chorea. Guidelines for the molecular genetics predictive test in Huntington's disease. *Neurology*. 1994;44(8):1533–1536.

Klein C. Genetics in dystonia. *Parkinsonism Relat Disord*. 2014;20(suppl 1): S137–S142.

Korf BR, Rehm HL. New approaches to molecular diagnosis. *JAMA*. 2013;309(14):1511–1521.

Singleton AB, Farrer MJ, Bonifati V. The genetics of Parkinson's disease: progress and therapeutic implications. *Mov Disord*. 2013;28(1):14–23.

SECTION IV: CEREBROVASCULAR DISEASES

Section Editor: *Stephan A. Mayer*

Acute Ischemic Stroke 35

*Charles C. Esenwa, Barry M. Czeisler,
and Stephan A. Mayer*

INTRODUCTION

Ischemic stroke is defined as an episode of neurologic dysfunction caused by vascular stenosis or occlusion leading to focal cerebral, spinal cord, or retinal infarction within a specific vascular territory. With the development of acute reperfusion therapies, streamlined algorithms for management of acute ischemic stroke (AIS) are necessary for effective treatment. Management revolves around the processes of (1) early diagnosis, including early stroke recognition and notification of emergency medical services (EMS); (2) rapid clinical and radiologic assessment; (3) early administration of intravenous (IV) thrombolytic therapy; (4) consideration for advanced reperfusion techniques; and (5) specialized post-stroke management in either a stroke unit or neurologic intensive care unit (neuro-ICU).

EPIDEMIOLOGY

An estimated 650,000 AIS occur each year in the United States alone. The most significant individual risk factors for ischemic stroke include hypertension, diabetes mellitus, cigarette smoking, poor nutrition, physical inactivity, cardiac dysrhythmia, alcohol consumption, and obesity. In-hospital mortality after AIS is comparatively rare, occurring in approximately 5% of cases, and is associated with increasing age, stroke severity, history of atrial fibrillation, previous stroke, carotid stenosis, diabetes mellitus, and history of coronary artery disease. Functional disability and morbidity from post-stroke complications occur much more commonly, affecting the majority of patients. As a result, only half of AIS patients are discharged home, whereas the remainder requires further care in skilled nursing facilities, rehabilitation, or palliative care centers.

PATHOBIOLOGY

Despite making up only 2% of total body weight, the brain consumes 20% of the body's total energy and relies on a constant supply of glucose and oxygen to maintain function and structural integrity. Each minute, nearly 1 L of blood is supplied to the brain through the carotid arteries and, to a lesser extent, the vertebrobasilar system. To ensure a constant cerebral blood flow (CBF) across a range of blood pressures and metabolic states, cerebral vessels constrict or dilate in response to changes in the concentration of carbon dioxide, oxygen, and vessel wall shear stress related to velocity of blood flow. The primary mediator of vasodilation is nitric oxide, which is released by endothelial cells and acts to relax the circumferential smooth muscle cells in the tunica media.

CEREBRAL BLOOD FLOW REDUCTION

When cerebral perfusion pressure falls below approximately 60 mm Hg due to either systemic hypotension or local arterial blockage, autoregulatory vasodilation cannot compensate leading to decreased CBF from its normal range of 50 to 60 mL/100g/min (Fig. 35.1). When CBF falls below 30 mL/100g/min, regional exchange of nutrients and oxygen fails within the neurovascular unit (endothelial cell, surrounding pericytes, basement membrane, perivascular astrocytes, and adjoining neurons) resulting in pathologic depolarization of neurons and glia and suppression of the normal electrical activity as evidenced by slowing and attenuation of the electroencephalographic background (Fig. 35.2). Sustained severe hypoperfusion, with CBF levels falling below 20 mL/100g/min, triggers a cascade of ischemic injury that can lead to irreversible neuronal necrosis and cerebral infarction.

INFARCT CORE AND PENUMBRA

With decreases in CBF below 20 mL/110g/min, assuming a normal rate of neuronal metabolism, brain tissue progresses from a state of reversible electrical dysfunction to a "penumbral" state of excitotoxic damage and programmed cell death (apoptosis). *Penumbra* is an ancient Latin term that refers to the shadow that advances across the land in advance of the complete darkness of a solar eclipse. In modern stroke therapy, penumbral tissue is brain tissue in the shadow of death.

Failure of the sodium/potassium transmembrane adenosine triphosphate (ATP) pump occurs first, causing neurons and glia

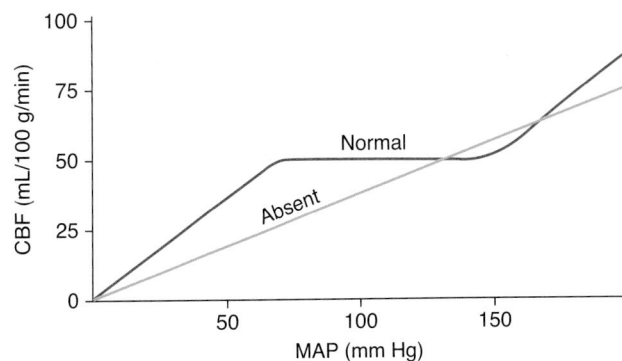

FIGURE 35.1 Cerebral autoregulation. With autoregulation intact (*red line*), CBF begins to fall below a normal range of 60 mL/100g/min and hits a critical ischemic level of approximately 20 mL/100g/min. When autoregulation is impaired or absent (*green line*), CBF can fall to critical levels when MAP is as high as 50 mm Hg. MAP, mean arterial pressure. CBF, cerebral blood flow.

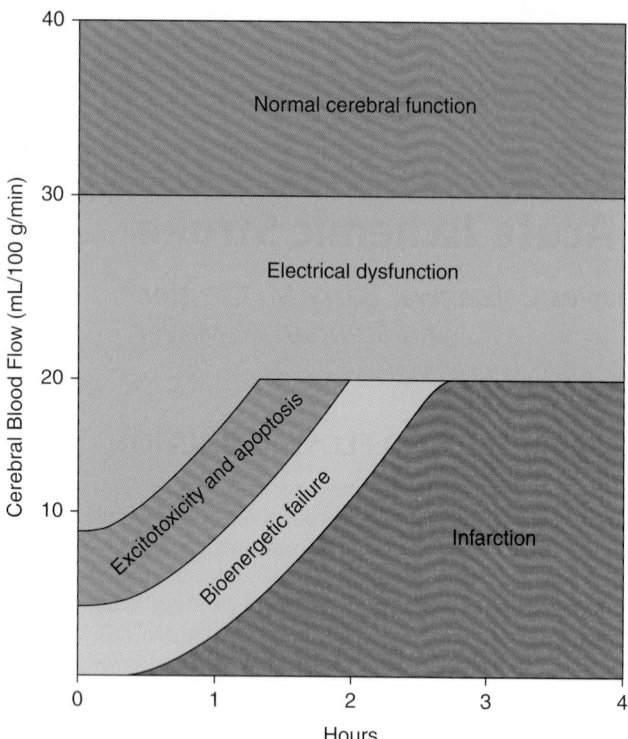

FIGURE 35.2 Progression of ischemic tissue to infarction over time as a function of CBF. A CBF level below 20 mL/100g/min is the level below which tissue progresses through a phase of reversible ischemic injury to infarction. Lower CBF produces more intense ischemia and faster progression to infarction.

to depolarize. Widespread depolarization causes uncontrolled release of excitatory neurotransmitters such as glutamate, which in turn leads to an intracellular influx of calcium and sodium. Once the phase of excitotoxicity and apoptosis has set in, a phase of bioenergetic failure occurs with ionic pump dysfunction and loss of normal transmembrane sodium and calcium gradients.

In the infarct core, where the bioenergetic failure is greatest, these massive electrolyte shifts cause water to passively follow its

osmotic gradient resulting in cellular swelling and eventual lysis. The resultant edema, termed *cytotoxic edema* as it results from intracellular swelling, manifests within minutes of the initial insult and can be detected with magnetic resonance imaging (MRI) as hyperintensity on diffusion-weighted imaging (DWI) sequences.

The core of the infarct is surrounded by an area of relative hypoperfusion, the ischemic penumbra, in which CBF is sufficient to temporarily support cell survival but insufficient to maintain normal cellular function indefinitely (Fig. 35.3). Penumbral tissue may be salvageable if adequate perfusion to the territory can be restored in a timely fashion, which is the basis for all AIS reperfusion therapies. Penumbral tissue, however, is inherently unstable and commonly will progress to completed infarction over time, making *time to reperfusion* the most important therapeutic factor for improving neurologic outcome and preventing mortality after AIS.

COMPLETED INFARCTION

It is estimated from human and experimental studies that the time from vessel occlusion to fully completed infarction in most cases ranges from 3 to 6 hours depending on the quality of collateral flow. Once the tissue becomes necrotic and infarcted, it is easily visible on both computed tomography (CT) and fluid-attenuated inversion recovery (FLAIR) MRI images. CBF is maintained at near normal levels up to the margin of a completed infarct where it rapidly drops to undetectable levels as long as the affected vessel remains occluded. Over the next several days, the infarct progressively swells. Ischemic cells that progress to frank tissue infarction release various proinflammatory cytokines and proteases that disrupt the architecture and function of the neurovascular unit, increasing permeability of the blood–brain barrier. Apoptosis is triggered through the function of various inflammatory processes, including the receptor/ligand combination of the CD95 receptor and tumor necrosis factor–related apoptosis-inducing ligand (TRAIL) and mitochondrial membrane release of cytochrome *c* oxidase, both of which lead to activation of the intrinsic programmed cell death cascade and delayed cell death. This delayed neurologic injury could in theory be prevented with neuroprotective agents, although none has proven to be of use in clinical trials.

The parenchymal inflammatory response results from upregulation of endothelial cell leukocyte adhesion receptors that cause

Dynamics of Infarct Core and Penumbra Topography Over Time

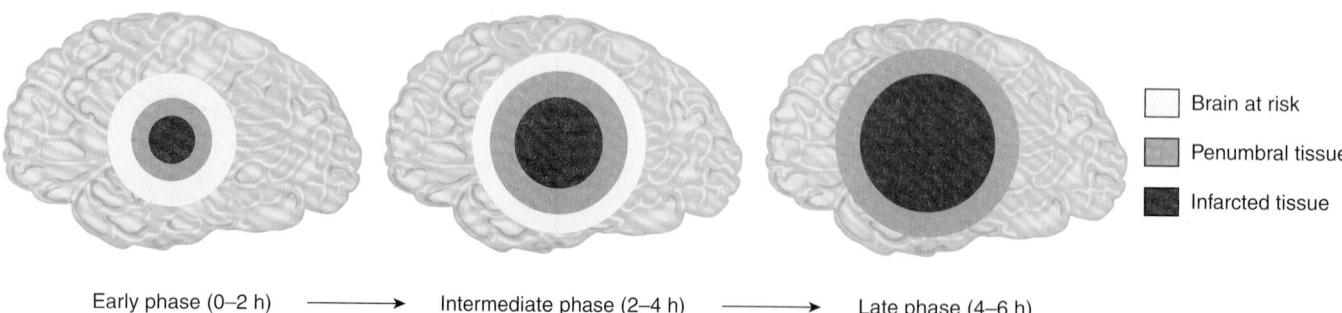

FIGURE 35.3 Dynamics of infarct core and penumbra topography over time in focal ischemia. In the earliest minutes to hours, only a portion of the total brain territory at risk is ischemic as a small core of infarct begins to form. Between 2 and 4 hours, the penumbra moves peripherally in a dynamic fashion around a progressively infarct core and collateral failure may lower CBF in some of the outermost regions of the territory at risk to ischemic levels. Beyond 4 hours, the penumbra evolves into a relatively thin rim of ischemic tissue around a large core of infarcted tissue making reperfusion less effective, as amount of salvageable tissue dwindles and the risk of hemorrhagic infarction increases.

leukocyte adhesion and transmigration into the affected tissue and is responsible for the prolonged process of tissue inflammation and remodeling after an infarct is completed, as the swelling resolves and the involved regions convert to gliotic scar tissue.

ETIOLOGY OF ISCHEMIC STROKE

The microscopic process of acute cerebral infarction is preceded by macrovascular occlusion of the territory in question. Accurate classification of AIS etiology is important to understand post-stroke prognosis, quantify the risk of recurrence, and guide strategies for secondary stroke prevention. Although imperfect, the Trial of Organon in Acute Stroke Treatment (TOAST) classification criteria is the most widely accepted ischemic stroke classification system and includes the following five subtypes: large artery atherosclerosis (15% to 40%), cardioembolic (15% to 30%), small-vessel occlusion or "lacunar" (15% to 30%), cryptogenic (up to 40%), and "other" cause (<5%) (Fig. 35.4).

LARGE-ARTERY ATHEROSCLEROSIS

Atherosclerotic plaque may develop at any point along the extracranial or intracranial arterial tree but is usually seen at vessel-branch points where turbulent flow occurs, most commonly at the common carotid bifurcation, vertebral artery origin, vertebrobasilar junction, or the origin of the middle or anterior cerebral arteries. Atherosclerotic plaque causes ischemic stroke by one of two mechanisms: hypoperfusion across a region of critical stenosis or, more commonly, plaque rupture leading to thrombus formation and subsequent distal embolization of thrombus or plaque fragments.

Artery-to-artery embolism occurs when fragments of atherosclerotic plaque or fresh thrombus formed on top of the plaque embolize to occlude a distal vessel. Plaques with a lipid-rich necrotic core and thin fibrous cap pose a risk of spontaneous rupture and activation of the coagulation cascade leading to superimposed thrombus formation. Biomechanical forces induced by turbulent blood flow along this irregular portion of vessel can act to destabilize the cholesterol plaque or dislodge a superimposed thrombus. When this happens, the thrombus may rapidly dissolve causing the clinical symptoms to be fleeting or absent, or it may persistently occlude a distal vessel leading to lasting symptoms of AIS.

Clinically, ischemia from large-artery atherosclerosis is difficult to distinguish from stroke originating from the heart (cardioembolic stroke). Favoring the former are repeated transient ischemic attacks or completed infarcts within the same vascular territory, the best example of which is repeated episodes of painless *transient monocular blindness* related to ipsilateral carotid artery atherosclerosis. This condition, known as *amaurosis fugax*, results from cholesterol embolism from the carotid plaque causing occlusion of the central retinal artery or one of its branches. When the lumen of the carotid artery is nearly occluded, transient attacks can also be due to retinal hypoperfusion, clinically manifesting as vision loss with exposure to bright light. Similarly, repeated episodes of vertigo, diplopia, hemiparesis, hemianesthesia, gait unsteadiness, and even loss of consciousness can be a sign of high-grade vertebral or basilar artery stenosis.

CARDIOEMBOLIC STROKE

Cardioembolic stroke includes all strokes caused by a cardiac source of thromboembolism. Most commonly, cardioembolism occurs from thrombus formed in the left atrial appendage of the heart in patients with atrial fibrillation, but cardioembolism can also result from a diseased native or prosthetic heart valve or ventricular wall thrombus resulting from recent myocardial infarction or severe dilated cardiomyopathy. Cardioembolic strokes can also result from neoplastic causes, such as atrial myxoma or marantic endocarditis, or infectious causes such as infectious endocarditis. Radiologically, scattered strokes at the gray–white matter junction that occur in both hemispheres, or in both the anterior and posterior circulation, are most commonly cardioembolic in origin. However, strokes that appear in association with proximal large-vessel

FIGURE 35.4 Stroke subtypes. This figure shows the TOAST classification criteria for ischemic stroke and the estimated relative distribution of stroke within each category.

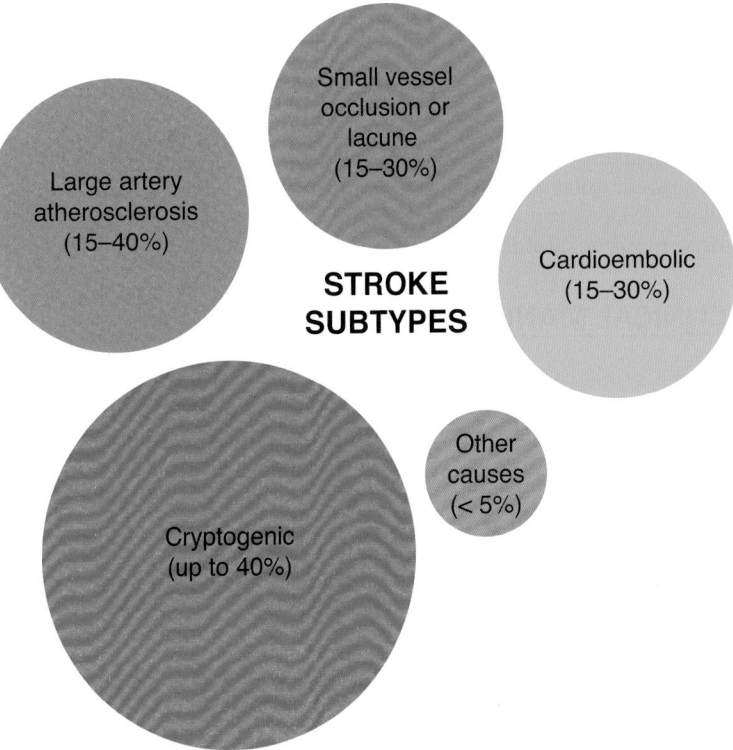

occlusions or that appear most consistent with small-vessel infarction can also be seen after cardioembolism.

SMALL-VESSEL INFARCTION

Lacunar strokes from small-vessel occlusion are clinically defined by five general subtypes: (1) pure motor hemiparesis, (2) pure sensory syndrome, (3) mixed sensorimotor syndrome, (4) ataxic hemiparesis, and (5) clumsy-hand dysarthria, although various other manifestations can occur depending on the territory of the vessel involved. These strokes result from blockage of small perforating arteries arising from the middle cerebral artery (lenticulostriate), the posterior cerebral or posterior communicating arteries (tuberothalamic, paramedian, posterior choroidal, inferolateral), and basilar artery (pontine perforators). These vessels are prone to segmental arterial wall disorganization and fibrosis, a process known as *lipohyalinosis*, and microatheroma formation. Over time, the arterial wall thickens and the vessel lumen is compromised causing a region of acute ischemia that is usually smaller than 1.5 cm in diameter. Hypertension is the greatest risk factor, although diabetes, age, and smoking may contribute as well. Lacunar infarction occurs most commonly in the basal ganglia, thalamus, internal capsule, corona radiata, and pons. Imaging helps distinguish lacunar stroke from other types of stroke by their subcortical location and relatively small size.

UNDETERMINED CAUSE OF STROKE

The etiology of up to 40% of strokes remains *cryptogenic*, or undetermined, even after extensive laboratory and radiologic investigation. However, many of these patients may in fact have undiagnosed atrial fibrillation with studies showing that 10% to 20% of "cryptogenic" stroke patients are found to have occult atrial fibrillation after prolonged cardiac monitoring. Although patent foramen ovale (PFO) and atrial septal defect are also associated with cryptogenic stroke in younger patients, PFO closure is not yet of proven efficacy for the prevention of stroke recurrence.

OTHER CAUSES OF STROKE

The "other" causes of stroke category makes up less than 5% of AIS, and it is defined by a specific disease process that is shown to have a temporal relationship or association to the stroke. In addition, diagnostic investigation should not reveal any other more-common mechanism. Examples include stroke due to hematological disorders (e.g., hypercoagulability, sickle cell anemia), infectious or inflammatory disease, intrinsic disease of the arterial wall (i.e., vasculopathy), vessel dissection, migraine-associated infarction, genetic disorders, or iatrogenic causes.

CLINICAL MANIFESTATIONS

Ischemic strokes can be defined clinically by the nature of the associated neurologic deficit with signs and symptoms fitting into defined syndromes representing specific vascular territories (Fig. 35.5). Knowledge of the following major stroke syndromes can oftentimes accurately predict the territory of infarction and specific vessel involved (Table 35.1). Exceptions arise when there is underlying preexisting CNS injury, presence of collateral circulation, or variations in the vascular or brain anatomy that can produce atypical or unexpected clinical presentations.

MIDDLE CEREBRAL ARTERY INFARCTION

Infarction of the middle cerebral artery (MCA) produces clinical syndromes that depend on the extent of the infarct and the side and level

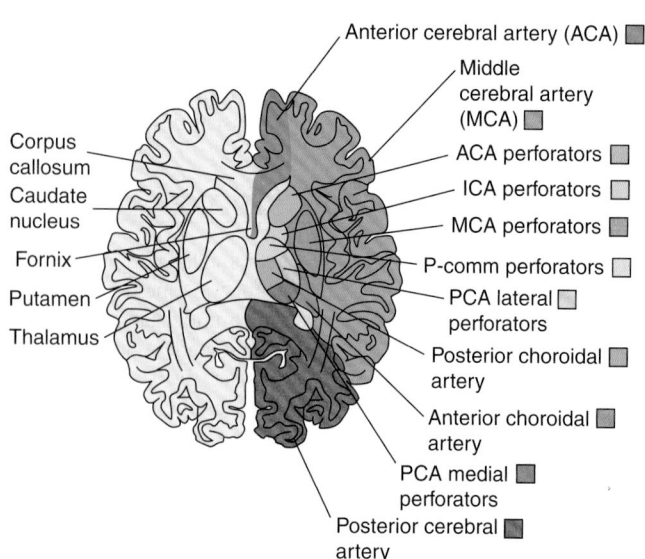

FIGURE 35.5 Cerebral vascular supply. ICA, internal carotid artery; posterior cerebral artery.

of vessel occlusion. Proximal, or branch MCA occlusion, can affect both the deep and the cortical hemispheric structures or deep structures only when there is robust collateral vascularization supplying the cortex. Isolated ischemia of the deep cerebral structures—mainly the internal capsule, basal ganglia, and corona radiata—occurs due to blockage of the lenticulostriate artery origins causing contralateral hemiparesis and possibly hemisensory loss that often is indistinguishable from a lacunar syndrome. Larger deep infarcts ("striatocapsular infarction") that affect cortical connections to the thalamus and optic radiations can cause the cortical syndromes of hemineglect, aphasia, and homonymous hemianopia or quadrantanopia.

Cortical ischemia in the MCA territory is encountered in isolation when vessel occlusion is localized to the superior or inferior MCA divisions (the number and location of these branch arteries can vary). Damage to either hemispheric cortex can cause contralateral limb weakness, contralateral sensory loss, astereognosia (inability to identify objects using touch), agraphesthesia (inability to recognize writing traced on the skin), diminished two-point discrimination, contralateral visual field deficits, and gaze deviation towards the damaged side. Ideational apraxia (inability to understand the purpose of an object or manipulate it) follows left-sided or bilateral hemispheric damage.

Syndromes resulting from a dominant (usually left) hemispheric lesion include aphasia (language dysfunction), bilateral ideomotor apraxia (inability to perform learned motor tasks), and buccolingual apraxia (inability to voluntarily direct mouth and tongue movements). The type and severity of aphasia depends on the location and size of the infarct. A superior MCA branch occlusion will affect the anterior perisylvian cortex and specifically the inferior frontal gyrus to produce Broca (expressive) aphasia that is characterized by decreased or absent word fluency and inability to write but with preserved comprehension. When aphasia is expressive or global, hemiparesis is also usually present and severe. Inferior branch MCA occlusion, affecting the posterior perisylvian cortex and specifically the superior temporal gyrus and temporoparietal junction, produces Wernicke (receptive) aphasia, which is characterized by preserved fluency and prosody but incomprehensible content, semantic and phonemic paraphasic errors, impaired comprehension, and inability to read, name, or repeat.

TABLE 35.1 Syndromes of Cerebral Infarction

Arterial Distribution	Subdivision	Syndrome
Middle cerebral	Main trunk	Variable combination of hemiplegia, hemianesthesia, gaze deviation/preference, hemianopia and global aphasia (dominant hemisphere), or profound multimodal hemineglect (nondominant hemisphere)
	Upper division	Variable combination of hemiparesis, hemianesthesia, gaze deviation, and expressive (Broca) aphasia (dominant hemisphere) or hemineglect (nondominant)
	Lower division	Variable combination of hemianopia or quadrantanopia, mild or absent hemiparesis, receptive (Wernicke) aphasia (dominant hemisphere), or hemineglect and behavior disorder (nondominant)
	Perforating branches	Contralateral hemiparesis occasionally seen in combination with ataxia or dysarthria
Internal carotid		Can be asymptomatic or cause any of the following: ipsilateral monocular blindness, transient limb shaking, or a combination of middle cerebral and anterior cerebral artery syndromes
Anterior cerebral		Variable combination of hemiparesis and sensory loss of the contralateral leg more than the arm, transcortical motor aphasia (dominant hemisphere), motor neglect (nondominant hemisphere), impaired responsiveness ("abulia"), gait apraxia, ideomotor apraxia, or tactile anomia (nondominant hemisphere)
Posterior cerebral	Main trunk	Variable combination of hemianopia or quadrantanopia, alexia, color anomia, inability to perceive parts of an objects as a whole ("simultanagnosia"), face blindness ("prosopagnosia"), amnesia, agitated delirium (especially when bilateral), or cerebral blindness (with bilateral injury)
	Perforating branches	*Thalamus*: pure sensory stroke that may leave a residual pain syndrome ("thalamic pain syndrome"), ataxia, aphasia (dominant), hemineglect (nondominant), visual field deficits, memory loss, or behavioral disturbances *Subthalamic nucleus*: hemiballism *Midbrain*: various eye movement abnormalities, depressed level of arousal, hemianesthesia, hemiparesis, hemiataxia, hemiparkinsonism

Receptive aphasia is often associated with a homonymous hemianopia or quadrantanopia, but hemiparesis can be mild or even absent. Gerstmann syndrome (left–right confusion, finger agnosia, acalculia, and agraphia) follows infarction of the dominant angular gyrus.

Infarction of the nondominant (usually right) parietal lobe produces contralateral hemispatial neglect or an inattention to sensory inputs or motor outputs to the contralateral half of the environment or body. Specific findings include visual neglect (that can involve the entire contralateral visual field or be specific to various objects), anosognosia (lack of awareness of neurologic deficits), asomatognosia (inability to recognize one's limb on the affected side), and allochiria (spatial transposition resulting in the patient attending to the ipsilateral hemispace when presented with a stimulus on the neglected contralateral side). Constructional apraxia (inability to assemble or draw objects) may result from damage to either hemisphere but is more obvious in nondominant hemispheric lesions. Although speech content or the propositional aspect of speech is preserved, a nondominant hemispheric lesion may cause deficits in the pragmatics, or sociolinguistic aspects of speech, involving tone and inferred intent.

ANTERIOR CEREBRAL ARTERY INFARCTION

Anterior cerebral artery (ACA) infarction most commonly causes contralateral leg hemiparesis and/or hemisensory loss, although many other features may also be seen. Similar to watershed infarcts, ACA territory infarcts can cause transcortical aphasia of the motor type. *Motor neglect*, or a disinclination to use the contralateral limb despite the absence of weakness, is often encountered and is due to dysfunction of the prefrontal supplementary motor cortex. Bilateral ACA infarction often results in executive dysfunction with motor inertia and *abulia* (paucity of spontaneous behaviors) or even *akinetic mutism* (awake unresponsiveness). *Gait apraxia*, although typical of bilateral lesions, can also result from unilateral strokes. *Alien hand syndrome* (unwilled motor activity) or hemiballism of the contralateral arm can result from injury to the anterior corpus callosum or medial frontal cortex. *Utilization* and *imitation behavior* are neurobehavioral syndromes that can occur with unilateral prefrontal infarcts. With utilization behavior, the patient automatically and impulsively grabs objects that appear within visual field and are within reach. Imitation behavior is automatic and involuntary imitation of the examiner's movements.

Occlusion of the recurrent artery of Heubner, a large perforating artery arising from the proximal ACA, leads to infarction of the head of the caudate, anterior internal capsule, and anterior putamen. Common clinical features include dysarthria, motor perseveration, contralateral hemiparesis, abulia, and incontinence.

INTERNAL CAROTID ARTERY INFARCTION

Acute carotid occlusion causes acute hemispheric hypoperfusion that, in the absence of a patent circle of Willis, can manifest as seizure, contralateral limb shaking, or holohemispheric infarction of both the ACA and MCA territories. Occasionally, and especially in the presence of a robust circle of Willis, occlusion of the internal carotid artery (ICA) spares the ACA and produces a clinical scenario indistinguishable from branch MCA infarction. If collateral flow across the posterior communicating artery, anterior communicating artery, or pial arteries is adequate, the occlusion can be clinically silent or only affect smaller susceptible areas. By contrast, ICA occlusion with poor collateral or a distal ICA "T occlusion" can lead to catastrophic holohemispheric infarction with sparing of only the posterior cerebral artery (PCA) territory (thalamus and medial temporal and occipital lobes).

BORDER ZONE INFARCTION

Border zone (or watershed) territories occur at the boundaries between the anterior, middle, and posterior cerebral arteries and are susceptible to ischemia in acute carotid occlusion or global hypoperfusion. *Superficial border zone infarction* occurs high along the convexity of the corona radiata between the deep and cortical structures anteriorly between the ACA and MCA territories or posteriorly between the MCA and PCA territories (Fig. 35.6). This pattern of infarction occurs when collateral flow is able to supply the majority of the involved territories but is unable to "meet" between territories. Resulting symptoms form a combination of weakness, hemisensory loss, and cortical signs. Transcortical aphasia of the expressive or receptive type with relatively preserved ability to repeat is also common. ACA–MCA watershed infarcts primarily cause arm weakness because the affected region corresponds anatomically with neurons in the motor strip that innervate the upper extremities. When bilateral, as occurs with cardiac arrest, ACA–MCA watershed infarctions result in *man-in-the-barrel syndrome* characterized by proximal bilateral arm and leg weakness with relative preservation of facial and distal extremity strength.

Internal border zone infarction (see Fig. 35.6) can occur with total ICA occlusion or with large MCA branch occlusions. Noncollateralized deep penetrating arteries that descend from the cortex to the lateral wall of the ventricles represent the most hemodynamically vulnerable "distal field" in this scenario. The result is a pattern of multiple small deep infarcts involving the deep white matter of the corona radiata and centrum semiovale.

ANTERIOR CHOROIDAL ARTERY INFARCTION

The anterior choroidal artery is the last branch of the ICA originating just proximal to the ACA–MCA bifurcation. It traverses posteriorly to supply a number of structures, including the internal capsule, lateral thalamus, and the lateral geniculate body or optic radiations. Thus, occlusion of the anterior choroidal artery results in the classic syndrome of contralateral hemiparesis, hemianesthesia, and homonymous hemianopia. Occasionally, cortical symptoms such as aphasia or hemineglect can result from disruption of thalamocortical white matter tracts.

POSTERIOR CEREBRAL ARTERY

Occlusion of the PCA will cause infarction of the occipital and inferior temporal lobes. The usual presentation is sudden onset of a contralateral homonymous hemianopia. Bilateral occipital lobe lesions can cause Anton syndrome (cortical blindness unrecognized by the patient). Charles Bonnet syndrome, or release visual hallucinations, can also be seen in cortical blindness from bilateral occipital lobe injury. Balint syndrome is seen in bilateral parietooccipital junction infarcts and is characterized by simultanagnosia (inability to perceive parts of an object as a whole), oculomotor apraxia (incoordination of gaze), and optic ataxia (poor hand coordination using visual guidance). Hemineglect, although uncommon with occipital lesions, can be seen when the injury extends to the parietal lobe. Left PCA infarcts that involve either the deep white matter of the temporoparietal junction or the splenium of the corpus callosum may cause alexia without agraphia, a type of disconnection syndrome between the nondominant occipital cortex and the language processing area in the dominant parietotemporal cortex. Inferomedial temporal lobe infarction may cause agitated delirium or global amnesia.

Proximal PCA infarction affecting the thalamic perforating arteries will lead to infarction of the thalamus or midbrain. If the ventral posterior nucleus of the thalamus is preferentially affected, the patient will have contralateral hemianesthesia. Hyperpathia may subsequently develop in a condition called the *Dejerine–Roussy* or *thalamic pain syndrome*. As the thalamus serves as a relay to the cortex, thalamic infarction can also cause a variety of atypical symptoms such as ataxia, aphasia (dominant), hemineglect (nondominant), visual field deficits, memory loss, or behavioral disturbances.

Lethargy or coma can result if the reticular activating system in the midbrain or thalami is affected and will often be accompanied by a combination of oculomotor abnormalities. Alterations in consciousness are especially common in the presence of an anatomically variant artery, termed the *artery of Percheron*, which supplies the bilateral medial thalami and rostral midbrain from a single vessel originating on a unilateral PCA. Midbrain lesions, when posterior, cause Parinaud syndrome characterized by sustained conjugate downgaze, upgaze paralysis, convergence or retraction nystagmus, lid retraction or Collier sign, and pupillary light-near dissociation.

VERTEBROBASILAR TERRITORY INFARCTION

The basilar artery is the main conduit to supply the PCA arteries and basilar thrombosis can manifest with a combination of medullary, pontine, midbrain, and posterior cortical signs. Basilar throm-

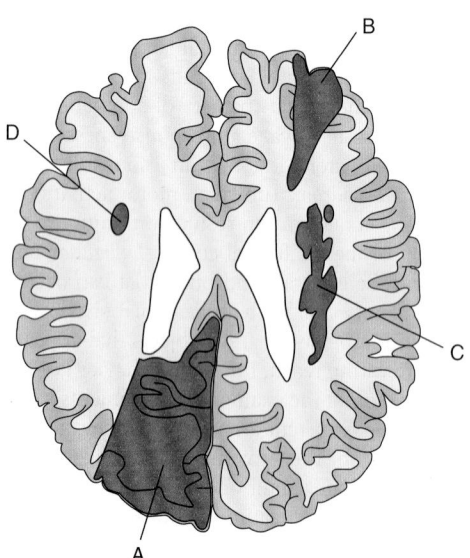

FIGURE 35.6 Schematic representation of different topographic patterns of cerebral infarction. (*A*) Territorial infarction (from PCA occlusion). (*B*) Watershed border-zone infarction (between the territories of the ACA and the MCA). (*C*) Internal border zone infarction (deep MCA territory). (*D*) Lacunar infarction (lenticulostriate-penetrating artery occlusion). (Adapted from Marshall R, Mayer S. *On Call Neurology*. 3rd ed. Philadelphia: Saunders; 2007.)

bosis leading to infarction of the anterior pons bilaterally causes "locked-in" syndrome: complete bilateral face, arm, and leg paralysis with isolated preservation of vertical eye movements and preservation of consciousness (see Chapter 18). Infarcts resulting from small-vessel thrombosis of the pontine perforating arteries cause a combination of cranial nerve dysfunction, long tract signs including weakness, reflexive posturing or hyperreflexia, sensory loss, and/or cerebellar findings. Small anterior pontine strokes can also produce lacunar syndromes without cranial nerve deficits that are clinically indistinguishable from anterior circulation lacunes. Oculomotor or gaze palsies, including internuclear ophthalmoplegia and skew deviation, or nystagmus, are also common. "Top of the basilar" syndrome refers to occlusion of bilateral distal basilar and proximal PCA thalamic and midbrain penetrating arteries from embolism. The result is a pattern of bilateral small-vessel infarcts involving the midbrain and thalami with asymmetric vertical gaze abnormalities and skew deviation, changes in level of consciousness, and variable bilateral motor and sensory deficits.

Infarction of the lateral medulla occurs when the posterior inferior cerebellar artery or a branch of the vertebral artery is af-fected. What results is a lateral medullary or *Wallenberg syndrome*, which is characterized by vertigo, ipsilateral ataxia, loss of pain and temperature sense in the ipsilateral face and the contralateral arm and leg, dysphagia, and ipsilateral oculosympathetic syndrome (Horner syndrome). Other brain stem infarct syndromes are described in Table 35.2.

DIAGNOSIS

SYMPTOM RECOGNITION

Delay in prehospital recognition of stroke symptoms is the greatest barrier to prompt treatment and a major factor in explaining why only 6% of patients with AIS receive fibrinolytic therapy. Despite the established benefit of timely assessment and the potential for neurologic recovery with early treatment, only approximately 20% of patients present within 2 hours of symptom onset and approximately 25% within the therapeutic window of 4.5 hours. Limited insight and lack of community-level awareness to the time-sensitive nature of treatment are partly to blame, with studies suggesting that only 5%

TABLE 35.2 Syndromes of Brain Stem Infarction

Syndrome		Artery Affected	Structure Involved	Manifestations
Medial syndromes	Medulla	Paramedian branches of basilar artery	Emerging fibers of 12th nerve	Ipsilateral paralysis of tongue
			Corticospinal tract	Contralateral limb paresis/paralysis
			Medial lemniscus	Contralateral hemianesthesia
	Inferior pons	Paramedian branches of basilar artery	Pontine gaze center, near or in nucleus of sixth nerve	Paralysis of gaze to side of lesion
			Emerging fibers of sixth nerve	Ipsilateral abduction paralysis
			Corticospinal tract	Contralateral limb paresis/paralysis
	Superior pons	Paramedian branches of basilar artery	Medial longitudinal fasciculus	Internuclear ophthalmoplegia
Lateral syndromes	Medulla	Posterior inferior cerebellar artery or vertebral artery branches	Emerging fibers of ninth and 10th nerves	Dysphagia, hoarseness, ipsilateral paralysis of vocal cord; ipsilateral loss of pharyngeal reflex
			Vestibular nuclei	Vertigo, nystagmus
			Descending tract and nucleus of fifth nerve	Ipsilateral facial analgesia
			Solitary nucleus and tract	Taste loss on ipsilateral half of tongue posteriorly
			Spinothalamic tract	Contralateral sensory loss
			Hypothalamospinal tract	Ipsilateral oculosympathetic dysfunction ("Horner syndrome")
	Inferior pons	Anterior inferior cerebellar artery	Emerging fibers of seventh nerve	Ipsilateral facial paralysis
			Solitary nucleus and tract	Taste loss on ipsilateral half of tongue anteriorly
			Cochlear nuclei	Hearing loss, tinnitus
			Spinothalamic tract	Contralateral sensory loss
	Mid-pons	Anterior inferior cerebellar artery and circumferential branches of basilar	Motor nucleus of fifth nerve	Ipsilateral jaw weakness
			Emerging sensory fibers of fifth nerve	Ipsilateral facial numbness

Modified from Rowland LP. Clinical syndromes of the spinal cord and brain stem. In: Kandel ER, Schwartz JH, Jessell T, eds. *Principles of Neural Science.* 3rd ed. New York: Elsevier; 1991:711–730.

TABLE 35.3 Prehospital Stroke Scales

Cincinnati Prehospital Stroke Scale/FAST	Yes	No
Facial droop?	☐	☐
Arm drift?	☐	☐
Speech abnormal?	☐	☐

POSITIVE SCREEN if any questions are positive

Los Angeles Motor Scale	Points		
	0	1	2
Facial strength	Normal	Droop	—
Arms outstretched	Normal	Drifts down	Falls rapidly
Grip strength	Normal	Weak grip	No grip

POSITIVE SCREEN for stroke with high likelihood of large vessel occlusion for a score of 2 or more.

of people in an urban population have knowledge of at least three stroke symptoms. The mnemonic FAST (face, arm, speech, time to call 911) has been disseminated using multiple community education efforts, in efforts to raise awareness about stroke symptoms and the urgent nature of seeking medical care. Public education efforts such as this play a critical role in increasing the proportion of patients who present within the therapeutic time window.

Once EMS is activated, first responders must quickly and accurately characterize the symptoms of a stroke. Prehospital stroke scales should be used to assist in the screening and rapid triage process [**Level 1**].[1] The most widely used are the Cincinnati Prehospital Stroke Scale, the Los Angeles Prehospital Stroke Screen, and the Face Arm Speech Test (FAST) (Table 35.3). Rapid stroke assessment should be followed by activation of the acute stroke chain of care beginning with prehospital notification, which has been shown to increase the use of intravenous tissue plasminogen activator (IV tPA) and decrease the time from symptom onset to treatment [**Level 1**].[1]

INITIAL HOSPITAL EVALUATION

The American Heart Association and American Stroke Association (AHA/ASA) guidelines recommend that all patients suspected of having an acute stroke be brought to stroke-certified centers to ensure a standardized level of care [**Level 1**].[1] On arrival to the emergency department, the patient must undergo rapid clinical and diagnostic evaluation in preparation for potential treatment. Initial history should be directed at defining the deficit and specific time of onset or last known time when the patient was seen normal. The clinician must then perform a rapid neurologic assessment using the National Institutes of Health Stroke Scale (NIHSS). The NIHSS (see Table 15.3) ranges from 0 to 42 with higher scores signifying greater neurologic deficit.

IMAGING

Computed Tomography

Noncontrast head computed tomography (NCHCT) is widely available, rapid, and extremely sensitive for detecting acute blood products (see also Chapter 20). Its value in distinguishing cere-

bral hemorrhage from presumed ischemia has made obtaining a NCHCT a vital and necessary step in the assessment of acute stroke. Early CT findings in AIS include loss of gray–white differentiation (seen first in the insular cortex), obscuration of gray matter in the basal ganglia, and acute thrombus visualized in the proximal MCA, also known as the *dense MCA* sign (Fig. 35.7A). However, CT findings in AIS are not reliably seen until after 6 hours from stroke onset, thus normal imaging in the setting of a clinical stroke syndrome suggests an ischemic etiology. The Alberta Stroke Programme Early CT Score (ASPECTS) can be helpful in quantifying signs of acute ischemia on NCHCT (see Fig. 15.3). The ASPECTS and NIHSS scores can help predict functional outcome and response to treatment.

Magnetic Resonance Imaging

Although CT is the most sensitive imaging modality for acute hemorrhagic stroke, MRI, and specifically DWI, is the most sensitive modality for detecting ischemic stroke within the first 6 hours of onset (Fig. 35.7D). Despite its superior sensitivity, however (see also Chapter 21), the use of MRI in the acute management of AIS is limited due to its relative unavailability in most emergency departments and the prolonged time necessary for image acquisition. Despite its superior sensitivity, small infarcts and those in the posterior circulation may not be seen on DWI, especially in the early hours after infarction. Although these issues limit its utility in the acute setting, obtaining an MRI after treatment decisions are made can be helpful in confirming the presence of ischemic stroke, identifying the specific stroke location, and helping to diagnose the stroke etiology.

Vascular Imaging

Computed tomography angiography (CTA) allows for acute evaluation of the cervical and cerebral vessels by opacifying the vasculature with IV contrast delineating any irregularities, stenoses, or occlusions (Fig. 35.7B). Magnetic resonance angiography (MRA) detects flow within blood vessels allowing for visualization of vasculature and any "flow voids" that occur within them but, similar to MRI, is limited by the time necessary for image acquisition. Special MRI techniques such as vessel wall imaging and arterial spin labeling can show details of the vessel wall and flow dynamics within the vessel, but their role in the clinical setting remains investigational. Ultrasound evaluation of the carotid arteries or the proximal intracranial vasculature can provide information about the direction of blood flow and define sites of arterial stenosis or occlusion. Although vessel imaging is not recommended for all cases of AIS, its use in select patients may help in planning for interventional therapies.

Perfusion Imaging

A computed tomography perfusion (CTP) study can be performed along with CTA measuring the time to arrival and volume of contrast arriving in various areas of the brain by repeatedly scanning during a timed IV contrast injection (Fig. 35.7C). The opposite hemisphere is used for comparison, and images are created to show relative amounts of CBF, cerebral blood volume (CBV), and mean transit time (MTT) of contrast. Perfusion imaging may help differentiate the penumbra from core infarct. The penumbra retains cerebrovascular autoregulation and experiences vasodilation and recruitment of collateral vessels in response to relative hypoperfusion. It is defined by a low CBF and prolonged MTT with a compensatory increase in CBV caused

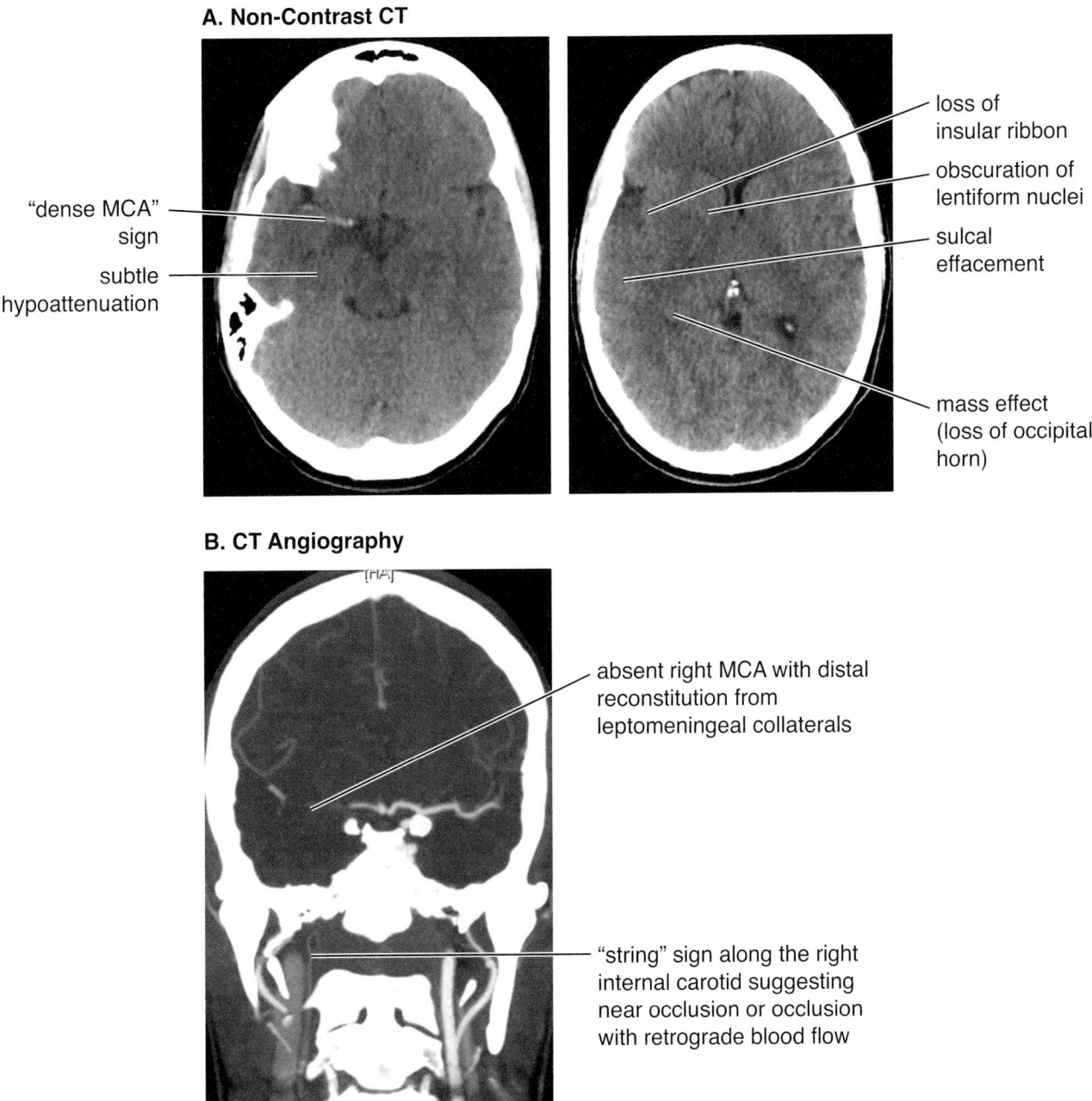

A. Non-Contrast CT

"dense MCA" sign

subtle hypoattenuation

loss of insular ribbon

obscuration of lentiform nuclei

sulcal effacement

mass effect (loss of occipital horn)

B. CT Angiography

absent right MCA with distal reconstitution from leptomeningeal collaterals

"string" sign along the right internal carotid suggesting near occlusion or occlusion with retrograde blood flow

FIGURE 35.7 Acute ischemic stroke imaging. This figure shows the stepwise imaging approach for a patient presenting with acute onset of left-sided weakness and right gaze deviation. The initial NCHCT **(A)** shows early infarct signs in the right hemisphere. CTA **(B)** shows an absent right ICA and right MCA. *(continued)*

by vasodilation. The ischemic core, in contrast, loses its physiologic ability to autoregulate and therefore has blood shunted away from it creating a relative deficit in CBV. If the penumbra further destabilizes, autoregulation fails and the area with low CBV expands.

Magnetic resonance perfusion (MRP) imaging is similar to CTP and can distinguish infarcted from at-risk tissue by comparing perfusion imaging to DWI sequences, but it is more time consuming than CTP. Despite their theoretical value, studies using perfusion techniques to guide the need and timing for reperfusion therapies have not shown an improvement in clinical outcomes. The use of perfusion imaging is therefore not routinely recommended,

although it can be employed to answer specific clinical questions on a case-by-case basis.

ACUTE TREATMENT

Estimations based on mathematical modeling suggest that 1.9 million neurons and 14 billion synapses are lost for every minute of ischemia in a large-vessel AIS. Stroke expansion is usually complete within 4 to 6 hours of onset, at which point all potentially salvageable areas of penumbra are irreversibly infarcted. Emergency treatment with IV tissue-plasminogen activator (tPA) is

C. CT Perfusion

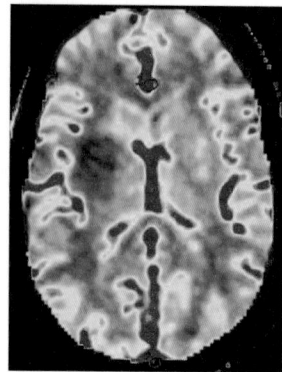 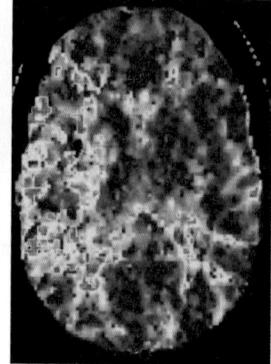 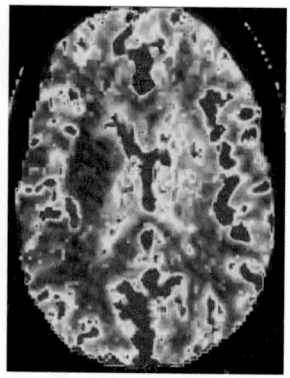

Cerebral blood volume (CBV) – decreased in the deep right MCA territory

Mean transit time (MTT): prolonged in the entire right MCA territory

Cerebral blood flow (CBF): Decreased in a large portion of the right MCA territory

FIGURE 35.7 *(continued)* CT perfusion **(C)** shows an area of core infarct defined by a low CBV, prolonged MTT, and decreased CBF surrounded by a widespread area of tissue at risk defined by relatively stable CBV, prolonged MTT, and decreased CBF. On MRI, the DWI sequence in the acute setting and the FLAIR sequence 1 year later **(D)** confirmed that only the presumed core area had infarcted and not the hemisphere as a whole, probably due to good leptomeningeal collaterals. CT, computed tomography; MRI, magnetic resonance imaging.

D. MRI

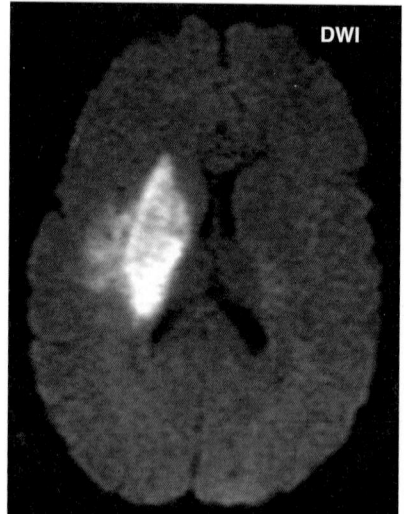 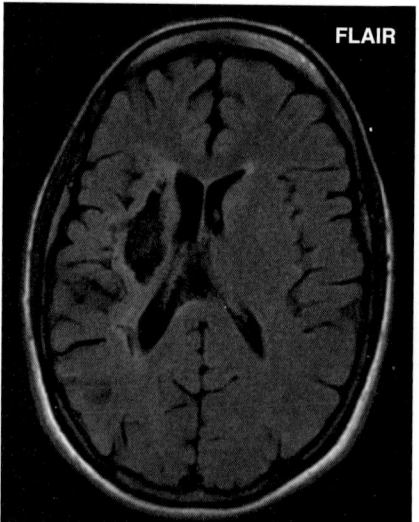

Diffusion weighted imaging (DWI): hyperintensity in the deep right MCA territory signifying acute infarct

Fluid attenuated inversion recovery (FLAIR): one year follow up showing chronic infarct in the deep structures with relative preservation of the cortex

the fundamental therapy used to achieve reperfusion for AIS. Benefit directly correlates with time to treatment with a linear relationship between shorter onset-to-needle time and improved 3-month functional outcome. Benefit levels off after 4.5 hours and soon after the risk of reperfusion causing hemorrhagic transformation exceeds the ability to rescue penumbral tissue at risk. Rapid onset-to-treatment time will always remain the most important factor in the treatment of AIS.

INTRAVENOUS THROMBOLYSIS

The only currently U.S. Food and Drug Administration (FDA)–approved medical treatment for AIS is IV tPA. As onset-to-treatment time increases, the effectiveness of tPA diminishes and the risk of hemorrhage increases. Optimal treatment involves the administration of tPA as quickly as possible up to 3 hours from symptom onset for most patients and 4.5 hours in a select group of patients [**Level 1**].[2,3] The original 3-hour time window is largely based

on the National Institute of Neurological Disorders and Stroke (NINDS) trial from 1995, which showed that administration of IV tPA within 3 hours of symptom onset led to an improved clinical outcome at 3 months with a 13% absolute increase in good functional recovery compared to placebo despite an approximate 6% absolute risk increase in symptomatic intracerebral hemorrhage (ICH) with IV tPA. This translates to a number needed to treat of eight patients to achieve good recovery in one patient who would have otherwise had a poor outcome.

A pooled analysis of the Alteplase Thrombolysis for Acute Noninterventional Therapy in Ischemic Stroke (ATLANTIS), European Cooperative Acute Stroke Study (ECASS) I and II, and NINDS trials showed that administration of tPA up to 4.5 hours after symptom onset appeared beneficial, which prompted the ECASS III trial. ECASS III excluded patients older than age 80 years, those with a baseline NIHSS score higher than 25, those with a history of diabetes and prior ischemic stroke, and those on anticoagulation regardless of international normalized ratio (INR) values. A benefit was seen for tPA administration within the 3- to 4.5-hour range, albeit milder than that seen in the original NINDS trial. The AHA/ASA therefore recommends the use of IV tPA up to 4.5 hours after ischemic stroke symptom onset in patients younger than 80 years of age who are not on anticoagulation and do not have both comorbid diabetes and history of stroke [**Level 1**].[3] A practical protocol and checklist for IV tPA use is provided in Chapter 15.

Contraindications to Intravenous Thrombolysis

Current contraindications for IV tPA are based on the inclusion criteria used in the original NINDS trial. However, these rigorous contraindications may not necessarily define the full population of patients who might benefit from tPA. Table 15.5 shows the relative strength of various contraindications to tPA therapy based on published experience since the original NINDS trials.

WEAK TO MODERATE RELATIVE CONTRAINDICATIONS

Minor symptoms, a rapidly resolving deficit, seizures, and hypo- or hyperglycemia at presentation are examples of relative contraindications. Despite these initial relative exclusions, most patients with minor or resolving deficits should in fact be considered for IV tPA treatment, as a subanalysis of the NINDS trial confirmed the benefit of tPA administration in this population. Seizure at time of presentation is also considered by most experts to be a relative rather than an absolute contraindication. The main concern here is treating a stroke mimic, although data suggests that the rate of hemorrhagic complications in stroke mimics treated with IV tPA is very low. Onset seizures are rare in AIS but do not increase the risk of hemorrhagic conversion per se. Blood glucose should be measured and corrected in all patients because hypo- or hyperglycemia can lead to neurologic deficits mimicking acute stroke, and hyperglycemia has been associated with an increased risk of hemorrhagic conversion after thrombolysis. Nonetheless, it may be reasonable to give IV tPA if the index of suspicion for a true stroke is high and glucose levels can be readily normalized during and after the treatment period.

Blood pressure higher than 185/110 mm Hg is a moderate relative contraindication to treatment. In most cases, blood pressure can be quickly controlled with a continuous IV infusion of nicardipine or clevidipine (see Table 38.3 for dosing) and IV tPA given once blood pressure is successfully lowered.

ABSOLUTE TO STRONG RELATIVE CONTRAINDICATIONS

The presence of cerebral hemorrhage on initial head CT, early infarction already involving greater than one-third of the MCA territory, or treatment beyond the 4.5-hour time window are absolute contraindications to IV thrombolysis (see Table 15.5). A weak level of anticoagulation with warfarin (INR 1.7–2.0) or stable mild thrombocytopenia (platelet count 50,000 to 100,000) are strong relative contraindications to IV tPA; in the proper circumstances, it might be reasonable to treat as long as a relative increment in hemorrhagic conversion is recognized and accepted. The use of novel anticoagulants, including dabigatran, rivaroxaban, and apixaban are more problematic because they do not produce reliable changes in prothrombin time (PT)/INR or partial thromboplastin time (PTT), and other assays are not readily available. The current consensus is to avoid using IV tPA and seek intra-arterial reperfusion strategies in patients who have taken a novel oral anticoagulant within 48 hours of presentation. It is important to note that tPA should never be delayed while waiting for a platelet count or INR in a patient with no suspicion of having a coagulation disturbance by history. Studies have shown that the

risk of encountering clinically significant thrombocytopenia or coagulopathy in tPA candidates in whom the history did not suggest a possible abnormality was only 0.2% to 0.3%.

As many as one-third of dissection patients can present with acute neurologic symptoms from ischemic stroke. Suspected aortic dissection is an absolute contraindication to thrombolysis, as IV tPA can worsen the dissection and prove fatal. Patients with characteristic chest or back pain should therefore be screened with urgent CTA of the chest to rule out aortic dissection prior to further consideration of thrombolysis.

Complications of Thrombolysis

HEMORRHAGIC CONVERSION

Hemorrhagic conversion of the infarcted tissue bed is a known complication after stroke, and risk is significantly increased in patients treated with IV tPA. Hemorrhagic conversion is classified as hemorrhagic infarction or parenchymal hematoma (PH) depending on radiologic characteristics. Hemorrhagic infarction is defined by hemorrhagic petechiae within the stroke bed and is not associated with a worsened outcome, whereas PH is defined by blood occupying either less than 30% of the stroke bed with mild space-occupying effect (PH1) or over 30% with significant mass effect (PH2). Only PH2 is as associated with an increase in mortality. Hemorrhagic conversion usually manifests with headache, nausea, vomiting, worsened neurologic deficit, and/or altered level of consciousness. Risk factors for hemorrhagic conversion after thrombolysis include advanced age, increased onset-to-treatment times, higher NIHSS (stroke severity), hyperglycemia, and hypertension before or after tPA administration. The SEDAN score (Table 35.4) is a well-validated tool that can help to identify IV tPA candidates with greater than the normal 3% risk of symptomatic hemorrhagic conversion.

ANGIOEDEMA

tPA-associated angioedema and/or anaphylaxis occurs in 1% to 5% of cases usually beginning 30 to 120 minutes after tPA infusion. Patients taking angiotensin-converting enzyme (ACE) inhibitors are at higher risk, but all patients receiving tPA should be monitored closely for signs of angioedema and airway compromise.

TABLE 35.4	The SEDAN Score for Predicting Risk of Hemorrhagic Conversion with IV tPA
Sugar (blood glucose level)	
• 145–216 mg/dL	+1
• >216 mg/dL	+2
Early infarct signs	+1
Dense MCA (or other vessel) sign on admission CT	+1
Age older than 75 yr	+1
NIHSS >9 points	+1
TOTAL	0–6

Total scores range from 0 to 6. The approximate risk of symptomatic hemorrhagic conversion for a score of 0, 1, 2, 3, 4, or 5+, respectively, are 1%, 3%, 6%, 10%, 20%, and 30%.

IV tPA, intravenous tissue plasminogen activator; MCA, middle cerebral artery; NIHSS, National Institutes of Health Stroke Scale.

From Strbian D, Engelter S, Michel P, et al. Symptomatic intracranial hemorrhage after stroke thrombolysis: the SEDAN score. *Ann Neurol.* 2012;71:634–641.

Should angioedema occur, administration of steroids, antihistamines, and/or epinephrine can be considered depending on severity and comorbidities.

ENDOVASCULAR THERAPIES

Successful recanalization after large-vessel occlusion is associated with improved prognosis, and early reperfusion has been consistently shown to result in better long-term functional outcome than later reperfusion. Unfortunately, IV tPA leads to recanalization less than 50% of the time in large-vessel occlusion on average, with smaller and more distal clots responding more favorably compared with the large proximal clots that cause massive infarcts. One study using transcranial Doppler after IV tPA found recanalization rates for distal MCA, proximal MCA, and distal ICA locations to be 44%, 29%, and 10%, respectively. Recanalization after tPA is also dependent on clot length, with lower rates of recanalization seen for clots greater than 8 mm in length. Due to the relatively low recanalization rates seen with IV tPA in large proximal vascular occlusions, intra-arterial thrombolysis with tPA (IA tPA), mechanical thrombectomy, and sonothrombolysis with high-frequency ultrasound have all been proposed as viable adjuncts to tPA in large-vessel occlusion.

Intra-arterial Thrombolysis

The first endovascular therapy developed for treatment of ischemic stroke was intra-arterial (IA) delivery of thrombolytics beginning in the 1990s. Initial studies showed favorable recanalization rates, which prompted the Prolyse in Acute Cerebral Thromboembolism (PROACT) II trial. In this study, 180 patients with proximal MCA occlusion within 6 hours of symptoms onset were randomized to IA prourokinase plus IV heparin versus IV heparin alone. Recanalization rates were 66% in the study group compared to 18% in the control group. Although mortality was similar in both, good functional outcome at 3 months was seen in 40% of the endovascular therapy group compared to 25% in the placebo group despite a higher rate of symptomatic ICH in the prourokinase group (10% vs. 2%). Mechanical thrombectomy devices have proven to be more effective at achieving recanalization than IA tPA, although IA thrombolysis continues to be used in adjunct to these newer devices.

Mechanical Thrombectomy

The Merci device was the first cerebral clot extraction device approved for use in acute large-vessel occlusion. Initial small and uncontrolled studies of this corkscrew-like device demonstrated recanalization in 40% to 60% of patients, with recanalization rates improving to 70% when thrombectomy was combined with IA tPA. The second available device was Penumbra, a suction device that showed recanalization rates of up to 80% within 8 hours of stroke in the Penumbra Pivotal Stroke Trial. The newest and most effective clot extraction devices are the intrathrombus retrievable stent devices. The Trevo and Solitaire intrathrombus "stentriever" devices were individually tested head-to-head with the Merci device and showed significantly higher rates of recanalization.

TRIALS OF CORKSCREW AND SUCTION DEVICES

Despite evidence showing increased recanalization rates with use of endovascular techniques of mechanical thrombectomy and or administration of IA tPA, the first randomized controlled trials evaluating the efficacy of endovascular therapies for improving neurologic outcome after AIS were not published until 2013. The Interventional Management of Stroke III (IMS III) Trial randomized patients who had already received IV tPA within 3 hours of stroke onset to additional endovascular therapy beginning within 5 hours of onset versus no additional treatment (IV tPA alone). The study did not show a benefit in functional outcomes at 3 months for tPA plus adjunctive endovascular therapy administered within 5 hours of stroke onset compared to tPA administration alone. The Local Versus Systemic Thrombolysis for Acute Ischemic Stroke (SYNTHESIS) trial randomized patients within 4.5 hours of stroke onset to IV tPA alone or within 6 hours of onset to endovascular intervention alone. Good functional recovery at 3 months was seen in 35% of the IV tPA group compared to 30% in the endovascular intervention group. The Mechanical Retrieval and Recanalization of Stroke Clots Using Embolectomy (MR-RESCUE), published concurrently with IMS III and SYNTHESIS, also failed to show benefit of endovascular intervention compared to IV tPA in patients with perfusion deficits determined by MR or CTP imaging.

The negative results in these trials prompted questions regarding optimal timing of therapy, patient selection, and the role of thrombectomy devices. In IMS III, for example, the mean time from stroke onset to start of endovascular therapy was longer than 4 hours and although not reported, time to recanalization likely exceeded the 4.5 hours that is accepted as beneficial for IV thrombolysis. Similarly, in SYNTHESIS, the endovascular group received intervention 1 hour later than the group receiving IV tPA, and in MR-RESCUE, the mean time from stroke onset to groin puncture was greater than 6 hours. IMS III and SYNTHESIS also did not confirm large-vessel occlusion prior to intervention, and consequently, nearly 25% of patients in IMS III randomized to the intervention group did not actually receive any intervention. For SYNTHESIS, if no large-vessel occlusion was seen on angiography, IA tPA was infused into the suspected vascular territory based on clinical exam, which is not likely to be an effective therapy. Finally, the newest retrievable stent devices were used infrequently in these trials because they were not yet available when the trials began, making it more difficult to achieve high rates of recanalization. Only 30% to 40% of patients in the intervention groups in IMS III and MR-RESCUE attained greater than 50% recanalization in affected territory compared with expected recanalization rates of 60% to 80% with the stent retriever devices.

STENTRIEVER TECHNOLOGY

In 2014, a well-designed randomized trial—Multicenter Randomized Clinical Trial of Endovascular Treatment for Acute Ischemic Stroke in the Netherlands (MR CLEAN)—employed more accurate patient selection measures than IMS III and SYNTHESIS, and unlike these two trials used retrievable stent thrombectomy devices. The proportion of patients with minimal or no disability at 90 days was 33% in those treated with IA therapy and tPA compared to 19% with tPA alone: a number needed to treat of seven patients to prevent one outcome of moderate or severe disability (Table 35.5). There was no effect on mortality. Mean time from stroke onset to IV tPA was 1 hour and 15 minutes and to groin puncture was 4 hours and 20 minutes. Follow-up CTA showed no residual large-vessel occlusion in 75% of the IA + tPA group and 33% of the tPA-only group.

In the spring of 2015, the Endovascular Treatment for Small Core and Anterior Circulation Proximal Occlusion with Emphasis on Minimizing CT to Recanalization Times (ESCAPE), SWIFT PRIME, and four additional randomized controlled trials comparing mechanical thrombectomy to tPA alone reported superior outcomes with intra-arterial treatment (Table 35.5). The preponderance of evidence supporting endovascular "bridging" therapy after administration of IV tPA will likely result in national recommendations for endovascular treatment as (1) an adjunctive treatment in patients with documented large-vessel occlusion of onset less than

TABLE 35.5 Recent Trials of Intra-Arterial Therapy for Acute Ischemic Stroke

Trial	N	Imaging Selection*	NIHSS	Time Window for IAT	TICI 2B-3 for IAT group	mRS 0-2 (%)				Mortality (%)		
						IAT[†]	Control	NNT	OR [95% CI]	IAT	Control	OR [95% CI]
MR CLEAN[4]	500	LVO	≥2	≤ 6 h	59%	33%	19%	7	2.1 [1.4 to 3.4]	21%	22%	NS
EXTEND-IA[5]	70	LVO and favorable CT perfusion	None	≤ 6 h	86%	71%	40%	3	4.2 [1.4 to 12]	9%	20%	NS
ESCAPE[6]	315	LVO and favorable collaterals on multiphase CTA	≥6	≤ 12 h	72%	53%	29%	4	1.7 [1.3 to 2.2]	10%	19%	0.5 [0.3 to 0.8]
REVASCAT[7]	206	LVO	≥6	≤ 8 h	66%	44%	28%	6	2.0 [1.1 to 3.5]	18%	15%	NS
SWIFT-PRIME[8]	196	LVO and favorable CT perfusion	10-30	≤ 6 h	83%	60%	35%	4	1.7 [1.2 to 2.3]	9%	12%	NS
THRACE[9]	395	LVO (including basilar)	10-25	≤ 5 h	NA	54%	42%	8	NA	13%	13%	NS
THERAPY[‡10]	108	LVO with clot length >8mm on NCHCT	≥8	≤ 4.5 h	NA	38%	34%	NS	NS	12%	24%	NS

*All studies except for THERAPY used CT angiography for confirmation of LVO.

[†]Treatment arms were IAT +/- IV tPA (if eligible) vs. Best Medical Management except for EXTEND-IA and SWIFT-PRIME which required IV tPA in the interventional group.

[‡]THERAPY trial terminated early due to other positive trials (planned enrollment of 692 patients) and was therefore underpowered to show significant results for this outcome.

mRS, modified Rankin scale; IAT, intra-arterial therapy; TICI, Thrombolysis in Cerebral Infarction score; LVO, large vessel occlusion; CTA, CT angiography; NCHCT, noncontrast head CT; tPA, tissue-plasminogen activator; NA, not available; NS, non-significant.

6 hours who have already received IV tPA or (2) sole treatment for patient with large vessel occlusion of less than 6 hours who have contraindications for IV tPA or are out of the 4.5-hour time window for IV tPA [**Level 1**].[4–10]

COMPLICATIONS

Like IV tPA, endovascular therapy carries an increased risk of symptomatic ICH that varies depending on the technique used and timing of intervention. Although earlier IA thrombolysis studies like PROACT II reported a rate of 10%, recent studies report rates of symptomatic ICH of around 6%. Asymptomatic hemorrhage is much more common and may even signify adequate reperfusion within the ischemic territory. Other complications of endovascular therapy include thrombus fragmentation with distal embolization, device malfunction, groin hematoma, and the rare vessel rupture.

CRITICAL CARE OF STROKE

Intensive care of stroke depends on a team approach and adherence to protocols that support best practices. Closed ICUs that provide around-the-clock availability of neurointensivists are important because this model has been shown to reduce costs, improve outcomes, and decrease hospital length of stay. These benefits may be the result of (1) organizational improvements, including the development of urgent interhospital transfer systems; (2) the uniform institution of best medical practices; (3) improved access to specialized neuroimaging, monitoring, and therapeutic techniques; and (4) the creation of physician and nursing care teams with special expertise in caring for neurologic patients. The use of checklists (Table 35.6) has been shown to improve outcome in stroke units and neurocritical care units.

TABLE 35.6 Stroke Unit Checklist

☐ BP goal <180/105 mm Hg for 24 h if IV tPA was given
☐ BP goal <220/120 mm Hg if no IV tPA was used
☐ Serial monitoring of vital signs
☐ Serial monitoring of neurologic deficits
☐ Dysphagia screen
☐ Aspirin (PO or rectal)[a]
☐ Enoxaparin 40 mg SC daily (heparin 5,000 units t.i.d. if renal dysfunction)[a]
☐ Place sequential compression device
☐ High-dose statin
☐ Neurovascular work-up: Carotid and intracranial Dopplers, CTA or MRA
☐ Cardiac workup: ECG, serial troponins, telemetry, echocardiogram
☐ Screen: hemoglobin A1c, lipid panel, toxicology, urinalysis
☐ Remove Foley

[a]Contraindicated in the first 24 hours after thrombolysis.

BP, blood pressure; PO, by mouth; SC, subcutaneous; ECG, electrocardiogram.

A systematized and multidisciplinary approach to poststroke management initiated in a specialized stroke unit or neuro-ICU has been shown to minimize common complications after stroke and should be used whenever possible [**Level 1**].[1] Aside from the prevention of poststroke complications, evaluation for stroke etiology and management aimed at limiting stroke recurrence should ensue in the period immediately following AIS. For details, refer to the chapter on secondary stroke prevention.

CLINICAL SYNDROMES

Malignant Middle Cerebral Artery Infarction

Large hemispheric or *malignant MCA* infarction is a massive stroke that occurs as a result of ICA or proximal MCA occlusion resulting in cerebral edema that leads to herniation and death in 40% to 80% of patients without treatment. Malignant MCA infarction is essentially a hemispheric compartment syndrome, in which swelling and increased local tissue pressure leads to extension of the ischemic territory, herniation, and compressive injury of the brain stem. Patients with acute infarction involving over half of the MCA territory are at risk, whereas 95% of those with infarction affecting more than two-thirds of the MCA territory will progress to herniation. Imaging, including CT and MRI, can be used as early as 6 hours after infarction to predict malignant evolution. These patients should be managed in a neuro-ICU to allow for detecting of early neurologic deterioration and prompt treatment of cerebral edema if it occurs. Monitoring of intracranial pressure (ICP) is not useful because the swelling is focal, and patients can herniate from cerebral edema without developing a rise in ICP. The definitive treatment to prevent herniation and mortality is hemicraniectomy, but bolus osmotherapy with hypertonic saline and mannitol are effective temporizing measures. Therapeutic hypothermia has been tested as a treatment for malignant cerebral edema but has not been shown to improve outcome. In most patients, medical therapies should be used as a bridge to decompressive surgery and not as standalone therapy.

Three trials for decompressive hemicraniectomy in malignant MCA infarction have been performed, although all were underpowered to show efficacy. As they used similar inclusion criteria, a prespecified combined analysis of these trials was performed and showed an absolute risk reduction of 51% for death or severe disability and a 23% absolute increase in the proportion of patients who were alive and able to walk independently at 6 months compared with conservative medical management. These results corresponded to a number needed to treat of two patients to prevent one death and four patients to turn what would have been one death to a patient living with a moderate level of functional disability but still able to walk independently. As a result, hemicraniectomy is recommended for the treatment of malignant MCA infarction in patients younger than 60 years of age when the procedure is in line with the wishes of the patient or the patient's family [**Level 1**].[5] None of the three trials included patients older than age 60 years, but a subsequent study, the Decompressive Surgery for the Treatment of Malignant Infarction of the Middle Cerebral Artery (DESTINY) II trial, showed a mortality reduction from 70% to 33% of patients, but with worsened neurologic outcomes compared to younger patients. There was not a significant increase in the survivors with mild or moderate disability, as nearly all of the survivors were bedbound or unable to walk independently. This expected prognosis for older patients should be discussed with family members prior to making any treatment decisions.

Cerebellar Infarction

Cerebellar infarction represents approximately 3% of total ischemic strokes. In cases of a large cerebellar infarction, cytotoxic edema in the limited compartment of the posterior fossa can lead to brain stem compression, hydrocephalus from obstruction of the fourth ventricle, and tonsillar or upward herniation. The peak period of deterioration is 72 hours, although patients may deteriorate earlier or as many as 10 days after the ischemic insult. Signs of worsening edema include drowsiness, gaze disturbance, hemiparesis, and hyperreflexia. The onset of these clinical signs is often insidious, and coma can develop rapidly without intervention, necessitating that all patient with large cerebellar infarction be closely monitored in an intensive care setting. In cases where brain stem compression or hydrocephalus appear, posterior fossa craniectomy is highly effective at preventing mortality and allowing for good functional outcome, although randomized trials have not been performed. Management with an external ventricular drain (EVD) or excision of the infarcted tissue can also effectively alleviate compression but carries the risk of upward herniation by lowering the supratentorial pressure. Thus, decompressive surgery should be the initial intervention considered in most cases.

Basilar Artery Occlusion

Basilar artery occlusion carries a mortality of up to 90% without treatment. Those who survive are often left with significant functional deficits ranging from ataxia or weakness to *locked-in* syndrome. Given its poor natural history, aggressive attempts at reperfusion, even beyond the accepted range of therapy for ischemic stroke in other locations, are often considered. Although IV tPA within 4.5 hours remains the only proven treatment option, anecdotal data shows potential benefit of IA thrombolysis or mechanical thrombectomy as long after stroke onset as 24 hours. For patients with mild to moderate symptoms, IV tPA and close monitoring may be sufficient. However, for those who present with severe symptoms, IV tPA, IA tPA, and/or mechanical thrombectomy are all appropriate considerations.

Cervical Artery Dissection

Carotid and vertebral artery dissections are uncommon etiologies of stroke causing only 2% of all cases. However, they account for a much higher proportion of AIS in young patients causing 10% to 25% of all strokes in this population. The most common risk factor is cervical twisting or trauma, but presentations can be spontaneous or resulting from an underlying arteriopathy such as fibromuscular dysplasia, Marfan syndrome, or Ehlers–Danlos syndrome type IV. Clinical presentations of internal carotid dissection include facial pain, headache, neck pain, an incomplete oculosympathetic syndrome (Horner syndrome with preserved sweat response), and contralateral stroke symptoms, such as hemiparesis or aphasia. When strokes occur, they most often result from artery-to-artery embolism but can also occur in a watershed territory from arterial narrowing or occlusion of the dissected vessel.

Although no randomized trials have been done comparing management options in acute cervical artery dissection, several meta-analyses have shown no difference in mortality or stroke occurrence in patients treated with antiplatelet agents versus those treated with anticoagulation. Nevertheless, anticoagulation is often used in patients with evidence of multiple infarcts, those with a free-floating thrombus within the lumen of the vessel, or in those with microemboli demonstrated by transcranial Doppler. In contrast, patients with large infarcts or intracranial extension of their dissection should be treated with antiplatelet agents due to an increased risk of bleeding with anticoagulation.

COMPLICATIONS OF STROKE

Neurologic Deterioration

Neurologic deterioration occurs in up to 40% of patients in the first 24 hours after AIS and is associated with a history of diabetes, high blood glucose concentrations, stroke severity, and early signs of edema on imaging. Although most forms of deterioration are due to progressive extension of the infarct core into surrounding penumbra, the causes of neurologic worsening are diverse and often require further investigation. All patients should undergo general and neurologic examination to determine the nature and extent of clinical change. Vital signs are important, especially because fever can cause deterioration and changes in blood pressure in either direction can have deleterious effects.

If neurologic worsening directly coincides with relative hypotension, trials of increasing cerebral perfusion can be used to confirm the presence of a blood pressure–dependent deficit. Administration of IV fluids, positioning the patient in the Trendelenburg position, or infusion of a vasopressor such as phenylephrine (starting at 20 μg/min, titrated upward to raise blood pressure by 20%) can be trialed followed by a repeat neurologic examination. If there is clinical improvement correlating to a higher mean arterial pressure, a blood pressure goal can be maintained using vasopressor agents administered under close observation in an intensive care setting. Vascular and perfusion imaging with CT or MRI may be useful at this point to evaluate for high-grade vascular stenosis and downstream perfusion/infarction mismatch.

Patients with large infarcts are more likely to develop hemorrhagic conversion, which, when symptomatic, usually presents with relatively abrupt changes in clinical signs and may be accompanied by symptoms of headache, nausea, and vomiting. Noncontrast head CT is indicated in such settings to evaluate for signs of hemorrhage. If a hemorrhage with associated mass effect is found, the clinician should reverse any form of anticoagulation or antiplatelet therapy (see Table 15.4).

If preliminary evaluations with examination, vital signs, and imaging do not reveal an etiology for neurologic worsening with depressed level of consciousness, EEG may be considered to evaluate for nonconvulsive seizure activity. Early seizures after AIS occur in approximately 5% of cases and are more common in cortical infarcts but can also occur after subcortical strokes. Although primary seizure prophylaxis is not recommended, treatment with antiepileptic agents is warranted after a seizure has occurred.

Blood Pressure Management

A *U-shaped* relationship exists between blood pressure on admission and clinical outcome, with both extremes conferring a poor outcome. The optimal blood pressure goal in AIS remains undefined. However, studies have consistently found that an acute fall in blood pressure, specifically a systolic decrease of higher than 20 mm Hg, is associated with poor functional outcome and increased mortality. Hypotension should be avoided in the acute phase of stroke, and any attempts at lowering blood pressure should be done slowly.

Current practice for those who have not received thrombolytic therapy is to allow permissive hypertension of up to 220/120 mm Hg for 24 to 48 hours, after which point antihypertensive therapy is started and slowly titrated to an extended goal toward normotension. This upper limit should be adjusted accordingly for patients with heart failure, valvular heart disease, or coronary artery disease in order to prevent any cardiac injury or complications. Similarly, in patients with hemorrhagic conversion or brain edema, blood pressure targets should be individualized at lower levels. A strict blood pressure goal of lower than 180/105 mm Hg should be maintained for 24 hours in those treated with IV tPA in order to limit secondary ICH [**Level 1**].[1]

Infectious Complications

ASPIRATION PNEUMONIA

Dysphagia occurs in nearly 40% of stroke patients and is associated with a significant increase in the incidence of pneumonia. Of all the medical complications after stroke, pneumonia carries the highest proportion of attributable risk for mortality. All stroke patients should undergo an early dysphagia screen using an objective test, such as a simple bedside water swallow test. Comprehensive evaluation by a speech–language pathologist followed by barium esophagography or videofluoroscopy may be necessary. Early recognition of dysphagia can lead to prevention techniques and therapies, such as maintaining patients in a sitting position after feeding and providing oral care, which may reduce morbidity and mortality associated with aspiration-related pneumonia. When necessary, a nasogastric or nasoduodenal feeding tube should be placed for nutritional support and medication administration. If prolonged dysphagia is expected, a percutaneous endoscopic gastrostomy allows for extended nutritional support.

URINARY TRACT INFECTION

Urinary tract infection occurs in 10% to 15% of stroke-related hospitalizations and is associated with worsened neurologic and functional outcomes. Risk factors for urinary tract infection include increasing age, female sex, poststroke disability, urinary retention, and, most importantly, urinary catheterization. Avoiding urinary catheterization and early removal of urinary catheters reduces the risk of catheter-associated urinary tract infections.

Venous Thromboembolism

Patients with stroke are at high risk for developing deep vein thrombosis (DVT) due to hemiparesis and immobility. Studies done in the absence of pharmacologic DVT prophylaxis suggest that DVT occurs in as many as 40% to 50% of hemiplegic patients within 2 weeks of stroke onset. The associated risk of pulmonary embolism is 15% in untreated patients, which can lead to early death following AIS.

Although unfractionated heparin has been proven effective for DVT prophylaxis, the Prevention of VTE After Acute Ischemic Stroke with Low-Molecular Weight Heparinoid Enoxaparin (PREVAIL) trial showed that enoxaparin 40 mg daily (q.d.) was more effective at preventing DVT than unfractionated heparin administered twice daily. Pneumatic sequential compression devices are also effective when used independently and provide an added benefit when used in addition to pharmacologic DVT prophylaxis. Early mobilization is also effective in preventing DVT and provides added benefits in functional recovery. Current guidelines recommend pharmacologic DVT prophylaxis in all stroke patients, unless there is a substantial risk of bleeding that would outweigh the potential benefits, in which case nonpharmacologic options should be employed [**Level 1**].[12] Pharmacologic DVT prophylaxis should also be held for 24 hours after tPA administration.

TABLE 35.7	Risk Factors for Death or Poor Functional Outcome after Ischemic Stroke

- Patient age
- Female gender
- Prestroke functional baseline
- NIHSS
- Infarct volume
- Diabetes mellitus
- Fever
- Heart failure

NIHSS, National Institutes of Health Stroke Scale.

STROKE OUTCOMES

Outcome after stroke is defined as the level of functional impairment or death months to years after the insult. Stroke is the third leading cause of death and the leading cause of disability among adults. Accurately predicting a patient's outcome can aid the clinician decide the best management approach and help the patient, and their family, establish appropriate expectations for quality of life. Using retrospective data from various cohorts, a number of prediction models have been established to predict long-term stroke outcomes at the time of the acute stroke. Stroke severity, which can be assessed with the NIHSS, and patient age have consistently proven predictive of outcome. Specific exam features that have been cited include upper extremity plegia and inability to walk independently. Others frequently cited factors include infarct volume, fever, diabetes, and congestive heart failure (Table 35.7). Outcome after ischemic stroke can be improved by care in a dedicated stroke unit, using a systematic approach to minimizing preventable medical complications, and instituting early rehabilitation (see Chapter 152).

LEVEL 1 EVIDENCE

1. Jauch EC, Saver JL, Adams HP Jr, et al. Guidelines for the early management of patients with acute ischemic stroke: a guideline for healthcare professionals from the American Heart Association/American Stroke Association. *Stroke.* 2013;44(3):870–947.
2. Tissue plasminogen activator for acute ischemic stroke. The National Institute of Neurological Disorders and Stroke rt-PA Stroke Study Group. *N Engl J Med.* 1995;333(24):1581–1587.
3. Del Zoppo GJ, Saver JL, Jauch EC, et al; American Heart Association Stroke Council. Expansion of the time window for treatment of acute ischemic stroke with intravenous tissue plasminogen activator: a science advisory from the American Heart Association/American Stroke Association. *Stroke.* 2009;40(8):2945–2948.
4. Berkhemer OA, Fransen PS, Beumer D, et al. A randomized trial of intraarterial treatment for acute ischemic stroke. *N Engl J Med.* 2015;372(1):11–20.
5. Campbell BCV, Mitchell PJ, Kleinig TJ, et al. Endovascular therapy for ischemic stroke with perfusion-imaging selection. *N Engl J Med.* 2015;372(11):1009–1018.
6. Goyal M, Demchuk AM, Menon BK, et al. Randomized assessment of rapid endovascular treatment of ischemic stroke. *N Engl J Med.* 2015;372(11):1019–1030.
7. Jovin TG, Chamorro A, Cobo E, et al. Thrombectomy within 8 hours after symptom onset in ischemic stroke. *N Engl J Med.* 2015. Epub ahead of print. doi: 10.1056/NEJMoa1503780.
8. Saver JL, Goyal M, Bonafe A, et al. Stent-retriever thrombectomy after intravenous t-PA vs. t-PA alone in stroke. *N Engl J Med.* 2015. Epub ahead of print. doi: 10.1056/NEJMoa1415061.
9. Trial and Cost Effectiveness Evaluation of Intra-Arterial Thrombectomy in Acute Ischemic Stroke (THRACE). Presented at the meeting of the European Stroke Organisation, April 2015; Glasgow, UK.
10. Assess the Penumbra System in the Treatment of Acute Stroke (THERAPY). Presented at the meeting of the European Stroke Organisation, April 2015; Glasgow, UK.
11. Vahedi K, Hofmeijer J, Juettler E, et al. for the DECIMAL, DESTINY, and HAMLET investigators. Early decompressive surgery in malignant infarction of the middle cerebral artery: a pooled analysis of three randomized controlled trials. *Lancet Neurol.* 2007;6:315–322.
12. Qaseem A, Chou R, Humphrey LL, et al; Clinical Guidelines Committee of the American College of Physicians. Venous thromboembolism prophylaxis in hospitalized patients: a clinical practice guideline from the American College of Physicians. *Ann Intern Med.* 2011;155(9):625–632.

SUGGESTED READINGS

Adams HP Jr, Bendixen BH, Kappelle LJ, et al. Classification of subtype of acute ischemic stroke. Definitions for use in a multicenter clinical trial. TOAST. Trial of Org 10172 in Acute Stroke Treatment. *Stroke.* 1993;24(1):35–41.

Ahmed N, Wahlgren N, Brainin M, et al. Relationship of blood pressure, antihypertensive therapy, and outcome in ischemic stroke treated with intravenous thrombolysis: retrospective analysis from Safe Implementation of Thrombolysis in Stroke-International Stroke Thrombolysis Register (SITS-ISTR). *Stroke.* 2009;40(7):2442–2449.

Aslanyan S, Weir CJ, Diener HC, et al. Pneumonia and urinary tract infection after acute ischaemic stroke: a tertiary analysis of the GAIN International trial. *Eur J Neurol.* 2004;11(1):49–53.

Ay H, Furie KL, Singhal A, et al. An evidence-based causative classification system for acute ischemic stroke. *Ann Neurol.* 2005;58(5):688–697. doi:10.1002/ana.20617.

Barlinn K, Tsivgoulis G, Barreto AD, et al. Outcomes following sonothrombolysis in severe acute ischemic stroke: subgroup analysis of the CLOTBUST trial. *Int J Stroke.* 2014;9(8):1006–1010. doi:10.1111/ijs.12340.

Benninger DH, Georgiadis D, Kremer C, et al. Mechanism of ischemic infarct in spontaneous carotid dissection. *Stroke.* 2004;35(2):482–485.

Bernhardt J, Collaboration AT. Early mobilization testing in patients with acute stroke. *Chest.* 2012;141(6):1641–1642; author reply 2–3.

Bhatia R, Hill MD, Shobha N, et al. Low rates of acute recanalization with intravenous recombinant tissue plasminogen activator in ischemic stroke: real-world experience and a call for action. *Stroke.* 2010;41(10):2254–2258.

Bose A, Henkes H, Alfke K, et al. The penumbra system: a mechanical device for the treatment of acute stroke due to thromboembolism. *AJNR Am J Neuroradiol.* 2008;29(7):1409–1413.

Broderick JP, Palesch YY, Demchuk AM, et al. Endovascular therapy after intravenous t-PA versus t-PA alone for stroke. *N Engl J Med.* 2013;368(10):893–903. doi:10.1056/NEJMoa1214300.

Castano C, Dorado L, Guerrero C, et al. Mechanical thrombectomy with the Solitaire AB device in large artery occlusions of the anterior circulation: a pilot study. *Stroke.* 2010;41(8):1836–1840.

Castillo J, Leira R, Garcia MM, et al. Blood pressure decrease during the acute phase of ischemic stroke is associated with brain injury and poor stroke outcome. *Stroke.* 2004;35(2):520–526.

Chan DK, Cordato D, O'Rourke F, et al. Comprehensive stroke units: a review of comparative evidence and experience. *Int J Stroke.* 2013;8(4):260–264.

Christensen LM, Krieger DW, Hojberg S, et al. Paroxysmal atrial fibrillation occurs often in cryptogenic ischaemic stroke. Final results from the SURPRISE study. *Eur J Neurol.* 2014;21(6):884–889.

Ciccone A, Valvassori L, Nichelatti M, et al. Endovascular treatment for acute ischemic stroke. *N Engl J Med*. 2013;368(10):904–913.

CLOTS (Clots in Legs Or sTockings after Stroke) Trials Collaboration; Dennis M, Sandercock P, et al. Effectiveness of intermittent pneumatic compression in reduction of risk of deep vein thrombosis in patients who have had a stroke (CLOTS 3): a multicentre randomised controlled trial. *Lancet*. 2013;382(9891):516–524.

del Zoppo GJ, Higashida RT, Furlan AJ, et al. PROACT: a phase II randomized trial of recombinant pro-urokinase by direct arterial delivery in acute middle cerebral artery stroke. PROACT Investigators. Prolyse in Acute Cerebral Thromboembolism. *Stroke*. 1998;29(1):4–11.

Dirnagl U, Iadecola C, Moskowitz MA. Pathobiology of ischaemic stroke: an integrated view. *Trends Neurosci*. 1999;22(9):391–397.

Dundar Y, Hill R, Dickson R, et al. Comparative efficacy of thrombolytics in acute myocardial infarction: a systematic review. *QJM*. 2003;96(2):103–113.

Dzialowski I, Hill MD, Coutts SB, et al. Extent of early ischemic changes on computed tomography (CT) before thrombolysis: prognostic value of the Alberta Stroke Program Early CT Score in ECASS II. *Stroke*. 2006;37(4):973–978. doi:10.1161/01.STR.0000206215.62441.56.

Edlow JA, Newman-Toker DE, Savitz SI. Diagnosis and initial management of cerebellar infarction. *Lancet Neurol*. 2008;7(10):951–964.

Engelter ST, Brandt T, Debette S, et al. Antiplatelets versus anticoagulation in cervical artery dissection. *Stroke*. 2007;38(9):2605–2611.

Fiorelli M, Bastianello S, von Kummer R, et al. Hemorrhagic transformation within 36 hours of a cerebral infarct: relationships with early clinical deterioration and 3-month outcome in the European Cooperative Acute Stroke Study I (ECASS I) cohort. *Stroke*. 1999;30(11):2280–2284.

Fisher CM. Concerning recurrent transient cerebral ischemic attacks. *Can Med Assoc J*. 1962;86:1091–1099.

Fonarow GC, Smith EE, Saver JL, et al. Improving door-to-needle times in acute ischemic stroke: the design and rationale for the American Heart Association/American Stroke Association's Target: Stroke initiative. *Stroke*. 2011;42(10):2983–2989.

Furlan A, Higashida R, Wechsler L, Gent M, Rowley H, Kase C, et al. Intra-arterial prourokinase for acute ischemic stroke. The PROACT II study: a randomized controlled trial. Prolyse in Acute Cerebral Thromboembolism. *JAMA*. 1999;282(21):2003–2011.

Gaul C, Dietrich W, Friedrich I, et al. Neurological symptoms in type A aortic dissections. *Stroke*. 2007;38(2):292–297.

Go AS, Mozaffarian D, Roger VL, et al. Heart disease and stroke statistics—2014 update: a report from the American Heart Association. *Circulation*. 2014;129(3):e28–e292.

Hacke W, Donnan G, Fieschi C, et al. Association of outcome with early stroke treatment: pooled analysis of ATLANTIS, ECASS, and NINDS rt-PA stroke trials. *Lancet*. 2004;363(9411):768–774.

Hacke W, Kaste M, Bluhmki E, et al. Thrombolysis with alteplase 3 to 4.5 hours after acute ischemic stroke. *N Engl J Med*. 2008;359(13):1317–1329.

Harrigan MR, Leonardo J, Gibbons KJ, et al. CT perfusion cerebral blood flow imaging in neurological critical care. *Neurocrit Care*. 2005;2(3):352–366.

Hemmen TM, Meyer BC, McClean TL, et al. Identification of nonischemic stroke mimics among 411 code strokes at the University of California, San Diego, Stroke Center. *J Stroke Cerebrovasc Dis*. 2008;17(1):23–25.

Heuschmann PU, Kolominsky-Rabas PL, Misselwitz B, et al. Predictors of in-hospital mortality and attributable risks of death after ischemic stroke: the German Stroke Registers Study Group. *Arch Intern Med*. 2004;164(16):1761–1768.

Hill MD, Lye T, Moss H, et al. Hemi-orolingual angioedema and ACE inhibition after alteplase treatment of stroke. *Neurology*. 2003;60(9):1525–1527.

Ihle-Hansen H, Thommessen B, Wyller TB, et al. Risk factors for and incidence of subtypes of ischemic stroke. *Funct Neurol*. 2012;27(1):35–40.

Ingeman A, Andersen G, Hundborg HH, et al. In-hospital medical complications, length of stay, and mortality among stroke unit patients. *Stroke*. 2011;42(11):3214–3218.

Jauss M, Krieger D, Hornig C, et al. Surgical and medical management of patients with massive cerebellar infarctions: results of the German-Austrian Cerebellar Infarction Study. *J Neurol*. 1999;246(4):257–264.

Johnston SC, Mendis S, Mathers CD. Global variation in stroke burden and mortality: estimates from monitoring, surveillance, and modelling. *Lancet Neurol*. 2009;8(4):345–354. doi:10.1016/S1474-4422(09)70023-7.

Kamran SI, Downey D, Ruff RL. Pneumatic sequential compression reduces the risk of deep vein thrombosis in stroke patients. *Neurology*. 1998;50(6):1683–1688.

Kase CS, Albers GW, Bladin C, et al. Neurological outcomes in patients with ischemic stroke receiving enoxaparin or heparin for venous thromboembolism prophylaxis: subanalysis of the Prevention of VTE after Acute Ischemic Stroke with LMWH (PREVAIL) study. *Stroke*. 2009;40(11):3532–3540.

Katzan IL, Cebul RD, Husak SH, et al. The effect of pneumonia on mortality among patients hospitalized for acute stroke. *Neurology*. 2003;60(4):620–625.

Kidwell CS, Jahan R, Gornbein J, et al. A trial of imaging selection and endovascular treatment for ischemic stroke. *N Engl J Med*. 2013;368(10):914–923.

Kidwell CS, Starkman S, Eckstein M, et al. Identifying stroke in the field. Prospective validation of the Los Angeles prehospital stroke screen (LAPSS). *Stroke*. 2000;31(1):71–76.

Koennecke HC, Belz W, Berfelde D, et al. Factors influencing in-hospital mortality and morbidity in patients treated on a stroke unit. *Neurology*. 2011;77(10):965–972.

Kothari RU, Pancioli A, Liu T, et al. Cincinnati Prehospital Stroke Scale: reproducibility and validity. *Ann Emerg Med*. 1999;33(4):373–378.

Krieger DW, Demchuk AM, Kasner SE, et al. Early clinical and radiological predictors of fatal brain swelling in ischemic stroke. *Stroke*. 1999;30(2):287–292.

Latchaw RE, Alberts MJ, Lev MH, et al. Recommendations for imaging of acute ischemic stroke: a scientific statement from the American Heart Association. *Stroke*. 2009;40(11):3646–3678.

Lees KR, Bluhmki E, von Kummer R, et al. Time to treatment with intravenous alteplase and outcome in stroke: an updated pooled analysis of ECASS, ATLANTIS, NINDS, and EPITHET trials. *Lancet*. 2010;375(9727):1695–1703.

Leonardi-Bee J, Bath PM, Phillips SJ, et al; IST Collaborative Group. Blood pressure and clinical outcomes in the International Stroke Trial. *Stroke*. 2002;33(5):1315–1320.

Lucas C, Moulin T, Deplanque D, et al. Stroke patterns of internal carotid artery dissection in 40 patients. *Stroke*. 1998;29(12):2646–2648.

Lyrer P, Engelter S. Antithrombotic drugs for carotid artery dissection. *Cochrane Database Syst Rev*. 2010;(10):CD000255.

Moser DK, Kimble LP, Alberts MJ, et al. Reducing delay in seeking treatment by patients with acute coronary syndrome and stroke: a scientific statement from the American Heart Association Council on Cardiovascular Nursing and Stroke Council. *J Cardiovasc Nurs*. 2007;22(4):326–343.

Mullins ME, Schaefer PW, Sorensen AG, et al. CT and conventional and diffusion-weighted MR imaging in acute stroke: study in 691 patients at presentation to the emergency department. *Radiology*. 2002;224(2):353–360.

Nogueira RG, Lutsep HL, Gupta R, et al. Trevo versus Merci retrievers for thrombectomy revascularisation of large vessel occlusions in acute ischaemic stroke (TREVO 2): a randomised trial. *Lancet*. 2012;380(9849):1231–1240.

Potter J, Mistri A, Brodie F, et al. Controlling hypertension and hypotension immediately post stroke (CHHIPS)—a randomised controlled trial. *Health Technol Assess*. 2009;13(9):iii, ix–xi, 1–73.

Riedel CH, Zimmermann P, Jensen-Kondering U, et al. The importance of size: successful recanalization by intravenous thrombolysis in acute anterior stroke depends on thrombus length. *Stroke*. 2011;42(6):1775–1777.

Saqqur M, Uchino K, Demchuk AM, et al. Site of arterial occlusion identified by transcranial Doppler predicts the response to intravenous thrombolysis for stroke. *Stroke*. 2007;38(3):948–954.

Saver JL. Time is brain—quantified. *Stroke*. 2006;37(1):263–266.

Saver JL, Fonarow GC, Smith EE, et al. Time to treatment with intravenous tissue plasminogen activator and outcome from acute ischemic stroke. *JAMA*. 2013;309(23):2480–2488.

Saver JL, Jahan R, Levy EI, et al. SOLITAIRE with the intention for thrombectomy (SWIFT) trial: design of a randomized, controlled, multicenter study comparing the SOLITAIRE Flow Restoration device and the MERCI Retriever in acute ischaemic stroke. *Int J Stroke*. 2014;9(5):658–668.

Schievink WI. Spontaneous dissection of the carotid and vertebral arteries. *N Engl J Med*. 2001;344(12):898–906.

Schneider AT, Pancioli AM, Khoury JC, et al. Trends in community knowledge of the warning signs and risk factors for stroke. *JAMA*. 2003;289(3):343–346.

Schonewille WJ, Wijman CA, Michel P, et al. Treatment and outcomes of acute basilar artery occlusion in the Basilar Artery International Cooperation Study (BASICS): a prospective registry study. *Lancet Neurol.* 2009;8(8): 724–730.

Silver B, Lu M, Morris DC, et al. Blood pressure declines and less favorable outcomes in the NINDS tPA stroke study. *J Neurol Sci.* 2008;271(1–2):61–67.

Singer OC, Humpich MC, Fiehler J, et al. Risk for symptomatic intracerebral hemorrhage after thrombolysis assessed by diffusion-weighted magnetic resonance imaging. *Ann Neurol.* 2008;63(1):52–60.

Smith WS, Sung G, Saver J, et al. Mechanical thrombectomy for acute ischemic stroke: final results of the Multi MERCI trial. *Stroke.* 2008;39(4):1205–1212.

Sussman E, Kellner C, McDowell M, et al. Endovascular thrombectomy following acute ischemic stroke: a single-center case series and critical review of the literature. *Brain Sci.* 2013;3(2):521–539.

The Publications Committee for the Trial of ORG 10172 in Acute Stroke Treatment Investigators. Low molecular weight heparinoid, ORG 10172 (danaparoid), and outcome after acute ischemic stroke: a randomized controlled trial. *JAMA.* 1998;279(16):1265–1272.

Tong D, Reeves MJ, Hernandez AF, et al. Times from symptom onset to hospital arrival in the Get with the Guidelines—Stroke Program 2002 to 2009: temporal trends and implications. *Stroke.* 2012;43(7):1912–1917.

Tsivgoulis G, Frey JL, Flaster M, et al. Pre-tissue plasminogen activator blood pressure levels and risk of symptomatic intracerebral hemorrhage. *Stroke.* 2009;40(11):3631–3634.

Weil AG, Rahme R, Moumdjian R, et al. Quality of life following hemicraniectomy for malignant MCA territory infarction. *Can J Neurol Sci.* 2011; 38(3):434–438.

Wessels T, Wessels C, Ellsiepen A, et al. Contribution of diffusion-weighted imaging in determination of stroke etiology. *AJNR Am J Neuroradiol.* 2006;27(1):35–39.

Wilson RD. Mortality and cost of pneumonia after stroke for different risk groups. *J Stroke Cerebrovasc Dis.* 2012;21(1):61–67.

Transient Ischemic Attack 36

Randolph S. Marshall

INTRODUCTION

Transient ischemic attack (TIA) describes neurologic symptoms of ischemic origin that last less than 24 hours. In fact, most attacks last only a few minutes to an hour. Often called a *mini-stroke*, a TIA may have ominous implications. About one in three people who have stroke risk factors and experience an authentic TIA will eventually have a stroke during their lifetime, with about half occurring within a year of the initial TIA.

PATHOBIOLOGY

TIAs have more than one mechanism. When severe carotid or vertebrobasilar stenosis is present, transient ischemia can be caused by low flow distally; such TIAs are typically brief and stereotyped, presenting with repeated episodes of the same syndrome. TIAs of this hemodynamic type may occur only during upright posture or during transient hypotension or cardiac arrhythmia. When TIAs are caused by embolism—from the heart, aorta, or proximal large-vessel atherosclerotic plaque or dissection—they may last longer, as the embolus transiently occludes a distal arterial branch before spontaneously dissolving. Less commonly, permanent small-vessel occlusion with evidence of a small infarct on magnetic resonance (MR) diffusion-weighted imaging (DWI) can result in a transient deficit lasting up to 24 hours before resolving ("cerebral infarction with transient symptoms"). A newer "tissue-based" definition of TIA restricts the diagnosis to brief episodes of focal neurologic dysfunction—typically less than 1 hour—without imaging evidence of acute infarction on computed tomography (CT) or MR imaging.

Small-vessel TIAs may result from lipohyalinosis and arteriolosclerosis of small penetrating vessels, such as the lenticulostriate branches of the middle cerebral artery, or penetrators of the vertebral and basilar arteries. Intracranial or extracranial arterial dissection may produce hemodynamic compromise or embolism. Fibromuscular dysplasia and Ehlers–Danlos type IV predispose to dissection. Vasospasm-related TIA may respond to calcium channel blockers.

TIAs have also been associated with hyperviscosity—polycythemia, sickle cell anemia, and thrombocythemia as well as with cerebral venous thrombosis, bacterial endocarditis, and temporal arteritis—and may clear with correction of these underlying disorders. TIAs in cocaine users may be the result of drug-induced cerebral vasospasm.

CLINICAL MANIFESTATIONS

Symptoms vary with the arterial territory involved. *Transient monocular blindness* (TMB or *amaurosis fugax*) due to ischemia in the territory of the central retinal artery consists of blurring or darkening of vision, peaking within a few seconds (sometimes as if a curtain had descended) and usually clearing within minutes. The most important cause of TMB is proximal internal artery stenosis producing either hemodynamic compromise or embolism. Hollenhorst plaques resulting from cholesterol microemboli may be seen in retinal artery branches.

Carotid territory TIAs that involve the brain produce varying combinations of limb weakness and sensory loss, aphasia, or hemineglect. Posterior circulation TIAs cause symptoms referable to the cerebrum (visual field loss or cortical blindness), brain stem (cranial nerve and long-tract symptoms, sometimes crossed or bilateral), and cerebellum. Some TIAs produce transient "lacunar syndromes" such as pure hemiparesis or pure hemisensory loss. TIAs can cause paroxysmal dyskinesias, including tremor, ataxia, limb dystonia, and myoclonic jerking. Coarse irregular shaking of an arm or leg lasting seconds to a minute, so-called limb-shaking TIA, and sometimes precipitated by a change to upright posture, is often associated with critical carotid artery stenosis or occlusion. Although rare, high-grade stenosis or complete occlusion of both internal carotid arteries and the proximal basilar artery can lead to "drop attacks."

In the *subclavian steal syndrome*, stenosis of the subclavian or innominate artery proximal to the origin of the vertebral artery leads to brain stem, cerebellar, or even cerebral symptoms, often manifested during exertion and sometimes accompanied by symptoms of arm claudication. The syndrome results from diversion of anterograde flow via the patent vertebral artery retrograde down the contralateral vertebral artery distal to the occlusion, depriving the basilar artery of blood flow.

Recurrent TIAs of the same type are more likely to be the result of perfusion failure due to critical narrowing or occlusion of the involved artery than of embolism.

DIAGNOSIS

The diagnosis of TIA may be difficult to ascertain when symptoms are ambiguous (e.g., staggering or drop attacks; dizziness, lightheadedness, or syncope; vertigo; fleeting diplopia; transient amnesia; atypical visual disturbance in one or both eyes such as flashes, distortions, or tunnel vision; a heavy sensation or "tiredness" in one or more limbs; or paresthesias in an area of fixed sensory loss or briefly affecting only one limb). The differential diagnosis of TIAs includes migraine, cardiac arrhythmia, seizures, hypoglycemia, compressive neuropathy, conversion, and neurosis. Multiple stereotyped current focal deficits with complete recovery between events should in particular raise the question of recurrent focal seizures.

Although TIAs are defined in terms of their clinical reversibility and are presumed to signify ischemia too brief or incomplete to cause infarction, imaging frequently demonstrates appropriately located infarcts. DWI-detected abnormalities are especially likely when symptoms last more than an hour, and those lasting longer than 3 hours show infarcts in 70% of cases. This is supported by evidence that neurologic deficits reemerged upon giving intravenous midazolam to TIA patients whose initial deficits had resolved and who did not have evidence of infarction on DWI, suggesting that TIA may cause a structural lesion.

TABLE 36.1	Diagnostic Tests for the Evaluation of Transient Ischemic Attack

In most patients

✓ Electrocardiogram

✓ Carotid imaging (Doppler, MR, or CT angiography)

✓ Transthoracic echocardiography

In selected patients

✓ Portable cardiac rhythm monitoring (Holter or event-loop monitoring)

✓ Erythrocyte sedimentation rate (rule out giant cell arteritis)

✓ Toxicology screen

✓ Hypercoagulable workup (see Chapter 118)

Patients with a documented small infarct or compelling history of TIA should undergo a standard ischemic stroke workup to identify a potentially treatable cause of recurrent stroke (Table 36.1).

TREATMENT

Prevention of subsequent stroke is the primary concern in a patient diagnosed with TIA. Treatment is identical to secondary prevention in patients diagnosed with acute ischemic stroke, as discussed in Chapter 35.

OUTCOME

Authentic TIAs are associated with a high risk of subsequent stroke. In 1,707 patients presenting with TIA to an emergency department, 10% had a stroke within the next 90 days, and in half, the stroke occurred within the first 48 hours of the TIA. Retinal TIAs had about half this rate of stroke (5% within 90 days). In four European studies combining 2,416 patients who presented with ischemic stroke, 15% to 26% of ischemic strokes were preceded by a TIA and 43% of TIAs occurred within 7 days of the stroke.

The best validated tool for assessing the risk of stroke after TIA is the "ABCD[2]" score, in which points are assigned for particular risk factors and presenting features of the TIA, with scores ranging from 0 to 7. A higher score implies a higher 90-day risk of stroke. For each score, the risk of subsequent stroke is consistently greater if an acute infarct identified on CT or MR is associated with the syndrome (Table 36.2).

Since initial publication of the ABCD[2] score, attempts to add additional scale items have been added, including the presence of more than one TIA (ABCD[3]), DWI-positive image, or the presence of greater than 50% carotid stenosis (ABCD[3]-I) or intracranial arterial stenosis (ABCD[3]-I[c/i]). Each of these scores adds a small degree of incremental predictive value compared to the original ABCD[2] score at the expense of simplicity. For clinical use and ease of communication, we recommend use of the standard ABCD[2] score while recognizing that multiple TIA events, cerebral infarction with transient symptoms, or evidence of significant extracranial or intracranial stenosis further increases the 90-day stroke risk.

Crescendo TIAs—two or more attacks within 24 hours—should be considered a medical emergency. Particularly concerning is the *capsular warning syndrome*: multiple brief attacks of motor impairment due to disease involving small lenticulostriate or basilar penetrating arteries. Asymptomatic coronary artery disease is especially common in patients with carotid stenosis and should be checked for. The overall risk of stroke, myocardial infarction, and vascular death remains high for at least 10 to 15 years in patients with a history of TIA.

TABLE 36.2	ABCD[2] Score	
FEATURES		**POINTS**
A	Age: 60 years or older	1
B	Blood pressure: ≥140 mm Hg systolic or ≥90 mm Hg diastolic or history of hypertension	1
C	Clinical: speech impairment without weakness (1 point) or unilateral weakness (2 points)	1 or 2
D	Duration: 10–59 min (1 point), ≥60 min (2 points)	1 or 2
D	Diabetes: a history of diabetes mellitus (1 point)	1

90-Day Stroke Risk	With Infarction	Without Infarction
≥6	19%	6%
6	17%	3%
4	8%	2%
3	4%	2%
2	4%	≤1%
≤1	<1%	≤1%

Data from Giles MF, Albers GW, Amarenco P, et al. Early stroke risk and ABCD2 score performance in tissue- vs time-defined TIA. A multicenter study. *Neurology.* 2011;77:1222–1228.

SUGGESTED READINGS

Adams RJ, Chimowitz MI, Alpert JS, et al. Coronary risk evaluation in patients with transient ischemic attack and ischemic stroke: a scientific statement for healthcare professionals from the Stroke Council and the Council on Clinical Cardiology of the American Heart Association/American Stroke Association. *Stroke.* 2003;34:2310–2322.

Albers GW, Caplan LR, Easton JD, et al. Transient ischemic attack—proposal for a new definition. *N Engl J Med.* 2002;347:1713–1716.

Alvarez-Sabin J, Lozano M, Sastre-Garriga J, et al. Transient ischemic attack: a common initial manifestation of cardiac myxomas. *Eur Neurol.* 2001;45:165–170.

Benavente O, Eliasziw M, Streifler JY, et al. Prognosis after transient monocular blindness associated with carotid-artery stenosis. *N Engl J Med.* 2001;345:1084–1090.

Blaser T, Hofmann K, Buerger T, et al. Risk of stroke, transient ischemic attack, and vessel occlusion before endarterectomy in patients with symptomatic severe carotid stenosis. *Stroke.* 2002;33:1057–1062.

Clark TG, Murphy MF, Rothwell PM. Long-term risks of stroke, myocardial infarction, and vascular death in "low risk" patients with a non-recent transient ischemic attack. *J Neurol Neurosurg Psychiatry.* 2003;74:577–580.

Coutts SB, Modi J, Patel SK, et al. CT/CT angiography and MRI findings predict recurrent stroke after transient ischemic attack and minor stroke: results of the prospective CATCH study. *Stroke.* 2012;43:1013–1017.

Crisostamo RA, Garcia MM, Tong DC. Detection of diffusion-weighted MRI abnormalities in patients with transient ischemic attack; correlation with clinical characteristics. *Stroke*. 2003;34:932–937.

Demirkaya S, Topcuoglu MA, Vural D. Fibromuscular dysplasia of the basilar artery: a case presenting with vertebrobasilar TIAs. *Eur J Neurol*. 2001;8: 89–90.

Gerstner E, Liberato B, Wright CB. Bi-hemispheric anterior cerebral artery with drop attacks and limb shaking TIAs. *Neurology*. 2005;65:174.

Giles MF, Albers GW, Amarenco P, et al. Early stroke risk and ABCD2 score performance in tissue- vs time-defined TIA. A multicenter study. *Neurology*. 2011;77:1222–1228.

Johnston SC, Gress DR, Browner WS, et al. Short-term prognosis after emergency department diagnosis of TIA. *JAMA*. 2000;284:2901–2906.

Johnston SC, Rothwell PM, Nguyen-Huynh MN, et al. Validation and refinement of scores to predict very early stroke risk after transient ischaemic attack. *Lancet*. 2007;369:283–292.

Johnston SC, Sidney S, Bernstein AL, et al. A comparison of risk factors for recurrent TIA and stroke in patients diagnosed with TIA. *Neurology*. 2003;60:280–285.

Kidwell CS, Alger JR, Di Salle F, et al. Diffusion MRI in patients with transient ischemic attacks. *Stroke*. 1999;30:2762.

Kiyohara T, Kamouchi M, Kumai Y, et al. ABCD3 and ABCD3-I scores are superior to ABCD2 score in the prediction of short- and long-term risks of stroke after transient ischemic attack. *Stroke*. 2014;45:418–425.

Klempen NL, Janardhan V, Schwartz RB, et al. Shaking limb transient ischemic attacks: unusual presentation of carotid artery occlusive disease. Report of two cases. *Neurosurgery*. 2002;51:483–487.

Lazar RM, Fitzsimmons BF, Marshall RS, et al. Midazolam challenge reinduces neurological deficits after transient ischemic attack. *Stroke*. 2003;34:794–796.

Lovett JK, Dennis MS, Sandercock PA, et al. Very early risk of stroke after a first transient ischemic attack. *Stroke*. 2003;34(suppl):e138–e140.

Merwick A, Albers GW, Amarenco P, et al. Addition of brain and carotid imaging to the ABCD² score to identify patients at early risk of stroke after transient ischaemic attack: a multicentre observational study. *Lancet Neurol*. 2010;9(11):1060–1069.

Poisson SN, Nguyen-Huynh MN, Johnston SC, et al. Intracranial large vessel occlusion as a predictor of decline in functional status after transient ischemic attack. *Stroke*. 2011;42:44–47.

Prabhakaran S. Reversible brain ischemia: lessons from transient ischemic attack. *Curr Opin Neurol*. 2007;20:65–70.

Rovira A, Rovira-Gols A, Pedraza S, et al. Diffusion-weighted MR imaging in the acute phase of transient ischemic attacks. *Am J Neuroradiol*. 2002;23:77–83.

Shah KH, Kleckner K, Edlow JA. Short-term prognosis of stroke among patients diagnosed in the emergency department with a transient ischemic attack. *Ann Emerg Med*. 2008;51:316–323.

Wu CM, McLaughlin K, Lorenzetti DL, et al. Early risk of stroke after transient ischemic attack: a systematic review and meta-analysis. *Arch Intern Med*. 2007;167:2417–2422.

Hypoxic–Ischemic Encephalopathy 37

Alexandra S. Reynolds and Sachin Agarwal

INTRODUCTION

Hypoxic–ischemic encephalopathy (HIE) is a term used to describe cerebral dysfunction after a global insult to the brain. Mechanisms of such damage include prolonged interruption of blood flow and/or oxygen, most commonly after cardiac arrest.

EPIDEMIOLOGY

Approximately 630,000 cardiac arrests occur in the United States per year with an overall 14% survival to discharge. Despite an increased survival from all-rhythm cardiac arrest, the mortality is at least 50% in those who have survived to the hospital admission and overall disease-specific mortality is around 90%. Brain injury alone is the primary cause in 68% of patients. Among all out-of-hospital cardiac arrest patients between 2000 and 2006, patients who found in asystolic arrest had the worst outcomes (1% survival to discharge and 0.5% 30-day survival), whereas those with shockable initial rhythm (ventricular fibrillation [VF] or pulseless ventricular tachycardia) had the best outcomes (15%–20% survival to discharge). Those with pulseless electrical activity (PEA) fell somewhere in the middle (5%–8% survival to discharge). In general, the faster the return to spontaneous circulation (ROSC), the better the outcome.

These numbers do not capture the neurologic morbidity associated with cardiac arrest. Those who survive may still have significant neurologic deficits including personality changes and problems with memory. Further, a proportion of patients will ultimately remain in minimally conscious or persistent vegetative states. The true proportions are unknown because of high rates of withdrawal of care in patients who remain comatose after a cardiac arrest leading to a "self-fulfilling prophecy."

PATHOBIOLOGY: CAUSES OF HYPOXIC–ISCHEMIC ENCEPHALOPATHY

CARDIAC ARREST

Cardiopulmonary arrest is a complex process that causes diffuse damage to the brain. The initial mechanisms of damage include hypoxemia and hypoperfusion due to circulatory arrest. However, as the cardiac arrest progresses, damage is caused by resultant hypoglycemia, acidosis, and toxin accumulation (see following text). The model of cardiac arrest resuscitation involves three time-sensitive ischemic–reperfusion phases, including electrical, circulatory, and metabolic. Although rapid reperfusion is needed after ischemia, it can also paradoxically contribute to tissue injury and destruction. Various mechanisms of cell death, including necrosis, apoptosis, and autophagy-associated cell death, have been implicated. Tissue necrosis results in swelling and this is exacerbated by rebound hyperemia from reperfusion as well as progression of the inflammatory cascade. On a molecular level, reintroduction of glucose causes formation of nitric oxide and oxygen free radicals that can induce DNA damage and consumption of NAD+ leading to a second round of cell death. Studies involving cellular, animal, and human models suggest that therapeutic hypothermia (TH) has the potential to mitigate these deleterious processes (Table 37.1) even after a period of ischemia. Models where hypothermia was initiated before reperfusion have resulted in the most cellular protection.

PROLONGED HYPOTENSION

Hypotension results in preferential injury to parts of the central nervous system that lie in between vascular distributions. Areas supplied by narrowed arteries are also at risk for hypoperfusion in low-flow states like carotid stenosis or in heart failure with low cardiac output. Low cerebral blood flow results in patchy ischemic infarctions. Watershed areas in the brain affected by hypotension include the cortical border zones between the anterior cerebral and middle cerebral arteries (ACA-MCA) and middle cerebral and posterior cerebral arteries (MCA-PCA) or internal border zone areas in the periventricular white matter or the deep structures supplied by the recurrent artery of Heubner and the anterior choroidal and

TABLE 37.1	Mechanisms of Neuroprotection with Therapeutic Hypothermia
Metabolic	Decreased cerebral metabolism (6%–10%/°C below 37°C)
	Inhibition of mitochondrial injury and dysfunction
	Decreased production of toxic metabolites and free radicals
Neuroinflammatory	Decreased generation of inflammatory proteins
	Decreased release of glutamate and decreased neuroexcitotoxicity
Vascular	Decreased vascular permeability and edema
	Decreased cerebral thermopooling, reducing local hyperthermia
Cellular	Decreased ion pump dysfunction and decreased intracellular calcium influx
	Decreased cell membrane leakage and cytotoxic edema
	Decreased apoptosis and proteolysis
Other	Decreased spreading depression-type depolarizations
	Suppression of epileptic activity
	Decreased coagulation activation with formation of fewer microthrombi

lenticulostriate arteries. In the spinal cord, the anterior portion of the midthoracic distribution is considered to be the watershed region; however, one study showed disproportionate damage to the lumbosacral spinal cord after prolonged hypotension and/or cardiac arrest.

HYPOXIA

Pure hypoxic hypoxia can occur in the absence of circulatory breakdown, in the case of aspiration, hanging/strangulation, or drowning. Hypoxic damage to the brain occurs solely due to decreased partial pressure of blood oxygen and results in a lesser degree of injury than combined hypoxic-ischemia. However, prolonged hypoxia will progress to cardiac arrest. Once oxygen supply to the brain is interrupted, adenosine triphosphate (ATP) stores only last for minutes. After energy-dependent membrane ion transport starts to fail, damaged cells release excitotoxic glutamate, intracellular calcium begins to accumulate and activates proteases and phospholipases, and damage is propagated via inflammatory cascades. Intracellular influx of calcium in surrounding areas leads to diffuse cell death. The areas particularly susceptible to hypoxic damage are hippocampal CA1 neurons, thalami, cerebellar Purkinje cells, and cortical pyramidal cells in layers 3, 5, and 6. Among the cortical areas, perirolandic areas are most vulnerable because of the high concentration of N-methyl-D-aspartate (NMDA) receptors. White matter injury also occurs because of damage to oligodendroglial cells.

CARBON MONOXIDE POISONING

Carbon monoxide (CO) primarily exerts harmful effects to the brain by causing hypoxemia in a so-called anemic–histotoxic hypoxia. As in hypoxic hypoxia, preservation of circulation portends a lesser damage to the brain. CO preferentially binds to heme proteins and displaces bound oxygen because of its greater affinity for hemoglobin. CO thus limits oxygen-carrying capacity of blood and impairs mitochondrial function of the tissues attempting to use oxygen, resulting in a hypoxic and acidotic state. Ultimately, CO poisoning causes intravascular and intracellular oxidative stress, inflammation, and apoptosis. The cortical laminae and basal ganglia are particularly prone to damage. Additional reports of delayed demyelination in the centrum semiovale have been published. In severe cases, cardiac toxicity can occur resulting in hypotensive brain injury as well.

CYANIDE POISONING

Cyanide poisoning causes metabolic failure by inhibiting oxidative phosphorylation. It results in direct metabolic damage to the brain but ultimately causes mixed injury due to early cardiac failure. Cyanide impairs oxidative phosphorylation by inhibiting the mitochondrial cytochrome oxidase a_3 complex. Mitochondria are unable to produce ATP and increased glycolysis occurs, quickly resulting in a metabolic acidosis as pyruvate is reduced to lactate. Coronary artery vasoconstriction occurs and cardiac output decreases suddenly, causing hypotension and cardiac shock. The brain is damaged not only from this hypotension but also from metabolic failure on a cellular level.

PROFOUND HYPOGLYCEMIA

Glucose is the primary source of energy for the brain in both adults and in infants, and prolonged or repeated hypoglycemic episodes can therefore cause significant injury to the brain. Concurrent hypoglycemia also exacerbates the damage caused by hypoxemia. Brain damage usually occurs once serum glucose levels fall below 20 mg/dL. Mechanisms of cell death with hypoglycemia are similar to hypoxia, including excitotoxic glutamate and aspartate release and involvement of NMDA receptors. More recent studies have shown that activation of poly (ADP ribose) polymerase-1 (PARP-1), release of zinc from nerve terminals, and activation of calcium-dependent protease calpain also contribute to neuronal death. Further, depolarization of the mitochondrial membrane leads to apoptosis. The parts of the brain most sensitive to low-glucose levels are the hippocampus (CA1, CA3, and dentate gyrus), caudate, putamen, and insular cortex.

Damage from hypoxic–ischemic injury also changes as the brain matures. In neonates, HIE often results in parietooccipital and thalamic damage, whereas in infants, basal ganglia damage is more frequent and in children, parietotemporal changes are seen.

CLINICAL FEATURES

The clinical manifestations of HIE can range from mild changes in cognition to coma. Damage to the hippocampus can result in memory deficits. Damage to the basal ganglia can present as a variety of movement disorders. Thalamic damage can result in a wide variety of symptoms from sensory changes to dementia or coma. Damage to the Purkinje cells results in cerebellar dysfunction. Cortical damage can result in inattentiveness, executive dysfunction, or aphasia. Because of the resistance of the deep gray matter of the brain stem to anoxic injury compared with the neocortex, HIE often results in coma with preservation of brain stem reflexes. However, brain death can occur with prolonged hypoxic–ischemic injury.

Watershed injury in the brain can manifest as proximal greater than distal extremity weakness and ultimately spasticity ("man-in-a-barrel syndrome"). Watershed injury to the spinal cord results in an "anterior cord syndrome" or Beck syndrome, including motor paralysis below the level of the lesion, loss of pain and temperature but intact proprioception and vibratory sensation, and loss of bowel and/or bladder control.

Lance-Adams syndrome, or posthypoxic action myoclonus, can occur several days after recovery from hypoxic injury to the brain.

The rare syndrome of delayed posthypoxic leukoencephalopathy (DPHL) following seemingly full recovery from a comatose state can occur days to weeks after the initial insult. The onset is usually insidious and can manifest as personality changes, irritability, inattentiveness, confusion, and memory problems. This can progress to include extrapyramidal motor symptoms and, in some cases, eventually coma or death. Those patients who survive stabilize to one of two ultimate syndromes: either parkinsonism with hallucinations or odd behaviors, or akinetic mutism. DPHL may occur as a result of any cause of HIE mentioned earlier but is most often seen in cases of acute CO poisoning or opioid overdose. The main histopathologic patterns seen in this syndrome are demyelination in the centrum semiovale and necrosis of the cortical laminae and basal ganglia, which correlate with brain magnetic resonance imaging (MRI) features. Severity and persistence of DPHL sequelae have been correlated to the presence and persistence of low signal intensity on the apparent diffusion coefficient (ADC) map on cranial MRI.

DIAGNOSIS

IMAGING

CT head is usually normal immediately after hypoxic–ischemic insult. In severe injury, there can be evidence of loss of the gray–white junction within hours (Fig. 37.1A). After 24 to 48 hours, linear hyperdensities outlining the cortex develop, corresponding to laminar necrosis of the cortex. After days, the "reversal sign" develops where cerebral white matter appears hyperdense than cortical gray matter. Pseudosubarachnoid hemorrhage can also occur when the falx cerebri and tentorium cerebelli appear hyperdense as compared to the adjacent injured parenchyma (see Fig. 37.1B).

MRI brain is the earliest way to visualize damage, as early cytotoxic edema can be visualized on diffusion-weighted imaging (DWI) and can be quantified using the ADC (see Fig. 37.1C–G). Importantly, DWI and ADC changes may not be apparent early on and thus early imaging may underestimate the injury burden. Moreover, there may be attenuation of ADC values for every 1°C decrease in body temperature. DWI sequences can pseudonormalize by seven days but T2 hyperintensities on fluid-attenuated inversion recovery (FLAIR) sequences develop after the first week. The damage is most often symmetric and corresponds in location to the neuronal subtypes that are preferentially damaged (see pathobiology section). With time, focal laminar necrosis can be seen due to deposition of blood products (see Fig. 37.1E). In one small study, changes occurring over time within the same patient were analyzed. The location of the injury shifts with time from the initial hypoxic–ischemic event, starting in the cerebellum and basal ganglia in days 1 and 2, moving to the cortex around days 3 to 5, and involving subcortical white matter on days 6 to 12. Pronounced hippocampal abnormalities on DWI—the so-called bright hippocampus sign—has been associated with extremely poor outcomes (see Fig. 37.1C,D). In the case of DPHL, MRI findings are pathognomonic, with diffuse T2 hyperintensities predominantly in the dorsal frontal and parietal lobes.

SOMATOSENSORY-EVOKED POTENTIALS

A noninvasive way to evaluate the functioning of the somatosensory system in a comatose patient is by performing evoked potentials. There are multiple types of evoked potentials including auditory and visual; however, somatosensory-evoked potentials (SSEPs) are most commonly used after a hypoxic–ischemic event or cardiac arrest. SSEPs are done by providing a transcutaneous electrical stimulation along a peripheral nerve, most commonly the median nerve. The impulse is then tracked as it travels up the peripheral nerve to the elbow (N5), Erb point in the brachial plexus (N9), the posterior column of the midcervical cord (N13), and ultimately to the contralateral primary sensory cortex (N20). In cases of significant cortical damage, the N20 can be absent (Fig. 37.2).

ELECTROENCEPHALOGRAPHY

The 2006 AAN practice parameters emphasized the importance of identifying electrographic seizures and burst suppression for prognostication, but minimal data was available at that time. In last few years, there have been many studies describing the evo-

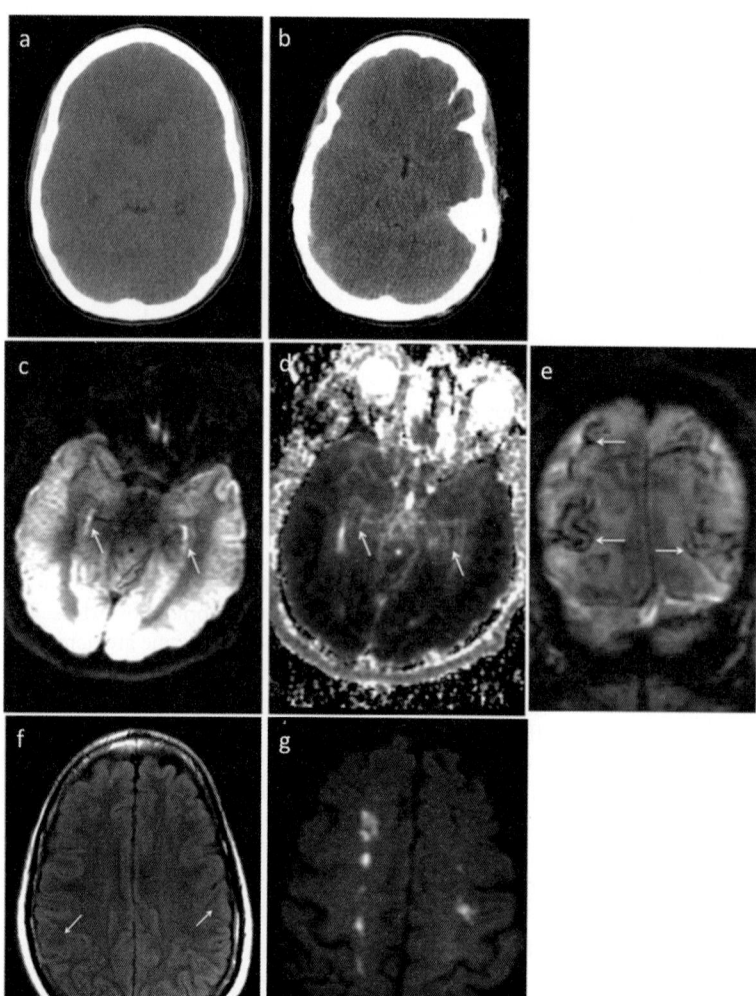

FIGURE 37.1 Imaging findings after HIE. CT scan done **(A)** 12 hours and **(B)** 10 days after a near-drowning episode. **A:** There is diffuse loss of gray–white matter differentiation and severe global cerebral edema. There are bilateral, but right greater than left, hypodensities of the basal ganglia. **B:** The diffusely attenuated white and gray matter result in a pseudosubarachnoid hemorrhage appearance of the relatively hyperdense dura. DWI **(C)** and ADC **(D)** sequences of an MRI done 2 days after a primary respiratory arrest showing restricted diffusion in the bilateral hippocampi (*arrows*) and diffusely throughout the cortex. **E:** Susceptibility-weighted imaging (SWI) sequence in coronal section done 7 days after a PEA arrest showing areas of laminar necrosis in the posterior parietal lobes (*arrows*). **F:** FLAIR sequence 10 days after cardio-pulmonary arrest only showing mild swelling and indistinctness of the gray–white junction in the bilateral parietal lobes (*arrows*). **G:** DWI sequence of an MRI done 11 days after a PEA arrest resulting from a type A aortic dissection. There are scattered foci of restricted diffusion along the ACA-MCA and MCA-PCA border zones, more prominent on the right, consistent with watershed infarct.

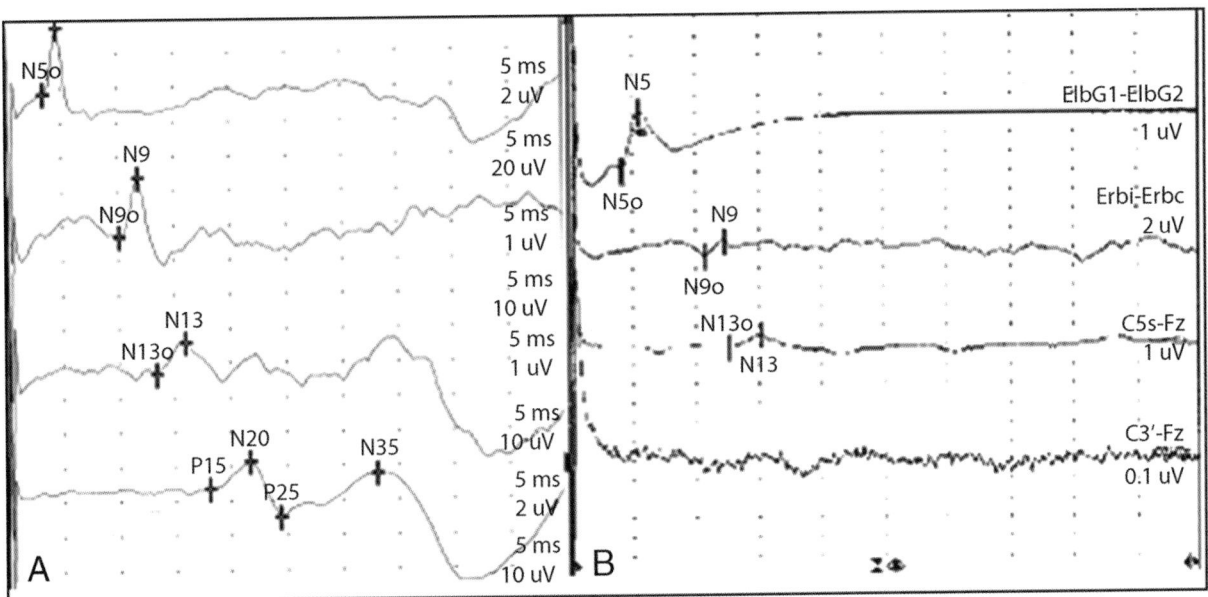

FIGURE 37.2 Median nerve somatosensory-evoked potentials. **A:** The normal SSEP tracing including the N5 waveform at the elbow, N9 at Erb point, N13 at the cervical cord, and N20 at the contralateral sensory cortex. **B:** An absent N20 after hypoxic–ischemic injury from cardiac arrest. (Chiota NA, Freeman WD, Barrett KM. Hypoxic-ischemic brain injury and prognosis after cardiac arrest. *Continuum Lifelong Learning Neurol.* 2011;17(5):1094–1118.)

lution of electroencephalography (EEG) during hypothermia and after rewarming. The occurrence of seizures more in the first 24 hours, that is, during hypothermia phase, was to be an unexpected observation. Therefore, many experts recommend early and prolonged EEG monitoring. Most studies have confirmed an incidence of seizures in 25% of patients, and status epilepticus at any point during the hospital course is thought to be a bad prognostic indicator. However, patients have achieved good outcomes after seizures were detected and treated aggressively. The most common finding on EEG is generalized periodic discharges that are also known to be a precursor of seizures and thus poor outcomes, but more systematic evaluation of different patterns needs to be done. EEG background features like continuity and reactivity have also been shown to be predictive of outcomes, i.e., persistence of continuous background and EEG reactivity in first few days of the event is associated with good recovery. Further research in this area is warranted and eventually inclusion of appropriate, well-studied EEG patterns should be a part of multimodal prognostication paradigm.

TREATMENT

GENERAL CONCEPTS

Intracranial pressure (ICP) can increase after cardiac arrest both because of reflex hyperemia post arrest and because of global cerebral edema in cases of significant global injury. High ICP and low cerebral perfusion pressures (CPP) are associated with poor outcomes. ICP also increases with seizure activity.

Hyperoxia is correlated with worse outcomes in humans. Each 100 mm Hg increase in PaO_2 above the normal level of 100 mm Hg is associated with 24% increased risk of mortality. Unnecessary increases in the fraction of inspired oxygen should be avoided. The goal for $PaCO_2$ should be on the higher end of normocapnia, as lower ends of the threshold are associated with decreased cerebral blood flow (CBF).

SEIZURES

With cortical damage comes the potential for development of complex, evolving epileptiform discharges and/or seizures. Early detection and treatment of seizures is paramount to prevent further brain damage. Myoclonic status epilepticus, characterized as a poor prognostic marker in pre-TH era, has been questioned by more recent small studies and case reports. The definition involved spontaneous, unrelenting, generalized, multifocal myoclonus involving face, limbs, and axial musculature but no EEG correlate was needed for the diagnosis. EEG monitoring with a trial of paralytic to remove muscle artifact, if necessary, should be attempted and if the patient is found to be in electrographic status epilepticus, they should be treated aggressively.

THERAPEUTIC HYPOTHERMIA

Beginning in the 1950s, cardiothoracic surgeons used moderate hypothermia (28°C to 32°C) during cardiac surgery to prevent brain ischemia. The idea of cooling after unexpected cardiac arrest and subsequent resuscitation, however, was not seriously pursued until the early 1990s, when animal studies became popular. In 2002, two randomized controlled trials were published suggesting that patients in cardiac arrest with an initial rhythm of VF who remained comatose after ROSC had better outcomes after mild TH to 32°C to 33°C for 12 to 24 hours [**Level 1**].[1,2] More recently, it was shown that there is no benefit to cooling to 33°C when compared to 36°C [**Level 1**].[3] It is recommended that all comatose survivors of cardiac arrest be cooled, despite there being a dearth of data supporting cooling after PEA or asystole. TH is neuroprotective in many ways (see Table 37.1). The hypothermia protocol is complex (Table 37.2) and requires close monitoring for shivering via the Bedside Shivering Assessment Scale (BSAS) (Table 37.3). Sometimes, EEG can detect microshivering that is not palpable on the neck or thorax. Shivering must be treated aggressively, as it increases metabolic demand, raises the patient's core temperature, causes tachycardia, and can increase ICP.

TABLE 37.2   Hypothermia Checklist

Contraindications

Absolute contraindications:

- Refractory bleeding at a noncompressible site or uncontrollable bleeding
- Severe and recurrent symptomatic bradycardia requiring pacing or continuous medial therapy

Relative contraindications (consider cooling to 36°C instead of 33°C):

- Acute multisystem organ failure due to prolonged arrest
- Hemodynamic instability requiring more than two vasopressors and/or recurrent cardiac arrests
- Mild bradycardia
- Concurrent meningitis
- Severe systemic infection and/or sepsis
- Significant trauma with high risk of internal bleeding
- Severe baseline neurologic or medical disorders
- Pregnancy or postpartum patient
- Head trauma with intracranial bleeding

Induction of Hypothermia

- Immediate initiation of cooling with ice packs, infusion of cold saline, and cooling blanket (protecting the skin from direct contact)
- Use of one of the following devices: Arctic Sun (superficial cooling pads) or Alsius or Innercool (intravascular temperature modulation devices)
- Administration of one-time paralytic dose for expediting cooling with rocuronium or vecuronium
- Central temperature monitoring with bladder or esophageal probe
- Maintain temperature for 24 hours after initiation of hypothermia.

Shivering

- cEEG to detect microshivering
- Goal Bedside Shivering Assessment Scale (BSAS) ≤1
- Acetaminophen 650 q4h standing
- Buspar 30 mg PO q8 standing
- Meperidine 25 mg IV q6h PRN shivering
- BAIR hugger set at 43°C for skin counterwarming
- If shivering refractory, can start Mg gtt at 0.5–1 g/h with goal Mg level 3–4 mEq/L
- If shivering still refractory, can add fentanyl, propofol, or dexmedetomidine gtts
- If shivering remains refractory to sedation, start neuromuscular blockade (must be on sedation) with vecuronium 0.1mg/kg IV qh or rocuronium or cisatracurium gtts.

Seizures and Myoclonus

- Continuous EEG to identify seizures
- Treat seizures aggressively with phenytoin, valproic acid, levetiracetam, or benzodiazepines.
- Noncortical myoclonus (i.e., Lance–Adams syndrome) has no effect on outcome but can be treated for comfort with levetiracetam, valproic acid, gabapentin, or benzodiazepines.

Rewarming to Normothermia

- Rewarm at 0.1 to 0.2°C/h to a goal of 37°C.
- Shivering is most common during rewarming and should be treated aggressively.

Other Monitoring

- Electrolytes should be monitored and repleted to a goal of K = 3.0 mEq/L, as overrepletion can result in hyperkalemia during rewarming.
- Platelets should be transfused for goal >20,000 or >50,000 if active bleeding.
- Send serum NSE daily for 3 days.

cEEG, continuous electroencephalography; PO, by mouth; IV, intravenous; PRN, as needed; Mg, magnesium; gtt, drip; EEG, electroencephalography; NSE, neuron-specific enolase.

TABLE 37.3   Bedside Shivering Assessment Scale

Score		Location of Shivering
0	None	None detected on palpation of masseter, neck, and chest muscles
1	Mild	Shivering localized to neck and thorax only
2	Moderate	Shivering involves gross movement of the arms and trunk.
3	Severe	Shivering involves gross movement of the arms, legs, and trunk.

OUTCOME

In 2006, the American Academy of Neurology published guidelines for prognostication in comatose survivors of cardiac arrest after an exhaustive review of the literature (Fig. 37.3). Features that nearly guaranteed poor outcome were early clinical (not electrographic) myoclonic status epilepticus, absent N20 responses on SSEPs in the first 72 hours after arrest, absent corneal or pupillary reflexes or extensor or absent motor response to pain at 72 hours, and serum neuron-specific enolase (NSE) greater than 33 μg/L. Subsequent studies looking at routine use of hypothermia in comatose patients post arrest have revealed an unacceptably high false-positive rate of almost every feature (see Fig. 37.3). These findings have prompted further studies on prognostic factors that may be valid for use in the posthypothermia era.

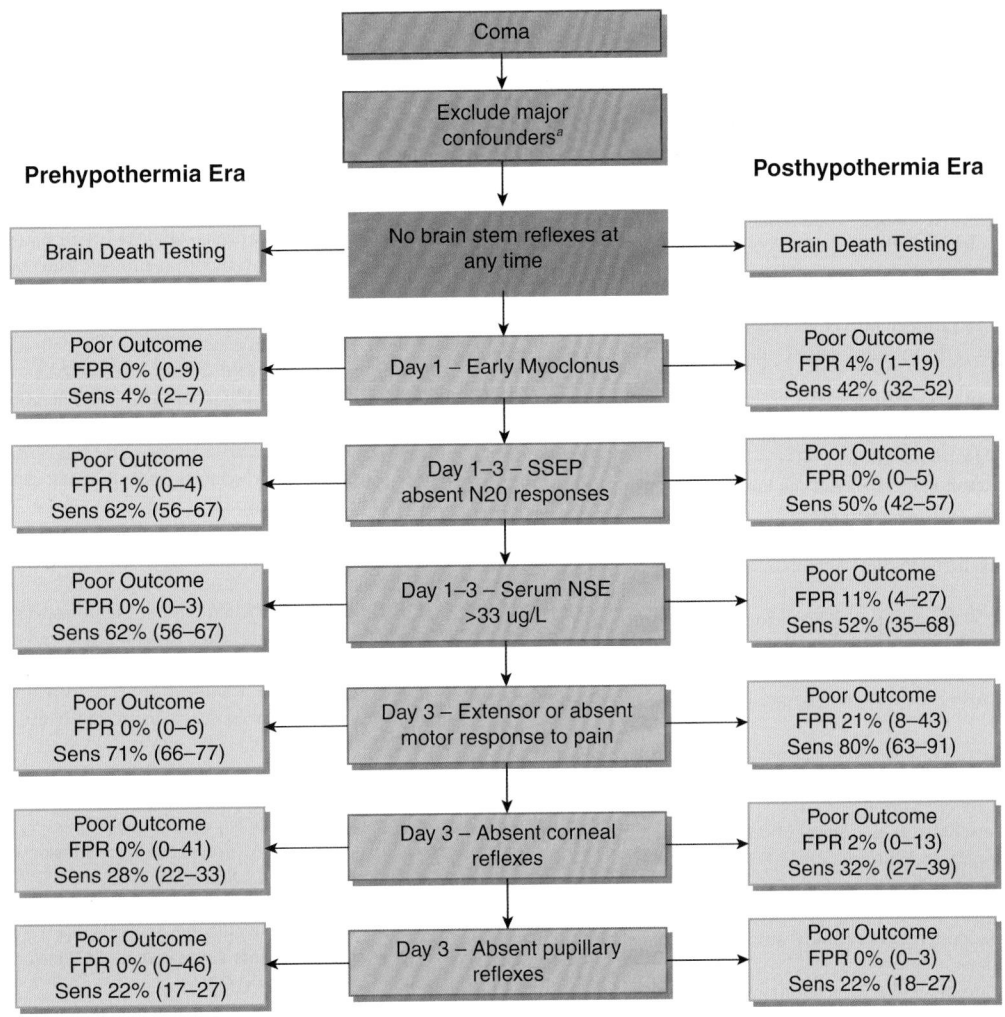

FIGURE 37.3 Prognostication algorithm in comatose survivors of cardiac arrest. On the *left* appear false-positive rate (FPR) and sensitivity of each feature in the prehypothermia era, on the *right* in the posthypothermia era. For posthypothermia era, in cases of multiple studies, the data from the study with the largest number of subjects were used. ªMajor confounders at the time of examination include hypothermia, sedatives/hypnotics, and paralytics. (Adapted from Wijdicks EF, Hijdra A, Young GB, et al. Practice parameter: prediction of outcome in comatose survivors after cardiopulmonary resuscitation [an evidence-based review]: report of the Quality Standards Subcommittee of the American Academy of Neurology. *Neurology.* 2006;67:203–210.)

Other biomarkers being studied as predictors of clinical outcome include brain-specific markers such as S100-B and micro-RNAs, inflammatory markers including C-reactive protein and the interleukins, and neurohormonal markers such as copeptin. The role of imaging in prognostication is also being studied. In particular, MRI has been studied in an attempt to quantify extent of cerebral damage on ADC. Ultimately, there may be a combination of biomarker and imaging data that may aid in prognostication when the patient's outcome is otherwise indeterminate based on clinical exam, NSE, and SSEP.

It is important to keep in mind the so-called self-fulfilling prophecy that occurs in clinical practice and is a limitation in many studies on outcome after cardiac arrest. There is always a temptation to prognosticate earlier and earlier due to scarcity of resources, anxious families, and astronomical health care costs. Additionally, results of tests that may not accurately predict outcome in the post-TH era can influence clinician decision making.

These tests are studied as predictors of outcome but often directly affect the clinician's decision making and counseling to families—thereby confounding any study of outcome. Moving forward, outcome measures need to be changed from survival to degree of neuropsychological impairment in survivors.

LEVEL 1 EVIDENCE

1. Hypothermia after Cardiac Arrest Study Group. Mild therapeutic hypothermia to improve the neurologic outcome after cardiac arrest. *N Engl J Med.* 2002;346:549–556.
2. Bernard SA, Gray TW, Buist MD, et al. Treatment of comatose survivors of out-of-hospital cardiac arrest with induced hypothermia. *N Engl J Med.* 2002;346:557–563.
3. Nielsen N, Wetterslev J, Cronberg T, et al. Targeted temperature management at 33°C versus 36°C after cardiac arrest. *N Engl J Med.* 2014;369:2197–2206.

SUGGESTED READINGS

Adrie C, Adib-Conquy M, Laurent I, et al. Successful cardiopulmonary resuscitation after cardiac arrest as a "sepsis-like" syndrome. *Circulation*. 2002; 106:562–568.

Arbelaez A, Castillo M, Mukherji SK. Diffusion-weighted MR imaging of global cerebral anoxia. *AJNR Am J Neuroradiol*. 1999;20:999–1007.

Bettermann K, Patel S. Neurologic complications of carbon monoxide intoxication. In: Biller J, Ferro JM, eds. *Neurologic Aspects of Systemic Disease Part II—Handbook of Clinical Neurology*. 3rd series. Amsterdam, The Netherlands: Elsevier; 2014:971–979.

Bouwes A, Binnekade JM, Kuiper MA, et al. Prognosis of coma after therapeutic hypothermia: a prospective cohort study. *Ann Neurol*. 2012;71: 206–212.

Daubin C, Quentin C, Allouche S, et al. Serum neuron-specific enolase as predictor of outcome in comatose cardiac-arrest survivors: a prospective cohort study. *BMC Cardiovasc Disord*. 2011;11:48.

Duggal N, Lach B. Selective vulnerability of the lumbosacral spinal cord after cardiac arrest. *Stroke*. 2002;33:116–121.

Els T, Kassubek J, Kubalek R, et al. Diffusion-weighted MRI during early global cerebral hypoxia: a predictor for clinical outcome? *Acta Neurol Scand*. 2004;110:361–367.

Fugate JE, Wijdicks EF, Mandrekar J, et al. Predictors of neurologic outcome in hypothermia after cardiac arrest. *Ann Neurol*. 2010;68:907–914.

Go AS, Mozaffarian D, Roger VL, et al. Heart disease and stroke statistics—2014 update: a report from the American Heart Association. *Circulation*. 2014;129: e28–e292.

Greer DM, Rosenthal ES, Wu O. Neuroprognostication of hypoxic-ischaemic coma in the therapeutic hypothermia era. *Nat Rev Neurol*. 2014;10: 190–203.

Greer D, Scripko P, Bartscher J, et al. Clinical MRI interpretation for outcome prediction in cardiac arrest. *Neurocrit Care*. 2012;17:240–244.

Jarnum H, Knutsson L, Rundgren M, et al. Diffusion and perfusion MRI of the brain in comatose patients treated with mild hypothermia after cardiac arrest: a prospective observational study. *Resuscitation*. 2009;80: 425–430.

Kamps MJ, Horn J, Oddo M, et al. Prognostication of neurologic outcome in cardiac arrest patients after mild therapeutic hypothermia: a meta-analysis of the current literature. *Intensive Care Med*. 2013;39:1671–1682.

Kilgannon JH, Jones AE, Parrillo JE, et al. Relationship between supranormal oxygen tension and outcome after resuscitation from cardiac arrest. *Circulation*. 2011;123:2717–2722.

Kim F, Nichol G, Maynard C, et al. Effect of prehospital induction of mild hypothermia on survival and neurological status among adults with cardiac arrest: a randomized clinical trial. *JAMA*. 2014;311:45–52.

Kim J, Choi BS, Kim K, et al. Prognostic performance of diffusion-weighted MRI combined with NSE in comatose cardiac survivors treated with mild hypothermia. *Neurocrit Care*. 2012;17:412–420.

Languren G, Montiel T, Julio-Amilpas A, et al. Neuronal damage and cognitive impairment associated with hypoglycemia: an integrated view. *Neurochem Int*. 2013;63:331–343.

Muttikkal TJ, Wintermark M. MRI patterns of global hypoxic-ischemic injury in adults. *J Neuroradiol*. 2013;40:164–171.

Oksanen T, Tiainen M, Skrifvars MB. Predictive power of serum NSE and OHCA score regarding 6-month neurologic outcome after out-of-hospital ventricular fibrillation and therapeutic hypothermia. *Resuscitation*. 2009;80: 165–170.

Polderman KH. Mechanisms of action, physiologic effects, and complications of hypothermia. *Crit Care Med*. 2009;37:S186–S202.

Pynnönen L, Falkenbach P, Kämäräinen A, et al. Therapeutic hypothermia after cardiac arrest—cerebral perfusion and metabolism during upper and lower threshold normocapnia. *Resuscitation*. 2011;82:1174–1179.

Rossetti AO, Oddo M, Logroscino G, et al. Prognostication after cardiac arrest and hypothermia: a prospective study. *Ann Neurol*. 2010;67:301–307.

Rossetti AO, Urbano LA, Delodder F, et al. Prognostic value of continuous EEG monitoring during therapeutic hypothermia after cardiac arrest. *Crit Care*. 2010;14:R173.

Rundgren M, Karlsson T, Nielsen N, et al. Neuron specific enolase and S-100B as predictors of outcome after cardiac arrest and induced hypothermia. *Resuscitation*. 2009;80:784–789.

Samaniego EA, Mlynash M, Caulfield AF, et al. Sedation confounds outcome prediction in cardiac arrest survivors treated with hypothermia. *Neurocrit Care*. 2011;15:113–119.

Satran R. Spinal cord infarction. *Stroke*. 1988;19:529–532.

Shprecher D, Mehta L. The syndrome of delayed post-hypoxic leukoencephalopathy. *NeuroRehabilitation*. 2010;26:65–72.

Singhal AB, Topcuoglu MA, Koroshetz WJ. Diffusion MRI in three types of anoxic encephalopathy. *J Neurol Sci*. 2002;196:37–40.

Steffen IG, Hasper D, Ploner CJ, et al. Mild therapeutic hypothermia alters neuron specific enolase as an outcome predictor after resuscitation: 97 prospective hypothermia patients compared to 133 historical non-hypothermia patients. *Crit Care*. 2010;14:R69.

Weaver LK. Clinical practice. Carbon monoxide poisoning. *N Engl J Med*. 2009;360:1217–1225.

Weisfeldt ML, Becker LB. Resuscitation after cardiac arrest: a 3-phase time-sensitive model. *JAMA*. 2002;288:3035–3038.

Wijman CA, Mlynash M, Caulfield AF, et al. Prognostic value of brain diffusion weighted imaging after cardiac arrest. *Ann Neurol*. 2009;65:394–402.

Wu O, Sorensen AG, Benner T, et al. Comatose patients with cardiac arrest: predicting clinical outcome with diffusion weighted MR imaging. *Radiology*. 2009;252:173–181.

38

Intracerebral Hemorrhage

Stephan A. Mayer, Fred Rincon, and J. P. Mohr

INTRODUCTION

Intracerebral hemorrhage (ICH) is defined as the acute spontaneous bleeding into the brain parenchyma (Fig. 38.1). Primary ICH results from microscopic small artery degeneration in the brain, caused either by chronic, poorly controlled hypertension (80% of cases) or amyloid angiopathy (20% of cases). Secondary ICH refers to intraparenchymal bleeding from a diagnosable anatomic vascular lesion or cause of coagulopathy (Table 38.1).

EPIDEMIOLOGY

The overall incidence of ICH is estimated to be 12 to 15 cases per 100,000/yr. As the least treatable and most devastating form of stroke, ICH is a leading cause of mortality, morbidity, and disability in the United States and worldwide, accounting for 10% to 30% of all stroke hospital admissions. Many ICH patients require long-term health care, and only 20% of patients regain functional independence. About 40% to 80% of ICH patients die within the first 30 days, and half of all deaths occur within the first 48 hours.

RISK FACTORS

Hypertension and older age are the strongest predictors of incident ICH. Studies have shown that noncompliance with antihypertensive medications increases the risk of ICH, and control of blood pressure has been shown to reduce this risk. Chronic hypertension causes a small-vessel vasculopathy characterized by fragmentation, degeneration, and the eventual rupture of small penetrating vessels within the brain termed *lipohyalinosis*. Commonly affected structures include the basal ganglia and thalamus (50%), lobar regions (33%), and brain stem and cerebellum (17%). On pathologic examination, the pattern of small-vessel damage is characterized by (1) degeneration of medial smooth muscle cells; (2) small miliary aneurysms associated with thrombosis and microhemorrhages; (3) accumulation of nonfatty debris; and (4) hyalinization of the intima, preferentially at bifurcation points and distal portions of the vessel. It is unclear why some patients develop deep brain infarcts and others develop hemorrhages, but some have implicated the sudden rupture of microaneurysms, also known as Charcot–Bouchard microaneurysms, as the basis for ICH. Other nonmodifiable risk factors for ICH include male gender and African-American or Japanese race/ethnicity.

Low cholesterol levels have been implicated as a risk factor for primary ICH, although there is controversy regarding this association, as the results from case-control and cohort studies and prospective randomized trials of cholesterol reduction have yielded conflicting results. Heavy alcohol intake has been implicated as a risk factor for ICH in several studies. In theory, alcohol may affect platelet function and coagulation physiology and enhance vascular fragility.

Cerebral amyloid angiopathy (CAA) is an important risk factor for ICH in the elderly (Fig. 38.2). CAA is characterized by the deposition of β-amyloid protein in small- to medium-sized blood vessels of the brain and leptomeninges, which may undergo

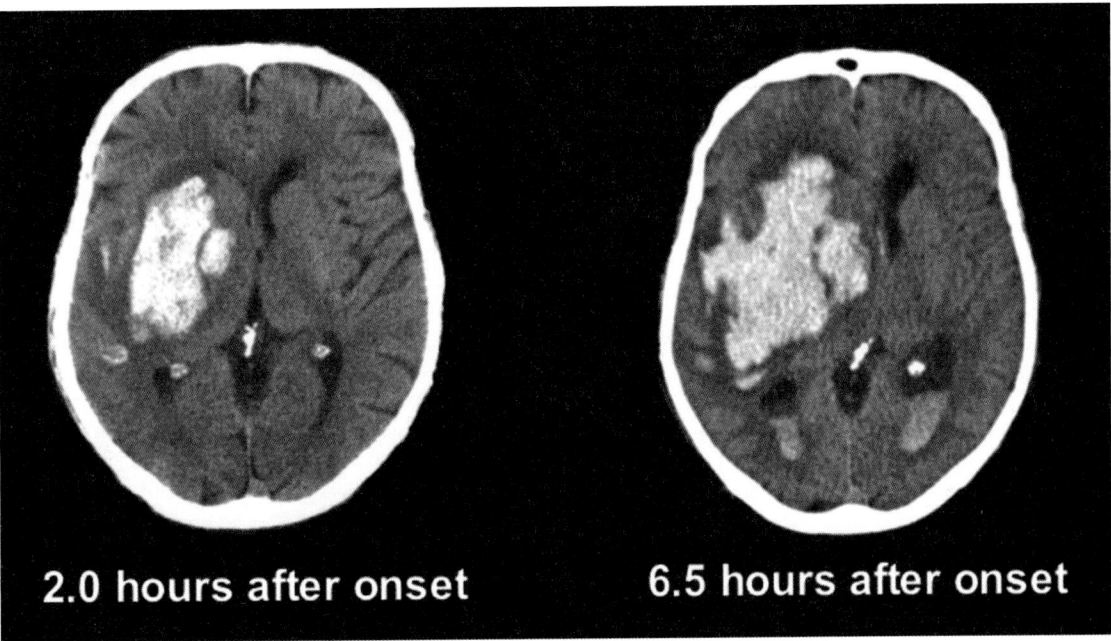

FIGURE 38.1 Basal ganglia ICH with hematoma followed by expansion and IVH.

TABLE 38.1	Etiologic Factors for Intracerebral Hemorrhage

Risk Factors for Primary Intracerebral Hemorrhage
Demographic
Age
Black race/ethnicity
Vascular risk factors
Chronic hypertension (small-vessel disease)
Alcohol
Smoking
Low cholesterol
Vascular pathology
Amyloid angiopathy (including hereditary forms)

Risk Factors for Secondary Intracerebral Hemorrhage
Brain infarction
Hemorrhagic transformation of subacute ischemic lesion
Cerebral venous/sinus thrombosis
Preexisting vascular lesions
Cavernous angioma
Arteriovenous malformation
Malignancies
Brain tumor
Cerebral metastasis
Inflammatory
Vasculitis
Endocarditis (mycotic aneurysm)
Hematologic
Coagulopathy
Thrombocytopenia
Iatrogenic
Anticoagulants
Fibrinolysis
Toxic
Cocaine
Amphetamines

fibrinoid necrosis. It can occur as a sporadic disorder, in association with Alzheimer disease, or with certain familial syndromes (apolipoprotein E2 and E4 allele). Brain tumors, sympathomimetic drugs, coagulopathies, cavernomas, and arteriovenous malformations also cause brain hemorrhages. Further differential diagnoses of underlying pathologies are summarized in Table 38.1. Although treatment with anticoagulants or fibrinolytic agents entails a higher risk of hemorrhage with increasing doses, the role of aspirin intake in this context is controversial. The detection of microbleeds in gradient echo magnetic resonance imaging (MRI) implies that aspirin is a risk factor for hemorrhage in patients on anticoagulant therapy; MRI evidence of microhemorrhages should prompt reconsideration of the indications for anticoagulation.

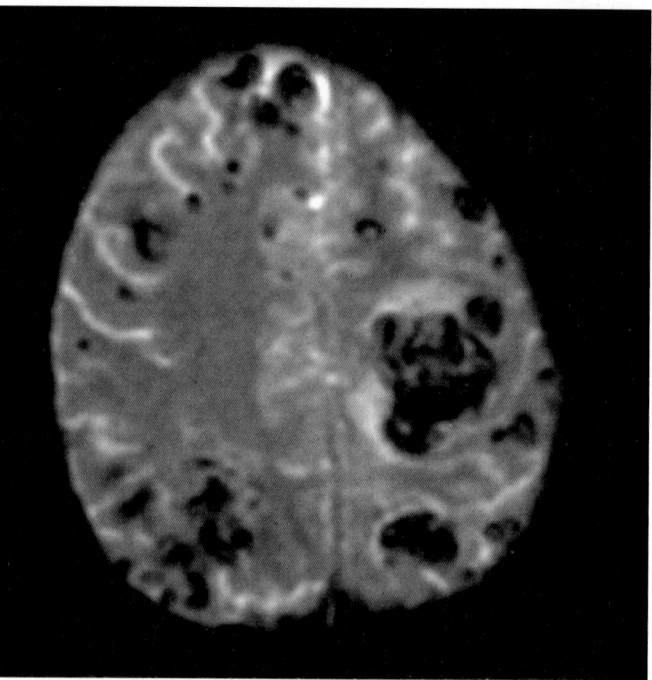

FIGURE 38.2 Gradient echo (GRE, T2*) MRI sequence showing multiple chronic cortical microbleeds, diagnostic of amyloid angiopathy.

PATHOBIOLOGY

Abrupt arterial rupture leads to rapid accumulation of blood within the brain parenchyma and increase in local tissue pressure followed by the abrupt onset of shearing forces and physical destruction. In addition to the relative mass effect, the hematoma itself induces three early pathophysiologic changes in the surrounding brain tissue: (1) neuronal and glial cell death due to apoptosis and inflammation, (2) vasogenic edema, and (3) breakdown of the blood–brain barrier (BBB).

Hematoma expansion is an important cause of early neurologic deterioration, and ICH volume is a powerful predictor of outcome after primary ICH. An expanding hematoma may result from persistent bleeding and/or rebleeding from a single arteriolar rupture. Some studies have reported evidence of ICH growth from bleeding into an ischemic penumbra zone surrounding the hematoma, but studies have not confirmed the existence of ischemia in the hypoperfused area in the periphery of the hematoma. Because ischemia does not explain the changes and degree of neurologic dysfunction that occurs after the hemorrhage, neurotoxic and inflammatory mechanisms have more recently been implicated in the pathogenesis of perihemorrhagic tissue damage.

Peri-ICH edema may be produced by local and systemic inflammatory mediators that enhance tissue damage either directly or indirectly by the activation of leukocytes, generation of prostaglandins and leukotrienes, and activation of the complement. Intracerebral blood is in part directly responsible for the formation of local edema after ICH.

CLINICAL MANIFESTATIONS

Because most spontaneous hemorrhages arise from tiny vessels, the accumulation of a hematoma takes time and explains the smooth onset of the clinical syndrome over minutes or hours.

The progressive course, frequent vomiting, and headache are major points that help to differentiate hemorrhage from infarction.

The *putamen* is the site most frequently affected. When the expanding hematoma involves the adjacent internal capsule, there is a contralateral hemiparesis, usually with hemianesthesia and hemianopia and, in large hematomas, aphasia or impaired awareness of the disorder. However, small self-limiting hematomas close to the capsular region may occasionally mimic lacunar syndromes featuring pure motor or sensory deficits. When the hemorrhage arises in the *thalamus*, hemianesthesia precedes the hemiparesis. Once contralateral motor, sensory, and visual field signs are established, the main points that distinguish the two sites are (1) conjugate horizontal ocular deviation in putaminal hemorrhage and (2) impaired upward gaze in thalamic hemorrhage. *Pontine* hemorrhage usually plunges the patient into coma with quadriparesis and grossly disconjugate ocular motility disorders, although small hemorrhages may mimic syndromes of infarction. Primary spontaneous hemorrhages within the *mesencephalon* or the *medulla* remain objects of debate and are rare curiosities. When they occur, the anatomic involvement is usually secondary to hemorrhage originating in neighboring diencephalic, cerebellar, or pontine regions. In the *cerebral lobes*, there is an as-yet-unexplained predilection for hemorrhages to occur within the posterior two-thirds of the brain. When they affect one or more cerebral lobes, the syndrome is difficult to distinguish, clinically, from infarction because progressive evolution and vomiting are much less frequent in infarction; also, lobar white matter hematomas often result from arteriovenous malformations, amyloid angiopathy, tumors, or other causes that only uncommonly affect the basal ganglia, thalamus, and pons.

Cerebellar hemorrhage warrants separate description because the mode of onset differs from that of cerebral hemorrhage and because it often necessitates surgical evacuation. The syndrome usually begins abruptly with vomiting and severe ataxia (which usually prevents standing and walking); it is occasionally accompanied by dysarthria, adjacent cranial nerve (mostly sixth and seventh) affection, and paralysis of conjugate lateral gaze to one side, findings that may mislead clinicians into thinking the disease is primarily in the brain stem. However, a cerebellar origin is suggested by the lack of changes in the level of consciousness and lack of focal weakness or sensory loss.

Enlargement of the mass does not change the clinical picture until there is enough brain stem compression to precipitate coma, at which point it is too late for surgical evacuation of the hemorrhage to reverse the disorder. This small margin of time between an alert state and an irreversible coma makes it imperative to consider the diagnosis in all patients with this clinical syndrome and is a reason to have patients who present in the emergency room with vomiting of undetermined origin attempt to stand and walk.

DIAGNOSTIC STUDIES

Nonenhanced computed tomography (CT) scan of the brain is the method of choice to evaluate the presence of ICH (see Fig. 38.1). CT scan evaluates the size and location of the hematoma, extension into the ventricular system, degree of surrounding edema, and anatomic disruption. Hematoma volume, a powerful predictor of 30-day mortality, can be easily calculated from CT scan images by use of the ABC ÷ 2 method, which involves multiplying the diameter of the hematoma in three dimensions and dividing by two (Fig. 38.3). CT angiography may reveal secondary ICH due to an aneurysm or arteriovenous malformation, or active contrast extravasation into the clot ("spot sign"), which implies an increased risk

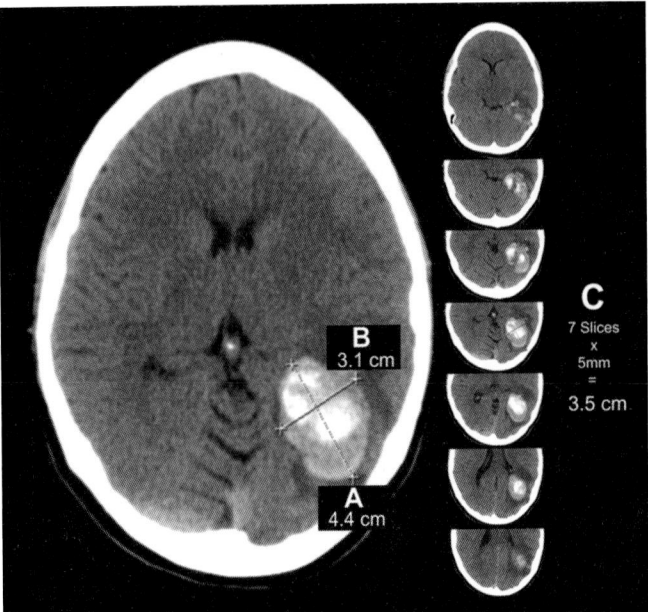

FIGURE 38.3 ICH volume measurement. (*A*) Largest hemorrhage axial diameter. (*B*) Largest axial diameter perpendicular to *A* on same slice. (*C*) Vertical hemorrhage diameter (number of slices with hemorrhage multiplied by slice thickness). For this example, ABC/2 = (4.4 cm × 3.1 cm × 3.5 cm)/2 = 23.9 cm³. (From Beslow LA, Ichord RN, Kasner SE, et al. ABC/XYZ estimates intracerebral hemorrhage volume as a percent of total brain volume in children. *Stroke*. 2010;41:691–694, with permission.)

of early hematoma growth when identified soon after the onset of symptoms. MRI techniques such as gradient echo (GRE, T2*) are highly sensitive for the diagnosis of ICH as well (see Fig. 38.2). MRI in patients with atypical ICH patterns on CT may disclose a cause of secondary ICH (i.e., tumor, arteriovenous malformation, or hemorrhagic infarction up to 20% of cases). Conventional diagnostic cerebral angiography should be reserved for patients in whom secondary causes of ICH are suspected, such as aneurysms, arteriovenous malformations, cortical vein or dural sinus thrombosis, or vasculitis. Findings on CT scan or MRI that should prompt angiographic study include the presence of subarachnoid hemorrhage (SAH), intraventricular hemorrhage (IVH), underlying calcification, or lobar hemorrhage in nonhypertensive younger patients. Diagnostic catheter angiography should be strongly considered in all patients with primary IVH and younger nonhypertensive patients with lobar ICH.

MEDICAL MANAGEMENT

Prehospital care of ICH follows similar guidelines as for other types of stroke, where the objective is to provide rapid access to medical facilities capable of dealing with stroke patients. In the emergency department, ICH patients should be triaged rapidly with CT scans to access stroke units or intensive care units (ICUs). Observation in an ICU or a similar setting is strongly recommended for at least the first 24 hours because the risk of neurologic deterioration is highest during this period and because the majority of patients with brain stem or cerebellar hemorrhage have depressed level of consciousness requiring ventilatory support. A protocolized checklist for care in the ICU is recommended to ensure standardization of best practices (Table 38.2).

TABLE 38.2	Medical Management Checklist for Acute Intracerebral Hemorrhage
Blood pressure	• Maintain mean arterial pressure <140 mm Hg with continuous infusion labetalol (2–10 mg/min) or nicardipine (5–15 mg/h)
	• If stuporous or comatose, measure ICP and maintain CPP >70 mm Hg.
Reversal of anticoagulation	• For elevated INR: vitamin K 10 mg IVP and 4F-PCC
	• INR 2 to <4: 25 U/kg; not to exceed 2,500 units
	• INR 4–6: 35 U/kg; not to exceed 3,500 units
	• INR >6: 50 U/kg; not to exceed 5,000 units
	• For heparin: protamine sulfate 10–50 mg slow IVP (1 mg reverses approximately 100 units of heparin)
	• For thrombocytopenia or platelet dysfunction: desmopressin 0.3 μg/kg IVP and/or transfuse 6 units of platelets
	• Expedited INR reversal for lifesaving neurosurgical intervention: recombinant activated factor VII 40–80 μg/kg (approximately 3.0–6.0 mg) IVP
Intracranial hypertension	• Elevate head of bed to 30 degrees
	• Mannitol 1.0–1.5 g IV
	• Hyperventilate to PCO_2 of 30 mm Hg
Fluids and nutrition	• Normal (0.9%) saline at 1.0 mL/kg/h
	• Begin enteral feeding via nasoduodenal tube within 24 hours.
Seizure prophylaxis	• For coma with intracranial hypertension or acute seizures: fosphenytoin (15–20 mg/kg) followed by 300 mg IV daily or levetiracetam 1,000 mg b.i.d. for 7 days
Physiologic homeostasis	• Cooling blankets to maintain T ≤37.5°C
	• Insulin drip to maintain glucose 120–180 mg/dL

4F-PCC, four-factor prothrombin complex concentrate containing factors II, VII, IX, and X.

EMERGENCY REVERSAL OF ANTICOAGULATION

Hemostatic abnormalities should be corrected as rapidly as possible. Patients at risk include those on oral anticoagulants (OACs) for several indications, antiplatelet agents, and congenital or acquired factor or platelet deficiencies. The incidence of ICH related to OACs has increased over the last decade. Vitamin K antagonists (VKAs) are the most commonly prescribed OACs, but new novel oral anticoagulant (NOAC) agents that inhibit thrombin or factor Xa such as dabigatran, rivaroxaban, and apixaban are increasingly being offered.

Patients with ICH receiving warfarin should be reversed immediately with a four-factor prothrombin complex concentrate (PCC) (25 to 50 U/kg depending on the baseline international normalized ratio [INR] level) and vitamin K 10-mg intravenous push (IVP). Four-factor PCCs contain vitamin K–dependent coagulation factors II, VII, IX, and X; normalize the INR more rapidly than fresh frozen plasma (FFP); and can be given in much smaller volumes much more rapidly [Level 1].[1] Treatment should never be delayed in order to check coagulation tests when a patient has acute ICH and a stated history of OAC use. Recent reports have also described the use of recombinant activated factor VIIa (rFVIIa), a powerful prohemostatic agent, to speed the reversal of warfarin anticoagulation in ICH patients. A single intravenous dose of rFVIIa can normalize the INR within minutes, with larger doses producing a longer duration of effect. A typical dose for reversing warfarin is 4 mg. rFVIIa has the drawback of a 5% risk of thromboembolic complications (ischemic stroke or myocardial infarction) and thus is only used to expedite lifesaving neurosurgical intervention.

Patients with ICH who have been anticoagulated with unfractionated or low molecular weight heparin should be reversed with protamine sulfate, and patients with thrombocytopenia or platelet dysfunction can be treated with a single dose of desmopressin (DDAVP) 0.3 μg/kg, platelet transfusions (6 to 8 units), or both (see Table 38.2). Newer agents such as direct thrombin inhibitors and factor Xa inhibitors provide a new challenge for the reversal of coagulopathy-related ICH, as no antidote currently exists. In the case of recent dabigatran ingestion, hemodialysis has been suggested. Potential reversal strategies included factor VIII inhibitor bypassing activity (FEIBA), PCCs, or rFVIIa. In this setting, consultation with a hematologist is also indicated.

BLOOD PRESSURE CONTROL

Acute ICH often leads to extreme arterial hypertension. Excessive reduction in blood pressure (BP) after ICH in the setting of impaired autoregulation can result in exacerbation of ischemic injury, whereas lack of BP control can theoretically exacerbate early hematoma growth and vasogenic edema. Single-center studies and a systematic review have reported an increased risk of deterioration, death, or dependency with extremely high or low admission BP after ICH. Although current American Heart Association (AHA) guidelines recommend a systolic BP (SBP) target of less than 180 mm Hg and mean BP target of less than 130 mm Hg, a recent phase 3 trial showed that lowering of SBP to less than 140 mm Hg compared to less than 180 mm Hg within 6 hours of onset resulted in no difference in mortality and borderline improvement in the extent of disability among survivors [Level 1].[2] Eligible patients in this study included patients with mild ICH (median Glasgow Coma Scale [GCS] 14, interquartile range [IQR] 12 to 15) and small ICH volumes (median volume 11, IQR 6 to 20 mL). Therefore, the results cannot be extrapolated to all subpopulations of ICH patients, particularly more severe critically ill ICH patients with comorbidities and larger hematomas with impaired autoregulation. Current AHA guidelines suggest that intracranial pressure (ICP) monitoring should be used in patients with large hematomas and depressed level of consciousness to ensure that cerebral perfusion pressure (CPP) is maintained above 60 mm Hg. A more recent study of 18 comatose ICH patients using brain multimodality monitoring showed that CPP levels greater than 80 mm Hg were associated with a reduced risk of critical brain tissue hypoxia, which in turn was associated with increased mortality. The Antihypertensive Treatment in Acute Cerebral Hemorrhage (ATACH) trial also confirmed the feasibility and safety of early rapid BP reduction in ICH. Both Intensive Blood Pressure Reduction in Acute Cerebral Haemorrhage Trial (INTERACT-II) and ATACH have shown that although early and intensive BP lowering is clinically feasible, for eligible patients, there is no clear effect on mortality.

Given the need to precisely control BP levels in the setting of impaired autoregulation, use of fast-acting continuous infusion agents with intra-arterial monitoring is recommended. Preferred agents are β-blockers (intravenous [IV] labetalol) and calcium channel blockers (nicardipine and clevidipine) (Table 38.3). Use of nitroprusside has drawbacks because this agent is associated with higher rate of medical complications and may exacerbate cerebral edema and ICP. Clevidipine, an ultra-short-acting, dihydropyridine L-type calcium channel blocker with rapid onset and offset of action, has also recently been approved for the reduction of BP. Comparative studies have demonstrated that clevidipine is as safe and effective as nitroglycerin, sodium nitroprusside, or nicardipine for reducing BP but has greater ability to maintain a given target range. Oral and sublingual agents are not preferred because of the need for immediate and precise BP control. Although no prospective study has addressed the timing of conversion from IV to oral antihypertensive management, this process can generally be started between 24 and 72 hours as long as the patient's critical condition has been stabilized.

CEREBRAL EDEMA

Large-volume ICH carries the risk of developing cerebral edema (Chapter 107) and elevated ICP. Brain swelling can progress for many days after the onset of ICH but most often drives neurologic deterioration within the first 72 hours in patients with hemorrhages exceeding 30 mL in volume. The presence of IVH further increases ICP and the risk of mortality. This effect is primarily related to the development of obstructive hydrocephalus and alterations of normal cerebrospinal fluid (CSF) flow dynamics. Patients with large-volume ICH, intracranial mass effect, and coma may benefit from ICP monitoring, although this intervention has not been proven to benefit outcomes after ICH.

TABLE 38.3 Parenteral Vasoactive Agents in Neurologic Emergencies: Preferred Antihypertensives and Vasopressors

Drug	Mechanism	Dose	Onset	Duration	Common Adverse Effects	Cautions
Labetalol	α1, β1, β2 antagonist	20–80 mg bolus every 10 min, up to max 300 mg; 0.5–2 mg/min infusion	5–10 min	3–6 h	Bradycardia (heart block), dizziness, nausea, vomiting, scalp tingling, bronchospasm, orthostatic hypotension, hepatic injury	Asthma, COPD, LV failure, second- or third-degree AV block
Esmolol	β1 antagonist	500 μg/kg bolus, 50–300 μg/kg/min infusion	1–2 min	10–30 min	Bradycardia (heart block), hypotension, nausea, bronchospasm	Asthma, COPD, LV failure, second- or third-degree AV block
Nicardipine	L-type CCB (dihydropyridine)	5–15 mg/h infusion	5–10 min	30 min to 4 h	Reflex tachycardia, headache, nausea, flushing, local phlebitis	LV failure, severe AS, cardiac ischemia
Enalaprilat	ACE inhibitor	0.625 mg bolus, then 1.25–5 mg every 6 h	15–30 min	6–12 h	Variable response, precipitous fall in BP in high-renin states headache, cough	Acute MI, h/o hypersensitivity
Fenoldopam	DA-1 agonist	0.1–0.3 μg/kg/min infusion	5–15 min	30 min to 4 h	Tachycardia, headache, nausea, dizziness, flushing	Glaucoma, liver disease (cirrhosis with portal HTN)
Clevidipine	L-type CCB (dihydropyridine)	1–2 mg/h infusion	2–4 min	5–15 min	Headache, nausea, vomiting	Soybean allergy
Nitroprusside[a]	Nitrovasodilator (arterial and venous)	0.25–10 μg/kg/min infusion	Immediate	1–4 min	Nausea, vomiting, muscle twitching, sweating, thiocyanate and cyanide intoxication	Coronary artery disease, elevated ICP

COPD, chronic obstructive pulmonary disease; LV, left ventricle; AV, atrioventricular; CCB, calcium channel blocker; AS, aortic stenosis; ACE, angiotensin-converting enzyme; MI, myocardial infarction; HTN, hypertension.

[a]Nitroprusside is becoming less favored for use in neurologic emergencies (see text).

Data from Rose JC, Mayer SA. Optimizing blood pressure in neurological emergencies. *Neurocrit Care.* 2004;1;287–299.

Management of cerebral edema should be guided by measurement of ICP with an external ventricular drainage or parenchymal monitor, with efforts directed at maintaining ICP less than 20 mm Hg and CPP greater than 70 mm Hg. Therapy should be directed by an algorithm that includes sedation, BP optimization, bolus osmotherapy, controlled hyperventilation, mild hypothermia, and, as a last resort, salvage hemicraniectomy in selected younger patients (see Chapter 107 for a detailed protocol). Empiric ICP therapy in the emergency department typically starts with 1.0 to 1.5 g/kg of 20% mannitol solution via a peripheral IV. Placement of a central venous line also allows administration of hypertonic saline solution, such as 30 to 60 mL of 23.4% saline solution given as a slow IVP over 10 to 20 minutes. Qureshi et al. demonstrated the effectiveness of 23.4% saline solution over 10% saline and mannitol during imminent transtentorial herniation in a canine model of ICH. Apart from a negative trial of glycerol given within 48 hours of ICH onset, no prospective randomized control trials have compared the effectiveness of the different osmotic agents available for the management of increased ICP in ICH. Effectiveness of hyperosmolar therapy for control of ICP depends on rapid institution of therapy and achieving higher differences in baseline osmolarity. Corticosteroids such as dexamethasone do not improve the outcome of ICH and are not indicated for the treatment of cerebral edema associated with this condition [**Level 1**].[3]

SEIZURES

Twelve percent of ICH patients experience convulsive seizures during their hospitalization; the risk is increased with lobar location. Seizure activity in ICH patients should aggressively be diagnosed and treated. Patients with ICH may benefit from prophylactic antiepileptic therapy (antiepileptic drugs [AEDs]), but no randomized trial has addressed the use of AEDs in the setting of ICH so current guidelines do not endorse the use of AEDs for ICH patients without seizures. Continuous electroencephalographic (EEG) monitoring is recommended in all comatose patients in order to detect convulsive seizures or status epilepticus. Even with anticonvulsant therapy, continuous EEG monitoring reveals electrographic seizure activity in 20% of comatose patients. It is unclear whether midazolam infusion or other aggressive measures to eliminate these seizures can improve outcome. If seizures have not occurred, anticonvulsants should be discontinued at discharge because they can hamper neurologic recovery during rehabilitation.

MEDICAL SUPPORT

For patients requiring ventilatory support, maintain normoxia, avoid routine hyperoxygenation, and prevent ventilator-associated infections. Additional measures in the stroke unit or ICU include evaluation and assessment of speech and swallowing for nutritional support, maintenance of normoglycemia (goal <180 mg/dL), gastrointestinal prophylaxis for intubated patients, and deep venous thrombosis prophylaxis, which can be safely started 48 hours after ICH onset. Early enteral feeding should be initiated via a nasoduodenal feeding tube within inpatients who lack the capacity to swallow to combat malnutrition and muscle wasting. Body temperature should be maintained at normal with antipyretics and surface cooling as needed.

SURGICAL MANAGEMENT

The most urgent treatment consideration for ICH is often whether to proceed emergently with surgical evacuation or ventricular drain placement. Owing to the irreversible nature of secondary brain injury related to herniation and ICP, results are always better when definitive measures to reverse these processes are performed as soon as possible. Delayed surgical intervention triggered by clinical deterioration must always be tempered by realization that an earlier procedure would have been the better plan.

VENTRICULAR DRAINAGE

External ventricular drainage is indicated in all stuporous or comatose patients with IVH and ventricular enlargement in whom aggressive support is indicated. This lifesaving procedure, which can be performed at the bedside, decompresses the intracranial vault and arrests the process of downward brain stem herniation by allowing drainage of bloody CSF into a drainage receptacle. Connecting the drainage system to a pressure transducer also allows measurement of ICP.

CRANIOTOMY

Apart from cases suffering cerebellar hemorrhage, any decision on whether, how, and when to intervene neurosurgically after ICH is subject to intense debate and awaits further data from ongoing prospective trials. To date, all clinical trial attempts have failed to show a superiority of hematoma evacuation over medical therapy for supratentorial ICH [**Level 1**].[4,5] However, these trials did not enroll patients if the investigator felt that emergency surgery was clearly a lifesaving intervention, leading to inclusion bias. Many experts feel that urgent craniotomy can improve the outcome of younger patients with large lobar hemorrhages and a deteriorating course due to mass effect.

In contrast to supratentorial ICH, it is widely accepted that patients with cerebellar hemorrhages exceeding 3 cm in diameter benefit from emergent surgical evacuation. Abrupt and dramatic deterioration to coma can occur within the first 24 hours of onset in these patients. For this reason, it is generally unwise to defer surgery in these patients until further clinical deterioration occurs.

As emergent craniotomy has been unable to improve neurologic outcome after ICH, the role of other surgical techniques such as minimally invasive surgery (MIS) has gained importance over the last decade. The advantages of MIS over conventional craniotomy include reduced operative time, the possibility of performance under local anesthesia, and reduced surgical trauma. Additional strategies currently under extensive research are thrombolytic therapy and surgical removal of hematomas, intraventricular administration of thrombolytics for IVH, and hemicraniectomy with duraplasty (Fig. 38.4).

SECONDARY PREVENTION

The risk of recurrent ICH is 2% per year in patients with chronic hypertension, and in those patients with diastolic BP higher than 90 mm Hg, the rate of recurrence is as high as 10% per year. BP reduction significantly decreases the risk of ICH and other forms of stroke and is unequivocally the most effective method for primary and secondary prevention of ICH. In the Perindopril Protection Against Recurrent Stroke Study (PROGRESS) trial, a BP regimen perindopril, an angiotensin-converting enzyme inhibitor, was found to be more effective than placebo for preventing recurrent stroke among both hypertensive and nonhypertensive individuals following incident stroke or TIA [**Level 1**].[6] Survivors of lobar ICH

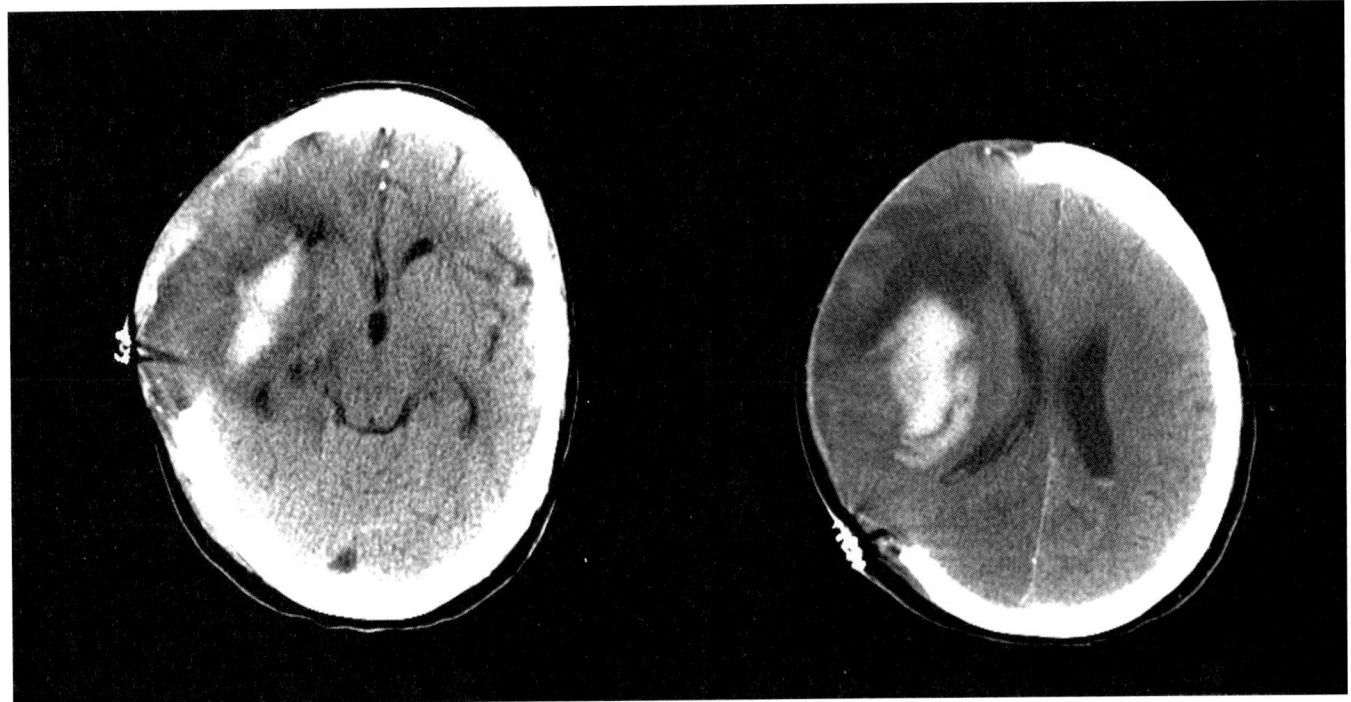

FIGURE 38.4 Lifesaving hemicraniectomy in a patient with lobar ICH considered otherwise lethal.

and most patients with deep hemispheric ICH who have history of atrial fibrillation should not be offered long-term anticoagulation therapy. Conversely, patients with high risk of thromboembolic events and low recurrent risk of ICH may benefit from long-term anticoagulation therapy.

TABLE 38.4	Determination of the Intracerebral Hemorrhage Score	
Component	**Score Points**
Glasgow Coma Scale score	
3–4	2
5–12	1
13–15	0
ICH volume (cm³)	
≥30	1
<30	0
IVH	
Yes	1
No	0
Infratentorial ICH	
Yes	1
No	0
Age (yr)	
≥80	1
<80	0

From Hemphill JC III, Bonovich DC, Besmertis L, et al. The ICH score: a simple, reliable grading scale for intracerebral hemorrhage. *Stroke.* 2001;32(4):891–897.

PROGNOSIS

The mortality of ICH is 35% to 50% at 30 days and 47% at 1 year. Factors that consistently predict mortality or adverse outcomes in ICH have been studied extensively. Independent predictors for 30-day and 1-year mortality include Glasgow Coma Scale and/or depressed level of consciousness, age, ICH volume, presence of IVH, and infratentorial origin. A simple clinical grading scale, the *ICH Score* (Table 38.4), permits calculation of mortality, allowing use of uniform terms and enhancing communication between physicians. The mortality rates for scores of 0, 1, 2, 3, 4, and 5 are 0%, 13%, 26%, 72%, 97%, and 100%, respectively. Additional factors associated with high mortality after ICH include the presence of SAH, wide pulse pressure, history of coronary artery disease, and hyperthermia. Factors associated with good outcomes include a low National Institutes of Health Stroke Scale (NIHSS) score and low temperature on admission.

Except in the most severe cases, caution is warranted when communicating a hopeless prognosis before aggressive efforts have been made to resuscitate victims of ICH. It has become increasingly evident that physicians tend to underestimate the chances of a good outcome and that many poor outcomes result from self-fulfilling prophesies of doom. Mortality after ICH is reduced in patients cared for in a specialty neurologic ICU. This is presumably the result of adherence to best medical practices, early transition to rehabilitation, and being cared for by a team or health care professionals who take an active interest in promoting survival and recovery.

LEVEL 1 EVIDENCE

1. Sarode R, Milling TJ, Refaai MA, et al. Efficacy and safety of a 4-factor prothrombin complex concentrate in patients on vitamin k antagonists presenting with major bleeding: a randomized, plasma-controlled, phase IIIb study. *Circulation.* 2013;128:1234–1243.

2. Anderson CS, Heeley E, Huang Y, et al. Rapid blood-pressure lowering in patients with acute intracerebral hemorrhage. *N Engl J Med.* 2013;368:2355–2365.

3. Poungvarin N, Bhoopat W, Viriyavejakul A, et al. Effects of dexamethasone in primary supratentorial intracerebral hemorrhage. *N Engl J Med.* 1987;316(20):1229–1233.

4. Mendelow AD, Gregson BA, Fernandes HM, et al. Early surgery versus initial conservative treatment in patients with spontaneous supratentorial intracerebral haematomas in the International Surgical Trial in Intracerebral Haemorrhage (STICH): a randomised trial. *Lancet.* 2005;365(9457):387–397.

5. Mendelow AD, Gregson BA, Rowan EN, et al; for the STICH II Investigators. Early surgery versus initial conservative treatment in patients with spontaneous supratentorial lobar intracerebral haematomas (STICH II): a randomised trial. *Lancet.* 2013;382(9890):397–408.

6. PROGRESS Collaborative Group. Randomised trial of a perindopril-based blood-presure-lowering regimen among 6105 individuals with previous stroke or transient ischaemic attack. *Lancet.* 2001;358:1033–1041.

SUGGESTED READINGS

Becker KJ, Baxter AB, Bybee HM, et al. Extravasation of radiographic contrast is an independent predictor of death in primary intracerebral hemorrhage. *Stroke.* 1999;30(10):2025–2032.

Brott T, Broderick J, Kothari R, et al. Early hemorrhage growth in patients with intracerebral hemorrhage. *Stroke.* 1997;28:1–5.

Diringer MN, Edwards DF. Admission to a neurologic/neurosurgical intensive care unit is associated with reduced mortality rate after intracerebral hemorrhage. *Crit Care Med.* 200 1;29:635–640.

Felberg RA, Grotta JC, Shirzadi AL, et al. Cell death in experimental intracerebral hemorrhage: the "black hole" model of hemorrhagic damage. *Ann Neurol.* 2002;51(4):517–524.

Goldstein JN, Fazen LE, Snider R, et al. Contrast extravasation on CT angiography predicts hematoma expansion in intracerebral hemorrhage. *Neurology.* 2007;68(12):889–894.

Greenberg SM. Cerebral amyloid angiopathy: prospects for clinical diagnosis and treatment. *Neurology.* 1998;51:690–694.

Hemphill JC III, Bonovich DC, Besmertis L, et al. The ICH score: a simple, reliable grading scale for intracerebral hemorrhage. *Stroke.* 2001;32(4):891–897.

Inaji M, Tomita H, Tone O, et al. Chronological changes of perihematomal edema of human intracerebral hematoma. *Acta Neurochir Suppl.* 2003;86:445–448.

Kothari RU, Brott T, Broderick JP, et al. The ABCs of measuring intracerebral hemorrhage volumes. *Stroke.* 1996;27(8):1304–1305.

Mayer SA, Kurtz P, Wyman A, et al. Clinical practices, complications, and mortality in neurological patients with acute severe hypertension: the Studying the Treatment of Acute hyperTension registry. *Crit Care Med.* 2011;39(10):2330–2336.

Mayer SA, Sacco RL, Shi T, et al. Neurologic deterioration in noncomatose patients with supratentorial intracerebral hemorrhage. *Neurology.* 1994;44(8):1379–1384.

Morgenstern LB, Hemphill JC III, Anderson C, et al; American Heart Association Stroke Council and Council on Cardiovascular Nursing. Guidelines for the management of spontaneous intracerebral hemorrhage: a guideline for healthcare professionals from the American Heart Association/American Stroke Association. *Stroke.* 2010;41:2108–2129.

Naidech AM, Maas MB, Levasseur-Franklin KE, et al. Desmopressin improves platelet activity in acute intracerebral hemorrhage. *Stroke.* 2014;45:2451–2453.

Ott KH, Kase CS, Ojemann RG, et al. Cerebellar hemorrhage: diagnosis and treatment. *Arch Neurol.* 1974;31:160–167.

Qureshi AI, Suri MF, Ringer AJ, et al. Regional intraparenchymal pressure differences in experimental intracerebral hemorrhage: effect of hypertonic saline. *Crit Care Med.* 2002;30(2):435–441.

Rincon F, Mayer SA. The epidemiology of intracerebral hemorrhage in the United States from 1979 to 2008. *Neurocrit Care.* 2013;19(1):95–102.

Vespa PM, O'Phelan K, Shah M, et al. Acute seizures after intracerebral hemorrhage: a factor in progressive midline shift and outcome. *Neurology.* 2003;60(9):1441–1446.

Wijman CA, Venkatasubramanian C, Bruins S, et al. Utility of early MRI in the diagnosis and management of acute spontaneous intracerebral hemorrhage. *Cerebrovasc Dis.* 2010;30(5):456–463.

Zazulia AR, Diringer MN, Videen TO, et al. Hypoperfusion without ischemia surrounding acute intracerebral hemorrhage. *J Cereb Blood Flow Metab.* 2001;21(7):804–810.

Subarachnoid Hemorrhage 39

*Stephan A. Mayer, Gary L. Bernardini,
and Robert A. Solomon*

INTRODUCTION

Subarachnoid hemorrhage (SAH) accounts for 5% of all strokes; it affects nearly 30,000 people each year in the United States, with an annual incidence of 1 per 10,000. Saccular (or berry) aneurysms at the base of the brain cause 80% of all cases of SAH. Nonaneurysmal causes of SAH are listed in Table 39.1. SAH most frequently occurs between ages 40 and 60 years, and women are affected more often than men.

SAH due to the rupture of an intracranial aneurysm is a devastating event; approximately 12% of patients die before receiving medical attention, and another 20% die after admission to the hospital. Of the two-thirds of patients who survive, approximately one-half remain permanently disabled, primarily due to neurocognitive deficits and depression. Advances in neurosurgery and intensive care, including an emphasis on early aneurysm clipping and aggressive therapy for vasospasm, have led to improved survival over the last three decades, with a reduction in overall case fatality from approximately 50% to 20% in high-volume centers.

PATHOLOGY AND EPIDEMIOLOGY OF INTRACRANIAL ANEURYSMS

Saccular aneurysms most often occur at the circle of Willis or its major branches, especially at bifurcations. They arise where the arterial elastic lamina and tunica media are defective and tend to enlarge with age. The typical aneurysm wall is composed only of intima and adventitia and can become paper thin. Many aneurysms, particularly those that rupture, are irregular and multilobulated, and larger aneurysms may be partially or completely filled with an organized clot, which occasionally is calcified. The point of rupture is usually through the dome of the aneurysm.

TABLE 39.1	Nonaneurysmal Causes of Subarachnoid Hemorrhage

- Trauma
- Idiopathic perimesencephalic SAH
- Arteriovenous malformation
- Intracranial arterial dissection
- Cocaine and amphetamine use
- Mycotic aneurysm
- Pituitary apoplexy
- Moyamoya disease
- Central nervous system vasculitis
- Sickle cell disease
- Coagulation disorders
- Primary or metastatic neoplasm

SAH, subarachnoid hemorrhage.

Eighty-five percent to 90% of intracranial aneurysms are located in the anterior circulation, with the three most common sites being the anterior communicating artery complex (approximately 40%), the junction of the posterior communicating and internal carotid artery (approximately 30%), and the middle cerebral artery at the first major branch point in the sylvian fissure (approximately 20%). Posterior circulation aneurysms most often occur at the apex of the basilar artery or at the junction of the vertebral and posteroinferior cerebellar artery. Saccular aneurysms of the distal cerebral arterial tree are rare. Nearly 20% of patients have two or more aneurysms; many of these are "mirror" aneurysms on the same vessel but on the contralateral side.

Intracranial aneurysms are uncommon in children but occur with a frequency of 2% in adults, suggesting that approximately 2 to 3 million Americans have an aneurysm. However, more than 90% of these are small (<10 mm) and remain asymptomatic throughout life. The annual risk of rupture of an asymptomatic intracranial aneurysm is approximately 0.7%. Important risk factors for the initial rupture of an aneurysm include increasing size, prior SAH from a separate aneurysm, and basilar apex and posterior communicating artery location (Table 39.2). The most powerful of these risk factors is size: for example, internal carotid artery aneurysms <7 mm in diameter bleed at a rate of approximately 0.1% per year, compared to an annual rate of 8% for those >25 mm in size. Other risk factors for aneurysm rupture in approximate order of importance include cigarette smoking, aneurysm-related headache or cranial nerve compression, heavy alcohol use, a family history of SAH, female sex (especially when postmenopausal), multiple aneurysms, hypertension, and exposure to cocaine or other sympathomimetic agents. In deciding whether to treat an unruptured intracranial aneurysm, the risks associated with repair should always be balanced against the patient's estimated lifetime risk of hemorrhage without repair.

The prevalence of aneurysms increases with age and is higher in patients with atherosclerosis, a family history of intracranial aneurysm, or autosomal dominant polycystic kidney disease (PCKD). Intracranial aneurysms have also been associated with Ehlers–Danlos syndrome, Marfan syndrome, pseudoxanthoma elasticum, coarctation of the aorta, and sickle cell disease. Screening for unruptured intracranial aneurysms with magnetic resonance angiography (MRA) is indicated in patients with PCKD and in family members who have two or more first-degree relatives with intracranial aneurysms; testing is positive in 5% to 10% of these individuals.

CLINICAL FEATURES

SAH usually commences with an explosive "thunderclap" headache followed by stiff neck. The pain is often described as "the worst headache of my life." The headache is usually generalized, but focal pain may refer to the site of aneurysmal rupture (e.g., periorbital pain related to an ophthalmic artery aneurysm). Commonly

TABLE 39.2   Five-Year Cumulative Hemorrhage Rates of Unruptured Aneurysms According to Size and Location

| | <7 mm | | 8–12 mm | 13–25 mm | ≥25 mm |
	No Prior SAH	Prior SAH[a]			
Cavernous carotid artery (N = 210)	0	0	0	3.0%	6.4%
ACA, MCA, ICA (not intracavernous) (N = 1,037)	0	1.5%	2.6%	14.5%	40%
Posterior circulation or P-comm (N = 445)	2.5%	3.4%	14.5%	18.4%	50%

[a]Refers to prior subarachnoid hemorrhage from a separate intracranial aneurysm.

SAH, subarachnoid hemorrhage; ACA, anterior communicating or anterior cerebral artery; MCA, middle cerebral artery; ICA, internal carotid artery; P-comm, posterior communicating artery.

From Wiebers DO, Whisnant JP, Huston J III, et al; International Study of Unruptured Intracranial Aneurysms Investigators. Unruptured intracranial aneurysms: natural history, clinical outcome, and risks of surgical and endovascular treatment. *Lancet.* 2003;362:103–110.

associated symptoms include loss of consciousness, nausea and vomiting, back or leg pain, and photophobia. In patients who lose consciousness, tonic posturing may occur and may be difficult to differentiate from a seizure. Although aneurysmal rupture often occurs during periods of exercise or physical stress, SAH can occur at any time, including sleep.

More than one-third of patients give a history of suspicious symptoms days or weeks earlier, including headache, stiff neck, nausea and vomiting, syncope, or disturbed vision. These prodromal symptoms are often due to minor leaking of blood from the aneurysm and are therefore referred to as "warning leaks" or "sentinel headaches." Initial misdiagnosis of SAH occurs in approximately 15% of patients, and those with the mildest symptoms are at greatest risk. Approximately 40% of misdiagnosed patients experience subsequent neurologic deterioration due to rebleeding, hydrocephalus, or vasospasm before reaching medical attention, with increased morbidity and mortality.

Stiff neck and the Kernig sign are hallmarks of SAH. However, these signs are not invariably present, and confusion and low back pain are sometimes more prominent than headache. Preretinal or subhyaloid hemorrhages—large, smooth-bordered, and on the retinal surface—occur in up to 25% of patients and are practically pathognomonic of SAH.

The most important determinant of outcome after SAH is the patient's neurologic condition on arrival at the hospital. Alterations in mental status are the most common abnormality; some patients remain alert and lucid; others are confused, delirious, amnestic, lethargic, stuporous, or comatose. The modified Hunt and Hess grading scale serves as a means for risk stratification for SAH based on the first neurologic examination (Table 39.3). Patients classified as grade I or II SAH have a relatively good prognosis, grade III carries an intermediate prognosis, and grades IV and V have a poor prognosis. Focal neurologic signs occur in a minority of patients but may point to the site of bleeding; hemiparesis or aphasia suggests a middle cerebral artery aneurysm, and paraparesis or abulia suggests an aneurysm of the proximal anterior cerebral artery. These focal signs are sometimes due to a large hematoma, which may require emergency evacuation.

In 10% of patients with nontraumatic SAH and in two-thirds of those with negative angiography, computed tomography (CT) reveals blood confined to the perimesencephalic cisterns, with the center of bleeding adjacent to the midbrain and pons (Fig. 39.1). Patients with "perimesencephalic" SAH always have normal findings on neurologic examination and a benign clinical

course; rebleeding and symptomatic vasospasm or hydrocephalus almost never occur. The source of hemorrhage in these patients is presumably venous.

Symptoms and signs of an unruptured intracranial aneurysm may result from compression of adjacent neural structures or thromboembolism. These aneurysms are often, but not always, large or giant (>25 mm). Aneurysms of the posterior communicating artery frequently compress the oculomotor nerve (almost always affecting the pupil). Aneurysms of the intracavernous segment of the internal carotid artery may damage the third, fourth, fifth, or sixth cranial nerves, and their rupture can lead to formation of a carotid–cavernous fistula. Less often, large aneurysms compress the cortex or brain stem, causing focal neurologic signs or seizures. Thrombosis within the aneurysmal sac occasionally sends emboli to the artery's distal territory, causing transient ischemic attacks or infarction. In the absence of SAH, some patients experience sudden, severe headache without nuchal

TABLE 39.3   Mortality according to the Hunt–Hess Grading Scale for Aneurysmal Subarachnoid Hemorrhage

| | | Hospital Mortality (%) | |
Grade	Clinical Findings	1968	2012
I	Asymptomatic or mild headache	11	3
II	Moderate to severe headache or oculomotor palsy	26	3
III	Confused, drowsy, or mild focal signs	37	9
IV	Stupor (localizes to pain)	71	24
V	Coma (posturing or no motor response to pain)	100	71
TOTAL		35	20

Data are from 275 patients reported by Hunt and Hess in 1968 and 1,200 patients treated at Columbia University Medical Center between 1996 and 2012.

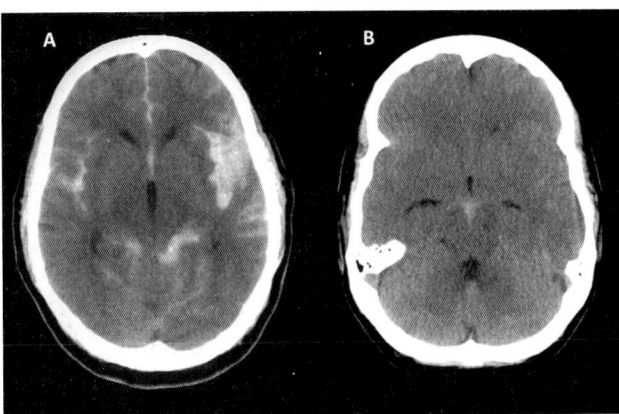

FIGURE 39.1 Two CT images of SAH. **A:** Diffuse thick SAH is seen in the anterior interhemispheric and bilateral sylvian fissures and the quadrigeminal cistern. A left middle cerebral artery aneurysm was identified. **B:** Perimesencephalic SAH; only a small focus of blood in the interpeduncular cistern is identified. No aneurysm was identified.

rigidity, perhaps related to aneurysmal enlargement, thrombosis, or meningeal irritation; these symptoms can clear with aneurysm clipping.

DIAGNOSIS

COMPUTED TOMOGRAPHY

CT should be the first diagnostic study for establishing the diagnosis of SAH because it is readily available and interpretation is straightforward. When SAH is misdiagnosed, the most common error is failure to obtain a CT scan. CT most commonly demonstrates diffuse blood in the basal cisterns (see Fig. 39.1); with more severe hemorrhages, blood extends into the sylvian and interhemispheral fissures, ventricular system, and over the convexities. The distribution of blood can provide important clues regarding the location of the ruptured aneurysm. CT may also demonstrate a focal intraparenchymal or subdural hemorrhage, ventricular enlargement,

a large thrombosed aneurysm, or infarction due to vasospasm. The sensitivity of CT for SAH is 90% to 95% within 24 hours, 80% at 3 days, and 50% at 1 week. Accordingly, a normal CT never rules out SAH, and a lumbar puncture should always be performed in patients with suspected SAH and negative CT. Magnetic resonance imaging (MRI) can also be used to make the initial diagnosis of SAH or can be used to detect a completely thrombosed aneurysm if the initial angiogram is negative.

LUMBAR PUNCTURE

The cerebrospinal fluid (CSF) is usually grossly bloody. SAH can be differentiated from a traumatic tap by a xanthochromic (yellow-tinged) appearance of the supernatant fluid after centrifugation. However, xanthochromia may take up to 12 hours to appear. The CSF pressure is nearly always high and the protein elevated. Initially, the proportion of CSF leukocytes to erythrocytes is that of peripheral blood, with a usual ratio of 1:700; after several days, a reactive pleocytosis and low glucose levels may arise from a sterile chemical meningitis caused by the blood. Red blood cells and xanthochromia disappear in about 2 weeks, unless hemorrhage recurs.

ANGIOGRAPHY

Cerebral angiography is the definitive diagnostic procedure for detecting intracranial aneurysms and defining their anatomy (Fig. 39.2). Although the increasing availability and image quality of CT and MRA has allowed some centers to use these tests to make the initial diagnosis, a four-vessel (bilateral internal carotid and vertebral artery injections) angiogram is mandatory when those tests are negative. Moreover, angiography performed during coiling or after surgical clipping is generally advisable to evaluate the adequacy of aneurysmal repair and to screen for smaller secondary aneurysms that may be missed by CT or MRA. Vasospasm, local thrombosis, or poor technique can lead to a false-negative angiogram. For this reason, patients with a negative angiogram at first should have a follow-up study 1 to 2 weeks later; an aneurysm will be demonstrated in about 5% of these cases. The exception to this rule is found in patients with "perimesencephalic" SAH who usually do not require follow-up angiography.

FIGURE 39.2 Lateral view of a left common carotid angiogram demonstrates a bilobed aneurysm of the left internal carotid artery at the level of the posterior communicating artery. (Courtesy of Dr. S. Chan.)

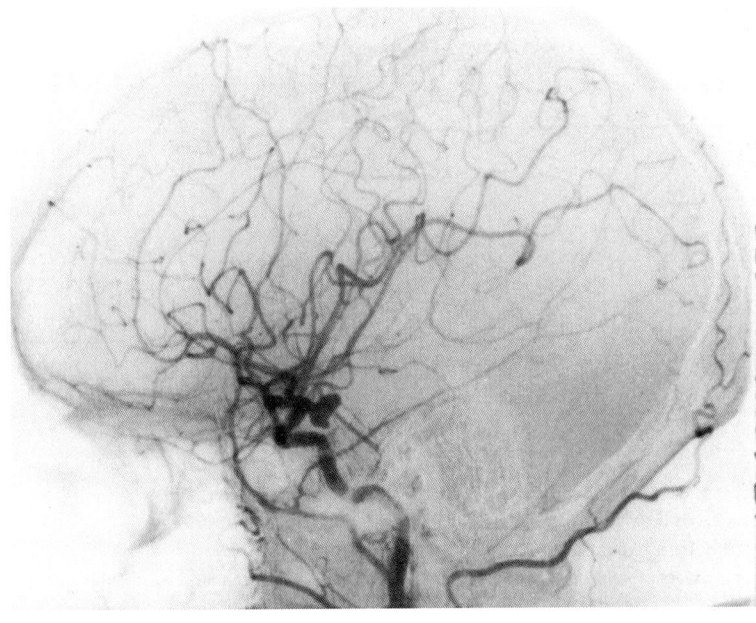

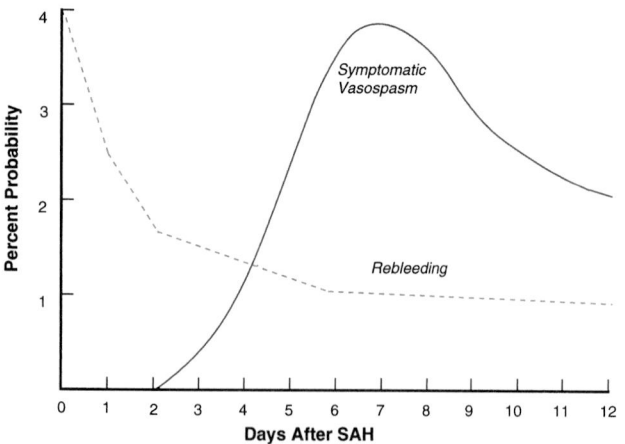

FIGURE 39.3 The daily percentage probability for the development of symptomatic vasospasm (*solid line*) or rebleeding (*dashed line*) after SAH. Day 0 denotes day of onset of SAH. SAH, subarachnoid hemorrhage.

COMPLICATIONS OF ANEURYSMAL SUBARACHNOID HEMORRHAGE

REBLEEDING

Aneurysmal rebleeding is a dreaded complication of SAH. The risk of rebleeding is highest within the first 24 hours after the initial aneurysmal rupture (4%) and remains elevated (approximately 1% to 2% per day) for the next 4 weeks (Fig. 39.3). The cumulative risk of rebleeding in untreated patients is 20% at 2 weeks, 30% at 1 month, and 40% at 6 months. After the first 6 months, the risk of rebleeding is 2% to 4% annually. Poor clinical grade and larger aneurysm size are the strongest risk factors for in-hospital rebleeding. The prognosis of patients who rebled is poor; approximately 50% die immediately, and another 30% die from subsequent complications. Although rebleeding is often attributed to uncontrolled hypertension, elevated blood pressure has not been convincingly linked to an increased risk of aneurysm rebleeding. Endogenous fibrinolysis of clot around the rupture point of the aneurysm may be a more important causative mechanism.

VASOSPASM

Delayed cerebral ischemia (DCI) from vasospasm accounts for a large proportion of morbidity and mortality after SAH. Progressive arterial narrowing develops after SAH in approximately 70% of patients, but delayed ischemic deficits develop in only 20% to 30%. The process begins 3 to 5 days after the hemorrhage, becomes maximal at 5 to 14 days, and gradually resolves over 2 to 4 weeks. Accordingly, deterioration attributable to vasospasm never occurs before the third day after SAH and occurs with peak frequency between 5 and 7 days (see Fig. 39.3). There is a strong relationship between the amount of cisternal blood seen on initial CT and the risk for development of symptomatic ischemia; for uncertain reasons, the presence of large amounts of blood in the lateral ventricles adds to this risk (Table 39.4). Symptomatic vasospasm usually involves a decrease in level of consciousness, hemiparesis, or both, and the process is usually most severe in the immediate vicinity of the aneurysm. In more severe cases, the symptoms develop earlier after aneurysm rupture, and multiple vascular territories are involved.

Although thick subarachnoid blood is the principal precipitating factor, the precise cause of arterial narrowing after SAH is poorly understood. Vasospasm is not simply due to vascular smooth muscle contraction, and changes in vessel caliber develop slowly over several days. Inflammatory arteriopathic changes are seen in the vessel wall, including subintimal edema and infiltration of leukocytes. The prevailing view is that substances released from the blood clot interact with the vessel wall to cause inflammatory arterial spasm. Putative mediators with intrinsic vasoconstrictive properties include oxyhemoglobin, hydroperoxides and leukotrienes, free radicals, prostaglandins, thromboxane A2, serotonin, endothelin, platelet-derived growth factor, and other inflammatory mediators. Cortical spreading depression may further contribute to DCI after SAH by creating prolonged neuronal depolarization in conjunction with a paradoxical reduction in local cerebral blood flow.

HYDROCEPHALUS

Acute symptomatic hydrocephalus occurs in 15% to 20% of patients with SAH and is primarily related to the volume of intraventricular and subarachnoid blood. In mild cases, hydrocephalus causes lethargy, psychomotor slowing, and impaired short-term memory. Additional findings may include limitation of upward

			Frequency of	
Grade	Criteria	Percentage of Affected Patients	Delayed Cerebral Ischemia	Infarction
0	No SAH or IVH	5%	0%	0%
1	Minimal/thin SAH, no biventricular IVH	30%	12%	6%
2	Minimal/thin SAH, *with* biventricular IVH	5%	21%	14 %
3	Thick SAH, no biventricular IVH	43%	19%	12%
4	Thick SAH, *with* biventricular IVH	17%	40%	28%
	All patients	100%	20%	12%

TABLE 39.4 Modified Fisher Computed Tomography Rating Scale for the Prediction of Symptomatic Vasospasm

Thick SAH is defined as completely filling at least one cistern or fissure.

SAH, subarachnoid hemorrhage; IVH, intraventricular hemorrhage.

From Claassen J, Bernardini GL, Kreiter K, et al. Effect of cisternal and ventricular blood on risk of delayed cerebral ischemia after subarachnoid hemorrhage: the Fisher scale revisited. *Stroke.* 2001;32:2012–2020.

gaze, sixth cranial nerve palsies, and lower extremity hyperreflexia. In more severe cases, acute obstructive hydrocephalus leads to elevated intracranial pressure and stupor or coma. Progressive brain stem herniation eventually results from continued CSF production unless a ventricular catheter is inserted.

Delayed hydrocephalus may develop 3 to 21 days after SAH. The clinical syndrome is that of normal pressure hydrocephalus, with failure to fully recover and prominent symptoms of dementia, gait disturbance, and urinary incontinence. The clinical response to ventriculoperitoneal shunting is usually excellent. Overall, 20% of SAH survivors require shunting for chronic hydrocephalus.

GLOBAL CEREBRAL EDEMA AND EARLY BRAIN INJURY

CT often demonstrates a characteristic form of global brain edema after poor-grade SAH (Fig. 39.4). This finding is most common in patients who experience loss of consciousness at the onset of bleeding, suggesting a transient episode of intracranial circulatory arrest with subsequent reperfusion injury to the brain. Global cerebral edema after SAH has been linked to an increased risk of mortality, disability, and cognitive dysfunction among survivors. MRI performed within 72 hours shows a distinctive pattern of symmetric ischemic injury in 70% of Hunt–Hess grade IV or V patients, most often involving the anterior cerebral artery territories, a process termed *early brain injury*. The relative contribution of acute ischemia, reperfusion injury, microvascular dysfunction, and inflammation in early brain injury remains poorly understood.

SEIZURES

Clinically obvious tonic–clonic seizures occur in 5% of SAH patients during hospitalization and in another 10% in the first year after discharge. Seizures after SAH are related primarily to focal pathology, including large subarachnoid clots, subdural hematoma, or cerebral infarction. Ictal events at the onset of bleeding do not portend an increased risk of late seizures. With continuous electroencephalographic monitoring, nonconvulsive seizures or status epilepticus can be detected in up to 20% of poor-grade patients and has become increasingly recognized as a cause of

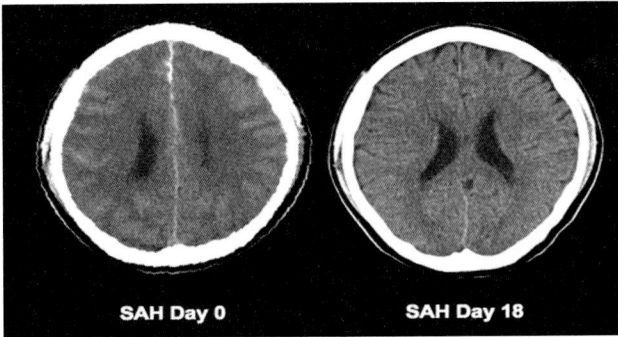

FIGURE 39.4 Global edema on the admission CT scan (SAH day 0) in a 55-year-old man with a Hunt–Hess grade V SAH from a left anterior communicating artery aneurysm which was clipped. Note the complete effacement of all convexity sulci and presence of "fingerlike" extensions of white matter lucencies to the cortical surface. A follow-up scan on SAH day 18 showed complete normalization of the CT findings. SAH, subarachnoid hemorrhage. (From Claassen J, Carhuapoma JR, Kreiter KT, et al. Global cerebral edema after subarachnoid hemorrhage: frequency, predictors, and impact on outcome. *Stroke*. 2002;33:1225–1232.)

otherwise unexplained clinical deterioration after SAH, with ominous implications for prognosis.

FLUID AND ELECTROLYTE DISTURBANCES

Hyponatremia and intravascular volume contraction frequently occur after SAH and reflect homeostatic derangements that favor excessive free-water retention and sodium loss. Hyponatremia occurs in 5% to 30% of patients after SAH and is usually related to inappropriate secretion of antidiuretic hormone and free-water retention. This process may be further exacerbated by excessive natriuresis that occurs after SAH ("cerebral salt wasting"), related to elevations of atrial natriuretic factor and the glomerular filtration rate. Whereas hyponatremia after SAH is usually asymptomatic, untreated sodium losses resulting in intravascular volume contraction can increase the risk of DCI in the presence of vasospasm. To minimize the development of hypovolemia and hyponatremia after SAH, patients should be given large volumes of isotonic crystalloid, with restriction of other potential sources of free water.

NEUROGENIC CARDIAC AND PULMONARY DISTURBANCES

Severe SAH is typically associated with a surge in catecholamine levels and sympathetic tone, which in turn can lead to neurogenic cardiac dysfunction, neurogenic pulmonary edema, or both (see also Chapter 115). Transient electrocardiographic abnormalities occur in 50% to 100% of SAH patients but usually do not produce symptoms. In some poor-grade patients, however, cardiac enzyme release and a reversible form of neurogenic "stunned myocardium" can occur. Hypotension, hypoxia, and reduction of cardiac output may occur acutely, leading to impaired cerebral perfusion in the face of increased intracranial pressure or vasospasm. Neurogenic pulmonary edema, characterized by increased permeability of the pulmonary vasculature, may occur in isolation or in combination with neurogenic cardiac injury.

FEVER

Fever develops in 80% of SAH patients at some time and may result from infection or "central" fever. Poor-grade patients with intraventricular blood often experience sustained fever that can lead to worsening of level of consciousness and exacerbation of ischemic injury caused by vasospasm. For these reasons, aggressive fever control in SAH patients with surface or intravascular cooling systems are recommended.

ANEMIA

SAH leads to a contraction of red blood cell mass. Combined with phlebotomy and volume resuscitation, all patients become progressively anemic during the first 10 days after SAH, and 20% to 40% require blood transfusions. With symptomatic vasospasm, even mild anemia (serum hemoglobin <10 mg/dL) can cause reduced oxygen delivery to ischemic brain tissue and should be avoided.

TREATMENT

The initial goal of treatment is to prevent rebleeding by excluding the aneurysmal sac from the intracranial circulation while preserving the parent artery and its branches. Once the aneurysm has been secured, the focus shifts toward monitoring and treating vasospasm and other secondary medical complications of SAH. This is best performed in an intensive care unit (ICU).

EMERGENCY MANAGEMENT

The diagnosis of SAH is almost always made in the emergency department. Management at this juncture should focus on (1) minimizing ongoing brain injury in poor-grade patients with mental status changes and (2) reducing the risk of aneurysm rebleeding prior to an effective repair procedure. In Hunt–Hess grades IV and V patients, the immediate concern is ensuring adequate perfusion and oxygenation of the brain. Patients with impaired ability to protect the airway should be intubated, supplemental oxygen should be given as needed, and hypotension should be treated aggressively with fluids and vasopressors to maintain a mean arterial pressure of 90 mm Hg. Stuporous or comatose patients with extensive SAH or intraventricular blood on CT should be empirically treated for intracranial hypertension with 1.0 g/kg of 20% mannitol prior to placement of an external ventricular drain. Medical interventions that may reduce the risk of acute aneurysm rebleeding include control of arterial hypertension (systolic blood pressure <160 mm Hg), intravenous (IV) loading with an antifibrinolytic agent (epsilon aminocaproic acid 4 g followed by 1 g/h until 4 hours prior to angiography, for a maximum of 72 hours after SAH onset) [**Level 1**][1], and administration of an anticonvulsant to minimize the risk of acute seizure activity (phenytoin 20 mg/kg IV is most commonly used).

SURGICAL MANAGEMENT

In the 1980s, neurosurgeons began to abandon the traditional practice of delaying surgery until several weeks after aneurysmal rupture, in favor of early clipping within 48 to 72 hours. This change in practice became feasible with safer microsurgical techniques. Nonetheless, surgery still remains hazardous, with a 5% to 10% risk of major morbidity or mortality in most cases; smaller aneurysms have a lower risk of procedural complications than larger aneurysms. Besides preventing early rebleeding, early surgery also permits aggressive treatment of vasospasm with hypertensive hypervolemic therapy, which can be dangerous with an unprotected aneurysm. Although early surgery was at one time reserved for patients in good clinical condition (Hunt–Hess grades I to III), this approach has been extended to all but the most moribund patients. The advent of endovascular coil embolization has been a major advance because it is a treatment option for high-risk patients who are not good candidates for early surgery.

The management of asymptomatic unruptured aneurysms is controversial. Most neurosurgeons recommend surgery for aneurysms larger than 5 mm, as long as the hoped-for benefit of surgery

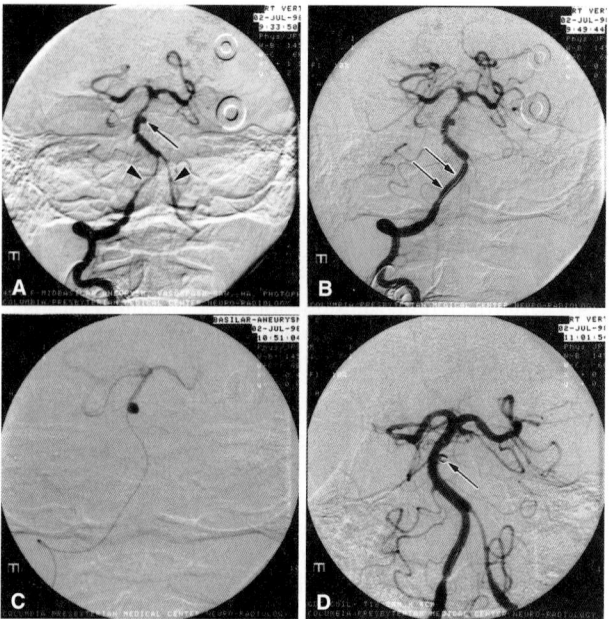

FIGURE 39.5 A: Cerebral angiogram demonstrates a left-pointing, 3-mm, midbasilar aneurysm (*closed arrow*) and vasospasm of both vertebral arteries (*open arrows*), the distal basilar artery, and the proximal right posterior cerebral artery. **B:** Significant increase in luminal diameter of the right vertebral artery after balloon angioplasty (*arrows*). **C:** Microcatheter positioned at the neck of the midbasilar aneurysm. **D:** Midbasilar aneurysm (*arrow*) with no residual filling after packing with a single platinum detachable coil. (Courtesy of Dr. Huang Duong.)

(reduced lifetime risk of bleeding) outweighs the risks. In good hands, the risk of major morbidity or mortality from clipping of an unruptured aneurysm is 2% to 5%; the risk is highest for large aneurysms and for aneurysms of the basilar artery.

ENDOVASCULAR THERAPY

Endovascular coil embolization, introduced in the early 1990s, is a safe and effective alternative to surgical clipping for treating ruptured intracranial aneurysms. Endovascular packing of aneurysms (Fig. 39.5) with soft, thrombogenic detachable platinum

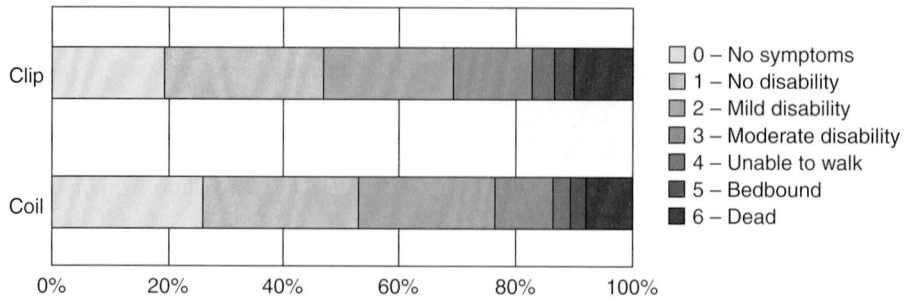

FIGURE 39.6 Distribution of modified Rankin Scale (mRS) outcome scores in the ISAT trial, which compared surgical clipping to endovascular coiling as the primary treatment for SAH due to ruptured intracranial aneurysm. The results showed that 190 of 801 (23.7%) patients allocated to coil treatment were dependent or dead at 1 year (mRS 3 to 6), compared with 243 of 793 (30.6%) allocated neurosurgical clipping (*P* = .0019).

coils leads to nearly complete obliteration of smaller aneurysms (<12 mm in diameter) in 80% to 90% of cases, with an acceptable complication rate of approximately 9% (see also Chapter 24). The long-term risk of postprocedural rebleeding is minimal after successful clipping or coiling, and there is fairly compelling evidence that the less invasive coiling procedure is safer. In the International Study of Aneurysm Treatment (ISAT), 2,134 SAH patients with predominantly small (<10 mm) anterior circulation aneurysms were randomly assigned to clip or coil therapy. Those treated with coils were 23% less likely to be dead or disabled 1 year later (Fig. 39.6) [**Level 1**].[2] Reasons for the observed improvement in outcome with coils are unclear but may include lower risk of perioperative rebleeding, reduced physical manipulation of the brain, less delayed ischemia from vasospasm, or other unidentified factors. Aneurysms with wide necks are less amenable to coil embolization because it is harder for the aneurysmal sac to contain the coil; in some cases, it is necessary to place a stent in the parent vessel across the aneurysm neck and deploy coils through the stent. The main disadvantage of endovascular treatment is the requirement for periodic reevaluation to ensure durable occlusion of the aneurysm. Approximately 5% of coiled patients develop recurrent dilatation at the neck of the original aneurysm and that requires repeat coil embolization or delayed surgical clipping.

Large, expanding aneurysms of the intracavernous internal carotid artery can be treated with proximal endovascular occlusion. Before permanent occlusion, a trial balloon occlusion is performed to determine whether there is adequate collateral flow through the circle of Willis to prevent symptomatic ischemia in the ipsilateral hemisphere. If the test occlusion is negative, an extracranial–intracranial bypass procedure may be considered before permanent occlusion is attempted.

INTENSIVE CARE MANAGEMENT

A suggested algorithm for the postoperative management of SAH is outlined in Table 39.5. All patients with SAH should be monitored in an ICU, where neurologic examinations can be performed frequently. Blood pressure control can be liberalized once the aneurysm has been repaired and brain perfusion becomes the dominant

TABLE 39.5	Critical Care Management Protocol for Acute Subarachnoid Hemorrhage
Blood pressure	• Control elevated blood pressure during the preoperative phase (systolic BP <160 mm Hg) with IV labetalol, nicardipine, or clevidipine to prevent rebleeding.
Rebleeding prophylaxis	• Epsilon aminocaproic acid 4 g IV upon diagnosis followed by 1 g/h until aneurysm repair, for a maximum of up to 72 h after ictus
IV hydration	• Normal (0.9%) saline or a balanced isotonic solution (i.e., Plasma-Lyte) at 1.0–1.5 mL/kg/h
Laboratory testing	• Periodically check complete blood count and electrolytes.
	• Obtain serial ECGs and check admission cardiac troponin I (cTI) to evaluate for cardiac injury; perform echocardiography in patients with abnormal ECG findings or cTI elevation.
Seizure prophylaxis	• Fosphenytoin (15–20 mg/kg) or levetiracetam 1g IV; discontinue on postop day 1 unless patient has seized, is poor grade, or has focal cortical pathology or is otherwise unstable
Vasospasm prophylaxis	• Nimodipine 60 mg PO every 4 hours until day SAH 21 or discharge
Physiologic homeostasis	• Cooling blankets to maintain T ≤37.5°C
	• Insulin drip to maintain glucose 120–180 mg/dL
	• Transfuse to maintain hemoglobin >7.0 g/dL (in the absence or active cerebral or cardiac ischemia).
Ventricular drainage	• Emergent external ventricular drain (EVD) placement in all stuporous/comatose patients (Hunt–Hess IV/V), as well as lethargic patients with hydrocephalus
	• Begin trials of clamping external ventricular drain and monitoring ICP on day 3 after placement.
	• Perform ventriculoperitoneal shunting during subacute phase of illness in patients with persistent cognitive dysfunction and ventriculomegaly
Vasospasm diagnosis	• Transcranial Doppler sonography every 1–2 days until the 10th day after SAH
	• CT angiography on days 4–8 after SAH if high risk
Therapy for symptomatic vasospasm	• Place patient in Trendelenberg (head down) position.
	• Infuse 500 mL 5% albumin or 1 L of 0.9% saline over 30 minutes.
	• If the deficit persists, raise the systolic BP with phenylephrine or norepinephrine until the deficit resolves (target 180–220 mm Hg).
	• If refractory, monitor cardiac output and add dobutamine or milrinone to maintain cardiac index ≥4.0 L/min/m².
	• Transfuse to maintain hemoglobin >10.0 g/dL.
	• Emergency angiogram for intra-arterial verapamil or cerebral angioplasty unless the patient responds well to the above measures

Adapted from Komotar R, Schmidt JM, Starke RM, et al. Resuscitation and critical care of poor grade subarachnoid hemorrhage. *Neurosurgery.* 2009;64(3):397–410.

consideration. Anticonvulsants are discontinued on the first postoperative day in good-grade patients who have not had a seizure; anticonvulsant prophylaxis is continued for approximately 1 week in poor-grade patients.

Most centers advocate the use of aggressive fluid resuscitation with isotonic crystalloid (with or without additional colloids) to prevent volume contraction, although this has not been proven to reduce the risk of symptomatic ischemia from vasospasm. A central venous or pulmonary artery catheter is used in high-risk patients to guide fluid administration on the basis of target cardiac filling pressures. The calcium channel blocker nimodipine reduced the frequency of delayed ischemic deterioration by about 30% in several clinical trials; this effect was attributed to reduction of calcium entry into ischemic neurons or by improvement in microcollateral flow because no effect on angiographic spasm was demonstrated [**Level 1**].[3]

Use of dexamethasone in acute SAH is controversial; it is often used in the perioperative period for brain relaxation. No specific evidence suggests that it is beneficial, although it may reduce the headache sometimes associated with vasospasm. Externalized ventricular drains are used to treat obstructive hydrocephalus in patients who are stuporous or comatose, but these devices carry a risk of infection (10% overall) and therefore should be removed once intracranial pressure is stable during a 24-hour clamping trial. Serial lumbar puncture is used to treat hydrocephalus in patients who are following commands.

Transcranial Doppler (TCD) ultrasonography is widely used to diagnose vasospasm of the larger cerebral arteries after SAH. Accelerated blood flow velocities, which occur as flow is maintained through narrowed arteries, have a sensitivity and specificity of 90% for angiographic vasospasm of the proximal middle cerebral artery, but they are less sensitive for detecting spasm of the anterior cerebral or basilar arteries. Increased TCD velocity does not imply increased likelihood of developing ischemia from vasospasm. For this reason, a CT perfusion scan is obtained between SAH days 4 and 8 to determine whether cerebral blood flow is regionally compromised.

Treatment of acute symptomatic vasospasm relies on increasing blood volume, blood pressure, and cardiac output in an attempt to improve cerebral blood flow through arteries in spasm that have lost the capacity to autoregulate. Crystalloid or colloid solutions are given to maintain pulmonary artery diastolic pressure greater than 14 mm Hg or central venous pressure greater than 8 mm Hg. Pressors such as norepinephrine or phenylephrine are used to elevate systolic blood pressure to levels as high as 180 to 220 mm Hg. Hypertensive–hypervolemic–hemodilution ("triple-H therapy") of this type results in clinical improvement in about 70% of patients; cerebral angioplasty can lead to dramatic improvement in patients with severe deficits that are refractory to hemodynamic augmentation (see Fig. 39.4).

Vasospasm can lead to clinically "silent" brain infarction in poor-grade patients who are stuporous or comatose and require sedation to assist in mechanical ventilation. To detect ischemia at its earliest stages, many centers rely on continuous EEG and invasive monitoring of brain tissue oxygen and cerebral blood flow to provide real-time information about the adequacy of cerebral perfusion and autoregulatory capacity (see also Chapter 33). Trends indicating a reduction in brain perfusion generally trigger a trial of induced hypertension or urgent referral for angiography.

OUTCOME

Approximately 20% of SAH patients treated at high-volume centers do not survive to discharge. In contrast to older patients indicating that delayed ischemia from vasospasm is the major cause of death and disability after SAH, most mortality today is related to the acute effects of hemorrhage in poor-grade patients (Fig. 39.7). Important risk factors for mortality or poor functional recovery after SAH include poor clinical grade, advanced age, large aneurysm size, aneurysm rebleeding, cerebral infarction from vasospasm, and global cerebral edema. Medical complications such as fever, hyperglycemia, and anemia have also been linked to poor outcome.

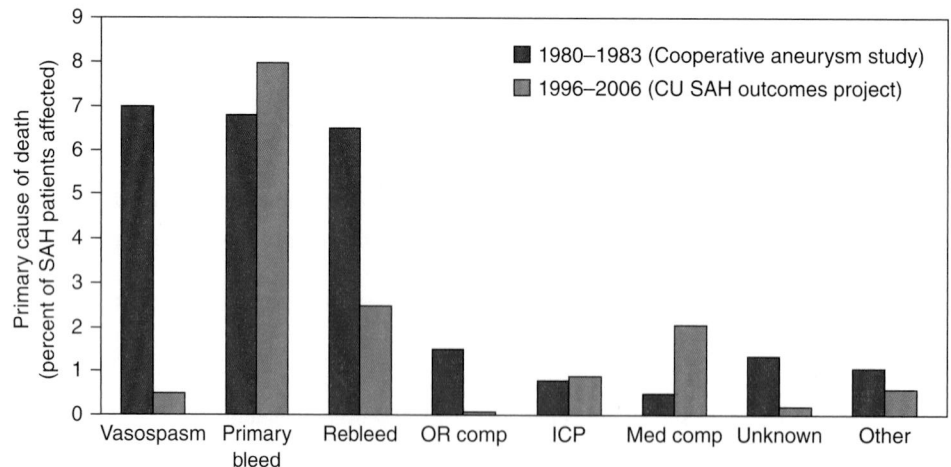

FIGURE 39.7 Mortality after SAH according to the primary cause of death or neurologic devastation leading to withdrawal of support. Data are from 3,521 patients enrolled in the Cooperative Aneurysm Study between 1980 and 1983 and 1,019 patients enrolled in the Columbia University Outcomes Project between 1996 and 2006. Numbers represent the percentage of all SAH patients who died as a direct consequence of the listed variable. (From Komotar R, Schmidt JM, Starke RM, et al. Resuscitation and critical care of poor grade subarachnoid hemorrhage. *Neurosurgery.* 2009;64[3]:397–410.)

In contrast to the focal neurologic deficits that typically follow ischemic stroke, survivors of SAH are disabled primarily by cognitive impairment. Neuropsychological testing reveals long-term problems in memory, concentration, psychomotor speed, visuospatial skills, or executive function in 60% to 80% of SAH patients. Depression and anxiety are also common. These disturbances do not lead to the outward appearance of disability but can affect work, relationships, and quality of life; about 50% of SAH patients do not return to their previous level of employment. Cognitive and physical rehabilitation are essential for maximizing recovery in severely affected patients.

OTHER KINDS OF MACROSCOPIC ANEURYSMS

FUSIFORM OR DOLICHOECTATIC ANEURYSMS

These circumferential vessel dilatations usually involve the carotid, basilar, or vertebral arteries. Atherosclerosis probably plays a role in their formation, but a developmental defect of the wall may be present in some. Fusiform aneurysms seldom become occluded with thrombus and rarely rupture. If bleeding occurs, treatment often requires proximal vessel occlusion.

MYCOTIC ANEURYSM

Mycotic aneurysms are caused by septic emboli, which are most often formed by bacterial endocarditis (Chapter 61). They are usually only a few millimeters in size and tend to occur on distal branches of pial vessels, especially those of the middle cerebral artery. Mycotic aneurysms have been reported in up to 10% of endocarditis patients, but arteriography is not routinely performed, and the incidence is probably underestimated. Pyogenic segmental arteritis from septic emboli in the absence of frank aneurysm formation can also lead to intracranial hemorrhage. Because rupture is fatal in 80% of patients with mycotic aneurysms, cerebral arteriography should be performed when endocarditis is accompanied by suspicious headaches, stiff neck, seizure, focal neurologic symptoms, or CSF pleocytosis. Although mycotic aneurysms occasionally disappear radiographically with antimicrobial therapy, the outcome cannot be predicted, and the aneurysm should be treated surgically as soon as possible.

PSEUDOANEURYSM

Dissection of an intracranial vessel, which usually results from trauma, can lead to extension of blood from the false lumen through the entire vessel wall. The extravasated blood is contained by either a thin layer of adventitia or the surrounding tissues and does not have a true aneurysmal wall, hence the designation *pseudoaneurysm*. If a vessel traversing the subarachnoid space is affected, SAH can result. Treatment may require endovascular or surgical vessel occlusion or trapping, or angioplasty and stenting of the involved segment.

VASCULAR (ARTERIOVENOUS) MALFORMATIONS

Vascular malformations account for less than 5% of all cases of SAH (see also Chapter 41). Intracranial and spinal vascular malformations can be classified into five main types: (1) arteriovenous malformations (AVMs), which are high-flow and most often symptomatic; (2) dural arteriovenous fistulas; (3) cavernous malformations; (4) capillary telangiectasias; and (5) venous malformations.

More than 90% of vascular malformations are asymptomatic throughout life. Bleeding may occur in patients at any age but is most likely to occur in patients younger than 40 years. They are occasionally familial, and in 7% to 10% of cases, AVMs coexist with saccular aneurysms.

AVMs are a conglomerate of abnormal arteries and veins with intervening gliotic brain tissue; they resemble a "bag of worms." When bleeding from an AVM occurs, reported initial mortality has ranged from 4% to 20%. Early rebleeding is far less likely than after aneurysm rupture, but recurrent hemorrhage occurs in 8% to 18% of patients annually over the next several years. For patients without hemorrhage, the risk of bleeding is 2% to 4% per year. Besides prior hemorrhage, risk factors for bleeding from an AVM include deep location and exclusively venous drainage, small size, a single draining vein, and high feeding-artery pressure.

The diagnosis of an AVM is made by MRI and arteriography. Small or thrombosed AVMs, especially in the brain stem, are occasionally missed by arteriography but detected by MRI, which better demonstrates the relationship of the malformation to surrounding brain and identifies its nidus. MRI is the preferred screening procedure for detecting vascular malformations; if surgery is contemplated, conventional angiography is required to delineate the vascular supply. Dural and spinal cord AVM should be kept in mind in patients with radiographically unexplained SAH.

Treatment depends on the location of the AVM and the age and condition of the patient. Direct surgical resection, endovascular glue embolization, and directed-beam radiation therapy with a linear accelerator or Gamma Knife are the main treatment modalities. The long-term value of these treatments is unclear. Embolization is most useful for shrinking the malformation before surgery or radiation; it is occasionally curative as a single mode of therapy.

LEVEL 1 EVIDENCE

1. Hillman J, Fridriksson S, Nilsson O, et al. Immediate administration of tranexamic acid and reduced incidence of early rebleeding after aneurysmal subarachnoid hemorrhage: a prospective randomized study. *J Neurosurg*. 2002;97:771–778.
2. Molyneux AJ, Kerr RS, Yu LM, et al. International subarachnoid aneurysm trial (ISAT) of neurosurgical clipping versus endovascular coiling in 2143 patients with ruptured intracranial aneurysms: a randomised comparison of effects on survival, dependency, seizures, rebleeding, subgroups, and aneurysm occlusion. *Lancet*. 2005;366:809–817.
3. Feigin VL, Rinkel GJ, Algra A, et al. Calcium antagonists in patients with aneurysmal subarachnoid hemorrhage: a systematic review. *Neurology*. 1998;50:876–883.

SUGGESTED READINGS

Broderick JP, Brott TG, Duldner JE, et al. Initial and recurrent bleeding are the major causes of death following subarachnoid hemorrhage. *Stroke*. 1994;25:1342–1347.

Brust JCM, Dickinson PCT, Hughes JEO, et al. The diagnosis and treatment of cerebral mycotic aneurysms. *Ann Neurol*. 1990;27:238–246.

Claassen J, Bernardini, GL, Kreiter K, et al. Effect of cisternal and ventricular blood on risk of delayed cerebral ischemia after subarachnoid hemorrhage: the Fisher scale revisited. *Stroke*. 2001;32:2012–2020.

Connolly ES Jr, Rabinstein AA, Carhuapoma JR, et al. Guidelines for the management of aneurysmal subarachnoid hemorrhage: a guideline for healthcare professionals from the American Heart Association/American Stroke Association. *Stroke*. 2012;43:1711–1737.

Crowley RW, Medel R, Dumont AS, et al. Angiographic vasospasm is strongly correlated with cerebral infarction after subarachnoid hemorrhage. *Stroke.* 2011;42:919–923.

Diringer MN, Bleck TP, Claude Hemphill J III, et al. Critical care management of patients following aneurysmal subarachnoid hemorrhage: recommendations from the Neurocritical Care Society's Multidisciplinary Consensus Conference. *Neurocrit Care.* 2011;15:211–240.

Fisher CM, Kistler JP, Davis JM. Relation of cerebral vasospasm to subarachnoid hemorrhage visualized by computerized tomographic scanning. *Neurosurgery.* 1980;6:1–9.

Hop JW, Rinkel GJE, Algra A, et al. Case-fatality rates and functional outcome after subarachnoid hemorrhage: a systematic review. *Stroke.* 1997;28:660–664.

Juvela S, Porras M, Heiskanen O. Natural history of unruptured intracranial aneurysms: a long-term follow-up study. *J Neurosurg.* 1993;79:174–182.

Komotar R, Schmidt JM, Starke RM, et al. Resuscitation and critical care of poor grade subarachnoid hemorrhage. *Neurosurgery.* 2009;64:397–411.

Kowalski RG, Claassen J, Kreiter KT, et al. Initial misdiagnosis and outcome after subarachnoid hemorrhage. *JAMA.* 2004;291:866–869.

Longstreth WT Jr, Nelson LM, Koepsell TD, et al. Clinical course of spontaneous subarachnoid hemorrhage: a population-based study in King County, Washington. *Neurology.* 1993;43:712–718.

Mast H, Young WL, Koennecke HC, et al. Risk of spontaneous hemorrhage after diagnosis of cerebral arteriovenous malformation. *Lancet.* 1997;350:1065–1068.

Mayer SA, Fink ME, Homma S, et al. Cardiac injury associated with neurogenic pulmonary edema following subarachnoid hemorrhage. *Neurology.* 1994;44:815–820.

Rinkel GJE, Djibuti M, Algra A, et al. Prevalence and risk of rupture of intracranial aneurysms: a systematic review. *Stroke.* 1998;29:251–256.

Perry JJ, Stiell IG, Sivilotti ML, et al. Clinical decision rules to rule out subarachnoid hemorrhage for acute headache. *JAMA.* 2013;310:1248–1255.

Schmidt JM, Ko SB, Helbok R, et al. Cerebral perfusion pressure thresholds for brain tissue hypoxia and metabolic crisis after poor-grade subarachnoid hemorrhage. *Stroke.* 2011;42(5):1351–1356.

Sehba FA, Pluta RM, Zhang JH. Metamorphosis of subarachnoid hemorrhage research: from delayed vasospasm to early brain injury. *Mol Neurobiol.* 2001;43(1):27–40.

Suarez JI, Tarr RW, Selman WR. Aneurysmal subarachnoid hemorrhage. *New Engl J Med.* 2006;354:387–396.

Vergouwen MD, Ilodigwe D, Macdonald RL. Cerebral infarction after subarachnoid hemorrhage contributes to poor outcome by vasospasm-dependent and -independent effects. *Stroke.* 2011;42(4):924–929.

Viñuela G, Duckwiler G, Mawad M. Guglielmi detachable coil embolization of acute intracranial aneurysm: perioperative anatomical and clinical outcome in 403 patients. *J Neurosurg.* 1997;86:475–482.

Wartenberg KE, Schmidt JM, Claassen J, et al. Medical complications after subarachnoid hemorrhage: frequency and impact on outcome. *Crit Care Med.* 2006;34:617–623.

Wiebers DO, Whisnant JP, Huston J III, et al; International Study of Unruptured Intracranial Aneurysms Investigators. Unruptured intracranial aneurysms: natural history, clinical outcome, and risks of surgical and endovascular treatment. *Lancet.* 2003;362:103–110.

Woitzik J, Dreier JP, Hecht N, et al. Delayed cerebral ischemia and spreading depolarization in absence of angiographic vasospasm after subarachnoid hemorrhage. *J Cereb Blood Flow Metab.* 2011;32:203–212.

Zaroff JG, Leong J, Kim H, et al. Cardiovascular predictors of long-term outcomes after non-traumatic subarachnoid hemorrhage. *Neurocrit Care.* 2012;17(3):374–381.

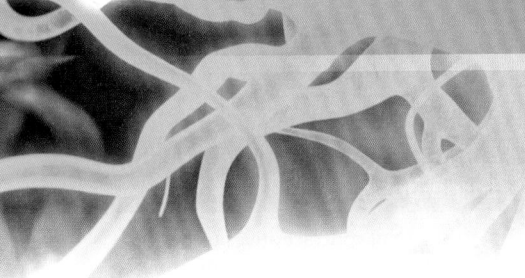

Natalie Organek and Jennifer A. Frontera

INTRODUCTION

Cerebral venous thrombosis (CVT) is thrombosis of the venous channels that drain blood from the brain (Fig. 40.1). Often, it is associated with other conditions causing thrombi, but not infrequently, its cause remains unknown. CVT commonly presents with isolated headache but also must be kept on the differential for causes of cerebral ischemia, hemorrhage, and even coma. CVT image findings may be subtle but are important because overlooking them can have catastrophic consequences. Treatment recommendations for CVT had been controversial for many years, although anticoagulation remains the mainstay of treatment. Overall, the outcome for CVT is positive; if it is treated early, recurrence rates are low.

EPIDEMIOLOGY

CVT is an uncommon disorder affecting a variable patient population. CVT in adults is thought to affect about 5 people per 1 million every year. Most accounts estimate that CVT represents slightly less than 1% of all strokes. The International Study on CVT (ISCVT), the largest multicenter collaboration of consecutively enrolled symptomatic CVT patients older than 15 years with imaging confirmation, collected data on 624 patients from 24 countries and 89 centers and found the following epidemiologic data for CVT: median age was 37 years (age range 16 to 86 years), 74% of enrollees were female. These data is in keeping with the general belief that, although it can affect any age or sex, in the adult population, CVT is largely a disorder of young to middle-aged females.

The Canadian Pediatric Ischemic Stroke Registry (CPISR) is one of the largest pediatric CVT registries and involved 16 pediatric tertiary care centers in Canada collecting data on 160 consecutive cases of radiologically confirmed CVT in children 0 to 18 years old. These data demonstrated an incidence of pediatric CVT to be about 6.7 per 1 million people, slightly more common than adult CVT. Among the 160 children enrolled, 54% were younger than 1 year old (with 43% younger than 1 month of age) and 54% were male. This follows the general understanding that the pediatric CVT population largely involves very young children and the female preponderance seen in adult CVT is not present in pediatric CVT populations.

FIGURE 40.1 Cerebral venous anatomy. (Reprinted with permission, Cleveland Clinic Center for Medical Art & Photography © 2014–2015. All Rights Reserved.)

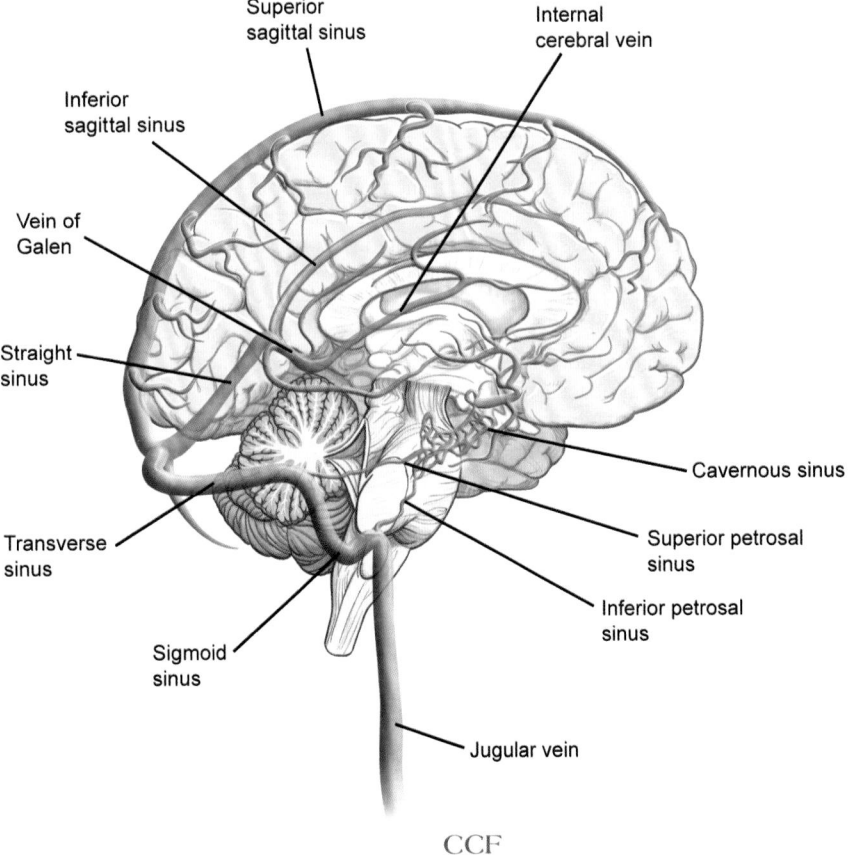

PATHOBIOLOGY

CVT has been attributed to numerous causes, yet even after extensive workup, almost 30% of CVT diagnoses remain idiopathic. ISCVT found that thrombophilia (34.1%) and oral contraception (54%, overall data corrected for females of childbearing age) accounted for a significant portion of the causes of CVT. Other important causes of CVT were puerperium (14%, overall data corrected for females of childbearing age) and pregnancy (6%, overall data corrected for females of childbearing age). Additionally, infection (especially of the ear, sinus, mouth, face, and neck) contributed to 12% of CVT cases in their data set, and malignancy (within and outside of the central nervous system [CNS], both solid tumor and hematologic) was found to have caused 7% of CVT in the ISCVT population. Regarding genetic causes, Marjot et al. performed a meta-analysis of 26 studies: This included 1,183 CVT patients, explored six genes, and demonstrated a statistically significant association between CVT and two genes: factor V Leiden (OR = 2.40; 95% CI, 1.75 to 3.30; $P <.00001$) and prothrombin gene mutation (OR = 5.48; 95% CI, 3.88 to 7.74; $P <.00001$). Finally, more than 44% of subjects were found to have more than one cause of CVT, an important fact to remember when exploring causes of CVT in hopes of preventing reoccurrence. Table 40.1 summarizes common causes of CVT.

In contrast to adult data, the most common cause of CVT in children is infection. In the CPISR data, acute infection was most commonly found in neonates (children younger than 1 month; 84%). Perinatal complications (51%) and dehydration (30%) were also common causes of CVT in the neonatal population. In older children (older than 1 month but younger than 18 years), chronic illness was the most common risk factor, especially connective tissue disorders (23%), hematologic disease (20%), and cancer (13%). Similar to the adult data, the CPISR data found prothrombotic states to be an important cause of CVT in neonates (20%) and children (54%).

CLINICAL FEATURES

The variable clinical presentation is one of the challenges of CVT. In adults, the disorder typically presents with symptoms attributed to increased intracranial pressure (ICP) associated with inability to drain the thrombosed vessel or focal neurologic disease ascribed to cerebral venous ischemia or hemorrhage.

Diffuse progressive headache over hours to days is the most common presentation in patients with CVT, although thunderclap and migrainous-type headache have also been described. Importantly, isolated headache without other neurologic findings or signs of elevated ICP occurred in 25% of confirmed CVT in the ISCVT cohort.

When CVT does cause an increase in ICP, patients commonly present with the following neurologic signs: papilledema, diplopia (most commonly due to sixth nerve palsy), headache which worsens with recumbency, nausea/vomiting, and encephalopathy. In addition to signs of increased ICP, focal neurologic deficits following cerebral ischemia or hemorrhage are also important clinical presentations in patients with CVT. The actual signs of the focal brain injury are attributed to the site of venous ischemia and are therefore variable but include focal weakness, sensory changes, visual field deficits, and aphasias. Further confounding this picture in CVT, the superior sagittal sinus, the most commonly involved cerebral venous structure in CVT, drains both cerebral hemispheres and therefore when thrombosed can cause bilateral

TABLE 40.1	Common Causes of Cerebral Sinus Thrombosis
Drugs	Oral contraceptives (especially in combination with tobacco and/or prothrombotic disease), hormone replacement therapy, asparaginase chemotherapy, tamoxifen, steroids, androgens
Hematologic diseases	Polycythemia, thrombocythemia, paroxysmal nocturnal hemoglobinuria
Hypercoagulable state	Protein C, S, or antithrombin III deficiency; factor V Leiden mutation; prothrombin gene mutation; antiphospholipid syndrome (lupus anticoagulant/anticardiolipin antibody); nephrotic syndrome; hyperhomocysteinemia
Infections	Encephalitis; cerebritis; meningitis; mastoiditis; otitis; sinusitis; infections of the mouth, face, and neck
Inflammatory diseases	Vasculitis, lupus, Wegener granulomatosis, inflammatory bowel disease, Behçet disease, thromboangiitis obliterans, sarcoidosis
Malignancy	CNS tumors with invasion of the venous sinus, hematologic cancers, hypercoagulable state due to malignancy
Obstetric	Pregnancy and puerperium
Trauma (including iatrogenic)	Head injury, lumbar puncture, neurosurgical procedures

CNS, central nervous system.
Adapted from Frontera J, ed. *Decision Making in Neurocritical Care.* New York: Thieme; 2009.

deficits complicating neurologic localization. A small yet clinically important subset of CVT patients are those with deep CVT. CVT affecting the basal ganglia or thalamus is commonly bilateral and can lead to venous ischemia or hemorrhages. CVT affecting the deep parts of the brain tend to be more severe and quickly results in profound deficits including altered mental status and coma.

The cavernous sinuses are a unique set of cerebral sinuses. They are deep bilateral structures at the base of the cerebrum that house the internal carotid artery, ophthalmic vein, branches of the sphenoid and superficial middle cerebral veins, as well as cranial nerves III, IV, V1, V2, and VI. Venous thrombosis affecting the cavernous sinuses are associated with palsies affecting these cranial nerves as well as pain, ptosis, chemosis, and proptosis. Increased intraocular pressure due to poor venous drainage can lead to loss of visual acuity. Most cavernous sinus thromboses are related to infection, typically due to *Staphylococcus aureus*, although *Streptococcus pneumoniae*, gram-negative rods, anaerobes, and occasionally fungal infections may be culprits. Spread of symptoms to the contralateral eye via the intracavernous sinuses may occur within 24 to 48 hours of the initial presentation and is pathognomonic for cavernous sinus thrombosis. Table 40.2 summarizes common syndromes associated with CVT.

TABLE 40.2	Common Cerebral Venous Thrombosis Syndromes
CVT Location	**Symptoms**
Superior sagittal sinus	Large vein, symptoms depend on location affected
	Motor deficits (can be bilateral due to central location)
	Psychiatric symptoms (when affecting the frontal lobes)
	Seizures due to cortical location
Transverse sinus	Aphasias when they affect areas of speech
Cerebral cortical vein	Deficit varies depending on location of CVT
	Seizures due to cortical location
Deep venous system	Change in mental status
	Coma
	Bilateral deficits due to central location
Cavernous sinus	Palsies affecting cranial nerves III, IV, V1, V2, or VI
	Orbital pain

CVT, cerebral venous thrombosis. Adapted from Frontera J, ed. *Decision Making in Neurocritical Care*. New York: Thieme; 2009.

Clinical presentation for CVT in children is similar to adults except in neonates where seizure is more common. In the CPISR database, 71% of neonates (children younger than 1 month old) with CVT had seizure attributed to CVT, in contrast to only 48% of non-neonate CPISR children and 44% of CVT patients older than 15 years.

DIAGNOSIS

CVT is a pathology known for its infrequent as well as variable clinical presentation both of which can complicate diagnosis. Delays in diagnosis of CVT are not uncommon; therefore, a high level of suspicion must be maintained in the proper clinical context. Diagnosing CVT begins with a thorough patient history and physical examination. Elements discovered in these investigations help to determine the necessary laboratory and radiologic evaluation.

The key to diagnosis in CVT is direct imaging of the cerebral venous system. Both computed tomography venography (CTV) and magnetic resonance venography (MRV) have been studied in CVT; they have been found to be equivalent imaging techniques in CVT. Figure 40.2A demonstrates CVT in the torcula on T2 magnetic resonance imaging (MRI) and in the left transverse sinus on MRV (Fig. 40.2B, *white arrows*). Drawbacks associated with CTV include radiation exposure, contrast allergy, and limited use in renal failure. MRV is limited in patients with pacemakers and requires significant time that is typically unavailable in urgent neurologic evaluations. Distinguishing thrombosis from venous hypoplasia can complicate interpretation of MRV and CTV imaging. Parenchymal MR imaging sequences can be useful in making this distinction (Table 40.3) and is particularly useful for diagnosing cavernous sinus thrombosis.

Conventional digital subtraction angiography was the gold standard for the diagnosis of CVT for many years, although, for the most part, it is currently reserved for inconclusive CTV or MRV imaging or when endovascular intervention is required. In patients with persistent symptoms or those with previously diagnosed CVT and a change in symptoms, repeat imaging should be considered to evaluate for new CVT as well as propagation of known thrombus.

In 2011, the American Heart Association (AHA) and the American Stroke Association (ASA) created the statement for health care professional on the diagnosis and management of

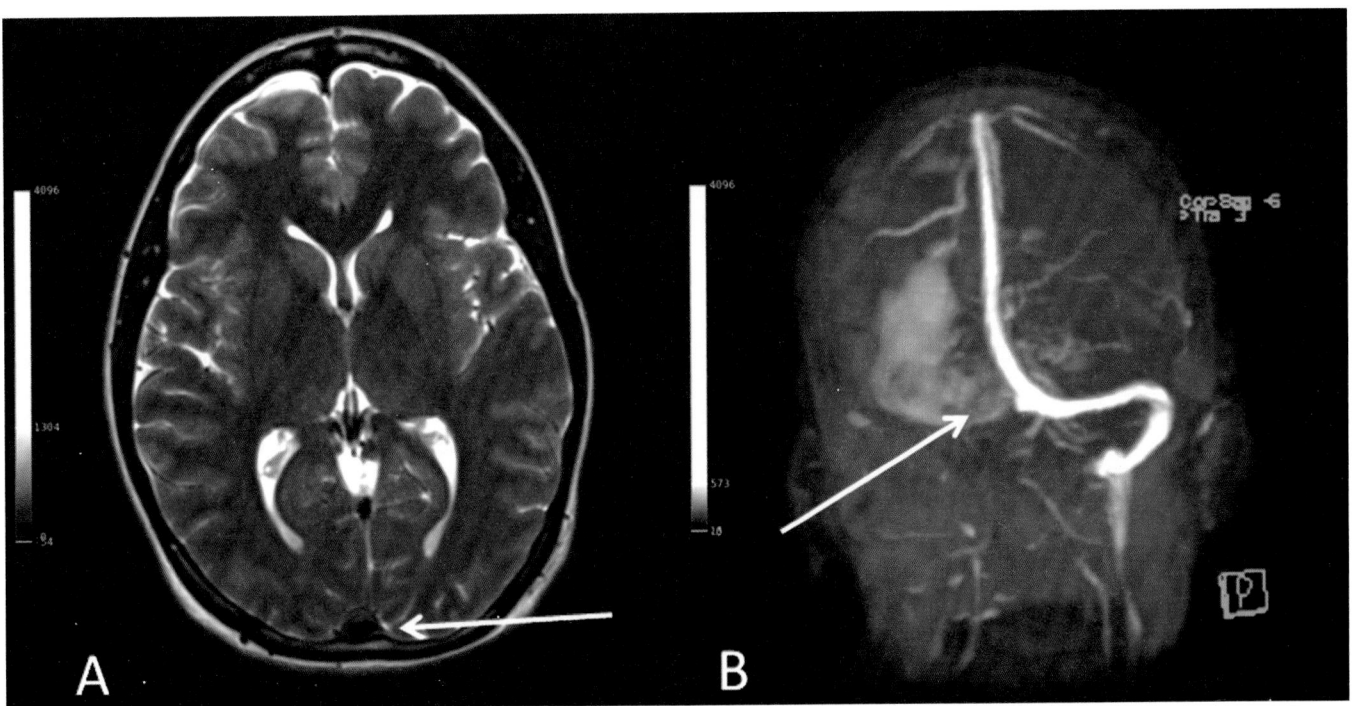

FIGURE 40.2 Axial T2 MRI **(A)** and coronal MRV **(B)** demonstrating a thrombus at the torcula (*white arrow* in **A**) and at the transverse sinus (*white arrow* in **B**).

TABLE 40.3 Using Magnetic Resonance Imaging to Age Cerebral Blood

Phase	Time	T1	T2	Hemoglobin
Acute	1–3 days	Isodense	Dark	Deoxyhemoglobin
Early subacute	3–7 days	Bright	Dark	Methemoglobin
Late subacute	7–14 days	Bright	Bright	Methemoglobin
Chronic	>14 days	Dark	Dark	Hemosiderin

Adapted from Frontera J, ed. *Decision Making in Neurocritical Care*. New York: Thieme; 2009.

cerebral venous thrombosis [**Level 1**],[2] which reviewed, among other topics, invasive and noninvasive CVT diagnostic imaging modalities. In the AHA/ASA review, noncontrast CT of the brain was the most common imaging modality for patients with new neurologic symptoms. Noncontrast head CT is often unremarkable but may demonstrate subtle signs suggestive of the CVT, namely, hyperdensities in the cerebral veins. This finding is present in only about one-third of patients. The most well-known noncontrast head CT finding in CVT is the dense triangle found in the posterior sagittal sinus called the *filled delta* sign. There is often a delay in visualization of this sign for days, but once present, it typically persists for weeks, which make it likely to be most helpful with late presentation of CVT. More often, noncontrast head CT demonstrates nonspecific indirect signs of CVT including CT hypodensities and a decrease in ventricular size both associated with parenchymal edema. Nonenhanced head CT is also helpful in demonstrating cerebral venous infarctions or intracerebral hemorrhage (ICH), which characteristically are in vascular distributions inconsistent with more common arterial disease. Perhaps most importantly, noncontrast CT is helpful in ruling out other causes for the clinical presentation. In CVT, contrast-enhanced CT may demonstrate the "empty delta sign" wherein the thrombus creates a filling defect in the cerebral venous system and, therefore, becomes "empty." Finally, as with most cerebrovascular disease, MRI of the brain can be helpful in demonstrating earlier signs of venous infarct associated with CVT.

CVT laboratory workup is focused on determining the cause and should include basic labs as well as an evaluation for hypercoagulability. Anticoagulation can affect the outcome of the hypercoagulable labs, and therefore, these should be examined prior to initiating anticoagulation treatment for CVT. Table 40.4 lists laboratory workup for CVT.

TABLE 40.4 Laboratory Workup for Cerebral Venous Thrombosis

Basic labs	CBC, chemistry, liver function testing, antinuclear antibody
Hypercoagulable workup (test prior to starting anticoagulation)	Coagulation studies, homocysteine, factor V Leiden mutation, prothrombin gene mutation, antiphospholipid and anticardiolipin antibodies, lupus coagulant, protein C and S, antithrombin III, fibrinogen
Specific testing (patient specific)	Urine protein (if nephrotic syndrome is suspected)

CBC, complete blood count.

D-dimer has been explored as a possible diagnostic marker for CVT, but high pretest probability remains paramount. Meng et al. performed a prospective study of confirmed CVT in 94.1% of patients who had elevated D-dimer and during the acute phase, the sensitivity and specificity of predicting CVT with D-dimer were 94.1% and 97.5%. Similarly, in a meta-analysis of 1,134 CVT cases by Dentali et al., D-dimer was found to have a mean sensitivity of 93.9% and mean specificity of 89.7%. The AHA/ASA CVT statement [**Level 1**][2] reviewed sensitivity and specificity of a number of studies exploring D-dimer and CVT and suggests D-dimer may be helpful in those with very low suspicion of CVT but cannot be used to preclude further evaluation in patients in whom there is a strong clinical suspicion.

Diagnosis of CVT in children is similar to adults in that, most importantly, although CVT is rare and has a nonspecific presentation, it must not be left off a comprehensive differential in children with appropriate neurologic symptoms. As described earlier, this may be especially challenging in neonates who more commonly present with seizure but have otherwise nonspecific presentation. In general, CVT imaging is very similar in children and adults, but neonatal physiologic differences must be considered. The hypointensity of the immature unmyelinated brain as well as the hyperintensity of physiologic polycythemia associated with neonates can mimic the "delta sign" and is therefore known as the *pseudodelta sign*. This CVT mimic in neonates is easily clarified with administration of contrast material. Additionally, in neonates, transfontanellar ultrasound has been explored for CVT diagnosis but was generally found unreliable especially in nonocclusive thrombus and therefore has limited use in neonatal CVT without confirmation with other imaging modalities.

TREATMENT

CVT treatment is typically trimodal: The mainstay of treatment is (1) anticoagulation, (2) treatment of the underlying etiology when appropriate (i.e., antimicrobial for cases involving infection) and (3) symptomatic treatment (headache management, addressing increased ICP). In patients who present with seizure, antiepileptic drugs (AEDs) are indicated.

Anticoagulation is essential for preventing CVT propagation and to prevent systemic thrombosis in those with underlying hypercoagulable states. Einhäupl et al. studied 20 patients with CVT (confirmed on imaging) who were randomized to intravenous unfractionated heparin (UFH) versus placebo. The study was stopped prematurely due to the obvious benefit of treatment with anticoagulation. Additionally, this group documented two ICHs, both in the placebo group (none among the anticoagulation treatment group). Subsequently, in a study by de Bruijn et al. [**Level 1**],[1] 59 patients with CVT were randomized to low molecular weight heparin

(LMWH) versus placebo. The placebo group was more likely to have a poor outcome compared with the treatment group, and no ICHs occurred in either group. The current AHA guidelines for CVT recommend initial anticoagulation with UFH or weight-based LMWH in full doses followed by vitamin K antagonists regardless of the presence of ICH [**Level 1**].[2] It is important to note that anticoagulation *should be administered for CVT even in the context of intracranial hemorrhage*. Concurrent with the present AHA recommendations, the ISCVT investigators compared the outcomes of CVT patients treated with UFH and LMWH and found a better efficacy and safety for LMWH. Additionally, a randomized controlled trial of 66 CVT patients also explored treatment with UFH and LMWH and found LMWH to have a significantly lower mortality in CVT compared to UFH [**Level 1**].[3] Most recently, in 2012, the American College of Chest Physicians formally recommended initial treatment for CVT with either dose-adjusted heparin or LMWH followed by oral anticoagulation for 3 to 6 months for most patients and lifelong anticoagulation for CVT patients with permanent risk factors for recurrent events [**Level 1**].[4] Finally, women of childbearing age with CVT present a unique challenge. In women with a history of CVT, oral contraceptives should generally be avoided and in pregnant women with a history of CVT, prophylaxis with LMWH during future pregnancies and in the postpartum period may be reasonable [**Level 1**].[5]

The data for endovascular invasive therapy, including direct endovascular thrombolysis and thrombectomy, to this point has not proven to provide greater benefit than anticoagulation alone except for case reports and small case series in patients with CVT who clinically deteriorate while on anticoagulation and in those who have an absolute contraindication to anticoagulation (such as hemodynamically significant hemorrhage or allergy to anticoagulation agents). Options for endovascular treatment include local infusion of recombinant tissue plasminogen activator as well as mechanical thrombolysis using balloons and rheolytic catheters. Thrombolysis adds the additional risks of parenchymal and systemic hemorrhage beyond the risks incurred by heparin or LMWH alone. In light of the recent advances in endovascular therapy, open surgical treatment for CVT is limited mostly to those patients with large cerebral venous infarcts who develop clinical and radiologic signs of herniation and may benefit from decompressive hemicraniectomy.

In patients with symptomatic intracranial hypertension, efforts to lower ICP should be considered. Elevation of the head of the bed with the head midline to promote venous drainage, osmotic therapy, and management of hypermetabolic states (shivering, fever, seizure, agitation) should be considered as part of routine intracranial hypertension management.

In patients with seizure related to CVT, AEDs should be administered [**Level 1**][2]; however, prophylactic AED use is not advised. Optimum duration of treatment with AEDs in CVT patients with seizure remains unknown.

There is a dearth of data regarding treatment of CVT in children; treatment guidelines are largely extrapolated from adult data. AHA/ASA [**Level 1**][2] current recommendations for treating CVT in children older than 1 month of age align with adult recommendations for treatment with anticoagulation even in the context of ICH. Treatment recommendations for children younger than 1 month of age remain controversial and variable. Neonates should be treated with anticoagulation for 6 weeks to 3 months with close imaging follow-up to assess for recanalization with low threshold for stopping anticoagulation at 6 weeks if the venous system recanalizes [**Level 1**].[2] AED recommendations in children (and neonates) are similar to that of adults.

OUTCOME

Overall, the outcome for most patients with CVT is positive, but there remains an important minority in whom the disease causes significant morbidity and mortality. According to ISCVT data, about 87% of CVT patients had complete recovery, but about 8% had significant morbidity with an additional mortality rate of about 5%. Similarly, Borhani Haghighi et al. investigated a national cohort of almost 3,500 CVT patients had a mortality rate of 4.39%. Certain characteristics have been found to be associated with poor outcome in CVT including male gender, age older than 37 years, those with significant neurologic deficit and coma, as well as those who develop seizure. In the acute phase of CVT, brain herniation attributed to CVT remains the most common cause of death; in the late stages, mortality associated with CVT is mostly related to the underlying cause of the thrombosis. Rates of CVT recurrence range from 2% to 4%.

In childhood, CVT coma has been shown to predict mortality, but overall, few studies have followed children for more than 2 years after CVT. In the CPISR data (with only over 2 years of follow-up), approximately 75% of neonates and approximately 50% of nonneonates were neurologically normal.

LEVEL 1 EVIDENCE

1. de Bruijn SF, Stam J. Randomized, placebo-controlled trial of anticoagulant treatment with low-molecular-weight heparin for cerebral sinus thrombosis. *Stroke*. 1999;30(3):484–488.
2. Saposnik G, Barinagarrementeria F, Brown RD Jr, et al. Diagnosis and management of cerebral venous thrombosis: a statement for healthcare professionals from the American Heart Association/American Stroke Association. *Stroke*. 2011;42(4):1158–1192.
3. Misra UK, Kalita J, Chandra S, et al. Low molecular weight heparin versus unfractionated heparin in cerebral venous sinus thrombosis: a randomized controlled trial. *Eur J Neurol*. 2012;19(7):1030–1036.
4. Lansberg MG, O'Donnell MJ, Khatri P, et al. Antithrombotic and thrombolytic therapy for ischemic stroke: antithrombotic therapy and prevention of thrombosis, 9th ed: American College of Chest Physicians evidence-based clinical practice guidelines. *Chest*. 2012;141(2)(suppl):e601S–e636S.
5. Bushnell C, McCullough LD, Awad IA, et al. Guidelines for the prevention of stroke in women: a statement for healthcare professionals from the American Heart Association/American Stroke Association. *Stroke*. 2014;45(5):1545–1588.

SUGGESTED READINGS

Borhani Haghighi A, Edgell RC, Cruz-Flores S, et al. Mortality of cerebral venous-sinus thrombosis in a large national sample. *Stroke*. 2012;43(1):262–264.

Bousser MG, Ferro JM. Cerebral venous thrombosis: an update. *Lancet Neurol*. 2007;6(2):162–170.

Canhão P, Falcão F, Ferro JM. Thrombolytics for cerebral sinus thrombosis: a systematic review. *Cerebrovasc Dis*. 2003;15(3):159–166.

Canhão P, Ferro JM, Lindgren AG, et al. Causes and predictors of death in cerebral venous thrombosis. *Stroke*. 2005;36(8):1720–1725.

Coutinho JM, Ferro JM, Canhão P, et al. Unfractionated or low-molecular weight heparin for the treatment of cerebral venous thrombosis. *Stroke*. 2010;41(11):2575–1580.

Dentali F, Squizzato A, Marchesi C, et al. D-dimer testing in the diagnosis of cerebral vein thrombosis: a systematic review and a meta-analysis of the literature. *J Thromb Haemost*. 2012;10(4):582–589.

deVeber G, Andrew M, Adams C, et al. Cerebral sinovenous thrombosis in children. *N Engl J Med.* 2001;345(6):417–423.

Einhäupl K, Bousser MG, de Bruijn SF, et al. EFNS guideline on the treatment of cerebral venous and sinus thrombosis. *Eur J Neurol.* 2006;13(6):553–559.

Einhäupl KM, Villringer A, Meister W, et al. Heparin treatment in sinus venous thrombosis. *Lancet.* 1991;338(8767):597–600.

Ferro JM, Canhão P, Stam J, et al; for ISCVT Investigators. Prognosis of cerebral vein and dural sinus thrombosis: results of the International Study on Cerebral Vein and Dural Sinus Thrombosis (ISCVT). *Stroke.* 2004;35(3):664–670.

Lee EJ. The empty delta sign. *Radiology.* 2002;224(3):788–789.

Marjot T, Yadav S, Hasan N, et al. Genes associated with adult cerebral venous thrombosis. *Stroke.* 2011;42(4):913–918.

Martinelli I, Bucciarelli P, Passamonti SM, et al. Long-term evaluation of the risk of recurrence after cerebral sinus-venous thrombosis. *Circulation.* 2010;121(25):2740–2746.

Meng R, Wang X, Hussain M, et al. Evaluation of plasma D-dimer plus fibrinogen in predicting acute CVST. *Int J Stroke.* 2014;9(2):166–173.

Yang JY, Chan AK, Callen DJ, et al. Neonatal cerebral sinovenous thrombosis: sifting the evidence for a diagnostic plan and treatment strategy. *Pediatrics.* 2010;126(3):e693–e700.

Vascular Malformations 41

J. P. Mohr and John Pile-Spellman

INTRODUCTION

This chapter deals with a heterogeneous group of central nervous system (CNS) vascular lesions, including true vascular malformations such as arteriovenous malformations (AVMs) and cavernous malformations, acquired fistulas, vascular neoplasms, and other rare vascular disorders.

ARTERIOVENOUS VASCULAR MALFORMATIONS

AVMs are the most common of these rare disorders. They are thought to be congenital, arising in the prenatal period but do not present clinically until middle life. A few are caused by brain contusions which enlarge the normal tiny arteriovenous shunts. Although many remain static anomalies, others enlarge in size and proliferate in vascular complexity, driven by incompletely understood pathophysiologic forces, in animal models related to Notch4 dysgenetic effects.

EPIDEMIOLOGY

AVMs are rare, occurring with a prevalence of 18 per 100,000 individuals. Every year, about 1 out of every 100 people with an AVM will experience a hemorrhage. Current population studies indicate an incident discovery rate of 1.5 per 100,000. The majority of AVMs are thought to remain asymptomatic throughout life. AVM symptoms tend to occur early in life; two-thirds of AVMs become symptomatic before age 40 years.

PATHOBIOLOGY

AVMs are not neoplasms. Most of them are thought to arise in the prenatal period but not present clinically until middle life. A few are caused by brain contusions which enlarge the normal tiny arteriovenous shunts. Although many remain static anomalies, others enlarge in size and proliferate in vascular complexity, driven by incompletely understood pathophysiologic forces, in animal models related to Notch4 dysgenetic effects.

Whether congenital or acquired, AVMs are anatomically limited to the brain, spinal cord, or dura. Those embedded in the brain are most common. Lacking capillaries at the main site of linkage between the arteries and veins, the nidus is a tangle of irregularly sized vascular channels lacking the expected media of arteries, often so thin walled they barely satisfy criteria for veins. Their location varies widely; some limited to the surface of a cerebral hemisphere, fed by a single small artery and draining to the single small vein. At the opposite extreme, others form a huge wedge from the brain surface through the white matter to the ventricular wall (schizencephalic AVM); some so large they occupy a large portion of one hemisphere. A few lie in the subsurface white matter, others limited to deep structures (e.g., basal ganglia, thalamus), brain stem, or spinal cord. Those on the brain surface lying in the border zone between the major cerebral arteries typically have a higher incidence of seizures but a lower hemorrhage rate than those deeper in the brain. Collateral from the adjacent dura may occur. Those that penetrate to the ventricular wall often draw collaterals from the deep vasculature supplying the basal ganglia. Venous drainage may be by superficial or the deep venous systems.

CLINICAL FEATURES

AVMs present most often with bleeding, less often with headaches or seizures, and occasionally with progressive gait disturbance, focal neurologic deficit, or cognitive decline. When hemorrhage occurs, it affects the following regions: intracerebral (30%), subarachnoid (15%), intraventricular (30%), and various combinations (25%). AVMs are the second most identifiable cause of subarachnoid hemorrhage (SAH) after brain aneurysms, accounting for 5% of all cases of SAH.

The most feared complication of AVMs by far is hemorrhage. Yet compared with aneurysmal rupture, the morbidity of AVM hemorrhage is far less serious; some barely symptomatic, few devastating. The hemorrhage usually arises within the nidus and when limited in volume, displaces adjacent healthy brain with varying degrees of symptoms and signs. For those AVMs that drain to the ventricular wall, bleeding may originate from the venous aspect of the malformation and extend mainly into the ventricle, which presents as intraventricular hemorrhage with hydrocephalus and only minor injury to adjacent brain structures. Larger hemorrhages escape the nidus and dissect into healthy brain tissue like any primary brain hematoma. Arteries feeding the AVM nidus may develop flow-related aneurysms, which may bleed separately, typically causing SAH syndromes.

The risk of an unruptured AVM bleeding on average is closer to 1% than the previously quoted 4% per year. Death from the first hemorrhage ranges between 5% and 20%, depending primarily on the size of the hemorrhage and the presence of ventricular extension. When hemorrhage occurs, some destabilization of the fistula occurs, and it sets the stage for recurrent hemorrhage. Once a bleeding event has occurred, an AVM is more than 5 times more likely to bleed again during the first year, but recurrent hemorrhage occurs in 8% to 18% of patients annually over the next several years. Besides prior hemorrhage, important risk factors for bleeding from an AVM include deep location, small size, and a single draining vein.

AVMs are less often associated with seizures or headaches. No distinctive features separate either the seizures or the types of headache (including migraine) from non-AVM causes (Figs. 41.1–41.3).

DIAGNOSIS

The diagnosis of AVM is made by magnetic resonance imaging (MRI) (Chapter 21) and angiography (Chapter 24) (see Fig. 41.1), less easily by computed tomography (CT) scan and—unless calcified—scarcely even by plan skill films. These tests can be repeated to analyze a change in the size of the AVM, recent bleeding, or the

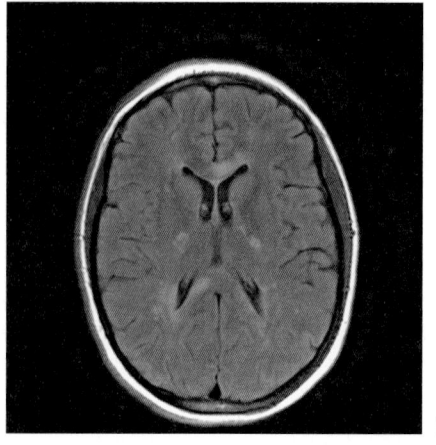
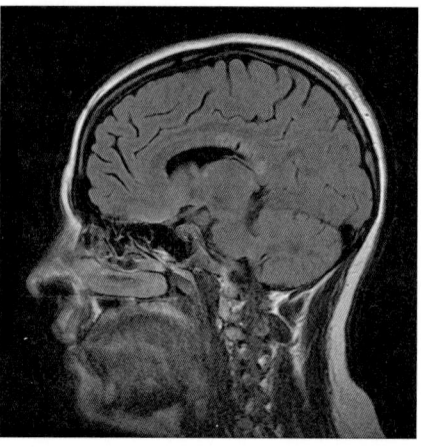
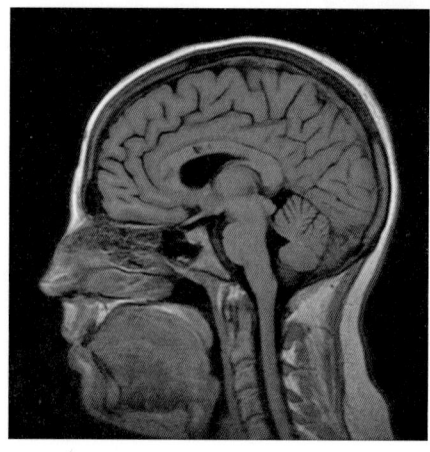

FIGURE 41.1 Left parietal AVM. Anteroposterior **(A)** and lateral **(B)** subtraction films in the arterial phase of a left internal carotid injection show the anterior cerebral artery supply and early superficial venous drainage of a left parietal AVM. Coronal **(C)** and axial **(D)** T2-weighted magnetic resonance images of the same patient show a serpiginous pattern of signal void representing flow in vascular structures. (Courtesy of Drs. J. A. Bello and S. K. Hilal.)

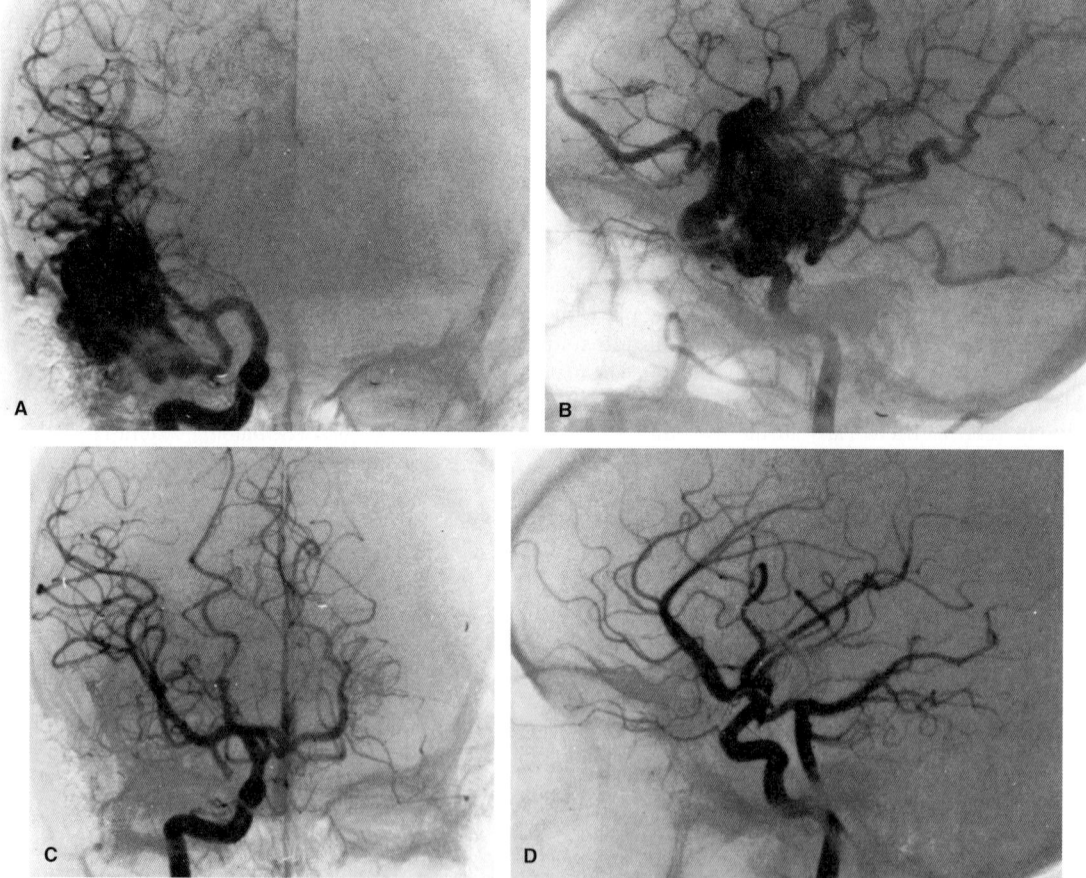

FIGURE 41.2 Right temporal AVM. **A:** Anteroposterior view from arterial phase of right internal carotid arteriogram shows a large enhancing vascular lesion in right temporal region supplied by enlarged branches of right middle cerebral artery. **B:** Lateral view demonstrates prominent early draining cortical veins emanating from AVM. Postembolization anteroposterior **(C)** and lateral **(D)** views of right internal carotid arteriogram show interval disappearance of right temporal AVM with multiple metallic coils seen within right middle cerebral arterial feeders. Note normal filling of both anterior and posterior cerebral arteries, thereby confirming increase in blood flow to normal brain structures. Patient did well after embolization with no complications. Follow-up definitive surgery found no evidence of flow within AVM, and the nidus was removed to prevent recurrence. (Courtesy of Drs. S. Chan and S. K. Hilal, Columbia University College of Physicians and Surgeons, New York, NY.)

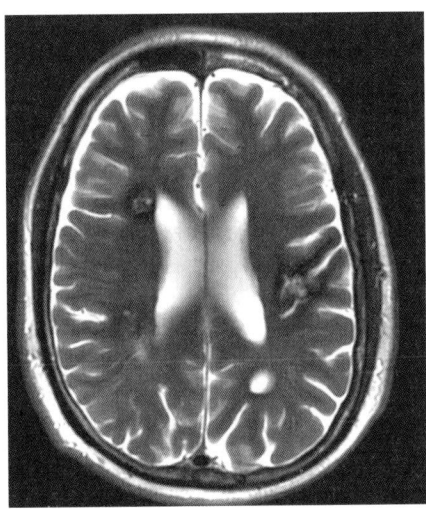

FIGURE 41.3 MRI scan showing the characteristic "target" lesion of a cavernous malformation.

TABLE 41.1	Spetzler–Martin Grading Scale

	Grade
Size of Nidus	
Small (<3 cm)	1
Medium (3–6 cm)	2
Large (>6 cm)	3
Eloquence of Adjacent Brain	
Noneloquent	0
Eloquent[a]	1
Venous Drainage	
Superficial only	0
Deep	1

[a]Scores are used only to estimate the risk of surgical AVM resection. Scores range from 1 to 5. Score of 1 denotes low risk of surgical morbidity (approximately 5%). AVMs with a score of 5 are considered inoperable, with a surgical risk approaching 50% or more.

appearance of new lesions. Small or thrombosed AVMs, especially in the brain stem, are occasionally missed by arteriography but detected by MRI, which better demonstrates the relationship of the malformation to surrounding brain and identifies its nidus. If surgery is contemplated, conventional angiography is required to delineate the vascular supply. Dural and cervical spinal cord AVM should be kept in mind in patients with radiographically unexplained SAH, requiring examination of the external carotid arterial supply and cervical vertebral arteries.

TREATMENT

Treatment depends on the location of the AVM and the age and condition of the patient. Direct *microsurgical resection, endovascular glue embolization,* and *directed-beam radiation therapy* with a linear accelerator or Gamma Knife are the main treatment modalities.

With the advent of MRI, asymptomatic AVMs or those presenting only with headaches or seizures have become increasingly prevalent. The increasing discovery of these conditions before bleeding occurs long posed a management dilemma—whether to take risks of eradicating the lesion, embedded as it is in brain, or await the natural history of hemorrhage, hoping that if it occurs, it will not much damage the adjacent tissues. The recently completed A Randomized trial of Unruptured Brain AVMs (ARUBA) trial indicates that the safer course appears to be delaying intervention unless hemorrhage occurs [**Level 1**].[1] The *Spetzler–Martin grading scale* is used to stratify the risk of death or major complications from surgery (Table 41.1).

Decision making for intervention is complex and relies on clinical expertise, the specifics of the anatomy of the AVM, and the wishes of the patient. Surgery remains the most effective means of eradicating AVMs. For larger or more complex lesions, intravascular occlusive therapy using quick-acting glues can obliterate some AVM feeders, shrinking the malformation before surgery or radiation; it is occasionally curative as a single mode of therapy (see Fig. 41.2). For the deeply lying lesions not suitable for embolization or surgery, focused-beam radiotherapy (radiosurgery) is an alternative therapy. Complete eradication of an AVM is documented with loss of any evidence of early venous filling during the arterial phase of angiography. Despite complete eradication documented by angiogram, a small number of lesions recur.

Vein of Galen malformations are a special AVM associated with the deep venous system, often with marked aneurysmal dilatation of the vein of Galen region. The arterial supply may be complex and difficult to occlude by intravascular or surgical techniques. Most present in neonates or young children. Arteriovenous shunting leads to cardiac failure and compression of the midbrain, which causes hydrocephalus. The currently accepted treatment of these lesions is embolization, occasionally followed by surgery.

OUTCOME

Former estimates of morbidity and mortality from AVM hemorrhage have been revised downward. Widely cited annual rates of 4% per year documented in some publications applied predominantly in those with large, complex AVMs who have bled in the past and whose AVM was deemed too daunting for attempted removal. For 49% of those presenting with first hemorrhage at a large referral institution, their morbidity documented by the modified Rankin Scale was one (no significant disability) and showed significantly better outcomes that those with primary brain hemorrhage not from AVM. Hemorrhages arising from venous aspect of the AVM into the ventricle may present with a spectacular-appearing hemohydrocephalus but experience as satisfactory outcome.

DURAL ARTERIOVENOUS FISTULAS

These shunts linking an arterial source directly to a dural sinus arise from a combination of factors: some traumatic, others from venous thrombosis, and some for reasons still not understood. They account for some 10% to 15% of intracranial vascular malformations.

Current classifications cite three types based on the site of venous drainage, presence of cortical venous reflux, and the number of fistulae. The site most affected are the transverse-sigmoid sinus, tentorial, and anterior cranial fossa (including the cavernous sinus) and less often the spinal system or foramen magnum.

Thrombosis of a large vein or sinus may be a more common cause. Current understanding is that the venous thrombosis creates a high-enough resistance to normal arterial flow as to force creation of new pathways. Closed head injury with trauma to the brain surface—commonly lateral temporal lobe—appears to join or enlarge the existing 90 μm arteriovenous shunts known to exist in the cerebral vasculature. Once having developed, these fistulas presumably lose their capacity for autoregulation and appear subject to the same forces for enlargement of arteriovenous links elsewhere.

Hemorrhage is the presenting symptom in 20%. Many other dural arteriovenous fistulas present with unusual syndromes of local brain edema, among them complex aphasia and visual disturbances. For fistulas affecting the cavernous sinus, the clinical spectrum is broad: A link to the venous system from a small arterial source may create diagnostic problems suggesting myasthenia gravis or ocular myopathy, less dramatic than the rapidly developing bulging erythematous eye in carotid-cavernous sinus fistula that was created by trauma.

When pursued by angiogram, there is usually delayed filling of the carotid or vertebrobasilar arteries, and those branches having access to a patent vein or sinus (meningeal and other dural arteries) can be dilated and convoluted to a degree seen in AVMs. Treatment is by transarterial or transvenous endovascular methods. Persistence in efforts is often required. Some reports document spontaneous regression.

CAVERNOUS MALFORMATIONS

Cavernous malformations are low-flow, highly focal vascular anomalies; most of them are less than 1 cm in size. They may occur anywhere in the brain. Histologically, they show a distinct cluster of tiny vessels of uniform size, hence the name *cavernous*. The individual vessels and even the cluster are too small to be seen on angiogram and are rarely documented by CT scan but are easily seen on MRI (see Fig. 41.3), thanks to the hemosiderin–iron composition from the slow flow through the lesion or from asymptomatic hemorrhages. Multiple lesions—some numbering in the many dozens—have been documented in families. Although they may be mistaken for a vascular tumor on imaging, there is no displacement of the surrounding structure.

Approximately two-thirds of cavernous malformations are diagnosed when patients with symptoms of hemorrhage, seizures, headaches, or vague neurologic symptoms occur. The risk of hemorrhage is 6% annually in patients who have already experienced a bleeding event, and the risk gradually goes down with time. The median interval from primary to a repeat hemorrhage is 8 months. The risk of bleeding in patients presenting with symptoms unrelated to hemorrhage is 2% annually. Of the one-third of patients who present with an incidentally discovered cavernous malformation, the bleeding risk is only 0.3% per year.

The bleeding events themselves tend to be low-impact, compatible with gradual breakdown of the malformation and "oozing" of blood over period of hours, in contrast with the violent bleeding events that can occur with rupture of a lenticulostriate artery in the setting of hypertensive intracerebral hemorrhage (see Chapter 38). The clinical effects of hemorrhage are accordingly usually limited, often causing no or minimal symptoms. Serious deficits are generally restricted to patients with malformations in the brain stem. If hemorrhage has occurred and the lesion is readily accessible, surgery is usually recommended.

VENOUS MALFORMATIONS

Venous malformations (also deep venous anomalies) have no apparent arterial supply. They are not an AVM, only anomalous venous drainage from normal arterial vessels. They may cause headaches, seizures, or, rarely, hemorrhage (Fig. 41.4). They generally lie in the deep white matter and portions of the brain stem and cerebellum and often have spiderlike venous branches into the adjacent parenchyma (so-called caput medusa). They are easily recognized using CT because of their contrast enhancement. Because they also serve as the venous draining system for the adjacent brain, they are not amenable to obliteration by occlusion of the arterial supply or surgical resection. They generally follow a benign course.

TELANGIECTASIAS

Telangiectasias are collections of engorged capillaries or cavernous spaces separated by relatively normal brain tissue. They are usually small and poorly circumscribed. Although found in any portion of the CNS, they have a propensity for the cerebral white matter. In the Rendu–Osler–Weber syndrome, brain telangiectasias are associated with similar lesions of the skin (mucous membranes, respiratory, gastrointestinal, and genitourinary tracts). Those occurring in the lung may provide a path for septic material for brain abscess formation. The fistulas are usually tiny, and some are not demonstrated despite angiography. Major hemorrhage is rare. Interest in genetic mapping for the remarkable variety of telangiectasias has increased greatly and may well lead to a total reclassification of these lesions separate from the classical clinical description.

STURGE–WEBER DISEASE

The main features of this rare disorder, also known as *Krabbe–Weber–Dimitri disease*, are localized atrophy and calcification of the

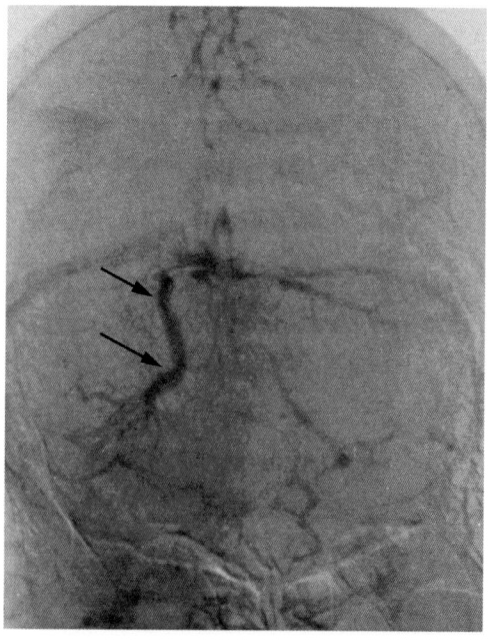

FIGURE 41.4 Subtraction posterior fossa angiogram, venous phase. In this anteroposterior view, the characteristic venous malformation is demonstrated (*arrows*).

cerebral cortex associated with *capillary malformations*. Any portion of the cerebral cortex may be affected by the atrophic process, but the occipital and parietal regions are most commonly involved. Usually also present is an ipsilateral port-wine–colored facial nevus, usually in the distribution of the first division of the trigeminal nerve. Included among the clinical features may be angiomatous malformations in the meninges, ipsilateral exophthalmos, glaucoma, buphthalmos, angiomas of the retina, optic atrophy, and dilated vessels in the sclera.

In the atrophic cortical areas, there is a loss of nerve cells and axons and a proliferation of the fibrous glia. The small vessels are thickened and calcified, particularly in the second and third cortical layers. Small calcium deposits are also present in the cerebral substance, and rarely, there are large calcified nodules. When an angioma is present, it is limited to the meninges overlying the area of shrunken cortex. Although the combination of a port-wine facial nevus and localized cortical atrophy may exist without clinical symptoms, convulsive seizures are usually present from infancy. Mental retardation, glaucoma, contralateral hemiplegia, and hemianopia are also present in most cases.

Sturge–Weber disease can be diagnosed without difficulty from the clinical syndrome. The presence of the cortical lesion can be demonstrated in most cases by the appearance of characteristic shadows in the radiographs. The treatment of Sturge–Weber disease is essentially symptomatic. Anticonvulsive drugs are given for the seizures. Radiation therapy has been recommended, but there is no evidence that it is of any benefit.

SINUS PERICRANII

The disorder is a combination of thin-walled vascular spaces interconnected by numerous anastomoses that protrude from the skull and communicate with the superior longitudinal sinus. The malformation is usually evident in infancy, soft and compressible; it increases in size when the venous pressure in the head is raised by coughing, straining, or lowering the head. It may enlarge slowly over a period of years. The external protuberance may be seen at any portion of the midline of the skull, including the occiput, but is most often found in the midportion of the forehead. Imaging shows a defect of the underlying bone, through which the lesion communicates with the longitudinal sinus.

VASCULAR TUMORS

These three forms of neoplastic lesions may be variations of the same tumor. Histologically, they are indistinguishable but share similar clinical features.

HEMANGIOBLASTOMAS

Hemangioblastomas are composed of primitive vascular elements and are rare, accounting for 1% to 2% of all intracranial neoplasms. They occur at all ages, but young and middle-aged adults are more frequently afflicted. In children, they are almost as common in the posterior fossa as are meningiomas. Symptoms are generally present for approximately a year before the diagnosis is made. Male incidence predominates. *Von Hippel–Lindau disease* is defined by the coexistence of hemangioblastoma and multiple angiomatoses of the retina, cysts of the kidney and pancreas, and, occasionally, renal cell carcinomas, and capillary nevi of the skin. There is a familial incidence in 20% of cases. Only 10% to 20% of the hemangioblastomas, however, are associated with the systemic signs known as the *Lindau syndrome*. All gradations of clinical expression between the full syndrome and incomplete manifestations may be seen in the same family. Associated with these disorders are pheochromocytoma, syringomyelia, and polycythemia (which disappear after resection of the neoplasm but returns with recurrence).

Hemangioblastomas occur predominantly in the cerebellum and are often associated with large cysts that are surrounded by a glial wall containing yellow proteinaceous fluid, the result of secretion, and hemorrhage from the tumor. It resembles the cyst and mural nodule of the cystic cerebellar astrocytoma but has a distinctive vascular appearance on an angiogram. They may be multiple, in which case difficulty in achieving a cure or total removal of the lesion may be encountered. They have no dural attachment.

Hemangioblastoma can also occur in the spinal cord or in the medulla in the area postrema. They rarely occur in the supratentorial area, where they may be confused with angioblastic meningiomas.

Clinical features of the hemangioblastoma of the cerebellum are symptoms typical of any cerebellar mass, such as headache, papilledema, and ataxia. When the tumor is multiple, lesions may involve the brain stem and upper cervical cord as well. Spinal cord hemangioblastomas are often associated with syrinx formation. Hemangioblastoma of the cerebellum can be diagnosed without difficulty with MRI and angiography. The diagnosis is even more certain when the tumor is associated with angiomas of the retina and polycythemia. Treatment is surgical, with evacuation of the cyst and removal of the mural nodule; 85% of all patients who undergo this treatment are alive and well 5 to 20 years after surgery. There is a high incidence of recurrence, however, if the tumor is partially removed or is associated with multiple tumors.

ANGIOBLASTIC MENINGIOMA AND HEMANGIOPERICYTOMA

Angioblastic meningioma is grossly identical to other meningiomas but has a significant dural attachment and is located either above or below the tentorium. *Hemangiopericytoma* originates in other areas of the body, presumably from blood vessel elements.

LEVEL 1 EVIDENCE

1. Mohr JP, Parides MK, Stapf C, et al; for the international ARUBA investigators. Medical management with or without interventional therapy for unruptured brain arteriovenous malformations (ARUBA): a multicentre, non-blinded, randomised trial. *Lancet.* 2014;383:614–621.

SUGGESTED READINGS

Brancati F, Valente EM, Tadini G, et al. Autosomal dominant hereditary benign telangiectasia maps to the CMC1 locus for capillary malformation on chromosome 5q14. *J Med Genet.* 2003;40:849–853.

Choi JH, Mast H, Sciacca RR, et al. Clinical outcome after first and recurrent hemorrhage in patients with untreated brain arteriovenous malformation. *Stroke.* 2006;37(5):1243–1247.

Comi AM. Pathophysiology of Sturge–Weber syndrome. *J Child Neurol.* 2003;18:509–516.

Cushing H, Bailey P. *Tumors Arising from the Blood Vessels of the Brain.* Springfield, IL: Charles C Thomas; 1928.

Eerola I, Boon LM, Mulliken JB, et al. Capillary malformation-arteriovenous malformation, a new clinical and genetic disorder caused by RASA1 mutations. *Am J Hum Genet.* 2003;73:1240–1249.

Flemming KD, Link MJ, Christianson TJH, et al. Prospective hemorrhage risk of intracerebral cavernous malformations. *Neurology.* 2012;78:632–636.

Guttmacher AE, Marchuk DA, White RI Jr. Hereditary hemorrhagic telangiectasia. *N Engl J Med.* 1995;333:918–924.

Hacein-Bey L, Konstas AA, Pile-Spellman J. Natural history, current concepts, classification, factors impacting endovascular therapy, and pathophysiology of cerebral and spinal dural arteriovenous fistula. *Clin Neurol Neurosurg.* 2014;121:64–75.

Hartmann A, Mast H, Choi JH, et al. Treatment of arteriovenous malformations of the brain. *Curr Neurol Neurosci Rep.* 2007;7(1):28–34.

Kruse F Jr. Hemangiopericytomas of the meninges (angioblastic meningioma of Cushing and Eisenhardt). Clinico-pathologic aspects and follow-up studies in 8 cases. *Neurology.* 1961;11:771–777.

Lasjaunias P. *Vascular Diseases in Neonates, Infants and Children. Interventional Neuroradiology Management.* Berlin, Germany: Springer-Verlag; 1997.

Naff NJ, Wemmer J, Hoenig-Rigamonti K, et al. A longitudinal study of venous malformations: documentation of a negligible risk and benign natural history. *Neurology.* 1998;50:1709–1714.

Neumann HP, Lips CJ, Hsia YE, et al. Von Hippel–Lindau syndrome. *Brain Pathol.* 1995;5:181–193.

Romanowski CA, Cavallin LI. Tuberous sclerosis, von Hippel–Lindau disease, Sturge–Weber syndrome. *Hosp Med.* 1998;59:226–231.

Sahlein DH, Mora P, Becske T, et al. Features predictive of brain arteriovenous malformation hemorrhage: extrapolation to a physiologic model. *Stroke.* 2014;45(7):1964–1970.

Sheu M, Fauteux G, Chang H, et al. Sinus pericranii: dermatologic considerations and literature review. *J Am Acad Dermatol.* 2002;46(6):934–941.

Slater A, Moore NR, Huson SM. The natural history of cerebellar hemangioblastomas in von Hippel–Lindau disease. *Am J Neuroradiol.* 2003;24:1570–1574.

Spetzler RF, Martin NA. A proposed grading system for arteriovenous malformations. *J Neurosurg.* 1986;65(4):476–483.

Stieg PE, Batjer HH, Samson D. *Intracranial Arteriovenous Malformations.* New York: Informa Healthcare; 2007.

Sung DI, Thang CH, Harisiadis L. Cerebellar hemangioblastomas. *Cancer.* 1982;49:553–555.

Tang SC, Jeng JS, Liu HM, et al. Diffuse capillary telangiectasia of the brain manifested as a slowly progressive course. *Cerebrovasc Dis.* 2003;15:140–142.

Central Nervous System Vasculitis 42

Fawaz Al-Mufti and Stephan A. Mayer

INTRODUCTION

Vasculitis affecting the central or peripheral nervous system often presents major diagnostic and therapeutic challenges for physicians because of its variable clinical manifestations and the lack of specific diagnostic tests other than biopsy. Central nervous system (CNS) vasculitis comprises a heterogeneous group of inflammatory diseases that affect leptomeningeal and parenchymal blood vessels of the brain with different but frequently overlapping clinical and pathologic manifestations.

The histopathologic changes of CNS vasculitis essentially consist of an inflammatory infiltrate within the vessel wall associated with necrosis, vessel occlusion and infarction, and in some cases, hemorrhage. The cases of CNS vasculitis are protean: It may occur as an idiopathic primary autoimmune process or within the context of systemic to autoimmune disease, as a reaction to an infection such as varicella-zoster or a neurodegenerative process such as amyloid angiopathy, after drug exposure (e.g., cocaine), as a manifestation of radiation exposure, and in the setting of malignancy. Although the precise pathogenesis often remains obscure, in all cases, the immune system plays a central role, and immunosuppressive agents are the cornerstones of treatment.

There are several different classifications for CNS vasculitis. Some classifications are based on the size of the affected vessels (small, medium, large), whereas other classifications are based on histologic features (e.g., granulomatous, lymphomatous, or leukocytoclastic inflammation) or immunologic markers (e.g., the association with antineutrophil cytoplasmic antibodies, or ANCAs, with some forms of vasculitis). CNS vasculitis can also be further broadly classified into primary and secondary vasculitis depending on whether the process is confined to the CNS or is part of a systemic illness.

In 2012, the International Chapel Hill Consensus Conference proposed a revised nomenclature system that groups different vasculitides by taking in consideration multiple factors including size of vessels and whether the vasculitis involves a single organ or is part of a more systemic condition (Table 42.1).

PRIMARY ANGIITIS OF THE CENTRAL NERVOUS SYSTEM

Primary angiitis of the central nervous system (PACNS) is associated with select inflammation and destruction of small- and medium-sized arteries of the brain parenchyma, spinal cord, and leptomeninges, resulting in symptoms and signs of CNS dysfunction. The term *angiitis* is synonymous with vasculitis and refers to involvement of blood vessels on both the arterial and venous sides of the circulation. PACNS is also frequently referred to as *primary central nervous system vasculitis*.

EPIDEMIOLOGY

The annual incidence rate of PACNS is 2.4 cases per 1 million person-years. The disease affects patients of all ages, peaking at 50 years of age, with a 2:1 male predominance.

PATHOBIOLOGY

The etiology and pathogenesis of PACNS is unknown. Infectious agents such as herpes zoster virus, West Nile virus, and varicella-zoster virus have been proposed as possible causes or triggers.

Three main histopathologic patterns are generally seen: granulomatous, lymphocytic, and necrotizing vasculitis. In lymphocytic PACNS, immunohistochemical staining reveals predominant infiltration by memory T cells in and around small cerebral vessels, signifying an antigen-specific immune response occurring in the wall of cerebral arteries.

CLINICAL FEATURES

Due to diffuse involvement of the CNS, the clinical manifestations are variable and nonspecific, with a clinical course ranging from hyperacute to stepwise to chronic and insidious. Mental obtundation and decreased cognition are the most frequent clinical presentations, usually evolving subacutely as a progressive encephalopathy. Other symptoms may include headaches, seizures, and focal neurologic deficits due to ischemic stroke or cerebral hemorrhage. Signs and symptoms of systemic vasculitis, such as peripheral neuropathy, fever, weight loss, or rash, are by definition lacking in PACNS.

DIAGNOSIS

On the basis of clinical experience and evidence from published work, Calabrese and Mallek proposed a set of criteria for the diagnosis of PACNS; the diagnosis is established when all three of the following criteria are met (Table 42.2).

There is no specific laboratory diagnostic test for PACNS, although routine laboratory testing, serologic evaluations, lumbar puncture results, neuroimaging studies, cerebral angiography, and brain biopsy may all have roles in the evaluation (Table 42.3). Acute phase reactants such as the erythrocyte sedimentation rate (ESR) and C-reactive protein (CRP) are usually normal in PACNS; elevated levels should raise suspicion of systemic involvement by either an infectious, malignant, or inflammatory process. Both serologic testing and analyses of the cerebrospinal fluid (CSF) are important for excluding secondary causes of CNS dysfunction that may mimic PACNS. Nonspecific abnormalities, primarily leukocyte and protein elevations, are seen on CSF analysis in 80% to 90% of patients with pathologically documented disease.

Magnetic resonance imaging (MRI) typically shows multifocal small-vessel infarcts and hemorrhages of varying age (Fig. 42.1). These vascular lesions often involve structures that are not typically involved in conventional cerebrovascular disease, such as the corpus callosum. In some cases, large-vessel infarcts, convexity subarachnoid hemorrhage, or small foci of gadolinium enhancement can occur. It is extremely rare for PACNS to cause advanced disease with severe symptoms with a normal MRI.

The gold standard for the detection of vascular abnormalities is digital subtraction angiography. In PACNS, cerebral angiography

TABLE 42.1   Vasculitis Syndromes: 2012 International Chapel Hill Consensus Conference

Syndromes	Pathologies
Large-Vessel Vasculitis	
Giant cell (temporal) arteritis	Granulomatous arteritis of aorta and its major branches; predilection for extracranial branches of carotid artery; often involves temporal artery; patients older than 50 years with polymyalgia rheumatica
Takayasu arteritis	Granulomatous arteritis of aorta and major branches; patients younger than age 50 years
Medium-Sized Vessel Vasculitis	
Polyarteritis nodosa	Necrotizing inflammation of medium- or small-sized arteries; no glomerulonephritis or vasculitis of arterioles, capillaries, venules
Kawasaki disease	Arteritis of large, medium-sized, small arteries plus mucocutaneous-lymph node syndrome; coronary arteries often involved; aorta and veins may be involved; usually in children
Small-Vessel Vasculitis	
Granulomatosis with polyangiitis (GPA) (Wegener granulomatosis)	Granulomatous inflammation including respiratory tract and necrotizing vasculitis of small to medium vessels (capillaries, venules, arterioles, arteries); necrotizing glomerulonephritis common
Eosinophilic granulomatosis with polyangiitis (EGPA) (Churg–Strauss syndrome)	Eosinophil-rich granulomatous inflammation of respiratory tract and necrotizing vasculitis of small- to medium-sized vessels; with asthma and eosinophilia
Microscopic polyangiitis (MPA)	Necrotizing vasculitis with few or no immune deposits; affects small vessels (capillaries, venules, arterioles); may involve small- and medium-sized arteries; common features: necrotizing glomerulonephritis and involvement of pulmonary capillaries
IgA vasculitis (IgAV) (Henoch–Schönlein purpura)	Vasculitis with IgA-dominant immune deposits on small vessels (capillaries, venules, arterioles); affects skin, gut, and glomeruli plus arthritis or arthralgia
Cryoglobulinemic vasculitis	Vasculitis with immune deposits on small vessels (capillaries, venules, arterioles); cryoglobulins in serum; skin and glomeruli often involved
Variable-Vessel Vasculitis (VVV)	
Behçet disease (BD)	Vasculitis that can affect arteries or veins accompanied by cutaneous, ocular, articular, gastrointestinal, and/or central nervous system inflammatory lesions
Cogan syndrome (CS)	Arteritis (affecting small, medium, or large arteries), aortitis, aortic aneurysms, and aortic and mitral valvulitis accompanied by ocular inflammatory lesions, including interstitial keratitis, uveitis, and episcleritis, and inner ear disease, including sensorineural hearing loss and vestibular dysfunction
Vasculitis associated with systemic disease	Vasculitis that is associated with and may be secondary to (caused by) a systemic disease (e.g., rheumatoid vasculitis, lupus vasculitis)
Vasculitis associated with probable etiology	Vasculitis that is associated with a probable specific etiology (e.g., hydralazine-associated microscopic polyangiitis, hepatitis B virus–associated vasculitis, hepatitis C virus–associated cryoglobulinemic vasculitis, etc.)

IgA, immunoglobulin A.

Modified from Jennette JC, Falk RJ, Bacon PA, et al. 2012 revised International Chapel Hill Consensus Conference nomenclature of vasculitides. *Arthritis Rheum.* 2013;65(1):1–11.

TABLE 42.2   Diagnostic Criteria for Primary Angiitis of the Central Nervous System

- History or clinical findings of an acquired neurologic deficit of unknown origin after a thorough initial basic assessment

- Cerebral angiography reveals classic features of vasculitis, or a CNS biopsy sample shows vasculitis.

- There is no evidence of systemic vasculitis or any other disorder to which the angiographic or pathologic features can be attributed to.

CNS, central nervous system.

may show areas of ectasia and stenosis referred to as *beading circumferential* or *eccentric vessel irregularities* with sharp cutoffs, delayed arterial emptying, small arteriovenous anastomotic channels, and rarely, microaneurysms (Fig. 42.2). The main condition that PACNS must be differentiated from a patient with beading on diagnostic angiography is reversible cerebral vasoconstriction syndrome (RCVS), a much more benign condition discussed later in this chapter (see also Chapter 43). About 4% of patients with primary CNS vasculitis present with a solitary tumorlike mass lesion due to brain tissue inflammation. Given the poor resolution of computed tomography (CT) and magnetic resonance (MR) angiography for distal medium and small blood vessels, these tests have limited sensitivity for diagnosing PACNS.

TABLE 42.3	Suggested Laboratory Testing for Central Nervous System Vasculitis

Basic Laboratory Testing

Complete blood count with differential

Serum urea nitrogen and creatinine

Serum aspartate and alanine aminotransferases

ESR and C-reactive protein

Urinalysis

CSF Studies

Cell count (mild to moderate CSF pleocytosis)

CSF protein (range 44–1,034 mg/dL) CSF glucose (usually normal)

Oligoclonal bands

Gram stain and cultures

Cytology and flow cytometry when malignancy is suspected

PCR and IgG, IgM directed at infectious sources (below)

Specialized Laboratory Testing

Antinuclear antibodies

Rheumatoid factor

Antibodies to the Ro/SSA, La/SSB, Sm, and RNP antigens

Antibodies to double-stranded DNA

Antineutrophil cytoplasmic antibodies (ANCA)

Serum C3 and C4

Serum cryoglobulins

Serum and urine protein electrophoresis with immune electrophoresis

Quantitative immunoglobulin levels (IgG, IgM, IgA)

Infectious Etiologies (in appropriate circumstances as indicated)

Bacterial—*Mycoplasma* PCR and serology, antistreptolysin O test (ASOT), syphilis serology, Mantoux skin test

Viral—serology for hepatitis B and C, parvovirus B19, HIV, herpes simplex virus, Epstein–Barr virus (EBV), cytomegalovirus (CMV), varicella

Fungal culture (*Aspergillus*, *Coccidioides*, and *Histoplasma* species)

Parasite: serum anticysticercal antibodies demonstrated by immunoblot assay and CSF ELISA for detection of anticysticercal antibodies or cysticercal antigens

Thrombophilia Investigations

Prolonged activated partial thromboplastin time (aPTT), which does not correct with mixing

Screening for lupus anticoagulant

Anticardiolipin antibody by ELISA

Anti–β2-microglobulin-1 antibody by ELISA

ESR, erythrocyte sedimentation rate; CSF, cerebrospinal fluid; PCR, polymerase chain reaction; IgG, immunoglobulin G; IgM, immunoglobulin M; IgA, immunoglobulin A; ELISA, enzyme-linked immunosorbent assay.

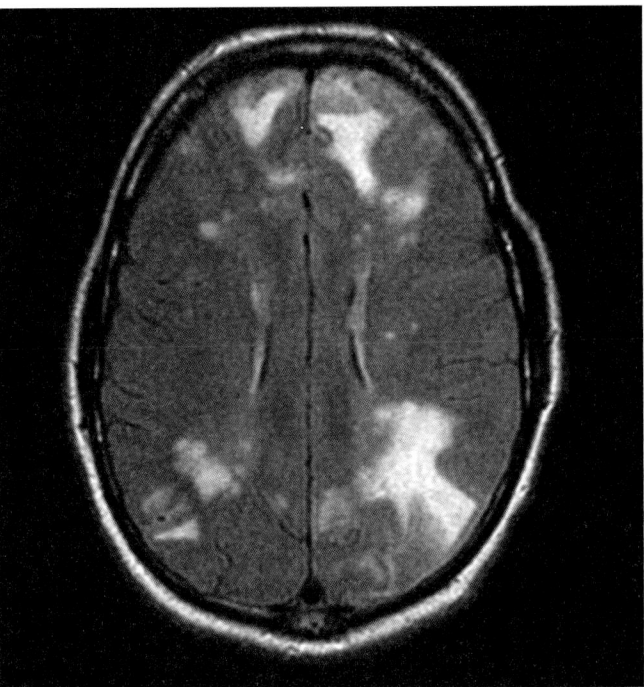

FIGURE 42.1 Fluid-attenuated inversion recovery (FLAIR) MRI showing multifocal infarcts in a patient with biopsy-proven PACNS.

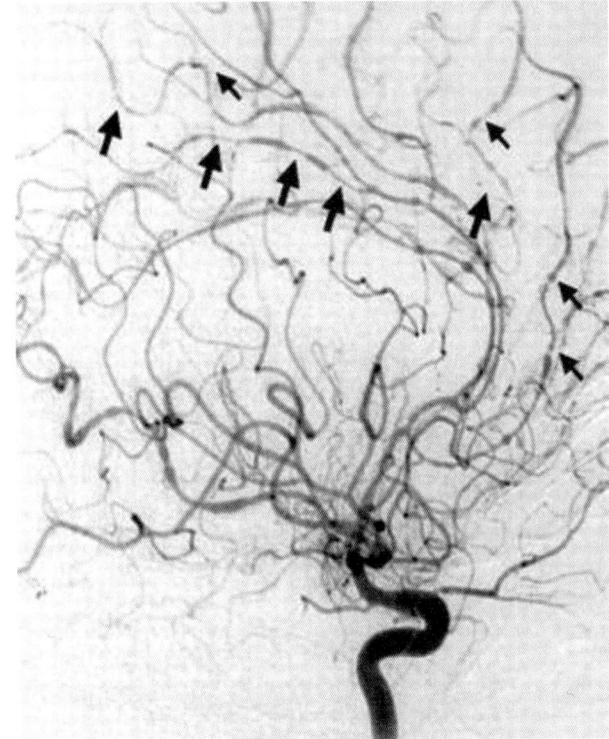

FIGURE 42.2 Typical angiographic findings in a patient with central nervous system vasculitis. *Arrows* point to areas of alternating stenosis and ectasia. (From Hajj-Ali RA, Ghamande S, Calabrese LH, et al. Central nervous system vasculitis in the intensive care unit. *Crit Care Clin.* 2002;18:897–914).

Arteries with diameter below 0.4 mm, arterioles, and capillaries are beyond the resolution of conventional angiography, and because PACNS often involves small blood vessels, the sensitivity of angiography in biopsy-proven PACNS cases is only 60%. Thus, a negative angiogram cannot exclude the diagnosis of PACNS. Furthermore, cerebral angiography has limited specificity since not infrequently, patients with angiographic findings interpreted as being positive for vasculitis are not found to have vasculitic changes at brain biopsy. It should be noted that normal biopsy specimens may reflect sample error due to the patchy distribution of inflammation. The false-negative rate of an initial biopsy is 25%; in some cases, two or more biopsies are necessary to establish the diagnosis. The yield of biopsy is improved with larger tissue blocks (i.e., 1 cm^3) with inclusion of the overlying meninges and when areas affected with enhancement on MRI are targeted.

TREATMENT

No randomized clinical trials of medical management for PACNS exist. First-line therapy usually starts with glucocorticoids. Fulminant PACNS in hospitalized patients usually starts with empiric intravenous *methylprednisolone*, 15 mg/kg/day for 3 to 5 days, followed by *prednisone*, 1 mg/kg/day to a maximum of 100 mg/day. Less severe disease in outpatients can be started on *prednisone* alone. Glucocorticoids should be continued at the initial dose for 4 to 6 weeks after which a slow taper should be initiated.

Patients with biopsy-confirmed granulomatous variant PACNS should be started on a combination of glucocorticoids and *cyclophosphamide*. *Cyclophosphamide* is given in order to induce remission in either a daily oral regimen (1.5 to 2 mg/kg/day) or a monthly intravenous regimen (600 to 750 mg/m^2, infused once a month). After induction of remission, typically in 3 to 6 months, *cyclophosphamide* therapy is switched to maintenance therapy with other agents such as mycophenolate mofetil or azathioprine.

In patients with lymphocytic variant PACNS or those in whom the diagnosis is performed by cerebral angiogram and not confirmed by biopsy, an initial glucocorticoid treatment is only followed by *cyclophosphamide* if the neurologic decline is progressive. As a general rule, chemotherapeutic immunosuppressant therapy should only be given to patients with biopsy-proven PACNS.

Treatment response is monitored by periodic reassessment of symptoms and neuroimaging abnormalities. A follow-up MRI should be obtained 4 to 6 weeks after beginning treatment, then every 3 to 6 months throughout therapy, and subsequently according to the evolution of the disease to assess for progression of the disease.

OUTCOME

Earlier descriptions characterized PACNS as a fatal disease, and most cases were diagnosed at autopsy. With better understanding of the disease and with aggressive immunosuppression, more favorable outcomes and improving mortality rate have been reported. Recent reports indicate that the short-term mortality rate is 10% and that 20% suffer severe functional impairment. Mild cognitive deficits and reduced energy level remain common among those with a good functional recovery. Approximately 30% of patients experience a relapse of the disease after going into remission, which requires reescalation of immunosuppression.

AMYLOID β–RELATED ANGIITIS

Amyloid β–related angiitis (ABRA) is a form of CNS vasculitis in which perivascular β-amyloid is thought to act as a trigger

for inflammation mediated by CD68+ macrophages and CD3+ T lymphocytes. The condition develops in patients with symptomatic or asymptomatic amyloid angiopathy (see also Chapter 38), which presents as dementia, gait disorder, and progressive brain hemorrhages (both microbleeds and parenchymal intracerebral hemorrhage). Patients with ABRA often exhibit altered mental status and respond to immunosuppressive treatment. Common CSF findings include an elevated protein and a lymphocytic pleocytosis. MRI often demonstrates T2 hyperintense lesions extending through the cortical white matter and often gray matter, suggestive of breakdown of the blood–brain barrier and a reversible leukoencephalopathy. Cerebral angiography shows beading in a minority of patients, perhaps due to involvement of exclusively medium- and small-sized vessels. In every case on brain biopsy, microglia, macrophages, and T cells surround amyloid-laden vessels. After initiating anti-inflammatory treatment consisting of steroids or *cyclophosphamide* for a duration ranging from 2 weeks to several months, a majority of patients with ABRA show improvement. However, some patients relapse, and other patients do not improve or progressively decline.

CENTRAL NERVOUS SYSTEM VASCULITIS ASSOCIATED WITH SYSTEMIC VASCULITIS

GIANT CELL (TEMPORAL) ARTERITIS

Giant cell arteritis (GCA), also known as *temporal arteritis* because of its predilection for superficial temporal artery involvement, is a large-vessel granulomatous vasculitis. The disease usually affects the aorta or its major branches, with a predilection for the branches of the cervical internal and external carotid arteries and the vertebral arteries. The intracranial vessels are generally spared. GCA is often linked with polymyalgia rheumatica in terms of its systemic manifestations, ESR elevation, and response to steroid therapy.

Epidemiology

GCA has an annual incidence that is highest among white individuals, ranging between 10 and 20 cases per 100,000 among persons older than 50 years of age. The incidence is markedly lower in persons of Asian or African descent in the range of 1 case per 100,000. Although GCA almost never occurs before age 50 years, the incidence increases thereafter, reaching its peak incidence between the ages of 70 and 80 years.

Pathobiology

Although the etiology of GCA is unknown, there appears to be an interplay between increasing age, a genetic predisposition, and infectious triggers that involves both the cellular and humoral immune system, resulting in an acute vascular inflammatory state. Current literature regarding the molecular basis of GCA suggests that activated dendritic cells, residing in the vessel wall, play an important role in the pathophysiology by initiating the pathogenic cascade, recruiting T cells and macrophages to form granulomatous infiltrates.

GCA is a panarteritis, including all the arterial layers. Thrombosis may develop at sites of active inflammation. Fibrosis, scarring, and narrowing or occlusion of the arteries develops secondary to the inflammation, tissue injury, and repair process.

Clinical Manifestations

GCA is classically characterized by a combination of five features:

1. Age older than 50 years,
2. A localized new-onset headache,

3. Tenderness over the temporal artery,
4. An elevated ESR (>50 mm/h), and
5. Biopsy revealing a necrotizing arteritis with a predominance of mononuclear cells or a granulomatous process with multinucleated giant cells.

The presence of three of the above five criteria is associated with 94% sensitivity and 91% specificity for the diagnosis of GCA. GCA typically presents with a constellation of constitutional symptoms, headache and tenderness over the temporal artery, jaw claudication, visual symptoms, and symptoms of polymyalgia rheumatica (diffuse myalgias and body aches). Because intracranial vascular involvement is rare in GCA, transient ischemic attacks (TIAs) and stroke are usually secondary to embolism or flow failure related to cervical vertebral or internal carotid lesions.

Neurologic manifestations arise in approximately 30% of patients, with more than half being peripheral neuropathies, followed by one-third with TIA or stroke, one-third with ophthalmologic symptoms, and one-fifth with neuro-otologic syndromes. Ophthalmologic symptoms can include transient monocular blindness (i.e., retinal TIA or amaurosis fugax) due to internal carotid artery stenosis or sustained unilateral visual loss due to anterior ischemic optic neuropathy or occlusion of the central retinal artery (see also Chapter 9).

Diagnosis

Tests to rule out CNS vasculitis should be performed as delineated in Table 42.3. The classic diagnostic screening test is an ESR, which is elevated in nearly all patients. CRP levels are also elevated, and CRP tends to correlate than ESR with GCA disease activity. Interleukin-6 levels may be used to evaluate disease progression, although this is investigational at this point.

Temporal artery biopsy, evidencing vasculitis with predominance of mononuclear cell infiltration or granulomatous inflammation, usually with multinucleated giant cells, is the gold standard for the diagnosis of GCA. A negative initial temporal artery biopsy may be present and occurs in up to 40% of patients with suspected of GCA. This may be due to sampling error due to skip lesions, biopsy, or attainment of too small a specimen (<2 cm). In the presence of a high index of suspicion, a contralateral biopsy should be performed if the first biopsy is negative. If bilateral temporal artery biopsies are negative, alternate artery biopsy sites should be considered.

Treatment

Treatment recommendations for GCA are based on clinical experience rather than the results of randomized controlled trials with most cases being managed effectively with glucocorticoid monotherapy. Induction therapy with *prednisone* at a dose of 1 mg/kg of body weight per day (maximum of 60 mg/day) is initiated in patients who lack symptoms or signs of ischemic organ damage (e.g., visual loss).

Patients with signs and symptoms suggestive of compromised blood flow to the eyes or the CNS should be managed with *methylprednisolone* at a dose of 1,000 mg/day for 3 consecutive days to more rapidly induce immunosuppression. This is then followed by oral therapy with 1 mg per kilogram of body weight per day (maximum of 60 mg/day) as recommended earlier for uncomplicated GCA. Once tissue necrosis occurs (e.g., optic nerve ischemia with blindness for several hours), it is irreversible.

Treatment initiation for suspected GCA with neurologic involvement should never be delayed until the biopsy is obtained because resolution of the inflammation occurs slowly after the start of treatment and a confirmed pathologic diagnosis can take several weeks or even months to attain.

Despite lack of prospective trials, anecdotal reports suggest some beneficial effects with glucocorticoid-sparing therapies such as *methotrexate*, *cyclophosphamide*, and *tocilizumab* (interleukin-6 receptor antagonist). These therapies may be considered in patients at highest risk of experiencing glucocorticoid-related side effects.

Once clinical signs have subsided and laboratory values have normalized, steroids can be tapered by 10 mg/kg every 2 to 4 weeks, with a substantial slowing of the taper to 1 mg decrements per month once the daily dose of 10 mg is reached. Expert consensus also recommends the addition of *acetylsalicylic* acid (ASA) (75 to 150 mg/day) to reduce the risk of ischemic complications such as visual loss, TIAs, or stroke.

Outcome

GCA tends to run a self-limited course over several months to several years. Rapid clinical improvement following the initiation of treatment is typical. The glucocorticoid dose can eventually be reduced or discontinued with the average duration of treatment being 2 to 3 years. Fatalities are rare.

POLYARTERITIS NODOSA

Polyarteritis nodosa (PAN) is a systemic necrotizing small- and medium-sized arteritis sparing the arterioles, capillaries, and venules. ANCAs are typically negative in PAN; this is important in differentiating it from ANCA-associated vasculitis, which can present almost indistinguishably, both clinically and pathologically.

Epidemiology

PAN is a rare disease occurring in two per million people, with about 25% of cases involving the CNS. Men and women are affected equally. The disease may occur at any age, but the peak incidence is in the fourth to sixth decades of life. With the advent of hepatitis B vaccination, the incidence of hepatitis B virus (HBV)–associated PAN is declining.

Pathobiology

The etiology of PAN remains unknown; immune complex deposition, antigen-specific T-cell–mediated immune responses and reactions to bacterial or viral infection have been postulated. Hepatitis B has been identified as one of the most common triggers for a subset of PAN; this form of arteritis may be monophasic with a good prognosis. PAN has also been reported with hepatitis C virus (HCV), cytomegalovirus (CMV), HIV, and parvovirus B19.

Vascular inflammatory lesions in PAN are segmental and predominate in branching points of small- and medium-sized arteries. Small vessels, including arterioles, capillaries, and venules, are characteristically spared, as are large vessels (the aorta and its major branches). Consequently, glomerulonephritis is not part of the spectrum of PAN. Vessel inflammation starts in the adventitia and vasa vasorum may subsequently progress to include the entire arterial wall, resulting in fibrinoid necrosis. At bifurcations and branch points, multiple small aneurysms can form, and at later stages, angiogenesis becomes apparent. As these lesions progress, they may rupture or occlude the vessel, resulting in hemorrhage or infarction. Vessel biopsies typically show acute necrotizing lesions intermixed with more chronic fibrotic or healing changes, representing different stages of the inflammatory process.

Clinical Manifestations

The ubiquitous nature of PAN allows for the diverse clinical manifestations, ranging from more chronic, insidious symptoms to acute, life-threatening complications. Nonspecific constitutional manifestations are common early in the course.

Peripheral neuropathy, in the form of mononeuritis multiplex or diffuse sensorimotor peripheral neuropathy, is the most common neurologic disorder. Involvement of the CNS occurs in fewer than 10% of patients with PAN. CNS manifestations range from headache, retinopathy, and encephalopathy with seizures and cognitive decline to cerebral infarction and intracerebral hemorrhage due to involvement of medium-sized vessels. Other symptoms may arise from affection of the cranial nerves or the spinal cord.

Cutaneous hemorrhages, tender erythematous eruptions, subcutaneous nodules, and necrotic ulcers may appear on the trunk or limbs. Variable degrees of renal insufficiency and hypertension may develop secondary to tissue infarction and hematoma formation secondary to rupture of renal microaneurysms. Furthermore, gastrointestinal, hepatic, testicular, or cardiac symptoms may develop.

Diagnosis

The diagnosis of PAN should be considered in all patients with an obscure febrile illness marked by systemic symptoms and chronic peripheral neuropathy. According to the American College of Rheumatology 1990 consensus criteria for the classification of PAN, the diagnosis is 82% sensitive and 87% specific in a patient with systemic vasculitis if there are more than 3 of the following 10 criteria: weight loss ($\geq$4 kg), livedo reticularis, testicular pain or tenderness, myalgia, mononeuritis multiplex or other polyneuropathy, hypertension, azotemia, HBV antibody, angiographic occlusion of visceral arteries, or biopsy evidence of granulocytes in vessel wall.

The diagnosis can often be established by biopsy of sural nerve, muscle, or testicle. A high index of suspicion is crucial to diagnose PAN. Basic laboratory tests, liver function studies, and hepatitis (HBV and HCV) serologies help rule out potential etiologies and ascertain the extent of organs affected and their degree of involvement. Acute-phase proteins are typically elevated. There is a leukocytosis with inconstant eosinophilia. Additional specialized autoimmune laboratory testing is valuable in narrowing the differential diagnosis (see Table 42.3). The presence of myeloperoxidase (MPO) ANCA or proteinase 3 (PR3) ANCA antibodies strongly argues against PAN and in favor of one of the ANCA-associated vasculitides.

Treatment

There is no specific therapy. Treatment varies according to the severity of the disease state ranging from high doses of corticosteroids in milder disease forms to a combination of corticosteroids and immunosuppressive drugs (*azathioprine, methotrexate,* or *cyclophosphamide*). Patients with mild PAN and evidence of infection with HBV or HCV should receive antivirals, whereas those with severe hepatitis virus–associated PAN, short-term treatment corticosteroids, and plasma exchange maybe considered until antiviral therapy becomes effective. Plasma exchange may have a role in the acute management of HBV-associated PAN.

Outcome

Untreated PAN is associated with a poor prognosis. The French Vasculitis Study Group described the 1- and 5-year relapse rates for patients with non–HBV-associated PAN as 9.2% and 24%, respectively; the relapse rates for HBV-associated PAN were lower.

Most deaths occur within 18 months of disease onset primarily due to renal failure and mesenteric, cardiac, or cerebral infarctions.

BEHÇET SYNDROME

Behçet syndrome is a chronic, multisystem vessel vasculitis that has no predilection to the type or size of vessel. Neurologic involvement occurs in about one in five patients.

Epidemiology

Behçet syndrome is most common in the Middle East and Eastern Asia with prevalence ranges from 13.5 to 35 per 100,000. In North American and Northern European countries, the prevalence is from 1 to 7 per 100,000. There is no gender predilection; the disease typically affects young adults 20 to 40 years of age.

Pathobiology

The exact cause is unknown, but there is increasing evidence that an underlying immune-mediated vasculitis underlies the mucocutaneous lesions. Although vasculitic changes may not be demonstrated in all lesions, the classic finding is a necrotizing leukocytoclastic obliterative perivasculitis with fibrinoid necrosis of postcapillary venules. Venous thrombosis with lymphocytic infiltration of capillaries, veins, and arteries of all sizes may also be visible. It has been reported that those with active Behçet syndrome have elevated serum levels of several proinflammatory cytokines, perhaps as a result of an aberrant immune reaction due to infectious or environmental pathogens. Numerous reports have found a strong genetic predisposition to develop Behçet disease among those with the HLA-B51 major histocompatibility complex subtype.

Clinical Manifestations

Behçet syndrome is characterized by uveitis and recurrent oral and genital aphthous ulcers. Other manifestations include ocular, cutaneous, joint, gastrointestinal, or CNS inflammatory lesions. Small-vessel vasculitis, thromboangiitis, vessel thrombosis, arteritis, and arterial aneurysms may occur. CNS involvement is present in 20% of patients and can be subdivided into parenchymal (inflammation of the CNS tissue) or nonparenchymal (vascular neuro-Behçet).

Parenchymal disease may be due to lesions in the corticospinal tract, periventricular white matter, basal ganglia, brain stem, and spinal cord. Clinical presentations are often subacute and manifestations may include headache, behavior changes, encephalopathy, acute meningeal syndromes, hemiparesis, hemisensory loss, seizures, cranial neuropathies, cerebellar dysfunction, alterations in mental status, and optic neuropathy. Spinal cord lesions may occur in isolation. Vascular manifestations may include diffuse vasculitis, venous sinus thrombosis, and uncommonly stroke due to arterial thrombosis, dissection, or aneurysm. In contrast to other systemic vasculitides, peripheral neuropathy is not commonly seen in Behçet syndrome.

Diagnosis

Due to the lack of a specific diagnostic laboratory test, the diagnosis is made based on clinical criteria. The Behçet International Study Group (ISG) criteria and the International Criteria for Behçet's Disease (ICBD) both require the presence of recurrent oral ulcers in addition to a constellation of recurrent genital ulcers, eye lesions (anterior or posterior uveitis or retinal vasculitis), or skin lesions (including erythema nodosum, pseudovasculitis, papulopustular lesions, or acneiform nodules consistent with Behçet). The ICBD also adds the presence of vascular lesions (superficial phlebitis, deep vein thrombosis, arterial thrombosis, or aneurysm formation) to the diagnostic criteria. Nonspecific markers of inflammation such as proinflammatory cytokines, circulating immune complexes, CSR, and the ESR may be elevated.

Treatment

Treatment is dependent on the severity of the disease and the organ systems involved. Glucocorticoids or other immunosuppressive agents should be considered for treatment of erythema nodosum and pyoderma gangrenosum. Posterior uveitis and neurologic involvement requires prompt treatment with both high-dose glucocorticoids and a second immunosuppressive agent (*azathioprine*, *tumor necrosis factor [TNF]-alpha inhibitors*, *cyclosporine*, *interferon* α, *cyclophosphamide*, and *methotrexate*).

Outcome

Behçet syndrome typically has a relapsing and remitting course. Delay in diagnosis and treatment increases morbidity and mortality. The greatest morbidity and mortality comes from neurologic, ocular, and large-vessel arterial or venous disease. Mucocutaneous, articular, and ocular diseases are often at their worst in the early years of disease; CNS and large-vessel involvement tends to develop later in the disease course. Patients with parenchymal CNS involvement have a worse outcome than patients with nonparenchymal vascular involvement, with more frequent recurrent disease, disability, and premature death.

THE ANTINEUTROPHIL CYTOPLASMIC ANTIBODY–POSITIVE VASCULITIDES

ANCA vasculitis is a group of necrotizing small-vessel vasculitides predominantly affecting small vessels (i.e., capillaries, venules, arterioles, and small arteries). ANCA antibodies (usually immunoglobulin G [IgG]) react against antigens in the cytoplasm of neutrophil granulocytes. Specific subtypes of ANCA are based on immunofluorescence patterns and target antigens. Cytoplasmic antineutrophil cytoplasmic antibody (c-ANCA) is directed specifically at proteinase 3 (PR3). Perinuclear antineutrophil cytoplasmic antibody (p-ANCA) antigens include MPO and bacterial permeability increasing (BPI) factor.

The ANCA-associated vasculitides include the following:

1. Granulomatosis with polyangiitis (formerly known as *Wegener granulomatosis*),
2. Microscopic polyangiitis,
3. Eosinophilic granulomatosis with polyangiitis (formerly *Churg–Strauss syndrome*),
4. Renal-limited vasculitis, and
5. Drug-induced vasculitis.

All are associated with ANCAs and a focal necrotizing, often crescentic, pauci-immune glomerulonephritis. The presence or absence of ANCA antibodies does not indicate presence or absence of disease. ANCA is highly correlated with the conditions described in the following sections, but not all patients with the condition test positive for the antibody. The association of ANCA positivity and disease activity remains controversial; however, the reappearance of ANCA after treatment can indicate a relapse.

Granulomatosis with Polyangiitis

The hallmarks of granulomatosis with polyangiitis (GPA), formerly known as *Wegener granulomatosis*, are necrotizing granulomatous inflammation involving the upper and lower respiratory tract, necrotizing glomerulonephritis, and systemic necrotizing vasculitis affecting predominantly small to medium vessels (e.g., capillaries, venules, arterioles, arteries, and veins).

EPIDEMIOLOGY

The annual incidence of GPA is 5 to 10 cases per million population equally affecting males and females between the ages of 65 and 70 years. GPA affects Caucasians more than Asians, Africans, and the Afro-Caribbean and African-American populations.

PATHOBIOLOGY

The immunopathobiology of GPA is complex and involves the generation of ANCA against PR3 in approximately 50% to 80% of GPA patients and against MPO in approximately 10% to 18% of GPA patients. GPA is believed to develop following exposure to infectious (bacterial, mycobacterial, fungal, or viral infections of the upper respiratory tract), environmental, chemical, toxic, or pharmacologic triggers in genetically predisposed individuals who lack tolerance to ANCA self-antigens.

CLINICAL MANIFESTATIONS

Prodromal symptoms may last for weeks to months with constitutional symptoms including fever, migratory arthralgias, malaise, anorexia, and weight loss. GPA has a predilection for the respiratory system and kidneys. According to criteria of the American Academy of Rheumatology, the diagnosis can be made if there are two of the following four criteria:

1. Oral ulcers or purulent bloody nasal discharge;
2. Abnormal chest film showing nodules, fixed infiltrates, or cavities;
3. Microscopic hematuria; or
4. Biopsy evidence of granulomatous inflammation in the wall of an artery or perivascular tissue.

As with other vasculitic syndromes, GPA affects the peripheral nervous system in the form of a sensorimotor peripheral neuropathy (mononeuritis multiplex) more than the CNS. The CNS is affected in less than 10% of patients. In such cases, intracranial granuloma may arise following direct invasion from the nasal cavity and in turn involvement of the basal cranial nerves. Additionally, aseptic meningeal necrotizing granulomas, encephalopathy, or vasculitis with secondary stroke or venous sinus thrombosis may occur.

DIAGNOSIS

Approximately 90% of patients are ANCA positive and 10% of patients are ANCA negative. The definitive diagnosis is made by biopsy of an affected organ (generally skin, kidney, or lung).

In patients with neurologic manifestations, involvement of the dura with pachymeningitis may be detected on MRI after contrast administration. Because the caliber of the affected vessels may be beyond the spatial resolution of digital subtraction angiography, radiologic confirmation of CNS vasculitis in Wegener granulomatosis is rare. Nerve biopsies may show arteritis in patients with polyneuropathy and no signs of systemic disease.

TREATMENT

Patients should be treated empirically if the clinical suspicion for ANCA vasculitis is high and a tissue diagnosis cannot be obtained in a timely manner. Therapy of GPA has two components: induction of remission and maintenance using immunosuppressive therapy. Patients with mild disease lacking active glomerulonephritis and organ-threatening or life-threatening manifestations may be treated with a regimen of glucocorticoids in combination with *methotrexate*. Patients with moderate to severe disease who are at imminent risk for organ damage or who have life-threatening manifestations should receive a regimen consisting of glucocorticoids in combination with either *cyclophosphamide* (oral or intravenous) or *rituximab*. Plasma exchange is reserved for patients with GPA or microscopic polyangiitis who have one or more of the following: pulmonary hemorrhage, a positive antiglomerular basement membrane antibody, a serum creatinine more than 5.7 mg/dL, and/or requiring dialysis.

OUTCOME

Long-term survival with GPA is improved with immunosuppression, and the natural history of this disease has transformed from being an imminently life-threatening condition to a chronic condition prone to relapse throughout life. Left untreated, approximately 90% of patients will experience severe morbidity or mortality within 2 years. Even with aggressive treatment, GPA continues to be associated with morbidity due to chronic renal, pulmonary, or CNS failure, which affects 12% to 25% of patients within 10 years. Death is generally due to irreversible organ dysfunction and progressive renal failure.

Microscopic Polyangiitis

In microscopic polyangiitis (MPA), a necrotizing vasculitis with few or no immune deposits predominantly affects small vessels (i.e., capillaries, venules, or arterioles) throughout the body. Necrotizing glomerulonephritis is very common, pulmonary capillaritis is common, and neurologic involvement occurs in about half of cases. Granulomatous inflammation is absent.

EPIDEMIOLOGY

The exact incidence and prevalence of MPA are unknown, although the incidence has been estimated to be in the range of six cases per million population affecting men slightly more than women, with an age range of 60 to 65 years.

PATHOBIOLOGY

As with GPA, the immunopathobiology of MPA is complex; there is increasing evidence that MPA is an autoimmune disease, with ANCA antibodies positive in 95% of cases. The pathophysiology involves the generation of ANCA against MPO in approximately 70% and against PR3 in 30% of MPA patients. ANCA, directed against MPO and PR3, activates neutrophils to produce reactive oxygen species and release lytic enzymes causing the detachment and destruction of endothelial cells contributing to the pathophysiology.

CLINICAL MANIFESTATIONS

As with all other systemic vasculitides, multiple organs are affected with MPA, primarily the kidneys in 90% of cases and less frequently the lungs. Renal involvement is manifested by microscopic hematuria and rapidly progressive glomerulonephritis; 10% progress to end-stage renal disease requiring renal replacement therapy. Pulmonary manifestations range from dyspnea, cough, and hemoptysis to pulmonary hemorrhages, secondary to pulmonary capillaritis, which can be life threatening. In contrast to GPA, MPA lacks granulomatous inflammation and involvement of the upper respiratory tract. The nervous system is involved in

50% of cases, with polyneuropathy or mononeuritis multiplex being the most common manifestation. Cerebral vasculitis resulting in tissue ischemia, hemorrhage, encephalopathy, and generalized or focal seizures can also occur.

DIAGNOSIS

Tests to rule out CNS vasculitis should be performed as delineated in Table 42.3. Microscopic hematuria with cellular casts in the urine in addition to proteinuria may be demonstrated on urinalysis. An important diagnostic test is the presence of p-ANCA against with MPO or PR3. In patients with neuropathy, an electromyogram (EMG) may reveal a sensorimotor peripheral neuropathy.

TREATMENT AND OUTCOME

The treatment and outcome of MPA is generally the same as that for GPA, as described earlier.

Eosinophilic Granulomatosis with Polyangiitis

Eosinophilic granulomatosis with polyangiitis (EGPA), previously known as *Churg–Strauss syndrome*, is a multisystem disorder due to small-vessel vasculitis characterized by eosinophil-rich and necrotizing granulomatous inflammation often involving the respiratory tract and necrotizing vasculitis predominantly affecting small to medium blood vessels. Asthma and peripheral blood eosinophilia are other prominent features. Mononeuritis multiplex is the most common form of neurologic involvement.

EPIDEMIOLOGY

The exact incidence and prevalence of EGPA is unknown but it is rare: Estimates are in the range of 10 to 13 cases per million population. The mean age at diagnosis is 48 years without clear gender predominance. There is a higher incidence among asthmatics.

PATHOBIOLOGY

EGPA is classified among the ANCA-positive vasculitides with several characteristics pointing to an immunologic etiology, which include the presence of elevated Th1 and Th2 lymphocyte function, increased eosinophil recruitment, decreased eosinophil apoptosis, and altered humoral immunity in the form of hypergammaglobulinemia and rheumatoid factor positivity. Genetic factors appear to play a role in the pathogenesis as implicated by the association with HLA class and certain interleukin-10 polymorphisms. Histopathologically, EGPA was originally described as a pathologic triad consisting of (1) necrotizing giant cell vasculitis, (2) eosinophilic tissue infiltration, and (3) extravascular necrotizing granuloma formation, but these characteristics rarely coexist in any one patient. Nerve biopsy may demonstrate epineural necrotizing vasculitis with accompanying eosinophil and lymphocyte infiltrates.

CLINICAL MANIFESTATIONS

The American Academy of Rheumatology established six criteria for the diagnosis of EGPA in patients with documented vasculitis. These included the presence of (1) asthma, (2) eosinophilia, (3) a mononeuropathy or polyneuropathy, (4) migratory transient pulmonary opacities detected radiographically, (5) paranasal sinus abnormalities, and (6) biopsy containing a blood vessel showing eosinophil infiltrates in extravascular areas. The presence of four or more of these criteria had a sensitivity of 85% and a specificity of 99% for EGPA.

A peripheral neuropathy, usually mononeuritis multiplex, associated with severe neuropathic pain is seen in up to 75% of patients; other neurologic manifestations may include subarachnoid and intracerebral parenchymal hemorrhage and cerebral infarction but these are rare.

DIAGNOSIS

A high index of suspicion is necessary for the diagnosis of EGPA. Tests to rule out CNS vasculitis should be performed (see Table 42.3). Most patients with EGPA have peripheral blood eosinophilia, although this may be obscured by use of systemic glucocorticoids to control asthma. ANCAs are noted in 40% to 60% of EGPA patients with the majority being MPO ANCA. Typical findings on chest high-resolution CT include patchy parenchymal consolidation or ground-glass opacification; nodules may also be noted.

TREATMENT

Systemic glucocorticoids are the cornerstone in EGPA therapy and are usually continued for 6 to 12 weeks and then gradually tapered. *Prednisone* 60 mg daily is a typical starting dose. Patients with severe disease with CNS or cardiac involvement require induction with *cyclophosphamide* in combination with systemic glucocorticoid therapy. Induction is followed by a transition to maintenance therapy with azathioprine or methotrexate and leflunomide to induce disease remission over 12 to 18 months; longer courses are necessary for patients with multiple relapses.

OUTCOME

With the use of systemic glucocorticoids and immunomodulatory medication, the prognosis of EGPA has improved dramatically from a 50% mortality rate among untreated patients within 3 months of onset to a 70% to 90% 5-year survival rate with aggressive therapy.

Death usually occurs secondary to cardiac failure, myocardial infarction, renal failure, cerebral hemorrhage, gastrointestinal bleeding, or status asthmaticus.

MISCELLANEOUS CAUSES AND MIMICS OF CENTRAL NERVOUS SYSTEM VASCULITIS

REVERSIBLE CEREBRAL VASOCONSTRICTION SYNDROME

Formerly known as *Call–Fleming syndrome*, RCVS is a monophasic self-limited acute cerebral vasoconstriction syndrome (see Chapter 43 for a full discussion). Patients typically present with headache and may develop minor neurologic deficits related to vasogenic edema or small infarcts, seizures, or convexity subarachnoid hemorrhage. Classic beading is seen on digital subtraction angiography that can be indistinguishable from PACNS. The important differences between RCVS and PACNS are that the former syndrome tends to be much more benign and self-limited. Misdiagnosis of RCVS as PACNS (Table 42.4) and treatment with immunosuppressive agents is not warranted because the condition results from myogenic arterial spasm rather than an autoimmune process causing intramural vessel inflammation. Apart from use of calcium channel blockers such as oral nimodipine 60 mg every 4 hours, treatment is supportive and spontaneous recovery over several weeks is the rule.

INTRAVASCULAR LARGE CELL LYMPHOMA

Intravascular large B-cell lymphoma (IVLBCL) is a rare type of non-Hodgkin lymphoma classified by the World Health Organization as an extranodal diffuse large B-cell lymphoma (LBCL) characterized

TABLE 42.4	Differentiating Primary Angiitis of the Central Nervous System (PACNS) and Reversible Cerebral Vasoconstriction Syndrome (RCVS)	
	PACNS	**RCVS**
Gender predominance and mean age at onset	Male, 50 yr	Female, 40 yr
Onset and clinical presentation	Insidious with subacute to chronic onset of headache with focal and nonfocal deficit	Acute onset of thunderclap headache with or without neurologic deficit
Clinical course	Chronic, relapsing	Remission within 1 month, monophasic
Headache	Progressive, dull aching	Severe, throbbing, often thunderclap
CSF findings	Abnormal lymphocytic pleocytosis and elevated protein levels	Normal to near normal
Diagnosis	Leptomeningeal and brain parenchymal tissue biopsy necessary	No biopsy indicated
Common neuroimaging findings	Ischemic, high-intensity T2/FLAIR lesions abnormal MRI images in 100 % of cases	Ischemic, edema, convexity subarachnoid hemorrhage, ICH normal MRI images in 20% of cases
Vascular findings	Normal in one-third of cases. Diffuse abnormalities are often indistinguishable from RCVS; irregular and asymmetric arterial stenoses or multiple occlusions are more suggestive of PCNSV; abnormalities might be irreversible.	Abnormal in all cases; strings of beads appearance of cerebral arteries; abnormalities reversible within 6–12 wk
Histologic findings	Vasculitic changes	Normal
Drug treatment	Glucocorticoids with or without cytotoxic agents	Nimodipine; no glucocorticoids
Immunosuppressive therapy	Essential	Not indicated
Prognosis	Improved with immunosuppressive therapy	Excellent

CSF, cerebrospinal fluid; FLAIR, fluid-attenuated inversion recovery; MRI, magnetic resonance imaging; ICH, intracranial hemorrhage; RCVS, reversible cerebral vasoconstriction syndrome; PCNSV, primary central nervous system vasculitis.

by the selective growth of neoplastic lymphocytes within blood vessel lumina of small vessels, particularly capillaries and venules. This type of lymphoma has also been described as *intravascular lymphomatosis, angiotropic large cell lymphoma,* and *malignant lymphangioendotheliomatosis.* IVLBCL is not a form of vasculitis per se but is often included in the differential diagnosis of PACNS because it can cause a rapidly progressive pattern of widespread brain infarction in a patient without risk factors for cerebrovascular disease.

Epidemiology

The incidence of IVLBCL is unknown; the median age at diagnosis is in the sixth to seventh decades with no gender predilection.

Pathobiology

The diagnosis of IVLBCL is made by demonstrating large lymphoid cells with high mitotic activity within small to medium blood vessels.

Clinical Manifestations

The clinical presentation is varied and often includes symptoms related to organ dysfunction caused by occlusion of small blood vessels. Constitutional symptoms are seen in 55% to 85 % of patients. IVLBCL is considered a disseminated disease at diagnosis frequently manifesting with CNS and cutaneous symptoms in Western countries or with hemophagocytic syndromes in Asian countries. Rapidly progressive, recurrent ischemic strokes and peripheral neuropathies are frequently seen. CNS symptoms may include progression from lethargy to coma, focal neurologic deficits, seizures, or central hyperventilation. Neurologic symptoms are less commonly seen in patients of Asian descent who frequently present with involvement of the bone marrow, spleen, and liver.

Diagnosis

A wide range of laboratory abnormalities may be seen, ranging from elevated lactate dehydrogenase, β2-microglobulin, and ESR levels to abnormal liver, renal, or thyroid function tests; anemia; thrombocytopenia; and hypoalbuminemia. CSF analysis only rarely demonstrates malignant cells but CSF cytology and flow cytometry should be obtained. IVLBCL is not typically associated with an obvious extravascular tumor mass, adenopathy, or detectable circulating lymphoma cells in the peripheral blood.

Brain biopsy or deep skin biopsy including the subcutaneous tissues is necessary to confirm the diagnosis. The bone marrow, lymph nodes, peripheral blood, and CSF are often uninvolved. Cerebral MRI findings include infarctions when occlusions occur in small arteries, patchy foci of white matter hyperintensities when the pathology involves the capillaries, mass-like lesions, and thickening of the meningeal vessels with meningeal or focal parenchymal enhancement.

Treatment and Outcome

Accurate and timely diagnosis of IVLBCL is still a problematic issue, and many cases are diagnosed at autopsy. However, in recent years, the heightened awareness of IVLBCL with appropriate investigations has resulted in more patients being diagnosed during life. Treatment of patients with IVLBCL includes a combination of *cyclophosphamide, doxorubicin, vincristine,* and *prednisone* with *rituximab,* a recombinant anti-CD20 monoclonal antibody (R-CHOP).

The addition of *rituximab* has been shown to improve progression-free 2-year survival from 27% to 56%.

INFECTIOUS CENTRAL NERVOUS SYSTEM VASCULITIS

Infection is a well-recognized cause of CNS vasculopathy that can mimic autoimmune PACNS. The spectrum of infections that can cause segmental vascular inflammation of the cerebral arteries ranges includes viruses (e.g., varicella-zoster virus or hepatitis C; see Chapter 66), bacterial meningitis, or endocarditis (see Chapters 61 and 63); chronic meningitis due to tuberculosis, spirochete infection (e.g., neurosyphilis), or fungal infection (e.g., *Aspergillus, Cryptococcus;* see Chapter 64); rickettsial infection (e.g., Rocky Mountain spotted fever; see Chapter 63); and parasites (see Chapter 65). In most cases, the process is believed to be due to direct invasion and proliferation of pathogens in vessel walls with resultant inflammation, although some may develop as a result of an autoimmune response initiated by exposure to a pathogen (e.g., cryoglobulinemic vasculitis in the setting of HCV infection).

Varicella-zoster virus is a frequent cause of viral CNS vasculitis affecting large vessels in immunocompetent hosts while causing a more extensive protracted disease in immunocompromised individuals by affecting small vessels. Hepatitis C has been associated with small-vessel vasculitis related to mixed cryoglobulinemia, which accounts for the majority of cases, or a small- to medium-vessel vasculitis similar to PAN.

Bacterial cerebral vasculitis usually starts as purulent infection at the base of the brain progressing to inflammatory cell infiltration of vessel walls, with subsequent septic thrombosis and thrombophlebitis manifesting clinically as ischemic stroke and hemorrhages. Syphilitic vasculitis usually occurs as part of tertiary syphilis and occurs for 10% to 40% of untreated cases. Diffuse syphilitic vasculitis preferentially involves the cortical arteries and veins, whereas the gummatous vasculitis usually affects proximal middle cerebral artery (MCA) branches. Classic angiographic findings include narrowing of the proximal portions of the cerebral arteries with distal beading due to alternating segmental stenoses and dilatations.

CNS tuberculosis is frequently associated with segmental infectious vasculitis, secondary aneurysm formation, and thromboses causing infarctions of the basal ganglia, cerebral cortex, brain stem, and cerebellum in patients with CNS tuberculosis.

DRUG-INDUCED CENTRAL NERVOUS SYSTEM VASCULITIS

Although the exact incidence and pathobiology is unknown, there is ample evidence that some illicit and therapeutic drugs can result in either a self-limited or more protracted form of cerebral vasculitis. The pathogenesis is likely multifactorial. Drugs with sympathomimetic activity (*amphetamines, cocaine, phenylpropanolamine*) have been frequently implicated in causing biopsy-proven inflammatory cerebral vasculitis, as well as ischemic stroke precipitated by noninflammatory cerebral vasoconstriction.

The clinical diagnosis is one of exclusion based on the temporal relationship between the administration of the offending drugs and clinically evident vasculitis. Management is generally supportive in addition to removal of the instigating agent, which alone is often sufficient to induce prompt resolution of clinical manifestations. There is little data to guide management of severe cases where there is vital organ involvement.

SUGGESTED READINGS

Al-Araji A, Kidd DP. Neuro-Behcet's disease: epidemiology, clinical characteristics, and management. *Lancet Neurol.* 2009;8(2):192–204.

Benamour S, Naji T, Alaoui FZ, et al. Neurological involvement in Behcet's disease. 154 cases from a cohort of 925 patients and review of the literature [in French]. *Rev Neurol (Paris).* 2006;162(11):1084–1090.

Booth AD, Almond MK, Burns A, et al. Outcome of ANCA-associated renal vasculitis: a 5-year retrospective study. *Am J Kidney Dis.* 2003;41(4):776–784.

Cacoub P, Saadoun D, Limal N, et al. Hepatitis C virus infection and mixed cryoglobulinaemia vasculitis: a review of neurological complications. *AIDS (London, England).* 2005;19(suppl 3):S128–S134.

Calabrese LH, Duna GF, Lie JT. Vasculitis in the central nervous system. *Arthritis Rheum.* 1997;40(1189):201.

Caselli RJ, Hunder GG. Neurologic complications of giant cell (temporal) arteritis. *Semin Neurol.* 1994;14(4):349–353.

Chan KH, Cheung RT, Lee R, et al. Cerebral infarcts complicating tuberculous meningitis. *Cerebrovas Dis.* 2005;19(6):391–395.

Chen M, Kallenberg CG. ANCA-associated vasculitides—advances in pathogenesis and treatment. *Nat Rev Rheumatol.* 2010;6(11):653–664.

Czarnecki EJ, Spickler EM. MR demonstration of Wegener granulomatosis of the infundibulum, a cause of diabetes insipidus. *AJNR Am J Neuroradiol.* 1995;16(4)(suppl):968–970.

Falk RJ, Jennette JC. ANCA small-vessel vasculitis. *J Am Soc Nephrol.* 1997;8(2):314–322.

Ferreri AJ, Dognini GP, Govi S, et al. Can rituximab change the usually dismal prognosis of patients with intravascular large B-cell lymphoma? *J Clin Oncol.* 2008;26(31):5134–5136.

Finkielman JD, Lee AS, Hummel AM, et al. ANCA are detectable in nearly all patients with active severe Wegener's granulomatosis. *Am J Med.* 2007;120(7):643.e9–e14.

Gayraud M, Guillevin L, le Toumelin P, et al. Long-term followup of polyarteritis nodosa, microscopic polyangiitis, and Churg-Strauss syndrome: analysis of four prospective trials including 278 patients. *Arthritis Rheum.* 2001;44(3):666–675.

Giang DW. Central nervous system vasculitis secondary to infections, toxins, and neoplasms. *Semin Neurol.* 1994;14(4):313–319.

Guillevin L, Cohen P, Gayraud M, et al. Churg-Strauss syndrome. Clinical study and long-term follow-up of 96 patients. *Medicine (Baltimore).* 1999;78(1):26–37.

Guillevin L, Durand-Gasselin B, Cevallos R, et al. Microscopic polyangiitis: clinical and laboratory findings in eighty-five patients. *Arthritis Rheum.* 1999;42(3):421–430.

Han S, Rehman HU, Jayaratne PS, et al. Microscopic polyangiitis complicated by cerebral haemorrhage. *Rheumatol Int.* 2006;26(11):1057–1060.

Hattori N, Ichimura M, Nagamatsu M, et al. Clinicopathological features of Churg-Strauss syndrome-associated neuropathy. *Brain.* 1999;122(pt 3):427–439.

Hunder GG, Bloch DA, Michel BA, et al. The American College of Rheumatology 1990 criteria for the classification of giant cell arteritis. *Arthritis Rheum.* 1990;33(8):1122–1128.

International Study Group for Behcet's Disease. Criteria for diagnosis of Behcet's disease. *Lancet.* 1990;335(8697):1078–1080.

Ito Y, Suzuki K, Yamazaki T, et al. ANCA-associated vasculitis (AAV) causing bilateral cerebral infarction and subsequent intracerebral hemorrhage without renal and respiratory dysfunction. *J Neurol Sci.* 2006;240(1–2):99–101.

Jennette JC, Falk RJ, Bacon PA, et al. 2012 revised International Chapel Hill Consensus Conference nomenclature of vasculitides. *Arthritis Rheum.* 2013;65(1):1–11.

Kalra S, Silman A, Akman-Demir G, et al. Diagnosis and management of neuro-Behcet's disease: international consensus recommendations. *J Neurol.* 2014;261(9):1662–1676.

Kelley RE. CNS vasculitis. *Front Biosci.* 2004;9:946–955.

Leavitt RY, Fauci AS, Bloch DA, et al. The American College of Rheumatology 1990 criteria for the classification of Wegener's granulomatosis. *Arthritis Rheum.* 1990;33(8):1101–1107.

Lhote F, Cohen P, Guillevin L. Polyarteritis nodosa, microscopic polyangiitis and Churg-Strauss syndrome. *Lupus.* 1998;7(4):238–258.

Lie JT. Primary (granulomatous) angiitis of the central nervous system: a clinicopathologic analysis of 15 new cases and a review of the literature. *Hum Pathol.* 1992;23:164–171.

Mahr A, Moosig F, Neumann T, et al. Eosinophilic granulomatosis with polyangiitis (Churg-Strauss): evolutions in classification, etiopathogenesis, assessment and management. *Curr Opin Rheumatol.* 2014;26(1):16–23.

Miller DV, Salvarani C, Hunder GG, et al. Biopsy findings in primary angiitis of the central nervous system. *Am J Surg Pathol.* 2009;33(1):35–43.

Moosig F, Bremer JP, Hellmich B, et al. A vasculitis centre based management strategy leads to improved outcome in eosinophilic granulomatosis and polyangiitis (Churg-Strauss, EGPA): monocentric experiences in 150 patients. *Ann Rheum Dis.* 2013;72(6):1011–1017.

Morrow PL, McQuillen JB. Cerebral vasculitis associated with cocaine abuse. *J Forensic Sci.* 1993;38(3):732–738.

Mouthon L, Dunogue B, Guillevin L. Diagnosis and classification of eosinophilic granulomatosis with polyangiitis (formerly named Churg-Strauss syndrome). *J Autoimmun.* 2014;48–49:99–103.

Mukhtyar C, Guillevin L, Cid MC, et al. EULAR recommendations for the management of primary small and medium vessel vasculitis. *Ann Rheum Dis.* 2009;68(3):310–317.

Pagnoux C, Cohen P, Guillevin L. Vasculitides secondary to infections. *Clin Exp Rheumatol.* 2006;24(2)(suppl 41):S71–S81.

Pagnoux C, Seror R, Henegar C, et al. Clinical features and outcomes in 348 patients with polyarteritis nodosa: a systematic retrospective study of patients diagnosed between 1963 and 2005 and entered into the French Vasculitis Study Group Database. *Arthritis Rheum.* 2010;62(2):616–626.

Pezzini A, Gulletta M, Pinelli L, et al. Meningovascular syphilis: a vascular syndrome with typical features? *Cerebrovasc Dis.* 2001;11(4):352–353.

Ponzoni M, Ferreri AJ, Campo E, et al. Definition, diagnosis, and management of intravascular large B-cell lymphoma: proposals and perspectives from an international consensus meeting. *J Clin Oncol.* 2007;25(21):3168–3173.

Pozzi M, Roccatagliata D, Sterzi R. Drug abuse and intracranial hemorrhage. *Neurol Sci.* 2008;29(suppl 2):S269–S270.

Provenzale JM, Allen NB. Neuroradiologic findings in polyarteritis nodosa. *AJNR Am J Neuroradiol.* 1996;17(6):1119–1126.

Saadoun D, Terrier B, Semoun O, et al. Hepatitis C virus-associated polyarteritis nodosa. *Arthritis Care Res.* 2011;63(3):427–435.

Salvarani C, Brown RD Jr, Calamia KT, et al. Primary central nervous system vasculitis: analysis of 101 patients. *Ann Neurol.* 2007;62(5):442–451.

Salvarani C, Brown RD Jr, Calamia KT, et al. Primary central nervous system vasculitis: comparison of patients with and without cerebral amyloid angiopathy. *Rheumatology (Oxford).* 2008;47(11):1671.

Salvasari C, Brown RD Jr, Hunder GG. Adult primary central nervous system vasculitis. *Lancet.* 2012;380(9843):767–777.

Samson M, Puéchal X, Devilliers H, et al. Long-term outcomes of 118 patients with eosinophilic granulomatosis with polyangiitis (Churg-Strauss syndrome) enrolled in two prospective trials. *J Autoimmun.* 2013;43:60–69.

Siva A, Saip S. The spectrum of nervous system involvement in Behcet's syndrome and its differential diagnosis. *J Neurol.* 2009;256(4):513–529.

Tamargo RJ, Connolly ES Jr, McKhann GM, et al. Clinicopathological review: primary angiitis of the central nervous system in association with cerebral amyloid angiopathy. *Neurosurgery.* 2003;53(1):136–143; discussion 143.

Watts RA, Mooney J, Skinner J, et al. The contrasting epidemiology of granulomatosis with polyangiitis (Wegener's) and microscopic polyangiitis. *Rheumatology (Oxford).* 2012;51(5):926–931.

Weyand CM, Goronzy JJ. Clinical practice. Giant-cell arteritis and polymyalgia rheumatica. *N Engl J Med.* 2014;371(1):50–57.

Weyand CM, Goronzy JJ. Immune mechanisms in medium and large-vessel vasculitis. *Nat Rev Rheumatol.* 2013;9(12):731–740.

Williams RL, Meltzer CC, Smirniotopoulos JG, et al. Cerebral MR imaging in intravascular lymphomatosis. *AJNR Am J Neuroradiol.* 1998;19(3):427–431.

Wolf J, Bergner R, Mutallib S, et al. Neurologic complications of Churg-Strauss syndrome—a prospective monocentric study. *Eur J Neurol.* 2010;17(4):582–588.

Yamamoto A, Kikuchi Y, Homma K, et al. Characteristics of intravascular large B-cell lymphoma on cerebral MR imaging. *AJNR Am J Neuroradiol.* 2012;33(2):292–296.

Younger DS. Vasculitis of the nervous system. *Curr Opin Neurol.* 2004;17(3):317–336.

Posterior Reversible Encephalopathy Syndrome and Other Cerebrovascular Syndromes

Sara K. Rostanski, Fawaz Al-Mufti, Claire S. Riley, and Joshua Z. Willey

POSTERIOR REVERSIBLE ENCEPHALOPATHY SYNDROME

The posterior reversible encephalopathy syndrome (PRES) has been evolving as a clinical entity for the last 10 years. Several terms have now been used interchangeably to define PRES, including reversible posterior leukoencephalopathy syndrome (RPLS), or by naming the underlying clinical cause. PRES is now recognized as a clinicoradiologic syndrome rather than a distinct disease entity with multiple different etiologies, which share several common features with the reversible cerebral vasoconstriction syndrome.

EPIDEMIOLOGY

Limited data exist to describe the epidemiology of this condition. The literature has mostly been centered around case reports and case series.

PATHOBIOLOGY

Disorders that cause PRES have in common cerebral injury due to failure of the cerebral vasculature to adapt to changes in blood pressure or cerebral hemodynamics or an excessive vascular reactivity in cerebral arterioles. The hallmark clinical entities that most often cause PRES are hypertensive encephalopathy and eclampsia (see also Chapter 124). A focal process that may share some features of this condition is cerebral hyperperfusion syndrome occurring after carotid endarterectomy. In patients with chronic hemodynamic failure, distal arterioles tend to dilate to reduce cerebral vascular resistance; in clinical scenarios of a sudden increase in cerebral blood flow, these maximally dilated cerebral arteries may not be able to adapt further to changes in cerebral blood flow, leading to cerebral edema and hemorrhage. In addition to impaired autoregulation in the face of hypertension and hyperperfusion, in many cases, PRES is also associated with abnormal capillary permeability in the brain and large-vessel proximal vasoconstriction detectable by angiography. Up to 87% of patients with PRES have diffuse vasoconstriction if studied with angiography, hence, PRES and reversible cerebral vasoconstriction syndrome (discussed later) often overlap and are felt in many cases to share a common pathogenesis. The result is vasogenic edema that preferentially affects the posterior hemispheres of the brain and the white matter more than the gray matter. Interspersed in this picture are scattered microinfarcts and microhemorrhages. The most severe cases can manifest as massive global cerebral edema with transtentorial herniation or larger infarcts or hemorrhages.

CLINICAL FEATURES

The clinical syndrome associated with PRES is dependent on the underlying cause, although regardless of underlying etiology, common clinical symptoms include headache, seizures, loss of visual acuity including blindness, nonlocalizing confusion, and

TABLE 43.1	Approximate Frequency of Clinical Features of Posterior Reversible Encephalopathy Syndrome
Clinical Feature	**Frequency**
Hypertension	80%
Consciousness impairment	75%
Seizures	70%
Headaches	40%
Visual abnormalities	30%
Nausea and vomiting	20%

somnolence (Table 43.1). The neurologic examination will not reveal localizing findings on the mental status, although cases of cortical blindness and Balint syndrome may occur due to involvement of the occipital lobes (Fig. 43.1). Other described findings include visual field cuts, loss of visual acuity, papilledema, and mild hemiparesis. More prominent bulbar and cerebellar symptoms have been described in case series where the pathology is restricted to the brain stem. A larger variety of clinical syndromes, which can be localized anywhere in the cerebral hemisphere occurs in the context of severe cases with cerebral infarction or hemorrhage. PRES leading to edema primarily involving the brain stem has also been described (Fig. 43.2).

DIAGNOSIS

Neuroimaging is essential in the diagnosis of this condition, with magnetic resonance imaging (MRI) providing greater clinical information than computed tomography (CT). The "classical" description in this condition is white matter hyperintensities seen on fluid-attenuated inversion recovery (FLAIR) sequences representing vasogenic edema (see also Chapter 21). The FLAIR changes have a predilection to occipital lobes and adjacent posterior temporal and parietal regions and are not typically associated with cerebral microhemorrhages, infarction, or involvement of gray matter structures. A hallmark of this condition is that these clinical findings improve with treatment of the underlying condition, along with the cerebral vasogenic edema. To some degree, however, the term *posterior reversible encephalopathy syndrome* may be a misnomer, as in several cases, the changes seen clinically or on imaging are neither posterior predominant nor reversible. Common underlying predisposing conditions include hypertensive emergency/malignant hypertension, eclampsia, and medication toxicity (notably FK-506 in prevention of transplant organ rejection). Table 43.2 describes a variety of underlying etiologies for PRES.

The differential diagnosis of PRES includes conditions which have a predilection for causing bilateral involvement of the hemispheres, particularly the white matter, or that affect watershed

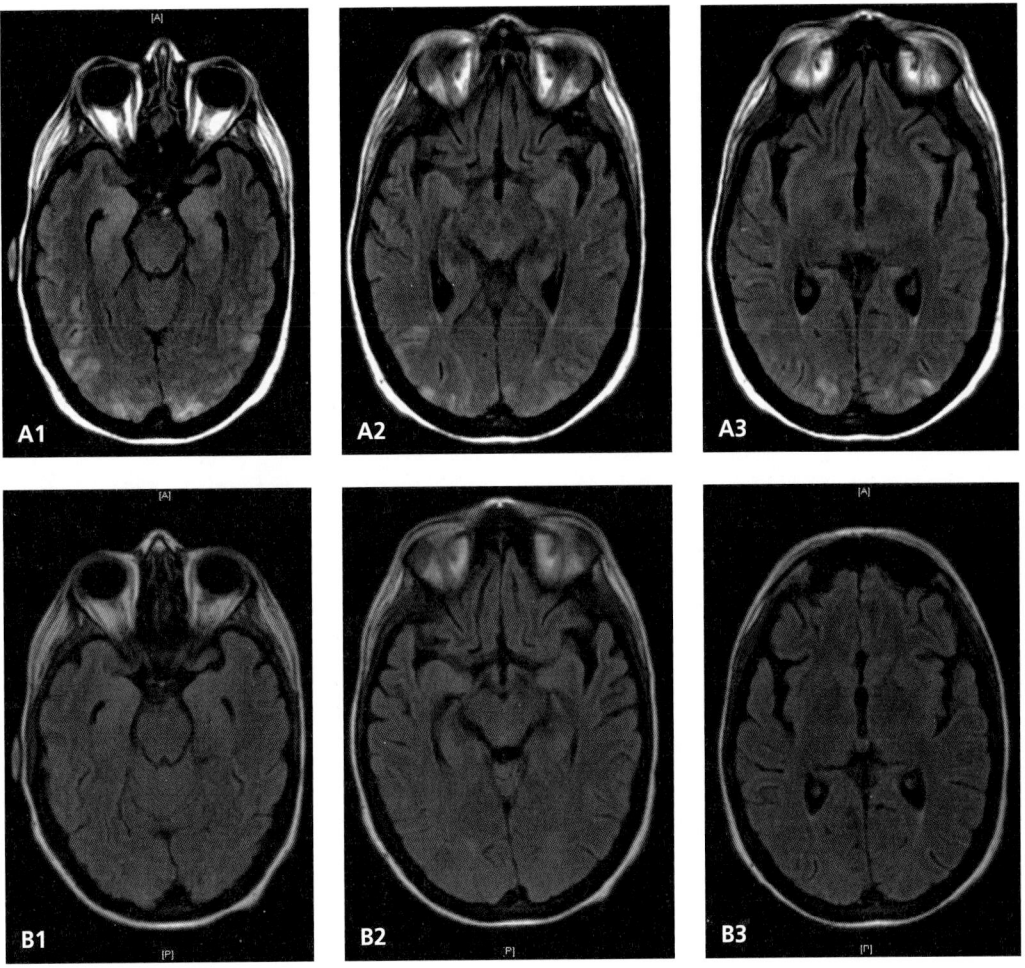

FIGURE 43.1 Magnetic resonance FLAIR image of posterior reversible encephalopathy syndrome on admission **(A)** and 2 weeks after stopping inciting medication **(B)**.

regions between the major vascular territories. These include progressive multifocal leukoencephalopathy, encephalitis, vasculitis, and watershed infarction from cardiac arrest, among others.

TREATMENT

Management of PRES begins with a careful review of medications and discontinuation of any potential inciting agent. Patients with PRES require the symptomatic measures usually taken in the intensive care unit (ICU). The need for upper airway protection should be evaluated continuously in patients with marked consciousness impairment or seizure activity.

Control of hypertensive emergency, if present, is an important part of the symptomatic management. The aim is not to normalize the blood pressure but rather to decrease the mean arterial pressure (MAP) by 20% to 25% within the first 2 hours and to bring the blood pressure down to 160/100 mm Hg within the first 6 hours. More rapid blood pressure reduction is not recommended because it can aggravate the cerebral perfusion pressure alterations and promote ischemia. Continuous infusion of intravenous (IV) antihypertensive agents is preferred to allow for precise blood pressure control within a tight range. The most commonly used agents include *labetalol*, *nicardipine*, or *clevidipine* if available (see Table 38.3).

Antiepileptic treatment should be initiated on an emergency basis for treatment of clinical or electrographic seizures or status epilepticus (see also Chapter 6). All comatose patients should undergo 48 hours of surveillance continuous electroencephalogram (EEG) monitoring in the ICU given the high risk of nonconvulsive seizures. Active seizures should be treated with a full loading dose of lorazepam 0.1 mg/kg IV. Once controlled, patients should be loaded with an IV anticonvulsant such as phenytoin 20 mg/kg IV, followed by 300 mg daily, or valproic acid, 45 mg/kg, followed by 500 mg IV every 6 hours. Refractory status epilepticus after treatment with a full loading dose of a benzodiazepine and IV antiepileptic agent should be treated with midazolam infusion (0.2 mg/kg IV load, followed by a starting dose of 0.2 mg/kg/h), which mandates continuous EEG monitoring and endotracheal intubation.

Patients with PRES due to eclampsia should also be started on magnesium infusion (1 to 2 g/h targeting a serum magnesium level of 2.0 to 3.5 to 4 mmol/L) [**Level 1**].[1] Magnesium infusion is also recommended for any PRES patient with hypomagnesemia.

REVERSIBLE CEREBRAL VASOCONSTRICTION SYNDROME

In 2007, the term *reversible cerebral vasoconstriction syndrome* (RCVS) was proposed to encompass several previously described miscellaneous cerebral vasculitic disorders, which included

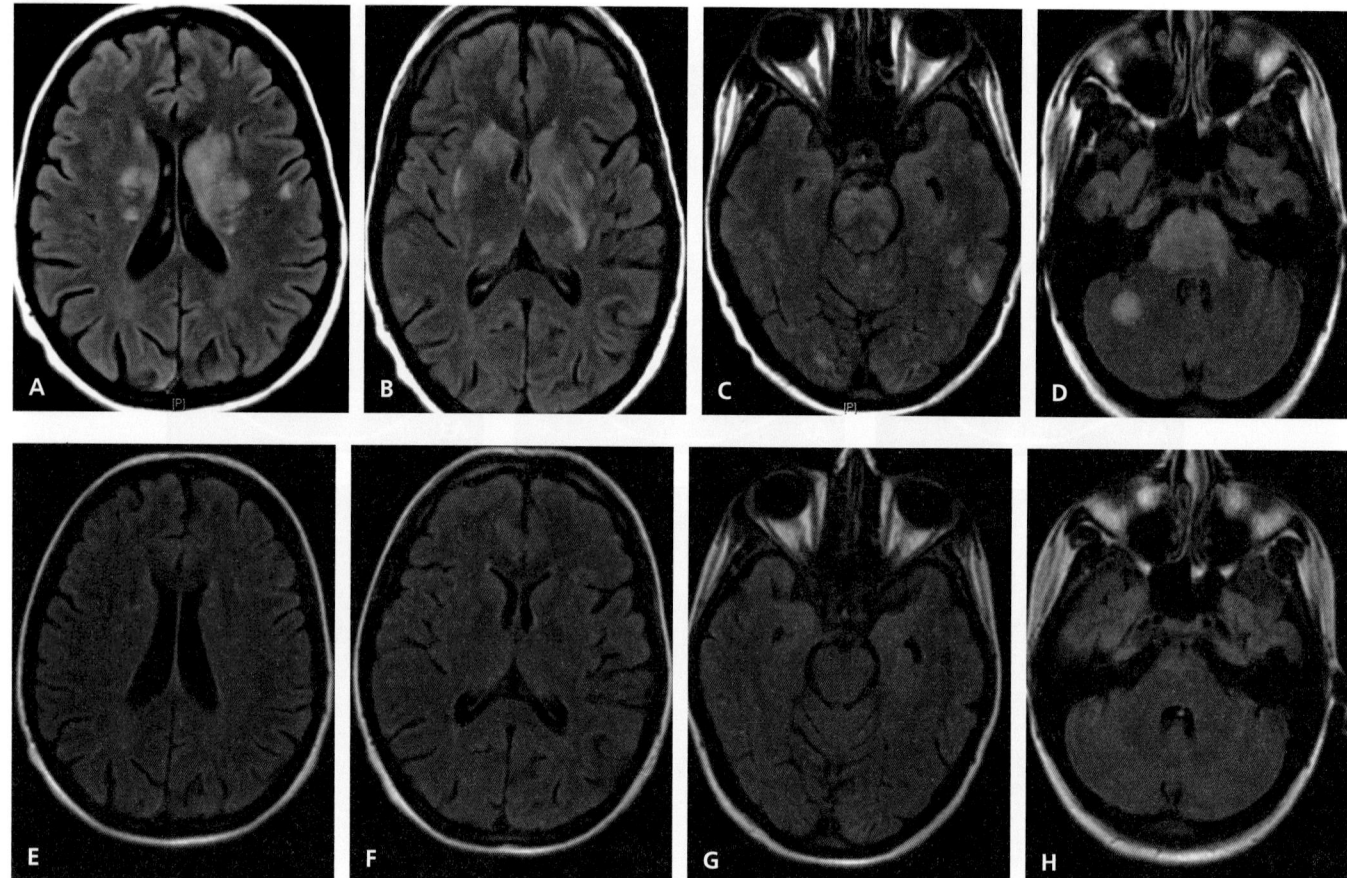

FIGURE 43.2 FLAIR images of posterior reversible encephalopathy syndrome presenting with prominent brain stem involvement **(A–D)**. Nine days later, the lesions had significantly resolved **(E–H)**.

Call–Fleming syndrome, thunderclap headache–associated vasoconstriction, postpartum angiopathy, migraine angiitis, and cerebral vasospasm caused by cocaine, amphetamines, sumatriptan, and other serotonergic and sympathomimetic drugs.

RCVS is characterized by a monophasic course of diffuse segmental constriction of cerebral arteries that resolves spontaneously within weeks to months. Although the angiographic findings may be indistinguishable from primary angiitis of the central nervous system (PACNS), RCVS is not a chronic condition that requires long-term immunosuppression. RVCS is not a form of vasculitis because vessel wall inflammatory infiltrates do not occur, although the angiographic findings are similar. The cerebrospinal fluid (CSF) is normal, and the clinical course tends to be benign given the marked and extensive angiographic abnormalities that can occur.

EPIDEMIOLOGY

Due to the lack of epidemiologic studies, the true incidence of RCVS has not been estimated. Since 2007, there has been a surge in the number of RCVS-related publications likely due to increased awareness.

PATHOBIOLOGY

Other than vasoconstriction, there is no known unifying pathologic mechanism that underlies RCVS because it is a syndrome rather than a distinct disease entity. An aberrant sympathetic response of cerebral vasculature is one of the preferred hypotheses resulting in an unpredictable and short-lived failure of normal regulation

of cerebral arterial tone. This leads to segmental vasoconstriction and vasodilatation in small cerebral vessels, often triggering thunderclap headaches due to stretching of vasa nervorum within the vessel walls.

RCVS appears to be an intrinsic process that can be triggered by a wide variety of pharmacologic and physical stimuli (Table 43.3). Different precipitating factors, including vasoconstrictive drug exposure (serotonergic or adrenergic agents), recreational drugs, and postpartum state are associated with RCVS in around 50% of cases. Head injuries and neurosurgical interventions have also been associated with RCVS.

PRES occurs in a substantial proportion of patients with RCVS. Hence, a shared pathophysiology between these two overlapping syndromes is highly probable. Severe forms of RCVS are likely to lead to PRES. In the past, it is likely that many of the cases termed *central nervous system vasculitis* and *benign angiitis of the central nervous system* may have actually referred to RCVS.

CLINICAL FEATURES

RCVS affects mainly women, with a mean age at onset of 40 years. In over 80% of cases, patients present with a sudden onset of single or recurrent thunderclap headaches. These headaches differ from those associated with aneurysmal subarachnoid hemorrhage (SAH) because they are usually short lived and intermittent, whereas SAH causes unremitting headaches that persist for days with prominent meningismus. Seizures occur and transient focal deficits in the form of visual, sensory, dysphasic, or motor deficits occur in

TABLE 43.2	Etiologies of Posterior Reversible Encephalopathy Syndrome

Malignant hypertension

Eclampsia

Immunosuppressants

- Tacrolimus (FK-506)
- Cyclosporine A
- Mycophenolate mofetil

Autoimmune disease

- Systemic lupus erythematosus
- Polyarteritis nodosa
- Wegener granulomatosis
- Systemic sclerosis

Chemotherapy drugs

- Cytarabine
- Gemcitabine
- Methotrexate
- Cisplatin
- Carboplatin

Biologic agents

- Erythropoietin (in end-stage renal disease)
- Immunomodulatory cytokines (interferon-α, interleukin-2)
- Monoclonal antibodies (rituximab, infliximab)
- Antiangiogenic agents (bevacizumab)
- Antilymphocyte globulin
- Intravenous immunoglobulins (IVIG)

Sepsis

Blood transfusion

Other agents

- Antiretroviral agents
- Linezolid
- Cocaine
- Ephedra
- IV contrast agents
- Carbamazepine

IV, intravenous.

TABLE 43.3	Precipitants of Reversible Cerebral Vasoconstriction Syndrome

Vasoactive drugs	Illicit drugs: cocaine, amphetamines, lysergic acid diethylamide (LSD), 3,4-methylenedioxymethamphetamine (MDMA, also known as *ecstasy*)
	Antidepressants: selective serotonin reuptake inhibitors, serotonin–noradrenaline reuptake inhibitors
	α-sympathomimetics agents: phenylpropanolamine, pseudoephedrine, ephedrine)
	Other: triptans, ergot alkaloid derivatives, ginseng
Catecholamine-secreting tumors	Pheochromocytoma
	Bronchial carcinoid tumor
Immunosuppressants or blood products	Intravenous immunoglobulin
	Tacrolimus
	Cyclophosphamide
	Erythropoietin
	α-Interferon
	Red blood cell transfusion
Metabolic abnormalities	Hypercalcemia
	Porphyria
	Phenytoin intoxication
	Binge drinking
Neurologic pathologies	Traumatic brain injury
	Neurosurgical interventions, for example, post carotid endarterectomy
	Subdural spinal hematoma
	Cerebral venous thrombosis
	CSF hypotension
	Autonomic dysreflexia/paroxysmal sympathetic hyperactivity
Pregnancy and puerperium	Usually peripartum or postpartum
	Associated with eclampsia or preeclampsia

CSF, cerebrospinal fluid.

Modified from Ducros A. Reversible cerebral vasoconstriction syndrome. *Lancet Neurol.* 2012;11(10):906–917.

approximately 20% of patients at some point during the course of the illness, either alone or in combination. The focal deficits usually last minutes to hours but in some cases are persistent and associated with focal infarction. Blood pressure surges occur in 40% of patients; it is unclear if these elevations are related to the primary condition or are a reaction to pain or neurologic injury. Rupture or reperfusion injuries involving small leptomeningeal arteries may cause convexity SAHs.

DIAGNOSIS

Calabrese et al. have proposed diagnostic criteria for RCVS that encompass clinical, radiographic, and CSF findings. Because RCVS can mimic PACNS, differentiation is crucial because management is extremely different (Table 43.4). Basic hematologic and meta-

bolic tests, including ESR and liver and renal function tests, are typically normal in RCVS. Tests to rule out CNS vasculitis should be performed as delineated in Table 42.3, but in addition, urine toxicology screens and urinary concentrations of vanillylmandelic acid and 5-hydroxyindoleacetic acid should be measured if pheochromocytoma is suspected.

A normal CSF profile is the rule, although mild abnormalities in the CSF can be present when subarachnoid or intracerebral hemorrhages exist. If the white blood cell count exceeds 10 cells/μL or the protein concentration exceeds 80 mg/dL, analysis of CSF should be repeated after a few weeks to ensure that these abnormalities have normalized.

Up to 50% of patients had a normal initial CT or MRI scan despite the presence of diffuse vasoconstriction on concomitant cere-

TABLE 43.4	**Summary of Critical Elements for the Diagnosis of Reversible Cerebral Vasoconstriction Syndrome**

A. Transfemoral angiography or indirect computed tomography angiography or magnetic resonance angiography documenting multifocal segmental cerebral artery vasoconstriction

B. No evidence for aneurysmal subarachnoid hemorrhage

C. Normal or near-normal cerebrospinal fluid analysis (protein level <80 mg/dL, leukocytes <10–15/mm³ and normal glucose level)

D. Severe, acute headaches with or without additional neurologic signs or symptoms

E. Monophasic course without new symptoms more than 1 mo after clinical onset

F. Reversibility of angiographic abnormalities within 12 wk after onset. If death occurs before the follow-up studies are completed, autopsy rules out such conditions as vasculitis, intracranial atherosclerosis, and aneurysmal subarachnoid hemorrhage, which can also manifest with headache and stroke.

Adapted from the International Headache Society criteria for acute reversible cerebral angiopathy and the criteria proposed in 2007 by Calabrese. Headache Classification Subcommittee of the International Headache Society. The international classification of headache disorders. *Cephalalgia.* 2004;24:1–160; Calabrese LH, Dodick DW, Schwedt TJ, et al. Narrative review: reversible cerebral vasoconstriction syndromes. *Ann Intern Med.* 2007;146(1):34–44.

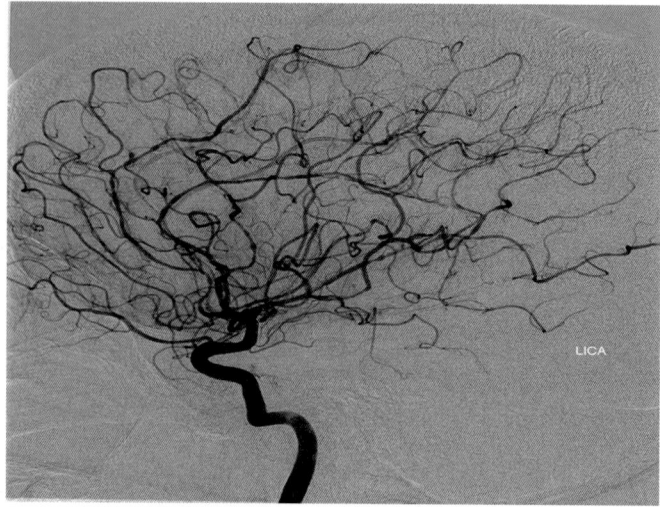

FIGURE 43.3 Multifocal beading of the cerebral vasculature, characteristic of reversible cerebral vasoconstriction syndrome. (From Neil WP, Dechant V, Urtecho J. Pearls and oy-sters: reversible cerebral vasoconstriction syndrome precipitated by ascent to high altitude. *Neurology.* 2011;76:e7–e9.)

bral angiography. By the end of the clinical course, 80% of patients eventually develop lesions on MRI. Common findings include convexity SAH, small discrete intracerebral hemorrhages, and infarcts.

Digital subtraction angiography (DSA) is he preferred method for demonstrating multifocal segmental vessel constriction. As is the case with PACNS, CT and magnetic resonance angiography (MRA) do not have sufficient resolution of the distal vasculature to demonstrate small-vessel "beading," although they can demonstrate spasm of the larger proximal vessels (Fig. 43.3). Findings on angiography maybe dynamic, with repeat scans demonstrating resolution of some abnormalities and new vasoconstriction of others. Initial angiography might be normal if performed very early in the course of the disease. Repeat angiography is sometimes useful if the diagnosis remains unclear days to weeks after the performance of an initial study. The onset of headache and cortical SAH may precede the development of vasospasm on vascular imaging, and indeed, elevated flow velocities on transcranial Doppler may predict the small minority of patients who are at risk for developing subsequent ischemic stroke due to severe vasospasm.

TREATMENT

Treatment of RCVS is largely supportive; there are no proven effective pharmacologic agents that can reverse the vasoconstriction, although *nimodipine* 60 mg every 4 hours, *verapamil* 60 mg every 6 hours, and *magnesium sulfate* 1 to 2 g/h IV have all been tried. Prospective and retrospective studies indicate that *nimodipine* 60 mg every 4 hours may help reduce the frequency and severity of headaches, but there is no evidence that it affects vasospasm or outcome. Management focuses on discontinuation or avoidance of precipitating agents, pain control, blood pressure control, antiepileptic drugs for seizure control, and admission to an ICU of

neurologic monitoring in severe cases. Steroids are not indicated, as they do not seem to prevent clinical deterioration and may be harmful with regard to side effects such as immunosuppression, hyperglycemia, and psychosis. Intra-arterial vasodilators and balloon angioplasty have been used in severe cases.

OUTCOME

RCVS is generally considered a monophasic, self-limiting condition with a good long-term prognosis. Headaches usually resolve within 3 weeks, and no new symptoms occur more than 1 month after presentation. The angiographic and parenchymal findings typically resolve within 12 weeks. Less than 5% of patients develop fulminant disease with multiple strokes and global cerebral edema. The vast majority of patients make a complete functional recovery. The case fatality rate is less than 1%.

FIBROMUSCULAR DYSPLASIA

Fibromuscular dysplasia (FMD) is a noninflammatory, nonatherosclerotic arteriopathy of medium-sized vessels of unknown cause. Although it can affect any vascular bed, the renal and cervicocranial carotid and vertebral arteries are most commonly involved.

EPIDEMIOLOGY

Cervicocranial FMD is a rare condition, with one autopsy study citing an overall prevalence of 0.02%. Rates for renovascular FMD are higher, with prevalence estimates of up to 4% shown in several studies. In confirmed FMD cases, renal involvement is generally seen in up to 65% of cases, with cerebrovascular involvement in 25% to 30% of cases. In a series of 1,100 FMD patients, women were twice as frequently affected as men with Caucasians disproportionately affected. The mean age of diagnosis in patients with cerebrovascular involvement is 50 years, older than for renovascular involvement. Approximately 10% of cases are felt to be familial. Diagnosis is frequently delayed, with up to 9 years elapsing from initial symptoms to diagnosis.

PATHOBIOLOGY

There are three types of FMD, characterized by arterial layer of involvement: intimal fibroplasia, medial dysplasia, and adventitial fibroplasia. Intimal fibroplasia occurs in up to 10% of cases and results from accumulation of abnormal subendothelial mesenchymal cells, which project into the vessel lumen. This commonly results in areas of smooth, focal stenosis or long tubular stenosis. Adventitial fibroplasia, where the fibrous adventitia is replaced by collagen, is very rare.

Medial dysplasia is the most common, with three distinct subtypes recognized: medial fibroplasia, perimedial fibroplasia, and medial hyperplasia. Medial fibroplasia is the most common and accounts for up to 80% of cases.

The main histologic hallmark is disruption of smooth muscle cells, which are replaced by fibroblasts and collagen. There is frequently secondary disruption of the internal elastic lamina, which may lead to aneurysm formation. The alternating areas of medial disruption give rise to the commonly seen "string of beads" radiographic appearance, where areas of stenosis are admixed with dilated areas that are of larger caliber than the original vessel. Perimedial fibroplasia results from abnormal collagen deposition between the media and adventitia, leading to areas of stenosis with preserved internal elastic lamina. Radiographic appearance may be similar to medial fibroplasia, but the "beads" are of smaller diameter than the original vessel.

Although the etiology is unknown, FMD is associated with a variety of diseases including alpha-1 antitrypsin deficiency, Marfan syndrome, and Alport syndrome. Given the female preponderance, hormonal links have been posited, although evidence is lacking. Ischemia at the level of the vasa vasorum has been suggested as a possible underlying factor, although this remains unproven.

CLINICAL FEATURES

Cervicocranial FMD is frequently an incidental finding and rates of neurologic symptoms vary. Neurologic complications mainly arise due to ischemic or hemorrhagic symptoms that result from stenosis, thrombosis, dissection, or aneurysmal formation. Carotid–cavernous fistulas have also been described. Severe stenosis can cause distal hypoperfusion. Thrombotic occlusion of a stenotic vessel or distal embolism can lead to hemispheric ischemic symptoms. SAH can result from intracranial aneurysm rupture. Spontaneous cervical dissection can also occur, and headache, dizziness, carotidynia, pulsatile tinnitus, and Horner syndrome are all symptoms commonly seen with cervicocranial FMD. Dissection may be more common in Asian populations.

DIAGNOSIS

The gold standard for diagnosis remains catheter-based angiography. Noninvasive imaging modalities such as Doppler ultrasound and MRA may also detect FMD, but because lesions most commonly occur in the middle to distal carotid artery near C1–C2, adequate visualization with Doppler may be limited. Based on the underlying histology, a string of beads appearance due to medial fibroplasia is most commonly seen. Aneurysmal dilatation and areas of smooth tubular stenosis may also be present (Fig. 43.4). When cervicocranial disease is discovered, intracranial vessels should be imaged to evaluate for aneurysms and renal vessels for renovascular disease that may predispose to hypertension. The main differential diagnoses to consider are vasculitis and atherosclerotic disease.

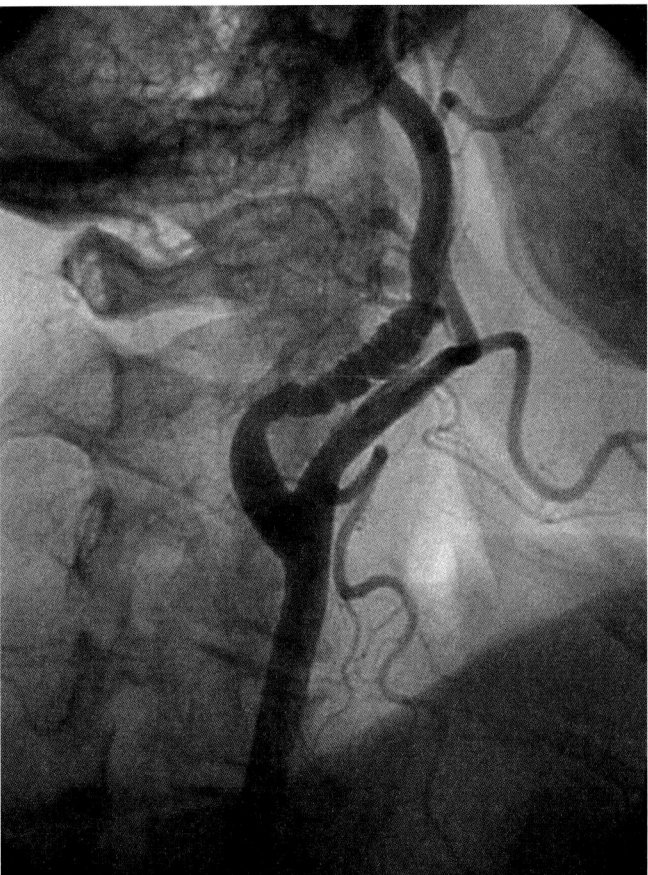

FIGURE 43.4 Angiogram of fibromuscular dysplasia in a 43-year-old female patient with multiple transient ischemic attacks. Note the multiple saccular dilatations of the internal carotid artery between the first and second cervical vertebrae.

TREATMENT

No trial data exist to guide treatment. Antiplatelet therapy is generally used when FMD is diagnosed to prevent thrombotic complications, although some practitioners institute therapy only when symptoms occur. In cases of dissection, a short course of anticoagulation is generally followed by long-term antiplatelet therapy in accordance with general practice. For patients with recurrent symptomatic ischemia refractory to medical treatment, percutaneous angioplasty is the treatment of choice, with stent placement reserved for those cases with concurrent dissection. Surgical intervention is reserved for rare, highly refractory cases. In addition to surgical dilatation, the two approaches generally used are resection with end-to-end anastomosis or carotid–middle cerebral artery (MCA) bypass. It should be emphasized that surgery is vanishingly rare in the era of percutaneous treatment. When intracranial aneurysms are present, treatment is based on size. Both endovascular coil embolization and microsurgical clipping via craniotomy are viable definitive treatment options.

OUTCOME

Although outcome data is limited to case series, in general, the course of cervicocranial FMD is fairly benign. Many patients who are asymptomatic at the time of diagnosis remain so at follow-up several years later. Angioplasty generally has excellent results in symptomatic patients, although true rates of recurrent ischemia are difficult to ascertain.

MOYAMOYA DISEASE

Moyamoya disease (MMD) is a chronic, progressive steno-occlusive arteriopathy of unclear etiology that affects the distal supraclinoid internal carotid artery (ICA) and/or proximal anterior and middle cerebral arteries. Chronic occlusive disease is believed to result in ischemia with subsequent neovascular proliferation of small, fragile, collateral vessels at the base of the brain. It is the hazy, fluffy angiographic appearance of this fine collateral network from which the name derives, as moyamoya means "puff of smoke" in Japanese. An essential distinction is between moyamoya disease and syndrome, where the latter refers to vessel stenosis and subsequent collateralization owing to a clearly identifiable underlying provoking condition. Commonly recognized causes of moyamoya syndrome include sickle cell disease, neurofibromatosis, advanced atherosclerosis, intracranial radiation, Down syndrome, autoimmune disease, and meningitis. The following discussion will focus on idiopathic MMD.

EPIDEMIOLOGY

Worldwide incidence and prevalence data is limited. MMD was initially described in Japan and incidence is generally felt to be highest in East Asia. Overall, worldwide incidence appears to be rising, although epidemiologic studies are limited by differences in data collection methods. Ascertainment bias due to increased disease awareness is also possible. Literature originating from East Asia reports incidence rates of 0.54 per 100,000 to 2.3 per 100,000 depending on the country, with higher rates reported in later reports and generally a higher female preponderance. There are far fewer North American and European epidemiologic studies. One that is oft quoted comes from Washington and California where the overall incidence was .086 per 100,000, again with a female majority. In terms of ethnicity-specific incidence, in this series, rates were highest in Asians and lowest in Hispanics. When patients with sickle cell disease were excluded, incidence rates in African-American and Caucasian patients were similar. General epidemiologic studies from Europe are lacking, although in a recently completed large case series from the Mayo clinic, there was significant predominance of moyamoya syndrome among women of European descent in their fourth decade of life with a significant prevalence of autoimmune diseases (notably Graves and Hashimoto disease and type 1 diabetes mellitus). A bimodal distribution of age of onset is generally demonstrated across studies, and although the average ages vary somewhat by country and study, the initial peak is generally in the first decade of life with the second in the fourth or fifth decade. Indeed, MMD is the most common cause of pediatric stroke in Asia. Clustering of MMD within families has been recognized, with rates as high as 15% in studies from Japan, consistent with an autosomal dominant trait with incomplete penetrance. Genetic heterogeneity is demonstrated by at least four documented linked loci; one site is located at 17q25.3 but no culprit gene has been identified.

PATHOBIOLOGY

The etiology of MMD remains unknown. Histopathologic studies have shown the stenotic vessels to have a severely thickened intima, primarily driven by smooth muscle proliferation, with luminal thrombosis and duplication and tortuosity of the internal elastic lamina frequently demonstrated on autopsy specimens. Signs of vascular inflammation are distinctly absent. Moyamoya vessels, the medium-sized dilated vessels originating from the distal ICA or proximal circle of Willis vessels, form complex networks, which anastomose with distal anterior cerebral artery (ACA) and/or MCA, with small, fragile, dilated vessels that penetrate the base of the brain. Pathologic evaluation has shown these dilated vessels to either have a very thin wall, prone to microaneurysm formation, or to be thick-walled with significant luminal stenosis and thrombosis.

Based on identification of a familial predisposition of 15% in Asia, recent genetic linkage studies identified the first susceptibility gene for MMD: RNF213 on chromosome 17, with the p.R4810K mutation demonstrating a high prevalence among East Asians. Although the exact etiologic role in MMD remains unknown, RNF213 is known to mediate vascular development in zebrafish, and its role in MMD is under active investigation. Interestingly, the p.R4810K mutation has not been found in European origin populations.

CLINICAL FEATURES

The main clinical manifestations relate to ischemia in the territory of the stenotic vessel, most often due to hemodynamic flow failure (rather than artery-to-artery embolus) or hemorrhage from the fragile neovascular lenticulostriate vessels that characterize the disease. Both intracerebral and subarachnoid hemorrhage can occur. Among adults, hemorrhage is more common in Asia than in North America and is infrequent in pediatric cases. When present intraparenchymally, hemorrhage is most often in the basal ganglia or thalamus with frequent intraventricular extension. This is presumably due to either rupture of microaneurysms or simply rupture of the fragile vessel wall in the setting of persistent hemodynamic stress. SAH is most commonly due to saccular aneurysm rupture at the circle of Willis frequently affecting the posterior circulation (most commonly the basilar bifurcation) because it is placed under increased stress given its role in providing collateral blood flow. Convexity SAH has also been observed in the setting of dilated pial collaterals, which are subsequently more prone to rupture.

Ischemia is the most common presentation in children and in adults in most studies. Ischemic symptoms are frequently hemispheric, with either a transient or fixed deficit depending on duration of ischemia, and are attributable to hemodynamic failure. Some patients may develop ischemic symptoms exclusively in deep hemispheric structures with relative sparing of cortical function. Cerebral infarction due to embolism or in situ thrombosis of a stenotic vessel is uncommon. In children, symptoms are frequently provoked by maneuvers that lead to hyperventilation and thus vasoconstriction, such as crying or inflating a balloon. Exercise-induced symptoms are another possible manifestation of chronic hemodynamic failure.

Other common manifestations of MMD include refractory migraine-like headache, thought to be due to dilation of meningeal and leptomeningeal vessels with subsequent activation of dural nociceptive receptors, as well as seizures. Some patients present primarily with cognitive or psychiatric symptoms from hypoperfusion, most commonly when bilateral frontal lobes are involved. Cognitive profiles of children with MMD reveal lower intelligence quotients independently of the incidence of stroke. Less common presentations include a choreiform movement disorder, particularly in children, resulting from the presence of dilated moyamoya vessels within the basal ganglia.

DIAGNOSIS

Diagnosis rests on angiographic demonstration of stenosis or occlusion of the bilateral supraclinoid ICAs and/or proximal ACA/MCAs with resulting proliferation of a small, fine network of collateral vessels originating just distal to the site of stenosis. The determination of MMD versus syndrome is incumbent upon exclusion of underlying conditions, which could predispose to the arterial narrowing. Recently, diagnostic guidelines have acknowledged that MRI and MRA can be used in lieu of conventional angiography if bilateral distal ICA stenoses on MRA are accompanied by abnormal vascular networks within the basal ganglia, frequently described as two or more flow voids (Fig. 43.5). In children, if the collateralization is present unilaterally but bilateral ICAs are stenotic, the condition is considered "definite" MMD, but when adults present with unilateral features, they are termed *probable moyamoya disease*. In some case series, up to 50% of patients will start with unilateral involvement, although in fact, many unilateral cases at 5 years of follow-up will demonstrate bilateral involvement. Posterior circulation involvement may be present in up to 10% of patients.

Disease severity on angiography is graded using the Suzuki classification, a scheme with six phases denoting increasing disease

TABLE 43.5	Suzuki Scale for Severity of Moyamoya Disease	
	Suzuki Stage	**Angiographic Description**
1	Narrowing of distal carotid	No other angiographic abnormalities aside from carotid narrowing
2	Initiation of the moyamoya	First signs of fine collateral networks become apparent
3	Intensification of the moyamoya	Collaterals become more pronounced, MCA and ACA may start to become obscured
4	Minimization of the moyamoya	First signs of external carotid artery (ECA) collaterals are apparent, moyamoya collaterals start to thin
5	Reduction of the moyamoya	Moyamoya collaterals further regress, carotid occlusion progresses proximally
6	Disappearance of the moyamoya	Only intracranial blood flow is via collaterals from the ECA; no angiographic evidence of distal carotid or moyamoya collaterals at the base of the brain

MCA, middle cerebral artery; ACA, anterior cerebral artery.

Adapted from Suzuki J, Takaku A. Cerebrovascular "moyamoya" disease. Disease showing abnormal net-like vessels in base of brain. *Arch Neurol.* 1969;20:288–299.

progression (Table 43.5). Level 1 denotes bilateral ICA stenosis in the absence of lenticulostriate collaterals and level 6 denotes complete carotid occlusion in which the distal internal carotid territory is exclusively supplied by the external carotid. Intermediate levels track the gradual progression and subsequent disappearance of lenticulostriate neovascularization as the disease progresses to complete internal artery occlusion. MMD can progress to any stage without further progression; only a minority of patients progress to stage 6.

In addition to angiographic severity, assessment of hemodynamic status may provide further insight into the clinical severity of MMD. One such method is via single-photon emission computed tomography (SPECT; see Chapter 22) or computed tomography perfusion (CTP; see Chapter 20) imaging, whereby the territory of decreased cerebral blood flow (CBF) can be imaged, measured consistent with a perfusion defect. CTP also allows assessment of vascular reserve by allowing evaluation of cerebral blood volume (CBV): As the severity of stenosis progresses, the distal arteries vasodilate, producing an increase in CBV. SPECT can also be used to assess vascular reserve by measuring changes in CBF before and after administration of acetazolamide, a carbonic anhydrase inhibitor that induces a transient metabolic acidosis in the brain, resulting in vasodilation. Failure to augment CBF in an area of reduced perfusion after acetazolamide implies that the distal vascular territory is already maximally dilated and hence at greater risk for progression to infarction. Transcranial Doppler ultrasonography (see Chapter 23) can also measure cerebrovascular reserve by comparing flow velocities before and after induced hypercapnia after inhalation of 5% carbon dioxide via face mask. Failure to augment CBF velocity by 5% implies a stake of maximal vasodilation and greater risk. Many centers will use degree of impaired vascular reserve to both risk stratify patients prior to surgery and to predict clinical improvement following intervention.

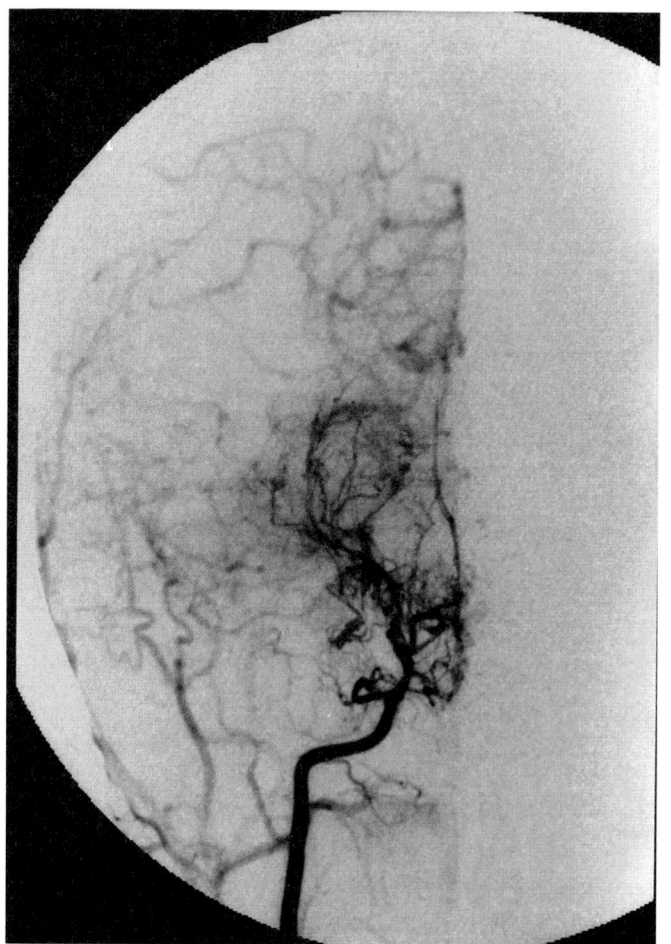

FIGURE 43.5 Internal carotid artery angiogram demonstrating moyamoya disease. (From Yomauchi T, Tada M, Houkin K, et al. Linkage of familial moyamoya disease [spontaneous occlusion of the circle of Willis] to chromosome 147q25. *Stroke.* 2000;31:930–935, with permission.)

An additional diagnostic finding of interest in children relates to characteristic EEG changes seen in MMD. Whereas in normal children, hyperventilation leads to high-amplitude slow waves which disappear once hyperventilation ceases (so-called buildup phenomenon); in children with MMD, these slow waves reappear, an occurrence termed *re-buildup*, which is thought to be due to posthyperventilation hypoxia and decreased CBF.

TREATMENT

Treatment revolves around various revascularization strategies that promote flow to distal territories, with the ultimate goal of reducing hemodynamic stroke and abnormal angiogenesis. Bypass surgery is generally recommended in patients who have had ischemic symptoms. Alternatively, both SPECT and transcranial Doppler have been used to stratify patients such that surgery is reserved for patients without stroke or transient ischemic attack (TIA) with evidence of hemodynamic failure and brain at risk. There are multiple revascularization strategies, generally divided into direct and indirect approaches. No randomized controlled trials have directly compared these techniques, with choice of method generally left to the discretion of the treating surgeon.

The direct approach is an anastomosis between the intracranial and extracranial circulation, which is most commonly achieved by connecting the superficial temporal artery (STA) to a branch of the MCA on the cortical surface. With this procedure, revascularization is immediate. Downsides include an increased risk of perioperative stroke or hemorrhage and the frequent occurrence (up to 25% in some studies) of the cerebral hyperperfusion syndrome, owing to the immediate revascularization in the setting of altered hemodynamics. The main symptoms of this syndrome include hemorrhage, seizures, and focal neurologic deficits from vasogenic cerebral edema.

There are two main indirect approaches: encephalomyosynangiosis (EMS) and encephaloduroarteriosynangiosis (EDAS). In the EMS procedure, a vascularized portion of the temporalis muscle is placed in direct apposition to the cortical surface, with dura closed around the muscle. In the EDAS procedure, a superficial artery, generally the STA, is placed on the cortical surface through a dural defect, sometimes with removal of intervening arachnoid (a modification termed *pial synangiosis*). Both of these techniques rely on the induced angiogenesis that naturally occurs between the underlying ischemic cortex and the apposed tissue or vessel. A third procedure is burr hole placement (with stripping of the underlying dura) in the vicinity of ischemic cortex, whereby scalp vessels grow through the burr holes to form collaterals with vessels on the cortical surface.

It is generally accepted that children achieve greater collateralization from indirect bypass than adults do, whereas direct bypass is more technically challenging in children given the smaller caliber of their vessels. An additional downside of indirect revascularization is that collateral formation may take weeks to months, a time during which repeat ischemic events may occur.

Less data exists on the prevention of hemorrhagic stroke among patients with MMD. The most exciting new development in the field of MMD is the completion of the Japanese Adult Moyamoya (JAM) trial, which offers the first prospective look at bypass as a means of reducing recurrent hemorrhage risk. This prospective randomized trial compared direct bypass to conservative management in a group of 80 patients with hemorrhage within 1 year prior to randomization. The recurrent hemorrhage rate was 11.9% in the surgical group compared with 31.6% in the conservative group (an annualized risk of 2.7% vs. 7.6% per year; $P = .04$)

[**Level 1**].[2] Further trials are needed to better define population subgroups who would most benefit from surgery to reduce ischemic symptoms.

Medical management of MMD has not been formally evaluated in clinical trials, although in case series, antiplatelet therapy may be effective at significantly reducing recurrent ischemic events, presumably by preventing microthrombus generation. Aspirin 81 to 325 mg daily is the most reasonable starting dose in MMD patients with no history of bleeding events. Anticoagulation is generally avoided given the attendant increased risk of hemorrhage on the setting of fragile vessels. When patients with MMD present acutely with ischemic symptoms, the focus of management should be on maintaining cerebral perfusion by avoiding hypotension and hyperventilation and ensuring adequate intravascular volume. There is insufficient evidence to guide whether MMD patients should be treated with recombinant tissue plasminogen activator within the treatment window because there is a theoretical increased risk of hemorrhage. Induced hypertension with phenylephrine starting at 20 µg/min, titrated to clinical effect, is a treatment option in the ICU for patients with a fluctuating neurologic deficit due to perfusion failure, but care should be taken to avoid surges in blood pressure that might provoke neovascular vessel bleeding.

OUTCOME

Data on the natural course of MMD in adults is not well known. Adults are generally felt to display less progression of proximal occlusion than children with lower recurrent stroke rates. Much of the data on progression in adults is from Japan, where a 5-year rate of progression of proximal stenosis as high as 20% has been shown in the affected vessel. Other studies have shown recurrent ipsilateral stroke rates over 5 years to be as high 65% in the absence of surgery. Female sex is generally the main identified risk factor for disease progression. Even in asymptomatic patients, disease activity is apparent, as seen from a Japanese study where 20% of asymptomatic patients had imaging evidence of infarction, whereas 40% had evidence of impaired cerebral hemodynamics. The annual rate of stroke in this asymptomatic population was 3.2%.

As stated previously, no randomized data exist to support one form of surgery over another for reducing ischemic symptoms; however, results from experienced centers have been overwhelmingly excellent in terms of decreasing recurrent ischemic stroke risk following revascularization in both children and adults. This type of data is subject to reporting bias, however. Low baseline degree of disability, a small extent of existing infarction, and the presence of collaterals are some of the factors that may predict good outcome after revascularization surgery.

BINSWANGER DISEASE

Binswanger disease (BD) refers to a progressive subcortical dementia with white matter degeneration of small-vessel etiology also known as *subcortical arteriosclerotic leukoencephalopathy*. It is not a well-defined disease entity, and in fact, the clinical picture in BD is similar to the subcortical dementia seen in other small-vessel angiopathies, for example, cerebral autosomal dominant arteriopathy with subcortical infarcts and leukoencephalopathy (CADASIL), which is discussed later in this chapter. In general, the term *Binswanger disease* is appropriately used when subcortical dementia is present in the setting of vascular risk factors with evidence of extensive deep and periventricular ischemic leukoencephalopathy on neuroimaging without an alternative explanatory cause.

EPIDEMIOLOGY

BD can be considered a subset of vascular dementia (VaD) (see Chapter 53). Given the extensive overlap between cerebrovascular disease and Alzheimer disease and other dementing pathologies, clinical diagnosis of "pure" VaD is fraught with challenges and prevalence estimates are highly variable. Estimating the true prevalence of BD within the context of VaD subtypes is therefore challenging. Although exact numbers are not known, BD in its classical form likely accounts for a minute portion of these "pure" VaD cases, as demonstrated by a 1987 literature review which found only 47 clinicopathologically confirmed BD cases over a period of 75 years.

PATHOBIOLOGY

The general pathologic picture is one of roughly symmetric degeneration of central white matter with myelin pallor and multiple lacunes. The term *incomplete white matter infarction* has been used to describe the pathology of BD. The degree of demyelination is heterogeneous with some areas demonstrating extensive demyelination and gliosis admixed with relatively normal-appearing white matter. Axonal loss is variable, there is no inflammatory cell infiltrate, and cortical atrophy is minimal, if not wholly absent. Although the arcuate fibers and anterior commissure are usually spared, central white matter from the periventricular region to the centrum semiovale, extending from frontal to occipital lobes, is involved to varying degrees. In addition to frequent lacunes, other hallmarks include dilated perivascular spaces, so-called état criblé, and moderately enlarged lateral and third ventricles. The vascular hallmarks are small, penetrating vessels with hyalinized, thickened walls with focal fibrinoid necrosis, notably without occlusion. Generally, there is some degree of atherosclerosis in large, proximal intracerebral arteries. Interestingly, perfusion studies have shown the areas of white matter hyperintensities to have lower CBF, suggesting chronic hypoperfusion and ischemic damage due to the small-vessel changes may be the pathophysiologic mechanism of the white matter degeneration.

CLINICAL FEATURES

The clinical manifestations of BD owe mainly to the disruption of white matter tracts interconnecting primary processing areas of the brain, theorized in particular to those specifically subserving the frontal cortices. Main signs include those that tend to localize to the frontal lobe, including slowed information processing, memory disturbances, and visuospatial deficits and executive dysfunction; the latter includes impaired initiation, planning, and goal-directed activity. Behavioral disturbances are frequent. Varying degrees of pyramidal and extrapyramidal dysfunction may be present in addition to pseudobulbar signs, parkinsonism, and gait abnormalities. Focal neurologic deficits may be present at the onset or during the disease course, owing to acute lacunar infarction.

DIAGNOSIS

No consensus guidelines exist for the diagnosis for BD. In general, the diagnosis is made when subcortical dementia is found in the presence of vascular risk factors, notably hypertension, with neuroimaging evidence of white matter disease. Other causes of leukoencephalopathy such as acute disseminated encephalomyelitis (ADEM) or progressive multifocal leukoencephalopathy must be absent. In general, patients with a known small-vessel arteriopathy and associated dementia, such as CADASIL, are not considered under the umbrella term of BD.

The white matter degeneration is best seen on MRI but is also present on CT where confluent, symmetric hypodense areas throughout the central white matter are apparent. On MRI, areas of white matter degeneration appear bright on T2 (white matter hyperintensities) and are best seen on FLAIR sequences where CSF is suppressed. The lesions are generally large and rather than being isolated to the immediate periventricular region, extend throughout the corona radiata and centrum semiovale. Scattered lacunes are frequently seen, both throughout the white and deep gray matter.

TREATMENT

Given most patients with BD have evidence of lacunar infarcts, treatment is directed at secondary stroke prevention, that is, modification of vascular risk factors and introduction of antiplatelets and statins. Control of hypertension is essential, in addition to aggressive diabetes management and smoking cessation. There is no evidence that hypertension control leads to reversal of white matter changes. Supportive care for patients with severe cognitive impairment is often necessary.

OUTCOME

In one series of clinicopathologically confirmed cases, clinical course took one of three patterns: gradual progression punctuated by acute focal deficits, gradual worsening not punctuated by acute focal deficits, and multiple acute focal deficits without progression.

SUSAC SYNDROME

Susac syndrome comprises a triad of encephalopathy, branch retinal artery occlusion (BRAO), and hearing loss. It is thought to be an autoimmune microangiopathic endotheliopathy that affects brain, retina, and cochlea. The disease, which was first described in 1977 by John O. Susac after he encountered two young women with personality changes, including paranoia and hostile behavior, hearing loss, and visual disturbances, is also termed *retinocochleocerebral vasculopathy* and is frequently misdiagnosed as multiple sclerosis (MS) or ADEM.

EPIDEMIOLOGY

Susac syndrome typically begins in the third or fourth decade but may occur during childhood or after age 70 years. There is 3:1 female predominance but no racial predilection. The true incidence and prevalence of the disease are unknown. About 100 cases have been reported but diagnostic confusion abounds and the condition is likely underdiagnosed.

PATHOBIOLOGY

Susac syndrome is thought to be an immune-mediated endotheliopathy of unknown etiology. Antiendothelial cell antibodies either play a pathogenic role or arise from endothelial damage caused by other immune mechanisms. Histopathologic examination of brain biopsy samples usually reveals microinfarcts in the cerebral cortex and white matter. Areas of demyelination along with axonal and neuronal damage are also seen. Pauci-inflammatory endothelial cell injury in small arterioles, capillaries, and venules is observed.

Muscle biopsy in patients with Susac syndrome shows abnormal endothelial cells, some swollen to the point of occluding small arterioles. Muscle inflammation is subclinical, unlike dermatomyositis,

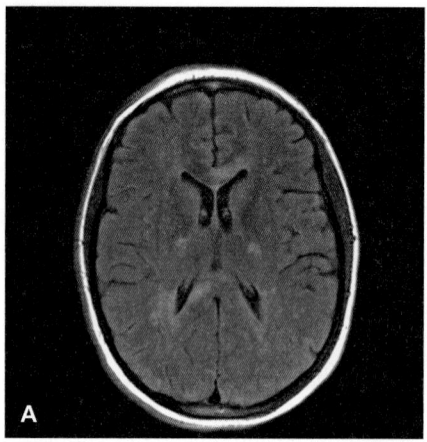
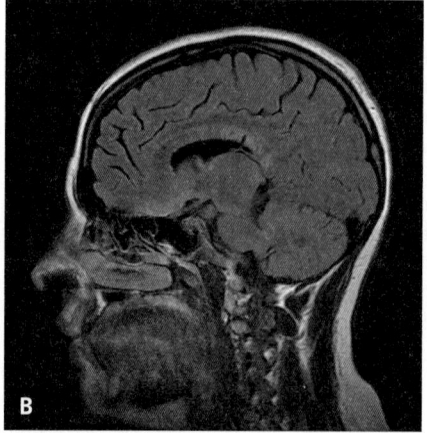
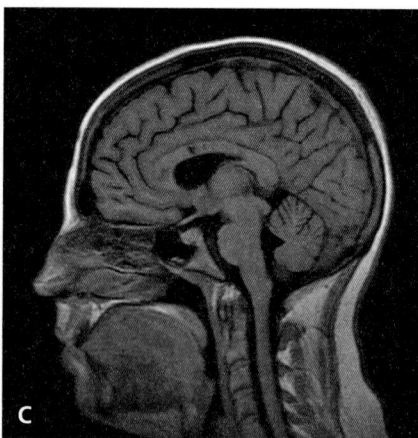

FIGURE 43.6 Susac syndrome findings on MRI. Axial FLAIR image **(A)** shows nonspecific lesions in the cerebral hemispheres. Sagittal FLAIR **(B)** and T1-weighted **(C)** images show the characteristic central "snowball lesions" and "punched out holes," respectively.

although the pathology is virtually identical, including endothelial cell degeneration and necrosis, as well as thickening, reduplication, and lamellation of the basement membrane.

CLINICAL FEATURES

Encephalopathy may be manifested by psychiatric symptoms, confusion, memory loss, or simply dulling of cognitive function. BRAO, which may occur before, during, or after the encephalopathy, may cause a scotoma or photopsia. Migrainous headaches often precede other symptoms, and the association with visual symptoms may be misleading. Hearing loss may be difficult to assess, depending on the degree of encephalopathy. It frequently affects the lower tones first, which implies microinfarction of the cochlear apex, a particularly vulnerable territory. The speed and severity of hearing loss varies from profound and precipitous, with loss of hearing in one ear and the other days to weeks thereafter, to slow and insidious or fluctuating as in Ménière disease. Hearing loss may be accompanied by nausea, vertigo, tinnitus, or gait ataxia.

DIAGNOSIS

Diagnosis requires a high index of suspicion because it is uncommon for the entire clinical triad to be present at the time of the first encounter with a physician. Furthermore, encephalopathic patients may not complain of hearing loss or visual problems. Brain

MRI, dilated funduscopic examination, and retinal fluorescein angiography are the most useful diagnostic tests.

Brain MRI reveals multiple small (typically 1 to 7 mm) white matter lesions in the cerebral hemispheres. The corpus callosum is involved in 88% to 100% of patients (Fig. 43.6). The callosal lesions that occur with acute encephalopathy are centrally located and have a "snowball" appearance. Basal ganglia, thalamic, brain stem, cerebellar, and gadolinium-enhancing lesions are common. Leptomeningeal enhancement is occasionally observed. Arteriography is typically normal because the affected arterioles are too small to be seen in angiography.

Although the MRI findings may lead to an incorrect diagnosis of MS or ADEM, the morphology and central location of the acute callosal lesions and their evolution into hypointense holes on T1-weighted imaging are characteristic findings in Susac syndrome and atypical of MS lesions, which are smaller and involve the callosal–septal interface.

Dilated funduscopic examination and retinal fluorescein angiography may reveal retinal infarcts and BRAO (Fig. 43.7). Audiometry may detect sensorineural hearing loss. Examination of the CSF during the acute encephalopathy typically reveals a mild lymphocytic pleocytosis. The protein content is often more than 100 mg/dL, an uncommon finding in MS. However, the occasional presence of oligoclonal bands or an elevated immunoglobulin G index may lead to further diagnostic confusion.

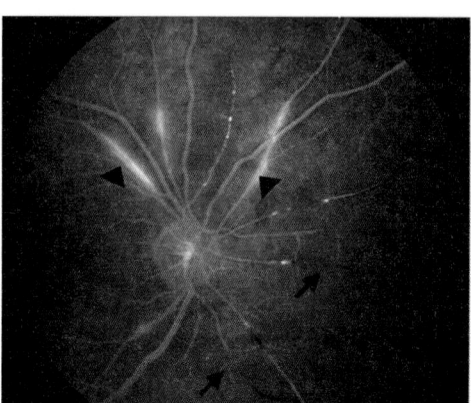
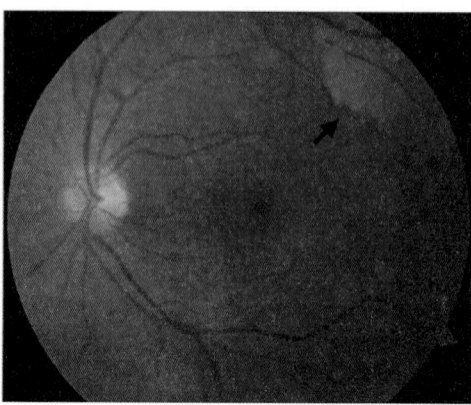

FIGURE 43.7 Left: Retinal abnormalities in Susac syndrome demonstrating hyperfluorescence of the arteriolar walls (*arrowheads*). **Right:** Retinography of the left eye shows retinal infarct (*arrow*). (Images courtesy of Zachary Grinspan, MD.)

TREATMENT

There have been no controlled therapeutic trials in Susac syndrome, but many different approaches have been explored. Treatment recommendations are largely based on anecdotes. Although the disease often enters spontaneous remission, treatment is recommended to try to prevent irreversible disability.

Prednisone monotherapy, pulses of methylprednisolone, or a combination of corticosteroids and IV immunoglobulin appears to be beneficial in some patients. More severe cases may respond to *cyclophosphamide* or *mycophenolate* mofetil. Plasma exchange has been used in refractory cases. The use of *rituximab* in dermatomyositis, a humorally mediated autoimmune vasculopathy that shares immunopathogenic features with Susac syndrome, has raised interest in B-cell depletion as a treatment strategy for Susac syndrome. Low-dose aspirin therapy is often added in attempt to forestall microinfarcts. Although aggressive treatment is often indicated, the disease is often self-limited and may remit spontaneously after several years, so tapering of immunotherapy should be attempted judiciously.

OUTCOME

Three major clinical courses have been described: monocyclic, polycyclic, and chronic continuous. Most patients with symptomatic encephalopathy follow a monocyclic course in which the disease remits spontaneously after 1 to 2 years and does not return. The polycyclic course includes variable periods of remission separating disease activity and may persist for many years. The chronic continuous syndrome shows variations in severity of symptoms but no clear remissions, even though a slow remission may eventually occur. Case reviews suggest that those with prominent encephalopathy are more likely to have a monocyclic course, whereas those with BRAO and hearing loss may be more likely to develop prolonged polycyclic disease.

The disease usually lasts 2 to 4 years with the chronic continuous course being the least common form of the illness. Although 50% of patients are able to lead a basically normal life, most are left with varying degrees of bilateral hearing loss, and 35% to 50% have residual cognitive dysfunction, which prevents some from returning to work. Asymptomatic visual field defects are much more common than symptomatic visual loss. Treatment with immunosuppressive chemotherapy may result in infertility.

SNEDDON SYNDROME

The association between livedo reticularis, a lacy erythematous or purplish rash on the anterior legs, and ischemic stroke was first described in 1965 by Dr. Ian Sneddon, a British dermatologist, and has subsequently been termed *Sneddon syndrome*. The exact underlying pathophysiology remains unknown and whether this entity is distinct from, or lies on a spectrum with, the antiphospholipid antibody syndrome remains to be clarified.

EPIDEMIOLOGY

Two forms of Sneddon syndrome (SS) are generally recognized: those associated with the presence of antiphospholipid antibodies and those that are not, so-called seronegative cases. This is a rare disease, with the overall annual incidence estimated at 4 per million and with women predominantly affected. In general, first clinical stroke is evident by the mid-40s.

PATHOBIOLOGY

Livedo reticularis (LR) is a dermatologic condition that refers to the lacy, mesh-like appearance of blood within the cutaneous venous system. Two general forms are recognized: "physiologic" LR or cutis marmorata, which occurs in the setting of cold temperatures and disappears when the affected limb is warmed, and "secondary" LR due to an underlying condition. Many disease states are associated with secondary LR, where either venous stasis or significant deoxygenation of blood within the cutaneous venous plexus gives the stereotypical appearance. In SS, it is subcutaneous arteriolar occlusion leading to decreased oxygenation of venous blood that causes LR, generally present over a large area. The trunk and limbs are usually involved, with the violaceous rings appearing irregular and broken.

Pathologic series of skin biopsy specimens of seronegative SS patients have shown that it is the small- to medium-sized arteries at the dermis–subcutaneous border that are affected. These vessels undergo four stages of involvement. Initially, there is endothelial disruption and lymphocyte infiltration, which is followed by partial vascular occlusion by stimulated monocytes that trap erythrocytes and fibrin, associated with a perivascular lymphohistiocytic infiltrate. Later stages are characterized by reorganization of this plug associated with subendothelial proliferation of smooth muscle cells and resolution of the perivascular infiltrate. The final stage is characterized by proliferation of fibroblasts and collagen, where completely occluded, shrunken vessels are apparent without inflammatory infiltrate. Following the discovery of an initial so-called endotheliitis stage, the presence of antiendothelial antibodies has been found in SS patients with one series showing up to 35% of patients harboring these antibodies. Whether they play a pathophysiologic role remains uncertain.

Unlike skin vessels, pathologic studies of cerebral vessels are limited. Stroke in SS patients most commonly affects the cortex and subcortical white matter, with some series showing frequent small, multifocal ischemic lesions within the deep white matter, a nonspecific finding that is seen in many disorders affecting small arteries including hypertension.

DIAGNOSIS

Diagnosis is made by the presence of skin biopsy–confirmed LR with the aforementioned pathologic features in the presence of focal neurologic deficit and imaging-confirmed cerebral infarction. Other conditions associated with LR should be ruled out to make the diagnosis of SS, for example, systemic lupus erythematosus and polyarteritis nodosa. The presence of antiphospholipid antibodies is not essential for the diagnosis, as up to 60% of cases are considered seronegative.

CLINICAL MANIFESTATIONS

In general, the first manifestations of SS are frequently nonspecific neurologic symptoms such as dizziness and headache. These are followed by LR, which in turn is followed by stroke. On average, symptoms evolve over 9 years. Patients seronegative for antiphospholipid antibodies generally have a wider area of LR and are less likely to have seizures compared to patients with antiphospholipid antibodies. Seropositive patients are more likely to have thrombocytopenia, in keeping with coexistent systemic lupus erythematosus and other autoimmune disease. SS is rare enough, however, that studies showing differences between seronegative and positive patients are inconsistent.

Multiple MRI patterns in patients with SS have been described. Some studies describe prominent infarcts affecting cortical–subcortical region, whereas others find FLAIR lesions in the deep periventricular white matter, suggesting small-vessel infarct. Scattered punctate subcortical T2 hyperintensities are also commonly seen in addition to confluent areas of mild FLAIR hyperintensity within central white matter. Although the majority of lesions are supratentorial, infratentorial lesions in cerebellar and medullary white matter occasionally are present. Basal ganglia lesions are notably infrequent.

Some studies have also shown an increased incidence of hypertension and cardiac valvular abnormalities (thickening and calcification) in SS patients in keeping with comorbid autoimmune disease, but this is not consistently observed across case series.

TREATMENT

No randomized trials on treatment in SS exist. In general, seronegative patients are generally treated with antiplatelets agents such as aspirin 325 mg daily, whereas seropositive patients are anticoagulated with warfarin (5 mg daily titrated to maintain the international normalized ratio between 2.0 and 3.0), along current antiphospholipid syndrome guidelines. Immunosuppressive regimens may be used for coexistent autoimmune disease.

OUTCOME

Given its low incidence, large longitudinal studies are lacking, which make accurate predictions about outcome challenging. In one study, only one patient became functionally impaired as a consequence of neurologic disease burden, whereas in another, up to 50% of patients had some degree of disability. Some studies have shown a correlation between disability and MRI lesion burden, whereas others have not. In general, individual infarcts in SS tend to be small and thus associated with a low degree of disability.

MARANTIC ENDOCARDITIS

Nonbacterial thrombotic endocarditis (NBTE) refers to sterile valvular vegetations made up of fibrin and platelets, which are found in association with many underlying conditions. Perhaps the most prominent association is with malignancy, where NBTE is termed *marantic* (or "wasted") *endocarditis*, and systemic lupus erythematosus (SLE), where the verrucous vegetations are termed *Libman–Sacks endocarditis* (LSE). NBTE can also be found in primary antiphospholipid syndrome (APS) and is increasingly recognized in a host of other systemic illnesses including sepsis, advanced AIDS, cirrhosis, and extensive burns. It has been hypothesized that hypercoagulability is a common link.

EPIDEMIOLOGY

The most common underlying tumors include mucin-producing adenocarcinomas of the colon, pancreas, ovary, and lung in addition to hematologic malignancies. Autopsy studies have put the incidence of NBTE in the general population at 1% with studies of SLE patients showing rates upwards of 30% and as high as 19% among cancer patients, although other series indicate lower rates among cancer patients. Specific features of SLE that predispose to LSE have not been consistent with some studies showing an increased risk in the presence of antiphospholipid antibodies, whereas others have not confirmed this association.

PATHOBIOLOGY

Despite the underlying cause, the pathology is generally the same: superficial bland vegetations affixed to a valve with preserved underlying architecture. The vegetations generally consist of a fibrin core with aggregated platelets, without any demonstrable evidence of infectious organisms or inflammatory reaction. Vegetations are generally found on left-sided valves, with the mitral valve most commonly affected. Vegetations have a predilection for the atrial side of the mitral valve and ventricular side of the aortic valve and are generally at the contact margins of the valve leaflets, perhaps due to the highest turbulence of blood at these locations with resulting microtrauma to the underlying valve. An underlying immune-mediated destructive process has also been hypothesized in addition to an underlying hypercoagulable state. NBTE vegetations span a range of sizes, from submillimeter to over 1 cm, with the lesions generally consisting of single or multiple mobile verrucae. It is thought that the lack of inflammatory reaction and attendant cellular organization makes these lesions particularly friable.

Although the underlying valve architecture is generally preserved in NBTE, one large echocardiographic study did find that a majority of patients had some degree of valvular dysfunction, most commonly regurgitation. Mitral and aortic valves were also diffusely thickened, demonstrating frequent calcification of the mitral valve annulus and chordae.

CLINICAL MANIFESTATIONS

Although NBTE rarely causes hemodynamically significant valvular dysfunction, the consequence of importance is systemic embolism, of which stroke is the most clinically apparent. In fact, it has been estimated that up to one-third of patients with NBTE have evidence of thromboembolic ischemic stroke, with rates as high as 55% noted in autopsy studies of cancer patients and between 10% and 20% in patients with SLE. One study on the brain MRI findings of NBTE patients (all with underlying adenocarcinoma) found that all cases showed evidence of numerous small- and medium-sized (1 to 3 cm) ischemic lesions in multiple vascular territories. This was in contrast to infective endocarditis patients, where diverse diffusion-weighted imaging (DWI) findings (single lesion, multiple lesions within one vascular territory, multiple punctate disseminated lesions) were seen in addition to hemorrhage. No reliable differences in presenting neurologic symptoms have been demonstrated between NBTE and infective endocarditis patients, with both focal deficits and diffuse encephalopathy described.

DIAGNOSIS

Because the lesions are generally smaller and not associated with underlying valvular dysfunction, cardiac murmurs are infrequent. Identifying NBTE is often more difficult than infective endocarditis and requires a high index of clinical suspicion, such as multiple infarcts in the setting of systemic malignancy or autoimmune disease in the absence of other explanations. Transesophageal echocardiography (TEE) is often needed, as the small size makes transthoracic echocardiography (TTE) evaluation insensitive. Indeed, one series demonstrated over twice the diagnostic yield of TEE compared with TTE in cancer patients with NBTE. Diagnosis rests on excluding an underlying infection, thus serial blood cultures in addition to a thorough systemic infectious evaluation is necessary. The distinction from culture-negative infective endocarditis may be particularly challenging because patients with malignancy and autoimmune disease often present with fever. In general, it is reasonable to consider NBTE in cryptogenic stroke patients with embolic-appearing infarcts when there is a concern for an underlying malignancy or rheumatologic disease.

TREATMENT

Although no trial data exists on treatment for NBTE, anticoagulation is generally recommended in those with marantic endocarditis and evidence of thromboembolic stroke. Heparinoids are preferred to warfarin given the superiority of the former in preventing venous thromboembolism in cancer patients. When NBTE is identified in patients with primary or secondary APS with evidence of stroke, anticoagulation with warfarin is generally recommended per APS treatment guidelines. The case of SLE with LSE is less clear, and in general, antiplatelet agents are recommended if there is no evidence of thromboembolism, with anticoagulation considered if strokes occur. No data exists on improvement in LSE lesions with immunologic therapy.

An additional concern is the potential for NBTE lesions to get secondarily infected; thus, antibiotic prophylaxis may be warranted in certain situations, for example, prior to high-risk dental procedures or surgery. Although rare, in severe cases with multiple strokes refractory to anticoagulation, surgical mitral valve replacement has been used.

OUTCOME

The outcome of NBTE generally depends on the underlying disease process. Echocardiography-based studies of patients with LSE have shown that during follow-up between 1 and 5 years, vegetations persisted, regressed, or appeared, making the course highly unpredictable. In marantic endocarditis, prognosis often depends on the underlying malignancy, with anticoagulation somewhat effective in preventing recurrent stroke although refractory cases have been reported.

CEREBRAL AUTOSOMAL DOMINANT ARTERIOPATHY WITH SUBCORTICAL INFARCTS AND LEUKOENCEPHALOPATHY (CADASIL)

CADASIL is one of the few single-gene disorders that causes stroke as a major manifestation. Patients present with multiple subcortical infarcts, progressive dementia and gait disorder, migraine headaches with aura, and psychiatric manifestations such as depression and psychosis. Common stroke risk factors, such as hypertension and diabetes mellitus, are conspicuously absent. The median age of the first stroke is 50 years, although the strokes may occur as early as 19 years of age. MRI findings include a widespread leukoencephalopathy, and the findings are virtually pathognomonic when involvement of the anterior temporal lobes and extreme capsule is seen. A phenotypic variant of CADASIL has been identified by familial clustering of hemiplegic migraine and labeled CADASILM ("M" for migraine.)

CADASIL is a protein elimination failure angiopathy, similar to amyloid angiopathy (see Chapter 38). The genetic defect is a mutation on chromosome 19p, in the *NOTCH3* gene, a highly conserved gene regulating development. The protein is a transmembrane receptor involved in intercellular communication, and it is found on vascular smooth muscle cells. Diagnosis is made by genetic testing, which can detect 70% of the clustering mutations causing the disease, or skin biopsy, in which the presence of granular osmiophilic material (GOM) between smooth muscle cells and the basement membrane or immunostaining for the NOTCH3 protein is seen. The mechanism by which the smooth muscle cell pathology leads to vasculopathy and stroke remains uncertain, but

it does not appear to be a thrombotic disorder. Apart from antiplatelet therapy with aspirin, clopidogrel, or a similar agent, there is no known treatment. The mean survival time is 20 years from onset of symptoms.

LEVEL 1 EVIDENCE

1. Altman D, Carroli G, Duley L, et al; Magpie Trial Collaborative Group. Do women with pre-eclampsia, and their babies, benefit from magnesium sulfate? The Magpie Trial: a randomised placebo-controlled trial. *Lancet.* 2002;359:1877–1890.
2. Miyamoto S, Yoshimoto T, Hashimoto N, et al. Effects of extracranial–intracranial bypass for patients with hemorrhagic moyamoya disease results of the Japan Adult Moyamoya Trial. *Stroke.* 2014;45(5):1415–1421.

SUGGESTED READINGS

Posterior Reversible Encephalopathy Syndrome
Bartynski WS, Boardman JF, Zeigler ZR, et al. Posterior reversible encephalopathy syndrome in infection, sepsis, and shock. *Am J Neuroradiol.* 2006;27(10): 2179–2190.
Casey SO, Sampaio RC, Michel E, et al. Posterior reversible encephalopathy syndrome: utility of fluid-attenuated inversion recovery MR imaging in the detection of cortical and subcortical lesions. *Am J Neuroradiol.* 2000;21(7):1199–1206.
Fugate JE, Claassen DO, Cloft HJ, et al. Posterior reversible encephalopathy syndrome: associated clinical and radiologic findings. *Mayo Clin Proc.* 2010;85(5): 427–432.
Hinchey J, Chaves C, Appignani B, et al. A reversible posterior leukoencephalopathy syndrome. *N Engl J Med.* 1996;334(8):494–500.
Staykov D, Schwab S. Posterior reversible encephalopathy syndrome. *J Intensive Care Med.* 2012;27(1):11–24.

Reversible Cerebral Vasoconstriction Syndrome
Calabrese LH, Dodick DW, Schwedt TJ, et al. Narrative review: reversible cerebral vasoconstriction syndromes. *Ann Intern Med.* 2007;146:34–44.
Chen SP, Fuh JL, Chang FC, et al. Transcranial color Doppler study for reversible cerebral vasoconstriction syndromes. *Ann Neurol.* 2008;63(6):751–757.
Chen SP, Fuh JL, Wang SJ, et al. Magnetic resonance angiography in reversible cerebral vasoconstriction syndromes. *Ann Neurol.* 2010;67(5):648–656.
Ducros A, Boukobza M, Porcher R, et al. The clinical and radiological spectrum of reversible cerebral vasoconstriction syndrome. A prospective series of 67 patients. *Brain.* 2007;130:3091–3101.

Fibromuscular Dysplasia
Corrin LS, Sandok BA, Houser OW. Cerebral ischemic events in patients with carotid artery fibromuscular dysplasia. *Arch Neurol.* 1981;38(10):616–618.
Mettinger KL. Fibromuscular dysplasia and the brain. II. Current concept of the disease. *Stroke.* 1982;13:53–58.
Olin JW, Gornick HL, Bacharach JM. Fibromuscular dysplasia: state of the science and critical unanswered questions. *Circulation.* 2014;129:1048–1078.
Schievink WI, Bjornsson J. Fibromuscular dysplasia of the internal carotid artery: a clinicopathological study. *Clin Neuropathol.* 1996;15:2–6.
Slovut DP, Olin JW. Fibromuscular dysplasia. *Curr Treat Options Cardiovasc Med.* 2005;7:159–169.
Slovut DP, Olin JW. Fibromuscular dysplasia. *N Engl J Med.* 2004;350(18): 1862–1871.

Moyamoya Disease
Ahn IM, Park D, Hann HJ. Incidence, prevalence and survival in moyamoya disease in Korea. *Stroke.* 2014;45:1090–1095.
Fukui M. Guidelines for the diagnosis and treatment of spontaneous occlusion of the circle of Willis ("moyamoya" disease). Research Committee on Spontaneous Occlusion of the Circle of Willis (Moyamoya Disease) of the Ministry of Health and Welfare, Japan. *Clin Neurol Neurosurg.* 1997;99:S238.

Kim S, Cho B, Phi JH, et al. Pediatric moyamoya disease: an analysis of 410 consecutive cases. *Ann Neurol.* 2010;68:92–101.

Kleinloog R, Regli L, Rinkel GJE, et al. Regional differences in incidence and patient characteristics of moyamoya disease: a systematic review. *J Neurol Neurosurg Psychiatry.* 2012;83:531–536.

Kuroda S, Hashimoto N, Yoshimoto T, et al. Radiological findings, clinical course, and outcome in asymptomatic moyamoya disease: results of multicenter survey in Japan. *Stroke.* 2007;38(5):1430–1435.

Kuroda S, Houkin K. Moyamoya disease: current concepts and future perspectives. *Lancet Neurol.* 2008;7:1056–1066.

Liu W, Morito D, Takashima S, et al. Identification of RNF213 as a susceptibility gene for moyamoya disease and its possible role in vascular development. *PLoS One.* 2011;6:e22542.

Miyamoto S, Yoshimoto T, Hashimoto N, et al. Effects of extracranial-intracranial bypass for patients with hemorrhagic moyamoya disease: results of the Japan adult moyamoya trial. *Stroke.* 2014;45:1415–1421.

Scott MR, Smith ER. Moyamoya disease and moyamoya syndrome. *N Engl J Med.* 2009;360:1226–1237.

Starke RM, Komotar RJ, Connolly ES. Optimal surgical treatment for moyamoya disease in adults: direct versus indirect bypass. *Neurosurg Focus.* 2009;26:E9.

Suzuki J, Takaku A. Cerebrovascular "moyamoya" disease. *Arch Neurol.* 1969; 20:288–299.

Binswanger Disease

Babikian V, Ropper AH. Binswanger's disease: a review. *Stroke.* 1987;18:2–12.

Caplan LR, Gomes JA. Binswanger disease—an update. *J Neurol Sci.* 2010;299 (1–2):9–10.

Farkas E, de Vos RA, Donka G, et al. Age-related microvascular degeneration in the human cerebral periventricular white matter. *Acta Neuropathol.* 2006; 111:150–157.

Fisher CM. Binswanger's encephalopathy: a review. *J Neurol.* 1989;236:65–79.

Fitzpatrick AL, Kuller LH, Lopez OL, et al. Survival following dementia onset: Alzheimer's disease and vascular dementia. *J Neurol Sci.* 2005;(229–230): 43–49.

Jellinger KA. Pathology and pathogenesis of vascular cognitive impairment—a critical update. *Front Aging Neurosci.* 2013;5(17):1–19.

Susac Syndrome

Aubart-Cohen F, Klein I, Alexandra JF, et al. Long-term outcome in Susac syndrome. *Medicine.* 2007;86:93–102.

García-Carrasco M, Mendoza-Pinto C, Cervera R. Diagnosis and classification of Susac syndrome. *Autoimmun Rev.* 2014;13(4):347–350.

Magro CM, Poe JC, Lubow M, et al. Susac syndrome an organ-specific autoimmune endotheliopathy syndrome associated with anti–endothelial cell antibodies. *Am J Clin Pathol.* 2011;136(6):903–912.

Martinet N, Fardeau C, Adam R, et al. Fluorescein and indocyanine green angiographies in Susac syndrome. *Retina.* 2007;27(9):1238–1242.

Mateen FJ, Zubkov AY, Muralidharan R, et al. Susac syndrome: clinical characteristics and treatment in 29 new cases. *Eur J Neurol.* 2012;19(6):800–811.

Rennebohm RM, Susac JO. Treatment of Susac's syndrome. *J Neurol Sci.* 2007; 257:215–220.

Susac JO, Hardman JM, Selhorst JB. Microangiopathy of the brain and retina. *Neurology.* 1979;29:313–316.

Susac JO, Murtagh FR, Egan RA, et al. MRI findings in Susac's syndrome. *Neurology.* 2003;61:1783–1787.

Sneddon Syndrome

Boesch SM, Plorer AL, Auer AJ, et al. The natural course of Sneddon syndrome: clinical and magnetic resonance imaging findings in a prospective six-year observation study. *J Neurol Neurosurg Psychiatry.* 2003;74:542–544.

Francès C, Le Tonquèze M, Salohzin KV, et al. Prevalence of anti-endothelial cell antibodies in patients with Sneddon's syndrome. *J Am Acad Dermatol.* 1995;33(1):64–68.

Francès C, Piette JC. The mystery of Sneddon syndrome: relationship with antiphospholipid syndrome and systemic lupus erythematosus. *J Autoimmun.* 2000;15(2):139–143.

Sneddon IB. Cerebro-vascular lesions and livedo reticularis. *Br J Dermatol.* 1965;77(4):180.

Wohlrab J, Frances C, Sullivan KE. Strange symptoms in Sneddon's syndrome. *Clin Immunol.* 2006;119:13–15.

Marantic Endocarditis

Dutta T, Karas MG, Segal AZ, et al. Yield of transesophageal echocardiography for nonbacterial thrombotic endocarditis and other cardiac sources of embolism in cancer patients with cerebral ischemia. *Am J Cardiol.* 2006;97 (6):894–898.

Greaves M, Cohen H, Machin SJ, et al. Guidelines on the investigation and management of the antiphospholipid syndrome. *Br J Haematol.* 2000;109(4): 704–715.

Katsouli A, Massad MG. Current issues in the diagnosis and management of blood culture-negative infective and non-infective endocarditis. *Ann Thorac Surg.* 2013;95(4):1467–1474.

Lee A, Levine MN, Baker RI. Low-molecular-weight heparin versus a coumarin for the prevention of recurrent thromboembolism in patients with cancer. *New Engl J Med.* 2003;349:146–153.

Moustafa S, Patton DJ, Balon Y, et al. Mitral valve surgery for marantic endocarditis and multiple cerebral embolisation. *Heart Lung Circ.* 2013;7(22): 545–547.

Reisner SA, Brenner B, Haim N, et al. Echocardiography in nonbacterial thrombotic endocarditis: from autopsy to clinical entity. *J Am Soc Echocardiogr.* 2000;13:876–881.

Roldan CA, Shively BK, Crawford MH. An echocardiographic study of valvular heart disease associated with systemic lupus erythematosus. *N Engl J Med.* 1996;335:1424–1430.

Singhal AB, Topcuoglu MA, Buonanno FS. Acute ischemic stroke patterns in infective and nonbacterial thrombotic endocarditis: a diffusion-weighted magnetic resonance imaging study. *Stroke.* 2002;33:1267–1273.

CADASIL

Carare RO, Hawkes CA, Jeffrey M, et al. Review: cerebral amyloid angiopathy, prion angiopathy, CADASIL and the spectrum of protein elimination failure angiopathies (PEFA) in neurodegenerative disease with a focus on therapy. *Neuropathol Appl Neurobiol.* 2013;39(6):593–611.

Ciolli LF, Pescini E, Salvadori A, et al. Influence of vascular risk factors and neuropsychological profile on functional performances in CADASIL: results from the MIcrovascular LEukoencephalopathy Study (MILES). *Eur J Neurol.* 2014;21(1):65–71.

Joutel A. Pathogenesis of CADASIL. *Bioessays.* 2011;33(1):73–80.

Pescini F, Nannucci S, Bertaccini B, et al. The Cerebral Autosomal-Dominant Arteriopathy With Subcortical Infarcts and Leukoencephalopathy (CADASIL) scale: a screening tool to select patients for NOTCH3 gene analysis. *Stroke.* 2012;43(11):2871–2876.

Primary and Secondary Stroke Prevention

44

Charles C. Esenwa and Mitchell S. V. Elkind

INTRODUCTION

Prevention of stroke can be divided into three types: (1) primordial prevention, which focuses on improving community-wide health behaviors, such as diet, exercise, and smoking; (2) primary prevention, which attempts to mitigate an individual's stroke risk factors; and (3) secondary prevention, which targets risk of stroke recurrence in those who have already suffered a stroke or transient ischemic attack (TIA).

Risk factors are generally classified as either nonmodifiable or modifiable. Nonmodifiable risk factors, although they cannot be altered, remain important in quantifying a patient's future risk of stroke. Examples include age, sex, family history, ethnicity, and race. Modifiable risk factors allow for intervention to decrease future risk of stroke.

Although primordial prevention deals with population-level risk of cardiovascular disease, individualized prevention measures require a careful history and tailored diagnostic evaluation to stratify stroke risk and guide the appropriate prevention strategy. Primary and secondary prevention methods both focus on improving the individual's risk factor profile, and secondary prevention methods further depend on the mechanism of the stroke. For ischemic stroke, these mechanisms include atherothrombotic, small vessel (or "lacunar"), cardioembolic, and cryptogenic; the last is responsible for up to 40% of strokes. Several randomized controlled trials have been conducted over the past four decades that have determined optimal therapy for stroke prevention and treatment, especially for atherothrombotic and cardioembolic stroke subtypes.

Hemorrhagic strokes account for 15% to 20% of all strokes and are further divided into subarachnoid hemorrhage (SAH) and intracerebral hemorrhage. Causes of SAH include trauma, berry or congenital aneurysms, and less often arteriovenous malformations. Intracerebral hemorrhage is most commonly caused by hypertension. Appropriate classification of a stroke and its etiology aids the clinician in determining the most effective prevention strategy.

The INTERSTROKE case-control study among 22 countries determined that 10 risk factors accounted for nearly 90% of strokes. Listed in order of significance, they are as follows: hypertension, cardiac disease, current smoking, waist-to-hip ratio, poor diet, sedentary lifestyle, excessive alcohol intake, diabetes mellitus, depression, and psychosocial stress. The highest burden of stroke in the United States falls in the so-called stroke belt located in the southeast, where high prevalences of diabetes, hypertension, and obesity remain likely important drivers of cerebrovascular disease.

PRIMORDIAL STROKE PREVENTION

DIET

The Mediterranean diet may protect against cardiovascular disease, including stroke. It is characterized by high intake of fruits, vegetables, and legumes; olive oil as the principal source of fat; moderate consumption of fish and poultry, with minimal intake of red meat and dairy; and an option of mild to moderate consumption of red wine, mostly with meals. Compared to a low-fat diet, this complex combination of nutrients decreased 5-year stroke risk by approximately 30% in a prospective study. In general, any diet aimed at promoting cardiovascular health, such as the Mediterranean diet or the Dietary Approach to Stop Hypertension (DASH) diet, revolves around the central notions of a high intake of plant-based nutrients, low-salt intake, and a curbing of saturated fats and simple sugars.

SMOKING

Tobacco use is strongly discouraged and among smokers, cessation of smoking leads to a reduction in stroke risk to levels similar to nonsmokers by 5 years.

EXERCISE

Physical activity is associated with a reduced risk of stroke and, importantly, several studies provide evidence that only a moderate level of activity is required, and so physical activity should be encouraged even among the elderly. A sedentary lifestyle, in combination with consumption of simple carbohydrates, has contributed to one-third of Americans becoming obese and to even more becoming overweight. Obesity is an independent risk factor for stroke, even after adjusting for physical activity and diet. Obesity is comorbid with diabetes, hypertension, and heart disease, moreover.

PRIMARY STROKE PREVENTION

Like primordial stroke prevention, primary stroke prevention aims to limit the risk of first-time stroke, but instead of dealing with groups of people, the health care provider focuses on each individual separately. Specific targets for intervention are a person's major modifiable risk factors including hypertension, diabetes mellitus, hypercholesterolemia, atrial fibrillation, and medication use. Several randomized trials have demonstrated the benefits of specific interventions to prevent a first stroke among patients with certain stroke risk factors (Table 44.1).

TABLE 44.1	Evidence-Based Primary Stroke Prevention
Risk Factor	**Treatment**
Hypertension	Antihypertensive
Myocardial infarction	HMG-CoA reductase inhibitor
Hyperlipidemia	HMG-CoA reductase inhibitor
Atrial fibrillation	Warfarin or oral anticoagulants
DM/vascular disease	ACE inhibitor
Asymptomatic carotid stenosis (60%–99%)	Consider carotid endarterectomy.
"High-risk" populations	HMG-CoA reductase inhibitor

HMG-CoA, hydroxymethylglutaryl-coenzyme A; DM, diabetes mellitus; ACE, angiotensin-converting enzyme.

HYPERTENSION

Blood pressure is the most important contributor to stroke incidence, increasing the risk of stroke in a linear fashion. High blood pressure accounts for 35% of all strokes. β-Blockers, thiazide diuretics, angiotensin-converting enzyme inhibitors (ACEIs), angiotensin II receptor blockers (ARBs), and calcium channel blockers are the most widely studied agents in stroke prevention. Although calcium channel blockers may provide the greatest neurovascular protection, they are also associated with an increased risk of heart failure. The general consensus is that protection against stroke depends on the level of blood pressure control rather than on the specific class of medication used. Blood pressure reductions of 10 mm Hg systolic or 5 mm Hg diastolic have been shown to reduce risk of first-time stroke by more than 40% [**Level 1**].[1] In the United States, efforts targeting hypertension have contributed to the steady decline in stroke incidence and stroke-related mortality in the last half century.

The effects of adequate blood pressure management may be more robust in those with diabetes mellitus. ACEIs and ARBs are recommended because they have been proven renoprotective and also effective in reducing cardiovascular events and specifically stroke in those with diabetes mellitus.

DIABETES MELLITUS

Epidemiologic studies show a positive relationship between hyperglycemia and stroke incidence, but aggressive management of hyperglycemia may actually be harmful. The Action to Control Cardiovascular Risk in Diabetes (ACCORD) study compared intensive glucose-lowering therapy with a goal glycated hemoglobin level below 6% versus glycated hemoglobin goals of 7% to 7.9% and found no difference in stroke incidence with a slight, but statistically significant, increase in overall mortality in the group undergoing tight control. Similarly, postprandial hyperglycemia and glycemic variability have both been associated with increased cardiovascular disease burden in epidemiologic studies, but prospective studies have not shown any benefit. Current recommendations are for a glycated hemoglobin goal of less than 7%.

The presence of diabetes also has ramifications for the management of other risk factors, specifically low-density lipoprotein (LDL) cholesterol. Diabetes is considered a cardiovascular disease equivalent and those 40 to 75 years of age with diabetes should be placed on a hydroxymethylglutaryl-coenzyme A (HMG-CoA) reductase inhibitor or statin, unless there is a contraindication.

HYPERCHOLESTEROLEMIA

Large epidemiologic studies, such as the Multiple Risk Factor Intervention Trial (MRFIT) that included over 350,000 men, have shown a positive association between death from ischemic stroke and increased cholesterol levels. There has also been evidence of a relationship between hemorrhagic strokes and low cholesterol levels. In line with the MRFIT data, trials using HMG-CoA reductase inhibitors among cardiac and other high–vascular disease risk patients have demonstrated benefits in terms of stroke risk reduction, in addition to the effects on cardiac event rates. The effect on stroke risk is more modest, however, probably reflecting the fact that stroke is more heterogeneous than heart disease and less strongly linked to elevated cholesterol levels.

In the Heart Protection Study (HPS), a randomized multicenter, placebo-controlled trial of simvastatin therapy, there was a 25% risk reduction for stroke (from 5.7% to 4.3%; P <.0001), without an increase in risk of hemorrhagic stroke over a 5-year period. Importantly, these benefits remained in those with LDL less than 100 mg/dL.

Evidence suggests that the optimal way to think about cholesterol goals within the context of primary stroke prevention is to consider the individual's long-term absolute risk of combined cardiovascular events. The Pooled Cohort Risk Assessment Equations was developed by the American College of Cardiology and American Heart Association using data from several large epidemiologic studies to predict a 10-year risk of cardiovascular events and identify appropriate candidates for statin therapy. Those with a high risk of cardiovascular events (considered to be at least 7.5% over 10 years) should be placed on cholesterol-lowering therapy, independent of specific risk factors. Other high-risk groups that should receive statin therapy are individuals with an LDL greater than 190 mg/dL and those aged 40 to 75 years with comorbid diabetes mellitus [**Level 1**].[2]

ATRIAL FIBRILLATION

Atrial fibrillation is the most important cause of embolic stroke. Anticoagulation is effective in preventing both incident and recurrent strokes in patients with atrial fibrillation [**Level 1**].[3] In the Stroke Prevention in Atrial Fibrillation (SPAF) study, anticoagulation reduced stroke recurrence substantially, even in patients older than the age of 75 years. Chance of embolization is associated with the following risk factors: age older than 75 years, previous embolization, sustained hypertension, and congestive heart failure. With one risk factor, the stroke incidence is nearly 3% per year and increases to 18% when all are present.

Warfarin, a vitamin K antagonist, is associated with a 60% to 70% relative risk reduction in stroke. More recently, two other classes of anticoagulant therapies have been employed: direct thrombin inhibitors and factor Xa inhibitors. Large randomized clinical trials that have compared warfarin to either dabigatran, rivaroxaban, or apixaban have shown similar or slightly better efficacy with the newer agents. Some of the trials also indicate a lowered risk of intracranial hemorrhage with less need for serum monitoring, although the role of serum monitoring for some agents is still under investigation. There are two deterrents to physicians routinely prescribing the newer agents, however. The first is the lack of a standardized clotting assay, such as the international normalized ratio (INR) for warfarin, that allows for rapid evaluation of level of anticoagulation, and the second is the lack of an effective antidote, such as fresh frozen plasma and vitamin K, that can be employed when major bleeding occurs. Current research is directed at addressing these concerns.

CAROTID STENOSIS

Another major source of preventable cerebral infarction is large-vessel atherosclerotic disease and specifically internal carotid artery stenosis. In asymptomatic patients with greater than 60% carotid stenosis and low perioperative risk, carotid endarterectomy (CEA) should be considered with the expectation that approximately 20 procedures must be performed to prevent one stroke over a 5-year period. Men are much more likely to benefit than women, which, along with the patient-specific perioperative risk, helps the clinician decide whether or not to recommend surgery. Although CEA is the gold standard, carotid artery stenting (CAS) is an alternative and may be employed if the anatomy is unfavorable to surgical intervention. There is no benefit of either procedure in patients with less than 50% stenosis or in chronic carotid occlusion.

SECONDARY STROKE PREVENTION

Once a stroke or TIA has occurred, the goals of the clinician are to minimize long-term disability and direct management to prevent another stroke (Fig. 44.1). Secondary stroke prevention measures do not alter progression of the initial stroke, but research has shown that initiating preventive therapy in the acute setting after stroke increases the likelihood of preventive therapy being in place in the long term.

STROKE MECHANISM AND EVALUATION

Therapies aimed at limiting risk of recurrence depend in large part on the mechanism of the stroke, its severity, and the individualized modifiable risk factor profile. Because the risk of a repeat stroke is highest in the first 2 weeks after the initial event, a comprehensive evaluation must be employed as soon as possible to determine stroke mechanism and quantify the underlying risk factors. The importance of a good history and physical examination cannot be overstated and should be followed by hypothesis-driven diagnostic testing. Magnetic resonance imaging (MRI) of the brain visualizes acute ischemic injury and can aide in determining the mechanism. Although lacunar strokes, or deep punctate infarcts within the white matter, predominantly occur from small-vessel disease, for example, large wedge-shaped infarcts or multifocal infarcts are more consistent with embolism. Extracranial vessel imaging specifically looking at the patency of the carotid arteries is a crucial step in the diagnostic algorithm, whereas intracranial vessel imaging in the form of magnetic resonance angiography (MRA) or computed tomography angiography (CTA) may be useful to identify intracranial stenosis. The gold standard for carotid imaging is digital subtraction angiography, but it is impractical for screening purposes. Carotid Doppler has therefore become the main screening test for carotid atherosclerosis, whereas the widespread availability of MRA and CTA provide alternatives to be used at the clinician's discretion and to confirm the findings on ultrasound.

Transthoracic echocardiography is used to assess structural cardiac abnormalities that predispose to cardioembolism. In cases with a high pretest probability of embolism, transesophageal echocardiogram can be used to better visualize the left atrium and cardiac valves, looking for intra-atrial thrombus, cardiac myxoma, or valvular vegetations. A second arm of the cardiac evaluation assesses the cardiac rhythm for evidence of atrial fibrillation. Electrocardiography and cardiac telemetry are used in screening, whereas prolonged monitoring for several weeks to months can be very helpful in capturing occult atrial fibrillation. Measuring LDL, high-density lipoprotein, hemoglobin A1c, and in appropriate or otherwise unexplained cases, erythrocyte sedimentation rate (ESR), C-reactive protein (CRP), or rapid plasma reagin (RPR) allow for proper management and prevention of recurrent stroke.

PREVENTION EARLY AFTER ACUTE STROKE

It is important to recognize that TIAs call for the same urgency in evaluation as MRI-proven strokes. Johnston et al. showed that

FIGURE 44.1 Effect of secondary stroke prevention measures on stroke recurrence. Estimated absolute risk reductions in stroke of various secondary stroke prevention therapies compared to placebo or in some cases, standard management. [a]Refers to symptomatic carotid stenosis of 70% to 99%. [b]Warfarin or direct oral anticoagulants. [c]Compared to single antiplatelet agent and not including dual antiplatelet therapy initiated in the acute setting after stroke.

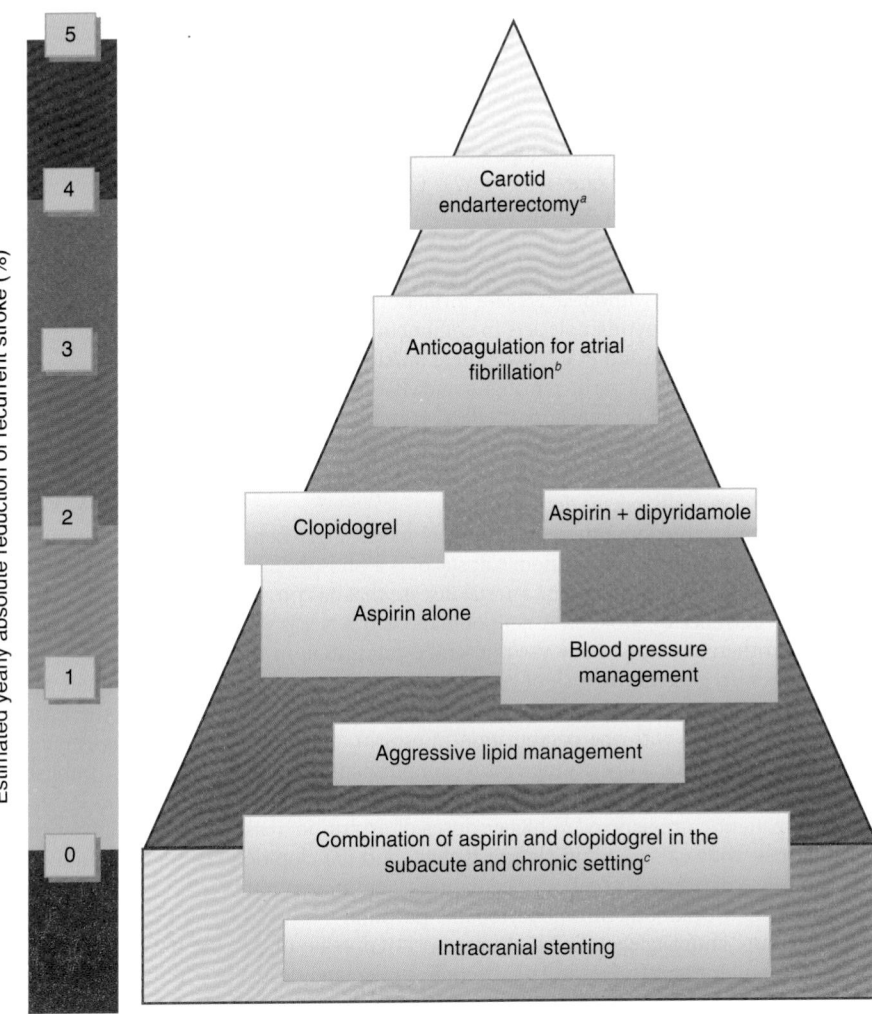

the risk of stroke after TIA is about 5% in the first 2 days and 10% within 90 days. Further, 1 in 20 individuals will suffer a fatal or disabling stroke within 90 days after TIA. Recent trials proved that urgent evaluation and directed management of TIA or minor stroke dramatically decreases the recurrence rate of stroke.

Early interventions aimed at stroke prevention revolve around mitigating high-risk situations, such as moderate to high-grade carotid stenosis and atrial fibrillation. In general, dual antiplatelet therapy in the realm of stroke prevention has been reserved for cases of atrial fibrillation in which a contraindication for anticoagulation exists, but one recent study challenged this notion. The Clopidogrel in High-risk Patients with Acute Nondisabling Cerebrovascular Events (CHANCE) trial found that a 21-day course of dual antiplatelet therapy with aspirin and clopidogrel among Chinese patients with TIA and minor stroke, given within 24 hours of symptom onset, lowered the 3-month stroke recurrence rate. A short course of aspirin and clopidogrel in the early period may therefore be considered but cannot be recommended for all patients until further studies replicate these findings. Short-term subcutaneous heparin is not effective in preventing stroke recurrence compared to aspirin, according to the International Stroke Trial (IST), which enrolled nearly 20,000 ischemic stroke patients; similar findings were seen in the Chinese Acute Stroke Trial (CAST) with nearly the same number of patients.

ANTIPLATELET THERAPY

All patients with ischemic stroke without a definite indication for anticoagulation, and in whom no contraindication is present, should receive long-term antiplatelet therapy. Aspirin monotherapy, the combination of aspirin with extended-release dipyridamole, or clopidogrel, are all acceptable options for initial therapy in the secondary prevention of noncardioembolic stroke [**Level 1**].[4]

The action of aspirin is to irreversibly acetylate and inhibit platelet cyclooxygenase-1, which stops synthesis of the powerful platelet aggregant thromboxane A2 (TXA2). Lower doses of aspirin have the advantage of minimizing inhibition of endothelial cell production of prostacyclin (PGI2), the powerful platelet antiaggregant. The concept of a balance between TXA2 and PGI2 in the normal circulation without aggregate formation won Sir John Vane a Nobel Prize. Dipyridamole acts in conjunction with aspirin by increasing adenosine and PGI2, two potent antiaggregants. The optimum dose of daily aspirin remains somewhat controversial, but doses as low as 30 mg daily appear effective and have less side effects such as gastrointestinal bleeding. The U.S. Food and Drug Administration (FDA) currently recommend doses between 50 and 325 mg daily for stroke prevention.

Clopidogrel, a thienopyridine derivative, is increasingly being used for secondary stroke prevention. Cilostazol is a phosphodiesterase 3 inhibitor used in peripheral arterial disease that has proven to reduce recurrence of stroke in Asian populations but is less well studied and therefore not widely used in stroke prevention in the United States. In general, the risk of adverse events with standard antiplatelet agents is very low, but a few points need to be considered: (1) treating with the combination of aspirin and dipyridamole requires twice daily dosing and is complicated by a high rate of secondary headache and gastrointestinal symptoms, thus reducing patient compliance; (2) higher doses of aspirin increase bleeding risk without providing clinical benefit; and (3) clopidogrel can cause diarrhea, thrombocytopenia, rash, and in very rare circumstances, thrombotic thrombocytopenic purpura.

As a group, antiplatelets offer an absolute risk reduction of 2% in yearly vascular events (myocardial infarction, stroke, and death), with a 0.1% to 0.2% increase in major extracranial hemorrhages

(number needed to harm is 500 to 1,000 to cause one major extracranial hemorrhage). There may also be a modest benefit of clopidogrel, or aspirin with dipyridamole, over aspirin alone for prevention of recurrent strokes, according to some meta-analyses. Aspirin with dipyridamole compared to aspirin alone produced an approximate annual absolute risk reduction of 1% in two large clinical trials. On the other hand, clopidogrel and the combination of aspirin with dipyridamole produced nearly identical results in one study. Choice of antiplatelet depends on the setting, comorbidities, and access to health care, but aspirin is the most widely studied and least expensive medication, making it ideal for large-scale use especially in developing countries where the number treated is usually determined by the cost of therapy. Clopidogrel and aspirin with dipyridamole are reasonable alternatives as first-line therapy or second-line therapy in those who have suffered a stroke while on aspirin.

More recently, dual antiplatelet therapy with clopidogrel and aspirin, compared to aspirin alone, has been investigated in secondary prevention after lacunar stroke in the Secondary Prevention of Small Subcortical Strokes (SPS3) trial. There was no evidence of a reduction in risk of stroke recurrence, despite an increase in risk of bleeding and mortality, among those treated with dual antiplatelet therapy. There are several reasons that may account for the difference in results between the CHANCE trial described earlier and SPS3: (1) CHANCE studied acute therapy, within 24 hours of stroke onset, with half of the participants randomized within 12 hours; (2) CHANCE included only patients with mild stroke and TIA, isolating a group with low risk of hemorrhagic conversion; and (3) CHANCE used dual antiplatelet agents for only 3 weeks, whereas SPS3 enrolled patients within 6 months of stroke onset and used dual antiplatelet therapy for the duration of the trial. The majority of the benefit from dual antiplatelet therapy in CHANCE occurred within the first week of treatment. This immediate reduction in recurrent vascular events is a phenomenon echoed in trials that studied dual antiplatelet agents within 24 hours of cardiac ischemia.

ANTICOAGULATION

Anticoagulation with warfarin is indicated in patients with definite cardioembolic sources of stroke such as mechanical valves or left ventricular thrombus. In patients with atrial fibrillation, anticoagulation with warfarin or one of the newer anticoagulants (described earlier) is indicated.

CAROTID ENDARTERECTOMY, ANGIOPLASTY, AND STENTING

In good surgical candidates, the treatment of choice for stroke and TIA caused by carotid stenosis of equal to, or greater than, 70% of the vessel diameter is CEA by a skilled surgeon with an acceptable complication rate (<5%) combined with optimal medical management, as demonstrated by three prospective studies: the North American Symptomatic Carotid Endarterectomy Trial (NASCET), the European Carotid Surgery Trial (ECST), and the U.S. Veterans Affairs Cooperative Study (VACS) on CEA [**Level 1**].[4] The first published case of successful CEA was performed by DeBakey in 1954, but it wasn't until 1991 that these studies confirmed its benefits. In those with high-grade carotid stenosis, CEA yields a number needed to treat of 16 to prevent one stroke over a 1-year period. There is also a benefit, albeit more modest, of CEA in symptomatic patients with moderate carotid stenosis (50% to 69%). Post hoc analysis has also demonstrated that the greatest value of CEA is within 2 weeks of the event, and contemporary literature argues for intervention as soon as is medically possible.

More recently, CAS has been compared to CEA in three large trials: Stent-Protected Angioplasty versus Carotid Endarterectomy (SPACE), International Carotid Stenting Study (ICSS), and the Carotid Revascularization Endarterectomy versus Stenting Trial (CREST). Results have been consistent in showing a slight increase in periprocedural stroke (30 days) with CAS compared to CEA. In SPACE and CREST, combined adverse outcomes over a 2-year period were similar, whereas ICSS showed that CEA was superior in combined outcomes both in the acute and long-term settings. Although CEA remains the treatment of choice for symptomatic high-grade carotid stenosis, CAS is an alternative that can be employed in high-risk surgical patients or those with unsuitable anatomy.

There have been a number of trials looking at strategies for preventing stroke from intracranial stenotic lesions that are not readily accessible to surgeons. Stroke distal to a 50% to 99% vascular stenosis carries a recurrence rate of 15% in the first year. The comparison of Warfarin and Aspirin for Symptomatic Intracranial Stenosis (WASID) trial studied aspirin versus warfarin in patients with symptomatic intracranial stenosis 50% to 99%. The study was stopped because of a high rate of adverse events in the warfarin group, leading researchers to conclude that warfarin provides no benefit over aspirin in patients with intracranial stenosis. Despite the negative primary result, the study provided the important finding that risk was highest in patients with greater than 70% stenosis, a group that had a 25% stroke recurrence rate in the first year. The subsequent Stenting versus Aggressive Medical Therapy of Intracranial Atherosclerotic Stenosis (SAMMPRIS) trial thus targeted patients with recent stroke and high-grade intracranial stenosis (>70%), comparing percutaneous transluminal angioplasty and stenting with best medical management with aggressive risk factor control. Both groups received dual antiplatelet therapy with aspirin and clopidogrel for 3 months. There was also aggressive management of risk factors including hypertension, lipids, diabetes, and tobacco use. The primary end point of recurrent stroke or death was reached in 20% of the stenting group as opposed to 12% in the medical management group. Interestingly, the medical group had a lower than expected stroke recurrence rate compared to the 25% risk predicted by the WASID study. The results suggested that aggressive medical therapy is superior to intervention for high-grade intracranial stenosis with currently available technology.

CARDIAC ABNORMALITIES

Treatment of cardiogenic emboli depends on the offending pathology: Infected prosthetic valves need replacement, and myxomatous emboli require surgical removal of the tumor (Table 44.2).

TABLE 44.2 Cardioembolic Sources of Stroke

High-Risk	Low-Risk/Unknown Risk
Atrial fibrillation	Cardiomyopathy
Mechanical prosthetic valve	Aortic arch atheroma
Recent myocardial infarction	Patent foramen ovale
Left ventricular thrombus	Atrial septal aneurysm
Rheumatic heart disease	Mitral valve strands
Marantic endocarditis	
Atrial myxoma	
Infective endocarditis	

The role of anticoagulation among patients with possible paradoxical embolism through a patent foramen ovale (PFO) is unclear, and current guidelines support the use of antiplatelet agents for secondary prevention in this setting. Whether closure of PFOs using transcardiac devices can reduce secondary stroke, risk has been investigated in three large prospective trials comparing closure to medical therapy. None of them were able to show benefit of PFO closure when compared to medical therapy alone. The risk of recurrent stroke is low among patients with stroke likely due to PFO but closure may still be considered on an individualized basis.

Aortic arch atheromatous plaque is another condition associated with increased risk of stroke, with retrospective case-control studies consistently showing an association. Complex plaques, defined by a protruding component greater than 4 mm, presence of a mobile component, or intraplaque ulceration, are deemed high risk for embolization. Despite the known association, a causal relationship between aortic arch atheroma and stroke has never been proven, mirroring the uncertainty in therapeutic recommendations. There is no clear evidence to support use of anticoagulation, even in complex plaques. Statins are recommended because of their potential to remodel and cause regression in atheromatous plaques, along with standard antiplatelet therapy for secondary stroke prevention.

MODIFIABLE RISK FACTOR MANAGEMENT

Hypertension

Recent studies have provided evidence for increased use of antihypertensive agents in patients with stroke and TIA. Despite evidence of the efficacy of blood pressure reduction in reducing risk of a first stroke, concerns about lowering blood pressure in patients with existing cerebrovascular disease remained due to the theoretical possibility that in patients with arterial disease of cerebral vessels, a reduction in blood pressure could worsen perfusion and precipitate clinical events or affect cognition.

Much has been made of the potential benefits of ACEIs or ARBs in stroke prevention. This has been an attractive hypothesis, but the data does not provide an entirely convincing picture regarding the privileged position of ACEIs and ARBs among antihypertensive agents, particularly after stroke. Although diabetics should probably receive these medications for prevention of progression of renal disease, it is not clear that this therapy dramatically reduces the incidence of stroke beyond what would be expected from reducing the blood pressure to a similar degree using other agents. The PROGRESS (Perindopril Protection against Recurrent Stroke Study) trial was designed and conducted in large part to address these concerns. PROGRESS was a randomized, double-blind, placebo-controlled trial of antihypertensive therapy among 6,105 patients with a history of hemorrhagic or ischemic stroke or TIA. Patients were enrolled independent of hypertension status, and 52% were nonhypertensive—considered to be systolic blood pressure 160 mm Hg or lower and diastolic blood pressure 90 mm Hg or lower—the blood pressure thresholds in use at the time the study started. Active treatment used the ACEI perindopril, with or without the thiazide diuretic indapamide. Active therapy led to a mean blood pressure reduction of 9/4 mm Hg compared with placebo, with a statistically significant 28% relative risk reduction in recurrent stroke or an absolute risk reduction of 4%. Of particular interest, the benefit of combination therapy was of a similar magnitude among hypertensive and nonhypertensive patients and was of greater benefit for those with initial hemorrhagic stroke (relative risk reduction 49%) than for those with ischemic stroke (relative risk reduction 26%), likely reflecting the even stronger association of blood pressure with hemorrhagic stroke risk. PROGRESS has therefore been interpreted as indicating a benefit for blood pressure reduction among patients with cerebrovascular disease, independent of a history of hypertension.

The SPS3 study, aside from studying the effect of dual antiplatelet therapy, also examined the role of strict versus standard blood pressure management (systolic <130 mm Hg vs. 130 to 149 mm Hg) on the outcome of stroke recurrence and showed a trend toward benefit in stroke recurrence in the lower blood pressure group (hazard ratio 0.81, confidence interval 0.63 to 1.03). Current guidelines recommend blood pressure lowering based on individualized targets, but it is reasonable to use a systolic blood pressure goal of less than 140 mm Hg and diastolic less than 90 mm Hg [**Level 1**].[5] Reducing daily salt intake to 2 g, engaging in regular physical activity, and losing weight in overweight or obese patients may also have substantial benefits on blood pressure levels, apart from use of pharmacologic therapy.

Hyperlipidemia

Hyperlipidemia is another important modifiable risk factor for vascular disease, although its relationship to stroke is less clear than that for heart disease. The Stroke Prevention by Aggressive Reduction in Cholesterol Levels (SPARCL) trial provides direct evidence of the benefit of statin therapy in secondary prevention of stroke among patients presenting with stroke or TIA. SPARCL enrolled 4,731 patients with stroke or TIA within the previous 6 months, and at least 30 days, after stroke. Patients were required to have baseline LDL cholesterol levels between 100 and 190 mg/dL. Those with atrial fibrillation, cardioembolism, and SAH were excluded and patients were randomized to atorvastatin 80 mg daily or to placebo. Over a median duration of follow-up of nearly 5 years, atorvastatin reduced the risk of recurrent stroke from 13.1% to 11.2%. Effects on other cardiovascular outcomes were slightly greater, but there was no effect on overall mortality.

Because lipids are not thought to contribute significantly to stroke risk, some of this benefit may derive from the anti-inflammatory or other effects of statins. Other putative mechanisms through which they exert their effects include effects on blood flow and vascular endothelial function, inflammation, free radical scavenging, hemostasis, and others.

Statins are the mainstay in lipid reduction therapy and aggressive lipid-lowering treatment should be employed after a stroke or TIA [**Level 1**].[2]

Diabetes Mellitus

Although glycemic control has been shown to reduce risks of microvascular complications, the benefit in reducing macrovascular complications, such as stroke, is less certain. In one trial, tight glycemic control of a prospective cohort of newly diagnosed diabetics was not found to significantly reduce stroke risk. Nonetheless, among sufferers of stroke who have concomitant diabetes, diet and exercise, oral hypoglycemic drugs, and insulin are recommended to obtain appropriate glycemic control.

Lifestyle Modification

Behavioral risk factors may be most difficult to control, but physicians should endeavor to educate patients about their importance. Smoking is addictive, and cessation may necessitate psychological counseling and medical aids, such as nicotine patches or varenicline. Physical activity should be encouraged, as a sedentary lifestyle is

associated with elevations in blood pressure and stroke risk. Alcohol consumption in excess of two drinks daily should be discouraged, although there is evidence that moderate alcohol consumption may actually have protective effects against stroke risk. However, proof that control of these risk factors reduces stroke risk is difficult to obtain from randomized trials. Patient education regarding behavioral risk factor control is extremely important and is similar for both primary and secondary stroke prevention [**Level 1**].[3]

HEMORRHAGIC STROKE

INTRACEREBRAL HEMORRHAGE

Intracerebral hemorrhage (ICH) accounts for approximately 10% to 15% of all strokes in the United States and carries a 1-year mortality close to 60%. Other than hypertension, spontaneous ICH can be caused by cerebral amyloid angiopathy, anticoagulation therapy, vascular malformations, brain tumors, cavernous angiomas, aneurysms, cerebral vein thrombosis, illicit drugs or alcohol abuse, pathologic coagulopathy, and genetic vasculopathies. Massive ICHs of more than 60 mL in volume are usually lethal because vital structures are irreversibly damaged, whereas smaller hemorrhages may be treated with supportive care. Given the dismal 1-year prognosis even with small- to moderate-sized hemorrhage, primary prevention of ICH is of the upmost importance.

Hypertension

As with ischemic stroke, first-time ICH can in many cases be avoided through identification and management of specific risk factors. Hypertension is the most important modifiable risk factor and doubles the risk of first-time spontaneous ICH. Blood pressure control lowers the risk of ICH recurrence by nearly 50%. Annual recurrence is high and occurs in 2% of those with a deep location and as high as 4% of those with a lobar localization. The higher risk of recurrence with lobar hemorrhage likely represents the occurrence of cerebral amyloid angiopathy in lobar vascular territories.

Cerebral Amyloid Angiopathy

Cerebral amyloid angiopathy (CAA) is not yet a modifiable risk factor but is helpful when assessing risk of recurrent ICH. CAA-associated microhemorrhages and microinfarcts are much more common than clinically evident bleeds, occurring one and eight times per year, respectively. The biggest risk factors for recurrent CAA-associated hemorrhages are age, the number of microbleeds present at baseline, and the presence of the apolipoprotein E E2 or E4 alleles.

Amyloid-depleting therapy is currently not available, limiting attempts at secondary prevention. The PROGRESS trial, discussed earlier, studied a subset of patients with recurrent ICH and determined that blood pressure lowering by systolic/diastolic of 9/4 mm Hg decreased risk of cumulative ICH by 50% and over 70% in those with presumed CAA, establishing the viability of a traditional risk prevention approach in those with CAA-related hemorrhage.

Patients with a history of symptomatic hemorrhage thought to be related to CAA carry a relative contraindication for chronic anticoagulation. Many studies reported an association of HMG-CoA reductase inhibitors with an increased risk of ICH, but that was ultimately refuted by a large meta-analysis that included over 40 trials with nearly 250,000 individuals. Nonetheless, there is no benefit for statins in the prevention of ICH, although they may be used in those with previous ICH who have other indications, such as cardiovascular disease or ischemic stroke.

Arteriovenous Malformations

Bleeding from arteriovenous malformations (AVMs) is the most common cause of ICH in those younger than 45 years of age. The Medical Management with or without Interventional Therapy for Unruptured Brain Arteriovenous Malformations (ARUBA) trial evaluated interventional therapy versus medical therapy alone as management of previously unruptured AVMs. The study was stopped early because those in the medical therapy group had a lower risk of stroke or death compared to the intervention group. It is therefore prudent to manage unruptured AVMs conservatively. AVMs that have ruptured are more likely to rebleed, and surgery, embolization, or stereotactic radiotherapy may be considered when anatomically feasible.

ANEURYSMAL SUBARACHNOID HEMORRHAGE

Extirpation of the aneurysm is the definitive therapy for aneurysms causing SAH and may be accomplished surgically or with balloons, coils, or embolic material deposited in the aneurysm. When it comes to prevention of aneurysmal rupture, knowing the projected natural history of the aneurysm and risk of intervention are the two most important factors driving the decision to intervene or to watch and wait. The International Study of Unruptured Intracranial Aneurysms (ISUIA) defined yearly risk of aneurysmal rupture by site and size of the aneurysm in question. The PHASES score was established in 2014 using a pooled analysis of six prospective trials, including over 8,000 individuals, to further help predict risk of aneurysmal rupture. It recognizes seven factors (hypertension, age, history of SAH, anatomic location, size, and geographical location of residence) as predictors of aneurysmal rupture that when combined into a single score, could more accurately quantify future risk of rupture and help determine the need for intervention. The risk of rupture must be weighed against the risks of the surgery, which are determined by the patient's comorbidities and the historical periprocedural risk of the institution.

STROKE REHABILITATION

A team approach for stroke rehabilitation, starting from a stroke recovery unit with experienced physiatrists and physical therapists, has proven beneficial for the optimum recovery of patients. This approach is particularly helpful in averting various complications from strokes, such as infections, contractures, and decubitus ulcers and in maximizing independence for patients with hemiplegia/paresis by teaching them to transfer effectively from bed to wheelchair. Activities of daily living (ADLs) may be optimized for personal hygiene, dressing, and feeding as well. Speech and occupational therapists should be consulted to help patients improve their communication skills and ADL skills.

Depression is a frequent accompaniment of stroke, partially not only because the reality of a physical disability exists but also because there is altered brain chemistry, which may respond well to selective serotonin reuptake inhibitors (SSRIs) and tricyclic antidepressants. One randomized trial found that escitalopram administered prophylactically to stroke patients was effective in preventing the development of depression. A Cochrane review of SSRIs in the poststroke setting showed them efficacious in improving not only depression but also stroke-related dependence as well as disability. Further studies will be needed to determine whether there is a benefit to prophylactic treatment of depression compared to treatment initiated at the time of diagnosis.

LEVEL 1 EVIDENCE

1. Law MR, Morris JK, Wald NJ. Use of blood pressure lowering drugs in the prevention of cardiovascular disease: meta-analysis of 147 randomised trials in the context of expectations from prospective epidemiological studies. *BMJ*. 2009;338:b1665.
2. Stone NJ, Robinson JG, Lichtenstein AH, et al. 2013 ACC/AHA guideline on the treatment of blood cholesterol to reduce atherosclerotic cardiovascular risk in adults: a report of the American College of Cardiology/American Heart Association Task Force on Practice Guidelines. *J Am Coll Cardiol*. 2014;63(25, pt B):2889–934.
3. Goldstein LB, Bushnell CD, Adams RJ, et al. Guidelines for the primary prevention of stroke: a guideline for healthcare professionals from the American Heart Association/American Stroke Association. *Stroke*. 2011;42(2):517–584.
4. Kernan WN, Ovbiagele B, Black HR, et al. Guidelines for the prevention of stroke in patients with stroke and transient ischemic attack: a guideline for healthcare professionals from the American Heart Association/American Stroke Association. *Stroke*. 2014;45(7):2160–2236.
5. James PA, Oparil S, Carter BL, et al. 2014 evidence-based guideline for the management of high blood pressure in adults: report from the panel members appointed to the Eighth Joint National Committee (JNC 8). *JAMA*. 2014;311(5):507–520.

SUGGESTED READINGS

Amarenco P, Bogousslavsky J, Callahan A III, et al. High-dose atorvastatin after stroke or transient ischemic attack. *N Engl J Med*. 2006;355(6):549–559.

Arima H, Tzourio C, Anderson C, et al. Effects of perindopril-based lowering of blood pressure on intracerebral hemorrhage related to amyloid angiopathy: the PROGRESS trial. *Stroke*. 2010;41(2):394–396.

Bailey RD, Hart RG, Benavente O, et al. Recurrent brain hemorrhage is more frequent than ischemic stroke after intracranial hemorrhage. *Neurology*. 2001;56(6):773–777.

Boden-Albala B, Cammack S, Chong J, et al. Diabetes, fasting glucose levels, and risk of ischemic stroke and vascular events: findings from the Northern Manhattan Study (NOMAS). *Diabetes Care*. 2008;31(6):1132–1137.

Chimowitz MI, Lynn MJ, Howlett-Smith H, et al. Comparison of warfarin and aspirin for symptomatic intracranial arterial stenosis. *N Engl J Med*. 2005;352(13):1305–1316.

Connolly SJ, Ezekowitz MD, Yusuf S, et al. Dabigatran versus warfarin in patients with atrial fibrillation. *N Engl J Med*. 2009;361(12):1139–1151.

DeBakey ME. Successful carotid endarterectomy for cerebrovascular insufficiency. Nineteen-year follow-up. *JAMA*. 1975;233(10):1083–1085.

Derdeyn CP, Chimowitz MI, Lynn MJ, et al. Aggressive medical treatment with or without stenting in high-risk patients with intracranial artery stenosis (SAMMPRIS): the final results of a randomised trial. *Lancet*. 2014;383(9914):333–341.

Eckstein HH, Ringleb P, Allenberg JR, et al. Results of the Stent-Protected Angioplasty versus Carotid Endarterectomy (SPACE) study to treat symptomatic stenoses at 2 years: a multinational, prospective, randomised trial. *Lancet Neurol*. 2008;7(10):893–902.

Ederle J, Dobson J, Featherstone RL, et al. Carotid artery stenting compared with endarterectomy in patients with symptomatic carotid stenosis (International Carotid Stenting Study): an interim analysis of a randomised controlled trial. *Lancet*. 2010;375(9719):985–997.

Elkind MS. Implications of stroke prevention trials: treatment of global risk. *Neurology*. 2005;65(1):17–21.

Elkind MS, Sacco RL, Macarthur RB, et al. High-dose lovastatin for acute ischemic stroke: results of the phase I dose escalation neuroprotection with statin therapy for acute recovery trial (NeuSTART). *Cerebrovasc Dis*. 2009;28(3):266–275.

Estruch R, Ros E, Martinez-Gonzalez MA. Mediterranean diet for primary prevention of cardiovascular disease. *N Engl J Med.* 2013;369(7):676–677.

Granger CB, Alexander JH, McMurray JJ, et al. Apixaban versus warfarin in patients with atrial fibrillation. *N Engl J Med.* 2011;365(11):981–992.

Greving JP, Wermer MJ, Brown RD Jr, et al. Development of the PHASES score for prediction of risk of rupture of intracranial aneurysms: a pooled analysis of six prospective cohort studies. *Lancet Neurol.* 2014;13(1):59–66.

Hackam DG, Woodward M, Newby LK, et al. Statins and intracerebral hemorrhage: collaborative systematic review and meta-analysis. *Circulation.* 2011;124(20):2233–2242.

Halkes PH, van Gijn J, Kappelle LJ, et al. Medium intensity oral anticoagulants versus aspirin after cerebral ischaemia of arterial origin (ESPRIT): a randomised controlled trial. *Lancet Neurol.* 2007;6(2):115–124.

Iso H, Jacobs DR Jr, Wentworth D, et al. Serum cholesterol levels and six-year mortality from stroke in 350,977 men screened for the multiple risk factor intervention trial. *N Engl J Med.* 1989;320(14):904–910.

Johnston SC, Gress DR, Browner WS, et al. Short-term prognosis after emergency department diagnosis of TIA. *JAMA.* 2000;284:2901–2906.

Lackland DT, Roccella EJ, Deutsch AF, et al. Factors influencing the decline in stroke mortality: a statement from the American Heart Association/American Stroke Association. *Stroke.* 2014;45(1):315–353.

LaRosa JC, Grundy SM, Waters DD, et al. Intensive lipid lowering with atorvastatin in patients with stable coronary disease. *N Engl J Med.* 2005;352(14): 1425–1435.

Lavallee PC, Meseguer E, Abboud H, et al. A transient ischaemic attack clinic with round-the-clock access (SOS-TIA): feasibility and effects. *Lancet Neurol.* 2007;6(11):953–960.

Luengo-Fernandez R, Gray AM, Rothwell PM. Effect of urgent treatment for transient ischaemic attack and minor stroke on disability and hospital costs (EXPRESS study): a prospective population-based sequential comparison. *Lancet Neurol.* 2009;8(3):235–243.

Mantese VA, Timaran CH, Chiu D, et al; CREST Investigators. The Carotid Revascularization Endarterectomy versus Stenting Trial (CREST): stenting versus carotid endarterectomy for carotid disease. *Stroke.* 2010;41(10)(suppl):S31–S34.

Meier B, Frank B, Wahl A, et al. Secondary stroke prevention: patent foramen ovale, aortic plaque, and carotid stenosis. *Eur Heart J.* 2012;33(6):705–713, 713a, 713b.

Mohr JP, Parides MK, Stapf C, et al. Medical management with or without interventional therapy for unruptured brain arteriovenous malformations (ARUBA): a multicentre, non-blinded, randomised trial. *Lancet.* 2014;383(9917):614–621.

Mohr JP, Thompson JL, Lazar RM, et al. A comparison of warfarin and aspirin for the prevention of recurrent ischemic stroke. *N Engl J Med.* 2001;345(20):1444–1451.

Patel MR, Mahaffey KW, Garg J, et al. Rivaroxaban versus warfarin in nonvalvular atrial fibrillation. *N Engl J Med.* 2011;365(10):883–891.

PROGRESS Collaborative Group. Randomised trial of a perindopril-based blood-pressure-lowering regimen among 6,105 individuals with previous stroke or transient ischaemic attack. *Lancet.* 2001;358(9287):1033–1041. doi:10.1016/S0140-6736(01)06178-5.

Rengifo-Moreno P, Palacios IF, Junpaparp P, et al. Patent foramen ovale transcatheter closure vs. medical therapy on recurrent vascular events: a systematic review and meta-analysis of randomized controlled trials. *Eur Heart J.* 2013;34(43):3342–3352.

Ridker PM, Cook NR, Lee IM, et al. A randomized trial of low-dose aspirin in the primary prevention of cardiovascular disease in women. *N Engl J Med.* 2005;352(13):1293–1304.

Robinson RG, Jorge RE, Moser DJ, et al. Escitalopram and problem-solving therapy for prevention of poststroke depression: a randomized controlled trial. *JAMA.* 2008;299(20):2391–2400.

Sacco RL, Chong JY, Prabhakaran S, et al. Experimental treatments for acute ischaemic stroke. *Lancet.* 2007;369(9558):331–341.

Sacco RL, Diener HC, Yusuf S, et al. Aspirin and extended-release dipyridamole versus clopidogrel for recurrent stroke. *N Engl J Med.* 2008;359(12): 1238–1251.

Standl E, Schnell O, Ceriello A. Postprandial hyperglycemia and glycemic variability: should we care? *Diabetes Care.* 2011;34(suppl 2):S120–S127.

Viswanathan A, Greenberg SM. Cerebral amyloid angiopathy in the elderly. *Ann Neurol.* 2011;70(6):871–880.

Wang Y, Wang Y, Zhao X, et al. Clopidogrel with aspirin in acute minor stroke or transient ischemic attack. *N Engl J Med.* 2013;369(1):11–19.

Wiebers DO, Whisnant JP, Huston J III, et al. Unruptured intracranial aneurysms: natural history, clinical outcome, and risks of surgical and endovascular treatment. *Lancet.* 2003;362(9378):103–110.

Wolf SL, Winstein CJ, Miller JP, et al. Effect of constraint-induced movement therapy on upper extremity function 3 to 9 months after stroke: the EXCITE randomized clinical trial. *JAMA.* 2006;296(17):2095–2104.

Concussion 45

James M. Noble and John F. Crary

INTRODUCTION

Concussion is a mild traumatic brain injury that has been recognized for centuries as an entity in accidents, battle, and sport. The visibility of higher profile cases of recurrent concussion in contact sports and growing concern of the potentially long-term impact of concussion, particularly among potentially vulnerable youth with developing brains, have brought concussion to the fore in recent years and perhaps rightfully so. In reflection of increasing concern, awareness, and research in the field, this chapter is the first version to appear into this established textbook.

DEFINITION

Concussion is a mild traumatic brain injury defined by a typically transient appearance of neurologic signs and symptoms, including headache, dizziness, imbalance, tiredness and fatigue, light and sound sensitivity, concentration difficulties, and memory impairment (often described as a brain "fog"), sleep disturbance, or mood disorder, following either a direct or indirect rapid movement in the brain causing extreme rotational or translational brain acceleration or deceleration injury. Loss of consciousness at the time of impact is not required to make a diagnosis of concussion. Additional symptoms of the time of impact may include transient visual disturbances or spontaneous visual hallucinations, commonly described to "seeing stars."

Concussion can occur by any traumatic etiology including falls from a sufficient height, motor vehicle accidents, nonpenetrating blast injuries in the field of combat, domestic violence, or other physical traumatic events. *Sport-related concussion* (SRC) is defined as a concussion that occurs coincidentally during the play of a contact sport with a high risk of concussion (i.e., American football, soccer [European football], hockey, lacrosse, basketball, wrestling, and rugby, among others) or during combat sports, which are distinguished by having the specific goal of inducing a concussion in the opponent (boxing, mixed martial arts, and related sports). Regardless of the etiology of concussion, the symptoms are largely indistinguishable but may have differing psychosocial factors associated with recovery.

In contrast to other more advanced forms of traumatic brain injury, concussion lacks defining neuroradiologic features such as hemorrhage or other obvious abnormalities on conventional neuroimaging such as computed tomography (CT) or magnetic resonance imaging (MRI). Although several fluid-based biomarkers and electroencephalogram approaches are currently under study, none is presently used in part of standard of care practice. High-field MRI sequences including diffusion tensor imaging and functional MRI (fMRI), among others, hold promise in establishing the diagnosis of concussion or perhaps even subconcussive injuries in serially monitored individuals but these too are not part of current standard of care practice. Given substantial differences in these MRI sequences between individuals, the comparison of an individual against normative values has substantial limitations and thus currently limits the use of diffusion tensor imaging and fMRI principally to research rather than clinical practice.

EPIDEMIOLOGY

The lifetime incidence of single and repeat concussion is not well known but is thought to occur in several million individuals annually in the United States alone. The epidemiology follows a trimodal pattern over lifetime with peaks in the first few months of life, followed by adolescence, and followed by a third peak in the elderly. Contributions to concussion etiology among the very young and very old likely principally relate to accidental falls, whereas concussions in adolescents may relate to risk-taking behaviors involving driving, exposure to violence, as well as exposure to increasingly competitive athletics. The annual incidence of SRC is at least 300,000 in the United States alone, although this is likely an underestimate given poor recognition by affected players. The epidemiology of recurrent concussion is not well described but is thought to happen in a small proportion of players previously affected by SRC.

PATHOBIOLOGY

Given that concussion patients generally have no evidence of structural brain injury using conventional neuroimaging with MRI or CT, concussion has historically been considered a physiologic alteration, but this has become a matter of some debate. Concussion may reflect substantial physiologic disturbance with significant microstructural axonal disruption, which remains difficult to detect but nonetheless occurs. These injuries may be widespread or alternatively relatively focal but involving pathways with major widespread clinical implications. Experimental models suggest metabolic changes including elevated tissue lactate, which peaks over the course of several days followed by gradual recovery of cerebral blood flow within the affected tissues, with most demonstrable changes resolving by 7 to 10 days. In response to rotational or translational shear physical stress, animal histopathologic models of concussion demonstrate disruption of the viscoelastic properties of axons with rare disruption or lysis of axons themselves (Fig. 45.1).

When considering an individual experiencing a single concussion, injury thresholds required to cause concussion are not well understood but are thought to occur following at least 60 g of

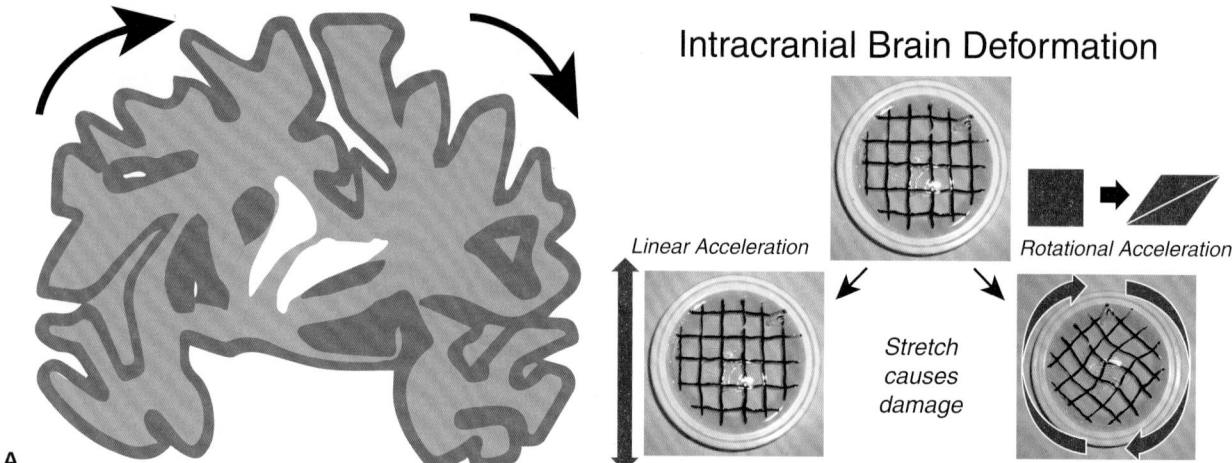

FIGURE 45.1 A: Conceptualized diagram of a human brain in coronal plane demonstrating brain inertia and distortion typical of rotational forces applied to the brain here during blunt impact to the lateral head causing rightward translational and rotational movement (*curved arrowheads* depict rotational force applied to the brain). Among myriad circumstances of brain injury, this example could occur during a hit to the left side of the head in the course of contact sports play. **B:** Physical simulations of intracranial brain deformation in response to linear versus rotational accelerations using 1% gelatin as a brain simulant, which has similar mechanical properties as brain. Linear accelerations cause very little deformation, whereas rotational accelerations induce marked central distortion. (Courtesy of Barclay Morrison, Associate Professor of Biomedical Engineering, Columbia University.)

linear acceleration or at least 2,000 to 4,000 rad/s² rotational acceleration; these forces are seldom if ever experienced in the course of normal daily life outside of recognized physically traumatic events experienced by the affected individuals. At present, risks for concussion occurrence, severity, and recurrence are not well understood but suggest prior traumatic brain injury raises the risk of subsequent concussion. The highly variable nature of concussion expression and recovery raises the possibility of an unrecognized gene–environment risk profile.

DIAGNOSIS

All 50 states of the United States mandate that every individual having experienced a possible or suspected SRC must be evaluated by a licensed practitioner prior to returning to play. In contrast to SRC, in which players in conjunction with team coaches and athletic trainers bring the diagnosis to attention, concussion experienced in other contexts such as motor vehicle accidents or other causes of trauma are often diagnosed at the time that the individual is brought to attention for other matters related to bodily trauma. Although many concussion screening rubrics have been proposed, fundamentally, the diagnosis is based on a clinician's suspicion that concussion has occurred based on neurologic symptoms, which should be typically without significant focal neurologic findings on examination. Any localizing or lateralizing signs or symptoms should prompt a clinician to consider neuroimaging, such as CT if the patient is suspected of having urgently declining neurologic condition or MRI if the patient is being assessed in a nonurgent setting or experiencing unexpectedly prolonged recovery of signs or symptoms following injury.

A number of devices and tools have been suggested to comprise concussion monitoring strategies, including questionnaires, complemented by a range of tests from simple reaction time to automated neuropsychological testing to more formal/conventional neuropsychological testing.

With the exception of formal neuropsychological testing, which has a significant disadvantage as a screening tool given its cost and time required, most if not all, other tests in this field were developed as a tool to assist in sideline assessments by nonmedical staff, with the intention of screening to limit the risk of prematurely returning a player to contact sport. However, they must be interpreted with substantial caution because they cannot supplant formal neurologic evaluation, which may capture subtleties not otherwise recognized on these screening assessments. Current consensus guidelines advocate the use of a standardized screening assessment, such as the Sideline Concussion Assessment Tool (third version) in the context of game play, but the validity of this and other screening tools in clinical contexts remain uncertain, and a comprehensive neurologic assessment should be pursued whenever concussion is suspected. Moreover, some screening assessments are considered normal within a relatively large range of values, are prone to retest bias, and may have limited generalizability beyond a relatively small reference population. Finally, most tests used in serial concussion monitoring programs are susceptible to "gaming" or "sandbagging" by a player eager to return to play, with baseline assessments purposefully performed poorly such that postconcussion assessments may not substantially differ.

TREATMENT

At present, there are no rigorously studied or U.S. Food and Drug Administration–approved medical therapies or physical therapy treatments, which have been clearly proven to hasten recovery following a single concussion or improve lingering postconcussion symptoms. Empiric approaches to concussion treatment among non–sport-related concussion are based on approaches developed for SRC recovery. For SRC, current empirically based guidelines recommend at least 24 hours removal from contact sport following any suspected concussion. Thereafter, players experience a graduated, patient-centered return to play protocol beginning with slow introduction of aerobic, followed by anaerobic exercise leading into full contact drills. Although some practitioners previously advocated for prolonged rest and removal from any potentially cognitively or physically engaging scenarios, such an approach may be more harmful from a psychosocial perspective for young individuals. A return-to-play protocol typically takes place over the course of at least a week following a suspected concussion, predicated on a player not reexperiencing symptoms of concussion as each threshold of activity is gradually approached. Only when a player is symptom-free and off all medications potentially providing a clinical advantage or benefit (including those used for pain relief) is the player considered to have recovered from a concussion.

In addition to strategies to reengage the athlete to playing the sport, a significant amount of attention is placed on young individuals attempting to reengage with the academic and other scholarly activities. This often involves a multimodal treatment approach involving the players, school, and parents in a process referred to as *return to learn*. At each point of contact with a young individual having experienced concussion, clinicians should attempt to assess the player's current level of stamina for athletic and/or cognitively stimulating activities as well as potentially aggravating symptoms such as screen time in the course of computer or cellular telephone use typically used in social and academic settings. These guidelines provide a tool to monitor progress and encourage the individual to be an active participant in the recovery. Approaches to patients affected by concussion in nonsport contexts should follow similar threshold-based, gradual, patient-centered approaches to return to work, social, and professional life.

Retirement from sport or a risky behavior associated with recurrent concussions in an individual patient may be considered in some scenarios; in the context of SRC, this concept is called *medical retirement*. Such a discussion is done in a highly individualized and often challenging manner, balancing factors of patient and family motivation, potential scholarship, or other fiscal incentive to continue playing against an uncertain and highly variable neurologic prognosis. However, this may be an appropriate decision among players who demonstrate progressively lower thresholds of injury required to express concussion, progressively longer neurologic recovery periods following successive concussions, and declining scholarly, neuropsychological, or athletic performance.

OUTCOME

The natural history of a single uncomplicated concussion is not well understood. Based on SRC studies of high school and collegiate athletes involved in contact sports, approximately 80% to 90% of all persons with single uncomplicated concussions will fully recover within several days to 2 weeks. In the short term, approximately 10% to 20% of individuals with concussion will have a prolonged recovery—longer than 1 to 2 weeks and occasionally up to several months. Symptoms lingering beyond this time frame raise the possibility of a preexistent or superimposed neuropsychological condition including a mood disorder or premorbid migraine headaches. Some studies have suggested that recurrent concussions portend to a more prolonged recovery, with decreasing threshold of injury in some being associated with subsequent concussion.

Following head trauma of any kind, including concussion, patients may be more likely to express migraine headaches, mood disorders, or benign paroxysmal positional vertigo, given likely contribution of the impact to canalithiasis. At present, no evidence exists to treat these individuals any differently than would a patient

be treated with these diagnoses as primary or nontraumatic disorders. However, some patients experiencing several lingering symptoms or syndromes may be best served by using therapies which offer treatment impact in multiple modalities through a relatively simple regimen.

The long-term risks and outcomes associated with single uncomplicated concussion are not well known but are thought to be associated with an increased risk of dementia if concussion is associated with loss of consciousness, particularly among apolipoprotein E4 carriers. Studies of apolipoprotein E4 are limited but have not identified differences in concussion risk or recovery based on carrier status. Although single uncomplicated concussion is considered a mild traumatic brain injury, recurrent concussions have been associated with significantly increased likelihood of developing major neuropsychiatric disorders associated with aging, including depression, dementia, Parkinson disease, amyotrophic lateral sclerosis, and erratic psychosocial behaviors including drug abuse and suicide, thus significantly impacting the quality of life of many affected individuals and their families.

One reason for the mandatory removal from play for a suspected concussion and graduated return to play thereafter is based on concern for a rare yet clearly defined neurologic syndrome called *second impact syndrome*. The disease has been identified exclusively among individuals who have returned to sports or had a second concussion prior to complete recovery from the first concussion, even if the two events are separated by days. The pathophysiology of second impact syndrome is not well understood but appears to involve severe, aggressive, and often medically refractory focal or whole brain edema following the second concussion.

CHRONIC TRAUMATIC ENCEPHALOPATHY

Chronic traumatic encephalopathy (CTE) is a term used to describe the long-term neurodegenerative syndrome that arises following mild yet repetitive traumatic brain injury. CTE was initially called *punch drunk* and later *dementia pugilistica* in light of its long established association with boxing. CTE can arise in any individual with repetitive concussive or subconcussive injuries (e.g., victims of domestic violence and psychiatric patients exhibiting head-banging behavior), but athletes who have participated in contact and/or combat sports have received the most attention. Military veterans represent another at risk population that has been increasingly studied. Furthermore, some veterans with a clinical diagnosis of posttraumatic stress disorder have been found to have CTE at autopsy, suggesting a potential overlap between these conditions.

CTE is associated with a spectrum of personality and behavioral changes, depression, increased suicidal behavior, memory loss, and cognitive dysfunction. The clinical spectrum of CTE is broad, and the full extent of the symptomatology awaits larger autopsy series, but recent research suggests that CTE has two clinical variants. The first is a *behavioral/mood variant* with features that develop at a younger age. The other is a *cognitive variant* that arises at an older age. Movement disorders, including parkinsonism, are also common. Further, it is not uncommon to observe motor neuron disease in CTE patients; this is referred to as *chronic traumatic encephalomyelopathy*. Dementia, parkinsonism, and motor neuron disease can occur singly or collectively in a single patient. Cognitive decline may be similar clinically to Alzheimer disease or frontotemporal dementia. Suicide has emerged as a cause of death among several former elite athletes, including in a period prior to recently increased CTE awareness, yet its epidemiology is not well understood.

Most CTE cases are thought to progress over decades. Manifestations of neurologic decline typically begin years after cessation of exposure to high-risk sports or recognized head injury, although some athletes have quit after developing chronic cognitive problems in the context of ongoing competitive play. Whether these changes signal active clinical manifestations of CTE is of great debate because no validated in vivo biomarkers currently exist.

The epidemiology of chronic traumatic encephalopathy is not well established given the lack for formalized diagnostic criteria and the similarities with other sporadic neurodegenerative diseases. This is even so in known high-risk combat sports such as boxing where to date, only case series have been published, followed by more recent series involving participants in contact sports such as football, hockey, baseball, and soccer as well as combat military veterans. Case reports also exist among domestic violence victims. A recent case series of professional football players from a highly selected population of families and individuals concerned about major neurobehavioral changes identified CTE in the vast majority of subjects. Despite potential for bias, for all known professional American football brain autopsies in 2011, all 12 exhibited neuropathologic signatures of CTE. Thus, among a total of 321 professional football player deaths in the same year, most presumably without dementia, a minimum of 3.7% had neuropathologic defined CTE at death. Several young football players with neuropathologically defined early-stage CTE, who died for unrelated causes, have had no recognizable neurologic or psychiatric symptoms. However, a growing concern is that it may have substantial clinical sequelae when advanced neuropathologic changes are present. To date, the disease has not been recognized in the absence of head trauma, although the threshold of risk (how much and how severe injury is required to cause CTE) remains uncertain. Also, whether a single traumatic brain injury can trigger CTE is not known.

The pathogenesis of CTE is currently under investigation. Physical trauma is thought to lead to mechanical stress in the acute setting, shearing cellular structures (e.g., axons, dendrites, synaptic connections, glial processes, and blood vessels), resulting in cognitive impairment, or postconcussive syndrome. Associated molecular changes with acute trauma include elevation of amyloid precursor protein and other proteins. Repetitive injury may progress to neurodegeneration, sometimes many years later. Gross brain changes are nonspecific but include brain atrophy and a cavum septum pellucidum. Microscopically, CTE patients exhibit massive accumulation of abnormal aggregates containing hyperphosphorylated forms of the microtubule-associated protein tau. Tau pathology is present in neurons and glia. As many as 85% of CTE patients also exhibit accumulation of 43 kDa TAR DNA–binding protein, the primary disease protein in amyotrophic lateral sclerosis. Amyloid plaques that are characteristic of Alzheimer disease and α-synuclein–positive inclusions of Parkinson disease can also be observed but are not prominent. The abnormal tau inclusions develop in a distinctive pattern that reflects the biomechanical characteristics of the injury, including focally in perivascular spaces and at the recess of sulci, a region that can display injury acutely in traumatic brain injury (Fig. 45.2). Additional findings include subcortical axonal varicosities and axonal loss.

Finally, given the distinctly known and highly preventable risk factor of head injury leading to concussion and presumably CTE in combat sports and perhaps also in contact sports, a substantial ethical and moral dilemma is raised by this spectrum of disease. Although many professional groups, including neurologists, have advocated for banning boxing, most likely public interest in these

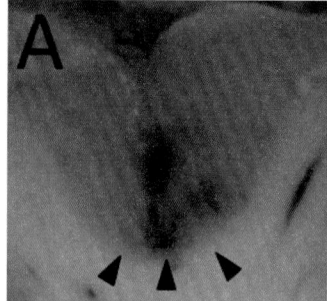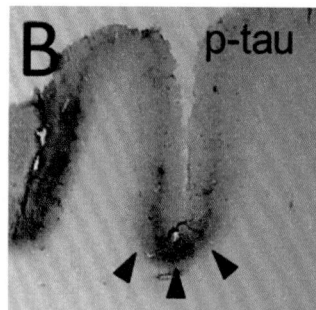

FIGURE 45.2 Regional vulnerability following traumatic brain injury. **A:** Contusions can be demonstrated grossly in the depths of the neocortical sulci after acute traumatic brain injury (*arrowheads*). **B:** Immunohistochemistry using antisera that specifically target abnormal hyperphosphorylated tau reveals a predilection for the neocortical sulci (*arrowheads*) in a retired professional football player with chronic traumatic encephalopathy. (B courtesy of Dr. Ann McKee, Boston University.)

sports will persist. Historical accounts suggest an increased risk of death during time periods when sports like these are banned yet persist in an underground or unsanctioned manner without the involvement of neurologists or colleagues in supervision or consultation. Until such time that the appetite of the general public wanes to the point of self-discontinuation of these sports, neurologists will continue to have an important role in combat sports and high-risk contact sports in helping shape public knowledge and better understanding near and long-term personalized risks for the individual athlete.

SUGGESTED READINGS

Breedlove EL, Robinson M, Talavage TM, et al. Biomechanical correlates of symptomatic and asymptomatic neurophysiological impairment in high school football. *J Biomech.* 2012;45(7):1265–1272.

Bruns J Jr, Hauser WA. The epidemiology of traumatic brain injury: a review. *Epilepsia.* 2003;44(suppl 10):2–10.

Cantu RC. The role of the neurologist in concussions: when to tell your patient to stop. *JAMA Neurol.* 2013;70(12):1481–1482.

Centers for Disease Control and Prevention. Nonfatal traumatic brain injuries related to sports and recreation activities among persons aged ≤19 years—United States, 2001–2009. *MMWR Morb Mortal Wkly Rep.* 2011;60(39):1337–1342.

Corsellis JA, Bruton CJ, Freeman-Browne D. The aftermath of boxing. *Psychol Med.* 1973;3(3):270–303.

Gavett BE, Stern RA, McKee AC. Chronic traumatic encephalopathy: a potential late effect of sport-related concussive and subconcussive head trauma. *Clin Sports Med.* 2011;30(1):179–188.

Giza CC, Hovda DA. The neurometabolic cascade of concussion. *J Athl Train.* 2001;36(3):228–235.

Giza CC, Kutcher JS, Ashwal S, et al. Summary of evidence-based guideline update: evaluation and management of concussion in sports: report of the Guideline Development Subcommittee of the American Academy of Neurology. *Neurology.* 2013;80(24):2250–2257.

Guskiewicz KM, Register-Mihalik J, McCrory P, et al. Evidence-based approach to revising the SCAT2: introducing the SCAT3. *Br J Sports Med.* 2013;47(5):289–293

Halstead ME, McAvoy K, Devore CD, et al. Returning to learning following a concussion. *Pediatrics.* 2013;132(5):948–957.

Holbourn AHS. Mechanics of head injuries. *Lancet.* 1943;242(6267):438–441.

Institute of Medicine, National Research Council. *Sports-Related Concussions In Youth: Improving The Science, Changing The Culture*. Washington, DC: The National Academies Press; 2013.

Lehman EJ, Hein MJ, Baron SL, et al. Neurodegenerative causes of death among retired National Football League players. *Neurology*. 2012;79(19):1970–1974.

Martland HS. Punch drunk. *JAMA*. 1928;91(15):1103–1107.

Martland HS, Beling CC. Traumatic cerebral hemorrhage. *Arch NeurPsych*. 1929;22(5):1001–1023.

Mayeux R, Ottman R, Maestre G, et al. Synergistic effects of traumatic head injury and apolipoprotein-epsilon 4 in patients with Alzheimer's disease. *Neurology*. 1995;45(3, pt 1):555–557.

McCrory P, Meeuwisse WH, Aubry M, et al. Consensus statement on concussion in sport: the 4th International Conference on Concussion in Sport held in Zurich, November 2012. *Br J Sports Med*. 2013;47(5):250–258.

McKee AC, Stern RA, Nowinski CJ, et al. The spectrum of disease in chronic traumatic encephalopathy. *Brain*. 2013;136(pt 1):43–64.

Moeller JJ, Tu B, Bazil CW. Quantitative and qualitative analysis of ambulatory electroencephalography during mild traumatic brain injury. *Arch Neurol*. 2012;68(12):1595–1598.

Murugavel M, Cubon V, Putukian M, et al. A longitudinal diffusion tensor imaging study assessing white matter fiber tracts after sports related concussion. *J Neurotrauma*. 2014;31(22):1860–1871.

Noble JM, Hesdorffer DC. Sport-related concussions: a review of epidemiology, challenges in diagnosis, and potential risk factors. *Neuropsychol Rev*. 2013;23(4):273–284.

Rigg JL, Mooney SR. Concussions and the military: issues specific to service members. *PM R*. 2011;3(10)(suppl 2):S380–S386.

Rowson S, Duma SM, Beckwith JG, et al. Rotational head kinematics in football impacts: an injury risk function for concussion. *Ann Biomed Eng*. 2012;40(1):1–13.

SCAT3. *Br J Sports Med*. 2013;47(5):259.

Shahim P, Tegner Y, Wilson DH, et al. Blood biomarkers for brain injury in concussed professional ice hockey players. *JAMA Neurol*. 2014;71(5):684–692.

Weinstein E, Turner M, Kuzma BB, et al. Second impact syndrome in football: new imaging and insights into a rare and devastating condition. *J Neurosurg Pediatr*. 2013;11(3):331–334.

Zhang L, Yang KH, King AL. A proposed injury threshold for mild traumatic brain injury. *J Biomech Eng*. 2004;126(2):226–236.

Traumatic Brain Injury 46

Neeraj Badjatia, Gunjan Y. Parikh, and Stephan A. Mayer

EPIDEMIOLOGY

Traumatic brain injury (TBI) is a modern scourge of industrialized society. It is a major cause of death, especially in young adults, and a major cause of disability. The costs in human misery and dollars are exceeded by few other conditions.

More than 2 million patients with head injuries are seen annually in U.S. emergency rooms, and 25% of these patients are admitted to a hospital. In general, total combined rates for TBI-related emergency department (ED) visits, hospitalizations, and deaths have increased over the past decade. Almost 10% of all deaths in the United States are caused by injury, and about half of the traumatic deaths involve the brain. In the United States, a head injury occurs every 7 seconds and a death every 5 minutes. About 200,000 people are killed or permanently disabled annually as a result.

Brain injuries occur at all ages, but the peak is in young adults between the ages of 15 and 24 years. Head injury is the leading cause of death among people younger than the age of 24 years. There is, however, a trend toward an increase of mortality rates from TBI among populations aged older than 65 years over the past decade. It is anticipated that this trend will continue as the overall population ages. Men are affected three or four times as often as women. The major causes of brain injury differ in different parts of the United States; in all areas, motor vehicle accidents are prominent, and in metropolitan areas, personal violence is prevalent.

PATHOBIOLOGY

SKULL FRACTURES

Skull fractures may be divided into linear, depressed, or comminuted types. If the scalp is lacerated over the fracture, it is considered an open or *compound fracture*. Skull fractures are important markers of a possibly serious injury but rarely cause problems by themselves; prognosis depends more on the nature and severity of injury to the brain than on the severity of injury to the skull.

About 80% of fractures are linear. They occur most commonly in the temporoparietal region, where the skull is thinnest. Detection of a linear fracture often raises the suspicion of serious brain injury, but computed tomography (CT) in most patients is otherwise normal. Nondisplaced, linear skull fractures generally do not require surgery and can be managed conservatively.

In *depressed fracture* of the skull, one or more fragments of bone are displaced inward, compressing the underlying brain. In comminuted fracture, there are multiple, shattered bone fragments, which may or may not be displaced. In 85% of cases, depressed fractures are open (or "compound") and liable to become infected or leak cerebrospinal fluid (CSF). Even when closed, most depressed or comminuted fractures require surgical exploration for debridement, elevation of bone fragments, and repair of dural lacerations.

The underlying brain is injured in many cases. In some patients, depressed skull fractures are associated with tearing, compression, or thrombosis of underlying venous dural sinuses.

Basilar skull fractures may be linear, depressed, or comminuted. They are frequently missed by standard skull x-rays and are best identified by CT bone windows. There may be associated cranial nerve injury or a dural tear adjacent to the fracture site, which may lead to delayed meningitis if bacteria enter the subarachnoid space. Signs that lead the physician to suspect a fracture of the petrous portion of the temporal bone include hemotympanum or tympanic perforation, hearing loss, CSF otorrhea, peripheral facial nerve weakness, or ecchymosis of the scalp overlying the mastoid process (Battle sign). Anosmia, bilateral periorbital ecchymosis, and CSF rhinorrhea suggest possible fracture of the sphenoid, frontal, or ethmoid bones.

CEREBRAL CONCUSSION AND AXONAL-SHEARING INJURY

Loss of consciousness at the moment of impact is caused by acceleration–deceleration movements of the head, which result in the stretching and shearing of axons. When the alteration of consciousness is brief (e.g., <6 hours), the term *concussion* is used. These patients may be completely unconscious or remain awake but appear dazed; most recover within seconds or minutes, rather than hours, and some have retrograde or anterograde amnesia surrounding the event.

The mechanism by which concussion leads to loss of consciousness is believed to be transient functional disruption of the reticular activating system caused by rotational forces on the upper brain stem. Experimentally, sudden and violent head rotation may produce concussion without impact to the head. Most patients with concussion have normal CT or magnetic resonance imaging (MRI) findings because concussion results from physiologic, rather than structural, injury to the brain. Only 5% of patients who have sustained a concussion and are otherwise intact have an intracranial hemorrhage on CT.

The term *diffuse axonal injury* (DAI) is applied to traumatic coma lasting more than 6 hours. In these cases, when no other cause of coma is identified by CT or MRI, it is presumed that widespread microscopic and macroscopic axonal-shearing injury has occurred. Coma of 6 to 24 hours duration is deemed mild DAI; coma lasting more than 24 hours is considered moderate or severe DAI, depending on the absence or presence of brain stem signs, such as decorticate or decerebrate posturing (Table 46.1).

Autonomic dysfunction (e.g., hypertension, hyperhidrosis, hyperpyrexia) is common in patients with acute severe DAI and may reflect brain stem or hypothalamic injury. Patients may remain unconscious for days, months, or years, and those who recover may be left with severe cognitive and motor impairment, including spasticity and ataxia. DAI is considered the single most important cause of persistent disability after traumatic brain damage.

TABLE 46.1 Clinical Characteristics and Outcome of Diffuse Brain Injuries

	Mild Concussion	Cerebral Contusion	Diffuse Axonal Injury		
			Mild	Moderate	Severe
Loss of consciousness	None	Immediate	Immediate	Immediate	Immediate
Length of unconsciousness	None	<6 h	6–24 h	>24 h	Days to weeks
Decerebrate posturing	None	None	Rare	Occasionally	Present
Posttraumatic amnesia	Minutes	Minutes to hours	Hours	Days	Weeks
Memory deficit	None	Mild	Mild to moderate	Mild to moderate	Severe
Motor deficits	None	None	None	Mild	Severe
Outcome at 3 mo (%)					
Good recovery	100	95	63	38	15
Moderate deficit	0	5	15	21	13
Severe deficit	0	0	6	12	14
Vegetative	0	0	1	5	7
Death	0	0	15	24	51

Adapted from Gennarelli TA. Cerebral concussion and diffuse brain injuries. In: Cooper PR, ed. *Head Injury*. 3rd ed. Baltimore: Williams & Wilkins; 1993:140.

Axonal-shearing injury tends to be most severe in specific brain regions that are anatomically predisposed to maximal stress from rotational forces. Macroscopic tissue tears, best visualized by MRI, tend to occur in midline structures, including the dorsolateral midbrain and pons, posterior corpus callosum, parasagittal white matter, periventricular regions, and internal capsule. Microscopic damage occurs more diffusely, as manifested by axonal retraction bulbs throughout the white matter of the cerebral hemispheres. Prolonged loss of consciousness from DAI tends to be associated with bilateral, asymmetric, focal lesions of the midbrain tegmentum, a region densely populated with reticular activating system neurons. Small hemorrhages, known as *gliding contusions*, are sometimes associated with focal-shearing lesions (Fig. 46.1).

Axonal shearing is thought to initiate a dynamic sequence of pathologic events that evolve over days to weeks. Initially, injury causes physical transection of some neurons and internal axonal damage to many others. In both cases, the process of axoplasmic transport continues, and materials flow from the cell body to the site of damage. These materials accumulate and may lead to secondary axonal transection, with formation of a "retraction ball" from 12 hours to several days after the injury. Membrane channels may open to admit toxic levels of calcium. If the patient survives, MRI may demonstrate chronic atrophy of involved white matter tracts (wallerian degeneration) and gliosis.

BRAIN SWELLING AND CEREBRAL EDEMA

Brain swelling after head injury is a poorly understood phenomenon that may result from several different mechanisms. Posttraumatic brain swelling may result from *cerebral edema* (e.g., an increase in the content of extravascular brain water), an increase in cerebral blood volume (CBV) resulting from abnormal vasodilatation, or both. Cerebral edema may be further classified as cytotoxic, vasogenic, or interstitial (see Chapter 107). The swelling may be diffuse or focal, adjacent to a parenchymal or extradural hemorrhage, or related to contusion or infarction.

Brain swelling may follow any type of head injury. Curiously, the magnitude of swelling does not always correlate well with the severity of injury. In some cases, particularly in young people, severe diffuse brain swelling that may be fatal occurs minutes to hours after a minor concussion. Abnormal dilation of the cerebral blood vessels is thought to lead to increased CBV, hyperperfusion, and increased vascular permeability, resulting in secondary leakage of plasma and vasogenic cerebral edema. Cerebral blood flow studies indicate that after an initial period of hypoperfusion within the first 24 hours, hyperemia occurs in nearly all patients 1 to 3 days after severe head injury, followed less commonly by arterial vasospasm between days 4 and 7. Severe brain swelling may be related to local endothelial and microcirculatory dysfunction or from damage to cerebral vasomotor regulatory centers in the brain stem.

PARENCHYMAL CONTUSION AND HEMORRHAGE

Cerebral *contusions* are focal parenchymal hemorrhages that result from scraping and bruising of the brain as it moves across the inner surface of the skull. The inferior frontal and temporal lobes, where brain tissue comes in contact with irregular protuberances at the base of the skull, are the most common sites of traumatic contusion (Fig. 46.2). Linear tears of the meninges or cerebral tissue, usually a result of cuts from the sharp edges of depressed skull fragments, are called *lacerations*.

Hemorrhagic contusions may occur at the site of a skull fracture but more often occur without a fracture and with the overlying pia and arachnoid left intact. In most patients, contusions are small and multiple. With lateral forces, contusions may occur at the site of the blow to the head (coup lesions) or at the opposite pole as the brain impacts on the inner table of the skull (contrecoup lesions). Contusions frequently enlarge over 12 to 24 hours, especially in the setting of coagulopathy. In some cases, contusions appear in delayed fashion 1 or more days after injury.

When rotational forces lead to tearing of small- or medium-sized vessels within the parenchyma, an intracerebral *hematoma* may occur (Fig. 46.3). Hematomas are focal collections of blood clots that displace the brain, in contrast to contusions, which resemble bruised and bloodied brain tissue (Fig. 46.4). Most

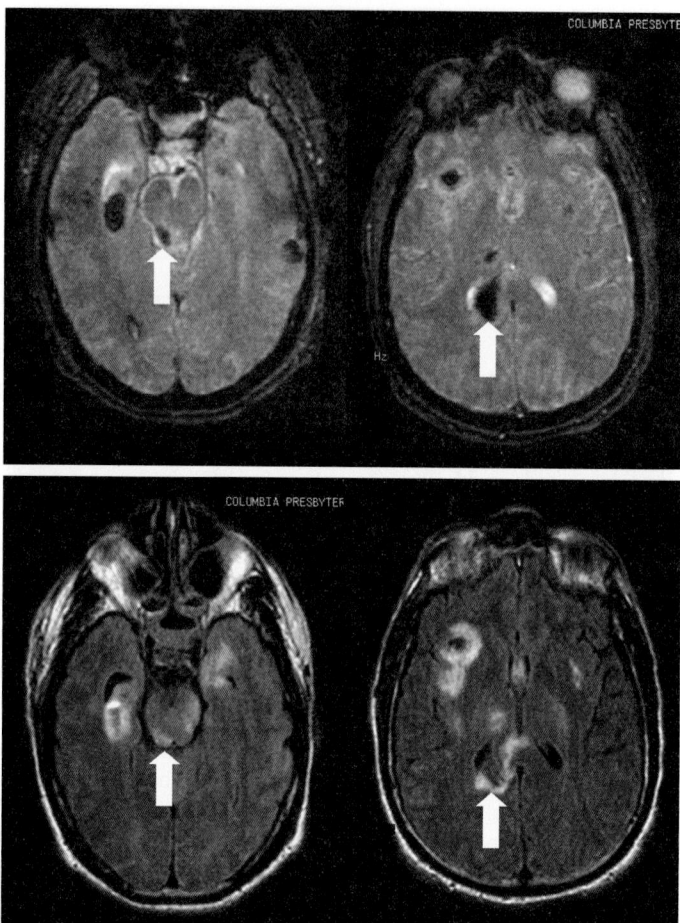

FIGURE 46.1 Focal MRI findings characteristic of diffuse axonal-shearing injury after neurotrauma. **Top:** Gradient echo (T2*) images demonstrating hemorrhagic lesions (gliding contusions) of the right dorsolateral midbrain and splenium of the corpus callosum. **Bottom:** FLAIR images showing edema in these regions.

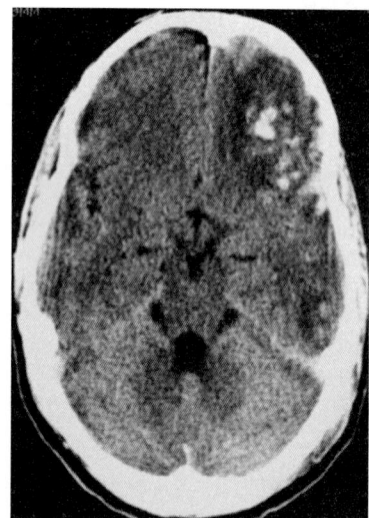

FIGURE 46.2 Traumatic contusions. Axial noncontrast view demonstrates areas of contusion with small focal hemorrhages involving the lower poles of the left frontal and temporal lobes adjacent to the rough cranial vault. (Courtesy of Drs. S. K. Hilal, J. A. Bello, and T. L. Chi.)

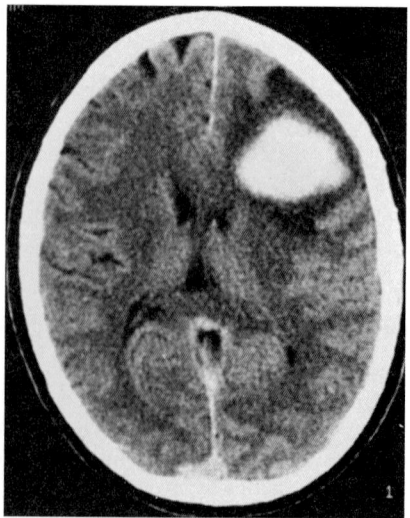

FIGURE 46.3 Traumatic intracerebral hemorrhage, frontal lobe. Axial noncontrast computed tomography demonstrates left frontal lobe density (hemorrhage), surrounding lucency (edema), and mass effect (sulcal and ventricular effacement). (Courtesy of Drs. S. K. Hilal and J. A. Bello.)

FIGURE 46.4 Pathologic specimen demonstrating traumatic contusions in the temporal lobes.

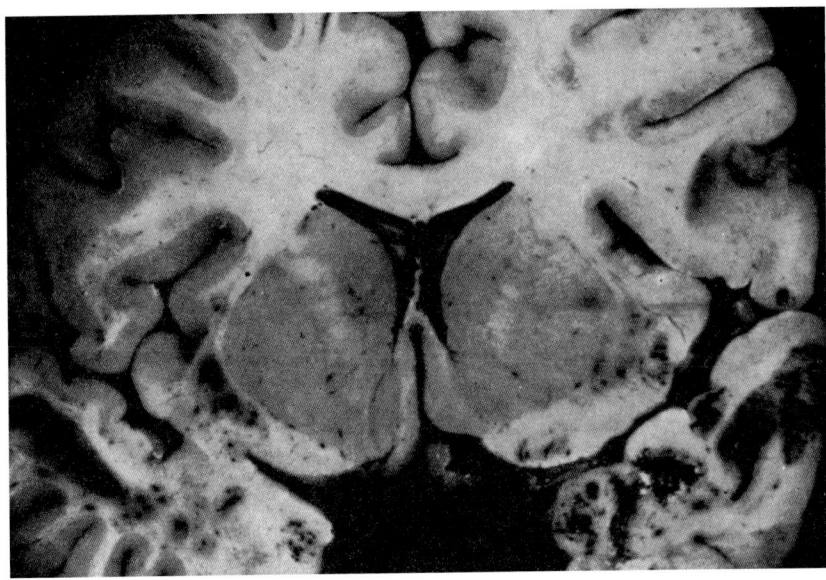

parenchymal hematomas are located in the deep white matter, in contrast to contusions, which tend to be cortical.

If there is no DAI, brain swelling, or secondary hemorrhage, recovery from one or more small contusions may be excellent. Healed contusions are often found at autopsy of people with no clinical evidence of permanent brain damage. Large, parenchymal hematomas with mass effect may require surgical evacuation.

Contusions are often managed conservatively unless they lead to significant symptomatic mass effect because they often consist of hemorrhagic or ecchymotic (but potentially viable) brain tissue.

SUBDURAL HEMATOMA

Subdural hematomas usually arise from a venous source, with blood filling the potential space between the dural and arachnoid membranes. In most cases, the bleeding is caused by movements of the brain within the skull that leads to stretching and tearing of "bridging" veins that drain from the surface of the brain to the dural sinuses.

Most subdural hematomas are located over the lateral cerebral convexities, but subdural blood may also collect along the medial surface of the hemisphere, between the tentorium and occipital lobe, between the temporal lobe and the base of the skull, or in the posterior fossa. CT usually reveals a high-density, crescentic collection across the entire hemispheric convexity (Fig. 46.5).

Elderly or alcoholic patients with cerebral atrophy are particularly prone to subdural bleeding; in these patients, large hematomas may result from trivial impact or even from pure acceleration–deceleration injuries, such as whiplash. Coagulopathy, including the use of oral anticoagulants, is another important risk factor for subdural hematoma and is associated with increased mortality.

Acute subdural hematomas, by definition, are symptomatic within 72 hours of injury, but most patients have neurologic symptoms from the moment of impact. They may occur after any type of head injury but seem to be less common after vehicular trauma and relatively more common after falls or assaults. Half of all patients with an acute subdural hematoma lose consciousness at the time of injury; 25% are in coma when they arrive at the hospital, and half of those who awaken lose consciousness for a second time after a "lucid interval" of minutes to hours as the subdural hematoma grows in size. Hemiparesis and pupillary abnormalities are the most common focal neurologic signs, each occurring in one-half

to two-thirds of patients. The usual picture is ipsilateral pupillary dilation and contralateral hemiparesis. However, so-called false localizing signs are common with acute subdural hematoma because uncal herniation may lead to compression of the contralateral cerebral peduncle or third cranial nerve against the tentorial edge (*Kernohan notch*).

Chronic subdural hematomas become symptomatic after 21 days. They are more likely to occur in patients after age 50 years. In 25% to 50% of cases, there is no recognized episode of head injury. Risk factors for chronic subdural hematomas include cerebral atrophy, alcoholism, bleeding disorders or use of anticoagulant medication, and overdrainage of a ventriculoperitoneal shunt.

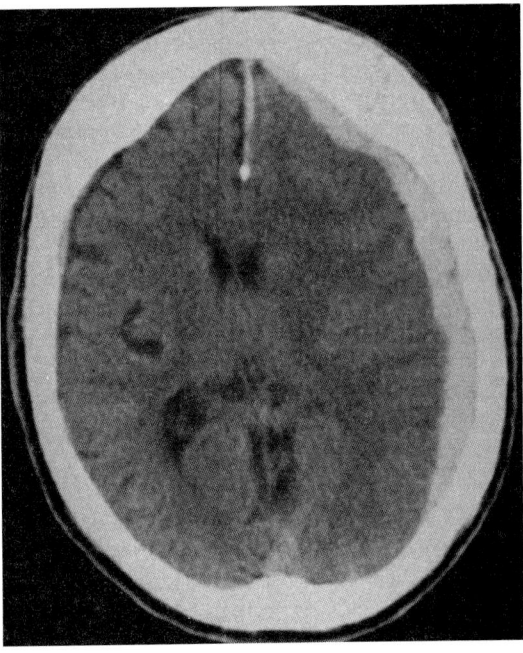

FIGURE 46.5 Acute subdural hematoma. Noncontrast axial CT demonstrates a hyperdense, crescent-shaped, extra-axial collection showing mass effect (sulcal and ventricular effacement) and midline shift from left to right. (Courtesy of Drs. J. A. Bello and S. K. Hilal.)

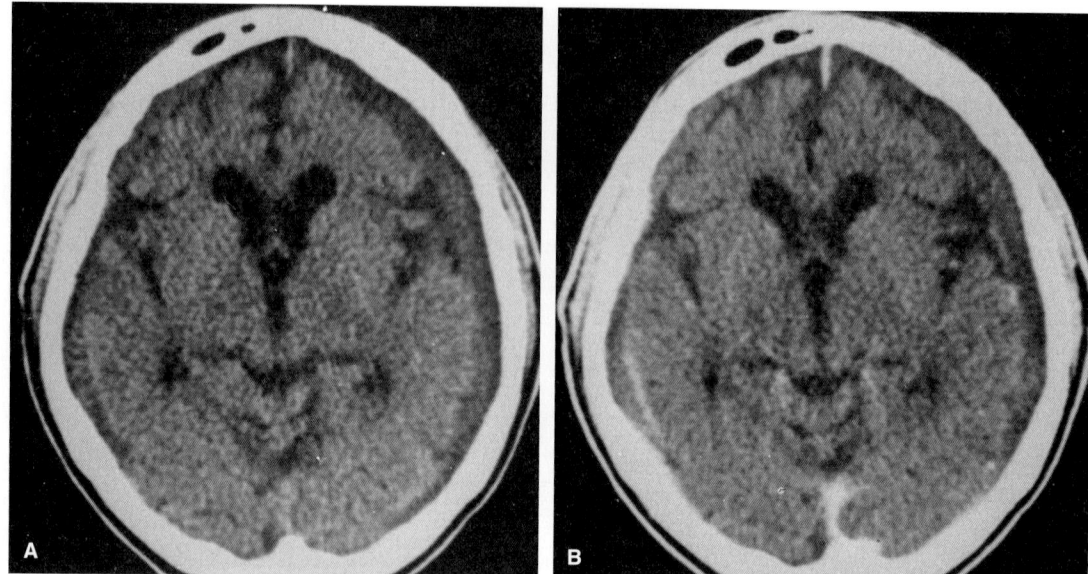

FIGURE 46.6 Bilateral chronic subdural hematoma. **A:** Noncontrast axial CT shows bilateral isodense extra-axial collections, larger on the left. **B:** These are better demonstrated on the postcontrast scan, in which enhancing membranes, typical of the subacute phase, may be seen. (Courtesy of Drs. J. A. Bello and S. K. Hilal.)

In many cases of chronic subdural hematoma, bleeding results from trivial trauma, and symptoms are minimal because the brain accommodates the gradual buildup of mass effect. After 1 week, fibroblasts on the inner surface of the dura form a thick outer membrane; after 2 weeks, a thin inner membrane develops, resulting in encapsulation of the clot, which eventually liquefies into a *hygroma*. Enlargement of the hematoma may then result from recurrent bleeding (acute-on-chronic subdural hematoma) or because of osmotic effects related to a high-protein content of the fluid. Symptoms may be restricted to altered mental status, a syndrome sometimes mistaken for dementia. CT typically shows an isodense or hypodense, crescent-shaped mass that deforms the surface of the brain, and the membranes may enhance with intravenous (IV) contrast (Fig. 46.6).

Symptomatic acute and chronic subdural hematomas with significant mass effect should be evacuated. Surgical evacuation of the thick, clotted blood that constitutes an acute subdural hematoma usually requires a large-window craniotomy. Outcome after surgical evacuation depends primarily on the severity of the initial deficit and the interval from injury to surgery. Liquefied chronic subdural hematomas are usually evacuated with drainage of the collections via a series of burr holes. Reoperations for acute and chronic subdural hematomas are required in about 15% of cases. Steroids have no role in the conservative management of smaller, minimally symptomatic, subdural hematomas.

EPIDURAL HEMATOMA

Epidural hematoma is a rare complication of head injury. It occurs in less than 1% of all cases but is found in 5% to 15% of autopsy series, attesting to the potential seriousness of this complication.

Bleeding into the epidural space is generally caused by a tear in the wall of one of the meningeal arteries, usually the middle meningeal artery, but in 15% of patients, the bleeding arises from a dural sinus. Seventy-five percent of patients are associated with a skull fracture. The dura is separated from the skull by the extravasated blood, and the size of the clot increases until the ruptured vessel is compressed or occluded by the hematoma.

Most epidural hematomas are located over the convexity of the hemisphere in the middle cranial fossa, but occasionally, hemorrhages may be confined to the anterior fossa, possibly as a result of tearing of anterior meningeal arteries. Extradural hemorrhage in the posterior fossa may occur when the torcular herophili is torn. In most cases, the hematoma is ipsilateral to the site of impact.

Epidural hematoma is primarily a problem of young adults; it is rarely seen in the elderly because the dura becomes increasingly adherent to the skull with advanced age. The clinical course, in one-third of patients, proceeds from an immediate loss of consciousness caused by concussion to a lucid interval and then to a relapse into coma, with hemiplegia as the epidural hematoma expands. The ipsilateral pupil loses reactivity to light because the third cranial nerve is stretched as the midbrain is displaced contralaterally. Later, it becomes fixed and dilated as the third nerve is compressed by the hippocampal gyrus as it herniates over the free edge of the tentorium.

As with acute subdural hematomas, false localizing signs may occur. The presence of cerebellar signs, nuchal rigidity, and drowsiness, together with a fracture of the occipital bone, should prompt suspicion of a clot in the posterior fossa.

Epidural blood takes on a bulging convex pattern on CT (Fig. 46.7) because the collection is limited by firm attachments from the dura to the cranial sutures. Progression to herniation and death may occur rapidly because the bleeding is arterial. The mortality rate approaches 100% in untreated patients and ranges from 5% to 30% in treated patients. As the interval between injury and surgical intervention decreases, survival improves. If there is little coexisting brain damage, functional recovery may be excellent.

TRAUMATIC SUBARACHNOID HEMORRHAGE

Some extravasation of blood into the subarachnoid spaces is to be expected in any patient with head injury. In most cases, subarachnoid blood is detected only by CSF examination and is of little clinical importance. With more serious injuries, when larger vessels traversing the subarachnoid space are torn, focal or diffuse

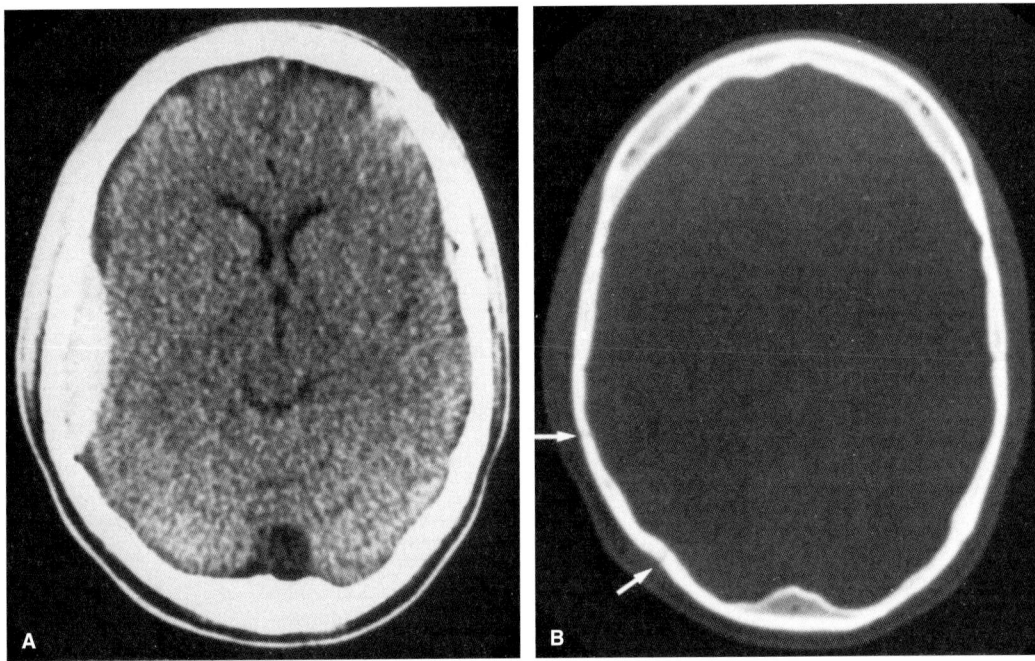

FIGURE 46.7 A: Epidural hematoma is evident on CT. **B:** CT with bone windows shows two adjacent fractures (*arrows*); the anterior fracture is at the site of the groove for the middle meningeal artery.

subarachnoid hemorrhage may be detected by CT. In most cases, traumatic subarachnoid hemorrhage is distributed over the convexities. By contrast, spontaneous aneurysmal rupture results in bleeding into the basal cisterns. Although the presence of a large amount of subarachnoid blood is a poor prognostic sign, delayed complications of aneurysmal subarachnoid hemorrhage, such as hydrocephalus and ischemia from vasospasm, are unusual after traumatic subarachnoid hemorrhage.

INITIAL ASSESSMENT AND STABILIZATION

On admission to the emergency room, resuscitation measures, history taking, and examination should begin simultaneously. The immediate goals of management are to assess and stabilize the airway, breathing, circulation, and disability (ABCD). The immediate goals of the initial neurologic assessment are to (1) perform a rapid screening neurologic examination; (2) classify the severity of the head injury as low, moderate, or high risk; (3) stabilize and rule out a fracture of the cervical spine; (4) begin empiric treatment for increased intracranial pressure (ICP) if it is suspected; and (5) perform an emergency CT scan of the head and neck to rule out bony fractures or intracranial bleeding. Careful screening at this time is also required to identify significant extracranial injuries.

CARDIOPULMONARY RESUSCITATION

Hypoxia and *hypotension* have a devastating effect on head-injured patients. If the patient is hypoxic (arterial oxygen saturation level <90%), in respiratory distress, or comatose and unable to protect his or her airway, endotracheal intubation should be performed urgently to be certain that the spine is immobilized during the procedure. Two doses of peri-intubation cefuroxime (1.5 g) may reduce the risk of subsequent pneumonia. Minute ventilation should initially be set to maintain a tidal volume of 6 mL/kg and rate of 8 to 12 breaths per minute, with the goal of maintaining the PCO_2 between 30 and 40 mm Hg. The fraction of inspired oxygen can

be quickly reduced from 100% to 40% as long as oxygen saturation levels are above 95%. Prophylactic aggressive hyperventilation (PCO_2 <25 mm Hg) during the acute stage of injury may cause excessive vasoconstriction and aggravation of ischemic injury and is contraindicated.

Hypotension (systolic blood pressure [BP] <90 mm Hg) should be corrected with large-volume IV infusions of isotonic fluids such as normal saline or lactated Ringer solution (10 to 40 mL/kg) and blood transfusions or vasopressors as needed. Systolic BP during the stabilization phase should be maintained above 90 mm Hg to ensure adequate cerebral blood flow. If the patient is hypotensive, bleeding into the abdomen, thorax, retroperitoneal space, or tissues surrounding a long-bone fracture should be excluded by CT. Hypotension may also reflect *spinal shock* related to a coexisting spinal cord injury (see Chapter 47). Hypertension associated with wide pulse pressure and bradycardia (Cushing reflex) may reflect increased ICP or focal brain stem injury.

INITIAL NEUROLOGIC ASSESSMENT AND STABILIZATION

A baseline neurologic evaluation should be performed immediately while airway, respiration, and circulation are assessed. Injuries may be ranked as low, moderate, or high risk according to risk factors and a rapid initial neurologic assessment (Table 46.2). The skull should be palpated for fractures, hematomas, and lacerations. A step-off or palpable bony shelf is presumed to be a depressed skull fracture. A hard neck collar should be in place for all patients with any history of concussion, whiplash, or trauma above the level of the clavicles.

The Glasgow Coma Scale (GCS; Table 46.3) is based on eye opening and the patient's best verbal and motor responses; these three individual scores should be recorded separately. The GCS is widely used as a semiquantitative clinical measure of the severity of brain injury; it also provides a guide to prognosis (Table 46.4). Patients who are comatose (GCS score ≤8), or

TABLE 46.2 Risk Stratification of Patients with Head Injury

Risk Category	Characteristics
Mild	• Normal neurologic examination
	• No concussion
	• No drug or alcohol intoxication
	• May complain of headache and dizziness
	• May have scalp abrasion, laceration, or hematoma
	• Absence of moderate or severe injury criteria
Moderate	• Glasgow Coma Scale score of 9–14 (confused, lethargic, stuporous)
	• Concussion
	• Posttraumatic amnesia
	• Vomiting
	• Seizure
	• Signs of possible basilar or depressed skull fracture of serious facial injury
	• Alcohol or drug intoxication
	• Unreliable or no history of injury
	• Age younger than 2, older than 65
Severe	• Glasgow Coma Scale score of 3–8 (comatose)
	• Progressive decline in level of consciousness ("talked and deteriorated")
	• Focal neurologic signs
	• Penetrating skull injury or palpable depressed skull fracture

Adapted from Masters SJ, McClean PM, Arcarese JS, et al. Skull x-ray examinations after head trauma. Recommendations by a multidisciplinary panel and validation study. *N Engl J Med.* 1987;316(2):84–91.

TABLE 46.3 Glasgow Coma Scale

Activity/Response	Score[a]
Eye opening	
Spontaneous	4
To voice	3
To pain	2
None	1
Best motor response	
Obeys commands	6
Localizes to pain	5
Withdraws to pain	4
Flexor posturing	3
Extensor posturing	2
None	1
Best verbal response	
Conversant and oriented	5
Conversant and disoriented	4
Inappropriate words	3
Incomprehensible sounds	2
None	1

[a]Total score = sum of the score for each of the three components.

From Teasdale G, Jennett B. Assessment of coma and impaired consciousness. A practical scale. *Lancet.* 1974;2:81–83.

RADIOGRAPHY AND IMAGING

CT is the emergency imaging method of choice for head and cervical spine injury. CT is more informative than standard skull radiographic films for detecting skull or neck fractures and provides unsurpassed sensitivity for detecting intracranial blood. In general, all patients with a head injury should have CT, except for those who are classified as low risk (e.g., without concussion; with no neurologic abnormalities on examination; and with no evidence or suspicion of a skull fracture, alcohol or drug intoxication, or other moderate-risk criteria) (see Table 46.2). The likelihood of detecting intracranial hemorrhage by CT in these patients is only 1 in 10,000. MRI is better for detecting subtle injury to the brain, particularly for focal lesions related to DAI, but is generally not used for emergency evaluations unless it is rapidly and readily available.

CT images of the head should be assessed for evidence of the presence of epidural or subdural hematoma, subarachnoid or intraventricular blood, parenchymal contusions and hemorrhages, cerebral edema, and gliding contusions related to DAI. With bone window settings, fractures, sinus opacification, and pneumocephalus may be identified. Axial CT images of the entire cervical spine should also be obtained in all patients. If traumatic arterial dissection is possible, CT angiography of the head and neck is indicated.

SECONDARY NEUROLOGIC EVALUATION

On arrival at the intensive care unit (ICU), more detailed physical and neurologic examinations should be performed (the "secondary survey"). The patient should again be examined for external signs of trauma to the neck, chest, back, abdomen, and limbs. A bloody

who show clinical signs of herniation, require emergency interventions to reduce ICP, including 30 degrees of head elevation, hyperventilation to a target arterial PCO_2 of 30 mm Hg, and 20% mannitol solution at a dose of 0.5 to 1.0 g/kg via rapid IV infusion (Table 46.5).

HISTORY

The circumstances of the accident and the clinical condition of the patient before admission to the emergency room should be ascertained from records of the emergency medical services, the patient (if possible), and eyewitnesses. The force and location of head impact should be determined as precisely as possible. Specific inquiry should be made about concussion; because patients are amnesic during the concussion, only an eyewitness may accurately gauge the duration of loss of consciousness.

Patients who have "talked and deteriorated" should be assumed to have an expanding intracranial hematoma until proven otherwise. Reports of headache, nausea, vomiting, confusion, or seizure activity must be noted. A medical history, including medications and drug and alcohol use, should be obtained. Recent drug and alcohol use occurs in many trauma patients.

TABLE 46.4 Estimated Mortality Based on Various Features of Head Injury	
	Mortality (%)
Glasgow Coma Scale score	
15	<1
11–14	3
8–10	15
6–7	20
4–5	50
3	80
Age (yr), among comatose patients	
16–35	30
36–45	40
46–55	50
56 or older	80
CT abnormalities, among comatose patients	
None	10
Intracranial pathology without diffuse swelling or midline shift	15
Intracranial pathology with diffuse swelling (cisterns compressed or absent)	35
Intracranial pathology with midline shift (>5 mm)	55
Intracranial pressure, among comatose patients	
<20 mm Hg	15
>20 mm Hg, reducible	45
>20 mm Hg, not reducible	90
Pathologic entity	
Epidural hematoma	5–15
Gunshot wound	55
Acute subdural hematoma	
Simple	20–25
Complicated	40–75
Bilateral	75–100

CT, computed tomography.

Percentages are adapted from several sources and have been rounded. Data are based on historical cohort studies and may not reflect current outcomes with aggressive surgical and critical care management.

From Greenberg J, Brawanaki A. Cranial trauma. In: Hacke W, ed. *Neurocritical Care*. New York: Springer-Verlag; 1994:705; Vollmer DG, Torner JC, Jane LA, et al. Age and outcome following traumatic coma: why do older patient's fare worse? *J Neurosurg*. 1991;75(suppl 1):S37–S49; Marshall LF, Gautille T, Klauber MR, et al. The outcome of severe closed head injury. *J Neurosurg*. 1991;75(suppl 1):S28–S36; Miller JD, Becker DP, Ward JD, et al. Significance of intracranial hypertension in severe head injury. *J Neurosurg*. 1977;47:503–516.

TABLE 46.5 Emergency Measures for Intracranial Pressure Reduction in an Unmonitored Patient with Clinical Signs of Herniation
1. Elevate head of bed 15–30 degrees.
2. Normal saline (0.9%) at 80–100 mL/h (avoid hypotonic fluids)
3. Intubate and hyperventilate (target PCO_2 = 28–32 mm Hg)
4. Mannitol 20% 1–1.5 g/kg via rapid IV infusion
5. Foley catheter
6. Neurosurgical consultation

IV, intravenous.

From Mayer SA, Chong J. Critical care management of increased intracranial pressure. *J Intensive Care Med*. 2002;17:55–67.

centration is 30 mg/dL or more, whereas lacrimal secretions and nasal mucus usually contain less than 5 mg/dL glucose.

After determining the patient's level of consciousness (e.g., alert, lethargic, stuporous, or comatose), a focused mental status examination should be performed if the patient is conversant. Particular attention should be paid to attention capabilities, concentration (e.g., counting backward from 20 to 1 or reciting the months in reverse), orientation, and memory, including assessment for retrograde and anterograde amnesia.

Eye movements, pupillary size and shape, and reactivity to light should be noted. A sluggishly reactive or dilated pupil suggests transtentorial herniation with compression of the third cranial nerve. A mid position, poorly reactive, irregular pupil may result from injury to the oculomotor nucleus in the midbrain tegmentum. Nystagmus often follows a concussion. In comatose patients, the oculocephalic and oculovestibular reflexes should be tested (see Chapter 18).

Motor examination should focus on identifying asymmetric weakness or posturing. Spontaneous movements should be assessed for preferential use of the limbs on one side. If the patient is not fully cooperative, lateralized weakness may be detected by assessment of an asymmetry in tone or tendon reflexes or by the presence of an arm drift, preferential localizing response to sternal rub, or extensor plantar reflex. Noxious stimuli, such as pinching the medial arm or applying nail bed pressure, may reveal subtle motor posturing in a limb that otherwise moves purposefully. *Decorticate posturing* (i.e., flexion of arms, extension of legs) results from injury to the corticospinal pathways at the level of the diencephalon or upper midbrain. *Decerebrate posturing* (i.e., extension of legs and arms) implies injury to the motor pathways at the level of the lower midbrain, pons, or medulla.

Gait is particularly important to check in low-risk patients who are treated and scheduled for release without CT. Balance and equilibrium, tested by tandem heel-to-toe walking, are frequently impaired after a concussion.

TREATMENT

ADMISSION TO THE HOSPITAL

Low-risk Group

Low-risk patients who meet all criteria described in Table 46.2, generally, may be discharged from the emergency room without CT, so long as a responsible person is available to observe the patient for the next 24 hours. In general, these are patients who

discharge from the nose or ear may indicate leakage of CSF; bloody CSF may be differentiated from blood by a positive halo test (i.e., a halo of CSF forms around the blood when dropped on a white cloth sheet). If there is no admixture of blood, CSF may be distinguished from nasal secretions because the CSF glucose con-

TABLE 46.6	Criteria for Hospital Admission after Head Injury

- Intracranial blood or fracture identified on head CT
- Confusion, agitation, or depressed level of consciousness
- Focal neurologic signs or symptoms
- Posttraumatic seizure
- Alcohol or drug intoxication
- Significant comorbid medical illness
- Lack of a reliable home environment for observation

CT, computed tomography.

did not sustain a concussion and have normal findings on neurologic examination. Patients are given a checklist of symptoms (e.g., headache, vomiting, confusion) and instructed to return immediately to the emergency room if any occur.

Moderate-risk Group

Among patients who have had a concussion, a normal GCS score of 15 (e.g., alert, fully oriented, and following commands) and normal CT eliminate the need for hospital admission. These patients may be discharged to home for observation with a warning card, even in the presence of headache, nausea, vomiting, dizziness, or retrograde amnesia, because the risk of a significant intracranial lesion developing thereafter is minimal. Criteria for hospital admission for patients with head injury are listed in Table 46.6.

Patients with mild to moderate neurologic deficits (generally corresponding to GCS scores of 9 to 14) and CT findings that do not require neurosurgical intervention should be admitted to an intermediate care unit or ICU for observation. Follow-up CT at 24 hours is often helpful to check for progression of bleeding.

High-risk Group

All patients with a serious head injury are admitted to the hospital. An early neurosurgical consultation is crucial because once the patient has been stabilized, assessed, and imaged, the immediate consideration is whether emergency surgery is indicated. If the decision is made to operate, surgery should proceed immediately because delays only increase the likelihood of further brain damage during the waiting period. Medical management of severe-injury patients should take place in an ICU. Although little may be done about the brain damage that occurs on impact, ICU care may play a major role in reducing secondary brain injury that develops over hours or days.

SURGICAL INTERVENTION

Simple wounds of the scalp should be thoroughly cleaned and sutured. Compound fractures of the skull should be completely debrided. Operative treatment of compound fractures should be performed as soon as possible but may be delayed for 24 hours until the patient is transported to a hospital equipped for this purpose or until the patient is hemodynamically stable. Elevation of small, depressed fractures need not be performed immediately, but the depressed fragments should be elevated before the patient is discharged from the hospital, particularly if the inner table of the skull is involved.

The treatment of massive acute subdural, epidural, or parenchymal hematomas with mass effect is *craniotomy* and surgical removal of the clot. Results from a large randomized clinical trial

indicate that decompressive *craniectomy*—removal of a large lateral portion of the skull—is not indicated emergently **[Level 1]**.[1] The bleeding point should be identified and either ligated or clipped. The operative results depend to a great extent on the degree of associated brain damage. In the absence of coexisting brain injury, remarkable improvement may occur after evacuation of a subdural or epidural hematoma, with disappearance of the hemiplegia or other focal neurologic signs.

Burr-hole or *twist-drill* evacuation is insufficient for acute, large, subdural, and epidural hematomas, but for liquefied, chronic, subdural hematomas, it is associated with better outcomes than craniotomy. A plastic catheter (e.g., Jackson-Pratt drain) is usually placed in the subdural space for several days until the drainage subsides.

INTRACRANIAL PRESSURE MANAGEMENT

As a general rule, an ICP monitor should be placed in all head-injured patients who are comatose (i.e., GCS score of 8) after resuscitation. Intracranial hypertension occurs in more than 50% of comatose patients with CT evidence of mass effect from intracranial hemorrhage or cerebral edema and in 10% to 15% of patients with normal imaging. A ventricular catheter or fiberoptic parenchymal monitor may be used. Ventriculostomy has the advantage of allowing CSF drainage to reduce ICP but has a high risk of infection (approximately 12%). The risk of infection or hemorrhage is substantially lower with parenchymal ICP monitors (approximately 1% to 2%).

Normal ICP is less than 15 mm Hg, or 20 cm H_2O. Cerebral perfusion pressure (CPP) is routinely monitored in conjunction with ICP because it is an important determinant of cerebral blood flow; CPP is defined as mean arterial BP minus ICP. The goal of ICP management after head injury is to maintain ICP less than 20 mm Hg and CPP greater than 60 mm Hg. The magnitude and duration of derangements beyond these targets is highly correlated with poor outcome after severe TBI.

Treatment of elevated ICP is most successful when a preestablished protocol is used. The Columbia University Medical Center stepwise management protocol for treating ICP elevations in monitored ICU patients is shown in Table 46.7 (see also Chapter 107).

An acute, severe increase in ICP always prompts a repeat CT to assess the need for a definitive neurosurgical procedure. If the

TABLE 46.7	Stepwise Treatment Protocol for Elevated Intracranial Pressure (>20 mm Hg for >10 min) in a Monitored Patient

1. Consider repeat CT and surgical intervention (ventricular drainage, craniotomy, or hemicraniectomy).

2. IV sedation to attain a motionless quiet state

3. Pressor infusion if CPP <60 mm Hg or reduction of blood pressure if CPP remains >110 mm Hg

4. Mannitol 0.25–1.5 g/kg IV every 2–6 h as needed

5. Hyperventilation to PCO_2 levels of 28–32 mm Hg

6. Systemic hypothermia (T = 33°C)

7. High-dose pentobarbital therapy (load with 5–20 mg/kg, maintain with 1–4 mg/kg/h)

See text for details.

CT, computed tomography; IV, intravenous; CPP, cerebral perfusion pressure.

Adapted from Mayer SA, Chong J. Critical care management of increased intracranial pressure. *J Intensive Care Med.* 2002;17:55–67.

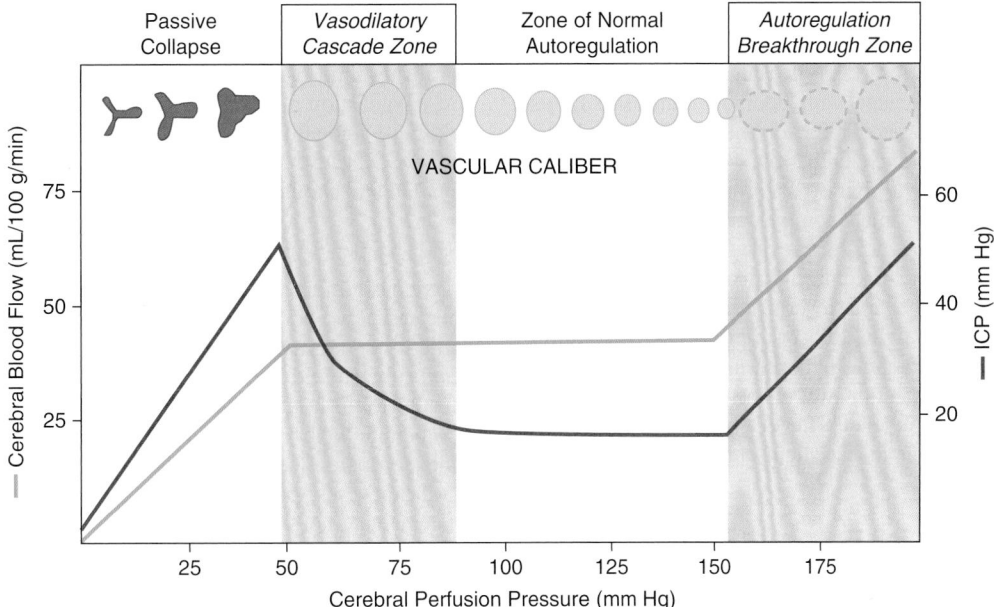

FIGURE 46.8 Relationship between extremes of CPP and ICP in states of reduced intracranial compliance. In the vasodilatory cascade zone, CPP insufficiency and intact pressure autoregulation leads to reflex cerebral vasodilation and increased ICP; the treatment is to raise CPP. In the autoregulation breakthrough zone, pressure and volume overload, which overwhelms the brain's capacity to autoregulate, leads to increased CBV and ICP; the treatment is to lower CPP. (Adapted from Rose JA, Mayer SA. Optimizing BP in neurological emergencies. *Neurocrit Care*. 2004;1:287–299, with permission.)

patient is agitated or appears to be fighting the ventilator, a short-acting IV sedative agent, such as propofol, or analgesic, such as fentanyl, should be given alone or in combination to attain a quiet, motionless state. Thereafter, if CPP is less than 60 mm Hg, vasopressors may lead to reduction of ICP by decreasing cerebral vasodilation that occurs in response to inadequate perfusion. Alternately, if CPP exceeds 120 mm Hg, BP reduction with IV labetalol or nicardipine may sometimes lead to a parallel decrease of ICP. The relationship between extremes of CPP and ICP in states of reduced intracranial compliance is shown in Figure 46.8.

Mannitol and hypertonic saline are used only after all surgical options have been exhausted and sedation and CPP optimization fail to normalize ICP. Mannitol, an osmotic diuretic, lowers ICP via its cerebral dehydrating effects. The initial dose of mannitol 20% solution is 0.5 to 1.0 g/kg, followed by doses of 0.25 to 1.0 g/kg as needed. Further doses should be given individually based on ICP measurements rather than on a standing basis. Mannitol boluses may also be used to reverse acute herniation syndromes (i.e., a blown pupil) resulting from compartmental mass effect and ICP gradients. The effect of mannitol is maximal when given rapidly; ICP reduction occurs within 10 to 20 minutes and may last for 2 to 6 hours. Serum osmolality should be monitored closely and the osmolar gap calculated by subtracting the measured osmolality from the calculated osmolality. Should the osmolar gap increase to greater than 15 mOsm/L, then there is a greater likelihood of mannitol leading to renal failure. Urinary losses should be compensated for with IV normal saline to avoid secondary hypovolemia. Assessment of intravascular volume status with a combination of invasive monitoring and ultrasound is generally recommended. More recently, hypertonic saline in the form of a 3% sodium chloride/acetate continuous infusion, or 10% or 23.4% NaCl as an alternative to mannitol bolus therapy, has been advocated for the treatment of intracranial hypertension and herniation syndromes. Studies

evaluating equiosmolar doses of mannitol and hypertonic saline indicate that in most cases, hypertonic saline is at least equivalent, if not superior, to mannitol for lowering ICP in terms of the rapidity, extent, and duration of ICP reduction. The exception is in the prehospital setting where empiric administration with hypertonic saline failed to improve outcomes after TBI [**Level 1**].[2] As a general rule in the critical care setting, hypertonic saline is generally preferred in patients who are hypotensive or hypovolemic, whereas mannitol is preferable for patients who are volume overloaded or who have congestive heart failure (CHF).

Hyperventilation lowers ICP by inducing cerebral alkalosis and reflex vasoconstriction, with a concomitant reduction of CBV. Hyperventilation to PCO_2 levels of 28 to 32 mm Hg may lower ICP within minutes, although the effect gradually diminishes over as little as 1 to 3 hours, as acid–base buffering mechanisms correct the alkalosis within the CNS. Additionally, prophylactic hyperventilation has been shown to lead to detrimental outcomes [**Level 1**],[3] and overly aggressive hyperventilation to PCO_2 levels less than 26 mm Hg may potentially exacerbate cerebral ischemia and, in general, should be avoided unless jugular venous oxygen saturation or brain tissue oxygen monitoring is available to ensure that cerebral hypoxia does not occur.

High-dose barbiturate therapy with pentobarbital given in doses equivalent to those used for general anesthesia (5 to 20 mg/kg as a loading dose, followed by 1 to 4 mg/kg/h) effectively lowers ICP in most patients who are refractory to the steps outlined earlier. It can be dosed as either a continuous infusion or given as bolus injection as needed for ICP control (50 to 200 mg every 15 minutes). The effect of pentobarbital is multifactorial but most likely stems from a coupled reduction in cerebral metabolism, blood flow, and blood volume. Pentobarbital may cause profound hypotension and usually requires the use of vasopressors to maintain CPP of at least 60 mm Hg. The other major side effect of pentobarbital is prolonged immobilization and ventilator dependence, which increases the risk of nosocomial infection and exposure to other iatrogenic complications. In a clinical trial, the prophylactic use of pentobarbital was associated with poor outcome, and its use currently is reserved for cases of refractory raised ICP [Level 1].[4]

Mild to moderate systemic hypothermia (33°C) has been shown to reduce ICP in patients with refractory intracranial hypertension. The application of hypothermia is complex and requires a management protocol that emphasizes the use of agents such as meperidine, fentanyl, or dexmedetomidine and neuromuscular blocking agents, if necessary, to prevent shivering that increases cerebral and metabolic stress and fights the cooling process. The routine application of mild to moderate hypothermia within 8 hours of TBI, as a form of neuroprotection, was tested in a large clinical trial and was shown not to be of benefit [Level 1].[5,6] For this reason, its use should be limited to the management of refractory intracranial hypertension.

INTENSIVE CARE UNIT MANAGEMENT OF SEVERE HEAD INJURY

Patients with severe head injuries are best treated in an ICU. In some hospitals, patients with head injuries are treated in a special neurologic or neurosurgical ICU. A time-coded flow sheet is helpful to allow for meticulous, continuous updating of the patient's clinical, neurologic, and physiologic status.

Serial Neurologic Evaluation

The patient should be examined repeatedly to evaluate level of consciousness and the presence or absence of signs of injury to the brain or cranial nerves. Variations in level of consciousness, reflected by changes in the GCS score or the appearance of hemiplegia or other focal neurologic signs, should prompt repeat CT.

Airway and Ventilation

In general, patients who are unable to protect their airways because of depressed levels of consciousness should be intubated with an endotracheal tube. Routine hyperventilation is not recommended; in the absence of increased ICP, ventilatory parameters should be set to maintain PCO_2 at 30 to 40 mm Hg and PO_2 at 90 to 100 mm Hg.

Blood Pressure Management

If the patient shows signs of hemodynamic instability, a radial artery catheter should be placed to monitor BP. Because cerebral blood flow autoregulation is frequently impaired in acute head injury, mean BP (or CPP if ICP is being monitored) must be carefully regulated to avoid hypotension that may lead to cerebral ischemia or hypertension that may exacerbate cerebral edema. Continuous infusion, short-acting vasopressors (e.g., phenylephrine and norepinephrine), and antihypertensive agents (e.g., labetalol and nicardipine) are preferable because of their abilities to stabilize BP within a narrow therapeutic range. Sodium nitroprusside should be avoided because it may dilate cerebral vessels and raise ICP.

Fluid Management

Only isotonic fluids, such as 0.9% (i.e., normal) saline or plasmalyte solution, should be administered to head-injured patients because the extra free water in half-normal saline or D5W may exacerbate cerebral edema. Hypertonic saline (i.e., 3% sodium chloride/ acetate solution) with a target osmolality of 300 to 320 mOsm/L

may be used as an alternative in patients with significant brain edema, and may reduce the number of ICP elevations, at the risk of causing fluid overload and pulmonary edema if volume status and oxygenation are not carefully monitored. CVP monitoring is helpful to guide fluid management in hypotensive or hypovolemic patients. Negative fluid balance is associated with poor outcome after TBI and should be avoided.

Nutrition

Severe head injury leads to a generalized hypermetabolic and catabolic response, with caloric requirements that are 50% to 100% higher than normal. Enteral feedings via a nasogastric or nasoduodenal tube should be instituted as soon as possible (e.g., usually after 24 to 48 hours). Early enteral feeding on day 1 after injury is generally well tolerated and has been shown to improve outcome compared with delayed feeding. Parenteral nutrition carries significant risks, primarily those of infection and electrolyte derangements, and should be used only if enteral feeding may not be tolerated.

Analgosedation

Patients may be agitated or delirious, which may lead to self-injury, forcible removal of monitoring devices, systemic and cerebral hypermetabolism, and increased ICP. Intubated patients may be sedated using a continuous IV infusion of a rapid-acting sedative agent, such as propofol, fentanyl, or remifentanil, that may be turned off periodically to allow neurologic assessments. Pain control should always be the first consideration when using analgosedation. Daily interruption of sedation in mechanically intubated patients allows for improved sensitivity to changes in neurologic status, more appropriate titration of sedation, and reduced duration of mechanical ventilation. Nonintubated patients with delirium may be treated with haloperidol 2 to 10 mg every 4 hours as needed, quetiapine 25 to 50 mg orally every 6 to 8 hours, or a similar agent.

Temperature Management

Fever (>38.3°C) is common after TBI and may be the result of infection or of central fever. Even small temperature elevations may exacerbate TBI and ischemic brain injury and should be aggressively treated. Newer cooling devices using adhesive cooling pads or intravascular heat-exchange catheters are superior to standard water-circulating cooling blankets for maintaining normothermia in comatose brain-injured patients.

Anticonvulsants

Phenytoin or fosphenytoin (15 to 20 mg/kg loading dose, then 300 mg/day) reduced the frequency of early (i.e., first week) posttraumatic seizures from 14% to 4% in a clinical trial of patients with intracranial hemorrhage but did not prevent later seizures [Level 1].[7] IV valproic acid or levetiracetam is an acceptable alternative for patients with phenytoin allergy. If the patient has not had a seizure, prophylactic anticonvulsants should be discontinued after 7 days. Anticonvulsant serum levels of head-injured patients should be monitored closely because subtherapeutic levels frequently result from drug hypermetabolism, particularly in younger men. Nonconvulsive seizures and status epilepticus, which are diagnosable only with continuous electroencephalogram (EEG) monitoring, occur in over 10% to 20% of comatose TBI patients, are associated with poor outcome, and generally warrant aggressive treatment with continuous infusion midazolam or similar agents.

Intensive Insulin Therapy

Continuous insulin infusion therapy to control blood glucose to between 100 and 180 mg/dL in hyperglycemic patients reduces mortality in critically ill surgical patients and is increasingly being adopted as a practice option in the ICU management of severe TBI. Meticulous attention, including hourly blood glucose monitoring, must be paid to avoid excessive hypoglycemia with continuous insulin infusion.

Steroids

Glucocorticoids have been used to treat cerebral edema for years but have not been shown to favorably alter outcomes or lower ICP in head-injured patients. A large randomized controlled trial demonstrated an increased rate of death in patients given high-dose steroids during the first week after TBI [Level 1].[8] This was probably attributable to increased risk of infection, hyperglycemia, or other complications. For these reasons, dexamethasone and other steroids are absolutely contraindicated for use in patients with head injury.

Deep Vein Thrombosis Prophylaxis

Patients with head injury who are immobilized are at high risk for deep vein thrombosis in the legs and pulmonary thromboembolism. Pneumatic compression boots should be used routinely to protect against this risk, and patients should also be given subcutaneous heparin 5,000 units every 8 hours or enoxaparin 40 mg daily. Low-dose anticoagulants to prevent thromboembolic disease can safely be added within 48 hours after injury, even in the presence of intracranial hemorrhage, so long as hematoma expansion is not noted on serial imaging.

Gastric Stress Ulcer Prophylaxis

Patients on mechanical ventilation or with coagulopathy are at increased risk of gastric stress ulceration and should receive pantoprazole 40 mg daily intravenously; famotidine 20 mg intravenously, every 12 hours; or sucralfate 1 g, orally, every 6 hours.

Antibiotics

The routine use of prophylactic antibiotics in patients with open skull injuries is controversial, and opinions are sharply divided. Prophylactic antibiotics with gram-positive activity, such as oxacillin, are often used to reduce the risk of meningitis in patients with CSF otorrhea, rhinorrhea, or intracranial air; however, these agents may increase the risk of infection with more virulent or resistant organisms. A single dose of an antibiotic with activity against gram-positive bacteria such as oxacillin of cefazolin should be administered immediately prior to the insertion of an intracranial monitor.

ACUTE COMPLICATIONS OF HEAD INJURY

CEREBROSPINAL FLUID FISTULA

CSF fistulas result from tearing of the dura and arachnoid membranes. They occur in 3% of patients with closed head injury and in 5% to 10% of those with basilar skull fractures. They are usually associated with fractures of the ethmoid, sphenoid, or orbital plate of the frontal bone.

CT may demonstrate pneumocephalus (air in the subarachnoid space). Clinical manifestations include obvious leakage of CSF from a scalp laceration, the nose, or the ear. CSF leakage ceases after head elevation alone for a few days in 85% of cases. If it persists, the insertion of a lumbar drain may lower CSF pressure, reduce flow through the fistula, and hasten spontaneous closure of the dural tear. Patients with dural leaks are at increased risk for meningitis, and although the use of prophylactic antibiotics is controversial, most physicians use them. Persistent CSF otorrhea or rhinorrhea for more than 2 weeks calls for surgical repair, as does recurrent meningitis. If there is a leak and the site of the fracture is not evident, a metrizamide CT study is the diagnostic method of choice.

CAROTID–CAVERNOUS FISTULA

Carotid–cavernous fistulae are characterized by the clinical triad of pulsating exophthalmos, ocular chemosis, and orbital bruit. They result from traumatic laceration of the internal carotid artery as it passes through the cavernous sinus; approximately 20% of cases are nontraumatic, and most of these are related to spontaneous rupture of an intracavernous internal carotid artery aneurysm. Other symptoms may include distended orbital and periorbital veins and paralysis of the cranial nerves (e.g., III, IV, V, and VI) that pass through or within the wall of the cavernous sinus.

Traumatic carotid–cavernous fistulae may develop immediately or within days after injury. Angiography is required to confirm the diagnosis (see Fig. 46.7). Endovascular treatment, with a balloon placed through the defect in the arterial wall into the venous side of the fistula, is the most effective means of repair and may prevent permanent visual loss caused by venous retinal infarction if performed as soon as possible after injury.

TRAUMATIC ARTERIAL DISSECTION AND VASCULAR INJURIES

Traumatic injuries may be associated with dissections of the extracranial or intracranial internal carotid or vertebral arteries, which may lead to thrombosis at the site of the intimal flap and stroke resulting from distal thromboembolism. The gold standard for diagnosis is conventional angiography, but CT and magnetic resonance (MR) angiography are often used to screen for arterial dissections. Anticoagulation with unfractionated heparin is the primary strategy to prevent intravascular thrombosis and thromboembolism. However, anticoagulation poses risks when there is evident intracranial hemorrhage or coexisting intracranial dissection with pseudoaneurysm formation. Treatment decisions must be individualized.

Basilar skull fractures are sometimes associated with thrombosis of adjacent dural sinuses; the sphenoid and transverse sinuses are most commonly involved. Symptoms are related to increased ICP or associated venous infarction. The diagnosis is established by angiography or MR venography, and anticoagulation is the treatment of choice (see Chapter 43).

In patients with large epidural or subdural hematomas and subfalcine herniation, secondary cerebral infarction may sometimes result from compression of the ipsilateral anterior cerebral artery against the falx or posterior cerebral artery against the tentorium. Urgent neurosurgical decompression to prevent these infarcts is the only effective management strategy.

CRANIAL NERVE INJURY

Injury to the cranial nerves can occur with basilar skull fractures (see Chapter 48). The facial nerve is the most commonly injured nerve in these cases, complicating 0.3% to 5% of all head injuries.

Occasionally, the paralysis may not develop until several days after the injury. Partial or complete recovery of function is the rule with traumatic injuries to the cranial nerves, with the exception of injury to the first or second cranial nerve.

INFECTIONS

Infections within the intracranial cavity after head injury may be extradural (e.g., osteomyelitis), subdural (e.g., empyema), subarachnoid (e.g., meningitis), or intracerebral (e.g., abscess). These infections usually develop in the first few weeks after injury but may be delayed. Diagnosis is suggested by CT or MRI and confirmed by culture of the infected tissue. Treatment includes surgical debridement and administration of antibiotics.

Meningitis may follow any type of open fracture associated with tearing of the dura, including compound skull fractures, penetrating missile injury, or linear fractures that extend into the nasal sinuses or the middle ear. Meningitis occurs in as few as 2% and as many as 22% of patients with basilar skull fractures. Cases of meningitis that develop within a few days after injury are almost always caused by pneumococcus or other gram-positive bacteria, but any pathogenic organism may be the cause. Diagnosis depends on the CSF findings after lumbar puncture. The principles of treatment are those recommended for meningitis in general (Chapter 61). The presence of a persistent CSF fistula with rhinorrhea or otorrhea favors the recurrence of meningitis; as many as seven or eight attacks have been reported. Treatment in such cases may require surgical closure of the fistula.

OUTCOMES

Outcomes that may be expected after head injury are often matters of great concern, particularly in those with serious injuries. *Depth of coma, CT findings,* and *age* of the patient are the variables most predictive of late outcome. Other factors of prognostic importance include the absence of pupillary responses, hypotension or hypoxemia on admission, specific patterns of injury noted on admission CT scan, persistently elevated ICP, hyperthermia, and critically reduced (<10 mm Hg) brain tissue oxygen levels. Functional outcomes from severe TBI have improved markedly over the past 20 years, although mortality remains constant at approximately 30%.

Severity of coma may be quantified using the admission GCS score (see Table 46.3), which has substantial prognostic value. Historically, patients scoring 3 or 4 (deep coma) have an 85% chance of dying or remaining vegetative, whereas these outcomes occur in only 5% to 10% of patients scoring 12 or more. In general, elderly patients do very poorly. In one series of comatose patients older than 65 years of age, only 10% survived, and only 4% regained functional independence. Death may result from progression to brain death or refractory medical complications but most often is the consequence of decisions to limit life support because poor functional recovery is anticipated. It is increasingly recognized, however, that caregivers tend to underestimate capacity for recovery from severe brain injury, and some fatal outcomes may be the result of self-fulfilling prophecy. Attempts to make a firm prognosis in severe head injuries, especially in the early stages, are hazardous because the outcome depends on so many variables. Some indices, however, are valuable as prognostic indicators (see Table 46.4).

In general, the prospects of recovery from trauma-induced coma are better than recovery from coma by other causes. Fifty percent of adults and 60% of children who experience trauma-induced coma for 30 days will recover consciousness within 1 year compared with 15% of patients in coma from nontraumatic causes. Recovery of consciousness is operationally defined as the ability to follow verbal commands convincingly and consistently. *Unresponsive wakefulness,* rather than the former used term *persistent vegetative state,* refers to a state of eyes open coma with no external signs of consciousness. The *minimally conscious state* refers to a transitional state between coma and full consciousness. Patients exhibit the capacity to understand and obey commands and make some purposeful behaviors but otherwise demonstrate a paucity of spontaneous thought and activity.

Cognitive impairment is by far the most common and disabling problem among survivors of head injury. During the acute phase, disorientation and agitation are particularly common. In addition to cognitive and motor deficits, headache, dizziness, vomiting, or vertigo may be present in the immediate posttraumatic period. These symptoms usually disappear in a few weeks but may persist for months. Common chronic cognitive problems include impaired short- and long-term memory, attention, and concentration; slowing of psychomotor speed and mental processing; and changes in personality. There may be loss of memory for the events that occurred in the immediate period after recovery of consciousness (i.e., *posttraumatic amnesia*) and a similar amnesia for the events immediately preceding the injury (i.e., *pretraumatic amnesia*). These periods of amnesia may encompass days, weeks, or years. Depression occurs in up to 40% of TBI survivors during the first year of recovery and is highly amenable to medical therapy. With time, there is usually considerable improvement in the signs and symptoms of brain damage, but permanent sequelae are common.

Early cognitive, physical, and occupational therapy is an important part of optimizing recovery after TBI. Physical therapy, including range-of-motion exercises to prevent limb contractures, may begin even while patients are still in the ICU. Once the patients are stabilized, they can be transferred to an acute or subacute rehabilitation facility. Whether cognitive rehabilitative measures truly improve neuropsychological outcome remains to be established.

In a study of patients with moderate or severe injuries, only 46% returned to work 2 years later, and most of those who did return to work did not go back to their original work. Only 18% were financially independent, inducing considerable stress on the family. Vocational training may play a key role in helping patients reintegrate into the workforce.

POSTCONCUSSION SYNDROME

About 40% of patients who have sustained minor or severe injuries to the head complain of dizziness, fatigue, insomnia, irritability, restlessness, and inability to concentrate. Often, there is overlap with anxiety and depression. This group of symptoms, which may be present for only a few weeks or may persist for years, is known as *postconcussion syndrome* (see also Chapter 45).

Postconcussion syndrome is somewhat misleadingly named because affected individuals need not have suffered loss of consciousness. There are no criteria to define the role of either physiologic or psychological factors in the etiology of postconcussion syndrome. Patients may be severely disabled yet have normal findings on neurologic examination and no MR evidence of brain injury. The correlation between the severity of the original injury and the severity and duration of later symptoms is poor. For instance, the incidence of postconcussion syndrome is not related to the duration of retrograde amnesia, coma, or posttraumatic amnesia. In some patients, symptoms may be related to the brain damage; in others, they seem to be entirely psychogenic. In practice, it is often difficult to sort out the complicated origins of this disorder.

Posttraumatic symptoms may develop in patients who had previously shown normal adjustment but are more likely to occur in patients who had psychiatric symptoms before the injury. Factors such as domestic or financial difficulties, unrewarding occupations, and the desire to obtain compensation, financial or otherwise, tend to produce and may prolong the symptoms once they have developed.

The prognosis of the postconcussion syndrome is uncertain. In general, progressive improvement may be expected. The duration of symptoms is not related to the severity of the injury. In some patients with only mild injuries, symptoms continue for long periods, whereas patients with severe injuries may have only mild or transient symptoms. By and large, however, it is a matter of 2 to 6 months before the headache and dizziness, and the more definite mental changes, show much improvement. Treatment for postconcussion syndrome is based on psychotherapy, cognitive and occupational therapy, vocational rehabilitation, and treatment with antidepressant or antianxiety agents.

SEIZURES AND POSTTRAUMATIC EPILEPSY

Posttraumatic seizures may be immediate (i.e., within 24 hours), early (i.e., within the first week), or late (i.e., occurring after the first week).

The exact incidence of seizures after head injury is unknown, but figures in the literature vary from 2.5% to 40%. As a rule, the more severe the injury, the greater the likelihood that seizures will develop. The overall incidence of seizures is about 25% in those with brain contusion or hematoma and as high as 50% in those with penetrating head injury.

Immediate seizures are infrequent; they are risk factors for further early seizures but not for late seizures. Early seizures occur in 3% to 14% of patients with head injury who are admitted to the hospital. Risk factors include depressed skull fracture, penetrating head injury, intracranial hemorrhage (i.e., epidural, subdural, or intraparenchymal), prolonged unconsciousness (i.e., more than 24 hours), coma, and immediate seizures; the risk of early seizures in patients with any of these risk factors is 20% to 30%. Children are more likely to develop early posttraumatic seizures than are adults. Patients who experience early seizures remain at risk for late seizures and should be maintained on anticonvulsants after discharge from the hospital.

The overall incidence of late seizures (e.g., posttraumatic epilepsy) after closed-head injury is 5%, but the risk is as high as 30% among patients with intracranial hemorrhage or a depressed skull fracture and 50% among patients who have experienced early seizures. About 60% of patients experience their initial seizures during the first year, but the risk of seizures remains increased for up to 15 years after a severe head injury. Because 25% of patients have only a single late seizure, many practitioners begin anticonvulsants only after a second seizure occurs. Therapy of posttraumatic epilepsy is discussed further in Chapter 58.

POSTTRAUMATIC MOVEMENT DISORDERS

Movement disorders are rare sequelae of head injury. Action tremor is most common, although its pathogenesis remains obscure. Cerebellar ataxia, rubral tremor, and palatal myoclonus have been described in patients with focal shearing injuries of the superior cerebellar peduncle, midbrain, and dentato-rubro-olivary triangle, respectively. Parkinsonism and other basal ganglia syndromes have been reported after a single episode of head trauma.

PEDIATRIC TRAUMA

Injuries are the leading cause of death in children, and brain injury is the most common cause of pediatric traumatic death. Motor vehicle accidents account for the largest number of severe injuries in children, but children are also prone to unique forms of injury, such as birth injury and child abuse. Children are more likely than adults to experience brain swelling and seizures after head injury and, in general, make better recoveries than do adults.

MISSILE-RELATED CEREBRAL BLAST INJURY

Historically, penetrating military missile and blast injuries to the brain have led to a uniformly fatal outcome. With improvements in body armor and helmet construction, however, a previously unrecognized syndrome of cerebral *blast injury* has been described in soldiers injured in the United States–Iraq conflict. The syndrome is produced by explosive devices that propel a blast wave and a shower of metallic fragments. In addition to producing concussion, DAI, and the typically encountered forms of acute intracranial bleeding, cerebral blast injury is manifest as massive brain swelling and diffuse arterial vasospasm that begins within several days and resolves on average of 2 weeks after the injury. The syndrome is attributed to diffuse high-frequency shock wave–mediated tissue injury at the time of impact. Hemicraniectomy is often used as a lifesaving procedure because standard measures to reduce brain edema and control ICP often fail despite absence of data regarding its efficacy. Arterial vasospasm, which can result in delayed cerebral infarction, can be treated successfully with balloon angioplasty.

LEVEL 1 EVIDENCE

1. Cooper DJ, Rosenfeld JV, Murray L, et al; for the DECRA Trial Investigators and the Australian and New Zealand Intensive Care Society Clinical Trials Group. Decompressive craniectomy in diffuse traumatic brain injury. *N Engl J Med.* 2011;364(16):1493–1502.
2. Muizelaar JP, Marmarou A, Ward JD, et al. Adverse effects of prolonged hyperventilation in patients with severe head injury: a randomized clinical trial. *J Neurosurg.* 1991;75(5):731–739.
3. Cooper DJ, Myles PS, McDermott FT, et al; for the HTS Study Investigators. Prehospital hypertonic saline resuscitation of patients with hypotension and severe traumatic brain injury: a randomized controlled trial. *JAMA.* 2004;291(11):1350–1357.
4. Ward JD, Becker DP, Miller JD, et al. Failure of prophylactic barbiturate coma in the treatment of severe head injury. *J Neurosurg.* 1985;62(3):383–388.
5. Clifton GL, Miller ER, Choi SC, et al. Lack of effect of induction of hypothermia after acute brain injury. *N Eng J Med.* 2001;344(8):556–563.
6. Clifton GL, Valadka A, Zygun D, et al. Very early hypothermia induction in patients with severe brain injury (the National Acute Brain Injury Study: Hypothermia II): a randomised trial. *Lancet Neurol.* 2011;10(2):131–139.
7. Temkin NR, Dikmen SS, Wilensky AJ, et al. A randomized, double-blind study of phenytoin for the prevention of posttraumatic seizures. *N Engl J Med.* 1990;323(8):497–502.
8. Roberts I, Yates D, Sandercock P, et al. Effect of intravenous corticosteroids on death within 14 days in 10008 adults with clinically significant head injury (MRC CRASH trial): randomised placebo-controlled trial. *Lancet.* 2004;364(9442);1321–1328.

SUGGESTED READINGS

Head Injury, General Considerations

Adams JH, Graham DI, Gennarelli TA, et al. Diffuse axonal injury in non-missile head injury. *J Neurol Neurosurg Psychiatry.* 1991;54:481–483.

Armonda RA, Bell RS, Vo AH, et al. Wartime traumatic cerebral vasospasm: recent review of combat casualties. *Neurosurgery.* 2006;59(6):1215–1225.

Brain Trauma Foundation. Guidelines for the management of severe traumatic brain injury. *J Neurotrauma.* 2007;24(suppl 1):s87–s90.

Cruz J, Minoja G, Okuchi K, et al. Successful use of the new high-dose mannitol treatment in patients with Glasgow Coma Scale scores of 3 and bilateral abnormal pupillary widening: a randomized trial. *J Neurosurg.* 2004;100:376–383.

Diringer MN, Zazulia AR. Osmotic therapy: fact and fiction. *Neurocrit Care.* 2004;1(2):219–233.

Eisenberg HM, Frankowski RF, Contant CF, et al. High-dose barbiturate control of elevated intracranial pressure in patients with severe head injury. *J Neurosurg.* 1988;69:15–23.

Ghajar J. Traumatic brain injury. *Lancet.* 2000;356:923–929.

Graham DI, Ford I, Adams JH, et al. Ischaemic brain damage is still common in fatal non-missile head injury. *J Neurol Neurosurg Psychiatry.* 1989;52:346–350.

Ibanez J, Arikan F, Pedraza S, et al. Reliability of clinical guidelines in the detection of patients at risk following mild head injury: results of a prospective study. *J Neurosurg.* 2004;100(5):825–834.

Jane JA, Anderson DK, Torner JC, et al. *Central Nervous System Trauma Status Report—1991.* New York: Mary Ann Liebert; 1992.

Lingsma H, Yue JK, Maas A, et al. Outcome prediction after mild and complicated mild traumatic brain injury: external validation of existing models and identification of new predictors using the TRACK-TBI pilot study. *J Neurotrauma.* 2015;32(2):83–94.

Marshall LF, Marshall SB, Klauber MR, et al. A new classification of head injury based on computerized tomography. *J Neurosurg.* 1991;75(suppl 1): S14–S20.

Martin NA, Patwardhan RV, Alexander MJ, et al. Characterization of cerebral hemodynamic phases following severe head trauma: hypoperfusion, hyperemia, and vasospasm. *J Neurosurg.* 1997;87:9–19.

Mayer SA, Chong J. Critical care management of increased intracranial pressure. *J Intensive Care Med.* 2002;17:55–67.

Merritt HH. Head injury. *War Med.* 1943;4:61–82.

Oertel M, Kelly DF, McArthur D, et al. Progressive hemorrhage after head trauma: predictors and consequences of the evolving injury. *J Neurosurg.* 2002;96:109–116.

Pearl GS. Traumatic neuropathology. *Clin Lab Med.* 1998;18:39–64.

Smith M. Monitoring intracranial pressure in traumatic brain injury. *Anesth Analg.* 2008;106(1):240–248.

Stiell IG, Wells GA, Vandemheen K, et al. The Canadian CT head rule for patients with minor head injury. *Lancet.* 2001;357:1391–1396.

Symonds C. Concussion and its sequelae. *Lancet.* 1962;1:1–5.

Tawil I, Stein DM, Mirvis SE, et al. Posttraumatic cerebral infarction: incidence, outcome, and risk factors. *J Trauma.* 2008;64(4):849–853.

Taylor SJ, Fettes SB, Jewkes C, et al. Prospective, randomized, controlled trial to determine the effect of early enhanced enteral nutrition on clinical outcome in mechanically ventilated patients suffering head injury. *Crit Care Med.* 1999;27:2525–2531.

Teasdale G, Jennett B. Assessment of coma and impaired consciousness. A practical scale. *Lancet.* 1974;2:81–83.

Teasdale GM, Murray G, Anderson E, et al. Risks of acute traumatic intracranial hematoma in children and adults: implications for management of head injuries. *BMJ.* 1990;300:363–367.

Valadka AB, Robertson CS. Surgery of cerebral trauma and associated critical care. *Neurosurgery.* 2007;61(1)(suppl):203–220.

Vespa PM, Nuwer MR, Nenov V, et al. Increased incidence and impact of nonconvulsive and convulsive seizures after traumatic brain injury as detected by continuous electroencephalographic monitoring. *J Neurosurg.* 1999;91: 750–760.

Vialet R, Albanese J, Thomachot L, et al. Isovolume hypertonic solutes (sodium chloride or mannitol) in the treatment of refractory posttraumatic intracranial hypertension: 2 mL/kg 7.5% saline is more effective than 2 mL/kg 20% mannitol. *Crit Care Med.* 2003;31:1683–1687.

Imaging

Bigler ED. Neuroimaging in pediatric traumatic head injury: diagnostic considerations and relationships to neurobehavioral outcome. *J Head Trauma Rehab.* 1999;14:406–423.

Eierud C, Craddock RC, Fletcher S, et al. Neuroimaging after mild traumatic brain injury: review and meta-analysis. *Neuroimage Clin.* 2014;4:283–94.

Glauser J. Head injury: which patients need imaging? Which test is best? *Cleveland Clinic J Med.* 2004;71(4):353–357.

Jeret JS, Mandell M, Anziska B, et al. Clinical predictors of abnormality disclosed by computed tomography after mild head trauma. *Neurosurgery.* 1993;32:9–16.

Schaefer PW, Huisman TA, Sorensen AG, et al. Diffusion-weighted MR imaging in closed head injury: high correlation with initial Glasgow coma scale score and score on modified Rankin scale at discharge. *Radiology.* 2004;233(1):58–66.

Schenarts PJ, Diaz J, Kaiser C, et al. Prospective comparison of admission computed tomographic scan and plain films of the upper cervical spine in trauma patients with altered mental status. *J Trauma Injury Infect Crit Care.* 2001;51:663–668.

Zee CS, Go JL. CT of head trauma. *Neuroimaging Clin N Am.* 1998;8:525–539.

Epidural Hematoma

Borzone M, Rivano C, Altomonte M, et al. Acute traumatic posterior fossa haematomas. *Acta Neurochir.* 1995;135:32–37.

Bricolo AP, Pasut LM. Extradural hematoma: toward zero mortality. *Neurosurgery.* 1984;14:8–12.

Bullock R, Smith RM, van Dellen JR. Nonoperative management of extradural hematoma. *Neurosurgery.* 1985;16:602–606.

Dhellemmes P, Lejeune JP, Christiaens JL, et al. Traumatic extradural hematomas in infancy and childhood. *J Neurosurg.* 1985;62:861–865.

Lobato RD, Rivas JJ, Cordobes F, et al. Acute epidural hematoma: an analysis of factors influencing the outcome of patients undergoing surgery in coma. *J Neurosurg.* 1988;68(1):48–57.

Subdural Hematoma

Bender MB. Recovery from subdural hematoma without surgery. *J Mt Sinai Hosp N Y.* 1960;26:52–58.

Bershad EM, Farhadi S, Suri MF, et al. Coagulopathy and inhospital deaths in patients with acute subdural hematoma. *J Neurosurg.* 2008;109:664–669.

Lee KS. The pathogenesis and clinical significance of traumatic subdural hygroma. *Brain Inj.* 1998;12:595–603.

Liu W, Bakker NA, Groen RJ. Chronic subdural hematoma: a systematic review and meta-analysis of surgical procedures. *J Neurosurg.* 2014;121(3): 665–673.

Munro D, Merritt HH. Surgical pathology of subdural hematoma. *Arch Neurol Psychiatry.* 1936;35:64–78.

Munro PT, Smith RD, Parke TR. Effect of patients' age on management of acute intracranial haematoma: prospective national study. *BMJ.* 2002;325:1001.

Rohde V, Graf G, Hassler W. Complications of burr-hole craniostomy and closed-system drainage for chronic subdural hematomas: a retrospective analysis of 376 patients. *Neurosurg Rev.* 2002;25:89–94.

Weigel R, Schmiedek P, Krauss JK. Outcome of contemporary surgery for chronic subdural haematoma: evidence based review. *J Neurol Neurosurg Psychiatry.* 2003;74:937–943.

Complications of Head Injury

Bell RB, Dierks EJ, Homer L, et al. Management of cerebrospinal fluid leak associated with craniomaxillofacial trauma. *J Oral Maxillofacial Surg.* 2004;62(6):676–684.

Chesnut RM. Intracranial pressure monitoring: headstone or a new head start. The BEST TRIP trial in perspective. *Intensive Care Med.* 2013;39(4): 771–774.

D'Ambrosio R, Perucca E. Epilepsy after head injury. *Curr Opin Neurol.* 2004;17(6):731–735.

Davis JM, Zimmerman RA. Injury to the carotid and vertebral arteries. *Neuroradiology.* 1983;25:55–70.

Dott NM. Carotid-cavernous arteriovenous fistula. *Clin Neurosurg.* 1969;16:17–21.

Friedman AP, Merritt HH. Damage to cranial nerves resulting from head injury. *Bull Los Angel Neurol Soc.* 1944;9:135–139.

Hemphill JC III, Gress DR, Halbach VV. Endovascular therapy of traumatic injuries of the intracranial cerebral arteries. *Crit Care Clin*. 1999;15:811–829.

Klisch J, Huppertz HJ, Spetzger U, et al. Transvenous treatment of carotid cavernous and dural arteriovenous fistulae: results for 31 patients and review of the literature. *Neurosurgery*. 2003;3(4):836–856.

Luo CB, Teng MM, Yen DH, et al. Endovascular embolization of recurrent traumatic carotid-cavernous fistulas managed previously with detachable balloons. *J Trauma*. 2004;56(6):1214–1220.

Morgan MK, Besser M, Johnston I, et al. Intracranial carotid artery injury in closed head trauma. *J Neurosurg*. 1987;66:192–197.

Scott BL, Jancovic J. Delayed-onset progressive movement disorders after static brain lesions. *Neurology*. 1996;46:68–74.

Stocchett N, Mass AIR. Traumatic intracranial hypertension. *N Engl J Med*. 2014;370:2121–2130.

Yuh EL, Hawryluk GW, Manley GT. Imaging concussion: a review. *Neurosurgery*. 2014;75(suppl 4):S50–S63.

Pediatric Trauma

Adelson PD, Kochanek PM. Head injury in children. *J Child Neurol*. 1998;13:2–15.

Carbaugh SF. Understanding shaken baby syndrome. *Adv Neonatal Care*. 2004;4(2):105–114.

Duhaime AC, Christian CW, Rorke LB, et al. Nonaccidental head injury in infants—the "shaken baby syndrome." *N Engl J Med*. 1998;338:1822–1829.

Schutzman SA, Barnes P, Duhaime AC, et al. Evaluation and management of children younger than two years old with apparently minor head trauma: proposed guidelines. *Pediatrics*. 2001;107:983–993.

Squier W. Shaken baby syndrome: the quest for evidence. *Dev Med Child Neurol*. 2008;50(1):10–14.

Ward JD. Pediatric issues in head trauma. *New Horiz*. 1995;3:539–545.

Outcome

Anderson VA, Morse SA, Catroppa C, et al. Thirty month outcome from early childhood head injury: a prospective analysis of neurobehavioural recovery. *Brain*. 2004;127(pt 12):2608–2620.

Annegers JF, Grabow JD, Groover RV, et al. Seizures after head trauma: a population study. *Neurology*. 1980;30:683–689.

Brooke OG. Delayed effects of head injuries in children. *BMJ*. 1988;296:948.

Cifu DX, Kreutzer JS, Marwitz JH, et al. Functional outcomes of older adults with traumatic brain injury: a prospective, multicenter analysis. *Arch Phys Med Rehabil*. 1996;77:883–888.

Dennis M, Levin HS. New perspectives on cognitive and behavioral outcome after childhood closed head injury. *Dev Neuropsychol*. 2004;25(1–2):1–3.

Englander J, Bushnik T, Duong TT, et al. Analyzing risk factors for late posttraumatic seizures: a prospective, multicenter investigation. *Arch Phys Med Rehabil*. 2003;84:365–373.

Gordon E, von Holst H, Rudehill A. Outcome of head injury in 2298 patients treated in a single clinic during a 21-year period. *J Neurosurg Anesthesiol*. 1995;7:235–247.

Jiang JY, Gao GY, Li WP, et al. Early indicators of prognosis in 846 cases of severe traumatic brain injury. *J Neurotrauma*. 2002;19(7):869–874.

Klonoff H, Clark C, Klonoff PS. Long-term outcome of head injuries: 23-year follow-up of children. *J Neurol Neurosurg Psychiatry*. 1993;56:410–415.

Levin HS, Amparo E, Eisenberg HM, et al. MRI and CT in relation to the neurobehavioral sequelae of mild and moderate head injuries. *J Neurosurg*. 1987;66:706–713.

Levin HS, Gary HS Jr, Eisenberg MM, et al. Neurobehavioral outcome one year after severe head injury: experience of the Traumatic Coma Data Bank. *J Neurosurg*. 1990;73:699–709.

Lishman WA. Physiogenesis and psychogenesis in the "postconcussional" syndrome. *Br J Psychiatry*. 1988;153:460.

Macciocchi SN, Barth JT, Littlefield LM. Outcome after mild head injury. *Clin Sports Med*. 1998;17:27–36.

Pohlmann-Eden B, Bruckmeir J. Predictors and dynamics of posttraumatic epilepsy. *Acta Neuro Scand*. 1997;95:257–262.

Rovlias A, Kotsou S. Classification and regression tree for prediction of outcome after severe head injury using simple clinical and laboratory variables. *J Neurotrauma*. 2004;21(7):886–893.

Sakas DE, Bullock MR, Teasdale GM. One-year outcome following craniotomy for traumatic hematoma in patients with fixed dilated pupils. *J Neurosurg*. 1995;82:961–965.

Silverberg N, Gardner AJ, Brubacher J, et al. Systematic review of multivariable prognostic models for mild traumatic brain injury [published online ahead of print September 15, 2014]. *J Neurotrauma*.

Temkin NR, Holubkov R, Machamer JE, et al. Classification and regression trees (CART) for prediction of function 1 year following head trauma. *J Neurosurg*. 1995;82:764–771.

Traumatic Spinal Cord Injury 47

Christopher E. Mandigo, Michael G. Kaiser,
and Peter D. Angevine

INTRODUCTION

Traumatic spinal cord injury (SCI) is a sudden event with possibly catastrophic effects that may create a medical, financial, and social burden for the individual and society. Adequate management of these patients requires knowledge of SCI, including epidemiology and pathophysiology, acute and chronic medical complications, and long-term rehabilitation and social needs.

ETIOLOGY AND EPIDEMIOLOGY

Epidemiologic data can guide the use of resources for treating and preventing SCI. The best source of this information for the United States is the National Spinal Cord Injury Database (NSCID), which has been collecting information from facilities that have participated in the Model Spinal Cord Injury System (MSCIS) since 1973. This database includes data from an estimated 13% of new SCI cases each year and has information on over 25,000 people with SCI. SCI occurs in the United States in approximately 40 per 1 million people per year, which results in about 12,000 new cases annually. This figure does not include injuries that result in fatality before hospital arrival, which may double the number of injuries. Currently, 225,000 to 300,000 people are living with SCI.

SCI primarily affects young adults aged between 16 and 30 years, but the average is increasing. The average age in the 1970s was 28.7 years; in the period 2005 to 2008, it was 39.5 years. The median age is 27 years, and 65% of SCI patients are younger than 35 years. The highest incidence occurs between ages 20 and 24 years. The most significant changes between the 1970s and 2005 to 2008 have occurred at the extremes of age. The proportion of patients older than 65 years has increased from 5% to 11%, and the proportion of children from birth to 15 years has decreased from 6% to 2%. The increasing age could arise from data collection bias, improved survival of older patients in the acute period of SCI,

or in age-specific incidence rates. That is, the larger population of elderly patients requires special consideration for medical, surgical, and rehabilitative care.

Seventy-eight percent of SCI patients are male. Among those injured after 2000, 63% were white, 23% were African-American, 12% were Hispanic, and 2% were from other racial or ethnic groups.

Motor vehicle accidents account for approximately 42% of cases, a relatively steady figure for 30 years. Falls account for 27% of all and are the most common cause in patients older than age 65 years. Work-related injury (10%), sports (7%), and violence, typically gunshot wounds (15%), account for most of the remaining causes of SCI. Most injuries occur on the weekends and during the summer months.

Since 2000, the most frequent neurologic category at discharge is incomplete tetraplegia (34%), followed by complete paraplegia (23%), complete tetraplegia (18%), and incomplete paraplegia (19%). Less than 1% of persons experienced complete neurologic recovery by hospital discharge. The average length of hospital stay for a patient with SCI was 15 days in 2005, and the length of rehabilitation stay was 36 days. As one might expect, length of stay for patients with neurologically complete injuries is significantly longer. The Life expectancy for patients with SCI is significantly less than those for uninjured people. Mortality rates are significantly higher during the first year after injury than during subsequent years. As shown in Table 47.1, adapted from the NSCID Web site, life expectancy rates for SCI are directly related to the severity of injury.

There are profound sociologic and economic effects from SCI. About 57% of people with SCI were employed at the time of their injury. Ten years after injury, only 32% of persons with paraplegia and 24% with tetraplegia are employed. About 80% to 90% of patients with SCI are eventually discharged to a private residence, and only 6% are discharged to nursing homes. The rest are discharged to hospitals, group living situations, or other destinations.

TABLE 47.1 Life Expectancy after Spinal Cord Injury

Age at Injury (yr)	No SCI	For Persons Who Survive the First 24 h					For Persons Surviving at Least 1 yr Postinjury				
		Motor Functional at Any Level	Para	Low Tetra (C5–C8)	High Tetra (C1–C4)	Ventilator Dependent at Any Level	Motor Functional at Any Level	Para	Low Tetra (C5–C8)	High Tetra (C1–C4)	Ventilator Dependent at Any Level
20	58	53	45	40	36	17	53	46	41	37	24
40	40	34	28	23	20	7	35	28	24	21	11
60	22	18	13	10	8	2	18	13	10	9	3

Life expectancy in years based on age and injury severity.
SCI, spinal cord injury.

Most SCI patients (53%) are single at the time of injury, and those who are married, or become married, are slightly more likely to become divorced than uninjured individuals. The average yearly and lifetime costs of SCI patients are directly related to the severity and level of injury. For example, patient with high tetraplegia (injury at C1–C4) is estimated to have expenses totaling $775,000 in the first year and $140,000 for each subsequent year. A 25-year-old with a C1–C4 injury will have a lifetime expense of $3 million, and a 50-year-old will have an expense of $1.8 million. A patient with low tetraplegia (injury at C5–C8) will have expenses of $500,000 in the first year and about $55,000 for each subsequent year. Paraplegics and incomplete motor injuries cost from $225,000 to $300,000 for the first year and $15,000 to $30,000 for each subsequent year. These numbers do not reflect the additional indirect costs that relate to unemployment and loss in productivity, which average another $60,000 per year per patient.

Nontraumatic SCI affects a large number of people and can result from a number of etiologies (see Chapter 111). These include multiple sclerosis (MS), neoplastic diseases, vascular disease, inflammatory disease, infections, and degenerative spinal stenosis. This population of patients more commonly presents with incomplete lesions and over a subacute or chronic period. The extent of injury at presentation, the response to treatment, and the prognosis of the underlying disease process will guide medical therapy and the ultimate rehabilitation goals.

MECHANISM OF INJURY

It is generally accepted that acute SCI is a two-step process that involves primary and secondary mechanisms. The primary mechanism results from the initial mechanical injury due to local deformation and energy transformation, whereas the secondary mechanisms encompass a cascade of biochemical and cellular processes that are initiated by the primary process and cause ongoing cellular damage and death.

Primary SCI is most commonly a combination of the initial impact as well as subsequent persisting compression. The most frequent primary mechanism of SCI is impact of bone and ligament against the spinal cord from high translational forces, such as that generated by flexion, extension, axial rotation, or vertebral compression. These motions may result in a variety of vertebral column injuries, which can be identified through imaging studies such as plain radiographs, computed tomography (CT) scans, or magnetic resonance imaging (MRI) scans. The spinal cord may consequently be compressed, stretched, or crushed by fracture or dislocations, burst fractures of the vertebral body, or acutely ruptured intervertebral disks. Injury can result from only the initial impact without ongoing compression. These may occur from severe ligamentous injuries in which the spinal column dislocates and then spontaneously reduces or when there is preexisting cervical spondylosis or spinal stenosis. In this circumstance, a trivial injury may cause major neurologic damage even without obvious fracture or dislocation after the event.

Similarly, SCI from sharp bone fragments or stabbing or missile injuries can produce a mixture of spinal cord laceration, concussion, contusion, and/or compression. Direct injuries, like indirect injuries, may be partial or complete in their destruction of the cord.

An understanding of the mechanism of injury and the radiographic findings can provide insight into the biomechanical stability of the vertebral column after SCI. For example, flexion injuries, particularly in the cervical and thoracic regions, may cause anterior compression fractures of vertebral bodies and unilateral or bilateral facet joint dislocation, which can cause spinal cord compression and spinal instability. Severe axial loading can cause complete fracture of the vertebral body with displacement of bony fragments and disk material into the spinal canal and SCI. Any combination of forces may occur in a single case. Understanding the mechanism of injury permits a more complete assessment of the underlying cord injury and the instability of the spinal column.

Secondary mechanisms that result from biochemical cascades that occur after the initial event are a source of ongoing SCI and neurologic deterioration. These cause damage to neural tissue on the cellular level and include the pathologic effects of microvascular changes, excitatory amino acids, cell membrane destabilization, free radicals, inflammatory mediators, and neuroglia apoptosis.

PATHOBIOLOGY

GROSS PATHOLOGY

The pathology of SCI has been divided into four relatively simple groups based on gross findings: solid cord injury, contusion/cavity, laceration, and massive compression. Solid cord injury refers to a cord that grossly appears normal without evidence of softening, discoloration, or cavity formation. However, damage to the cord can be clearly seen on histologic examination. Contusion or cavity injuries have no breach or disruption in the surface anatomy, and there are no dural adhesions. Areas of hemorrhage and necrosis (eventually evolving into cysts) are readily identified in the cord parenchyma. In many instances, these lesions taper rostrally and caudally in a cone-like fashion along the ventral regions of the posterior columns. Lacerations result in clear-cut disruption of the surface anatomy. This type of injury is most often caused by penetrating missiles or sharp fragments of bone. The lesions are characterized by a break in the glia limitans, with damage to the underlying cord parenchyma. The epicenter of the injury generally shows minimal to no evidence of cavity formation; rather, the lesion is dominated by the deposition of a variable amount of collagenous connective tissue that, in most cases, is adherent to the overlying meninges. With massive compression injury, the cord is macerated or pulpified to a varying degree. This lesion is often accompanied by severe vertebral body fractures or dislocations. In many instances, the epicenter of this lesion is replaced by connective tissue scar and fragments of nerve roots. The tissue response is similar to that seen with laceration injuries where extensive fibrous scarring occurs over time.

There are additional anatomic characteristics of SCI worth noting. The lesion may be surprisingly small and may involve no more than a single spinal cord segment. There may be multiple lesions, especially with gunshot wounds. It is also rare to observe a complete transection of the spinal cord; on close examination, there is almost always a small amount of residual tissue traversing the cord.

HISTOPATHOLOGY

The histologic changes in SCI can be divided into immediate, acute, intermediate, and late phases.

Immediate Phase (Initial 1 to 2 Hours)

The immediate event, presumably arising from the primary injury, consists of the actual mechanical disruption of tissue that occurs at the time of injury, such as tears, compression, and distortions.

Vascular changes are commonly found and are characterized by vasodilatation, congestion (hyperemia), and petechial hemorrhages. In many cases, however, no abnormalities are observed during this early time period, particularly in the absence of a massive compression or laceration injury. This lack of pathologic changes in the early period reflects the observation that the pathology of SCI is also due to secondary phenomena, which include progressive edema, ischemia, hemorrhage, inflammation, hyperthermia, as well as calcium–, free radical–, nitric oxide–, and glutamate-mediated cell injury.

Acute Phase (Hours to 1 to 2 Days)

Vascular changes, edema, hemorrhage, inflammation, and neuronal and myelin changes characterize this phase. Edema may be vasogenic or cytotoxic. Vasogenic edema is leakage of plasma fluid into the extracellular space from breakdown of the blood–brain barrier (BBB). Cytotoxic edema results from intracellular swelling after cell death. Edema from either mechanism may result in pressure-induced ischemia caused by diminished blood flow to the injured region. Edema is seen from 3 hours to 3 days after injury. In addition to creating pressure effects, cell swelling may also alter astroglial functions.

Injury to vessels may lead to hemorrhage, which occurs primarily in the gray matter following contusion injury. Hemorrhages are primarily due to rupture of postcapillary venules or sulcal arterioles, either from mechanical disruption by the trauma or from intravascular coagulation leading to venous stasis and distention.

The inflammatory response that follows early after injury is a complex process involving vascular changes, cellular responses, and chemical mediators. There is a mild influx of neutrophils within 1 day, a peak at 2 days, and most are gone by 3 days. It is likely that the neutrophilic response is neurotoxic in nature, as these cells normally act to eradicate infection through the release of free radicals.

Neurons are very vulnerable to injury following SCI. Most neurons die from necrosis, but neuronal apoptosis also has been observed. Acute injury is characterized by axonal swelling, manifested as retraction balls or spheroids. Myelin breakdown occurs early following SCI. It is characterized initially by swelling of myelin sheaths and ultimately by its fragmentation and phagocytosis by macrophages. The loss of myelin occurs with the destructive process and is almost always associated with axonal pathology. Oligodendrocytes, like neurons, are exquisitely sensitive to SCI and undergo necrosis and apoptosis. It is likely that the death of oligodendrocytes contributes significantly to the process of wallerian degeneration.

Intermediate Phase (Days to Weeks)

Over the ensuing days and weeks, there are prominent glial responses with the elimination of necrotic debris, the beginning of astroglial scarring, the resolution of edema, the revascularization of tissue, and restoration of the BBB.

Late Phase (Weeks to Months/Years)

The later phases of SCI are characterized by wallerian degeneration, astroglial and mesenchymal scar formation, development of cysts and syrinx, and schwannosis.

Wallerian degeneration is the anterograde disintegration of axons and their myelin sheaths that have been transected following injury. It is characterized by distorted and fragmented myelin sheaths with absent or malformed axons. An astroglial "scar,"

which comprises tightly interwoven astrocyte processes and extracellular matrix, eventually replaces the destroyed myelinated axon. Wallerian degeneration is a protracted process and may take more than a year to complete. The spinal cord may also be replaced by fibrous connective tissue and collagen. This occurs particularly after lacerating-type injuries and is stimulated by violation of the glia limitans. This abnormal healing coupled with astroglial scarring are thought to create physical and biochemical barriers to axonal migration and spinal cord healing.

Another late finding is the formation of cysts and syrinxes, which may be single, multiple, or multiloculated. Cysts and syrinxes are surrounded by an astrogliotic wall and represent the final "healing" phase of the necrotic process. These cavities are filled with extracellular fluid and commonly contain residual macrophages, small bands of connective tissue, and blood vessels. These cavities typically do not create a clinical problem, except that they do not provide a good substrate for regeneration.

Schwannosis is an aberrant intra- and extramedullary proliferation of Schwann cells with associated axons. It is similar, if not identical, to traumatic neuromas that occur in injured peripheral nerves. Varying amounts of spinal cord tissue may be replaced by schwannosis. The Schwann cells are introduced into the spinal cord after penetrating injuries. The incidence of schwannosis in human SCI is very high and directly correlates with time after injury, suggesting an ongoing mechanism. Its clinical significance is unclear. The prolific schwannosis may be a physical barrier to spinal cord healing. The aberrant axons that are part of this process may have untoward physiologic consequences and potentially contribute to pain, spasticity, and other abnormal responses observed in the chronically injured patient with SCI.

In general, the morphologic responses in human SCI are stereotyped and follow discernible patterns. Early glial (astrocytic and microglial) responses may greatly influence the outcome of SCI.

DIAGNOSIS, NEUROLOGIC ASSESSMENT, AND CLASSIFICATION

CLINICAL EVALUATION

The diagnosis and initial management in patients with SCI often are intertwined, as a large percentage of patients present acutely, often with multisystem trauma, and require rapid assessment and medical intervention.

Prehospital trauma protocols are critical to prevent further injury to the spinal cord, particularly by modifying factors that contribute to secondary spinal cord damage. *Any patient with suspected SCI should be immobilized with a hard cervical collar and/or a rigid head-strap/backboard until definitive neurosurgical assessment can take place.* Treatment of hypoxia and hypotension, proper monitoring of vital signs, and transfer to an appropriate trauma center will affect ultimate outcomes positively.

On arrival to the trauma center, a rapid assessment should be undertaken to assess the status of the airway, respiratory, and circulatory (ABC) systems. In addition, a cursory assessment of the neurologic status ("disability") and removal of all clothing with attention to possible injuries missed on the primary survey ("exposure") are now included in the initial steps of trauma protocols. Clinical signs of shock and hypoxia require immediate attention and appropriate therapy.

Specific diagnosis of SCI requires a more comprehensive neurologic exam as outlined later in the text with the steps necessary to determine the exact spinal cord impairment. Concomitant with the

TABLE 47.2	**High-Risk Criteria for Patients Who Clearly Need C-Spine Imaging**

- Altered mental status (GCS <15)
- Neurologic deficit (i.e., limb weakness or paralysis, numbness, tingling)
- Distracting injuries present
- Neck pain or tenderness present
- Decreased range of motion of the cervical spine

GCS, Glasgow Coma Scale.

physical exam, complete and accurate imaging studies of the spinal column are necessary if SCI is suspected. These can enhance the accuracy of diagnosis and determine the extent of spinal column injury, especially in a comatose, confused, or uncooperative patient. Imaging studies are not necessary when patients are awake, are alert and cooperative without evidence of intoxication, do not have evidence of neurologic injury, and have no pain or tenderness along the spine to palpation and no associated injuries distracting from the general evaluation.

IMAGING STUDIES

Risk Stratification

Trauma patients typically arrive with neck collars. Some patients are clearly at high risk, whereas other can be cleared clinically in the emergency department or intensive care unit (ICU) without imaging. The cervical collar and spinal precautions should remain in place, and cervical spine imaging is clearly necessary; when clear symptoms, neck pain, or distracting conditions exist, clinical conditions are met (Table 47.2). National Emergency X-Radiography Utilization Study (NEXUS) criteria (Table 47.3) address the question of who does not require imaging after presenting with head or neck trauma. *A patient who meets all five NEXUS criteria is deemed to have a low probability of injury to the cervical spine and can be cleared clinically without imaging because the risk of significant injury is miniscule* [**Level 1**].[1] The Canadian C-spine rule offers even slightly better sensitivity and specificity for identifying low-risk patients but is a bit more complicated to use.

Cervical X-rays

Anteroposterior (AP) and lateral x-rays can be taken of the appropriate spinal region as directed by the clinical evaluation. AP and

TABLE 47.3	**NEXUS Criteria for Low-Risk Patients Who Do Not Require Imaging after Head or Neck Injury[a]**

1. No tenderness at the posterior midline of the cervical spine
2. No focal neurologic deficit
3. Normal level of alertness
4. No evidence of intoxication
5. No clinically apparent, painful injury that might distract the patient from the pain of a cervical spine injury

[a]In these patients, the neck collar can be removed and the patient cleared clinically after demonstrating full range of motion with no neck pain or point tenderness.

NEXUS, National Emergency X-Radiography Utilization Study.

lateral x-rays of the cervical spine, visualizing the superior part of the first thoracic vertebral body, and open-mouth, odontoid radiographic views can form part of the initial radiologic survey. However, due to its ease of use and superior sensitivity, most centers go directly to cervical spine CT as the initial imaging study of choice. When CT scanning is available, plain x-rays contribute no additional information and need not be obtained.

Upright flexion and extension films, when appropriate, are useful for assessing biomechanical instability due to ligamentous injury. In suspected thoracic and lumbar injuries, AP, lateral, oblique, upright, and dynamic (flexion/extension) views may be necessary. Indications for thoracolumbar x-rays include falls greater than 6 ft, expulsion from motor vehicles, complaints of back pain, associated injuries, and altered mental status with an unknown mechanism of injury.

Cervical Computed Tomography

High-resolution CT scanning (see Chapter 20) with sagittal and coronal reconstruction is the best procedure for evaluating uncertain findings seen on x-rays as well as for detecting bone pathology (Fig. 47.1). The study should be performed from the occiput to T1 with three-dimensional sagittal and coronal reformats. Three-dimensional reconstructions allow for visualization in the coronal, sagittal, and axial planes and provide superior injury detection compared with plain x-ray. The main limitation of CT rests in its relative inability to detect changes in soft tissues including the spinal cord and ligamentous structures.

Whether it is safe to remove a neck collar in a comatose or obtunded patient with a normal neck CT has long remained a vexing clinical conundrum. In the past, it was felt that it was necessary to obtain a cervical MRI within 72 hours in order to rule out possible ligamentous injury, which appears as swelling or thickening of the interspinal ligaments. More recent data indicates that in obtunded or intubated patients, the use of modern CT alone is sufficient to exclude unstable cervical spine injuries. The complete absence of any sign of fracture or misalignment of the bony structures indicates a less than 0.1% chance of the patient harboring a clinically significant unstable cervical spine injury [**Level 1**].[2]

MRI (see Chapter 21) is the best technique for imaging the spinal cord itself. Specific indications for MRI scanning include a neurologic deficit with normal x-rays, lack of correlation between a neurologic deficit and x-ray findings, deterioration following closed reduction, and failed attempts at closed reduction. Multiplanar, high-resolution MRI with T1-weighted and gradient echo or T2-weighted imaging is the most specific and sensitive technique for assessing soft-tissue paraspinal lesions, disk herniation, spinal cord hemorrhage, spinal cord edema, and intra- or extradural hemorrhage (Fig. 47.2). The ability to adequately monitor the critically injured must be a priority when MRI is considered. If MRI is not available or possible, CT myelography is the current best alternative.

NEUROLOGIC ASSESSMENT AND CLASSIFICATION

The most widely accepted, standardized method of classifying SCI is the *International Standards for Neurological and Functional Classification of Spinal Cord Injury* published jointly by the American Spinal Injury Association (ASIA) and the International Medical Society of Paraplegia (IMSOP). It is more commonly known as the ASIA Impairment Scale. This is an excellent guide for clinical

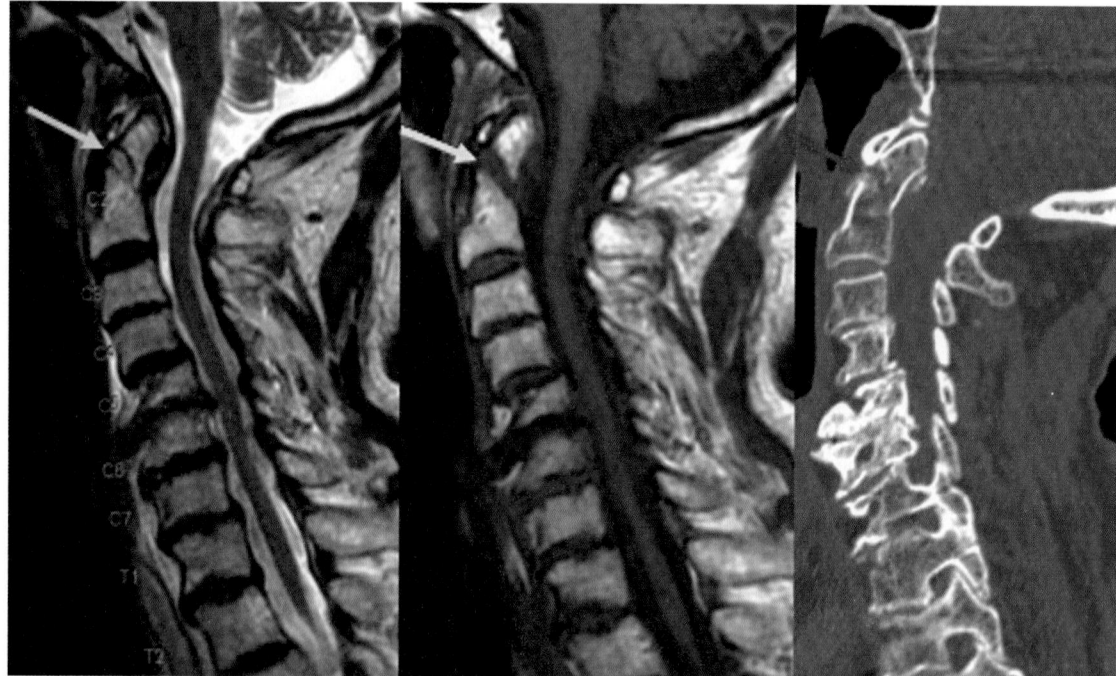

FIGURE 47.1 Type 2 acute dens fracture (*blue arrow* and *green arrow*) on sagittal T1- **(left)** and T2 **(center)**-weighted MRI and a CT sagittal reconstruction (*red arrow*) **(right)**. (Images courtesy of Dr. Alexander Khandji.)

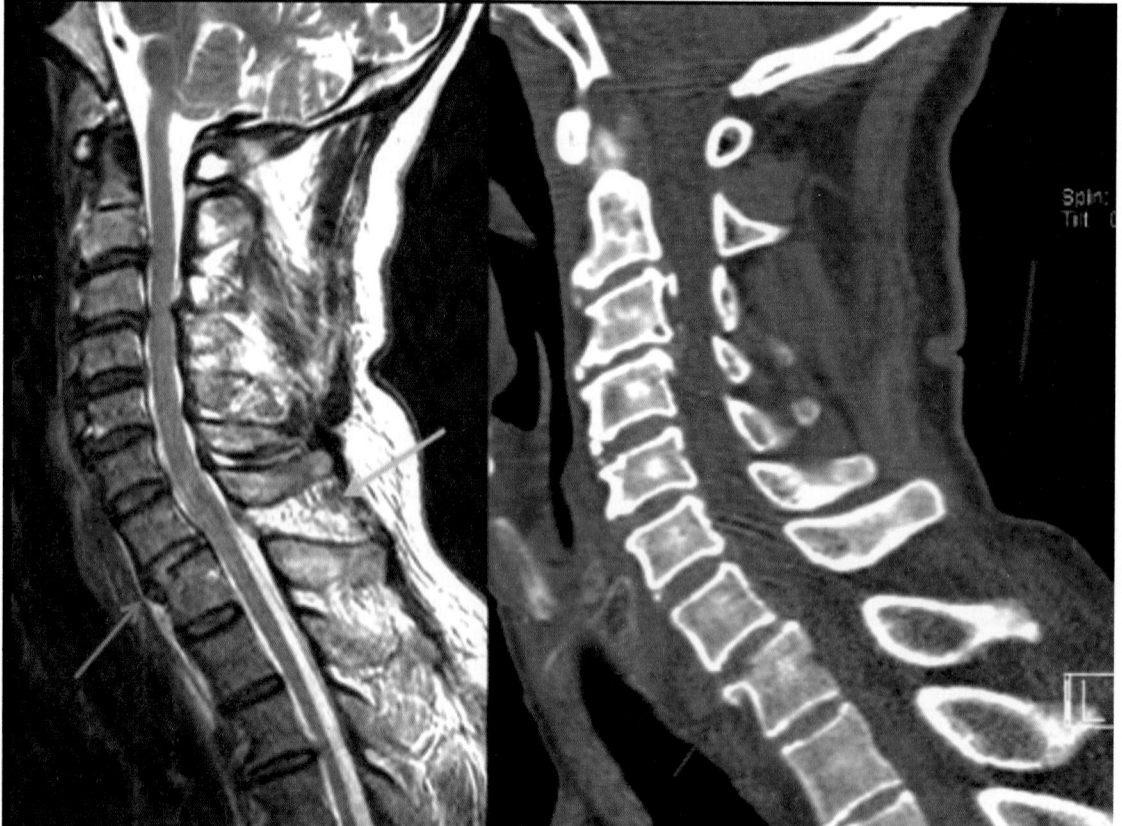

FIGURE 47.2 **Left:** Non–fat-saturated T2 image showing anterior subluxation of C7 on T1 (with anterior tear drop fracture of T1 *blue arrow*) and widened interspinous space C7–T1 posteriorly (*green arrow*). **Right:** Sagittal CT reconstruction demonstrating anterior teardrop fracture of T1 (*red arrow*). (Images courtesy of Dr. Alexander Khandji.)

TABLE 47.4	American Spinal Injury Association (ASIA) Impairment Scale	
A	Complete	No sensory or motor function preserved in the lowest sacral segments (S4/S5)
B	Sensory incomplete	Sensory but no motor function preserved below the neurologic level, including the sacral segments
C	Motor incomplete	Motor function is preserved below the neurologic level, and more than half of the key muscles below the level have a grade <3, and there is some sacral sensory and/or motor sparing.
D	Motor incomplete	Motor function is preserved below the neurologic level, and more than half of the key muscles below the level have a grade ≥3, and there is some sacral sensory and/or motor sparing.
E	Normal	Sensory and motor functions are normal. There can be reflex abnormalities.

evaluation and neurologic assessment and allows uniform comparisons among clinicians and researchers.

The ASIA Impairment Scale is scored from A to E and is detailed in Table 47.4. The steps to classify injury severity in a patient with SCI are described in Table 47.5. There are some terms that require clear definitions for categorizing impairments within the ASIA scoring system. The motor level is the most caudal key muscle group that is graded 3/5 or greater, with the segments cephalad to that level graded normal strength (5/5). The sensory level is the most caudal dermatome to have normal light touch and pinprick sensation on both sides. The neurologic level of injury is the most caudal level at which both motor and sensory modalities are intact. A complete injury is the absence of motor and sensory function in the lowest sacral segments. An incomplete injury has preservation of motor or sensory function below the neurologic level of injury that includes the lowest sacral segments. A zone of partial preservation describes all segments below the neurologic level of injury that have preserved motor or sensory findings; this is used only in complete injuries.

TABLE 47.5	Physical Examination Steps for Classifying Spinal Cord Injury
1.	Perform sensory examination in 28 dermatomes bilaterally for pinprick and light touch, including the S4/S5 dermatome, and test for anal sensation.
2.	Determine sensory level (right and left).
3.	Perform motor examination in the 10 key muscle groups, including anal contraction.
4.	Determine motor level (right and left).
5.	Determine neurologic level of injury.
6.	Classify injury as complete or incomplete.
7.	Categorize ASIA Impairment Scale (A–E).
8.	Determine zone of partial preservation if ASIA A.

ASIA, American Spinal Injury Association.

A subset of SCIs has been grouped by their specific clinical features into six clinical syndromes: Brown-Séquard, central cord, anterior cord, posterior cord, conus medullaris, and cauda equina.

Brown-Séquard Syndrome

This syndrome is characterized anatomically by a hemicord injury with ipsilateral proprioceptive and motor loss and contralateral pain and temperature sensation loss below the level of the lesion. The pattern of neurologic deficits observed in Brown-Séquard injuries result from the local spinal cord anatomy. Pain and temperature fibers cross to the opposite side of the spinal cord at the level of nerve root entry, whereas the proprioception and motor fibers decussate at the level of the brain stem. Brown-Séquard accounts for 1% to 5% of all traumatic SCIs. The most common presentation is the Brown-Séquard plus syndrome, which refers to a relative ipsilateral hemiplegia with a relative contralateral hemianalgesia. Although Brown-Séquard traditionally has been associated with stab or missile injuries, a variety of etiologies may cause this syndrome. Brown-Séquard has the best prognosis for ambulation of the SCI clinical syndromes, as 75% to 90% of patients ambulate independently in long-term follow-up.

Central Cord Syndrome

This lesion is characterized by disproportionately more motor impairment of the upper than the lower extremities, bladder dysfunction, and varying degrees of sensory loss below the level of the lesion. The most common presentation occurs in older patients with preexisting cervical spondylosis who experience hyperextension injuries of the cervical spine. Cord compression occurs between osteophyte–disk complexes anteriorly and infolded ligamenta flava posteriorly. Studies have reported falls as the most common etiology, followed by motor vehicle accidents. Recent evidence from clinical–pathologic studies using MRI scans has demonstrated that this clinical pattern likely results from injury to the corticospinal tract in the cervical spine, which affects the distal, more than proximal, limb musculature and not the specific somatotopic representation within the corticospinal tract. It is considered the most common of the SCI syndromes, accounting for approximately 9% of all traumatic SCIs. Central cord syndrome generally has a favorable prognosis for functional recovery, especially in younger patients with good hand function, evidence of early motor recovery, and absence of lower extremity impairment.

Anterior Cord Syndrome

This syndrome results from a lesion that affects the anterior two-thirds of the spinal cord with preservation of the posterior columns. It is characterized by complete paralysis and loss of pain and temperature sensation below the level of the lesion, accompanied by preservation of touch and proprioception. It occurs in 3% of all traumatic SCIs. It can result from flexion injuries, direct damage from bony fragments or disk compression, or secondary to occlusion of the anterior spinal artery. This syndrome carries a poor prognosis for functional improvement.

Posterior Cord Syndrome

This is the least common of the clinical syndromes and has an incidence of less than 1%. It is a lesion of the posterior columns with resultant loss of touch and proprioception below the level of injury and preservation of pain and temperature sensation and motor strength. It can be caused by hyperextension, posterior spinal artery occlusion, or nontraumatic etiologies such as tumors or vitamin B_{12} deficiency.

Conus Medullaris and Cauda Equina Syndromes

Conus medullaris syndrome is an injury of the caudal spinal cord (conus) and its associated sacral nerve roots within the spinal canal. The conus typically sits at the level between the first and second lumbar vertebrae. This condition is characterized by a combination of upper and lower motor neuron signs. Findings include saddle anesthesia, areflexic bladder and bowel, and variable degrees of lower extremity weakness and sensory loss.

Cauda equina syndrome results from an injury to the lumbosacral nerve roots within the neural canal below the conus medullaris and presents with saddle anesthesia, bladder and bowel dysfunction, and variable lower extremity involvement. The difference from the conus medullaris syndrome is the absence of upper motor neuron signs, and it is usually characterized by asymmetric lower extremity weakness and reflex changes. It is believed to have a better prognosis for neurologic recovery than SCI because nerve roots have the ability to regenerate. Important predictors for favorable outcome from cauda equina are early diagnosis and surgical decompression.

ACUTE MEDICAL MANAGEMENT

The acute management of patients with SCI is primarily directed at medical stabilization to prevent secondary injury and to permit the accurate clinical and radiographic diagnosis of spinal cord and column pathology. The specifics of initial management have been detailed to some degree in the earlier section covering diagnosis of SCI, as the acute management and evaluation of SCI are intertwined.

GENERAL TRAUMA CARE

In general, patients should be managed at a trauma center, preferably level 1, with SCI experience. If an appropriate trauma center is not immediately available, transfer to a trauma center as soon as possible is advocated. Emergency medical services in urban areas should preferentially take patients to level 1 centers, potentially bypassing nearer hospitals. Level 1 centers are required to have in-house neurosurgical consultation for rapid evaluation. The patient should be immobilized with a cervical collar and backboard/head-strap as soon as possible. The backboard can be removed after radiographic studies are completed and interpreted. The cervical collar should be maintained until the cervical spine has been clinically and/or radiographically cleared. Neurosurgical evaluation should happen as soon as possible; neural element decompression and spinal stabilization within 24 hours may improve neurologic recovery in patients with deficits and spinal cord compression, but the clinical data are inadequate to advocate this as a standard of care. It is important to note that there has been no demonstrated increased risk of neurologic deterioration from early surgery.

STEROIDS

High-dose methylprednisolone has long been considered a potential neuroprotective agent in SCI, with the potential of reducing tissue injury by inhibiting lipid peroxidase and free radical production. Methylprednisolone therapy was evaluated in 487 SCI patients in the National Acute Spinal Cord Injury Study II (NASCIS

II), trial in 1990. Patients were given a bolus of 30 mg/kg of methylprednisolone over 15 minutes, followed by a 5.4-mg/kg infusion over 23 hours. The authors reported a mean improvement of 5 points in motor score (total possible score = 50) and 4 points in sensory scores (total possible score = 58) for patients treated with methylprednisolone compared to controls at 6 months, but only if they received the drug within 8 hours of injury. Although NASCIS II was initially reported as a positive trial, re-analysis has showed that the strength of the evidence generated is weakened by omission of data from publication, the arbitrary assignment of an 8-hour therapeutic window, the inconsistency of reported benefit, and the absence of functional outcome measures. Accordingly, the beneficial results of NASCIS II have been downgraded to Class III medical evidence. Due to a trend towards more serious complications associated with steroid use, current guidelines do not recommend administration of methylprednisolone (MP) for the treatment of acute SCI [**Level 1**].[3]

AUTONOMIC DYSFUNCTION AND BLOOD PRESSURE MANAGEMENT

Autonomic dysfunction with hypotension can occur acutely in SCI, especially in patients with cervical injuries. Autonomic dysfunction may result from a variety of reasons including the following: spinal shock, neurogenic shock, hypovolemia, bradycardia, sepsis, and cardiogenic shock. Hypotension is a common contributor to secondary neurologic injury and should be avoided; its treatment can involve careful volume resuscitation, vasopressors, and diagnostic maneuvers such as an arterial line, a central venous catheter, and noninvasive continuous cardiac output assessment. *Current SCI guidelines recommend maintenance of mean arterial pressure at a minimum value of 85 to 90 mm Hg for the first 7 days after injury.* This has limited supporting clinical data, but hypotension clearly should be avoided. Occasionally, intravenous (IV) atropine sulfate may be necessary to counter unopposed parasympathetic activity. Vasomotor paralysis may also cause loss of thermal control and lead to poikilothermy, which usually may be treated by the appropriate use of warming blankets. Acute cervical SCI is also associated with a risk of cardiac arrhythmia due to excess vagal tone, as well as complicating hypoxia, hypotension, and fluid and electrolyte imbalances.

CRITICAL CARE

After complete medical stabilization, neurologic assessment, and spinal column stabilization and/or bracing within the initial 24 to 48 hours, attention is paid to the prevention of common medical problems in patients with acute SCI. Prophylactic treatment for deep venous thrombosis should begin no later than 72 hours after SCI. The first-line therapy is subcutaneous injection of low molecular weight heparin (enoxaparin 40 mq SC QD), and second-line therapy is subcutaneous injection of unfractionated heparin (5000 U SC BID or TID). In patients with contraindications to anticoagulation, an inferior vena cava filter should be placed to prevent pulmonary embolism. Lower extremity sequential compression devices should also be employed when feasible. Stress ulceration should be prevented with proton pump inhibitors or H2 blockers with a minimum of 4 weeks of therapy after SCI. Nutritional support, via feeding tubes or parental nutrition if appropriate, is suggested to begin with 72 hours after SCI. Pressure ulcers of the occiput, sacrum, and heels should be prevented through manual or automatic turning every 2 hours without lateral sliding to prevent sacral shearing. Rehabilitation maneuvers should begin as soon as possible and should include passive and active range-of-motion (ROM) activities, bowel and bladder programs (e.g., chronic intermittent catheterizations), pulmonary programs (mechanical ventilation, manually assisted cough), and dysphagia evaluations.

SURGICAL TREATMENT

After control of the acute medical issues and accurate neurologic and radiographic diagnosis of SCI, attention is directed toward treating instability of the vertebral column and neural element compression, if present. This is directed by neurosurgical or orthopedic caregivers. There are currently no standards and no evidence-based guidelines regarding the role and method of decompression in acute SCI. In a recent prospective randomized trial, decompression of cervical spinal cord injuries within 24 hours of injury was found to be safe and associated with improved neurologic outcome at 6 months follow-up when compared to more delayed surgical intervention [**Level 1**].[4] The management of cervical, thoracic, and lumbar spine and spinal cord injuries depends mainly on the particular injury but also on a surgeon's personal experience and practice norms in his or her center. The options include closed reduction via traction and open surgical procedures. The overall goals are to decompress the spinal cord and nerve roots, to restore the spinal alignment, and to prevent progressive deformity.

Cervical spine fracture or dislocations may be treated with closed reduction through the use of traction. Thoracic and lumbar fractures cannot be corrected with this treatment. Traction uses skull tongs or the headpiece of a halo attached to a system to apply rostral force, usually with rope, a pulley, and weights. An initial weight of 5 to 15 lb is applied and a lateral x-ray is obtained. Weight can be increased at 5-lb increments, and a neurologic exam and lateral x-ray should be obtained after each adjustment. The maximum weight applied relates to the level of injury. A general rule of 3 to 5 lb per vertebral level is used. We suggest that after 35 lb is applied, patients be observed for at least an hour with repeat cervical spine x-rays before the weight is cautiously increased further. Muscle relaxants and analgesics may help facilitate reduction.

Cervical spine surgery is indicated for injuries that are not amenable or do not respond to closed reduction. These include unstable cervical fractures and cord compression with an incomplete neurologic deficit. Patients without neurologic deficits are often treated nonoperatively with bracing unless there is evidence of instability. Some penetrating injuries may require surgical exploration to ensure that there are no foreign bodies imbedded in the tissue and also to clean the wound to prevent infection.

Thoracolumbar injuries do not lend themselves to external traction, and accordingly, surgical repair is typically achieved through open reduction followed by stabilization. There are a variety of anterior and posterior approaches that employ metallic implants such as interbody cages, pedicle screws, laminar wires or hooks, and connecting rods.

In clinical studies, surgery has little effect on the neurologic outcome of the primary injury. When cord compression is evident, or the initial neurologic deficit progresses, immediate decompression (i.e., 1 to 2 hours after injury) may halt or reverse the process. There are no set rules for determining appropriate selection of early or late surgical intervention. Individual patient factors and clinical judgment continue to direct the surgical timing in each case.

CHRONIC MEDICAL MANAGEMENT

Chronic medical therapy is directed at preventing and treating the common, and often severe, medical complications of SCI. SCI produces a wide variety of changes in systemic physiology that can lead to a number of complications, which rival the impact of neurologic deficits on function and quality of life. In the MSCI database, rehospitalizations occurred in 55% of patients in the first year after SCI and continued at a stable rate of about 37% per year over the next 20 years. Factors contributing to the risk of rehospitalization included increased age and severity of SCI. Genitourinary problems, respiratory complications, and pressure ulcers were the most common reasons for hospitalization. As mentioned earlier, life expectancy is reduced among patients with SCI. The mortality rates are highest during the first year. Higher injury levels, more severe injury, and older age correlate with higher mortality. The most common causes of death are respiratory diseases and cardiovascular events.

AUTONOMIC DYSREFLEXIA

Injuries above T6 may be complicated by autonomic dysreflexia, which results from the loss of coordinated autonomic responses to physiologic stimuli. Uninhibited or exaggerated sympathetic responses to noxious stimuli can lead to extreme hypertension through vasoconstriction. The parasympathetic system will respond with vasodilation and bradycardia above the level of the lesion, but it is not sufficient to correct the elevated blood pressure (BP). SCIs below T6 do not produce dramatic effects as the intact splanchnic innervation allows for compensatory dilatation of the splanchnic vascular bed.

Typical stimuli producing autonomic dysreflexia include bladder distention, bowel impaction, pressure sores, bone fractures, or occult visceral disturbances.

Common clinical manifestations are hypertension, bradycardia, headache, and sweating. Attacks have a range of severity from asymptomatic hypertension to hypertensive crisis with possible cardiac arrest from bradycardia and intracranial hemorrhage. The severity of attacks correlates with the severity of the SCI. The management of acute autonomic dysreflexia involves monitoring BP, removing tight-fitting garments, and searching for sources of noxious stimuli, including bladder distension and fecal impaction. Reduction of elevated BP can be achieved with sitting the patient upright and with rapid-acting antihypertensives with short half-lives. Sublingual or oral nitrates and IV β-blockers, calcium channel blockers, or angiotensin-converting enzyme (ACE) inhibitors are often used. Recognition and avoidance of inciting stimuli are important in preventing attacks.

Orthostatic hypotension can also affect patients with SCI. Treatment involves the implementation of temporary maneuvers, such as gradual position changes, compression stockings, and abdominal binders until the body adapts to the loss of peripheral tone. Medical therapy, if necessary, can include salt tablets to increase blood volume, α-adrenergic agonists, such as midodrine, or mineralocorticoid supplements, such as fludrocortisone.

CORONARY ARTERY DISEASE

Coronary artery disease (CAD) is a prominent complication of SCI with long-term survivors. Patients with SCI are more likely to acquire CAD risk factors than the average population secondary to loss of muscle mass, inactivity, and increased body fat. CAD is

3 to 10 times more likely in patients with chronic SCI, and SCI patients have higher mortality rates with CAD-related events. This is partly explained by abnormal presentations that occur in patients with lesions higher than T5 and the higher likelihood of episodic autonomic dysreflexia.

PULMONARY DISEASE

Cervical and high thoracic SCI will affect respiration. The severity of respiratory failure and need for assisted ventilation is directly related to the level and severity of SCI. Patients have impaired cough strength and difficulty mobilizing lung secretions and are at increased risk for pneumonia, especially during the first year following injury (see also Chapter 116). Prevention of pneumonia includes chest physiotherapy and pneumococcal vaccination. Deep venous thrombosis and pulmonary embolism are common early complications of SCI. Prophylactic use of low molecular weight heparin is the treatment of choice for most patients with SCI; treatment should be continued for at least 3 months after SCI, after which the risk appears to approximate that of the general population.

GENITOURINARY COMPLICATIONS

SCI produces bladder dysfunction, often referred to as the *neurogenic bladder* (see also Chapter 121). Other complications can result from this, including infections, vesicoureteral reflux, renal failure, and nephrocalculi. Urologic evaluation with regular follow-up is recommended for patients after SCI. Genitourinary complications may not produce symptoms and, if untreated, can have serious consequences. The frequency and specific testing involved (serum creatinine, cystoscopy, urodynamic studies, renal ultrasound) are not well defined but depend in part on the nature of the patient's urologic problems and other risk factors.

After SCI, the sensation for bladder fullness as well as motor control of bladder and sphincter function can be impaired. Depending on the timing, the level, and the severity of injury, one of several types of bladder dysfunction can occur. These include bladder hyperactivity with reflexive bladder emptying, sphincter hyperactivity with impaired emptying of the bladder, detrusor-sphincter dyssynergia leading to uncoordinated bladder contractions, bladder flaccidity with urinary retention, and overflow incontinence.

Clean intermittent catheterization (CIC) programs achieve the goal of preserving renal function while eliminating urine at regular and socially acceptable times. This avoids high bladder pressures, retention, incontinence, and infection. This should be initiated as early as possible after SCI. Catheterization is performed approximately every 4 hours and is adjusted as necessary. Often, patients have a fluid intake restriction of 2 L to prevent bladder overdistention. After ruling out an infection and adjusting the frequency of CIC and fluid intake, medications targeting the sympathetic and parasympathetic receptors are employed depending on the specific bladder condition.

Urinary tract infections (UTIs) are common in SCI and are the most frequent source of septicemia in SCI patients. Asymptomatic UTIs are not generally treated, and prophylactic antibiotics are not used for prevention.

Sexual dysfunction has a high prevalence in SCI; dysfunction in males can exceed 75% and is related to the severity of injury. There are a variety of treatment options for men with SCI, which include medicines for erectile dysfunction and surgically implanted prosthetics. Sexual responses in women may also be impaired after SCI, but ovulation and fertility are generally unaffected. Pregnancy with

SCI is considered high risk because of the high rate of complications secondary to infections and autonomic dysreflexia.

GASTROINTESTINAL DYSFUNCTION

Bowel dysfunction is very common after SCI and can significantly affect quality of life. There are no evidence-based recommendations for clinical management of this problem. A structured bowel regimen employing a regular diet, 2 to 3 L of fluid/day, 30 g of fiber, and chemical and mechanical stimulation is often employed to achieve predictable bowel evacuation to avoid fecal incontinence and impaction.

ABNORMAL BONE METABOLISM

Osteoporosis can affect the bones below the level of SCI, most likely secondary to disuse, and may predispose to fractures. Bone resorption in the first few months after SCI can lead to symptomatic hypercalcemia. Treatment can involve the use of hydration with IV fluids, loop diuretics, and IV bisphosphonate therapy.

Heterotopic ossification, the deposition of bone within the soft tissue around peripheral joints, can also occur in SCI. This occurs in up to half of SCI patients but is symptomatic, as evidenced by pain and inflammation in the affected joints, in 10% to 20% of patients. Treatment involves passive ROM exercise, oral bisphosphonates, nonsteroidal anti-inflammatory drugs (NSAIDs), and, in some cases, delayed surgery.

SPASTICITY

Spasticity results from the disruption of the descending inhibitory pathways, with a concomitant increase in the excitability of spinal reflexes and resting muscle tone. Spasticity can negatively affect quality of life through pain, decreased mobility, muscle spasms, and ultimately, contractures. Prevention of contractures involves proper positioning, passive ROM exercises, appropriate splinting, and treatment of spasticity. However, the increased tone can also make some activities easier, such as standing and transfers. Treatment can include physical therapy, passive ROM exercises, oral medications (baclofen, tizanidine, valium, etc.), and surgical interventions (intrathecal baclofen pumps, rhizotomies, etc.).

PSYCHIATRIC COMPLICATIONS

Psychiatric disorders associated with SCI include depression, suicide, and drug addiction. Approximately a third of patients with SCI will be depressed within the first year after SCI; this is not closely associated with severity of injury. Suicide occurs at a rate four to five times higher in patients with SCI and is the leading cause of death in patients with SCI younger than the age of 55 years. Patients should be regularly screened for symptoms of depression, and symptoms should be treated immediately.

CONCLUSION

SCI remains a difficult medical, social, and financial problem. A more clear understanding of the pathophysiology and resultant medical complications has resulted in improved long-term survival and functional status. However, the unsolved problem of SCI repair remains. It is worth remembering that the best treatment is prevention. Nationwide educational programs should be concerned with combating the causes of SCI: motor vehicle safety, water and occupational safety, eliminating drunk driving, adhering to speed limits, and mandatory use of seatbelts and other protective gear.

LEVEL 1 EVIDENCE

1. Hoffman JR, Mower WR, Wolfson AB, et al. Validity of a set of clinical criteria to rule out injury to the cervical spine in patients with blunt trauma. *N Engl J Med*. 2000;343:94–99.

2. Panczykowski DM, Tomycz ND, Okonkwo DO. Comparative effectiveness of using computed tomography alone to exclude cervical spine injuries in obtunded or intubated patients: meta-analysis of 14,327 patients with blunt trauma. *J Neurosurg*. 2011; 115:541–549.

3. Hurlburt RJ, Hadley MN, Walters BC, et al. Pharmacological therapy for acute spinal cord injury. *Neurosurgery*. 2013;72: 93–105.

4. Fehlings MG, Vaccaro A, Wilson JR, et al. Early versus delayed decompression for traumatic cervical spinal cord injury: results of the surgical timing in acute spinal cord injury study (STASCIS). *PLoS ONE*. 2012;7(2):e32037. doi:10.1371/journal .pone.0032037.

SUGGESTED READINGS

Bracken MB. Methylprednisolone and spinal cord injury. *J Neurosurg*. 2002;96:140–141.

Inoue T, Manley GT, Patel N, et al. Medical and surgical management after spinal cord injury: vasopressor usage, early surgerys, and complications. *J Neurotrauma*. 2014;31:284–291.

Jackson AB, Dijkers M, Devivo MJ, et al. A demographic profile of new traumatic spinal cord injuries: change and stability over 30 years. *Arch Phys Med Rehabil*. 2004;85:1740–1748.

Kong CY, Hosseini AM, Belanger LM, et al. A prospective evaluation of hemodynamic management in acute spinal cord injury patients. *Spinal Cord*. 2013;51:466–471.

Maynard FM Jr, Bracken MB, Creasey G, et al. International standards for neurological and functional classification of spinal cord injury. American Spinal Injury Association. *Spinal Cord*. 1997;35:266–274.

McKinley W, Santos K, Meade M, et al. Incidence and outcomes of spinal cord injury clinical syndromes. *J Spinal Cord Med*. 2007;30:215–224.

Stiell IG, Clement C, McKnight RD, et al. The Canadian C-spine rule versus the NEXUS low-risk criteria in patients with trauma. *N Engl J Med*. 2003;349:2510–2158.

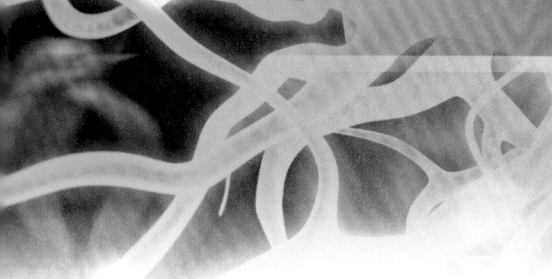

Traumatic Cranial and Peripheral Nerve Injuries 48

Jennifer F. Russo, Charles B. Mikell,
and Christopher J. Winfree

INTRODUCTION

Traumatic injury to peripheral nerves is associated with significant disability and decreased quality of life. In this chapter, we discuss the classification, pathophysiology, evaluation, and treatment of peripheral nerve injuries, as well as the clinical manifestations of common peripheral and cranial nerve lesions. Understanding of the principles described in this chapter, by clinicians, is important for timely diagnosis and treatment of these common clinical entities.

EPIDEMIOLOGY

It has been estimated that approximately 3% to 10% of all patients presenting to a level 1 trauma center present with injury to a peripheral nerve. Motor vehicle accidents are most commonly cited as the leading cause, whereas industrial accidents, recreational vehicle use, falls, gunshot and stab wounds, as well as iatrogenic injuries also contribute. The potential economic and social impact of these injuries is compounded by the fact that they occur most commonly within the productive age range, with highest incidence reported between 20 and 40 years of age. Males are affected more often than females, and injury to the nerves of the upper extremity occur more commonly than do those to the nerves of the lower extremity. Peripheral nerve injuries are also commonly comorbid with traumatic injury to the brain, which can result in delayed diagnosis and intervention.

PATHOBIOLOGY

ANATOMY AND PHYSIOLOGY

Evaluation of traumatic peripheral nerve injury requires understanding of nerve structure. Peripheral nerves consist of a mixture of myelinated and unmyelinated, somatic and autonomic, nerve fibers. Each fiber is surrounded by an endoneurial sheath, which provides some tensile strength. Multiple fibers, of various types, are grouped together into fascicles and surrounded by the perineurium, a specialized structure composed of perineurial cells and collagen that serves to maintain homeostasis of the endoneurial fluid that surrounds individual fibers. This perineural sheath provides most of the tensile strength and elasticity of the nerve and provides a diffusion barrier that resists and maintains intrafascicular pressure. Multiple fasciculi, in turn, are embedded in a connective tissue matrix called the *epineurium*, which protects the nerve from compression. The most superficial layer of the epineurium condenses to form an external epineural sheath, which gives the nerve a cord-like appearance on gross examination.

Both within and between nerve fibers, the number, size, and organization of fascicles varies significantly. As fascicles branch, split, and rejoin continuously along their course, sections through the nerve may alternatively reveal plexiform and cable-like structure, which has implications for both clinical presentation of nerve injuries, as well

as surgical repair and functional regeneration. Further, variability in internal organization is partially responsible for observed differences in the prevalence of particular nerve injuries. That is, peripheral nerves with a higher proportion of epineural tissue to fasciculi may be more resistant to compression injuries, whereas peripheral nerves with greater numbers of fasciculi have greater tensile strength.

MECHANISMS OF INJURY

Traumatic nerve injuries may be acute or chronic and iatrogenic or idiopathic. They result from the application of kinetic energy to a nerve, which is transformed into damaging compressive or tensile forces. Chronic traumatic nerve injuries most often result from anatomic nerve entrapment leading to well-described clinical entities, such as carpal tunnel syndrome. These chronic syndromes, requiring unique medical and surgical treatment approaches, are discussed more thoroughly in Chapter 87.

Acute traumatic nerve injuries occur, most commonly, from traction/stretch, compression, contusion, laceration, or ischemia. Injury is derived primarily from direct application of mechanical forces and secondarily from vascular compromise. Multiple mechanisms of injury may be present, particularly when the lesion occurs during a catastrophic event, such as a motor vehicle accident. Identifying the type of insult incurred, when possible, is important for treatment planning, as various types of forces result in different patterns of injury.

INJURY CLASSIFICATION

Two major classifications systems are used most commonly to describe peripheral nerve injuries. The injury categories defined by these systems each have unique diagnostic characteristics, prognoses, and therapeutic approaches.

The classification system used most commonly in clinical settings was proposed by Seddon in 1942. Seddon's system divides injuries into three main categories delineated by the extent of disruption to the structure of the nerve. The three categories are *neurapraxia*, *axonotmesis*, and *neurotmesis* (Table 48.1).

Neurapraxia is the least severe of the three injury types. It most commonly is caused by a mild insult resulting in focal demyelination with no associated axonal degeneration. It is characterized by transient focal conduction block across the lesion. The axon distal to the site of injury remains intact and the nerve remains in continuity. Clinically, this class of injury may manifest as weakness or sensory loss in the anatomic distribution of the affected nerve. Prognosis for this type of injury is excellent, with spontaneous recovery occurring within hours to, in the most severe cases, a few months. No specific therapeutic intervention is required.

Axonotmesis occurs most commonly during crush, stretch, or percussive injuries, such as gunshot wounds where injury is most commonly caused by indirect heat and shock wave from the bullet rather than transection. These injuries result in irreversible damage to axonal elements including the myelin sheath, leading to distal degeneration. Supporting structures such as the epineurium, perineurium, and, at times, the endoneurium remain intact.

TABLE 48.1 Seddon's Nerve Injury Classifications and Prognosis

Class	Pathology	Mechanism	Treatment	Prognosis	Time Course
Neurapraxia	Demyelination	Compression Ischemia	Medical Physical therapy	Excellent	Hours to 3 mo
Axonotmesis	Axonal disruption Distal degeneration Epineurium intact	Crush Stretch Percussion	Variable: may require surgery	Variable: good to poor	Weeks to years
Neurotmesis	Complete loss of continuity Transection Distal degeneration	Sharp injuries Traction	Surgical: end-to-end neurorrhaphy, grafting or neurotization	Poor/nil without repair	Months to years with surgery No spontaneous recovery

Prognosis for axonotmetic injuries depends on several factors. These factors include the degree of disruption of the internal structure of the nerve, as well as distance from the end organ and the particular characteristics of the injured nerve. Spontaneous recovery is possible after axonotmetic injury, but the time course is considerably greater than that of neurapraxic lesions. Recovery is more commonly partial than complete.

Neurotmesis is defined by complete loss of continuity of the nerve. All connective tissue layers, the axon, and the myelin sheath are irreversibly damaged. Surgical intervention is required, as no spontaneous recovery is possible. The timing of surgery is dependent on the mechanism of injury, as blunt injuries continue to evolve through an inflammatory process over a period of weeks. Prognosis after surgery is variable but is generally poorer than that of spontaneous recovery.

A second important peripheral nerve injury classification system was proposed by Sunderland in 1951 (Table 48.2). Expanding on the work of Seddon, he described five classes of nerve injury, with class I describing neurapraxic lesions and class V equivalent to neurotmesis. For classes II to IV, Sunderland subdivided axonotmesis into three levels, of increasing severity and worsening prognosis, based on the extent of internal disruption, from axon only in class II to endoneurial sheath in class III and perineurium in class IV. Although this additional level of detail is helpful in a research setting, the clinical use is more limited, as all classes II to IV will require the same initial therapeutic approach. Nevertheless, this classification scheme highlights the importance of internal nerve structure for spontaneous recovery and functional regeneration.

REPAIR AND REGENERATION

Characteristic pathologic changes in the nerve occur as a result of traumatic insult. In the mildest form, demyelination is observed at the injury site. When trauma results in axonal disruption, the distal nerve undergoes a process of degeneration that extends to the end organ. The duration of the degenerative process is dependent on the distance of the injury from the end organ. Morphologic and functional changes also take place within the proximal stump adjacent to the injury site.

In the initial period immediately following injury, acute axonal degeneration, extending approximately 300 mm proximally and distally from the lesion site, is triggered by an influx of extracellular calcium. On electron microscopy, vacuoles resembling autophagosomes accumulate in the axon ends. Swelling and disruption of neurofilaments is observed.

These immediate changes are followed by fragmentation and phagocytosis of the myelin sheath. Within 2 days, whorls of myelin debris and small lipid droplets may be observed within the Schwann cells. Circulating macrophages are recruited and enter

TABLE 48.2 Sunderland's Classification of Peripheral Nerve Injuries

Class	Pathology	Mechanism	Treatment	Prognosis	Time Course
I	Demyelination	Compression Ischemia	Medical Physical therapy	Excellent	Hours to 3 mo
II	Axonal disruption Distal degeneration	Crush Stretch Percussion	Variable	Good	Months to years
III	II + endoneurial disruption	Crush Stretch Percussion	Variable	Moderate	Months to years
IV	III + perineurial disruption	Crush Stretch Percussion Traction	Variable	Poor without repair	Months to years
V	Complete transection	Sharp injury Traction	Surgery	Poor/nil without repair	Months to years with surgery No spontaneous recovery

the distal stump. Loss of axonal contact and the presence of macrophages stimulate Schwann cell proliferation and dedifferentiation. These dedifferentiated Schwann cells line up along the basal lamina to form bands of Büngner, which will act as guides to regenerating nerve axons.

Reinnervation occurs via two main mechanisms: collateral axonal sprouting from uninjured axons and axonal regeneration, which occurs spontaneously from the proximal stump following degeneration. Collateral sprouting is an early mechanism of functional motor recovery. It occurs with incomplete lesions, in which some of the axons remain intact. New axonal outgrowths are noted to arise from both nearby nodes and terminal branches. These fine axonal extensions travel along the remaining nerve structures to provide partial reinnervation to nearby motor targets. Generally, collateral sprouting is not sufficient to restore full power to the muscle but may be responsible for some early functional recovery.

Axonal regeneration is the primary mechanism by which reinnervation occurs, following distal degeneration, in axonotmetic and neurotmetic lesions. Regeneration begins from the proximal stump and extends along intact basal lamina toward the end organ at a variable rate of approximately 1 to 2 mm/day. Once the target organ has been reached, a process of maturation occurs to reestablish functional connection. The appearance of clinical evidence of reinnervation reflects both the distance from injury site to the end organ and the maturation process. Rate of regeneration appears to be slower for transected lesions than for crush injuries.

Successful regeneration and functional recovery rely on a number of factors. Inflammation and scar tissue provide major barriers to axonal growth. Gap lengths that are too long result in disorganized and highly tortuous axonal paths, which may coalesce within scar tissue to form a nonfunctional and potentially painful bulb referred to as a *neuroma*.

Even when regeneration does occur successfully, functional recovery is not guaranteed. Regenerating sprouts must be able to form mature connections with appropriate motor or sensory targets in order for recovery to occur. In highly mixed nerves, with an approximately equal amount of sensory and motor fibers, some regenerating motor fibers may be lost to sensory targets or vice versa. Nerves that contain one predominant modality generally have a better prognosis for functional recovery.

Finally, sensory targets maintain viability for a much longer period of time than does muscle tissue. Within 12 to 18 months, fibrotic changes take place in denervated muscle that make successful reinnervation unlikely. Sensory targets, on the other hand, maintain viability for up to 2 to 3 years. Therefore, patients may continue to experience recovery of sensation well beyond the period of motor recovery.

CLINICAL FEATURES

The clinical manifestation of traumatic peripheral nerve injury depends on the mode, location, and extent of the injury sustained. Signs and symptoms reflect both the location and severity of the lesion, as well as the composition of the injured nerve. Injury to a nerve that consists predominantly of motor fibers will manifest as weakness or paralysis and atrophy in the corresponding myotomal distribution. Injury to a predominantly sensory nerve, on the other hand, will present with sensory alteration or loss in the corresponding dermatomes. Autonomic and trophic function may also be affected resulting in decreased sweating, hair loss, and skin changes in the affected region. Partial lesions and faulty regeneration may result in the development of difficult to treat pain, often

described as "pins and needles," stabbing or burning in character. For some patients, a debilitating symptom complex called *complex regional pain syndrome II*, also referred to as *causalgia*, may develop, which is characterized by allodynia, autonomic dysregulation, and maladaptive neuroplastic changes in central nervous system (CNS) response to and processing of pain signals. This syndrome often does not respond well to conventional pain management strategies.

Some common associations are seen between various injury mechanisms and specific peripheral nerves. Awareness by clinicians, of these associations, may contribute to the earlier identification and treatment of potentially disabling injuries. Some of these common associations and their clinical presentations are discussed in the following section.

CRANIAL NERVE LESIONS

Acute injury to cranial nerves often accompanies trauma to the head and neck. Significant injury may occur even with mild head trauma. One study by Coello and colleagues that evaluated cranial nerve function in 16,440 mild head trauma patients, defined by a Glasgow Coma Scale score of 14 or 15 at the time of presentation, over a period of 6 years, found a prevalence of associated cranial nerve injury of 0.3%, with the olfactory nerve being the most commonly affected, followed by the facial nerves and the nerves responsible for ocular movement. Injury to the lower cranial nerves (IX to XII) was noted to occur less frequently as a consequence of head trauma but to be more closely associated with iatrogenic injury during various medical and surgical interventions. The prevalence, location, and type of cranial nerve injuries observed most frequently result from the specific anatomic vulnerabilities of the affected nerve.

Cranial Nerve I: The Olfactory Nerve

The olfactory nerve, responsible for our ability to detect and distinguish smells, is one of the most commonly cited cranial nerves to be injured as a result of head trauma. Olfactory dysfunction has been reported to occur in up to 4% to 7% of all cases of head trauma. Injury may occur at multiple sites along the olfactory pathway. It is most often associated with acceleration–deceleration forces, such as those generated during motor vehicle accidents. Common injury sites include the olfactory nerve filaments as they cross the cribriform plate and are subject to shearing forces; the olfactory bulb, which may be contused against the frontal bone; and the cortical olfactory tracts, which may be damaged by edema, hemorrhage, or ischemic injury of the orbitofrontal and temporal lobes. *Anosmia*, the complete loss of odor detection, is the most common clinical finding, but *parosmia*, a decrease in olfaction acuity, is also observed, particularly with injury to the temporal lobe. The perception of taste, which is reliant on olfaction, is also commonly impaired in patients with injury to the olfactory nerve, and it is this symptom for treatment of which most patients present.

Despite the relative frequency with which injury to the olfactory nerve occurs following head trauma, deficits are rarely identified in the acute period. This may be because of the fact that trauma patients present with multiple injuries of varying severity and immediacy that require disproportionate allocation of resources. Nevertheless, loss of olfaction may have significant impact on quality of life, resulting in diminishment of enjoyment of food and other sensual experiences reliant on smell; loss of employment, when dependent on the sense of smell or taste; and decreased ability to detect environmental cues that may signal danger, such as the odor of volatile gas or fire. Awareness by clinicians of the association of head trauma with cranial nerve I dysfunction is important for early detection and diagnosis.

Cranial Nerve II: The Optic Nerve

Traumatic optic neuropathy, which may result in complete or partial loss of visual acuity in the affected eye, has been reported to occur in 1.4% to 5% of head trauma cases. Injury may be *direct*, resulting from anatomic disruption of nerve fibers by fracture fragments, penetrating trauma, or hematoma within the nerve sheath, or *indirect*, reflecting the transmission of forces to the optic canal during blunt head trauma. Early decompressive surgery may be required to prevent irreversible vision loss.

Additionally, injury to the optic nerve is recognized as a potential complication of facial fracture repair in patients with maxillofacial trauma, with a reported incidence of 0.3%. Mechanisms include direct intraoperative nerve injury, retinal vascular occlusion from orbital edema, and increased intraorbital pressure in the optic canal resulting in indirect injury to the nerve. This complication is most often reported after surgical intervention of the orbital floor, and ischemia is the most common final pathway leading to injury.

Unlike skeletal tissues, the optic nerve and retinal tissues are extremely sensitive to hypoxia and pressure, with irreversible ischemic damage occurring within 60 minutes to 2 hours. Because of this sensitivity, prompt identification of even subtle changes in visual acuity by the clinician is essential to provide potentially vision-sparing interventions in a timely manner.

Cranial Nerve III, IV, VI: The Oculomotor, Trochlear, and Abducens Nerve

Together, the oculomotor, trochlear, and abducens nerves innervate the muscles responsible for ocular movements. Damage to these nerves is a common complication of closed head injury. It may result in diplopia, impairments in eye movement, and ocular deviation. Injury to the nerves may occur at the nuclei in the brain stem, as the nerve exits the brain stem, and at the point where it pierces the dura mater. The site of injury reflects both the injury mechanism and the anatomic characteristics of the nerve. One or all of the nerves for oculomotor control may be affected, and clinical presentation will vary accordingly.

Cranial nerve III, the oculomotor nerve, innervates many of the muscles responsible for eye movement, including the medial rectus, superior rectus, inferior rectus, inferior oblique, levator palpebrae superior, and the pupillary constrictor. Additionally, the oculomotor nerve carries parasympathetic fibers to the eye. Complete lesion of this nerve results in a "down and out" deviation of the eye, ptosis, dilation of the pupil, and loss of pupillary constriction to light but not accommodation. Partial lesions may result in any combination of these findings, depending on the specific nerve fibers affected. Because the parasympathetic fibers run along the outside of the nerve, compressive lesions, such as an expanding hematoma or progressive uncal herniation secondary to intracranial hemorrhage or edema, tend to present with pupillary changes first, which may progress to oculomotor palsy with increasing pressure. Aneurysms of the posterior communicating artery may also compress the third cranial nerve and should be considered when evaluating a patient with oculomotor nerve palsy. Injuries that cause third nerve ischemia, on the other hand, are more likely to affect the motor fibers before disrupting the parasympathetic components. This distinction may help the clinician to identify the etiology of idiopathic third nerve palsy.

The trochlear nerve provides innervation to the superior oblique muscle. Lesion of this nerve results in an inability to move the eye medially and inferiorly. The resulting diplopia may be resolved by inclining the head toward the unaffected eye. Trochlear nerve palsies occurring in isolation have been observed following dorsal midbrain hemorrhage and as a complication of dental anesthesia during upper molar surgery but are extremely rare. Generally, injury to the fourth cranial nerve is accompanied by other oculomotor and neurologic deficits.

The abducens nerve innervates the lateral rectus muscle, which is responsible for abduction of the eye. Injury to this nerve results in severe double vision in almost all gaze directions and medial deviation. Traumatic injury to the sixth cranial nerve has been associated with cranial base fracture and the development of clival epidural hematoma, as well as cervical hyperextension, atlanto-occipital dislocation, and hyperflexion. The sixth cranial nerve vulnerability to injury is thought to be a result of its long and delicate intracranial source. After exiting the pons, it ascends vertically within the subarachnoid space for 15 mm before piercing the dura mater. From there, the nerve travels over the ridge of the petrous bone, change directions abruptly at a 120-degree angle to enter Dorello canal, a triangular space defined by the apex of the petrous bone, the posterior clinoidal process, and a thickened portion of the dura mater, which connects the two, referred to as *Gruber ligament*. The nerve is tethered by the dura on either side of the canal. From Dorello canal, the nerve passes through the cavernous sinus and the superior orbital fissure to reach the lateral rectus muscle. Traumatic injury to the abducens nerve is thought to occur most commonly by downward displacement against the petrous ridge at the point at which it turns to enter the canal.

Cranial Nerve V: The Trigeminal Nerve

The trigeminal nerve supplies sensation to the face through three major peripheral branches, the ophthalmic (VI), maxillary (V2), and mandibular (V3) nerves. V1 and V2 are purely sensory, whereas V3 also carries motor fibers to the muscles of mastication. V1 is also responsible for the corneal reflex. Traumatic injury to the branches of the trigeminal nerve is uncommon but may result from dental or cranial trauma or as a side effect of dental and surgical procedures in the region. Several cases of damage to the lingual nerve, which is a branch of the mandibular division, which provides sensation to the anterior two-thirds of the tongue, and which is joined by the chorda tympani from cranial nerve VII, have been reported with the use of supraglottic airway devices. Compression of the nerve branch by the device results in temporary loss of sensation and taste (from the gustatory fibers of cranial nerve VII) in the anterior tongue, which, although potentially upsetting to the patient, generally resolves spontaneously within 6 to 9 weeks. The patient experiencing these symptoms postoperatively should be reassured regarding chance of recovery.

Cranial Nerve VII: The Facial Nerve

The facial nerve provides most of the motor innervation for the muscles of expression in the face. It also, via the nervus intermedius, relays afferent taste sensation from the anterior two-thirds of the tongue and carries sympathetic fibers to the lacrimal and salivary glands. Depending on the location of the injury, motor, autonomic, and gustatory deficits may be seen. Lesions of the intracranial portion of the nerve near the origin or close to the geniculate ganglion by the internal acoustic meatus, may affect all three components, whereas those in the facial canal of the temporal bone between the geniculate ganglion and the origin of the chorda tympani near the stylomastoid foramen may spare lacrimation. Lesions occurring after the stylomastoid process in the extracranial portion of the nerve result primarily in motor deficits. Symptoms may be mild to severe depending on the severity of injury.

Injury to the facial nerve may present as complete paralysis of the facial muscles, with flattening of the facial folds around the nose, lips, and forehead; widening of palpebral fissures; and incomplete closure of the eyelid on the affected side, which can result in corneal scarring from desiccation particularly if the injury also affects lacrimation. Decreased salivation and loss of taste in the anterior two-thirds of the tongue may also be present if the chorda tympani is affected. Less commonly, patients with seventh nerve injuries may experience sensitivity to loud sounds, or hyperacusis, as the facial nerve supplies motor input to the stapedius muscle, which has a dampening effect on the tympanic membrane. During regeneration, *synkinesis* may develop, which is the movement of unrelated facial muscles during attempts at isolated muscle movements, such as lip twitch with blinking, if aberrant reinnervation occurs. Importantly, lesions of the peripheral facial nerve can be distinguished from central motor pathway lesions by assessing involvement of the forehead. Central lesions spare forehead motion due to bilateral representation in the CNS, whereas peripheral lesions do not.

Traumatic injury to the facial nerve may result from temporal bone fracture, penetrating injuries, such as knife or gunshot wounds, as a result of surgery for other indications, including resection of acoustic neuroma, or in the neonate at the time of delivery by the application of forceps. The superficial peripheral branches are particularly vulnerable to injury. Studies suggest that approximately 7% to 10% of temporal bone fractures result in facial nerve dysfunction. Trauma to the temporal bone may result in both an initial direct injury to the nerve followed by a secondary ischemic injury, as edema causes increased pressure in the fallopian canal containing the nerve. Decompressive surgery may be necessary to prevent progression of injury and should be undertaken as early as possible. Likewise, penetrating injuries most often result in nerve transection and early surgical exploration is desirable. Surgical approach is dependent on the location of the injury.

Cranial Nerve IX: The Glossopharyngeal Nerve

Trauma to cranial nerves IX, X, XI, and XII is most often iatrogenic. The glossopharyngeal nerve carries both sensory and motor fibers. The sensory fibers transmit information from the upper part of the pharynx and taste from the posterior one-third of the tongue. The motor component innervates the constrictor muscles of the pharynx and the stylopharyngeus as well as secretory glands in the pharyngeal mucosa. Traumatic injury to the nerve occurs most commonly with fractures through the jugular foramen where it exits the skull together with the vagus and accessory nerves. Lesions resulting from trauma are rarely isolated and occur most commonly with injuries of the X and XI cranial nerves. Clinically, glossopharyngeal dysfunction presents with diminished taste in the posterior one-third of the tongue and loss of gag reflex on the side of the lesion. The presence of dysphagia or dysarthria may signal concomitant injury to the vagus nerve, as these symptoms are rarely present in isolated glossopharyngeal injuries.

Cranial Nerve X: The Vagus Nerve

The vagus nerve provides motor, sensory, and autonomic innervation to a wide variety of targets. Motor fibers originating in the nucleus ambiguous in the brain stem innervate the somatic muscles of the pharynx and larynx, which coordinate the initial phase of swallowing. Autonomic fibers from the dorsal motor nucleus provide innervation to the heart, lungs, esophagus, and stomach. Sensory fibers from the upper gastrointestinal tract and oropharynx

travel within the vagus nerve to the spinal nucleus, and sensation from the thoracic and abdominal organs is transmitted to the tractus solitarius. Dysarthria and dysphagia may occur with injury, and the palate on the affected side will be low at rest. Deviation of the uvula toward the unaffected side with phonation may be observed as the unopposed contralateral muscles contract.

Individual branches of the vagus nerve may be injured during surgical intervention on the head and neck. Careful physical examination aids injury localization, as clinical presentation varies with site of lesion. Injury to the pharyngeal branches of the vagus nerve will present with dysphagia, which may be mild or severe. The superior laryngeal nerve, which carries sensory fibers from the larynx and provides motor innervation to the cricothyroid muscle, will present with anesthesia of the larynx and paralysis of the cricothyroid muscle. Injury to the recurrent laryngeal nerve leads to vocal cord paralysis, resulting in hoarseness and dysphonia. The voice may sound breathy or harsh during speech production. Bilateral injury results in complete vocal cord paralysis, which can be distinguished by the presence of dyspnea, inspiratory stridor, and an inability to phonate, *aphonia*. Lesions of the pharyngeal and superior laryngeal nerves may also produce vocal abnormalities, resulting in a voice that is weak and easily fatigable.

Cranial Nerve XI: The Spinal Accessory Nerve

The spinal accessory nerve, unlike the other cranial nerves, originates from the C2, C3, and C4 in the upper cervical spinal cord. It enters the skull through the foramen magnum and then travels back out through the jugular foramen with cranial nerves IX and X. Like the glossopharyngeal and vagus nerves, the spinal accessory nerve may be damaged by trauma that results in fracture through the jugular foramen. Iatrogenic injury has also been observed during lymph node biopsy, internal jugular central venous line placement, and carotid endarterectomy. In these instances, injury generally occurs extracranially as the nerve passes through the posterior triangle in the neck.

The spinal accessory nerve carries motor fibers to the sternocleidomastoid muscle and the upper portion of the trapezius. Lesions of this nerve result in atrophy of the upper trapezius, inability to shrug the affected shoulder, and impairment in rotation of head to the contralateral side. Winging of the scapula at rest, which is worsened by abduction, may be present. The scapular winging that results from upper trapezius weakness may be distinguished from that associated with long thoracic nerve injury and anterior serratus weakness by the position of the scapula at rest. When the anterior serratus is affected, winging will be minimal at rest and increase with shoulder flexion.

Cranial Nerve XII: The Hypoglossal Nerve

The hypoglossal nerve originates from the medulla and exits the skull through the hypoglossal foramen in the posterior fossa. It carries motor fibers to the muscles of the tongue and is particularly important for articulation. Injury to this nerve produces dysarthria and atrophy with deviation of the tongue on protrusion toward the side of the lesion due to the action of the unopposed contralateral muscles. Trauma to the hypoglossal nerve has been reported with many surgical interventions including carotid endarterectomy, endotracheal intubation, and supraglottic airway device usage. Cranial nerve XII compression during head turning has also been observed to result from medially oriented, elongated, styloid processes with associated ossification of the stylohyoid ligament. During acute head trauma, hypoglossal nerve injury may be associated with fracture of the occipital condyle. Presence of a 12th nerve palsy after trauma should prompt a magnetic resonance imaging (MRI) of the cervical spine to assess spinal stability. Urgent decompression may be necessary to prevent irreversible injury to the spinal cord.

UPPER EXTREMITY NERVE LESIONS

The peripheral nerves of the upper extremity are vulnerable to traumatic injury by compression and stretch, lacerating and penetrating wounds, fracture and dislocation of nearby bones and joints, and ischemic and iatrogenic insults of various etiologies. Trauma, resulting in injury, may be either acute or chronic. Carpal tunnel syndrome and cubital tunnel syndrome are two examples of chronic entrapment syndromes, in which the application of chronic traumatic compressive forces result in impaired nerve function. These and other common entrapment syndromes will be discussed in detail in subsequent chapters. This section will focus on common acute upper extremity traumatic peripheral nerve injuries and their mechanisms.

Brachial Plexus Injuries

Injury to the brachial plexus, which supplies much of the motor, sensory, and vasomotor innervation of the upper limb and shoulder, can be severely disabling, particularly as traumatic injury to the brachial plexus tends to occur most frequently within the productive age groups. Recovery is often incomplete, resulting in lasting disability, which may negatively affect quality of life. The superficial location, large size, and position between two highly mobile structures (the neck and the arm) make the brachial plexus vulnerable to traumatic injury. Although brachial plexopathies will be discussed in greater detail elsewhere in this book, it is important for the clinician to be aware of common traumatic mechanisms and presentations of brachial plexus injury.

The brachial plexus, which travels from the spinal cord to the axilla, is derived from the nerve roots of C5–T1. It is progressively divided into five roots, three trunks (upper, middle, lower), six divisions (three anterior, three posterior), three cords (lateral, posterior, and medial), and several terminal branches which provide motor, sensory, and sympathetic innervation to the upper limb. C5 and C6 contain the largest number of motor fibers, whereas C7 and T1 contain the least. C7 contains the largest amount of sensory fibers followed in descending order by C6, C8, T1, and C5. These relative sensory and motor distributions have implications for both injury presentation and chance of spontaneous functional recovery, as nerves with greater proportion of either sensory or motor fibers have a greater likelihood of having regenerating axons make appropriate end-organ connections, as compared to mixed nerves.

Injury to the plexus occurs commonly with stretch from extreme positioning associated with falls, direct lacerating or penetrating trauma, dislocation of the shoulder, traction during birth, and stretch or compression during surgical positioning. Injury may be classified as *supraclavicular* (affecting roots and trunks), *retroclavicular* (divisions), or *infraclavicular* (trunks and terminal nerves) with deficit pattern reflecting the site of injury. Supraclavicular lesions result in motor and sensory loss in myotomal and dermatomal distributions associated with the affected roots, whereas infraclavicular injuries tend to have deficits limited to the territories of the terminal branches. Infraclavicular injuries are more commonly seen with penetrating injuries, whereas high-velocity injuries, as occur with motor vehicle accidents, are more likely to result in closed traction supraclavicular injury patterns.

Additionally, injuries may be classified as *upper* (C5–C6), *lower* (C8–T1), or *panplexal* (C5–T1) with implications for both presentation and prognosis. The presence of Horner syndrome or involvement of proximal branches such as the dorsal scapular, which provides motor innervation to the rhomboids, or latissimus dorsi dysfunction due to long thoracic nerve injury, indicates a proximal injury and carries a poorer prognosis. Dysautonomic features such as vasomotor abnormalities or skin changes may be observed in the affected limb. Severe pain in an anesthetic limb may be suggestive of root avulsion, in which the nerve roots are torn from their attachment to the spinal cord by the force of the injury. Avulsion generally requires a different surgical approach than more distal nerve injuries and may carry a worse prognosis. In acute trauma, the position of the arm at time of impact, as well as the associated injuries, may provide clues to the clinician about possible plexus injuries.

The upper plexus is the most common site of injury. Injury to this region results from closed traction, which occurs when the shoulder is forcibly separated from the head. This injury pattern is common in contact sports, as well as postoperatively as a result of prolonged positioning with contralateral rotation of the head or upper extremity abduction greater than 90 degrees. It may also result from the application of excessive traction to the plexus during delivery and is referred to as *Erb palsy* (C5–C6) or *Erb palsy plus* (C5–C7), depending on the roots involved. Weakness or paralysis of the deltoid, biceps, brachioradialis, pectoralis major, supraspinatus, infraspinatus, subscapularis, and teres major results in the classic "waiter's tip" position, with internal rotation of the arm, extension and pronation of the forearm, and flexion of the wrists and fingers. The biceps reflex is absent and sensory loss incomplete, with hypesthesia on the outer surface of the arm and forearm. Contracture may result if passive range-of-motion exercises are not undertaken early. Prognosis for upper plexus injuries associated with birth trauma is generally very good, with 90% chance of spontaneous recovery reported most often in the literature, although controversy remains regarding the optimal timing of surgical intervention in these patients. Generally, the watchful waiting period of 3 to 6 months in adults with closed nerve injuries is extended to 9 months in children.

Traumatic lower plexopathies, affecting C8–T1 nerve roots, are less common than upper plexus injuries but have been associated with thoracic surgery requiring median sternotomy, cervical rib and band syndrome, obstetrical trauma, and the presence of a Pancoast tumor by compression or direct tumor invasion. The resulting syndrome is referred to as *Klumpke palsy*. It presents with isolated hand paralysis and ipsilateral Horner syndrome. This clinical presentation mimics that of a combined median and ulnar lesion. Sensory loss is observed on the medial arm and forearm and the ulnar side of the hand. Atrophy of the intrinsic hand muscles occurs and the triceps reflex is lost. The anatomic particularities of the C8 and T1 nerve roots make the lower plexus more susceptible to avulsion than the upper and middle plexus. The greater vulnerability to avulsion results in a poorer prognosis for lower plexus injuries.

Isolated middle plexus injury, affecting nerve root C7 or the middle trunk, is the least common form of traumatic brachial plexopathy. These lesions cause paralysis in a primarily radial distribution with sparing of the brachioradialis. Due to extensive dual innervation, sensory loss is minimal and may be limited hypesthesia over the dorsal surface of the hand and forearm.

A complete lesion of the brachial plexus results in a flail arm with or without ipsilateral Horner syndrome. Complete plexus injuries carry the worst prognosis and extensive surgical intervention, including amputation, may be required to restore function and alleviate pain.

Proximal Nerve Injuries

The *long thoracic nerve* is a purely motor nerve that arises from the ventral rami of C5–C7. It provides motor innervation to the serratus anterior muscle which stabilizes, protracts, and upwardly rotates the scapula to abduct the arm over the head. Weakness or paralysis of this nerve results in winging of the scapula, which is particularly notable during abduction and forward flexion. Very little winging is observed at rest, which distinguishes long thoracic palsy from injury to the spinal accessory nerve. Abduction between 90 and 180 degrees may be limited.

Injury to this nerve is usually isolated and may result from blunt trauma to the thorax or forceful depression of the shoulder girdle, as may occur during a fall. It commonly occurs during participation in contact sports. Iatrogenic injury has been associated with first rib resection and radical mastectomy. Long thoracic nerve palsy may also result from carrying heavy loads on the shoulder. Fortunately, as most injuries to the long thoracic nerve are neurapraxic, spontaneous recovery is expected and prognosis is good.

The *suprascapular nerve* branches from the upper trunk and is derived of fibers mostly from C5. It provides motor innervation to the supraspinatus and the infraspinatus muscles, as well as sensory and sympathetic innervation to two-thirds of the shoulder capsule, the glenohumeral, and the acromioclavicular joints. Weakness of the supraspinatus muscle results in difficulty in initiating shoulder abduction, particularly through the first 15 to 30 degrees, after which the deltoid takes over. The infraspinatus externally rotates the shoulder, and weakness may be observed with external rotation as a result of suprascapular nerve injury. Isolated injury is rare with shoulder trauma, although chronic trauma from entrapment by the suprascapular ligament has been reported. Compression by tumors and ganglion cysts may also occur.

Median Nerve

The median nerve derives from the C6–T1 nerve roots. In the forearm, it provides motor innervation to the pronator teres, the flexor carpi radialis, palmaris longus, and flexor digitorum superficialis muscles before branching into the purely motor anterior interosseous nerve and the main branch. The main branch passes through the carpal tunnel and then gives off the recurrent thenar nerve to provide innervation to the abductor and lateral flexor pollicis brevis and the opponens brevis. It terminates in the palm where it supplies innervation to lumbricals I and II. The median nerve is therefore involved with pronation of the forearm, wrist flexion, thumb, index and middle finger flexion, and opposition of the thumb.

Additionally, the median nerve provides sensation to the radial palm, ventral thumb, index, middle fingers, and the radial half of the ring finger. The dorsal surfaces of the distal phalanx of the thumb and the terminal phalanges of the index and middle fingers are also supplied by the median nerve.

Injury to the median nerve may occur at multiple points along its course as a result of trauma. Median nerve palsy has been associated with stabbing injuries to the brachial plexus, crush injury from prolonged crutch or tourniquet usage, fracture of the distal humerus, anterior shoulder dislocation, and Colles fracture of the wrist, although chronic trauma due to entrapment is the most common median nerve injury observed clinically. The nerve may become entrapped within the carpal tunnel or between the heads of the pronator teres in the forearm. Chronic entrapment within the carpal tunnel results in pain and sensory loss in the distal median distribution with wasting and weakness of the thenar muscles and lumbricals I and II. Direct traumatic injury to the median nerve has also been reported secondary to poorly placed steroid injections for treatment of carpal tunnel syndrome. Histologic examination in several cases revealed the presence of white crystals with the median nerve sheath suggesting that aberrant injection directly into the nerve was the likely mechanism of injury. Carpal tunnel syndrome is discussed more thoroughly in subsequent chapters.

Radial Nerve

The radial nerve arises from the posterior cord and contains elements from C5–T1 nerve roots. It is composed of primarily motor fibers and provides innervation to the wrist, forearm, and finger extensors. It passes through the axilla to supply the triceps and then winds around the posterior humerus, descending in the spiral groove. The nerve innervates the brachioradialis and extensor carpi radialis longus muscles before branching into the superficial radial nerve, which carries sensory information from the dorsoradial aspect of the distal forearm and the dorsal surface of the hand and the posterior interosseous nerve, which supplies motor innervation to the remaining forearm, wrist, and finger extensors as well as the supinator.

The clinical presentation of traumatic injury to the radial nerve will vary with the level at which the injury occurs. Several common injury mechanisms have been identified that are associated with lesions at various levels. Injury to the nerve in the axilla, resulting from the use of crutches that are too long, causes extensor weakness and numbness in the radial distribution described earlier. Midshaft humeral fracture or external compression, referred to commonly as *Saturday night palsy* when it occurs after a particularly heavy night's sleep on an extended arm, causes weakness of forearm and wrist extensors with wrist drop and weakness of finger extensors. Elbow extension is preserved.

Iatrogenic trauma to the radial nerve has also been reported in the literature to have occurred with peripheral venous cannulation and arterial monitoring at the wrist, blood pressure cuffs at the midhumeral shaft, and rarely, with vaccine administration in the upper arm. Prognosis is generally good due to the predominant motor component of the radial nerve limiting motor/sensory cross-reinnervation and synergy between radial nerve innervated muscles.

Ulnar Nerve

The ulnar nerve is a terminal branch of the medial cord of the plexus and contains fibers from C8 to T1 nerve roots. It descends between the biceps and triceps before moving posteriorly to pass behind the medial epicondyle and through the cubital tunnel to the forearm. It provides motor fibers to the flexor carpi ulnaris and flexor digitorum profundus II before passing through Guyon canal into the hand. The ulnar nerve terminates as a superficial sensory branch, which supplies the palmar and dorsal sides of the ulnar part of the hand and the palmar and dorsal surfaces of the little finger and the medial half of the ring finger. A deep motor branch supplies the abductor, opponens, and flexor digiti minimi medially and the adductor pollicis and the medial half of the flexor pollicis brevis laterally. It is responsible for many of the fine motor manipulations of the hand, and injury can be quite disabling.

The superficial course of the ulnar nerve behind the medial epicondyle makes this nerve vulnerable to injury by external compression. Ulnar nerve palsy is one of the most commonly reported postoperative peripheral nerve complications and may result from poor positioning, insufficient padding around the elbow, or from external pressure by surgical instruments and personnel. Entrapment of the ulnar nerve may also occur at the elbow in the ulnar groove, distal to the elbow as it traverses the cubital tunnel, or within Guyon canal at the wrist. Several cases of ulnar nerve palsy at the wrist have been reported to result from ganglion cysts within Guyon canal, leading to weakness and atrophy of the intrinsic muscles of the hand. Injury to the ulnar nerve may also be seen with articular fractures of the distal humerus. Prolonged denervation may result in clawing of the little and ring finger and atrophy of hypothenar and interosseous muscles.

The likelihood of functional recovery after traumatic injury is lower for the ulnar nerve than for either the median or the radial nerve. This inequity is attributed to the ulnar nerves innervation of muscles responsible for fine movement in the hand, which require greater specificity in reinnervation to regain useful function.

Axillary Nerve

The axillary nerve arises as a terminal branch of the posterior cord with fibers originating from C5 to C6 nerve roots. The axillary nerve crosses anterior to the subscapularis before entering the quadrilateral space and dividing into two main trunks. The posterior branch supplies motor innervation to the teres minor and posterior deltoid before terminating as the superior lateral brachial cutaneous nerve, whereas the anterior branch travels within the deltoid muscle providing motor innervation to the middle and anterior deltoid muscle.

Traumatic injury to the nerve is associated with glenohumeral dislocation, proximal humeral fracture, and direct blow to the deltoid muscle, as can occur during sports events. Compression can also occur within the quadrilateral space, resulting in deltoid muscle weakness and diffuse pain over the posterior shoulder. Compression is thought to be secondary to the development of abnormal fibrous bands and hypertrophy of the muscles forming the boundaries of the anatomic space. The axillary nerve is vulnerable to iatrogenic injury during surgery involving the shoulder and glenohumeral joint, including shoulder arthroscopy during portal placement. Clinically, injury to the axillary nerve may present with weakness of shoulder abduction and paresthesia over the lateral arm. Prognosis for axillary nerve injury is generally good, although it varies with injury mechanism and severity.

LOWER EXTREMITY NERVE LESIONS

Lumbosacral Plexus

The nerve supply to the pelvis and lower limbs originates from the lumbosacral plexus. Functionally and anatomically, the lumbosacral plexus can be divided into two major divisions, the lumbar and sacral plexuses.

The lumbar plexus is formed within the psoas major muscle and is derived from the nerve roots of L2–L4. The lumbar plexus gives rise to the *femoral nerve*, which passes along the lateral border of the psoas major, under the inguinal ligament, to the anterior leg where it supplies motor innervation to the pectineus, sartorius, rectus femoris, vastus lateralis, vastus intermedius, and vastus medialis muscles. The femoral nerve then terminates as the saphenous nerve, providing sensation to the medial lower leg.

The *obturator nerve* also arises from the anterior branches of L2, L3, and L4. It passes through the obturator canal in the pelvis and gives off anterior branches that supply the adductors. It also may provide sensation to the inner thigh and knee, although cutaneous innervation in this area is highly variable.

A number of smaller sensory nerves also arise from the lumbar plexus. These nerves include the *iliohypogastric*, the *ilioinguinal*, the *genitofemoral*, and the *lateral femoral cutaneous nerve*. Lesions of these nerves is discussed individually in the following text, but traumatic injury is most often iatrogenic or anatomic and rarely the result of acute trauma.

The sacral plexus is formed from the nerve roots of L5, S1, and S2 with variable contribution from L4. The sacral plexus supplies motor innervation to the gluteus minimus, gluteus medius, and tensor fascia lata via the *superior gluteal nerve*, which contains fibers from L4 to S1, whereas the *inferior gluteal nerve*, derived from L5 to S1, supplies the gluteus maximus.

The *sciatic nerve* forms from the posterior divisions of L4–S1. It exits the pelvis through the greater sciatic foramen and through the piriformis muscle, which can act as a site of compression when hypertrophied. The sciatic nerve travels down the posterior leg as two anatomically approximated but functionally distinct components: the lateral peroneal portion and the medial tibial portion. In the posterior thigh, the lateral peroneal portion of the sciatic nerve provides motor innervation to the short head of the biceps femoris, whereas the medial tibial division supplies the long head of the biceps femoris, the semitendinosus, and the semimembranosus. The lateral position of the peroneal portion increases its vulnerability to injury, particularly from penetrating and concussive forces. At the level of the posterior knee, the sciatic nerve divides into the common peroneal and tibial nerves.

Traumatic injury to the lumbosacral plexus is uncommon, although injury has been observed to occur secondary to gynecologic surgery and normal labor due to compression by fetal presenting part or instrumentation used in vaginal delivery. Hematoma, abscess, and tumor may all present with lumbosacral plexopathy. Clinical presentation varies with the site and severity of injury, although damage to the plexus may be distinguished form more peripheral injury if dysfunction of the anal sphincter is present.

The Obturator Nerve

Traumatic injury of the obturator nerve is uncommon; compression may result from expanding pelvic masses such as hematomas, tumors, or abscesses or from compression by the presenting part of the fetus during labor. Clinically, injury to the obturator nerve manifests as abnormal gait due to adductor weakness. Internal and external rotation of the thigh may also be affected.

The Iliohypogastric Nerve

The iliohypogastric nerve is derived from the upper portion of the lumbar plexus. It provides sensation to the upper buttocks and the lower abdomen as well as supplying some motor innervation to the internal oblique and transversus abdominis muscle. Traumatic injury to this nerve is most commonly reported as an iatrogenic complication of surgery. Aberrant suture or staple placement, development of painful neuroma, or entrapment of the nerve in fibrous adhesions can cause anesthesia, pain, and paresthesia that is refractory to most conventional pain management strategies. Entrapment in mesh used for hernia repair has also been reported. In cases of nerve injury uncomplicated by pain, lesion to this nerve may produce minimal deficits with anesthesia over a small strip of skin as the primary manifestation.

The Ilioinguinal Nerve

The ilioinguinal nerve provides sensation to the pubic region, the upper inner thigh, and the external genitalia. Injury to the ilioinguinal nerve often accompanies injury to the iliohypogastric nerves and is associated with similar traumatic mechanisms.

The Genitofemoral Nerve

The genitofemoral nerve is a sensory nerve that derives from the L2 nerve root. It provides sensation to the scrotum and a portion of the inner thigh. Traumatic injury of this nerve is rare.

The Lateral Femoral Cutaneous Nerve

The lateral femoral cutaneous nerve is derived from nerve fibers between L2 and L3. This sensory nerve travels beneath the fascia of the iliacus and emerges at the anterior superior iliac spine. It divides into two branches: a posterior branch, which provides sensation to the external buttock, and an anterior branch, which provides sensation to the outer lateral thigh. A syndrome called *meralgia paresthetica*, which consists of dysesthesia and sensory loss along the lateral thigh, occurs with compression of the anterior branch. Compression may result as a consequence of tight-fitting belts and pants, lumbar hyperlordosis resulting from pregnancy, prolonged maintenance of the lithotomy position during surgery, or extreme hip flexion during vaginal delivery. Hypertrophy of the iliopsoas, as can occur with dancers who repeatedly maintain the leg in greater than 90 degrees of flexion, has also been reported as a cause of lateral cutaneous femoral neuropathy. Complete examination should be undertaken to rule out more potentially dangerous causes of lateral thigh pain, such as malignancy.

The Femoral Nerve

Traumatic injury to the femoral nerve is less common than injury to the sciatic, common peroneal, or tibial nerves, although injury may result from femur and pubic ramus fractures. More commonly, injury to the femoral nerve is derived from compression within the pelvis by tumor, abscesses, and other space-occupying lesions such as enlarged lymph nodes. Spontaneous hematoma within the iliacus or retroperitoneal space, associated classically with hemophilia and more recently with the use of anticoagulation medication, has also been described in the literature as a cause of femoral neuropathy. In hemophiliacs, it has been shown that bleeding into the iliacus muscle, which occupies a nondistensible space between the pelvic bone and the iliac fascia, raises the pressure within the compartment, compressing the femoral nerve as it travels between the iliacus and psoas muscles. A second mechanism has also been proposed based on more recent anatomic studies, which suggests that blood within the iliac fascia traps the femoral nerve at the point at which it passes beneath the inguinal ligament. In this model, hemorrhagic dissection down to the level of the inguinal ligament is necessary for compression to occur and may explain why femoral neuropathy generally presents in isolation.

Injury to the femoral nerve results in weakness of the iliopsoas, paralysis of the quadriceps femoris, and hypesthesia over the anteromedial leg in the distribution of the saphenous nerve. Patellar reflex is lost and the leg is often held in flexed, abducted, and externally rotated position. Severe abnormalities in gait may be observed, particularly when attempting to walk on an incline or upstairs, as both hip flexion and knee extension are affected.

The Sciatic Nerve

Lesions of the sciatic nerve comprise the largest subset of lower extremity traumatic injuries. At the level of the buttocks, injection injury is the most common cause of traumatic nerve lesion with hip fracture/dislocation; hip arthroplasty; fall-related contusion; gunshot wounds; laceration, such as from a boat propeller; and compression from prolonged immobilization following in descending order. In the thigh, gunshot wounds, followed by stretch injury associated with femoral shaft fracture, and laceration in the posterior thigh were the most common mechanisms of traumatic injury. In all locations, injury to the common peroneal division of the sciatic nerve occurs more frequently than injury of the tibial division. This is hypothesized to be the result of the lateral position of the peroneal division.

Complete lesion of the sciatic nerve is rare. Clinically, it presents as weakness of knee flexion as well as complete paralysis of all movements of the ankles and toes. Ankle reflex is lost and foot drop is observed on the affected side. Gait is characterized by a circular swinging motion of the hip during leg advancement as patients attempt to compensate for the loss of ankle dorsiflexion. Sensation is altered on the outer surface of the lower leg, over the toes, and on the instep and sole of the foot. *Sciatica*, or pain extending from the low back to the toes following the course of the nerves that is associated with foot drop and weakness in ankle eversion, suggests compression at the level of the L5–S1 nerve roots and should warrant imaging evaluation of the lumbar spine.

The Common Peroneal Nerve

The common peroneal nerve is particularly vulnerable to traumatic injury. Its anatomic course around the fibular head makes it susceptible to stretch, contusion, and compression forces around the knee, as well as to laceration resulting from fibular fracture. Compressive trauma may occur with leg crossing, squatting, or prolonged lateral decubitus position with insufficient padding while sleeping, unconscious, or anesthetized. Injury to the common peroneal nerve results in footdrop and weakness in ankle eversion. Patients may be unable to extend the toes. Depending on the level of injury, sensory loss may occur over the outer leg, shin, instep, and dorsal surface of the four small toes.

Injuries to the common peroneal nerve carry a worse prognosis than do injuries to other nerves of the lower leg. This is thought to be due to a number of factors including the distance from target end organs, the mixed nature of the nerve, the risk for more severe injury associated with the nerve's lateral location, and the characteristics of the target muscles which require coordinated input for effective contraction. Distal injuries tend to have a better chance of recovery than do their proximal counterparts.

The Tibial Nerve

Injury to the tibial nerve occurs significantly less frequently than injury to the common peroneal, and it carries a much better prognosis. Contusion with fracture, laceration, and gunshot wounds are the most common mechanisms of traumatic injury. As the tibial nerve provides motor innervation to the gastrocnemius and soleus, complete lesion of the nerve leads to paralysis of plantar flexion and inversion of the foot as well as flexion and abduction of the toes. Sensory loss occurs over the plantar aspect of the foot and plantar reflex is lost.

A syndrome of chronic trauma by entrapment, called *tarsal tunnel syndrome*, has also been described as occurring within the flexor retinaculum in proximity to the medial malleolus. This syndrome produces a variable pain over the tarsal tunnel behind the medial malleolus with radiation to the plantar aspect of the foot, heel, and arch, which may be described as burning, tingling, or numbness. Discomfort is often exacerbated by prolonged weight-bearing activity and may be present at night. Bifurcation of the tibial nerve into the medial and lateral plantar nerves proximal to the tunnel is thought to be an anatomically predisposing factor for the development of the syndrome.

Prognosis after tibial nerve injury is favorable as compared to that of the common peroneal nerve. This is attributed to several factors intrinsic to the nerve including a greater connective tissue to fascicle ratio, with increased shock-absorbing capabilities; a singular fixation point, which provides more elasticity and protection from stretch; a better blood supply to minimize secondary ischemic damage; and closer proximity to end-organ targets. Additionally, functional recovery is aided by the size and biomechanical characteristics of the gastrocnemius and soleus muscles, which require relatively little innervation for contraction to be effective.

DIAGNOSIS

The initial diagnosis of traumatic nerve injury is clinical; it relies primarily on a thorough physical examination and the identification of a history that is suggestive of acute or chronic trauma. The mechanism of trauma, along with the presence of injuries to other structures, such as skeletal fractures or lacerations that are commonly associated with injury to peripheral nerves, may help focus the clinician's initial examination on those areas most likely to be effected, although a full cranial and peripheral nerve examination should be undertaken whenever possible. Evaluation may be complicated by injuries that require immediate lifesaving therapeutic intervention, as well as by alterations in level of consciousness in a multi-injury trauma patient.

Once a peripheral nerve injury has been identified by clinical evaluation, additional information should be sought regarding pathophysiology and extent of the injury, as these factors will influence the timing and type of treatment provided. Several laboratory and imaging tools are available to aid in classification, including electrodiagnostic studies, ultrasound, MRI, magnetic resonance neurography, and somatosensory-evoked potentials.

ELECTRODIAGNOSTIC FINDINGS IN PERIPHERAL NERVE INJURY

Electrodiagnostic evaluation, consisting primarily of electromyography (EMG) and nerve conduction studies, is critical for establishing the severity, location, and prognosis of peripheral nerve lesions. Properly timed examination seeks to answer four important questions: (1) localization of the injury, (2) pathophysiology, (3) severity of resultant dysfunction, and (4) progress of reinnervation and likelihood of spontaneous recovery. More detailed information regarding the administration and general characteristics of these tests is provided in Chapter 26. In this section, we focus on the electrophysiologic characteristics associated with each of Seddon's nerve injury types and their impact on surgical planning.

Neurapraxia

Neurapraxic lesions are characterized by focal conduction block at the site of the lesion with no loss of conduction in the distal segment. The injury, which is usually the result of direct compression or ischemia, results in focal demyelination with no associated axonal loss. On nerve conduction studies, this is reflected by maintenance of the compound muscle action potential (CMAP) and sensory nerve action potential (SNAP) on stimulation distal to the lesion site when recording from distal nerve targets. When stimulation is applied proximal to the lesion, CMAP recordings might show loss of amplitude, slowing of conduction velocity, and change in morphology. SNAP will demonstrate a similar pattern, although interpretation of SNAPs is somewhat more complicated,

as amplitude is also affected by distance between the stimulating and recording electrodes. Abnormalities are expected to resolve with remyelination, although some conduction slowing may persist permanently, as remyelination results in shorter and thinner internodes than previously present, with slightly decreased conduction capability.

Needle EMG of neurapraxic lesions is characterized by loss of motor unit action potentials that are under voluntary control and abnormal patterns of motor unit recruitment. In incomplete lesions in which some proportion of axons are blocked, rendering some motor units ineffective, remaining unaffected motor units must increase the rate of firing to generate the same amount of force. On EMG, this abnormal recruitment results in a decreased number of motor unit action potentials (MUAPs) of normal morphology, amplitude, and duration, firing rapidly. No MUAPs will be observed with complete neurapraxic lesions. Resolution of these findings will occur with remyelination.

Axonotmesis

In axonotmesis, unlike neurapraxia, injury to the nerve produces complete or partial axonal disruption, resulting in progressive degeneration of the distal stump. The time to completion of the degenerative process depends on the length of the distal stump, as well as on fiber composition, but is generally completed within 10 to 14 days. The time required to complete this process is reflected in the evolution of the electrodiagnostic picture, and studies carried out in the acute traumatic period will not adequately distinguish neurapraxic from axonotmetic and neurotmetic lesions.

Generally, on nerve conduction studies, upon completion of the degenerative process, CMAP and SNAP, distal to the injury, will show a decrease in amplitude that is proportional to the degree of axonal loss. Motor fibers degenerate quicker with completion experimentally determined to occur around 5 to 8 days and complete loss of amplitude observed around 9 days. Sensory fibers require more time and complete loss is generally observed at day 11. Comparison of CMAP amplitude in the injured limb may be made to that of the unaffected side to approximate the degree of axonal loss. Comparison of distal to proximal CMAP amplitude within the affected limb may estimate the amount of demyelination present.

Needle EMG provides a measure of end-organ denervation. Fibrillation potentials and sharp waves are markers of denervation resulting from axonal degeneration in complete lesions. Their appearance distinguishes neurapraxic lesions from axonotmesis and neurotmesis, although the timing of their appearance is dependent on the distance from the injury site. Proximal muscles may begin to show fibrillation potentials at 10 to 14 days, whereas distal muscles may require 3 to 4 weeks. Incomplete lesions will show firing patterns similar to that of neurapraxia.

As regeneration progresses, motor units will remodel. Surviving MUAPs will become increasingly complex and "nascent units" will develop. Nascent units are characteristically of small amplitude, polyphasic, and with a rapid firing rate. These early MUAPs will develop into fully reinnervated units, which exhibit large amplitude, increased duration, and polyphasia, indicating increased motor unit territory. Evidence of such reinnervation, from local sources, may appear as early as 3 weeks, indicating the possibility of spontaneous recovery, although generally axonal reinnervation requires 3 to 4 months before adequate assessment can be made. Serial examinations may be used to follow the progress of reinnervation. If no evidence of regeneration is found within 3 to 6 months, surgical exploration may be appropriate.

Neurotmesis

Neurotmetic lesions are by definition complete lesions, resulting from transection of all structural nerve elements. Initial electrodiagnostic studies will follow the same pattern of progressive degeneration as occurs in axonotmesis. Unlike axonotmesis, no evidence of reinnervation will be apparent on follow-up examinations, as fully transected nerves are not capable of undergoing functional spontaneous regeneration. Surgical intervention with grafting or tension-free reapproximation is required.

TIMING OF STUDIES

Some debate exists regarding the optimal timing of electrodiagnostic evaluations. Conventional teaching is that initial evaluation should be performed no earlier than 3 weeks to allow for degeneration to be completed. Immediate evaluation, within 7 days of the injury, on the other hand, has been proposed as a potentially valuable tool both in lesion localization and to determine whether a lesion is complete or incomplete. Detection of conduction block precisely identifies the location of the injury, which may be particularly helpful in the setting of extensive or anatomically distorting trauma. Incomplete lesions carry a better prognosis and are less likely to need early surgical intervention.

In general, the timing of studies should reflect the clinical setting and questions to be answered, with the following guidelines applicable: (1) Studies performed within 1 week provide information regarding completeness of lesion and location; (2) at 1 to 2 weeks, neurapraxia can be separated from axonotmesis and neurotmesis; (3) evaluation at 3 weeks provides the most information regarding lesion type and prognosis; and (4) by 3 to 4 months evidence of reinnervation should be present.

ROLE IN SURGICAL PLANNING

EMG is also an important tool for surgical planning. In thinking about nerve repair and functional recovery, consideration must be given to the time required for regenerating axons to reach the target tissues and establish mature connections. This thought is particularly important for motor recovery, as irreversible changes are observed to occur in muscle within 12 to 18 months, rendering innervation after that point ineffectual. Regeneration, after either grafting or direct anastomosis, occurs at a rate of approximately 1 inch per month. Surgery must be timed to allow for the appropriate period of regeneration to occur. EMG assists in this planning by monitoring the progression of reinnervation. By measuring the distance from the injury site to the most proximal muscle and calculating the time needed for reinnervation to occur based on regeneration rate, EMG evaluation can be planned to assess for spontaneous recovery within a timeframe that would still facilitate successful surgical intervention. Surgery may provide some benefit when performed outside the ideal window, as sensory targets remain viable for up to 2 to 3 years and reestablishment of protective sensation may be achieved.

TREATMENT

The timing and technique of surgical intervention is dependent on the mechanism and characteristics of the nerve injury. Injuries may be classified as either open or closed, depending on the status of the associated cutaneous tissue (Figs. 48.1 and 48.2).

Closed peripheral nerve injuries occur most commonly as a result of stretching, contusion, or compression and are more likely to be in continuity. Transection is rare, and neurapraxic and axonotmetic injuries predominate. Lesions of this sort rarely require immediate surgical intervention and should be managed conservatively for a period of at least 3 months to allow for spontaneous recovery.

Open injuries, which result from lacerations, are more frequently associated with neurotmetic lesions and may require early surgery. In general, prognosis for functional recovery is better if

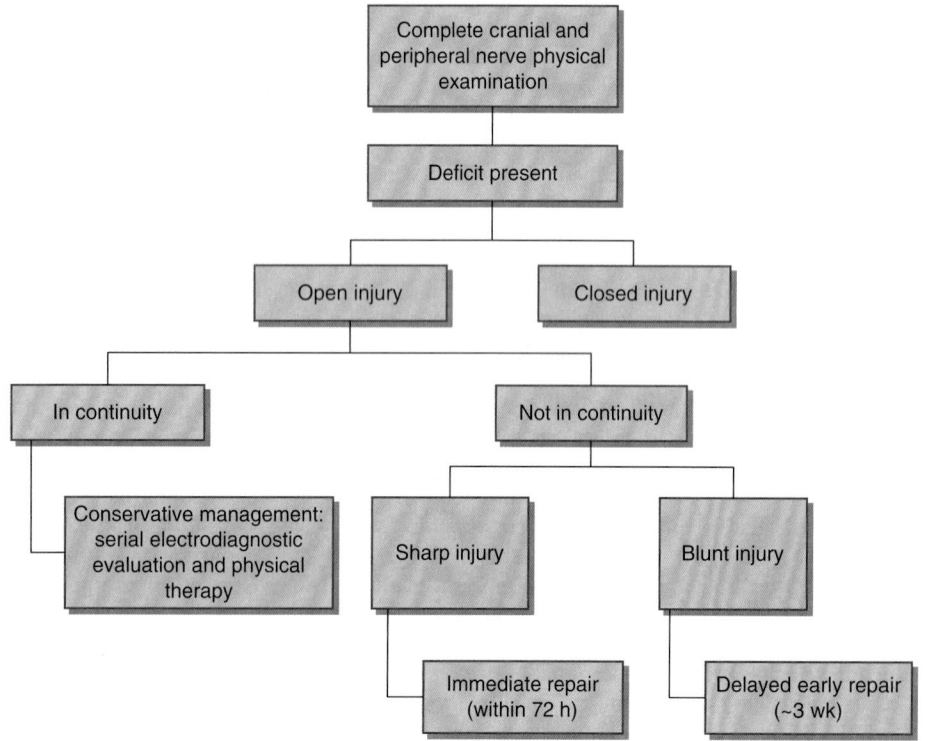

FIGURE 48.1 Initial evaluation of open nerve injury.

Complete cranial and peripheral nerve physical examination

Deficit present

Open injury — Closed injury

In continuity — Not in continuity

Conservative management: serial electrodiagnostic evaluation and physical therapy

Sharp injury — Blunt injury

Immediate repair (within 72 h)

Delayed early repair (~3 wk)

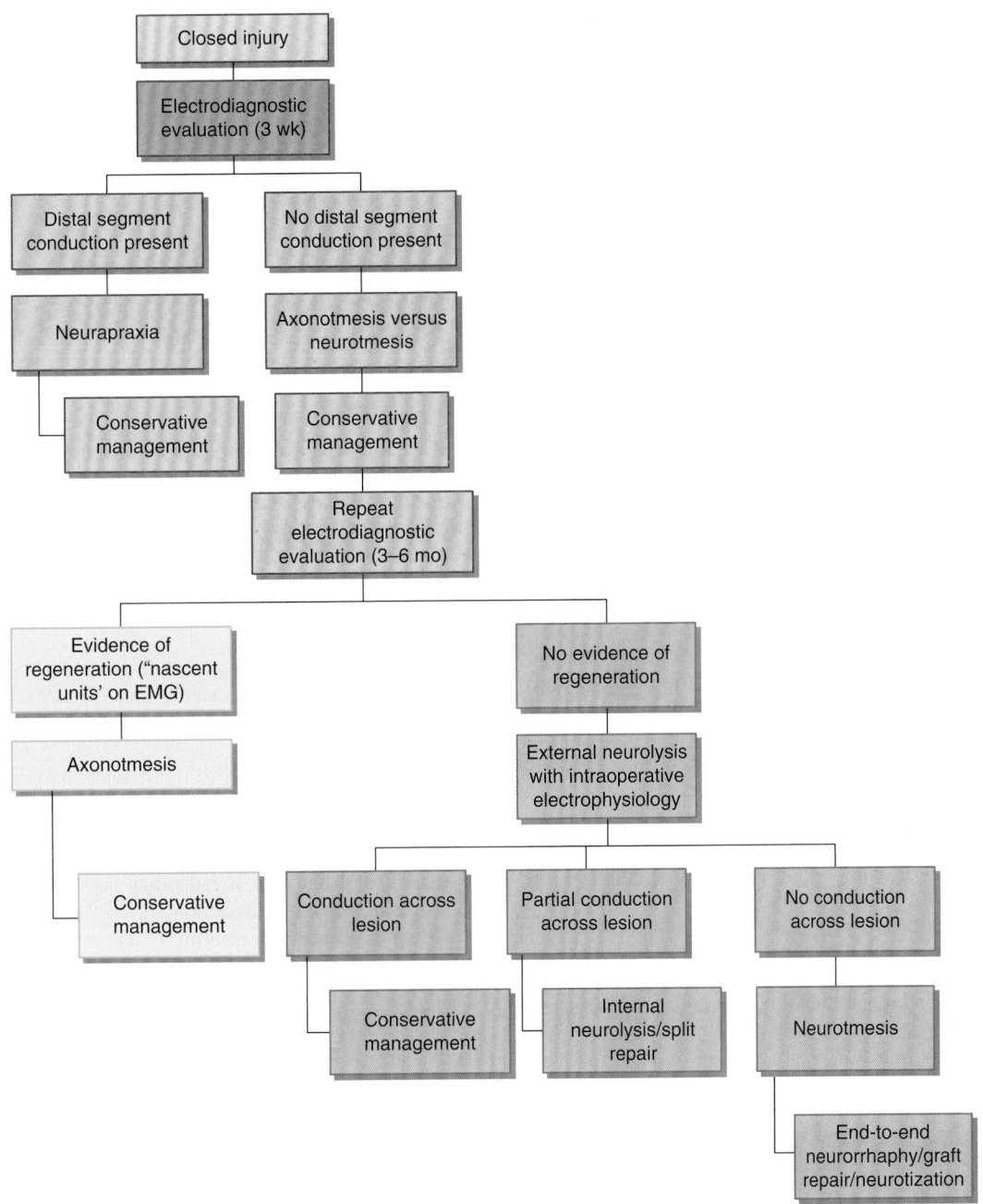

FIGURE 48.2 Closed nerve injury management.

spontaneous regeneration is able to occur. Therefore, open injuries with a nerve in continuity may be treated conservatively, with medical management, early mobilization and physical therapy, and serial electrodiagnostic studies to monitor progress. If no evidence of reinnervation is found within 3 months, surgical exploration may be appropriate. On the other hand, for open injuries with evidence of nerve transection, early surgical exploration is preferred. The timing and extent of the surgery will differ according to the mechanism of injury.

Sharp injury to a nerve, as is seen most commonly with knife or scalpel wounds, results in clean transection with minimal trauma to adjacent nerve tissue and no inflammation. Sharp injuries should be repaired promptly, ideally within the first 3 days after injury, and are usually able to be directly reapproximated with tension-free suture. Prognosis is generally good in these cases.

Blunt transections that are often associated with boat propeller accidents have significant inflammation and damage to surrounding tissues. Inflammatory changes in the blunt ends continue to evolve over a period of 3 weeks, and surgical repair should be delayed. Ongoing inflammation can disrupt the repair. Direct reapproximation is less likely to be successfully performed, as the contused areas must be trimmed back to the point of healthy tissue, lengthening the gap. Nerve grafting may be necessary. Prognosis is poorer after grafting than direct termino-terminal *neurorrhaphy* but good functional recovery may still be achieved.

Nerve injuries sustained as a result of gunshot wounds require special consideration. Most lesions caused by gunshot wounds are the result of indirect heat and shock waves generated by the bullet, rather than transection. As continuity is usually preserved, spontaneous recovery may be achieved. Further, damage to surrounding tissues may limit the success of early repairs. Therefore, surgical exploration and repair should be delayed for 3 to 4 months postinjury.

INDICATIONS FOR EARLY OPERATIVE MANAGEMENT

Early operative management may be indicated in certain settings. As discussed earlier, sharp transections, in which transected ends are not significantly contused, benefit from surgery performed within 3 days. Progressive nerve deficit suggests the presence of associated vascular injury or abnormality. Evidence of an expanding hematoma, pseudoaneurysm, or other compressive lesion should prompt early surgical intervention to alleviate compression.

SURGICAL TECHNIQUES

The goal of surgical repair is to restore functional connectivity across the site of lesion and to alleviate neural pain. This may be accomplished by the removal of scar tissue, reapproximation and direct suturing of transected nerve ends, or through the interposition of graft material. The type and extent of surgical intervention is dependent on lesion characteristics.

Neurolysis

The term *neurolysis* refers to the exposure of a peripheral nerve and dissection free of surrounding tissues. External or internal neurolysis may be performed.

External neurolysis is the first step of all surgical peripheral nerve interventions. During this step, the nerve is freed from surrounding tissue and mobilized (Fig. 48.3). Thickened and scarred areas of the endoneurium are removed as the surgeon progresses from normal to abnormal tissue, distal and proximal to the lesion. Careful dissection seeks to minimize disruption to vasculature that could slow healing or cause secondary injury.

For lesions in continuity, upon completion of external neurolysis, intraoperative stimulation and electrophysiologic recording is employed to assess functional connectivity. An electric stimulus is applied proximal to the lesion and response is recorded distally (Fig. 48.4). If a measurable response is present in the distal segment, external neurolysis may be sufficient to relieve pain and

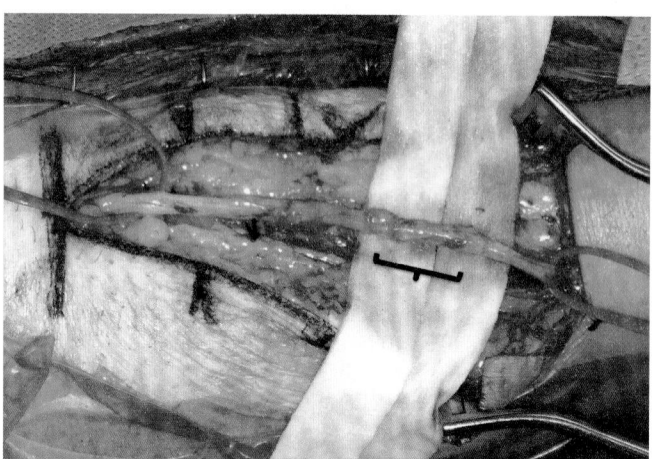

FIGURE 48.3 Intraoperative photo demonstrating a sural nerve injury that occurred during an Achilles tendon repair. External neurolysis across the injured segment reveals a traumatic neuroma marked by the *black bracket*. The nerve is in continuity.

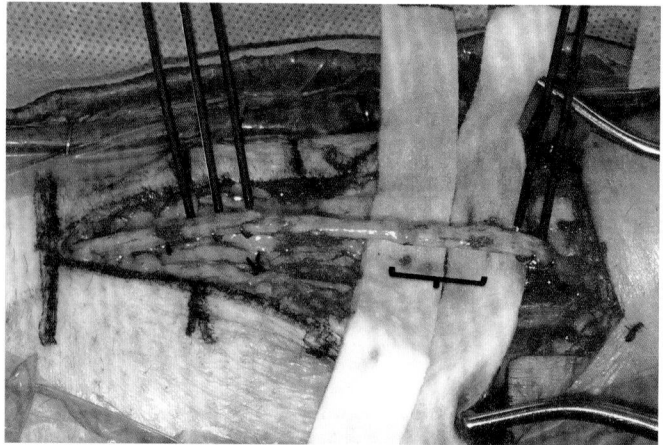

FIGURE 48.4 Intraoperative photo demonstrating a sural nerve neuroma-in-continuity marked with the *black bracket*. Intraoperative nerve action potential (NAP) recording using the hook electrodes reveal no conduction across the injured segment. Therefore, the neuroma is excised, and a conduit repair is performed.

support healing. If no response is noted, resection and repair may be warranted. Performing external neurolysis prior to intraoperative electrophysiologic evaluation allows more accurate placement of electrodes.

Internal neurolysis refers to the dissection and mobilization of individual nerve fascicles for evaluation and scar tissue removal. It is indicated for use with incomplete lesions that are associated with pain refractory to conventional medical therapy. Removal of scar tissue from around individual fascicles may help alleviate neuropathic pain, but dissection within the nerve sheath has the potential to damage regenerating axons. Internal neurolysis is also performed as part of a split repair, described in the following text.

Split Repair

Split repair is an operative technique that is used when electrophysiologic examination reveals conductive heterogeneity around the circumference of a nerve. After internal neurolysis is complete, individual fascicles can be tested and preserved if conductance across the lesion is achieved. Those fascicles that do not conduct will undergo resection and repair with either direct end-to-end neurorrhaphy or with grafts. The benefit of the split repair technique is that it allows uninjured fascicles to undergo spontaneous regeneration, which generally is more successful than either direct suturing or graft interposition.

End-to-End Neurorrhaphy

End-to-end neurorrhaphy refers to the reapproximation and suturing together of transected nerve ends. It is commonly used to repair sharp transections and generally carries a better prognosis than grafting. The use of this technique is limited by the size of the gap created after resection of injured tissue. Excessive tension at the suture line can increase scar formation and impede functional recovery. External neurolysis and mobilization of the nerve stumps may help to decrease the gap length. Transposition of some nerves, such as the ulnar nerve at the elbow, may also provide more length. Groups of fascicles may be individually reapproximated and sutured to help minimize formation of neuroma and maximize chance of regeneration. As the composition of fascicles changes every 1 to 2 mm, various techniques have been developed to try to match fascicles by predominant component, motor or sensory, to improve the chance of proper end-organ target reinnervation.

Graft Repair

For nerve gaps that are too long to be directly sutured without excessive tension, nerve graft repair is indicated. Longer gap lengths are commonly seen as a result of blunt transections, which damage tissue surrounding the lesion, and moderate to long complete lesions in continuity, which require resection. Although autografts are used most commonly today, cadaveric nerve grafts and specialized hollow tubes have also been used to restore continuity of the nerve.

For this procedure, the sural, antebrachial cutaneous, or superficial sensory radial nerve is harvested from the patient. Damaged nerve tissue is removed from the lesion site proximally and distally until normal fascicular structure is identified. Groups of fascicles are carefully separated and small-caliber donor nerve grafts are sutured to the healthy nerve tissue. The ends of the grafts are "fish-mouthed" or spread to increase the surface area. Good results can be achieved with this technique, although controversy exists regarding the maximum length for which grafts are successful. An inverse relationship has been observed between graft length and prognosis.

Nerve Transfer

Nerve transfer is an additional option for restoring function to an injured limb, particularly when the nerve lesion cannot be repaired by the techniques described earlier. This technique, which is variably referred to as *neurotization*, *nerve crossing*, and *heterotopic nerve suture*, is used most commonly to treat avulsive injuries of the brachial plexus. In this surgical technique, an uninjured nerve is used as a substitute for one that is no longer working. Transfers may be single or dual, in which either one or two nerve transfers are used to restore function. Nerves may be coapted end-to-end or end-to-side in which the proximal end of the recipient nerve is sutured to an epineural window in the intact, donor nerve. Generally, end-to-end direct neurorrhaphy is preferred. The term *neurotization*, commonly seen in the literature, is reserved for cases of nerve transfer in which a donor nerve is directly implanted into a muscle. The benefit of nerve transfer is that the time for regeneration and reinnervation is shortened by shortening the distance over which a nerve must regenerate. The primary goals of these surgeries include restoration of elbow flexion, shoulder abduction, and protective hand sensation.

The most commonly used procedure for restoration of elbow flexion was described by Oberlin and colleagues in 1994. During the Oberlin procedure, one or two fascicles from the ulnar nerve branch are transferred directly to the motor branch of the biceps. Intraoperative stimulation may be employed to identify fascicles of the ulnar nerve that innervate the flexor carpi ulnaris to minimize resulting deficit. Direct transfer of the ulnar fascicles to the biceps motor branch reduces sensory/motor cross-reinnervation by limiting aberrant motor reinnervation of the sensory territory of the lateral antebrachial cutaneous nerve. A second common procedure used to reestablish elbow flexion is transfer of a group of intercostal nerves to the musculocutaneous nerve. This transfer may be used when the Oberlin procedure is not available. Because the intercostal nerve is not a native elbow flexor, a period of retraining, which can extend from 12 to 24 months, may be necessary to restore function.

Similar procedures are used to restore shoulder abduction and external rotation, which are important for shoulder stability. The most commonly used procedure to restore shoulder abduction is the transfer of the spinal accessory nerve to the suprascapular nerve. In this procedure, distal fascicles of the spinal accessory nerve are directly sutured to the suprascapular nerve, which provides motor innervation to the supraspinatus. Superior branches of the spinal accessory nerve, which innervate the trapezius, are left intact to preserve function. An additional strategy to restore shoulder abduction is transfer of the triceps branch of the radial nerve to the axillary nerve, which innervates the deltoids. Nerve branches of the long, medial or lateral head of the triceps may be used. This procedure may be combined with spinal accessory transfer to maximize chance of functional recovery. In all cases, the choice of intervention derives from the needs and functional status of the individual patient.

Tendon Transfer

A final option for restoring some function and stability for patients who present for late treatment, when successful reinnervation is less likely, is tendon transfer. Tendon transfer consists of the transfer of an entire functioning muscle, with its innervation, to replace the actions of one that is paralyzed and thereby restore some motion across a joint. Tendon transfers are generally the last resort before fusion options are considered.

OUTCOMES

Functional restoration is dependent on both injury and patient-specific factors. Age, mechanism and type of injury, location, and timing of intervention all influence the final outcome. The interaction of these complex clinical characteristics makes prognostication difficult.

In general, neurapraxic lesions have the best prognosis with functional recovery apparent within weeks to a few months. Axonotmetic injuries recover more slowly, requiring several months for regeneration to occur. Neurotmetic lesions carry the worse prognosis with chance of recovery closely related to timing and type of surgical intervention. These lesions will not recover spontaneously. Sensory restoration can continue for a period of up to 3 years, whereas muscle targets are no longer viable after 12 to 18 months. Spontaneous recovery always carries a better prognosis than surgical reapproximation, and clinical recovery may be followed for up to 3 years.

SUGGESTED READINGS

Ali ZS, Bakar D, Li YR, et al. Utility of delayed surgical repair of neonatal brachial plexus palsy. *J Neurosurg Pediatrics*. 2014;13(4):462–470.

Antoniadis G, Kretschmer T, Pedro M, et al. Iatrogenic nerve injuries: prevalence, diagnosis and treatment. *Dtsch Arztebl Int*. 2014;111(16):273–279.

Bodine-Fowler SC, Allsing S, Botte MJ. Time course of muscle atrophy and recovery following a phenol-induced nerve block. *Muscle Nerve*. 1996;19:497–504.

Brecknell JE, Fawcett JW. Axonal regeneration. *Biol Rev*. 1996;71:227–255.

Brown M, Holland R, Hopkins W. Motor nerve sprouting. *Ann Rev Neurosci*. 1981;4:17–42.

Burnett MG, Zager EL. Pathophysiology of peripheral nerve injury: a brief review. *Neurosurg Focus*. 2004;16(5):E1.

Chaudhry V, Cornblath DR. Wallerian degeneration in human nerves: serial electrophysiological studies. *Muscle Nerve*. 1992;15:687–693.

Dejerine-Klumpke A. The classic: Klumpke's paralysis 1859–1927. *Clin Orthopaed Rel Res*. 1999;368:3–4.

Dorfman LJ. Quantitative clinical electrophysiology in the evaluation of nerve injury and regeneration. *Muscle Nerve*. 1990;13:822–828.

Dubuisson AS, Kline DG. Brachial plexus injuries: a survey of 100 consecutive cases from a single service. *Neurosurgery.* 2002;51(3):673–683.

Elhassan B, Bishop A, Shin A, et al. Shoulder tendon transfer options for adult patients with brachial plexus injury. *J Hand Surg.* 2010;35A:1211–1219.

Giuffre JL, Kakar S, Bishop AT, et al. Current concepts of the treatment of adult brachial plexus injuries. *J Hand Surg.* 2010;35A:678–688.

Gunasekera SM, Wijesekara RL, Sesath HG. Proximal axonal changes after peripheral nerve injury in man. *Muscle Nerve.* 2011;43(3):425–431.

Guth L. Neuromuscular function after regeneration of interrupted nerve fibers into partially denervated muscle. *Experimental Neurol.* 1962;6:129–141.

Irgit KS, Cush G. Tendon transfers for peroneal nerve injuries in the multiple ligament injured knee. *J Knee Surg.* 2012;25(4):327–333.

Kim DH. Mechanisms of injury in operative brachial plexus lesions. *Neurosurg Focus.* 2004;16(5):E2.

Kim DH, Cho YJ, Tiel RL, et al. Outcomes of surgery in 1019 brachial plexus lesions treated at Louisiana State University Health Sciences Center. *J Neurosurg.* 2003;98(5):1005–1016.

Kline DG. Surgical repair of peripheral nerve injury. *Muscle Nerve.* 1990;13:843–852.

Kline DG, Kim D, Midha R, et al. Management and results of sciatic nerve injuries: a 24-year experience. *J Neurosurg.* 1998;89:13–23.

Lee SK, Wolfe SW. Nerve transfers for the upper extremity: new horizons in nerve reconstruction. *J Am Assoc Orthoped Surg.* 2012;20(8):506–517.

Murovic JA. Lower-extremity peripheral nerve injuries: a Louisiana State University Health Sciences Center Literature Review with comparison of the operative outcomes of 806 Louisiana State University Health Sciences Center sciatic, common peroneal, and tibial nerve lesions. *Neurosurgery.* 2009;65(suppl 4):A18–A23.

Murovic JA. Upper-extremity peripheral nerve injuries: a Louisiana State University Health Sciences Center literature review with comparison of the operative outcomes of 1837 Louisiana State University Health Sciences Center median, radial, and ulnar nerve lesions. *Neurosurgery.* 2008;65(4):A11–A17.

Navarro X, Vivo M, Valero-Cabre A. Neural plasticity after peripheral nerve injury and regeneration. *Progress Neurobiol.* 2007;82:163–201.

Seddon H. A classification of nerve injuries. *Br Med J.* 1942;2(4260):237–239.

Seiler JG III, Desai MJ, Payne SH. Tendon transfers for radial, median, and ulnar nerve palsy. *J Am Acad Orthop Surg.* 2013;21(11):675–684.

Stewart JD. Peripheral nerve fascicles: anatomy and clinical relevance. *Muscle Nerve.* 2003;28:525–541.

Sunderland S. A classification of peripheral nerve injuries producing loss of function. *Brain.* 1951;74(4):491–516.

Sunderland S. The anatomy and physiology of nerve injury. *Muscle Nerve.* 1990;13:771–784.

Winfree CJ, Kline DG. Intraoperative positioning nerve injuries. *Surg Neurol.* 2005;63:5–18.

Wong CA. Nerve injuries after neuraxial anaesthesia and their medicolegal implications. *Best Pract Res Clin Obstet Gynaecol.* 2010;24:367–381.

Yang LJ, Chang KW, Chung KC. A systematic review of nerve transfer and nerve repair for the treatment of adult upper brachial plexus injury. *Neurosurgery.* 2012;71(2):417–429; discussion 429.

Mild Cognitive Impairment 49

Lawrence S. Honig

INTRODUCTION

Cognitive complaints are common in the population. In many such cases, history and examination reveal significant impairment in more than one cognitive domain and concomitant functional decline—and in these cases the findings provide for a diagnosis of dementia (see Chapter 11). However, in many other cases, there may be involvement of just one cognitive domain and/or lack of any clear functional decline, and diagnosis of dementia may not be warranted. An "intermediate state," neither representing dementia proper nor normality, must exist in the gradually progressive transition from normal brain health to dementia. There needs to be some means to categorize such a state as a diagnostic entity, even though it may simply be early stage of a degenerative brain disease. In the 20th century, a variety of nonspecific terms were invoked to describe this intermediate state, including "pure amnestic disorder," "age-related memory impairment (ARMI)," "age-associated memory impairment (AAMI)," "questionable dementia (QD)," "cognitive impairment no dementia (CIND)," and "prodromal dementia." Originally, such terms were predicated on the idea that perhaps this change was to be expected during normal aging. With the increased understanding of the biologic underpinnings of cognitive disorders, this view became less tenable. Thus for individuals with impairment not meeting dementia criteria, the term *mild cognitive impairment* or MCI was coined. The original clinical definition of MCI was memory-based and required a subjective memory complaint, a documented objective deficit in memory, overall normal general cognitive function, and a lack of "significant" functional impairment precluding a diagnosis of dementia. This was codified by the American Academy of Neurology in 2001. A large proportion of these cases ultimately develop dementia, mostly due to Alzheimer disease, at a rate of between 7% and 20% per year, although over a few years, some persons remain relatively stable, nonprogressive, or even improve. The definition of MCI has been broadened to domains other than memory to reflect non-Alzheimer dementias, (Table 49.1). These other types of MCI include single domain amnestic, amnestic multidomain, nonamnestic single domain, and nonamnestic multidomain impairments (Table 49.2).

MCI has also been codified by the committees of the American Psychiatric Association in 2013. The formulation of the diagnostic criteria of *Diagnostic and Statistical Manual of Mental Disorders*, 5th edition (*DSM-5*), recognizes that for each dementing disorder, there must be a state in which the impairment does not reach the level of dementia. Thus, each dementing disorder is categorized as a "major neurocognitive disorder" or "minor neurocognitive disorder." For example, Alzheimer dementia is "major," whereas amnestic MCI is "minor." For Alzheimer disease, which is the likely outcome for most amnestic MCI patients, biomarkers have allowed segmentation of the relatively slow neurodegenerative process into different diagnostic phases. The National Institute on Aging and Alzheimer's Association workgroup in 2011 divided the Alzheimer neurodegenerative spectrum into three phases: "preclinical" disease in which persons are

TABLE 49.1 Broad Definition of Mild Cognitive Impairment

Core Criteria	Examples
Subjective (self-reported or informant-reported) cognitive complaint	• Forgetfulness about events, appointments, or items of information • Forgetfulness regarding date or time • Misplacing or "losing" objects • Word-finding problems, such as "forgetting words" • Spatial disorientation, such as becoming lost
Objective evidence of cognitive dysfunction on testing	• Decreased performance on standardized testing of cognitive domains, including memory, language, visuospatial, attentional, or executive functions or skills[a]
Preservation of functional activities	• Essentially normal function in living activities[b]
Absence of diagnosis of dementia	• Diagnosis of dementia is exclusionary.[c]

[a]Various cutoffs have been used for the objective tests, including 1.5 standard deviations below age- and sex-adjusted norms on one or more tests within a particular cognitive domain.

[b]Functional preservation is the most problematic of the three core inclusionary features because function may depend on living situation and demands.

[c]Diagnosis of MCI and dementia are mutually exclusionary, but diagnosis of dementia is not independent from the criteria in the table.

TABLE 49.2   Classification of Types of Mild Cognitive Impairment

MCI Type	Domains Affected	Possible Prodromal Disease
Amnestic single domain	Memory alone	Alzheimer disease
Amnestic multidomain	Memory PLUS one or more other domain: language, attention, executive, or visuospatial dysfunction	Alzheimer disease
Nonamnestic single domain	Language, attention, executive, or visuospatial dysfunction	Frontotemporal dementia, Lewy body dementia, vascular dementia, posterior cortical atrophy, hydrocephalus
Nonamnestic multidomain	Memory not affected but more than one domain affected: language, attention, executive, or visuospatial dysfunction	Frontotemporal dementia, Lewy body dementia, vascular dementia, posterior cortical atrophy, hydrocephalus

Different types of MCI, left-most column, may ultimately more likely represent, as shown in right-most column, prodromal states of different dementia disorders. MCI, mild cognitive impairment.

asymptomatic but have biomarker evidence of an early Alzheimer process, a "symptomatic predementia phase" synonymous with MCI, and then the actual symptomatic dementia phase of Alzheimer disease (Table 49.3 and Fig. 49.1). In summary, *mild cognitive impairment* is a diagnostic term referring to a cognitively impaired state of less extent or severity than a dementia. MCI is generally, but not always, an early symptomatic state of a neurodegenerative process.

EPIDEMIOLOGY

Both incidence and prevalence of MCI increase with age. Prevalence estimates vary widely depending on the exact definition of MCI. Subjective memory or other cognitive complaints (e.g., word finding) that are elicited upon interview are extremely common in the elderly, although they depend on the population examined; in the United States, there is a prevalence of about 80% in persons older than age 70 years. However, most such persons will not have MCI when using objective neuropsychological testing measures to confirm memory or other cognitive dysfunction. Only a proportion of persons with subjective memory or cognitive complaints present for neurologic or medical attention. Of those who do present for medical evaluation, yet do not have diagnosable dementia, a high proportion (as many as 85%) will indeed meet MCI criteria.

MCI, defined as involving reasonably preserved function but combined subjective memory or cognitive change and objective memory or cognitive impairment (see Table 49.1), is not as common as subjective memory complaints. The prevalence and incidence rates depend on the population assessed, including age, education, and cultural milieu, and the exact diagnostic criteria. Thus in persons older than age 60 years, prevalence estimates for overall MCI have varied from as low as 1% to 5% to as high as 30% to 40%. Studies of populations older than age 75 years in North America and Europe suggest a convergent estimate of prevalence of about 20%, most of which MCI is amnestic or amnestic multidomain. Incidence rates of overall MCI vary in different reports from as low as 10 to as high as 200 cases per 1,000 person-years, depending on exact age range of elderly, the population studied, the numbers of years followed, and the exact criteria applied.

Risk factors for MCI appear to be the same as the risk factors for dementia conditions, notably Alzheimer disease (see Chapter 50). Age is the dominant risk factor. Gender has not proven to be a risk factor when controlling for age. Lower education has generally been found to be a risk factor, as sometimes has ethnicity, medical illnesses including cardiovascular disease, and genetic factors, including apolipoprotein E (APOE) $\varepsilon 4$ allele. If a case of MCI ultimately progresses to a particular dementia, then retrospectively, it is found that the risk factors for that form of MCI were those for the dementia disorder. However, for the MCI patients who improve

TABLE 49.3   Stages of Alzheimer Disease

Stage of Alzheimer Disease	Cognitive Signs and Symptoms	Functional Impairment	Biomarker Status
No disease	None	None	Negative
Presymptomatic disease (preclinical Alzheimer)	None	None	Positive
Symptomatic predementia (mild cognitive impairment)	Single or multidomain	Not significant	Positive
Symptomatic dementia (Alzheimer disease)	Multiple domains	Definite Impairment	Positive

This formulation is the result of the National Institute on Aging and Alzheimer's Association workgroups, as published in 2011. Biomarkers include structural MRI (regional hippocampal atrophy), PET metabolic imaging (bitemporoparietal hypometabolism), PET amyloid imaging (evidence of amyloid), and cerebrospinal fluid (low β-amyloid-42, high tau, and high phospho-tau).

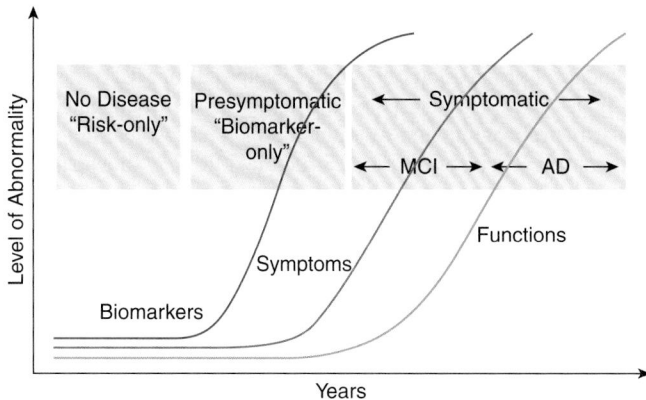

FIGURE 49.1 MCI on the spectrum of neurodegeneration. The figure shows schematic increases over time in brain biomarkers (*red line*), symptoms (*blue line*), and functional deficits (*green line*). For Alzheimer disease, biomarkers include (1) evidence for fibrillar β-amyloid accumulation in the brain through florbetapir, florbetaben, or flutemetamol imaging or because of low cerebrospinal fluid β-amyloid-42 and (2) evidence of neurodegeneration indicated by decreased hippocampal volume, decreased gray matter gyral thickness, or increased tau and/or phospho-tau in the cerebrospinal fluid. Symptoms would include memory, language, visuospatial, or executive dysfunction confirmed on neuropsychological testing. A disease-free (*at risk*) period is followed by an asymptomatic but biomarker-positive period (*presymptomatic*), followed by a *symptomatic* period. This latter period consists of an intermediate, earlier time period marked by cognitive symptoms without significant effect on function (*MCI*) and a later time period in which cognitive symptoms are more evident and there is concomitant functional impairment (*dementia*).

over 1 to 3 years, or stay stable, and do not progress to dementia, the major risk factors, in retrospect, are psychiatric illnesses, including depression and anxiety, and reversible medical conditions.

Overall, younger persons, younger than age 50 to 60 years, presenting with subjective memory complaints, with or without objective confirmation, are more likely to have an underlying psychiatric basis to their dysfunction than are elderly persons. This is likely due to both the fact that early dementia is less common in the younger population and because anxiety and depression more often present in the younger population than present de novo in the elderly.

Most studies with strict criteria for objective dysfunction show that MCI subtypes of amnestic or amnestic multidomain are more common. Nonamnestic single or multidomain subtypes are less common. This might be expected from the relative prevalences of the underlying dementia disorders (see Table 49.2).

MCI is not a pathologically specific diagnosis, so the epidemiology of progression to dementia is important. It is clear that the majority of persons meeting criteria for MCI do progress to dementia over a period of 5 to 10 years. Both the rate of such progression and the particular dementia to which there is progression vary, in part depending on severity and in part depending on the type of MCI. Overall, amnestic MCI and amnestic multidomain MCI both most frequently progress to Alzheimer disease at generally reported rates of 10% to 20% per year. Some other less common forms of MCI, such as single-domain visuospatial, may upon progression best fit the clinical syndromatic diagnosis of posterior

cortical atrophy, which, however, usually still reflects underlying Alzheimer disease pathology. Even persons who "revert" from MCI to normal cognition are at higher future risk of dementia. However, some persons remain stable with a diagnosis of MCI for many years, and the underlying basis of their dysfunction is unclear, as is their ultimate prognosis.

PATHOBIOLOGY

The pathobiology of MCI is that of the disorders for which it is a precursor state. Thus, if MCI is an early form of Alzheimer disease, then Alzheimer pathology is the substrate. Correspondingly, if the MCI is a precursor to frontotemporal dementia (FTD), then the pathology is that of FTD. Thus the condition, as presently defined, is not a homogeneous clinicopathologic entity. The reader is referred to Chapter 11 on the dementias and the individual chapters on Alzheimer disease (see Chapter 50) and other dementias.

CLINICAL FEATURES, DIAGNOSIS, AND PROGNOSIS

MCI manifestations are subjective and objective cognitive impairment (see Table 49.1), but each of the cardinal aspects of MCI has interpretative leeway. Generally, a diagnosis of MCI requires a "consistent" symptomatology, not single disturbing events. Corroboration of a patient's symptoms by a knowledgeable informant also increases likelihood that the symptoms represent abnormal cognition. Assessment of objective memory and cognitive impairment depends on the exact domains (memory, language, attention, executive and visuospatial function), the tests used for each domain, and the criteria for abnormality. Different standards have been used, including 1, 1.5, or 2 standard deviations below the normative mean, without formal consensus or agreement on which of these is most appropriate.

Assuming the unequivocal presence of subjective and objective cognitive changes, often the most diagnostically difficult criteria to assess is that of relative preservation of function. Particularly in the elderly, depending on their spousal or family support and on their residential environment, the patient may not be expected or in the habit of performing routine functions commonly performed earlier in life. Bills may be prearranged; meals may be preprepared; and travel may be circumscribed or always accompanied. In these settings, it is often difficult to assess what is evidence of significant functional decline. Even persons engaged in their occupation may have a narrow range of responsibilities and well-learned skills in their occupational field that makes decline in function inevident.

The first criteria for MCI were developed during the 1990s. In 2001, the American Academy of Neurology encoded the criteria (see Table 49.1) without specifying exact measures for impairments. More recently in 2011, consensus panels sponsored by the National Institute on Aging and the Alzheimer's Association have provided criteria for MCI with accompanying criteria for preceding (presymptomatic) and frequent subsequent (Alzheimer dementia) conditions. These National Institute on Aging and Alzheimer's Association criteria are consistent with current biomarker evidence that MCI is the middle part of a spectrum (see Table 49.3 and Fig. 49.1). This spectrum comprises persons without disease but with a risk factor for dementia such as family history or APOE ε4 genotype, persons who are presymptomatic (showing evidence of early disease biomarkers accumulation such as cerebral amyloidosis), early symptomatic individuals with MCI, and later symptomatic individuals with Alzheimer disease or another dementia.

DIAGNOSTIC TESTING

Diagnostic testing of persons with MCI should consist of testing to exclude reversible causes of cognitive impairment. Thus, in most cases, the evaluation should proceed similarly to the evaluation of the patient with dementia. Neuropsychological testing may have even greater use in the case of suspected MCI than in dementia. Psychometric test results can be helpful in establishing the extent of cognitive impairment, the domains affected, and the degree to which there is impairment, in comparison to a normative sample of others with comparable age, sex, and education. Such testing provides strong assistance in the diagnosis of MCI and also provides a baseline for subsequent evaluations.

Laboratory and imaging studies have two potential roles. The first role is to exclude nonneurodegenerative medical conditions not evident on the clinical examination that might be responsible for the cognitive impairment and might be reversible with known therapies. The second reason is to discern biomarkers whether in cerebrospinal fluid or on brain imaging that might be of value in assessing the prognosis of the MCI state and whether it is more or less likely to progress to a dementing disorder.

Exclusionary tests are those used in Alzheimer disease and include blood laboratory testing to assess the presence of renal or hepatic dysfunction, B_{12} deficiency, thyroid deficiency, and in some cases, infectious diseases such as Lyme disease, syphilis, or HIV infection. Routine neuroimaging using magnetic resonance imaging (MRI) is often reasonable to exclude structural disorders representing infections, tumors, traumatic, hydrocephalic, or vascular injuries and may also provide information on pattern of brain atrophy indicative of an underlying process (see the following text). Electroencephalography (EEG) or other neurophysiologic measures are rarely needed, unless there is the suggestion of some episodic nature to the symptoms suggesting the possibility of complex partial seizures. EEG would typically be normal or show nonspecific mild temporal slowing or diffuse background rhythm slowing. Cerebrospinal fluid testing is optional. Like MRI, it may rarely reveal the unlikely presence of an unsuspected contributory condition that might have its own specific therapeutic approach. Such disorders include central nervous system (CNS) inflammatory, infectious, or neoplastic disorders, including neurosyphilis, neurosarcoidosis, or meningeal carcinomatosis.

To determine the etiology of MCI and assist prognostically, a number of tests have been shown to be of value in assessing the likelihood of progression of cognitive symptoms of MCI to dementia (Table 49.4). These tests include structural neuroimaging, molecular neuroimaging, and examination of cerebrospinal fluid biomarkers and genetic biomarkers. Structural MRI may show patterns of cerebral atrophy, which can be suggestive of the presence of a particular neurodegenerative disorder. Early Alzheimer disease is marked by temporal lobe and parietal lobe gyral atrophy and cortical thinning. Studies show that temporal lobe atrophy is associated with a greater risk of progression of memory symptoms and development of Alzheimer dementia. FTD is more often marked by asymmetric or symmetric frontal and anterior temporal atrophy (see Chapter 51). Molecular neuroimaging using positron emission tomography (PET) imaging tracers for amyloid such as florbetapir, florbetaben, or flutemetamol may show the early deposition of fibrillar β-amyloid indicative of the presence of neuritic plaques. Positive amyloid imaging is a strong risk for progression of MCI to Alzheimer disease dementia, and negative amyloid imaging makes it less likely to predict AD, although various cutoffs for imaging have been used. Likewise, cerebrospinal fluid biomarkers, particularly, the presence of low β-amyloid-42 but also likely the presence of high tau and phospho-tau, are associated with MCI progression to Alzheimer disease. Genetic testing for *APOE* genotype is not recommended, but there is evidence that particularly in those older than age 65 years, the presence of one or two *APOE* ε4 alleles is associated with a higher risk of progression to Alzheimer disease. The combinations of these factors in which multiple markers indicate the same incipient disease process are likely of even greater prognostic value, although correspondingly, the presence of discordant biomarkers makes prognostication of progression less clear.

TREATMENT

Because many cases of MCI, particularly amnestic MCI, develop into Alzheimer disease over time, a number of investigations have examined whether any of the four commonly used disease-specific treatments available for Alzheimer disease are of any benefit in either improving cognition or delaying the time period to

---

TABLE 49.4 Biomarkers Useful in Prognostication for Mild Cognitive Impairment

Biomarker	Result	Prognostic Implications
Brain MRI	Focal decreased hippocampal volume, parietal gyral atrophy, or cortical thinning	Likely AD
Fluorodeoxyglucose PET imaging	Bitemporoparietal hypometabolism Frontal or anterior temporal hypometabolism Occipital hypometabolism	Likely AD Suggestive of FTD Suggestive of PCA or DLB
Florbetapir, florbetaben, or flutemetamol PET imaging	Positive signal for fibrillar amyloid	Suggestive of AD with or without involvement of DLB
Ioflupane SPECT imaging	Decreased unilateral or bilateral striatal uptake	Suggestive of DLB
Cerebrospinal fluid biomarker analysis	Low β-amyloid-42 High phospho-tau	Suggestive of AD
Apolipoprotein E genotyping	ε4 Allele present	Suggestive of underlying AD
Glucocerebrosidase (GBA) genotyping	Presence of a GBA mutation	Suggestive of possible DLB

MRI, magnetic resonance imaging; AD, Alzheimer disease; PET, positron emission tomography; FTD, frontotemporal dementia; PCA, posterior cortical atrophy; DLB, dementia with Lewy bodies; SPECT, single-photon emission computed tomography.

conversion to dementia[1]. The three cholinesterase inhibitors donepezil, galantamine, and rivastigmine have all been the subjects of trials in MCI. Only donepezil (10 mg/day) showed some mild evidence [**Level 1**][1] of efficacy in delaying progression to a diagnosis of Alzheimer disease (sometimes termed *conversion*). Galantamine trials showed a small degree of increased mortality in drug treatment compared to placebo, but it is suspected that this was a statistical finding, not necessarily indicative of an injurious effect of this drug in MCI. The sole approved noncholinesterase inhibitor Alzheimer medication memantine has been tried in MCI and mild AD and has been found to be inefficacious.

Disease-modifying treatments are not yet available for MCI or Alzheimer disease. The wide presumption is that if a medication is shown to slow the progression of Alzheimer disease, that treatment at the MCI stage would be even more useful than treatment of mild AD. Even if a drug worked equally effectively at different stages of the disease, slowing progressive disease earlier would be more beneficial than slowing it later. Thus, increasingly prospective investigational therapies for Alzheimer disease are also being tested in subject populations with MCI. Such approaches include immune therapies designed to clear β-amyloid monomers or polymers, including active immunogens or passive monoclonal antibodies, β- or γ-secretase inhibitors designed to decrease intracerebral generation of β-amyloid, and other potential treatments that have been proposed to lessen tau aggregation or decrease synaptic or neuronal injury. However, when treating persons with MCI as if they have early Alzheimer disease, it is important to be certain that indeed this disease is the underlying pathologic process. For this reason including imaging biomarkers for β-amyloid and tau, cerebrospinal fluid biomarkers for β-amyloid, tau, phospho-tau, synuclein, and others and genetic markers including APOE genotype may be useful in predicting which persons with MCI are most likely to be in the early phases of Alzheimer disease and thus warrant therapies designed to deter progression of the Alzheimer disease process.

MCI also frequently involves concurrent anxiety or depression. In some cases, as mentioned earlier, the primary etiology of the MCI state may be depression. Thus, for any individual with anxiety or depression, consideration should be given to treatment of the psychiatric symptoms with antidepressants, most commonly selective serotonin reuptake inhibitors such as fluoxetine, sertraline, paroxetine, citalopram, or escitalopram.

LEVEL 1 EVIDENCE

1. Lu PH, Edland SD, Teng E, et al; Alzheimer's Disease Cooperative Study Group. Donepezil delays progression to AD in MCI subjects with depressive symptoms. *Neurology.* 2009;72:2115–2121.

SUGGESTED READINGS

Albert MS, DeKosky ST, Dickson D, et al. The diagnosis of mild cognitive impairment due to Alzheimer's disease: recommendations from the National Institute on Aging-Alzheimer's Association workgroups on diagnostic guidelines for Alzheimer's disease. *Alzheimers Dement.* 2011;7:270–279.

Albert M, Soldan A, Gottesman R, et al. Cognitive changes preceding clinical symptom onset of mild cognitive impairment and relationship to ApoE genotype. *Curr Alzheimer Res.* 2014;11:773–784.

Bondi MW, Edmonds EC, Jak AJ, et al. Neuropsychological criteria for mild cognitive impairment improves diagnostic precision, biomarker associations, and progression rates. *J Alzheimers Dis.* 2014;42:275–289.

Delrieu J, Piau A, Caillaud C, et al. Managing cognitive dysfunction through the continuum of Alzheimer's disease: role of pharmacotherapy. *CNS Drugs.* 2011;25:213–226.

Dukart J, Mueller K, Villringer A, et al; Alzheimer's Disease Neuroimaging Initiative. Relationship between imaging biomarkers, age, progression and symptom severity in Alzheimer's disease. *Neuroimage Clin.* 2013;3:84–94.

Farlow MR. Treatment of mild cognitive impairment (MCI). *Curr Alzheimer Res.* 2009;6:362–367.

Ferman TJ, Smith GE, Kantarci K, et al. Nonamnestic mild cognitive impairment progresses to dementia with Lewy bodies. *Neurology.* 2013;81:2032–2038.

Fleisher AS, Chen K, Liu X, et al. Using positron emission tomography and florbetapir F18 to image cortical amyloid in patients with mild cognitive impairment or dementia due to Alzheimer disease. *Arch Neurol.* 2011;68:1404–1411.

Jack CR Jr, Albert MS, Knopman DS, et al. Introduction to the recommendations from the National Institute on Aging-Alzheimer's Association workgroups on diagnostic guidelines for Alzheimer's disease. *Alzheimers Dement.* 2011;7:257–262.

Karow DS, McEvoy LK, Fennema-Notestine C, et al; Alzheimer's Disease Neuroimaging Initiative. Relative capability of MR imaging and FDG PET to depict changes associated with prodromal and early Alzheimer disease. *Radiology.* 2010;256:932–942.

Kemppainen NM, Scheinin NM, Koivunen J, et al. Five-year follow-up of 11C-PIB uptake in Alzheimer's disease and MCI. *Eur J Nucl Med Mol Imaging.* 2014;41:283–289.

Knopman DS, Petersen RC. Mild cognitive impairment and mild dementia: a clinical perspective. *Mayo Clin Proc.* 2014;89:1452–1459.

Landau SM, Harvey D, Madison CM, et al; Alzheimer's Disease Neuroimaging Initiative. Comparing predictors of conversion and decline in mild cognitive impairment. *Neurology.* 2010;75:230–238.

Lim YY, Maruff P, Pietrzak RH, et al; AIBL Research Group. Effect of amyloid on memory and non-memory decline from preclinical to clinical Alzheimer's disease. *Brain.* 2014;137:221–231.

Mattsson N, Tosun D, Insel PS, et al; Alzheimer's Disease Neuroimaging Initiative. Association of brain amyloid-β with cerebral perfusion and structure in Alzheimer's disease and mild cognitive impairment. *Brain.* 2014;137:1550–1561.

McKhann GM, Knopman DS, Chertkow H, et al. The diagnosis of dementia due to Alzheimer's disease: recommendations from the National Institute on Aging-Alzheimer's Association workgroups on diagnostic guidelines for Alzheimer's disease. *Alzheimers Dement.* 2011;7:263–269.

Pagani M, Dessi B, Morbelli S, et al. MCI patients declining and not-declining at mid-term follow-up: FDG-PET findings. *Curr Alzheimer Res.* 2010;7:287–294.

Petersen RC, Aisen P, Boeve BF, et al. Mild cognitive impairment due to Alzheimer disease in the community. *Ann Neurol.* 2013;74:199–208.

Petersen RC, Caracciolo B, Brayne C, et al. Mild cognitive impairment: a concept in evolution. *J Intern Med.* 2014;275:214–228.

Petersen RC, Smith GE, Waring SC, et al. Mild cognitive impairment: clinical characterization and outcome. *Arch Neurol.* 1999;56:303–308.

Prestia A, Caroli A, van der Flier WM, et al. Prediction of dementia in MCI patients based on core diagnostic markers for Alzheimer disease. *Neurology.* 2013;80:1048–1056.

Roberts R, Knopman DS. Classification and epidemiology of MCI. *Clin Geriatr Med.* 2013;29:753–772.

Roberts RO, Knopman DS, Mielke MM, et al. Higher risk of progression to dementia in mild cognitive impairment cases who revert to normal. *Neurology.* 2014;82:317–325.

Rowe CC, Bourgeat P, Ellis KA, et al. Predicting Alzheimer disease with β-amyloid imaging: results from the Australian imaging, biomarkers, and lifestyle study of ageing. *Ann Neurol.* 2013;74:905–913.

Sperling RA, Aisen PS, Beckett LA, et al. Toward defining the preclinical stages of Alzheimer's disease: recommendations from the National Institute on Aging-Alzheimer's Association workgroups on diagnostic guidelines for Alzheimer's disease. *Alzheimers Dement.* 2011;7:280–292.

Tricco AC, Soobiah C, Berliner S, et al. Efficacy and safety of cognitive enhancers for patients with mild cognitive impairment: a systematic review and meta-analysis. *CMAJ.* 2013;185:1393–1401.

van de Pol LA, Korf ES, van der Flier WM, et al. Magnetic resonance imaging predictors of cognition in mild cognitive impairment. *Arch Neurol.* 2007;64:1023–1028.

Ward A, Arrighi HM, Michels S, et al. Mild cognitive impairment: disparity of incidence and prevalence estimates. *Alzheimers Dement.* 2012;8:14–21.

Alzheimer Disease 50

Lawrence S. Honig, Scott A. Small, and
Richard Mayeux

INTRODUCTION

The most common dementia is Alzheimer disease. The disease was first named by Emil Kraepelin in 1910, after Alois Alzheimer, who in 1906 had described the clinical features and pathologic manifestations of dementia in a 51-year-old woman. For some decades, Alzheimer disease was considered a presenile form of dementia, affecting individuals with symptoms beginning before age 65 years. But the mid-20th century brought the understanding that the same clinical, pathologic, ultrastructural, and biochemical features of presenile Alzheimer disease are shared by those with the more common "senile" (older than age 65 years) dementia. The disease is commonly sporadic, although susceptibility relates to a variety of genetic risk factors. Uncommonly, the disease has an autosomal dominant inheritance pattern, particularly in younger persons. In a look back to the past, an analysis of the DNA of Alois Alzheimer's first described case, nearly 100 years after her evaluation, revealed that her condition resulted from a mutation (F176L) in exon 6 of one of these autosomal dominant genes, presenilin 1.

EPIDEMIOLOGY

Alzheimer disease is a chronic disease of aging, and both the incidence and prevalence of disease increase with age. Prevalence estimates reveal that fewer than 1% of persons younger than age 65 years are clinically affected, but about 5% are affected at age 65 to 75 years, about 20% at age 75 to 85 years, and likely over 50% at age 85 years and older. The increasing prevalence with age is because the age-specific incidence, or the number of new cases arising over a specific period of time, rises steeply from less than 1% per year before age 65 years to about 6% per year for individuals aged 85 years and older. The average duration of symptoms from first noticeable symptoms until death is typically from 10 to 20 or more years.

It is presumed that both environmental and genetic factors are involved in the risk of the disease. But extensive investigations, as to environmental risk factors other than age, have not resulted in clear risk factors for Alzheimer disease itself. Late-life depression is associated with Alzheimer disease, although the direction of causality is unclear—it is likely that depressive symptoms are often early manifestations of this dementing disorder. Traumatic head injury has been associated with increased risk of dementia, but it is not clear that trauma is a risk for Alzheimer disease itself versus other dementias. Likewise, diabetes and cardiovascular and cerebrovascular disorders have been associated with increased risk of dementia, but these may be due to additive ischemic injury to the brain, rather than a true increase in Alzheimer disease. Studies of identical twins show that they are not necessarily concordantly affected, so almost certainly there are some factors other than classic genetic ones. However, the main risk factors for development of Alzheimer disease, each small in and of itself, appear to be the members of a growing long list of genetic variations (Table 50.1).

GENETIC BASIS OF ALZHEIMER DISEASE

Most Alzheimer disease is "sporadic" rather than a mendelian dominant or recessive condition. However, a small proportion of the total number of persons with Alzheimer disease (<0.5%) have disease that is transmitted as an autosomal dominant identified monogenic familial disorder, commonly, but not always, with onset before age 65 years. Mutations in three genes, the amyloid precursor protein (APP) gene on chromosome 21, the presenilin 1 (PSEN1) gene on chromosome 14, and the presenilin 2 (PSEN2) gene on chromosome 1, result in such autosomal dominant forms of the disease beginning as early as the third decade of life, with essentially complete penetrance (see Table 50.1). In addition, trisomy 21, or Down syndrome, results in near certainty of Alzheimer disease pathology by age 50 years and in symptoms of the disease in those who survive long enough. Finally, there is a mutation in APP (the "Icelandic" allele, A673T) which is highly correlated with protection from Alzheimer disease. There are at least 204 described different pathogenic mutations in PSEN1, and it is the most common form of familial early-onset Alzheimer disease. Mutations in these three genes account for as many as half of the familial forms of early-onset Alzheimer disease and may be considered deterministic because of nearly complete correspondence between the genotype and phenotype. Mutations in these three genes seem to lead to increased production of amyloid-β (Aβ) or specifically the Aβ42 peptide.

There is a higher risk of Alzheimer disease in first-degree relatives of persons with Alzheimer disease. Siblings of patients have about twice the expected lifetime risk of developing the disease. Monozygotic twins have significantly higher concordance of Alzheimer disease than do dizygotic twins. Some of the genetic risk relates to the ε4 polymorphism of the APOE gene on chromosome 19, which shows a strong association with onset of Alzheimer disease in the age range of 60 to 80 years. The ε4 polymorphism of APOE is a normally occurring variant of the gene present in about one-third of the unaffected American population but present in about two-thirds of those with late-onset Alzheimer disease. APOE has been called a *susceptibility* gene because possession of the ε4 allele, a polymorphism, does not always lead to Alzheimer disease. One APOE-ε4 allele is associated with about a 2- to 3-fold increased risk, whereas having two copies is associated with a 5- to 10-fold increased risk. The population attributable risk associated with APOE-ε4 is approximately 20%, making it one of the most important risk factors for the disease.

A large number of gene variants have now been identified, that each conveys a smaller risk of Alzheimer disease than that of APOE-ε4 (see Table 50.1). About 20 such genes are currently identified including some involved in lipid biology, intracellular processing, or endosomal pathways (e.g., SORL1) and others involved in inflammation or the immune response, cell migration, cytoskeleton, axonal transport, and microglial cell function. Other genes will likely be identified adding to the already complex genetic architecture of this disease.

TABLE 50.1   Chromosomal Loci and Genes Related to Alzheimer Disease

Chromosome Locus	Gene/Candidate	Genetic Inheritance	Possible Mechanism
14q24.13	PSEN1	Autosomal dominant	Increased generation of Aβ42
1q31.42	PSEN2	Autosomal dominant	Increased generation of Aβ42
21q21.3	APP	Autosomal dominant	Increased Aβ42 or Aβ42 aggregation
21q21.3	APP(A673T)	Protective factor	Decreased generation of Aβ42
19q13.2	APOE	Risk factor	Decreased clearance of Aβ42
11q23.3	SORL1	Risk factor	Lipid/protein endocytosis/trafficking
2q14.3	BIN1	Risk factor	Lipid/protein endocytosis/trafficking
6p12.3	CD2AP	Risk factor	Lipid/protein endocytosis/trafficking
11q14.2	PICALM	Risk factor	Lipid/protein endocytosis/trafficking
19p13.3	ABCA7	Risk factor	Lipid/protein endocytosis/trafficking
8p21.1	CLU	Risk factor	Lipid/protein endocytosis/chaperone
1q32.2	CR1	Risk factor	Cell adhesion to particles/complexes
19q13.3	CD33	Risk factor	Cell adhesion/immune response
18q12.1	DSG2	Risk factor	Cell adhesion
14q22.1	FERMT2	Risk factor	Cell adhesion/cytoskeletal function
20q13.31	CASS4	Risk factor	Cell adhesion/cytoskeletal function
7p14.1	NME8	Risk factor	Cytoskeletal function
6p21.3	HLA-DRB5/1	Risk factor	Immune response/trafficking
5q14.3	MEF2C	Risk factor	Immune response/synaptic function
2q37.1	INPP5D	Risk factor	Immune response/signaling
11q12.1	MS4A6A	Risk factor	Signal transduction
7q34	EPHA1	Risk factor	Receptor tyrosine kinase/signaling
8p21.2	PTK2B	Risk factor	Receptor tyrosine kinase/signaling
14q32.12	SLC24A4-RIN3	Risk factor	Cation exchange transporter
7q22.1	ZCWPW1	Risk factor	Regulation gene expression
11p11.2	CELF1	Risk factor	Regulation gene expression (splicing)
6p21.1	TREM2(R47H)	Risk factor	Immune response/Aβ42 clearance
6p21.1	TREML2(S144G)	Protective factor	Immune response/Aβ42 clearance

List of genetic markers related to risk of Alzheimer disease. PSEN1, PSEN2, and APP are genes for which mutations can lead to autosomal dominant inherited Alzheimer disease, although a particular mutation in APP can also be protective against Alzheimer disease. APOE, SORL1, and the other genes listed all have been shown to have allelic variation that affects risk of Alzheimer disease.

PATHOBIOLOGY

Alzheimer disease pathology is marked by two specific neuropathologic features (Table 50.2; Fig. 50.1): extracellular amyloid plaques molecularly consisting in large part of a fibrillar aggregation of the 40 and 42 amino acid peptides Aβ40 and Aβ42 and intracellular neurofibrillary tangles, which consist of paired helical filamentous polymers of hyperphosphorylated tau protein. Although these specific features permit pathologic diagnosis of Alzheimer disease, it is likely that the symptoms of the disease relate primarily to extensive synaptic losses and later to frank neuronal losses. Much of the earliest brunt of this injury is borne by the entorhinal region of the medial temporal lobe.

The senile neuritic plaques are spherical microscopic lesions with a core of extracellular Aβ infiltrated and surrounded by abnormal nerve fibers (neurites). The Aβ40 and Aβ42 peptides are derived from the APP, a transmembrane protein present in most tissues.

A region of the APP resides within an intramembranous domain of intracellular organelles in neurons, and several proteolytic enzyme activities, known as *secretases*, are responsible for cleavage of the protein. When cleaved by α-secretase, a soluble peptide derivative of amyloid is formed. However, when the APP is cleaved by β-secretase, and subsequently by γ-secretase, the peptides Aβ40 and Aβ42 are generated. These Aβ peptide monomers aggregate, forming oligomers, and ultimately large polymers, a process that can be demonstrated in vitro and presumably results in the amyloid plaques observed histologically. It is thus not surprising that the three autosomal dominant genes for Alzheimer disease are the APP gene itself and the PSEN1 and PSEN2 genes, which contribute to γ-secretase activity. Although there is little doubt as to a pathologic role of APP products, it is not clear which products might be most responsible for presumed neurotoxicity and synaptic losses: monomers, oligomers, polymers, or even other more soluble fragments. In addition to the parenchymal deposition of amyloid in

TABLE 50.2	Pathologic Hallmarks of Alzheimer Disease	
Macroscopic/Regional	**Clinical Implications**	
Hippocampal atrophy	Memory impairment	
Parietotemporal atrophy	Dysnomia/visuospatial impairment	
Nucleus basalis cell loss	Attentional impairment	
Microscopic	**Molecular Concomitant**	
Neuritic plaques	Aβ42 and Aβ40 fibrillar aggregates with associated neuritic changes	
Diffuse plaques	Aβ42 and Aβ40 fibrillar aggregates	
Neurofibrillary tangles	Paired helical filamentous aggregates of phosphorylated tau protein	
Synaptic loss	Not known—but accompanied by decreases in various neurotransmitters	
Neuronal loss	Not known	
Granulovacuolar degeneration	Intraneuronal vesicular changes	

List of pathologic hallmarks of Alzheimer disease, including macroscopic/regional changes and microscopic changes and their clinical and molecular correlates.

Alzheimer disease, there is in nearly all cases amyloid angiopathy, which is amyloid deposition around meningeal and cerebral vessels. This condition is of varying severity and import in different patients but is accompanied by a propensity for hemorrhages, which may be microscopic, although visible on T2*-weighted gradient echo magnetic resonance imaging (MRI), or macroscopic, with medium or large lobar hemorrhages. In a small proportion of patients, acute localized or diffuse brain edema may occur, now known as *amyloid-related imaging abnormality edema* or ARIA-E, either spontaneously or after delivery of investigational antiamyloid therapies.

Neurofibrillary tangles are fibrillary intracytoplasmic structures within the neurons. Electron microscopy shows paired helical filaments of the microtubule-associated protein, known as *tau protein*. Normally, tau is a protein responsible in part for the axonal cytoskeleton, participating in microtubule assembly. In Alzheimer disease, hyperphosphorylated tau aggregates form, which are recognized in the electron microscope as twisted paired helical filaments and recognized in the light microscope as neurofibrillary tangles. Neurofibrillary tangles are not specific to Alzheimer disease, but in this disease, they occur first in the hippocampal formation and later are seen throughout the cerebral cortex. This apparent topographic spread of tangles has been codified as a staging system by Braak and Braak, including involvement of entorhinal (stages 1 and 2), hippocampal (stages 3 and 4), and neocortical (stages 5 and 6) regions. Tangles seem to increase in severity and extent with

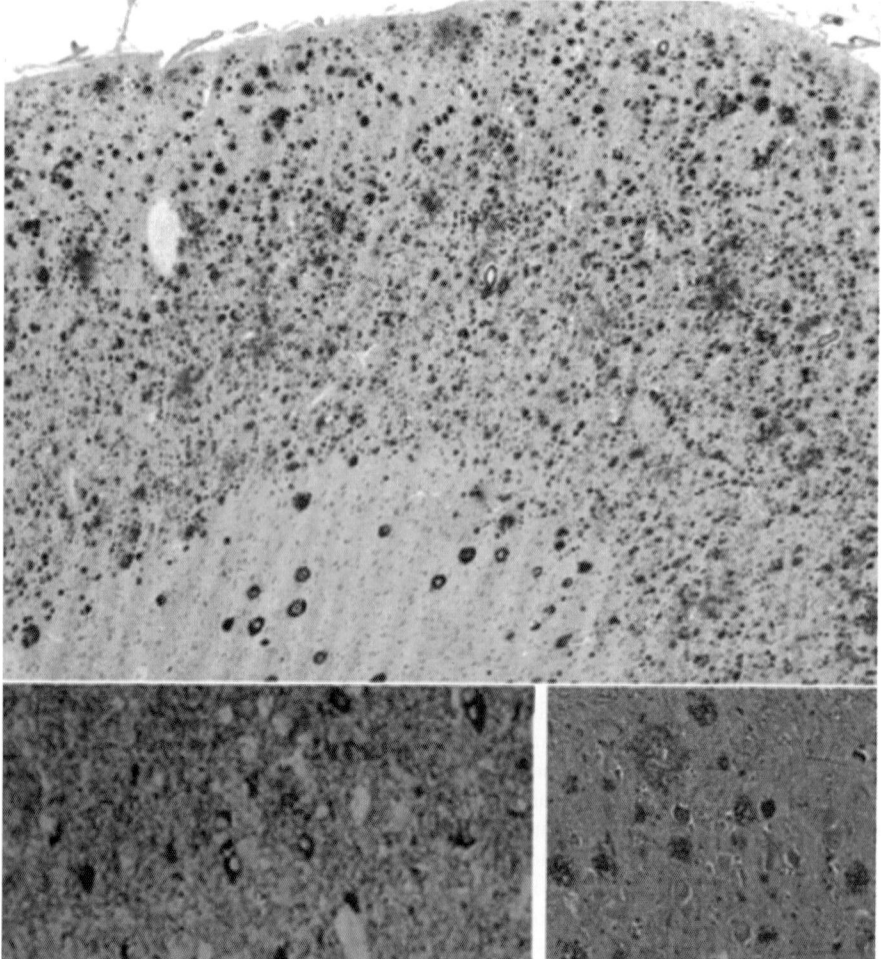

FIGURE 50.1 **Top panel** shows a cortical brain section immunohistochemically stained with antibody to β-amyloid. There are extensive stained extracellular deposits, which include plaques and also blood vessel staining in the white matter (amyloid angiopathy). **Bottom left panel** shows section stained with antibody specific for phosphorylated tau protein, and the intracellular stained deposits are neurofibrillary tangles. **Bottom right panel** shows a histochemical stained section (silver stained with the Bielschowsky method), visualizing both plaques and tangles.

disease progression. This is more evident than is the case for amyloid plaques, which latter are often present even before symptoms and do not appear to correlate so highly with disease severity in autopsy tissues. Recent human in vivo imaging evidence suggests that amyloid deposition does indeed increase with disease, but it may "saturate" earlier than the formation of tangles. The relative injurious basis of these two hallmark pathologies is still not clear.

An important but nonspecific pathologic feature of Alzheimer disease is widespread, regionally specific losses of synapses and ultimately losses of neurons. Synaptic losses are accompanied by a wide variety of neurotransmitter deficits. These include particular decline in cholinergic terminals in the hippocampus and cortex, which apparently owes to early and prominent degenerative involvement of the nucleus basalis of Meynert, whose large cholinergic neurons project widely. It is this cholinergic deficit that informs the basis for treatment of Alzheimer disease with drugs that increase cholinergic tone. Alzheimer disease is also variably marked by granulovacuolar degeneration of hippocampal pyramidal cells, which is a poorly understood pathologic feature, amyloid deposition in blood vessels, and glial changes. Finally, it is common in Alzheimer to have coexistent pathologies such as intracytoplasmic inclusions of α-synuclein known as *Lewy bodies* or *Lewy neurites*. Lewy bodies are discussed in Chapters 52 and 83, as they represent pathologic hallmarks of Parkinson spectrum disease. They are present in as many as 35% of Alzheimer disease brains and even present in brains of persons with early-onset autosomal dominant Alzheimer disease, for example due to PSEN1 mutations. The reason for the common co-occurrence of these two degenerative pathologies is uncertain. Vascular lesions, in addition to amyloid angiopathy (discussed earlier), are another common coexistent pathology, occurring in 30% to 50% brains of persons with Alzheimer disease. These include microinfarcts, microhemorrhages, and lacunar or large-artery infarcts. It is likely that, when present, Lewy body pathology and vascular pathologies contribute to the phenotype in Alzheimer disease, leading to the term *mixed dementia*. However, most studies show that the burden of plaques and tangles is best correlated with the progressive dementia in Alzheimer disease.

CLINICAL FEATURES

The signs and symptoms of Alzheimer disease present and evolve variably, with the most common early signs being subjectively and objectively impaired memory (see Chapter 11). Overall, there is slow progressive cognitive impairment, eventually affecting many cognitive domains. When persons live long enough, this disease process results in complete incapacity, and ultimately death, from conditions associated with severe cognitive dysfunction. Course from first symptoms to death is often as long as 20 years, although typically, diagnosis is not made until the disease is well established on a molecular basis (evident through molecular changes in cerebrospinal fluid [CSF] or neuroimaging). Although it is likely that the disease progresses at different rates in different persons, it is unlikely that there is truly any "plateau" or temporary cessation of progression.

Cognitive impairment is the hallmark of Alzheimer disease. Memory impairment is the most common presenting symptom, present in over 90% of affected patients. The difficulty with memory is most prominent for newly acquired information, so-called short-term memory, whereas immediate, or "working" memory, is typically unaffected. "Long-term memory" for remote events is relatively unimpaired in the early phases of the illness but ultimately is also severely affected. As the disease progresses, impairments in language and visuospatial function

typically become more prominent (Fig. 50.2), as well as impairments in abstract reasoning and executive function or decision making. The increasing impairment in language and visuospatial function may be particularly evident on serial office testing (see Fig. 50.2). In some, language dysfunction may be the earliest subjective symptom or objective sign, and this syndrome of primary progressive aphasia (PPA), often of a "logopenic" variety (lvPPA), is often due to Alzheimer disease and is discussed in Chapter 51. In other persons, visuospatial impairment, which may progress to the extent of complete cortical blindness, may be the presenting symptom of Alzheimer disease, and this syndrome is termed *posterior cortical atrophy* (PCA).

Behavioral dysfunction is present at some point in the course of most patients with Alzheimer disease. The most common symptoms are depressive, with apathy and anhedonia, but irritability, agitation, insomnia, hypersomnia, decreased or increased food intake, dependency, disinhibition, repetitive or compulsive activities, all may occur. These symptoms in some cases likely relate to neuroanatomic changes but in other cases may represent reactive changes to cognitive incapacities. Psychotic symptoms including delusions and auditory or visual hallucinations may occur. Delusions frequently have paranoid ideation regarding theft or infidelity and also may involve misidentification of place or person; they are much more common than hallucinations. Indeed, the presence of detailed visual hallucinations, in the absence of concomitant primary visual system disease, should be a clue as to involvement of Lewy body dementia (see Chapter 52) as primary (diffuse Lewy body disease) or contributing (Lewy body variant of Alzheimer disease) dementia disorders.

Functional decline results from both cognitive and behavioral features. Loss of employment, financial difficulties, marital or other family dysfunction, driving difficulties, and difficulties learning new technologies such as automobile controls, home entertainment device remote controls, computers, or home security systems are frequent.

Examination of the patient with Alzheimer disease typically reveals only impairments in mental state. The remainder of the neurologic examination is usually normal, especially in the mild to moderate stages. In the later stages of the disease, extrapyramidal signs, including rigidity, bradykinesia, shuffling gait, and postural change, are not uncommon. These features may in some cases be solely a consequence of Alzheimer disease but in other cases may relate to concomitant involvement of Lewy body dementia (see Chapter 52). Primary motor and sensory functions are typically spared. Early symptoms of seizures or falling or early signs of cortical motor or sensory dysfunction, cranial or motor neuropathies, or cerebellar dysfunction, should all strongly raise the possibility of some other form of dementia (see Chapter 11).

DIAGNOSIS

The first organized criteria for clinical diagnosis of Alzheimer disease were established in 1984 by a joint effort of the National Institute of Neurological and Communicative Disorders and Stroke and the Alzheimer's Association (previously known as *the Alzheimer's Disease and Related Disorders Association*). These criteria, the NINCDS–ADRDA criteria, consisted of three levels of clinical certainty: definite, reserved only for autopsy-confirmed cases, probable, and possible. The criteria included a history of progressive deterioration in cognitive ability, not explicable by other known disorders, involving memory and at least one other cognitive domain, and causing some significant disturbance of functioning in the patient. These criteria were endorsed by the American Academy

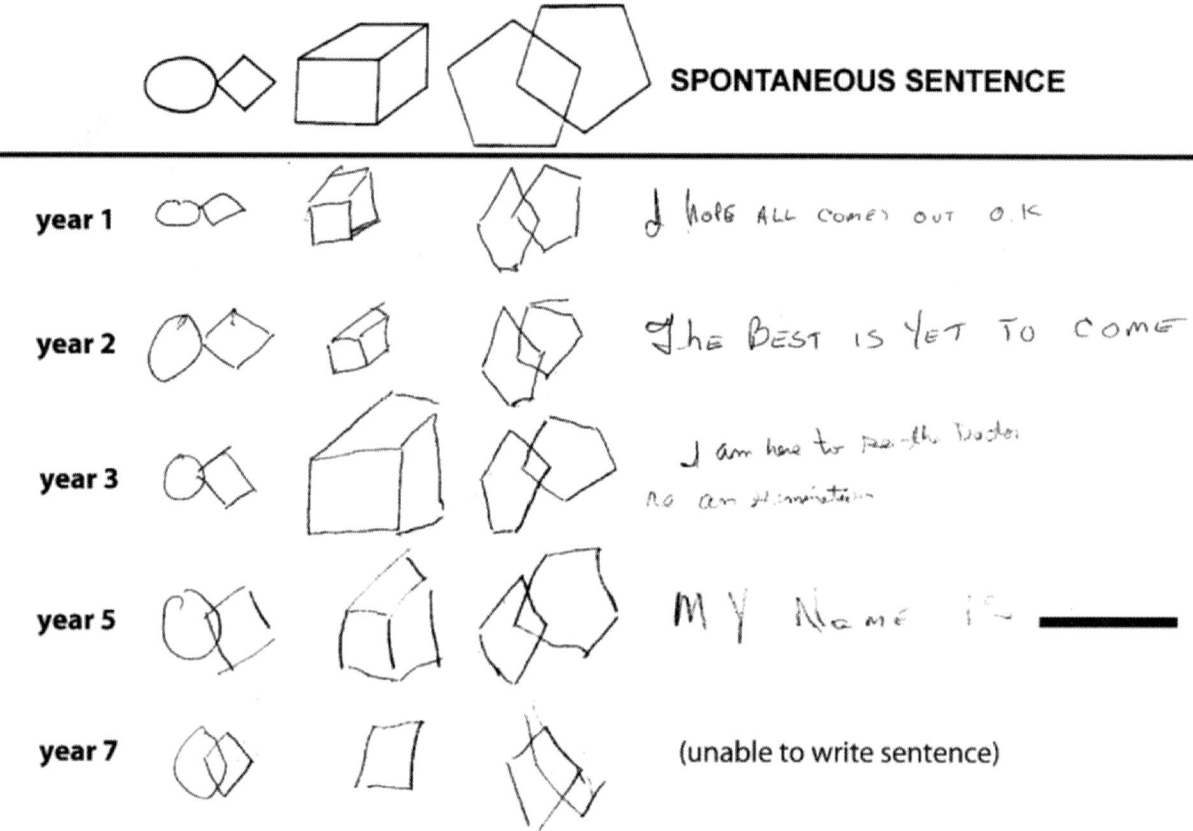

FIGURE 50.2 Mental status testing in a patient with memory problems, for whom a diagnosis of Alzheimer disease was made in year 1. Over a 7-year period, the drawings show increasing impairment in constructional praxis—the ability to copy figures. *Top row* shows example provided to the patient, and subsequent rows are the patient's performance initially and in succeeding years. The patient was also asked each visit to write a full sentence of his or her choice. There is increasing difficulty with both penmanship and content.

of Neurology in 2001, with the additional provision of preferred laboratory tests, such as computed tomography (CT) or MRI, and optional laboratory tests, such as serologic testing for syphilis. However, over time, it became clear that these criteria were inadequate due to the requirements for memory involvement, functional disturbance, and the lack of reference to more modern and specific biologic imaging and fluid marker tests, referred to in the following text. New sets of criteria have been developed by consensus sponsored by the National Institute on Aging and the Alzheimer's Association, and these NIA-AA criteria provide for preclinical diagnosis, early symptomatic diagnosis without functional impairment (see Chapter 49), and presymptomatic diagnosis.

DIAGNOSTIC TESTING

Neuropsychological testing is useful in establishing the extent of cognitive impairment in terms of domains affected and in terms of degree of affectation compared to persons of comparable age, sex, and education (normative results). Examination of test results in comparison to persons of a similar group allows for better assessment than results on an absolute basis because of the general wide variation in performance on these tests, which relate in large part to education (see Chapter 30). Such testing can also be very useful in following progression of disease. Routine laboratory examinations of blood, urine, and CSF are unremarkable in Alzheimer disease. Electroencephalography and other neurophysiologic measures are

nonspecific, revealing background rhythm slowing or other changes not diagnostic of any particular brain condition. Likewise, routine imaging by CT or MRI does not reveal gross structural abnormalities other than atrophy, particularly early in the course of the disease. Later in the disease, significant cortical and subcortical atrophy, although not entirely specific, is typically observed (Fig. 50.3). Most importantly, it has become clear that both CSF and functional brain imaging can show relatively sensitive and specific markers of Alzheimer disease (see Chapter 11, see the following text, and Fig. 50.4) and can be of use in the differential diagnosis of this disorder. Genetic tests are generally not recommended for diagnosis of Alzheimer disease. However, selected testing may be useful in the diagnosis in families with the rare early-onset autosomal dominant forms of Alzheimer disease. For sporadic or familial late-onset Alzheimer disease (LOAD), the $\varepsilon4$ polymorphism of the apolipoprotein E (*APOE*) gene is associated with a higher risk of the disease, but because at least one-third of persons with Alzheimer have no $\varepsilon4$ alleles, and because some persons with even two $\varepsilon4$ alleles are symptom free even in their 10th decade of life, the test does not provide sufficient sensitivity or specificity to be used for diagnosis and is not recommended.

Measurements of CSF proteins (see Chapter 31) are established to be of use in the diagnosis of Alzheimer disease. Typically in Alzheimer disease, Aβ42 is decreased in concentration, perhaps related in part to deposition of amyloid in the brain. Total tau

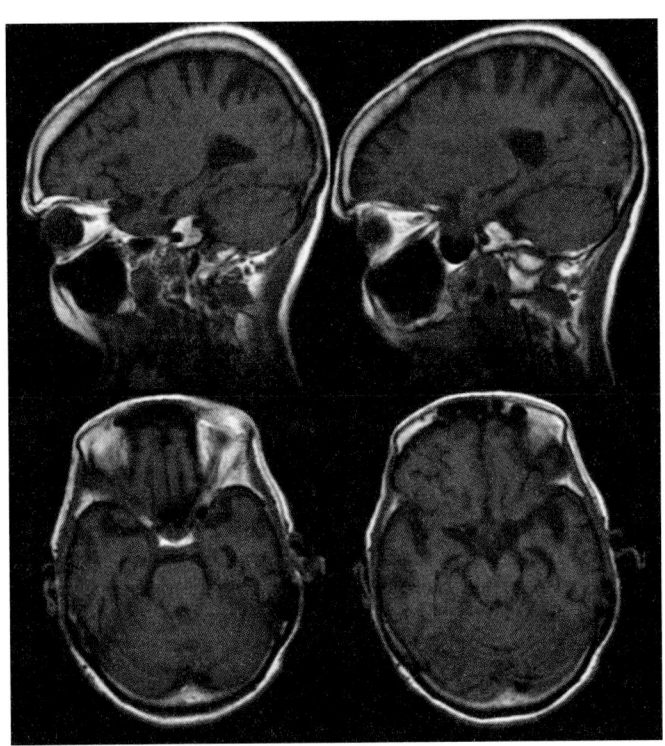
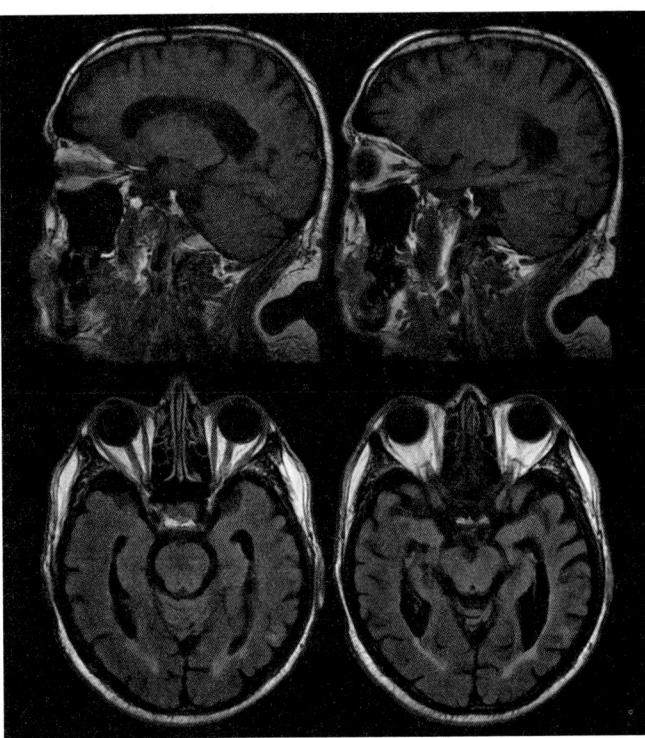

FIGURE 50.3 MRI T1-weighted structural images from two patients (**A** and **B**) with Alzheimer disease, including in each patient selected sagittal (*top rows*) and axial (*bottom rows*) images. **A** shows a pattern of atrophy most prominent in parietal regions. **B** shows a pattern of atrophy more prominent in temporal regions.

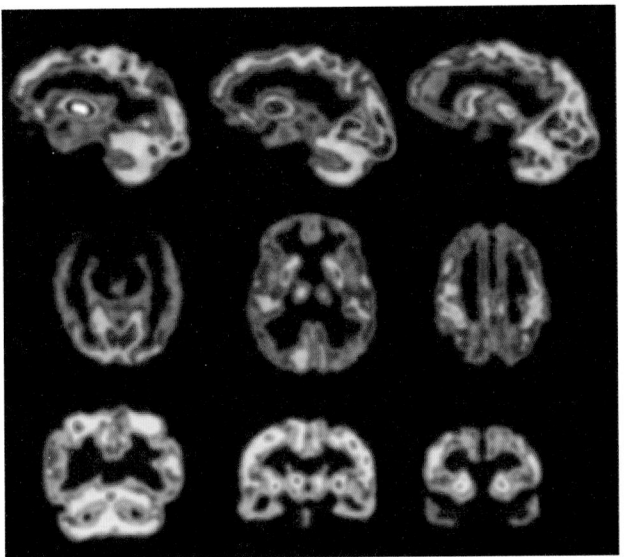
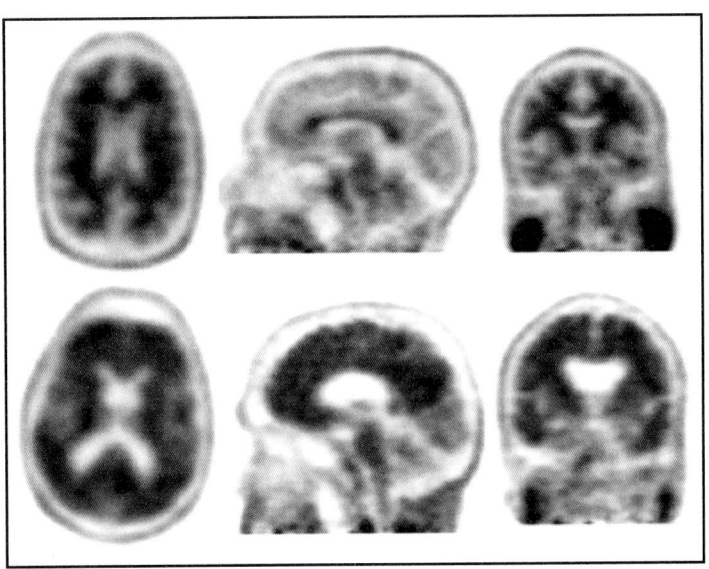

FIGURE 50.4 **A** shows images from a single patient who underwent an ^{18}F-fluorodeoxyglucose PET scan. *Top row* shows sagittal sections, *middle row* axial sections, and *bottom row* coronal sections. The images demonstrate decreased brain metabolic activity in bilateral parietal, temporal, and to a lesser extent frontal regions. Note that in this color coding scheme, "cooler" colors such as green and blue are lower activity, and "hotter" colors such as yellow, red, and white are higher activity. **B** shows ^{18}F-florbetapir PET scan in two individuals, with a black and white image display scheme, in which blacker represents higher uptake of florbetapir. Each row shows an example of an axial, sagittal, and coronal brain imaging slice. The *top row* is of a normal control individual who shows cerebral uptake of the radioligand only in the white matter. The *bottom* row shows the images of patient with Alzheimer disease, who shows extensive gray matter uptake of the radioligand throughout cerebral cortex including frontal, temporal, and parietal regions, and basal ganglia.

protein is typically elevated, relating presumably to neurodegeneration and loss of axonal integrity. Phosphorylated tau (phospho-tau) is also elevated and more specific for Alzheimer disease because in this disorder, the tau protein is abnormally phosphorylated. Combined measures of the concentrations of these three biomarkers results in sensitivity and specificity each in the range of 90%. Of note, it is clear that changes in $A\beta42$, tau, and phosphorylated tau can precede clinical symptoms and diagnosis of disease by up to 15 years. Blood analytes in serum or plasma including $A\beta40$, $A\beta42$, and proteomic and lipodomic panels have not yet proven to be of use in the diagnosis of Alzheimer disease.

Brain imaging has become important in diagnosis of Alzheimer disease, can aid in early detection of disease, and may be helpful in research studies following treatment of the disease. Brain imaging includes "structural" imaging, "functional" imaging, and "molecular" imaging. Structural imaging techniques including CT and MRI are used to exclude other causes of dementia, such as tumors or strokes. However, in Alzheimer disease, structural imaging typically reveals dilatation of the lateral ventricles and widening of the cortical sulci, particularly in temporal and parietal regions (see Fig. 50.3). Such cortical atrophy is not specific for Alzheimer disease, as it can be seen in some older individuals who function normally by clinical and neuropsychological testing. During the last decade, MRI approaches have been developed to measure precise volumetric changes in the brain, and these can be useful in differentiating Alzheimer disease from frontotemporal dementia and have been used in monitoring therapies with investigational drugs (see Chapter 21). Functional brain imaging techniques include single-photon emission computed tomography (SPECT), positron emission tomography (PET), and functional magnetic resonance imaging (fMRI) (see Chapters 21 and 22). Although using different technologies, functional imaging techniques hold in common a sensitivity to brain metabolism—either glucose uptake in the case of ^{18}F-fluorodeoxyglucose-PET or the closely correlated blood flow measures examined by ^{99}mTc hexamethyl-propylene-aminoxime (HMPAO)-SPECT or fMRI. Studies using PET or SPECT reveal a characteristic pattern of hypometabolism and hypoperfusion in the mesial temporal and posterior parietal lobes, with preservation of function of the deep gray nuclei and the primary sensory and motor cortices (see Fig. 50.4A). With the superior spatial resolution afforded by fMRI, studies have begun to map patterns of dysfunction in smaller brain subregions of the medial temporal lobe, the general area where the disease is thought to begin. Within the hippocampal formation, high-resolution fMRI has shown that, in contrast to the early stages of Alzheimer disease that target the entorhinal cortex, normal aging involves the dentate gyrus, a neighboring hippocampal subregion. Finally, the most recent development in brain imaging is being able to detect the molecular features of Alzheimer disease: amyloid-containing plaques and neurofibrillary tangles. The first such molecular imaging reagent for detecting neuritic plaques in vivo was "Pittsburgh compound B" (PIB, whose chemical formulation is ^{11}C-6-OH-benzothazole-1), but there are currently three approved ^{18}F-labeled reagents: florbetapir, florbetaben, and flutemetamol, all of which have been shown through clinical and autopsy studies to show cortical binding of radioligand in Alzheimer disease (see Fig. 50.4B). The absence of cortical binding is inconsistent with Alzheimer disease. However, as might be expected for a disease that starts with small amounts of asymptomatic $A\beta42$ deposition, a substantial fraction of clinically normal elders (e.g., about 25% of those older than age 65 years, with increasing proportions in older age groups) do have some binding, consistent with the possibility that they may later develop Alzheimer disease. New investigational radioligands for aggregated tau, as well as SPECT and PET radiopharmaceutical reagents to examine dopaminergic systems, promise a greater armamentarium of advanced molecular imaging biomarkers that may assist in early diagnosis and assessment of disease.

TREATMENT

Therapies for Alzheimer disease are currently symptomatic, as there are no proven disease-modifying treatments. Nonspecific treatments for secondary symptoms of Alzheimer disease can be useful. These include treatment of depressive symptomatology with antidepressants including selective serotonin reuptake inhibitors. Likewise, treatment of psychotic symptoms such delusions and hallucinations, as well as agitation and irritability can be managed with judicious use of antipsychotic medications. Side effects of these medications can be impairing, including drug-induced parkinsonism. Neuroleptics have, in some studies but not others, been associated with small increases in mortality from various causes. Anxiolytics such as benzodiazepines may also be used but are generally avoided due to adverse effects on cognition. Despite potential risks, pharmacologic treatment of behavioral symptoms with neuroleptics can be of major help to patients and their caregivers.

There are five disease-specific treatments available for Alzheimer at this time. These five medications are symptomatic and do not appear to modify disease course but have received U.S. Food and Drug Administration (FDA) approval for specific treatment of the disease (Table 50.3) on the basis of level 1 randomized

TABLE 50.3	Treatments of Alzheimer Disease	
Medication	Dosages	Presumed Mechanism
Tacrine hydrochloride	40–160 mg/day oral	Cholinesterase inhibition
Donepezil hydrochloride	5–10 mg/day PR or 23 mg/day ER oral	Cholinesterase inhibition
Galantamine hydrobromide	8–24 mg/day PR or ER oral	Cholinesterase inhibition
Rivastigmine tartrate	3–12 mg/day oral or 4.5–13.3 mg/day transdermal	Cholinesterase inhibition
Memantine hydrochloride	5–20 mg/day PR or 7–28 mg/day ER oral	NMDA receptor inhibition

List of the five medications approved by the U.S. Food and Drug Administration (FDA) specifically for Alzheimer disease. Tacrine is rarely used due to dosing schedule and required laboratory monitoring. Donepezil and rivastigmine are labeled for use in mild, moderate, and severe disease; galantamine is labeled for use in mild and moderate disease; memantine is labeled for use only in moderate and severe disease.

ER, extended release; PR, prompt release; NMDA, *N*-methyl-D-aspartate.

placebo-controlled trials. Four of these are cholinesterase inhibitors, which effectively increase synaptic levels of brain acetylcholine through inhibition of synaptic acetylcholinesterase, which normally hydrolyzes acetylcholine released from the presynaptic neuron into the synaptic cleft. Tacrine was the first such drug [**Level 1**],[1] but it is no longer in common use due to four times daily dosing and hepatotoxicity. The three cholinesterase inhibitors currently in common use are donepezil [**Level 1**],[2–4] rivastigmine [**Level 1**],[5] and galantamine [**Level 1**].[6] The evidence is that these three have similar mild efficacy in improving cognition and may also cause small improvements in behavior and function in patients with mild, moderate, or severe Alzheimer disease (see Level 1 Evidence in the following section). One other drug, memantine, has been approved for treatment only of moderate to severe Alzheimer disease, for which there is level 1 evidence [**Level 1**],[7,8] whereas such evidence is lacking for mild disease. Memantine is an activity-dependent N-methyl-D-aspartate receptor antagonist and provides an independent modest benefit in cognition, behavior, and function in persons with moderate to severe disease. This benefit occurs in both settings of monotherapy [**Level 1**][7] and concomitant therapy with cholinesterase inhibitors [**Level 1**][8] in such patients.

Disease-modifying treatments are not yet available. However, the increasing understanding of Alzheimer disease as a disorder characterized by accumulation of β-amyloid, and tau aggregates has given rise to a significant number of experimental drugs that have been studied or are currently under investigation. Current approaches to potentially ameliorating the course of Alzheimer disease include monoclonal antibodies or active immunizations designed to clear amyloid protein from the brain, β-secretase inhibitors designed to decrease intracerebral generation of β-amyloid, and other therapies proposed to deter tau aggregation or neuronal dysfunction.

LEVEL 1 EVIDENCE

1. Davis KL, Thal LJ, Gamzu ER, et al. A double-blind, placebo-controlled multicenter study of tacrine for Alzheimer's disease. The Tacrine Collaborative Study Group. *N Engl J Med.* 1992;327:1253–1259.
2. Rogers SL, Friedhoff LT. The efficacy and safety of donepezil in patients with Alzheimer's disease: results of a US Multicentre, Randomized, Double-Blind, Placebo-Controlled Trial. The Donepezil Study Group. *Dementia.* 1996;7:293–303.
3. Rogers SL, Doody RS, Mohs RC, et al. Donepezil improves cognition and global function in Alzheimer disease: a 15-week, double-blind, placebo-controlled study. Donepezil Study Group. *Arch Intern Med.* 1998;158:1021–1031.
4. Winblad B, Engedal K, Soininen H, et al; Donepezil Nordic Study Group. A 1-year, randomized, placebo-controlled study of donepezil in patients with mild to moderate AD. *Neurology.* 2001;57:489–495.
5. Rösler M, Anand R, Cicin-Sain A, et al. Efficacy and safety of rivastigmine in patients with Alzheimer's disease: international randomised controlled trial. *BMJ.* 1999;318:633–638.
6. Wilkinson D, Murray J. Galantamine: a randomized, double-blind, dose comparison in patients with Alzheimer's disease. *Int J Geriatr Psychiatry.* 2001;16:852–857.
7. Reisberg B, Doody R, Stöffler A, et al; Memantine Study Group. Memantine in moderate-to-severe Alzheimer's disease. *N Engl J Med.* 2003;348:1333–1341.
8. Tariot PN, Farlow MR, Grossberg GT, et al; Memantine Study Group. Memantine treatment in patients with moderate to severe Alzheimer disease already receiving donepezil: a randomized controlled trial. *JAMA.* 2004;291:317–324.

SUGGESTED READINGS

Albert MS, DeKosky ST, Dickson D, et al. The diagnosis of mild cognitive impairment due to Alzheimer's disease: recommendations from the National Institute on Aging-Alzheimer's Association workgroups on diagnostic guidelines for Alzheimer's disease. *Alzheimers Dement.* 2011;7:270–279.
Bertram L, Tanzi RE. The genetics of Alzheimer's disease. *Prog Mol Biol Transl Sci.* 2012;107:79–100.
Blennow K, Zetterberg H. The application of cerebrospinal fluid biomarkers in early diagnosis of Alzheimer disease. *Med Clin North Am.* 2013;97:369–376.
Carrillo MC, Rowe CC, Szoeke C, et al; NIA/Alzheimer Association and International Working Group. Research and standardization in Alzheimer's trials: reaching international consensus. *Alzheimers Dement.* 2013;9:160–168.
Chouraki V, Seshadri S. Genetics of Alzheimer's disease. *Adv Genet.* 2014;87:245–294.
Farina N, Isaac MG, Clark AR, et al. Vitamin E for Alzheimer's dementia and mild cognitive impairment. *Cochrane Database Syst Rev.* 2012;11:CD002854.
Frisoni GB, Bocchetta M, Chételat G, et al. Imaging markers for Alzheimer disease: which vs how. *Neurology.* 2013;81:487–500.
Hardy J, Bogdanovic N, Winblad B, et al. Pathways to Alzheimer's disease. *J Intern Med.* 2014;275:296–303.
Henriksen K, O'Bryant SE, Hampel H, et al; Blood-Based Biomarker Interest Group. The future of blood-based biomarkers for Alzheimer's disease. *Alzheimers Dement.* 2014;10:115–1131.
Hill DL, Schwarz AJ, Isaac M, et al. Coalition Against Major Diseases/European Medicines Agency biomarker qualification of hippocampal volume for enrichment of clinical trials in predementia stages of Alzheimer's disease. *Alzheimers Dement.* 2014;10:421–429.
Honig LS. Translational research in neurology: dementia. *Arch Neurol.* 2012;69:969–977.
Honig LS, Boyd CD. Treatment of Alzheimer's disease: current management and experimental therapeutics. *Curr Transl Geriatr Exp Gerontol Rep.* 2013;2:174–181.
Hyman BT, Phelps CH, Beach TG, et al. National Institute on Aging-Alzheimer's Association guidelines for the neuropathologic assessment of Alzheimer's disease. *Alzheimers Dement.* 2012;8:1–13.
Jack CR Jr, Barrio JR, Kepe V. Cerebral amyloid PET imaging in Alzheimer's disease. *Acta Neuropathol.* 2013;126:643–657.
Jack CR Jr, Holtzman DM. Biomarker modeling of Alzheimer's disease. *Neuron.* 2013;80:1347–1358.
Jonsson T, Atwal JK, Steinberg S, et al. A mutation in APP protects against Alzheimer's disease and age-related cognitive decline. *Nature.* 2012;488:96–99.
Kantarci K. Molecular imaging of Alzheimer disease pathology. *AJNR Am J Neuroradiol.* 2014;35:S12–S17.
Karch CM, Cruchaga C, Goate AM. Alzheimer's disease genetics: from the bench to the clinic. *Neuron.* 2014;83:11–26.
Klunk WE. Amyloid imaging as a biomarker for cerebral β-amyloidosis and risk prediction for Alzheimer dementia. *Neurobiol Aging.* 2011;32(suppl 1):S20–S36.
Koyama A, Okereke OI, Yang T, et al. Plasma amyloid-β as a predictor of dementia and cognitive decline: a systematic review and meta-analysis. *Arch Neurol.* 2012;69:824–831.
Lambert JC, Ibrahim-Verbaas CA, Harold D, et al. Meta-analysis of 74,046 individuals identifies 11 new susceptibility loci for Alzheimer's disease. *Nat Genet.* 2013;45:1452–1458.
Lannfelt L, Relkin NR, Siemers ER. Amyloid-β-directed immunotherapy for Alzheimer's disease. *J Intern Med.* 2014;275:284–295.
Lyketsos CG, Carrillo MC, Ryan JM, et al. Neuropsychiatric symptoms in Alzheimer's disease. *Alzheimers Dement.* 2011;7:532–539.
Mayeux R, Schupf N. Blood-based biomarkers for Alzheimer's disease: plasma Aβ40 and Aβ42, and genetic variants. *Neurobiol Aging.* 2011;32(suppl 1):S10–S19.

Mayeux R, Stern Y. Epidemiology of Alzheimer disease. *Cold Spring Harb Perspect Med.* 2012;2:a006239.

McKhann G, Drachman D, Folstein M, et al. Clinical diagnosis of Alzheimer's disease: report of the NINCDS-ADRDA Work Group under the auspices of Department of Health and Human Services Task Force on Alzheimer's Disease. *Neurology.* 1984;34:939–944.

McKhann GM, Knopman DS, Chertkow H, et al. The diagnosis of dementia due to Alzheimer's disease: recommendations from the National Institute on Aging-Alzheimer's Association workgroups on diagnostic guidelines for Alzheimer's disease. *Alzheimers Dement.* 2011;7:263–269.

Morris JC, Blennow K, Froelich L, et al. Harmonized diagnostic criteria for Alzheimer's disease: recommendations. *J Intern Med.* 2014;275:204–213.

Müller U, Winter P, Graeber MB. A presenilin 1 mutation in the first case of Alzheimer's disease. *Lancet Neurol.* 2013;12:129–130.

Nelson PT, Alafuzoff I, Bigio EH, et al. Correlation of Alzheimer disease neuropathologic changes with cognitive status: a review of the literature. *J Neuropathol Exp Neurol.* 2012;71:362–381.

Reitz C, Mayeux R. Alzheimer disease: epidemiology, diagnostic criteria, risk factors and biomarkers. *Biochem Pharmacol.* 2014;88:640–651.

Ryman DC, Acosta-Baena N, Aisen PS, et al; Dominantly Inherited Alzheimer Network. Symptom onset in autosomal dominant Alzheimer disease: a systematic review and meta-analysis. *Neurology.* 2014;83:253–260.

Schellenberg GD, Montine TJ. The genetics and neuropathology of Alzheimer's disease. *Acta Neuropathol.* 2012;124:305–323.

Schneider LS, Mangialasche F, Andreasen N, et al. Clinical trials and late-stage drug development for Alzheimer's disease: an appraisal from 1984 to 2014. *J Intern Med.* 2014;275:251–283.

Small SA. Imaging Alzheimer's disease. *Curr Neurol Neurosci Rep.* 2003;3:385–392.

Sperling RA, Aisen PS, Beckett LA, et al. Toward defining the preclinical stages of Alzheimer's disease: recommendations from the National Institute on Aging-Alzheimer's Association workgroups on diagnostic guidelines for Alzheimer's disease. *Alzheimers Dement.* 2011;7:280–292.

Steinerman JR, Honig LS. Laboratory biomarkers in Alzheimer disease. *Curr Neurol Neurosci Reports.* 2007;7:381–387.

Vellas B, Carrillo MC, Sampaio C, et al; EU/US/CTAD Task Force Members. Designing drug trials for Alzheimer's disease: what we have learned from the release of the phase III antibody trials: a report from the EU/US/CTAD Task Force. *Alzheimers Dement.* 2013;9:438–444.

Verghese PB, Castellano JM, Holtzman DM. Apolipoprotein E in Alzheimer's disease and other neurological disorders. *Lancet Neurol.* 2011;10:241–252.

Weintraub S, Wicklund AH, Salmon DP. The neuropsychological profile of Alzheimer disease. *Cold Spring Harb Perspect Med.* 2012;2:a006171.

Wisniewski T, Goñi F. Immunotherapy for Alzheimer's disease. *Biochem Pharmacol.* 2014;88:499–507.

Frontotemporal Dementia 51

Edward D. Huey and Stephanie Cosentino

INTRODUCTION

Frontotemporal dementia (FTD) is the most common clinical presentation of frontotemporal lobar degeneration (FTLD). Two main FTD phenotypes are seen. One form is primarily a disorder of behavior and executive function (bvFTD), and the second, less frequent form is primarily a disorder of language, termed *primary progressive aphasia* (PPA) and defined by predominant language impairment for at least 2 years. Classifications of PPA include nonfluent/agrammatic (naPPA), semantic variant (svPPA), and logopenic variant (lvPPA). Combinations of behavioral and language symptoms that do not fit clearly into defined clinical subtypes reflect overlapping distributions of neuropathology in prefrontal and anterior temporal regions and can be present at disease onset but typically become more frequent with advancing disease severity.

EPIDEMIOLOGY

Overall, FTD is the fourth most common dementia (behind Alzheimer disease [AD], vascular dementia, and dementia with Lewy bodies), affecting 1% to 16% of all people with dementia; FTD is the most common cause of dementia prior to age 60 years and approaches the prevalence of AD prior to age 65 years. Approximately 60% of cases occur in individuals aged 45 to 64 years. Although we do not yet have definitive epidemiologic studies, the estimated point prevalence of FTD within this age range, based on studies primarily including Caucasians in North America and Europe, is 15 to 22/100,000. Most studies implicate an equal distribution by gender.

PATHOBIOLOGY

At autopsy, gross frontal and temporal lobe atrophy is usually evident, with histopathology revealing neuronal loss and gliosis affecting superficial cortical lamina of these same cortical regions, along with absence of the typical pathologic findings of AD. FTLD encompasses several different pathologies, including neuronal inclusions containing TAR DNA binding protein (TDP-43), tau isoforms, and fused in sarcoma (FUS) protein. Some patients have evidence of amyotrophic lateral sclerosis (ALS). As demonstrated in Figure 51.1, several gene mutations associated with FTD result in specific neuropathologies and sometimes specific clinical presentations. Therefore, for some patients, the clinician can infer the neuropathology based on some (e.g., FTD-ALS), but not other (e.g., behavioral variant FTD), clinical presentations.

Only fewer than half of all FTD patients will demonstrate prominent tau aggregates, whereas approximately half will stain for ubiquitin, a nonspecific marker of cell death, although the breakdown of pathologies across subtypes differs (Fig. 51.2). A major FTLD subtype associated with tau aggregates is Pick disease. First described by Alois Alzheimer, Pick disease is characterized by argyrophilic cytoplasmic tau inclusions (Pick bodies) and swollen neurons (Pick cells). Ubiquitin-positive cases of FTLD were recently discovered to be characterized by inclusions composed

FIGURE 51.1 Association between pathologic, genetic, and clinical variants of FTD. CBD, corticobasal degeneration; PSP, progressive supranuclear palsy.

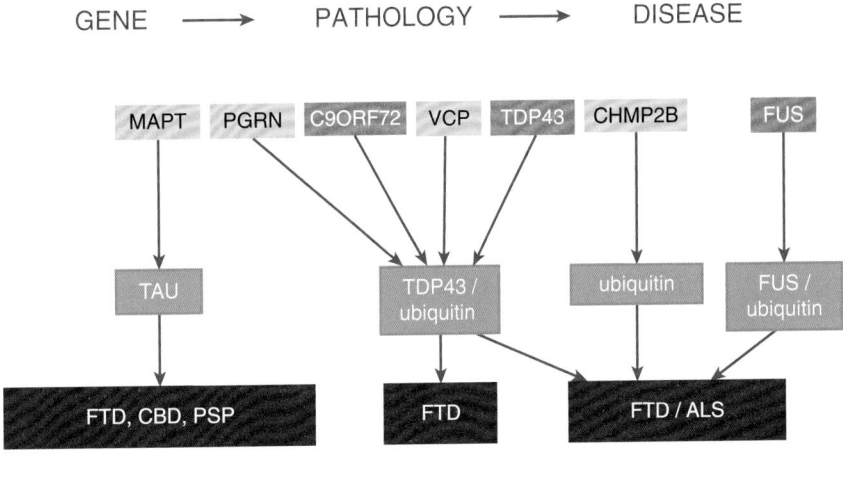

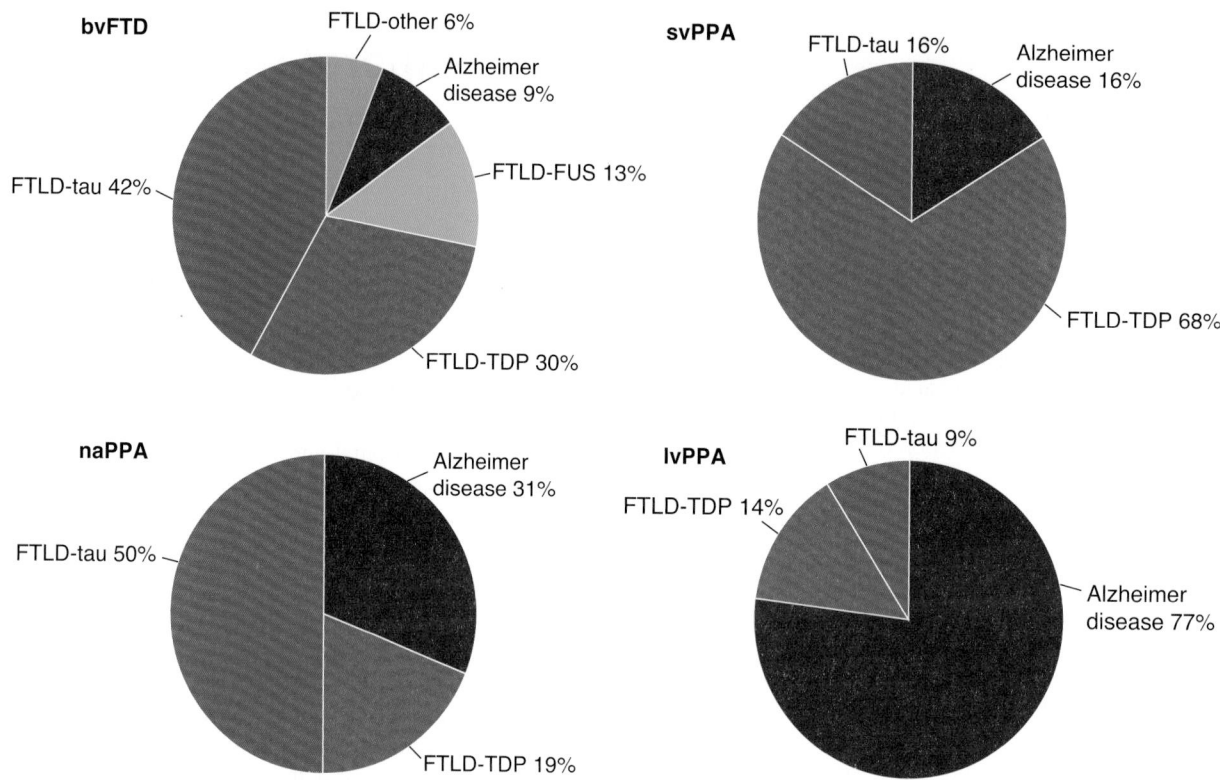

FIGURE 51.2 Distribution of neuropathology across clinical subtypes of FTD. (Permission to reproduce this figure granted by Dr. Glenda Halliday, University of New South Wales, Sydney, Australia. Chare L, Hodges JR, Leyton CE, et al. New criteria for frontotemporal dementia syndromes: clinical and pathological diagnostic implications. *J Neurol Neurosurg Psychiatry*. 2014;85[5]:865–870.)

of aggregates of TDP-43 and more rarely FUS. The clinical presentation of FTD-ALS is associated with TDP-43 positive FTLD (see Fig. 51.1).

GENETICS

An estimated 40% of cases of FTLD are familial, but only 10% follow a clear autosomal dominant pattern. Mutations in three genes account for the great majority of cases of FTD with an identified genetic cause (see Fig. 51.1). The most common genetic cause of both FTD and ALS appears to be the recently identified hexanucleotide repeat expansion in *C9ORF72* on chromosome 9. This expansion accounts for approximately 34% of familial ALS, 6% of sporadic ALS, 26% of familial FTD (with or without ALS), and 5% of sporadic FTD. The discovery of *C9ORF72* links FTD and ALS with several other neurologic disorders involving repeat expansions including Huntington disease, fragile X syndrome, myotonic dystrophy, and some of the spinocerebellar ataxias. The phenotype associated with *C9ORF72* expansions can be FTD, ALS, or combined FTD-ALS.

The two other known major genetic causes of FTD are mutations in the *MAPT* (tau) and *GRN* genes. Tau binds to microtubules, and it exists in isoforms of three and four microtubule-binding domains generated by alternate splicing of exon 10. Deposition of three-repeat tau is associated with Pick disease, whereas four-repeat tau is associated with CBD and PSP. *GRN* is an oncogene that codes for the protein granulin, which is a growth factor involved in wound healing. Reduced levels of granulin are associated with FTD, but elevated levels of granulin are associated with certain tumors including teratomas and breast, esophageal, and liver cancers.

This is similar to another FTD/oncogene, FUS. Rare other genetic causes of FTD include mutations in valosin-containing protein, *TDP-43*, and *CHMP2B*. Clinical genetic testing can be considered with the guidance of a genetic counselor. Until recently, it was generally thought that an FTD patient should have a first-degree relative with FTD or a related illness to be offered clinical genetic testing. However, genetic testing of cases of FTD-ALS without a family history for *C9ORF72* should be considered. Clinical presentation and pathology in family members can guide genetic testing and whether to test only for known mutations or to sequence the gene.

CLINICAL MANIFESTATIONS

BEHAVIORAL VARIANT

The ventral prefrontal cortex is usually involved in bvFTD and appears to play an important role in social cognition and behavior. Alteration in personality and behavior, reflecting impaired judgment of social norms, is a hallmark feature of bvFTD. Patients display a loss of social graces, generally characterized by decreased empathy, diminished reactions to emotional events, excessive familiarity with strangers or acquaintances, inappropriate jocularity, and a general lack of self-consciousness. Distractibility, impulsivity, and apathy are also components of bvFTD. Such symptoms may be subtle at onset. The apathetic and amotivational aspect of bvFTD may initially be mistaken for depressed mood; however, it is relatively rare for patients with bvFTD to endorse feelings of sadness or hopelessness. Patients may also present with stereotyped behaviors, involving movement, language, or more complex behaviors. Increased appetite and hyperphagia, particularly for sweets, and hyperorality can also occur. Patients with bvFTD frequently demonstrate reduced awareness of or lack of concern for their symptoms.

PRIMARY PROGRESSIVE APHASIA

The three PPA phenotypes reflect disruption to different components of the language network, with naPPA reflecting left frontal perisylvian involvement, svPPA reflecting anterior temporal involvement, and lvPPA associated with left posterior temporoparietal compromise. naPPA patients generally demonstrate reduced speech output that is both effortful and dysgrammatic. Such symptoms may be preceded by anomia, subtle deficits in sentence construction, as well as apraxia of speech (i.e., impaired motor planning and sequencing of the movements required for correct speech production). Comprehension is generally preserved, although patients may have difficulty decoding syntactically complex phrases. In contrast, svPPA is a fluent aphasia, with normal prosody and tempo, but patients have progressive loss of semantic knowledge (i.e., understanding and recognizing the meaning of words and/or objects). Anomia and single-word comprehension deficits are the core diagnostic criteria. Surface dyslexia, the phonologic decoding or "regularization" of irregularly spelled words (e.g., *sue* for *sew*), is also a feature of svPPA, reflecting loss of item-specific knowledge. Patients with svPPA are also described to present with fixations on and/or frequent questions about the meaning of a word (e.g., "What is a comb?"). Behavioral changes are also typical of svPPA, including obsessive-compulsiveness and socioemotional changes characterized by indifference and lack of warmth particularly with differential right hemisphere involvement. There is evidence that the behavioral syndrome associated with svPPA overlaps with, but differs in some ways from, the behavioral symptoms in bvFTD. Additional signs of compromise to right anterior temporal regions include prosopagnosia (inability to recognize faces) and loss of semantic knowledge for other visual stimuli. Finally, lvPPA is characterized by slow spontaneous speech, with frequent word finding pauses and difficulty naming, phonologic paraphasias (i.e., use of an incorrect word that is phonologically related to the intended word), as well as sentence repetition errors. Repetition errors are generally seen for sentences of increasing length and complexity rather than for single words or simple phrases and appear to reflect limited auditory short-term memory capacity. lvPPA is most often associated with AD pathology but reflects FTD pathology in approximately one-third of cases.

In addition to the primary behavioral and language phenotypes described earlier, patients with FTD may present with or develop various movement abnormalities. Approximately 15% of patients with bvFTD exhibit signs of motor neuron disease consistent with ALS, whereas 20% to 30% of all patients with FTD display parkinsonism at some point. There are also an increasing number of reports of patients who present with psychosis, most frequently in the case of *C9ORF72* or *GRN* mutations.

DIAGNOSIS

Rapidly developing knowledge regarding the phenotypes associated with FTLD has resulted in recent revisions to the diagnostic criteria in 2011. The new bvFTD criteria allow for heterogeneous presentation of disease as well as levels of diagnostic certainty (i.e., possible, probable, definite), whereas the new PPA criteria include lvPPA as a third variant. In one neuropathologic case series, addition of the lvPPA diagnostic category resulted in reclassification of approximately half of cases that had been previously diagnosed as naPPA and improved separation of FTD versus AD pathology.

The diagnostic probability of FTD is heightened in those younger than 65 years and in those with an autosomal dominant pattern of inheritance. The diagnostic workup for FTD begins with cognitive and behavioral assessment. Formal neuropsychological testing can identify subtle language or executive dysfunction that aid in the differential diagnosis of FTD from other dementias as well as in the characterization of the FTD phenotype. Regarding the cognitive profile of FTD versus AD, a common differential diagnosis, visuospatial functions are generally well preserved in FTD. Moreover, although the retrieval of information from memory may be equally impaired in both groups, it is generally the case that the ability to store new information in long-term memory is preserved in FTD as compared to AD. Indeed, the integrity of memory storage, measured through recognition testing and proportion of information retained after a delay, has traditionally served as a critical variable for differentiating AD from FTD. However, it is increasingly recognized that poor performance on these metrics may be more common in FTD than initially appreciated. New diagnostic criteria for bvFTD (2011) allow for inclusion of individuals with atypical cognitive presentations such as those with severe amnesia or spatial disorientation. Finally, it is possible that objectively measured cognition can be within normal limits in patients with bvFTD despite marked behavioral changes in everyday life, or alternatively, performance may be globally impaired secondary to apathy, inattention, or automatic responding.

Magnetic resonance imaging (MRI) in FTD often reveals cortical volume loss in the frontal and anterior temporal lobes with relative sparing of posterior parietal and occipital cortices (Figs. 51.3 and 51.4). Functional neuroimaging (18-fluoro-deoxy-glucose positron emission tomography [FDG-PET] or technetium-99m hexamethylpropyleneamine oxime single-photon emission computed tomography [HMPAO-SPECT]) often reveals frontotemporal hypometabolism. naPPA is associated with left-sided frontal perisylvian involvement and svPPA with anterior temporal involvement. Cerebrospinal fluid (CSF) findings include normal cell counts and protein. CSF tau and Aβ42 levels have not demonstrated sufficiently

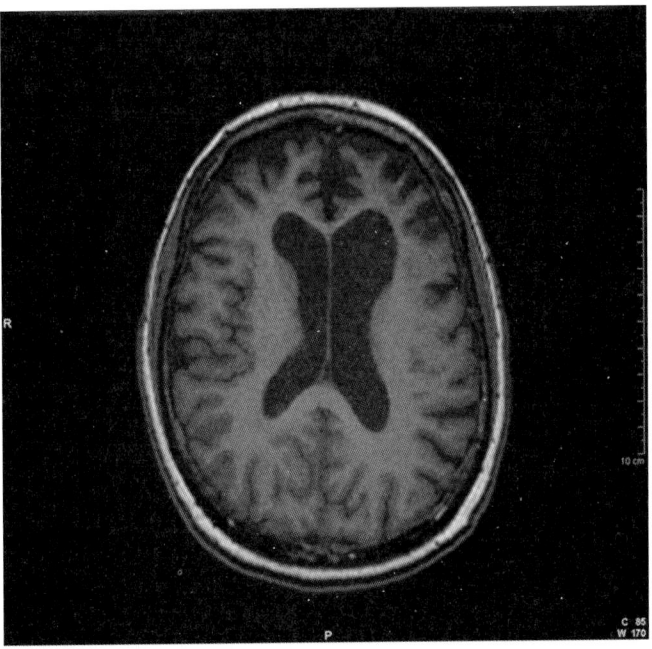

FIGURE 51.3 MRI demonstrating frontal atrophy in a patient with behavioral variant FTD.

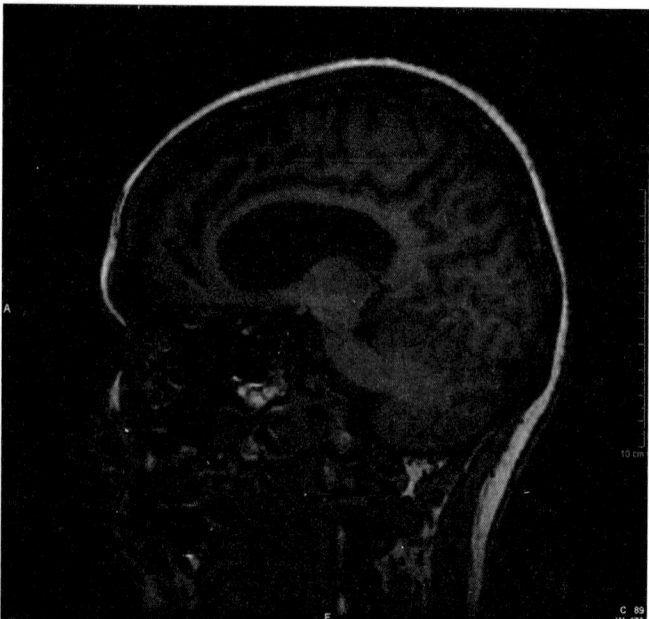

FIGURE 51.4 Sagittal brain magnetic resonance image of the patient shown in Figure 51.3.

reliable differences from controls to use as a diagnostic test for FTD, but these protein levels can be useful to distinguish FTD and AD, as patients with AD will usually show elevated levels of tau and phosphorylated tau and reduced levels of Aβ42 compared to controls and patients with FTLD. These tests can be helpful when AD and FTLD are in the differential diagnosis and to determine the neuropathologic process associated with certain clinical presentations such as logopenic PPA. The differential diagnosis for FTD can contain both neurodegenerative and psychiatric illnesses. The development of motor symptoms can elucidate the underlying pathology with symptoms of corticobasal syndrome or progressive supranuclear palsy associated with underlying tau pathology and symptoms of ALS associated with underlying TDP-43 pathology.

TREATMENT

Currently, we do not have medications that have been shown to be disease-modifying therapies for FTD. Cholinesterase inhibitors do not appear to help (level 2 studies). Serotonergic antidepressants show some efficacy reducing certain behavioral symptoms including agitation and repetitive behaviors in level 1 and 2 studies [**Level 1**].[1] Atypical antipsychotic medications are also often used to attempt to reduce behavioral symptoms in FTD. Cognitive deficits and apathy generally do not improve with medication treatment. Memantine has not demonstrated efficacy for the treatment of FTD [**Level 1**].[2]

Management of FTD relies in large part on nonpharmacologic interventions. Foremost of these is patient and family education. At diagnosis, patients and families will want to know what to expect in the years to come. Genetic counselors can be useful for education about genetic testing. Referral to local support groups and to nationwide organizations such as the Association for Frontotemporal Degeneration can be helpful. A symptom diary can be a useful tool to track symptoms, especially behavioral symptoms, as the disease progresses, and to see the effects of therapeutic interventions as they are introduced. Environmental modifications, including locking doors and removing visible food, can be helpful for wandering

behavior and hyperphagia. Providing only small portions on plates can also be useful. Wander bracelets can improve safety and now can be equipped with GPS to help in finding the patient. Physicians should continually assess if the level of assistance provided to the caregiver is sufficient. The behavioral symptoms of bvFTD can put family members of patients at risk for physical injury or sexually inappropriate behavior toward minors. Children are often at greater risk for exposure to behavioral symptoms in FTD than in other types of dementia because the patients are often younger, more likely to have young children at home, and more mobile. These behaviors will likely necessitate placement out of the home. In the later stages of the illness, palliative care and hospice referrals can be helpful in managing symptoms.

OUTCOME

Knowledge on the natural history of FTD is limited to epidemiologic studies drawn from dementia specialty centers. The median time from first symptom onset to death ranges from 9 years for bvFTD (range 3 to 16 years), to 9.5 years for PPA (range 3 to 12 years), to 12 years for semantic dementia (range 6 to 18 years). Comorbid motor neuron disease shortens life span, with median survival of 5 years from symptom onset (range 3 to 12 years). The ways in which people die from FTD are similar to other types of dementia and include infection, often related to decreased mobility, aspiration, or incontinence, and decreased oral intake of food and water leading to dehydration and malnutrition.

LEVEL 1 EVIDENCE

1. Huey ED, Putnam KT, Grafman J. A systematic review of neurotransmitter deficits and treatments in frontotemporal dementia. *Neurology.* 2006;66:17–22.
2. Boxer AL, Knopman DS, Kaufer DI, et al. Memantine in patients with frontotemporal lobar degeneration: a multicentre, randomised, double-blind, placebo-controlled trial. *Lancet Neurol.* 2013;12:149–156.

SUGGESTED READINGS

Chare L, Hodges JR, Leyton CE, et al. New criteria for frontotemporal dementia syndromes: clinical and pathological diagnostic implications. *J Neurol Neurosurg Psychiatry.* 2014;85(8):865–870.

Davies RR, Kipps CM, Mitchell J, et al. Progression in frontotemporal dementia: identifying a benign behavioral variant by magnetic resonance imaging. *Arch Neurol.* 2006;63:1627–1631.

DeJesus-Hernandez M, Mackenzie IR, Boeve BF, et al. Expanded GGGGCC hexanucleotide repeat in noncoding region of C9ORF72 causes chromosome 9p-linked FTD and ALS. *Neuron.* 2011;72:245–256.

Goldman JS. New approaches to genetic counseling and testing for Alzheimer's disease and frontotemporal degeneration. *Curr Neurol Neurosci Rep.* 2012;12:502–510.

Gorno-Tempini ML, Brambati SM, Ginex V, et al. The logopenic/phonological variant of primary progressive aphasia. *Neurology.* 2008;71:1227–1234.

Gorno-Tempini ML, Hillis AE, Weintraub S, et al. Classification of primary progressive aphasia and its variants. *Neurology.* 2011;76:1006–1014.

Harciarek M, Cosentino S. Language, executive function and social cognition in the diagnosis of frontotemporal dementia syndromes. *Int Rev Psychiatry.* 2013;25:178–196.

Hornberger M, Piguet O, Kipps C, et al. Executive function in progressive and non-progressive behavioral variant frontotemporal dementia. *Neurology.* 2008;71:1481–1488.

Hornberger M, Shelley BP, Kipps CM, et al. Can progressive and non-progressive behavioural variant frontotemporal dementia be distinguished at presentation? *J Neurol Neurosurg Psychiatry.* 2009;80:591–593.

Khan BK, Yokoyama JS, Takada LT, et al. Atypical, slowly progressive behavioural variant frontotemporal dementia associated with C9ORF72 hexanucleotide expansion. *J Neurol Neurosurg Psychiatry.* 2012;83:358–364.

Knopman DS, Roberts RO. Estimating the number of persons with frontotemporal lobar degeneration in the US population. *J Mol Neurosci.* 2011;45:330–335.

Onyike CU, Diehl-Schmid J. The epidemiology of frontotemporal dementia. *Int Rev Psychiatry.* 2013;25:130–137.

Park HK, Chung SJ. New perspective of parkinsonism in frontotemporal lobar degeneration. *J Mov Disord.* 2013;6:1–8.

Rascovsky K, Hodges JR, Knopman D, et al. Sensitivity of revised diagnostic criteria for the behavioural variant of frontotemporal dementia. *Brain.* 2011;134:2456–2477.

Renton AE, Majounie E, Waite A, et al. A hexanucleotide repeat expansion in C9ORF72 is the cause of chromosome 9p21-linked ALS-FTD. *Neuron.* 2011;72:257–268.

Rosen HJ, Allison SC, Ogar JM, et al. Behavioral features in semantic dementia vs other forms of progressive aphasias. *Neurology.* 2006;67:1752–1756.

Seeley WW, Bauer AM, Miller BL, et al. The natural history of temporal variant frontotemporal dementia. *Neurology.* 2005;64:1384–1390.

Shinagawa S, Nakajima S, Plitman E, et al. Psychosis in frontotemporal dementia. *J Alzheimers Dis.* 2014;42:485–499.

Snowden JS, Thompson JC, Neary D. Knowledge of famous faces and names in semantic dementia. *Brain.* 2004;127:860–872.

Thompson SA, Patterson K, Hodges JR. Left/right asymmetry of atrophy in semantic dementia: behavioral-cognitive implications. *Neurology.* 2003;61:1196–1203.

Van Blitterswijk M, DeJesus-Hernandez M, Rademakers R. How do C9ORF72 repeat expansions cause amyotrophic lateral sclerosis and frontotemporal dementia: can we learn from other noncoding repeat expansion disorders? *Curr Opin Neurol.* 2012;25:689–700.

Lewy Body Dementias 52

Sarah C. Janicki and Karen S. Marder

INTRODUCTION

Dementia with Lewy bodies (DLB) and Parkinson disease dementia (PDD) share many clinical and pathologic features. They are therefore discussed together and referred to as Lewy body dementias (LBD). Whether DLB and PDD are distinct disorders, or whether they represent different presentations of the same disease, is an area of ongoing investigation. Symptoms of each disorder may arise from variations in regional and temporal onset of neural dysfunction and degeneration. By consensus, when cognitive impairments are coincident with or appear within 1 year of the motor signs, DLB is diagnosed; the term *Parkinson disease dementia* is used when decline occurs in the course of well-established Parkinson disease (PD). Pathologically, both conditions are characterized by the presence of Lewy bodies, intraneuronal inclusions containing α-synuclein and ubiquitin in the brain stem, limbic area, forebrain, and neocortex.

EPIDEMIOLOGY

DLB and PDD are relatively common conditions, together affecting an estimated 1.3 million individuals in the United States.

DEMENTIA WITH LEWY BODIES

DLB is considered to be a common cause of dementia, with an estimated worldwide population prevalence of 4.2% to 7.5% and incidence of 3.8% in those newly diagnosed with dementia; however, the actual prevalence and incidence rates may be much higher due to the clinical difficulty of diagnosing DLB. Men may be more susceptible to DLB and have a worse prognosis than women.

PARKINSON DISEASE DEMENTIA

The estimated prevalence of PDD among the general population is 2% to 3%. Among patients diagnosed with PD, the prevalence of dementia is more than 30%, with a lifetime incidence of up to 80% of individuals with PD who reach the age of 90 years. Although the majority of PD patients will eventually develop dementia, the time from the onset of motor symptoms to dementia varies markedly. Few prospective biomarker studies exist to assist in prediction of patients' clinical course. Risk factors for dementia in PD include older age, age at onset of PD 60 years or older, duration of PD, and severity of parkinsonism, particularly the postural instability gait difficulty (PIGD) subtype. However, even patients with mild PD may have symptoms of cognitive impairment that does not meet criteria for dementia (mild cognitive impairment in Parkinson disease [PD-MCI]). PD-MCI may occur in up to one-quarter of patients at the time of initial PD diagnosis.

PATHOBIOLOGY

NEUROPATHOLOGY

Common pathologic findings of LBD are illustrated in Figure 52.1. Lewy body (LB) pathology, particularly in the cortex, is the most important factor in the development of both DLB and PDD. There have been few comparative neuropathologic studies to determine whether the neuropathology of PDD differs from DLB or whether both conditions exist on a continuum. Neuronal loss in the substantia nigra may be more extensive in PDD than in DLB; other features including cortical LB and Alzheimer pathology have not been found to differ in PDD and DLB.

Dementia with Lewy Bodies

Pathologic features associated with DLB are summarized in Table 52.1. LBs are the only essential feature in the pathologic diagnosis of DLB; other features are apparent in most but not all cases.

LEWY BODIES

LBs are eosinophilic intracytoplasmic neuronal inclusion bodies and are found in both the subcortical regions and brain stem as well as in the cortex in DLB (see Fig. 52.1A). Brain stem LB occurs in the substantia nigra and locus coeruleus. The term *cortical Lewy body* refers to less well-defined spherical inclusions seen in cortical neurons (see Fig. 52.1B). In some individuals, proper identification of cortical LB may be overshadowed by the coincidence of severe Alzheimer changes; in other individuals, limitations in sampling may lead to an underidentification of cortical LB.

LEWY NEURITES

Lewy neurites (LN) are neurofilament abnormalities and a distinctive part of LB pathology in which proteins cluster into diffuse aggregates (see Fig. 52.1C and D). They occur in the hippocampus (cornu ammonis two-third region), amygdala, nucleus basalis of Meynert, dorsal vagal nucleus, and other brain stem nuclei.

ALZHEIMER PATHOLOGY

Most cases of DLB demonstrate comorbid Alzheimer disease (AD) pathology including amyloid plaques and neurofibrillary tangles. Plaque types in DLB are classified as either diffuse/immature plaques with tau-positive neurites or diffuse/immature plaques with tau-negative, ubiquitin-positive neurites.

SPONGIFORM CHANGE/MICROVACUOLATION

This is a feature of some DLB cases and occurs mainly in temporal cortex. It may relate to the severity of the disease. Although similar to spongiform change in Creutzfeldt–Jakob and prion-related diseases, there is no evidence that DLB is a transmissible disorder or linked to abnormal prion protein.

Parkinson Disease Dementia

Although PD often coexists with other common causes of dementia, such as AD, neuropathologic studies have found that the degree of LB pathology (including LB and LN) may have a closer correlation with cognitive decline and dementia in PD than does the degree of AD pathology.

FIGURE 52.1 Pathology of Lewy body dementias. **A:** Pars compacta of the substantia nigra: two pigmented neurons each one including two Lewy bodies. Subcortical Lewy bodies have a basophilic central core or are eosinophilic depending on the plane of section and are surrounded by a pale, narrow halo. **B:** Occipitotemporalis gyrus, fifth layer including a cortical Lewy body–containing neuron. Cortical Lewy bodies are ill defined and diffusely eosinophilic. The nuclear chromatin of cortical Lewy body–containing neurons is often vesiculated. **C:** Nucleus coeruleus. **D:** Substantia innominata or nucleus of Meynert. Both **C** and **D** exhibit α-synuclein–labeled Lewy bodies and Lewy neurites. (**A** and **B,** Luxol fast blue counterstained with hematoxylin and eosin; **C** and **D,** α-synuclein. Original magnification: **A,** 400×; **B,** 630×; **C** and **D,** 200×. Courtesy of JP Vonsattel, MD.)

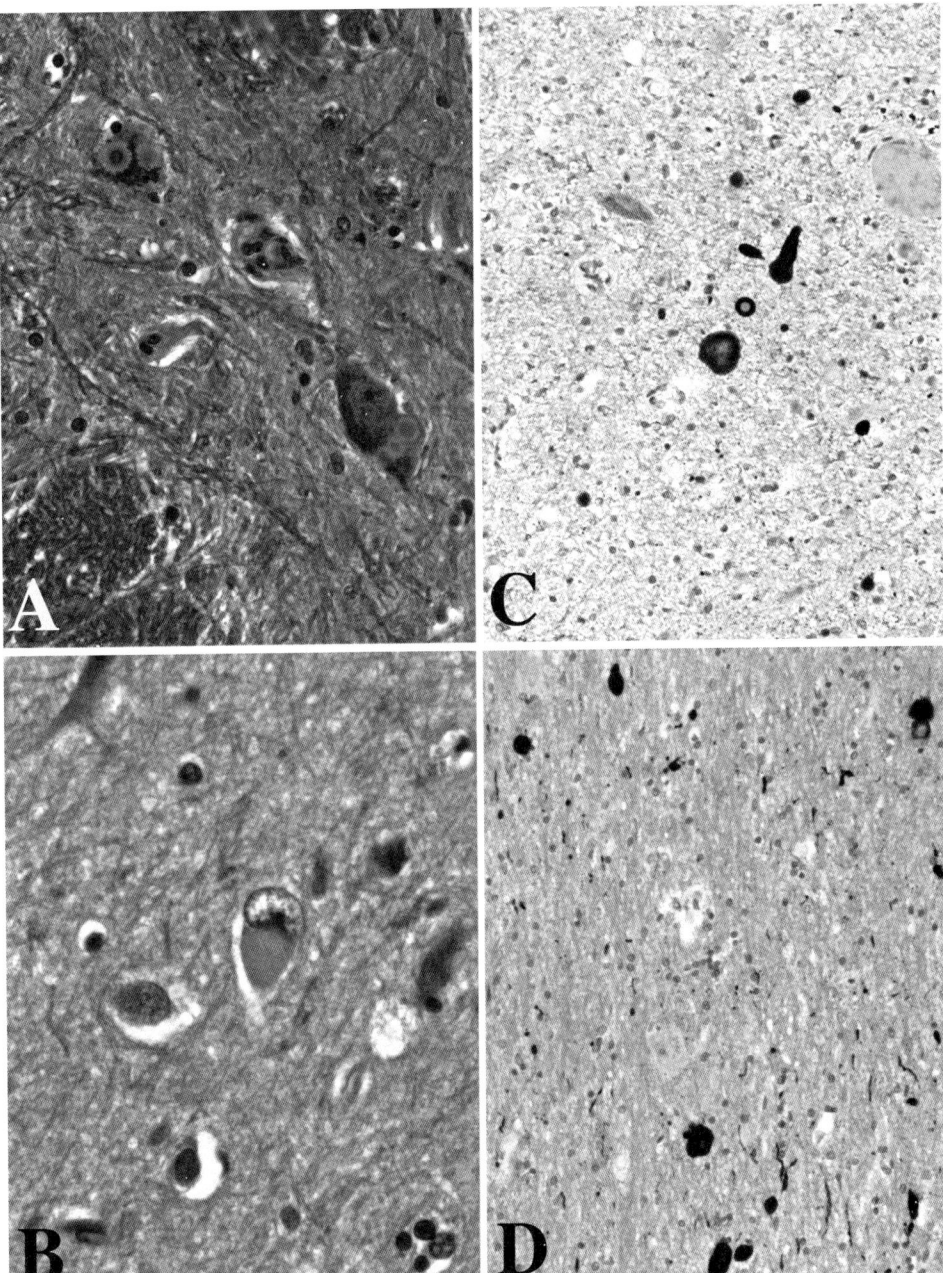

A possible synergistic role between AD and PD pathology needs further research. A few studies have found that reduced amyloid β_{1-42} in the cerebrospinal fluid is associated with cognitive decline in patients with PD, as it is in patients with AD alone. Other data suggest that that α-synuclein deposition promotes the intracellular aggregation of tau and β-amyloid in cell models and that there is a more rapid disease progression in PDD cases with coexistent AD. It is likely that given the substantial prevalence of both AD and PD, at least some patients with PD may have cognitive decline that is attributed to or exacerbated by AD.

NEUROTRANSMITTER SYSTEMS

The exact mechanisms leading to dementia in DLB and PDD are unknown. However, there is an association between structural neuropathologic findings in LBD; dopamine depletion; and noradrenergic, serotonergic, and cholinergic dysfunction. LBs have a predilection for the substantia nigra, and both PDD and DLB are characterized by dopaminergic changes in the striatum and frontal cortex, leading to parkinsonism. In addition to motor control, dopamine is involved in a range of nonmotor behaviors such as cognition, motivation, sleep, and mood. The cholinergic nucleus basalis is another LB predilection site, leading to widespread and severe cortical cholinergic deficits. LBD pathology may also affect brain stem nuclei such as the locus coeruleus, which receives noradrenergic activation, and the serotonergic raphe nuclei. All of these areas are known to be involved in modulation of cognitive and psychiatric symptoms.

GENETIC RISK FACTORS

Although large genome-wide association studies (GWAS) have identified a variety of genes contributing to sporadic PD, similar large studies have not been published yet for PDD, and only one

TABLE 52.1 Pathologic Features Associated with Dementia with Lewy Bodies

Essential for diagnosis of DLB:

- Lewy bodies

Associated but not essential for diagnosis of DLB:

- Lewy-related neurites
- Plaques (all morphologic types)
- Neurofibrillary tangles
- Regional neuronal loss, especially in the brain stem (including the substantia nigra and the locus coeruleus) and the nucleus basalis of Meynert
- Microvacuolation (spongiform changes) and synapse loss
- Reduced concentrations of choline acetyltransferase (ChAT) in neocortex

DLB, dementia with Lewy bodies.

GWAS study has been done in DLB. However, the importance of genetic factors for these diseases has begun to be established.

Glucocerebrosidase

Several individual studies and an international multicenter collaborative study have demonstrated that patients with PD who carried mutations for the lysosomal enzyme glucocerebrosidase (*GBA1*) have a higher incidence of PD-MCI and PDD. Other multicenter autopsy studies have demonstrated that subjects with DLB were more than eight times more likely to carry a *GBA1* mutation than were controls. Further analyses indicate that *GBA1* mutations are also significantly associated with earlier age at onset and death in DLB. Although mechanisms underlying *GBA1*-associated parkinsonism and dementia are still not completely understood, accumulating evidence suggests that impairment of the aging lysosome, enhanced by deficient or mutant glucocerebrosidase, can affect α-synuclein degradation.

Leucine-Rich Repeat Kinase 2

To date, cross-sectional studies have not identified specific cognitive dysfunction associated with mutations in leucine-rich repeat kinase 2 (*LRRK2*), a common cause of genetic PD. Of note, *LRRK2* G2019S carriers are more likely to have the PIGD phenotype, which is more likely to be associated with cognitive impairment. The PIGD phenotype, however, has not been associated with cognitive impairment in cross-sectional studies of *LRRK2* G2019S carriers.

Apolipoprotein E

Although cross-sectional studies have yielded disparate results, two prospective cohort studies found no association between *APOE* ε4 genotype and the development of PDD or rate of change on the MMSE in patients with PD. One study examined rate of change on the Mattis Dementia Rating Scale (MDRS) over time and showed that the ε4 allele was associated with a more rapid decline in MDRS scores (3 points per year; hazard ratio 2.8). In contrast, a recent large multinational case-control genetic association study using pathologically diagnosed samples demonstrated that the *APOE* ε4 allele was a strong genetic risk factor for DLB.

CLINICAL MANIFESTATIONS

DEMENTIA WITH LEWY BODIES

The core diagnostic criteria for probable and possible DLB as proposed by the third report of the DLB consortium, and as commonly used in clinical practice, are included in Table 52.2 [**Level 1**].[1] These core criteria have a sensitivity of 83% and a specificity of 95% for the presence of neocortical LBs at autopsy. However, these core criteria are more predictive of the relatively rare "pure" form of DLB rather than the more common findings of mixed DLB and AD pathology.

Supportive clinical features include repeated falls, syncope, transient loss of consciousness, severe autonomic dysfunction, depression, systematized delusions, or hallucinations in other sensory and perceptual modalities. The presence of low uptake in a myocardial scintigraphy study has been included as a supportive feature in recently revised criteria for diagnosis of DLB. Although these features may support the clinical diagnosis, they lack diagnostic specificity of the core features and can be seen in other neurodegenerative disorders.

PARKINSON DISEASE DEMENTIA

The diagnosis of PDD requires a clinical diagnosis of PD accompanied by cognitive impairment of sufficient magnitude to interfere with social or occupational function and the criteria for diagnosis as outlined by the International Parkinson and Movement Disorder Society are presented in Table 52.3. Criteria for diagnosis of PD-MCI have also been established (Table 52.4). It is estimated that PD-MCI occurs in up to 25% of nondemented individuals with PD and predicts a more rapid cognitive decline and shorter time to dementia.

TABLE 52.2 Diagnostic Criteria for Dementia with Lewy Bodies

Core features of DLB

- Fluctuating attention and concentration
- Recurrent well-formed visual hallucinations
- Spontaneous parkinsonism

Suggestive features of DLB

- Rapid eye movement (REM) behavior disorder
- Severe neuroleptic sensitivity
- Low dopamine transporter uptake in the basal ganglia demonstrated by ioflupane I-123 dopamine transporter SPECT imaging (DaTscan)

Probable DLB: dementia *plus*

- Two core features OR
- One core feature AND one suggestive feature

Possible DLB: dementia *plus*

- One core feature OR
- One suggestive feature

DLB, dementia with Lewy bodies; SPECT, single-photon emission computed tomography.

Data from McKeith IG, Dickson DW, Lowe J, et al. Diagnosis and management of dementia with Lewy bodies: third report of the DLB Consortium. *Neurology.* 2005;65:1863–1872.

TABLE 52.3 Criteria for Parkinson Disease Dementia

	Core Features	Associated Features	Exclusions
Probable PDD	• PD diagnosis • Slowly progressive dementia	• Cognitive deficits in two of four domains (attention, executive function, visuospatial function, and free recall) • At least one behavioral symptom (apathy, depression/anxiety, hallucinations, delusions, or excessive daytime sleepiness)	• Vascular disease on imaging or other abnormality that may cause cognitive impairment but not dementia • Unknown time interval between motor and cognitive symptoms • Acute confusion resulting from systemic diseases or abnormalities or drug intoxication • Features compatible with probable vascular dementia
Possible PDD	• PD diagnosis • Slowly progressive dementia	• Atypical cognitive deficits in one or more domain (fluent aphasia or storage-failure amnesia) with preserved attention OR • Vascular disease on imaging or other abnormality that may cause cognitive impairment, but not dementia, and/or unknown time interval between motor and cognitive symptoms	• Acute confusion resulting from systemic diseases or abnormalities or drug intoxication • Features compatible with probable vascular dementia

PDD, Parkinson disease dementia; PD, Parkinson disease.

Data from Emre M, Aarsland D, Brown R, et al. Clinical diagnostic criteria for dementia associated with Parkinson's disease. *Movement Disorders*. 2007;22: 1689–1707.

Important clinical features of DLB and PDD are discussed in more detail in the following text.

COGNITIVE IMPAIRMENT

Early signs of cognitive impairment in patients with LBD include executive dysfunction, visuospatial impairment, and deficits in verbal memory. Executive dysfunction is a hallmark feature of LBD and includes impairment in set shifting, attention, and planning. Memory deficits in LBD are to be related to retrieval of learned information, which is improved by cuing.

PSYCHIATRIC SYMPTOMS

Depression, anxiety, apathy, and fatigue commonly occur in LBD and are closely associated with cognitive decline. Detailed visual

TABLE 52.4 Criteria for Mild Cognitive Impairment in Parkinson Disease

	Inclusion	Exclusion
PD-MCI, single domain	• PD diagnosis • Gradual cognitive decline • Cognitive deficits on testing (two tests in a single domain) • Cognitive deficits not sufficient to interfere significantly with functional independence	• PDD diagnosis • Other primary explanation for cognitive impairment (delirium, stroke, depression, metabolic abnormalities, medication effects, or head trauma) • Other PD-associated comorbid conditions (motor impairment, severe anxiety, depression, excessive daytime sleepiness, or psychosis) that significantly influence cognitive testing
PD-MCI, multiple domain	• PD diagnosis • Gradual cognitive decline • Cognitive deficits on testing (at least one test in two or more domains) • Cognitive deficits not sufficient to interfere significantly with functional independence	• PDD diagnosis • Other primary explanation for cognitive impairment (delirium, stroke, depression, metabolic abnormalities, medication effects, or head trauma) • Other PD-associated comorbid conditions (motor impairment, severe anxiety, depression, excessive daytime sleepiness, or psychosis) that significantly influence cognitive testing

PD-MCI, mild cognitive impairment in Parkinson disease; PD, Parkinson disease; PDD, Parkinson disease dementia.

Data from Litvan I, Goldman JG, Troster AI, et al. Diagnostic criteria for mild cognitive impairment in Parkinson's disease: Movement Disorder Society Task Force Guildelines. *Movement Disorders*. 2012;27:349–356.

hallucinations frequently occur in both conditions as well. There is often overlap between visual hallucinations and other disorders of visual perception, including misidentification syndromes and visual agnosias. Auditory, tactile, or gustatory hallucinations may also occur but are less common. Visual hallucinations and delusions occur in up to 50% of patients with PDD, and their presence is strongly associated with cognitive dysfunction. Several drugs used in the treatment of PD, including anticholinergic agents, dopaminergic agents, and amantadine can exacerbate psychotic symptoms. In nondemented PD patients, those with hallucinations are more likely to develop dementia than are patients without this symptom.

PARKINSONISM

The most common extrapyramidal findings on examination in LBD are rigidity and bradykinesia, whereas other common signs are hypophonic speech, masked facies, stooped posture, and shuffling gait. Resting tremor is less common in DLB than in PDD, especially in older individuals. In PDD, motor signs predate dementia by 10 years on average. Patients with tremor-dominant PD are less likely to develop cognitive impairment than are those with more prominent PIGD.

SLEEP DISORDERS

Sleep disorders in patients with LBD include sleep fragmentation, nightmares, and rapid eye movement behavior disorder (RBD). Recent research has shown that RBD may occur decades prior to the onset of cognitive and motor symptoms in patients with LBD. RBD is somewhat more common in DLB but occurs in 15% to 30% of patients with PD and is associated with an increased risk of future cognitive impairment or dementia.

AUTONOMIC DYSFUNCTION

Dysautonomias including orthostatic hypotension, erectile dysfunction, and constipation occur an average of 5 years prior to the onset of cognitive or motor symptoms in patients with LBD. Several studies have also shown that LBD patients have an increased prevalence of cardiac abnormalities, particularly prolonged QT syndrome, even in patients who have never complained of chest pain or other cardiovascular problems.

FLUCTUATING ATTENTION AND CONCENTRATION

Significant fluctuations in cognition are one of three core features in DLB but rarely occur in PDD. Patients may show episodic deficits in cognition that alternate with periods of normal or near-normal performance. Excessive daytime sleepiness with confusion on awakening occurs frequently and may be accentuated by an unstimulating environment. Fluctuations may include both rapid (lasting minutes or hours) as well slower (weekly or monthly) variations in alertness. As a result, changes in mental status and behavior may be seen within a single clinical interview as well as between consecutive examinations. Caregivers are the most reliable source of information regarding the presence of fluctuations.

DIAGNOSIS

A diagnosis of DLB or PDD is based on thorough history and neurologic examination, with documentation of findings as previously described. A careful search for extrapyramidal features should be part of a general neurologic examination. The use of a standardized assessment for parkinsonian features may be particularly useful for research purposes. The Mini-Mental State Examination (MMSE) is less sensitive to the earliest cognitive changes in LBD due to its reliance on memory and language performance and its weakness in assessment of executive dysfunction. Alternative generic tests such as Dementia Rating Scale and Montreal Cognitive Assessment (MoCA) and PD-specific scales such as Parkinson Disease-Cognitive Rating Scale have shown higher sensitivity in PD and have been recommended for use in LBD. Because of the frequent comorbidity of depression in PD, screening for depression as an alternative cause or a contributor to cognitive impairment is recommended.

Medications should be carefully reviewed, and those with potential cognitive side effects, particularly anticholinergic agents, should be eliminated if possible. Laboratory workup is also advised to exclude other potentially reversible causes of symptoms including infection, metabolic derangement, vitamin B_{12} deficiency, or thyroid disease. Ancillary evaluations may include neuropsychologic testing and neuroimaging.

NEUROPSYCHOLOGIC TESTING

To most thoroughly assess for associated cognitive changes in PDD, formal neuropsychologic testing is recommended. Comparison of neuropsychologic test profiles among patients with AD, DLB, and PDD revealed no differences between DLB and PDD. Although patients with PDD and DLB were more likely to have visuospatial and attentional deficits, AD patients were more likely to have significant impairment on memory testing, particularly memory encoding; however, there is a subset of PDD patients who have prominent verbal memory impairment as a presenting sign. The presence of prominent deficits on tests of executive function and problem solving, such as the Wisconsin Card Sorting Test (WCST), the Trail Making Test (TMT), and verbal fluency for categories and letters, may be useful clinical diagnostic indicators of LBD, as may pronounced impairment on tests of visuospatial performance such as block design, clock drawing, or figure copy tests. With the progression of dementia, the selectivity of this pattern for LBD versus AD may be lost. As a result, making an accurate differential diagnosis during the later stages of dementia using clinical presentation and neuropsychologic testing alone becomes increasingly difficult, as the cognitive deficits demonstrated in advanced LBD frequently overlap with those seen in AD. For such patients, functional neuroimaging may assist in diagnosis.

NEUROIMAGING

Magnetic Resonance Imaging

A structural imaging study, including computed tomography (CT) of the head without contrast or magnetic resonance imaging (MRI), should be obtained on patients without recent brain imaging to assess for alternative structural abnormalities that may be contributing to or causing patients' complaints, including localized neoplasms, infections, strokes, or diffuse subcortical cerebrovascular disease. However, CT or MRI as isolated studies have limited diagnostic use. Generalized atrophy and white matter hyperintensities are nonspecific findings in dementia, and MRI may play a limited role in differentiating between types of dementia. Several studies indicate that MRI coronal sections through the hippocampi usually show a greater degree of hippocampal atrophy in AD compared with DLB. Volumetric analyses of MRI scans have also suggested atrophy of the putamen and dorsal mesopontine gray matter in

DLB compared with AD. There is insufficient evidence for use of MRI to differentiate DLB from PDD. Despite the changes in the occipital lobe on functional imaging as described in the following text, regional occipital atrophy is generally not observed on MRI in DLB or PDD.

Functional Brain Imaging

On single-photon emission computed tomography (SPECT) and positron emission tomography (PET) scans, DLB, and PDD patients show decreased perfusion and metabolism in the lateral frontal, temporoparietal, and occipital lobes, respectively. These occipital lobe findings have potential diagnostic use in distinguishing DLB from AD, with a sensitivity and specificity for SPECT of 65% and 87% and for PET of 90% and 80%. Some imaging studies find that mediotemporal glucose metabolism is decreased in DLB and AD but preserved in PDD.

Using specific ligands for the dopamine transporter, ioflupane I-123 dopamine transporter SPECT imaging (DaTscan) demonstrates reduced striatal dopaminergic activity in DLB and PDD. These findings are also seen in PD, multiple systems atrophy, and progressive supranuclear palsy but not in AD. A study in 326 patients with dementia reported a sensitivity of 78% and a specificity of 90% for DLB versus AD using DaTscan. A positive DaTscan result is considered a suggestive feature in the diagnosis of probable or possible DLB.

Amyloid Imaging

The high frequency of concomitant AD pathology in LBD has prompted investigations in amyloid imaging, although it is not commonly used in the clinical setting at the current time. Most studies demonstrate higher amyloid binding in DLB compared with PDD and in PDD compared with PD and controls. According to a recent meta-analysis, about 57%, 35%, 13%, and 21% of amyloid scans in DLB, PDD, PD, and controls, respectively, have positive amyloid imaging findings. The pattern of amyloid tracer binding in positive scans in DLB and PDD is very similar to that seen in AD, with preferential binding in the frontal lobes, posterior cingulate and precuneus, temporoparietal region, and striatum.

AUTONOMIC TESTING

Autonomic studies may be useful in distinguishing between DLB and AD. Patients with DLB may have abnormal cardiac 123I-meta-iodobenzylguanidine (MIBG) uptake, vagal dysfunction, and abnormal skin reflexes on sudomotor testing.

DIFFERENTIAL DIAGNOSIS

In practice, alternative diagnostic considerations are AD (with co-existing parkinsonism or prominent psychiatric features) and vascular dementia.

Although subtle extrapyramidal signs may be present in early stages of AD, notable parkinsonism does not develop until late-stage AD. Alternatively, AD may develop in a patient with PD, as the two disorders are common. This might be difficult to distinguish from PDD early on, but the early appearance of cortical dysfunction, such as aphasia or apraxia, or profound early memory loss usually suggests the presence of concomitant AD. Given that the pathologic changes of AD and DLB often occur together, it can be particularly difficult to clinically differentiate these diagnoses particularly in later stages. In these cases, functional neuroimaging may provide some indication of underlying pathologic etiology.

Infarctions in multiple vascular territories affecting periventricular and subcortical white matter, basal ganglia, and brain stem can produce dementia and vascular parkinsonism. A history of vascular risk factors, abrupt onset of symptoms with stepwise progression over time, focal neurologic signs, and evidence of diffuse vascular disease on neuroimaging suggest this alternate diagnosis.

A broader differential diagnosis includes Parkinson-plus syndromes including corticobasal syndrome (CBS) and progressive supranuclear palsy (PSP). Alternately, cognitive and behavioral decline may be related to depression or medication effects, and delirium may be caused by metabolic or systemic disorders.

TREATMENT

The treatment of patients with LBD is clinically challenging and limited to symptomatic management. Because medications may be poorly tolerated, patient and caregiver education regarding risks, benefits, and limitations of treatment is important. Although common treatment regimens can be followed for several LBD symptoms, management of parkinsonism and psychosis varies subtly between DLB and PDD.

COGNITIVE SYMPTOMS

The first step in the treatment of cognitive decline in patients with LBD should be elimination of medications with detrimental cognitive effects, including anticholinergic medications.

The cholinesterase inhibitor rivastigmine (9.5 mg/day by transdermal patch or 6 to 12 mg/day orally) is U.S. Food and Drug Administration (FDA) approved for the symptomatic treatment of cognitive impairment in PDD [**Level 1**].[2] Although there are no FDA-approved treatments for DLB, the use of rivastigmine is supported by meta-analysis as well as by report of benefit in open-label studies and two randomized, controlled trials. Rivastigmine treatment has been shown to improve neuropsychologic test performance as well as function in activities of daily living (ADLs) in LBD patients. It may also reduce psychiatric and motor symptoms, although benefits for visual hallucinations and delusions have not been demonstrated. There have been case reports of worsening cognitive function, rapid eye movement sleep disorder, or parkinsonism with cholinesterase inhibitors, so patients should be followed carefully while using these drugs. These medications also carry risk of gastrointestinal side effects including nausea, vomiting, or diarrhea, although risk appears to be minimized through transdermal delivery. If cholinesterase inhibitors are discontinued, they should be tapered as opposed to abruptly stopped in order to minimize risk of sudden cognitive and behavioral worsening.

Studies of the effects of memantine (10 mg orally twice per day) in LBD are inconsistent, but some limited trials demonstrate benefit on cognition, sleep, motor symptoms, and quality of life. However, other studies have noted that memantine may worsen delusions and hallucinations in patients with LBD.

MOTOR SYMPTOMS

Given patients' risk of falls and fluctuations in alertness, clinicians should encourage caregivers to take preventative steps to improve safety in the home environment. Physical therapy and mobility aids may help in the management of motor symptoms.

Parkinson Disease Dementia

Treatment of motor symptoms is similar in PD with and without dementia. However, patients with PDD may be particularly susceptible to the neuropsychiatric side effects of dopaminergic medications, which may limit dosage level or require concomitant use of antipsychotic agents. Anticholinergic agents frequently worsen cognitive impairment and should be avoided in patients with PDD. Patients with PDD are generally excluded from consideration for deep brain stimulation (DBS) therapy due to poor outcome.

Dementia with Lewy Bodies

Dopaminergic therapy is less effective in treating motor symptoms in DLB than in PDD. There is open-label evidence supporting the use of carbidopa/levodopa in DLB but with a risk for worsening of psychotic symptoms. Carbidopa/levodopa may be more effective than dopamine agonists in DLB and causes fewer side effects. A suggested initial dose is one tablet of carbidopa/levodopa 25/100 mg daily, titrated upward over several weeks to one tablet three times per day as tolerated and according to clinical response.

PSYCHOSIS

Parkinson Disease Dementia

Visual hallucinations and delusions can be treated with atypical antipsychotic agents. Caution should be used with these agents because of the risk of motor side effects. Severe side effects, although not as common as in DLB, do occur in a substantial portion of patients with PDD. Doses should be started at the lowest possible and titrated upward gradually.

Among the atypical antipsychotic agents, clozapine has the best established use [**Level 1**],[3] with an extremely low risk of exacerbating parkinsonism; however, it has a risk of fatal agranulocytosis and requires close monitoring of white blood cell count. Quetiapine is also effective and has a more favorable side effect profile; however, patients and caregivers must be educated about its association with increased risk of cardiac morbidity and mortality and stroke in elderly patients with dementia. Conventional antipsychotic agents are much more likely to exacerbate motor parkinsonism and should be avoided in PDD.

Dementia with Lewy Bodies

Because patients with DLB can be very sensitive to neuroleptic agents, older conventional antipsychotics should be avoided. It is estimated that almost 60% of patients with DLB may exhibit exaggerated extrapyramidal signs, sedation, immobility, or neuroleptic malignant syndrome (NMS) with fever, generalized rigidity and muscle breakdown following exposure to neuroleptics. Passive observation of visual hallucinations and delusions can be considered if these symptoms are not causing significant disruption. If a patient experiences severe, disabling psychosis, a trial of a cholinesterase inhibitor or lowering the dose of dopaminergic medications should be considered first. Randomized, placebo-controlled studies suggest that antipsychotic agents have limited efficacy in patients with in DLB. If antipsychotic therapy is required, only atypical neuroleptics, in particular quetiapine or clozapine, should be used in the smallest doses possible and patients and caregivers should be warned about the possibility of severe side effects. If clinical response is not seen from one medication, it should be discontinued and another agent tried, rather than escalating the dose of the first agent.

MOOD DISORDERS

Selective serotonin reuptake inhibitors (SSRIs) may be effective in treating anxiety and depression in patients with LBD; however, more research needs to be performed on the safety of these medications in these patient populations. Electroconvulsive therapy (ECT) has been successfully used to treat depression. Benzodiazepines should be avoided (except in RBD), especially for long-term use, because of the potential for worsening confusion, gait disorder, and paradoxical agitation. Tricyclic antidepressants should be avoided due to their anticholinergic effects.

SLEEP

Proper sleep hygiene is important in optimizing the sleep–wake cycle. Maintaining a daily routine, exposure to natural light during the daytime hours, eliminating daytime naps, and elimination of late-day caffeine consumption are important recommendations.

If RBD is present, clonazepam (0.25 to 1.5 mg orally before bed) or melatonin (3 mg orally before bed) can be used to effectively treat symptoms. Nonpharmacologic treatments may include the placement of the mattress on the floor, padding the corners of furniture, and removing potentially dangerous objects from the bedroom.

AUTONOMIC SYMPTOMS

Use of fludrocortisone (initial dosage 0.1 mg orally daily), midodrine (10 mg orally three times per day), or a combination of the two can improve symptoms of orthostatic hypotension. Nonpharmacologic treatment may include use of compression stockings and salt tablets. Stool softeners can be considered for constipation, and adult diapers can be used for urinary incontinence.

OTHER CONSIDERATIONS

In addition to symptomatic treatment, it is important to discuss management of finances and medications with patients and caregivers. Cognitive impairment and parkinsonism associated with LBD place patients at higher risk for driving impairment. A formal driving evaluation should be considered in patients with DLB who wish to continue driving.

FUTURE DIRECTIONS

No clinical trials published to date have investigated disease-modifying agents in PDD or DLB. Future clinical trial investigations in LBD may include stimulation of endogenous neurotrophic factors, reduction of α-synuclein aggregation, immune-modulating therapies, and inflammatory inhibitors.

OUTCOME

DEMENTIA WITH LEWY BODIES

There is no cure or disease-modifying therapy for DLB. Psychotic symptoms, particularly visual hallucinations, persist over time. Parkinsonism also worsens over time, especially in patients for whom this is an early symptom. Although some studies have reported that the rates of cognitive decline are similar for AD and DLB, others report a disparity. In one study, survival time in DLB was 7.7 years from onset of cognitive symptoms versus 9.3 years for patients with AD, a finding supported in another cohort. Other studies have found that patients with DLB progress to institutionalization earlier than patients with other types of dementia, perhaps due to earlier development of parkinsonism and daytime somnolence. Survival after nursing home placement is significantly impacted by the presence of depression and parkinsonism, including rigidity and gait abnormalities.

PARKINSON DISEASE DEMENTIA

Dementia in PD is associated with reduced patient and caregiver quality of life, reduced survival, and increased risks of nursing home admission. Incident dementia in PD has been associated with a twofold increase in mortality over a 4-year time period, even after controlling for severity of motor symptoms.

LEVEL 1 EVIDENCE

1. McKeith IG, Dickson DW, Lowe J, et al. Diagnosis and management of dementia with Lewy bodies: third report of the DLB Consortium. *Neurology.* 2005;65:1863–1872.
2. Maidment I, Fox C, Boustani M. Cholinesterase inhibitors for Parkinson's disease dementia. *Cochrane Database Syst Rev.* 2006;(1):CD004747.
3. The Parkinson Study Group. Low-dose clozapine for the treatment of drug-induced psychosis in Parkinson's disease. *N Engl J Med.* 1999;340:757–763.

SUGGESTED READINGS

Aarsland D, Brønnick K, Ehrt U, et al. Neuropsychiatric symptoms in patients with Parkinson's disease and dementia: frequency, profile and associated care giver stress. *J Neurol Neurosurg Psychiatry.* 2007;78:36–42.

Aarsland D, Brønnick K, Larsen JP, et al. Cognitive impairment in incident, untreated Parkinson disease: the Norwegian ParkWest study. *Neurology.* 2009;72:1121–1126.

Aarsland D, Bronnick K, Williams-Gray C, et al. Mild cognitive impairment in Parkinson disease: a multicenter pooled analysis. *Neurology.* 2010;75:1062–1069.

Aarsland D, Perry R, Brown A, et al. Neuropathology of dementia in Parkinson's disease: a prospective, community-based study. *Ann Neurol.* 2005;58:773–776.

Aarsland D, Perry R, Larsen JP, et al. Neuroleptic sensitivity in Parkinson's disease and parkinsonian dementias. *J Clin Psychiatry.* 2005;66:633–637.

Aarsland D, Zaccai J, Brayne C. A systematic review of prevalence studies of dementia in Parkinson's disease. *Mov Disord.* 2005;20:1255–1263.

Ballard C, Holmes C, McKeith I, et al. Psychiatric morbidity in dementia with Lewy bodies: a prospective clinical and neuropathological comparative study with Alzheimer's disease. *Am J Psychiatry.* 1999;156:1039–1045.

Beyer MK, Larsen JP, Aarsland D. Gray matter atrophy in Parkinson disease with dementia and dementia with Lewy bodies. *Neurology.* 2007;69:747–754.

Boeve BF, Silber MH, Ferman TJ, et al. Association of REM sleep behavior disorder and neurodegenerative disease may reflect an underlying synucleinopathy. *Mov Disord.* 2001;16:622–630.

Buter TC, van den Hout A, Matthews FE, et al. Dementia and survival in Parkinson disease: a 12-year population study. *Neurology.* 2008;70:1017–1022.

Dalrymple-Alford JC, MacAskill MR, Nakas CT, et al. The MoCA: well-suited screen for cognitive impairment in Parkinson disease. *Neurology.* 2010;75:1717–1725.

Ehrt U, Broich K, Larsen JP, et al. Use of drugs with anticholinergic effect and impact on cognition in Parkinson's disease: a cohort study. *J Neurol Neurosurg Psychiatry.* 2010;81:160–165.

Ferman TJ, Boeve BF, Smith GE, et al. Inclusion of RBD improves the diagnostic classification of dementia with Lewy bodies. *Neurology.* 2011;77:875–882.

Kantarci K, Ferman TJ, Boeve BF, et al. Focal atrophy on MRI and neuropathologic classification of dementia with Lewy bodies. *Neurology.* 2012;79:553–560.

Klatka LA, Louis ED, Schiffer RB. Psychiatric features in diffuse Lewy body disease: a clinicopathologic study using Alzheimer's disease and Parkinson's disease comparison groups. *Neurology.* 1996;47:1148–1152.

Kövari E, Gold G, Herrmann FR, et al. Lewy body densities in the entorhinal and anterior cingulate cortex predict cognitive deficits in Parkinson's disease. *Acta Neuropathol.* 2003;106:83–88.

Levy G, Tang MX, Louis ED, et al. The association of incident dementia with mortality in PD. *Neurology.* 2002;59:1708–1713.

Lippa CF, Duda JE, Grossman M, et al. DLB and PDD boundary issues: diagnosis, treatment, molecular pathology, and biomarkers. *Neurology.* 2007;68:812–819.

Lobotesis K, Fenwick JD, Phipps A, et al. Occipital hypoperfusion on SPECT in dementia with Lewy bodies but not AD. *Neurology.* 2001;56:643–649.

Louis ED, Schupf N, Manly J, et al. Association between mild parkinsonian signs and mild cognitive impairment in a community. *Neurology.* 2005;64:1157–1161.

McKeith I, O'Brien J, Walker Z, et al. Sensitivity and specificity of dopamine transporter imaging with 123I-FP-CIT SPECT in dementia with Lewy bodies: a phase III, multicentre study. *Lancet Neurol.* 2007;6:305–313.

Minoshima S, Foster NL, Sima AA, et al. Alzheimer's disease versus dementia with Lewy bodies: cerebral metabolic distinction with autopsy confirmation. *Ann Neurol.* 2001;50:358–365.

Morley JF, Xie SX, Hurtig HI, et al. Genetic influences on cognitive decline in Parkinson's disease. *Mov Disord.* 2012;27:512–518.

O'Brien JT, McKeith IG, Walker Z, et al. Diagnostic accuracy of 123I-FP-CIT SPECT in possible dementia with Lewy bodies. *Br J Psychiatry.* 2009;194:34–39.

Oda H, Ishii K, Terashima A, et al. Myocardial scintigraphy may predict the conversion to probable dementia with Lewy bodies. *Neurology.* 2013;81:1741–1745.

Parsons TD, Rogers SA, Braaten AJ, et al. Cognitive sequelae of subthalamic nucleus deep brain stimulation in Parkinson's disease: a meta-analysis. *Lancet Neurol.* 2006;5:578–588.

Raskin SA, Borod JC, Tweedy J. Neuropsychological aspects of Parkinson's disease. *Neuropsychol Rev.* 1990;1:185–221.

Ravina B, Putt M, Siderowf A, et al. Donepezil for dementia in Parkinson's disease: a randomised, double blind, placebo controlled, crossover study. *J Neurol Neurosurg Psychiatry.* 2005;76:934–939.

Stern Y, Marder K, Tang MX, et al. Antecedent clinical features associated with dementia in Parkinson's disease. *Neurology.* 1993;43:1690–1692.

Svenningsson P, Westman E, Ballard C, et al. Cognitive impairment in patients with Parkinson's disease: diagnosis, biomarkers, and treatment. *Lancet Neurol.* 2012;11:697–707.

Vendette M, Gagnon JF, Décary A, et al. REM sleep behavior disorder predicts cognitive impairment in Parkinson disease without dementia. *Neurology.* 2007;69:1843–1849.

Walker Z, Costa DC, Walker RW, et al. Differentiation of dementia with Lewy bodies from Parkinson's disease using a dopaminergic presynaptic ligand. *J Neurol Neurosurg Psychiatry.* 2002;73:134–140.

Yoshita M, Taki J, Yokoyama K, et al. Value of 123I-MIBG radioactivity in the differential diagnosis of DLB from AD. *Neurology.* 2006;66:1850–1854.

Nikolaos Scarmeas

INTRODUCTION

During much of the 20th century, it was assumed that most dementia of the elderly was vascular in origin, an assumption challenged during the last few decades after the recognition and importance of Alzheimer-type pathologic changes. Nevertheless, with wider use of modern sophisticated neuroimaging techniques and accumulation of more knowledge on cerebral microinfarcts, interest in the role of vascular disease on cognitive decline reemerged and the clinical importance of vascular lesions in cognitive performance has been a new focus of attention lately.

Brain injury caused by stroke can undoubtedly contribute to dementia and intellectual impairment. Vascular dementia is a progressive cognitive dysfunction caused by stroke, often ischemic, but also hemorrhagic cerebrovascular disease as well as ischemic white matter disease or sequelae of hypotension or hypoxia.

Diagnosis of vascular dementia has been controversial, and its definition has been unsettled despite numerous attempts at clarification. Unlike other neurodegenerative dementias, there are no specific pathologic criteria. Cerebrovascular disease is itself a heterogeneous disorder, with a variety of pathophysiologic mechanisms and clinical manifestations, and correspondingly, vascular dementia manifests also as a heterogeneous syndrome. Vascular dementia can result from a variety of mechanisms (Table 53.1 and Figs. 53.1–53.3).

There are many criteria for the clinical diagnosis of "vascular dementia," some not adequately validated, many inconsistently applied and in general lacking satisfactorily high sensitivity and specificity. In terms of terminology, the concept of "vascular cognitive impairment" has been also recently proposed; a more general term referring to "cognitive impairment that is caused by or associated with vascular factors" and includes severity stages corresponding to either dementia or mild cognitive impairment.

Overall, as a practical rule, a diagnosis of vascular dementia requires (1) clinically (symptoms/signs) and radiologically ascertained strokes (see Figs. 53.1–53.3), (2) dementia, and (3) a clear temporal relationship between stroke(s) and dementia.

EPIDEMIOLOGY

As many as 15% to 20% of patients with acute ischemic stroke older than age 60 years have dementia at the time of the stroke,

TABLE 53.1 Proposed Types of Vascular Dementia Based on Localization and Pathophysiologic Mechanism	
Vascular Dementia Subtype	**Comments/Additional Information for Each Subtype, Including Localization, and Mechanisms**
Critically located (strategic "single") infarcts	Bilateral frontal infarctions from anterior cerebral artery occlusions
	Bilateral thalamic infarction from posterior cerebral artery occlusions
	Middle cerebral artery occlusions leading to frontal/parietal infarcts, etc.
Multiple ischemic infarcts affecting large vessels	Not necessarily in critical locations but leading to significant parenchymal volume loss
Small-vessel disease	Multiple lacunar infarcts in the basal ganglia
	Multiple lacunar infarcts in subcortical or periventricular white matter leading to a more widespread, patchy pattern often described as leukoaraiosis in brain imaging studies (*Binswanger disease*)
Hemorrhagic infarcts	Intraparenchymal hemorrhages due to chronic vascular damage from hypertension
	Amyloid angiopathy
	Intracerebral or subdural hematomas or subarachnoid hemorrhage
Hypoperfusion	Due to systemic causes such as heart failure, hypotension, bypass surgery, cardiac arrest, medications, or other systemic conditions
Other mechanisms	Combinations of the above
	Cerebral autosomal dominant arteriopathy with subcortical infarcts and leuko-encephalopathy (CADASIL), an autosomal dominant form of cerebrovascular dementia (and also migraines and psychiatric symptoms) related to mutations in the *notch3* gene on chromosome 19
	Mitochondrial encephalomyopathy with lactic acidosis and stroke-like episodes (MELAS)

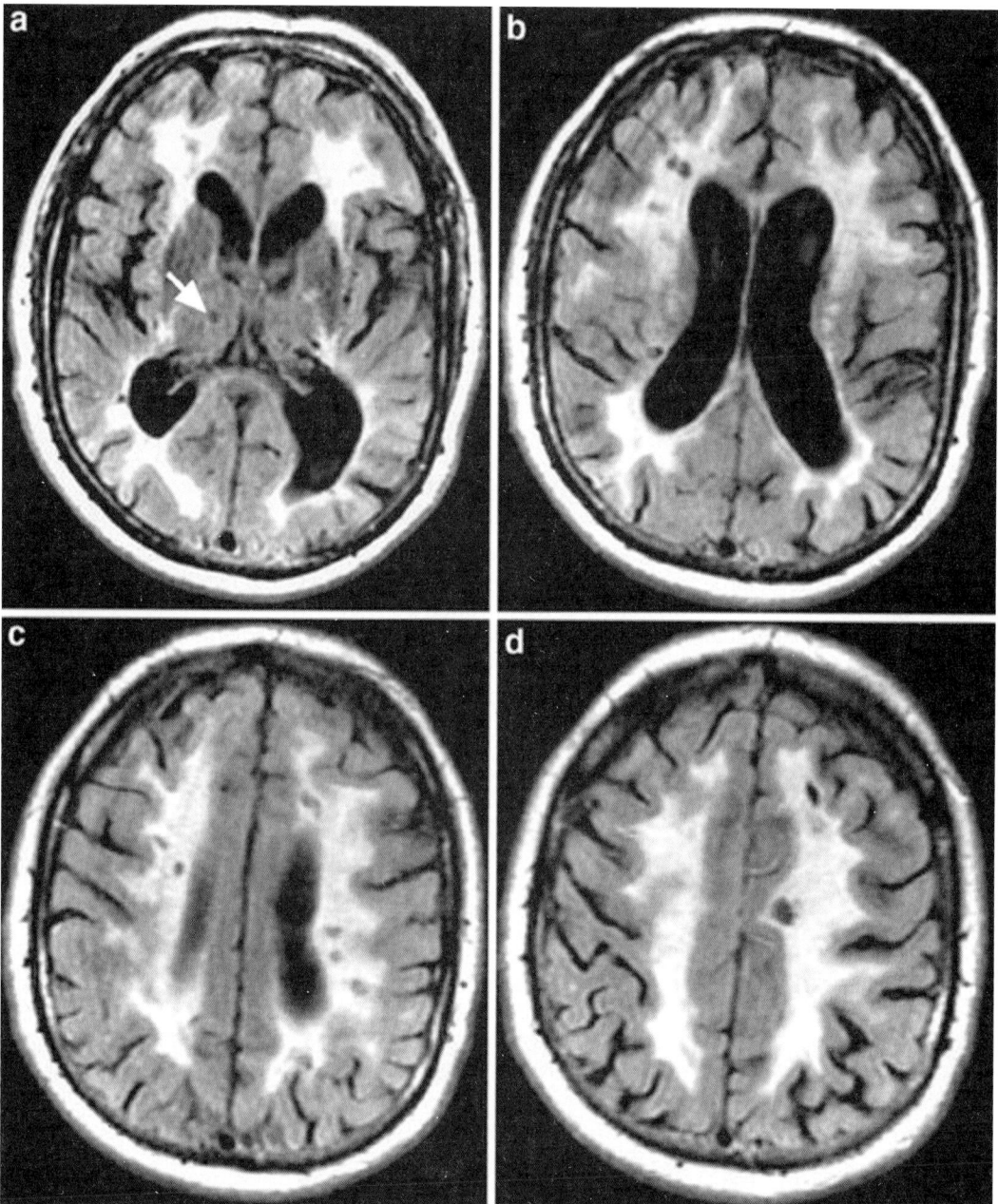

FIGURE 53.1 Binswanger disease in an 85-year-old man with dementia. **A–D:** Axial fluid-attenuated inversion recovery magnetic resonance images show extensive symmetric hyperintensity involving periventricular and lobar white matter. These lesions have a rather sharp outer border and show sparing of the U-fibers. This diffuse involvement was considered more than 25% of the total white matter. There are also a lacunar right thalamic infarct (*arrow*), several bilateral hypointense lesions within the periventricular hyperintensity representing lacunar infarcts and an important global cerebral atrophy. (From Guermazi A, Miaux Y, Rovira-Cañellas A, et al. Neuroradiological findings in vascular dementia. *Neuroradiology.* 2007;49[1]:1–22.)

and 5% per year become demented thereafter. On a clinical basis, vascular dementia has been long considered as the second (after Alzheimer disease) or even the third (after Alzheimer and dementia with Lewy bodies) most frequent cause of dementia. Considering pathologic series data and related clinical–pathologic correlations makes the issue quite more complex.

Although the vast majority of elderly demented patients have Alzheimer-type pathologic changes (70% to 80%), approximately half of them have coexisting cerebrovascular infarctions

too, whereas only about 30% have "pure" Alzheimer only pathology. Therefore, the majority of demented subjects have mixed Alzheimer and vascular pathologic changes. Adding to the argument of higher contribution rates of vascular dementia is the fact that most pathologic studies consider only larger infarcts, whereas microinfarcts (if time and resources permit their identification) are extremely common and diffuse in the brain. Finally, many white matter abnormalities visualized on brain magnetic resonance imaging are often undetectable by

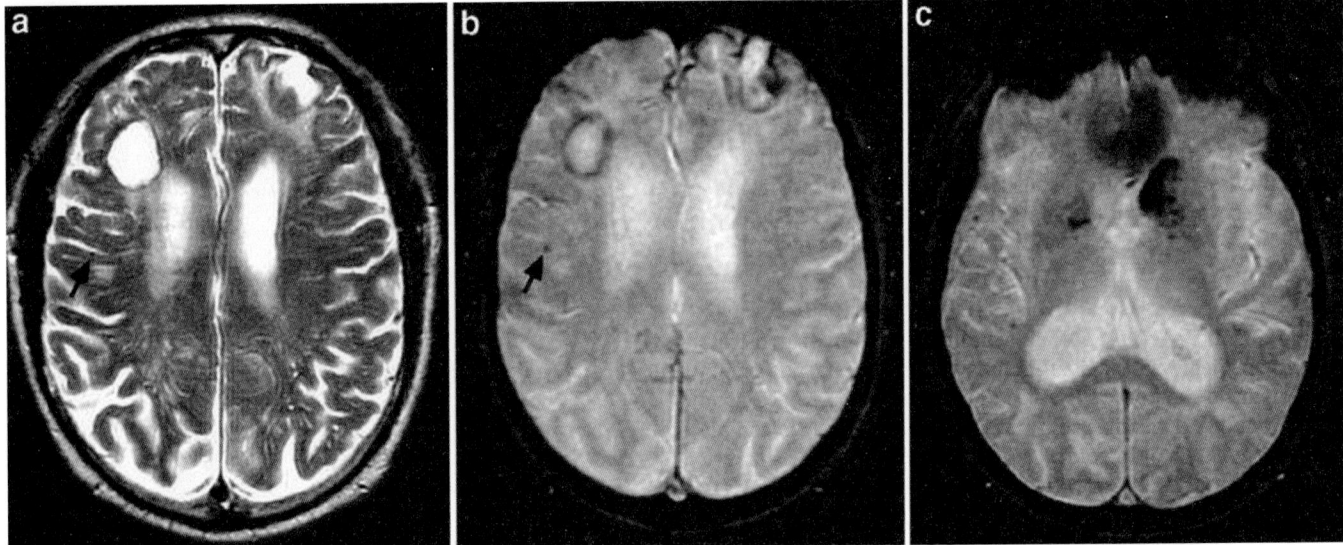

FIGURE 53.2 Amyloid angiopathy in a 66-year-old man with dementia. **A:** Axial spin-echo T2-weighted MR image shows bilateral large frontal hemorrhages surrounded by a rim of hypointensity due to hemosiderin deposition. There is also another right frontal punctate hypointense lesion (*arrows*), best seen on **B**, the axial gradient echo T2-weighted MR image. **C:** Axial gradient echo T2-weighted MR image caudal to **B** shows additional hypointensities bilaterally in the basal ganglia and the right parietal lobe (From Guermazi A, Miaux Y, Rovira-Cañellas A, et al. Neuroradiological findings in vascular dementia. *Neuroradiology.* 2007;49[1]:1–22.)

standard neuropathologic examinations performed on autopsy, suggesting limited sensitivity of neuropathology for detection of cerebrovascular damage.

On the counterargument, the clinical salience of such micro-infarcts on cognitive function has not been convincingly demonstrated. Additionally, dementia due to infarcts solely without significant pathologic contributions of the Alzheimer or Lewy body type (i.e., pure vascular dementia) is strikingly uncommon with

estimated rates between 2% and 10% of dementias (not more than 5% of dementias in the United States).

PATHOBIOLOGY: CAUSES OF VASCULAR DEMENTIA

Overall, strokes themselves and factors that predispose to cerebrovascular disease are considered risk factors for vascular dementia.

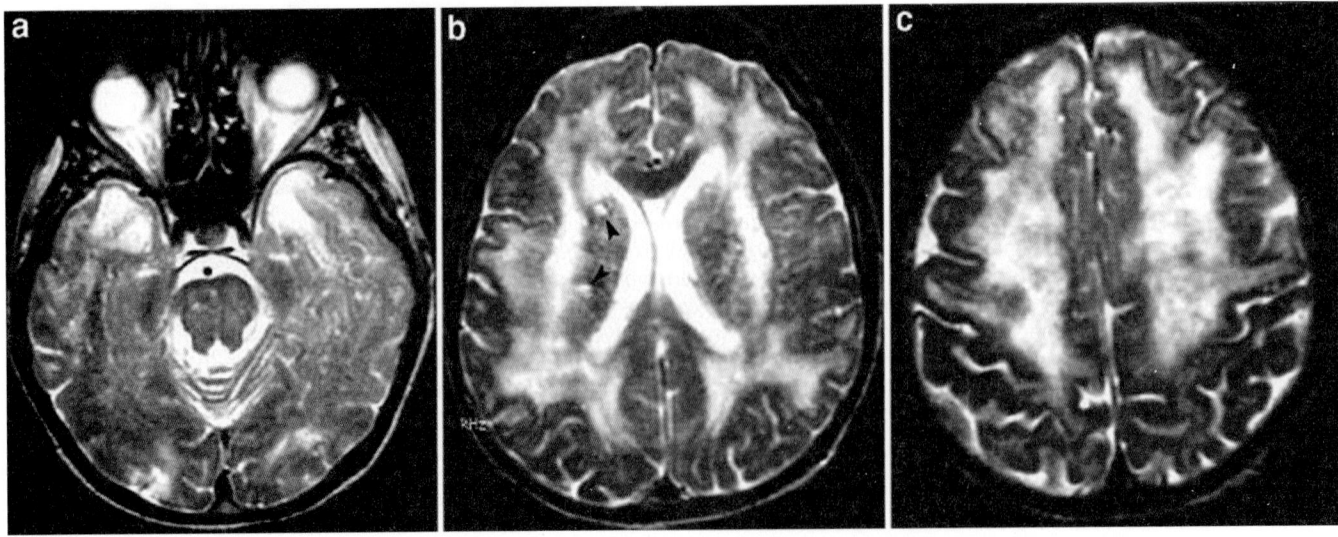

FIGURE 53.3 CADASIL in a 57-year-old man with cognitive impairment. **A:** Axial spin-echo T2-weighted MR images show an extensive white matter abnormalities with characteristic symmetric involvement of the anterior part of the temporal lobes and **(B)** external and extreme capsules without involvement of the internal capsules. They also show **(C)** extensive white matter changes in the centrum ovale, extending toward the cortex in some places. There are also two small lacunar infarcts in the right basal ganglia (*arrowheads*). (From Guermazi A, Miaux Y, Rovira-Cañellas A, et al. Neuroradiological findings in vascular dementia. *Neuroradiology.* 2007;49[1]:1–22.)

Predisposing conditions for cerebral infarcts are numerous and should be included in patients' workups. Patients with vascular dementia are usually old and may suffer from cardiovascular disease, including heart attacks, cardiac arrhythmias, congestive heart failure, or from diabetes, hypertension, dyslipidemia, with eventual damage in many organs. Beyond genetic susceptibility to strokes, rare genetic causes of vascular dementia include cerebral autosomal dominant arteriopathy with subcortical infarcts and leukoencephalopathy and mitochondrial encephalomyopathy with lactic acidosis and stroke-like episodes.

Whether Alzheimer-type pathologic changes induce cerebrovascular damage or whether brain infarcts promote Alzheimer neuropathology is not settled. Overall, there is a complex interaction between stroke, vascular risk factors, and Alzheimer disease, although the exact nature of this interaction remains unknown.

CLINICAL MANIFESTATIONS

The symptoms and signs of vascular dementia may include impairment in acquiring and remembering new information, impaired reasoning, judgment and handling of complex tasks, deficits in visual spatial abilities, problems with language function (comprehension, expression, etc.), and changes in personality or behavior. The exact mix of the aforementioned in each case depends on cerebral localization of infarcts. If for example, the temporal lobe neural circuits responsible for memory functions are less affected, amnesic deficits, a key feature in Alzheimer disease, may be less prominent in vascular dementia. Focal noncognitive deficits related to vascular dementia causing strokes may also coexist.

A more "cortical" version with more clear stepwise deterioration including focal motor or sensory symptoms and signs, aphasia, neglect, abulia, apraxia, agnosia, amnesia, etc. resulting from repeated distinct strokes may be present. However, vascular dementia often presents as a more "subcortical" syndrome that is characterized by apathy, inertia, bradyphrenia, deficits in attention and concentration, executive disfunction (problems with organization, planning, and strategy), often abnormal gait (which may mimic apraxic or magnetic or that of lower body parkinsonism), urinary urgency or incontinence, depression as well as emotional incontinence ("pseudobulbar affect"), including inappropriate crying or laughing.

In general, in the differential diagnosis from Alzheimer disease, features that would favor the diagnosis of vascular dementia would include (to a certain extend temporally and clinically relating to cerebral infarcts) an abrupt onset of dementia, a stepwise deterioration and a fluctuating course.

DIAGNOSIS

There are no diagnostic tests specific for vascular dementia.

Clinical presence of stroke documented by either history (symptoms) or neurologic examination (residual signs), although not entirely required, enhances specificity of vascular dementia diagnosis.

Presence of infarcts in brain imaging studies is a requirement. Their nature (hemorrhagic, ischemic), size (small, large), number (one strategic, many), or location (cortical, subcortical, different brain structures) can widely vary. Widespread, confluent white matter disease often called *leukoaraiosis* can be noted.

Evaluation to define a specific stroke subtype and etiology should be definitely included.

Deficits may be detected in neuropsychological evaluation, but their nature is also nonspecific because they depend on stroke local-ization that may vary from patient to patient. However, deficits in frontal function, including difficulties with attention–concentration, slow speed of processing, difficulties with initiation, and executive dysfunction may be prominent. Particularly in subcortical forms of vascular dementia, amnestic deficits may be characterized by difficulties in free recall with relative improvement in recognition (i.e., when aided with various strategy cues).

TREATMENT

Because stroke is the cause of vascular dementia, primary prevention of stroke may reduce vascular dementia rates and treatment of already existing stroke—secondary preventions of stroke recurrence are central to vacular dementia course and prognosis. For example, smoking cessation, control-treatment of hypertension, diabetes, dyslipidemia, obesity, etc. are indicative preventive strategies. Similarly, antiplatelets, anticoagulants, and carotid endarterectomy (whenever indicated according to specific stroke characteristics) are examples of stroke recurrence prevention approaches. Stroke treatment and stroke preventative strategies are discussed in more detail in Chapters 35 and 44.

The efficacy of cholinesterase inhibitors and memantine, proven therapies for dementia of the Alzheimer type, is not that extensively studied in vascular dementia. In general, efficacy of all these medications—medication classes has been demonstrated in mixed (Alzheimer and vascular) dementia and not in pure vascular dementia [Level 1].[1-7] Given that such mixed dementia is quite common and that it is clinically often hard to exclude coexisting Alzheimer pathologic changes in many patients diagnosed with vascular dementia, it stands to reason to offer cholinesterase inhibitors and memantine therapy to such patients. Initiation with one of the three cholinesterase inhibitors subsequently followed by addition of memantine is the common practice. The doses commonly prescribed and corresponding titration schedules toward the maximum dose (occurring during the course of weeks/months depending on the particular medication) are those used for Alzheimer dementia, the main official indication for such treatments (Table 53.2).

OUTCOME

Prognosis in vascular dementia is more variable than that of Alzheimer disease because it is largely dependent on coexisting strokes. If, particularly with modification of cerebrovascular disease

TABLE 53.2	Medications Commonly Prescribed for Vascular Dementia		
Medication – Active Substance	Route	Targeted Maximum Daily Dose	Frequency of Administration
Donepezil	Oral	10 mg	Once a day
Rivastigmine	Oral	12 mg	6 mg twice a day
Rivastigmine	Transdermal	13.3 mg	Once a day
Galantamine	Oral	24 mg	Once a day
Memantine	Oral	20 mg	10 mg twice a day
Memantine	Oral	28 mg	Once a day

risk factors, none or only a limited number of future strokes occur, the cognitive deficits can remain relatively static for protracted periods or until death. For other vascular dementia patients who continue to suffer from additional cerebral infarcts, a progressive cognitive decline and dementia deterioration is usually noted.

LEVEL 1 EVIDENCE

1. Black S, Roman GC, Geldmacher DS, et al. Efficacy and tolerability of donepezil in vascular dementia: positive results of a 24-week, multicenter, international, randomized, placebo-controlled clinical trial. *Stroke*. 2003;34:2323–2330.
2. Wilkinson D, Doody R, Helme R, et al. Donepezil in vascular dementia: a randomized, placebo-controlled study. *Neurology*. 2003;61:479–486.
3. Erkinjuntti T, Kurz A, Gauthier S, et al. Efficacy of galantamine in probable vascular dementia and Alzheimer's disease combined with cerebrovascular disease: a randomised trial. *Lancet*. 2002;359:1283–1290.
4. Auchus AP, Brashear HR, Salloway S, et al. Galantamine treatment of vascular dementia: a randomized trial. *Neurology*. 2007;69:448–458.
5. Orgogozo JM, Rigaud AS, Stoffler A, et al. Efficacy and safety of memantine in patients with mild to moderate vascular dementia: a randomized, placebo-controlled trial (MMM 300). *Stroke*. 2002;33:1834–1839.
6. Wilcock G, Mobius HJ, Stoffler A. A double-blind, placebo-controlled multicentre study of memantine in mild to moderate vascular dementia (MMM500). *Int Clin Psychopharmacol*. 2002;17:297–305.
7. Kumar V, Anand R, Messina J, et al. An efficacy and safety analysis of Exelon in Alzheimer's disease patients with concurrent vascular risk factors. *Eur J Neurol*. 2000;7:159–169.

SUGGESTED READINGS

Breteler MM. Vascular risk factors for Alzheimer's disease: an epidemiologic perspective. *Neurobiol Aging*. 2000;21:153–160.

Chui HC, Mack W, Jackson JE, et al. Clinical criteria for the diagnosis of vascular dementia: a multicenter study of comparability and interrater reliability. *Arch Neurol*. 2000;57:191–196.

Chui HC, Zheng L, Reed BR, et al. Vascular risk factors and Alzheimer's disease: are these risk factors for plaques and tangles or for concomitant vascular pathology that increases the likelihood of dementia? An evidence-based review. *Alzheimers Res Ther*. 2012;4:1.

Erkinjuntti T. Subcortical vascular dementia. *Cerebrovasc Dis*. 2002;13(suppl 2): 58–60.

Gold G, Giannakopoulos P, Montes-Paixao Junior C, et al. Sensitivity and specificity of newly proposed clinical criteria for possible vascular dementia. *Neurology*. 1997;49:690–694.

Hachinski V, Iadecola C, Petersen RC, et al. National Institute of Neurological Disorders and Stroke-Canadian Stroke Network vascular cognitive impairment harmonization standards. *Stroke*. 2006;37:2220–2241.

Hachinski VC, Lassen NA, Marshall J. Multi-infarct dementia. A cause of mental deterioration in the elderly. *Lancet*. 1974;2:207–210.

Jellinger KA. The pathology of ischemic-vascular dementia: an update. *J Neurol Sci*. 2002;203–204:153–157.

Kalaria RN, Ballard C. Overlap between pathology of Alzheimer disease and vascular dementia. *Alzheimer Dis Assoc Disord*. 1999;13(suppl 3):S115–S123.

Kalmijn S, Foley D, White L, et al. Metabolic cardiovascular syndrome and risk of dementia in Japanese-American elderly men. The Honolulu-Asia aging study. *Arterioscler Thromb Vasc Biol*. 2000;20:2255–2260.

Kavirajan H, Schneider LS. Efficacy and adverse effects of cholinesterase inhibitors and memantine in vascular dementia: a meta-analysis of randomised controlled trials. *Lancet Neurol*. 2007;6:782–792.

Langa KM, Foster NL, Larson EB. Mixed dementia: emerging concepts and therapeutic implications. *JAMA*. 2004;292:2901–2908.

Launer LJ, Hughes TM, White LR. Microinfarcts, brain atrophy, and cognitive function: the Honolulu Asia Aging Study Autopsy Study. *Ann Neurol*. 2011;70:774–780.

Libon DJ, Heilman KM. Assessing the impact of vascular disease in demented and nondemented patients. *Stroke*. 2008;39:783–784.

Lobo A, Launer LJ, Fratiglioni L, et al. Prevalence of dementia and major subtypes in Europe: a collaborative study of population-based cohorts. Neurologic Diseases in the Elderly Research Group. *Neurology*. 2000;54:S4–S9.

Lopez OL, Kuller LH, Becker JT. Diagnosis, risk factors, and treatment of vascular dementia. *Curr Neurol Neurosci Rep*. 2004;4:358–367.

Lopez OL, Kuller LH, Becker JT, et al. Classification of vascular dementia in the Cardiovascular Health Study Cognition Study. *Neurology*. 2005;64: 1539–1547.

Marchant NL, Reed BR, Sanossian N, et al. The aging brain and cognition: contribution of vascular injury and abeta to mild cognitive dysfunction. *JAMA Neurol*. 2013;70:488–495.

Moorhouse P. Rockwood K. Vascular cognitive impairment: current concepts and clinical developments. *Lancet Neurol*. 2008;7:246–255.

O'Brien JT, Erkinjuntti T, Reisberg B, et al. Vascular cognitive impairment. *Lancet Neurol*. 2003;2:89–98.

Reed BR, Marchant NL, Jagust WJ, et al. Coronary risk correlates with cerebral amyloid deposition. *Neurobiol Aging*. 2012;33:1979–1987.

Reed BR, Mungas DM, Kramer JH, et al. Profiles of neuropsychological impairment in autopsy-defined Alzheimer's disease and cerebrovascular disease. *Brain*. 2007;130:731–739.

Regier DA, Kuhl A, Kupfer DJ. The DSM-5: classification and criteria changes. *World Psychiatry*. 2013;12:92–98.

Roman GC. Vascular dementia: distinguishing characteristics, treatment, and prevention. *J Am Geriatr Soc*. 2003;51:S296–S304.

Roman GC, Sachdev P, Royall DR, et al. Vascular cognitive disorder: a new diagnostic category updating vascular cognitive impairment and vascular dementia. *J Neurol Sci*. 2004;226:81–87.

Roman GC, Tatemichi TK, Erkinjuntti T, et al. Vascular dementia: diagnostic criteria for research studies. Report of the NINDS-AIREN International Workshop. *Neurology*. 1993;43:250–260.

Sonnen JA, Larson EB, Crane PK, et al. Pathological correlates of dementia in a longitudinal, population-based sample of aging. *Ann Neurol*. 2007;62:406–413.

Tomlinson BE, Blessed G, Roth M. Observations on the brains of demented old people. *J Neurol Sci*. 1970;11:205–242.

Troncoso JC, Zonderman AB, Resnick SM, et al. Effect of infarcts on dementia in the Baltimore longitudinal study of aging. *Ann Neurol*. 2008;64:168–176.

Westover MB, Bianchi MT, Yang C, et al. Estimating cerebral microinfarct burden from autopsy samples. *Neurology*. 2013;80:1365–1369.

Wetterling T, Kanitz RD, Borgis KJ. Comparison of different diagnostic criteria for vascular dementia (ADDTC, DSM-IV, ICD-10, NINDS-AIREN). *Stroke*. 1996;27:30–36.

Zheng L, Mack WJ, Chui HC, et al. Coronary artery disease is associated with cognitive decline independent of changes on magnetic resonance imaging in cognitively normal elderly adults. *J Am Geriatr Soc*. 2012;60:499–504.

Primary and Secondary Headache Syndromes 54

Peter J. Goadsby and Denise E. Chou

ANATOMY AND PHYSIOLOGY OF HEADACHE

Headache is one of the most common symptoms evaluated by neurologists and bears a vast differential diagnosis. The successful management of both primary and secondary headache disorders requires an understanding of the relevant neuroanatomy and underlying physiology.

Pain typically occurs when peripheral nociceptors are stimulated in response to factors such as tissue injury or visceral distension. In this setting, pain perception is a normal physiologic response mediated by a healthy nervous system. However, pain can also occur from damage or inappropriate activation of pain-producing pathways of the peripheral or central nervous system. Headache may result from either or both of these mechanisms. There are relatively few pain-generating cranial structures, which include the scalp, falx cerebri, dural sinuses, and proximal segments of the large pial arteries. The majority of the brain parenchyma, ventricular ependyma, choroid plexus, and pial veins are not thought to be capable of producing pain.

The key structures involved in primary headache appear to be the following:

- the large intracranial vessels, dura mater, and the peripheral terminals of the trigeminal nerve that innervate these structures
- the caudal portion of the trigeminal nucleus, which extends into the dorsal horns of the upper cervical spinal cord and receives input from the first and second cervical nerve roots (the trigeminocervical complex)
- rostral pain-processing regions, such as the ventroposteromedial thalamus and the cortex
- pain modulatory systems in the brain that modulate input from trigeminal nociceptors at all levels of the pain-processing pathways and influence vegetative functions, such as hypothalamus and brain stem structures

The innervation of the large intracranial vessels and dura mater by the trigeminal nerve is referred to as the *trigeminovascular system*. Cranial autonomic symptoms, such as *lacrimation, conjunctival injection, nasal congestion, rhinorrhea, periorbital swelling, aural fullness,* and *ptosis,* are prominent in the trigeminal autonomic cephalalgias (TACs) and may also be seen in migraine. Such autonomic symptoms result from activation of cranial parasympathetic pathways; functional imaging studies also suggest that vascular changes in migraine and cluster headache, when present, are similarly driven by these cranial autonomic systems. These symptoms can often be mistaken for signs of sinus inflammation, frequently resulting in inappropriate management. Migraine and other primary headache syndromes are not primarily "vascular headaches" as was once thought; these disorders do not reliably demonstrate vascular changes, and treatment outcomes cannot be predicted by vascular effects. Migraine is fundamentally a brain disorder and should be understood and treated as such.

CLINICAL EVALUATION OF HEADACHE DISORDERS

The differential diagnosis of a new, severe headache is quite different from a chronic, recurrent headache. There is a greater likelihood of finding a potentially serious cause with new-onset and severe headache than with recurrent headache over years. Life-threatening headache is relatively uncommon, but vigilance is required in order to recognize and appropriately treat such patients. Serious causes to be considered include meningitis, subarachnoid hemorrhage, epidural or subdural hematoma, glaucoma, tumor, and purulent sinusitis. The approach to the patient presenting with severe, new-onset headache is also discussed in Chapter 7.

A classification system for headache disorders has been established by the International Headache Society (IHS)—the International Classification of Headache Disorders, now in its third edition. The most recent version divides headache disorders into *primary syndromes* (in which the headache and associated features constitute the disorder itself) and *secondary disorders* (in which the headache results from exogenous causes).

SECONDARY HEADACHE

Concerning underlying conditions that are associated with headache are described in the following text and detailed further in Chapter 7; however, it should be noted that the vast majority of patients presenting with severe headache have a benign cause. The management of secondary headache focuses on diagnosis and treatment of the underlying cause.

- **Meningitis:** Acute, severe headache with fever and stiff neck suggests meningitis (see Chapter 61). Often, there is significant worsening of pain with eye movement. Lumbar puncture is necessary for diagnosis. Meningitis can be easily mistaken for migraine in that the cardinal symptoms of pounding headache, photophobia, nausea, and vomiting are frequently present, perhaps reflecting the underlying physiology in some of these cases.
- **Subarachnoid hemorrhage:** Acute, severe headache with stiff neck but without fever suggests subarachnoid hemorrhage (see Chapter 39). A ruptured aneurysm, arteriovenous malformation, or intraparenchymal hemorrhage may also present with headache alone. In rare cases (particularly if the hemorrhage is small or below the foramen magnum), head computed tomography (CT) can be normal. Thus, lumbar puncture may be required for definitive diagnosis of a subarachnoid hemorrhage.

- **Brain tumor:** Brain tumor is a rare cause of headache and even less commonly a cause of severe pain. The head pain is generally nondescript—an intermittent deep, dull ache of moderate intensity, which may worsen with exertion or change in position and may be associated with nausea and vomiting. Such symptoms are caused by migraine far more often than from brain tumor. The headache of brain tumor awakens patients from sleep in about 10% of cases. Vomiting that precedes the development of headache by weeks is highly characteristic of posterior fossa brain tumors. Head pain triggered by Valsalva maneuvers such as bending, lifting, or coughing can be due to a posterior fossa mass. De novo headache in a patient with known malignancy may suggest cerebral metastases and/or carcinomatous meningitis.

- **Temporal arteritis:** Temporal (giant cell) arteritis is an inflammatory disorder of arteries that frequently involves the extracranial carotid circulation. The average age of onset is 70 years, and women account for 65% of cases. About half of patients with untreated temporal arteritis develop blindness due to involvement of the ophthalmic artery and its branches. Because treatment with glucocorticoids is effective in preventing this complication, prompt recognition of the disorder is important. Headache is the dominant symptom and often appears in association with malaise and myalgias. Head pain may be unilateral or bilateral and is located temporally in 50% of patients but may involve any and all aspects of the cranium. The quality is almost always described as dull and boring, with superimposed episodic stabbing pains and exquisite scalp tenderness. Patients often describe a superficial origin of their headache (external to the skull, rather than originating deep within the head as in migraine). Headache is usually worse at night and often aggravated by exposure to cold. Additional findings may include reddened, tender nodules or red streaking of the skin overlying the temporal arteries and tenderness of the temporal or, less commonly, the occipital arteries. The management of temporal arteritis is further discussed in Chapters 7 and 42.

- **Glaucoma:** Glaucoma may present with a prostrating headache associated with nausea and vomiting. The headache often starts with severe eye pain. On physical examination, the eye is often red with a fixed, moderately dilated pupil.

PRIMARY HEADACHE SYNDROMES

Primary headache syndromes are disorders in which the headache and associated features occur in the absence of exogenous etiologies. The most common are migraine, tension-type headache, and the TACs, notably cluster headache; the complete list is in Table 54.1.

MIGRAINE

EPIDEMIOLOGY

Migraine is the second most common cause of headache and ranks among the top 20 causes of disability worldwide by the World Health Organization. It afflicts approximately 12% of the population annually (15% of women and 6% of men over a 1-year period). Migraine is a recurring syndrome of head pain along with symptoms of neurologic dysfunction, such as sensitivity to sensory stimuli (light, sound, smell, or movement); nausea and vomiting often accompany the headache.

The migraine brain is particularly sensitive to environmental and sensory stimuli; migraine-prone patients do not habituate easily to sensory input. Headache can be initiated or amplified by various triggers, including bright lights, sounds, smells, or other afferent stimulation; hunger; stress or the let down from stress; physical exertion; stormy weather, altitude, or barometric pressure changes; hormonal fluctuations during menses; lack of or excess sleep; and alcohol or other chemicals, such as nitrates. Identifying a patient's susceptibility to specific triggers can be useful in advising lifestyle adjustments as part of the treatment plan.

PATHOPHYSIOLOGY

The sensory sensitivity that is characteristic of migraine is probably due to dysfunction of monoaminergic sensory control systems located in the brain stem and diencephalon. Activation of cells in the trigeminal nucleus results in the release of vasoactive neuropeptides, particularly calcitonin gene–related peptide (CGRP), at vascular terminations of the trigeminal nerve and within the trigeminal nucleus. Centrally, second-order trigeminal neurons cross the midline and project to ventrobasal and posterior nuclei of the thalamus for further processing. There are additional projections to the periaqueductal gray and hypothalamus, from which reciprocal descending systems have established antinociceptive effects. Other brain stem regions likely to be involved in descending modulation of trigeminal pain include the nucleus locus coeruleus in the pons and the rostroventromedial medulla.

Pharmacologic and other data implicate the involvement of the neurotransmitter 5-hydroxytryptamine (5-HT or serotonin) in migraine. The *triptans* were designed to selectively stimulate subpopulations of 5-HT receptors; at least 14 different 5-HT receptors have been identified in humans. The triptans are potent agonists of 5-HT_{1B} and 5-HT_{1D} receptors, and some are active at the 5-HT_{1F} receptors (agonists of the latter are called *ditans*). Triptans arrest nerve signaling in the nociceptive pathways of the trigeminovascular system, at least in the trigeminal nucleus caudalis and trigeminal sensory thalamus, in addition to cranial vasoconstriction. *Ditans*, recently shown to be effective in acute migraine, act only at neuronal targets. An interesting range of neural targets is now being actively pursed for the acute and preventive management of migraine.

Data also support a role for dopamine in the pathophysiology of migraine. The majority of migraine symptoms can be induced by dopaminergic stimulation. Moreover, there is dopamine receptor hypersensitivity in migraineurs, as demonstrated by the induction of yawning, nausea, vomiting, hypotension, and other symptoms of a migraine attack by dopaminergic agonists at doses that do not affect nonmigraineurs. Dopamine receptor antagonists are effective therapeutic agents in migraine, especially when given parenterally or concurrently with other antimigraine agents. Moreover, hypothalamic activation, anterior to that seen in cluster headache, has now been shown in the premonitory phase of migraine using functional imaging and this may hold a key to understanding some part of the role of dopamine in the disorder.

Migraine genes have been identified by studying families with familial hemiplegic migraine (FHM) and reveal involvement of ion channels, suggesting that alterations in membrane excitability can predispose to migraine. Mutations involving the $\text{Ca}_v 2.1$ (P/Q)–type voltage-gated calcium channel *CACNA1A* gene are now known to cause FHM-1; this mutation is responsible for about 50% of cases of FHM. Mutations in the $\text{Na}^+\text{-K}^+\text{ATPase}$ *ATP1A2* gene, designated FHM-2, are responsible for about 20% of FHM.

TABLE 54.1   Primary Headache Disorders

Migraine	1.1 Migraine without aura	**Tension-type headache**	2.1 Infrequent episodic tension-type headache
	1.2 Migraine with aura		2.2 Frequent episodic tension-type headache
	1.2.1 Migraine with typical aura		2.3 Chronic tension-type headache
	1.2.1.1 Typical aura with headache	**Trigeminal autonomic cephalalgias**	3.1 Cluster headache
	1.2.1.2 Typical aura without headache		3.1.1 Episodic cluster headache
	1.2.2 Migraine with brain stem aura		3.1.2 Chronic cluster headache
	1.2.3 Hemiplegic migraine		3.2 Paroxysmal hemicrania
	1.2.3.1 Familial hemiplegic migraine (FHM)		3.2.1 Episodic paroxysmal hemicrania
	1.2.3.1.1 Familial hemiplegic migraine type 1		3.2.2 Chronic paroxysmal hemicrania
	1.2.3.1.2 Familial hemiplegic migraine type 2		3.3 Short-lasting unilateral neuralgiform headache attacks
	1.2.3.1.3 Familial hemiplegic migraine type 3		3.3.1 Short-lasting unilateral neuralgiform headache attacks with conjunctival injection and tearing (SUNCT)
	1.2.3.2 Sporadic hemiplegic migraine		3.3.2 Short-lasting unilateral neuralgiform headache attacks with cranial autonomic symptoms (SUNA)
	1.2.4 Retinal migraine		3.4 Hemicrania continua
	1.3 Chronic migraine	**Other primary headache disorders**	4.1 Primary cough headache
	1.4 Complications of migraine		4.2 Primary exercise headache
	1.4.1 Status migrainosus		4.3 Primary headache associated with sexual activity
	1.4.2 Persistent aura without infarction		4.4 Primary thunderclap headache
	1.4.3 Migrainous infarction		4.5 Cold-stimulus headache
	1.4.4 Migraine aura-triggered seizure		4.5.1 Headache attributed to external application of a cold stimulus
	1.5 Probable migraine		4.5.2 Headache attributed to ingestion or inhalation of a cold stimulus
	1.5.1 Probable migraine without aura		4.6 External-pressure headache
	1.5.2 Probable migraine with aura		4.6.1 External-compression headache
	1.6 Episodic syndromes that may be associated with migraine		4.6.2 External-traction headache
	1.6.1 Recurrent gastrointestinal disturbance		4.7 Primary stabbing headache
	1.6.1.1 Cyclical vomiting syndrome		4.8 Nummular headache
	1.6.1.2 Abdominal migraine		4.9 Hypnic headache
	1.6.2 Benign paroxysmal vertigo		4.10 New daily persistent headache (NDPH)
	1.6.3 Benign paroxysmal torticollis		

Modified from Headache Classification Committee of the International Headache Society. The International Classification of Headache Disorders, 3rd edition (beta version). *Cephalalgia*. 2013;33:629–808.

Mutations in the neuronal voltage-gated sodium channel *SCN1A* cause FHM-3.

DIAGNOSIS AND CLINICAL FEATURES

Diagnostic criteria for migraine headache are summarized in Table 54.2. Migraine has several forms that have been defined: migraine with and without aura, episodic migraine, and chronic migraine (see Table 54.1). The migraine aura, such as the visual disturbances with flashing lights or zigzag lines moving across the vi-

sual field or other neurologic symptoms, is reported in only 20% to 25% of patients. Patients with episodes of migraine that occur on 15 or more days per month are considered to have chronic migraine. Most patients with disabling headache likely have migraine, as opposed to tension-type headache, which is the most common primary headache disorder (discussed later in this chapter).

Patients with acephalgic migraine (typical aura without headache, 1.2.1.2) experience recurrent neurologic symptoms, frequently with nausea or vomiting, but with little or no headache. Vertigo can be prominent; it has been estimated that one-third of

TABLE 54.2	Simplified Diagnostic Criteria for Migraine

Repeated attacks of headache lasting 4–72 h in patients with a normal physical examination, no other reasonable cause for the headache, and

At Least Two of the Following Features	Plus at Least One of the Following Features
Unilateral pain	Nausea/vomiting
Throbbing pain	Photophobia and phonophobia
Aggravation by movement	
Moderate or severe intensity	

Adapted from Headache Classification Committee of the International Headache Society. The International Classification of Headache Disorders, 3rd edition (beta version). *Cephalalgia.* 2013;33:629–808.

patients referred for vertigo or dizziness have a primary diagnosis of migraine. Migraine aura can have prominent brain stem symptoms (such as diplopia, ataxia, altered consciousness, dysarthria, tinnitus, and vertigo) and the terms *basilar artery* and *basilar-type migraine* have now been replaced by *migraine with brain stem aura* (see Table 54.1).

TREATMENT OF MIGRAINE

Once a diagnosis of migraine has been established, it is important to assess the extent of a patient's disease and level of functional impairment. The Migraine Disability Assessment Score (MIDAS) is a well-validated, easy-to-use tool. A headache diary also helps assess disability as well as the frequency of abortive medication use. Patient education is an important aspect of migraine management. It is useful for patients to understand that migraine is an inherited vulnerability for head pain and associated neurologic symptoms and that although the disorder cannot be "cured," migraine can be modified and managed by lifestyle adjustments and medications. Furthermore, patients should be reassured that migraine is generally not associated with serious or life-threatening illnesses.

Nonpharmacologic Management

Migraine can often be managed at least in part by a variety of nonpharmacologic approaches. Many benefit by identifying and avoiding specific headache triggers. A regulated lifestyle is important, including a healthy diet (with a regular eating schedule), exercise, routinized sleep patterns, avoidance of excess caffeine and alcohol, and minimizing acute changes in stress levels (such as through biofeedback, meditation, or yoga). Lifestyle modifications that are effective in reducing headache frequency should be maintained on a routine basis, as these provide a simple, cost-effective approach to migraine management. If these measures fail to prevent an attack, abortive pharmacologic measures are then needed.

Pharmacologic Treatment

ABORTIVE (ACUTE ATTACK) THERAPIES

Table 54.3 summarizes the commonly used medications for acute migraine, which include the nonsteroidal anti-inflammatory drugs (NSAIDs), 5-HT$_{1B/1D}$ receptor agonists, and dopamine receptor

antagonists [**Level 1**].[1–16] Selecting the optimal regimen for an individual patient depends on several factors, the most important of which is the severity of the attack. Mild migraine attacks can usually be managed by oral agents, with an average efficacy rate of 50% to 70%. Severe migraine attacks may require intranasal or parenteral treatments for faster onset. In general, an adequate dose of the selected medication should be used as soon as possible after the onset of an attack. If additional medication is required within 1 hour due to persistence or recurrence of symptoms, the initial dose should be increased or a different class of rescue therapy should be taken. Migraine therapy must be individualized; a standardized approach for all patients is not feasible. Furthermore, a treatment regimen may need to be frequently revised until a successful plan is reached that provides rapid, complete, and consistent relief with minimal side effects (Table 54.4).

NONSTEROIDAL ANTI-INFLAMMATORY DRUGS

NSAIDs can significantly reduce the severity and duration of a migraine attack and are most effective when taken early in the attack. However, these agents alone may not completely abort a moderate or severe migraine attack. The combination of aspirin and metoclopramide has been shown to be comparable to a single dose of oral sumatriptan. Important side effects of NSAIDs include dyspepsia and gastrointestinal irritation, as well as potential cardiovascular and renal effects (particularly with frequent or long-term use).

5-HYDROXYTRYPTAMINE$_{1B/1D}$ RECEPTOR AGONISTS (TRIPTANS)

Stimulation of 5-HT$_{1B/1D}$ receptors can abort an acute migraine attack. Ergotamine and dihydroergotamine are nonselective receptor agonists, whereas the triptans are selective 5-HT$_{1B/1D}$ receptor agonists. A variety of triptans, 5-HT$_{1B/1D}$ receptor agonists—sumatriptan, almotriptan, eletriptan, frovatriptan, naratriptan, rizatriptan, and zolmitriptan—are now available for the acute treatment of migraine. Each drug in the triptan class has similar pharmacologic properties but varies slightly in terms of clinical efficacy. Rizatriptan and eletriptan are the most likely to be efficacious. Sumatriptan and zolmitriptan have similar rates of efficacy as well as time to onset, with an advantage of having different routes of administration. Almotriptan has a similar rate of efficacy to sumatriptan but is better tolerated, whereas frovatriptan and naratriptan are somewhat slower in onset yet have milder side effect profiles. Clinical efficacy appears to be related more to the t_{max} (time to peak plasma level) than to the potency, half-life, or bioavailability. This observation is consistent with various studies indicating that faster acting analgesics are more effective than slower acting agents.

Unfortunately, monotherapy with oral triptan therapy does not yield rapid, consistent, and complete relief of migraine in all patients. Triptans may not be effective in migraine with aura unless taken after completion of the aura and initiation of the headache; recurrence of headache is another limitation of triptan use. Evidence from randomized controlled trials demonstrates that coadministration of a longer acting NSAID (such as naproxen 500 mg) with sumatriptan will augment the initial effect of sumatriptan and, importantly, reduce rates of headache recurrence. Side effects of triptans include nausea, chest tightness, dizziness, asthenia, and flushing. 5-HT$_{1B/1D}$ agonists are contraindicated in individuals with a history of cardiovascular or cerebrovascular disease.

Nasal formulations of dihydroergotamine (Migranal), zolmitriptan (Zomig nasal), or sumatriptan can be useful in patients

TABLE 54.3 Acute Treatment of Migraine Attacks

Drug	Trade Name	Dosage
NSAIDs		
Naproxen[a]	Aleve, Anaprox, generic	220–550 mg PO b.i.d.
Ibuprofen[a]	Advil, Motrin, Nuprin, generic	400–800 mg PO q6–8h
Acetylsalicylic acid[a]	Aspirin, generic	500–1,000 mg PO b.i.d.
Tolfenamic acid	Clotam Rapid	200 mg PO; may repeat × 1 after 1–2 h
Diclofenac potassium[a]	Cambia, generic	50 mg PO with water
Compound Analgesics		
Acetaminophen, aspirin, caffeine[a]	Excedrin Migraine	Two tablets or caplets q6h (max 8 per day)
5-HT$_1$ B/1D Agonists		
Oral		
Naratriptan[a]	Amerge, generic	2.5-mg tablet at onset; may repeat once after 4 h
Rizatriptan[a]	Maxalt, generic Maxalt-MLT	5–10-mg tablet at onset; may repeat after 2 h (max 30 mg/day)
Sumatriptan[a]	Imitrex, generic	50–100-mg tablet at onset; may repeat after 2 h (max 200 mg/day)
Frovatriptan[a]	Frova	2.5-mg tablet at onset, may repeat after 2 h (max 5 mg/day)
Almotriptan[a]	Axert	6.25–12.5-mg tablet at onset, may repeat after 2 h (max 25 mg/day)
Eletriptan[a]	Relpax	20–40-mg mg tablet at onset (max 80 mg/day)
Zolmitriptan[a]	Zomig, generic Zomig Rapimelt	2.5–5-mg tablet at onset; may repeat after 2 h (max 10 mg/day)
Nasal		
Dihydroergotamine[a]	Migranal Nasal Spray	Prior to nasal spray, the pump must be primed four times; 1 spray (0.5 mg) is administered, followed in 15 min by a second spray
Sumatriptan[a]	Imitrex Nasal Spray	5–20-mg intranasal spray as four sprays of 5 mg or a single 20-mg spray (may repeat once after 2 h, not to exceed a dose of 40 mg/day)
Zolmitriptan[a]	Zomig	2.5–5 mg intranasal spray as one spray (may repeat once after 2 h, not to exceed a dose of 10 mg/day)
Parenteral		
Dihydroergotamine[a]	DHE-45	1 mg IV, IM, or SC at onset and q1h (max 3 mg/day, 6 mg/week)
Sumatriptan[a]	Imitrex injection, generic Alsuma Sumavel DosePro	6 mg SC at onset (may repeat once after 1 h for max of two doses in 24 h)
Dopamine Receptor Antagonists		
Oral		
Metoclopramide	Reglan,[b] generic[b]	5–10 mg/day
Prochlorperazine	Compazine,[b] generic[b]	1–25 mg/day
Promethazine	Phenergan,[b] generic[b]	25–50 mg/day
Chlorpromazine	Thorazine,[b] generic[b]	25–50 mg/day
Parenteral		
Metoclopramide[a]	Reglan,[b] generic	10 mg IV
Prochlorperazine[a]	Compazine,[b] generic[b]	10 mg IV
Chlorpromazine[a]	Thorazine,[b] generic[b]	12.5–25 mg IM or IV (0.1 mg/kg IV at 2 mg/min)
Promethazine	Phenergan,[b] generic[b]	12.5–25 mg IM or IV (slow)

Antiemetics (e.g., domperidone 10 mg or ondansetron 4 or 8 mg) or prokinetics (e.g., metoclopramide 10 mg) are sometimes useful adjuncts.

[a]Supported by level 1 evidence.

[b]Not all drugs are specifically indicated by the FDA for migraine. Local regulations and guidelines should be consulted.

NSAIDs, nonsteroidal anti-inflammatory drugs; PO, by mouth; 5-HT, 5-hydroxytryptamine; IV, intravenous; IM, intramuscular; SC, subcutaneous.

TABLE 54.4	Clinical Stratification of Acute Specific Migraine Treatments
Clinical Situation	**Treatment Options**
Failed NSAIDS/analgesics	**First tier**
	Sumatriptan 50–100 mg PO
	Almotriptan 12.5 mg PO
	Rizatriptan 10 mg PO
	Eletriptan 40 mg PO
	Zolmitriptan 5 mg PO
	Slower effect/better tolerability
	Naratriptan 2.5 mg PO
	Frovatriptan 2.5 mg PO
Early nausea or difficulty taking tablets	Zolmitriptan 5 mg nasal spray
	Sumatriptan 20 mg nasal spray
	Rizatriptan 10 mg MLT wafer
	Zolmitriptan 5 mg ZMT Rapimelt
Early vomiting	Zolmitriptan 5 mg nasal spray
	Sumatriptan 6 mg SC
Headache recurrence	Naratriptan 2.5 mg PO
	Almotriptan 12.5 mg PO
	Eletriptan 40 mg PO
Tolerating acute treatments poorly due to side effects	Naratriptan 2.5 mg PO
	Almotriptan 12.5 mg PO
Menstrual-associated headache	Frovatriptan 2.5 mg with Naprosyn 500 mg around menses
Rapidly developing symptoms	Zolmitriptan 5 mg nasal spray
	Sumatriptan 6 mg SC
	Dihydroergotamine 1 mg IM

NSAIDs, nonsteroidal anti-inflammatory drugs; PO, by mouth; SC, subcutaneous; IM, intramuscular.

requiring a nonoral route of administration (e.g., due to nausea/vomiting). Intranasal administration can result in substantial blood levels within 30 to 60 minutes. Although nasal sprays in theory might provide faster and more effective relief than oral formulations, their reported efficacy is only 50% to 60%. Studies with a new inhalational formulation of dihydroergotamine indicate that its absorption problems can be overcome to produce rapid onset of action with good tolerability.

Sumatriptan and dihydroergotamine are also available in injection formulations. Sumatriptan 4 to 6 mg subcutaneously (SC) is effective in approximately 50% to 80% of patients. Peak plasma levels of dihydroergotamine are achieved 3 minutes after intravenous (IV) dosing, 30 minutes after intramuscular (IM) dosing, and 45 minutes after SC dosing. If an attack has not already reached peak, SC or IM administration of 1-mg dihydroergotamine can be effective in about 80% to 90% of patients.

DOPAMINE RECEPTOR ANTAGONISTS

Oral or parenteral dopamine receptor antagonists can be considered as adjunctive acute migraine treatments. Drug absorption is impaired during migraine due to reduced gastrointestinal motility (even in the absence of nausea) and is related to the severity of the attack, rather than duration. Therefore, when oral NSAIDs and/or triptans fail, the addition of a dopamine receptor antagonist (such as metoclopramide 10 mg) should be considered to enhance gastric absorption, as well as to decrease nausea/vomiting. Certain phenothiazine drugs (such as promethazine, prochlorperazine, or chlorpromazine) can also independently improve headache pain, particularly when given parenterally, although may be sedating due to their antihistamine properties.

OTHER MEDICATIONS FOR ACUTE MIGRAINE

Opioids are modestly effective in the acute treatment of migraine and are commonly administered in the emergency room. Such agents can "help" in the sense that the pain of migraine is eliminated or reduced. However, this regimen is suboptimal for patients with recurrent headache. Opioids do not treat the underlying headache pathophysiology; rather, they act to alter the sensation of pain, and there is evidence that they can render other migraine medications (such as triptans) less effective. Moreover, frequent opioid use can result in medication overuse headache and result in physical dependence or addiction; opioid craving and/or withdrawal can in turn worsen migraine. Therefore, it is recommended that opioid use in migraine be restricted to patients with severe, but infrequent, headaches that are unresponsive to other pharmacologic approaches or who have contraindications to other treatments.

Butalbital-containing compounds (such as Fioricet or Fiorinal) are also frequently given for acute migraine treatment. Although these medications may provide analgesic relief, there is a high potential for dependence and the development of medication overuse headache (also known as *rebound headache*), which is a state of refractory daily or near-daily headache. This condition is likely not a separate headache entity but a reaction of the migraine patient to a particular medicine. Butalbital-containing medications have been banned in some countries and although still available in the United States, should be avoided.

PREVENTIVE TREATMENTS FOR MIGRAINE

Patients who experience an increasing frequency of migraine attacks or attacks that are poorly responsive to abortive medications, warrant preventive therapy. In general, a preventive medication should be considered for patients with four or more attacks a month; however, the decision of when to start a preventive agent may also depend on the severity and duration of attacks. Many of these medications have significant side effects, and the therapeutic dose can vary significantly among individual patients. The mechanism of action of these drugs is not entirely known; it is likely that they modify the brain sensitivity that underlies migraine. Patients are usually started on a low dose of the selected medication; the dose is then gradually titrated up to a reasonable maximum to achieve clinical response. A preventive medication must be taken daily, and there is usually a lag of at least 2 to 12 weeks before benefit may be seen.

Commonly used medications for the prevention of migraine are listed in Table 54.5 [**Level 1**].[17–39] The drugs that have been approved by the U.S. Food and Drug Administration (FDA) for the prophylactic treatment of migraine include propranolol, timolol, sodium valproate, topiramate, and methysergide (not available in the United States). In addition, a number of other drugs appear to display prophylactic efficacy. This includes amitriptyline, nortriptyline, candesartan, flunarizine, phenelzine, gabapentin, and cyproheptadine. Onabotulinum toxin type A has been shown

TABLE 54.5 Preventive Treatments in Migraine[a]

Drug	Dose	Selected Side Effects
β-Blockers		Fatigue, postural symptoms, bradycardia, depression, nightmares
Propranolol[b]	40–120 mg b.i.d.	Caution in patients with asthma
Metoprolol[b]	25–100 mg b.i.d.	—
Timolol[b]	5–10 mg b.i.d.	—
Atenolol	25–100 mg q.d.	—
Nadolol	40–240 mg divided b.i.d. or t.i.d.	—
Anticonvulsants		
Topiramate[b]	25–200 mg/day	Paresthesias, cognitive impairment, weight loss, nausea, fatigue, glaucoma, and metabolic acidosis; caution with nephrolithiasis
Valproate[b]	400–600 mg b.i.d.	Drowsiness, weight gain, hair loss, tremor, hematologic or liver abnormalities, fetal abnormalities
Gabapentin	900–3,600 mg q.d.	Dizziness, sedation, weight gain
Antidepressants		
Amitriptyline	10–100 mg at night	Drowsiness, dry mouth, constipation, blurred vision, postural hypotension, weight gain
Nortriptyline	10–100 mg at night	*Note:* Some patients may only need a total dose of 10 mg, although generally, 1–1.5 mg/kg body weight is required.
Doxepin	10–75 mg at night	Sedation, dry mouth, weight gain
Venlafaxine[b]	75–150 mg q.d.	Nausea, insomnia, dizziness, fatigue, nervousness
Serotonergic drugs		
Methysergide[c]	1–4 mg q.d.	Drowsiness, leg cramps, hair loss, retroperitoneal fibrosis (1-month drug holiday is required every 6 mo)
Other Classes		
Flunarizine[c] (calcium channel blocker)	5–15 mg q.d.	Drowsiness, weight gain, depression, parkinsonism
Candesartan (ARB inhibitor)	16 mg q.d.	Dizziness, hypotension
Pizotifen[c]	0.5–2 mg q.d.	Weight gain, drowsiness
Onabotulinum toxin type A[b] (Botox)	155 units divided in 31 sites (PREEMPT protocol)	Loss of brow furrow, ptosis, pain at injection sites, neck stiffness
Complementary Agents		
Petasites (butterbur)[b]	75 mg b.i.d.	Stomach upset
Riboflavin (vitamin B2)	400 mg q.d.	Urine discoloration
Magnesium	500–600 mg q.d.	Increased bowel motility
Feverfew (MIG-99)	6.25 mg t.i.d.	Stomach upset, nausea

[a]Commonly used preventives are listed with typical doses and common side effects. Not all listed medicines are approved by the FDA; local regulations and guidelines should be consulted.

[b]Supported by level 1 evidence.

[c]Not available in the United States.

ARB, angiotensin II receptor blocker; PREEMPT, Phase III Research Evaluating Migraine Prophylaxis Therapy protocol.

to be effective in placebo-controlled studies for the prevention of chronic migraine but not of episodic migraine. The probability of success with any one of these medications is approximately 50% to 75%. Once effective stabilization is achieved, the drug is continued for approximately 6 to 12 months and then slowly tapered to assess whether continuation is needed. Many patients are able to wean off prophylactic medications successfully, with fewer and milder attacks for long periods, suggesting that these drugs may alter the natural history of migraine.

TENSION-TYPE HEADACHE

CLINICAL FEATURES

Tension-type headache (TTH) is the most common primary headache disorder, although patients rarely present to the clinic due to the low level of associated disability. TTH is characterized by bilateral tight, bandlike head discomfort of mild to moderate severity. The pain usually progresses slowly, fluctuates in severity, and may persist more or less continuously for many days. The headache may be episodic or chronic (present on 15 or more days per month). Unlike migraine, TTH is otherwise featureless and lacks accompanying features such as nausea, vomiting, photophobia, phonophobia, osmophobia, throbbing, and aggravation with movement.

PATHOPHYSIOLOGY

The pathophysiology of TTH is incompletely understood. It seems likely that TTH is due to a primary disorder of central nervous system pain modulation alone, unlike migraine, which involves a more generalized disturbance of sensory modulation. Data suggest a genetic contribution to TTH, although this may not be a valid finding, as these studies likely included many migraine patients. The name *tension-type headache* implies that pain is a product of *nervous tension*; however, there is no clear evidence for tension as an etiology. Muscle contraction has been considered to be a feature that distinguishes TTH from migraine, but there appear to be no differences in contraction between the two headache types.

TREATMENT

The pain of TTH usually responds to simple analgesics such as acetaminophen, aspirin, or other NSAIDs. Behavioral approaches including relaxation can also be effective. Clinical studies have demonstrated that triptans in pure TTH are not helpful, although triptans are effective in TTH when the patient also has migraine. For chronic TTH, amitriptyline (10 to 100 mg/day) is the only proven treatment; other tricyclics, selective serotonin reuptake inhibitors,

and the benzodiazepines have not been shown to be effective. There is no evidence for the efficacy of acupuncture. Placebo-controlled trials of onabotulinum toxin type A in chronic TTH have been negative.

TRIGEMINAL AUTONOMIC CEPHALALGIAS

The TACs describe a group of primary headaches including cluster headache, paroxysmal hemicrania, SUNCT (short-lasting unilateral neuralgiform headache attacks with conjunctival injection and tearing)/SUNA (short-lasting unilateral neuralgiform headache attacks with cranial autonomic symptoms), and hemicrania continua (see Table 54.1). The TACs are characterized by relatively short-lasting attacks of head pain associated with cranial autonomic symptoms, such as lacrimation, conjunctival injection, or nasal congestion (Table 54.6). Pain is usually severe and may occur more than once a day. Because of the associated nasal congestion or rhinorrhea, patients are often misdiagnosed with "sinus headache" and treated with decongestants, which are ineffective. The key feature of this class of headaches is the lateralized nature of symptoms (e.g., side-locked head pain and ipsilateral cranial autonomic features).

TACs must be differentiated from short-lasting headaches that do not have prominent cranial autonomic syndromes, notably trigeminal neuralgia, primary stabbing headache, and hypnic headache. The cycling pattern and length, frequency, and timing of attacks are useful in classifying patients. Patients with TACs should undergo pituitary imaging and pituitary function tests, as there is an excess of TAC presentations in patients with pituitary tumor–related headache.

TABLE 54.6 Clinical Features of the Trigeminal Autonomic Cephalalgias

	Cluster Headache	Paroxysmal Hemicrania	SUNCT/SUNA
Gender pain	M > F	F = M	F ~ M
Type	Stabbing, boring	Throbbing, boring, stabbing	Burning, stabbing, sharp
Severity	Excruciating	Excruciating	Severe to excruciating
Site	Orbit, temple	Orbit, temple	Periorbital
Attack frequency	1/alternate day–8/day	1–20/day (>5/day for more than half the time)	3–200/day
Duration of attack	15–180 min	2–30 min	5–240 s
Autonomic features	Yes	Yes	Yes (prominent conjunctival injection and lacrimation)[a]
Migrainous features[b]	Yes	Yes	Yes
Alcohol trigger	Yes	No	No
Cutaneous triggers	No	No	Yes
Indomethacin effect	—	Yes[c]	—
Abortive treatment	Sumatriptan injection or nasal spray Oxygen	No effective treatment	Lidocaine (IV)
Prophylactic treatment	Verapamil Methysergide Lithium	Indomethacin	Lamotrigine Topiramate Gabapentin

[a]If conjunctival injection and tearing not present, consider SUNA.

[b]Nausea, photophobia, or phonophobia; photophobia and phonophobia are typically unilateral on the side of the pain.

[c]Indicates complete response to indomethacin.

SUNCT, short-lasting unilateral neuralgiform headache attacks with conjunctival injection and tearing; SUNA, short-lasting unilateral neuralgiform headache attacks with cranial autonomic features; M, male; F, female; IV, intravenous.

CLUSTER HEADACHE

CLINICAL FEATURES

Cluster headache is a rare primary headache syndrome with a population frequency of approximately 0.1%, affecting men more than women at a ratio of 3:1. The pain is deep, usually retroorbital, often excruciating in intensity, nonfluctuating, and explosive in quality. A core feature of cluster headache is periodicity. At least one of the daily attacks of pain recurs at about the same hour each day for the duration of a cluster bout. Onset is nocturnal in about 50% of patients. The typical cluster headache patient has daily bouts of one or two attacks of relatively short-duration unilateral pain for 8 to 10 weeks a year; this is usually followed by a pain-free interval that averages a little less than 1 year. Cluster headache is characterized as chronic when there is less than 1 month of sustained remission without treatment. Patients with cluster headache tend to be restless during attacks and may pace, rock, or rub their head for relief; some may even become aggressive during attacks. This is in sharp contrast to patients with migraine who prefer to remain motionless during attacks.

PATHOPHYSIOLOGY

Cluster headache is likely to be a disorder involving central pacemaker neurons in the posterior hypothalamic region, thus accounting for its periodicity. Other hallmark features of cluster headache include the ipsilateral symptoms of cranial parasympathetic autonomic activation: conjunctival injection or lacrimation, rhinorrhea or nasal congestion, or cranial sympathetic dysfunction such as ptosis. The sympathetic deficit is peripheral and likely due to parasympathetic activation with injury to ascending sympathetic fibers surrounding a dilated carotid artery as it passes into the cranial cavity. When present, photophobia and phonophobia are far more likely to be unilateral and on the same side of the pain, rather than bilateral, as is seen in migraine. This phenomenon of unilateral photophobia/phonophobia is characteristic of TACs.

TREATMENT

As with migraine, there are both abortive (acute) medications and preventive therapies that can be used during a cluster bout [**Level 1**].[40-48]

ABORTIVE TREATMENT

Cluster headache attacks peak rapidly, and thus a treatment with quick onset is required. Many patients with acute cluster headache respond very well to oxygen inhalation. This should be given as 100% oxygen at 10 to 12 L/min for 15 to 20 minutes at the onset of the attack. Sumatriptan 6 mg SC is rapid in onset and will usually shorten an attack to 10 to 15 minutes; there is no evidence of tachyphylaxis. Sumatriptan (20 mg) and zolmitriptan (5 mg) nasal sprays are also both effective in acute cluster headache. Oral sumatriptan is not effective for either prevention or acute treatment of cluster headache.

PREVENTIVE TREATMENTS

Table 54.7 summarizes commonly used treatments for the prevention of cluster headache. The choice of a preventive treatment in cluster headache depends in part on the length of the bout. Patients with long bouts or those with chronic cluster headache require medicines that are safe when taken for long periods. For patients with relatively short bouts, limited courses of oral glucocorticoids can be very useful. A 10-day course of prednisone, beginning at 60

TABLE 54.7	Preventive Management of Cluster Headache	
Short-Term Prevention	**Long-Term Prevention**
Episodic Cluster Headache	Episodic Cluster Headache and Prolonged Chronic Cluster Headache
Prednisone 1 mg/kg up to 60 mg q.d, tapering over 21 days	Verapamil 160–960 mg/day (*immediate-release formulation, divided b.i.d. or t.i.d.*)
Verapamil 160–960 mg/day	Lithium 400–800 mg/day
Greater occipital nerve injection[a]	Topiramate[b] 100–400 mg/day
	Gabapentin[b] 1,200–3,600 mg/day
	Melatonin[b] 9–12 mg/day

[a]Supported by level 1 evidence.
[b]Unproven but of potential benefit.

mg daily for 7 days and followed by a rapid taper, can also help to interrupt the cycle. Lithium (400 to 800 mg/day) appears to be particularly useful for the chronic form of the disorder.

Many experts favor verapamil as the first-line preventive treatment for patients with chronic cluster headache or prolonged bouts. Although verapamil compares favorably with lithium in practice, some patients require verapamil doses far in excess of those administered for cardiac disorders. The initial dose range is 40 to 80 mg twice daily; effective doses may be as high as 960 mg/day. Side effects include constipation and lower extremity edema. Of greater concern is the cardiovascular safety of verapamil, particularly at high doses. Verapamil can induce heart block by slowing conduction in the atrioventricular node and thus requires close monitoring of the PR interval with serial electrocardiograms (ECGs). Approximately 20% of patients treated with verapamil develop ECG abnormalities, which can occur at doses as low as 240 mg/day; these abnormalities can worsen over time in patients on stable doses. A baseline ECG is recommended for all patients. The ECG is then repeated 10 days after a dose change in those patients whose dose is being increased above 240 mg daily. Dose increases are usually made in 80-mg increments. Patients on long-term verapamil should have ECG monitoring every 6 months.

NEUROSTIMULATION THERAPY

When medical therapies fail in chronic cluster headache, neurostimulation strategies can be considered. Deep brain stimulation of the region of the posterior hypothalamic gray matter has proven successful in a substantial proportion of patients, although with its morbidity and possible mortality, it is not recommended prior to less invasive approaches. Favorable results have also been reported with the less invasive approach of occipital nerve stimulation and sphenopalatine ganglion stimulation, as well as with a noninvasive vagal nerve stimulator.

PAROXYSMAL HEMICRANIA

Paroxysmal hemicrania (PH) is characterized by unilateral, severe, short-lasting attacks (2 to 45 minutes) of head pain that are frequent (more than five times per day). Like cluster headache, the pain tends to be retroorbital but also may be experienced in other regions of the head and is associated with ipsilateral cranial autonomic phenomena such as lacrimation and nasal congestion. However, unlike cluster headache, which predominantly affects males, the male-to-female ratio in PH is close to 1:1. Episodic PH is characterized by periods of remission, whereas the nonremitting form is termed *chronic PH*. The course of PH is typically rapid (<72 hours) and is marked by an excellent response to indomethacin (25 to 75 mg t.i.d.), which can completely suppress attacks. Although therapy may be complicated by indomethacin-induced gastrointestinal side effects, currently, there are no consistently effective alternatives. Topiramate (50 to 300 mg/day) has been reported to be helpful in some cases, as has piroxicam (20 to 40 mg/day), although not to the same extent as indomethacin. Verapamil, an effective treatment for cluster headache, does not appear to be useful for PH. In occasional patients, PH can coexist with trigeminal neuralgia (PH-tic syndrome); similar to cluster-tic syndrome, each component may require separate treatment.

Secondary PH has been reported from lesions in the region of the sella turcica, including arteriovenous malformation, cavernous sinus meningioma, pituitary pathology, and epidermoid tumors. Secondary PH is more likely if the patient requires high doses (>200 mg/day) of indomethacin. In patients with apparent bilateral PH, raised cerebrospinal fluid (CSF) pressure should be suspected. It is important to note that indomethacin reduces CSF pressure. When a diagnosis of PH is considered, as with other TACs, magnetic resonance imaging (MRI) is indicated to exclude a pituitary lesion.

SUNCT/SUNA

CLINICAL FEATURES

SUNCT is a rare primary headache syndrome characterized by severe, unilateral orbital or temporal pain that is stabbing or throbbing in quality. Diagnosis requires at least 20 attacks, lasting for 5 to 240 seconds; ipsilateral conjunctival injection and lacrimation should be present. In some patients, conjunctival injection or lacrimation is missing, and the diagnosis of SUNA can be made.

The pain of SUNCT/SUNA is unilateral and may be located anywhere in the head. Three basic patterns can be seen: *single stabs*, which are usually short-lived; *groups of stabs*; or a longer attack consisting of many stabs between which the pain does not completely resolve, thus yielding a *"sawtooth" pattern* with attacks lasting many minutes. Each pattern may be seen in the context of an underlying continuous head pain. Characteristics that lead to a suspected diagnosis of SUNCT are the cutaneous (or other) triggerability of attacks, a lack of refractory period to triggering between attacks, and the lack of a response to indomethacin. Apart from trigeminal sensory disturbance, the neurologic examination is normal in primary SUNCT.

The diagnosis of SUNCT is often confused with trigeminal neuralgia (TN) particularly in first-division TN (as discussed in Chapter 55). Minimal or no cranial autonomic symptoms and a clear refractory period to triggering indicate a diagnosis of TN. Secondary SUNCT can be seen with posterior fossa or pituitary lesions. All patients with SUNCT/SUNA should be evaluated with pituitary function tests and a brain MRI with pituitary views.

TREATMENT

Abortive therapy is not practical in SUNCT/SUNA because the attacks are of such short duration. The main goal of treatment is long-term prevention to minimize disability. The most effective prophylactic medication is lamotrigine at doses of 200 to 400 mg/day. Topiramate (50 to 300 mg/day) and gabapentin (800 to 2,700 mg/day) may also be effective. Carbamazepine (400 to 600 mg/day) has been reported by some to be moderately helpful. Surgical approaches such as microvascular decompression or destructive trigeminal procedures are seldom useful and often cause long-term complications such as permanent numbness and anesthesia doloroso. Greater occipital nerve blocks may yield limited benefit in some patients. Occipital nerve stimulation is probably helpful in a subgroup of patients with SUNCT/SUNA. For intractable cases, short-term prevention with IV lidocaine, which can arrest symptoms rapidly, can be useful.

HEMICRANIA CONTINUA

The essential features of hemicrania continua are moderate and continuous unilateral pain with superimposed exacerbations of severe pain, which may be associated with cranial autonomic features and photophobia/phonophobia on the affected side. The age of onset ranges from 11 to 58 years; women are affected twice as often as men. The cause is unknown, although as with other TAC syndromes, pituitary pathology has been associated with HC.

As with PH, definitive treatment is indomethacin (25 to 75 mg t.i.d.); other NSAIDs appear to be of little or no benefit. Indomethacin should be initiated at 25 mg PO t.i.d., then increased to 50 mg t.i.d. if no effect, and further to 75 mg t.i.d. if needed. Up to 2 weeks at the maximal dose may be necessary to assess whether a dose has a useful effect. Topiramate can be helpful in some patients, as can greater occipital nerve blocks. Occipital nerve stimulation probably has a role in patients with hemicrania continua who are unable to tolerate indomethacin.

OTHER PRIMARY HEADACHES

PRIMARY COUGH HEADACHE

Primary cough headache is a generalized headache that begins suddenly, lasts for several minutes, sometimes up to a few hours, and is precipitated by coughing; it is preventable by avoiding coughing or other precipitating events, which can include sneezing, straining, laughing, or stooping. In all patients with this syndrome, serious etiologies must be excluded before a diagnosis of "benign" primary cough headache can be established (as discussed earlier in this chapter and also in Chapter 7). Benign cough headache can resemble benign exertional headache (in the following text), but patients with the former condition are typically older.

Indomethacin 25 to 50 mg two to three times daily is the treatment of choice. Some patients with cough headache obtain complete cessation of their attacks with lumbar puncture; this is a simple option when compared to prolonged use of indomethacin, and it is effective in about one-third of patients. The mechanism of this response is unclear.

PRIMARY EXERTIONAL HEADACHE

Primary exertional headache (PEH) has features resembling both cough headache and migraine. It may be precipitated by any form of exercise and often has the pulsatile quality of migraine. The pain, which can last from 5 minutes to 24 hours, is bilateral and throbbing at onset; migrainous features may develop in patients susceptible to migraine. When seen, it tends to be shorter in adolescents. PEH can be prevented by avoiding excessive exertion, particularly in hot weather or at high altitude.

The mechanism of PEH is unclear. Acute venous distension may account for the acute onset of headache with straining and breath holding. As with primary cough headache, serious underlying conditions must be excluded. Pain from angina may be referred to the head, probably by central connections of vagal afferents, and may present as exertional headache (cardiac cephalgia) upon exercising. Other potential causes include pheochromocytoma, intracranial lesions, and carotid artery stenosis.

Treatment for benign PEH includes indomethacin (25 to 150 mg/day) and modification of one's exercise regimen. Propranolol may also provide prophylactic benefit. Indomethacin (50 mg), ergotamine (1 mg orally), or dihydroergotamine (2 mg intranasally) taken 30 to 45 minutes before exercise can be helpful as prophylaxis.

PRIMARY HEADACHE ASSOCIATED WITH SEXUAL ACTIVITY

The pain of primary sex headache usually begins as a dull, bilateral headache that suddenly becomes intense at orgasm. The headache can be prevented or eased by ceasing sexual activity before orgasm. Three types of sex headache are reported: a dull ache in the head and neck that intensifies as sexual excitement increases; a sudden, severe, explosive headache occurring at orgasm; and a postural headache developing after coitus that resembles the headache of low CSF pressure. The latter arises from vigorous sexual activity and is a form of low CSF pressure headache. Headaches developing at the time of orgasm are not always benign; 5% to 12% of cases of subarachnoid hemorrhage are precipitated by sexual intercourse. Sex headache is reported by men more often than women and may occur at any time during the years of sexual activity. It may develop on several occasions in succession and then disappear, even without an obvious change in sexual activity. In patients who stop sexual activity when headache is first noticed, the pain may subside within a period of 5 minutes to 2 hours. In about half of patients, sex headache will self-remit within 6 months. About half of patients with sex headache have a history of exertional headaches, and comorbid migraine is also more likely in this population.

Treatment includes reassurance (once serious causes have been excluded) and advising patients to cease sexual activity if a "warning" headache develops. If the headache occurs regularly, propranolol can be used for prevention (40 to 200 mg/day) or alternatively diltiazem (60 mg t.i.d.). Ergotamine (1 mg) or indomethacin (25 to 50 mg) taken about 30 to 45 minutes prior to sexual activity can also be helpful.

PRIMARY STABBING HEADACHE

Primary stabbing headache (PSH) is characterized by stab-like pains in the head or, rarely, the face, lasting from one to many seconds or minutes and occurring as a single stab or a series of stabs, absence of associated cranial autonomic features, absence of cutaneous triggering of attacks, and a pattern of recurrence at irregular intervals (hours to days). The pains have been variously described as *ice pick pains* or *jabs and jolts* and are more common in patients with other primary headaches, such as migraine and the TACs. If pain is frequent, indomethacin (25 to 50 mg b.i.d. or t.i.d.) can be used for prophylaxis.

NUMMULAR HEADACHE

The pain in nummular headache is localized to a round or elliptical focus that is fixed in place, ranging in size from 1 to 6 cm and may be continuous or intermittent. In rare cases, it may be multifocal. Nummular headache is usually continuous with exacerbations, although can be episodic. There may be focal sensory disturbances, such as allodynia or hypesthesia. The pathophysiology is unknown, although a focal neuropathic disorder has been suggested. Local dermatologic or bony lesions must be excluded by examination and investigation. Treatment includes tricyclics, such as amitriptyline, or anticonvulsants, such as topiramate, valproate, or gabapentin; however, the condition may be difficult to treat.

HYPNIC HEADACHE

Hypnic headache is marked by occurrence after a few hours following sleep onset. The headache lasts from 15 to 30 minutes and is typically generalized and moderate in severity, although can also be unilateral and throbbing. Photophobia or phonophobia and nausea are usually absent. Attacks can occur up to three times throughout the night, and daytime naps can also precipitate head pain. Most patients are female, and the onset is usually after age of 60 years. The major secondary consideration in this headache type is poorly controlled hypertension; 24-hour blood pressure monitoring is recommended in such cases.

Patients with hypnic headache usually respond to lithium carbonate (200 to 600 mg nightly). For those intolerant of lithium, verapamil (160 mg) or indomethacin (25 to 75 mg) may be tried. One to two cups of coffee or oral caffeine (60 to 100 mg) at bedtime may be effective in approximately one-third of patients. Case reports suggest that melatonin and flunarizine (5 mg nightly) can also be helpful.

NEW DAILY PERSISTENT HEADACHE

New daily persistent headache (NDPH) is a clinically distinct syndrome, characterized by daily headache from onset for at least 3 months. The patient with NDPH can clearly recall the exact date and moment of onset. The headache usually begins abruptly, although onset may be more gradual in some cases; evolution over 3 days has been proposed as the upper limit for this syndrome. Antecedent illness (such as an upper respiratory infection or viral prodrome) has been reported in about one-third of patients with NDPH in one series. However, often there is no remarkable triggering event. The first priority is to distinguish between a primary and a secondary cause of this syndrome. Subarachnoid hemorrhage is the most serious of the secondary causes and must be excluded either by history or appropriate investigation. Other causes include chronic meningitis, as well as abnormalities of CSF pressure (see Chapter 7).

Primary NDPH can be of the migrainous type or can be appear featureless, appearing as new-onset TTH. Migrainous features are common and include unilateral headache and throbbing pain; nausea, photophobia, and/or phonophobia occur in about half of patients. Some patients have a previous history of episodic migraine. Treatment of migrainous-type primary NDPH consists of using standard migraine preventive therapies (see earlier discussion). Featureless NDPH tends to be most refractory to treatment—although conventional headache preventive therapies (such as tricyclic antidepressants and anticonvulsants) can be offered, most are ineffective.

POSTTRAUMATIC HEADACHE

A traumatic event can trigger a headache process that lasts for many months or years after the event. The term *trauma* is used here very broadly: Headache can develop following an injury to the head (including after neurosurgical; dental; or ear, nose, and throat procedures), but it can also develop after an infectious episode such as with viral meningitis or a flulike illness. The underlying theme appears to be that a traumatic event involving the pain-producing meninges can trigger a headache process that lasts for many years. Complaints of dizziness, vertigo, and impaired memory can accompany the headache. Symptoms may remit after several weeks or persist for months and even years after the injury. Typically, the neurologic examination is normal and CT or MRI studies are unrevealing. However, serious underlying causes must be ruled out, such as chronic subdural hematoma, subarachnoid hemorrhage, and carotid dissection.

LEVEL 1 EVIDENCE

1. Silberstein SD. Practice parameter: evidence-based guidelines for migraine headache (an evidence-based review): report of the Quality Standards Subcommittee of the American Academy of Neurology. *Neurology.* 2000;55:754–762.

2. Kloster R, Nestvold K, Vilming ST. A double-blind study of ibuprofen versus placebo in the treatment of acute migraine attacks. *Cephalalgia.* 1992;12:169–171; discussion 128.

3. Johnson ES, Ratcliffe DM, Wilkinson M. Naproxen sodium in the treatment of migraine. *Cephalalgia.* 1985;5:5–10.

4. Lipton RB, Grosberg B, Singer RP, et al. Efficacy and tolerability of a new powdered formulation of diclofenac potassium for oral solution for the acute treatment of migraine: results from the International Migraine Pain Assessment Clinical Trial (IMPACT). *Cephalalgia.* 2010;30(11):1336–1345.

5. Tokola RA, Kangasniemi P, Neuvonen PJ, et al. Tolfenamic acid, metoclopramide, caffeine and their combinations in the treatment of migraine attacks. *Cephalalgia.* 1984;4:253–263.

6. Lipton RB, Stewart WF, Ryan RE Jr, et al. Efficacy and safety of acetaminophen, aspirin, and caffeine in alleviating migraine headache pain: three double-blind, randomized, placebo-controlled trials. *Arch Neurol.* 1998;55:210–217.

7. Thorlund K, Mills EJ, Wu P, et al. Comparative efficacy of triptans for the abortive treatment of migraine: a multiple treatment comparison meta-analysis. *Cephalalgia.* 2014;34(4):258–267.

8. Ferrari MD, Roon KI, Lipton RB, et al. Oral triptans (serotonin 5-HT(1B/1D) agonists) in acute migraine treatment: a meta-analysis of 53 trials. *Lancet.* 2001;358(9294):1668–1675.

9. Tfelt-Hansen P, De Vries P, Saxena PR. Triptans in migraine: a comparative review of pharmacology, pharmacokinetics, and efficacy. *Drugs.* 2000;60(6):1259–1287.

10. Silberstein SD, Elkind AH, Schreiber C, et al. A randomized trial of frovatriptan for the intermittent prevention of menstrual migraine. *Neurology.* 2004;63:261–269.

11. Brandes JL, Poole A, Kallela M, et al. Short-term frovatriptan for the prevention of difficult-to-treat menstrual migraine attacks. *Cephalalgia.* 2009;29:1133–1148.

12. Dihydroergotamine Nasal Spray Multicenter Investigators. Efficacy, safety, and tolerability of dihydroergotamine nasal spray as monotherapy in the treatment of acute migraine. *Headache.* 1995;35:177–184.

13. Callaham M, Raskin N. A controlled study of dihydroergotamine in the treatment of acute migraine headache. *Headache.* 1986;26:168–171.

14. Colman I, Brown MD, Innes GD, et al. Parenteral metoclopramide for acute migraine: meta-analysis of randomised controlled trials. *BMJ.* 2004;329(7479):1369–1373.

15. Kelly AM, Walcynski T, Gunn B. The relative efficacy of phenothiazines for the treatment of acute migraine: a meta-analysis. *Headache.* 2009;49(9):1324–1332.

16. Bigal ME, Bordini CA, Speciali JG. Intravenous chlorpromazine in the emergency department treatment of migraines: a randomized controlled trial. *J Emerg Med.* 2002;23(2):141–148.

17. Silberstein S, Holland S, Freitag F, et al. Evidence-based guideline update: pharmacologic treatment for episodic migraine prevention in adults: report of the Quality Standards Subcommittee of the American Academy of Neurology and the American Headache Society. *Neurology.* 2012;78:1337–1345.

18. Holland S, Silberstein S, Freitag F, et al. Evidence-based guideline update: NSAIDs and other complementary treatments for episodic migraine prevention in adults: report of the Quality Standards Subcommittee of the American Academy of Neurology and the American Headache Society. *Neurology.* 2012;78:1346–1353.

19. Borgesen SE, Nielsen JL, Moller CE. Prophylactic treatment of migraine with propranolol. A clinical trial. *Acta Neurol Scand.* 1974;50:651–656.

20. Forssman B, Henriksson KG, Johannsson V, et al. Propranolol for migraine prophylaxis. *Headache.* 1976;16:238–245.

21. Pradalier A, Serratrice G, Collard M, et al. Long-acting propranolol in migraine prophylaxis: results of a double-blind, placebo-controlled study. *Cephalalgia.* 1989;9:247–253.

22. Tfelt-Hansen P, Standnes B, Kangasneimi P, et al. Timolol vs propranolol vs placebo in common migraine prophylaxis: a double-blind multicenter trial. *Acta Neurol Scand.* 1984;69:1–8.

23. Briggs RS, Millac PA. Timolol in migraine prophylaxis. *Headache.* 1979;19:379–381.

24. Stellar S, Ahrens SP, Meibohm AR, et al. Migraine prevention with timolol. A double-blind crossover study. *JAMA.* 1984;252:2576–2580.

25. Andersson PG, Dahl S, Hansen JH, et al. Prophylactic treatment of classical and non-classical migraine with metoprolol—a comparison with placebo. *Cephalalgia.* 1983;3:207–212.

26. Kangasniemi P, Andersen AR, Andersson PG, et al. Classic migraine: effective prophylaxis with metoprolol. *Cephalalgia.* 1987;7:231–238.

27. Steiner TJ, Joseph R, Hedman C, et al. Metoprolol in the prophylaxis of migraine: parallel-groups comparison with placebo and dose-ranging follow-up. *Headache.* 1988;28:15–23.

28. Diener HC, Bussone G, Van Oene JC, et al. Topiramate reduces headache days in chronic migraine: a randomized, double-blind, placebo-controlled study. *Cephalalgia.* 2007;27:814–823.

29. Storey JR, Calder CS, Hart DE, et al. Topiramate in migraine prevention: a double-blind, placebo-controlled study. *Headache.* 2001;41:968–975.

30. Brandes JL, Saper JR, Diamond M, et al; MIGR-002 Study Group. Topiramate for migraine prevention: a randomized controlled trial. *JAMA.* 2004;291:965–973.

31. Mei D, Capuano A, Vollono C, et al. Topiramate in migraine prophylaxis: a randomised double-blind versus placebo study. *Neurol Sci.* 2004;25:245–250.

32. Silberstein SD, Neto W, Schmitt J, et al; MIGR-001 Study Group. Topiramate in migraine prevention: results of a large controlled trial. *Arch Neurol.* 2004;61:490–495.

33. Freitag FG, Collins SD, Carlson HA, et al. A randomized trial of divalproex sodium extended-release tablets in migraine prophylaxis. *Neurology.* 2002;58:1652–1659.

34. Ozyalcin SN, Talu GK, Kiziltan E, et al. The efficacy and safety of venlafaxine in the prophylaxis of migraine. *Headache.* 2005;45:144–152.

35. Diener HC, Dodick DW, Aurora SK, et al. Onabotulinum-toxinA for treatment of chronic migraine: results from the double-blind, randomized, placebo-controlled phase of the PREEMPT 2 trial. *Cephalalgia*. 2010;30:804–814.
36. Aurora SK, Dodick DW, Turkel CC, et al. Onabotulinum-toxinA for treatment of chronic migraine. Results from the double-blind, randomized, placebo-controlled phase of the PREEMPT 1 trial. *Cephalalgia*. 2010;30:793–803.
37. Dodick DW, Turkel CC, DeGryse RE, et al. Onabotulinum-toxinA for treatment of chronic migraine: pooled results from the double-blind, randomized, placebo-controlled phases of the PREEMPT clinical program. *Headache*. 2010;50:921–936.
38. Lipton RB, Göbel H, Einhäupl KM, et al. Petasites hybridus root (butterbur) is an effective preventive treatment for migraine. *Neurology*. 2004;63:2240–2244.
39. Maizels M, Blumenfeld A, Burchette R. A combination of riboflavin, magnesium, and feverfew for migraine prophylaxis: a randomized trial. *Headache*. 2004;44:885–890.
40. Ekbom K, Monstad I, Prusinski A, et al. Subcutaneous sumatriptan in the acute treatment of cluster headache: a dose comparison study. *Acta Neurol Scand*. 1993;88:63–69.
41. The Sumatriptan Cluster Headache Study Group. Treatment of acute cluster headache with sumatriptan. *N Engl J Med*. 1991;325:322–326.
42. van Vliet JA, Bahra A, Martin V, et al. Intranasal sumatriptan in cluster headache. *Neurology*. 2003;60:630–633.
43. Rapoport AM, Mathew NT, Silberstein SD, et al. Zolmitriptan nasal spray in the acute treatment of cluster headache. *Neurology*. 2007;69:821–826.
44. Cittadini E, May A, Straube A, et al. Effectiveness of intranasal zolmitriptan in acute cluster headache. *Arch Neurol*. 2006;63:1537–1542.
45. Bahra A, Gawel MJ, Hardebo JE, et al. Oral zolmitriptan is effective in the acute treatment of cluster headache. *Neurology*. 2000;54:1832–1839.
46. Fogan L. Treatment of cluster headache: a double blind comparison of oxygen v. air inhalation. *Arch Neurol*. 1985;42:362–363.
47. Cohen A, Burns B, Goadsby P. High flow oxygen for treatment of cluster headache. *JAMA*. 2009;302:2451–2457.
48. Ambrosini A, Vandenheede M, Rossi P, et al. Suboccipital injection with a mixture of rapid and long-acting steroids in cluster headache: a double-blind placebo-controlled study. *Pain*. 2005;118:92–96.

SUGGESTED READINGS

Akerman S, Holland P, Goadsby PJ. Diencephalic and brainstem mechanisms in migraine. *Nat Rev Neurosci*. 2011;12:570–584.

Cittadini E, Goadsby PJ. Hemicrania continua: a clinical study of 39 patients with diagnostic implications. *Brain*. 2010;133:1973–1986.

Cittadini E, Matharu MS, Goadsby PJ. Paroxysmal hemicrania: a prospective clinical study of 31 cases. *Brain*. 2008;131:1142–1155.

Cohen AS, Matharu MS, Goadsby PJ. Short-lasting unilateral neuralgiform headache attacks with conjunctival injection and tearing (SUNCT) or cranial autonomic features (SUNA). A prospective clinical study of SUNCT and SUNA. *Brain*. 2006;129:2746–2760.

Goadsby PJ. Therapeutic prospects for migraine: can paradise be regained? *Ann Neurol*. 2013;74:423–434.

Goadsby PJ, Dodick D, Silberstein SD. *Chronic Daily Headache for Clinicians*. Hamilton, Canada: BC Decker; 2005.

Headache Classification Committee of the International Headache Society. The International Classification of Headache Disorders, 3rd edition (beta version). *Cephalalgia*. 2013;33:629–808.

Lance JW, Goadsby PJ. *Mechanism and Management of Headache*. 7th ed. New York: Elsevier; 2005.

Lipton RB, Bigal M. *Migraine and Other Headache Disorders*. New York: Marcel Dekker, Taylor & Francis Books; 2006.

Lipton RB, Bigal ME, Diamond M, et al. Migraine prevalence, disease burden, and the need for preventive therapy. *Neurology*. 2007;68:343–349.

Maniyar FH, Sprenger T, Monteith T, et al. Brain activations in the premonitory phase of nitroglycerin triggered migraine attacks. *Brain*. 2014;137:232–241.

Murray CJ, Vos T, Lozano R, et al. Disability-adjusted life years (DALYs) for 291 diseases and injuries in 21 regions, 1990-2010: a systematic analysis for the Global Burden of Disease Study 2010. *Lancet*. 2012;380:2197–2223.

Olesen J, Tfelt-Hansen P, Ramadan N, et al. *The Headaches*. Philadelphia: Lippincott Williams & Wilkins; 2005.CLUSTER HEADACHE

Cranial Neuralgias and Facial Pain Disorders 55

Marianna Shnayderman Yugrakh and Denise E. Chou

INTRODUCTION

Facial pain can originate from various facial structures and includes pain due to disorders of the sinuses, ears, and nose, temporomandibular disorders (TMD), dental and oral pathologies, and various ophthalmologic problems, all of which can activate nociceptive pathways via infection, inflammation, trauma, or malignancy. Primary nervous system disorders causing facial pain span the breadth of the neuraxis and include cranial neuralgias, small fiber neuropathies, primary headache disorders, and central pain disorders involving the spinothalamocortical system. Facial pain may be perceived away from a region of pathology (referred pain) due to the complex sensory innervation of the face (including cranial nerves V, VII, IX, and X, with overlapping innervation of the ear), dural innervation from branches of the trigeminal and vagus nerves, as well as proximity of the spinal trigeminal nucleus to upper cervical afferent pathways. Sensory input convergence in the spinal trigeminal nucleus is one of the mechanisms of referred pain. Table 55.1 highlights etiologies of facial pain including the peripheral nervous system and the tissues innervated. Primary pain syndromes can be recognized and treated only after a workup for secondary etiologies. The general principle for the diagnosis of secondary facial pain disorders, based on the *International Classification of Headache Disorders*, 3rd edition (*ICHD-3*), is establishment of a causal relationship between pain and a disorder of facial or cranial structures with respect to chronology, congruous exacerbation, and improvement in symptoms, and signs of the primary pathology evoking pain on physical examination.

FACIAL PAIN DUE TO DISORDERS OF SINUSES, EARS, AND NOSE

RHINOSINUSITIS

Epidemiology and Pathobiology

Rhinitis and sinusitis are not uncommon causes of facial pain and may exacerbate a primary headache disorder. However, the term *sinus headache* is frequently misused to describe facial and head pain (which in actuality is most often migraine) incorrectly denoting that underlying sinus pathology is the etiology of pain. This attribution of head and facial pain to sinus pathology may have two causes: (1) migraine is a disorder associated with increased parasympathetic outflow with nasal congestion and lacrimation, and (2) the causality between headache and inflammatory changes in the nasal sinuses is difficult to establish, as the latter is highly prevalent and can be asymptomatic. Nasal mucosal changes (particularly in the ethmoid and maxillary sinuses), which may be signs of acute or chronic rhinosinusitis, can be identified in almost 50% of adults who undergo magnetic resonance imaging (MRI) testing for suspected intracranial disease. Although acute rhinosinusitis has long been considered a cause of facial and head pain, only the 3rd edition of the *ICHD* from 2013 has included chronic rhinosinusitis

as a potential etiology. This revision was based on findings from recent studies, such as the American Migraine Prevalence and Prevention (AMPP) study, which reported that patients with chronic rhinitis were one-fourth more likely to be of higher headache frequency categories.

Nasal and sinus mucosa are innervated by the first and second divisions of the trigeminal nerve. The first division innervates the frontal and anterior ethmoid sinuses, whereas the second carries nociceptive signals from the maxillary, sphenoid, and posterior ethmoid sinuses. Infectious or allergic triggers result in release of inflammatory mediators that activate nociceptive neurons in the spinal trigeminal nucleus, signaling local facial pain and additionally may produce referred head pain. More frequent or persistent referred pain may result from peripheral and central sensitization of the trigeminal system.

Clinical Manifestations and Diagnosis

Acute rhinosinusitis symptoms include rhinorrhea and purulence, fever, hyposmia, halitosis, and symptoms akin to an upper respiratory tract infection. Acute sinusitis pain can be localized, described as deep pressure, congestion, or fullness felt in the face and teeth, and is often exacerbated by lying down. Pain may be facial but can also be referred posteriorly. Frontal sinusitis pain is typically behind the eyes and around the center of the forehead, with the frontal region being sensitive to percussion and associated with supraorbital nerve sensitivity. In ethmoid sinusitis, pain is also retroorbital and may radiate to the temples, with eye sensitivity to pressure. Maxillary sinusitis pain is appreciated over the cheeks, but can radiate to the ear or teeth, with sensitivity of teeth to percussion. Isolated sphenoid sinusitis is a relatively rare, serious disorder with the potential complication of cavernous sinus thrombophlebitis. It most commonly presents with refractory nonlocalizing headache, followed by visual complaints and cranial nerve palsies. Because of its deep location, tenderness on exam is not appreciable. Computed tomography (CT), MRI, or endoscopic techniques allow for the diagnosis.

ICHD-3 diagnostic criteria for headache or facial pain attributed to acute rhinosinusitis requires clinical, nasal endoscopic, and/or imaging evidence of acute rhinosinusitis, and two of the following: (1) establishment of a temporal relation of pain to onset of rhinosinusitis, (2) either improvement or worsening of pain symptoms paralleling improvement or worsening of rhinosinusitis symptoms, (3) pain exacerbated by pressure applied over the paranasal sinuses, and (4) pain localized ipsilateral in the case of unilateral rhinosinusitis. Headache or facial pain attributed to chronic rhinosinusitis is diagnosed based on evidence of current or past infection, and evidence of causation as discussed earlier.

Treatment and Outcome

Infectious rhinosinusitis may be treated with antibiotics, depending on patient risk profile for bacterial infection. Facial pressure and pain caused by inferior and middle nasal turbinate congestion can

TABLE 55.1   Etiologies of Facial Pain Including the Peripheral Nervous System and Tissues Innervated

Nerve and Sensory Distribution	Primary PNS Disorders	Disorders Outside of the Nervous System	
Trigeminal nerve, ophthalmic division	Classical TN (idiopathic or with vascular loop) Painful trigeminal neuropathies: • Symptomatic TN (tumor, vascular malformation, multiple sclerosis plaque at dorsal root entry zone) • Herpes zoster ophthalmicus and postherpetic trigeminal neuropathy • Posttraumatic (anesthesia dolorosa) Paratrigeminal oculosympathetic syndrome (Raeder syndrome)	Eyes[a]:	acute angle-closure glaucoma, iritis, uveitis, scleritis, conjunctivitis, trochleitis
		Sinuses (frontal and anterior ethmoid):	acute rhinosinusitis, septal deflections, hypertrophic turbinates, nasal spurs
		Arteries:	giant cell arteritis (temporal arteritis)
Trigeminal nerve, maxillary division	Classical TN Painful trigeminal neuropathies: • Symptomatic TN • Acute herpes zoster and postherpetic trigeminal neuropathy • Posttraumatic (anesthesia dolorosa)	Maxillary teeth:	pulpitis, cracked tooth syndrome, dentine sensitivity, dental abscess
		Oral cavity:	mucosal malignancies, infections, inflammation, blockage of a major salivary gland duct
		Sinuses (maxillary, sphenoid, posterior ethmoid):	acute rhinosinusitis, chronic rhinosinusitis
Trigeminal nerve, mandibular division	Classical TN Painful trigeminal neuropathies: • Symptomatic TN • Acute herpes zoster and postherpetic trigeminal neuropathy • Posttraumatic (anesthesia dolorosa) Auriculotemporal syndrome (Frey syndrome) Burning mouth syndrome	Mandibular teeth, oral cavity, tongue:	as per maxillary teeth and oral cavity
		Temporomandibular joint:	temporomandibular disorders: arthritic and degenerative joint disease, disk displacement, myalgia and myofascial pain
		External auditory meatus, anterior pinna:	laceration and tumors of pinna: external otitis, foreign bodies, squamous cell and basal cell carcinomas, adenocarcinoma
		Arteries:	giant cell arteritis (temporal arteritis)
Facial nerve, nervus intermedius branch	Nervus intermedius neuralgia Trigeminal neuropathies: • Herpes zoster (Ramsey-Hunt syndrome) and postherpetic neuralgia Acoustic neuroma	Mastoid cells and skin overlying the mastoid process:	otitis media, mastoiditis
		External auditory meatus, lateral pinna:	external otitis, foreign bodies, local tumors
		Nasopharynx, palate:	local/infiltrative tumors, inflammation

(continued)

TABLE 55.1	Etiologies of Facial Pain Including the Peripheral Nervous System and Tissues Innervated (continued)		
Nerve and Sensory Distribution	**Primary PNS Disorders**	**Disorders Outside of the Nervous System**	
Glossopharyngeal nerve and vagal nerve	Glossovagopharyngeal neuralgia Nerve compression by elongated styloid process (Eagle syndrome)	External ear canal and tympanic membrane: Upper pharynx, posterior tonsils, base of tongue, soft palate:	external otitis, foreign bodies, squamous cell and basal cell carcinomas, adenocarcinoma, tympanic membrane perforation local tumors, inflammation, infection

Pain in a specific distribution should warrant consideration of the various etiologies listed in addition to consideration of central nervous system causes.
[a]Eye pain without ophthalmoplegia.
PNS, peripheral nervous system; TN, trigeminal neuralgia.

be relieved with a nasal corticosteroid spray, such as mometasone furoate, or systemic decongestants. Allergic rhinitis treatment involves identifying the allergens and desensitization, or antihistamine use during seasonal episodes, and topical steroids. If aggressive medical therapy fails, surgical approaches targeting nasal anatomic abnormalities predisposing recurrent infection may be considered.

FACIAL PAIN ATTRIBUTED TO DISORDERS OF THE NOSE AND MUCOSAL CONTACT POINTS

Other conditions that may cause facial pain and headache include nasal passage abnormalities due to septal deflections, hypertrophic turbinates, and nasal septal spurs. Mucosal contact points are defined as two structures in the nasal cavity that remain in contact after decongestion therapy, and have been cited as an etiology of facial pain; several surgical outcomes series indicate that patients obtain relief from headache and facial pain after endoscopic endonasal surgery. On the other hand, a large cohort study of consecutive patients in a rhinology clinic identified equal prevalence of nasal mucosal contact points in patients with and without facial pain, and yet another study found presence of contact points on CT imaging in 55% of patients without correlation to facial or head pain, both suggesting that their coexistence is coincidental. The causality of mucosal contact points and facial pain requires further investigation.

OTALGIA ATTRIBUTED TO DISORDER OF EARS AND REFERRED PAIN

Otalgia is diagnosed based on the identification of a primary ear disorder and evidence of causation. Ear pain can be dull, aching, or stabbing; may radiate to the temples; and may be associated with ear fullness, tenderness, burning, or itching. Primary disorders of the ear by compartment are listed in Table 55.1. About half of all earaches are due to structural lesions of the external or middle ear; the rest are due to referred pain from remote structures. This is due to overlapping sensory innervation in this small region: branches of the mandibular division of V and branches of C2 and C3 to the pinna; mandibular division branches of V as well as VII, IX, and X branches to the external auditory canal and the tympanic mem-

brane; and branches of VII to the middle ear. Etiologies of referred otalgia are also summarized in Table 55.1.

FACIAL PAIN DUE TO TEMPOROMANDIBULAR DISORDERS AND DISORDERS OF THE TEETH OR MOUTH

Dental pain, frequently poorly localized, has several major causes as summarized in Table 55.1. Nondental intraoral pain can be secondary to oral mucosa malignancies, inflammatory and infectious disorders, or blockage of a major salivary gland duct with pain that is predominantly preprandial. Periodontal disorders involve bone and periodontal ligament; these are associated with clearly localized pain and are typically managed with conventional dental treatments. Atypical odontalgia, or posttraumatic trigeminal neuropathic pain that is localized to an area where a tooth has previously been extracted, is a subtype of persistent idiopathic facial pain discussed later in the chapter.

TEMPOROMANDIBULAR JOINT DISORDERS (TMD)
Epidemiology and Pathobiology

TMDs encompass pathologies related to the joint and/or to the muscles and constitute one of the most common causes of orofacial pain, affecting 10% to 15% of the population. The temporomandibular joint (TMJ) is composed of an upper and lower compartment separated by a fibrocartilaginous disk allowing rotary and translational movement of the mandible. Dysfunction may be secondary to trauma, changes in occlusion, and behavioral influences including clenching and grinding of the teeth. Other risk factors include asymmetry in joints, poor posture causing muscle strain, and female gender. Joint disorders associated with pain include arthritis, degenerative disk disease, and joint dysfunction such as disk–condyle incoordination or articular disk displacement. Pain is mediated via the pain-sensitive joint capsule and posterior disk attachment, with nociceptive signals transmitted via the mandibular branch of the trigeminal nerve. The pathophysiology of primary muscle pain, including myalgia and myofascial pain with referral is poorly understood.

Pressure on tender trigger points, or nodular bands under the skin in muscles, tendons, or fascia, can cause pain locally or in other parts of the body via referral patterns. Initial muscle aggravation may be associated with oral habits or postural abnormalities.

Clinical Manifestations and Diagnosis

Common symptoms of TMD, in addition to jaw pain, include discomfort with biting or chewing, clicking or popping sounds when opening or closing the mouth, markedly limited mouth opening (<40 mm) if a disk becomes permanently displaced relative to the joint, and crepitus with mandibular movements in degenerative joint disease. MRI is the gold standard for imaging soft tissues and disk position, whereas CT can identify degenerative changes. The evidence-based diagnostic protocol and classification system for TMD, updated in 2014, combines clinical and radiologic findings. Pain originating in the TMJ may be aching, throbbing, sharp, or a tightening sensation, present at rest or provoked with movement in the ramus of the mandible, temporal area, and pre- and postauricular areas. Myofascial pain is described as dull or achy, associated with the presence of trigger points which may involve the masseters or temporalis muscles directly or refer pain to the preauricular area, temporal region, ear, or head. Facial pain or headache secondary to TMD is diagnosed based on evidence of causation including temporal relationship of pain to the disorder, exacerbation of pain by movement or pressure on the joint or muscles, and same laterality.

Treatment and Outcome

Temporomandibular disorders are usually self-limiting and few require therapeutic interventions. Management includes patient education about avoiding clenching behaviors and chewy foods, performing jaw stretching exercises, progressive relaxation, and biofeedback. Physical therapy for posture training and joint mobility, as well as stabilization devices and anterior positioning appliances can reduce TMD-related pain. Nonsteroidal anti-inflammatory drugs, particularly naproxen [**Level 1**],[1] and muscle relaxants are first-line pharmacologic treatments, followed by tricyclic antidepressants, which have been used extensively for chronic musculoskeletal pain and facial pain as well as high-dose gabapentin, around 3,400 mg/day [**Level 1**].[2]

TRIGEMINAL AND OTHER CRANIAL NEURALGIAS

Compression or traction on several cranial nerves by a structural lesion may lead to paroxysms of stabbing pain in the innervated region, or *neuralgia*. In trigeminal neuralgia, the most common of the neuralgias, the majority of cases involve lesions affecting the dorsal root entry zone without compromising the function of the nerve. In this region, myelin is generated by astrocytes, rather than Schwann cells, and is more vulnerable to compression than the nerve in its more peripheral course, suggesting susceptibility to ephaptic transmission with crossed modality activation, or allodynia, and hyperexcitability. In some cases, an underlying vascular loop can be identified on imaging or intraoperatively as a cause of compression. In other cases, bilateral vascular loops are incidentally identified in symptomatic patients or in up to 8% of asymptomatic patients who obtain imaging for other reasons, making it difficult to determine if the neuralgia is primary or secondary. For this reason, the *ICHD-3* and current literature use the terms *classical neuralgia* to diagnose the syndrome where a structural lesion such as a vascular loop may exist but has not been identified yet, and *symptomatic neuralgia* or *painful neuropathy* for the syndrome with an identified lesion other than vascular loops.

TRIGEMINAL NEURALGIA
Epidemiology and Pathobiology

Classical trigeminal neuralgia (TN) is characterized by severe, lancinating pain strictly limited to the distribution of one or more divisions of the trigeminal nerve. There is typically a refractory period up to minutes, during which usual triggers cannot provoke another attack. TN is relatively rare, with a prevalence of 0.07% to 0.3%. It is more common among individuals older than 60 years of age, with a female-to-male ratio of approximately 2:1. Classical TN is idiopathic or caused by compression or stretching of the nerve roots by arteries (particularly the superior cerebellar artery) or veins. Tumors, including meningiomas and neuromas, cysts, and vascular malformations can produce identical symptoms if there is only distention of the trigeminal roots without invasion.

Although pain is typically discrete during bouts, a period of days to years of atypical continuous pain termed *pretrigeminal neuralgia* as well as background pain between attacks have been reported. Trigeminal neuralgia with concomitant persistent facial pain is often referred to as *atypical TN* or *TN type 2*, and central sensitization is thought to account for the interictal pain. In this variant, neurovascular compression is less likely to be identified.

Clinical Manifestations and Diagnosis

The pain of TN is severe in intensity, electrical shock–like or stabbing in quality, and lasts seconds to a few minutes but can become prolonged over time. Although not every attack need be provoked, at least three should be precipitated to meet diagnostic criteria for typical TN. Mechanical stimulation in the trigeminal distributions (or trigger zones) may set off pain, including otherwise innocuous stimuli such as breeze or wind, brushing teeth, chewing, and combing hair. Diagnosis requires that the pain be limited to one or more divisions of the trigeminal nerve, typically unilateral, with no radiation beyond the trigeminal distribution. Mild ipsilateral parasympathetic symptoms including facial flushing, lacrimation, and conjunctival injection may also accompany the pain.

The differential for TN includes short-lasting unilateral neuralgiform headache attacks with conjunctival injection and tearing (SUNCT) or short-lasting unilateral neuralgiform headache attacks with cranial autonomic symptoms (SUNA) syndrome (discussed previously in Chapter 54). Although attacks in TN and SUNCT/SUNA have phenotypic overlap, including trigger areas, length, and quality of pain, the two conditions can be distinguished by a refractory period (present in TN and often absent in SUNCT/SUNA), extent of associated cranial autonomic features (prominent in SUNCT/SUNA and less so in TN), and treatment response (described in the following text). It is crucial to differentiate these syndromes in order to institute appropriate first-line medical therapy early and to avoid unnecessary surgical interventions for vascular abnormalities that may be incidentally identified in patients with a SUNCT or SUNA phenotypes, although a few cases of successful microvascular decompression have been described. Functional MRI may also be of diagnostic use, as ipsilateral hypothalamic activation may be seen in SUNCT and not in TN.

The presence of bilateral symptoms and trigeminal sensory deficits may suggest symptomatic TN, although the absence of such features does not necessarily exclude an underlying structural or systemic disorder. Electromyogram (EMG) trigeminal reflex testing is sensitive and specific for identifying symptomatic TN and is a reasonable early diagnostic test. Additionally, all patients with TN symptomatology should undergo brain imaging to evaluate for secondary causes, as well as compressive vascular lesions (as in classical TN). Different MRI sequences have been used to optimize visualization of veins and arteries surrounding the trigeminal nerve. If standard T1-weighted MRI does not provide sufficient visualization of the trigeminal nerve, axial fast imaging employing steady-state acquisition (FIESTA) and three-dimensional (3D)-spoiled gradient echo (SPGR) multiplanar reconstruction sequences with and without contrast may be used. Standard MRI sequences can identify other secondary causes of TN including tumors and multiple sclerosis (MS) plaques, particularly in the cases of bilateral TN. Painful trigeminal neuropathy from demyelinating lesions can present with all the characteristics of classical TN and affects up to 5% of patients with MS. If there is hypoesthesia in the affected trigeminal distribution, a more extensive workup for the etiology of nerve damage is warranted, as detailed in Chapter 86.

Treatment and Outcome

Medical treatment, summarized in Table 55.2, is aimed at reducing attack frequency and severity over time and is effective for approximately 70% to 80% of patients with classical TN. Several randomized controlled trials (RCTs) have demonstrated efficacy of carbamazepine [**Level 1**],[3] with 58% to 100% of patients achieving near-complete pain control and treatment response beginning as soon as 2 days after initiation. Other RCTs have shown probable efficacy of oxcarbazepine and possible effectiveness of baclofen and lamotrigine. Additionally, smaller studies suggest that gabapentin,

valproate, and levetiracetam, as well as phenytoin and tizanidine (although both with rapidly diminishing effects over time), may have benefit in TN. Type 2 TN is less likely to respond to any of the aforementioned treatments. OnabotulinumtoxinA [**Level 1**],[4] injected to the affected skin or mucosal region, has also been recently shown to be effective in reducing pain severity and attack frequency in a double-blind, saline injection placebo-controlled trial, although side effects included facial asymmetry lasting up to 7 weeks.

If medical therapy fails or is poorly tolerated, interventional treatments can be considered. Microvascular decompression (MVD) involves craniotomy and repositioning of vessels out of contact from the trigeminal nerve. Up to 80% of patients become pain-free following the procedure, with 73% maintaining pain freedom at 5 years; however, there are multiple risks of serious complications, as well as sensory loss in 7% of patients and hearing loss in up to 10% of patients. Gamma knife radiosurgery, in which a beam of radiation is focused at the trigeminal root, has been reported to result in pain freedom in 69% of patients after 1 year, with the number falling to 52% at 3 years. Complications include sensory loss or paresthesias in 6% to 13% of patients. Finally, percutaneous procedures on the Gasserian ganglion, or rhizotomies, involve penetration of the foramen ovale and lesioning of the trigeminal ganglion and/or its roots via glycerol injection, radiofrequency thermocoagulation, or mechanical compression. In a few studies using independent outcome measures, pain freedom was attained in 90% of patients immediately following rhizotomy, but dropped to 54% to 64% after 3 years. Adverse effects are frequent, with sensory loss occurring in almost half of cases, dysesthesias in 6%, masticatory difficulties in up to 50%, and anesthesia

TABLE 55.2	**Medications Commonly Used in Cranial Neuralgias**		
Medication	**Maintenance Dose**	**Side Effects**	**Additional Considerations**
Carbamazepine	300–1,600 mg/day	Sedation, dizziness, cognitive impairment, hyponatremia, rash, aplastic anemia	• Multiple drug interactions (CYP450 inducer) • Response can be seen within 48 h.
Oxcarbazepine	600–1,800 mg/day	Less severe than with carbamazepine but include sedation, dizziness, hyponatremia, rash	• Cross-allergy with carbamazepine in 25% of cases • Equally effective to carbamazepine
Gabapentin	600–2,400 mg/day	Sedation, peripheral edema	• Extra doses can be used for acute treatment.
Lamotrigine	150–400 mg/day	Stevens–Johnson syndrome, sedation, dizziness	• Very slow dose uptitration necessary
Baclofen	30–80 mg/day	Sedation, ataxia, fatigue	• Risk of seizures if stopped rapidly
Phenytoin	200–400 mg/day	Sedation, ataxia, cognitive impairment, rash	• Multiple drug interactions (CYP450 inducer) • Used as an initial intravenous treatment but therapeutic effect lost quickly
Tizanidine	12 mg/day	Sedation, dizziness, orthostatic hypotension	• Therapeutic effects are lost within 1–3 mo.
Levetiracetam	3–4 g/day	Irritability, depression	• Used as an add-on therapy
OnabotulinumtoxinA	75 units	Facial weakness, transient edema	• 5 units (0.1 mL) injected in 15 points in epidermis/dermis or submucosally to region affected

Evidence for use derived from trigeminal neuralgia clinical studies.

dolorosa, or painful numbness that can develop 3 to 6 months after the procedure, in about 4%. Peripheral techniques involving interruption of the trigeminal nerve have only been reported in case series, and to date, there are no direct comparative studies of procedural therapies for TN.

GLOSSOPHARYNGEAL NEURALGIA

Glossopharyngeal neuralgia, also known as *vagoglossopharyngeal neuralgia*, is characterized by paroxysms of severe stabbing pain in the ear, base of tongue, and/or tonsils. These regions are innervated by the auricular and pharyngeal branches of the glossopharyngeal nerve and by the vagus nerve. Neurovascular compression of the glossopharyngeal nerve, particularly by the posterior inferior cerebellar artery lying anteriorly to the nerve root entry zone, may be demonstrated on imaging or intraoperatively. Annual incidence rates for the disorder are 0.4 to 0.8 per 100,000 person-years. Diagnostic criteria are similar to TN, with attacks precipitated by talking, coughing, yawning, or swallowing. Weight loss may be seen in such cases due to avoidance of eating. Symptoms can be bilateral in up to 12% of patients, and nearly 75% experience remissions. Interestingly, up to 11% of patients with glossopharyngeal neuralgia may have comorbid TN. Paroxysms can occur in association with vagal symptoms of bradycardia and syncope, as well as hoarseness. There are also reports of symptomatic neuralgia, or glossopharyngeal neuropathy, caused by multiple sclerosis, Arnold-Chiari malformation, cerebellopontine angle tumors, as well as local tumors in the regions of pain. Treatment options are drawn from experience in TN, Table 55.2. Surgical treatments include ablation or decompression of both glossopharyngeal and vagal nerve roots, with microvascular decompression and intracranial sectioning of nerve rootlets or rhizotomy having more favorable outcomes than either radiofrequency neurolysis or gamma knife radiosurgery.

NERVUS INTERMEDIUS NEURALGIA

Facial nerve, or nervus intermedius, neuralgia is characterized by paroxysms of severe lancinating pain deep in the auditory canal. The nervus intermedius is a sensory branch of the facial nerve that innervates the external auditory canal, middle ear, nasopharynx, and palate. Diagnostic criteria are similar to that of TN, except pain can be precipitated by stimulation of the pinna or posterior wall of the external auditory canal. There is often tenderness in this region and there may be associated lacrimation or excessive salivation. Unlike in TN and glossopharyngeal neuralgia, neurovascular compression is rarely visualized on MRI because the nervus intermedius is less than 0.5 mm in diameter and variable in course. Nervus intermedius neuropathy may be due to acute herpes zoster, or Ramsay Hunt Syndrome, which is further described in Chapter 86. Pharmacotherapy is similar to TN, and surgical management, which typically targets branches of the glossopharyngeal and vagal nerves, can also be considered.

IDIOPATHIC FACIAL PAIN

BURNING MOUTH SYNDROME

Burning or dysesthesia of the mouth or tongue without evidence of oral mucosal diseases is referred to as *burning mouth syndrome* (BMS). It is more common among women, particularly after the fourth decade of life. The diagnosis requires having constant daily pain for a minimum of 3 months, lasting at least for several hours per day. Pain is described as burning and is felt superficially in the oral mucosa, often affecting tip and anterior tongue bilaterally. Other symptoms include dysgeusia and sensation of dryness. The underlying pathophysiology has not been fully elucidated, although trigeminal small-fiber sensory neuropathy with loss of epithelial and subpapillary nerve fibers (akin to the burning feet syndrome) has been demonstrated. Increased expression of TRPV1, a heat- and capsaicin-activated cation channel that is upregulated in several chronic hypersensitivity and pain disorders, has also been noted in patients with BMS. Possible central pathways include abnormalities in tonic inhibition of sensory pathways due to dysfunctional gustatory signaling, as well as changes in central pain modulation with reduced endogenous dopamine levels in the putamen and dysfunction of the nigrostriatal dopaminergic pathway.

Workup includes evaluation for secondary causes of oral mucosal pain, including candidiasis and lichen planus, disorders of salivation and xerostomia due to medications or Sjögren syndrome, hormonal disturbances, hematologic disorders, nutritional deficiencies, and diabetes mellitus. No clinical abnormalities in oral mucosa have been identified on morphologic evaluation, except for increased keratin marker expression suggesting epithelial differentiation and proliferation. Treatment options evaluated in randomized clinical trials include topical clonazepam, selective serotonin reuptake inhibitors, topical and systemic capsaicin (although poorly tolerated), and alpha-lipoic acid. Based on expert opinion, current understanding of the pathophysiology, and common clinical practice, a trial of tricyclic antidepressants should also be considered.

PERSISTENT IDIOPATHIC FACIAL PAIN

Previously called *atypical facial pain*, persistent idiopathic facial pain (PIFP) is a diagnosis of exclusion that is denoted by facial pain lacking characteristics of cranial neuralgias and is not associated with any physical signs or evidence of primary pathology. This syndrome is rare, with an estimated prevalence of 0.03% and usually affecting the middle-aged demographic. The pathogenesis of the disorder is not understood; similar mechanisms have been implicated as in burning mouth syndrome. Patients frequently attribute their pain to an antecedent event, such as a dental procedure or minor trauma to the face, although symptoms may persist long after the initial injury has healed without any residual local pathology. Atypical odontalgia may be a subtype of PIFP, referring to pain in one or more teeth following root canal treatment or in tooth sockets after extraction and deafferentation of trigeminal nerve fibers, without evidence of persistent etiology. Psychological distress is an important factor in the evaluation and treatment of patients with persistent facial pain; although causation is not established, anxiety disorders as well as affective and somatoform disorders are is highly prevalent in this population.

Patients with PIFP describe daily unremitting pain that does not localize to a nerve distribution; quality is dull, aching, or nagging but may present with sharp exacerbations. There are no associated symptoms or neurologic deficits and for diagnosis, a dental cause is excluded by appropriate investigations. The diagnosis of PIFP is made after 3 months of persistent daily pain lasting several hours per day. Treatment options are based on expert opinion rather than controlled studies and include amitriptyline, gabapentin, venlafaxine, and topiramate.

PRIMARY HEADACHE DISORDERS PRESENTING AS FACIAL PAIN

A subset of patients with migraine may experience pain in facial areas, referred to as *facial migraine* or *lower half headache* in the literature. The prevalence of facial pain in a population of 517 migraineurs was estimated to be nearly 9%, and patients with facial pain experienced more cranial autonomic symptoms than those without facial pain. Carotidynia is also frequently reported and/or noted on physical examination (with tenderness on gentle palpation of the carotid artery). Facial-only migraine otherwise shares similar characteristics to traditional migraine regarding pain quality and associated features as well as treatment response to oral triptans. Similarly, cluster headache and paroxysmal hemicrania can also present as pain in the orofacial area without associated headache. Recognizing that facial pain may be a manifestation of a primary headache syndrome can prevent unnecessary interventions, workup, and delays in appropriate therapy.

LEVEL 1 EVIDENCE

1. Ta LE, Dionne RA. Treatment of painful temporomandibular joints with a cyclooxygenase-2 inhibitor: a randomized placebo-controlled comparison of celecoxib to naproxen. *Pain*. 2004;111:13–21.
2. Kimos P, Biggs C, Mah J, et al. Analgesic action of gabapentin on chronic pain in the masticatory muscles: a randomized controlled trial. *Pain*. 2007;127:151–160.
3. Campbell FG, Graham JG, Zilkha KJ. Clinical trial of carbamazepine (Tegretol) in trigeminal neuralgia. *J Neurol Neurosurg Psychiatry*. 1966;29:265–267.
4. Wu CJ, Lian YJ, Zheng YK, et al. Botulinum toxin type A for the treatment of trigeminal neuralgia: results from a randomized, double blind, placebo-controlled trial. *Cephalalgia*. 2012;32: 443–450.

SUGGESTED READINGS

Headache Classification Committee of the International Headache Society. The International Classification of Headache Disorders, 3rd edition, (beta version). *Cephalalgia*. 2013;33:629–808.

Shephard MK, MacGregor A, Zakrzewsa JM. Orofacial pain: a guide for the headache physician. *Headache*. 2014;54:22–39.

Facial Pain due to Disorders of Sinuses, Ears, and Nose

Aaseth K, Grande RB, Kvaerner K, et al. Chronic rhinosinusitis gives a ninefold increased risk of chronic headache. The Akershus study of chronic headache. *Cephalalgia*. 2009;30:152–160.

Abu-Bakra M, Jones NS. Prevalence of nasal mucosal contact points in patients with facial pain compared with patients without facial pain. *J Laryngol Otol*. 2001;115:629–631.

Bieger-Farhan AK, Nichani J, Willatt DJ. Nasal septal mucosal contact points: associated symptoms and sinus CT scan scoring. *Clin Otolaryngol*. 2004;29:165–168.

Cady RK, Dodick DW, Levine HL, et al. Sinus headache: a neurology, otolaryngology, allergy, and primary care consensus on diagnosis and treatment. *Mayo Clin Proc*. 2005;80:908–916.

Göbel H, Baloh RW. Disorder of ear, nose, and sinus. In: Olesen J, Goadsby PJ, Ramadan NM, et al, eds. *The Headaches*. 3rd ed. Philadelphia: Lippincott Williams & Wilkins; 2006:1019–1027.

Iwabuchi Y, Hanamure Y, Ueno K, et al. Clinical significance of asymptomatic sinus abnormalities on magnetic resonance imaging. *Arch Otolaryngol Head Neck Surg*. 1997;123:602–604.

Lawson W, Reinero AJ. Isolated sphenoid sinus disease: an analysis of 132 cases. *Laryngoscope*. 1997;107:1590–1595.

Martin VT, Fanning KM, Serrano D, et al. Chronic rhinitis and its association with headache frequency and disability in persons with migraine: results of the American Migraine Prevalence and Prevention (AMPP) study. *Cephalalgia*. 2014;34:336–348.

Facial Pain due to Temporomandibular Disorders and Disorders of Teeth or Mouth

Fricton J, Look JO, Wright E, et al. Systematic review and meta-analysis of randomized controlled trials evaluating intraoral orthopedic appliances for temporomandibular disorders. *J Orofac Pain*. 2010;24:237–254.

Graff-Radford SB, Canavan DW. Headache attributed to orofacial/temporomandibular pathology. In: Olesen J, Goadsby PJ, Ramadan NM, et al, eds. *The Headaches*. 3rd ed. Philadelphia: Lippincott Williams & Wilkins; 2006: 1029–1035.

Mujakperuo HR, Watson M, Morrison R, et al. Pharmacological interventions for pain in patients with temporomandibular disorders. *Cochrane Database Syst Rev*. 2010;10:CD004715.

Rizzatti-Barbosa CM, Nogueira MT, de Andrade ED, et al. Clinical evaluation of amitriptyline for the control of chronic pain caused by temporomandibular joint disorders. *Cranio*. 2003;21:221–225.

Schiffman E, Ohrbach R, Truelove E, et al. Diagnostic criteria for temporomandibular disorders (DC/TMD) for clinical and research applications: recommendations of the International RDC/TMD Consortium Network and Orofacial Pain Special Interest Group. *J Orofacial Pain Headache*. 2014;28:6–27.

Sharav Y, Singer E, Schmidt E, et al. The analgesic effect of amitriptyline on chronic facial pain. *Pain*. 1987;31:199–209.

Trigeminal and Other Cranial Neuralgias

Bruyn GW. Nervus intermedius neuralgia (Hunt). *Cephalalgia*. 1984;4:71–78.

Cruccu G, Biasiotta A, Di Rezze S, et al. Trigeminal neuralgia and pain related to multiple sclerosis. *Pain*. 2009;143:186–191.

Dieleman JP, Kerklaan J, Huygen FJ, et al. Incidence rates and treatment of neuropathic pain conditions in the general population. *Pain*. 2008;137: 681–688.

Favoni V, Grimaldi D, Pierangeli G, et al. SUNCT/SUNA and neurovascular compression: new cases and critical literature review. *Cephalalgia*. 2013;33: 1337–1348.

Fromm GH. Graff-Radford SB, Terrance CF, et al. Pre-trigeminal neuralgia. *Neurology*. 1990;40:1493–1495.

Gronseth G, Cruccu G, Alksne J, et al. Practice parameter: the diagnostic evaluation and treatment of trigeminal neuralgia (an evidence-based review): report of the Quality Standards Subcommittee of the American Academy of Neurology and the European Federation of Neurological Societies. *Neurology*. 2008;71;1183–1190.

Kandan SR, Khan S, Jeyaretna DS, et al. Neuralgia of the glossopharyngeal and vagal nerves: long-term outcome following surgical treatment and literature review. *Br J Neurosurg*. 2010;24:441–446.

Katusic S, Williams DB, Beard CM, et al. Incidence and clinical features of glossopharyngeal neuralgia, Rochester, Minnesota, 1945–1984. *Neuroepidemiology*. 1991;10:266–275.

Love S, Cakham HB. Trigeminal neuralgia pathology and pathogenesis. *Brain*. 2001;124:2347–2360.

MacDonald BK, Cockerel OC, Sander JW, et al. The incidence and lifetime prevalence of neurological disorders in a community-based study in the UK. *Brain*. 2000;123:665–676.

Meaney JF, Eldridge PR, Dunn LT, et al. Demonstration of neurovascular compression in trigeminal neuralgia with magnetic resonance imaging. Comparison of surgical findings in 52 consecutive operative cases. *J Neurosurg*. 1995; 83:799–805.

Nurmikko TJ, Jansen TS. Trigeminal neuralgia and other facial neuralgias. In: Olesen J, Goadsby PJ, Ramadan NM, et al, eds. *The Headaches*. 3rd ed. Philadelphia: Lippincott Williams & Wilkins; 2006:1053–1062.

Rushton JG, Stevens JC, Miller RH. Glossopharyngeal (vagoglossopharyngeal) neuralgia: a study of 217 cases. *Arch Neurol*. 1981;38:201–205.

Saers SJ, Han KS, de Ru JA. Microvascular decompression may be an effective treatment for nervus intermedius neuralgia. *J Laryngol Otol*. 2011;125: 520–522.

Zakrzewska JM. Diagnosis and differential diagnosis of trigeminal neuralgia. *Clin J Pain*. 2002;18:14–21.

Idiopathic and Primary Facial Pain Disorders

Bittar G, Graff-Radford SB. A retrospective study of patients with cluster headache. *Oral Surg Oral Med Oral Pathol.* 1992;73:519–525.

De Moraes M, do Amaral Bezerra BA, da Rocha Neto PC, et al. Randomized trials for the treatment of burning mouth syndrome: an evidence-based review of the literature. *J Oral Pathol Med.* 2012;41:281–287.

Hagelberg N, Forssell H, Rinne JO, et al. Striatal dopamine D1 and D2 receptors in burning mouth syndrome. *Pain.* 2003;101:149–154.

Lauria G, Majorana A, Borgna M, et al. Trigeminal small-fiber sensory neuropathy causes burning mouth syndrome. *Pain.* 2005;115:332–337.

Mueller D, Obermann M, Yoon MS, et al. Prevalence of trigeminal neuralgia and persistent idiopathic facial pain: a population-based study. *Cephalalgia.* 2011;31:1542–1548.

Obermann M, Mueller D, Yoon MS, et al. Migraine with isolated facial pain: a diagnostic challenge. *Cephalalgia.* 2007;27:1278–1282.

Patton LL, Siegel MA, Benoliel R, et al. Management of burning mouth syndrome: systematic review and management recommendations. *Oral Surg Oral Med Oral Path Oral Radiol Endod.* 2007;103:e1–e13.

Sardella A, Demarosi F, Barbieri C, et al. An up-to-date view on persistent idiopathic facial pain. *Minerva Stomatol.* 2009;58:289–299.

Yoon MS, Mueller D, Hansen N, et al. Prevalence of facial pain in migraine: a population-based study. *Cephalalgia.* 2010;30:92–96.

Yilmaz Z, Renton T, Yiangou Y, et al. Burning mouth syndrome as a trigeminal small fiber neuropathy: increased heat and capsaicin receptor TRPV1 in nerve fibres correlates with pain score. *J Clin Neurosci.* 2007;14:864–871.

Complex Regional Pain Syndrome 56

Michael L. Weinberger and Thomas H. Brannagan III

INTRODUCTION

The complex regional pain syndrome has a long and changing history in medical practice. Veldman suggested that Ambrose Pare, in 1598, may have been the first to describe the syndrome of widespread limb pain with swelling, discoloration, and temperature change. Silas Weir Mitchell, a civil war era physician, discussed the relationship of the central and peripheral mechanisms and "reflex transfers" in the spinal cord along with his description of causalgia in soldiers who had intense nerve pain and autonomic dysregulation after gunshot wounds in battle. The term *causalgia* is attributed to Mitchell and the term *reflex sympathetic dystrophy* to Evans 80 years later. Other terms include the hand–shoulder syndrome, sympathalgia, algodystrophy, and Sudeck dystrophy. A consensus conference in 1993 led to a redefinition as the "complex regional pain syndrome" (CRPS). CRPS type 1 was intended to replace reflex sympathetic dystrophy (RSD) and CRPS type 2 to replace "causalgia." These changes were an attempt to eliminate the implication that the sympathetic nervous system is involved in generating pain while agreeing that sympathetically maintained pain is a symptom.

EPIDEMIOLOGY

In two population-based studies, the incidence of CRPS was 5.46 to 26.2 per 100,000 person-years. The prevalence was estimated at 20.57 per 100,000 in Olmsted County. Women are three times more likely to be affected and postmenopausal women have the highest risk. The mean age at onset is 46 years, with the highest incidence between ages 61 and 70 years.

CLINICAL MANIFESTATIONS

CRPS 1 is a disorder with pain out of proportion to the severity of the injury, allodynia, vasomotor disturbances, motor disturbances, and trophic changes in the skin. Allodynia is defined as "pain resulting from a stimulus (such as a light touch of the skin) that would not normally provoke pain." The symptoms typically follow trauma, which may be mild, but can occur after a myocardial infarction or varicella-zoster infection. A bone fracture is a common preceding event in about 45% of all patients. The arm is affected more commonly than the leg.

The pain is described as deep, sharp, sensitive, and hot. Patients are often sensitive to cold sensations and often guard their limbs to avoid physical contact. Swelling, edema, heat, and color changes occur in the affected limb, followed by osteoporosis and changes in hair, skin, and nail growth. The pain does not conform to nerve or root distribution and usually spreads beyond the area of injury. Some patients with CRPS 1 have dystonic postures of a hand or foot. Features similar to psychogenic movement disorders have been noted by some authors, including the difficulty initiating movement, abrupt onset, and dystonia at rest.

PATHOLOGY

CRPS 2 is defined by the presence of a nerve injury. In a single autopsy case of a CRPS 1 patient, pathologic changes included loss of posterior horn cells and activation of microglia and astrocytes. These changes were most prominent at the site of injury but extended throughout the length of the spinal cord. A study of amputated limbs noted microvascular changes with thickened basal membranes in capillaries in muscle and the loss of C fibers in some patients. In skin biopsy, CRPS 1, defined by the absence of an identified nerve injury, may show fewer small sensory epidermal nerve fibers than controls. Functional magnetic resonance imaging (fMRI) has demonstrated cortical reorganization with shrinkage of the contralateral primary somatosensory cortex, which can be reversed with pain relief.

PATHOBIOLOGY

There is little information about the pathophysiology of CRPS. Both peripheral and central neural mechanisms have been proposed. Human leukocyte antigen (HLA) associations have been described but not confirmed. Theories of the pathogenesis have centered on central sensitization, oxidative damage, and inflammation. After an injury, an initial barrage of C fiber afferent activity may result in central sensitization (see Chapter 57) of dorsal horn neurons, resulting in allodynia and expansion of the distribution of pain. Patients with CRPS have increased levels of proinflammatory cytokines and markers of glial cell activation in the cerebrospinal fluid (CSF). They also have increased markers for oxidative damage, including malondialdehyde. Loss of inhibitory dorsal horn neurons may be evident. More recently, an autoimmune mechanism has been proposed. Studies have demonstrated autoantibodies to autonomic nervous system autoantigens in 30% to 40% of CRPS patients but not in controls or neuropathy patients. Immunoglobulin G (IgG) antibodies to autonomic receptors ($\beta2$ adrenergic receptor and muscarinic-2 receptor) has been demonstrated. Also, $\alpha1$ adrenoreceptors on nociceptive afferents has been shown to be upregulated in dermal nerves and epidermal cells, which may augment pain and neuroinflammation in CRPS.

DIAGNOSTIC CRITERIA

In addition to the changes in terminology, diagnostic criteria have also evolved. Early attempts to define diagnostic criteria were based on anecdotal accumulation of signs and symptoms. Kozin et al. established diagnostic criteria in 1976, including categories for definite, probable, and doubtful RSD. Gibbons proposed a diagnostic scale based on clinical signs and symptoms and laboratory tests including response to sympathetic nerve block. Blumberg proposed a numeric grading scale based on autonomic symptoms, motor symptoms, and sensory symptoms.

The International Association for the Study of Pain (IASP) diagnostic criteria for CRPS from Merskey and Bogduk (1994) include the following:

1. The presence of an initiating noxious event or a cause of immobilization
2. Continuing pain, allodynia, or hyperalgesia with which the pain is disproportionate to any inciting event
3. Evidence at some time of edema, changes in skin blood flow, or abnormal sudomotor activity in the region of pain
4. This diagnosis is excluded by the existence of conditions that would otherwise account for the degree of pain and dysfunction: type 1: without evidence of major nerve damage; type 2: with evidence of major nerve damage.

A consensus workshop in 2003 proposed changes because of the concern that the aforementioned criteria lack specificity in the face of high sensitivity. Validation studies of these criteria suggest that overdiagnosis may be a problem and the inclusion of objective data beyond the subjective and historic data currently called for may improve specificity with modest diminishment in sensitivity.

The Budapest criteria have been accepted by the IASP for the third revision of formal taxonomy and diagnostic criteria of pain states. Clinical diagnostic criteria for CRPS include an array of painful conditions characterized by continuing (spontaneous or evoked) regional pain that is seemingly disproportionate in time or degree to the usual course of any known trauma or other lesion. The pain is regional (not in a specific nerve territory or dermatome) and usually shows distal predominance of abnormal sensory, motor, sudomotor vasomotor, or trophic findings, all with variable progression over time.

CLINICAL DIAGNOSTIC CRITERIA

1. *Continuing pain disproportionate to an inciting event*
2. *Must include at least one symptom in three of the four following categories:*
   a. Sensory: hyperesthesia, allodynia, or both
   b. Vasomotor: temperature asymmetry, skin color changes, skin color asymmetry, or all of these
   c. Sudomotor/edema: edema, sweating, sweating asymmetry, or all three
   d. Motor/trophic: decreased range of motion, motor dysfunction (weakness tremor, dystonic posture), trophic changes (hair, nail, skin), or all three
3. *Must display at least one sign at the time of evaluation in two or more categories:*
   a. Sensory: hyperalgesia (to pinprick), allodynia (to light touch, temperature sensation, or deep somatic pressure or joint movement), or combinations of these
   b. Vasomotor: evidence of temperature asymmetry ($>1°C$), skin color changes or asymmetry, or combinations
   c. Sudomotor/edema: edema, sweating changes, or sweating asymmetry
   d. Motor/trophic: decreased range of motion, motor dysfunction (weakness, tremor, dystonia), or trophic changes (hair, skin, nails)
4. *No other diagnosis better explains the sign and symptoms.*

These criteria have no implications of etiology or pathophysiology. Tests of these criteria demonstrated lower rates of overdiagnosis with little loss of sensitivity.

Published data report that the clinical criteria result in a sensitivity of 85% and sensitivity of 69% and the research criteria, 70% and 96%, respectively.

Other diagnostic tests have included thermography, bone scans, and quantitative sensory testing. Schurmann et al. studied patients with acute radial fracture who met the 1994 IASP criteria and the 1999 Bruehl research criteria. They found a high specificity but low sensitivity for bone scans. Thermography demonstrated poor sensitivity and specificity. Magnetic resonance imaging (MRI) showed high specificity but poor sensitivity. Plain x-rays showed high specificity but low sensitivity with a positive predictive value of 58% and a negative predictive value of 86%. The authors suggest that these tests are not useful for screening but bone scan and MRI have high specificity; however, clinical criteria are still the gold standard.

Historically, three stages of CRPS have been described. Recent analyses have not supported this theory but have suggested three possible subtypes: (1) limited syndrome with predominance of vasomotor signs, (2) limited syndrome with predominance of neuropathic pain/sensory abnormalities, and (3) full blown CRPS with greatest degree of motor/trophic and disuse-related changes.

TREATMENT

Because the etiology of CRPS is uncertain and treatment proposals for CRPS have been untested in placebo-controlled trials but based on historic precedent and anecdotal reports, therapy is debated. Physical therapy and functional restoration have played a major role in the treatment of CRPS. Current guidelines have been developed by consensus. The focus is gradual and progressive movement and use of the limb with increased load bearing as well as desensitization to sensory stimuli. Nerve block, psychotherapy, cognitive behavioral techniques, and pharmacotherapy are added to allow a patient to participate in occupational and physical therapy. Edema must also be addressed with active motion or special garments. The goal is to progress through desensitization, increasing flexibility, edema control, increased range of motion, stress loading, normal postures and balance, and then to normal usage, with vocational and functional rehabilitation.

Few placebo-controlled randomized trials of drug therapy for CRPS have been carried out, and current therapy is largely based on treatment of neuropathic pain. *Biphosphonates*, including clodronate and alendronate, have been shown to provide effective pain relief in placebo-controlled trials (Table 56.1) [Level 1].[1,2] IV ketamine in anesthetic doses over 5 to 10 days has also been reported in open-label controlled trials to be effective in producing symptom reduction or remission in a subgroup of patients refractory to other therapies [Level 1].[3,4] A study of subanesthetic doses of ketamine in refractory CRPS patient was not effective [Level 1].[5] A recent Cochrane Review concluded that there is moderate to low quality evidence supporting its use in the treatment of CRRPS [Level 1].[1] Oral steroids (*methylprednisolone* 32 mg for 2 weeks, then tapering off for 2 weeks or *prednisone* 30 mg for 12 weeks) have been reported to be more effective than placebo, but the weight of current evidence indicates that overall there is no evidence for their effectiveness [Level 1].[1,3] Intravenous (IV) phentolamine (0.5 g/kg) has shown no significant pain relief but sympatholytic agents (also including phenoxbenzamine and clonidine) have been used despite lack of supportive data from clinical

TABLE 56.1	Therapies with Evidence of Efficacy for Pain Relief in Complex Regional Pain Syndrome	
Strong Level of Evidence		
Biphosphonates		
IV Pamidronate	60 mg IV single dose	
IV Alendronate	7.5 mg QD IV x 3 days	
PO Alendronate	40 mg QD x 8 weeks	
IV Clodronate	300 mg QD IV x 10 days	
Moderate Level of Evidence		
IV Ketamine	Up to 0.35 mg/kg/hr[a]	
Limited level of Evidence		
PO Tadalafil	20 mg QD x 12 weeks	
IV immunoglobulin	0.4 g/kg over 5 days	
IV Bretylium	1.5 mg/kg (with lidocaine 0.5 mg/kg)	
Epidural clonidine	300 µg via intrathecal injection	

[a]Infusion can be given continuous for up to 4 days, or over 4 hours per day over 10 days.

Adapted from Complex regional pain syndrome: concise guidance to good practices. *Clin Med.* 2011;11(6):596–600.

studies. Other treatments that have been used without clear evidence of efficacy include topical agents such as *dimethyl sulfoxide* (DMSO) and *lidocaine*, *thalidomide* (doses ranging from 50 mg twice a week to 400 mg a day), calcitonin, and *gabapentin* (600 mg titrated up to 1,800 mg a day).

Other recommended drugs are those used for neuropathic pain conditions such as peripheral diabetic neuropathy and postherpetic neuralgia. Antidepressants such as *amitriptyline* or *nortriptyline* (10 mg titrating up to 150 mg) with secondary consideration of *venlafaxine* (75 mg titrating up as needed to 225 mg), *duloxetine* (20 mg titrating up to 60 to 120 mg q.d.), and *bupropion* (150 to 300 mg q.d.) should be considered. Anticonvulsants beyond gabapentin may also be helpful, despite evidence supporting their use. *Carbamazepine* (50 mg titrating up to maximum of 1,600 mg q.d.) has been used as an add-on included with spinal cord stimulation in CRPS patients. Opioids may also be considered. The diversity of recommendations is a measure of the lack of efficacy.

Interventional techniques include sympathetic block for differentiating sympathetically maintained versus independent pain. There is limited evidence for the efficacy of stellate and lumbar sympathetic blocks for CRPS. IV regional anesthesia with guanethidine or reserpine has failed but bretylium and clonidine have been reported to show efficacy. Epidural infusions with a local anesthetic alone or with opioid or clonidine have all been reported to provide pain relief. Neurolytic sympathetic techniques have been used since 1889. Open surgical sympathectomy was replaced by endoscopic procedures and radiofrequency has been used. Radiofrequency ablation has been advocated.

Spinal cord stimulation improved pain and quality of life in a randomized controlled trial by Kemler et al. Intrathecal drugs have been given by implantable pump, including morphine, bupivacaine, clonidine, ziconotide, and baclofen. Intrathecal baclofen has

also been used for CRPS-related dystonia. The diversity of recommended therapies is an indication that none is generally more effective than any other.

LEVEL 1 REFERENCES

1. Complex regional pain syndrome: concise guidance to good practices. *Clin Med.* 2011;11(6):596–600.
2. Adami S, Fossaluzza V, Gatti D, et al. Bisphosphonate therapy of reflex sympathetic dystrophy syndrome. *Ann Rheum Dis.* 1997;56:201–204.
3. Connolly SB, Prager JP, Harden RN. A systematic review of ketamine for complex regional pain syndrome [published online ahead of print January 15, 2013]. *Pain Med.* 2015;16(5):943–969. doi:10.1111/pme.12675.
4. Kiefer RT, Rohr P, Ploppa A, et al. Efficacy of ketamine in anesthetic dosage for the treatment of refractory complex regional pain syndrome: an open label phase II study. *Pain Med.* 2008;9:1173–1201.
5. Kiefer RT, Rohr P, Ploppa A, et al. A pilot open-label study of the efficacy of subanesthetic isomeric S(+)-ketamine in refractory CRPS patient. Pain Med. 2008;9:44–54.
6. Christensen K, Jensen EM, Noer I. The reflex dystrophy syndrome response to treatment with systemic corticosteroids. *Acta Chir Scand.* 1982;148:653–655.

SUGGESTED READINGS

Albrecht PJ, Hines S, Eisenberg E, et al. Pathologic alterations of cutaneous innervation and vasculature in affected limbs from patients with complex regional pain syndrome. *Pain.* 2006;120:244–266.

Alexander GM, Perreault MJ, Reichenberger ER, et al. Changes in immune and glial markers in the CSF of patients with complex regional pain syndrome. *Brain Behav Immun.* 2007;21:668–676.

Bennett DS, Brookoff D. Complex regional pain syndromes (reflex sympathetic dystrophy and causalgia) and spinal cord stimulation. *Pain Med.* 2006;7(suppl):S64–S96.

Bhatia KP, Bhatt MH, Marsden CD. The causalgia–dystonia syndrome. *Brain.* 1993;116:843–851.

Birklein F, O'Neill D, Schlereth T. Complex regional pain syndrome: an optimistic perspective. *Neurology.* 2015;84:89–96.

Blumberg H. A new clinical approach for diagnosing reflex sympathetic dystrophy. In: Bond MR, Charlton JE, Woolf CJ, eds. *Proceedings of the 6th World Congress on Pain, Pain Research and Clinical Management.* Vol 4. Amsterdam, The Netherlands: Elsevier; 1991:455–481.

Breuhl S, Harden RN, Galer BS, et al. External validation of the IASP criteria for complex regional pain syndrome and proposed research diagnostic criteria. *Pain.* 1999;81:147–154.

Burton AW, Lubenow TR, Raj PR. Traditional interventional therapies. In: *CRPS: Current Diagnosis and Therapy (Progress in Pain Research and Management).* Vol 32. Seattle, WA: IASP Press; 2005.

Cepeda MS, Lau J, Carr DB. Defining the therapeutic role of local anesthetic sympathetic blockade in complex regional pain syndrome: a narrative and systematic review. *Clin J Pain.* 2002;18:216–233.

Cooper DE, DeLee JC, Ramamurthy S. Reflex sympathetic dystrophy of the knee. Treatment using continuous epidural anesthesia. *J Bone Joint Surg Am.* 1989;71:365–369.

de Mos M, de Bruijn AGJ, Huygen FJPM, et al. The incidence of complex regional pain syndrome: a population-based study. *Pain.* 2007;129:12–20.

Del Valle L, Schwartzman RJ, Alexander G. Spinal cord histopathological alterations in a patient with long standing complex regional pain syndrome. *Brain Behav Immun.* 2008;23:85–91.

Devers A, Galer BS. Topical lidocaine patch relieves a variety of neuropathic conditions: an open label study. *Clin J Pain.* 2000;16:205–208.

Eisenberg E, Shtahl S, Geller R, et al. Serum and salivary oxidative analysis in complex regional pain syndrome. *Pain.* 2008;138:226–232.

Evans J. Reflex sympathetic dystrophy. *Surg Clin North Am.* 1946;26:780–790.

Galer BS, Bruehl S, Harden RN. IASP diagnostic criteria for complex regional pain syndrome: a preliminary empirical validation study. *Clin J Pain.* 1998; 14:48–54.

Gibbons J, Wilson PR. RSD score: criteria for the diagnosis of reflex sympathetic dystrophy and causalgia. *Clin J Pain.* 1992;8:260–263.

Gobelet C, Waldburger M, Meier JL. The effect of adding calcitonin to physical therapy on reflex sympathetic dystrophy. *Pain.* 1992;48:171–175.

Harden RN, Bruehl SP. Diagnosis of complex regional pain syndrome: signs, symptoms, and new empirically derived diagnostic criteria. *Clin J Pain.* 2006;22(5):415–419.

Harden RN, Bruehl S, Stanton-Hicks M, et al. Proposed new diagnostic criteria for complex regional pain syndrome. *Pain Med.* 2007;8:326–331.

Harden RN, Swan M, King A, et al. Treatment of complex regional pain functional restoration. *Clin J Pain.* 2006;22:420–424.

Harke H, Gretenkort P, Ladleif HU, et al. The response of neuropathic pain and pain in complex regional pain syndrome I to carbamazepine and sustained-release morphine in patients pretreated with spinal cord stimulation: a double blind randomized study. *Anesth Analg.* 2001;92:488–495.

Hord AH, Rooks MD, Stephens BO, et al. Intravenous regional bretylium and lidocaine for the treatment of reflex sympathetic dystrophy: a randomized, double-blind study. *Anesth Analg.* 1992;7:818–821.

Kemler MA, De Vet HC, Barendse GA, et al. The effect of spinal cord stimulation in patients with chronic reflex sympathetic dystrophy: two years' follow up of the randomized controlled trial. *Ann Neurol.* 2004;55:13–18.

Kiefer RT, Rohr P, Ploppa A, et al. Efficacy of ketamine in anesthetic dosage for the treatment of refractory complex regional pain syndrome: an open label phase II study. *Pain Med.* 2008;9:1173–1201.

Kohr D, Singh P, Tschernatsch M, et al. Autoimmunity against the β2 adrenergic receptor or muscarinic-2 receptor in complex regional pain syndrome. *Pain.* 2011;152:2690–2700.

Kozin F, Ryan LM, Carerra GF, et al. The reflex sympathetic dystrophy syndrome (RSDS). III. Scintigraphic studies further evidence for the therapeutic efficacy of systemic corticosteroids and proposed diagnostic criteria. *Am J Med.* 1981; 70(1):23–30.

Lang A, Fahn S. Movement disorder of RSD. *Neurology.* 1990;40:1476–1478.

Lee GW, Weeks PM. The role of bone scintigraphy in diagnosing reflex sympathetic dystrophy. *J Hand Surg Am.* 1995;20:458–463.

Lubenow TR, Buvanendran A, Stanton-Hicks M. Implanted therapies. In: *CRPS: Current Diagnosis and Therapy (Progress in Pain Research and Management).* Vol 32. Seattle, WA: IASP Press; 2005.

Merskey H, Bogduk N, eds. *Classification of Chronic Pain: Descriptions of Chronic Pain Syndromes and Definitions of Pain Terms.* 2nd ed. Seattle, WA: IASP Press; 1994.

Mitchell SW. *Injuries of the Nerves and Their Consequences.* New York: Dover; 1865.

Oaklander AL, Rissmiller JG, Gelman LB, et al. Evidence of focal small-fiber axonal degeneration in complex regional pain syndrome—I. *Pain.* 2006; 120:235–243.

O'Connell NE, Wand BM, McAuley J, et al. Interventions for treating pain and disability in adults with complex regional pain syndrome. *Cochrane Database Syst Rev.* 2013;4:CD009416.

Perez RS, Zuurmond WW, Bezemer PD, et al. The treatment of complex regional pain syndrome type I with free radical scavengers: a randomized controlled study. *Pain.* 2003;102:297–307.

Rauck RL, Eisenach JC, Jackson K, et al. Epidural clonidine treatment for refractory reflex sympathetic dystrophy. *Anesthesiology.* 1993;79:1163–1169.

Sandroni P, Benrud-Larson LM, McClelland RL, et al. Complex regional pain syndrome type I: incidence and prevalence in Olmsted County, a population-based study. *Pain.* 2003;103:199–207.

Schurmann M, Zaspel J, Lohr P, et al. Imaging in early posttraumatic complex regional pain syndrome: a comparison of diagnostic methods. *Clin J Pain.* 2007;23:449–457.

Schwartzman RJ, Kerrigan J. The movement disorder of reflex sympathetic dystrophy. *Neurology.* 1990;40:57–61.

Stude P, Enax-Krumova EK, Lenz M, et al. Local anesthetic sympathectomy restores fMRI cortical maps in CRPS I after upper extremity stellate blockade: a prospective case study. *Pain Physician.* 2014;17:E637–E644.

Van de Beek WJ, Schwartzman RJ, Van Nes SI, et al. Diagnostic criteria used in studies of reflex sympathetic dystrophy. *Neurology.* 2002;26:522–526.

Van de Vusse AC, Stomp-van den Berg SG, Kessels AH, et al. Randomised controlled trial of gabapentin in complex regional pain syndrome type 1 [ISRCTN84121379]. *BMC Neurol.* 2004;4:13.

Van der Laan L, ter Laak HJ, Gabreëls-Festen A, et al. Complex regional pain syndrome type I (RSD). Pathology of skeletal muscle and peripheral nerve. *Neurology.* 1998;51:20–25.

Van Hilten BJ, van de Beek WJT, Hoff JL, et al. Intrathecal baclofen for the treatment of dystonia in patients with reflex sympathetic dystrophy. *N Engl J Med.* 2000;343:625–630.

Varenna M, Zucchi F, Ghiringhelli D, et al. Intravenous clodronate in the treatment of reflex sympathetic dystrophy syndrome. A randomized, double blind, placebo controlled study. *J Rheumatol.* 2000;27:1477–1483.

Veldman PHJM, Reynen HM, Arntz I, et al. Signs and symptoms of reflex sympathetic dystrophy: prospective study of 829 patients. *Lancet.* 1993;342:1012–1016.

Verdugo RJ, Campero M, Ochoa JL. Phentolamine sympathetic block in painful polyneuropathies. II. Further questioning of the concept of "sympathetically maintained pain." *Neurology.* 1994;44:1010–1014.

Verdugo RJ, Ochoa JL. "Sympathetically maintained pain." 1. Phentolamine block questions the concept. *Neurology.* 1994;44:1003–1010.

Werner R, Davidoff G, Jackson MD, et al. Factors affecting the sensitivity and specificity of the three-phase technetium bone scan in the diagnosis of reflex sympathetic dystrophy in the upper extremity. *J Hand Surg Am.* 1989;14:520–523.

Wilkinson HA. Percutaneous radiofrequency upper thoracic sympathectomy. *Neurosurgery.* 1996;38:715–725.

Wilson PR, Bogduk N. Retrospection, science and epidemiology of CRPS. In: *CRPS: Current Diagnosis and Therapy (Progress in Pain Research and Management).* Vol 32. Seattle, WA: IASP Press; 2005.

Zuniga RE, Perera S, Abram SE. Intrathecal baclofen: a useful agent in the treatment of well established complex regional pain syndrome. *Reg Anesth Pain Med.* 2002;27:90–93.

Thomas H. Brannagan III

INTRODUCTION

In addition to numbness, neuropathic pain may result from damage to any level of the sensory pathway, from the small nerve fibers to the sensory cortex. This large category includes some of the most agonizing of human afflictions. This chapter reviews the normal neurologic processing of pain, the mechanisms underlying neurogenic pain, its clinical features, and the broad range of its pharmacologic therapies, with a particular emphasis on painful polyneuropathy.

DEFINITIONS

See the glossary in Table 57.1.

Pain is an unpleasant sensory and emotional experience associated with actual or potential tissue damage or described in terms of such damage. Pain can be classified broadly as nociceptive or neuropathic. Nociceptive pain clearly serves a protective function, warning of the presence of injury and is frequently the decisive factor prompting a patient to seek medical care. Sensitization of peripheral nociceptors and central nervous system (CNS) changes occur, protecting the damaged area, by avoiding contact. Neuropathic pain is a maladaptive pain, which results from nervous system damage and pain in the absence of nociceptor stimulation or an inappropriate

| TABLE 57.1 | Glossary of Neuropathic Pain Terms |

Allodynia: occurs when a nonnociceptive stimulus is perceived as painful

Central sensitization: an abnormal sensitivity with a spread of hypersensitivity to uninjured sites and pain resulting from stimulation of low-threshold Aβ mechanoreceptors. Central sensitization follows a brief high-frequency input, and the increased response to subsequent inputs may be prolonged after the high-frequency input ceases.

Neuralgia: pain in the distribution of a single peripheral nerve

Neuropathic pain: pain resulting from noninflammatory dysfunction of the peripheral nervous system or CNS, without peripheral nociceptor stimulation or trauma

Nociceptive pain: pain that is protective and arises when the process injuring tissue stimulates pain receptors.

Pain: an unpleasant sensory and emotional experience associated with actual or potential tissue damage or described in terms of such damage

Windup: results from repetitive C-fiber firing at low frequencies that results in a progressive buildup of the amplitude of the response of the dorsal horn neuron, only during the repetitive train

CNS, central nervous system.

response to nociceptor stimulation. Nociceptive and neuropathic pains are not synonymous with acute and chronic pain. Rheumatoid arthritis, for example, is a chronic pain, which is nociceptive. A herniated disk may acutely cause radicular pain, which is neuropathic.

Neuropathic pain is defined as pain resulting from noninflammatory dysfunction of the peripheral nervous system or CNS, without peripheral nociceptor stimulation or trauma. It must be distinguished from primary nociceptive pain, which arises when the process injuring the tissue stimulates pain receptors. *Deafferentation pain* follows interruption of the primary afferent nociceptive pathways at any point, although this term most often refers to syndromes following CNS injury.

Neuropathic pain often refers to pain associated with injury to the peripheral nervous system. This general term is often used, synonymously, with *painful polyneuropathy*, although it also encompasses pain syndromes that follow focal peripheral nerve injury. *Neuralgia* refers more specifically to pain in the distribution of a single peripheral nerve.

Other clinical syndromes with neurogenic pain include the *complex regional pain syndrome* (CPRS). CPRS I was formerly known as *reflex sympathetic dystrophy*, and CPRS II was formerly *causalgia*.

Some neurogenic pain syndromes are so unique that they have individual designations, including thalamic pain syndrome, trigeminal neuralgia, and postherpetic neuralgia.

NORMAL PROCESSING OF PAIN

PERIPHERAL NOCICEPTION

Following noxious chemical, mechanical, or thermal stimulation, transduction occurs at the peripheral sensory nerve terminal through a poorly understood process, causing depolarization of the distal nerve fibers and transmission of nociceptive impulses up the sensory axons to the dorsal root ganglion (DRG) and dorsal nerve roots. Axons carrying nociceptive information are divided into three primary groups: (1) the heavily myelinated, rapidly conducting, intermediate-diameter beta fibers; (2) the finely myelinated, slower conducting, small-diameter A-delta fibers; and (3) the unmyelinated, very slowly conducting, very-small-diameter C fibers. Local factors at the site of injury may sensitize nociceptors and cause hyperalgesia, including potassium leaked from damaged cells, histamine, and bradykinin, whereas prostaglandin and leukotriene formation concurrently cause vasodilatation, local edema, and erythema.

A normally propagated nociceptive action potential may also rebound antidromically through other axonal branches at a site of injury, resulting in the release of substance P from the distal sensory nerve terminal. Substance P activates other C fibers and contributes to the release of histamine, further promoting nociception, vasodilation, and enlarging the region of hypersensitivity. Substance P also acts as a nociceptive neurotransmitter in the dorsal horn of the spinal cord, exciting the relay neurons that modulate pain transmission.

CENTRAL NOCICEPTION

Sensory axons carrying nociceptive impulses project to the spinal cord via the DRG and terminate in the dorsal horn. There, Rexed laminae I, II, and V play a role in modulating nociceptive transmission. Layer I, the marginal zone, caps the top of the dorsal horn and the A-delta nociceptors largely terminate here. Most lamina I cells are nociceptive-specific, responding only to noxious stimuli, and ultimately project to the contralateral midbrain and thalamus. The majority of C-fiber nociceptors terminate in lamina II (i.e., substantia gelatinosa). Very few laminae-II neurons project to sites rostral to the spinal cord, instead forming interneuronal connections that modify input from the primary sensory neurons. Lamina V receives some direct input from the A-delta neurons, but the receptive fields of the neurons in this lamina are larger than those in the lamina I, suggesting more neuronal convergence at this level, and some dendrites from laminae V extend dorsally into laminae I and II. Cells in the deeper layers of the spinal cord gray matter have extremely complex receptive fields and wide areas of cutaneous input, with some input from deeper tissues.

Many nociceptive impulses ultimately pass contralaterally, across the spinal cord through the anterior commissure, to the spinothalamic tract, before ascending to brain stem targets, including the reticular formation in the rostral medulla and the periaqueductal gray matter in the dorsal midbrain. Most of the spinothalamic neurons ultimately ascend to the ventroposterolateral nucleus of the thalamus, although they may branch to provide input to these brain stem targets. However, some axons terminate solely in these bulbar regions, which then send projections to thalamic nuclei.

The periaqueductal gray matter, the reticular formation, and the raphe magnus nucleus also harbor neurons containing endorphins or having endorphin receptors. *Endorphins* are endogenous chemical transmitters whose receptors may also be activated by morphine and other exogenous narcotics; this collection of neurons is known as the *enkephalinergic system*. After synapsing in the thalamus, a final group of neurons convey primary nociceptive information through the posterior limb of the internal capsule to the postcentral gyrus. Many nociceptive axons also project to a much wider area, the full range of which has not been fully defined.

The sensation and the subjective experience of pain are produced by a complex series of interactions. Transmission of nociception in spinal neurons depends not only on input from peripheral nociceptive neurons but also on input from nonnociceptive primary afferents as well as modulation at several levels. Enkephalinergic neurons play a critical role in the modulation of nociceptive input, extending from the cortex and hypothalamus through the periaqueductal gray matter of the midbrain and the rostral medulla to the dorsal horn of the spinal cord. Nociceptive, cortical, and other inputs activate neurons in the reticular formation and the raphe magnus, which then descend to the substantia gelatinosa (Rexed lamina II) in the dorsal horn of the spinal cord, to inhibit nociceptive input from peripheral neurons, thereby diminishing pain.

Unlike the discriminative somatosensory experience, the affective component of pain varies considerably between individuals and may help explain the substantial differences in pain tolerance in the general population. Central pathways proposed as mediators of the affective experience of pain include the reticular formation and its projections to the thalamus as well as the medial thalamic nuclei and their projections to the frontal lobes. The discharge of neurons within the reticular formation correlates with escape behavior in animals, and frontal lobe lesions (e.g., frontal lobotomy) as well as bilateral medial thalamic lesions produce subjective indifference to pain in humans, despite normal somatosensory discrimination. Psychological factors, including the anxiety level, unpleasant memories of physically painful experiences, the anticipation of imminent physical injury or possible death, and others may also bear on our perception of pain. Both psychological factors and the physiologic modulation of the nociceptive impulse are influenced by changes in serotonergic activity.

PATHOBIOLOGY OF NEUROPATHIC PAIN

PERIPHERAL MECHANISMS

Transection of a peripheral nerve induces retrograde shrinkage of both myelinated and unmyelinated axons and reduced conduction velocities. Axonal sprouting from the proximal nerve stump is a normal reaction to such injury, and these sprouts grow toward the distal nerve stump in an attempt to restore axonal continuity. Within 1 to 2 days, multiple unmyelinated sprouts appear and grow from transected axons. If these sprouts fail to enter a Schwann cell tube in the distal nerve segment, they curl to form a mass containing fibrous tissue, blood vessels, clusters of unmyelinated axons, and Schwann cells, known as a *neuroma*. Division of an entire nerve trunk with prevention of regeneration (e.g., amputation) yields a nerve-end neuroma, whereas total division with partial regeneration (e.g., surgical nerve repair) may create a neuroma-in-continuity at the site of the anastomosis. Trauma over the length of a nerve, even without transection (e.g., stretch injury), may damage small axon fascicles or individual axons at multiple levels, creating disseminated microneuromas. Neuromas may also appear following crush injury. Unfortunately, neuroma formation favors nociceptive afferents.

Neuromas are a source of both spontaneous and evoked electrical discharges, as indicated by recording from dorsal root filaments with the injured nerve at rest. These discharges increase with mechanical stimulation at the site of the neuroma and are more likely to affect sensory rather than motor or autonomic fibers. Chronic discharges, particularly, appear to originate primarily in the C fibers. Ectopic neuropacemakers remain near thresholds for repetitive firing and often generate repetitive afterdischarges following a single depolarization. This activity may be due to the high density of sodium channels, originally destined for the transected distal axon, that accumulate in the stump neuroma, enhancing sodium influx and chronically lowering the membrane potential toward the depolarization threshold. Close contact between the disorganized axonal sprouts within the neuroma may also cause current to be passed laterally from one axon to another, a short circuit called *ephaptic transmission*. Recurrent after discharges and other sustained activity may also result from the cyclic passage of current back and forth in a loop between two ephapses (i.e., *circus propagation*, as seen in some cardiac arrhythmias).

Faulty axonal regeneration and ephapse formation may also appear in nerves chronically injured by demyelination or axonal degeneration, in the absence of external trauma. Spontaneous discharges may be induced not only by mechanical stimulation but also by heat, cold, ischemia, chemical irritation, and metabolic stimuli. Mechanical stimulation may induce a burst of discharges and afterdischarges, and heating and cooling modulate discharge rates and patterns. Peptides and other neuroactive substances, especially α-adrenergic agonists, increase activity in experimental neuromas.

Ectopic pacemaker activity has been recorded in the phantom limb syndrome and may explain the hypersensitivity to heat and cold in that syndrome. Many of the core features of painful neuropathy and neuralgia, such as spontaneous electric, burning, and aching dysesthesias and hyperesthesia, could also be related to ectopic discharges. Sensitivity to mechanical stimulation in neuralgia or compressive mononeuropathy, which may provoke pain long outlasting the inciting stimulus, may result from the repetitive discharges and afterdischarges provoked by neuroma compression.

CENTRAL MECHANISMS

Although the aforementioned peripheral mechanisms play a role in neuropathic pain, central mechanisms are also important and may predominate in chronic peripheral nerve injury. The failure of measures designed to interrupt peripheral input from the painful region to fully relieve the pain of phantom limb syndrome, including pharmacologic blockade of the damaged nerve proximal to the site of injury, dorsal rhizotomy, and even spinal and other CNS block illustrates the confounding influence of central mechanisms. After peripheral nerve injury, the aberrant rerouting of impulses within the brain and spinal cord may result in the diversion of impulses from nonnociceptive pathways to nociceptive pathways. This has been demonstrated experimentally in mapping studies of the spinal cord and brain, done before and after transection of a single peripheral nerve in one limb. Initially, the central pain pathways serving the denervated area fall silent, but electrical activity gradually resumes within a few days. Some of this activity may be induced by nonnociceptive stimulation of areas supplied by an uninjured nerve that is remote from the dermatomes supplied by the injured nerve, suggesting spread of nonnociceptive impulses from normal routes into nociceptive pathways that were previously supplied by the injured nerve.

This phenomenon, known as *somatotopic reorganization*, could result from limited axonal sprouting over short distances within the spinal cord, and the formation of new synapses, prompted when primary sensory input is interrupted. Another explanation is that the loss of primary afferent input to a central spinal pathway following peripheral nerve injury may unmask previously quiescent synapses. These synapses, supplied by nearby spinal axons serving sensation in other regions, enable surreptitious stimulation of the denervated pathway, and produce phantom sensations, including pain.

Afferent fiber discharges may trigger cell death of neurons in the dorsal horn, where inhibitory interneurons are concentrated, possibly through an excitotoxic mechanism. This may result in increased pain transmission.

C-fiber afferents release glutamate and synapse on second-order neurons in the dorsal horn to have excitatory effects on glutamate synapses at AMPA receptors, which results in depolarization of the membrane. This depolarization releases the inhibition of the NMDA receptor by the magnesium ion, and there is an influx of calcium. Second-order neurons are gradually depolarized and responses are amplified, changing the response of neurons to subsequent input.

Two processes that are distinct occur at the dorsal horn, which are designated "windup" and "central sensitization." Windup results from repetitive C-fiber firing at low frequencies that results in a progressive buildup of the amplitude of the response of the dorsal horn neuron, only during the repetitive train. Central sensitization is an abnormal sensitivity with a spread of hypersensitivity to uninjured sites and pain resulting from stimulation of low-threshold $A\beta$ mechanoreceptors. Central sensitization follows a brief high-frequency input, and the increased response to subsequent inputs may be prolonged, after the high-frequency input ceases. Both can

be blocked by NMDA receptor antagonists. Central sensitization can result from windup. This is a result of the calcium influx through the NMDA receptor following depolarization of the dorsal horn membrane. The intracellular calcium activates a number of kinases, among which protein kinase C (PKC) is likely important. PKC enhances the NMDA receptor, which results in subsequent glutamate binding of the NMDA receptor generating an inward current. Although windup can result in central sensitization, it is not necessary for central sensitization to occur.

Similar observations were noted long ago by Denny-Brown, who described an enlarged and hypersensitive dermatomal region in primates after severance of the surrounding nerve roots distal to the DRG, compared to section proximal to the DRG. This suggested plasticity of the dorsal horn neurons secondary to input from the DRG.

Mapping CNS pathways during selective stimulation of cutaneous fields demonstrates wide-ranging synaptic inputs that reach well beyond their normal functional boundaries within the spinal cord. Similar phenomena have also been demonstrated at more rostral levels of the nervous system, including the thalamic nuclei. These phenomena could explain the phantom limb syndrome, in which a patient has the sensation that an amputated limb is still present. They may also play a role in some of the features of neuropathic pain, including the perception of one type of stimulus as another (i.e., *allesthesia*), when touch is perceived as heat, or when a nonnociceptive stimulus is perceived as painful (i.e., *allodynia*).

CLINICAL MANIFESTATIONS

Neuropathic pain is estimated to affect up to 1% of the population and is even more prevalent in the elderly. It affects 10% of people with diabetic neuropathy and is often the complication having the greatest impact on the quality of life for the patient with diabetes. The repertoire of agents effective for the control of this potentially debilitating symptom has expanded considerably in the last decade.

Trauma to the peripheral nervous system can take a variety of forms; it may be predominantly axonal or predominantly demyelinating and may disproportionately affect the sensory or motor nerves, or the small or large nerve fibers. It may begin acutely or chronically, depending on the cause. Small-fiber dysfunction classically causes loss of temperature and pain sensation, with subjective feelings of numbness, most often starting in a distal, symmetric pattern in the feet, with gradual ascension. However, pure small-fiber injury often presents with paresthesias (e.g., tingling, cold, or burning sensations) and neuropathic pain (e.g., electric, lancinating, stabbing, or aching quality). Patients may also complain of allodynia and are particularly bothered by contact of the feet and bedsheets. Unlike large-fiber, sensory nerve injury, tendon reflexes may be preserved in these patients. The most common cause is diabetes mellitus, but the many other causes include Sjögren syndrome, alcohol or drug toxicity, HIV, hyperlipidemia, amyloidosis, Tangier disease, and Fabry disease (see Table 87.1).

Large-fiber, sensory nerve injury typically causes loss of vibration and position sense, with subjective numbness. Also, it usually begins in a distal symmetric pattern, affecting the feet and gradually ascending. With sufficient progression, it causes lower limb incoordination and unsteadiness of gait. Tendon reflexes are diminished or absent, and motor nerve involvement may produce weakness. Neuropathic pain may follow injury to the large sensory fibers, although concurrent small-fiber injury is also present in most of these cases. Patients with symptoms suggesting painful polyneuropathy must undergo a thorough neurologic evaluation, including detailed history, physical examination, electrophysiologic studies, imaging, and serum studies (see Chapter 87). Other, nonneurogenic causes of pain must be excluded. Patients with pure small-fiber neuropathy, however, may have normal electrophysiologic studies. A skin biopsy to count epidermal nerve fiber density can be used to confirm the diagnosis (see Fig. 87.11). Epidermal nerve fiber density less than the 5th percentile of normal is considered abnormal. Treatment of these patients focuses on the cause of nerve injury, if reversible.

TREATMENT

GENERAL PRINCIPLES

Patients with neuropathic pain vary more in response to treatments than patients with other disorders and the course of neuropathic pain may be difficult to predict, with unexpected exacerbations and spontaneous remissions. The therapeutic goal of treatment is to return the patient to normal functioning, with reduction of pain to tolerable levels. The patient should understand and accept this goal at the outset and not expect complete elimination of pain. Furthermore, the patient should also understand that numbness, weakness, and other neuropathic symptoms would not be improved by these medications. Patients often benefit from physical therapy, regular exercise, and constructive activity. Refractory symptoms may lead to treatment by a multidisciplinary team in a reputable pain clinic. This team should include not only a physician specialist but also a psychiatrist or psychologist trained in pain management who may assist with analysis of the affective component of the symptoms and issues such as secondary gain as well as with conditioning and psychotherapy. Some patients may also benefit from adjunctive (i.e., complementary) biofeedback and meditation methods.

PHARMACOLOGIC THERAPY

A summary of the major drugs evaluated for the treatment of neuropathic pain, along with their efficacy, is presented in Table 57.2.

Antinociceptive Agents

Unlike primary nociceptive pain, neuropathic pain is often resistant to traditional analgesic therapy, including that of NSAIDs such as ibuprofen and aspirin. Acetaminophen is generally minimally effective. Opioid analgesics are also less likely to provide chronic relief than in other pain states, although they may be useful as part of a multimodal regimen in refractory patients. They have been shown in short-term, placebo-controlled, double-blind randomized trials to be beneficial in neuropathic pain. Physicians regularly employing opioids for the treatment of neuropathic pain should be trained in chronic use and must be vigilant in monitoring patients' patterns of drug consumption and response to avoid addictive patterns. Patients taking opioid therapy may benefit from a referral to a pain clinic for appropriate long-term monitoring and evaluation of tolerance, dependence, and drug abuse, when appropriate.

TRAMADOL HYDROCHLORIDE

Tramadol hydrochloride, unlike most other analgesics, has been proved effective for the treatment of painful neuropathy in a placebo-controlled, double-blind, randomized trial [Level 1].[1] It is a weak inhibitor of norepinephrine and serotonin reuptake and has low affinity for the μ-opioid receptors (i.e., approximately one-tenth the strength of codeine). The beneficial effects in neuropathic pain are attributed to serotonergic modulation of pain transmission within the brain and spinal cord. It is well-tolerated but may cause mild constipation, headache, or sedation. Therapy is usually initiated at 50 mg/day, gradually increasing on a weekly schedule to 150 to 200 mg/day, or the maximal effective dose, whichever is lower. Some relief may appear almost immediately, but maximal benefit may not be seen for 1 to 2 weeks after initiation or dosage change.

Anticonvulsants

The antiexcitatory properties of the antiepileptic drugs (AEDs) make them attractive agents for the suppression of the spontaneous neuronal discharges underlying neuropathic pain. Early trials of phenytoin gave conflicting results, but carbamazepine was effective in two placebo-controlled and one comparative study (vs. tricyclic antidepressants [TCAs]) at doses of 300 to 1,000 mg/day. Common adverse effects of carbamazepine include somnolence, dizziness, and gait disturbances, and rarely, leucopenia, hepatotoxicity, and inappropriate secretion of antidiuretic hormone. Oxcarbazepine may also be effective, with fewer side effects.

Gabapentin and pregabalin are effective AEDs for suppressing neuropathic pain, proven in placebo-controlled trials for painful diabetic neuropathy, postherpetic neuralgia, and other neuropathic pain syndromes [Level 1].[2,3] They act by modulating the alpha 2 delta subunit of the calcium channel, which has been shown to be upregulated after nerve injury. Side effects are generally mild, although sedation is often a limiting factor in the elderly. Ankle swelling and weight gain occur in some patients. Initial doses of pregabalin are 150 mg/day, in two divided doses, are gradually increased to efficacy over several weeks; the slow increase may prevent excessive sedation.

Lamotrigine, a voltage-dependent sodium channel blocker, proved effective in treating the pain of HIV neuropathy and in trigeminal neuralgia but was negative in a large neuropathic pain trial [Level 1].[4] In those studies demonstrating efficacy, doses of 50 to 400 mg/day were used. The most concerning side effect of lamotrigine is a Stevens–Johnson rash; to avoid the rash, a slow titration is used typically starting at 25 mg/day. Zonisamide, a sodium and T-type calcium channel blocker and enhancer of GABA release, tiagabine, and topiramate may have a role in the treatment of neuropathic pain.

Lacosamide, a medication that enhances slow inactivation of voltage-gated sodium channels, reduced diabetic neuropathy pain in double-blind, randomized, placebo-controlled trials, at a dose of 400 mg a day.

Tricyclic Antidepressants

Amitriptyline was one of the first agents proven effective for the treatment of painful neuropathy. The TCAs block serotonin and noradrenalin reuptake and modulate pain transmission within the CNS. They may also inhibit sodium channel function, and the pain relief they provide is independent of any effect on mood. Amitriptyline has been effective in numerous double-blind, placebo-controlled trials [Level 1].[5] Other TCAs, such as desipramine and nortriptyline may also be effective and may sometimes work when amitriptyline does not [Level 1].[6] Unfortunately, the TCAs have anticholinergic effects including sedation, orthostatic hypotension, and urinary retention that often limit their use in diabetic and elderly subjects. Sedation during initial therapy may improve over 1 or 2 weeks.

TABLE 57.2 Medications Used to Treat Neuropathic Pain

Medication	Starting Doses	Maintenance Doses	Data Supporting the Use	Selected Side Effects
Antidepressants				
Duloxetine	20–30 mg q.d.	60–120 mg/day	PCT—diabetic neuropathy	Diarrhea, nausea, dizziness
Amitriptyline	10–25 mg q.h.s.	50–150 mg/day	PCT—diabetic neuropathy	Arrhythmia, urinary retention, sexual dysfunction
Nortriptyline	10–25 mg q.h.s.	50–150 mg/day	Anecdotal reports	Less somnolence and orthostatic hypotension than amitriptyline
Venlafaxine	37.5 mg q.d.	150–375 mg/day	Anecdotal reports—neuropathy, postherpetic neuralgia	Hypertension, sexual dysfunction, nausea
Bupropion SR	150 mg q.d.	150 mg b.i.d.	PCT—neuropathic pain	Dry mouth, headache, insomnia, dizziness
Anticonvulsants				
Pregabalin	75 mg b.i.d.	150–300 mg b.i.d.	PCT—diabetic neuropathy, postherpetic neuralgia	Somnolence, fatigue, pedal edema, weight gain
Gabapentin	100 mg t.i.d.	300 mg t.i.d.–1,200 mg q.i.d.	PCT—diabetic neuropathy, postherpetic neuralgia	Somnolence, fatigue, pedal edema
Lamotrigine	25 mg q.d.	100–250 mg b.i.d.	PCT—HIV neuropathy, diabetic neuropathy	Stevens–Johnson rash
Oxcarbazepine	75 mg q.h.s.	300–1,200 mg b.i.d.	Anecdotal reports—trigeminal neuralgia	Gastrointestinal ataxia, hyponatremia, rash
Topiramate	15–25 mg q.h.s.	100–400 mg b.i.d.	Anecdotal reports—diabetic neuropathy, neuropathic pain	Somnolence, word-finding difficulties, kidney stones
Lacosamide	100 mg q.d.	400 mg q.d.	PCT—diabetic neuropathy	Dizziness, nausea
Other Medications				
Mexiletine	150 mg daily	600–1,200 mg daily	Anecdotal, subgroup analysis of PCT	Nausea/vomiting, palpitations, chest pain
Tramadol	25 mg daily	200–400 mg daily	PCT—diabetic neuropathy	Seizures, nausea, headache, constipation, somnolence
CR-oxycodone	10 mg q.d.	40 mg q.d.	PCT—diabetic neuropathy	Constipation, somnolence, nausea, dizziness, vomiting
Tapentadol ER	50 mg b.i.d.	100–250 mg b.i.d.	PCT—diabetic neuropathy [Level 1][9]	Constipation, somnolence, dizziness, nausea, vomiting, fatigue
Tizanidine	1 mg daily	4–36 mg daily	Open label studies in neuropathic pain	Dizziness, drowsiness, fatigue, liver damage
Methadone	5 mg daily	10–20 mg daily	PCT—neuropathic pain	Nausea, dizziness, constipation
Capsaicin 8% patch	1 patch	1 patch q12wk	PCT—postherpetic neuralgia, HIV neuropathy	Application site reactions, including increase in pain, nausea
Lidocaine patch 5%	1 patch for 12 h	1–3 patches for 12 h	PCT—postherpetic neuralgia	Application site reactions

PCT, placebo-controlled trials; SR, sustained release; CR, controlled release; ER, extended release.

Typical starting doses are 10 to 25 mg at bedtime, gradually increasing every 2 weeks to effect or maximally tolerated dose (i.e., not more than 150 mg/day). If no benefit appears after 4 to 6 weeks at maximally tolerated doses, another agent should be tried.

Selective Serotonin Reuptake Inhibitors

Selective serotonin reuptake inhibitors (SSRIs) have not been studied as extensively as the TCAs in the treatment of neuropathic pain.

However, paroxetine and citalopram were more effective than placebo but less effective than the TCAs in treating neuropathic pain, whereas fluoxetine has not been effective in the limited studies performed thus far.

Serotonin–Norepinephrine Reuptake Inhibitors

Duloxetine is beneficial for diabetic neuropathy pain, with efficacy demonstrated in double-blind, placebo-controlled trials [Level 1].[7]

The typical starting dose is 20 to 30 mg/day, which is titrated up to 60 mg/day. Some patients have an improved response to 120-mg dose. Nausea and dizziness are the most common side effects. Venlafaxine is a serotonin and weak noradrenalin reuptake inhibitor that demonstrated efficacy equivalent to imipramine in a randomized trial.

Other Drugs

Both intravenous lidocaine and its oral conjoiner, mexiletine, (150 to 1,200 mg) have great potential, theoretically, for the suppression of aberrant neuronal excitation, but results have been inconsistent. The lidocaine patch delivers topical agent to an affected area, decreasing spontaneous discharge in cutaneous nerves. It may reduce regional pain in severely affected areas, such as the soles of the feet. Capsaicin (0.075%) cream, which depletes substance P from the cutaneous sensory nerves with chronic topical use, is effective. However, patients find this drug inconvenient because topical application is required three times per day. It is caustic and irritates any mucous membranes it may contact (e.g., eye and mouth, after accidental transfer from the hand during application). It also actually increases neuropathic pain during the initial 1 to 2 weeks of therapy (i.e., the early depletion phase), before producing relief. A high-concentration capsaicin (8%) patch results in prolonged pain relief with a single application for up to 12 weeks [**Level 1**].[8]

LEVEL 1 EVIDENCE

1. Harati Y, Gooch CL, Swenson M, et al. A double-blind, randomized trial of tramadol for treatment of the pain of diabetic neuropathy. *Neurology.* 1998;50:1842–1846.
2. Backonja M, Beydoun A, Edwards KR, et al. Gabapentin for the symptomatic treatment of painful neuropathy in patients with diabetes mellitus: a randomized controlled trial. *JAMA.* 1998;280:1831–1836.
3. Lesser H, Sharma U, LaMoreaux L, et al. Pregabalin relieves symptoms of painful diabetic peripheral neuropathy: a randomized controlled trial. *Neurology.* 2004;63:2104–2110.
4. Simpson DM, Olney R, McArthur JC, et al. A placebo-controlled trial of lamotrigine for painful HIV-associated neuropathy. *Neurology.* 2000;54:2115–2119.
5. Max MB, Culnane M, Schafer SC, et al. Amitriptyline relieves diabetic neuropathy pain in patients with normal or depressed mood. *Neurology.* 1987;37(4):589–596.
6. Max MB, Lynch SA, Muir J, et al. Effects of desipramine, amitriptyline, and fluoxetine on pain in diabetic neuropathy. *N Engl J Med.* 1992;326:1250–1256.
7. Wernicke JF, Pritchett YL, D'Souza DN, et al. A randomized controlled trial of duloxetine in diabetic peripheral neuropathic pain. *Neurology.* 2006;67:1411–1420.
8. Irving GA, Backonja MM, Dunteman E, et al. A multicenter, randomized, double-blind, controlled study of NGX-4010, a high-concentration capsaicin patch, for the treatment of postherpetic neuralgia. *Pain Med.* 2011;12:99–109.
9. Vinik AI, Shapiro DY, Rauschkolb C, et al. A randomized withdrawal, placebo-controlled study evaluating the efficacy and tolerability of tapentadol extended release in patients with chronic painful diabetic peripheral neuropathy. *Diabetes Care.* 2014;37:2302–2309.

SUGGESTED READINGS

Neuropathic Pain

Cohen SP, Mao J. Neuropathic pain: mechanisms and their clinical implications. *BMJ.* 2014;348:f7656.

Costigan M, Scholz J, Woolf CJ. Neuropathic pain: a maladaptive response of the nervous system to damage. *Annu Rev Neurosci.* 2009;32:1–32.

Treede RD, Jensen TS, Campbell JN, et al. Neuropathic pain: redefinition and a grading system for clinical and research purposes. *Neurology.* 2008;70: 1630–1635.

Ulane CM, Brannagan TH III. Neuropathies: DPN, HIV, idiopathic. In: Brummett, CM, Cohen SP, eds. *Managing Pain.* Oxford, England: Oxford University Press; 2013.

Treatment of Neuropathic Pain

Bril V, England J, Franklin GM. Evidence-based guideline: treatment of painful diabetic neuropathy: report of the American Academy of Neurology, the American Association of Neuromuscular and Electrodiagnostic Medicine, and the American Academy of Physical Medicine and Rehabilitation. *Neurology.* 2011;76:1758–1765.

The Capsaicin Study Group. Treatment of painful diabetic neuropathy with topical capsaicin: a multicenter, double-blind, vehicle-controlled study. *Arch Intern Med.* 1991;151:2225–2229.

Dejgård A, Petersen P, Kastrup J. Mexiletine for treatment of chronic painful diabetic neuropathy. *Lancet.* 1988;1:9–11.

Errington AC, Stohr T, Heers C, et al. The investigational anticonvulsant lacosamide selectively enhances slow inactivation of voltage-gated sodium channels. *Mol Pharmacol.* 2008;73:157–169.

Foley KM. Opioids and chronic neuropathic pain. *N Engl J Med.* 2003;348: 1279–1281.

Gomez-Perez FJ, Choza R, Rios JM, et al. Nortriptyline–fluphenazine vs. carbamazepine in the symptomatic treatment of diabetic neuropathy. *Arch Med Res.* 1996;27:525–529.

Heit HA. Addiction, physical dependence, and tolerance: precise definitions to help clinicians evaluate and treat chronic pain patients. *J Pain Palliat Care Pharmacother.* 2003;17:15–29.

Kastrup J, Petersen P, Dejgård A, et al. Intravenous lidocaine infusion—a new treatment of chronic painful diabetic neuropathy? *Pain.* 1987;28:69–75.

McCleane G. 200 mg daily of lamotrigine has no analgesic effect in neuropathic pain: a randomised, double-blind placebo controlled trial. *Pain.* 1999;83:105–107.

Morley JS, Bridson J, Nash TP, et al. Low-dose methadone has an analgesic effect in neuropathic pain: a double-blind randomized controlled crossover trial. *Palliat Med.* 2003;17:576–587.

Oskarsson P, Ljunggren JG, Lins PE. Efficacy and safety of mexiletine in the treatment of painful diabetic neuropathy. *Diabetes Care.* 1997;20:1594–1597.

Rauck RL, Shaibani A, Biton V, et al. Lacosamide in painful diabetic peripheral neuropathy: a phase 2 double-blind placebo-controlled study. *Clin J Pain.* 2007;23:150–158.

Saudek DC, Werns S, Reidenberg MM. Phenytoin in the treatment of diabetic symmetrical polyneuropathy. *Clin Pharmacol Ther.* 1977;22(2):196–199.

Simpson DM, Brown S, Tobias J. Controlled trial of high-concentration capsaicin patch for treatment of painful HIV neuropathy. *Neurology.* 2008;70:2305–2313.

Sindrup SH, Bach FW, Madsen C, et al. Venlafaxine versus imipramine in painful polyneuropathy. *Neurology.* 2003;60:1284–1289.

Stracke H, Meyer UE, Schumacher HE, et al. Mexiletine in the treatment of diabetic neuropathy. *Diabetes Care.* 1992;15:1550–1555.

Tandan R, Lewis GA, Krusinski PB, et al. Topical capsaicin in painful diabetic neuropathy: controlled study with long-term follow-up. *Diabetes Care.* 1992;15:8–14.

Wright JM, Oki JC, Graves L III. Mexiletine in the symptomatic treatment of diabetic peripheral neuropathy. *Ann Pharmacother.* 1997;31:29–34.

Zakrzewska JM, Chaudhry Z, Nurmikko TJ, et al. Lamotrigine (Lamictal) in refractory trigeminal neuralgia: results from a double-blind placebo-controlled crossover trial. *Pain.* 1997;73:223–230.

Zhou M, Chen N, He L, et al. Oxcarbazepine for neuropathic pain. *Cochrane Database Syst Rev.* 2013;3:CD007963.

Epilepsy 58

Carl W. Bazil, Shraddha Srinivasan, and Timothy A. Pedley

INTRODUCTION

An epileptic seizure is the result of a temporary physiologic dysfunction of the brain caused by an abnormal, self-limited, and hypersynchronous electrical discharge of cortical neurons. There are many different kinds of seizures, each with characteristic behavioral changes and electrophysiologic disturbances that can usually be detected in scalp electroencephalography (EEG) recordings. The particular manifestations of any single seizure depend on several factors: whether most or only a part of the cerebral cortex is involved at the beginning, the functions of the cortical areas where the seizure originates, the subsequent pattern of spread of the electrical ictal discharge within the brain, and the extent to which subcortical and brain stem structures are engaged.

A seizure is a transient epileptic event, a symptom of disturbed brain function. Although seizures are the cardinal manifestation of epilepsy, not all seizures imply epilepsy. For example, seizures may be self-limited in that they occur only during the course of an acute medical or neurologic illness such as metabolic disarray or drug intoxication; they do not persist after the underlying disorder has resolved. Some people, for no discoverable reason, have a single unprovoked seizure. These kinds of seizures are not epilepsy.

Epilepsy is a chronic disorder, or group of chronic disorders, in which the indispensable feature is recurrence of seizures that are typically unprovoked and usually unpredictable. About 50 million people are affected worldwide. Each distinct form of epilepsy has its own natural history and response to treatment. This diversity presumably reflects the fact that epilepsy can arise from a variety of underlying conditions and pathophysiologic mechanisms, although most cases are classified as idiopathic (of presumed genetic origin) or cryptogenic (arising from a past injury that is not defined).

CLASSIFICATION OF SEIZURES AND EPILEPSY

Accurate classification of seizures and epilepsy is essential for understanding epileptic phenomena, developing a rational plan of investigation, making decisions about when and for how long to treat, choosing the appropriate antiepileptic drug (AED), and conducting scientific investigations that require delineation of clinical and EEG phenotypes.

CLASSIFICATION OF SEIZURES

The classification that is still followed today is the 1981 classification of epileptic seizures developed by the International League Against Epilepsy (ILAE; Table 58.1). This system classifies seizures by clinical symptoms supplemented by EEG data.

TABLE 58.1 International League Against Epilepsy Classification of Epileptic Seizures

I. Partial (focal) seizures

  A. Simple partial seizures (consciousness not impaired)

    1. With motor signs (including jacksonian, versive, and postural)

    2. With sensory symptoms (including visual, somatosensory, auditory, olfactory, gustatory, and vertiginous)

    3. With psychic symptoms (including dysphasia, dysmnesic, hallucinatory, and affective changes)

    4. With autonomic symptoms (including epigastric sensation, pallor, flushing, pupillary changes)

  B. Complex partial seizures (consciousness is impaired)

    1. Simple partial onset followed by impaired consciousness

    2. With impairment of consciousness at onset

    3. With automatisms

  C. Partial seizures evolving to secondarily generalized seizures

II. Generalized seizures of nonfocal origin (convulsive or nonconvulsive)

  A. Absence seizures

    1. With impaired consciousness only

    2. With one or more of the following: atonic components, tonic components, automatisms, autonomic components

  B. Myoclonic seizures

    Myoclonic jerks (single or multiple)

  C. Tonic–clonic seizures (may include clonic–tonic–clonic seizures)

  D. Tonic seizures

  E. Atonic seizures

III. Unclassified epileptic seizures

From the Commission on Classification and Terminology of the International League Against Epilepsy. Proposal for revised clinical and electroencephalographic classification of epileptic seizures. *Epilepsia.* 1981;22:489–501.

Inherent in the ILAE classification are two important physiologic principles. First, seizures are fundamentally of two types: those with onset limited to a part of one cerebral hemisphere (*partial* or *focal* seizures) and those that seem to involve the brain diffusely from the beginning (*generalized* seizures). Second, seizures are dynamic and evolving; clinical expression is determined as much by the sequence of spread of electrical discharge within the brain as by the area where the ictal discharge originates. Variations in the seizure pattern exhibited by an individual imply variability in the extent and pattern of spread of the electrical discharge. Both generalized and partial seizures are further divided into subtypes. For partial seizures, the most important subdivision is based on consciousness, which is preserved in *simple* partial seizures or lost in *complex* partial seizures. Simple partial seizures may evolve into complex partial seizures, and either simple or complex partial seizures may evolve into secondarily generalized seizures. In adults, most generalized seizures have a focal onset whether or not this is apparent clinically. For generalized seizures, subdivisions are based mainly on the presence or absence and character of ictal motor manifestations.

The initial events of a seizure, described by either the patient or an observer, are usually the most reliable clinical indication to determine whether a seizure begins focally or is generalized from the moment of onset. Sometimes, however, a focal signature is lacking for several possible reasons:

1. The patient may be amnesic after the seizure, with no memory of early events.
2. Consciousness may be impaired so quickly or the seizure may generalize so rapidly that early distinguishing features are blurred or lost.
3. The seizure may originate in a brain region that is not associated with an obvious behavioral function. Thus, the seizure becomes clinically evident only when the discharge spreads beyond the ictal-onset zone or becomes generalized.

In 2010, the ILAE published a proposal for a revised classification of the epilepsies based on "terminology and concepts for organization." As many epilepsy syndromes include both focal and generalized seizures, the classification distinguishing focal from generalized epilepsies was abandoned. In addition, a focal seizure was conceptualized as originating at some point within networks limited to one hemisphere. In contrast, a generalized seizure was conceptualized as originating at some point within, and then rapidly involving, networks distributed bilaterally. The three broad etiologic categories became genetic, structural/metabolic, and unknown, instead of cryptogenic, symptomatic, and idiopathic.

Partial Seizures

Simple partial seizures result when the ictal discharge occurs in a limited and often circumscribed area of cortex, the *epileptogenic focus*. Almost any symptom or phenomenon can be the subjective (aura) or observable manifestation of a simple partial seizure, varying from elementary motor (jacksonian seizures, adversive seizures) and unilateral sensory disturbance to complex emotional, psychoillusory, hallucinatory, or dysmnesic phenomena. Especially common auras include an epigastric rising sensation, fear, a feeling of unreality or detachment, déjà vu and jamais vu experiences, and olfactory hallucinations. Patients can interact normally with the environment during simple partial seizures except for limitations imposed by the seizure on specific localized brain functions.

Complex partial seizures, on the other hand, are defined by impaired consciousness and imply bilateral spread of the seizure discharge at least to basal forebrain and limbic areas. In addition to loss of consciousness, patients with complex partial seizures usually exhibit automatisms, such as lip smacking, repeated swallowing, clumsy perseveration of an ongoing motor task, or some other complex motor activity that is undirected and inappropriate. Postictally, patients are confused and disoriented for several minutes,

and determining the transition from ictal to postictal state may be difficult without simultaneous EEG recording. Of complex partial seizures, 70% to 80% arise from the temporal lobe; foci in the frontal and occipital lobes account for most of the remainder.

Generalized Seizures

Generalized tonic–clonic (grand mal) seizures (Video 58.1) are characterized by abrupt loss of consciousness with bilateral tonic extension of the trunk and limbs (*tonic phase*), often accompanied by a loud vocalization as air is forcedly expelled across contracted vocal cords (*epileptic cry*), followed by synchronous muscle jerking (*clonic phase*). In some patients, a few clonic jerks precede the tonic–clonic sequence; in others, only a tonic or clonic phase is apparent. Postictally, patients are briefly unarousable and then lethargic and confused, often preferring to sleep. Many patients report inconsistent nonspecific premonitory symptoms (*epileptic prodrome*) for minutes to a few hours before a generalized tonic–clonic seizure. Common symptoms include ill-defined anxiety, irritability, decreased concentration, and headache or other uncomfortable feelings; these are not auras.

Absence (petit mal) seizures are momentary lapses in awareness that are accompanied by motionless staring and arrest of any ongoing activity. Absence seizures begin and end abruptly; they occur without warning or postictal period. Mild myoclonic jerks of the eyelid or facial muscles, variable loss of muscle tone, and automatisms may accompany longer attacks. When the beginning and end of the seizure are less distinct, or if tonic and autonomic components are included, the term *atypical absence* seizure is used. Atypical absences are seen most often in children with epilepsy who are developmentally delayed or in epileptic encephalopathies, such as the Lennox–Gastaut syndrome (defined later in the chapter). *Myoclonic* seizures are characterized by rapid brief muscle jerks that can occur bilaterally, synchronously or asynchronously, or unilaterally. Myoclonic jerks range from isolated small movements of face, arm, or leg muscles to massive bilateral spasms simultaneously affecting the head, limbs, and trunk.

Atonic (astatic) seizures, (Video 58.2) also called *drop attacks*, are characterized by sudden loss of muscle tone, which may be fragmentary (e.g., head drop) or generalized, resulting in a fall. When atonic seizures are preceded by a brief myoclonic seizure or tonic spasm, an acceleratory force is added to the fall, thereby contributing to the high rate of self-injury with this type of seizure.

CLASSIFICATION OF EPILEPSY (EPILEPTIC SYNDROMES)

Attempting to classify the kind of epilepsy a patient has is often more important than describing seizures because the formulation includes other relevant clinical information of which the seizures are only a part. The other data include historical information (e.g., a personal history of brain injury or family history of first-degree relatives with seizures); findings on neurologic examination; and results of EEG, brain imaging, and biochemical studies.

The ILAE classification separates major groups of epilepsy first on the basis of whether seizures are partial (*localization-related epilepsies*) or generalized (*generalized epilepsies*) and second by cause (*idiopathic, symptomatic,* or *cryptogenic epilepsy*). Subtypes of epilepsy are grouped according to the patient's age and, in the case of localization-related epilepsies, by the anatomic location of the presumed ictal-onset zone.

Classification of the epilepsies has been less successful and more controversial than the classification of seizure types. A basic problem is that the classification scheme is empiric, with clinical and EEG data traditionally emphasized over anatomic, pathologic, or specific etiologic information. This classification is useful for some reasonably well-defined syndromes, such as *infantile spasms* or *benign partial childhood epilepsy with central–midtemporal spikes*, especially because of the prognostic and treatment implications of these disorders. On the other hand, few epilepsies imply a specific disease or defect. A further drawback to the ILAE classification is that the same epileptic syndrome (e.g., infantile spasms or Lennox–Gastaut syndrome) may be "symptomatic" of a specific disease (e.g., tuberous sclerosis), considered "cryptogenic" on the basis of nonspecific imaging abnormalities, or categorized as "idiopathic." Another biologic incongruity is the excessive detail in which some syndromes are identified, with specific entities culled from what are more likely simply different biologic expressions of the same abnormality (e.g., childhood and juvenile forms of absence epilepsy). As a result, a new classification of epilepsy syndromes has been proposed and is presently under discussion (Engel, 2006).

With the foregoing reservations, there is little question that defining common epilepsy syndromes has practical value. Table 58.2 gives a modified version of the current ILAE classification.

TABLE 58.2 Modified Classification of Epileptic Syndromes

I. Idiopathic epilepsy syndromes (focal or generalized)

  A. Benign neonatal convulsions

    1. Familial

    2. Nonfamilial

  B. Benign childhood epilepsy

    1. With central–midtemporal spikes

    2. With occipital spikes

  C. Childhood/juvenile absence epilepsy

  D. Juvenile myoclonic epilepsy (including generalized tonic–clonic seizures on awakening)

  E. Idiopathic epilepsy, otherwise unspecified

II. Symptomatic epilepsy syndromes (focal or generalized)

  A. West syndrome (infantile spasms)

  B. Lennox–Gastaut syndrome

  C. Early myoclonic encephalopathy

  D. Epilepsia partialis continua

    1. Rasmussen syndrome (encephalitic form)

    2. Restricted form

  E. Acquired epileptic aphasia (Landau–Kleffner syndrome)

  F. Temporal lobe epilepsy

  G. Frontal lobe epilepsy

  H. Posttraumatic epilepsy

  I. Other symptomatic epilepsy, focal or generalized, not specified

III. Other epilepsy syndromes of uncertain or mixed classification

  A. Neonatal seizures

  B. Febrile seizures

  C. Reflex epilepsy

  D. Other unspecified

SELECTED GENERALIZED EPILEPSY SYNDROMES

INFANTILE SPASMS (WEST SYNDROME)

The term *infantile spasms* denotes a unique age-specific form of generalized epilepsy that may be either idiopathic or symptomatic. When all clinical data are considered, including results of imaging studies, only about 15% of patients are now classified as idiopathic. Symptomatic cases result from diverse conditions, including cerebral dysgenesis, tuberous sclerosis, phenylketonuria, intrauterine infections, or hypoxic–ischemic injury.

Seizures are characterized by sudden flexor or extensor spasms that simultaneously involve the head, trunk, and limbs. The attacks usually begin before 6 months of age. The EEG is grossly abnormal, showing chaotic high-voltage slow activity with multifocal spikes, a pattern termed *hypsarrhythmia*. The treatment of choice is corticotropin or prednisone; spasms are notoriously refractory to conventional AEDs. Exceptions are topiramate and zonisamide, which have been shown to be an effective alternative to corticotropin in selected cases. Vigabatrin is also effective, especially in children with tuberous sclerosis. Patients on this drug must be monitored for visual field deficits. Although treatment with corticotropin, vigabatrin, zonisamide, or topiramate usually controls spasms and reverses the EEG abnormalities, it has little effect on long-term prognosis. Only about 5% to 10% of children with infantile spasms have normal or near-normal intelligence, and more than 66% have severe disabilities.

CHILDHOOD ABSENCE (PETIT MAL) EPILEPSY

This disorder begins most often between the ages of 4 and 12 years and is characterized predominantly by recurrent absence seizures, which, if untreated, can occur literally hundreds of times each day. EEG activity during an absence attack is characterized by stereotyped, bilateral, 3-Hz spike-wave discharges. Generalized tonic–clonic seizures also occur in 30% to 50% of cases. Most children are normal, both neurologically and intellectually. Ethosuximide and valproate are equally effective in treating absence seizures, but valproate or lamotrigine are preferable if generalized tonic–clonic seizures coexist. Topiramate, levetiracetam, and zonisamide may also be effective in generalized-onset seizures.

LENNOX–GASTAUT SYNDROME

This term is applied to a heterogeneous group of childhood epileptic encephalopathies that are characterized by mental retardation, uncontrolled seizures, and a distinctive EEG pattern. The syndrome is not a pathologic entity because clinical and EEG manifestations result from brain malformations, perinatal asphyxia, severe head injury, central nervous system (CNS) infection, or, rarely, a progressive degenerative or metabolic syndrome. A presumptive cause can be identified in 65% to 70% of affected children. Seizures usually begin before age 4 years, and about 25% of children have a history of infantile spasms. No treatment is consistently effective, and 80% of children continue to have seizures as adults. Best results are generally obtained with broad-spectrum AEDs, such as valproate, clobazam, lamotrigine, topiramate, or zonisamide. Rufinamide may be particularly effective for atonic seizures associated with this syndrome. Despite the higher incidence of severe side effects, felbamate is often effective when these other agents do not result in optimal seizure control. Refractory cases may be considered for vagus nerve stimulation or anterior corpus callosotomy. Both of these are palliative procedures, and complete seizure control is rare.

JUVENILE MYOCLONIC EPILEPSY

The juvenile myoclonic epilepsy (JME) subtype of idiopathic generalized epilepsy most often begins in otherwise healthy individuals between the ages of 8 and 20 years. The fully developed syndrome comprises morning myoclonic jerks, generalized tonic–clonic seizures that occur just after waking, normal intelligence, a family history of similar seizures, and an EEG that shows generalized spikes, 4- to 6-Hz spike waves, and multiple spike (polyspike) discharges. The myoclonic jerks vary in intensity from bilateral massive spasms and falls to minor isolated muscle jerks that many patients consider nothing more than "morning clumsiness." Linkage studies have produced conflicting results with different groups reporting susceptibility loci on chromosomes 6p, 5q, and 15q. A mutation in the α-1 subunit of the γ-aminobutyric acid (GABA)$_A$ receptor has been found in a large French Canadian family with JME but not in individuals with the common sporadic form of JME. Valproate is the treatment of choice and controls seizures and myoclonus in more than 80% of cases. Lamotrigine, zonisamide, levetiracetam, and topiramate can be equally effective in many patients, although lamotrigine sometimes exacerbates myoclonus.

SELECTED LOCALIZATION-RELATED EPILEPSY SYNDROMES

BENIGN FOCAL EPILEPSY OF CHILDHOOD

Several "benign" focal epilepsies occur in children, of which the most common is the syndrome associated with central–midtemporal spikes on EEG. This form of idiopathic focal epilepsy, also known as *benign rolandic epilepsy*, accounts for about 15% of all pediatric seizure disorders.

Onset is between 4 and 13 years of age; children are otherwise normal. Most children have attacks mainly or exclusively at night. Sleep promotes secondary generalization, so that parents report only generalized tonic–clonic seizures; any focal manifestations go unobserved. In contrast, seizures that occur during the day are clearly focal, with twitching of one side of the face; speech arrest; drooling from a corner of the mouth; and paresthesias of the tongue, lips, inner cheeks, and face. Seizures may progress to include clonic jerking or tonic posturing of the arm and leg on one side. Consciousness is usually preserved.

The interictal EEG abnormality is distinctive and shows stereotyped diphasic or triphasic sharp waves over the central–midtemporal (rolandic) regions. Discharges may be unilateral or bilateral. They increase in abundance during sleep and, when unilateral, switch from side to side on successive EEGs. In about 30% of cases, generalized spike-wave activity also occurs. The EEG pattern is inherited as an autosomal dominant trait with age-dependent penetrance. The inheritance pattern of the seizures, although clearly familial, is probably multifactorial and less well understood. More than half the children who show the characteristic EEG abnormality never have clinical attacks. Linkage has been reported in some families to chromosome 15q14.

The prognosis is uniformly good. Seizures disappear by mid to late adolescence in all cases. Seizures in many children appear to be self-limited, and not all children need AED treatment. Treatment can usually be deferred until after the second or third attack. Because seizures are easily controlled and self-limited, drugs with the fewest adverse effects, such as carbamazepine, oxcarbazepine, or gabapentin, should be used. Low doses, often producing subtherapeutic blood concentrations, are generally effective. Polytherapy should be avoided.

TEMPORAL LOBE EPILEPSY

This is the most common epilepsy syndrome of adults. In most cases, the epileptogenic region involves mesial temporal lobe structures, especially the hippocampus, amygdala, and parahippocampal gyrus. Seizures usually begin in late childhood or adolescence, and a history of febrile seizures is common. Virtually all patients have complex partial seizures, some of which secondarily generalize. Auras are frequent; visceral sensations are particularly common. Other typical behavioral features include a motionless stare, loss of awareness that may be gradual, and oral–alimentary automatisms, such as lip smacking (Video 58.3). A variable but often prolonged period of postictal confusion is the rule. Interictal EEGs show focal temporal slowing and epileptiform sharp waves or spikes over the anterior temporal region. AEDs are usually successful in suppressing secondarily generalized seizures, but most patients continue to have partial attacks. When seizures persist, anterior temporal lobe resection or selective amygdalohippocampectomy is the treatment of choice. For appropriate patients with mesial temporal sclerosis, ablation with laser or Gamma Knife has also been used, although it is not known whether these are as effective as more traditional resection in the long term. The results of a randomized controlled trial comparing seizure outcomes in patients treated either medically or surgically were striking: 58% of surgically treated patients were seizure free at 1 year compared with 8% of medically treated patients. Other series have shown that temporal lobe resection for refractory medial temporal lobe epilepsy associated with hippocampal sclerosis results in complete seizure control for at least 1 year in over 80% of patients. More controversial is the need for long-term anticonvulsant drug treatment after successful operation; a minority of patients may relapse several years later.

FRONTAL LOBE EPILEPSY

The particular pattern of the many types of frontal lobe seizures depends on the specific location where the seizure discharge originates and on the pathways subsequently involved in propagation. Despite this variability, the following features, when taken together, suggest frontal lobe epilepsy:

1. Brief seizures that begin and end abruptly with little, if any, postictal period
2. A tendency for seizures to cluster and to occur at night
3. Prominent, but often bizarre, motor manifestations, such as asynchronous thrashing or flailing of arms and legs; pedaling leg movements; pelvic thrusting; and loud, sometimes obscene, vocalizations, all of which may suggest psychogenic seizures (Video 58.4)
4. Minimal abnormality on scalp EEG recordings
5. A history of status epilepticus

Frontal lobe epilepsy occurs in some families as an autosomal dominant syndrome. In these patients, seizures almost always occur during sleep. Most patients respond well to medication.

POSTTRAUMATIC SEIZURES

Seizures occur within 1 year in about 7% of civilian and in about 34% of military head injuries. The differences relate mainly to the much higher proportion of penetrating wounds in military cases. The risk of developing posttraumatic epilepsy is directly related to the severity of the injury and also correlates with the total volume of brain lost as measured by computed tomography (CT). Depressed skull fractures may or may not be a risk; the rate of posttraumatic epilepsy was 17% in one series but not increased above control levels in another. Head injuries are classified as *severe* if they result in brain contusion, intracerebral or intracranial hematoma, unconsciousness, or amnesia for more than 24 hours or in persistent neurologic abnormalities, such as aphasia, hemiparesis, or dementia. *Mild* head injury (brief loss of consciousness, no skull fracture, no focal neurologic signs, no contusion or hematoma) does not increase the risk of seizures significantly above general population rates.

Nearly 60% of those who have seizures have the first attack in the first year after the injury. In the Vietnam Head Injury Study, however, more than 15% of patients did not have epilepsy until 5 or more years later. Posttraumatic seizures are classified as *early* (within the first 1 to 2 weeks after injury) or *late*. Only recurrent late seizures (those that occur after the patient has recovered from the acute effects of the injury) should be considered *posttraumatic epilepsy*. Early seizures, however, even if isolated, increase the chance of developing posttraumatic epilepsy. About 70% of patients have partial or secondarily generalized seizures. *Impact seizures* occur at the time of or immediately after the injury. These attacks are attributed to an acute reaction of the brain to trauma and do not increase the risk of later epilepsy.

Overt seizures should be treated according to principles reviewed later in this chapter. The most controversial issue concerns the prophylactic use of AEDs to retard or abort the development of subsequent seizures. Based on the data of Temkin et al. (1990), we recommend treating patients with severe head trauma, as just defined, with an antiepileptic medication for the first week after injury to minimize complications from seizures occurring during acute management. If seizures have not occurred, we do not continue medication beyond the initial 1 to 2 weeks because evidence does not show that longer treatment prevents the development of later seizures or of posttraumatic epilepsy. Data suggest that valproate is less effective than phenytoin in suppressing acute seizures and is also ineffective in preventing the development of posttraumatic epilepsy.

EPILEPSIA PARTIALIS CONTINUA

Epilepsia partialis continua (EPC) refers to unremitting motor seizures involving part or all of one side of the body. They typically consist of repeated clonic or myoclonic jerks that may remain focal or regional or may march from one muscle group to another, with the extent of motor involvement waxing and waning in endless variation (Video 58.5). In adults, EPC occurs in diverse settings, such as with subacute or chronic inflammatory diseases of the brain (Kozhevnikov Russian spring–summer encephalitis, Behçet disease) or with acute strokes, metastases, and metabolic encephalopathies, especially hyperosmolar nonketotic hyperglycemia.

The most distinctive form of EPC, known as the *Rasmussen syndrome*, occurs in children; it usually begins before the age of 10 years. The underlying disorder is chronic focal encephalitis, although an infectious agent has not been identified consistently. About two-thirds of patients report an infectious or inflammatory illness 1 to 6 months before onset of EPC. Generalized tonic–clonic seizures are often the first sign and appear before the EPC establishes itself. About 20% of cases begin with an episode of convulsive status epilepticus. Slow neurologic deterioration inevitably follows, with development of hemiparesis, mental impairment, and, usually, hemianopia. If the dominant hemisphere is affected, aphasia occurs. EEGs are always abnormal, but findings are not specific, and they frequently do not correlate with clinical manifestations. Magnetic resonance imaging (MRI) may be normal early but later shows unilateral cortical atrophy and signal changes consistent with gliosis. Autoantibodies to the GluR3 protein of the glutamate receptor have been found in some patients, suggesting that autoimmunity may

play a role in the pathogenesis of the disorder in some patients, and immunotherapy is sometimes beneficial. AEDs are usually ineffective in controlling seizures and preventing progression of the disease, as are corticosteroids and antiviral agents. When seizures have not spontaneously remitted by the time there is a severe degree of hemiparesis, functional hemispherectomy can control seizures and leads to substantial intellectual improvement in many patients. Controversy arises in the decision about the best time for hemispherectomy, for example, whether it should be performed earlier before there is serious motor or language impairment.

EPIDEMIOLOGY

In the United States, about 6.5 persons per 1,000 population are affected with recurrent unprovoked seizures, so-called active epilepsy. Based on 1990 census figures, age-adjusted annual incidence rates for epilepsy range from 31 to 57 per 100,000 in the United States (Fig. 58.1). Incidence rates are highest among young children and the elderly; epilepsy affects males 1.1 to 1.5 times more often than females.

Complex partial seizures are the most common seizure type among newly diagnosed cases, but age-related variability occurs in the proportions of different seizure types (Fig. 58.2). The cause of epilepsy also varies somewhat with age. Despite advances in diagnostic capabilities, however, the "unknown" etiologic category remains larger than any other for all age groups (Fig. 58.3). Cerebrovascular disease, associated developmental neurologic disorders (e.g., cerebral palsy and mental retardation), and head trauma are the other most commonly identified causes.

Although defined genetic disorders account for only about 1% of epilepsy cases, heritable factors are important. Monozygotic twins have a much higher concordance rate for epilepsy than do dizygotic twins. By age 25 years, nearly 9% of children of mothers with epilepsy and 2.4% of children of affected fathers develop epilepsy. The reason for an increased risk of seizures in children of women with epilepsy is not known.

Some forms of epilepsy are more heritable than others. For example, children of parents with absence seizures have a higher risk of developing epilepsy (9%) than do offspring of parents with other types of generalized seizures or partial seizures (5%). As a general rule, though, even offspring born to a high-risk parent have a 90% or greater chance of being unaffected by epilepsy.

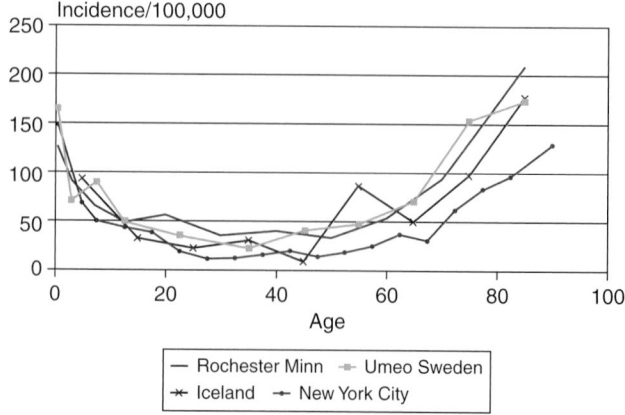

FIGURE 58.1 Age-specific incidence of epilepsy in Rochester, Minnesota, 1935–1984. (From Hauser WA, Annegers JF, Kurland LT. Incidence of epilepsy and unprovoked seizures in Rochester, Minnesota: 1935-1984. *Epilepsia.* 1993;34(3): 453-468.)

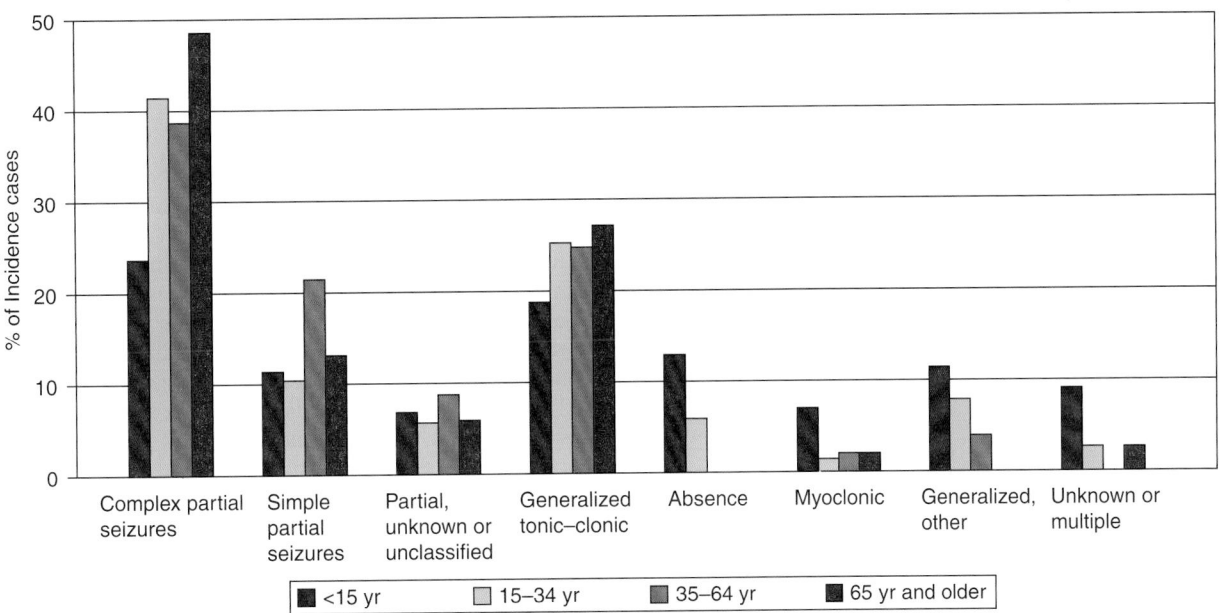

FIGURE 58.2 Proportion of seizure types in newly diagnosed cases of epilepsy in Rochester, Minnesota, 1935–1984. (From Hauser WA, Annegers JF, Kurland LT. Incidence of epilepsy and unprovoked seizures in Rochester, Minnesota: 1935-1984. *Epilepsia*. 1993;34(3):453-468.)

Many persons who experience a first unprovoked seizure never have a second. By definition, these people do not have epilepsy and generally do not require long-term drug treatment. Unfortunately, our ability to identify such individuals with accuracy is imperfect. Treatment decisions must be based on epidemiologic and individual considerations. Some seizure types, such as absence and myoclonic, are virtually always recurrent by the time the patient is seen by a physician. On the other hand, patients with convulsive seizures may seek medical attention after a first occurrence because of the dramatic nature of the attack. Prospective studies of recurrence after a first seizure indicate a 2-year recurrence risk of about 40%, which is similar in children and adults. The risk is lowest in people with an idiopathic generalized first seizure and normal EEG (about 24%), higher with idiopathic generalized seizures and an abnormal EEG (about 48%), and highest with symptomatic (i.e., known preceding brain injury or neurologic syndrome) seizures and an abnormal EEG (about 65%). Epileptiform, but not nonepileptiform, EEG abnormalities impart a greater risk for recurrence. If the first seizure is a partial seizure, the relative risk of recurrence is also increased. The risk for further recurrence after a second unprovoked seizure is greater than 80%; a second unprovoked seizure is, therefore, a reliable marker of epilepsy.

About 4% of persons living to age 74 years have at least one unprovoked seizure. When provoked seizures (i.e., febrile seizures or those related to an acute illness) are included, the likelihood of experiencing a seizure by age 74 years increases to at least 9%. The risk of developing epilepsy is about 3% by age 74 years.

Of persons with epilepsy, 60% to 70% achieve remission of seizures with AED therapy. Factors that favor remission include an idiopathic (or cryptogenic) form of epilepsy, normal findings on neurologic examination, and onset in early to middle childhood (except neonatal seizures). Unfavorable prognostic factors include partial seizures, an abnormal EEG, and associated mental retardation or cerebral palsy (Table 58.3). Those who fail to achieve remission have drug-resistant epilepsy and may be candidates for alternative therapies, including surgery or devices as well as additional drug treatment. Drug-resistant epilepsy is defined by the ILAE as "failure of adequate trials of two tolerated and appropriately used antiepileptic drugs to achieve sustained seizure freedom."

FIGURE 58.3 Etiology of epilepsy in all cases of newly diagnosed seizures in Rochester, Minnesota, 1935–1984. (From Hauser WA, Annegers JF, Kurland LT. Incidence of epilepsy and unprovoked seizures in Rochester, Minnesota: 1935-1984. *Epilepsia*. 1993;34(3):453-468.)

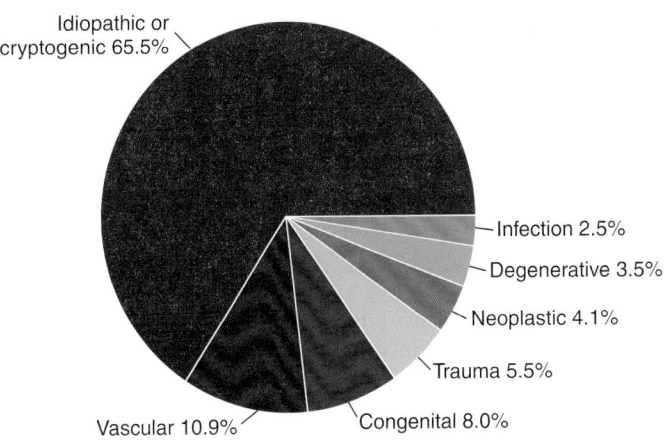

TABLE 58.3	*Predictors of Intractable Epilepsy*
Very young at onset (<2 yr)	
Frequent generalized seizures	
Failure to achieve control readily	
Evidence of brain damage	
A specific cause of the seizures	
Severe EEG abnormality	
Low IQ	
Atonic atypical absence seizures	

EEG, electroencephalogram.

Mortality is increased in persons with epilepsy, but the risk is incurred mainly by symptomatic cases in which higher death rates are related primarily to the underlying disease rather than to epilepsy. Accidental deaths, especially drowning, are more common, however, in all patients with epilepsy. Sudden unexplained death is nearly 25 times more common in patients with epilepsy than in the general population; estimates of incidence rates range from 1 in 500 to 1 in 2,000 per year. Severe epilepsy, uncontrolled generalized convulsions, especially nocturnal, and need for multiple AEDs are risk factors.

INITIAL DIAGNOSTIC EVALUATION

The diagnostic evaluation has three objectives: to determine if the patient has epilepsy; to classify the type of epilepsy and identify an epilepsy syndrome, if possible; and to define the specific underlying cause. Accurate diagnosis leads directly to proper treatment and formulation of a rational plan of management. The differential diagnosis is considered in Section II, Chapter 5.

Because epilepsy comprises a group of conditions and is not a single homogeneous disorder and because seizures may be symptoms of both diverse brain disorders and an otherwise normal brain, it is neither possible nor desirable to develop inflexible guidelines for what constitutes a standard or minimal diagnostic evaluation. The clinical data from the history and physical examination should allow a reasonable determination of probable diagnosis, seizure and epilepsy classification, and likelihood of underlying brain disorder. Based on these considerations, diagnostic testing should be undertaken selectively.

HISTORY AND EXAMINATION

A complete history is the cornerstone for establishing a diagnosis of epilepsy. Because patients frequently have no or only limited recall of their attacks, it is important to obtain additional information from family members or friends who have witnessed seizures. An adequate history should provide a clear picture of the clinical features of the seizures and the sequence in which manifestations evolve; the course of the epileptic disorder; seizure precipitants, such as alcohol or sleep deprivation; risk factors for seizures, such as abnormal gestation, febrile seizures, family history of epilepsy, head injury, encephalitis or meningitis, and stroke; and response to previous treatment. In children, developmental history is important.

In describing the epileptic seizure, care should be taken to elicit a detailed description of any aura. The aura was once considered to be the warning of an impending attack, but it is actually a simple partial seizure made apparent by subjective feelings or experiential phenomena observable only by the patient. Auras precede many complex partial or generalized seizures and are experienced by 50% to 60% of adults with epilepsy. Auras confirm the suspicion that the seizure begins locally within the brain; they may also provide direct clues about the location or laterality of the focus. Information about later events in the seizure usually are obtained from an observer because of the patient's impaired awareness or frank loss of consciousness or because of postictal amnesia, even though responses to questions during the seizure indicate preserved responsiveness.

The nature of repetitive automatic or purposeless movements (automatisms), sustained postures, presence of myoclonus, and the duration of the seizure help to delineate specific seizure types or epileptic syndromes. Nonspecific postictal findings of lethargy and confusion must be distinguished from focal neurologic abnormalities, such as hemiparesis or aphasia, which could point to the hemisphere of seizure onset.

Information about risk factors (Fig. 58.4) may suggest a particular cause and assist in prognosis. In addition to these risk factors, migraines with auras and depression have been reported to be independent risk factors for unprovoked seizures. Discussion of risk factors with parents may be necessary because children or adults

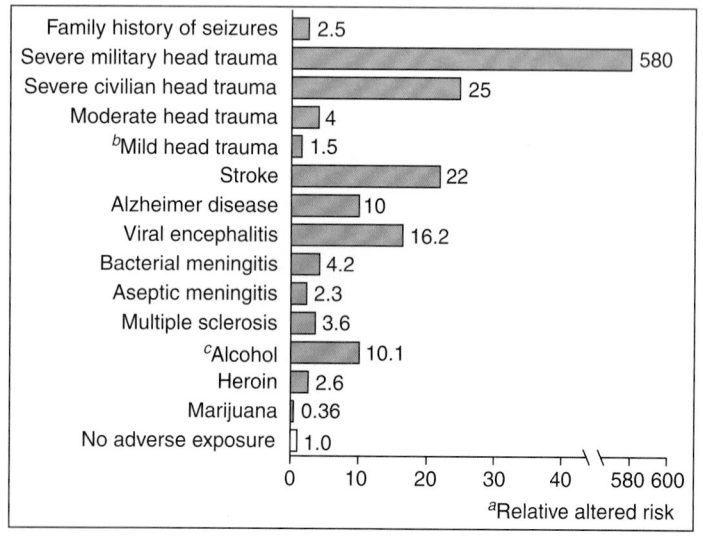

FIGURE 58.4 Risk factors for epilepsy. [a]Relative to people without these adverse exposures. [b]Not statistically significant. [c]One pint of 80 proof, 2.5 bottles of wine. (From Hauser WA, Hesdorffer DC. *Epilepsy: Frequency, Causes and Consequences.* New York: Demos; 1990.)

may be uninformed about, or may not recall, early childhood events, such as perinatal encephalopathy, febrile seizures, brain infections, head injuries, or intermittent absence seizures. Age at seizure onset and course of the seizure disorder should be clarified because these features differ in the various epilepsy syndromes.

Findings on neurologic examination are usually normal in patients with epilepsy but occasionally may provide etiologic clues. Focal signs indicate an underlying cerebral lesion. Asymmetry of the hand or face may indicate localized or hemispheric cerebral atrophy contralateral to the smaller side. Phakomatoses are commonly associated with seizures and are suggested by café au lait spots, facial angioma, conjunctival telangiectasia, hypopigmented macules, fibroangiomatous nevi, or lumbosacral shagreen patches.

ELECTROENCEPHALOGRAPHY

Because epilepsy is fundamentally a physiologic disturbance of brain function, the EEG is the most important laboratory test in evaluating patients with seizures. The EEG helps both to establish the diagnosis of epilepsy and to characterize specific epileptic syndromes. EEG findings may also help in management and in prognosis.

Epileptiform discharges (spikes and sharp waves) are highly correlated with seizure susceptibility and can be recorded on the first EEG in about 50% of patients. Similar findings are recorded in only 1% to 2% of normal adults and in a somewhat higher percentage of normal children. When multiple EEGs are obtained, epileptiform abnormalities eventually appear in 60% to 90% of adults with epilepsy, but the yield of positive studies does not increase substantially after three or four tests. Prolonged ambulatory or inpatient recordings increase the yield of interictal epileptiform abnormalities both because of the longer sampling times but also because complete sleep–wake cycles are included. It is important to remember, therefore, that 10% to 40% of patients with epilepsy do not show epileptiform abnormalities on routine EEG. Thus, a normal or nonspecifically abnormal EEG never excludes the diagnosis. Sleep, hyperventilation, photic stimulation, and special electrode placements are routinely used to increase the probability of recording epileptiform abnormalities. Different and distinctive patterns of epileptiform discharge occur in specific epilepsy syndromes as summarized in Chapter 25.

BRAIN IMAGING

MRI should be performed in all patients older than age 18 years and in children with abnormal development, abnormal findings on physical examination, or seizure types that are likely to be manifestations of symptomatic epilepsy. CT will often miss common epileptogenic lesions such as hippocampal sclerosis, cortical dysplasia, and cavernous malformations. Because CT is very sensitive for detecting brain calcifications, a noncontrast CT (in addition to MRI) may be helpful in patients at risk for neurocysticercosis.

Routine imaging is not necessary for children with idiopathic epilepsy, including the benign focal epilepsy syndromes (see section "Benign Epilepsy Syndromes"). Brain MRI, although more costly, is more sensitive than CT in detecting potentially epileptogenic lesions, such as cortical dysplasia, hamartomas, differentiated glial tumors, and cavernous malformations. Both axial and coronal planes should be imaged using both T1 and T2 sequences. Gadolinium injection does not increase the sensitivity for detecting cerebral lesions but may assist in differentiating possible causes.

Imaging in the coronal plane perpendicular to the long axis of the hippocampus and other variations in technique have improved the detection of hippocampal atrophy and gliosis, findings that are highly correlated with mesial temporal sclerosis (Fig. 58.5) and an epileptogenic temporal lobe. An even more sensitive measure of hippocampal atrophy is MRI measurement of the volume of the hippocampus. Hippocampal volume measurements in an individual patient then can be compared with those of normal control subjects. In patients being considered for surgery, interictal

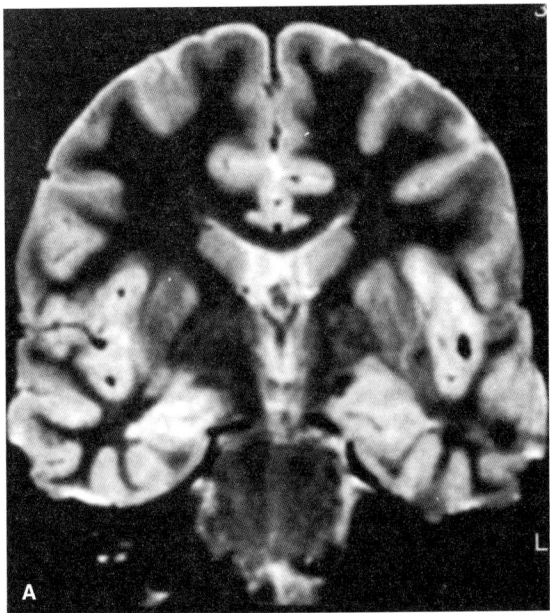 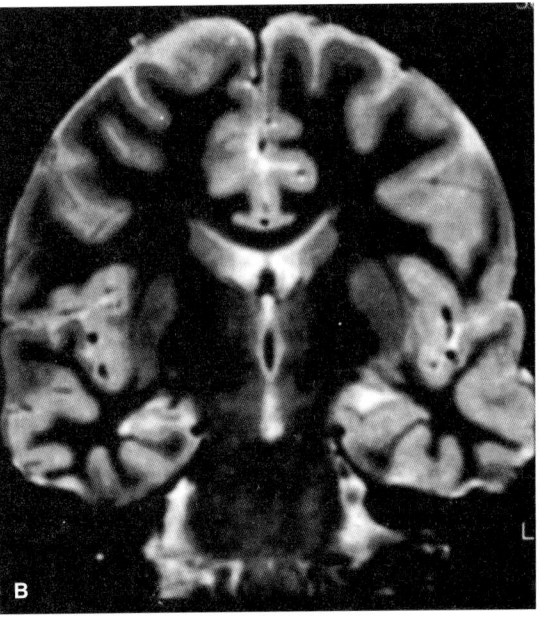

FIGURE 58.5 Mesial temporal sclerosis. **A,B:** Short-tau inversion recovery (STIR) coronal magnetic resonance images through the temporal lobes show increased signal and decreased size of right hippocampus as compared with left. These findings are characteristic of mesial temporal sclerosis. Note incidental focal dilatation of left choroid fissure, which represents a choroid fissure cyst and is a normal variant. (Courtesy of Dr. S. Chan, Columbia University College of Physicians and Surgeons, New York, NY.)

positron emission tomography (PET) scans can add valuable localizing information, especially when the MRI scan is negative. Single-photon emission computed tomography (SPECT) scans are also used, although resolution is less than either MRI or PET. Subtraction ictal SPECT co-registered with MRI (SISCOM) is also helpful in localizing the epileptogenic brain region in some cases.

OTHER LABORATORY TESTS

Routine blood tests are necessary in newborns and in older patients with acute or chronic systemic disease to detect abnormal electrolyte, glucose, calcium, or magnesium values or impaired liver or kidney function that may contribute to seizure occurrence. They are rarely diagnostically useful in healthy children or adults. Serum electrolytes, liver function tests, and a complete blood count (CBC) should be obtained when infectious or metabolic abnormalities are suspected, but they are useful mainly as baseline studies before initiating AED treatment.

Any suspicion of meningitis or encephalitis mandates lumbar puncture. Urine or blood toxicologic screens should be considered when otherwise unexplained new-onset generalized seizures occur.

LONG-TERM MONITORING

The most direct and convincing evidence of an epileptic basis for a patient's episodic symptoms is the electrographic recording of a seizure discharge during a typical behavioral attack. Such recordings are especially necessary if the history is ambiguous, EEGs are repeatedly normal or nonspecifically abnormal, and reasonable treatment has failed. Because most patients have seizures infrequently, routine EEG rarely records an attack. Long-term monitoring permits continuous EEG recording for extended periods, thus increasing the likelihood of recording seizures or interictal epileptiform discharges. Two methods of long-term monitoring are now widely available: simultaneous closed-circuit television (CCTV) and EEG (CCTV/EEG) monitoring and ambulatory EEG. Both have greatly improved diagnostic accuracy and the reliability of seizure classification, and both provide continuous recordings through one or more complete sleep–wake cycles, which increases the likelihood of capturing actual ictal events. Each has its own specific advantages and disadvantages. The method chosen depends on the question posed by a particular patient.

Long-term monitoring using CCTV/EEG, usually in a specially designed hospital unit, is the procedure of choice to document psychogenic seizures and other nonepileptic paroxysmal events. It can also establish electrical–clinical correlations, confirm seizure type, and direct further treatment including the localization of epileptogenic foci for possible resective surgery. The emphasis in monitoring units is usually on behavioral events, not interictal EEG activity. The availability of full-time technical or nursing staff ensures high-quality recordings and permits examination of patients during clinical events. AEDs can be discontinued safely to facilitate seizure occurrence. Computerized detection programs are used to screen EEG continuously for epileptiform abnormalities and subclinical seizures.

Ambulatory EEG is another method for long-term monitoring that is designed for outpatient use in the patient's home, school, or work environment. This is often especially helpful in evaluating children who are usually more comfortable in their familiar and unrestricted home environments. The major limitations of ambulatory monitoring are the variable technical quality resulting from lack of expert supervision and maintenance of electrode integrity, frequent distortion of EEG data by environmental contaminants,

and the absence of video documentation of behavioral changes. Ambulatory monitoring is most useful in documenting interictal epileptiform activity when routine EEGs have been repeatedly negative or in recording ictal discharges during typical behavioral events. It may also reveal the presence of unrecognized electrographic seizures (particularly absences) if frequent. At the present time, however, ambulatory EEG is not a substitute for CCTV/EEG monitoring, especially when psychogenic seizures are an issue or when patients are being evaluated for epilepsy surgery.

MEDICAL TREATMENT

Therapy of epilepsy has three goals: (1) to eliminate seizures or reduce their frequency to the maximum extent possible, (2) to avoid side effects associated with long-term treatment, and (3) to assist the patient in maintaining or restoring normal psychosocial and vocational adjustment. No medical treatment now available can induce a permanent remission ("cure") or prevent development of epilepsy by altering the process of epileptogenesis.

The decision to institute AED therapy should be based on a thoughtful and informed analysis of the issues involved. Isolated infrequent seizures, whether convulsive or not, probably pose little medical risk to otherwise healthy persons. However, even relatively minor seizures, especially those associated with loss or alteration of alertness, can be associated with many psychosocial, vocational, and safety ramifications. Finally, the probability of seizure recurrence varies substantially among patients, depending on the type of epilepsy and any associated neurologic or medical problems. Drug treatment, on the other hand, carries a risk of adverse effects, which approaches 30% after initial treatment. Treatment of children raises additional issues, especially the unknown effects of long-term AED use on brain development, learning, and behavior.

These considerations mean that although drug treatment is indicated and is beneficial for most patients with epilepsy, certain circumstances call for AEDs to be deferred or used only for a limited time. As a rule of thumb, AEDs should be prescribed when the potential benefits of treatment clearly outweigh possible adverse effects of therapy.

ACUTE SYMPTOMATIC SEIZURES

These seizures are caused by, or associated with, an acute medical or neurologic illness (see Chapter 6). A childhood febrile seizure is the most common example of an acute symptomatic seizure, but other frequently encountered causes include metabolic or toxic encephalopathies, head trauma, and acute brain infections. Prophylactic phenytoin has been shown to reduce the frequency of seizures in patients with severe traumatic brain injury from 14% to 4% during the first week after injury [**Level 1**].[2] To the extent that these conditions resolve without permanent brain damage, seizures are usually self-limited. The primary therapeutic concern in such patients should be identification and treatment of the underlying disorder. If AEDs are needed to suppress seizures acutely, they generally do not need to be continued after the patient recovers.

THE SINGLE SEIZURE

About 25% of patients with unprovoked seizures come to a physician after a single attack, nearly always a generalized tonic–clonic seizure. Most of these people have no risk factors for epilepsy, have normal findings on neurologic examination, and have a normal first EEG. Only about 25% of such patients later develop epilepsy. For this group, the need for treatment is questionable. For many years, no convincing data indicated any beneficial effect of treatment on preventing recurrence. In 1993, a large multicenter randomized study from Italy convincingly demonstrated that AEDs reduce the risk of relapse after the first unprovoked convulsive seizure. Among nearly 400 children and adults, treatment within 7 days of a first seizure was followed by a recurrence rate of 25% at 2 years. In contrast, untreated patients had a recurrence rate of 51%. When patients with previous "uncertain spells" were excluded from the analysis, treatment benefit was still evident, but the magnitude of the effect was reduced to a recurrence rate of 30% in the treated group and 42% in untreated patients.

Although treatment of first seizures reduces the relapse rate even in low-risk patients, there is no evidence that such treatment alters long-term prognosis. In 2015, a new evidence-based guideline for management of adults with a first unprovoked seizure identified the following risk factors for progression to epilepsy: a prior brain insult, an EEG with epileptiform abnormalities, a significant brain-imaging abnormality, and a nocturnal seizure [Level 1].[2] Clinicians' recommendations whether to initiate immediate AED treatment after a first seizure should be based on individualized assessments that weigh the risk of recurrence against the potential side effects of AED therapy and consider patient preferences. Immediate treatment will not improve the long-term prognosis for seizure remission but will reduce seizure risk over the subsequent 2 years. In most patients with idiopathic epilepsy, deferring treatment until a second seizure occurs is a reasonable and often preferable decision.

BENIGN EPILEPSY SYNDROMES

Several electroclinical syndromes begin in childhood and are associated with normal development, normal findings on neurologic examination, and normal brain imaging studies. They have a uniformly good prognosis for complete remission in mid to late adolescence without long-term behavioral or cognitive problems. The most common and best characterized of these syndromes is benign partial epilepsy of childhood with central–midtemporal sharp waves (rolandic epilepsy). Most seizures occur at night as secondarily generalized convulsions. Focal seizures occur during the day and are characterized by twitching of one side of the face, anarthria, salivation, and paresthesias of the face and inner mouth followed variably by hemiclonic movements or hemitonic posturing. Other generally benign syndromes include childhood epilepsy with occipital paroxysms and benign epilepsy with affective symptoms.

Because of the good prognosis, the sole goal of treatment in such cases is to prevent recurrence. Because many children, especially those who are older, tend to have only a few seizures, treatment is not always necessary. AEDs are usually reserved for children whose seizures are frequent or relatively severe or whose parents, or the children themselves, are frightened at the prospect of future attacks. With these considerations in mind, only about half the children with benign partial epilepsy require treatment.

ANTIEPILEPTIC DRUGS

Selection of Antiepileptic Drugs

Two nationwide collaborative Veterans Administration Cooperative Studies (1985 and 1992) compared the effectiveness of the then available major AEDs. In the 1985 study, carbamazepine, phenytoin, primidone, and phenobarbital were equally effective in controlling complex partial and secondarily generalized seizures [Level 1].[3] In the 1992 study, carbamazepine was slightly more effective than valproate in treating complex partial seizures, but both drugs were of equal efficacy in controlling secondarily generalized seizures [Level 3].[4] These studies also demonstrated that despite their relatively uniform ability to suppress seizures, the drugs had different risks of adverse effects. More recently, there have been randomized trials in patients with partial seizures comparing the effectiveness of gabapentin, lamotrigine, topiramate, or oxcarbazepine to that of carbamazepine and phenytoin. None has shown definite superiority, although many have demonstrated that the newer agents have improved tolerability. *A survey of epilepsy experts in North America found that carbamazepine remains the drug of first choice for partial seizures when both efficacy and tolerability are considered.* Gabapentin, pregabalin, lamotrigine, topiramate, oxcarbazepine, levetiracetam, and phenytoin remain reasonable alternatives for many patients. The SANAD trial, a large open-label study, randomized patients with focal epilepsy to carbamazepine, lamotrigine, oxcarbazepine, or topiramate. Lamotrigine had a slight advantage in time to treatment failure, but as in previous comparative studies, the differences among agents in terms of effectiveness were minimal [Level 1].[5] Many smaller trials have directly compared various drugs against each other with similar findings; although there may be differences in tolerability, there are no clear advantages in efficacy when an appropriate agent is used at a therapeutic dose [Level 1].[6]

In general, valproate is the drug of choice for generalized-onset seizures and can be used advantageously as monotherapy when several generalized seizure types coexist (Table 58.4). Lamotrigine, levetiracetam, topiramate, and zonisamide are suitable alternatives if valproate is ineffective or not tolerated. A second arm of the SANAD trial compared the effectiveness of valproate, lamotrigine, and topiramate in patients with all types of generalized or unclassified seizures. Valproate was found to be slightly more effective overall, especially for idiopathic epilepsy, although the differences were minimal [Level 1].[7] Phenytoin, carbamazepine, and oxcarbazepine are useful in suppressing generalized tonic–clonic seizures, but the response is less predictable than that with valproate. Carbamazepine, phenytoin, gabapentin, and lamotrigine can aggravate myoclonic seizures; all of these except lamotrigine also sometimes exacerbate absence seizures. Tiagabine can aggravate or induce absence

TABLE 58.4	Drugs Used in Treating Different Types of Seizures
Type of Seizure	**Drugs[a]**
Localization related epilepsy	
Simple and complex partial; secondarily generalized	Carbamazepine, lamotrigine, topiramate, levetiracetam, lacosamide, oxcarbazepine, pregabalin, valproate, gabapentin, zonisamide, phenytoin, primidone, phenobarbital, perampanel, ezogabine, clobazam
Primary generalized seizures	
Tonic–clonic	Valproate, lamotrigine, topiramate, levetiracetam, zonisamide, carbamazepine, oxcarbazepine, phenytoin
Absence	Valproate, lamotrigine, ethosuximide, zonisamide
Myoclonic	Valproate, clonazepam, levetiracetam
Tonic	Valproate, felbamate, clonazepam, zonisamide, rufinamide

[a]Not all drugs have FDA approval for listed uses.

seizures. Ethosuximide is as effective as valproate in controlling absence seizures and has fewer side effects. Ethosuximide is ineffective against tonic–clonic seizures, however, so its main use is as an alternative to valproate in patients who have only absence seizures.

Many of the newer AEDs have been shown to be effective as adjunctive or add-on therapy for patients with seizures that are refractory to a single medication. Gabapentin can be effective for the treatment of mixed seizure disorders, and gabapentin, lamotrigine, oxcarbazepine, and topiramate for the treatment of refractory partial seizures in children. Evidence also suggests that lamotrigine and topiramate are also effective for adjunctive treatment of idiopathic generalized epilepsy in adults and children, as well as treatment of the Lennox Gastaut syndrome [**Level 1**].[8]

Clobazam was recently U.S. Food and Drug Administration (FDA) approved for add-on therapy in severe epilepsies such as Lennox–Gastaut syndrome. It is also effective in focal epilepsies that are refractory to other medications and has been widely prescribed worldwide for this indication. Vigabatrin was approved by the FDA for treating infantile spasms in children 1 month to 2 years of age.

Of the more recently introduced antiepileptic medications, lacosamide, ezogabine, and perampanel have been approved for use in focal epilepsies refractory to other medications, and rufinamide was additionally approved to treat seizures associated with Lennox–Gastaut syndrome.

Elderly patients with epilepsy require special consideration because of age-related changes in both pharmacokinetic profiles and pharmacodynamic characteristics. Relevant physiologic changes include decreased hepatic metabolism and plasma protein binding, decreased renal clearance, and slower gastrointestinal motility and absorption. There is greater sensitivity to both desirable and undesirable effects on brain function. Additionally, concurrent medical illnesses are common, and as a result, most elderly patients take multiple drugs, which increase the likelihood of clinically significant drug interactions. Several clinical trials involving elderly patients, including a large Veterans Administration cooperative study, have found that lamotrigine and gabapentin are better tolerated than carbamazepine, although, as in younger patients, differences in effectiveness, if any, are small.

Adverse Effects of Antiepileptic Drugs

All AEDs have undesirable effects in some patients. Although interindividual variation occurs, most adverse drug effects are mild and dose related. Many are common to virtually all AEDs, especially when treatment is started. These include sedation, mental dulling, impaired memory and concentration, mood changes, gastrointestinal upset, and dizziness. The incidence of particular adverse effects varies with the individual agent. In general, sedation and cognitive effects are less likely with lamotrigine or gabapentin than with older agents, especially in elderly persons. Some adverse effects are relatively specific for particular drugs.

DOSE-RELATED SIDE EFFECTS

These typically appear when a drug is first given or when the dosage is increased. They usually, but not always, correlate with blood concentrations of the parent drug or major metabolites (Table 58.5). Dose-related side effects are always reversible on lowering the dosage or discontinuing the drug. An exception to this is the peripheral vision loss with vigabatrin, which may progress despite stopping the drug. Adverse effects frequently determine the limits of treatment with a particular drug and have a major influence on compliance with the prescribed regimen. Because dose-related side effects are broadly predictable, they are often the major differentiating feature in choosing among otherwise equally effective therapies.

IDIOSYNCRATIC SIDE EFFECTS

Idiosyncratic responses account for most serious and virtually all life-threatening adverse reactions to AEDs. Many AEDs can cause similar serious side effects (see Table 58.5), but with the exception of rash, these are fortunately rare. For example, the risk of carbamazepine-induced agranulocytosis or aplastic anemia is about 2 per 575,000; with felbamate, the risk of aplastic anemia may be as high as 1 per 5,000. Idiosyncratic reactions are not dose related; rather they arise either from an immune-mediated reaction to the drug or from poorly defined individual factors, largely genetic, that convey an unusual sensitivity to the drug. An example of the genetic mechanism is valproate-induced fatal hepatotoxicity. Valproate, like most AEDs, is metabolized in the liver, but several biochemical pathways are available to the drug. Clinical and experimental data indicate that one of these pathways results in a hepatotoxic compound that may accumulate and lead to microvesicular steatosis with necrosis. The extent to which this pathway is involved in biotransformation is age dependent and promoted by concurrent use of other drugs that are eliminated in the liver. Thus, most patients who have had fatal hepatotoxicity were younger than 2 years of age and treated with polytherapy (Table 58.6). In addition, most had severe epilepsy associated with mental retardation, developmental delay, or congenital brain anomalies. No hepatic deaths have occurred in persons older than 10 years treated with valproate alone.

No laboratory test, certainly not untargeted routine blood monitoring, identifies individuals specifically at risk for valproate hepatotoxicity or any other drug-related idiosyncratic reaction. Clinical data, however, permit identification of groups of patients at increased risk for serious adverse drug reactions, including patients with known or suspected metabolic or biochemical disorders, a history of previous drug reactions, and medical illnesses affecting hematopoiesis or liver and kidney function.

Rash can occur with virtually any drug, and rarely, this results in Stevens–Johnson syndrome. The frequency of severe rash is about the same with carbamazepine, phenytoin, phenobarbital, and (if started slowly over several weeks) lamotrigine. There is some cross-reactivity among these drugs, so that a patient who develops a rash with one has a slightly increased risk of developing a rash with another. Rash is unusual with valproate, gabapentin, pregabalin, or levetiracetam. To date, life-threatening idiosyncratic effects have not been reported with gabapentin, pregabalin, topiramate, oxcarbazepine, tiagabine, or levetiracetam.

Antiepileptic Drug Pharmacology

Table 58.7 provides summary information about dose requirements, pharmacokinetic properties, and therapeutic concentration ranges for the major AEDs available in the United States. Of patients with epilepsy, 60% to 70% achieve satisfactory control of seizures with currently available AEDs, but fewer than 50% of adults achieve complete control without drug side effects. Many patients continue to have frequent seizures despite optimal medical therapy.

Treatment should start with a single AED chosen according to the type of seizure or epilepsy syndrome and then be adjusted as necessary, by considerations of side effects, required dosing schedule, and cost. Phenytoin, phenobarbital, gabapentin, and levetiracetam can be loaded acutely. There is evidence either from comparative or dose-controlled trials that gabapentin, lamotrigine, topiramate,

TABLE 58.5 Toxicity of Antiepileptic Drugs

Dose-Related Adverse Effects
Systemic Toxicity
Gastrointestinal (dyspepsia, nausea, diarrhea; esp. valproate, zonisamide)
Benign elevation in liver enzymes (esp. valproate, phenobarbital, phenytoin, carbamazepine, oxcarbazepine)
Benign leukopenia (esp. carbamazepine)
Gingival hypertrophy (esp. phenytoin)
Weight gain (esp. valproate, gabapentin, pregabalin)
Anorexia and weight loss (esp. felbamate, topiramate, zonisamide)
Hair loss, change in hair texture (esp. valproate)
Hirsutism (esp. phenytoin, valproate)
Hyponatremia (esp. carbamazepine, oxcarbazepine)
Coarsening of facial features (esp. phenytoin)
Dupuytren contracture, frozen shoulder
Osteoporosis (esp. phenytoin, carbamazepine, valproate)
Impotence (esp. phenobarbital, carbamazepine)
Neurologic Toxicity
Drowsiness, sedation
Impaired cognition (memory, concentration; esp. topiramate)
Depression and mood changes (esp. phenobarbital, levetiracetam, topiramate)
Irritability, hyperactivity
Insomnia (esp. felbamate)

Dose-Related Adverse Effects
Neurologic Toxicity (continued)
Peripheral visual field restriction (vigabatrin)
Dizziness/vertigo
Nystagmus, diplopia
Ataxia
Tremor, asterixis
Dyskinesias, dystonia, myoclonus
Dysarthria
Headache
Sensory neuropathy
Systemic Toxicity
Rash (rare with valproate, gabapentin, levetiracetam, pregabalin)
Exfoliative dermatitis
Erythema multiforme
Stevens–Johnson syndrome (esp. lamotrigine)
Agranulocytosis
Aplastic anemia (esp. felbamate)
Hepatic failure (esp. felbamate, valproate)
Pancreatitis
Connective tissue disorders
Thrombocytopenia (esp. valproate)
Pseudolymphoma syndrome

and oxcarbazepine have efficacy as monotherapy in newly diagnosed adolescents and adults with either partial or mixed seizure disorders. There is also evidence that lamotrigine is effective for newly diagnosed absence seizures in children. In the absence of status epilepticus (Chapter 6), AEDs should be started at low dosages to minimize acute toxicity. They can then be increased according to the patient's tolerance and the drug's pharmacokinetics. The initial target dose should produce a serum concentration in the low to mid therapeutic range. Further increases can then be titrated according to the patient's clinical progress, which is measured mainly by seizure frequency and the occurrence of drug side effects. A drug should not be judged a failure unless seizures remain uncontrolled at the maximal tolerated dosage, regardless of the blood level.

TABLE 58.6 Effect of Age and Treatment on Risk of Developing Fatal Valproate Hepatotoxicity

Age	Monotherapy	Polytherapy
<2 yr	1/7,000	1/500
>2 yr	1/80,000	1/25,000

Modified from Dreifuss FE, Santilli N, Langer DH, et al. *Neurology.* 1987;37:379–385.

Dosage changes generally should not be made until the effects of the drug have been observed at steady-state concentrations (a time about equal to five drug half-lives). If the first drug is ineffective, an appropriate alternative should be gradually substituted (see Table 58.4). Combination treatment using two drugs should be attempted only when monotherapy with primary AEDs fails. Combination therapy is sometimes effective, but the price of improved seizure control is often additional drug toxicity. Sometimes, combination therapy with relatively nonsedating drugs (e.g., carbamazepine, lamotrigine, gabapentin, or valproate) is preferable to high-dose monotherapy with a sedating drug (e.g., phenobarbital or primidone). When used together, carbamazepine and lamotrigine result in a pharmacodynamic interaction that often produces neurotoxicity at dosages that are usually well tolerated when either drug is used alone.

Dosing intervals should usually be less than one-third to one-half the drug's half-life to minimize fluctuations between peak and trough blood concentrations. Large fluctuations can result in drug-induced side effects at peak levels and in breakthrough seizures at trough concentrations. Sometimes, however, a drug has a relatively long pharmacodynamic half-life, so that twice a day dosing is reasonable even if the pharmacokinetic half-life is short. This is typically the case with valproate, tiagabine, pregabalin, gabapentin, and levetiracetam. Extended-release formulations of most commonly used AEDs are available, which allow less frequent dosing and decreased peak and trough levels, thereby potentially

TABLE 58.7 Antiepileptic Drugs: Dosage and Pharmacokinetic Data

Drug	Usual Adult Dose 24 h (mg)	Half-life (h)	Usually Effective Plasma Concentration (µg/mL)	Time-to-Peak Concentration (h)	Bound Fraction (%)
Phenytoin	300–400	22	10–20	3–8	90–95
Carbamazepine	800–1,600	8–22	8–12	4–8	75
Phenobarbital	90–180	100	15–40	2–8	45
Valproate	1,000–3,000	15–20	50–120	3–8	80–90
Ethosuximide	750–1,500	60	40–100	3–7	<5
Felbamate	2,400–3,600	14–23	20–140	2–6	25
Gabapentin	1,800–3,600	5–7	4–16[a]	2–3	<5
Lamotrigine	100–500	12–60[b]	2–16[a]	2–5	55
Topiramate	200–400	19–25[b]	4–10[a]	2–4	9–17
Vigabatrin	1,000–3,000	5–7	NE	1–4	5
Tiagabine	32–56	5–13	NE	1	95
Levetiracetam	1,000–3,000	6–8	5–45[a]	1	<10
Oxcarbazepine	900–2,400	8–10[c]	10–35[a]	3–13	40[c]
Zonisamide	100–600	24–60[b]	10–40[a]	2–6	40
Pregabalin	150–600	5–7	NE	1	<5
Lacosamide	200–400	12–16	NE	1–4	<15
Rufinamide	2,400–3,200	6–10	NE	4–6	34
Clobazam	10–40	36–42	NE	0.5–4	80–90
Ezogabine	600–1,200	7–11	NE	0.5–2	80
Perampanel	8–12	105	NE	0.5–2.5	95

[a]Not established; corresponds to usual range in patients treated with recommended dose.
[b]Highly dependent on concurrently administered drugs.
[c]Of metahydroxy derivative, the active metabolite.
NE, not established.

improving tolerability and compliance. Bioavailability is not necessarily equivalent to immediate-release formulations, and different extended-release delivery systems with alternate manufacturers of the same drug can also create variation in peak and trough levels, as well as total absorption.

Therapeutic drug monitoring has greatly improved the care of patients with epilepsy, but published therapeutic ranges are only guidelines. Most patients whose drug concentrations are within a standard therapeutic range usually achieve adequate seizure control with minimal side effects, but notable exceptions occur. Some patients develop unacceptable side effects at "subtherapeutic" concentrations; others benefit from "toxic" concentrations without adverse effects.

Determining serum drug concentrations when seizure control has been achieved or when side effects appear can assist future management decisions. Drug levels are also useful in documenting compliance and in assessing the magnitude and significance of known or suspected drug interactions. Therapeutic drug monitoring is an essential guide to treating neonates, infants, young children, elderly persons, and patients with diseases (e.g., liver or kidney failure) or physiologic conditions (e.g., pregnancy) that alter drug pharmacokinetics. Although the total blood concentrations that are routinely reported are satisfactory for most indications, unbound (free) concentrations are useful when protein binding is altered, as in renal failure, pregnancy, extensive third-degree burns,

and combination therapy using two or more drugs that are highly bound to serum proteins (e.g., phenytoin, valproate, tiagabine).

Specific Drugs

Phenytoin is unique among AEDs because it exhibits nonlinear elimination at therapeutically useful serum concentrations. That is, hepatic enzyme systems metabolizing phenytoin become increasingly saturated at plasma concentrations greater than 10 to 12 µg/mL, and metabolic rate approaches a constant value at high concentrations. With increasing doses, phenytoin plasma concentrations rise exponentially (Fig. 58.6), so that steady-state concentration at one dose cannot be used to predict directly the steady-state concentration at a higher dose. Clinically, this requires cautious titration within the therapeutic range, using dose increments of 30 mg to avoid toxic effects.

Carbamazepine induces activation of the enzymes that metabolize it. The process, termed *autoinduction*, is time dependent. When carbamazepine is first introduced, the half-life approximates 30 hours. With increasing hepatic clearance in the first 3 to 4 weeks of therapy, however, the half-life shortens to 11 to 20 hours. As a result, the starting dose should be low and then increased gradually, and dosing should be frequent (three or four times daily). Extended-release formulations permit twice a day administration. The principal metabolite is carbamazepine-10,11-epoxide, which is pharmacologically active. Under certain circumstances (e.g., when

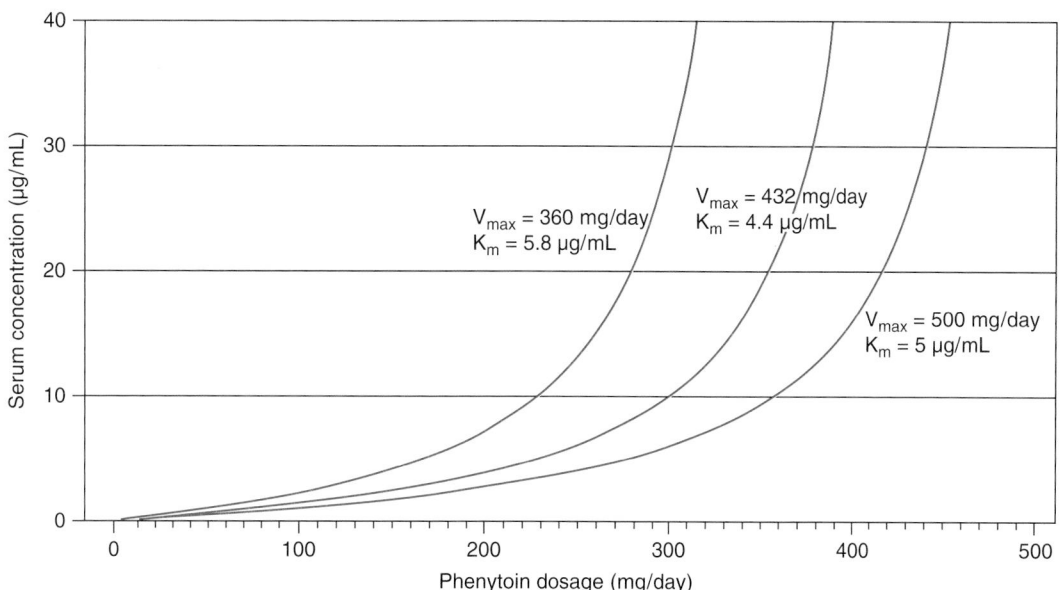

FIGURE 58.6 Phenytoin dose concentration curves from three representative adult patients. Note the markedly nonlinear relationship in the 200- to 400-mg dose range. Careful dose titration is necessary in this portion of the curve to avoid neurotoxicity. K_m, Michaelis–Menten constant; V_{max}, maximum elimination rate.

coadministered with valproate or felbamate), the epoxide metabolite accumulates selectively, thereby producing neurotoxic effects even though the plasma concentration of the parent drug is in the therapeutic range or even low.

Valproate is highly bound to plasma proteins, but the binding is concentration dependent and nonlinear. The unbound fraction increases at plasma concentrations greater than 75 μg/mL because protein-binding sites become saturated. For example, doubling the plasma concentration from 75 to 150 μg/mL can result in a more than sixfold rise in concentration of free drug (from 6.5 to 45 μg/mL). Therefore, as the dose of valproate is increased, side effects may worsen rapidly because of the increasing proportion of unbound drug. Furthermore, adverse effects may vary in the course of a single day or from day to day because concentrations of unbound drug fluctuate despite seemingly small changes in total blood levels. Additionally, circulating fatty acids displace valproate from protein-binding sites. If fatty acid levels are high, the amount of unbound valproate increases. Lamotrigine and felbamate prolong the half-life of valproate and therefore a reduced dosage is typically necessary when these drugs are added.

Gabapentin requires an intestinal amino acid transport system for absorption. Because the transporter is saturable, the percentage of drug that is absorbed after an oral dose decreases with increasing dosage. More frequent dosing schedules using smaller amounts may therefore be necessary to increase blood levels. When dosages above 3,600 mg/day are used, blood levels can be helpful in demonstrating that an increase in dosage is reflected in an increased serum concentration. Gabapentin does not interact to any clinically significant degree with any other drugs, which makes it especially useful when AED polytherapy is necessary and in patients with medical illnesses that also require drug treatment. It is not metabolized in the liver, but as it is excreted unchanged by the kidneys, dose adjustment is required in patients with renal failure. *Pregabalin* is structurally and mechanistically similar to gabapentin but does not show dose-dependent absorption. It has increased potency compared with gabapentin and can be effective with twice-daily dosing.

Lamotrigine is highly sensitive to coadministration of many other AEDs. Enzyme-inducing agents, such as phenytoin and carbamazepine, decrease the half-life of lamotrigine from 24 to 16 hours (or less) as do oral contraceptive agents. In contrast, enzyme inhibition by valproate increases the half-life of lamotrigine to 60 hours. Therefore, lamotrigine dosing depends very much on whether it is used as monotherapy or in combination with other AEDs. Lamotrigine concentrations are also lowered by administration of oral contraceptives, and levels can decrease dramatically during the latter months of pregnancy requiring frequent monitoring and dose adjustment. Lamotrigine has little or no effect on other classes of drugs. Rash occurs in about 10% of patients; it is more common in children and rarely leads to Stevens–Johnson syndrome. The incidence of rash can be minimized by slow titration schedules.

Levetiracetam, like gabapentin, has no appreciable interactions with other drugs and therefore has advantages in medically complicated patients. The plasma half-life is 6 to 8 hours, but clinical trials support twice-daily dosing, possibly owing to a longer pharmacodynamic half-life. Metabolism occurs in the liver, and there is also renal clearance. Adverse effects are generally mild and self-limited, although mood changes and even psychosis occur in a small subset of patients. No life-threatening idiosyncratic reactions have yet been described.

Oxcarbazepine is structurally similar to carbamazepine, but it is metabolized by a different pathway. As a result, there is no epoxide metabolite that is responsible for some of the adverse effects of carbamazepine. Although individual patients may tolerate oxcarbazepine better than carbamazepine, the overall profiles of the two drugs are similar, including development of leukopenia (usually transient, asymptomatic, and benign), mild increase in hepatic enzymes, and hyponatremia. Pharmacologic half-life of the active metabolite, a metahydroxy derivative (MHD), is 8 to 10 hours. Clinical studies support twice-daily dosing, although peak toxicity can occur when this is done at higher dosages.

Topiramate is affected by other AEDs taken concurrently. Carbamazepine, phenytoin, and phenobarbital shorten its half-life;

valproate has little effect. Topiramate does not affect most other drugs, although phenytoin blood levels may increase by 25%. Adverse cognitive effects, especially word-finding difficulty and impaired memory, frequently limit the dosage patients can tolerate. These are usually dose dependent and can be minimized with slow titration schedules. Cognitive effects are also less common in monotherapy. Glaucoma, anhydrosis, and renal stones occur rarely. Doses above 400 mg/day do not usually lead to better seizure control but are associated with an increasing incidence of side effects.

Tiagabine is highly bound to serum proteins and will therefore displace other drugs (e.g., phenytoin, valproate) that are also protein bound. Other drugs do not affect tiagabine's metabolism significantly. Gastrointestinal side effects usually limit the rate at which the dosage may be increased.

Zonisamide is affected by other drugs that induce hepatic enzymes. As monotherapy, zonisamide's half-life is about 60 hours. When coadministered with enzyme-inducing drugs, its half-life can be reduced to 24 hours. In either case, once-daily dosing is appropriate. Although its metabolism occurs primarily in the liver, zonisamide itself does not appear to affect other drugs. Rash, renal stones, and anhydrosis are rare side effects.

Felbamate has a much higher risk of serious adverse reactions, including aplastic anemia and hepatic failure, than other AEDs. The actual risk has been difficult to estimate but is probably between 1 per 5,000 and 1 per 20,000 exposures. For this reason, its use is currently restricted to patients who are refractory to other agents and in whom the risk of continued seizures outweighs the risk of side effects. Use of felbamate is also limited by other common but less serious adverse effects, including anorexia, weight loss, insomnia, and nausea, and by numerous complex drug interactions. Nonetheless, felbamate remains useful in cases of severe epilepsy such as Lennox–Gastaut syndrome.

Lacosamide enhances the slow inactivation of sodium channels without affecting fast inactivation. It may prolong the PR interval, which can result in cardiac conduction problems. A baseline electrocardiogram (ECG) is suggested prior to initiating this drug.

Rufinamide is a triazole derivative whose exact mechanism is unknown. *In vitro* prolongs the inactive state of the sodium channels, thereby limiting repetitive firing of Na^+-dependent action potentials mediating anticonvulsant effects. Its use is limited largely to refractory generalized epilepsies, especially in controlling tonic seizures.

Clobazam has been used in many countries around the world, but it was only recently FDA approved in the United States for adjunctive treatment of Lennox–Gastaut syndrome. It is widely used off-label as adjunctive treatment for partial seizures. In catamenial epilepsy, it can be prescribed in doses of 20 to 30 mg daily for 10 days during the perimenstrual period. Serious reactions including Stevens–Johnson syndrome and toxic epidermal necrolysis (TEN) have been reported.

Ezogabine is FDA approved as an adjunctive medicine in patients with partial seizures. All patients starting on this medication should undergo a baseline and periodic eye exams every 6 months including dilated funduscopy and visual acuity testing. Blue discoloration of the skin, especially of the lips and nail bed, has been reported. QT prolongation has also been observed, warranting monitoring with ECG especially in patients with electrolyte and cardiac abnormalities. This medicine can cause urinary retention and therefore is better avoided in elderly male patients with prostate enlargement.

Perampanel, which is FDA approved as an adjunctive medication in partial seizures, has a unique mechanism of action in that it is the first noncompetitive antagonist of the AMPA glutamate receptor. It comes with a boxed warning of dose-related serious neuropsychiatric events including homicidal thoughts and aggression. Being both an inducer and a substrate of the CYP3A4 enzymes, drug interactions with other antiseizure medications exist.

Discontinuing Antiepileptic Drugs

Epidemiologic studies indicate that 60% to 70% of patients with epilepsy become free of seizures for at least 5 years within 10 years of diagnosis. Similarly, prospective clinical trials of treated patients whose seizures were in remission for 2 years or more showed that a nearly identical percentage of patients remained seizure free after drug withdrawal [**Level 1**].[9] Chance of recurrence continues to decline with seizure freedom for 2 to 5 years. These studies also identified predictors that permit patients to be classified as being at low or high risk for seizure relapse after drug therapy ends. The risk of relapse was high if patients required more than one AED to control seizures, if seizure control was difficult to establish, if the patient had a history of generalized tonic–clonic seizures, and if the EEG was significantly abnormal when drug withdrawal was considered. Continued freedom from seizures is favored by longer seizure-free intervals (>4 years) before drug withdrawal is attempted, few seizures before remission, monotherapy, normal EEG, and no difficulty establishing seizure control.

All benign epilepsy syndromes of childhood carry an excellent prognosis for permanent drug-free remission. In contrast, JME has a high rate of relapse when drugs are discontinued, even in patients who have been seizure free for years. The prognosis for most other epilepsy syndromes is largely unknown.

Discontinuing AED therapy in appropriate patients can be considered when they have been seizure free for at least 2 years. The most powerful argument for stopping AEDs is concern about long-term systemic and neurologic toxicity, which can be insidious and not apparent for many years after a drug has been introduced. On the other hand, however, is the concern of the patient or family about seizure recurrence. Even a single seizure can have disastrous psychosocial and vocational consequences, particularly in adults. Therefore, the decision to withdraw drugs must be weighed carefully in the light of individual circumstances. If a decision is made to discontinue AEDs, we favor slow withdrawal, over 3 to 6 months, but this recommendation is controversial because few studies of different withdrawal rates have been conducted.

REPRODUCTIVE HEALTH ISSUES

Gender-based differences in AED pharmacokinetics, sex steroid hormones, and reproductive life events raise special issues for women with epilepsy. The management of pregnancy in a woman with epilepsy is discussed in detail in Chapter 124. This section focuses on the effects of reproductive hormones on seizures and on the effects of seizures and AEDs on reproductive health.

Although the prevalence of epilepsy is not higher in women, epilepsy in women can be specially affected by changes in reproductive steroids. Estrogen is a proconvulsant drug in animal models of epilepsy, whereas progesterone and its metabolites have anticonvulsant effects. Ovarian steroid hormones act at the neuronal membrane and on the genome to produce immediate and long-lasting effects on excitability. Estrogen reduces GABA-mediated inhibition, whereas progesterone enhances GABA effects. Estrogen also potentiates the action of excitatory neurotransmitters in some brain regions and increases the number of excitatory synapses. These dynamic and significant changes in neuronal excitability are observed with changes in estrogen and progesterone concentrations similar to those observed in the human menstrual cycle.

Approximately one-third of women with epilepsy report patterns of seizure occurrence that relate to phases of the menstrual cycle (*catamenial seizures*). Women with catamenial seizures indicate that seizures are more frequent, or more severe, just before menstruation and during the time of menstrual flow. In some women, seizures also increase at ovulation. These are times in the menstrual cycle when estrogen levels are relatively high and progesterone concentration is relatively low. Several small clinical trials have described benefit from chronic progesterone therapy in women with catamenial seizure patterns. Changes in seizures related to puberty and menopause are not well understood.

The pharmacokinetics of some AEDs can complicate epilepsy management in women. AEDs that induce activity of the cytochrome P-450 enzyme system (carbamazepine, phenytoin, phenobarbital, primidone, and, to a lesser extent, topiramate and oxcarbazepine) interfere with the effectiveness of estrogen-based hormonal contraception. In women taking these drugs, the metabolism and binding of contraceptive steroids is enhanced, thus reducing the biologically active fraction of steroid hormone. The failure rate of oral contraceptive pills exceeds 6% per year in women taking enzyme-inducing AEDs, in contrast to a failure rate of less than 1% per year in medication-compliant women without epilepsy. A woman motivated to avoid pregnancy should consider using a contraceptive preparation containing 50 μg or more of an estrogenic compound or using an additional barrier method of contraception. Alternatively, she should discuss with her physician the possibility of selecting an AED that does not alter steroid metabolism or binding.

Reproductive health may be compromised in both women and men with epilepsy. Fertility rates for men and women with epilepsy are one-third to two-thirds those of men and women without epilepsy. Lower birth rates cannot be explained on the basis of lower marriage rates because marriage rates for women with epilepsy are now similar to those of nonepileptic women. Reduced fertility appears to be the direct result of a disturbance in reproductive physiology.

Men and women with epilepsy show a higher than expected frequency of reproductive endocrine disturbances. These include abnormalities both in the cyclic release and concentration of pituitary luteinizing hormone and prolactin and in the concentration of gonadal steroid hormones. Some of these abnormalities are likely to be a consequence of seizure activity. AEDs can also alter concentrations of gonadal steroids by affecting steroid hormone metabolism and binding. AEDs that increase steroid metabolism and binding reduce steroid hormone feedback at the hypothalamus and pituitary. AEDs that inhibit steroid metabolism (e.g., valproate) increase concentrations of steroid hormones, particularly androgens.

The polycystic ovary syndrome (PCOS) is a gynecologic disorder affecting approximately 7% of reproductive-age women. Women with epilepsy are at risk for developing features of this syndrome. Diagnostic requirements for PCOS are phenotypic or serologic evidence for hyperandrogenism and anovulatory cycles (Morrell, 2003). Phenotypic signs of hyperandrogenism include hirsutism, truncal obesity, and acne. Hirsutism presents as increased facial and body hair, coarsening of pubic hair with extension down the inner thigh, and male pattern scalp hair loss—temporal recession and thinning over the crown. Health consequences of PCOS include infertility, accelerated atherosclerosis, diabetes, and endometrial carcinoma, underscoring the importance of detection and treatment. As many as 30% of cycles in women with epilepsy are anovulatory, and anovulatory cycles appear to be most frequent in women receiving valproic acid (VPA). Women with epilepsy are more likely

to have polycystic-appearing ovaries, which along with hyperandrogenism occur in as many as 40% of women with epilepsy receiving VPA. The long-term consequences of PCOS in women with epilepsy are unknown. Data such as these suggest that epilepsy and some AEDs individually affect fertility and that these effects may be additive. This implies that optimal therapy for epilepsy will consider disease–treatment effects on reproductive health.

Sexual dysfunction affects about one-third of men and women with epilepsy. Men report low sexual desire, difficulty achieving or maintaining an erection, or delayed ejaculation. Women with epilepsy can experience painful intercourse because of vaginismus and lack of lubrication. Although there are certainly psychosocial reasons for sexual dysfunction in some people with epilepsy, physiologic causes are demonstrable in others. Physiologic causes of sexual dysfunction include disruption of brain regions controlling sexual behavior by epileptogenic discharges, abnormalities of pituitary and gonadal hormones, and side effects of AEDs.

Although no anticonvulsant drug is free of teratogenic effects, the risk is low and generally less than that of uncontrolled seizures during pregnancy. The exceptions to this are valproate and topiramate, both of which are associated with increased risk of congenital malformations in prospective monotherapy studies. Valproate has also been shown to carry a dose-dependent risk of decreased IQ compared with phenytoin, carbamazepine, and lamotrigine. In all cases, the lowest effective dose should be used, and polypharmacy should be avoided [**Level 1**].[10] Women with epilepsy who have difficulty conceiving, irregular or abnormal menstrual cycles, midcycle menstrual bleeding, sexual dysfunction, obesity, or hirsutism should be referred for a reproductive endocrine evaluation. Men with sexual dysfunction or difficulty conceiving should also have an endocrine evaluation and semen analysis. All the reproductive disorders seen in people with epilepsy are potentially treatable.

BONE HEALTH

Persons with epilepsy are at greater risk for bone disease, which typically presents as pathologic fractures. Bone biochemical abnormalities described in people with epilepsy include hypocalcemia, hypophosphatemia, elevated serum alkaline phosphatase, elevated parathyroid hormone (PTH), and reduced levels of vitamin D and its active metabolites (Pack & Morrell, 2004). The most severe bone and biochemical abnormalities are found in patients receiving AED polytherapy and in those who have taken AEDs for a longer time. Effects are more pronounced with enzyme-inducing AEDs, especially phenytoin.

SURGICAL TREATMENT

Surgery should be considered when seizures are uncontrolled by optimal medical management and when they disrupt the quality of life. Quantifying these issues, however, has defied strict definition, perhaps deservedly, because intractability is clearly more than continued seizures. Only patients know how their lives differ from what they would like them to be; the concept of *disability* includes both physical and psychological components. Some patients with refractory seizures suffer little disability; others, for whatever reason, find their lives severely compromised by infrequent attacks. Still, others have had their seizures completely cured by surgery but are still disabled and incapable of functioning productively. Determining which patients are "medically refractory" and which are "satisfactorily controlled" can always be argued in the abstract.

Fortunately in practice, there is usually general agreement about which patients should be referred for surgical evaluation.

Patients are less likely to benefit from further attempts at medical treatment if seizures have not been controlled after two trials of high-dose monotherapy using two appropriate drugs and one trial of combination therapy. These therapeutic efforts can be accomplished within 1 to 2 years; the detrimental effects of continued seizures or drug toxicity warrant referral to a specialized center after that time.

There are few blanket contraindications to epilepsy surgery today, although patients with severe concurrent medical illness and progressive neurologic syndromes are usually excluded. Some centers prefer not to operate on patients with psychosis or other serious psychiatric disorder, those older than 60 years, and those with an IQ of less than 70. Patients in these categories, however, must be considered individually. Many patients who undergo corpus callosum section for atonic seizures associated with Lennox–Gastaut syndrome have IQs less than 70. Although surgery for epilepsy is increasingly performed in children, functional resections in infancy remain controversial for several reasons: the uncertain natural history of seizures in many of these patients; the unknown effects of surgery on the immature brain; and the lack of data about long-term neurologic, behavioral, and psychological outcomes.

Because of technical advances in imaging and electrophysiologic monitoring, epilepsy surgery is no longer automatically contraindicated in patients with multifocal interictal epileptiform abnormalities or even foci near language or other eloquent cortical areas.

RESECTIVE PROCEDURES

Focal brain resection is the most common type of epilepsy surgery. Resection is appropriate if seizures begin in an identifiable and restricted cortical area, if the surgical excision will encompass all or most of the epileptogenic tissue, and if the resection will not impair neurologic function. These criteria are met most often by patients with temporal lobe epilepsy, but extratemporal resections are increasingly common.

ANTERIOR TEMPORAL LOBE RESECTION

This resective procedure is the most common, but the operation varies in what is considered "standard," especially with regard to how much lateral neocortical and mesial limbic structures are removed. The traditional operation is Spencer's 1991 anteromedial temporal lobe resection, which includes removal of the anterior middle and inferior temporal gyri, parahippocampal gyrus, 3.5 to 4 cm of hippocampus, and a variable amount of amygdala. For nondominant foci, this approach may be slightly modified to include the anterior superior temporal gyrus as well. Increasingly, some centers (including ours) are using selective amygdalohippocampectomy, a smaller resection with similar efficacy. Patients with medial temporal lobe epilepsy associated with hippocampal sclerosis are ideal candidates for either operation because over 80% will become seizure free, with the remainder having substantial improvement. Results of a large multi-center study in the United States were reported by Spencer et al. in 2003, confirming the high rates of complete seizure control following temporal lobe resection [**Level 1**].[11] A randomized controlled Canadian trial has demonstrated clear superiority of surgery over medical management in patients with medial temporal lobe epilepsy [**Level 1**].[12] Other methods of mesial temporal ablation have been reported, including Gamma Knife radiation and localized laser ablation. Although preliminary results are encouraging, it is not known whether these methods are as effective at seizure control as traditional resection or if there are differences in adverse effect outcomes.

Lesionectomy

Well-circumscribed epileptogenic structural lesions (cavernous angiomas, hamartomas, gangliogliomas, and other encapsulated tumors) can be removed by stereotactic microsurgery. The extent to which tissue margins surrounding the lesion are included in the resection depends on how the margins are defined (radiologic, visual, electrophysiologic, or histologic inspection) and the surgeon's preference. Seizures are controlled by this method in 50% to 60% of patients. A lesion involving the cerebral cortex should always be considered the source of a patient's seizures, unless compelling EEG evidence suggests otherwise.

Nonlesional Cortical Resections

When a lesion cannot be visualized by MRI, it is difficult to demonstrate a restricted ictal-onset zone outside the anterior temporal lobe. Although alternative imaging (PET or SPECT scan) may help identify the seizure-onset zone, this situation almost always requires placement of intracranial electrodes to map the extent of epileptogenic tissue and to determine its relation to functional brain areas. Outcome after nonlesional cortical resections is not as good as with anterior temporal lobectomy or lesionectomy, mainly because the boundaries of epileptogenic cortical areas often cannot be delineated precisely, and removal of all the epileptogenic tissue often is not possible.

CORPUS CALLOSOTOMY

Section of the corpus callosum disconnects the two hemispheres and is indicated for treatment of patients with uncontrolled atonic or tonic seizures in the absence of an identifiable focus suitable for resection. Leaving the posterior 20% to 30% of the corpus callosum intact seems to reduce complications. Most patients referred for corpus callosotomy have severe and frequent seizures of multiple types, usually with mental retardation and a severely abnormal EEG (the Lennox–Gastaut syndrome).

Unlike resective surgery, corpus callosotomy is palliative, not curative. Nonetheless, it can be strikingly effective for generalized seizures, with 80% of patients experiencing complete or nearly complete cessation of atonic, tonic, and tonic–clonic attacks. This outcome is often remarkably beneficial because it eliminates falls and the associated self-injury. The effect on partial seizures, however, is inconsistent and unpredictable. Complex partial seizures are reduced or eliminated in about half the patients, but simple or complex partial seizures are exacerbated in about 25%. Therefore, refractory partial seizures alone are not an indication for corpus callosotomy. Similarly, absence, atypical absence, and myoclonic seizures either do not benefit or show an inconsistent response.

HEMISPHERECTOMY

Removal (hemispherectomy) or disconnection (functional hemispherectomy) of large cortical areas from one side of the brain is indicated when the epileptogenic lesion involves most or all of one hemisphere. Because hemispherectomy guarantees permanent hemiplegia, hemisensory loss, and usually hemianopia, it can be considered only in children with a unilateral structural lesion that has already resulted in those abnormalities and who have refractory unilateral seizures. Examples of conditions suitable for hemispherectomy include infantile hemiplegia syndromes, Sturge–Weber disease, Rasmussen syndrome, and severe unilateral developmental anomalies, such as hemimegalencephaly. In appropriate patients, the results are dramatic. Seizures cease, behavior improves, and development accelerates (Table 58.8).

TABLE 58.8 **Outcome after Epilepsy Surgical Procedures**

Procedure	Seizure Free (%)	Improved (%)	Not Improved (%)	n
Anterior temporal lobectomy	69	22	9	3,579
Lesionectomy	67	22	12	293
Nonlesional extratemporal neocortical resection	45	35	20	805
Hemispherectomy	67	21	12	190
Corpus callosum section	8	61	31	563

Modified from Engel J Jr. *Surgical Treatment of the Epilepsies.* 2nd ed. New York: Raven; 1993.

PREOPERATIVE EVALUATION

The objective in evaluating patients for focal resection is to demonstrate that all seizures originate in a limited cortical area that can be removed safely. This determination requires more extensive evaluation than is necessary in the routine management of patients with epilepsy. The different tests used provide complementary information about normal and epileptic brain functions.

CCTV/EEG monitoring is necessary to record a representative sample of the patient's typical seizures to confirm the diagnosis and classification and also to localize the cortical area involved in ictal onset. Volumetric or other special MRI techniques may demonstrate unilateral hippocampal atrophy or other anatomic abnormalities that may be epileptogenic. PET and ictal SPECT are useful in demonstrating focal abnormalities in glucose metabolism or cerebral blood flow that correspond to the epileptogenic brain region. Neuropsychological testing is useful in demonstrating focal cognitive dysfunction, especially language and memory. Intracarotid injection of amobarbital (the *Wada test*) to determine hemispheric dominance for language and memory competence is generally considered necessary before temporal lobectomy, but the implications of a failed test are uncertain. Although functional MRI (fMRI) reliably lateralizes language, determining memory competence of one temporal lobe has not yet been reliably established.

Intracranial electrodes are necessary if noninvasive methods do not unequivocally localize the epileptogenic area or if different noninvasive tests give conflicting results. Intracranial electrode placement is also necessary when vital brain functions (language, motor cortex) must be mapped in relation to the planned resection.

NEUROSTIMULATION IN DRUG-RESISTANT EPILEPSY

When epilepsy surgery is not possible due to multiple foci of seizure onset or seizure onset in eloquent cortex that is not resectable, neurostimulation has emerged as an alternative to failed drug therapy.

Vagus Nerve Stimulation

This is the first FDA-approved device for the treatment of medically refractory partial seizures. Like corpus callosotomy, vagus nerve stimulation (VNS) is a palliative procedure because very few patients become seizure free. VNS is delivered via a stimulating lead attached to the left vagus nerve. The stimulus generator is implanted in the upper left chest. The device is usually programmed to give a 30-second electrical pulse every 5 minutes, although stimulus parameters can be adjusted to the requirements of an individual patient. In patients with aura, a magnetic wand can be used to deliver VNS on demand, which may abort seizure progression. About 55% of children have at least a 50% reduction in seizure frequency, which compares favorably with the efficacy of new AEDs [**Level 1**].[13] VNS may be considered for seizures in children, for Lennox Gastaut associated seizures, and for improving mood in adults with epilepsy (Level C). VNS may be considered to have improved efficacy over time. Children should be carefully monitored for site infection after VNS implantation. Chronic adverse effects include hoarseness and difficulty swallowing, both of which increase at the time of stimulation.

Because VNS became FDA approved, several other therapies using neurostimulation have been developed, including responsive neurostimulation, deep brain stimulation of the anterior nucleus of the thalamus, trigeminal nerve stimulation, and transcutaneous VNS.

Deep Brain Stimulation

The anterior nucleus of the thalamus, a core component of the Papez circuit, serves as a relay station that can amplify and synchronize seizure discharges from the hippocampus and the thalamus. Therefore, its inhibition by electrical stimulation is thought to abort or prevent seizures. Multicontact depth electrodes are implanted bilaterally into the anterior nuclei using a stereotactic approach. In the pivotal DBS study, depression (14.8% in active treatment vs. 1.8% in controls) and memory impairment (13% in active treatment vs. 1.8% in controls) were the most common adverse events. Asymptomatic hemorrhages occurred in 4.5% of subjects, but no disability or death was attributed to the hemorrhages.

Responsive Neurostimulation

The responsive neurostimulation (RNS) is now FDA approved as of November 2013 and commercially available as the NeuroPace device for individuals 18 years of age or older with drug-resistant epilepsy and partial-onset seizures that localize to no more than two epileptogenic foci. The NeuroPace responsive neurostimulation system consists of a pulse generator, seizure detection software, and recording and stimulating intracranial electrodes. Unlike the other systems described earlier which deliver a preprogrammed stimulation to prevent seizures, the RNS system works by detecting a seizure and then delivering a stimulus to terminate the electrical component of the seizure at its point of origin. In the pivotal trial which was randomized, prospective, double-blind, sham stimulation controlled, there was no difference in the rate of adverse events between the active and sham stimulation groups. However, the study demonstrated that patients with the device turned on had a 38% reduction in the average number of seizures per month, compared to a 17% reduction in the sham group. The depth or subdural strip electrodes are placed in close proximity to the seizure focus that is predetermined by surface/depth electrode video EEG evaluation. Hence, patients who are a high surgical risk cannot receive this device.

Once the device is implanted, patients cannot have an MRI, electroconvulsive therapy, transcranial magnetic stimulation, and diathermy procedures. Status epilepticus is covered in Section II, Chapter 6.

GENE MUTATIONS IN EPILEPSY

Genetic factors are implicated strongly in several epilepsy syndromes, and twin studies have confirmed important genetic determinants in both localization-related and generalized types of seizure disorders. The concordance rate for monozygotic twins with idiopathic generalized epilepsy is well over 75%. Hereditary aspects are easiest to discern in childhood absence epilepsy, JME, benign rolandic epilepsy, and idiopathic grand mal seizures. Some inherited disorders, such as tuberous sclerosis and neurofibromatosis, are associated with brain lesions that in turn give rise to symptomatic epilepsies. In most cases of epilepsy, however, the role of genetic factors is complex because there are multiple interacting genes that convey varying degrees of seizure susceptibility and also affect the brain's response to environmental influences. In any given patient, the relative contribution from genetic or acquired factors determines whether the epilepsy presents as an idiopathic syndrome or as a symptomatic disorder. In addition, however, there also seems to be some degree of sharing of genetic susceptibilities in both the idiopathic and symptomatic epilepsies because children of parents with either localization-related or generalized epilepsy develop seizures at increased rates, although the difference is greatest in families with idiopathic generalized epilepsy. Thus, a major challenge facing investigators today is to clarify how different genes alter an individual's susceptibility to seizures and epilepsy in the presence of acquired brain pathology or as a reaction to acute or subacute cerebral dysfunction. This is no easy task, however, because the number of genes that encode molecules that regulate cortical excitability directly through membrane and synaptic functions and the second messenger cascades that indirectly regulate membrane proteins involved in signal transduction is very large.

A number of causative genes have been identified in idiopathic epilepsies with a monogenic mode of inheritance (Table 58.9). Mutations in two voltage-gated potassium channel genes, *KCNQ2* (chr 20q13) and *KCNQ3*, (chr 8q24), cause benign familial neonatal convulsions. Autosomal dominant frontal lobe epilepsy is caused by mutations in two cholinergic receptor genes, the *CHRNA4* (chr 20q13) and *CHRNB2* (chr 1q). A syndrome of generalized epilepsy with febrile seizures (GEFS$^+$) has been related to mutations in three Na$^+$ channel subunits: *SCN1B* (chr 19q13), *SCN1A* (2q24), and *SCN2A* (2q24). A similar syndrome has also been seen in families with mutations in the γ2 subunit gene (*GABRG2* on chr 5q34) of the GABA$_A$ receptor. De novo mutations in the α1 subunit of the Na$^+$ channel also cause severe myoclonic epilepsy of infancy (Dravet syndrome). Mutations in the *CLCN2* gene encoding a Cl$^-$ channel have recently been described in three families with idiopathic generalized epilepsies of heterogeneous phenotype. An autosomal dominant form of JME occurring in a French Canadian family is associated with a mutation in the α1 subunit of the GABA receptor (*GABRA1*). A mutation in the leucine-rich glioma inactivated (*LCI1*) gene on chromosome 10q22-24 causes an autosomal dominant form of partial epilepsy with auditory features.

TABLE 58.9	Genes Identified in Idiopathic Human Epilepsies	
Gene	**Syndrome**	**Chromosome**
Na$^+$ Channels		
SCN1A	Generalized epilepsy with febrile seizures plus (GEFS$^+$)	2q24
SCN1A	Severe myoclonic epilepsy of infancy	2q
SCN2A	Benign familial neonatal seizures and GEFS$^+$	2q24
SCN1B	GEFS$^+$	19q13
K$^+$ Channels		
KCNQ2	Benign familial neonatal seizures	20q13
KCNQ3	Benign familial neonatal seizures	8q24
Cl$^-$ Channels		
CLN2	Idiopathic generalized epilepsy (heterogeneous)	3q26
Ca^{2+} Channels		
CACNA1A (P/Q)	Absence epilepsy and cerebellar ataxia	19q
CACNB4	Idiopathic generalized epilepsy (heterogeneous)	2q22–23
Nicotinic AChR		
CHRNA4	Autosomal dominant nocturnal frontal lobe epilepsy	20q13
CHRNB2	Autosomal dominant nocturnal frontal lobe epilepsy	1q
GABA$_A$ Receptor		
GABRG2	GEFS$^+$	5q34
GABRA1	Juvenile myoclonic epilepsy (French Canadian family)	
Other		
LGI1	Autosomal dominant partial epilepsy with auditory features	10q22–24

AChR, acetylcholine receptor; GABA, γ-aminobutyric acid.

PSYCHOSOCIAL AND PSYCHIATRIC ISSUES

The impact of epilepsy on the quality of life is usually greater than the limitations imposed by the seizures alone. The diagnosis of epilepsy frequently carries other consequences that can greatly alter the lives of many patients. For adults, the most important problems are discrimination at work and driving restrictions, which lead to loss of mobility and independence. Children and adults alike may be shunned by uninformed friends. Patients must learn to avoid situations that precipitate seizures, and a change in lifestyle may be necessary. Common factors that increase the likelihood of seizure occurrence include sleep deprivation (whether due to lifestyle

TABLE 58.10	Factors that Lower the Seizure Threshold	
Common	**Occasional**
Sleep deprivation	Barbiturate withdrawal
Alcohol withdrawal	Hyperventilation
Stress	Flashing lights
Dehydration	Diet and missed meals
Drugs and drug interactions	Specific "reflex" triggers
Systemic infection	
Trauma	
Malnutrition	
Noncompliance	

or to coexisting sleep disorders), alcohol (and other drugs), and emotional stress (Table 58.10). Compliance with AED treatment is often an issue, especially with adolescents. Psychiatric symptoms, especially depression, may complicate management.

Some restrictions are medically appropriate, at least for limited times. For example, when seizures impair consciousness or judgment, driving and certain kinds of employment (working at exposed heights or with power equipment) and a few other activities (swimming alone) should be interdicted. On the other hand, legal prohibitions on driving vary in different states in the United States and in different countries and are often not medically justified. Employers frequently have unrealistic fears about the physical effects of a seizure, the potential for liability, and the impact on insurance costs. In fact, the Americans with Disabilities Act prohibits denying employment to persons with disability if the disability does not prevent them from meeting job requirements.

Children have special problems because their seizures affect the entire family. Parents may, with the best of intentions, handicap the child by being overly restrictive. The necessary and special attention received by the "sick" child may encourage passive manipulative behavior and overdependence while unintentionally exacerbating normal sibling rivalries.

The physician must be sensitive to these important quality of life concerns, even when they are not raised spontaneously by the patient or family. In fact, psychosocial issues often become the major focus of follow-up visits after the diagnosis has been made, the initial evaluation completed, and treatment started. We cannot emphasize too much the physician's responsibility to educate society to counter misperceptions and prejudices and to separate myth from medical fact. The Epilepsy Foundation (Landover, MD; 1-800-332-1000; www.epilepsyfoundation.com) and its nationwide system of affiliates have a wealth of materials about epilepsy suitable for patient, family, and public education.

Depression is common in people with epilepsy: Over half of patients with uncontrolled seizures are depressed. Even patients with well-controlled seizures have higher rates of depression than the general population. Suicide rates are tripled, with the highest rates seen in the 6 months after diagnosis. Patients should be observed for signs of depression and queried specifically about their mood, with attention to the potential need for psychiatric referral and initiation of antidepressant drugs. A simple screening tool developed specifically for use in people with epilepsy appears to allow rapid and accurate recognition of major depression. The FDA recently released an advisory indicating an increased risk of

suicidal thoughts in patients enrolled in clinical trials (0.43% in patients adding any additional agent vs. 0.22% for those adding placebo). The significance for newly diagnosed patients is unclear, but it seems prudent to observe patients starting new AEDs closely for mood changes.

Treatment of depression begins with optimal treatment of the seizure disorder. Barbiturate and succinimide drugs may adversely affect mood, inducing symptoms that mimic endogenous depression. Topiramate and levetiracetam seem to cause depression in a small minority of patients, whereas lamotrigine can occasionally improve depression. Levetiracetam has also been associated with rare psychosis. Although tricyclic antidepressants reduce the seizure threshold in experimental models of epilepsy, this is not a practical concern because they only rarely trigger seizures or increase seizure frequency in humans. Monoamine oxidase (MAO) inhibitors neither induce seizures nor increase seizure frequency. Modern electroconvulsive therapy does not worsen epilepsy. We have used all available selective serotonin reuptake inhibitors (SSRIs) without exacerbating seizures.

Anxiety disorders are also common in epilepsy patients. When present, some AEDs can exacerbate the condition, mainly levetiracetam, topiramate, and zonisamide. Other agents (including gabapentin, pregabalin, and benzodiazepines) can improve anxiety. Of the benzodiazepines, only clonazepam and clobazam are used for chronic treatment of epilepsy.

The relation between psychosis and epilepsy is controversial. No convincing evidence shows that interictal psychosis is a manifestation of epilepsy, but some demographic features are overrepresented in patients with epilepsy. Postictal psychosis is, however, a well-recognized and self-limited complication of epilepsy. Its cause is unknown, but it may represent a behavioral analog of Todd paresis. Symptoms typically appear 24 to 72 hours after a lucid interval following a prolonged seizure or cluster of seizures and are more common in patients with a history of encephalitis or a family history of neuropsychiatric problems. Postictal psychosis is more common with ambiguous localization on monitoring suggesting that broad, bilaterally distributed epileptogenic networks may be a risk factor. Delusions and paranoia are common. The psychosis is self-limited, usually to a few days, although symptoms occasionally last as long as 1 to 2 weeks. Treatment with haloperidol or risperidone is usually effective. In cases where postictal psychosis regularly follows clusters of seizures, chronic treatment with low-dose risperidone can be helpful. Long-term emphasis should be on improving seizure control. Phenothiazines, butyrophenones, and clozapine lower seizure threshold in experimental animals and occasionally seem to induce seizures in nonepileptic patients. Most occurrences have been associated with high drug doses or a rapid increase in dose. With the possible exception of clozapine, however, little evidence supports the notion that reasonable and conservative use of antipsychotic medications increases seizure frequency in patients with epilepsy.

Interictal aggressive behavior is not more common in people with epilepsy. Directed aggression during seizures occurs in less than 0.02% of patients with severe epilepsy; it is almost certainly less common in the general epilepsy population. Undirected pushing or resistance occasionally occur postictally when attempts are made to restrain confused patients.

COMPLIANCE

The most common cause of breakthrough seizures is noncompliance with the prescribed therapeutic regimen. Only about 70% of patients take antiepileptic medications as prescribed. For phenytoin or carbamazepine, noncompliance can be inferred when sequential blood levels vary by more than 20%, assuming similarly timed samples and unchanged dosage. Persistently low AED levels in the face of increasing dosage also generally imply poor compliance. Caution is warranted with phenytoin, however, because as many as 20% of patients have low levels as a result of poor absorption or rapid metabolism.

Noncompliance is especially common in adolescents and elderly persons, when seizures are infrequent or not perceived as disabling, when AEDs must be taken several times each day, and when toxic effects persist. Compliance can be improved by patient education, by simplifying drug regimens (using less frequent dosing with extended-release preparations when appropriate), and by tailoring dosing schedules to the patient's daily routines. Pillbox devices that alert the patient to scheduled doses can be useful.

PSYCHOGENIC SEIZURES

Psychogenic nonepileptic seizures (PNES) are diagnosed in 20% to 30% of patients who present to epilepsy centers for difficult to control seizures. They are often misdiagnosed as epileptic seizures and are treated with antiseizure medications without adequate investigation, quite often resulting in significant morbidity. The estimates of prevalence of concurrent epilepsy among patients with PNES vary from 5% to 56%. They are believed to be a manifestation of an underlying psychological stress and are classified under conversion disorders, which are a type of somatoform disorder. A specific traumatic event at any point of time in the patient's life, including physical or sexual abuse, death of a loved one, divorce, or other similar loss may be identified in patients with PNES. The diagnosis of PNES can be challenging, as the presentation of these seizures is very diverse; they can range from mimicking a generalized convulsion to less often, an atonic event. Although no single semiologic feature is specific for diagnosing PNES, the motor manifestations usually are more asynchronous, variable, and fluctuating in intensity, and specific movements such as writing, thrashing, pelvic thrusting, opisthotonus, and jactitation are more suggestive of PNES (Video 58.6). Ictal stuttering, weeping, and eye closure are relatively uncommon in epileptic seizures and are suggestive of, but not diagnostic of, PNES. In one study, the occurrence of an episode in the doctor's examination room was estimated to have a 75% predictive value for PNES. Video-EEG evaluation is almost always required to verify the diagnosis, as descriptions of patients and onlookers are invariably incomplete, and even trained medical personnel cannot reliably distinguish epileptic from nonepileptic seizures by visualization alone. PNES also can occur in patients with concurrent epilepsy, further confounding accurate diagnosis of each event. Even with video-EEG recording, some frontal lobe seizures with bizarre semiologies can be misdiagnosed as PNES and often do not have an ictal EEG correlate. The key challenge is in presenting the diagnosis to patients, as acceptance of the diagnosis is a very important factor in response to treatment and counseling. Psychiatric intervention is the mainstay of treating PNES and is individualized according to the underlying psychiatric comorbidity. Ideally after diagnosis, the patients should be followed by a neurologist and a psychiatrist with close dialogue between the two, and cautious discontinuation of the antiseizure medication should be coordinated, where applicable. Neurologic follow-up should be maintained after the diagnosis, until the patient has been fully transitioned to psychiatric care.

Videos can be found in the companion e-book edition. For a full list of video legends, please see the front matter.

LEVEL 1 REFERENCES

1. Krumholz A, Wiebe S, Gronseth GS, et al. Evidence-based guideline: management of an unprovoked first seizure in adults. Report of the Guideline Development Subcommittee of the American Academy of Neurology and the American Epilepsy Society. *Neurology.* 2015;84:1705–1713.
2. Temkin NR, Dikmen SS, Wilensky AJ, et al. A randomized, double-blind study of phenytoin for the prevention of post-traumatic seizures. *N Engl J Med.* 1990;323:497–502.
3. Mattson RH, Cramer JA, Collins JF, et al. A comparison of carbamazepine, phenobarbital,phenytoin, and primidone in partial and secondarily generalized tonic–clonic seizures. *N Engl J Med.* 1985;313:145–151.
4. Mattson RH, Cramer JA, Collins JF. Comparison of valproate with carbamazepine for the treatment of complex partial seizures and secondarily generalized tonic–clonic seizures in adults. *N Engl J Med.* 1992;327:765–771.
5. Marson AG, Al-Kharusi AM, Alwaidh M, et al. The SANAD study of effectiveness of carbamazepine, gabapentin, lamotrigine, oxcarbazepine, or topiramate for treatment of partial epilepsy: an unblinded randomised controlled trial. *Lancet.* 2007;369(9566):1000–1015.
6. French J, Kanner AM, Bautista J. Efficacy and tolerability of the new antiepileptic drugs. I. Treatment of new onset epilepsy. *Neurology.* 2004;62:1252–1260.
7. Marson AG, Al-Kharusi AM, Alwaidh M, et al. The SANAD study of effectiveness of valproate, lamotrigine, or topiramate for generalised and unclassifiable epilepsy: an unblinded randomised controlled trial. *Lancet.* 2007;369(9566):1016–1026.
8. French J, Kanner AM, Bautista J. Efficacy and tolerability of the new antiepileptic drugs. II. Treatment of refractory epilepsy. *Neurology.* 2004;62:1261–1273.
9. Medical Research Council Antiepileptic Drug Withdrawal Study Group. Randomised study of antiepileptic drug withdrawal in patients in remission. *Lancet.* 1991;337:1175–1180.
10. Harden CL, Meador KJ, Pennell PB, et al. Practice Parameter update: management issues for women with epilepsy—focus on pregnancy (an evidence-based review): teratogenesis and perinatal outcomes. Report of the Quality Standards Subcommittee and Therapeutics and Technology Assessment Subcommittee of the American Academy of Neurology and American Epilepsy Society. *Neurology.* 2009;73:133–141.
11. Spencer SS, Berg AT, Vickrey BG, et al. Initial outcomes in the multicenter study of epilepsy surgery. *Neurology.* 2003;61:1680–1685.
12. Wiebe S, Blume WT, Girvin JP, et al. A randomized, controlled trial of surgery for temporal-lobe epilepsy. *N Engl J Med.* 2001;345:311–318.
13. Morris GL, Gloss D, Buchhalter J, et al. Evidence-based guideline update: vagus nerve stimulation for the treatment of epilepsy. Report of the Guideline Development Subcommittee of the American Academy of Neurology. *Neurology.* 2013;81:1453–1459.

SUGGESTED READINGS

Alper K, Kuzniecky R, Carlson C, et al. Postictal psychosis in partial epilepsy: a case–control study. *Ann Neurol.* 2008;63(5):602–610.

Bazil CW. *Living Well with Epilepsy.* New York: HarperCollins, Inc.; 2004.

Bazil CW, Malow BA, Sammaritano MR, eds. *Sleep and Epilepsy: The Clinical Spectrum.* New York: Elsevier; 2002.

Bazil CW, Pedley TA. Clinical pharmacology of antiepileptic drugs. *Clin Neuropharmacol*. 2003;26:38–52.

Beghi E. Overview of studies to prevent posttraumatic epilepsy. *Epilepsia*. 2003;44(suppl 10):21–26.

Benardo LS. Prevention of epilepsy after head trauma: do we need new drugs or a new approach? *Epilepsia*. 2003;44(suppl 10):27–33.

Benbadis SR. Nonepileptic behavioral disorders: diagnosis and treatment. *Continuum (Minneap Minn)*. 2013;19(3 Epilepsy):715–729.

Berg AT, Shinnar S. The risk of seizure recurrence following a first unprovoked seizure: a quantitative review. *Neurology*. 1991;41:965–972.

Brodie MJ, French JA. Management of epilepsy in adolescents and adults. *Lancet*. 2000;356:323–329.

Cendes F. Febrile seizures and mesial temporal sclerosis. *Curr Opin Neurol*. 2004;17:161–164.

Christensen J, Vestergaard M, Mortensen PB, et al. Epilepsy and risk of suicide: a population-based case–control study. *Lancet Neurol*. 2007;6:693–698.

Commission on Classification and Terminology of the International League Against Epilepsy. Proposal for revised clinical and electroencephalographic classification of epileptic seizures. *Epilepsia*. 1981;12:489–501.

DeLorenzo RJ, Pellock JM, Towne AR, et al. Epidemiology of status epilepticus. *J Clin Neurophysiol*. 1995;12:316–325.

Engel J Jr. ILAE classification of epilepsy syndromes. *Epilepsy Res*. 2006;70(suppl 1):S5–S10.

Engel J Jr. *Surgical Treatment of the Epilepsies*. 2nd ed. New York: Raven Press; 1993.

Engel J Jr, Pedley TA, eds. *Epilepsy: A Comprehensive Textbook*. Philadelphia: Lippincott Williams & Wilkins; 1998.

First Seizure Trial Group. Randomized clinical trial on the efficacy of antiepileptic drugs in reducing the risk of relapse after a first unprovoked tonic–clonic seizure. *Neurology*. 1993;43:478–483.

Fisher R, Salanova V, Witt T, et al. Electrical stimulation of the anterior nucleus of thalamus for treatment of refractory epilepsy. *Epilepsia*. 2010;51(5):899–908.

Gilliam FG, Barry JJ, Hermann BP, et al. Rapid detection of major depression in epilepsy: a multicentre study. *Lancet Neurol*. 2006;5(5):399–405.

Gourfinkel-An I, Baulac S, Nabbout R, et al. Monogenic idiopathic epilepsies. *Lancet Neurol*. 2004;3:209–218.

Granata T, Fusco L, Gobbi G, et al. Experience with immunomodulatory treatments in Rasmussen's encephalitis. *Neurology*. 2003;61:1807–1810.

Gutierrez-Delicado E, Serratosa JM. Genetics of the epilepsies. *Curr Opin Neurol*. 2004;17:147–153.

Hauser WA, Hesdorffer DC. *Epilepsy: Frequency, Causes and Consequences*. New York: Demos; 1990.

Hauser WA, Rich SS, Lee JR, et al. Risk of recurrent seizures after two unprovoked seizures. *N Engl J Med*. 1998;338:429–434.

Hirsch LJ, Hauser WA. Can sudden unexplained death in epilepsy be prevented? *Lancet*. 2004;364(9452):2157–2158.

Jackson GD, Berkovic SF, Tress BM, et al. Hippocampal sclerosis can be reliably detected by magnetic resonance imaging. *Neurology*. 1990;40:1869–1875.

Kanner AM, Nieto JC. Depressive disorders in epilepsy. *Neurology*. 1999;53:S26–S32.

Karceski S, Morrell M, Carpenter D. The Expert Consensus Guideline Series. Treatment of epilepsy. *Epilepsy Behav*. 2001;2:A1–A50.

Kwan P, Brodie MJ. Early identification of refractory epilepsy. *N Engl J Med*. 2000;342:314–319.

Mendez MF, Cummings JL, Benson DF. Depression in epilepsy. Significance and phenomenology. *Arch Neurol*. 1986;43:766–770.

Morrell MJ. Reproductive and metabolic disorders in women with epilepsy. *Epilepsia*. 2003;44(suppl 4):11–20.

Morrell MJ. Responsive cortical stimulation for the treatment of medically intractable partial epilepsy. *Neurology*. 2011;77(13):1295–1304.

Morrell MJ, Flynn K, eds. *Women with Epilepsy*. Cambridge, United Kingdom: Cambridge University Press; 2003.

Musicco M, Beghi E, Solari A, et al. Treatment of first tonic–clonic seizure does not improve the prognosis of epilepsy. *Neurology*. 1997;49:991–998.

Nguyen DK, Spencer SS. Recent advances in the treatment of epilepsy. *Arch Neurol*. 2003;60:929–935.

Noebels JL. The biology of epilepsy genes. *Annu Rev Neurosci*. 2003;26:599–625.

Ottman R, Winawer MR, Kalachikov S, et al. LGI1 mutations in autosomal dominant partial epilepsy with auditory features. *Neurology*. 2004;62(7):1120–1126.

Pack AM, Morrell MJ. Epilepsy and bone health in adults. *Epilepsy Behav*. 2004;5(suppl 2):S24–S29.

Pedley TA, Hauser WA. Sudden death in epilepsy: a wake-up call for management. *Lancet*. 2002;359:1790–1791.

Pellock JM, Willmore LJ. A rational guide to routine blood monitoring in patients receiving antiepileptic drugs. *Neurology*. 1991;41:961–964.

Salazar AM, Jabbari B, Vance SC, et al. Epilepsy after penetrating head injury. I. Clinical correlates: a report of the Vietnam Head Injury Study. *Neurology*. 1985;35:1406–1414.

Scheffer IE, Berkovic SF. The genetics of human epilepsy. *Trends Pharmacol Sci*. 2003;24:428–433.

Sheen VL, Walsh CA. Developmental genetic malformations of the cerebral cortex. *Curr Neurol Neurosci Rep*. 2003;3:433–441.

Sillanpaa M, Jalava M, Kaleva O, et al. Long-term prognosis of seizures with onset in childhood. *N Engl J Med*. 1998;338:1715–1722.

Spencer SS, Berg AT, Vickrey BG, et al; Multicenter Study of Epilepsy Surgery. Predicting long-term seizure outcome after resective epilepsy surgery: the multicenter study. *Neurology*. 2005;65(6):912–918.

Sperling MR, Feldman H, Kirman J, et al. Seizure control and mortality in epilepsy. *Ann Neurol*. 1999;46:45–50.

Sullivan JE, Dlugos DJ. Idiopathic generalized epilepsy. *Curr Treat Options Neurol*. 2004;6:231–242.

Treiman DM, Meyers PD, Walton NY, et al. A comparison of four treatments for generalized convulsive status epilepticus. *N Engl J Med*. 1998;339:792–798.

U.S. Food and Drug Administration. *Information for Healthcare Professionals: Suicidality and Antiepileptic Drugs*. Rockville, MD: U.S. Food and Drug Administration; 2008.

Wyllie E, ed. *The Treatment of Epilepsy*. 3rd ed. Philadelphia: Lippincott Williams & Wilkins; 2001.

Zahn CA, Morrell MJ, Collins SD, et al. Management issues for women with epilepsy: a review of the literature. *Neurology*. 1998;51:949–956.

Ménière Syndrome, Benign Paroxysmal Positional Vertigo, and Vestibular Neuritis

59

Ian S. Storper

INTRODUCTION

Three of the most common causes of peripheral vertigo are Ménière syndrome, benign paroxysmal positional vertigo, and vestibular neuritis. Each syndrome has its own distinct type of vertigo. The purpose of this chapter is to explain the clinical presentation and current treatment principles of each syndrome to aid the clinician in diagnosis and management.

MÉNIÈRE DISEASE

Although Ménière disease was described over 140 years ago, little about it is understood. The condition is often progressive; with medical and surgical treatment options, however, disability may be averted or ameliorated. A recent study using health claims data from 60 million patients in the United States reports prevalence as 190 per 100,000 with a female-to-male ratio of 1.89:1 [Level 1].[1] The prevalence increases with age.

This disease was first reported by Prosper Ménière in Paris in 1861 [Level 1].[13] As described, patients typically suffered recurrent attacks of vertigo lasting from hours to days. Coincident with the attacks were episodes of unilateral hearing loss and roaring tinnitus. At first, the hearing loss and tinnitus occurred only with the attacks, but as the disease progressed, they became permanent. In 1943, Cawthorne added a fourth symptom: fullness in the affected ear. Table 59.1 lists the clinical features of Ménière disease. Although the cause of Ménière disease still remains unknown, it was postulated by Knapp in 1871 that symptoms were caused by dilatation of the endolymphatic compartment of the inner ear during attacks and renormalization afterward [Level 1].[11] This idea is still widely accepted, as the vast majority of patients respond to sodium management.

DEFINITIONS

Ménière disease is defined as the *idiopathic* occurrence of attacks of vertigo, hearing loss, tinnitus, or fullness in the affected ear. If a cause is assumed, the term is *Ménière syndrome*. The causes of Ménière syndrome are listed in Table 59.2.

Episodes typically last from hours to days. After an attack, the patient often feels "foggy" or tired. Initially, only one or two symptoms may be present; for example, a patient may experience only episodic vertigo; the hallmark is fluctuation. In the early stages,

TABLE 59.1	Ménière Disease Clinical Features

Episodes of the following:

- Unilateral hearing loss
- Tinnitus in affected ear
- Vertigo
- Fullness in affected ear

TABLE 59.2	Some Causes of Ménière Syndrome

- Trauma or trauma or rupture of the inner ear membranes (perilymphatic fistula)
- Postinfectious: labyrinthitis, meningitis, Lyme disease, or otosyphilis
- Congenital anatomic abnormality
- Tumor, e.g., vestibular Schwannoma pressing on the eighth nerves
- Vertebrobasilar insufficiency—central signs and symptoms are also seen

patients are often asymptomatic between attacks. With progression, low-frequency hearing loss can become permanent and may progress to all frequencies. Tinnitus is usually loud and roaring. Vertigo can be severe, a true spinning sensation of the patient or surroundings. Nausea, vomiting, sweating, and pallor are typical, as the vertigo arises in the inner ear rather than in the brain. Some describe a linear motion or feel as if they are on a boat. Rarely, vertigo is noted only with change of position, mimicking benign paroxysmal positional vertigo. It is distinguishable because positional vertigo of Ménière disease occurs in attacks. If left untreated, disequilibrium may persist between attacks of vertigo. Most Ménière sufferers are women, attributable to hormonal causes of increased water retention. Symptoms may be worse prior to the menstrual cycle.

Typically, attacks become less frequent and less severe over time, with or without medical management. Within about 2 years of diagnosis, more than half of all patients are better, even without treatment. Treatment decreases the frequency and severity of attacks and minimizes permanent hearing or balance loss. Only 5% of medically treated patients progress to surgery.

About 10% of patients never experience vertigo; their disorder is termed *cochlear Ménière disease*. Ten percent of patients never experience auditory symptoms. The term *burned out Ménière disease* applies to the patient who has totally lost auditory and vestibular function. There is no loss of consciousness during Ménière attacks; if it occurs, neurologic disease is likely. A rare entity associated with Ménière disease is referred to as *drop attack* or *crisis of Tumarkin*; the patient suddenly drops to the ground. Head injury may ensue.

DIAGNOSIS

Ménière disease is diagnosed clinically; no test has sufficient sensitivity and specificity to be pathognomonic. Tests are used to rule out other disorders and to help confirm the diagnosis. Careful history and physical examination are essential. Ménière disease should be considered in any patient without other obvious cause who suffers episodic vertigo, hearing loss, tinnitus, or fullness in the ear. Ménière disease is not diagnosed unless symptoms have occurred at least twice. Between attacks, the examination is often normal, especially early in the disease. During an attack, a patient typically appears acutely vertiginous, with horizontal nystagmus beating toward the affected ear. If nystagmus is vertical, central nervous system (CNS) disease is considered.

Tests that aid in the diagnosis of Ménière disease include audiometry (complete audiologic evaluation [CAE]), videonystagmography (VNG), and magnetic resonance imaging (MRI). If the symptoms are bilateral, blood tests for autoimmune inner ear disease and infections are ordered. Early in the disease, the CAE is often normal. Later, low-frequency sensorineural hearing loss can develop. Ultimately, hearing loss may also involve high frequencies. Rarely, the hearing asymmetries may be in the high frequencies rather than the low frequencies. During an attack, there may be hearing loss in the affected ear, which may resolve afterward. If conductive hearing loss is found, other diagnoses, such as superior semicircular canal dehiscence or cholesteatoma, should be considered.

Early in Ménière disease, the VNG is usually normal because vestibular function recovers between attacks. As the disease progresses, caloric testing often yields a unilateral vestibular weakness. If testing is inadvertently performed during an attack, hyperfunction of the affected ear is usually seen. In end-stage disease, there is complete weakness (100%) in the affected ear. If central pathology is the cause of vertigo, caloric test results are usually normal. Gaze and positional testing, as well as optokinetic nystagmus testing, are often abnormal.

MRI is recommended for every patient with recurrent vertigo, asymmetric sensorineural hearing loss, or unilateral constant tinnitus. The study should include the brain and internal auditory canals, with and without gadolinium. This test evaluates intracranial pathology such as vestibular Schwannoma, stroke, or demyelination, which can cause these symptoms. If symptoms begin after age 60 years, Doppler examinations are performed to evaluate possible cerebrovascular disease. Electrocochleography is helpful in diagnosing Ménière disease. The test demonstrates high ratios of the summating potential/action potential in Ménière patients; sensitivity and specificity are not high enough for routine use. Once other causes are excluded, the most accurate way to establish the diagnosis is to determine whether it responds to treatment.

MEDICAL TREATMENT

Therapy begins with diet and medication. Approximately 85% of patients respond very well, with significant decrease in frequency and severity of attacks. About 5% of patients find that therapy with diet and medication is inadequate and requires middle ear injections or surgery.

The standard for medical management is a low-sodium diet and thiazide diuretic. First, it should be ascertained that this is safe for the patient by consultation with their internist. A new patient should be started on a diuretic between attacks of vertigo. Diet should be a strict 1,500 mg/day sodium regimen; the patient should be informed that this requires checking labels carefully. If patients eat outside the home, it should be in places where they can limit the amount of sodium. Sodium intake should be even with each meal to avoid surges in pressure. Patients are advised to drink copious amounts of water to help flush out the sodium and maintain blood pressure. They are urged to avoid caffeine and alcohol, which are thought to aggravate symptoms. Emotional stress can also aggravate Ménière disease, and psychiatric consultation may be necessary.

Because sodium levels are hormonally regulated, adding a diuretic is useful. Typically, the patient is started on hydrochlorothiazide 37.5 mg/triamterene 25 mg once daily. This diuretic sheds sodium well and is required only once daily. Triamterene typically protects the potassium level. Electrolyte levels and renal function should be monitored periodically while this diuretic is being taken. Discontinuation

TABLE 59.3	Medical Treatment of Ménière Disease
• 1,500 mg/day sodium diet and increased water intake
• Thiazide diuretic
• Vestibular suppressants
• Anticholinergics
• Antihistamines
• Benzodiazepines
• Corticosteroids

or dose adjustment may be required. Patients should be advised that it can take a few weeks to know if this regimen is beneficial.

Vestibular suppressants can help control vertigo during attacks. Anticholinergic drugs are useful because they are not severely sedating. The author prefers glycopyrrolate 2 mg by mouth (PO) twice daily as needed during attacks. An alternative is meclizine 12.5, 25, or 50 mg PO up to three times daily. Although meclizine is effective, it is sedating. Benzodiazepines are also vestibular suppressants. Diazepam 5 mg PO three times daily during attacks can be useful but is also sedating and habit forming. It should be used with caution if vertigo does not respond to the other drugs mentioned. Corticosteroids may also be beneficial. Table 59.3 summarizes medical treatment of Ménière disease.

In the event of intractable vertigo with nausea and vomiting, an emergency room visit may be necessary. Intravenous hydration should be administered, being careful not to overload the patient with sodium. Promethazine 75 mg intramuscularly or droperidol 0.625 mg intravenously are useful for emergencies, but both are heavily sedating.

SURGICAL MANAGEMENT

Surgical treatments for Ménière disease may be destructive or conservative. In all cases, these operations are performed only if symptoms persist despite medical optimization.

Conservative Procedures

ENDOLYMPHATIC SHUNT

These procedures are designed to decrease the pressure in the endolymphatic compartment by shunting the fluid out of it. Current shunting procedures are performed under general anesthesia by drilling medially through the mastoid cortex down to the endolymphatic sac, opening it, and allowing the fluid to drain into the mastoid cavity.

In the past, shunts were controversial. The controversy arose in the 1980s when a Danish group found similar vertigo control in patients who had undergone endolymphatic shunts to those who had undergone only mastoidectomy ("sham procedures") [Level 1].[17] However, the same data were reevaluated in 2000 by Welling and Nagaraja [Level 1].[18] In comparing the shunt group to the sham group, vertigo control was significantly better in the shunt group, nausea and vomiting were significantly less in the shunt group, and tinnitus was significantly less in the shunt group. Sood et al. in 2014 published a meta-analysis of all articles citing results from this operation according to current guidelines from 1970 to 2013. They report that endolymphatic shunt controls vertigo effectively in 75% of patients who failed medical treatment [Level 1].[16] Complications of shunt procedures are rare and do not differ significantly from those of mastoidectomy. It is a reasonable first procedure for patients with good hearing and mild to moderate vertigo.

VESTIBULAR NEURECTOMY

The vestibular nerve can be separated from the cochlear nerve and sectioned. Although the vestibular nerve is cut, this procedure is generally considered a conservative procedure because hearing is preserved. The risks of craniotomy must be considered, and the indications are more stringent. Patient selection criteria for vestibular neurectomy include episodic disabling vertigo owing to Ménière disease, serviceable hearing in the affected ear, and failure of medical management. Moreover, there must be unilateral vestibular weakness in the affected ear on caloric testing but not 100%. This procedure should not be performed on the side of an only hearing or significantly better hearing ear. The results of vestibular neurectomy are excellent [**Level 1**].[3,12] Vertigo is controlled in 94% of patients. Hearing loss, tinnitus, and fullness are unaffected; the patient must continue on low-sodium diet and diuretic. Complications include sensorineural hearing loss in 2% to 3% of patients, cerebrospinal fluid (CSF) leak in 5% to 12%, temporary unsteadiness in up to 25%, headache in 10%, and tinnitus in 7%. It should be performed in patients with disabling episodic vertigo or in those who have failed shunt surgery.

DESTRUCTIVE PROCEDURES: LABYRINTHECTOMY

In this operation, the vestibular portion of the inner ear is destroyed and all five end organs are removed. Because the hearing in the operated ear is destroyed, this procedure is limited to patients with no serviceable hearing in the affected ear; who suffer from episodic, disabling vertigo; and in whom medical management has failed. This is the standard for vertigo control in patients with no hearing. Vestibular weakness must be shown in the affected ear on caloric testing but not 100%. Labyrinthectomy typically eradicates attacks of vertigo about 95% of the time. Aside from temporary postoperative unsteadiness in 10% of patients, the risks of this procedure do not differ significantly from those of mastoidectomy. Table 59.4 lists surgical options for Ménière disease.

OTHER TREATMENT METHODS

Intratympanic Corticosteroids

Intratympanic dexamethasone given at regular intervals has been described as a method of controlling episodes of Ménière disease which continue despite adherence to low sodium diet and diuretic therapy [**Level 1**].[20] Typically three perfusions of dexamethasone 24 mg/ml separated by 10 minutes are performed for a total of 1 ml. Repeat injections may be necessary for recurrent symptoms.

Intratympanic Gentamicin

Gentamicin is instilled into the middle ear, which provides a pathway into the inner ear via the round window. This aminoglycoside preferentially destroys vestibular hair cells over cochlear hair cells. Results vary. Vertigo control is about 80%, but there is significant incidence of sensorineural hearing loss. In one study, it was found that patients given intratympanic gentamicin had a statistically significant decrease in pure tone average and speech discrimination scores but that patients undergoing vestibular neurectomy did not. Vertigo control was achieved in 80% of patients given gentamicin and in 95% of patients with neurectomy. In another

TABLE 59.4 *Surgical Options for Ménière Disease*

- Endolymphatic shunt
- Vestibular neurectomy
- Labyrinthectomy

study, 90% of patients had complete initial control of vertigo after gentamicin, but 29% had recurrence after 4 months. In a third more recent study, 85% of patients had complete control of vertigo from gentamicin perfusion, but hearing was decreased in 25.6% [**Level 1**].[8,9,19] Gentamicin is less effective for vertigo control than surgery. There is risk of postprocedure long-term unsteadiness. In 2014, Casani et al. demonstrated less long-term unsteadiness and hearing loss using a lower dose regimen [**Level 1**].[4]

Meniett Device

This device delivers pressure pulses to the inner ear via a tympanostomy tube to generate gradients in the endolymphatic compartment via the round window. The device is worn for 5 minutes three times per day. Significant benefit from the use of this device has not been clearly demonstrated.

Streptomycin

This drug has been banned by the U.S. Food and Drug Administration (FDA) because of its inner ear toxicity. However, it is useful for end-stage patients with bilateral Ménière disease who still have attacks of vertigo and no hearing. The drug is administered intramuscularly, in regular doses, until caloric responses disappear. The drug eradicates the remaining vestibular function.

BENIGN PAROXYSMAL POSITIONAL VERTIGO

Benign paroxysmal positional vertigo (BPPV) has been described as the most common cause of peripheral vertigo with prevalence from 10.7 to 64 cases per 100,000 and prevalence over a lifetime of 2.4% [**Level 1**].[10] The average age of onset is from 50 to 60 years, with a 2 to 3:1 female-to-male ratio. It was first described by Barany in 1921 [**Level 1**].[2] Patients report episodic vertigo sensations, which are caused by head motion; often, patients describe it as being aggravated by arising from or getting into bed or tossing during sleep. These episodes can be intense and can cause a fall. Characteristically, there is no vertigo if there is no head motion. Each episode typically lasts for less than a minute. There is no hearing loss, tinnitus, or fullness in the ear associated with this condition. The incidence increases with age and there is a slight female-to-male predominance. Approximately half of cases occur after head trauma.

This disorder is thought to be caused by dislodgement of otoconia—calcium carbonate crystals normally present in the utricle or saccule—into the semicircular canals. These crystals add inertia to the torsion-pendulum model of semicircular canal activation. When there is a mismatch of inertia between the two ears, there is disagreeing signal sent along the right and left vestibular nerves, resulting in nystagmus and a sensation of vertigo until the inner ear motion has stopped. This condition is self-limited; it, however, can be present for an extended period of time prior to dissipating. This condition most commonly occurs in the posterior semicircular canal and occasionally the horizontal semicircular canal; it rarely occurs in the superior semicircular canal.

Diagnosis is established by provocative positional maneuvers. For posterior canal BPPV, the Dix–Hallpike maneuver is performed, where the patient's head is turned toward the affected side and they lie back quickly, extending the neck [**Level 1**].[15] If the maneuver is positive, vertical–torsional nystagmus is seen for a number of seconds, with latency and fatigability. For horizontal canal BPPV, diagnosis is established by seeing horizontal nystagmus with latency and fatigability when rolling the head to the affected side in the supine position. Diagnosing superior canal BPPV involves eliciting vertical nystagmus and central lesions need to be excluded. These maneuvers should not be performed unless neurovascular problems have been excluded first.

Treatment involves canalith repositioning maneuvers, thought to dislodge the crystals and allow them to drop out into a safe compartment of the inner ear. Although there are a numerous maneuvers, the most common ones are those described by Epley in 1992 [**Level 1**].[6] For posterior semicircular canal BPPV, the maneuver consists of five steps: (1) Dix–Hallpike maneuver; (2) turning the head to the opposite side; (3) rolling over onto the opposite side, head downward; (4) sitting up and then turning the head forward; and (5) tucking the chin. The maneuver is repeated until nystagmus dissipates. The patient is instructed to keep their head level for the next 48 hours. This maneuver is highly successful but sometimes has to be repeated over multiple sessions. Physical therapists can be consulted. For severe, recalcitrant cases, singular neurectomy can be offered.

VESTIBULAR NEURITIS

Vestibular neuritis (or vestibular neuronitis) was described by Dix and Hallpike in 1952. It is a clinical syndrome where a patient develops severe vertigo, often associated with nausea, vomiting, and/or prostration, which resolves over a period of days to weeks. There are no other neurologic deficits and there is no loss of consciousness. In general, older age portends a prolonged and possibly incomplete recovery. Vestibular neuritis has an incidence of about 3.5 cases per 100,000 persons [**Level 1**].[15] Typical age of onset is between 30 and 60 years and there is no gender difference. Approximately 30% of affected individuals suffered an upper respiratory infection preceding their symptoms.

The cause of this condition has been postulated to be reactivation of herpes simplex or other neurotropic virus, but this has not been proven. Histologic findings performed postmortem on individuals who have suffered this condition have shown an atrophic superior vestibular nerve and ganglion [**Level 1**].[14]

Treatment is supportive. Hydration may be required and during the intense period, vestibular suppressants are helpful. They should be discontinued as soon as reasonable as they can prolong recovery time. Imaging studies such as MRI and computed tomography angiography (CTA) are typically ordered to rule out neurovascular or other central causes. Patients usually exhibit nonfatigable horizontal nystagmus at presentation. After the initial severe vertigo has dissipated, recovery time can be prolonged in some individuals whence vestibular rehabilitation can be beneficial. A recent study showed that corticosteroids administered over the first 3 weeks after onset improved symptoms more quickly than vestibular rehabilitation but that long-term results were similar [**Level 1**].[7]

CONCLUSION

The clinical syndromes of three of the most common types of peripheral vertigo have been discussed. It should be remembered that there are numerous other causes of peripheral and central vertigo to be considered when evaluating patients.

LEVEL 1 EVIDENCE

1. Alexander TH, Harris JP. Current epidemiology of Meniere's syndrome. *Otolaryngol Clin North Am.* 2010;43:965–970.
2. Barany R. Diagnose von krankheitserscheinungen im bereiche des Otolithenapparates. *Acta Otolaryngol.* 1921;2:434–437.
3. Brackmann DE. Surgical treatment of vertigo. *J Laryngol Otol.* 1990;104:849–859.
4. Casani AP, Cerchiai N, Navari E, et al. Intratympanic gentamicin for Ménière disease: short- and long-term followup of two regimens of treatment. *Otolaryngol Head Neck Surg.* 2014;150:847–852.
5. Dix M, Hallpike C. The pathology, symptomatology and diagnosis of certain common disorders of the vestibular system. *Proc R Soc Med.* 1952;45:341–354.
6. Epley JM. The canalith repositioning procedure: for treatment of benign paroxysmal positional vertigo. *Otolaryngol Head Neck Surg.* 1992;107:399–404.
7. Goudakis JK, Markou KD, Psillas G, et al. Corticosteroids and vestibular exercises in vestibular neuritis: single-blind randomized clinical trial. *JAMA Otolaryngol Head Neck Surg.* 2014; 140:434–440.
8. Hillman TA, Chen DA, Arriaga MA. Vestibular neurectomy vs intratympanic gentamicin for Meniere's disease. *Laryngoscope.* 2004;114:216–222.
9. Kaplan DM, Nedzelski JM, Chen JM, et al. Intratympanic gentamicin for treatment of unilateral Meniere's disease. *Laryngoscope.* 2000;110:1298–1305.
10. Kim J-S, Zee DS. Benign paroxysmal positional vertigo. *NEJM.* 2014;370:1138–1147.
11. Knapp H. A clinical analysis of the inflammatory affections of the inner ear. *Arch Ophthalmol.* 1871;2:204–283.
12. McKenzie KG. Intracranial division of the vestibular portion of the auditory nerve for Meniere's disease. *CMAJ.* 1936;34: 369–381.
13. Ménière P. Memoire sur des lesions de l'orielle interne donnant lieu a des symptoms de congestion cerebrale apoplectiforme. *Gaz Med Paris.* 1861;16:597–601.
14. Richard C, Linthicum FH. Vestibular neuritis: the vertigo disappears, the histological traces remain. *Otol Neurotol.* 2012;33: e59–e60.
15. Sekitani T, Imate Y, Noguchi T, et al. Vestibular neuritis epidemiological survey by questionnaire in Japan. *Acta Otolaryngol Suppl.* 1993;503:9–12.
16. Sood AJ, Lambert PR, Nguyen SA, et al. Endolymphatic sac surgery for Ménière disease: a systematic review and meta-analysis. *Otol Neurotol.* 2014;35(6):1033–1045.
17. Thomsen J, Bretlau P, Tos M, et al. Placebo effect in surgery for Meniere's disease. *Arch Otolaryngol.* 1981;107:271–277.
18. Welling DB, Nagaraja HN. Endolymphatic mastoid shunt: a reevaluation of efficacy. *Otolaryngol Head Neck Surg.* 2000;122: 340–345.
19. Wu IC, Minor LB. Long term hearing outcome in patients receiving gentamicin for Meniere's disease. *Laryngoscope.* 2003; 113:815–820.
20. McRackan TR, Best J, Pearce EC, et al. Intratympanic dexamethasone as a symptomatic treatment for Meniere's Disease. *Otol Neurotol.* 2014;35:1638–1640.

SUGGESTED READINGS

Coelho DH, Lalwani AK. Medical management of Ménière's disease. *Laryngoscope.* 2008;118(6):1099–1108.

Gates GA, Green JD. Intermittent pressure therapy of intractable Meniere's disease using Meniett device: a preliminary report. *Laryngoscope.* 2002; 112:1489–1493.

Paparella MM, Hanson DG. Endolymphatic sac drainage for intractable vertigo (method and experiences). *Laryngoscope.* 1976;86:697–703.

Parry RH. A case of tinnitus and vertigo treated by division of the auditory nerve. *J Laryngol Otol.* 1904;19:402–406.

Portmann G. Vertigo: surgical treatment by opening the saccus endolymphaticus. *Arch Otolaryngol.* 1927;6:309–319.

Storper IS, Spitzer JB, Scanlan M. Use of glycopyrrolate in the treatment of Ménière's disease. *Laryngoscope.* 1998;108:1442–1445.

Thirlwall AS, Kundu S. Diuretics for Ménière's disease or syndrome. *Cochrane Database Syst Rev.* 2006;3:CD003599.

INTRODUCTION

Transient global amnesia (TGA) is characterized by sudden inability to form new memory traces (*anterograde amnesia*) in addition to retrograde memory loss for events of the preceding days, weeks, or even years.

EPIDEMIOLOGY

Patients are usually middle aged or elderly and otherwise healthy. Recurrent attacks occur in 15% to 30% of cases, and fewer than 3% have more than three attacks. Intervals between attacks range from 1 month to 19 years.

PATHOBIOLOGY

The cause of TGA is uncertain. Case-control series and anecdotal reports variably implicate seizures, stroke, or migraine. Against an epileptic basis for TGA are the infrequency of recurrence, absence of other seizure phenomena, and normal electroencephalogram (EEG) even during attacks. In transient epileptic amnesia (TEA), attacks are usually less than an hour in duration, tend to occur on awakening, are often accompanied by other ictal symptoms, and are likely to recur; ictal and interictal EEG abnormalities are often present, and symptoms respond to anticonvulsant therapy.

TGA has been anecdotally described in association with carotid artery occlusion and amaurosis fugax, with infarction of the inferomedial temporal lobe, the cingulate gyrus, or the retrosplenial corpus callosum and with cerebral angiography (especially vertebral). In large series, however, major risk factors for stroke (hypertension, diabetes mellitus, tobacco, ischemic heart disease, atrial fibrillation, and past stroke or transient ischemic attack [TIA]) are no more common among patients with TGA than in age-matched controls, and TGA is not a risk factor for stroke. Studies addressing a possible association of TGA with cardiac valvular disease or patent foramen ovale have been inconsistent. Patients with amnestic stroke owing to documented posterior cerebral artery occlusion do not report previous TGA; their neurologic signs usually include more than simple amnesia (e.g., visual impairment), and they do not exhibit repetitive queries. Reduced blood flow to the thalamus or temporal lobes has been documented during attacks of TGA but could be secondary to neuronal dysfunction rather than its cause.

Valve incompetence of the internal jugular vein is present in many patients with TGA, raising the possibility of cerebral venous congestion during Valsalva-like activities. Intracranial venous reflux during Valsalva maneuver could not be demonstrated in the same patients, however, and such a mechanism is unlikely to explain symptoms that last hours and seldom recur.

Epidemiologic studies confirm an association of TGA with migraine, even though in most migraine patients, headache attacks are recurrent, whereas attacks of TGA are not. Sometimes, both amnestic and migrainous attacks (including visual symptoms and vomiting) occur simultaneously or follow one another. A case report described a man with repeated episodes of TGA associated with sexual activity whose spells cleared as long as he took the β-blocker metoprolol. Cortical spreading depression (possibly the pathophysiologic basis of cerebral symptoms of migraine) could, by affecting the hippocampus, explain some cases of TGA.

CLINICAL MANIFESTATIONS

During attacks, which affect both verbal and nonverbal memory, there is often bewilderment or anxiety and a tendency to repeat one or several questions (e.g., "Where am I?"). Physical and neurologic examinations, including mental status, are otherwise normal. Immediate registration of events (e.g., serial digits) is intact, and self-identification is preserved. Attacks last minutes or hours, rarely longer than a day, with gradual recovery. Retrograde amnesia clears in a forward fashion, often with permanent loss for events occurring within minutes or a few hours of the attack; there is also permanent amnesia for events during the attack itself. Headache frequently accompanies attacks; less often, there is nausea, dizziness, chills, flushing, or limb paresthesias. TGA is frequently precipitated by physical or emotional stress, such as sexual intercourse, driving an automobile, pain, photogenic events, or swimming in cold water. Because amnesia can accompany a variety of neurologic disturbances, such as head trauma, intoxication, partial complex seizures, or dissociative states, criteria for diagnosing TGA should include observation of the attack by others.

Permanently impaired memory following an acute attack is rare, although subtle defects have been reported.

DIAGNOSIS

Diffusion-weighted magnetic resonance imaging (MRI) detected highly focal lesions in the CA1 field of the hippocampus in 70% of TGA patients, bilaterally in only 12%, appearing 24 to 48 hours after TGA onset (i.e., not during the acute memory impairment) and disappearing over several weeks. Magnetic resonance (MR) spectroscopy identified reversible lactate peaks within the same lesions, consistent with ischemia. Functional MRI during the acute phase of amnesia identified reversible reduced functional connectivity bilaterally in hippocampi and other temporolimbic regions considered part of an "episodic memory network."

TREATMENT

A study of 142 cases plus literature review suggested three subgroups of TGA (excluding patients with epilepsy or TIA). In women, TGA was mainly associated with an emotional precipitating event and a history of anxiety or depression. In men, attacks are more often followed a physical precipitating event perhaps associated with a Valsalva maneuver. In younger patients, an association with migraine was most prominent. Thus, even when strict diagnostic criteria are applied, TGA probably has diverse origins. In patients in whom epilepsy and migraine can be excluded and who have risk factors for cerebrovascular disease, antiplatelet drugs should be considered, but the benign natural history makes it difficult to evaluate any preventive treatment.

SUGGESTED READINGS

Agosti C, Akkawi NM, Borroni B, et al. Recurrency in transient global amnesia: a retrospective study. *Eur J Neurol.* 2006;13:986–989.

Baracchini C, Tonello S, Farina F, et al. Jugular veins in transient global amnesia: innocent bystanders. *Stroke.* 2012;43:2289–2292.

Bartsch T, Alke K, Deuschl G, et al. Evolution of hippocampal CA-1 diffusion lesions in transient global amnesia. *Ann Neurol.* 2007;62:475–480.

Bartsch T, Altke K, Wolff S, et al. Focal MR spectroscopy of hippocampal CA-1 lesions in transient global amnesia. *Neurology.* 2008;70:1030–1035.

Bartsch T, Butler C. Transient amnestic syndromes. *Nat Rev Neurol.* 2013;9: 86–97.

Berlit P. Successful prophylaxis of recurrent transient global amnesia with metoprolol. *Neurology.* 2000;55:1937–1938.

Bilo L, Meo R, Ruosi P, et al. Transient epileptic amnesia: an emerging late-onset epileptic syndrome. *Epilepsia.* 2009;50(suppl 5):58–61.

Chen ST, Tang LM, Lee TH, et al. Transient global amnesia and amaurosis fugax in a patient with common carotid artery occlusion—a case report. *Angiology.* 2000;51:257–261.

Eustache F, Desgranges B, Laville P, et al. Episodic memory in transient global amnesia: encoding, storage, or retrieval deficit? *J Neurol Neurosurg Psychiatry.* 1999;66:148–154.

Gallardo-Tur A, Romero-Godoy J, de la Cruz A, et al. Transient global amnesia associated with an acute infarction at the cingulate gyrus. *Case Rep Clin Med.* 2014;2014:418180. doi:10.1155/2014/418180.

LaBar KS, Gitelman DR, Parrish TB, et al. Functional changes in temporal lobe activity during transient global amnesia. *Neurology.* 2002;58:638–641.

Lin KH, Chen YT, Fuh JL, et al. Migraine is associated with a higher risk of transient global amnesia: a nationwide cohort study. *Eur J Neurol.* 2014;21: 718–724.

Maalikjy AN, Agosti C, Anzola GP, et al. Transient global amnesia: a clinical and sonographic study. *Eur Neurol.* 2003;49:67–71.

Mangla A, Navi BB, Layton K, et al. Transient global amnesia and the risk of ischemic stroke. *Stroke.* 2014;45:389–393.

Peer M, Nitzan M, Goldberg I, et al. Reversible functional connectivity disturbances during transient global amnesia. *Ann Neurol.* 2014;75:634–643.

Quinette P, Guillery-Girard B, Dayan J, et al. What does transient global amnesia really mean? Review of the literature and thorough study of 142 cases. *Brain.* 2006;129:1640–1658.

Romero JR, Mercado M, Beiser AS, et al. Transient global amnesia and neurological events: the Framingham Heart Study. *Front Neurol.* 2013;4:47. doi:10.3389//fneur.2013.00047.

Sedlaczek O, Hirsch JG, Grips E, et al. Detection of delayed focal MR changes in the lateral hippocampus in transient global amnesia. *Neurology.* 2004;62(12): 2165–2270.

Toledo M, Pujadas F, Grivé E, et al. Lack of evidence for arterial ischemia in transient global amnesia. *Stroke.* 2008;39:476–479.

Acute Bacterial Meningitis and Infective Endocarditis 61

Burk Jubelt and Barnett R. Nathan

INTRODUCTION

The parenchyma, coverings, and blood vessels of the nervous system may be invaded by virtually any pathogenic microorganism. It is customary, for convenience of description, to divide the syndromes produced according to the initial site of involvement. This division is arbitrary because the inflammatory process frequently involves more than one of these structures.

Involvement of the meninges by pathogenic microorganisms is known as *leptomeningitis* when the infection and inflammatory response are confined to the subarachnoid space and the arachnoid and pia. Cases are divided into acute, subacute, and chronic meningitis according to the rapidity with which the inflammatory process develops. This rate of development, in part, is related to the nature of the infecting organism. Chronic meningitis is discussed in Chapter 64. In some cases, acute bacterial meningitis can be complicated by focal purulent abscesses of the central nervous system (CNS) (Fig. 61.1) or its surrounding structures (empyema). These focal bacterial infections are discussed in Chapter 62.

Acute bacterial meningitis presents as a neurologic emergency and often overlaps with sepsis, and the principles of therapy are the same: early initiation of broad-spectrum antibiotics, volume resuscitation and vasopressors in the face of hypotension, and careful attention to airway control and oxygenation.

ACUTE BACTERIAL MENINGITIS

Bacteria may gain access to the ventriculosubarachnoid space by way of the blood, in the course of septicemia, or as a metastasis from infection of the heart, lung, or other viscera. The meninges may also be invaded by direct extension from a septic focus in the skull, spine, or parenchyma of the nervous system (e.g., sinusitis, otitis, osteomyelitis, brain abscess). Organisms may also gain entrance to the subarachnoid space through compound fractures of the skull and fractures through the nasal sinuses or mastoid or after neurosurgical procedures. Pathogen introduction by lumbar puncture is rare. The pathologic background, symptoms, and clinical course of most patients with acute purulent meningitis are similar

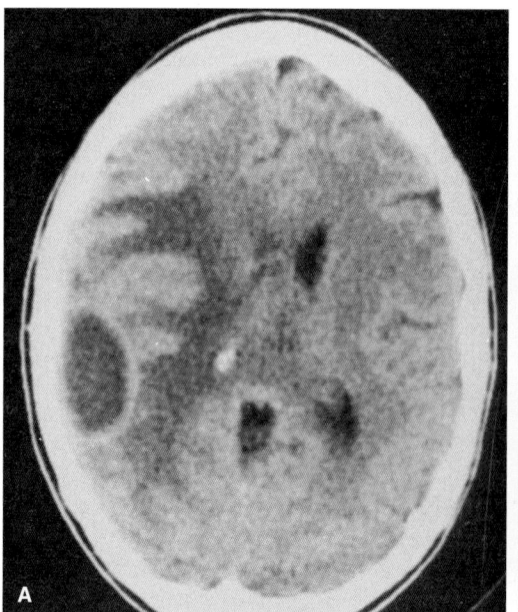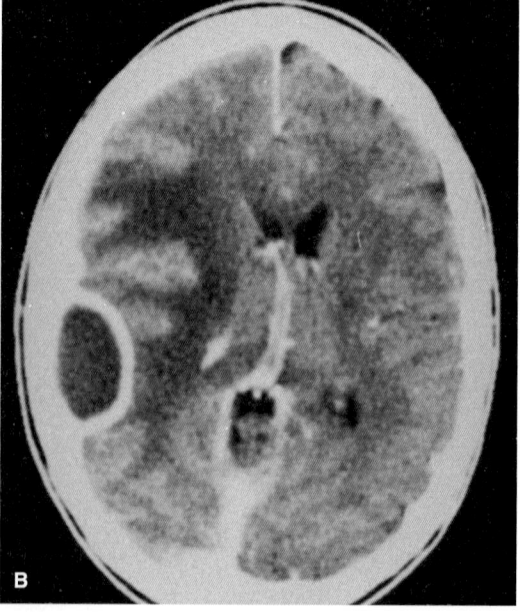

FIGURE 61.1 Epidural abscess. **A:** Axial, noncontrast CT demonstrates a right posterior temporal lucent epidural collection with prominent white matter edema in the underlying cerebral parenchyma. Calcified choroid in the effaced atrium of the right lateral ventricle is shifted anteromedially. **B:** Postcontrast scan at this same level demonstrates abnormal dural enhancement and shift of the internal cerebral veins owing to the mass effect. (Courtesy of Drs. J. A. Bello and S. K. Hilal.)

FIGURE 61.2 Management algorithm for adults with suspected acute bacterial meningitis. CNS, central nervous system; STAT, immediately; CSF, cerebrospinal fluid; CT, computed tomography. (From Tunkel AR, Hartman BJ, Kaplan SJ, et al. Practice guidelines for the management of bacterial meningitis. *Clin Infect Dis.* 2004;39:1267–1284.)

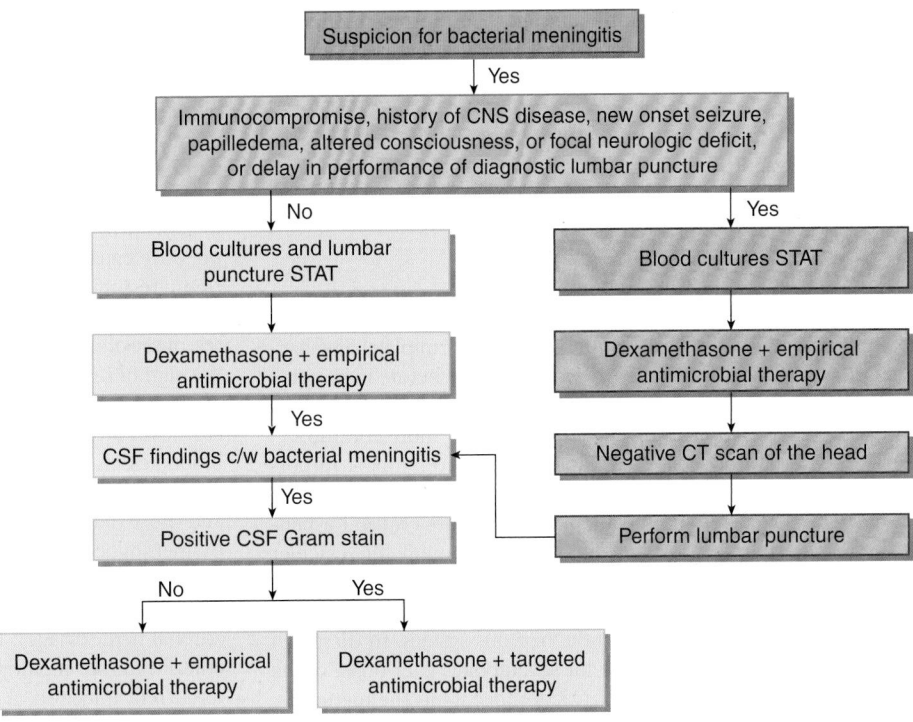

regardless of the causative organism. The classic triad of fever, neck stiffness, and altered mental status occurs in less than half of all patients, but 95% have at least two of four symptoms of fever, neck stiffness, altered mental status, and headache. Empiric therapy depends on age, whether the infection is community or nosocomially acquired, and other risk factors (head trauma or surgery, crowded living conditions, and underlying illnesses [e.g., diabetes, alcoholism, hematologic and immunologic disorders]). Diagnosis and therapy depend on the isolation and identification of the organism and determination of the source of the infection (Fig. 61.2).

Acute purulent meningitis may be the result of infection with almost any pathogenic bacteria. Isolated examples of infection by uncommon forms are recorded in the literature. In the United States, *Streptococcus pneumoniae* now accounts for about one-half of cases when the infecting organism is identified, and *Neisseria meningitidis* accounts for about one-fourth of the total cases (Table 61.1).

In the neonatal period, group B streptococci and *Escherichia coli* are the most common causative agents. Approximately 60%

of the postneonatal bacterial meningitis of children used to be caused by *Haemophilus influenzae*. Introduction of the *H. influenzae* type B vaccine was followed by a 100-fold decrease in incidence. However, the peak incidence still occurs in children younger than 2 months of age. Overall fatality rate from bacterial meningitis is now about 15%. Many deaths occur during the first 48 hours of hospitalization.

MENINGOCOCCAL MENINGITIS

Meningococcal meningitis occurs in sporadic form and at irregular intervals in epidemics. Epidemics are especially likely to occur during large shifts in population, and crowding as in a time of war, and in college dormitories.

Epidemiology

Meningococcus is the causative organism in about 25% of all cases of bacterial meningitis in the United States. Serogroup B is now the most commonly reported serotype (50%). Children and

---

TABLE 61.1 Causes of Bacterial Meningitis in the United States

Organism	Adults (18 Yr and Older)		Children (17 Yr and Younger)	
	No. of Cases Reported	Percentage of Total	No. of Cases Reported	Percentage of Total
Haemophilus influenzae	65	6%	47	8%
Streptococcus pneumoniae	769	71%	200	34%
Neisseria meningitidis	130	12%	106	18%
Group B *Streptococcus*	76	7%	223	38%
Listeria monocytogenes	46	4%	12	2%
Total	1,086	100%	588	100%

Data from Thigpen MC, Whitney CG, Messonnier NE, et al. Bacterial meningitis in the United States, 1998–2007. *N Engl J Med.* 2011;364(21):2016–2025.

young adults are predominantly affected. The normal habitat of the meningococcus is the nasopharynx, and the disease is spread by colonized individuals. A polysaccharide vaccine for groups A, C, Y, and W-135 meningococci has reduced the incidence of meningococcal infection among military recruits. The vaccine also has been used for control of serogroup C outbreaks in schools and on college campuses and for children with increased risk of infection (asplenia, HIV infection, complement deficiencies).

Pathobiology

Meningococci (*N. meningitidis*) may gain access to the meninges directly from the nasopharynx through the cribriform plate. The bacteria, however, are usually recovered from blood before meningitis commences, indicating that colonization of the nasopharynx with subsequent bacteremia and spread to the CNS is more common.

The bacterial polysaccharide capsule seems to be most important in attachment and penetration to gain access to the body. Elements in the bacterial cell wall (pili, fimbria) are critical for penetration into the cerebrospinal fluid (CSF) through the vascular endothelium and in induction of the inflammatory response.

In acute fulminating cases, death may occur before there are any significant pathologic changes in the nervous system. In the usual case, when death does not occur for several days after onset of the disease, an intense inflammatory reaction occurs in the meninges. The inflammatory reaction is especially severe in the subarachnoid space over the convexity of the brain and around the cisterns at the base of the brain. It may extend along the Virchow–Robin perivascular spaces into the brain and spinal cord. Meningococci, both intra- and extracellular, are found in the meninges and CSF. With progression of the infection, the pia–arachnoid becomes thickened and adhesions may form. Inflammatory reaction and fibrosis of the meninges along the roots of the cranial nerves are thought to cause the cranial nerve palsies that are seen occasionally.

Damage to the auditory nerve often occurs suddenly, and the resulting hearing loss is usually permanent. The damage may result from extension of the infection to the inner ear or from thrombosis of the nutrient artery. Signs and symptoms of parenchymal damage (e.g., hemiplegia, aphasia, and cerebellar signs) are caused by infarcts resulting from thrombosis of inflamed arteries or veins.

In the past, the inflammation in meningitis had been attributed mainly to the toxic effects of bacteria. In all types of meningitis, the contribution to the inflammatory process of cytokines released by phagocytic and immunoactive cells, particularly interleukin 1 and tumor necrosis factor, has been recognized. These studies have formed the basis for the use of anti-inflammatory corticosteroids in the treatment of meningitis.

Clinical Manifestations

The onset of meningococcal meningitis is similar to that of other forms of meningitis and is accompanied by chills and fever, headache, nausea and vomiting, pain in the back, stiffness of the neck, and prostration. The occurrence of a petechial or hemorrhagic skin rash is a manifestation of meningococcemia. At the onset of meningitis, the patient is irritable. In children, there is frequently a characteristic sharp, shrill cry (meningeal cry). With progress of the disease, the sensorium becomes clouded and stupor or coma may develop. Occasionally, the onset may be fulminant and accompanied by deep coma. Convulsive seizures are often an early symptom, especially in children, but focal neurologic signs are uncommon in the initial presentation.

The patient appears acutely ill and may be confused, stuporous, or obtunded. The temperature is elevated at 101°F to 103°F, but it

may occasionally be normal at the onset. The pulse is usually rapid and the respiratory rate is increased. Blood pressure is normal except in acute fulminating cases when there may be profound hypotension. A petechial rash may be found in the skin, mucous membranes, or conjunctiva in meningococcemia but never in the nail beds. It usually fades in 3 or 4 days. There is rigidity of the neck with Kernig and Brudzinski signs. These signs may be absent in newborn, elderly, or comatose patients. Increased intracranial pressure causes bulging of an unclosed anterior fontanelle and periodic respiration. Cranial nerve palsies and focal neurologic signs are uncommon and usually do not develop until several days after the onset of infection. The optic discs are normal, but papilledema is a sign of increased intracranial pressure.

Complications and sequelae include those commonly associated with any inflammatory process in the meninges and cerebral blood vessels (i.e., convulsions, cranial nerve palsies, focal cerebral lesions, damage to the spinal cord or nerve roots, hydrocephalus) and those that are due to involvement of other portions of the body by meningococci (e.g., panophthalmitis and other types of ocular infection, arthritis, purpura, pericarditis, endocarditis, myocarditis, pleurisy, orchitis, epididymitis, albuminuria or hematuria, adrenal hemorrhage). Disseminated intravascular coagulation may complicate the meningitis. Complications may also arise from intercurrent infection of the upper respiratory tract, middle ear, and lungs. Any of these complications may leave permanent residua, but the most common sequelae are due to injury of the nervous system. These include deafness, ocular palsies, blindness, changes in cognitive functioning, convulsions, and hydrocephalus. With the available methods of treatment, complications and sequelae of meningeal infection are rare, and the complications due to the involvement of other parts of the body by the meningococci or other intercurrent infections are more readily controlled.

Diagnosis

The white blood cell count is increased, usually in the range of 10,000/mm³ to 30,000/mm³, but occasionally may be normal or higher than 40,000/mm³. The urine may contain albumin, casts, and red blood cell (RBC). Meningococci may be cultured from the nasopharynx in most cases, from the blood in more than 50% of the cases in the early stages, and from skin lesions when these are present.

The CSF is under increased pressure, usually between 200 and 500 mm H_2O. The fluid is cloudy (purulent) because it contains a large number of cells, predominantly polymorphonuclear leukocytes. The cell count in the fluid is usually between 2,000/mm³ and 10,000/mm³. Occasionally, it may be less than 100/mm³ and infrequently, more than 20,000/mm³. The protein concentration is increased. The glucose concentration is decreased usually to levels below 20 mg/dL. Gram-negative diplococci may be seen intra- and extracellularly in stained smears of the fluid, and meningococci may be cultured in more than 90% of untreated patients. Meningococcal meningitis may be diagnosed with certainty only by the isolation of the organism from the CSF. The diagnosis may be made, however, with relative certainty before the organisms are isolated in a patient with headache, vomiting, chills and fever, neck stiffness, and a petechial cutaneous rash, especially if there is an epidemic of meningococcal meningitis or if there has been exposure to a known case of meningococcal meningitis.

To establish the diagnosis of meningococcal meningitis, cultures should be made of skin lesions, nasopharyngeal secretions, blood, and CSF. The diagnosis may be established in many cases by examination of smears of the sediment of the CSF after application of the Gram stain.

Treatment

Antibiotic therapy for bacterial meningitis usually commences before the causative organism is confirmed (empiric therapy). Therefore, the initial regimen should be appropriate for most likely organisms, the determination of which depends to some extent on the patient's age and the predisposing and associated conditions. Third- or fourth-generation cephalosporins, usually ceftriaxone or cefotaxime, in combination with vancomycin have become the first choice of treatment for bacterial meningitis (Table 61.2). Their spectrum is broad, and they have become particularly useful since the occurrence of S. pneumoniae strains that are resistant to penicillin or ampicillin and amoxicillin. Once the result of culture and sensitivities is known, antibiotic therapy is modified accordingly (Table 61.3). Unless a dramatic response to therapy occurs, the CSF should be examined 24 to 48 hours after the initiation of treatment to assess the effectiveness of the antibiotic. Posttreatment examination of the CSF is not a meaningful criterion of recovery, and the CSF does not need to be reexamined if the patient is clinically well. The recommended duration of treatment is 7 days.

Several studies have suggested an improved outcome with the use of corticosteroids particularly if dexamethasone 6 mg every 6 hours is given shortly before the initiation of antibiotic treatment and continued for 4 days [**Level 1**].[1] Corticosteroids are beneficial in treating children with acute bacterial meningitis, especially in preventing hearing loss. Data in adults confirmed meningococcal meningitis favor steroid therapy to prevent hearing loss and decrease morbidity for those living in high-income countries. The lack of benefit in low-income countries may be due to the length of time between symptom onset and medical care, as well as poor nutrition and other comorbidities.

TABLE 61.2	Recommended Empiric Antibiotics for Suspected Bacterial Meningitis according to Age or Predisposing Factors
Age or Predisposing Feature	**Antibiotics**
Age 0–4 wk	Ampicillin plus either cefotaxime or an aminoglycoside[a]
Age 1 mo–50 yr	Vancomycin plus cefotaxime or ceftriaxone[b]
Age older than 50 yr	Vancomycin plus ampicillin plus ceftriaxone or cefotaxime plus vancomycin[b]
Impaired cellular immunity	Vancomycin plus ampicillin plus either cefepime or meropenem
Recurrent meningitis	Vancomycin plus cefotaxime or ceftriaxone
Basilar skull fracture	Vancomycin plus cefotaxime or ceftriaxone
Head trauma, neurosurgery, or CSF shunt	Vancomycin plus ceftazidime, cefepime, or meropenem

[a]Usually gentamycin 50 to 100 mg/kg.
[b]Add ampicillin if Listeria monocytogenes is a suspected pathogen.
CSF, cerebrospinal fluid.
From van de Beek D, Brouwer MC, Thwaites GE, et al. Advances in treatment of bacterial meningitis. Lancet. 2012;380(9854):1693–1702.

TABLE 61.3	Dosing of Empiric Antibiotics for Acute Bacterial Meningitis
Medication	**Dosing**
Pediatric Dosing[a]	
Cefotaxime	50 mg/kg IV every 6 h up to 12 g/day
Ceftriaxone	75 mg/kg initially, then 50 mg/kg every 12 h, up to 4 g/day
Vancomycin	15 mg/kg IV every 8 h
Ampicillin	50 mg/kg IV every 6 h
Penicillin G	250,000 to 400,000 U/kg/day in four to six divided doses
Gentamycin	2.5 mg/kg IV every 8 h
Adult Dosing	
Cefotaxime	2 g IV every 4 h
Ceftriaxone	2 g IV every 12 h
Cefepime	2 g every 8 h
Vancomycin	750–1,000 mg IV every 12 h or 10–15 mg/kg IV every 12 h
Ampicillin	2 g IV every 4–6 h
Penicillin G	4 million units IV every 4 h
Meropenem	2 g IV every 8 h

[a]Older than 1 month of age.
IV, intravenous.

Dehydration is common in this condition, and fluid balance should be monitored carefully to avoid hypovolemic shock. Hyponatremia frequently occurs and may be caused either by overzealous free-water replacement, cerebral salt wasting, or inappropriate antidiuretic hormone (ADH) secretion. Heparinization should be considered if disseminated intravascular coagulation occurs. Anticonvulsants should be used to control recurrent seizures. Cerebral edema may require the use of osmotic diuretics, corticosteroids, and hyperventilation.

Meningococcus can be highly contagious and is spread by droplets. Persons who have had intimate contact with patients with acute meningococcal meningitis should be given oral (PO) rifampin (children: 20 mg/kg/day; adults: 600 mg/day) as a prophylactic measure.

Outcome

The mortality rate of meningococcal meningitis has historically ranged 50% to 90%. With present-day therapy, however, the overall mortality rate is about 10%, and the incidence of complications and sequelae is low. Features of the disease that influence the mortality rate are the age of the patient, bacteremia, rapidity of treatment, complications, and general condition of the individual. The lowest fatality rates are seen in patients aged between 5 and 10 years. The highest mortality rates occur in infants, in elderly, in debilitated individuals, and in those with extensive hemorrhages into the adrenal gland.

PNEUMOCOCCAL MENINGITIS

Pneumococcus (S. pneumoniae) is about twice as frequent as the meningococcus as a cause of meningitis.

Epidemiology

S. pneumoniae accounts for about 50% of all bacterial meningitis. The infection may occur at any age, but more than 50% of the patients are younger than 1 year or older than 50 years. The frequency should begin to decline with vaccination of children between 2 and 23 months of age and the elderly. Clinical symptoms, physical signs, and laboratory findings in pneumococcal meningitis are similar to those in other forms of acute purulent meningitis.

Pathobiology

Meningeal infection is usually a complication of infections of the lungs, otitis media, mastoiditis, sinusitis, fractures of the skull, CSF fistulas, and upper respiratory infections. Alcoholism, surgical or functional asplenism, sickle cell disease, and cochlear implants predispose patients to developing pneumococcal meningitis.

Diagnosis

Diagnosis is usually made without difficulty because the CSF contains many organisms. Gram-positive diplococci are seen in smears of the CSF or its sediment and identified in CSF and blood cultures.

Treatment

The prevalence of penicillin- and cephalosporin-resistant *S. pneumoniae* has made a third- or fourth-generation cephalosporin plus vancomycin the initial treatment for *S. pneumoniae* meningitis until sensitivities are known (see Table 61.2). Treatment should be continued for 2 weeks. The use of corticosteroids, especially dexamethasone 6 mg every 6 hours, for the first 4 days of illness, started before antibiotics, significantly decreases mortality, hearing loss, and morbidity in adults from high-income countries [**Level 1**].[1] Any primary focus of infection should be eradicated by surgery if necessary. Persistent CSF fistulas after fractures of the skull must be closed by craniotomy and suturing of the dura. Otherwise, the meningitis will almost certainly recur.

Outcome

Before the introduction of sulfonamide antibiotics, the mortality rate in pneumococcal meningitis was almost 100%. It is now approximately 20% to 25%. The prognosis for recovery is best in cases that follow fractures of the skull and those with no known source of infection. About 30% of survivors have permanent sequelae. The mortality rate is especially high when the meningitis follows pneumonia, empyema, or lung abscess or when a persisting bacteremia indicates the presence of an endocarditis. The triad syndrome of pneumococcal meningitis, pneumonia, and endocarditis (Austrian syndrome) has a particularly high fatality rate.

HAEMOPHILUS INFLUENZAE MENINGITIS

Infections of the meninges by *H. influenzae* were historically a disease of infants and children until the introduction of the *H. influenzae* vaccine. Now, meningitis due to *H. influenzae* is more common in adults.

Epidemiology

In the United States and other countries where *H. influenzae* type B vaccination is widespread, the incidence of meningitis due to this organism in children is now negligible. It remains an important disease elsewhere, however. Where the vaccine is not available, *H. influenzae* meningitis is predominantly a disease of infancy and early childhood; more than 50% of the cases occur within the first 2 years of life and 90% before the age of 5 years. In the United States, *H. influenzae* meningitis is now more common in adults.

Pathobiology

In adults, *H. influenzae* meningitis is more commonly secondary to acute sinusitis, otitis media, or fracture of the skull. It is associated with CSF rhinorrhea, immunologic deficiency, diabetes mellitus, and alcoholism. Currently, cases tend to occur in the autumn and spring, with fewest occurring in the summer months. The pathology of *H. influenzae* meningitis does not differ from that of other forms of acute purulent meningitis. In patients with a protracted course, localized pockets of infection in the meninges or cortex, hydrocephalus, cranial nerve palsies, and cerebrovascular complications may occur.

Clinical Features

The symptoms and signs of *H. influenzae* meningitis are similar to those of other forms of acute bacterial meningitis.

Diagnosis

The CSF abnormalities are similar to those described for the other acute meningitides. The organisms may be identified by Gram stain and cultured from the CSF. Blood cultures are often positive early in the illness.

Treatment

Because of resistance to ampicillin, third- or fourth-generation cephalosporins are used in initial therapy of *H. influenzae* meningitis and are effective. Further treatment can be directed by culture and sensitivities. A total duration of 7 days of treatment is usually sufficient. Recent studies have indicated that treatment with dexamethasone (6 mg every 6 hours, for the first 4 days of illness, started before antibiotics) may reduce the frequency of sequelae, including hearing loss and morbidity [**Level 1**].[1]

Outcome

Antibiotic treatment has reduced the mortality rate to less than 10%, but sequelae are not uncommon. These include paralysis of extraocular muscles, deafness, blindness, hemiplegia, recurrent convulsions, and cognitive impairment. Subdural effusion, which may occur in infants with any form of meningitis, is most commonly seen with *H. influenzae* meningitis. These typically resolve without therapy.

STAPHYLOCOCCAL MENINGITIS

Staphylococci (*Staphylococcus aureus* and coagulase-negative staphylococci) are a relatively infrequent cause of meningitis. Meningitis may develop as a result of spread from furuncles on the face or from staphylococcal infections elsewhere in the body. Staphylococcal meningitis can be a complication of endocarditis, epidural or subdural abscess, and neurosurgical procedures involving shunting to relieve hydrocephalus. Intravenous treatment with either penicillinase-resistant penicillin (nafcillin) or vancomycin is the preferred treatment. Complications, such as ventriculitis, arachnoiditis, and hydrocephalus, may occur. The original focus of infection should be eradicated. Laminectomy should be performed immediately when a spinal epidural abscess is present, and a cranial subdural abscess should be drained through craniotomy openings.

STREPTOCOCCAL MENINGITIS

Infection with streptococcal strains other than *S. pneumoniae* account for less than 5% of all cases of meningitis. The symptoms are the same as for other forms of meningitis. Treatment is the same as outlined for the treatment of pneumococcal meningitis together with surgical eradication of the primary focus.

LISTERIA MONOCYTOGENES

Meningitis caused by *Listeria monocytogenes* occurs in the elderly, infants, or adults with chronic diseases (e.g., renal disease with dialysis or transplantation, cancer, connective tissue disorders, chronic alcoholism). It may occur, however, without any predisposing factor, and the incidence of such cases appears to be increasing. *L. monocytogenes* is a gram-positive, facultative anaerobic bacterium. The primary disease processes to which it is associated are sepsis and meningitis.

Epidemiology

The estimated incidence is 0.2 cases per 100,000 adults per year in developed countries. The highest incidence occurs in neonates and adults older than 60 years of age. *Listeria* is the third most frequent cause of community-acquired bacterial meningitis after *S. pneumoniae* and *N. meningitidis*.

Pathobiology

Listeriosis, both sporadic and epidemic, is primarily food-borne disease. Milk products have historically been associated with *Listeria*; however, the contamination is not just associated with dairy. There have been reports of vegetable, meat, and cold cuts. Additionally, it is reported in as many as 3% of hospital-acquired meningitis.

Clinical Manifestations

Symptoms and signs of patients presenting with *L. monocytogenes* meningitis are not significantly different from those found in the general population of patients with community-acquired bacterial meningitis. In a prospective study of patients with *L. monocytogenes* meningitis, the prevalence of the classic triad of fever, neck stiffness, and altered mental status was 43%, and almost all patients presented with at least two of the four classic symptoms of headache, fever, neck stiffness, and altered mental status. Similar presentations have been reported in other types of community-acquired bacterial meningitis. The disease, however, can be more subacute than other causes of bacterial meningitis, with a large proportion of patients having days of symptoms prior to presentation. Occasionally, *L. monocytogenes* meningitis occurs with prominent brain stem findings (rhombencephalitis).

Diagnosis

Diagnostic workup of listeria meningitis should include a CSF examination. A higher number of patients will have atypical CSF findings (normal in up to 25%) than other types of bacterial meningitis, although the majority will still have an elevated CSF white blood cell count, elevated protein, and low glucose. Gram stain of the CSF is typically negative, although a laboratory report of "diphtheroids" seen on Gram stain can occur. Blood cultures for *L. monocytogenes* are positive in up to half of the cases of meningitis. A high number of patients develop hyponatremia.

Treatment

Ampicillin is the drug of choice for *L. monocytogenes* because the bacterium is resistant to cephalosporins. If *Listeria* is considered a reasonable possibility, ampicillin 2 g IV q4 to 6 hours should be added to the initial therapy (see Table 61.3 for empiric antibiotic regimens and dosing). Trimethoprim/sulfisoxazole 10 to 20 mg/kg daily divided q6 to 12 hours is an acceptable alternative. Because most cases occur in patients with an already abnormal immune system, corticosteroids should probably not be used as adjunctive therapy.

Outcome

Even with appropriate antibiotic therapy, listeria meningitis has one of the highest mortalities of all causes of community-acquired bacterial meningitis ranging from 30% to 40%. Neurologic sequelae occur in approximately 15% of survivors.

ACUTE MENINGITIS CAUSED BY OTHER BACTERIA

Meningitis in the newborn infant is most often caused by group B β-hemolytic streptococci. Coliform gram-negative bacilli especially *E. coli* are also common. Meningitis due to these organisms often accompanies septicemia. The infant shows irritability, lethargy, anorexia, and bulging fontanelles. Meningitis caused by gram-negative enteric bacteria also occurs in immunosuppressed or chronically ill, hospitalized adult patients, and in persons with penetrating head injuries, neurosurgical procedures, congenital defects, or diabetes mellitus. In these circumstances, meningitis may be difficult to recognize because of altered consciousness related to the underlying illness.

A third- or fourth-generation cephalosporin is typically used for treatment of gram-negative meningitis. If *Pseudomonas aeruginosa* is present or suspected, ceftazidime or meropenem is preferred. Care also must be taken to ensure that the organism is sensitive to the agents chosen.

ACUTE PURULENT MENINGITIS OF UNKNOWN CAUSE

Patients may have clinical symptoms indicative of an acute purulent meningitis but with atypical CSF findings. These patients have usually manifested nonspecific symptoms and have often been treated for several days with some form of antimicrobial therapy in dosages sufficient to modify the CSF abnormalities but not sufficient to eradicate the infection. In these cases, the CSF pleocytosis is usually only moderate (500 to 1,000 cells/mm^3 with predominance of polymorphonuclear leukocytes), and the glucose concentration is normal or only slightly decreased. Organisms are not seen on stained smears and are cultured with difficulty. Repeated lumbar puncture may be helpful in arriving at the correct diagnosis. CSF polymerase chain reaction (PCR) tests may identify the organism when cultures are negative.

Antibiotics should be selected on the basis of epidemiologic or clinical factors. The age of the patient and the setting in which the infection occurred are the primary considerations. In patients with partially treated meningitis and in those with meningitis of unknown etiology, third- or fourth-generation cephalosporins and vancomycin are the antibiotics of choice for initial therapy. Ampicillin should be added in neonates or if *L. monocytogenes* is a possibility. Therapy should be modified based on antimicrobial sensitivity testing. The mortality and frequency of neurologic complications of these patients are similar to those of patients in whom the responsible bacteria have been identified.

RECURRENT BACTERIAL MENINGITIS

Repeated episodes of bacterial meningitis signal a host defect, either in local anatomy or in antibacterial and immunologic defenses. Recurrent bacterial meningitis usually follows trauma; several years may pass between the trauma and the first bout of meningitis. *S. pneumoniae* is the most common pathogen accounting for about a third of cases. Bacteria may enter the subarachnoid space through the cribriform plate, a basilar skull fracture, erosive bony changes in the mastoid, congenital dermal defects along the craniospinal axis, penetrating head injuries, or neurosurgical procedures. CSF rhinorrhea or otorrhea is often present but may be transient. It may be detected by testing for a significant concentration of glucose in nasal or aural secretions. Cryptic CSF leaks may be demonstrated by monitoring the course of radioiodine-labeled albumin instilled intrathecally or by CT after intrathecal injection of water-soluble contrast material.

Treatment of culture-documented recurrent meningitis is similar to that for first bouts. Patients with recurrent pneumococcal meningitis should be vaccinated with pneumococcal vaccine. Surgical closure of CSF fistulas is indicated to prevent further episodes of meningitis.

ENDOCARDITIS AND SEPTIC EMBOLISM

Infective endocarditis (IE) is a systemic disease with a multitude of manifestations. Of these, perhaps none is more devastating than the effects on the brain. Cerebrovascular complications have been reported to occur in 25% to 80% in the case of IE, although most studies hover around 30%.

EPIDEMIOLOGY

The etiology of IE has changed remarkably in the antibiotic era. Rheumatic heart disease now accounts for fewer than 25% of cases, whereas it once accounted for nearly 75%. At the present time, endocarditis is secondary to prosthetic valves, intravenous drug use, and degenerative cardiac disease related to aging. Congenital heart abnormalities remain an important cause, especially in children. Unfortunately, morbidity and mortality rates have not been affected much by these etiologic changes and the use of antibiotics, thus probably reflecting more severe infections at the present time. In the past, the terms *acute* or *subacute* were used to describe IE. These subdivisions, however, are artificial; the underlying cause of the endocarditis and the specific organism involved are more useful considerations when determining prognosis and treatment.

PATHOBIOLOGY

S. aureus and viridans streptococci are the most common causative organisms of endocarditis and its associated cerebrovascular complications.

CLINICAL MANIFESTATIONS

Neurologic complications of IE are important because of their frequency and severity. They may be the first manifestation of the underlying intracardiac infection. *Cerebral infarcts*, either bland, or less often hemorrhagic are most common. Infarcts of cranial or peripheral nerves and of the spinal cord rarely occur. *Intracranial hemorrhages* caused by focal segmental infectious vasculitis, mycotic aneurysms, or, rarely, brain abscess also are frequent. These complications presumably result from emboli of infective material from the heart. Inflammatory arteritis also has been implicated as a cause particularly of intracranial hemorrhage when no mycotic aneurysm is apparent. An encephalopathy, sometimes with prominent psychiatric features, may occur and may be related to microemboli with or without microabscess formation, vasculitis, toxic effects of medications, or metabolic abnormalities associated with the illness occurring either individually or concurrently. Seizures may occur in association with any of the cerebral complications.

IE always should be considered in sudden neurologic vascular events, particularly when known predisposing factors exist, such as cardiac disease, intravenous drug use, fever, or infection elsewhere in the body. The frequency of neurologic events is between 20% and 40% in most reported series of endocarditis. As might be anticipated, neurologic complications are more frequent in endocarditis that affects the left side of the heart. The type of organism is also important in determining the frequency of neurologic events. *S. aureus* in particular is associated with a high risk of nervous system complications.

DIAGNOSIS

The identification of the infecting organism of endocarditis is made by blood cultures. Always draw at least two sets of blood cultures. Two sets of blood cultures have greater than 90% sensitivity when bacteremia is present. Three sets of cultures improve sensitivity and may be useful when antibiotics have been administered previously. For diagnosing subacute IE, draw at least three sets of blood cultures over 24 hours. This can detect up to 98% of cases in patients who have not recently received antibiotics. In the case of acute IE, three sets may be drawn over 30 minutes (with separate blood draws). Transthoracic echo is a good screening tool for identifying a cardiac vegetation. Sensitivity is even greater with transesophageal echocardiography. Evidence suggests that the diagnosis and treatment regimen are changed in about 15% of cases when a transesophageal echo is used.

Diagnostic evaluation of neurologic events depends in part on whether the presence of IE already has been established. Imaging studies are important to define the nature of lesions that have focal neurologic findings. Differentiation of infarcts from hemorrhages or abscesses may be accomplished by either computed tomography (CT) or magnetic resonance imaging (MRI). On occasion, both techniques may be necessary to clearly define the nature of the lesion. Analysis of the CSF is mandatory in cases of meningitis regardless of whether the diagnosis of IE has already been made. Such analysis also is useful in encephalopathic conditions to evaluate for low-grade meningitic infection. Lumbar puncture should be considered strongly when stroke is associated with fever, even if endocarditis is not yet documented. Lumbar puncture is probably not useful in known cases of IE with focal CNS presentations where a clearly defined lesion has been identified with imaging studies. Demonstration of suspected mycotic aneurysms may be made by arteriography, magnetic resonance angiography (MRA) or CT angiography. However, some practitioners have advocated arteriography in all cases of IE. No controlled studies have been done. In a retrospective analysis, hemorrhage was less likely to occur if surgery was postponed until MRI contrast enhancement around small hemorrhage, microbleeds, or small infarcts had resolved.

TREATMENT

Management of the neurologic complications of IE includes early antibiotic therapy directed empirically at the appropriate organism and then focused once the organism has been identified and sensitivities documented. Early diagnosis and antibiotic treatment does help reduce neurologic sequela. Although there are no randomized trials investigating the role of thrombolysis, heparin anticoagulation, or antiplatelet agents in acute ischemic stroke secondary to IE, case series suggest that there is a high risk of hemorrhagic conversion when using these agents. Prolonged antibiotic treatment is required, and surgical replacement of infected valves may be necessary. Brain abscesses that do not resolve rapidly with systemic antibiotics should be aspirated. Mycotic aneurysms are typically managed by endovascular therapy, such as coiling and embolization.

SEPSIS-ASSOCIATED ENCEPHALOPATHY

Sepsis-associated encephalopathy (SAE) or septic encephalopathy is broadly described as the alteration in level of consciousness that is frequently seen in association with sepsis and systemic inflammatory response syndrome (SIRS). Sepsis is broadly defined as an infection with the addition of SIRS. The criteria for SIRS include increased or decreased body temperature ($>38°C$ or $<36°C$), tachycardia (>90 beats per minute), tachypnea (respiratory rate >20 breaths per min or an arterial partial pressure of carbon dioxide <32 mm Hg), and abnormally low or high white blood cell count ($>12,000$ or $<4,000$ cells/μL). The diagnosis of SAE is essentially a diagnosis of exclusion. It is not attributed to medications, direct CNS injury or infection, hepatic or renal encephalopathy, seizures, and not directly attributed to infection (i.e., not from septic emboli). SAE presents with altered mental status and without focal neurologic deficits. There can be mild delirium to coma and it frequently precedes diagnosis of sepsis by 24 to 48 hours.

The incidence of SAE is difficult to ascertain, as it is a diagnosis of exclusion. There are no diagnostic tests and most studies are retrospective. Sepsis and SIRS are common; it is estimated that there are over 1 million cases per year in the United States or 50 to 100 cases per 100,000. It is estimated that over 50% of septic patients are delirious, with SAE as the single most likely cause of delirium in the intensive care unit (ICU). Additionally, delirious patients in the ICU have a higher mortality than those without mental status changes. Of those septic patients developing SAE, their mortality is also significantly higher than those who do not develop SAE (56% vs. 35%).

There are numerous proposed mechanisms for the development of SAE. These include the release of inflammatory cytokines, damage to the blood–brain barrier, development of microscopic brain injury and altered cerebral metabolism, microcirculation, and neurotransmitters. Treatment of SAE mostly involves stopping or eliminating confounders that may be contributing to the encephalopathy and treating the sepsis and organ failure. Withdrawal of sedative medications (particularly benzodiazepines) is crucial. Dexmedetomidine may be useful adjunct to decrease encephalopathy, ventilator days, and duration of ICU stay in patients with septic encephalopathy [**Level 1**].[2]

ASEPTIC MENINGEAL REACTION

Aseptic meningeal reaction refers to those cases with evidence of a meningeal reaction in the CSF in the absence of any infecting organism. These conditions are discussed in this chapter because the main differential diagnosis is bacterial meningitis.

Aseptic or noninfectious meningeal inflammation results from four general causes: (1) in reaction to a parameningeal focus of infection or necrosis focus within the skull or spinal canal, (2) introduction of foreign substances (e.g., air, dyes, drugs, blood) into the subarachnoid space, (3) connective tissue disorders, and (4) systemically administered medications (e.g., trimethoprim/sulfoxazole, nonsteroidal anti-inflammatory agents, intravenous immunoglobulin (IVIG), isoniazid, carbamazepine, OKT3 monoclonal antibodies).

The symptoms present in the patients in the first group are associated with the infection or morbid process in the skull or spinal cavity. Only occasionally are there any symptoms and signs of meningeal irritation.

In the second group of patients, where the meningeal reaction is the result of the introduction of foreign substances into the subarachnoid space, fever, headache, and stiffness of the neck may occur. The appearance of these symptoms leads to the suspicion that an actual infection of the meninges has been produced by the inadvertent introduction of pathogenic organisms. The normal glucose concentration of the CSF and the absence of organisms in culture establish the nature of the meningeal reaction.

An aseptic meningeal reaction may complicate the course of systemic lupus erythematosus (SLE) and other collagen-vascular diseases. In certain instances, the meningeal reaction in patients with SLE may be induced by nonsteroidal anti-inflammatory drugs or azathioprine.

The findings in the CSF characteristic of an aseptic meningeal reaction are an increase in pressure, a varying degree of pleocytosis (10 to 4,000 cells/mm^3), a slight or moderate increase in the protein concentration, normal glucose concentration, and the absence of organisms in culture. Exceptionally, and without explanation, the aseptic meningeal reaction of SLE may be accompanied by low CSF glucose concentrations. With a severe degree of meningeal reaction, the CSF may be purulent in appearance and may contain several thousand cells per cubic millimeter with a predominance of polymorphonuclear leukocytes. With a lesser degree of meningeal reaction, the CSF may be normal in appearance or only slightly cloudy and may contain a moderate number of cells (10 to several hundred cells per cubic millimeter), with lymphocytes being the predominating cell type in the CSF.

The pathogenesis of the changes in the CSF is not clearly understood. The septic foci in the head, more commonly associated with an aseptic meningeal reaction, are septic thrombosis of the intracranial venous sinuses; osteomyelitis of the spine or skull; extradural, subdural, or intracerebral abscesses; or septic cerebral emboli. Nonseptic foci of necrosis are accompanied only rarely by an aseptic meningeal reaction. Occasionally, patients with an intracerebral tumor or cerebral hemorrhage located near the ventricular walls may show similar changes in the CSF.

The diagnosis of an aseptic meningeal reaction in patients with a septic or necrotic focus in the skull or spinal cord is important in that it directs attention to the presence of this focus and the necessity for appropriate surgical and medical therapy before the meninges are actually invaded by the infectious process or before other cerebral or spinal complications develop.

LEVEL 1 EVIDENCE

1. Brouwer MC, McIntyre P, Prasad K, et al. Corticosteroids for acute bacterial meningitis. *Cochrane Database Syst Rev*. 2013;6: CD004405. doi:10.1002/14651858.CD004405.pub4.

2. Pandharipande PP, Pun BT, Herr DL, et al. Effect of sedation with dexmedetomidine vs lorazepam on acute brain dysfunction in mechanically ventilated patients: the MENDS randomized controlled trial. *JAMA.* 2007;298(22):2644–2653.

SUGGESTED READINGS

Acute Bacterial Meningitis

Amaya-Villar R, García-Cabrera E, Sulleiro-Igual E, et al. Three-year multicenter surveillance of community-acquired *Listeria monocytogenes* meningitis in adults. *BMC Infect Dis.* 2010;10:324.

Brouwer MC, Tunkel AR, van de Beek D. Epidemiology, diagnosis, and antimicrobial treatment of acute bacterial meningitis. *Clin Microbiol Rev.* 2010; 23(3):467–492.

Brouwer MC, van de Beek D, Heckenberg SG, et al. Community-acquired *Listeria monocytogenes* meningitis in adults. *Clin Infect Dis.* 2006;43(10): 1233–1238.

Durand ML, Calderwood SB, Weber DJ, et al. Acute bacterial meningitis in adults: a review of 493 episodes. *N Engl J Med.* 1993;328:21–28.

Erdem H, Elaldi N, Oztoprak N, et al. Mortality indicators in pneumococcal meningitis: therapeutic implications. *Int J Infect Dis.* 2014;19:13–19.

Lai WA, Chen SF, Tsai NW, et al. Non-cephalosporin-susceptible, glucose nonfermentative Gram-negative bacilli meningitis in post-neurosurgical adults: clinical characteristics and therapeutic outcome. *Clin Neurol Neurosurg.* 2014;116:61–66.

Lorber B. *Listeria monocytogenes.* In: Mandell GL, Bennet JE, Dolin R, eds. *Principles and Practice of Infectious Diseases.* Philadelphia: Churchill Livingstone; 2005:2478–2484.

Mylonakis E, Hohmann EL, Calderwood SB. Central nervous system infection with *Listeria monocytogenes.* 33 years' experience at a general hospital and review of 776 episodes from the literature. *Medicine (Baltimore).* 1998;77(5): 313–336.

Pintado V, Pazos R, Jimenez-Mejias ME, et al. Methicillin-resistant *Staphylococcus aureus* meningitis in adults: a multicenter study of 86 cases. *Medicine.* 2012; 91(1):10–17.

Pomar V, Benito N, Lopez-Contreras J, et al. Spontaneous gram-negative bacillary meningitis in adult patients: characteristics and outcome. *BMC Infect Dis.* 2013;13:451.

Prouox N, Frechette D, Toye B, et al. Delays in the administration of antibiotics are associated with mortality from adult acute bacterial meningitis. *QJM.* 2005;98:291–198.

Stockmann C, Ampofo K, Byington CL, et al. Pneumococcal meningitis in children: epidemiology, serotypes, and outcomes from 1997–2010 in Utah. *Pediatrics.* 2013;132(3):421–428.

Tacon CL, Flower O. Diagnosis and management of bacterial meningitis in the paediatric population: a review. *Emerg Med Int.* 2012;2012:320309.

Thigpen MC, Whitney CG, Messonnier NE, et al. Bacterial meningitis in the United States, 1998–2007. *N Engl J Med.* 2011;364(21):2016–2025.

Tunkel AR, Hartman BJ, Kaplan SJ, et al. Practice guidelines for the management of bacterial meningitis. *Clin Infect Dis.* 2004;39:1267–1284.

van de Beek D, Brouwer MC, Thwaites GE, et al. Advances in treatment of bacterial meningitis. *Lancet.* 2012;380(9854):1693–1702.

van de Beek D, de Gans J, Spanjaard L, et al. Clinical features and prognostic factors in adults with bacterial meningitis. *N Engl J Med.* 2004;35:1849–1859.

van de Beek D, de Gans J, Tunkel AR, et al. Community acquired bacterial meningitis in adults. *N Engl J Med.* 2006;354:44–53.

van de Beek D, Drake JM, Tunkel AR. Nosocomial bacterial meningitis. *N Engl J Med.* 2010;362(2):146–154.

van de Beek D, Farrar JJ, de Gans J, et al. Adjunctive dexamethasone in bacterial meningitis: a meta-analysis of individual patient data. *Lancet Neurol.* 2010;9(3):254–263.

Weisfelt M, de Gans J, van de Beek D. Bacterial meningitis: a review of effective pharmacotherapy. *Expert Opin Pharmacother.* 2007;8:1493–1504.

Weisfelt M, van de Beek D, Spanjaard L, et al. Clinical features, complications, and outcomes in adults with pneumococcal meningitis: a prospective case series. *Lancet Neurol.* 2006;5:123–129.

Infective Endocarditis

Brust J, Dickinson P, Hughes J, et al. The diagnosis and treatment of cerebral mycotic aneurysms. *Ann Neurol.* 1990;27:238–246.

Calza L, Manfredi R, Chiodo F. Infective endocarditis: a review of the best treatment options. *Expert Opin Pharmacother.* 2004;5:1899–1916.

Chapot R, Houdart E, Saint-Maurice JP, et al. Endovascular treatment of cerebral mycotic aneurysms. *Radiology.* 2002;222(2):389–396.

Giulieri S, Meuli RA, Cavassini M. Complications of infective endocarditis. In: Scheld WM, Whitley RJ, Marra CM, eds. *Infections of the Central Nervous System.* 4th ed. Philadelphia: Lippincott Williams & Wilkins; 2014: 579–607.

Gregoratos G. Infective endocarditis in the elderly: diagnosis and management. *Am J Geriatr Cardiol.* 2003;12:183–189.

Kang DH, Kim YJ, Kim SH, et al. Early surgery versus conventional treatment for infective endocarditis. *N Engl J Med.* 2012;366(26):2466–2473.

Kannoth S, Thomas SV. Intracranial microbial aneurysm (infectious aneurysm): current options for diagnosis and management. *Neurocrit Care.* 2009;11(1): 120–129.

Kin H, Yoshioka K, Kawazoe K, et al. Management of infectious endocarditis with mycotic aneurysm evaluated by brain magnetic resonance imaging. *Eur J Cardiothorac Surg.* 2013;44(5):924–930.

Lee M-R, Chnagw S-A, Choi S-H, et al. Clinical features of right-sided infective endocarditis occurings in non-drug users. *J Korean Med Sci.* 2014;29: 776–781.

Lee SJ, Oh SS, Lim DS, et al. Clinical significance of cerebrovascular complications in patients with acute infective endocarditis: a retrospective analysis of a 12-year single-center experience. *BMC Neurol.* 2014;14:30.

Morris NA, Matiello M, Lyons JL, et al. Neurologic complications in infective endocarditis: identification, management, and impact on cardiac surgery. *Neurohospitalist.* 2014;4(4):213–222.

Mourvillier B, Trouillet JL, Timsit JF, et al. Infective endocarditis in the intensive care unit: clinical spectrum and prognostic factors in 228 consecutive patients. *Intensive Care Med.* 2004;30(11):2046–2052.

Prendergast BD. Diagnostic criteria and problems in infective endocarditis. *Heart (British Cardiac Society).* 2004;90(6):611–613.

Rizzi M, Ravasio V, Carobbio A, et al; Investigators of the Italian Study on Endocarditis. Predicting the occurrence of embolic events: an analysis of 1456 episodes of infective endocarditis from the Italian Study on Endocarditis (SEI). *BMC Infect Dis.* 2014;14:230.

Tunkel AR, Pradhan SK. Central nervous system infections in injection drug users. *Infect Dis Clin North Am.* 2002;16:589–605.

Valencia E, Miro J. Endocarditis in the setting of HIV infection. *Mayo Clin Proc.* 2004;79(5):682–686.

Walker KA, Sampson JB, Skalabrin EJ, et al. Clinical characteristics and thrombolytic outcomes of infective endocarditis-associated stroke. *Neurohospitalist.* 2012;2(3):87–91.

Septic Encephalopathy

Gofton TE, Young GB. Sepsis-associated encephalopathy. *Nat Rev Neurol.* 2012; 8(10):557–566.

Martin GS. Sepsis, severe sepsis and septic shock: changes in incidence, pathogens and outcomes. *Expert Rev Anti Infect Ther.* 2012;10(6):701–706.

Zhang LN, Wang XT, Ai YH, et al. Epidemiological features and risk factors of sepsis-associated encephalopathy in intensive care unit patients: 2008–2011. *Chin Med J (Engl).* 2012;125(5):828–831.

Aseptic Meningeal Reaction

Alexander EL, Alexander GE. Aseptic meningoencephalitis in primary Sjögren's syndrome. *Neurology.* 1983;33:593–598.

Canoso JJ, Cohen AS. Aseptic meningitis in systemic lupus erythematosus. *Arthritis Rheum.* 1975;18:369–374.

Kampylafka EI, Alexopoulos H, Kosmidis ML, et al. Incidence and prevalence of major central nervous system involvement in systemic lupus erythematosus: a 3-year prospective study of 370 patients. *PloS One.* 2013;8(2):e55843.

Repplinger MD, Falk PM. Trimethoprim-sulfamethoxazole-induced aseptic meningitis. *Am J Emerg Med.* 2011;29(2):242.e3–e5.

Roos KL. Mycobacterium tuberculosis meningitis and other etiologies of the aseptic meningitis syndrome. *Semin Neurol.* 2000;20:329–335.

Gary L. Bernardini

BRAIN ABSCESS

A brain abscess is a focal purulent infection within the brain parenchyma. A brain abscess starts as a localized area of cerebritis; abscesses vary in size from a microscopic collection of inflammatory cells to an area of purulent necrosis presenting as a mass lesion.

Advances in the diagnosis and treatment of brain abscesses have been achieved with the use of computed tomography (CT), magnetic resonance imaging (MRI), magnetic resonance spectroscopy (MRS), stereotactic brain biopsy and aspiration, and newer broad-spectrum antibiotics.

EPIDEMIOLOGY

A brain abscess is two to three times more common in males than in females, with the highest morbidity in fourth decade of life. Over the past 30 years, advances in management of brain abscesses have resulted in a significant decline in mortality from 30% to 50% before 1980, to 4% to 20% today. Up to 25% of all cases occur in children younger than 15 years old, with a cluster in the 4- to 7-year-old age group, usually the result of cyanotic congenital heart disease or an otic infection.

ETIOLOGY

A brain abscess is classified based on the likely source of infection. A brain abscess may develop from any of the following predisposing or associated conditions: (1) direct extension of cranial infection, ethmoid or frontal sinusitis, subacute or chronic otitis media, or mastoiditis; (2) hematogenous dissemination of infection from elsewhere in the body (e.g., lung abscess, bacterial endocarditis, intra-abdominal infections, dental infections, congenital heart disease); and (3) direct inoculation via wounds, fracture of the skull, or neurosurgical procedures.

Infection in the middle ear or mastoid may spread to the cerebellum or temporal lobe through involvement of bone and meninges or by seeding of bacteria through valveless emissary and sinus veins that drain these regions. Infection may originate from tonsils or abscessed teeth, or frontal, ethmoid, or rarely the maxillary sinuses, with sinus infections often spreading to frontal lobes through erosion of the skull.

For hematogenous spread, cerebral lesions are found in distal territories of the middle cerebral artery and frequently are multiple, often seen at the junction of gray-white matter. Potential sources for hematogenous spread of infection include upper respiratory tract (lung abscess or empyema), bacterial endocarditis, skin infections, intra-abdominal, or pelvic infections. Twenty percent to 30% of brain abscesses have no obvious source, and are so-called cryptogenic brain abscesses. In some cases, cryptogenic brain abscess may have a cardiac or lung source. For example, congenital cardiac defects and pulmonary arteriovenous malformations (e.g., hereditary hemorrhagic telangiectasia) predispose to brain abscess. In these two disorders, infected emboli bypass pulmonary filtration system and gain access to the cerebral arterial system. Similarly, cases of cryptogenic brain abscess caused by vegetations on patent foramen ovale (PFO) or right-to-left shunting via PFO have been reported. In infants and children, congenital heart disease is a common predisposing factor for brain abscess. The predisposing conditions of hereditary hemorrhagic telangiectasia or Rendu-Osler-Weber disease can be the source of a brain abscess via paradoxical septic emboli from lung.

A brain abscess can occur following penetrating head injury or neurosurgical procedures, although occurrence of abscesses after penetrating brain injury is low. In children, penetration of a lead pencil tip through the thin squamous portion of the temporal bone has resulted in abscess formation. Finally, brain abscess is almost never a consequence of bacterial meningitis, except in infants.

CAUSATIVE ORGANISMS OF BRAIN ABSCESS

The infecting organism may be any of the common pyogenic bacteria depending on the site of entry; the most common are *Staphylococcus aureus*, streptococci (anaerobic, aerobic, or microaerophilic species), *Enterobacteriaceae*, *Pseudomonas* spp., and anaerobes such as *Bacteroides* spp. (Table 62.1). In infants, gram-negative organisms are the most frequent isolates. In adult patients with direct spread of infection from an otogenic source, the most common organisms are streptococci, *Bacteroides* spp., *Pseudomonas* spp., *Enterobacteriaceae*, and *Haemophilus*. Other causative organisms from oral or hematogenous spread include streptococci, *S. aureus*, *Bacteroides* spp., and *Fusobacterium* spp. After penetrating head injury or neurosurgical procedure, abscess formation is usually due to *S. aureus* (methicillin-resistant *Staphylococcus aureus* or MRSA), *Staphylococcus epidermidis*, streptococci, *Enterobacteriaceae*, *Pseudomonas*, or *Clostridium* spp. Brain abscesses as a complication of bacterial endocarditis are due to streptococci, MRSA, and *Serratia marcescens*. In the immunocompromised host, *Toxoplasma*, *Listeria*, *Nocardia*, *Aspergillus*, *Cryptococcus*, *Coccidioidomycosis*, *Mycobacterium tuberculosis*, *Enterobacteriaceae*, and other fungal pathogens are causative organisms of brain abscess. Brain abscess may be due to a parasitic infection such as *Entamoeba histolytica*, cysticercosis, *Schistosoma*, or toxocariasis. Following liver transplantation, invasive pulmonary aspergillosis can be a source of brain abscesses. Cultures may be sterile in patients who have received antimicrobial therapy before biopsy but any material obtained should be sent to the laboratory. A positive Gram stain guides therapy even when the culture is negative. In a study of 90 patients with diagnosis of brain abscess, microbiologic diagnosis was obtained in 83% of cases. More than one pathogen was found in 23% of cases.

PATHOBIOLOGY

The pathologic changes in brain abscesses are similar regardless of the origin: direct extension to the brain from a contiguous site of infection, retrograde thrombosis of veins, or hematogenous dissemination (Fig. 62.1).

TABLE 62.1 Brain Abscess

Source	Pathogen
Oral cavity, hematogenous spread (intra-abdominal/pelvic infections), otitis, mastoiditis, paranasal sinusitis	Streptococci spp. (aerobic and anaerobic), *Staphylococcus aureus, Bacteroides* spp., *Pseudomonas* spp., *Haemophilus* spp., *Enterobacteriaceae, Prevotella melaninogenica, Fusobacterium*
Trauma/neurosurgical procedure	*Staphylococcus aureus* or *Staphylococcus epidermidis, Streptococcus* spp., *Enterobacteriaceae, Pseudomonas* spp., *Clostridium* spp.
Pyogenic lung infections	Streptococci, staphylococci, *Bacteroides* spp., *Fusobacterium* spp., *Enterobacteriaceae*
Cardiac origin (e.g., cyanotic heart disease, right-to-left shunts, bacterial endocarditis)	*Streptococcus* spp., *Serratia marcescens*, methicillin-resistant *Staphylococcus aureus* (MRSA)
Immunocompromised	*Pseudomonas, Toxoplasma, Listeria, Nocardia, Aspergillus, Cryptococcus, Coccidioides, Mycobacterium tuberculosis, Enterobacteriaceae*, other fungal pathogens
Parasitic infections	*Cysticercosis, Entamoeba histolytica, Schistosoma, Paragonimus*

Four stages of maturation of brain abscess are recognized: (1) within the first 3 days, suppurative inflammation of brain tissue is characterized by *early cerebritis*, appearing as either a patchy or nonenhancing hypodensity on CT or MRI; (2) *late cerebritis* (days 4 to 9) with an area of central necrosis, edema, and ring enhancement on CT and MRI; (3) *early capsule formation* (days 10 to 14); and (4) *final maturation* of the capsule, which takes about 2 weeks. When host defenses control the spread of the infection, macroglia and fibroblasts proliferate in an attempt to surround the infected and necrotic tissue, and granulation tissue and fibrous encapsulation develop. The developing capsule around the abscess formed by the inflammatory response is thicker on the cortical surface than on the ventricular side. If the capsule ruptures, purulent material is released into the ventricular system, a process associated with a high mortality rate. Edema surrounding a brain abscess is common.

Two signal-mediated CNS immune responses to invading pathogens that may be important in the developing abscess include the Toll-like and Nod-like receptors (TLR and NLR, respectively) systems. Activation of TLR by invading pathogens leads to a complex array of immune-mediated response including control of infection burden, immune infiltrates, and inflammatory mediators. Likewise, NLR activates a number of immune-specific interleukins responsible for bacterial recognition and subsequent cytokine release that acts to restrict bacterial spread during abscess formation.

CLINICAL MANIFESTATIONS

The symptoms of a brain abscess are typical of an expanding mass lesion in the brain with elevated intracranial pressure (ICP) and include headache with or without fever as the initial symptoms, followed by nausea, vomiting, lethargy, and focal neurologic deficits. Fever is present in approximately 50% of patients; however, the combination of fever and leukocytosis is present in over 50% cases of brain abscess. Sudden worsening of preexisting headache, new-onset nuchal rigidity, and seizures may herald rupture of brain

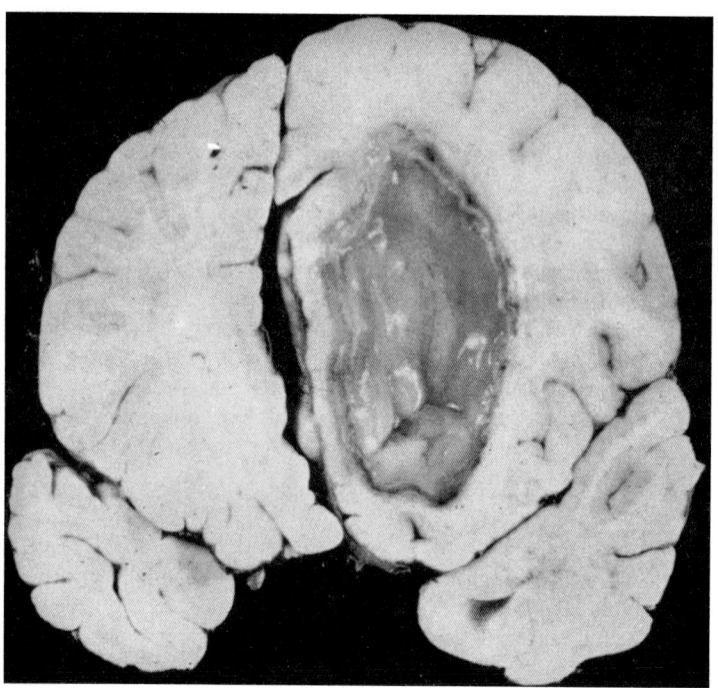

FIGURE 62.1 Brain abscess. Abscess in frontal lobe secondary to pulmonary infection. (Courtesy of Dr. Abner Wolf.)

abscess into the ventricular space. The abrupt onset of a severe headache is less common with abscess and is more often associated with acute bacterial meningitis or subarachnoid hemorrhage. Seizures, focal or generalized, are common with abscess.

Focal neurologic deficits develop in approximately 50% of patients, depending on abscess location. Hemiparesis, apathy, and confusion may be seen with lesions of the frontal lobe, hemianopia, and aphasia, particularly anomia, with abscesses in the temporal or parietooccipital lobes and ataxia, intention tremor, nystagmus, with cerebellar abscess (Fig. 62.2). The presence of papilledema and/or third or sixth cranial nerve palsies may be due to increased ICP.

Abscesses in the brain stem are rare. The classic findings of brain stem syndromes are often lacking because abscess tends to expand longitudinally along fiber tracts rather than transversely. Subdural or, rarely, epidural infections in the frontal regions may present with the same signs and symptoms as those of an abscess in the frontal lobe. Fever and focal seizures favor the diagnosis of subdural rather than intraparenchymal abscess, although these findings are not specific.

Transverse sinus thrombosis often follows middle ear or mastoid infection (see Fig. 62.2) and may be accompanied by seizures and signs of increased ICP, making the clinical differentiation between this condition and abscess of the temporal lobe or hemispheres difficult. With transverse sinus thrombosis, papilledema may result from blockage of venous drainage from the brain. Focal neurologic signs favor the diagnosis of abscess.

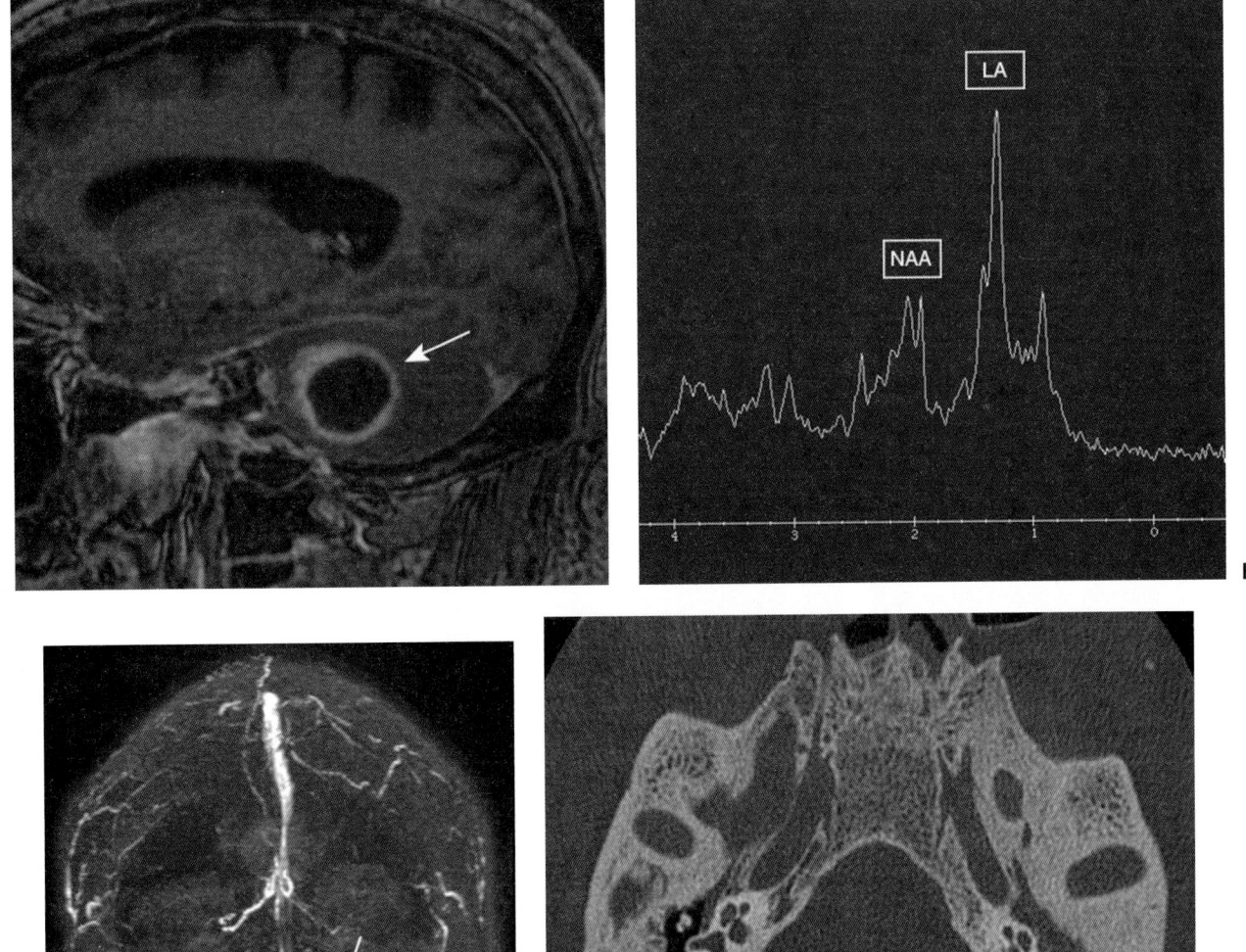

FIGURE 62.2 Cerebellar abscess with mastoiditis. **A:** Sagittal MRI T1-weighted image after gadolinium administration demonstrates ring enhancement (*white arrow*) of cerebellar abscess. **B:** MRI spectroscopy demonstrating characteristic lactate "peak" associated with necrotic tissue of abscess. **C:** Complication of mastoiditis with bilateral transverse sinus thrombosis (*arrows*). **D:** CT bone windows demonstrating sclerotic change of the right mastoid sinus (*left arrow*), consistent with chronic mastoiditis. (Courtesy of Dr. William Wagle.)

DIAGNOSTIC TESTING

Brain abscess should be suspected when seizures, focal neurologic signs, or increased ICP develop in a patient with known acute or chronic infection in the middle ear, mastoid, nasal sinuses, heart, or lungs and in those with congenital heart disease. Neuroimaging by CT or MRI is essential to making the diagnosis.

Although CT scan can be useful, MRI neuroimaging is the neuroimaging study of choice, both for diagnosis and treatment of brain abscess. MRI with gadolinium is more sensitive and specific than contrast CT in diagnosing early cerebritis. On neuroimaging, abscesses are frequently found in the gray–white junction in watershed regions between vascular territories. Serial MRI permits accurate localization of cerebritis or abscess and serial assessment of the size of the lesion, its demarcation, the extent of surrounding edema, and total mass effect and allows for staging of the abscess. MRS may help differentiate brain abscesses based on metabolic patterns of lactate, amino acids, or acetate from other similar appearing lesions (e.g., tumor). The presence of lactate, amino acids, acetate, and succinate on MRS is considered specific for brain abscess (see Fig. 62.2). With a mature encapsulated abscess, both contrast CT and MRI with gadolinium reveal the ring-enhancing mass with surrounding vasogenic edema. Additional MRI sequences with fluid-attenuated inversion recovery (FLAIR), T2- and diffusion-weighted images show characteristic changes (Fig. 62.3).

The differential diagnosis, based on the appearance of lesions seen on CT or MRI, includes glioblastoma, metastatic tumor, infarct, arteriovenous malformation, resolving hematoma, and granuloma. Features supporting the diagnosis of brain abscess include gas within the center of a ring-enhancing lesion, a thinner enhancing rim (<5 mm) than with brain tumors, more regular borders with ringlike enhancement, and ependymal enhancement associated with ventriculitis or ventricular rupture (see Fig. 62.3). MRI with diffusion-weighted image (DWI) and calculation of the apparent diffusion coefficient (ADC) may aid in differentiating tumor from abscess. With brain abscess, MRI DWI signal is hyperintense with associated low ADC values, compared to brain tumor with similar DWI appearance but high ADC. Thallium-201 brain single-photon emission computerized tomography (SPECT) may differentiate intracerebral lymphoma from *Toxoplasma* encephalitis in patients with AIDS. Unlike pyogenic brain abscesses, the signal of *Toxoplasma* abscesses may not be hyperintense on DWI MRI. Often, empiric treatment for *Toxoplasma* can be initiated with evaluation for responsiveness to treatment using follow-up MRI imaging several weeks later.

Either CT or MRI may distinguish abscess from mycotic aneurysms or herpes encephalitis, each of which may cause similar symptoms and signs. Mycotic aneurysm, usually in the distribution of the middle cerebral arteries, may be accompanied by meningitis

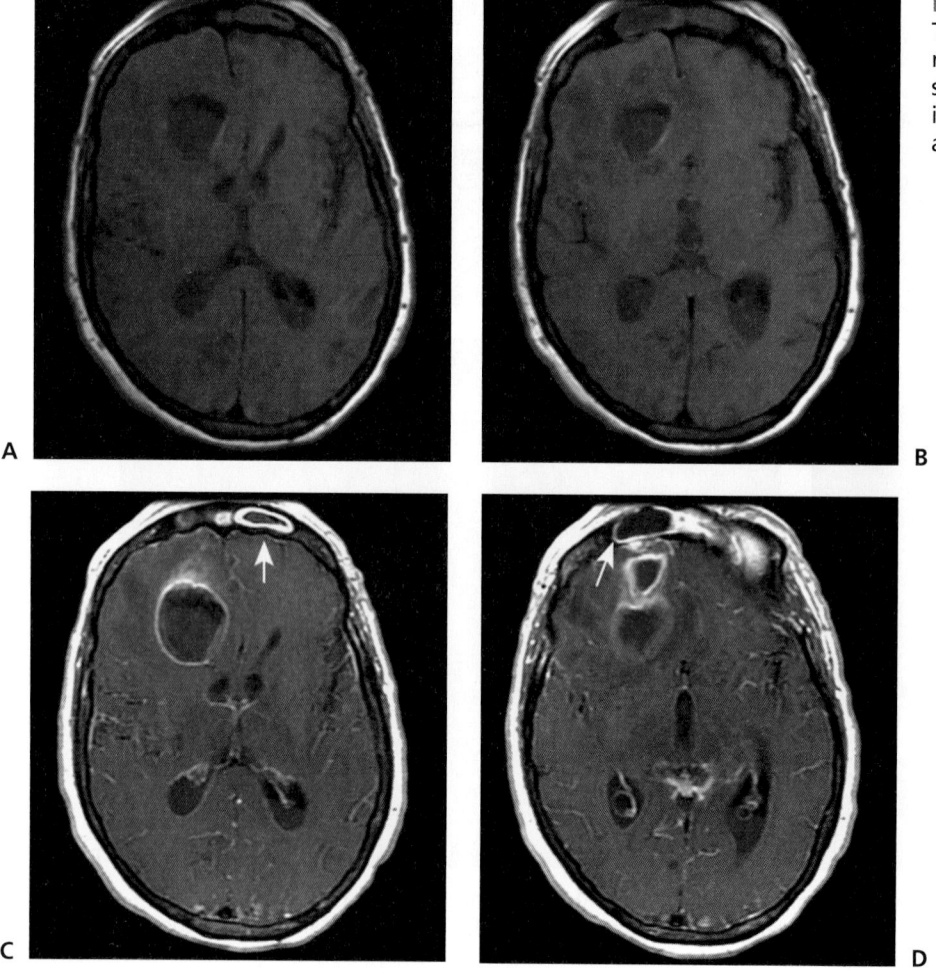

A

B

C

D

FIGURE 62.3 **Brain abscesses. A–I:** MRI T1-weighted images **(A and B)** show right frontal lobe abscess with adjacent, smaller anterior-located abscess with typical ring enhancement after gadolinium administration **(C and D).** *(continued)*

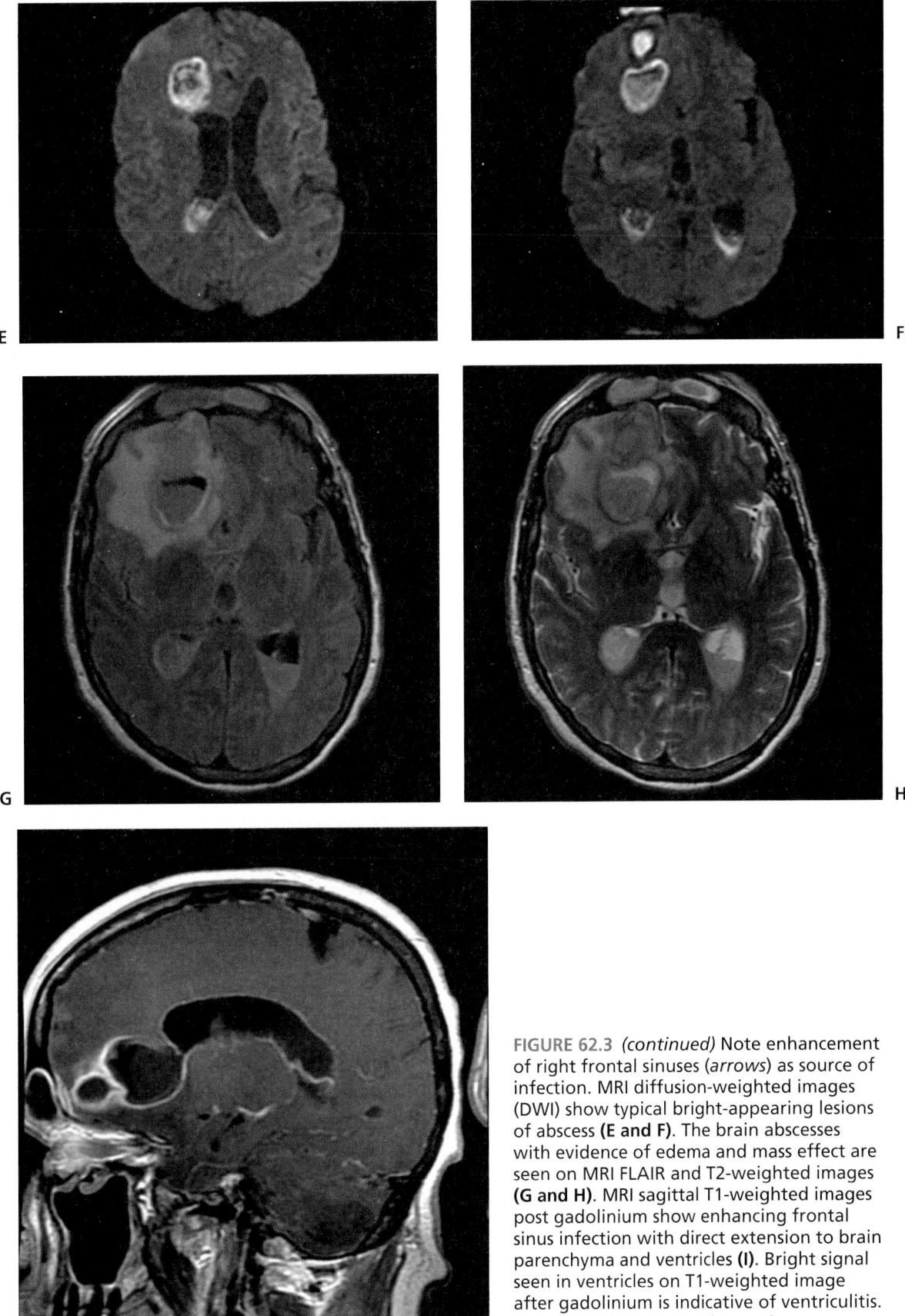

FIGURE 62.3 *(continued)* Note enhancement of right frontal sinuses *(arrows)* as source of infection. MRI diffusion-weighted images (DWI) show typical bright-appearing lesions of abscess **(E and F)**. The brain abscesses with evidence of edema and mass effect are seen on MRI FLAIR and T2-weighted images **(G and H)**. MRI sagittal T1-weighted images post gadolinium show enhancing frontal sinus infection with direct extension to brain parenchyma and ventricles **(I)**. Bright signal seen in ventricles on T1-weighted image after gadolinium is indicative of ventriculitis. (Courtesy of Dr. James Thomas.)

in bacterial endocarditis. CT or MRI may exclude abscess, but CT angiography is often necessary to identify the aneurysm before rupture. Herpes simplex encephalitis presents with headache, fever, and an acute temporal lobe or frontal lobe syndrome. On CT or MRI, the temporal lobe is swollen, with irregular lucency and patchy contrast enhancement.

Lumbar puncture is contraindicated in patients suspected of having a brain abscess because of the clear risk of transtentorial herniation.

Both erythrocyte sedimentation rate (ESR) and C-reactive protein (CRP) may be elevated in patients with brain abscess. Blood cultures are positive in patients with hematogenous dissemination as the source of infection.

Extension of the abscess to the meninges or ventricles is accompanied by findings associated with acute meningitis or ventriculitis. Rupture of an abscess into the ventricles is signaled by a sudden rise in ICP and the presence of free pus, with marked increases in CSF cell count to levels of 20,000/mm^3 to 50,000/mm^3. A decrease in glucose content below 40 mg/dL indicates that the meninges have been invaded by bacteria. Only rarely are CSF cultures positive.

TREATMENT

The introduction of CT revolutionized the management of brain abscess. Now with MRI, it is possible to diagnose and localize cerebritis or abscess, dictate choice of treatment, and monitor patient response. Current recommended treatment for most brain abscesses is stereotactic aspiration to obtain specimens for culture and special studies, and guide treatment with appropriate antimicrobial therapy.

Surgical treatment in the past included open evacuation and excision or freehand needle aspiration through burr hole. Currently, most surgeons prefer CT-guided stereotactic aspiration and drainage. This method is the treatment of choice for most abscesses, particularly those that are deep-seated, multiple, or located in eloquent areas of the brain. Empiric antimicrobial therapy is based on Gram stain results from the specimen obtained by stereotactic aspiration and on the presumptive source of the abscess. Open craniotomy with excision is now performed infrequently and is reserved for patients with multiloculated abscesses, those with antimicrobial-resistant pathogens, abscesses due to *Nocardia*, abscesses containing gas resistant to antibiotics, and posttraumatic abscesses containing foreign bodies or contaminated bone fragments.

Choosing the appropriate antimicrobial therapy depends on the ability of the drug to penetrate the abscess cavity and its activity against the suspected pathogen. Penicillin and chloramphenicol was the standard therapy for brain abscesses at one time but is rarely used today. These have been replaced by vancomycin, third- and fourth-generation cephalosporins (e.g., cefotaxime, ceftriaxone, ceftazidime, and cefepime), metronidazole, and meropenem (Table 62.2). Combination therapy with third- or fourth-generation cephalosporins and vancomycin appears to be highly effective for empiric treatment of a brain abscess. Metronidazole is added when otitis, mastoiditis, or paranasal sinusitis is the suspected source of infection. Additional antibiotic coverage may be needed for some organisms (e.g., *Actinomyces* species) when the abscess is secondary to dental procedures or dental abscess. Special consideration of antimicrobial coverage must be given for *Enterobacteriaceae* or *Pseudomonas aeruginosa* particularly when an otogenic source of brain abscess is suspected. Vancomycin plus a third-generation cephalosporin may be given initially in cases of brain abscess from neurosurgical procedures, while awaiting final culture results. Vancomycin is also used in cases of MRSA abscesses. The rare

TABLE 62.2	Specific Intravenous Antimicrobials for Treatment of Brain Abscess
Vancomycin[a]	45–60 mg/kg/day, q6–12h
Meropenem	2 g q8h (used as first-line or second-line therapy)
Cefotaxime	2 g q4–8h (maximum 12 g/day)
Ceftriaxone	2 g q12h (maximum 4 g/day)
Ceftazidime	1–2 g q4–8h (maximum 6 g/day)
Cefepime	2 g q8h (maximum 6 g/day)
Metronidazole	500 mg q6h (1,500–2,000 mg/day)
Voriconazole	Loading dose of 6 mg/kg q12h × 2, followed by 4 mg/kg q12h

[a]Doses adjusted based on serum peak and trough levels; adjusted based on creatinine clearance.

tuberculosis abscesses can be treated with combination of isoniazid, rifampin, ethambutol, and pyrazinamide for 2 to 4 months, and thereafter isoniazid and rifampin are given for at least 1 year. Aspergillosis abscesses are most effectively treated with voriconazole. Amphotericin B may be considered if voriconazole cannot be given. It is generally recommended that parenteral antibiotics for most abscesses be given for a total of 6 to 8 weeks, followed by an additional 2- to 3-month course of oral antibiotic therapy.

Clinical improvement and CT or MRI s are used to monitor the effectiveness of antibiotic treatment. Follow-up CT may show a small area of residual enhancement even after adequate antimicrobial therapy. Occasionally, previous ring-enhancing lesion on CT disappears with medical management, suggesting that these reversible lesions are forms of suppurative cerebritis.

Seizures may occur in up to 50% of patients with brain abscess, early in the course. However, one large retrospective study found seizures in only 16% of patients with brain abscess. Anticonvulsants may be administered for prophylaxis or to prevent the recurrence of seizures. Newer agents such as levetiracetam are as effective as other anticonvulsants (e.g., phenytoin or carbamazepine) that have been used in the past. Generally, these agents are given for at least 3 months after surgery for abscess and electroencephalogram (EEG) may be useful to help guide duration of therapy.

The use of corticosteroids for these patients is controversial. In patients with life-threatening cerebral edema, midline shift, or impending herniation, a short course of high-dose corticosteroids may be appropriate. Further deterioration with severe brain edema may require intubation with intensive care management to control elevated ICP. Hemicraniectomy may be considered in cases of increased ICP refractory to medical therapy. Prolonged use of corticosteroids is not recommended because the steroids may interfere with granulation tissue formation and reduce the concentration of antibiotics within the infected tissue.

OUTCOME

The outcome of untreated brain abscess is, with rare exceptions, death. Mortality in pre-CT series varied from 35% to 55%. In the era of advanced neuroimaging with CT and MRI, the mortality rate of brain abscesses is 0% to 30%. Overall morbidity and mortality of brain abscess is related to delayed diagnosis, presence of single or multiple abscesses, intraventricular rupture, presence of coma or rapidly declining neurologic status at the time of diagnosis, or fungal infections. Patients with depressed level of consciousness on admission tend to do poorly. Intraventricular rupture of a brain abscess and posterior fossa location are associated with mortality rates exceeding 80%. In a univariate analysis of mortality, Glasgow Coma Scale score on admission of less than or equal to 9 was an independent predictor of in-hospital mortality in one study. Immunocompromised individuals have worse outcomes and higher mortality rates. The highest death rate is found when the primary infection is in the lungs.

Sequelae of brain abscess include recurrence of the abscess or the development of new abscesses if the primary focus persists. Residual neurologic sequelae with hemiparesis, seizures, or intellectual or behavioral impairment are seen in 30% to 56% of patients.

SUBDURAL EMPYEMA

A subdural empyema is a collection of loculated pus in the subdural space. The symptoms are similar to those of a brain abscess. A subdural infection in adults usually arises from a contiguous spread of infection; paranasal sinusitis is the most common source. Otitis, head trauma, and neurosurgical procedures are other sources of infection. The most common pathogen in subdural empyema are anaerobic and microaerophilic streptococci. In a minority of cases, S. aureus and multiple organisms, including gram-negative organisms such as Escherichia coli and anaerobic organisms, such as Bacteroides, may be present. P. aeruginosa or S. epidermidis may be found in cases following neurosurgical procedures. In addition, Clostridium perfringens subdural empyemas can occur from the site of recent surgical wound or trauma.

The infection spreads to the subdural space through retrograde thrombophlebitis via venous sinuses or direct extension through bone and dura. Once the infection develops, it may spread over the convexities and along the falx, although characteristic loculation is common. Associated complications include septic cortical vein thrombosis, brain or epidural abscess, and meningitis. Subdural empyema typically presents with focal headache, fever, and in 80% to 90% of patients, focal neurologic signs. The combination of fever, rapidly progressive neurologic deterioration, and focal seizures is particularly suggestive of this disorder. Symptoms of subdural empyema may begin 1 to 2 weeks after a sinus infection. Infratentorial empyema is a rare complication of bacterial meningitis and can present with nonlocalizing symptoms of neck stiffness and decreased level of consciousness.

DIAGNOSIS

Neuroimaging with either CT or MRI reveals a typical crescent-shaped area of hypodensity over a hemisphere, along the dura, or adjoining the falx, with enhancement of the margins around the empyema after administration of contrast. However, the diagnostic test of choice is MRI with gadolinium enhancement for the delineation of the presence and extent of the subdural empyema and to identify concurrent intracranial infections. CT may miss some lesions that can be detected by MRI. Lumbar puncture is contraindicated for the same reason it is with brain abscess, i.e., because of mass effect and potential for herniation.

TREATMENT

Treatment of nearly all cases of subdural empyema is immediate surgical drainage and antibiotic therapy. Intravenous antibiotics are given depending on the organism identified, or if unknown, empiric treatment with antibiotics similar to those used in brain abscess based on predisposing or associated conditions. Anticonvulsants

are frequently required. There is controversy about which type of neurosurgical technique is useful for drainage of subdural empyema. CT accurately localizes the pus collection, and some advocate drainage through selective burr holes. Others prefer open craniotomy for more complete removal of the infection, especially when the empyema is loculated. Limited craniotomy is also used for placement of a drain into the subdural space and for local infusion of antibiotics. Use of either burr hole or craniotomy for drainage of subdural empyema is individualized. Neuroendoscopic technique for drainage of both brain abscess and subdural empyema is an alternative to surgical treatment. In cases of fulminant subdural empyema, decompressive craniectomy, irrigation of the empyema, and subdural drainage may be required. The recommended duration of antibiotic therapy is 3 to 4 weeks after surgical drainage.

SPINAL EPIDURAL ABSCESS

Spinal epidural abscess is infection in the epidural space around the spinal cord and may arise from hematogenous spread from a distant site, direct inoculation, or contiguous spread from skin, soft tissue, or bone infection. Typically, spinal epidural abscess is associated with diabetes, trauma, intravenous drug use, alcohol, age, or immunosuppression with the single most important risk factor being diabetes. The most important pathogen for spinal epidural abscess is S. aureus found in over 60% of cases. Most common sources of infection are skin abscesses and bony infections involving the spine. The most common location of spinal epidural abscesses is in dorsal epidural space, although one 10-year study found up to 30% may be located in the ventral epidural space.

The clinical presentation of spinal epidural abscess is back pain and fever; these symptoms commonly are followed by focal neurologic deficits of radiculitis, then paraparesis, sensory level, bladder or bowel dysfunction, and eventual para- or quadriplegia.

DIAGNOSIS

As with brain abscess, both ESR and CRP are invariably elevated. Complete blood count and blood cultures should be obtained. Lumbar puncture is contraindicated, as it can lead to introduction of infection into subarachnoid space. Magnetic resonance imaging is more sensitive than CT with contrast in identifying spinal epidural abscess, with MRI approaching 90% sensitivity in some studies. Additional benefits of MRI include the ability to detect cord involvement (swelling or necrosis), diskitis, and osteomyelitis (Fig. 62.4).

TREATMENT

Treatment for spinal epidural abscess includes surgery (e.g., decompression with laminectomy) and antibiotics. Initial antimicrobial therapy should include antibiotics for MRSA and gram-negative bacilli. A combination of a third- or fourth-generation cephalosporin and vancomycin are recommended. Once the specific organism is identified from surgical specimen and antimicrobial sensitivity, then antibiotic therapy is modified accordingly. Some reports suggest spinal epidural abscess can be successfully treated with antibiotics alone (before neurologic symptoms appear); however, surgical decompression and drainage remains the mainstay of treatment in most cases.

OUTCOME

The prognosis in spinal epidural abscess is dependent on the mechanism causing the neurologic deficits. Compression of the cord can be helped by surgery, but deficits due to vascular ischemia,

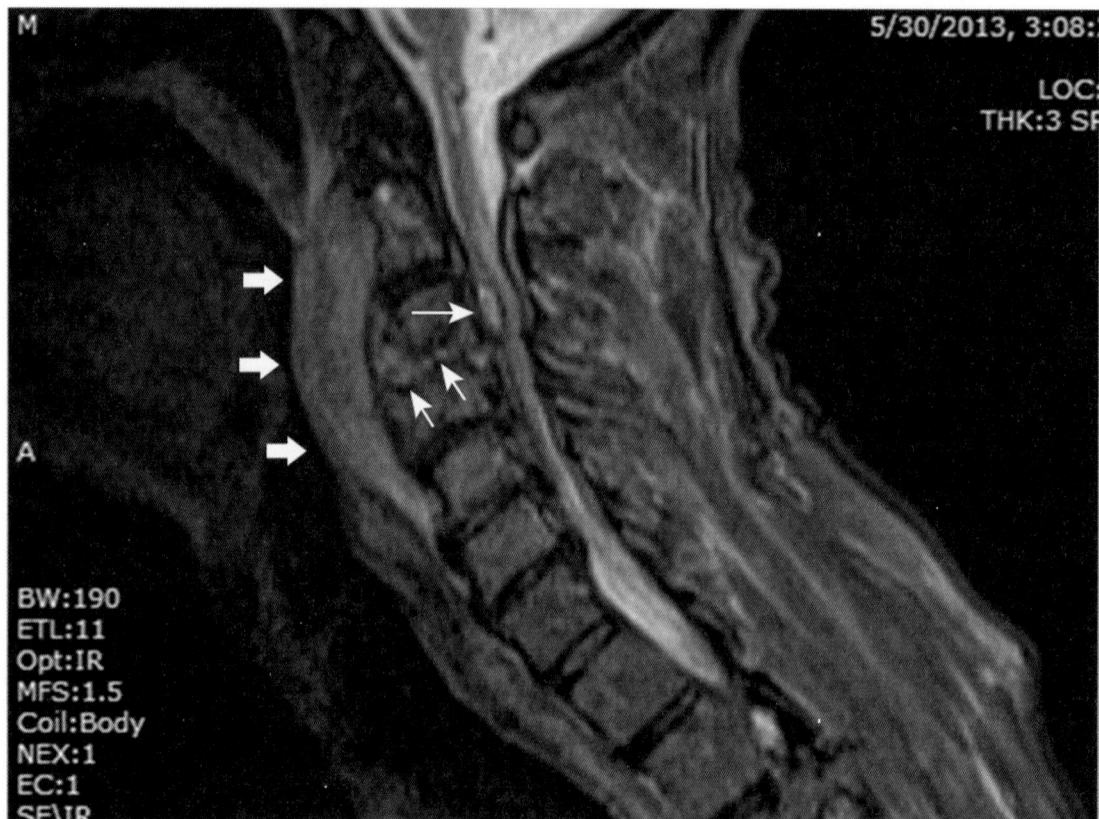

FIGURE 62.4 Spinal epidural abscess. MRI T2-weighted image showing increased signal in anterior epidural space at C3 spinal level (*large arrow*) consistent with abscess. Prevertebral soft-tissue infection (*three solid arrowheads*) is the source of infection. Evidence of osteomyelitis and involvement of intervertebral disk with diskitis at C3 vertebral body (*two small arrows*). (Courtesy of Dr. Karen Roos.)

with thrombosis or thrombophlebitis involving surrounding leptomeningeal vessels, or inflammatory response of glial cells, are not improved by surgery. Rehabilitation can significantly affect outcome in spinal epidural abscess.

MALIGNANT OTITIS EXTERNA

Malignant (necrotizing) otitis externa is an invasive infection of the external auditory canal and skull base; it penetrates epithelium and spreads to surrounding soft tissue to cause cellulitis and abscess. If untreated, the infection may extend to the temporomandibular joint, mastoid, or more commonly to soft tissues below the temporal bone. The syndrome occurs more frequently in elderly diabetic patients and immunocompromised persons (e.g., patients with HIV, chemotherapy, or organ transplantation) than in immunocompetent individuals.

Common symptoms of malignant otitis externa are severe otalgia that worsens at night, purulent otorrhea, and painful swelling of surrounding tissues. Conductive hearing loss may result from obstruction of the external auditory canal. Trismus may indicate irritation of the masseter muscles or involvement of the temporomandibular joint. Owing to its anatomic location in the temporal bone and petrous apex, the facial nerve may be affected as the first symptom in up to 30% of patients. Facial nerve involvement is most common, followed (in order) by glossopharyngeal, vagal, and spinal accessory nerves at the jugular foramen; hypoglossal nerve as it exits the hypoglossal canal; and trigeminal and abducens nerves at the petrous apex. Olfactory, oculomotor,

and trochlear nerves are spared. Rarely, dysphagia results from lesions of cranial nerves IX through XII, and the findings may be mistaken for laryngeal carcinoma. Fever and weight loss are uncommon. Mastoid tenderness is evident on examination. The diagnostic finding of granulation tissue, stemming from extension of infection to the cartilaginous portion of the ear canal, may be seen on otoscopic examination. In rare cases, meningitis, brain abscess, and dural sinus thrombophlebitis can occur and are often fatal.

DIAGNOSIS

The diagnosis of malignant otitis externa is often initially missed but can be made by combination of clinical, laboratory, and radiologic findings. General laboratory testing is invariably normal with the exception of ESR and CRP, which are elevated. The ESR is almost always elevated in greater than 50 mm/h. Both ESR and CRP can be useful in monitoring disease activity.

Neuroimaging

CT is most useful in showing the location and extent of disease and evaluating evidence of bony erosion but may appear normal early in the illness. Initial CT can help predict severity of disease course based on early findings of extension of infection beyond the external auditory canal. The presence of bone erosion along with soft tissue abnormalities in the subtemporal area is almost pathognomonic for the disease. MRI with and without gadolinium is the study of choice, but it is not useful in detecting bony changes. However, MRI can provide useful information regarding the extent of skull-base and intracranial soft-tissue involvement. Bone scanning with technetium-99 (scans) methylene diphosphonate can be very sensitive but not specific. Gallium-67 SPECT may be more sensitive and accurate in early detection of malignant external otitis, sensitive in measuring ongoing infectious process, and beneficial in monitoring response to therapy. However, it remains less frequently used compared to serial CT scanning.

Biopsy

The differential diagnosis of malignant otitis externa includes squamous cell carcinoma of the temporal bone. Radiologic testing cannot differentiate tumor from necrotizing infection of malignant otitis externa and biopsy is often necessary to distinguish between these two processes. Findings of positive culture for *Pseudomonas* spp. along with elevated ESR and CRP confirm the diagnosis of malignant otitis externa.

ETIOLOGY

In most cases, *P. aeruginosa* is the causative organism. Less often, cases of malignant otitis externa have been reported due to *Klebsiella, S. aureus, Proteus mirabilis,* and other *Pseudomonas* spp. In HIV-positive individuals or in AIDS, either *P. aeruginosa* or the fungus *Aspergillus fumigatus* may be isolated. In some patients with AIDS, *Streptococcus, Staphylococcus,* and *Proteus* spp. may be isolated as mixed or sole pathogens. Interestingly, ear irrigation with water contaminated with *Pseudomonas* spp. is often the causative event leading to malignant otitis externa.

TREATMENT

Antipseudomonal agents are the agents of choice for treatment of malignant otitis externa (Table 62.3). Rare cases of fungal (e.g., *Aspergillus* species) malignant external otitis do exist. In the preantibiotic era, mortality rates were greater than 50%, and surgical debridement was the treatment of choice. Likewise, standard treatment with intravenous antibiotics consisted of an antipseudomonal penicillin for 4 to 8 weeks, combined with an aminoglycoside for at least 2 weeks, or if tolerated, 4 to 6 weeks. Current successful treatment is based on single-drug therapy. Advantages of quinolones include low toxicity, excellent penetration into bone, and no dosage adjustment required in the elderly patient with renal impairment. Double-antibiotic therapy may be considered with more extensive lesions. Fluoroquinolone-resistant strains exist so alternative therapy must be considered. Such alternative treatment includes antipseudomonal beta-lactams, including piperacillin, combination piperacillin-tazobactam, ceftazidime, and cefepime. In some drug-resistant cases, use of cephalosporins

TABLE 62.3	Antimicrobial Agents for Treatment of Malignant Otitis Externa
Antipseudomonal agents	Ciprofloxacin 400 mg IV q8h
	Levofloxacin 750 mg IV daily
	Ceftazidime 2 g IV q8h
	Cefepime 2 mg IV q8h
Antimicrobials for *Aspergillus* species	Voriconazole 4–6 mg/kg IV q12h
	Liposomal amphotericin B 5–7.5 mg/kg/day IV
	Amphotericin B + itraconazole 5 mg/kg/day + 600 mg oral daily

and antipseudomonal penicillins in combination with debridement may be necessary. Rare complications of retropharyngeal abscesses are drained surgically. If *Aspergillus* species is causative agent, voriconazole has been successful as first-line treatment and shown superiority to amphotericin B in a randomized trial. Despite these newer treatments, the mortality rate is still 10% to 20% and may be as high as 50% if treatment is delayed.

Hyperbaric oxygen therapy efficacy remains unproven and is rarely now used for refractory cases of malignant otitis externa. Recent studies suggest that facial cranial nerve involvement may be a marker for extension of disease but by itself not an adverse prognostic factor. If untreated or inadequately treated, malignant external otitis may result in osteomyelitis of the base of the skull, sigmoid sinus thrombosis, abscess formation, meningitis, and death.

OSTEOMYELITIS OF THE SKULL BASE

Osteomyelitis of the base of the skull is a rare complication of malignant external otitis, chronic mastoiditis, or paranasal sinus infection. As with malignant otitis, the patients are usually elderly, diabetic, or immunocompromised. Symptoms include headache, otalgia, hearing loss, and otorrhea, but patients are frequently without fever. Osteomyelitis may occur in conjunction with otitis but usually appears weeks or months after starting antibiotics. As the process spreads, cranial nerves may be affected, especially the VII and VIII nerves. Extension of skull base osteomyelitis to the jugular foramen or hypoglossal canal may affect cranial nerves IX through XII, leading to dysphagia. In advanced cases, spread to the petrous pyramid may affect III, IV, V, and VI cranial nerves to cause ocular palsies or trigeminal neuralgia.

DIAGNOSIS

Laboratory abnormalities include a normal or slightly elevated white blood cell (WBC) count and high ESR. In general, leukocytosis is not common and not useful to diagnosis and management. The use of thin-cut CT sections through the skull base and temporal bones to visualize bony involvement plays an important role in the diagnosis of osteomyelitis and in assessing extent of disease. However, because more than 30% of affected bone needs to be demineralized to appear eroded on CT, early disease may escape detection by CT.

MRI is useful in delineating soft-tissue involvement but has not proved beneficial for initial diagnosis or determining efficacy of treatment for skull-base osteomyelitis. Technetium bone scanning is a sensitive indicator of osteomyelitis but is not helpful in determining resolution of disease. Technetium uptake is nonspecific and may be seen in a number of conditions such as infection, trauma, neoplasm, and postoperatively. Gallium-67 citrate scans may be useful in tracking resolution of disease over time. Neither bone nor gallium scans are useful in determining the exact extent of the infection. Unlike technetium-99 scans, gallium-67 scans return to normal sooner once the infection is resolved and can be useful to signal clearing of infection. *S. aureus* is now the most common isolated organism in osteomyelitis. Other potential causative agents include *P. aeruginosa, S. epidermidis, Proteus, Salmonella, Mycobacterium, Aspergillus,* and *Candida.*

TREATMENT

Therapy for osteomyelitis consists of intravenous administration of antibiotics, usually a combination of an antipseudomonal penicillin or cephalosporin. Ciprofloxacin, with its strong bone penetration, has been effective when used alone or with other antibiotics. Ceftazidime has bactericidal activity against *Pseudomonas* and has been used successfully as monotherapy. The disease is usually extensive, and conservative management of skull-base osteomyelitis is still an extended course of therapy. In rare cases of *Aspergillus* osteomyelitis, surgical debridement with radical mastoidectomy is usually required, in addition to long-term antifungal therapy. Monthly gallium scans may help to determine the response and duration of antibiotic therapy. In refractory cases, hyperbaric oxygen has been used as adjuvant therapy. Antibiotics should be continued for at least 1 week after the gallium scan becomes normal. Duration of antibiotic therapy varies but is usually for at least 1 month and, in some cases, may extend up to 6 months after diagnosis. Follow-up gallium scans may be performed 1 week after completion of antibiotic therapy to detect early recurrence and at 3 months for late recurrence. Mortality rates of 40% have been reported, but with prolonged antibiotic therapy, complete cure may be achieved. Recurrences may manifest up to 1 year later; true cure is considered when the patient is disease-free for a year after the treatment is begun.

SUGGESTED READINGS

Brain Abscess, Subdural Empyema, and Spinal Epidural Abscess

Alderson D, Strong AJ, Ingham HR, et al. Fifteen-year review of the mortality of brain abscess. *Neurosurgery.* 1981;8:1–6.

Auvichayapat N, Auvichayapat P, Aungwarawong S. Brain abscesses in infants and children: a retrospective study of 107 patients in northeast Thailand. *J Med Assoc Thai.* 2007;90:1601–1607.

Baggish AL, Nadiminti H. Intracranial abscess from embolic *Serratia marcescens* endocarditis. *Lancet Infect Dis.* 2007;7:630.

Balasubramaniam P, Madakira PB, Ninan A, et al. Response of central nervous system aspergillosis to voriconazole. *Neurol India.* 2007;55:301–303.

Bernardini GL. Diagnosis and management of brain abscess and subdural empyema. *Curr Neurol Neurosci Rep.* 2004;4(6):448–456.

Carpentier PA, Duncan DS, Miller SD. Glial toll-like receptor signaling in central nervous system infection and autoimmunity. *Brain Behav Immun.* 2008;22:140–147.

Chen FC, Tseng YZ, Wu SP, et al. Vegetation on patent foramen ovale presenting as a cryptogenic brain abscess. *Int J Cardiol.* 2008;124:e49–e50.

Chong-Han CH, Cortez SC, Tung GA. Diffusion-weighted MRI of cerebral *Toxoplasma* abscess. *AJR Am J Roentgenol.* 2003;181:1711–1714.

Courville CB, Nielsen JM. Fatal complications of otitis media: with particular reference to intracranial lesions in a series of 10,000 autopsies. *Arch Otolaryngol.* 1934;19:451–501.

Cunha BA, Krol V, Kodali V. Methicillin-resistant *Staphylococcus aureus* (MRSA) mitral valve acute bacterial endocarditis (ABE) in a patient with Job's syndrome (hyperimmunoglobulin E syndrome) successfully treated with linezolid and high-dose daptomycin. *Heart Lung.* 2008;37:72–75.

de Falco R, Scarano E, Cigliano A, et al. Surgical treatment of subdural empyema: a critical review. *J Neurosurg Sci.* 1996;40:53–58.

Dill ST, Cobbs CG, McDonald CK. Subdural empyema: analysis of 32 cases and review. *Clin Infect Dis.* 1995;20:372–386.

Finsterer J, Hess B. Neuromuscular and central nervous system manifestations of *Clostridium perfringens* infections. *Infection.* 2007;35:396–405.

Garg M, Gupta RK, Husain M, et al. Brain abscesses: etiologic categorization with in vivo proton MR spectroscopy. *Radiology.* 2004;230:519–527.

Greenlee JE. Subdural empyema. *Curr Treat Options Neurol.* 2003;5:13–22.

Guzman R, Barth A, Lovblad KO, et al. Use of diffusion-weighted magnetic resonance imaging in differentiating purulent brain processes from cystic brain tumors. *J Neurosurg.* 2002;97:1101–1107.

Hakan T, Ceran N, Erdem I, et al. Bacterial brain abscesses: an evaluation of 96 cases. *J Infect.* 2006;52:359–366.

Harvey FH, Carlow TJ. Brainstem abscess and the syndrome of acute tegmental encephalitis. *Ann Neurol.* 1980;7:371–376.

Heilpern KL, Lorber B. Focal intracranial infections. *Infect Dis Clin North Am.* 1996;10:879–898.

Jaggi RS, Husain M, Chawla S, et al. Diagnosis of bacterial cerebellitis: diffusion imaging and proton magnetic resonance imaging. *Pediatr Neurol.* 2005;32:72–74.

Jansson AK, Enblad P, Sjolin J. Efficacy and safety of cefotaxime in combination with metronidazole for empirical treatment of brain abscesses in clinical practice: a retrospective study of 66 consecutive cases. *Eur J Clin Microbiol Infect Dis.* 2004;23:7–14.

Kaushik K, Karade S, Kumer S, et al. Tuberculous brain abscess in a patient with HIV infection. *Indian J Tuberc.* 2007;54:196–198.

Kawamata T, Takeshita M, Ishizuka N, et al. Patent foramen ovale as a possible risk factor for cryptogenic grain abscess: report of two cases. *Neurosurgery.* 2001;49:204–206.

Kielian T. Microglia and chemokines in infectious diseases of the nervous system. Views and reviews. *Front Biosci.* 2004;9:732–750.

Lefebvre L, Metellus P, Dufour H, et al. Linezolid for treatment of subdural empyema due to *Streptococcus*: case reports. *Surg Neurol.* 2009;71(1):89–91; discussion 91.

Lu CH, Chang WN, Lui CC. Strategies for the management of bacterial brain abscess. *J Clin Neurosci.* 2006;13:979–985.

Macewen W. *Pyogenic Infective Diseases of the Brain and Spinal Cord: Meningitis, Abscess of Brain, Infective Sinus Thrombosis.* Glasgow, United Kingdom: James Maclehose & Sons; 1893.

Mathisen GE, Johnson JP. Brain abscess. *Clin Infect Dis.* 1997;25:763–779.

Menon S, Bharadwaj R, Chowdhary A, et al. Current epidemiology of intracranial abscesses: a prospective 5 year study. *J Med Microbiol.* 2008;57:1259–1268.

Merritt HH, Fremont-Smith F. *The Cerebrospinal Fluid.* Philadelphia: WB Saunders; 1938.

Miranda HA, Castellar-Leones SM, Elzain MA, et al. Brain abscess: current management. *J Neurosci Rural Pract.* 2013:4:S67–S81.

Mueller-Mang C, Castillo M, Mang TG, et al. Fungal versus bacterial brain abscesses: is diffusion-weighted MR imaging a useful tool in the differential diagnosis? *Neuroradiology.* 2007;49:651–657.

Muthusamy KA, Waran V, Puthucheary SD. Spectra of central nervous system melioidosis. *J Clin Neurosci.* 2007;14:1213–1215.

Muzumdar D, Jhawar S, Goel A. Brain abscess: an overview. *Int J Surg.* 2011;9:136–144.

Nathoo N, Nadvi SS, Narotam PK, et al. Brain abscess: management and outcome analysis of a computed tomography era experience with 973 patients. *World Neurosurg.* 2011;75:716–726.

Rosenblum ML, Hoff JT, Norman D, et al. Decreased mortality from brain abscesses since the advent of computerized tomography. *J Neurosurg.* 1978;49:658–668.

Seydoux C, Francioli P. Bacterial brain abscesses: factors influencing mortality and sequelae. *Clin Infect Dis.* 1992;15:394–401.

Shaw MDM, Russell JA. Cerebellar abscess: a review of 47 cases. *J Neurol Neurosurg Psychiatry.* 1975;38:429–435.

Tattevin P, Bruneel F, Clair B, et al. Bacterial brain abscesses: a retrospective study of 94 patients admitted to an intensive care unit (1980 to 1999). *Am J Med.* 2003;115:143–146.

Ulivieri S, Oliveri G, Filosomi G. Brain abscess and Rendu–Osler–Weber disease. Care report and review of the literature. *J Neurosurg Sci.* 2007;51:77–79.

Van de Beek D, Campeau NG, Wijdicks EF. The clinical challenge of recognizing intratentorial empyema. *Neurology.* 2007;69:477–481.

Wada Y, Kubo T, Asano T, et al. Fulminant subdural empyema treated with a wide decompressive craniectomy and continuous irrigation—case report. *Neurol Med Chir.* 2002;42:414–416.

Weingarten K, Zimmerman RD, Becker RD, et al. Subdural and epidural empyemas: MR imaging. *AJR Am J Roentgenol.* 1989;152:615–621.

Weisberg LA. Nonsurgical management of focal intracranial infection. *Neurology.* 1981;31:575–580.

Wispelwey B, Dacey RG Jr, Scheld WM. Brain abscess. In: Scheld WM, Whitley RJ, Durack DT, eds. *Infections of the Central Nervous System.* New York: Raven Press; 1991:457–486.

Yadav YR, Sinha M, Neha, et al. Endoscopic management of brain abscesses. *Neurol India.* 2008;56:12–16.

Zia WC, Lewin JJ. Advances in the management of central nervous system infections in the ICU. *Crit Care Clin.* 2007;22:661–694.

Zimmerman RA. Imaging of intracranial infections. In: Scheld WM, Whitley RJ, Durack DT, eds. *Infections of the Central Nervous System.* New York: Raven Press; 1991:887–908.

Malignant External Otitis and Osteomyelitis

Bernstein JM, Holland NJ, Porter GC, et al. Resistance of *Pseudomonas* to ciprofloxacin: implications for the treatment of malignant otitis externa. *J Laryngol Otol.* 2007;121:118–123.

Dinapoli RP, Thomas JE. Neurologic aspects of malignant external otitis: report of three cases. *Mayo Clin Proc.* 1971;46:339–344.

Grandis JR, Curtin HD, Yu VL. Necrotizing (malignant) external otitis: prospective comparison of CT and MRI in diagnosis and follow-up. *Radiology.* 1995;196:499–504.

Herbrecth R, Denning DW, Patterson TF, et al. Voriconazole versus amphotericin B for primary therapy of invasive aspergillosis. *N Engl J Med.* 2002;347:408–415.

Hern JD, Almeyda J, Thomas DM, et al. Malignant otitis externa in HIV and AIDS. *J Laryngol Otol.* 1996;110:770–775.

Ismail H, Hellier WP, Batty V. Use of magnetic resonance imaging as the primary imaging modality in the diagnosis and follow-up of malignant external otitis. *J Laryngol Otol.* 2004;118:576–579.

Karantanas AH, Karantzas G, Katsiva V, et al. CT and MRI in malignant external otitis: a report of four cases. *Comput Med Imaging Graph.* 2003;27:27–34.

Kondziella D, Skagervik I. Malignant external otitis with extensive cranial neuropathy but no facial paralysis. *J Neurol.* 2007;254:1298–1299.

Mani N, Sughoff H, Rajagopal S, et al. Cranial nerve involvement in malignant external otitis: implications for clinical outcome. *Laryngoscope.* 2007;117:907–910.

Mardinger O, Rosen D, Minkow B, et al. Temporomandibular joint involvement in malignant external otitis. *Oral Surg Med Oral Pathol Radiol Endod.* 2003;96:398–403.

Meyers BR, Mendelson MH, Parisier SC, et al. Malignant external otitis. Comparison of monotherapy vs combination therapy. *Arch Otolaryngol Head Neck Surg.* 1987;113:974–978.

Narozny W, Kuczkowski J, Stankiewicz C, et al. Value of hyperbaric oxygen in bacterial and fungal malignant external otitis treatment. *Eur Arch Otorhinolaryngol.* 2006;263:680–684.

Nicolai P, Lombardi D, Berlucchi M, et al. Drainage of retro-parapharyngeal abscess: an additional indication for endoscopic sinus surgery. *Eur Arch Otorhinolaryngol.* 2005;262:722–730.

Okpala NC, Siraj QH, Nilssen E, et al. Radiological and radionuclide investigation of malignant otitis externa. *J Laryngol Otol.* 2005;119:71–75.

Peleg U, Perez R, Berelowitz D, et al. Stratification for malignant external otitis. *Otolaryngol Head Neck Surg.* 2007;137:301–305.

Parize P, Chandesris MO, Laternier F, et al. Antifungal therapy of *Aspergillus* invasive otitis externa: efficacy of voriconazole and review. *Antimicrob Agents Chemother.* 2009;53:1048–1053.

Ress BD, Luntz M, Telischi FF, et al. Necrotizing external otitis in patients with AIDS. *Laryngoscope.* 1997;107:456–460.

Rubin GJ, Branstetter BF IV, Yu VL. The changing face of malignant (necrotizing) external otitis: clinical, radiological, and anatomic correlations. *Lancet Infect Dis.* 2004;4:34–39.

Soudry E, Joshua BZ, Sulkes J, et al. Characteristics and prognosis of malignant external otitis with facial paralysis. *Arch Otolaryngol Head Neck Surg.* 2007;133:1002–1004.

Sreepada GS, Gangadhar S, Kwartler JA. Skull base osteomyelitis secondary to malignant otitis externa. *Curr Opin Otolaryngol Head Neck Surg.* 2003;11:316–323.

Sudhoff H, Rajagopal S, Mani N, et al. Usefulness of CT scans in malignant external otitis: effective tool for the diagnosis, but of limited value in predicting outcome. *Eur Arch Otorhinolaryngol.* 2008;265:53–56.

Tierney MR, Baker AS. Infections of the head and neck in diabetes mellitus. *Infect Dis Clin North Am.* 1995;9:195–216.

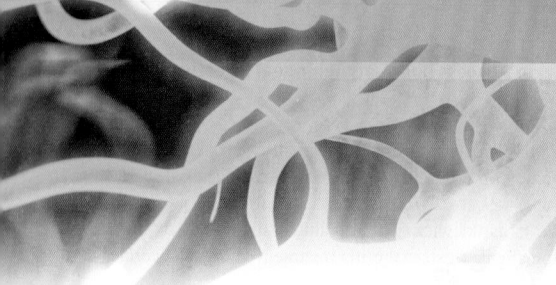

Other Bacterial Central Nervous System Infections and Toxins 63

Barnett R. Nathan and Burk Jubelt

INTRODUCTION

Acute bacterial meningitis (see Chapter 61) occurs when bacteria invade and infect the leptomeninges, causing an acute clinical syndrome of fever, headache, meningismus, and neurologic dysfunction with polymorphonuclear pleocytosis in the cerebrospinal fluid (CSF). This chapter discusses a wide variety of less common bacterial infections that can either infect the central nervous system (CNS) directly, cause parainfectious central or peripheral neurologic syndromes, or create toxins that lead to neurologic dysfunction.

RICKETTSIAL INFECTIONS

Rickettsiae are obligate, intracellular pleomorphic coccobacilli. Each *Rickettsia* pathogenic for humans is capable of multiplying in arthropods and in animals and humans. They have a gram-negative cell wall and an internal structure similar to that of bacteria (i.e., with a prokaryotic DNA arrangement and ribosomes). Diseases due to rickettsiae are divided into five groups on the basis of their biologic properties and epidemiologic features: typhus, spotted fever, scrub typhus, Q fever, and trench fever. Invasion of the nervous system is common only in infections with organisms of the first three groups. Infection with Rocky Mountain spotted fever is the most important rickettsial infection currently in the United States. A sixth group of rickettsiae in the genus *Ehrlichia* have come to be recognized as significant pathogens in humans in the past 15 years. Ehrlichial infections have also been associated with CNS symptoms, but the frequency of nervous system infection is still not certain.

ROCKY MOUNTAIN SPOTTED FEVER

Rocky Mountain spotted fever (RMSF) is an acute endemic febrile disease due to infection with *Rickettsia rickettsii. R. rickettsii* is a gram-negative, obligate intracellular bacterium. It is transmitted to humans by various ticks, the most common of which are the *Dermacentor andersoni* (wood tick), which is found in western region of the United States, and the *Dermacentor variabilis* (dog tick), which is found in the East and South. *Rhipicephalus sanguineus* (brown dog tick) is also a vector for RMSF in the southwestern United States. Rabbits, squirrels, and other small rodents serve as hosts for the ticks and are responsible for maintaining the infection in nature. Diseases of the RMSF group are present throughout the world. Because this is a tick-borne disease, it has a seasonal variation, with the summer months having the greatest number of reports.

Epidemiology

The disease has been reported from almost all states and from Canada, Mexico, and South America. Approximately 1,000 to 2,000 cases are reported annually in the United States, mostly from rural areas of southwestern and south-central states. Most cases are seen during the period of maximal tick activity—the late spring and early summer months. Men are more commonly affected than women, and cases are most frequently reported in those older than 40 years.

Preventative measures include personal care and vaccination. Tick-infested areas should be avoided. If exposure is necessary, high boots, leggings, or socks should be worn outside the trouser legs. Body and clothing should be inspected after exposure, and attached ticks should be removed with tweezers. Hands should be carefully washed after handling the ticks. Workers whose occupations require constant exposure to tick-infested regions should be vaccinated yearly just before the advent of the tick season.

Pathobiology

The agent has a tropism for vascular endothelial cells. Thus, any organ can be infected. The pathologic changes are most severe in the skin, but the heart, lungs, and CNS are also involved. The brain is edematous, and minute petechial hemorrhages are present. The characteristic microscopic lesions are small, round nodules composed of elongated microglia, lymphocytes, and endothelial cells. These are scattered diffusely through the nervous system in close relationship to small vessels. Vessels in the center of the lesions show severe degeneration. The endothelial cells are swollen, and the lumen may be occluded. Minute areas of focal necrosis are common as the result of thrombosis of small arterioles. Some degree of perivascular infiltration without the presence of nodules may be seen in both the meninges and the brain parenchyma.

Clinical Manifestations

A history of tick bite is elicited in about 70% of patients. The incubation period varies from 3 to 12 days. The onset is usually abrupt, with severe headache, fever, chills, myalgias, arthralgias, restlessness, prostration, anorexia, nausea, vomiting, and at times, delirium and coma. A rose-red maculopapular rash appears between the second and sixth day (usually on the fourth febrile day) on the wrists, ankles, palms, soles, and forearms. The rash rapidly spreads to the legs, arms, and chest. The rash becomes petechial and fails to fade on pressure by about the fourth day. Although cardiac, pulmonary, hepatic, and renal involvement can occur, they are less frequent than neurologic disease.

Neurologic symptoms occur early and are frequently a prominent feature. CNS signs and symptoms affect 20% to 25% of patients. Headache, restlessness, insomnia, and neck and back stiffness are common. Delirium, lethargy, or coma alternating with restlessness is present during the height of the fever. Tremors, athetoid movements, convulsions, opisthotonos, and muscular rigidity may occur. Retinal venous engorgement, retinal edema, papilledema, retinal exudates, and choroiditis may occur. Deafness, visual disturbances, slurred speech, and confusion may be present and may persist for a few weeks following recovery. Encephalitis is the most common major complication. Other major complications include adult respiratory distress, syndrome, cardiac arrhythmias, pulmonary edema, skin necrosis, gastrointestinal bleeding, and coagulopathies.

Diagnosis

The white cell count (WBC) is either normal or mildly elevated. Thrombocytopenia may develop and is common. Proteinuria, hematuria, and oliguria commonly occur. Hyponatremia is also common. CSF pressure and glucose concentration are usually normal. The CSF is clear, but a slight lymphocytic pleocytosis and a slight increase in the protein concentration may occur. Eosinophilic meningitis has been reported.

The diagnosis is made on the basis of the development of the characteristic rash and other symptoms of the disease after exposure to ticks. Clinical distinction from typhus fever may be impossible. The onset of the rash in distal parts of the limbs favors a diagnosis of RMSF. In rare instances, however, neurologic signs may occur before the rash appears.

Diagnosis of RMSF is best performed by indirect immunofluorescence assay (IFA) with *R. rickettsii* antigen performed on two-paired serum samples to demonstrate a significant (fourfold) rise in antibody titers. The first titer, taken in the first week of the disease, will typically be very low or absent. After 2 to 4 weeks, those with disease should have a fourfold rise in antibody titer. Immunoglobulin (Ig) G titers are more specific than IgM. Unfortunately, because the organism is an obligate intercellular bacterium which resides in the endothelial cells, blood for polymerase chain reaction (PCR) is typically low yield. Nonspecific testing including blood work may demonstrate a leukocytosis (with left shift), thrombocytopenia, hyponatremia, and elevated liver function tests. In patients with neurologic involvement, CSF may be normal but may also develop a lymphocytic or neutrophilic pleocytosis (1 to 200 WBC) and a mild to moderate protein elevated in 30% to 50%. Neuroimaging is nonspecific with cerebral or spinal cord edema, white matter lesions, and at times microhemorrhages.

Treatment

Doxycycline 100 mg twice a day for 7 to 14 days is the first-line treatment for adults and children of all ages and should be initiated immediately whenever RMSF is suspected.

Tetracycline 500 mg four times a day can also be used. There may be value to ciprofloxacin or chloramphenicol in patients unable to tolerate tetracycline or doxycycline. In children, chloramphenicol is the alternative to doxycycline to avoid tooth discoloration caused by tetracyclines. Any patient seriously considered to have RMSF should be treated promptly while diagnostic tests proceed.

Other spotted fever group rickettsiae in the United States that rarely cause an RMSF picture are *Rickettsia akari* (causes rickettsialpox), *Rickettsia parkeri* (eschars and a maculopapular or vesiculopapular rash), and *Rickettsia felis* (cat fleas). Except for some variation in their incubation times, the pathology and clinical picture are similar to those of RMSF. All such infections respond to tetracyclines (doxycycline) or chloramphenicol.

Outcome

There has been a dramatic fall in the mortality rate, decreasing from 28% in 1944 to less than 1% in 2001. In patients who recover, the fever is over by the end of the third week, although mild cases may become afebrile before the end of the second week. Convalescence may be slow, and neurologic sequelae may persist for several months. Long-term prognosis depends on the severity of the infection, host factors (e.g., age, the presence of other illness), and the promptness with which antimicrobial treatment is started.

EPIDEMIC TYPHUS

Three types of infection with rickettsiae of the typhus group are recognized: primary louse-borne epidemic typhus; its recrudescent form, Brill–Zinsser disease; and flea-borne endemic murine typhus.

Epidemiology

Since its recognition in the 16th century, typhus has been known as one of the great epidemic diseases of the world. It is especially prevalent in times of war or whenever there is a massing of people in camps, prisons, or ships.

Epidemic typhus (caused by *Rickettsia prowazekii*) is spread among humans by the human body louse (*Pediculus humanus corporis*). Outbreaks of epidemic typhus last occurred in the United States in the 19th century. Freedom from lice explains the absence of epidemics in the United States. Sporadic cases in the United States have been associated with flying squirrel contact. The location of epidemic disease is now limited to the Balkans, the Middle East, North Africa, Asia, Russia, and the Andes. All age groups are affected.

Rickettsiae may remain viable for as long as 20 years in the tissues of recovered patients without manifesting symptoms. Brill–Zinsser disease is a recrudescence of epidemic typhus that occurs years after the initial attack and may cause a new epidemic.

Murine typhus (*Rickettsia typhi*) is worldwide in distribution and is spread to humans by fleas. In the United States, the disease is most prevalent in southeastern and Gulf Coast states and southern California, among individuals whose occupations bring them into rat-infested areas. The disease is most common in the late summer and fall months.

Diagnosis

A presumptive diagnosis of typhus fever may be made on the basis of the characteristic skin rash and signs of involvement of the nervous system. The diagnosis is established by serology. Antibodies to specific rickettsiae may be detected.

Clinical Manifestations

The course of typhus fever usually extends over 2 to 3 weeks. Death from epidemic typhus usually occurs between the 9th and 18th day of illness. In patients who recover, the temperature begins to fall after 14 to 18 days and reaches normal levels in 2 to 4 days. Complications include bronchitis and bronchopneumonia; myocardial disease; gangrene of the skin or limbs; and thrombosis of large abdominal, pulmonary, or cerebral vessels. Common neurologic manifestations include confusion, drowsiness, seizures, focal deficits, and coma.

Treatment

Treatment is with doxycycline, clarithromycin, or chloramphenicol, as with RMSF.

Outcome

The prognosis of epidemic typhus depends on the patient's age and immunization status. The disease is usually mild in children younger than 10 years. After the third decade, mortality increases steadily with each decade. Death is usually due to the development of pneumonia, circulatory collapse, and renal failure. The mortality rate for murine typhus in the United States is low (<1%). There are no neurologic residua in patients who recover.

SCRUB TYPHUS

Scrub typhus is an infectious disease caused by *Orientia tsutsugamushi* (previously called *Rickettsia tsutsugamushi*), which is transmitted to humans by the bite of larval trombiculid mites (chiggers). It resembles the other rickettsial diseases and is characterized by sudden onset of fever, cutaneous eruption, and the presence of an ulcerative lesion (eschar) at the site of attachment of the chigger.

Epidemiology

The disease is limited to eastern and southeastern Asia, India, and northern Australia and adjacent islands.

Clinical Manifestations

The disease begins abruptly after an incubation period of 10 to 12 days, with fever, chills, and headache. The headache increases in intensity and may become severe. Conjunctival congestion, moderate generalized lymphadenopathy, deafness, apathy, and anorexia are common symptoms. In one series, meningitis and encephalitis occurred in 15%. Delirium, coma, restlessness, and muscular twitchings are also present in severe cases. A primary lesion (the eschar) is seen in nearly all cases and represents the former site of attachment of the infected mite. There may be multiple eschars. The cutaneous rash appears between the fifth and eighth day of the disease. The eruption is macular or maculopapular and nonhemorrhagic. The trunk is involved first with later extension to the limbs.

Diagnosis

The diagnosis is made on the basis of the development of typical symptoms, the presence of the characteristic eschar, and serology. Sensitive PCR techniques are becoming available. Elevation of hepatic enzymes and creatinine as well as thrombocytopenia is common with severe illness.

Treatment and Outcome

In patients who recover, body temperature begins to fall at the end of the second or third week. Permanent residua are not common, but the period of convalescence may extend over several months. In fatal cases, death usually occurs in the second or third week as a result of pneumonia, cardiac failure, or cerebral involvement. In the preantibiotic era, mortality could reach 60% depending on geographic locale and virulence of the strain. Deaths are rare with appropriate antibiotic treatment, which is similar to the treatment for RMSF (doxycycline).

EHRLICHIOSIS AND ANAPLASMOSIS

Ehrlichiosis or anaplasmosis are tick-borne diseases with the preponderance of disease occurring in the summer months. They are small, gram-negative, obligate intracellular bacteria that infect leukocytes. Three forms of human infection have been identified in the United States. One species, *Ehrlichia chaffeensis*, is associated with human monocytotropic ehrlichiosis (HME), and the organism may be preferentially found in these cells. Human granulocytotropic ehrlichiosis (HGE) is also referred to as *human granulocytotropic anaplasmosis* (HGA). HGE is caused by *Anaplasma phagocytophilum*. Both human infections are detectable in the appropriate cells as coccobacillary forms. It has become possible to cultivate the organisms, and PCR reactions are increasingly available. Most diagnostic studies still rely on antibody detection. HME is transmitted by *Amblyomma americanum* (lone star tick) and possibly other ticks, whereas HGE is transmitted by ixodid ticks and probably *D. andersoni*. A third agent, *Ehrlichia ewingii*, causes canine granulocytic ehrlichiosis. It is transmitted by *A. americanum*.

Epidemiology

The epidemiologic range for both agents appears to be extending. In 2010, Unites States cases attributed to *E. chaffeensis* declined almost 22% (944 to 740 cases), whereas those cases attributed to *A. phagocytophilum* increased by 52% (1,161 to 1,761 cases). HME is more common in the states in the South and Southeast region, whereas HGE was first found in the Midwest. Now, cases are regularly reported from New England, all Atlantic Coast states, south-central states, and California. Coinfection of HGE with *Borrelia burgdorferi* and HME with RMSF has been reported. *E. ewingii* is found in south-central, southeastern, mid-Atlantic, and coastal states.

Clinical Manifestations

Infection usually presents as a febrile, systemic process often associated with myalgia and headache. CNS complications occur in 20% to 35% of infected patients. Changes in mental status, meningitis, meningoencephalitis, seizures, cranial nerve palsies, and ataxia have also been noted and are correlated with more serious illness. Cardiac and respiratory failure can occur. Rashes have been reported in about 20% of cases. This makes it difficult to distinguish the illness from RMSF, whose distribution overlaps with *E. chaffeensis*. *E. ewingii* is more likely to occur in immunocompromised hosts. Children tend to have more severe disease.

Diagnosis

Because of the nonspecific nature of the symptoms and signs, a high index of suspicion is required. A history of exposure to ticks may be helpful, but epidemiologic studies have shown that serologic evidence of infection usually is not correlated with known tick bites. Lymphopenia is often a feature of *E. chaffeensis* infection, whereas granulocytopenia is usually noted with the HGE infection. Thrombocytopenia and leukopenia are seen with *E. ewingii* infection. Elevated hepatic enzymes are usually present. Microscopic blood examination with a Wright–Giemsa stain may reveal the classic intraleukocytic morula. CSF pleocytosis and an increased protein concentration have been reported and appear to correlate with altered mental status. The most widely available diagnostic test remains a fourfold rise in antibody titer. Confirmation of the diagnosis can be attained by immunofluorescent detection of the intracellular organisms. PCR is available for both HME and HGA, although this test has yet to be standardized and not always readily available. Culturing of the causative organisms is now also possible but is not as sensitive as PCR.

Treatment and Outcome

Complete understanding of the course of ehrlichiosis has yet to be achieved. Initially, a high proportion of reported cases was fatal in both HME and HGE. However, serologic studies indicate that asymptomatic or minor infections are common. Currently reported case fatality rates are 3% to 10%. Clinically, it has also been found that some cases may be self-limited even without treatment. Treatment with doxycycline 100 mg twice a day for 7 days often results in rapid improvement. Therefore, prognosis seems to be good if accurate diagnosis is made and treatment started promptly.

BRUCELLOSIS

Brucellosis (undulant fever) is a disease with protean manifestations, resulting from infection with short, slender, rod-shaped, gram-negative microorganisms of the genus *Brucella*. The infection is transmitted to humans from animals (cattle, pigs, sheep, goats, and others). The illness is prone to occur in slaughterhouse workers, livestock producers, veterinarians, and persons who ingest unpasteurized milk or milk products.

PATHOBIOLOGY

The two major species that can infect humans are *Brucella suis* from swine and *Brucella abortus* from cattle. Inoculation is via the skin, inhalation, or ingestion. It is a slow-growing organism having an incubation time of up to 2 to 3 weeks.

CLINICAL MANIFESTATIONS

There is a broad clinical spectrum from asymptomatic to fatal disease. An acute, febrile illness is characteristic of the early stages of the disease. The common symptoms include chills, night sweats, fever, weakness, and generalized malaise; 70% of patients experience body aches and nearly 50% complain of headache. Other symptoms on presentation can include anorexia, nausea and vomiting, arthritis, endocarditis, malodorous sweat, or orchitis. Early constitutional symptoms are followed by the subacute and chronic stages in about 15% to 20% of patients with localized infection of the bones, joints, lungs, kidneys, liver, lymph nodes, and other organs. Neurologic complications have been reported in up to 25% but are more likely much less common occurring in about 5% of cases. These complications can include meningitis, encephalitis, myelitis, radiculitis, neuritis, and meningovasculitis. Nonspecific neurologic signs and symptoms may include seizures, cranial neuropathies, gait disturbances, hemiparesis and hemisensory disturbance, and mental status changes.

DIAGNOSIS

Diagnosis is made with culture. This is a slow-growing organism and may take up to 30 days to grow. Blood, CSF, or bone marrow can be cultured. Additionally, PCR may be helpful. Screening blood work may demonstrate a pancytopenia. Lumbar puncture may reveal a mildly increased opening pressure and a lymphocytic pleocytosis (<500 WBC), slightly elevated protein, and a small decrease in the glucose concentration. The CSF has increased gamma globulin levels and often contains *Brucella*-agglutinating antibodies. Neuroimaging may demonstrate white matter changes in the brain, particularly in a periventricular distribution. These white matter lesions are seen best with fluid-attenuated inversion recovery (FLAIR) sequences and can enhance with gadolinium.

TREATMENT AND OUTCOME

Treatment likely requires multiple antibiotics for multiple months, although there has been success with monotherapy with doxycycline 100 mg orally (PO) twice a day (b.i.d.) for 45 days, with fewer recurrences than a 30-day course [Level 1].[1] Treatment of systemic disease is with doxycycline plus an aminoglycoside (intramuscular streptomycin or intravenous [IV] gentamicin), rifampin, or ofloxacin [Level 1].[2,3] Trimethoprim/sulfisoxazole is an alternative to the tetracyclines. Neurologic disease is treated with triple therapy with the addition of trimethoprim–sulfamethoxazole or ceftriaxone to one of the aforementioned regimens.

ANTHRAX

Bacillus anthracis is a large endospore-forming, aerobic, gram-positive nonmotile bacterium that produces a black, eschar-like cutaneous lesion after cutaneous inoculation.

EPIDEMIOLOGY

Anthrax is primarily a disease of herbivores; however, it causes cutaneous lesions as well as respiratory and gastrointestinal infections in humans. Anthrax is one of the oldest documented infectious diseases. It may have caused two Egyptian plagues in 1491 BC. Inhalational anthrax occurred in England in the 19th century as woolsorter's disease, and in Germany, it became known as *ragpicker's disease* as a result of the infection of mill workers with anthrax spores from contaminated fibers from goats. Prior to the 2001 bioterrorism-related outbreak of 11 inhalational cases and 12 suspected or confirmed cases of cutaneous anthrax, there had been only 18 sporadic cases total in the United States during the 20th century, with the last case in 1976. Therefore, other than bioterrorist attacks or laboratory accidents, the populations most at risk for anthrax are individuals who work closely with domesticated animals. Countries such as Turkey have much higher incidences of anthrax than the United States.

CLINICAL MANIFESTATIONS

Anthrax meningitis can be acquired via the cutaneous or the inhalation route. Infection via cutaneous inoculation is most common, comprising upwards of 90% of cases. Inhalation accounts for only 5% of cases. *B. anthracis* CNS complications follow skin or inhalation of the spores by 3 days to a week. Meningitis develops as a result of lymphohematogenous spread from the primary lesions. The disease is primarily a hemorrhagic meningoencephalitis and is fulminant and rapidly progressive.

DIAGNOSIS

The CSF profile is typical of meningitis, with thousands of WBC (neutrophilic), low-glucose, and high-protein concentration. Red blood cells in large numbers are seen in the CSF as well as gram-positive organisms. Computed tomography (CT) and magnetic resonance imaging (MRI) may demonstrate leptomeningeal enhancement and parenchymal or subarachnoid blood and may show basal ganglia enhancement.

TREATMENT AND OUTCOME

Although the cutaneous forms of anthrax can be self-limiting, the hemorrhagic meningoencephalitis has a near 100% mortality rate. Treatment of the meningitis should include a fluoroquinolone plus one or two additional agents with good CSF penetration such as penicillin or ampicillin, meropenem, rifampicin, or vancomycin. Corticosteroids should be considered in cases with severe cerebral edema.

BARTONELLA

Bartonella henselae, the etiologic agent for catscratch disease (CSD), is a motile, flagellated, gram-negative, intracellular bacterium that is related to *Brucella* and *Rickettsia*. As the name suggests, this agent is common in cats. There is a bacteremia in close to 70% of infected cats. In up to 90% of human disease, there is a history of exposure to cats.

EPIDEMIOLOGY

The disease in humans is globally endemic, most common in autumn and winter in the United States. Children and young adults are most likely to contract CSD. The disease is likely spread to humans via scratches of domestic or feral cats, particularly kittens. There is also some evidence that suggests that CSD may be transmitted directly to humans by the bite of infected cat fleas, although this has not been proven. Incidence is in the range of 9 to 10 per 100,000 in the United States with 2% to 4% developing encephalopathy (500 to 1,000 cases per year) in the United States.

CLINICAL MANIFESTATIONS

The clinical syndrome of CSD typically begins with a papule or pustule developing at the scratch site approximately 1 week after contact with a cat (usually a kitten). This progresses over the course of 1 to 7 weeks to a painful regional lymphadenopathy. Fever, sometimes relapsing, malaise, fatigue, and headache are common systemic signs and symptoms. In the rare case where encephalopathy develops, this typically follows the painful adenopathy. Of those that advance to CNS disease, 50% to 80% can present with focal or generalized seizures or status epilepticus. Focal deficits such as aphasia, hemiplegia, cranial nerve palsies, ataxia, delirium, and coma can also occur. Ocular findings such as neuroretinitis, optic neuritis, and papillitis can also be commonly seen.

DIAGNOSIS

IFA testing and enzyme-linked immunosorbent assay (ELISA) are used to detect serum antibody to *B. henselae*. A titer greater than 1:64 suggests recent *Bartonella* infection. A fourfold or greater increase (6 weeks later) is confirmatory. The IFA shows cross-reactivity between *Bartonella* species, Epstein–Barr virus, cytomegalovirus, *Toxoplasma gondii*, and *Streptococcus pyogenes*. About 84% of patients have positive titers within 1 to 2 weeks of clinical CSD, and 16% develop positive titers 4 to 8 weeks later. Nonspecific findings include a peripheral leukocytosis and CSF with a mild lymphocytic pleocytosis and elevated protein concentration (seen in only about one-third of patients). Less than 20% of patients with CNS CSD have neuroimaging findings. Those that have been reported have included cerebral white matter lesions, basal ganglia and thalamic lesions, and rarely, cortical lesions.

TREATMENT AND OUTCOME

CSD is usually self-limited, resolving in 2 to 4 months. It is unclear as to the best treatment for CSD. Many cases including those with CNS involvement are self-limited and require no antibiotic treatment. Most studies of antibiotic treatment are retrospective and small. A randomized controlled trial using azithromycin demonstrated efficacy in reducing lymph node size [**Level 1**].[4] Other antibiotics that have shown efficacy in retrospective studies include doxycycline, rifampin, trimethoprim–sulfamethoxazole, and ciprofloxacin. Prognosis is typically good, although some with CNS involvement may develop epilepsy and cognitive deficits.

WHIPPLE DISEASE

Tropheryma whipplei is a rod-shaped, gram-positive bacterium. It was finally isolated in eukaryotic cells in the year 2000 and propagated in culture at 37°C but was believed to resist culturing for a long time. Now it is known that it can only be cultured if part of its eukaryotic host is present.

EPIDEMIOLOGY

T. whipplei is believed to have an environmental derivation because its closest known relatives, Actinobacteria, originated from the soil. However, *T. whipplei* actually is completely dependent on humans for growth. Whipple disease is caused by *T. whipplei*. This is a rare disease, and although there is no current estimate on its incidence, there are only about 1,000 cases reported in the literature. Classic Whipple disease is most common in middle-aged white men, although it can affect any sex, age, and race.

CLINICAL MANIFESTATIONS

The signs and symptoms of classic disease are primarily gastrointestinal. The disease has a prodromal stage with a wide variety of nonspecific symptoms and also arthralgias and arthritis. After the prodromal stage comes the steady-state stage. The time between the stages can be quite long, averaging 6 years. In the steady-state stage, diarrhea and weight loss are the classic symptoms. Neurologic involvement occurs in 6% to 63% of patients with classic Whipple disease. The most common signs and symptoms of CNS Whipple are alterations in cognition and supranuclear gaze palsy, myoclonus, ataxia, hypothalamic dysfunction, and altered level of consciousness. Abnormal movement of the eye muscles, termed *oculomasticatory* or *oculofacioskeletal myorhythmia*, is considered pathognomonic for Whipple disease. Isolated CNS Whipple disease (without gastrointestinal involvement) has been reported in 32 patients. In these cases, the disease progression is more fulminant, with about a third dying from the disease (vs. about 25% with classic Whipple with CNS involvement).

DIAGNOSIS

Laboratory workup for Whipple disease should include routine blood work. Although nonspecific, many with the disease have acute-phase reactants, anemia, leukocytosis, thrombocytosis, and evidence of malnutrition. Thrombocytopenia and eosinophilia have also been reported. The classic diagnostic test is periodic acid–Schiff (PAS) staining of small-bowel biopsy specimens, which on light microscopy shows magenta-stained inclusions within macrophages of the lamina propria. There is also a PCR test for *T. whipplei*, which should be used in conjunction with the PAS staining.

TREATMENT AND OUTCOME

Treatment for CNS Whipple disease is long-term antibiotic treatment (up to a year). Antibiotics that have had some success with classic Whipple disease include tetracycline, penicillin, trimethoprim–sulfamethoxazole, and ceftriaxone. There have never been any randomized trials, however. Based on in vitro data, a potential regimen for CNS Whipple disease is doxycycline and hydroxychloroquine plus a high dose of sulfamethoxazole or sulfadiazine. Chronic neurologic sequelae are common with CNS involvement.

MYCOPLASMA PNEUMONIAE

Mycoplasmas, originally called *pleuropneumonia-like organisms*, lack a cell wall. Individual mycoplasmas are bound by a unit membrane that encloses the cytoplasm, DNA, RNA, and other cellular components. They are the smallest free-living organisms and are resistant to penicillin and other cell wall–active antimicrobials. Of mycoplasmas that infect humans, *Mycoplasma pneumoniae* is the only species that has been clearly shown to be a significant cause of disease.

PATHOBIOLOGY

M. pneumoniae is spread from person to person by infected respiratory droplets. It is a major cause of acute respiratory disease, including pneumonia. Prior to neurologic involvement, an antecedent respiratory illness often occurs. A variety of neurologic conditions has been described *in association with M. pneumoniae* infection: meningitis, encephalitis, postinfectious leukoencephalitis, acute cerebellar ataxia, transverse myelitis, ascending polyneuritis, radiculopathy, cranial neuropathy, and acute psychosis. The most common neurologic condition appears to be meningoencephalitis with alterations in mental status that is a parainfectious immune-mediated disorder rather than infectious disorder. The neurologic features associated with *M. pneumoniae* infection, however, are so diverse that the correct diagnosis may not be made on clinical grounds alone. MRI is usually normal. Focal or diffuse edema is occasionally seen. If postinfectious demyelinating encephalitis occurs, white matter lesions will be seen on FLAIR and T2 images. The CSF usually contains polymorphonuclear leukocytes and mononuclear cells in varying proportions. The CSF has normal or mildly elevated protein concentration and a normal glucose concentration. Bacterial, viral, and mycoplasma cultures of the CSF are usually sterile.

DIAGNOSIS

Retrospective diagnosis may be made by cold isohemagglutinins for human type O erythrocytes. These may be detected in about 50% of patients during the second week of illness; they are the first antibodies to disappear. Specific antibodies may also be demonstrated by enzyme immunoassay and are more accurate. PCR is now being used to on blood and CSF.

TREATMENT AND OUTCOME

Doxycycline (not in children) and the macrolides azithromycin and clarithromycin are the drugs of choice for *M. pneumoniae* infections. It appears that corticosteroids may be beneficial along with antibiotics in severe cases that may be postinfectious. There are no controlled studies.

LEGIONELLA PNEUMOPHILA

Legionella pneumophila is a poorly staining gram-negative bacterium that either does not grow or grows very slowly on most artificial media. The organism was first isolated from fatal cases of pneumonia among persons attending an American Legion Convention in Philadelphia in 1976. The bacterium is acquired by inhalation of contaminated aerosols or dust from air-conditioning systems, water, or soil.

CLINICAL MANIFESTATIONS

Pneumonia is the most typical systemic manifestation of infection. Upper respiratory infection, a severe influenza-like syndrome (Pontiac fever), and gastrointestinal disease may also occur. Several neurologic conditions have been described in association with *L. pneumophila* infection (Legionnaires disease or legionellosis): acute encephalomyelitis, severe cerebellar ataxia, chorea, and peripheral neuropathy. Confusion, delirium, and hallucinations are common symptoms. The pathophysiology of these syndromes is unclear because bacteria have rarely been demonstrated in

the CNS. Myoglobinuria and elevated serum creatine kinase levels also have been reported.

DIAGNOSIS

L. pneumophila is rarely recovered from pleural fluid, sputum, or blood; it frequently may be isolated from respiratory secretions by transtracheal aspiration or bronchoalveolar lavage and lung biopsy tissue. Urinary antigen detection methods appear to be very sensitive. A retrospective diagnosis may be made by a significant rise in specific serum antibodies. The CSF, CT, and MRI are usually normal. The electroencephalograph frequently reveals diffuse slowing.

TREATMENT AND OUTCOME

The treatment of choice is azithromycin or clarithromycin. Quinolones (levofloxacin) are equally effective. Relapses are uncommon if treatment is continued for 14 days. When relapses occur, they usually respond to a second course of the antibiotic. The true incidence of neurologic involvement in Legionnaires disease is still unknown. The neurologic deficit is known to be reversible, but little exact information about recovery is available.

BACTERIAL TOXINS: DIPHTHERIA, TETANUS, AND BOTULISM

Clostridium tetani, *Clostridium botulinum*, and *Corynebacterium diphtheriae* each produce toxins that affect the nervous system. In the case of *Corynebacterium diphtheriae*, the toxin produced causes a peripheral (cranial nerve) neuropathy, the toxin of *Clostridium botulinum* affects the neuromuscular junction, and that of *Clostridium tetani* affects the CNS.

DIPHTHERIA

C. diphtheriae is a nonmotile, noncapsulated, club-shaped, gram-positive bacillus. Diphtheria is most commonly an infection of the upper respiratory tract and causes fever, sore throat, and malaise. A thick, gray-green fibrin membrane, the pseudomembrane, often forms over the site(s) of infection as a result of the combined effects of bacterial growth, toxin production, necrosis of underlying tissue, and the host immune response. Recognition that the systemic organ damage was due to the action of diphtheria toxin led to the development of both an effective antitoxin-based therapy for acute infection and a highly successful toxoid vaccine.

The exotoxin of *C. diphtheriae* inhibits protein synthesis in mammalian cells by inactivation of transfer RNA (tRNA) translocase. It is composed of two segments: one necessary for binding to the cell and a shorter portion that then is cleaved and enters the cell. The specificity of the exotoxin for heart and peripheral nerve is attributed to receptor-binding affinity at the cell surface. The development of neuropathy is proportional to the severity of the primary infection. In the pharyngeal infections, palatal and pharyngo–laryngo–esophageal paralysis are early and prominent features. Other than these manifestations and the common ciliary paralysis, the resistance of other cranial nerves and the brain to these effects is unexplained.

BOTULISM

Botulism is a rare and potentially fatal paralytic illness caused by a toxin produced by the bacteria *C. botulinum*. The most common mode of transmission is ingestion of toxic spores produced by the bacteria in contaminated food.

Pathobiology

C. botulinum is a large, usually gram-positive strictly anaerobic bacillus, which forms a subterminal spore. The species is divided into four physiologic groups. Each strain produce slightly different toxins. A single strain almost always produces only one toxin type. *C. botulinum* spores are found worldwide and inhabit soil samples and marine sediments. These spores are able to tolerate 100°C at 1 atm for several hours; because boiling renders solutions more anaerobic, it may actually favor the growth of *C. botulinum*. Proper preparation of food in a pressure cooker (>1 atm) will kill spores. Botulinum toxin is synthesized as a single polypeptide chain of low potency. It is then nicked by a bacterial protease to produce two chains, with the light chain constituting approximately one-third of the total mass. The nicked toxin type A is, on a molecular weight basis, the most potent toxin found in nature. In contrast to the spores, high temperatures destroy the toxin. Once present at the synapse, the toxin ultimately prevents the release of acetylcholine. The toxin enters the cell by receptor-mediated endocytosis. The result is that stimulation of the presynaptic cell (e.g., the alpha motor neuron) fails to produce transmitter release, thus producing paralysis in the motor system or autonomic dysfunction when parasympathetic nerve terminals or autonomic ganglia are involved. The toxins only affect the free proteins; once vesicular and synaptic proteins have formed a complex to cause transmitter release, they are not subject to attack. Once damaged, the synapse is permanently affected. The recovery of function requires sprouting of the presynaptic axon and the subsequent formation of a new synapse.

In food-borne botulism, toxin is ingested with the food in which it was produced. It is absorbed primarily in the duodenum and jejunum and passes into the bloodstream by which it reaches peripheral cholinergic synapses (including the neuromuscular junction). In cases of wound botulism, spores are introduced into a wound, where they germinate and produce toxin. Infant botulism, and probably adult botulism of unknown etiology, follows ingestion of spores, with subsequent bacterial colonization of the small intestine. Gastric acid–lowering agents and antibiotic use may predispose to gastrointestinal colonization with *C. botulinum*.

Clinical Manifestations

The clinical manifestations of botulism depend on the type of toxin produced, rather than the site of its production. The classic presentation of botulism is that of a patient who develops acute, bilateral cranial neuropathies associated with symmetric descending weakness. *Food-borne* botulism usually develops between 12 and 36 hours after toxin ingestion. The initial complaints are nausea and a dry mouth and sometimes diarrhea. Cranial nerve dysfunction most commonly starts with the eyes, including blurred vision due to pupillary dilation (reflecting parasympathetic dysfunction) or diplopia (reflecting dysfunction of nerves III, IV, or VI). Pupils are either dilated or unreactive in less than 50% of patients. The absence of these signs in no way diminishes the likelihood of botulism. Lower cranial nerve dysfunction manifests as dysphagia, dysarthria, and hypoglossal weakness. Weakness then spreads to the upper extremities, the trunk, and the lower extremities. Respiratory dysfunction and failure may result from either upper airway obstruction from a weakened glottis or diaphragmatic weakness. Autonomic problems may include gastrointestinal dysfunction, alterations in resting heart rate, loss of responsiveness to hypotension or postural change, hypothermia, or urinary retention, although these are not usually as common or severe as that seen in tetanus. Recovery may not begin for up to 100 days.

Infantile botulism presents with constipation, which may be followed by feeding difficulties, hypotonia, increased drooling, and a weak cry (see also Chapter 136). Upper airway obstruction may be the initial sign and is the major indication for intubation. In severe cases, the condition progresses to include cranial neuropathies and respiratory weakness, with ventilatory failure occurring in about 50% of diagnosed patients. The condition progresses for 1 to 2 weeks and then stabilizes for another 2 to 3 weeks before recovery starts.

Wound botulism lacks the prodromal gastrointestinal disorder of the food-borne form but is otherwise similar in presentation. Fever, if present, reflects wound infection rather than botulism. The wound itself may rarely appear to be healing well while neurologic manifestations are occurring. The incubation period varies from 4 to 14 days.

Diagnosis

Laboratory evaluation includes anaerobic cultures and toxin assays of serum, stool, and the implicated food if available. Confirmation and toxin typing is obtained in almost 75% of cases. Early cases are more likely to be diagnosed by the toxin assay, whereas those studied later in the disease are more likely to have a positive culture than a positive toxin assay. Specimens should be obtained and sent in consultation with the appropriate officials (in the United States, the Centers for Disease Control and Prevention [CDC]). Toxin excretion may continue up to 1 month after the onset of illness, and stool cultures may remain positive for a similar period.

Electrophysiologic studies reveals normal nerve conduction velocities; the amplitude of compound muscle action potentials is reduced in 85% of cases, although not all motor units may demonstrate this abnormality. Repetitive nerve stimulation at high rates (≥20 Hz, compared with the 4 Hz rate employed in the diagnosis of myasthenia gravis) may reveal a small increment in the motor response.

Management

Patients who receive appropriate airway and ventilator management should recover unless there are other complications (see Chapter 116). There have been increasing survival rates in patients with botulism that follow the improvement in critical care medicine, particularly in the arena of ventilatory support. The decision to intubate is similar to most cases of neuromuscular respiratory failure (i.e., Guillain–Barré, myasthenia gravis) and should be based on (1) assessment of upper airway competency and (2) changes in vital capacity (in general, <12 mL/kg or a rapidly declining vital capacity suggests the need to intubate). Do not wait for the PCO_2 to rise or the oxygen saturation to fall before intubating the patient. If contaminated food may still reside in the gastrointestinal tract, purgatives may be useful unless ileus has occurred, in which case gastric lavage may prove valuable. Patients should be given botulinum antitoxin. In the United States, equine bivalent (A and B) antitoxin is available from the CDC or some state health departments. Monovalent type E antitoxin should be added when type E exposure is suspected. The role of antibiotic treatment is untested, but penicillin G, 10 to 20 million units daily, is frequently recommended. Metronidazole may be an effective alternative. The use of local antibiotics, such as penicillin G or metronidazole, may be helpful in eradicating *C. botulinum* in wound botulism. Antibiotic use, however, is not recommended for infant botulism because cell death and lysis may result in the release of more toxin. Aminoglycoside antibiotics and tetracyclines, in particular, may increase the degree of neuromuscular blockade by impairing neuronal calcium entry. This effect has not been reported in adult cases but should be considered when gastrointestinal botulism is encountered.

TETANUS

Tetanus is an infectious toxidrome characterized by a prolonged contraction of skeletal muscles. The syndrome is caused by *tetanospasmin*, a toxin produced by *Clostridium tetani*. *C tetani* is a slender, obligately anaerobic bacillus and although it is classified as a gram-positive organism, it may stain variably, especially in tissue or older cultures. Most strains are slightly motile and they have abundant flagellae during growth. The mature organism loses its flagellae and forms a spherical terminal spore, producing a profile such as that of a tennis racket.

Pathobiology

Tetanospasmin spores resist extremes of temperature and moisture, are stable at atmospheric oxygen tension, and can survive indefinitely and are viable after exposure to ethanol, phenol, or formalin. Death of the spores can be accomplished by exposure to 100°C for 4 hours, autoclaving at 121°C, and 103 kPa (15 psi) for 15 minutes or with exposure to iodine, glutaraldehyde, or hydrogen peroxide. Spores can be isolated from animal feces and therefore are ubiquitous in the environment. The spores of *C. tetani* will germinate and the bacteria proliferate when the oxygen tension of the tissue is low. Once growing, two exotoxins are produced: tetanospasmin and tetanolysin. Tetanospasmin, or "tetanus toxin," is felt to cause all the typical clinical manifestations of tetanus. It is synthesized as a single 151-kDa (1315 amino acid) chain. This molecule is then cleaved by a bacterial protease into a heavy chain and a light chain connected by a disulfide bridge. The disulfide bridge is necessary for the activity of the toxin. The DNA for this polypeptide resides on a single plasmid; strains of *C. tetani*, which do not have this plasmid, have no toxogenic properties.

Tetanospasmin inhibits neurotransmitter release at the presynaptic nerve terminal and this is what accounts for the clinical presentation of tetanus. The toxin first binds to the presynaptic membrane and then must pass through the cell membrane and into the cytoplasm. Once in the cytoplasm of the presynaptic terminal, tetanospasmin inactivates synaptobrevin, a neuronal protein that "docks" the neurotransmitter filled vesicle to the membrane. Because synaptobrevin is inactivated, the vesicle is unable to fuse with the membrane and neurotransmitter cannot be released. Tetanospasmin travels via retrograde transport back to the cell body and can then cross several orders of synaptically connected neurons. This process allows the toxin to move from the neuromuscular junction of alpha motor neurons to the spinal cord and ultimately to the brain. This explains the effects of tetanospasmin on the neuromuscular junction, autonomic function, and the CNS. Tetanospasmin also is hematogenously spread but ultimately must still enter the nervous system via neurons and retrograde transport.

Once transported to the spinal cord, tetanospasmin primarily affects the inhibitory neurons. These inhibitory neurons use either glycine or γ-aminobutyric acid (GABA) as neurotransmitters. Without these neurons, the motor neuron increases its firing rate, ultimately causing rigidity of the muscle innervated by this neuron. More clinically relevant is the fact that without this inhibition, the normal inhibition of antagonist muscles is impaired, and in response to movement or stimulation, the characteristic tetanic spasm occurs.

Clinical Manifestations

Tetanus is classified into four clinical types: generalized, localized, cephalic, and neonatal. These four clinical subtypes represent the site of toxin action either predominantly at the neuromuscular junction or inhibition in the CNS. Incubation time (the time from spore inoculation to first symptoms) for all clinical types depends on severity and distance of injury or inoculum site to the CNS, with more severe disease developing more quickly and mild disease taking longer.

Generalized tetanus is the most commonly recognized form of the disease with trismus, or lockjaw, as the most common presenting sign. Trismus is caused by rigidity of the masseter muscles that in turn prevent the opening of the mouth. The more severe it is, the smaller the opening between the upper and lower jaw. Trismus results in a facial expression called *risus sardonicus*, which consists of lateral extension of the corners of the mouth, raised eyelids, and wrinkling of the forehead. These facial features may at times be subtle. Involvement of other muscle groups can then follow the onset of trismus, first the neck, then the thorax and abdomen, and finally the extremities.

Tetanospasms, or generalized spasms that superficially resemble opisthotonos, decerebrate posturing, or seizures are elicited by either external or internal stimuli. Because full consciousness is retained, the spasms are extremely painful. This maintenance of consciousness helps to differentiate them from seizures or decerebrate posturing. Respiratory compromise, due to spasm of the glottis, diaphragm, or abdominal muscles, is the most serious early problem in generalized tetanus.

Later in the illness, defects in autonomic dysfunction, usually as manifested by increased sympathetic tone, are frequently noted in patients with severe tetanus. Autonomic dysfunction is now the leading cause of death in tetanus patients. It is characterized by labile hypertension (and sometimes hypotension) and tachycardia, arrhythmias, peripheral vascular constriction, diaphoresis, pyrexia, increased carbon dioxide output, and increased urinary catecholamine excretion. The progression of the disease may last for 10 to 14 days. This reflects the time it takes for the toxin to be transported to the CNS. Recovery may take 4 weeks or more. Without antitoxin, the disease persists for as long as the toxin is produced, and because toxin is produced in insufficient quantities to stimulate an immune response, recurrent tetanus is documented.

Neonatal tetanus is a generalized form of the disease and is far more common in underdeveloped countries than in the developed world. It is the leading cause of neonatal mortality in many parts of the world, and of the diseases which can be vaccinated against, it is second only to measles as a cause of childhood death. It usually follows an infection of the umbilical stump, often because of improper wound care. A lack of maternal immunity to tetanus is also necessary for the development of this disease. The incubation period is anywhere between 1 to 10 days postpartum. The infants usually present with weakness, irritability, and inability to suck. Tetanic spasms occur later, and the opisthotonic posturing can be confused with neonatal seizures or other metabolic or congenital abnormalities which cause posturing in this age group. The hypersympathetic state described earlier is also common and is frequently the cause of death. The mortality rate is up to 90% and developmental retardation is common in those who survive.

Localized and *cephalic* tetanus is characterized by fixed rigidity of the muscles at or near the site of injury. This may be mild or painful and may persist for months, sometimes resolving spontaneously. Partial immunity to the toxin may be mechanism responsible for preventing further spread and generalized tetanus; however, unless treated, localized tetanus can evolve into the generalized form. The cephalic form is an unusual type of localized tetanus and occurs with injuries to the head or at times is associated with *C. tetani* infections of the middle ear. Patients on presentation have weakness of the facial musculature, dysphagia, and extraocular muscle involvement. Both cephalic and localized forms of tetanus can spread to become the generalized form.

Diagnosis

The diagnosis of tetanus is primarily clinical. A clinical picture of trismus, muscle rigidity, stimulus-induced tetany, and a history of a wound or injury within the last 3 weeks is highly suggestive of generalized tetanus. Likewise, a newborn with a poor suck and increased muscle rigidity and spasms, in the setting of poor umbilical hygiene and a mother with no immunization history, likely has neonatal tetanus. *C. tetani* is rarely cultured from the wound, and in any case, a positive culture does not prove the presence of the disease nor does a negative culture disprove it. Blood and serum studies are usually normal or nonspecific and CSF is usually normal.

Treatment

A patient with generalized tetanus or neonatal tetanus will require the facilities and the expertise of an intensive care unit to survive. A review of 335 consecutive tetanus patients revealed that survival drastically improved after the development of intensive care units (44% mortality vs. 15%) and that the major improvement came from the prevention of death from respiratory failure (Table 63.1).

Treatment of generalized tetanus should begin with administration of human tetanus immunoglobulin (HTIG) to neutralize the tetanospasmin, which has not yet entered neurons. A single dose of 500 IU is as effective as higher doses ranging from 3,000 to 5,000 IU. Equine antitetanus serum may be more readily available, particularly in underdeveloped regions; however, it has a much higher incidence of adverse reactions such as anaphylaxis and serum sickness. It is dosed at 10,000 to 1,000,000 units intramuscularly. Debriding the portal of entry does not change the course of the disease, although it may help prevent secondary infection.

Antibiotic treatment should be initiated at the outset, although it likely plays a minor role in the treatment of the disease. In an open study comparing metronidazole and penicillin, *metronidazole* 500 mg IV every 6 hours for 7 to 10 days was superior with significantly less progression of the disease, shorter hospitalization, and improved survival.

Muscle relaxation is best accomplished with benzodiazepines or baclofen. Very large doses are required to control spasms. Continuous magnesium infusion (2 to 4 g/h, targeted to serum magnesium levels of 2 to 4 mg/dL) can also aid in reducing neuronal excitability and spasms. If GABA receptor upregulation with benzodiazepines or baclofen is unsuccessful in controlling the muscle spasms, then neuromuscular blockade with vecuronium or rocuronium may be necessary. Control of autonomic instability, primarily sympathetic storming, can be achieved with a variety of agents. IV labetalol,

a combined α- and β-blocker, is the first-line treatment of choice. Clonidine and dexmedetomidine are α-2 receptor agonists that reduce basal sympathetic tone and may be helpful in suppressing sympathetic surges. There is no agreed upon specific regimen for the treatment of neonatal tetanus; however, it is treated much like generalized variety.

LEVEL 1 EVIDENCE

1. Solera J, Geijo P, Largo J, et al. A randomized, double-blind study to assess the optimal duration of doxycycline treatment for human brucellosis. *Clin Infect Dis.* 2004;39(12):1776–1782.
2. Saltoglu N, Tasova Y, Inal AS, et al. Efficacy of rifampicin plus doxycycline versus rifampicin plus quinolone in the treatment of brucellosis. *Saudi Med J.* 2002;23(8):921–924.
3. Roushan MR, Amiri MJ, Janmohammadi N, et al. Comparison of the efficacy of gentamicin for 5 days plus doxycycline for 8 weeks versus streptomycin for 2 weeks plus doxycycline for 45 days in the treatment of human brucellosis: a randomized clinical trial. *J Antimicrob Chemother.* 2010;65(5):1028–1035.
4. Bass JW, Freitas BC, Freitas AD, et al. Prospective randomized double blind placebo-controlled evaluation of azithromycin for treatment of cat-scratch disease. *Pediatr Infect Dis J.* 1998; 17(6):447–452.

SUGGESTED READINGS

Rickettsia

Bleck TP. Central nervous system involvement in rickettsial diseases. *Neurol Clin.* 1999;17:801–812.

Buckingham SC, Marshall GS, Schutze GE, et al. Clinical and laboratory features, hospital course, and outcome of Rocky Mountain spotted fever in children. *J Pediatr.* 2007;150(2):180–184, 184.e1.

Chapman AS, Bakken JS, Folk SM, et al; Tickborne Rickettsial Disease Working Group; Centers for Disease Control and Prevention. Diagnosis and management of tick-borne rickettsial diseases: Rocky Mountain spotted fever, ehrlichiosis, and anaplasmosis—United States: a practical guide for physicians and other health-care and public health professionals. *MMWR Recomm Rep.* 2006;55(RR-4):1–27.

Chen LF, Sexton DJ. What's new in Rocky Mountain spotted fever? *Infect Dis Clin North Am.* 2008;22(3):415–432, vii–viii.

Cunha BA. Clinical features of Rocky Mountain spotted fever. *Lancet Infect Dis.* 2008;8(3):143–144.

Hamburg BJ, Storch GA, Micek ST, et al. The importance of early treatment with doxycycline in human ehrlichiosis. *Medicine (Baltimore).* 2008;87:53–60.

Kim DE, Lee SH, Park KI, et al. Scrub typhus encephalomyelitis with prominent neurological signs. *Arch Neurol.* 2000;57:1770–1772.

Lai CH, Huang CK, Weng HC, et al. Clinical characteristics of acute Q fever, scrub typhus, and murine typhus with delayed defervescence despite doxycycline treatment. *Am J Trop Med Hyg.* 2008;79(3):441–446.

Lee N, Ip M, Wong B, et al. Risk factors associated with life-threatening rickettsial infections. *Am J Trop Med Hyg.* 2008;78(6):973–978.

Ratnasamy N, Everett ED, Roland WE, et al. Central nervous system manifestations of human ehrlichiosis. *Clin Infect Dis.* 1996;23:314–319.

Spach DH, Liles WC, Campbell GL, et al. Tick-borne diseases in the United States. *N Engl J Med.* 1993;329:936–947.

Stone JH, Dierberg K, Aram G, et al. Human monocytic ehrlichiosis. *JAMA.* 2004;292:2263–2270.

Brucellosis

Akdeniz H, Irmak H, Anlar O, et al. Central nervous system brucellosis: presentation, diagnosis and treatment. *J Infect.* 1998;36(3):297–301.

Al-Nakshabandi NA. The spectrum of imaging findings of brucellosis: a pictorial essay. *Can Assoc Radiol J.* 2012;63(1):5–11.

TABLE 63.1	Mainstays of Treatment for Severe Tetanus

- Neutralizing existing toxin before it enters the nervous system
- Inhibition of further production of tetanus toxin
- Muscle relaxation and sedation
- Management of autonomic instability
- Ventilator, nutritional, and general ICU support

ICU, intensive care unit.

Erdem H, Ulu-Kilic A, Kilic S, et al. Efficacy and tolerability of antibiotic combinations in neurobrucellosis: results of the Istanbul study. *Antimicrob Agents Chemother.* 2012;56(3):1523–1528.

Gul HC, Erdem H, Gorenek L, et al. Management of neurobrucellosis: an assessment of 11 cases. *Intern Med.* 2008;47(11):995–1001.

McLean DR, Russell N, Khan MY. Neurobrucellosis: clinical and therapeutic features. *Clin Infect Dis.* 1992;15:582–590.

Mousa AR, Koshy TS, Araj GF, et al. *Brucella* meningitis: presentation, diagnosis and treatment—a prospective study of ten cases. *Q J Med.* 1986;60: 873–885.

Shakir RA, Al-Din AS, Araj GF, et al. Clinical categories of neurobrucellosis. A report on 19 cases. *Brain.* 1987;110:213–223.

Young EJ. An overview of human brucellosis. *Clin Infect Dis.* 1995;21(2): 283–289.

Anthrax

Leblebicioglu H, Turan D, Eroglu C, et al. A cluster of anthrax cases including meningitis. *Trop Doct.* 2006;36(1):51–53.

Meyer MA. Neurologic complications of anthrax: a review of the literature. *Arch Neurol.* 2003;60(4):483–488.

Sejvar JJ, Tenover FC, Stephens DS. Management of anthrax meningitis. *Lancet Infect Dis.* 2005;5(5):287–295.

Shafazand S, Doyle R, Ruoss S, et al. Inhalational anthrax: epidemiology, diagnosis, and management. *Chest.* 1999;116(5):1369–1376.

Yildirim H, Kabakus N, Koc M, et al. Meningoencephalitis due to anthrax: CT and MR findings. *Pediatr Radiol.* 2006;36(11):1190–1193.

Bartonella

Nervi SJ, Ressner RA, Drayton JR, et al. Catscratch disease. Medscape Web site. http://emedicine.medscape.com/article/214100-overview. Accessed January 25, 2015.

Seah AB, Azran MS, Rucker JC, et al. Magnetic resonance imaging abnormalities in cat-scratch disease encephalopathy. *J Neuroophthalmol.* 2003;23(1): 16–21.

Vermeulen MJ, Verbakel H, Notermans DW, et al. Evaluation of sensitivity, specificity and cross-reactivity in *Bartonella henselae* serology. *J Med Microbiol.* 2010;59(pt 6):743–745.

Whipple Disease

Crapoulet N, Barbry P, Raoult D, et al. Global transcriptome analysis of *Tropheryma whipplei* in response to temperature stresses. *J Bacteriol.* 2006; 188(14):5228–5239.

Fenollar F, Puéchal X, Raoult D. Whipple's disease. *N Engl J Med.* 2007; 356(1):55–66.

Louis ED, Lynch T, Kaufmann P, et al. Diagnostic guidelines in central nervous system Whipple's disease. *Ann Neurol.* 1996;40(4):561–568.

Mycoplasma

Bitnum A, Ford-Jones EL, Petric M, et al. Acute childhood encephalitis and *Mycoplasma pneumoniae. Clin Infect Dis.* 2001;32:1674–1684.

Gorman MP, Rincon SP, Pierce VM. Case records of the Massachusetts General Hospital. Case 19-2014. A 19-year-old woman with headache, fever, stiff neck, and mental-status changes. *N Engl J Med.* 2014;370(25):2427–2438.

Huber BM, Strozzi S, Steinlin M, et al. *Mycoplasma pneumoniae* associated opsoclonus-myoclonus syndrome in three cases. *Eur J Pediatr.* 2010;169(4):441–445.

Lin JJ, Hsia SH, Wu CT, et al. *Mycoplasma pneumoniae*-related postencephalitic epilepsy in children. *Epilepsia.* 2011;52(11):1979–1985.

Sotgiu S, Pugliatti M, Rosati G, et al. Neurological disorders associated with *Mycoplasma pneumoniae* infection. *Eur J Neurol.* 2003;10:165–168.

Tsiodras S, Kelesidis I, Kelesidis T, et al. Central nervous system manifestations of *Mycoplasma pneumoniae* infections. *J Infect.* 2005;51:343–354.

Legionella

de Lau LM, Siepman DA, Remmers MJ, et al. Acute disseminating encephalomyelitis following legionnaires disease. *Arch Neurol.* 2010;67(5):623–626.

Johnson JD, Raff MJ, Van Arsdall JA. Neurologic manifestations of Legionnaires' disease. *Medicine (Baltimore).* 1984;63:303–310.

Morelli N, Battaglia E, Lattuada P. Brainstem involvement in Legionnaires' disease. *Infection.* 2006;34(1):49–52.

Pendelbury WW, Perl DP, Winn WC Jr, et al. Neuropathologic evaluation of 40 confirmed cases of *Legionella* pneumonia. *Neurology.* 1983;33:1340–1344.

Shelburne SA, Kielhofner MA, Tiwari PS. Cerebellar involvement in legionellosis. *South Med J.* 2004;97:61–64.

Bacterial Toxins

Ahmadsyah I, Salim A. Treatment of tetanus: an open study to compare the efficacy of procaine penicillin and metronidazole. *Br Med J (Clin Res Ed).* 1985;291(6496):648–650.

Anlar B, Yalaz K, Dizmen R. Long-term prognosis after neonatal tetanus. *Dev Med Child Neurol.* 1989;31(1):76–80.

Bleck TP. Pharmacology of tetanus. *Clin Neuropharmacol.* 1986;9(2):103–120.

Centers for Disease Control and Prevention. Progress towards the global elimination of neonatal tetanus, 1989-1993. *MMWR Morb Mortal Wkly Rep.* 1994;43(48):885–887, 893–894.

Centers for Disease Control and Prevention. Rocky Mountain spotted fever: symptoms, diagnosis, and treatment. Centers for Disease Control and Prevention Web site. http://www.cdc.gov/rmsf/symptoms/index.html. Accessed January 1, 2015

Centers for Disease Control and Prevention. Rocky Mountain spotted fever (RMSF): statistics and epidemiology. Centers for Disease Control and Prevention Web site. http://www.cdc.gov/rmsf/stats/. Accessed January 1, 2015

Cherington M. Electrophysiologic methods as an aid in diagnosis of botulism: a review. *Muscle Nerve.* 1982;5(9S):S28–S29.

Colebatch JG, Wolff AH, Gilbert RJ, et al. Slow recovery from severe foodborne botulism. *Lancet.* 1989;2(8673):1216–1217.

Kimura F, Sasaki N, Uehara H. Long-term recurrent infection of tetanus in an elderly patient. *Am J Emerg Med.* 2001;19(2):168.

Murphy JR. *Corynebacterium diphtheriae.* In: Baron S, ed. *Medical Microbiology.* Galveston, TX: University of Texas Medical Branch; 1996.

Tacket CO, Rogawsk MA. Botulism. In: Simpson LL, ed. *Botulinum Neurotoxin and Tetanus Toxin.* San Diego, CA: Academic Press; 1989:351–378.

Trujillo MH, Castillo A, España J, et al. Impact of intensive care management on the prognosis of tetanus. Analysis of 641 cases. *Chest.* 1987;92(1):63–65.

Vita G, Girlanda P, Puglisi RM, et al. Cardiovascular-reflex testing and single-fiber electromyography in botulism. A longitudinal study. *Arch Neurol.* 1987;44(2):202–206.

INTRODUCTION

Chronic meningitis is commonly defined as inflammation of the meninges, most often accompanied by a pleocytosis of greater than 5 white blood cells per microliter in the cerebrospinal fluid (CSF), that has persisted for at least 1 month without spontaneous resolution. Clinical presentation often includes headache, nausea, vomiting, cranial neuropathies, symptoms of elevated intracranial pressure, or focal neurologic deficits (Table 64.1). The most common etiologies of chronic meningitis fall into three broad categories: infectious, autoimmune, and neoplastic. This chapter will focus on the most common infectious etiologies of chronic meningitis. Fungal, bacterial, and parasitic pathogens can invade the central nervous system and present clinically as chronic meningitis. Increasing use of immunosuppressant medications for autoimmune disease and posttransplantation immunosuppression, as well as predisposing conditions, such as impaired cellular and humoral immunity, have led to a larger population at risk for infectious causes of chronic meningitis.

Despite an increasing array of diagnostic assays, there remain a large proportion of patients with chronic meningitis who remain without a definitive pathogen identified. A thorough history and skillful physical examination is the key to guide further diagnostic testing (Table 64.2) and management (Table 64.3). When history, examination, CSF analysis, and imaging fail to yield an etiology, biopsy is required to establish a definitive diagnosis.

FUNGAL MENINGITIS

Fungi exist in two forms, molds and yeasts. Molds are the tubular form, consisting of hyphae that can be branched or contain a single filament. Yeasts are thick-walled, single-celled organisms that live inside cells. Dimorphic yeasts assume tubular forms at lower temperature but become encapsulated at temperatures above 35°C. Either fungal form can infect the nervous system, producing meningitis, vasculitis, abscess, granulomas, or encephalitis.

Fungi are universal saprophytic organisms found as spores in soil, on the skin of mammals and birds, and in bat or bird guano. They commonly enter the body through inhalation; direct invasion through the skin, mucus membranes, or sinuses; or via penetrating wounds. Although invasive fungal disease typically affects immunocompromised individuals, some organisms such as *Coccidioides* spp. and *Cryptococcus* spp. can also affect immunocompetent individuals. Fungal infections of the nervous system mainly occur in the presence of immunosuppression as a consequence of AIDS, cancer, hematologic malignancy, hereditary immune defects, organ or stem cell transplantation, or other conditions requiring therapeutic immunosuppression.

CRYPTOCOCCAL MENINGITIS

Epidemiology and Pathobiology

Cryptococcal meningitis is most often caused by the encapsulated yeast *Cryptococcus neoformans*, but other cryptococcal species, such as *Cryptococcus gattii*, are emerging as pathogens that affect immunocompetent individuals. With a worldwide distribution, *C. neoformans* is ubiquitous, found primarily in bird droppings, soil, and citrus peel. *C. gattii* is more commonly associated with the bark of several tree species. Infection usually occurs through inhalation of the organism, followed by a respiratory infection and dissemination. Cryptococcal meningitis is most common in people with impaired cell-mediated immunity, especially those with HIV infection, hematologic malignancies, solid organ transplant recipients, and patients on chronic corticosteroids or other immunosuppressive therapy. In patients immunocompromised due to HIV infection, cryptococcal meningitis is the most common systemic fungal infection and a frequent etiology of central nervous system (CNS) infection, with a prevalence varying from 10% in the United States to as high as 30% in sub-Saharan Africa.

Clinical Features

CRYPTOCOCCUS GATTII

This is a rare pathogen, with disease confined to tropical and subtropical climates, particularly the highly endemic regions of Australia and Papua New Guinea. In 2004, an outbreak of *C. gattii* infections was documented in the United States Pacific Northwest states of Oregon and Washington. A large retrospective review of the Pacific Northwest *C. gattii* infections revealed important clinical differences between *C. gattii* infections in the United States Pacific Northwest and historically endemic areas. Although *C. gattii* in historically endemic areas has been reported to infect primarily immunocompetent persons, causing meningoencephalitis, *C. gattii* infections in Oregon and Washington State occurred frequently in immunocompromised persons and presented most often as respiratory illness. Time from symptom onset to diagnosis of *C. gattii* infection was significantly longer among patients with pulmonary infections (50 days) than those with either CNS (24 days) or bloodstream infections (27 days). There were no differences in immune status between patients with bloodstream infections and either pulmonary or CNS infections.

CRYPTOCOCCUS NEOFORMANS

The clinical manifestations of *C. neoformans* infection depends largely on the host immune status. Severity of infection varies from asymptomatic incidental pulmonary nodules to widely disseminated disease. HIV-infected patients with CD4+ counts of less than 50 cells/μL are especially vulnerable to disseminated infection and meningitis. Cryptococcal meningitis typically begins insidiously, with 75% of patients developing headache and fever over a 2- to 4-week period. As the infection evolves, 50% of people develop nausea, vomiting, and altered mental status. Visual symptoms and seizures are also common. Over half of immunocompromised patients develop intracranial hypertension; this is even more common in immunocompetent hosts. As increased intracranial pressure develops, patients become obtunded, and without intervention, herniation will follow.

TABLE 64.1	Neurologic and Systemic Symptoms and Imaging Characteristics of Chronic Infectious Meningitis		
Condition	**Neurologic Presentation**	**Systemic Symptoms**	**Neuroimaging**
Cryptococcosis	Headache and fever (75%), nausea and vomiting (50%), altered mental status (50%), visual symptoms, seizures	Pulmonary, multiorgan involvement	Hydrocephalus, cerebral edema, leptomeningeal enhancement, and cryptococcomas
Coccidioidomycosis	Headache (75%); nausea and vomiting (40%); altered mental status (39%–73%); focal neurologic deficits, including ataxia, gait disturbance, diplopia, or facial palsies (33%–80%); and nuchal rigidity (20%)	Pulmonary, lymph nodes, skin	Hydrocephalus, meningeal enhancement, nodular enhancement, basilar meningitis, cerebral infarction
Blastomycosis	Focal neurologic deficits, seizures, and altered mental status Less common: fever, headache, and meningismus	Pulmonary, verrucous or fungating skin lesions, bones, joints, genitourinary system	Single or multiple abscesses, granuloma, meningeal enhancement, epidural extensions, and overlying osteomyelitis
Histoplasmosis	Headache and altered mental status	Acute pulmonary infection with fever, chills, and pulmonary opacities Multiorgan including bone marrow	Normal, granuloma, meningeal enhancement
Aspergillosis	Solitary mass lesion, cavernous sinus thrombosis, multiple intracranial abscesses, acute or chronic basilar meningitis, vasculitis, or myelitis	Pulmonary, sinusitis, multiorgan involvement	Multiple abscesses, meningeal enhancement, infarction, hemorrhage, sinusitis with extension
Tuberculosis	Headache, vomiting, meningeal signs, focal deficits, vision loss, cranial nerve palsies	Pulmonary, malaise, anorexia, fatigue, weight loss, fever, myalgia	Enhancement of the basilar meninges, thick exudates, obstructive hydrocephalus, miliary pattern, tuberculoma, and periventricular infarcts
Syphilis	Meningitis (headache, photophobia, nausea and vomiting, cranial nerve deficits), general paresis, psychiatric illness, cognitive decline, tabes dorsalis, or vascular disease	Genital ulcers, fever, lymphadenopathy, headache, malaise, myalgia, and a macular or pustular rash of the palms and soles Multiorgan involvement	Leptomeningeal enhancement, white matter disease in the brain and posterior columns, ischemic stroke
Borreliosis	Early: septic lymphocytic meningitis, cranial neuritis, or painful polyradiculitis Late: myelitis, encephalitis, and neurobehavioral changes	Rash, fever, diffuse aches and pains, headaches, malaise, fatigue, carditis	White matter edema with enhancement

Diagnosis

The diagnosis of cryptococcal meningitis should be considered in patients presenting with a subacute presentation of headache and fever, especially in the setting of HIV infection or immunosuppression. Computerized tomography (CT) and magnetic resonance imaging (MRI) are nonspecific for the diagnosis of cryptococcal meningitis but may reveal hydrocephalus, cerebral edema, leptomeningeal enhancement, or cryptococcomas. Classic MRI findings for fungal meningitis are shown in Figure 64.1. Lumbar puncture, the diagnostic procedure of choice, demonstrates an increased opening pressure, a mild mononuclear pleocytosis, increased protein, and low glucose concentrations. Patients with severe immunosuppression may lack this typical CSF appearance. The cryptococcal capsular polysaccharide antigen (CrAg) assay is both sensitive and specific for detecting *C. neoformans* in CSF samples

and can be quantitated for prognostication. The CrAg titer is not reliable for determining response to therapy. Although a positive CrAg assay in serum cannot confirm the diagnosis of cryptococcal meningitis, a negative CrAg assay virtually excludes the diagnosis. Because the CrAg lateral flow assay (LFA) has nearly 100% sensitivity and specificity on CSF samples, it is considered the optimal point-of-care diagnostic assay for cryptococcal meningitis. In areas where CrAg is not available, direct CSF examination with India ink preparation is often used. Fungal culture for the organism is 90% sensitive and can also be useful for speciation, although it typically requires days for culture to grow. *C. neoformans* cultured from CSF, blood, or other sites produces white mucoid (depending on the capsule thickness) colonies, usually within 48 to 72 hours, on most bacterial and fungal media. Although *C. neoformans* grows at 37°C, a temperature of 30°C to 35°C is optimal.

TABLE 64.2   Cerebrospinal Fluid Characteristics and Serum Diagnostics for Chronic Infectious Meningitis

Condition	Microscopic Appearance	LP Opening Pressure	CSF WBC	CSF Differential	CSF Glucose	CSF Protein	CSF Diagnostics	Serum Diagnostics
Cryptococcosis	Encapsulated fungi; yeast-like cells with budding daughter cells; capsule visualized by India ink (halo effect)	High	High or normal	Mononuclear	Low	High	Fungal smear, fungal culture, India ink stain, CrAg lateral flow assay (LFA)	Blood culture
Coccidioidomycosis	Yeast form endosporulating spherules; branched septate hyphae with alternating arthroconidia	Normal	High	Early PMN, lymphocytic, eosinophilic (70%)	Low	High	Fungal culture, microscopy, complement fixation antibody assay, PCR	Microscopy from bronchoalveolar lavage (BAL) fluid, or other body fluid, or a positive culture from any location
Blastomycosis	Mycelium at room temperature; yeast phase at 37°C. Conidia, yeast cells with multinucleate broad budding.	High	High	Early PMN, lymphocytic	Low	High	Fungal culture, biopsy of involved tissue with micro	Direct visualization of the organism via microscopy
Histoplasmosis	Hyphae large macroconidia and smaller infectious microconidia. At temperatures <35°C yeast form. Hyphal elements possible.	Normal	High	Mononuclear	Low	High	Fungal smear and culture, antigen titers	Fungal culture from involved organ, antigen titers
Aspergillosis	Septate hyphae branched at 45-degree angles with conidiophores. Hyphae develop terminal buds forming small conidia.	Normal	High	Early neutrophil, lymphocytic	Low	High	Fungal culture, biopsy of affected tissue with micro, PCR	Galactomannan and beta-D-glucan. Microscopy, culture, or PCR from bronchoalveolar lavage or affected tissue.
Tuberculosis	Intracellular aerobic gram-positive acid-fast pleomorphic bacillus	High	High or normal	Mixed pleocytosis	Low	High	AFB smear and culture, PCR; GeneXpert, MODS	QuantiFERON, PPD, BAL for AFB smear and culture
Syphilis	Spirochetal bacterium	Normal	High or normal	Lymphocytic	Normal	High or normal	Darkfield microscopy, VDRL, PCR	RPR, VDRL, (FTA-ABS) and *Treponema pallidum* particle agglutination tests (MHA-TP)
Borreliosis	Spirochetal bacterium	Normal	High	Lymphocytic	Normal	High or normal	Darkfield microscopy, IgG and IgM antibody index, PCR	Two-tier testing (ELISA and IgM/IgG immunoblot)

LP, lumbar puncture; CSF, cerebrospinal fluid; WBC, white blood cell; CrAg, cryptococcal capsular polysaccharide antigen; PMN, polymorphonuclear; PCR, polymerase chain reaction; AFB, acid-fast bacillus; MODS, microscopic observation drug susceptibility; PPD, purified protein derivative; VDRL, Venereal Disease Research Laboratory; RPR, rapid plasma reagin; FTA-ABS, fluorescent treponemal antibody absorption; Ig, immunoglobulin; ELISA, enzyme-linked immunosorbent assay.

TABLE 64.3 Treatment of Chronic Infectious Meningitis

Condition	Treatment	Alternatives and Other Considerations
Cryptococcosis	Amphotericin B (AmB) 0.7–1 mg/kg/day IV plus flucytosine 100 mg/kg/day × 14 days then fluconazole 400 mg PO daily × 8 wk then fluconazole 200 mg daily lifelong	Repeat LP to keep opening pressures in normal range; CSF shunting when needed.
Coccidioidomycosis	Induction therapy with oral fluconazole 400–800 mg/day, followed by 200–400 mg/day indefinitely	Itraconazole 400–600 mg/day or amphotericin B 0.5–0.7 mg/kg/day. Intrathecal amphotericin B in addition to an azole. Shunting for hydrocephalus when needed.
Blastomycosis	Liposomal amphotericin B, 5 mg/kg/day for 4–6 wk, followed by an oral azole. Possible options for azole therapy include fluconazole (800 mg/day), itraconazole (200 mg two or three times per day), or voriconazole (200–400 mg twice per day) for at least 12 months and until resolution of CSF abnormalities.	Surgical drainage of any epidural abscess
Histoplasmosis	Liposomal amphotericin B (5.0 mg/kg daily for a total of 175 mg/kg given over 4–6 wk). Fluconazole (800 mg/day) should be continued for 9–12 mo.	Chronic fluconazole maintenance therapy (800 mg/day) in relapsing patients. Intrathecal amphotericin B.
Aspergillosis	Voriconazole 6 mg/kg IV twice a day on day 1 followed by 4 mg/kg IV twice daily. Followed by maintenance therapy of voriconazole 200 mg every 12 h.	Voriconazole plus caspofungin for invasive disease
Tuberculosis	Intensive four-drug regimen × 2 mo then continuation two-drug regimen × 10 mo based on resistance patterns	Choice of treatment should be directed by resistance patterns. Steroids should be considered for meningitis.
Syphilis	Aqueous penicillin G 18–24 million U/day administered as 3–4 million units IV every 4 h or as continuous infusion for 10–14 days	Procaine penicillin 2.4 million units IM daily with probenecid 500 mg orally four times daily for 10–14 days
Borreliosis	Ceftriaxone 2 g IV daily for 14 days	IV cefotaxime or IV penicillin G. Oral doxycycline.

IV, intravenous; PO, by mouth; LP, lumbar puncture; CSF, cerebrospinal fluid; IM, intramuscular.

Treatment

A combination of antifungal medication and aggressive management of hydrocephalus is integral to the successful treatment of patients with cryptococcal meningitis. Amphotericin B (AmB) plus flucytosine, as compared with AmB alone, is associated with improved survival of patients with cryptococcal meningitis. Elevated intracranial pressure (ICP) can be managed through a variety of treatments. Patients should initially undergo daily lumbar punctures to reduce opening pressure until normal opening pressure is consistently maintained; some patients may require multiple daily lumbar punctures. For patients requiring frequent lumbar punctures, placement of a lumbar drain or ventriculostomy can provide a temporary means for controlling ICP. Ventriculoperitoneal shunt can be considered for patients with persistently elevated ICP. A recent retrospective study of elevated ICP in patients with cryptococcal meningitis determined by aggressive management of ICP during the initial 5 days of illness was associated with lower mortality than initial antifungal management alone.

Although guidelines for treatment of cryptococcal disease are based primarily on data from *C. neoformans* infections in HIV and solid organ transplant patients, these guidelines are intended to apply to patients with *C. neoformans* or *C. gattii* infections. A limited number of *C. gattii*–specific recommendations were included for the first time in the 2010 Infectious Diseases Society of America guidelines and are based on data from *C. gattii* infections in historically endemic areas. These recommendations pertain mainly to patients with cryptococcomas, which previous data have suggested are more common in patients infected with *C. gattii* than *C. neoformans*, and include consideration of surgery for patients with large cryptococcomas, increased radiologic and follow-up evaluations for those with cryptococcomas or hydrocephalus, and possible use of amphotericin B/5 flucytosine (AmB/5FC) in patients with large and/or multiple pulmonary cryptococcomas.

Outcomes

Poor prognostic factors include low CSF glucose concentration, high CSF cryptococcal antigen titer (>1:1,024), high CSF lactate level, altered level of consciousness, hydrocephalus, and elevated ICP.

COCCIDIOIDOMYCOSIS

Epidemiology and Pathobiology

Coccidioides immitis is a fungus endemic to the southwestern United States, Northern Mexico, and areas of South America. The mycelial phase of *Coccidioides* spp. is able to withstand extreme desert climates and after rainfalls will multiply to form arthroconidia. Infection in humans occurs when aerosolized arthroconidia are inhaled. Once inhaled, *C. immitis* usually results in a self-limited respiratory infection, commonly known as *valley fever*. In susceptible populations, a pulmonary infection can progress to severe disseminated disease. Dissemination is more likely to occur in patients of African or Asian descent, pregnant women, and people who are immunocompromised, especially due to HIV infection or long-term immunosuppressive therapy.

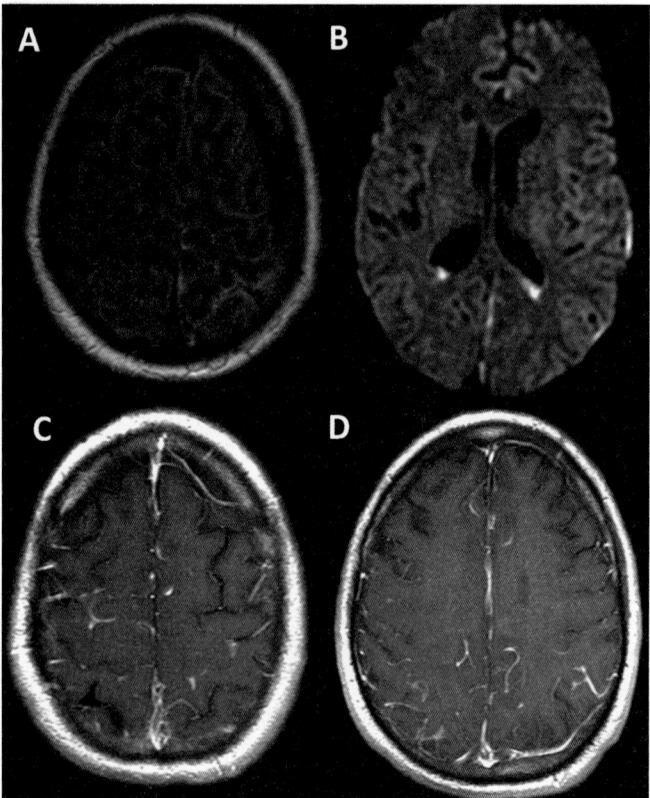

FIGURE 64.1 Axial brain MRI. **A:** T2 fluid-attenuated inversion recovery (FLAIR) with leptomeningeal hyperintensity in the posterior frontal lobe. **B:** Diffusion-weighted imaging (DWI) demonstrating pus in the posterior horn of the lateral ventricle. **C and D:** T1 post contrast with avid leptomeningeal enhancement.

Clinical Features

Similar to tuberculosis, chronic meningitis due to *C. immitis* classically involves the basilar meninges. The most common symptom is headache, which is present in over 75% of patients. Other presenting signs and symptoms are related to elevated ICP and include nausea and vomiting (40%); altered mental status (39% to 73%); focal neurologic deficits, including ataxia, gait disturbance, diplopia, or facial palsies (33% to 80%); and nuchal rigidity (20%).

In patients with HIV infection, coccidioidomycosis can resemble *Pneumocystis jiroveci* pneumonia, producing a unique reticulonodular diffuse infiltrative pulmonary disease and constitutional symptoms of dyspnea, fever, and night sweats. Coccidioidomycosis frequently disseminates in patients with HIV infection, with common sites of dissemination including the meninges, lymph nodes, and skin. Although patients who are HIV-positive can present with unique symptoms, most HIV-infected patients present with symptoms similar to those seen in immunocompetent patients. Hydrocephalus, cerebral infarction, and vasculitis are potential complications of *C. immitis* meningitis. Communicating hydrocephalus is a well-known complication of basilar meningitis, secondary to obstruction of arachnoid villi blocking reabsorption of CSF and may develop during the initial or later stages of the infection. Hydrocephalus develops in about 20% to 50% of patients with *C. immitis* meningitis and is associated with a 12-fold increased risk of mortality. Cerebral infarction, as well as venous and dural

thrombosis, has been reported during the initial and later stages of infection. Perivascular inflammation is typically associated with infarction of the basal ganglia, thalamus, and cerebral white matter.

Diagnosis

Coccidioidomycosis can be diagnosed using serologic testing, histopathology, or culture of tissue or fluid from the infected site. Identification of *C. immitis* spherules in tissue, sputum, and bronchoalveolar lavage (BAL) fluid, or a positive culture from any location in the body, is diagnostic of coccidioidal infection. Definitive diagnosis of *C. immitis* meningitis requires identification or culture of the organism from the brain or CSF. Unfortunately, CSF culture is often negative and presumptive diagnosis is typically made through a combination of CSF and serologic testing. CSF is typically abnormal, with a lymphocytic pleocytosis with early neutrophil predominance, and low glucose concentration. Of note, this pathogen may cause a CSF eosinophilia in up to 70% of patients with meningitis, a finding that is relatively uncommon with other fungal pathogens. Detection of antibodies to *C. immitis* in the CSF using the complement fixation antibody assay is the most sensitive test for confirming meningeal infection. Repeated CSF sampling is sometimes required to confirm the diagnosis, as antibody test results can be negative early during the course of infection (71% to 94% sensitive). Enzyme immunoassay for IgM and IgG and latex agglutination tests are less sensitive in CSF samples. Although polymerase chain reaction (PCR) assays have been used to detect *C. immitis* infection, they are not routinely available.

Treatment

Oral fluconazole is recommended for the treatment of *C. immitis* meningitis. Practice guidelines recommend high-dose induction therapy with oral fluconazole 400 mg/day to 800 mg/day, followed by 200 mg/day to 400 mg/day indefinitely. Itraconazole, administered in dosages of 400 to 600 mg/day, has been reported to be comparably effective. Some physicians also initiate therapy with intrathecal AmB in addition to an azole based on their belief that responses are more prompt with this approach.

Hydrocephalus nearly always requires a neurosurgical shunt for decompression. Patients who do not respond to fluconazole or itraconazole are candidates for intrathecal AmB therapy with or without continuation of azole treatment. The most common life-threatening complication of coccidioidal meningitis is CNS vasculitis leading to cerebral ischemia, infarction, and hemorrhage. Some physicians endorse the use of concomitant high-dose, intravenous, short-term corticosteroids, but larger randomized studies are lacking.

Outcomes

Approximately 66% to 80% of patients treated with oral azoles alone achieved initial clinical improvement or remission of meningitis. However, up to 75% of patients relapse; therefore, lifelong prophylaxis with fluconazole 400 mg/day is recommended. Without treatment, the frequency of relapse is high and outcome poor.

BLASTOMYCOSIS AND HISTOPLASMOSIS

Epidemiology

Blastomyces dermatitidis and *Histoplasma capsulatum* are dimorphic fungi endemic to the Mississippi and Ohio river valleys. Although isolated cases of infection have been reported outside this geographic area, most patients reside within these areas. *Histoplasma* and *Blastomyces* species are ubiquitous environmental organisms, existing in the mycelial phase and then converting to the yeast phase at body temperature. Both organisms produce a large spectrum of disease, ranging from subclinical infection to disseminated disease.

Pathobiology

B. dermatitidis, a thick-walled yeast with broad-based budding daughter cells, is endemic to the Great Lakes and Mississippi and Ohio river valleys. Like histoplasmosis, infection with blastomycosis is acquired via inhalation of spores into the lung and can manifest as pulmonary or extrapulmonary disease. Chest radiographs commonly demonstrate nodular or lobar infiltrates with cavitations. If the organism evades nonspecific host defense mechanisms in the lungs, it will convert into the yeast phase and multiply. The organism then spreads hematogenously to other organs. Cutaneous involvement is seen in 60% of patients with blastomycosis, manifesting as verrucous or fungating lesions with irregular borders. Other sites less frequently involved include bones, joints, genitourinary system, and the CNS.

H. capsulatum, like *B. dermatitidis*, is primarily found in the Mississippi and Ohio river valleys, and infection is acquired via inhalation. Histoplasmosis may produce an acute pulmonary infection with fever, chills, and pulmonary opacities. Patients with impaired cellular immunity, such as HIV-infected individuals, typically present with chronic pulmonary symptoms with progression to severe disseminated disease. Infection disseminates hematogenously to distant sites, such as the liver, spleen, and CNS. Bone marrow involvement is common and often manifests as thrombocytopenia, anemia, or leukopenia.

Clinical Features

CNS infection with blastomycosis occurs in less than 10% of people with disseminated disease and manifests as solitary or multiple abscesses and acute or chronic meningitis. Unlike other fungal CNS infections, blastomycosis is more likely to present with focal neurologic deficits, seizures, and altered mental status, whereas symptoms of fever, headache, and meningismus are less common. Although intracranial infection results most frequently from hematogenous seeding of the brain parenchyma from the lungs, epidural extension from overlying vertebral or skull osteomyelitis have been described.

Most patients with pulmonary histoplasmosis are asymptomatic and have resolution of the infection without therapy. It is common for individuals in the Mississippi and Ohio river valleys to have asymptomatic pulmonary nodules. Dissemination occurs during both primary infection and reactivation of latent infection. CNS involvement occurs in less than 20% of patients with disseminated infection and most frequently affects patients with severely impaired cellular immunity, such as people who are HIV-infected. Presenting symptoms typically include headache and altered mental status; although less common, patients may also present with focal neurologic deficits, seizures, ischemic stroke, and mass lesions.

Diagnosis

Direct visualization of blastomycosis via microscopy is the only method of rapid diagnosis but has variable sensitivity. Lumbar puncture typically reveals elevated opening pressure, and CSF is notable for elevated protein concentration, low glucose concentration, and a pleocytosis with neutrophilic predominance early in the disease course followed by a lymphocytic predominance. The gold standard for diagnosis remains CSF culture, which is positive in 70% of patients with blastomycosis. Growth of *B. dermatitidis* on culture media can occur within 5 to 10 days but may take

2 to 4 weeks for definitive identification of the organism. More invasive procedures, such as brain biopsy and ventricular sampling of CSF, are more likely to provide sufficient material for definitive diagnosis and are often needed for diagnosing intracranial disease. The use of CSF and serum antigen titers and antibodies are useful, although as with histoplasmosis, significant cross-reactivity occurs with other dimorphic fungi.

In histoplasmosis meningitis, CSF frequently demonstrates a mononuclear pleocytosis, increased protein concentration, and decreased glucose concentration. CSF culture is not sensitive for diagnosing histoplasmosis. The use of CSF and serum antigen titers and antibodies are useful, although as with blastomycosis, significant cross-reactivity occurs with other dimorphic fungi. Because meningitis is typically the result of disseminated infection, testing for the organism in the blood or bone marrow should also be considered.

Treatment

AmB should be given for blastomycosis infection as a lipid formulation at a dosage of 5 mg/kg/day for 4 to 6 weeks, followed by an oral azole. Possible options for azole therapy include fluconazole (800 mg/day), itraconazole (200 mg two or three times per day), or voriconazole (200 to 400 mg twice per day) for at least 12 months and until resolution of CSF abnormalities. Patients with immunodeficiency due to HIV or immunosuppressive therapy have high rates of relapse and should be maintained on long-term secondary prophylaxis with fluconazole indefinitely. For selected patients with neurologic dysfunction caused by focal CNS blastomycosis, surgery may be beneficial. Surgical drainage of an epidural abscess may be necessary for reducing morbidity and mortality from this disorder.

Treatment of CNS histoplasmosis is challenging. Despite treatment with AmB, mortality ranges from 20% to 40% of patients with meningitis, and up to half of responders relapse after therapy is discontinued. The optimal treatment for *H. capsulatum* meningitis is liposomal AmB (5.0 mg/kg daily for a total of 175 mg/kg given over 4 to 6 weeks). To reduce the risk of relapse, fluconazole (800 mg/day) should be continued for 9 to 12 months after completion of AmB. Chronic fluconazole maintenance therapy (800 mg/day) should be considered for patients who relapse after completing a full course of therapy. Itraconazole, although more active against *H. capsulatum* in animal models, does not cross the blood–brain barrier in adequate amounts to treat CNS infection. Intrathecal administration of amphotericin directly into the ventricles, cisterna magna, or lumbar arachnoid space should be reserved for severe infections that do not respond to conventional therapy.

ASPERGILLOSIS

Epidemiology and Pathobiology

Aspergillus species are ubiquitous soil inhabitants that grow and survive on organic debris. This organism sporulates abundantly, releasing conidia into the atmosphere in large quantities. The conidia are small in diameter, making it possible to reach smaller areas of the lung, including the alveoli. Although humans inhale several hundred conidia per day, inhalation of organisms rarely results in disease because the conidia are efficiently eliminated by host immune mechanisms. Alveolar macrophages and neutrophils constitute the first line of host defense against aerosolized conidia.

Historically, disease was limited to individuals with repetitive exposure to pathogens, producing a mild condition known as *farmer's lung*. *Aspergillus* spp. can also produce lung aspergillomas, characterized as an overgrowth of fungus in preexisting cavitary lung lesions. More recently, the incidence and severity of *Aspergillus* spp. infections has increased due to a growing number of people living with immunosuppression, leading to the disease known as *invasive aspergillosis*. Populations significantly at risk for invasive aspergillosis include patients undergoing treatment for hematologic malignancies, recipients of allogeneic hematopoietic stem cell transplant and solid organ transplant, people who are HIV infected, and individuals with chronic granulomatous disease.

Clinical Features

Cerebral aspergillosis occurs in approximately 10% to 20% of patients with invasive disease and results from hematogenous dissemination of the organism or via direct extension from rhinosinusitis. CNS infection can present as a solitary mass lesion, cavernous sinus thrombosis, multiple intracranial abscesses, acute or chronic basilar meningitis, vasculitis, or myelitis. Pathologically, cerebral aspergillosis has a propensity for vascular invasion, infarction, hemorrhage, and aneurysm formation; as a result, the clinical presentation may mimic cerebral vasculitis, ischemic or hemorrhagic infarction, or subarachnoid hemorrhage. In patients with suspected cerebral aspergillosis, it is important to examine the lungs and sinuses for evidence of infection and potential sites for obtaining biopsy or culture material.

Diagnosis

Diagnosis of aspergillosis in immunocompromised patients remains difficult. As with many invasive fungal CNS infections, diagnosis is often achieved through examination of the primary entry site of infection. Thus, in patients with suspected CNS aspergillosis, it is important to examine the lungs and sinuses for evidence of infection and potential sites for obtaining biopsy or culture material. MRI of the brain typically reveals a manifestation of infection, such as cerebral infarction, hemorrhagic lesions, solid-enhancing aspergillomas, or ring-enhancing abscesses. Dural enhancement is usually seen in lesions adjacent to infected paranasal sinuses and indicates direct extension of disease.

Several serum laboratory markers can aid in the diagnosis of invasive aspergillosis. Enzyme-linked immunosorbent assay (ELISA) testing for the fungal cell wall constituents galactomannan and beta-D-glucan should be considered. CSF galactomannan assay using latex agglutination or ELISA may be a useful adjunct to serum testing; however, data is limited to small sample sizes with variable performance and reliability (sensitivity of 70% to 90%). Several PCR assays can detect *Aspergillus* spp. in blood and BAL fluid samples; a recent study to detect *Aspergillus* spp. in fresh tissue and BAL fluid reported a sensitivity and specificity of 86% and 100%, respectively. Experience with PCR to detect *Aspergillus* spp. in CSF samples is limited.

Treatment

Unfortunately, cerebral aspergillosis, especially in an immunocompromised patient, is difficult to treat and has a high mortality rate. The use of voriconazole, a newer antifungal agent, has reduced the mortality of an infection that was previously associated with almost universal mortality. Clinical trials have demonstrated that voriconazole is more effective than AmB as initial therapy for invasive aspergillosis and is associated with significantly improved survival (71% vs. 58%, respectively). *In vitro* studies evaluating combination therapy with voriconazole and caspofungin for *Aspergillus* spp. have provided promising results in patients with invasive aspergillosis.

TUBERCULOSIS

EPIDEMIOLOGY AND PATHOBIOLOGY

Mycobacterium tuberculosis is an intracellular aerobic gram-positive acid-fast pleomorphic bacillus that can cause chronic meningitis. Transmission occurs primarily by inhalation of airborne droplet nuclei into the lungs. *M. tuberculosis* multiplies in alveolar macrophages, and within weeks, the bacilli can hematogenously disseminate to extrapulmonary sites, including the meninges and adjacent brain parenchyma. Tuberculous meningitis is an aggressive form of extrapulmonary disease that is more common in patients infected with HIV.

CLINICAL FEATURES

Meningitis is typically preceded by nonspecific symptoms of malaise, anorexia, fatigue, weight loss, fever, myalgia, and headache. In immunocompetent patients, headache, vomiting, meningeal signs, focal deficits, vision loss, cranial nerve palsies, and raised ICP are characteristic clinical features. Cerebral vessels may be affected by adjacent meningeal inflammation, producing vasospasm, constriction, and eventually thrombosis with cerebral infarction. As the disease progresses, the patient will become comatose from elevated ICP and obstructive hydrocephalus.

DIAGNOSIS

Despite its many limitations, tuberculin skin testing remains in widespread use. The Centers for Disease Control and Prevention (CDC), the American Thoracic Society, and the Infectious Diseases Society of America's guidelines recommend that one should not obtain a tuberculin skin test unless treatment would be offered in the event of a positive test result. Negative results from the purified protein derivative test do not rule out tuberculosis (TB); if the 5-tuberculin skin test result is negative and suspicion for TB is high, the test can be repeated with the 250-tuberculin test. Note that this test is often nonreactive in persons with tuberculous meningitis.

Diagnosing tuberculous meningitis can be difficult and typically involves a combination of neuroimaging, serologic studies, and CSF analysis. Meningitis in the setting of concomitant pulmonary TB is highly suggestive of tuberculous meningitis. Both CT and MRI of the brain are valuable for diagnosing TB meningitis and evaluating for complications. The hallmark pathologic feature of tuberculous meningitis is the presence of a thick exudate most prominent in the basilar meninges. Characteristic abnormalities include enhancement of the basilar meninges, thick exudates, obstructive hydrocephalus, and periventricular infarcts. Characteristic imaging abnormalities for TB meningitis can be found in Figure 64.2. Chest CT is sensitive for detecting pulmonary abnormalities in patients with tuberculous meningitis. Mediastinal and hilar lymphadenopathy, miliary pattern, and bronchopneumonic infiltrate are frequently noted.

Characteristic CSF abnormalities include a mononuclear pleocytosis, low glucose concentration, and elevated protein concentration. CSF pleocytosis can be lower in HIV-infected patients. Of note, 16% of patients with confirmed cryptococcal meningitis, 5% with TB, and 4% with bacterial meningitis will have normal CSF cell counts and biochemistry. Although CSF acid-fast bacillus

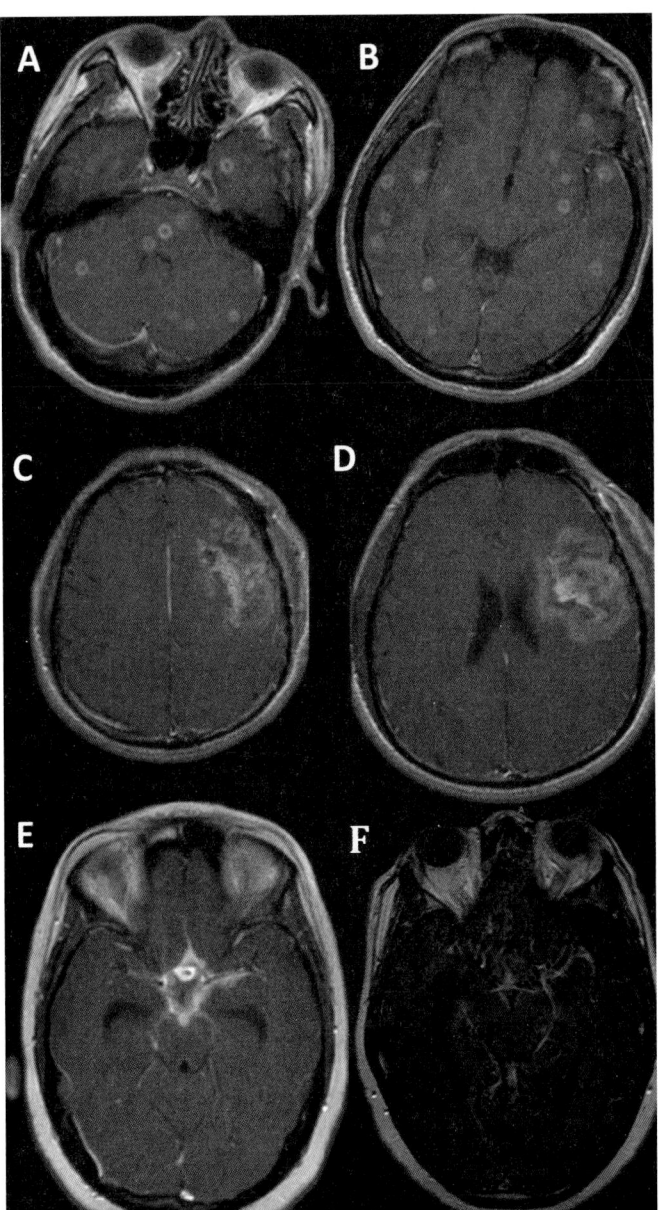

FIGURE 64.2 Axial brain MRI. **A and B:** T1 post contrast with multiple ring-enhancing lesions seen in miliary TB. **C and D:** T1 post contrast with large L frontal tuberculoma. **E and F:** T1 post contrast demonstrating avid basilar meningitis with leptomeningeal enhancement.

(AFB) smear and culture are crucial for making a diagnosis of tuberculous meningitis, there is a wide range of reported sensitivities for AFB smear; sensitivities can reach as high as 52% when large volume CSF samples (>6 mL) are evaluated by microscopy for at least 30 minutes. Conventional CSF culture for *M. tuberculosis* on Lowenstein–Jensen medium is positive in approximately 45% to 90% of cases but usually takes several weeks for a positive result. Detection of *M. tuberculosis* DNA in CSF by PCR assay is a useful ancillary diagnostic test, with nearly 100% specificity, but sensitivity varies between 30% and 50%, thus limiting its usefulness. Other assays that may prove more sensitive include detection of intracellular bacteria by a modified Ziehl–Neelsen stain and early secretory antigen target (ESAT)-6 in CSF leukocytes. In addition,

the World Health Organization has concluded that tests such as GeneXpert and microscopic observation drug susceptibility (MODS) assay are useful for the diagnosis of TB. The GeneXpert relies on DNA-PCR technique for detection of TB and rifampicin resistance while producing results in only 3 hours. The MODS was recently endorsed for rapid screening of multidrug-resistant TB. This technology uses an inverted light microscope to examine liquid culture for growth of the characteristic "cord"-like structures of TB. This can be completed in 7 to 10 days, compared to conventional solid culture that takes several weeks.

TREATMENT

Empiric treatment should be initiated when tuberculous meningitis is initially suspected, as the organism grows slowly, speciation can take weeks, and earlier treatment is associated with better outcomes. First-line antituberculous medications include rifampicin, isoniazid, pyrazinamide, ethambutol (RIPE), and streptomycin. Most first-line antituberculosis drugs (except ethambutol) achieve satisfactory levels in the CSF. Multidrug-resistant and extremely drug-resistant (XDR) TB pose a serious growing problem, and treatment should be individualized based on sensitivity testing. Adjunctive corticosteroids significantly reduce death and disabling residual neurologic deficits and should be used regardless of HIV status, although evidence for added benefit for HIV-infected patients is inconclusive.

NEUROSYPHILIS

Neurosyphilis has played an important role in the evolution of modern neurology. Paretic neurosyphilis was the first psychiatric disorder for which a specific cerebral pathology and treatment was reported. Erb described spinal syphilis tabes dorsalis in 1892. Quincke introduced lumbar puncture, and CSF examination was used to diagnose infection, even in asymptomatic people. *Treponema pallidum* was identified in the brain by Noguchi and Moore in 1913. The first effective treatment came in 1918 when Wagner-Jaurregg gave fever therapy for paresis. He was the first neurologist to win the Nobel Prize. Then came arsenical chemotherapy, the first planned use of a drug that would attack the organism without harming host tissues; this was Ehrlich's concept of "the magic bullet." Safer and more effective therapy came in 1945 with the introduction of penicillin, which has been in use since and has revolutionized the disease. Following the introduction of penicillin in the 1940s and 1950s, the incidence of neurosyphilis declined for two main reasons: (1) Fewer people spread the disease because those affected were being identified and treated and (2) many neurosyphilis infections were prevented because penicillin was being used to treat gonorrhea and other infections. For instance, the frequency of neurosyphilis as a cause of first admission to a psychiatric hospital plummeted from 5.9 cases per 100,000 population in 1942 to 0.1 cases per 100,000 in 1965. New cases became so rare that many hospitals discarded routine testing to detect syphilis.

During the next few decades, some investigators detected a shift in clinical patterns, but this finding was debated. The population at highest incidence was young homosexual men. Finally, in 1981, the AIDS epidemic occurred. The incidence of primary and secondary syphilis rose from 13.7 cases per 100,000 in 1981 to 18.4 cases per 100,000 in 1989, an increase of 34%. In the ensuing years, the incidence of syphilis declined. In 1997, fewer than 8,000 cases of early syphilis were reported in the United States, the lowest rate in 38 years and a sixfold decline from 1990. In addition to this alarming increase in the incidence of syphilis in industrialized countries, syphilis, like HIV, is an enormous health problem in developing countries. For instance, syphilis seropositivity among pregnant women in sub-Saharan Africa may be higher than 10%. Since 2000, there has been an unexpected increase in new cases of primary and secondary syphilis in the United States. Trends in Western Europe, Brazil, and Canada were similar, presumably because of a resurgence of unsafe sexual practices. Even before the HIV era, there had been a shift in clinical manifestations because of the widespread use of antibiotics. Previously common parenchymal forms became rare, whereas the incidence of meningeal (including meningitis, radiculitis, and cranial neuritis) and vascular syndromes have increased.

EPIDEMIOLOGY AND PATHOBIOLOGY

Syphilis is caused by the thin, motile corkscrew bacterium *T. pallidum*. This organism cannot be routinely cultured in the laboratory and is difficult to visualize using traditional light microscopy. Transmission is primarily via sexual contact with an infected individual or by vertical transmission from mother to fetus. Without treatment, the disease will inevitably progress through a series of clinical stages. In general, syphilis can be classified as early or late infection. Early infection encompasses primary, secondary, and early latent syphilis. Late infection refers to tertiary syphilis.

CLINICAL FEATURES

After sexual exposure to the organism, an asymptomatic incubation period of approximately 3 weeks occurs, followed by the development of a painless genital ulceration or chancre. If left untreated, the chancre will resolve in 3 to 5 weeks and the disease will progress to secondary syphilis. Secondary syphilis is a syndrome of fever, lymphadenopathy, headache, malaise, myalgia, and a macular or pustular rash of the palms and soles. During this stage, involvement of other organ systems produces clinical symptoms, including mucosal lesions, renal failure, hepatitis, and neurologic symptoms. The signs and symptoms of secondary syphilis typically resolve in 4 to 10 weeks, and the patient is deemed latently infected. About one-third of patients with untreated latent syphilis will progress to develop late or tertiary syphilis, which can affect any organ in the body, particularly the nervous system, manifesting with a variety of symptoms.

T. pallidum spreads hematogenously to the CNS early in the course of disease, and clinical signs and symptoms are not limited to stage of disease. Patterns of meningitis or vascular disease may be more common earlier in disease, whereas late disease presents as parenchymal or spinal cord pathologies. Although neurosyphilis can produce a wide variety of manifestations, including general paresis, psychiatric illness, cognitive decline, tabes dorsalis, or vascular disease, this section will limit the discussion to syphilitic meningitis.

Syphilitic meningitis typically presents in the secondary stage of syphilis within 2 years of acquiring infection. Although meningitis is less common than other forms of neurosyphilis, abnormal CSF with pleocytosis and elevated protein concentration occurs in up to 25% of patients. The most common presenting symptoms include headache, photophobia, nausea and vomiting, meningismus, and cranial nerve deficits. Although any cranial nerve can be affected, cranial nerves VII and VIII are most commonly affected.

DIAGNOSIS

The diagnosis of neurosyphilis is typically made through a combination of history, physical examination, and results of serologic and CSF analyses. The first step in diagnosis is performing serologic testing for syphilis using Venereal Disease Research Laboratory (VDRL) and rapid plasma reagin assays. These assays detect IgG and IgM antibodies to a cardiolipin-lecithin cholesterol antigen and remain positive in patients who have had syphilis, regardless of treatment. Treponemal assays, including the fluorescent treponemal antibody absorption (FTA-ABS) and *T. pallidum* particle agglutination tests (MHA-TP) measure treponemal antibodies and are used for confirming infection. Treponemal assays should also be positive in patients with neurosyphilis. The sensitivities of treponemal-specific tests (TST), although in the range of 80% for primary syphilis, are believed to be nearly 100% in cases of secondary syphilis. False-positive TST are infrequent.

In syphilitic meningitis, CSF typically has a mononuclear-predominant pleocytosis, elevated protein concentration (>45 mg/dL), and normal or decreased glucose concentration. Although CSF immunologic tests, such as VDRL, are usually abnormal in syphilitic meningitis (70% sensitivity), a negative result does not rule out neurosyphilis. More recently, PCR assays have been developed to detect *T. pallidum* in the CSF, but 50% of patients with syphilitic involvement of the CNS have a negative PCR. Other new techniques include using CSF-FTA and percentage of CSF B cells when CSF-VDRL is negative to aid in establishing the diagnosis of neurosyphilis.

TREATMENT

Penicillin is the first-line therapy for neurosyphilis. The CDC recommends 18 million units to 24 million units of aqueous penicillin G per day administered as 3 million units to 4 million units intravenous (IV) every 4 hours or as continuous infusion for 10 to 14 days. An alternative is procaine penicillin 2.4 million units intramuscular (IM) daily with probenecid 500 mg orally 4 times daily for 10 to 14 days [**Level 1**].[1]

LYME DISEASE

EPIDEMIOLOGY

Lyme disease is the most common tickborne infection in the United States. The CDC reports that 300,000 cases of Lyme disease are diagnosed in the United States each year, with 96% of cases concentrated in 13 states (Connecticut, Delaware, Maine, Maryland, Massachusetts, Minnesota, New Hampshire, New Jersey, New York, Pennsylvania, Vermont, Virginia, and Wisconsin). In humans, the signs and symptoms of Lyme borreliosis most frequently appear in spring, summer, and early autumn, coinciding with the activity of nymphs and with the increasing recreational use of tick habitats by the public.

PATHOBIOLOGY

North American Lyme borreliosis, or Lyme disease, is caused by *Borrelia burgdorferi*, which is transmitted by specific *Ixodes* spp. ticks. In Europe, at least five species of Lyme *Borrelia* (*Borrelia afzelii*, *Borrelia garinii*, *B. burgdorferi*, *Borrelia spielmanii*, and *Borrelia bavariensis*) can cause the disease, leading to a wider variety of possible clinical manifestations in Europe than in North America. Transmission of the organism occurs through injection of tick saliva during feeding. A feeding period of more than 36 hours is usually required for transmission of *B. burgdorferi* by *Ixodes scapularis* or *Ixodes pacificus*. In North America, the only species of Lyme *Borrelia* known to cause human disease is *B. burgdorferi*.

CLINICAL FEATURES

Initial infection is typically manifested by a skin lesion known as *erythema migrans*. Erythema migrans consists of an area of erythroderma that enlarges over days to weeks, often reaching several inches in diameter. Spirochetes initially proliferate at the site of the tick bite. When sufficiently numerous, they slowly migrate centrifugally from the site of inoculation, typically for up to 30 days after the bite. Depending on the location on the body, the rash may be round or elliptical. Central pallor may be present.

Early disseminated disease is usually characterized by a multifocal rash, with each new focus representing a nidus of spirochetes that spread hematogenously from the initial site. The bacterial dissemination is accompanied by the usual host inflammatory reaction to bacteremia: fever, diffuse aches and pains, headaches, malaise, fatigue. Up to 5% of infected individuals develop heart block, known as *Lyme carditis*, sometimes requiring a temporary pacemaker. Early dissemination affects the nervous system in 10% to 15% of patients, primarily in the first few months after the initial infection, during what is often termed *acute disseminated infection*. Most commonly, patients present with an aseptic lymphocytic meningitis, cranial neuritis, or painful polyradiculitis. First described in Europe, Garin-Bujadoux-Bannwarth syndrome is now considered to include all or part of a classic triad: lymphocytic meningitis, cranial neuritis, and polyradiculitis. Cranial and peripheral nerve involvement can occur anywhere along the course of affected nerves, not preferentially in the subarachnoid space. Approximately three-fourths of patients with Lyme-associated cranial neuropathies present with a facial nerve palsy. Early studies suggested this could be bilateral in up to one quarter of cases.

Late Lyme disease can manifest as arthritis or the skin disorder known as *acrodermatitis chronica atrophicans*, a tissue paper thinning of the skin. Neurologic manifestations of late Lyme disease include myelitis, encephalitis, and neurobehavioral changes. Much attention has focused on patients who have persistent fatigue and cognitive difficulty after receiving treatment for Lyme disease with regimens that should be highly effective even for severe infections, a disorder often referred to as *post–Lyme syndrome*. This topic is controversial and is beyond the scope of this chapter.

DIAGNOSIS

Typical erythema migrans is usually sufficiently distinctive to allow a clinical diagnosis in the absence of a supporting laboratory test. Serologic assays for antibodies to Lyme *Borrelia* are positive infrequently at this stage, and thus should be obtained only in atypical cases, and then in conjunction with convalescent phase serologic testing 2 to 6 weeks after obtaining the acute sample. Treatment at this stage will prevent progression to neurologic Lyme disease.

The majority of patients with early Lyme disease are seropositive on serum two-tier testing (ELISA and IgG immunoblot). Those who are seronegative at presentation will convert in 2 weeks after acute phase. CSF testing for intrathecal antibody production and lumbar puncture showing lymphocytic meningitis are useful to confirm diagnosis. CSF PCR is insensitive for the diagnosis of neurologic Lyme disease and should not be routinely used. Late neurologic Lyme disease requires a positive serum two-tier (ELISA and IgG immunoblot) seropositivity and evidence of intrathecal antibody. CSF examination generally supports an active infection with a lymphocytic meningitis, elevated protein concentration, and normal glucose concentration.

TREATMENT

For adult patients with early Lyme disease and the acute neurologic presentation of meningitis or radiculopathy, ceftriaxone 2 g IV daily for 14 days is recommended [**Level 1**].[2] Parenteral therapy with cefotaxime or penicillin G may be acceptable alternatives

[**Level 1**].[2] Oral doxycycline has good oral absorption and CNS penetration and may also be an alternative. Late neurologic Lyme disease may present as encephalomyelitis, peripheral neuropathy, or encephalopathy. These patients should be treated with ceftriaxone 2 g IV once daily for 2 to 4 weeks. Cefotaxime or penicillin G may be acceptable alternatives. Retreatment is not indicated for persistent or recurrent symptoms.

LEVEL 1 EVIDENCE

1. Centers for Disease Control and Prevention. 2010 guidelines for treatment of sexually transmitted diseases. *MMWR Morb Mortal Wkly Rep.* 2010;59(RR-12):1–110.
2. Wormser GP, Dattwyler RJ, Shapiro ED, et al. The clinical assessment, treatment, and prevention of Lyme disease, human granulocytic anaplasmosis, and babesiosis: clinical practice guidelines by the Infectious Diseases Society of America. *Clin Infect Dis.* 2006;43(9):1089–1134.

SUGGESTED READINGS

Ackermann R, Rehse-Kupper B, Gollmer E, et al. Chronic neurologic manifestations of erythema migrans borreliosis. *Ann N Y Acad Sci.* 1988;539:16–23.

Alspaugh JA, Perfect JR. Fungal infections of the central nervous system. In: Roos KL, ed. *Principles of Neurologic Infectious Disease.* New York: McGraw-Hill; 2005:175.

Ampel NM. Coccidioidomycosis in persons infected with HIV type 1. *Clin Infect Dis.* 2005;41(8):1174–1178.

Arsura EL, Johnson R, Penrose J, et al. Neuroimaging as a guide to predict outcomes for patients with coccidioidal meningitis. *Clin Infect Dis.* 2005; 40(4):624–627.

Blair JE. Coccidioidal meningitis: update on epidemiology, clinical features, diagnosis, and management. *Curr Infect Dis Rep.* 2009;11(4):289–295.

Bush JW, Wuerz T, Embil JM, et al. Outcomes of persons with blastomycosis involving the central nervous system. *Diagn Microbiol Infect Dis.* 2013;76(2): 175–181.

Cecchini D, Ambrosioni J, Brezzo C, et al. Tuberculous meningitis in HIV-infected and non-infected patients: comparison of cerebrospinal fluid findings. *Int J Tuberc Lung Dis.* 2009;13(2):269–271.

Chapman SW, Dismukes WE, Proia LA, et al. Clinical practice guidelines for the management of blastomycosis: 2008 update by the Infectious Diseases Society of America. *Clin Infect Dis.* 2008;46:1801–1812.

Day J. Cryptococcal meningitis. *Pract Neurol.* 2004;4:274–285.

Day JN, Chau TTH, Wolbers M, et al. Combination antifungal therapy for cryptococcal meningitis. *New Engl J Med.* 2013;368(14):1291–1302.

de Vedia L, Arechavala A, Calderón MI, et al. Relevance of intracranial hypertension control in the management of *Cryptococcus neoformans* meningitis related to AIDS. *Infection.* 2013;41(6):1073–1077.

Diekema DJ, Messer SA, Hollis RJ, et al. Activities of caspofungin, itraconazole, posaconazole, ravuconazole, voriconazole, and amphotericin B against 448 recent clinical isolates of filamentous fungi. *J Clin Microbiol.* 2003; 41(8):3623–3626.

Drake KW, Adam RD. Coccidioidal meningitis and brain abscesses: analysis of 71 cases at a referral center. *Neurology.* 2009;73(21):1780–1786.

Ellner JJ, Bennett JE. Chronic meningitis. *Medicine.* 1976;55:34.

Feng GD, Shi M, Ma L, et al. Diagnostic accuracy of intracellular *Mycobacterium tuberculosis* detection for tuberculous meningitis. *Am J Respir Crit Care Med.* 2014;189(4):475–481.

Flood JM, Weinstock HS, Guroy ME, et al. Neurosyphilis during the AIDS epidemic, San Francisco 1985–1992. *J Infect Dis.* 1998;177(4):931–940.

Galgiani JN, Ampel NM, Blair JE, et al. Coccidioidomycosis. *Clin Infect Dis.* 2005;41(9):1217–1223.

Garcia-Monco JC. CNS tuberculosis and mycobacteriosis. In: Roos KL, ed. *Principles of Neurologic Infectious Disease.* New York: McGraw-Hill; 2005:195.

Graybill JR, Sobel J, Saag M, et al. Diagnosis and management of increased intracranial pressure in patients with AIDS and cryptococcal meningitis. The NIAID Mycoses Study Group and AIDS Cooperative Treatment Groups. *Clin Infect Dis.* 2000;30(1):47–54.

Halerin JJ. Lyme disease: a multisystem infection that affects the nervous system. *Continuum (Minneap Minn).* 2012;18(6):1338–1350.

Halperin JJ. Lyme disease: neurology, neurobiology, and behavior. *Clin Infect Dis.* 2014;58(9):1267–1272.

Halperin JJ, Logigian EL, Finkel MF, et al. Practice parameters for the diagnosis of patients with nervous system Lyme borreliosis (Lyme disease). *Neurology.* 1996;46:619–627.

Herbrecht R, Denning DW, Patterson TF, et al. Voriconazole versus amphotericin B for primary therapy of invasive aspergillosis. *N Engl J Med.* 2002;347(6):408–415.

Hook EW, Chansolme DH. Neurosyphilis. In: Roos KL, ed. *Principles of Neurologic Infectious Disease.* New York: McGraw-Hill; 2005:215.

Jain KK, Mittal SK, Kuman S, et al. Imaging feature of central nervous system fungal infections. *Neurol India.* 2007;55(3):214–250.

Kabanda T, Siedner MJ, Klausner JD, et al. Point-of-care diagnosis and prognostication of cryptococcal meningitis with the cryptococcal antigen lateral flow assay on cerebrospinal fluid. *Clin Infect Dis.* 2014;58(1):113–116.

Kalina P, Decker A, Kornel E, et al. Lyme disease of the brainstem. *Neuroradiology.* 2005;47:903–907.

Kleinschmidt-DeMasters BK. Central nervous system aspergillosis: a 20-year retrospective series. *Hum Pathol.* 2002;33(1):116–124.

Latge JP. *Aspergillus fumigatus* and aspergillosis. *Clin Microbiol Rev.* 1999;12(2):310–350.

Lemos LB, Guo M, Baliga M. Blastomycosis: organ involvement and etiological diagnosis. A review of 123 patients from Mississippi. *Ann Diagn Pathol.* 2000;4(6):391–406.

Lu CH, Chang WN, Chang HW, et al. The prognostic factors of cryptococcal meningitis in HIV-negative patients. *J Hosp Infect.* 1999;42(4):313–320.

Macsween KF, Bicanic T, Brouwer AE, et al. Lumbar drainage for control of raised cerebrospinal fluid pressure in cryptococcal meningitis: case report and review. *J Infect.* 2005;51(4):e221–e224.

Mamidi A, DeSimone JA, Pomerantz RJ. Central nervous system infections in individuals with HIV-1 infection. *J Neurovirol.* 2002;8(3):158–167.

Marra CM, Tantalo LC, Maxwell CL, et al. Alternative cerebrospinal fluid tests to diagnose neurosyphilis in HIV-infected individuals. *Neurology.* 2004;63(1):85–88.

Marra CM, Tantalo LC, Maxwell CL, et al. The rapid plasma reagin test cannot replace the venereal disease research laboratory test for neurosyphilis diagnosis. *Sex Transm Dis.* 2012;39(6):453–457.

Mitchell TG, Perfect JR. Cryptococcosis in the era of AIDS: 100 years after the discovery of *Cryptococcus neoformans*. *Clin Microbiol Rev.* 1995;8(4):515–548.

Moore DA, Evans CA, Gilman RH, et al. Microscopic-observation drug-susceptibility assay for the diagnosis of TB. *N Engl J Med.* 2006;355(15):1539–1550.

Moore JE, Hopkins HH. Asymptomatic neurosyphilis: VI. The prognosis of early and late asymptomatic neurosyphilis. *JAMA.* 1930;95(22):1637–1641.

Powderly WG. Current approach to the acute management of cryptococcal infections. *J Infect.* 2000;41(1):18–22.

Prasad K, Singh MB. Corticosteroids for managing tuberculous meningitis. *Cochrane Database Syst Rev.* 2008;(1):CD002244.

Ragland AS, Arusa E, Ismail Y, et al. Eosinophilic pleocytosis in coccidioidal meningitis: frequency and significance. *Am J Med.* 1993;95(3):254–257.

Reinwald M, Spiess B, Heinz WJ, et al. Aspergillus PCR-based investigation of fresh tissue and effusion samples in patients with suspected invasive aspergillosis enhances diagnostic capabilities. *J Clin Microbiol.* 2013;51(12):4178–4185.

Roos KL, Bryan JP, Maggio WW, et al. Intracranial blastomycoma. *Medicine (Baltimore).* 1987;66(3):224–235.

Saccente M, Woods GL. Clinical and laboratory update on blastomycosis. *Clin Microbiol Rev.* 2010;23(2):367–381.

Segal BH, Walsh TJ. Current approaches to diagnosis and treatment of invasive aspergillosis. *Am J Respir Crit Care Med.* 2006;173(7):707–717.

Smith JE, Aksamit AJ Jr. Outcome of chronic idiopathic meningitis. *Mayo Clin Proc.* 1994;69(6):548–556.

Smith RM, Mba-Jonas A, Tourdjman M, et al. Treatment and outcomes among patients with *Cryptococcus gattii* infections in the United States Pacific Northwest. *PLoS One.* 2014;9(2):e88875.

Solomons RS, van Elsland SL, Visser DH, et al. Commercial nucleic acid amplification tests in tuberculous meningitis-a meta-analysis. *Diagn Microbiol Infect Dis.* 2014;78(4):398–403.

Stanek G, Wormser GP, Gray J, et al. Lyme borreliosis. *Lancet.* 2012;379:461–473.

Stewart SM. The bacteriological diagnosis of tuberculous meningitis. *J Clin Pathol.* 1953;6(3):241–242.

Targeted tuberculin testing and treatment of latent tuberculosis infection. *Am J Respir Crit Care Med.* 2000;161(4, pt 2):S221–S247.

Thwaites GE, Chau TT, Farrar JJ. Improving the bacteriological diagnosis of tuberculous meningitis. *J Clin Microbiol.* 2004;42(1):378–379.

Van der Horst CM, Saag MS, Cloud GA, et al. Treatment of cryptococcal meningitis associated with the acquired immunodeficiency syndrome. National Institute of Allergy and Infectious Diseases Mycoses Study Group and AIDS Clinical Trials Group. *New Engl J Med.* 1997;337(1):15–21.

Walusimbi, Bwanga F, De Costa A, et al. Meta-analysis to compare the accuracy of GeneXpert, MODS and the WHO 2007 algorithm for diagnosis of smear-negative pulmonary tuberculosis. *BMC Infect Dis.* 2013;13:507.

Wheat LJ, Freifeld AG, Kleiman MB, et al. Clinical practice guidelines for the management of histoplasmosis: 2007 update by the Infectious Diseases Society of America. *Clin Infect Dis.* 2007;45:807–825.

Woodworth GF, McGirt MJ, Williams MA, et al. The use of ventriculoperitoneal shunts for uncontrollable intracranial hypertension without ventriculomegaly secondary to HIV-associated cryptococcal meningitis. *Surg Neurol.* 2005;63(6):529–531.

INTRODUCTION

Parasitic infections are a tremendous public health burden in tropical and subtropical regions. Parasitic tropical diseases of the nervous system can be found anywhere in the world due to the exponential increase in international travel, tourism, and migration. One important factor is the disregard of tourists and business travelers for the prophylactic measures recommended before traveling to parts of the world where potential exposure to endemic parasitic diseases may occur. When travel history precedes the onset of the disease, neurologists should have a high index of suspicion based on basic knowledge of the most common parasitic neurologic diseases (Table 65.1) in order to diagnose and treat these exotic conditions.

Parasitic diseases are divided into *protozoan infections* caused by unicellular organisms (malaria, trypanosomiasis, amebiasis) and *metazoan infections* caused by worms (helminths), mainly cestodes or tapeworms (cysticercosis), nematodes or round worms (larva migrans, baylisascariasis, gnathostomiasis, strongyloidiasis), and trematodes or flukes (paragonimiasis). Not included in this chapter are neurologic diseases transmitted by ectoparasites, such as ticks and other arthropods, including Lyme disease (a spirochetal infection caused by *Borrelia burgdorferi*) (see Chapter 64); other forms of borreliosis presenting as relapsing fevers transmitted to humans by lice or ticks (see Chapter 64); and gram-negative bacterial infections, such as the Rickettsial typhus group (caused by *Rickettsia prowazekii* and *Rickettsia typhi*, transmitted respectively by the body louse *Pediculus humanus* and the rat flea *Xenopsylla cheopis*), as well

TABLE 65.1 Parasitic Infections of the Nervous System

Name	Agent	Reservoir	Transmission
Metazoan Infections			
Neurocysticercosis	*Taenia solium*	Pigs, humans	Human *Taenia* carriers
Gnathostomiasis	*Gnathostoma spinigerum*	Fish, poultry, dogs, cats	Undercooked fish, poultry
Hydatid cysts	*Echinococcus* species	Dogs, foxes, sheep, cows	Dogs' feces
Larva migrans	*Toxocara canis, Toxocara cati, Ascaris* species	Dogs, cats	Dogs' and cats' feces
Baylisascariasis	*Baylisascaris procyonis*	Raccoon (*Procyon lotor*)	Raccoons' feces
Paragonimiasis	*Paragonimus westermani*	Fresh water crustaceans, snails	Eating uncooked crustaceans
Schistosomiasis/ bilharziasis	*Schistosoma* species	Fresh water snails	Skin penetration by larval forms (cercariae) in infected water
Sparganosis	*Spirometra mansoni*	Reptiles, amphibians	Eating uncooked frogs or snakes
Strongyloidiasis	*Strongyloides stercoralis*	Human	Infected soil contact
Trichinosis	*Trichinella spiralis*	Pigs	Eating undercooked pork
Protozoan Infections			
African trypanosomiasis Sleeping sickness	*Trypanosoma brucei*	Ungulates	Tsetse flies (*Glossina*)
American trypanosomiasis Chagas disease	*Trypanosoma cruzi*	Opossum, dogs	Triatomine bugs
Amebiasis	*Entamoeba histolytica*	Human	Ingestion of food contaminated with feces
Primary amebic meningoencephalitis	*Naegleria* species	Warm fresh water ponds	Nasal route while swimming
Granulomatous amebic encephalitis	*Acanthamoeba* species	Fresh and brackish water	Nasal route while swimming
Cerebral malaria	*Plasmodium falciparum*	Human	*Anopheles* mosquitoes
Toxoplasmosis	*Toxoplasma gondii*	Cat	Cats' feces in contaminated soil or vegetables

as the spotted fevers transmitted by ticks and caused by *Rickettsia rickettsii* (see Chapter 63). *Toxoplasma gondii* infection is discussed in the context of HIV infection (see Chapter 67).

PROTOZOAN INFECTIONS OF THE NERVOUS SYSTEM

CEREBRAL MALARIA

Cerebral malaria is an acute encephalopathy caused by *Plasmodium falciparum*, the most virulent of the four *Plasmodium* species that infect humans when a female *Anopheles* mosquito inoculates the protozoan parasites through the skin. Parasites are carried to the liver where they mature and multiply to enter the red cells in the bloodstream.

According to the Centers for Disease Control and Prevention (CDC), malaria causes 660,000 deaths each year, mainly among young children in sub-Saharan Africa. In 2011, the number of malaria cases reported in the United States was the largest since 1971, representing a 48% increase from 2008. Most malaria infections occurred among travelers to regions with active malaria transmission.

Clinical Features

Malaria presents with typical bouts of intermittent fever with chills, rigors, and anemia. Cerebral malaria may be heralded by headache, vomiting, and a clinical picture of encephalopathy developing over days in a febrile patient, accompanied by confusion, decreased responsiveness, and somnolence rapidly progressing to stupor and coma. Psychomotor agitation and psychiatric manifestations may precede cerebral malaria. Focal findings are uncommon, except when stroke occurs. In children, tonic–clonic seizures occur, followed by postictal unresponsiveness.

In adults, cerebral malaria may occur in the setting of severe malaria presenting with acute respiratory distress; pulmonary edema; acute renal failure and hemoglobinuria ("blackwater fever"); jaundice and liver failure; severe anemia; thrombocytopenia; disseminated intravascular coagulation; and bleeding complications, including intracranial hemorrhages. Severe hypoglycemia must be assumed to be present in children with cerebral malaria and should be treated promptly and aggressively.

Retinal hemorrhages and exudates are usually seen on funduscopic examination and reflect the cerebral small-vessel vasculopathy. Meningeal signs do not occur and cerebrospinal fluid (CSF) is normal; however, spinal tap is mandatory to exclude other causes of encephalopathy. Brain imaging may show evidence of brain swelling and herniation or small hemorrhages.

Treatment

The drugs of choice for treatment of cerebral malaria are the derivatives of artemisinin, such as artesunate, artemether, or arteether. Quinine is an equivalent alternative for cerebral malaria. Development of drug resistance to artemisinin derivatives has occurred and combination therapy for *P. falciparum* malaria with other antimalarial drug is recommended. Cerebral malaria is a critical condition and requires intensive care treatment; complications such as hypoglycemia, respiratory distress syndrome, and acute renal and liver failure must be promptly recognized and treated. Severe anemia or bleeding diathesis may require blood transfusions. Steroids are not recommended in cerebral malaria. Despite treatment, the mortality is over 25%, but survivors usually recover without sequelae; however, residual hemiplegia, extrapyramidal symptoms, blindness, psychiatric symptoms, and epilepsy may occur.

There is intensive research on the immune mechanisms of cerebral malaria leading to vascular occlusion by parasitized erythrocytes, vasoconstriction, and alterations of the blood–brain barrier with decreased cerebral blood flow, edema, demyelination, ischemia, hypoxia, acidosis, and death. Potential therapies based on nitric oxide bioavailability, high levels of endothelin-1, and angiopoietin dysfunction appear promising.

Malaria prevention relies on avoiding exposure to mosquitoes using repellents and insecticide-treated bed nets and prophylactic use of antimalarial drugs prior to, during, and after travel to endemic malaria regions. A viable malaria vaccine is yet to succeed.

TRYPANOSOMIASIS

Two human infections with protozoa of the genus *Trypanosoma* have neurologic importance: African trypanosomiasis (sleeping sickness) and American trypanosomiasis (Chagas disease); both are transmitted by infected arthropods, the tsetse fly (*Glossina* species) in Africa, and triatomine (reduviid) bugs in South America.

African Trypanosomiasis

This fatal encephalitis is caused by infection with *Trypanosoma brucei rhodesiense* and *Trypanosoma brucei gambiense*, endemic respectively to East and West Africa. Tsetse fly infests one-third of Africa's landmass representing a problem of appalling magnitude. African trypanosomiasis or *sleeping sickness* is a chronic encephalitis, with diencephalic involvement resulting in disruption of the circadian sleep/wake cycle manifested by excessive daytime sleepiness, sleep attacks similar to those of narcolepsy, and nocturnal insomnia. There are also psychiatric manifestations, seizures, coma, and finally death. CSF shows lymphocytic pleocytosis and moderate increase in protein concentration and immunoglobulins (Ig), especially intrathecal IgM. African trypanosomes can be identified by fine needle aspirate of enlarged cervical lymph nodes, as well as in blood and CSF. The combination of nifurtimox and eflornithine appears to be a promising treatment.

American Trypanosomiasis

Human infection with *Trypanosoma cruzi* (Chagas disease) affects an estimated 10 million people in Latin America causing about 50,000 annual deaths. Presence of infected asymptomatic blood donors in the United States led blood banks to perform routine trypanosome screening with radioimmunoprecipitation.

Acute infection following the triatomine bite causes subcutaneous swelling typically located in the orbital region (Romaña sign), cervical lymph node enlargement, and acute myocarditis or encephalitis. A striking feature of Chagas disease is the selective neuronal destruction with denervation of the myenteric plexus of the intestine causing megaesophagus and megacolon and denervation of the ganglionar neurons in the conduction system of the heart leading to a chronic dilated cardiomyopathy. The dilated heart becomes an important cause of embolic stroke. At autopsy, one-third of patients with chronic Chagas disease have left ventricular thrombi.

T. cruzi can be demonstrated in blood or CSF or by serologic testing. Treatment of acute disease or reactivations includes nifurtimox, benznidazole, or itraconazole. There is no effective therapy for chronic Chagas disease. Secondary prevention of stroke with long-term anticoagulation is recommended.

AMEBIC MENINGOENCEPHALITIS

Primary amebic meningoencephalitis is due to infection with the free-living ameba *Naegleria fowleri*. Infection is acquired by swimming in warm bodies of natural or man-made fresh water.

The organisms penetrate the cribriform plate and reach the brain causing acute meningoencephalitis and brain abscess. The clinical presentation is typical of purulent meningitis. The organisms are seldom isolated. Treatment with intravenous and intrathecal amphotericin B, intravenous and intrathecal miconazole, and oral rifampin should be started based on clinical suspicion in patients with meningitis and history of swimming in warm fresh waters.

A chronic granulomatous form of amebic meningoencephalitis often accompanied by cutaneous infection and keratitis is caused by infection with the opportunistic free-living amebae *Balamuthia mandrillaris* and by several species of *Acanthamoeba* affecting immunosuppressed patients, transplant recipients, or malnourished individuals. Treatment is often unsuccessful.

METAZOAN INFECTIONS OF THE NERVOUS SYSTEM

NEUROCYSTICERCOSIS

Neurocysticercosis is the human infection with larval forms (cysticerci) of the pig tapeworm *Taenia solium*. Neurocysticercosis is the most common neurologic infection caused by helminthes (cestodes) in humans. Contrary to common belief, consumption of poorly cooked pork infected with *T. solium* cysticerci does not cause neurocysticercosis but results in intestinal tapeworm infection or human taeniasis. Neurocysticercosis occurs from human-to-human transmission of fertilized *T. solium* eggs from a human carrier of intestinal *Taenia*. Humans become intermediate hosts in the life cycle of *T. solium* by ingesting *Taenia* eggs due to fecal contamination of water or food. Failure of intestinal *Taenia* carriers to wash their hands after defecation is the most common source of infection.

Pathobiology

Ingested eggs hatch in the intestine, enter the bloodstream, and are carried into the host tissues including heart, muscles, and the brain and spinal cord where cysticerci develop into cystic forms called *Cysticercus racemosus* (Latin *racemus*, bunch of grapes). Neurocysticercosis can be prevented with hand washing, clean water, and environmental sanitation.

Cysticerci are found in the brain parenchyma, the subarachnoid spaces, the ventricular system, the eye, the spinal cord and intrathecal nerve roots, as well as in the heart, the muscles, and subcutaneous tissues. Although many cysticerci fail to elicit a foreign body reaction, inflammation around each cysticercus eventually develops, accompanied by edema, reactive gliosis, and formation of dense exudates in the subarachnoid space composed of collagen, lymphocytes, multinucleated giant cells, eosinophils, and hyalinized parasitic membranes found in parenchymal lesions but also causing eosinophilic meningitis, ventriculitis, and radiculitis. Stroke may result from involvement of the blood vessels by the inflammation. Even calcified lesions may develop perilesional edema associated with seizure activity.

Clinical Features

Neurocysticercosis is the most common cause of epilepsy in tropical areas of Latin America, Africa, and Asia. It results in 50,000 deaths per year and is a frequent cause of chronic neurologic disorders due to irreversible brain or spinal cord damage. Neurocysticercosis is becoming increasingly prevalent in industrialized countries because of travel and migration. In the United States, 1,494 patients with

neurocysticercosis were reported between 1980 and 2004, making it the most common imported disease of the nervous system.

Cysticercosis is a pleomorphic disease capable of producing epilepsy, stroke with focal neurologic deficits, intracranial hypertension, and reversible dementia. Diagnostic criteria have been clearly established. Reported cases in the United States presented with seizures (66%), hydrocephalus (16%), and headaches (15%) due to parenchymal neurocysticercosis brain lesions (91%); the remainder had ventricular cysts (6%), subarachnoid cysts (2%), and spinal cord lesions (0.2%).

Diagnosis

The diagnosis of neurocysticercosis is based on clinical findings, a history of travel to endemic regions or potential exposure to *Taenia* carriers, and immunologic tests. The possibility that a patient harbors an intestinal *Taenia* should be explored with repeated examinations of stools for ova and parasites. On neuroimaging, parenchymal neurocysticercosis shows single or multiple cysts in the parenchyma, with the typical "hole-in-donut" appearance with presence of the radiodense scolex of the parasite. In subarachnoid neurocysticercosis, there is abnormal enhancement of the leptomeninges, hydrocephalus, and cystic lesions located at the sylvian fissure or basal cisterns. Multiple calcified lesions ("starry sky") on computed tomography (CT) indicate spontaneous resolution. CSF usually shows lymphocytic pleocytosis, presence of eosinophils, increased protein (up to 2,000 mg/dL), and normal glucose. Serum immunoblot and CSF enzyme-linked immunosorbent assay (ELISA) are useful confirmatory tests.

Treatment

The recommended treatment for patients with viable subarachnoid or parenchymal cysts is albendazole for 8 to 15 days, usually in combination with dexamethasone to avoid the risk of stroke or brain edema. Dexamethasone administration should begin prior to the start of albendazole therapy and should be prolonged for several days. Isolated intraventricular cysts in the fourth ventricle are best treated with endoscopic surgery. Shunt placement must be considered before the start of albendazole in patients with hydrocephalus.

LARVA MIGRANS AND EOSINOPHILIC MENINGITIS

Infection of the nervous system by nematodes or roundworms occurs when humans become hosts to the parasite and the moving worms migrate producing the clinical syndrome called *larva migrans* usually accompanied by eosinophilic meningitis. The severity of the infection depends mainly on the size and vitality of the parasite, ranging from the severe meningoencephalitis or myelitis caused by the tracts of the spike-covered worm *Gnathostoma spinigerum* in Thailand or the highly motile *Ascaris* of the North American raccoon *Baylisascariasis procyonis* or by to the relatively benign eosinophilic meningitis caused in Southeast Asia by *Angiostrongylus cantonensis*, the rat lungworm.

Pathobiology

A history of travel is usually elicited because humans become hosts to the parasite by ingestion of contaminated Japanese-style raw fish, such as sushi and sashimi, and consumption of natural and exotic foods, such as raw mollusks, shrimp, freshwater crustaceans, snails, snakes, frogs, or insufficiently cooked chicken or duck contaminated with the infective larvae of the parasite. Once ingested, the highly motile larvae cross the intestinal wall and migrate to subcutaneous tissues causing cutaneous larva migrans,

TABLE 65.2	Nematode (Round Worm) Infections of the Nervous System Causing Larva Migrans Syndrome and Eosinophilic Meningitis		
Name	**Agent**	**Geographic Location**	**Clinical Presentation**
Angiostrongyliasis Eosinophilic meningitis	*Angiostrongylus cantonensis*	China, Southeast Asia, Taiwan, Thailand, Vietnam, Australia, South Pacific islands	Eosinophilic aseptic meningitis
	Angiostrongylus costaricensis	Costa Rica, Central America	
Gnathostomiasis	*Gnathostoma spinigerum*	Southeast Asia	Meningoencephalitis, myelitis, eosinophilic meningitis, cutaneous and visceral larva migrans
Baylisascariasis	*Baylisascaris procyonis*	North America	Meningoencephalitis, myelitis, eosinophilic meningitis, eye involvement, cutaneous larva migrans
Toxocariasis Larva migrans	*Toxocara canis, Toxocara cati* *Ascaris* spp.	Worldwide	Eosinophilic meningitis, eye involvement, myelitis, encephalitis, cutaneous larva migrans

continuing to visceral larva migrans with involvement of internal organs, skeletal muscles, the eye, and the nervous system. Table 65.2 summarizes the main geographic forms of the larva migrans syndromes and eosinophilic meningitis.

These conditions usually present with eosinophilic pleocytosis in the CSF demonstrated with the use of the Giemsa or Wright stain showing greater than 10 eosinophils per mL or more than 10% of the total CSF leukocyte count. Eosinophils are effectors of the adaptive immune response (helper T cell type 2) directed against destruction of metazoan multicellular parasites.

Clinical Features

Neurologic forms of presentation include the relatively benign eosinophilic meningitis of angiostrongyliasis to the more severe cases with encephalitis, transverse myelitis, seizures, meningitis, subarachnoid hemorrhage, and focal neurologic deficits associated with parenchymal brain hemorrhages that occur with larger parasites causing gnathostomiasis and baylisascariasis.

Diagnosis

CSF examination may range from the normal appearance and mild eosinophilic meningitis of angiostrongyliasis to the usually bloody and xanthochromic CSF of gnathostomiasis and baylisascariasis, with severe eosinophilic pleocytosis (up to 3,000 cells/mm^3), mild increase in protein concentration, and normal glucose concentration. Blood eosinophilia is usually present. Neuroimaging shows the tracts of the parasites as long or multiple parenchymal brain hemorrhages or evidence of multiple foci of myelitis. Diagnosis is confirmed by identification of the larvae in CSF or tissue samples.

Treatment

The recommended treatment of eosinophilic meningomyelitis is a combination of antihelmintics and intravenous corticosteroids, such as albendazole with intravenous dexamethasone.

SCHISTOSOMIASIS (BILHARZIA)

Human schistosomiasis is a parasitic disease caused by trematode flukes of the genus *Schistosoma*. Some 230 million people worldwide are infected with *Schistosoma* spp. The geographic

distribution of different agents of schistosomiasis is summarized in Table 65.3. Parasitic adult worms remain in the venous circulation for years, evading the immune system and excreting over 100,000 fertile eggs daily. Immune responses of the host to the parasites' eggs explain the pathology of schistosomiasis. Some *Schistosoma* species cause chronic liver damage with portal hypertension, whereas others produce bladder and urogenital lesions in chronic carriers.

Pathobiology

Neurologic involvement occurs during the early postinfective stage when *Schistosoma japonicum* eggs reach the brain causing meningoencephalitis; infection with *Schistosoma mansoni* and *Schistosoma haematobium* produce preferential involvement of the spinal cord (myelitis and myeloradiculitis), particularly of the conus medullaris, cauda equina, or the spinal cord. *Schistosoma* ectopic eggs reach the central nervous system (CNS) through retrograde venous flow into the Batson venous plexus. This parasitic myelopathy can be manifested as an acute painful flaccid paraplegia with areflexia, sphincter dysfunction, urinary incontinence, impotence, and sensory disturbances; acute transverse myelitis, spastic paraplegia, painful lumbosacral radiculopathy with backache, and cauda equina syndrome also occur.

Diagnosis

The diagnosis must be suspected on the basis of a clinical presentation of acute painful lumbosacral myelopathy or conus medullaris syndrome with imaging findings suggestive of bilharziasis in a patient with history of travel or exposure to *Schistosoma* cercariae after swimming in fresh water. The diagnosis is confirmed by demonstration of *Schistosoma* antibodies in serum and/or CSF and presence of *Schistosoma* eggs in biopsy of rectal mucosa or in stools and urine.

Treatment

Schistosomal myelitis usually responds to treatment with the schistosomicidal drug praziquantel in combination with steroids; other schistosomicidal drugs are oxamniquine and metrifonate. Surgery with decompressive laminectomy and debridement is usually

TABLE 65.3   Clinical Syndromes and Geographic Distribution of Schistosomiasis

Clinical Syndromes	Agent	Geographic Location
Parasitic myelitis (conus medullaris)	*Schistosoma mansoni*	Africa, Middle East, Caribbean, Brazil, Venezuela, Suriname
Intestinal schistosomiasis	*Schistosoma japonicum*	
Liver fibrosis with portal hypertension		China, Indonesia, Philippines
Meningoencephalitis	*Schistosoma haematobium*	Africa, Middle East
Urogenital schistosomiasis	*Schistosoma intercalatum*	West Africa
Squamous cell carcinoma of the bladder	*Schistosoma guineensis*	East Africa
	Schistosoma mekongi	Mekong river basin

reserved for cases of acute myelitis that deteriorate despite intensive schistosomicidal treatment. Preventive measures in countries affected include the use of chemotherapy, snail control measures, and behavioral modification.

SUGGESTED READINGS

Akpek G, Uslu A, Huebner T, et al. Granulomatous amebic encephalitis: an under-recognized cause of infectious mortality after hematopoietic stem cell transplantation. *Transpl Infect Dis.* 2011;13:366–373.

Babokhov P, Sanyaolu AO, Oyibo WA, et al. A current analysis of chemotherapy strategies for the treatment of human African trypanosomiasis. *Pathog Glob Health.* 2013;107:242–252. doi:10.1179/2047773213Y.0000000105.

Baird RA, Wiebe S, Zunt JR, et al. Evidence-based guideline: treatment of parenchymal neurocysticercosis: report of the Guideline Development Subcommittee of the American Academy of Neurology. *Neurology.* 2013;80:1424–1429.

Bauer C. Baylisascariasis—infections of animals and humans with "unusual" roundworms. *Vet Parasitol.* 2013;193:404–412.

Carabin H, Ndimubanzi PC, Budke CM, et al. Clinical manifestations associated with neurocysticercosis: a systematic review. *PLoS Negl Trop Dis.* 2011;5(5):e1152. doi:10.1371/journal.pntd.0001152.

Carod-Artal FJ. American trypanosomiasis. *Handb Clin Neurol.* 2013;114: 103–123. doi:10.1016/B978-0-444-53490-3.00007-8.

Carod-Artal FJ, Gascon J. Chagas disease and stroke. *Lancet Neurol.* 2010;9:533–542.

Carvalho LJ, Moreira A, Daniel-Ribeiro CT, et al. Vascular dysfunction as a target for adjuvant therapy in cerebral malaria. *Mem Inst Oswaldo Cruz (Rio de Janeiro).* 2014;109(5):577–588. doi:10.1590/0074-0276140061.

Centers for Disease Control and Prevention. Travelers' health yellow book. http://wwwnc.cdc.gov/travel/page/yellowbook-home-2014. Accessed June 2014.

Colley DG, Bustinduy AL, Secor WE, et al. Human schistosomiasis. *Lancet.* 2014;383:2253–2264.

Cook GC, ed. *Manson's Tropical Diseases.* 20th ed. London, United Kingdom: WB Saunders; 1996.

Del Brutto OH, Garcia HH. Neurocysticercosis. *Handb Clin Neurol.* 2013;114: 313–325.

Del Brutto OH, Rajshekhar V, White AC, et al. Proposed diagnostic criteria for neurocysticercosis. *Neurology.* 2001;57:177–183.

Garcia HH, Tanowitz HB, Del Brutto OH, eds. *Neuroparasitology and Tropical Neurology. Handbook of Clinical Neurology.* Vol. 114 (3rd series). Amsterdam, The Netherlands: Elsevier B.V.; 2013.

Graeff-Teixeira C, da Silva AC, Yoshimura K. Update on eosinophilic meningoencephalitis and its clinical relevance. *Clin Microbiol Rev.* 2009;22: 322–348.

Hannisch W, Hallagan LF. Primary amebic meningoencephalitis: a review of the clinical literature. *Wilderness Environ Med.* 1997;8:211–213.

Harvey K, Esposito DH, Han P, et al; Centers for Disease Control and Prevention. Surveillance for travel-related disease—GeoSentinel Surveillance System, United States, 1997–2011. *MMWR Surveill Summ.* 2013;62:1–23.

Higgins SJ, Kain KC, Liles WC. Immunopathogenesis of falciparum malaria: implications for adjunctive therapy in the management of severe and cerebral malaria. *Expert Rev Anti Infect Ther.* 2011;9:803–819. doi:10.1586/eri.11.96.

Kennedy PG. The continuing problem of human African trypanosomiasis (sleeping sickness). *Ann Neurol.* 2008;64:116–127.

Lejon V, Bentivoglio M, Franco JR. Human African trypanosomiasis. *Handb Clin Neurol.* 2013;114:169–181.

Lorenz V, Karanis G, Karanis P. Malaria vaccine development and how external forces shape it: an overview. *Int J Environ Res Public Health.* 2014;11:6791–6807. doi:10.3390/ijerph110706791.

Lv S, Zhang Y, Steinmann P, et al. Helminth infections of the central nervous system occurring in Southeast Asia and the Far East. *Adv Parasitol.* 2010;72: 351–408.

Marks M, Gupta-Wright A, Doherty JF, et al. Managing malaria in the intensive care unit. *Br J Anaesth.* 2014;113(6):910–921. doi:10.1093/bja/aeu157.

Marquez JM, Arauz A. Cerebrovascular complications of neurocysticercosis. *Neurologist.* 2012;18:17–22.

Nash TE, Pretell EJ, Lescano AG, et al. Perilesional brain oedema and seizure activity in patients with calcified neurocysticercosis: a prospective cohort and nested case-control study. *Lancet Neurol.* 2008;7:1099–1105.

Noubiap JJN. Shifting from quinine to artesunate as first-line treatment of severe malaria in children and adults: saving more lives. *J Infect Public Health.* 2014;7(5):407–412. doi:10.1016/j.jiph.2014.04.007.

Pittella JE. Pathology of CNS parasitic infections. *Handb Clin Neurol.* 2013;114:65–88. doi:10.1016/B978-0-444-53490-3.00005-4.

Postels DG, Birbeck GL. Cerebral malaria. *Handb Clin Neurol.* 2013;114:91–102.

Roggelin L, Cramer JP. Malaria prevention in the pregnant traveller: a review. *Travel Med Infect Dis.* 2014;12:229–236. doi:10.1016/j.tmaid.2014.04.007.

Román GC. The neurology of parasitic diseases and malaria. *Continuum (Minneap Minn).* 2011;17(1. Neurologic Complications of Systemic Disease):113–133. doi:10.1212/01.CON.0000394678.13115.ad.

Román GC. Tropical myelopathies. *Handb Clin Neurol.* 2014;121:1521–1548. doi:10.1016/B978-0-7020-4088-7.00102-4.

Sarkar PK, Ahluwalia G, Vijayan VK, et al. Critical care aspects of malaria. *J Intensive Care Med.* 2010;25:93–103.

Schmutzhard E. Eosinophilic myelitis, a souvenir from South East Asia. *Pract Neurol.* 2007;7:48–51.

Shikani HJ, Freeman BD, Lisanti MP, et al. Cerebral malaria: we have come a long way. *Am J Pathol.* 2012;181:1484–1492.

Visvesvara GS. Infections with free-living amebae. *Handb Clin Neurol.* 2013;114: 153–168.

World Health Organization; Centers for Disease Control and Prevention. Severe falciparum malaria. *Trans Roy Soc Trop Med Hyg.* 2000;94(suppl 1):S1–S90.

Viral Infections 66

Shibani S. Mukerji and Jennifer L. Lyons

> *"The single biggest threat to man's continued dominance on the planet is a virus."*
>
> – Joshua Lederberg, Nobel Prize winner

INTRODUCTION

Viral infections of the central nervous system (CNS) are a diverse group of diseases that have plagued mankind for centuries. Infections can occur in the spinal cord (myelitis), cerebrum (encephalitis), meninges (meningitis), brain stem (rhombencephalitis), or any of these in combination. Additionally, viral infections at disparate sites may damage the CNS indirectly through a misguided immune response. This chapter highlights the common causes of CNS viral infections (aside from HIV, which is discussed in a separate chapter), discusses the clinical manifestations and the methods of detection, and when applicable, reviews treatment options.

Viruses invade humans by a variety of mechanisms. This can include skin penetration, infection of mucosal membranes, such as in respiratory or gastrointestinal epithelium, or by direct inoculation into the bloodstream. After primary inoculation, neurotropic viruses gain entry into the CNS by one of a number of mechanisms.

Experiments with several viral strains show that replication occurring in tissue, such as skeletal muscle or skin, allows access to peripheral nerve endings. Some neurotropic viruses are able to infect nerves and then spread by retrograde transport to the sensory ganglia. Characteristic of this is the herpes simplex virus, which replicates in the skin and infects adjacent sensory nerve endings. The virus is then able to tether its capsid onto the host's transport complex, travel toward the dorsal root ganglia, and establish latency.

On the other hand, infection within the bloodstream is dependent on the site of inoculation and ability to infect endothelial cells or cell populations within plasma (e.g., HIV infection of T lymphocytes). Once in the blood, a virus must cross the blood–brain barrier (BBB) to spread into brain parenchyma. In cases like HIV, when infected inflammatory cells, such as lymphocytes or macrophage mononuclear cells cross the BBB, the virus gains entry in a process termed the *Trojan horse*. In other cases, high viremic loads lead to passive transport into the brain or spinal cord. Individual viruses can use multiple mechanisms of viral CNS entry, and in fact, many viruses are able to spread to the CNS using both neural and hematogenous pathways as will be discussed with poliovirus and varicella-zoster virus (VZV).

The widespread availability of viral nucleic acid amplification has revolutionized diagnostics in CNS viral infections and reduced the need to perform open brain biopsies. The polymerase chain reaction (PCR) technique is ideally suited for organisms that are difficult to culture and can retain its sensitivity even after small doses of antiviral therapies. However, this technique relies on a viral load high enough for detection by PCR, a factor not always present in cerebrospinal fluid (CSF), leading to false negatives.

False negatives also occur when heme breakdown from a bloody lumbar puncture interferes with nucleic acid detection. False-positive CSF PCR results occur with viruses that associate themselves with peripheral blood cells and enter the CNS during an inflammatory process but are themselves not the source of the CNS disorder. This phenomenon occurs with Epstein–Barr virus (EBV), as peripheral blood mononuclear cells are latently infected. EBV's relevance as a pathologic agent in the CSF can be unclear and is discussed further in this chapter.

Additional diagnostic methods for CNS viral infections include detection of virus-specific immunoglobulin (Ig) M that relies on the host's ability to mount an immunologic response to the infecting agent. The detection of virus-specific antibodies requires a competent immune system and sufficient time to develop antibodies. Interpretation of antibody levels can be confusing, as some serum antibodies last for months or even years after infection that is often asymptomatic, as seen in West Nile virus where IgM-specific antibodies can persist for months and is not reflective of acute infection. Occasionally, antibody cross-reactivity can also lead to false-positive detection. In contrast to serum antibodies, the presence of virus-specific IgM antibodies in CSF is indicative of intrathecal synthesis and diagnostic of neuroinvasive disease.

Serum virus-specific IgG can be helpful when a corresponding rise in titer between acute and convalescent phases occurs. One limitation here is in the setting of postinfectious complications, where antibody detection in the acute phase was not pursued. Isolated IgG detection, especially in infections that are common and usually asymptomatic, is of limited use.

Antiviral agents are few in number, and treatment in many cases of CNS viral infections remains supportive. Herpes simplex virus, VZV, cytomegalovirus, HIV, and influenza have targeted therapies with varying efficacy. The lack of options in many cases leads physicians to focus on managing the complications of these diseases, often including use of anti-inflammatory agents, such as corticosteroids, to suppress immune-mediated injury. As seen in almost every aspect of medicine, prevention is the best approach to combatting viral diseases and requires comprehensive vaccination programs, mosquito repellents, appropriate protective gear, animal surveillance programs, and education.

PICORNAVIRUS

Picornaviruses are some of the oldest and most diversified viruses to cause human disease. The picornavirus family has four primary groups resulting in human pathogenesis: enteroviruses (e.g., polioviruses, coxsackieviruses, and echoviruses), rhinoviruses (RV), hepatoviruses (e.g., hepatitis A), and parechoviruses. These viruses are nonenveloped, single-stranded RNA viruses. It is estimated that the majority of viral meningitis cases globally are caused by picornaviruses, specifically enteroviruses, as are most cases of acute flaccid paralysis.

ENTEROVIRUSES

Poliomyelitis

Poliomyelitis is a disease that plagued the world in the late 19th and early 20th century, as widespread epidemics resulted in paralysis or death. The name poliomyelitis is derived from two Greek words, *polios* ("gray") and *meylon* ("marrow" or "spinal cord"). The control of polio following the development of both the inactivated polio vaccine (IPV) and live-attenuated oral vaccines (OPV) is a remarkable achievement in science. In the United States, the last case of naturally occurring polio was in 1979. There continues to be endemic areas, namely in Afghanistan, Nigeria, and Pakistan, with additional occasional outbreaks elsewhere. The worldwide eradication of polio is the goal of the World Health Organization (WHO) and many countries, as well as nonprofit organizations.

PATHOBIOLOGY

Poliomyelitis virus is an enterovirus whose main route of human infectivity is via the gastrointestinal tract. There are three serotypes (types 1, 2, and 3), with all serotypes being neurotropic. Poliovirus type 1 is the most frequently encountered in human infections around the world. Although the disease occurs in all age groups, it is rarely seen before 6 months of age. Infections are spread via the fecal–oral route and are highly influenced by hygiene standards. The virus replicates initially in the gastrointestinal tract's lymphatic system (Peyer patches), followed by viremia and immune activation. How the virus gains access to the nervous system remains uncertain. One hypothesis is the poliomyelitis virus, which is able to replicate in skeletal muscles, can spread into peripheral motor axons, and access anterior horn cells of the spinal cord via retrograde transport. This hypothesis has been tested in mouse models with expression of transgenic poliomyelitis virus receptor. A second hypothesis is by direct spread from the blood due to a breakdown in the BBB. These mechanisms for CNS entry are not mutually exclusive.

CLINICAL MANIFESTATIONS

Although CNS complication is the most feared outcome of polio infection, it is a not a common occurrence when evaluating poliomyelitis infections as a whole. Nearly 90% of infections are asymptomatic and recognized only by isolation of the virus from the oropharynx or in feces. Approximately 4% to 8% of those infected will have a minor, self-limited illness similar to other enteroviral infections with headache, anorexia, abdominal pain, and a sore throat. These cases are typically identified during epidemics. In 1% to 2% of infected individuals, there are the more severe clinical manifestations of fever, headache, and evidence of meningismus. Frank paralysis occurs in only 0.1% of all poliovirus infections, and the clinical course can be divided into two phases. A prodromal phase of sore throat, fever, and symptoms suggestive of upper respiratory infection is most common in young patients. Mild abdominal upset and meningeal irritation are more common in adults. There is a short recovery period for 2 to 3 days before an abrupt onset of fever, chills, myalgias, headache, and symptoms consistent with meningitis. Paresthesias and muscle fasciculations can precede muscle weakness and paralysis. When paralysis occurs, it is typically asymmetric, and the lower extremities are more commonly involved than the upper extremities. When quadriplegia occurs, it is more frequently seen in adults than infants. Paralysis of the diaphragm and intercostal muscles in spinal poliomyelitis occurs more often in young adults than in the extreme age groups. Bulbar paralysis is due to weakness of muscle groups innervated by cranial nerves, and in polio, the glossopharyngeal and vagus nerves are most commonly affected, followed by the oculomotor nerve. Older adults are more likely to have medullary involvement, and these patients are at high risk for aspiration and need for mechanical ventilation.

DIAGNOSIS

The diagnosis of paralytic polio is clinically suspected with the development of asymmetric acute flaccid paralysis following a febrile illness. It is more likely to be suspected in those who are unvaccinated coming from endemic countries or those with immunodeficiencies. Other viruses to consider in the differential are other enteroviruses, especially enterovirus 71, and arboviral infections, such as West Nile virus (discussed later in the chapter).

CSF pleocytosis is evident as early as meningeal symptoms are present, with an initial polymorphonuclear profile that eventually shifts to a lymphocytic predominance. An increased protein concentration is most prominently seen if there is severe paralysis. These abnormalities are not distinguishable from other viral causes of aseptic meningitis and thus, identification of the poliomyelitis virus is necessary to confirm the diagnosis. Isolation of poliomyelitis virus by CSF culture is challenging and is not typically performed. Polio is more easily isolated from oral secretions and feces, and with rapid identification of polioviruses by genomic amplification using PCR, clinicians can distinguish poliomyelitis viral infections from other enteroviruses or other infectious causes.

TREATMENT

There are no antiviral drugs for treatment of poliomyelitis, and symptom management is the primary focus. Respiratory muscle paralysis or cases of bulbar poliomyelitis frequently require mechanical ventilation and aggressive management of secretions. Bowel function also requires special attention in spinal poliomyelitis. Long-term management of physical and psychiatric sequelae obliges a comprehensive team of both physical and occupational therapy along with orthopedic services and psychiatry.

The inactivated and oral poliomyelitis vaccinations have been used effectively for controlling paralytic poliomyelitis but differ in terms of asymptomatic viral shedding and risk of contracting vaccine-related disease. IPV is an injectable preparation containing antigen units for all three polio serotypes. In the United States, the IPV is the only version administered and is typically given with other childhood vaccines at 2, 4, 6 to 18 months, and 4 to 6 years. Children develop little to no secretory antibody response to the IPV. If exposed to live polioviruses, these children are more likely to have asymptomatic infections but still shed virus in their feces, exposing nonimmunized contacts. Most oral poliomyelitis vaccine (OPV) preparations also immunize against all three serotypes. The prevalence of poliomyelitis-specific antibody to all three serotypes following three doses of OPV is approximately 96%. Nonimmune OPV recipients will shed vaccine viruses in feces and the oropharynx that can be spread to nonimmunized children. This aspect can be advantageous in poorly vaccinated communities, as children can develop OPV-specific antibodies despite not having received the vaccine. A rare event is the development of vaccine-associated paralytic poliomyelitis, an occurrence in 1 per 2.6 million vaccine doses and is only associated with OPV. The WHO still recommends the use of the trivalent OPV in underdeveloped nations because of cost, ease of administration, and greater secretory immunity in the gastrointestinal tract.

OUTCOME

The prognosis of paralytic poliomyelitis depends on age (infants and children are more likely to recover) and severity of paralysis (i.e., partial vs. complete paralysis). Permanent weakness from polio paralytic infections occurs in approximately two-thirds of patients. Complete recovery is unlikely in cases with severe acute flaccid paralysis or in those requiring mechanical ventilation. Increased mortality is typically seen in those with polio encephalitis, bulbar involvement due to glossopharyngeal and/or vagus nerve impairment, and/or respiratory muscle paralysis.

Following the epidemics in the early 20th century, some individuals with partial or full recovery from paralytic polio experienced a new onset of neuromuscular weakness, pain, and fatigue. In such cases, muscle weakness and atrophy were identified in muscles that had been previously affected. These symptoms have been collectively called the *postpolio syndrome* and, in those with slowly progressive weakness, atrophy, and fasciculations, termed *postpolio progressive muscular atrophy* (PPMA; discussed separately).

Enteroviruses 70 and 71

Acute hemorrhagic conjunctivitis was first recognized in 1970 and is the result of either enterovirus 70 or an antigenic variant of coxsackievirus A24. The disease is characterized by the rapid onset of painful conjunctivitis and subconjunctival hemorrhage. Complete recovery is typically seen within 1 to 2 weeks. Epidemics predominantly occur in tropical and subtropical regions lasting several months and will affect large populations.

Neurologic complications of acute hemorrhagic conjunctivitis primarily include an asymmetric acute flaccid paralysis. Those affected appear clinically similar to those with spinal poliomyelitis except for the preceding association with acute hemorrhagic conjunctivitis. Prodromal symptoms for acute hemorrhagic conjunctivitis–associated paralysis include fever and malaise then an acute, severe radicular pain. This is followed by flaccid, asymmetric weakness of the legs with proximal muscles (e.g., quadriceps muscle) more affected. Reflexes are diminished or absent. Permanent paralysis or residual weakness is present in over half the cases. The virus is difficult to isolate in the CSF by PCR when neurologic symptoms arise, but high titers of virus-specific antibodies are typically detectable in the CSF in those with paralysis.

Enterovirus 71 has been the etiologic agent responsible for several encephalitis epidemics throughout the world, resulting in substantial mortality and morbidity. The largest enterovirus 71 epidemic occurred in Taiwan in 1988, resulting in 1.5 million people affected, of which 405 children developed serious neurologic complications with 78 deaths. Every 2 to 3 years, large enterovirus 71 outbreaks occur around the Asia–Pacific rim, affecting thousands. As such, enterovirus 71 is now recognized as an emerging neurotropic virus. Enterovirus 71 can cause hand-foot-and-mouth disease as well as upper respiratory infections and gastroenteritis. In those affected neurologically, manifestations include myoclonic jerks, tremors, ataxia, cranial nerve palsy, meningitis, and meningoencephalitis. Polio-like flaccid paralysis occurs in about 10% of patients. Fulminant neurogenic pulmonary edema and apnea from rhombencephalitis occurred in epidemics affecting children in Taiwan and Malaysia, and these disease manifestations are the primary cause of death in enterovirus 71–infected individuals. Most of the patients had magnetic resonance imaging (MRI) T2-weighted high-intensity lesions in the brain stem. Diagnosis may be made by virus isolation from throat, feces, or vesicles; by antibody studies; and CSF reverse transcriptase polymerase chain reaction (RT-PCR).

COXSACKIEVIRUS AND ECHOVIRUSES

Neurologic manifestations of human viral infections caused by group A and group B coxsackieviruses and echoviruses primarily are meningitides. Historically, group B coxsackieviruses and echoviruses are the most frequently implicated serotypes in meningitis; exceptions include when a single serotype causes a widespread outbreak. For example, coxsackievirus A9 was responsible for most cases in an outbreak in the Gansu Province, China in 2005 and Alberta, Canada in 2010.

The symptoms and signs of meningeal involvement of coxsackieviruses and echoviruses are similar to other viruses that cause meningitis. The severity of disease varies, with the extremes of life having the more severe meningitis. Headache is frequent, and if meningismus is present, it can vary in severity and typically begins 24 to 48 hours following onset of symptoms. In infants, the dominant symptoms are fever and irritability, with less than 10% having evidence of meningeal irritation. Frequently, there is a prodromal or associated upper respiratory tract infection or symptoms. Acute CNS complications include febrile seizures, elevated intracranial pressure, and coma. When considering alternate diagnoses for enterovirus meningitis, bacterial meningitis needs to be considered and should be treated empirically with broad-spectrum antibiotics. Arboviruses, acute HIV, herpesviruses, Lyme borreliosis, leptospirosis, and lymphocytic choriomeningitis virus are other infectious etiologies in the differential.

CSF analysis typically demonstrates clear fluid with normal to mildly elevated pressure. There is a mild to moderate pleocytosis that ranges from 10 to 500/mm^3 and rarely exceeds 1,000/mm^3. Initial differential cell counts demonstrate a high percentage of neutrophils but an eventual shift to a lymphocytic predominance. The CSF glucose concentration is generally normal and protein concentrations are normal to slightly elevated. PCR is the primary means of virus detection with greater than 95% sensitivity and specificity. Viral cultures are infrequently used, as they are insensitive and can take days for results to return.

Treatment is largely symptom management. Containment during outbreaks is critical, with good hygiene practices and protective equipment for high-risk groups. The broad-spectrum antipicornaviral agent pleconaril is an orally administered inhibitor of enterovirus replication. There have been two placebo-controlled clinical trials that showed a shortened course of illness compared to placebo, but the benefit was modest. The drug has not been approved for use in the United States.

Although encephalitis is not commonly caused by coxsackievirus or echovirus (with the exception of enterovirus 71), it can occur in immunocompromised patients. The severity of encephalitis is variable, with seizures, hemichorea, and acute cerebellar ataxia being described. In patients with agammaglobulinemia, hematopoietic transplantation, or B-cell depletion with immunotherapy agents, enterovirus can cause a chronic, severe, and fatal meningitis and encephalitis. In such cases, enterovirus can be recovered in the CSF by PCR at different time points throughout the disease course. Intravenous immunoglobulin (IVIg) and pleconaril have been used with some success.

Sporadic cases of acute flaccid paralysis have been seen with coxsackieviruses and are typically less severe than in poliovirus-associated disease. For example, in an 11-year program monitoring of acute flaccid paralysis in the Slovak Republic as part of the WHO strategy for polio eradication, coxsackievirus B and echoviruses were the most common etiologies for acute flaccid paralysis in the post–polio vaccine era. These viruses are also reported etiologies for oculomotor palsies, Guillain–Barré syndrome (GBS), opsoclonus–myoclonus, and transverse myelitis.

ARBOVIRUSES

Arboviruses comprise a group of viruses from four genera that all have in common transmission to humans via arthropods: alphaviruses, flaviviruses, bunyaviruses, and reoviruses. Human infection due to arboviruses follows patterns of vector activity. That is to say that seasons and years when the insects are most abundant logically see higher rates of infections. Most arboviruses have vertebrate reservoirs, such as birds or small mammals, and are transmitted by mosquitoes or ticks. Continuation of the life cycle relies on a constant interaction between hosts (e.g., birds, mammals) and vectors (e.g., ticks, mosquitoes). Animals that act as hosts maintain high enough levels of viremia and are able to retransmit infections back to arthropods when bitten. However, humans and horses are "dead-end" hosts, as they are not able to sustain elevated levels of viremia without succumbing to disease. Endemicity varies widely, as do outcomes. Figure 66.1 demonstrates highly endemic areas for many encephalitis-associated viruses.

Arboviruses are important causes of encephalitis worldwide, and neuroinvasion is usually coupled with an intense inflammatory reaction and/or edema, the effects of which can be devastating. Alternatively, neurologic disease can occur as a parainfectious inflammatory disorder in the setting of systemic disease without specific evidence of nervous system infection per se. Fortunately, for the most part, exposure leads to asymptomatic seroconversion or a mild self-limited illness; typically, only a fraction progress to severe neurologic disease and/or death.

Acute arboviral infections are diagnosed typically by serum and/or CSF antibody detection via enzyme-linked immunosorbent assay (ELISA) for virus-specific IgM antibodies. Given the high prevalence of asymptomatic infection and potential for persistence of IgM in serum, antibody detection must be confirmed with a fourfold titer increase in IgG between the acute and convalescent phase (4 weeks post the acute phase). In general, though, the presence of CSF virus-specific IgM antibodies is indicative of intrathecal synthesis and is diagnostic for neuroinvasive disease. CSF RNA detection is highly specific for active infection, but its sensitivity in arboviral infections is not nearly as high as seen in herpes simplex DNA detection. CSF PCR can be especially helpful in immunocompromised people who are unable to mount or have a delayed antibody response. Culturing arboviruses is not routinely performed, as they are difficult to isolate due to low levels of viremia in humans. There are no specific antiviral therapies for the treatment of neuroinvasive arboviral infections and the focus remains on supportive care and exposure prevention.

FLAVIVIRUSES

Flaviviruses are positive-sense, single-stranded, enveloped viruses with icosahedral capsids. Many have the capability of neuroinvasion and severe damage throughout the neuraxis. Inflammatory reactions accompany infection. Table 66.1 outlines the most consistently described statistics for flaviviruses that cause neurologic disease.

Dengue

There are four serotypes of this flavivirus, and infection with one does not confer protection from infection with the others. Dengue is carried by the *Aedes* mosquito and can be acquired throughout Central and South America, Puerto Rico, Africa and the Middle East, Southeast Asia and the Pacific, and Australia (see Fig. 66.1A). The southern United States occasionally sees cases as well. Millions are infected each year. Vertical transmission is also known, as is spread through infected blood and organ donation.

PATHOBIOLOGY

As with other flaviviruses, inoculation proceeds to local immune cell infection and carriage to a lymph center, where replication occurs and viremia results. The virus makes its way to the CNS, although mechanisms of infection are not well understood. Virus is detected in the CNS, although it is not known if this occurs passively across an altered BBB or as an active infection. Vasogenic edema results, and a systemic inflammatory response can elicit immune-mediated damage of multiple organs and the neuraxis.

CLINICAL MANIFESTATIONS

After exposure and subsequent incubation of several days to just over a week, those who are symptomatic will experience fever, myalgias, and malaise most commonly, occasionally with a rash. Severe systemic disease can follow over a matter of days, characterized by thrombocytopenia, multifocal hemorrhage, shock, and death. Neurologic manifestations can accompany severe disease and range from encephalopathy to direct nervous system infection accompanied by an inflammatory response causing meningoencephalitis and/or myelitis to a parainfectious immune diseases

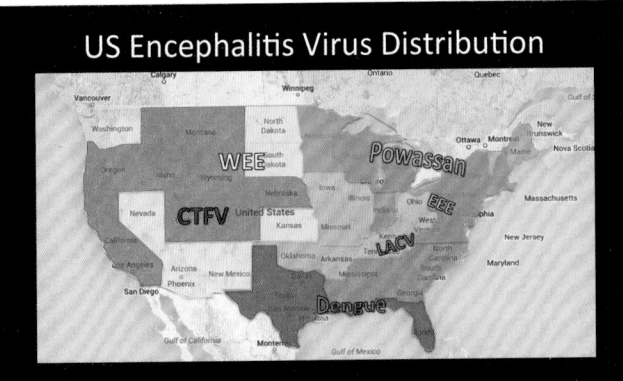

FIGURE 66.1 A: Global distribution of viral etiologies of encephalitis. Herpesviruses and rabies are excluded, as these are all ubiquitous around the globe. United States and Canada are endemic to multiple viruses but most vary by region. **B:** Distribution of nonherpes, non-WNV, and non-SLE viral encephalitis viruses in the United States. WNV has been reported from all continental states, and St. Louis has only not been seen in New England.

TABLE 66.1 Nervous System Disease Caused by Flaviviruses

Virus	Endemic Locale	No. of Infections Annually	Systemic Symptomatic Disease (% of Infections)	Neurologic Disease (% Symptomatic Infections)	Neurologic Manifestations	Case Fatality Rate	Long-term Sequelae	Preventive Strategies
Japanese encephalitis virus	Southeast Asia, Japan, Pacific Islands	30,000–50,000	0.30	0.001–0.02	Encephalitis with brain stem and occasionally spinal cord involvement	25%	30%	Vector control, vaccine
West Nile virus	Africa, Middle East, Continental United States, Puerto Rico	~150,000 (United States)	20	1	Meningoencephalitis and/or acute flaccid paralysis	10% overall, 15%–30% in age older than 70 yr	50%	Vector control, blood and organ donation restrictions
Dengue virus	Central and South America, Puerto Rico, Africa, Middle East, India, Southeast Asia, Pacific Islands, Northern Australia	50–400 million	0.5–1	4–50	Meningoencephalitis, ADEM, GBS, CNS hemorrhage	4%–5%	~25%	Vector control
Murray Valley encephalitis virus	Northern Australia, New Guinea	Occurs in outbreaks	Outbreaks of 21–114 cases	0.1–0.7 of all infections	Meningoencephalitis	20%–40%	30%–50%	Vector control
Tick-borne encephalitis virus	Europe, Southern Russia, East Asia	~35,000	2–33	25–30	Meningoencephalitis	1%–2% (Western Europe) 30%–40% (Eastern Russia)	35%–60%	Vector control, vaccine
Kunjin virus	Northern Australia, New Guinea	Occurs in outbreaks	Minority	Minority	Mild meningoencephalitis or encephalomyelitis	<1%	NA	Vector control
St. Louis encephalitis virus	Continental United States	~1,000; higher in outbreaks	<1	>60	Meningoencephalitis	5%–15%	Up to 50%	Vector control
Powassan virus	Canada, Northern United States, Russia	NA; seroprevalence 0%–5% in endemic areas	Minority	NA; <50 cases reported 2001–2012 but incidence rising	Meningoencephalitis and/or encephalomyelitis	10%	50%	Vector control

ADEM, acute disseminated encephalomyelitis; GBS, Guillain–Barré syndrome; CNS, central nervous system; NA, not applicable.

such as GBS and acute disseminated encephalomyelitis (ADEM). Up to 50% of those who are symptomatic will develop neurologic complications. Risk factors for developing severe disease include young age, certain HLA genotypes, female gender, and superinfection with a second serotype. Serotypes 2 and 3 are associated more so with neuroinvasive disease than are the others.

DIAGNOSIS

Given the protean neurologic complications, there is no specific neuroimaging finding related to dengue, and computed tomography (CT) or MRI of the brain may be entirely normal. Similarly, CSF may be normal or only demonstrate elevated protein concentration; this appears to relate to the type of neurologic complication present. Opening pressures can also be elevated. If there is a pleocytosis, it is generally lymphocytic. If caught early, RNA can be detected from the blood and/or CSF; otherwise, antibody detection from blood and/or CSF demonstrating active or recent production is diagnostic. In endemic areas, a tourniquet test to assess capillary fragility can be performed at the bedside in the appropriate clinical context to make a presumptive diagnosis.

TREATMENT

No vaccine or specific therapies exist for dengue infection, although aggressive supportive treatment early on, with platelet transfusions, rehydration, and management of elevated intracranial pressure, may improve survival. Case fatality rate is 4% to 5%, although some 25% of survivors will suffer residual neurologic deficits (see Table 66.1).

Tick-Borne Encephalitis Virus

Tick-borne encephalitis virus is carried by the *Ixodes* tick. It is found across Europe and Asia and is responsible for thousands of infections each year (see Fig. 66.1A). Men are more commonly affected than women. Viral infection results in replication in lymphatic cells, vascular dispersion, and entry into brain parenchyma by means of brain microvascular endothelial cells. Viral presence in the brain incites an inflammatory reaction that precipitates widespread damage throughout the cerebrum, cerebellum, brain stem, and sometimes the spinal cord. After an incubation period of about a week, patients develop a fever that lasts several days and then progresses to headache, nausea, and occasionally meningismus. They can further develop encephalopathy and brain stem dysfunction several days later, and in the most severe cases, severe back pain and upper more so than lower extremity paresis can occur. Diagnosis is best made by demonstration of intrathecal tick-borne encephalitis virus–specific antibody production; serum antibodies can be useful in the patient who has never received vaccination. CSF usually shows a modest lymphocytic pleocytosis and elevated protein concentration, although in some cases, a polymorphonuclear pleocytosis has been demonstrated.

Treatment of tick-borne encephalitis virus is supportive. Mortality varies by location, at 1% to 2% for Western Europe but up to 40% for Eastern Russia (see Table 66.1). Long-term neuropsychiatric sequelae occur in more than half of the survivors. An effective vaccine exists, but for a variety of reasons, vaccination rates overall remain low.

Japanese Encephalitis Virus

Japanese encephalitis virus is transmitted by the *Culex* mosquito. It was first identified in Japan in 1871 but now includes much of Southeast Asia (see Fig. 66.1A). Like its sibling flaviviruses, initial replication is in lymphoid tissue followed by transient viremia that carries the virus to the brain; once inside the CNS, it imparts damage both by infection and reactive inflammation.

Most Japanese encephalitis virus infections are asymptomatic; about 1 in 300 is clinically apparent. Somewhere between 1 and 20 in 1,000 produce neuroinvasive disease. This translates, though, into some 50,000 cases of encephalitis a year, with a mortality rate of about 25%. Children and young adults are at highest risk.

In symptomatic cases, after an incubation period of a little over a week, fever sets in, along with chills, myalgias, and occasionally meningismus. In children, abdominal pain and nausea are common. Symptoms can quickly progress to limb weakness and extrapyramidal signs and subsequently to coma and death. Imaging and pathologic specimens show thalamic and cerebral peduncular involvement, but viral involvement is typically widespread throughout the brain and even into the spinal cord occasionally. CSF typically shows a lymphocytic pleocytosis of up to 1,000 cells/μL and a modestly increased protein concentration. Diagnosis is usually by antibody detection from CSF or by serologic increases between acute and convalescent phases; RNA isolation from CSF is diagnostic, as well. As with other flavivirus infections that are usually asymptomatic and/or have vaccines available, a single positive IgG in endemic areas may not indicate active disease.

Treatment is supportive, keeping in mind that death commonly is secondary to cerebral edema and increased intracranial pressure. Of those who survive, about 30% will have long-term deficits (see Table 66.1), again making prevention strategies key. These include vector control and vaccination; there is a highly effective vaccine for Japanese encephalitis virus, but vaccination campaigns are unfortunately currently lacking.

West Nile Virus and Kunjin Virus

West Nile virus was originally isolated in Africa but since introduction to New York in 1999 has been endemic in the United States (see Fig. 66.1A). Its vector is the *Culex* mosquito, although infected donated blood has been another mode of transmission. As of 2012, all 48 contiguous states in the United States had reported cases. Most cases of West Nile virus are asymptomatic and go unreported; there were an estimated 1.8 million infections in North America between 1999 and 2010. Hundreds to thousands of symptomatic cases are reported to the Centers for Disease Control and Prevention (CDC) each year. As such, seroprevalence of West Nile virus IgG in endemic areas is actually quite high. Of the symptomatic cases, the most common symptoms are fever and malaise. Less than 1% will go on to develop what is considered neuroinvasive disease: meningitis, encephalitis, or myeloradiculitis. Risk factors for developing neuroinvasive disease are age older than 50 years, immune suppression, homelessness, chronic renal disease, hepatitis C infection, and CCR5 mutations.

PATHOBIOLOGY

West Nile virus has an incubation period of 2 to 14 days, after which replication occurs in lymph tissue, followed by viremia and carriage to the CNS, where it infects neurons and anterior horn cells. How it does so remains elusive, as receptors have not been identified. Nor is it known how the virus crosses the BBB. As with many viral CNS diseases, though, its mechanism of neuronal injury and death is not only directly related to viral infection but also to the intense inflammatory reaction that imparts bystander damage to the delicate resident cells in the brain and spinal cord.

CLINICAL MANIFESTATIONS

West Nile virus neuroinvasive disease presentation depends on the part of the neuraxis that is involved. Fever, headache, meningismus, and encephalopathy herald meningoencephalitis, whereas radicular pain and flaccid asymmetric limb paralysis accompany anterior horn cell infection. New parkinsonism points to basal ganglia involvement.

DIAGNOSIS

Diagnosis can be made by detection of West Nile virus RNA in the CSF, although this is fleeting and insensitive after about 48 hours, or by CSF IgM or by a fourfold increase in antibody titers from acute to convalescent phase. CSF otherwise should demonstrate a lymphocytic pleocytosis with moderately elevated protein concentration and normal glucose concentration; however, neutrophilic predominance can also be seen. Although West Nile virus RNA can be detected in urine, use of this assay in acute disease is not standard. Neuroimaging may be normal or may demonstrate leptomeningeal enhancement; radicular enhancement; and/or T2 hyperintensities in the subcortical white matter, deep gray matter structures, and/or the spinal cord parenchyma.

TREATMENT

As with many viruses, West Nile virus is a monophasic illness for which there is no proven specific therapy other than supportive therapy. IVIg, West Nile virus–specific IgG, and ribavirin all have been not clearly beneficial, but corticosteroids are commonly used to modulate inflammation. Long-term sequelae are the rule for survivors of neuroinvasive disease, and about 10% die (see Table 66.1), making prevention of mosquito bites the most logical management strategy.

Kunjin is a subtype of West Nile virus isolated in northern Australia that primarily causes disease in horses; human disease has been reported and is similar to but much milder than West Nile virus neuroinvasive disease (see Fig. 66.1A). It can be transmitted to humans, also by the *Culex* mosquito, and occurs typically in small outbreaks (see Table 66.1).

Murray Valley Encephalitis Virus

Murray Valley encephalitis virus is carried by the *Culex* mosquito and is endemic to Northern Australia and Guinea (see Fig. 66.1A). It mostly has occurred in outbreaks with case numbers in the teens to low hundreds, making it much less of a threat than most other flaviviruses. Four outbreaks may have occurred in the early part of the 20th century under the moniker "Australian X" disease, and in 1951, the virus was isolated during the first documented Murray Valley encephalitis virus outbreak. Subsequent outbreaks occurred in 1956, 1974, and 2011. There have been sporadic cases additionally. A study conducted immediately after the 2011 outbreak demonstrated 2.2% seroprevalence in endemic areas, with higher numbers coming from those born before 1974.

Incubation time averages 2 weeks. The vast majority of cases are asymptomatic or gives rise to a mild febrile illness with headache that does not come to medical attention. About 1 out of 150 to 1,000 infections develop more severe symptoms several days later of lethargy, encephalopathy, and occasionally seizures that can progress to brain stem symptoms, flaccid paralysis due to myelitis, and death. The case fatality rate is 15% to 30%, and about 30% to 50% suffer long-term neurologic deficits (see Table 66.1).

In severe cases, T2-weighted MRI of the brain shows bilateral thalamic and brain stem hyperintensities. Pathologically, virus has been recovered from brain tissue, and additionally, there is a striking widespread reactive inflammatory infiltrate throughout the gray matter.

Diagnosis is often by serology, suggesting that specific Murray Valley encephalitis virus IgM appears several days after infection and persists for months. Antibodies can also be evaluated in CSF, as well, and there are Murray Valley encephalitis virus RNA assays for detection in serum. Management is supportive.

St. Louis Encephalitis Virus

St. Louis encephalitis virus is carried by *Culex* species mosquitoes and is a cause of epidemic encephalitis in both North and South America but mostly in the United States (see Fig. 66.1B). Epidemics typically occur during the summer season. The vast majority of individuals have asymptomatic infections. Otherwise, presenting symptoms mimic a flulike illness and include fever, headache, and lethargy. Neurologic features can include seizures, ataxia, confusion, hemiparesis, and myoclonus.

CSF analysis demonstrates a predominantly lymphocytic pleocytosis. St. Louis encephalitis virus is rarely isolated from blood or serum and diagnosis largely requires demonstration of St. Louis encephalitis virus–specific CSF IgM. MRI can show T2-hyperintensities in the basal ganglia and in some cases, abnormal signal is seen within the substantia nigra. Pathology in St. Louis encephalitis virus cases includes perivascular, meningeal, and capillary lymphocytic infiltrates and activated microglia in gray and white matter. There are widespread neuronal degenerative changes, more obvious in cortex, basal ganglia, and cerebellum. A few St. Louis encephalitis virus cases have evidence of inflammation and neuronal loss in the spinal cord.

Treatment is supportive. Mortality varies considerably in case series and has been reported as high as 20%; long-term morbidity occurs in up to 50% of cases (see Table 66.1). Prognosis is worse with those who develop seizures.

Powassan Virus

This flavivirus is carried by the *Dermacentor* spp. and *Ixodes* ticks and is endemic in Canada, the northern United States, and parts of Russia (see Fig. 66.1B). It derives its name from the town in Canada where disease was first identified in 1958. Like Murray Valley encephalitis virus and St. Louis encephalitis virus, its epidemiologic significance pales in comparison to other flaviviruses.

Symptoms occur after an incubation period of 1 to 4 weeks and begin with malaise, fever, and pharyngitis but can progress to hemiplegia, vomiting, marked brain stem dysfunction, coma, and death. CSF studies, as with nearly all viral encephalitides, usually demonstrate a moderate lymphocytic pleocytosis and modestly elevated protein concentration. RNA and antibodies can be detected in blood and/or CSF, although the tests are not widely available; referral to state laboratories in the United States is advised.

Pathologic studies demonstrate intense lymphocytic infiltrates and necrosis of gray matter mostly in the basal ganglia, thalamus, and mesial temporal lobes, although involvement is widespread. Neuronal cells demonstrate eosinophilic inclusion bodies. There is no specific therapy for this disease, and treatment is supportive. About half of the survivors suffer permanent sequelae (see Table 66.1).

BUNYAVIRUSES

Bunyaviruses are negative-sense, single-stranded helical RNA viruses that are encapsulated. Although some are arboviruses, several are spread by rodents and are not associated with significant neurologic disease. Those that do result in encephalitis have less epidemiologic significance than most of the flaviviruses, which are found in densely populated areas, are widespread globally, and/or are much more neurovirulent.

Lacrosse Virus

Lacrosse virus is transmitted by the *Aedes triseriatus* mosquito. Lacrosse virus is endemic to the United States, and symptomatic cases are most commonly seen across the Ohio River Valley, mid-Atlantic, and Midwest. In these areas, the incidence is about 10 to 30 per 100,000 population but only about 0.3% to 4% are symptomatic. Most cases are reported in children, with only about 3% occurring beyond the age of 20 years.

Initial infection causes viral replication in muscle followed by viremia and CNS invasion. The mechanism of entry into the CNS is unknown, but neurons and glial cells in the frontal, temporal, and parietal lobes are mostly affected. Presentation is of headache and fever, which progresses over days to seizures and encephalopathy about 25% to 50% of the time. CSF demonstrates a lymphocytic pleocytosis with modestly elevated protein concentration, although results can be entirely normal. Lacrosse virus IgM in CSF is diagnostic; otherwise, diagnosis comes from fourfold increase in IgG antibody titers from acute to convalescent phase. Alternatively, antigen detection on biopsy specimen provides the diagnosis. Treatment is supportive and the disease monophasic; mortality is less than 1%.

Jamestown Canyon Virus

This virus infects many species of mosquitoes and flies and is found throughout the United States into Canada. It is an extremely rare cause of mild meningoencephalitis, with less than a score of cases reported. However, seroprevalence has been reported as high as 27%, suggesting neurovirulence is very low. Symptoms mirror those of other arboviruses, with onset of a mild febrile illness followed by severe headaches. Serologic studies are diagnostic when a fourfold rise in IgG is seen between acute and convalescent phases; treatment is supportive.

REOVIRUSES

Reoviruses are a family of double-stranded, nonenveloped RNA viruses with icosahedral capsids. As with bunyaviruses, these infections are considerably more isolated than most flavivirus infections.

This Reoviridae genus includes Colorado tick fever virus, California hare coltivirus, Salmon River virus, and the European Eyach virus. All are associated with human disease, but Colorado tick fever virus causes the majority of human infections. It is carried by *Dermacentor andersoni* ticks and is mostly seen in the Rocky Mountains and western United States into Canada at elevations of 4,000 to 10,000 feet. Men are more often infected than women, likely due to lifestyle characteristics leading to exposure. There have been some 200 to 300 cases reported, but the incidence is likely much higher, as most infections are thought to be asymptomatic. Presentation after an incubation period of about 3 to 5 days is of acute fever, headache, nausea, myalgias, and in some, a maculopapular rash. About a week later, a meningoencephalitis may develop (mostly children). There can be additional systemic involvement of the heart, liver, testes, epididymis, and lungs. Only a couple of deaths have been reported, and these have been due to hemorrhagic shock complicating disease. This monophasic illness resolves after another week.

CSF often shows a lymphocytic pleocytosis and modestly elevated protein concentration. Diagnosis is made by viral isolation

from blood or CSF or serologies and treatment is supportive, with special care to avoid antiplatelet agents given the potential for hemorrhagic complications.

TOGAVIRUSES

Togaviruses are positive-sense, single-stranded, enveloped viruses with icosahedral capsids. There are two genera: *Alphavirus* and *Rubivirus*. *Alphavirus* species are arboviruses, whereas *Rubivirus* contains rubella, which is transmitted via droplet or mother–child transmission.

Alphavirus (Equine Encephalitis)

There are three types of equine encephalitis, all belonging to the genus *Alphavirus*, that occur in the Americas (see Fig. 66.1A): Eastern equine encephalitis (EEE), Western equine encephalitis (WEE), and Venezuelan equine encephalitis (VEE). These viruses affect horses primarily but in 1938 were found to cause human disease in those having close contact with affected animals.

Equine encephalitides are rare human infections and occur either in isolated cases or in short-lived epidemics when environmental conditions favor viral amplification. WEE and EEE are seen on the western and eastern coasts of the United States and into Canada with some overlap into the Midwest and Great Lakes regions (see Fig. 66.1B). VEE occurs throughout Central America into the northern part of South America.

EEE is the most severe of the equine encephalitides, frequently progressing to coma and death. The disease begins with a short prodrome (~5 days) of a flulike illness: fever, headache, malaise, nausea, and vomiting. This quickly is followed by confusion, stupor or coma, and possibly seizures. Focal neurologic signs can be present, including tremor, cranial nerve palsies, and plegia. In a recent case series, the median CSF white blood cell count was 370 cells/mm³ (median 70% neutrophils). The median total protein concentration was 97 mg/dL, and the CSF glucose concentration was normal. Diagnosis of EEE encephalitis relies on the detection of IgM antibodies in the serum and/or CSF. PCR and genomic amplification is available for EEE, and virus isolation from CSF or brain remains the diagnostic gold standard. The majority of those with EEE and neurologic symptoms have abnormal brain MRI. Lesions are best seen on T2-weighted sequences with the basal ganglia and thalamus most affected (Fig. 66.2).

Pathologic findings on gross examination in EEE are notable for diffuse cerebral edema. There is typically acute or chronic perivascular and meningeal inflammation seen within the basal ganglia, thalamus, cortex, brain stem, and spinal cord. Inflammatory infiltrates, neuronal death, and rarefied tissue can correlate to changes seen on MRI. EEE immunohistochemistry has shown clusters of infected cells primarily in gray matter with neurons as the predominant cell type affected (Fig. 66.3). In cases of myelitis, anterior horn cells are affected.

Estimates of case fatalities of EEE range from 30% to 70%. In children, length of prodrome was statistically associated with clinical outcome at the time of discharge, with longer prodromes having more favorable outcomes. This relationship is not as clear in adults, although patients with more favorable outcomes tended to have longer prodromes. In patients who recover, the morbidity from EEE is high, with sequelae ranging from intellectual disabilities, cranial nerve palsies, hemiplegia, aphasia, and seizures.

WEE and VEE infections are less severe. The vast majority of children and adults have a flulike illness with fever and malaise lasting up to 2 weeks. The extremes of age are at risk for neuroinvasive disease but less than 10% progress to coma. Hemiparesis,

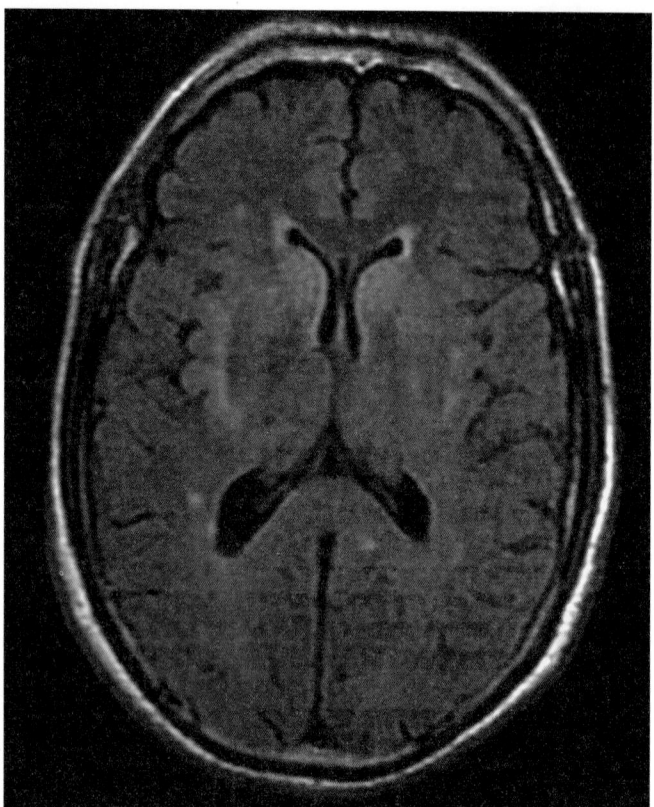

FIGURE 66.2 Axial T2 fluid-attenuated inversion recovery (FLAIR)–weighted MRI in a patient with encephalitis due to EEE shows hyperintensities in the basal ganglia bilaterally.

tremors, and cranial nerve palsies may occur with long-term sequelae that include cognitive decline and intellectual disabilities.

Rubivirus

RUBELLA

Rubella, also known as the *German measles*, is caused by a positive sense, single-stranded RNA virus. The name *rubella* is derived from Latin, meaning "little red," as it generally produces a mild exanthematous disease in children and adults. However, infection occurring during pregnancy, particularly in the first trimester, can result in severe consequences including miscarriage, stillbirth, or infants born with congenital malformations and severe neurologic deficits, known as *congenital rubella syndrome*. Rubella also produces a rare chronic form of progressive encephalitis termed *progressive rubella panencephalitis*, which can be seen in children with congenital rubella syndrome or those with postnatal infections.

In the 1970s, rubella infections occurred in epidemics in the United States approximately every 6 to 9 years prior to licensing of the rubella vaccine. The last U.S. epidemic in 1964 to 1965 resulted in over 12.5 million cases of rubella, with 20,000 infants born with congenital rubella syndrome. In 2004, after implementation of a universal vaccination program, elimination of endemic rubella virus transmission was documented in the United States. Rubella infections are still prevalent worldwide, as the virus continues to circulate where vaccination programs have not been established. Transmission of the virus is by the respiratory route and replication occurs in the nasopharynx and lymph nodes.

There can be severe neurologic morbidity from rubella arising when a pregnant woman is infected. The frequency of congenital defects is highest in the first trimester of pregnancy and falls as gestation advances. For a long time after birth, infants with congenital rubella syndrome may shed virus from the nasopharynx, eye, or CSF, producing a chronic, persistent infection in the fetus. Neurologic abnormalities are observed by 18 months of age. Infants with rubella encephalitis are hypotonic, inactive, and irritable with a typically full anterior fontanel. Eventually, opisthotonic posturing, rigidity, paresis, seizures, and developmental delays can occur. The syndrome includes sensorineural hearing loss, cardiovascular anomalies, congestive heart failure (CHF), cataracts, thrombocytopenia, and areas of hyperpigmentation about the navel, forehead, and cheeks.

In postnatal infections, rubella results in a mild systemic illness with an incubation of period of 2 to 3 weeks. Lymphadenopathy is often the initial clue with a subsequent erythematous rash on the face and trunk. The neurologic symptoms are rare, occurring in less than 0.1% of rubella cases. Rubella can produce

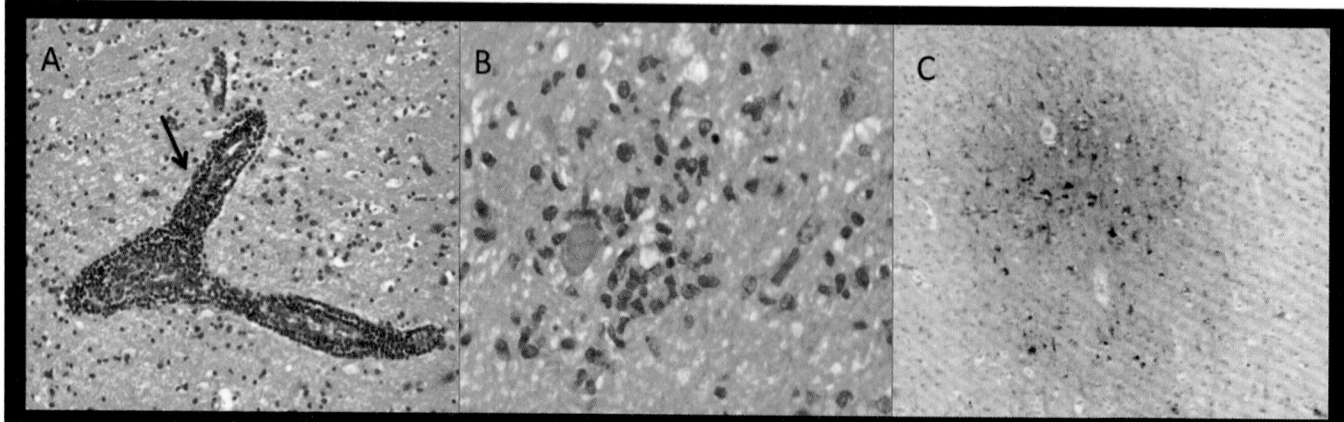

FIGURE 66.3 Histopathologic features in EEE. **A:** Hematoxylin and eosin–stained section of thalamus showing perivascular cuffing (*arrow*) (magnification ×20). **B:** Hematoxylin and eosin–stained section showing neuronal degeneration and inflammation. **C:** EEE virus–specific antibody stained section of frontal cortex. (Courtesy of Dr. Pedro Ciarliani.)

an encephalitis, meningitis, or myelitis. There are sporadic case reports of GBS following the presence of rash.

Serum abnormalities seen with rubella infections include leukopenia with atypical lymphocytosis or thrombocytopenia. The CSF in postnatal rubella or in congenital rubella syndrome contains a lymphocytic pleocytosis and moderately increased protein concentration. Diagnosis of rubella is supported by detecting rubella-specific IgM and confirmed by detecting rubella virus in throat washings or rubella virus RNA in CSF or urine by using RT-PCR. Rubella virus can be recovered from the CSF of approximately 25% of patients and may persist in the CSF for more than 1 year after birth. On MRI of the brain in congenital rubella syndrome, there are basal ganglia, periventricular and cortical calcifications, multifocal T2-hyperintensities, and evidence of delayed myelination.

Prevention is the primary method of combating rubella. The rubella vaccine is a live attenuated virus that is usually given as part of the MMR (measles, mumps, and rubella) vaccine. Due to risk of congenital rubella syndrome, rubella vaccination is particularly important for nonimmune women who may become pregnant.

PROGRESSIVE RUBELLA PANENCEPHALITIS

Progressive rubella panencephalitis is an extremely rare and fatal neurodegenerative disorder that can follow either congenital or postnatal rubella infections. The insidious development of neurologic deterioration following years after a rubella infection was first described in the *New England Journal of Medicine* in two consecutive papers in 1975. Several clinical and neuropathologic features seen in progressive rubella panencephalitis mirror that of subacute sclerosing panencephalitis following measles infections (SSPE; discussed under "Measles Encephalitis"). Progressive rubella panencephalitis is typically seen in the second decade of life. The syndrome begins with a dementing illness and ataxia, the latter being the most consistent neurologic sign in progressive rubella panencephalitis. As the disease progresses, the ataxia worsens with dysmetria, dysdiadochokinesia, and truncal titubation. Dysarthria is prominent. The development of pyramidal tract involvement, retinopathy, seizures, and multifocal myoclonus can occur over a protected period of time over 8 to 10 years. Headache and meningismus are not seen.

Progressive rubella panencephalitis and SSPE occur in people who have elevated antiviral antibodies and apparent intact cellular immunity. In the cases reported of progressive rubella panencephalitis, there were high titers of rubella-specific IgG in CSF and sera. The high ratio of CSF-to-sera of rubella-specific antibodies suggests intrathecal synthesis. The rubella virus is rarely isolated. In these cases, it is important to rule out the presence of measles-specific antibodies given the similarity in presentations. Electroencephalogram (EEG) reveals diffuse slowing but without the characteristic pattern in SSPE.

The neuropathologic features of progressive rubella panencephalitis on gross examination show atrophy of the rhombencephalon, centrum semiovale, and basal ganglia with ventricular dilatation, particularly in the fourth ventricle. Microscopically, the cerebellum has atrophy of all cell layers. Neuronal loss is present and widespread. Inclusion bodies seen in SSPE are not present in progressive rubella panencephalitis. There is evidence of chronic inflammation and demyelination with diffuse astrogliosis of the white matter with perivascular lymphocytic and plasma cell infiltrates. Progressive rubella panencephalitis produces a picture consistent with vasculitis. There are IgG deposits in cerebral vessels as well as

the presence of multinucleated giant cells and lymphocytes in vessel walls. Most of the extracted IgG is specific to rubella.

The diagnosis of progressive rubella panencephalitis is easier in children with congenital rubella syndrome. In those who had postnatal rubella infections, the differential should include SSPE as well as dementing illness of childhood. However, with the onset of ataxia, the diagnosis is clearer and demonstration of CSF and sera rubella-specific antibodies is diagnostic. The emphasis remains on preventative measures through vaccination programs, as there are no specific treatments.

ORTHOMYXOVIRUSES: INFLUENZA VIRUS

Influenza is a negative-sense RNA virus with three subtypes (A, B, and C). Further delineation is based on hemagglutinins (H) and neuraminidases (N). The majority of symptomatic infections result in a monophasic, febrile, respiratory illness, but certain hemagglutinin and neuraminidase types confer particularly severe virulence, raising morbidity and mortality.

Neurologic complications are most severe with influenza A and are more commonly seen in children but overall are rare. Additionally, direct CNS infection by influenza is rare, and parainfectious or postinfectious autoimmune and toxin-mediated diseases are the most common neurologic complications. Febrile seizures, encephalopathy, Reye syndrome, GBS, and encephalitis have all been described. Encephalopathy and encephalitis may be clinically indistinguishable and as such are typically described interchangeably, although the pathophysiology of these two entities differs greatly.

Influenza is seen worldwide, but the most commonly reported neurologic complications of encephalopathy/encephalitis come from Japan, where the usual population affected is children younger than 5 years old. This age group accounts for some 80% of influenza-associated encephalopathies. Fatality rate is about 25% to 35%, and another 20% to 40% have residual neurologic deficits after convalescence.

The pathophysiology of influenza-associated encephalopathy is unknown. Virus can be recovered from brain tissue or CSF occasionally, but this is rare. More plausible is a scenario of overwhelming cytokine production, inciting edema and necrosis involving the brain stem and deep gray matter structures of the cerebrum. CT and MRI frequently demonstrate abnormalities in these regions or more widespread edema; it is uncommon in influenza-associated encephalopathy for neuroimaging to be normal.

Influenza-associated encephalopathy typically presents early in the course of the respiratory disease about 1 to 2 days after fever onset. Depressed level of consciousness is invariable. Seizure occurs some 80% of the time, and EEG is abnormal. Symptoms can progress to coma and death. For neurologic complications, neuraminidase inhibitors are used, but again because these are thought not to be directly due to viral invasion of the brain, this approach is to minimize the complicating triggers. Treatment for the neurologic complications is aimed at reducing inflammation and edema.

PARAMYXOVIRUSES

HENIPAVIRUSES

Hendra virus and Nipah virus are single-stranded, enveloped, negative-sense RNA paramyxoviruses. In the CNS, they cause encephalitis. Their reservoir is the *Pteropus* fruit bat, which resides in Southeast Asia, Madagascar, India, and northern Australia (see Fig. 66.1A). These are primarily nonhuman viruses: Hendra is an equine virus and Nipah a swine virus, but human transmission has occurred due to both exposure to the fruit bat and exposure to infected animals, usually via saliva. This is extremely rare.

Pathogenesis in the CNS is related both to parenchymal infection and widespread, severe vasculitis. Initial invasion of the CNS seems to occur in a retrograde fashion through the trigeminal nerve or directly across the BBB.

Presentation of Hendra or Nipah virus infection is that of a rapidly progressive encephalitis occurring 1 to 2 weeks after exposure, starting as a fever perhaps with myalgias progressing to confusion, seizure, coma, and death over the course of several days. Mortality rate is 40% to 75%, and no definitive treatment exists.

MEASLES ENCEPHALITIS

Measles virus is a small single-stranded RNA virus belonging to the genus *Morbillivirus* of the family Paramyxoviridae. Measles virus is highly infectious, spreading rapidly between individuals primarily through aerosolized respiratory droplets over short distances. Measles virus can also be suspended in the air for long periods of time via small-particle aerosols. Infection spread can occur swiftly in a sparsely vaccinated population due to poor herd immunity. The most common manifestation of measles is a febrile childhood exanthem.

Infection with measles virus is associated with a robust cell-mediated immune response and downstream upregulation of cytokines. The virus does not usually replicate extensively in brain tissue, and it is thought that key mutations may be needed to confer a neurovirulent phenotype. Hypothesized viral routes to CNS include migration of infected leukocytes through the BBB, via endothelial cells, or through neuronal viral transport. The virus and subsequent immune response can result in severe brain injury.

There are three main neurologic complications that can arise from measles infections: post measles encephalomyelitis (PME), measles inclusion body encephalitis (MIBE), and SSPE. Toxic encephalopathy and acute infantile hemiplegia rarely occur with measles infections and are more likely related to complications of severe febrile illnesses of childhood and are not specific to measles.

PME is akin to ADEM and is seen weeks after a measles infection. Symptoms include headaches, changes in mental status, and seizures, and most PME cases had preceding morbilliform rash and fever that are typically seen with measles virus. In patients with myelitis, back pain with bladder and bowel dysfunction is prominent. CSF analysis can show a mild lymphocytic pleocytosis and elevated protein concentrations. MRI scans demonstrate T2 hyperintensities in the white matter of the brain and spinal cord. In histopathologic studies of the brain, there is evidence of inflammation and demyelination; however, measles virus is not present, suggesting that PME is likely a postviral autoimmune phenomenon.

MIBE, also known as *immunosuppressive measles encephalitis*, typically occurs months after a measles infection and affects immunocompromised individuals who are unable to clear measles virus. The disease has been described in those with hematologic malignancies, HIV, and solid organ and stem cell transplantation. Nearly all reported MIBE cases have altered mental status and seizures. The seizures are typically refractory focal motor seizures, but generalized seizures and epilepsia partialis continua have been reported. Focal motor deficits, speech impairment, and visual symptoms are also seen. There is progressive deterioration in the level of consciousness typically leading to coma and death in weeks to months. CSF analysis is usually normal, but a mild pleocytosis and elevated protein concentration may be seen. Brain biopsy is necessary to establish a definitive diagnosis. Measles hemagglutinin and matrix proteins can be visualized by immunohistochemical staining, and intranuclear and intracytoplasmic paramyxovirus particles are seen in neurons, glia, and endothelial cells with electron microscopy. In cases of MIBE and SSPE, it is thought that the virus is likely replication-defective making culturing measles virus difficult and the presence of measles is best demonstrated by RT-PCR. The measles vaccine has been implicated as a cause in immunocompromised patients with MIBE.

General supportive measures are the primary treatment. The role of postexposure Ig prophylaxis is unclear. In several patients, intravenous ribavirin treatment has resulted in temporary improvement but is not approved for the treatment of measles. The measles vaccine has been successfully used without serious complications in many immunocompromised patients including those with HIV who do not have evidence of severe immunosuppression.

SUBACUTE SCLEROSING PANENCEPHALITIS

SSPE is a rare, slowly progressive, fatal disease of the CNS typically occurring in children and young adults. SSPE develops in immunocompetent persons after a prolonged latent period following a measles infection. There is a higher risk of SSPE associated with a measles infection before the age of 2 years. The disease follows a stereotypic pattern beginning with behavioral changes after a period of weeks to months. Eventually, there is the appearance of myoclonus and focal deficits (speech disorder, ataxia, paresis, or vision loss). If epilepsy is present, generalized tonic–clonic seizures are the most common. As the disease progresses, there is increased pyramidal and extrapyramidal tone and whole-body myoclonic jerks. There have been very few reports of remission; the disease is typically prolonged over months to years and ends in death.

The presence of periodic complexes on EEG is classic for SSPE, with a spike and delta wave component of 0.5- to 3-second duration and intercomplex intervals of 4 to 30 seconds. These complexes are recognizable in the early stages. Those affected with SSPE have elevated levels of measles-specific IgG antibodies in the CSF and serum, unlike in MIBE. There are no specific MRI findings for SSPE. Striking histologic features of SSPE are hypertrophic astrocytes and microglial proliferation. A perivascular infiltration occurs in the cortex and white matter with plasma and other mononuclear cells. Patchy areas of demyelination and gliosis occur in the white matter and deeper layers of the cortex. The neurons of the cortex, basal ganglia, pons, and inferior olives show degenerative changes. Intranuclear and intracytoplasmic eosinophilic inclusion bodies contain measles virus nucleocapsids. The measles virus extracted from brain tissue in SSPE is highly defective due to lack of membrane protein production, which renders the virus incapable of being fully assembled and shed from the cell surface.

No drug treatments are available to clear the persistent measles virus from the CNS. Intraventricular interferon with intravenous or intraventricular ribavirin has resulted in clinical improvement or stopped progression in case reports but has not cured the disease. No controlled studies have been performed for SSPE. The focus remains on symptomatic and supportive treatments including treatment of myoclonus and seizures, but the disease and its sequelae are entirely preventable by maintaining measles immunization rates greater than 90% in populations.

RHABDOVIRUS: RABIES

Rabies is one of the most deadly and feared viruses with fatality rates essentially at 100%. The disease is present in all continents, except in Antarctica, with the predominant burden of illness in Asia and Africa. It has a variable incubation period followed by pain or paresthesia at the site of the bite and ultimately a progressive encephalomyelitis and death.

EPIDEMIOLOGY

Rabies is underreported in many areas around the world. The estimated worldwide mortality from rabies is approximately 60,000 per year, which is more than any other single zoonotic disease. The route of transmission is typically via the bite of an infected animal, allowing breakdown of the dermal barrier and deposition of the virus into tissues. Dogs remain the principle vector for human rabies, and dog bites are responsible for over 95% of cases. During 2012, the United States and its territories reported 6,162 rabid animals to the CDC, including raccoons, bats, skunks, foxes, cats, cattle, and dogs. Humans are considered dead-end hosts, with human-to-human transmissions occurring only in rare circumstances, such as in transplantations. Airborne transmission of rabies has been reported in spelunkers of bat-infested caves and laboratory workers with no known bat bites.

PATHOBIOLOGY

Rabies is derived from a negative sense, single-stranded RNA virus belonging to the genus *Lyssavirus*. The virus is enveloped and bacilliform (bullet-shaped). Once transcribed by the host, viral replication and transcription occur in cytoplasmic inclusions within neuronal cells termed *Negri bodies*. The virus then is able to use the host cell machinery to travel retrograde by axonal transport mechanisms to the dorsal root ganglia or cell bodies in the spinal cord or brain stem. In the CNS, viral replication is enhanced and clinical disease develops.

CLINICAL FEATURES

There are two clinical forms of rabies traditionally described: encephalitic (furious) and paralytic (dumb) (Table 66.2). The earliest symptom reported is pain or paresthesia at the site of infection in about half of patients due to viral replication in the local dorsal root ganglia. Other symptoms include fever, headache, and lethargy. The encephalitic course is heralded by hypersalivation, alternating patterns of agitation and lucidity, and hydrophobia leading to pharyngeal spasms, all ultimately leading to coma and death. The paralytic form classically begins with limb weakness early; there are no convulsions or laryngeal spasms. The paralysis results in flaccid tone and can spread to involve other limbs. The paralytic form of rabies has a longer prodromal period and a more protracted course. The typical incubation period is 1 to 6 months. Longer incubations of up to 8 years post exposure have been reported with evidence of genetic data to exclude the possibility of reexposure.

DIAGNOSIS

Diagnostic tests rely on the widespread dissemination of the virus. MRI of the affected brain shows a pattern of mild T2 hyperintensities primarily in the brain stem, hippocampus, thalamus, and cerebral white matter (Fig. 66.4). Postcontrast enhancement in the brain is observed late in the course. In paralytic rabies, the brachial plexus can enhance in the prodromal phase. The MRI changes seen in rabies are preferential to the brain stem.

The diagnosis can be made by fluorescent antibody staining of corneal smears or nuchal skin biopsies, although both false-negative and false-positive results occur, and/or by the detection of viral nucleic acid using RT-PCR in biologic fluids including saliva and CSF. Although viral shedding in saliva is used for testing, sensitivity on single sample testing can be as low as 70%. This is attributed to intermittent shedding, and thus multiple successive saliva samples or skin biopsies reach sensitivities greater than 95%.

Histopathologic diagnosis of rabies was for many years dependent on visualization of Negri bodies in infected neurons on biopsies. These are inclusions, which are classically round or ovoid eosinophilic bodies with basophilic stippling. Negri bodies are most prominent in the brain stem, hippocampus, and in Purkinje cells but can been seen in cortical neurons and spinal ganglia. A histologic picture of encephalitis and/or myelitis can occur but is not universal, as considerable variability in the inflammatory response may be due to differences in the infecting rabies virus strain. Perivascular lymphocytic inflammation and microglial activation are typically found in the brain stem and spinal cord but can be widespread. In paralytic rabies, inflammation is most evident in the anterior horn. Rabies viral antigen is frequently identified in cases where Negri bodies are absent and can be shown in non-CNS tissue including the cornea and nasal mucosa.

TREATMENT

No effective therapies exist for rabies after the development of symptoms. Of the individuals who have survived, one received preexposure immunization and eight received postexposure prophylaxis prior to the onset of symptoms. There has been a single case of a 15-year-old girl who was in contact with a bat 1 month prior to symptom onset and did not receive postexposure prophylaxis who survived after treatment with a combination of medical therapies, which included therapeutic coma with ribavirin, amantadine, benzodiazepines, and ketamine, dubbed the "Milwaukee protocol." This paradigm with case-by-case modifications for the treatment of rabies remains controversial, as at least 26 subsequent cases have failed to repeat this isolated success. Additional therapies for rabies, including Ig plus vaccination, ribavirin, and interferon α, have not been successful to date. Thus, the best approach to rabies is exposure avoidance and vaccinating those anticipating potential exposure. Access to postexposure prophylaxis may be lifesaving for those who do become exposed.

ARENAVIRUSES

This is a large family of negative-sense RNA viruses that infect rodents asymptomatically. Human contact with the animal or its excrement results in viral transmission. "Old world" arenaviruses include Lassa virus, found in Africa, and lymphocytic choriomeningitis virus, found throughout the world. "New world" arenaviruses include Whitewater Arroyo virus found in North America, Junin virus found in Argentina, and Machupo virus found in Bolivia and parts of Paraguay. Lymphocytic choriomeningitis virus causes a variety of neurologic manifestations described in the following section. Lassa, Whitewater Arroyo virus, Junin, and Machupo all cause hemorrhagic fever, with mortality rates of 15% to 35%. Infection is via droplet inhalation, escort by alveolar macrophages to lymph nodes, subsequent replication, and dissemination. Symptoms start as a febrile illness that can progress

TABLE 66.2 **Features of Furious versus Paralytic Symptoms in Patients Infected with Rabies Virus**

	Furious	Paralytic
General Features in Patients Infected with Dog RABV Variants		
Prevalence	2/3 (67%)	1/3 (33%)
Average survival without intensive care support	5–7 days ($n = 80$)	11 days ($n = 35$)
Location of bite and relation to unsuccessful immunization	Anywhere; not related	Anywhere; not related
Prodromal symptoms	Nonspecific with local neuropathic pain in a third of patients	Nonspecific with local neuropathic pain in a third of patients
Rabies characteristics[a]	Present but might not be seen at all stages	None or minimal, phobic spasms in only half, inspiratory spasms might not be obvious due to weakness of neck muscles and diaphragm; percussion myoedema at deltoids and chest wall (in the absence of hyponatremia, renal failure, hypothyroidism, and severe cachexia)
Sensory deficits	At bitten segment due to ganglionitis; loss of pinprick sensation followed by loss of joint position sense	At bitten segment due to ganglionitis; loss of pinprick sensation followed by loss of joint position sense
Flaccid weakness with areflexia	Appears only when comatose	Ascending pure motor weakness, predominantly involving proximal and facial musculature as initial manifestation, whereas consciousness is fully preserved
Electrophysiologic features	Subclinical anterior horn cell dysfunction; sensory neuronopathy in patients with local neuropathic symptoms	Evidence of peripheral demyelination or axonopathy; sensory neuronopathy in patients with local neuropathic symptoms
MRI Findings in Patients Infected with Dog RABV Variants		
Prodromal phase	Enhancing hypersignal T2 changes along the brachial plexus and associated spinal nerve roots at levels corresponding with the bitten extremity; nonenhancing ill-defined mild hypersignal T2 changes of the spinal cord, temporal lobe cortices, hippocampal gyri, and cerebral white matter	Enhancing hypersignal T2 changes along the brachial plexus and associated spinal nerve roots at levels corresponding with the bitten extremity; nonenhancing ill-defined mild hypersignal T2 changes of the spinal cord, temporal lobe cortices, hippocampal gyri, and cerebral white matter
Acute neurologic (noncomatose) phase	Progression of abnormal hypersignal T2 changes	Progression of abnormal hypersignal T2 changes
Comatose phase	Moderate gadolinium enhancement, especially in limbic structures, thalamus, substantia nigra, tectal plates, brain stem, deep gray matter, cranial nerve nuclei, spinal cord, and cranial and spinal nerve roots	Moderate gadolinium enhancement, especially in limbic structures, thalamus, substantia nigra, tectal plates, brain stem, deep gray matter, cranial nerve nuclei, spinal cord, and cranial and spinal nerve roots
General Features of Early-Stage Rabies in Naturally Infected Dogs		
Viral load in brain structures	Several times greater than paralytic at all 12 regions examined	Several times lower than furious at all 12 regions examined
Cytokine or chemokine mRNA transcripts	Barely detected; TNF-α detectable but at nonsignificant concentration	TNF-α, interferon γ, and interleukin 1β
FLAIR signal abnormality indicative of macrocellular damage revealed by MRI	Faint signal in cervical cord, brain stem, temporal lobes, and cerebral hemispheres	Moderate to intense signal in hypothalamus, brain stem, cervical cord, and temporal lobes
Blood–brain barrier status (examined by presence or absence of contrast-enhanced lesion)	Intact; no contrast-enhanced lesion	Intact; no contrast-enhanced lesion
Neuropathology	Caudal-rostral polarity of viral antigen; greater viral antigen reported in many regions, including frontal and occipital cortices and most spinal cord levels; inflammation generally mild throughout the CNS	Prominent inflammation in brain stem, in association with lower extent of viral antigen; caudal-rostral polarity of viral antigen

[a]Change in consciousness, phobic spasms, spontaneous inspiratory spasms, and autonomic dysfunctions.
RABV, rabies virus; MRI, magnetic resonance imaging; TNF-α, tumor necrosis factor-alpha; FLAIR, fluid-attenuated inversion recovery; CNS, central nervous system.
From Hemachudha T, Ugolini G, Wacharapluesadee S, et al. Human rabies: neuropathogenesis, diagnosis, and management. *Lancet Neurol.* 2013;12(5):498–513.

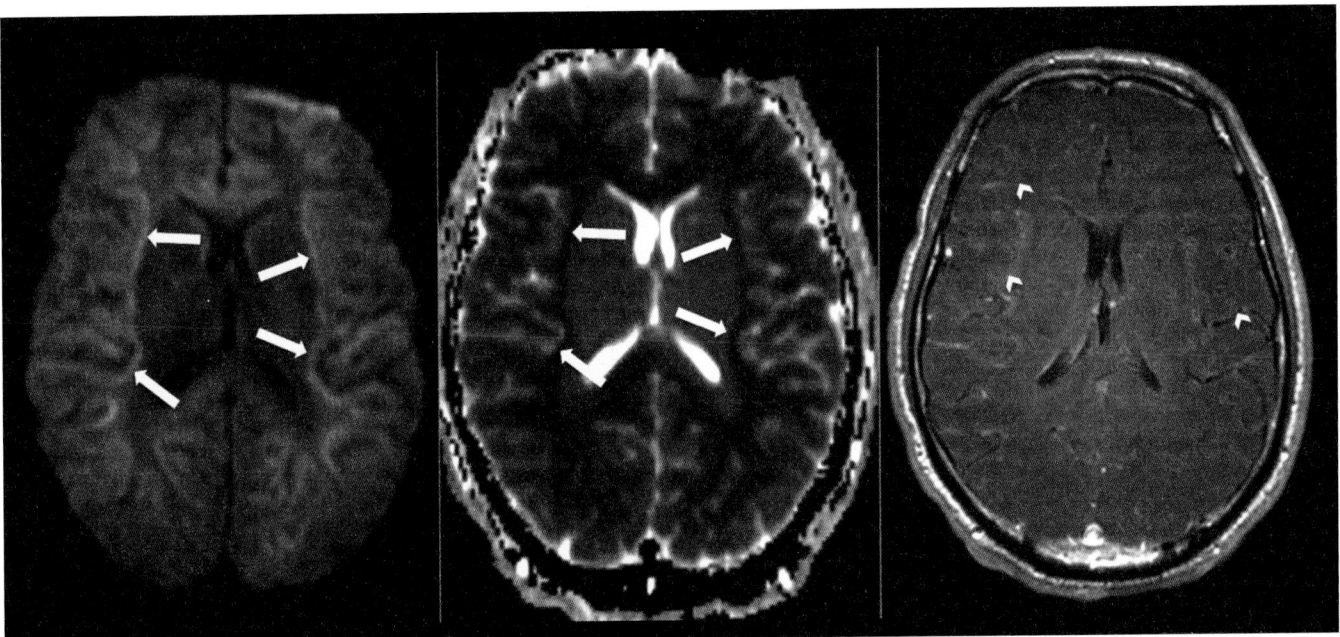

FIGURE 66.4 Axial diffusion-weighted imaging **(far left)**, apparent diffusion coefficient **(middle)**, and T1-weighted MRI after administration of gadolinium **(right)** at the level of the caudate heads in a patient with rabies encephalitis demonstrate diffusion restriction within the subcortical white matter (*arrows*) and diffuse leptomeningeal enhancement (*arrowheads*). The white matter diffusion restriction is thought secondary to wallerian degeneration and leptomeningeal enhancement to leptomeningitis.

to encephalopathy and severe thrombocytopenia and platelet aggregation inhibition, resulting in multifocal hemorrhage. These infections tend to occur in outbreaks, and men are more frequently affected than women, a feature thought to be related to exposure patterns.

LYMPHOCYTIC CHORIOMENINGITIS VIRUS

Of the arenaviruses, lymphocytic choriomeningitis virus can be found throughout the world. In addition to murine transmission, outbreaks in the setting of solid organ transplantation have also been reported, albeit rarely, but with uniformly fatal outcomes. Vertical transmission is also known to occur. The more common mode of infection is via exposure to infected rodent excrement, and most often the infection is asymptomatic if the host is immune competent. Indeed, the donors of those solid organ transplant recipients who died from infection were unaware of their infection, and one even had a lymphocytic choriomeningitis virus–infected pet hamster.

Initial incubation time is 1 to 3 weeks. Lymphocytic choriomeningitis virus is neurotropic, and viremia results in carriage of virus to brain. The most common neurologic complication is viral meningitis that is self-limited; more severe encephalitis is rare, although in a study of undiagnosed encephalitides, 2.3% were found to be due to lymphocytic choriomeningitis virus, suggesting potential underdiagnosis. Other complications include orchitis, arthritis, pericarditis, and pancreatitis. CSF studies in the immunocompromised may be acellular, but in cases of viral meningitis, there is usually a strongly predominantly lymphocytic pleocytosis and elevated protein concentration. Lymphocytic choriomeningitis virus RNA can occasionally be detected in blood or CSF, but diagnosis is more reliably made by serology in the correct clinical setting. Treatment is supportive.

Lymphocytic choriomeningitis virus has also been reported as an important teratogen, and many of the cases reported have been in the United States. About half of the mothers had symptomatic infection and one-third had rodent exposures, which suggests an education potential for prevention purposes. Children born to these mothers suffered chorioretinitis, hydrocephalus, and/or periventricular calcifications.

ADENOVIRUS

Adenovirus is a nonenveloped, double-stranded DNA virus with an icosahedral capsid belonging to the family Adenoviridae. Infection primarily occurs in mucoepithelial cells of the respiratory tract, conjunctiva, and gastrointestinal tracts, followed by lymphoid tissue replication and subsequent viremia. Infections can be monophasic, but the virus can alternatively establish latency and oncologic transformation.

Adenovirus infection of the nervous system is rare and described in terms of case reports. Most are in the setting of bone marrow transplant. Adenovirus infection occurs in both children and adults; case reports have additional commonalities of immune suppression and co-occurring CSF virus detection. Presentation is of meningoencephalitis that may progress to involve the spinal cord. Encephalopathy, headache, and fever are present initially with progression to stupor, coma, and death. CSF may just show elevated protein concentration and detectable adenovirus DNA. Pathology demonstrates adenovirus widespread gliosis, neuronal loss, and adenoviral neuronal inclusions most prominent in the brain stem and diencephalon, with the posterior horns predominantly affected in myelitis. T2-weighted MRI of the brain demonstrates hyperintensities predominantly in the brain stem and deep gray matter structures. Reported outcomes have been dismal, but no reliable epidemiologic data exists.

HERPESVIRUSES

The human herpesvirus group consists of neurotropic viruses that establish latent infections within the nervous system for the lifetime of their host. These viruses contain double-stranded DNA molecules. The family consists of eight members: herpes simplex virus 1 and 2 (HSV-1, HSV-2), VZV, cytomegalovirus, EBV, and human herpesvirus 6, 7, and 8 (HHV-6, HHV-7, HHV-8). These are pleiotropic viruses that are capable of causing tissue injury, vasculitis, angiogenesis, and tumorigenesis.

HERPES SIMPLEX VIRUS 1 AND 2

The herpes simplex virus (HSV) is a common virus with two closely related types, HSV-1 and HSV-2, sharing 70% genomic homology. HSV-1 and HSV-2 establish latent infections in dorsal root ganglia and can reactivate years later, causing meningitis (HSV-2) or encephalitis (HSV-1 primarily). In adults, seroprevalence for HSV-1 and HSV-2 is 50% to 90% and 4% to 40%, respectively.

Herpes Simplex Virus Encephalitis

Herpes simplex virus encephalitis (HSE) is the most commonly identified cause of sporadic encephalitis in the United States, Europe, and Australia. The incidence is estimated at about three cases per million population but with bimodal age distribution. The majority of patients are younger than 20 years old or older than 50 years, with a peak incidence between 60 and 64 years of age. There is no sex preference or seasonal variability. In immunocompetent adults, more than 90% of cases are due to HSV-1. HSV-2 can be responsible for HSE and is typically seen in immunosuppressed individuals or in neonates. The pathogenesis for HSE is either reactivation within the trigeminal ganglion with axonal spread into the frontal and temporal lobes, reactivation of latent virus within the CNS, or a primary infection of the CNS. These are not mutually exclusive.

CLINICAL MANIFESTATIONS

The clinical presentations of HSE is headache and fever, with personality or behavioral changes, disorientation, and/or seizures. The combination of fever and headache with personality changes or confusion is seen in the majority of cases, although only rarely will an individual have the complete triad of symptoms.

DIAGNOSIS

The CSF is abnormal in more than 95% of HSE patients, revealing a moderate pleocytosis with predominately mononuclear cells. Red blood cells are frequently present. There can be a moderate increase in CSF protein concentration, whereas hypoglycorrhachia is seen only occasionally and not expected. PCR for HSV-1 is 98% sensitive and 94% specific. False-negative results can be seen during the first 72 hours of illness and testing can turn positive 1 to 2 days later. PCR results can remain positive even while on treatment in 40% of HSE patients, although by and large, these statistics do not come from therapy with acyclovir. The CSF white blood cell count in immunocompromised hosts may not be elevated, and in general, immunocompromised patients have lower white blood cell count numbers in comparison to those with healthy immune systems. EEG changes are nonspecific and classically demonstrate periodic lateralized epileptiform discharges or seizures. MRI is the superior imaging modality, demonstrating abnormalities 24 to 48 hours earlier than CT. The diagnosis of HSE is supported by T2 hyperintensities in cortical and subcortical regions of the medial temporal lobes, insula, orbitofrontal, and cingulate gyri (Fig. 66.5).

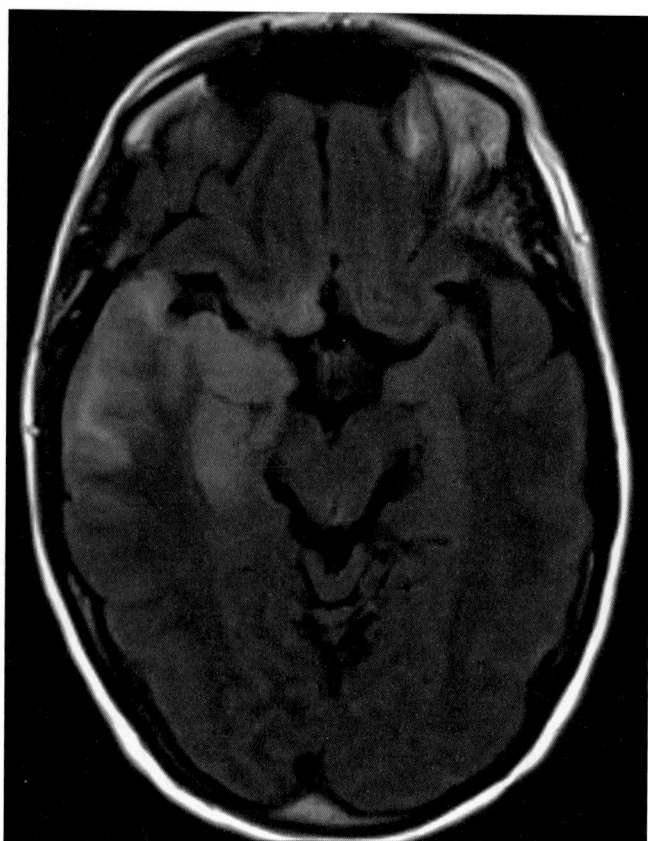

FIGURE 66.5 Axial T2-weighted FLAIR MRI at the level of the superior cerebellar peduncle and tentorium cerebelli in a patient with limbic encephalitis due to HSV-1 demonstrates T2 hyperintensity and edema in the anterior temporal lobe on the right.

There may be additional evidence of subacute hemorrhages within edematous brain tissue. Restricted diffusion correlates with cytotoxic edema and is present early in disease.

TREATMENT

The introduction of acyclovir in 1984, which prevents viral replication by DNA polymerase inhibition, resulted in dramatically reduced mortality rates from HSE. Acyclovir for HSE is dosed at 10 mg/kg every 8 hours for 21 days in patients with normal renal function; relapse is an issue in undertreated patients. If the patient is not clinically improving, foscarnet can be substituted for acyclovir.

Resistance to acyclovir is very uncommon in treatment-naïve patients, with overall prevalence of resistant HSV-1 estimated to be about 0.3%. Acyclovir resistance stems from viral thymidine kinase mutations in 95% of cases or in viral DNA polymerase genes. These mutations result in decreased or absent HSV thymidine kinase production, altered affinity of the thymidine kinase, or HSV DNA polymerase for the active phosphorylated acyclovir. In immunocompromised people who are receiving long-term prophylactic acyclovir, the risk of acyclovir-resistant HSV and VZV increases. In these patients, treatment with foscarnet and cidofovir are second-line agents.

OUTCOME

HSE is a medical emergency, as prognosis is dependent on early initiation of treatment. Despite highly favorable results with acyclovir, treatment initiation continues to be delayed primarily due to failure to recognize the disease early, and predictors of adverse outcomes despite treatment include age (older than 30 years old), Glasgow Coma Scale score less than 6, and duration of symptoms prior to starting acyclovir.

Neonatal Herpes Simplex Virus 2 Encephalitis

Neonatal HSV infections are some of the most life-threatening infections in newborns. In the United States, neonatal HSV encephalitis affects approximately 1,500 to 2,220 babies per year. HSV-2 accounts for 70% of these cases. The majority of infected infants acquire HSV in the peripartum period during delivery.

HSV infections in infants are grouped into three categories: disseminated disease, CNS involvement, and limited disease to the skin, eyes, and/or mouth. This classification system is predictive of morbidity and mortality. Factors influencing outcomes in neonatal HSE include prematurity, seizures, and multiple dermatologic infections of the skin. Almost one-third of neonates with HSV infection have CNS disease. The clinical manifestations include nonspecific signs of encephalitis/meningitis such as lethargy, poor feeding, labile temperature, seizures, opisthotonus, and bulging fontanels. The median age of presentation for HSV-2 encephalitis is day 16 to 19 of life.

Neonatal CSF HSV PCR is highly sensitive and specific for herpes DNA. HSV DNA is detectable in the first week of illness even while on antiviral therapy. Initiation of acyclovir before the development of CNS disease, disseminated disease, or depressed consciousness improves outcomes. The first-line treatment for neonatal HSE is intravenous acyclovir at 60 mg/kg/day divided three times a day for 21 days. It is recommended to obtain a repeat CSF HSV PCR at the end of therapy and if HSV DNA is still present, to continue therapy. There is higher morbidity and mortality associated with prolonged HSV infection despite therapy. Mortality in the era of antiviral therapy is 4% for CNS HSV disease at 1 year. Long-term neurologic consequences include cerebral palsy, intellectual disabilities, attention deficits, and epilepsy.

Benign Recurrent Lymphocytic Meningitis

A syndrome of recurrent episodes of benign, self-limited, sterile meningitis were first described by Mollaret in 1944. For years, the condition was referred to as *Mollaret meningitis.*

PATHOBIOLOGY

Benign recurrent lymphocytic meningitis is a syndrome that appears to be related to infection with a variety of herpes simplex viruses. In recent years, detection of herpes simplex virus type 2 genome by PCR has been most often, but not uniformly, reported. Other cases have been linked to varicella-zoster infection. CNS epidermoid cysts can give rise to Mollaret meningitis especially with surgical manipulation of cyst contents. A familial association, where more than one family member had Mollaret, has been documented.

CLINICAL MANIFESTATIONS

The syndrome is characterized by repeated, short-lived, spontaneous, remitting attacks of headache and nuchal rigidity. Between attacks, the patient enjoys good health. The meningitic episodes usually last 2 or 3 days. Most are characterized by mild meningitis without associated neurologic abnormalities. The patient's body temperature is moderately elevated with a maximum of 104°F (40°C). Neck stiffness and the signs of meningeal irritation are present. The first attack may appear at any age between childhood and late adult years. Both sexes are equally affected. The episodes usually recur for 3 to 5 years.

DIAGNOSIS

During the attacks, there is CSF pleocytosis and slight elevation of the protein concentration. The CSF glucose concentration is normal. The cell count ranges from 200 to several thousand cells per cubic millimeter; most cells are mononuclear. Large, fragile endothelial cells are found in the CSF in the early phases of the disease; their presence is variable and is not considered essential for the diagnosis.

DIAGNOSIS AND TREATMENT

Patients with Mollaret meningitis always recover rapidly and spontaneously without specific therapy. There is no effective therapy for shortening the attack or preventing additional attacks, although in some anecdotal reports, acyclovir was beneficial.

VARICELLA-ZOSTER VIRUS

VZV is a human herpesvirus that causes both a primary infection (chickenpox) and can reactivate, producing shingles (zoster), meningitis, and encephalitis. After primary infection, the virus persists in a latent form within cranial nerve or dorsal root ganglia and has intermittent periods of reactivation and shedding. VZV reactivation primarily occurs from the spinal ganglia, with the thorax being the most common site of latent infection, followed by lumbar, cervical, and then sacral regions.

VZV encephalitis is more common in those with immunodeficiency or immunosenescence (waning T-cell immunity to varicella). Encephalitis can occur in the absence of a rash. Diagnosis is confirmed with either VZV DNA or anti-VZV IgM detection in the CSF. Intravenous acyclovir 10 to 15 mg/kg every 8 hours for 10 to 14 days is the generally recommended treatment.

Symptomatic ataxia can occur with primary varicella infections and is traditionally seen in children. Acute cerebellar ataxia is due to either direct viral infection of the cerebellum or is a parainfectious process. Ataxia can be antecedent to or present up to 14 days after the onset of a primary varicella rash. In one of the largest series of children with acute cerebellar ataxia due to viral causes, boys are more likely to be affected than girls and have worse gait disturbances and associated cranial nerve involvement. Those with varicella-related acute cerebellar ataxia tended to have worse ataxia than seen in other viral syndromes but have more rapid rates of recovery with good neurologic outcomes.

Herpes Zoster

Herpes zoster primarily is seen in healthy individuals older than age 50 years and in immunocompromised people, particularly those with HIV or recipients of bone marrow transplant. The incidence rate of zoster ranges between 3 and 5 per 1,000 person-years in North America, Europe, and Asia. There is an age-specific rise in incidence rates in those older than age 80 years to 8 to 12 per 1,000 person-years. It is estimated the number of zoster infections worldwide is rising because the general population is aging, the availability of antiviral treatment has had the effect of more people being diagnosed, and because those who are immunocompromised are living longer.

Pain typically heralds the onset of zoster. The pain of zoster is described as severe, sharp, lancinating, radicular pain in the distribution of the affected nerve root. The pain can be associated with pruritus and paraesthesia. A unilateral dermatomal vesicular rash in the area supplied by the affected root or roots typically follows days later. The vesicles are usually clustered and contain clear fluid, which then desquamate and scab within 5 to 10 days. Occasionally, the pain is present without the ensuing rash in a condition known as *zoster sine herpete*. Treatment choices for uncomplicated zoster include oral acyclovir, valacyclovir, or famciclovir with preferential use of valacyclovir or famciclovir due to similar dosing and better CNS pharmacokinetics. A 7- to 10-day course of antiviral therapy is recommended.

Cranial ganglia are affected in approximately 20% of people. In those with cranial nerve involvement, the trigeminal nerve is most often affected. Zoster ophthalmicus, within the V1 distribution of the trigeminal nerve, is often accompanied by keratitis and can lead to blindness. A vesicular rash at the tip of the nose (Hutchinson sign) is a strong predictor of ocular involvement, indicating involvement of the nasociliary branch of V1, which also supplies the cornea and conjunctiva. A herpes zoster rash can precede optic neuritis or ophthalmoplegia. The combination of facial palsy and vesicles in the external auditory canal, tympanic membrane, or on the ipsilateral anterior tongue or hard palate is termed *Ramsay Hunt syndrome*. This syndrome is an indicator of zoster involvement of the facial nerve. The facial palsy in Ramsay Hunt can be severe and those affected are less likely to recover.

The most common complication of zoster is the development of postherpetic neuralgia (PHN). The definition of PHN varies but is generally defined as continued pain in the affected dermatome that persists beyond 4 to 6 weeks after resolution of a rash. The risk of developing PHN varies and is highest in the elderly as well as those who are immunocompromised. Several prospective studies report that 30% to 50% of patients with PHN experience pain lasting over 1 year and with some experiencing pain lasting up to 10 years. The central mechanisms for PHN remain unknown. Treatment of PHN is difficult, and pain can be refractory to multiple analgesics. Combinations of topical treatments (lidocaine or capsaicin) and oral analgesics (tricyclic antidepressants, anticonvulsants, and opioids) are typically used. Interventions such as sympathetic nerve blocks, epidural injections of lidocaine or steroids, or pulsed radiofrequency have either failed to demonstrate benefit or the data is not robust to recommend these procedures.

VZV infection can rarely result in muscle weakness affecting bulbar, limb, or truncal muscles and is typically within the distribution predicted by the rash. For example, peripheral facial weakness is seen with VZV oticus or unilateral diaphragmatic paresis when affecting the cervical myotomes. Neurogenic bladder and loss of anal sphincter control can follow sacral herpes zoster. Segmental zoster paresis is highly associated with PHN. In patients with postganglionic lesions, an MRI can show T2 signal hyperintensity within the affected plexus or nerve, enlargement of the nerve, or enhancement.

Additionally, the VZV is emerging as a relevant ischemic and hemorrhagic stroke risk factor. Large population studies in the United Kingdom and Taiwan show an increase in the incidence of stroke or transient ischemic attack (TIA) the year following herpes zoster, with a greater relative risk (4.5-fold higher) after herpes zoster ophthalmicus. In pediatric populations, nearly one-third of ischemic arteriopathies are associated with varicella infections.

The hypothesis is that reactivation from ganglia results in viral spread to the adventitia of local blood vessels and eventual transmural migration into the media. Inflammatory cells including neutrophils in early VZV vasculopathy and T cells are directed to the infected sites secreting inflammatory factors that result in remodeling of the vessel. Pathology demonstrates evidence of multinucleated giant cells, Cowdry A inclusion bodies, and herpesvirus in arteries. VZV vasculopathy affects small and large arteries with an emphasis on small artery involvement. In contrast, immunocompromised hosts can develop the entire spectrum of small, large, and mixed artery involvement with VZV vasculopathy.

Those affected with VZV vasculopathy do not necessarily have a history of zoster or varicella rash. In cases when a zoster rash is present, there was often a time delay of an average of 4 months between the rash and neurologic symptoms. Anti-VZV IgM in the CSF is more sensitive than CSF VZV DNA for detecting VZV-associated vasculopathy. When VZV vasculopathy is suspected or confirmed, treatment with intravenous acyclovir for a minimum of 14 days is suggested based on category 3 evidence (expert opinion). Oral prednisone at 1 mg/kg for 5 days without taper has been given as an adjuvant to suppress the inflammatory response in arteries, but this dosing is arbitrary.

Myelitis may complicate acute varicella infection or can be a consequence of reactivation. Clinical features include paraparesis with a sensory level approximately 1 to 2 weeks following a dermatomal rash. MRI T2-weighted images can show focal areas of hyperintense lesions (Fig. 66.6). Immunocompromised hosts have a more progressive, insidious course that can be ultimately fatal. Gross histopathology shows areas of necrosis and inflammation

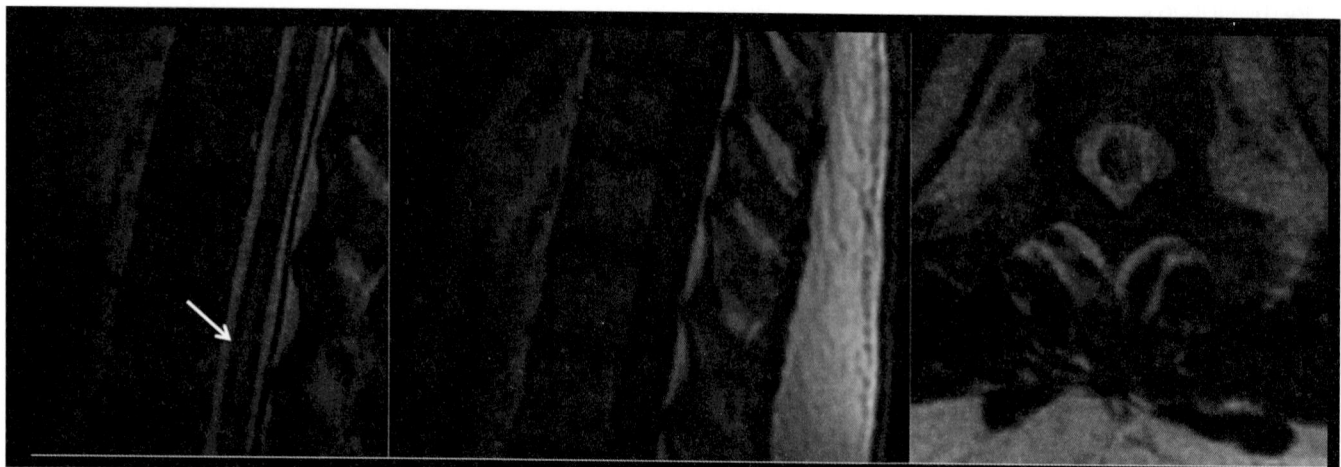

FIGURE 66.6 Midsagittal T2-weighted **(far left)** and postcontrast T1-weighted **(middle)** of the thoracic spine from a patient with varicella-zoster myelopathy show multiple levels of intrinsic cord T2 hyperintensity **(left)** with patchy enhancement **(middle)** from T10 to T12 (*arrow*); axial T2-weighted image at the level of T12 demonstrates both white and gray matter involvement by the lesion.

with invasion of the spinal cord by VZV. Diagnosis is confirmed by presence of VZV DNA and/or anti-VZV IgM in the CSF. Aggressive treatment with intravenous acyclovir and consideration of corticosteroids may produce a favorable response, although evidence is lacking.

In the United States, the herpes zoster vaccine has been licensed since 2006 for use in patients older than the age 60 years without primary or acquired immunodeficiency. The attenuated VZV vaccine reduces the incidence of HZ and can reduce the severity of complications including PHN.

EPSTEIN–BARR VIRUS

EBV is a double-stranded, helical DNA gamma herpesvirus that infects B lymphocytes primarily and subsequently establishes latency. In the nervous system, primary infection is associated with meningitis, encephalitis, myelitis, radiculitis, cerebellar ataxia, GBS, and ADEM. These entities and associations are rare. CNS disease due to reactivation is primarily seen in the setting of profound immune suppression, whereby primary CNS lymphoma is precipitated by EBV-mediated B-cell transformation; this is most closely associated with advanced HIV infection. However, there are case reports of meningoencephalomyelitis occurring in the setting of apparent reactivation.

EBV is one of the most common infections worldwide. Primary inoculation occurs usually by adolescence through infected saliva transfer. The virus replicates in the pharyngeal tonsils and transforms short-lived B lymphocytes to prevent their apoptosis. Primary infection is usually asymptomatic, but infectious mononucleosis can also occur about a month into infection. This is characterized by profound fatigue, lymphadenopathy, splenomegaly, and fever. The nervous system complications mentioned earlier rarely follow. In ADEM or GBS, pathophysiology is due to parainfectious inflammation. For the other entities, there is at least a component of inflammation, and the degree of direct viral pathogenesis is unknown but likely small if any.

Diagnosis of primary EBV infection is by serology. The detection of viral capsid antigen (VCA) IgM indicates recent infection; in chronic/latent infection, this antibody wanes in favor of VCA IgG and EBV nuclear antigen. EBV DNA can be detected in blood and CSF as well, but this does not necessarily indicate pathogenic connection to the disease at hand. Treatment is supportive aside from EBV-associated primary CNS lymphoma, which is treated as a neoplasm with chemotherapy and/or radiation. In the setting of primary infection nervous system complications, treatment often involves corticosteroids, IVIg, and/or plasmapheresis.

Pathologic studies of CNS EBV infections unrelated to primary CNS lymphoma are lacking. Although the virus is detectable in CSF, its positive predictive value is actually quite low. Furthermore, replication can occur in the setting of other infections or illnesses, which makes caution in interpreting results of paramount importance, as this finding could very well be an epiphenomenon. In AIDS-related disease, however, detection of EBV DNA from CSF has a very high sensitivity and specificity for CNS lymphoma.

CYTOMEGALOVIRUS

Cytomegalovirus (CMV) is a common cause of viral opportunistic infections in persons who are immunocompromised from either HIV (CD4 counts <50 cells/mm^3) or those who have undergone transplantation. CMV is also the most common cause of congenital viral infection resulting in neurologic impairments. In the general population, CMV seroprevalence varies considerably, ranging from 50% to 80% in sexually active adults. It is seen in almost all homosexual men with HIV. Symptomatic CMV infections of the nervous system in adults can result in retinitis, encephalitis, polyradiculitis (usually of the lumbosacral nerve roots), myelitis, or vasculitic mononeuritis multiplex. Since the advent of antiretroviral therapy, the incidence of CMV infections affecting the CNS has decreased considerably.

CMV encephalitis clinically presents as a subacute encephalopathy with features of disorientation, lethargy, apathy, and possibly fever. Focal neurologic deficits include seizures and cranial nerve palsies. Clinical signs of brain stem or cerebellar involvement occur in about 30% of those affected. MRI of the brain can show periventricular enhancement or increased T2 hyperintensity on the ependymal surfaces or can be entirely normal. CSF pleocytosis is rare, and if present, it is a mild lymphocytic pleocytosis with an elevation in CSF protein concentration. The diagnosis in the correct clinical setting is strongly supported by a positive CSF CMV PCR (sensitivity 60% to 100%; specificity 89% to 100%).

Additionally, CMV can produce a lumbosacral polyradiculopathy that is often associated with concurrent infection elsewhere. Those with polyradiculopathy develop subacute lower extremity weakness, paresthesia, and lumbar pain with progression to flaccid paraplegia and areflexia. Ascending sensory loss is often asymmetric. Sacral involvement includes urinary retention and fecal incontinence. If perianal anesthesia is present, there is likely anal sphincter dysfunction and conus medullaris involvement, similar to Elsberg syndrome most commonly seen in the setting of HSV-2 reactivation. CSF studies typically reveal a high polymorphonuclear pleocytosis, elevated protein concentration, and hypoglycorrhachia. CSF RT-PCR is positive for CMV in many cases. In the absence of therapy, progressive rubella panencephalitis is a progressive illness and is fatal.

Anti-CMV treatments can be effective if given early in the disease course. The treatment guidelines for CMV infections affecting the nervous system in the adult suggest combination therapy with IV ganciclovir 5 mg/kg and IV foscarnet 90 mg/kg twice daily to stabilize disease. The duration is continued until neurologic improvement is evident which can take weeks to months. Oral valganciclovir is recommended for CMV infections as maintenance therapy for life or until evidence of immune recovery (i.e., >100 cells/μL for at least 3 to 6 months) with antiretroviral therapy is demonstrated. Oral agents for active CNS infection are unlikely to be effective.

Congenital CMV infections are largely asymptomatic, with 10% to 15% of infants presenting with symptoms. The incidence varies in different populations around the world with rates ranging from 0.2% to 3% of all births. Vertical CMV transmission can result from primary maternal infection in pregnancy, can follow reactivation of a previous infection, or can be seen by reinfection with a new strain. Long-term sequelae include sensorineural hearing loss, microcephaly, chorioretinitis and/or optic atrophy, seizures, and a wide range of intellectual developmental disorders. Therapeutic interventions preventing fetal CMV infections with proven efficacy in cases of documented maternal infection are lacking, and no preventive vaccine exists.

HUMAN HERPESVIRUS 6

HHV 6 (Roseolovirus) is a double-stranded, enveloped DNA betaherpesvirus that has two subtypes: A and B. Exanthem subitum is caused by type B. Primary infection typically occurs in childhood, and latency is established in lymphocytes.

Neurologic complications of HHV 6 only occur in the setting of immune suppression. The most frequent scenario is after hematopoietic cell transplantation, when the virus reactivates and causes a limbic encephalitis and occasionally myelitis. Mori (2010) found an incidence of about 4% after first transplantation and 11% in the setting of a second transplant.

Patients with HHV 6 encephalitis will develop headaches and encephalopathy, usually consisting of disorientation, short-term memory dysfunction, seizure, and depressed consciousness, which in the scenario of immune suppression should always raise red flags toward intracranial pathology. HHV 6 replication can be detected in CSF, and especially when disparate to that in blood, this along with characteristic neuroimaging and clinical scenario support the diagnosis. The caveat is that HHV 6 reactivation is common in this setting, and so isolated detection of viral DNA is not unilaterally diagnostic.

Neuroimaging typically demonstrates bilateral mesial temporal hyperintensities perhaps with extension into the thalamus; pathologic examination has correlated increased HHV 6 DNA to these areas. Antiviral treatment, typically with foscarnet and/or ganciclovir, can reduce viral burden and prevent mortality, although long-term deficits frequently remain.

POLYOMAVIRUS

JOHN CUNNINGHAM VIRUS

John Cunningham virus (JCV) is a double-stranded, circular DNA polyomavirus with an icosahedral capsid and no envelope. It is ubiquitous throughout the world and only infects human cells, making animal study a challenge. There are seven types and multiple subtypes of JCV, all originating in Africa, resulting in trackable migration patterns.

Pathobiology

Initial infection is usually asymptomatic and usually occurs in the first two decades of life. By adulthood, nearly 80% of any given population is seropositive. Latency is subsequently established in kidneys or peripheral blood mononuclear cells, although periodic viral shedding in urine is known to occur. Reactivation is precipitated in the setting of immune compromise, and the virus makes its way to the brain parenchyma, where it productively infects oligodendroglial cells and produces the pathologic entity that is known as *progressive multifocal leukoencephalopathy* (PML).

The predisposing immune suppression for PML since the 1980s is most commonly in the setting of advanced HIV infection with a CD4 count of less than 200. However, the original cases of PML were described in lymphoproliferative disorders, and this still occurs. Additionally, certain biologic agents used to treat autoimmune disease and even autoimmune diseases in and of themselves have been associated with immune suppression sufficient to trigger JCV reactivation and PML. A diagram of such predisposing factors and their relative risk can be found in Figure 66.7. Notably, natalizumab and other immunomodulating agents used in the treatment of multiple sclerosis, although far behind HIV-related cases to date, is an important scenario in which PML occurs.

JCV entry into the brain is not well understood. If indeed the latency is in peripheral blood mononuclear cells, these may be chaperoned across the BBB to their target glial cells. Once across this immunologic barrier, the virus binds cell surface glycoproteins and secondarily serotonin (5HT2A) receptors to gain entry. Clathrin-coated vesicles initiate transport into the cell, where virus travels in a retrograde fashion to the nucleus in order to establish productive infection. As mentioned earlier, oligodendrocytes are the primary targets of infection in the brain, but certain variants have the capability to infect cerebellar granule cells or pyramidal neurons in the cortex. These latter two types of infection are very rare. By and large, productive infection leads to cell destruction, demyelination, and macrophage infiltration to mop up the debris. This occurs at multiple foci in the brain initially, but as the infection spreads, plaques form and coalesce, thus making the descriptor PML apropos.

Clinical Features

Clinically, symptoms manifest with dependence on localization of demyelination. Typical presentations are that of a subacute process over several weeks. Cortical weakness and ataxia are common, but language disturbance, visual disturbance, hemispatial neglect, and impaired gait are also well described. Headache is a common accompaniment, but notably absent are signs/symptoms localizable to the spinal cord, which is spared in this entity.

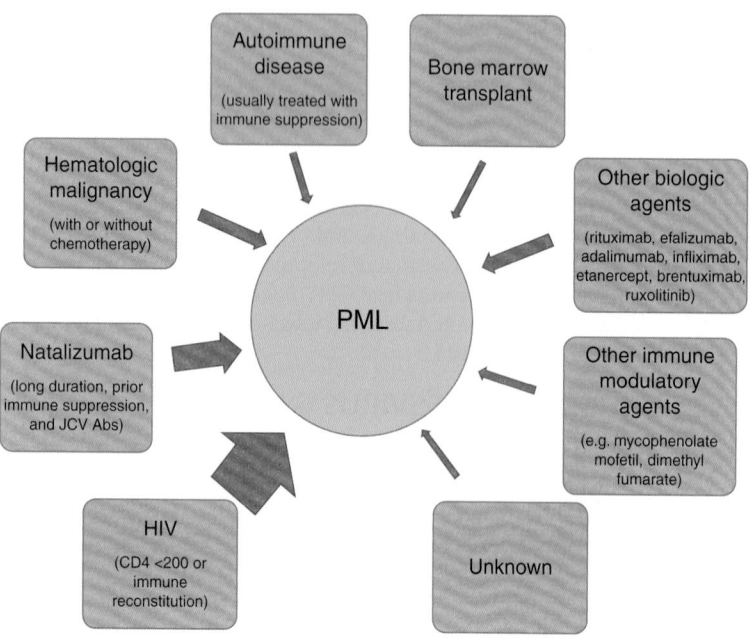

FIGURE 66.7 Predisposing factors for PML. Relative number of cases is depicted by arrow size. By far, advanced HIV infection or immune reconstitution has been the most frequent predisposing factor. Natalizumab therapy for the treatment of multiple sclerosis has emerged in the 21st century as an important risk factor, with duration of treatment, prior immune suppression, and JCV antibody positivity on treatment conferring highest risk. Hematologic malignancy has been the longest standing risk factor. Autoimmune diseases, bone marrow transplant, and other biologic or immune modulatory agents predispose as well, although autoimmune disease contribution unilaterally is controversial, as patients with PML in this setting are nearly always treated with corticosteroids or immune modulatory agents. Finally, some cases are idiopathic.

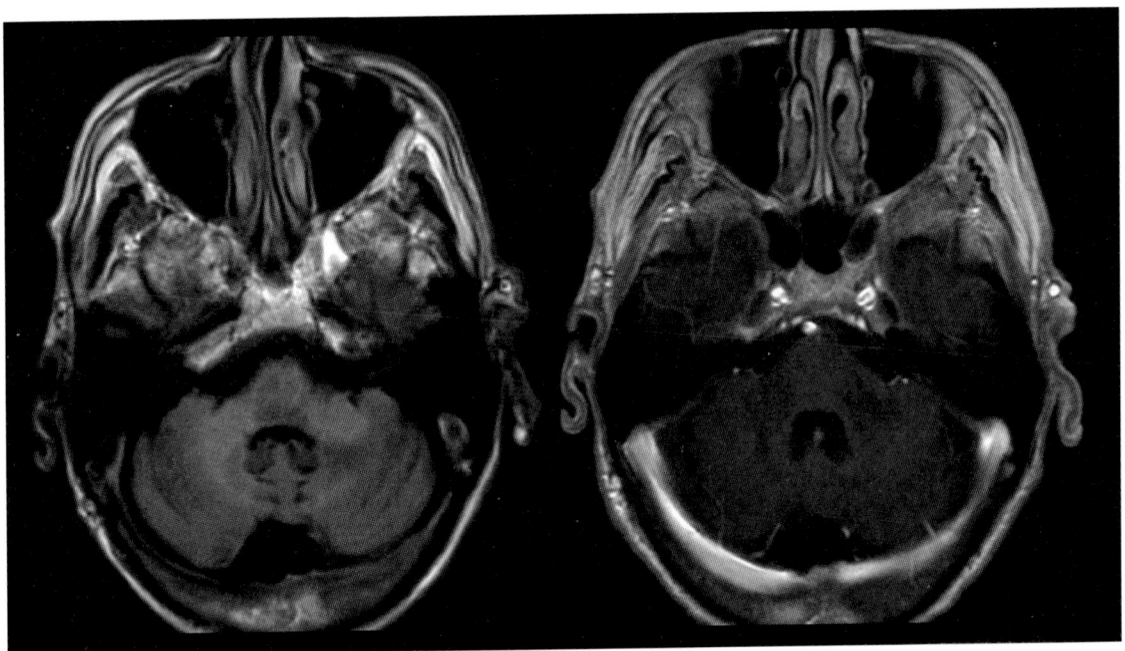

FIGURE 66.8 Axial T2-weighted FLAIR **(left)** and T1-weighted MRI after administration of gadolinium **(right)** at the level of the middle cerebellar peduncles in a patient with PML in the setting of advanced HIV demonstrate T2 hyperintensity and T1 hypointensity within the pons extending into the middle cerebellar peduncles bilaterally.

JCV is a known precipitant of the immune reconstitution inflammatory syndrome (IRIS) seen with rapid viral clearance upon initiation of combination antiretroviral therapy (cART) in advanced HIV infection (also in the setting of natalizumab withdrawal). This entity is rare in the CNS but occurs in about 1% of treated HIV infections; when opportunistic infection is present at the time of HIV diagnosis, reduction in antigen load prior to initiation of cART is one strategy to prevent IRIS. In the setting of PML IRIS, however, this is not possible, as there are no known treatments available for reducing antigen burden. As such, there is no good way to prevent PML IRIS at this time. If it does occur, treatment is supportive and most commonly albeit counterintuitively involves corticosteroids to manipulate the intracranial inflammatory response.

Diagnosis

Diagnosis of PML has evolved from pathologic to laboratory and imaging-based. That is to say, although biopsy is gold standard, this is now reserved for cases whose imaging or laboratory data are unclear. Biopsy will show enlarged, bizarre astrocytes, multifocal but coalescent demyelination, and oligodendroglial nuclear inclusions that stain for JCV by immunohistochemistry. However, more commonly, the combination of brain MRI and CSF detection of JCV DNA in the correct clinical context clinch the diagnosis. In fact, if JCV DNA is not detected but the imaging and scenario are highly suspicious, repeat testing should be performed. CSF studies otherwise can be normal or can show a modest lymphocytic pleocytosis with normal or slightly elevated protein concentration. These findings notably are all but indistinguishable from acute or chronic HIV meningitis. Hypoglycorrhachia is not found. MRI shows multiple T1-weighted hypointense and T2-weighted hyperintense plaques in the subcortical white matter that involve the subcortical U-fibers but do not involve the cortical ribbon. Middle cerebellar peduncular involvement is common (Fig. 66.8). In the setting of immune compromise, gadolinium enhancement is seen only about 15% of the time, whereas in the setting of immune reconstitution, this number increases but only to about 40%.

Treatment

There are no specific treatments for PML except to reconstitute the immune system. Potential viral-targeted therapies have included 5HT2A antagonists; mefloquine; and antivirals such as acyclovir, cidofovir, zidovudine, vidarabine, and cytarabine. These have largely been evaluated separately and have failed. In natalizumab-associated PML, plasmapheresis has been used to rapidly remove drug from the system. In HIV, cART has changed the epidemiology from 1-year survival of less than 10% to greater than 50%. Those with higher CD4 counts at diagnosis have more favorable outcomes.

SUGGESTED READINGS

Achard JM, Lallement PY, Veyssier P. Recurrent aseptic meningitis secondary to intracranial epidermoid cyst and Mollaret's meningitis: two distinct entities or a single disease? A case report and a nosologic discussion. *Am J Med.* 1990;89:807–810.

Adams JM. Persistent or slow viral infections and related diseases. *West J Med.* 1975;122(5):380–393.

Aicardi J, Goutieres F, Arsenio-Nunes ML, et al. Acute measles encephalitis in children with immunosuppression. *Pediatrics.* 1977;59(2):232–239.

Anders HJ, Goebel FD. Cytomegalovirus polyradiculopathy in patients with AIDS. *Clin Infect Dis.* 1998;27(2):345–352.

Anders HJ, Weiss N, Bogner JR, et al. Ganciclovir and foscarnet efficacy in AIDS-related CMV polyradiculopathy. *J Infect.* 1998;36(1):29–33.

Anlar B, Aydin OF, Guven A, et al. Retrospective evaluation of interferon-beta treatment in subacute sclerosing panencephalitis. *Clin Ther.* 2004;26(11):1890–1894. doi:10.1016/j.clinthera.2004.11.002.

Armstrong PM, Andreadis TG. Eastern equine encephalitis virus—old enemy, new threat. *N Engl J Med.* 2013;368(18):1670–1673. doi:10.1056/NEJMp1213696.

Aurelius E, Johansson B, Sköldenberg B, et al. Rapid diagnosis of herpes simplex encephalitis by nested polymerase chain reaction assay of cerebrospinal fluid. *Lancet*. 1991; 337(8735):189–192.

Benson CA, Kaplan JE, Masur H, et al. Treating opportunistic infections among HIV-infected adults and adolescents: recommendations from CDC, the National Institutes of Health, and the HIV Medicine Association/Infectious Diseases Society of America. *MMWR Recomm Rep*. 2004;53(RR-15):1–112.

Benson PC, Swadron SP. Empiric acyclovir is infrequently initiated in the emergency department to patients ultimately diagnosed with encephalitis. *Ann Emerg Med*. 2006;47(1):100–105. doi:10.1016/j.annemergmed.2005.07.019.

Berger JR, Aksamit AJ, Clifford DB, et al. PML diagnostic criteria: consensus statement from the AAN Neuroinfectious Disease Section. *Neurology*. 2013;80:1430–1438.

Bitnun A, Shannon P, Durward A, et al. Measles inclusion-body encephalitis caused by the vaccine strain of measles virus. *Clin Infect Dis*. 1999;29(4):855–861. doi:10.1086/520449.

Black EM, Lowings JP, Smith J, et al. A rapid RT-PCR method to differentiate six established genotypes of rabies and rabies-related viruses using TaqMan technology. *J Virol Methods*. 2002;105(1):25–35.

Boland TA, McGuone D, Jindal J, et al. Phylogenetic and epidemiologic evidence of multiyear incubation in human rabies. *Ann Neurol*. 2014;75(1):155–160. doi:10.1002/ana.24016.

Bonthius DJ, Stanek N, Grose C. Subacute sclerosing panencephalitis, a measles complication, in an internationally adopted child. *Emerg Infect Dis*. 2000;6(4):377–381. doi:10.3201/eid0604.000409.

Bradley H, Markowitz LE, Gibson T, et al. Seroprevalence of herpes simplex virus types 1 and 2—United States, 1999–2010. *J Infect Dis*. 2014;209(3):325–333. doi:10.1093/infdis/jit458.

Buchanan R, Bonthius DJ. Measles virus and associated central nervous system sequelae. *Semin Pediatr Neurol*. 2012;19(3):107–114. doi:10.1016/j.spen.2012.02.003.

Centers for Disease Control and Prevention. Notes from the field: acute hemorrhagic conjunctivitis outbreaks caused by coxsackievirus A24v—Uganda and southern Sudan, 2010. *MMWR Morb Mortal Wkly Rep*. 2010;59(32):1024.

Centers for Disease Control and Prevention. Rubella and congenital rubella syndrome control and elimination—global progress, 2000–2012. *MMWR Morb Mortal Wkly Rep*. 2013;62(48):983–986.

Cerna F, Mehrad B, Luby JP, et al. St. Louis encephalitis and the substantia nigra: MR imaging evaluation. *AJNR Am J Neuroradiol*. 1999;20(7):1281–1283.

Chopra JS, Banerjee AK, Murthy JM, et al. Paralytic rabies: a clinico-pathological study. *Brain*. 1980;103(4):789–802.

Chopra JS, Sawhney IM, Dhand UK, et al. Neurological complications of acute haemorrhagic conjunctivitis. *J Neurol Sci*. 1986;73(2):177–191.

Connolly AM, Dodson WE, Prensky AL, et al. Course and outcome of acute cerebellar ataxia. *Ann Neurol*. 1994;35(6):673–679. doi:10.1002/ana.410350607.

Conomy JP, Leibovitz A, McCombs W, et al. Airborne rabies encephalitis: demonstration of rabies virus in the human central nervous system. *Neurology*. 1977;27(1):67–69.

Cui A, Yu D, Zhu Z, et al. An outbreak of aseptic meningitis caused by coxsackievirus A9 in Gansu, the People's Republic of China. *Virol J*. 2010;7:72. doi:10.1186/1743-422X-7-72.

Dacheux L, Reynes JM, Buchy P, et al. A reliable diagnosis of human rabies based on analysis of skin biopsy specimens. *Clin Infect Dis*. 2008;47(11):1410–1417. doi:10.1086/592969.

Dalakas MC, Elder G, Hallett M, et al. A long-term follow-up study of patients with post-poliomyelitis neuromuscular symptoms. *N Engl J Med*. 1986;314(15):959–963. doi:10.1056/NEJM198604103141505.

Debiasi RL, Tyler KL. Molecular methods for diagnosis of viral encephalitis. *Clin Microbiol Rev*. 2004;17(4):903–925, table of contents. doi:10.1128/CMR.17.4.903-925.2004.

Demir N, Cokar O, Bolukbasi F, et al. A close look at EEG in subacute sclerosing panencephalitis. *J Clin Neurophysiol*. 2013;30(4):348–356. doi:10.1097/WNP.0b013e31829ddcb6.

Deresiewicz RL, Thaler SJ, Hsu L, et al. Clinical and neuroradiographic manifestations of eastern equine encephalitis. *N Engl J Med*. 1997;336(26):1867–1874. doi:10.1056/NEJM199706263362604.

Desmond MM, Wilson GS, Melnick JL, et al. Congenital rubella encephalitis. Course and early sequelae. *J Pediatr*. 1967;71(3):311–331.

Desmond RA, Accortt NA, Talley L, et al. Enteroviral meningitis: natural history and outcome of pleconaril therapy. *Antimicrob Agents Chemother*. 2006;50(7):2409–2414. doi:10.1128/AAC.00227-06.

Dittmar S, Harms H, Runkler N, et al. Measles virus-induced block of transendothelial migration of T lymphocytes and infection-mediated virus spread across endothelial cell barriers. *J Virol*. 2008;82(22):11273–11282. doi:10.1128/JVI.00775-08.

Domingues RB, Fink MC, Tsanaclis AM, et al. Diagnosis of herpes simplex encephalitis by magnetic resonance imaging and polymerase chain reaction assay of cerebrospinal fluid. *J Neurol Sci*. 1998;157(2):148–153.

Duckworth JL, Hawley JS, Riedy G, et al. Magnetic resonance restricted diffusion resolution correlates with clinical improvement and response to treatment in herpes simplex encephalitis. *Neurocrit Care*. 2005;3(3):251–253. doi:10.1385/NCC:3:3:251.

Dworkin RH, O'Connor AB, Kent J, et al; International Association for the Study of Pain Neuropathic Pain Special Interest Group. Interventional management of neuropathic pain: NeuPSIG recommendations. *Pain*. 2013;154(11):2249–2261. doi:10.1016/j.pain.2013.06.004.

Dyer JL, Wallace R, Orciari L, et al. Rabies surveillance in the United States during 2012. *J Am Vet Med Assoc*. 2013;243(6):805–815. doi:10.2460/javma.243.6.805.

Earnest MP, Goolishian HA, Calverley JR, et al. Neurologic, intellectual, and psychologic sequelae following western encephalitis. A follow-up study of 35 cases. *Neurology*. 1971;21(9):969–974.

Farazmand P, Woolley PD, Kinghorn GR. Mollaret's meningitis and herpes simplex virus type 2 infections. *Int J STD AIDS*. 2011;22(6):306–307.

Ferris BG Jr, Auld PA, Cronkhite L, et al. Life-threatening poliomyelitis, Boston, 1955. *N Engl J Med*. 1960;262:371–380. doi:10.1056/NEJM196002252620801.

Figueiredo CA, Klautau GB, Afonso AM, et al. Isolation and genotype analysis of rubella virus from a case of Guillain-Barre syndrome. *J Clin Virol*. 2008;43(3):343–345. doi:10.1016/j.jcv.2008.07.015.

Fooks AR, Banyard AC, Horton DL, et al. Current status of rabies and prospects for elimination. *Lancet*. 2014;384(9951):1389–1399. doi:10.1016/S0140-6736(13)62707-5.

Frederiks JAM, Bruyn GW. Mollaret's meningitis. In: Vinken PJ, Bruyn GW, Klawans HL, et al, eds. *Handbook of Clinical Neurology*. Vol. 56. New York: Elsevier Science Publishing; 1989:627–635.

Freeman AF, Jacobsohn DA, Shulman ST, et al. A new complication of stem cell transplantation: measles inclusion body encephalitis. *Pediatrics*. 2004;114(5):e657–e660. doi:10.1542/peds.2004-0949.

Frey TK. Neurological aspects of rubella virus infection. *Intervirology*. 1997;40(2–3):167–175.

Fu YC, Chi CS, Jan SL, et al. Pulmonary edema of enterovirus 71 encephalomyelitis is associated with left ventricular failure: implications for treatment. *Pediatr Pulmonol*. 203;35(4):263–268. doi:10.1002/ppul.10258.

Gilden D. Efficacy of live zoster vaccine in preventing zoster and postherpetic neuralgia. *J Intern Med*. 2011;269(5):496–506. doi:10.1111/j.1365-2796.2011.02359.x.

Gilden D. Varicella zoster virus and central nervous system syndromes. *Herpes*. 2004;11(suppl 2):89A–94A.

Gilden DH, Beinlich BR, Rubinstien EM, et al. Varicella-zoster virus myelitis: an expanding spectrum. *Neurology*. 1994;44(10):1818–1823.

Gilden DH, Kleinschmidt-DeMasters BK, LaGuardia JJ, et al. Neurologic complications of the reactivation of varicella-zoster virus. *N Engl J Med*. 2000;342(9):635–645. doi:10.1056/NEJM200003023420906.

Gnann JW Jr. Varicella-zoster virus: atypical presentations and unusual complications. *J Infect Dis*. 2002;186(suppl 1):S91–S98. doi:10.1086/342963.

Greenlee JE. The equine encephalitides. *Handb Clin Neurol*. 2014;123:417–432. doi:10.1016/B978-0-444-53488-0.00019-5.

Greer DM, Robbins GK, Lijewski V, et al. Case records of the Massachusetts General Hospital. Case 1-2013. A 63-year-old man with paresthesias and difficulty swallowing. *N Engl J Med*. 2013;368(2):172–180. doi:10.1056/NEJMcpc1209935.

Griffin DE, Ward BJ, Jauregui E, et al. Immune activation in measles. *N Engl J Med*. 1989;320(25):1667–1672. doi:10.1056/NEJM198906223202506.

Griffiths P. Cytomegalovirus infection of the central nervous system. *Herpes.* 2004;11(suppl 2):95A–104A.

Guess HA, Broughton DD, Melton LJ III, et al. Population-based studies of varicella complications. *Pediatrics.* 1986;78(4, pt 2):723–727.

Hall WW, Choppin PW. Measles-virus proteins in the brain tissue of patients with subacute sclerosing panencephalitis: absence of the M protein. *N Engl J Med.* 1981;304(19):1152–1155. doi:10.1056/NEJM198105073041906.

Hardie DR, Albertyn C, Heckmann JM, et al. Molecular characterisation of virus in the brains of patients with measles inclusion body encephalitis (MIBE). *Virol J.* 2013;10:283. doi:10.1186/1743-422X-10-283.

Hardy GE Jr, Hopkins CC, Linnemann CC Jr, et al. Trivalent oral poliovirus vaccine: a comparison of two infant immunization schedules. *Pediatrics.* 1970;45(3):444–448.

Hemachudha T, Ugolini G, Wacharapluesadee S, et al. Human rabies: neuropathogenesis, diagnosis, and management. *Lancet Neurol.* 2013;12(5):498–513. doi:10.1016/S1474-4422(13)70038-3.

Herrmann KL. Rubella in the United States: toward a strategy for disease control and elimination. *Epidemiol Infect.* 1991;107(1):55–61.

Herzon H, Shelton JT, Bruyn HB. Sequelae of western equine and other arthropod-borne encephalitides. *Neurology.* 1957;7(8):535–548.

Holland NR, Power C, Mathews VP, et al. Cytomegalovirus encephalitis in acquired immunodeficiency syndrome (AIDS). *Neurology.* 1994;44(3, pt 1):507–514.

Hopkins CC, Hollinger FB, Johnson RF, et al. The epidemiology of St. Louis encephalitis in Dallas, Texas, 1966. *Am J Epidemiol.* 1975;102(1):1–15.

Horstmann DM. Clinical aspects of acute poliomyelitis. *Am J Med.* 1949;6(5):592–605.

Houff SA, Sever JL. Slow virus diseases of the central nervous system. *Dis Mon.* 1985;31(8):1–71.

Jackson AC, Warrell MJ, Rupprecht CE, et al. Management of rabies in humans. *Clin Infect Dis.* 2003;36(1):60–63. doi:10.1086/344905.

Jensenius M, Myrvang B, Storvold G, et al. Herpes simplex virus type 2 DNA detected in cerebrospinal fluid of 9 patients with Mollaret's meningitis. *Acta Neurol Scand.* 1998;98:209–212.

Johnson RT, Griffin DE, Hirsch RL, et al. Measles encephalomyelitis—clinical and immunologic studies. *N Engl J Med.* 1984;310(3):137–141. doi:10.1056/NEJM198401193100301.

Jones LK Jr, Reda H, Watson JC. Clinical, electrophysiologic, and imaging features of zoster-associated limb paresis. *Muscle Nerve.* 2014;50(2):177–185. doi:10.1002/mus.24141.

Kang JH, Ho JD, Chen YH, et al. Increased risk of stroke after a herpes zoster attack: a population-based follow-up study. *Stroke.* 2009;40(11):3443–3448. doi:10.1161/STROKEAHA.109.562017.

Kawai K, Gebremeskel BG, Acosta CJ. Systematic review of incidence and complications of herpes zoster: towards a global perspective. *BMJ Open.* 2014;4(6):e004833. doi:10.1136/bmjopen-2014-004833.

Kimberlin DW. Advances in the treatment of neonatal herpes simplex infections. *Rev Med Virol.* 2001;11(3):157–163.

Kimberlin DW. Neonatal herpes simplex infection. *Clin Microbiol Rev.* 2004;17(1):1–13.

Kimberlin DW, Lakeman FD, Arvin AM, et al. Application of the polymerase chain reaction to the diagnosis and management of neonatal herpes simplex virus disease. National Institute of Allergy and Infectious Diseases Collaborative Antiviral Study Group. *J Infect Dis.* 1996;174(6):1162–1167.

Kimberlin DW, Lin CY, Jacobs RF, et al; Infectious Diseases Collaborative Antiviral Study Group. Natural history of neonatal herpes simplex virus infections in the acyclovir era. *Pediatrics.* 2001;108(2):223–229.

Kimberlin DW, Lin CY, Jacobs RF, et al; Infectious Diseases Collaborative Antiviral Study Group. Safety and efficacy of high-dose intravenous acyclovir in the management of neonatal herpes simplex virus infections. *Pediatrics.* 2001;108(2):230–238.

Klement C, Kissova R, Lengyelova V, et al. Human enterovirus surveillance in the Slovak Republic from 2001 to 2011. *Epidemiol Infect.* 2013;141(12):2658–2662. doi:10.1017/S0950268813000563.

Kupila L, Vuorinen T, Vainionpaa R, et al. Etiology of aseptic meningitis and encephalitis in an adult population. *Neurology.* 2006;66(1):75–80. doi:10.1212/01.wnl.0000191407.81333.00.

Langan SM, Minassian C, Smeeth L, et al. Risk of stroke following herpes zoster: a self-controlled case-series study. *Clin Infect Dis.* 2014;58(11):1497–1503. doi:10.1093/cid/ciu098.

Laothamatas J, Sungkarat W, Hemachudha T. Neuroimaging in rabies. *Adv Virus Res.* 2011;79:309–327. doi:10.1016/B978-0-12-387040-7.00014-7.

Mandell GL, Bennett, JE, Dolin R. *Mandell, Douglas, and Bennett's Principles and Practice of Infectious Diseases.* 7th ed. Philadelphia: Churchill Livingstone/Elsevier; 2010.

Mani J, Reddy BC, Borgohain R, et al. Magnetic resonance imaging in rabies. *Postgrad Med J.* 2003;79(932):352–354.

Mease PJ, Ochs HD, Wedgwood RJ. Successful treatment of echovirus meningoencephalitis and myositis-fasciitis with intravenous immune globulin therapy in a patient with X-linked agammaglobulinemia. *N Engl J Med.* 1981;304(21):1278–1281. doi:10.1056/NEJM198105213042107.

Miller E, Cradock-Watson JE, Pollock TM. Consequences of confirmed maternal rubella at successive stages of pregnancy. *Lancet.* 1982;2(8302):781–784.

Modlin JF, Dagan R, Berlin LE, et al. Focal encephalitis with enterovirus infections. *Pediatrics.* 1991;88(4):841–845.

Modlin JF, Jabbour JT, Witte JJ, et al. Epidemiologic studies of measles, measles vaccine, and subacute sclerosing panencephalitis. *Pediatrics.* 1977;59(4):505–512.

Mori Y, Miyamoto T, Nagafuji K, et al. High incidence of human herpesvirus 6-associated encephalitis/myelitis following a second unrelated cord blood transplantation. *Biol Blood Marrow Transplant.* 2010;16(11):1596–1602.

Moturi EK, Porter KA, Wassilak SG, et al. Progress toward polio eradication—worldwide, 2013-2014. *MMWR Morb Mortal Wkly Rep.* 2014;63(21):468–472.

Mulder DW, Parrott M, Thaler M. Sequelae of western equine encephalitis. *Neurology.* 1951;1(4):318–327.

Mustafa MM, Weitman SD, Winick NJ, et al. Subacute measles encephalitis in the young immunocompromised host: report of two cases diagnosed by polymerase chain reaction and treated with ribavirin and review of the literature. *Clin Infect Dis.* 1993;16(5):654–660.

Nagel MA, Gilden D. Complications of varicella zoster virus reactivation. *Curr Treat Options Neurol.* 2013;15(4):439–453. doi:10.1007/s11940-013-0246-5.

Nau R, Lantsch M, Stiefel M, et al. Varicella zoster virus-associated focal vasculitis without herpes zoster: recovery after treatment with acyclovir. *Neurology.* 1998;51(3):914–915.

Ohya T, Yamashita Y, Shibuya I, et al. A serial (18)FDG-PET study of a patient with SSPE who had good prognosis by combination therapy with interferon alpha and ribavirin. *Eur J Paediatr Neurol.* 2014;18(4):536–539. doi:10.1016/j.ejpn.2014.03.001.

Oldstone MB, Lewicki H, Thomas D, et al. Measles virus infection in a transgenic model: virus-induced immunosuppression and central nervous system disease. *Cell.* 1999;98(5):629–640.

Omland LH, Vestergaard BF, Wandall JH. Herpes simplex virus type 2 infections of the central nervous system: a retrospective study of 49 patients. *Scand J Infect Dis.* 2008;40(1):59–62.

O'Neil KM, Pallansch MA, Winkelstein JA, et al. Chronic group A coxsackievirus infection in agammaglobulinemia: demonstration of genomic variation of serotypically identical isolates persistently excreted by the same patient. *J Infect Dis.* 1988;157(1):183–186.

Pabbaraju K, Wong S, Chan EN, et al. Genetic characterization of a Coxsackie A9 virus associated with aseptic meningitis in Alberta, Canada in 2010. *Virol J.* 2013;10:93. doi:10.1186/1743-422X-10-93.

Pahud BA, Glaser CA, Dekker CL, et al. Varicella zoster disease of the central nervous system: epidemiological, clinical, and laboratory features 10 years after the introduction of the varicella vaccine. *J Infect Dis.* 2011;203(3):316–323. doi:10.1093/infdis/jiq066.

Peckham CS, Chin KS, Coleman JC, et al. Cytomegalovirus infection in pregnancy: preliminary findings from a prospective study. *Lancet.* 1983;1(8338):1352–1355.

Peters AC, Vielvoye GJ, Versteeg J, et al. ECHO 25 focal encephalitis and subacute hemichorea. *Neurology.* 1979;29(5):676–681.

Phuapradit P, Roongwithu N, Limsukon P, et al. Radiculomyelitis complicating acute haemorrhagic conjunctivitis. A clinical study. *J Neurol Sci.* 1976;27(1):117–122.

Pierelli F, Tilia G, Damiani A, et al. Brainstem CMV encephalitis in AIDS: clinical case and MRI features. *Neurology.* 1997;48(2):529–530.

Pottage JC Jr, Kessler HA. Herpes simplex virus resistance to acyclovir: clinical relevance. *Infect Agents Dis.* 1995;4(3):115–124.

Quartier P, Foray S, Casanova JL, et al. Enteroviral meningoencephalitis in X-linked agammaglobulinemia: intensive immunoglobulin therapy and sequential viral detection in cerebrospinal fluid by polymerase chain reaction. *Pediatr Infect Dis J.* 2000;19(11):1106–1108.

Rabenau HF, Buxbaum S, Preiser W, et al. Seroprevalence of herpes simplex virus types 1 and type 2 in the Frankfurt am Main area, Germany. *Med Microbiol Immunol.* 2002;190(4):153–160.

Reda H, Watson JC, Jones LK Jr. Zoster-associated mononeuropathies (ZAMs): a retrospective series. *Muscle Nerve.* 2012;45(5):734–739. doi:10.1002/mus.23342.

Reilly GS, Shin RK. Teaching NeuroImages: herpes zoster ophthalmicus-related oculomotor palsy accompanied by Hutchinson sign. *Neurology.* 2010;74(15):e65. doi:10.1212/WNL.0b013e3181d8c1f6.

Ren R, Racaniello VR. Poliovirus spreads from muscle to the central nervous system by neural pathways. *J Infect Dis.* 1992;166(4):747–752.

Reyes MG, Gardner JJ, Poland JD, et al. St Louis encephalitis. Quantitative histologic and immunofluorescent studies. *Arch Neurol.* 1981;38(6):329–334.

Roos RP, Graves MC, Wollmann RL, et al. Immunologic and virologic studies of measles inclusion body encephalitis in an immunosuppressed host: the relationship to subacute sclerosing panencephalitis. *Neurology.* 1981;31(10):1263–1270.

Rorabaugh ML, Berlin LE, Heldrich F, et al. Aseptic meningitis in infants younger than 2 years of age: acute illness and neurologic complications. *Pediatrics.* 1993;92(2):206–211.

Rotbart HA, Webster AD, Pleconaril Treatment Registry Group. Treatment of potentially life-threatening enterovirus infections with pleconaril. *Clin Infect Dis.* 2001;32(2):228–235. doi:10.1086/318452.

Sabin AB. Pathogenesis of poliomyelitis; reappraisal in the light of new data. *Science.* 1956;123(3209):1151–1157.

Sauerbrei A, Bohn K, Heim A, et al. Novel resistance-associated mutations of thymidine kinase and DNA polymerase genes of herpes simplex virus type 1 and type 2. *Antiviral Therapy.* 2011;16(8):1297–1308. doi:10.3851/IMP1870; 10.3851/IMP1870.

Schultz DR, Barthal JS, Garrett G. Western equine encephalitis with rapid onset of parkinsonism. *Neurology.* 1977;27(11):1095–1096.

Silverman MA, Misasi J, Smole S, et al. Eastern equine encephalitis in children, Massachusetts and New Hampshire, USA, 1970–2010. *Emerg Infect Dis.* 2013;19(2):194–201, quiz 352. doi:10.3201/eid1902.120039.

Spinsanti LI, Diaz LA, Glatstein N, et al. Human outbreak of St. Louis encephalitis detected in Argentina, 2005. *J Clin Virol.* 2008;42(1):27–33. doi:10.1016/j.jcv.2007.11.022.

Tan IL, McArthur JC, Venkatesan A, et al. Atypical manifestations and poor outcome of herpes simplex encephalitis in the immunocompromised. *Neurology.* 2012;79(21):2125–2132. doi:10.1212/WNL.0b013e3182752ceb.

Thomas SL, Minassian C, Ganesan V, et al. Chickenpox and risk of stroke: a self-controlled case series analysis. *Clin Infect Dis.* 2014;58(1):61–68. doi:10.1093/cid/cit659.

Tomoda A, Nomura K, Shiraishi S, et al. Trial of intraventricular ribavirin therapy for subacute sclerosing panencephalitis in Japan. *Brain Dev.* 2003;25(7):514–517.

Townsend CL, Forsgren M, Ahlfors K, et al. Long-term outcomes of congenital cytomegalovirus infection in Sweden and the United Kingdom. *Clin Infect Dis.* 2013;56(9):1232–1239. doi:10.1093/cid/cit018.

Townsend JJ, Baringer JR, Wolinsky JS, et al. Progressive rubella panencephalitis. Late onset after congenital rubella. *N Engl J Med.* 1975;292(19):990–993. doi:10.1056/NEJM197505082921902.

Townsend JJ, Stroop WG, Baringer JR, et al. Neuropathology of progressive rubella panencephalitis after childhood rubella. *Neurology.* 1982;32(2):185–190.

Tunkel AR, Glaser CA, Bloch KC, et al. The management of encephalitis: clinical practice guidelines by the Infectious Diseases Society of America. *Clin Infect Dis.* 2008;47(3):303–327. doi:10.1086/589747.

Turner KM, Lee HC, Boppana SB, et al. Incidence and impact of CMV infection in very low birth weight infants. *Pediatrics.* 2014;133(3):e609–e615. doi:10.1542/peds.2013-2217.

Tyler KL, McPhee DA. Molecular and genetic aspects of the pathogenesis of viral infections of the central nervous system. *Crit Rev Neurobiol.* 1987;3(3):221–243.

Wacharapluesadee S, Phumesin P, Supavonwong P, et al. Comparative detection of rabies RNA by NASBA, real-time PCR and conventional PCR. *J Virol Methods.* 2011;175(2):278–282. doi:10.1016/j.jviromet.2011.05.007.

Wadia NH, Katrak SM, Misra VP, et al. Polio-like motor paralysis associated with acute hemorrhagic conjunctivitis in an outbreak in 1981 in Bombay, India: clinical and serologic studies. *J Infect Dis.* 1983;147(4):660–668.

Wasay M, Diaz-Arrastia R, Suss RA, et al. St Louis encephalitis: a review of 11 cases in a 1995 Dallas, Tex, epidemic. *Arch Neurol.* 2000;57(1):114–118.

Weil ML, Itabashi H, Cremer NE, et al. Chronic progressive panencephalitis due to rubella virus simulating subacute sclerosing panencephalitis. *N Engl J Med.* 1975;292(19):994–998. doi:10.1056/NEJM197505082921903.

Weinstein L, Shelokov A, Seltser R, et al. A comparison of the clinical features of poliomyelitis in adults and in children. *N Engl J Med.* 1952;246(8):297–302.

Whitley RJ, Alford CA, Hirsch MS, et al. Vidarabine versus acyclovir therapy in herpes simplex encephalitis. *N Engl J Med.* 1986;314(3):144–149. doi:10.1056/NEJM198601163140303.

Whitley R, Arvin A, Prober C, et al. A controlled trial comparing vidarabine with acyclovir in neonatal herpes simplex virus infection. Infectious Diseases Collaborative Antiviral Study Group. *N Engl J Med.* 1991;324(7):444–449. doi:10.1056/NEJM199102143240703.

Whitley R, Arvin A, Prober C, et al. Predictors of morbidity and mortality in neonates with herpes simplex virus infections. The National Institute of Allergy and Infectious Diseases Collaborative Antiviral Study Group. *N Engl J Med.* 1991;324(7):450–454. doi:10.1056/NEJM199102143240704.

Williams KH, Hollinger FB, Metzger WR, et al. The epidemiology of St. Louis encephalitis in Corpus Christi, Texas, 1966. *Am J Epidemiol.* 1975;102(1):16–24.

Willoughby RE Jr, Tieves KS, Hoffman GM, et al. Survival after treatment of rabies with induction of coma. *N Engl J Med.* 2005;352(24):2508–2514. doi:10.1056/NEJMoa050382.

Winkler WG, Fashinell TR, Leffingwell L, et al. Airborne rabies transmission in a laboratory worker. *JAMA.* 1973;226(10):1219–1221.

Wolinsky JS, Waxham MN, Hess JL, et al. Immunochemical features of a case of progressive rubella panencephalitis. *Clin Exp Immunol.* 1982;48(2):359–366.

Wood MJ, Johnson RW, McKendrick MW, et al. A randomized trial of acyclovir for 7 days or 21 days with and without prednisolone for treatment of acute herpes zoster. *N Engl J Med.* 1994;330(13):896–900. doi:10.1056/NEJM199403313301304.

Yamashita Y, Matsuishi T, Murakami Y, et al. Neuroimaging findings (ultrasonography, CT, MRI) in 3 infants with congenital rubella syndrome. *Pediatr Radiol.* 1991;21(8):547–549.

Yan JJ, Wang JR, Liu CC, et al. An outbreak of enterovirus 71 infection in Taiwan 1998: a comprehensive pathological, virological, and molecular study on a case of fulminant encephalitis. *J Clin Virol.* 20;17(1):13–22.

Yawn BP, Saddier P, Wollan PC, et al. A population-based study of the incidence and complication rates of herpes zoster before zoster vaccine introduction. *Mayo Clin Proc.* 2007;82(11):1341–1349.

Kiran Thakur, Ned Sacktor, Carolyn Barley Britton,
and Barbara S. Koppel

INTRODUCTION

Acquired immunodeficiency syndrome (AIDS) is the most devastating pandemic of the 20th and early 21st centuries. It was first recognized in 1981 through a growing number of reports of rare opportunistic infections, including *Pneumocystis carinii* pneumonia (PCP), and malignancies, such as Kaposi sarcoma, occurring in previously healthy gay men. Similar cases were discovered in intravenous (IV) drug users, and in 1982, the Centers for Disease Control and Prevention (CDC) proposed epidemiologic surveillance criteria. In 1983, human immunodeficiency virus (HIV) type 1 was isolated from human peripheral blood lymphocytes, and shortly thereafter, this retrovirus was established as the cause of AIDS. As the worldwide magnitude of the HIV pandemic became clear, the pace of research grew. The virus was sequenced and its structure elucidated by x-ray crystallography. The life cycle of the HIV, with the discovery of binding to the CD4 glycoprotein receptor, leading to the immune dysregulation was discovered soon after initial viral identification. Further understanding of the mechanisms of human infection and pathogenesis and development of successful drug therapies occurred. Central nervous system (CNS) complications due to infection by HIV-1 were first described early in the epidemic, when severe neurocognitive disease attributable to the virus was common in individuals with profound immunodeficiency.

CLASSIFICATION OF HIV DISEASE

In 1986, the CDC proposed staging criteria for HIV infection. These were modified in 1987 to include HIV-associated dementia and myelopathy among the 23 AIDS-defining illnesses. Revisions, in 1993, added three laboratory categories that are stratified by CD4 cell numbers and three clinical categories (Table 67.1).

AIDS-defining illnesses were expanded to include positive HIV serology and pulmonary tuberculosis (TB), recurrent bacterial pneumonia, invasive cervical carcinoma, or a CD4 lymphocyte count less than 200 cells/mm³. These revisions define the end stage of HIV infection and clarify the relationship of specific clinical syndromes, especially those affecting the nervous system that are not themselves diagnostic of AIDS, to advanced immunosuppression. In contrast to the CDC system, the World Health Organization (WHO) Clinical Staging and Disease Classification System revised in 2006 can be used readily in resource-constrained settings without access to CD4 cell count measurements or other diagnostic and laboratory testing methods (Table 67.2).

The WHO system classified HIV disease on the basis of clinical manifestations that can be recognized and treated by clinicians in diverse settings and by clinicians with varying levels of HIV expertise and training. This classification system guides medical management of HIV-infected persons. CD4 lymphocyte count levels and viral load assays have mostly supplanted staging criteria for decisions about antiretroviral therapy. Staging is still useful for prognosis and decisions about opportunistic infection prophylaxis and identifying patients most at risk for opportunistic infections and malignancy.

EPIDEMIOLOGY

HIV infection is still an enduring pandemic affecting virtually all population groups and countries. According to the 2013 UNAIDS report, in 2012, there were 35 million people worldwide living with HIV infection. Among these HIV-positive individuals, 25 million (71%) are living in sub-Saharan Africa and 1.3 million live in North America. HIV-2 is restricted to West Africa and those countries with historical and socioeconomic ties to the region and commonly co-occurs with HIV-1. Retrospective analysis of banked blood showed that HIV was present in the United States in the 1970s. In 2013, the CDC estimated the prevalence of HIV/AIDS at 1.1 million Americans (Table 67.3). Estimates were that 16% of infected individuals were unaware of their HIV status. Cumulative deaths due to AIDS totaled 636,000, with 15,529 deaths in 2010.

In 2000, AIDS became the leading cause of death among African-American men aged 35 to 44 years and women aged 25 to 34 years. The disproportionate representation of African-American and Hispanic men is related to IV drug use: African-Americans represent approximately 12% of the U.S. population

TABLE 67.1	1992 Centers for Disease Control and Prevention Classification of HIV Infection
Laboratory Categories	
Category 1—CD4 lymphocyte count >500 cells/mm³	
Category 2—CD4 lymphocyte count from 200 through 499 cells/mm³	
Category 3—CD4 lymphocyte count <200 cells/mm³	
Clinical Categories	
Category A—asymptomatic infection, persistent generalized lymphadenopathy, and acute primary HIV infection	
Category B—symptomatic conditions not included in the CDC 1987 surveillance case definition of AIDS that are judged by a physician to be HIV related or where medical management is complicated by HIV infection (e.g., sepsis, bacterial endocarditis, pulmonary TB, cervical dysplasia or carcinoma, vulvovaginal candidiasis)	
Category C—any of the 23 conditions listed in CDC 1987 case definition for AIDS	

CDC, Centers for Disease Control and Prevention; TB, tuberculosis.
Adapted from United States Congress, Office of Technology Assessment. *The CDC's Case Definition of AIDS: Implications of the Proposed Revisions- Background Paper.* Washington, DC: US Government Printing Office; 1992.

TABLE 67.2	World Health Organization Clinical Staging of Established HIV Infection	
HIV-Associated Symptoms	**WHO Clinical Stage**	
Asymptomatic	1	
Mild symptoms	2	
Advanced symptoms	3	
Severe symptoms	4	

Adapted from World Health Organization. *WHO Case Definitions of HIV for Surveillance and Revised Clinical Staging and Immunological Classification of HIV-Related Disease in Adults and Children*; 2007.

but accounted for an estimated 44% of new HIV infections in 2009. African-Americans also accounted for 44% of individuals living with HIV infection in 2009. Hispanic/Latinos represent 16% of the U.S. population but accounted for 19% of individuals living with HIV infection in 2009. Although affected by drug use, unprotected heterosexual activity has become the predominant transmission risk for minority women. There has also been a significant increase in the incidence of HIV infection among the elderly. By 2015, it is anticipated that 50% of HIV-seropositive individuals will be older than age 50 years.

The introduction of combination antiretroviral therapy (cART) in 1996 profoundly changed HIV/AIDS epidemiology in the United States and other resource-rich countries. Since the introduction of cART, there has been a 38% decline in incident AIDS cases and a 67% decline in deaths from AIDS in the United States. Progress in

TABLE 67.3	Epidemiology of HIV/AIDS: United States and Global Data: 2012 and 2013	
United States—through 2012		
Adults/adolescents	1,144,500	
Pediatric (<13 yr)	10,834	
Total	1,155,334	
Demographics (Adult)		
Race		
African-American	44%	
Non-Hispanic white	34%	
Hispanic	21%	
Gender		
Men	75%	
Women	25%	
Global—2008		
Total cases through 2012	35,300,000	
Sub-Saharan Africa	25,500,000	
South and Southeast Asia	3,900,000	
Number of new HIV infections in 2007	2,300,000	
Deaths due to AIDS in 2012	1,600,000	
Children with AIDS (<15 yr) in 2012	3,300,000	

Adapted from Centers for Disease Control and Prevention. www.cdc.gov. 2013; 2013 World Health Statistics. World Health Organization. www.who.int.

some developing countries remains hampered by limited access to formal cART programs. Through the U.S. President's Emergency Plan for AIDS Relief (PEPFAR), UNAIDS, the WHO, as well as nongovernmental organizations and local ministries of health, there has been an increase in formal cART programs in many developing regions, with the hopes of disease stabilization in the next 5 to 10 years.

The major routes of HIV transmission include sexual contact, mother-to-child, injection drug use with contaminated needles, and exposure to infected blood or blood products, with sexual transmission being the most common route of exposure worldwide. Worldwide, heterosexual activity is the most common mode of transmission. In the United States, homosexual activity is the most common risk behavior (45%) followed by high-risk heterosexual behavior (27%) and injection drug use (22%). The fastest-growing populations with AIDS in the United States are women (who account for 26% of cases), African-American and Hispanic minorities, and IV drug users.

Recipients of blood products or clotting factor for hemophilia, or other coagulation/blood disorders, account for less than 1% of adult AIDS cases. In the United States, routine testing of blood products has largely eliminated this source of infection. Occupational exposure with validated transmission and seroconversion is well documented but rare. Most percutaneous or mucocutaneous exposures have been to blood or bloody fluid. Prospective studies of known exposures estimate the average risk for HIV transmission following percutaneous exposure ("needlestick") to be approximately 0.3% and after mucous membrane exposure, 0.09%.

AIDS IN CHILDREN

This topic is discussed more fully in Chapter 147. By the end of 2012, nearly 4,500 children in North America younger than the age of 15 years were living with HIV infection. Most children are infected perinatally. Since 1992, perinatal transmission in the United States has declined sharply, from a peak of 1,000 to 2,000 cases annually to only 38 cases in 2006 resulting from successful implementation of CDC guidelines for maternal counseling, testing, and antiretroviral treatment.

Worldwide, however, perinatal transmission continues to post a large burden on worldwide incidence of HIV infection. There are an estimated 3.3 million HIV infections in children in 2012, with 260,000 new infections in 2012. Among these new infections in children, 88% of them are in sub-Saharan Africa. Perinatal infection of children depends on maternal viral load and the stage of pregnancy during which the infection is acquired. After delivery, a substantial number of children return to seronegative status.

Hallmarks of early infection include developmental delay and cognitive dysfunction, loss of previously acquired milestones, and vasculopathy that can cause stroke or hemorrhage. In Africa, some studies show no difference in neuropsychological measures and school success in HIV-positive children compared with HIV-negative controls who have similar nutritional and socioeconomic status. However, a mortality rate of 61% by age 4 years for very ill children must qualify such a comparison.

ETIOLOGY

HIV is an enveloped RNA lentivirus. It contains an RNA-dependent DNA polymerase (reverse transcriptase) that produces a provirus capable of integrating into host cell DNA. In the target cell, the virus exists in both free and integrated states.

Human HIV infection is considered a cross-species (zoonotic) infection, arising from monkeys infected with simian immunodeficiency virus (SIV) through multiple independent transmissions. Of the two recognized viral species, HIV-1 is found worldwide and is more prevalent, whereas HIV-2 is found in Western Africa and in Europe among African immigrants and their sexual partners. Sporadic cases of HIV-2 occur in the United States, but they are rare in comparison to HIV-1. A variety of evidence suggests that the AIDS pandemic most likely originated in equatorial Western Africa. HIV-1 is characterized by extensive genetic diversity and can be divided into three classes: group M (major), group O (outlier), and group N (new, non-M, and non-O). Group M is responsible for 90% of cases of HIV infection globally and is represented by nine major subtypes or clades. The HIV-1 subtypes in the United States and Europe differ from the subtypes seen elsewhere in the world. In the United States and Europe, clade B is the predominant subtype, whereas in sub-Saharan Africa, clades A, C, and D are predominant subtypes.

PATHOBIOLOGY

The primary infectious event includes breach of a mucosal barrier, enhancing viral entry. Viremia drives infection and massive depletion of CD4 T cells, particularly in the gut-associated lymphoid tissue (GALT). The immune reaction to the virus causes activation of CD8 T cells and virus-specific antibody production, which in turn promotes rebound of CD4 T cells and slowed viral replication, although importantly the mucosal lymph system does not recover to its preinfective condition. Progression of HIV is caused in part by this constant immune activation that detrimentally affects the immune system through a combination of direct loss of infected CD4 T lymphocytes and bystander cell killing. Infection of CD4 lymphocytes by HIV, mediated by viral attachment to the cell surface CD4 receptor, leads to cell death. In humans, the CD4 receptor is expressed on several cell types, including neurons and glia in the brain, but there is no evidence of viral replication in cells other than lymphocytes, macrophages, monocytes, and their derivatives. In 1996, a chemokine receptor was identified as a coreceptor that is necessary for viral entry into cells. In acute and early HIV infection, an M-tropic viral strain that prefers to replicate in macrophages with the chemokine receptor CCR5 predominates (R5 strain). In advanced infection, a T-tropic viral strain that prefers T cells with the chemokine receptor CXCR4 evolves and becomes predominant (X4 virus). Genetic variation in the chemokine receptor may affect susceptibility to HIV infection. Relative resistance to infection is observed in individuals who are homozygous for a 32 base-pair deletion in CCR5. Progression rates in AIDS may be affected by changes in the presentation of viral epitopes by infected cells to cytotoxic T lymphocytes. Accelerated progression to AIDS is associated with a single amino acid substitution in the HLA-B35 allele (HLA-B*35-Px). However, the predictive value of observations about the effect of HLA polymorphisms on disease progression might be restricted to specific populations. Primary HIV infection can be asymptomatic or, in 50% to 70% of the cases, results in an acute, self-limited mononucleosis-like illness with fever, headache, myalgia, malaise, lethargy, sore throat, lymphadenopathy, and maculopapular rash. Painful ulceration of the buccal mucosa may impede swallowing (odynophagia).

Acute infection is characterized by viremia, high viral replication rates (up to 1 million RNA molecules per milliliter), viral isolation from peripheral blood lymphocytes, and high serum levels of a viral-core antigen, p24. Cytotoxic lymphocytes and soluble factors from CD8 lymphocytes are effective in reducing viral load to a set point that differs for each individual. Despite the effective early immune response, there is almost simultaneous immune dysfunction. Neutralizing antibodies, initially immunoglobulin (Ig) M and later IgG, appear in 2 to 6 weeks, resulting in clearance of viremia and a decrease in serum p24 levels. Rarely, antibodies do not appear for several months or, exceptionally, not at all.

Adverse immunologic effects occur early and are more severe in symptomatic persons. An early absolute lymphopenia affects both CD4 helper and CD8 suppressor cells with lymphocyte hyporesponsiveness to mitogens and antigens and thrombocytopenia. Lymphocytosis, especially of CD8 lymphocytes, usually follows with inversion of the CD4/CD8 ratio. Atypical lymphocytes are sometimes seen. Early changes in the CD4/CD8 ratio are usually transient, but reversion to more normal values is accompanied by persistent functional abnormalities. Cutaneous anergy is a direct result of the viral effects on CD4 cells.

After acute infection and seroconversion, clinical latency may last several years before onset of symptoms due to development of secondary infection, malignancy, or neurologic disease. There is no biologic latency, however. HIV infection is a chronic, persistent infection of variable viral replication rate.

The viral load set point after acute infection correlates with rate of progression to symptomatic infection or AIDS. Several proprietary assays provide quantitative measurement of plasma HIV RNA. The branched (b)DNA assay detects as few as 20 to 50 copies per milliliter. Recognition of acute infection is important because early antiretroviral treatment may prevent extensive seeding of lymphoid tissues or even eliminate infection. Without treatment, viral replication is robust and even in the absence of a decline in CD4 count may cause cardiovascular disease, nephropathy, and non–AIDS-related cancers.

It is estimated that 10 billion virions enter the plasma daily in untreated people. Virus is found mainly in tissues, not plasma; total lymphoid viral burden is three times that of plasma, the majority in follicular dendritic cells within germinal centers, where virus is passively adherent. The total body viral load is 100 billion HIV RNA copies. Approximately 10% of latently infected cells contain replication-competent provirus. Cellular destruction of lymphoid tissue is mediated by direct HIV-cytopathic effects, autoimmunity, and other mechanisms. Eventually, the lymphoid system is overwhelmed by the viral burden, which increases with advancing disease and culminates in AIDS.

Other factors that may augment HIV replication and the onset of symptoms include the following: the biologic variability of HIV and the appearance of increasingly virulent strains; host immunogenetics; and interactions with concomitant infection by cytomegalovirus (CMV), herpes simplex virus, hepatitis B and C viruses, human herpesvirus (HHV)-6, and human T-lymphotropic virus type 1 (HTLV-1) that upregulate expression of HIV and cell-killing ability by cytokines. Cytokines and chemokines are released by immune cells in response to infection and may upregulate or downregulate viral replication.

Other immunologic abnormalities in AIDS are caused by effects of HIV on B cells or macrophages, which result in hypergammaglobulinemia, impaired antibody responses to new antigens (including encapsulated bacteria), and increased levels of immune complexes. Antibodies to platelets may cause thrombocytopenia.

cART and specific prophylaxis have reduced the incidence of AIDS-related opportunistic infections and neoplasms in the United

States and other countries where treatment is readily available. cART refers to the use of three or more antiretroviral drugs from two antiretroviral drug classes. The major classes of antiretroviral drugs include nucleotide reverse transcriptase inhibitors, nonnucleotide reverse transcriptase inhibitors, protease inhibitors, integrase inhibitors, entry inhibitors, and fusion inhibitors. These antiretroviral drug classes interfere with different stages of HIV replication. The types of infections or neoplasms that complicate HIV infection have not changed and are similar worldwide, with varying frequencies depending on local factors. In untreated HIV infection, PCP is the most common opportunistic pathogen. Other opportunistic infections are often multiple and include fungal, viral, bacterial, and parasitic organisms. Many of these infections involve the CNS, usually secondarily but sometimes as the primary infection. For example, the papovavirus that causes progressive multifocal leukoencephalopathy causes a primary brain infection. Infections that are common in developing countries, such as trypanosomiasis, cysticercosis, and malaria, are sometimes seen in recent immigrants to the United States. Hepatitis B and C infections are important comorbid conditions, especially among those who acquire HIV from injection drug use. Kaposi sarcoma (an AIDS defining erythematous macular or nodular patch typically involving the face, oral mucosa, or upper trunk), Hodgkin and non-Hodgkin lymphoma, and cervical cancer, the most commonly encountered neoplasms related to immunosuppression, have become very rare in the setting of effective antiretroviral treatment. Non–AIDS-defining malignancies are now more common in treated populations, including anal cancer, lung cancer, liver cancer, and cancers of the head and neck. With the use of cART, HIV-positive individuals live significantly longer, and indeed more than 75% of HIV-positive individuals older than 50 years of age now die from non–HIV-related causes.

CENTRAL NERVOUS SYSTEM PATHOGENESIS

HIV enters the CNS at the time of primary infection and can result in no apparent disease, in acute self-limited syndromes, or in chronic disorders. Neurologic disorders are found in up to 70% of patients in clinical series, and more than 80% of autopsy series, of AIDS patients. In 10% to 20% of patients, the neurologic disorder is the first manifestation of AIDS. Uncommonly, a neurologic disorder is the sole evidence of chronic HIV infection and the cause of death. A high prevalence of neurologic disorders is observed in all populations studied, including those in sub-Saharan Africa and Asian regions bordering the Pacific Ocean. Despite the reduction in incidence of primary HIV-related syndromes, autopsy series of cART-treated patients who died of AIDS or unrelated causes show abnormalities in most brains, which in some cases were the cause of death. Cognitive impairment or HIV-associated neurocognitive disorder (HAND) is the most important HIV-related clinical syndrome.

Evidence of early CNS invasion includes isolation of virus from cerebrospinal fluid (CSF) or neural tissue (brain, spinal cord, peripheral nerve) and intrathecal production of antibodies to HIV. How HIV enters the CNS is not known. Possible mechanisms include intracellular transport across the blood–brain barrier within infected macrophages, as free-virus seeding of the leptomeninges, or as free virus after replication within the choroid plexus or vascular epithelium. In vitro studies using a proteomic platform suggest that HIV-1-infected monocyte-derived macrophages upregulate a large number of human brain microvascular endothelial cells, causing blood–brain barrier dysfunction that facilitates the development of CNS disease. Chemokines seem to play an important

role in enhanced transmigration of HIV-infected lymphocytes across the blood–brain barrier. In vitro studies show enhanced HIV-infected leukocyte transmigration in response to the chemokine CCL2 (monocyte chemoattractant protein [MCP]-1) with disruption of the blood–brain barrier, enhanced permeability, reduction of tight junction proteins, and expression of the matrix metalloproteinases MMP-2 and MMP-9. In the brain, viral infection is detected only in microglial cells or macrophages by in situ hybridization techniques; it is not found in neurons or glial cells, even though these cells have CD4 and chemokine receptors.

The high frequency of neurologic disorders in HIV infection has led to the designation of HIV as a *neurotropic virus*. The term *neurotropic* implies selective vulnerability and targeting of brain by the virus. Alternatively, the high frequency of neurologic disorders may be explained by the chronicity of infection, which results in continued seeding of the CNS and chronic immune activation. Specific neurotropism is not needed for continued accrual of neurologic damage. It has been difficult to establish correlation of neurologic syndromes with productive viral replication in the affected tissue. There is, however, an increase in the viral burden or viral load with advancing disease that parallels dementia and other neurologic syndromes. The mechanism of neurologic injury is believed to be indirect. Potential mechanisms include immune-mediated indirect injury; restricted persistent cellular infection; cellular injury due to cytokines released by infected monocytes and macrophages; excitotoxic amino acid injury; voltage-mediated increase of intracellular calcium; free radical damage; potentiation of inflammatory damage by chemokines and lipid inflammatory mediators (arachidonic acid and platelet-activating factor); direct cellular toxicity of HIV gene products, such as the envelope gp120, tat, and gp41; and cross-reacting antibody to an HIV glycoprotein binding a cell membrane epitope, resulting in cell receptor blockade. Studies show the involvement of double-stranded RNA-activated protein kinase in apoptotic neuronal death due to HIV-gp120. This enzyme is elevated in brain tissue of patients with HIV dementia. More than one mechanism may be important. Genetic changes in the virus in the host may result in noncytopathic CNS virus with enhanced replicative capacity in monocytes and macrophages, leading to a greater viral burden in the CNS than is apparent in the periphery. Phenotypic and viral load discordance is documented in several studies of plasma and CSF.

This compartmentalization of virus may explain the occurrence of neurologic syndromes when peripheral viral replication appears to be well controlled.

CLINICAL MANIFESTATIONS

HIV-RELATED SYNDROMES

Neurologic disorders may occur at any stage from seroconversion to AIDS. Dementia and myelopathy are diagnostic of AIDS even without opportunistic infections; neuropathy is the most common direct HIV-related neurologic disease. All levels of the neuraxis may be affected, including multisystem disorders. Neurologic disorders are likely to be transient in early HIV infection, but they become progressive or chronic with persistent infection and worsening immunosuppression.

The neurologic syndromes in early HIV infection are indistinguishable from disorders that occur with infection by other viruses (Table 67.4). These include aseptic meningitis, reversible encephalopathy, leukoencephalitis, seizures, transverse myelitis, cranial and peripheral neuropathy (Bell palsy, Guillain–Barré

TABLE 67.4	Primary HIV-Related Neurologic Syndromes: Acute Infection
Acute aseptic meningitis	
Acute encephalopathy	
Leukoencephalitis	
Seizures, generalized or focal	
Transverse myelitis	
Cranial and peripheral neuropathies	
Bell palsy	
Acute inflammatory demyelinating polyneuropathy of the Guillain–Barré type	
Polymyositis	
Myoglobinuria	

TABLE 67.5	Primary HIV-Related Neurologic Syndromes: Chronic Infection
Persistent or recurrent meningeal pleocytosis with or without meningeal symptoms	
Diffuse and focal cerebral syndromes	
Dementia, static or progressive with or without motor signs	
Mild cognitive impairment, neuropsychological test criteria only	
Organic psychiatric disorder	
Cerebrovascular syndromes	
Cerebellar ataxia	
Seizure disorder	
Multisystem degeneration	
Chronic progressive myelopathy	
Cranial and peripheral neuropathies	
Bell palsy	
Hearing loss	
Phrenic nerve paralysis	
Lateral femoral cutaneous nerve	
Chronic inflammatory demyelinating polyneuropathy	
Distal symmetric sensory neuropathy	
Mononeuritis multiplex	
Autonomic neuropathy	
Myopathy	

syndrome), polymyositis, and myoglobinuria. Brachial neuritis and ganglioneuritis have been reported only rarely. The course is typically self-limited, and patients often experience full neurologic recovery. A recent study from the Multicenter AIDS Cohort Study suggests that older HIV-positive individuals in the cART era experience a higher incidence of neurologic disease compared to age-matched HIV-negative individuals. In addition, HIV-positive individuals experience neurologic diagnoses at an earlier age compared to HIV-negative individuals. Excess neurologic disease was found in the categories of nervous system infections, dementia, seizures/epilepsy, and peripheral nervous system disorders in this study.

CSF abnormalities (pleocytosis up to 200 cells/mm^3 and oligoclonal bands) differentiate HIV syndromes from postinfectious disorders. Tests for HIV antibody may be negative because these syndromes may precede or accompany seroconversion, and the tests must be repeated in several weeks. If acute HIV infection is strongly suspected, p24 antigen and viral load assay should be considered if serology is negative. Hepatitis B and hepatitis C serology should be determined in all HIV-seropositive patients. Early antiretroviral therapy may be offered to decrease the high viral load typical of acute infection quickly, thereby lowering the viral load set point. No specific treatment is indicated for these self-limited disorders except that plasmapheresis or immunoglobulin is used in cases of Guillain–Barré syndrome and steroids for polymyositis.

In chronic HIV infection, neurologic disorders may accompany systemic HIV disease or secondary disorders (Table 67.5).

Chronic or recurrent CSF pleocytosis sometimes occurs with meningeal symptoms but is often asymptomatic. Chronic pleocytosis does not predict any specific neurologic complication. Ascribing CSF pleocytosis to HIV infection requires exclusion of secondary pathogens or tumor. In a cross-sectional study, HIV-related CSF pleocytosis was uncommon in individuals with blood CD4 counts below 50 cells/µL or in those on effective antiretroviral therapy.

HIV-Associated Neurocognitive Disorder

Cognitive impairment is a well-recognized complication of chronic HIV infection in all populations; it can range from mild to severe (Table 67.6). Its prevalence may be underestimated in resource-limited settings. Despite some success, there are enormous challenges to developing special dementia scales for use in resource-limited settings, including multiple languages, regional dialects, and low formal education rates. The International HIV Dementia Scale is a brief screening test that can be performed by

nonneurologists and has been validated as a potential screening test for dementia in HIV-positive individuals in resource-limited settings. There are several scales for classification of HIV cognitive impairment, including revision of the AIDS Task Force of the American Academy of Neurology (AAN) criteria.

Minor motor signs, usually motor slowness or tremor, may be present. HIV-associated dementia, known variously as *HIV-1–associated dementia complex*, *HIV dementia*, or *AIDS dementia complex*, is diagnostic of AIDS. Older designations are subacute encephalitis, subacute encephalopathy, or HIV encephalitis. HIV dementia refers to HIV-positive individuals with moderate to severe cognitive impairment on neuropsychological testing and marked difficulties in activities of daily living due to the cognitive impairment. In the pre-cART era, HIV dementia, the most severe stage of HAND, was a common stage of cognitive impairment among HIV-positive individuals with advanced immunosuppression. In HIV-positive individuals on cART, HIV dementia is rarely seen, and less severe stages of HAND such as HIV-associated mild

TABLE 67.6	HIV-1–Associated Neurocognitive Disorder
Severe Manifestations	
HIV-1–associated dementia	
Mild Manifestations	
HIV-1–associated mild neurocognitive disorder	
Asymptomatic neuropsychological impairment	

neurocognitive disorder (MND) are the most common clinically recognized stage of cognitive impairment. HAND including all three stages (asymptomatic neuropsychological impairment [ANI], MND, and HIV dementia) may be seen in 40% to 50% of HIV-positive individuals with advanced infection in some studies, with ANI and MND being the most common stages. Peripheral neuropathy coexists in 25% of patients.

HIV dementia in the absence of cART is an insidiously progressive subcortical dementia. Early symptoms include apathy, social withdrawal, diminished libido, slow thinking, poor concentration, and forgetfulness. Psychiatric syndromes, such as psychosis, depression, or mania, are sometimes profound and may be the first manifestation of HIV infection. Motor signs include slow movements, tremor, parkinsonian features, leg weakness, and gait ataxia. There may also be headaches, seizures, or frontal release signs. Although the disorder is usually progressive in HIV-positive individuals not on cART, some patients on cART develop a static level of disability, and others may improve in response to medical treatment for HIV or complicating disorders. When progressive, the disease culminates in akinetic mutism, an immobile bedridden state with global cognitive impairment and urinary incontinence.

In children, there may be a similar static or progressive encephalopathy. Most affected children meet criteria for AIDS, but progressive encephalopathy can occur before immunologic dysfunction is severe. Neurologic findings include intellectual deterioration, microcephaly, loss of developmental milestones, and progressive motor impairment that may culminate in spastic quadriparesis and pseudobulbar palsy. Seizures are usually due to fever. Myoclonus and extrapyramidal rigidity are rare.

The CSF is usually normal or shows mild pleocytosis, protein elevation, and oligoclonal bands. Virus can be cultured from CSF. In HIV-positive individuals not on cART, both CSF and plasma viral load correlate with occurrence of dementia but may be discordant in some cases where CSF load is greater than plasma. In HIV-positive individuals on cART, CSF and plasma viral load do not correlate with HAND stage. CSF markers of immune activation, HIV p24 antigen, β_2-microglobulin, tumor necrosis factor, and antimyelin basic protein in cART-treated HIV-positive individuals do not correlate with severity of dementia. None of these markers is predictive of, or specific for, dementia. CSF and serum markers such as neopterin and tryptophan levels and CSF serotonin metabolites and quinolinic acid levels lack predictive value or specificity but can correlate with severity of dementia. Elevated levels of CSF neurofilament protein, a marker of axonal injury, are found in HIV-infected patients with dementia. Levels decline in individuals who have a clinical response to antiretroviral therapy, suggesting its possible use as an indicator of drug efficacy. Efforts to identify markers for progression to dementia have been disappointing. A recent study suggested that increased levels of sphingomyelin and ceramide and the accumulation of lipid peroxidation products are associated with declining cognitive status. Further studies are needed to confirm these findings.

In adults, computed tomography (CT) or magnetic resonance imaging (MRI) scans show cortical atrophy and ventricular dilatation, sometimes with white matter changes. On CT, there is attenuation of white matter; MRI shows hyperintense white matter lesions on T2-weighted and proton density sequences ranging from discrete foci to large confluent periventricular lesions (Fig. 67.1).

CT in children shows basal ganglia calcification and cerebral atrophy. MRI white matter changes may not correlate with dementia and may disappear spontaneously or with antiretroviral therapy.

Abnormalities in functional neuroimaging are detected in HIV-infected individuals whether they have dementia or not. The abnormalities become worse or change with progressive cognitive

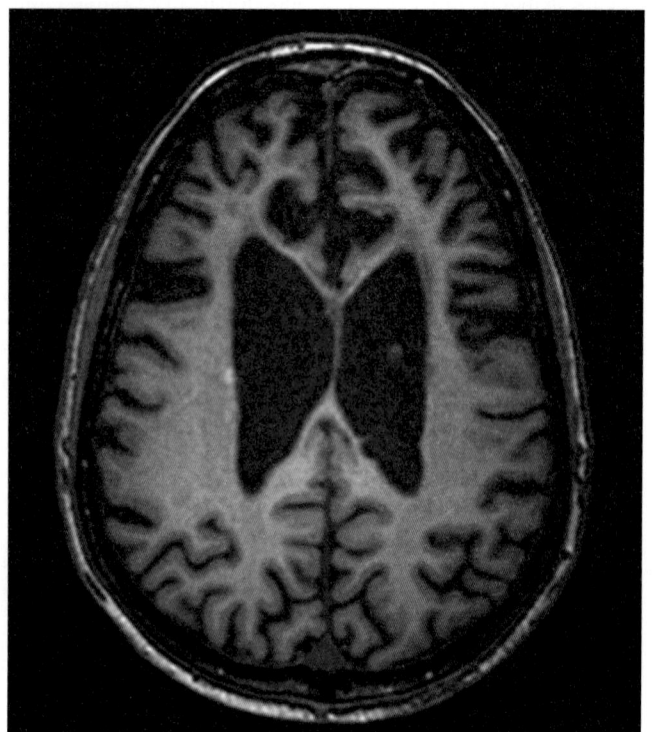
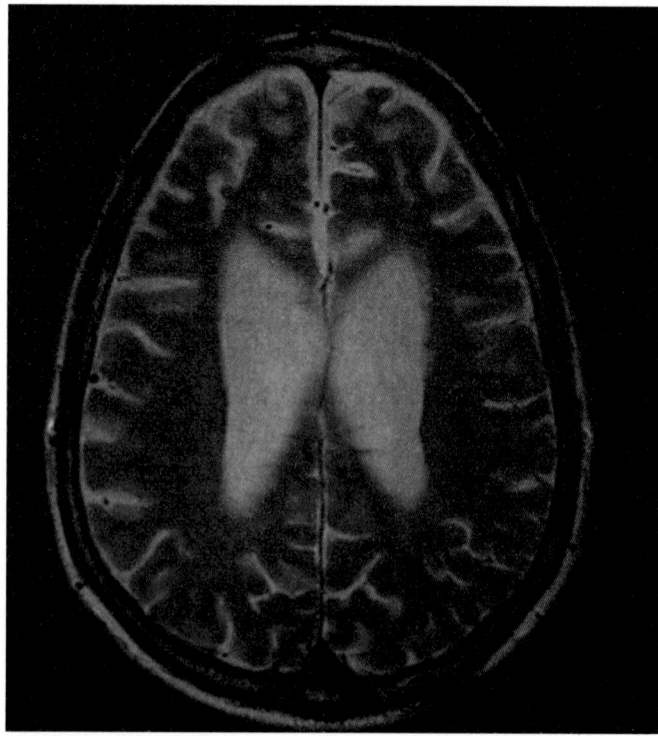

A   **B**

FIGURE 67.1 HIV-positive subject with progressive dementia. **A:** T1-weighted and **(B)** T2-weighted MRI scans show ventricular enlargement and cortical atrophy, particularly in the frontal lobe. There is also some mild periventricular T2 hyperintensity.

impairment. ^{18}F-fluorodeoxyglucose-positron emission tomography (PET) shows relative hypermetabolism in the thalamus and basal ganglia in HIV-infected individuals. Progressive dementia is accompanied by cortical and subcortical hypometabolism. Single-photon emission computed tomography (SPECT) shows multifocal cortical perfusion deficits in the frontal lobes, worse in those with dementia. Cerebral metabolite abnormalities demonstrated by magnetic resonance spectroscopy (MRS) include elevated myoinositol and choline levels in frontal white matter indicative of glial proliferation in patients with mild cognitive impairment. Severe dementia is associated with decreased levels of N-acetylaspartate, a neuronal marker. Dynamic cerebral blood volume (CBV) studies by functional MRI show increased CBV in deep and cortical gray matter in HIV-positive individuals and even greater increases in the deep gray matter of those with dementia. Continuous arterial spin label MRI showed reduced caudate blood flow and volume in patients with cognitive impairment. Abnormalities may improve with antiretroviral treatment.

Pathologic abnormalities in brain include microglial nodules, multinucleated giant cells, focal perivascular demyelination and gliosis, and neuronal loss in frontal cortex. Although there is often no correlation between the severity of these pathologic changes and the severity of dementia, recent studies suggest that neuronal injury may be missed by standard pathologic survey techniques. In a prospective study, severity of neurocognitive impairment was correlated with microneuroanatomic injury to dendritic structures that resulted in dendritic simplification but not to viral burden or presence of microglial nodules and multinucleated giant cells. Astrocyte cell death through apoptotic mechanisms may reduce the neuroprotective functions of this cellular population. In vitro studies show that soluble Fas ligand (sFasL) from HIV-infected macrophages triggers apoptosis of uninfected astrocytes. A study of pre-cART HIV-infected patients with dementia showed elevated CSF sFasL levels in this group compared with HIV-negative controls and HIV-positive nondemented patients. More prospective data are needed to understand the role of apoptosis in HIV dementia and the use of markers for apoptosis as predictors of dementia.

The incidence of HIV dementia is lower than the frequency with which pathologic abnormalities are found. The CDC reported a prevalence of 7.3% for the diagnosis of HIV encephalopathy in 1987 through 1991. The Multicenter AIDS Cohort Study Group reported a 4% prevalence of dementia diagnosis, with a 7% annual rate and 15% overall probability of dementia before death. There are increased mortality rates among demented patients. A subset of individuals may show clinical progression in their HAND stage. Some HIV-positive individuals on cART may demonstrate ongoing CNS changes as identified by subcortical atrophy on MRI studies in the absence of clinical changes. Other HIV-positive individuals may show clinical deterioration on neuropsychological testing. Some HIV-positive individuals may show clinical improvement which is sustained. Additional HIV-positive individuals with HAND may have a fluctuating course from abnormal to normal and then abnormal neuropsychological test performance again. HIV dementia now is rarely seen in the United States where cART is commonly used. However, in resource-limited countries, many HIV-positive individuals are not on cART. In 2012, according to UNAIDS, around 9.7 million people living with HIV infection had access to antiretroviral therapy in low- and middle-income countries. This number represents 61% of people eligible for treatment under the 2010 WHO guidelines and only 34% of people eligible under the 2013 WHO guidelines. In sub-Saharan Africa, where 70% of the world's HIV-positive population resides because HIV-

positive individuals are frequently not on cART, the frequency of HIV dementia may be much higher than the prevalence in the United States. Studies in Uganda suggest that the frequency of HIV dementia among antiretroviral-naïve HIV-positive individuals presenting to an infectious disease clinic may be as high as 31% to 41%. If this proportion is seen throughout resource-limited countries, then HIV dementia may be among the most common forms of dementia globally along with Alzheimer disease and vascular dementia. The question of whether specific HIV subtypes are associated with an increased risk of dementia is unresolved, with some studies showing an increased risk for dementia in HIV subtype D–infected individuals compared to HIV subtype A–infected individuals in Uganda, whereas other studies show no association of HIV subtype with risk of dementia. Similarly, initial studies suggested that HIV subtype C may have a decreased risk of dementia compared to subtype B, but recent studies suggest no difference between HIV subtypes B and C and risk of dementia.

The diagnosis of HIV-associated dementia requires exclusion of secondary opportunistic infections or neoplasms. Other confounding variables include drug use, vitamin B_{12} deficiency, metabolic disorders, concurrent infections such as hepatitis C infection, CNS side effects of medications (e.g., efavirenz, which can cause CNS side effects in 50% of HIV-positive individuals after initiation), and age-related comorbidities in an aging HIV-infected population due to successful antiretroviral treatment. Older survivors of HIV are at risk for vascular disease and degenerative disorders associated with dementia such as Alzheimer disease. In most studies, antiretroviral therapy reduces the incidence and mortality of AIDS dementia. In general, the prevalence of HAND in HIV is expected to increase with longer survival and the aging of HIV-positive individuals. The primary treatment for HAND is cART, which is associated with cognitive improvement in the majority of antiretroviral-naïve HIV-positive individuals. Treatment of comorbid conditions frequently associated with HAND such as depression is also beneficial. Clinical trials of adjunctive therapies such as selegiline, a monoamine oxidase type B inhibitor, and minocycline have showed no benefit. Antioxidants and agents that block gp120 are ineffective. Neuropsychological test abnormalities can accrue with advancing disease. Those showing a decline in neuropsychological test performance, however, have an increased risk of death. In an early multicenter study of 19,462 HIV-infected people, the strongest predictors of significant dementia were CD4+ T-lymphocyte counts of less than 100 cells/μL, anemia, and an AIDS-defining infection or neoplasm (18.6% to 24.9% risk in 2 years). In the post–highly active antiretroviral therapy (HAART) era, HAND is often independent of advanced immunosuppression.

Antiretroviral therapy using drugs with good CNS penetration may benefit the symptomatic patient with CNS virologic escape, but some studies suggest that the beneficial effect of treatment is independent of CNS penetration. A randomized clinical trial of cART with good CNS penetration compared to cART with poor CNS penetration showed no clinical benefit for the group randomized to cART with good CNS penetration. Suppression of viral replication in both the blood and CSF is critical for effective treatment of HAND. Initiation of cART is usually associated with immune system recovery and cognitive benefits. However, some HIV-positive individuals after initiation of cART may experience clinical deterioration despite recovery of the immune system from immunodeficiency, a condition known as *immune reconstitution inflammatory syndrome* (IRIS). When IRIS involves the CNS, opportunistic infections of the CNS such as cryptococcal meningitis or progressive multifocal leukoencephalopathy may present.

In addition, an acute syndrome of fulminant HIV encephalitis can occur in rare cases in which cognition worsens despite virologic suppression and immune system recovery. Risk factors for IRIS include a low CD4 nadir at initiation of cART, the presence of an underlying opportunistic infection, and a sharp decline in viral load after starting cART. Corticosteroids have been used in HIV-positive individuals with noninfectious encephalitis after cART initiation, with clinical improvement in some cases. Additional studies of the role of corticosteroids for the treatment of IRIS are needed.

Further work is needed to understand the pathogenesis and risk for HAND in the post-cART era.

Stroke

Most studies show an association with stroke incidence and HIV status in the post-cART era that extends beyond traditional risk factors including hypertension, dyslipidemia, diabetes mellitus, and smoking. Although modification of these risk factors is an important strategy to decrease stroke risk among HIV-infected individuals, studies have demonstrated an excess risk of stroke in HIV infection. Multiple mechanisms unique to HIV infection may cause an increased stroke risk. Impaired fibrinolysis resulting in a hypercoagulable state may occur. Intracranial vasculopathy has been described in untreated, severely immunocompromised HIV infected individuals with and without strokes, often in combination with aneurysmal arteriopathy and, at times, with concomitant infections including varicella-zoster virus and CMV. Marked clinical and radiographic improvement of vasculopathy documented after initiation of cART suggests that this mechanism is likely of considerably less clinical relevance for virologically suppressed individuals on cART. In addition, cumulative exposure to cART may lead to a rise in vascular risk over time. Impaired glucose metabolism due to antiretroviral therapy may also add to stroke risk. In addition, stroke syndromes may follow secondary infections or neoplasms, such as cryptococcus or other fungi, toxoplasmosis, TB, herpes zoster, CMV, syphilis, or lymphoma. Other causes include HIV-related vasculitis, cardiogenic emboli, thrombogenic conditions such as hyperviscosity, disseminated intravascular coagulation, and the presence of lupus anticoagulant. Cerebral hemorrhage may follow HIV-associated thrombocytopenia or toxoplasmosis.

Evaluation of cerebrovascular syndromes includes screening for classical risk factors including high blood pressure, impaired glucose tolerance, and hyperlipidemia. Additional studies that should be obtained include imaging; CSF examination; cultures for viruses, bacteria, mycobacteria, and fungi; serum and CSF antibodies for cryptococcus, syphilis, and toxoplasmosis; plasma and CSF HIV viral load; polymerase chain reaction (PCR) of CSF for suspect pathogens; echocardiography; carotid Doppler; lipid profiles; coagulation profiles; platelet count; and determination of procoagulants. If vasculitis is suspected, angiography or brain or meningeal biopsy may be useful. Management is directed to the underlying mechanism and may include a change in antiretroviral therapy.

Seizures

Seizure activity complicating HIV infection should raise the suspicion for an underlying structural brain lesion, especially in the setting of focal seizure activity, in patients whose CD4 counts are less than 400 cells/μL, and if focal neurologic signs are present on examination. If seizures are generalized, common etiologies include an underlying metabolic derangement or diffuse meningoencephalitis. Underlying infectious and noninfectious causes to consider, especially in those patients with low CD4 counts, include toxoplasmosis, cryptococcoma, primary CNS lymphoma, and progressive multifocal

leukoencephalopathy. In a study of 100 consecutive cases, secondary pathogens were identified in 53% and HIV encephalopathy in 24%; there was no identified cause in 23%. In another study, status epilepticus was associated with CNS infection in a third of patients, most commonly toxoplasmosis. Seizures in HIV-infected patients have been reported in 4% to 14% of patients and are a common disease-defining presentation. The diagnosis of seizures in HIV patients includes basic laboratory parameters, drug levels if available, neuroimaging, lumbar puncture, and electroencephalogram (EEG). If antiepileptics are indicated, one should consult recent guidelines for the initiation of antiepileptic medications and dosage adjustments of antiretroviral drugs due to antiepileptic drug–antiretroviral drug interactions by a joint panel of the AAN and the International League Against Epilepsy.

Leukoencephalopathy

Leukoencephalopathies in acute or chronic HIV infection include acute fulminating and fatal leukoencephalitis, multifocal vacuolar leukoencephalopathy presenting as rapid dementia, and a relapsing–remitting leukoencephalitis that may simulate multiple sclerosis. The pathogenesis of these syndromes is uncertain. A severe demyelinating leukoencephalopathy with intense perivascular infiltration by HIV-gp41 immunoreactive monocytes/macrophages and lymphocytes is described in patients who failed HAART treatment despite good virologic response in one case. Some speculate this illness is a form of IRIS.

Movement Disorders

Movement disorders in patients with HIV infection were frequently described in the pre-cART era, including patients presenting with tremors, chorea, dyskinesias, and athetosis, most commonly associated with opportunistic infections such as toxoplasmosis. In the post-cART era, movement disorders can also be present, specifically tremors and parkinsonism, which may arise as a consequence of primary infection or side effects of medications. In the current cART era, movement disorders are most commonly described in the setting of HAND. Cognitive decline typically precedes tremor and gait disturbance. Interestingly, there appears to be a greater susceptibility to drug-induced parkinsonism in HIV-infected patients likely related to dopaminergic neuron dysfunction from primary HIV infection which occurs early in infection. Movement disorders related to peripheral neuropathy have also been frequently described in HIV, including restless legs syndrome as well as painful legs and moving toes syndrome.

Myelopathy

Chronic progressive myelopathy, an AIDS-defining illness, is characterized by progressive spastic paraparesis, ataxia, and sphincter dysfunction. Vascular myelopathy presents with a subacute onset of clinical signs and symptoms, developing over weeks to months. Common symptoms include bilateral lower extremity weakness with spasticity. Patients also experience bowel, bladder, and erectile dysfunction with variable sensory disturbances. Deep tendon reflexes are hyperactive with an extensor plantar response. Pathologic findings are similar to those of subacute combined degeneration due to vitamin B_{12} deficiency and include vacuolar change with intramyelin swelling or demyelination that is most severe in the lateral and posterior columns. Microglial nodules and giant cells are sometimes seen, and HIV can be sometimes cultured or detected by hybridization techniques. Pathologic abnormalities are more common than clinical symptoms. Diagnosis requires ruling out causes by measuring serum vitamin B_{12} levels, copper levels, rapid plasma reagin (RPR), and HTLV-1 antibodies before making the diagnosis. Lumbar puncture should be performed to rule out infection with herpes simplex virus, varicella-zoster virus, CMV, and neurosyphilis. In HIV-associated vacuolar myelopathy, the CSF may be normal, or it may show mild pleocytosis with mild elevation in protein. Neuroimaging should be performed, although it is important to note that the spinal MRI may be normal or it may show spinal atrophy or patchy abnormalities on T2-weighted images. Somatosensory evoked potentials (SEP) help to confirm myelopathy, whereas nerve conduction studies can detect coexistent neuropathy if present. No specific treatment is available for myelopathy. The impact of cART is unknown. Antispasticity drugs such as baclofen or bladder relaxants such as imipramine must be used cautiously to avoid sedation or exacerbating weakness.

Motor Neuron Disease

Several cases of an amyotrophic lateral sclerosis (ALS)–like illness have been reported as the initial neurologic syndrome in patients with varying degrees of immunosuppression, ranging from profoundly reduced to near-normal CD4 lymphocyte levels. Clinically, HIV-associated ALS differs from sporadic ALS in that the patients present with symptoms at a younger age, have a more rapid progression, have a high CSF protein, and may recover after initiation of cART. Electromyographic (EMG) features have been shown to be consistent with ALS in one series of six patients. It is important to note that because of the potential reversibility of ALS-like symptoms in HIV infection, testing for HIV infection is generally recommended in younger patients presenting with motor neuron symptoms.

Peripheral Neuropathy

Distal sensory polyneuropathy (DSPN) is the most common neurologic manifestation of HIV infection, with more than 50% of patients with advanced HIV having evidence of DSPN on neurologic examination. Risk factors for development of sensory neuropathy include advanced age, lower CD4 nadir, current ART use, and past "D-drug" use (specific dideoxynucleoside analog antiretrovirals, that is, ddI [didanosine], ddC [zalcitabine], and d4T [stavudine]). Overall, the incidence of neuropathy has increased because of the longer survival of HIV-infected patients, likely related to comorbidities including diabetes mellitus, alcohol abuse, and vitamin B_{12} deficiency. Symptoms are typically symmetric, predominantly distal and sensory. Patients may experience numbness, tightness, pain, burning, or hyperalgesia in the feet. Signs include stocking-glove sensory loss, mild muscle wasting and weakness, and loss of ankle jerks. Conduction studies show sensorimotor neuropathy with mixed axonal and demyelinating features. Clinically, HIV-related DSPN is indistinguishable from the neuropathy due to nucleoside reverse transcriptase inhibitors. Pathologic findings include axonal degeneration, loss of large myelinated fibers, and variable inflammatory cell infiltration. CSF may be normal or show mild pleocytosis and elevated protein. HIV can rarely be cultured from nerve, but the cellular localization of the virus is not known. The neuropathy may be mediated by the binding of gp120 envelope viral glycoprotein to sensory ganglion cells.

Neuropathic pain is associated with significant disability in daily activities, unemployment, and overall reduced quality of life. It is sometimes responsive to anticonvulsants (gabapentin, pregabalin, lamotrigine), tricyclic antidepressants, selective serotonin-norepinephrine reuptake inhibitors (duloxetine), topical anesthetic patches or creams, high-concentration capsaicin patch, and nonsteroidal or narcotic analgesics. Immune globulin is sometimes used in refractory cases, but reports of success are only anecdotal. Clinical trials have shown that recombinant human nerve growth factor is effective, but it is currently unavailable. There are also reports that smoked cannabis is effective for pain but may be associated with CNS side effects.

Other clinical manifestations of HIV infection include mononeuropathies, mononeuritis multiplex, inflammatory demyelinating polyneuropathy, and ganglioneuritis. Inflammatory demyelinating polyneuropathy may occur in its acute form early in the course of disease as part of the acute retroviral syndrome. Chronic inflammatory demyelinating polyneuropathy may also occur early in infection when there is immune dysregulation. It is distinguished from Guillain–Barré syndrome by a subacute or progressive course and variable response to corticosteroids, intravenous immunoglobulin (IVIG), or plasmapheresis. Electrodiagnostic studies show demyelination with variable axonal damage. Histopathologic studies reveal epineurial inflammatory cell infiltrates, demyelination, and axonal degeneration. CSF may show a pleocytosis, but findings are nondiagnostic. Mononeuropathies due to entrapment neuropathies are also commonly seen in patients with HIV infection. It is important to note that focal cranial neuropathies warrant further evaluation including neuroimaging and CSF analysis. Mononeuropathy multiplex due to peripheral nerve infarction associated with vasculitis is rarely described secondary to primary HIV infection and is more frequently described with CMV opportunistic infection as described later in this chapter.

Myopathy

HIV-associated myopathy may range from mild symptoms to severe rhabdomyolysis, with HIV-associated polymyositis being the most frequent clinical syndrome. HIV-associated polymyositis is clinically and pathologically similar to autoimmune polymyositis and is characterized by proximal limb weakness, mild creatine kinase elevation, and myopathic features on EMG. The mechanism by which HIV leads to inflammatory myopathy is not fully understood, but a T-cell–mediated and MHC I–restricted cytotoxic process triggered by HIV has been proposed. HIV-associated myopathy has also been described as part of an IRIS. Although treatment is not established in HIV-associated myopathy, patients may respond to steroids or IVIG. Other differentials to consider include myopathies related to cART or infectious etiologies. Stavudine (d4T) can cause HIV-associated neuromuscular weakness syndrome (HANWS) which is characterized by a rapidly progressive weakness, resembling Guillain–Barré syndrome, with associated lactic acidosis due to mitochondrial dysfunction. Zidovudine may also cause a clinically similar myopathy due to its effects on mitochondria. Muscle biopsies show ragged red fibers and deficient cytochrome oxidase. Some patients respond well to steroid therapy without accelerated progression of HIV disease.

OPPORTUNISTIC INFECTIONS

The spectrum of viral, bacterial, and fungal opportunistic infections, well described for their devastating consequences prior to the cART era, remain prevalent in many countries where cART medications remain poorly accessible, in patients not adherent to their HIV drug regimen, and as immune reconstitution phenomenon (Table 67.7).

Meningitis may be caused by such viruses including herpes simplex virus, varicella-zoster virus, CMV, and Epstein–Barr virus (EBV); fungi (*Cryptococcus, Histoplasma, Coccidioides, Candida*); bacteria

TABLE 67.7	Secondary Neurologic Syndromes in HIV Infection and AIDS: Opportunistic Infections and Neoplasms
Leptomeninges	
Viral	CMV, HSV, VZV, EBV, hepatitis B
Fungal	*Cryptococcus, Histoplasma, Coccidioides, Candida*
Bacterial	*Listeria, Treponema pallidum*, pyogenic bacteria (*Salmonella, Staphylococcus aureus*), atypical or conventional mycobacteria
Neoplasm	Lymphoma
Cerebral Syndromes	
Diffuse Encephalopathy or Encephalitis	
Viral	CMV, HSV, VZV, hepatitis C
Bacterial	Atypical mycobacteria
Parasitic	*Acanthamoeba, Toxoplasma*
Neoplasm	Lymphoma
Focal Cerebral Syndromes	
Viral	HSV, VZV, PML
Fungal	Abscess due to *Cryptococcus, Candida, Zygomycetes, Histoplasma, Aspergillus*
Bacterial	Abscess due to pyogenic bacteria, mycobacteria (tuberculoma), *Listeria, Nocardia*
Parasitic	*Trypanosoma cruzi, Taenia solium, Toxoplasma*
Neoplasm	Primary or metastatic lymphoma, glioma, metastatic Kaposi sarcoma
Cerebrovascular Syndromes and Seizures	
Viral	VZV, HSV, rarely PML
Fungal	*Cryptococcus, Aspergillus*
Bacterial	*T. pallidum, Mycobacterium tuberculosis*
Parasitic	*Toxoplasma*
Neoplasm	Lymphoma, lymphomatoid granulomatosis, metastatic Kaposi sarcoma
Other	Cerebral hemorrhage, cardiac emboli, vasculitis
Movement Disorders	
Viral	PML, HIV
Bacterial	CNS Whipple disease
Parasitic	*Toxoplasma*
Spinal Cord Syndromes	
Viral	VZV, CMV, HSV, HTLV-1
Bacterial	Mycobacteria, myogenic bacteria, *T. pallidum*
Parasitic	Toxoplasmosis
Neoplasm	Lymphoma, Kaposi sarcoma
Cranial and Peripheral Neuropathy	
Viral	CMV (retinitis, polyradiculitis, mononeuritis multiplex)
Fungal	*Candida* (retinitis)
Parasitic	*Toxoplasma* (retinitis)
Myositis	
Bacterial	*S. aureus*, mycobacteria
Parasitic	*Toxoplasma*

CMV, cytomegalovirus; HSV, herpes simplex virus; VZV, varicella-zoster virus; EBV, Epstein–Barr virus; PML, progressive multifocal leukoencephalopathy; CNS, central nervous system; HTLV-1, human T-lymphotropic virus type 1.

(*Listeria*, *Treponema pallidum*, atypical or conventional mycobacteria, pyogenic bacteria such as *Salmonella*, *Staphylococcus aureus*); and neoplasm (carcinomatous meningitis due to lymphoma).

Focal brain syndromes may be caused by *Toxoplasma*, progressive multifocal leukoencephalopathy, abscesses related to *Nocardia*, *Listeria*, *Taenia solium*, *Candida*, *Cryptococcus*, *Histoplasma*, *Aspergillus*, *Coccidioides*, *Mycobacterium tuberculosis*, atypical mycobacteria, and pyogenic bacteria.

VIRAL INFECTIONS

The pattern of opportunistic viral infection associated with AIDS has changed since the introduction of effective HIV therapy. Early in the AIDS epidemic, syndromes such as shingles or recurrent aseptic meningitis raised suspicion of an immunodeficient state, and the encephalitis eventually attributed to HIV itself was initially attributed to CMV infection. In contrast, contemporary concerns include facilitation of HIV spread by simultaneous herpes genital infection, use of vaccinations in households of AIDS patients, and other epidemiologic considerations. However, in severely immunosuppressed patients, viral infections of the nervous system remain prominent. For further information about viral infections, see Chapter 66.

Progressive Multifocal Leukoencephalopathy

Progressive multifocal leukoencephalopathy (PML) was recognized early in the HIV pandemic as a complication of AIDS in profoundly immunosuppressed patients. PML is caused by JC virus (JCV), which is a ubiquitous polyomavirus. CNS disease is characterized by lytic infection of oligodendrocytes, causing demyelination. Clinically, patients develop a subacute neurologic decline with focal neurologic symptoms and signs. Localization is hemispheric in 85% to 90% of cases; the posterior fossa is affected in the remainder. Focal or generalized seizures occur in 6% of patients. Imaging shows hypodense subcortical lesions on CT and T2-hyperintense lesions on MRI that spare the cortical gray matter (Fig. 67.2). In PML-IRIS, MRI may show contrast enhancement on T1 postgadolinium sequences, most commonly associated pathologically with CD8+ T cells infiltrating the perivascular spaces. CSF analysis should be performed for JCV detectable on PCR, although a negative study does not exclude the diagnosis, and repeat testing is often recommended if clinical and radiographic imaging is consistent with the diagnosis.

In AIDS patients, PML lesions may stabilize spontaneously, and they may also respond to antiretroviral therapy. cART has led to significant improvement in survival, although patients are often left with serious neurologic sequelae. Despite anecdotal reports of efficacy, clinical trials have not shown any benefit from IV or intrathecal cytosine arabinoside, topotecan, and cidofovir. Immune reconstitution following antiretroviral therapy favorably impacts the clinical course in some but not all patients with PML. This may be explained by a selective loss of JCV-specific CD4 cells. The IRIS with either emergence or clinical progression of PML has been reported. When PML is the AIDS-defining illness, improved prognosis is associated with CD4 cell counts greater than 300 cells/μL, evidence of inflammatory response indicated by gadolinium enhancement on MRI, and reduction in the JCV viral load in CSF.

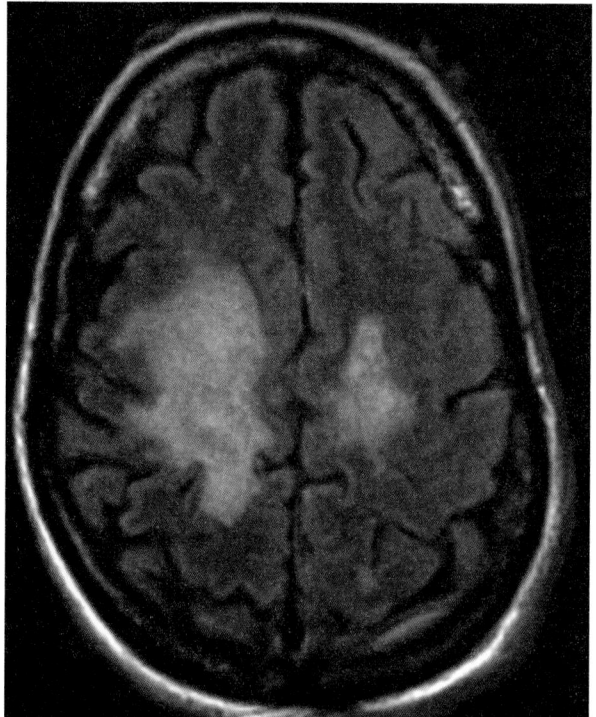
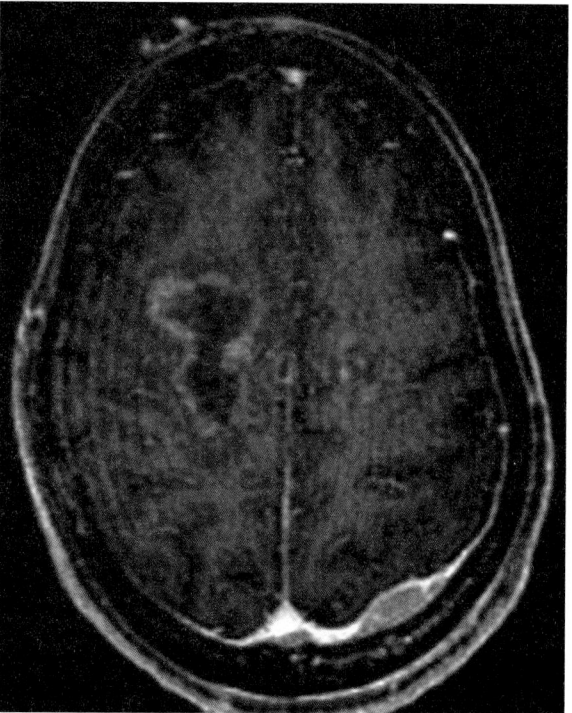

A

B

FIGURE 67.2 A 38-year-old woman with a history of HIV/AIDS recently resumed antiretroviral medication with CD4 count rising from 23 to 78 cells/μL in 2 months, viral load of 340,000, presenting with left-sided weakness that became worse after 2 weeks, and diagnosed with PML as a complication of IRIS. **A:** Fluid-attenuated inversion recovery (FLAIR) hyperintense lesions in bilateral frontoparietal white matter extending to the subcortical regions, larger on the right than left, associated with **(B)** irregular peripheral enhancement. (Courtesy of Dr. Doris Lin, Department of Radiology, Johns Hopkins University School of Medicine.)

Varicella-Zoster Virus

Varicella-zoster virus (VZV), the causative agent of varicella (chickenpox) and herpes zoster (shingles), is common in the general population with a lifetime prevalence of 15% to 30%. A ubiquitous latent virus, VZV remains dormant in the dorsal root ganglia after primary infection, characterized by fever and vesicular rash, most commonly occurring in early childhood. In severely immunosuppressed patients, the infection is reactivated, leading, in some cases, to disseminated diseases with manifestations including pneumonia, diffuse rash, and visceral involvement. Neurologic syndromes resulting from reactivation of VZV in the immunocompromised patient also include shingles, transverse myelitis, meningoencephalitis, and vasculitis.

Shingles beginning with painful dysesthesias or paresthesias (often described as itching) is followed in 7 to 10 days by a contagious vesicular rash that eventually crusts. The acute phase lasts up to a month and may be followed by chronic neuralgic pain for years, although this is less likely if effective antiviral treatment is started promptly. Location is most commonly thoracic, followed by cervical and trigeminal dermatomal distributions. Neurologic complications in addition to postherpetic neuralgia include large- or small-vessel stroke due to vasculitis induced in the vessel wall by the virus, myelitis, segmental myoclonus, and meningitis or encephalitis. Zoster ophthalmicus, which involves the first division of the trigeminal nerve, can lead to blindness from corneal scarring.

Diagnosis is made by CSF PCR analysis or antibody detection. VZV antibodies can be detected in 2.5% to 7% of HIV-infected patients with meningitis, encephalitis, myelitis, or retinitis who have a history of shingles. MRI of the brain or spinal cord may show focal or meningeal enhancement. In patients with encephalitis, CSF shows a mononuclear pleocytosis, increased protein, and, sometimes, low glucose.

Treatment of VZV complications with acyclovir or famciclovir should be started within 72 hours of the rash to prevent pain. Vaccination with two doses of live attenuated virus is recommended even in HIV-infected patients if their CD4 cell count is greater than 200 cells/μL, as this may decrease future complications.

Herpes Simplex Viruses

Herpes simplex virus (HSV) is a neurotropic virus, causing encephalitis in both immunocompetent and immunosuppressed patients. The virus targets structures of the mesial temporal lobe, producing symptoms including headache, fever, confusion, language and memory impairment, and, in severe cases, depressed consciousness and status epilepticus. In those who are immunosuppressed, a more indolent course may present due to the limited inflammatory response that can be mounted. Diagnosis is made with multiplex PCR on CSF instead of brain biopsy, although false-negative CSF PCR has occurred. It is important to note that CSF pleocytosis may be absent in HIV-positive patients. Quantifying the viral load offers prognostic information: Mortality is 22% in patients who have greater than 100,000 copies per microliter, whereas sequelae are mild to moderate (seizures, permanent memory impairment) in those with fewer viral copies. Neuroimaging may show edema and hemorrhagic necrosis in the temporal lobes and basal frontal lobes, reflecting the path of viral entry from its latent presence in the trigeminal nerve. In a retrospective analysis, immunocompromised adults had more extensive involvement of the brain with involvement of the brain stem, cerebellum, and atypical regions including scattered lesions in the cerebrum, sometimes in the absence of temporal lobe involvement. EEG shows focal slowing, often with periodic complexes or other epileptiform discharges in the same areas. Abundant viral inclusions (Cowdry type A bodies) can be seen in patients without necrosis or hemorrhage on pathologic examination. Serum antibodies to herpes simplex 1 are present in up to 70% of the general population and to herpes simplex 2 in 16% to 33%. Because of this, the presence of antibodies does not help in diagnosis. Morbidity and mortality of HSV encephalitis in HIV patients remain high despite acyclovir, as patients may present atypically and may have associated acyclovir resistance.

HHV-6 and HHV-7 are important causes of encephalitis, meningitis, and myelitis in patients with AIDS that also have predilection for the temporal lobes. HHV-8 is responsible for Kaposi sarcoma, which rarely involves the CNS.

Cytomegalovirus

CMV is typically a manifestation of severe immunocompromised state (CD4 count <50 cells/μL) and most commonly presents with retinitis and gastrointestinal symptoms but may also present with a primary neurologic syndrome including rhombencephalitis, ventriculitis, or polyradiculopathy. CMV-associated polyradiculopathy is a common neurologic presentation with rapid development of flaccid paraplegia, urinary retention, and pain radiating into the lumbar and sacral root distributions. CMV encephalitis may present with subcortical diffuse white matter abnormalities and may be clinically difficult to differentiate from HIV-associated encephalopathy. A neuropathology study of HIV-infected patients reported 28 (17%) cases of CMV encephalitis, most of them with premortem diagnosis of HIV-associated cognitive decline.

Diagnostic workup should include ophthalmologic examination, as 30% of patients with neurologic CMV complications present with concomitant CMV retinitis, and CSF should be tested for CMV-PCR. Treatment recommendations for neurologic CMV complications vary and include ganciclovir, foscarnet, or both. Induction therapy is recommended for at least 4 weeks, with maintenance therapy for at least 6 months with monitoring of CSF PCR and immune reconstitution.

Human T-Lymphotropic Virus Types 1 and 2

HTLV is also neurotropic and a member of the same family of retroviruses as HIV. There is conflicting evidence on whether HTLV-1 coinfection accelerates or slows HIV infection and whether HIV coinfection predisposes to clinical manifestations of tropical spastic paraparesis. HTLV-1 causes a chronic spastic paraparesis with gradual onset, and its most frequent symptoms are gait disturbance and urinary symptoms. Contrary to the conflicting evidence of HTLV-1 coinfection, it is generally accepted that HTLV-2 coinfection exerts a negative effect on HIV-1 replication by modulating the cellular microenvironment, favoring its own viability and inhibiting HIV-1 progression. Therapy for HTLV-1/2 remains symptomatic using medications to improve spasticity. Treatment with cART including zidovudine/lamivudine may decrease HTLV-1 viral load and improve neurologic function, although no randomized control trials have been conducted.

Hepatitis B and C

Due to shared mode of transmission, coinfection of HIV and HBV is common, with an estimated 4 million people worldwide being coinfected. Neurologic conditions caused primarily by hepatitis B infection including peripheral neuropathy and encephalopathy related to hyperammonemia may increase the severity of cognitive decline and peripheral neuropathy symptoms seen with primary HIV infection. HIV and hepatitis C virus (HCV) share large worldwide populations as well with an estimated 25% to 40% of individuals being coinfected in the United States, with the highest number in those who are IV drug users. HCV alone is known to be neurotoxic, and there is evidence that with coinfection, the neurotoxic effects of HCV and HIV infection are additive, although one of the major issues in studying this population is the many confounders including history of IV drug use, sex, and educational status. In one study, clinically significant HIV-associated neurocognitive decline and peripheral neuropathy are not exacerbated by active HCV infection in the setting of optimally treated HIV infection, although the long-term consequences of HCV coinfection remain important and incompletely understood. HCV coinfection has been also correlated with an increased risk of primary intracranial hemorrhage, although the role for HCV coinfection in the risk of ischemic stroke is less well-defined.

FUNGAL INFECTIONS

Fungal infections and their treatment are discussed in detail in Chapter 64, so only those aspects important for HIV-infected patients are presented here.

Cryptococcosis

Cryptococcal infection, the most common cause of meningitis in AIDS, was a presenting illness in 25% to 50% of AIDS patients in older clinical series and remains prevalent in many regions worldwide. The yeast is a ubiquitous environmental encapsulated fungus found in soil and bird feces and enters the body via inhalation. CNS involvement emerges from latent infection most commonly when CD4 counts fall below 100 cells/μL. Cryptococcal meningitis most commonly presents as a subacute meningitis or meningoencephalitis. Some patients demonstrate more severe symptoms such as seizures, lethargy, and coma resulting from elevated intracranial pressure (ICP). In protracted meningeal infection, small cryptococcomas can be found, and stroke may occur due to vasculitis. CT and MRI can be normal early on but show hydrocephalus and meningeal enhancement as the infection evolves. Cryptococcomas can be visualized near the ventricles and adjacent to subarachnoid spaces. CSF should be tested for cryptococcal antigen and cultured for fungus. In resource-limited settings, India ink staining is frequently used, as cryptococcal antigen testing may not be available. CSF opening and closing pressure should be measured, as it is elevated in the majority of patients with cryptococcal meningitis. The principles of treatment for patients with cryptococcal meningitis include (1) antifungal therapy, (2) lowering elevated ICP, (3) initiating or optimizing antiretroviral therapy to improve immune function, and (4) management of immune reconstitution if it develops. Induction therapy includes amphotericin B plus flucytosine. Fluconazole is the basis of maintenance therapy and must be continued until there is recovery of immune function. Patients with elevated opening pressure should undergo daily therapeutic lumbar punctures with measurement of closing pressures until pressures have normalized.

Primary prophylaxis using fluconazole or another azole may be instituted if the CD4 count falls below 200 cells/μL. Early initiation of antiretroviral therapy in the setting of cryptococcal meningitis has been shown to increase mortality, and treatment is typically delayed for at least a few weeks after treatment of fungal infection.

Candidiasis

Candida is a rare cause of meningitis in severely immunosuppressed patients. Autopsies have occasionally shown *Candida* in brain parenchyma. Resistant organisms may emerge in patients who have been treated with fluconazole for primary prophylaxis.

Coccidioidomycosis

Coccidioidomycosis is endemic to the southwestern United States and certain areas of Mexico and Central and South America. Immunosuppressed patients more commonly develop disseminated infection, although rarely present with CNS involvement. Basilar meningitis is the most common presentation in those with neurologic involvement, which is typically accompanied by a reticulonodular diffuse infiltrative pneumonia. As the organism is often difficult to grow on CSF culture, presumptive diagnosis is often made through identification of *Coccidioides immitis* spherules in tissue, sputum, bronchoalveolar lavage (BAL) fluid, or other body fluid. Chronic meningitis due to *C. immitis* occurs in about 10% of patients from endemic areas with CD4 counts less than 200 cells/μL. The most common symptoms are headache and slowly worsening mental status changes. Symptoms are usually severe only in patients who develop endarteritis obliterans or hydrocephalus. Treatment of disseminated coccidioidomycosis includes systemic antifungal therapy with amphotericin B or azoles. Amphotericin B remains the drug of choice for life-threatening disease.

Histoplasmosis

Histoplasma capsulatum var capsulatum (*H. capsulatum*) primarily affects those living in the valleys of the Ohio and Mississippi rivers in the United States and those living in Latin America. *H. capsulatum var duboisii* is described only in Africa and is a common endemic mycosis in HIV-positive patients. In patients with advanced HIV infection, histoplasmosis typically manifests with disseminated disease, as opposed to the asymptomatic or limited pulmonary infection observed in the majority of healthy individuals exposed to *H. capsulatum*. Neurologic symptoms include headache and encephalopathy, with findings of a lymphocytic meningitis and focal parenchymal lesions in the brain or spinal cord.

Aspergillosis

Aspergillus fumigatus is a rare cause of brain abscess in HIV patients. *Aspergillus* is an angiotropic fungus that causes a necrotizing angiitis in the brain. Secondary thrombosis and hemorrhage can occur, with the anterior and middle cerebral arteries being most commonly involved. Evolving hemorrhagic infarcts convert into septic infarcts with associated abscesses and cerebritis. Mycotic aneurysms may develop, or intra-arterial thrombosis may present with subarachnoid hemorrhage. Intracranial spread of *Aspergillus* infection occurs less frequently through direct or contiguous spread. Direct extension from the sinuses or orbit has been reported, causing abscess formation in the frontal lobes. Meningitis, less frequent than abscess, tends to involve the base of the brain. *Aspergillus*, myelitis, and invasion of the cavernous sinus have all been reported in AIDS patients. *Mucorales* can cause a similar picture, but this organism is not increased in frequency in AIDS patients.

Neuroimaging should be obtained prior to lumbar puncture to determine whether there is abscess formation. Organisms are rarely found in CSF, and surgical removal of *Aspergillus* abscesses may be the only manner of diagnosis. Amphotericin B combined with flucytosine and treatment of the source of infection is the treatment of choice.

PARASITIC INFECTIONS

The geographic and patient ecologies of parasitic and HIV infections intersect in many areas including the tropical environments of sub-Saharan Africa, Central and South America, Thailand, and

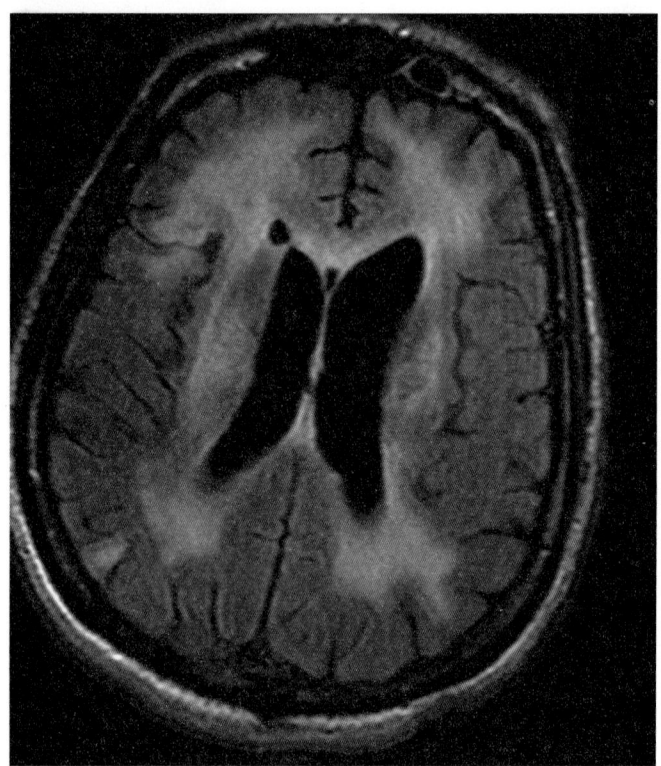
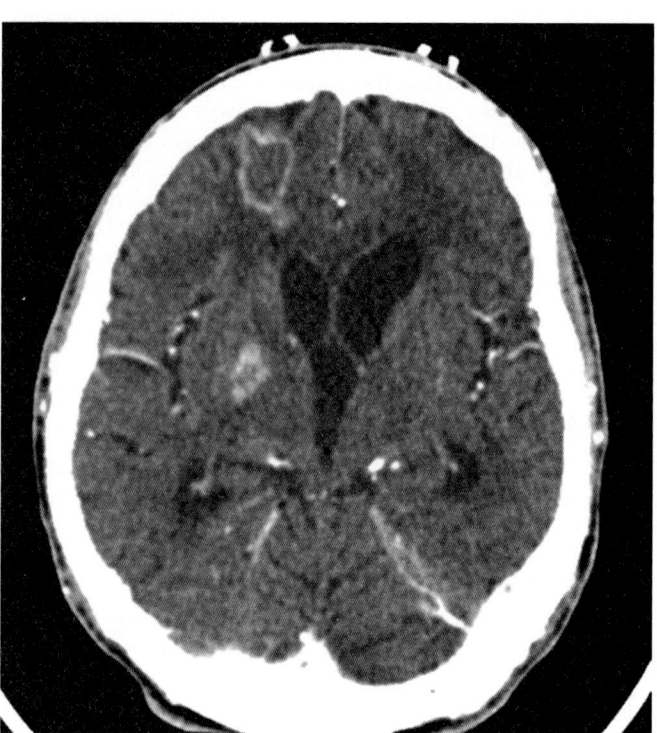

FIGURE 67.3 A: FLAIR MRI and **(B)** contrast-enhanced CT in an HIV-positive patient with toxoplasmosis. Extensive bilateral white matter T2 hyperintensity and multiple contrast-enhancing lesions are present.

India, which foster the presence of malaria and other parasitic infections. Discussion in the following sections focuses on the interaction of parasitic infections in HIV-positive patients.

Toxoplasmosis

For many years, toxoplasmosis was the most common cause of brain lesions in patients with AIDS and a frequent cause of death. Today, *Toxoplasma gondii* accounts for less than 2% of AIDS deaths in the United States, although it remains a major contributor to death in HIV-positive patients worldwide. Most of this gain is due to effective antiretroviral treatment, but effective and well-tolerated drugs for both treatment and prophylaxis of toxoplasmosis infection have also contributed. Although 95% of cases represent reactivation of latent infection, seronegative patients should avoid consumption of raw meat, unpasteurized milk, and exposure to cats and cat litter. Neurologic symptoms are referable to the sites of mass lesions. These most often occur at the gray–white junction and in the thalamus or basal ganglia. With multiple lesions, the clinical picture may appear nonfocal with seizures and signs of increased ICP. Meningitis, ventriculitis, and hydrocephalus have been described in the AIDS population, although they are less common presentations than focal mass lesions. Fever and headache are present in up to 70% of patients. CT and MR scans demonstrate ring-enhancing or nodular lesions with marked surrounding edema. With MRI, lesions have decreased signal with T1-weighted sequences but increased signal on T2-weighted images (Fig. 67.3). Multiple lesions are seen in 60% of cases. Thallium brain SPECT shows decreased uptake with a toxoplasmosis abscess which can be helpful in distinguishing CNS toxoplasmosis from primary CNS lymphoma, which shows increased uptake. A radiologic and clinical response to treatment should be seen in 7 to 10 days after the initiation of treatment. As a result, most cases are now diagnosed by therapeutic response

rather than brain biopsy. Because severe immunosuppression may result in a false-negative response, *Toxoplasma* serology should be obtained as soon as a diagnosis of HIV infection is made. PCR for *Toxoplasma* can be done on CSF, but it has a low yield.

Treatment is with sulfadiazine or sulfadoxine and pyrimethamine. Folinic acid should be given to avoid vitamin B deficiency in the patient. Inadvertent substitution of folic acid will allow survival of the parasite. Patients allergic to sulfa can undergo desensitization or receive atovaquone, clindamycin plus pyrimethamine, or cotrimoxazole, which can also be used for primary prophylaxis. Maintenance therapy can be stopped when the CD4 cell count exceeds 100 cells/μL.

Malaria

Malaria is widespread in many of the same areas where HIV is prevalent, although the effects of coinfection are poorly understood. Patients at highest risk for cerebral manifestations of malaria include those with a lack of acquired immunity toward *Plasmodium falciparum*. When it involves the brain, *P. falciparum* infection causes seizures, including status epilepticus; cerebral edema; alteration of consciousness and coma; and signs of brain stem dysfunction. The pathogenesis of cerebral malaria remains incompletely understood, but key factors include cerebral capillary blockade and parasitized red blood cell (pRBC) sequestration, the host's immunologic status and immunologic response to infection, and pathogen-related antigen expression and release of toxins that interact with cerebral endothelial structure and may contribute to secondary parenchymal changes. In children, sequelae in severe cases include developmental delay, cognitive dysfunction, epilepsy, attention deficit disorder, and poor school performance. Prevention includes reducing opportunities for exposure to mosquitos using insecticides and protective netting as well as prophylactic drug regimens determined by local sensitivity patterns. Treatment includes parental antimalarial treatment, preferably with IV artesunate as well as supportive management.

Trypanosomiasis

Infection by *Trypanosoma brucei gambiense* or *rhodesiense* causes sleeping sickness in Africa, and *Trypanosoma cruzi* causes Chagas disease in South America; in AIDS patients, it may rarely lead to mass lesions or meningoencephalitis.

Cysticercosis

Immunosuppression does not affect the virulence and prevalence of *Taenia solium* infection, but neurocysticercosis should be considered in the differential of an HIV-positive patient from a region endemic for cysticerci. Lesions are most often calcified, although cysts containing live organisms in the larval state are occasionally seen. Anticonvulsant drugs are necessary to treat seizures, but antiparasitic agents, such as praziquantel and albendazole, are rarely needed.

BACTERIAL AND MYCOBACTERIAL INFECTION

Syphilis

Neurosyphilis, which is caused by *T. pallidum*, occurs with greater frequency in individuals coinfected with HIV. Although not an opportunistic infection, syphilitic infection behaves differently in the presence of AIDS, and genital syphilis facilitates acquiring HIV infection. About 15% of patients with primary syphilis are seropositive for HIV. Conversely, positive serology for syphilis may occur in over 35% of some HIV-infected populations. Progression from primary syphilis (painless chancre) to later stages is typically more rapid in HIV-infected patients with lower CD4 counts. Syphilis can affect many parts of the nervous system including the meninges, brain, brain stem, spinal cord, nerve roots, and cerebral and spinal blood vessels. Syndromes of early neurosyphilis are more common than late syndromes (general paresis and tabes dorsalis). Syphilitic meningitis is the earliest neurologic complication of syphilis and is caused by invasion of the meninges by the spirochete. These can sometimes lead to cerebral vasculitis and stroke, most commonly involving the middle cerebral artery (MCA). Late stages of neurosyphilis include meningovascular involvement of the medium and large vessels as well as parenchymatous disease. Parenchymatous neurosyphilis is typified by tabes dorsalis, involving the dorsal roots and posterior columns, and general paresis. All patients who are HIV positive and also seropositive for syphilis require an analysis of CSF to detect and treat neurosyphilis before it has permanent and disabling consequences. Although a positive CSF serology using fluorescent treponemal antibody (FTA) or Venereal Disease Research Laboratory (VDRL) is enough to initiate treatment, the CSF in neurosyphilis also usually contains white blood cells (WBCs) (usually mononuclear) and may also have increased protein. CSF VDRL, however, may be negative. Treatment with IV penicillin or 4 weeks of doxycycline or minocycline should be continued until there is a fourfold drop in serum titers. Ceftriaxone has a 23% failure rate, so its use is not recommended. HIV patients should have serology tested monthly for 3 months and at 3-month intervals thereafter. Lumbar puncture should be repeated after 6 months to ensure an adequate response to treatment. If serologic titers remain stable or rise, retreatment is indicated. Complete normalization of CSF VDRL reactivity is less likely in those with higher baseline values and peripheral blood CD4 counts less than 200 cells/μL.

Mycobacteria

MYCOBACTERIUM AVIUM-INTRACELLULARE

Mycobacterium avium-intracellulare was one of the earliest opportunistic infections described in patients with AIDS, although neurologic involvement was usually detected only at autopsy. The organism has been responsible for cases of immune reconstitution syndrome when antiviral treatment is started. Patients with disseminated *M. avium-intracellulare* may develop meningoencephalitis, cranial neuropathies, and epidural abscess, but defining neurologic syndromes due to *M. avium-intracellulare* has been difficult due to coinfection with several opportunistic organisms.

MYCOBACTERIUM TUBERCULOSIS

Worldwide, over 14 million people are coinfected with TB and HIV. In 2012, an estimated 1.3 million died of TB, including 320,000 coinfected with HIV. Tuberculous meningitis (TBM), which is the most deadly form of the disease, is five times more frequent in HIV-positive patients. The elevated risk of TB in HIV-infected persons is due in part to impairment of T-cell–mediated immunity, with TB risk increasing as CD4 cell count declines. In addition, the Beijing strain of TB, which has particularly high virulence, is associated with HIV infection and multidrug resistance.

The Beijing genotype *Mycobacterium tuberculosis* is significantly associated with HIV infection and multidrug resistance in cases of TBM.

CNS manifestations of TB occur from hematogenous dissemination of the bacteria from primary lung involvement, with formation of small subpial and subependymal foci. In HIV-positive patients, clinical presentation is typically similar to those who are HIV negative, although those who have very low CD4 counts can present atypically with more disseminated disease and altered consciousness. The most common presentation is meningitis, which is frequently a subacute or chronic presentation, followed by tuberculomas. Meningitis preferentially involves the basilar meninges and is associated with hydrocephalus, multiple cranial neuropathies, and ischemic stroke. TB may also present with spine disease, affecting the vertebral bodies (Pott disease) or the spinal cord. Diagnosis can be particularly challenging, as the clinical picture often mimics other opportunistic infections, including cryptococcal meningitis. CSF may show an early neutrophilic response followed by lymphocytic predominance, low glucose, and elevated protein, although studies have shown that there is a reduced CSF WBC count in HIV-infected adults not receiving cART compared to HIV-uninfected adults. CSF protein has also been noted to be normal in HIV-positive patients. When cultured from CSF, the organism takes 3 to 4 weeks to grow and can be difficult to detect. AFB can also be detected by PCR, although the sensitivity is low. Recent discovery of the use of CSF gene expert may be particularly beneficial in TBM, although ongoing studies are needed to determine its sensitivity and specificity in the HIV-positive population. Treatment for TBM is extrapolated from clinical trials for pulmonary TB and includes rifampicin, isoniazid (INH), pyrazinamide, and streptomycin (or ethambutol) for intensive phase followed by rifampicin and INH for maintenance along with adjunctive corticosteroids. Recent studies have shown that high-dose rifampicin and a fluoroquinolone early in treatment may decrease mortality. It is important to note that there is an increased risk for drug resistance to INH and rifampicin in HIV-positive patients with TB, causing further challenges to treatment. For those who are cART naïve, delay in treatment initiation is recommended.

NEOPLASMS

Lymphoma incidence has declined markedly, from a range of 0.6% to 3% of patients in pre-cART clinical series to rare or no occurrence in post-cART series. Clinical signs are nonspecific and include focal neurologic signs, seizures, cranial neuropathy, and headache. CT may be normal or show hypodense lesions as well as single or multiple lesions with patchy or nodular enhancement. Thallium SPECT shows increased uptake in lymphoma, which aids in distinguishing it from toxoplasmosis which shows decreased uptake. EBV DNA is found in PCR studies of CSF but is not predictive of the diagnosis. Brain biopsy is required for diagnosis. Response to therapy with radiation and chemotherapy is improved by current antiretroviral regimens, with longer survivals and reports of complete tumor regression, although this is rare. Opportunistic infections may coexist with tumor and should be excluded by appropriate studies.

Other neoplasms reported rarely in AIDS patients include metastatic Kaposi sarcoma (associated with HHV-8) and primary glial tumors, but their incidence has also been dramatically decreased by cART. Non–AIDS-defining malignancies are now more important in the treated HIV population and occur with increased frequency compared with the uninfected population. An elevated risk is reported for the following cancers: anal, vaginal, Hodgkin lymphoma, liver, lung, melanoma, oropharyngeal, leukemia, colorectal, and renal. Routine cancer screening and smoking cessation are therefore important in this population.

NUTRITIONAL AND METABOLIC CONSEQUENCES

Nutritional deficiency may result from inadequate amounts of thiamine, vitamin B$_{12}$, folic acid, and glutathione which in turn may cause encephalopathy, dementia, neuropathy, or spinal cord disorders. Metabolic abnormalities often occur in late-stage disease and are reversible causes of encephalopathy. Testosterone deficiency is increasingly recognized in long survivors and may contribute to encephalopathy.

DIAGNOSTIC EVALUATION

The diagnostic evaluation of patients with a suspected HIV-related illness includes an enzyme-linked immunosorbent assay (ELISA) for HIV serology. Positive results are confirmed by Western blot. Depending on local laws, serologic tests may require informed consent and counseling. In patients with otherwise typical viral syndromes, such as aseptic meningitis or transverse myelitis, HIV infection must be suspected even in the absence of known high-risk behavior. Absence of antibodies during the acute illness does not negate the diagnosis because these disorders typically occur at the time of seroconversion. Other helpful diagnostic studies include determination of CD-lymphocyte subset ratio, plasma HIV viral load, serum protein electrophoresis, quantitative immunoglobulins, and platelet count.

Evaluation for specific neurologic syndromes should be preceded by a general physical examination to assist in excluding opportunistic infections or tumor. Evaluation may require biopsy of skin, lymph nodes, or bone marrow as well as chest radiography. Blood culture for viruses and fungi may also prove necessary.

Accurate neurologic diagnosis requires systematic evaluation, including assessment for the possibility of multiple diseases. Thorough neurologic examination should be performed. CSF is most helpful in syphilis, viral, and fungal infections. PCR of CSF can be helpful for pathogenic diagnosis of HSV, VZV, CMV, toxoplasma, and PML, but negative results do not exclude infection. CSF abnormalities are common in asymptomatic HIV infection and must be interpreted with caution in considering other possible conditions. CT and, especially, MRI are useful in distinguishing focal from diffuse brain lesions. MRS and thallium SPECT can help in distinguishing tumor from infection. Proton MRS and other functional imaging may also be useful in HIV-associated cognitive impairment. Brain biopsy may be required for differential diagnosis. Stereotactic biopsy is a low-risk procedure in experienced hands. For solitary lesions not causing herniation, it is reasonable to treat for toxoplasmosis. Biopsy is reserved for patients who do not respond to appropriate treatment and for PCR and seronegative cases.

Myelopathy is evaluated by MRI with gadolinium to exclude a compressive lesion. CSF is a useful adjunct test to rule out infectious etiologies. EMG and nerve conduction studies are useful in evaluating chronic inflammatory demyelinating polyneuropathy, anterior horn cell disease, polyradiculopathy, peripheral neuropathy, and myopathy. Nerve or muscle biopsy may be required.

TREATMENT, COURSE, AND OUTCOME

Potent cART has transformed the course of AIDS from a fatal disease to a chronic illness. Even before cART, prophylactic treatment of common opportunistic infections had reduced AIDS deaths. Improved medical care has also reduced the need for hospital admissions in this population.

Antiretroviral drugs improve morbidity due to HIV and extend survival. More than 40 drugs in 7 classes, including combination drugs, have been approved for use, and more are in clinical trials or development (Table 67.8). New drugs are in development that target various phases of the viral cycle and include attachment inhibitors and chemokine receptor inhibitors.

Current recommendations regarding initiation of cART include starting antiretroviral therapy for all HIV-positive patients with a CD4 count ≤500 cells/mm^3. Deliberately delaying initiation of antiviral treatment (e.g., until the CD4 count is below 500 cells/mm^3) contributes to non-AIDS events, such as cardiovascular, renal, and hepatic disease, that can occur as a result of an infection's ongoing inflammatory effects and is associated with higher mortality.

ADVERSE NEUROLOGIC EFFECTS OF DRUG TREATMENT FOR HIV INFECTION

The most important adverse effect of initiation of cART in an immunosuppressed patient is immune reconstitution syndromes.

Vaccination of patients with HIV infection (or their household contacts) is considered worth the risk if the percentage of CD4 lymphocytes is above 15% in children, or greater than 200 cells/mm^3. With varicella vaccine, clinicians should be prepared to use acyclovir if symptoms of varicella infection develop. Measles vaccine has rarely led to subacute sclerosing panencephalitis. Other antimicrobials used for prevention or maintenance therapy of fungal and parasitic infections can have neurologic side effects, such as testosterone deficiency with azole use, neuropathy with INH if supplemental vitamin B$_6$ is not given, and seizures from ganciclovir. Increased sensitivity to psychotropic drugs leading to prominent extrapyramidal effects is seen in AIDS patients. As new medications with different mechanisms of action are introduced, it is important that any adverse effects be reported using systems such as the U.S. Food and Drug Administration (FDA's) Sentinel

TABLE 67.8 Categories of Drugs Used to Treat HIV

Name	Former Name	Brand Name	Side Effect	Year Introduced
Nucleoside Reverse Transcriptase Inhibitors				
Abacavir	—	Ziagen	Cognitive, myopathy, seizures	1998
Didanosine	DDI	Videx	Neuropathy, myopathy	1991
Lamivudine	<3TC>	Epivir	Neuropathy, lactic acidosis	1995
Stavudine[a]	<d4T>	Zerit	Neuropathy, myopathy	1994
Zalcitabine[a]	<ddC>	Hivid	Neuropathy	1992
Zidovudine	<AZT>	Retrovir	Neuropathy, myopathy, cognitive, seizures	1987
Nucleotide Reverse Transcriptase Inhibitors				
Emtricitabine	<FTC>	Emtriva	Lactic acidosis	2003
Tenofovir	—	Viread	Encephalopathy	2001
Nonnucleoside Reverse Transcriptase Inhibitors				
Delavirdine	—	—	Rescriptor	1997
Efavirenz	—	Sustiva	Cognitive, insomnia, hallucinations	1998
Etravirine	<TMC-125>	Intelence	—	2008
Nevirapine	—	Viramune	—	1996
Rilpivirine	—	Edurant	—	2011
Protease Inhibitors				
Amprenavir[a]	—	Agenerase	Lipodystrophy, metabolic syndrome, myopathy (if combined with statins)	1999
Atazanavir	—	Reyataz	Same	2003
Darunavir	—	Prezista	Same	2006
Fosamprenavir	—	Lexiva	Same	2007
Indinavir[a]	—	Crixivan	Same plus neuropathy	1996
Nelfinavir	—	Viracept	Same plus visual symptoms	1997
Ritonavir	—	Norvir	Same plus neuropathy and visual symptoms	1996
Saquinavir	—	Invirase	Same plus neuropathy	1995
Tipranavir	—	Aptivus	Same plus neuropathy	2006
Integrase Inhibitors				
Raltegravir	—	Isentress	Muscle necrosis	2007
Dolutegravir	—	Tivicay	—	2013
Entry Inhibitors				
Maraviroc	—	Selzentry	—	2008
Fusion Inhibitors				
Enfuvirtide	—	Fuzeon	Sleep disruption	2007
Combination Drugs				
Lamivudine/zidovudine	—	Combivir	See above	1997
Abacavir/lamivudine	—	Epzicom	See above	2005
Abacavir/lamivudine/zidovudine	—	Trizivir	See above	2000
Emtricitabine/tenofovir	—	Truvada	Lactic acidosis	2004
Emtricitabine/tenofovir/efavirenz	—	Atripla	Insomnia, hallucinations	2006
Lopinavir/ritonavir	—	Kaletra	Same as above	2000
Emtricitabine/rilpivirine/tenofovir	—	Complera	See above	2011
Elvitegravir, cobicistat, emtricitabine, tenofovir	—	Stribild	See above	2012

[a]Rarely used in the United States.

Initiative to detect trends that will allow practitioners to best balance risks and benefits in treating HIV infection.

Table 67.8 lists medications in current use by class, with neurologic toxicities. The following is a brief summary of the most important toxicities.

Zidovudine causes a mitochondrial myopathy with ragged red fibers with muscle energy failure. Severe anemia (which can be corrected using erythropoietin growth factor) also contributes to fatigue.

The "D-drugs," didanosine (ddI), zalcitabine (ddC), and stavudine (d4T), cause a sensory neuropathy that is often painful and sometimes difficult to distinguish from the neuropathy caused by HIV itself. D-drugs are now rarely used because of the risk of sensory neuropathy.

Efavirenz, a nonnucleoside reverse transcriptase inhibitor, causes sleep disruption and nightmares that can lead to its discontinuation by patients.

Protease inhibitors (Pis) such as ritonavir and nelfinavir cause lipodystrophy. The cosmetic consequences often result in patients avoiding these drugs. The associated metabolic syndrome contributes to higher rates (16% per year) of myocardial infarction and, presumably, other vascular disease in long-term users. Some PIs, including indinavir, saquinavir, and ritonavir, are also associated with neuropathy, probably resulting from effects on dorsal root ganglia.

Muscle necrosis with myoglobinuria has been reported with raltegravir, an integrase inhibitor. Lactic acidosis is associated with some nucleoside reverse transcriptase inhibitors.

PRECAUTIONS FOR CLINICAL AND LABORATORY SERVICES

Strict observation of contamination management procedures or universal precautions is mandatory. Hospital patients with known or suspected HIV infection are not isolated unless they have respiratory infection, such as TB, or severe neutropenia. Strict precautions should be observed in handling all waste, body fluids, and surgical specimens. Gloves must be worn to prevent skin and mucocutaneous contact with blood, excretions, secretions, and tissues of infected patients. Goggles or glasses should be used if heavy aerosol contamination with blood or other secretions is anticipated (e.g., in the operating room). Masks are not needed unless the patient requires respiratory isolation for other reasons. Needles and other sharp instruments in contact with infected blood should be disposed of in proper safety containers. Health care workers should not recap needles to avoid needlestick injury.

The risks to health care workers are small but real. HIV seroconversion has been documented following needlestick injury or mucocutaneous exposure. The converse risk to patients from infected workers is exceedingly small, but HIV-positive workers should not perform or assist with invasive procedures in which cuts may occur. Postexposure prophylaxis with two drugs is recommended for HIV exposure through percutaneous or mucosal routes and with three drugs for significant blood exposure (visibly contaminated needle or device with deep penetration). HIV and hepatitis B and C serologies should be determined immediately. Problems encountered with postexposure prophylaxis include side effects of therapy, lack of efficacy, and false-positive HIV tests on rapid screening assays. Postexposure treatment is estimated to reduce HIV transmission risk by 80%.

HIV is readily inactivated by heat and standard sterilization solutions, including 70% alcohol. Special sterilization procedures may not be necessary but are often used.

OUTCOME

HIV-infected patients treated optimally can survive more than 20 years. They may die of HIV infection, causes unrelated to HIV infection, or of complications related to treatment. All patients need rigorous evaluation for systemic and neurologic syndromes irrespective of the stage of infection because of the risk for multiple, coexistent, or sequential problems, including disorders unrelated to HIV.

FUTURE DIRECTIONS

Great strides have been made in the medical management of HIV infection, with the prevalence of some neurologic sequelae seen with profound immunosuppression reduced. Nonetheless, HIV infection remains a serious diagnosis with common neurologic manifestations and is rapidly fatal in countries where access to effective treatment is limited. Therapy does not eliminate latent provirus and may fail if resistant mutants arise. Candidate vaccines are in clinical trials in areas of high seroprevalence and seroconversion. The complex biology of the virus and the host immunogenetic response to infection pose significant challenges to successful vaccine development. Additional strategies to "cure" HIV infection include the "shock and kill" strategy, which uses drugs to "shock" latent HIV virus into replicating, and then the active virus and cells producing the active virus would be "killed" by antiretroviral therapy, normal immune system processes, or other interventions designed to kill infected cells. Elimination of viral reservoirs including the CNS remains as potential problems to this strategy for "cure" and is a subject of significant active investigation.

SUGGESTED READINGS

Alfahad T, Nath A. Retroviruses and amyotrophic lateral sclerosis. *Antiviral Res.* 2013;99:180–187.

Antinori A, Arendt G, Becker JT, et al. Updated nosology for HIV-associated neurocognitive disorders. *Neurology.* 2007;69:1789–1799.

Behar R, Wiley C, McCutchan JA. Cytomegalovirus polyradiculoneuropathy in acquired immune deficiency syndrome. *Neurology.* 1987;37:557–561.

Bicanic T, Brouwer A, Meintjes G, et al. Relationship of cerebrospinal fluid pressure, fungal burden and outcome in patients with cryptococcal meningitis undergoing serial lumbar punctures. *AIDS.* 2009;23(6):701–706.

Birbeck GL, French JA, Perucca E, et al. Antiepileptic drug selection for people with HIV/AIDS: evidence-based guidelines from the ILAE and AAN. *Epilepsia.* 2012;53:207–214.

Boisse L, Gill MJ, Power C. HIV infection of the central nervous system: clinical features and neuropathogenesis. *Neurol Clin.* 2008;26:799–819.

Bozzette SA, Ake CF, Tam HK, et al. Cardiovascular and cerebrovascular events in patients treated for human immunodeficiency virus infection. *N Engl J Med.* 2003;348:702–710.

Centers for Disease Control and Prevention. Updated U.S. Public Health Service guidelines for the management of occupational exposures to HIV and recommendations for postexposure prophylaxis. *MMWR Recomm Rep.* 2005;54(RR-9):1–17.

Centers for Disease Control and Prevention. Racial/ethnic disparities in diagnoses of HIV/AIDS—33 states, 2001–2005. *MMWR Morb Mortal Wkly Rep.* 2007;56:189–193.

Cherry CL, Skolasky RL, Lal L, et al. Antiretroviral use and other risks for HIV-associated neuropathies in an international cohort. *Neurology.* 2006;66:867–873.

Chetty R. Vasculitides associated with HIV infection. *J Clin Pathol.* 2001;54:275–278.

Chow FC, Regan S, Feske S, et al. Comparison of ischemic stroke incidence in HIV-infected and non-HIV-infected patients in a US health care system. *J Acquir Immune Defic Syndr.* 2012;60:351–358.

Cornblath DR, McArthur JC, Kennedy PG, et al. Inflammatory demyelinating peripheral neuropathies associated with human T-cell lymphotropic virus type III infection. *Ann Neurol.* 1987;21:32–40.

De Clerq E. Emerging antiviral drugs. *Expert Opin Emerg Drugs.* 2008;13:393–416.

Durand M, Sheehy O, Baril JG, et al. Risk of spontaneous intracranial hemorrhage in HIV-infected individuals: a population-based cohort study. *J Stroke Cerebrovasc Dis.* 2013;22:e34–e41.

Eilbott DJ, Peress N, Burger H, et al. Human immunodeficiency virus type 1 in spinal cords of acquired immunodeficiency syndrome patients with myelopathy: expression and replication in macrophages. *Proc Natl Acad Sci USA.* 1989;86:3337–3341.

Ellis RJ, Rosario D, Clifford DB, et al. Continued high prevalence and adverse clinical impact of human immunodeficiency virus-associated sensory neuropathy in the era of combination antiretroviral therapy: the CHARTER Study. *Arch Neurol.* 2010;67:552–558.

Epstein LG, Gendelman HE. Human immunodeficiency virus type 1 infection of the nervous system: pathogenetic mechanisms. *Ann Neurol.* 1993;33:429–436.

Epstein LG, Sharer LR, Oleske JM, et al. Neurologic manifestations of human immunodeficiency virus infection in children. *Pediatrics.* 1986;78:678–687.

Gray F, Chretien F, Vallat Decouvelaere V, et al. The changing pattern of HIV neuropathology in the HAART era. *J Neuropathol Exp Neurol.* 2003;62:429–440.

Hammer SM, Eron JJ Jr, Reiss P, et al. Antiretroviral treatment of adult HIV infection: 2008 recommendations of the International AIDS Society-USA panel. *JAMA.* 2008;300:555–570.

Hollander H, Stringari S. Human immunodeficiency virus-associated meningitis. Clinical course and correlations. *Am J Med.* 1987;83:813–816.

Illa I, Nath A, Dalakas M. Immunocytochemical and virological characteristics of HIV-associated inflammatory myopathies: similarities with seronegative polymyositis. *Ann Neurol.* 1991;29:474–481.

Kwan CK, Ernst JD. HIV and tuberculosis: a deadly human syndemic. *Clin Microbiol Rev.* 2011;24:351–376.

Letendre SL, Cherner M, Ellis RJ, et al. The effects of hepatitis C, HIV, and methamphetamine dependence on neuropsychological performance: biological correlates of disease. *AIDS.* 2005;19(suppl 3):S72–S78.

Liner KJ, Hall CD, Robertson KR. Impact of human immunodeficiency virus (HIV) subtypes on HIV-associated neurological disease. *J Neurovirol.* 2007;13:291–304.

Luft BJ, Haffner R, Korzun AH, et al. Toxoplasmic encephalitis in patients with the acquired immunodeficiency syndrome. *N Engl J Med.* 1993;329:995–1000.

Makadzange AT, Ndhlovu CE, Takarinda K, et al. Early versus delayed initiation of antiretroviral therapy for concurrent HIV infection and cryptococcal meningitis in sub-saharan Africa. *Clin Infect Dis.* 2010;50:1532–1538.

Manabe YC, Campbell JD, Sydnor E, et al. Immune reconstitution inflammatory syndrome: risk factors and treatment implications. *J Acquir Immune Defic Syndr.* 2007;46:456–462.

Mateen F, Shinohara R, Carone M, et al. Neurologic disorders incidence in HIV+ vs HIV- men: Multicenter AIDS Cohort Study, 1996-2011. *Neurology.* 2012;79:1873–1880.

Modi G, Modi M, Martinus I, et al. New-onset seizures associated with HIV infection. *Neurology.* 2000;55:1558–1561.

Morgello S, Estanislao L, Simpson D, et al. HIV-associated distal sensory polyneuropathy in the era of highly active antiretroviral therapy: the Manhattan HIV Brain Bank. *Arch Neurol.* 2004;61:546–551.

Moulignier A, Moulonguet A, Pialoux G, et al. Reversible ALS-like disorder in HIV infection. *Neurology.* 2001;57:995–1001.

Murdoch DM, Venter WDF, Feldman C, et al. Incidence and risk factors for the immune reconstitution inflammatory syndrome in HIV patients in South Africa: a prospective study. *AIDS.* 2008;22:601–610.

Nath A, Jankovic J, Pettigrew LC. Movement disorders and AIDS. *Neurology.* 1987;37:37–41.

Navia BA, Cho ES, Petito CK, et al. The AIDS dementia complex: part II. Neuropathology. *Ann Neurol.* 1986;19:525–535.

Navia BA, Jordan BD, Price RW. The AIDS dementia complex: part I. Clinical features. *Ann Neurol.* 1986;19:517–524.

Ovbiagele B, Nath A. Increasing incidence of ischemic stroke in patients with HIV infection. *Neurology.* 2011;76:444–450.

Park MK, Hospenthal DR, Bennett JE. Treatment of hydrocephalus secondary to cryptococcal meningitis by use of shunting. *Clin Infect Dis.* 1999;28:629–633.

Petito CK, Navia BA, Cho ES, et al. Vacuolar myelopathy pathologically resembling subacute combined degeneration in patients with the acquired immunodeficiency syndrome. *N Engl J Med.* 1985;312:874–879.

Postels DG, Birbeck GL. Cerebral malaria. *Handb Clin Neurol.* 2013;114:91–102.

Price RW, Spudich S. Antiretroviral therapy and central nervous system HIV type 1 infection. *J Infect Dis.* 2008;197(3):S294–S306.

Rosso AL, Mattos JP, Correa RB, et al. Parkinsonism and AIDS: a clinical comparative study before and after HAART. *Arq Neuropsiquiatr.* 2009;67:827–830.

Rozenberg F, Deback C, Agut H. Herpes simplex encephalitis: from virus to therapy. *Infect Disord Drug Targets.* 2011;11:235–250.

Sacktor N, Skolasky RL, Tarwater PM, et al. Response to systemic HIV viral load suppression correlates with psychomotor speed performance. *Neurology.* 2003;61:567–569.

Sacktor NC, Wong M, Nakasujja N, et al. The International HIV Dementia Scale: a new rapid screening test for HIV dementia. *AIDS.* 2005;19:1367–1374.

San-Andres FJ, Rubio R, Castilla J, et al. Incidence of acquired immunodeficiency syndrome-associated opportunistic diseases and the effect of treatment on a cohort of 1115 patients infected with human immunodeficiency virus, 1989–1997. *Clin Infect Dis.* 2003;36:1177–1185.

Sanchez-Ramos JR, Factor SA, Weiner WJ, et al. Hemichorea-hemiballismus associated with acquired immune deficiency syndrome and cerebral toxoplasmosis. *Mov Disord.* 1989;4:266–273.

Satishchandra P, Sinha S. Seizures in HIV-seropositive individuals: NIMHANS experience and review. *Epilepsia.* 2008;49(suppl 6):33–41.

Schiffito G, McDermott MP, McArthur JC, et al. Incidence and risk factors for HIV-associated distal sensory polyneuropathy. *Neurology.* 2002;58:1764–1768.

Sellier P, Monsuez JJ, Evans J, et al. Human immunodeficiency virus-associated polymyositis during immune restoration with combination antiretroviral therapy. *Am J Med.* 2000;109:510–512.

Sevigny JJ, Albert SM, McDermott MP, et al. An evaluation of neurocognitive status and markers of immune activation as predictors of time to death in advanced infection. *Arch Neurol.* 2007;64:97–102.

Simpson DM, Bender AN. Human immunodeficiency virus-associated myopathy: analysis of 11 patients. *Ann Neurol.* 1988;24:79–84.

Sloan D, Dlamini S, Paul N, et al. Treatment of acute cryptococcal meningitis in HIV infected adults, with an emphasis on resource-limited settings. *Cochrane Database Syst Rev.* 2008;4:CD005647.

Smyth K, Affandi JS, McArthur JC, et al. Prevalence and risk factors for HIV-associated neuropathy in Melbourne, Australia 1993–2006. *HIV Med.* 2007;8:362–373.

Tan IL, McArthur JC, Venkatesan A, et al. Atypical manifestations and poor outcome of herpes simplex encephalitis in the immunocompromised. *Neurology.* 2012;79:2125–2132.

Thurnher MM, Post JD, Rieger A, et al. Initial and follow-up MR imaging findings in AIDS-related progressive multifocal leukoencephalopathy treated with highly active antiretroviral therapy. *AJNR Am J Neuroradiol.* 2001;22:977–984.

Valcour VG, Shikuma CM, Watters MR, et al. Cognitive impairment in older HIV-1 seropositive individuals: prevalence and potential mechanisms. *AIDS.* 2004;18(suppl 1):S79–S86.

Venkataramana A, Pardo CA, McArthur JC, et al. Immune reconstitution inflammatory syndrome in the CNS of HIV-infected patients. *Neurology.* 2006;67:383–388.

Wiley CA, Schrier RD, Nelson JA, et al. Cellular localization of human immunodeficiency virus infection within the brains of acquired immune deficiency syndrome patients. *Proc Natl Acad Sci U S A.* 1986;83:7089–7093.

Wong MH, Robertson K, Nakasujja N, et al. Frequency of and risk factors for HIV dementia in an HIV clinic in sub-Saharan Africa. *Neurology.* 2007;68:350–355.

World Health Organization. *Consolidated Guidelines on the Use of Antiretroviral Drugs for Treating and Preventing HIV Infection: Recommendations for a Public Health Approach.* Geneva, Switzerland: World Health Organization; 2013.

Prion Diseases 68

Lawrence S. Honig

INTRODUCTION

Prion diseases are a less common group of neurodegenerative disorders. There are several disorders distinguished by clinical presentation and pathoetiologic basis but marked by spongiform neurodegeneration and an unusual protein-based molecular pathogenesis. The particular agents responsible for the diseases are not nucleic acids, viruses, or living organisms but rather "*protein-aceous infectious* particles" or *prion* molecules, a concept developed and established through the groundbreaking research of Stanley Prusiner, who was awarded a Nobel Prize for this work. The prion protein is a specific, relatively small translational product of just over 200 amino acids length. This neuronal protein (prion protein [PrP]) is present in cells in its usual, "normal" cellular conformation (known as PrP^C) with a protein secondary structure consisting of about 45% alpha helical segments and very little beta sheet internal structure. However, in prion diseases, there is an abnormal "scrapies" or protease-resistant conformation (known as PrP^{Sc} or PrP^{res}), which is marked by 40%, beta-pleated sheet molecular architecture and has only about 30% alpha helical structure. In the prion diseases, there is an accumulation of the abnormally folded PrP^{res} protein causing nervous system dysfunction and destruction, through protein–protein interactions presumably within cells but ultimately spreading between cells. Specifically, misfolded copies of the protein cause conformation changes in normal PrP^C, converting it, in turn, to the abnormal form. There is an exponential increase in brain accumulation of abnormal prion protein, leading to rapidly escalating progressive nervous system destruction.

Prion diseases have a plural epidemiology: They may occur in both sporadic, nongenetic forms and genetic, familial forms, like many neurodegenerative disorders, but they may also occur as "acquired diseases," through transmission by iatrogenic, surgical, or cannibalistic exposures of persons to nervous system tissue of affected individuals. Hence, they are also known as *transmissible*

spongiform encephalopathies. The archetypical and most common of these uncommon disorders is Creutzfeldt–Jakob disease (CJD), named after two neurologists who described some cases of rapidly progressive dementia in the early part of the 20th century (which may not necessarily all have represented prion disorders). Although prion disease is sometimes easily recognizable, the differential diagnosis is often broad, particularly early in the course of the disease. The rapidity of symptom progression, together with the fact that different alternative diagnoses may have specific effective treatments, makes expeditious recognition and diagnosis particular important for this set of disorders.

EPIDEMIOLOGY

Prion diseases can be classified by their clinical-epidemiologic bases. Prion diseases may occur as sporadic genetic or acquired forms (Table 68.1). The hallmark of sporadic CJD (sCJD) is generally a rapidly progressive dementia, typically with gait dysfunction, although there are other rarer clinical phenotypes such as sporadic fatal insomnia (sFI). There are three distinct clinical forms of genetic prion diseases: Familial CJD (fCJD) clinical presentation is like that of sCJD; Gerstmann–Sträussler–Scheinker (GSS) disease is typically marked more by ataxia; and familial fatal insomnia is marked by severe insomnia and autonomic changes. Acquired CJD, transmitted through exposure to prions, was first described in the disease Kuru, discovered in New Guinea during the mid-20th century. Transmitted by ritual cannibalism, this disease has fortunately since vanished. Other forms of acquired disease include iatrogenic CJD (iCJD) transmitted through medical products, grafts, or transplants and variant CJD transmitted via consumption of tissues of cows who had bovine prion disease.

CJD occurs across all human populations, with an incidence of about 1.5 cases per million individuals per year, or about 400 persons per year in the United States. It is an uncommon

TABLE 68.1 Prion Disease Classification

Category	Name of Disorder or Syndrome	Abbreviation	Subtypes
Sporadic	Sporadic Creutzfeldt–Jakob disease	sCJD	Includes Heidenhain and Brownell–Oppenheimer variants
	Sporadic fatal insomnia	sFI	—
	Variable protease-sensitive prionopathy	VPSPr	—
Genetic	Familial CJD	fCJD	Missense, octapeptide repeat mutations
	Gerstmann–Sträussler–Scheinker syndrome	GSS	—
	Fatal familial insomnia	FFI	—
Acquired	Variant CJD	vCJD	—
	Kuru	Kuru	—
	Iatrogenic CJD	iCJD	Human growth hormone, dural and corneal transplants, reused depth electrodes

dementia. Compared to the approximately 1.5 per thousand individuals per year (500,000 in the United States) who develop Alzheimer disease, CJD is a condition with a thousandfold less common incidence. However, because the survival after a diagnosis of CJD is typically less than 1 year, whereas that for Alzheimer disease may be 20 years, the prevalence of CJD among living persons is still rarer. Among the 6 million Americans with dementia, the large majority of whom have Alzheimer disease, only about a few hundred have CJD, or about 1 in 20,000. Conversely, because of the short survival time for CJD, a higher proportion, nearly 1 in 1,000 deaths of persons with dementia each year are due to CJD. As a proportion of the total number of deaths in the nation, CJD represents about 1 in 10,000 deaths, despite having an incidence of only about 1.5 in a million. There has been increased attention and interest in the prion disorders, but there is no evidence that sCJD has had increased incidence over the decades. There has been a mildly increasing secular trend in the annual death rate in the United States over the past 30 years from about 0.9 cases per million to about 1.5 cases per million population, but this is almost certainly due to increased ascertainment rather than increased disease incidence.

SPORADIC CREUTZFELDT–JAKOB DISEASE

sCJD represents approximately 85% to 90% of prion disease. This disorder occurs without any known risk factor other than age. sCJD is very uncommon before the fourth decade of life and is principally found in the age range of 50 to 80 years. However, it is likely that the disease is clinically overlooked in the extreme elderly, so although it is clear that the age-specific incidence increases in the middle years, from age 30 to 60 years, it is not certain that the age-specific incidence declines among the older old (e.g., older than age 80 years). CJD incidence and prevalence are equal regarding gender, affecting males and females equally. U.S. statistics do show a somewhat higher rate of CJD in whites than African-Americans, but this may be due to disparities in dementia care and diagnosis. Because there are no known environmental risk factors, it is not known why individuals develop sCJD, but presumably the disease represents the consequence of a stochastic accident in which there was age-dependent initial abnormal folding of prion protein, leading to inexorable disease. There is a single nucleotide polymorphism at the prion protein codon 129, with alleles coding for either methionine (M) or valine (V), which does affect risk. CJD is more common among codon 129 homozygotes (MM or VV) than heterozygotes (MV). In the North American and European populations, only about 50% of the individuals are homozygotes at codon 129, whereas over 80% of sCJD cases are homozygous at codon 129. Thus, there is some protection for persons from being heterozygous at the codon 129 polymorphism.

PRION DISEASE OF GENETIC ORIGIN

Whether presenting as dementia (fCJD) or ataxia (GSS), genetically transmitted prion disease represents only about 10% to 15% of prion disease cases. In genetic or familial prion disease, there is a mutation in the prion protein gene (PRNP) which causes with very high likelihood the eventual production of misfolded prion proteins leading to the progressive spongiform disease. There are about 30 such mutations, nearly all missense mutations and there is one portion of the gene which has an octapeptide repeat of variable length. Penetrance of the prion mutations is usually complete. The clinical expression of fCJD is less affected by codon 129 homozygosity, but for certain mutations, the clinical phenotype may depend on the cis-genotype at codon 129. Overall, the phenotype of fCJD is similar to sCJD, but onset is often at an earlier age (e.g., 30 to 50 years) and the disease course for some mutations may be more protracted in duration—up to more than 20 years.

ACQUIRED CREUTZFELDT–JAKOB DISEASE

iCJD in which CJD is acquired through transmission of infective prions via medical substances or procedures is very uncommon, currently representing less than 1% of prion disease in the United States. Rare events of transmission of CJD by exposure to contaminated neurosurgical instruments, electroencephalography (EEG) depth electrodes, or corneal transplants have been described. The vast majority of iCJD occurred as a consequence of administration of human-derived pituitary growth hormones, before modern recombinant DNA-based pharmaceutical production, and from the neurosurgical use of human dural grafts. Since the understanding of these risks, iCJD has nearly vanished. Human-to-human transmissibility of prion disease was first evident in the disease kuru, a predominantly ataxic disorder in certain tribal regions of New Guinea. This disorder arose in the 1950s, reaching a prevalence in certain tribes as high as 2% but has now been eliminated, with the recognition that this disorder was due to exposure of individuals to brain tissue prepared because of ritual cannibalistic practices, since discontinued. There is no demonstrated risk of CJD transmission from saliva, tears, urine, or feces. Blood has not shown any transmissibility for sCJD, although there is evidence that variant CJD can be transmitted through blood transfusions. Studies have not shown any increased risk of CJD to medical personnel.

VARIANT CREUTZFELDT–JAKOB DISEASE

Variant CJD disorder typically affects younger persons. It first appeared in the United Kingdom in the 1990s and was rapidly linked to the immediately prior epidemic in the same nation of prion disease in cows, known as *bovine spongiform encephalopathy* (BSE). It is clear that exposure of people to abnormal cow prions, almost certainly through the human gastrointestinal tract, caused a tiny proportion of individuals so exposed to develop a lethal prion disease, originally known as *new variant CJD*, now known as *variant CJD* (vCJD). Initially, there were enormous fears that this disease might spread widely. However, over the past 20 years, this epidemic of disease has been small, amounting to a world total of less than 300 cases, including about 200 in the United Kingdom, and scattered cases elsewhere in the world. There has not been one "endogenous" case in the United States, that is, in persons who have not also lived in affected regions such as the United Kingdom. The incidence of vCJD in the United Kingdom rose to as high as 20 to 30 persons per year but is now less than 1 person per year. The epidemiology of this disorder was different from sCJD, in that the disease affected younger persons, almost all between the ages of 10 and 50 years and only affected persons homozygous at prion codon 129, with apparent complete protection by heterozygosity (MV genotype) at codon 129.

PRION DISEASES IN OTHER SPECIES

Scrapie, a disease of sheep and goats, has likely been known since biblical times. Cows can develop BSE. Other ungulate mammals also have prion disease, including deer, elk, and moose, which develop the cervid disorder, chronic wasting disease (CWD). Experimentally, or through consumption of prion disease-affected animal tissues, prion disease can be seen in a numerous species. These diseases include transmissible mink encephalopathy (TME), feline spongiform encephalopathy (FSE), and exotic ungulate spongiform encephalopathy (EUE) in nyala, oryx, and greater kudu.

PATHOBIOLOGY

Prion protein is a normal cellular protein, which is most expressed in the nervous system, and localizes to the synaptic regions, although its function is unknown. Prion protein belongs to the larger family of genes known as *cluster of differentiation* (CD) genes, many of whose members are found in cells of the immune lineage and whose functions may include cell–cell interactions and signaling. Presence of prion protein in various other bodily tissues likely relates to expression in cells of lymphatic lineage. The relative paucity of prion protein in non-neural tissues likely explains the confinement of prion disease symptoms to the nervous system. It also explains the lack of any demonstrable transmission from person to person, other than through exposure to nervous system tissues (which have included brain, pituitary, dura, and cornea). It is likely that in individuals developing sCJD, chance explains a rare spontaneous conversion of PrP^C to PrP^{res}. However, once PrP^{res} is formed, there is an escalating production of more PrP^{res} through the process of protein–protein induced conformational change mentioned earlier. This process can be shown to occur in vitro, in culture, and in animal models.

A number of observations have established the protein-based nature of the disease process. Injection of PrP^{res} into experimental animals in their brains or even elsewhere (in sufficient quantities) results in prion degenerative brain disease. The transmissible agents are not destroyed by nuclease enzymes that inactivate DNA or RNA nor by ultraviolet or X-irradiation and because of its folded state, is resistant to proteases. However, prions are inactivated by destructive/denaturing agents such as concentrated formic acid, phenol, bleach, or sodium hydroxide (lye) as well as by extreme dry heat (600°C). Although injected PrP^{res} causes prion degeneration and death in normal mice, mice that are genetic knockouts for the prion gene do not have prion degeneration, regardless of the amount of PrP^{res} they are administered, because they have no PrP^C which can be converted.

Prion proteins are highly conserved, but interspecies differences do provide a barrier to transmissibility. Exposure to or consumption tissues from sheep with prion disease (scrapies) has never been associated with human prion disease. In addition, in experimental animal systems, it can be shown that there is a greater barrier to transmission if the prion agent is from a molecularly more distant species. However, it is clear that bovine prion protein is sufficiently similar to human prions, as to allow transmission of BSE to humans. The small but prolonged epidemic of vCJD resulted from a preceding epidemic of BSE in cattle. Evidence to date indicates that in some persons, consumption of bovine material, likely containing nervous system tissue, led to vCJD, through a process of transluminal gastrointestinal lymphatic-mediated transmission to the nervous system. In vCJD, but not sCJD or fCJD, abnormal prion protein can be shown to be present in lymphoid-containing extraneural tissues, including blood, tonsils, and appendix.

CLINICAL MANIFESTATIONS

SPORADIC CREUTZFELDT–JAKOB DISEASE

The classic clinical manifestations of CJD are the triad of rapidly progressive dementia, myoclonus, and ataxia. At earliest presentation, only one or none of these symptoms may be present. However, in any patient with rapid appearance of one of these symptoms, without other obvious explanation, particularly in the age range of 40 to 80 years, the possibility of prion disease should be considered. The most important clinical manifestation is unexplained rapid but incremental (noncatastrophic) progressive cognitive or motoric impairment over a period of weeks to months. However, the earliest symptoms may be very vague, constitutional (fatigue, insomnia, anorexia), or neuropsychiatric (apathy, depression, anxiety, personality change, or emotional lability).

Symptoms

The dementia of sporadic and fCJD is typically "cortical" with impairments in memory, concentration, language, praxis, or visuoperception. However, true episodic memory impairment, as seen in Alzheimer disease, is usually less evident until later in the disease. Psychiatric abnormalities, including various behavior changes, and psychotic symptoms including hallucinations and delusions are not uncommon. Focal neurologic deficits including visual disturbances, focal weakness or sensory symptoms, and ataxia are common. Ataxia is usually of a cerebellar type, with gait imbalance more common than appendicular or ocular signs. Myoclonus is a striking sign, particularly as the rapid development of this movement disorder is uncommon in the absence of metabolic or drug effects. A particularly prominent feature in the later stages of CJD is startle myoclonus, in which an auditory or other sensory stimulus results in more or less generalized myoclonic movement. By the later stages of disease, myoclonus is present in more than 80% of patients.

Clinical Course

Neurologic deterioration proceeds with increasing rapidity in CJD. Caregivers often describe day-by-day deterioration, and physicians can observe this in hospitalized patients. Rapid evaluation is mandatory for anyone with suspected CJD. Ultimately, the entire course of disease from first symptoms to spastic quadriparesis, akinesia, and mutism and then to death, typically occurs within 6 to 12 months. It is not uncommon for it to occur in 2 to 6 months. In general, the clinical manifestations of sCJD and fCJD are similar, with similar disease courses. fCJD may present at earlier ages. For many mutations, the course from symptom onset to death is equally brief as for sCJD, but for some mutations, there may be more prolonged course that can range to as long as more than 20 years from symptom onset to death. Recent years have also identified a form of sCJD due to "variably protease resistant prion protein," and this form of disease may also have more protracted course than the more common sCJD due to completely protease resistant prion protein accumulation.

Variant Presentations

Distinctive clinical "variant" presentations of sCJD have been described according to the dominant symptoms at presentation, but these varieties of sCJD should not be confused with vCJD, a transmissible disorder related to BSE. The Heidenhain variant is marked by initial symptoms that are primarily visuoperceptual, including visual hallucinations or illusions, and/or the rapidly progressive development of cortical blindness. It is not uncommon for persons to have ophthalmologic evaluations and/or cataract procedures due to misdiagnosis of the symptoms as ocular rather than cerebral. Cerebral involvement of the occipital cortex is responsible for these symptoms. The Brownell-Oppenheimer variant is marked by prominent cerebellar symptoms, including ataxia of gait, and reflects greater early cerebellar involvement. Some clinicians refer to other variants of disease based on initial symptoms as "cognitive" or "affective" variants.

KURU

Kuru was the first transmissible neurodegenerative disease to be identified in humans. This condition, and its transmissible nature, was elucidated after its identification as an increasing epidemic among the Fore tribal peoples of Papua New Guinea in the mid-20th century. Carleton Gajdusek, who received a Nobel Prize for his discovery, showed with colleagues that the disease was spread through brain tissue and that it could be experimentally transmitted to primates. Kuru was marked by an asymptomatic incubation period of years to decades, followed by rapidly progressive symptoms of ataxia, gait disorder, instability, anorexia, and "shivering" (tremors and myoclonus). Subsequent progression included dysarthria progressive to muteness, dysphagia, urinary and bowel incontinence, and increasing cognitive impairment and dementia. Total duration of disease typically was about 1 to 2 years after symptom onset. The disease was disproportionate in women and children. It became evident that the disease was transmitted from person to person during the preparation, manipulation, and presumed consumption of human brain tissue from deceased individuals as part of ritualistic mortuary practices. These practices were eliminated after increasing Western exposure, and the disease slowly disappeared.

VARIANT CREUTZFELDT–JAKOB DISEASE

vCJD was first recognized in 1996 in Great Britain when cases of young-onset spongiform disease were identified. Typical symptoms differ from those of other prion disorders. Age of onset is typically age 10 to 40 years, almost nonoverlapping with sCJD. Painful sensory symptoms including lancinating paresthesias are common. Psychiatric symptoms including apathy, depression, and psychosis are common, occurring in nearly 90% of individuals at presentation. Neurologic symptoms develop, including increasing cognitive impairment, cerebellar ataxia, and often abnormal movements including dystonia, chorea, and myoclonus. Progressive neurologic deterioration results in death often 1 to 2 years after onset but sometimes with much greater duration of disease of some years. With the appropriate symptoms, vCJD should be suspected particularly in individuals who lived in the United Kingdom or other European countries between 1980 and the present, but the worldwide incidence is now less than five cases per year. All affected persons with vCJD are homozygous for methionine at codon 129. Other than the effects of age and codon 129 genotype, it is unclear why so few persons in the United Kingdom developed vCJD, given the very large exposure of the population to cows affected by BSE. There were hundreds of thousands of affected cows, and there was likely much exposure prior to recognition of BSE, its hazards, and control of the bovine epidemic, through elimination of ruminant tissues from cow food stocks and aggressive herd culling. There is frequent confusion by the public between sCJD and vCJD, known popularly as *mad cow disease*. Although vCJD does represent the only known trans-species transmission to humans of neurodegenerative disease, there has not yet been documented an endogenous case in the United States, originating from exposure to U.S. bovine products.

FAMILIAL CREUTZFELDT–JAKOB DISEASE

fCJD may present identically to sCJD. The presence of a family history, and/or an earlier age of onset, may be the only clinical indication. Genetic testing can confirm the familial, inherited basis. Familial disease is present in the United States and worldwide in about 10% to 15% of cases of CJD, but certain ethnic groups have increased prevalence of mutations. Specific mutations may present with particular phenotypes. For many fCJD cases, symptoms and duration of disease may be much like that of sCJD, although

as mentioned, age of onset may be earlier, and sometimes duration of disease may be longer. GSS syndrome is a rare prion disease characterized by ataxia and spasticity. Representing less than 5% of CJD cases (or an incidence less than 5 cases per 100 million), most cases are associated with mutations in codons 102, 105, 117, or 198 of the PRNP gene, which have 100% penetrance. Typically, individuals carrying a GSS mutation develop symptoms at age 40 to 70 years, and despite dominance of ataxia, there is heterogeneity of symptoms, partly depending on the mutation. In the most common form (codon 102 mutation), cerebellar ataxia and gait disturbance (ataxia, spasticity, rigidity) are the predominant symptoms, with dementia occurring later in disease, and myoclonus less common. In other forms, spasticity (codon 105 mutation), dementia (codon 117 mutation), or parkinsonism (codon 117 and 198 mutations) may be more prominently discriminating features. Typically, GSS is a slower prion illness, with duration of disease of 5 to 10 years before death.

FATAL FAMILIAL INSOMNIA

This very rare disease is transmitted through an autosomal dominant mutation occurring at PRNP codon 178 in the setting of a cis-methionine at codon 129. Age of onset is typically 40 to 60 years. Symptoms include progressive sleep disturbance and dysautonomia. Over the course of months to years, ataxia and dementia ensue. The sleep disturbance is characterized by a loss of normal circadian sleep–activity patterns. In addition to decreased sleep duration, dreamlike confusional states may occur during waking hours. Autonomic dysfunctions may include irregular blood pressure and heart rate, hyperthermia, hyperhidrosis, and excessive lacrimation. Pathologically, thalamic involvement is prominent.

DIAGNOSIS

Diagnosis of CJD or other prion diseases is based on clinical history and examination. Rapidly progressive neurologic symptoms without clear metabolic, infectious, or inflammatory cause should always prompt consideration of this category of disease. Although the triad of rapidly progressive dementia, ataxia, and myoclonus may be highly suspicious for prion disease, there are other disorders that can present similarly and prion diseases may present atypically without the classic set of progressive symptoms. Thus, paraclinical imaging and laboratory studies can be very useful.

DIFFERENTIAL DIAGNOSIS

Prion disease should be considered in the differential diagnosis of all rapidly progressive neurologic disorders. Demographic information can be useful in assessing the likelihood of sCJD because this disease is more common above age 40 to 50 years. Family history is key in ascertaining the likelihood of fCJD or GSS, which may present in the third or fourth decade of life. Typically, the history of acuity and symptom onset is most important. Although CJD presents with rapid deterioration, with a typical history of the patient being completely normal some months prior, there are other neurodegenerative disease that may have the appearance of rapidity, including Lewy body degeneration, which may be marked by fluctuations, and even unrecognized Alzheimer disease. However, more commonly, the diagnostic possibilities include neurodegenerative disease due to CJD versus some infectious or inflammatory condition. Although herpes or rabies encephalitis, or tuberculous, HIV, fungal, or other meningoencephalitides should be in the differential diagnosis, they are usually most easily diagnostically established or eliminated from consideration by history, blood tests, and, most importantly, cerebrospinal fluid examination. Most challenging in the differential diagnosis of rapid progressive neurodeterioration are the immune-mediated and other inflammatory encephalitis (see Chapter 71). N-methyl-D-aspartate (NMDA)-receptor antibody encephalitis typically occurs in persons younger than the age of 30 years so is uncommonly a strong consideration, depending on symptoms. However, voltage-gated potassium channel antibody encephalitis and other immune-mediated syndromes marked by antineuronal antibodies may strongly be in the differential. In rare cases, epileptic syndromes with persistent subclinical activity or syndromes of ischemic or metabolic changes may mimic CJD. Appropriate use of biomarker and imaging studies is key to rapid and accurate diagnosis; judicious use of brain biopsy may be extremely helpful.

CEREBROSPINAL FLUID ANALYSIS

Lumbar puncture classically was the first diagnostic test performed when the possibility of prion disease was considered. This is because so many other rapidly progressive dementias are marked by the presence of a pleocytosis or other signs of infection or inflammation. In addition, the presence of significant white cells in the cerebrospinal fluid (CSF) is virtually exclusionary of prion disease (unless a concomitant condition is present). In prion disorders, the CSF cell counts are normal, as is glucose level. Protein level may be normal or mildly elevated. A variety of biomarker proteins may be elevated in the CSF of patients with prion disease, relating to the ongoing acute neurodegeneration. Specifically, elevations of CSF 14-3-3 protein and tau protein, both neuronal proteins, may support the diagnosis of CJD

if used in the proper clinical setting. However, the levels of these proteins increase in CSF following acute neuronal damage of various causes, including infectious, inflammatory, traumatic disorders. These biomarker proteins are not the prion proteins themselves, and presence of abnormal levels of these proteins does not exclude other diagnoses, nor do normal levels exclude diagnosis of CJD. These CSF tests are much less sensitive, and may be normal in vCJD, and in more indolent cases of CJD including GSS, fCJD, and iCJD. Other marker proteins including neuron-specific enolase (NSE) are even less useful. Newly developed tests such as the real-time quaking-induced conversion (RTQuIC) assay attempt to actually assay extremely low levels of prions in CSF or other fluids such as urine or nasal mucosal brushings but are still unproven in both sensitivity and specificity. For the differential diagnosis of the patient with dementia, it is notable that typically in CJD, beta-amyloid 42 may be low, along with high total tau levels—thus, the pattern of these two markers may be similar to that of Alzheimer disease. However, usually tau levels in CJD are much higher than in Alzheimer disease, and phosphorylated tau is not elevated in CJD (unless there is concomitant Alzheimer disease).

ELECTROENCEPHALOGRAPHY

Abnormal EEG findings typically occur during the course of disease, but even "typical" abnormalities are not specific for prion disease. In sCJD, nonspecific background slowing is often seen early in the disease. Periodic, or pseudoperiodic, synchronous, biphasic or triphasic sharp wave complexes are common features (Fig. 68.1). They may be seen in the middle to late stages of the disease in up to

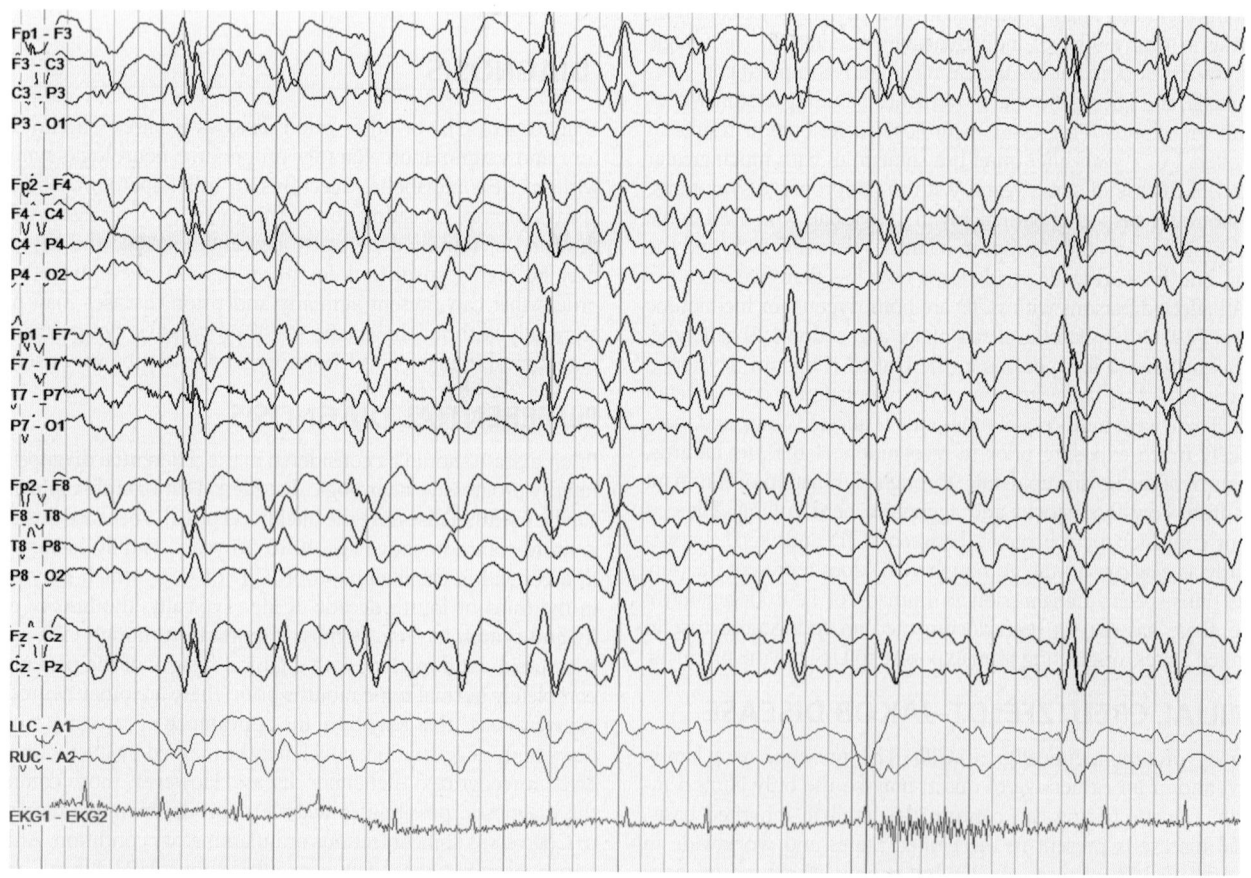

FIGURE 68.1 EEG tracings show pseudoperiodic generalized paroxysmal discharges. The EEG montage shows generalized paroxysmal discharges with a sharp, often triphasic, morphology that occur in a nearly periodic fashion of about one per second. Amplitude is somewhat greater in the frontal regions.

75% of patients. A slow background rhythm is noted universally in the terminal stages but is nonspecific. In the proper clinical setting, presence of periodic sharp wave complexes may strongly support the diagnosis of sCJD, although apparently identical-appearing complexes can appear in hepatic encephalopathy, herpes encephalitis, and rabies encephalitis, among other acute brain illnesses. Periodic sharp wave complexes are infrequently seen in iCJD and fCJD, and usually not observed in vCJD.

NEUROIMAGING

Magnetic resonance imaging (MRI) has become the most reliable marker of prion disease. Abnormal diffusion-weighted imaging (DWI) signal occurs in the majority of cases at disease presentation. The particular appearance of increased DWI signal abnormality with regional abnormalities in the cortical ribbon, and commonly, concomitant signal increased in the deep gray nuclei including caudate, putamen, and thalami may be quite characteristic (Fig. 68.2). Typically, there is little or no increased signal on corresponding T2-weighted images, particularly as seen on fluid-attenuated inversion recovery (FLAIR) sequences. Although, particularly later in disease, there may be some increased FLAIR signal in addition to the abnormal DWI signal. Despite the sensitivity of these signal abnormalities, they are not completely specific, with a variety of other ischemic, encephalitic, or epileptic conditions able to produce similar gray matter DWI signal abnormalities without significant T2 signal change. Thus, although MRI has become the marker most used for diagnosis of CJD, interpretation requires the appropriate clinical situation, and MRI does not alleviate the need for additional testing.

BRAIN BIOPSY

Biopsy has the potential to provide definitive diagnosis of prion disorders. Because of the transmissibility of prions, biopsy is done under general anesthesia, through an open, not stereotactic, neurosurgical approach through a small skull opening, using nonreusable equipment and full operating room infection control precautions. Risk of patient morbidity or mortality from brain biopsy is low and relates principally to general anesthesia and respiratory status. The histopathologic examination of brain biopsy tissue may not be definitive. Like for CSF, the presence of a robust inflammatory picture, including lymphocytic, microglial, or macrophage accumulations, strongly militates against a diagnosis of CJD. The typical findings in CJD may range from subtle to prominent—with spongiform change, including a diffuse vacuolation of the neuropil, as well as variable degrees of astrocytic gliosis and neuronal loss (Fig. 68.3). Prion-containing amyloid plaques consisting of aggregated prion

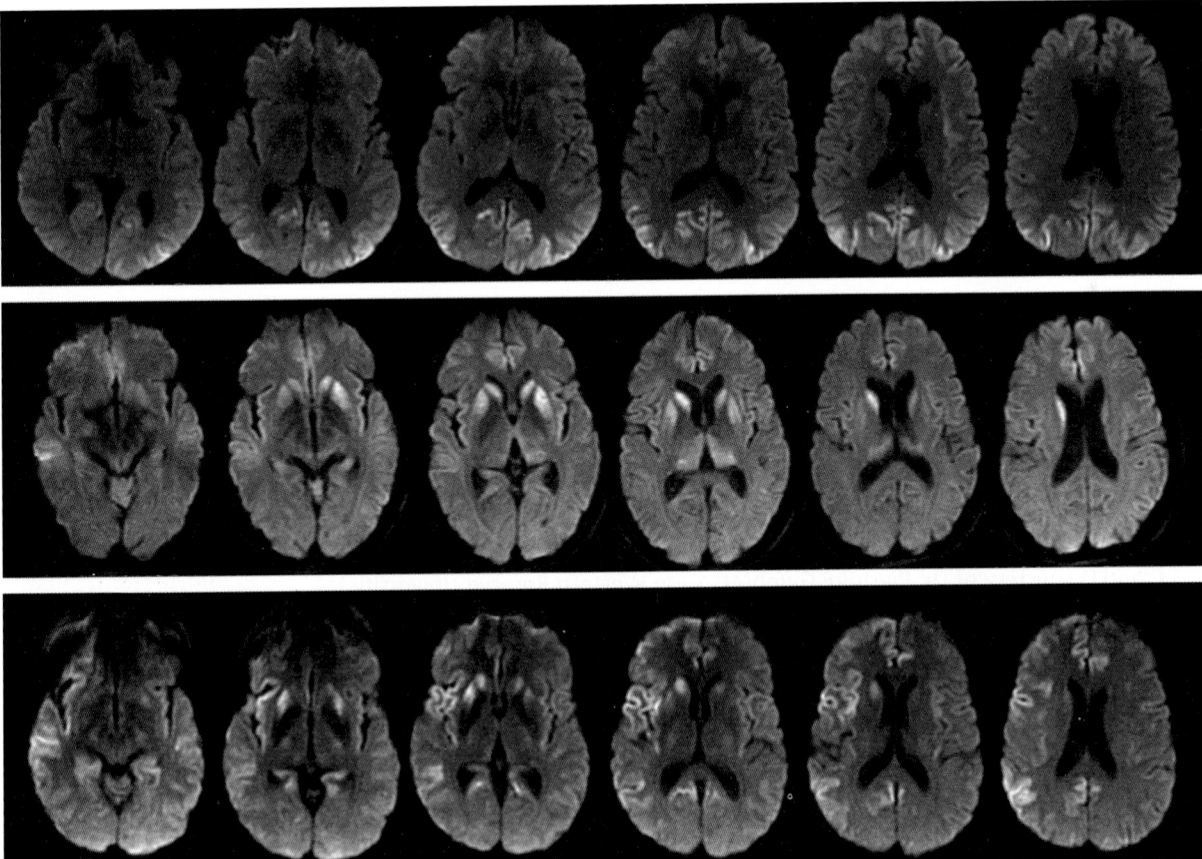

FIGURE 68.2 The three rows shown are from three different patients, each with definite CJD, having pathologic confirmation of CJD. These rows show the variable involvement of cortex and basal ganglia in different affected individuals. Each row shows six contiguous axial slices obtained using a DWI sequence. In the patient imaged in the *top row*, prominent increased signal can be seen in the parietooccipital cortical ribbon bilaterally, but there is no clear signal abnormality in the basal ganglia. In the patient imaged in the *middle row*, there is prominent DWI signal abnormality in the basal ganglia and thalami bilaterally but much less so in the cortical ribbon. In the *bottom row*, the patient's images show significant abnormalities in both basal ganglia and cortical ribbon.

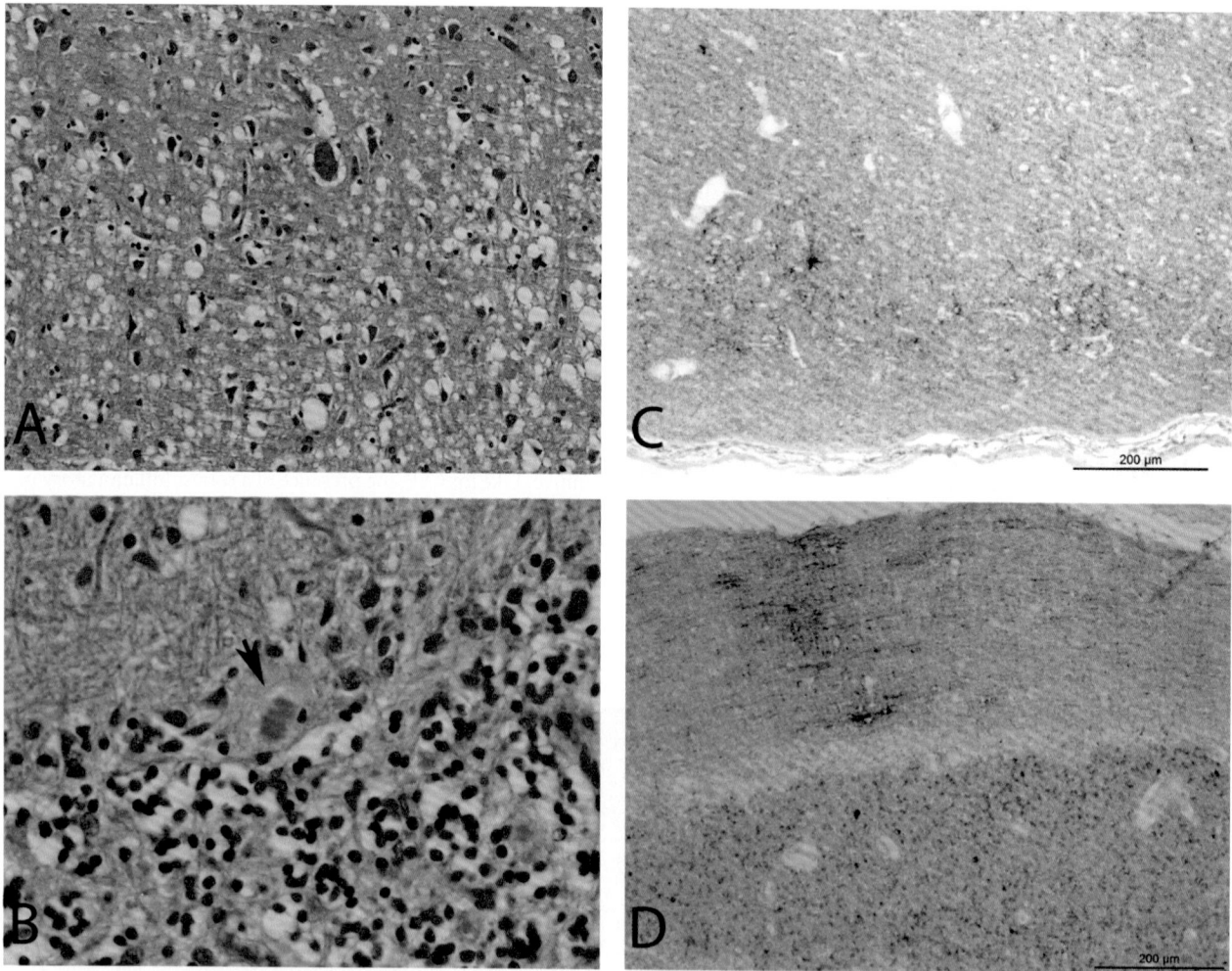

FIGURE 68.3 **A** and **B** show stained histologic sections of frontal cortex and cerebellar cortex, respectively, stained with hematoxylin, eosin, and Luxol fast blue. **C** and **D** show immunohistochemically stained sections of frontal cortex and cerebellar cortex, respectively, stained with monoclonal antibody 3F4, specific for PrP^res. **A** and **C** are oriented with white matter up and pial surface downward. **A** shows prominent vacuolation of the gray matter more than the white matter, typical of prion-related spongiform change. **C** shows brown staining of granular deposits of abnormal prion protein, variably aggregated but more prominent in gray matter than white matter. **B** and **D** are oriented with cerebellar molecular layer up and granular cell layer downward. **B** shows minimal spongiform change but a prominent kuru plaque (*arrow*). **D** shows brown staining of granular deposits of abnormal prion protein in the molecular layer. (A and B courtesy of Dr. Jean Paul Vonsattel, Columbia University; C and D courtesy of Dr. Pierluigi Gambetti, Case Western Reserve University.)

protein may rarely be seen. However, despite the lack a robust histopathologic readout, the availability of biochemical tests on biopsy brain tissue has resulted in near elimination of any "false-negative" biopsy results. Biochemical tests on biopsy brain tissue, including electrophoretic Western blot testing and immunohistochemistry for PrP^res are highly sensitive and completely specific for CJD and also enable molecular "typing" of the condition. In the United States, the National Prion Disease Pathology Surveillance Center performs Western immunoblot analysis to detect the presence of abnormal PrP. Different electrophoretic banding patterns have been elucidated through the work of Pierluigi Gambetti and colleagues in the United States and John Collinge and colleagues in the United Kingdom based on electrophoretic mobility due to the glycosylation status of PrP. These gel-visualized subtypes can be combined with codon 129 genotype (MM, MV, or VV) to further molecularly categorize the prion disorder. Different subtypes have somewhat

different histopathologies, brain regional predilections, and clinical course, especially duration. The advantage of brain biopsy is that a definitive diagnosis of CJD may be made, or alternatively, an alternate diagnosis may be established. The disadvantage of biopsy is that it is a surgical procedure with low, but some attendant risk, and that it is quite possible that a diagnosis will be made for which there are no disease-modifying treatment options. However, the value of a definitive diagnosis should not be underestimated because it obviates the need for any further clinical evaluations and investigations and gives certainty to families and medical professionals.

GENETIC TESTING

Genetic tests have the ability to definitively diagnose prion disorders only in those cases in which there is a familial inherited prion disease. Furthermore, despite increased speeds in genetic testing, it is not uncommon to have a patient die of disease before the genetic results are available. Thus, barring a completely clear family history of a known mutation, with clear clinical syndrome, other testing should still be pursued. Even in persons without family history, it is possible due to early parental demises from other causes, uncertain parentage, or even spontaneous mutation, that a genetic form of prion disease might be present. Thus, it is reasonable to offer all patients and their families, the option of genetic testing of the affected patient, after full genetic counseling of family members. Genetic testing can most conveniently be performed on DNA from blood leukocytes but can also be performed on biopsy or autopsy tissue to examine the PRNP gene for polymorphisms or mutations. For patients with a known family history of CJD, the presence of a known pathogenic mutation in the symptomatic patient is diagnostic.

TREATMENT AND OUTCOME

Prion disease is particular feared, perhaps more than possibly any medical disorder, because of its combination of rapidity and inevitable lethality. The disease is not cataclysmic, in that death can be anticipated over a period of weeks to months. However, it is so rapid that usually neither patients nor families have time to reflect, arrange affairs, or fully anticipate the disease progress and mortal outcome. Arriving at a definitive diagnosis during life, through brain biopsy, or in the case of familial disorders through genetic testing, can be helpful to patients and families, in obviating guilty thoughts regarding potentially missed avenues of investigation or treatment. Once a diagnosis of prion disease is well-established, there is no legitimate medical role for non-indicated medications such as antivirals, antibiotics, glucocorticoids, or plasma exchange. It is clear that such treatments never provide benefit, and indeed, they may often provide risk of side effects, in addition to being medically inappropriate.

Supportive care is important. This includes social support, with appropriate dissemination of information, and involvement of hospice services, whether at home or institutional. Medical supportive care includes physical aspects such as wheelchairs, hospital beds, and hoists as well as pharmacologic interventions including anticonvulsants such as levetiracetam or valproate to treat seizures or myoclonus, benzodiazepines to treat anxiety and myoclonus, neuroleptics to assist in agitation and insomnia, glycopyrrolate to treat excessive secretions, and other comfort measures. Discussion of end-of-life issues should not be ignored. It is important to address family concerns regarding nutrition, and to discuss for this disorder, the lack of any clear medical benefit in enteral feeding, and the futility of resuscitative measures in the face of accelerating catastrophic nervous system failure. Although the wishes of patients and their families are paramount, adequate educational efforts are important for optimal medical care. Prion diseases are, in most jurisdictions, illnesses that have mandated reporting to the public health authorities. Brain autopsy is encouraged because of its benefits with regard to disease categorization, surveillance, and confirmation of cases for families and physicians, particularly when biopsy has not been performed during life. Brain autopsy is also an important tool in the research and study of these diseases. Genetic counseling should be provided in families for whom the disease has a suspected familial or genetic basis.

There are no drugs or treatments proven to affect the outcome of established prion disease in either animals or humans. It can be theoretically proposed that disease-modifying treatment might be based on (1) preventing abnormal prion conformational change, (2) preventing prion–prion interactions, (3) removing abnormal prion proteins from the nervous system, or (4) alleviating the deleterious effects of abnormal prion protein. To date, a few small trials have been based on in vitro and animal model data suggesting that heterocyclic compounds might impede abnormal prion folding or induced conformational changes. Two trials of quinacrine, a drug, which may impede abnormal prion protein folding, have failed to show any evident beneficial effect on human prion diseases. Similarly, trials of tetracycline drugs have also not shown evidence of efficacy. There is substantial interest in the possibility of clearing prion protein through immunization strategies, as is being tested in other neurodegenerative diseases such as Alzheimer disease. In prion disease, to date, such investigations are preclinical, using animal models.

SUGGESTED READINGS

Aguzzi A, Nuvolone M, Zhu C. The immunobiology of prion diseases. *Nat Rev Immunol*. 2013;13:888–902.

Alcalde-Cabero E, Almazan-Isla J, Brandel JP, et al. Health professions and risk of sporadic Creutzfeldt-Jakob disease, 1965 to 2010. *Euro Surveill*. 2012;17(15):3.

Barash JA. Clinical features of sporadic fatal insomnia. *Rev Neurol Dis*. 2009;6: E87–E93.

Carswell C, Thompson A, Lukic A, et al. MRI findings are often missed in the diagnosis of Creutzfeldt-Jakob disease. *BMC Neurol*. 2012;12:153.

Chitravas N, Jung RS, Kofskey DM, et al. Treatable neurological disorders misdiagnosed as Creutzfeldt-Jakob disease. *Ann Neurol*. 2011;70:437–444.

Chohan G, Pennington C, Mackenzie JM, et al. The role of cerebrospinal fluid 14-3-3 and other proteins in the diagnosis of sporadic Creutzfeldt-Jakob disease in the UK: a 10-year review. *J Neurol Neurosurg Psychiatry*. 2010;81:1243–1248.

Colby DW, Prusiner SB. Prions. *Cold Spring Harb Perspect Biol*. 2011;3(1): a006833.

Collinge J, Gorham M, Hudson F, et al. Safety and efficacy of quinacrine in human prion disease (PRION-1 study): a patient-preference trial. *Lancet Neurol*. 2009;8:334–344.

Gambetti P, Dong Z, Yuan J, et al. A novel human disease with abnormal prion protein sensitive to protease. *Ann Neurol*. 2008;63:697–708.

Gambetti P, Kong Q, Zou W, et al. Sporadic and familial CJD: classification and characterisation. *Br Med Bull*. 2003;66:213–239.

Gambetti P, Parchi P, Chen SG. Hereditary Creutzfeldt-Jakob disease and fatal familial insomnia. *Clin Lab Med*. 2003;23:43–64.

Geschwind MD, Kuo AL, Wong KS, et al. Quinacrine treatment trial for sporadic Creutzfeldt-Jakob disease. *Neurology*. 2013;81:2015–2023.

Head MW. Human prion diseases: molecular, cellular and population biology. *Neuropathology*. 2013;33:221–236.

Head MW, Ironside JW. Review: Creutzfeldt-Jakob disease: prion protein type, disease phenotype and agent strain. *Neuropathol Appl Neurobiol*. 2012;38:296–310.

Head MW, Yull HM, Ritchie DL, et al. Variably protease-sensitive prionopathy in the UK: a retrospective review 1991–2008. *Brain*. 2013;136: 1102–1115.

Heath CA, Cooper SA, Murray K, et al. Diagnosing variant Creutzfeldt-Jakob disease: a retrospective analysis of the first 150 cases in the UK. *J Neurol Neurosurg Psychiatry*. 2011;82:646–651.

Heath CA, Cooper SA, Murray K, et al. Validation of diagnostic criteria for variant Creutzfeldt-Jakob disease. *Ann Neurol*. 2010;67:761–770.

Ironside JW. Variant Creutzfeldt-Jakob disease: an update. *Folia Neuropathol*. 2012;50:50–56.

Johnson RT, Gibbs CJ Jr. Creutzfeldt-Jakob disease and related transmissible spongiform encephalopathies. *N Engl J Med*. 1998;339:1994–2004.

Kretzschmar H, Tatzelt J. Prion disease: a tale of folds and strains. *Brain Pathol*. 2013;23:321–332.

Liberski PP, Sikorska B, Lindenbaum S, et al. Kuru: genes, cannibals and neuropathology. *J Neuropathol Exp Neurol*. 2012;71:92–103.

Lloyd SE, Mead S, Collinge J. Genetics of prion diseases. *Curr Opin Genet Dev*. 2013;23:345–351.

Macfarlane RG, Wroe SJ, Collinge J, et al. Neuroimaging findings in human prion disease. *J Neurol Neurosurg Psychiatry*. 2007;78:664–670.

McGuire LI, Peden AH, Orrú CD, et al. Real time quaking-induced conversion analysis of cerebrospinal fluid in sporadic Creutzfeldt-Jakob disease. *Ann Neurol*. 2012;72:278–285.

Muayqil T, Gronseth G, Camicioli R. Evidence-based guideline: diagnostic accuracy of CSF 14-3-3 protein in sporadic Creutzfeldt-Jakob disease: report of the guideline development subcommittee of the American Academy of Neurology. *Neurology*. 2012;79:1499–1506.

Parchi P, Saverioni D. Molecular pathology, classification, and diagnosis of sporadic human prion disease variants. *Folia Neuropathol*. 2012;50:20–45.

Prusiner SB. Biology and genetics of prions causing neurodegeneration. *Annu Rev Genet*. 2013;47:601–623.

Prusiner SB. Prions. *Proc Natl Acad Sci U S A*. 1998;95:13363–13383.

Prusiner SB. Prions: novel infectious pathogens. *Adv Virus Res*. 1984;29:1–56.

Puoti G, Bizzi A, Forloni G, et al. Sporadic human prion diseases: molecular insights and diagnosis. *Lancet Neurol*. 2012;11:618–628.

Roettger Y, Du Y, Bacher M, et al. Immunotherapy in prion disease. *Nat Rev Neurol*. 2013;9:98–105.

Sikorska B, Knight R, Ironside JW, et al. Creutzfeldt-Jakob disease. *Adv Exp Med Biol*. 2012;724:76–90.

Talbott SD, Plato BM, Sattenberg RJ, et al. Cortical restricted diffusion as the predominant MRI finding in sporadic Creutzfeldt-Jakob disease. *Acta Radiol*. 2011;52:336–339.

Thomas JG, Chenoweth CE, Sullivan SE. Iatrogenic Creutzfeldt-Jakob disease via surgical instruments. *J Clin Neurosci*. 2013;20:1207–1212.

Wadsworth JD, Asante EA, Collinge J. Review: contribution of transgenic models to understanding human prion disease. *Neuropathol Appl Neurobiol*. 2010;36:576–597.

Will RG, Ward HJ. Clinical features of variant Creutzfeldt-Jakob disease. *Curr Top Microbiol Immunol*. 2004;284:121–132.

Zerr I, Kallenberg K, Summers DM, et al. Updated clinical diagnostic criteria for sporadic Creutzfeldt-Jakob disease. *Brain*. 2009;132:2659–2668.

Zou WQ, Puoti G, Xiao X, et al. Variably protease-sensitive prionopathy: a new sporadic disease of the prion protein. *Ann Neurol*. 2010;68:162–172.

Multiple Sclerosis and Allied Demyelinating Diseases 69

Claire S. Riley

INTRODUCTION

Among demyelinating diseases, multiple sclerosis (MS) is the most common and widely recognized. It is the leading cause of nontraumatic neurologic disability in young people. The identification of a pathologic autoantibody has definitively separated neuromyelitis optica (NMO) from MS, where it was previously considered an MS subtype. Marchiafava–Bignami disease, a rare demyelinating condition often associated with alcoholism, is discussed here as well, although the mechanism is thought to be toxic rather than inflammatory. The discussion that follows considers each disease state separately with the unifying pathophysiology of demyelination.

MULTIPLE SCLEROSIS

MS is a chronic inflammatory demyelinating disease of the central nervous system (CNS) of unknown cause. The course is extremely variable, but most patients initially experience relapses with complete or near-complete recovery interspersed with periods of clinical remission. Although a minority of patients has only minimal symptoms, many become disabled in time as a result of incomplete recovery from relapses or conversion to a progressive form of the disease.

EPIDEMIOLOGY

MS affects approximately 400,000 people in the United States and 2.5 million worldwide. It is a leading cause of nontraumatic disability in young adults. The disease typically begins between the ages of 20 and 40 years. The first symptoms rarely occur before age 10 years or after age 60 years. Women are affected approximately twice as often as men except in individuals with the primary progressive form of the disease where there is no gender preponderance.

PATHOBIOLOGY

The etiology of MS is unknown. It probably results from complex interactions between environmental factors and susceptibility genes, which lead to an aberrant immune response and damage to the myelin sheath, oligodendrocytes, axons, and neurons.

Studies in a mouse model of MS, experimental autoimmune encephalomyelitis (EAE), histopathologic studies of MS lesions, and immunologic markers in serum and cerebrospinal fluid (CSF) of MS patients suggest that MS is an immune-mediated disease. A virus, bacterium, or other environmental toxin might induce an immune response in genetically susceptible persons. Antigen-presenting cells (APCs) provide relevant antigens to CD4+ T-helper cells in the periphery, which lead to their activation and the subsequent generation of autoreactive proinflammatory T-helper (Th) 1 and

17 subsets. B cells and monocytes are also activated. These autoreactive T cells interact with adhesion molecules on the endothelial surface of CNS venules and, with antibodies and monocytes, cross the disrupted blood–brain barrier with the aid of proteases (e.g., matrix metalloproteinases) and chemokines. Within the CNS, target antigens are recognized (putative antigens include myelin basic protein, myelin-associated glycoprotein, myelin-oligodendrocyte glycoprotein, proteolipid protein [PLP], αB-crystallin, phosphodiesterases, and S-100 protein), T cells are reactivated, and the immune response is amplified. Proinflammatory T-helper cells proliferate and B cells continue their maturation to antibody-secreting plasma cells, whereas monocytes become activated macrophages. Together, these immune cells produce inflammatory cytokines (e.g., interleukin [IL]-12, IL-23, interferon γ, tumor necrosis factor [TNF]-α), proteases, free radicals, antibodies, nitric oxide, glutamate, and other stressors that collectively lead to damage of myelin and oligodendrocytes. In the appropriate cytokine milieu, CD4+ Th2 cells proliferate and secrete anti-inflammatory cytokines (e.g., IL-4, Il-5, IL-13, and transforming growth factor-β) that suppress the immune response. Depending on the location and extent of damage, demyelination may impair or block nerve conduction and result in neurologic symptoms. With a loss of trophic support from oligodendrocytes, axons may degenerate to cause irreversible neurologic deficits. Spontaneous improvement of symptoms is attributed to resolution of inflammation, adaptive mechanisms (e.g., reorganization of sodium channels), or remyelination.

It had long been thought that Th1 and Th2 subsets arose from the terminal differentiation of the CD4+ T cells. However, a third pathway has been identified, induced by IL-1, IL-6, and transforming growth factor-β, and then expanded and maintained by IL-23, which is secreted by APCs. This third subset, a proinflammatory T-helper cell, is known as *Th17* because it produces IL-17. Th17 cells secrete a number of cytokines, including TNF-α and granulocyte macrophage colony stimulating factor (GM-CSF), which are critical for the development of EAE. MS patients have monocyte-derived dendritic cells that secrete higher levels of IL-23 than healthy controls. Higher levels of IL-17 mRNA-bearing mononuclear cells are found in the serum of MS patients having relapses than in patients in remission.

Although MS is typically considered a T-cell–mediated disease, a growing body of evidence supports a pathogenic role of B cells, including the frequent observation of intrathecal production of immunoglobulin in MS patients, identification of antibodies that react to specific myelin antigens within MS lesions, a pathologic pattern of MS characterized by antibody-associated demyelination (see the following text), and the discovery of B-cell follicles in the meninges of patients with secondary progressive MS. Pathologic studies have shown that B-cell clones are shared between the meninges and parenchyma of individual MS patients. Furthermore, B cells are efficient APCs and B-cell depletion is a promising therapeutic approach in MS.

Chronic demyelinating plaques appear translucent, sharply demarcated, and are most frequently found in the periventricular white matter, brain stem, cerebellum, and spinal cord. Lesions are characterized by extensive demyelination, gliosis, variable axonal loss, and a minimal inflammatory infiltrate consisting of T lymphocytes and macrophages. Demyelination accompanied by a perivascular infiltrate consisting predominantly of T cells, lipid-laden macrophages, and prominent reactive astrocytes are typical features of actively demyelinating lesions. Although demyelination with relative preservation of axons is often considered the pathologic hallmark of MS, axonal transection is common, especially in areas of active inflammation and demyelination. In autopsies of 52 MS cases, prominent cortical demyelination was seen with a mild but diffuse inflammatory infiltrate with microglial activation in normal-appearing white matter of patients with secondary or primary progressive MS. Cortical demyelination was rare in patients with relapsing–remitting MS.

Lucchinetti and colleagues identified four distinct pathologic patterns in an immunohistopathologic study of actively demyelinating MS lesions in 83 cases (51 biopsies and 32 autopsies). All four patterns contained an inflammatory infiltrate consisting of T lymphocytes and macrophages. The most common type, pattern II, was characterized by the deposition of immunoglobulin and complement. Pattern I was characterized by macrophage-associated demyelination. In patterns III and IV, demyelination was due to an oligodendrogliopathy. Pattern III was differentiated from pattern IV by a preferential loss of myelin-associated glycoprotein. Multiple active lesions were discovered in 27 autopsy cases. The same lesion pattern was observed within each patient, but there was marked heterogeneity between patients, suggesting that MS might have multiple pathogenic mechanisms. However, the results of this study were challenged by another autopsy series of 12 relapsing–remitting MS patients who died in the setting of an acute relapse. Most cases, including one who died 17 hours after an exacerbation, included lesions characterized by extensive oligodendrocyte apoptosis with intact myelin sheaths and slight or no inflammatory infiltrate. More than one of the aforementioned patterns were observed in some patients. The investigators concluded that pattern III lesions represent an early stage of lesion formation that precedes inflammation and demyelination. However, biopsy and some autopsy studies are susceptible to inherent selection bias and the findings may not be representative of typical MS.

Genetic Risk Factors

The strongest known genetic factor influencing MS susceptibility is the human leukocyte antigen (HLA)-DRB1*1501 haplotype. However, it is not essential for the development of MS, increases the risk two- to fourfold, and is present in 20% to 30% of normal individuals. Linkage and association analysis of 931 family trios (individuals with MS and their parents) screened 300,000 single-nucleotide polymorphisms and identified two genes outside of the HLA region, interleukin-2 receptor alpha gene (IL2RA) and interleukin-7 receptor alpha gene (IL7RA), which also increase the risk of MS. IL2RA encodes the alpha chain of the IL-2 receptor, which is essential for regulation of T-cell responses and has been implicated in the pathogenesis of other autoimmune diseases, including Graves disease and type 1 diabetes mellitus. IL7RA encodes the alpha chain of the IL-7 receptor. IL-7 functions in the homeostasis of memory T cells and may play a role in the generation of autoreactive T cells in MS patients. The effect of these allelic variants on overall MS risk is small but statistically significant. Additional genome-wide association studies have identified 110 MS risk variants in 103 loci, which are not within the major histocompatibility complex.

Additional evidence for a genetic predisposition includes increased risk in some ethnic groups (e.g., Caucasians of northern European ancestry) and decreased risk in others (e.g., Native Americans), varying prevalence rates among different racial groups in the same geographic location, a 20% to 40% increased risk of MS in first-degree relatives, whereas adopted children of MS patients have a risk similar to the general population, and 25% to 30% concordance in monozygotic twins compared to 5% in dizygotic twins. However, 70% of identical twins are discordant for MS, so environmental factors and other unknown influences must contribute to susceptibility.

Environmental Influences

In general, there is a latitudinal gradient with an increased prevalence of MS further from the equator in both hemispheres. Large differences in the frequency of MS are observed in some homogenous populations living at different latitudes. Several regions with similar latitude have vastly different MS prevalence rates, which in some instances can be accounted for by differences in ethnic susceptibility (e.g., Great Britain and Japan lie at the same latitude, but the prevalence in Britain is approximately 60 times more than in Japan).

Further evidence of an environmental effect comes from migration studies and apparent epidemics and disease clusters. In general, immigrants who move from one area to another before the age of 15 years acquire the MS prevalence rate of the new region. The altered risk develops gradually and may be imperceptible in the immigrants themselves but is obtained by their children. Notable exceptions include Israeli-born children of European and American immigrants who have a frequency of MS similar to that of their parents. Therefore, genetics may sometimes be more important than the environment. Migrating after age 15 years does not affect the risk of MS.

Apparent MS epidemics occurred in Iceland and the Faroe Islands after World War II, suggesting an infectious or other environmental cause. The arrival of British troops to the Faroe Islands in 1940 also brought the first neurologist to the islands, so that increased awareness of the disease and better case ascertainment may have led to the apparent "epidemic." However, the onset of the disease occurred after 1942 in all of the identified cases except for a few who had spent time away from the islands.

More than the expected number of MS cases has been reported in several areas, including Key West, Florida; Orange County, California; Los Alamos County, New Mexico; Hordaland, Norway; and Colchester County, Nova Scotia, raising the possibility of a shared environmental exposure causing the disease. Mercury toxicity, zinc, viruses, and other toxins have been suggested but no credible evidence has explained these clusters, which may have occurred by chance.

Multiple environmental factors may influence the risk of MS, including vitamin D, which has emerged as one compelling possibility. The active form of vitamin D, 1,25-dihydroxyvitamin D_3, has immunomodulatory properties and can prevent or ameliorate experimental allergic encephalomyelitis (EAE), a mouse model of MS. Numerous studies have found an inverse correlation between sunlight exposure (the most common source of vitamin D) and dietary intake of vitamin D and the risk of MS. The relationship to sunlight exposure may help explain the latitudinal variation of MS prevalence. Furthermore, a study of U.S. military personnel found that higher serum levels of 25-hydroxyvitamin D_3 (25[OH] D_3) were associated with a lower risk of MS. Similar findings in the

Netherlands were reported, but only in women, as well as a negative correlation between 25(OH)D$_3$ levels and disability. However, it is not known whether vitamin D supplementation modifies the disease in people already diagnosed with MS.

High-salt diet has been shown to increase severity of EAE and induce pathogenic TH17 cells in humans and mice *in vitro*. This has been hypothesized to explain in part the increasing incidence of MS and other autoimmune diseases in countries with "Western diet."

Among the possible infectious causes, the case for EBV is of interest. The frequency of MS is low in people who are seronegative for EBV, but the risk is increased in those who have had infectious mononucleosis. The evidence for other microbial agents is less compelling, but it is possible that a number of viruses or bacteria might act as a nonspecific trigger of MS in genetically susceptible individuals.

Physical trauma or psychological stress might precede the onset of either MS or MS exacerbations. Although temporal associations are common, a clear causal relationship is lacking. The Therapeutics and Technology Assessment Subcommittee of the American Academy of Neurology concluded that there is no significant association between trauma and MS onset or exacerbation. The committee also concluded that, although possible, there is no clear relationship between antecedent psychological stress and the onset of MS or exacerbations. However, a study in Israel concluded that stress associated with the 2006 war between Israel and Lebanon increased exacerbations in civilians with MS.

CLINICAL MANIFESTATIONS

A clinically isolated syndrome (e.g., optic neuritis, transverse myelitis, or a brain stem or cerebellar syndrome) heralds the onset of the disease in approximately 85% to 90% of all cases. A relapsing–remitting course ensues and is often followed by a progressive phase of the disease. Symptoms, which depend on lesion location and extent of tissue destruction, range from mild and intermittent to severe and persistent or progressive (Table 69.1). The disease begins insidiously and gradually worsens in the remaining 10% to 15% of patients, termed *primary progressive multiple sclerosis*.

Acute optic neuritis is one of the most common manifestations. Patients typically note unilateral visual loss that evolves over a few days and is preceded or accompanied by orbital pain that occurs with or is exacerbated by eye movement. Progressive visual failure over many years is uncommon. On examination, visual loss varies from mild to severe. Visual acuity of 20/200 or worse is found in about 33% of patients, but complete loss of vision is rare. Dyschromatopsia and a central scotoma or other visual field defects are common. A relative afferent pupillary defect (RAPD), which may be the only clinical evidence of optic neuritis, is invariably present unless there is a prior history of or current optic neuritis in the opposite eye. The absence of a RAPD in a person with acute visual loss raises the possibility of uveitis, which occurs with increased frequency in MS. Funduscopy in optic neuritis is often normal, but swelling of the optic disc is observed in 35% of patients. Retinal hemorrhages and exudates are uncommon.

Spontaneous recovery of vision usually occurs within the first month, even when visual loss is severe. Lack of improvement suggests an alternative diagnosis because 98% of patients with visual acuity 20/50 or worse improve at least three lines on a Snellen letter chart within 6 months after the onset of symptoms. Optic atrophy is frequently found after the acute episode resolves.

Temporary worsening of vision with physical activity was originally described by Uhthoff in 1890. Uhthoff phenomenon now refers to new or worsening neurologic symptoms that occur in some patients with elevations in temperature (often during exercise or a hot shower). Symptoms are transient and attributed to reversible conduction block along demyelinated nerve fibers.

Oculomotor abnormalities are common. Diplopia usually results from a sixth nerve palsy or internuclear ophthalmoplegia. Other forms of nystagmus (e.g., gaze-evoked or pendular) are also common. Smooth pursuit and saccadic eye movement abnormalities may be observed. Third or fourth nerve palsies, the one-and-a-half syndrome (reflecting damage to the parapontine reticular formation or the sixth nerve nucleus causing ipsilateral gaze palsy as well as impaired adduction in contralateral gaze due to damage to the medial longitudinal fasciculus), opsoclonus, and symptomatic homonymous field defects are rare.

TABLE 69.1 Classic Signs and Symptoms of Relapsing Multiple Sclerosis

Symptom	Sign	Localization
Blurred vision	Relative afferent pupillary defect	Optic nerve
	Disc pallor	
	Papillitis	
	Red desaturation	
Diplopia	Nystagmus	III, IV, and VI nerve nuclei and outflow tracts
	Internuclear ophthalmoplegia	MLF
	One-and-a-half syndrome	PPRF
Vibratory or electrical sensation with neck flexion	None—"Lhermitte sign" is a symptom	Cervical spine
Paroxysmal dystonia	Brief, often painful, usually unilateral muscle spasms	Corticospinal tracts
	May manifest as paroxysmal dysarthria or facial spasms	
Pseudobulbar affect	Laughing or crying uncontrollably without emotional congruence with the displayed affect	Brain stem, also frontal and parietal subcortical white matter

MLF, medial longitudinal fasciculus; PPRF, paramedian pontine reticular formation.

Facial numbness and vertigo can be difficult to distinguish from peripheral vestibular dysfunction, or facial weakness that is usually of the upper motor neuron type, but may mimic an idiopathic Bell palsy. Sudden hearing loss is uncommon and should raise the possibility of Susac syndrome. Intractable hiccups are rare but may result from lesions in the medulla or upper cervical spine. Intractable hiccups or vomiting should raise the possibility of NMO. Dysphagia is uncommon except in advanced MS. Limb weakness is common in MS and may occur during an acute exacerbation or incomplete recovery from an acute attack. The legs are more often affected than the arms and hands.

Approximately 70% of patients have some spasticity, which most commonly involves the legs. Spasticity is often accompanied by painful spasms and upper motor neuron signs. Spasticity often impairs mobility and activities of daily living and disrupts sleep. Gait abnormalities are common and usually a result of ataxia, weakness, or spasticity. However, in some instances, spasticity of the leg extensors permits weight bearing and improves gait. In nonambulatory patients, spasticity may interfere with transfers and personal hygiene.

An extensor plantar response is seldom the only evidence of corticospinal tract dysfunction. Demyelinating lesions in the anterior horn cells and dorsal root entry zones occasionally result in atrophy and hyporeflexia.

Paresthesias, dysesthesias, hypesthesia, or the Lhermitte sign (whereby neck flexion generates an electric sensation that usually radiates from the back of the neck to the lower back and possibly into one or more limbs) are common initial manifestations of MS and occur in most patients at some time.

An action tremor of the arms is common in MS patients. It is often accompanied by other signs of cerebellar disease, including gait ataxia, dysmetria, dysdiadochokinesia, and dysarthria. Tremor of the head, trunk, and legs is much less frequent. Incapacitating tremor, scanning speech, and truncal ataxia are seen in advanced disease.

Paroxysmal symptoms in MS are brief, repetitive, stereotyped attacks of neurologic dysfunction that are thought to result from ephaptic spread of abnormal electrical discharges from partially demyelinated nerve fibers ("cross-talk"). These discharges can arise from areas with acute inflammation and demyelination or chronic tissue damage. The symptoms usually last a few seconds to a few minutes and may occur anywhere from a few to 200 times per day. Attacks may occur spontaneously or be provoked by sudden noises, emotion, movement, hyperventilation, or tactile stimulation. The most common symptoms are trigeminal neuralgia and tonic spasms. Paroxysmal dysarthria, ataxia, diplopia, itching, paresthesias, pain, hemifacial spasm, and glossopharyngeal neuralgia are less frequent.

Trigeminal neuralgia occurs in about 2% of MS patients. The character and quality of the pain is usually indistinguishable from idiopathic trigeminal neuralgia. However, trigeminal neuralgia in MS is more likely to involve both sides of the face and is often accompanied by trigeminal neuropathy or other signs of brain stem dysfunction.

Paroxysmal dystonia, or tonic spasms, the second most common movement disorder in MS (only tremor occurs more frequently), are stereotyped, sometimes painful attacks of unilateral dystonic posturing of the limbs. They are occasionally bilateral and rarely involve the face. The attacks last between 30 seconds and 2 minutes and can occur up to 60 times a day. Tonic spasms are probably caused by demyelinating lesions involving the corticospinal tract. However, they are not pathognomonic for MS and are occasionally seen in patients with cerebral ischemia or spinal cord trauma.

Pseudobulbar affect is characterized by episodes of laughing or crying that do not coincide with the individual's emotional state.

This can cause significant emotional distress to both patients and caregivers.

Fatigue is one of the most common and disabling MS symptoms. It is out of proportion to physical activities and is typically worse in the afternoon. Fatigue may precede the first clinical demyelinating event by months or years in one-third of patients. The etiology of MS-related fatigue is poorly understood. No association exists between fatigue and disease course; disability; brain volume; or MRI lesion load, location, or activity.

Bladder dysfunction, which can result in failure to store or empty urine, or a combination of the two, affects approximately 75% of patients. In 15%, symptoms are severe enough to prevent the patients from leaving home or attending social activities. Demyelinating lesions above the level of the pons may result in detrusor hyperreflexia with uninhibited bladder contractions, which causes urinary urgency that is often accompanied by frequency, nocturia, and urge incontinence. Lesions involving the reticulospinal pathways above S2 and below the pons may also lead to involuntary bladder contractions or cause simultaneous contraction of the bladder wall and urethra, a condition known as *detrusor-sphincter dyssynergia*. Patients with detrusor-sphincter dyssynergia have storage and emptying dysfunction and a combination of urgency, frequency, difficulty initiating voiding, incomplete emptying, and incontinence. Damage to the upper urinary tract and kidneys as a result of increased intravesicular pressure is rare. Hypocontractility and failure of the bladder to empty properly occurs with demyelination of the lower sacral anterior horn cells. Complete inability to void is uncommon.

Bowel dysfunction often coexists with bladder dysfunction and is present in up to 70% of patients. Constipation, which may be caused by immobility, decreased fluid intake, or medication side effects (especially those used to treat bladder dysfunction), is common.

Sexual dysfunction is present in up to 90% of patients. It is most likely to occur in progressive MS but affects up to two-thirds of patients with relapsing–remitting disease. The most common symptoms among men are erectile and ejaculatory dysfunction. Women have difficulties achieving orgasm, decreased vaginal lubrication, and reduced vaginal sensation. Both men and women may have reduced libido. Physiologic (e.g., fatigue, weakness, spasticity, pain, hypesthesia) and psychological factors (e.g., depression, anxiety about bladder and bowel dysfunction) may interfere with sexual activity. Many of the medications commonly used to treat other MS symptoms, including anticholinergics, antidepressants, and baclofen, can adversely affect sexual function.

Depression is clearly the most common affective disorder in MS with a lifetime prevalence of 50% before age 60 years. Some patients experience depressive symptoms but do not meet diagnostic criteria for major depression. The etiology of depression is likely multifactorial with psychosocial and biologic factors contributing to such a high frequency. There is concern that the β-interferons may cause or exacerbate depression. Episodes of major depression may occur during periods of exacerbations, remission, or disease progression. Although much less common than depression, bipolar disorder, anxiety, pseudobulbar affect, and euphoria are also prevalent in patients with MS.

Cognitive impairment occurs in up to 65% of patients with MS. Short-term memory, attention, concentration, verbal intelligence, visuospatial skills, and information processing are the domains most commonly affected. Disturbances of language and immediate and long-term memory occur less frequently. Disability and disease duration are generally poor predictors of cognitive dysfunction, which can occur early in the course of MS. However, cognitively impaired patients have more lesions, more severe tissue damage, and smaller brain volumes than unimpaired patients as measured by conventional and nonconventional MRI techniques. Changes detected by magnetization transfer imaging in normal-appearing brain tissue may have a stronger correlation with cognitive dysfunction than T1 or T2 lesion load.

In most patients, cognitive dysfunction is subtle and goes undetected in the neurologist's office. The Mini-Mental State Examination is not useful because it may fail to identify nearly 75% of MS patients deemed to be cognitively impaired by detailed neuropsychological testing.

Approximately 70% of patients experience pain at some time. Pain can occur during an acute exacerbation (e.g., ocular pain with optic neuritis or dysesthesias with demyelinating plaques involving spinal cord), but almost half of MS patients have chronic pain. It is not a major problem for most, but 20% have severe pain. In addition to painful muscle spasms, paroxysmal phenomena, and the sensory symptoms discussed earlier, MS patients are more likely to have joint, muscular, and extremity pain than age- and sex-matched controls. Many patients also complain of neck and back pain, which may be due to posture or gait abnormalities.

Disease Course

No biologic markers or MRI features distinguish the several forms of MS. The current classification system is based on consensus and relies on the clinical course (Fig. 69.1). Appropriate classification

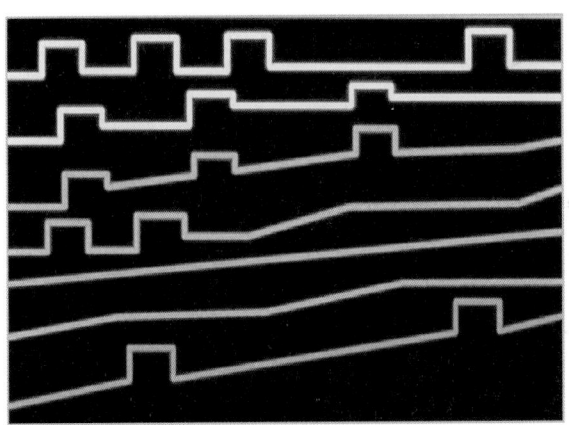

FIGURE 69.1 The course of MS has been divided into four subtypes based on consensus of specialists. Most patients begin with a relapsing–remitting course (RRMS). Many of these eventually follow a secondary progressive pattern (SPMS). Approximately 10% to 15% of patients have primary progressive disease (PPMS), whereas the progressive relapsing form (PRMS) is very uncommon. The *top two lines* show that disease is labeled as RRMS irrespective of whether recovery from relapses is complete (*first line*) or incomplete (*second line*), as long as a stable baseline is reestablished. The *next two lines* demonstrate that disease is called *secondary progressive multiple sclerosis* irrespective of whether relapses continue, as long as the disease is gradually worsening either between attacks or in the absence of attacks. The *next two lines* show that disease may steadily worsen (*first line*) or there may be periodic plateaus (*second line*). The *bottom line* shows progression from onset followed by the development of relapses. (Reprinted with permission from Lublin FD, Reingold SC. Defining the clinical course of multiple sclerosis: results of an international survey. *Neurology.* 1996;46:907–911.)

of patients is imperative for appropriate treatment with the disease-modifying drugs (see the following text).

Relapsing–remitting MS is the initial form of the disease in 85% to 90% of patients. It is characterized by acute relapses interspersed with clinical remissions. Symptoms from a relapse typically evolve over several days to a week before reaching a nadir. Recovery is variable, but approximately 40% of relapses result in persistent neurologic deficit and patients may accumulate disability in a stepwise fashion. When left untreated, most patients with relapsing–remitting MS ultimately enter the secondary progressive phase of MS, which is characterized by gradual deterioration with or without occasional superimposed relapses.

Ten percent to 15% of patients have primary progressive MS, which is characterized by continuous and usually gradual deterioration of neurologic function (e.g., a slowly progressive monoparesis). There may be plateaus and slight fluctuations, but relapses do not occur. Fifteen percent to 40% of patients who start with the primary progressive form later have an acute relapse, which may not occur for many years after the original symptoms. This type of MS is referred to as *progressive relapsing multiple sclerosis* and is the least common form.

Different mechanisms may be responsible for symptomatic worsening. An inflammatory component may result in relapses, whereas neurodegeneration may be responsible for progressive disease.

Pregnancy

Pregnancy is protective in MS, particularly during the third trimester when there is a 70% reduction in the annualized relapse rate compared with the year prior to pregnancy. However, when MS is left untreated, about 30% of women have a relapse in the first 3 months postpartum before the risk returns to the prepregnancy rate 4 to 6 months after delivery. These effects may be the result of changes in Th1 and Th2 immune responses mediated by estriol or vitamin D, both of which are markedly elevated during the final trimester of pregnancy and fall abruptly after delivery; other hormonal changes that occur during pregnancy may also play a role.

Women with relapses during pregnancy or in the year prior to pregnancy are more likely to have a relapse in the first 3 months postpartum than women without relapses during these periods, but it is impossible to accurately predict who will have a relapse. In an uncontrolled study, intravenous immunoglobulin (IVIG) ameliorated the increased risk of postpartum exacerbations. However, the results of a subsequent randomized, double-blind trial were not as encouraging. Furthermore, there is now good evidence from well-designed, large, placebo-controlled trials that IVIG is an ineffective therapy for relapsing–remitting and secondary progressive MS. Breastfeeding does not affect the postpartum course of MS.

Vaccination

Infections, including minor upper respiratory infections, increase the risk of MS exacerbations. Strategies that minimize the risk of infection should be incorporated. Concerns that vaccinations may trigger MS exacerbations are based on anecdotes. However, a prospective, randomized, double-blind, placebo-controlled trial, showed that influenza immunization does not increase the risk of relapse or disease progression and patients should be routinely vaccinated. Hepatitis B, tetanus, and varicella vaccines appear to be safe in MS patients. There are few data regarding the safety of other vaccines in MS, but patients who meet the CDC guidelines should be advised to have them. Patients treated with fingolimod or mitoxantrone should not receive live attenuated vaccines, as there is some risk of developing the infection the vaccine is meant to prevent, or they may have an attenuated response to the vaccination. It is probably best to delay immunizations for 4 to 6 weeks in the setting of an MS relapse because the goal of relapse management is to diminish the immune system's reactivity, and vaccination has the opposite effect.

DIAGNOSIS

The diagnosis of MS is established based on clinical criteria usually in combination with MRI. Examination of the CSF may be helpful. However, no single test result is pathognomonic of MS.

Imaging

Brain MRI abnormalities are present in more than 95% of recently diagnosed MS patients. Five to 10 new or enlarging gadolinium-enhancing or T2 brain lesions are identified for every one clinical exacerbation in patients with relapsing MS. Spinal cord lesions are detected by MRI in 75% to 90% of those with established MS.

Fifty percent to 70% of clinically isolated syndrome patients have asymptomatic T2 brain lesions, and 27% to 42% have clini-

cally silent spinal cord lesions. However, conventional MRI lacks pathologic specificity, and areas of edema, demyelination, axonal damage, gliosis, and remyelination all appear as T2 hyperintensities. Furthermore, there is poor correlation between disability and T2-weighted abnormalities. Nonconventional MRI techniques, including diffusion tensor imaging, magnetic transfer imaging, and proton magnetic resonance spectroscopy (MRS), have more pathologic specificity than conventional MRI and can detect and quantify tissue damage within visible T2 lesions and normal-appearing brain tissue. These techniques may enhance the ability to monitor disease evolution and understanding of the mechanisms that lead to irreversible disability.

On T2-weighted imaging, brain lesions are typically 3 to 15 mm in diameter, round or ovoid, and located in the periventricular white matter, corpus callosum, centrum semiovale, juxtacortical regions, pons, floor of the fourth ventricle, cerebellar peduncles, or cerebellar hemispheres (Figs. 69.2 and 69.3). Larger lesions in the cerebral hemispheres associated with mass effect, edema, or ring enhancement, which resemble tumors and are known as

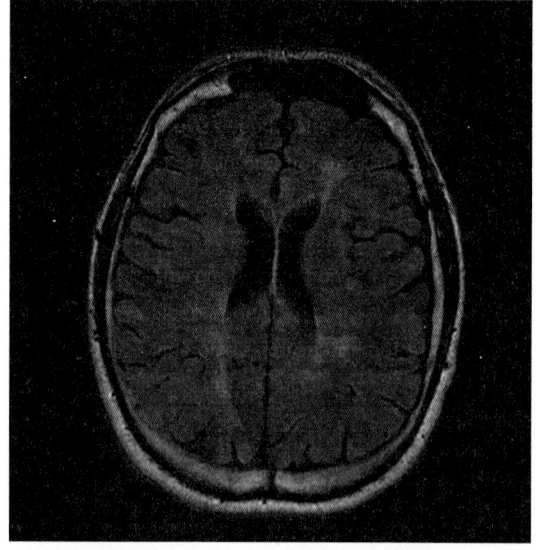

A

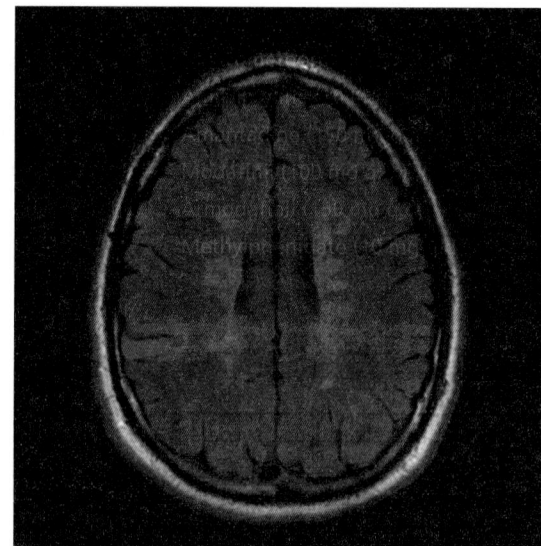

B

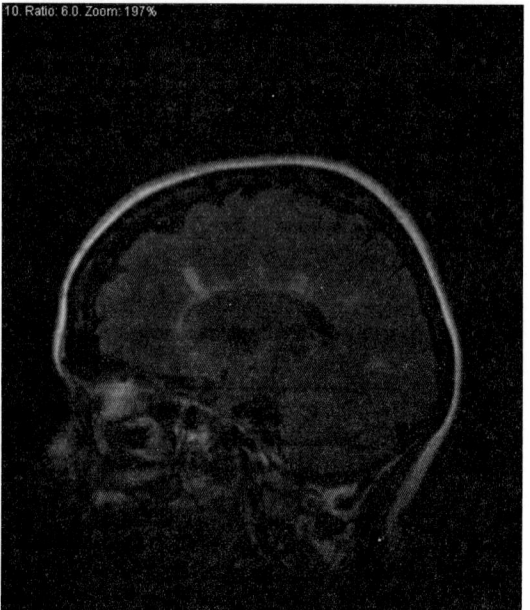

C

FIGURE 69.2 Brain MRI from relapsing–remitting MS patients. Axial **(A and B)** and sagittal **(C)** fluid-attenuated inversion recovery (FLAIR) images demonstrate multiple periventricular white matter lesions. Many of the lesions are oriented perpendicular to the lateral ventricles and are the MRI correlate of "Dawson fingers," which was originally a pathologic description of MS plaques. Also note the juxtacortical lesion in the right parietal lobe **(A)**. The location and morphology of the lesions is characteristic of MS.

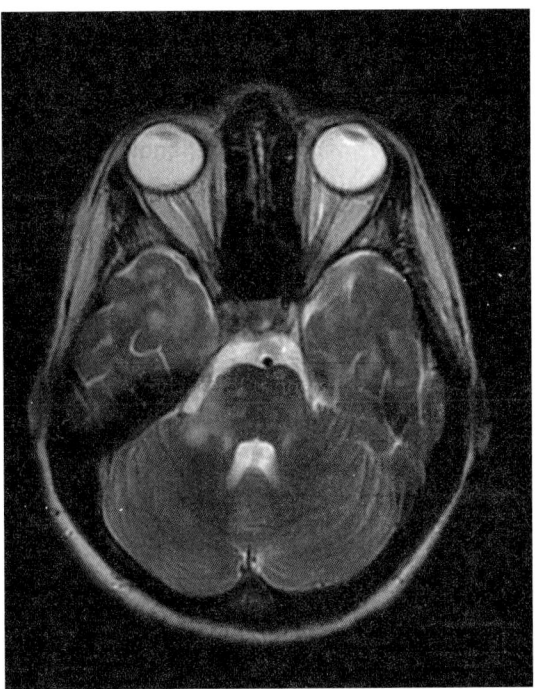
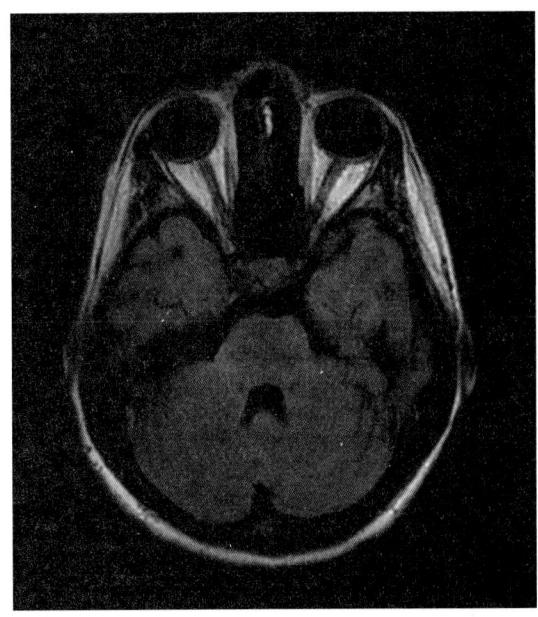

A   **B**

FIGURE 69.3 Brain MRI of the posterior fossa in an MS patient. An axial T2-weighted image **(A)** reveals multiple infratentorial lesions consistent with MS. The lesions are not well visualized on the FLAIR image **(B)**. Although FLAIR is a more sensitive sequence than T2 for demonstrating supratentorial lesions, it is suboptimal for detecting infratentorial lesions.

tumefactive lesions, are occasionally observed (Fig. 69.4). Cortical lesions are not well visualized by standard MRI techniques.

In patients with relapsing MS, gadolinium enhancement, which represents active inflammation and disruption of the blood–brain barrier, is the earliest phase of lesion development seen on conventional MRI (Fig. 69.5). Almost all new brain T2 lesions demonstrate enhancement on postgadolinium T1-weighted imaging, and 65% to 80% are hypointense on the corresponding pregadolinium T1-weighted sequence. Gadolinium enhancement typically resolves after 2 to 4 weeks. Persistent enhancement raises

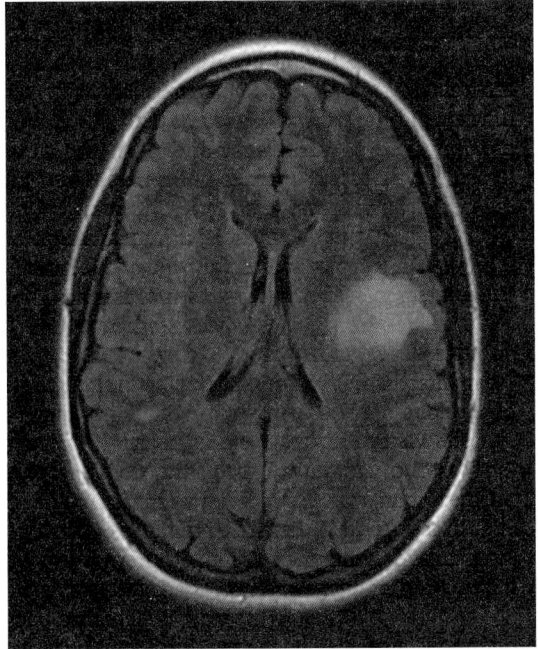
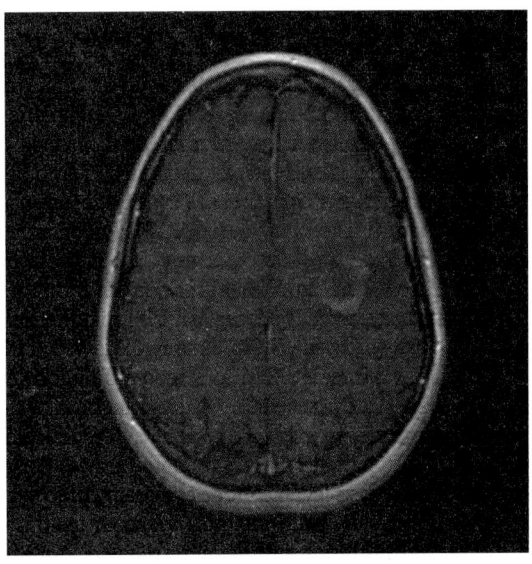

A   **B**

FIGURE 69.4 Brain MRI from a patient with relapsing–remitting MS. Axial FLAIR **(A)** and postgadolinium T1-weighted **(B)** images reveal a large ring-enhancing mass-like lesion with surrounding vasogenic edema in the left hemisphere. There is also a much smaller nonenhancing lesion in the right hemisphere. The findings are consistent with tumefactive MS.

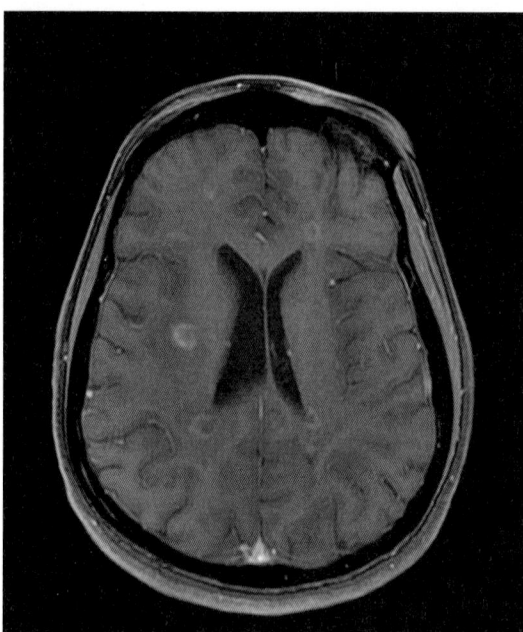

FIGURE 69.5 Brain MRI from a relapsing–remitting MS patient. A postcontrast T1-weighted image reveals multiple gadolinium-enhancing lesions. Gadolinium enhancement, which represents disruption of the blood–brain barrier and active inflammation, is the earliest phase of lesion development that can be detected on conventional MRI.

the possibility of neurosarcoidosis or neoplasm because only 3% to 5% of MS lesions enhance for more than 8 weeks. T2 lesions may become smaller, but they rarely disappear, whereas the majority of T1-hypointense lesions become isointense in 6 to 12 months, presumably as a result of resolution of edema and remyelination. However, 30% to 45% of hypointense lesions remain hypointense

and are called *chronic black holes* (Fig. 69.6). Chronic black holes represent areas of extensive demyelination and axonal damage and have a much better correlation with disability than T2 lesions, especially in patients with secondary progressive MS.

Spinal cord lesions are more common in the cervical than thoracic spine, appear hyperintense on T2-weighted imaging, and have a predilection for the white matter in the lateral and posterior columns. Adjacent gray matter is commonly involved. Lesions typically occupy less than half of the cross-sectional area of the cord and extend fewer than two vertebral segments (Fig. 69.7). Hypointense lesions on T1-weighted spinal cord MRI are uncommon in MS patients. Unlike gadolinium-enhancing brain lesions, active spinal cord lesions are frequently accompanied by clinical symptoms. However, asymptomatic spinal cord lesions are also common. Clinically silent spinal cord lesions are particularly useful for diagnosing MS in patients with vague neurologic symptoms and nonspecific findings on brain MRI because intramedullary cord lesions are rare in healthy people.

In general, relapsing–remitting MS patients have more gadolinium-enhancing lesions than those with progressive disease. Patients with secondary progressive MS tend to have more chronic black holes than those with the relapsing–remitting or primary progressive disease. Primary progressive MS patients are more likely to have few T2 brain lesions and diffuse spinal cord abnormalities. However, MRI characteristics are not diagnostic of the subtypes of MS—these remain clinically based.

Biomarkers

Examination of the CSF can aid in the diagnosis of MS and helps to exclude alternative diagnoses. CSF contains fewer than six white blood cells (WBCs) per cubic millimeter and normal protein content in most patients with a clinically isolated syndrome or established MS. A mild lymphocytic pleocytosis or elevated protein level is seen in about 35%. More than 50 WBCs per cubic millimeter or a protein content over 100 mg/dL are rarely observed and raise the possibility of an alternative diagnosis.

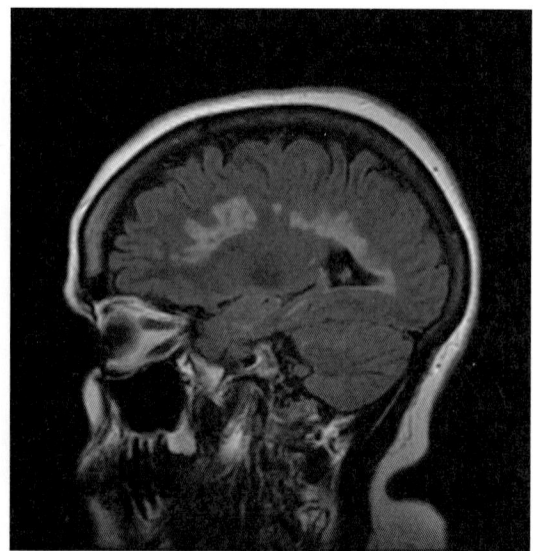
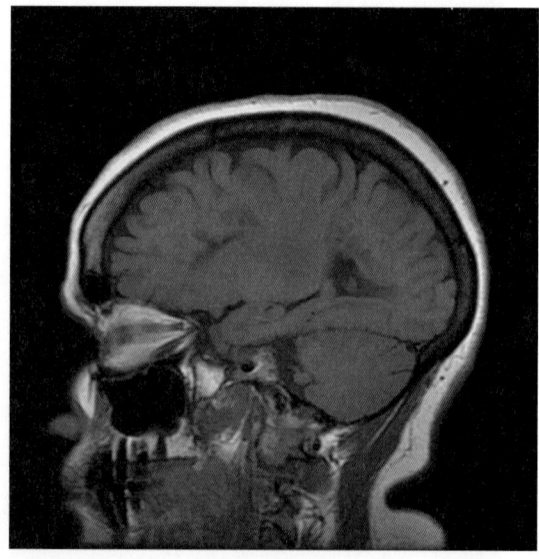

A   **B**

FIGURE 69.6 Brain MRI from a patient with secondary progressive MS. A sagittal FLAIR image **(A)** reveals multiple periventricular white matter lesions consistent with MS. Note that many of the lesions are hypointense on the pregadolinium T1-weighted image **(B)**. Persistent T1-hypointense lesions ("black holes") represent areas of significant demyelination and axonal damage and have a stronger correlation with disability than T2-hyperintense lesions, especially in patients with secondary progressive MS.

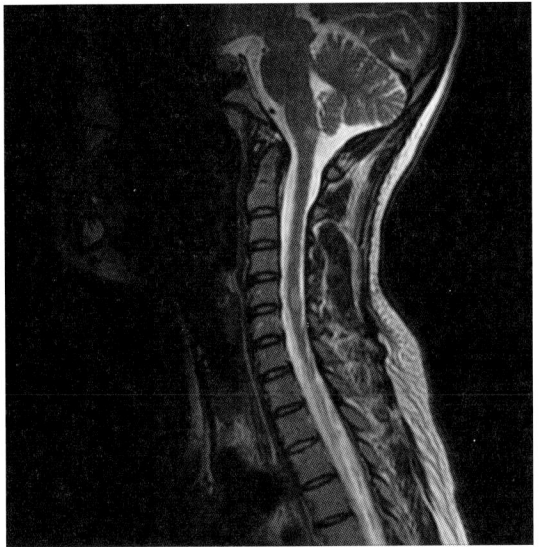
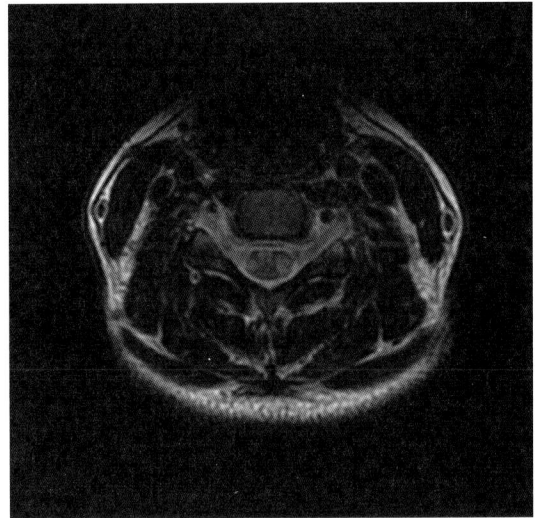

A   **B**

FIGURE 69.7 Cervical spine MRI from a relapsing–remitting MS patient. Axial **(A)** and sagittal **(B)** T2-weighted images reveal intramedullary lesions at C5–C6 consistent with demyelination. Also note the lesion at the cervicomedullary junction.

CSF immunoglobulin abnormalities are common. The immunoglobulin (Ig) G index, which measures intrathecal production of IgG, is elevated in 70% to 85% of MS patients. Isoelectric focusing followed by immunoblotting detects oligoclonal bands (OCBs) in more than 95% of patients (two or more bands detected in the CSF that are not present in the serum are considered abnormal). Unfortunately, many U.S. clinical laboratories use older and less sensitive methods to identify OCBs. Treatment with corticosteroids lowers the IgG index but has no effect on OCBs. An elevated IgG index and the presence of OCBs are not restricted to MS and are observed in 20% to 40% of patients with other inflammatory, demyelinating, or infectious diseases and occasionally other neurologic disorders, including the Guillain–Barré syndrome and other peripheral neuropathies. Therefore, CSF abnormalities should always be considered in conjunction with the clinical and MRI findings.

A single immunoglobulin band restricted to the CSF is of unclear significance and may be found in healthy individuals, as well as a variety of illnesses, including clinically isolated syndromes, MS, infectious and inflammatory diseases, CNS lymphoma, peripheral neuropathy, or migraine headaches. However, when the CSF is reexamined after an average of 6 months, one-third of patients, the majority of whom have demyelinating disease, show a change from a monoclonal to oligoclonal pattern.

A high CSF level of myelin basic protein indicates damage to myelin and is not useful in differentiating MS from other illnesses, including cerebrovascular disease, infections, neoplasms, or inflammatory diseases.

Visual-evoked potentials (VEPs) are sensitive for detecting clinically silent lesions in the anterior visual pathways although they are no longer included in the MS diagnostic criteria. VEPs are abnormal (prolonged P100 latency or greater than 6 milliseconds interocular difference if the latencies are normal) in approximately 30% of patients with clinically isolated syndromes other than optic neuritis and more than 50% of MS patients without a history of visual symptoms or clinical evidence of optic nerve dysfunction. However, abnormal VEPs may be observed in patients with other disorders, including compressive lesions of the optic nerve or chiasm, glaucoma, retinal disease, vitamin B_{12} deficiency, infectious

diseases (e.g., neuroborreliosis, neurosyphilis), systemic lupus erythematosus (SLE), and neurosarcoidosis.

VEPs are prolonged in almost all patients with a recent episode of optic neuritis, and routine testing for diagnostic purposes is not indicated. However, latencies shorten (presumably as a result of remyelination or ion channel reorganization) between 3 months and 2 to 3 years after acute optic neuritis and return to normal in about 25% of patients, so normal responses do not exclude the possibility of prior optic neuritis. Multifocal VEPs, which simultaneously record responses from multiple regions of the visual field are more sensitive than conventional VEPs but are not currently widely available.

MRI has largely supplanted the use of somatosensory and brain stem auditory-evoked potentials, which are rarely useful for identifying patients at increased risk for developing MS and are not included in the MS diagnostic criteria.

Optical coherence tomography (OCT) is a noninvasive technique that uses low-frequency infrared light to measure retinal nerve fiber layer thickness (RNFL) and macular volume. OCT, which has been used by ophthalmologists since 1990 to monitor glaucoma, is now used in MS. Thinning of the RNFL occurs after optic neuritis as a result of loss of retinal axons. The eyes of MS patients without a history of optic neuritis also undergo thinning of the RNFL. OCT is used as a secondary and tertiary outcome measure in clinical trials and by some neurologists and ophthalmologists to follow patients with or without a history of optic neuritis.

Diagnostic Criteria

New MS diagnostic criteria, referred to as the *McDonald criteria* (after the late Ian McDonald), were established in 2001 and revised in 2005 and 2010 (Table 69.2). MRI abnormalities may be used to demonstrate dissemination in space and time, provided an individual has had one episode of neurologic dysfunction consistent with demyelinating disease (see the following text). This has allowed for an earlier diagnosis. Eighty percent of patients diagnosed with MS based on MRI criteria will develop *clinically definite multiple sclerosis* (CDMS), a term formerly used to indicate two clinical demyelinating attacks separated in time and space, within 3 years if they

TABLE 69.2	Multiple Sclerosis Diagnostic Criteria
Clinical Presentation	**Additional Data Required for MS Diagnosis**
Two or more attacks with objective evidence of two or more lesion on clinical examination or objective clinical evidence of one lesion with reasonable historical evidence of a prior attack	None
Two or more attacks with objective evidence of one lesion on clinical examination	Dissemination in space demonstrated by one of the following: a. DIS on MRI[a] b. Second clinical attack
One attack with objective evidence of two or more lesions on clinical examination	Dissemination in time demonstrated by one of the following: a. MRI[b] b. Second clinical attack
One attack with objective evidence of one lesion on clinical examination	Dissemination in space demonstrated by one of the following: a. MRI[a] b. Second clinical attack *and* Dissemination in time demonstrated by one of the following: a. DIT criteria for MRI[b] b. Second clinical attack
Insidious neurologic progression suggestive of MS (i.e., a clinical presentation consistent with primary progressive MS)	One year of disease progression *and* two of the following: a. Dissemination in space in brain according to 2010 McDonald criteria b. Spinal cord MRI with two T2 lesions c. Positive CSF[c]

If all criteria are fulfilled and alternative diagnoses have been excluded, the diagnosis is MS. If there is a suspicion of MS but only some of the criteria are met, the diagnosis is "possible MS."

[a]See Table 69.3 for MRI criteria for dissemination in space.

[b]See Table 69.4 for MRI criteria for dissemination in time.

[c]Positive CSF: two or more oligoclonal bands detected in the CSF that are not present in the serum or an elevated IgG index.

MS, multiple sclerosis; DIS, dissemination in space; MRI, magnetic resonance imaging; DIT, dissemination in time, CSF, cerebrospinal fluid.

Adapted from Polman CH, Reingold SC, Banwell B, et al. Diagnostic criteria for multiple sclerosis: 2010 revisions to the "McDonald Criteria." *Ann Neurol.* 2011;69:292–302.

are left untreated. Early diagnosis is of great importance because MS disease-modifying drugs seem to be most effective when given early in the disease and a delay in treatment can result in irreversible neurologic damage.

The diagnosis of relapsing–remitting MS requires at least one episode of neurologic dysfunction consistent with inflammation and demyelination occurring in the absence of fever or infection and lasting at least 24 hours along with objective evidence of lesions disseminated in space and time. Dissemination in space may be demonstrated by two anatomically distinct lesions on examination that are consistent with CNS demyelination (e.g., an extensor plantar response and optic atrophy) or a focal lesion on examination along with MRI evidence of dissemination in space (Tables 69.2 and 69.3). In the absence of two clinical attacks, dissemination in time may be demonstrated by subclinical disease evolution on MRI (Table 69.4). The diagnosis of primary progressive MS requires at

TABLE 69.3	Magnetic Resonance Imaging Criteria for Dissemination in Space

T2 lesion in at least two of the four following areas:

- Periventricular
- Juxtacortical
- Infratentorial
- Spinal cord

If brain stem or spinal cord lesion is symptomatic, it is excluded from lesion count for DIS.

Adapted from Polman CH, Reingold SC, Banwell B, et al. Diagnostic criteria for multiple sclerosis: 2010 revisions to the "McDonald Criteria." *Ann Neurol.* 2011;69:292–302.

TABLE 69.4	Magnetic Resonance Imaging Criteria for Dissemination in Time

One of the following:

- One new T2 and/or contrast-enhancing lesion on any follow-up MRI
- Presence of asymptomatic gadolinium-enhancing and nonenhancing lesions at any one time

MRI, magnetic resonance imaging

Adapted from Polman CH, Reingold SC, Banwell B, et al. Diagnostic criteria for multiple sclerosis: 2010 revisions to the "McDonald Criteria." *Ann Neurol.* 2011;69:292–302.

TABLE 69.5	Radiologically Isolated Syndrome

CNS white matter abnormalities meet the following criteria:

- Ovoid well circumscribed and homogeneous foci with or without involvement of corpus callosum
- T2 hyperintensities >3 mm^2 and meeting three of four Barkhof criteria for dissemination in space
- CNS anomalies to not fit vascular pattern

No history of remitting clinical symptoms consistent with neurologic dysfunction

MRI anomalies do not account for clinically apparent impairments

MRI anomalies not related to toxic substances or medical condition

MRI anomalies not better accounted for by another disease

Exclusion of MRI phenotypes of leukoaraiosis or extensive white matter involvement without involvement of corpus callosum

CNS, central nervous system; MRI, magnetic resonance imaging.

Adapted from Okuda D, Mowry EM, Beheshtian A, et al. Incidental MRI anomalies suggestive of multiple sclerosis: the radiologically isolated syndrome. *Neurology.* 2009;72(9):800–805.

least 1 year of insidious neurologic progression combined with a variety of MRI and CSF abnormalities (see Table 69.2).

Characteristic MS lesions are occasionally discovered on MRI in individuals with no history of neurologic symptom and a normal examination. In the absence of clinical evidence of demyelination, even if MRI abnormalities are accompanied by the presence of CSF OCBs, an elevated IgG index, and delayed VEPs, a diagnosis of MS cannot be established. Formal criteria for this, termed *radiologically isolated syndrome*, were established in 2009 (Table 69.5).

DIFFERENTIAL DIAGNOSIS

In the absence of a definite diagnostic test, MS remains a diagnosis of exclusion. Most of the disorders that may mimic MS can be excluded by a detailed history, thorough examination, and appropriate laboratory tests and diagnostic studies.

Infections that may mimic MS include neuroborreliosis, neurosyphilis, and rarely progressive multifocal leukoencephalopathy. Human T-lymphotropic virus type-1 (HTLV-1) and HIV should be considered in patients with a progressive myelopathy. Acute disseminated encephalomyelitis may be impossible to distinguish from a first attack of MS. However, it is more likely to follow an infection or vaccination; more common in children; and generally includes encephalopathy, which is a rare manifestation of MS. Although patients with sarcoidosis may initially present with neurologic symptoms, evaluation usually reveals evidence of systemic sarcoidosis. Other autoimmune diseases that should be considered include Behçet syndrome, Sjögren syndrome, SLE, vasculitis, and the antiphospholipid antibody syndrome. Susac syndrome is an autoimmune microangiopathic endotheliopathy that affects brain, retina, and cochlea and results in encephalopathy, hearing loss, and branch retinal artery occlusions. It may be mistaken for MS because of prominent white matter lesions that are observed on brain MRI. Drug-induced demyelination is a strong possibility in patients with Crohn disease or rheumatoid or psoriatic arthritis treated with antitumor necrosis factor therapies. NMO and the NMO spectrum of disorders may be difficult to distinguish from MS, particularly early in the disease, in patients with recurrent optic neuritis and minimally abnormal brain MRI, or in patients with brain MRI findings more characteristic of MS. NMO-IgG seropositivity may help differentiate the diseases. Neoplasms (especially primary CNS lymphoma and gliomas) occasionally enter the differential diagnosis. Hyperacute onset of symptoms suggests stroke. Primary lateral sclerosis may simulate primary progressive MS but does not relapse and is monosymptomatic. MRI and CSF analysis usually help differentiate the two diseases. Hereditary spastic paraparesis should be considered in patients with a progressive spastic paraparesis, especially if there is a family history of similar illness. Other causes of a progressive myelopathy that should be considered in patients suspected of having progressive MS include adrenomyeloneuropathy, vitamin B_{12} deficiency, copper deficiency, spondylotic myelopathy, spinal cord tumors, and a spinal dural arteriovenous fistula.

TREATMENT

Therapy for MS consists of treatment of acute exacerbations, disease-modifying drugs, and symptomatic therapies. Optimal management often requires a multidisciplinary approach with pharmacologic and nonpharmacologic measures.

Treatment of Acute Exacerbations

High-dose intravenous (IV) corticosteroids hasten recovery from acute exacerbations but do not seem to affect the degree of recovery. A typical regimen consists of a 3- to 5-day course of 1,000 mg of IV methylprednisolone with or without an oral prednisone taper. Some patients with severe attacks seem to respond better to an additional 2 to 5 days of treatment. Because treatment does not seem to affect long-term outcome, not every MS exacerbation (e.g., mild sensory symptoms) requires treatment. In the Optic Neuritis Treatment Trial, patients who received oral prednisone 1 mg/kg/day did not improve any faster than the placebo-treated group. Furthermore, treatment with oral prednisone was associated with an increased risk of subsequent optic neuritis. Therefore, there does not appear to be a role for low-dose oral corticosteroids in the treatment of MS acute exacerbations [Level 1].[1]

Fever and infections, including asymptomatic urinary tract infections, can cause transient worsening of MS symptoms without a corresponding worsening of the underlying disease. This is known as a *pseudoexacerbation*. Infections should be excluded in the setting of new or worsening symptoms before treatment with corticosteroids is initiated and fevers should be treated aggressively.

Plasma exchange may be warranted for the treatment of acute relapses that result in significant residual disability despite high-dose IV corticosteroid therapy. In a small, but well-designed study, 42% of patients with severe demyelinating events that did not respond to high-dose IV corticosteroids had marked functional improvement after seven plasma exchanges. Patients who responded were treated an average of more than 40 days after the onset of symptoms. The investigators of a larger retrospective study reported similar results and concluded that plasma exchange may be effective when initiated more than 60 days after the onset of an acute demyelinating event.

Disease-modifying Drugs

The β-interferons and glatiramer acetate are commonly used relapsing–remitting MS therapies. They are modestly effective in reducing relapses and have positive effects on a variety of disability and MRI measures [Level 1].[2–6] Studies have also shown that these agents are effective (and possibly even more so) when initiated at the time of an initial clinical demyelinating event in patients with at least two or three asymptomatic brain lesions (i.e., prior to an MS diagnosis), and delaying treatment results in irreversible neurologic deficit [**Level 1**].[7–10] The interferons and glatiramer acetate clearly alter the short-term course of MS. Anecdotes along with retrospective and prospective open-label studies suggest a long-term treatment benefit, but controlled studies are lacking.

In head-to-head studies, the clinical effectiveness of glatiramer acetate was similar to the high-dose interferons (i.e., interferon β-1b 250 μg administered subcutaneously every other day and interferon β-1a 44 μg administered subcutaneously thrice weekly) in patients with relapsing–remitting MS.

The advent of oral therapies for relapsing MS, with the U.S. Food and Drug Administration (FDA) approval of fingolimod in 2010, followed by teriflunomide and dimethyl fumarate in 2012 and 2013, respectively, dramatically increased the options, with 10 therapies approved for the most common form of MS as of 2014. Table 69.6 summarizes available therapies for relapsing forms of MS.

The therapeutic effects of interferon may be due to its antiproliferative action, downregulation of costimulatory molecules, decrease of proinflammatory cytokines, or through effects on matrix metalloproteinases and adhesion molecules, which reduce the permeability of the blood–brain barrier and limit trafficking of T lymphocytes into the CNS. The beneficial effects of glatiramer acetate, a synthetic polypeptide composed of the four amino acids L-alanine, L-glutamic acid, L-lysine, and L-tyrosine, may result

TABLE 69.6	Overview of Disease-Modifying Therapies for Relapsing Forms of Multiple Sclerosis		
Treatment	**Dosage**	**Potential Side Effects**	**Monitoring**
IFNβ-1b	250 μg SC q.o.d.	Flulike symptoms	CBC
IFNβ-1a	30 μg IM q.wk.	LFT abnormalities	LFTs
IFNβ-1a	22 μg or 44 μg SC t.i.w.	Leukopenia	TFTs
		Neutralizing antibodies	
		Depression	
		Injection site necrosis (rare)	
Glatiramer acetate	20 mg SC daily	Site reactions	None
	or	Lipoatrophy	
	40 mg SC t.i.w.	Immediate postinjection reactions	
Mitoxantrone	12 mg/m² IV q12wk	Heart failure	MUGA scan annually after completion, assess ejection fraction prior to each dose.
		Promyelocytic leukemia	
		Bone marrow suppression	CBC
		Alopecia	Lifetime maximum dose: 140 mg/m²
Natalizumab	300 mg IV q4wk	Progressive multifocal leukoencephalopathy	JCV Ab
		LFT abnormalities	MRI brain
		Hypersensitivity reaction	LFTs
Fingolimod	0.5 mg PO daily	Bradycardia at first dose	First-dose observation with ECG before and 6 h after dosing and hourly vital signs, VZV immunity, baseline macula exam with follow-up eye exam 3–4 mo after initiation
		LFT abnormalities	
		Lymphopenia	
		Macular edema	
		Reactivation of herpes virus (zoster, oral or genital herpes)	
Teriflunomide	7 mg or 14 mg PO daily	Gastrointestinal side effects	Monthly LFTs for 6 mo after starting treatment
		Hair thinning	
		LFT abnormalities (black box warning: hepatic failure)	Quantiferon gold or TB skin test
		Hypertension	
		Tuberculosis reactivation	
Dimethyl fumarate	240 mg PO b.i.d.	Gastrointestinal upset	CBC with differential
		Flushing	LFT
		LFT abnormalities	
		Lymphopenia	

IFNB, interferon β; SC, subcutaneous; IM, intramuscular; LFT, liver function test; CBC, complete blood count; TFT, thyroid function test; IV, intravenous; MUGA, multigated acquisition; JCV, John Cunningham virus; MRI, magnetic resonance imaging; ECG, electrocardiogram; VZV, varicella-zoster virus; PO, by mouth.

from reactive Th2 cells that cross the blood–brain barrier and increase the secretion of suppressor-type cytokines and downregulate inflammatory activity within the CNS, a process known as *bystander suppression*.

Natalizumab is a humanized monoclonal antibody that is highly effective for reducing relapse rate and new T2 and contrast-enhancing lesions on MRI in relapsing MS [**Level 1**].[11,12] However, because it is associated with a low risk of progressive multifocal leukoencephalopathy (PML), it is used in conjunction with antibody testing for John Cunningham virus to predict risk of PML. Natalizumab likely exerts its therapeutic effects by blocking the binding of the α4-subunit of α4β1 integrin expressed on the surface of activated T cells with its receptor vascular cell receptor molecule-1 (VCAM-1) on the vascular endothelial surface at the blood–brain barrier. The interaction between α4 and VCAM-1 is critical in order for T cells to gain access into the CNS.

Fingolimod is a functional antagonist of the sphingosine 1 phosphate receptor, which prevents egress of lymphocytes from peripheral lymph nodes. Reduction in relapse rate and MRI outcomes was significant compared to placebo and to weekly intramuscular interferon β-1a in two large randomized, double-blind, placebo-controlled trials [**Level 1**].[13,14] Teriflunomide is a pyrimidine synthesis inhibitor, which slows expansion of activated lymphocytes. Modest efficacy in relapse rate reduction as well as reduction in sustained disability production was shown in large double-blind placebo-controlled trials [**Level 1**].[15,16] Dimethyl fumarate is a fumaric acid ester shown to be effective in reducing relapse frequency and MRI activity in relapsing forms of MS [**Level 1**].[17,18] Mechanism of action is hypothesized to be related to scavenging free radicals and acting through modulation of NF-kB and Nrf2 pathways.

Initial treatment decisions should be individualized and based on a combination of efficacy, route of administration, and potential side effects particularly related to concomitant medical issues.

Neutralizing antibodies (NAbs) develop in 15% to 25% of patients treated with interferon β-1a 44 μg subcutaneously three times a week and 25% to 40% treated with interferon β-1b. Interferon β-1a 30 μg administered intramuscularly is clearly less immunogenic with NAbs occurring in only 2% of patients. NAbs typically develop between 6 and 18 months after the initiation of treatment and only rarely after more than 2 years of therapy. Although they may be transient, persistent high-titer NAbs (>100 NU/mL) are associated with a reduced therapeutic effect. Six percent of patients develop persistent anti-natalizumab antibodies, which are associated with a clear loss of efficacy and an increased risk of infusion-related hypersensitivity reactions.

Secondary progressive MS is more difficult to treat than the relapsing–remitting form of the disease. The high-dose interferons and a double dose of once-weekly intramuscular interferon β-1a reduce the number of relapses and MRI activity but do not have a consistent effect on disability progression. Patients with superimposed relapses, gadolinium-enhancing lesions, or rapidly accumulating disability may be most likely to respond to treatment. In a small study, glatiramer did not prevent progression of disability in patients with primary or secondary progressive MS.

Periodic pulses of IV methylprednisolone are not effective in preventing disability in patients with secondary progressive MS. However, in one study of patients with mild relapsing–remitting MS, they had a favorable effect on disability, brain atrophy, and T1-hypointense lesions.

Mitoxantrone is an anthracenedione with immunosuppressive and immunomodulatory properties and the only FDA-approved therapy for secondary progressive MS. However, its effects are modest and safety is a concern, so risks and benefits need to be carefully considered before treatment is initiated. Mitoxantrone is also effective in highly active relapsing MS. Six monthly infusions of 20 mg of mitoxantrone combined with 1 g of IV methylprednisolone dramatically reduce gadolinium-enhancing brain lesions and seem to decrease relapses and disability in patients with rapidly worsening relapsing–remitting and secondary progressive MS and active brain MRI.

There are no proven therapies for primary progressive MS. Mitoxantrone and interferon appear to be ineffective. Glatiramer acetate was evaluated in a large clinical trial, but the study was stopped prematurely because of futility. A trial with rituximab, a monoclonal antibody directed against the CD20 antigen on the surface of B cells, also yielded negative results. However, post hoc analyses of the two studies suggest that glatiramer acetate may be beneficial in men and a possible treatment effect with rituximab in several subgroups, including patients younger than age of 51 years and in those with baseline gadolinium-enhancing lesions.

Symptom Management

Therapies to alleviate the daily symptoms of MS are integral part of patient care. Successful treatment often involves a combination of pharmacotherapy with nonpharmacologic measures, such as rehabilitation, exercise, or lifestyle and environmental modifications. See Table 69.7 for an overview of symptomatic management of common MS symptoms.

Management of spasticity includes evaluation and treatment of potentially exacerbating factors. Once exacerbating factors are minimized, a combination of physical therapy interventions and pharmacologic management is optimal. The most commonly used agents are baclofen and tizanidine alone or in combination. Common adverse effects of baclofen include limb weakness, sedation, and confusion. At higher doses, weakness may negate the benefit of spasticity reduction. Abrupt discontinuation of baclofen can result in seizures, confusion, hallucinations, and a marked increase in muscle tone. The use of tizanidine is mainly limited by drowsiness. Increased weakness is usually not a problem. Gabapentin may also be effective. The use of benzodiazepines has largely been supplanted by baclofen and tizanidine, which are better tolerated. Botulinum toxin may be effective for focal spasticity. Intrathecal baclofen may be beneficial for patients with severe leg spasticity that does not respond to oral agents at the highest tolerable dose.

Occupational and physical therapy are the mainstays of treatment for motor impairment. The potassium channel blocker dalfampridine, which is a sustained release formulation of 4-aminopyridine, enhances conduction across demyelinated nerve fibers. It improved leg strength and walking speed in some patients with relapsing and progressive forms of MS in two therapeutic trials. Dalfampridine increases the risk of seizures, especially at higher doses, and is contraindicated in those with history of seizures or impaired kidney function. The risk of seizure appears to be low with the effective dose of dalfampridine, which is 10 mg twice daily [**Level 1**].[19]

Depression responds well to psychotherapy and antidepressants, alone or in combination. Amitriptyline is effective for pseudobulbar affect (pathologic laughing or crying), as is a mixture of dextromethorphan and quinidine [**Level 1**].[20]

To date, there is no clearly effective treatment for MS-related cognitive impairment. Some patients may benefit from cognitive remediation and strategies to compensate for deficits. Donepezil improved memory in one small, controlled trial in MS patients

TABLE 69.7 Management of Multiple Sclerosis Symptoms

Symptom	Nonpharmacologic Approaches	Pharmacologic Approaches (Starting Dosage)
Spasticity	Physical and occupational therapy Exercise Evaluation of aggravating factors which may include the following: • Urinary tract infection • Decubitus ulcers • Pain • Constipation • Tight-fitting garments • Interferon β	Baclofen (oral 10 mg t.i.d. or intrathecal) Tizanidine (4 mg q.h.s.) Benzodiazepines (varies) Botulinum toxin Gabapentin (300 mg t.i.d.)
Weakness	Physical and occupational therapy	Dalfampridine (10 mg b.i.d.)
Depression	Psychotherapy Support groups	Selective serotonin reuptake inhibitors Serotonin–norepinephrine reuptake inhibitors
Pseudobulbar affect	Psychotherapy to manage triggers	Dextromethorphan/quinidine (20/10 mg b.i.d.) Amitriptyline (10 mg q.h.s.)
Fatigue	Improve sleep habits Energy conservation techniques Evaluation of other causes of fatigue including the following: • Anemia • Thyroid dysfunction • Sleep apnea • Side effects of other medications • Elevated core body temperature	Amantadine (150 mg b.i.d.) Modafinil (100 mg q.d.) Armodafinil (150 mg q.d.) Methylphenidate (10 mg q.d.)
Sexual dysfunction	Psychotherapy and relationship counseling to help couples manage sexual difficulties Mechanical vibrators and vacuum devices to enhance blood flow, increase lubrication, and stimulate orgasm	Selective phosphodiesterase 5 inhibitors for erectile dysfunction Estrogen creams for vaginal dryness
Cognitive impairment	Neuropsychological testing to define areas of deficit, identify areas of relative strength for compensatory strategies Cognitive remediation	No clearly effective pharmacotherapy
Urinary dysfunction	Urodynamic studies to define specific type of dysfunction—failure to store or empty Biofeedback Evaluate for infection Clean intermittent catheterization	Anticholinergics Mirabegron (25 mg q.d.) α-Adrenergic antagonist Botulinum toxin Desmopressin for nocturia 0.1 mg q.h.s.
Bowel dysfunction	Biofeedback Dietary changes to increase fiber Increase water intake for constipation Scheduled defecation	Stool softener Stimulant laxative Osmotic laxative
Tremor	Deep brain stimulation	Primidone (25 mg q.h.s.) Propranolol (20 mg b.i.d.) Clonazepam (0.5 b.i.d.) Ondansetron (8 mg b.i.d.)

TABLE 69.7	Management of Multiple Sclerosis Symptoms *(continued)*	
Symptom	**Nonpharmacologic Approaches**	**Pharmacologic Approaches (Starting Dosage)**
Paroxysmal symptoms (trigeminal neuralgia, paroxysmal dystonia)	Avoidance of triggers	Carbamazepine (100 mg b.i.d.)
		Acetazolamide (250 mg b.i.d.)
		Phenytoin (100 mg t.i.d.)
		Lamotrigine (100 mg q.d.)
		Baclofen (10 mg t.i.d.)
Pain	Avoidance of triggers	Gabapentin (300 mg t.i.d.)
		Pregabalin (75 mg b.i.d.)
		Amitriptyline (25 mg q.h.s.)
		Duloxetine (30 mg daily)
		Venlafaxine (37.5 mg b.i.d.)

with mild to moderate cognitive impairment. In an open-label pilot study, donepezil was also effective in improving attention, memory, and executive functioning in severely cognitively impaired patients with MS who were residents of a long-term care facility. In another randomized, double-blind trial, low-dose (4.5 mg daily) naltrexone, an opioid receptor antagonist, improved self-reported cognitive function in MS patients. Disease-modifying drugs that minimize lesion development, tissue destruction, or brain atrophy may limit cognitive decline.

Bladder dysfunction in MS can be well characterized by a urologic evaluation and urodynamic studies. A combination of anticholinergic therapy and an α-adrenergic antagonist (doxazosin, prazosin, tamsulosin, terazosin) may facilitate emptying in individual with sphincter detrusor dyssynergia. Clean intermittent catheterization combined with an anticholinergic agent may be necessary for some patients. Those unable to tolerate medications or perform self-catheterization may require an indwelling catheter. Catheterization is the mainstay of therapy in patients with detrusor hypocontractility and emptying difficulties. Patients with good upper extremity function are usually able to perform clean intermittent catheterization. An indwelling catheter may be necessary for patients who cannot perform self-catheterization because long-term intermittent catheterization by a caregiver is usually not practical. Urologic follow-up is necessary for patients with a chronic indwelling catheter to monitor for the development of urinary tract and genital complications.

Numerous medications have been reported to be successful in treating MS tremor, including carbamazepine, clonazepam, gabapentin, levetiracetam, primidone, ondansetron, propranolol, and tetrahydrocannabinol. However, these agents are rarely effective and tremor can be the most difficult MS symptom to treat. Thalamic deep brain stimulation may result in dramatic improvement. Stable MS patients with disabling tremor for at least 1 year despite medical therapy who have no significant cognitive dysfunction, speech or swallowing problems, or other deficits in the affected limbs may be good candidates.

If treatment is warranted, dysesthesias and pain usually respond to anticonvulsants and antidepressants, either used alone or in combination. Gabapentin, pregabalin, amitriptyline, nortriptyline, and duloxetine commonly provide relief. Myelopathic pain responds to opioids, which may be necessary in some patients.

Referral to a pain specialist may be helpful for patients with refractory pain.

OUTCOME

MS is an extremely variable illness. Therefore, counseling patients with clinically isolated syndromes and early MS poses a major challenge for clinicians. However, brain MRI abnormalities after an initial clinical demyelinating event provide important prognostic information regarding the development of MS. Fifty-one percent of patients who initially have optic neuritis and at least three brain MRI T2-hyperintense lesions develop CDMS within 5 years compared to only 16% who have normal brain MRI. CDMS develops within 20 years in 82% of CIS patients with at least one brain MRI T2 lesion compared with 21% with a normal baseline brain MRI. Forty-one percent to 50% of placebo-treated patients in the interferon β or glatiramer acetate clinically isolated syndrome trials, which required at least two or three asymptomatic brain lesions for entry, developed CDMS within 2 to 3 years. In those studies, the risk of MS at 18 to 24 months was greatest in patients with more than eight T2-hyperintense lesions or at least one gadolinium-enhancing lesion on a baseline brain MRI.

In general, the larger the number of baseline brain MRI lesions at the time of a clinically isolated syndrome, the greater the risk of long-term disability. There is also a modest correlation between the change in MRI T2 lesion volume in the first 5 years and long-term disability. However, possible outcomes are wide ranging. In one natural history study, 45% of those with at least 10 lesions on initial brain MRI had reached Expanded Disability Status Scale (EDSS) 6 after 20 years, but 35% had only mild disability.

Although the course of MS is essentially impossible to predict in an individual patient, female sex, younger age at onset, and little disability 5 years after onset are generally favorable prognostic signs. Male sex, older age at onset, frequent attacks early in the course of the disease, a short interval between the first two attacks, incomplete recovery from the first attack, rapidly accumulating disability, cerebellar involvement as a first symptom, and progressive disease from onset are associated with worse outcome. Optic neuritis as a first attack is associated with a favorable short- and intermediate-term outcome, but 20-year disability is similar among patients who present with optic neuritis, brain stem, or spinal cord syndromes. African-Americans have a lower prevalence of MS than whites but tend to accumulate disability more rapidly.

In one natural history study, 24% of patients with a clinically isolated syndrome who were followed for an average of 4 years reached an EDSS score of 6 or more (EDSS 6 is defined as unable to walk 100 m without unilateral assistance) and 40% of those followed for 6 to 15 years entered the secondary progressive phase of the disease. In another study, the natural course of the disease was less aggressive with only 24% of patients reaching EDSS of 6 or more and 39% developing secondary progressive MS 20 years after the onset of their first clinical demyelinating event.

Some patients have a very mild form of relapsing–remitting MS with minimal or no disability at least 10 years after disease onset, which is often referred to as *benign multiple sclerosis*. Although natural history studies have yielded conflicting results, most suggest that many of these patients will develop significant disability and enter the secondary progressive phase of the disease within 20 years. There are no reliable predictors to identify which patients will continue to have a mild course. Furthermore, neuropsychological testing reveals cognitive impairment in approximately 20% to 45% of patients considered to have benign MS. Therefore, the diagnosis of benign MS should include an assessment of cognitive function and only be considered in retrospect and after prolonged follow-up.

The Marburg variant of MS is a rare, fulminant, and usually monophasic illness that typically results in death within 1 year. It can be difficult to differentiate from severe acute disseminated encephalomyelitis. Pathologically, it is characterized by robust macrophage infiltrate and destruction of axons as well as demyelination and prominent tissue necrosis.

Schilder disease, or myelinoclastic diffuse sclerosis, is a vanishingly rare pediatric form of demyelinating disease characterized by formation of bilateral plaques in the centrum semiovale with pathology consistent with MS without additional lesions in the CNS in the setting of normal peripheral nervous system function, normal adrenal function, and no deficit in very long-chain fatty acids. A handful of cases have been reported since the original description by Schilder in 1912. There is controversy regarding the potential contamination of case series with children eventually found to have adrenoleukodystrophy.

NEUROMYELITIS OPTICA SPECTRUM DISORDER

Neuromyelitis optica spectrum disorder (NMOSD) is a severe inflammatory demyelinating disease of the CNS that is distinct from MS. Originally considered a monophasic illness characterized by the co-occurrence of acute or subacute optic neuritis and transverse myelitis, it is now recognized that NMOSD patients typically have recurrent attacks, and the disease is not always limited to the optic nerves and spinal cord. Although there is overlap with the presentation of MS, the disease has a distinct pathologic antibody and the features of the optic neuritis and myelitis are distinct from MS. The most common clinical syndrome is longitudinally extensive transverse myelitis, as opposed to the relatively short segments of spinal cord that tend to be involved in MS myelitis. Optic neuritis may be unilateral or bilateral and is often severe with poor recovery. A third clinical hallmark is intractable nausea, vomiting, or hiccups.

EPIDEMIOLOGY

The true incidence and prevalence of NMOSD are unknown. However, the disease is much less common than MS; estimated prevalence rate is about 1% to 2% that of MS in the United States. NMOSD usually begins late in the fourth decade, but the onset may occur during childhood or after age 70 years. Women are affected four to nine times as often as men, and nonwhite individuals are more commonly affected than whites.

PATHOBIOLOGY

Aquaporin 4-IgG is both a sensitive and highly specific serum autoantibody that is present in about 70% of NMOSD patients in either serum or CSF. Pathogenicity of the aquaporin 4-IgG has been demonstrated by passive transfer in animal models.

Acute NMO lesions are characterized by extensive demyelination and axonal damage and contain an inflammatory infiltrate consisting mainly of macrophages, B lymphocytes, eosinophils, and granulocytes. T lymphocytes are sparse. Immunoglobulin and products of complement activation are deposited in a distinctive perivascular rim and rosette pattern. Intramedullary lesions typically extend over several spinal levels, involve both gray and white matter, and are often necrotic. Gliosis, cystic degeneration, cavitation, and atrophy are typical of chronic spinal cord and optic nerve and chiasmal lesions.

Aquaporin-4 (AQP4), which is the main water channel in the CNS, is the target antigen in NMOSD. AQP4 is located primarily in perivascular and subpial astrocytic foot processes and expressed in high levels within the optic nerves, hypothalamus, brain stem, periventricular regions, and gray matter of the spinal cord. AQP4 loss may impair water homeostasis and glutamate transport and lead to oligodendrocyte injury, demyelination, and axonal damage. The circumventricular organs around the third and fourth ventricles contain high density of AQP4 and this may explain the presentations of intractable nausea, vomiting, hiccups, as well as hypothalamic dysfunction.

A marked loss of AQP4 immunoreactivity is observed in all NMO demyelinating lesions regardless of location, stage, or degree of necrosis and occurs in regions with extensive vasculocentric immunoglobulin and complement deposition.

CLINICAL MANIFESTATIONS

Patients typically experience frequent and severe exacerbations of optic neuritis or myelitis interspersed with periods of remissions. See Table 69.8 for a description of classic NMOSD presentations. A secondary progressive course with continuous worsening between exacerbations is uncommon, occurring in only 2% of patients.

At onset, patients usually present with unilateral optic neuritis or myelitis. In approximately 50% of patients, the initial attack is severe with visual acuity reduced to finger counting or worse or Medical Research Council (MRC) grade 3 or 4 weakness in at least one extremity. There is often considerable improvement after the

TABLE 69.8	Classic Presentations of Neuromyelitis Optica Spectrum Disorder	
Symptom	Sign	Localization
Blurred vision	Relative apparent pupillary defect	Optic nerve
Pain with eye movement	Red desaturation	
Leg weakness	Paraparesis or monoparesis	Spinal cord
Intractable vomiting or hiccups		Area postrema

first attack, but a second episode occurs in 55% of patients within 1 year and in 90% within 5 years.

Disease outside of the spinal cord and optic nerves occurs in 10% to 15% of patients. Symptoms include vomiting, intractable hiccups, narcolepsy, facial weakness or numbness, diplopia, vertigo, dysarthria, trigeminal neuralgia, tremor, ataxia, hearing loss, hemiparesis, and encephalopathy.

The prognosis of untreated NMOSD is poor, with the potential for profound visual loss and weakness developing early in the course of the disease as a result of incomplete recovery from attacks. Myelopathic pain, spasticity, dysesthesias, tonic spasms, as well as bowel and bladder dysfunction are common. In a cohort of patients seen at the Mayo Clinic, 60% were legally blind in at least one eye and more than 50% had either a mono- or paraplegia within 8 years of disease onset. The 5-year survival rate was only 68%, and all deaths were attributable to respiratory failure from acute intramedullary cervical spine lesions.

DIAGNOSIS

The diagnosis of NMO is established by clinical features that are supported by MRI and, sometimes, serologic findings. A new set of diagnostic criteria for NMOSD has been proposed by an expert consensus panel and is likely to be published in 2014. Current diagnostic criteria are listed in Table 69.9. In a patient with a history of optic neuritis, myelitis extending over three or four spinal cord segments, and an unremarkable brain MRI, the diagnosis is usually straightforward. However, diagnostic uncertainty often exists when patients initially present with severe optic neuritis and a normal or minimally abnormal brain MRI or a longitudinally extensive transverse myelitis. The latter may be defined as NMOSD after infectious and collagen-vascular diseases, sarcoidosis, tumors, and vascular myelopathies are excluded. These patients have a *form fruste* of the disease with optic neuritis or longitudinally extensive transverse myelitis and unremarkable brain MRI.

Initial brain MRI is normal or reveals fewer than three or four white matter lesions in 97% of patients. If not already present, subsequent imaging often reveals clinically silent nonspecific white matter lesions. However, at least 10% of patients eventually develop lesions characteristic of MS.

Approximately 7% of AQP4-IgG seropositive patients develop brain lesions that are considered characteristic of NMO but atypical of MS. These lesions tend to occur in the hypothalamus, thalamus, brain stem, and around the third and fourth ventricles, which are all sites of high AQP4 expression. Large lesions in the cerebral hemispheres are occasionally observed.

In the setting of a recent myelitis, spinal cord MRI is the most sensitive diagnostic test for NMO. Longitudinally extensive T2

TABLE 69.9	Neuromyelitis Optica Diagnostic Criteria

Required criteria:

1. Optic neuritis

2. Acute myelitis

At least two of three supportive criteria:

1. Spinal cord MRI lesion extending three or more contiguous vertebral segments

2. Initial brain MRI with fewer than four white matter lesions or three lesions if one is periventricular

3. NMO-IgG seropositivity

MRI, magnetic resonance imaging; NMO-IgG, neuromyelitis optica immunoglobulin G.

Adapted from Wingerchuk DM, Lennon VA, Pittock SJ, et al. Revised diagnostic criteria for neuromyelitis optica. *Neurology.* 2006;66:1485–1489.

lesions involving more than three vertebral segments, and frequently more than six, are characteristic of NMO (Fig. 69.8). Preferential central gray matter involvement as well as gadolinium enhancement and spinal cord swelling are common. Lesions often become smaller over weeks to months, either spontaneously or in response to corticosteroids, and spinal cord atrophy may develop.

The morphology of acute NMO spinal cord lesions is unlike MS lesions, which rarely involve more than one-and-a-half vertebral segments or gray matter. Although characteristic of NMO, longitudinally extensive lesions are not specific and are seen in a variety of illnesses, including infectious and other inflammatory diseases, as well as in patients with vascular lesions and tumors (Fig. 69.9).

Biomarkers

AQP4-IgG is detected in 73% of patients with NMO and has a 91% specificity in differentiating NMO from MS patients who present with myelitis and optic neuritis. The antibody appears to be even more specific in distinguishing NMO from classic MS and a variety of other autoimmune and inflammatory neurologic disorders.

In patients with a history of optic neuritis, a longitudinally extensive myelitis, and a minimally abnormal brain MRI, AQP4-IgG testing is not necessary to establish a diagnosis of NMO, as negative serology does not exclude it. Serologic testing may be most useful in patients who have a history consistent with NMO but atypical brain lesions or MRI findings characteristic of MS.

AQP4-IgG is also detected in 45% of patients at high risk for developing NMO (i.e., patients with recurrent optic neuritis or

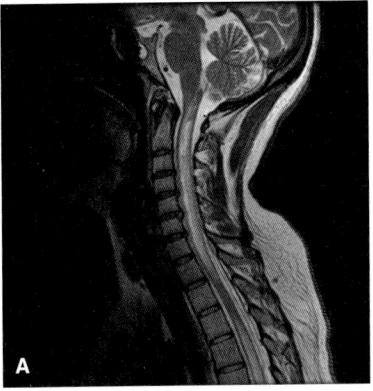
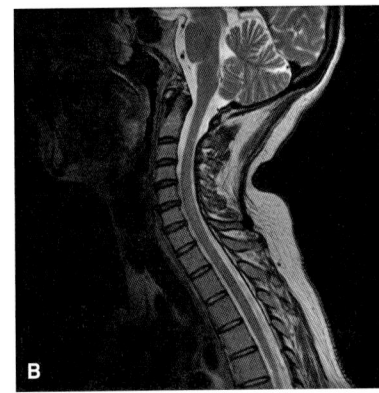

FIGURE 69.8 NMOSD patient with an acute myelitis. Sagittal T2-weighted image **(A)** of the cervical spine shows an intramedullary lesion extending from C1 to T1 accompanied by spinal cord swelling. A second lesion is seen in the visualized portion of the upper thoracic spine. A follow-up MRI **(B)** 8 months later shows marked improvement.

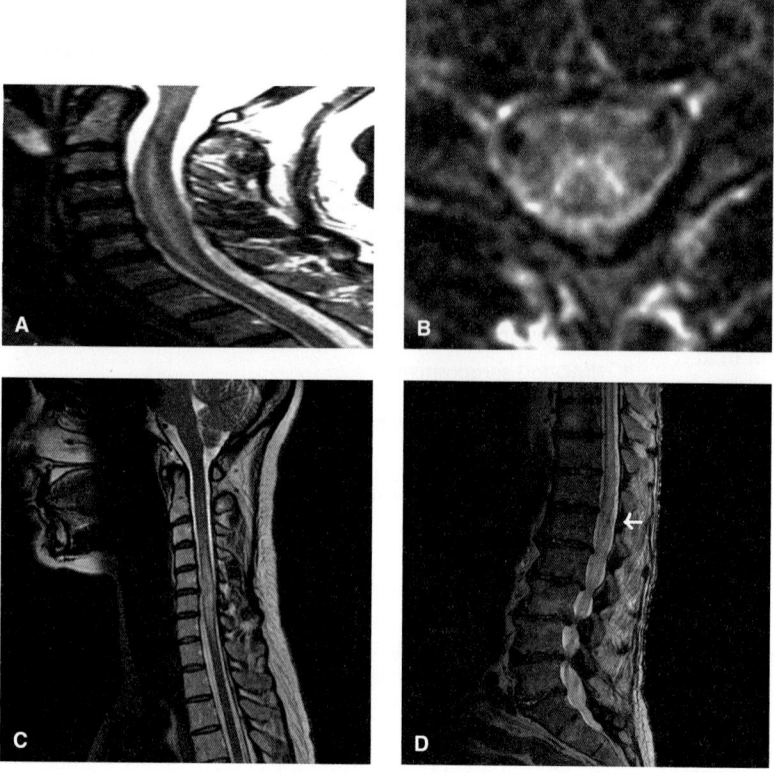

FIGURE 69.9 Longitudinally extensive spinal cord lesions in other diseases. Sagittal **(A)** and axial **(B)** T2-weighted images of the cervical spine show an intramedullary lesion predominantly involving gray matter from C2 to C6 in a patient with neuroborreliosis. A sagittal T2-weighted image **(C)** of the cervical spine shows an intramedullary lesion extending from C4 to T1 and spinal cord swelling at C5–C6 in a patient with neurosarcoidosis. A sagittal T2-weighted image **(D)** of the distal spinal cord and conus medullaris shows increased signal in the lower thoracic spinal cord, a small hemorrhage (*arrow*) at the conus tip, and numerous flow voids along the posterior spinal cord surface in a patient with a dural arteriovenous fistula.

longitudinally extensive transverse myelitis and brain MRI findings that do not fulfill criteria for MS). Seropositivity predicts the development of NMO or recurrent longitudinally extensive transverse myelitis and provides the rationale for AQP4-IgG testing in these individuals.

Although not part of the current NMO diagnostic criteria, CSF analysis may be informative in some patients and useful to exclude alternative diagnoses. When examined within 4 weeks of the onset of an exacerbation, the CSF typically reveals a mild pleocytosis and an elevated protein. However, approximately 35% of patients have greater than 50 WBC per cubic millimeter and there may be more than 1,000 WBC per cubic millimeter. In addition, more than 5 neutrophils per cubic millimeter are present in the CSF in up to 60% of patients. Neutrophilic pleocytosis or more than 50 WBC per cubic millimeter in the CSF are uncommon findings in MS. Oligoclonal bands are present in about 20% to 30% of NMO patients and are not useful in differentiating NMO from MS.

Serum non–organ-specific autoantibodies, especially antinuclear or extractable nuclear antibodies, are frequently detected in NMO patients. Rheumatoid factor or double-stranded DNA antibodies are less commonly observed. The clinical significance of these antibodies is unclear, as the coexistence of NMO with SLE, Sjögren syndrome, or other autoimmune diseases with the exception of thyroid disease, is rare. However, their presence is another indication of aberrant humoral immunity.

TREATMENT

NMO exacerbations are usually treated with intravenous methylprednisolone 1 g daily for 5 to 7 days. Plasma exchange, which is indicated for severe exacerbations that do not respond to high-dose intravenous corticosteroids, results in functional improvement in up to 60% of patients.

There are ongoing early phase controlled therapeutic trials in NMO with monoclonal antibodies including the complement inhibitor eculizumab and the IL-6 receptor inhibitor, tocilizumab. Level 1 treatment evidence is lacking in NMO and NMOSD. Treatment with immunosuppressive or immunomodulatory therapies aimed at altering the course of the disease is based on anecdotes and small open-label studies. Interferon-β and glatiramer acetate appear to worsen the course of NMOSD. Mycophenolate mofetil or the combination of prednisone and azathioprine may be beneficial in some patients. Mitoxantrone was reported to have some benefit in a study of five patients, but treatment is limited to 2 to 3 years due to dose-related irreversible cardiotoxicity. Treatment-associated leukemia is also a concern, as it is in MS. The results of an open-label study with rituximab, a monoclonal antibody directed against the CD20 antigen on the surface of B cells, are encouraging. However, B-cell depletion does not prevent severe disease activity and a randomized controlled trial is needed.

Therapies aimed at treating spasticity, pain, sphincter dysfunction, and other chronic NMOSD symptoms play an integral part in patient management and are similar to the ones used to treat some of the daily symptoms of MS.

MARCHIAFAVA–BIGNAMI DISEASE

Primary degeneration of the corpus callosum is characterized clinically by altered mental status, seizures, and multifocal CNS signs. Demyelination of the corpus callosum without inflammation is the primary pathologic feature but other areas of the CNS may be involved. The disease was first described by Marchiafava and Bignami in 1903 in three Italian red wine drinkers.

EPIDEMIOLOGY

A few hundred cases have been described in the world's literature, but the disease is probably more common. Before the advent of modern imaging, however, the diagnosis was rarely made before

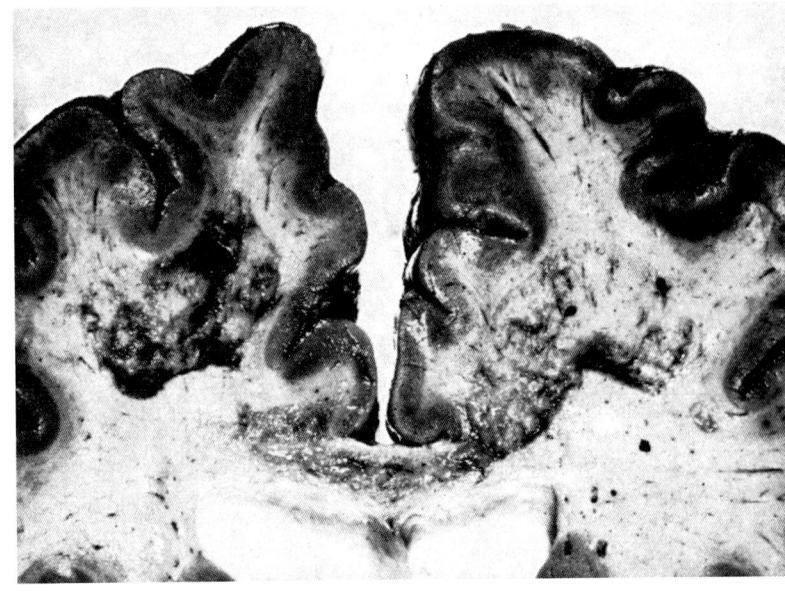

FIGURE 69.10 Marchiafava–Bignami disease. Acute necrosis of corpus callosum and neighboring white matter of the frontal lobes. (From Merritt HH, Weisman AD. Primary degeneration of the corpus callosum [Marchiafava-Bignami's disease]. *J Neuropathol Exp Neurol.* 1945;4:155–163.)

death because the symptoms and findings are nonspecific. Genetic susceptibility has been suspected because of the frequency of reports in Italian men. Onset is usually in middle age or later.

PATHOBIOLOGY

The cause is not known. The condition was first noted in middle-aged and elderly Italian men who consumed red wine. It has been described worldwide, however, and is not confined to red wine. In some cases, alcohol consumption was not a factor. Nutritional deficiencies have also been implicated. The syndrome is rare, however, even in severe malnutrition. Toxic factors have been suggested, but no agent has been implicated.

The sine qua non is necrosis of the medial zone of the corpus callosum. The dorsal and ventral rims are spared. The necrosis varies from softening and discoloration (Fig. 69.10) to cavitation and cyst formation. Usually, all stages of degeneration are found. In most cases, the rostral position of the corpus callosum is affected first. The lesions arise as small symmetric foci that extend and become confluent. Although medial necrosis of the corpus callosum is the principal finding, there also may be degeneration of the anterior commissure (Fig. 69.11), posterior commissure, centrum semiovale, subcortical white matter, long association bundles, and middle cerebellar peduncles. All these lesions have a constant bilateral symmetry. Usually spared are the internal capsule, corona radiata, and subgyral arcuate fibers. The gray matter is not grossly affected.

Few diseases have such a well-defined pathologic picture. The corpus callosum may be infarcted as a result of occlusion of the anterior cerebral artery, but the symmetry of the lesions, sparing of the gray matter, and occurrence of similar lesions in the anterior commissure, long association bundles, and cerebellar peduncles are found only in Marchiafava–Bignami disease. The microscopic alterations are the result of a sharply defined necrotic process with loss of myelin but relative preservation of axis cylinders in the periphery of the lesions. There is usually no evidence of inflammation aside from a few perivascular lymphocytes. In most cases, fat-filled phagocytes are common. Gliosis is usually not well advanced. Capillary endothelial proliferation may be present in the affected

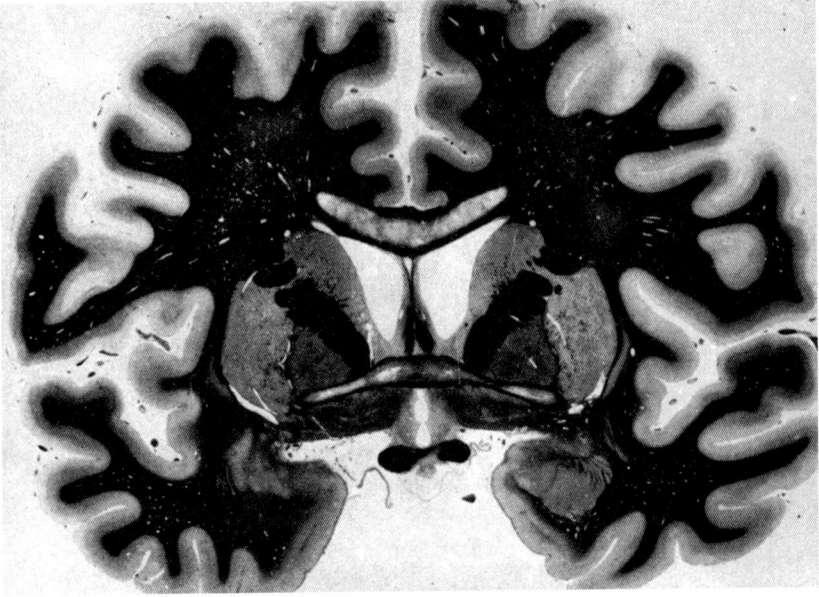

FIGURE 69.11 Marchiafava–Bignami disease. Medial necrosis of the corpus callosum and anterior commissure with sparing of the margins. (Courtesy of Dr. P. I. Yakovlev.)

area, but no thrombi are seen. The disease has been reported with central pontine myelinolysis or Wernicke encephalopathy in alcoholics and in nonalcoholic persons, thus suggesting a possible common pathogenesis.

CLINICAL MANIFESTATIONS

The onset is usually insidious, and the first symptoms are so nonspecific that the time of onset is difficult to determine. There is a mixture of focal and diffuse signs of cerebral disease. In addition to memory loss and confusion, manic, paranoid, or delusional states may occur. Depression and extreme apathy are typical.

DIAGNOSIS

Marchiafava–Bignami disease is suspected when insidiously developing dementia, multifocal neurologic signs, and seizures occur in elderly men, particularly alcohol abusers. CT and MRI are accurate in diagnosis, but MRI is preferred in showing the callosal lesions and symmetric demyelinating lesions in subcortical white matter. In the original reports, status epilepticus was prominent and, in modern times, an acute form may be seen. The differential diagnosis includes Wernicke encephalopathy, which may occur simultaneously, manifested by ataxia, ophthalmoplegia, and nystagmus as well as dementia or delirium.

In a review of 153 cases reported between 1981 and 2012, CSF pleocytosis was reported in 0% of the confirmed minimal brain damage (MBD) cases. Elevated CSF protein was found in only 8%.

TREATMENT

Generally, the outlook for recovery is poor. However, spontaneous recovery has been reported, and some patients improve with thiamine or corticosteroid therapy. Metabolic recovery may be documented by MRS.

OUTCOME

The disease is slowly progressive and results in death within 3 to 6 years. Rarely, fever lasts days or weeks, or a temporary remission may be seen.

LEVEL 1 EVIDENCE

1. Beck RW, Cleary PA, Anderson MM Jr, et al. A randomized, controlled trial of corticosteroids in the treatment of acute optic neuritis. The Optic Neuritis Study Group. N Engl J Med. 1992;326:581–588.
2. Interferon beta-1b is effective in relapsing–remitting multiple sclerosis. I. Clinical results of a multicenter, randomized, double-blind, placebo-controlled trial. The IFNB Multiple Sclerosis Study Group. Neurology. 1993;43:655–661.
3. Clanet M, Radue EW, Kappos L, et al. A randomized, double-blind, dose-comparison study of weekly interferon beta-1a in relapsing MS. Neurology. 2002;59:1507–1517.
4. Randomised double-blind placebo-controlled study of interferon beta-1a in relapsing/remitting multiple sclerosis. PRISMS (Prevention of Relapses and Disability by Interferon beta-1a Subcutaneously in Multiple Sclerosis) Study Group. Lancet. 1998;352:1498–1504.
5. Comi G, Filippi M, Wolinsky JS. European/Canadian multicenter, double-blind, randomized, placebo-controlled study of the effects of glatiramer acetate on magnetic resonance imaging-measured disease activity and burden in patients with relapsing multiple sclerosis. European/Canadian Glatiramer Acetate Study Group. Ann Neurol. 2001;49:290–297.
6. Johnson KP, Brooks BR, Cohen JA, et al. Copolymer 1 reduces relapse rate and improves disability in relapsing–remitting multiple sclerosis: results of a phase III multicenter, double-blind placebo-controlled trial. The Copolymer 1 Multiple Sclerosis Study Group. Neurology. 1995;45:1268–1276.
7. Jacobs LD, Beck RW, Simon JH, et al. Intramuscular interferon beta-1a therapy initiated during a first demyelinating event in multiple sclerosis. CHAMPS Study Group. N Engl J Med. 2000;343:898–904.
8. Kappos L, Freedman MS, Polman CH, et al. Effect of early versus delayed interferon beta-1b treatment on disability after a first clinical event suggestive of multiple sclerosis: a 3-year follow-up analysis of the BENEFIT study. Lancet. 2007;370:389–397.
9. Kappos L, Polman CH, Freedman MS, et al. Treatment with interferon beta-1b delays conversion to clinically definite and McDonald MS in patients with clinically isolated syndromes. Neurology. 2006;67:1242–1249.
10. Comi G, Martinelli V, Rodegher M, et al. Effect of glatiramer acetate on conversion to clinically definite multiple sclerosis in patients with clinically isolated syndrome (PreCISe study): a randomised, double-blind, placebo-controlled trial. Lancet. 2009;374(9700):1503–1511.
11. Polman CH, O'Connor PW, Havrdova E, et al. A randomized, placebo-controlled trial of natalizumab for relapsing multiple sclerosis. N Engl J Med. 2006;354:899–910.
12. Rudick RA, Stuart WH, Calabresi PA, et al. Natalizumab plus interferon beta-1 for relapsing multiple sclerosis. N Engl J Med. 2006;354:911–923.
13. Kappos L, Radue EW, O'Connor P, et al. A placebo-controlled trial of oral fingolimod in relapsing multiple sclerosis. New Engl J Med. 2010;362(5):387–401.
14. Cohen JA, Barkhof F, Comi G, et al. Oral fingolimod or intramuscular interferon for relapsing multiple sclerosis. New Engl J Med. 2010;362(5):402–415.
15. O'Connor P, Wolinsky J, Confavreux C, et al. Randomized trial of oral teriflunomide for relapsing multiple sclerosis. N Engl J Med. 2011;365:1293–1303.
16. Confavreux C, O'Connor P, Comi G, et al. Oral teriflunomide for patients with relapsing multiple sclerosis (TOWER): a randomised, double-blind, placebo-controlled, phase 3 trial. Lancet Neurol. 2014;13:247–256.
17. Gold R, Kappos L, Arnold DL, et al. Placebo-controlled phase 3 study of oral BG-12 for relapsing multiple sclerosis. N Engl J Med. 2012;367(12):1098–1107.
18. Fox RJ, Miller DH, Phillips JT, et al. Placebo-controlled phase 3 study of oral BG-12 or glatiramer in multiple sclerosis. N Engl J Med. 2012;367(12):1087–1097.
19. Goodman AD, Brown TR, Krupp LB, et al. Sustained-release oral fampridine in multiple sclerosis: a randomised, double-blind, controlled trial. Lancet. 2009;373(9665):732–738.
20. Panitch HS, Thisted RA, Smith RA, et al. Randomized, controlled trial of dextromethorphan/quinidine for pseudobulbar affect in multiple sclerosis. Ann Neurol. 2006;59(5):780–787.

SUGGESTED READINGS

Multiple Sclerosis
Antel J, Bar-Or A. Roles of immunoglobulins and B cells in multiple sclerosis: from pathogenesis to treatment. J Neuroimmunol. 2006;180:3–8.

Ascherio A, Munger KL. Environmental risk factors for multiple sclerosis. Part I: the role of infection. *Ann Neurol.* 2007;61:288–299.

Ascherio A, Munger KL. Environmental risk factors for multiple sclerosis. Part II: noninfectious factors. *Ann Neurol.* 2007;61:504–513.

Bakshi R, Thompson AJ, Rocca MA, et al. MRI in multiple sclerosis: current status and future prospects. *Lancet Neurol.* 2008;7:615–625.

Barkhof F, Rocca M, Francis G, et al. Validation of diagnostic magnetic resonance imaging criteria for multiple sclerosis and response to interferon beta1a. *Ann Neurol.* 2003;53:718–724.

Barnett MH, Prineas JW. Relapsing and remitting multiple sclerosis: pathology of the newly forming lesion. *Ann Neurol.* 2004;55:458–468.

Bitsch A, Kuhlmann T, Stadelmann C, et al. A longitudinal MRI study of histopathologically defined hypointense multiple sclerosis lesions. *Ann Neurol.* 2001;49:793–796.

Bosca I, Pascual AM, Casanova B, et al. Four new cases of therapy-related acute promyelocytic leukemia after mitoxantrone. *Neurology.* 2008;71:457–458.

Brooks BR, Thisted RA, Appel SH, et al; AVP-923 ALS Study Group. Treatment of pseudobulbar affect in ALS with dextromethorphan/quinidine: a randomized trial. *Neurology.* 2004;63(8):1364–1370.

CHAMPS Study Group. MRI predictors of early conversion to clinically definite MS in the CHAMPS placebo group. *Neurology.* 2002;59:998–1005.

Cohen JA, Cutter GR, Fischer JS, et al. Benefit of interferon beta-1a on MSFC progression in secondary progressive MS. *Neurology.* 2002;59:679–687.

Cole SR, Beck RW, Moke PS, et al. The predictive value of CSF oligoclonal banding for MS 5 years after optic neuritis. Optic Neuritis Study Group. *Neurology.* 1998;51:885–887.

Confavreux C, Hutchinson M, Hours MM, et al. Rate of pregnancy-related relapse in multiple sclerosis. Pregnancy in Multiple Sclerosis Group. *N Engl J Med.* 1998;339:285–291.

Confavreux C, Suissa S, Saddier P, et al. Vaccinations and the risk of relapse in multiple sclerosis. Vaccines in Multiple Sclerosis Study Group. *N Engl J Med.* 2001;344:319–326.

Cotton F, Weiner HL, Jolesz FA, et al. MRI contrast uptake in new lesions in relapsing–remitting MS followed at weekly intervals. *Neurology.* 2003;60:640–646.

Durelli L, Verdun E, Barbero P, et al. Every-other-day interferon beta-1b versus once-weekly interferon beta-1a for multiple sclerosis: results of a 2-year prospective randomised multicentre study (INCOMIN). *Lancet.* 2002;359:1453–1460.

Dyment DA, Ebers GC, Sadovnick AD. Genetics of multiple sclerosis. *Lancet Neurol.* 2004;3:104–110.

Edan G, Miller D, Clanet M, et al. Therapeutic effect of mitoxantrone combined with methylprednisolone in multiple sclerosis: a randomised multicentre study of active disease using MRI and clinical criteria. *J Neurol Neurosurg Psychiatry.* 1997;62:112–118.

Fazekas F, Barkhof F, Filippi M, et al. The contribution of magnetic resonance imaging to the diagnosis of multiple sclerosis. *Neurology.* 1999;53:448–456.

Fazekas F, Lublin FD, Li D, et al. Intravenous immunoglobulin in relapsing–remitting multiple sclerosis: a dose-finding trial. *Neurology.* 2008;71:265–271.

Fazekas F, Sorensen PS, Filippi M, et al. MRI results from the European Study on Intravenous Immunoglobulin in Secondary Progressive Multiple Sclerosis (ESIMS). *Mult Scler.* 2005;11:433–440.

Fisniku LK, Brex PA, Altmann DR, et al. Disability and T2 MRI lesions: a 20-year follow-up of patients with relapse onset of multiple sclerosis. *Brain.* 2008;131:808–817.

Francis GS, Rice GP, Alsop JC. Interferon beta-1a in MS: results following development of neutralizing antibodies in PRISMS. *Neurology.* 2005;65:48–55.

Frohman EM, Racke MK, Raine CS. Multiple sclerosis—the plaque and its pathogenesis. *N Engl J Med.* 2006;354:942–955.

Ghalie RG, Edan G, Laurent M, et al. Cardiac adverse effects associated with mitoxantrone (Novantrone) therapy in patients with MS. *Neurology.* 2002;59:909–913.

Ghalie RG, Mauch E, Edan G, et al. A study of therapy-related acute leukaemia after mitoxantrone therapy for multiple sclerosis. *Mult Scler.* 2002;8:441–445.

Golan D, Somer E, Dishon S, et al. Impact of exposure to war stress on exacerbations of multiple sclerosis. *Ann Neurol.* 2008;64:143–148.

Goodin DS, Ebers GC, Johnson KP, et al. The relationship of MS to physical trauma and psychological stress: report of the Therapeutics and Technology Assessment Subcommittee of the American Academy of Neurology. *Neurology.* 1999;52:1737–1745.

Goodkin DE, Kinkel RP, Weinstock-Guttman B, et al. A phase II study of i.v. methylprednisolone in secondary-progressive multiple sclerosis. *Neurology.* 1998;51:239–245.

Haas J. High dose IVIG in the post partum period for prevention of exacerbations in MS. *Mult Scler.* 2000;6(suppl 2):S18–S20.

Haas J, Hommes OR. A dose comparison study of IVIG in postpartum relapsing–remitting multiple sclerosis. *Mult Scler.* 2007;13:900–908.

Hafler DA, Compston A, Sawcer S, et al. Risk alleles for multiple sclerosis identified by a genomewide study. *N Engl J Med.* 2007;357:851–862.

Harris JO, Frank JA, Patronas N, et al. Serial gadolinium-enhanced magnetic resonance imaging scans in patients with early, relapsing–remitting multiple sclerosis: implications for clinical trials and natural history. *Ann Neurol.* 1991;29:548–555.

Hartung HP, Gonsette R, Konig N, et al. Mitoxantrone in progressive multiple sclerosis: a placebo-controlled, double-blind, randomised, multicentre trial. *Lancet.* 2002;360:2018–2025.

Hauser SL, Waubant E, Arnold DL, et al. B-cell depletion with rituximab in relapsing–remitting multiple sclerosis. *N Engl J Med.* 2008;358:676–688.

Hawkins SA, McDonnell GV. Benign multiple sclerosis? Clinical course, long term follow up, and assessment of prognostic factors. *J Neurol Neurosurg Psychiatry.* 1999;67:148–152.

Hogancamp WE, Rodriguez M, Weinshenker BG. The epidemiology of multiple sclerosis. *Mayo Clin Proc.* 1997;72:871–878.

Hommes OR, Sorensen PS, Fazekas F, et al. Intravenous immunoglobulin in secondary progressive multiple sclerosis: randomised placebo-controlled trial. *Lancet.* 2004;364:1149–1156.

International Multiple Sclerosis Genetics Consortium; Beecham AH, Patsopoulos NA, et al. Analysis of immune-related loci identifies 48 new susceptibility variants for multiple sclerosis. *Nat Genet.* 2013;45(11):1353–1360.

Jacobs LD, Cookfair DL, Rudick RA, et al. Intramuscular interferon beta-1a for disease progression in relapsing multiple sclerosis. The Multiple Sclerosis Collaborative Research Group (MSCRG). *Ann Neurol.* 1996;39:285–294.

Kappos L, Polman C, Pozzilli C, et al. Final analysis of the European multicenter trial on IFNbeta-1b in secondary-progressive MS. *Neurology.* 2001;57:1969–1975.

Kappos L, Weinshenker B, Pozzilli C, et al. Interferon beta-1b in secondary progressive MS: a combined analysis of the two trials. *Neurology.* 2004;63:1779–1787.

Keegan M, Pineda AA, McClelland RL, et al. Plasma exchange for severe attacks of CNS demyelination: predictors of response. *Neurology.* 2002;58:143–146.

Kikly K, Liu L, Na S, et al. The IL-23/Th(17) axis: therapeutic targets for autoimmune inflammation. *Curr Opin Immunol.* 2006;18:670–675.

Kleinewietfeld M, Manzel A, Titze J, et al. Sodium chloride drives autoimmune disease by the induction of pathogenic TH17 cells. *Nature.* 2013;496(7446):518–522.

Kragt J, van AB, Killestein J, et al. Higher levels of 25-hydroxyvitamin D are associated with a lower incidence of multiple sclerosis only in women. *Mult Scler.* 2009;15:9–15.

Krapf H, Morrissey SP, Zenker O, et al. Effect of mitoxantrone on MRI in progressive MS: results of the MIMS trial. *Neurology.* 2005;65:690–695.

Kutzelnigg A, Lucchinetti CF, Stadelmann C, et al. Cortical demyelination and diffuse white matter injury in multiple sclerosis. *Brain.* 2005;128:2705–2712.

Lincoln MR, Montpetit A, Cader MZ, et al. A predominant role for the HLA class II region in the association of the MHC region with multiple sclerosis. *Nat Genet.* 2005;37:1108–1112.

Link H, Huang YM. Oligoclonal bands in multiple sclerosis cerebrospinal fluid: an update on methodology and clinical usefulness. *J Neuroimmunol.* 2006;180:17–28.

Lovato L, Willis SN, Rodig SJ, et al. Related B cell clones populate the meninges and parenchyma of patients with multiple sclerosis. *Brain.* 2011;134:534–541.

Lublin FD, Baier M, Cutter G. Effect of relapses on development of residual deficit in multiple sclerosis. *Neurology.* 2003;61:1528–1532.

Lublin FD, Reingold SC. Defining the clinical course of multiple sclerosis: results of an international survey. National Multiple Sclerosis Society (USA) Advisory Committee on Clinical Trials of New Agents in Multiple Sclerosis. *Neurology.* 1996;46:907–911.

Lucchinetti CF, Bruck W, Lassmann H. Evidence for pathogenic heterogeneity in multiple sclerosis. *Ann Neurol.* 2004;56:308.

Lucchinetti CF, Gavrilova RH, Metz I, et al. Clinical and radiographic spectrum of pathologically confirmed tumefactive multiple sclerosis. *Brain.* 2008;131:1759–1775.

Magliozzi R, Howell O, Vora A, et al. Meningeal B-cell follicles in secondary progressive multiple sclerosis associate with early onset of disease and severe cortical pathology. *Brain.* 2007;130:1089–1104.

Manzel A, Muller D, Hafler D, et al. Role of "western diet" in inflammatory autoimmune diseases. *Curr Allergy Asthma Rep.* 2014;14(1):404.

McFarland HF, Martin R. Multiple sclerosis: a complicated picture of autoimmunity. *Nat Immunol.* 2007;8:913–919.

Mikol DD, Barkhof F, Chang P, et al. Comparison of subcutaneous interferon beta-1a with glatiramer acetate in patients with relapsing multiple sclerosis (the REbif vs Glatiramer Acetate in Relapsing MS Disease [REGARD] study): a multicentre, randomised, parallel, open-label trial. *Lancet Neurol.* 2008;7:903–914.

Miller AE, Morgante LA, Buchwald LY, et al. A multicenter, randomized, double-blind, placebo-controlled trial of influenza immunization in multiple sclerosis. *Neurology.* 1997;48:312–314.

Miller DH, Weinshenker BG, Filippi M, et al. Differential diagnosis of suspected multiple sclerosis: a consensus approach. *Mult Scler.* 2008;14:1157–1174.

Munger KL, Levin LI, Hollis BW, et al. Serum 25-hydroxyvitamin D levels and risk of multiple sclerosis. *JAMA.* 2006;296:2832–2838.

Oksenberg JR, Barcellos LF. Multiple sclerosis genetics: leaving no stone unturned. *Genes Immun.* 2005;6:375–387.

Panitch H, Goodin DS, Francis G, et al. Randomized, comparative study of interferon beta-1a treatment regimens in MS: The EVIDENCE Trial. *Neurology.* 2002;59:1496–1506.

Panitch H, Miller A, Paty D, et al. Interferon beta-1b in secondary progressive MS: results from a 3-year controlled study. *Neurology.* 2004;63:1788–1795.

Panitch HS, Thisted RA, Smith RA, et al; Psuedobulbar Affect in Multiple Sclerosis Study Group. Randomized, controlled trial of dextromethorphan/quinidine for pseudobulbar affect in multiple sclerosis. *Ann Neurol.* 2006;59(5):780–787.

Paty DW, Li DK. Interferon beta-1b is effective in relapsing–remitting multiple sclerosis. II. MRI analysis results of a multicenter, randomized, double-blind, placebo-controlled trial. UBC MS/MRI Study Group and the IFNB Multiple Sclerosis Study Group. *Neurology.* 1993;43:662–667.

Polman CH, Reingold SC, Edan G, et al. Diagnostic criteria for multiple sclerosis: 2005 revisions to the "McDonald criteria." *Ann Neurol.* 2005;58:840–846.

Poser CM, Goutieres F, Carpentier MA, et al. Schilder's myelinoclastic diffuse sclerosis. *Pediatrics.* 1986;77(1):107–112.

PRISMS Study Group and the University of British Columbia MS/MRI Analysis Group. PRISMS-4: long-term efficacy of interferon-beta-1a in relapsing MS. *Neurology.* 2001;56:1628–1636.

Pu{licken} M, Gordon-Lipkin E, Balcer LJ, et al. Optical coherence tomography and disease subtype in multiple sclerosis. *Neurology.* 2007;69:2085–2092.

Rudick RA, Cookfair DL, Simonian NA, et al. Cerebrospinal fluid abnormalities in a phase III trial of Avonex (IFNbeta-1a) for relapsing multiple sclerosis. The Multiple Sclerosis Collaborative Research Group. *J Neuroimmunol.* 1999;93:8–14.

Rutschmann OT, McCrory DC, Matchar DB. Immunization and MS: a summary of published evidence and recommendations. *Neurology.* 2002;59:1837–1843.

Sayao AL, Devonshire V, Tremlett H. Longitudinal follow-up of "benign" multiple sclerosis at 20 years. *Neurology.* 2007;68:496–500.

Secondary Progressive Efficacy Clinical Trial of Recombinant Interferon-beta-1a in MS (SPECTRIMS) Study Group. Randomized controlled trial of interferon-beta-1a in secondary progressive MS: clinical results. *Neurology.* 2001;56:1496–1504.

Simon JH, Jacobs LD, Campion M, et al. Magnetic resonance studies of intramuscular interferon beta-1a for relapsing multiple sclerosis. The Multiple Sclerosis Collaborative Research Group. *Ann Neurol.* 1998;43:79–87.

Sorensen PS, Koch-Henriksen N, Ross C, et al. Appearance and disappearance of neutralizing antibodies during interferon-beta therapy. *Neurology.* 2005;65:33–39.

The 5-year risk of MS after optic neuritis. Experience of the optic neuritis treatment trial. Optic Neuritis Study Group. *Neurology.* 1997;49:1404–1413.

Tintore M, Rovira A, Rio J, et al. New diagnostic criteria for multiple sclerosis: application in first demyelinating episode. *Neurology.* 2003;60:27–30.

Trapp BD, Peterson J, Ransohoff RM, et al. Axonal transection in the lesions of multiple sclerosis. *N Engl J Med.* 1998;338:278–285.

Tullman MJ. Symptomatic therapy in multiple sclerosis. *Continuum: Mult Scler.* 2004;10(6):142–172.

van Waesberghe JH, Kamphorst W, De Groot CJ, et al. Axonal loss in multiple sclerosis lesions: magnetic resonance imaging insights into substrates of disability. *Ann Neurol.* 1999;46:747–754.

Vukusic S, Hutchinson M, Hours M, et al. Pregnancy and multiple sclerosis (the PRIMS study): clinical predictors of post-partum relapse. *Brain.* 2004;127:1353–1360.

Weinshenker BG, Bass B, Rice GP, et al. The natural history of multiple sclerosis: a geographically based study. I. Clinical course and disability. *Brain.* 1989;112(pt 1):133–146.

Weinshenker BG, Bass B, Rice GP, et al. The natural history of multiple sclerosis: a geographically based study. 2. Predictive value of the early clinical course. *Brain.* 1989;112(pt 6):1419–1428.

Weinshenker BG, O'Brien PC, Petterson TM, et al. A randomized trial of plasma exchange in acute central nervous system inflammatory demyelinating disease. *Ann Neurol.* 1999;46:878–886.

Wolinsky JS, Narayana PA, O'Connor P, et al. Glatiramer acetate in primary progressive multiple sclerosis: results of a multinational, multicenter, double-blind, placebo-controlled trial. *Ann Neurol.* 2007;61:14–24.

Zivadinov R, Rudick RA, De MR, et al. Effects of IV methylprednisolone on brain atrophy in relapsing–remitting MS. *Neurology.* 2001;57:1239–1247.

Neuromyelitis Optica

Cree B. Neuromyelitis optica: diagnosis, pathogenesis and treatment. *Curr Neurol Neurosci Rep.* 2008;8:427–433.

Cree BA, Lamb S, Morgan K, et al. An open label study of the effects of rituximab in neuromyelitis optica. *Neurology.* 2005;64:1270–1272.

de Seze J, Lebrun C, Stojkovic T, et al. Is Devic's neuromyelitis optica a separate disease? A comparative study with multiple sclerosis. *Mult Scler.* 2003;9:521–525.

Jarius S, Paul F, Franciotta D, et al. Mechanisms of disease: aquaporin-4 antibodies in neuromyelitis optica. *Nat Clin Pract Neurol.* 2008;4:202–214.

Lennon VA, Kryzer TJ, Pittock SJ, et al. IgG marker of optic-spinal multiple sclerosis binds to the aquaporin-4 water channel. *J Exp Med.* 2005;202:473–477.

Lennon VA, Wingerchuk DM, Kryzer TJ, et al. A serum autoantibody marker of neuromyelitis optica: distinction from multiple sclerosis. *Lancet.* 2004;364:2106–2112.

Lucchinetti CF, Mandler RN, McGavern D, et al. A role for humoral mechanisms in the pathogenesis of Devic's neuromyelitis optica. *Brain.* 2002;125:1450–1461.

Mandler RN, Ahmed W, Dencoff JE. Devic's neuromyelitis optica: a prospective study of seven patients treated with prednisone and azathioprine. *Neurology.* 1998;51:1219–1220.

Mandler RN, Davis LE, Jeffery DR, et al. Devic's neuromyelitis optica: a clinicopathological study of 8 patients. *Ann Neurol.* 1993;34:162–168.

Matiello M, Lennon VA, Jacob A, et al. NMO-IgG predicts the outcome of recurrent optic neuritis. *Neurology.* 2008;70:2197–2200.

Mealy MA, Wingerchuk DM, Greenberg BM, Levy M. Epidemiology of neuromyelitis optica in the United States: a multicenter analysis. *Arch Neurol.* 2012;69(8):1039–1043.

O'Riordan JI, Gallagher HL, Thompson AJ, et al. Clinical, CSF, and MRI findings in Devic's neuromyelitis optica. *J Neurol Neurosurg Psychiatry.* 1996;60:382–387.

Pittock SJ. Neuromyelitis optica: a new perspective. *Semin Neurol.* 2008;28:95–104.

Pittock SJ, Lennon VA, de Seze J, et al. Neuromyelitis optica and non organ-specific autoimmunity. *Arch Neurol.* 2008;65:78–83.

Pittock SJ, Lennon VA, Krecke K, et al. Brain abnormalities in neuromyelitis optica. *Arch Neurol.* 2006;63:390–396.

Pittock SJ, Weinshenker BG, Lucchinetti CF, et al. Neuromyelitis optica brain lesions localized at sites of high aquaporin 4 expression. *Arch Neurol.* 2006;63:964–968.

Roemer SF, Parisi JE, Lennon VA, et al. Pattern-specific loss of aquaporin-4 immunoreactivity distinguishes neuromyelitis optica from multiple sclerosis. *Brain.* 2007;130:1194–1205.

Takahashi T, Fujihara K, Nakashima I, et al. Anti-aquaporin-4 antibody is involved in the pathogenesis of NMO: a study on antibody titre. *Brain.* 2007;130:1235–1243.

Weinshenker BG, Wingerchuk DM, Vukusic S, et al. Neuromyelitis optica IgG predicts relapse after longitudinally extensive transverse myelitis. *Ann Neurol.* 2006;59:566–569.

Wingerchuk DM. Neuromyelitis optica: effect of gender. *J Neurol Sci.* 2009;286 (1–2):18–23.

Wingerchuk DM, Hogancamp WF, O'Brien PC, et al. The clinical course of neuromyelitis optica (Devic's syndrome). *Neurology.* 1999;53:1107–1114.

Wingerchuk DM, Lennon VA, Pittock SJ, et al. Revised diagnostic criteria for neuromyelitis optica. *Neurology.* 2006;66:1485–1489.

Wingerchuk DM, Pittock SJ, Lucchinetti CF, et al. A secondary progressive clinical course is uncommon in neuromyelitis optica. *Neurology.* 2007; 68:603–605.

Marchiafava–Bignami

Aggunlu L, Oner Y, Kocer B, et al. The value of diffusion-weighted imaging in the diagnosis of Marchiafava–Bignami disease: apropos of a case. *J Neuroimaging.* 2008;18(2):188–190.

Berek K, Wagner M, Chemelli AP, et al. Hemispheric disconnection in Marchiafava–Bignami disease: clinical, neuropsychological and MRI findings. *J Neurol Sci.* 1994;123:2–5.

Celik Y, Temizoz O, Genchellac H, et al. A non-alcoholic patient with acute Marchiafava–Bignami disease associated with gynecologic malignancy: paraneoplastic Marchiafava–Bignami disease? *Clin Neurol Neurosurg.* 2007; 109(6):505–508.

Heinrich A, Runge U, Khaw AV. Clinicoradiologic subtypes of Marchiafava–Bignami disease. *J Neurol.* 2004;251(9):1050–1059.

Hillbom M, Saloheimo P, Fujioka S, et al. Diagnosis and management of Marchiafava-Bignami disease. *J Neurol Nuerosurg Psychiatry.* 2014;85: 168–173.

Ironside R, Bosanquet FD, McMenemey WH. Central demyelination of the corpus callosum (Marchiafava–Bignami disease). *Brain.* 1961;84: 212–230.

Kawarabuki K, Sakakibara T, Hirai M, et al. Marchiafava–Bignami disease: magnetic resonance imaging findings in corpus callosum and subcortical white matter. *Eur J Radiol.* 2003;48(2):175–177.

Marchiafava E, Bignami A. Sopra un'alterazione del corpo calloso osservata in soggetti alcoolisti. *Riv Patol Nerv Ment.* 1903;8:544–549.

Rusche-Skolarus LE, Lucey BP, Vo KD, et al. Transient encephalopathy in a postoperative non-alcoholic female with Marchiafava–Bignami disease. *Clin Neurol Neurosurg.* 2007;109(8):713–715.

Tao H, Kitagawa N, Kako Y, et al. A case of anorexia nervosa with Marchiafava–Bignami disease that responded to high-dose intravenous corticosteroid administration. *Psychiatry Res.* 2007;156(2):181–184.

Pontine and Extrapontine Myelinolysis 70

Gary L. Bernardini and Elliott L. Mancall

INTRODUCTION

In 1959, Adams, Victor, and Mancall described a distinctive, previously unrecognized disease characterized primarily by the symmetric destruction of myelin sheaths in the basis pontis. They called it *central pontine myelinolysis* (CPM). The general term *myelinolysis* may be more appropriate because the condition affects extrapontine brain areas as well. The term *osmotic demyelination syndrome* has also been applied. CPM can occur alone or in combination with extrapontine myelinolysis (EPM) in 10% to 20% of cases; isolated EPM may also be found.

Myelinolysis is a neurologic complication that can develop after too rapid correction of hyponatremia to normal or supranormal levels. Chronic alcoholism and undernutrition are frequently associated with this condition. Pontine myelinolysis has been seen, however, in hyponatremic nonalcoholic patients, including conditions of dehydration resulting from vomiting, diarrhea, or diuretic therapy, with postoperative overhydration or with psychogenic water intoxication. Severe malnutrition, including that resulting from extensive burn injuries, may be a predisposing condition. In addition, pontine myelinolysis occurs in chronic alcohol users with profound hypophosphatemia. There may also be an association between hyponatremia and hypokalemia in some cases. Some reports of myelinolysis have been in patients with alcoholic cirrhosis or after interferon therapy who had normal serum sodium. However, in most cases, the main factor underlying development of myelinolysis appears to be too rapid correction of serum sodium levels. Correction after hypernatremia rather than hyponatremia has also been encountered. The condition has been described with increasing frequency in patients undergoing orthotopic liver transplantation. Pontine myelinolysis is found in 0.28% to 9.8% of these cases. In liver failure, lack of sufficient energy for adequate glial cell function, deficiency of important organic osmolytes such as myoinositol to protect the brain from sudden changes in serum osmolality, or negative nitrogen balance decreasing amount of amino acids to form essential organic osmolytes are possibilities that predispose these patients to develop CPM. Similarly, rapid correction of hyponatremia has led to myelinolysis in the uremic patient on hemodialysis. However, a more benign form of pontine myelinolysis may occur without hyponatremia in alcoholic binge drinkers or some with anorexia nervosa. This syndrome has good clinical outcome, and magnetic resonance imaging (MRI) abnormalities disappear. EPM incidence appears to be increasing possibly due to sensitivity in detection through improved quality MRI.

EPIDEMIOLOGY

Predisposing factors associated with CPM include alcoholism, chronic malnutrition, and sodium imbalances. In large case series of patients with CPM, Lampl and Yazdi found that 39.4% were alcoholics, 21.5% had too rapid correction of hyponatremia, and 17.4% were liver transplant recipients. Studies have reported CPM

to occur in cases of rapid correction of hyponatremia *or* hypernatremia. In addition, the incidence of CPM increases in alcoholic patients even with normonatremia. An association of hypokalemia with hyponatremia has been implicated in this disease, with suggestion of correcting hypokalemia prior to correcting low sodium levels in treating these patients.

CLINICAL MANIFESTATIONS

The clinical manifestations vary from asymptomatic to comatose, although patients may present with generalized encephalopathy associated with low levels of serum sodium. Neurologic signs and symptoms of myelinolysis usually appear within 2 to 3 days after rapid correction of sodium levels. Classically, initial symptoms of dysarthria and dysphagia with initial flaccid quadriplegia (later to become spastic) can be seen on examination after correction of hyponatremia. Other findings are mutism, behavioral abnormalities, frank psychosis, ophthalmoparesis, bulbar and pseudobulbar palsy, hyperreflexia, seizures, and coma. Typically, rapidly progressive corticobulbar and corticospinal syndrome may be noted in debilitated patient, often during an acute illness with associated electrolyte imbalance and correction or overcorrection of hyponatremia. Although the patients are mute, coma is unusual. The patients may be "locked in," and communication by eye blinking can sometimes be established. The course is rapid, and death generally ensues within days or weeks after onset of symptoms.

EPM can lead to ataxia, irregular behavior, visual field deficits, parkinsonism, choreoathetosis, dystonia, or paroxysmal kinesigenic dyskinesias. The movement disorders can appear with or without radiographic evidence of EPM. Movement disorders as result of EPM may represent treatable form with some improvement noted after dopaminergic therapy. In EPM, bilateral symmetric involvement may affect white matter of basal ganglia (caudate/putamen), cerebellum, thalamus, midbrain (substantia nigra), corpus callosum, subcortical white matter, claustrum, hypothalamus, lateral geniculate bodies, amygdala, subthalamic nuclei, or medial lemnisci with sparing of the pons and globus pallidus.

DIAGNOSIS

Although historically, most cases have been diagnosed only at autopsy, the syndrome can now be diagnosed in life through neuroimaging along with clinical presentation. Computed tomography (CT) scans may be normal, especially early in the course, but CT abnormalities include symmetric areas of hypodensity in the basis pons and extrapontine regions without associated mass effect. MRI is more sensitive and typically shows symmetric increased signal intensity in the central pons (described as *trident-shaped*) on T2-weighted and fluid-attenuated inversion recovery (FLAIR) images; lesions appear hypointense on T1-weighted images and typically do not enhance (Fig. 70.1). MRI diffusion-weighted imaging (DWI) may be even more sensitive testing because it

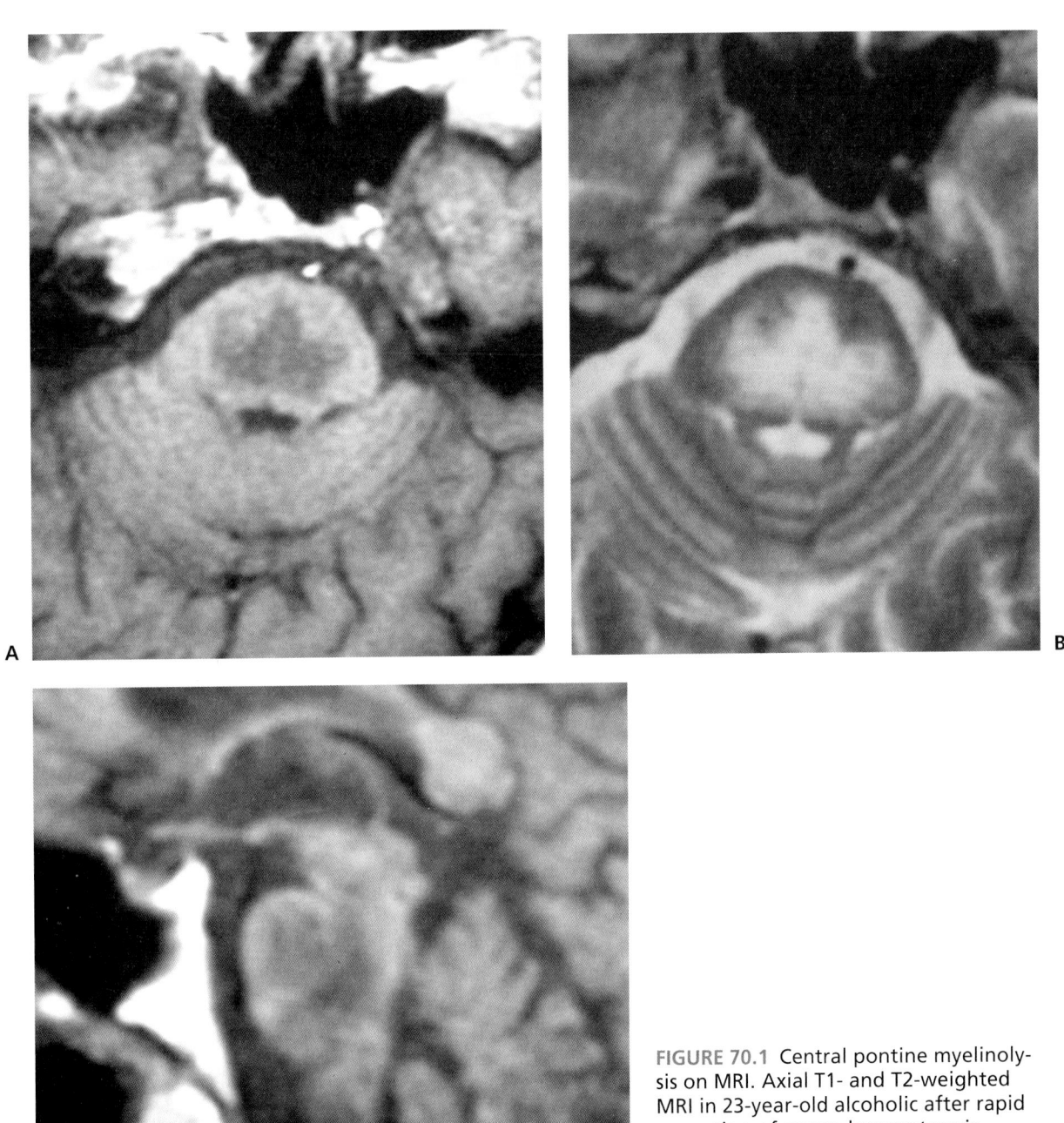

FIGURE 70.1 Central pontine myelinolysis on MRI. Axial T1- and T2-weighted MRI in 23-year-old alcoholic after rapid correction of severe hyponatremia, showing hypointense **(A)** and hyperintense **(B)** "trident-shaped" basis pontine lesion consistent with pontine myelinolysis. **C:** Sagittal T1-weighted MRI showing hypointensity in area of pons consistent with demyelination. (Courtesy of Dr. William Wagle.)

demonstrates increased signal of restricted diffusion of water in the central pons within 24 hours of onset of symptoms of myelinolysis. Lesions seen within the basis pons typically spare the tegmentum and may extend to ventral midbrain but rarely involve medulla.

Even though conventional imaging with CT and MRI may lag behind clinical manifestations by up to 2 weeks, MRI DWI remains the most sensitive technique for early diagnosis. However, in clinically suspicious cases with initial negative neuroimaging, repeat MRI is recommended within 2 weeks of symptom onset. Other studies with magnetic resonance spectroscopy, with decreased N-acetylaspartate (NAA)/creatine (Cr) ratio, increased choline (Cho)/Cr ratio may be helpful in the acute phase with diagnosis of CPM. Brain stem auditory–evoked responses may demonstrate prolonged III to V and I to V latencies consistent with bilateral pontine lesions. An electroencephalogram (EEG) may show slowing and low voltage. Cerebrospinal fluid (CSF) levels of protein and myelin basic protein may be elevated.

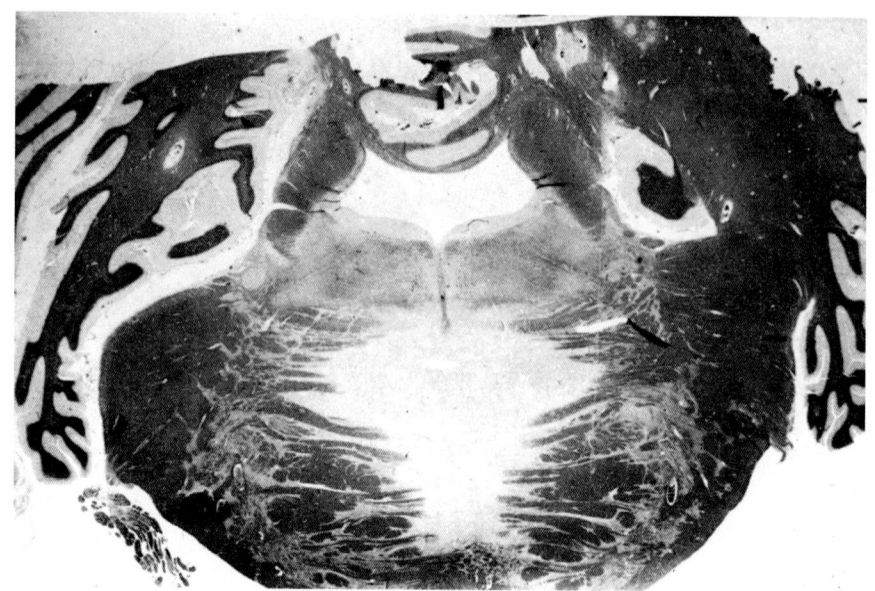

FIGURE 70.2 Central pontine myelinolysis. Histologic section through rostral pons showing characteristic lesion. (Courtesy of Dr. J. Kepes.)

PATHOBIOLOGY

The principal pathologic change is demyelination; within affected areas, there is degeneration with loss of oligodendrocytes but nerve cells and axon sheaths are spared, blood vessels are unaffected, and there is no inflammation. The pathophysiology seems caused by physiologic imbalance of osmoles in the brain. Apoptosis may deplete supply of energy to glial cells and Na^+/K^+ adenosine triphosphatase (ATPase) pumps, thus impairing cellular adaptation to osmotic stress. In animal studies, the initial event after administration of hypertonic saline in hypotonic rats seems to be opening of the blood–brain barrier, followed sequentially by swelling of the inner loop of the myelin sheath, oligodendrocyte degeneration, and release of macrophage-derived factors leading to the eventual breakdown of myelin. Histologically, the lesion begins in the median raphe and may involve all or part of the base of the pons (Fig. 70.2). The lesion may spread into the pontine tegmentum or superiorly into the mesencephalon or involve bilateral extrapontine areas with or without concurrent basis pontis lesions. Microscopically, lesions resemble those of Marchiafava–Bignami disease (demyelination of corpus callosum and other commissural fibers, commonly seen in the context of chronic alcoholism and malnutrition).

The exact cause of myelinolysis is uncertain. In those with hyponatremia that has been rapidly corrected to normal or supranormal levels, it is not clear whether the low sodium, the rate of correction, or absolute change in serum sodium content is causative factor. However, symptoms are more likely to develop with rapid correction of chronic (>48 hours) rather than acute hyponatremia. In experimental animals, pontine myelinolysis developed in hyponatremic rats, rabbits, or dogs treated rapidly with hypernatremic saline. Animals left with untreated hyponatremia did not develop neuropathologic changes. Therefore, attention has focused on rate of correction of the hyponatremia rather than on hyponatremia itself as inciting mechanism of myelinolysis. A recent study has suggested loss of activity of brain aquaporins (specifically aquaporins 1 and 4) affecting redistribution of water and osmolytes across various brain compartments may be seen in pontine myelinolysis.

PREVENTION AND TREATMENT

Prevention of myelinolysis includes judicious correction of hyponatremia with normal saline and free-water restriction, discontinuation of diuretic therapy, and correction of associated metabolic abnormalities and medical complications. At present, there are no clinical trials providing Level 1 evidence for the appropriate treatment of CPM. Hyponatremic patients who are asymptomatic may not require saline infusion. Those with agitated confusion, seizures, or coma should be treated with normal saline until the symptoms improve. Caution should be used in giving hypertonic saline to patients with symptomatic hyponatremia; frequent laboratory evaluations of serum sodium should be used as a guide to avoid too rapid correction of low sodium levels.

Stepwise correction of hyponatremia is shown in Table 70.1. Some have reported success in treating CPM with high-dose pulse therapy with methylprednisolone (1 g/day for 5 days), plasmapheresis, or immunoglobulins. Based on clinical data and animal studies, there is low incidence of myelinolysis if increase in serum sodium is less than or equal to 12 mmol/L in 24 hours. Late appearance of tremor, dystonia, or cognitive and

TABLE 70.1 **Stepwise Correction of Hyponatremia**
1. **Calculate total sodium deficit.** Sodium deficit = (140 − serum sodium) × total body water (TBW = 0.6 [men] or 0.5 [women] × kg lean body mass)
2. **Determination of rate of sodium infusion** Depending on desired rate of increased serum sodium (i.e., ≤12 mmol/L/day) and effect of 1 L of any infusate on serum sodium levels Use the formula: change in serum sodium = (infusate sodium + infusate potassium) − serum sodium/TBW + 1
3. **Maximum desired sodium increase over 24 h: ≤12 mmol/L**

TBW, total body water.

behavioral changes has been reported in survivors. Prognostics factors that are favorable for recovery include absence of coexisting hypokalemia, less severe hyponatremia, and less severe clinical syndrome on admission and discharge. Full recovery has also been seen.

SUGGESTED READINGS

Adams RD, Victor M, Mancall EL. Central pontine myelinolysis: a hitherto undescribed disease occurring in alcoholic and malnourished patients. *AMA Arch Neurol Psychiatry.* 1959;81:154–172.

Adrogue HJ, Madias NE. Hyponatraemia. *N Engl J Med.* 2000;342:1581–1589.

Ashrafian H, Davey P. A review of the causes of central pontine myelinolysis: yet another apoptotic illness? *Eur J Neurol.* 2001;8:103–109.

Ayus JC, Krothpalli RK, Arieff AI. Treatment of symptomatic hyponatremia and its relation to brain damage. *N Engl J Med.* 1987;317:1190–1195.

Baba Y, Wszolek ZK, Normand MM. Paroxysmal kinesigenic dyskinesia associated with central pontine myelinolysis. *Parkinsonism Relat Disord.* 2003;10:113.

Brunner JE, Redmond JM, Haggar AM, et al. Central pontine myelinolysis and pontine lesions after rapid correction of hyponatremia: a prospective magnetic resonance imaging study. *Ann Neurol.* 1990;27:61–66.

Donahue SP, Kardon RH, Thompson HS. Hourglass-shaped visual fields as a sign of bilateral lateral geniculate myelinolysis. *Am J Ophthalmol.* 1995;119:378–380.

Guo Y, Hu JH, Lin W. Central pontine myelinolysis after liver transplantation: MR diffusion, spectroscopy and perfusion findings. *Magn Reson Imaging.* 2006;24:1395–1398.

Hadfield MG, Kubal WS. Extrapontine myelinolysis of the basal ganglia without central pontine myelinolysis. *Clin Neuropathol.* 1996;15:96–100.

Harris CP, Townsend JJ, Baringer JR. Symptomatic hyponatremia: can myelinolysis be prevented by treatment? *J Neurol Neurosurg Psychiatry.* 1993;56:626–632.

Heng AE, Vacher P, Aublet-Cuvelier B, et al. Centropontine myelinolysis after correction of hyponatremia: role of associated hypokalemia. *Clin Nephrol.* 2007;67:345–351.

Huang WY, Weng WC, Peng TI, et al. Central pontine and extrapontine myelinolysis after rapid correction of hyponatremia by hemodialysis in a uremic patient. *Ren Fail.* 2007;29:635–638.

Kallakatta RN, Radhakrishnan A, Fayaz RK, et al. Clinical and functional outcome and factors predicting prognosis in osmotic demyelination syndrome (central pontine and/or extrapontine myelinolysis) in 25 patients. *J Neurol Neurosurg Psychiatry.* 2011;82:326–331.

Kleinschmidt-Demasters BK, Norenberg MD. Rapid correction of hyponatremia causes demyelination: relation to central pontine myelinolysis. *Science.* 1981;211:1068–1070.

Lampl C, Yazdi K. Central pontine myelinolysis. *Eur Neurol.* 2002;47:3–10.

Lee TM, Cheung CC, Lau EY, et al. Cognitive and emotional dysfunction after central pontine myelinolysis. *Behav Neurol.* 2003;14:103–107.

Lim L, Krystal A. Psychotic disorder in a patient with central and extrapontine myelinolysis. *Psychiatry Clin Neurosci.* 2007;61:320–322.

Lohr JW. Osmotic demyelination syndrome following correction of hyponatremia: association of hypokalemia. *Am J Med.* 1994;96:408–413.

Martin RJ. Central pontine and extrapontine myelinolysis: the osmotic demyelination syndromes. *J Neurol Neurosurg Psychiatry.* 2004;75(suppl 3):iii22–iii28.

Mascarenhas JV, Jude EB. Central pontine myelinolysis: electrolytes and beyond. *BMJ Case Rep.* 2014;28:1–3.

Mitchell AW, Burn DJ, Reading PJ. Central pontine myelinolysis temporally related to hypophosphatemia. *J Neurol Neurosurg Psychiatry.* 2003;74:820.

Morlan L, Rodriguez E, Gonzales J, et al. Central pontine myelinolysis following correction of hyponatremia: MRI diagnosis. *Eur Neurol.* 1990;30:149–152.

Popescu BF, Bunyan RF, Guo Y, et al. Evidence for aquaporin involvement in human central pontine myelinolysis. *Acta Neuropathol Commun.* 2013;1:40.

Rojiani AM, Cho ES, Sharer L, et al. Electrolyte-induced demyelination in rats. 2. Ultrastructural evolution. *Acta Neuropathol.* 1994;88:293–299.

Ruzek KA, Campeau NG, Miller GM. Early diagnosis of central pontine myelinolysis with diffusion-weighted imaging. *AJNR Am J Neuroradiol.* 2004;25:210–213.

Sakamoto E, Hagiwara D, Morishita Y, et al. Complete recovery of central pontine myelinolysis by high dose pulse therapy with methylprednisolone [in Japanese]. *Nihon Naika Gakkai Zasshi.* 2007;96:2291–2293.

Salerno SM, Kurlan R, Joy SE, et al. Dystonia in central pontine myelinolysis without evidence of extrapontine myelinolysis. *J Neurol Neurosurg Psychiatry.* 1993;56:1221–1223.

Saner FH, Koeppen S, Meyer M, et al. Treatment of central pontine myelinolysis with plasmapheresis and immunoglobulins in liver transplant patient. *Transpl Int.* 2008;21:390–391.

Schrier RW. Treatment of hyponatremia. *N Engl J Med.* 1985;312:1121–1123.

Snell DM, Bartley C. Osmotic demyelination syndrome following rapid correction of hyponatraemia. *Anaesthesia.* 2008;63:92–95.

Thompson DS, Hutton JT, Stears JC, et al. Computerized tomography in the diagnosis of central and extrapontine myelinolysis. *Arch Neurol.* 1981;38:243–246.

Uchino A, Yuzuriha T, Murakami M, et al. Magnetic resonance imaging of sequelae of central pontine myelinolysis in chronic alcohol abusers. *Neuroradiology.* 2003;45:877–880.

Wadhwa J, Ananthakrishnan R, Sadashiv S, et al. Extrapontine myelinolysis: rare manifestation of a well-known disorder. *BMJ Case Rep.* 2013.

Wright DG, Laureno R, Victor M. Pontine and extrapontine myelinolysis. *Brain.* 1979;102:361–385.

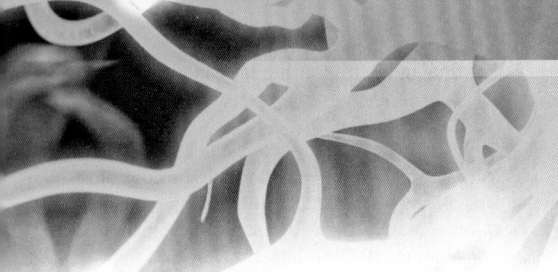

Autoimmune Meningitis and Encephalitis 71

Lawrence S. Honig

INTRODUCTION

Meningitis and encephalitis are defined as inflammatory conditions of the meninges or brain, and often occur together as meningoencephalitis, affecting both meninges and cerebrum. Meningitis may present with various symptoms including headache, fever, painful eye movements, neck stiffness, and cranial or limb radiculopathies. However, it is specifically defined by evidence of cellular infiltration of the meninges. As such, it is generally evident through laboratory testing, finding abnormal numbers of white blood cells in the cerebrospinal fluid (CSF), and sometimes also evident radiologically through abnormal densities or enhancements of the meninges. Encephalitis is more difficult to define clinically, as the symptoms may include varying degrees and regional involvements of brain dysfunction. Indeed, many disorders are described as encephalitis even when they may involve a subacute injurious process to the brain that does not specifically include inflammation per se. (These include toxic, metabolic, mitochondrial, prion, or neoplastic disorders discussed in other chapters that best would be termed *encephalopathies*, rather than encephalitides.) The gold standard for defining encephalitis is brain biopsy, but this is required infrequently. Encephalitis can generally be inferred by the presence of abnormal clinical findings referable to the brain, with accompanying evidence of inflammation of the brain, often by neuroimaging. Supportive features can include electroencephalographic findings suggesting acute brain injury, and accompanying meningitis. Classically, meningitis and encephalitis were perceived as attributable to infectious etiologies. Causative organisms included more or less relatively identifiable typical or atypical bacteria, fungi, or parasites or often less identifiable viruses. However, recent decades have brought with them the advent of increasing general good health, decreasing infectious causes of these disorders, and increasingly potent molecular tools allowing better diagnosis. Thus, it has become clear that a significant fraction of meningitis and encephalitis, particularly after the period of infancy, and particularly in the developed world, has no apparent infectious cause. In recent years, a number of inflammatory syndromes without known external organismal causative underpinnings have been defined as clinicopathologic entities. The acute multiple sclerosis–like syndrome, involving mostly white matter, called *acute disseminated encephalomyelitis* (ADEM), still has no clear pathoetiology. However, improvements of molecular assay techniques have led to the categorization of a number of other clinical encephalitis syndromes, mostly involving cerebral gray matter, through identification of the presence in serum and/or CSF of characteristic antibodies to nervous system proteins. The antigens to which these antibodies are directed include intraneuronal proteins (Hu, Yo, Ma), synaptic proteins, and cell surface proteins. The cell surface antigens are actually the most common and most notably include the voltage-gated potassium channel complex (VGKCC) receptor and glutamate N-methyl-D-aspartate receptor (NMDAR). Despite incomplete understanding of their pathogenic basis, these various encephalitic disorders characterized by presence of antineuronal antibodies are best termed the *immune-mediated encephalitides*. They may be further categorized as being of autoimmune idiopathic nature or autoimmune and associated with a neoplasm. These latter are termed *paraneoplastic syndromes*. However, because so many of the same syndromes occur in the presence or absence of a neoplasm, it is most useful to consider these disorders as immune-mediated, with or without an identified underlying associated factor such as a malignancy.

EPIDEMIOLOGY

The incidence and prevalence of encephalitis is not well established due to differences in populations, diagnosis, and reporting. Recent studies suggest an overall incidence rate across all age ranges of about 50 cases of all-cause encephalitis per million persons. Of these, about 40% are infectious, 40% unknown cause, 10% ADEM, and 5% each are NMDAR and VGKCC antibody encephalitis. A number of studies have suggested that, excluding infants and excluding epidemics, NMDAR encephalitis is more common than any other single sporadic viral encephalitic etiology. Thus in adults, the incidence of VGKCC and NMDAR antibody disorders probably is each somewhat similar to that of Creutzfeldt–Jakob disease with an incidence rate of about two per million persons per year. VGKCC antibody encephalitis occurs more often in persons older than the age of 50 years and affects men more than women (about 65% men). NMDAR encephalitis is increasingly recognized in the pediatric population, and more than half of cases occur in children. A series of about 500 cases has shown a median age of onset of 21 years with a range of 8 months to 85 years. There is a strong female predominance (81%), but among patients younger than 12 years, or older than 45 years, as many as 40% of cases are male. Only about 40% of patients have tumors, but of those with tumors, more than 95% are women. Tumors are more common among patients of Asian or African ancestry. Individuals with tumors that are resected improve more quickly, require less treatment, and are much less likely to relapse. With or without tumor, 2 years after treatment, there is a good outcome in 80% of cases, with independent living, without disability, or only mild symptoms or disability. However, there is also a fatality rate of about 5%.

PATHOBIOLOGY

The general defining feature of the immune-mediated meningoencephalitides are the presence of specific autoantibodies directed toward nervous system antigens. It is not entirely clear that the antibodies themselves are pathogenic, and some have suggested that they might be bystanders in disease pathogenesis. For the antibodies directed toward intraneuronal antigens, evidence is indeed weak that the antigen relates to the syndromes and that the antibodies themselves are pathogenic; perhaps cytotoxic T cells are more responsible for disease pathogenesis and neural destruction. For the cell surface antigens, a variety of observations are suggestive that the antibodies themselves may play an important part in the pathogenesis of the disorders. Antibody levels may correlate with disease activity; procedures to reduce immune response may result in clinical improvement; and in some cases, animal models have been developed mimicking the effects of antigen depletion. The genesis of these disorders is generally conceptualized as beginning with the development of an immune response to an autoantigen in the nervous system, either spontaneously due to exposure of the immune system to antigens displayed by a tumor, virus, or microbe or due to unmasking of otherwise privileged nervous system antigens due to brain injury or infection. The antigen provoking the response may be the actual neural antigen or a cross-reacting closely related molecule due to "molecular mimicry." Once an immune response has occurred, there is immune-mediated attack on normal nervous system tissue. Such attack may occur after any inciting infection or injury has already resolved.

Immune-mediated encephalitides may be associated with antibodies to cell surface proteins, such as the VGKCC, NMDAR, α-amino-3-hydroxy-5-methyl-4-isoxazolepropionic acid (AMPA) receptor, or to γ-aminobutyric acid-B (GABA$_B$) or glycine (GLY) receptors or may be associated with antibodies to synaptic proteins such as glutamic acid decarboxylase (GAD) or amphiphysin or may be associated with intraneuronal proteins such as Hu, Yo, Ma, or Ri (Table 71.1). Any of these syndromes may occur in the context of paraneoplasia, in which presumably some onconeural antigen on the tumor prompted the immune response, or "spontaneously" without the presence of a tumor. In general, the presumed deleterious effects of an antibody may relate simply to interference with neural transmission or to the development of immune-mediated attack on the patients neural tissue. NMDAR encephalitis is associated with the presence of anti-NR1 subunit antibodies, which apparently bind the NMDAR causing internalization of these receptors important for neurotransmission, particularly in the hippocampus. Pathologic studies of biopsies performed on patients with NMDAR antibody encephalitis often additionally show mild inflammation with perivascular infiltrates, which likely brings to the region injurious cytokines, but neurons and their connections are often intact. To the extent that there is only loss of neurotransmitter function and/or presence of noxious inflammatory molecules, elimination of the injurious antibody and the inflammatory response can allow for cellular production of new receptor proteins providing for complete recovery of function. To the extent that there is an immune attack on neurons, recovery is unlikely. In paraneoplastic cerebellar degeneration due to anti-Yo, pathologic studies show complete destructive depletion of all Purkinje cells, severely, and permanently impairing cerebellar function. Likewise in anti-Hu syndrome, there appears to be hippocampal atrophy with loss of neurons.

CLINICAL MANIFESTATIONS

The clinical hallmarks of the immune-mediated meningoencephalitides are subacute deterioration of central nervous system function, accompanied typically by some evidence of an inflammatory process in the central nervous system on CSF testing and/or neuroimaging. It is often the speed, rather than the particular clinical characteristics that indicates an immune-mediated meningoencephalitis. Rapidly progressive central neurologic dysfunction, in the face of no clear evidence of toxic, vascular, neoplastic, or infectious nervous system involvement, should promptly raise the suspicion of an immune-mediated or prion-mediated (see Chapter 68) disorder.

Diagnostic testing, reviewed in the following text, is essential to interpret the clinical findings. Magnetic resonance imaging (MRI) of the brain in these immune-mediated disorders may show MRI signal abnormalities in gray or white matter on T2-weighted or fluid-attenuated inversion recovery (FLAIR) imaging sequences. Signal abnormalities may also be seen on diffusion-weighted imaging (DWI) of the cortical ribbon and deep nuclei, similar to changes seen in prion diseases or ischemic disorders. However,

TABLE 71.1   Immune-mediated Meningoencephalitides

Antigen Category	Antigen	Syndrome	Tumor	Reversible
Cell surface protein	VGKCC (LGI1, CASPR2, contactin-2)	LE, hyponatremia	Lung, thymus, thyroid, ovary, kidney	+
	NMDA receptor	LE, oral dyskinesias	Teratoma	+
	AMPA receptor	LE	Lung, breast, thymus	+
	GABA$_B$ receptor	LE	SCLC	+
	mGluR5 receptor	LE	Lymphoma	+
	GLY receptor	LE, SPS	Thymus, lymphoma	+/−
	Ganglionic AChR	Dysautonomia, LE?, Cblm?	Breast, others	+/−
Synaptic protein	GAD	LE, SPS, Cblm	Various	+/−
	Amphiphysin	LE, SPS	Breast, SCLC	+/−
Intraneuronal antigen	Hu	LE, sensory ataxia	SCLC, others	−
	Yo	Cblm	Breast, ovary	−
	Ri	LE, Cblm, myoclonus, opsoclonus	Breast, SCLC	−
	CRMP5/CV2	LE, Cblm, uveitis	SCLC, thymus	+/−
	Ma2 (Ma/Ta)	LE, opsoclonus	Testes	+/−
Other antigens	P/Q calcium channel	LE?	SCLC	+
	Thyroglobulin, microsomal	Meningoencephalitis?		+

LE, limbic encephalitis; SPS, stiff person syndrome; SCLC, small cell lung cancer; Cblm, cerebellar disorder.

the distinguishing feature of the immune-mediated disorders is inflammation. Even if DWI signal abnormalities are seen, they are accompanied by more extensive FLAIR or T2-weighted imaging abnormalities not common in prion disease. And contrast-enhanced imaging may show areas of breakdown of the blood–brain barrier, definitely inconsistent with prion disease but common in inflammatory disease. But it is CSF and blood studies that best help define the immune-mediated disorders. CSF may show evidence of central nervous system inflammation such as the presence of pleocytosis and elevated protein. Cellular fluid is not characteristically seen in prion disease. Blood and CSF studies may identify marker antibodies that characterize distinct clinicopathologic entities with characteristic diagnostic, prognostic, and therapeutic features. Some of these immune syndromes are sufficiently recognizable disorders through their clinical phenotype, even though it may take some days to weeks to confirm an immune-mediated disorder with an antibody test. Other syndromes may not be as easily recognized but nonetheless may show a somewhat consistent epidemiology and clinical presentation.

LIMBIC ENCEPHALITIS

Limbic encephalitis is a syndrome in which there is subacute affliction that principally involves the deeper, medial forebrain structures of the temporal, and to a lesser extent frontal and parietal, lobes, specifically the hippocampal formation and amygdala, parahippocampal regions, and insular and cingulate cortices. Clinical symptoms of limbic encephalitis are subacute, over days to weeks to months. Typically, decline in memory is a predominant feature, with confusion and disorientation, occurring over a less prolonged time period than typical for mild cognitive impairment (MCI) and neurodegenerative disorders such as Alzheimer disease. Memory dysfunction is often lateralized and may be more verbal, involving left hippocampus, or more visual, involving right hippocampus. Patients may repeat themselves and may have confusional episodes but often neuropsychiatric symptoms are more noticeable to friends and relatives. Personality and/or behavioral changes, including depression, apathy, irritability, aggression, disinhibition, and impulsiveness, are common, as well as frank psychosis with delusions and paranoia. These symptoms reflect involvement of the limbic structures. Seizures are common. Indeed, frequently, the first clinical feature that prompts consideration of organic neurologic disease, as opposed to psychiatric interpretation, may be new onset of complex partial or generalized seizures. Changes in eating habits and sexual desire may also occur as well as sleep disturbance. Limbic encephalitis was first described in the last two decades of the 20th century as relating to antibodies to intraneuronal antigens such as Hu, Ma, or Yo and often associated with a cancer. Thus, limbic encephalitis almost became synonymous with paraneoplastic encephalitis. However, during the first decade of the 21st century, a whole new family of limbic encephalitis disorders was described, in which the antibodies are specific for neuronal cell surface antigens (see Table 71.1). These syndromes, associated with antibodies to cell surface antigens, are more common than the prior family. The antigens are usually expressed throughout the nervous system but tend to be particularly enriched in the hippocampus, and in some cases the cerebellum, and thus are associated with limbic encephalitis and sometimes cerebellar dysfunction. The cell surface antigens include those of the VGKCC, which includes antigens LGI1 (leucine-rich glioma inactivated 1 protein also known as *epitempin*), CASPR2 (contactin-associated protein 2) and contactin-2, to glutamate receptors including the NR1 subunit of the NMDAR or the GluR1 or GluR2 subunits of the AMPA

receptor or to GABA$_B$ or GLY receptors. Each syndrome tends to have its own symptomatology, although symptoms overlap. The two most important such entities, each relatively recognizable from their clinical syndromes, are VGKCC antibody encephalitis and NMDAR antibody encephalitis.

Voltage-gated Potassium Channel Complex Encephalitis

This typically affects individuals older than age 50 years and typically is a relatively "pure" limbic encephalitis that affects both mesial temporal lobes but is usually asymmetric in presentation, affecting one cerebral hemisphere more than the other. There are several clinical presentations. One common presentation involves clinical hallmarks of memory loss with occasional generalized seizures and sometimes brief seizures lasting only 1 to 2 seconds and involving speech arrest or brief facial contortion. Typically, patients and/or observers may be aware of these spells, but other than a brief interruption of activities, the spells themselves may not significantly impede patient function. Initially, unilateral hippocampal involvement is most common but usually progresses to involve both hippocampi clinically and by imaging. These patients may also have significant neuropsychiatric symptoms including personality change or apathy or aggression. Another archetypical presentation is with faciobrachial seizures or spasms, which typically last 2 to 5 seconds and involve unilateral grimacing and dystonic or mild myoclonic movements of the ipsilateral arm in addition to the face. With this presentation, most often the motor symptoms are first noted before informants report marked memory or personality changes. Subsequently, memory is involved. Serum is usually positive for antibody specific to LGI1, part of the VGKCC. Frequently, electroencephalography may be abnormal with slowing but does not show any electroencephalogram (EEG) surface sharp waves even during these clinically seizure-like events. A psychiatric cause is often posited because of the bizarre nature of the events, without surface electrode-based electrographic concomitant. However, the spells are quite responsive to anticonvulsants, particularly phenytoin. Generalized convulsive seizures may also occur but are less common. The third, least common presentation of VGKCC encephalitis is one of Morvan syndrome, frequently associated with the CASPR2 antibody, with severe sleep disturbance, most marked by insomnia but also by daytime sleep attacks. Other features include confusion and hallucinations, and autonomic disturbances including tachycardia, hypertension, incontinence, constipation, and hyperhidrosis. Rash may occur and peripheral nervous system features including stiffness and muscle twitching that represents neuromyotonia. Although these three presentations may recognizably occur, some patients have overlapping features. Another common feature of VGKCC encephalitides is hyponatremia. Serum sodium levels in the 120 to 130 mEq/L range, or occasionally lower, are common, occurring in 60% of cases. This electrolyte abnormality can itself exacerbate the cognitive symptomatology and decrease seizure threshold. Typically, oral sodium chloride supplementation is required to maintain adequate serum sodium levels. MRI typically (i.e., in 80% of cases) shows T2 and T2 FLAIR hyperintensity, usually without marked DWI signal abnormality nor necessarily any contrast enhancement upon delivery of gadolinium contrast agents. Lumbar puncture typically (i.e., in 80% of cases) shows at least a mild pleocytosis, with cell counts ranging from 5 to 100 white blood cells/μL but absent red blood cells and normal or only mildly elevated protein and normal glucose. The differential diagnosis often includes herpes encephalitis, and clues that herpes family virus is not the etiology include the somewhat more subacute history of weeks to months (rather than days), the characteristic brief EEG-negative seizures if present, the lack of red blood cells in CSF or hemorrhage by MRI, and the frequently relatively "inactive" EEG (often without frank epileptiform activity). Nonetheless, antiviral therapy for herpes simplex virus (HSV) is appropriate until CSF is proven negative for HSV DNA by rapid polymerase chain reaction (PCR) testing. Presence of VGKCC antibody should prompt search for a tumor, particularly in the lungs, although only about 10% of cases are tumor-associated. Immune treatments are often very effective, commonly with significant or complete neurologic recovery from limbic encephalitis due to VGKCC antibody. Disease relapses, depending on definition, are infrequent, occurring in at most 5% to 10% of cases, but in some cases, a propensity for seizures may persist, requiring continued treatment with antiepileptic agents.

N-methyl-D-aspartate Receptor Antibody Encephalitis

This presents as a subacute encephalopathy, sometimes preceded by a prodromal nonspecific or "viral" illness but then developing prominent neuropsychiatric symptoms. Symptoms of psychosis, with disorganized or paranoid thoughts, atypical behavior, and social withdrawal may occur early on. This disorder occurs principally in young women, although now recognized in both children and men. Because of these demographics, it is common for the disorder to first be the subject of psychiatric investigations and treatment; a diagnosis of "catatonia" is often tendered. Development of more profound confusion, motor symptoms including focal dystonia, weakness, ataxia, tremors, myoclonus, and chorea, and onset of seizures prompts neurologic evaluation. Frequently, the nonepileptic motor symptoms are confused for seizures, but seizures are also common, and the seizures of this disorder do typically have an EEG correlate, although not usually classic spike and wave discharges. EEG also frequently shows characteristic abnormalities such as the "extreme delta-brush" pattern in adults, which are almost pathognomonic for this disorder. MRI is abnormal only in about half of cases and may show focal areas of T2 or FLAIR signal abnormality in limbic regions, or cortical regions, and sometimes areas of frank inflammation with contrast enhancement. CSF typically shows a pleocytosis, commonly with 5 to 100 white blood cells/μL, and sometimes mildly elevated protein and oligoclonal bands. Respiratory depression, sometimes requiring mechanical ventilation, may occur in up to half of cases, and the disease may progress to coma. Autonomic dysregulation is common, with persistent tachycardia, punctuated by episodic bradycardia and sinus pauses (asystole up to 10 seconds), the latter often in the context of nasogastric tube placement, orotracheal suctioning, or other vagal stimulatory maneuvers. Flushing, sweating, and urinary and bowel changes may also occur. The most pathognomonic clinical finding is oral, buccal, lingual, and facial dyskinesias, which may occur in fragmentary and intermittent fashion or may be nearly continuous. Often there is a rhythmic, myoclonic nature to these movements. They can also be extremely intense, with injuries to tongue and lips from biting. Any case of N-methyl-D-aspartate receptor antibody encephalitis (NMDARAE) should prompt immediate search for a teratoma. In women, ovarian teratomas occur in about 50% of cases, and prompt removal of a discovered tumor is generally the most effective therapy. The encephalitic illness can be extremely prolonged, even with aggressive treatments. However, it is common to have marked or complete recovery over a period of 4 to 12 months, although cases have been described with recovery proceeding over years. Relapses, depending on the definition, occur

in up to 25% of cases, often in the first year; cases associated with tumors that are resected extremely rarely relapse, absent a diagnosis of additional tumor.

Other Neuronal Cell Surface Receptor Antibody Encephalitides

These are less common than those associated with antibody to VGKCC or NMDAR. But limbic encephalitides with some similarity to VGKCC-associated disorders may be marked by antibodies to non-NMDA glutamate receptor such as the AMPA, GABA$_B$, or GLY receptors. These disorders do not have as consistent phenotypes as VGKCC antibody encephalitis but also typically involve memory dysfunction, behavioral dysfunction, and epileptic seizures. Seizures may be complex partial or generalized convulsive seizures. Unexplained new-onset epilepsy in a younger or middle-aged patient, somewhat more commonly female than male, age 30 to 60 years, is a not uncommon presentation of these rarer disorders.

Limbic Encephalitis Associated with the Antineuronal Anti-Hu Antibody

This typically presents with subacute memory disorder. Generally, the course is one of several months, sometimes associated with behavior change but less commonly with seizures. Sensory ataxia due to proprioceptive losses, due to dorsal root ganglionopathy, occurs commonly in about half of cases. Other symptoms can include cerebellar dysfunction, brain stem signs, and autonomic symptoms including gastrointestinal pseudo-obstruction. In about 90% of cases, there is an associated tumor, which is usually a lung tumor, and is often small cell lung cancer. The neurologic syndrome virtually always precedes the discovery of the tumor, and the tumor may often be quite small and limited. Tumor removal more often than not does result in stabilization of the neurologic symptoms, particularly if there is complete tumor resection. However, limited recovery occurs in only about a third of cases, and significant improvement is very rare.

SUBACUTE CEREBELLAR DEGENERATION

This is a clinically recognizable disorder in which over a period of days to weeks or several months, there is increasingly severe ataxia. Gait ataxia, appendicular ataxia with intention tremor, and dysarthria are all common features. Other brain stem signs such as nystagmus, diplopia, oscillopsia, hyperreflexia, and nausea and vomiting may occur. Serum testing reveals antibodies directed against cerebellar neuronal antigens, typically the anti-Yo antibody, although anti-Ri, anti-Hu, anti-Ma, anti-GAD, anti-PCA-2, and other antibodies have been identified less commonly. Anti-Ri syndrome usually is marked by opsoclonus. The CSF may have evidence of pleocytosis and high protein, and in such cases, steroid treatment may be more useful. Search for a tumor is mandatory. In women, more than 80% of cases have a carcinoma of breast or ovary, or occasionally other locations. Like anti-Hu encephalitis, tumors in anti-Yo encephalitis are often small, more limited, and usually not identified until neurologic presentation and associated investigations. Like anti-Hu syndrome, stabilization may occur with tumor removal. However, meaningful recovery does not occur.

OTHER IMMUNE-RELATED MENINGOENCEPHALITIDES

These are associated with antineuronal antibodies in subacute retinal degeneration due to CAR antibody and syndromes associated with antibodies to Ma2 (Ma/Ta), ganglionic acetylcholine receptors, mGluR5 receptor, and CRMP5/CV2. Antibodies to synaptic antigens such as GAD and amphiphysin likewise are associated with encephalitides. Hashimoto encephalitis is a meningoencephalitic illness presenting with confusion, headaches, and seizures and marked by antimicrosomal and antithyroglobulin antibodies. This controversial entity is now referred to as *steroid-responsive encephalitis* because the condition often responds markedly to steroid therapy. CSF typically shows mild evidence of meningitis, often with high CSF protein, and sometimes pleocytosis. The role of thyroid antibodies is unclear. Other meningoencephalitic disorders that appear immune-mediated relate to systemic inflammatory conditions including Behçet disease, Vogt–Koyanagi syndrome, systemic lupus, and other disorders. Acute disseminated encephalomyelitis, postinfectious and postvaccination inflammatory disorders, and unidentifiable aseptic meningitides, and the syndromes of new-onset refractory status epilepticus (NORSE) or febrile infection-related epilepsy syndrome (FIRES) also bear similarities to the disorders described earlier but are generally not accompanied by sensitive or specific disease biomarkers.

DIAGNOSIS

The diagnosis of immune-mediated encephalitides starts with clinical history and examination. Typically, the disorder is subacute to acute but sometimes the disorders may develop over a background of some mild, nonspecific, and not clearly related symptoms ongoing for some years. More commonly, there is an escalating course de novo and rapidly, of cognitive, behavioral, and/or epileptic dysfunction without metabolic, infectious, or systemic inflammatory causes. Typically, this rapid progression of symptoms should prompt an aggressive diagnostic evaluation to provide the information required for appropriate categorization of the disorder. This is because the various disorders, although poorly understood, still have particular empirically established treatment options. Although imaging is often helpful in localization, and neurophysiologic studies are helpful in assessing the contributions of epileptic activities, it is laboratory studies of blood and CSF that may be most useful.

Blood testing can be of great diagnostic use. Antibody tests for VGKCC antibodies or other antibodies termed *paraneoplastic* (see Table 71.1) can often be highly sensitive and specific. The major limitation of these tests is that reporting of results may take some days to weeks.

It is essential to also perform CSF analysis to assess for the presence of inflammation; the results of this are available within hours. CSF cell counts are informative as to whether there is an inflammatory cellular component. Cytologic examination permits exclusion of neoplastic cell involvement. Microbiologic and serologic tests allow for determination of whether bacterial or viral infectious elements are present. Antibody panels may be used, particularly for NMDARAE. Of the immune-mediated encephalitides, most disorders are most easily diagnosed in the blood, although the NMDA disorder may present with antibodies only evident in the CSF. For monitoring purposes, CSF antibodies may have use, whereas blood NMDAR antibody levels do not seem to correlate with symptoms and improvement. Thus, CSF is diagnostically important but also the ability to follow CSF cell counts and protein and antibody levels in the case of NMDAR antibody provide key metrics for monitoring the status of treatment.

Electroencephalography (EEG) is important to exclude the possibility that subclinical epileptic activity is responsible for abnormalities in mental status or motoric function. EEG provides help when there are frequent subclinical seizures in assisting the choice and dosage of antiepileptic medications.

Neuroimaging has become a somewhat reliable marker for limbic encephalitis, particular in the mid to late stages of VGKCC disorders (Fig. 71.1). Frequently, there are T2 and T2 FLAIR abnormalities in hippocampal or other limbic regions, and in some cases evidence of restricted diffusion on DWI imaging, indicating water content changes associated with presumed acute injury. NMDAR encephalitis is less likely to show MRI abnormalities, although in some cases, there are clear areas of injury. For some of the encephalitides, there may be imaging evidence of meningitis and/or evidence of inflammatory cortical or subcortical lesions, which may show contrast enhancement. When abnormalities are present, their evolution can be used as a gauge of the progress of treatment. Nuclear medicine metabolic (fluorodeoxyglucose positron emission tomography [PET]) or perfusion ([99mTc]-hexamethyl propylene amine oxime [HMPAO] or [99mTc]-ethyl cysteine dimer [EDC] single-photon emission computed tomography [SPECT]) scans of patients with limbic encephalitides may be normal or show areas of decreased metabolism/perfusion but more often show hypermetabolism and hyperperfusion in the affected temporal lobes, presumably due to overactivity.

Systemic body imaging can become important in the diagnostic evaluation of these disorders because of the possibility of a distant tumor prompting an antibody response, which then is associated with nervous system dysfunction. The presence of VGKCC, NMDAR, or anti-Hu antibodies should respectively prompt thorough examination of the lungs, ovaries, or breasts and ovaries.

Brain biopsy has the potential to provide specific pathoetiologic information in cases where blood and CSF studies are noninformative. In particular, some infectious processes, including viral and other infectious disorders can be detected on brain biopsy. If prion disease, such as Creutzfeldt–Jakob disease, is within the differential diagnosis, then brain biopsy is valuable in establishing or excluding that diagnosis. However in general, brain biopsy is often diagnostically unrevealing in the immune-mediated encephalitides. Biopsy may reveal lymphocytic infiltrates in the parenchyma, vasculocentric involvement, and may confirm the presence and relative involvement of gray and white matter. However, lacking an infectious organism, these pathologic findings are usually insufficiently specific to be helpful. Thus, specific settings in which brain biopsy should be considered are as follows: (1) Prion disease is within the differential diagnosis; (2) infectious disease not otherwise discoverable is being considered; and (3) inflammatory disease is strongly suspected but it is not clear if there is active disease or a burned out process. In this latter situation, the limitation is that a brain biopsy, even if directed at a neuroimaged lesional area, may not be representative of other areas.

TREATMENT AND OUTCOME

Treatment of the immune-mediated encephalitides includes both symptomatic treatment for seizures and immune-related therapies. Immunomodulatory therapies are warranted in this family of syndromes, but in general, only the cell surface antibody-mediated syndromes, such as VGKCC, NMDAR, and related antibody-mediated encephalitides are highly responsive. The syndromes associated with intraneuronal antigens, such as anti-Hu, usually show little benefit from treatment.

Immune treatments include "first-line treatments," which consist of high-dose intravenous corticosteroids, intravenous immunoglobulin infusions, and plasma exchange. Second-line treatments comprise more potent immunosuppressive therapies, including rituximab, mycophenolate, azathioprine, and cyclophosphamide.

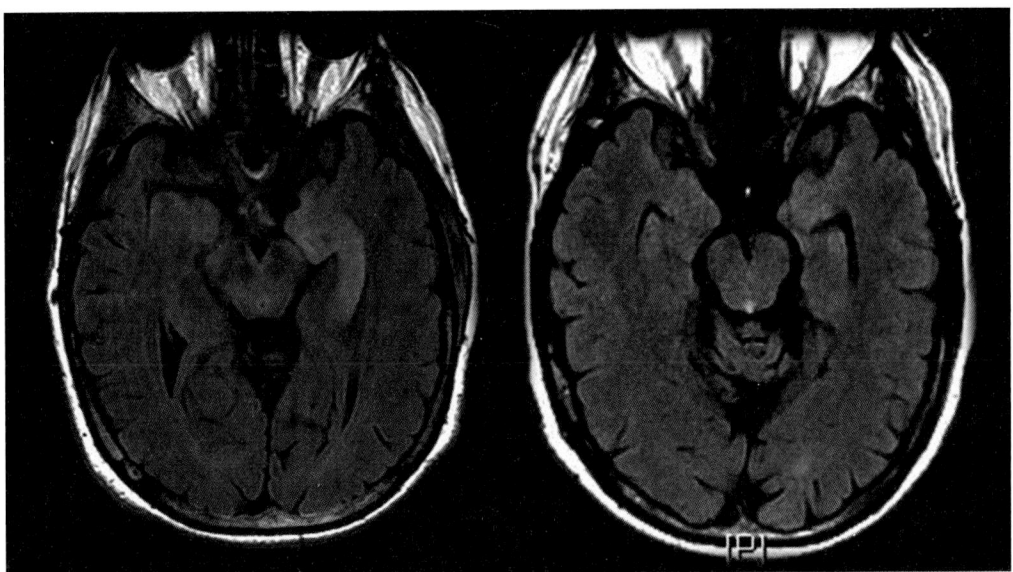

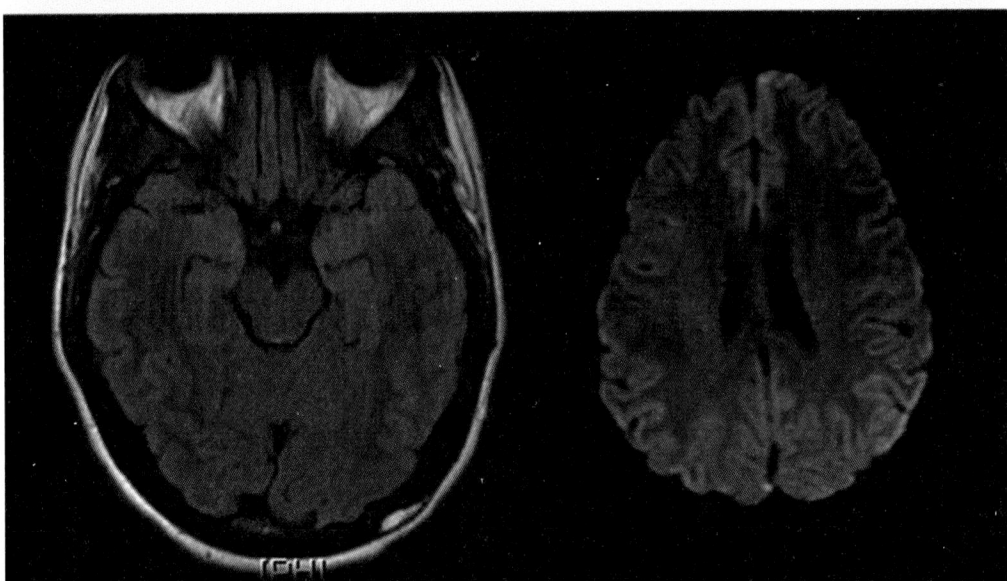

FIGURE 71.1 Neuroimaging in immune-mediated encephalitis. **Top row** shows MRI imaging of a patient with VGKCC encephalitis with T2 FLAIR sequences 1 month after onset of symptoms (*top left*) and 5 months later after treatment. Prominent left hippocampal hyperintensity and swelling on initial image has essentially resolved after treatment. **Bottom row** shows two patients with NMDAR encephalitis. *Bottom left* shows essentially normal MRI imaging on T2 FLAIR sequence of patient with severe symptoms. *Bottom right* shows DWI sequence on a different patient, showing subtle increased signal on left greater than right parietal cortical ribbon.

There are to date no published controlled trials of these various therapeutic approaches, so all such therapies are both empiric and off-label (unapproved) at this time. Complicating interpretation of therapeutic interventions are the fact that a number of the immune-mediated encephalitides may have a monophasic course and eventually, even if only after months or years, show spontaneous recovery without specific therapy (e.g., NMDARAE) and the fact that the different antibody syndromes do appear to have different responsiveness to different therapeutic interventions.

Corticosteroid course is frequently the first treatment for these disorders and presumably acts both by decreasing the inflammatory response and decreasing antibody production. Steroid actions start within hours but also cease within hours to days of termination of therapy. It is particularly useful for limbic encephalitis associated with VGKCC antibodies and some of the other cell surface antibodies. It is less obviously efficacious in NMDARAE, particularly when there is not such an inflammatory component (e.g., in individuals with little degree of pleocytosis). Typical steroid dosages are 1,000 mg methylprednisolone intravenously daily for 5 days. For VGKCC encephalitis, intravenous steroids are followed by oral treatment, often with a relatively prolonged taper. Prednisone at doses of about 1 mg/kg can be given, with a taper over months. If there is no reemergence of symptoms, patients may be able to have complete discontinuation of steroids by 4 to 12 months, although some patients require chronic treatment with either steroids or second-line agents discussed in the following text. Chronic steroid treatment is not of evident use in NMDARAE. Side effects of steroids may be limiting even in the acute setting, including behavioral dysfunction, euphoria, and insomnia. Side effects of chronic treatment must also be monitored, including weight gain, facial plethora, diabetes, and fungal and other infections.

Intravenous human immunoglobulin (IVIG) infusion is the other first treatment for these disorders. Presumed mechanism of action is interference through competition or binding with circulating pathogenic antibodies and/or immunoregulatory effects. Typical dosage is 0.4 g/kg for 5 days, for a total dosage of 2 g/kg. IVIG has a plasma half-life of about 28 days and therapeutic span of weeks to months. Frequently, cotreatment with both methylprednisolone and IVIG is performed as first-line treatment. Retreatment with IVIG for relapses may be performed after 1 or more months.

Plasma exchange (plasmapheresis) is another putative first-line treatment for immune-mediated disorders. Exchange in five plus sessions over 2 weeks may have some use. Most often considered in persons presenting with respiratory failure, this intervention is less often used for several reasons. For NMDARAE, antibody production is apparently principally in the central nervous system, so it is theoretically, as well as practically less clear that removal of plasma antibody is effective. Other reasons why plasma exchange is less used, include that it is less expeditious, requiring multiple treatments over many days, and more arduous for the patient requiring large venous cannulas in persons who may be agitated. Furthermore, if IVIG infusion is contemplated, then plasmapheresis would be counterproductive, removing the infused therapeutic immunoglobulin.

Second-line treatments for these disorders are generally used either as steroid-sparing agents in cases that appear to be steroid-dependent or IVIG-dependent or in cases where steroids and/or IVIG treatment is not accompanied by evidence of recovery over about 4 weeks. These second-line treatments include targeted specific immunosuppression with rituximab or nonspecific immunosuppression with mycophenolate, azathioprine, or cyclophosphamide. Rituximab is a chimeric mouse/human monoclonal antibody directed against the human lymphocyte cell surface antigen CD20. It eliminates B cells and is a proven treatment for lymphopoietic malignancies, as well as proven treatment by randomized controlled trials in the nonmalignant inflammatory disease rheumatoid arthritis. In nonmalignant conditions, a single infusion of 1,000 mg, given with appropriate premedications and monitoring, over hours results in near certain complete elimination of all B lymphocytes. This elimination typically occurs within several days. Although the half-life of the drug is only weeks, the B-cell depletion last months (typically 6 to 9 months, particularly after first treatment, although in a small percentage of patients up to several years). This results in substantial reductions in antibody-producing cells. The advantage of the treatment is that, aside from occasional infusion reactions, this focused immunosuppression is well tolerated and easily monitored (by counts of peripheral CD19-positive B cells). The therapy is not reversible, except through passage of time. However, if neurologic recovery is incomplete, or if there is a relapse, retreatment with rituximab will again deplete any recovered B cells. In many cases, a single treatment is adequate, presumably because the body's repopulated antibody-producing cells do not include the clones producing the pathogenic antibody. Experience seems to indicate that rituximab may be particularly successful second-line treatment for NMDARAE, with beginning of improvement in symptoms often occurring some weeks following

therapeutic infusion. Side effects of rituximab can include potentially serious or even lethal infusion reactions (which however are very uncommon in nonmalignant conditions), chronic immunosuppression, and in rare cases progressive multifocal leukoencephalopathy. Mycophenolate and azathioprine can also be used as more general immunosuppressants following steroids and/or IVIG. Mycophenolate levels can be monitored, and white blood cell counts can be monitored during treatment with these drugs. Cyclophosphamide is a more toxic chemotherapeutic agent that can be used to achieve a higher degree of immunosuppression in refractory cases. There are no large therapeutic series with these agents.

SUGGESTED READINGS

Bataller L, Dalmau J. Neuro-ophthalmology and paraneoplastic syndromes. *Curr Opin Neurol.* 2004;17:3–8.

Bien CG, Vincent A. Immune-mediated pediatric epilepsies. *Handb Clin Neurol.* 2013;111:521–531.

Boronat A, Sabater L, Saiz A, et al. GABA(B) receptor antibodies in limbic encephalitis and anti-GAD-associated neurologic disorders. *Neurology.* 2011;76:795–800.

Chong JY, Rowland LP, Utiger RD. Hashimoto encephalopathy: syndrome or myth? *Arch Neurol.* 2003;60:164–171.

Dalmau J, Tüzün E, Wu HY, et al. Paraneoplastic anti-N-methyl-D-aspartate receptor encephalitis associated with ovarian teratoma. *Ann Neurol.* 2007;61:25–36.

Dayalu P, Teener JW. Stiff person syndrome and other anti-GAD-associated neurologic disorders. *Semin Neurol.* 2012;32:544–549.

Gable MS, Sheriff H, Dalmau J, et al. The frequency of autoimmune N-methyl-D-aspartate receptor encephalitis surpasses that of individual viral etiologies in young individuals enrolled in the California Encephalitis Project. *Clin Infect Dis.* 2012;54:899–904.

Graus F, Dalmau J. Paraneoplastic neurological syndromes. *Curr Opin Neurol.* 2012;25:795–801.

Graus F, Saiz A, Dalmau J. Antibodies and neuronal autoimmune disorders of the CNS. *J Neurol.* 2010;257:509–517.

Hoffmann LA, Jarius S, Pellkofer HL, et al. Anti-Ma and anti-Ta associated paraneoplastic neurological syndromes: 22 newly diagnosed patients and review of previous cases. *J Neurol Neurosurg Psychiatry.* 2008;79:767–773.

Irani SR, Bien CG, Lang B. Autoimmune epilepsies. *Curr Opin Neurol.* 2011;24:146–153.

Irani SR, Pettingill P, Kleopa KA, et al. Morvan syndrome: clinical and serological observations in 29 cases. *Ann Neurol.* 2012;72:241–255.

Irani SR, Stagg CJ, Schott JM, et al. Faciobrachial dystonic seizures: the influence of immunotherapy on seizure control and prevention of cognitive impairment in a broadening phenotype. *Brain.* 2013;136:3151–3162.

Jones KC, Benseler SM, Moharir M. Anti-NMDA receptor encephalitis. *Neuroimaging Clin N Am.* 2013;23:309–320.

Jubelt B, Mihai C, Li TM, et al. Rhombencephalitis/brainstem encephalitis. *Curr Neurol Neurosci Rep.* 2011;11:543–552.

Leypoldt F, Wandinger KP. Paraneoplastic neurological syndromes. *Clin Exp Immunol.* 2014;175:336–348.

Lang B, Dale RC, Vincent A. New autoantibody mediated disorders of the central nervous system. *Curr Opin Neurol.* 2003;16:351–357.

Malter MP, Helmstaedter C, Urbach H, et al. Antibodies to glutamic acid decarboxylase define a form of limbic encephalitis. *Ann Neurol.* 2010;67:470–478.

Melzer N, Meuth SG, Wiendl H. Paraneoplastic and non-paraneoplastic autoimmunity to neurons in the central nervous system. *J Neurol.* 2013;260:1215–1233.

Merchut MP. Management of voltage-gated potassium channel antibody disorders. *Neurol Clin.* 2010;28:941–959.

Moscato EH, Peng X, Jain A, et al. Acute mechanisms underlying antibody effects in anti-N-methyl-D-aspartate receptor encephalitis. *Ann Neurol.* 2014;76:108–119.

Peery HE, Day GS, Doja A, et al. Anti-NMDA receptor encephalitis in children: the disorder, its diagnosis, and treatment. *Handb Clin Neurol.* 2013;112:1229–1233.

Petit-Pedrol M, Armangue T, Peng X, et al. Encephalitis with refractory seizures, status epilepticus, and antibodies to the GABAA receptor: a case series, characterisation of the antigen, and analysis of the effects of antibodies. *Lancet Neurol.* 2014;13:276–286.

Posner JB. Anti-Hu autoantibody associated sensory neuropathy/encephalomyelitis: a model of paraneoplastic syndrome. *Perspect Biol Med.* 1995;38:167–181.

Prüss H, Voltz R, Gelderblom H, et al. Spontaneous remission of anti-Ma associated paraneoplastic mesodiencephalic and brainstem encephalitis. *J Neurol.* 2008;255:292–294.

Rosenblum MK. Paraneoplasia and autoimmunologic injury of the nervous system: the anti-Hu syndrome. *Brain Pathol.* 1993;3:199–212.

Rosenfeld MR, Titulaer MJ, Dalmau J. Paraneoplastic syndromes and autoimmune encephalitis: five new things. *Neurol Clin Pract.* 2012;2:215–223.

Schiess N, Pardo CA. Hashimoto's encephalopathy. *Ann N Y Acad Sci.* 2008;1142:254–265.

Serratrice G, Serratrice J. Continuous muscle activity, Morvan's syndrome and limbic encephalitis: ionic or non ionic disorders? *Acta Myol.* 2011; 30:32–33.

Titulaer MJ, McCracken L, Gabilondo I, et al. Late-onset anti-NMDA receptor encephalitis. *Neurology.* 2013;81:1058–1063.

Titulaer MJ, McCracken L, Gabilondo I, et al. Treatment and prognostic factors for long-term outcome in patients with anti-NMDA receptor encephalitis: an observational cohort study. *Lancet Neurol.* 2013;12:157–165.

Turner MR, Irani SR, Leite MI, et al. Progressive encephalomyelitis with rigidity and myoclonus: glycine and NMDA receptor antibodies. *Neurology.* 2011;77:439–443.

Vernino S. Paraneoplastic cerebellar degeneration. *Handb Clin Neurol.* 2012;103:215–223.

Vincent A, Bien CG, Irani SR, et al. Autoantibodies associated with diseases of the CNS: new developments and future challenges. *Lancet Neurol.* 2011;10:759–772.

Wandinger KP, Saschenbrecker S, Stoecker W, et al. Anti-NMDA-receptor encephalitis: a severe, multistage, treatable disorder presenting with psychosis. *J Neuroimmunol.* 2011;231:86–91.

Neurosarcoidosis 72

John C. M. Brust

INTRODUCTION

Sarcoidosis is a multisystem, granulomatous disease of unknown cause. Sarcoid granulomas resemble those of tuberculosis but lack tubercle bacilli or caseation, although central necrosis is sometimes seen. Active lesions contain epithelioid and multinucleate giant cells; such lesions may resolve but more often become fibrotic.

EPIDEMIOLOGY

Sarcoidosis occurs worldwide, with estimated incidence ranging from 3 to 50 cases per 100,000 population. Incidence is especially high among African-Americans, in whom the disease is more likely to be chronic and severe. Susceptibility to sarcoidosis is polygenetically influenced, and different polymorphisms involving the major histocompatibility complex predict the severity of disease. Onset is most often in the third or fourth decade, but the disease also affects children and the elderly. Sarcoid granulomas are attributed to heightened immune responses to unidentified exogenous antigens. An infectious cause remains elusive. Sarcoidosis is described in patients with HIV infection treated with highly active antiretroviral therapy (HAART), reflecting what is known as the *immune reconstitution inflammatory syndrome*. Sarcoidosis has also developed following interferon alpha therapy for hepatitis C.

PATHOBIOLOGY

The disorder is mediated primarily by CD4+ T-helper 1 (Th1) cells and mononuclear phagocytes, with participation of numerous cytokines and chemokines that include interleukins, adhesion molecules, interferon gamma, tumor necrosis factor (TNF)-alpha, and transforming growth factor-beta. Lesions may affect any organ, especially lungs, lymph nodes, skin, bones, eyes, and salivary glands. Although nearly 20% of patients with neurosarcoidosis lack systemic symptoms or signs, workup reveals systemic sarcoidosis in as many as 97%. When nervous system disease complicates systemic sarcoidosis, it usually does so within 2 years of onset.

In the central nervous system (CNS), sarcoid granulomas most often involve the meninges, especially at the base of the brain, with secondary infiltration of cranial nerves and obstruction of cerebrospinal fluid (CSF) flow. Lesions tend to be perivascular and thereby may spread intraparenchymally, frequently affecting the hypothalamus and, less often, other CNS structures, including the spinal cord. Granulomas also occur in peripheral nerves and muscle.

CLINICAL MANIFESTATIONS

Given the unpredictable dispersal of lesions, sarcoidosis is a clinically protean disease systemically and neurologically. Nearly 50% of patients with neurosarcoidosis have more than one neurologic complication, with relative frequencies varying among different clinical series (Table 72.1).

TABLE 72.1	Symptoms and Signs in Neurosarcoidosis
Signs and Symptoms	(%)
Cranial neuropathy	50–75
Aseptic meningitis	10–20
CNS parenchymal disease	5–15
Peripheral neuropathy	5–10
Myopathy	10
Hydrocephalus	10

CNS, central nervous system.

Although any cranial nerve may be affected, the most frequently affected is the seventh, sometimes in association with uveitis and parotitis (uveoparotid fever) but usually alone, thus suggesting Bell palsy. Facial weakness may be bilateral and either simultaneous or sequential and may recur after recovery. Eighth nerve involvement, the second most common cranial neuropathy in sarcoidosis, causes deafness (often bilateral) and vestibular symptoms. Optic nerve involvement causes papillitis or retrobulbar neuritis and eventually optic atrophy. Trigeminal nerve involvement causes either sensory loss or neuralgia.

Granulomas involve the hypothalamus more often than the pituitary, thereby producing combinations of endocrinologic and nonendocrinologic symptoms that include diabetes insipidus, decreased libido, galactorrhea, amenorrhea, abnormal sleep patterns, altered appetite, temperature dysregulation, and abnormal behavior. Cerebral granulomas may be scattered diffusely, with some too small to be detected on computed tomography (CT) or magnetic resonance imaging (MRI), or they may consist of one or larger masses that mimic a brain neoplasm. Seizures are common in such patients. Cognitive and behavioral symptoms include dementia, depression, psychosis, hallucinations, and delirium. Rarely, sarcoid vasculitis causes cerebral infarction (or even intracranial hemorrhage) in a pattern clinically and pathologically indistinguishable from what is commonly called *granulomatous angiitis* of the nervous system. Autoantibodies to endothelial cells have been identified in patients with neurosarcoidosis.

Intraparenchymal or extraparenchymal spinal cord lesions can cause back pain, radiculopathy, and spastic paraparesis. Intramedullary lesions are often discontinuous and span several spinal segments.

Meningeal infiltration may be asymptomatic or may produce symptomatic aseptic meningitis, cauda equina signs, hydrocephalus (which can rapidly and fatally decompensate), and ependymitis with encephalopathy. Meningeal or dural mass lesions can be mistaken for meningiomas. Skull base lesions can mimic an acoustic or trigeminal schwannoma.

Peripheral nerve lesions cause mononeuropathy; mononeuropathy multiplex; and sensory, motor, or sensorimotor polyneuropathy, either chronically progressive or resembling Guillain–Barré neuropathy. Most common is a chronic axonal sensorimotor neuropathy. Small-fiber sensory and autonomic neuropathy is also described.

A positive muscle biopsy has been reported in as many as 75% of patients with sarcoidosis, and muscle granulomas may be seen on MRI. Muscle granulomas are usually asymptomatic, although they sometimes cause palpable nodules or progressive diffuse polymyositis.

DIAGNOSIS

In patients known to have sarcoidosis, the appearance of neurologic symptoms usually poses no diagnostic problem, but alternative possibilities must be kept in mind. The differential diagnosis of neurosarcoidosis includes infection, autoimmune and inflammatory disorders, neoplasm, and demyelinating disease (Table 72.2). Altered mental status could be caused by hypercalcemia, corticosteroid effects, or systemic organ involvement and metabolic derangement. Progressive multifocal leukoencephalopathy has been reported in at least 30 patients with sarcoidosis. Patients with neurologic symptoms require both systemic and neurologic investigation. CNS granulomas, symptomatic or asymptomatic, are apparent on either T2-weighted or contrast-enhanced MRI; they are sometimes calcified. Leptomeningeal MRI enhancement is common, and imaging may reveal hydrocephalus and spinal cord, cauda equina, or optic nerve involvement.

Multiple periventricular and white matter lesions on T2 and fluid-attenuated inversion recovery (FLAIR) MRI may suggest multiple sclerosis. Multiple sclerosis plaques do not enhance with gadolinium beyond the acute inflammatory stage; sarcoid granulomas may not enhance in patients receiving corticosteroids. These lesions might represent either granulomas or small infarcts secondary to granulomatous vasculitis. Consistent with the latter is occasional contrast enhancement along nearby blood vessels. The CSF may contain as many as a few thousand white blood cells (WBCs) (usually with lymphocytic preponderance), as well as elevated protein levels, low sugar content, elevated immunoglobulin G (IgG) and IgG index, oligoclonal bands, elevated angiotensin-converting enzyme (ACE) levels (neither sensitive nor specific), and an elevated CD4+-to-CD8+ cell ratio.

Other studies, tailored to need with individual patients, include chest radiographs (revealing either asymptomatic hilar adenopathy or, more ominously, fibronodular disease and abnormal in nearly 90% of patients with sarcoidosis), pulmonary function studies, identification of a high ratio of CD4+-to-CD8+ T cells on bronchiolar lavage, serum calcium (elevated in about 20% of patients with sarcoidosis), urinary calcium (elevated in 50% of patients), serum ACE (elevated in 65% of patients), serum gamma globulin (elevated in 50% of patients), serum sodium, and endocrinologic studies (thyroid function tests, cortisol, gonadotropins, testosterone or estradiol, and prolactin). Serum-soluble interleukin-2 receptor levels are also nonspecific but have been found to correlate with disease activity.

About two-thirds of patients are anergic to tuberculin-purified protein derivative, mumps, and other antigens, and those who are positive are usually only weakly so. Ophthalmologic or otolaryngologic consultation may disclose unsuspected lesions. Systemic or brain gallium scanning may be positive but is nonspecific. Whole-body 2-fluoro-1-deoxyglucose positron emission tomography (PET) may identify sites of inflammation not seen on MRI or with gallium scanning.

Diagnosis ultimately depends on histology; biopsy sites include lymph nodes (including transbronchial), salivary glands, conjunctiva, skin, liver, and, as a last resort, meninges or brain.

COURSE AND TREATMENT

About two-thirds of patients with neurosarcoidosis have a self-limited monophasic illness; the rest have a chronic, remitting–relapsing course. With treatment, death from neurologic disease is unusual. Although controlled studies are lacking, corticosteroids appear to reduce symptoms and size of granulomas; it is unclear whether they affect the natural history. Their use depends on the clinical setting. Short-term therapy may be given to patients with aseptic meningitis or isolated facial palsy. Long-term treatment is often necessary for intraparenchymal lesions, hydrocephalus, optic or other cranial nerve involvement, peripheral neuropathy, or symptomatic myopathy. A daily dose of 40 to 80 mg prednisone may be given for a few weeks and then slowly tapered, either to a lowest possible maintenance dose or, if possible, to discontinuation. Higher initial doses may be necessary in some patients. Anecdotally reported adjunctive immunosuppressive treatment for refractory patients includes mycophenolate mofetil, azathioprine, methotrexate, cyclophosphamide, rituximab, thalidomide, cyclosporine, chloroquine, hydroxychloroquine, and the TNF-alpha antagonists infliximab and adalimumab. Radiation therapy has been used but with uncertain benefit.

Surgery should be considered a last resort for patients with intracranial mass lesions unresponsive to pharmacotherapy or with hydrocephalus.

SUGGESTED READINGS

Almeida FA Jr, Sager JS, Eiger G. Coexistent sarcoidosis and HIV infection: an immunological paradox? *J Infect.* 2006;52:195–201.

Berger C, Sommer C, Meinck HM. Isolated sarcoid myopathy. *Muscle Nerve.* 2002;26:553–556.

Carlson ML, White JR Jr, Espahbodi M, et al. Cranial base manifestations of neurosarcoidosis: a review of 305 patients. *Otol Neurotol.* 2015;36(1):156–166.

Colover JJ. Sarcoidosis with involvement of the nervous system. *Brain.* 1948;71:451–475.

Dubey N, Miletich RS, Wasey M, et al. Role of fluorodeoxyglucose positron emission tomography in the diagnosis of neurosarcoidosis. *J Neurol Sci.* 2002;205:77–81.

Grutters JC, Fellrath JM, Mulder L, et al. Serum soluble interleukin-2 receptor measurement in patients with sarcoidosis: a clinical evaluation. *Chest.* 2003;124:186–195.

Hoitsma E, Faber CG, Drent M, et al. Neurosarcoidosis: a clinical dilemma. *Lancet Neurol.* 2004;3(7):397–407.

TABLE 72.2	Differential Diagnosis for Sarcoidosis
CNS infection, especially tuberculous and fungal meningitis	
CNS neoplasm, especially carcinomatous and lymphomatous meningitis	
Demyelinating disease	
Vasculitis	
Peripheral neuropathy, including mononeuropathy multiplex	
Myopathy	

CNS, central nervous system.

Jamilloux Y, Néel A, Lecouffe-Desprets M, et al. Progressive multifocal leukoencephalopathy in patients with sarcoidosis. *Neurology*. 2014;82:1307–1313.

Krumholz A, Stern BJ. Neurologic manifestations of sarcoidosis. *Handb Clin Neurol*. 2014;119:305–333.

Metyass S, Tawadrous M, Yeter KC, et al. Neurosarcoidosis mimicking multiple sclerosis successfully treated with methotrexate and adalimumab. *Int J Rheum Dis*. 2014;17:214–216.

Moller DR. Treatment of sarcoidosis—from a basic science point of view. *J Intern Med*. 2003;253:31–40.

Nowak DA, Widenka DC. Neurosarcoidosis: a review of its intracranial manifestation. *J Neurol*. 2001;248:363–372.

Nozaki K, Judson MA. Neurosarcoidosis: clinical manifestations, diagnosis, and treatment. *Presse Med*. 2012;41:e331–e348.

O'Dwyer JP, Al-Moyeed BA, Farrall MA, et al. Neurosarcoidosis-related intracranial haemorrhage: three new cases and a systematic review of the literature. *Eur J Neurol*. 2013;20:71–78.

Pereira J, Anderson NE, McAuley D, et al. Medically refractory neurosarcoidosis treated with infliximab. *Intern Med J*. 2011;41:354–357.

Quinones-Hinojosa A, Chang EF, Khan SA, et al. Isolated trigeminal nerve sarcoid granuloma mimicking trigeminal schwannoma: case report. *Neurosurgery*. 2003;52:700–705.

Said G. Sarcoidosis of the peripheral nervous system. *Handb Clin Neurol*. 2013;115:485–495.

Scott TF, Yandora K, Valeri A, et al. Aggressive therapy for sarcoidosis. Long-term follow-up of 48 treated patients. *Arch Neurol*. 2007;64:691–696.

Sohn M, Culver DA, Judson MA, et al. Spinal cord neurosarcoidosis. *Am J Med Sci*. 2014;347(3):195–198.

Spencer TS, Campellone JV, Maldonado I. Clinical and magnetic resonance imaging manifestations of neurosarcoidosis. *Semin Arthritis Rheum*. 2005;34:649–661.

Tobias S, Prayson RA, Lee JH. Necrotizing neurosarcoidosis of the cranial base resembling an en plaque sphenoid wing meningioma: case report. *Neurosurgery*. 2002;51:1290–1294.

Essential Tremor 73

Elan D. Louis

INTRODUCTION

Essential tremor (ET) is a chronic, progressive neurologic disease. The hallmark motor feature is a 4- to 12-Hz kinetic tremor (tremor occurring during voluntary movements, such as writing or eating) that involves the arms and hands (Fig. 73.1). Tremor may eventually spread to involve the head (i.e., the neck), voice, and jaw. Given the presence of etiologic, clinical, and pharmacologic response profile and pathologic heterogeneity, there is growing support for the notion that ET may be a family of diseases whose central defining feature is kinetic tremor of the arms and which might more accurately be referred to as *the essential tremors*.

EPIDEMIOLOGY

ET is among the most prevalent adult-onset movement disorders, although it may occur at any age, and pediatric cases, with age of onset in the first decade of life, have been reported. In a recent meta-analysis of data from 28 population-based prevalence studies in 19 countries, the pooled prevalence of ET across all ages was 0.9%. The prevalence increases markedly with age and especially with advanced age. In the meta-analysis, prevalence among persons aged 65 years and older was 4.6%, and in some studies, the prevalence among persons aged 95 years and older reached values in excess of 20%. The rate at which new ET cases arise (i.e., the incidence rate) has been estimated as 619 per 100,000 person-years among individuals age 65 years and older; this incidence rises with age. Established risk factors for ET include older age and family history of ET.

ETIOLOGY

Both genetic and environmental (i.e., toxic) factors are likely contributors to disease etiology. Many large kindreds show an autosomal dominant pattern of inheritance, and first-degree relatives of ET patients are approximately 5 times more likely to develop the disease than are members of the population and 10 times more likely if the proband's tremor began at an early age.

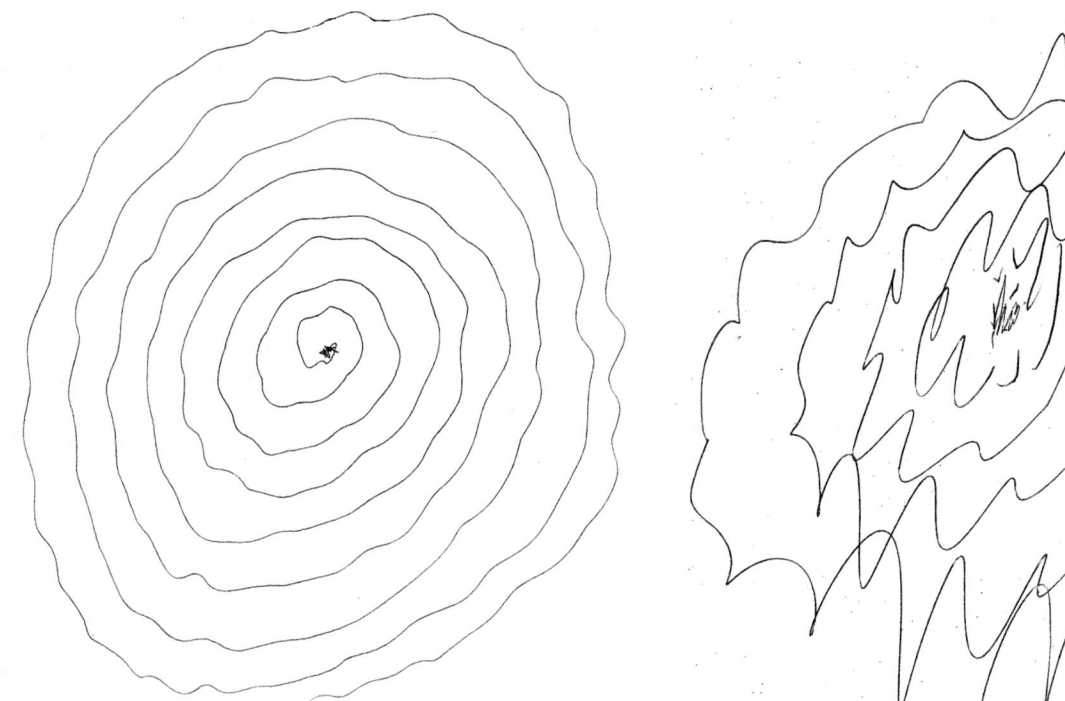

A

B

FIGURE 73.1 Spirals drawn by patients with ET who have moderate arm tremor **(A)** and severe arm tremor **(B)**.

The prevalence of a family history of ET is high in ET patients seen in neurologic clinics and even higher in younger onset than older onset ET cases. A variant in the Lingo-1 gene has been most consistently associated with ET; however, no major causal genes have been identified so far, and this is likely due to phenocopies, incomplete penetrance, bilineal inheritance, or possibly other modes of inheritance. The existence of sporadic cases (i.e., cases without apparent family history), variability in age at onset in familial cases, and lack of complete disease concordance in monozygotic twins all argue for nongenetic (i.e., environmental) causes as well. A number of environmental toxins are under investigation, including β-carboline alkaloids (e.g., harmane, a dietary toxin) and lead. One epidemiologic study indicated a possible protective role of cigarette smoking and another suggested that higher levels of premorbid ethanol consumption raise the risk of developing ET with the presumed mechanism being Purkinje cell toxicity. The identification of modifiable risk factors would have important implications in terms of disease prevention.

PATHOBIOLOGY

The olivary model of ET, first proposed in the early 1970s, posited that a tremor pacemaker in the inferior olivary nucleus was driving the tremor in ET. However, there are major problems with this model, including the absence of direct empirical support and, therefore, there has been trend to move away from this model. In more recent years, mechanistic research on ET has focused more on the cerebellum and the role it seems to play in the biology of ET. Interest in the cerebellum was initially motivated by

neuroimaging studies, which strongly implicate the importance of this brain region in ET, and clinical studies, which frequently note the presence of cerebellar signs in patients with ET. More recently, controlled postmortem studies have revealed an array of degenerative changes in the cerebellar cortex, primarily involving the Purkinje cells and surrounding neuronal populations, in the majority of ET cases (Fig. 73.2). In some studies, there is actual Purkinje cell loss. A smaller group of ET cases demonstrates a pattern of Lewy bodies that are relatively restricted to the locus ceruleus. Of mechanistic interest is that the noradrenergic neurons of the locus ceruleus project to the cerebellum and synapse with Purkinje cells. Hence, there is growing support for the notion that the cerebellum may be central to disease pathobiology and that the pathobiology is neurodegenerative.

CLINICAL MANIFESTATIONS

Symptoms and signs of ET can begin at any age, and about 5% begin in childhood, although the incidence increases markedly with advancing age, and most prevalent cases are age 60 years or older.

The cardinal feature of ET is kinetic tremor, evidenced during a variety of activities on neurologic examination (e.g., finger–nose–finger maneuver, spiral drawing) (Video 73.1). The tremor is generally mildly asymmetric, affecting one arm more than the other, with on average an approximate 30% difference between sides; in approximately 5% of patients, the tremor is markedly asymmetric or even unilateral. In approximately 50% of patients, the tremor has an intentional component, worsening on finger–nose–finger maneuver as the patient approaches the target. Intention tremor is not limited

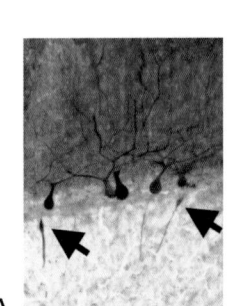
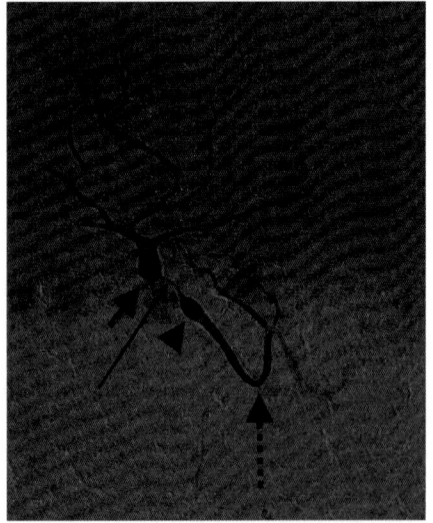
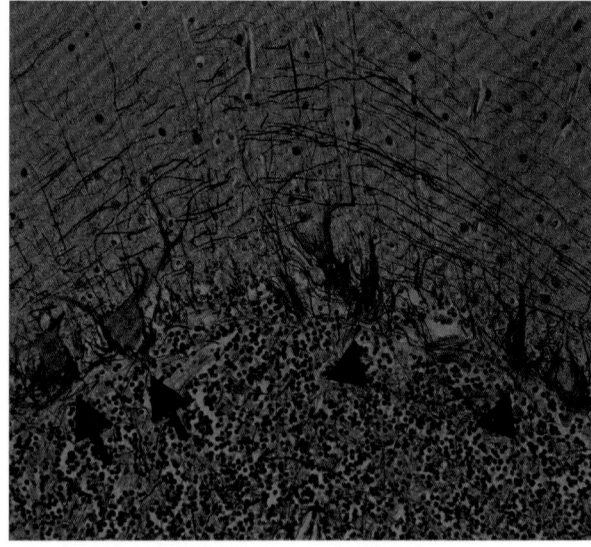

FIGURE 73.2 A: Calbindin-stained section of the cerebellar vermis of an ET case (100×). Torpedoes (two *arrows*, ovoid swellings of the proximal portion of the Purkinje cell axon) occur in significantly greater numbers in ET cases than controls and are markers of an abnormal Purkinje cell biology. **B:** Calbindin-stained section of the cerebellar cortex of an ET case (200×). From left to right, one can see the Purkinje cell body (*arrow*), the normal thin initial axonal segment (*long, thin arrow*), the torpedo (*arrowhead*), and the thickened axon with recurrent collateral formation (*dotted arrow*) and terminal branching of the Purkinje axon. These morphologic changes occur to a greater degree in ET cases than controls and are markers of an abnormal Purkinje cell biology. **C:** Calbindin-stained section of the cerebellar cortex of an ET case (200×). Hypertrophy of the basket cell processes is seen (two *arrows*, "hairy baskets"); in some instances, there is Purkinje cell loss and the baskets are empty (two *arrowheads*). These changes occur to a greater degree in ET cases than controls and are markers of both an abnormal Purkinje cell biology and reactive changes in the surrounding neuronal populations.

to the arms; in 10% of patients, it is detectable in the head when the patient's head approaches a target (e.g., while drinking from a cup or a spoon). Postural tremor also occurs in patients with ET and is generally worse in the wing-beat position than when the arms are held straight in front of the patient. The tremor in the two arms is generally out of phase, creating a seesaw effect when the arms are held in a wing-beat position and contributing to the observation that functionality may improve when two rather than one hand is used (e.g., while holding a cup). The postural tremor of ET is generally greatest in amplitude at the wrist joint rather than more proximal or distal joints and generally involves wrist flexion extension rather than wrist rotation supination. As a rule, the amplitude of kinetic tremor exceeds that of postural tremor, and the converse pattern should raise questions about the diagnosis. Tremor at rest, without other cardinal features of parkinsonism, occurs in approximately 20% of patients with ET attending a specialty clinic, but in contrast to that of Parkinson disease (PD), it is a late feature and it has only been observed in the arm rather than the arm and leg. Another motor feature of ET, aside from tremor, is gait ataxia, which is in excess of that seen in similarly aged controls. In most patients, this is mild, although in some, it may be of moderate severity. There is some evidence that gait ataxia is more pronounced in patients with midline cranial tremors (e.g., neck, jaw, voice). Saccadic eye movement abnormalities have also been detected in ET patients in several physiologic studies, although these are of a subclinical nature.

Recent years have witnessed an increasing appreciation of the presence of nonmotor features in ET patients, which may broadly be classed into cognitive, psychiatric, and sensory. Cognitive changes are in excess of those seen in similarly aged controls and range from mild changes across several domains, but especially executive function, to mild cognitive impairment and dementia, both of which occur to a greater extent than in age-matched controls. The pathobiology of these cognitive changes is unclear at present. Psychiatric manifestations include secondary anxiety and depression. The presence of a primary mood disturbance, which precedes the motor manifestations, is supported by at least one prospective study. A harm avoidant personality has been reported in studies that have assessed personality traits in ET, and this may be one feature, which makes patients reluctant to undergo therapeutic surgery even in the setting of severe and disabling tremor. Sensory changes include diminished hearing in excess of that seen in age-matched controls and a mild olfactory deficit in some although not all studies.

Initially, the tremor may be mild and asymptomatic and it may not worsen for years, but in most individuals, the tremor worsens over time. Several patterns of progression have been described (Fig. 73.3). The two most common are (1) late life onset and (2) early life onset with mild, stable tremor for many years and then a late life worsening. The least common pattern is that of early life onset with marked worsening over the ensuing years to decade. There are few prospective, longitudinal natural history studies, but the best estimates of rate of change indicate that arm tremor worsens by 2% to 5% per year. With the progression of time, there is a tendency for the spread of tremor beyond the arms, such that patients develop cranial tremors (neck, voice, jaw), particularly in women with ET, among whom the risk of neck tremor is several-fold higher than that of men with ET. The prevalence of neck tremor is the highest of these, with voice tremor being less so and jaw tremor being even less so. Neck tremor is generally of a "no-no" (i.e., horizontal) variety but can also be a "yes-yes" (i.e., vertical) tremor or a more complex tremor with a rotatory component. Unless severe, the neck tremor, which is a postural tremor, should subside and resolve when the patient is recumbent. Isolated neck

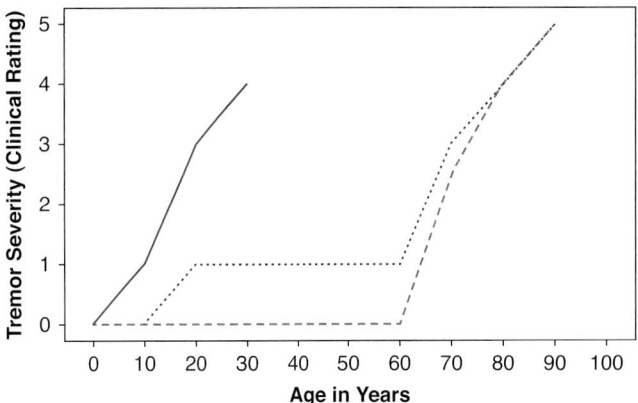

FIGURE 73.3 Three patterns of progression in ET. The two most common are (1) late life onset (*blue dashed line*) and (2) early life onset with mild, stable tremor for many years followed by late life worsening (*purple dotted line*). The least common pattern is that of (3) early life onset with marked worsening over the ensuing years to decade (*red solid line*).

tremor, with minimal or no accompanying arm tremor, is extremely rare and should raise suspicion that the diagnosis is dystonia rather than ET. A curious feature of the neck tremor is that patients are often unaware of its presence, particularly when it is mild. The presence of dystonic postures in ET cases is controversial, although it is likely that the presence of mild dystonia in some cases does not preclude a diagnosis of ET, especially when the dystonia is a late finding in a case with long-standing and severe ET.

Although in the past ET was often viewed as a "benign" problem, the term *benign essential tremor* is no longer considered appropriate. Indeed, the majority of patients have tremor-related disability, and 15% to 25% are sufficiently motorically disabled by high-amplitude shaking that they cannot continue to work.

ET patients have about a fourfold increased risk of developing incident PD, thereby developing what is referred to as *essential tremor–Parkinson disease* (ET-PD). The pathobiology of this connection is not fully understood.

DIAGNOSIS

Thirty percent to 50% of "ET" cases are misdiagnosed and do not have ET, with many of these cases having dystonia or PD. Differentiation may be made readily, however, by the absence of rigidity or bradykinesia or other signs of parkinsonism (e.g., hypomimia) in these cases. The characteristics of the tremor are also important in distinguishing an ET patient from one with PD (Table 73.1). The presence of isolated postural tremor (with minimal kinetic tremor), a postural tremor involving the metacarpophalangeal joints rather than the wrist, and a postural tremor characterized by greater wrist rotation than flexion and extension are all indicators that the likely diagnosis is emerging PD rather than ET (see Table 73.1). Reemergent tremor is a postural tremor that commences after a brief latency, rather than immediately, and is a feature of PD. Dystonia in the arm is characterized by dystonic posturing (e.g., "spooning of the fingers" [i.e., the tendency during arm extension to flex the wrist and hyperextend the metacarpophalangeal and phalangeal joints]) and the presence of a tremor that is neither rhythmic nor oscillatory. The possibility of neck dystonia should be assessed and is characterized by head tilt or rotation with head tremor,

TABLE 73.1	Clinical Examination Features that Help Distinguish Essential Tremor from Parkinson Disease	
	ET	PD
Rest tremor (arms)	+[a]	+
Rest tremor (legs)	−[a]	+
Kinetic tremor (arms)	+	+[b]
Postural tremor (arms)	+	+[c]
Intention tremor (arms)	Common	Rare
Reemergent tremor		+
Head tremor	Common	Rare
Jaw tremor	+[d]	+
Voice tremor	+	−
Rigidity	−[e]	+
Bradykinesia	−[f]	+
Hypomimia	−	+
Tachyphemia	−	+

[a]When present, rest tremor generally occurs in ET cases with disease of longer duration and greater severity rather than mild cases of short duration. It is restricted to the arms.

[b]The kinetic tremor of ET is generally of higher amplitude than that of PD, although this is not always the case.

[c]A postural tremor involving the metacarpophalangeal joints rather than the wrist and a postural tremor characterized by greater wrist rotation than flexion and extension are both indicators that the likely diagnosis is emerging PD rather than ET. An isolated postural tremor (with minimal or no kinetic tremor) is a feature of PD rather than ET. The presence of flexed posturing of the wrist and/or fingers is often a sign of PD.

[d]The jaw tremor in ET generally occurs when the mouth is open (e.g., while talking or while saying "ahhhhh"); in PD, it generally occurs while the mouth is closed.

[e]During passive movement, the movement may be ratchety, with cogwheeling, but there should be no rigidity.

[f]Older ET patients may have ratings of 1 on the motor portion of the Unified Parkinson's Disease Rating Scale.

+, present; −, absent; ET, essential tremor; PD, Parkinson disease.

hypertrophy of the sternocleidomastoid muscle, the presence of a tremor null point, and a sensory trick by history (Table 73.2). Absence of cerebellar speech (i.e., either scanning or dysarthric) and nystagmus distinguishes ET from the spinocerebellar ataxias. Hyperthyroidism or the use of medications such as lithium or valproate is usually excluded by clinical history. A difficult differential is between a mild case of ET and enhanced physiologic tremor, although the presence of neck tremor should exclude the latter. Computerized tremor analysis, with inertial loading, can assist with this differential. In patients with a tremor of central origin (ET), the primary tremor frequency should not change with inertial loading.

TREATMENT

The tremor may be severe enough to result in embarrassment and functional disability, and these are the main motivations for treatment. β-Blockers (especially propranolol) [**Level 1**][1] and primidone [**Level 1**],[2] alone or in combination, are the most effective pharmacologic therapies, although many patients chose to discontinue these medications due to their limited efficacy. Propranolol has been used in doses up to 360 mg daily, although doses in excess of 100 mg are rarely tolerated in the elderly. Asthma is a relative

TABLE 73.2	Clinical Examination Features that Help Distinguish Essential Tremor from Dystonia	
	ET	Dystonia
Rhythmic and oscillatory tremor	+	+/−
Tremor has a directional quality	−[a]	+
Tremor null point	−[b]	+
Head tremor resolves while supine	+	−
Head tremor with little or no arm tremor	−[c]	+
Head tilt or rotation	−	+
Hypertrophy of the sternocleidomastoid or other neck muscles	−	+
Voice breaks with voice tremor	−	+/−
Dystonic posturing in hands (e.g., "spooning")	−	+

[a]Dystonic tremor often has a directional quality seeming to move in one direction more than the opposite.

[b]Tremors, in general, are very positionally dependent in ET, but this should not be confused with a null point.

[c]Isolated head tremor should be a clue that the diagnosis is likely to be dystonia rather than ET.

+, present; −, absent; ET, essential tremor.

contraindication to the use of propranolol but is not an absolute contraindication and must be assessed on a case-by-case basis. Primidone is given in doses up to 1,500 mg daily, although lower doses are often effective. An acute nausea and/or ataxia is observed in approximately 25% of patients who are prescribed this medication, and preloading the patient with phenobarbital (e.g., 30 mg twice a day [b.i.d.] for 3 days) is one method that is used to avoid this unwanted side effect. These drugs reduce the amplitude of tremor in 30% to 70% of patients, but they do not abolish it unless the tremor is mild. Other agents that have been used include topiramate [**Level 1**],[3] gabapentin [**Level 1**],[4] and benzodiazepines (alprazolam or clonazepam) [**Level 1**].[5] Many patients note that tremor is temporarily suppressed by drinking ethanol, but a rebound exacerbation sometimes follows the next day. High-frequency thalamic stimulation markedly reduces the severity of the tremor and has replaced stereotactic thalamotomy as the treatment of choice for severe pharmacologically refractory tremor. Several other emerging surgical therapies are currently under evaluation.

Videos can be found in the companion e-book edition. For a full list of video legends, please see the front matter.

LEVEL 1 EVIDENCE

1. Winkler GF, Young RR. Efficacy of chronic propranolol therapy in action tremors of the familial, senile or essential varieties. *N Engl J Med.* 1974;290(18):984–988.

2. Findley LJ, Cleeves L, Calzetti S. Primidone in essential tremor of the hands and head: a double blind controlled clinical study. *J Neurol Neurosurg Psychiatry.* 1985;48(9):911–915.

3. Ondo WG, Jankovic J, Connor GS, et al; Topiramate Essential Tremor Study Investigators. Topiramate in essential tremor: a double-blind, placebo-controlled trial. *Neurology.* 2006;14;66(5):672–677.

4. Gironell A, Kulisevsky J, Barbanoj M, et al. A randomized placebo-controlled comparative trial of gabapentin and propranolol in essential tremor. *Arch Neurol.* 1999;56(4):475–480.

5. Gunal DI, Afsar N, Bekiroglu N, et al. New alternative agents in essential tremor therapy: double-blind placebo-controlled study of alprazolam and acetazolamide. *Neurol Sci.* 2000;21(5):315–317.

SUGGESTED READINGS

Babij R, Lee M, Cortés E, et al. Purkinje cell axonal anatomy: quantifying morphometric changes in essential tremor vs. control brains. *Brain.* 2013;136(pt 10):3051–3061.

Benito-León J, Louis ED, Bermejo-Pareja F. Population-based case–control study of cognitive function in essential tremor. *Neurology.* 2006;66(1):69–74.

Bermejo-Pareja F. Essential tremor—a neurodegenerative disorder associated with cognitive defects? *Nat Rev Neurol.* 2011;7(5):273–282.

Bermejo-Pareja F, Louis ED, Benito-León J. Risk of incident dementia in essential tremor: a population-based study. *Mov Disord.* 2007;22(11):1573–1580.

Bermejo-Pareja F, Puertas-Martín V. Cognitive features of essential tremor: a review of the clinical aspects and possible mechanistic underpinnings. *Tremor Other Hyperkinet Mov (N Y).* 2012;2.

Cerasa A, Messina D, Nicoletti G, et al. Cerebellar atrophy in essential tremor using an automated segmentation method. *AJNR Am J Neuroradiol.* 2009;30(6):1240–1243.

Critchley M. Observations on essential (heredofamial) tremor. *Brain.* 1949;72(pt 2):113–139.

Diaz NL, Louis ED. Survey of medication usage patterns among essential tremor patients: movement disorder specialists vs. general neurologists. *Parkinsonism Relat Disord.* 2010;16(9):604–607.

Elias WJ, Huss D, Voss T, et al. A pilot study of focused ultrasound thalamotomy for essential tremor. *N Engl J Med.* 2013;369(7):640–648.

Erickson-Davis CR, Faust PL, Vonsattel JGV, et al. "Hairy baskets" associated with degenerative Purkinje cell changes in essential tremor. *J Neuropathol Exp Neurol.* 2010;69:262–271.

Gitchel GT, Wetzel PA, Baron MS. Slowed saccades and increased square wave jerks in essential tremor. *Tremor Other Hyperkinet Mov (N Y).* 2013;3.

Helmchen C, Hagenow A, Miesner J, et al. Eye movement abnormalities in essential tremor may indicate cerebellar dysfunction. *Brain.* 2003;126(pt 6):1319–1332.

Hubble JP, Busenbark KL, Pahwa R, et al. Clinical expression of essential tremor: effects of gender and age. *Mov Disord.* 1997;12(6):969–972.

Jiménez-Jiménez FJ, Alonso-Navarro H, Garcia-Martín E, et al. Update on genetics of essential tremor. *Acta Neurol Scand.* 2013;128(6):359–371.

Kuhlenbäumer G, Hopfner F, Deuschl G. Genetics of essential tremor: meta-analysis and review. *Neurology.* 2014;82(11):1000–1007.

LaRoia H, Louis ED. Association between essential tremor and other neurodegenerative conditions: what is the epidemiological evidence? *Neuroepidemiology.* 2011;37(1):1–10.

Louis ED. "Essential tremor" or "the essential tremors": is this one disease or a family of diseases? *Neuroepidemiology.* 2014;42(2):81–89.

Louis ED. From neurons to neuron neighborhoods: the rewiring of the cerebellar cortex in essential tremor. *Cerebellum.* 2014;13(4):501–512.

Louis ED. Re-thinking the biology of essential tremor: from models to morphology. *Parkinsonism Related Disord.* 2014;20(suppl 1):S88–S93.

Louis ED. The primary type of tremor in essential tremor is kinetic rather than postural: cross-sectional observation of tremor phenomenology in 369 cases. *Eur J Neurol.* 2013;20(4):725–727.

Louis ED, Agnew A, Gillman A, et al. Estimating annual rate of decline: prospective, longitudinal data on arm tremor severity in two groups of essential tremor cases. *J Neurology Neurosurg Psychiatry.* 2011;82(7):761–765.

Louis ED, Faust PL, Vonsattel JP, et al. Neuropathological changes in essential tremor: 33 cases compared with 21 controls. *Brain.* 2007;130(pt 12):3297–3307.

Louis ED, Ferreira JJ. How common is the most common adult movement disorder? Update on the worldwide prevalence of essential tremor. *Mov Disord.* 2010;25(5):534–541.

Louis ED, Ford B, Frucht S, et al. Risk of tremor and impairment from tremor in relatives of patients with essential tremor: a community-based family study. *Ann Neurol.* 2001;49(6):761–769.

Louis ED, Galecki M, Rao AK. Four essential tremor cases with moderately impaired gait: how impaired can gait be in this disease? *Tremor Other Hyperkinet Mov (N Y).* 2013;3.

Louis ED, Jiang W, Pellegrino KM, et al. Elevated blood harmane (1-methyl-9h-pyrido[3,4-b]indole) concentrations in essential tremor. *Neurotoxicology.* 2008;29(2):294–300.

Louis ED, Rios E, Henchcliffe C. How are we doing with the treatment of essential tremor (ET)? Persistence of ET patients on medication: data from 528 patients in three settings. *Eur J Neurol.* 2010;17(6):882–884.

Ondo WG, Sutton L, Dat Vuong K, et al. Hearing impairment in essential tremor. *Neurology.* 2003;61(8):1093–1097.

Pagan FL, Butman JA, Dambrosia JM, et al. Evaluation of essential tremor with multi-voxel magnetic resonance spectroscopy. *Neurology.* 2003;60(8):1344–1347.

Passamonti L, Cerasa A, Quattrone A. Neuroimaging of essential tremor: what is the evidence for cerebellar involvement? *Tremor Other Hyperkinet Mov (N Y).* 2012;2.

Phibbs F, Fang JY, Cooper MK, et al. Prevalence of unilateral tremor in autosomal dominant essential tremor. *Mov Disord.* 2009;24(1):108–111.

Schrag A, Münchau A, Bhatia KP, et al. Essential tremor: an overdiagnosed condition? *J Neurol.* 2000;247(12):955–959.

Stefansson H, Steinberg S, Petursson H, et al. Variant in the sequence of the LINGO1 gene confers risk of essential tremor. *Nat Genet.* 2009;41(3):277–279.

Zappia M, Albanese A, Bruno E, et al. Treatment of essential tremor: a systematic review of evidence and recommendations from the Italian Movement Disorders Association. *J Neurol.* 2013;260(3):714–740.

Zesiewcz TA, Elble RJ, Louis ED, et al. Evidence-based guideline update: treatment of essential tremor: report of the Quality Standards subcommittee of the American Academy of Neurology. *Neurology.* 2011;77(19):1752–1755.

Tics and Tourette Syndrome 74

Stanley Fahn and Daphne Robakis

INTRODUCTION

Tics are brief, sudden, repetitive movements (motor tics) or utterances (phonic or vocal tics) that are temporarily suppressible and are usually preceded by a strong urge to perform the tic. The distinction between motor and vocal tics is somewhat arbitrary because production of vocal tics requires the involvement of facial, oropharyngeal, or diaphragmatic musculature. The Gilles de la Tourette syndrome, named after the author of the seminal description and commonly shortened to *Tourette syndrome* (TS), is the most well-described tic disorder.

TS is a neurobehavioral disorder consisting of both multiple motor and phonic tics (not necessarily concurrently) that change in character over time, beginning before 18 years of age, and with symptoms that wax and wane but last more than 1 year. For the diagnosis of TS, these motor and phonic tics are not caused by exogenous factors such as cocaine or a medical condition such as encephalitis or trauma. Although the earlier definition as proposed by the American Psychiatric Association in its *Diagnostic and Statistical Manual of Mental Disorders*, 5th edition (*DSM-5*), is a useful criterion for research on the disorder, it excludes chronic tics in the motor or vocal domains alone, which are likely milder expressions of the same condition (Table 74.1). Other causes of ticlike syndromes include neuroacanthocytosis, encephalitis, prior neuroleptic use, and head trauma. Many patients with TS have a behavioral component of obsessive–compulsive disorder (OCD), attention deficit disorder (ADD), anxiety, or poor impulse control. These behavioral features usually impose more disability than do the tics.

Primary tics not part of TS may be classified under chronic motor/vocal tic disorder, in which tics persist beyond 1 year, or transient motor/vocal tic disorder, in which tics last less than 1 year, the latter being the most common tic disorder in children. Most adults with tics had idiopathic tics as children, but primary or secondary tic disorders can develop in adulthood. Insult to the basal ganglia by diverse mechanisms including stroke, infection, trauma, autoimmune process, or neurodegenerative disease can cause the appearance of tics, possibly via disruption of dopamine circuits. Similar to tardive dyskinesias, tardive tics may appear after varying lengths of treatment with antipsychotics or as a consequence of discontinuation of treatment. Substances such as caffeine, stimulants, and certain antiepileptics (carbamazepine, lamotrigine) have been reported to exacerbate or provoke the emergence of tics. Tics generally follow an anatomic distribution more heavily weighted toward the craniocervical regions than the trunk and limbs. Tics are rarely of psychogenic origin but due to similar clinical features are often difficult to differentiate from organic tics.

EPIDEMIOLOGY

Estimates of prevalence rates of tics have varied broadly, depending on clinical definitions, the age range of participants, and other features of study design. Studies of children yield higher prevalence estimates than do studies of adolescents and adults, as tics typically attenuate in severity or remit entirely by young adulthood. Conservative estimates for lifetime prevalence rates are 1 per 1,000 in boys and 2 per 10,000 in girls. On average, tics begin around age 5 years and increase in severity, reaching a most intense period around age 10 years. After that, tics usually decline in severity until, by age 18 years, nearly half of the patients are virtually free of tics.

PATHOBIOLOGY

Research into the pathobiology of tics has focused mainly on Tourette but the causes of TS are still unknown. The search for genetic mutations has yielded modest evidence for linkage to chromosome 11q23 in a large French Canadian family and to 11q23–q24, 2p11, and 8q22 in Afrikaner families, although these findings generally have yet to be replicated. A de novo chromosomal inversion on chromosome 13q31.1 in a child with TS led to identification of a frameshift mutation in *SLITRK1*, a gene that promotes dendritic growth, as one rare cause of TS. Although early family studies suggested that the genetic transmission of TS is autosomal dominant with a strong sex-specific difference in penetrance, more recent studies have indicated that the mode of inheritance is more complicated than this, appearing semidominant and semirecessive and having greater penetrance in homozygotes than in heterozygotes.

Anatomic MRI has documented reduced volumes of the basal ganglia, particularly the caudate nucleus, as well as thinning of sensorimotor, primary motor, and premotor cortices in persons with TS. These findings are thought to represent hypoplasia in motor portions of the cortical–basal ganglia circuits, and these developmental disturbances contribute to the genesis of tic behaviors. Preliminary postmortem studies suggest the presence of reduced GABAergic interneurons in the basal ganglia, possibly contributing to excess excitability of these motor circuits. Separate circuits within the prefrontal and parietal cortices, and in the hippocampus, are thought to help modulate tic-generating activity in the basal ganglia and motor cortices, producing an activity-dependent hypertrophy of these brain regions. Although dopamine receptor–blocking drugs can suppress tics and have long suggested the presence of supersensitive

TABLE 74.1	Tourette Syndrome—Diagnostic Criteria
Both multiple motor and one or more vocal tics (not necessarily concurrently)	
The tics may increase or decrease in frequency but have persisted for more than 1 yr since first onset.	
Onset before age 18 yr	
No other direct causes, such as drugs, encephalitis, or neurodegenerative disorders	

Data from American Psychiatric Association. *Diagnostic and Statistical Manual of Mental Disorders*. 5th ed. Arlington, VA: American Psychiatric Association; 2013.

dopamine receptors, postmortem binding studies of dopamine receptors failed to provide support for this hypothesis. Positron emission tomography (PET) studies have provided inconsistent evidence for increased dopamine storage and release in striatum.

An immune hypothesis proposes that TS is sometimes caused by infection with β-hemolytic *Streptococcus*, as seen in children who develop Sydenham chorea. Known as a *pediatric autoimmune neuropsychiatric disorder associated with streptococcus infections* (PANDAS), evidence for this proposed etiology for a small minority of TS patients has been inconsistent and controversial.

CLINICAL FEATURES

As defined by *DSM-5*, a tic is a sudden, rapid, recurrent, nonrhythmic motor movement or vocalization. Tics range from intermittent simple brief jerks (simple tics) to a complex pattern of rapid, coordinated, involuntary movements (complex tics) arising abruptly from a background of normal activity and often preceded by a vague, unpleasant sensation that is relieved by the movement (Video 74.1). Although tics usually can be suppressed for a short time, the inner sensation builds relentlessly, producing a burst of tic behavior when the patient stops suppressing them. Tics usually begin in the face (eye blinking, grimacing), neck (head shaking), and shoulders (shrugging), but they can also begin with sounds (sniffing, throat clearing, barking, words, or parts of words). They can progress to involve the thorax and limbs and foul utterances (coprolalia). Repeating sounds (echolalia) or movements (echopraxia) are sometimes seen. The speed of tics ranges from very fast (clonic tics) to sustained contractions (dystonic tics). Simple clonic tics resemble essential myoclonus, and the two conditions are difficult to distinguish. Dystonic tics need to be differentiated from primary torsion dystonia. Sydenham chorea is distinct in manifesting as a continuous restless type of movement pattern, and it is self-limited. Premonitory sensations, intermittency, and suppressibility help distinguish tics from most other movement disorders.

Behavioral or psychiatric symptoms are present in 90% of patients with TS and may be considered part of the clinical syndrome. Impulse control problems are common and can present as aggressivity, rage attacks, antisocial or inappropriate sexual behavior, or self-injury. Obsessive–compulsive symptoms associated with tics overlap with those seen in non–tic-related OCD but are less likely to manifest as compulsive washing or cleaning rituals and more likely to be characterized by obsessions with symmetry, the need to do and redo activities, and "just right" perceptions. Some complex tics can resemble compulsions. Attentional difficulties often precede the appearance of tics by several years and usually reflect coexisting Attention deficit hyperactivity disorder (ADHD) but may also be attributable to other factors such as cognitive fatigue from the effort to suppress tics, obsessions like mental counting, or mood disorders. TS patients have higher rates of sleep disturbances including difficulty falling asleep and staying asleep and have increased sleep latencies and arousals on polysomnography. Tics can persist during sleep, in contrast to most other hyperkinetic movement disorders, usually in an attenuated form. Alterations in sleep and wakefulness patterns may be intrinsic to the disease itself or may be caused by medications used to treat tics and comorbid conditions.

TREATMENT

In evaluating patients with tics, assessing the influence of tics on the person's emotional, social, scholastic, and occupational functioning is of central importance in deciding whether and when to intervene therapeutically. In TS, identifying and treating psychiatric comorbidities is often of greatest help, as frequently the symptoms OCD, ADD, depression, and anxiety are more disabling than are the tics. Treatment is aimed at achieving a tolerable degree of tic suppression. A supportive, individualized, multidisciplinary approach that involves neurology, psychiatry, and psychology, as well as education of the patient, parents, and teachers about the natural history of TS and its comorbidities, is usually indispensable to effective treatment.

When tics are mild and not socially or academically disabling, no treatment may be required. When they are more severe, the frequency and forcefulness of motor and phonic tics can sometimes be reduced with clonazepam, clonidine, or guanfacine [Level 1].[1,2] Dopamine antagonists and depletors are more effective but often have more adverse effects [Level 1],[3–7] including tardive dystonia, and thus are often reserved for second- or third-line treatments. Habit reversal therapy (HRT) and comprehensive behavioral intervention for tics (CBIT), which is based on HRT, have been used successfully as first-line treatments or in combination with pharmacotherapy [Level 1].[8–12] OCD, ADHD, depression, and anxiety disorders, if present, all require specific therapies, including psychotherapies, behavioral therapies, and medication [Level 1].[13,14] Pharmacologic options are listed in Table 74.2.

TABLE 74.2	Medications Used in the Treatment of Tourette Syndrome and Its Most Common Co-occurring Illness	
Medication Type	**Medication**	**Dose**
Tics		
α-Agonists	Clonidine	0.1–0.3 mg/day
	Guanfacine	1–6 mg/day
Catecholamine depletors	Tetrabenazine	12.5–300 mg/day
Dopamine-blocking agents	Risperidone	0.5–6 mg/day
	Ziprasidone	20–100 mg/day
	Aripiprazole	2–30 mg/day
	Fluphenazine	50–400 mg/day
	Pimozide	1–6 mg/day
	Haloperidol	0.5–10 mg/day
	Thioridazine	150–300 mg/day
	Trifluoperazine	2–10 mg/day
	Thiothixene	1–15 mg/day
	Olanzapine	5–20 mg/day
Other	Clonazepam	1–4 mg/day
	Baclofen	30–60 mg/day
OCD		
SSRIs	Fluoxetine	20–60 mg/day
	Sertraline	50–200 mg/day
	Paroxetine	20–50 mg/day
	Fluvoxamine	100–300 mg/day
	Clomipramine	100–200 mg/day
ADHD		
Stimulants	Methylphenidate	10–60 mg/day
	Amphetamine	10–40 mg/day
	Atomoxetine	40–80 mg/day

OCD, obsessive–compulsive disorder; SSRI, selective serotonin reuptake inhibitors; ADHD, attention deficit hyperactivity disorder.

Neurosurgery, using deep brain stimulation, is being applied to patients with severe and intractable tics that cause great disability [**Level 1**].[15,16] Different targets in the brain are being tested, but no consensus has been reached as to the best target. Botulinum toxin may be helpful in patients with focal simple motor and vocal tics and for dystonic tics [**Level 1**].[17]

OUTCOME

Primary tic disorders including TS are not neurodegenerative diseases and do not worsen after reaching maximum severity in the preteen years. Rather, the motor and phonic tics have disappeared by adulthood in the majority of patients. In some cases, tics will wax and wane in severity throughout life. It remains controversial whether factors such as tic severity or dysfunction caused by tics correlate with long-term outcomes, and therefore, individual outcomes cannot be reliably predicted. The prognosis for secondary tic disorders varies according to the underlying condition. For those who continue to manifest tics all their life, almost all with persistent tics have learned to live a normal life. In a few individuals, tics can remain a social embarrassment or occupational problem, such as those in acting or politics. Such individuals may require tic-suppressing medication and if that fails, be candidates for neurosurgical intervention. TS patients who suffer from significant social dysfunction often do so as a result of their behavioral symptoms rather than the tics. However, the combination of tics and comorbid psychiatric conditions can be debilitating and remain a challenge for many TS patients throughout their lives.

Videos can be found in the companion e-book edition. For a full list of video legends, please see the front matter.

LEVEL 1 EVIDENCE

1. Scahill L, Chappell PB, Kim YS, et al. A placebo-controlled study of guanfacine in the treatment of children with tic disorders and attention deficit hyperactivity disorder. *Am J Psychiatry*. 2001;158(7):1067–1074.
2. Du YS, Li HF, Vance A, et al. Randomized double-blind multicentre placebo-controlled clinical trial of the clonidine adhesive patch for the treatment of tic disorders. *Aust N Z J Psychiatry*. 2008;42(9):807–813.
3. Yoo HK, Joung YS, Lee JS, et al. A multicenter, randomized, double-blind, placebo-controlled study of aripiprazole in children and adolescents with Tourette's disorder. *J Clin Psychiatry*. 2013;74(8):e772–e780.
4. Scahill L, Leckman JF, Schultz RT, et al. A placebo-controlled trial of risperidone in Tourette syndrome. *Neurology*. 2003;60(7):1130–1135.
5. Pringsheim T, Marras C. Pimozide for tics in Tourette's syndrome. *Cochrane Database Syst Rev*. 2009;(2):Cd006996.
6. Onofrj M, Paci C, D'Andreamatteo G, et al. Olanzapine in severe Gilles de la Tourette syndrome: a 52-week double-blind cross-over study vs. low-dose pimozide. *J Neurol*. 2000;247(6):443–446.
7. Dion Y, Annable L, Sandor P, et al. Risperidone in the treatment of Tourette syndrome: a double-blind, placebo-controlled trial. *J Clin Psychopharmacol*. 2002;22(1):31–39.
8. Deckersbach T, Rauch S, Buhlmann U, et al. Habit reversal versus supportive psychotherapy in Tourette's disorder: a randomized controlled trial and predictors of treatment response. *Behav Res Ther*. 2006;44(8):1079–1090.

9. McGuire JF, Piacentini J, Brennan EA, et al. A meta-analysis of behavior therapy for Tourette syndrome. *J Psychiatr Res*. 2014;50:106–112.
10. Piacentini J, Woods DW, Scahill L, et al. Behavior therapy for children with Tourette disorder: a randomized controlled trial. *JAMA*. 2010;303(19):1929–1937.
11. Wilhelm S, Deckersbach T, Coffey BJ, et al. Habit reversal versus supportive psychotherapy for Tourette's disorder: a randomized controlled trial. *Am J Psychiatry*. 2003;160(6):1175–1177.
12. Wilhelm S, Peterson AL, Piacentini J, et al. Randomized trial of behavior therapy for adults with Tourette syndrome. *Arch Gen Psychiatry*. 2012;69(8):795–803.
13. Bloch MH, Panza KE, Landeros-Weisenberger A, et al. Meta-analysis: treatment of attention-deficit/hyperactivity disorder in children with comorbid tic disorders. *J Am Acad Child Adolesc Psychiatry*. 2009;48(9):884–893.
14. Tourette's Syndrome Study Group. Treatment of ADHD in children with tics: a randomized controlled trial. *Neurology*. 2002;58(4):527–536.
15. Maciunas RJ, Maddux BN, Riley DE, et al. Prospective randomized double-blind trial of bilateral thalamic deep brain stimulation in adults with Tourette syndrome. *J Neurosurg*. 2007;107(5):1004–1014.
16. Ackermans L, Duits A, van der Linden C, et al. Double-blind clinical trial of thalamic stimulation in patients with Tourette syndrome. *Brain*. 2011;134(pt 3):832–844.
17. Marras C, Andrews D, Sime E, et al. Botulinum toxin for simple motor tics: a randomized, double-blind, controlled clinical trial. *Neurology*. 2001;56(5):605–610.

SUGGESTED READINGS

Abelson JF, Kwan KY, O'Roak BJ, et al. Sequence variants in SLITRK1 are associated with Tourette's syndrome. *Science*. 2005;310:317–320.
Albin RL, Koeppe RA, Bohnen NI, et al. Increased ventral striatal monoaminergic innervation in Tourette syndrome. *Neurology*. 2003;61:310–315.
Albin RL, Mink JW. Recent advances in Tourette syndrome research. *Trends Neurosci*. 2006;29:175–182.
American Psychiatric Association. *Diagnostic and Statistical Manual of Mental Disorders*. 5th ed. Arlington, VA: American Psychiatric Association; 2013.
Bronfeld M, Bar-Gad I. Tic disorders: what happens in the basal ganglia? *Neuroscientist*. 2013;19(1):101–108.
Church AJ, Dale RC, Lees AJ, et al. Tourette's syndrome: a cross sectional study to examine the PANDAS hypothesis. *J Neurol Neurosurg Psychiatry*. 2003;74:602–607.
Cohen DJ, Jankovic J, Goetz CG, eds. *Tourette Syndrome*. Philadelphia: Lippincott Williams & Wilkins; 2001.
Deng H, Gao K, Jankovic J. The genetics of Tourette syndrome. *Nat Rev Neurol*. 2012;8(4):203–213.
Diaz-Anzaldua A, Joober R, Riviere JB, et al. Tourette syndrome and dopaminergic genes: a family-based association study in the French Canadian founder population. *Mol Psychiatry*. 2004;9:272–277.
Fahn S. Motor and vocal tics. In: Kurlan R, ed. *Handbook of Tourette's Syndrome and Related Tic and Behavioral Disorders*. 2nd ed. New York: Marcel Dekker; 2005:1–14.
Gilbert D. Treatment of children and adolescents with tics and Tourette syndrome. *J Child Neurol*. 2006;21:690–700.
Gilles de la Tourette G. Étude sur une affection nerveuse caracterisée par de l'incoordination motrice accompagnée d'echolalie et de copralalie. *Arch Neurol*. 1885;9:19–42, 158–200.
Harris K, Singer HS. Tic disorders: neural circuits, neurochemistry, and neuroimmunology. *J Child Neurol*. 2006;21:678–689.
Jankovic J. Tourette's syndrome. *N Engl J Med*. 2001;345:1184–1192.

Kalanithi PS, Zheng W, Kataoka Y, et al. Altered parvalbumin-positive neuron distribution in basal ganglia of individuals with Tourette syndrome. *Proc Natl Acad Sci U S A.* 2005;102:13307–13312.

Kenney C, Jankovic J. Tetrabenazine in the treatment of hyperkinetic movement disorders. *Expert Rev Neurother.* 2006;6:7–17.

Knight T, Steeves T, Day L, et al. Prevalence of tic disorders: a systematic review and meta-analysis. *Pediatr Neurol.* 2012;47(2):77–90.

Leckman JF, Zhang HP, Vitale A, et al. Course of tic severity in Tourette syndrome: the first two decades. *Pediatrics.* 1998;102:14–19.

Lerner A, Bagic A, Simmons JM, et al. Widespread abnormality of the γ-aminobutyric acid-ergic system in Tourette syndrome. *Brain.* 2012;135 (pt 6):1926–1936.

Loiselle CR, Wendlandt JT, Rohde CA, et al. Antistreptococcal, neuronal, and nuclear antibodies in Tourette syndrome. *Pediatr Neurol.* 2003;28:119–125.

Merette C, Brassard A, Potvin A, et al. Significant linkage for Tourette syndrome in a large French Canadian family. *Am J Hum Genet.* 2000;67: 1008–1013.

Minzer K, Lee O, Hong JJ, et al. Increased prefrontal D2 protein in Tourette syndrome: a postmortem analysis of frontal cortex and striatum. *J Neurol Sci.* 2004;219:55–61.

Peterson BS, Cohen DJ. The treatment of Tourette's syndrome: a multimodal developmental intervention. *J Clin Psychiatry.* 1998;59(suppl 1):62–72.

Pourfar M, Feigin A, Tang CC, et al. Abnormal metabolic brain networks in Tourette syndrome. *Neurology.* 2011;76(11):944–952.

Scahill L, Woods DW, Himle MB, et al. Current controversies on the role of behavior therapy in Tourette syndrome. *Mov Disord.* 2013;28(9):1179–1183.

Scharf JM, Yu D, Mathews CA, et al. Genome-wide association study of Tourette's syndrome. *Mol Psychiatry.* 2013;18(6):721–728.

Schrock LE, Mink JW, Woods DW, et al; Tourette Syndrome Association International Deep Brain Stimulation Database and Registry Study Group. Tourette syndrome deep brain stimulation: a review and updated recommendations. *Mov Disord.* 2015;30(4):448–471. doi:10.1002/mds.26094.

Simonic I, Nyholt DR, Gericke GS, et al. Further evidence for linkage of Gilles de la Tourette syndrome (GTS) susceptibility loci on chromosomes 2p11, 8q22, and 11q23-24 in South African Afrikaners. *Am J Med Genet.* 2001;105:163–167.

Singer HS. Tourette's syndrome: from behaviour to biology. *Lancet Neurol.* 2005;4:149–159.

Singer HS, Loiselle CR, Lee O, et al. Anti-basal ganglia antibodies in PANDAS. *Mov Disord.* 2004;19:406–415.

Singer HS, Szymanski S, Giuliano J, et al. Elevated intrasynaptic dopamine release in Tourette's syndrome measured by PET. *Am J Psychiatry.* 2002;159:1329–1336.

Sowell ER, Kan E, Yoshii J, et al. Thinning of gray matter in the sensorimotor cortices of children with Tourette syndrome. *Nat Neurosci.* 2008;11:637–639.

Spessot AL, Peterson BS. Tourette syndrome: a multifactorial, developmental psychopathology. In: Dante Cicchetti, Cohen DJ, eds. *Manual of Developmental Psychopathology.* Vol 3. 2nd ed. New York: John Wiley; 2006:436–469.

Tourette Syndrome Classification Study Group. Definitions and classification of tic disorders. *Arch Neurol.* 1993;50:1013–1016.

Wijemanne S, Wu LJ, Jankovic J. Long-term efficacy and safety of fluphenazine in patients with Tourette syndrome. *Mov Disord.* 2014;29(1):126–130.

Restless Legs Syndrome 75

William G. Ondo

INTRODUCTION

Restless legs syndrome (RLS), also known as *Willis–Ekbom disease* (WED), is clinically defined by the presence of four positive criteria: (1) an urge to move the limbs with or without sensations, (2) worsening at rest, (3) improvement with activity, and (4) worsening in the evening or night. The diagnosis of RLS is exclusively based on those symptoms. The diagnostic criterion for children relies mostly of description from the child's perspective, family history of RLS, and sleep disturbance. There is also an expanding literature linking RLS in children to attention deficit disorders.

Patient subjective semantic descriptions can be quite varied and tend to be suggestible and education dependent. The sensation is always unpleasant but not necessarily painful. It is usually deep within the legs and commonly between the knee and ankle. The key is to rephrase their description into a question asking if that sensation makes you want to move your legs. Essentially, all patients report transient symptomatic improvement from walking, although other movements also help. In general, harsh sensory stimuli can also mitigate RLS. Other clinical features typical for RLS include the tendency for symptoms to gradually worsen with age, improvement with dopaminergic treatments, a positive family history, and periodic limb movements while asleep (PLMS). Traditionally, the neurologic examination is normal in RLS; however, leg/feet stereotypies are sometimes present later in the day although usually suppressible.

In most cases, only a simple evaluation is justified for clinically typical RLS. Serum ferritin and iron-binding saturation for serum iron deficiency and electrolytes for renal failure should be obtained. It should be noted that severe iron deficiency may exist in the setting of a normal ferritin level because it is an acute phase reactant and increases with age. Nerve conduction velocities may be performed in atypical presentations (i.e., sensations beginning in the feet or superficial pain) or when physical symptoms and signs are consistent with a peripheral neuropathy. Polysomnographic evaluation is not generally needed. Several confounding diagnosis need to be considered (Table 75.1).

EPIDEMIOLOGY

Studies in predominantly Caucasian populations consistently show that between 5% and 15% of people have RLS, which is clinically significant in 2% to 3%. In general, northern European countries demonstrated the highest prevalence, followed by Germanic/Anglo-Saxon, then Mediterranean countries. The prevalence tends to decline the farther east one progresses, with lower rates in Asia. People from Africa have never been specifically studied but anecdotally, African-Americans only rarely present with RLS. Women usually have higher RLS rates; however, this female predisposition is lost in nulliparous women.

TABLE 75.1	Differential Diagnosis of Restless Legs Syndrome
Condition	**How Different from RLS**
Akathisia	Whole body urge to move, associated with dopamine blockers, not as circadian
Cramp	Chaotic visible/palpable muscle contraction, can be stopped by stretching muscle, no urge to move
Myalgia	Muscle ache, may be worse at night but no true urge to move
Neuropathic pain	Usually superficial, burning, electric, feet most involved
Radiculopathy	Usually asymmetric, more position dependent but not urge to move other than to move from painful position
Body positional discomfort	Can't get comfortable in any position but not a true urge to move
Moving toes, painful legs	Slow writhing dystonic movement of toes/feet, not suppressible

RLS, restless legs syndrome.

PATHOBIOLOGY

Pathophysiologic studies show a number of objective abnormalities in RLS; however, our understanding is incomplete. The most robust observation is reduced central nervous system (CNS) iron stores, even in the setting of normal systemic iron studies. RLS patients show reduced cerebrospinal fluid CSF) ferritin, reduced iron on magnetic resonance imaging (MRI), especially in the striatum and red nucleus, reduced iron on CNS ultrasonography in the substantia nigra, and most importantly, reduced iron and iron-related proteins at autopsy, including reduced H-ferritin staining, iron staining, and increased transferrin stains, but also reduced transferrin receptors. Researches also demonstrate reduced Thy-1 expression, which is regulated by iron levels. Substantia nigra dopaminergic cells are neither reduced in number nor are there markers associated with neurodegenerative diseases, such as tau or α-synuclein abnormalities.

Brain dopaminergic systems are also implicated in RLS by the dramatic improvement from dopaminergics. However, dopaminergic brain imaging studies are inconsistent and show modest or no abnormalities in a pattern that defies simple explanation and is interpreted by some to actually suggest increased dopamine turnover.

Iron and dopamine are intricately related. Although a number of theories explain the relationship, human data is lacking. The neural localization of RLS is also unknown. Functional involvement of the medial thalamus, cerebellum, and brain stem has been implicated using functional MRI techniques. Spinal cord lesions often result in RLS and PLMS and animal models that lesion the diencephalospinal dopaminergic (A11) nucleus, which descends the spinal cord, mimic features of RLS in mice and rats, mostly increasing locomotor activity. Iron deprivation augments the phenotype.

Opioid pathways are implicated by clinical improvement seen with narcotics and pathologic data that shows reduced beta-endorphin–positive cells and Met-enkephalin–positive cells in six RLS patients compared to six controls. Glutaminergic activity is increased in the thalamus of RLS patients and correlates with arousal but not PLMS. Afferent systems are also implicated as shown by increased sensitivity to pinprick pain ratings (static hyperalgesia). These researchers felt this type of hyperalgesia was probably mediated by central sensitization to A-delta fiber high-threshold mechanoreceptor input, a hallmark sign of the hyperalgesia type of neuropathic pain.

In 40% to 60% of cases, a family history of RLS can be found, although this is often not initially reported by the patient. Twin studies also show a very high concordance rate. Many linkages have been identified in traditional familial studies but in no case has a specific gene mutation been identified. To date, six risk factor genes identified through genome-wide association studies have been published. The most robust associations include BTBDP, MEIS1, and PTPRD.

The most common diseases associated with RLS include renal failure, systemic iron deficiency, neuropathy, myelinopathy, pregnancy, multiple sclerosis, and possibly Parkinson disease and essential tremor. There are reports associating RLS with many other conditions.

TREATMENT

The development of validated rating scales and standardized diagnostic criteria have vastly improved the quality of RLS treatment trials. Multiple medications have demonstrated efficacy in well-designed class I trials, especially dopaminergics, alpha-2 delta ligands, opioids, and iron (Table 75.2). With the possible exception of iron, all are felt to provide only symptomatic relief,

TABLE 75.2 Medications and Doses Used for Restless Legs Syndrome

Drug	Amount per Dose (mg)	Duration of Effect (h)	Comment
Dopaminergics: immediate effect, considered first-line therapy			
L-Dopa	100–250	2–6	Positive class 1 trials, fast onset, can use PRN, highest augmentation rates
Pramipexole	0.125–1	5–12	Positive class 1 trials, commonly used, slower onset but longer duration, extended release available
Ropinirole	0.25–4	4–8	Positive class 1 trials, extended release preparations available
Rotigotine	1–4	24	Positive class 1 trials, commonly used patch preparation
Pergolide	0.125–1	6–14	Well studied (class 2) but seldom used due to risk of cardiac valve fibrosis and other possible ergot adverse events (AE)
Apomorphine	1–3	1	Injection of short-acting powerful drug, anecdotal PRN use
Cabergoline	0.25–2	>24	Longest acting but may have same AEs as other ergot DAs
Bromocriptine	5–20	4–6	Rarely used in RLS
Opioids: Numerous opioids are used.			
Methadone	2–15	8–12	Open label data only, very good long-term tolerability and efficacy, several-day latency to benefit
Hydrocodone	5–10	4–10	Faster acting, shorter duration
Oxycodone	5–20	5–10	Best studied opioid
Alpha-2 delta blockers			
Gabapentin	300–1,200	4–8	Small controlled trials, may help painful component of RLS
Pregabalin	50–300	6–12	Positive class 1 and 2 trials, not approved
Gabapentin enacarbil	600–1,800	8–16	Gabapentin prodrug with better absorption/bioavailability; positive class 1 trials, approved in the United States
Benzodiazepines: more beneficial for sleep than RLS, can be used in combination with other RLS medications. Clonazepam (0.5–2.0 mg) is traditionally used.			
Oral iron	>50	?	No specific iron salt superior, titrate up as tolerated; minimal data of efficacy
IV iron	1,000	?	Usually not repeated before 3 months, several-day latency to benefit, long-term safety unknown, patients with normal serum ferritin equally responsive. Anecdotal evidence favors iron dextran preparations.

PRN, as necessary; DAs, dopamine agonists; RLS, restless legs syndrome; IV, intravenous.

rather than any curative effect. Therefore, treatment should only be initiated when the benefits are felt to justify any potential side effects and costs. Over time, both dosing and drug changes may be required to maximize benefit and minimize the risk of side effects.

Dopamine agonists (DA) are the most best investigated consistently effective treatments for RLS. The improvement is immediate and often very dramatic. DA consistently demonstrate dramatic improvement in PLMS but modest or no improvement in other sleep parameters. No direct evidence favors any particular DA. Rotigotine patch, pramipexole, and ropinirole are best studied and all have class A evidence supporting their use. The dopamine precursor levodopa also effectively treats RLS and may have a more rapid onset of action. However, several comparative studies have favored DA over levodopa.

Immediate-release oral DA work best if administered at least 90 minutes before the onset of symptoms. The effect is immediate, so titration to the smallest effective dose can be fairly rapid. Based on pharmacokinetics, many people may benefit from more than one dose, despite the formal indications, which recommend dosing 1 to 3 hours before bed. Extended-release preparations of pramipexole and ropinirole are also very effective but have not been formally studied. Nausea, sedation, and impulse control disorders can occur but hallucinations and hypotension rarely occur in RLS, making these drugs better tolerated in RLS compared to Parkinson disease.

The long-term use of DA for RLS is more problematic because some subjects develop tolerance, and others can develop augmentation. Augmentation is defined by an earlier phase shift of symptom onset, an increased intensity of symptoms, increased anatomic involvement, or less relief with movement. Levodopa has the worst augmentation, whereas augmentation with DA is modest at 1 year (2% to 9%) but seems to increase linearly over time. Risk factors for augmentation have been inconsistent but include lower serum ferritin, higher dose of a dopaminergic, worse RLS, a family history of RLS, and absence of neuropathy.

Drugs that bind to the alpha-2 delta subunit of the voltage-dependent calcium channel also improve RLS. As a class, they seem to improve International Restless Legs Scale (IRLS) scores similarly to DA; however, sleep studies show less improvement in PLMS but better sleep architecture. Gabapentin is the least studied but shows benefit. The gabapentin enacarbil sustained release tablet is a novel preparation that is absorbed much more effectively in the gastrointestinal tract and can achieve higher and more sustained serum levels of gabapentin. Multiple large class I trials have demonstrated efficacy, and the drug is approved for use in multiple countries. Pregabalin is also proven effective in high-quality studies but is not approved by regulatory agencies.

Opioid medications, also known as *narcotics*, have long been known to successfully treat RLS. Open-label trials consistently demonstrate good initial and long-term results, with relatively little tolerance, dependence, or addiction. Low-dose methadone especially shows excellent long-term efficacy and tolerability. However, only oxycodone has been evaluated in a placebo-controlled multicenter trial.

Although open-label oral iron supplementation has been reported to improve RLS, the only controlled study of oral iron supplementation failed to improve RLS symptoms. Oral iron, however, has numerous limitations related to absorption and tolerance. In contrast, the administration of high-dose (1 g) intravenous iron can dramatically increase serum ferritin levels. Clinical studies with different iron preparations have shown mixed but mostly favorable results.

Numerous other agents including other antiepileptic medications, benzodiazepines, clonidine, baclofen, tramadol, and magnesium have been reported to help RLS but suffer from limited data and cannot be recommended as either first- or second-line therapy. Physical measures that increase activity or create a sensory stimulus can also improve RLS but are often problematic when one desires sleep.

SUGGESTED READINGS

Allen RP, Barker PB, Horská A, et al. Thalamic glutamate/glutamine in restless legs syndrome: increased and related to disturbed sleep. *Neurology.* 2013; 80(22):2028–2034.

Allen RP, Barker PB, Wehrl F, et al. MRI measurement of brain iron in patients with restless legs syndrome. *Neurology.* 2001;56(2):263–265.

Allen RP, Chen C, Garcia-Borreguero D, et al. Comparison of pregabalin with pramipexole for restless legs syndrome. *N Engl J Med.* 2014;370(7):621–631.

Allen RP, Picchietti D, Hening WA, et al. Restless legs syndrome: diagnostic criteria, special considerations, and epidemiology. A report from the restless legs syndrome diagnosis and epidemiology workshop at the National Institutes of Health. *Sleep Med.* 2003;4(2):101–119.

Beneš HD, García-Borreguero D, Ferini-Strambi L, et al. Augmentation in the treatment of restless legs syndrome with transdermal rotigotine. *Sleep Med.* 2012;13(6):589–597.

Connor JR, Wang XS, Patton SM, et al. Decreased transferrin receptor expression by neuromelanin cells in restless legs syndrome. *Neurology.* 2004;62(9):1563–1567.

Earley CJ, Connor JR, Beard JL, et al. Abnormalities in CSF concentrations of ferritin and transferrin in restless legs syndrome. *Neurology.* 2000;54(8): 1698–1700.

Earley CJ, Kuwabara H, Wong DF, et al. Increased synaptic dopamine in the putamen in restless legs syndrome. *Sleep.* 2013;36(1):51–57.

Furudate NY, Komada Y, Kobayashi M, et al. Daytime dysfunction in children with restless legs syndrome. *J Neurol Sci.* 2014;336(1–2):232–236.

García-Borreguero D, Högl B, Ferini-Strambi L, et al. Systematic evaluation of augmentation during treatment with ropinirole in restless legs syndrome (Willis-Ekbom disease): results from a prospective, multicenter study over 66 weeks. *Mov Disord.* 2012;27(2):277–283.

Garcia-Borreguero D, Kohnen R, Silber MH, et al. The long-term treatment of restless legs syndrome/Willis-Ekbom disease: evidence-based guidelines and clinical consensus best practice guidance: a report from the International Restless Legs Syndrome Study Group. *Sleep Med.* 2013;14(7):675–684.

Godau JU, Klose U, Di Santo A, et al. Multiregional brain iron deficiency in restless legs syndrome. *Mov Disord.* 2008;23(8):1184–1187.

Högl B, Garcia-Borreguero D, Kohnen R, et al. Progressive development of augmentation during long-term treatment with levodopa in restless legs syndrome: results of a prospective multi-center study. *J Neurol.* 2010;257(2):230–237.

Hornyak MH, Scholz H, Kohnen R, et al. What treatment works best for restless legs syndrome? Meta-analyses of dopaminergic and non-dopaminergic medications. *Sleep Med Rev.* 2014;18(2):153–164.

Merlino GA, Serafini A, Young JJ, et al. Gabapentin enacarbil, a gabapentin prodrug for the treatment of the neurological symptoms associated with disorders such as restless legs syndrome. *Curr Opin Investig Drugs.* 2009;10(1):91–102.

Ondo WG, He Y, Rajasekaran S, et al. Clinical correlates of 6-hydroxydopamine injections into A11 dopaminergic neurons in rats: a possible model for restless legs syndrome. *Mov Disord.* 2000;15(1):154–158.

Ondo W, Romanyshyn J, Voung KD, et al. Long-term treatment of restless legs syndrome with dopamine agonists. *Arch Neurol.* 2004;61(9):1393–1397.

Picchietti DL, Bruni O, de Weerd A, et al. Pediatric restless legs syndrome diagnostic criteria: an update by the International Restless Legs Syndrome Study Group. *Sleep Med.* 2013;14(12):1253–1259.

Schormair BD, Kemlink D, Roeske D, et al. PTPRD (protein tyrosine phosphatase receptor type delta) is associated with restless legs syndrome. *Nat Genet.* 2008;40(8):946–948.

Silber MH, Becker PM, Earley C, et al. Willis-Ekbom Disease Foundation revised consensus statement on the management of restless legs syndrome. *Mayo Clin Proc.* 2013;88(9):977–986.

Silver N, Allen RP, Senerth J, et al. A 10-year, longitudinal assessment of dopamine agonists and methadone in the treatment of restless legs syndrome. *Sleep Med.* 2011;12(5):440–444.

Stiasny-Kolster K, Pfau DB, Oertel WH, et al. Hyperalgesia and functional sensory loss in restless legs syndrome. *Pain.* 2013;154(8):1457–1463.

Walters AS, Ondo WG, Zhu W, et al. Does the endogenous opiate system play a role in the restless legs syndrome? A pilot post-mortem study. *J Neurol Sci.* 2009;279(1–2):62–65.

Winkelmann J, Schormair B, Lichtner P, et al. Genome-wide association study of restless legs syndrome identifies common variants in three genomic regions. *Nat Genet.* 2007;39(8):1000–1006.

Yeh P, Walters AS, Tsuang JW. Restless legs syndrome: a comprehensive overview on its epidemiology, risk factors, and treatment. *Sleep Breath.* 2012;16(4):987–1007.

INTRODUCTION

After parkinsonism, dystonia is the most common movement disorder encountered in movement disorder clinics. The term *dystonia* was coined by Oppenheim in 1911 to indicate that the disorder he was describing manifested hypotonia at one occasion and tonic muscle spasms at another, usually but not exclusively elicited on volitional movements. Although the term *dystonia* has undergone various definitions since 1911, the most recent definition is: "Dystonia is a movement disorder characterized by sustained or intermittent muscle contractions causing abnormal, often repetitive, movements, postures, or both. Dystonic movements are typically patterned, twisting, and may be tremulous. Dystonia is often initiated or worsened by voluntary action and associated with overflow muscle activation."

Limb, axial, and cranial voluntary muscles can all be affected by dystonia. The abnormal movements are often exacerbated during voluntary movements, so-called action dystonia.

If the dystonic contractions appear only with a specific action, it is referred to as *task-specific dystonia* (e.g., writer's cramp and musician's cramp). As the dystonic condition progresses, voluntary movements in parts of the body not affected with dystonia can induce dystonic movements of the involved body part, so-called overflow. Talking is a common activity that causes overflow dystonia in other body parts. With further progression, the affected part can develop dystonic movements while at rest, and sustained abnormal postures may be the eventual outcome.

Dystonic movements tend to increase with fatigue, stress, and emotional states; they tend to be suppressed with relaxation, hypnosis, and sleep. Dystonia often disappears during deep sleep, unless the movements are extremely severe. A characteristic and almost unique feature of dystonic movements is that they can be diminished by tactile or proprioceptive "sensory tricks" (gestes antagoniste). For example, patients with cervical dystonia (torticollis) often place a hand on the chin or side of the face to reduce nuchal contractions, and orolingual dystonia is often helped by touching the lips or placing an object in the mouth. Lying down may reduce truncal dystonia; walking backward or running may reduce leg dystonia.

Rapid muscle spasms that occur in a repetitive pattern may be present in torsion dystonia; when rhythmic, the term *dystonic tremor* is applied. Rarely, some children and adolescents with primary or secondary dystonia may experience a crisis, a sudden increase in the severity of dystonia, which has been called *dystonic storm* or *status dystonicus*. This can cause myoglobinuria with a threat of death by renal failure. These patients require treatment in an intensive care unit (ICU) using sedating agents such as propofol and midazolam, intrathecal baclofen, and in some cases, emergency deep brain stimulation of the internal globus pallidus.

EPIDEMIOLOGY

Epidemiologic studies in dystonia typically segregate patients with dystonia into primary (no known cause or no known lesion) and secondary (an environmental or hereditary lesion in the brain) and into focal, segmental, and generalized forms of dystonia. An epidemiologic study of primary dystonia in the population living in Rochester, Minnesota, found the prevalence of generalized dystonia to be 3.4 per 100,000 population and the prevalence of focal dystonia to be 30 per 100,000. The frequency of primary dystonia in the Ashkenazi Jewish population is much higher (between 1/6,000 and 1/2,000) because this population descends from a limited group of founders of the DYT1 mutation. The origin of the mutation was traced to the northern part of the historic Jewish Pale of settlement (Lithuania and Byelorussia) approximately 400 years ago. Focal dystonia is more common than segmental dystonia, and generalized dystonia is very infrequent, about one-tenth as common as focal dystonia. The prevalence rate of focal dystonias varies in different countries, being slightly lower in Japan (between 6 and 14 per 100,000) than in Western Europe (between 11 and 14 per 100,000).

PATHOBIOLOGY

PATHOLOGY

Dystonia is considered a disorder of the central nervous system, with neuropathology showing structural lesions in degenerative forms of dystonia (e.g., Wilson disease and neurodegenerations with brain iron accumulation) and static lesions (e.g., post stroke, post trauma) and those with no structural lesion in the primary dystonias, some metabolic disorders (e.g., dopa-responsive disorder due to genetic mutations causing reduced synthesis of dopamine), and tardive dystonia (due to a persistent complication of dopamine receptor–blocking agents; see Chapter 80). When structural lesions are found in the brain associated with degenerative diseases and environmental insults, the putamen or its connections (including thalamus and cerebral cortex) are the regions affected.

ETIOLOGY

Dystonia can be caused by genetic mutations (inherited dystonia, discussed in the following section) and environmental insults (acquired dystonia), but by far, the most common are dystonias without a known cause (idiopathic dystonia). The last group makes up the majority of focal dystonias. The acquired dystonias are listed in Table 76.1. Most of the causes in this table result in structural lesions, but two do not—drug-induced and psychogenic dystonia.

GENETICS

A large number of gene mutations have been discovered to cause both primary (nonstructural) dystonia and degenerative dystonia. Table 76.2 lists the heredodegenerative dystonias. These are divided into autosomal dominant, autosomal recessive, X-linked, and mitochondrial disorders. Typically, these diseases result in progressive degenerative changes in the basal ganglia and their connections. These can usually be detected by magnetic resonance

TABLE 76.1 Causes of Acquired Dystonia

1. Perinatal cerebral injury
   a. Athetoid cerebral palsy
   b. Delayed-onset dystonia
2. Encephalitis, infections, and post infections
   a. Poststreptococcal
   b. Subacute sclerosing leukoencephalopathy
   c. Progressive multifocal leukoencephalopathy
   d. Creutzfeldt–Jakob disease
   e. HIV/AIDS
   f. Abscess
3. Head trauma
4. Paraneoplastic syndromes
5. Primary antiphospholipid syndrome
6. Focal cerebral vascular injury
7. Arteriovenous malformation
8. Hypoxia
9. Brain tumor
10. Multiple sclerosis
11. Cervical cord injury or lesion
12. Lumbar canal stenosis
13. Peripheral injury
14. Electrical injury
15. Drug-induced
    a. Levodopa
    b. Dopamine D2 receptor–blocking agents
       i. Acute dystonic reaction
       ii. Tardive dystonia
    c. Ergotism
    d. Anticonvulsants
16. Toxins—Mn, CO, carbon disulfide, cyanide, methanol, disulfiram, 3-nitroproprionic acid
17. Metabolic—hypoparathyroidism
18. Psychogenic

Mn, manganese; CO, carbon monoxide.

TABLE 76.2 Heredodegenerative Diseases (Typically Not Pure Dystonia)

Autosomal dominant
   a. Huntington disease
   b. Machado–Joseph disease (SCA3)
   c. Other SCA subtypes (e.g., SCA2, 6, 17)
   d. Familial basal ganglia calcification (Fahr disease)
   e. Frontotemporal dementia (FTD)
   f. Dentatorubropallidoluysian atrophy (DRPLA)
   g. NBIA3/neuroferritinopathy

Autosomal recessive
   a. Juvenile parkinsonism (*parkin*)
   b. Wilson disease
   c. Glutaric acidemia
   d. NBIA1/pantothenic kinase associated neurodegeneration (PKAN)
   e. NBIA2/infantile neuroaxonal dystrophy (INAD)/PLAN for phospholipase A2 deficiency
   f. NBIA4/mitochondrial membrane protein–associated neurodegeneration (MPAN)
   g. NBIA6/coenzyme A synthase protein–associated neurodegeneration (CoPAN)
   h. Aceruloplasminemia (one of the NBIAs)
   i. Fatty acid hydroxylase neurodegeneration (FAHN) (one of the NBIAs)
   j. Gangliosidoses (GM1, GM2)
   k. Dystonic lipidosis/Niemann–Pick, type C (NPC1)
   l. Juvenile neuronal ceroid–lipofuscinosis
   m. Metachromatic leukodystrophy
   n. Homocystinuria
   o. Propionic acidemia
   p. Methylmalonic aciduria
   q. Hartnup disease
   r. Ataxia telangiectasia
   s. Ataxia with vitamin E deficiency
   t. Ataxia with ocular apraxia type 2
   u. Neuroacanthocytosis
   v. Neuronal intranuclear inclusion disease
   w. Friedreich ataxia

X-linked recessive and dominant
   a. Lubag (X-linked dystonia–parkinsonism; DYT3)
   b. Pelizaeus–Merzbacher disease
   c. Deafness/dystonia syndrome
   d. Lesch–Nyhan syndrome
   e. Rett syndrome
   f. NBIA5/beta-propeller protein–associated neurodegeneration (BPAN)

imaging (MRI) and a metabolic workup. Neurodegenerations with brain iron accumulations (NBIAs) are clinically detected by the presence of high iron content in the globus pallidus and other brain regions where there is decreased signal intensity T2-weighted images. Table 76.3 lists the gene mutations in the NBIAs.

The majority of patients with dystonia are without structural lesions in the brain. These so-called primary dystonias can be genetic or idiopathic. The genetic forms began to be classified by geneticists with a DYT1 label. But the labeling has become a mixed bag with both primary dystonias and one heredodegenerative dystonia being in this list. Unfortunately, the paroxysmal dyskinesias were also classified with a DYT label, when in fact these disorders should have been labeled as a separate entity. Table 76.4 provides the DYT classification.

TABLE 76.2 Heredodegenerative Diseases (Typically Not Pure Dystonia) *(continued)*

Mitochondrial

a.	Leigh disease
b.	Leber disease
c.	MERRF/MELAS

Complex etiology (multifactorial)

a.	Parkinson disease
b.	Progressive supranuclear palsy
c.	Multiple system atrophy
d.	Cortical–basal degeneration

SCA, spinocerebellar ataxia; NBIA, neurodegeneration with brain iron accumulation; PLAN, PLA2G6-associated neurodegeneration; MERRF, myoclonic epilepsy with ragged red fibers; MELAS, myopathy, encephalopathy, lactic acidosis, and stroke-like episodes.

Adapted and updated from Fahn S, Bressman SB, Marsden CD. Classification of dystonia. *Adv Neurol.* 1998;78:1–10.

PATHOPHYSIOLOGY

In the absence of overt evidence of neurodegeneration, investigation has turned to functional studies to better understand the pathophysiology of primary dystonia. Positron emission tomography (PET) has identified a range of changes including increased resting glucose metabolism in the premotor cortex and lentiform nucleus and decreased D2 dopamine receptor binding in the putamen. In DYT1 dystonia, two patterns of abnormal metabolic activity have been found. In nonmanifesting carriers and resting affected carriers, there is hypermetabolism of the lentiform

nucleus, cerebellum, and supplementary motor cortex. On the other hand, in DYT1 patients having active muscle contractions, metabolic activity is increased in the thalamus, cerebellum, and midbrain.

Although standard MRIs have not revealed structural pathology, diffusion tensor imaging (DTI) has shown subtle abnormalities in sensorimotor circuitry of dystonia patients. In DYT1 mutation carriers, there is reduced fractional anisotropy (FA) in subgyral white matter of the primary sensorimotor cortex, and in gene carriers manifesting dystonia, FA is also reduced in the pons in the region of the left superior cerebellar peduncle. Abnormal FA has also been observed in the lentiform nucleus and in white matter adjacent to this nucleus in patients with focal dystonia. Human and animal models of DYT1 dystonia reveal that a cerebellar outflow tract disruption between cerebellum and thalamus is associated with disease manifestations, provided that the remainder of the cerebellothalamocortical pathway is intact. In contrast, nonmanifesting DYT1 gene carriers have an additional disruption in this pathway between thalamus and cerebral cortex.

Neurophysiologic studies demonstrate a variety of changes consistent with abnormalities in inhibitory control, sensorimotor integration, and brain plasticity. The electromyogram (EMG) in the dystonias shows cocontraction of agonist and antagonist muscles with prolonged bursts and overflow to extraneous muscles. Spinal and brain stem reflex abnormalities, including reduced reciprocal inhibition and protracted blink reflex recovery, indicate a reduced presynaptic inhibition of muscle afferent input to the inhibitory interneurons as a result of defective descending motor control. The sensorimotor cerebral cortex shows increased and disorganized receptive fields, and sensory temporal discrimination thresholds are increased in DYT1 mutation carriers with and without clinical dystonia. Further, tests probing brain plasticity, such as paired associated stimulation, reveal increased long-term potentiation.

TABLE 76.3 The Neurodegenerations with Brain Iron Accumulation

Label	Acronym	Gene	Chromosome	MRI	Protein
NBIA1	PKAN	*PANK2*	20p13	GP, "eye of the tiger"	PANK2
NBIA2	PLAN; PARK14	*PLA2G6*	22q13.1	GP± SN	
NBIA3	Neuroferritinopathy	*FTL1*	19q13.33	CN, GP, SN, putamen, RN	Ferritin light-chain polypeptide
NBIA4	MPAN	C19orf12	19q12	GP, SN	Mitochondrial protein
NBIA5	BPAN; SENDA	*WDR45*	Xp11.23 dominant	GP, SN halo; white matter	β-propellar protein
NBIA6	CoPAN	*COASY*	17q21.2	GP, SN, putamen, thalamus, tiger eye	Coenzyme A synthase
NBIA	Aceruloplasminemia	*CP*	3q24-q25	BG, dentate, thalamus, Cx	Ceruloplasmin
NBIA; SPG35	FAHN	*FA2H*	16q23.1	GP, white matter	FA 2-hydroxylase
PARK9	Kufor-Rakeb	*ATP13A2*	1p36.13	Putamen, CN	ATP13A2
Late onset	Woodhouse–Sakati syndrome	C2orf27; CDAF17	2q31.1	GP, SN, white matter	Nucleolar transmembrane protein

MRI, magnetic resonance imaging; NBIA, neurodegeneration with brain iron accumulation; GP, globus pallidus; PLAN, PLA2G6-associated neurodegeneration; MPAN, mitochondrial membrane protein–associated neurodegeneration; SN, substantia nigra; BPAN, beta-propeller protein–associated neurodegeneration; SENDA, static encephalopathy of childhood with neurodegeneration in adulthood; CoPAN, coenzyme A synthase protein–associated neurodegeneration; BG, basal ganglia; Cx, cortex; FAHN, fatty acid hydroxylase–associated neurodegeneration; CN, caudate nucleus; FA, fatty acid.

TABLE 76.4 DYT Gene Nomenclature for the Dystonias

Name	Locus	Inheritance Pattern	Phenotype	Gene, Product
DYT1	9q34.11	AD	Early onset, limb onset (Oppenheim dystonia)	*TOR1A*, torsinA
DYT2	Unknown	AR	Early onset	Unknown
DYT3	Xq13.1	XR	Filipino, X-linked dystonia–parkinsonism (lubag)	*TAF1*
DYT4	19p13.3	AD	Generalized dystonia with spasmodic dysphonia	*TUBB4A*, beta-tubulin 4a
DYT5a	14q22.2	AD	DRD (Segawa disease)	*GCH1*, GTP cyclohydrolase 1
DYT5b	11p15.5	AR	DRD, infantile parkinsonism	TH, tyrosine hydroxylase
DYT6	8p11.21	AD	Mixed type, onset often with spasmodic dysphonia, Amish Mennonite and others	*THAP1*
DYT7	18p	AD	Adult cervical	Unknown
DYT8	2q35	AD	Paroxysmal nonkinesigenic dyskinesia (Mount–Rebak)	Formerly called *myofibrillogenesis regulator 1*, now *PNKD*, PNKD protein
DYT9	1p34.2	AD	Paroxysmal choreoathetosis with episodic ataxia and spasticity	Now known to be the gene for GLUT1; same as DYT18
DYT10	16p11.2	AD	Paroxysmal kinesigenic dyskinesia (PKD) (EKD1)	*PRRT2* gene, proline rich transmembrane protein 2
DYT11	7q21.3	AD	Myoclonus–dystonia	*SGCE*, ε-sarcoglycan
DYT12	19q13.2	AD	Rapid-onset dystonia–parkinsonism (RDP)	*ATP1A3*, Na$^+$/K$^+$-ATPase alpha 3 subunit
DYT13	1p36	AD	Cervical–cranial–brachial	Unknown
DYT15	18p11	AD	Myoclonus–dystonia	Unknown
DYT16	2q31.2	AR	Early-onset dystonia–parkinsonism	PRKRA
DYT17	20p11.2-q13	AR	Juvenile onset with torticollis, spreading to segmental and generalized dystonia	Unknown
DYT18	1p34.2	AD	Paroxysmal exertional dyskinesia (PED)	*SLC2A1*, glucose transporter 1 (GLUT1)
DYT19	16q13-q21	AD	Paroxysmal kinesigenic dyskinesia without epilepsy (EKD2)	Unknown
DYT20	2q31	AD	Paroxysmal nonkinesigenic dyskinesia (PNKD2)	Unknown
DYT21	2q14.3-q21.3	AD	Adult-onset mixed dystonia, only in Sweden, so far	Unknown
DYT23	9q34.11	AD	Cervical dystonia	*CIZ1* (CDKN1A-interacting zinc finger protein 1)
DYT24	11p14.2	AD	Cervical–cranial–brachial dystonia (jerky torticollis)	*ANO3* (anoctamin 3)
DYT25	18p11.21	AD	Cervical–cranial dystonia	*GNAL* (guanine nucleotide–binding protein alpha-activating)

Genetic nomenclature is presented in the chronologic order named. The DYT1 gene has a deletion of one of a sequential pair of GAG triplets. DYT2 was set aside for any possible autosomal recessive forms of primary dystonia. DYT3 is associated with X-linked dystonia–parkinsonism, also known as *lubag*, and encountered in Filipino males and appears to be caused by mutations that lead to reduced expression of the transcription factor TATA-box binding protein–associated factors 1. It is the only disorder in this table that is a neurodegenerative disease. The other conditions in the table have not been associated with degeneration yet. DYT4 was labeled for an Australian family with dystonia, including a whispering dysphonia. DYT5a is for the GTP cyclohydrolase I gene mutations causing autosomal dominant DRD. DYT5b is for autosomal recessive DRD and infantile parkinsonism associated with mutations in the gene for tyrosine hydroxylase. DYT6 is the gene causing an adult- and childhood-onset dystonia of cranial, cervical, and limb muscles (mixed) initially discovered in a large Amish Mennonite kindred but now known to be worldwide. DYT7 is for familial torticollis in a family from northwest Germany. DYT8 to 10 are for paroxysmal dyskinesias: 8 is for nonkinesigenic type (PNKD) known as the *Mount–Rebak syndrome*; 9 is for a family with episodic choreoathetosis and spasticity, now recognized to be the same as DYT18; 10 is for PKD on chromosome 16. The same gene mutation can cause episodic ataxia and hemiplegic migraine. DYT11 has been named for mutations in the ε-sarcoglycan gene that causes myoclonus–dystonia. DYT12 is for the Na$^+$/K$^+$-ATPase alpha 3 subunit gene mapped to chromosome 19q causing rapid-onset dystonia–parkinsonism. Speech is often involved. This gene mutation also can cause alternating hemiplegia of childhood. DYT13 is for gene mapped to 1p36 causing cervical–cranial–brachial dystonia in a family in Italy. DYT15 is for a myoclonus–dystonia family mapped to 18p11. DYT16 is for the stress response gene, PRKRA, which encodes the protein kinase, interferon-inducible double-stranded RNA-dependent activator identified in Brazilian families with early-onset dystonia–parkinsonism. DYT17 is for juvenile-onset cervical dystonia that can become generalized; DYT18 as PED due to a gene mutation in the glucose transporter. DYT19 causes another form of PKD without epilepsy. DYT20 causes a second form of PNKD. DYT21 was found in a Swedish family with dystonia. DYT23 causes familial cervical dystonia. DYT24 causes jerky torticollis. DYT25 results in cervical–cranial segmental dystonia.

AD, autosomal dominant; AR, autosomal recessive; DRD, dopa-responsive dystonia; M-D, myoclonus–dystonia; RDP, rapid-onset dystonia–parkinsonism; XR, X-linked recessive.

The functional and microstructural changes described earlier, although not always found in all forms of primary dystonia, point to altered motor control that may begin with abnormal inhibition or abnormal brain plasticity enhanced by feedback mechanisms. Because primary dystonia is etiologically heterogeneous, there are probably several different (possibly converging) pathways that lead to these changes, producing a common clinical picture of dystonic muscle contractions.

CLASSIFICATION OF TORSION DYSTONIA

To emphasize the twisting quality of the abnormal movements and postures, the term *torsion* is often placed in front of the word dystonia. An updated classification of torsion dystonia organizes the dystonias into two major axes: clinical features and etiology. The clinical features axis has five sections, and the etiology axis has two sections (Table 76.5). Within the clinical features axis are age at onset, body distribution, temporal pattern, presence of other movement disorders, and presence of systemic manifestations.

Age at onset is the most important factor related to prognosis of primary dystonia. As a general rule, the younger the age at onset, the more likely the dystonia will become severe and spread to multiple parts of the body. In contrast, the older the age at onset, the more likely dystonia will remain focal. Onset of dystonia in a leg is the second most important predictive factor for a more rapidly progressive course.

Because dystonia usually begins in a single body part, and because dystonia either remains focal or spreads to other body parts, it is useful to classify dystonia according to anatomic distribution. *Focal dystonia* affects only a single area. Frequently seen types of focal dystonia have specific labels: blepharospasm, torticollis, oromandibular dystonia, spastic dysphonia, writer's cramp, or occupational cramp. If dystonia spreads, it usually affects a contiguous body part. When dystonia affects two or more contiguous parts of the body, it is *segmental dystonia*. *Generalized dystonia* is a combination of trunk plus at least two other parts of the body. *Multifocal dystonia* fills a gap in the preceding designations, describing involvement of two or more noncontiguous parts. Dystonia affecting one-half of the body

---

TABLE 76.5 Classification of Torsion Dystonia

Clinical Features

1. Age at onset

Infancy (birth to 2 yr)	Typically a metabolic disorder
Childhood (3–12 yr)	Commonly general or segmental, isolated or combined, inherited
Adolescence (13–20 yr)	Commonly general or segmental, isolated or combined, inherited
Early adulthood (21–40 yr)	Commonly segmental or focal, idiopathic or inherited
Late adulthood (older than 40 yr)	Commonly focal, idiopathic

2. Body distribution
- Focal (single body region)
- Segmental (two or more contiguous regions)
- Multifocal (two noncontiguous or more regions)
- Generalized (trunk + two or more other regions)
- Hemidystonia (unilateral arm + leg ± face)

3. Temporal pattern

Persistent	Can be inherited, idiopathic, secondary
Action-induced	Common onset of inherited and idiopathic (includes task-specific)
Diurnal	May be present in DRD
Paroxysmal	Paroxysmal dyskinesias

4. Associated features (other movement disorders are present in addition to dystonia)

Isolated dystonia	Dystonia is the only motor feature, with the exception of tremor.
Combined dystonia	Dystonia is combined with other movement disorders (such as myoclonus, parkinsonism, etc.).

5. Other neurologic or systemic manifestations
Examples: cognitive impairment in degenerative dystonia; psychiatric symptoms in Wilson disease

Etiology

Neuropathology

   Degenerations

   Static lesions

   No structural lesion

Inherited or Acquired

   Inherited

   Acquired

   Idiopathic

DRD, dopa-responsive dystonia.
Data from Albanese A, Bhatia K, Bressman SB, et al. Phenomenology and classification of dystonia: a consensus update. *Mov Disord.* 2013;28(7):863–873.

is *hemidystonia*, which is usually symptomatic rather than primary. Adult-onset dystonia is often much more focal than generalized.

The most common focal dystonia is cervical dystonia (torticollis), followed by dystonias of cranial muscles: blepharospasm, spasmodic dysphonia, or oromandibular dystonia. Less common is arm dystonia, such as writer's cramp. The most common segmental dystonia involves the cranial muscles (Meige syndrome) or cranial and neck muscles (cranial–cervical dystonia).

The temporal pattern feature distinguishes between the great majority of dystonias that are continual even when the affected body part is at rest from the dystonia that appears only when that body part is voluntarily in motion. A diurnal pattern may be seen in dopa-responsive dystonia, being mild or absent in the morning and worsening as the day goes on. Paroxysmal dystonia is classified as part of a separate movement disorder, paroxysmal dyskinesias.

The associated features category separates those dystonias which are isolated (no other movement disorder present, with the exception of tremor) and those dystonias which are combined with other movement disorders, the most common being parkinsonism and myoclonus. Parkinsonism is commonly seen in DYT3, DYT5a, DYT5b, DYT12, and DYT16; myoclonus is present in DYT11 and DYT15 (see Table 76.4). Myoclonic jerks are sometimes seen in DYT1 and in tardive dystonia.

The etiologic classification includes pathology. Both pathology and etiology have been discussed earlier and in Tables 76.1 to 76.4.

CLINICAL MANIFESTATIONS

CARDINAL MOTOR FEATURES

Some clinical motor features of dystonia were described in the "Introduction." There are four more that are typical in dystonia. Dystonic contractions are (1) of relatively long duration (compared to myoclonus and chorea), although short-duration contractions can occur in dystonia; (2) there is simultaneous contractions of agonist and antagonist muscles affecting the involved body part; (3) dystonic contractions usually result in a twisting of the affected body part (rather than simply flexion or extension); and (4) they involve the same muscle groups repetitively (called *patterned movements*). Myoclonus also has a patterned involvement, but chorea tends to flow from one body part to another. The speed of dystonic contractions can be slow or fast, even reaching the speed of myoclonus. The dystonia usually is activated or made worse when the involved body part moves voluntarily. But the voluntary movement can be highly selective. For example, a child with DYT1 dystonia may manifest twisting and elevation of a leg when walking forward but not when walking backward or running (or sitting or lying). As the disorder worsens, there is less selectivity, and the muscles can be involved even while at rest. Body position is another important factor. Dystonia may be absent when the patient is sitting and appear when the patient stands up. Dystonic tremor is usually not completely rhythmic, compared to parkinsonian tremor or essential tremor. Cervical dystonia is often associated with arrhythmic tremor of the neck; the tremor is always in the horizontal plane. Some patients with primary dystonia may manifest tremor of the arms and hands that resemble essential tremor.

When evaluating a patient with dystonia, the first question is "Is dystonia present, or is the involved muscle tight because of guarding from pain or is it rigidity?" Then, determine if it is isolated dystonia (no other movement disorder present) or combined dystonia (another movement disorder present, often parkinsonism or myoclonus). This step will then focus the diagnosis to a considerable degree. The presence or absence of other neurologic signs is equally important because this would direct one into considering an acquired or neurodegenerative diagnosis. Then other features, such as age at onset, family history, rate of progression, body parts involved, and MRI results will guide the evaluator to a differential diagnosis. Some genes are available for testing commercially, and this should be pursued when those gene mutations are within the differential diagnosis. There are specific syndromes of various types of dystonia, and their patterns will help lead one to the correct diagnosis. These are discussed next.

OPPENHEIM DYSTONIA (DYT1)

The gene at the DYT1 locus has been identified and causes the dystonia described by Oppenheim. In most patients with DYT1 dystonia, symptoms begin in childhood or adolescence, and the mean age at onset is 13 years. Symptoms rarely begin after age 26, although onset as late as the seventh decade may occur. In most patients, first symptoms involve an arm or a leg (Video 76.1), with rare cases beginning in the cervical or cranial muscles. About 65% of all DYT1 patients progress to a generalized or multifocal distribution, but the proportion progressing is even higher for those with childhood onset. About 10% have segmental dystonia and 25% only focal involvement. Most of those with focal dystonia have writer's cramp, but isolated cervical (torticollis) and upper facial (blepharospasm) dystonias have been reported. In terms of body regions ultimately involved, one or more limbs are affected in the vast majority, with over 95% having an affected arm. The trunk and neck are affected in 25% to 35% of cases, and they may be the regions producing the greatest disability; the cranial muscles are less likely to be involved. Also, there may be great intrafamilial variability, ranging from no dystonia (70% of gene carriers have no dystonia) to mild writer's cramp to severe generalized dystonia. When dystonia begins in a leg, it usually starts as an action dystonia resulting in a peculiar twisting of the leg when the child walks forward, even though walking backward, running, or dancing may still be normal. Bizarre stepping or a bowing gait may be noted when the dystonic movements affect proximal muscles of the leg. Difficulty in placing the heel on the ground is evident when distal muscles are affected. As the disorder progresses, the movements may appear when the leg is at rest; the foot may be plantar flexed and ankle everted or inverted; the knee and hip often assume a flexed posture.

With arm involvement, action dystonia may interfere with writing; the fingers curl, the wrist flexes and pronates, the triceps contract, and the elbow elevates. Dystonic tremor of the arm is common, with features of both postural and action tremors. With progression, other activities of the arm are impaired; the arm often moves backward behind the body when the patient walks. Later, dystonia may be present when the arm is at rest.

As the dystonia becomes worse, the contractions become constant so that instead of moving, the body part remains in a fixed twisted posture. The trunk may develop wiggling movements and fixed scoliosis, lordosis, and tortipelvis. The neck may become involved with torticollis, anterocollis, retrocollis, or head tilt and shift. Facial grimacing and difficulties in speech may occur but are much less common. Although muscle tone and power seem normal, the involuntary movements interfere and make voluntary activity extremely difficult. In general, mental activity is normal, and there are no alterations in tendon reflexes or sensation. The rate of progression of this type of dystonia is extremely variable; in most cases, generalized spread occurs within the first 5 to 10 years followed by a static phase, but late worsening, especially more forceful contractions in a body region already affected, may occur. The continuous spasms result in marked distortion of the body to a degree rarely seen in any other disease. With active treatment, it is now uncommon to encounter the severe deformities seen before the 1980s.

Oppenheim dystonia is an autosomal dominant disorder with markedly reduced penetrance of 30% to 40%. The DYT1 gene is localized to chromosome 9q34.1 and encodes the protein torsinA. To date, there is only one clearly pathogenic DYT1 mutation, namely, a GAG deletion in exon 5 of the TOR1A gene. The deletion results in the loss of a glutamic acid residue at position 302 or 303 in the 332-amino acid protein. There are several other coding variants in TOR1A, and one of these, a single nucleotide polymorphism (SNP) that results in coding for either aspartic or histidine at position 216, has recently been identified to modify clinical expression in DYT1 GAG mutation carriers. The histidine allele, present in about 12% of the population, when inherited in trans, protects an individual carrying the GAG deletion from expressing dystonia.

TorsinA is a member of the AAA+ superfamily (ATPases Associated with a variety of cellular Activities). This family of proteins has many functions that are critical to assembly, disassembly, and operation of protein complexes. TorsinA is widely distributed in the brain; it is restricted to neurons and normally associated with the endoplasmic reticulum (ER). In cellular models, mutated torsinA relocates from the ER to the nuclear envelope (NE). Mutant torsinA expression is also associated with abnormal morphology and apparent thickening of the NE including altered connections between the inner and outer membranes, as well as generation of whorled membrane inclusions, which appear to "spin off" the ER/NE. Its aberrant localization and interactions may result in stress-induced abnormalities, including impaired dopamine release. It has also been shown that mutant torsinA interferes with cytoskeletal events, which may affect development of neuronal pathways in the brain.

Oppenheim dystonia affects most ethnic groups but is particularly prevalent in the Ashkenazi Jewish population, in which the prevalence is about 1 per 6,000, as mentioned in the epidemiology section.

Because all DYT1 cases, Jewish and non-Jewish, have one recurring mutation, screening for the mutation is straightforward. Genetic testing is recommended for all patients with primary dystonia with an onset before age 26 years regardless of family history. It is also advised for those with later onset who have a relative with early onset. Genetic counseling should accompany testing; DYT1 has low penetrance, which is affected by the presence of the histidine substitution described earlier. Further, there is variable expression, and importantly, DYT1 does not account for all genetic causes of primary dystonia, even among those with early onset; these complex issues require discussion with patients and their family members.

OTHER EARLY-ONSET NON-DYT1 PRIMARY DYSTONIAS

DYT1 accounts for most childhood- and adolescent-onset primary dystonia in Ashkenazi Jews but only about 30% to 50% in non-Jews. Although some families are clinically similar to DYT1, other families have autosomal dominant inheritance of a somewhat different family phenotype. Dystonia begins on average several years later with a higher proportion having adult onset, and there is greater involvement of muscles in the cranial–cervical region. In two large related Amish Mennonite families with this phenotype, a gene locus (DYT6) was mapped to chromosome 8p and then the mutated gene identified as THAP1. A heterozygous 5bp (GGGTT) insertion followed by

a 3 bp deletion (AAC) in exon 2 of the gene was detected in this large family. The mutation causes a frame shift at amino acid position number 44 of the protein resulting in a premature stop codon at position 73. THAP1 is a member of a family of cellular factors sharing a highly conserved THAP domain, which is an atypical zinc finger. Associated with its DNA binding domain, THAP1 regulates endothelial cell proliferation. In addition to the THAP domain at the N-terminus, THAP1 possesses a nuclear localization signal at its C-terminus. One proposed disease mechanism is that DYT6 mutations disrupt DNA binding and produce transcriptional dysregulation. Although this gene was initially thought to have a limited role, restricted to related Amish Mennonite families, different THAP1 mutations in families with diverse ancestries have now been identified. Despite the diversity of mutation types and ancestries, a similar phenotype has been observed thus far: with relatively early-onset (although the range is wide with a significant proportion having onset after 18 years) and commonly occurring cranial muscle involvement causing speech abnormalities. Many affected individuals in this kindred are disabled by dysphonia, dysarthria, and cervical dystonia.

ADULT-ONSET PRIMARY DYSTONIA

Most primary dystonias are of adult onset with estimates of prevalence ranging from 11.7 to 49 per 100,000. The adult dystonias usually remain localized to the muscles (and immediately contiguous muscles) first involved (i.e., focal and segmental dystonias). Common sites are neck (cervical dystonia), face (blepharospasm), jaw (oromandibular dystonia), vocal cords (spasmodic dysphonia), and arm (writer's cramp).

Family studies have demonstrated an increased rate of dystonia among family members, suggesting a genetic etiology. With equal rates in parents, offspring, and siblings, the pattern of transmission is consistent with autosomal dominant inheritance; however, it seems to be much less penetrant than childhood-onset dystonia, with penetrance rates of only 10% to 15% rather than 30% to 40% and few with higher penetrance. In one such family with cervical dystonia, a locus, DYT7 on chromosome 18p, was mapped. This locus has been excluded in other adult-onset families, so its role in primary dystonia is not known. Because the majority of adult-onset dystonia patients do not have many affected relatives, association studies using cases and controls have been employed to find genetic risk factors. Adult-onset focal dystonias have been associated with polymorphisms in the D5 dopamine receptor gene and also with a DYT1 haplotype, but these findings have not been consistently replicated.

Cervical dystonia, commonly known as *spasmodic torticollis* or *wry neck*, is the most common focal dystonia (Video 76.2). It occurs at any age, usually beginning between ages 20 and 60 years, and is more frequent in women. Any combination of neck muscles can be involved, especially the sternocleidomastoid, trapezius, splenius capitis, levator scapulae, and scalenus muscles. Sustained turning, tilting, flexing, or extending of the neck or shifting of the head laterally or anteriorly can result. Frequently, the shoulder is elevated and anteriorly displaced on the side to which the chin turns. Instead of sustained head deviation, some patients have jerking movements of the head. Neck pain occurs in about two-thirds of patients with cervical dystonia and usually responds successfully to injections of botulinum toxin at the site of the pain. A common sensory trick to relieve cervical dystonia is to place one hand on the back of the head or chin. About 10% of patients with cervical dystonia have a remission, usually within a year of onset; most remissions are followed by a relapse years later.

Some patients with torticollis have a horizontal head tremor that may be impossible to distinguish from essential tremor. Other considerations in the differential diagnosis of dystonic torticollis are congenital contracture of the sternocleidomastoid muscle, which can be treated with surgical release. In young boys after a full meal, extreme head tilt may be caused by gastroesophageal reflux (*Sandifer syndrome*), which can be treated either medically or by plication surgery. Other diagnostic considerations are trochlear nerve palsy; Arnold–Chiari malformation; malformations of the cervical spine, such as Klippel–Feil fusion or atlantoaxial subluxation; cervical infections; and spasms from cervical muscle shortening.

Blepharospasm is caused by contraction of the orbicularis oculi muscles. It usually begins with increased frequency of blinking, followed by closure of the eyelids, and then more firm and prolonged closure of the lids, which may produce functional blindness if untreated. Blinking and lid closure can be intermittent and are often temporarily suppressed by talking, humming, singing, or looking down. The condition is worsened by walking and by bright light. A common sensory trick that relieves contractions is placing of a finger just lateral to the orbit. Blepharospasm is usually accompanied by cocontraction of lower facial muscles, such as the platysma and risorius. This type of focal dystonia sometimes becomes segmental by spreading to other cranial targets, such as the jaw (Video 76.3), tongue, vocal cords, or cervical muscles. The combination of blepharospasm with cervical or other cranial dystonias is called *craniocervical segmental dystonia* or *Meige syndrome*. Blepharospasm occurs more often in women than in men, usually beginning after age 50 years, although younger people may be affected. Abnormalities of the blink reflex have been found with blepharospasm and with other cranial or cervical dystonias.

The differential diagnosis of blepharospasm includes *hemifacial spasm*, which is unilateral. Rarely, hemifacial spasm is bilateral, but the contractions on the two sides of the face are not synchronous as they are in blepharospasm. *Blinking tics* can resemble blepharospasm, but tics almost always begin in childhood. *Sjögren syndrome* of dry eyes often causes the eyelids to close, but testing for tear production usually distinguishes this disorder. Injections of botulinum toxin into the contracting muscles are effective in more than 80% of patients with blepharospasm.

Writer's cramp of adult onset usually remains limited to one limb, often the dominant side (Video 76.4). In about one-third of cases, it spreads to the other arm. When it affects only writing, the patient may learn to write with the nondominant hand. For bilateral involvement or for dystonia that affects other activities (buttoning, shaving, or playing a musical instrument), carefully placed injections of botulinum toxin may be effective.

Dystonia of the vocal cords occurs in two forms. The more common type is *spasmodic adductor dysphonia*, in which the vocalis muscles contract, bringing the vocal cords together and causing the voice to be restricted, strangled, and coarse, often broken up with pauses. *Breathy (whispering) dysphonia* (spasmodic abductor dysphonia) is caused by contractions of the posterior cricoarytenoids (abductor muscles of the vocal cords) so that the patient cannot talk in a loud voice and tends to run out of air while trying to speak. Spasmodic dysphonia is often associated with tremor of the vocal cords. Essential tremor (with vocal cord tremor) is an important differential diagnosis; the presence of tremor in the hands or neck leads to such diagnosis. Injections of botulinum toxin can be dramatically effective for spasmodic adductor dysphonia but are less certain for breathy dysphonia. For each type, a physician must be experienced with the procedure of injecting the correct muscle. Some patients with the strangulated voice of adductor dysphonia will compensate by speaking in a whisper, which could confuse the examiner into misdiagnosing abductor dysphonia. When encountering a patient with supposed breathy dysphonia, the examiner needs to inquire if whispering is done purposefully in order to talk fluently.

COMBINED DYSTONIA SYNDROMES

This category includes nondegenerative disorders in which parkinsonism (dopa-responsive dystonia and rapid-onset dystonia–parkinsonism) or myoclonus (myoclonus–dystonia) coexists with dystonia.

Dopa-Responsive Dystonia

A small minority of patients with childhood-onset dystonia have the autosomal dominant disorder dopa-responsive dystonia (DRD), sometimes called *Segawa disease*. Distinguishing DRD from primary isolated dystonia is important because DRD responds so well to treatment. It differs from primary dystonia by the signs of parkinsonism, which may be subtle. These include bradykinesia, cogwheel rigidity, and impaired postural reflexes. Other distinguishing features include diurnal fluctuations with improvement after sleep and worsening as the day wears on; a peculiar "spastic" straight-legged gait, with a tendency to walk on the toes; hyperreflexia, particularly in the legs and sometimes with Babinski signs; and a remarkable therapeutic response to low doses of levodopa that is sustained without the development of long-term fluctuations observed in Parkinson disease.

DRD usually begins between ages 6 and 16 years but can appear at any age. When it begins in infants, it resembles cerebral palsy. When it begins in adults, it often manifests as pure parkinsonism, mimicking Parkinson disease, responding to levodopa, and having a generally benign course. DRD affects girls more often than boys, has a worldwide distribution, and is not known to have a higher prevalence in any specific ethnic group. Mutations in the gene for GTP cyclohydrolase 1 (*GCH1*) located at 14q22.2 are responsible for the majority of DRD. More than 60 different mutations have been reported; they are thought to have a dominant negative effect on enzyme activity. In some patients, other genetic etiologies can be found (e.g., recessively inherited mutations in tyrosine hydroxylase), but in others, no genetic cause can be identified.

GCH1 catalyzes the first and rate-limiting step in the biosynthesis of tetrahydrobiopterin (BH4), the cofactor required for the enzymes tyrosine hydroxylase, phenylalanine hydroxylase, and tryptophan hydroxylase. These hydroxylase enzymes add an –OH group to the parent amino acid and are required for the synthesis of biogenic amines. The genetic label for DRD owing to GCH1 mutations is DYT5a.

Pathologic investigations of DRD revealed no loss of neurons within the substantia nigra pars compacta, but the cells are immature with little neuromelanin. Neuromelanin synthesis requires dopamine (or other monoamines) as the initial precursor. Biochemically, there is marked reduction in dopamine concentration and tyrosine hydroxylase activity within the striatum in DRD.

Aside from mutations in GCH1, DRD can rarely be caused by mutations in other enzymes involved in dopamine synthesis including tyrosine hydroxylase and pterin synthesis deficiencies. DRD owing to tyrosine hydroxylase deficiency (DYT5b) is an autosomal recessive disorder that begins in infancy or early childhood. The phenotype may mimic DRD, but clinical features range from a mild syndrome of spastic paraparesis to severe parkinsonism, dystonia, and oculogyric crises. The pterin deficiency syndromes can include other features such as ptosis, miosis, rigidity, hypokinesia, chorea, myoclonus, seizures, temperature disturbance, and hypersalivation. These latter features represent deficiencies of norepinephrine and serotonin in addition to dopamine; hyperphenylalaninemia is present, and the disorder may respond partially to levodopa.

Another disorder of infants is the autosomal recessive deficiency of the enzyme aromatic L-amino acid decarboxylase, which catalyzes the transformation of levodopa to dopamine. Levodopa is ineffective in this disorder, but patients respond partially to dopamine agonists coupled with a monoamine oxidase inhibitor.

The most important differential diagnosis of DRD is juvenile parkinsonism, a progressive nigral degenerative disorder usually caused by homozygous or compound heterozygous mutations in the *parkin* gene (PARK2). In this disorder, dystonia often precedes the parkinsonian features, which become the major clinical feature. Distinguishing laboratory tests include fluorodopa PET and β-CIT single-photon emission computed tomography (SPECT), which are normal in DRD but abnormal in juvenile parkinsonism, showing marked reduction in uptake in the striatum. Other differential features of DRD from juvenile parkinsonism and Oppenheim dystonia are listed in Table 76.6.

One may also suspect DRD if a young patient with dystonia responds dramatically to low doses of anticholinergic agents. However, the most effective agent is levodopa. The suggested starting dose of carbidopa/levodopa for DRD is 12.5/50 mg two or three times a day, a dose low enough to avoid acute dyskinesias, which may sometimes occur if therapy is started with higher doses. The usual maintenance dose is 25/100 mg two or three times a day.

Rapid-onset Dystonia–Parkinsonism

Rapid-onset dystonia–parkinsonism (RDP) is a rare combined dystonia syndrome that begins during childhood or early adulthood. It is characterized by both dystonia and parkinsonism that usually begins suddenly, over hours to days, and may be associated with physical or emotional stress. Symptoms may, however, begin more insidiously and then have a period of rapid worsening. After the period of worsening, symptoms tend to stabilize, although improvement may occur. The phenotype resembles dystonic–parkinsonian Wilson disease, with prominent bulbar signs (including risus sardonicus), relatively sustained dystonic limb posturing, waxy effortful rapid successive movements, and postural instability. Inheritance is autosomal dominant, and de novo mutations have

TABLE 76.6 Differential Features between Dopa-Responsive Dystonia, Oppenheim Torsion Dystonia, and Juvenile Parkinson Disease

Features	DRD	DYT1	JPD
Average age at onset (range)	6 yr (infancy—sixth decade)	13 yr (4 yr—seventh decade)	Adolescence (7 yr—sixth decade)
Gender	Female > male	Female = male	Male = female
Initial signs	Leg > arm or trunk action dystonia, abnormal gait (scissoring, toe walking)	Arm or leg action dystonia, occasionally trunk or neck	Foot/leg > hand/arm dystonia, rest tremor (especially legs), akinesia/rigidity
Diurnal fluctuations	Often prominent	Rare	May occur
Bradykinesia	Yes (may be mild)	No	Yes
Postural instability	Occurs	No	Occurs
Response to L-dopa			
Initial	Excellent to very low to low dose	Inconsistent and usually not dramatic	Excellent to low to moderate dose
Long term	Excellent		Dyskinesias, may fluctuate
CSF			
HVA	↓	Normal	↓
Biopterin	↓	Normal	↓
Neopterin	↓↓	Normal	↓
F-DOPA PET	Normal or slightly reduced without worsening over time	Normal	Decreased and worsens over time
Inheritance	AD, reduced penetrance	AD, reduced penetrance	AR
Gene	Heterozygous mutations in *GCH1* in many, rarely recessive *GCH1* or *TH*	Heterozygous GAG deletion in DYT1	Homozygous or compound heterozygous *parkin* mutations
Testing	Screening for *GCH1* mutations in select labs	Commercially available	Commercially available
Prognosis	Return to near normal with treatment in most	Progresses at first, then tends to stabilize after several years	Slow to moderate progression

DRD, dopa-responsive dystonia; DYT1, Oppenheim torsion dystonia; JPD, juvenile Parkinson disease; CSF, cerebrospinal fluid; HVA, homovanillic acid; ↓, decreased; AD, autosomal dominant; AR, autosomal recessive.

been observed. The responsible gene, which maps to chromosome 19q13 (classified as DYT12), has been identified; it codes for Na$^+$/K$^+$-ATPase a3, a catalytic subunit of the sodium–potassium pump that functions to maintain an electrochemical gradient across the plasma membrane. In RDP patients, the cerebrospinal fluid (CSF) homovanillic acid concentration is low, there are no imaging abnormalities, and in two autopsies, no neurodegeneration was detected. However, subsequent cases in one family were found with changes in some subcortical regions. There is no effective treatment. The mutated gene has also been found to cause the disorder known as *alternating hemiplegia of childhood.*

Myoclonus–Dystonia

Although lightning-like movements occasionally occur in Oppenheim dystonia, they are a prominent feature in a distinct autosomal dominant disorder known as *myoclonus–dystonia* (M-D). In families with M-D, affected individuals have myoclonus as the primary sign, and it may occur with or without dystonia; rarely, dystonia is the only feature as writer's cramp or torticollis. Symptom onset is usually in the first or second decade; males and females are equally affected in most, but not all, families, and the pattern of inheritance appears autosomal dominant with reduced penetrance that is dependent on the transmitting parent. That is, most affected individuals inherit the disorder through their father, a finding consistent with a maternal imprinting mechanism. The neck and arms are involved most commonly, followed by the trunk and bulbar muscles, with less common involvement of the legs. The disorder tends to plateau in adulthood, and affected adults often report that the muscle jerks respond dramatically to alcohol. Also, there appears to be an excess of psychiatric symptoms, including obsessive–compulsive disorder (OCD), in family members, even those not affected with motor signs of M-D.

A large proportion of familial M-D is owing to mutations in the ε-sarcoglycan gene mapped to chromosome 7q21.3 (DYT11). The sarcoglycans are a family of genes that encode components of the dystrophin–glycoprotein complex, and mutations in α-, β-, γ-, and Δ-sarcoglycan produce recessive muscular limb-girdle dystrophy. ε-Sarcoglycan, however, is expressed widely in brain, is located at the plasma membrane, and is imprinted. In a cellular model, the mutant protein is retained intracellularly, becomes polyubiquitinated, and is rapidly degraded by the proteasome. Furthermore, torsinA binds to and promotes the degradation of ε-sarcoglycan mutants when both proteins are coexpressed.

ε-Sarcoglycan mutations do not account for all familial M-D and probably are not responsible for most sporadic M-D. There is at least one other gene locus for M-D; in one family with M-D, a locus on 18p (DYT15) was mapped.

SECONDARY DYSTONIA

Secondary dystonia can occur as the result of an environmental injury (acquired dystonia) or a heredodegenerative disorder (inherited degenerative or dystonia) that affects the brain, especially the basal ganglia. Spinal cord injury and peripheral injury are also recognized causes of dystonia. Examples of acquired dystonia include levodopa-induced dystonia in the treatment of parkinsonism; acute and tardive dystonia owing to dopamine receptor–blocking agents; and dystonias associated with cerebral palsy, cerebral hypoxia, cerebrovascular disease, cerebral infectious and postinfectious states, brain tumor, and toxicants such as manganese, cyanide, and 3-nitroproprionic acid. Other acquired causes include psychogenic disorders, peripheral trauma followed by focal dystonia in the affected region, head injury, and delayed-onset dystonia

after cerebral infarct or other cerebral insult. Prior history of one of these insults suggests the correct diagnosis, as does neuroimaging that shows a lesion in the basal ganglia or their connections.

A more complete listing of secondary dystonias was presented in Tables 76.1, 76.2 and 76.3. A number of disorders in this group, such as the infectious and toxicant-induced neurodegenerations, are not limited to pure dystonia but show a mixture of other neurologic features, often the parkinsonian features bradykinesia and rigidity. *Tardive dystonia*, a persistent complication of agents that block dopamine receptors, is a common form of secondary dystonia. Tardive dystonia is usually focal or segmental, affecting the cranial structures in adults; in children and adolescents, however, it can be generalized, involving the trunk and limbs. It often is associated with features of tardive dyskinesia, especially oral–buccal–lingual movements (see Chapter 80). Clues suggesting a secondary dystonia are listed in Table 76.7.

NBIAs were discussed in the section on genetics and are listed in Table 76.3. An X-linked recessive disorder causing dystonia and parkinsonism affects young adult Filipino men. The Filipino name for the condition is *lubag*. It has been designated as DYT3. It can begin with dystonia in the feet or cranial structures; lingual and oromandibular dystonias are common, sometimes with stridor. With progression, generalized dystonia often develops. Many patients develop parkinsonism; in some patients, the sole manifestation may be progressive parkinsonism. The abnormal gene is localized to the centromeric region of the X chromosome, and disease-specific mutations have been identified, which lead to a reduced expression of the general transcription factor TATA-box binding protein–associated factor 1 (*TAF1*). Pathologic study reveals a mosaic pattern of gliosis in the striatum. Patients respond only partially to levodopa, anticholinergics, baclofen, clonazepam, or zolpidem.

Psychogenic dystonia can be considered within the secondary dystonia category. For many decades, Oppenheim dystonia was considered psychogenic because of the bizarre nature of the symptoms, exaggeration in periods of stress, variability, and suppression by sensory tricks. This misdiagnosis often led to a long delay in identification of the nature of the disorder and to prolonged periods of needless psychotherapy. Awareness of the capricious nature of the disorder and serial observation of patients can avoid this pitfall. On the other hand, psychogenic dystonia does occur but in less than 5% of patients who otherwise would be considered

---

TABLE 76.7 Clues Suggestive of Symptomatic Dystonia

1. History of possible etiologic factor, for example, head trauma, peripheral trauma, encephalitis, toxin exposure, drug exposure, perinatal anoxia

2. Presence of neurologic abnormality aside from dystonia, for example, parkinsonism, dementia, seizures, ocular, ataxia, neuropathy, spasticity

3. Onset of dystonia at rest (instead of action)

4. Early onset of speech involvement

5. Leg involvement in an adult

6. Hemidystonia

7. Abnormal routine brain imaging

8. Abnormal laboratory workup

9. Presence of false weakness or sensory exam or other clues of psychogenic etiology (see Table 76.8)

TABLE 76.8	Clues Suggestive of Psychogenic Dystonia

Clues relating to the movements

1. Abrupt onset

2. Inconsistent movements (changing characteristics over time)

3. Incongruous movements and postures (movements do not fit with recognized patterns or with normal physiologic patterns)

4. Presence of additional types of abnormal movements that are not consistent with the basic abnormal movement pattern or are not congruous with a known movement disorder, particularly rhythmic shaking, bizarre gait, deliberate slowness carrying out requested voluntary movement, bursts of verbal gibberish, and excessive startle (bizarre movements in response to sudden unexpected noise or threatening movement)

5. Spontaneous remissions

6. Movements disappear with distraction

7. Response to placebo, suggestion, or psychotherapy

8. Present as a paroxysmal disorder

9. Dystonia beginning as a fixed posture

10. Twisting facial movements that move the mouth to one side or the other (Note: Organic dystonia of the facial muscles usually does not move the mouth sideways.)

Clues relating to other medical observations

1. False (give-way) weakness

2. False sensory complaints

3. Multiple somatizations or undiagnosed conditions

4. Self-inflicted injuries

5. Obvious psychiatric disturbances

6. Employment in the health profession or in insurance claims field

7. Presence of secondary gain, including continuing care by a "devoted" spouse

8. Litigation or compensation pending

TABLE 76.9	Other Movement Disorders in Which Dystonia May Be Present

Tic disorders with dystonic tics

Paroxysmal dyskinesias with dystonia

    Paroxysmal kinesigenic dyskinesia

    Paroxysmal nonkinesigenic dyskinesia

    Paroxysmal exertional dyskinesia

    Benign infantile paroxysmal dyskinesias

Hypnogenic dystonia (sometimes these are seizures)

they are often mistaken for dystonia. However, these contractions are secondary to either a peripheral or a reflex mechanism or as a reaction to some other problem. For example, Sandifer syndrome is a result of gastroesophageal reflux, with apparent reduction in the gastric contractions when the head is tilted to the side; Isaacs syndrome is a result of continuous peripheral neural firing; orthopedic disease causes a number of postural changes; and seizures can result in sustained twisting postures.

TREATMENT

After levodopa therapy has been tested to be certain that DRD has not been overlooked, other oral medications may be effective and should be tried in people with dystonia not amenable or not adequately responding to botulinum toxin injections. The following

TABLE 76.10	Pseudodystonias (Not Classified as Dystonia but Can Be Mistaken for Dystonia because of Sustained Postures)

Sandifer syndrome

Stiff person syndrome

Isaacs syndrome

Satoyoshi syndrome

Rotational atlantoaxial subluxation

Soft-tissue nuchal mass

Bone disease

Ligamentous absence, laxity, or damage

Congenital muscular torticollis

Congenital postural torticollis

Juvenile rheumatoid arthritis

Ocular postural torticollis

Congenital Klippel–Feil syndrome

Posterior fossa tumor

Syringomyelia

Arnold–Chiari malformation

Trochlear nerve palsy

Vestibular torticollis

Seizures manifesting as sustained twisting postures

Inflammatory myopathy

to have primary torsion dystonia. Clues suggestive of psychogenic dystonia are listed in Table 76.8.

OTHER MOVEMENT DISORDERS WITH DYSTONIA

Dystonia can appear in disorders not ordinarily considered to be part of torsion dystonia (Table 76.9). These include dystonic tics that are more conveniently classified with tic disorders (see Chapter 74), paroxysmal dyskinesias more conveniently classified with paroxysmal dyskinesias, and hypnogenic dystonia that can be either paroxysmal dyskinesias or seizures.

PSEUDODYSTONIA

To complete the classification, Table 76.10 lists disorders that can mimic torsion dystonia but are not generally considered to be true dystonias. These disorders typically manifest themselves as sustained muscle contractions or abnormal postures, which is why drugs have been reported to be effective in dystonia: high-dose anticholinergics (e.g., trihexyphenidyl), high-dose baclofen, benzodiazepines (clonazepam, diazepam), and antidopaminergics (tetrabenazine, dopamine receptor blockers).

Test one drug at a time. The procedure can take months before a combination of medications can be found that are beneficial. Anticholinergics may be the most effective and is the only class of drugs other than botulinum toxin shown to be effective in a controlled clinical trial [Level 1].[1] Trihexyphenidyl is better tolerated in children than in adults. In both groups, start with a small dose (1 mg three times a day [t.i.d.]) and if tolerated, increase after 1 week to 2 mg t.i.d. The dose can be increased weekly at that rate until benefit or side effects are seen. The most common anticholinergic side effect is dry mouth and blurred vision due to dilated pupils. There could also be constipation and difficulty initiating a urinary stream. If a patient has glaucoma, pilocarpine eye drops need to be applied, and one should work with an ophthalmologist. Pilocarpine eye drops (1/4%) is also useful to overcome blurred vision due to dilated pupils. Dry mouth can be relieved with drinking more fluids or sucking on sugar-free hard candies. For urinary or bowel symptoms, adding pyridostigmine starting at 30 mg twice a day (b.i.d.) and increasing the dose to obtain relief often helps. A side effect that limits the use of anticholinergics is forgetfulness or short-term memory loss. The only relief is to lower the dose or discontinue the drug. The dose of trihexyphenidyl could reach over 120 mg/day in children. Adults may not tolerate more than 30 mg/day. Building the dosage up very slowly is the only way to achieve the effective high doses. If side effects occur, one can reduce the dose to the point at which the adverse effects have cleared while still achieving some benefit. If side effects occur without ever achieving benefit, it is best to titrate the dose downward over several days and eliminate it.

After the optimum dose of the anticholinergic agent has been reached, a second drug can be added. Baclofen, beginning at 10 mg at bedtime (h.s.), can be increased weekly by 10 mg until 10 mg four times a day (q.i.d.) is reached. If no adverse effects or benefit is seen, continue to increase the dose. As much as 90 to 120 mg/day may be necessary to see benefit. A major limitation is drowsiness, and a high dose may not be reached. If some benefit is seen, continue using it at a dose that is tolerated and then add a third medication. Clonazepam, diazepam, and tetrabenazine can all be tried using the same principle of starting with a low dose and building it up gradually until either side effects or benefit is seen.

For focal dystonias, such as blepharospasm, torticollis, oromandibular dystonia, and spastic dysphonia, local injections of botulinum toxin are beneficial [Level 1].[2–6] This agent also can be used to treat generalized dystonia, with injections limited to the most severely affected focal site. This muscle-weakening agent can be effective for about 3 months before a repeat injection is needed. Current batches of the toxin contain less antigenic protein than the original batch, making it less likely that patients will develop antibodies to botulinum toxin, which would render that particular strain of toxin ineffective.

Stereotactic brain surgery may ameliorate dystonia and can be considered if medical therapies fail. Deep brain stimulation has mostly replaced ablative surgery, which had been thalamotomy and especially pallidotomy. The main target for deep brain stimulation is the globus pallidus interna. Bilateral deep brain stimulation of the pallidum appears to provide moderate to marked improvement for generalized primary dystonia without the high risk for dysarthria that occurs after bilateral thalamotomy, but dysarthria and other neurologic complications can sometimes occur. The subthalamic nucleus is being evaluated as another target for deep brain stimulation.

Videos can be found in the companion e-book edition. For a full list of video legends, please see the front matter.

LEVEL 1 EVIDENCE

1. Burke RE, Fahn S, Marsden CD. Torsion dystonia: a double-blind, prospective trial of high-dosage trihexyphenidyl. *Neurology.* 1986;36:160–164.
2. Comella CL, Jankovic J, Shannon KM, et al; for Dystonia Study Group. Comparison of botulinum toxin serotypes A and B for the treatment of cervical dystonia. *Neurology.* 2005;65:1423–1429.
3. Truong D, Comella C, Fernandez HH, et al; for Dysport Benign Essential Blepharospasm Study Group. Efficacy and safety of purified botulinum toxin type A (Dysport) for the treatment of benign essential blepharospasm: a randomized, placebo-controlled, phase II trial. *Parkinsonism Relat Disord.* 2008;14:407–414.
4. Charles D, Brashear A, Hauser RA, et al; for CD 140 Study Group. Efficacy, tolerability, and immunogenicity of onabotulinumtoxina in a randomized, double-blind, placebo-controlled trial for cervical dystonia. *Clin Neuropharmacol.* 2012;35(5):208–214.
5. Comella CL, Jankovic J, Truong DD, et al; for U.S. XEOMIN Cervical Dystonia Study Group. Efficacy and safety of incobotulinumtoxinA (NT 201, XEOMIN®, botulinum neurotoxin type A, without accessory proteins) in patients with cervical dystonia. *J Neurol Sci.* 2011;308(1–2):103–109.
6. Jankovic J, Comella C, Hanschmann A, et al. Efficacy and safety of incobotulinumtoxinA (NT 201, Xeomin) in the treatment of blepharospasm-a randomized trial. *Mov Disord.* 2011;26(8):1521–1528.

SUGGESTED READINGS

Albanese A, Bhatia K, Bressman SB, et al. Phenomenology and classification of dystonia: a consensus update. *Mov Disord.* 2013;28(7):863–873.

Argyelan M, Carbon M, Niethammer M, et al. Cerebellothalamocortical connectivity regulates penetrance in dystonia. *J Neurosci.* 2009;29(31):9740–9747.

Asmus F, Zimprich A, Tezenas du Montcel S, et al. Myoclonus-dystonia syndrome: epsilon-sarcoglycan mutations and phenotype. *Ann Neurol.* 2002;52:489–492.

Brandfonbrener AG, Robson C. Review of 113 musicians with focal dystonia seen between 1985 and 2002 at a clinic for performing artists. *Adv Neurol.* 2004;94:255–256.

Brashear A, Dobyns WB, de Carvalho Aguiar P, et al. The phenotypic spectrum of rapid-onset dystonia-parkinsonism (RDP) and mutations in the ATP1A3 gene. *Brain.* 2007;130(3):828–835.

Breakefield XO, Blood AJ, Li Y, et al. The pathophysiological basis of dystonias. *Nat Rev Neurosci.* 2008;9:222–234.

Bressman SB, Sabatti C, Raymond D, et al. The DYT1 phenotype and guidelines for diagnostic testing. *Neurology.* 2000;54(9):1746–1752.

Charlesworth G, Bhatia KP, Wood NW. The genetics of dystonia: new twists in an old tale. *Brain.* 2013;136(pt 7):2017–2037.

Chuang C, Fahn S, Frucht SJ. The natural history and treatment of acquired hemidystonia: report of 33 cases and review of the literature. *J Neurol Neurosurg Psychiatry.* 2002;72:59–67.

Dauer WT, Burke RE, Greene P, et al. Current concepts on the clinical features, aetiology and management of idiopathic cervical dystonia. *Brain.* 1998;121:547–560.

de Carvalho Aguiar P, Sweadner KJ, Penniston JT, et al. Mutations in the Na+/K+-ATPase alpha3 gene ATP1A3 are associated with rapid-onset dystonia parkinsonism. *Neuron.* 2004;43(2):169–175.

Eidelberg D, Moeller JR, Antonini A, et al. Functional brain networks in DYT1 dystonia. *Ann Neurol.* 1998;44:303–312.

Frucht SJ, Fahn S, Greene PE, et al. The natural history of embouchure dystonia. *Mov Disord.* 2001;16:899–906.

Fuchs T, Gavarini S, Saunders-Pullman R, et al. Mutations in the THAP1 gene are responsible for DYT6 primary torsion dystonia. *Nat Genet.* 2009;41:286–288.

Fung VS, Jinnah HA, Bhatia K, Vidailhet M. Assessment of patients with isolated or combined dystonia: an update on dystonia syndromes. *Mov Disord.* 2013;28(7):889–898.

Geyer HL, Bressman SB. The diagnosis of dystonia. *Lancet Neurol.* 2006;5:780–790.

Goodchild RE, Kim C, Dauer WT. Loss of the dystonia-associated protein torsinA selectively disrupts the nuclear envelope. *Neuron.* 2005;48:923–932.

Grattan-Smith PJ, Wevers RA, Steenbergen-Spanjers GC, et al. Tyrosine hydroxylase deficiency: clinical manifestations of catecholamine insufficiency in infancy. *Mov Disord.* 2002;17:354–359.

Greene P, Kang UJ, Fahn S. Spread of symptoms in idiopathic torsion dystonia. *Mov Disord.* 1995;10:143–152.

Groen JL, Kallen MC, van de Warrenburg BP, et al. Phenotypes and genetic architecture of focal primary torsion dystonia. *J Neurol Neurosurg Psychiatry.* 2012;83(10):1006–1011.

Hayflick SJ, Westaway SK, Levinson B, et al. Genetic, clinical, and radiographic delineation of Hallervorden–Spatz syndrome. *N Engl J Med.* 2003;348(2):33–40.

Holton JL, Schneide SA, Ganessharajah T, et al. Neuropathology of primary adult-onset dystonia. *Neurology.* 2008;70:695–699.

Klein C, Fahn S. Translation of Oppenheim's 1911 paper on dystonia. *Mov Disord.* 2013;28(7):851–862.

Kumar KR, Lohmann K, Masuho I, et al. Mutations in GNAL: a novel cause of craniocervical dystonia. *JAMA Neurol.* 2014;71(4):490–494.

Kuoppamaki M, Bhatia KP, Quinn N. Progressive delayed-onset dystonia after cerebral anoxic insult in adults. *Mov Disord.* 2002;17:1345–1349.

Liang CC, Tanabe LM, Jou S, et al. TorsinA hypofunction causes abnormal twisting movements and sensorimotor circuit neurodegeneration. *J Clin Invest.* 2014;124(7):3080–3092.

Lohmann K, Klein C. Genetics of dystonia: what's known? What's new? What's next? *Mov Disord.* 2013;28(7):899–905.

McNaught KS, Kapustin A, Jackson T, et al. Brainstem pathology in DYT1 primary torsion dystonia. *Ann Neurol.* 2004;56(4):540–547.

Muller J, Wissel T, Masuhr F, et al. Clinical characteristics of the geste antagoniste in cervical dystonia. *J Neurol.* 2001;248:478–482.

Nutt JG, Muenter MD, Aronson A, et al. Epidemiology of focal and generalized dystonia in Rochester, Minnesota. *Mov Disord.* 1988;3:188–194.

Nygaard TG, Trugman JM, de Yebenes JG, et al. Dopa-responsive dystonia: the spectrum of clinical manifestations in a large North American family. *Neurology.* 1990;40:66–69.

Oblak AL, Hagen MC, Sweadner KJ, et al. Rapid-onset dystonia-parkinsonism associated with the I758S mutation of the ATP1A3 gene: a neuropathologic and neuroanatomical study of four siblings. *Acta Neuropathol.* 2014;128(1):81–98.

Opal P, Tintner R, Jankovic J, et al. Intrafamilial phenotypic variability of the DYT1 dystonia: from asymptomatic TOR1A gene carrier status to dystonic storm. *Mov Disord.* 2002;17:339–345.

Oppenheim H. Über eine eigenartige Krampfkrankheit des kindlichen und jugendlichen alters (dysbasia lordotica progressiva, dystonia musculorum deformans). *Neurol Centrabl.* 1911;30:1090–1107.

Quartarone A, Hallett M. Emerging concepts in the physiological basis of dystonia. *Mov Disord.* 2013;28(7):958–967.

Risch N, Bressman S, Senthil G, et al. Intragenic cis and trans modification of genetic susceptibility in DYT1 torsion dystonia. *Am J Hum Genet.* 2007;80:1188–1193.

Risch N, De Leon D, Ozelius L, et al. Genetic analysis of idiopathic torsion dystonia in Ashkenazi Jews and their recent descent from a small founder population. *Nat Genet.* 1995;9:152–159.

Saunders-Pullman R, Fuchs T, San Luciano M, et al. Heterogeneity in primary dystonia: lessons from THAP1, GNAL, and TOR1A in Amish-Mennonites. *Mov Disord.* 2014;29(6):812–818.

Saunders-Pullman R, Shriberg J, Heiman G, et al. Myoclonus dystonia—possible association with obsessive-compulsive disorder and alcohol dependence. *Neurology.* 2002;58:242–245.

Schneider SA, Dusek P, Hardy J, et al. Genetics and pathophysiology of neurodegeneration with brain iron accumulation (NBIA). *Curr Neuropharmacol.* 2013;11(1):59–79.

Segawa M, Hosaka A, Miyagawa F, et al. Hereditary progressive dystonia with marked diurnal fluctuation. *Adv Neurol.* 1976;14:215–233.

Thenganatt MA, Fahn S. Botulinum toxin for the treatment of movement disorders. *Curr Neurol Neurosci Rep.* 2012;12(4):399–409.

Uluğ AM, Vo A, Argyelan M, et al. Cerebellothalamocortical pathway abnormalities in torsinA DYT1 knock-in mice. *Proc Natl Acad Sci U S A.* 2011;108(16):6638–6643.

Vidailhet M, Vercueil L, Houeto JL, et al. Bilateral, pallidal, deep-brain stimulation in primary generalised dystonia: a prospective 3 year follow-up study. *Lancet Neurol.* 2007;6:223–229.

Volkmann J, Mueller J, Deuschl G, et al. Pallidal neurostimulation in patients with medication-refractory cervical dystonia: a randomised, sham-controlled trial. *Lancet Neurol.* 2014;13(9):875–884.

Zimprich A, Grabowski M, Asmus F, et al. Mutations in the gene encoding epsilon-sarcoglycan cause myoclonus-dystonia syndrome. *Nat Genet.* 2001;29(1):66–69.

Paul Greene

INTRODUCTION

In hemifacial spasm (HFS) there are involuntary contractions on one side of the face in muscles innervated by the facial nerve (cranial nerve VII) (Figs. 77.1 and 77.2). According to Digre and Corbett, the condition was first described in 1875 by Schultze but was first separated from other forms of facial twitching by Gowers in 1888. HFS is rare in this country. The age-adjusted incidence was 0.78 per 100,000 per year in Olmsted County, Minnesota, only 3% of the incidence of Bell palsy.

PHENOMENOLOGY

The contractions in HFS usually start as individual muscle twitches in the eyelids. Over time, twitches spread to other facial nerve–innervated muscles including the frontalis, paranasal muscles, zygomaticus major, perioral muscles, platysma, and occasionally, the periauricular muscles. Trains of twitches may develop and, when severe, there may be periods of sustained muscle contraction causing complete eye closure. Pain in HFS is very rare, usually from patients with concurrent involvement of the trigeminal nerve producing tic douloureux (the combination is called *tic convulsive*). Contractions in HFS diminish, but do not disappear, during sleep and patients often report worsening with stress. This is surprising for what is usually presumed to be a peripheral nerve disease (see the following discussion). HFS usually progresses slowly if at all but may produce facial weakness in patients with long duration of disease. About 1% of reported cases of HFS are bilateral (with twitching that is asynchronous from side to side). The majority of cases of HFS are sporadic, although there are occasional reports of familial cases (Video 77.1).

DIFFERENTIAL DIAGNOSIS

There are few other diseases that produce twitches, trains of twitches, and occasionally, episodes of sustained muscle contraction (Table 77.1). Facial dystonia is usually more sustained and bilateral and muscle contractions are not usually synchronous. The rippling movements of facial myokymia are often unilateral but are slow and asynchronous. Motor tics in the face may be unilateral and rapid, but there is usually a warning sensation before the movements and the movements are usually suppressible, at least briefly. Synkinesis after Bell palsy or other cause produces synchronous contractions but only during blinking or voluntary movement. However, some patients develop HFS in addition to a synkinesis after nerve injury. Epilepsia partialis continua does mimic the movements of HFS precisely but usually involves the masseters (cranial nerve VII) and is rarely limited to the face.

PATHOGENESIS

The pathogenesis of HFS is thought to be compression of the facial nerve where it exits the brain stem (the root exit zone), usually by an aberrant artery, such as the anterior inferior cerebellar artery, posterior inferior cerebellar artery, or internal auditory artery, or a normal vein. Irritation of the nerve at this site is felt to generate spontaneous electrical activity, causing muscle contractions, and "cross-talk" or simultaneous activation of axons going to different parts of the face. However, other causes of compression at the root exit zone besides normal arteries rarely occur, such as draining veins of arteriovenous malformations (AVMs), aneurysms, tumors, or plaques of multiple sclerosis in the central myelin at the root

FIGURE 77.1 The anterior inferior cerebellar artery (*A*) runs between cranial nerves *VII* and *VIII* and compresses nerve VII. (From Ma Z, Li M, Cao Y, et al. Keyhole microsurgery for trigeminal neuralgia, hemifacial spasm and glossopharyngeal neuralgia. *Eur Arch Otorhinolaryngol.* 2010;267:449–454.)

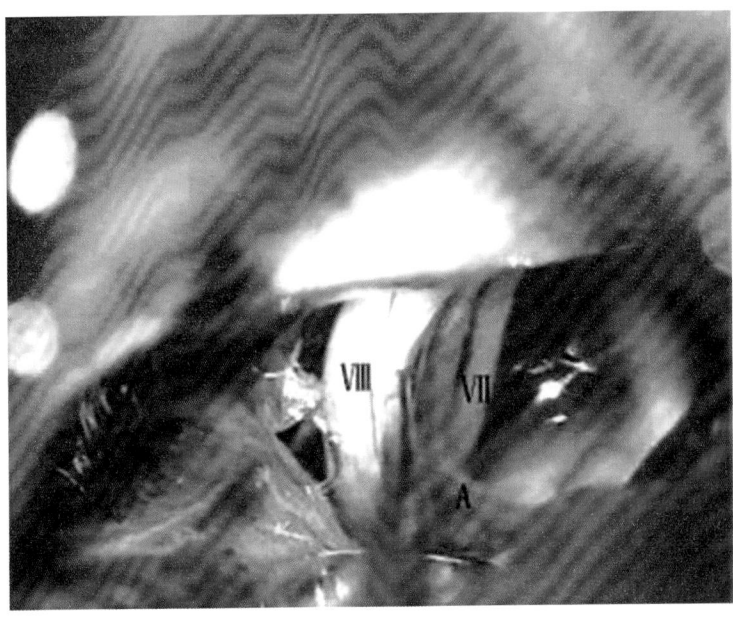

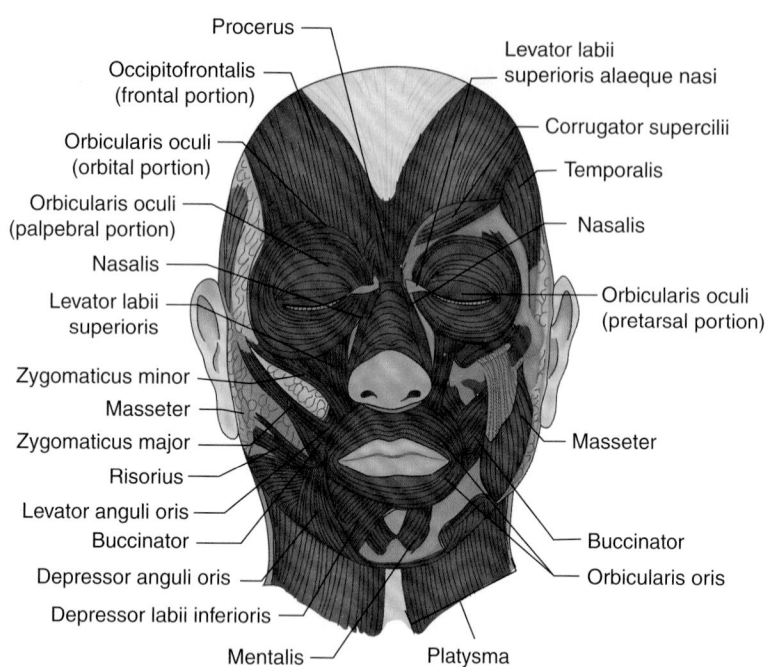

Procerus — Occipitofrontalis (frontal portion) — Orbicularis oculi (orbital portion) — Orbicularis oculi (palpebral portion) — Nasalis — Levator labii superioris — Zygomaticus minor — Masseter — Zygomaticus major — Risorius — Levator anguli oris — Buccinator — Depressor anguli oris — Depressor labii inferioris — Mentalis — Platysma

Levator labii superioris alaeque nasi — Corrugator supercilii — Temporalis — Nasalis — Orbicularis oculi (pretarsal portion) — Masseter — Buccinator — Orbicularis oris

FIGURE 77.2 Muscles innervated by the facial nerve.

exit zone of the facial nerve. For this reason, all patients with HFS should have a magnetic resonance imaging (MRI) with attention to the posterior fossa. If compression by aberrant arteries is the most common cause for HFS, it would be reasonable that arterial hypertension causing ectatic vessels might be a risk factor for HFS. Older studies suggested this, but recent carefully controlled studies failed to find such an association.

Occasionally, HFS has been seen after Bell palsy, bony overgrowth as in Paget disease pinching the stylomastoid foramen, and other peripheral lesions of the facial nerve. This has led to speculation that facial nerve compression induces a change in the facial nucleus, which is necessary for HFS to occur. The likelihood of such a facial nucleus change would increase as the site of compression gets closer to the nucleus. This alternative hypothesis is strengthened by the small number of cases of HFS associated with central lesions at the site of the facial nerve nucleus. In addition, there is evidence in HFS suggesting hyperexcitability of the facial nerve nucleus, including enhancement of F waves and other findings.

TREATMENT

HFS can be treated with medications, botulinum toxin (BTX) injections, or by craniectomy and separation of an arterial loop from the root exit zone of the facial nerve (microvascular decompression). Medications are generally the least successful treatment. There is a single controlled study suggesting benefit from orphenadrine and dimethylaminoethanol, but this was never repeated and this treatment is rarely used today. Successful treatment of HFS in small numbers of patients has been reported with carbamazepine, clonazepam, baclofen, gabapentin, and felbamate but improvement was "rare" in several hundred patients treated with anticonvulsants in one large series. Even when spasms improve with medications, the improvement is usually temporary.

BTX has proved extremely useful in treating HFS, especially for orbicularis oculi contractions, for which most series report an almost 100% success rate (Table 77.2). The success rate is lower for lower facial muscles (although this is rarely reported) due to the

TABLE 77.1 Differential Diagnosis of Hemifacial Spasm

Condition	Similarities to HFS	Differences from HFS
Facial dystonia	May include rapid contractions	Very rarely unilateral. Mostly slower contractions. Spasms not usually synchronous in different facial muscles.
Myokymia	May be unilateral	Slower contractions. Spasms usually asynchronous in different muscles.
Motor tics	May be rapid, unilateral, and synchronous in different muscles	Usually an inner sensation before the movements. Movements usually suppressible at least briefly.
Synkinesis (e.g., after Bell palsy)	May be rapid, unilateral, and synchronous in different muscles	Spasms only occur with blinking or voluntary movement.
Epilepsia partialis continua (EPC)	May be rapid, unilateral, and synchronous in different muscles	Unlike HFS, may involve the masseter muscle. Usually involves extracranial muscles.

HFS, hemifacial spasm.

TABLE 77.2 Botulinum Toxin Treatment of Hemifacial Spasm

A. Some people have dramatically different sensitivity to BTX, so initially inject just the muscle causing the most troublesome symptom (usually the orbicularis oculi [Oo]).

B. Optimal concentration of toxin, volume per injection, and number of sites per muscle are not known for most muscles (including the Oo). Most people use concentrations of 5–10 U/0.1 mL. The general rule is as follows: Use more dilute toxin to get a greater effect and use more concentrated toxin to get less spread to nearby muscles.

C. Major side effects are as follows:

Ptosis (from leakage to the Levator palpebrae)

Ecchymoses

Dermatochalasis (usually in the lower lid)

Xerophthalmia or epiphora (usually short lasting)

Excess weakness of the injected muscle (not usually the Oo)

Diplopia (uncommon)—from lateral canthus injections

Entropion (rare)—from lower lid injections

D. In the Oo, avoid injecting the upper lid in the midline (to minimize the risk of ptosis). Lower lid injections are always necessary; injections in the orbital portion of the Oo are sometimes necessary.

E. Start with a small dose and increase the dose gradually to minimize side effects. Some reasonable starting doses are as follows:

Orbicularis oculi—2.5 units per site with one site in the lower lid, lateral canthus, medial and lateral pretarsal components of the Oo, and orbital component of the Oo

Frontalis—2.5 units in two or three sites

Nasalis—2.5 units

Zygomaticus major—1 unit in one site

Depressor anguli oris, depressor labii inferioris, mentalis—2.5 units, one site in each

Platysma—2.5 units in three or four sites

F. Instruct patients to always notify you about problems arising after BTX injections: Patients may coincidentally develop an unrelated problem in the weeks following a BTX injection.

BTX, botulinum toxin.

development of facial weakness before resolution of the spasms in some patients. Excess weakness of the orbicularis oculi is very rare, although leakage to the levator palpebrae causing ptosis is common. The risk of ptosis depends on the volume of toxin injected (greater volume produces greater risk) and the injection site (closer to the insertion of the levator at the middle of the upper lid increases the risk). Other less common side effects include ecchymoses at the injection site, entropion of the lower lid, dry eye, excess tearing, and bagginess under the eye. Diplopia occasionally occurs, probably from spread of toxin to one or both lateral recti. All side effects from BTX injections are transient and there is no evidence that chronic BTX injections induce any permanent change. Benefit from BTX injections for HFS lasts 3 to 6 months, after which symptoms return and repeat injections are required.

Microvascular decompression, first popularized by Jannetta in the 1970s, appears to be the definitive treatment for HFS. When a vessel is compressing the facial nerve, a sponge is placed between the nerve and the vessel. In a large series, 1,327 patients were followed for up to 3 years and 90.5% were felt to have an excellent outcome after the first surgery. There were 2.3% of patients who did not improve and had a second surgery (in the opinion of the surgeons, the wrong vessel had been decompressed) and 90% of these were felt to have an excellent response. However, up to about 10% of patients experience return of spasms and require repeat operation, possibly when the sponge is dislodged. Serious complications (death, stroke, or cerebellar hematoma) occur in less than 1% in most series. Permanent facial weakness or hearing loss are uncommon, occurring in about 5%. Other rare surgical complications including wound infection or hematoma, cerebrospinal fluid leak (CSF), bacterial meningitis, and pseudomeningocele are also possible. However, vascular compression of the root exit zone of the facial nerve is not found in all cases, and current MRI techniques are not yet sufficient to guarantee that an offending vessel will be found. For all these reasons, many patients prefer to avoid surgery if possible, and BTX injections are the treatment of first choice for most patients.

Videos can be found in the companion e-book edition. For a full list of video legends, please see the front matter.

SUGGESTED READINGS

Auger RG, Whisnant JP. Hemifacial spasm in Rochester and Olmsted County, Minnesota, 1960 to 1984. *Arch Neurol.* 1990;47:1233–1234.

Barker FG, Jannetta PJ, Bissonette DJ, et al. Microvascular decompression for hemifacial spasm. *J Neurosurg.* 1995;82:201–210.

Colosimo C, Chianese M, Romano S, et al. Is hypertension associated with hemifacial spasm? *Neurology.* 2003;61:587.

Digre K, Corbett JJ. Hemifacial spasm: differential diagnosis, mechanism, and treatment. *Adv Neurol.* 1988;49:151–176.

Ehni G, Woltman HW. Hemifacial spasms: review of one hundred and six cases. *Arch Neurol Psychiatry.* 1945;53:205–211.

Ferguson JH. Hemifacial spasm and the facial nucleus. *Ann Neurol.* 1978;4:97–103.

Gowers WR. *A Manual of Disease of the Nervous System.* Philadelphia: P Blakiston; 1888.

Hughes EC, Brackmann DE, Weinstein RC. Seventh nerve spasm: effect of modification of cholinergic balance. *Otolaryngol Head Neck Surg.* 1980;88:491–499.

Ishikawa M, Ohira T, Namiki J, et al. Electrophysiological investigation of hemifacial spasm after microvascular decompression: F waves of the facial muscles, blink reflexes, and abnormal muscle responses. *J Neurosurg.* 1997;86:654–661.

Jannetta PJ, Abbasy M, Maroon JC, et al. Etiology and definitive microsurgical treatment of hemifacial spasm. *J Neurosurg.* 1977;47:321–328.

Leonardos A, Greene PE, Weimer LH, et al. Hemifacial spasm associated with intraparenchymal brain stem tumor. *Mov Disord.* 2011;26:2325–2326.

Martinelli P, Giuliani S, Ippoliti M. Hemifacial spasm due to peripheral injury of facial nerve: a nuclear syndrome? *Mov Disord.* 1992;7:181–184.

Miwa H, Mizuno Y, Kondo T. Familial hemifacial spasm: report of cases and review of literature. *J Neurol Sci.* 2002;193:97–102.

Nielsen VK. Pathophysiology of hemifacial spasm: I. Ephaptic transmission and ectopic excitation. *Neurology.* 1984;34:418–426.

Schultze F. Linksseitiger facialiskrampf in folge eines aneurysma der arteria vertebralis sinistra. *Archiv f Pathol Anat.* 1875;65:385–391.

Wang L, Hu X, Dong H, et al. Clinical features and treatment status of hemifacial spasm in China. *Chin Med J.* 2014;127(5):845–849.

Yaltho TC, Jankovic J. The many faces of hemifacial spasm: differential diagnosis of unilateral facial spasms. *Mov Disord.* 2011;26:1582–1592.

Zhong J, Li ST, Zhu J, et al. A clinical analysis on microvascular decompression surgery in a series of 3000 cases. *Clin Neurol Neurosurg.* 2012;114:846–851.

INTRODUCTION

Myoclonus is characterized by lightning-like muscle jerks. Electrophysiologically, these jerks are associated with electromyographic discharges that are relatively short in duration compared to voluntary jerks. Myoclonic jerks may be positive due to active muscle contractions, or negative in which jerks occur due to lapses of postural tone (the classic example of this is asterixis).

EPIDEMIOLOGY

Myoclonus has a prevalence rate of 8.6 per 100,000, based on a study in Olmsted County published in 1999.

PATHOBIOLOGY

Although the electrophysiology of myoclonus is well understood, the actual pathophysiology is not. Myoclonus can be classified based on either anatomic localization or etiology. Anatomically, myoclonus can originate from either the central or peripheral nervous system. In the central nervous system, the location is further subdivided into cortical, subcortical, brain stem, and spinal cord origin.

Myoclonus is usually classified based on anatomic localization (Table 78.1). The etiology and clinical characteristics of myoclonus from each anatomic location will be discussed in the following text.

CORTICAL MYOCLONUS

Myoclonus originating in the cortex has unique electrophysiologic features, as described in Table 78.2. The first three are unique to cortical myoclonus and are not seen in subcortical or spinal myoclonus.

Back-averaging by electroencephalography (EEG) is very helpful in identifying cortical spikes prior to the jerks, but the technique is not routinely available. It is done by averaging at least 150 to 200 myoclonic jerks and capturing their preceding *cortical spikes*. A short duration between the spike and the jerk indicates fast conduction from the cortex to the muscles via the corticospinal pathway, usually less than 50 milliseconds.

Giant somatosensory-evoked potentials (SEPs) are very large cortical potentials seen by SEP recording techniques such as by stimulation of the median nerve while recording EEG. A typical SEP has a negative (upward) phase followed by positive (downward) and negative phases, respectively. Only positive and the second negative phases are enlarged in cortical myoclonus. These phases are motor volleys, as compared to the first negative phase which is a sensory volley.

The *C-reflex* is a form of a long-latency reflex. When we stimulate muscle fibers, the afferent pathway is conducted through Ia sensory fibers, spinal cord, nucleus cuneatus, or gracilis and

TABLE 78.1	Classification of Myoclonus		
Clinical	**Anatomic**		**Etiology**
1. **At rest**	1. **Cortical**		1. **Physiologic**
Action	Focal		2. **Essential**
Reflex	Multifocal		3. **Epileptic**
2. **Focal**	Generalized		4. **Symptomatic**
Axial	Epilepsia partialis continua		Storage diseases
Multifocal	2. **Thalamic**		Cerebellar degenerations
Generalized	3. **Brain stem**		Basal ganglia degenerations
3. **Irregular**	Reticular		Dementias
Oscillatory	Startle		Infectious encephalopathy
Rhythmic	Palatal		Metabolic encephalopathy
	4. **Spinal**		Toxic encephalopathy
	Segmental		Hypoxia
	Propriospinal		Focal damage
	5. **Peripheral**		

Myoclonus can be classified according to clinical features, by anatomic origin of the pathophysiology of the jerks, and by etiology.

TABLE 78.2 Characteristic Electrophysiologic Features of Myoclonus from Different Anatomic Origins

Cortical Myoclonus	Spinal Myoclonus
• Focal spikes or sharp waves of 10–40 ms duration preceding the jerk on back-averaged EEG	• EMG burst durations are typically longer than 100 ms.
• Giant SEPs	• *Spinal segmental myoclonus*
• Enhanced C-reflexes	• Recruitment pattern: Jerks start from one or two spinal segments and spread up and down along spinal segments. For example, jerking in the upper extremity from a structural lesion in the C7 spinal segment could be identified by an initial jerk of the ipsilateral triceps muscles with possible upward spreading to biceps and trapezius muscles and simultaneous downward spreading to C8-innervated intrinsic hand muscles.
• EMG burst duration typically shorter than in subcortical or spinal myoclonus; <100 ms and usually 20–50 ms in duration	
• Rostrocaudal recruitment pattern on polymyography with very fast spreading (jerks may appear almost at the same time on regular polymyography)	• Velocity of spread is slower than in cortical myoclonus because it is not via fast-conducting corticospinal pathways.
Subcortical Myoclonus Including Brain Stem Myoclonus	• *Propriospinal myoclonus*
• EMG burst durations vary among subtypes, generally longer than that seen in cortical myoclonus, as long as 100 ms.	• Typical recruitment pattern up and down along axial muscles on polymyography. For example, jerks can originate in T12 rectus abdominis muscles and spread up and down to axial muscles above and below, respectively (e.g., up to higher level rectus abdominis and down to iliopsoas).
• Typical recruitment pattern:	
• *Reticular reflex myoclonus* typically originates in the lower brain stem, most commonly CN XI–innervated muscles such as SCM. It spreads up to CNs VII– and V–innervated muscles and simultaneously down to muscles in the upper cervical levels.	• Slow velocity of spread as it is conducted through the slow propriospinal fibers (slowest among all forms of myoclonus described above).
• *Hyperekplexia* spreads between CN-innervated muscles. It can start from CN in the midbrain such as orbicularis oculi then spreading down to lower CN-innervated muscles. Jerks occur after somesthetic (touch), auditory, or, less commonly, visual stimuli.	

EEG, electroencephalography; SEP, somatosensory-evoked potential; EMG, electromyography; CN, cranial nerve; SCM, sternocleidomastoid muscles.

ultimately to the primary sensory cortex. Then, the efferent pathway is conducted through the corticospinal tract to the alpha-motoneuron. This typically takes about 40 to 50 seconds in the upper extremities. Therefore, when one electrically stimulates a muscle, the C-reflex will be seen on electromyography (EMG) recording about 40 to 50 milliseconds after the stimulation. C-reflexes are typically enhanced in cortical myoclonus.

Multichannel EMG recording, also called *polymyography*, can also be helpful in visualization of patterns of spread from one muscle to another, called the *recruitment pattern*. Typical recruitment patterns in cortical myoclonus are described in Table 78.2.

It is worth mentioning the Bereitschaftspotentials (BPs) here. The BP is a form of voluntary, movement-related potential seen on back-averaging EEG technique. It is also called a *premovement* or *readiness potential*. It is helpful in differentiating organic from psychogenic myoclonus; BPs are present in psychogenic movements but not in organic myoclonus.

SUBCORTICAL INCLUDING BRAIN STEM MYOCLONUS

The three main types of brain stem myoclonus are reticular reflex myoclonus, hyperekplexia, and palatal myoclonus. Myoclonus–dystonia syndrome or essential myoclonus also has a subcortical origin, as does myoclonus occurring after thalamic stroke (typically negative myoclonus or asterixis affecting one arm). The electrophysiologic findings are described in Table 78.2.

Hyperekplexia, or exaggerated startle, has the nucleus gigantocellularis as a generator. It shows recruitment patterns, as described

in Table 78.2. Lack of habituation is a feature of hyperekplexia: After repetitive stimuli, jerks will be less frequent and less severe clinically and electrophysiologically in the normal startle response but may fail to habituate in hyperekplexia.

SPINAL MYOCLONUS

Two major forms of spinal myoclonus exist: spinal segmental and propriospinal myoclonus. The typical recruitment pattern and the velocity of spread are described in Table 78.2.

Spinal segmental myoclonus typically originates within a few or several adjacent spinal segments, typically cervical or lumbar.

Propriospinal myoclonus refers to axial jerks that originate in spinal cord segments, with spread up and down along the longitudinal axis of spinal cord. The very slow-conducting propriospinal pathway helps coordinate forelimb and hind limb movements in animals, such as cats, but the role of this pathway in humans is unclear.

It has been reported in the literature that BPs are associated with propriospinal myoclonus, and thus, a psychogenic cause has been proposed. However, there is evidence that there is disruption of fiber tracts in spinal cord seen on diffusion tensor imaging in patients with propriospinal myoclonus, suggesting that some forms of propriospinal myoclonus are organic.

PERIPHERAL MYOCLONUS

A typical example of peripheral myoclonus is hemifacial spasm, but peripheral myoclonus can also occur from irritation of spinal nerve roots, plexus, or peripheral nerves. The EMG burst duration varies, and there is lack of electrophysiologic patterns described earlier.

CLINICAL MANIFESTATIONS

When myoclonus is observed, one should attempt to answer the following questions in order to elucidate the cause:

1. What is the distribution of myoclonus? What body part(s) is(are) affected? Is it focal, segmental (affecting multiple contiguous body regions), multifocal (multiple noncontiguous body regions), or generalized?
2. Is myoclonus positive or negative (due to lapse of muscle tone)? The classic example of negative myoclonus is asterixis, seen in hepatic encephalopathy or uremia. Negative myoclonus of the legs when standing can be seen in patients with posthypoxic myoclonus (Lance–Adams syndrome), producing a so-called bouncing gait.
3. Is myoclonus spontaneous (occurring at rest), action-induced, stimulation-induced, or reflex-induced? One example of stimulation-induced myoclonus is hyperekplexia, which is typically induced by somesthetic (typically in mantle area including forehead and nose), auditory and, less commonly, visual stimuli. Reflex-induced myoclonus (a hallmark of cortical myoclonus) can be tested by using the examiner's finger to tap a body region, such as a patient's finger, hand, or arm, which then would produce a myoclonic jerk. The latency between reflex stimuli and myoclonic jerks in cortical myoclonus is relatively short, suggesting efferent conduction via the corticospinal pathway. Longer latency would suggest slower conducting pathways such as the propriospinal pathway.
4. Is the myoclonus rhythmic or nonrhythmic? Is it synchronous?
5. Are there any other associated phenomena such as dystonia or ataxia?

CORTICAL MYOCLONUS

Cortical myoclonus can be focal, multifocal, or generalized. If it is focal, it usually affects the distal limbs such as the hands and fingers. It can be positive or negative, may occur either at rest or with action, and is often stimulus-sensitive. It can be continuous and rhythmic, for example, *epilepsia partialis continua* in which patients have myoclonic jerks on one side of the body (Video 78.1). Cortical myoclonus may occur as a fragment of epilepsy (epileptic myoclonus, see "Diagnosis" section). Posthypoxic myoclonus is typically generalized, nonrhythmic, synchronous, and stimulus-sensitive (to tactile or auditory stimuli) but can also occur at rest (Video 78.2).

Familial cortical myoclonic tremor with epilepsy (FCMTE; also called *benign adult familial myoclonic epilepsy* [BAFME]) is a rare autosomal dominant genetic condition, characterized by small-amplitude myoclonic jerks in distal limbs that may look like and be misdiagnosed as essential tremor.

SUBCORTICAL MYOCLONUS

Subcortical myoclonus can originate from subcortical regions or the brain stem. *Myoclonus–dystonia syndrome*, previously called *essential myoclonus*, is a form of subcortical myoclonus (Video 78.3). Patients typically have myoclonic jerks mixed with dystonia, in the same or adjacent body regions. Myoclonus usually involves the neck and upper body such as the shoulders, arms, or hands. Dystonia seen in this condition also has similar involvement in the upper body such as the neck or hands (e.g., patients can present with writer's cramp).

Brain stem myoclonus, a form of subcortical myoclonus, includes hyperekplexia, reticular reflex myoclonus, and palatal myoclonus.

Hyperekplexia typically does not occur at rest, induced instead by a typical stimulus (Video 78.4). Patients typically do not habituate to repeated stimuli. Nevertheless, we do not recommend examining patients with hyperekplexia with repetitive stimuli because repeated nose taps can lead to severe body stiffness especially in infants.

In *reticular reflex myoclonus*, patients usually have myoclonic jerks involving the sternocleidomastoid and facial and neck muscles with the pattern of spread correlating with electrophysiologic recruitment, usually rostral and caudal.

We describe the clinical features of *palatal myoclonus* in the "Diagnosis" section.

SPINAL MYOCLONUS

Spinal myoclonus includes spinal segmental myoclonus and propriospinal myoclonus.

In *spinal segmental myoclonus*, muscles in one or two adjacent spinal segments are typically affected. It can occur at rest or with action, may be rhythmic or nonrhythmic, but is usually not reflex-induced. When patients present with myoclonic jerks in one limb, one should always think about possible pathology in the spinal cord, such as a primary spinal cord malignancy.

Propriospinal myoclonus typically presents with axial jerks (Video 78.5). Patients typically have truncal flexion, usually nonrhythmic, at rest or with action or reflex-induced, with a relatively long latency due to slow conduction via propriospinal pathways. The differential diagnosis of axial jerks includes propriospinal myoclonus and reticular reflex myoclonus, but in the latter form, it usually involves a higher truncal region than propriospinal myoclonus.

PERIPHERAL MYOCLONUS

Peripheral myoclonus from nerve root, plexus, or peripheral nerve involvement typically affects a limb in the distribution corresponding to neural structures that are innervated. It usually occurs at rest and does change with action. Sometimes, it is difficult to differentiate from spinal segmental myoclonus, and spine imaging is required to rule out spinal pathology. *Hemifacial spasm* is a form of peripheral myoclonus (Video 78.6). It is characterized by clonic, sometimes tonic contraction of cranial nerve (CN) VII–innervated muscles, most commonly the orbicularis oculi, zygomaticus, and frontalis.

DIAGNOSIS

After one characterizes myoclonus phenomenologically, the next step is to identify the etiology. The etiologic classification of myoclonus of C. David Marsden, S. Fahn, and H. Shibasaki is most commonly used; *physiologic, essential, epileptic,* and *symptomatic myoclonus.* Here, we will integrate neuroanatomic classification with etiologic classification to show the correlation between these approaches.

PHYSIOLOGIC MYOCLONUS

Examples of physiologic myoclonus are jerks during sleep (hypnic jerks) and hiccups (diaphragmatic myoclonus).

CORTICAL MYOCLONUS

Cortical myoclonus can be epileptic or symptomatic. *Epileptic myoclonus* is fragments of epilepsy or myoclonic epilepsy and is cortical in origin. *Epilepsia partialis continua* can occur from a focal structural lesion typically seen in *Rasmussen encephalitis*, an autoimmune disorder leading to gliosis and hemiatrophy of one cerebral hemisphere (see Video 78.1).

The differential diagnosis of progressive myoclonic epilepsy is described in Table 78.3. EEG is helpful in identifying epileptiform discharges. Investigations to confirm the diagnosis depend on the specific etiology, for example, a skin biopsy to search for Lafora bodies in Lafora body disease, or a muscle biopsy to look for ragged red fibers in myoclonic epilepsy with ragged red fibers (MERRF). Genetic testing with appropriate genetic counseling is also used to confirm these entities.

Cortical myoclonus may be symptomatic, secondary to systemic or heredodegenerative disorders, for example, storage diseases or mitochondrial disorders mentioned previously. On the other hand, symptomatic myoclonus may be either cortical, brain stem, spinal, or peripheral in origin. The list of symptomatic myoclonus disorders is lengthy and further workup depends on the suspected location and etiology. Patients with *posthypoxic myoclonus* have a history of mainly respiratory rather than cardiac arrest. Anoxic brain damage can be seen on neuroimaging. *Subacute sclerosing panencephalitis (SSPE)* is another example of symptomatic cortical myoclonus. EEG typically reveals generalized periodic discharges every 4 to 14 seconds. *Dentatorubral-pallidoluysian atrophy* (DRPLA) or Haw River syndrome, an autosomal dominant disorder of CAG repeat expansions,

is another example in which patients can have cortical myoclonus associated with chorea, ataxia, dementia, and epilepsy. It was originally described in Japanese populations but is also found in other ethnic groups. The differential diagnoses of myoclonus associated with dementia also include *Creutzfeldt–Jakob disease* (CJD), *corticobasal syndrome*, and *Alzheimer disease*, among others. Myoclonus can also be seen in *spinocerebellar ataxia type 14 (SCA14)*.

SUBCORTICAL MYOCLONUS

Subcortical myoclonus includes myoclonus–dystonia syndrome, hyperekplexia, and palatal myoclonus, among others. Here, we will also mention opsoclonus–myoclonus, which is due to dysfunction of brain stem and cerebellum.

Myoclonus–dystonia syndrome is also known as *essential myoclonus* or *DYT 11*. It is a form of subcortical myoclonus caused by a mutation in the *SCGE* gene (epsilon–sarcoglycan gene). This gene has maternal imprinting, that is, maternal allele does not express, and the abnormal gene is typically inherited from the father. In one rare condition, Russell–Silver syndrome where there is uniparental disomy, both alleles are from the mother, and therefore, both

---

TABLE 78.3 Differential Diagnosis of Myoclonus Classified by Anatomic Localization

Cortical Myoclonus	Subcortical Myoclonus Including Brain Stem Myoclonus
• Epileptic	• Subcortical
• Epilepsy partialis continua: Etiology can be Rasmussen encephalitis or focal cortical lesion.	• Myoclonus–dystonia syndrome (essential myoclonus)
• Progressive myoclonic epilepsy	• Brain stem
• Unverricht–Lundborg syndrome (Baltic myoclonus, *EPM1* mutation, encoding for cystatin B)	• Physiologic
• Lafora body disease (autosomal recessive, *EPM2A* mutation, encoding for laforin)	• Hypnic jerks
• Neuronal ceroid lipofuscinosis (NCL or Batten disease)	• Hiccups
• Sialidosis	• Hyperekplexia
• Myoclonic epilepsy with ragged red fibers (MERRF, mitochondrial disorder)	• Variants include progressive encephalomyelitis, rigidity and myoclonus (PERM), and excessive startle syndromes.
• Symptomatic	• Palatal myoclonus
• Posthypoxic myoclonus	• Essential palatal myoclonus
• Secondary to systemic diseases or metabolic causes	• Symptomatic palatal myoclonus
• Renal or hepatic failure	• Opsoclonus–myoclonus (brain stem and cerebellum)
• Infection-related	• Symptomatic: secondary to structural lesions in brain stem
• Subacute sclerosing panencephalitis (SSPE), Creutzfeldt–Jakob disease (CJD)	**Spinal Myoclonus**
• Myoclonus associated with neurodegenerative disorders	• Spinal segmental myoclonus
• Dentatorubral-pallidoluysian atrophy (DRPLA), corticobasal syndrome, and Alzheimer disease	• Symptomatic: secondary to structural lesions in spinal cord
• Heredodegenerative disorders	• Propriospinal myoclonus
• Storage diseases	**Peripheral Myoclonus**
• Mitochondrial disorders	• Hemifacial spasm
• Spinocerebellar ataxia (SCA), such as SCA14	• Symptomatic
	• Secondary to nerve root, plexus, or peripheral nerve lesions

This table lists the differential diagnoses of myoclonus, primarily classified by anatomic locations. We also integrate the original etiologic classification of C. David Marsden, S. Fahn, and H. Shibasaki, with the anatomic locations. Note that the list of symptomatic cortical myoclonus is extensive, and we include only examples. Symptomatic myoclonus (such as myoclonus from focal structural lesion) can occur anywhere within the neuraxis.

copies of the normal *SCGE* gene are imprinted leading to a lack of expression of one normal allele. This can cause the phenotype of myoclonus–dystonia syndrome. Symptoms of myoclonus–dystonia syndrome are usually relieved by alcohol and associated neuropsychiatric features such as anxiety and obsessive–compulsive disorder are common.

Hyperekplexia, a form of brain stem myoclonus, may be hereditary or secondary. The genetics of hyperekplexia is complex: There are autosomal dominant and recessive forms. One of the well-known hereditary forms is autosomal dominant, caused by mutations in the glycine receptor gene, but other genes have also been reported. Secondary (i.e., symptomatic) hyperekplexia has been reported due to brain stem encephalitis from an autoimmune or paraneoplastic process. Sometimes, it can be associated with severe muscle rigidity and stiffness, also called *progressive encephalomyelitis, rigidity, and myoclonus* (PERM).

Certain excessive startle syndromes may be culturally related and also can manifest as echolalia and automatic obedience. These syndromes are known by colorful regional names, such as *The Jumping Frenchmen of Maine* (Quebec), *myriachit* (Siberia), *Latah* (Indonesia, Malaysia), and *Ragin' Cajun* (Louisiana). These syndromes are not true forms of myoclonus because the movements are more prolonged in duration and subject to conscious suppression.

Palatal myoclonus is another form of subcortical myoclonus, with rhythmic jerky movements of the soft palate at the rate of 2 to 2.5 Hz. There are two forms of palatal myoclonus, essential and symptomatic. In essential palatal myoclonus (EPM), patients have ear clicks from contraction of the tensor veli palatini leading to movements of the opening of the eustachian tube. Symptomatic palatal myoclonus (SPM) is a delayed phenomenon that usually occurs weeks or months after a lesion in Guillain–Mollaret triangle, which is defined by the line between dentate nucleus, contralateral red nucleus, and contralateral inferior olivary nucleus (Fig. 78.1). The central tegmental tract runs between red nucleus and inferior olivary nucleus, which then sends fibers to contralateral dentate nucleus through the inferior cerebellar peduncle. Then, the dentate nucleus sends a projection to the red nucleus via the superior cerebellar peduncle. Lesions in this triangle may be ischemic, demyelinating, infectious, or postinfectious, among others. Hypertrophy and hyperintensity of the inferior olivary nucleus on T2 image on magnetic resonance imaging (MRI) can be seen in SPM. Unlike EPM, patients do not usually have ear clicks. Pendular nystagmus can also be seen in SPM. *Progressive ataxia with palatal tremor* (PAPT) is a syndrome that when seen suggests the possibility of adult-onset Alexander disease, a disorder caused by *GFAP* gene mutations. Sagittal view of the MRI in adult-onset Alexander disease can reveal atrophy of the spinal cord from the cervical portion down, giving the so-called tadpole sign. Diagnosis is confirmed by genetic testing.

Opsoclonus–myoclonus–ataxia syndrome (OMAS) (Kinsbourne disease) is diagnosed by a constellation of opsoclonus, myoclonus, and ataxia. In children, it can occur as a paraneoplastic process, typically seen with neuroblastoma associated with anti-Ri antibody, and abdominal imaging is required to screen for this cancer. In adults, it is associated with postinfectious (such as postviral), autoimmune, or paraneoplastic processes affecting the brain stem. Neuroimaging, cerebrospinal fluid (CSF) studies including paraneoplastic panel in blood and CSF are helpful in diagnosis. A course of steroids and/or intravenous immunoglobulin (IVIG) is warranted.

SPINAL MYOCLONUS

Spinal myoclonus includes spinal segmental myoclonus and propriospinal myoclonus. *Spinal segmental myoclonus is symptomatic*

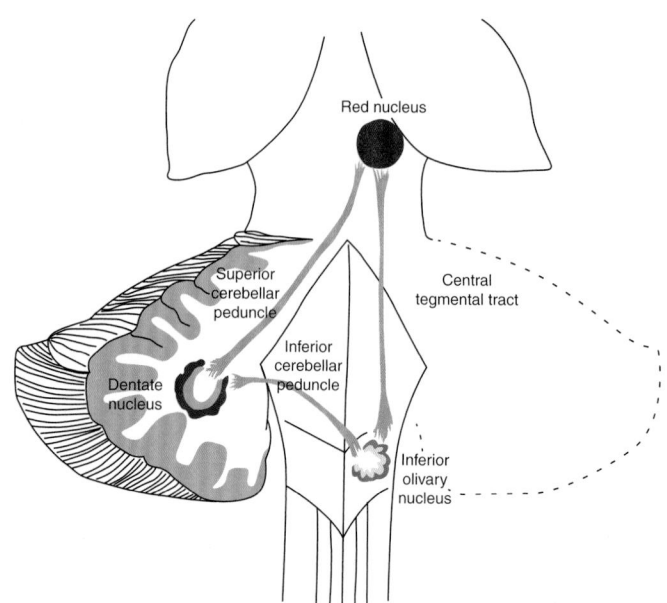

FIGURE 78.1 Guillain–Mollaret triangle. Red nucleus, inferior olivary nucleus, and dentate nucleus on contralateral sides form the three corners of this triangle. The central tegmental tract runs from the red nucleus to the inferior olivary nucleus, which sends the projection to the dentate nucleus via the inferior cerebellar peduncle. Dentate nucleus sends the projection through the red nucleus via superior cerebellar peduncle. Lesions in this triangle can lead to palatal myoclonus. (Courtesy of Thananan Thammongkolchai, MD.)

until proven otherwise; therefore, neuroimaging of the spine at appropriate levels is needed. In *propriospinal myoclonus*, we also suggest obtaining neuroimaging of the spine to rule out a structural lesion. There is controversy about a psychogenic versus organic origin of propriospinal myoclonus.

PERIPHERAL MYOCLONUS

Peripheral myoclonus of the limbs requires workup such as nerve conduction studies and EMG to confirm the location of the lesions, that is, neural structure involved or myotomal level. In hemifacial spasm, an MRI with visualization of the facial nerve and nearby vascular structures should be obtained. Sometimes, a vascular loop can be seen abutting the facial nerve.

TREATMENT

Specific treatment of myoclonus depends on the etiologic diagnosis, for example, treatment of hepatic encephalopathy in asterixis or employing antiepileptic agents in myoclonic epilepsy. If specific treatment is not available, symptomatic treatment can be pursued. Pharmacologic treatments commonly employed are clonazepam, levetiracetam, and valproic acid. There are no clear guidelines regarding which medication should be initiated, although anatomic localization guides treatment. The treatment is shown in Table 78.4.

OUTCOME

The prognosis and natural history of myoclonus depend on its specific etiology. For example, prognosis is good after treating an

TABLE 78.4 Treatment of Myoclonus

Specific treatment depending on the etiologies

Symptomatic treatment

- Pharmacologic treatment
  - Levetiracetam (preferred in cortical myoclonus rather than subcortical or spinal); 1,000–3,000 mg/day divided twice a day; dose up to 4,000 mg/day has been used.
  - Clonazepam (can be used in cortical, subcortical, and spinal myoclonus); starting dose 0.5–1 mg/day; typical dose 3 mg/day or more; sometimes up to 15 mg/day
  - Valproic acid; typical dose 1,000–1,500 mg/day
  - Zonisamide or primidone (used less commonly when the aforementioned conventional medications fail); dosing for zonisamide 100–200 mg/day; for primidone 500–750 mg/day but usually poorly tolerated at such high doses
  - Others (nonconventional treatments)
    - Sodium oxybate in some forms of myoclonus that responds to alcohol such as myoclonus–dystonia syndrome and posthypoxic myoclonus; average dose 6.5 mg/day, maximum 9 mg/day
    - 5-Hydroxytryptophan in posthypoxic myoclonus
- Botulinum toxin injection
  - Hemifacial spasm (treatment of choice)
- Deep brain stimulation (DBS)
  - Pallidal DBS has been reported to improve both dystonia and myoclonus in myoclonus–dystonia syndrome, compared to Vim DBS, which improves only myoclonus but not dystonia. Data remains limited.

Specific treatment of myoclonus depends on the etiologic diagnosis. If specific treatment is not available, symptomatic treatment can be pursued.
Vim DBS, ventrointermediate nucleus deep brain stimulation.

underlying systemic disorder, removing a structural lesion, or treating an underlying autoimmune or paraneoplastic process. The outcome of other forms of myoclonus is variable.

Videos can be found in the companion e-book edition. For a full list of video legends, please see the front matter.

SUGGESTED READINGS

Agarwal P, Frucht SJ. Myoclonus. *Curr Opin Neurol.* 2003;16:515–521.

Bakker MJ, van Dijk JG, van den Maagdenberg AM, et al. Startle syndromes. *Lancet Neurol.* 2006;5:513–524.

Brown P, Thompson PD, Rothwell JC, et al. Axial myoclonus of propriospinal origin. *Brain.* 1991;114(pt 1A):197–214.

Caviness JN. Pathophysiology and treatment of myoclonus. *Neurol Clin.* 2009;27:757–777, vii.

Caviness JN. Treatment of myoclonus. *Neurotherapeutics.* 2014;11:188–200.

Caviness JN, Alving LI, Maraganore DM, et al. The incidence and prevalence of myoclonus in Olmsted County, Minnesota. *Mayo Clin Proc.* 1999;74:565–569.

Chang VC, Frucht SJ. Myoclonus. *Curr Treat Options Neurol.* 2008;10:222–229.

Deuschl G, Mischke G, Schenck E, et al. Symptomatic and essential rhythmic palatal myoclonus. *Brain.* 1990;113(pt 6):1645–1672.

Deuschl G, Wilms H. Clinical spectrum and physiology of palatal tremor. *Mov Disord.* 2002;17(suppl 2):S63–S66.

Dreissen YE, Bakker MJ, Koelman JH, et al. Exaggerated startle reactions. *Clin Neurophysiol.* 2012;123:34–44.

Erro R, Bhatia KP, Edwards MJ, et al. Clinical diagnosis of propriospinal myoclonus is unreliable: an electrophysiologic study. *Mov Disord.* 2013;28:1868–1873.

Fahn S, Marsden CD, Van Woert MH. Definition and classification of myoclonus. *Adv Neurol.* 1986;43:1–5.

Franceschetti S, Michelucci R, Canafoglia L, et al. Progressive myoclonic epilepsies: definitive and still undetermined causes. *Neurology.* 2014;82:405–411.

Ghosh D, Indulkar S. Primary myoclonus-dystonia: a diagnosis often missed in children. *J Child Neurol.* 2013;28:1418–1422.

Gorman MP. Update on diagnosis, treatment, and prognosis in opsoclonus-myoclonus-ataxia syndrome. *Curr Opin Pediatr.* 2010;22:745–750.

Guettard E, Portnoi MF, Lohmann-Hedrich K, et al. Myoclonus-dystonia due to maternal uniparental disomy. *Arch Neurol.* 2008;65:1380–1385.

Ikeda A, Kakigi R, Funai N, et al. Cortical tremor: a variant of cortical reflex myoclonus. *Neurology.* 1990;40:1561–1565.

Klaas JP, Ahlskog JE, Pittock SJ, et al. Adult-onset opsoclonus-myoclonus syndrome. *Arch Neurol.* 2012;69:1598–1607.

Lance JW, Adams RD. The syndrome of intention or action myoclonus as a sequel to hypoxic encephalopathy. *Brain.* 1963;86:111–136.

Raymond D, Ozelius L. Myoclonus-dystonia. In: Pagon RA, Adam MP, Ardinger HH, et al, eds. *GeneReviews®.* Seattle, WA: University of Washington, Seattle; 1993.

Roze E, Bounolleau P, Ducreux D, et al. Propriospinal myoclonus revisited: clinical, neurophysiologic, and neuroradiologic findings. *Neurology.* 2009;72:1301–1309.

Rughani AI, Lozano AM. Surgical treatment of myoclonus dystonia syndrome. *Mov Disord.* 2013;28:282–287.

Samuel M, Torun N, Tuite PJ, et al. Progressive ataxia and palatal tremor (PAPT): clinical and MRI assessment with review of palatal tremors. *Brain.* 2004;127:1252–1268.

Turner MR, Irani SR, Leite MI, et al. Progressive encephalomyelitis with rigidity and myoclonus: glycine and NMDA receptor antibodies. *Neurology.* 2011;77:439–443.

van der Salm SM, Tijssen MA, Koelman JH, et al. The Bereitschaftspotential in jerky movement disorders. *J Neurol Neurosurg Psychiatry.* 2012;83:1162–1167.

van Rootselaar AF, van Schaik IN, van den Maagdenberg AM, et al. Familial cortical myoclonic tremor with epilepsy: a single syndromic classification for a group of pedigrees bearing common features. *Mov Disord.* 2005;20:665–673.

Hereditary and Acquired Ataxias 79

Rachel Saunders-Pullman, Susan B. Bressman,
and Roger N. Rosenberg

INTRODUCTION

Ataxia is characterized by incoordination, and herein we describe ataxias that are due to lesions in the cerebellum and efferent or afferent connections. Cerebellar ataxias may be subdivided into three categories: acquired, nondegenerative ataxias; nonhereditary, degenerative ataxias; and hereditary ataxias. Hereditary ataxias can be further divided by mechanism of inheritance into those that are autosomal dominant, autosomal recessive, X-linked, and due to mitochondrial mutations.

The first autosomal recessive (AR) ataxias were described by Friedreich in the 1860s with clinical features including areflexia. In the early 1900s, cases that varied slightly from Friedreich ataxias (FRDA) were classified as *atypical FRDA*. Nosology was primarily based on pathologic features. Patients with markedly different clinical features might be diagnosed with "Marie" ataxia (retained reflexes and later onset than FRDA) or "Menzel" ataxia (olivopontocerebellar atrophy [OPCA] in autosomal dominant [AD] ataxia). Often, olivopontocerebellar atrophy was the term used for any non-FRDA cases as well as sporadic, late-onset ataxias. It was not until the later 20th century that Harding introduced firm clinical classification schema for hereditary ataxias. With the subsequent development of molecular genetics, loci for AR, AD, X-linked, and mitochondrial DNA mutations were discovered and added another level to classification. However, in population-based studies, 33% to 92% of families with AD ataxias and 40% to 46% of families with AR ataxias remained without genetic diagnoses after systematic testing.

Prevalence estimates of ataxia depend on whether a clinical or genetic definition is proposed. Even when considering the rubric of clinical ataxia, worldwide prevalence is highly variable and difficult to determine because of region-specific genetic population effects, regional differences in testing and diagnosis, and limited reports from some countries. AD ataxias are the most prevalent hereditary ataxias, with a range of 0.0 to 5.6 per 100,000 and an average of 2.7 cases per 100,000. Spinocerebellar ataxia type 3 (SCA3)/Machado–Joseph disease is the most common AD ataxia, followed by SCA2 and SCA6. The prevalence of AR ataxias ranges from 0.0 to 7.2 per 100,000 with an average of 3.3 per 10,000. Among AR ataxias, Friedreich ataxia is the most frequent followed by ataxia with oculomotor apraxia or ataxia-telangiectasia.

This chapter will focus primarily on the hereditary ataxias, although the acquired ataxias will be covered in brief.

ACQUIRED ATAXIAS

Acquired etiologies of ataxia should be sought in all cases that are not clearly hereditary. Treatment for acquired ataxias is highly directed by etiology, and therefore etiologies of sporadic-appearing ataxias should be interrogated. Ataxia may be stable, progressive, or intermittent. The differential can be considered relative to rapidity of onset and includes exogenous or endogenous causes.

Acute-onset ataxia is more likely to be due to vascular disease, trauma, toxins (such as alcohol, toluene), multiple sclerosis and other demyelinating diseases, thiamine deficiency, cerebellitis (especially in children), and primary/metastatic tumor or paraneoplastic disease. It may be subacute or chronic, including due to tumor as well as paraneoplastic cerebellar degeneration (especially associated with ovary, breast, or lung neoplasm), thyroid disease, other immune-related diseases (including steroid-responsive encephalopathy thyroiditis), anti–glutamic acid decarboxylase (anti-GAD) ataxia, gluten enteropathy, vitamin E deficiency (which may be secondary to a malabsorption syndrome), toxins (including alcohol, mercury, and medications such as phenytoin), infections (including prion disease, HIV, and Whipple), leptomeningeal metastasis, vitamin B_{12} deficiency, and multiple system atrophy (a prominent cause of sporadic ataxia in adults associated with alpha-synuclein deposition in the pathognomonic glial cytoplasmic inclusions). In children with acquired ataxia, special concern must be given to intoxication (especially antiepileptics, lead, and alcohol), infectious or postinfectious cerebellitis (often attributable to enteroviral, picornavirus, or Epstein–Barr virus [EBV]), tumor, vascular disease, brain stem encephalitis, migraine, and hypothyroidism.

The first step in assessment for all ataxias should include neuroimaging with magnetic resonance imaging (MRI) to evaluate the cerebellum as well as additional structures and to determine the extent and etiology of cerebellar and noncerebellar disease. If acquired ataxias are not consistent with vascular, traumatic, or demyelinating disease, additional evaluation includes assessment of thyroid function, vitamin E and B_1, anti-GAD antibodies, and paraneoplastic antibodies. If suspicion of paraneoplastic etiology is present, additional work-up for assessment of a primary tumor should be considered, even in the absence of paraneoplastic antibodies. Most patients with gluten-related neurologic disease do not have associated gastrointestinal symptoms; therefore, assessment for gluten-related ataxia in an individual includes testing anti-gliadin immunoglobulin (Ig) A and IgG, antitransglutaminase-2 (anti-TG-2) and, if possible, TG-6 antibodies.

HEREDITARY ATAXIAS

Hereditary ataxias are generally progressive, although there is a subgroup of episodic hereditary ataxias, which is separately discussed. The hereditary ataxias comprise heterogeneous disorders that share three features: ataxia, pathology involving the cerebellum or its connections, and heritability. The pathology usually affects more than the cerebellum, including also the posterior columns, pyramidal tracts, pontine nuclei, and basal ganglia, with corresponding additional neurologic signs. Clinical features may include ataxic gait and arm movements, as well as dysarthria, nystagmus, and signs of neuropathy. Within a family, clinical and pathologic features may differ and the heterogeneity creates problems for classification. Because the phenotypic range of hereditary ataxias is broad, with some family members demonstrating ataxia and other different movement disorders or parts of a syndrome—such as mental retardation in a child in proband with fragile X tremor ataxia syndrome (FXTAS)—determination of family history should query for symptoms or diagnosis of chorea, dystonia, parkinsonism, tremor, mental retardation, neuropathy, epilepsy, visual loss, diabetes, and deafness.

Ataxia is often classified based on mode of inheritance, with broad separation between the autosomal dominant cerebellar ataxias (ADCAs), the AR ataxias, and those that are X-linked and mitochondrial. However, the mode of inheritance is not always clear, owing to variable penetrance, anticipation, new mutations, small family sizes, and nonpaternity. Hereditary ataxias should be considered in apparently sporadic cases without known etiology as well. Although cases with parent–child transmission are either dominant or (if maternally inherited) mitochondrial, those with only an affected sibling may be recessive, dominant, or mitochondrial.

AR ataxias are often of early onset, and dominant ataxias are of later onset. However, as many of one-third of individuals with FRDA, the most common recessive ataxia, may have late-onset disease, among the common ADCAs, especially SCA7, but also SCA1–3, 8, and 13 may begin in childhood or even infancy. Dominant ataxias are more often associated with DNA trinucleotide repeats, but FRDA is also a trinucleotide repeat disorder. Whereas the dominant ataxias are usually believed to be due to toxic gain-of-function events, it is believed that AR ataxias are due to decreased translation and loss of functional protein. Both dominant and recessive ataxias may show cerebellar and extracerebellar neurologic features; however, nonneurologic manifestations, such as cardiomyopathy and diabetes (FRDA) and immunodeficiency (ataxia-telangiectasia [AT]), are more frequent in the recessive forms.

AUTOSOMAL DOMINANT ATAXIAS

Classification

In 1893, Marie applied the term *hereditary cerebellar ataxia* to syndromes that differed from Friedreich ataxia in their later-onset autosomal dominant inheritance, hyperactive tendon reflexes, and, frequently, ophthalmoplegia. Classification of ADCAs has been the subject of controversy since this time because nosology was based on pathology with poor clinical–pathologic correlation even within a single family. Harding challenged these confusing pathology-based schemes, lumping ADCAs, and then dividing them into clinical groups. With the mapping and cloning of autosomal dominant ataxia genes, emphasis has shifted to a genetic classification, incorporating clinical features when possible. A broad separation exists between those disorders that are chronic and progressive (the spinocerebellar ataxias, the SCAs) and those with primarily episodic appearance of ataxia (the episodic ataxias). Registration of SCA genes with the Human Genome Organization (HUGO) has led to a sequential numbering system of autosomal SCA loci, with 33 SCA loci and 21 known genes (Table 79.1). However, the numbering is based on the temporal order when SCA numbers were assigned and does not have clinical or pathologic significance. SCAs may be further subclassified into genetic groups (polyglutamine cytosine–adenine–guanine [CAG] repeat disorders, noncoding repeat expansions, and others), although the SCAs show tremendous clinical overlap. Nonetheless, for some SCAs, there are characteristic features which, when present, may be highly suggestive of a particular SCA. For example, seizures are prominent in SCA10, retinopathy in SCA7, and later age of onset and slower progression in SCA6 (see Table 79.1).

Epidemiology

Worldwide, ADCAs occur with a frequency of 1 to 5:100,000. Frequencies of specific SCAs vary by geographic region and this is attributed to founder effects in the populations. The most common ADCA worldwide is SCA3 (21%), then SCA2 and SCA6 (15% each), SCA1 (6%) and SCA7 (2%), and SCA8 (2–5%). The United States frequency pattern is very similar to that worldwide and SCA13 and SCA17 are also seen (less frequently than SCA8). SCA2 is common in Koreans. SCA3 is more common in Portugal, Japan, and Germany than in the United Kingdom. Dentatorubral-pallidoluysian atrophy (DRPLA) accounts for 20% of autosomal dominant SCA in Japan but is uncommon in the United States, where most cases are of African-American origin. SCA12 is common in eastern India but rare elsewhere.

Etiologic and Genetic Features

Although some distinct features can be discerned, most SCAs have many characteristics in common, and classification is complicated by intra- and interfamilial variation. Symptoms usually begin in early- or mid-adult years, but the age at onset varies from childhood to the eighth decade (see Table 79.1). The first and generally most prominent sign is gait ataxia, occasionally starting with sudden falls. Limb ataxia and dysarthria are also early symptoms. Hyperreflexia may be present initially, but tendon reflexes may later be depressed, and vibration and proprioception may be lost. Eye signs include nystagmus, slow saccades, and abnormal pursuit. Dementia, dystonia, parkinsonism, tremor, fasciculations, neuropathy, and distal wasting may occur, although the frequency of these features differs among the various SCAs. Anticipation and potentiation, earlier onset, and more severe symptoms in succeeding generations are observed in most of the SCAs (most dramatically in SCA7 and DRPLA but not in SCA6), and the majority are severely disabled 10 to 20 years after symptom onset (see Table 79.1). Some advocate classification of the ADCA by pathogenesis in those with known genes, dividing into those caused by (1) unstable CAG trinucleotide repeats in the protein-coding region leading many (poly) glutamine repeats (these include SCA1, 2, 3, 6, 7, and 17 and DRPLA); (2) noncoding repeat expansions (SCA8, 10, 12, 31, and 36); and (3) those caused by more traditional genetic mechanisms, including single gene deletions (SCA15 and 16), duplications (SCA20), and point mutations (SCA5, 11, 13, 14, 23, 27, 28, and 35). Among this last class are genes associated with glutamate signaling (SCA5), tau regulation (SCA11 and 27), ion channel functions (SCA13 and 14), mitochondrial activity (SCA28), and calcium signaling (SCA15/16). Whereas ADCAs are generally progressive, the subgroup of episodic ataxias is predominantly intermittent. It is associated with mutations in ion channel genes (EA1, 2, and 5) or signaling (glutamate, EA6) and is separately discussed, although there is overlap with the other ADCAs, as SCA6 is due to CAG repeats in the calcium channel gene CACNA1A. In SCAs with repeat expansions, paternal and maternal transmissions differ, and in all but SCA8, there is a greater tendency for an increase in repeat size in paternally transmitted disease chromosomes. As a result, anticipation is more pronounced in paternally transmitted disease. In SCA8, most expansions occur during maternal transmission.

Coding CAG and Polyglutamine Disorders (Spinocerebellar Ataxia Types 1, 2, 3, 6, 7, and 17 and Dentatorubral-Pallidoluysian Atrophy)

SCA1, SCA2, SCA3, SCA6, and SCA7 are the most frequent etiologies of ADCAs in families worldwide, together accounting for 50% to 60%. As in other dominant disorders with trinucleotide

TABLE 79.1 Autosomal Dominant Ataxias

Disorder	Gene (Mutation Type/Locus)	Gene Product	Phenotype: Age of Onset (Years, Range) Some Typical Features[a]
SCA1	SCA1 (CAG repeat)	Ataxin-1	30s (childhood to older than 60) **Young adult onset; pyramidal signs;** extrapyramidal signs; dysphagia; **ophthalmoparesis;** neuropathy; **tongue atrophy, facial fasciculations**
SCA2	SCA2 (CAG repeat)	Ataxin-2	20s–30s (infancy to 67) **Young adult onset; very slow saccades;** neuropathy; hyporeflexia; dementia; **extrapyramidal signs; pyramidal signs rare; tongue atrophy, facial fasciculation**
SCA3	MJD (CAG repeat)	Machado–Joseph disease protein 1	30s (6–70) **Young adult onset; ophthalmoparesis;** pyramidal and extrapyramidal signs; amyotrophy; sensory loss; **very slow saccades**
SCA4	SCA4 (chromosome 16q22.1)		30s (19–59) **Sensory axonal neuropathy;** deafness; pyramidal signs; **generalized areflexia**
SCA5	SCA5 (nonrepeat mutations)	Spectrin β chain, brain 2	30s (10–68) **Slowly progressive**
SCA6	CACNA1A (CAG repeat)	Voltage-dependent calcium channel α1A subunit	48 (19–75) **Older onset; slowly progressive; sometimes episodic; downbeat nystagmus**
SCA7	SCA7 (CAG repeat)	Ataxin-7	30s (infancy to 60) **Visual loss with optic atrophy and pigmentary retinopathy;** ophthalmoparesis; pyramidal signs; extreme anticipation
SCA8	SCA8 (CAG-CTG)	Kelch-like 1	39 (18–65) **Slowly progressive;** hyperreflexia, decreased vibratory sense; **maternal bias for transmission**
SCA10	SCA10 (ATTCT repeat)	Ataxin-10	36 **Seizures;** polyneuropathy
SCA11	SCA11 (nonrepeat mutations)	—	30 (15–70) Slowly progressive; hyperreflexia; vertical nystagmus
SCA12	PPP2R2B (CAG repeat)	Serine/threonine protein phosphatase	33 (8–55) **Early tremor; bradykinesia;** dystonia; **dementia;** dysautonomia; hyperreflexia
SCA13	SCA13 (nonrepeat mutations)	—	Childhood **Slowly progressive; mental retardation; short stature**
SCA14	PRKCG (nonrepeat mutations)	Protein kinase C gamma	28 (12–42) Early axial **myoclonus**
SCA15/16	SCA15 (deletion of the 5′ part of gene)	Inositol triphosphate receptor	Childhood to teen (childhood to 66) **Slowly progressive;** dysarthria (pure ataxia); **head tremor;** nystagmus
SCA17	TBP (CAA/CAG repeat mutation)	TATA-box–binding/transcription initiation (TFIID)	6–34 **Dementia; parkinsonism;** dystonia; chorea; myoclonus; seizures; cerebral and cerebellar atrophy on MRI
SCA18	7q22-q32	—	Teen Motor/sensory neuropathy
SCA19/22	1p21-q21	—	10–46 **Slowly progressive; tremor;** myoclonus; cognitive impairment
SCA20	— (260-kb duplication)	—	46 (19–64) Palatal tremor/myoclonus; dysarthria; hypermetric saccades; pyramidal signs; dentate calcification on CT
SCA21	—	—	6–30 Akinesia; rigidity; **tremor;** cognitive impairment

TABLE 79.1   Autosomal Dominant Ataxias *(continued)*

Disorder	Gene (Mutation Type/Locus)	Gene Product	Phenotype: Age of Onset (Years, Range) Some Typical Features[a]
SCA23	—	—	40–60 Dysarthria; abnormal eye movements; reduced vibration and position sense
SCA25	—	—	1–39 Sensory neuropathy
SCA26	—	—	(26–60) Dysarthria; irregular visual pursuits
SCA27	—	FGF14/fibroblast growth factor 14	11 (7–20) Early-onset **tremor**; dyskinesia; **dementia/cognitive deficits**
SCA28	—	—	19 (12–36) Nystagmus; ophthalmoparesis; ptosis; hyperreflexia
SCA29	—	—	Childhood Learning deficits
DRPLA	DRPLA (CAG repeat)	Atrophin-1–related protein	30s (childhood to 70) **Early-onset myoclonus and epilepsy; late-onset chorea; dementia in both**
Episodic Ataxias			
EA1	KCNA 1	Voltage-gated potassium channel protein Kv1.1	Childhood (2–15) **Exercise- or startle-induced ataxia**; myokymia (attack duration: seconds to minutes); no vertigo
EA2	CACNA1A (nonrepeat mutations)	Voltage-dependent P/Q-type calcium channel subunit	Childhood (3–52) **Stress- or fatigue-induced episodic ataxia** (attack duration: minutes to hours); **downbeat nystagmus**; later permanent ataxia; acetazolamide responsive
EA5	CACNB4	Dihydropyridine-sensitive calcium channel subunit	—

[a]Ataxia including dysarthria is common for all; features suggesting diagnosis are bolded.

SCA, spinocerebellar ataxia; MRI, magnetic resonance imaging; CT, computed tomography; DRPLA, dentatorubral-pallidoluysian atrophy; EA, episodic ataxia.

expansions (e.g., Huntington disease, DRPLA), there is generally an inverse relationship between repeat size and age at onset, with a threshold of expanded alleles needed for disease. However, in some of these there is an intermediate range of alleles, whereby the upper limit of normal overlaps with the lower range of abnormal repeats. These are now separated into "mutable normal" alleles where they are not disease causing but with transmission expand to cause disease and "reduced penetrance" alleles that may or may not cause disease. Another feature of the trinucleotide expansion disorders is meiotic instability and anticipation. In a parent–child transmission, the size of the repeat may change, either expanding or contracting; with expansion, there may be earlier onset or worse severity in subsequent generations (anticipation).

The CAG expansions result in an expanded polyglutamine tract because CAG codes for glutamine. Unlike the FRDA triplet expansion in the recessive Friedreich ataxia, which causes disease by inducing frataxin deficiency, the dominant SCA triplet expansions cause disease by altering the protein, a toxic gain of function. Polyglutamine protein inclusions are postulated due to impaired protein clearance and transcriptional dysregulation. As each polyglutamine disorder has distinctive clinical–pathologic features, some other feature, in addition to the polyglutamine, must play a role.

SPINOCEREBELLAR ATAXIA TYPE 1

The first ADCA locus, SCA1, was mapped to the short arm of chromosome 6 in 1974, and in 1993, the SCA1 mutation was identified as due to a trinucleotide (CAG) repeat expansion. The expansion was specifically sought because of the known anticipation in SCA1 families and the earlier identification of expanded trinucleotide repeats and anticipation in Huntington disease. The protein encoded by SCA1 is called *ataxin-1* (ATXN1), a ubiquitously expressed protein of unknown function. Mutated ATXN1 accumulates in the nucleus into aggregates, termed *nuclear inclusions*. These inclusions include ubiquitin, chaperones, and proteasomal subunits that are important for protein refolding and degradation, and abnormal protein clearance thus may mediate SCA1 pathogenicity.

Different trinucleotide repeats, those with cytosine–adenine–thymine (CAT), serve to stabilize the polyglutamine repeat from expanding. Normal SCA1 alleles have 6 to 44 CAG repeats, and the repeat configuration is interrupted by one to three CAT repeats when the allele contains 21 or more repeats. Abnormal alleles have 39 or more repeats without the CAT interruption. Mutable normal (intermediate) alleles are those with 36 to 38 CAG repeats without the CAT interruption. Intermediate alleles appear to have no associated clinical signs but on transmission to offspring can expand to the abnormal range. As with other polyglutamine disorders, the repeat size is overall associated with earlier age of onset and severity of disease, but approximately half of the variance in age at onset is not fully explained by repeat size alone; therefore, additional mechanisms are involved.

The prevalence of SCA1 is estimated at 1 to 2 per 100,000, varying in different populations. It is estimated to be responsible for 6% of ADCAs in North America, approximately 30% in Italy, England, and Serbia, and 40% in South Africa. SCA1 rarely accounts for ataxia in singleton or apparently recessive cases.

Typically, SCA1 starts in the third to fourth decade, but the range at onset is 6 years of age to late adulthood. Gait ataxia predominates and is often the first sign, usually with mild dysarthria, hypermetric saccades, nystagmus, and hyperreflexia. With progression, nystagmus may disappear and saccadic abnormalities and ophthalmoparesis (particularly upgaze) develop. Worsening limb, gait, and speech ataxia evolve. Hypotonia with decreased tendon reflexes and sensory loss are common later. Although mild dysphagia may occur early, bulbar manifestations including lingual atrophy, fasciculations, and severe dysphagia usually present late in the disease. Optic atrophy, dementia, personality change, dystonia, and chorea are less common. Maculopathy, more common in SCA7, has also been reported. Classically, SCA1 is more rapidly progressive than other SCAs, with progression to death in 10 to 30 years and early-onset disease more rapidly progressive. Late-onset disease may be restricted to a pure cerebellar disorder, as is seen in SCA6.

The pathology includes neuronal loss in the cerebellum, brain stem, spinocerebellar tracts, and dorsal columns with rare involvement of the substantia nigra and basal ganglia. Purkinje cell loss and severe neuronal degeneration in the inferior olive are seen; degeneration is also seen in the cranial nerve nuclei, restiform body, brachium conjunctivum, dorsal and ventral spinocerebellar tracts, posterior columns, and, rarely, the anterior horn cells. MRI shows atrophy of the brachia pontis and anterior lobe of the cerebellum and enlargement of the fourth ventricle, and spinal cord atrophy may be present.

SPINOCEREBELLAR ATAXIA TYPE 2

Mapped in ataxic patients from the Holguin province of Cuba who descended from an Iberian founder, SCA2 families were subsequently found in Italy, Germany, French Canada, Tunisia, and Japan. The SCA2 gene encodes the protein ataxin-2.

Normal individuals have 31 or fewer CAG repeats (with most containing 22), with 32 repeats of uncertain significance and CAG expansions of 33 or more associated with disease. Repeat length closely correlates with age at onset and severity. SCA2 may have marked anticipation, instability, and expansions. Large expansions over 200 and homozygosity are associated with retinitis pigmentosa, myoclonic encephalopathy, and early-onset parkinsonism. Intermediate length expansions may increase the risk of amyotrophic lateral sclerosis (ALS) and the atypical parkinsonism, progressive supranuclear palsy (PSP), and repeats of 33 or more or with a preserved CAA interruption may manifest as ALS or levodopa-responsive parkinsonism. The function of *ataxin-2*, the protein encoded by SCA2, is not known, but in normal and SCA2 brains, it is localized in the cytoplasm of neurons, especially Purkinje cells. Immunocytochemical studies suggest that the protein is associated with endoplasmic reticulum and may be involved in processing of mRNA and/or regulation of translation, and elevated repeats lead to aggregation of disease protein. Further, ataxin-2 knockout models suggest that it may play a role in modification

of other neurodegenerative diseases, including not only ALS but SCA1 and 3 as well.

SCA2 is a relatively frequent cause of ADCA worldwide, ranging from 14% to 18% in German and American ADCA families, to 37% to 47% in Italian and English families, and more than 30% in ADCA families from eastern India. Rarely, it is found in families with apparent recessive inheritance (i.e., siblings but not parents affected) or in sporadic cases, and some of this may be attributed to the tremendous anticipation whereby the child with markedly more repeats presents prior to the parent with fewer, albeit pathologic, repeats.

SCA2 usually begins in the third to fourth decade, but onset varies from infancy to the seventh decade. The most common clinical features are progressive gait and limb ataxia and dysarthria (Video 79.1). SCA2 is often described as a cerebellar-plus disorder, as other accompanying features are common and include depressed or absent tendon reflexes, slow saccades, kinetic or postural arm tremor, fasciculations, ophthalmoparesis, vibratory and position sensory loss, and sleep disturbances. Chorea and dystonia have been reported in 38% of cases and dementia in 37%. Less common features are leg cramps and leg hyperreflexia. Although levodopa-responsive parkinsonism is classically associated with SCA3, it may be present in SCA2 as well. Nystagmus is an initial feature that tends to disappear as slow saccades emerge. Although other SCA subtypes include these features, patients with SCA2 are most likely to have slow saccades and hyporeflexia. Many show electrophysiologic evidence of axonal neuropathy with severe involvement of sensory fibers. The highly variable phenotype occasionally seems to "breed true" in families (e.g., kindreds with dementia and extrapyramidal signs or with moderate ataxia, facial fasciculations, prominent eye signs that include lid lag, and retinitis). Abnormal motor control with periodic leg movements during sleep and rapid eye movement (REM) sleep without atonia are common.

Pathology, like clinical signs, is variable. Usually, there is severe neuronal loss in the inferior olive, pons, and cerebellum (OPCA). However, there may also be degeneration of the substantia nigra, dorsal columns, and anterior horn cells. Degeneration is rarely restricted to the cerebellum.

As with other SCAs, because there are overlapping clinical features, molecular genetic testing is necessary to confirm the diagnosis.

SPINOCEREBELLAR ATAXIA TYPE 3/MACHADO–JOSEPH DISEASE

Machado–Joseph disease (MJD) was first described in families of Azorean Portuguese descent, also seen in German, Dutch, African-American, and Japanese families, and eventually linked to chromosome 14q24.3-q32. Subsequent linkage to the same region was found in French families that were clinically similar to SCA1 or SCA2, and the locus was numbered SCA3. Because these French families were not of Azorean descent, and because there were several clinical differences (lack of dystonia and facial fasciculations), it was uncertain whether MJD and SCA3 were owing to different genes, different mutations in the same gene, or the varying phenotypic expressions of the same mutation in individuals with different ancestry. In 1994, an expanded and unstable CAG repeat was found in the coding region of the MJD gene and all 14q-linked families have the same unstable CAG repeat within the SCA3/MJD gene, so that now SCA3 and MJD are viewed as a single genetic disorder with a wide clinical spectrum. SCA3 is the most common ADCA worldwide. As with the other ADCA genes, there may be intrafamilial genetic modifiers (including differences within the SCA3/MJD gene) that influence the phenotype.

The normal repeat number is up to 43, and disease alleles in affected individuals range from 52 to 89 repeats. Intermediate allele size is between 48 and 54 repeats, is associated with meiotic instability and pathologic expansion in subsequent generations, and infrequently may manifest with restless legs syndrome, dysautonomia, and/or polyneuropathy. As in other CAG repeat diseases, there is a strong inverse correlation between the length of the repeat and age at onset, and there is instability in paternal meioses. Some, but not all, homozygous SCA3 individuals have early-onset severe disease, suggesting a gene dosage effect.

The SCA3/MJD gene encodes *ataxin-3*, a protein not related to ataxin-1 or ataxin-2. It binds and cleaves ubiquitin chains, suggesting that it may be a mixed linkage, ubiquitin chain–editing or regulatory enzyme linked to quality control and endoplasmic reticulum–associated protein degradation. It is ubiquitously expressed in the cytoplasm of cell bodies and processes. In SCA3/MJD brain, there is aberrant nuclear localization and accumulation of ubiquitinated nuclear inclusions. The sites and burden of brain degradation in SCA3 is similar to SCA2.

Common signs, regardless of age at onset, include limb and gait ataxia, dysarthria, and progressive ophthalmoplegia. Findings that are more dependent on age at onset include pyramidal signs, dystonia and rigidity, amyotrophy, facial and lingual fasciculations, and lid retraction with bulging eyes. Four clinical subclasses have been proposed:

1. Adolescent or young adult onset: rapidly progressive with spasticity, rigidity, bradykinesia, weakness, dystonia, and ataxia
2. Mid-adult onset (ages 30 to 50 years): moderate progression of ataxia
3. Late-adult onset (ages 40 to 70 years): slower progression of ataxia, prominent peripheral nerve signs, and few extrapyramidal findings
4. Adult onset: parkinsonism and peripheral neuropathy

The pathology had been considered distinct with primarily spinopontine atrophy and involvement of pontine nuclei, spinocerebellar tracts, Clarke column, anterior horn cells, substantia nigra, and basal ganglia; the inferior olives and cerebellar cortex were thought to be always spared. With mutation screening, however, it is now evident that the olives and cerebellar cortex may be involved.

SCA3 is the most common cause of ADCA in many but not all populations. In the United States, about 21% of ADCA families have SCA3; in a study of mixed populations, 41% were SCA3, but this dropped to 17% when Portuguese families were excluded. SCA3 is common in Germany (accounting for 50% of ADCA cases), China, and Japan but uncommon in England and rare in Italy (Figs. 79.1 and 79.2).

SPINOCEREBELLAR ATAXIA TYPE 6

The SCA6 gene maps to chromosome 19p13 and encodes for an α1A voltage-dependent calcium channel subunit (CACNA1A). It differs from other polyglutamine SCAs in the following: (1) Pathology is associated with a lower number of CAG repeats; (2) repeat is stable during transmission and anticipation is generally not observed; (3) there is a later onset, less severely progressive course, and the disorder tends to be more purely cerebellar; and (4) it is allelic with other generally nonprogressive channelopathies. There are three distinct phenotypes associated with different CACNA1A mutations. The SCA6 symbol is reserved for an adult-onset cerebellar syndrome with CAG repeat expansions. SCA6 CAG repeats are 20 to 33, with an average disease-causing length of 22. Normal expansions are 4 to 18, and 19 repeats are considered intermediate.

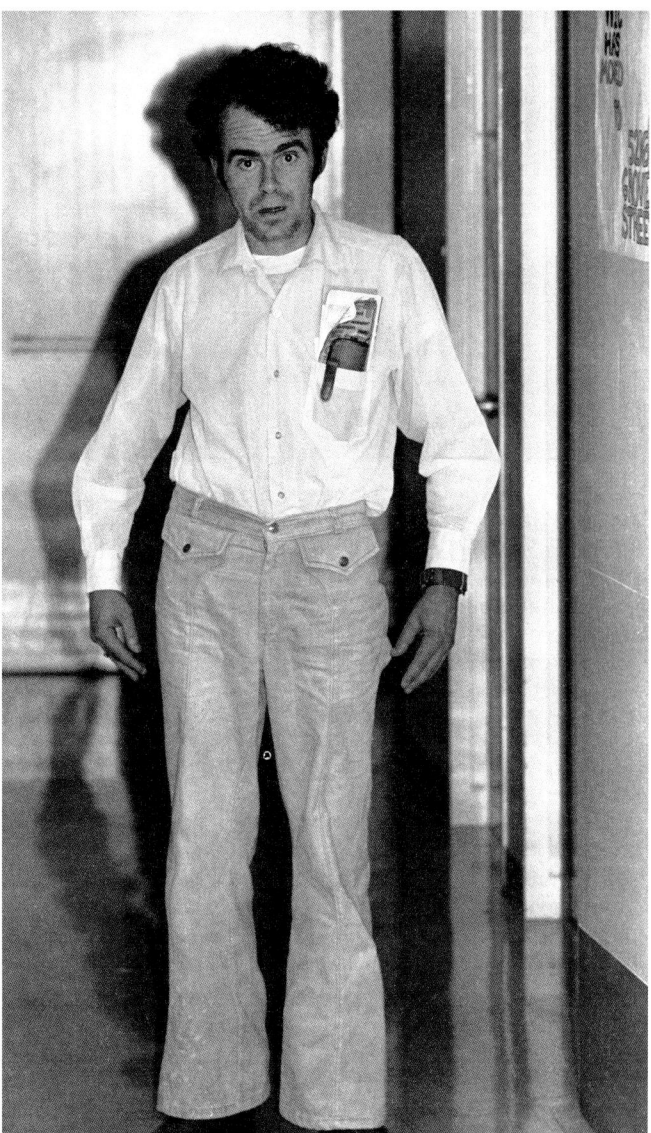

FIGURE 79.1 Patient JM of the Joseph family who, at age 38 years, shows dystonic posturing of his head, arms, trunk, and legs in association with prominent spasticity of his extremities. He has been symptomatic for 12 years. (From Rosenberg RN, Nyhan WL, Coutinho P, et al. Joseph's disease: an autosomal dominant neurological disease in the Portuguese of the United States and the Azores Islands. *Adv Neurol.* 1978;21:33–57.)

The two other phenotypes associated with CACNA1A mutations are familial hemiplegic migraine (FHM) and episodic ataxia type 2 (EA2). EA2 is caused by CACNA1A mutations that predict protein truncation, abnormal splicing, or, rarely, missense mutations, and about 50% of FHM is associated with CACNA1A missense mutations. In addition, a CACNA1A missense mutation, G293R, causes a more severe SCA6-like phenotype. Although most families "breed true" as SCA6, FHM, or EA2, phenotypic overlap may occur. SCA6 patients may also have episodes of ataxia. One family with CAG expansions had members with episodic ataxia and others with progressive ataxia and another with EA2 had members with hemiplegia or migraine during episodes of ataxia. The correlation between number of SCA6 repeats and age at onset is quite loose; 22 repeats, the most common expansion, is associated with

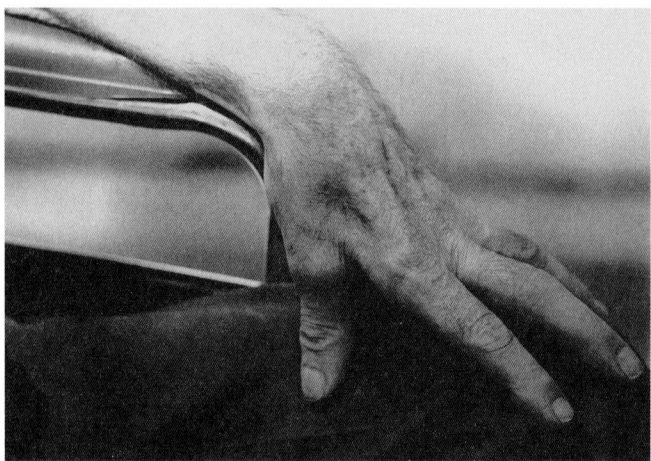

FIGURE 79.2 A 74-year-old man and grandson of the Joseph proband showed progressive disease for 12 years with truncal ataxia, cerebellar dysarthria, areflexia, distal sensory deficits, and distal atrophy. The degree of atrophy of the intrinsic hand muscles can be seen. Thus, he manifests a neurologic syndrome of late onset and, as a direct descendant of Antone Joseph, he suggests the possibility of a wide spectrum of disease. (From Rosenberg RN, Nyhan WL, Coutinho P, et al. Joseph's disease: an autosomal dominant neurological disease in the Portuguese of the United States and the Azores Islands. *Adv Neurol.* 1978;21:33–57.)

range of age at onset, even within sibships. Like MJD, the phenotype is more severe in homozygous individuals.

The molecular basis of disease is unknown, and thus far, studies suggest that expanded CAG repeats do not affect the functioning of the voltage-gated calcium channels but rather reflect a gain of function of the protein, although this remains an area of active research.

The clinical picture of SCA6 is fairly uniform. The average age at onset is somewhat older than other SCAs, about 45 to 50 years (range, 20 to 75 years). The first symptom is usually unsteady gait. Dysarthria, leg cramps, and diplopia can also be early symptoms. Occasionally, patients describe positional vertigo or nausea. Cerebellar signs include gait and limb ataxia (especially leg), cerebellar dysarthria, saccadic pursuit, and dysmetric saccades. Horizontal and downbeat nystagmus (most prominent on lateral gaze) are common eye signs, but very slow saccades are not observed. Noncerebellar signs occur with less frequency and usually less clinical impact than in other SCA disorders but include hyperreflexia, decreased vibration and position sense, impaired upgaze, and parkinsonism. Onset of ataxia may be episodic or apoplectic and resembles EA2 with attacks of unsteadiness, vertigo, and dysarthria that last for hours; between attacks, there are few if any symptoms or signs. The attacks may occur for years before progressive cerebellar signs emerge.

The course is slowly progressive, the least progressive of the SCAs and generally does not shorten life span. After 10 to 15 years, most affected individuals are no longer able to walk without assistance. MRI shows cerebellar atrophy but little brain stem or cortical atrophy. Pathologically, there is cerebellar atrophy with loss of Purkinje and granule cells and limited involvement of the inferior olives.

In the United States and Germany, SCA6 accounts for 10% to 15% of ADCA families. It is more common in Japan (30%) and is uncommon in France, where only 1% of ADCA families harbor the mutation. Five percent to 6% of sporadic ataxia patients demonstrate SCA6 expansions. Some are new mutations, but it is also likely that some appear sporadic because of the late age at onset and relatively indolent course.

SPINOCEREBELLAR ATAXIA TYPE 7

SCA7 differs from other forms of ADCA by the associated severe retinal photoreceptor degeneration producing cone-rod dystrophy and is notable for unstable repeat length during meiosis. It is a result of the expansion of a coding sequence CAG repeat in ataxin-7, an integral component of the transcription coactivator complex involved in regulation of transcription. Normal alleles have up to 29 repeats. Abnormal alleles have from 36 to more than 450 repeats. Intermediate repeats are between 30 and 35. Alleles in this range are considered to be unstable, producing an increased risk of having a child with an abnormal repeat length but are not convincingly associated with a phenotype. Dramatic examples of anticipation, especially with paternal transmission, are due to repeat instability, which exceeds any other CAG repeat SCA, and is related to age at onset, rate of progression, and clinical signs.

SCA7 age at onset ranges from infancy to the seventh decade and averages around 30 years. The course varies with age at onset. A severe infantile form occurs with large expansions (>200) that are paternally inherited. These infants have hypotonia, dysphagia, visual loss, cerebellar and cerebral atrophy, and congestive heart failure with cardiac anomalies. This differs from childhood and adult forms, which are marked by early visual loss, moderately progressive limb and gait ataxia, dysarthria, ophthalmoparesis, and Babinski signs. In late-onset cases (fourth to sixth decade), ataxia may occur in isolation or it may precede visual symptoms (see Table 79.1). Affected individuals all have abnormal yellow–blue color discrimination (which in the mildest forms may be asymptomatic), and clinically, there is often optic disc pallor with granular and atrophic changes in the macula.

Degeneration affects the cerebellum, basis pontis, inferior olive, and retinal ganglion cells. Neuronal intranuclear inclusions containing the expanded polyglutamine tract are found in many brain regions, most frequently in the inferior olive. SCA7 accounts for almost all families with both ADCA and retinal degeneration and about 5% of all ADCA families.

SPINOCEREBELLAR ATAXIA TYPE 17

Initially described in a Japanese patient with childhood-onset ataxia and no family history, SCA17 has now been reported in Japanese and European kindreds. Age at onset ranges from 19 to 48 years, starting with gait ataxia and dementia. Psychiatric features sometimes precede the motor disorder. Limb ataxia, hyperreflexia, chorea, dystonia, myoclonus, parkinsonism (including tremor, bradykinesia, postural instability, and rigidity, sometimes mimicking MSA-C), as well as epilepsy have also been reported. MRI is notable for both cerebral and cerebellar atrophy. SCA17 is secondary to a CAG repeat expansion in the TATA-binding protein (TBG) gene, a transcription-initiating factor (TFIID). Normal repeat length is 29 to 42, and patients have 44 to 63 CAG repeats. Similar to SCA6, repeats are generally stable in subsequent generations. Neuropathology demonstrates Purkinje cell loss and intranuclear inclusions with polyglutamine expansions.

DENTATORUBRAL-PALLIDOLUYSIAN ATROPHY

DRPLA is most common in Japan where it constitutes 10% to 20% of ADCA families. Rare cases have been described in other groups. The pathology involves the dentate, red nucleus, subthalamic nucleus, and the external globus pallidus; the posterior columns may be involved. The phenotype includes ataxia and dementia but varies in other features depending on age at onset. Early-onset cases (before age 20 years) tend to show severe and rapid progression of myoclonus, epilepsy, and cognitive decline, whereas later onset cases display ataxia, chorea, dementia, and psychiatric problems (resembling Huntington disease; see Table 79.1). Anticipation is evident, and paternal transmission is associated with more severe early-onset disease. One clinical variant, the *Haw River syndrome*, was described in an African-American family in North Carolina. This variant includes all the aforementioned symptoms except for myoclonic seizures, and additional features include basal ganglia calcification, neuroaxonal dystrophy, and demyelination of the central white matter. MRI may show atrophy of the cerebral cortex, cerebellum, and pontomesencephalic tegmentum, with high signal in white matter of the cerebrum and brain stem.

The disorder is a result of an expansion of a CAG repeat in the DRPLA gene, which maps to chromosome 12p. There is an inverse relationship between repeat size and age at onset; normal subjects have up to 35 repeats and disease alleles have 48 or more (see Table 79.1). The gene is expressed in all tissues, including brain. The DRPLA gene product, *atrophin-1*, is found in neuronal cytoplasm. Ubiquinated intranuclear inclusions are seen in neurons and to a lesser extent in glia. The neuronal inclusions are concentrated in the striatum, pontine nuclei, inferior olive, cerebellar cortex, and dentate.

Spinocerebellar Ataxias due to Noncoding Repeat Expansions (Spinocerebellar Ataxia Types 8, 10, 12, 31, and 36)

In contrast to the polyglutamine disorders, these SCAs are due to repeat expansions, usually trinucleotide, pentanucleotide, or hexanucleotide, which are transcribed to RNA but are not translated into protein.

SPINOCEREBELLAR ATAXIA TYPE 8

SCA8 has a slowly progressive course that begins at a mean of 39 years (range 1 to 65 years). The common initial findings include limb and gait ataxia and dysarthria and, compared to other SCAs, severe scanning dysarthria, truncal titubation, and leg ataxia are more common. Severely affected individuals are not able to walk by the fourth decade. Hyperreflexia, Babinski signs with spasticity, and ophthalmoplegia may also occur.

SCA8 is unique among the ataxia trinucleotide repeat disorders for several reasons: (1) The trinucleotide repeat is a cytosine–thymine–guanine (CTG) repeat rather than a CAG repeat, (2) the repeat length does not necessarily correlate with severity, (3) abnormal allele length has been reported in other ataxias as well as normal controls, and (4) allele expansion occurs with maternal transmission and contraction with paternal transmission. It is similar to SCA12 (a CAG trinucleotide repeat) but differs from other trinucleotide repeat disorders in that the product is a noncoding RNA. Abnormal CTG expansions (>44 repeats) have been reported in healthy and disease controls. The SCA8 transcript may downregulate the adjacent gene Kelch-like 1 (KLHL1), leading to neurodegeneration. However, initial studies with transgenic mice suggest that CTG expansions produce an ataxic phenotype.

SPINOCEREBELLAR ATAXIA TYPE 10

SCA10 is caused by a large ATTCT pentanucleotide repeat expansion in intron 9 of *ataxin-10*, a new type of dynamic repeat

expansion. Although the normal repeat range is 10 to 22 alleles, affected individuals have 800 to 4,500 repeats. The expanded repeat alleles are unstable with paternal transmission, and there is an inverse correlation between the repeat number and age at onset. An association between ataxia or seizure phenotype and allele size has not been established.

In 1999, two independent groups mapped this locus to chromosome 22q. The phenotype is marked by pure cerebellar signs and seizures. Most families are of Mexican or Brazilian ancestry suggesting a common, possibly Native American, founder population. Age at onset ranges from 12 to 48 years, with evidence of anticipation. There is slowly progressive ataxia with eventual difficulty sitting. Scanning dysarthria, dyscoordination of oral muscles, upper limb incoordination, and abnormal tracking eye movements also develop in most patients. Although seizures may be infrequently associated with SCA2 and SCA17, they are a prominent feature in SCA10: between 20% and 100% of patients have recurrent partial complex and generalized motor seizures. Seizures usually start after the gait ataxia and are well controlled with anticonvulsants. Mild cognitive disorders, mood disorders, mild pyramidal signs, behavioral disturbances, and peripheral neuropathy may occur. Furthermore, nonneurologic features of hepatic failure, anemia, and/or thrombocytopenia were reported in one family. MRI demonstrates progressive pancerebellar atrophy, and interictal electroencephalogram shows evidence of cortical dysfunction with or without focal epileptiform discharges in some.

SPINOCEREBELLAR ATAXIA TYPE 12

SCA12 has been described in American European and Indian Asian families. It starts between ages 8 and 55 years, usually in the mid-30s. It differs clinically from other ADCAs with its frequent action tremor. The slowly progressive ataxia may not be disabling. Other features include hyperreflexia, subtle parkinsonism, focal dystonia, dysautonomia, dementia, and psychiatric features. MRI shows cerebral as well as cerebellar atrophy. Although the disorder is due to CAG repeat expansions, they are not translated and it is not believed to cause polyglutamine-related toxicity. Normal repeat length is 7 to 28 repeats, whereas it is greater than 65 repeats in affected individuals.

SPINOCEREBELLAR ATAXIA TYPE 13

SCA31 is due to a pentanucleotide repeat (TGGAA)n insertion in the intron of BEAN/TK2. It is most frequently seen in those of Japanese descent and has been less frequently seen in individuals of East Asian background, including Korea and China. It is clinically characterized by pure cerebellar ataxia and pathologically by halo-like structures surrounding the degenerating Purkinje cells, attributed to nuclear deformity and Golgi fragmentation. Because of its late age at onset, often in the 60s, and its pure cerebellar features, it is most compared to SCA6.

SPINOCEREBELLAR ATAXIA TYPE 36

SCA36 is also characterized by a late-onset slowly progressive ataxia in the 50s (range 29 to 65 years) and often with preserved gait even after 10 years but is a cerebellar plus syndrome. First symptoms are often balance difficulties, and dysarthria and appendicular cerebellar features are almost universal. SCA36 is associated with sensorineural hearing loss. There may be overlap with motor neuron disease, with muscle atrophy and denervation including lingual, often causing dysphagia. Frontal–subcortical cognitive impairment may emerge. There is rare associated dystonia and parkinsonism. SCA36 is due to a hexanucleotide GGCCTG repeat expansion in NOP56. Six hundred fifty repeats or greater are associated with symptoms. Cases have been reported in Japan, Spain, and Italy, including singleton cases. Therefore, in areas with a founder mutation and the clinical features, molecular genetic testing may be considered even without a family history.

Spinocerebellar Ataxias due to Traditional Conventional Genetic Mechanism

These include point mutations (5, 11, 13, 14, 27, 28, 35, and 38), single gene deletions (SCA15/16), and duplications (SCA20).

SPINOCEREBELLAR ATAXIA TYPE 5

This locus was mapped to the pericentromeric region of chromosome llq in a kindred descended from the paternal grandparents of President Abraham Lincoln. The affected gene β-III spectrin (SPTBN2) is highly expressed in Purkinje cells and is involved in glutamate signaling. Symptoms of this relatively benign, slowly progressive, cerebellar syndrome appear at 10 to 68 years with anticipation (see Table 79.1). All four juvenile-onset patients (10 to 18 years) resulted from maternal transmission rather than the paternal pattern seen in the other SCA syndromes. The juvenile-onset patients showed cerebellar and pyramidal tract signs, as well as bulbar dysfunction.

SPINOCEREBELLAR ATAXIA TYPE 11

SCA11 has been reported in four families, including those with British, Pakistani British, French, and German ancestry. It presents with young onset, average age of 25 years (range 11 to 70 years), benign slowly progressive gait and limb ataxia, and with a normal life expectancy. It is primarily cerebellar except for mild pyramidal signs, although dystonia and peripheral neuropathy may be present. It is due to mutations in TTBK2, a gene that is widely expressed in the brain but particularly in Purkinje cells, granular cell layer, hippocampus, and midbrain, including substantia nigra. It phosphorylates tau protein and stabilizes Purkinje cells.

SPINOCEREBELLAR ATAXIA TYPE 13

SCA13 was initially observed in French and Filipino families and is due to mutations in the voltage-gated potassium channel KCNC3. It is present in both early-onset infantile and adult-onset forms. When onset is in infancy, it is characterized by cognitive impairment, severe cerebellar atrophy, and ataxia and motor deficits. Adult-onset cases are primarily characterized by progressive ataxia and cerebellar degeneration. Nystagmus and pyramidal features were also noted as well as, infrequently, seizures. Most adult-onset cases have mild progression.

SPINOCEREBELLAR ATAXIA TYPE 14

Initially described in a single Japanese family, individuals with early- (<27 years) and late-onset ataxia were described; those with early onset also have intermittent axial myoclonus, whereas those with late onset had pure ataxia. The gene was mapped to 19q13, and later an American family with overlapping linkage, but without any members demonstrating axial myoclonus, was reported. Mutations affect the protein kinase C gamma gene in American and Japanese families.

SPINOCEREBELLAR ATAXIA TYPES 19/22

This locus overlaps with SCA22 and was initially mapped through identification of the KCND3 gene in a Dutch family with slowly progressive mild ataxia, nystagmus, infrequent cognitive impairment, myoclonus, sensory neuropathy, and irregular postural tremor (SCA19). Age of onset ranged from 20 to 45 years. MRI showed marked cerebellar hemispheric atrophy with mild vermian and cerebral atrophy. KCND3 mutations are believed to cause ataxia through impairment of protein maturation and/or channel dysfunction.

SPINOCEREBELLAR ATAXIA TYPE 23

SCA23 is mapped to 20p13-p12.23 and was originally described in Dutch family. Age of onset ranged from 43 to 56 years and disease duration from 1 to 23 years. A classic pattern of gait difficulty, limb ataxia, and dysarthria was present. Neuropathology of one individual revealed pronounced Purkinje cell loss, especially in the vermis, dentate nuclei, and inferior olives. It is due to heterozygous mutation in the PDYN gene.

SPINOCEREBELLAR ATAXIA TYPE 27

Missense mutations in the gene encoding fibroblast growth factor 14 on chromosome 13q34 have been described in a Dutch pedigree with SCA27. Childhood-onset postural tremor and slowly progressive ataxia began in young adulthood.

SPINOCEREBELLAR ATAXIA TYPE 28

SCA28 is a slowly progressive disorder described primarily in Italian and French families. Mean age at onset is 30 years with ataxia, and there are frequent ophthalmologic features including slow saccades, ophthalmoparesis, and ptosis. It is caused by heterozygous mutation in the AFG3L2 gene, which is hypothesized to lead to protection of the cerebellum from degeneration and is allelic to the SPAX gene.

SPINOCEREBELLAR ATAXIA TYPE 35

SCA35 was described in two Chinese families with slowly progressive ataxia, generally affecting gait first with pyramidal signs in the legs, with onset in the 40s, and also associated with tremor, cervical dystonia, and ocular dysmetria. However, there was tremendous phenotypic variation in a third described family that included childhood onset of disease and mental retardation. SCA35 is due to missense mutations in transglutaminase 6 (TMG6).

SPINOCEREBELLAR ATAXIA TYPE 38

SCA38 is due to mutations in the ELOV5 gene, whose product is highly expressed in Purkinje cells and is involved in the synthesis of polyunsaturated fatty acids. Recently determined, missense mutations have been reported in Italian and French families. Ataxia is characterized as primarily slowly progressive cerebellar phenotype with onset in the 40s but with the majority also demonstrated mild to moderate axonal sensory neuropathy.

SPINOCEREBELLAR ATAXIA TYPES 15/16

SCA15 is characterized by late-onset slowly progressive cerebellar ataxia, action and postural tremor, dorsal column involvement, gaze impairment, overall slow progression, and vermian atrophy on MRI. It is due to a heterozygous deletion of the inositol 1,4,5,-triphosphate receptor type 1 (ITPR1) and resultant haploinsufficiency (although one missense mutation has been reported). This signaling protein has been proposed as a unifying feature in cerebellar ataxias. The previously denoted SCA16 has now been merged with SCA15.

Duplications:

SPINOCEREBELLAR ATAXIA TYPE 20

This syndrome was identified in an Australian family of Anglo-Celtic descent and is due to duplications on chromosome 11q12. Age at onset is 9 to 64 years with a mean of 47 years. Slowly progressive dysarthria and gait ataxia were typical. Most patients have a 2-Hz palatal tremor with some spread to lips and pharynx as well as dysphonia. Mild pyramidal features and hypermetric saccades are seen. MRI demonstrates dentate nucleus calcification. Two of nine individuals with imaging also had pallidal calcification and two had olivary calcification. Hence, pathology in the Mollaret triangle may account for the palatal tremor. No calcium metabolic etiology has been identified, and the syndrome differs from familial idiopathic brain calcification.

Additional Spinocerebellar Ataxias

Additional SCAs whose loci have been mapped but for which no gene has been determined include SCA4, 18, 21, 25, 26, and 30.

SPINOCEREBELLAR ATAXIA TYPE 4

SCA4 maps to chromosome 16q. The phenotype consists of late-onset (19 to 59 years) ataxia, prominent sensory axonal neuropathy, normal eye movements in most, and pyramidal tract signs and deafness in some.

SPINOCEREBELLAR ATAXIA TYPE 18

SCA18 is a syndrome of ataxia and hereditary sensorimotor neuropathy reported in an American family of Irish ancestry. Onset is usually in adolescence. All affected individuals developed gait ataxia, dysmetria, and nystagmus. This condition exemplifies the overlap between hereditary sensory neuropathies and the SCAs because sensory loss, pyramidal tract signs, and muscle weakness were also seen. In some patients, nerve conduction studies showed sensory axonal neuropathy, and muscle biopsy revealed neurogenic atrophy. MRI demonstrated mild cerebellar atrophy. Linkage to 7q22-q32 was demonstrated.

SPINOCEREBELLAR ATAXIA TYPE 21

SCA21 is mapped to 7p15-21 and has been described in one French family. Age of onset ranged from 6 to 30 years with an average of 17 years. It is characterized by slowly progressive gait and limb ataxia and hyporeflexia, as well as parkinsonian features of akinesia, rigidity, tremor, or mild cognitive impairment.

SPINOCEREBELLAR ATAXIA TYPE 25

Localized to chromosome 2p, SCA25 was reported in a French family with ataxia and sensory neuropathy. Age at onset was 17 months to 39 years. Most patients had prominent ataxia, but some had a purely sensory neuropathy with minimal cerebellar involvement, and gastrointestinal symptoms were often present. The condition may mimic FRDA. Linkage to chromosome 2p was identified, and missense mutations affecting the potassium channel KCNC3 function have been identified, although the causative gene is not clear.

SPINOCEREBELLAR ATAXIA TYPE 26

Localized to chromosome 19p13.3, this disorder was reported in a Norwegian family. All affected members had a slowly progressive cerebellar ataxia, with age at onset ranging from 26 to 60 years and atrophy confined to the cerebellum.

SPINOCEREBELLAR ATAXIA TYPE 37

SCA37 is mapped to 1p32 and characterized by abnormal vertical eye movements.

Other Unmapped Autosomal Dominant Cerebellar Ataxias

The mapped and cloned SCA genes account for as much as 60% to 90% of ADCAs, depending on geographic region. Other loci for ADCA remain to be identified.

Genetic Testing for Autosomal Dominant Disorders

Genetic testing for a SCA is usually considered if the family history is consistent with dominant inheritance. Rarely, sporadic cases, especially SCA6 and SCA2, may be due to a SCA. Before embarking on SCA screening in a sporadic case, however, imaging and evaluation of acquired causes should be performed; if these are unrevealing, FRDA should be screened first, as this is a more likely cause than any SCA.

Consent for genetic testing is the patient's decision. Counseling is a critical part of the testing process so that patients and family members can learn the complexities of both positive and negative results. For example, comprehensive commercial ataxia testing does not screen for about 40% of genetic causes of ataxia; a negative result in these screens does not exclude genetic causation.

Molecular genetic clinical testing is now available for many of the SCAs, including DRPLA. Because testing all genes is expensive, clinicians may choose to prioritize tests on the basis of clinical features, such as retinopathy for SCA7, action tremor for SCA12, seizures for early-onset DRPLA or SCA10, and on ethnicity (see Table 79.1). However, there are often no distinguishing features to help choose the most likely SCA. Whole-panel testing may then be a reasonable alternative, or clinicians may choose a mini-panel with the most common disorders (which are also trinucleotide repeat disorders) SCA1, 2, 3, 6, and 7.

EPISODIC OR PAROXYSMAL ATAXIAS

Episodes of ataxia can be the first manifestation of metabolic disorders such as multiple carboxylase deficiencies or aminoacidurias. However, the term *episodic* or *paroxysmal ataxia* is generally applied when the major manifestations are self-limited episodes of cerebellar dysfunction with little evidence of fixed or progressive neurologic dysfunction. Two major clinical–genetic subtypes are described: episodic ataxia with myokymia (EA1/myokymia) and episodic ataxia with nystagmus (EA2/nystagmus). Additional episodic ataxia genes have also been described but are less common than EA1 and EA2.

In EA1/myokymia, the attacks usually last a few minutes; they can occur spontaneously but are also provoked by startle, sudden movement, or change in posture and exercise (especially if the subject is excited, anxious, or fatigued). Usually, these are one or a few attacks each day. Onset is in childhood or adolescence; the disorder is not associated with neurologic deterioration, but myokymia appears around the eyes and in the hands. The Achilles tendon may be shortened and there may be a tremor of the hands. The attacks are often heralded by an aura of weightlessness or weakness; an attack comprises ataxia, dysarthria, shaking tremor, and twitching. In some families, acetazolamide (1,000 mg/day) reduces the frequency of attacks; phenytoin and other anticonvulsants may reduce myokymia. This disorder is caused by missense point mutations in the potassium voltage-gated channel gene KCNA1 on chromosome 12p (see Table 79.1).

EA2/nystagmus attacks last longer, usually hours or even days. Attacks are provoked by stress, exercise, fatigue, caffeine, fever, alcohol, and phenytoin. They do not generally occur more than once per day. Age at onset varies from infancy to 40 years and typically starts in childhood or adolescence. Unlike EA1/myokymia, the cerebellar syndrome may progress with increasing ataxia and dysarthria. Even when there is no progressive cerebellar syndrome, interictal nystagmus is often seen (see Table 79.1). During an attack, associated symptoms include headache, diaphoresis, nausea, vertigo, ataxia, dysarthria, tinnitus, ptosis, and ocular palsy. Acetazolamide is usually effective in reducing attacks. Most families with EA2 harbor mutations in the gene for brain-specific CACNA1A. In one family, the dihydropyridine-sensitive L-type calcium channel β-4 subunit was involved.

Different mutations in CACNA1A can also produce SCA6 or hemiplegic migraine, and some families have overlapping phenotypes. Most EA2 mutations are nonsense changes that result in truncated proteins and reduction in P/Q channel activity.

SPORADIC CEREBELLAR ATAXIA OF LATE ONSET

Many patients with ataxia beginning after age 40 years have no affected relatives. Some apparent sporadic cases with late-onset ataxia are a result of SCA mutations. Compared with ADCA, sporadic cases begin later (in the sixth decade), have a more rapid course, and are less likely to have ophthalmoplegia, amyotrophy, retinal degeneration, or optic atrophy. However, many of these patients have parkinsonism and upper motor neuron signs. Some also have autonomic dysfunction and are classified as having multisystem atrophy of the olivopontocerebellar type (MSA-C).

AUTOSOMAL RECESSIVE ATAXIAS

AR inheritance is usually suspected when siblings or cousins are affected but parents are not, in cases with parental consanguinity, or from populations with a founder mutation. Apparently, sporadic cases may also have AR inheritance.

Classification of recessive ataxias may be made on a pathogenic etiology, leading to a separation between those ataxias presumed related to (1) oxidative stress and mitochondria dysfunction, such as FRDA, ataxia with vitamin E deficiency (AVED), abetalipoproteinemia, Refsum disease, and others; (2) impaired DNA repair, such as AT, ataxia with oculomotor apraxia type 1 (AOA1) and type 2 (AOA2); (3) metabolic storage disorders (e.g., lysosomal) and others (Table 79.2); and (4) abnormal protein folding and degradation, such as autosomal recessive spastic ataxia of Charlevoix–Saguenay (ARSACS) and Marinesco–Sjögren syndrome (MSS). These groups also differ by phenotype: Among the disorders of mitochondrial dysfunction and oxidative stress, sensory loss and areflexia are prominent, but little cerebellar atrophy is seen. In contrast, in the disorders of defective DNA repair, cerebellar dysfunction is the primary source of the ataxia, and oculomotor apraxia is common. Additional ataxias with different or unknown pathogenic mechanisms are listed in Table 79.2 and include early-onset cerebellar ataxia with retained tendon reflexes, which is the second most common AR ataxia.

Classification

There are multiple potentially treatable forms of AR ataxia which, although uncommon, should be considered because of their potential response to dietary or other therapy. Additionally, these forms usually decline without treatment. These include any of the vitamin E–related ataxias, Refsum disease (which may be treated with a diet low in phytanic acid), other mild peroxisomal disorders (including that due to mutations in PEX10), biotinidase deficiency, cerebrotendinous xanthomatosis, possibly coenzyme 10 deficiency, and inborn errors of metabolism that may present with intermittent ataxia, including late-onset maple syrup urine disease, urea cycle defects, organic acidurias, Hartnup disease, pyruvate dehydrogenase deficiency, and glucose transporter type 1 (GLUT1) deficiency.

Epidemiology

The frequency and most common causes of AR ataxias vary with the ethnicity and geographic origin of the population studied. For example, FRDA, with a prevalence of 1 in 30,000 to 50,000 people is the most common form of hereditary ataxia in the United States and Europe but is not common in Mexico, China, and Japan. In Europe overall, ataxia with oculomotor apraxia type 2 (AOA2) is the second most frequent AR ataxia after FRDA. However, among AR ataxias in Portugal, the frequency of FRDA is 38% and AOA1 is 21%. AOA1 is the most common cause of AR ataxia in Japan. In the United States, there are few reports of AOA1 and AOA2, yet the frequency of AT is approximately 1 in 40,000 births.

Ataxias Associated with Oxidative Stress and Mitochondrial Dysfunction

Friedreich ataxia (FRDA), first described in 1863, is the most common early-onset ataxia and comprises a large proportion of the AR ataxias. The typical clinical features are juvenile onset (starting around puberty and usually by age 25 years) with progressive ataxia of gait and limbs, absent or hypoactive tendon reflexes in the legs, and extensor plantar responses. Other common features are dysarthria, corticospinal tract deficits, proprioceptive and vibratory sensory loss in the legs, and scoliosis. Approximately two-thirds have cardiomyopathy, up to 30% have diabetes mellitus with impaired glucose tolerance in another large proportion, and obstructive sleep apnea is present in about 20%. With the identification of the FRDA gene, FTX, and the ability to test a range of cases, it has become clear that there is an "atypical" phenotype as well: 25% of the cases have later age at onset, often with preserved tendon reflexes or slower course.

The prevalence of FRDA in North America and Europe is about 1 to 2 per 50,000, with a carrier frequency of about 1:60 to 1:120. Boys and girls are equally affected. Because the disorder is AR, parents are asymptomatic, and consanguinity is found in 5.6% to 28% of affected families. The risk for siblings is 25% and, in small families, only one person may be affected.

FXN maps to 9q and encodes a highly conserved, mitochondrial protein, frataxin. Ninety-six percent of FRDA patients are homozygous for an expansion of a GAA triplet repeat in the first intron of FXN, leading to a deficiency in the frataxin protein. About 4% are compound heterozygotes, with a GAA intronic expansion in one allele and an inactivating mutation in the other allele. Some, but not all, compound heterozygotes have milder disease.

Normal chromosomes have fewer than 34 triplets, and disease chromosomes have 66 to more than 1,700 repeats with the majority having between 600 and 1,200. Repeats in normal chromosomes

TABLE 79.2 Other Hereditary Ataxias

Disorder	Gene (Mutation Type/Locus)	Gene Product	Phenotype: Age of Onset (Years, Range) Some Typical Features[a]
Autosomal Recessive Ataxias			
FRDA	*FXN* 9q13	Frataxin	Childhood to teen (infancy to 40) **Hyporeflexia; proprioceptive loss; sensory loss; visual loss (optic atrophy, retinopathy); neuropathy**; dysarthria; Babinksi signs; cardiomyopathy; scoliosis; may be manifest by late-onset **spastic paraparesis** without much or any ataxia
AVED	*TTPA* 8q13.1-3	α-Tocopherol transferase protein	Childhood to teen (2–52) FRDA-like head titubation; **retinitis pigmentosa; sensory neuropathy; acanthocytes**
AT	*ATM* 11q22.3	Serine protein kinase ATM	Early childhood (infancy to 27) **Oculocutaneous telangiectasia**; immunodeficiency; **elevated AFP**; malignancy; **oculomotor apraxia; chorea; athetosis**
AOA1	*APTX* 9p13.3	Aprataxin	7 (2–16) Dysarthria; dysmetria; axonal neuropathy with areflexia; chorea; dystonia; **oculomotor apraxia; low serum albumin and total cholesterol**
AOA2	*SEXT* 9q34	Senataxin	15 (10–25) **Sensory motor neuropathy; oculomotor apraxia**; chorea; dystonia; **elevated AFP; low serum albumin**
ARSACS	*SACS* 13q12	Sacsin	Childhood **Retinal striations; spasticity**; peripheral neuropathy
IOSCA	*IOSCA* 10q24	Twinkle, Twinky	Infancy Peripheral neuropathy; chorea; optic atrophy; hearing loss
Marinesco–Sjögren	*MSS*	—	Infancy Cataracts, mental retardation, hypotonia, myopathy
Additional Autosomal Recessive Ataxias			
Abetalipoproteinemia (**severe sensory neuropathy, GI biopsy**) and hypobetalipoproteinemia			
Aminoacidurias			
Ataxia-telangiectasia variant (ATV1)/Nijmegen breakage syndrome			
Autosomal recessive cerebellar ataxia type 1 (ARCA1/SYNE related)			
Biotinidase deficiency			
Carboxylase deficiencies			
Cerebrotendinous xanthomatosis (**cataracts**)			
Ceroid lipofuscinosis			
Childhood ataxia with CNS hypomyelination/vanishing white matter (CACH) (**MRI and transthyretin isoelectric focusing**)			
Cockayne syndrome			
Hexosaminidase deficiency			
Hypoceruloplasminemia with ataxia and dysarthria (onset in 40s)			
Late-onset Tay–Sachs disease			
Leigh (also mitochondrial inheritance)			
Leukodystrophies			
Mitochondrial recessive ataxia syndrome (MIRAS)			
Other recessive ataxias with hypogonadism, myoclonus, optic atrophy and mental retardation, deafness			
Refsum disease			
Sialidosis			
Spinocerebellar ataxia with neuropathy (SCAN1) (**sensory motor neuropathy**)			

Disorder	Gene (Mutation Type/Locus)	Gene Product	Phenotype: Age of Onset (Years, Range) Some Typical Features[a]
Additional Autosomal Recessive Ataxias			
Urea cycle defects			
Wilson disease (**parkinsonism, tremor, dystonias, ceruloplasmin**)			
Xeroderma pigmentosum			
X-linked Ataxias			
Ataxia with spasticity, mental retardation, deafness			
Fragile X–associated tremor/ataxia syndrome (FXTAS)			
Uncomplicated ataxia			
X-linked sideroblastic anemia with ataxia			
Mitochondrial Inheritance Ataxias			
CoQ10 deficiency (**muscle biopsy, CoQ measurement**)			
Leigh syndrome (also autosomal recessive)			
Mitochondrial encephalomyopathies (MERRF, NARP, KSS)			

[a]Ataxia including dysarthria is common for all; onset usually before age 20 years, although some have late-onset forms; features suggesting diagnosis are bolded. FRDA, Friedreich ataxia; AVED, ataxia with vitamin E deficiency; AT, ataxia-telangiectasia; AFP, α-fetoprotein; AOA1, ataxia with oculomotor apraxia type 1; AOA2, ataxia with oculomotor apraxia type 1; ARSACS, autosomal recessive spastic ataxia of Charlevoix–Saguenay; IOSCA, infantile-onset spinocerebellar ataxia; GI, gastrointestinal; CNS, central nervous system; MRI; magnetic resonance imaging; MERRF; myoclonus epilepsy and ragged red fibers; NARP, neuropathy, ataxia, retinitis pigmentosa; KSS, Kearns–Sayre syndrome.

are stable when transmitted from parent to child, but expanded GAA repeats show meiotic instability, usually contracting after paternal transmission and either expanding or contracting with maternal transmission. Repeats of 34 to 65, which are rare, are termed *premutation alleles* because they may expand during parental transmission to produce causal mutations. Anticipation is generally not associated with FRDA. Alleles containing 44 to 66 GAA repeats can cause clinical but milder later onset disease, if the other allele is fully expanded to the disease range. The mechanism is thought to be somatic instability in the proportion of cells having 66 or more repeats.

The FTX expansion interferes with frataxin transcription and is associated with a great reduction of normally spliced FTX mRNA. Larger repeats more profoundly inhibit frataxin transcription and cause earlier onset and more severe symptoms. The amount of residual mRNA and thus the age at onset correlates with the shorter of the two expanded repeats. Cardiac disease and diabetes are also at increased frequency in patients with larger repeat size (>500).

The pathology in FRDA is attributed to the deficiency of functional frataxin. Tissues with high levels of frataxin expression, such as heart, liver, skeletal muscle, pancreas, and spinal cord, are affected. Frataxin localizes to the inner mitochondrial membrane and is directly involved in regulating iron homeostasis. The absence of normal frataxin causes defects of mitochondrial oxidative phosphorylation. This ultimately leads to susceptibility to increased oxidative stress, mitochondrial iron accumulation, and lower levels of iron–sulfur proteins. Decreases in complex I to III activity and altered heme synthesis lead to reduced oxidative phosphorylation and accumulation of free radicals. Iron deposits have been demonstrated in the cardiac tissue of FRDA patients, consistent with defective responses to oxidative stress, including damage to iron–sulfur cluster respiratory enzymes.

In FRDA patients, the spinal cord may be thinner than normal. Degeneration and sclerosis are seen in the posterior columns, spinocerebellar tracts, and corticospinal tracts. Nerve cells are lost in the dorsal root ganglia and Clarke column. Peripheral nerves are involved, with fewer large myelinated axons. The brain stem, cerebellum, and cerebrum are normal except for mild degenerative changes of the pontine and medullary nuclei, optic tracts, and Purkinje cells in the cerebellum. Cardiac muscle, nerves, and ganglia are also involved.

Clinical features vary by age at onset and can be divided into early-onset FRDA, late-onset Friedreich ataxia (LOFA), and very late-onset Friedreich ataxia (VLOFA). Symptoms usually begin between ages 8 and 15 years but may start in infancy or after age 50 years. Like other triplicate repeat disorders, there is a correlation between the GAA repeat size and clinical features, particularly age at onset and rate of progression. However, the age at onset correlates with the shorter of the two alleles because FRDA, unlike other triplicate repeat disorders, is recessive (with expanded repeats in both alleles) and is a result of loss of frataxin function. The GAA size, however, does not entirely account for the variability in age at onset or clinical progression; somatic mosaicism and other genetic or environmental modifiers also play a role.

In typical early-onset FRDA, gait ataxia is the most common symptom and is usually the first. Although the gait disorder may be seen in children who have been walking normally, it is more common that children are slow to walk, the gait is clumsy and awkward, and they are less agile than other children. Within a few years, ataxia appears in the arms and trunk, a combination of cerebellar asynergia and loss of proprioceptive sense. Movements are jerky, awkward, and poorly controlled. Intention tremor, most common in the arms, may affect the trunk. Frequent repositioning or pseudoathetosis and true generalized chorea may occur. Speech becomes explosive or slurred and finally unintelligible. Dysphagia is present in over 90%. Limb weakness is common, sometimes leading to paraplegia.

Vibratory loss is an early sign. Frequently, position sense is impaired in the legs and later in the arms. Loss of two-point discrimination, partial astereognosis, and impaired appreciation of pain, temperature, or tactile sensation are occasionally seen. Loss of leg reflexes and the presence of Babinski signs were once considered necessary for diagnosis; almost all patients with typical recessive or sporadic early-onset ataxia with these features have the *FXN* hyperexpansion.

Ocular movements are usually abnormal; fixation instability and square wave jerks are the most common abnormalities. Also frequent are jerky pursuit, ocular dysmetria, and failure of fixation suppression of the vestibular ocular reflexes. Nystagmus and optic atrophy are each seen in about 25% of patients, but severely reduced visual acuity is rare. Sensorineural hearing loss occurs in about 10%. Sphincter impairment may occur, especially when patients are bedridden; dementia and psychosis are unusual, and although motor planning is often impaired, the condition is not incompatible with a high degree of intellectual development. Worse cognition is correlated with larger GAA repeats. Skeletal abnormalities are common. Scoliosis or kyphosis, usually in the upper thoracic region, affects more than 75%. Pes cavus and equinovarus deformities occur in more than 50%. Restless legs syndrome is reported in 30% to 50%.

Cardiac disease is found in more than 85%, with hypertrophic cardiomyopathy in two-thirds of patients. The electrocardiogram (ECG) most commonly shows ST-segment changes and T-wave inversions. Congestive heart failure occurs late and may be precipitated by atrial fibrillation. Diabetes mellitus is found in 10% to 30%.

The course is progressive, and most patients cease walking by 15 years after onset of symptoms. Life expectancy appears to be changing with more advanced management and recognition of milder phenotypes. Although older studies reported mean age at death in the mid-30s, resulting from infection or cardiac disease, in more recent studies, the average interval from symptom onset to death was 36 years.

Late-onset Friedreich Ataxia, Very Late-onset Friedreich Ataxia

With the advent of FRDA testing in large populations, it has become evident that the spectrum of FRDA includes slowly progressive disease, late-onset (after age 25 years, often with less than 500 GAA repeats), very late-onset (>40 years at onset, often with less than 300 GAA repeats), FRDA with retained reflexes (FARR), spastic paraparesis without ataxia, and FRDA without cardiomyopathy. The oldest age of onset reported is 80 years. In one study of ataxic subjects who were clinically thought not to have FRDA, 10% of those with recessive disease and 5% with sporadic disease had homozygous GAA hyperexpansions. To some extent, this variability, especially between families, is explained by the length of the GAA expansion. However, GAA expansion does not account for all the variation, particularly with repeat sizes above 500. For example, Acadian FRDA patients descend from a single founder and have the typical homozygous hyperexpansion with repeat lengths similar to those of other FRDA patients, but they have milder symptoms and cardiopathy is rare.

Clinical testing is currently available to screen for the GAA expansions, which in the homozygous form, account for 96% of cases. In cases with only a single expanded allele, further screening may identify deleterious mutations (nonsense or frameshift mutations that result in premature termination of translation or missense mutations in the highly conserved carboxy terminus) on the other allele.

Laboratory findings include characteristic ECG changes and echocardiogram evidence of concentric ventricular hypertrophy or, less commonly, asymmetric septal hypertrophy. Normal peripheral nerve conduction studies with absent or markedly reduced sensory nerve action potentials distinguish FRDA from Charcot–Marie–Tooth disease. Other common abnormalities are reduced amplitude of visual-evoked responses and small or absent somatosensory-evoked potentials recorded over the clavicle and delayed dispersed potentials at the sensory cortex. Computed tomography and MRI of the brain are usually normal in the early stages but may show cerebellar atrophy, especially with advanced or late-onset disease. Cervical spinal cord atrophy can often be detected on MRI. The cerebrospinal fluid is normal. Vitamin E levels should be assessed, as vitamin E deficiency is an important and treatable differential diagnosis and may mimic FRDA.

Specific treatment for FRDA includes physical therapy and walking aids, speech therapy, psychological support, and treatment of associated cardiac disease (cardiac arrhythmia is a major cause of death) and diabetes. Genetic counseling should be offered. No specific pharmaceutical for FRDA has yet been developed, although there is a range of studies underway.

Ataxias Related to Vitamin E Deficiency

Two forms of vitamin E–related ataxia are widely recognized, ataxia with vitamin E deficiency and abetalipoproteinemia. A third, Cayman ataxia, is likely due to the absence of binding to vitamin E–like compounds.

Ataxia with vitamin E deficiency (AVED) is an AR disorder characterized by progressive ataxia, proprioceptive loss, and areflexia. Additionally, decreased visual acuity due to retinitis pigmentosa, head titubation, Babinski sign, and dystonia may be present. Most individuals with AVED present in adolescence. AVED mimics FRDA clinically; however, later onset, prominent titubation (28% of cases) and dystonia are more common than with FRDA.

Plasma vitamin E (α-tocopherol) is markedly reduced in the setting of a normal lipid and lipoprotein profile; as the normal range of vitamin E is very laboratory dependent, no universal normal range is given, but generally, the level is less than 4.0 μmol/L. Care should be taken in the preparation of the sample, as oxidation in room air may invalidate the results. Malabsorption can be excluded by normal vitamin A and D levels.

Deleterious mutations are found in the α-tocopherol transfer protein (*TTPA*) gene, which maps to chromosome 8q13. Mutation leads to impaired incorporation of α-tocopherol into very low-density lipoprotein (VLDL), which is needed for the efficient recycling of vitamin E. A milder phenotype, including retained reflexes and later onset, may occur with missense mutations that allow some residual TTP activity.

Treatment is with lifelong large-dose oral vitamin E replacement. It is believed that early treatment is associated with better outcome. Siblings should be evaluated for vitamin E deficiency, as presymptomatic treatment may prevent development of symptoms.

Abetalipoproteinemia (Bassen–Kornzweig) and cholestatic liver disease are also associated with vitamin E deficiency. In contrast to AVED, there is often malabsorption, and there are acanthocytes on peripheral smear.

Mitochondrial-Associated Ataxias

Nuclear mutations that encode mitochondrial proteins and mutations in mitochondrial-encoded proteins may also cause ataxia. Other ataxias such as Refsum disease may have mechanisms postulated to impair mitochondrial function.

Mitochondrial recessive ataxias include SANDO (sensory-ataxic neuropathy, dysarthria, and ophthalmoparesis) and *infantile-onset spinocerebellar ataxia* (IOSCA) and are due to mutations in genes for the nuclear-encoded mitochondrial enzymes DNA-polymerase gamma (POLG) and the mitochondrial helicase twinkle (c10orf2), respectively. IOSCA is a rare infantile-onset AR disorder, which was first mapped to chromosome 10q24 in Finnish families. Affected children develop ataxia, athetosis, and loss of tendon reflexes before age 2 years. This is followed by hypotonia, optic atrophy, ophthalmoplegia, deafness, and sensory neuropathy. Missense mutations in POLG cause predominantly sensory axonal neuropathy and ataxia, which is juvenile or adult in onset. There may be associated myoclonus, epilepsy, ophthalmoparesis, cognitive decline, cardiomyopathy, or liver failure.

Mitochondrial disorders due to mutations of the mitochondrial genome also account for progressive ataxia, particularly in children. Mitochondrial encephalomyopathy with ragged red fibers (MERRF) is characterized by ataxia, myoclonus, seizures, myopathy, and hearing loss. Maternal relatives may be asymptomatic or have partial syndromes, including a characteristic "horse collar" distribution of lipomas. Other mitochondrially inherited disorders, including coenzyme Q10 (CoQ10) deficiency; neurogenic muscle weakness, ataxia, and retinitis pigmentosa (NARP); Kearns–Sayre syndrome (KSS); and Leigh syndrome are described in Chapter 139.

Refsum disease is a childhood-onset ataxia syndrome characterized by sensory loss, areflexia, and absence of cerebellar atrophy. Other features include anosmia, early-onset retinitis pigmentosa with variable combinations of neuropathy, deafness, and ichthyosis. Mutations in the *PHYH* and *PEX7* genes cause changes in the phytanoyl-coenzyme A hydroxylase, and peroxisomal biogenesis factor-7 proteins, respectively. These lead to accumulation of phytanic acid and disturbance of peroxisomal function and mitochondrial dysfunction. This may be treated in part with a diet low in phytanic acid.

Ataxia-Telangiectasia and Other Ataxias Associated with Defective DNA Repair

Among AR ataxias, several have prominent oculomotor apraxia and are associated with impaired DNA repair. These encompass AT, where cerebellar degeneration is the most prominent feature, as well as ataxia with oculomotor apraxia, AOA1 and AOA2. These differ from FRDA and AVED, where the posterior columns and the spinocerebellar tracts are the major sites of degeneration, and the cerebellum is not primarily involved. Other AR ataxias associated with DNA repair malfunction, ataxia-like disorder (ATLD), spinocerebellar ataxia with axonal neuropathy (SCAN1), Cockayne syndrome, and xeroderma pigmentosum will also be briefly discussed.

Although AT, AOA1, and AOA2 are also childhood-onset disorders with prominent ataxia-like FRDA, they generally differ from FRDA in several ways: (1) There is prominent oculomotor apraxia in all three conditions but not in FRDA; (2) movement disorders—particularly dystonia and chorea—are frequent in these syndromes and less common in FRDA; and (3) cerebellar abnormalities are prominent, whereas in FRDA, MRI shows only mild cerebellar atrophy until late in the course of disease. Further, upper motor neuron features are uncommon in these conditions, except rarely in AOA1 and AOA2, whereas these are more frequent in FRDA. These conditions are also associated with abnormalities in α-fetoprotein (AFP) (increased in AT and AOA2), Igs (decreased in AT, may be increased in AOA2), carcinoembryonic antigen (CEA) (increased in AT), and albumin (decreased in AOA1).

Ataxia-telangiectasia is an early-onset AR ataxia that affects multiple body systems but whose hallmark feature is cerebellar degeneration. It is due to loss of function of the nuclear protein kinase, ataxia-telangiectasia mutated (ATM), which mediates the cellular repair response to double-stranded (DS) DNA breaks.

AT is characterized by progressive cerebellar ataxia starting at ages 1 to 4 years, oculomotor apraxia, and dysarthria. Later onset is uncommon, although cases with onset in early adulthood have been described. Although clinical symptoms and signs may vary, truncal ataxia in infancy, which becomes more obvious when the child learns to walk, is typical. With progression, the ataxia becomes more appendicular as well. Prominent oculomotor abnormalities include difficulty generating saccades, dependence on head thrusts to fixate, ocular dysmetria, and nystagmus. Facial hypomimia, chorea, dystonia, drooling, dysarthria, myoclonus, and peripheral neuropathy may appear in later childhood or in adolescence. Most AT patients require a wheelchair by their teens. Mild mental retardation has been reported in some cases.

Nonneurologic symptoms usually also appear. Cutaneous telangiectasias are characteristic but are not always present and generally do not appear in the first years of life; hence, they may come after the first neurologic symptoms. Telangiectasias involve the conjunctivae, face, ears, and flexor creases. Growth retardation and delayed sexual development may occur. Immune dysfunction is typical and includes recurrent respiratory and cutaneous infections, lymphopenia, and decreased concentrations of IgA and IgG. There may be progeria and premature graying. About 38% of patients develop malignancies, most frequently leukemia or lymphoma at a young age and epithelial malignancies at a later age. Increased sensitivity to ionizing radiation is a characteristic feature. The rate of cancer in heterozygote carriers is also increased.

The disease is progressive; with supportive care, most patients now live beyond age 20 years, and some live to the fifth or sixth decade. Ten percent to 15% of cases in a United Kingdom sample were noted to have a milder phenotype with later onset and slower course of neurologic deterioration. Therefore, AT may infrequently account for later onset progressive ataxia. Milder phenotypes with late onset or less progressive disease are generally attributable to mutations that permit some residual ATM kinase activity. However, cases with late-onset and absent protein have been reported, suggesting that genetic modifiers may also play a role in affecting the neurologic phenotype of AT. More slowly progressive "variant AT" with preservation of gait but prominent dystonia, myoclonus, and chorea has also been reported.

The gene *ATM* maps to chromosome 11 (see Table 79.2) and encodes the protein kinase ATM, a serine/threonine kinase that affects multiple substrates. Classic AT is usually caused by compound heterozygosity or homozygosity for null *ATM* alleles that truncate or severely destabilize the ATM protein. Most mutations are truncating or splice mutations, and approximately 10% are missense mutations that inactivate the protein. Mutations may occur throughout the gene. "Leaky" splice mutations or presumed promoter deficits, associated with residual functional ATM protein, are usually associated with a milder phenotype and may contribute to some but not all of the phenotypic variability. ATM is a key regulator of multiple signaling cascades that respond to DSDNA breaks induced by damaging agents or by normal processes, such as meiotic recombination. The altered responses involve failure to activate cell checkpoints and repair DNA at G1, S, and G2/M. Molecular studies suggest that ATM is quickly engaged after DSDNA breaks are detected, and it phosphorylates multiple substrates involved in the response to DNA damage. The MRE11–RAD50–NBS1 (MRN) complex is one of the initial sensors that detects the breaks and hence triggers ATM and the DNA repair response.

Insults that may cause DNA breaks are varied, including environmental triggers of ionizing and nonionizing radiation and radiomimetic chemicals, but it has also been hypothesized that the endogenous oxidative stress associated with the high metabolic demands of neurons may contribute to DNA damage and subsequent cell death in ATM-deficient neurons.

Mutations in the MRE11 nuclease, which is the first part of the MRN complex, may cause AT-like disease, and mutations in the NBS1 component of the MRN complex are associated with Nijmegen breakage syndrome (see later in the text).

Pathologically, loss of Purkinje cells is seen in the cerebellum with less prominent changes in the granule cell layer, dentate and inferior olivary nuclei, ventral horns, and spinal ganglia. MRI demonstrates cerebellar atrophy. Other laboratory abnormalities include elevated AFP (observed in >95% of patients), elevated CEA, decreased serum concentrations of IgA, IgE, and IgG2 (with normal to increased IgM), cytogenetic abnormalities including a 7;14 reciprocal chromosome translocation, decreased or absent ATM protein on immunoblotting, abnormal sensitivity to ionizing radiation and radiomimetic chemicals, and mutations in the ATM gene.

One percent of the population is heterozygous for an ATM mutation. As noted, there is genetic heterogeneity that contributes to AT. Population screening for the mutation is difficult because the gene is large and there are many different mutations; however, among different ethnic groups, founder effects lead to a small number of alleles accounting for most causal mutations and facilitates molecular genetic testing in those groups. In other individuals, which constitute the majority of patients, clinical functional assays for putative ATM problems are performed prior to mutation screening. After establishment of cell lines, immunoblotting for ATM protein can determine whether any or trace ATM protein is present. An assessment of protein levels may be difficult to quantify, so colony survival assay (CSA) is usually performed in addition. The CSA is a radiosensitivity assay performed on cultured cells, which assesses lymphoblastoid survival after irradiation. Although no treatment is curative, supportive treatment including caution about doses of ionizing radiation used, physical therapy, monitoring for malignancy and treatment of infection, and genetic counseling is beneficial. Multiple therapies are currently under investigation.

Ataxia-Telangiectasia–Like Disorders

SYNDROMES WITH ABNORMALITIES IN THE MRE11–RAD50–NBS1 COMPLEX

Ataxia-telangiectasia–like disorders (ATLD) resembles mild AT in that it is associated with later age of onset and a milder clinical course of disease. ATLD is caused by hypomorphic mutations in the MRE11 gene, which is part of the MRN complex described in the earlier text. ATLD patients have normal ATM levels but decreased amounts of the MRE11 protein.

Although *Nijmegen breakage syndrome*, also known as *AT variant 1*, is due to a deficiency in another part of the MRN complex, its neurologic manifestations are very different from AT, with microcephaly and mental retardation but not ataxia, ocular apraxia, or telangiectasia. Interestingly, the cellular manifestations mimic that of AT, with radiosensitivity and chromosome 7;14 translocations.

There are several AR ataxias presumed due to deficiencies in single-strand DNA (SSDNA) repair. Unlike AT and disorders of DSDNA repair, these do not appear to be associated with predisposition to cancer and, hence, are felt to attack primarily nondividing cells.

ATAXIA WITH OCULOMOTOR APRAXIA 1

AOA resembles AT and can be divided into two subtypes, AOA1 and AOA2. AOA1, also known as *hereditary motor and sensory neuropathy associated with cerebellar atrophy* (HMSNCA) and as early-onset ataxia with oculomotor apraxia and hypoalbuminemia, is characterized by slowly progressive childhood-onset ataxia with subsequent oculomotor apraxia and a severe axonal motor neuropathy. The mean age at onset is 4 to 7 years and typically ranges from 2 to 16 years. The disease begins with gait instability, which is followed by dysarthria and appendicular ataxia and tremor. The oculomotor apraxia presents with limitation of ocular movements on command, abnormal fixation and head movement which precede eye contraversion, and hypometric saccades. This usually progresses to external ophthalmoplegia with vertical gaze lost first. The neuropathy begins with generalized areflexia and then proceeds to weakness followed by quadriplegia, wasting, and loss of ambulation. Usually, hands and feet are short and atrophic, and pes cavus is present in approximately 30%. Chorea is very common (approximately 80% of cases) and often regresses. Arm dystonia is present in approximately 50% of cases. Although cognition is normal in some, in others, there may be late cognitive decline. This has been described as a dysexecutive syndrome due to frontocerebellar pathway dysfunction. Although most patients are no longer ambulatory after 11 years of disease, some patients have had the disease as long as 20 years before needing a wheelchair. There are also occasional late-onset cases beginning at 28 and 29 years. There is generally a long life span, with survival to age 71 years.

Pathologically, there is cerebellar atrophy with marked significant Purkinje cell loss and posterior column and spinocerebellar tract degeneration as well as axonal neuropathy with marked loss of myelinated fibers. Hypoalbuminemia is present in 83% of individuals who have had the disease more than 10 to 15 years, and hypercholesterolemia is present in 70% of patients with disease of this duration. Milder forms with later age of onset, without apraxia and hypoalbuminemia and with pyramidal features, have been described. Diagnosis is based on MRI findings that demonstrate cerebellar atrophy in all and electromyogram (EMG)/nerve conduction (NC) studies that show axonal neuropathy, clinical features, and the exclusion of FRDA, AT, and AVED. In contrast to AT, AFP levels are normal.

The causative gene, *APTX*, encodes apraxin, which may play a role in the repair of SSDNA. SSDNA breaks are believed to be common and elicited by endogenous processes, occurring as metabolic intermediates or as sequelae of oxidative stress. Apraxin is a nuclear protein that catalyzes the hydrolysis of adenylate groups from 59 phosphate termini at nicks and gaps of SSDNA, thereby helping repair breaks. Unlike AT, the symptomatology is limited to the nervous system. Although the cells are not radiosensitive using the CSA for AT, they are sensitive to agents associated with SSDNA breaks, such as hydrogen peroxide. Most individuals have homozygous truncating mutations, although missense mutations have been reported, and these may be associated with later onset.

ATAXIA WITH OCULOMOTOR APRAXIA 2

A second form of AOA, AOA2 is associated with elevated AFP, like AT, but the increases are moderate (fivefold) compared with AT (10-fold increase). Symptoms of ataxia begin with gait imbalance and onset at a later age than AT and AOA1 (usually between 11 and 22 years, with mean age of onset of 15.6 years and a range of 3 to 30 years) and are the prominent cause of early disability. Oculomotor apraxia occurs frequently (approximately 47% of individuals) but less often than AOA1. Movement disorders, particularly arm dystonia, chorea, and head or arm tremor, are common, with dystonia or chorea in 40%. Unlike AOA1, these are less likely to regress. Later, axonal sensory neuropathy with pes cavus is frequent, occurring in over 90% of cases. It is usually moderate in severity, leading to less disability than in AOA1 but nonetheless affects function. No extraneurologic features except early menopause have been reported.

Elevated AFP is present in over 90% of cases. Serum cholesterol is elevated in approximately 50% of cases. Serum creatine kinase may be elevated, and increased IgG and IgA have been reported in some families. In contrast to AT, ATM protein levels are normal. MRI demonstrates marked cerebellar atrophy. EMG/NC show axonal sensorimotor neuropathy. Sural nerve biopsy demonstrates axonal neuropathy with preferential loss of large myelinated fibers. Cerebellar atrophy is most prominent in the vermis and anterior lobe and with gracile and cuneate demyelination.

AOA2 is secondary to mutations in the gene encoding senataxin, an ortholog of yeast RNA helicase. ALS4 (amyotrophic lateral sclerosis 4) is also due to mutations in *SETX*. The disease is attributed to faulty repair in SSDNA breaks.

SPINOCEREBELLAR ATAXIA WITH AXONAL NEUROPATHY

SCAN1 clinically mimics FRDA, with ataxia, axonal sensorimotor polyneuropathy, distal atrophy, and pes cavus. SCAN1 differs from other DNA repair disorders in that it is not associated with oculomotor apraxia. It was first reported in a Saudi Arabian family and is characterized by prominent ataxia and peripheral axonal and sensory neuropathy resembling Charcot–Marie–Tooth. Symptoms usually begin in the second decade (13 to 15 years) with slowly progressive cerebellar ataxia with gait imbalance. Subsequently, nystagmus and dysarthria develop. These are followed by areflexia and sensory loss, with pain and touch involved initially, and later loss of vibratory sense ensues. Steppage gait develops, and most patients become wheelchair dependent. Mild hypoalbuminemia and mild hypercholesterolemia may occur. Like AOA1, pathology is limited to the nervous system, and there is no associated cancer predisposition. SCAN1 is caused by homozygous mutation in the *TDP1* gene, which is integral for TDP1 function to remove DNA-bound topoisomerase 1 and is important in SSDNA repair.

Finally, other AR ataxias which are associated with DNA repair include Cockayne syndrome and xeroderma pigmentosum.

Other Autosomal Recessive Ataxias

Autosomal recessive cerebellar ataxia 1 (ARCA1), described in a French Canadian cohort, is characterized by dysarthria, cerebellar atrophy, slow saccades in approximately 30%, and brisk reflexes. Age of onset is older than most AR ataxias, with mean age of 30 years (range 17 to 46 years), and it has slow progression. It is due to mutations in the *SYNE* gene, which encodes synaptic nuclear envelope protein, believed responsible for cytoskeleton integrity, and which may alter glutamate signaling.

ARSACS is phenotypically similar to the hereditary spastic paraplegias. ARSACS is an early childhood-onset disorder (12 to 18 months) characterized by ataxia, spasticity, dysarthria, distal muscle wasting, distal sensorimotor neuropathy mainly in the legs, and horizontal gaze nystagmus. Yellow streaks of hypermyelination, known as *retinal striations*, are noted in Quebec-born patients. Although initially described in eastern Canada, families in Japan, Italy, and Tunisia have now been reported, and the gene may be responsible for more cases of childhood-onset ataxia than previously recognized. The gene encodes a novel protein, sacsin, which is similar to heat shock chaperone proteins, and although its

function is not well understood, it may play a role in chaperone-mediated protein folding.

Another early-onset recessive ataxia is the *Marinesco–Sjögren syndrome*, characterized by infantile onset, ataxia, bilateral cataracts, mental retardation, and short stature. It is due to mutations in *SIL1* encoding the SIL1 protein, which leads to disturbed chaperone dysfunction and disturbed protein folding. Other rare AR conditions include ataxia with pigmentary retinopathy, ataxia with deafness, and ataxia with hypogonadism.

The *Ramsay Hunt syndrome* is an etiologically heterogeneous syndrome characterized by myoclonus and progressive ataxia. It is most commonly a result of the mitochondrial syndrome MERRF.

The AR disorder Unverricht–Lundborg disease, or progressive myoclonus epilepsy (PME) type 1, which maps to chromosome 21q, may also cause Ramsay Hunt syndrome. The PME type 1 gene encodes cystatin B, which acts within cells to block the action of cathepsins, proteases that degrade other cell proteins.

Additional etiologies of AR ataxias are listed in Table 79.2.

X-linked Hereditary Ataxias

X-linked inherited ataxias are rare except for the FXTAS associated with premutation expansions (55 to 200 CGG repeats) in the fragile X mental retardation gene (*FMR1*), which causes fragile X syndrome in the full mutation range (>200 repeats). This late-onset disorder of adult male carriers of premutation alleles has the core features of ataxia and intention or postural tremor. Additionally, there may be short-term memory loss, executive functional deficits, parkinsonism, peripheral neuropathy, proximal leg weakness, and autonomic dysfunction. Patients present after the age of 50 years, with a mean age of 60 years. MRI for most patients shows increased T2 signal at the middle cerebellar peduncles (MCP sign). Cerebral and cerebellar atrophy as well as increased T2 signal in deep and subependymal white matter may also be seen. Intranuclear, neuronal, and astrocytic inclusions are present in the brain and brain stem.

Penetrance is age related with 75% of male carriers older than 80 years expressing signs. Penetrance in female carriers is much lower, with infrequent cases of neurologic dysfunction, although there is a high rate of premature ovarian failure. The frequency of premutation carriers is 1:259 in women and 1:813 in men. Because of the high prevalence, it has been suggested that FXTAS may be one of the leading causes of neurodegenerative disease in men. However, the phenotype appears one of primarily ataxia plus the other features rather than with parkinsonism or tremor as the predominant early feature.

Rare syndromes of pure ataxia and spastic paraparesis with ataxia beginning in childhood, adolescence, or early adult years have an X-linked recessive pattern. An infant-onset X-linked form includes ataxia, deafness, optic atrophy, and hypotonia. X-linked sideroblastic anemia and ataxia is due to a mutation in ABC7, a mitochondrial iron transport protein. It may result in a nonprogressive or slowly progressive ataxia in boys, and anemia may be asymptomatic.

Diagnostic Evaluation of Early-onset Recessive Ataxia

The diagnostic workup of a patient with early-onset recessive ataxia depends on the constellation of clinical features in the family. If FRDA genetic testing is negative, other causes of sporadic or recessive ataxia need to be considered (see Table 79.2). Peripheral blood evaluation includes assessment of vitamin E, AFP, hexosaminidase A, very long-chain fatty acids and lipids, Igs, lactate and pyruvate, ceruloplasmin, and thyroid function. Additional studies including screens for amino and organic acids, biotinidase, ammonia level, phytanic acid, electron microscopy (EM) for curvilinear bodies, and mitochondrial mutation screening may be indicated depending on clinical features. EMG/NC studies may help delineate the presence of a peripheral neuropathy and distinguish axonal from demyelinating neuropathy. Ophthalmologic evaluation may assist in diagnosis of retinitis pigmentosa, cataracts, and cherry-red spots. Depending on clinical features, skin or muscle biopsy may be warranted, for example targeting Niemann–Pick disease, type C (NPC), CoQ10 deficiency, and mitochondrial disorders. Finally, clinical molecular genetic testing is also available for AVED, abetalipoproteinemia, Refsum, AT, AOA1 and AOA2, POLG, and SACS, as well as the ADCA, which can occasionally present as sporadic or recessive disease.

OVERALL TESTING CONSIDERATIONS

Recommendations regarding testing include exclusion of acquired causes as noted earlier and focus depending on ethnicity, type of family history (dominant appearing, if parent–child inheritance, or recessive appearing if siblings only), age at onset of ataxia, and phenotype, especially features in addition to ataxia. Differences in ethnic groups, which are primarily due to founder mutations, are delineated in the suggested readings and may suggest prioritizing for particular genetic etiologies. Further, although some features strongly suggest certain etiologies, such as maculopathy in SCA7 and with prominent features described in Tables 79.1 and 79.2, there is tremendous overlap, and molecular genetic testing is often required for diagnosis. Clinical molecular genetic testing is available for the ADCAs for SCA1, SCA2, SCA3, SCA5, SCA6, SCA7, SCA8, SCA10, SCA11, SCA12, SCA13, SCA14, SCA17, and DRPLA; for the episodic ataxias: EA1, EA2, and EA5; and the AR ataxias: AT, FRDA, AOA1, AOA2, MSS, AVED, FXTAS, and ARSACS.

If there is a positive dominant-appearing family history, in general, screening should be considered for the more common ADCAs, SCA1, 2, 3, 6, and 7 and in those of Asian descent, DRPLA as well. For recessive-appearing family history, focus first on Friedreich, then ataxiatelangiectasia, ataxia due to vitamin E deficiency, mitochondrial etiology including POLG and ataxia with oculomotor apraxia (AOA) types 1 and 2, and ARSACS. With onset older than age 45 years, screening for fragile X mental retardation 1 FMR1 premutations should be considered (see also Chapter 34, Genetic Testing and DNA Diagnosis).

TREATMENT OF HEREDITARY ATAXIAS

Treatment of hereditary ataxias is focused on (1) treatment of identified deficits, such as vitamin E and biotin in AVED and biotinidase deficiency, and dietary restriction, such as of phytanic acid in Refsum; (2) supportive therapies for ataxia as well as comorbid features of a syndrome, such as lioresal for spasticity or botulinum toxin therapy for dystonia; (3) genetic counseling; (4) avoidance of toxins in certain conditions, such as unnecessary ionizing radiation in AT; and (5) pharmacotherapeutics directed to the ataxia, which are generally limited thus far.

Supportive therapies vary depending on the disorder but often include proper aids for mobility such as canes/walkers or wheelchairs as needed, ramps for wheelchairs, grab bars for safety, and weighted eating utensils. Physical therapy and occupational therapy may improve quality of life. In FRDA, orthopedic procedures are indicated for the relief of foot deformity. Speech and swallowing evaluations and therapy are usually indicated, including communication devices when needed. Additional supportive therapy includes treatment of conditions which may accompany the ataxia, including spasticity, movement disorders, bladder issues, depression, and pain. For example, levodopa may bring symptomatic relief of the parkinsonian features of rigidity, tremor, and bradykinesia; Lioresal or tizanidine may help spasticity. Doses are those used for respective treatment of parkinsonism and spasticity.

No specific pharmacologic treatments definitively benefit the hereditary ataxias. Symptomatic relief may occur for both riluzole (100 mg/day) and amantadine (300 mg/day), although level of evidence is not high (level B for riluzole and level C for amantadine). For FRDA, it has been suggested that antioxidant therapies may slow progression, especially cardiac manifestations, and, as noted, promising therapies are emerging but are not yet proven. Thus far, idebenone has not been demonstrated helpful. Varenicline (2 mg/day) may benefit SCA3 (level B evidence). Acetazolamide (1,000 mg/day) can control the attacks of the episodic paroxysmal cerebellar ataxias (EA1 and EA2), and phenytoin (200 mg/day) ameliorates the facial and hand myokymia associated with EA1. We can hope for novel specific therapies based on our increasing knowledge of the molecular mechanisms underlying the hereditary ataxias.

Videos can be found in the companion e-book edition. For a full list of video legends, please see the front matter.

SUGGESTED READINGS

Aicardi J, Barbosa C, Andermann E, et al. Ataxia-oculomotor apraxia: a syndrome mimicking ataxia-telangiectasia. *Ann Neurol.* 1988;24:497–502.

Alterman N, Fattal-Valevski A, Moyal L, et al. Ataxia-telangiectasia: mild neurological presentation despite null ATM and severe cellular phenotype. *Am J Med Genet A.* 2007;143A(16):1827–1834.

Ashizawa T, Figueroa KP, Perlman SL, et al. Clinical characteristics of patients with spinocerebellar ataxias 1, 2, 3 and 6 in the US; a prospective observational study. *Orphanet J Rare Dis.* 2013;8:177.

Ashley CN, Hoang KD, Lynch DR, et al. Childhood ataxia: clinical features, pathogenesis, key unanswered questions, and future directions. *J Child Neurol.* 2012;27:1095.

Bailus BJ, Segal DJ. The prospect of molecular therapy for Angelman syndrome and other monogenic neurologic disorders. *BMC Neuroscience.* 2014;15:76.

Benton CS, de Silva R, Rutledge SL, et al. Molecular/clinical studies in SCA 7 define a broad clinical spectrum and infantile phenotype. *Neurology.* 1998;51:1081–1085.

Bidichandani SI, Delatycki MB. Friedreich ataxia. GeneReviews Web site. http://www.ncbi.nlm.nih.gov/books/NBK1281/. Accessed April 28, 2015.

Biesecker LG, Green RC. Diagnostic clinical genome and exome sequencing. *N Engl J Med.* 2014;370:2418–2425.

Bird T. Hereditary ataxia overview. GeneReviews Web site. http://www.ncbi.nlm.nih.gov/books/NBK1138/. Accessed April 28, 2015.

Botez MI, Botez-Marquard T, Elie R, et al. Amantadine hydrochloride treatment in heredodegenerative ataxias: a double blind study. *J Neurol Neurosurg Psychiatry.* 1996;61:259–264.

Botez MI, Young SN, Botez T, et al. Treatment of heredo-degenerative ataxias with amantadine hydrochloride. *Can J Neurol Sci.* 1991;18:307–311.

Broccoletti T, Del Giudice E, Amorosi S, et al. Steroid-induced improvement of neurological signs in ataxia-telangiectasia patients. *Eur J Neurol.* 2008;15:223–228.

Bromley D, Anderson PC, Daggett V. Structural consequences of mutations to the α-tocopherol transfer protein associated with the neurodegenerative disease ataxia with vitamin E deficiency. *Biochemistry.* 2013;52:4264.

Brunt EP, van Weerden TW. Familial paroxysmal kinesigenic ataxia and continuous myokymia. *Brain.* 1990;113:1361–1382.

Brussino A, Brusco A, Durr A. Spinocerebellar ataxia type 28. GeneReviews Web site. http://www.ncbi.nlm.nih.gov/books/NBK54582/. Accessed April 28, 2015.

Campuzano V, Montermini L, Molto MD, et al. Friedreich's ataxia: autosomal recessive disease caused by an intronic triplet repeat expansion. *Science.* 1996;271:1374–1375.

Carlson KM, Andresen JM, Orr HT. Emerging pathogenic pathways in the spinocerebellar ataxias. *Curr Opin Genet Dev.* 2009;19:247.

Cavalier L, Ouahchi K, Kayden HJ, et al. Ataxia with isolated vitamin E deficiency: heterogeneity of mutations and phenotypic variability in a large number of families. *Am J Hum Genet*. 1998;62:301–310.

Chung MY, Soong BW. Reply to: SCA-19 and SCA-22: evidence for one locus with a worldwide distribution. *Brain*. 2004;127:E7.

Crosby AH, Patel H, Chioza BA, et al. Defective mitochondrial mRNA maturation is associated with spastic ataxia. *Am J Hum Genet*. 2010;87:655–660.

Da Pozzo P, Cardaioli E, Malfatti E, et al. A novel mutation in the mitochondrial tRNA(Pro) gene associated with late-onset ataxia, retinitis pigmentosa, deafness, leukoencephalopathy and complex I deficiency. *Eur J Hum Genet*. 2009;17:1092–1096.

Date H, Onodera O, Tanaka H, et al. Early-onset ataxia with ocular motor apraxia and hypoalbuminemia is caused by mutations in a new HIT superfamily gene. *Nat Genet*. 2001;29:184–188.

de Bot ST, Willemsen MA, Vermeer S, et al. Reviewing the genetic causes of spastic-ataxias. *Neurology*. 2012;79:1507–1514.

de Vries B, Mamsa H, Stam AH, et al. Episodic ataxia associated with EAAT1 mutation C186S affecting glutamate reuptake. *Arch Neurol*. 2009;66:97–101.

Delatycki MB, Corben LA. Clinical features of Friedreich ataxia. *J Child Neurol*. 2012;27:1133.

Depondt C, Donatello S, Simonis N, et al. Autosomal recessive cerebellar ataxia of adult onset due to STUB1 mutations. *Neurology*. 2014;82:1749–1750.

Di Gregorio E, Borroni B, Giorgio E, et al. ELOVL5 mutations cause spinocerebellar ataxia 38. *Am J Hum Genet*. 2014;95:209.

Di Prospero NA, Baker A, Jeffries N, et al. Neurological effects of high-dose idebenone in patients with Friedreich's ataxia: a randomized placebo controlled trial. *Lancet Neurol*. 2007;6:878–886.

Didelot A, Honnorat J. Paraneoplastic disorders of the central and peripheral nervous systems. *Handb Clin Neurol*. 2014;121:1159–1179.

Duarri A, Jezierska J, Fokkens M, et al. Mutations in potassium channel kcnd3 cause spinocerebellar ataxia type 19. *Ann Neurol*. 2012;72(6):870–880.

Dupre N, Gros-Louis F, Bouchard J, et al. SYNE1-related autosomal recessive cerebellar ataxia. GeneReviews Web site. http://www.ncbi.nlm.nih.gov/books/NBK1379/. Accessed April 28, 2015.

Durr A. Autosomal dominant cerebellar ataxias: polyglutamine expansions and beyond. *Lancet Neurol*. 2010;9:885–894.

Elsayed SM, Heller R, Thoenes M, et al. Autosomal dominant SCA5 and autosomal recessive infantile SCA are allelic conditions resulting from SPTBN2 mutations. *Eur J Hum Genet*. 2013;22:286–288.

Engert JC, Berube P, Mercier J, et al. ARSACS, a spastic ataxia common in northeastern Quebec, is caused by mutations in a new gene encoding an 11.5-kb ORF. *Nat Genet*. 2000;24:120–125.

Fernandez-Alvarez E, Perez-Duena B. Paroxysmal movement disorders and episodic ataxias. *Handb Clin Neurol*. 2013;112:847–852.

Finsterer J. Mitochondrial ataxias. *Can J Neurol Sci*. 2009;36:543–553.

Flanigan K, Gardner K, Alderson K, et al. Autosomal dominant spinocerebellar ataxia with sensory axonal neuropathy (SCA4): clinical description and genetic localization to chromosome 16q22.1. *Am J Hum Genet*. 1996;59:392–399.

Fogel BL. Childhood cerebellar ataxia. *J Child Neurol*. 2012;27:1138.

Friedreich N. Uber Ataxic mit besonderer Berucksichtigung der hereditaren Formen. *Virchows Arch Pathol Anat*. 1863;26:391–419, 433–459; 27:1–26.

Fujigasaki H, Martin JJ, De Deyn PP, et al. CAG repeat expansion in the TATA box-binding protein gene causes autosomal dominant cerebellar ataxia. *Brain*. 2001;124:1939–1947.

Fujioka S, Sundal C, Wszolek ZK. Autosomal dominant cerebellar ataxia type III: a review of the phenotypic and genotypic characteristics. *Orphanet J Rare Dis*. 2013;8:14.

Fukuhara N, Nakajima T, Sakajiri K, et al. Hereditary motor and sensory neuropathy associated with cerebellar atrophy (HMSNCA): a new disease. *J Neurol Sci*. 1995;133:140–151.

Gatti RA. Ataxia-telangiectasia. GeneReviews Web site. http://www.ncbi.nlm.nih.gov/books/NBK26468/. Accessed April 28, 2015.

Gomez CM. Spinocerebellar ataxia type 6. GeneReviews Web site. http://www.ncbi.nlm.nih.gov/books/NBK1140/. Accessed April 28, 2015.

Gotoda T, Arita M, Arai H, et al. Adult-onset spinocerebellar dysfunction caused by a mutation in the gene for the alpha tocopherol transfer protein. *N Engl J Med*. 1995;333:1313–1318.

Hadjivassiliou M, Duker AP, Sanders DS. Gluten-related neurologic dysfunction. *Handb Clin Neurol*. 2014;120:607–619.

Hall DA, O'Keefe JA. Fragile X-associated tremor ataxia syndrome: the expanding clinical picture, pathophysiology, epidemiology, and update on treatment. *Tremor Other Hyperkinet Mov*. 2012;2.

Harding AE. Clinical features and classification of inherited ataxias. *Adv Neurol*. 1993;61:1–14.

Harding AE. Friedreich's ataxia: a clinical and genetic study of 90 families with an analysis of early diagnostic criteria and intrafamilial clustering of clinical features. *Brain*. 1981;104:589–620.

Higgins JJ, Morton DH, Loveless JM. Posterior column ataxia with retinitis pigmentosa (AXPC1) maps to chromosome 1q31-q32. *Neurology*. 1999;52:146–150.

Ikeda Y, Dalton JC, Moseley ML, et al. Spinocerebellar ataxia type 8: molecular genetic comparisons and haplotype analysis of 37 families with ataxia. *Amer J Hum Gen*. 2004;75:3.

Ikeda Y, Dick KA, Weatherspoon MR, et al. Spectrin mutations cause spinocerebellar ataxia type 5. *Nat Genet*. 2006;38:184–190.

Ishiura H, Fukuda Y, Mitsui J, et al. Posterior column ataxia with retinitis pigmentosa in a Japanese family with a novel mutation in LVCR1. *Neurogenetics*. 2011;12:117–121.

Jacobi H, Bauer P, Giunti P, et al. The natural history of spinocerebellar ataxia type 1, 2, 3, and 6. *Neurology*. 2011;77:1035.

Jen JC, Graves TD, Hess EJ, et al. Primary episodic ataxias: diagnosis, pathogenesis and treatment. *Brain*. 2007;130:2484–2493.

Jodice C, Mantuano E, Veneziano L, et al. Episodic ataxia type 2 (EA2) and spinocerebellar ataxia type 6 (SCA6) due to CAG repeat expansion in the CACNA I A gene on chromosome l9p. *Hum Mol Genet*. 1997;11:1973–1978.

Johansson J, Forsgren L, Sandgren O, et al. Expanded CAG repeats in Swedish spinocerebellar ataxia type 7 (SCA7) patients: effect of CAG repeat length on the clinical manifestation. *Hum Mol Genet*. 1998;7:171–176.

Kearney M, Orrell RW, Fahey M, et al. Antioxidants and other pharmacological treatments for Friedreich ataxia. *Cochrane Database Syst Rev*. 2012;4:CD007791.

Kersten HM, Roxburgh RH, Danesh-Meyer HV. Ophthalmic manifestations of inherited neurodegenerative disorders. *Nature*. 2014;10:349.

Kim JY, Park SS, Joo SI, et al. Molecular analysis of spinocerebellar ataxias in Koreans: frequencies and reference ranges of SCA1, SCA2, SCA3, SCA6, and SCA7. *Mol Cells*. 2001;12:336–341.

Kinali M, Jungbluth H, Eunson LH, et al. Expanding the phenotype of potassium channelopathy: severe neuromyotonia and skeletal deformities without prominent episodic ataxia. *Neuromuscul Disord*. 2004;14:689–693.

Klein CH, Bird TD, Ertekin-Taner N, et al. DNMT1 mutation hot spot causes varied phenotypes of HSAN1 with dementia and hearing loss. *Neurology*. 2013;80:824–828.

Klockgether T. Sporadic adult-onset ataxia of unknown etiology. *Handb Clin Neurol*. 2012;103:253–262.

Klockgether T. Update on degenerative ataxias. *Curr Opin Neurol*. 2011;24:339–345.

Klockgether T, Ludtke R, Kramer B, et al. The natural history of degenerative ataxia: a retrospective study in 466 patients. *Brain*. 1998;121(pt 4):589–600.

Klockgether T, Paulson H. Milestones in ataxia. *Mov Dis*. 2011;26:1134.

Koeppen AH, Mazurkiewicz JE. Friedreich ataxia: neuropathology revised. *J Neuropath Exp Neurol*. 2013;72:78.

Kotagal V. Acetazolamide-responsive ataxia. *Semin Neurol*. 2012;32(5):533–537.

Kulkarni A, Wilson D. The involvement of DNA-damage and -repair defects in neurological dysfunction. *Am J Hum Genet*. 2008;82:539–566.

Lamperti C, Naini A, Hirano M, et al. Cerebellar ataxia and coenzyme Q10 deficiency. *Neurology*. 2003;60:1206–1208.

Le Ber I, Moreira MC, Rivaud-Pechoux S, et al. Cerebellar ataxia with oculomotor apraxia type 1: clinical and genetic studies. *Brain*. 2003;126:2761–2672.

Lhatoo SD, Rao DG, Kane NM, et al. Very late onset Friedreich's presenting as spastic tetraparesis without ataxia or neuropathy. *Neurology*. 2001;56:1776–1777.

Lin IS, Wu RM, Lee-Chen GJ, et al. The SCA17 phenotype can include features of MSA-C, PSP and cognitive impairment. *Parkinsonism Relat Disord*. 2007;13:246–249.

Mantuano E, Veneziano L, Jodice C, et al. Spinocerebellar ataxia type 6 and episodic ataxia type 2: differences and similarities between two allelic disorders. *Cytogenet Genome Res*. 2003;100:147–153.

Mariotti C, Solari A, Torta D, et al. Idebenone treatment in Friedreich patients: one-year-long randomized placebo-controlled trial. *Neurology*. 2003;60:1676–1679.

Martino D, Stamelou M, Bhatia KP. The differential diagnosis of Huntington's disease-like syndromes: "red flags" for the clinician. *J Neurol Neuro Psych*. 2013;84:650.

Matsuura T, Ranum LP, Volpini V, et al. Spinocerebellar ataxia type 10 is rare in populations other than Mexicans. *Neurology*. 2002;58:983–984.

Matsuura T, Yamagata T, Burgess DL, et al. Large expansion of the ATTCT pentanucleotide repeat in spinocerebellar ataxia type 10. *Nat Genet*. 2000;26:191–194.

Miyatake S, Osaka H, Shiina M, et al. Expanding the phenotypic spectrum of TUBB4A-associated hypomyelinating leukoencephalopathies. *Neurology*. 2014;82:2230–2237.

Miyoshi Y, Yamada T, Tanimura M, et al. A novel autosomal dominant spinocerebellar ataxia (SCA16) linked to chromosome 8q22.1-24.1. *Neurology*. 2001;57:96–100.

Mollet J, Delahodde A, Serre V, et al. CABC1 gene mutations cause ubiquinone deficiency with cerebellar ataxia and seizures. *Am J Hum Genet*. 2008;82:623–630.

Mondal B, Paul P, Paul M, et al. An update on spino-cerebellar ataxias. *Ann Indian Acad Neurol*. 2013;16:295–303.

Moreira MC, Barbot C, Tachi N, et al. The gene mutated in ataxia-ocular apraxia 1 encodes the new HIT/Zn-finger protein aprataxin. *Nat Genet*. 2001;29:189–193.

Moreira MC, Klur S, Watanabe M, et al. Senataxin, the ortholog of a yeast RNA helicase, is mutant in ataxia-ocular apraxia 2. *Nat Genet*. 2004;36:225–227.

Musselman KE, Stoyanov CT, Marasigan R, et al. Prevalence of ataxia in children: a systematic review. *Neurology*. 2014;82:80–89.

Németh AH, Kwasniewska AC, Lise S, et al. Next generation sequencing for molecular diagnosis of neurological disorders using ataxias as a model. *Brain*. 2013;136:3106–3118.

O'Hearn E, Holmes SE, Calvert PC, et al. SCA-12: tremor with cerebellar and cortical atrophy is associated with a CAG repeat expansion. *Neurology*. 2001;56:299–303.

Ophoff RA, Terwindt GM, Vergouwe MN, et al. Familial hemiplegic migraine and episodic ataxia type-2 are caused by mutations in the CA2+ channel gene CACNLIA4. *Cell*. 1996;87:543–552.

Orr HT. Cell biology of spinocerebellar ataxia. *J Cell Bio*. 2012;197:167.

Palhan VB, Chen S, Peng GH, et al. Polyglutamine-expanded ataxin-7 inhibits STAGA histone acetyltransferase activity to produce retinal degeneration. *Proc Natl Acad Sci U S A*. 2005;102:8472–8477.

Pandolfo M. Friedreich ataxia. *Arch Neurol*. 2008;65:1296–1302.

Panzer J, Dalmau J. Movement disorders in paraneoplastic and autoimmune disease. *Curr Opin Neur*. 2011;24:346.

Paulson H. Machado-Joseph disease/spinocerebellar ataxia type 3. *Handb Clin Neurol*. 2011;103:437.

Paulson HL, Perez MK, Trottier PY, et al. Intranuclear inclusions of expanded polyglutamine protein in spinocerebellar ataxia type 3. *Neuron*. 1997;19:333–344.

Pfeffer G, Blakely EL, Alston CL, et al. Adult-onset spinocerebellar ataxia syndromes due to MTATP6 mutations. *J Neurol Neurosurg Psychiatry*. 2012;83:883–886.

Potter NT, Nance MA. Genetic testing for ataxia in North America. *Mol Diagn*. 2000;5:91–99.

Priller J, Scherzer CR, Faber PW, et al. Frataxin gene of Friedreich's ataxia is targeted to mitochondria. *Ann Neurol*. 1997;42:265–269.

Rajakulendran S, Schorge S, Kullmann DM, et al. Episodic ataxia type 1: a neuronal potassium channelopathy. *Neurotherapeutics*. 2007;4:258–266.

Ranurn LP, Schut LJ, Lundgren JK, et al. Spinocerebellar ataxia type 5 in a family descended from the grandparents of President Lincoln maps to chromosome 11. *Nat Genet*. 1994;8:280–284.

Renaud M, Anheim M, Kamsteeg EJ, et al. Autosomal recessive cerebellar ataxia type 3 due to ANO10 mutations: delineation and genotype-phenotype correlation study. *JAMA Neurol*. 2014;71(10):1305–1310.

Ristori G, Romano S, Visconti A, et al. Riluzole in cerebellar ataxia: a randomized, double-blind, placebo-controlled pilot trial. *Neurology*. 2010;74:839–845.

Rosenberg R, Paulson H. The inherited ataxias. In: Rosenberg RN, Prusiner SB, DiMauro S, et al, eds. *The Molecular and Genetic Basis of Neurologic and Psychiatric Disease*. Philadelphia: Butterworth-Heineman; 2003:369–382.

Rosenberg RN, Nyhan WL, Bay C, et al. Autosomal dominant striatonigral degeneration: a clinical, pathologic and biochemical study of a new genetic disorder. *Neurology*. 1976;26:703–714.

Ruano L, Melo C, Silva MC, et al. The global epidemiology of hereditary ataxia and spastic paraplegia: a systematic review of prevalence studies. *Neuroepidemiology*. 2014;42:174–183.

Rüb U, Schöls L, Paulson H, et al. Clinical features, neurogenetics and neuropathology of the polyglutamine spinocerebellar ataxias type 1, 2, 3, 6 and 7. *Prog Neurobiol*. 2013;104:38–66.

Schelhaas HJ, Verbeek DS, Van de Warrenburg BP, et al. SCA19 and SCA22: evidence for one locus with a worldwide distribution. *Brain*. 2004;127:E6.

Schöls L, Amoiridis G, Przuntek H, et al. Friedreich ataxia: revision of the phenotype according to molecular genetics. *Brain*. 1997;120:2131–2140.

Schuelke M. Ataxia with vitamin E deficiency. GeneReviews Web site. http://www.ncbi.nlm.nih.gov/books/NBK1241/. Accessed April 28, 2015.

Seidel K, Siswanto S, Brunt ER, et al. Brain pathology of spinocerebellar ataxias. *Acta Neuropathol*. 2012;124:1–21.

Shakkottai VG, Fogel BL. Clinical neurogenetics: autosomal dominant spinocerebellar ataxia. *Neurol Clin*. 2013;31:987–1007.

Stevanin G, Bouslam N, Thobois S, et al. Spinocerebellar ataxia with sensory neuropathy (SCA25) maps to chromosome 2p. *Ann Neurol*. 2004;55:97–104.

Storey E, Bahlo M, Fahey M, et al. A new dominantly inherited pure cerebellar ataxia, SCA 30. *J Neurol Neurosurg Psychiatry*. 2009;80:408–411.

Subramony SH. Approach to ataxic diseases. *Handb Clin Neurol*. 2012;103:127–134.

Subramony SH. Overview of autosomal dominant ataxias. *Handb Clin Neurol*. 2012;103:389–398.

Subramony SH, Advincula J, Perlman S, et al. Comprehensive phenotype of the p.Arg420his allelic form of spinocerebellar ataxia type 13. *Cerebellum*. 2013;12:932.

Subramony SH, Ashizawa T. Spinocerebellar ataxia type 1. GeneReviews Web site. http://www.ncbi.nlm.nih.gov/books/NBK1184/. Accessed April 28, 2015.

Tezenas du Montcel S, Durr A, Bauer P, et al. Modulation of the age at onset in spinocerebellar ataxia by CAG tracts in various genes. *Brain*. 2014;137:2444–2455.

Toyoshima Y, Onodera O, Yamada M, et al. Spinocerebellar ataxia type 17. GeneReviews Web site. http://www.ncbi.nlm.nih.gov/books/NBK1438/. Accessed April 28, 2015.

van de Warrenburg BPC, van Gaalen J, Boesch S, et al. EFNS/ENS consensus on the diagnosis and management of chronic ataxias in adulthood. *Eur J Neurol*. 2014;21:552.

van Swieten JC, Brusse E, de Graaf BM, et al. A mutation in the fibroblast growth factor 14 gene is associated with autosomal dominant cerebral ataxia. *Am J Hum Genet*. 2003;72:191–199.

Verbeek DS. Spinocerebellar ataxia type 23: a genetic update. *Cerebellum*. 2009;8:104.

Vermeer S, van de Warrenburg BP, Kamsteeg E. ARSACS. GeneReviews Web site. http://www.ncbi.nlm.nih.gov/books/NBK1255/. Accessed April 28, 2015.

Waters MF, Minassian NA, Stevanin G, et al. Mutations in voltage-gated potassium channel KCNC3 cause degenerative and developmental central nervous system phenotypes. *Nat Genet*. 2006;38:447–451.

Winchester S, Sing P, Mikati MA. Ataxia. *Handb Clin Neurol*. 2013;112:1213–1217.

Winter N, Kovermann P, Fahlke C. A point mutation associated with episodic ataxia 6 increases glutamate transporter anion currents. *Brain*. 2012;135:3416–3425.

Wolf NI, Koenig M. Progressive cerebellar atrophy: hereditary ataxias and disorders with spinocerebellar degeneration. *Handb Clin Neurol*. 2013;113:1869–1878.

Zanni G, Bertini ES. X-linked disorders with cerebellar dysgenesis. *Orphanet J Rare Dis*. 2011;6:24.

Zesiewicz TA, Greenstein PE, Sullivan KL, et al. A randomized trial of varenicline (Chantix) for the treatment of spinocerebellar ataxia type 3. *Neurology*. 2012;78:545–550.

Zesiewicz TA, Sullivan KL. Treatment of ataxia and imbalance with varenicline (Chantix): report of 2 patients with spinocerebellar ataxia (types 3 and 14). *Clin Neuropharmacol*. 2008;31:363–365.

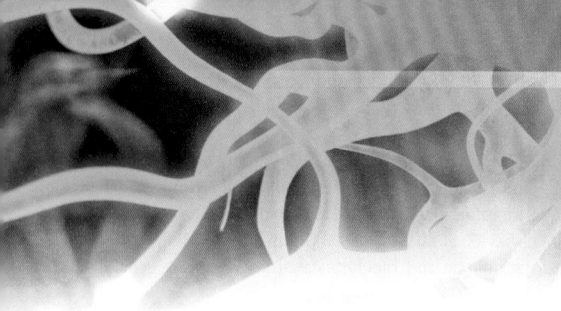

Tardive Dyskinesia and Other Neuroleptic-Induced Syndromes 80

Un Jung Kang, Robert E. Burke, and Stanley Fahn

INTRODUCTION

Antipsychotic drugs are commonly called *neuroleptics* because they often induce parkinsonism. They also cause other movement and sensory disorders, such as akathisia, acute dystonic reactions, neuroleptic malignant syndrome, and tardive dyskinesia syndromes, which are the most feared because they are persistent even after the offending drugs are discontinued (Table 80.1). The common pathophysiologic mechanism of neuroleptics is binding to and antagonizing dopamine D2 receptors. The dopamine receptor–blocking agents (DRBAs) are used not only as antipsychotic agents (e.g., the phenothiazines and the butyrophenones) but also for the treatment of gastrointestinal disorders (e.g., metoclopramide). Tardive and other neuroleptic-induced disorders are iatrogenic, and hence, the prescribing physician bears primary responsibility for causing these disorders. The physician to whom affected patients seek a consultation has the responsibility to make the diagnosis and institute appropriate treatment.

EPIDEMIOLOGY

The neuroleptic-induced neurologic complications are often referred to as *extrapyramidal syndromes* (EPS). Their prevalence ranges from 20% to 50% of exposed. Drug-induced parkinsonism is the most common form. Acute dystonic reactions occur in about 2% to 5% of patients, more commonly in younger patients and in males than females. Tardive syndromes may occur in about one-third of patients exposed to these drugs. Classic tardive dyskinesia is most common and estimates of prevalence range widely but mostly from 15% to 30% with an annual incidence rate of about 5% in the first 4 to 5 years. Prevalence and incidence increase with age; it is more severe among elderly women and more likely to occur with longer duration of exposure to antipsychotic drugs. Tardive dystonia is more rare than the classic type and is more common in younger patients. Other tardive syndromes, including tardive akathisia, account for about 10% of all tardive syndromes.

PATHOBIOLOGY

The pathogenesis of the tardive dyskinesia syndromes is not well understood. Dopamine receptor supersensitivity occurs with these agents, but other drugs that induce similar supersensitivity, such as dopamine-depleting drugs (e.g., reserpine and tetrabenazine), do not cause tardive dyskinesia. The DRBAs that bind most tightly to the receptors are the ones most likely to induce tardive dyskinesia. To explain its delayed onset and persistence, maladaptive synaptic plasticity has been proposed as an underlying mechanism. Others proposed a neurodegenerative process triggered by oxidative stress or by the drugs binding to neuromelanin with resulting internalization of the cell membrane, but all these hypotheses remain to be validated. Genetic polymorphism studies have noted association of variations of monoamine receptors or metabolism genes with tardive dyskinesia, but these findings have not been consistently replicated.

So-called atypical neuroleptics (also called *second-generation antipsychotics*) have been developed and were initially thought to reduce the incidence of the various movement disorders, but subsequent studies have noted similar incidence of these complications from both second- and first-generation antipsychotics. Some second-generation antipsychotics, however, are definitely atypical in that they have less propensity to produce these movement disorders. Clozapine (Clozaril), a drug that predominantly blocks the D4 receptor and serotonin receptor subtypes, is free of these complications, except for acute akathisia. Quetiapine is also relatively free from the adverse effects listed earlier. The dopamine-depleting drugs, reserpine and tetrabenazine, can induce acute akathisia and drug-induced parkinsonism. Tetrabenazine has also been implicated in acute dystonic reactions and neuroleptic malignant syndrome. But neither drug has been convincingly implicated in causing persistent dyskinesias. In addition, calcium channel blockers, such as flunarizine and cinnarizine, and rarely selective serotonin reuptake inhibitors and lithium can produce parkinsonism and tardive syndromes, and the mechanism by which these drugs produce these complications is not known.

CLINICAL MANIFESTATIONS

It is important to recognize the different phenomenologies caused by the DRBAs; each requires specific treatment.

TABLE 80.1	Adverse Neurologic Effects of D2 Receptor–Blocking Agents
Extrapyramidal Syndromes	
Acute dystonic reaction	
Oculogyric crisis	
Acute akathisia	
Drug-induced parkinsonism	
Neuroleptic malignant syndrome	
Tardive Dyskinesia Syndromes	
Withdrawal emergent syndrome	
Classic orobuccolingual dyskinesia (some use tardive dyskinesia to refer to the classic type)	
Tardive dystonia	
Tardive akathisia	
Tardive tics	
Tardive myoclonus	
Tardive tremor	

Acute dystonic reactions tend to occur within the first few days of exposure to the DRBA and predominantly affect children and young adults, males more than females. Severe sustained twisting and uncomfortable postures of limbs, trunk, neck, tongue, and face are dramatic. *Oculogyric crisis* is a form of dystonia in which the eyes are deviated conjugately in a fixed posture for minutes or hours. *Acute akathisia* occurs within the first few days or weeks of drug use. It may also appear later in treatment when dosage is being increased. Akathisia consists of a *subjective* sense of restlessness or aversion to being still and is associated with *motor* features of restlessness. These include frequent and repetitive stereotyped movements, such as pacing, repeatedly caressing the scalp, or crossing and uncrossing the legs. It can occur in subjects of any age. *Drug-induced parkinsonism* resembles idiopathic parkinsonism in manifesting all the cardinal signs of parkinsonism, including tremor.

The *neuroleptic malignant syndrome* is characterized by a triad of fever, signs of autonomic dysfunction (e.g., pallor, diaphoresis, blood pressure (BP) instability, tachycardia, pulmonary congestion, tachypnea), and a movement disorder (usually akinesia and rigidity). The level of consciousness may be depressed, eventually leading to stupor or coma; death may occur.

The *withdrawal emergent syndrome* may be a mild variant of tardive dyskinesia. "Emergent" implies that the symptoms emerge after abrupt cessation of the chronic use of an antipsychotic drug. The syndrome is primarily one of children, and it persists only for a few weeks before dissipating. The abnormal movements resemble those of Sydenham chorea; they are not stereotyped and repetitive, as seen in classic tardive dyskinesia.

The *persistent dyskinesia syndromes* are the most feared complications of antipsychotic medications because the symptoms are long-lasting and often permanent. *Classic tardive dyskinesia* consists of repetitive (stereotypic) movements. The lower part of the face is most often involved. This orobuccolingual dyskinesia resembles continual chewing movements, with the tongue intermittently darting out of the mouth (Video 80.1). Movements of the trunk may cause a repetitive pattern of flexion and extension (body rocking). The distal parts of the limbs may show incessant flexion–extension movements. The proximal muscles are usually spared, but respiratory dyskinesias may occur. If not accompanied by akathisia or dystonia, the patient may not be aware of the dyskinesia.

Several other important forms of tardive dyskinesia syndrome are now recognized. Unlike the classic oral dyskinesia described earlier, these other forms are frequently quite disabling. *Tardive dystonia* is a chronic dystonia caused by DRBAs (Video 80.2). Individuals of all ages are susceptible to tardive dystonia, and younger individuals are more likely to have a more severe generalized form. In older individuals, tardive dystonia is usually focal (affecting a single body part), often in the face or neck, and may remain confined to these regions or may spread to the arms and trunk. The legs are infrequently affected. Often, neck involvement consists of retrocollis and the trunk arches backward. The arms are typically rotated internally, the elbows extended, and the wrists flexed. The differential diagnosis includes all of the many causes of dystonia. Wilson disease, in particular, must be excluded specifically in any patient with psychiatric symptoms and dystonia.

Tardive akathisia is another important disabling variant of tardive dyskinesia. It is a chronic akathisia consisting of a subjective aversion to being still. Motor signs of restlessness include frequent, repeated, stereotyped movements, such as marching in place, crossing and uncrossing the legs, and repetitively rubbing the face or hair with the hand (Video 80.3). Patients may make moaning sounds. Patients may not use the word "restless" to describe their symptoms; instead, they may use expressions such as "going to jump out of my skin" or "jittery" or "exploding inside." Akathisia can be expressed as focal discomfort, such as pain. It can be an exceedingly distressing symptom. In contrast to acute akathisia, the delayed type tends to become worse when antipsychotic medication is withdrawn, similar to the worsening of classic tardive dyskinesia on discontinuance of these drugs. As with other types of tardive dyskinesia syndrome, tardive akathisia tends to persist. Usually, tardive akathisia is associated with classic oral dyskinesia. Classic tardive dyskinesia, tardive dystonia, and tardive akathisia may occur together. Less common variants of tardive dyskinesia include *tardive tics*, *tardive myoclonus*, and *tardive tremor*.

DIAGNOSIS

The diagnosis of tardive dyskinesia syndrome depends on the recognition of a typical pattern of abnormal involuntary movements or sensory symptoms plus documented use of the offending agents as discussed earlier. The symptoms should have either started while the patient was still taking the drug or within 3 months of discontinuing the drug.

Table 80.2 lists movement disorders affecting the face. Huntington disease causing chorea and oromandibular dystonia are the major differential diagnoses of the oral dyskinesias. Oromandibular dystonia is probably the most common form of spontaneous oral dyskinesia. Clinical features differentiating these disorders from classic tardive dyskinesia are presented in Table 80.3. Patients with Huntington disease are frequently treated with antipsychotic drugs; a resulting tardive dyskinesia may be superimposed on the chorea; the presence of akathisia or repetitive (stereotyped) involuntary movements suggests the additional diagnosis of tardive dyskinesia. Often, oromandibular dystonia takes the appearance of a repetitive opening and closing of the jaw as the patient attempts to overcome the muscle pulling. To discern if the repetitive movements are volitional or spontaneous, the examiner should ask the patient not to fight the movements but to let them come out as they want to. In dystonia, there will usually be a sustained contraction, such as jaw opening or clenching.

The diagnosis of drug-induced parkinsonism is based on the cardinal features of tremor at rest, bradykinesia, and rigidity, plus the history of current or recent discontinuation of a neuroleptic drug. In acute dystonic reactions, the features are sustained, twisting movements and postures of the cranial, cervical, and other body parts, plus the history of recent exposure to a DRBA. In neuroleptic malignant syndrome, the patient is usually rigid, obtunded, confused, and febrile, plus the history of recent exposure to a DRBA. Akathisia includes a sensory complaint, so the diagnosis depends on a description by the patient, plus the history of recent exposure to a DRBA. The most characteristic complaint is the inability to sit still. Often accompanying this complaint are some motor phenomenologies such as crossing and uncrossing legs, repetitive caressing of the scalp, and repetitive body rocking. The diagnosis of focal akathisia is often missed because the patient refers to the unpleasant symptom as pain. Painful or burning mouth or vagina is the most common focal akathitic complaint.

TREATMENT

Efforts should be made to prevent the tardive dyskinesia syndromes. Antipsychotic drugs should be given only when indicated, namely, to control psychosis or a few other conditions where no

TABLE 80.2 Movement Disorders Affecting Face

Chorea and Stereotypies

- **Encephalitis lethargica; postencephalitic**
- **Drug-induced**
  - Tardive dyskinesia (antipsychotics)
  - Levodopa
  - Anticholinergic drugs
  - Phenytoin intoxication
  - Antihistamines
  - Tricyclic antidepressants
- **Huntington disease**
- **Hepatocerebral degeneration**
- **Cerebellar and brain stem infarction**
- **Edentulous malocclusion**
- **Idiopathic**

Dystonia

- **Meige syndrome**
  - Complete: oromandibular dystonia plus blepharospasm
  - Incomplete syndromes
    - Mandibular dystonia
    - Orofacial dystonia
    - Lingual dystonia
    - Pharyngeal dystonia
    - Essential blepharospasm
- **Bruxism**
  - As part of a segmental or generalized dystonic syndrome

Myoclonus, Tics and Tremor

- **Facial tics**
- **Facial myoclonus of central origin**
- **Facial nerve irritability**
  - Hemifacial spasm
  - Myokymia
  - Faulty regeneration; synkinesis
- **Tremor**
  - Essential tremor of neck and jaw
  - Parkinsonian tremor of jaw, tongue, and lips
  - Idiopathic tremor of neck, jaw, tongue, or lips
  - Cerebellar tremor of neck

other effective agent has been helpful, as in some choreic disorders or tics. These drugs should not be used indiscriminately, and when they are used, the dosage and duration should be as low and as brief as possible. If the psychosis has been controlled, the physician should attempt to reduce the dosage and even try to eliminate the drug, if possible. In nonpsychotic disorders, such as tics, other drugs should be tried first, and only if they fail should a DRBA be used.

Acute dystonic reactions are easily reversible with parenteral administration of antihistamines (e.g., diphenhydramine, 50 mg intravenously), anticholinergic drugs (e.g., benztropine mesylate [Cogentin], 2 mg intramuscularly), or diazepam (5 to 7.5 mg intramuscularly). Acute akathisia disappears on discontinuance of the offending drug. Acute akathisia sometimes improves with the β-adrenergic blocker propranolol given in doses of 20 to 80 mg/day or mirtazapine (15 mg/day) [**Level 1**].[1] Drug-induced parkinsonism does not respond to levodopa, probably because the dopamine receptors are blocked and occupied by the antipsychotic agent. Oral anticholinergic drugs (trihexyphenidyl 2 to 15 mg/day) and amantadine (up to 300 mg/day) are effective. On withdrawal of the offending antipsychotic drug, the symptoms slowly disappear in weeks or months. For neuroleptic malignant syndrome, a potentially lethal condition, treatment needs to be started immediately with hospitalization, withdrawal of the antipsychotic medication, and initiating supportive therapy, including intravenous hydration and cooling. Although controlled trials have not been conducted, numerous reports suggest that dantrolene sodium, a muscle relaxant, and levodopa or direct-acting dopamine agonists may be beneficial. Carbamazepine is also effective. In most patients, the antipsychotic medication can be restarted later without recurrence of the syndrome. The withdrawal emergent syndrome is self-limiting but may take weeks to resolve. Reintroducing the antipsychotic drug and then slowly tapering the dosage can eliminate the choreic movements.

Once a tardive dyskinesia syndrome has appeared, the logical treatment approach calls for eliminating the causative agents, DRBAs, if possible. It is best to taper the offending antipsychotic drug slowly and then discontinue it rather than stopping the DRBA suddenly if tardive dyskinesia is suspected. Sudden discontinuation has often precipitated full-blown tardive dyskinesia. The dyskinesia and akathisia of tardive dyskinesia may slowly subside in months or years without need for further treatment. Although these drugs cause tardive dyskinesias, paradoxically, they also mask the movements due to their D2 receptor blockade. Reducing the dosage or discontinuing the offending drug can therefore unmask or worsen the disorder, and reinstituting the drug can suppress the movements. Tardive dyskinesias may increase transiently in the first few weeks after withdrawal. If the dyskinetic or akathitic symptoms are too distressing after stopping the DRBAs, treatment with dopamine-depleting drugs, such as tetrabenazine or reserpine, may suppress them.

If it is not possible to stop the drugs because of active psychosis, then increasing the dosage or adding a dopamine-depleting drug, such as reserpine (0.75 to 1.5 mg/day) or tetrabenazine (25 to 150 mg/day), may suppress the dyskinesia and akathisia. The dosage should be increased gradually to avoid their side effects. Addition of α-methyltyrosine (500 to 1,500 mg/day) may be necessary to relieve symptoms, but this combination is more likely to cause postural hypotension and parkinsonism. With time, these dopamine-depleting drugs may eventually be tapered and discontinued. Tardive dystonia may be treated by dopamine depletion, but unlike oral tardive dyskinesia and akathisia, it may also be treated with anticholinergic drugs. In some patients with focal tardive dystonia, treatment with botulinum toxin injections is an option.

OUTCOME

Neuroleptic-induced movement disorders improve with reduction or discontinuation of the neuroleptics. There are few published data on remission rate of tardive syndromes after complete withdrawal of DRBAs; the remission rate is low, ranging from 2% to 13%, and improvement is seen in about 20% to 30%. Those who remain

TABLE 80.3   Clinical Features of Classic Tardive Dyskinesia, Oromandibular Dystonia, and Huntington Disease

Clinical Signs	TD	OMD	HD
Type of Involuntary Movements	Stereotypic	Dystonic	Choreic
Flowing movements	0	0	+++
Repetitive movements	+++	+	±
Sustained contractions	+	+++	±
Movements of mouth	+++	+++	+
Blepharospasm	+	+++	+
Forehead chorea	±	±	++
Platysma	±	+++	±
Masticatory muscles	+++	+++	±
Nuchal muscles	+	++	±
Trunk, legs	++	0	+++
Akathisia	++	0	0
Marching in place	++	0	0
Truncal rocking	++	0	+
Motor impersistence (tongue, grip)	0	0	+++
Stuttering, ataxic gait	±	0	+++
Postural instability	0	0	+++
Effect of			
Antidopaminergics	Decrease	Decrease	Decrease
Anticholinergics	Increase	Decrease	±
Effect on			
Talking, chewing	±	+++	+
Swallowing	0	++	+++

0, not seen; ±, may be seen; +, occasionally seen; ++, usually seen; +++, almost always seen.

TD, tardive dyskinesia; OMD, oromandibular dystonia; HD, Huntington disease.

on the DRBAs may also show apparent disappearance of tardive dyskinesia in up to 60% of cases, but their symptoms are likely masked by DRBAs, and their improvement is often associated with worsening of drug-induce parkinsonism.

Videos can be found in the companion e-book edition. For a full list of video legends, please see the front matter.

LEVEL 1 EVIDENCE

1. Adler L, Angrist B, Peselow E, et al. A controlled assessment of propranolol in the treatment of neuroleptic-induced akathisia. *Br J Psychiatry.* 1986;149:42–45.

SUGGESTED READINGS

Bakker PR, de Groot IW, van Os J, et al. Long-stay psychiatric patients: a prospective study revealing persistent antipsychotic-induced movement disorder. *PLoS One.* 2011;6(10):e25588.

Bhidayasiri R, Fahn S, Weiner WJ, et al. Evidence-based guideline: treatment of tardive syndromes: report of the Guideline Development Subcommittee of the American Academy of Neurology. *Neurology.* 2013;81(5):463–469.

Burke RE, Kang UJ, Jankovic J, et al. Tardive akathisia: an analysis of clinical features and response to open therapeutic trials. *Mov Disord.* 1989;4:157–175.

Correll CU, Leucht S, Kane JM. Lower risk for tardive dyskinesia associated with second-generation antipsychotics: a systematic review of 1-year studies. *Am J Psychiatry.* 2004;161:414–425.

Dolder CR, Jeste DV. Incidence of tardive dyskinesia with typical versus atypical antipsychotics in very high risk patients. *Biol Psychiatry.* 2003;53:1142–1145.

Glazer WM, Morgenstern H, Schooler N, et al. Predictors of improvement in tardive dyskinesia following discontinuation of neuroleptic medication. *Br J Psychiatry.* 1990;157:585–592.

Henderson VW, Wooten GF. Neuroleptic malignant syndrome: a pathogenetic role for dopamine receptor blockade? *Neurology.* 1981;31:132–137.

Kenney C, Hunter C, Jankovic J. Long-term tolerability of tetrabenazine in the treatment of hyperkinetic movement disorders. *Mov Disord.* 2007;22(2):193–197.

Kane JM, Woerner M, Borenstein M, et al. Integrating incidence and prevalence of tardive dyskinesia. *Psychopharmacol Bull.* 1986;22:254–258.

Kang UJ, Burke RE, Fahn S. Natural history and treatment of tardive dystonia. *Mov Disord.* 1986;1:193–208.

Kimiagar I, Dobronevsky E, Prokhorov T, et al. Rapid improvement of tardive dyskinesia with tetrabenazine, clonazepam and clozapine combined: a naturalistic long-term follow-up study. *J Neurol.* 2012;4:660–664.

Kiriakakis V, Bhatia KP, Quinn NP, et al. The natural history of tardive dystonia: a long-term follow-up study of 107 cases. *Brain.* 1998;121:2053–2066.

Leucht S, Cipriani A, Spineli L, et al. Comparative efficacy and tolerability of 15 antipsychotic drugs in schizophrenia: a multiple-treatments meta-analysis. *Lancet.* 2013;382(9896):951–962.

Miller DD, Caroff SN, Davis SM, et al; Clinical Antipsychotic Trials of Intervention Effectiveness (CATIE) Investigators. Extrapyramidal side-effects of antipsychotics in a randomised trial. *Br J Psychiatry.* 2008;193(4):279–288.

Muscettola G, Barbato G, Pampallona S, et al. Extrapyramidal syndromes in neuroleptic-treated patients: prevalence, risk factors, and association with tardive dyskinesia. *J Clin Psychopharmacol.* 1999;19:203–208.

Oosthuizen PP, Emsley RA, Maritz JS, et al. Incidence of tardive dyskinesia in first-episode psychosis patients treated with low-dose haloperidol. *J Clin Psychiatry.* 2003;64:1075–1080.

Paulsen JS, Caligiuri MP, Palmer B, et al. Risk factors for orofacial and limbtruncal tardive dyskinesia in older patients: a prospective longitudinal study. *Psychopharmacology (Berl).* 1996;123:307–314.

Peña MS, Yaltho TC, Jankovic J. Tardive dyskinesia and other movement disorders secondary to aripiprazole. *Mov Disord.* 2011;26(1):147–152.

Poyurovsky M, Bergman J, Pashinian A, et al. Beneficial effect of low-dose mirtazapine in acute aripiprazole-induced akathisia. *Int Clin Psychopharmacol.* 2014;29(5):296–298.

Seeman P. Dopamine D2 receptors as treatment targets in schizophrenia. *Clin Schizophr Relat Psychoses.* 2010;4(1):56–73.

Seeman P, Tallerico T. Antipsychotic drugs which elicit little or no parkinsonism bind more loosely than dopamine to brain D2 receptors, yet occupy high levels of these receptors. *Mol Psychiatry.* 1998;3:123–134.

Seeman P, Tinazzi M. Loss of dopamine neuron terminals in antipsychotic-treated schizophrenia; relation to tardive dyskinesia. *Prog Neuropsychopharmacol Biol Psychiatry.* 2013;44:178–183.

Smith JM, Baldessarini RJ. Changes in prevalence, severity, and recovery in tardive dyskinesia with age. *Arch Gen Psychiatry.* 1980;37:1368–1373.

Choreas 81

Joseph Jankovic and Stanley Fahn

INTRODUCTION

Chorea is a hyperkinetic movement disorder characterized by continual, jerk-like movements that flow randomly from one body part to another. Patients may be able to partially suppress the involuntary movements or "camouflage" them by incorporating them into semipurposeful activities (parakinesia). As a result of chorea, patients have difficulty maintaining a sustained voluntary contraction, such as tongue protrusion or a persistent hand grip, resulting in intermittent contractions and relaxations (milkmaid grip). Chorea should be differentiated from "pseudochoreoathetosis" due to loss of proprioception. Choreic movements can be associated with many disorders; the most common are listed in Table 81.1.

SYDENHAM DISEASE AND OTHER CHILDHOOD CHOREAS

In 1686, Thomas Sydenham described the chorea now known by his name but originally called *St. Vitus dance*. His description was of children with a halting gait and jerky movements. Sydenham disease (acute chorea, St. Vitus dance, chorea minor, rheumatic chorea) is a disease of childhood characterized by chorea, which is often asymmetric or may be unilateral (hemichorea) in about 20% of the cases (Video 81.1). The abnormal movements give the child a restless appearance. The chorea, with some exceptions, is self-limited and fatalities are rare except as a result of cardiac complications. Because chorea is only one of many manifestations, including a variety of neurologic, psychiatric, cardiac, rheumatologic, and other problems, the term *Sydenham disease* is more appropriate than calling the disorder *Sydenham chorea*, an earlier term.

ETIOLOGY AND PATHOBIOLOGY

Sydenham disease is considered an autoimmune disorder, a consequence of infection with group A β-hemolytic *Streptococcus*. Unlike arthritis and carditis, which occur soon after the infection, chorea may be delayed for 6 months or longer. The *Streptococcus* is thought to induce antibodies that cross-react with neuronal cytoplasmic antigens of caudate and subthalamic nuclei, which apparently account for the symptoms characteristic of rheumatic chorea. These antineuronal antibodies are found in the serum of nearly all patients with Sydenham disease. Antibodies to cardiolipin, which have been found in chorea associated with lupus erythematosus, have not been found in Sydenham chorea. Postmortem changes in rare fatal cases that came to autopsy can be attributed to embolic phenomena due to associated carditis. A mild degree of inflammatory reaction has been found in a few patients.

Knowledge of the etiology and immunology of Sydenham chorea has spawned the concept of other pediatric autoimmune neuropsychiatric disorders associated with streptococcal infection (PANDAS) and pediatric acute-onset neuropsychiatric syndrome (PANS). There is, however, considerable debate among the experts about the pathophysiologic mechanisms of PANDAS and PANS and its possible relationship to other movement disorders, including tics.

INCIDENCE

The incidence of Sydenham disease had fallen dramatically with the introduction of antibiotics and with better sanitary conditions. It now is encountered infrequently in developed countries, but it is still common in developing countries. Acute chorea is almost exclusively a disease of childhood; over 80% of the cases occur in patients between the age of 5 and 15 years. Onset of the first attack after the age of 15 years is uncommon. After spontaneous remission, some female patients have a recurrence during pregnancy, so-called chorea gravidarum, or with the use of oral contraceptives in the late teens and early 20s. All races are affected. Girls are affected more than twice as frequently as boys. The disease occurs at all times of the year but seems to be less common in summer.

CLINICAL FEATURES

In addition to the choreic movements and accompanying motor impersistence (inability to sustain certain simple voluntary acts such as protruding the tongue), Sydenham disease is associated with a variety of neurobehavioral problems, such as irritability; emotional lability; anxiety; obsessive–compulsive behavior and other neuropsychiatric manifestations; speech impairment; and, more rarely, encephalopathy, reflex changes, weakness, gait disturbance, headache, seizures, and cranial neuropathy.

The clinical features of the chorea in Sydenham disease differ from chorea in patients with Huntington disease (HD). In Sydenham, the chorea is manifested by a restless-appearing motor behavior, whereas in HD, the chorea consists of more isolated, jerky movements that become more flowing as the chorea worsens. Physiologic recordings in Sydenham chorea reveal the bursts of electromyographic (EMG) activity to last more than 100 milliseconds and to occur asynchronously in antagonistic muscles. These findings are in contrast to the chorea associated with HD, in which more frequent and shorter EMG bursts of 10 to 30 milliseconds and 50 to 100 milliseconds occur.

COMPLICATIONS

Other manifestations of the rheumatic infection may occur during the course of the chorea or may precede or follow it. Cardiac complications, usually endocarditis, occur in approximately 20% of patients. Myocarditis and pericarditis are less common. Vegetative endocarditis and embolic phenomena may occur but are rare. A previous history of rheumatic polyarthritis is common, but involvement of the joints during the course of the chorea is rare. Other infrequent complications include subcutaneous rheumatic nodules, erythema nodosum, and purpura. Persistent mental and behavioral effects can also result from Sydenham disease.

TABLE 81.1 Differential Diagnosis of Chorea

Developmental choreas

Physiologic chorea of infancy

Chorea minima

Idiopathic choreas

Buccal–oral–lingual dyskinesia and edentulous orodyskinesia
In older adults, senile chorea (probably several causes)

Hereditary choreas

Huntington disease

Benign hereditary chorea (*TITF-1* gene)

Neuroacanthocytosis (*VPS13A* gene)

Other heredodegenerations: Huntington disease–like (HDL)
disorders (e.g., prion protein *PRNP*, *junctophilin*, or *JPH3*
genes), dentatorubral–pallidoluysian atrophy (*DRPLA* gene),
spinocerebellar ataxias (SCA2, SCA17), *C9orf72* expansions,
ataxia telangiectasia, ataxia with oculomotor apraxia type 1
(apraxin gene), ataxia with oculomotor apraxia type 2 (due
to mutations in the *senataxin* gene), tuberous sclerosis of
basal ganglia, pantothenate kinase associated neurodegeneration, other neurodegenerations with brain iron accumulation Wilson disease, neuroferritinopathy, infantile bilateral
necrosis

Neurometabolic disorders

Lesch–Nyhan syndrome, lysosomal storage disorders, amino acid
disorders, Leigh disease, porphyria

Drugs

Neuroleptics (tardive dyskinesia, withdrawal emergent syndrome), dopaminergic drugs, anticholinergics, amphetamines,
cocaine, tricyclics, oral contraceptives

Toxins

Alcohol intoxication and withdrawal, anoxia, carbon monoxide,
manganese, mercury, thallium, toluene

Metabolic and endocrine disorders

Hypernatremia, hyponatremia, hypomagnesemia, hypocalcemia, hypoglycemia, hyperglycemia (nonketotic)

Pregnancy (chorea gravidarum)

Acquired hepatocerebral degeneration

Renal failure

Nutritional (e.g., ketogenic diet, beriberi, pellagra, vitamin B_{12}
deficiency, particularly in infants)

Infectious and postinfectious

Sydenham chorea

Encephalitis lethargica

Various other infectious and postinfectious encephalitis,
Creutzfeldt–Jakob disease

Immunologic

Systemic lupus erythematosus, antiphospholipid syndrome, chorea gravidarum

Henoch–Schönlein purpura, NMDA antibody encephalitis

AIDS

Vascular

Infarction or hemorrhage

Arteriovenous malformation, moyamoya disease

Polycythemia rubra vera

Antiphospholipid syndrome

Migraine

Following cardiac surgery with hypothermia and extracorporeal
circulation in children (choreoathetosis and orofacial dyskinesia, hypotonia, and pseudobulbar signs or CHAP syndrome)

Tumors

Trauma

Other secondary choreas

Cerebral palsy (anoxic), kernicterus, sarcoidosis, MS disease,
Behçet disease, polyarteritis nodosa, mitochondrial disorders

Miscellaneous

Paroxysmal dyskinesias (choreoathetosis), familial dyskinesia, and
facial myokymia

NMDA, *N*-methyl-D-aspartate; MS, multiple sclerosis.
Modified from Fahn S, Jankovic J. *Principles and Practice of Movement Disorders.* Philadelphia: Churchill Livingstone/Elsevier; 2007.

DIAGNOSIS

The diagnosis is made without difficulty from the appearance of
the acute or subacute onset of characteristic choreic movements
in a child with relatively recent history of streptococcal infection,
although such a history may not be always elicited. Helpful for
diagnosis are the presence of associated behavioral changes and
diffuse slowing on the electroencephalogram. Although serum antistreptolysin O (ASO) titers may be elevated, this and other immunologic tests, including rheumatoid factor, antinuclear antibodies,
rheumatic B-cell alloantigen D8/17, and cerebrospinal fluid (CSF)
oligoclonal bands are often negative (although CSF pleocytosis has
been reported in a few cases). Magnetic resonance imaging (MRI)
is usually normal except for occasional selective enlargement of the
caudate, putamen, and globus pallidus. In contrast to many other
types of choreic disorders, positron emission tomography (PET)

scan in Sydenham disease reveals striatal hypermetabolism that returns to normal when the choreic movements abate.

Several other causes of symptomatic chorea presenting in
childhood should be considered in the differential diagnosis of
Sydenham disease (see Table 81.1). The *withdrawal emergent syndrome*, occurring in children when neuroleptic agents are suddenly
discontinued, closely resembles the type of chorea seen in Sydenham, but a history of having taken these drugs should make the
diagnosis rather easy. One condition that may be confused with
the chorea of Sydenham is benign hereditary chorea, a childhood-
onset, genetic, nonprogressive disorder (discussed later in the text).

Other dyskinesias in childhood also could present a problem in
differential diagnosis, but the clinical distinctions between these and
choreic movements should lead to the correct diagnosis. Tics may
offer some difficulty, but these movements are more stereotyped

rather than random; they are usually temporarily suppressible, often preceded by a premonitory sensation, and associated with noises or phonic tics. Some genetic forms of dystonia begin in childhood, but the sustained and twisting movements are quite distinct from choreic movements. However, some dystonic movements are more rapid and these have been mislabeled as chorea. Dystonic movements are typically patterned, affecting the same body parts repetitiously. Also, childhood dystonia persists and does not have the self-limiting characteristic of Sydenham disease. Myoclonus–dystonia, also called *essential hereditary myoclonus*, can begin in childhood and sometimes could be difficult to distinguish from chorea. In contrast to chorea, which produces a jerk-like movement that affects different body parts in a random fashion, myoclonus tends to be more predictable affecting the same group of muscles.

Athetosis, a form of slow chorea consisting of writhing, nonpatterned movements, when it occurs in childhood is often seen in the setting of static encephalopathy (cerebral palsy) or some metabolic diseases and usually occurs in the first few years of life. One cause of cerebral palsy, particularly in underdeveloped countries is kernicterus due to bilirubin encephalopathy associated with neonatal jaundice. Besides delayed developmental milestones and choreoathetotic movements, patients with kernicterus often exhibit vertical ophthalmoparesis, deafness, and dysplasia of the dental enamel (Fig. 81.1 and Video 81.2).

TREATMENT

There is no preventive treatment for the disease. Symptomatic therapy may be of great value in the control of the movements. When the severity of the movements interferes with proper rest, sedatives may be needed. If further treatment is necessary, a benzodiazepine, valproate, or corticosteroids may be effective. Although antidopaminergic drugs can suppress choreic movements, a dopamine receptor–blocking agent, such as a phenothiazine, should not be administered because of its potential to produce tardive dyskinesia

or tardive dystonia. If the chorea is particularly troublesome by impairing motor coordination or balance, dopamine-depleting drug tetrabenazine may be very effective in reducing the amplitude of the chorea. Treatment generally consists of a full 10-day course of oral penicillin V therapy or an injection of benzathine penicillin G. Prophylactic administration of penicillin for at least 10 years is recommended to prevent other manifestations of rheumatic fever, of which Sydenham disease may be its sole manifestation.

COURSE AND OUTCOME

Sydenham disease often is a benign condition, and complete recovery is the rule in uncomplicated cases. The mortality rate of approximately 2% is due to associated cardiac complications. The duration of the symptoms is quite variable. In the average case, the motor symptoms persist for 3 to 6 weeks, but the neuropsychiatric symptoms may persist for years or may even be lifelong. Occasionally, the course may be prolonged for several months, and it is not unusual for involuntary movements of a mild degree to persist for many months after recrudescence of the more severe movements. Recurrences after months or several years are reported in approximately a third of the cases.

Susceptibility to *chorea gravidarum*, chorea from oral contraceptives, and even topical vaginal creams containing estrogen and increased sensitivity to levodopa-induced chorea are possible sequelae of Sydenham disease. Some cases of chorea gravidarum may have serum antibasal ganglia antibodies, supporting an immunologic basis of this disorder. Because patients with chorea gravidarum often have a prior history of Sydenham disease, also frequently associated with the presence of antibasal ganglia antibodies, the two disorders may overlap pathogenically. The end of pregnancy and the discontinuation of oral contraceptives or estrogen provide relief from the involuntary movements. A postmortem examination of a case of chorea gravidarum revealed neuronal loss and astrocytosis in the striatum.

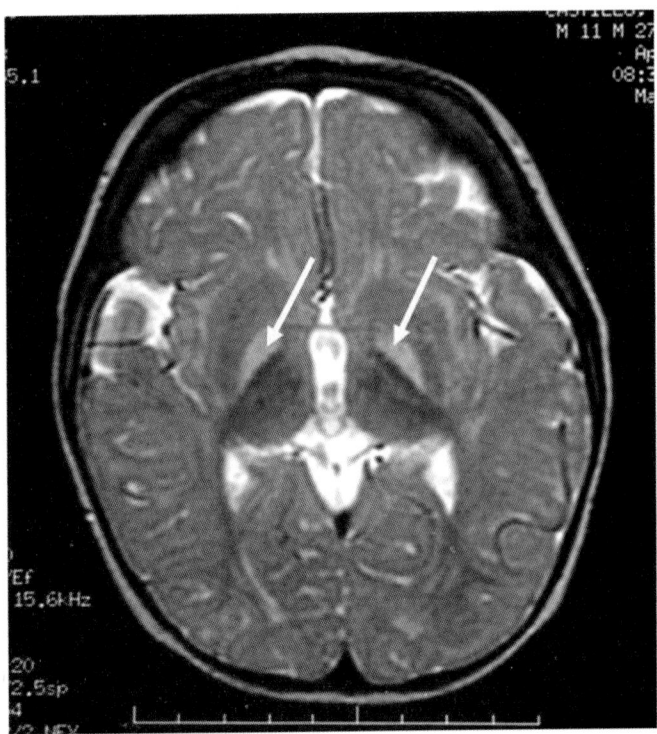

FIGURE 81.1 MRI of an 11-year-old boy with kernicterus. The T2-weighted image shows abnormal pallidal signal *(arrows)*. See also Video 81.2.

AUTOIMMUNE CHOREAS

Chorea in *systemic lupus erythematosus* (SLE), often fluctuating and intermittent, has been associated with the presence of serum antiphospholipid antibodies (lupus anticoagulant), a heterogeneous group of antibodies that can cause platelet dysfunction and result in thrombosis. PET has not found caudate hypometabolism in SLE, in contrast to many other choreas. Treatment with antidopaminergic agents has been successful.

The primary antiphospholipid antibody syndrome also causes chorea, particularly in young women. Systemically, patients may have migraine, spontaneous abortions, venous and arterial thromboses, thickened cardiac valves, livedo reticularis, and Raynaud phenomenon. The central nervous system is involved with strokes, multi-infarct dementia, and chorea. Activated partial thromboplastin time is prolonged because of the presence of lupus anticoagulant, and high titers of anticardiolipin antibodies exist. Anticoagulation, immunosuppressive drugs, and plasmapheresis have had variable success; it is difficult to interpret the effectiveness of therapeutic interventions because spontaneous remission occurs frequently. Striatal hypermetabolism may be documented by PET scan.

Chorea associated with anti–*N*-methyl-D-aspartate (NMDA) receptor encephalitis is particularly important to recognize because if the diagnosis and treatment are delayed, it can be fatal. Often presenting as a subacute neuropsychiatric disorder, anti-NMDA encephalitis is characterized by a variety of neurologic and movement disorders including chorea, stereotypy, dystonia, and myorhythmia. A search for ovarian teratoma or other benign tumors should be initiated because their removal is a critical part of the treatment. Immunoglobulin G antibodies against the NR1 subunit of the NMDA receptor are often identified.

VASCULAR CHOREA AND BALLISM

Choreic movements confined to the arm and leg on one side of the body (hemichorea, hemiballism) may develop abruptly in middle-aged or elderly patients. Ballistic movements are a more violent form of chorea and are characterized by large amplitude uncoordinated activity of the proximal appendicular muscles, so vigorous that the limbs are forcefully and aimlessly thrown about. Padding of the limbs or side rails may be necessary to prevent injury. The movements are present at rest and may be suppressed during voluntary limb movement.

The sudden onset suggests a vascular basis; indeed, it may be preceded by hemiplegia or hemiparesis. In such instances, the choreic or ballistic movements appear when motor function returns. This type of movement disorder is the result of a destructive lesion of the contralateral subthalamic nucleus or its connections. It has also been seen with scattered encephalomalacic lesions involving the internal capsule and basal ganglia. Vascular lesions, hemorrhagic or occlusive in nature, are the most common cause, but hemiballism has been found in association with tumors and plaques from multiple sclerosis (MS) in the subthalamic nucleus and has occasionally followed attempted thalamotomy when the target was missed. In general, the movements tend to diminish over time, but they may be persistent and require therapeutic intervention. The agents noted previously for the control of choreic movements in general have proved effective.

A not uncommon cause of hemiballism/hemichorea in patients with AIDS is a toxoplasmosis lesion involving the subthalamic nucleus, which can also respond to antidopaminergic medication.

Chorea-ballism is a common feature of hyperosmolar hyperglycemic nonketotic syndrome, which appears related to hypoperfusion in the striatum.

Choreoathetosis as a sequela to surgery for congenital heart disease appears to be associated with prolonged time on pump, deep hypothermia, and circulatory arrest. In most cases of postpump syndrome, the chorea persists, and fewer than 25% improve with antidopaminergic therapy.

NEUROACANTHOCYTOSIS

Perhaps the most common hereditary chorea after HD is neuroacanthocytosis, formerly called *chorea-acanthocytosis*. The chorea is typically less severe than that seen with HD but occasionally can be just as severe. In addition to chorea, patients with neuroacanthocytosis often have tics, stereotypies, seizures, cognitive decline, amyotrophy, dysphagia, absent tendon reflexes, high serum creatine kinase, feeding dystonia (tongue pushes food out of the mouth), and self-mutilation with lip and tongue biting. Age at onset is typically in adolescence and young adulthood, but the range is wide (8 to 62 years). Like HD, a young age at onset is more likely to produce parkinsonism or dystonia rather than chorea. The diagnosis depends on finding more than 10% spiky erythrocytes (acanthocytes) in blood smears. Some authorities have proposed that detection of acanthocytes can be enhanced if a wet smear of blood is diluted 1:1 with normal saline (Fig. 81.2). Occasionally, electron microscopy is needed to confirm the presence of acanthocytes.

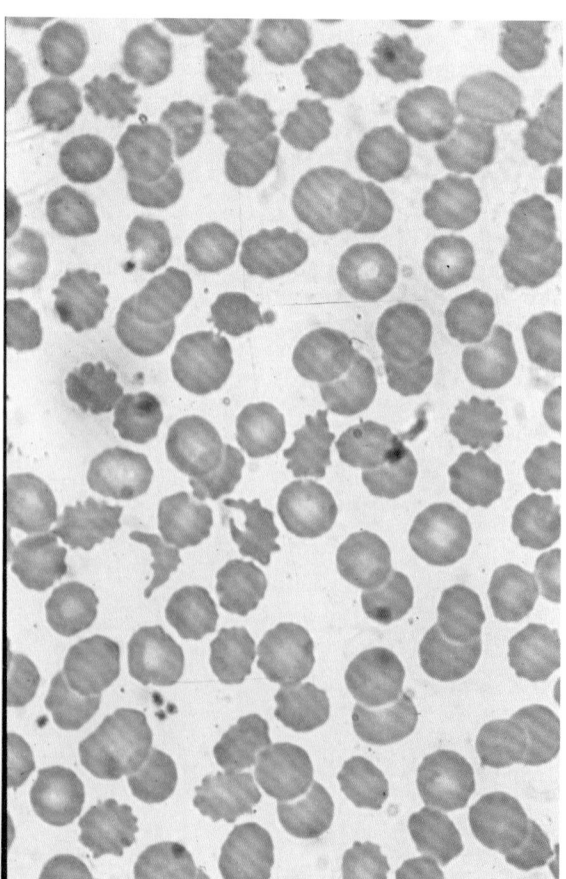

FIGURE 81.2 Acanthocytes in a patient with neuroacanthocytosis.

The cerebral pathology is similar to that of HD, with striatal degeneration causing caudate atrophy but without intranuclear inclusions immunostaining with antibodies against huntingtin protein. PET scan typically shows hypometabolism in the caudate nucleus as well as reduced fluorodopa uptake and decreased dopamine receptor binding in the striatum. Erythrocyte membrane lipids are altered. Tightly bound palmitic acid (C16:0) is increased, and stearic acid (C18:0) is decreased. Choline acetyltransferase and glutamic acid decarboxylase are normal in basal ganglia and cortex, substance P levels are low in the substantia nigra and striatum, and norepinephrine is elevated in the putamen and pallidum.

Neuroacanthocytosis has been found to be due to various mutations on the *CHAC* (chorea-acanthocytosis) gene, later renamed *VPS13A* on chromosome 9q21.2, coding for the protein named *chorein* (Fig. 81.3).

A rare patient with neuroacanthocytosis may have the McLeod phenotype, an X-linked (Xp21) form of acanthocytosis associated with chorea, seizures, neuropathy, liver disease, hemolysis, and elevated creatine kinase values.

DENTATORUBRAL–PALLIDOLUYSIAN ATROPHY

Once thought to be found mainly in the Japanese population, this autosomal dominant disorder is now known to be more widespread, thanks to discovery of expanded cytosine–adenine–guanine (CAG) repeats in the dentatorubral–pallidoluysian atrophy gene (*DRPLA* or *ATN1*) on chromosome 12p13.31 that codes for the atrophin-1 protein, which is phosphorylated by c-Jun NH-terminal kinase (JNK). The abnormal polyQ protein has reduced affinity for JNK. Also called the *Haw River syndrome* because of its occurrence in some African-Americans in North Carolina, DRPLA clinically overlaps with HD and manifests combinations of chorea, myoclonus, seizures, ataxia, and dementia. The phenotype varies according to triplet (CAG) repeat length, and anticipation and excess of paternal inheritance in younger onset cases with longer repeat lengths are seen. The neuropathologic spectrum is centered around the cerebellofugal and pallidofugal systems, but neurodegenerative changes can be found in many nuclei. In contrast to HD, DRPLA is typically associated with white matter degeneration.

HUNTINGTON DISEASE–LIKE SYNDROMES

In addition to neuroacanthocytosis and DRPLA, other syndromes that resemble HD have been reported, in which genetic linkage has been made to other gene markers. When the HD gene test is normal, one should consider these less common conditions. Huntington disease–like (HDL) 1 is an autosomal dominant disorder mapped to the prion protein gene (*PRNP*) on chromosome 20p with eight extra octapeptide repeats in the prion protein. The autosomal dominant HDL2 appears to be present exclusively or predominantly in individuals of African origin. It is due to cytosine–thymine–guanine (CTG) and CAG repeat expansions of the gene on chromosome 16q24.2, encoding junctophilin-3, a protein of the junctional complex linking the plasma membrane and the endoplasmic reticulum. HDL3, although labeled as such, is an autosomal recessive neurodegenerative disease beginning at 3 to 4 years of age. It is manifested by chorea, dystonia, ataxia, gait disorder, spasticity, seizures, mutism, intellectual impairment, and bilateral frontal and caudate atrophy. HDL3 has been linked to 4p15.3. Although labeled as a spinocerebellar degeneration, SCA17 can present with chorea and manifest with other features of HD. SCA17 is due to an expanded CAG repeat in the gene on chromosome 6q27 for the TATA-binding protein, which has a transcription initiation function. Another relatively common HD phenocopy is C9orf72 expansion at 9p21.2.

BENIGN HEREDITARY CHOREA

This rare, childhood-onset, choreic disorder is nonprogressive and may even lessen in severity over time. This autosomal dominant disorder is caused by mutations in the *NKX2-1* (previously called *TITF1*) gene on chromosome 14q13.3, coding for a transcription essential for the organogenesis of the lung, thyroid, and basal ganglia. This syndrome has been also described in patients with deletion of not only the *NKX2-1* gene but also the contiguous *PAX9* gene. These mutations should be considered in children and adults with chorea, slight motor delay, gait ataxia, dystonia, myoclonus, tics, intellectual impairment, congenital hypothyroidism, and chronic lung disease, hence the term *brain–thyroid–lung syndrome*. Brain MRI has been generally reported to be unremarkable but

FIGURE 81.3 Absence of chorein in patient (*155a*) with neuroacanthocytosis (Western blot). (Courtesy Dr. Benedikt Bader, Munich, Germany.)

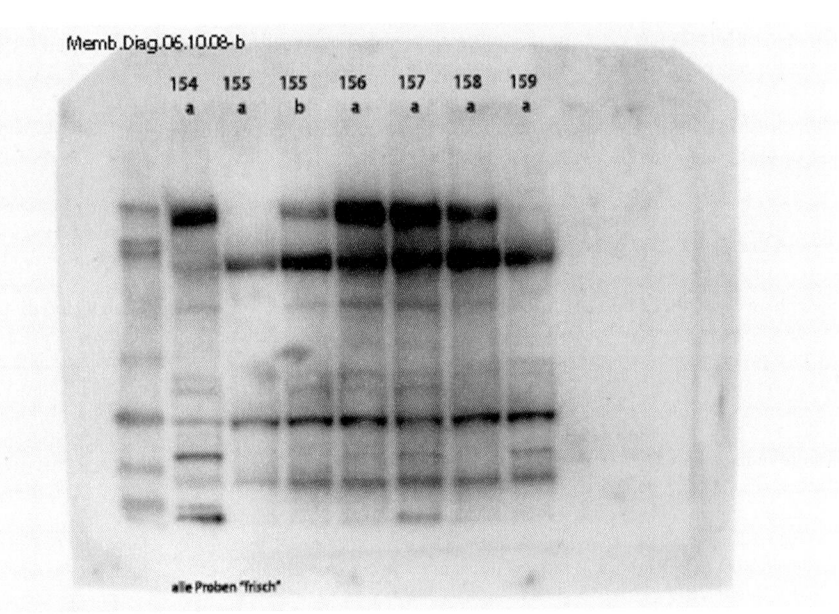

some cases showed hypoplastic pallida, lack of differentiation of medial and lateral components, and bilateral signal hyperintensities on T2-weighted MRI images. About half of the patients spontaneously improve in adulthood. Tetrabenazine and, paradoxically, levodopa improves troublesome chorea.

ESSENTIAL CHOREA

In the absence of a family history, a benign nonprogressive chorea without other neurologic features can be rarely encountered, so-called essential chorea. When it occurs in the elderly, the term *senile chorea* is sometimes used, but its nosology is uncertain, as some patients diagnosed with senile or essential chorea have been found to have a CAG expansion in the HD gene.

The movements usually begin insidiously, are mild, and usually involve the limbs. More complex movements of the lingual–facial–buccal regions, however, are on occasion encountered. Slow progression in the intensity and extent of the movements may occur. In addition to HD, many other cases have been later diagnosed with other disorders, such as the antiphospholipid antibody syndrome, hypocalcemia, tardive dyskinesia, and basal ganglia calcification. Still, a rare patient can remain undiagnosed despite extensive investigation and is left with the diagnosis of essential (senile) chorea. In such a case, pathologic changes are found in the caudate nucleus and putamen but not to the degree seen in HD. Significantly, degenerative changes in the cerebral cortex are absent. In general, the symptoms are mild and there is little need to resort to therapeutic measures. In those instances in which oral–facial and neck muscle involvement occurs, however, drugs used to control chorea as indicated previously may prove useful.

OTHER CHOREAS

It is beyond the scope of this review to describe all causes of choreas but the reader is directed to Table 81.1 and suggested readings for less common forms of choreic disorders.

Treatment of chorea should focus on identification of specific and potentially treatable cause, such as drugs and infectious and autoimmune or paraneoplastic etiologies. Symptomatic relief of chorea is similar to that in patients with HD and typically involves the use of tetrabenazine, a monoamine depletor. Rarely, if chorea is disabling, pallidal deep brain stimulation may be considered.

Videos can be found in the companion e-book edition. For a full list of video legends, please see the front matter.

SUGGESTED READINGS

Sydenham and Other Choreas of Childhood

Oosterveer DM, Overweg-Plandsoen WC, Roos RA. Sydenham's chorea: a practical overview of the current literature. *Pediatr Neurol.* 2010;43:1–6.

Paz JA, Silva CA, Marques-Dias MJ. Randomized double-blind study with prednisone in Sydenham's chorea. *Pediatr Neurol.* 2006;34:264–269.

Autoimmune Choreas

Baizabal-Carvallo JF, Bonnet C, Jankovic J. Movement disorders in systemic lupus erythematosus and the antiphospholipid syndrome. *J Neural Transm.* 2013;120(11):1579–1589.

Baizabal-Carvallo JF, Jankovic J. Movement disorders in autoimmune diseases. *Mov Disord.* 2012;27(8):935–946.

Baizabal-Carvallo JF, Stocco A, Muscal E, et al. The spectrum of movement disorders in children with anti-NMDA receptor encephalitis. *Mov Disord.* 2013;28(4):543–547.

Kurlan R, Johnson D, Kaplan EL; Tourette Syndrome Study Group. Streptococcal infection and exacerbations of childhood tics and obsessive—compulsive symptoms: a prospective blinded cohort study. *Pediatrics.* 2008;121:1188–1197.

Sanna G, D'Cruz D, Cuadrado MJ. Cerebral manifestations in the antiphospholipid (Hughes) syndrome. *Rheum Dis Clin North Am.* 2006;32:465–490.

Singer HS, Gause C, Morris C, et al; Tourette Syndrome Study Group. Serial immune markers do not correlate with clinical exacerbations in pediatric autoimmune neuropsychiatric disorders associated with streptococcal infections. *Pediatrics.* 2008;121:1198–1205.

Vascular Chorea-Ballism

Dobson-Stone C, Velayos-Baeza A, Filippone LA, et al. Chorein detection for the diagnosis of chorea-acanthocytosis. *Ann Neurol.* 2004;56(2):299–302.

du Plessis AJ, Bellinger DC, Gauvreau K, et al. Neurologic outcome of choreoathetoid encephalopathy after cardiac surgery. *Pediatr Neurol.* 2002;27:9–17.

Oh S-H, Lee K-Y, Im J-H, et al. Chorea associated with non-ketotic hyperglycemia and hyperintensity basal ganglia lesion on T1-weighted brain MRI study: a meta-analysis of 53 cases including four present cases. *J Neurol Sci.* 2002;200:57–62.

Neuroacanthocytosis

Mehanna R, Jankovic J. Movement disorders in cerebrovascular disease. *Lancet Neurol.* 2013;12(6):597–608.

Walker RH, Jung HH, Dobson-Stone C, et al. Neurologic phenotypes associated with acanthocytosis. *Neurology.* 2007;68:92–98.

Walterfang M, Looi JC, Styner M, et al. Shape alterations in the striatum in chorea-acanthocytosis. *Psychiatry Res.* 2011;192:29–36.

Dentatorubral–Pallidoluysian Atrophy

Munoz E, Campdelacreu J, Ferrer I, et al. Severe cerebral white matter involvement in a case of dentatorubropallidoluysian atrophy studied at autopsy. *Arch Neurol.* 2004;61:946–949.

Wardle M, Morris HR, Robertson NP. Clinical and genetic characteristics of non-Asian dentatorubral-pallidoluysian atrophy: a systematic review. *Mov Disord.* 2009;24:1636–1640.

Huntington Disease–like Syndromes

Greenstein PE, Vonsattel JP, Margolis RL, et al. Huntington's disease like-2 neuropathology. *Mov Disord.* 2007;22:1416–1423.

Hensman Moss DJ, Poulter M, Beck J, et al. C9orf72 expansions are the most common genetic cause of Huntington disease phenocopies. *Neurology.* 2014;82(4):292–299.

Rudnicki DD, Holmes SE, Lin MW, et al. Huntington's disease-like 2 is associated with CUG repeat-containing RNA foci. *Ann Neurol.* 2007;61:272–282.

Schneider SA, van de Warrenburg BP, Hughes TD, et al. Phenotypic homogeneity of the Huntington disease-like presentation in a SCA17 family. *Neurology.* 2006;67:1701–1703.

Schneider SA, Walker RH, Bhatia KP. The Huntington's disease-like syndromes: what to consider in patients with a negative Huntington's disease gene test. *Nat Clin Pract Neurol.* 2007;3:517–525.

Seixas AI, Holmes SE, Takeshima H, et al. Loss of junctophilin-3 contributes to Huntington disease-like 2 pathogenesis. *Ann Neurol.* 2012;71(2):245–257.

Benign Hereditary Chorea

Kleiner-Fisman G, Lang AE. Benign hereditary chorea revisited: a journey to understanding. *Mov Disord.* 2007;22:2297–2305.

Patel NJ, Jankovic J. NKX2-1-related disorders. GeneReviews Web site. http://www.ncbi.nlm.nih.gov/books/NBK185066/

Peall KJ, Lumsden D, Kneen R, et al. Benign hereditary chorea related to NKX2.1: expansion of the genotypic and phenotypic spectrum. *Dev Med Child Neurol.* 2014;56(7):642–648.

Essential Chorea

Ruiz PJG, Gomez-Tortosa E, Delbarrio A, et al. Senile chorea: a multicenter prospective study. *Acta Neurol Scand.* 1997;95:180–183.

Other Choreas and Related Topics

Cardoso F, Seppi K, Mair KJ, et al. Seminar on choreas. *Lancet Neurol.* 2006;5:589–602.

Colver A, Fairhurst C, Pharoah PO. Cerebral palsy. *Lancet.* 2014;383(9924): 1240–1249.

Edwards TC, Zrinzo L, Limousin P, et al. Deep brain stimulation in the treatment of chorea. *Mov Disord.* 2012;27(3):357–363.

Jankovic J, Roos RA. Chorea associated with Huntington's disease: to treat or not to treat? *Mov Disord.* 2014;29(11):1414–1418.

Jimenez-Shahed J, Jankovic J. Tetrabenazine for treatment of chorea associated with Huntington's disease. *Expert Opin Orphan Drugs.* 2013;1:423–436.

Ondo WG, Adam OR, Jankovic J, et al. Dramatic response of facial stereotype/ tic to tetrabenazine in the first reported cases of neuroferritinopathy in the United States. *Mov Disord.* 2010;25:2470–2472.

O'Toole O, Lennon VA, Ahlskog JE, et al. Autoimmune chorea in adults. *Neurology.* 2013;80(12):1133–1144.

Schneider SA, Dusek P, Hardy J, et al. Genetics and pathophysiology of neurodegeneration with brain iron accumulation (NBIA). *Curr Neuropharmacol.* 2013;11:59–79.

Shen V, Clarence-Smith K, Hunter C, et al. Safety and efficacy of tetrabenazine and use of concomitant medications during long-term treatment of chorea associated with Huntington's and other diseases. *Tremor Other Hyperkinetic Mov (N Y).* 2013;3. http://tremorjournal.org/article/view/191.

Waln O, Jankovic J. An update on tardive dyskinesia: from phenomenology to treatment. *Tremor Other Hyperkinet Mov (N Y).* 2013;3. pii:tre-03-161-4138-1.

Watchko JF, Tiribelli C. Bilirubin-induced neurologic damage—mechanisms and management approaches. *N Engl J Med.* 2013;369(21):2021–2030.

Huntington Disease 82

Karen S. Marder

INTRODUCTION

Huntington disease (HD) is an autosomal dominant neurodegenerative disorder caused by a cytosine–adenine–guanine (CAG) polyglutamine repeat expansion in exon 1 of the Huntington (HTT) gene on chromosome 4p16.3. The age of onset, defined based on the presence of a characteristic extrapyramidal movement disorder, is inversely related to CAG repeat length such that higher CAG repeat length is associated with earlier age at onset. HD is characterized by a triad of symptoms and signs including motor, cognitive, and psychiatric manifestations. Studies of premanifest HD have demonstrated changes in imaging biomarkers (putamen and caudate) that predate onset of motor signs more than 15 years prior to onset and cognitive changes that occur 10 years prior to motor onset. Symptomatic treatment for chorea but no disease-modifying therapy is currently available. The development of imaging, biofluid, and quantitative cognitive and motor testing will facilitate clinical trial development in prodromal HD.

EPIDEMIOLOGY

James Huntington provided the first comprehensive description of the disease and its inheritance pattern in 1872. Since that time, it has been described worldwide. Prevalence of HD based on a meta-analysis of 13 "service-based" studies was 2.71 per 100,000 (95% confidence interval [CI], 1.55 to 4.72). Prevalence was significantly lower in Asia 0.4 per 100,000 compared to Europe, North America, and Australia 5.7 per 100,000. Among people of European ancestry, 4 to 7 per 100,000 people have HD, with far lower prevalence among Asians and Black Africans. Incidence based on four studies was 0.38 per 100,000 per year (95% CI: 0.16, 0.94), with incidence much lower in Asia compared to those of European ancestry. Seven common haplotypes have been identified in the *HTT* gene, with a single ancestral haplotype accounting for 50% of all European chromosomes, supporting the theory that HD may have originated in Northern Europe and spread worldwide.

PATHOBIOLOGY

GENETICS

Age of onset of HD, defined by the presence of extrapyramidal motor signs, occurs most often between 40 and 50 years (mean age 45 years); however, cases have been reported as young as age 2 years and as old as 85 years. Between 5% and 10% develop HD before age 20 years (juvenile HD) and about 10% after age 60 years. CAG repeat length is inversely correlated with age at onset and accounts for 50% to 70% of the variance in age at onset. Repeat lengths of 26 or less are normal. Repeats between 27 and 35 are considered intermediate or "high normal" and represent 3% to 5% of all "normal" alleles. Although carriers of 27 to 35 repeats

will not develop manifest HD, this range confers meiotic instability, and parents, especially fathers, may transmit repeats to their children that are within the HD range. Carriers of 27 to 35 repeats may evidence subtle behavioral changes, an "endophenotype," although they do not have motor or cognitive impairment. Repeats between 36 and 39 are associated with incomplete or reduced penetrance, meaning that some individuals will develop HD, generally late onset, and others will not. Diagnosis of HD in the 36 to 39 repeat range may be difficult due to confounding with age-associated signs. Individuals with 40 or more repeats will develop HD (fully penetrant) if they live long enough. Most individuals with HD have between 40 and 50 repeats. Those with juvenile HD usually have greater than 50 repeats, although greater than 100 repeats have been reported.

There is a greater chance for CAG expansion in sperm than in ova, which explains the concept of "genetic anticipation," an earlier age at onset in the next generation. Mothers with HD pass on approximately the same number of repeats (± 3), whereas fathers with HD, because of meiotic instability, often pass on a higher CAG repeat length. Ninety percent of juvenile HD cases have inherited the disease from their fathers. Despite the inverse correlation with age, there is significant variability of age of onset of HD even among individuals with the same CAG repeat length.

NEUROPATHOLOGY

Neuronal loss begins in the striatum. A five-point grading system based on macroscopic and microscopic criteria correlates with the Shoulson–Fahn Total Functional Capacity scale (Fig. 82.1). The scale ranges from 0 (no pathology) to grade 4. The earliest changes are seen in the medial paraventricular portions of the caudate nucleus (50% of neurons are lost in grade 1), in the tail of the caudate, and in the dorsal putamen. Ninety-five percent of neurons are lost in grade 4. Astrocytes increase steadily from grade 2 to 4, with severe gliosis in stage IV. Although neuronal loss in the striatum is the hallmark of HD, extrastriatal involvement (globus pallidus, subthalamic nucleus, substantia nigra pars reticulata, thalamus, brain stem, and neocortex) occurs but is less severe than the striatum (see Fig. 82.1).

Microscopically, the caudate contains shrunken neurons and ubiquitinated, round intranuclear inclusions. These inclusions consist of large aggregates of abnormal huntingtin protein (HTT) (Fig. 82.2B). The normal function of HTT, a predominantly cytoplasmic protein, is not completely understood. HD is believed to arise primarily from a gain of toxic function from an abnormal conformation of mutant HTT; however, loss of function of HTT and toxicity from RNA may also contribute. HTT is essential for early embryonic development. Despite widespread expression of abnormal HTT, the striatum is relatively selectively vulnerable. Subcortical prefrontal white matter shows CD68-labeled microglial cells and macrophages, which probably reflects the slow ongoing widespread degenerative process involving the cortical neurons and their processes (Fig. 82.2A).

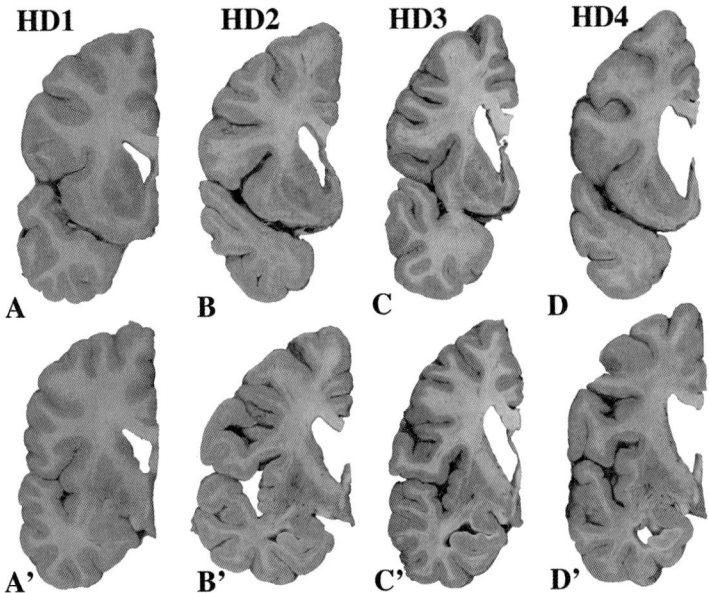

FIGURE 82.1 Gradations of Huntington disease pathology. Neuropathologic gradations of Huntington disease using a 5-point scale (0 to 4). **A–D:** Coronal sections passing through the nucleus accumbens including the head of the caudate nucleus and putamen. **A'–D':** Coronal sections passing through the globus pallidus including the putamen and caudal segment of the head of the caudate nucleus. **A and A':** Neuropathologic grade of severity 1 (HD1): (about 5% of all HD brains) there is minimal detectable change on gross examination at the sites shown in **A and A'**; however, the body and tail of the caudate nucleus are atrophic. **B and B':** Neuropathologic grade of severity 2 (HD2): (about 15% of HD brains) the volume loss of the neostriatum is moderate with relative preservation of its shape. The medial outline of the head of the caudate nucleus is only slightly convex, but it still bulges into the lateral ventricle **(B)**. The medial edge of the lenticular nucleus **(B')** lost its medial convexity. **C and C':** Neuropathologic grade of severity 3 (HD3): (about 50% of HD brains) the medial outline of the head of the caudate nucleus forms a straight line or is slightly concave medially **(C)**. The volume loss of the lenticular nucleus (putamen and globus pallidus) is discrete, and its medial outline is parallel to the anterior limb of internal capsule or is slightly concave medially **(C')**. **D and D':** Neuropathologic grade of severity 4 (HD4): (about 30% of HD brains) the striatum is severely atrophic. The medial contour of the head of the caudate nucleus is concave, as is the anterior limb of internal capsule **(D)**. (Courtesy of JP Vonsattel, MD.)

NEUROCHEMISTRY

Up to 95% of the GABAergic medium spiny neurons that project to the globus pallidus and the substantia nigra are lost, whereas large cholinergic interneurons are selectively spared. Loss of the medium spiny neurons may be due to excessive stimulation of excitatory amino acid receptors, especially N-methyl-D-aspartate (NMDA) receptors. Although dopamine, glutamate, and γ-aminobutyric acid (GABA) are thought to be most affected in HD and have been targets for therapy, multiple neurotransmitters and their receptors are involved. Cannabinoid and adenosine A2a receptor binding in the striatum and globus pallidus externa are affected early. There is typically loss of dopamine D1 receptors in the striatum as well as cannabinoid and D1 receptors in the substantia nigra as the disease progresses. Loss of substance P/dynorphin neurons occurs in the late stages and correlates clinically with dystonia.

CLINICAL MANIFESTATIONS

The triad of symptoms and signs associated with HD is an extrapyramidal movement disorder, cognitive impairment, and behavioral impairment (Table 82.1). Any one of the triad may occur first. Three carefully designed observational studies including individuals at risk for HD and early symptomatic HD (PHAROS, PREDICT HD, TRACK HD) have facilitated in-depth characterization of individuals followed longitudinally including the period of phenoconversion. The course of HD can be divided into several periods. During the premanifest period (from birth to approximately 10 to 15 years prior to phenoconversion), individuals are clinically indistinguishable from controls (presymptomatic phase). The prodromal phase, which follows, is characterized by subtle motor, cognitive, and psychiatric features leading up to phenoconversion. Phenoconversion is defined clinically, as unequivocally manifesting the extrapyramidal motor signs of HD, when HD is diagnosed.

MOTOR SIGNS

The extrapyramidal movement disorder is the defining feature of HD and is characterized by both involuntary movements (chorea, dystonia) and impairment in voluntary movements (eye movements, gait, swallowing). The Unified Huntington's Disease Rating Scale includes a 124-point assessment of the motor signs of HD including eye movements (reduced saccades and breakdown of smooth pursuit), fine motor coordination, chorea, dystonia, and gait and balance (Video 82.1). Chorea, derived from the Greek word "dance," is an involuntary movement that is brief but not as lightening-like as myoclonus. These random movements may be present in the limbs, face, or trunk (see Video 82.1). They are exacerbated with stress and are thought to disappear during sleep.

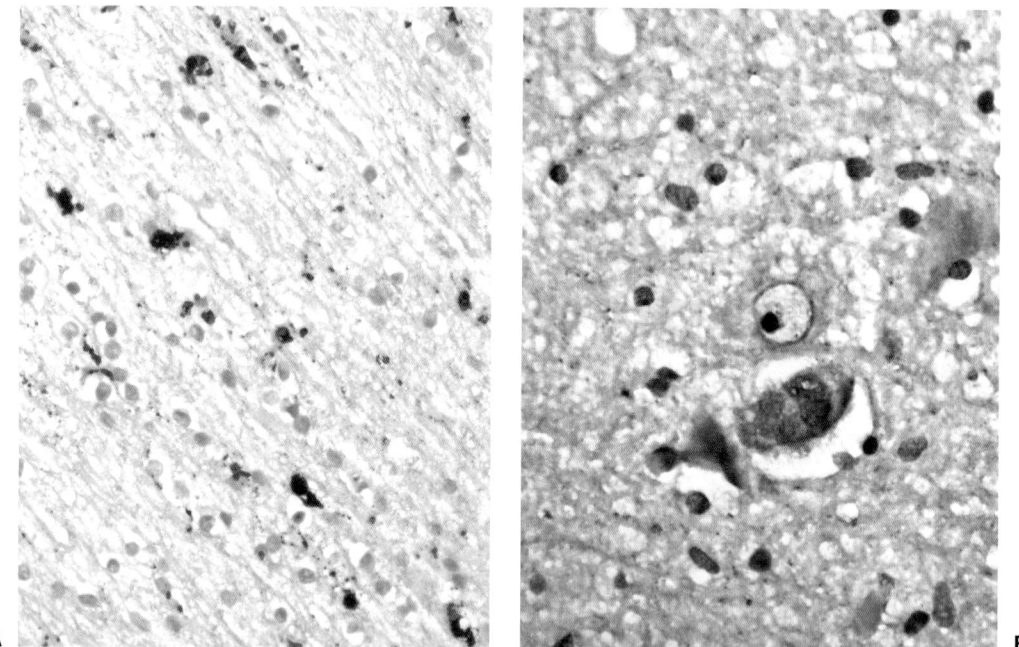

FIGURE 82.2 Neuronal intranuclear inclusion. **A:** The presence of CD68-labeled microglial cells and macrophages within the subcortical prefrontal white matter (Brodmann area [BA] 9) is shown. **B:** Two neurons from putamen (HD3-neuropathologic staging) are shown. One of them exhibits a ubiquitinated, round nuclear inclusion. The other neuron is shrunken and diffusely labeled with antibodies directed against ubiquitinated proteins. (Courtesy of JP Vonsattel, MD.)

Chorea tends to be present in the early symptomatic phase, peak mid disease, and decline or disappear in the late phase of the disease. In contrast, bradykinesia, dystonia, and rigidity increase, particularly during the late stages of the disease, and affect voluntary movements. Most individuals need some assistance with walking, for example, assistive devices, approximately 7 years from onset of motor signs. Falls and choking are frequent mid- to late-stage events that may be life threatening. In addition to chorea, other motor features include motor impersistence. Examples include the inability to maintain tongue protrusion for 10 seconds or to maintain voluntary contraction while gripping, colloquially known as *milkmaid grip*. Impairments in fine motor activity that may include slowing and irregularity can be measured clinically or with quantitative motor assessment including speed of finger tapping and paced tapping. Variability of the inter tap interval or the pace of walking are among the earliest detectable signs of motor impairment, at a time when impairment is not detectable on neurologic examination or recognized by the individual. The earlier the disease onset, the less likely there will be chorea. Children presenting with HD present with an akinetic rigid form of the disease. Stiffness in the legs may also be accompanied by scissoring of gait, bradykinesia, and clumsiness. Seizures occur in 25% of juvenile HD cases.

COGNITIVE IMPAIRMENT

Although HD is diagnosed based on the presence of an extrapyramidal motor disorder, numerous cross-sectional and longitudinal studies have documented impairment primarily in executive function and psychomotor slowing that may begin 10 to 15 years prior to motor onset during the prodromal phase. Deficits in executive function including the ability to plan, organize, and monitor behavior are particularly prominent. These cognitive domains have been closely associated with the frontal lobes and the frontostriatal circuits and are similar to the cognitive impairment seen in Parkinson disease or vascular dementia. Patients with HD do not have a primary disorder of memory retention but have difficulty acquiring information efficiently or consistently retrieving it. In contrast to patients with Alzheimer disease (AD), patients with HD show marked improvement in response to cued recall, similar to that in other patients with frontal lobe disease. Unlike the cortical dementias, such as AD, HD does not prominently involve language until late in the illness. Among individuals who are in the premanifest stage, deficits in motor planning/speed (e.g., paced tapping, two-choice reaction time) and sensory-perceptual processing (emotional recognition and University of Pennsylvania smell identification test) best predict time to diagnosis after motor symptoms and CAG repeat

TABLE 82.1	Clinical Manifestations of Huntington Disease
Clinical Domain	**Signs**
Motor	Involuntary movements • Chorea, dystonia, dysphagia, dysarthria Voluntary movements • Slow saccade initiation and interrupted pursuit • Finger tapping/pronation supination, gait and balance
Cognitive	Processing speed, executive function, visuospatial perception, episodic memory, smell identification
Psychiatric	Irritability, obsessive–compulsive symptoms, perseverative behavior, depression, apathy, anosognosia

Clinical manifestations in HD occur in three domains: motor (defining feature of the disease), cognitive, and psychiatric.

length and age. Using traditional neuropsychological tests, 40% of premanifest individuals meet criteria for mild cognitive impairment (MCI) (using cutoff scores 1.5 standard deviation [SD] below the mean of a comparison group in at least one domain) and displayed mild impairments in episodic memory, processing speed, executive functioning, and/or visuospatial perception. The prevalence of MCI increases over the 10 years prior to diagnosis, as individuals get closer to their estimated age at onset of diagnosis. The majority have nonamnestic MCI (18%), followed by amnestic MCI (7.5%) in premanifest HD. During the premanifest period, individuals may recognize subtle functional decline in capacity to perform their jobs and handle financial affairs. Children present a special case. They often have cognitive decline, manifesting as poor school performance, characterized by poor attention and may be misdiagnosed as attention deficit disorder.

BEHAVIORAL SIGNS

A range of psychiatric manifestations can be seen in both premanifest and manifest HD including most commonly irritability, obsessive–compulsive symptoms, depression (in up to 50%), and apathy. Apathy may increase significantly in premanifest HD and is associated with prediction of functional decline. Like apathy, obsessive–compulsive symptoms (OCS) are referable to frontostriatal circuits, in particular the orbitofrontal cortex. OCS also increase over time as the individual approaches phenoconversion. Perseverative behavior that is not ego dystonic, for example, getting stuck on an idea, may also be seen. Anosognosia is frequent in HD. Individuals with HD are less likely to report motor symptoms that are present on exam than Parkinson disease patients. Almost half of the participants in the PREDICT HD study who phenoconverted did not report motor symptoms, consistent with unawareness. Using the problem behavior assessment, three clusters of symptoms identified in manifest HD were depression, apathy, and irritability. Among HD patients, there is no clear relationship between psychiatric symptoms and disease progression, except for apathy, which correlates with disease duration. This may be due to the availability of effective treatment for affective symptoms and the episodic nature of these symptoms. Suicidal ideation and suicide are more common in HD compared to age-matched controls. Completed suicide has been reported to be 7- to 12-fold more common in HD than controls. Psychosis is rare. Critical periods for suicidal ideation have been identified close to the time of phenoconversion and early in the early symptomatic stage. In children, behavioral changes may include depression, aggression, impulsivity, and obsessions.

DIAGNOSIS

Diagnosis is based on the unequivocal presence of an extrapyramidal movement disorder in the setting an expanded CAG repeat or a family history of HD based on autopsy or a close family member who has undergone genetic testing. The differential diagnosis of chorea is presented in Chapter 81. Individuals from confirmed HD families who present with signs and symptoms of HD should undergo a careful history and physical examination. As in sporadic cases, there should be consideration of causes of chorea including thyroid function tests, B$_{12}$, antinuclear antibody, antistreptolysin O, and HIV. Because HD is the most likely etiology of the extrapyramidal movement disorder in a family with a documented HD family, genetic testing for the expanded CAG repeat is a more cost-effective approach. It is essential that any individual (symptomatic or presymptomatic) who is considering

genetic testing be offered genetic counseling performed according to published guidelines. A center specialized in HD with a team of professionals including a neurologist, psychiatrist, and a genetic counselor is preferable.

If there is no family history of HD, a careful medication history including dopamine antagonist exposure resulting in tardive dyskinesia should be sought. Additional tests would include complete blood count, thyroid function tests (hyperthyroidism), B$_{12}$ deficiency, a smear for acanthocytes and creatine phosphokinase to detect neuroacanthocytosis, a sedimentation rate (to rule out autoimmune disorders such as Sydenham chorea or lupus), and ceruloplasmin (for Wilson disease). Nonpaternity may also be an explanation for lack of a family history of HD.

There are several other causes of autosomal dominant slowly progressive chorea including HDL2 caused by a mutation in JPH3 which is located on chromosome 16q24.3. JPH3 that is responsible for making the protein junctophilin-3 and dentatorubral-pallidoluysian atrophy caused by a mutation in *ATN1* are reviewed in Chapter 81 along with a more complete differential diagnosis of chorea.

In individuals with HD, routine studies of blood, urine, and cerebrospinal fluid are normal. Structural magnetic resonance imaging (MRI) may show enlargement of the lateral ventricles due to atrophy of the caudate and putamen (Fig. 82.3). In a longitudinal study PREDICT HD, striatal volume decline was faster in premanifest and manifest HD compared to age-matched controls and was seen 10 years before diagnosis of "phenoconversion." Structural MRI measures of striatal atrophy may be the earliest changes referable to HD but are not sufficiently sensitive or specific as a diagnostic marker for an individual patient. Diffusion tensor imaging, functional MRI, and fluorodeoxyglucose positron emission tomography are used in research settings as potential surrogate markers, however, are not yet useful for diagnostic purposes. In longitudinal studies, these structural and functional imaging markers correlate with calculated time to disease onset based on CAG and age, motor, and cognitive function and may also independently predict phenoconversion. In manifest HD, measures of striatal volume correlates with motor and cognitive function.

TREATMENT

No disease-modifying therapies have been approved for HD. Disease-modifying therapies have been directed primarily at oxidative stress and mitochondrial mechanisms of action. A 5-year phase III study including 600 HD participants randomized to CoQ10 2,400 mg or placebo was stopped early because of futility in 2014. A 3-year phase III study of creatine 40 mg/day was also stopped early in 2014 for futility. Small fetal transplant trials have been conducted, and one multicenter longitudinal study is ongoing. Preparatory work on RNA interference and antisense oligonucleotide–based therapies could be particularly effective in a highly penetrant single gene disorder such as HD. The design of neuroprotective trials in premanifest individuals presents unique challenges associated with whether participants must know whether they have an expanded CAG repeat to participate and if not, whether it is ethical to randomize noncarriers to the active agent. A recent phase II study of 30 mg of creatine compared to placebo (PRECREST) demonstrated feasibility of randomizing both premanifest individuals who knew their mutation status as well as those who had not undergone clinical genetic testing in a prevention trial. This study also demonstrated the potential value of imaging as a more sensitive measure of change than clinical measures over an 18-month period [**Level 1**].[1–4]

Control

Prodromal HD

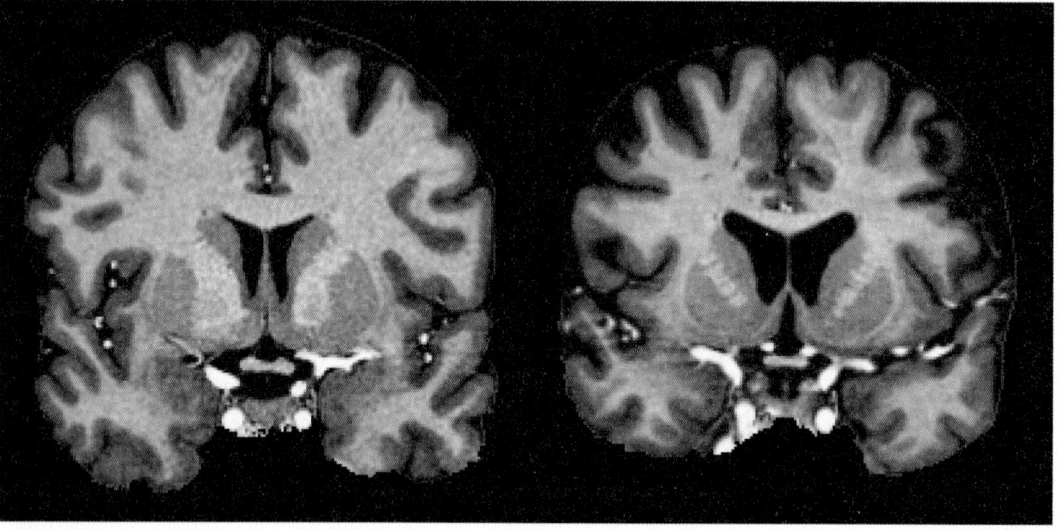

FIGURE 82.3 7T MP2RAGE images at 0.65-mm resolution showing striatal volume loss and brain shrinkage in other regions in prodromal HD (*right*, 38-year-old woman, 6.5 years to predicted onset vs. control; *left*, 38-year-old woman). (Courtesy of Christopher A. Ross, MD, PhD, and Jun Hua, PhD.)

TREATMENT OF MOVEMENT DISORDER

Antidopaminergic Agents for Chorea

About 90% of people with HD develop chorea, but treatment is advised only if it is functionally or emotionally disabling. Tetrabenazine (TBZ) [**Level 1**][5] is the only U.S. Food and Drug Administration (FDA)–approved medication for the symptomatic treatment of chorea. In a double-blind placebo-controlled study (class I) including 54 HD randomized to TBZ up to 100 mg and 30 to placebo, chorea was reduced by 23.5% after 12 weeks. TBZ reversibly inhibits the central vesicular monoamine transporter type 2 (VMAT2) and depletes presynaptic dopamine more selectively than norepinephrine and serotonin. The highest binding density for TBZ is in the caudate, putamen, and nucleus accumbens, where HD pathology is the greatest. Starting dose of TBZ is 12.5 mg daily titrated to three times daily with a maximum dose of 100 mg. At 50 mg, the FDA requires that CYP2D6 genotyping be done. Poor metabolizers of CYP2D6 should not exceed the 50-mg dose. Because it is metabolized by Cyp2D6, drug interactions that might raise TBZ need to be considered. It is generally well tolerated but dose-dependent side effects include worsening depression, fatigue, parkinsonism, and akathisia. Tardive dyskinesia is not described.

Neuroleptics and atypical neuroleptics that block postsynaptic D2 receptors have been studied in smaller trials but may be limited by side effects especially tardive dyskinesia and worsening gait and swallowing. Haloperidol, fluphenazine, and pimozide are high-potency atypical antipsychotics that can suppress chorea but do have dose-limiting side effects. Similarly, small trials of atypical neuroleptics such as olanzapine, risperidone, quetiapine, and ziprasidone have been performed with mixed results. Treatment with these typical and atypical antipsychotics rather than TBZ is advised if both motor and behavioral symptomatology is being addressed simultaneously.

Antiglutamatergic Therapy for Chorea

Glutamate toxicity resulting in degeneration of medium spiny striatal neurons is the concept behind treatment with NMDA receptor antagonists such as amantadine or compound that disrupt glutamate transmission such as riluzole. These have been shown to have none to minimal symptomatic or neuroprotective benefits in level 1 studies.

TREATMENT OF DYSTONIA

There have been no class 1 studies for dystonia in the setting of HD. Botulinum toxin injections can be also used for focal dystonia associated with HD.

TREATMENT OF VOLUNTARY MOTOR IMPAIRMENT (GAIT AND SWALLOWING)

There are no medical treatments for the voluntary motor impairments (gait, swallowing); however, physical, occupational, and swallowing therapy could provide benefit in terms of reduced fall risk and psychological well-being and increased caloric intake. There have been no randomized controlled trials of exercise in manifest or premanifest HD.

TREATMENT OF WEIGHT LOSS

Weight loss is also common as HD progresses. Increased caloric intake is necessary to maintain body mass index even in the presymptomatic state when there are no obvious movements to account for increased energy expenditure. In manifest HD, weight loss is correlated with rate of disease progression. Weight loss may not only be attributable to severity of the extrapyramidal movement disorder, decreased caloric intake due to dysphagia, or depression but may also be due to a hypermetabolic state associated with HD. Attention to increasing caloric intake to maintain weight, particularly as the disease progresses, is essential for well-being. Pureed foods and thickened liquids and frequent small meals may improve caloric intake. Feeding tube placement is an individual decision that should be discussed well before the need in the later stages of the disease.

TREATMENT OF COGNITIVE IMPAIRMENT

There are no approved treatments for cognitive impairment in HD. Small studies have been conducted with cholinesterase inhibitors including donepezil and rivastigmine with no significant improvement. A randomized controlled trial of citalopram in nondepressed HD patients showed no change in executive function after 20 weeks; however, there was improvement in mood suggesting an effect on subsyndromal depression [**Level 1**].[6] The largest study to date (class 1) included 403 HD participants at 64 centers followed for 6 months, randomized to latrepirdine (20 mg) versus placebo [**Level 1**].[7] This agent thought to be a mitochondrial stabilizer did not show a difference in performance on Mini-Mental Status Examination or Clinician Interview–Based Impression of Change.

TREATMENT OF PSYCHIATRIC SYMPTOMS

The FDA-approved medications for depression, irritability, obsessive–compulsive behaviors, and general anxiety and aggression have been used to treat individuals with HD. Data is confined to case series and small open-label studies. There are no class I studies specifically for the treatment of psychiatric symptomatology.

OUTCOME

The course of HD is generally 15 to 20 years from the time of diagnosis based on the presence of an extrapyramidal syndrome consistent with HD. The course of juvenile HD rarely exceeds 15 years. The most frequent cause of death is aspiration pneumonia, although accidents, especially subdural hematoma, are common. Increasing attention to the benefits of weight maintenance and balance training may be life prolonging. The completion of three well-designed observational studies of at risk and early symptomatic individuals (PHAROS, TRACK HD, and PREDICT HD) will facilitate the design of new clinical trials that are adequately powered to detect change at all stages of the illness.

Videos can be found in the companion e-book edition. For a full list of video legends, please see the front matter.

LEVEL 1 EVIDENCE

1. Armstrong MJ, Miyasaki JM; American Academy of Neurology. Evidence-based guideline: pharmacologic treatment of chorea in Huntington disease: report of the guideline development subcommittee of the American Academy of Neurology. *Neurology*. 2012;79(6):597–603.
2. Bonelli RM, Wenning GK. Pharmacological management of Huntington's disease: an evidence-based review. *Curr Pharm Des*. 2006;12(21):2701–2720.
3. Frank S, Jankovic J. Advances in the pharmacological management of Huntington's disease. *Drugs*. 2010;70(5):561–571.
4. Venuto CS, McGarry A, Ma Q, et al. Pharmacologic approaches to the treatment of Huntington's disease. *Mov Disord*. 2012;27:31–41. doi:10.1002/mds.23953.
5. Huntington Study Group. Tetrabenazine as antichorea therapy in Huntington disease: a randomized controlled trial. *Neurology*. 2006;66(3):366–372.
6. Beglinger LJ, Adams WH, Langbehn D, et al. Results of the citalopram to enhance cognition in Huntington disease trial. *Mov Disord*. 2014;29(3):401–405.
7. Kieburtz K, McDermott MP, Voss TS, et al; Huntington Disease Study Group DIMOND Investigators. A randomized, placebo-controlled trial of latrepirdine in Huntington disease. *Arch Neurol*. 2010;67(2):154–160.

SUGGESTED READINGS

Anderson K, Craufurd D, Edmondson MC, et al. An international survey-based algorithm for the pharmacologic treatment of obsessive-compulsive behaviors in Huntington's disease. *PLoS Curr*. 2011;3:RRN1261.

Dorsey ER; Huntington Study Group COHORT Investigators. Characterization of a large group of individuals with Huntington disease and their relatives enrolled in the COHORT study. *PLoS One*. 2012;7(2):e29522. doi:10.1371/journal.pone.0029522.

Duff K, Paulsen J, Mills J, et al; PREDICT-HD Investigators and Coordinators of the Huntington Study Group. Mild cognitive impairment in prediagnosed Huntington disease. *Neurology*. 2010;75(6):500–507. doi:10.1212/WNL.0b013e3181eccfa2.

Groves M, van Duijn E, Anderson K, et al. An international survey-based algorithm for the pharmacologic treatment of irritability in Huntington's disease. *PLoS Curr*. 2011;3:RRN1259.

Gusella JF, Wexler NS, Conneally PM, et al. A polymorphic DNA marker genetically linked to Huntington's disease. *Nature*. 1983;306:234–238.

Huntington Study Group PHAROS Investigators. At risk for Huntington disease: the PHAROS (Prospective Huntington At Risk Observational Study) cohort enrolled. *Arch Neurol*. 2006;63(7):991–996.

Killoran A, Biglan KM, Jankovic J, et al. Characterization of the Huntington intermediate CAG repeat expansion phenotype in PHAROS. *Neurology*. 2013;80(22):2022–2027. doi:10.1212/WNL.0b013e318294b304.

Lee JM, Gillis T, Mysore JS, et al. Common SNP-based haplotype analysis of the 4p16.3 Huntington disease gene region. *Am J Hum Genet*. 2012;90(3):434–444.

Paulsen JS, Langbehn DR, Stout JC, et al. Detection of Huntington's disease decades before diagnosis: the Predict-HD study. *J Neurol Neurosurg Psychiatry*. 2008;70:874–880.

Paulsen JS, Long JD, Johnson HJ, et al. Clinical and biomarker changes in premanifest Huntington disease show trial feasibility: a decade of the Predict-HD study. *Frontiers in Aging Neuroscience*. 2014;6:78. doi:10.3389/fnagi.2014.00078.

Pringsheim T, Wiltshire K, Day L, et al. The incidence and prevalence of Huntington's disease: a systematic review and meta-analysis. *Mov Disord*. 2012;27:1083–1091.

Quarrell OW, Rigby AS, Barron L, et al. Reduced penetrance alleles for Huntington's disease: a multi-centre direct observational study. *J Med Genet*. 2007;44:e68.

Rosas HD, Doros G, Gevorkian S, et al. PRECREST: a phase II prevention and biomarker trial of creatine in at-risk Huntington disease. *Neurology*. 2014;82(10):850–857. doi:10.1212/WNL.0000000000000187.

Ross CA, Tabrizi SJ. Huntington's disease: from molecular pathogenesis to clinical treatment. *Lancet Neurol*. 2011;10(1):83–98. doi:10.1016/S1474-4422(10)70245-3.

Shoulson I, Kurlan R, Rubin AJ, et al. Assessment of functional capacity in neurodegenerative movement disorders: Huntington's disease as a prototype. In: Munsat TL, ed. *Quantification of Neurological Deficit*. Boston, MA: Butterworth; 1989:271–283.

Stout JC, Paulsen JS, Queller S, et al. Neurocognitive signs in prodromal Huntington disease. *Neuropsychology*. 2011;25(1):1–14. doi:10.1037/a0020937.

Tabrizi SJ, Langbehn DR, Leavitt BR, et al. Biological and clinical manifestations of Huntington's disease in the longitudinal TRACK-HD study: cross-sectional analysis of baseline data. *Lancet Neurol*. 2009;8:791–801.

Tabrizi SJ, Scahill RI, Owen G, et al. Predictors of phenotypic progression and disease onset in premanifest and early-stage Huntington's disease in the TRACK-HD study: analysis of 36-month observational data. *Lancet Neurol*. 2013;12:637–649.

The Huntington's Disease Collaborative Research Group. A novel gene containing a trinucleotide repeat that is expanded and unstable on Huntington's disease chromosomes. *Cell*. 1993;72:971–983.

The Huntington Study Group. Unified Huntington's Disease Rating Scale: reliability and consistency. *Mov Disord*. 1996;11:136–142.

Vonsattel JP, DiFiglia M. Huntington disease. *J Neuropathol Exp Neurol*. 1998;57(5):369–384.

Vonsattel JP, Myers RH, Stevens TJ, et al. Neuropathological classification of Huntington's disease. *J Neuropathol Exp Neurol*. 1985;44(6):559–577.

Wexler NS, Lorimer J, Porter J, et al. Venezuelan kindreds reveal that genetic and environmental factors modulate Huntington's disease age of onset. *Proc Natl Acad Sci U S A*. 2004;101:3498–3503.

Parkinson Disease 83

Stanley Fahn and Un Jung Kang

INTRODUCTION

In 1817, James Parkinson described the major clinical motor features of what today is recognized as the symptom complex known as *parkinsonism*, manifested by any combination of six cardinal features: tremor at rest, rigidity, bradykinesia–hypokinesia, flexed posture, loss of postural reflexes, and the freezing phenomenon. At least two of these features, with at least one being either tremor at rest or bradykinesia, must be present for a clinical diagnosis of parkinsonism. The many causes of parkinsonism (Table 83.1) are divided into five categories—primary, symptomatic/secondary, Parkinson-plus syndromes, various heredodegenerative diseases in which parkinsonism is a manifestation, and parkinsonism with neurotransmitter enzyme deficit. An example of parkinsonism with dopamine enzyme deficit and a benign clinical course is the condition known as *dopa-responsive dystonia*, covered in the chapter on dystonia (see Chapter 76). Primary parkinsonism is known as *Parkinson disease* (PD), which can be sporadic or familial; it is the most common type of parkinsonism encountered by neurologists and is the second most common neurodegenerative disease after Alzheimer disease (AD). In addition to the motor features of PD, the importance of nonmotor features, ranging from fatigue, sleep, and behavioral disturbances to autonomic and sensory symptoms is increasingly appreciated as contributors to the overall disability of patients with PD.

The core biochemical pathology in parkinsonism is decreased dopaminergic neurotransmission in the basal ganglia. In most of the diseases in Table 83.1, degeneration of the nigrostriatal dopamine system results in marked loss of striatal dopamine content. In some, degeneration of the striatum with loss of dopamine receptors is present and is probably responsible for the lack of therapeutic effect by dopaminergic agents in these disorders. Drug-induced parkinsonism is the result of blockade of dopamine receptors or depletion of dopamine storage. It is not known how hydrocephalus or abnormal calcium metabolism produces parkinsonism. Physiologically, the decreased dopaminergic activity in the striatum leads to abnormal activities of the subthalamic nucleus and the globus pallidus interna (GPi), which is the predominant efferent nucleus in the basal ganglia. Understanding the biochemical pathology led to dopamine replacement therapy; understanding the physiologic change in brain network circuitry led to surgical interventions, such as deep brain stimulation of GPi, the subthalamic nucleus and ventrointermediate nucleus of the thalamus. Lesioning of these nuclei (pallidotomy, thalamotomy) is an alternative surgical technique. In addition, nondopaminergic system deficit is associated with many of the nonmotor symptoms.

EPIDEMIOLOGY

PD makes up approximately 80% of cases of parkinsonism listed in Table 83.1. The incidence and prevalence of PD increase with age. The mean age at onset is about 60 years. Onset at younger than 20 years is known as *juvenile parkinsonism*. Many cases are due to mutations in the *PRKN* gene, an autosomal recessive disorder without Lewy bodies in the degenerating substantia nigra. Some heredodegenerative diseases such as Huntington disease and Wilson disease can present as juvenile parkinsonism. Onset of primary parkinsonism between 20 and 40 years is defined as *young-onset PD*; some investigators extend the age to 50 years to account for higher genetic contribution than later onset cases. PD is more common in men, with a male-to-female ratio of 3:2. The prevalence of PD is approximately 160 per 100,000, and the incidence is about 20 per 100,000 per year. The prevalence and incidence increase exponentially with age, and at age 70 years, the prevalence is approximately 550 per 100,000, and the incidence is 120 per 100,000 per year.

PATHOBIOLOGY

PATHOLOGY

The pathology of PD is distinctive. Degeneration of the neuromelanin-containing neurons in the brain stem occurs, especially dopamine-containing neurons in the ventral tier of the pars compacta in the substantia nigra and in the noradrenergic-containing neurons in the locus ceruleus; many of the surviving neurons in these nuclei contain eosinophilic cytoplasmic proteinaceous inclusions known as *Lewy bodies*, the pathologic hallmark of the disease. The nigral dopaminergic neurons project to the neostriatum (nigrostriatal pathway). By the time symptoms appear, the substantia nigra already has lost about 60% of dopaminergic neurons and the dopamine content in the striatum is about 80% less than normal. Incidental Lewy bodies seen at neuropathologic examination in individuals without PD symptoms or signs are thought to represent presymptomatic individuals who would have ultimately developed clinical manifestations of PD. Lewy bodies and Lewy neurites (intra-axonal aggregates) contain the protein, α-synuclein, and are present both in PD and dementia with Lewy bodies, which is associated with wide spread cortical pathology. Other synucleinopathies include multiple system atrophy (MSA) with oligodendrocyte inclusions containing α-synuclein and some forms of neurodegeneration with brain iron accumulation (NBIA), which shows axonal spheroids with α-synuclein deposition.

Staining for Lewy bodies and neurites with antibodies to α-synuclein indicates that the aggregation of α-synuclein first occurs in the olfactory apparatus and in the caudal brain stem, especially the dorsal motor nucleus of the vagus in the medulla even in cases without involvement of substantia nigra pars compacta or clinical PD symptoms. Braak proposed a staging system for PD pathology and proposed a hypothesis that the Lewy-related pathology progressively spread rostrally up the brain stem and then into the telencephalon and cerebral cortex (Fig. 83.1). However, Lewy pathology does not correlate with actual cell loss or function and there are many cases that do not fit the pattern

TABLE 83.1 Classification of Major Parkinsonian Syndromes

Extrapyramidal Syndromes

- Parkinson disease—sporadic and familial

Secondary Parkinsonism

- Drug-induced: dopamine antagonists and depleters
- Hemiatrophy—hemiparkinsonism
- Hydrocephalus; normal pressure hydrocephalus
- Hypoxia
- Infectious; postencephalitic
- Metabolic; parathyroid dysfunction
- Toxin: Mn, CO, MPTP, cyanide
- Trauma
- Tumor
- Vascular; multi-infarct state

Parkinson-Plus Syndromes

- Corticobasal degeneration
- Dementia syndromes
  - Alzheimer disease
  - Dementia with Lewy bodies
  - Frontotemporal dementia
- Lytico–Bodig (Guam parkinsonism–dementia–ALS)
- Multiple system atrophy syndromes
  - Striatonigral degeneration (MSA-P)
  - Shy–Drager syndrome
  - Sporadic olivopontocerebellar degeneration (OPCA) (MSA-C)
  - Motor neuron disease–parkinsonism
- Progressive pallidal atrophy
- Progressive supranuclear palsy (PSP)

Heredodegenerative Diseases

- Neurodegeneration with brain iron accumulation (NBIA)
- Huntington disease (Westphal variant)
- Lubag (X-linked dystonia-parkinsonism)
- Mitochondrial cytopathies with striatal necrosis
- Neuroacanthocytosis
- Wilson disease

Parkinsonism with Neurotransmitter Enzyme Deficit

- Enzymatic deficiencies of dopamine synthesis

Mn, manganese; CO, carbon monoxide; MPTP, 1-methyl-4-phenyl-1,2,3,6-tetrahydropyridine; ALS, amyotrophic lateral sclerosis; MSA-P, multiple system atrophy with predominant parkinsonism; MSA-C, multiple system atrophy with cerebellar features.

of hypothesized progression. The susceptible neurons containing Lewy neurites belong to the class of projection neurons with an axon that is disproportionately long, thin, and poorly myelinated or unmyelinated.

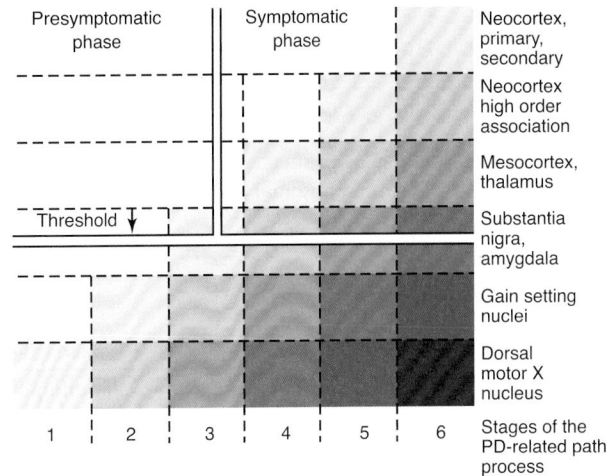

FIGURE 83.1 Six stages of PD based on distribution of Lewy neurites in the brain. Staining for α-synuclein in Lewy neurites reveals their distribution. The *darkest color* represents the most intense deposition of Lewy neurites and their earliest appearance, which is in the olfactory tubercle and dorsal motor nucleus of the vagus. The substantia nigra develops Lewy neurites at stage 3, following which symptoms of PD appear (Braak stage 4). The neocortex is involved in stages 5 and 6. The susceptible neurons belong to the class of projection neurons with an axon that is disproportionately long, thin, and poorly myelinated or unmyelinated. (From Braak H, Bohl JR, Müller CM, et al. Stanley Fahn lecture 2005: the staging procedure for the inclusion body pathology associated with sporadic Parkinson's disease reconsidered. *Mov Disord*. 2006;21[12]:2042–2051.)

ETIOLOGY

The cause of PD in the vast majority of patients is unknown. Research has discovered both environmental and genetic factors. The discovery that the chemical agent 1-methyl-4-phenyl-1,2,3,6-tetrahydropyridine (MPTP) can cause parkinsonism raised the possibility that PD might be caused by an environmental toxin. No single environmental factor has emerged as essential, but growing up in a rural farming environment has been disproportionately frequent in some studies, suggesting potential role of pesticides, some resembling MPTP in chemical structures. Exposure to excess levels of manganese may produce a neurobehavioral syndrome that shares some of the cognitive and motor features of PD, but whether it increases the risk of idiopathic PD is controversial. Interestingly, decreased risk of PD in those with high level of caffeine consumption or cigarette smoking has been consistently noted. High uric acid levels are also associated with decreased risk and slower progression of PD.

GENETICS

Contribution of genetic factors has been recognized only since late 1990s. Studies of twins showed that onset of PD before age 50 years has a higher likelihood of a genetic cause. The first genetic form of PD was discovered in 1997 and now more than 20 different genetic forms of parkinsonism, labeled as PARK, have been discovered. Many of them are Parkinson-plus syndromes, and pathology is variable including some without Lewy body and some as NBIAs. These are summarized in Table 83.2. We will discuss well-established genetic forms with typical PD clinical phenotypes here.

TABLE 83.2 The Most Definitive Genetic Forms of Parkinson Disease

Name and Locus	Gene	Mode of Inheritance	Pathologic and Clinical Features	Protein Function	Where Found
PARK1 and 4 4q22.1	SCNA	Autosomal dominant	Lewy bodies; earlier onset and more aggressive course; L-dopa–responsive parkinsonism, dementia, hallucinations, autonomic dysfunction	*α-Synuclein* possibly synaptic vesicle trafficking, elevated in bird song learning	Families in Germany, Italy, United States (Contoursi kindred), Greece, Spain
PARK8 12q12	LRRK2	Autosomal dominant	Pathologic pleomorphism; indistinguishable from idiopathic PD		Worldwide
PARK2 6q26	PRKN	Autosomal recessive	Often juvenile onset without Lewy bodies; slowly progressive; no dementia	Parkin, a ubiquitin E3 ligase, attaches short ubiquitin peptide chains to a range of proteins, likely to mark degradation; supports mitophagy	Ubiquitous, originally in Japan, very common in juvenile onset
PARK6 1p36.12	PINK-1	Autosomal recessive	Juvenile onset	Mitochondrial kinase, modulates mitochondrial dynamics; supports mitophagy	Families in Italy, Spain, Philippines, Taiwan, Israel, Japan, Ireland, and North America
PARK7 1p36.23	DJ-1	Autosomal recessive	Early onset	Possible atypical peroxiredoxin and may play a role in apoptosis	Families in Holland, Italy, Uruguay
Glucocerebrosidase 1q22	GBA	Autosomal dominant; susceptibility gene; low penetrance; most common genetic risk factor gene	Indistinguishable from idiopathic PD	Lysosomal enzyme	About 13% of sporadic PD in Ashkenazi Jews, found in all ethnic groups

PD, Parkinson disease.

The first genetic cause of PD (PARK1) was discovered to be mutations in *SNCA* gene located on chromosome 4q22.1 coding for the protein α-synuclein. α-Synuclein is an abundant presynaptic protein. The resulting parkinsonism transmits in an autosomal dominant pattern. It is rare, being reported only in a small number of families originating in Greece, Italy, Germany, and Spain. However, single nucleotide polymorphisms have been associated with sporadic PD and the protein α-synuclein is present in Lewy bodies, even in patients with PD without genetic mutations, suggesting potential pathophysiologic role of α-synuclein in sporadic form of PD. It is not known if Lewy bodies contribute to neuronal degeneration or are a protective mechanism to slow neuronal death. Duplication and triplication of the α-synuclein gene also cause familial parkinsonism (PARK4), suggesting that overexpression of the normal (wild-type) protein suffices to provoke dopaminergic neurodegeneration.

Another gene defect causing familial PD is PARK8, which has been mapped to chromosome 12q12 and encodes for a previously unknown protein named *leucine-rich repeat kinase-2* (LRRK2), also known as *dardarin*. This 2527 amino acid protein belongs to the family of the ROCO protein, contains a protein kinase domain, and is ubiquitously expressed in the central nervous system (CNS). About a dozen pathogenic *LRRK2* mutations have been identified, which have been found to be the most frequent genetic cause of

PD, accounting to up to 5% of familial cases in the Caucasian population. Some ethnic groups have a particularly high prevalence; the most common mutation, G2019S, has an increased frequency among Ashkenazi Jews (18.3% of those with PD) and North African Berbers (39% of those with PD). *LRRK2* mutations result in an autosomal dominant parkinsonism that resembles late-onset idiopathic PD. Genome-wide association studies have shown significance of *LRRK2* polymorphism in sporadic PD as well. Although the neuropathology associated with *LRRK2* mutations is highly variable with some with Lewy bodies and others with neurofibrillary tangles, degeneration of substantia nigra neurons has been observed consistently.

The most commonly occurring gene defect causing juvenile familial parkinsonism is PARK2 (*PRKN*) on chromosome 6q26, coding for the E2-dependent E3 ubiquitin-protein ligase, parkin. Mutations in the parkin gene result in an autosomal recessive parkinsonism that is slowly progressive, with onset usually before age 30 years and with sleep benefit; rest tremor can be present. This cause of PD has a better prognosis for both motor and cognitive outcomes than idiopathic PD. There is degeneration of substantia nigra neurons, but in most instances, no Lewy body inclusions are found. Some typical adult-onset PD patients have been found to have a single heterozygotic mutation of the *PRKN* gene and with Lewy bodies at autopsy. Other recessive forms with similar juvenile parkinsonism include those with PTEN-induced putative kinase 1 (*PINK1*; PARK6) and *DJ-1* (PARK7) mutations.

Glucocerebrosidase (*GBA*) gene mutations, when homozygous, cause autosomal recessive Gaucher disease. Heterozygous carriers are at increased risk for developing PD that is indistinguishable from idiopathic PD. PD patients with *GBA* mutations tend to have more cognitive problems, and about 13% of Ashkenazi Jews with PD have this mutation, but the same mutation causes PD in other ethnic groups as well.

PATHOGENESIS

Two major pathogenic hypotheses have emerged from epidemiologic and genetic evidences as well as postmortem examinations. One hypothesis proposes that mitochondrial dysfunction and oxidative stress are critical in the pathogenesis, whereas there is also evidence that misfolding and aggregation of proteins are instrumental in the PD neurodegenerative process. These two hypotheses are not mutually exclusive, and interactions among these pathogenic factors are likely to be important in understanding the mechanisms of neurodegeneration in PD.

Environmental toxins associated with PD risk can damage mitochondria and generate oxidative stress. Postmortem biochemical observations also show that complex I activity of mitochondria is reduced in substantia nigra of patients with PD. Such a defect would decrease the synthesis of ATP and also lead to the buildup of free electrons, thereby increasing oxidative stress. Substantia nigra in patients with PD shows severe depletion of reduced glutathione, the major substrate required for the elimination of reactive oxygen species. This change is also seen in brains with incidental Lewy bodies and therefore could be the one of the earliest biochemical abnormalities of PD. It is not known, however, if this change is the cause or the result of oxidative stress. Iron in the substantia nigra may also play a critical role because it can catalyze the formation of the highly reactive hydroxyl radical from hydrogen peroxide. Recessive genes such as *PRKN* and *PINK1* have been shown to have wide ranging effects on mitochondrial quality control such as regulating mitochondria biogenesis, maintaining fission–fusion balance to remove damaged mitochondria, transport of mitochondria, and turnover of damaged mitochondria by recruiting autophagic machinery. Another recessive gene, *DJ-1* is implicated in a pathway handling oxidative stress. Endogenous factors may also predispose melanin-containing monoaminergic neurons to neurodegeneration. Cellular oxidation reactions (such as enzymatic oxidation and auto-oxidation of dopamine and other monoamines) result in the formation of reactive oxygen species such as dopamine quinone and other metabolic products that can damage the monoamine neurons. In addition, dopaminergic neurons and other susceptible neurons such as noradrenergic neurons in locus ceruleus are autonomous pacemakers and have long highly arborized axons, thereby subjected to high metabolic demands. A presence of a particular calcium channel may predispose these neurons to basal metabolic stress.

Most of the genes involved in PD seem to have multiple cellular functions. Nonetheless, genes producing recessive forms of PD have been implicated more in mitochondrial and metabolic pathways as noted earlier, whereas genes associated with autosomal dominant forms of PD have been noted to be involved in protein degradation homeostasis. Whether the hallmark of PD pathology, the Lewy body, which contains α-synuclein contributes to the toxicity or is a protective mechanism is not known. Evidence points to toxicity of protofibrillar forms of α-synuclein, and intriguing experimental evidence suggests that abnormal forms of α-synuclein may have the prion-like property of propagating its abnormal conformation and spreading the pathology along the neuronal projections and across the synaptic connections. α-Synuclein is involved in vesicle recycling. LKKR2 plays a role in vesicular trafficking and cytoskeletal function. Another PD gene, vacuolar protein sorting 35 (*VPS35*) was identified to cause autosomal dominant PD with typical features and good response to levodopa. This gene encodes a subunit of the retromer complex involved in endosomes and vesicular recycling. α-Synuclein and LRRK2 affects protein degradation pathways, including autophagy, a process of cell degradation of dysfunctional cellular components by lysosomes. Glucocerebrosidase is a lysosomal enzyme.

CLINICAL MANIFESTATIONS

CARDINAL MOTOR FEATURES

The clinical features of tremor, bradykinesia, rigidity, loss of postural reflexes, flexed posture, and freezing are the six cardinal motor features of parkinsonism. Not all need to be present, but at least two should be seen, either rest tremor or bradykinesia, before parkinsonism is considered clinically probable. *Rest tremor* at a frequency of 4 to 5 Hz is present in the extremities, almost always distally; occasionally, the rest tremor occurs in the proximal part of the limb instead of distally. The classic "pill-rolling" tremor involves the thumb and forefinger. Rest tremor disappears with action but sometimes reemerges as the limbs maintain a posture (Video 83.1). Rest tremor is also common in the lips, chin, and tongue. Rest tremor of the hands increases with walking and may be an early sign when others are not yet present. Stress or excitement worsens the tremor. Some patients will have an action tremor instead of or in addition to rest tremor. The biggest differential diagnosis of parkinsonian tremor is essential tremor (ET). Ordinarily, these two causes of tremor are easy to distinguish. Tremor of PD is typically a rest tremor, whereas that of ET is a postural and action tremor. However, the manifestations of these tremors can overlap, with patients with severe ET having rest tremor. Not all patients with PD have tremor; when absent, the diagnosis is more difficult to make, and it usually takes longer after onset of symptoms to make a diagnosis. Eventually, bradykinesia worsens to the point of some disability, such as micrographia or dragging a leg when walking, that the patient seeks medical attention.

Akinesia is a paucity of spontaneous movement, but the term is often used interchangeably with *bradykinesia* and *hypokinesia*. Bradykinesia (slowness of movement, difficulty initiating movement, and loss of automatic movement) and hypokinesia (reduction in amplitude of movement, particularly with repetitive movements, so-called decrementing) are the most common features of parkinsonism, although they may appear after the tremor. Bradykinesia has many facets, depending on the affected body parts. The face loses spontaneous expression (masked facies, *hypomimia*) with decreased frequency of blinking. Poverty of spontaneous movement is characterized by loss of gesturing and by the patient's tendency to sit motionless. Speech becomes soft (*hypophonia*), and the voice has a monotonous tone with a lack of inflection (*aprosody*). Some patients do not enunciate clearly (*dysarthria*) and do not separate syllables clearly, thus running the words together (*tachyphemia*). Bradykinesia of the dominant hand results in small and slow handwriting (*micrographia*) and in difficulty shaving, brushing teeth, combing hair, buttoning, or applying makeup. Playing musical instruments is impaired. Walking is slow, with a shortened stride length and a tendency to shuffle with loss of heel strike; arm swing decreases and eventually is lost. Difficulty arising from a deep chair, getting out of automobiles, and turning in bed are symptoms of truncal/body bradykinesia. Drooling saliva results from failure to swallow spontaneously, a feature of bradykinesia, and is not caused by excessive production of saliva. The patients can swallow properly when asked to do so but only constant reminders allow them to keep swallowing saliva. Similarly, arm swing can be normal if the patient voluntarily, and with effort, wishes to have the arms swing on walking. Pronounced bradykinesia prevents a patient with parkinsonism from driving an automobile when foot movement from the accelerator to the brake pedal is too slow.

Bradykinesia is commonly misinterpreted by patients as weakness. Fatigue, a common complaint in PD, particularly in the mild stage of the disease before pronounced slowness appears, may be related to mild bradykinesia or rigidity or may be an independent feature. Subtle signs of bradykinesia can be detected even in the early stage of parkinsonism if one examines for slowness in shrugging the shoulders, lack of gesturing, decreased arm swing, and decrementing amplitude of rapid successive movements. With advancing bradykinesia, slowness and difficulty in the execution of activities of daily living increase. A meal normally consumed in 20 minutes may be only half eaten in an hour or more. Swallowing may become impaired with advancing disease, and choking and aspiration are concerns. Bradykinesia is manifested in many ways depending on the body part affected (Table 83.3).

Rigidity is an increase in muscle tone that is elicited when the examiner moves the patient's limbs, neck, or trunk. This increased resistance to passive movement is equal in all directions and usually is manifested by a ratchety "give" during the movement. This so-called cogwheeling is caused by the underlying tremor even in the absence of visible tremor. Cogwheeling also occurs in patients with ET. Rigidity of the passive limb increases while another limb is engaged in voluntary active movement ("Froment maneuver").

Flexed posture commonly begins in the arms and spreads to involve the entire body. The head is bowed; the trunk is bent forward; the back is kyphotic; the arms are held in front of the body; and the elbows, hips, and knees are flexed. Deformities of the hands include ulnar deviation of the hands, flexion of the metacarpophalangeal joints, and extension of the interphalangeal joints (striatal hand). Inversion of the feet is apparent, and the big toes may be dorsiflexed (striatal toe) and the other toes curled downward. Lateral tilting of the trunk commonly develops (Pisa syndrome), and extreme flexion of the trunk (camptocormia) is sometimes seen.

Loss of postural reflexes leads to falling and eventually to inability to stand unassisted. Postural reflexes are tested by the *pull test*, which is performed by the examiner, who stands behind the patient and gives a sudden firm pull on the shoulders after explaining the procedure and who checks for retropulsion (Videos 83.2 and 83.3). With advance warning, a normal person can recover within two steps. The examiner should always be prepared to catch the patient when this test is conducted; otherwise, a person who has lost postural reflexes could fall. The examiner should have a solid wall behind him or her in case a heavy patient falling backward also causes the examiner to fall backward. As postural reflexes are impaired, the patient collapses into the chair on attempting to sit down (sitting en bloc). Walking can be marked by festination, whereby the patient walks faster and faster, trying to move the feet forward to be under the flexed body's center of gravity and thus prevent falling.

The *freezing* phenomenon (motor block) is a transient inability to perform active movements. It most often affects the legs when walking but also can involve eyelid opening (known as *apraxia*

TABLE 83.3	Clinical Signs of Bradykinesia

Cranial

- Hypomimia (masked face)
- Staring expression with decreased blinking and retracted lids
- Hypometric saccades
- Impaired convergence
- Impaired upward gaze
- Hypophonia (soft voice)
- Aprosody of speech (loss of inflection of voice)
- Palilalia (repetition of first syllable)
- Sialorrhea (drooling of saliva)

Upper Limbs

- Reduced spontaneous movement (e.g., lack of gesturing)
- Decrementing amplitude with repetitive movements of opening and closing fists, pronating and supinating the forearms, and tapping a finger on the thumb
- Micrographia and slowness with handwriting
- Slowness in cutting food, dressing, and in hygienic care
- Decreased arm swing when walking

Lower Limbs

- Decrementing amplitude with repetitive movements of stomping feet or tapping toes
- Short, slow steps when walking
- Not elevating feet as high as normal when walking, tendency to shuffle
- Narrow base when walking
- Tendency to walk on toes; loss of heel strike

Body Bradykinesia

- Slowness in initiating movement on command
- Difficulty arising from a chair and turning in bed
- Difficulty carrying out two motor acts simultaneously
- Reduced shrugging of shoulders

of lid opening or levator inhibition), speaking (*palilalia*), and writing. Freezing occurs suddenly and is transient, lasting usually no more than several seconds with each occurrence. The feet seem as if "glued to the ground" and then suddenly become "unstuck," allowing the patient to walk again (Video 83.3). Freezing typically occurs when the patient begins to walk (start hesitation); turns while walking; or approaches a destination, such as a chair in which to sit (destination hesitation); it is often induced when the patient walks in crowded places (e.g., in the narrow confines of a theater row or when trying to go through a revolving door, or when suddenly confronted by a person coming into their path) and when there is a time restriction to the walking (e.g., trying to enter or exit an elevator before the door closes or when trying to cross a street before the traffic light turns to red). Freezing is often overcome by visual clues, such as having the patient step over objects, and is much less frequent when the patient is going up or down steps than when walking on level ground. The combination of freezing of gait and loss of postural reflexes is particularly devastating because it often leads to falls. Falling is responsible for the high incidence of hip fractures in parkinsonian patients.

SYMPTOMS AND SIGNS

The clinical signs and symptoms of PD can be divided into motor and nonmotor features of PD and those due to complications or adverse effects of the medications employed to treat the disease. The clinical motor features of PD are represented within the six cardinal features of parkinsonism discussed earlier. Of the six cardinal motor signs, tremor, bradykinesia, and rigidity occur early in the course of the disease, whereas flexed posture, loss of postural reflexes, and freezing of gait occur in more advanced stages. Falling is a late symptom. If these normally advanced signs and symptoms occur within 2 years of onset, one should suspect another cause of parkinsonism, such as progressive supranuclear palsy or MSA.

The onset of PD is insidious; tremor is the symptom first recognized in 70% of patients (Table 83.4). Symptoms often begin unilaterally; as the disease progresses, symptoms and signs become bilateral. The disease can remain confined to one side for several years before the other side becomes involved. The disease progresses slowly, and if untreated, the patient eventually becomes wheelchair-bound and bedridden. Despite having severe bradykinesia with marked immobility, patients, when presented with a sudden stimulus, may rise suddenly and move normally for a short burst of motor activity, so-called kinesia paradoxica. The Hoehn-Yahr clinical staging (Table 83.5) captures the progression of the motor features of PD, from unilateral to bilateral, to loss of postural reflexes to disability. Disability in carrying out activities of daily living is scored on

TABLE 83.4 Initial Symptoms in Parkinson Disease

Symptoms	No. of Cases (n = 183)	Percentage
Tremor	129	70.5
Stiffness or slowness of movement	36	19.7
Loss of dexterity and/or handwriting disturbance	23	12.6
Gait disturbance	21	11.5
Muscle pain, cramps, aching	15	8.2
Depression, nervousness, or other psychiatric disturbance	8	4.4
Speech disturbance	7	3.8
General fatigue, muscle weakness	5	2.7
Drooling	3	1.6
Loss of arm swing	3	1.6
Facial masking	3	1.6
Dysphagia	1	0.5
Paresthesia	1	0.5
Average number of initial symptoms per patient		**1.4**

TABLE 83.5 The Modified Hoehn and Yahr Staging Scale for Parkinson Disease

Stage 0	No signs of disease
Stage 1	Unilateral disease
Stage 1.5	Unilateral plus midline/axial involvement
Stage 2	Bilateral disease, without impairment of balance
Stage 2.5	Mild bilateral disease, with an abnormal pull test but with recovery to avoid falling
Stage 3	Mild to moderate bilateral disease; some postural instability (would fall on the pull test if not caught); physically independent
Stage 4	Severe disability; still able to walk or stand unassisted, but a walking aid is advisable to prevent falling
Stage 5	Wheelchair-bound or bedridden unless aided

From Fahn S, Elton RL, Members of the UPDRS Development Committee. The unified Parkinson's disease rating scale. In Fahn S, Marsden CD, Calne DB, et al, eds. *Recent Developments in Parkinson's Disease*. Vol. 2. Florham Park, NJ: Macmillan Healthcare Information; 1987:153–163, 293–304.

the Schwab-England scale. More detailed scoring of individual signs and symptoms of PD are captured in the Unified Parkinson's Disease Rating Scale (UPDRS) and its newer version that includes more nonmotor symptoms, the Movement Disorder Society (MDS)-UPDRS.

The nonmotor symptoms of PD (Table 83.6) can be more troublesome than the motor features of PD. Behavioral and personality changes include a reduced attention span, visuospatial impairment, and a personality that slowly becomes more dependent, fearful, indecisive, and passive. The spouse gradually makes more of the decisions and becomes the dominant partner. The patient speaks less spontaneously. The patient eventually sits much of the day and is inactive unless encouraged to exercise. Passivity and lack of motivation are common and are expressed by the patient's aversion to visiting friends. The patient is more reticent to participate in conversations. Depression is frequent in patients with PD, with about 25% to 50% prevalence. Anxiety may be even more common, often with depression.

Cognitive decline is not an early feature but can become pronounced as the patient ages. Memory impairment, in contrast to AD, is not a feature of early PD; rather, the patient is just slow in responding to questions, so-called bradyphrenia. The correct answer can be obtained if the patient is given enough time. Subtle signs of bradyphrenia include tip-of-the-tongue phenomena from diminished verbal fluency and the inability to change mental set rapidly. In a cross section of patients with PD, 15% to 20% have a more profound dementia, but as many as 75% will develop dementia in their late 70s. Most of these patients have developed Lewy bodies in cortical neurons (Parkinson disease dementia [PDD]), and some have developed concurrent AD. These disorders are not always distinguishable, but dementia with Lewy bodies is often characterized by fluctuating hallucinations.

Sensory symptoms are fairly common, but objective sensory impairment is not seen in PD. Symptoms of pain, burning, and tingling occur in the region of motor involvement. A patient may have dull pain in one shoulder as an early symptom of the disease, which often is misdiagnosed as arthritis or bursitis, and even before clear-cut signs of bradykinesia appear in that same arm. Akathisia (inability to sit still, restlessness) and the restless legs syndrome (RLS) occur in some patients with PD. In both syndromes, uncomfortable sensations disappear with movement, and sometimes, the two

TABLE 83.6   Nonmotor Features of Parkinson Disease

Personality and Behavior	Sensory
• Depression	• Pain
• Fearfulness	• Paresthesia, numbness
• Anxiety	• Burning
• Loss of assertive drive	• Akathisia
• Passivity	• Restless legs syndrome
• Greater dependence	• Hyposmia
• Inability to make decisions	**Autonomic**
• Loss of motivation, apathy	• Orthostatic hypotension
• Abulia	• Bladder problems
Cognition and Mental State	• Gastrointestinal; constipation
• Bradyphrenia	• Sexual dysfunction
• "Tip of the tongue" phenomenon	• Seborrhea
• Confusion	• Sweating
• Dementia	• Rhinorrhea
Sleep Problems	**Behavioral Problems due to Medications**
• Sleep fragmentation	• Hallucinations
• REM sleep behavior disorder	• Psychosis
• Excessive daytime sleepiness	• Punding
• Altered sleep–wake cycle	• Compulsive behaviors
• Drug-induced sleep attacks	• Nonmotor offs
	Other
	• Fatigue

REM, rapid eye movement.

conditions are difficult to distinguish. Akathisia, if present, is usually present most of the day; it may respond to levodopa but otherwise has not been treated successfully. The RLS develops late in the day with crawling sensations in the legs and may be associated with periodic movements in sleep, thereby disturbing sleep. Other sleep problems are fragmented sleep and rapid eye movement (REM) sleep behavior disorder (acting out one's dreams); the latter is usually successfully treated with clonazepam; melatonin may also provide relief. Other sleep problems are encountered with dopaminergic medications including excessive daytime sleepiness and sudden attacks of sleep without warning.

Autonomic disturbances also are encountered. The skin is cooler, constipation is a major complaint, bladder emptying is inadequate, erection may be difficult to achieve, and blood pressure may be low. Orthostatic hypotension is not uncommon and is made worse with dopaminergic medications. A major diagnostic consideration is the dysautonomia of MSA, which often has features of parkinsonism and cerebellar dysfunction. Seborrhea and seborrheic dermatitis are common but can be controlled with good hygiene and facial cleansing. Other nonmotor features of PD are reduced sense of smell (hyposmia), rhinorrhea, and excessive sweating.

Tendon reflexes are usually unimpaired in PD; an abnormal extensor plantar reflex suggests a Parkinson-plus syndrome, but an extension of the big toe "striatal toe" is seen in PD and can mimic a Babinski sign. More common is flexion of the toes on the involved side of the body; this can be the presenting complaint. An uninhibited glabellar reflex (Myerson sign) and palmomental reflexes are common, even early in the disease.

DIFFERENTIAL DIAGNOSIS

The diagnosis of PD is based on the clinical features of parkinsonism; insidious asymmetric onset; slow worsening of symptoms; and the lack of other findings in the history, examination, or laboratory tests that would point to some other cause of parkinsonism (see Tables 83.1 and 83.7). The presence of rest tremor and substantial benefit from levodopa strongly support the diagnosis of PD. One of the most common disorders mistaken for PD is ET (see Chapter 73), which is characterized by postural and kinetic tremor, and not rest tremor unless the disease is advanced. Some patients with ET eventually develop PD. MRI is normal in PD, unless dementia or some other disorder is present. Dopamine transporter (DAT) single-photon emission computed tomography (SPECT) or positron emission tomography (PET) and 3,4-dihydroxy-6-18F-fluoro-L-phenylalanine (FDOPA) PET correlate with decreased dopaminergic nerve terminals in the striatum; the caudal putamen is affected first. DAT SPECT is available in United States and in most of the rest of the world.

TABLE 83.7 Clues Indicate the Likely Type of Parkinsonism

Clinical	Alternative Diagnoses
Never responded to levodopa	Other than PD
Predominantly unilateral	PD; HP–HA syndrome; CBS
Symmetric onset	PD; most forms of parkinsonism
Presence of rest tremor	PD; secondary parkinsonism
Lack of rest tremor	PD; Parkinson-plus syndromes
History of encephalitis	Postencephalitic parkinsonism
History of toxin exposure	Parkinsonism caused by the toxin
Taking neuroleptics	Drug-induced parkinsonism
Shuffling gait much greater than upper limb bradykinesia	Normal pressure hydrocephalus; vascular parkinsonism
Severe unilateral rigidity	CBS
Cortical sensory signs	CBD
Unilateral cortical myoclonus	CBD
Unilateral apraxia	CBD
Alien limb	CBD
Early dementia	Dementia with Lewy bodies; AD; frontotemporal dementia
Psychotic sensitivity to levodopa	Dementia with Lewy bodies; AD
Early loss of postural reflexes	Progressive supranuclear palsy
Early falling	Progressive supranuclear palsy
Impaired downgaze	Progressive supranuclear palsy
MRI: caudate atrophy	HD; neuroacanthocytosis
MRI: decreased T2 signal in striatum	Multiple system atrophy
MRI: midbrain atrophy	Progressive supranuclear palsy
"Apraxia" of eyelid opening	Progressive supranuclear palsy
Deep nasolabial folds	Progressive supranuclear palsy
Furrowed forehead and eyebrows (quizzical look)	Progressive supranuclear palsy
Excessive hesitation between words when speaking	Progressive supranuclear palsy; CBD
Nuchal dystonia	Progressive supranuclear palsy
Abducted arms when walking	Progressive supranuclear palsy
Square wave jerks	Progressive supranuclear palsy; multiple system atrophy; CBS
Pure freezing	Progressive supranuclear palsy
Meaningful orthostatic hypotension	Multiple system atrophy
Urinary or fecal incontinence	Multiple system atrophy
Cerebellar dysarthria and dysmetria	Multiple system atrophy, SCA2, SCA3, SCA17
Laryngeal stridor (vocal cord paresis)	Multiple system atrophy
Lower motor neuron findings	Multiple system atrophy; neuroacanthocytosis
Upper motor neuron findings	Multiple system atrophy
Early orofacial dyskinesia with levodopa	Multiple system atrophy
Laboratory	
Fresh blood smear: acanthocytes	Neuroacanthocytosis
Grossly elevated creatine kinase	Neuroacanthocytosis
MRI: many lacunes	Vascular parkinsonism
MRI: "eye of the tiger" in pallidum	Pantothenate kinase–associated neurodegeneration (PKAN)
MRI: huge ventricles	Normal pressure hydrocephalus
Abnormal autonomic function tests	Multiple system atrophy
Denervation on sphincter EMG	Multiple system atrophy

PD, Parkinson disease; HP–HA, hemiparkinsonism–hemiatrophy; CBS, cortical-basal syndrome; CBD, cortical-basal degeneration; AD, Alzheimer disease; MRI, magnetic resonance imaging; HD, Huntington disease; SCA, spinocerebellar atrophy; EMG, electromyography.

It can be used to distinguish the diagnosis of PD from ET; the DAT scan is normal in ET. ^{18}F-fluorodeoxyglucose (FDG)-PET reveals hypermetabolism in the lentiform nucleus and a progressive metabolic network pattern that correlates with disease worsening. A different metabolic network pattern is associated with declining cognition in PD and also in Parkinson-plus syndromes.

Several clinical clues suggest that a patient with parkinsonism has some form of the syndrome other than PD itself (Table 83.7). In general, PD often presents with symptoms on only one side of the body, whereas patients with symptomatic parkinsonism or Parkinson-plus syndromes almost always have symmetric symptoms and signs (notable exceptions are cortical–basal syndrome and parkinsonism resulting from a focal brain injury, such as head trauma). Similarly, a rest tremor usually indicates PD because it much less often seen in symptomatic parkinsonism or Parkinson-plus syndromes, except in drug-induced and MPTP-induced parkinsonism, which do include rest tremor. The patient who does not have unilateral onset or rest tremor, however, still can have PD that begins symmetrically and without tremor. Perhaps the most important diagnostic aid is the response to levodopa. Patients with PD almost always have a clear-cut, satisfactory response to this drug. If a patient never responds to levodopa, the diagnosis of some other form of parkinsonism is likely. A response to levodopa, however, does not confirm the diagnosis of PD because many cases of symptomatic parkinsonism (e.g., MPTP, postencephalitic, reserpine induced) and many forms of Parkinson-plus syndromes in their early stages (e.g., MSA) also respond to levodopa. Table 83.7 provides a list of some helpful clues. Chapter 84 provides clinical descriptions of other parkinsonian disorders.

TREATMENT

At present, treatment is aimed at controlling motor and nonmotor symptoms of PD because no drug or surgical approach unequivocally prevents progression of the disease, although some clinical trials suggest that monoamine oxidase-B (MAO-B) inhibitors may slow clinical progression. Treatment is individualized because each patient has a unique set of symptoms; signs; response to medications; and a host of social, occupational, and emotional needs that must be considered. The goal is to keep the patient functioning independently as long as possible. Practical guides are the symptoms and degree of functional impairment and the expected benefits and risks of therapeutic agents. Much of the therapeutic effort in advanced PD involves controlling the motor adverse effects of levodopa, namely, dyskinesias and wearing-off.

Although pharmacotherapy is the basis of treatment, physiotherapy and exercise are also important [Level 1].[1] It involves patients participating actively in their own care, promotes exercise, keeps muscles active, preserves mobility, and improves balance. This approach is especially beneficial as parkinsonism advances because many patients tend to remain sitting and inactive. Psychiatric assistance may be required to deal with depression and anxiety and the social and familial problems that may develop with this chronic disabling illness. Electroconvulsive therapy may have a role in patients with severe intractable depression.

USEFUL DRUGS AND SURGICAL PROCEDURES

Table 83.8 lists the drugs useful in parkinsonism according to mechanisms of action. It also lists some of the surgical approaches available. Selection of the most suitable drugs for the individual

TABLE 83.8	**Therapeutic Choices for Parkinson Disease**
Medications	

- Dopamine precursor: levodopa ± carbidopa, standard and extended release
- Dopamine agonists: bromocriptine, pramipexole, ropinirole, apomorphine, cabergoline, rotigotine
- Catechol-O-methyltransferase inhibitors: entacapone and tolcapone
- Dopamine releaser: amantadine
- Glutamate antagonist: amantadine
- Monoamine oxidase type B inhibitors: selegiline and rasagiline
- Anticholinergics: trihexyphenidyl, benztropine, ethopropazine, biperiden, cycrimine, procyclidine. Weaker anticholinergics: diphenhydramine, orphenadrine, amitriptyline
- Muscle relaxants: cyclobenzaprine, diazepam, baclofen
- Peripheral antidopaminergic for nausea and anorexia: domperidone
- Antidepressants: amitriptyline and other tricyclics, fluoxetine and other serotonin uptake inhibitors
- Antianxiety agents: benzodiazepines
- Antipsychotics: clozapine, quetiapine
- Cholinesterase inhibitors for dementia: rivastigmine, donepezil
- REM sleep behavior disorder: clonazepam, melatonin
- Hypnotics: zolpidem, mirtazapine, amitriptyline, trazodone
- Antisoporific (daytime drowsiness): modafinil (Provigil), methylphenidate
- Anti–restless legs: dopamine agonists, pregabalin, gabapentin, opioids (e.g., propoxyphene, tramadol, oxycodone)
- Antisialorrhea: glycopyrrolate, propantheline, trospium (Sanctura), and other non–CNS-penetrating anticholinergics; botulinum toxin injection into salivary glands
- Antihypotensives: midodrine (ProAmatine), fludrocortisone, droxidopa
- Anticonstipation: high-fiber diet, polyethylene glycol (MiraLAX), and other laxatives

Surgery

- Ablative surgery
  - Thalamotomy
  - Pallidotomy
- Deep brain stimulation
  - Thalamic stimulation
  - Pallidal stimulation
  - Subthalamic stimulation

patient and deciding when to use them in the course of the disease are challenges for the treating clinician. Because PD is chronic and progressive, treatment is lifelong. Medications and their doses change with time as adverse effects and new symptoms are encountered. Tactical strategy is based on the severity of symptoms.

In Table 83.8, *carbidopa* is listed as the peripheral dopa decarboxylase inhibitor, but in many countries, *benserazide* is also available. These agents potentiate the effects of levodopa, thus allowing about a fourfold reduction in dosage to obtain the same benefit. Moreover, by preventing the formation of peripheral dopamine, which can act at the area postrema (vomiting center), they block the development of anorexia, nausea, and vomiting. *Domperidone* is a dopamine receptor antagonist that does not enter the CNS; it is used to prevent nausea not only from levodopa but also from dopamine agonists. Domperidone is not available in the United States. Providing larger doses of carbidopa may also reduce gastrointestinal adverse effects.

Of the listed dopamine agonists, bromocriptine, pramipexole, ropinirole, rotigotine, and apomorphine are available in the United States; they are reviewed in a later section. Pergolide and cabergoline affect heart valve serotonin (5-hydroxytryptamine) 2B (5HT2B) receptors and can cause a fibrotic valvulopathy. Pergolide is no longer available in the United States. Because it is not absorbed through the intestinal tract and it is water-soluble, apomorphine is used as an injectable, rapidly acting dopaminergic drug to overcome "off" states (rescue effect). Subcutaneous apomorphine infusions are available in Europe, as are lisuride and cabergoline. Catechol-*O*-methyltransferase (COMT) inhibitors extend the elimination half-life of levodopa. Entacapone has a very short half-life and is given with each dose of levodopa. Tolcapone is longer-acting but requires monitoring for hepatotoxicity.

Amantadine, selegiline, rasagiline, and the anticholinergics are reviewed in following sections. Because the anticholinergics can cause forgetfulness and even psychosis, they should be used cautiously in patients most susceptible (those older than 70 years). The antihistaminics, tricyclics, and cyclobenzaprine have milder anticholinergic properties that make them useful in PD, particularly in the older patient who should not take the stronger anticholinergics. A number of medications listed in Table 83.8 are used to treat the many nonmotor problems seen in PD; these are discussed in a later section. The surgical procedures are also covered separately.

Levodopa is uniformly accepted as the most effective drug available for symptomatic relief of many of the motor features of PD. If it were uniformly and persistently successful and also free of complications, new strategies for other treatment would not be needed. Unfortunately, 75% of patients have serious complications after 5 years of levodopa therapy (Table 83.9).

TABLE 83.9	Five Major Outcomes after More Than 5 Years of Levodopa Therapy (*n* = 330 Patients)[a]	
Smooth good response		*n* = 83 (25%)
Troublesome fluctuations		*n* = 142 (43%)
Troublesome dyskinesias		*n* = 67 (19%)
Toxicity at therapeutic or subtherapeutic dosages		*n* = 14 (4%)
Total or substantial loss of efficacy		*n* = 27 (8%)

[a]Thirty-six patients had both troublesome fluctuations and troublesome dyskinesias.
From Fahn S. Adverse effects of levodopa. In: Olanow CW, Lieberman AN, eds. *The Scientific Basis for the Treatment of Parkinson's Disease.* Carnforth, England: Parthenon; 1992:89–112.

TREATMENT ACCORDING TO THE STAGE OF PARKINSON DISEASE

EARLY STAGE

Authorities generally agree that in the early stage of PD when symptoms are noticed but not troublesome, symptomatic treatment is not necessary. All symptomatic drugs can induce side effects, and if a patient is not troubled socially or occupationally by mild symptoms, drug therapy can be delayed until symptoms become more pronounced. If disease-modifying therapies become available, they should be started at the time of diagnosis.

Selegiline delays the need for levodopa therapy by an average of 9 months. Because this MAO-B inhibitor provides a mild symptomatic effect, it has not been possible to conclude that selegiline also exerts a neuroprotective effect. However, a controlled study evaluating selegiline in the presence of levodopa therapy showed that those on selegiline performed better than subjects receiving placebo, including less development of the freezing phenomenon, thus, selegiline should be considered as a therapeutic option at the time the diagnosis of PD is made [**Level 1**].[2,3] Selegiline (dose: 5 mg with breakfast and lunch) has few adverse effects when given without levodopa, but when given concurrently with levodopa, it increases the dopaminergic effect, allows a lower dose of levodopa, and contributes to dopaminergic-induced dyskinesias and hallucinations. *Rasagiline,* another irreversible propargylamine MAO-B inhibitor, also provides mild symptomatic effect, and controlled studies suggest it might have some disease-modifying effect as well (dose: 1 mg per day) [**Level 1**].[4] Exenatide showed promise of slowing progression in a pilot trial [**Level 1**].[5]

STAGE WHEN SYMPTOMS AND SIGNS REQUIRE SYMPTOMATIC TREATMENT

Eventually, PD progresses and symptomatic treatment must be used. The most common problems that clinicians consider important in deciding to use symptomatic agents are the following: threat to employment; threat to ability to handle domestic, financial, or social affairs; threat to handle activities of daily living; and appreciable worsening of gait or balance. In clinical practice, a global judgment for initiating such therapy is made in discussions between the patient and the treating physician.

The major decision is when to introduce levodopa, the most effective drug. All patients are likely to develop complications associated with long-term use (see Table 83.9). Younger patients, in particular, are more likely to show response fluctuations and dyskinesias, so other antiparkinsonian drugs, including dopamine agonists, could be used first to delay the introduction of levodopa in patients younger than age 50 years. This approach is known as the *levodopa-sparing strategy.* When symptoms threaten quality of life, levodopa is needed and should be administered at the lowest effective dose. High doses are more likely to induce the motor complications of dyskinesias and wearing-off. Concern that levodopa may hasten nigral dopaminergic neuronal degeneration has been largely diminished because a controlled trial, the ELLDOPA (earlier vs. later levodopa therapy in PD) study, showed that those with levodopa treatment actually are less impaired even after stopping medication for a few weeks (Fig. 83.2). The mechanism for this long-lasting improvement is not known.

The drugs used in the levodopa-sparing strategy are discussed first, for these are tolerated in younger patients, who are most prone to develop motor complications from levodopa and who can often respond to these other drugs. For patients older than

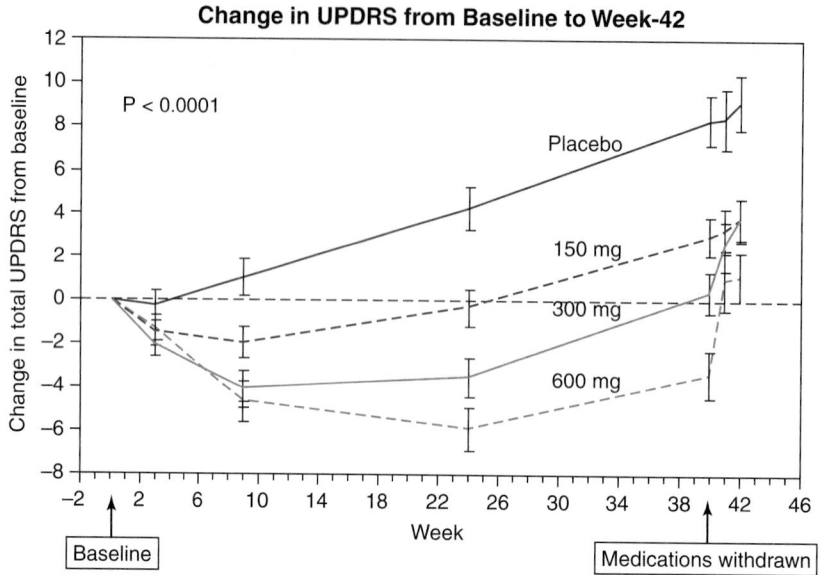

Change in UPDRS from Baseline to Week-42

P < 0.0001

Placebo

150 mg

300 mg

600 mg

Baseline

Medications withdrawn

FIGURE 83.2 Effect of different dosages of levodopa on the severity of PD based on changes in the Unified Parkinson's Disease Rating Scale (UPDRS). Data are from the ELLDOPA study in which subjects with early, untreated PD were randomized equally to one of three doses of levodopa (with carbidopa) or placebo. Treatment lasted 40 weeks, after which the medication was tapered to zero over 3 days, and the subjects were evaluated 7 and 14 days later. The changes in subjects treated with levodopa at different dosages or with placebo were determined on the basis of the total score of UPDRS. The scores were obtained by the blinded treating investigator who performed the evaluations before the morning dose of the daily dose of the study drug. The points on the curves represent mean changes from baseline in the total scores at each visit. Improvement in parkinsonism is represented by lower scores and worsening by higher scores. Negative scores on the curves indicate improvement from baseline. The bars indicate standard error. The last 2 weeks (weeks 40 to 42) allowed a return of symptoms and signs, but those on levodopa did not reach the same degree of worsening seen in those treated with placebo. (Data from Parkinson Study Group. Levodopa and the progression of Parkinson's disease. *N Engl J Med.* 2004;351[24]:2498–2508.)

70 years or those who have some cognitive impairment, levodopa is the preferred drug because it is the most effective with the least risk of inducing psychiatric adverse effects.

Amantadine

Amantadine is a mild indirect dopaminergic agent that acts by augmenting dopamine release at storage sites and possibly blocking reuptake of dopamine into the presynaptic terminals. It also has some anticholinergic and antiglutamatergic properties. In the early stages of PD, it is effective in about two-thirds of patients. A major advantage is that benefit, if it occurs, is seen in a couple of days. The effect can be substantial. Unfortunately, its benefit in more advanced PD is often short-lived, with patients reporting a fall-off effect after several months of treatment. A common adverse effect is livedo reticularis (a reddish mottling of skin) around the knees (these are not harmful); other adverse effects are ankle edema and visual hallucinosis. Sometimes, when the drug is discontinued, a gradual worsening of parkinsonian signs may follow, thus indicating that the drug has been helpful. The usual dose is 100 mg two times per day, but sometimes, a higher dose (up to 200 mg two times per day) may be required. Amantadine can be useful not only in the early phases of symptomatic therapy by forestalling use of levodopa or reducing the required dosage of levodopa but also in the advanced stages as an adjunctive drug to levodopa and the dopamine agonists. It can also reduce the severity of levodopa-induced dyskinesias, probably by its antiglutamatergic mechanism of action, and it is the most effective antidyskinetic drug available.

Anticholinergic (Antimuscarinic) Drugs

As a general rule, anticholinergic agents are less effective antiparkinsonian agents than are the dopamine agonists but may be more effective against tremor. The anticholinergic drugs are estimated to improve parkinsonism by about 20%. Many clinicians find that when tremor is not relieved by an agonist or levodopa, addition of an anticholinergic drug may be helpful. Trihexyphenidyl is a widely used anticholinergic agent. A common starting dose is 2 mg three times per day. It can be gradually increased to 15 mg or more per day.

Adverse effects from anticholinergic drugs are common, particularly in the age range of most patients with PD. Adverse cerebral effects are predominantly forgetfulness and decreased short-term memory. Occasionally, hallucinations and psychosis occur, particularly in the elderly patient; these drugs should be avoided in patients older than 70 years. If tremor is not relieved by dopaminergic drugs and one wishes to add an anticholinergic agent to the therapy for an elderly patient, amitriptyline, diphenhydramine, orphenadrine, or cyclobenzaprine is sometimes beneficial, with less CNS side effects of more potent agents. Diphenhydramine and amitriptyline can cause drowsiness and can be used as a hypnotic. For tremor control, the dose is increased gradually to 50 mg three times per day. A similar dose schedule is useful for orphenadrine. Cyclobenzaprine can be increased gradually until 20 mg three times per day is reached. Anticholinergics can reduce sialorrhea.

Peripheral side effects are common and are often the reason for discontinuing or limiting the dosage of anticholinergic drugs. Another approach is to treat peripheral adverse effects by appropriate antidotes. Pilocarpine eye drops can overcome dilated pupils that can cause blurred vision and can be useful if glaucoma is present. Pyridostigmine, up to 60 mg three times per day, can help to overcome dry mouth, urinary difficulties, and constipation.

Dopamine Agonists

Controlled trials comparing dopamine agonists and levodopa have been carried out [**Level 1**].[6,7] Dopamine agonists can be used as monotherapy in the early stage of the disease to delay introduction of levodopa or as conjunctive therapy with levodopa to potentiate an antiparkinsonian effect, to reduce the dosage needed for levodopa alone, and to overcome some of the adverse effects of long-term use of levodopa. Early use of dopamine agonists, by delaying the introduction of levodopa, delays the time to develop complications from chronic levodopa therapy such as motor fluctuations and dyskinesia. However, levodopa is added eventually for most patients on dopamine agonists and long-term follow-up studies show similar eventual prevalence of these complications in both groups [**Level 1**].[8]

The agonists are less effective than levodopa as antiparkinsonian agents, and most patients require the addition of levodopa within a couple of years. Bromocriptine, pergolide, lisuride, and cabergoline are ergot derivatives. As such, they could induce red inflamed skin (St. Anthony's fire), but this side effect is rare and is reversible on discontinuing the drug. Retroperitoneal, pleural, and pericardial fibrosis are more serious adverse, but also rare, events. Restrictive fibrotic cardiac valvulopathy may occur in up to one-third of patients taking pergolide (detected by echocardiography), due to its agonist effect on the heart valve 5HT2B receptors, and this drug is no longer available in the United States. The nonergoline agonists, pramipexole and ropinirole, are the most commonly used dopamine agonists. They can cause excessive daytime sleepiness and ankle edema (with redness of the skin). Sleep attacks, including falling asleep without warning when driving a vehicle, are infrequent problems with dopamine agonists, but drivers need to be cautioned about such a serious possibility. Observing sleep attacks at home when just sitting in a chair is a warning sign not to drive. Defensive methods, such as delaying a dose of agonist or taking a stimulant such as modafinil or methylphenidate before a long drive, may be reasonable, but studies on whether these approaches are effective have not been carried out. Besides sleep effects and ankle edema, dopamine agonists are more prone than levodopa to induce hallucinations, particularly in the elderly who already may have some cognitive impairment.

A serious behavioral adverse effect from dopamine agonists is the development of impulse control problems in approximately 17% of subjects. These consist of pathologic gambling, hypersexuality, impulsive binge eating with weight gain, compulsive shopping, and excessive generosity, such as charitable contributions. Patients and their care providers need to be warned about this potential risk and the dosage markedly reduced or discontinued at the first sign of such a complication. Fortunately, the impulse control problem is reversible but usually requires discontinuation of these agents. Rapid elimination can induce a withdrawal reaction, so a gradual taper of the drug is preferred.

All agonists can induce anorexia and nausea. Orthostatic hypotension tends to occur when the drug is first introduced. Afterward, this complication is much less common. Therefore, the best starting regimen is a small dose at bedtime for the first 3 days (bromocriptine 1.25 mg, pramipexole 0.125 mg, ropinirole 0.25 mg) and then a switch from bedtime to daytime regimens at this dose for the next few days. The daily dose can be increased gradually at weekly intervals to avoid adverse effects (bromocriptine 1.25 mg, pramipexole 0.25 mg, ropinirole 0.75 mg) until a benefit or a plateau dosage is reached (bromocriptine 5 mg three times per

day, pramipexole 0.5 mg three times per day, ropinirole 1 mg three times per day). If this plateau is not satisfactory, the dose either can be increased gradually until it is quadrupled or can be held constant while beginning carbidopa/levodopa. Extended-release tablets of pramipexole and ropinirole are also available and can be given once a day. The same total daily dose as the immediate release formulations provides similar effects.

Rotigotine is not absorbed via the intestinal tract but is absorbed transdermally. It is available as a dermal patch, with absorption over 24 hours. It is a weak dopamine agonist, but the once-a-day dermal patch application is convenient, and as such allows day-long plasma levels of the agonist, which theoretically could reduce wearing-off and nocturnal akinesia.

Besides the adverse effects listed earlier, there are subtle differences among the dopamine agonists. Cabergoline has the longest pharmacologic half-life and theoretically could be taken in once-a-day dosing, but valvulopathy is a risk. All agonists act at the D2 receptor, which may account for most, if not all, of their anti-PD activity (Table 83.10). Pergolide acts at both the D1 and D2 dopamine receptors. Bromocriptine is a partial D1 antagonist. Pergolide, pramipexole, and ropinirole also act at the D3 dopamine receptor, but it is not clear what effect this has clinically, but it is conceivable that the D2/D3 ratio may be instrumental in causing the impulse control problems seen with these drugs. All three appear to be equally effective against PD; bromocriptine appears to have the weakest anti-PD effect. Dopamine agonists, when used in the absence of levodopa, rarely induce dyskinesias. Whether this is because of their longer half-life and possibly more continuous dopaminergic receptor stimulation or because they exert a different receptor effect than that of levodopa is unknown. If the agonists alone are not sufficiently effective, carbidopa/levodopa is needed.

Levodopa

In controlled trials comparing levodopa and agonists as initial therapy, levodopa produced a superior clinical response but more fluctuations and dyskinesias as noted earlier. Some clinicians prefer to begin therapy with carbidopa/levodopa for early symptomatic treatment and to add an agonist after a small dose has been reached (e.g., 25/100 mg three times per day). This approach is particularly useful if a patient already has some disability. The advantage of using levodopa at this stage in preference to a dopamine agonist is that a therapeutic response is virtually guaranteed. Nearly all patients with PD respond to levodopa and do so quickly. In contrast, only some benefit derives adequately from a dopamine agonist alone, and it may take months to discover

TABLE 83.10	Effect on Receptors by Dopamine Agonists					
Agonist	D1	D2	D3	D4	D5	5-HT Receptor
Bromocriptine	−	+	+ +	+	+	0
Pergolide	+	+ +	+ + +	?	+	+ +
Pramipexole	−	+ +	+ + + +	+ +	?	?
Ropinirole	−	+ +	+ + + +	+	−	?
Cabergoline	−	+ + +	?	?	?	+ +
Lisuride	+	+ +	?	?	?	+

+, activates; −, inhibits; 0, no effect; ?, uncertain.

this because of a slower buildup of dosage. Therefore, if a definite response is needed quickly (e.g., to remain at work or to be self-sufficient), levodopa is preferable. On the other hand, if there is no particular urgency for a rapid clinical response and if the patient has no cognitive problems and is younger than 50 years of age, then beginning with a dopamine agonist allows one to use the levodopa-sparing strategy. Patients older than 70 years are less likely to develop response fluctuations with levodopa and more likely to develop confusion and hallucinations with dopamine agonists, so in this population, carbidopa/levodopa would be a good choice as a starting drug.

STAGE WHEN SYMPTOMS AND SIGNS REQUIRE TREATMENT WITH LEVODOPA

When other antiparkinsonian medications are no longer bringing about a satisfactory response, levodopa is required to reduce the severity of parkinsonism. Levodopa is the most potent anti-PD drug. In treating patients with PD, the rule of thumb has been to use the lowest dosage that can bring about adequate symptom reversal, not the highest dosage that the patient can tolerate. As previously mentioned, the longer the duration of disease and the higher the dose, the greater the likelihood motor complications will occur. After 5 years of levodopa therapy, about 75% of patients with PD have some form of troublesome complication (see Table 83.9). On the other hand, a dose-response study showed a clear-cut dose-related clinical benefit, which is an advantage with higher dosages (see Fig. 83.2) [**Level 1**].[9]

Combining levodopa with a peripheral dopa decarboxylase inhibitor (e.g., carbidopa) increases therapeutic potency and reduces gastrointestinal adverse effects, which can also be mitigated by increasing the dosage of levodopa slowly. A safe approach is to start with half tablet of 25/100 mg strength carbidopa/levodopa once a day. Continue for a week and weekly increase by another half tablet. By the sixth week, a plateau dose of 25/100 mg three times daily is reached. Giving levodopa with meals during this titration phase will reduce the risk for anorexia and nausea. If there is inadequate benefit, continue to increase the dose but at a faster rate. The 25/250-mg tablets can also be used, and a dose of 25/250 mg three or four times a day is common in patients with more advanced disease.

Extended-release forms of carbidopa/levodopa (Sinemet CR) and benserazide/levodopa (Madopar HBS) provide a longer half-life and a lower peak plasma level of levodopa. In the early stage of levodopa therapy, when complications have not yet developed, use of extended-release carbidopa/levodopa had not proven advantageous over the use of the standard preparation in a controlled trial because it did not delay motor fluctuations. However, it may be useful to start treatment with such an extended-release preparation in elderly patients to avoid too high a brain concentration of levodopa that might induce side effects such as drowsiness.

Once response fluctuations have developed, the extended-release preparation could reduce mild wearing-off. Also, a bedtime dose often allows more mobility during the night. Disadvantages are a delay in the response with each dose, less reliability of absorption, and the possibility of a late-in-the-day excessive dyskinesia response that can be prolonged. For a quick response on awakening, patients often take the standard (immediate release) preparation as the first morning dose in addition to the extended-release form. Some patients need a combination of standard and extended-release preparations of levodopa throughout the day to obtain a smoother response and minimize their motor complications.

The extended-release tablets of carbidopa/levodopa are available in two strengths: scored (50/200 mg, which can be broken in half) and unscored (25/100 mg). Neither should be crushed because the matrix of the tablet that delays solubilization would no longer be intact. When added to a dopamine agonist, a dose of 25/100 mg three to four times per day often suffices. When used alone, a starting dose of 25/100 mg three times per day often is necessary and can be increased as needed to 50/200 mg three or four times per day. For those desiring to produce a continuous dopaminergic stimulation effect, multiple dosing a day should be considered. If greater relief is required, a dopamine agonist or standard carbidopa/levodopa should be added.

It should be noted that the entire content of the extended-release formulation is not absorbed before the tablet passes through the duodenum and jejunum (the sites where levodopa is absorbed), so that an equivalent dose needs to be approximately 1.3 times greater than a dose of standard carbidopa/levodopa to achieve the same clinical efficacy. A combination of immediate and extended release carbidopa/levodopa in capsules (Rytary) has become available; it has a longer half-life and may offer advantages in some patients.

Some clinicians attempt to extend the plasma half-life of levodopa by adding a COMT inhibitor, such as entacapone, with each dose of levodopa. A clinical trial found such a combination resulted in earlier dyskinesias than levodopa alone.

INADEQUATE RESPONSE TO LEVODOPA TREATMENT

As a general rule, the single most important piece of information to help the differential diagnosis of PD and other forms of parkinsonism is the response to levodopa. If the response is nil or minor, the disorder probably is not PD. An adequate response, however, does not ensure the diagnosis of PD. All presynaptic disorders (e.g., reserpine-induced, MPTP-induced, postencephalitic parkinsonism) respond to levodopa. Also, a response to levodopa can occur in the early stages of MSA and progressive supranuclear palsy; only later, when striatal dopamine receptors are lost, is the response lost.

Before concluding that levodopa is without effect in a given patient, an adequate dose must be tested. Not every symptom has to respond, but bradykinesia and rigidity respond best, whereas tremor can be resistant. Therefore, if rest tremor is the only symptom, lack of improvement does not exclude the diagnosis of PD. Tremor may never respond satisfactorily, even if adjunctive antiparkinsonian drugs are also used. Before concluding that *carbidopa/levodopa* is ineffective, a dose up to 2,000 mg levodopa per day should be tried if tolerated. If anorexia, nausea, or vomiting prevent attainment of a therapeutic dosage, the addition of extra carbidopa (additional 25 mg four times per day) or domperidone (10 to 20 mg before each levodopa dose) is usually effective in overcoming the adverse effect. If other adverse effects (drug-induced dystonia, psychosis, confusion, sleepiness, postural hypotension) prevent attainment of an effective dose, uncertainty about the diagnosis of PD will continue. In particular, dystonia induced by low doses of levodopa suggests a diagnosis of MSA. Similarly, drug-induced psychosis suggests PDD, diffuse Lewy body disease, or accompanying AD. Clozapine or quetiapine may suppress psychosis and allow the use of levodopa.

COMPLICATIONS OF LONG-TERM LEVODOPA THERAPY

Response fluctuations (wearing-off), dyskinesias, and behavioral effects are the major problems encountered with long-term levodopa therapy (Tables 83.11 and 83.12). These problems are features of an advanced stage of PD.

FLUCTUATIONS

Response to dopaminergic drugs consists of the short-duration response (SDR) within the time frame of hours and the long-duration response (LDR) that develops more slowly over weeks or longer. When levodopa therapy is initiated, the benefit from levodopa is usually sustained, with general improvement throughout the day and no dose-timing variations; mostly consisting of LDR. Skipping a dose is usually without loss of effect, and the response is evident on arising in the morning despite the lack of medication throughout the night. The pharmacokinetics of levodopa show a short initial distribution phase with a half-life of 5 to 10 minutes, a peak plasma concentration in about 30 minutes, and an elimination phase of about 90 minutes. Brain levels follow plasma levels. The mechanism for the LDR of levodopa is not known. It cannot be explained by a prolonged storage of dopamine from exogenous levodopa in residual nigrostriatal nerve terminals, and basal ganglia circuitry plasticity is probably responsible for this phenomenon.

With chronic levodopa therapy, however, most patients, including all patients with onset before age 40 years, begin to experience fluctuations. At first, fluctuations take the form of wearing-off (also known as *end-of-dose deterioration*), which is defined as a return of parkinsonian symptoms in less than 4 hours after the last dose. Gradually, the duration of benefit shortens further and the "off" state becomes more profound. The magnitude of the SDR to levodopa in patients with fluctuations may increase because the loss of the LDR leads to worse "off" states and patients notice fluctuations more readily due to greater difference between "on" and "off" states.

In some patients, these fluctuations become more abrupt in onset and random in timing; the condition is then the "on–off" effect and cannot be related to the timing of the levodopa intake. Motor "offs" are often accompanied by changes in mood (depression, dysphoria), anxiety, thought (more bradyphrenia), sensory symptoms (pain, akathisia), and dysautonomia (excessive sweating, urgency). Such behavioral, sensory, and autonomic "offs" can occur in the absence of motor "offs" and then they are difficult to recognize. Patients, in order to eliminate these unpleasant sensations, often take more frequent doses of levodopa, which has led some clinicians to call this the *dopamine disequilibrium syndrome*.

The brief peripheral half-life of levodopa, by itself, is not likely to be responsible for fluctuations. The half-life, present from the

TABLE 83.12 Behavioral Adverse Effects with Levodopa

- Drowsiness
- Delusions
- Reverse sleep–wake cycle
- Paranoia
- Vivid dreams
- Confusion
- Benign hallucinations
- Dementia
- Malignant hallucinations
- Behavioral "offs"
  - Depression, anxiety, panic, pain, akathisia, dysphoria

beginning of treatment, does not change. Also, no difference exists in the pharmacokinetics in patients with early disease who show a stable response and in those with advanced disease and fluctuations. Loss of striatal storage sites of dopamine by itself is not the sole cause of fluctuations either. The central effects on basal circuitry are likely to be involved. Some hypothesize that intermittent (compared with continuous) administration of levodopa contributes to the development of motor complications. These peaks and valleys of brain dopamine levels are thought to alter the striatal dopaminoceptive medium spiny GABAergic neurons and their synaptic connections with other striatal interneurons and cortical afferents that provide glutamatergic input.

Once established, motor complications are seemingly irreversible. Substituting dopamine agonists for levodopa therapy or maintaining plasma concentrations at a constant therapeutic level by chronic infusion of levodopa diminishes the severity of the complications but does not eliminate them. Jejunal infusions of levodopa via a catheter inserted via the abdominal wall into the stomach and then passed into the jejunum, subcutaneous infusions of apomorphine, and hourly oral administration of liquefied levodopa have been used to "smooth out" the effect of levodopa. Selegiline, rasagiline, and COMT inhibitors are partially effective in treating mild wearing-off problems, probably by prolonging dopamine levels at the synapse [**Level 1**].[10] The addition of these drugs to patients taking levodopa, however, may lead to dopaminergic side effects, including increased dyskinesias, confusion, and hallucinations. Another approach is to combine the slow-release forms of carbidopa/levodopa (Sinemet CR) with the standard (immediate-release) form. Again, this approach is effective mainly on wearing-off problems and not on complicated on–off fluctuations. Furthermore, the sustained-release formulation results in less predictable plasma levels of levodopa and often increases dyskinesias. Standard carbidopa/levodopa can be given alone by shortening the interval between doses. For the more severe state of on–off phenomenon, a more rapid and more predictable response sometimes can be achieved by dissolving the levodopa tablet in carbonated water or ascorbic acid solution because an acidic solvent can both dissolve levodopa and prevent its auto-oxidation. Liquid levodopa enters the small intestine faster, is absorbed faster, and can be used to fine-tune dosing. Patients with fluctuations often develop delayed "ons" and dose failures resulting from delayed entry of levodopa into the small intestine. Liquefying or crushing levodopa by the patient's teeth can help resolve this problem.

TABLE 83.11 Major Fluctuations and Dyskinesias as Complications of Levodopa

Fluctuations (Offs)	Dyskinesias
• Slow "wearing-off"	• Peak-dose chorea and dystonia
• Sudden "off"	• Diphasic chorea and dystonia
• Random "off"	• "Off" dystonia
• Yo-yoing	• Myoclonus
• Episodic failure to respond (dose failures)	
• Delayed "on"	
• Weak response at end of day	
• Varied response in relationship to meals	
• Sudden transient freezing	

A large meal that slows gastric emptying and high-protein meals can cause dose failures in some patients. Levodopa is absorbed from the small intestine by the transport system for large neutral amino acids and thus competes with these other amino acids for this transport. Patients with this problem may benefit by taking levodopa before meals and also from special diets that contain little protein for the first two meals of the day, followed by a high-protein meal at the end of the day when they can afford to be "off."

Direct-acting dopamine agonists, with their biologic half-lives longer than that of levodopa, can be used in combination with standard or slow-release forms of levodopa. The agonists are useful for treating both wearing-off and on–off by reducing both the frequency and the depth of the "off" states. In yet another approach to treating on–offs, the patients inject themselves with apomorphine subcutaneously to quickly return to the "on" state. Trimethobenzamide or the peripheral dopamine receptor antagonist domperidone can be used to block nausea and vomiting from apomorphine.

DYSKINESIAS

Dyskinesias are commonly encountered with levodopa therapy but are often mild enough to be unnoticed by the patient. Severe forms, including chorea, ballism, dystonia, or combinations of these, can be disabling. The incidence and severity increase with duration and dosage of levodopa therapy, but they may appear early in patients with severe parkinsonism. Dyskinesias are divided into the following categories according to the timing of levodopa dosing:

1. Peak-dose dyskinesias appear at the height of antiparkinsonian benefit (20 minutes to 2 hours after a dose).
2. Diphasic dyskinesias, usually affecting the legs, appear at the beginning and end of the dosing cycle. Often, these may be mostly noticed by the patient at the end of the dose, blending into tremor that occurs during "off" state (see Video 83.4).
3. "Off" dystonia, which can be painful sustained cramps, appears during "off" states and may be seen at first as "early-morning dystonia" presenting as painful foot cramps; these are relieved by the next dose of levodopa.

Dyskinesias are usually seen in patients who have fluctuations, and some patients may move rapidly from severe peak-dose dyskinesias to severe "offs"; this process is known as *yo-yoing*. These patients may have only a brief "on" state. More commonly, they have good "ons" for parts of the day but are intermittently disabled by dyskinesias or "offs." These diurnal variations are major problems; patients with this combination have a narrow therapeutic window for levodopa. The mechanisms for dyskinesias, fluctuations, and good response that lead to "on" are not well understood, and they may have common pathways as well as differential ones. For example, those with dyskinesias are usually good responders to dopaminergic agents and many drugs that reduce dyskinesia may make parkinsonism worse. On the other hand, sensitivity to dyskinesias is not altered by chronic infusion of levodopa, whereas fluctuations are suppressed. Because dopamine agonists are much less likely to cause dyskinesias, which have much less activation of the D1 receptor, increased sensitivity and response of the D1 receptor by dopamine derived from levodopa are thought to play a role in the production of dyskinesias.

Amantadine can reduce the severity of dyskinesias, but a dosage of at least 400 mg/day is required, and it is not known how long the benefit may last. Treatment of peak-dose dyskinesias also includes reducing the size of each dose of levodopa. If doing so results in more wearing-off, the levodopa can be given more frequently with smaller dosages, or a dopamine agonist or inhibitor

of MAO-B or COMT can be added with the reduced dose of levodopa. Diphasic dyskinesias are more difficult to treat. Increasing the dosage of levodopa can eliminate this type of dyskinesia, but peak-dose dyskinesia usually ensues. A switch to a dopamine agonist as the major antiparkinsonian drug is more effective; low doses of levodopa are used as an adjunctive agent. The end-of-day dyskinesia is a part of the end-of-dose dyskinesia (part of diphasic dyskinesia). There is always a last dose of the day, and when that wears off, dyskinesias ensue. Medications such as amantadine and dopamine agonists rarely help end-of-day dyskinesias. Patients usually find that by taking the last dose of levodopa at home in the evening, and then allowing the dyskinesias to occur, lasting usually no more than 1 to 2 hours, the patient can live with this situation. Once the dyskinesia fades, the patient is then comfortable the rest of the evening. The principle of treating "off dystonia" is to try to keep the patient "on" most of the time. Here again, using a dopamine agonist as the major antiparkinsonian drug, with low doses of levodopa as an adjunct, can often be effective.

FREEZING

The freezing phenomenon is often listed as a type of fluctuation because of transient difficulty in initiating movement. But this phenomenon should be considered as distinct from the other types of fluctuations. "Off-freezing" must be distinguished from "on-freezing." Off-freezing, best considered a feature of parkinsonism itself, was encountered before levodopa was discovered. The treatment goal of off-freezing is to keep the patient from turning "off." On-freezing remains an enigma; it tends to be aggravated by increasing the dosage of levodopa or by adding direct-acting dopamine agonists or selegiline without reducing the dosage of levodopa. Rather, it may be lessened by reducing the dosage of levodopa. There is no satisfactory treatment for on-freezing. Both on- and off-freezing seem to correlate with both the duration of illness and the duration of levodopa therapy. Patients with a combination of complicated fluctuations, dyskinesias, and off-freezing may respond to subthalamic nucleus stimulation. On-freezing does not respond to surgical therapy.

MENTAL AND BEHAVIORAL COMPLICATIONS

The adverse effects of confusion, agitation, hallucinations, delusions, paranoia, and mania are probably related to activation of dopamine receptors in nonstriatal regions, particularly cortical and limbic structures. Both levodopa and dopamine agonists can cause these complications, with the latter more prone to do so. Elderly patients and those with diffuse Lewy body disease or concomitant AD are sensitive to small doses of these dopaminergics. But all patients with PD, regardless of age, can develop psychosis if they take excessive amounts of levodopa or agonists to overcome "off" periods. Patients with pronounced behavioral/sensory offs tend to take more and more levodopa.

Although antipsychotic drugs can reduce levodopa-induced psychosis, adding neuroleptics that block D2 dopamine receptors worsens parkinsonism. Rather, quetiapine or clozapine, antipsychotic agents that preferentially block the dopamine D4 and serotonin receptors, can often treat psychosis without worsening parkinsonism. These drugs easily induce drowsiness, and they should be given at bedtime, starting with a dose of 12.5 mg. The dose can be gradually increased if necessary. Start with quetiapine to avoid the biweekly blood counts required with clozapine. Quetiapine is much less effective than clozapine, and it is not uncommon that clozapine is required. Because clozapine induces agranulocytosis in 1% to 2% of patients, patients must have blood counts monitored biweekly, and the drug must be discontinued if leukopenia develops. If clozapine is not tolerated, other drugs, including small doses of olanzapine, molindone, pimozide, or other relatively weak antipsychotic drugs, can be used. If the antipsychotic drugs increase the parkinsonism, lowering the dosage of levodopa to avoid the psychosis is preferable to maintaining the antipsychotic agent at high dosage. Levodopa cannot be discontinued suddenly because the abrupt cessation may induce a neuroleptic malignant-like syndrome.

Impulse control problems (gambling, hypersexuality, excessive eating, and shopping) induced by dopamine agonists or less commonly by levodopa can be devastating to the patient and family. Patients and families need to be aware about these potential problems so they can inform the treating physician. Fortunately, these problems are eliminated by reducing the dosage but sometimes only by discontinuing the agonists. Levodopa would need to substitute for the agonists.

Punding is a behavioral disorder that has a resemblance to the impulse control problems discussed earlier. The term was first used in amphetamine abusers and refers to an abnormal motor behavior in which there is intense repetitive handling and examining of objects, such as picking at oneself, taking apart watches and radios, or sorting and arranging of common objects, such as lining up pebbles, rocks, or other small objects. Punding has been reported with levodopa and dopamine agonists. Treatment is problematic, but atypical antipsychotics have been suggested.

TREATING THE NONMOTOR PROBLEMS OF PARKINSON DISEASE

Although many nonmotor symptoms can appear before the classic cardinal motor features of PD (e.g., hyposmia, REM sleep behavior disorder, depression, anxiety, constipation), many do not appear until later in the disease. Cognitive decline occurs late and is probably the most devastating nonmotor problem. When dementia occurs, the patient is not able to tolerate dopaminergics because of the susceptibility for psychosis, especially hallucinations, but also paranoia. Treatment of psychosis was discussed in the preceding section. Dementia is difficult to treat, but some response can be seen with the cholinesterase inhibitors, rivastigmine 1.5 to 6 mg twice a day and donepezil 5 to 10 mg/day. Antidepressants are needed for treating depression. The serotonin uptake inhibitors are effective in treating depression of PD but may aggravate parkinsonism if antiparkinsonian drugs are not given concurrently. Tricyclics may be equally effective. Because of its anticholinergic and soporific effects, amitriptyline can be useful for these properties as well as for its antidepressant effect. Alprazolam, diazepam, and other benzodiazepines are usually well tolerated without worsening parkinsonism and can help to lessen tremor by reducing the reaction to stress that worsens tremor.

REM sleep behavior disorder, a condition where one moves while dreaming, is common in patients with PD. It is more troublesome for the bed partner than for the patient, but it can also cause the patient to fall out of bed and injure himself. It is extremely well treated with clonazepam at bedtime. Start with 0.5 mg and increase the dose if necessary. Sleep fragmentation is common in PD, and many patients have a difficult time falling back asleep after an arousal. A short-acting hypnotic given at that time (not at bedtime), such as zolpidem 5 mg, can provide relief. The other hypnotics listed in Table 83.8 can also be effective. If the patient requires an antipsychotic for vivid dreams, quetiapine or clozapine, which cause drowsiness, can be used instead of the hypnotics listed in the table. Excessive daytime sleepiness is another type of sleep problem

that is common in PD; it is due to medications. Dopamine agonists commonly cause drowsiness, and in older patients with cognitive problems, levodopa can cause drowsiness at the peak of the dose. Modafinil up to 200 mg morning and midafternoon or methylphenidate up to 10 mg three times a day may provide some relief.

Many patients with PD develop RLS, which consists of unpleasant crawling sensations in the legs, particularly when sitting and relaxing in the evening, and which disappear on walking. Whether RLS is an epiphenomenon of PD, because both conditions respond to dopaminergics, is not clear. It is possible that RLS is a result of the dopaminergic medications used to treat PD. Sporadic and familial RLS respond to dopamine agonists and levodopa, but these drugs can cause augmentation, a worsening of the restless legs symptoms—more severe unpleasant sensations, occurring earlier in the day and spreading to involve other body parts. Fortunately, pregabalin 300 mg/day is effective [**Level 1**].[11] Opioids are also effective in treating RLS and periodic movements in sleep, whether in patients with PD or those with sporadic and familial RLS. Tramadol 25 mg late in the day before the onset of symptoms is usually effective, and one can titrate up to 150 mg/day if necessary. Oxycodone 5 to 15 mg, methadone 5 to 20 mg, and codeine 30 to 60 mg are also effective.

The varied autonomic symptoms in PD need to be treated specifically. Orthostatic hypotension can respond to midodrine, starting with 10 mg/day and titrate up to three doses a day if necessary. If midodrine is not effective, fludrocortisone can be used as well as adding salt to the diet. Combinations of these agents may be needed. Supine hypertension can be an adverse effect, and the head of the bed may need to be elevated to avoid that. It is important that the patient's blood pressure, lying, sitting, and standing, be monitored by the family at home, reporting to the treating physician so the dosages of these agents can be properly adjusted. Droxidopa is a new agent approved for treating orthostatic hypotension. It is metabolized in the peripheral circulation to norepinephrine by the enzyme dopa decarboxylase. Thus, it will not be effective if more than 100 mg/day of carbidopa is being used.

Sialorrhea can be an annoying and embarrassing problem. Anticholinergics are effective, but most available agents are tertiary amines that enter the CNS and can impair memory or cause hallucinations in older patients. Quaternary amines, such as glycopyrrolate and propantheline, do not penetrate the CNS, and they are preferable. If such drugs are not completely effective, injections of botulinum toxin into the salivary glands can be attempted; an overdosage could impair swallowing, so an experienced physician should carry out the injections. Constipation is a common complaint. It should be treated with a high-fiber diet, supplemented by laxatives such as polyethylene glycol (MiraLAX).

SURGICAL THERAPY

Prior to the introduction of levodopa therapy, stereotactic surgery producing lesions in the thalamus or pallidum was common, resulting in reduction in tremor more than relief from other features of PD. Such surgery faded away after levodopa became available. But with the problems of motor complications from levodopa, there has been renewed interest in surgical therapy, mainly to treat these motor complications. The surgical approaches listed in Table 83.8 are not considered in the early stages of PD but are reserved for patients who respond to levodopa and who have developed intractable motor complications from it. Stereotaxic lesions have been largely replaced by high-frequency electrical stimulation at the same targets because of safety concerns. *Thalamotomy and thalamic stimulation* (the target for both is the ventral intermediate nucleus) are best for contralateral intractable tremor. Tremor can be relieved in at least 70% of cases. Although a unilateral lesion carries a small risk, bilateral operations result in dysarthria in 15% to 20% of patients. Thalamic stimulation seems to be safer and can be equally effective against tremor, but it runs the risks associated with foreign bodies and thin electronic wires that can break. *Pallidotomy and pallidal stimulation* (the target is the posterolateral part of the GPi) are most effective for treating contralateral dopa-induced dystonia and chorea but also have some benefit for bradykinesia and tremor. The target in the GPi is believed to be the site of afferent excitatory glutamatergic fibers coming from the subthalamic nucleus, which is overactive in PD.

Lesions of the subthalamic nucleus, although effective in relieving parkinsonism in animal models, are hazardous in humans because hemichorea or hemiballism may result. Instead, *stimulation of the subthalamic nucleus* is used and appears to be the most effective in reducing contralateral bradykinesia and tremor [**Level 1**].[12] Indeed, the most common type of surgery today is to use electrical stimulation of the subthalamic nucleus. Such deep brain stimulation (DBS) provides a reduction in not only tremor but also bradykinesia and rigidity, allowing a reduction in dosage of dopaminergic medication. The antiparkinsonian effect is never better than the best levodopa effect (except for tremor in which surgery seems superior). It is not effective against symptoms that do not respond to levodopa (with the exception of intractable tremor, which can respond to stimulation). Therefore, DBS can be useful in patients with a very good anti-PD response to levodopa but with uncontrollable response fluctuations. DBS has the potential to smooth out these fluctuations. This type of surgery often allows a marked reduction in levodopa dosage, thereby reducing dopa-induced dyskinesias as well as treating parkinsonian symptoms. The best results are seen with younger patients. DBS in the GPi is superior for controlling dyskinesias. The presence of cognitive problems and lack of benefit from levodopa are contraindications. Cognitive problems worsen with surgical penetration in the brain. DBS produces levodopa-like benefits probably by restoring the physiologic balance in the basal ganglia circuitry, bypassing the need to restore dopamine levels. In this concept, DBS could be considered an "electronic levodopa." Adverse effects from the surgery include brain hemorrhage (rare), infection from a foreign body, speech impairment, dystonia, and breakage of the wires. Unfortunately, even in young patients, there can be impaired cognition, dysarthria, depression with suicide attempts, and incomplete control of fluctuations and dyskinesias. Targeting the GPi results in less dysarthria, depression, and cognitive impairment than the subthalamic nucleus. Experienced neurosurgeons and accurate placement of the electrodes are most important, and follow-up programming of the stimulators is an ongoing process to reach the ideal electrical settings. Exposure of the metallic stimulators to diathermy can result in permanent brain injury.

Pilot trials suggest that stimulation of the pedunculopontine nucleus can reduce falling, but results have been inconsistent. Controlled trials are needed to determine if falling and freezing of gait respond to the stimulation of this target. Controlled surgical trials of *fetal dopaminergic tissue implants* have found the benefits to be less efficacious than initially reported in open-label investigations and have also led to the development of persistent dyskinesias. Until this problem can be solved, transplantation surgery is not a useful option. The same concern exists for the potential of cellular therapy with dopaminergic stem cells. On the other hand, intrajejunal infusion of levodopa is already available and it offers a smooth pharmacokinetic profile of levodopa that reduces clinical fluctuations and dyskinesias [**Level 1**].[13] Percutaneous catheterization of the stomach with the catheter advanced into the jejunum avoids intracerebral penetration with its potential adverse effects.

OUTCOME

PD, being a neurodegenerative disease, worsens with time. Before the introduction of levodopa, PD caused severe disability or death in 25% of patients within 5 years of onset, in 65% in the next 5 years, and in 89% in those surviving 15 years. The mortality rate from PD was three times that of the general population matched for age, sex, and racial origin. Although no definite evidence indicates that levodopa alters the underlying pathologic process or stems the progressive nature of the disease, indications exist of a major impact on survival time and functional capacity. The mortality rate has dropped 50%, and longevity is extended by several years.

A debated point in the treatment of PD is the cause of declining efficacy from continuing treatment with levodopa seen in many patients. End-stage PD is denoted when the response to levodopa is inadequate to allow patient-assisted activities of daily living. Progression of the illness with further loss of dopamine storage sites in the presynaptic terminals cannot be the explanation for this outcome because loss of these structures in postencephalitic parkinsonism results in greater, not lower, sensitivity to levodopa. Perhaps as PD progresses, it is associated with loss of striatal dopamine receptors and loss of the presynaptic dopaminergic neuron.

After about 15 years of disease, most patients are seriously disabled, and the mortality rate increases compared to an age- and gender-matched population. Despite very effective medications for the early symptoms of PD, the motor symptoms of bradykinesia return and loss of postural reflexes constantly worsen, limiting ambulation. Falling and incurring fractures are common. In stage 5, patients require a wheelchair. Dysphagia with choking and aspiration and immobility with decubitus ulcers are common events. Dementia develops in most patients, rendering patients susceptible to psychosis with hallucinations and paranoid ideation. Patients become dependent on others for activities of daily living, and many are placed in nursing homes. Such a course emphasizes the importance of better understanding the pathogenesis and the need for disease-modifying therapy.

Videos can be found in the companion e-book edition. For a full list of video legends, please see the front matter.

LEVEL 1 EVIDENCE

1. Corcos DM, Robichaud JA, David FJ, et al. A two-year randomized controlled trial of progressive resistance exercise for Parkinson's disease. *Mov Disord*. 2013;28(9):1230–1240.
2. Pålhagen S, Heinonen E, Hägglund J, et al. Selegiline slows the progression of the symptoms of Parkinson disease. *Neurology*. 2006;66(8):1200–1206.
3. Shoulson I, Oakes D, Fahn S, et al. Impact of sustained deprenyl (selegiline) in levodopa-treated Parkinson's disease: a randomized placebo-controlled extension of the deprenyl and tocopherol antioxidative therapy of parkinsonism trial. *Ann Neurol*. 2002;51:604–612.
4. Olanow CW, Rascol O, Hauser R, et al. A double-blind, delayed-start trial of rasagiline in Parkinson's disease. *N Engl J Med*. 2009;361(13):1268–1278.
5. Aviles-Olmos I, Dickson J, Kefalopoulou Z, et al. Exenatide and the treatment of patients with Parkinson's disease. *J Clin Invest*. 2013;123(6):2730–2736.

6. Parkinson Study Group. Pramipexole versus levodopa as the initial treatment for Parkinson's disease: a randomized controlled trial. *JAMA*. 2000;284:1931–1938.

7. Rascol O, Brooks DJ, Korczyn AD, et al. A five-year study of the incidence of dyskinesia in patients with early Parkinson's disease who were treated with ropinirole or levodopa. *N Engl J Med*. 2000;342:1484–1491.

8. PD MED Collaborative Group. Long-term effectiveness of dopamine agonists and monoamine oxidase B inhibitors compared with levodopa as initial treatment for Parkinson's disease (PD MED): a large, open-label, pragmatic randomised trial. *Lancet*. 2014;384(9949):1196–1205.

9. Parkinson Study Group. Levodopa and the progression of Parkinson's disease. *N Engl J Med*. 2004;351(24):2498–2508.

10. Rascol O, Brooks DJ, Melamed E, et al. Rasagiline as an adjunct to levodopa in patients with Parkinson's disease and motor fluctuations (LARGO, Lasting effect in Adjunct therapy with Rasagiline Given Once daily, study): a randomised, double-blind, parallel-group trial. *Lancet*. 2005;365(9463):947–954.

11. Allen RP, Chen C, Garcia-Borreguero D, et al. Comparison of pregabalin with pramipexole for restless legs syndrome. *N Engl J Med*. 2014;370:621–631.

12. Deuschl G, Schade-Brittinger C, Krack P, et al. A randomized trial of deep-brain stimulation for Parkinson's disease. *N Engl J Med*. 2006;355(9):896–908.

13. Olanow CW, Kieburtz K, Rascol O, et al. Factors predictive of the development of Levodopa-induced dyskinesia and wearing-off in Parkinson's disease. *Mov Disord*. 2013;28(8):1064–1071.

SUGGESTED READINGS

Alcalay RNE, Caccappolo H, Mejia-Santana MX, et al. Cognitive and motor function in long-duration PARKIN-associated Parkinson disease. *JAMA Neurol*. 2014;71(1):62–67.

Braak H, Bohl JR, Müller CM, et al. Stanley Fahn lecture 2005: the staging procedure for the inclusion body pathology associated with sporadic Parkinson's disease reconsidered. *Mov Disord*. 2006;21(12):2042–2051.

Burke RE, Dauer WT, Vonsattel JP. A critical evaluation of the Braak staging scheme for Parkinson's disease. *Ann Neurol*. 2008;64(5):485–491.

Fahn S. The history of dopamine and levodopa in the treatment of Parkinson's disease. *Mov Disord*. 2008;23(suppl 3):S497–S508.

Fahn S, Elton RL, Members of the UPDRS Development Committee. The unified Parkinson's disease rating scale. In: Fahn S, Marsden CD, Calne DB, et al, eds. *Recent Developments in Parkinson's Disease*. Vol 2. Florham Park, NJ: Macmillan Healthcare Information; 1987:153–163, 293–304.

Friedman J, Lannon M, Comella C, et al. Low-dose clozapine for the treatment of drug-induced psychosis in Parkinson's disease. *N Engl J Med*. 1999;340:757–763.

Giladi N, McDermott MP, Fahn S, et al. Freezing of gait in PD: prospective assessment in the DATATOP cohort. *Neurology*. 2001;56:1712–1721.

Goker-Alpan O, Lopez G, Vithayathil J, et al. The spectrum of parkinsonian manifestations associated with glucocerebrosidase mutations. *Arch Neurol*. 2008;65:1353–1357.

Healy DG, Falchi M, O'Sullivan SS, et al. Phenotype, genotype, and worldwide genetic penetrance of LRRK2-associated Parkinson's disease: a case–control study. *Lancet Neurol*. 2008;7(7):583–590.

Hely MA, Reid WG, Adena MA, et al. The Sydney multicenter study of Parkinson's disease: the inevitability of dementia at 20 years. *Mov Disord*. 2008;23(6):837–844.

Kempster PA, Williams DR, Selikhova M, et al. Patterns of levodopa response in Parkinson's disease: a clinico-pathological study. *Brain*. 2007;130(pt 8):2123–2128.

Klein C, Lohmann-Hedrich K, Rogaeva E, et al. Deciphering the role of heterozygous mutations in genes associated with parkinsonism. *Lancet Neurol*. 2007;6(7):652–662.

Krack P, Batir A, Van Blercom N, et al. Five-year follow-up of bilateral stimulation of the subthalamic nucleus in advanced Parkinson's disease. *N Engl J Med*. 2003;349:1925–1934.

Li F, Harmer P, Fitzgerald K, et al. Tai chi and postural stability in patients with Parkinson's disease. *N Engl J Med*. 2012;366(6):511–519.

Lippa CF, Duda JE, Grossman M, et al. DLB and PDD boundary issues: diagnosis, treatment, molecular pathology, and biomarkers. *Neurology*. 2007;68(11):812–819.

Miyasaki JM, Shannon K, Voon V, et al. Practice parameter: evaluation and treatment of depression, psychosis, and dementia in Parkinson disease (an evidence-based review). Report of the Quality Standards Subcommittee of the American Academy of Neurology. *Neurology*. 2006;66(7):996–1002.

Nalls MA, Pankratz N, Lill CM, et al. Large-scale meta-analysis of genome-wide association data identifies six new risk loci for Parkinson's disease. *Nat Genet*. 2014;46(9):989–993.

Nutt JG. Continuous dopaminergic stimulation: is it the answer to the motor complications of levodopa? *Mov Disord*. 2007;22(1):1–9.

Pahwa R, Factor SA, Lyons KE, et al. Practice parameter: treatment of Parkinson disease with motor fluctuations and dyskinesia (an evidence-based review). Report of the Quality Standards Subcommittee of the American Academy of Neurology. *Neurology*. 2006;66(7):983–995.

Poulopoulos M, Levy OA, Alcalay RN. The neuropathology of genetic Parkinson's disease. *Mov Disord*. 2012;27(7):831–842.

Rabinak CA, Nirenberg MJ. Dopamine agonist withdrawal syndrome in Parkinson disease. *Arch Neurol*. 2010;67(1):58–63.

Rascol O, Brooks DJ, Korczyn AD, et al. Development of dyskinesias in a 5-year trial of ropinirole and L-dopa. *Mov Disord*. 2006;21(11):1844–1850.

Sako W, Miyazaki Y, Izumi Y, et al. Which target is best for patients with Parkinson's disease? A meta-analysis of pallidal and subthalamic stimulation. *J Neurol Neurosurg Psychiatry*. 2014;85(9):982–986.

Scarffe LA, Stevens DA, Dawson VL, et al. Parkin and PINK1: much more than mitophagy. *Trends Neurosci*. 2014;37(6):315–324.

Sulzer D, Surmeier DJ. Neuronal vulnerability, pathogenesis, and Parkinson's disease. *Mov Disord*. 2013;28(6):715–724.

Tanner CM, Goldman SM. Epidemiology of Parkinson's disease. *Neuroepidemiology*. 1996;14:317–335.

Tanner CM, Ottman R, Goldman SM, et al. Parkinson disease in twins: an etiologic study. *JAMA*. 1999;281:341–346.

Thomas A, Iacono D, Luciano AL, et al. Duration of amantadine benefit on dyskinesia of severe Parkinson's disease. *J Neurol Neurosurg Psychiatry*. 2004;75(1):141–143.

Witt K, Daniels C, Reiff J, et al. Neuropsychological and psychiatric changes after deep brain stimulation for Parkinson's disease: a randomised, multicentre study. *Lancet Neurol*. 2008;7(7):605–614.

Zimprich A, Biskup S, Leitner P, et al. Mutations in LRRK2 cause autosomal dominant parkinsonism with pleomorphic pathology. *Neuron*. 2004;44:601–607.

Parkinson-Plus Syndromes 84

Paul Greene

INTRODUCTION

Parkinson disease (PD) is the most common cause for a dopamine deficiency syndrome, but other causes for this syndrome had been identified from a small number of pathologic examinations since the early 20th century. It was not until the introduction of levodopa to treat PD in the late 1950s and early 1960s that clinicians began to identify patients who had dopamine deficiency signs but, unlike patients with PD, had minimal or no improvement with levodopa. Because multiple causes for levodopa-unresponsive dopamine deficiency states were soon identified, such patients were said to have parkinsonism or Parkinson-plus syndromes.

PROGRESSIVE SUPRANUCLEAR PALSY, MULTIPLE SYSTEM ATROPHY, CORTICOBASAL DEGENERATION

The three most common Parkinson-plus syndromes are progressive supranuclear palsy (PSP), multiple system atrophy (MSA), and corticobasal degeneration (CBD).

HISTORY

Progressive Supranuclear Palsy

In 1964, Steele, Richardson, and Olszewski reviewed autopsies of patients who had a syndrome of pseudobulbar palsy, supranuclear ocular palsy (chiefly affecting vertical gaze), axial rigidity and dystonia, early loss of postural reflexes, and dementia. They found a pattern of neuronal degeneration and neurofibrillary tangles (NFTs), chiefly affecting the pons and midbrain. This condition became known as the *Steele–Richardson–Olszewski syndrome* or PSP. As more autopsies became available, it became clear that this characteristic pathology could also produce other patterns of initial symptoms in addition to the originally described disease now called *Richardson syndrome*. In progressive supranuclear palsy-parkinsonism (PSP-P), patients in the early stage of the disease resemble idiopathic PD. However, occasional patients with PSP pathology may also present with corticobasal syndrome (see the following text), progressive nonfluent aphasia (PNFA), akinesia with gait freezing, primarily ataxia, or even pure dementia.

Multiple System Atrophy

It was noticed as early as 1900 that some patients with parkinsonian signs had additional signs and symptoms referable to other brain systems: cerebellar dysfunction (called *olivopontocerebellar atrophy* or OPCA) or autonomic dysfunction (termed *Shy–Drager syndrome* or SDS). Another syndrome of rapidly progressive parkinsonism with neuronal loss and gliosis primarily in the putamen and substantia nigra but no Lewy bodies on autopsy was termed *striatonigral degeneration* (SND). It was eventually noticed that some patients had elements of all these syndromes, and that patients with one clinical syndrome might have pathology overlapping with the other syndromes. The term *multiple system atrophy* (MSA) was introduced to indicate that SND, SDS, and OPCA were all part of a single disease spectrum. The later identification of a common pathology (synuclein-containing glial cytoplasmic inclusions) confirmed the suspicion that these conditions represented one disease (Table 84.2). Some patients with MSA have upper motor neuron signs and one of the original SDS patients had lower motor signs as well. It is not clear how many patients with parkinsonism and motor neuron disease have the pathology of MSA, so that the current criteria for MSA do not include the parkinsonism–amyotrophy syndrome. Because most patients have some degree of autonomic dysfunction, the disease is now characterized according to the presenting motor dysfunction: MSA-P when parkinsonism dominates the picture and MSA-C when cerebellar dysfunction predominates.

Corticobasal Degeneration

Initially reported as corticodentatonigral degeneration with neuronal achromasia in 1967, this disorder was characterized clinically by a combination of levodopa-unresponsive parkinsonism with early loss of balance, severe unilateral limb dystonia, and almost any focal cortical deficit. The pathology was also characteristic: enlarged achromatic neurons in cortical areas (particularly parietal and frontal lobes) along with nigral and striatal neuronal degeneration without Lewy bodies. The syndrome, also called *cortical–basal ganglionic degeneration* in the past, is now usually called *corticobasal degeneration* (CBD). As with PSP, it is now recognized that this pathology can also present clinically in other ways: as a frontal behavioral-spatial syndrome, PNFA, a progressive supranuclear palsy-like syndrome (PSPS), and dementia without motor abnormalities. Because patients with the pathology of PSP may mimic CBD, the original clinical syndrome is now called *corticobasal syndrome*. The overlap in both pathology and clinical features between CBD and PSP has raised concerns that the two diagnoses may represent a spectrum of a single disease despite a small number of pathologic findings unique to each diagnosis.

EPIDEMIOLOGY

The reported prevalence of each syndrome varies dramatically. In part, this is because clinical studies tend to underestimate the prevalence, whereas autopsy studies tend to overestimate the prevalence (because unusual cases are more likely to come to autopsy). PSP is the most common, generally reported in clinical studies to have a prevalence of 1 to 20 per 100,000 (compared to 100 to 200 per 100,000 for PD). In a large autopsy study, of all patients diagnosed with parkinsonism, about 4% had a pathologic diagnosis of PSP, about 2% had MSA, and about 1% had CBD (compared with more than 60% with PD).

PATHOBIOLOGY

Progressive Supranuclear Palsy

Atrophy of the dorsal midbrain, globus pallidus, and subthalamic nucleus; depigmentation of the substantia nigra; and mild dilatation of the third and fourth ventricles and aqueduct are seen on gross visual inspection of the postmortem brain in typical PSP. Light microscopy shows neuronal loss with gliosis, numerous NFTs, and neuropil threads in many subcortical structures, including the subthalamic nucleus, pallidum, substantia nigra, locus ceruleus, periaqueductal gray matter, superior colliculi, nucleus basalis, inferior olive, red nucleus, oculomotor nuclei, and cerebral cortex, especially the prefrontal and precentral areas. The NFTs appear as skeins of fine fibrils, often globose in shape in brain stem neurons. Ultrastructurally, they are composed of short, straight 12- to 15-nm tubules arranged in circling and interlacing bundles containing neurofilament proteins and the neurotubule-associated protein tau. In PSP, inclusion of exon 10 of tau creates a predominance of four repeated microtubule-binding domains, compared with a mixture of three and four repeated domains in Alzheimer disease. The typical astrocytic lesion in PSP is the tufted astrocyte, in contrast to the astrocytic lesion in CBD, the astrocytic plaque (see following text). Coiled bodies consisting of NFTs are found in astrocytes in both PSP and CBD (Fig. 84.1).

Multiple System Atrophy

The full pathologic spectrum of MSA consists of neuronal loss and gliosis in the neostriatum, substantia nigra, globus pallidus, cerebellum, inferior olives, basis pontine nuclei, intermediolateral horn cells, corticospinal tracts, and, rarely, anterior horn cells. A characteristic pathologic feature is the presence of widespread glial cytoplasmic inclusions, particularly in oligodendroglia. These argyrophilic, α-synuclein–positive, perinuclear structures are primarily composed of straight microtubules containing ubiquitin and tau protein. In SND, nerve cell loss and gliosis are found predominantly in the substantia nigra and neostriatum. In SDS, the preganglionic sympathetic neurons in the intermediolateral horns are lost. In addition, other areas may be affected, particularly the substantia

nigra (to produce parkinsonism), the cerebellum (to cause ataxia), and the striatum (to cause lack of response to levodopa). In OPCA, there is degeneration of the olives, pons, and cerebellum as well as neuronal loss in the striatum and substantia nigra. Less often, the anterior horn cells are involved (to cause amyotrophy) (Fig. 84.2).

Corticobasal Degeneration

In CBD there is asymmetric atrophy usually most severe in the frontoparietal region with relative sparing of the occipital lobes. Swollen vacuolated neurons are found in the atrophic cortical areas and to a lesser degree in the affected subcortical regions. These swollen or ballooned neurons contain phosphorylated neurofilaments and sometimes tau and ubiquitin. There is neuronal loss and gliosis in affected cortex and in the globus pallidus, putamen, red nucleus, thalamus, subthalamic nucleus, substantia nigra, locus ceruleus, and to a lesser degree in the dentate nucleus. Remaining neurons in affected areas contain the globose tangles common in PSP, in this setting called *corticobasal bodies*. As in PSP, white matter is affected with a variety of abnormalities including tau-containing fibrils coiling around the nuclei of oligodendroglia (coiled bodies). The typical glial finding in CBD is not the tufted astrocyte common in PSP but tau-containing processes surrounding astrocytes called *astrocytic plaques*. As in PSP, 4-repeat tau predominates but the insoluble tau fragments in CBD have a different ultrastructure from the insoluble fragments of tau in PSP (Fig. 84.3).

SYMPTOMS AND SIGNS

Progressive Supranuclear Palsy

Patients with classical PSP or Richardson syndrome have an akinetic rigid Parkinson-like syndrome with early loss of postural reflexes, falls, and dementia and usually have a supranuclear palsy early in the course. Rest tremor, asymmetric onset, and improvement with levodopa are uncommon. Axial rigidity often exceeds limb rigidity, and the posture may be erect. Patients have facial dystonia with deep nasolabial folds and furrowed brow (Procerus sign), an appearance of surprise or concern. When the patient walks, the neck may be extended, the arms abducted at the shoulders and flexed

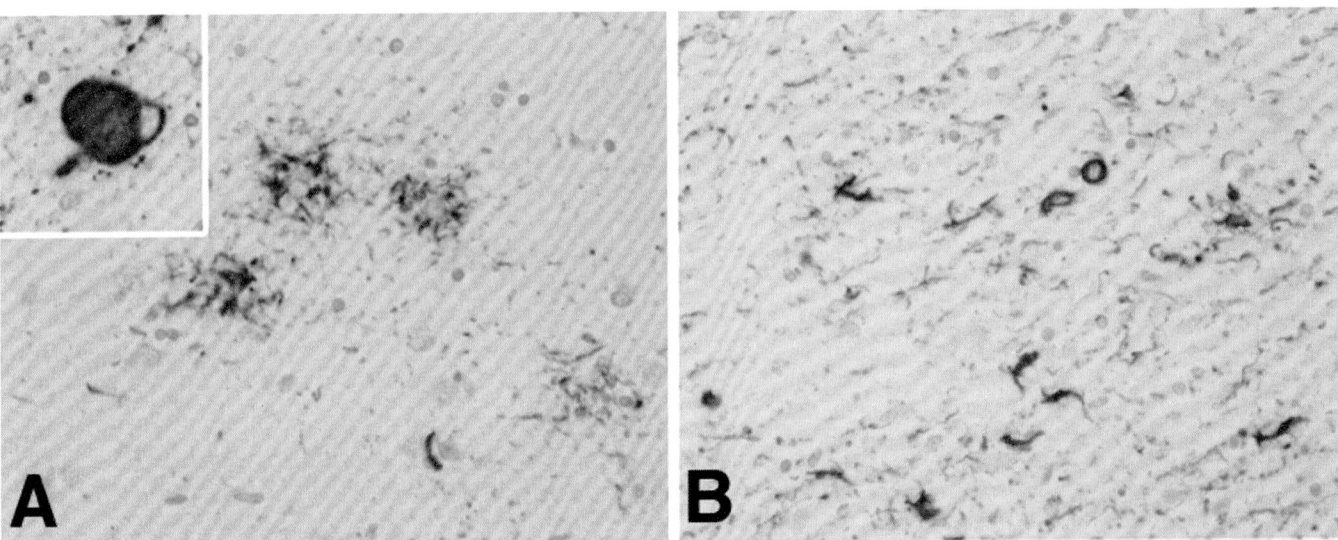

FIGURE 84.1 Pathology of PSP. The typical pathologic findings in PSP are tufted astrocytes **(A)**, globose NFT (*inset* in **A**), and coiled bodies **(B)**. (Modified from Dickson DW. Neuropathology of non-Alzheimer disease degenerative. *Int J Clin Exp Path*. 2010;3:1–23.)

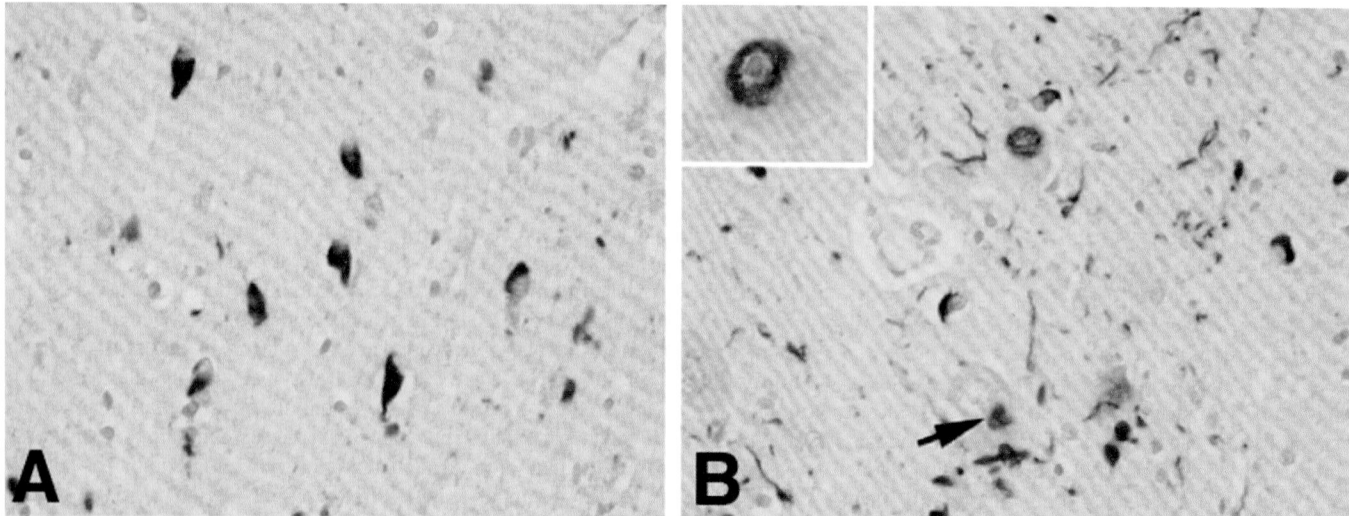

FIGURE 84.2 Pathology of MSA. The typical pathologic findings in MSA are glial cytoplasmic inclusions **(A)**, but they may be accompanied by neuronal inclusions (*arrow* in **B**) and α-synuclein–positive fibrillar neuronal inclusions (*inset* in **B**). (Modified from Dickson DW. Neuropathology of non-Alzheimer disease degenerative. *Int J Clin Exp Path*. 2010;3:1–23.)

at the elbows. Dysphagia and dysarthria usually appear early and become severe. The voice is slurred and hoarse, and some patients become anarthric as the disease progresses. Gait "freezing" may be prominent, and transient arrest of motor activity interrupts walking, speaking, and/or other actions.

The first visual symptoms in Richardson syndrome are failure to maintain eye contact in social interactions and difficulty with tasks requiring downgaze, such as reading, eating, or descending stairs. Hesitation on voluntary downgaze is found on examination accompanied by loss of vertical opticokinetic nystagmus on downward movement of the target. Patients often complain of diplopia, blurred vision, or difficulty reading. Disturbances of eyelid motility are also common, including lid retraction (resulting in a staring expression), blepharospasm, and apraxia of eyelid opening

or closing. Eyelid opening and closing apraxia (which are probably not true apraxia) are far more common in PSP than in any other extrapyramidal disorder. Fixation instability with coarse square-wave jerks and faulty suppression of the vestibulo–ocular reflex are common.

The cognitive impairment of PSP syndromes has been considered the archetype of subcortical dementia. The striking features are severe bradyphrenia (slowed thought), impaired verbal fluency, and difficulty with sequential actions or shifting from one task to another. Cognitive tests that depend on visual performance are especially affected. Apathy and disinhibition are common. Impulsiveness compounds postural instability and often leads to behavior that accentuates fall risk. Emotional incontinence is dominated by inappropriate weeping or, less frequently, laughing.

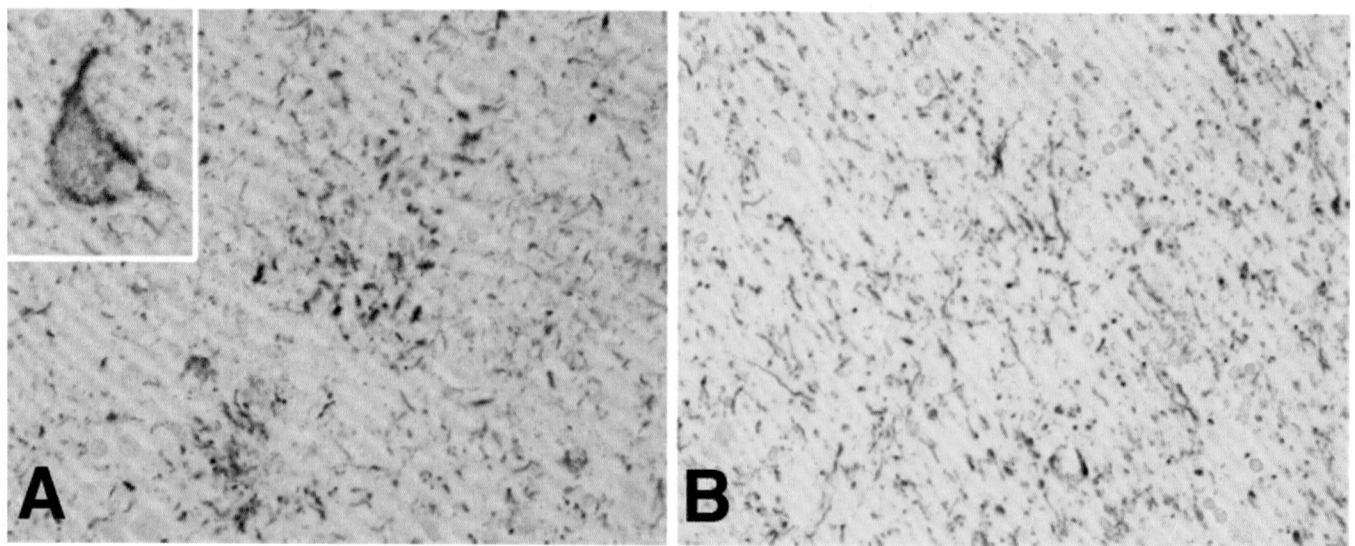

FIGURE 84.3 Pathology of CBD. The typical pathologic findings in CBD are astrocytic plaques (clusters of tau-positive processes around a central astrocyte) **(A)**, ballooned neurons (*inset* in **A**) and threadlike processes **(B)**. (Modified from Dickson DW. Neuropathology of non-Alzheimer disease degenerative. *Int J Clin Exp Path*. 2010;3:1–23.)

The course of PSP is aggressive; 3 to 4 years after onset, patients cannot walk without assistance and at a median of 5 years after onset, they are confined to bed and chair. They succumb to infection (from aspiration or pressure ulcers) or the sequelae of falls. The course varies according to the clinical syndrome, but Richardson syndrome has inexorable deterioration, culminating in death in 6 to 10 years in most cases.

In PSP-P, falls, dementia, and supranuclear palsy develop later and patients are more likely to have an asymmetric onset, rest tremor, and response to levodopa early in the course (although these usually do not persist). In some patients with PSP pathology, depending on the distribution of pathology, language difficulty may precede motor signs, presenting as a dysarthric, slow expressive aphasia (called *primary progressive aphasia* or *progressive nonfluent aphasia*). In a small number of patients, variation in pathology may produce other initial syndromes: freezing and balance difficulty without significant rigidity (akinesia with gait freezing), pure dementia without significant motor deficits, cerebellar syndrome, or corticobasal syndrome (see the following text) (Videos 84.1 and 84.2).

Multiple System Atrophy

The defining symptoms of SND are those of parkinsonism without tremor. Progression is usually rapid, and beneficial response to levodopa is absent or slight, presumably because striatal neurons containing dopamine receptors are usually lost. Dystonic reactions are common following low-dosage levodopa therapy. Orthostatic hypotension is a common presenting symptom of SDS syndrome (sometimes with labile blood pressure), but other dysautonomic symptoms are also troublesome, including impotence, urge incontinence, incomplete bladder emptying, and gastrointestinal (GI) motility disorders. Laryngeal stridor (often at night but sometimes during the day as well) strongly suggests SDS syndrome and can be life threatening. Other sleep symptoms include dysrhythmic breathing, sleep, and central apnea. OPCA is characterized by a mixture of parkinsonism and cerebellar syndrome, including gait ataxia, dysmetria, scanning speech, nystagmus, hypometric saccades, supranuclear upgaze impairment, and other cerebellar eye movement abnormalities. The least common presentation of MSA involves amyotrophy mimicking amyotrophic lateral sclerosis (ALS) (often combined with parkinsonism). Some patients with pathologic MSA may have pure autonomic failure for many years before developing other symptoms (and some may have the pathology and eventually develop symptoms of Lewy body disease). Dementia in MSA is rarely severe. As noted earlier, combinations of these symptoms often occur. Most patients progress rapidly and are in a wheelchair by a median 6 to 7 years after onset, although patients with cerebellar deficit predominance seem to progress more slowly. As in other Parkinson-plus syndromes, patients die from pulmonary, urinary tract and pressure ulcer infections, and complications of falls. Unlike the other syndromes, patients with MSA are also at risk for cardiopulmonary arrest due to autonomic dysfunction.

Corticobasal Degeneration

The onset of CBD is insidious and typically unilateral, with focal cortical deficits, and often marked rigidity–dystonia in the involved arm and/or leg. Sustained postures leading to contractures are common. Bradykinesia is usually present but may be hard to detect in the dystonic limb or limbs. Cortical signs of apraxia, alien limb phenomenon, cortical sensory loss, cortical reflex myoclonus, and occasionally aphasia are usually dramatic.

In addition to focal signs, global cortical dysfunction (dementia) is common. Speech is hesitant and dysarthric, gait is poor, and occasionally action tremor is evident. Falls usually occur shortly after onset of the disease. The disease usually spreads slowly to involve both sides of the body, and supranuclear gaze difficulties can occur late in the course. Patients with CBD pathology may present with several other syndromes. In the frontal behavioral-spatial syndrome, patients present with some combination of executive dysfunction, behavioral change, and visuospatial deficits. CBD at the onset may also look like PSP, PNFA, or a dementia without characteristic motor or focal cortical features (Video 84.3).

DIAGNOSIS

There have now been consensus criteria for the diagnosis of each of these syndromes. They were developed primarily for clinical research but are commonly used for clinical diagnosis as well (Tables 84.1 to 84.3).

Levodopa-unresponsive parkinsonism with early involvement of gait and balance suggests a Parkinson-plus syndrome, most commonly PSP, MSA, or CBD. There are two challenges: (1) Can we identify patients with signs and symptoms of one disease but the pathology of another? (2) Can we identify patients who seem to have idiopathic PD early in the course but actually have one of these syndromes?

It is not possible to predict the underlying pathology 100% of the time. Supranuclear vertical ophthalmoplegia suggests Richardson disease. Vertical eye movements are usually affected first in PSP whereas they develop late in CBD and are usually horizontal in MSA. Significant cerebellar deficits are most common in MSA but are rarely present in PSP. Autonomic failure is a hallmark of MSA and is uncommon in PSP and CBD but can be prominent in diffuse Lewy body disease (DLBD). Significant cognitive impairment is common is PSP and CBD but uncommon in MSA. Focal cortical deficits are a defining feature of CBD but occur in a minority of patients with PSP. Visual hallucinations and dopa-dyskinesias are more likely to be present in PD than in PSP-P or the other syndromes. Vascular parkinsonism often meets criteria for a Parkinson-plus syndrome and can be mistaken for PSP if eye movements are involved. Vascular parkinsonism can only be present with significant magnetic resonance imaging (MRI) abnormality, but white matter disease on MRI does not exclude PSP, MSA, or CBD. Frontotemporal lobar degeneration (FTLD)-parkinsonism can mimic any of these conditions, especially if the dementia lags behind the motor symptoms.

PSP or CBD may present as dementia without motor abnormalities or as levodopa-responsive parkinsonism without incompatible signs and there may be no clinical way to correctly identify the disease until it progresses. Any patient with symmetric parkinsonian signs or where the lower body is more affected than the upper body may eventually develop a Parkinson-plus syndrome but this is neither sensitive nor specific.

[18]F-fluorodeoxyglucose (FDG) positron emission tomography (PET) can accurately distinguish between PD and all Parkinson-plus syndromes but is not generally available. There are other imaging markers for each of these syndromes but none is yet accepted as sensitive and specific. Midbrain atrophy can be quantified on computed tomography or MRI and is often different for PSP, MSA, and CBD. Rostral midbrain atrophy greater than pons atrophy may resemble the beak of a hummingbird in PSP. There may be hyperintensity in the dorsolateral margin of the putamen

TABLE 84.1 Diagnostic Criteria for Progressive Supranuclear Palsy

Inclusion Criteria for Possible or Probable PSP

Gradually progressive disorder with age at or older than 40 yr

Exclusion Criteria for Possible or Probable PSP

Recent history of encephalitis

Alien limb syndrome

Cortical sensory deficits

Focal frontal or temporoparietal atrophy

Hallucinations or delusions unrelated to dopaminergic therapy

Cortical dementia of the Alzheimer type

Prominent, early cerebellar symptoms

Unexplained dysautonomia

Evidence of other conditions that might explain symptoms

Supportive Criteria for Possible or Probable PSP

Symmetric proximal > distal akinesia or rigidity

Abnormal neck posture, especially retrocollis

Poor or absent improvement with levodopa

Early dysphagia and dysarthria

Early onset of cognitive impairment, including two or more of the following:

* Apathy
* Impairment of abstract thought
* Decreased verbal fluency
* Use or imitation behavior
* Frontal release signs

Possible PSP

Either:

* Vertical supranuclear palsy
* Slowing of vertical saccades and postural instability with falls after less than 1 yr of disease

Probable PSP

Vertical supranuclear palsy and prominent postural instability with the tendency to fall within the first year of disease

Definite PSP

Meets all criteria for possible or probable PSP and histopathologic confirmation at autopsy

PSP, progressive supranuclear palsy.
Modified from Litvan I, Bhatia KP, Burn DJ, et al. SIC task force appraisal of clinical diagnostic criteria for parkinsonian disorders. *Mov Dis.* 2003;18:467–486.

TABLE 84.2 Diagnostic Criteria for Multiple System Atrophy

Possible MSA

Gradually progressive sporadic disease starting older than age 30 yr

* At least one feature suggesting autonomic dysfunction:
  * Unexplained urinary urgency, frequency, or incomplete bladder emptying
  * Erectile dysfunction in males
  * Significant orthostatic hypotension
* At least one additional feature of MSA (see below)
* Either:
  * Parkinsonism (bradykinesia with rigidity, tremor, or postural instability
  * Cerebellar syndrome (gait ataxia with cerebellar dysarthria, limb ataxia, cerebellar oculomotor dysfunction)

Probable MSA

Gradually progressive sporadic disease starting older than age 30 yr

* Autonomic failure with either:
  * Urinary incontinence (inability to control the release of urine from the bladder) with erectile dysfunction in men
  * Orthostatic decrease of blood pressure within 3 min of standing by at least 30 mm Hg systolic or 15 mm Hg diastolic
* Either:
  * Poorly levodopa-responsive parkinsonism (bradykinesia with rigidity, tremor, or postural instability)
  * Cerebellar syndrome (gait ataxia with cerebellar dysarthria, limb ataxia, cerebellar oculomotor dysfunction)

Additional Features of Possible MSA

* Possible MSA-P or MSA-C
  * Babinski sign with hyperreflexia
  * Stridor
* Possible MSA-P
  * Rapidly progressive parkinsonism
  * Poor response to levodopa
  * Postural instability within 3 yr of motor onset
  * Gait ataxia, cerebellar dysarthria, limb ataxia, or cerebellar oculomotor dysfunction
  * Dysphagia within 5 yr of motor onset
  * Atrophy on MRI of putamen, middle cerebellar peduncle, pons, or cerebellum
* Possible MSA-C
  * Parkinsonism (bradykinesia and rigidity)
  * Atrophy on MRI of putamen, middle cerebellar peduncle or pons
  * Hypometabolism on FDG-PET in putamen
  * Presynaptic nigrostriatal dopaminergic denervation on SPECT or PET

MSA, multiple system atrophy; MSA-P, MSA-parkinsonism; MSA-C, MSA-cerebellar dysfunction; MRI, magnetic resonance imaging; FDG-PET, ^{18}F-fluorodeoxyglucose-positron emission tomography; SPECT, single-photon emission computed tomography; PET, positron emission tomography.
Modified from Gilman S, Wenning GK, Low PA, et al. Second consensus statement on the diagnosis of multiple system atrophy. *Neurology.* 2008;71:670–676.

("putaminal slit" sign) and cruciform increased signal in the pons ("hot cross bun" sign) in MSA. Focal cortical atrophy suggests CBD. Autonomic failure in MSA affects preganglionic sympathetic neurons (plasma epinephrine is normal when the patient is supine but fails to rise when the patient stands), and this may differentiate it from orthostasis in DLBD.

TABLE 84.3 Diagnostic Criteria for Corticobasal Degeneration

Probable CBD	PSP Syndrome (PSPS)
• Insidious onset and gradual progression	Three of the following:
• Onset on or after age 50 yr, present for at least 1 yr, less than two affected relatives	• Axial or symmetric limb rigidity or akinesia
• Either:	• Postural instability or falls
• Probable CBS	• Urinary incontinence
• FBS	• Behavioral change
• NAV with at least one probable CBS feature (see below)	• Supranuclear vertical gaze palsy or decreased vertical saccade velocity
Probable CBS	**Possible CBD**
Asymmetric presentation of both:	• Insidious onset and gradual progression
• At least two of the following:	• Present for at least 1 yr
• Limb rigidity or akinesia	• Either:
• Limb dystonia	• Probable CBS
• Limb myoclonus	• NAV or FBS
• At least two of the following:	• PSPS with at least one possible CBS feature (see below)
• Orobuccal or limb apraxia	**Possible CBS**
• Cortical sensory deficit	Asymmetric or symmetric presentation of both:
• Alien limb (more than just overflow levitation)	• At least one of the following:
FBS Syndrome	• Limb rigidity or akinesia
Two of the following:	• Limb dystonia
• Executive dysfunction	• Limb myoclonus
• Behavioral or personality change	• At least one of the following:
• Visuospatial deficits	• Orobuccal or limb apraxia
Nonfluent/Agrammatic Variant (NAV) of Primary Progressive Aphasia	• Cortical sensory deficit
Effortful, agrammatic speech with at least one of the following:	• Alien limb (more than just overflow levitation)
• Impaired grammar/sentence comprehension with relatively preserved single word comprehension	
• Groping, distorted speech production (apraxia of speech)	

CBD, corticobasal degeneration; CBS, corticobasal syndrome; FBS, frontal behavioural-spatial syndrome; NAV, non-fluent/aggramatic variant of primary progressive aphasia; PSP, progressive supranuclear palsy.
Modified from Armstrong MJ, Irene Litvan I, Lang AE, et al. Criteria for the diagnosis of corticobasal degeneration. *Neurology.* 2013;80:496–503.

In the past, these syndromes were thought to be sporadic, but recently a small number of genetic conditions have been identified that may be clinically diagnosed as PSP, MSA, or CBD.

TREATMENT

The treatment of all Parkinson-plus syndromes is difficult and the approaches are similar in PSP, CBD, and MSA and so are discussed together. Medications are usually ineffective for parkinsonian symptoms in these conditions but are more likely to be effective in MSA-C when the striatum is relatively spared. Levodopa, however, can exaggerate orthostatic hypotension in MSA. Measures to overcome this problem include wearing support hose, ingesting salt, and taking fludrocortisone, midodrine, and other hypertensive agents. Patients can sleep with head elevated to avoid nocturnal hypertension and, if this is a problem, the dose of fludrocortisone should be kept to a minimum. If the striatum

becomes more involved, with presumed loss of dopamine receptors, the benefit of levodopa diminishes. Treatment with levodopa requires increasing the dose to the maximum-tolerated dose or up to 2 g/day (in the presence of carbidopa) to determine whether any therapeutic response can be obtained. Apraxia of eyelid opening (mainly in PSP) and painful dystonia or rigidity can be treated with botulinum toxin when the symptoms are relatively focal and the muscles can be located and injected. Tricyclic antidepressants or dextromethorphan/quinidine may suppress inappropriate crying or laughing. Anticholinergic drugs in modest doses or botulinum toxin injections may be useful in controlling drooling. Patients with Parkinson-plus syndromes are at high risk for swallowing difficulty, so botulinum toxin should be used with care. Antidepressants may be helpful for depression in all Parkinson syndromes (it is not known if some antidepressants are more effective than others), although most patients do not tolerate dopamine receptor–blocking agents that are sometimes used to treat depression. 1-Deamino-8-D-arginine vasopressin at bedtime may help avoid nocturnal incontinence (and also help orthostasis). Constipation is managed as with idiopathic PD but may be less responsive to treatment. As with other Parkinson-plus syndromes, painful cramps may respond to botulinum toxin injections. Some families use enteric feeding when there is risk of aspiration. Gastric tubes do not prevent regurgitation followed by aspiration. Duodenal tubes do prevent aspiration but require continuous feeding, not bolus feeding (Table 84.4).

DRUG/TOXIN-INDUCED PARKINSONISM

DOPAMINE RECEPTOR BLOCKING DRUGS

Drugs that block striatal dopamine D2 receptors (e.g., phenothiazines, butyrophenones, thioxanthenes, and other centrally acting dopamine receptor blockers including some antinausea medications and some calcium channel blockers) or deplete striatal dopamine (e.g., reserpine, tetrabenazine) can induce a parkinsonian state. It may take weeks to months for the parkinsonism to resolve after the offending agent is withdrawn. Parkinsonism that persists longer than 6 months after drug withdrawal is attributed to underlying PD that became evident during exposure to these antidopaminergic drugs. Anticholinergic drugs can ameliorate drug-induced parkinsonian signs and symptoms. The atypical antipsychotic agents, clozapine and quetiapine, are the antipsychotics least likely to induce or worsen parkinsonism.

1-METHYL-4-PHENYL-1,2,3,6-TETRAHYDROPYRIDINE

Although rare, parkinsonism induced by this toxin is important because it selectively destroys the dopamine nigrostriatal neurons, and the mechanism has been investigated intensively for possible clues to the etiology and pathogenesis of PD. 1-Methyl-4-phenyl-1,2,3,6-tetrahydropyridine (MPTP) is a protoxin, being converted to MPP$^+$ by the action of the enzyme monoamine oxidase type B. MPP$^+$ is taken up selectively by dopamine neurons and terminals via the dopamine transporter system. MPP$^+$ inhibits complex I in the mitochondria, depletes ATP, and increases the content of superoxide ion radicals. Superoxide in turn can react with nitric oxide to form the oxyradical peroxynitrite. MPTP-induced parkinsonism has occurred in drug abusers who used it intravenously and possibly also in some laboratory workers exposed to the toxin. The clinical syndrome is indistinguishable from PD and responds to levodopa. PET indicates that a subclinical exposure to MPTP results in a reduction of fluorodopa uptake in the striatum, thereby making the person liable to future development of parkinsonism.

OTHER DRUGS BESIDES DOPAMINE RECEPTOR BLOCKERS AND MPTP

Many other medications are occasionally reported to cause reversible parkinsonism, including antidepressants, anticonvulsants, antihypertensive medications, antiarrhythmics, immunosuppressants and others. In some cases, parkinsonism is relatively common; in others, parkinsonism is reported only rarely. In the rare cases, other medications known to cause parkinsonism may have also played a role and some may be coincidental idiopathic PD. For a partial list of drugs causing parkinsonism, see Table 84.5.

LYTICO–BODIG (PARKINSON–DEMENTIA–AMYOTROPHIC LATERAL SCLEROSIS COMPLEX OF GUAM)

Although not definitely a drug-induced disorder, epidemiologic evidence supports a probable environmental cause for Lytico–Bodig, with exposure occurring during adolescence or early adult years. Lytico–Bodig was identified when Chamorro natives on Guam in the Western Pacific were found to have a surprising incidence of parkinsonism, dementia, and motor neuron disease. The incidence has declined gradually with modernization of the culture. One hypothesis is that environmental exposure to the neurotoxin found in the seed of the plant *Cycas circinalis* was responsible for the neuronal degeneration. Natives on Guam used this seed to make flour in World War II. However, this hypothesis has been refuted. Besides parkinsonism, dementia, and motor neuron disease in various combinations, supranuclear gaze defects also appear. A characteristic pathologic finding is the presence of NFTs in the degenerating neurons, including the substantia nigra. Lewy bodies and senile plaques are absent.

TABLE 84.4	Treatment of Progressive Supranuclear Palsy, Multiple System Atrophy, and Corticobasal Degeneration	
Indication	**Treatment**	**Potential Side Effects**
Motor difficulty	Sinemet to tolerance	Orthostasis (esp. MSA), dystonia (esp. MSA), nausea, psychosis, others
Apraxia of eyelid opening (esp. PSP)	BTX injections	Ptosis, others
Depression	Antidepressants (except DRBA)	Lethargy, agitation, others
Drooling	Anticholinergics, BTX	Dry mouth, confusion (anticholinergics), dysphagia (esp. BTX)
Nocturnal incontinence	DDAVP	Hypertension
Constipation	As with PD	—
Painful muscle cramps	BTX	Excess muscle weakness
Aspiration	Gastric or duodenal tube	—

MSA, multiple system atrophy; PSP, progressive supranuclear palsy; BTX, botulinum toxin; DRBA, dopamine receptor–blocking agents; DDVAP, 1-deamino-8-D-arginine vasopressin; PD, Parkinson disease.

TABLE 84.5   Drugs Causing Drug-Induced Parkinsonism

Drugs/Indications	Mechanism of Action
High Risk of DIP	
First-generation antipsychotics: haloperidol, chlorpromazine, pimozide, thioxanthenes, trifluoperazine, others	Dopamine receptor blockade
Second-generation antipsychotics: risperidone, olanzapine, ziprasidone, aripiprazole	Dopamine receptor blockade
Dopamine depletors: tetrabenazine, reserpine	Dopamine depletion
Antiemetics: metoclopramide, prochlorperazine	Dopamine receptor blockade
Ca^{++} channel blockers: flunarizine, cinnarizine	Dopamine receptor blockade
MPTP	Destruction of dopamine-producing neurons
Intermediate Risk of DIP	
Atypical antipsychotics: quetiapine, clozapine	Dopamine receptor blockade
Ca++ channel blockers: diltiazem, verapamil	—
Antiepileptics: valproic acid, phenytoin, levetiracetam	—
Mood stabilizers: lithium	—
Low Risk of DIP	—
Antiarrhythmics: amiodarone	—
Immunosuppressants: cyclosporine	—
Antidepressants: SSRIs: fluoxetine, sertraline	—
MAO inhibitors: moclobemide, phenelzine	MAO inhibition
Antivirals: acyclovir, vidarabine, anti-HIV drugs	—
Statins: lovastatin	—
Antifungals: amphotericin B	—
Hormones: medroxyprogesterone, levothyroxine sodium	—
Cholinesterase inhibitors: donepezil, rivastigmine	—

Reports of parkinsonism in the low-risk category may be contaminated by coincidental idiopathic Parkinson disease or by polypharmacy.

DIP, drug-induced parkinsonism; MPTP, 1-methyl-4-phenyl-1,2,3,6-tetrahydropyridine; SSRIs, selective serotonin reuptake inhibitors; MAO, monoamine oxidase.

Data from Lopez-Sendon J, Mena MA, de Yebenes JG. Drug-induced parkinsonism. *Expert Opin Drug Saf*. 2013;12:487–496.

HEMIPARKINSONISM–HEMIATROPHY SYNDROME

This relatively benign syndrome consists of hemiparkinsonism in association with ipsilateral body hemiatrophy and/or contralateral brain hemiatrophy. The parkinsonism usually begins in young adults and may remain as hemiparkinsonism, sometimes with hemidystonia, or progress to generalized parkinsonism. It tends to be nonprogressive or slowly progressive compared with PD. The disorder is thought to result from brain injury early in life, possibly even perinatally. It sometimes responds to medications.

NORMAL PRESSURE HYDROCEPHALUS

The gait disorder in normal pressure hydrocephalus (see Chapter 106) resembles that of parkinsonism, with shuffling short steps and loss of postural reflexes and sometimes freezing. Features of urinary incontinence and dementia occur later. Tremor is rare. The grossly enlarged ventricles lead to the correct diagnosis, with the symptoms often improving on removal or shunting of CSF. The gait disorder is in striking contrast to the lack of parkinsonism in the upper part of the body. The major differential diagnoses for lower body parkinsonism include vascular parkinsonism and Parkinson-plus syndromes.

PARKINSON–DEMENTIA SYNDROMES

Although bradyphrenia is common in PD, dementia also occurs in over 30% of PD patients in clinics. The incidence of dementia increases with age, and those with dementia have a higher mortality rate. The two most common pathologic substrates for dementia in parkinsonism are pathologic changes typical of AD and the presence of Lewy bodies diffusely in the cerebral cortex. It is not known if the Alzheimer changes are coincidental because of the elderly population of affected individuals or whether AD and PD are somehow related. A clinical distinction has been made between patients who develop dementia before motor symptoms (or within a year of developing motor symptoms), labeled *DLBD* and those who develop dementia long after motor symptoms appear, labeled

Parkinson disease dementia (PDD). Because these conditions are similar in most other pathologic and clinical features, it is not known if these represent the spectrum of one disease or multiple separate diseases. Similarly, it is not known whether the spread of Lewy bodies into the cortex is a feature of progression of PD or a distinct entity.

POSTENCEPHALITIC PARKINSONISM

Although rarely encountered today, postencephalitic parkinsonism was common in the first half of the 20th century. Parkinsonism was the most prominent sequel of the pandemics of encephalitis lethargica (von Economo encephalitis) that occurred between 1919 and 1926. Although the causative agent was never established, it affected mainly the midbrain, thus destroying the substantia nigra. The pathology is distinctive because of the presence of NFTs in the remaining nigral neurons and absence of Lewy bodies. In addition to slowly progressive parkinsonism, with features similar to those of PD, oculogyric crises often occurred in which the eyes deviate to a fixed position for minutes to hours. Dystonia, tics, behavioral disorders, and ocular palsies may be present. Patients with postencephalitic parkinsonism are more sensitive to levodopa, with development of dyskinesias, mania, or hypersexuality at low dosages. Anticholinergics are tolerated and are effective against oculogyria.

VASCULAR PARKINSONISM

Vascular parkinsonism resulting from lacunar disease is not common but can be diagnosed by neuroimaging, with MRI evidence of hyperintense T2-weighted signals compatible with small infarcts. Hypertension is usually required for the development of this disorder. The onset of symptoms, usually with a gait disorder, is insidious, and the course is progressive. A history of a major stroke preceding the onset of parkinsonism is rare, although a stepwise course is sometimes seen. Gait is profoundly affected (lower body parkinsonism) with freezing and loss of postural reflexes. Tremor is rare. Response to the typical antiparkinsonian agents is usually minimal or absent.

Videos can be found in the companion e-book edition. For a full list of video legends, please see the front matter.

SUGGESTED READINGS

Armstrong MJ. Diagnosis and treatment of corticobasal degeneration. *Curr Treat Options Neurol.* 2014;16:282.

Cheyette SR, Cummings JL. Encephalitis lethargica: lessons for contemporary neuropsychiatry. *J Neuropsych Clin Neurosci.* 1995;7:125–134.

FitzGerald PM, Jankovic J. Lower body parkinsonism: evidence for vascular etiology. *Mov Disord.* 1989;4:249–260.

Friedman DI, Jankovic J, McCrary JA III. Neuro-ophthalmic findings in progressive supranuclear palsy. *J Clin Neuroophthalmol.* 1992;12:104–109.

Giladi N, Burke RE, Kostic V, et al. Hemiparkinsonism-hemiatrophy syndrome: clinical and neuroradiological features. *Neurology.* 1990;40:1731–1734.

Goetz CG, Emre M, Dubois B. Parkinson's disease dementia: definitions, guidelines, and research perspectives in diagnosis. *Ann Neurol.* 2008;64(suppl 2):S81–S92.

Gupta A, Lang AE. Potential placebo effect in assessing idiopathic normal pressure hydrocephalus. Case report. *J Neurosurg.* 2011;114:1428–1431.

Langston JW, Ballard P, Tetrud JW, et al. Chronic Parkinsonism in humans due to a product of meperidine-analog synthesis. *Science.* 1983;219:979–980.

Lanska DJ. The history of movement disorders. In: Finger S, Boller F, Tyler KL, eds. *Handbook of Clinical Neurology, History of Neurology.* Vol 95. Amsterdam, the Netherlands: Elsevier BV; 2010:501–546.

Lee SL. Guam dementia syndrome revisited in 2011. *Curr Opin Neurol.* 2011;24:517–524.

Lippa CF, Duda JE, Grossman M, et al. DLB and PDD boundary issues: diagnosis, treatment, molecular pathology, and biomarkers. *Neurology.* 2007;68:812–819.

Liscic RM, Srulijes K, Gröger A, et al. Differentiation of progressive supranuclear palsy: clinical, imaging and laboratory tools. *Acta Neurol Scand.* 2013;127:362–370.

Litvan I, Bhatia KP, Burn DJ, et al. SIC Task Force appraisal of clinical diagnostic criteria for Parkinsonian disorders. *Mov Disord.* 2003;18:467–486.

McGirt MJ, Woodworth G, Coon AL, et al. Diagnosis, treatment and analysis of long-term outcomes in idiopathic normal pressure hydrocephalus. *Neurosurg.* 2005;57:699–705.

Rebeiz JJ, Kolodny EH, Richardson EP Jr. Corticodentatonigral degeneration with neuronal achromasia: a progressive disorder in late adult life. *Trans Am Neurol Assoc.* 1967;92:23–26.

Seppi K, Poewe W. Brain magnetic resonance imaging techniques in the diagnosis of parkinsonian syndromes. *Neuroimag Clin N Am.* 2010;20:29–55.

Stamelou S, Quinn NP, Bhatia KP. "Atypical" atypical parkinsonism: new genetic conditions presenting with features of progressive supranuclear palsy, corticobasal degeneration, or multiple system atrophy—a diagnostic guide. *Mov Disord.* 2013;28:1184–1199.

Steele JC, Richardson JC, Olszewski J. Progressive supranuclear palsy: a heterogenous degeneration involving the brain stem, basal ganglia and cerebellum with vertical gaze and pseudobulbar palsy, nuchal dystonia and dementia. *Arch Neurol.* 1964;10:333–359.

Thobois S, Guillouet S, Broussolle E. Contributions of PET and SPECT to the understanding of the pathophysiology of Parkinson's disease. *Neurophysiol Clin.* 2001;31:321–340.

Wenning GK, Krismer F. Multiple system atrophy. *Handb Clin Neurol.* 2013;117:229–241.

Zijlmans JC, Daniel SE, Hughes AJ, et al. Clinicopathological investigation of vascular parkinsonism, including clinical criteria for diagnosis. *Mov Disord.* 2004;19:630–640.

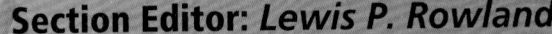

Amyotrophic Lateral Sclerosis and Motor Neuron Diseases 85

Rebecca Traub and Hiroshi Mitsumoto

INTRODUCTION

Several different diseases are characterized by progressive degeneration and loss of motor neurons in the spinal cord with or without similar lesions in the motor nuclei of the brain stem, the motor cortex, or both and by replacement of the lost cells by gliosis. All these can be considered *motor neuron diseases* (plural). The term *motor neuron disease* (singular), however, is used to describe an adult disease, *amyotrophic lateral sclerosis* (ALS), in which both upper and lower motor neurons are affected. (The terms *motor neuron disease* and *amyotrophic lateral sclerosis* have become equivalent in the United States.)

The term *spinal muscular atrophy* (SMA) refers to syndromes characterized solely by lower motor neuron signs. By conventional usage, the term *spinal muscular atrophy* is reserved for the childhood form, which is heritable, as described in Chapter 141.

Other motor neuron disease variants include progressive muscular atrophy, in which patients show only lower motor neuron signs; primary lateral sclerosis, in which patients show only upper motor neuron signs; progressive bulbar palsy, with weakness limited to bulbar muscles; and monomelic amyotrophy, in which the usual lower motor neuron findings are restricted to a single limb. These motor neuron disease subtypes are described more in detail in the following sections (Table 85.1).

It should be noted that there is some clinical overlap between motor neuron diseases, pure motor neuropathies (particularly those that are hereditary), and the hereditary spastic paraplegias (HSP). Distinguishing and classifying clinical phenotypes that lie in the overlap between these diagnoses often clinically challenging at present because of lack of diagnostic biomarkers.

TABLE 85.1 Motor Neuron Disease Variants

Amyotrophic lateral sclerosis (ALS)	Upper and lower motor neuron degeneration
Progressive muscular atrophy (PMA)	Purely lower motor neuron involvement
Primary lateral sclerosis (PLS)	Purely upper motor neuron involvement
Progressive bulbar palsy	Bulbar symptoms only or bulbar-onset ALS
Monomelic muscular atrophy	Lower motor neuron predominant, one arm
Bibrachial amyotrophy	Lower motor neuron predominant, both arms

AMYOTROPHIC LATERAL SCLEROSIS

DEFINITION

ALS is a disease of unknown cause and pathogenesis. It is defined pathologically as one in which there is degeneration of both upper and lower motor neurons. Charcot made the key clinical and pathologic descriptions, and the disease is named for him in Europe. In the United States, the disease is colloquially called *Lou Gehrig disease* after the famous baseball player who had the disease. Clinically, ALS is defined by evidence of both lower motor neuron disease (weakness, wasting, and fasciculation) and upper motor neuron disease (spasticity, hyperactive tendon reflexes, Hoffmann signs, Babinski signs, or clonus) in the same limbs. The accuracy of clinical diagnosis is assumed to be more than 95%, but that figure has not been formally tested. Nevertheless, the reliability of clinical diagnosis suffices to make the findings in the history and examination part of the definition.

EPIDEMIOLOGY

ALS is found worldwide in roughly the same prevalence (about 50×10^{-6}), with the exception of a few geographic areas with high prevalence of ALS, parkinsonism, and dementia complex, most notably on the island of Guam in the past. Case-control studies have not identified consistent risk factors related to occupation, diet, or socioeconomic status. There appears to be an increased risk of ALS among certain professional athletes and some suggestion that repeated head trauma may increase the risk for the disease.

The disease is generally of middle and late life. Only 10% of cases begin before age 40 years; 5% begin before age 30 years, with a greater proportion of those younger cases attributed to hereditary motor neuron diseases. An increase in age-adjusted incidence is seen in succeeding decades, except for a decrease after age 80 years. In most series, men are affected one to two times more often than women. There is no known ethnic predilection except slightly higher incidence in Norway because of some concentration of genetic mutations.

GENETICS

Approximately 5% to 10% of ALS cases are familial. Most are autosomal dominant in inheritance, but autosomal recessive and X-linked mutations have also been described. Increasingly recognized are "sporadic" ALS cases, which can be linked to specific genetic mutations, sometimes as a result of de novo mutations or incomplete penetrance. New mutations accounting for familial ALS continue to be described, and at the time of publication of this book, new mutations are likely to have been found not included in this chapter.

The two most common forms of autosomal dominant familial ALS are related to mutations in the C9ORF72 gene and the SOD1 gene. C9ORF72 repeat expansions are linked to both ALS, frontotemporal dementia (FTD), and often a combination of both clinical phenotypes. C9ORF72 mutations are currently the most common cause of familial ALS. Mutations in the SOD1 gene (ALS1) are the second most common cause of familial ALS. Many mutations in this gene have been described, and clinical phenotype is variable. Evidence suggests that mutant protein exerts its effects through accumulation of toxic protein. The SOD1 mutation has been used extensively in research as a model for studying pathology in ALS and identifying compounds for treatment trials.

Other familial ALS gene mutations have provided insight into potential pathogenic mechanisms in sporadic disease. Mutations in the fused in sarcoma (FUS) gene (ALS6) and TAR DNA-binding protein 43 (TDP-43) gene (ALS10) suggest a possible mechanism of RNA regulation and metabolism underlying sporadic disease. The pathogenic expansion in C9ORF72 familial ALS may also exert effects through RNA toxicity.

A list of the currently identified mutations in familial ALS at the time of publication of this text are listed in Table 85.2.

TABLE 85.2 Familial Amyotrophic Lateral Sclerosis

Name	Site	Gene	Inheritance	Comment
FTD–ALS	9p21	C9ORF72	AD	ALS and FTD Hexanucleotide expansion Most common cause of familial ALS
ALS1	21q22.1	SOD1	AD	Adult 15%–20% of familial ALS
ALS2	2q33	Alsin	AR	Juvenile; may resemble PLS
ALS3	18q21	—	—	—
ALS4	9q34	Senataxin (SETX)	AD	Juvenile; slow progression; allelic to CMT2
ALS5	15q15.1-q21.1	SPG11	AR	Juvenile Most common AR ALS Also seen in HSP
ALS6	16p11.2	Fused in sarcoma (FUS)	AD	Adult
ALS7	20p13	—	AD	Adult
ALS8	20q13.33	VAPB	AD	Adult
ALS9	14q11.2	ANG	AD	—
ALS10	1p36.22	TARDBP	AD	Some with FTD
ALS11	6q21	FIG4	AD	Allelic to CMT 4J (AR)
ALS12	10p13	OPTN	AD/AR	—
ALS13	12q24.12	ATXN2	AD	CAG expansions and increased ALS risk Expansions also seen with SCA2
ALS14	9p13.3	VCP	AD	Mutations also seen with IBMPFD
ALS15	Xp11.21	UBQLN2	X-linked	Reduced penetrance in women
ALS16	9p13.3	SIGMAR1	AR	Juvenile
ALS17	3p11.2	CHMP2B	AD	May cause FTD
ALS18	17p13.2	PFN1	AD	—
ALS19	2q34	ERBB4	AD	—
ALS20	12q13.13	HNRNPA1	AD	May cause multisystem proteinopathy
ALS21	5q31.2	MATR3	AD	Formerly distal myopathy 2, VCPDM

Other genes described and implicated in familial ALS–DAO, NEFH, HNRNPA2B1, SQSTM1.

FTD, frontotemporal dementia; ALS, amyotrophic lateral sclerosis; AD, autosomal dominant; AR, autosomal recessive; PLS, primary lateral sclerosis; HSP, hereditary spastic paraplegia; CMT 2, Charcot-Marie-Tooth hereditary neuropathy type 2; CMT 4J, Charcot-Marie-Tooth neuropathy type 4J; CAG, cytosine–adenine–guanine; SCA 2, spinocerebellar ataxia type 2; IBMPFD, inclusion body myopathy with Paget disease and frontotemporal dementia; VCPDM, vocal cord and pharyngeal dysfunction with distal myopathy.

X-LINKED RECESSIVE SPINOBULBAR MUSCULAR ATROPHY (KENNEDY DISEASE)

Although not typically included among the list of familial ALS, X-linked recessive spinobulbar muscular atrophy (Kennedy disease) should be included as a hereditary motor neuron disease. The gene maps to Xq11-q12, the site of the androgen receptor. The mutation is an expansion of a cytosine–adenine–guanine (CAG) repeat. Symptoms usually begin after age 40 years, with dysarthria and dysphagia with prominent tongue and mentalis fasciculations and with a slow course and limb weakness delayed for years. Upper motor neuron signs are often absent. In contrast to ALS, there is often an associated large-fiber sensory peripheral neuropathy. Gynecomastia is present in most but not all patients. Diagnostic clues include the characteristic distribution of signs, lack of upper motor neuron signs, slow progression, and a family history suggesting X-linked inheritance.

PATHOBIOLOGY

The cause of sporadic ALS is not known. The only established risk factors are age and family history. Environmental factors have been suspected, likely in combination with genetic susceptibility, but no clear risk exposures have been identified. There is increasing interest in repetitive head trauma and a link to chronic traumatic encephalopathy, although this link has yet to be well established. Theories regarding the cause of ALS have included infectious causes, including retroviruses, effects of excitotoxic amino acids, mitochondrial dysregulation, oxidative stress, and autoimmune causes, but little evidence conclusively supports one of these causes. Increasing evidence points to abnormal RNA processing and metabolism underlying ALS, although the exact mechanisms and triggers have yet to be elucidated.

PATHOLOGY

The pathology of ALS implies selective vulnerability of motor neurons, which show several neuronal inclusions that include ubiquitinated skeins or Lewy-like formations and Bunina bodies (Fig. 85.1). These structures are found in most patients with sporadic ALS. In some familial forms, a different form is the "hyaline conglomerate," which includes neurofilaments and does not contain ubiquitin. Authorities believe the cellular abnormalities identify a common basic mechanism for the syndromes of ALS, progressive muscular atrophy, primary lateral sclerosis, and amyotrophic lateral sclerosis–frontotemporal dementia (ALS–FTD).

The neuronal antigen in the inclusions recognized by antibodies to ubiquitin has been identified as TDP-43, and mutations in the TDP-43 gene are responsible for approximately 5% of familial ALS.

CLINICAL MANIFESTATIONS

Weakness may commence in the legs, hands, proximal arms, or bulbar muscles (with dysarthria and dysphagia). Often, the hands are affected first, usually asymmetrically, and with atrophy (Fig. 85.2). Progressive painless weakness is the typical primarily clinical feature of ALS. Gait is impaired because leg muscles are weak, and footdrop is characteristic, although

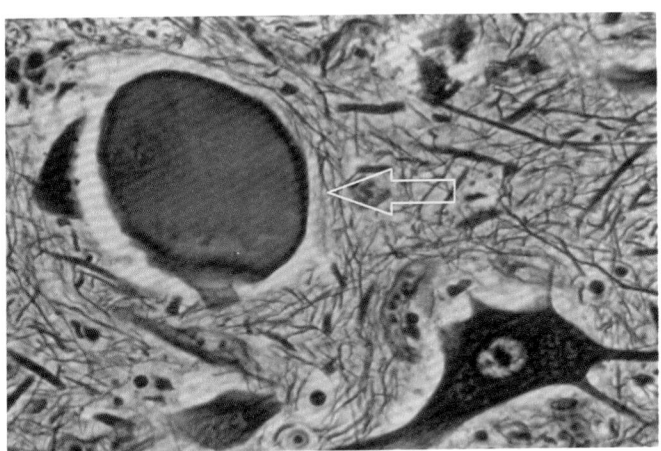

A

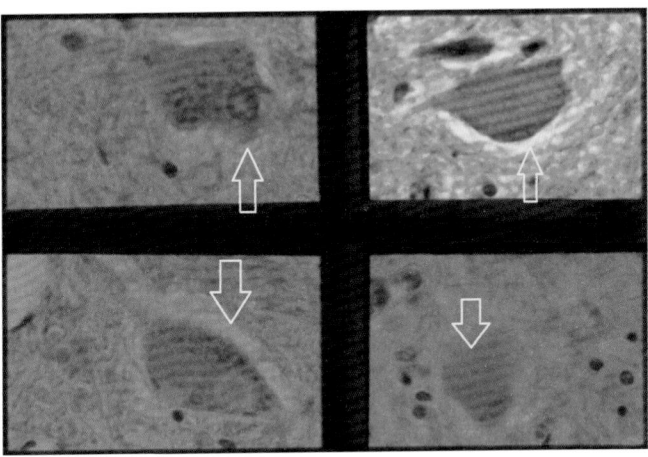

B

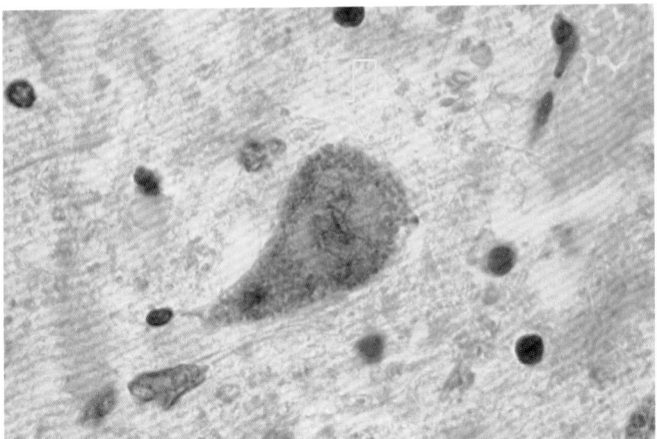

C

FIGURE 85.1 Pathologic findings in ALS. **A:** Axonal swelling and axonal spheroids (*arrow*) (Bodian silver stain, ×400 magnification). **B:** Motor neuron degeneration (*arrows*) (hematoxylin and eosin stain, ×400 magnification). **C:** Ubiquitinated skein-like inclusion (*arrow*) (ubiquitin immunoperoxidase stain, ×400 magnification).

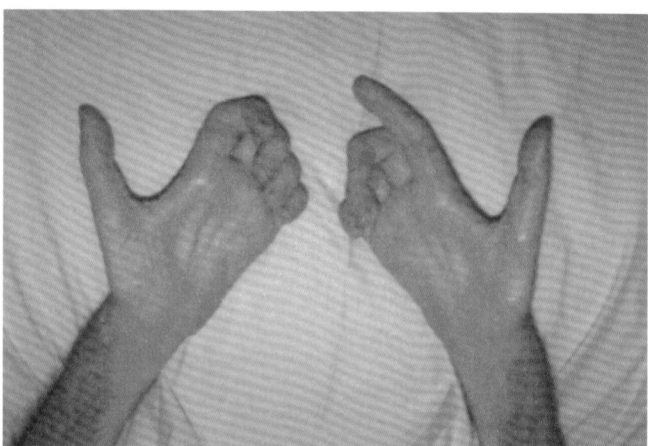

FIGURE 85.2 Hand atrophy in ALS.

| TABLE 85.3 | Typical Clinical Findings in Amyotrophic Lateral Sclerosis |

Upper Motor Neuron Symptoms and Signs
Spasticity
Hyperreflexia in deep tendon reflexes and/or clonus
Babinski sign/extensor plantar response
Hoffman sign
Increased jaw jerk
Spastic dysarthria
Pseudobulbar affect

Lower Motor Neuron Symptoms and Signs
Decreased muscle tone
Muscle atrophy
Fasciculations
Cramps
Hyporeflexia
Tongue atrophy and fasciculations
Facial weakness
Dysphagia
Dysarthria
Respiratory weakness
Neck weakness, head drop

proximal limb muscles are sometimes affected first. Alternatively, a spastic gait disorder may ensue. Slowly, the weakness becomes more severe, and more areas of the body are affected, leading to an increasing state of dependency. Muscle cramps (attributed to the hypersensitivity of denervated muscle) and weight loss (resulting from the combination of muscle wasting and dysphagia) are characteristic symptoms. Respiratory impairment is usually a late symptom but may, rarely, be an early or even the first manifestation; breathing is compromised by diaphragm and paresis of intercostal muscles, and dysphagia may lead to aspiration and pneumonitis, both of which can be the terminal event. Sensation is not clinically affected unless a preexisting neuropathy is present; pain and persistent paresthesias are atypical for this diagnosis, unless there is a complicating disease (e.g., diabetic neuropathy). Typically, bladder function is spared. The eye muscles are affected only exceptionally. Pain is not an early symptom but may occur later when limbs are immobile due to severe spasticity and joint contracture.

Lower motor neuron signs must be evident if the diagnosis is to be considered valid. Fasciculations may be seen in the tongue, even without dysarthria. If there is weakness and wasting of limb muscles, fasciculations are almost always seen. Tendon reflexes may be increased or decreased; the combination of overactive reflexes with Hoffmann signs in arms with weak, wasted, and fasciculating muscles is virtually pathognomonic of ALS. Unequivocal signs of upper motor neuron disorder are spasticity, Hoffmann or Babinski signs, and clonus. If a spastic gait disorder is seen without lower motor neuron signs in the legs, weakness in the legs may not be found, but incoordination is evident by clumsiness and slowness in the performance of alternating movements (Table 85.3).

The cranial nerve motor nuclei are implicated by dysarthria, lingual wasting and fasciculations, and impaired movement of the uvula (Fig. 85.3). Facial weakness and wasting can be discerned, especially in the mentalis muscle, but is usually not prominent. Dysarthria and dysphagia caused by upper motor neuron disease is made evident by movements of the uvula that are more vigorous on reflex innervation than on volition; that is, the uvula does not move well (or at all) on phonation, but a vigorous response is seen in the pharyngeal or gag reflex.

A common manifestation of pseudobulbar palsy is emotional lability with inappropriate laughing or, more often, crying, and that can be regarded erroneously as a reactive depression because of the diagnosis. Emotional lability is better regarded as a

release phenomenon of the complex reflexes involved in emotional expression.

The course is generally relentless and progressive without remissions, relapses, or even stable plateaus. Death results from respiratory failure, aspiration pneumonitis, or pulmonary embolism after prolonged immobility. The mean duration of symptoms is about 4 years; nearly 10% of patients live longer than 10 years. Once a tracheostomy has been placed, the patient may be kept alive for years, although totally paralyzed and unable to move anything other than the eyes; this condition can be a locked-in state, and even eye muscles are paralyzed. Exceptional patients die in the first year or live longer than 25 years.

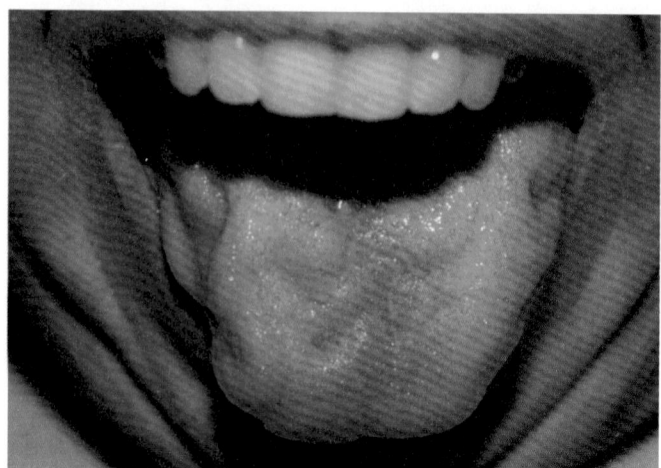

FIGURE 85.3 Tongue atrophy in ALS.

TABLE 85.4	Revised El Escorial Criteria for the Diagnosis of Amyotrophic Lateral Sclerosis

- Suspected ALS: a pure LMN syndrome in two or more regions

- Possible ALS: UMN and LMN signs present together in one region or UMN signs alone in two or more regions or LMN signs rostral to UMN signs

- Laboratory-supported ALS: UMN and LMN signs in one region or UMN signs alone in one region with LMN signs identified by EMG in two regions

- Probable ALS: UMN and LMN signs in more than two regions, and some UMN signs must be rostral to (above) LMN signs

- Definite ALS: UMN and LMN signs in three or more regions

All require absence of electrophysiologic or pathologic evidence of another disease process to explain clinical findings.

ALS, amyotrophic lateral sclerosis; LMN, lower motor neuron; UMN, upper motor neuron; EMG, electromyogram.

AMYOTROPHIC LATERAL SCLEROSIS DIAGNOSTIC CRITERIA

A number of different diagnostic criteria have been proposed for the clinical and research diagnosis of ALS. The most commonly used criteria are the revised El Escorial criteria (Table 85.4), which requires, for the diagnosis of definite ALS, the combination of upper and lower motor neuron findings in three of four potential anatomic regions (cranial, cervical, thoracic, and lumbosacral). The Awaji ALS criteria were developed in 2008 with the intention of including a greater number of ALS patients earlier in their clinical course through some adjustments to the electrodiagnostic and clinical criteria required (Table 85.5). These criteria are primarily designed for research uses, and many patients are diagnosed with and treated for ALS before they meet the complete criteria.

AMYOTROPHIC LATERAL SCLEROSIS AND FRONTOTEMPORAL DEMENTIA

About 10% of patients with ALS have associated dementia. The most common pathology is that of FTD; some show postmortem changes of Alzheimer disease and some show nonspecific pathology. The most common form of familial ALS, secondary to expansions in the C9ORF72 gene, often include both ALS and FTD within the same patient or family. Abnormalities in TDP-43 protein are also seen in both ALS and FTD pathology, linking the disorders. Why certain patients express more cognitive involvement and other more motor neuron pathology is not well understood.

MOTOR NEURON DISEASE VARIANTS

PROGRESSIVE MUSCULAR ATROPHY

Progressive muscular atrophy (PMA) is the term used to describe the lower motor neuron only form of motor neuron disease. Clinical findings and course are similar to ALS but without the associated upper motor neuron signs, such as hyperreflexia, Babinski or Hoffman signs, or spasticity. Many patients will have lower motor neuron predominant ALS, but pathologically true PMA probably accounts for less than 8% of cases. These patients usually live longer than ALS on average of 12 months.

TABLE 85.5	Awaji Criteria for the Diagnosis of Amyotrophic Lateral Sclerosis

The diagnosis of amyotrophic lateral sclerosis (ALS) requires the presence of the following:

- Evidence of lower motor neuron (LMN) degeneration by clinical, electrophysiologic, or neuropathologic examination

- Evidence of upper motor neuron (UMN) degeneration by clinical examination

- Progressive spread of symptoms or signs within a region or to other regions, as determined by history, physical examination, or electrophysiologic tests

The absence of the following:

- Electrophysiologic or pathologic evidence of other disease processes that might explain the signs of LMN and/or UMN degeneration

- Neuroimaging evidence of other disease processes that might explain the observed clinical and electrophysiologic signs

Diagnostic Categories

- Clinically definite ALS is defined by clinical or electrophysiologic evidence by the presence of LMN as well as UMN signs in the bulbar region and at least two spinal regions or the presence of LMN and UMN signs in three spinal regions.

- Clinically probable ALS is defined on clinical or electrophysiologic evidence by LMN and UMN signs in at least two regions with some UMN signs necessarily rostral to (above) the LMN signs.

- Clinically possible ALS is defined when clinical or electrophysiologic signs of UMN and LMN dysfunction are found in only one region, or UMN signs are found alone in two or more regions, or LMN signs are found rostral.

The diagnosis of PMA should always be made with caution, as it raises the question of a potentially treatable motor neuropathy, such as multifocal motor neuropathy. Diagnostic testing should include electrodiagnostic testing (electromyography and nerve conducting studies) with proximal stimulation on nerve conduction studies to exclude areas of conduction block and demyelinating findings, lab testing to evaluate for antibodies often seen in motor neuropathies, and consideration for spinal fluid testing to look for elevated protein. Magnetic resonance imaging (MRI) of the brain and transcranial magnetic stimulation can be used to look for subclinical upper motor neuron involvement.

PRIMARY LATERAL SCLEROSIS

Primary lateral sclerosis (PLS) refers to the clinical syndrome of progressive motor neuron disease affecting only upper motor neurons. As with PMA, there are often patients with upper motor neuron–dominant ALS, and true isolated upper motor neuron disease is uncommon, less than 5% of cases in autopsy series. The clinical symptoms and signs in PLS include spasticity and associated gait dysfunction, spastic dysarthria, and associated pathologic reflexes. Testing must include neuroimaging to exclude structural causes of upper motor neuron injury, lab testing to evaluate for metabolic disorders mimicking the clinical picture, and consideration for spinal fluid testing for infectious and inflammatory causes. Electrodiagnostic testing is critical for evaluating for lower motor neuron involvement, even in patients without clinical atrophy or fasciculations, and may need repeating over months to years to confirm the absence of denervation. It is generally agreed among experts that the diagnosis of PLS requires at least 4 years' observation. When spasticity and upper motor neuron findings are restricted to the legs or spare bulbar muscles, the clinician must consider the alternative diagnosis of HSP.

PROGRESSIVE BULBAR PALSY

The term *progressive bulbar palsy* has been used to describe motor neuron disease selectively affecting the bulbar muscles, causing dysarthria and dysphagia. This term is falling out of favor, as most of these patients do have at least some limb involvement, sometimes subclinical, at the time that bulbar symptoms begin. The term *bulbar-onset ALS* is more appropriate to describe those patients presenting with early or prominent bulbar symptoms.

MONOMELIC MUSCULAR ATROPHY

Monomelic muscular atrophy is a focal motor neuron disease restricted to one limb, usually an arm and a hand rather than a leg. Other names for the syndrome include *monomelic amyotrophy*, *benign focal amyotrophy*, *SMA of the unilateral upper extremity*, and *Hirayama syndrome*.

Monomelic muscular atrophy affects men 10 times more often than women and starts at about age 20 years, in contrast to typical sporadic ALS, which has a much older age of onset. The disease is most commonly seen in southeastern Asia, particularly Japan and India, although cases have been reported in Western countries. The weakness typically involves the hand and forearm, involving C7–T1 innervated muscles. Tendon reflexes are generally reduced in the affected arm. Upper motor neuron signs in other limbs are not seen. The condition progresses for 1 or 2 years and then seems to become arrested in most cases, although some have continued slow progression for many years. The origin of the disorder is not known, but most believe it is a focal motor neuron disorder or repetitive flexion–extension injury to the cervical spinal cord.

The differential diagnosis for monomelic muscular atrophy should include the initial onset of a more generalized ALS, multifocal motor neuropathy, or polio-like infectious syndromes, as in those seen with West Nile virus.

BIBRACHIAL AMYOTROPHY

A few percent of patients develop a lower motor neuron syndrome restricted to both arms. As in monomelic amyotrophy, it is more common in men than women, with a ratio of 8 to 9:1. It usually presents with proximal arm and shoulder muscle weakness. The progression is much slower than typical ALS. Arm posture is typically pronated and arms are dangling; sometimes it is called a *man-in-a-barrel*. Usually, lower motor neuron findings predominate, but sometimes upper motor neuron signs are present.

DIAGNOSTIC TESTING

ALS is primarily a clinical diagnosis, and electrodiagnostic, radiographic, and lab test results must be combined with the clinical picture to form the diagnosis. Ultimately, a clinical history and an attentive physical and neurologic exam are the most important diagnostic tools in ALS evaluation. The combination of typical upper and lower motor neuron findings in multiple limbs and affecting bulbar muscles has little differential diagnosis.

ELECTRODIAGNOSTIC TESTING

Electrodiagnostic testing including nerve conduction studies (NCS) and electromyography (EMG) are critical to confirming the lower motor neuron involvement in ALS and excluding motor

neuropathy mimics. NCS may show low motor amplitudes but may also be normal, particularly early in the course. NCS primarily are done to exclude findings suggestive of motor neuropathy, with conduction block or other demyelinating findings. Abnormal sensory responses should not be seen in ALS unless related to a pre-existing condition (e.g., diabetic neuropathy). Needle EMG should demonstrate evidence of active denervation (fibrillation and fasciculation potentials) and chronic denervation in three body segments (cranial, cervical, thoracic, and lumbosacral) to meet Awaji or El Escorial criteria. It should be noted that the electrodiagnostic findings must be combined with radiographic and clinical exam, as a severe polyradiculopathy or motor neuropathy might demonstrate similar EMG abnormalities.

Transcranial magnetic stimulation (TMS) is an electrodiagnostic method used to assess for upper motor neuron abnormalities in ALS, most useful when the predominant clinical picture is of lower motor neuron dysfunction. Stimulation over the motor cortex, cervical spine, and lumbar spine is performed with recording of a compound motor action potential (CMAP), assessing for delayed latency and central conduction. Unfortunately, it is done only at a few medical centers.

NEUROIMAGING

Imaging of the brain and spine, with MRI when possible, is typically recommended to exclude structural processes, most notably spinal stenosis, that might mimic ALS. Brain imaging occasionally demonstrates abnormalities in the corticospinal tracts that support the clinical findings of upper motor neuron disease or atrophy suggestive of an associated FTD. In most cases of ALS, neuroimaging is normal or demonstrates mild incidental abnormalities.

LAB TESTING

Spinal fluid studies are not required in the assessment of a patient with suspected ALS but should be considered in atypical cases, lower motor neuron (PMA) or upper motor neuron variants (PLS), or when there is concern for a motor neuropathy mimic, looking for elevation in protein, white blood cells, abnormal cytology, or elevated IgG synthesis.

Blood tests are recommended to evaluate for metabolic, endocrine, or inflammatory conditions that might mimic ALS. Testing for monoclonal gammopathy, antiganglioside antibodies, angiotensin-converting enzyme (ACE) levels, parathyroid hormone, and paraneoplastic markers rarely result in alternative diagnosis. Creatine kinase (CK) levels are often modestly elevated in ALS and are not inconsistent with the diagnosis. Genetic testing for familial ALS can be considered in cases in which there is a suggestive family history but is best performed with the help of a genetic counselor or physician experienced in genetic testing.

MUSCLE BIOPSY

Muscle biopsy is not routinely recommended in the evaluation of ALS and associated motor neuron disorders and typically demonstrates findings consistent with active and chronic denervation. The primary indication for muscle biopsy when considering a diagnosis of ALS is if there are clinical findings suggestive of inclusion body myositis, which may have some overlap in clinical presentation.

DIFFERENTIAL DIAGNOSES

Although the typical clinical picture of ALS is difficult to confuse with other neurologic disorders, cases occur which sometimes raise the question of other neuromuscular disorders with similar clinical phenotypes. Given that there is currently no disease-modifying treatment for ALS, the focus of testing when this diagnosis is considered is on excluding these other potentially treatable disorders (Table 85.6).

MULTIFOCAL MOTOR NEUROPATHY

Multifocal motor neuropathy (MMN) or multifocal motor neuropathy with conduction block (MMNCB) is a clinical syndrome of pure motor neuropathy, with conduction block in more than one nerve and not at sites of entrapment neuropathy. Anti-GM1 or other ganglioside antibodies are often associated. Symptoms often begin or predominate in the upper extremities. Although frank

TABLE 85.6	Differential Diagnosis of Motor Neuron Diseases
Multifocal motor neuropathy	• Primarily lower motor neuron syndrome but may have preserved reflexes • Conduction block on nerve conduction studies • Lab testing for GM1 antibodies
Chronic inflammatory demyelinating polyneuropathy	• Typically sensorimotor involvement clinically • Demyelinating findings on nerve conduction studies • Elevated CSF protein
Myasthenia gravis	• Typically more ocular symptoms, fluctuation, and fatigability • Decrement on repetitive stimulation with nerve conduction studies and no denervation on needle EMG • Acetylcholine receptor and muscle-specific kinase antibodies if clinically appropriate
Spinal stenosis	• Typically more pain and sensory symptoms • MRI or other imaging demonstrates structural abnormalities • No bulbar or facial involvement
Inclusion body myositis	• Typically affects quadriceps and finger flexors more severely • Needle EMG shows myopathic findings • Greater elevations in CK levels • Muscle biopsy to confirm diagnosis if clinical suspicion
Postpolio syndrome	• History of polio with later life decline in strength
Hereditary spastic paraparesis	• Upper motor neuron syndrome affecting primarily the legs • Family history may be useful • Genetic testing when clinically appropriate
Benign fasciculation syndrome/cramp fasciculation syndrome	• Absence of weakness, muscle wasting • Electrodiagnostics may show fasciculations but no other abnormalities
Paraneoplastic syndromes	• Paraneoplastic panel/antibody testing
Other systemic disorders	• Diabetes, sarcoidosis, parathyroid disease, hexosaminidase A deficiency

CSF, cerebrospinal fluid; EMG, electromyogram; MRI, magnetic resonance imaging; CK, creatinine kinase.

upper motor neuron findings should not be present, deep tendon reflexes are sometimes relatively preserved and muscle atrophy is often minimal given the degree of weakness. MMN is a potentially treatable autoimmune condition, treated with intravenous immunoglobulin (IVIG) or other immunosuppressing drugs, so the focus of NCS is often on assessing for this treatable diagnosis.

MYASTHENIA GRAVIS

Myasthenia gravis (MG) is a common cause of dysarthria and dysphagia in people who are in the age range of those afflicted with ALS and may be considered in the differential diagnosis when bulbar symptoms predominate. If there is concomitant ptosis or ophthalmoparesis, if diurnal fluctuation in severity is marked, or if remissions have occurred, MG is more likely. If there is suspicion for this diagnosis, testing should include blood testing of antibodies to acetylcholine receptor and muscle-specific tyrosine kinase (MuSK) and repetitive stimulation with NCS.

SPINAL STENOSIS

Although spinal disease should not cause bulbar symptoms, in patients with pure limb symptoms, cervical and lumbosacral polyradiculopathy due to spinal stenosis can cause a combination of upper and lower motor neuron symptoms and exam findings, which may be difficult to distinguish from limb-onset ALS. Spine imaging with MRI is thus recommended for all patients in whom the diagnosis of ALS is being considered.

MYOPATHY

Myopathy, most notably inclusion body myositis (IBM), may present with a clinical syndrome similar to ALS, with prominent arm weakness (typically affecting finger flexors and quadriceps disproportionately) and bulbar symptoms. Needle EMG testing is usually suggestive of a myopathic disorder, but sometimes neurogenic findings are seen. CK levels should be higher in IBM than in ALS. Fasciculations and upper motor neuron findings should not be seen in muscle disorders. Muscle biopsy is recommended when inflammatory myopathies are considered.

POSTPOLIO SYNDROME

Postpolio syndrome is a clinical worsening of weakness years after full or partial recovery from viral poliomyelitis. The consensus is that this syndrome is a residual effect in previously paralyzed muscles and that it is not a new motor neuron disease. Progression is slow and is limited to previously paralyzed muscles.

BENIGN FASCICULATIONS

Fasciculations, with or with muscle cramps, in the absence of weakness or upper motor neuron findings is nearly always a benign finding. There is no increased risk for future motor neuron disease in these patients. Electrodiagnostic testing may be useful to demonstrate no evidence of active or chronic denervation and reassure the patient regarding the diagnosis.

TREATMENT

Sadly, there is no effective drug therapy for disease modification in ALS. Therapeutic trials have shown no benefit from immunosuppression, immunoenhancement, plasmapheresis, lymph node irradiation, glutamate antagonists, nerve growth factors, antiviral agents, and numerous other categories of drugs.

Riluzole, a glutamate inhibitor, is the only drug approved by the U.S. Food and Drug Administration (FDA) for the treatment of ALS. In two randomized controlled trials, it was shown to improve 12- and 18-month survival, although the benefits were small [**Level 1**].[1,2] The usual dose is 50 mg twice daily. The most common side effects are nausea and dizziness, and hepatic function monitoring is recommended.

Treatment is therefore primarily symptomatic (Table 85.7), and emotional support is vitally important; management may be carried out most efficiently in a multidisciplinary ALS center, which is one of the few interventions shown to improve survival and quality of life [**Level 1**].[3] Early in the course, patients should try to continue to perform routine activities as long as they can. There is difference of opinion about exercising weak muscles, but physical therapy can help maintain function as long as possible. Drooling of saliva (sialorrhea) may be helped by atropine sulfate, glycopyrrolate, amitriptyline, or botulinum toxin injections into the salivary glands. Antispasticity agents have not been helpful in the spastic gait disorder, but intrathecal administration of baclofen might be considered in some patients, particularly those with PLS. Dysphagia leads to percutaneous gastrostomy to maintain nutrition; it does not prevent aspiration. Communication devices can ameliorate severe dysarthria. Noninvasive positive pressure ventilation has been used with increasing frequency to improve nocturnal dyspnea, insomnia, and overall respiratory discomfort, and it is likely not only to prolong life but also improve quality of life [**Level 1**].[4] Medications may also help with pseudobulbar symptoms, including the use of the combination drug dextromethorphan-quinidine [**Level 1**].[5]

The long-term care of patients with ALS has been addressed by evidence-based medicine recommendations made by a committee of the American Academy of Neurology. It is important for patients to be followed by one of the multidisciplinary ALS clinics because evidence shows that patients will have better symptomatic treatment, improved quality of life, and prolonged survival. The major decision concerns the use of tracheostomy and chronic mechanical ventilation, which can be done at home. In making the decision, patients should be informed fully about the long-term consequences of life without movement; they must decide whether they want to be kept alive or made as comfortable as possible—two choices that are not identical. Palliative care (relief of symptoms but not prolonging life) is becoming a standard option.

TABLE 85.7	Treatment for Amyotrophic Lateral Sclerosis and Motor Neuron Disorders

Disease Modifying

- Riluzole: only FDA-approved disease-modifying therapy for ALS

Improving Quality of Life and/or Survival

- Multidisciplinary ALS center care
- Noninvasive positive pressure ventilation/cough assist machine
- Physical therapy and rehabilitation
- Durable medical equipment and assistive devices to prevent falls and improve mobility
- Nutritional/calorie maintenance and percutaneous gastrostomy tube
- Tracheostomy and mechanical ventilation

Symptomatic Therapies

- Treatment of sialorrhea—atropine, glycopyrrolate, amitriptyline, botulinum toxin injections
- Treatment of spasticity—baclofen, cyclobenzaprine, benzodiazepines, intrathecal baclofen
- Communication devices
- Pseudobulbar symptom management—dextromethorphan-quinidine, selective serotonin reuptake inhibitors (SSRIs)
- Treatment of depression and associated mood disorders—SSRI, SNRI, tricyclic antidepressants
- Treatment of fatigue—modafinil, pyridostigmine
- Emotional support for patient and family caregivers

Comfort Measures, Pain Control, Palliative Care, and Hospice

FDA, U.S. Food and Drug Administration; ALS, amyotrophic lateral sclerosis; SNRI, serotonin–norepinephrine reuptake inhibitors.

LEVEL 1 EVIDENCE

1. Bensimon G, Lacomblez L, Meininger V. A controlled trial of riluzole in amyotrophic lateral sclerosis. ALS/Riluzole Study Group. *N Engl J Med.* 1994;330:585–591.
2. Lacomblez L, Bensimon G, Leigh PN, et al. Dose-ranging study of riluzole in amyotrophic lateral sclerosis. Amyotrophic Lateral Sclerosis/Riluzole Study Group II. *Lancet.* 1996;347:1425–1431.
3. Van den Berg JP, Kalmijn S, Lindeman E, et al. Multidisciplinary ALS care improves quality of life in patients with ALS. *Neurology.* 2005;65:1264–1267.
4. Bourke SC, Tomlinson M, Williams TL, et al. Effects of noninvasive ventilation on survival and quality of life in patients with amyotrophic lateral sclerosis: a randomised controlled trial. *Lancet Neurol.* 2006;5:140–147.
5. Brooks BR, Thisted RA, Appel SH, et al. Treatment of pseudobulbar affect in ALS with dextromethorphan/quinidine: a randomized trial. *Neurology.* 2004;63:1364–1370.

SUGGESTED READINGS

Andersen PM, Abrahams S, Borasio GD, et al. EFNS guidelines on the clinical management of amyotrophic lateral sclerosis (MALS)—revised report of an EFNS task force. *Eur J Neurol.* 2012;19:360–375.

Ashworth NL, Satkunam LE, Deforge D. Treatment for spasticity in amyotrophic lateral sclerosis/motor neuron disease. *Cochrane Database Syst Rev.* 2012;2:CD004156.

Baldinger R, Katzberg HD, Weber M. Treatment for cramps in amyotrophic lateral sclerosis/motor neuron disease. *Cochrane Database Syst Rev.* 2012;4:CD004157.

Blexrud MD, Windebank AJ, Daube JR. Long-term follow-up of 121 patients with benign fasciculations. *Ann Neurol.* 1993;34:622–625.

Brooks BR, Miller RG, Swash M, et al. El Escorial revisited: revised criteria for the diagnosis of amyotrophic lateral sclerosis. *Amyotroph Lateral Scler Other Motor Neuron Disord.* 2000;1:293–299.

Byrne S, Walsh C, Lynch C, et al. Rate of familial amyotrophic lateral sclerosis: a systematic review and meta-analysis. *J Neurol Neurosurg Psychiatry.* 2011;82:623–627.

Chancellor AM, Warlow CP. Adult onset motor neuron disease: worldwide mortality, incidence and distribution since 1950. *J Neurol Neurosurg Psychiatry.* 1992;55:1106–1115.

Dalakas MC, Elder G, Hallett M, et al. A long-term follow-up study of patients with post-poliomyelitis neuromuscular symptoms. *N Engl J Med.* 1986;314:959–963.

D'Amico E, Pasmantier M, Lee YW, et al. Clinical evolution of pure upper motor neuron disease/dysfunction (PUMMD). *Muscle Nerve.* 2013;47:28–32.

de Carvalho M, Dengler R, Eisen A, et al. Electrodiagnostic criteria for diagnosis of ALS. *Clin Neurophysiol.* 2008;119:497–503.

DeJesus-Hernandez M, Mackenzie IR, Boeve BF, et al. Expanded GGGGCC hexanucleotide repeat in noncoding region of C9ORF72 causes chromosome 9p-linked FTD and ALS. *Neuron.* 2011;72:245–256.

Dimos JT, Rodolfa KT, Niakan KK, et al. Induced pluripotent stem cells generated from patients with ALS can be differentiated into motor neurons. *Science.* 2008;321:1218–1221.

Donofrio PD, Berger A, Brannagan TH III, et al. Consensus statement: the use of intravenous immunoglobulin in the treatment of neuromuscular conditions report of the AANEM ad hoc committee. *Muscle Nerve.* 2009;40:890–900.

Floyd AG, Yu QP, Piboolnurak P, et al. Transcranial magnetic stimulation in ALS: utility of central motor conduction tests. *Neurology.* 2009;72:498–504.

Gordon PH, Cheng B, Katz IB, et al. Clinical features that distinguish PLS, upper motor neuron-dominant ALS, and typical ALS. *Neurology.* 2009;72:1948–1952.

Gordon PH, Cheng B, Katz IB, et al. The natural history of primary lateral sclerosis. *Neurology.* 2006;66:647–653.

Gourie-Devi M, Nalini A. Long-term follow-up of 44 patients with brachial monomelic amyotrophy. *Acta Neurol Scand.* 2003;107:215–220.

Hirayama K, Tokumaru Y. Cervical dural sac and spinal cord in juvenile muscular atrophy of distal upper extremity. *Neurology.* 2000;54:1922–1926.

Huang YC, Ro LS, Chang HS, et al. A clinical study of Hirayama disease in Taiwan. *Muscle Nerve.* 2008;37:576–582.

Ince PG, Evans J, Knopp M, et al. Corticospinal tract degeneration in the progressive muscular atrophy variant of ALS. *Neurology.* 2003;60:1252–1258.

Joint Task Force of the European Federation of Neurological Societies and the Peripheral Nerve Society. European Federation of Neurological Societies/Peripheral Nerve Society guideline on management of multifocal motor neuropathy. Report of a joint task force of the European Federation of Neurological Societies and the Peripheral Nerve Society—first revision. *J Peripher Nerv Syst.* 2010;15:295–301.

Kaufmann P, Pullman SL, Shungu DC, et al. Objective tests for upper motor neuron involvement in amyotrophic lateral sclerosis (ALS). *Neurology.* 2004;62:1753–1757.

Kim WK, Liu X, Sandner J, et al. Study of 962 patients indicates progressive muscular *Neurology.* 2009;73:1686–1692.

Lawyer T Jr, Netsky MG. Amyotrophic lateral sclerosis. *AMA Arch Neurol Psychiatry.* 1953;69:171–192.

Miller RG, Jackson CE, Kasarskis EJ, et al. Practice parameter update: the care of the patient with amyotrophic lateral sclerosis: drug, nutritional, and respiratory therapies (an evidence-based review): report of the Quality Standards Subcommittee of the American Academy of Neurology. *Neurology.* 2009;73:1218–1226.

Miller RG, Jackson CE, Kasarkis EJ, et al. Practice parameter update: the care of the patient with amyotrophic lateral sclerosis: multidisciplinary care, symptom management, and cognitive/behavioral impairment (an evidence-based review): report of the Quality Standards Subcommittee of the American Academy of Neurology. *Neurology.* 2009;73:1227–1233.

Miller RG, Mitchell JD, Moore DH. Riluzole for amyotrophic lateral sclerosis (ALS)/motor neuron disease (MND). *Cochrane Database Syst Rev.* 2012;3:CD001447.

Mitsumoto H, Chad D, Pioro E. *Amyotrophic Lateral Sclerosis.* Philadelphia: FA Davis; 1998.

Nagai M, Re DB, Nagata T, et al. Astrocytes expressing ALS-linked mutated SOD1 release factors selectively toxic to motor neurons. *Nat Neurosci.* 2007;10:615–622.

Pouget J, Trefouret S, Attarian S. Transcranial magnetic stimulation (TMS): compared sensitivity of different motor response parameters in ALS. *Amyotroph Lateral Scler Other Motor Neuron Disord.* 2000;1(suppl 2): S45–S49.

Re DB, Le Verche V, Yu C, et al. Necroptosis drives motor neuron death in models of both sporadic and familial ALS. *Neuron.* 2014;81:1001–1008.

Renton AE, Majounie E, Waite A, et al. A hexanucleotide repeat expansion in C9ORF72 is the cause of chromosome 9p21-linked ALS-FTD. *Neuron.* 2011;72:257–268.

Rosen DR, Siddique T, Patterson D, et al. Mutations in Cu/Zn superoxide dismutase gene are associated with familial amyotrophic lateral sclerosis. *Nature.* 1993;362:59–62.

Rowland LP. Diagnosis of amyotrophic lateral sclerosis. *J Neurol Sci.* 1998;160(suppl 1):S6–S24.

Rowland LP. Progressive muscular atrophy and other lower motor neuron syndromes of adults. *Muscle Nerve.* 2010;41:161–165.

Rowland LP, Shneider NA. Amyotrophic lateral sclerosis. *N Engl J Med.* 2001;344:1688–1700.

Wijesekera LC, Mathers S, Talman P, et al. Natural history and clinical features of the flail arm and flail leg ALS variants. *Neurology.* 2009;72:1087–1094.

Comana M. Cioroiu and Thomas H. Brannagan III

Isolated cranial neuropathies are not uncommon, the most frequently encountered of which is Bell palsy. These syndromes can be seen in both the inpatient and outpatient settings, and all have a very varied differential diagnosis. The cranial nerve examination is a crucial component of a complete neurologic exam. Cranial nerve injury can be implicated in various diseases with widespread neurologic involvement such as stroke, multiple sclerosis, and demyelinating neuropathies, particularly when other pathways and neuroanatomic regions are involved as well. Cranial neuropathies can occur together (with involvement of more than one nerve) or in isolation (with involvement of only one nerve). Multiple cranial neuropathies are most often caused by cancer, infarct, and trauma, and these etiologies must be considered and carefully excluded when evaluating these patients, with particular attention paid to the brain stem where several cranial nerves localize together. However, occasionally, there may be abnormal findings limited to one cranial nerve in isolation. In these instances of isolated cranial neuropathies, the differential diagnosis depends on the nerve involved and the clinical picture as a whole. This chapter will address common cranial mononeuropathies and their evaluation and management. Several of these are addressed in other chapters of this text and are referred to when appropriate.

THE OLFACTORY NERVE (CRANIAL NERVE I)

The ability to smell is a special quality relegated to the olfactory cells in the nasal mucosa. The molecular biology of smell is uncertain, but transcription-activating factors, such as Olf-1, found exclusively in neurons with olfactory receptors, probably direct cellular differentiation. Smell may be impaired after injury of the nasal mucosa, the olfactory bulb or its filaments, or central nervous system (CNS) connections. Nerve injury causes diminution or loss of the sense of smell. The most common complaint of patients with olfactory nerve injury, however, is not loss of smell but diminished taste; olfaction plays a key role in taste perception because of the volatile substances in many food and beverages. A loss of sense of smell may be congenital or acquired and occurs in various conditions (Table 86.1). The sense of smell is most commonly impaired, transiently, because of allergic nasal congestion or the common cold. The most common traumatic olfactory nerve injury occurs in head injury, usually of the acceleration–deceleration variety, including motor vehicle accidents. The delicate olfactory nerve filaments are sheared by the perforations of the cribriform plate. The olfactory bulb can also be contused or lacerated in head injuries. Leigh and Zee (2006) reported altered olfactory sense in 7.2% of patients with head injuries at a military hospital, with complete loss in 4.1% and partial loss in 3.1%. Recovery of smell occurred in only 6 of 72 patients. In a study of head injuries in civilians, Friedman and Merritt (1944) found that the olfactory nerve was damaged in 11 (2.6%) of 430 patients. In all patients, anosmia was bilateral. In three, the loss was transient and disappeared within 2 weeks of injury. *Parosmia* (i.e., perversion of sense of smell) was present in 12 patients.

Inflammatory or neuritic lesions of the bulb or tract are uncommon, but these structures are sometimes affected in meningitis or in mononeuritis multiplex. Rarely, patients with diabetes mellitus have impaired smell, sometimes stemming from olfactory nerve infarction. Hyposmia or anosmia is also common early in Refsum disease (an autosomal recessive disease leading to an overaccumulation of phytanic acid). Kallmann syndrome is an X-linked inherited disorder causing hypogonadism and anosmia due to olfactory tract hypoplasia. The olfactory bulb or tract may be compressed by meningiomas (particularly at the olfactory groove or sphenoidal ridge), metastatic tumors, or aneurysms in the anterior fossa or by infiltrating tumors of the frontal lobe. The Foster–Kennedy syndrome is a classic syndrome caused by a tumor invading the orbitofrontal region, leading to unilateral and ipsilateral optic atrophy, contralateral papilledema, and anosmia. Neurodegenerative diseases at times may be heralded by a loss of smell, and this is seen particularly with Parkinson disease, where loss of smell may be a presenting sign. Certain drugs are often implicated in a loss of smell, particularly cocaine when used intranasally, although other toxins such as cadmium and chemotherapeutic agents have been implicated as well.

Parosmia is not accompanied by impairment of olfactory acuity and is most commonly caused by lesions of the temporal lobe, although it has been reported with injury to the olfactory bulb or tract.

TABLE 86.1	Causes of Loss of Smell Related to Olfactory Nerve Injury
Congenital	Refsum disease
	Kallmann syndrome
	Congenital anosmia
Acquired	Inflammatory
	• Rhinitis
	• Meningitis
	• Mononeuritis multiplex
	Head trauma
	Tumor
	• Meningioma at olfactory groove
	• Frontal lobe glioma
	• Metastasis
	Neurodegenerative
	• Parkinson disease
	• Alzheimer disease
	Toxic
	• Cocaine
	• Cadmium
	• Smoking
	• Chemotherapeutic agents
	Vitamin deficiency
	• Thiamine (B_1)
	• B_{12}
	Psychiatric disease

Olfactory hallucinations may occur in psychosis or as a seizure aura that involves the hippocampal or uncinate gyrus; perceptions are described as strange, unpleasant, and ill-defined odors. Increased sensitivity to olfactory stimuli is generally rare, although it may occur in migraineurs and in patients with reactive airways disease, perhaps because of prior sensitization to olfactory triggers. Cases in which the sense of smell is so acute that it is a source of continuous discomfort, however, may be psychogenic.

THE OPTIC NERVE (CRANIAL NERVE II) AND CRANIAL NERVES III, IV, AND VI

Disorders of the visual system are described in Chapter 9.

THE TRIGEMINAL NERVE (CRANIAL NERVE V)

The fifth cranial nerve, or the trigeminal nerve, has both a large sensory component as well as a smaller motor component. The nerve has three major branches—the ophthalmic division (V1), the maxillary division (V2), and the mandibular division (V3). These three branches carry sensory information from distinct dermatomes of the face, head, and mucous membranes and converge on the trigeminal or gasserian ganglion located in Meckel's cave (which serves as the dorsal root ganglion). Sensory fibers from all three divisions ascend in the pons to terminate in the three parts of the trigeminal nucleus. The spinal trigeminal nucleus receives afferent fibers related to facial pain and temperature sensation, the principal sensory nucleus receives fibers related to light touch and mechanoreception, whereas the mesencephalic nucleus contains cell bodies with fibers carrying information regarding jaw proprioception. Motor branches originate in the motor nucleus of the trigeminal nerve and are distributed in the mandibular division to innervate the muscles of mastication.

Injury to the fifth cranial nerve causes loss of soft-tactile, thermal, and pain sensation in the face; loss of the corneal and sneezing (i.e., sternutatory) reflexes; and paralysis of the muscles of mastication. Lesions of the trigeminal pathways in the pons usually affect the motor and chief sensory nuclei causing paralysis of the muscles of mastication and loss of light touch perception in the face; lesions in the medulla affect only the descending tract and cause loss of facial light touch sensation. Brain magnetic resonance imaging (MRI) with contrast is often useful to search for mass lesions, ischemia, and inflammation, whereas electrophysiologic testing (e.g., blink reflex testing) may help quantitate both the afferent (i.e., trigeminal nerve) and efferent (i.e., facial nerve) components of the corneal reflex. The fifth nerve may be injured by trauma, neoplasm, aneurysm, or meningeal infection. Infarcts and other vascular lesions, as well as intramedullary tumors, may damage the sensory and motor nuclei in the pons and medulla. Isolated lesions of the descending tract may occur in syringobulbia or in multiple sclerosis. Common causes of trigeminal nerve injury with facial numbness include dental or cranial trauma, herpes zoster, head and neck tumors, intracranial tumors, and idiopathic trigeminal neuropathy. Less common causes include multiple sclerosis, systemic sclerosis, mixed connective tissue diseases, amyloidosis, and sarcoidosis. Isolated facial numbness may also occur without a clearly identifiable cause (i.e., *idiopathic trigeminal neuropathy*), but these patients must be carefully evaluated to ensure an occult process is not overlooked. Although restricted loss of sensation over the chin (i.e., the *numb chin syndrome*) usually is caused by dental trauma, dental or surgical procedures, or even poorly fitting dentures,

this syndrome is a recognized initial feature of a systemic malignancy such as lymphoma, metastatic breast carcinoma, melanoma, or prostate cancer. MRI of the mandible may help separate these disorders. Painful facial numbness may herald nasopharyngeal or metastatic carcinoma. Isolated weakness of the trigeminal innervated muscles of mastication may be seen in motor neuron disease where patients often develop jaw weakness and dysphagia. This can also be seen with diseases of the neuromuscular junction, that is, myasthenia gravis.

TRIGEMINAL NEURALGIA

Epidemiology and Pathobiology

Trigeminal neuralgia, also commonly known as *tic douloureux*, is a syndrome of extremely severe facial pain without numbness or objective findings in the fifth nerve distribution (see also Chapter 55). This disorder of the trigeminal nerve is characterized by recurrent paroxysms of sharp, stabbing pains in the distribution of one or more nerve branches. Unlike herpes zoster, the second and third divisions of the trigeminal nerve are the most commonly involved and the first is primarily affected in only less than 5% of patients. Onset is usually in middle or late life but may occur at any age. Typical trigeminal neuralgia occasionally affects children but rarely occurs before age 35 years— presentation at that age should prompt an investigation for demyelinating disease. The incidence of trigeminal neuralgia is slightly greater in women than in men and found to be about 12.6 per 100,000 people in some studies.

The cause remains unknown. In most cases, no organic disease of the fifth nerve or the CNS is identified. Degenerative or fibrotic changes in the gasserian ganglion have been described but are too variable to be considered causal. Trigeminal nerve compression related to an anomalous blood vessel, usually in the vicinity of the ganglion, is a long-standing but controversial etiology of the disorder. Most commonly, this is thought to be compression by a loop of either the anterior inferior cerebellar or superior cerebellar artery. Painful symptoms typical of trigeminal neuralgia occasionally occur with demyelinating brain stem lesions including those produced by multiple sclerosis, as well as vascular ischemia affecting the descending root of the fifth nerve. When trigeminal neuralgia has a known structural cause, it is categorized as symptomatic, as opposed to the idiopathic form that has no known etiology. Although trigeminal neuralgia usually follows other symptoms of multiple sclerosis rather than precedes them, up to 10% of patients may have facial pain as part of their initial presentation. Tumors invading the gasserian ganglion or the cerebellopontine angle may also cause symptoms of trigeminal neuralgia, although usually in the setting of an abnormal neurologic examination. The paroxysmal attacks of facial pain in trigeminal neuralgia may be related to excessive discharge within the descending nucleus of the nerve triggered by an influx of impulses. Relief of symptoms by section of the greater auricular or occipital nerves in some patients suggests a role for peripheral excitation, and interruption of an episode by intravenous phenytoin, as well as a general therapeutic response to antiepileptic agents, suggests aberrant neuronal discharge may also play an important part in the pathophysiology of this disorder. Trigeminal neuralgia is the most common of all neuralgias.

Clinical Manifestations and Diagnosis

The pain is extremely severe, is described by many patients as among the worst pain imaginable, and in severe and refractory cases, the risk of suicide is increased. The pain appears in paroxysms and typically lasts seconds, although episodes of up to 15 minutes can occur. Between episodes, the patient is free of symptoms, except for fear of an impending attack. The pain is searing or burning, coming in lightning-like jabs. The frequency of attacks varies from many times a day to a few times a month. The patient ceases to talk when the pain strikes and may rub or pinch the face; movements of the face and jaw may accompany the pain. Sometimes, ipsilateral lacrimation is prominent. No objective loss of cutaneous sensation is found during or after the paroxysms, but the patient may complain of facial hyperesthesia.

A characteristic feature in the presentation is the *trigger zone*, stimulation of which sets off a typical paroxysm of pain. This zone is a small area on the cheek, lip, or nose that may be stimulated by facial movement, chewing, brushing teeth, or touch. The patient may avoid making facial expressions during conversation, may go without eating for days, or may avoid the slightest breeze to prevent an attack. The pain is limited strictly to one or more branches of the fifth nerve and does not spread beyond the distribution of that nerve. The second division is involved more frequently than the third. Pain may spread to one or both of the other divisions. In cases of long duration, all three divisions are affected in 15% of patients. The pain is occasionally bilateral (5%) for some but rarely occurs at the same time. Bilateral trigeminal neuralgia is encountered most often in patients with multiple sclerosis. A new classification scheme differentiates classic trigeminal neuralgia with paroxysms of pain from a different form, in which the paroxysms are associated with a concomitant dull, constant facial pain.

The diagnosis of trigeminal neuralgia is usually made from the history. Neurologic examination in patients with trigeminal neuralgia is usually normal, although some patients may also have concurrent hemifacial spasm, and patients whose attacks are provoked by eating may appear thin or cachectic. The results of serum studies and other diagnostic evaluations are also normal. Characteristically, patients avoid touching the area of origin when asked to point it out, instead holding the tip of the index finger a short distance from the face. On examination, patients will show no clinical sensory or motor deficits in the trigeminal nerve distribution, although the affected area is often very sensitive. Computed tomography (CT) or MRI of the brain is reasonable to exclude structural causes and at times may demonstrate an aberrant vessel causing compression. However, the sensitivity and specificity of MRI for identifying neurovascular compression is variable and thus its role for this purpose is controversial. In 2008, the American Academy of Neurology put forth a practice parameter concerning the diagnosis and treatment of trigeminal neuralgia, which stated that electrodiagnostic evaluation of the trigeminal reflex is a reasonable first step in excluding symptomatic trigeminal neuralgia and can be considered before imaging.

Trigeminal neuralgia must be differentiated from other types of facial pain or headache, especially infections of the teeth and nasal sinuses. These pains are usually steady instead of episodic, are often throbbing, and persist for many hours. However, it is not uncommon for patients with trigeminal neuralgia to undergo surgical treatment of the sinuses and/or tooth extractions before the diagnosis is established. Conversely, patients with diseased teeth may be referred to neurology with a diagnosis of trigeminal neuralgia, although careful dental examination usually identifies the teeth as the source of pain in these patients.

Temporomandibular joint disease may also mimic trigeminal neuralgia, but the pain is not paroxysmal and, although exacerbated by eating, no trigger point may be identified and symptoms

are usually less severe between meals. Cluster headaches are another consideration but occur in protracted clusters rather than as brief events and are accompanied by ipsilateral nasal congestion, ipsilateral conjunctival injection and lacrimation, and an ipsilateral Horner syndrome. Atypical facial pain may have a trigeminal distribution but the individual paroxysms always last longer than a few seconds (usually minutes or hours). The pain itself is dull, aching, crushing, or burning. Surgical treatment is not effective in atypical facial pain and its etiology remains obscure, although it may be associated with depression.

A more detailed discussion of headache and facial pain syndromes can be found in Chapter 7.

Treatment and Outcome

Although surgical options now exist, medical therapy remains first line as far as treatment options. Trigeminal neuralgia is most effectively treated with carbamazepine at 800 mg/day to a maximum dose of 1,500 mg/day in four divided doses. A Cochrane Database review found carbamazepine to be consistently effective, with a number needed to treat of 1.8. However, dosing should be titrated to effect, and doses producing serum levels above the therapeutic range for seizure control may be needed as long as potentially dose-limiting side effects are tolerated. Overdosage is manifested by drowsiness, dizziness, ataxia, unsteady gait, and nausea. Hepatotoxicity may occur but is usually reversible with discontinuation. Another more rare but serious complication is aplastic anemia, and both periodic liver function testing and monitoring of the blood count are needed. In some patients, tolerance may develop over time. Baclofen is also effective in many cases in doses of 40 to 80 mg/day; phenytoin is less effective but may be used as adjunctive therapy. Some of the newer antiepileptic agents may also provide some relief, and oxcarbazepine, a derivative of carbamazepine, in doses of 400 to 1,200 mg/day is thought to be as effective as carbamazepine. Other medications which have been shown to be effective in some cases (although no controlled trials exist) include lamotrigine, gabapentin, pregabalin, sumatriptan, and topiramate. More recently, both intravenous lidocaine and onabotulism toxin A have been found to be successful in treating acute episodes of trigeminal neuralgia, although more rigorous trials are needed. Surgical procedures used to treat this condition include microvascular decompression, radiofrequency ablation, balloon microcompression, and chemical gangliolysis and rhizotomy. More recently, stereotactic radiosurgery using Gamma Knife has been used with noted improvements in pain scores. Of these methods, radiofrequency ablation has met with the greatest success in initial treatment, although recurrence rates have not been studied carefully. As compression of the trigeminal nerve by arterial loops may play a role in some cases, posterior fossa exploration with decompression has sometimes been used for refractory cases. Other chronic masses, such as arteriovenous malformation, aneurysm, and cholesteatoma, may also cause compression of the ganglion and may be more amenable to surgical correction.

THE FACIAL NERVE (CRANIAL NERVE VII)

The seventh cranial nerve (facial nerve), although predominantly motor, also serves an important parasympathetic and sensory function (Fig. 86.1). On exiting the brain stem ventrally via the internal acoustic meatus in the petrous part of the temporal bone near the pontomedullary junction, the facial nerve forms two divisions: the nervus intermedius and the motor root. The motor root is

THE FACIAL NERVE

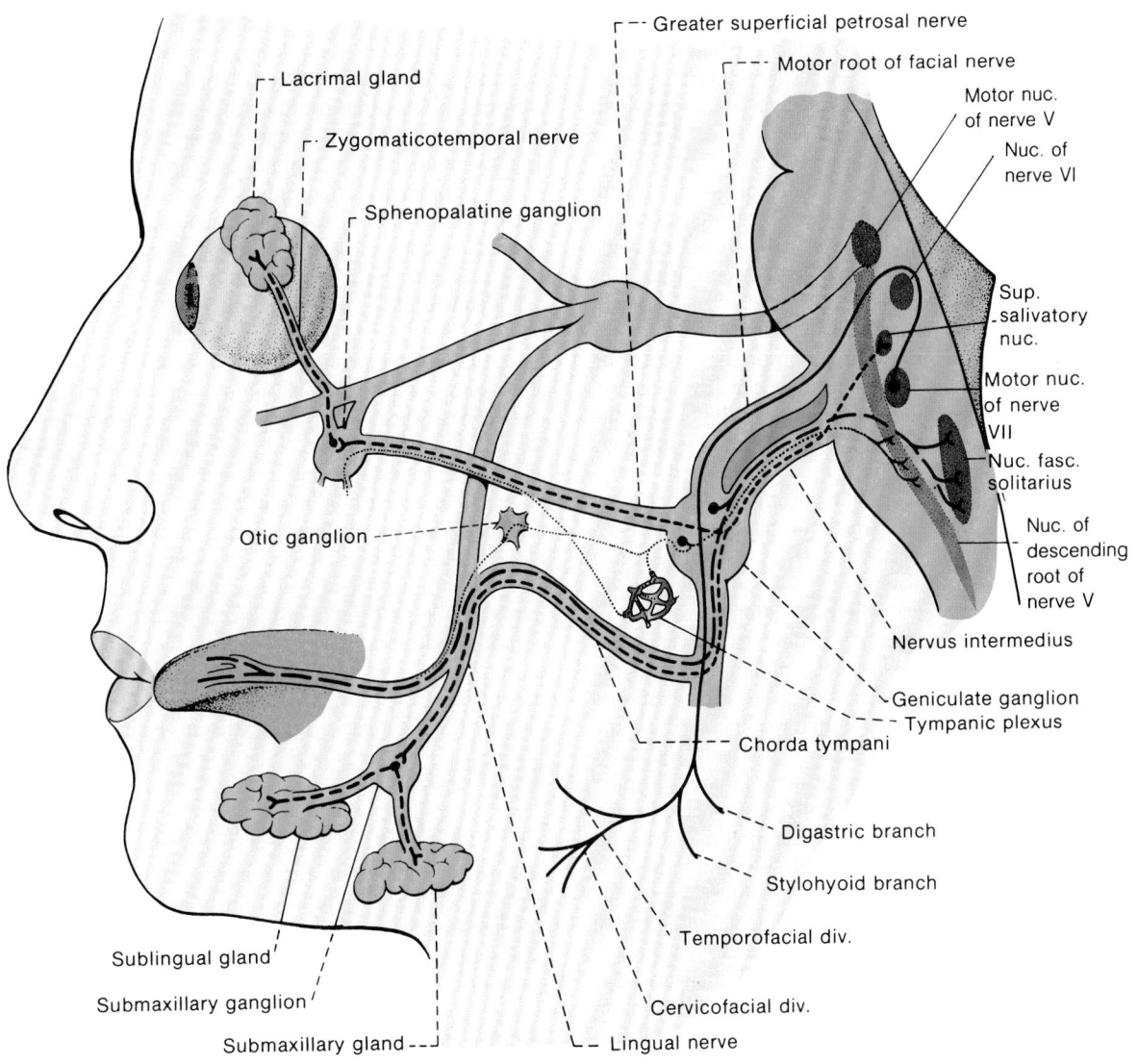

FIGURE 86.1 Anatomy of the facial nerve. (From Campbell WW. *DeJong's The Neurologic Examination.* 6th ed. Philadelphia: Lippincott Williams and Wilkins; 2005.)

composed of nerve fibers arising from the facial motor nucleus, and after exiting the nucleus, these axons travel dorsomedially in the pons to circle the abducens nucleus (thus forming the facial colliculus) and travel down to meet the nervus intermedius to form the facial nerve. The nervus intermedius arises from superior salivatory and lacrimal nuclei (eventually sending parasympathetic innervation to the salivary glands, specifically the submaxillary and sphenopalatine ganglia), the nucleus solitarius (fibers of which ultimately relays afferent taste sensation from the anterior two-thirds of the tongue), and the spinal trigeminal nucleus (carrying somatosensory afferent fibers to parts of the face and ear). The fibers of the seventh cranial nerve arising from the spinal trigeminal nucleus may also relay proprioceptive impulses from the facial muscles and cutaneous sensation from the posteromedial surface of the pinna and the external auditory canal. The fibers arising from the nucleus solitarius and spinal trigeminal nucleus together synapse in the geniculate ganglion in close proximity to the brain stem. Distal to the geniculate ganglion, the facial nerve forms several branches.

Axons from the superior lacrimal nucleus form the greater petrosal nerve, which synapses in the sphenopalatine ganglion prior to innervating the lacrimal glands. Fibers originating from the nucleus solitarius and the superior salivatory and nuclei travel further distally in the facial nerve prior to forming the chorda tympani, a branch of the nerve which crosses the middle ear and exits the skull to join the lingual nerve. Just prior to the chorda tympani, the facial nerve also gives off a motor branch to the stapedius muscle. Distal to the chorda tympani, the motor root of the facial nerve runs through the facial canal and exits the skull via the stylomastoid foramen. At this point, it gives rise to the posterior auricular nerve innervating the scalp and ear, as well as a motor branch to the stylohyoid muscle and digastric muscle. The nerve then continues on into the parotid gland, where it divides into its five major branches—temporal, zygomatic, buccal, marginal mandibular, and cervical.

Lesions near the origin of the nerve, or in the vicinity of the geniculate ganglion, are accompanied by loss of motor, gustatory, and autonomic functions. Lesions between the geniculate ganglion and the origin of the chorda tympani typically spare lacrimation, whereas lesions near the stylomastoid foramen spare taste and lacrimation, causing only ipsilateral facial paralysis of the upper and lower face. Lesions of the facial nerve nucleus in the brain stem also cause ipsilateral paralysis of all facial muscles, both upper and lower.

The pattern of peripheral or nuclear injury (the peripheral seventh nerve lesion) must be distinguished from that associated with central motor pathway lesions above the level of the nucleus, which cause weakness and paralysis in the lower half of the face while sparing forehead wrinkling because of redundancy of central pathways subserving upper face muscles (central facial weakness; supranuclear palsy). In supranuclear lesions, voluntary contractions of the face differ, being more or less intense, from those occurring during spontaneous emotional expression, particularly when accompanied by laughing or crying. Depending on the precise site and extent of associated injury within the CNS, other neurologic signs may also appear.

Owing to this anatomic organization, the signs of peripheral facial nerve injury are somewhat variable (Table 86.2). More severe injury produces obvious facial paralysis at rest with sagging of the muscles of the lower ipsilateral face. The normal folds and lines around the lips, nose, and forehead are attenuated; the palpebral fissure is wider than normal; and voluntary movement of the facial and platysmal muscles is absent. Smiling highlights the weakness by contrasting the normal and unaffected orbicularis oris with the droop of the affected side. Although weakness of both the upper and lower halves of the face is seen, occasionally, the lower muscles may be weaker than the upper, or more rarely, the upper muscles may be weaker than the lower, with partial nerve injury. Saliva may seep from the paralyzed side of the mouth at rest, and food or fluids may leak out when eating. Closure of the eyelid is incomplete, and the upward and inward deviation of the eye may be seen during examination when eye closure is attempted (Bell phenomenon). This common complication assumes great importance because early patching and lubrication of the affected eye after seventh nerve injury is critical to prevent corneal desiccation and potentially permanent scarring. Tear production is diminished only if the lesion is proximal to the geniculate ganglion. With lesions peripheral to the ganglion, lacrimation is spared but tears may still be sequestered in the conjunctival sac because incomplete eyelid closure no longer moves them effectively through the

lacrimal duct. The corneal reflex is also impaired by paralysis of the upper lid, although preservation of corneal sensation and the afferent portion of the reflex is confirmed by consensual blinking of the contralateral eyelid during corneal reflex testing. Decreased salivation and loss of taste in the anterior two-thirds of the tongue are present when the chorda tympani is affected. Loss of somatic sensation to the external auditory canal, however, is less common. The seventh nerve also supplies the stapedius muscle, and patients may develop increased sensitivity to loud sounds (i.e., hyperacusis) when the small muscle is paralyzed and its dampening effect on the tympanic membrane is lost. Recovery from facial paralysis depends on the severity of the lesion and the specific cause. If the nerve is completely crushed or severed, the chances of even partial recovery are remote, especially if the intraneural scaffolding necessary to guide axonal regeneration is lost. In contrast, in purely demyelinative lesions without axonal injury, excellent and often complete recovery is expected. When the facial nerve attempts to regenerate through proximal axonal growth across an injured segment, axonal extension sometimes results in aberrant reinnervation. This faulty circuit results in the movement of previously unrelated facial muscles when the patient attempts isolated activation of a separate muscle, a process known as *synkinesis*. In such patients, for example, lip movement may occur with each eye blink. Aberrant reinnervation may also cause excessive lacrimation during activation of the facial muscles or when the salivary glands are activated during eating (e.g., producing "crocodile tears"). In addition, some patients develop paroxysmal clonic contractions of the hemifacial muscles (i.e., hemifacial spasm) that may simulate focal seizures.

BELL PALSY

Epidemiology and Pathobiology

Bell palsy, named after the Scottish anatomist Charles Bell, is a common clinical syndrome of uncertain etiology in which acute, unilateral paresis or paralysis of muscles innervated by the facial nerve appears spontaneously, over hours to days, and is the most common cause of facial nerve injury and acute mononeuropathy. It occurs at all ages but is slightly more common in the third to fifth decades and is equally likely to affect the right or left sides. Bell palsy is the common cause of facial nerve paralysis and in one study accounted for 65% of cases of peripheral facial paralysis in a pediatric population (excluding congenital causes). Recurrence, either on the same or on the opposite side, is rare and raises the question of a more generalized disorder. Familial Bell palsy is reported but is also rare. Risk factors are not well defined, although some patients report exposure of the affected side to a steady breeze or fan for several hours just prior to onset. It has also found to be associated with diabetes mellitus, pregnancy, and hypertension. Some postulate that it may be caused by reactivation of a latent herpes simplex virus or varicella-zoster, and possibly human herpesvirus 6 (HHV-6). Lyme disease is also often implicated particularly in cases of bilateral facial palsy.

Clinical Features and Diagnosis

Pain is not typical except in the Ramsay Hunt syndrome (see the following section), which is caused by herpes zoster and is usually accompanied by vesicular eruption in the sensory distribution of the seventh nerve in the ipsilateral ear. Patients typically present with unilateral facial weakness or complete paralysis, which can be scored from 1 to 6 on the House–Brackmann scale which is determined by measurements of eyebrow and mouth movements. Facial weakness is associated with diminished lacrimation, impaired taste

TABLE 86.2	Clinical Manifestations of Lesions of the Facial Nerve		
Location of Lesion	Motor Function	Gustatory Sensation	Lacrimation
At facial nerve nucleus in pons	Impaired	Impaired	Impaired
Origin of nerve/ geniculate ganglion	Impaired	Impaired	Impaired
Between geniculate ganglion and chorda tympani	Impaired	Impaired	Spared
At stylomastoid foramen	Impaired	Spared	Spared

in the anterior two-thirds of the tongue on the affected side, and a weakened or absent blink reflex. Given the innervation of the stapedius muscle, there may be an increased sensitivity to noise on the affected side. There should not, however, be any impairment of eye movements, change in vision, or other bulbar symptoms such as dysphagia or facial numbness. When present, any of those signs or symptoms should prompt one to look for an alternative diagnosis. In 2013, the American Academy of Otolaryngology–Head and Neck Surgery Foundation (AAO-HNSF) published a new clinical practice guideline on the diagnosis and treatment of Bell palsy. Regarding appropriate diagnostic workup, it was concluded that in the appropriate clinical scenario following a complete history and examination, there is no role for laboratory investigation, diagnostic imaging, or electrodiagnostic testing (unless there is complete facial paralysis). Patients should, however, be referred to a specialist in cases of new or worsening findings, ocular symptoms, or incomplete recovery 3 months after onset. Nevertheless, nerve conduction studies (NCS) of the extracranial portion of the facial nerve are at times performed (particularly in cases of complete paralysis) along with needle recordings from its myotomes (e.g., facial muscle electromyography [EMG]) to help determine the nature and degree of injury. Injury to the intracranial portion may be detected by blink reflex testing.

Treatment and Outcome

Although permanent deficits may occur in severe cases, the vast majority of patients with Bell palsy experience full, functional recovery with minimal to no residual signs. Long-term prognosis is typically very favorable, although there is some recent limited evidence that these patients may be at a slightly higher risk for developing cancer (particularly oral cancer) and a slightly higher risk of stroke. Inflammation, herpes simplex virus infection, and swelling with compression may be involved in the pathogenesis of Bell palsy, so steroids, antiviral medication (acyclovir), and surgical decompression have been advocated as acute therapy. A large, randomized controlled study showed that 94% receiving prednisolone 25 mg b.i.d. for 10 days had a good recovery at 9 months compared with 82% who did not receive steroids. The same study showed no benefit for the antiviral agent acyclovir at doses of 400 mg five times per day for 10 days, although another large study showed benefit for valacyclovir at 1 g/day for 5 days. Surgical intervention has been looked at as well, and a recent Cochrane Database review found insufficient evidence to decide whether it is beneficial or harmful but given the generally good prognosis and spontaneous recovery is often not recommended. Early physical therapy may be beneficial particularly in cases of very severe paresis or complete paralysis. The 2013 AAO-HNSF practice guidelines recommend offering antiviral therapy in addition to oral steroids with 72 hours of symptom onset although made no recommendation regarding the use of physical therapy, acupuncture, or surgical referral. The American Academy of Neurology published an update regarding recommendations on steroids and antiviral therapy which stated that steroids should be offered to those with new-onset palsy and that antiviral may be offered although are likely to be of modest benefit at best. It is important that affected patients patch the weak eye overnight, as weakness of eye closure may lead to dry eyes and corneal abrasions. Eye drops such as artificial tears and lubricating ointments should be given as well. The prognosis of facial nerve injury after Bell palsy has also been the focus of much discussion. In general, preservation of motor amplitudes on NCS after 7 to 10 days supports retained axonal integrity and suggests a favorable prognosis for recovery. In contrast, rapid loss of motor amplitudes

suggests prominent axonal involvement, wallerian degeneration, and poorer chance for functional improvement. Needle EMG examination may also aid in detecting denervation change, further supporting axonal injury. Electroneurography (ENoG) has recently been looked at with regard to its prognostic value, and ENoG value was found to be positively correlated with a higher chance of recovery in both Bell palsy and Ramsay Hunt syndrome, although it is not commonly used in practice. In the long term, patients may develop synkinesis as described earlier.

RAMSAY HUNT SYNDROME

Ramsay Hunt syndrome, also known as *herpes zoster oticus*, is another cause of facial mononeuropathy although much less common than Bell palsy and tends to affect younger patients. Mean incidence is thought to be about five cases per 100,000 person-years. It is caused by a reactivation of a latent varicella-zoster virus infection affecting the geniculate ganglion leading to inflammation of the facial nerve and therefore is seen commonly in immunocompromised conditions (i.e., posttransplant, in the setting of malignancy). Typically, in addition to facial weakness, as in Bell palsy, there is associated hyperacusis, diminished taste, and impaired salivation and lacrimation. The degree of weakness in these patients is often more severe than in those with Bell palsy, and pain is a distinguishing factor. Pain is very common and can be in deep to the face; in the ear; or in the orbit, tongue, or palate (particularly if sensory fibers are involved). Most commonly, there is pain behind the ear on the affected side. On examination, one may see herpetic vesicles in the external auditory canal or behind the ear and at times may also be found on the neck and palate. However, a rash is not always seen (or may erupt after the onset of weakness) and one must have a high index of clinical suspicion based on the patient's history and presentation in order to consider this diagnosis rather than Bell palsy. Herpetic infection can spread to the eighth cranial nerve leading to complaints of nausea, tinnitus, and vertigo and infrequently to other cranial nerves as well.

Both steroids and antivirals have been used to treat Ramsay Hunt syndrome with varying degrees of success. Although there have been no randomized controlled trials, several studies have noted that early administration of steroids and antivirals (within 3 to 5 days) leads to improved facial and vestibulocochlear nerve recovery. Some suggest using intravenous methylprednisolone in those patients not improving or with poor prognostic factors. Overall, patients with Ramsay Hunt syndrome have an overall poorer prognosis than those with Bell palsy and often have an incomplete recovery.

OTHER CAUSES OF FACIAL NERVE INJURY

Many other processes may significantly damage the facial nerve. Intracranially, it may be injured by tumors, aneurysms, meningeal infections, leukemia, osteomyelitis, herpes zoster, Paget disease, sarcomas, and bony tumors, among others. It may also be damaged by leprous polyneuritis, Guillain–Barré syndrome, and diphtheritic polyneuropathy. Diabetic seventh nerve lesions may also occur but are less common than other cranial mononeuropathies in that disorder. The peripheral segment of the nerve may be compressed by tumors of the parotid gland, sarcoidosis, and more rarely, mumps. Bilateral facial palsy also may be caused by many of the same conditions producing unilateral paralysis but is most often seen in sarcoidosis, Guillain–Barré syndrome, leprosy, leukemia, and meningococcal meningitis. Sarcoid, in fact, can be implicated in most cranial neuropathies and a full discussion of neurosarcoidosis can be found in Chapter 72. *Melkersson–Rosenthal syndrome* is a syndrome presenting in childhood characterized by a constellation of clinical symptoms and signs including facial and lip edema, a furrowed and fissured tongue (lingua plicata), and recurrent attacks of facial weakness. Although there is no known etiology, it is thought to be familial in some instances. Other congenital causes of facial palsy include Möbius syndrome, in which facial weakness is associated with impaired lateral eye movement due to poor development of both the seventh and sixth cranial nerves. The facial nucleus, itself, may be damaged by vascular lesions, multiple sclerosis, intraparenchymal tumors, inflammatory lesions, and acute poliomyelitis, among others. The relatively superficial peripheral branches of the seventh nerve are vulnerable to stab and gunshot wounds, cuts, and in neonates, birth trauma. Occasionally, the nerve is also injured in surgeries involving the mastoid and parotid glands, acoustic neuroma resection, and trigeminal ganglion decompression, as well as in fractures of the temporal bone.

Cases of facial nerve injury with a specific, identifiable cause may require aggressive intervention. Microsurgical anastomosis may be performed in some cases of transection of the extracranial nerve or its branches. However, when the nerve is damaged proximal to the stylomastoid foramen, operative anastomosis becomes more difficult. Surgery may still be indicated, however, if a mass lesion is found before excessive damage is done. In cases of partial or inaccessible intracranial facial nerve injury, compensatory surgical reinnervation may be provided by suturing the distal portion of the 7th nerve to the central portion of either the 11th nerve or the 12th nerve. With rehabilitative training, these patients may learn to reroute impulses formerly destined for the sternocleidomastoid muscle, or half of the tongue, to the newly rewired facial musculature. However, use of the 11th nerve for this procedure causes permanent paralysis of the sternocleidomastoid and upper fibers of the trapezius muscle, whereas use of the 12th nerve causes atrophy and paralysis of one-half of the tongue. Anastomosis of the facial nerve with either the 11th or the 12th nerve should be performed as soon as possible following acute injury, such as with surgical misadventure by surgery of the mastoid or removal of an acoustic neuroma, for instance. In other situations, surgery may need to be delayed for up to 6 months or more to determine whether spontaneous regeneration occurs.

Hemifacial spasm is a disorder involving involuntary muscle contractions of facial muscles on one side of the face and is covered in detail in Chapter 77.

THE ACOUSTIC NERVE (CRANIAL NERVE VIII)

Eighth nerve disorders are described in Chapter 59.

THE GLOSSOPHARYNGEAL NERVE (CRANIAL NERVE IX)

The ninth cranial nerve contains both motor and sensory (general as well as taste) fibers. The motor fibers originating in the nucleus ambiguus supply the stylopharyngeus muscle and the constrictors of the pharynx, whereas other efferent fibers innervate secretory glands in the pharyngeal mucosa. The sensory fibers carry general sensation from the upper part of the pharynx (as well as the tonsil, tympanic membrane, and external ear) and the special sensation of taste from the posterior one-third of the tongue. The glossopharyngeal nerve also conveys sensory afferent fibers from

the carotid sinus and body by way of the nucleus solitarius and provides parasympathetic innervation to the parotid gland via the otic ganglion through the lesser petrosal nerve. Isolated lesions of the nerve, or its nuclei, are rare and are not accompanied by perceptible disability. Taste is lost on the posterior one-third of the tongue, and the gag reflex is absent on the side of the lesion. Injuries of the ninth nerve by infections or tumors are rarely isolated and are usually accompanied by signs of injury to nearby cranial nerves. As the 9th, 10th, and 11th nerves exit the jugular foramen together, tumors at that point produce multiple cranial nerve palsies (i.e., *jugular foramen syndrome*). Within the brain stem, the tractus solitarius receives taste fibers from both the seventh and the ninth nerves and is commonly injured by vascular or neoplastic lesions in the brain stem.

GLOSSOPHARYNGEAL NEURALGIA

Glossopharyngeal neuralgia (GN), also known as *tic douloureux* of the ninth nerve, is characterized by paroxysms of excruciating pain in the region of the tonsils, posterior pharynx, and back of the tongue with radiation to the middle ear. The cause of GN is unknown, and no significant pathologic changes occur in most cases. Idiopathic GN must be differentiated from pain in the distribution of the nerve following its injury in the neck by tumors. GN is rare, with a frequency of approximately 5% that of trigeminal neuralgia. Unlike trigeminal neuralgia, men and women are affected equally and GN is more likely to be bilateral than trigeminal neuralgia. The paroxysms consist of burning or stabbing pain and may occur spontaneously but are often precipitated by swallowing, talking, or touching the tonsils or posterior pharynx. The attacks usually last only a few seconds but sometimes may last several minutes, and they may occur many times daily or once every few weeks. Patients may become emaciated because of the fear that chewing each morsel of food will precipitate a pain paroxysm; general quality of life may be seriously affected, especially in severe cases. On occasion, attacks may lead to syncope, arrhythmia, or convulsions due to stimulation of the carotid sinus reflex.

The diagnosis of GN is best made by history and may be confirmed by provocative testing (e.g., precipitation by stimulation of the tonsils, posterior pharynx, or base of the tongue) or by transient relief of pain following the application of topical anesthetic to the ninth nerve dermatome. Following this procedure, the pain is no longer precipitated by stimulation, and the patient may swallow food and talk without discomfort until the anesthetic wears off. The differential diagnosis is limited but includes neuralgia of the mandibular branch of the fifth nerve. There may be long remissions, during which pain is no longer triggered. The pains usually recur, however, unless prevented by medical therapy or surgical resection of the nerve. Medications used to treat trigeminal neuralgia are equally effective with GN, and carbamazepine alone or in combination with phenytoin often provides effective control and induces a pharmacologic remission. Duloxetine as well as certain newer antiepileptic drugs such as pregabalin, gabapentin, topiramate, and lamotrigine might also be effective.

If medical therapy is unsuccessful and the pain is intractable, surgical interventions have been shown to be effective, including microvascular decompression, radiofrequency ablation, and Gamma Knife ablation. Intracranial transection of the nerve may also provide relief. Following this procedure, the mucous membrane supplied by the ninth nerve is permanently anesthetized, with ipsilateral loss of the gag reflex and ipsilateral loss of taste on the posterior one-third of the tongue. Motor symptoms, such as dysphagia or dysarthria, are not typical unless the 10th nerve is injured during surgery.

THE VAGUS NERVE (CRANIAL NERVE X)

Efferent fibers of the vagus nerve arise from both the nucleus ambiguus and the dorsal motor nucleus. Fibers from the nucleus ambiguus ultimately innervate the somatic muscles of the pharynx and larynx through the pharyngeal, superior laryngeal, and recurrent laryngeal nerves, whereas those from the dorsal motor nucleus supply autonomic innervation to the heart, lungs, esophagus, and stomach. The vagus nerve also relays sensory fibers from the mucosa in the oropharynx and upper part of the gastrointestinal tract to the spinal nucleus of the trigeminal nucleus and relays sensory fibers from the thoracic and abdominal organs to the tractus solitarius. Central lesions of the above nuclei in the brain stem cause a number of symptoms. Unilateral lesions of the nucleus ambiguus result in dysarthria and dysphagia, although rarely is the condition severe. However, because the nucleus has a considerable longitudinal extent in the medulla, such lesions may produce dysarthria without dysphagia or vice versa (i.e., caudal nuclear lesions cause dysphagia, whereas rostral lesions produce dysarthria). Hoarseness may also occur, but speech is usually intelligible. Dysphagia is usually slight, although occasionally, a more severe transient aphagia necessitates the use of a feeding tube for days to weeks. On examination, contraction of the palatal muscles is absent on the affected side during gag reflex testing. The palate on the affected side is lax at rest, and the uvula deviates to the opposite side on phonation, drawn away from the paralyzed muscles by normal, contralateral, palatal contraction (i.e., contralateral uvular deviation).

In contrast to the mild deficits typically seen with unilateral lesions, bilateral lesions of the nucleus ambiguus cause complete aphonia and aphagia. Focused bilateral injury of this type is rare but may be seen in advanced amyotrophic lateral sclerosis (ALS) in the setting of pseudobulbar palsy. Selective destruction of portions of the nucleus ambiguus may be produced by syringobulbia, intramedullary tumors, or ischemia and may cause a clinical syndrome of vocal cord paralysis during adduction. The patient may talk and swallow without difficulty, but inspiratory stridor and dyspnea may appear and progress sufficiently to require tracheotomy. Unilateral lesions of the dorsal motor nucleus are not accompanied by any significant symptoms, but bilateral lesions may produce life-threatening autonomic instability. The dorsal nucleus may be damaged by infection (e.g., acute poliomyelitis), intramedullary tumor, ischemia, and polyneuropathy, especially that associated with diphtheria and Guillain–Barré syndrome.

Individual branches of the vagus nerve are most amenable to injury in the neck, thorax, and, less commonly, the abdomen. Injury to the pharyngeal branches of the vagus nerve causes dysphagia, whereas lesions of the superior laryngeal nerve produce anesthesia of the upper part of the larynx and paralysis of the cricothyroid muscle. In these cases, the voice is weak and easily fatigable. Injury to a single, recurrent laryngeal nerve (i.e., frequently seen with aneurysms of the aorta, tumors or trauma of the neck, and occasionally after operations in the neck) causes unilateral paralysis of the vocal cords with hoarseness and dysphonia; bilateral injury causes complete vocal cord paralysis with aphonia and inspiratory stridor. Partial bilateral paralysis may produce a paralysis of both abductors, with severe dyspnea and inspiratory stridor, but does

not usually cause any alteration in the voice. Bilateral lesions of the vagus nerve invariably lead to death via cardiac arrhythmias, irregular respirations, gastrointestinal atonia, and complete paralysis of the pharynx and larynx.

THE SPINAL ACCESSORY NERVE (CRANIAL NERVE XI)

The spinal accessory nerve is composed of two primary branches—the first is a small accessory cranial branch contributing visceral efferent fibers to the vagus nerve, which emerges from the jugular foramen to blend with the vagus as it descends (primarily in the recurrent laryngeal nerve). The majority of the accessory nerve, the spinal portion, innervates the sternocleidomastoid and part or all of the trapezius muscles. Its fibers originate in the upper cervical spinal cord (C2, C3, and C4), enter the skull via the foramen magnum, and travel through the jugular foramen along the carotid artery to innervate the sternocleidomastoid (SCM) muscle. Another branch emerges in the mid-SCM at its posterior border and crosses the posterior triangle of the neck to innervate the upper trapezius. It is important to note that supranuclear efferents to the SCM are primarily ipsilateral, whereas inputs to the trapezius cross contralaterally from the motor cortex. Therefore, on examination, a lesion of the ipsilateral hemisphere or accessory spinal nerve will result in an inability to turn the head contralaterally (as the SCM turns the head in the opposite direction). Fibers of the spinal accessory nerve also travel in the medial longitudinal fasciculus, where they make connections with the oculomotor, trochlear, abducens, and vestibular nuclei and help coordinate eye movements with head motion in response to external stimuli.

Lesions of the spinal portion of the 11th nerve produce weakness and atrophy of the trapezius muscle and SCM, impairing rotary movements of the neck and chin to the opposite side, and weakness of shrugging movements of the shoulder. Weakness of the upper portion of the trapezius results in winging of the scapula, which must be differentiated from that produced by weakness of the serratus anterior. Scapular winging from weakness of the trapezius is present at rest (e.g., arms at side) and becomes worse on abduction of the shoulder. Scapular winging from weakness of the serratus anterior is negligible at rest and worsens during flexion of the shoulder (holding or pushing the arm forward). Bilateral paralysis of the trapezius may present with "dropped head syndrome" due to weakness of head extension. With unilateral SCM weakness, there is typically little head tilt, as there are contributions from several other muscles to head rotation, although the patient will have difficulty turning the head to the contralateral side. The accessory or cranial portion of the nerve originates in the nucleus ambiguus and passes through the jugular foramen with the 10th nerve, traveling with the spinal fibers (see earlier), eventually innervating the larynx, and functionally is considered by some to be a part of the vagus nerve complex.

The nucleus of the 11th nerve may be destroyed by infections and degenerative disorders in the medulla, such as syringobulbia or ALS. The nerve itself may be injured by polyneuropathy, meningeal infection, extramedullary tumor (e.g., meningioma and neurinoma), trauma (i.e., basilar skull fracture), or by destructive processes in the occipital bone. It is particularly vulnerable to damage along its course in the posterior triangle of the neck, for instance, during lymph node biopsy, radiation, cannulation of the internal jugular vein, or carotid endarterectomy. The SCM and trapezius are also often involved in cases of extrapyramidal dysfunction (discussed in later chapters), such as torticollis due to cervical dystonia. Idiopathic focal mononeuropathies of the spinal accessory nerve exists although are rare, and the nerve at times may be involved in cases of Parsonage–Turner syndrome. Primary diseases of muscle and the neuromuscular junction also commonly involve the muscles innervated by the 11th cranial nerve, such as in fascioscapulohumeral dystrophy, myotonic dystrophy, and myasthenia gravis. Diagnosis of a spinal accessory nerve palsy is made clinically but can be supported with imaging and electrodiagnostic testing. Recent reports point to a potential role for ultrasound in diagnosis and in determining etiology.

THE HYPOGLOSSAL NERVE (CRANIAL NERVE XII)

The hypoglossal nerve (a pure motor nerve) emerges from the medulla between the ventrolateral sulcus, between the olive and the pyramids, as a number of rootlets that converge into the hypoglossal nerve. The nerve then exits the cranium through the hypoglossal foramen in the posterior cranial fossa traveling close to cranial nerves IX, X, and XI and passing downward near the inferior ganglion of the vagus to lie between the internal carotid artery and internal jugular vein. It then crosses laterally to the bifurcation of the common carotid artery and loops above the hyoid bone before moving ventrally to supply the genioglossus (which has crossed supranuclear innervation) and other muscles of the tongue with the exception of the palatoglossus (innervated by the vagus nerve). The 12th nerve and its nucleus may be injured by most of the same processes that damage the 10th and 11th nuclei. Occlusions of the short branches of the basilar artery supplying the paramedian medulla cause paralysis of the tongue on one side and paralysis of the arm and leg on the opposite side (i.e., alternating hemiplegia). Unilateral injury to the nucleus results in atrophy and paralysis of the muscles of one-half of the tongue causing deviation toward the paralyzed side with protrusion.

Fibrillation of the muscles is seen with chronic injury to the hypoglossal nerve or its nucleus in syringobulbia or ALS and may be observed as miniscule twitching of the surface of the tongue on visual inspection. Bilateral paralysis of the nucleus or nerve produces atrophy of both sides of the tongue and paralysis of all movements with severe dysarthria and difficulty manipulating food in the mouth. The tongue is only rarely affected by supranuclear lesions within the CNS; unilateral weakness may accompany severe hemiplegia with slight deviation of the tongue to the paralyzed side when protruded. Moderate weakness of the tongue may accompany pseudobulbar palsy but is never as severe as that caused by destruction of both medullary nuclei. The hypoglossal nerve is susceptible to injury anywhere along its course (both intra and extramedullary) and can be involved in cases of meningitis, neoplastic infiltration, trauma, lymphadenopathy, radiation, and processes involving the skull base. Occasionally, muscle diseases may involve the tongue, such as in myotonic dystrophy where percussion of the tongue may cause a temporary contraction along the line of percussion.

SUGGESTED READINGS

Ashkan K, Marsh H. Microvascular decompression for trigeminal neuralgia in the elderly: a review of the safety and efficacy. *Neurosurgery.* 2004;55(4): 840–848.

Auger RG, Pipegras DG, Laws ER Jr. Hemifacial spasm: results of microvascular decompression of the facial nerve in 54 patients. *Mayo Clin Proc.* 1986;61: 640–644.

Boghen DR, Glaser JS. Ischemic optic neuropathy: the clinical profile and natural history. *Brain.* 1975;98:689–708.

Brin MF, Blitzer A, Stewart C, et al. Treatment of spasmodic dysphonia (laryngeal dystonia) with local injections of botulinum toxin: review and technical aspects. In: Blitzer A, Brin MF, Sasaki CT, et al, eds. *Neurological Disorders of the Larynx.* New York: Thieme Medical Publishers; 1992:214–218.

Brisman R. Repeat gamma knife radiosurgery for trigeminal neuralgia. *Stereotact Funct Neurosurg.* 2003;81(1–4):43–49.

Brisman R. Trigeminal neuralgia and multiple sclerosis. *Arch Neurol.* 1987;44: 379–381.

Ceylan S, Karakus A, Duru S, et al. Glossopharyngeal neuralgia: a study of 6 cases. *Neurosurg Rev.* 1997;20:196–200.

Cheuk AV, Chin LS, Petit JH, et al. Gamma knife surgery for trigeminal neuralgia: outcome, imaging, and brainstem correlates. *Int J Radiat Oncol Biol Phys.* 2004;60(2):537–541.

Dunphy EB. Alcohol-tobacco amblyopia: a historical survey. *Am J Ophthalmol.* 1969;68:569–578.

Eldridge PR, Sinha AK, Javadpour M, et al. Microvascular decompression for trigeminal neuralgia in patients with multiple sclerosis. *Stereotact Funct Neurosurg.* 2003;81(1–4):57–64.

Ford FR, Woodhall B. Phenomena due to misdirection of regenerating fibers of cranial, spinal and autonomic nerves: clinical observations. *Arch Surg.* 1938;36:480–496.

Friedman AP, Merritt HH. Damage to cranial nerves resulting from head injury. *Bull Los Angeles Neurol Soc.* 1944;9:135–139.

Fukuda H, Ishikawa M, Okumura R. Demonstration of neurovascular compression in trigeminal neuralgia and hemifacial spasm with magnetic resonance imaging: comparison with surgical findings in 60 consecutive cases. *Surg Neurol.* 2003;59(2):93–99.

Furuta Y, Fukuda S, Chida E, et al. Reactivation of herpes simplex virus type 1 in patients with Bell's palsy. *J Med Virol.* 1998;54:162–166.

Gouda JJ, Brown JA. Atypical facial pain and other pain syndromes: differential diagnosis and treatment. *Neurosurg Clin N Am.* 1997;8:87–100.

Hato N, Tamada H, Kohno H, et al. Valacyclovir and prednisolone treatment for Bell's palsy: a multicenter, randomized, place-controlled study. *Otol Neurotol.* 2007;28:408–413.

Jankovic J, Ford J. Blepharospasm and orofacial-cervical dystonia: clinical and pharmacological findings in 100 patients. *Ann Neurol.* 1983;13:402–411.

Jannetta P. Observations on the etiology of trigeminal neuralgia, hemifacial spasm, acoustic nerve dysfunction and glossopharyngeal neuralgia: definitive microsurgical treatment and results in 11 patients. *Neurochirurgie.* 1977;20:145–154.

Jitpimolmard S, Tiamkao S, Laopaiboon M. Long-term results of botulinum toxin type A (Dysport) in the treatment of hemifacial spasm: a report of 175 cases. *J Neurol Neurosurg Psychiatry.* 1998;64:751–757.

Juncos JL, Beal MF. Idiopathic cranial polyneuropathy: a 5-year experience. *Brain.* 1987;110:197–212.

Kalovidouris A, Mancuso AA, Dillon W. A CT-clinical approach to patients with symptoms related to the V, VII, IX–XII cranial nerves and cervical sympathetics. *Radiology.* 1984;151:671–676.

Keane JR. Mutiple cranial nerve palsies: analysis of 979 cases. *Arch Neurol.* 2005;62(11):1714–1717.

Kemp LW, Reich SG. Hemifacial spasm. *Curr Treat Options Neurol.* 2004;6(3):175–179.

Lecky BRF, Hughes RAC, Murray NMF. Trigeminal sensory neuropathy. *Brain.* 1987;110:1463–1486.

Leigh RJ, Zee DS. *The Neurology of Eye Movements.* 4th ed. Oxford, United Kingdom: Oxford University Press; 2006.

Lopez BC, Hamlyn PJ, Zakrzewska JM. Stereotactic radiosurgery for primary trigeminal neuralgia: state of the evidence and recommendations for future reports. *J Neurol Neurosurg Psychiatry.* 2004;75(7):1019–1024.

Lossos A, Siegal T. Numb chin syndrome in cancer patients: etiology, response to treatment, and prognostic significance. *Neurology.* 1992;42:1181–1184.

Ludlow CL, Naunton RF, Fujita M, et al. Effects of botulinum toxin injections on speech in adductor spasmodic dysphonia. *Neurology.* 1988;38: 1220–1225.

Majoie CB, Hulsmans FJ, Castelijns JA, et al. Symptoms and signs related to the trigeminal nerve: diagnostic yield of MR imaging. *Radiology.* 1998;209: 557–562.

Murakami S, Nakashiro Y, Mizobuchi M, et al. Varicella-zoster virus distribution in Ramsay Hunt syndrome revealed by polymerase chain reaction. *Acta Otolaryngol*. 1998;118:145–149.

Nadeau SE, Trobe JD. Pupil sparing in oculomotor palsy: a brief review. *Ann Neurol*. 1983;13:143–148.

Nielsen VK. Electrophysiology of the facial nerve in hemifacial spasm: ectopic/ephaptic excitation. *Muscle Nerve*. 1985;8:545–555.

Ozkale Y, Erol I, Saygı S, et al. Overview of pediatric peripheral facial nerve paralysis: analysis of 40 patients. *J Child Neurol*. 2015;30(2):193–199.

Pearce JM. Melkersson's syndrome. *J Neurol Neurosurg Psychiatry*. 1995;58:340.

Portenoy RK, Duma C, Foley KM. Acute herpetic and postherpetic neuralgia: clinical review and current management. *Ann Neurol*. 1986;20:651–664.

Rozen TD. Trigeminal neuralgia and glossopharyngeal neuralgia. *Neurol Clin*. 2004;22(1):185–206.

Rush JA, Younge BR. Paralysis of cranial nerves III, IV and VI: cause and prognosis in 1,000 cases. *Arch Ophthalmol*. 1981;99:76–79.

Searles RP, Mladinich K, Messner RP. Isolated trigeminal sensory neuropathy: early manifestations of mixed connective tissue disease. *Neurology*. 1978;28:1286–1289.

Shaya M, Jawahar A, Caldito G, et al. Gamma knife radiosurgery for trigeminal neuralgia: a study of predictors of success, efficacy, safety, and outcome at LSUHSC. *Surg Neurol*. 2004;61(6):529–534.

Spillane JD, Wells CEC. Isolated trigeminal neuropathy. *Brain*. 1959;82:391–416.

Stevens H. Melkersson's syndrome. *Neurology*. 1965;15:263–266.

Sullivan FM, Swan IR, Donnan PT, et al. Early treatment with prednisolone or acyclovir in Bell's palsy. *N Engl J Med*. 2007;357:1598–1607.

Tan EK, Chan LL. Clinico-radiologic correlation in unilateral and bilateral hemifacial spasm. *J Neurol Sci*. 2004;222(1–2):59–64.

Tankere F, Maisonobe T, Lamas G, et al. Electrophysiological determination of the site involved in generating abnormal muscle responses in hemifacial spasm. *Muscle Nerve*. 1998;21:1013–1018.

Tenser RB. Trigeminal neuralgia: mechanisms of treatment. *Neurology*. 1998;51:17–19.

Troost BT, Daroff RB. The ocular motor defects in progressive supranuclear palsy. *Ann Neurol*. 1977;2:397–403.

Van Zandycke M, Martin JJ, Vande Gaer L, et al. Facial myokymia in the Guillain-Barré syndrome: a clinicopathologic study. *Neurology*. 1982;32:744–748.

Victor M, Dreyfus PM. Tobacco-alcohol amblyopia: further comments on its pathology. *Arch Ophthalmol*. 1965;74:649–657.

Wang A, Jankovic J. Hemifacial spasm: clinical findings and treatment. *Muscle Nerve*. 1998;21:1740–1747.

Wartenberg R. *Hemifacial Spasm: A Clinical and Pathological Study*. London, United Kingdom: Oxford University Press; 1952.

Willoughby EW, Anderson NE. Lower cranial nerve motor function in unilateral vascular lesions of the cerebral hemisphere. *BMJ*. 1984;289:791–794.

Yoshino N. Akimoto H. Yamada I, et al. Trigeminal neuralgia: evaluation of neuralgic manifestation and site of neurovascular compression with 3D CISS MR imaging and MR angiography. *Radiology*. 2003;228(2):539–545.

Acquired Peripheral Neuropathies 87

Thomas H. Brannagan III and Kurenai Tanji

APPROACH TO PERIPHERAL NERVE DISORDERS

The peripheral nervous system is composed of multiple cell types and elements that subserve diverse motor, sensory, and autonomic functions. The clinical manifestations of neuropathies depend on the severity, distribution, and functions affected. *Peripheral neuropathy* and *polyneuropathy* are terms that describe syndromes resulting from diffuse lesions of peripheral nerves, usually manifested by weakness, sensory loss, pain, and autonomic dysfunction. *Mononeuropathy* indicates a disorder of a single nerve often resulting from local trauma, compression, or entrapment. *Mononeuropathy multiplex* signifies focal involvement of two or more nerves, usually as a result of a generalized disorder such as diabetes mellitus or vasculitis. This chapter discusses an approach to peripheral nerve disorders, mononeuropathies, including plexus disorders, and specific acquired polyneuropathies. Inherited neuropathies are discussed in Chapter 88.

EPIDEMIOLOGY

Peripheral neuropathy which includes polyneuropathies of various causes and mononeuropathies are common disorders. One mononeuropathy, carpal tunnel syndrome, is estimated to occur in 3% to 5.8% and is three times more common in women than men. A prevalence of 2% to 7% of symmetric polyneuropathy has been found in studies conducted around the world. Currently, the most common cause of peripheral neuropathy worldwide is diabetes, although prior to 1994, the most common cause of peripheral neuropathy worldwide was leprosy. The prevalence of peripheral neuropathy increases with age, affecting 15% of the population older than the age of 40 years and 24% older than the age of 70 years.

CLINICAL FEATURES

Polyneuropathy may occur at any age, although particular syndromes are more likely to occur in certain age groups. Charcot–Marie–Tooth (CMT) disease, for example, often begins in childhood or adolescence, whereas neuropathy associated with paraproteinemia is seen more frequently with increasing age. The onset and progression differ; the Guillain–Barré syndrome (GBS), tick paralysis, and porphyria begin acutely and may remit. Others, such as vitamin B_{12} deficiency or carcinomatous neuropathy, begin insidiously and progress slowly. Still others, such as chronic inflammatory demyelinating polyneuropathy, may begin acutely or insidiously and then progress with remissions and relapses.

The myelin sheaths or the motor or sensory axons or neurons themselves may be predominantly affected, or the neuropathy may be mixed, axonal, or demyelinating. Most polyneuropathies, especially those with primary demyelination, affect both motor and sensory functions. A predominantly motor polyneuropathy is seen in lead toxicity, dapsone or *n*-hexane intoxication, tick paralysis,

porphyria, some cases of GBS, and multifocal motor neuropathy. Sensory neuropathy is divided into loss of large-diameter and small-diameter nerve fibers, although a combination of fiber types is most typical. Predominantly small-fiber neuropathy, often with concomitant autonomic dysfunction, is seen in diabetes mellitus, amyloidosis, Fabry disease, and lepromatous leprosy. Less prevalent, predominant large-fiber neuropathy occurs with thallium poisoning, paraneoplastic ganglioneuritis, Sjögren disease, pyridoxine (vitamin B_6) toxicity, and syphilis. Predominant involvement of the autonomic system can be seen in acute or chronic autonomic neuropathy or in amyloidosis.

Symptoms of polyneuropathy include distal pain, paresthesias, weakness, and sensory loss. Pain may be spontaneous or elicited by stimulation of the skin and may be sharp or burning. Paresthesias are usually described as numbness (a dead sensation), tingling, buzzing, stinging, burning, or a feeling of constriction. Lack of pain perception may result in repeated traumatic injuries with degeneration of joints (*arthropathy* or *Charcot joints*) and in chronic ulcerations.

Weakness is greatest in distal limb muscles in most neuropathies; there may be paralysis of the intrinsic foot and hand muscles with footdrop or wrist-drop. Tendon reflexes are often lost, especially in demyelinating neuropathy. In severe polyneuropathy, the patient may become quadriplegic and respirator dependent. The cranial nerves may be affected, particularly in GBS and diphtheritic neuropathy. Cutaneous sensory loss appears in a stocking-and-glove distribution. All modes of sensation may be affected, or there may be selective impairment of "large" myelinated fiber functions (position and vibratory sense) or "small" unmyelinated fiber functions (pain and temperature perception). Often, detection of painful stimuli is impaired with a delayed and greater than normal reaction. Inappropriate pain perception is often paradoxically present despite loss of pain fibers.

Involvement of autonomic nerves may cause miosis (small pupil), Adie pupils, anhidrosis (impaired sweating), orthostatic hypotension, sphincter disturbance, gastrointestinal dysmotility, impotence, and vasomotor abnormalities; these may occur without other evidence of neuropathy but are more commonly seen in association with symmetric distal polyneuropathy. Diabetes mellitus is the most common cause. Amyloidosis causes notably severe autonomic neuropathy. The majority of neuropathy types produce distal impairment of sweating, vasomotor reflexes, and local influences that help produce the typical trophic signs in the feet of neuropathy patients. Distal loss of sweating may induce symptomatic excessive sweating proximally as a compensatory response.

In *mononeuropathy* or *mononeuropathy multiplex*, focal motor, sensory, and reflex changes are restricted to areas innervated by specific nerves. When multiple distal nerves are affected in mononeuropathy multiplex, the pattern may coalesce into more symmetric involvement suggesting polyneuropathy. The most frequent causes of mononeuropathy multiplex are vasculitic neuropathy, diabetes mellitus, rheumatoid arthritis, brachial neuropathy, leprosy, or sarcoidosis. Asymmetric neuropathy is also seen in multifocal motor neuropathy with conduction block, sometimes with increased anti-GM1 antibody titers, multifocal demyelinating sensory and motor neuropathy (Lewis–Sumner syndrome), and brachial neuritis.

Processes that affect nerve roots are termed *radiculopathies* and affect a single or multiple myotomes or dermatomes. Focal compression is most common, but other processes also target nerves at these proximal sites. Electric-like pain radiating down a specific segment is most characteristic; loss of sensation or strength in a specific territory occurs with more severe involvement. *Plexopathy* occurs with compromise of the brachial or lumbosacral plexus and often displays a pattern of multiple contiguous nerves or nerve root impairment.

Superficial cutaneous nerves may be thickened and visibly enlarged secondary to Schwann cell proliferation and collagen deposition from repeated episodes of segmental demyelination and remyelination or from amyloid or polysaccharide deposition in the nerves. Hypertrophic nerves may be observed or palpated in the demyelinating form of CMT disease (type I), Dejerine–Sottas neuropathy, Refsum disease, von Recklinghausen disease (neurofibromatosis), and various other disorders.

Fasciculations, or spontaneous contractions of individual motor units, are visible twitches of limb or cranial muscles. They are characteristic of anterior horn cell diseases but also occasionally occur in other chronic neuropathic conditions. *Fibrillation* potentials are discharges of denervated single muscle fibers and are not visible on the skin but are recordable during electromyography (EMG). *Myokymia* is worm-like muscle activity seen in limb muscles in a small number of disorders including radiation plexopathy, episodic ataxia type 1, and certain autoimmune channelopathies. Potassium channel antibodies or defects are implicated in some entities; facial myokymia is more common and less specific.

ETIOLOGY AND DIAGNOSIS

Peripheral nerve disorders may be divided into hereditary and acquired forms. The most common hereditary disorder is CMT type 1A (peroneal muscular atrophy), which is associated with duplication of the peripheral myelin protein 22 (*PMP22*) gene. Deletion of the same region produces hereditary neuropathy with liability to pressure palsies. The most commonly acquired neuropathies in the United States are associated with diabetes mellitus; selected other causes of polyneuropathy are listed in Table 87.1. Trauma, compression, and entrapment are considered in the differential diagnosis of mononeuropathies, especially median neuropathy at the wrist, ulnar nerve at the elbow, or fibular nerve across the fibular head. Patients with any form of polyneuropathy are more vulnerable to mechanical and toxic nerve injury; cachectic or immobile patients may develop focal neuropathy from pressure or trauma.

In the evaluation of a patient with peripheral neuropathy, a detailed family, social, and medical and medication history; neurologic examination; and electrodiagnostic and laboratory testing are usually necessary for diagnosis. The American Academy of Neurology has made recommendations for evaluation of distal symmetric polyneuropathy (Table 87.2). Well over 200 individual causes are known, many of which are evident from initial screening measures. Skin or nerve biopsy studies are indicated in some cases. Despite these efforts, the cause of a significant minority remains idiopathic after a comprehensive evaluation. A classification of the most common acquired and hereditary polyneuropathies and their laboratory evaluation are presented in Table 87.1.

TREATMENT

Treatment of patients with peripheral nerve disorders can be divided into two phases: removal or treatment of the inciting condition and symptomatic therapy. Specific treatments are considered in discussions of individual disorders.

Symptomatic treatment of polyneuropathy consists of general supportive measures, amelioration of pain, and physiotherapy. Tracheal intubation and respiratory support may be needed in GBS. The corneas are protected if significant eye closure weakness is present. The bed is kept clean and the sheets are kept smooth to prevent injury to the anesthetic skin; a special mattress can be used to prevent pressure sores. Chronic compression of vulnerable nerves (ulnar at the elbow and common fibular at the knee) is avoided. Paralyzed limbs are splinted to prevent contractures. Physical therapy includes massage and passive joint movement. In chronic polyneuropathy with footdrop, a foot orthosis often improves gait. Treatment of neuropathic pain (see Chapter 57) and autonomic failure (see Chapter 112) are discussed elsewhere in the book.

OUTCOME

Polyneuropathy may be progressive or remitting, and the prognosis is affected by the extent of nerve degeneration. With removal or treatment of the inciting cause, recovery is more rapid if macroscopic continuity of the nerves is maintained. Conversely, recovery may be delayed for many months or remain incomplete if significant wallerian degeneration occurs. Axonal regeneration proceeds at a rate of 1 to 2 mm/day and may be further delayed where the axons must penetrate scar tissue, injured nerve segments, or other barriers. Aberrant growth of axonal sprouts may lead to formation of persistent neuromas. After severe wallerian degeneration, there may be permanent weakness, muscular wasting, diminution of reflexes, and sensory loss. In demyelinating neuropathies, recovery is sometimes more rapid and complete because of remyelination or resolution of conduction block.

MONONEUROPATHIES AND COMPRESSION NEUROPATHIES

THE SPINAL ROOTS AND BRACHIAL PLEXUS

At each cervical spinal level, numerous rootlets containing both motor and sensory fibers join after leaving the spinal cord to form the spinal roots that exit the spinal canal through the intervertebral foramen of the spinal column, immediately branching into anterior and posterior rami. The nerve roots are commonly injured by degenerative joint disease and disk herniation at the cervical and lumbosacral levels. Importantly, the dorsal root ganglia (i.e., the cell bodies of the sensory nerves) are located outside the foramen and are spared in foraminal compression, meaning the remainder of the sensory nerve will remain viable and will appear normal on nerve conduction studies, even though it is disconnected from the central nervous system (CNS) and the patient reports numbness and pain. Before forming the brachial plexus, the C5 nerve root gives off a proximal branch, the *dorsal scapular nerve* (to the rhomboid muscles), whereas the C5, C6, and C7 roots give proximal branches that join to form the *long thoracic nerve*, supplying the serratus anterior muscle. The C5 and C6 roots then join to form the *upper trunk* of the brachial plexus, whereas the C7 root forms the *middle trunk*, and the C8 and T1

TABLE 87.1 Neuropathy Diagnosis and Laboratory Tests

Cause or Diagnosis	Manifestations	Laboratory Tests
Vitamin deficiency/excess	S, SM, SYM	Vitamins B_{12}, pyridoxine (B_6), B_1, folate, vitamin E, methylmalonic acid
Infectious		
Lyme disease	S, SM, SYM, MF, CN	Serology, PCR
HIV-1	S, SM, SYM, MF, CN	Serology, PCR
Hepatitis C	S, SM, SYM, MF, CN	Serology, PCR
Herpes zoster	S, radicular	Serology, PCR
CMV	SM, M, SYM, MF	Serology, PCR, culture
Immune mediated		
Guillain–Barré and variants	SM, S, M, SYM, MF, CN	IgG antiganglioside antibodies (GM1, GD1a, GQ1b, GD1b), urine porphyrins
IgM antibody associated	M, MF	IgM anti-GM1, GD1a
	S, SM, SYM	IgM anti-MAG, sulfatide, GD1b, GQ1b
Monoclonal gammopathy	M, S, SM, SYM, MF	Serum immunofixation electrophoresis, quantitative immunoglobulins
Autonomic neuropathy	Autonomic dysfunction	Antinicotinic acetylcholine receptor antibodies, anti-Hu
Vasculitis	SM, S, MF, SYM	ESR, cryoglobulins, hepatitis C serology, or PCR
Sarcoidosis	SM, S, MF, SYM	ACE, chest radiograph
Celiac disease	S, SM, MF, SYM	Antigliadin, endomysial, transglutaminase antibodies
Rheumatologic diseases	SM, S, MF, SYM	SSA-Ro, SSB-La antibodies
Sjögren syndrome	—	ANA, ANCA (PR3, myeloperoxidase), dsDNA, Ab, RNP, rheumatoid factor
Lupus	—	—
Wegener granulomatosis Rheumatoid arthritis	—	—
Paraneoplastic		
Lung cancer	S, SYM	Anti-Hu Ab, chest radiograph/CT
Waldenström syndrome	SM, S, M, SYM, MF	Serum immunofixation electrophoresis
Myeloma	SM, M, SYM, MF	Serum and urine immunofixation electrophoresis, skeletal survey
Hereditary		
CMT-1	Demyelinating, SM, SYM, MF	DNA tests for PMP-22, MPZ, EGR2, Cx32, others
CMT-2	Axonal, SM, SYM	DNA tests for NF-L, Cx32, MPZ, others
Mitochondrial	NARP, SM, MF	Serum lactate, thymidine phosphorylase, DNA testing
Other	Axonal, S, SM, amyloid, porphyria	DNA tests for transthyretin, periaxin, urine porphyrins
Metabolic/toxic		
Diabetes	S, SM, SYM, MF, CN	Fasting glucose, HgbA1c, glucose tolerance test
Renal failure	S, SM, SYM	Chem 7
Thyroid disease	S, SM, SYM, MF	TSH, T4
Heavy metal toxicity	S, SM, SYM, MF	Urine lead, mercury, arsenic, thallium

S, sensory; SM, sensorimotor; SYM, symmetric; MF, multifocal; CN, cranial nerves; PCR, polymerase chain reaction; CMV, cytomegalovirus; GM1, GD1a, ganglioside components of myelin; M, motor; MAG, myelin-associated glycoprotein; ESR, erythrocyte sedimentation rate; ACE, angiotensin-converting enzyme; SSA, SSB, antigens for Sjögren syndrome severe antibodies; ANA, antinuclear antibody; ANCA, antineutrophil cytoplasmic antibodies; RNP, ribonucleoprotein; CT, computed tomography; PMP, peripheral myelin protein; MPZ, myelin protein zero; NARP, neuropathy, ataxia, and retinitis pigmentosa; EGR, early growth response protein; Cx32, connexin; NF-L, neurofilament light chain; HgbA1c, hemoglobin A1c; TSH, thyroid-stimulating hormone.

TABLE 87.2 American Academy of Neurology Recommendations for Testing for Distal Symmetric Polyneuropathy

Basic Laboratory Evaluation for Distal Symmetric Neuropathy

CBC, ESR, or CRP

Vitamin B_{12}[a] and if B_{12} is low normal, metabolites, including methylmalonic acid and/or homocysteine.[a]

Comprehensive metabolic panel, including fasting blood glucose[a], glucose tolerance test[a] if indicated to look for impaired glucose tolerance

Serum protein immunofixation electrophoresis[a]

Urine analysis, urine electrophoresis

Inquire about drugs and toxins

Other Laboratory Testing that May Be Performed in Selected Patients

ANA, rheumatoid factor, anti-Ro/SSA, anti-LA/SSB, antineutrophil cytoplasmic antigen (ANCA) antibodies, cryoglobulins

Campylobacter jejuni, cytomegalovirus (CMV), hepatitis panel (B and C), HIV, Lyme antibodies, herpesviruses tests, West Nile virus tests, cerebrospinal fluid (CSF) analysis

Antigliadin; IgA transglutaminase antibodies; endomysial antibodies; vitamins E, B_1, and B_6

Serum angiotensin-converting enzyme (ACE), CSF analysis with CSF ACE

Arsenic, lead, mercury, thallium

Antiganglioside antibodies (GM1, GD1a, GD1b, GD3, GQ1b, GT1b), anti-MAG, paraneoplastic antibodies (anti-Hu, anti-CV2), CSF oligoclonal bands

Molecular tests for Charcot–Marie–Tooth, Hereditary neuropathy with tendency to pressure palsy (HNPP), familial amyloidosis

Skeletal survey; computed tomography or MRI of chest, abdomen, or pelvis; ultrasound of abdomen and pelvis; positron emission tomography (PET), CSF cytology

[a]Tests with highest yield.

CBC, complete blood count; ESR, erythrocyte sedimentation rate; CRP, C-reactive protein; IgA, immunoglobulin A; MAG, myelin-associated glycoprotein; MRI, magnetic resonance imaging.

Data from England JD, Gronseth GS, Franklin G, et al. Practice parameter: evaluation of distal symmetric polyneuropathy: role of laboratory and genetic testing (an evidence-based review). *Neurology.* 2009;72:185–192.

roots form the *lower trunk*. The upper trunk gives off a small branch, the *suprascapular* nerve, which supplies the supra- and infraspinatus muscles. All trunks pass through the supraclavicular fossa under the cervical and scalene muscles. Each trunk then forms two branches and these branches regroup to form new divisions, the cords, as they course through the *thoracic outlet*, between the first rib and the clavicle, along with the subclavian artery. The lateral branches of the upper and middle trunks contribute to the *lateral cord* (i.e., C5, C6, C7), whereas the medial branches join with the lateral branch of the lower trunk and move dorsally to form the *posterior cord* (i.e., C5, C6, C7, C8). Finally, the lower trunk gives rise to the *medial cord* (i.e., C8, T1). The *lateral and medial pectoral nerves* branch off near the juncture of the trunks and the lateral and medial cords, respectively, supplying the pectoralis major muscle.

The *thoracodorsal nerve* that supplies the latissimus dorsi and the *subscapular* nerve that supplies the teres major each branch medially off the posterior cord. The posterior cord persists distally, becoming the *radial nerve*, after giving off a smaller lateral branch, the *axillary nerve*, which supplies the deltoid. The lateral and medial cords then each contribute a branch to form the *median nerve*, composed of the medial branch of the lateral cord and the lateral branch of the medial cord, joined in the middle of the plexus. The lateral branch of the lateral cord persists distally, becoming the *musculocutaneous nerve*, whereas the medial branch of the medial cord becomes the *ulnar nerve* (Fig. 87.1; Tables 87.3 and 87.4).

The brachial plexus may be injured by traumatic, neoplastic, infectious, radiation, and other processes. Careful history and neurologic examination, in concert with a detailed understanding of plexus anatomy, is the first step in recognizing plexus injury and differentiating it from injury to the nerve roots or peripheral nerves. Electrophysiologic assessment with EMG and nerve conductions is often critical in confirming the diagnosis, and imaging studies may also be indicated. Mixed syndromes of radicular plexus and peripheral nerve injury may also occur, making localization even more challenging. The roots or trunks of the brachial plexus may be damaged by lacerations, gunshot wounds, or direct trauma. They may be compressed by tumors or aneurysms or stretched and torn by violent movements of the shoulder in falls, dislocation of the shoulder, carrying heavy loads on or over the shoulder, and by traction during birth. The syndromes of the roots and trunks cause deficits principally in the distribution of the affected nerve roots. Partial paralysis and incomplete sensory loss are common because many muscles of the arm receive innervation from two or more roots. Compression at the level of the thoracic outlet (*thoracic outlet syndrome*) is addressed separately in Chapter 78.

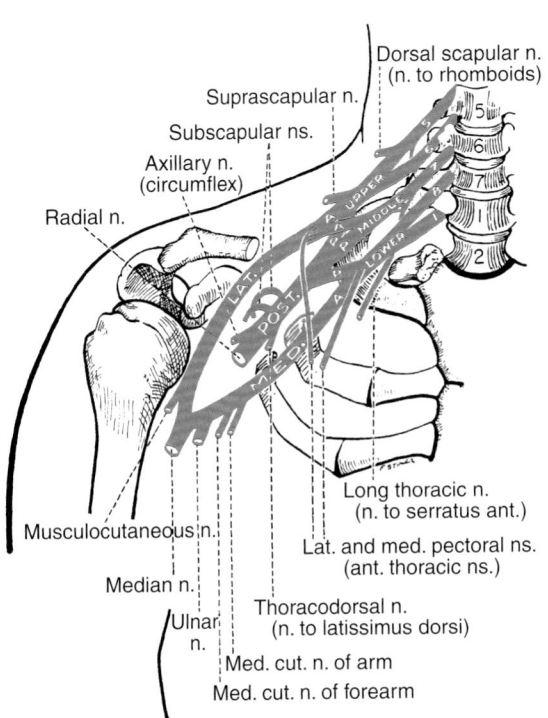

FIGURE 87.1 The brachial plexus. (From Haymaker W, Woodhall B. *Peripheral Nerve Injuries.* Philadelphia: WB Saunders; 1945.)

TABLE 87.3	Innervation of the Muscles of the Shoulder Girdle	
Muscle	**Nerve**	**Spinal Nerve Roots**
Sternocleidomastoid	Accessory	X1, C2, C3
Trapezius	Accessory	C3, C4
Serratus anterior	Long thoracic	C5, C7
Levator scapulae	Dorsal scapular	C5, C6
Rhomboideus major	Dorsal scapular	C5, C6
Rhomboideus minor	Dorsal scapular	C5, C6
Subclavius	Subclavian	C5, C6
Supraspinatus	Suprascapular	C5, C6
Infraspinatus	Suprascapular	C5, C6
Pectoralis major	Medial and lateral pectoralis	C5, C6
Pectoralis minor	Medial pectoralis	C5, C6
Teres major	Subscapular	C5, C6
Latissimus dorsi	Thoracodorsal	C6, C7
Subscapularis	Subscapular	C5, C6
Deltoid	Axillaris	C5, C6
Teres minor	Axillaris	C5, C6

TABLE 87.4	Innervation of Muscles of the Arm and Forearm	
Muscle	**Nerve**	**Root**
Biceps brachii Brachialis	Musculocutaneous	C5, C6
Triceps	Radialis	C7, C8
Anconeus	Radialis	C7, C8
Brachioradialis	Radialis	C5, C6
Extensor carpi radialis	Radialis	C6, C7
Pronator teres	Medianus	C6, C7
Flexor carpi radialis	Medianus	C7, C8
Palmaris longus	Medianus	C7, C8
Flexor digitorum sublimis	Medianus	C7, C8
Flexor digitorum profundus	Medianus, ulnaris	C7, C8
Flexor carpi ulnaris	Ulnaris	C7, C8
Supinator	Radialis	C7, C8
Extensor digitorum communis	Radialis	C7, C8
Extensor digiti minimi	Radialis	C7, C8
Extensor carpi ulnaris	Radialis	C7, C8
Abductor pollicis longus and brevis	Radialis	C7, C8
Extensor indicis proprius	Radialis	C7, C8

Trunk and Root Injury

UPPER RADICULAR SYNDROME

Upper radicular syndrome (Erb or Erb–Duchenne palsy) results from damage to the upper roots (C4, C5, or C6) or the upper trunk. Such lesions are most commonly the result of stretch injuries during difficult deliveries, especially when forceps are used, and cause paralysis of the deltoid, biceps, brachioradialis, pectoralis major, supraspinatus, infraspinatus, subscapularis, and teres major muscles in varying combinations. If the lesion is near the roots, the serratus anterior, rhomboids, and levator scapulae are also paralyzed. Clinically, this causes weakness of flexion at the elbow and of abduction and internal and external rotation of the arm. There is also weakness or paralysis of apposition of the scapula and backward–inward movements of the arm. Sensory loss is incomplete and consists of hypesthesia on the outer surface of the arm and forearm. The biceps reflex is absent. Unless treated by passive range-of-motion exercise, these patients may develop chronic contractures with the arm extended at the side, fully adducted, and pronated, with the hand flexed and facing rearward (e.g., the waiter's tip position).

MIDDLE RADICULAR SYNDROME

Middle radicular syndrome results from damage to the seventh cervical root (C7) or the middle trunk. Such lesions cause paralysis primarily of the muscles supplied by the radial nerve except the brachioradialis, which is entirely spared. Clinical weakness parallels that of injury to the radial nerve below the level of its branch to the brachioradialis. Sensory loss is variable and when present is limited to hypesthesia over the dorsal surface of the forearm and the external part of the dorsal surface of the hand.

LOWER RADICULAR SYNDROME (KLUMPKE PALSY)

Lower radicular syndrome (Klumpke palsy) results from injury to the lower trunk or lower roots (C7–T1), which causes paralysis of the flexor carpi ulnaris, the flexor digitorum, the interossei, and the thenar and hypothenar muscles. This pattern mimics a combined lesion of the median and ulnar nerves. Clinically, a flattened or simian hand is seen, with loss of all intrinsic hand musculature and with loss of sensation on the inner side of the arm and forearm and on the ulnar side of the hand. The triceps reflex is lost. If the communicating branch to the inferior cervical ganglion is injured, there is paralysis of the sympathetic nerves, causing a Horner syndrome.

Cord Injury

Lesions of the cords cause motor and sensory loss resembling that seen after injury to two or more peripheral nerves. *Lateral cord* injury causes weakness in the distribution of the musculocutaneous nerve and the lateral head of the median nerve, including weakness in the pronator teres, flexor carpi radialis, and flexor pollicis. *Posterior cord* injury causes weakness paralleling that resulting from combined damage to the radial and axillary nerves, whereas *medial cord* injury mimics combined damage to the ulnar nerve and the medial head of the median nerve (finger-flexion weakness).

Diffuse Plexus Injury

Generalized injury to the brachial plexus is usually unilateral but occasionally appears bilaterally. Such injury results from a more diffuse polyneuropathy, such as chronic inflammatory demyelinating neuropathy, or from multifocal motor neuropathy. A variety of insults may produce injury selectively affecting the brachial plexus, but tumor infiltration, radiation plexitis, and idiopathic plexitis are among the most important. Almost any neoplasm with a propensity for the chest may affect the plexus, but those cancers originating locally, such as lung and breast cancer, are most likely to cause injury. Such tumors may cause extrinsic compression of the plexus as they grow or may directly infiltrate the nervous tissue. Other neoplasms, such as lymphoma, may infiltrate the plexus and cause progressive deficits without any apparent mass effect or enlargement of the plexus itself in the initial stages. Magnetic resonance imaging (MRI) with contrast is the best way to confirm these lesions.

Idiopathic brachial plexitis (also known as the *Parsonage–Turner syndrome* or *neuralgic amyotrophy*) usually begins with a sudden, sharp pain affecting one shoulder, often with radiation down the ipsilateral arm, later followed by arm or shoulder weakness. The pain persists for hours or a few days with gradual improvement and usually resolves completely within days to weeks, leaving some sensory and motor dysfunction. It may be bilateral or asymmetric. Localization is often difficult, because plexus involvement ranges from diffuse to multifocal, and often includes patchy injury to the nerve branches off the plexus (e.g., the axillary nerve).

Electrodiagnostic studies, if performed at least 14 to 21 days after onset, usually localize the injury to the plexus but may demonstrate multifocal involvement. Patterns of both axonal and demyelination injury have been reported. The diversity of physiologic disorders in different nerves or even within the same nerve is attributed to involvement of the terminal nerve twigs or to patchy damage of discrete bundles of fibers within the cords or trunks of the brachial plexus or its branches. The long thoracic and anterior interosseous nerves are commonly affected. Autoimmune or infectious causes have been suggested, but the etiology is obscure. Some cases have occurred in small epidemics, and the disorder may follow intravenous heroin use, HIV seroconversion, surgery, and delivery.

There is no clear evidence that immunosuppressive therapy alters the course of the disease. However, short courses of tapering oral steroids are often prescribed if the patient presents shortly after symptom onset. Variants of this syndrome have also been described, including one with isolated, pure sensory injury affecting the lateral, antebrachial, cutaneous, and the median nerves.

A hereditary form that is frequently recurrent and bilateral is rarely encountered. Lumbosacral plexitis also occurs but much less frequently. Recovery depends on the severity of the initial insult. Although most patients recover well over 6 to 12 months, some are left with permanent disability. It is considered good in about 66%, fair in 20%, and poor in 14%. Clinical recovery may take 2 months to 3 years.

Thoracic Outlet Syndrome

The term *thoracic outlet syndrome* (TOS) encompasses different syndromes that arise from compression of the nerves in the brachial plexus or blood vessels (i.e., subclavian or axillary arteries, or veins in the same area). The putative compression sources are also diverse. How often these lesions are actually responsible for symptoms and how the symptoms should be treated are matters of intense debate. Studies done mainly by orthopedists, vascular surgeons, and neurosurgeons have included reports on several hundred patients who were treated surgically for this syndrome. When neurologists write about the neurogenic form of TOS, however, the tone is always skeptical, and the syndrome is described as exceedingly rare, with an annual incidence of about 1 per 1 million persons.

PATHOLOGY

The T1 and C8 nerve roots and the lower trunk of the brachial plexus are exposed to compression and angulation by anatomic anomalies that include cervical ribs and fibrous bands—of uncertain origin. Other nearby structures, such as scalene muscles, are dubious sources of compression. Cervical ribs are commonly found in asymptomatic people, and it is therefore difficult to assume that the presence of a cervical rib necessarily explains local symptoms. In addition to the neural syndromes, the same anomalies may compress local blood vessels and cause vascular syndromes, usually separated into arterial and venous entities. These conditions are also rare and may cause neurogenic symptoms by distal nerve ischemia but not pressure on the brachial plexus. Some cases follow local trauma.

CLINICAL FEATURES

Patients have pain in the shoulders, arms, and hands, or sometimes in all three locations. Hand pain is often most severe in the fourth and fifth fingers. The pain is aggravated by use of the arm and arm "fatigue" may be prominent, meaning local discomfort after brief effort. There may or may not be hypesthesia in the affected area.

Critics have divided cases into two groups: the *true* neurogenic TOS and the *disputed* syndrome. In the *true* syndrome, there are definite clinical and electrodiagnostic abnormalities. This disorder is rare and is almost always caused by a taut fibrous band extending from a cervical rib or abnormally elongated C7 transverse process; the band stretches the distal C8 and T1 roots or lower brachial plexus trunk. There is unequivocal wasting and weakness of hand muscles innervated by these segments. Changes are almost always unilateral.

EMG and nerve conduction studies demonstrate a pattern of low-amplitude median motor, ulnar sensory, and medial antebrachial cutaneous-evoked responses. Ulnar motor responses to hypothenar muscles may be involved to a lesser degree. EMG signs of active and chronic denervation are limited to involved muscles, most severely in the abductor pollicis brevis, and are attributed to a major contribution from T1.

In the *disputed* form, there are no objective motor or sensory signs or consistent laboratory abnormalities. Attempts to reproduce the syndrome by passive abduction of the arm (i.e., the Adson test) or other maneuvers have been cited, but the same abnormalities may be found in normal people and have no specific diagnostic value. The diagnosis is usually made by the treating surgeon; symptoms are frequently bilateral and complicated by legal or other nonmedical issues.

Similarly, studies of the application of electrodiagnostic techniques have not been blinded or controlled, so less specific abnormalities have been noted; the findings include isolated abnormalities of ulnar sensory nerve amplitude, conduction velocity after stimulation of the Erb point, ulnar F waves, and ulnar somatosensory-evoked potentials. MRI may show deviation or distortion of nerves or blood vessels, bands extending from the C7 transverse process, or other local anomalies. MRI quantitative estimates of the size of the thoracic outlet may show smaller than average dimensions, as were the cases in blinded reviews of series that compared vascular and neurogenic patients together with controls but do not prove that the differences are causative. Magnetic resonance angiography and Doppler ultrasonography may help assess possible vascular compression.

DIAGNOSIS AND TREATMENT

In cases of *true* TOS, diagnosis must exclude entrapment syndromes in the arm and compressive lesions in the cervical spine. The "upper limb tension test" is said to be comparable to straight leg raising, is carried out by abducting the arms to 90 degrees in external rotation, bringing on symptoms within 60 seconds. EMG, MRI, and sonography after raising the arm have been used to aid in diagnosis. However, warnings continue to appear about false-positive maneuvers to evoke pain. Danielson and Odderson injected botulinum toxin into the anterior scalene muscle under ultrasound guidance. Subclavian artery flow rates were measured with Doppler ultrasound. Three weeks later, symptoms had improved and blood flow in the artery, tested with the arm extended, had improved. A placebo-controlled formal study of this "scalene muscle chemodenervation" would help resolve the uncertainty of the procedure which could be used for diagnosis, treatment, and screening for surgery. However, no consensus has been achieved for the surgical procedure of choice, which may or may not include botulinum, rib resection, brachial plexus neurolysis, scalenectomy, or release of the subclavian artery and vein. Exercise programs have also been advocated.

In the *disputed* form, when no objective findings are noted on neurologic examination, there are problems. Each case must be evaluated separately, but caution is reasonable when symptoms are not accompanied by objective changes. Conservative therapy should be given an adequate trial; postural adjustments, passive exercise to increase mobility of shoulder muscles, and an exercise program have all been advocated. The results of surgery are difficult to evaluate without objective signs or diagnostic laboratory abnormalities to track; placebo effects are rarely considered in the evaluation of surgery. Symptomatic improvement also appears to be unrelated to the surgical procedure or the particular structure that has been excised or resected. Surgery is not without hazard; complications may include causalgia, injury of the long thoracic nerve, infection, and laceration of the subclavian artery.

THE SPINAL ROOTS AND LUMBAR AND SACRAL PLEXI

The Lumbar Plexus

The spinal roots at L2, L3, and L4 join to form the *lumbar plexus* in the psoas major muscle. This plexus gives off a number of principally sensory nerves, including the iliohypogastric, the ilioinguinal, the genitofemoral, and the lateral femoral cutaneous. The *femoral nerve* is derived from the L2, L3, and L4 roots, passing to the anterior leg along the lateral aspect of the psoas muscle (which it supplies); exiting the pelvis; and passing under the inguinal ligament to supply the pectineus, sartorius, rectus femoris, vastus lateralis, vastus intermedius, and vastus medialis muscles; and terminates as the pure sensory saphenous nerve in the medial lower leg.

The *obturator nerve* arises from anterior branches of the L2, L3, and L4 roots, forming in the psoas muscle and entering the pelvis anteriorly to the sacroiliac joint. It passes through the obturator canal, branching anteriorly to supply the adductor longus and brevis, and the gracilis, as well as posteriorly to supply the obturator externus, and half of the adductor magnus. It carries sensation from a small and variable area on the inner surface of the medial thigh, knee, and occasionally just below the medial knee.

The Sacral Plexus

The sacral plexus is formed from the L5, S1, and S2 roots, with variable contributions from L4. The *superior gluteal nerve* arises from the L4, L5, and S1 roots and supplies the gluteus medius and minimus and tensor fascia lata; the *inferior gluteal nerve* arises from the L5 and S1 roots and supplies the gluteus maximus.

The *sciatic nerve* is formed from the posterior fusion of the L4, L5, and S1 roots, exiting the pelvis via the greater sciatic foramen and passes through or under the piriformis muscle. It is functionally divided into a lateral fibular portion, which supplies the short head of the biceps femoris, and a medial tibial portion, which supplies the long head of the biceps femoris, the semitendinosus, and the semimembranosus. The nerve divides into the common fibular (formerly called the *peroneal*) and tibial nerves above the posterior knee.

The *common fibular nerve* branches laterally from the sciatic trunk in the popliteal fossa then moves superficially to wind around the head of the fibula. It then divides into the *superficial fibular nerve* to supply the peroneus longus and peroneus brevis and the *deep fibular nerve*, which supplies the tibialis anterior, extensor hallucis longus, peroneus tertius, and extensor digitorum brevis. The *tibial nerve* supplies the gastrocnemius and soleus, tibialis posterior, flexor digitorum longus, and flexor hallucis longus. It descends through the lower leg between the medial malleolus and the flexor retinaculum, dividing into the *medial plantar nerve* to supply the abductor hallucis, flexor digitorum brevis and flexor hallucis brevis, and the *lateral plantar nerve* to supply the abductor digiti minimi, flexor digiti minimi, abductor hallucis, and interosseous muscles. Both the tibial and fibular nerves supply sensory branches, which join to form the *sural nerve* below the popliteal space.

Radiation Plexopathy

Irradiation for carcinoma may damage nervous tissue, especially with high-voltage therapy. Brachial plexopathy is seen after radiotherapy for breast cancer; caudal roots and lumbosacral plexus are sometimes affected by radiation therapy for testicular cancer or Hodgkin disease. The first symptom is usually severe pain, followed by paresthesia and sensory loss. There may be a latent period of 12 to 20 months; in milder cases, several years may elapse before symptoms appear. Limb weakness peaks many months later. Latency intervals of up to 20 years have been reported. The damage may affect a single peripheral nerve initially and then progress slowly to involve others. Clinically, tendon reflexes disappear before weakness and atrophy becomes obvious; fasciculation and myokymia may be prominent. EMG and conduction studies reveal evidence of axonal damage; myokymic discharges are characteristic and can help differentiate plexopathy caused by radiation from plexopathy caused by tumor infiltration. High-resolution MRI is also potentially useful. No effective treatment is known. Radiation-induced fibrosis and microvascular injury are suspected mechanisms.

THE PROXIMAL NERVES OF THE ARM

The Axillary Nerve

The axillary nerve is the last branch of the posterior cord of the brachial plexus before forming the radial nerve. It arises from C5 and C6, supplies the deltoid and teres minor muscles, and transmits cutaneous sensation from a small patch on the lateral shoulder. Axillary neuropathy may be caused by trauma, fracture, humeral head dislocation, and brachial plexitis. Weakness of arm abduction after the first 15 to 30 degrees of movement is typical. Outward, backward, and forward movements of the arm are also weakened, although less dramatically. Sensory loss is limited to a small patch over the lateral deltoid.

The Long Thoracic Nerve

The long thoracic nerve arises from C5, C6, and C7 and supplies the serratus anterior muscle. This nerve is most commonly injured in isolation by forceful, downward pressure on the shoulder, which

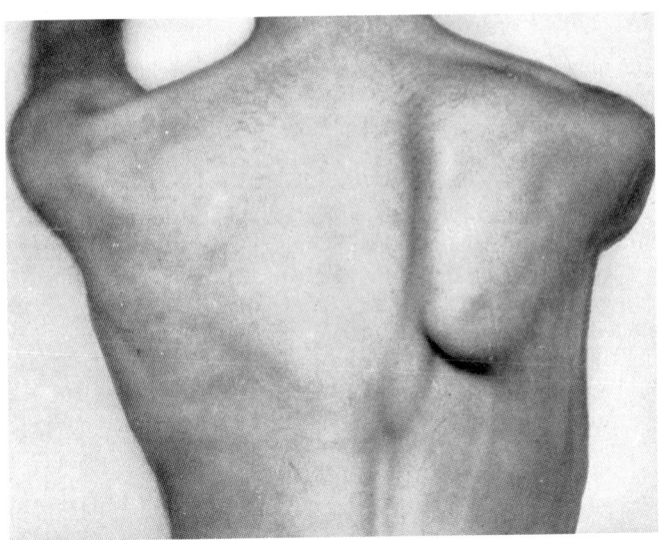

FIGURE 87.2 Paralysis of the serratus anterior muscle with winging of the scapula.

stretches and compresses it. Typically, such pressure is caused by carrying excessively heavy loads on the shoulder (e.g., furniture, carpets, heavy sacks, backpacks slung over one shoulder, etc.), although it may also appear after acute impact, such as that occurring while playing football. A more archaic term, although one still in use, is *hod-carrier's palsy*, in reference to the hod or container bricklayers formerly placed on the shoulder to carry bricks up to roof tops when constructing chimneys. Injury of this nerve destabilizes the scapula, causing winging, and prevents the rotation of the scapula needed to enable the last few degrees of abduction of the arm from 90 to 180 degrees over the head. Injury following acute or chronic trauma is characterized by weakness in elevation of the arm above the horizontal plane. Winging of the scapula is most prominent when the arm is fully abducted or elevated anteriorly (Fig. 87.2). Winging is often not readily apparent with the arm resting at the side.

The Brachial Cutaneous and Antebrachial Cutaneous Nerves

The brachial and antebrachial cutaneous nerves branch directly from the C8 to T1 plexus and provide sensation to the medial arm and upper two-thirds of the forearm. These nerves are usually injured in conjunction with the medial cord of the brachial plexus and are rarely injured in isolation.

The Suprascapular Nerve

The suprascapular nerve fibers arise from C5 and C6, ultimately branching from the upper trunk of the brachial plexus. The primarily motor nerve innervates the supraspinatus and infraspinatus muscles. Affected patients have difficulty moving the arm from the side through the first 15 to 30 degrees of abduction and with external shoulder rotation. Shoulder trauma or more diffuse brachial plexus injury is most common; isolated nerve injury is rare.

THE PERIPHERAL NERVES

The Radial Nerve

The radial nerve is a continuation of the posterior cord and contains elements of the C5, C6, C7, C8, and T1 nerve roots. It is predominantly a motor nerve and innervates the chief extensors of the forearm, wrist, and fingers. It descends through the axilla to supply the triceps, giving off three minor sensory branches to the upper arm, then winds posteriorly around the humerus in the *spiral groove*. After exiting the spiral groove, the nerve innervates the brachioradialis and extensor carpi radialis longus muscles then moves laterally to enter the forearm between the brachialis and brachioradialis muscles. There, it branches into a primary sensory component, the *superficial radial nerve*, which supplies sensation to the dorsoradial aspect of the distal forearm and the dorsal surface of the hand, and a motor component, the *posterior interosseous nerve*, which supplies all the remaining forearm extensor muscles and often the supinator as well (Table 87.5).

The clinical findings after radial nerve injury depend on the level of the lesion. Injury in the axilla, classically caused by improperly fitting crutches that are too long, causes triceps weakness as well as weakness of the remaining radial myotome and numbness in the radial dermatome. Injury in the spiral groove caused by humeral fracture or extrinsic compression (e.g., *Saturday night palsy*) causes weakness of the radial myotome below the elbow, with prominent wrist-drop, weakness of finger extension, and sensory loss in the distribution of the superficial radial nerve but preserved elbow extension. Mild elbow flexor weakness may be present as a result of involvement of the brachioradialis, which should be easy to distinguish on physical examination. The posterior interosseous branch may also be injured by entrapment as it passes through the supinator muscle in the tight space of the arcade of Frohse.

Injury of the posterior interosseous nerve spares the brachioradialis and the extensor carpi radialis longus, as well as the superficial radial nerve, causing radial deviation of the wrist with attempted wrist extension but no sensory loss (i.e., posterior interosseous neuropathy). Damage to the superficial radial branch may occur at the wrist as a result of tight-fitting jewelry or handcuffs, causing pure sensory loss over the dorsum of the hand without weakness. Evaluation of radial nerve injury often includes electrodiagnostic studies and may include imaging studies, depending on the site of the lesion. Treatment focuses on relieving the cause of compressive injury, if possible. Posterior interosseous nerve syndrome is sometimes treated with surgical release.

The Median Nerve

The median nerve derives from the C6 through T1 nerve roots, passing through the lateral and medial cords of the brachial plexus, which each contributes a segment to the nerve. The median nerve passes down the arm and through the two heads of the pronator teres at the level of the forearm, ultimately supplying the pronator teres as well as the flexor carpi radialis, palmaris longus, and flexor digitorum superficialis muscles. It then branches into the pure

TABLE 87.5	Muscles Innervated by the Radial Nerve	
Triceps	Extensor digiti minimi
Anconeus	Extensor carpi ulnaris
Brachioradialis	Abductor pollicis longus
Extensor carpi radialis longus and brevis	Extensor pollicis longus and brevis
Supinator	Extensor indicis proprius
Extensor digitorum communis	

TABLE 87.6	Muscles Innervated by the Median Nerve
Pronator teres	Pronator quadratus
Flexor carpi radialis	Abductor pollicis brevis
Palmaris longus	Opponens pollicis
Flexor digitorum sublimis	Flexor pollicis brevis
Flexor digitorum profundus	Lumbricales (digits one and two)
Flexor pollicis longus	

motor *anterior interosseous nerve*, which supplies the flexor pollicis longus, pronator quadratus, and flexor digitorum profundus I and II, and into a main branch, which passes through the carpal tunnel, further branching into the *recurrent thenar nerve*, supplying the abductor and the lateral flexor pollicis brevi and the opponens pollicis before terminating in the palm, where it supplies lumbricals I and II. Pronation is mediated by the pronator quadratus and pronator teres, wrist flexion by the flexor carpi radialis and palmaris longus, flexion of the thumb and the index and middle fingers by the superficial and deep flexors, and opposition of the thumb by the opponens pollicis (Table 87.6).

The median nerve supplies sensation to the radial side of the palm, the ventral thumb, index and middle fingers, the radial half of the ring finger, as well as the dorsal surfaces of the distal phalanx of the thumb, and the middle and terminal phalanges of the index and middle fingers. Isolated lesions of the median nerve cause weakness and sensory loss in the aforementioned distributions, but only a few movements are paralyzed because of the synergistic contributions of muscles innervated by other nerves to these movements. However, there may be absence of flexion in the index finger and near-complete paralysis of the opponens pollicis. The median nerve may be injured by trauma, ischemia, and other processes but most commonly is damaged by anatomic compression. It may be entrapped between the heads of the pronator teres muscle, causing weakness and sensory loss in the above distributions, with sparing of the pronator teres itself, which is innervated more proximally (i.e., the pronator teres syndrome).

Entrapment of the anterior interosseous nerve (i.e., the anterior interosseous neuropathy) often presents with pain but produces no sensory loss. Symptoms include weakness of the flexor pollicis longus, flexor digitorum profundus I and II, and the pronator quadratus. Attempts to make the "OK" sign with the thumb and index finger produces a triangle rather than a circle (e.g., the pinch sign). The most common of all the nerve entrapment syndromes is the *carpal tunnel syndrome*. This syndrome results from entrapment of the median nerve as it passes through the tunnel defined by the carpal bones and the transverse carpal ligament, resulting in pain and sensory loss in a distal median distribution; wasting and weakness of thenar muscles and median innervated lumbricals is seen in severe cases. Although the diagnosis is primarily clinical, electrophysiologic studies may confirm the lesion and provide information on severity. Conservative treatment with application of a neutral position wrist splint is often effective. More severe or refractory cases, especially when motor deficits appear or splinting or other conservative measures fail to provide relief, may be treated by surgical release of the carpal tunnel. Many underlying disorders may predispose to the condition including diabetes, uremia, hypothyroidism, amyloidosis, and pregnancy.

The Ulnar Nerve

The ulnar nerve arises from C8 to T1 roots and the medial cord of the brachial plexus. It passes between the biceps and triceps, moving posteriorly to pass behind the medial epicondyle in the ulnar groove. It enters the forearm through the cubital tunnel, supplying the flexor carpi ulnaris and the flexor digitorum profundus II and IV, then moves medially to enter the hand through Guyon canal, where it divides into a superficial sensory branch and a deep motor branch, which supplies the abductor, opponens, and flexor digiti minimi medially. It then moves laterally to the adductor pollicis and the medial half of the flexor pollicis brevis (Table 87.7).

The nerve supplies sensation to the palmar and dorsal surfaces of the little finger, the medial half of the ring finger, and both palmar and dorsal sides of the ulnar portion of the hand. Complete lesions of the proximal ulnar nerve are characterized by weakness of flexion and adduction of the wrist and of flexion of the ring and the little fingers, paralysis of abduction and opposition of the little finger, paralysis of adduction of the thumb, and paralysis of adduction and abduction of the fingers, along with atrophy of the hypothenar muscles and the interossei. Atrophy of the first dorsal interosseous is especially obvious on the dorsum of the hand between the thumb and the index finger. Sensory loss is greatest in the little finger and is present to a lesser extent on the inner side of the ring finger. Chronic lesions result in clawing of ulnar innervated fingers. The ulnar nerve may also be injured by trauma, ischemia, and other causes but similar to the median nerve, it is most commonly injured by compression. Entrapment primarily occurs in three locations. The most common site is at the elbow, in or just proximal to the ulnar groove. Just distal to the elbow, the nerve may become entrapped in the cubital tunnel, the tunnel formed by the aponeurosis connecting the two heads of the flexor carpi ulnaris. Proximal nerve injury causes weakness in the ulnar myotomes of the hand and may include the flexor carpi ulnaris (FCU) and flexor digitorum profundus (FDP) III and IV, depending on the precise site of the compression. The nerve is potentially compressed at the elbow by direct pressure from arms of chairs, table edges, and excessive elbow flexion. A protective elbow pad is useful in some cases. Various forms of surgical decompression are available for the most extreme cases. Guyon canal stenosis in the wrist, most commonly associated with a ganglion cyst, causes weakness and atrophy of intrinsic hand muscles. Sensory symptoms may be minimal, although nerve conduction studies to the digits are abnormal. However, the FCU and FDP III and IV are spared, in addition to sensation on the dorsal hand surface, which is innervated by the dorsal ulnar cutaneous nerve that arises in the distal forearm. The innervation of hand muscles is summarized in Table 87.4.

TABLE 87.7	Muscles Innervated by the Ulnar Nerve	
Flexor carpi ulnaris		Flexor digiti minimi
Flexor digitorum profundus (digits four and five)		All interossei
Palmaris brevis		Lumbricales (digits three and four)
Abductor digiti minimi		Flexor pollicis brevis
Opponens digiti minimi		

The Musculocutaneous Nerve

The musculocutaneous nerve originates from the C5 and C6 nerve roots and the main branch of the upper trunk of the brachial plexus. It provides innervation to the coracobrachialis, biceps brachii, and brachialis muscles and provides sensation to the ventrolateral forearm (lateral antebrachial sensory nerve), as well as to a small area on the dorsolateral outer surface of the forearm. Isolated injuries of the nerve are rare and it is not typically prone to focal compression. Lesions of the musculocutaneous nerve produce weakness of flexion and supination of the forearm, sensory loss in the musculocutaneous myotomes, and loss of the biceps reflex. Forearm flexion may still be performed by the brachioradialis muscle innervated by the radial nerve. However, because the bicep is the chief supinator of the forearm, this movement is paralyzed. Excessive windsurfing is associated with compression of the lateral antebrachial sensory branch.

THE NERVES OF THE LEG

The Obturator Nerve

Lesions of the obturator nerve are uncommon and may be caused by pelvic tumors, obturator hernias, and by passage of the head of the fetus during difficult labor. Injuries to the obturator nerve result in severe weakness of adduction and to a lesser extent, internal and external rotation of the thigh. Pain in the knee joint is sometimes caused by pelvic involvement of the geniculate branch of the obturator.

The Iliohypogastric Nerve

The iliohypogastric nerve is a predominately sensory nerve that originates from the uppermost part of the lumbar plexus. It provides sensation to the outer and upper parts of the buttocks and the lower part of the abdomen and supplies partial innervation to the internal oblique and transversalis muscles. Lesions of the iliohypogastric nerve are rare. It may be divided by incisions in kidney operations or together with the ilioinguinal nerve in operations in the inguinal region, such as hernia repair. Lesions of these nerves produce no significant motor loss and only a small area of cutaneous anesthesia.

The Ilioinguinal Nerve

The ilioinguinal nerve is also a branch of the upper lumbar plexus. It provides sensation to the upper inner portion of the thigh, the pubic region, and the external genitalia and supplies the transversalis, internal oblique, and external oblique muscles. The ilioinguinal nerve is usually injured in concert with the iliohypogastric nerve and is only rarely injured in isolation.

The Genitofemoral Nerve

This predominately sensory nerve originates from the second lumbar root and provides sensation to the scrotum and the contiguous area of the inner surface of the thigh. Lesions of the genitofemoral nerve are rare. Irritative lesions of the nerve in the abdominal wall are accompanied by painful hyperesthesia at the root of the thigh and the scrotum.

The Lateral Femoral Cutaneous Nerve of the Thigh

This nerve is formed by fibers from the second and third lumbar roots. It crosses beneath the fascia iliaca to emerge at the anterosuperior iliac spine, descends in the thigh beneath the fascia lata, and divides into two branches. The posterior branch passes obliquely backward through the fascia lata and provides sensation to the superior external buttock. The anterior branch, which is more important clinically, pierces the fascia lata through a small fibrous canal located about 10 cm below the ligament and provides sensation to the outer surface of the thigh.

Lesions to this nerve principally affect the anterior branch, causing the clinical syndrome of *meralgia paresthetica*, and includes dysesthesias and sensory loss along the lateral thigh. The use of tight, heavy, utility belts or corsets and religious talismans; obesity; weight loss; and pregnancy are implicated as possible contributors to compression. Pains in the lateral thigh may also be caused by spinal lesions or pelvic tumors, which must be excluded by appropriate diagnostic studies. The course of meralgia paresthetica is variable. Occasionally, symptoms disappear spontaneously. In most patients, removal of contributing factors aids in resolution of symptoms.

The Femoral Nerve

The femoral nerve may be compressed by tumors, other pelvic lesions, pubic ramus or femur fractures, as well as by ischemia in diabetic neuropathy and other conditions. Assessment of hip adduction helps to separate this condition from lumbar plexopathy or radiculopathy.

Injury to the nerve produces weakness of leg extension and thigh flexion. Walking on level ground is possible so long as the leg is extended, but if the slightest flexion occurs, the patient's knee may collapse. Climbing stairs or walking uphill is difficult or impossible. The quadriceps reflex is lost on the affected side. Saphenous sensory loss is also diagnostically useful. In severe cases, orthopedic appliances that fix the knee joint in extension or tendon transposition may be considered.

The Sciatic Nerve

The main trunk of the sciatic nerve is derived from the lower lumbosacral nerve roots and retains a strict segregation of fibular and tibial fibers. Total paralysis of muscles innervated by the sciatic nerve is rare. Even with a lesion in the thigh, the common fibular division is often more severely damaged than the tibial.

Important sources of injury include gunshot, shrapnel, or stab wounds to the leg or pelvis; fractures of the pelvis or femur; dislocations of the hip; pressure of the fetal head during delivery; or pelvic tumors. The nerve is sometimes inadvertently injured by intramuscular injection of drugs, especially in infants. Compression can occur in the posterior thigh by sharp chair edges or operating room tables. Injury by the piriformis muscle (*piriformis syndrome*) is controversial but very rare, but convincing cases are described. *Sciatica* is a term used to describe pain in the low back and in the leg along the course of the nerve, but the vast majority of these patients have nerve root injury at the L5–S1 level, often caused by intervertebral disk herniation. The clinical features of cervical and lumbar disk herniation are considered in Chapters 109 and 110.

Complete injury of the sciatic nerve causes paralysis of all the movements of the ankle and toes, as well as weakness or paralysis of knee flexion. Gait is marked by footdrop and the ankle jerk is lost, along with sensation on the outer surface of the leg, on the instep and sole of the foot, and over the toes.

The Common Fibular Nerve

The common fibular branch of the sciatic nerve is a mixed nerve innervating the extensor muscles of the ankle and toes and the foot evertors. It provides sensation from the outer side of the leg, the front of its lower one-third, the instep, and the dorsal surface of the four inner toes over their proximal phalanges. The common fibular nerve is highly subjected to trauma. It may be damaged by wounds near the knee. The nerve is readily compressed or stretched as it curves around the fibular head by leg crossing, squatting, or resting the edge of the leg against a hard surface while sleeping, intoxicated, or anesthetized. Ganglion cysts, sometimes palpable at the fibular head, are well described. Common fibular neuropathy results in foot drop and weak foot eversion. The patient may not dorsiflex the ankle, straighten or extend the toes, or evert the foot, and there is sensory loss in the nerve distribution. Recovery is dependent on the extent of injury, which usually correlates with the degree and duration of extrinsic compression. Ambulation in patients with footdrop may be greatly aided by ankle–foot orthoses.

The Tibial Nerve

Tibial neuropathy is uncommon. It may be injured by gunshot wounds or leg fractures. A complete lesion of the nerve produces paralysis of plantar flexion and inversion of the foot, flexion and separation of the toes, and sensory loss in the nerve distribution. The ankle jerk and plantar reflex are lost. Rarely, compression of the posterior tibial branch of the nerve at the medial malleolus produces pain and paresthesia in the soles of the feet in a manner similar to compression of the median nerve at the wrist (*tarsal tunnel syndrome*); however, this process is much less prevalent. Other conditions that produce foot pain and/or numbness, including digital neuropathy, focal disorders of the foot, plantar fasciitis, early polyneuropathy, and Morton neuroma that produce foot pain and numbness are all more frequent.

SPECIFIC ACQUIRED POLYNEUROPATHIES

GUILLAIN–BARRÉ SYNDROME

The GBS is characterized by acute onset of peripheral and cranial nerve dysfunction. Viral respiratory or gastrointestinal infection, immunization, or surgery often precedes neurologic symptoms by 5 days to 4 weeks. Symptoms and signs include rapidly progressive symmetric weakness, loss of tendon reflexes, facial diplegia, oropharyngeal and respiratory paresis, and impaired sensation in the hands and feet. The condition worsens for several days to 3 weeks, followed by a period of stability and then gradual improvement to normal or nearly normal function. Early plasmapheresis or intravenous immunoglobulin (IVIG) (2 g/kg in divided doses) accelerates recovery and diminishes the incidence of long-term neurologic disability.

In North America and Europe, acute inflammatory demyelinating polyneuropathy accounts for over 90% of GBS. GBS also includes acute motor axonal neuropathy (AMAN), acute motor and sensory axonal neuropathy (AMSAN), Miller Fisher syndrome, and acute autonomic and sensory neuropathies.

Etiology

The cause of GBS is incompletely understood. There is evidence that it is immune mediated. There is inflammatory pathology and patients improve with immunomodulatory therapy. A disease with similar clinical features (i.e., similar pathologic, electrophysiologic, and cerebrospinal fluid [CSF] alterations) can be induced in experimental animals by immunization with whole peripheral nerve, peripheral nerve myelin, or, in some species, peripheral nerve myelin P2 basic protein or galactocerebroside. An important first step in

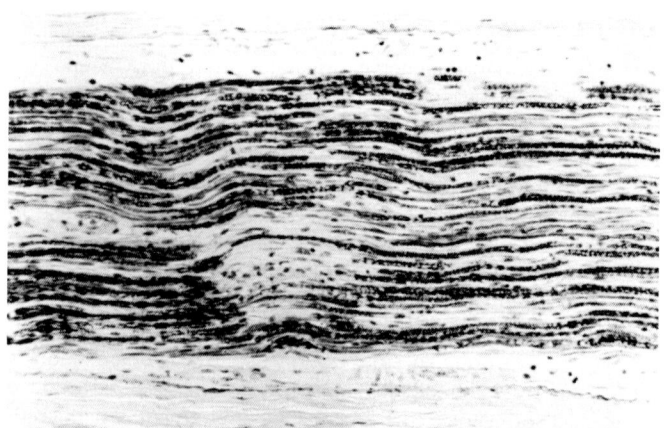

FIGURE 87.3 Focal demyelination in acute GBS. (Courtesy of Dr. Arthur Asbury.)

autoimmune disease is the impairment of self-tolerance, and there is evidence that this occurs by molecular mimicry in two forms of GBS, AMAN, and Miller Fisher syndrome, with cross-reactive epitopes between *Campylobacter jejuni* and peripheral nerve. When GBS is preceded by a viral infection, there is no evidence of direct viral infection of peripheral nerves or nerve roots.

Electrophysiology and Pathology

Nerve conduction velocities are reduced in GBS, but values may be normal early in the course. Distal motor latencies may be prolonged. Because of demyelination of nerve roots, minimal F-wave latency is often increased or responses are absent from proximal conduction block. Conduction slowing may persist for months or years after clinical recovery. In general, the severity of neurologic abnormality is not related to the degree of conduction slowing but is related to the extent of conduction block or axonal loss. Long-standing weakness is most apt to occur when compound motor action potential (CMAP) amplitudes are reduced to less than 20% of normal.

Histologically, GBS is characterized by focal segmental demyelination (Fig. 87.3) with perivascular and endoneurial infiltrates of lymphocytes and monocytes or macrophages (Fig. 87.4). These lesions are scattered throughout the nerves, nerve roots, and cranial nerves. In particularly severe lesions, there is both axonal degen-

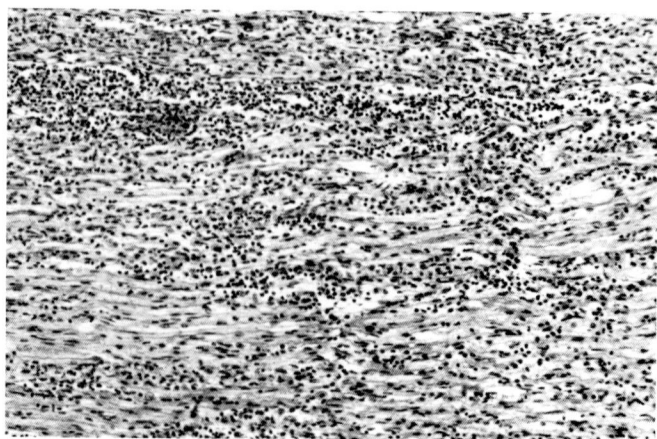

FIGURE 87.4 Diffuse mononuclear infiltrate in peripheral nerve in GBS. (Courtesy of Dr. Arthur Asbury.)

eration and segmental demyelination. During recovery, remyelination occurs, but the lymphocytic infiltrates may persist.

Incidence

GBS is the most frequently acquired demyelinating neuropathy, with an incidence of 0.6 to 1.9 cases per 100,000 population. The incidence increases gradually with age, but the disease may occur at any age. Men and women are affected equally. The incidence increases in patients with Hodgkin disease, as well as with pregnancy or general surgery.

Clinical Features

GBS often appears days to weeks after symptoms of a viral upper respiratory or gastrointestinal infection. Usually, the first neurologic symptoms are a result of symmetric limb weakness, often with paresthesia. In contrast to most other neuropathies, proximal muscles are sometimes initially affected more than distal muscles. Occasionally, facial, ocular, or oropharyngeal muscles are affected first; more than 50% of patients have facial diplegia, and dysphagia and dysarthria develop in a similar number. Some patients require mechanical ventilation. Tendon reflexes may be normal for the first few days but are then lost. The degree of sensory impairment varies. In some patients, all sensory modalities are preserved; others have marked diminution in perception of joint position, vibration, pain, and temperature in stocking-and-glove distribution. Patients occasionally exhibit papilledema, sensory ataxia, and transient extensor plantar responses. Autonomic dysfunction, including orthostatic hypotension, labile blood pressure, tachyarrhythmia, and bradyarrhythmia or resting tachycardia is frequent in more severe cases and an important cause of morbidity and mortality. Many have muscle tenderness, and the nerves may be sensitive to pressure, but there are no signs of meningeal irritation such as nuchal rigidity.

Variants

AMAN is a variant of GBS. There is motor axonal degeneration and little or no demyelination or inflammation. Despite the axonal involvement, recovery is similar to the demyelinating form. AMAN may follow infection with *C. jejuni*, *Mycoplasma pneumoniae*, or parenteral injection of gangliosides.

The *Miller Fisher syndrome* is characterized by gait ataxia, areflexia, and ophthalmoparesis; pupillary abnormalities are sometimes present. It is considered a variant of GBS because it is often preceded by respiratory infection, it progresses for weeks and then improves, and CSF protein content is increased. There is no limb weakness, however, and nerve conductions are generally normal; however, H reflexes may be affected. In some cases, MRI shows brain stem hyperintense lesions.

Other GBS variants include *AMSAN*, acute sensory neuropathy or neuronopathy, and acute autonomic neuropathy or pandysautonomia (see Chapter 112).

Laboratory Data

The CSF protein content is elevated in most patients with GBS but may be normal in the first few days after onset. The CSF cell count is usually normal, but some patients with otherwise typical GBS have 10 to 100 mononuclear cells/μL of CSF. Antecedent infectious mononucleosis, cytomegalovirus (CMV) infection, viral hepatitis, HIV infection, or other viral diseases may be documented by serologic studies. Increased titers of immunoglobulin G (IgG) or immunoglobulin A (IgA) antibodies to GM1 or GD1a gangliosides

may be found in the axonal form of GBS; anti-GQ1b antibodies are closely associated with the Miller Fisher syndrome.

Outcome

Symptoms are usually most severe within 1 week of onset but may progress for 3 weeks or more. Death is uncommon but may follow aspiration pneumonia, pulmonary embolism, intercurrent infection, or autonomic dysfunction. The rate of recovery varies. In some, it is rapid, with restoration to normal function within a few weeks. In most, recovery is slow and not complete for many months. Recovery is accelerated by early institution of plasmapheresis or IVIG therapy. In untreated series, about 35% of patients have permanent residual hyporeflexia, atrophy, and weakness of distal muscles or facial paresis. A biphasic illness, with partial recovery followed by relapse, is present in fewer than 10% of patients. Recurrence after full recovery occurs in about 2%.

Diagnosis and Differential Diagnosis

The characteristic history of subacute development of symmetric motor or sensorimotor neuropathy after a viral illness, delivery, or surgery, together with compatible electrophysiology and an elevated CSF protein content with normal cell count, defines GBS.

In the past, the principal diseases to be differentiated from GBS were diphtheritic polyneuropathy and acute poliomyelitis. Both are now rare in the United States. Diphtheritic polyneuropathy can usually be distinguished by the long latency period between the respiratory infection and onset of neuritis, the frequency of paralysis of accommodation, and the relatively slow evolution of symptoms. Acute anterior poliomyelitis was distinguished by asymmetry of paralysis, signs of meningeal irritation, fever, and CSF pleocytosis. Acute West Nile viral infection, however, can lead to a similar picture. Acute encephalitis is the most common West Nile neurologic manifestation, but an acute paralytic syndrome is the next most frequent. Asymmetric or monomelic weakness is characteristic, but some cases develop in a GBS-like manner. Some cases have a flulike prodrome without notable encephalitis. Occasionally, patients with HIV infection have a disorder identical to GBS. Porphyric neuropathy resembles GBS clinically but is differentiated by normal CSF protein, recurrent abdominal crisis, mental symptoms, onset after exposure to barbiturates or other drugs, and high urinary levels of δ-aminolevulinic acid and porphobilinogen. Development of a GBS-like syndrome during prolonged parenteral feeding should raise the possibility of hypophosphatemia-induced neural dysfunction. Toxic neuropathies caused by *n*-hexane inhalation or thallium or arsenic ingestion may begin acutely or subacutely. Botulism may be difficult to discriminate on clinical grounds from purely motor forms of GBS, but ocular muscles and the pupils are frequently affected. Electrophysiologic tests in botulism reveal normal nerve conduction velocities and a facilitating response to repetitive nerve stimulation. Tick paralysis, which occurs almost exclusively in children, should be excluded by careful scalp examination.

Treatment

Early plasmapheresis [**Level 1**][1,2] or IVIG [**Level 1**][3] therapy has proved useful in patients with GBS. Glucocorticoid administration does not shorten the course or affect the prognosis. Mechanically assisted ventilation is sometimes necessary, and precautions against aspiration of food or stomach contents must be taken if oropharyngeal muscles are affected. Exposure keratitis must be prevented in patients with facial diplegia.

CHRONIC INFLAMMATORY DEMYELINATING POLYNEUROPATHY

Chronic inflammatory demyelinating polyneuropathy (CIDP) may begin insidiously or acutely, as GBS, and then follow a chronic progressive or relapsing course. It often follows nonspecific viral infections, although less often than in GBS. Segmental demyelination and lymphocytic infiltrates are present in peripheral nerves, and a similar disease can be induced in experimental animals by immunization with peripheral nerve myelin. The CSF protein content is often increased but less consistently than in GBS. An infantile form of CIDP begins with hypotonia and delayed motor development. Optic neuritis has been noted in some patients. Nerves may become enlarged because of Schwann cell proliferation and collagen deposition after recurrent segmental demyelination and remyelination (Figs. 87.5 and 87.6).

In contrast to GBS, glucocorticoid therapy is often beneficial. CIDP is also responsive to plasmapheresis [**Level 1**][4] or IVIG [**Level 1**].[5] Immunosuppressive drug therapy may be effective in resistant cases. Research criteria for the diagnosis of CIDP have been recommended, but there is no specific test, and the diagnosis is often made on clinical grounds. A predominantly sensory or distal form of CIDP and a multifocal form (the Lewis–Sumner syndrome) have been described. Tests for HIV-1, monoclonal paraproteins, antibodies to myelin-associated glycoprotein (MAG), and occasionally, CMT disease type 1 or hereditary neuropathy with liability to pressure palsy are performed in suspected patients to evaluate possible causes of demyelinating neuropathy.

MULTIFOCAL MOTOR NEUROPATHY

Multifocal motor neuropathy (MMN) is a clinical syndrome of lower motor neuron dysfunction. Typically, there is weakness, wasting, and fasciculation with preserved or absent tendon reflexes. The findings are typically asymmetric and affect the arms and hands more than the legs. Electrophysiologic evidence of denervation is accompanied by the defining abnormality, physiologic evidence of multifocal motor conduction block, at sites other than typical compression sites. Other signs of demyelination are also described; conduction block is not present in all patients, including some with positive antibody titers. MMN is associated with increased titers of immunoglobulin M (IgM) anti-GM1 in approximately 60%

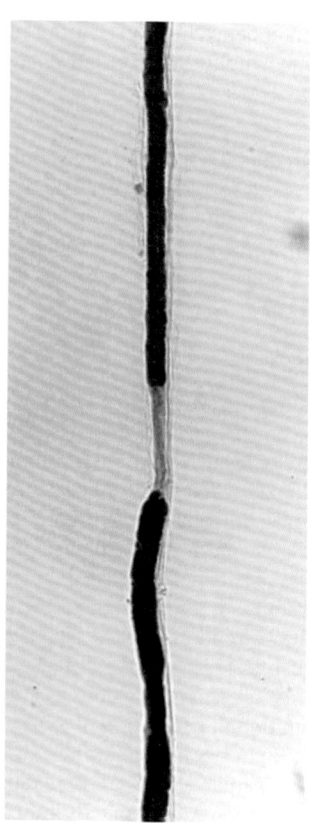

FIGURE 87.6 Teased fiber showing demyelination in a patient with CIDP (magnification ×400).

of patients; less frequently, anti-GD1a antibodies are found. The clinical syndrome also occurs in patients with normal anti-GM1 antibody titers. It is important to distinguish these patients from patients with typical motor neuron disease because the weakness of MMN is potentially reversible with IVIG [**Level 1**][6] or immunosuppressive drug therapy.

SENSORY NEURONOPATHY AND NEUROPATHY

Sensory neuropathy may result from primary involvement of the sensory root ganglia, as in ganglioneuritis or sensory neuronitis, or the nerve may be directly affected as in distal sensory neuropathy. *Ganglioneuritis* may be acute or subacute in onset and is characterized by numbness, paresthesia, and pain that can be distal or radicular or can involve the entire body, including the face. Ataxia and autonomic dysfunction may be evident. Small- or large-fiber sensation or both may be affected to varying degrees. Tendon reflexes may be present or absent, and strength is normal. The disease may be self-limiting or chronic, with relapses or slow progression. Motor nerve conduction velocities are normal or near normal, but sensory potentials are reduced in amplitude or absent. Routine electrophysiologic studies may be normal if the disease is mild or if only small fibers are affected. CSF protein content is normal or slightly elevated. Response to glucocorticoids or immunosuppressive therapy is variable. Pathologic studies of spinal root ganglia show inflammatory infiltrates with a predominance of T cells and macrophages. Some patients have sicca or Sjögren syndrome with anti-Ro (SSA) and anti-La (SSB) antibodies.

Several autoantibodies to peripheral nerve antigens are associated with sensory neuropathy. Some patients with sensory axonal

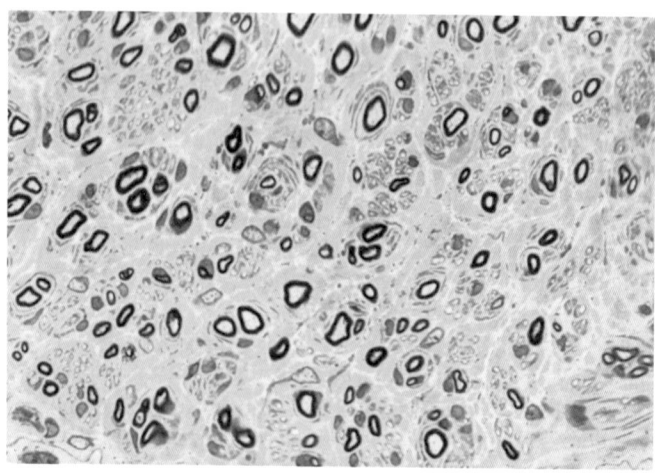

FIGURE 87.5 Semithin section showing multifocal thinly myelinated fibers in a patient with CIDP (magnification ×600).

neuropathies have monoclonal or polyclonal IgM antisulfatide antibodies, and monoclonal IgM autoantibodies with anti-GD1b and disialosyl ganglioside antibody activity have been associated with large-fiber sensory neuropathy. Other causes of sensory neuropathy include HIV-1 infection, vitamin B_6 deficiency or toxicity, celiac disease, paraneoplastic neuropathy, amyloidosis, and toxic neuropathy.

IDIOPATHIC AUTONOMIC NEUROPATHY

This condition is characterized by sympathetic, parasympathetic, or enteric nerve dysfunction. Acute, subacute, and chronic forms are known and discussed in Chapter 112.

VASCULITIC AND CRYOGLOBULINEMIC NEUROPATHIES

Vasculitic neuropathy is manifested as mononeuritis multiplex or distal symmetric polyneuropathy. Nerve conduction studies may show electrical inexcitability of nerve segments distal to an injury caused by vascular occlusion. If some nerve fascicles are spared, conduction proceeds at a normal rate, but summated response amplitude is diminished. The diagnosis of peripheral nerve involvement may be established by nerve and muscle biopsies (Fig. 87.7), which typically show inflammatory cell infiltrates and necrosis of blood vessel walls. The biopsy specimen, however, may show only axonal degeneration if vasculitis produced a nerve injury that is proximal to the biopsy site or if no affected vessels are encountered in the specimen.

Vasculitis may be confined to the peripheral nerves or may be associated with systemic disease, such as polyarteritis or cryoglobulinemia. The most common systemic cause of vasculitic neuropathy is polyarteritis nodosa, which may cause purpuric skin lesions, renal failure, Raynaud phenomenon, constitutional symptoms, and sometimes, mixed polyclonal cryoglobulinemia; hepatitis B or C virus (HBV or HCV) or HIV infection may be found. Cryoglobulins are immunoglobulins that precipitate in the cold and are classified as types I through III. Type I contains a monoclonal immunoglobulin only, type II contains both monoclonal and polyclonal immunoglobulins, and type III contains mixed polyclonal immunoglobulins. Types I and II are associated with plasma cell dyscrasia, and type III may be associated with polyarteritis nodosa and HBV or HCV infection. Cryoglobulin testing samples must be kept warm to prevent precipitation prior to laboratory analysis.

Other causes of vasculitic neuropathy include the Churg–Strauss syndrome with asthma and eosinophilia; Sjögren syndrome with xerophthalmia, xerostomia, and anti-Ro and anti-La antibodies; and Wegener granulomatosis with necrotizing granulomatous lesions in the upper or lower respiratory tract, glomerulonephritis, and antineutrophil cytoplasmic antigen antibodies. Less commonly, vasculitic neuropathy is seen in rheumatoid arthritis, systemic lupus erythematosus, and systemic sclerosis. Vasculitis may respond to therapy with prednisone (60 mg qd) and cyclophosphamide (1 g/m^2 every month × 6 months). Plasmapheresis is also useful in the treatment of cryoglobulinemia.

NEUROPATHIES ASSOCIATED WITH MYELOMA AND NONMALIGNANT IMMUNOGLOBULIN G OR IMMUNOGLOBULIN A MONOCLONAL GAMMOPATHIES

Peripheral neuropathy is found in approximately 50% of patients with osteosclerotic myeloma and IgG or IgA monoclonal gammopathies. Some patients have the POEMS syndrome (polyneuropathy, organomegaly, endocrinopathy, M protein, and skin changes) or Crow–Fukase syndrome with hyperpigmentation of skin, edema, excessive hair growth, hepatosplenomegaly, papilledema, elevated CSF protein content, hypogonadism, and hypothyroidism. POEMS syndrome is sometimes associated with nonosteosclerotic myeloma or with nonmalignant monoclonal gammopathy. The IgG or IgA light-chain type is almost always λ. Electrophysiologic and pathologic abnormalities are consistent with demyelination and axonal degeneration; the patterns may resemble CIDP.

Malignant or nonmalignant IgG or IgA monoclonal gammopathy may also be associated with neuropathy in primary amyloidosis, in which fragments of the monoclonal light chains are deposited as amyloid in peripheral nerve, and in types I and II cryoglobulinemia, in which the monoclonal immunoglobulins are components of the cryoprecipitates.

The significance of IgG or IgA monoclonal gammopathies is uncertain in the absence of myeloma, POEMS syndrome, amyloidosis, or cryoglobulinemia. Nonmalignant monoclonal gammopathies are found more frequently in patients with neuropathy of otherwise unknown etiology; however, they are also present in approximately 1% of normal adults, and the frequency increases with age or in chronic infections or inflammatory diseases, so the association with neuropathy in some cases could be coincidental. Other causes of neuropathy, particularly inflammatory conditions such as CIDP, should be considered. In cases of myeloma, irradiation, chemotherapy, or bone marrow transplantation may be beneficial. Some patients with neuropathy associated with IgG and IgA monoclonal proteins of undetermined significance (MGUS) improve with plasmapheresis.

NEUROPATHIES ASSOCIATED WITH IMMUNOGLOBULIN M MONOCLONAL ANTIBODIES THAT REACT WITH PERIPHERAL NERVE GLYCOCONJUGATE ANTIGENS

In several syndromes, peripheral neuropathy is associated with polyclonal or monoclonal IgM autoantibodies that react with glycoconjugates in peripheral nerve. IgM antibodies that react with MAG are associated with a chronic demyelinating sensorimotor neuropathy. Pathologic studies show deposits of the monoclonal IgM and complement on affected myelin sheaths, and passive transfer of the autoantibodies in experimental animals reproduces the neuropathy. Treatment consisting of plasmapheresis and che-

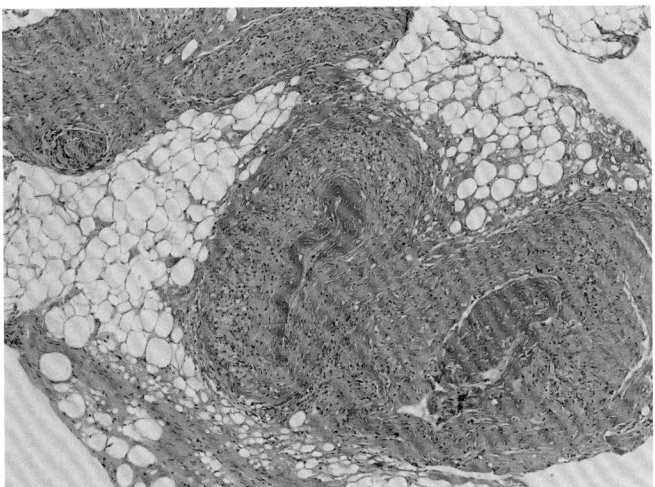

FIGURE 87.7 Necrotizing vasculitis (magnification ×200).

motherapy to reduce autoantibody concentrations, or IVIG, frequently results in clinical improvement.

Other syndromes associated with monoclonal or polyclonal IgM autoantibodies include the following: MMN or lower motor neuron syndrome–associated anti-GD1a ganglioside antibodies, large-fiber sensory neuropathy with anti-GD1b and disialosyl ganglioside antibodies, and axonal sensory neuropathy associated with antisulfatide antibodies. Antisulfatide antibodies typically are associated with small-fiber or small- and large-fiber neuropathy, but 25% of cases demonstrate a CIDP-like demyelinating neuropathy.

PROGRESSIVE INFLAMMATORY NEUROPATHY (AMONG SWINE SLAUGHTERHOUSE WORKERS)

Beginning in 2007, 24 patients who worked in three different pork-processing plants developed an inflammatory neuropathy that resembled CIDP. Those affected worked at the head table, where a compressed air device was used to extract pig brains. Patients had a polyradiculoneuropathy with weakness and pain. Some patients had facial neuropathy. The symptoms progressed from 8 to 213 days. The CSF protein was elevated in the majority from 63 to 210 mg/dL, with pleocytosis in only one patient. Nerve conduction studies showed demyelinating and axonal changes. Serum from the patients demonstrated IgG staining of neural tissue.

AMYLOID NEUROPATHY

Amyloid is an insoluble extracellular aggregate of proteins that forms in nerve or other tissues when any of several proteins is produced in excess. The two principal forms of amyloid protein that cause neuropathy are immunoglobulin light chains in patients with primary amyloidosis and plasma cell dyscrasias and transthyretin in hereditary amyloidosis. The syndrome is often that of a painful, small-fiber sensory neuropathy with progressive autonomic failure, symmetric loss of pain and temperature sensations with spared position and vibratory senses, carpal tunnel syndrome, or some combination of these symptoms. The diagnosis of amyloid neuropathy can be established by histologic demonstration of amyloid in nerve (Fig. 87.8),

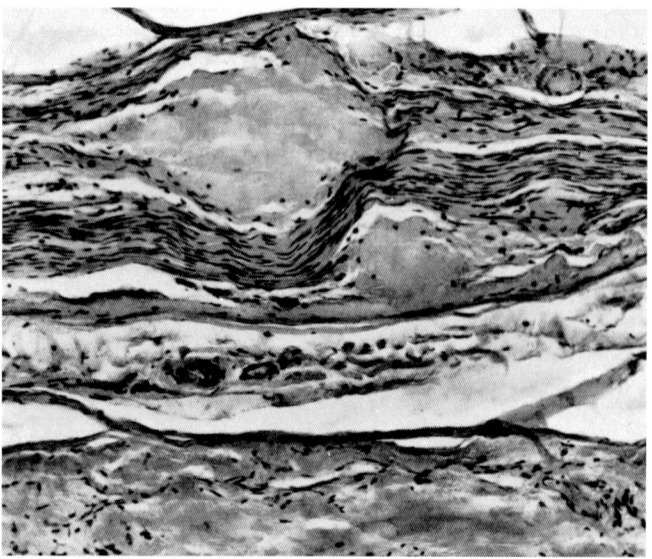

FIGURE 87.8 Amyloid neuropathy. Massive deposits of endoneurial amyloid compress nerve fiber bundles. (Courtesy of Dr. Arthur Asbury.)

followed by immunocytochemical characterization of the deposits with the use of antibodies to immunoglobulin light chains or transthyretin. Mutation of the transthyretin gene is detected by DNA analysis. Other hereditary amyloidosis causes, such as apolipoprotein A1 and gelsolin, lead to less severe and less frequent neuropathy. Electrophoresis of serum and urine with immunofixation can assist in the diagnosis of primary amyloid neuropathy. Prognosis is generally poor. Liver transplantation has been reported to be beneficial for hereditary amyloidosis, and high-dose chemotherapy followed by bone marrow transplantation has been reported to help some patients with primary amyloidosis. Medications that stabilize the transthyretin tetramer and decrease the formation of amyloid, including tafamidis 20 mg qd [**Level 1**][7] and diflunisal 250 mg qd [**Level 1**],[8] may improve the neuropathy. Also under development are RNA silencers, which block the production of transthyretin.

NEUROPATHY ASSOCIATED WITH CARCINOMA (PARANEOPLASTIC NEUROPATHY)

Both direct and indirect effects of malignant neoplasms on the peripheral nervous system are recognized. In some patients, the nerves or nerve roots are compressed or infiltrated by neoplastic cells. In others, there is no evidence of damage to the nerves by the neoplasm, and dietary deficiency or metabolic, toxic, or immunologic factors may be responsible.

The most characteristic paraneoplastic disorder is a sensory neuropathy of subacute onset associated with small cell carcinoma of the lung. Electrodiagnostic studies reveal loss of sensory-evoked responses. Autoantibodies against the Hu antigen (antineuronal nuclear or ANNA-1) are characteristic, and postmortem studies show loss of neurons, deposition of antibodies, and inflammatory cells in dorsal root ganglia.

Less consistently associated with carcinoma is a distal sensorimotor polyneuropathy without specific features. Nerve biopsy may reveal infiltration by tumor cells, axonal degeneration, or demyelination. A primarily motor syndrome of subacute onset rarely occurs in Hodgkin disease and other lymphomas. In these patients, the predominant lesion is degeneration of anterior horn cells, but demyelination, perivascular mononuclear cell infiltrates, and alterations in Schwann cell morphology in ventral roots are also observed.

The diagnosis of malignancy should be suspected in a middle-aged or elderly patient with a subacute sensory neuropathy or polyradiculopathy of obscure cause, particularly with weight loss. The course is often progressive unless the primary malignancy is successfully treated. CSF examination for malignant cells is valuable in the diagnosis of malignant meningeal infiltration. In some instances of meningeal infiltration, radiotherapy or intrathecal chemotherapy may be valuable.

HYPOTHYROID NEUROPATHY

Entrapment neuropathies are relatively common in patients with hypothyroidism, probably because acid mucopolysaccharide protein complexes (mucoid) are deposited in the nerve. Painful paresthesia in the hands and feet is the most common symptom of hypothyroidism. Weakness is not a feature. Tendon reflexes are reduced or absent and, when present, may show the characteristic delayed or "hung-up" response. Direct muscle percussion produces transient mounding of the underlying skin and muscle (myoedema). Nerve conduction studies show mild slowing of motor nerve conduction and decreased sensory response amplitude. Morphologic studies show evidence of demyelination, axonal loss, and excessive glycogen within Schwann cells. CSF protein content is often more than 100 mg/dL. Rarely, dysfunction of cranial nerves IX, X, and XII causes hoarseness and dysarthria, probably as a result of local myxedematous infiltration of the nerves. The peripheral neuropathy may occur before there is laboratory evidence of hypothyroidism. Once identified, thyroid replacement causes clinical, electrophysiologic, and morphologic improvement.

ACROMEGALIC NEUROPATHY

Entrapment neuropathy is also relatively common in patients with acromegaly. Rarely, acromegalic patients note distal paresthesia but in contrast to myxedematous patients, weakness may be severe and peripheral nerves may be palpable. There is a significant correlation between total exchangeable body sodium and the severity of the neuropathy. The nerves are enlarged because there is increased endoneurial and perineurial connective tissue, perhaps stimulated by increased levels of somatomedin C (IGF-1). Tendon reflexes are reduced. Nerve conduction velocities are mildly slow with low evoked response amplitudes.

HYPERTHYROID NEUROPATHY

Hyperthyroidism can produce a syndrome consisting of diffuse weakness and fasciculations with preserved or hyperactive tendon reflexes, resembling amyotrophic lateral sclerosis (ALS). However, the symptoms and signs disappear with treatment of the toxic state. No convincing pathologic studies have established the presence of chronic sensorimotor neuropathy with hyperthyroidism.

CELIAC NEUROPATHY

Celiac disease is a chronic inflammatory enteropathy with a prevalence of 1:250. Peripheral neuropathy is the most common neurologic condition associated with celiac disease. It is not thought to be a result of nutritional deficiency. In over half of patients with celiac neuropathy, gastrointestinal complaints are absent. Celiac disease is caused by exposure to ingested gluten, the storage proteins of wheat, and similar proteins found in barley and rye. Patients have specific HLA-DQ2 and HLA-DQ8 alleles.

The neuropathy is usually predominantly sensory. Multifocal involvement is frequent, with early involvement of the hands and face, although some have a length-dependent pattern. A small-fiber neuropathy is more common initially, but a sensorimotor polyneuropathy is also seen. Diagnosis is suspected with elevated gliadin or transglutaminase antibodies and confirmed by a duodenal biopsy demonstrating inflammation, crypt hyperplasia, and villous atrophy in the small intestine mucosa. Gastrointestinal symptoms improve with a gluten-free diet. The symptoms of peripheral neuropathy have improved in some, but not all, patients on a gluten-free diet. Only small amounts of gluten exposure can trigger an active immune response.

UREMIC NEUROPATHY

Peripheral neuropathy is only one of the neuromuscular syndromes associated with chronic renal failure. Restless legs, cramps, and muscle twitching may be early manifestations of peripheral nerve disease. Peripheral neuropathy is present in 70% of patients with chronic renal failure, but most are subclinical and are identified only by nerve conduction studies. Symptoms include painful dysesthesia and glove-stocking loss of sensation, as well as weakness of distal muscles. Electrodiagnostic studies show a sensorimotor neuropathy with axonal features. Pathologic studies confirm the axonopathy. Secondary demyelination may result from axonal loss. Dialysis rarely reverses the neuropathy but may stabilize symptoms; peritoneal dialysis is more effective than hemodialysis. Serial nerve conduction studies can measure the effectiveness of hemodialysis but is no longer routinely used. Renal transplantation often resolves the neuropathy following surgery.

Mononeuropathy, particularly carpal tunnel syndrome, often appears distal to an implanted arteriovenous fistula, suggesting ischemia as a possible mechanism. Distal ischemia from implanted bovine shunts may cause a more severe ischemic neuropathy in the median, ulnar, and radial nerves, possibly from excessive arteriovenous shunting. Chronic hemodialysis (>10 years) causes excessive accumulation of β_2-microglobulin (generalized amyloidosis), another possible cause of carpal tunnel syndrome and uremic polyneuropathy.

The cause of uremic neuropathy is uncertain. An accumulation of a toxic metabolite is most likely, but its identity is unknown. A 2- to 60-kDa molecular weight compound in the plasma of uremic patients induced an axonal neuropathy in experimental animals.

NEUROPATHY ASSOCIATED WITH HEPATIC DISEASE

Peripheral neuropathy is rarely associated with primary diseases of the liver. A painful sensory neuropathy is seen with primary biliary cirrhosis, probably caused by xanthoma formation in and around nerves. Electrodiagnostic studies may be normal, or the amplitude of the sensory-evoked response may be low or absent. Nerve biopsy shows loss of small-diameter nerve fibers. Sudanophilic material is seen in cells of the perineurium. Treatment is directed at pain control. Tricyclic antidepressants or anticonvulsants may relieve paresthesia.

Infectious diseases of the liver may also be associated with peripheral neuropathy. Viral hepatitis (especially hepatitis C associated with cryoglobulinemia), HIV or CMV infection, and infectious mononucleosis may be associated with acute demyelinating neuropathy (GBS), chronic demyelinating neuropathy, or mononeuropathy multiplex. Immunologically mediated diseases such as polyarteritis and sarcoidosis may also cause liver abnormalities and mononeuropathy multiplex.

Peripheral neuropathy is often seen with toxic liver disease or hepatic metabolic diseases such as acute intermittent porphyria and abetalipoproteinemia.

NEUROPATHIES ASSOCIATED WITH INFECTION

Neuropathy of Leprosy

Direct infiltration of small-diameter peripheral nerve fibers by *Mycobacterium leprae* causes the neuropathy of leprosy. It was formerly the most common neuropathy in the world, although it is now overtaken by diabetic neuropathy, largely because of a recent sharp decline in incidence in many endemic areas, especially India. From 2002 to 2007, the incidence globally had dramatically decreased at an average rate of nearly 20% per year based on WHO reports. In the United States, the disease is less endemic but is seen in immigrants from India, Southeast Asia, and Central Africa.

Peripheral nerves are affected differently in tuberculoid and lepromatous forms. In tuberculoid leprosy, there are small hypopigmented areas with superficial sensory loss, and the underlying subcutaneous sensory nerves may be visibly or palpably enlarged.

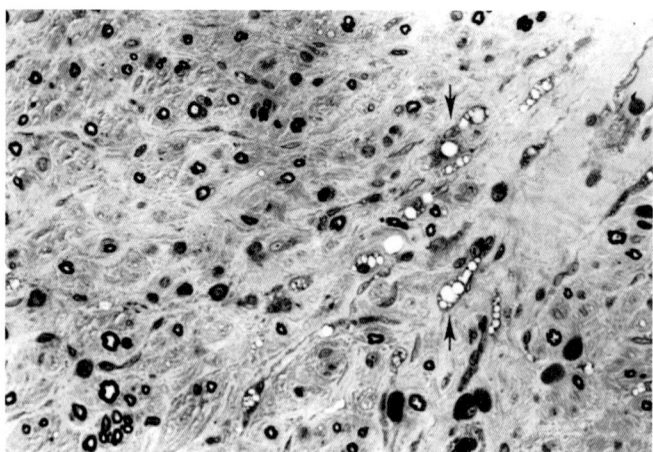

FIGURE 87.9 Lepromatous leprous neuritis. Few myelinated fibers are scattered in fibrotic endoneurium. Abundant foam cells (*arrows*) contain *M. leprae* bacilli when viewed at higher magnification. (Courtesy of Dr. Arthur Asbury.)

Large nerve trunks, such as the ulnar, fibular, facial, and posterior auricular nerves, may be enmeshed in granulomas and scar tissue. Endoneurial caseation necrosis may occur. The clinical picture is one of mononeuritis or mononeuritis multiplex.

In lepromatous leprosy, Hansen bacilli proliferate in large numbers within Schwann cells and macrophages in the endoneurium and perineurium of subcutaneous nerve twigs (Fig. 87.9), particularly in cool areas of the body (pinnae of the ears and dorsum of the hands, forearms, and feet). Loss of cutaneous sensibility is observed in affected patches; these may later coalesce to cover large parts of the body. Position sense may be preserved in affected areas, whereas pain and temperature sensibility is lost, a dissociation similar to that in syringomyelia. Tendon reflexes are preserved.

Acute mononeuritis multiplex may appear during chemotherapy of lepromatous leprosy in conjunction with erythema nodosum. This complication is treated with thalidomide, which is also associated with neuropathy.

Treatment is designed to eradicate the bacterium and to prevent secondary immune reactions that may damage nerves. Dapsone is effective but may cause toxic motor neuropathy. Because of the dense sensory loss, painless and inadvertent traumatic injuries, such as self-inflicted burns, may occur without extreme caution to avoid trauma to the anesthetic areas.

Diphtheritic Neuropathy

Although diphtheria itself is rare, diphtheritic neuropathy occurs in approximately 20% of infected patients. *Corynebacterium diphtheriae* infects the larynx and pharynx, as well as cutaneous wounds. The organisms release an exotoxin that causes myocarditis and, later, symmetric neuropathy. The neuropathy often begins with impaired visual accommodation and paresis of ocular and oropharyngeal muscles, and quadriparesis follows. Nerve conduction velocities are slow, reflecting the underlying demyelinating neuropathy. Diphtheria may be prevented by immunization, and if infection occurs, antibiotic therapy may be used. Recovery may be slow, and physiologic measures resolve after the clinical syndrome.

HIV-Related Neuropathies

Several neuropathies afflict patients infected with HIV, depending on the stage of the illness and the immunocompetence of the patient. An acute demyelinating neuropathy indistinguishable from sporadic GBS may occur early in the course of infection, often with no signs of immunodeficiency or at the time of seroconversion, as well as once AIDS develops. Sometimes a CSF pleocytosis is present, which is not typical of GBS in non–HIV-infected patients.

Subacute demyelinating neuropathy, clinically indistinguishable from idiopathic CIDP, is usually found in HIV-positive patients before there is evidence of immunodeficiency (AIDS). The CSF protein content is increased in both idiopathic CIDP and HIV-associated demyelinating neuropathy. Steroids, plasmapheresis, and IVIG therapy have been reported to be effective treatments.

In patients who fulfill diagnostic criteria for AIDS, there is frequently a distal sensorimotor polyneuropathy with axonal features. The syndrome is dominated by severe painful paresthesia most intensely affecting the feet. This painful neuropathy can be the most functionally disabling manifestation of AIDS. Nerve conduction studies may be normal, but reduced intraepidermal nerve fiber density is seen on skin biopsy. The exact mechanism is uncertain. HIV infection of dorsal root ganglion neurons has been demonstrated. Because of the scarcity of neuronal infection, other causes such as toxicity of activated macrophages and cytokines and viral protein toxicity have been considered. No treatment reverses the symptoms, but symptomatic medications, such as lamotrigine or gabapentin, may help. One form of neuropathy in HIV-infected patients is the diffuse infiltrative lymphocytosis syndrome (DILS), a hyperimmune reaction to HIV infection.

Mononeuropathy multiplex can occur in HIV-infected patients at any stage of the disease, sometimes with hepatitis. When CD4 cells number fewer than 50/mm^3, the likely cause of the mononeuropathy is CMV, and prompt treatment with ganciclovir sodium (Cytovene) may be lifesaving. CMV infection is also associated with polyradiculopathy.

The dideoxynucleotide antiretroviral medications, used to treat HIV infection, may cause painful sensory neuropathy, which is problematic to separate from primary painful HIV sensory neuropathy.

Neuropathy of Herpes Zoster

Varicella-zoster virus infection of the dorsal root ganglion produces radicular pain that may precede or follow the appearance of the characteristic skin eruption. Although primarily a sensory neuropathy, weakness from motor involvement occurs in 0.5% to 5% of infected patients. Herpes zoster (shingles) is a common phenomenon most frequent in elderly patients, cancer patients, or immunosuppressed patients. Postrash pain (postherpetic neuralgia) usually in the same distribution as the dermatomal rash occurs in a minority, but risk increases significantly with age (50% over 70 years). For diagnosis, pain should persist for 1 to 6 months after the rash disappears. Severe acute pain, more intense rash, scarring, sensory loss, and fever increase the risk of postherpetic neuralgia. Zoster infections are also associated with GBS and CSF pleocytosis. Zoster infection often occurs in patients with HIV infection; the combination of herpes infection and focal weakness in a young person should alert the clinician to the possibility of HIV infection.

Herpes zoster may affect any level of the neuraxis, but it most often involves thoracic dermatomes and cranial nerves with sensory ganglia (V and VII). Ophthalmic herpes infection characteristically involves the gasserian ganglion and the first division of the trigeminal nerve. There may be weakness of ocular muscles and ptosis. Infection of the geniculate ganglion of the facial (VII) nerve causes a vesicular herpetic eruption in the external auditory meatus, vertigo, deafness, and facial weakness (Ramsay Hunt syndrome). Pain is constant and burning and may include paroxysms of very severe pain.

Treatment with acyclovir (Zovirax), 4 g/day in five doses for 7 to 10 days or other antiviral agents decreases the incidence of segmental motor neuritis and sensory axonopathy. They may also reduce the incidence of postherpetic neuralgia. Tricyclic antidepressants, opioids, anticonvulsants (pregabalin), and lidocaine patches may show symptomatic benefit, some verified in randomized clinical trials. An attenuated varicella-zoster virus vaccine is recommended in adults 60 years and older, without contraindications, to prevent the development of herpes zoster.

SARCOID NEUROPATHY

Neurologic symptoms appear in 4% of patients with sarcoidosis. Most commonly, there are single or multiple cranial nerve palsies that fluctuate in intensity. Of the cranial nerves, the seventh is most commonly affected, and, as in diabetes mellitus, the facial nerve syndrome in sarcoidosis is indistinguishable from idiopathic Bell palsy. Some cranial neuropathies in sarcoidosis result from basilar meningitis. One distinguishing feature of sarcoid mononeuropathy is a large area of sensory loss on the trunk.

Patients with sarcoidosis occasionally experience symmetric polyneuropathy months or years after the diagnosis is established. The neuropathy may be the first manifestation before the diagnosis of sarcoidosis is made. The clinical syndromes may include GBS, lumbosacral plexopathy, mononeuritis multiplex, pure sensory neuropathy, and small-fiber and autonomic neuropathy. Cranial nerve symptoms are seen in close to one-half of patients.

Nerve biopsy shows a mixture of wallerian degeneration and segmental demyelination with sarcoid granulomas in endoneurium and epineurium (Fig. 87.10). Sarcoid neuropathy may respond to steroid therapy.

POLYNEUROPATHY ASSOCIATED WITH DIETARY STATES

Thiamine deficiency may cause two clinical syndromes: *wet beriberi*, in which congestive heart failure is the predominant syndrome, and *dry beriberi*, in which peripheral neuropathy is the predominant symptom. Patients with thiamine deficiency have severe

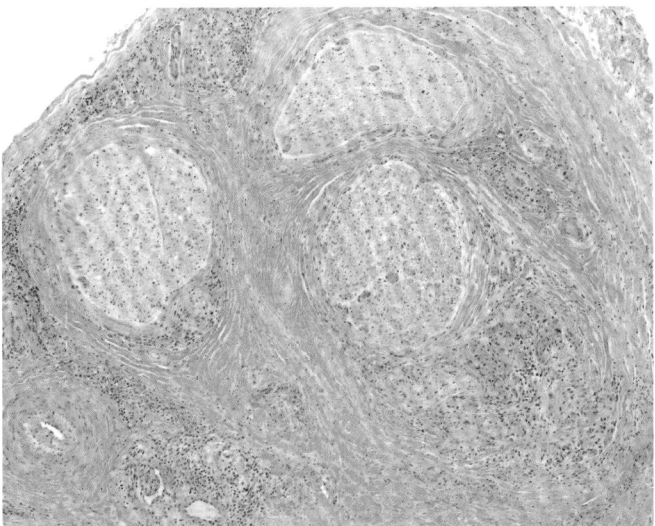

FIGURE 87.10 Nerve biopsy in patient with sarcoid neuropathy showing granuloma (magnification ×40).

burning dysesthesia in the feet more than in the hands, weakness and wasting of distal muscles more than of proximal muscles, trophic changes (shiny skin, hair loss), and distal sensory loss. EMG and nerve conduction studies reveal the presence of a diffuse sensorimotor peripheral neuropathy that is axonal. Axonal degeneration is also the principal finding seen on nerve biopsy specimens. Treatment of both beriberis should include parenteral B-complex vitamins followed by oral thiamine. Recovery is slow; there may be residual muscular weakness and atrophy.

Niacin (nicotinic acid) deficiency causes pellagra characterized by hyperkeratotic skin lesions. Peripheral neuropathy is usually present in niacin-deficient patients, but the neuropathy does not improve solely with niacin supplementation, likely because of multivitamin deficiency. Symptoms usually improve when additional thiamine and pyridoxine are added to the diet.

Vitamin B_{12} deficiency causes the classic clinical syndrome of subacute combined degeneration of the spinal cord. Separation of the peripheral neuropathic symptoms from spinal cord involvement is difficult. Painful paresthesias are present, but sensory ataxia with loss of vibration and joint position sense is most severe. Despite the myelopathy, tendon reflexes are often diminished or absent. B_{12}-deficiency neuropathy may be present with low normal B_{12} levels and can be established with measurement of the elevated metabolites methylmalonic acid and homocysteine.

Nitrous oxide also irreversibly inactivates cobalamin, producing the same syndrome. A single anesthetic dose in a vulnerable individual or chronic exposure usually with abuse of dental or medical sources or commercial propellants (whipped cream) may result in B_{12} deficiency. Hematologic abnormalities are usually absent in abuse cases.

Vitamin B_6 (pyridoxine) deficiency produces a peripheral neuropathy, and the most common cause of pyridoxine deficiency is ingestion of the antituberculous drug isoniazid. Isoniazid increases the excretion of pyridoxine. The resulting neuropathy affects sensory fibers more than motor fibers and is caused by axonal loss. Treatment consists of supplemental pyridoxine to compensate for the added excretion. The neuropathy can be prevented by prophylactic pyridoxine administration. Pyridoxine excess can lead to severe sensory neuropathy as well.

Vitamin E deficiency contributes to neuropathy in fat malabsorption syndromes—including abetalipoproteinemia, congenital biliary atresia, pancreatic dysfunction, and surgical removal of large portions of the small intestine. The clinical syndrome of vitamin E deficiency resembles spinocerebellar degeneration with ataxia, severe sensory loss of joint position and vibration, and hyporeflexia. Motor nerve conduction studies are normal, but sensory-evoked responses are of low amplitude or absent.

Somatosensory-evoked responses show a delay in central conduction. EMG is usually normal. Serum vitamin E levels can be measured. Repletion with large oral doses is often sufficient if initiated early in the disease course.

Copper deficiency can result in a neuropathy, which is often accompanied by a myelopathy and leukopenia. Some patients develop copper deficiency from excessive use of zinc. Copper supplementation stops the progression, although recovery is often not complete.

Strachan syndrome includes visual loss, oral ulcers, skin changes, and painful neuropathy. The syndrome was originally described in Jamaican sugar workers and caused an epidemic in Cuba in 1991. A nutrient-poor diet with deficient B vitamins has been implicated.

Gastric bypass surgery is associated with subacute and sometimes severe axonal neuropathy that accompanies the rapid postoperative weight loss. Vitamin deficiency of various types is to play a crucial role.

CRITICAL ILLNESS POLYNEUROPATHY

Severe sensorimotor peripheral neuropathy is seen in many patients who are critically ill, suffering from sepsis and multiple organ failure. The diagnosis may arise when a patient experiences difficulty being weaned from a ventilator after a bout of sepsis. Electrodiagnostic studies show a severe sensorimotor axonal neuropathy, but conventional studies may be unable to distinguish this entity from the more common critical illness myopathy, discussed in detail in Chapter 91. Recovery of neuronal function may occur if the underlying cause of multiple organ failure is treated successfully.

NEUROPATHIES CAUSED BY HEAVY METALS

Arsenic

Neuropathy may follow chronic exposure to small amounts of arsenic or ingestion or parenteral administration of a large amount. Chronic exposure may occur in industries in which arsenic is released as a byproduct, such as in copper or lead smelting. Because of the prevalence of these byproducts, arsenic neuropathy is the most common of all heavy metal–induced neuropathies. Acute gastrointestinal symptoms, vomiting, and diarrhea occur when a toxic quantity of arsenic is ingested, but these symptoms may be absent if the arsenic is given parenterally or taken in small amounts over long periods. Acute exposure may lead to encephalopathy or coma. The evolution of polyneuropathy is much slower in chronic arsenic poisoning. Sensory symptoms are prominent in the early stages. Pain and paresthesia in the legs may be present for several days or weeks before onset of weakness. The weakness may progress to complete flaccid paralysis of the legs and sometimes the arms, depending on the dosage. Cutaneous sensation is impaired in a stocking-and-glove distribution, with vibration and position sensation being most affected. Tendon reflexes are lost. Pigmentation and hyperkeratosis of the skin and changes in the nails (*Mees lines*) are frequently present. Arsenic is present in the urine in the acute stages of poisoning but is quickly cleared; levels persist in the hair and nails. Nerve conduction velocities may be normal or mildly diminished; the amplitude of sensory- and motor-evoked responses may be reduced. Pathologic examination of nerves shows axonal degeneration. Arsenic polyneuropathy is generally treated with a chelating agent, but the effectiveness is uncertain, given the rapid clearance in most patients.

Lead

Most toxic neuropathies cause symmetric weakness and loss of sensation in distal regions more than proximal regions, feet worse than legs. Lead neuropathy is atypical because of motor predominance and arm involvement.

Lead neuropathy occurs almost exclusively in adults. Infants poisoned with lead usually develop encephalopathy. Lead may enter the body through the lungs, skin, or gut. Occupational lead poisoning was common in earlier eras, notably in silver miners, but rarely is encountered in battery workers, painters, and pottery glazers. Accidental lead poisoning follows ingestion of lead in food or beverages or occurs in children who ingest lead paint. Lead poisoning may cause abdominal distress (lead colic). The classic description is focal wrist-drop in a radial neuropathy pattern; however, weakness is not generally limited to one nerve and produces bilateral arm weakness and wasting and lesser or later leg involvement. Footdrop is the most common leg sign. Sensory symptoms and signs are usually absent. Rarely, upper motor neuron signs occur with the lower motor neuron disorder and mimic ALS. Laboratory findings include anemia with basophilic stippling of the red cells, increased serum uric acid, and slight elevation of CSF protein content. Urinary lead excretion is elevated, particularly after administration of a chelating agent. Urinary porphobilinogen excretion is also elevated, but δ-aminolevulinic acid is normal. Primary therapy is prevention of further exposure to lead. With termination of exposure and use of chelation therapy, recovery is gradual over several months.

Mercury

Mercury is used in the electrical and chemical industries. There are two forms of mercury: elemental and organic. The organic form of mercury (methyl and ethyl mercury) is most toxic to the CNS, although distal paresthesia and sensory ataxia are prominent (presumably secondary to dorsal root ganglion degeneration). Ventral roots and motor function are spared. Inorganic mercury may be absorbed through the gastrointestinal tract, and elemental mercury may be absorbed directly through the skin or lungs (it is volatile at room temperature). Elemental mercury exposure is a rare cause of weakness and axonal motor and sensory fiber loss.

Thallium

This element is used as a rodenticide and in other industrial processes. Children exposed to thallium, as with lead, may develop encephalopathy, whereas neuropathy occurs in adults. In contrast to lead poisoning, thallium neuropathy primarily affects sensory and autonomic fibers. Severe disturbing dysesthesia appears acutely, and diffuse alopecia is a characteristic feature. Signs of cardiovascular autonomic neuropathy are sometimes delayed and recover slowly. Electrophysiologic findings are consistent with an axonal neuropathy.

Other Chemicals

Acrylamide monomer is used to prepare polyacrylamide. It is used in chemical laboratories and for the treatment of liquid sewage. Exposure to the monomer produces a distal sensorimotor neuropathy that may be associated with trophic skin changes and a mild dementia. Polyacrylamides, however, are not neurotoxic. Carbon disulfide (CS_2) is rarely inhaled in industrial settings. Exposure may lead to sensorimotor axonal neuropathy.

Many organophosphates, used in insecticides and rodenticides, are acetylcholinesterase inhibitors and may cause delayed neuropathy. The clinical and electrophysiologic features are similar to those of neuropathies caused by chemotherapeutics. Some, however, affect the CNS, as well as peripheral nerves, and some have certain specific features. *Triorthocresyl phosphate* (Jamaica ginger or jake), an adulterant used in illegal liquor (moonshine) and as a cooking oil contaminant, was responsible for neuropathy epidemics. *Dimethylaminopropionitrile*, which is used to manufacture polyurethane foam, causes urologic dysfunction and sensory loss localized to sacral dermatomes. Exposure to *methylbromide*, an insecticide, results in a mixture of pyramidal tract, cerebellar, and peripheral nerve dysfunction. Accidental ingestion of *pyriminil*, a rat poison marketed under the name Vacor, gives rise to an acute severe distal axonopathy with prominent autonomic involvement accompanied by acute diabetes mellitus secondary to necrosis of pancreatic β cells.

Drugs of abuse may lead to neuropathy, notably *n*-hexane and methyl-*N*-butyl ketone, found in widely available household solvents, fuels, and cleaning agents. Inhalation of these materials through the nose or mouth (huffing) occurs in teens and young adults. Axonal degeneration with sensory and motor impairment is seen, but focal conduction block associated with giant axonal swellings is also characteristic. The phenomenon is similar to the rare hereditary entity, giant axonal neuropathy, linked to a defect in the gigaxonin gene.

Ingested neurotoxins from various sea creatures harboring toxins can induce nerve dysfunction, mostly through sodium channel blockade and block in nerve conduction, mostly producing sensory neuropathy, cramps, diarrhea, and vomiting. Examples include ciguatera from reef fish exposed to a ciguatoxin-producing dinoflagellate, saxitoxin (paralytic shellfish poisoning), brevetoxin B (neurotoxic shellfish poisoning), and tetrodotoxin (puffer fish [fugu]). A number of insect venoms are also neurotoxic. Most cause neuromuscular junction blockade, but some, including tick paralysis and frog skin toxins, block sodium channels and peripheral nerve conduction.

NEUROPATHIES CAUSED BY THERAPEUTIC DRUGS

Many medications have been suspected of causing neuropathy, but relatively few have convincing clinical features, laboratory support, or reproduction in animal models. Different aspects of the problem are discussed in Chapters 105 and 128. Most of these neuropathies are dose related, presenting with predominantly sensory symptoms and signs or with a combination of sensory, motor, and autonomic involvement. Most cause toxicity by targeting the axon or dorsal root ganglion neurons directly, but toxicity to Schwann cells and myelin occurs with some agents as well. Pathogenic mechanisms are agent specific and varied. Identification of a toxic effect is most simple when symptoms occur soon after drug exposure or a change in dosage. Most patients fall into this category. In contrast, it is problematic to diagnose a slowly progressive neuropathy starting many months or years on a chronic agent. For example, statin drugs provide a case in point and are discussed later. "Coasting" is a phenomenon in which neuropathy may continue to progress, usually for 2 to 3 weeks, despite drug discontinuation. Improvement after drug cessation helps support the toxic effect, but recovery may be delayed for many months or be incomplete when significant axonal degeneration occurs. Discussion of all of the numerous substances temporally linked to neuropathy is outside the scope of this chapter, and the interested reader should consult comprehensive reviews cited in the "Suggested Readings" section. Some of the more important and best established causes are discussed.

Chemotherapy is an area in which some toxicity is tolerable assuming the agent is efficacious. The most commonly used antineoplastic agents linked with neuropathy are *vincristine*, *cisplatin* (Platinol), *carboplatin*, *oxaliplatin*, and *taxoids* (paclitaxel, docetaxel). Vincristine causes a dose-dependent, symmetric, progressive sensorimotor distal neuropathy that begins in the legs and is associated with areflexia. CMT type 1A patients are especially vulnerable, and treatment may unmask subclinical cases. In contrast, platin neuropathy is a purely sensory distal neuropathy with paresthesia, impaired vibration sense, and loss of ankle jerks, likely owing to toxicity and drug access to dorsal root ganglia but not α-motor neurons. The drug binds to and alters DNA and may trigger apoptosis if DNA repair fails. An additional acute, transient syndrome of cold-induced paresthesias, painful throat and jaw tightness, and occasionally focal weakness is associated with oxaliplatin infusion; peripheral nerve hyperexcitability has been demonstrated.

Paclitaxel (Taxol) is used to treat cancers of the breast, ovary, and lung. It causes a predominantly sensory neuropathy, but administration of a single high dose may affect motor and autonomic fibers as well. Disordered arrays of microtubules are induced.

Neuropathy is also a prominent feature in chemotherapy with suramin (axonal or demyelinating), bortezomib (Velcade), misonidazole, ixabepilone, and thalidomide (sensory). Many chemoprotectant agents to blunt the neurotoxic effects have been studied; none are routinely used in humans, but some show promise. Use of numerous other therapeutic drugs may produce neuropathy, including colchicine (myoneuropathy), gold salts, isoniazid (without B_6), metronidazole, nitrofurantoin, and podophyllotoxin resin. Amiodarone (Cordarone) may cause a severe symmetric distal sensorimotor neuropathy, an autonomic or demyelinating neuropathy resembling CIDP. Phenytoin (Dilantin) may produce minor distal sensory impairment and areflexia but mostly after long-standing high dosage and is likely overdiagnosed. The major toxicity of some nucleoside analog antiretroviral medications (didanosine [ddI], zalcitabine [ddC], and stavudine [d4T]) is peripheral neuropathy, which may be difficult to distinguish from HIV neuropathy. Others, such as azidothymidine (AZT), are not linked to neuropathy. A predominantly motor neuropathy has been related to disulfiram (Antabuse) and to dapsone. Statin use was associated with idiopathic neuropathy in a single large study, especially in those with definite neuropathy and longer term exposure. The methods of this study have been criticized, and the link remains controversial. Another large study in patients with diabetes mellitus found statin use protective against developing neuropathy.

ALCOHOLIC NEUROPATHY

Peripheral neuropathy in alcohol abusers is well known, but the cause is still debated. A widely held belief is that the neuropathy of alcoholism is owing entirely to nutritional deficiency, particularly vitamin B_1 (thiamine). Koike and colleagues, however, provide the best support for a direct toxic effect of ethanol. Alcoholics with normal thiamine levels develop predominantly small-fiber sensory neuropathy, the most frequent clinical type. More subacute onset with motor involvement is also seen in alcoholics with thiamine deficiency and nondrinkers with primary thiamine deficiency. Symptoms of small-fiber neuropathy, such as burning and pain, are common in chronic alcohol drinkers. Later, loss of vibration sense, proprioception, and tendon reflexes may occur. Sensory ataxia may be problematic to separate from alcoholic cerebellar degeneration. Abstinence can lead to meaningful recovery; vitamin supplements alone are not clearly effective but advised.

DIABETIC NEUROPATHY

Peripheral neuropathy occurs in approximately 50% of patients with diabetes mellitus, most commonly as a distal symmetric neuropathy. There are, however, several other distinct neuropathy syndromes that occur in patients with diabetes.

In one form, the symptoms and signs are transient; in the other, they progress steadily. The transient category includes acute painful neuropathies, mononeuropathies, and radiculopathies. The painful type starts abruptly with a disabling and continuous pain, often a burning sensation in a stocking distribution. Sometimes, the pain is localized to the thighs as a femoral neuropathy. The onset is often associated with weight loss. This disorder has been designated "diabetic neuropathic cachexia." The pain may last for months. Recovery from severe pain, however, is usually complete within 1 year, and the disorder does not necessarily progress to a conventional sensory polyneuropathy.

The progressive type comprises sensorimotor polyneuropathies with or without autonomic symptoms and signs. Although the actual cause of diabetic neuropathies is unknown, focal nerve involvement is considered to be immune mediated, and progressive symmetric polyneuropathy is probably owing to microvascular disease resulting from hyperglycemia. There may be as many causal factors as there are clinical pictures. There is evidence of oxidative damage and activation of protein kinase C β-activation in endothelial cells. However, it seems that hyperglycemic hypoxia is mainly responsible for the conduction changes seen in damaged diabetic nerves. Dysfunction of ion conductances, especially voltage-gated ion channels, could contribute to abnormalities in the generation and conduction of action potentials.

Impaired glucose tolerance is also associated with peripheral neuropathy. A 2-hour glucose tolerance test is the preferred method to screen for diabetes or impaired glucose tolerance in patients with neuropathy, being preferable to a fasting glucose or a hemoglobin A1c.

A syndrome recognized by a triad of pain; severe asymmetric muscle weakness; and wasting of the iliopsoas, quadriceps, and adductor muscles is named *diabetic amyotrophy* or *diabetic lumbosacral radiculoplexus neuropathy*. Onset is usually acute, but it may evolve over weeks. It occurs primarily in older non–insulin-dependent diabetics and is often accompanied by severe weight loss and (diabetic neuropathic cachexia). Knee reflexes are absent, but there is little or no sensory loss. Although long described as involving the proximal leg muscles, this syndrome can also involve the arms and even respiratory system. The condition improves spontaneously but may last 1 to 3 years with incomplete recovery.

Mononeuropathies

It is generally believed but incompletely proven that focal neuropathies are more frequent in diabetic patients than in the general population. The syndromes are usually localized to common sites of nerve entrapment or external compression and may imply an increased liability to pressure palsies. This applies to the median nerve at the carpal tunnel, the ulnar at the elbow, and the fibular at the fibular head. The electrophysiologic features are similar to those seen in nondiabetic patients with pressure palsies, except that abnormalities outside the clinically affected areas sometimes indicate that the palsies are superimposed on a generalized neuropathy. Cranial nerve palsies are most often localized to the third and sixth nerves. They start abruptly and usually spontaneously resolve completely within 6 months; relapses are rare.

Generalized Polyneuropathies

The most common diabetic neuropathy is a diffuse distal symmetric and predominantly sensory neuropathy with or without autonomic manifestations. Balance may be impaired from proprioceptive loss. Distal limb weakness is usually minimal. The neuropathy develops slowly and is related to the duration of the diabetes, but not all patients are so afflicted. Once present, it does not resolve or significantly recover. Intensive glucose control limited complications, including peripheral neuropathy, in the diabetes control and complication trial (DCCT) with significant differences in nerve conduction values between intensive and standard glucose control groups [**Level 1**].[9] Pain and temperature sensation transmitted through the smallest fibers may be affected before the large-fiber modalities (vibration, light touch, position sense). Small-fiber function can be evaluated by determining perception thresholds for warming and cooling or increasingly by assessment of epidermal nerve fiber density from skin biopsy samples (Fig. 87.11). Many patients with diabetic neuropathy do not have pain but do have numb or anesthetic feet. Diabetic neuropathy is the major predictor of foot ulcers and amputations.

The prevalence of diabetic autonomic neuropathy (DAN) may be underestimated because nonspecific symptoms are undiagnosed or

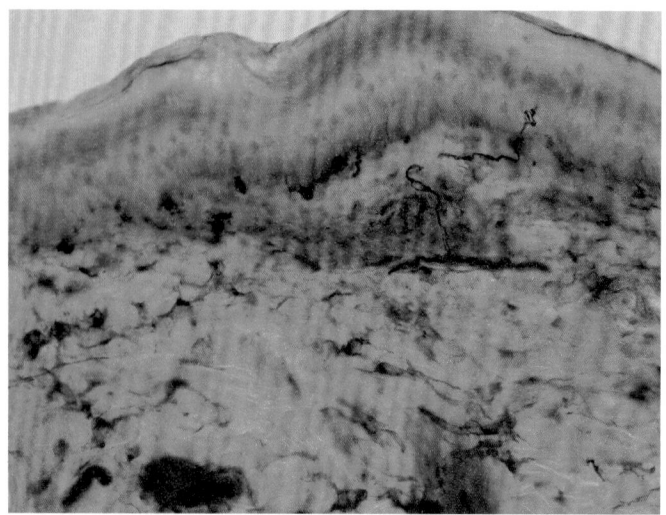

FIGURE 87.11 Skin biopsy with staining for PGP 9.5, which shows a reduced number of nerve fibers crossing the epidermal–dermal border (magnification × 400).

the condition may be asymptomatic. Symptoms appear insidiously after the onset of diabetes. The process progresses slowly and is usually irreversible. DAN is an important prognostic indicator with a mortality rate in diabetics without other initial complications of 23% at 8 years compared to 3% at 8 years in diabetics without DAN and similar disease duration. Noninvasive autonomic screening batteries can be performed, and dedicated autonomic testing laboratories are becoming widely available (see Chapter 112).

Mild slowing of motor and sensory conduction is a common finding in diabetics, even among those without overt neuropathy. It is generally attributed to axonal degeneration with secondary demyelination. Therapeutic attempts, including continuous subcutaneous insulin infusion to correct hyperglycemia to prevent the diabetic complications, have been unsuccessful in most instances. Although combined pancreas and kidney transplantation may halt the progression of diabetic polyneuropathy, the long-term effect is still doubtful. Patients with pain may benefit from duloxetine or pregabalin, but side effects may preclude treatment in some.

LYME NEUROPATHY

Lyme disease is commonly diagnosed in the United States and Europe. It is caused by a tick-borne spirochete, *Borrelia burgdorferi*. The most common clinical feature of neuroborreliosis is a painful sensory radiculitis, which may appear about 3 weeks after the erythema migrans. Pain intensity varies from day to day and is often severe, jumping from one area to another and often associated with patchy areas of unpleasant dysesthesia. Onset may be subacute potentially simulating GBS but with significant CSF pleocytosis and without clear signs of demyelination. Focal neurologic signs are common and may present as cranial neuropathy (61%), limb paresis (12%), or both (16%), but detailed electrodiagnostic signs often point to mononeuropathy multiplex. The clinical pattern may appear as a mononeuropathy, plexopathy, mononeuropathy multiplex, or distal symmetric polyneuropathy. The facial nerve is frequently affected; involvement is unilateral twice as often as bilateral. Ophthalmoparesis occasionally occurs. Myeloradiculitis and chronic progressive encephalomyelitis are rare. In some, the disorder is associated with dilated cardiomyopathy. Arthralgia is common among patients in the United States but rare among

Europeans (6%). The triad of painful radiculitis, predominantly cranial mononeuritis multiplex, and lymphocytic pleocytosis in the CSF is known as *Bannwarth syndrome* in Europe. Peripheral nerve biopsy shows perineurial and epineurial vasculitis and axonal degeneration. The diagnosis of neuroborreliosis is based on the presence of inflammatory CSF changes and specific intrathecal *B. burgdorferi* antibodies. In some infected patients, however, no free antibodies are detectable. Antigen detection in CSF is sometimes helpful. Polymerase chain reaction technique for detecting spirochetes or spirochetal DNA is less specific. The prognosis is good after high-dose penicillin or ceftriaxone treatment. Disabling sequelae are rare and occur mainly in patients with previous CNS lesions.

IDIOPATHIC NEUROPATHY

Patients with a peripheral neuropathy of undiagnosed cause may be later found to have an immune-mediated or hereditary neuropathy with more intensive evaluation. Even then, however, 10% to 35% of patients remain without an identified cause. Among those with painful sensory neuropathy involving the feet, this percentage is even higher. Although no cure is available for the neuropathy, treatment may include management of pain, physical therapy, and counseling related to prognosis. When there is no identifiable cause of a symmetric predominantly sensory neuropathy, after a thorough evaluation, the neuropathy rarely progresses to loss of ambulation or disability. Persistent pain is a frequent problem. Care must be taken to conduct an adequate search for treatable underlying disorders.

LEVEL 1 EVIDENCE

1. French Cooperative Group on Plasma Exchange in Guillain-Barré Syndrome. Plasma exchange in Guillain-Barré syndrome: one-year follow-up. *Ann Neurol.* 1992;32:94–97.
2. The Guillain-Barré Syndrome Study Group. Plasmapheresis and acute Guillain-Barré syndrome. *Neurology.* 1985;35:1096–1104.
3. Plasma Exchange/Sandoglobulin Guillain-Barré Syndrome Trial Group. Randomised trial of plasma exchange, intravenous immunoglobulin, and combined treatments in Guillain-Barré syndrome. *Lancet.* 1997;349:225–230.
4. Dyck PJ, Daube J, O'Brien P, et al. Plasma exchange in chronic inflammatory demyelinating polyradiculoneuropathy. *N Engl J Med.* 1986;314:461–465.
5. Hughes RA, Donofrio PD, Bril V, et al. Intravenous immune globulin (10% caprylate-chromatography purified) for the treatment of chronic inflammatory demyelinating polyradiculoneuropathy: a randomised placebo-controlled trial. *Lancet Neurol.* 2008;7:136–144.
6. Hahn AF, Beydoun SR, Lawson V, et al; IVIG in MMN Study Team. A controlled trial of intravenous immunoglobulin in multifocal motor neuropathy. *J Peripher Nerv Syst.* 2013;18:321–330.
7. Coelho T, Maia LF, Martins da Silva A, et al. Tafamidis for transthyretin familial amyloid polyneuropathy: a randomized, controlled trial. *Neurology.* 2012;79:785–792.
8. Berk JL, Suhr OB, Obici L, et al; Diflunisal Trial Consortium. Repurposing diflunisal for familial amyloid polyneuropathy: a randomized clinical trial. *JAMA.* 2013;310(24):2658–2667.
9. The Diabetes Control and Complications Trial Research Group. The effect of intensive diabetes therapy on the development and progression of neuropathy. *Ann Intern Med.* 1995;122:561–568.

SUGGESTED READINGS

General

Cashman CR, Höke A. Mechanisms of distal axonal degeneration in peripheral neuropathies [published online ahead of print January 21, 2015]. *Neurosci Lett.*

Cioroiu C, Brannagan TH III. Peripheral neuropathy. *Curr Geriatr Reports.* 2014;3:83–90.

Dyck PJ, Thomas PK, eds. *Peripheral Neuropathy.* Philadelphia: WB Saunders; 2005.

England JD, Gronseth GS, Franklin G, et al. Practice parameter: evaluation of distal symmetric polyneuropathy: role of laboratory and genetic testing (an evidence-based review). *Neurology.* 2009;72:185–192.

Martyn CN, Hughes RA. Epidemiology of peripheral neuropathy. *J Neurol Neurosurg Psychiatry.* 1997;62:310–318.

Brachial Neuritis

Evans BA, Stevens JC, Dyck PJ. Lumbosacral plexus neuropathy. *Neurology.* 1981;31:1327–1330.

Kuhlenbäumer G, Hannibal MC, Nelis E, et al. Mutations in SEPT9 cause hereditary neuralgic amyotrophy. *Nat Genet.* 2005;37:1044–1046.

Sumner AJ. Idiopathic brachial neuritis. *Neurosurgery.* 2009;65(4)(suppl):A150–A152.

van Alfen N, van Engelen BG, Hughes RA. Treatment for idiopathic and hereditary neuralgic amyotrophy (brachial neuritis). *Cochrane Database Syst Rev.* 2009;(3):CD006976.

Thoracic Outlet Syndrome

Cherrington M, Cherrington C. Thoracic outlet syndrome: reimbursement patterns and patient profiles. *Neurology.* 1992;42:943–945.

Danielson K, Odderson IR. Botulinum toxin type A improves blood flow in vascular thoracic outlet syndrome. *Am J Phys Med Rehabil.* 2008;87:956–959.

Demondion X, Bacqueville E, Paul C, et al. Thoracic outlet: assessment with MR imaging in asymptomatic and symptomatic populations. *Radiology.* 2003;227:461–468.

Gilliatt RW, Le Quesne PL, Logue V, et al. Wasting of the hand associated with a cervical rib or band. *J Neurol Neurosurg Psychiatry.* 1977;33:615–624.

Kothari MJ, Macintosh K, Heistand M, et al. Medial antebrachial cutaneous sensory studies in the evaluation of neurogenic thoracic outlet syndrome. *Muscle Nerve.* 1998;21:647–649.

Levin KH, Wilbourn AJ, Maggiano HJ. Cervical rib and median sternotomy-related brachial plexopathies: a reassessment. *Neurology.* 1998;50:1407–1413.

Nord KM, Kapoor P, Fisher J, et al. False positive rate of thoracic outlet syndrome diagnostic maneuvers. *Electromyogr Clin Neurophysiol.* 2008;48(2):67–74.

Roos DB. Thoracic outlet syndrome is underdiagnosed. *Muscle Nerve.* 1999;22:126–129.

Sanders RJ, Hammond SL, Rao N. Diagnosis of thoracic outlet syndrome. *J Vasc Surg.* 2007;46:601–604.

Simon NG, Ralph JW, Chin C, et al. Sonographic diagnosis of true neurogenic thoracic outlet syndrome. *Neurology.* 2013;81:1965.

Tsao BE, Ferrante MA, Wilbourn AJ, et al. The electrodiagnostic features of true neurogenic thoracic outlet syndrome. *Muscle Nerve.* 2014;49:724–727.

Wilbourn AJ. Thoracic outlet syndrome is overdiagnosed. *Muscle Nerve.* 1999;22:130–136.

Radiation Plexopathy

Dropcho EJ. Neurotoxicity of radiation therapy. *Neurol Clin.* 2010;28(1):217–234.

Foley KM, Woodruff JM, Ellis FT, et al. Radiation-induced malignant and atypical peripheral nerve sheath tumors. *Ann Neurol.* 1980;7:311–318.

Lalu T, Mercier B, Birouk N, et al. Pure motor neuropathy after radiation therapy: 6 cases. *Rev Neurol (Paris).* 1998;154:40–44.

Pradat PF, Delanian S. Late radiation injury to peripheral nerves. *Handb Clin Neurol.* 2013;115:743–758.

Mononeuropathies

Buchthal F, Rosenfalck A, Trojaborg W. Electrophysiological findings in entrapment of the median nerve at the wrist and elbow. *J Neurol Neurosurg Psychiatry.* 1974;37:340–360.

Stewart JD. *Focal Peripheral Neuropathies.* 4th ed. West Vancouver, Canada: JBJ Publishing; 2009.

Sunderland S. *Nerves and Nerve Injuries*. 2nd ed. Edinburgh, United Kingdom: Churchill Livingstone; 1979.

Yuen EC, Olney RK, So YT. Sciatic neuropathy: clinical and prognostic features in 73 patients. *Neurology*. 2004;44:1669–1674.

Guillain–Barré Syndrome and Variants

Al-Shekhlee A, Katirji B. Electrodiagnostic features of acute paralytic poliomyelitis associated with West Nile virus infection. *Muscle Nerve*. 2004;29:376–380.

De Sousa EA, Brannagan TH. Guillain–Barré syndrome. In: Kalman B, Brannagan TH, eds. *Neuroimmunology in Clinical Practice*. Blackwell: Oxford; 2008:117–122.

Feasby TE, Gilbert JJ, Brown WP, et al. An acute axonal form of Guillain–Barré polyneuropathy. *Brain*. 1986;109:1115–1126.

Hafer-Macko C, Hsieh ST, Li CY, et al. Acute motor axonal neuropathy: an antibody-mediated attack on axolemma. *Ann Neurol*. 1996;40:635–644.

Hughes RA, Cornblath DR. Guillain–Barré syndrome. *Lancet*. 2005;366:1653–1666.

Ropper AH, Wijdicks EF, Truax BT. *Guillain–Barré Syndrome*. Philadelphia: FA Davis; 1991.

van den Berg B, Walgaard C, Drenthen J, et al. Guillain-Barré syndrome: pathogenesis, diagnosis, treatment and prognosis. *Nat Rev Neurol*. 2014;10:469–482.

Van Koningsveld R, Schmitz PIM, van der Meché FGA, et al. Effect of methylprednisolone when added to standard treatment with intravenous immunoglobulin for Guillain–Barré syndrome. *Lancet*. 2004;373:192–196.

Wakerley BR, Uncini A, Yuki N; GBS Classification Group. Guillain-Barré and Miller Fisher syndromes—new diagnostic classification. *Nat Rev Neurol*. 2014;10:537–544.

Willison H, Scherer SS. Ranvier revisited: novel nodal antigens stimulate interest in GBS pathogenesis. *Neurology*. 2014;83:106–108.

Chronic Inflammatory Demyelinating Polyneuropathy

Ad Hoc Subcommittee of the American Academy of Neurology AIDS Task Force. Research criteria for diagnosis of chronic inflammatory demyelinating polyneuropathy (CIDP). *Neurology*. 1991;41:617–618.

Berger AR, Bradley WG, Brannagan TH, et al. Guidelines for the diagnosis and treatment of chronic inflammatory demyelinating polyneuropathy. *J Peripher Nerv Syst*. 2003;8:282–284.

Brannagan TH. Current diagnosis of CIDP: the need for biomarkers. *J Peripher Nerv Syst*. 2011;16(suppl):3–13.

Brannagan TH. Current treatments of chronic immune mediated demyelinating polyneuropathies. *Muscle Nerve*. 2009;39:363–378.

Dyck PJ, Lais AC, Ohta M, et al. Chronic inflammatory polyradiculoneuropathy. *Mayo Clin Proc*. 1975;50:621–637.

Latov N. Diagnosis and treatment of chronic acquired demyelinating polyneuropathies. *Nat Rev Neurol*. 2014;10:435–446.

Van Dijk GW, Notermans NC, Franssen H, et al. Response to intravenous immunoglobulin treatment in chronic inflammatory demyelinating polyneuropathy with only sensory symptoms. *J Neurol*. 1996;243:318–322.

Multifocal Motor Neuropathy

Joint Task Force of the EFNS and the PNS. European Federation of Neurological Societies/Peripheral Nerve Society guideline on management of multifocal motor neuropathy. Report of a joint task force of the European Federation of Neurological Societies and the Peripheral Nerve Society. *J Peripher Nerv Syst*. 2010;15:295–301.

Kinsella L, Lange D, Trojaborg T, et al. The clinical and electrophysiologic correlates of anti-GM1 antibodies. *Neurology*. 1994;44:1278–1282.

Idiopathic Sensory Neuronopathy or Ganglioneuritis

Griffin JW, Cornblath DR, Alexander E, et al. Ataxic sensory neuropathy and dorsal root ganglioneuritis associated with Sjögren's syndrome. *Ann Neurol*. 1990;27:304–315.

Quattrini A, Corbo M, Dhaliwal SK, et al. Anti-sulfatide antibodies in neurological disease: binding to rat dorsal root ganglia neurons. *J Neurol Sci*. 1992;112:152–159.

Sobue G, Yasuda T, Kachi T, et al. Chronic progressive sensory ataxic neuropathy: clinicopathological features of idiopathic and Sjögren's syndrome associated cases. *J Neurol*. 1993;240:1–7.

Willison HJ, O'Leary CP, Veitch J, et al. The clinical and laboratory features of chronic sensory ataxic neuropathy with anti-disialosyl IgM antibodies. *Brain*. 2001;124:1968–1977.

Windebank AJ, Blexrud MD, Dyck PJ, et al. The syndrome of acute sensory neuropathy. *Neurology*. 1990;40:584–589.

Idiopathic Autonomic Neuropathy

Mericle RA, Triggs WJ. Treatment of acute pandysautonomia with intravenous immunoglobulin. *J Neurol Neurosurg Psychiatry*. 1997;62:529–531.

Vernino S, Vernino S, Low PA, et al. Autoantibodies to ganglionic receptors in autoimmune autonomic neuropathies. *N Engl J Med*. 2000;343:847–855.

Vasculitic and Cryoglobulinemic Neuropathies

Brannagan TH. Retroviral-associated vasculitis of the nervous system. *Neurol Clin*. 1997;15:927–944.

Collins MP, Periquet MI, Mendell JR, et al. Nonsystemic vasculitic neuropathy: insights from a clinical cohort. *Neurology*. 2003;61:623–630.

Dyck PJ, Benstead TJ, Conn DL, et al. Nonsystemic vasculitic neuropathy. *Brain*. 1987;110:845–854.

Ferri C, La Civita L, Longombardo R, et al. Mixed cryoglobulinaemia: a cross-road between autoimmune and lymphoproliferative disorders. *Lupus*. 1998;7:275–279.

Gwathmey KG, Burns TM, Collins MP, et al. Vasculitic neuropathies. *Lancet Neurol*. 2014;13:67–82.

Nemni R, Corbo M, Fazio R, et al. Cryoglobulinemic neuropathy: a clinical, morphological and immunocytochemical study of 8 cases. *Brain*. 1988;111:541–552.

Said G, Lacroix-Ciaudo C, Fujimura H, et al. The peripheral neuropathy of necrotizing arteritis: a clinicopathological study. *Ann Neurol*. 1988;23:461–466.

Neuropathies Associated with Myeloma and Nonmalignant Immunoglobulin G or Immunoglobulin A Monoclonal Gammopathies

Dispenzieri A, Kyle RA, Lacy MQ, et al. POEMS syndrome: definitions and long-term outcome. *Blood*. 2003;101:2496–2506.

Dyck PJ, Low PA, Windebank AJ, et al. Plasma-exchange in polyneuropathy associated with monoclonal gammopathy of undetermined significance. *N Engl J Med*. 1991;325:1482–1486.

Kelly JJ Jr, Kyle RA, Latov N. *Polyneuropathies Associated with Plasma Cell Dyscrasias*. Boston, MA: Martinus-Nijhoff; 1987.

Motor, Sensory, and Sensorimotor Neuropathies Associated with Immunoglobulin M Monoclonal or Polyclonal Autoantibodies to Peripheral Nerve

Dalakas MC, Rakocevic G, Salajegheh M, et al. Placebo-controlled trial of rituximab in IgM anti-myelin-associated glycoprotein antibody demyelinating neuropathy. *Ann Neurol*. 2009;65:286–293.

Latov N. Pathogenesis and therapy of neuropathies associated with monoclonal gammopathies. *Ann Neurol*. 1995;37(suppl 1):S32–S42.

Pedersen SF, Pullman SL, Latov N, et al. Physiological tremor analysis of patients with anti-myelin-associated glycoprotein associated neuropathy and tremor. *Muscle Nerve*. 1997;20:38–44.

Quattrini A, Corbo M, Dhaliwal SK, et al. Anti-sulfatide antibodies in neurological disease: binding to rat dorsal root ganglia neurons. *J Neurol Sci*. 1992;112:152–159.

Renaud S, Gregor M, Fuhr P, et al. Rituximab in the treatment of polyneuropathy associated with anti-MAG antibodies. *Muscle Nerve*. 2003;27:611–615.

Progressive Inflammatory Neuropathy

Center for Disease Control and Prevention. Investigation of progressive inflammatory neuropathy among swine slaughterhouse worker—Minnesota, 2007–2008. *MMWR Morb Mortal Wkly Rep*. 2008;57:122–124.

Meeusen JW, Klein CJ, Pirko I, et al. Potassium channel complex autoimmunity induced by inhaled brain tissue aerosol. *Ann Neurol*. 2012;71:417–426.

Amyloid Neuropathy

Benson MD, Kincaid JC. The molecular biology and clinical features of amyloid neuropathy. *Muscle Nerve*. 2007;36:411–423.

Kelly JJ Jr, Kyle RA, O'Brien PC, et al. The natural history of peripheral neuropathy in primary systemic amyloidosis. *Ann Neurol.* 1979;6:1–7.

Planté-Bordeneuve V, Said G. Familial amyloid polyneuropathy. *Lancet Neurol.* 2011;10:1086–1097.

Quattrini A, Nemni R, Sferrazza B, et al. Amyloid neuropathy simulating lower motor neuron disease. *Neurology.* 1998;51:600–602.

Neuropathy Associated with Carcinoma (Paraneoplastic Neuropathy)

Camdessanche JP, Antoine JC, Honnorat J, et al. Paraneoplastic peripheral neuropathy associated with anti-Hu antibodies. A clinical and electrophysiologic study of 20 patients. *Brain.* 2002;125:166–175.

Dalmau J, Graus F, Rosenblum MK, et al. Anti-Hu associated paraneoplastic encephalomyelitis/sensory neuropathy: a clinical study of 71 patients. *Medicine.* 1992;71:59–72.

Graus F, Dalmau J. Paraneoplastic neuropathies. *Curr Opin Neurol.* 2013;26: 489–495.

Schold SC, Cho ES, Somasundaram M, et al. Subacute motor neuronopathy: a remote effect of lymphoma. *Ann Neurol.* 1979;5:271–287.

Hypothyroid Neuropathy

Dyck PJ, Lambert EH. Polyneuropathy associated with hypothyroidism. *J Neuropathol Exp Neurol.* 1970;9:631–658.

Misiunas A, Niepomniszcze H, Ravera B, et al. Peripheral neuropathy in subclinical hypothyroidism. *Thyroid.* 1995;5:283–286.

Nemni R, Bottacchi E, Fazio R, et al. Polyneuropathy in hypothyroidism: clinical, electrophysiological and morphological findings in four cases. *J Neurol Neurosurg Psychiatry.* 1987;50:1454–1460.

Acromegalic Neuropathy

Jamal GA, Kerr DJ, McLellaan AR, et al. Generalized peripheral nerve dysfunction in acromegaly: a study by conventional and novel neurophysiological techniques. *J Neurol Neurosurg Psychiatry.* 1987;50:885–894.

Khaleeli AA, Levy RD, Edwards RHT, et al. The neuromuscular features of acromegaly: a clinical and pathological study. *J Neurol Neurosurg Psychiatry.* 1984;47:1009–1015.

Low PA, McLeod JG, Turtle JR, et al. Peripheral neuropathy in acromegaly. *Brain.* 1974;97:139–152.

Celiac Neuropathy

Brannagan TH, Hays AP, Chin SS, et al. Small fiber neuropathy/neuronopathy associated with celiac disease: skin biopsy findings. *Arch Neurol.* 2005;62:1574–1578.

Chin RL, Sander HW, Brannagan TH, et al. Celiac neuropathy. *Neurology.* 2003;60:1581–1585.

Cicarelli G, Della Rocca G, Amboni M, et al. Clinical and neurological abnormalities in adult celiac disease. *J Neurol Sci.* 2003;24:311–317.

Cooke WT, Smith WE. Neurological disorders associated with adult coeliac disease. *Brain.* 1966;89:683–722.

Kaplan JG, Pack D, Horoupian D, et al. Distal axonopathy associated with chronic gluten enteropathy: a treatable disorder. *Neurology.* 1988;38:642–645.

Uremic Neuropathy

Bolton CF. Peripheral neuropathies associated with chronic renal failure. *Can J Neurol Sci.* 1980;7:89–96.

Cantaro S, Zara G, Battaggia C, et al. *In vivo* and *in vitro* neurotoxic action of plasma ultrafiltrate from uraemic patients. *Nephrol Dial Transplant.* 1998;13:2288–2293.

Neuropathy Associated with Hepatic Disease

Inoue A, Tsukada M, Koh CS, et al. Chronic relapsing demyelinating polyneuropathy associated with hepatitis B infection. *Neurology.* 1987;37: 1663–1666.

Taukada N, Koh CS, Inoue A, et al. Demyelinating neuropathy associated with hepatitis B virus infection: detection of immune complexes composed of hepatitis B virus antigen. *Neurol Sci.* 1987;77:203–210.

Zaltron S, Puoti M, Liberini P, et al. High prevalence of peripheral neuropathy in hepatitis C virus infected patients with symptomatic and asymptomatic cryoglobulinaemia. *J Gastroenterol Hepatol.* 1998;30:391–395.

Neuropathy of Leprosy

Nascimento OJ. Leprosy neuropathy: clinical presentations. *Arq Neuropsiquiatr.* 2013;71:661–666.

Rosenberg RN, Lovelace RE. Mononeuritis multiplex in lepromatous leprosy. *Arch Neurol.* 1968;19:310–314.

World Health Organization. Leprosy elimination. Leprosy today. World Health Organization Web site. http://www.who.int/lep/en. Accessed April 29, 2015.

Diphtheritic Neuropathy

Kurdi A, Abdul-Kader M. Clinical and electrophysiological studies of diphtheritic neuritis in Jordan. *J Neurol Sci.* 1979;42:243–250.

Solders G, Nennesmo I, Persson A. Diphtheritic neuropathy: an analysis based on muscle and nerve biopsy and repeated neurophysiological and autonomic function tests. *J Neurol Neurosurg Psychiatry.* 1989;52:876–880.

HIV-Related Neuropathies

Behar R, Wiley C, McCutchan JA. Cytomegalovirus polyradiculopathy in AIDS. *Neurology.* 1987;37:557–561.

Brannagan TH, Nuovo GJ, Hays AP, et al. Human immunodeficiency virus infection of dorsal root ganglion neurons detected by polymerase chain reaction in situ hybridization. *Ann Neurol.* 1997;42:368–372.

Brannagan TH, Zhou Y. HIV-associated Guillain–Barré syndrome. *J Neurol Sci.* 2003;208:39–42.

Cornblath DR, McArthur JC, Kennedy PGE, et al. Inflammatory demyelinating peripheral neuropathies associated with human T-cell lymphotropic virus type III infection. *Ann Neurol.* 1987;21:32–40.

Gherardi RK, Chretien F, Delfau-Larue MH, et al. Neuropathy in diffuse infiltrative lymphocytosis syndrome. *Neurology.* 1998;50:1041–1044.

Said G, Lacroix C, Chemouli P, et al. Cytomegalovirus neuropathy in acquired immunodeficiency syndrome: a clinical and pathological study. *Ann Neurol.* 1991;29:139–195.

Schütz SG, Robinson-Papp J. HIV-related neuropathy: current perspectives. *HIV AIDS.* 2013;5:243–251.

Neuropathy of Herpes Zoster

Denny-Brown D, Adams RD, Brady PJ. Pathologic features of herpes zoster: a note on "geniculate herpes." *Arch Neurol Psychiatry.* 1944;51:216–231.

Dubinsky RM, Kabbani H, El-Chami Z, et al. Practice parameter: treatment of postherpetic neuralgia: an evidence-based report of the Quality Standards Subcommittee of the American Academy of Neurology. *Neurology.* 2004;63:959–965.

Dworkin RH, Johnson RW, Breuer J, et al. Recommendations for the management of herpes zoster. *Clin Infect Dis.* 2007;44:S1–S26.

Hales CM, Harpaz R, Ortega-Sanchez I, et al; Centers for Disease Control and Prevention. Update on recommendations for use of herpes zoster vaccine. *MMWR Morb Mortal Wkly Rep.* 2014;63:729–731.

Mondelli M, Romano C, Passero S, et al. Effects of acyclovir on sensory axonal neuropathy, segmental motor paresis and postherpetic neuralgia in herpes zoster patients. *Eur Neurol.* 1996;36:288–292.

Raja SN, Haythornthwaite JA, Pappagallo M, et al. Opioids versus antidepressants in postherpetic neuralgia. A randomized placebo-controlled trial. *Neurology.* 2002;59:1015–1021.

Tick Paralysis

Swift TR, Ignacio OJ. Tick paralysis: electrophysiologic signs. *Neurology.* 1975;25:1130–1133.

Vedanarayanan VV, Evans OB, Subramony SH. Tick paralysis in children; electrophysiology and possibility of misdiagnosis. *Neurology.* 2002;59:1088–1090.

Sarcoid Neuropathy

Burns TM, Dyck PJ, Aksamit AJ, et al. The natural history and long-term outcome of 57 limb sarcoidosis neuropathy cases. *J Neurol Sci.* 2006;244:77–87.

Hoitsma E, Marziniak M, Faber CG, et al. Small fibre neuropathy in sarcoidosis. *Lancet.* 2002;359:2085–2086.

Said G. Sarcoidosis of the peripheral nervous system. *Handb Clin Neurol.* 2013;115:485–495.

Polyneuropathy Associated with Dietary States

Green R, Kinsella LJ. Current concepts in the diagnosis of cobalamin deficiency. *Neurology.* 1995;45:1435–1440.

Kumar N, Elliott MA, Hoyer JD, et al. "Myelodysplasia," myeloneuropathy, and copper deficiency. *Mayo Clin Proc.* 2005;80:943–946.

Parry GJ, Bredeson DE. Sensory neuropathy with low-dose pyridoxine. *Neurology.* 1985;35:1466–1468.

Saperstein DS, Wolfe GI, Gronseth GS, et al. Challenges in the identification of cobalamin-deficiency polyneuropathy. *Arch Neurol.* 2003;60:1296–1301.

Schaumburg H, Kaplan J, Windebank A, et al. Sensory neuropathy from pyridoxine abuse. A new megavitamin syndrome. *N Engl J Med.* 1983;309:445–448.

Sokol RJ, Guggenheim MA, Iannaccone ST, et al. Improved neurologic function after long-term correction of vitamin E deficiency in children with chronic cholestasis. *N Engl J Med.* 1985;313:1580–1586.

Victor M, Adams RD, Collins GH. *The Wernicke–Korsakoff Syndrome.* Philadelphia: FA Davis; 1971.

Critical Illness Polyneuropathy

Bolton CF, Laverty DA, Brown JD, et al. Critically ill polyneuropathy: electrophysiological studies and differentiation from Guillain–Barré syndrome. *J Neurol Neurosurg Psychiatry.* 1986;49:563–573.

Neuropathy Produced by Metals, Toxins, and Therapeutic Agents

Buchthal F, Behse F. Electromyography and nerve biopsy in men exposed to lead. *Br J Ind Med.* 1979;36:135–147.

Cavaletti G. Chemotherapy-induced peripheral neurotoxicity (CIPN): what we need and what we know. *J Peripher Nerv Syst.* 2014;19:66–76.

Chang AP, England JD, Garcia CA, et al. Focal conduction block in n-hexane polyneuropathy. *Muscle Nerve.* 1998;21:964–969.

Chaudhry V, Cornblath DR, Polydefkis M, et al. Characteristics of bortezomib- and thalidomide-induced peripheral neuropathy. *J Peripher Nerv Syst.* 2008;13:275–282.

Chen H, Clifford DB, Deng L, et al. Peripheral neuropathy in ART-experienced patients: prevalence and risk factors. *J Neurovirol.* 2013;19:557–564.

Chu CC, Huang CC, Ryu SJ, et al. Chronic inorganic mercury-induced peripheral neuropathy. *Acta Neurol Scand.* 1998;98:461–465.

Davis LE, Standefer JC, Kornfeld M, et al. Acute thallium poisoning: toxicological and morphological studies of the nervous system. *Ann Neurol.* 1981;10:38–44.

Davis TM, Yeap BB, Davis WA, et al. Lipid lowering therapy and sensory peripheral neuropathy in type 2 diabetes mellitus: the Fremantle Diabetes Study. *Diabetologia.* 2008;51:562–566.

Gaist D, Jeppesen U, Andersen M, et al. Statins and risks of polyneuropathy: a case-control study. *Neurology.* 2002;58:1333–1337.

Gignoux L, Cortinovis-Tourniaire P, Grimaud J, et al. A brachial form of motor neuropathy caused by lead poisoning. *Rev Neurol (Paris).* 1998;154:771–773.

Goebel HH, Schmidt PF, Bohl J, et al. Polyneuropathy due to acute arsenic intoxication: biopsy studies. *J Neuropathol Exp Neurol.* 1990;49:137–149.

Iñiguez C, Larrodé P, Mayordomo JI, et al. Reversible peripheral neuropathy induced by a single administration of high-dose paclitaxel. *Neurology.* 1998;51:868–870.

Koike H, Iijima M, Sugiura M, et al. Alcoholic neuropathy is clinicopathologically distinct from thiamine deficiency neuropathy. *Ann Neurol.* 2003;54:19–29.

Krarup-Hansen A, Reitz B, Krarup C, et al. Histology and platinum content of sensory ganglia and sural nerves in patients treated with cisplatin and carboplatin: an autopsy study. *Neuropathol Appl Neurobiol.* 1999;25:29–40.

Laquery A, Ronnel A, Vignolly B, et al. Thalidomide neuropathy: an electrophysiologic study. *Muscle Nerve.* 1986;9:837–844.

Lehky TJ, Leonard GD, Wilson RH, et al. Oxaliplatin-induced neurotoxicity: acute hyperexcitability and chronic neuropathy. *Muscle Nerve.* 2004;29:387–392.

Leis AA, Stokic DS, Olivier J. Statins and polyneuropathy: setting the record straight. *Muscle Nerve.* 2005;32:428–430.

Molloy FM, Floeter MK, Syet NA, et al. Thalidomide neuropathy in patients treated for metastatic prostate cancer. *Muscle Nerve.* 2001;24:1050–1057.

Nordentoft T, Andersen EB, Mogensen PH. Initial sensorimotor and delayed autonomic neuropathy in acute thallium poisoning. *Neurotoxicology.* 1998;19:421–426.

Oh S. Electrophysiological profile in arsenic neuropathy. *J Neurol Neurosurg Psychiatry.* 1991;54:1103–1105.

Pratt RW, Weimer LH. Medication and toxin-induced peripheral neuropathy. *Semin Neurol.* 2005;25:204–216.

Diabetic Neuropathy

Abbott CA, Vileikyte L, Williamson S, et al. Multicenter study of the incidence of predictive risk factors for diabetic neuropathic foot ulceration. *Diabetes Care.* 1998;21:1071–1075.

Asbury AK. Proximal diabetic neuropathy. *Ann Neurol.* 1977;2:179–180.

Behse F, Buchthal F, Carlsen F. Nerve biopsy and conduction studies in diabetic neuropathy. *J Neurol Neurosurg Psychiatry.* 1977;10:1072–1082.

Brannagan TH, Promisloff RA, McCluskey LF, et al. Proximal diabetic neuropathy presenting with respiratory weakness. *J Neurol Neurosurg Psychiatry.* 1999;67:539–541.

Dyck PJ, Albers JW, Andersen H, et al; Toronto Expert Panel on Diabetic Neuropathy. Diabetic polyneuropathies: update on research definition, diagnostic criteria and estimation of severity. *Diabetes Metab Res Rev.* 2011;27:620–628.

Dyck PJ, Giannini C. Pathologic alterations in the diabetic neuropathies of humans: a review. *J Neuropathol Exp Neurol.* 1996;55:1181–1193.

Dyck PJB, Windebank AJ. Diabetic and nondiabetic lumbosacral radiculoplexus neuropathies: new insights into pathophysiology and treatment. *Muscle Nerve.* 2002;25:477–491.

Hinder LM, Vincent AM, Burant CF, et al. Bioenergetics in diabetic neuropathy: what we need to know. *J Peripher Nerv Syst.* 2012;17(suppl 2):10–14.

Hur J, Sullivan KA, Callaghan BC, et al. Identification of factors associated with sural nerve regeneration and degeneration in diabetic neuropathy. *Diabetes Care.* 2013;36:4043–4049.

Llewelyn JG, Thomas PK, King RH. Epineurial microvasculitis in proximal diabetic neuropathy. *J Neurol.* 1998;245:159–165.

Navarro X, Sutherland DE, Kennedy WR. Long-term effects of pancreatic transplantation on diabetic neuropathy. *Ann Neurol.* 1998;44:149–150.

Said G, Elgrably F, Lacroix C, et al. Painful proximal diabetic neuropathy: inflammatory nerve lesions and spontaneous favorable outcome. *Ann Neurol.* 1997;41:762–770.

Smith AG. Impaired glucose tolerance and metabolic syndrome in idiopathic neuropathy. *J Peripher Nerv Syst.* 2012;17(suppl 2):15–21.

Lyme Neuropathy

Coyle PK, Deng Z, Schutzer SE, et al. Detection of *Borrelia burgdorferi* antigens in cerebrospinal fluid. *Neurology.* 1993;43:1093–1098.

Halperin JJ. Lyme disease and the peripheral nervous system. *Muscle Nerve.* 2003;28:133–143.

Halperin J, Luft BJ, Volkman DJ, et al. Lyme neuroborreliosis. Peripheral nervous system manifestations. *Brain.* 1990;11:1207–1221.

Hansen K, Lebech AM. The clinical and epidemiological profile of Lyme neuroborreliosis in Denmark 1985–1990: a prospective study of 187 patients with *Borrelia burgdorferi* specific intrathecal antibody production. *Brain.* 1992;115:399–423.

Pachner AR, Steere AC. The triad of neurologic manifestations of Lyme disease: meningitis, cranial neuritis, and radiculoneuritis. *Neurology.* 1985;35:47–53.

Idiopathic Neuropathy

Chia L, Fernandez A, Lacroix C, et al. Contribution of nerve biopsy findings to the diagnosis of disabling neuropathy in the elderly. A retrospective review of 100 consecutive patients. *Brain.* 1996;119:1091–1098.

De Sousa EA, Hays AP, Chin RL, et al. Characteristics of patients with sensory neuropathy diagnosed by abnormal small nerve fibres on skin biopsy. *J Neurol Neurosurg Psychiatry.* 2006;77:983–985.

Dyck PJ, Oviatt KF, Lambert EH. Intensive evaluation of referred unclassified neuropathies yields improved diagnosis. *Neurology.* 1981;10:222–226.

Notermans NC, Wokke JHJ, Franssen H, et al. Chronic idiopathic polyneuropathy presenting in middle or old age: a clinical and electrophysiological study of 75 patients. *J Neurol Neurosurg Psychiatry.* 1993;56:1066–1071.

Periquet MI, Novak V, Collins MP, et al. Painful sensory neuropathy: prospective evaluation using skin biopsy. *Neurology.* 1999;53:1641–1647.

Wolfe GI, Baker NS, Amato AA, et al. Chronic cryptogenic sensory polyneuropathy: clinical and laboratory characteristics. *Arch Neurol.* 1999;56:540–547.

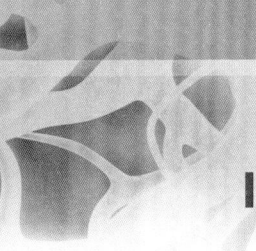

Inherited Peripheral Neuropathies 88

Chiara Pisciotta and Michael E. Shy

INTRODUCTION

Inherited neuropathies, collectively known as *Charcot–Marie–Tooth* (CMT) *disease*, are a group of genetically and phenotypically heterogeneous peripheral neuropathies associated with mutations or copy number variations in over 70 distinct genes. Named after the three neurologists who first described the condition in 1886, CMT is the most common inherited neuromuscular disease. CMT is a motor and sensory neuropathy (HMSN) that is closely related to two other rarer inherited neuropathies: distal hereditary motor neuropathy (dHMN), which has predominantly motor involvement, and hereditary sensory/autonomic neuropathy (HSN or HSAN), which involves only or predominantly sensory and autonomic nerves. These three disorders represent a continuum and are often collectively termed *Charcot–Marie–Tooth and related disorders*.

CMT is divided into different forms based on the pattern of inheritance and neurophysiologic studies. Autosomal dominant forms are subdivided into demyelinating (CMT1) and axonal (CMT2) forms. CMT4 and CMTX designate the autosomal recessive and X-linked forms, respectively. The term *Dejerine–Sottas neuropathy* (DSN) is currently used primarily to denote severe early-onset clinical phenotypes regardless of the inheritance pattern. The classification of CMT has been divided further into subtypes, identified by letters, as defined by the mutated gene (Table 88.1).

EPIDEMIOLOGY

The prevalence of CMT is about 1 in 2,500 people, with a global distribution and no ethnic predisposition. CMT1A, associated with 17p11.2 duplication in the region containing the peripheral myelin protein 22 gene (*PMP22*), is the most common form of CMT and accounts for 60% to 70% of demyelinating CMT patients (around 50% of all CMT cases). Mutations in the gap junction beta 1 gene (*GJB1*) causing CMTX result in approximately 10% to 20% of CMT cases and CMT1B associated with mutations in the myelin protein zero gene (*MPZ*) accounts for less than 5%. Patients with CMT2 are about 20% of all cases. The prevalence of hereditary neuropathy with liability to pressure palsies (HNPP) is not known, but about 85% of patients with clinical evidence of this syndrome have a chromosome 17p11.2 deletion.

PATHOBIOLOGY

A common feature of most genes mutated in CMT is the role they play in maintaining the structure or function of cellular components of the peripheral nervous system, myelinating Schwann cells, and the axons they ensheath (Fig. 88.1). Schwann cells and axons interact at multiple points along the peripheral nerve, including the adaxonal (opposing the axon) membrane, paranodal myelin loops, microvilli, and juxtaparanodal basal lamina. These interactions are mutually beneficial, providing trophic support to the axon and myelinating cues to the Schwann cell. An example

TABLE 88.1	Classification of Charcot–Marie–Tooth: Specific Genetic Types
Type	**Gene/Locus**
Autosomal Dominant CMT1 (ADCMT1)	
CMT1A	Dup 17p (PMP22)
CMT1B	MPZ
CMT1C	SIMPLE
CMT1D	EGR2
CMT1E	PMP22 point mutations
CMT1F	NEFL
Hereditary Neuropathy with Liability to Pressure Palsies	
HNPP	Del 17p/PMP22 point mutations
X-linked CMT	
CMTX1	GJB1
Autosomal Dominant CMT2 (ADCMT2)	
CMT2A	MFN2
CMT2B	RAB7
CMT2C	TRPV4
CMT2D	GARS
CMT2E	NEFL
CMT2F	HSP27 (HSPB1)
CMT2L	HSP22 (HSPB8)
CMT2K	GDAP1
Autosomal Recessive Demyelinating CMT (CMT4)	
CMT4A	GDAP1
CMT4B1	MTMR2
CMT4C	SH3TC2
CMT4F	PRX
CMT4J	FIG4
Autosomal Recessive Axonal CMT (AR-CMT2)	
AR-CMT2A	LMNA

AD, autosomal dominant; AR, autosomal recessive; CMT, Charcot–Marie–Tooth; Dup, duplication; MPZ, myelin protein zero; SIMPLE, small integral membrane protein of the lysosome/late endosome; EGR2, early growth response 2; PMP22, peripheral myelin protein 22; NEFL, neurofilament light chain; HNPP, hereditary neuropathy with liability to pressure palsies; Del, deletion; GJB1, gap junction protein beta1; MFN2, mitofusin 2; RAB7, RAB7, member RAS oncogene family; GARS, glycyl tRNA synthetase; HSP27, heat shock 27 kDa protein 1; HSP22, heat shock 22 kDa protein 8; GDAP1, ganglioside induced differentiation associated protein 1; MTMR2, myotubularin related protein 2; SH3TC2, SH3 domain and tetratricopeptide repeats 2; PRX, periaxin; FIG4, FIG4 homologue; LMNA, lamin A/C.

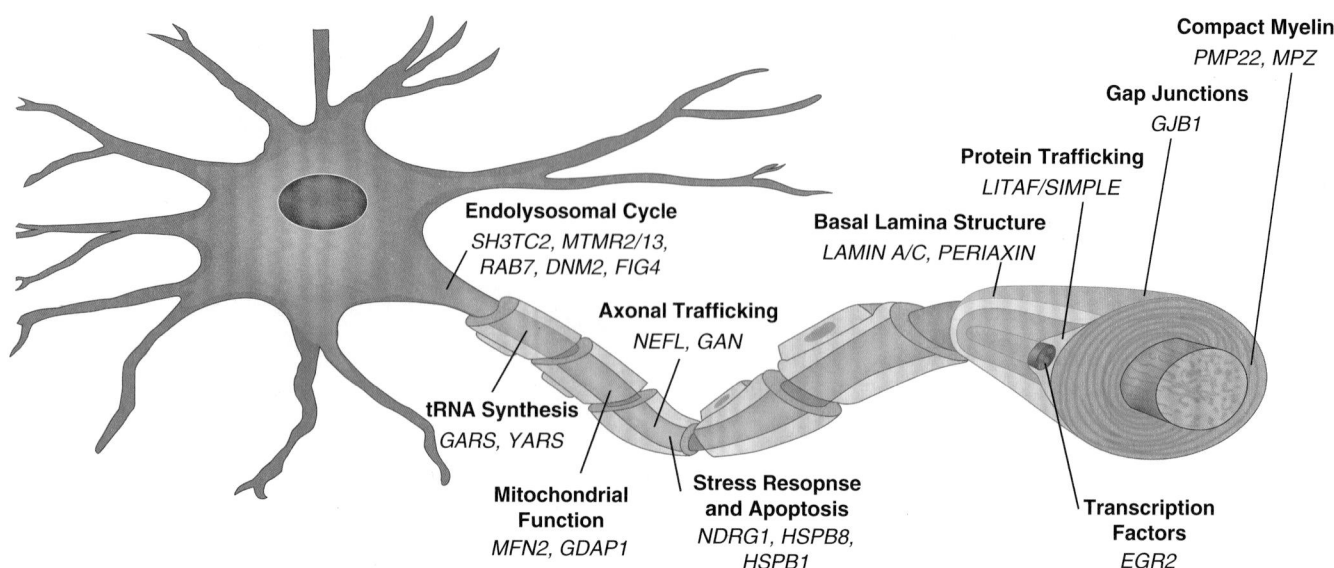

FIGURE 88.1 Schematic drawing of a neuron, its axon, and Schwann cells with the major genes associated with Charcot–Marie–Tooth disease represented along with their respective function and cellular compartment. (Adapted from Saporta MA, Shy ME. Inherited peripheral neuropathies. *Neurol Clin.* 2013;31:597–619.)

of this important interaction is the occurrence of secondary axonal degeneration in all forms of demyelinating CMT. Indeed, although the primary metabolic or structural defect often affects either the myelin or the axon, axonal degeneration represents the final common pathway in both forms of peripheral neuropathies. In demyelinating neuropathies, the secondary axonal degeneration presumably occurs because of inadequate Schwann cell support of the axon. In these neuropathies, secondary axonal degeneration may contribute more to clinical impairment than the primary demyelination. Impaired interactions between axons and mutant Schwann cells seem to be the common process linking all forms

of demyelinating CMT. Most cases of CMT1 are caused by mutations in myelin-specific genes including *PMP22* (CMT1A), *MPZ* (CMT1B) and *GJB1* (CMT1X), or other genes associated with Schwann cell function, including those that exert transcriptional control of myelination and intracellular trafficking. At a pathologic level, dysmyelination, demyelination, remyelination, and axonal loss are characteristic features of the various demyelinating forms of CMT1. In DSN, myelin may never have formed normally, which is referred to as *dysmyelination*. In CMT1, onion bulbs of concentric Schwann cell lamellae are usually present on nerve biopsies (Fig. 88.2), with loss of both small- and large-diameter myelinated

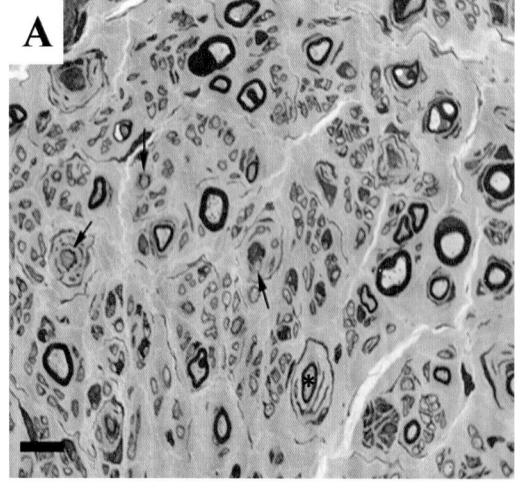
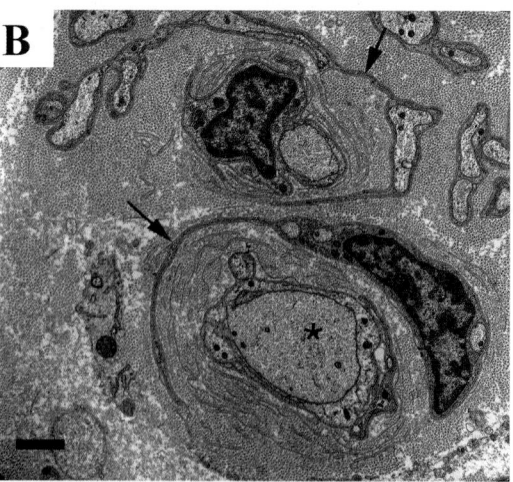

FIGURE 88.2 Pathologic findings in demyelinating Charcot–Marie–Tooth disease. **A:** Cross-section of a sural nerve biopsy of a patient with demyelinating CMT showing numerous demyelinated axons (*arrows*) and occasional classical onion bulbs (*asterisk*). Thionine and acridine orange stain. Bar = 10 μm. **B:** Electron micrograph showing a demyelinated axon (*asterisk*) surrounded by some excess basal lamina. The Schwann cells associated with small, unmyelinated axons are abnormally long and attenuated (*arrows*). Bar = 1 μm. (From Saporta MA, Shy ME. Inherited peripheral neuropathies. *Neurol Clin.* 2013;31:597–619.)

fibers and a decrease in the number of myelinated axons. Focal, sausage-like thickenings of the myelin sheath (tomacula) are characteristic of HNPP but may also be found in other forms of CMT1, particularly CMT1B. In CMT1, disability typically correlates better with secondary axonal degeneration than with demyelination itself, again demonstrating the importance of Schwann cell–axonal interactions in demyelinating disease.

Several recent studies have demonstrated a susceptibility of Schwann cells to mutations yielding misfolded proteins, as seen in certain *PMP22* and *MPZ* point mutations. Misfolded proteins may accumulate in the endoplasmic reticulum (ER) of Schwann cells inducing an unfolded protein response (UPR), a series of cellular events that help the ER to cope with the increased metabolic demand caused by retention of the misfolded protein. This, in turn, causes downregulation of the myelination program genes and dedifferentiation of Schwann cells, a toxic gain of function that worsens with the demyelination and is potentially amenable to therapeutic intervention.

Spinal motor neurons and dorsal root ganglion sensory neurons that are affected in CMT have particular challenges in maintaining homeostasis, as their axons extend up to 1 m distal from the cell body. Because the majority of neuronal proteins are synthesized in the cell body, intensive transport of proteins must occur between the soma and the axonal extremity via anterograde transport. Additionally, signals from the periphery containing toxic or prosurvival factors, as well as damaged proteins, return to the cell body via retrograde transport. Indeed, axonal trafficking is emerging as a common theme of various seemingly diverse genes that are associated with CMT type 2. Mutations in genes associated with axonal structure and function result in CMT2. Some examples include mutations in proteins of the neuronal cytoskeleton (neurofilament light chain-NEFL, CMT2E), proteins associated with axonal mitochondrial dynamics (mitofusin 2-MFN2, CMT2A and ganglioside-induced differentiation protein 1-GDAP1, CMT2K), and protein associated with regulation of membrane and intracellular trafficking (Ras-associated protein RAB7, CMT2B, for example). The pathologic hallmark of CMT2 is axonal degeneration with loss of all types of nerve fibers in the absence of onion bulb formation.

CLINICAL MANIFESTATIONS

Despite phenotypic variability, there are characteristic clinical patterns for many types of CMT (Table 88.2). The "classical" CMT phenotype consists of normal early milestones such as beginning to walk by a year of age. This is followed by gradually progressing weakness and sensory loss during the first two decades of life. The classic phenotype typically features a steppage gait, pes cavus, sensory loss in a stocking or glove distribution, inverted champagne bottle legs, and atrophy in the hands (Fig. 88.3). Although both motor and sensory nerves are usually affected, the more prominent phenotypic characteristic is related to motor difficulty in most cases. Physical examination shows decreased or absent deep tendon reflexes, often diffusely but always involving the Achilles tendon. Findings are usually symmetric. Pronounced asymmetries in symptoms suggest HNPP if they are episodic. Otherwise, they are more consistent with acquired disorders. Patients with classical CMT almost always have impaired proprioception with balance difficulty. Affected children are usually slow runners and have difficulty with activities that require balance (e.g., skating, walking along a log across a stream). Ankle–foot orthotics (AFOs) are frequently required by the third decade. Fine movements of the

hands for activities such as turning a key or using buttons and zippers may be impaired, but the hands are rarely as affected as the feet. Deep and superficial muscles that are innervated by the peroneal nerve, such as the tibialis anterior and peroneus brevis and longus muscles often cause more symptoms than do the plantar flexion muscles innervated by the tibial nerve, such as the gastrocnemius. As a result, tripping and spraining one's ankle are frequent symptoms. Most patients remain ambulatory throughout life and have a normal life span.

However, CMT, as well as genetically, may be clinically heterogenous, with variability in the age of onset, speed of progression, and electrophysiologic findings. Onset may differ depending on the genetic subtype, including early-onset, infantile forms with delayed milestones (historically designated DSN) and late-onset, adult forms. Symptoms are usually slowly progressive, especially for the classic and late-onset phenotype, but can be severe, particularly in early-onset forms.

ELECTROPHYSIOLOGY

Electrophysiologic studies allow for classification of CMT into demyelinating (CMT1) and axonal (CMT2) forms. The standard cutoff for demyelinating motor nerve conduction velocity (MNCV) is 38 m/s in the upper extremities. Axonal forms (CMT2) exhibit MNCVs greater than 45 m/s but a decrease in compound muscle action potential (CMAP) amplitudes. The dominant intermediate forms (I-CMT) show MNCVs between 25 and 45 m/s. Conduction velocities are performed in the upper limbs because CMAP amplitudes are often unobtainable in the legs, even for demyelinating forms of CMT, due to either conduction failure or secondary axonal degeneration.

The usual electrodiagnostic finding in demyelinated inherited neuropathies is widespread uniform slowing of conduction velocities, as opposed to the multifocal segmental slowing found in demyelinating acquired neuropathies in which temporal dispersion and conduction blocks are frequently seen. Exceptions to this rule are women with CMTX, patients with HNPP, and some CMT1B cases with specific *MPZ* mutations. In these cases, focal demyelination with temporal dispersion or conduction block can be seen. In other cases of CMT1, the finding of focal slowing should raise the possibility of a superimposed inflammatory neuropathy.

DIAGNOSIS

The first step is to determine whether the patient has a genetic neuropathy. Where there is an affected parent, either an autosomal dominant (AD) or X-linked (if there is no definite male-to-male transmission) inheritance is likely. If there are multiple affected siblings, no parents affected, and/or consanguineous parents, then autosomal recessive (AR) inheritance is likely. However, recognizing CMT can be challenging particularly when there is no family history or if families are small. Factors pointing to an inherited neuropathy in such circumstances include presentations in childhood, slow progression, the presence of foot deformities, and the lack of positive sensory symptoms (dysesthesias, paresthesias) in the presence of clear sensory signs. Patients may have undergone foot surgery in childhood or reported difficulties with sports at school.

Genetic testing is the "gold standard" for the diagnosis of inherited neuropathies. However, it is a challenge to keep the costs reasonable particularly because there are so many known genetic causes.

TABLE 88.2 Specific Phenotypes of Charcot–Marie–Tooth

Type	Specific Phenotype
CMT1	
CMT1A	Classic CMT phenotype with disease onset in the first two decades of life. Patients complain of walking difficulties, distal weakness associated with wasting, sensory loss, and foot deformities. Slow progression and AFOs often required. MNCVs are uniformly slow (mean range 17–21 m/s).
CMT1B	Associated with distinct phenotypes: late mild phenotype, adult-onset, and intermediate MNCVs; DSN with early infantile onset, severe phenotype, delayed walking, and MNCV <10 m/s; classic CMT phenotype (see CMT1A)
CMT1C	CMT1 (frequently resemble those with CMT1A)
CMT1D	Usually presents with DSN
CMT1E	Distinct phenotypes depending on the location and amino acid change: DSN with early onset, delay in walking, severe phenotype (deafness may also be present), very slow MNCVs; CMT1 with later onset and milder phenotype; HNPP
CMT1F	"Demyelinating" form of CMT2E with earlier onset (infancy or childhood), more severe phenotype (delayed motor milestones), and slower MNCVs
HNPP	Recurrent episodic painless mononeuropathies, typically at entrapment sites, in response to nerve injury from pressure or stretching. Superimposed, length-dependent, sensory-predominant neuropathy of large fibers.
X-linked CMT	
CMTX1	Males have a more severe phenotype than females. MNCVs in the intermediate range (male MNCVs < female MNCVs). Nerve conduction can be patchy with temporal dispersion and conduction blocks, especially in females.
CMT2	
CMT2A	Usually severe phenotype with onset in infancy or early childhood, progressive course, and predominant motor involvement with many patients requiring a wheelchair to ambulate by the age of 20 years. Rarely, later onset and milder phenotype. Additional clinical features may be present as optic atrophy or pyramidal signs.
CMT2B	Predominant sensory involvement with ulcerations, infections, and sometimes amputations. Patients usually have in addition the typical motor symptoms of CMT. Autonomic dysfunctions can be also observed.
CMT2C	Predominant motor involvement, vocal cord paralysis (hoarseness and stridor), and respiratory dysfunction. Other distinctive clinical features may include bone deformities such as scoliosis, short stature, and/or scapular winging. The age of onset is often in the first decade of life.
CMT2D	It usually presents in the second decade with more pronounced weakness and wasting of the distal upper extremities compared to the lower extremities. Sensory findings are usually mild and may even be absent. In this situation, the disorder has been classified as dHMN type V.
CMT2E	The age of onset ranges from infancy and childhood typically with severe impairment to adulthood with mild impairment. Weakness and wasting starts in the legs with all sensory modalities reported to be affected. MNCVs can be normal, intermediate, or slow (CMT1F).
CMT2F	Most patients have a dHMN phenotype (dHMN type IIB). Typically, this is a motor distal length-dependent neuropathy with slow progression proximally of symptoms. Sensory findings may be present, especially later in the disease course. The age of onset is typically late adolescence to early adulthood.
CMT2L	CMT2 or dHMN-IIA if sensory involvement is not present (see CMT2F)
CMT2K	Typically results in a much milder phenotype than the recessive form (CMT4A) with no vocal cord involvement and onset ranging from adolescence to adulthood
CMT4/AR-CMT2	
CMT4A	Infantile-onset, severe progressive neuropathy with a variable vocal cord involvement and diaphragm paralysis
CMT4B1	Infantile onset with severe phenotype (both proximal and distal) cranial nerve involvement, especially facial weakness. Wheelchair dependent by adulthood.
CMT4C	The phenotype can be severe with early and severe scoliosis. The onset is slightly later than other AR-CMT.
CMT4F	Severe early-onset neuropathy with prominent sensory involvement and ataxia.
CMT4J	Onset in early childhood with a severe motor phenotype, sometimes asymmetric. Rapid progression to a wheelchair has been described in adulthood.
AR-CMT2A	Severe axonal neuropathy with proximal involvement and rapid progression. Cardiomyopathy can be an associated feature. Onset usually in the second decade of life.

CMT1, autosomal dominant demyelinating Charcot–Marie–Tooth; AFOs, ankle–foot orthotics; MNCV, motor nerve conduction velocity; DSN, Dejerine–Sottas neuropathy; HNPP, hereditary neuropathy with liability to pressure palsies; CMT2, autosomal dominant axonal Charcot–Marie–Tooth; dHMN, distal hereditary motor neuropathy; CMT4, autosomal recessive demyelinating Charcot–Marie–Tooth; AR, autosomal recessive.

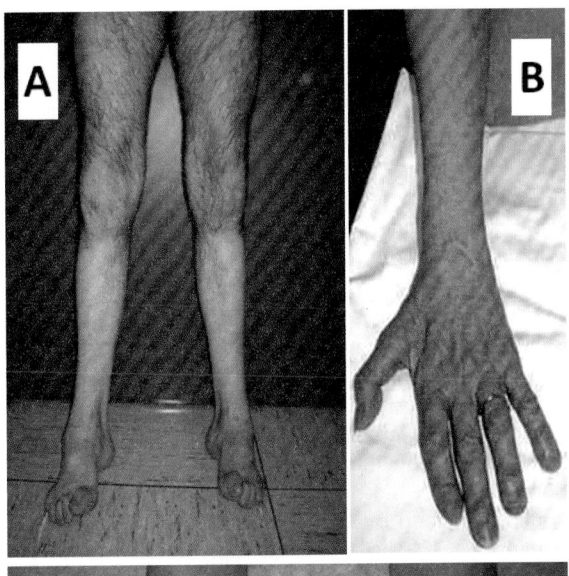

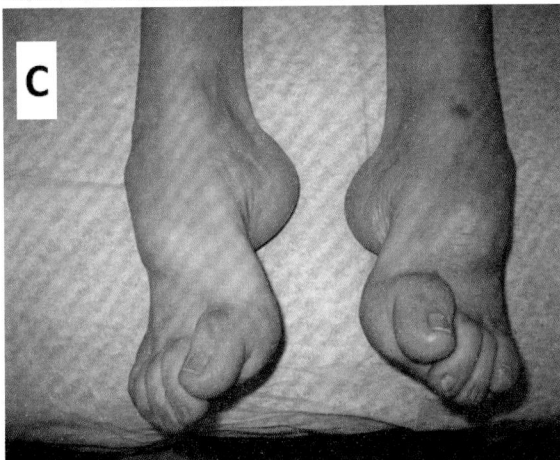

FIGURE 88.3 A: Wasting of distal muscles in lower limbs leading to inverted champagne bottle legs. **B:** Example of wasting of intrinsic muscles of the hands. **C:** Pes cavus with hammer toes.

Although there are many genes associated with CMT, in North America, mutations in only four genes (*PMP22* duplication/deletion, *GJB1*, *MPZ*, and *MFN2*) account for over 90% of CMT cases.

GENETIC TESTING STRATEGIES

Strategies for focusing genetic testing have been in place since at least 2011, with several groups suggesting algorithms guided by MNCV results and patterns of inheritance, as well as age of onset of symptoms. These algorithms rely on careful phenotyping and sequential Sanger sequencing of candidate genes. Although this approach is reasonably successful, with over 60% of patients with CMT achieving a genetic diagnosis, it is no longer the most efficient, rapid, or cost-effective method of achieving a molecular diagnosis, especially for CMT2, dHMN, and HSAN. In fact, diagnostic approaches are shifting to incorporate rapidly developing next-generation sequencing (NGS) techniques, as the cost of these drops below that of serial candidate gene screening.

However, the authors think it is still reasonable to provide some information about how to pursue genetic testing. Genetic testing strategies must take into account the frequency of the subtypes, the phenotype and electrophysiologic characteristics, and the inheritance pattern. This can be quite challenging, as the same gene can be involved in demyelinating, axonal, or intermediate forms and can display autosomal dominant or recessive inheritance depending on the nature and position of the mutation. Based on these elements, the clinician can address the molecular genetic investigations.

AGE OF ONSET AND PROGRESSION

Three different categories can be identified. Patients with a classical phenotype, who begin walking on time and develop weakness or sensory loss during the first two decades of life, belong to the first group. Impairment slowly increases and patients rarely require ambulation aids beyond ankle foot orthotics. The large majority of patients with CMT1A and males with CMTX fall into this category.

The second group is the early-onset phenotypes in which patients do not begin walking until they are at least 15 months of age. These patients are often severely affected and are likely to require above the knee bracing, walkers, or wheelchairs for ambulation by 20 years of age. The genetic spectrum of early-onset CMT is very heterogeneous, including both dominant and recessive forms. The majority of these represent demyelinating phenotypes with very slow MNCVs and the most common are CMT1A, CMT1B, and CMT1E for the dominant forms and CMT4A, CMT4C, and CMT4F for the recessive ones. In addition to the demyelinating phenotypes, severe early-onset axonal neuropathies can be due to *MFN2* (CMT2A) or *GDAP1* (AR-CMT2K) mutations. Patients with CMT2A are frequently severely affected in infancy and childhood and present with a predominant motor neuropathy.

The third phenotype is defined as adult onset, in which patients do not develop symptoms of CMT until adulthood, often not until approximately 40 years of age. A large group of patients with axonal CMT and patients with a later onset CMT1B fall into this group.

ASSOCIATED SYMPTOMS AND SIGNS

The recognition of additional symptoms and signs can lead to a better definition of the type of CMT. A recurrent nerve palsy history is typical of HNPP, which presents with transient focal motor and/or sensory deficits in the distribution of individual nerves or plexuses, usually precipitated by pressure. A split hand syndrome (the abductor pollicis brevis being more wasted and weaker than the first dorsal interosseus) is a distinctive sign of CMTX, especially males. Transient CNS dysfunction and stroke-like episodes characterized by dysarthria, episodic weakness, and ataxia are also rarely reported by patients with CMTX. Optic atrophy and pyramidal signs are occasionally observed in patients with *MFN2* mutations. Vocal cord paralysis is frequent in CMT2C, caused by mutations in *TRPV4* (transient receptor potential cation channel subfamily V member 4) gene, whereas tonic pupils can be an additional clinical feature of axonal late-onset form due to *MPZ* mutations. Amputations and skin ulcers are the main feature of CMT2B and other autonomic symptoms, as light-headedness or hypo-/hyperhidrosis, can be reported. Mutations in *SH3TC2* (SH3 domain and tetratricopeptide repeat domain 2) gene, causing CMT4C, are a frequent cause of severe scoliosis.

NEUROPHYSIOLOGIC PATTERN

As previously mentioned, CMT1 are characterized by MNCVs at upper limbs below 38 m/s. CMAP can be reduced in amplitude due to secondary axonal loss. In CMT1A, MNCVs are uniformly slow in all nerves with a mean range of 17 to 21 m/s. Very slow MNCVs (<10 m/s) are suggestive of early-onset CM1B, *PMP22* point mutations, or demyelinating recessive phenotypes (CMT4).

Preserved or mildly slowed MNCV (mostly >45 m/s at upper limbs) and reduced CMAP are in keeping with CMT2. Especially for severe phenotypes, in which CMAP and sensory nerve action potentials (SNAP) are unobtainable distally, it is recommended to perform nerve conductions on proximal nerves for a proper diagnostic workup to fully investigate the possibility of a severe demyelinating rather than an axonal pathology. Sensory nerve conduction evaluation is required to differentiate CMT2 from dHMN, and it should be performed especially at lower limbs because SNAP amplitude could be normal at upper limbs in mild phenotypes. Some forms of dHMN can have a minimal sensory impairment and in these cases, the discrepancy between CMAP and SNAP amplitude reduction should be taken into account for the differential diagnosis.

"Intermediate" MNCV, in the range of 25 to 45 m/s, is consistent with I-CMT. MNCVs are not uniformly slow and can differ among different nerves in the same individuals or among family members. Therefore, although a single nerve can be sufficient to make a diagnosis of CMT1, multiple nerve evaluation must be performed especially in these cases. Temporal dispersion and conduction blocks can also be present. The most common intermediate forms of CMT are due to *MPZ* and *GJB1* mutations. Focal slowing at typical sites of compression (median nerve at wrist, ulnar nerve at elbow, and peroneal nerve at fibular head) and a superimposed, diffuse, sensory neuropathy is suggestive of HNPP.

INHERITANCE PATTERN

The AD transmission is the most common pattern of inheritance in CMT with a vertical transmission from a generation to another. If there is no male-to-male transmission, X-linked inheritance should be taken into account, whereas in case of consanguinity, AR inheritance is likely. However, many patients present with no clear family history and these cases should be considered as sporadic cases due to de novo mutation, reduced penetrance/intrafamilial variability, or proband of an AR inheritance. So, the absence of a family history of neuropathy should not dissuade clinicians from considering an underlying genetic cause.

ETHNICITY

It is important to be aware of the specific mutation frequencies occurring in certain populations because some genetic mutations have been reported in specific ethnic groups. In northern Europe and the United States, AD inheritance is much more common than AR, which should be considered for those patients coming from countries where consanguinity is more frequent, such as Mediterranean and Middle Eastern populations.

Currently, genetic testing is in a transition phase with both traditional Sanger sequencing and NGS technology being used by most dedicated CMT clinics, and whole exome sequencing is not far behind. A review of these techniques is beyond the scope of this chapter but a reference is provided. Ensuring that genetic testing is focused and cost-effective is important for patients and their families.

SPECIFIC TYPES OF CHARCOT–MARIE–TOOTH

AUTOSOMAL DOMINANT DEMYELINATING CHARCOT–MARIE–TOOTH

CMT1 or AD demyelinating CMT includes types that are caused by mutations in genes involved in Schwann cell function and myelin sheath formation. This group includes the majority of patients with CMT.

CMT1A is the most common form of CMT1 and is caused by a 1.4 Mb 17p11.2 duplication including the *PMP22* gene, which should be checked first in any patient with demyelinating CMT, even if sporadic (approximately 10% of CMT1A cases). Patients affected by CMT1A usually have the "classic CMT phenotype" with disease onset in the first two decades of life. They complain of walking difficulties, distal weakness associated with wasting, sensory loss, and foot deformities. Patients progress very slowly and they often require AFOs. Inter- and intrafamilial variability is frequently observed.

HNPP is caused by the reciprocal deletion of the 1.4 Mb stretch of chromosome 17p11.2 containing the *PMP22* gene. A small percentage of people with HNPP have frameshift, splice site, or point mutation of the *PMP22* gene. The hallmark feature of HNPP is recurrent episodic focal numbness, tingling, and weakness in response to nerve injury from pressure or stretching. These individual mononeuropathies (characteristically painless) typically occur at entrapment sites, such as the carpal tunnel, ulnar groove, and fibular head, and the palsies may last hours, days, weeks, or occasionally longer. They are often superimposed on preexisting diffuse, length-dependent, sensory-predominant neuropathy of large fibers.

CMT1X is the second most common form of CMT and in families with no definite male-to-male transmission, mutations in *GJB1*, encoding the protein Cx32, should be investigated. Males have a more severe phenotype than females and their MNCVs are in demyelinating range but usually not uniform. Females present with a milder phenotype and MNCVs are in the intermediate or axonal range. Nerve conduction study can be patchy with temporal dispersion and conduction blocks mimicking inflammatory neuropathies. It has been assumed that the cause of the difference in phenotype observed in women is due to variable X-inactivation; however, there is no evidence as yet to support this theory.

CMT1B is caused by approximately 200 different mutations in the *MPZ* gene, which encodes for the major protein component of the myelin sheath. CMT1B is associated with two distinct phenotypes: (1) an early infantile-onset severe phenotype with delayed walking and MNCV less than 10 m/s often referred to as *DSN* or (2) a much later, milder phenotype with onset at around age 40 years and MNCV around 40 m/s. CMT1B can also cause the "classical CMT phenotype" in about 15% of total CMT1B cases. The phenotypes depend on the particular mutation.

CMT1E is caused by point mutations in the PMP22 gene. Depending on the location and amino acid change, these patients may have an earlier onset with a more severe phenotype than those with CMT1A caused by the duplication. These severe cases may also have deafness and much slower MNCVs compared to CMT1A patients who simply have a duplication in the *PMP22* gene. Onset within the first 2 years of life with a delay in walking is not uncommon; however, the clinical phenotype is variable and onset may be later. The disease severity depends on the particular *PMP22* mutation and some cases can be very mild or even resemble HNPP.

Mutations in *EGR2* (early growth response protein 2) (CMT1D) and *SIMPLE* (small integral membrane protein of the lysosome/late endosome) (CMT1C) are very rare (<1%). CMT1D patients usually present with DSN, whereas CMT1C patients frequently resemble those with CMT1A.

AUTOSOMAL DOMINANT AXONAL CHARCOT–MARIE–TOOTH

Phenotypic clues are helpful in guiding the diagnosis of patients with CMT2, which can be difficult to distinguish from an idiopathic axonal neuropathy when family history is negative. CMT2 may present with a "classical CMT phenotype" with lower limb symptoms (difficulty walking/foot deformity) with onset in the first two decades of life. However, these patients are often more severely affected compared to patients with CMT1A for example. Profound sensory impairment characterizes a second phenotype, as illustrated in CMT2B, and selective initial involvement of the upper limbs is distinctive of the third phenotype, typical of CMT2D. However, among patients with axonal neuropathy, genetic testing is less likely to be positive, as there are many genes known to cause axonal CMT with each gene accountable for only a very small proportion of cases with the exception of *MFN2* in northern Europe and the United States and *GDAP1* in southern Europe and Mediterranean area. However, with the advent of NGS, it is certain that the number of genetic causes of CMT2 will significantly increase over the next few years.

Mutations in the *MFN2* gene cause CMT2A. The phenotype is often severe with onset in infancy or early childhood, progressive course, and predominant motor involvement, with many patients requiring a wheelchair to ambulate by the age of 20 years. Rarely, some patients present later in life (during childhood, adolescence, or even adulthood) with a milder phenotype. Some additional clinical features such as optic atrophy or pyramidal signs are observed. Diagnosis can be difficult because there are already a number of benign polymorphisms reported with the gene.

CMT2B is caused by mutations in the *RAB7* gene. It is characterized by mild to moderate sensory loss that typically leads to ulcerations, infections, and sometimes amputations. Patients with CMT2B usually have in addition the typical motor symptoms of CMT. On occasion, the sensory loss can be severe and patients can be clinically indistinguishable from HSAN1. Autonomic dysfunctions can be also observed.

CMT2C, caused by mutations in the *TRPV4* gene, is characterized by a predominantly motor neuropathy with vocal cord and diaphragm paralysis, often presenting with hoarseness and stridor. Other distinctive clinical features may include bone deformities such as scoliosis, short stature, and/or scapular winging. The age of onset is often in the first decade of life but adolescent- and adult-onset forms have been reported with potentially marked intrafamilial variability.

CMT2D is a predominantly motor disorder associated with mutations in the *GARS* (glycyl tRNA synthetase) gene. It usually presents in the second decade with a distinct clinical phenotype characterized by more pronounced weakness and wasting of the distal upper extremities compared to the lower extremities. Patients may have a "split hand" appearance with wasting more obvious in the first dorsal interosseus and thenar eminence muscles compared to the hypothenar eminence muscles. Sensory findings are usually mild and may even be absent. In this situation, the disorder has been classified as dHMN type V.

CMT2E is caused by mutations in the *NEFL* gene. The age of onset ranges from infancy and childhood typically with severe impairment to adulthood with mild impairment. Weakness and wasting starts in the legs with all sensory modalities reported to be affected. Confusingly for the clinician, MNCVs can be in either the axonal or demyelinating range, probably due to the loss of large-diameter fibers. The "demyelinating" form is also termed *CMT1F*. Neurofilaments, however, are important cytoskeletal components of the axon and therefore, patients with *NEFL* mutations are referred as having an axonal neuropathy regardless of the MNCVs. Typically, those with slowed conductions present early either in infancy with delayed motor milestones or in late childhood/early adolescence.

CMT2F is caused by mutations in *HSPB1* gene, a member of the distal heat shock protein (HSP) superfamily and is also known as *HSP27*. Most patients with mutations in this gene have a dHMN phenotype (dHMN type IIB) with nerve conduction velocities in the axonal range. Sensory findings may be present, especially later in the disease course. Typically, this is a distal length-dependent neuropathy with slow progression proximally of symptoms. The age of onset is typically late adolescence to early adulthood. Mutations in the *HSPB8* gene (also known as *HSP22*), another member of the HSP superfamily, cause either CMT2L or dHMN type IIA. It is rarer and phenotypically indistinguishable from CMT2F/dHMN type IIB.

CMT2K is caused by mutations in the *GDAP1* gene. An autosomal recessive form also exists, CMT4A, and is more common than the autosomal dominant form, CMT2K. Although the recessive form may be quite severe with vocal cord paralysis, the dominant form typically results in a much milder phenotype with no vocal cord involvement and onset ranging from adolescence to even adulthood. A recent study found that *GDAP1* mutations accounted for 15% of CMT2 cases in southern Spain, suggesting, along with data from southern Italy, that this may be the most common form of CMT2 in the Mediterranean area. This again emphasizes the importance of considering a patient's ethnic background in guiding the diagnostic workup.

Mutations in *DNM2* (dynamin 2), *DYNC1H1* (cytoplasmic dynein heavy chain 1), and *AARS* (alanyl-tRNA synthetase) genes are very rare cause of CMT2.

AUTOSOMAL RECESSIVE DEMYELINATING CHARCOT–MARIE–TOOTH

CMT4 includes all forms of autosomal recessive CMT and are typically associated with demyelinating conduction velocities on electrophysiologic testing. CMT4 should be considered especially if there is a history of consanguinity. As a rule, AR-CMT present with an earlier onset and a more severe phenotype than the AD forms. Weakness often progresses to involve proximal muscles and results in early loss of ambulation. The most common forms of CMT4 are briefly mentioned.

CMT4A is caused by mutations in *GDAP1*, the same gene that cause CMT2K, both discussed previously. It is characterized by an infantile-onset and a severe progressive neuropathy with a variable vocal cord involvement.

Mutations in *MTMR2* (myotubularin-related protein 2), causing CMT4B1, are associated to infantile onset with proximal and distal weakness, cranial nerve involvement, especially facial weakness. The patients usually become wheelchair dependent by adulthood.

Mutation in *SH3TC2* is a frequent cause of CMT4 (CMT4C). The hallmark of this form is an early and severe scoliosis, and the onset is slightly later than other AR-CMT.

CMT4F is due to *PRX* (periaxin) mutations, which cause prominent sensory involvement with severe ataxia. Characteristically, patients have demyelinating conductions with a severe early-onset neuropathy. There are a particularly large number of polymorphisms in periaxin and care should be taken to ensure that mutations, either homozygous or compound heterozygous, segregate with the neuropathy in a family and that the phenotype is appropriate before concluding that mutations are disease causing.

CMT4J is caused by mutations in *FIG4* (factor-induced gene 4). Again, the onset here is early childhood with a severe motor phenotype, which is sometimes asymmetric. Rapid progression to a wheelchair in later adulthood has been described.

Nerve conductions are usually very slow and abnormalities on electromyography (EMG) may be similar to those seen in motor neuron disease (mutations in *FIG4* are also associated with amyotrophic lateral sclerosis type 11).

AR-CMT2 forms are very rare except for those associated with *LMNA* (lamin A/C) mutations, characterized by a severe axonal neuropathy with rapid progression, proximal weakness, and kyphoscoliosis. It most commonly presents in the second decade of life. Cardiomyopathy can be an associated feature.

DISTAL HEREDITARY MOTOR NEUROPATHY

The dHMNs are very similar to CMT in that they are inherited length-dependent slowly progressive neuropathies with onset usually starting in the first two decades. Clinically, however, they are defined by being exclusively motor in nature, even though many of them have minor sensory abnormalities and there is a degree of overlap between CMT2 and dHMN where the same mutation in the same gene can cause both phenotypes. Clinical examination confirms distal weakness and wasting with reduced or absent reflexes. Neurophysiology testing reveals reduced CMAP amplitudes with no or mild sensory abnormalities and EMG testing may reveal a predominantly distal pattern of denervation. For many dHMN, however, the exact genetic mutation remains to be elucidated and a report shows that 80% of tested dHMN patients with dominant inheritance has no positive genetic test. However, some dHMN disorders have signature clinical features that suggest specific genetic testing. Apart from the classic distal motor phenotype, typical of dHMN type 2A and 2B (discussed earlier), other clinical features may help in the selection of genetic testing in patients. Pyramidal tract signs of hyperreflexia and spasticity with distal motor weakness are likely associated with mutations in *SETX* (senataxin) or *BSCL2* (Berardinelli–Seip congenital lipodystrophy type 2). *SETX* mutations are also linked to the phenotypes diagnosed as juvenile amyotrophic lateral sclerosis (ALS4). Among patients with *BSCL2* mutations, the upper limbs may be the first involved with a variable degree of spastic paraplegia. The upper extremity onset without spasticity could also suggest mutations in *GARS* (previously described). Vocal cord involvement with scoliosis and skeletal dysplasias may suggest *TRPV4* mutations, which can present with phenotypes of scapuloperoneal spinal muscular atrophy, CMT2C, or dHMN.

HEREDITARY SENSORY AND AUTONOMIC NEUROPATHY

HSAN is a group of severe disorders affecting peripheral sensory and autonomic neurons with considerable clinical and genetic heterogeneity. A prominent hallmark of virtually all patients is the presence of prominent small-fiber sensory loss (Aδ and/or C-fibers). As a group, these patients tend to have more devastating handicaps compared with HMSN due to the frequent occurrence of ulcers, amputations, and variably severe autonomic dysfunction. Motor involvement can be present as well and it is important to realize that extremity weakness need not be excluded in consideration of these genetic disorders, as variable expression has been described. Generally, the sensory features are prominent. This is best illustrated in some HSAN1 patients with *SPTLC1* (serine palmitoyltransferase, long-chain base subunit 1) mutations, the most common AD form. This disease is very difficult to differentiate from CMT2B secondary to *RAB7* mutations, emphasizing the overlap between HMSN and related disorders. Unlike with HMSN, there is a much smaller set of known genes for HSAN. Classification within HSAN is based on the mode of inheritance and clinical

features and the genetic causes. HSAN1 varieties are dominantly inherited and have a juvenile or adult onset characterized by prominent sensory loss as well as autonomic disturbance. HSAN types 2 to 5 all have autosomal recessive inheritance and usually congenital onset. Mutations in each of these varieties are commonly seen in consanguineous families from founder mutations.

TREATMENT

Despite the great improvement in our biologic understanding of inherited neuropathies, derived mostly from developments in molecular biology and transgenic animal models in the last 25 years, there is still no treatment available for any type of CMT. Physical therapy, occupational therapy, and a few orthopedic procedures are still the cornerstone of CMT treatment (Table 88.3). A detailed family history and often examination of family members are required for prognosis and genetic counseling.

A dedicated, multidisciplinary rehabilitation team can significantly contribute to the management of patients with CMT and improve functionality and quality of life. Physical therapy strategies to maintain muscle strength and tone, prevent muscle contractures, and improve balance are a common need for most patients with CMT. Orthotics also are an important component of treating these patients, providing support and improving balance for ambulation. Occupational therapy focused on developing tools and strategies to help patients with activities of daily living will benefit patients with CMT, especially those with hand weakness. Tendon lengthening and tendon transfers can benefit a subset of CMT patients with muscle contractures and tendon shortening and patients with significant weakness in functionally relevant muscles, respectively; however, the optimal timing of such procedures is still controversial. Foot surgery is sometimes offered to correct inverted feet, pes cavus, and hammertoes. This surgical intervention may improve walking, alleviate pain over pressure points, and prevent plantar ulcers. However, foot surgery is generally unnecessary and does not improve weakness and sensory loss.

NORMALIZATION OF GENE DOSAGE

Reducing the expression of PMP22 in Schwann cells (hence treating the overexpression of PMP22) is a biologic strategy being tested

TABLE 88.3 Treatments and Aims	
Physical therapy	To maintain muscle strength and tone, prevent muscle contractures, and improve balance
Orthotics	To provide support and improve balance for ambulation
Occupational therapy	To provide tools and strategies for activities of daily living, especially for patients with hand weakness
Tendon lengthening	For patients with muscle contractures and tendon shortening
Tendon transfers	For patients with significant weakness in functionally relevant muscles
Foot surgery	To correct inverted feet, pes cavus, and hammer toes. It may improve walking and prevent plantar ulcers.

to treat CMT1A. High-dose ascorbic acid (vitamin C) was shown to decrease PMP22 levels and symptoms in mice with CMT1A, so that they were able to stay on a rotating rod longer, cross a beam more rapidly, and grip for longer than untreated mice. Several studies have been performed in humans with CMT1A, testing different doses of vitamin C (1 to 4 g/day) for up to 2 years. Unfortunately, all studies failed to meet their primary outcome measures and did not show a significant effect on phenotype.

Steroid hormones are epigenetic regulators of gene expression, and progesterone can stimulate PMP22 expression in cultured Schwann cells. Progesterone antagonists have been shown to decrease PMP22 expression in a rat model of CMT1A, improving their phenotype (specifically, the axonal loss seen during disease progression). Unfortunately, onapristone, the compound shown to have therapeutic effects in this study, do not have an appropriate safety profile to be administered in humans. Efforts to develop bioequivalent compounds with a better safety profile are ongoing.

NEUROTROPHIC SUPPORT

The growth factor neurotrophin 3 promotes nerve regeneration after injury and the survival of Schwann cells. Accordingly, injection of recombinant neurotrophin 3 improved regeneration and remyelination in animal models. A pilot study in eight patients with CMT1A resulted in an increase in myelinated fiber density, a reduction in the neurologic impairment score, and improved sensory modalities as compared with placebo controls, calling for a larger randomized controlled trial. An additional study provided preclinical data demonstrating efficacy of adeno-associated virus (AAV)–mediated neurotrophin 3 gene therapy in a mouse model of CMT1A.

REDUCTION OF NEUROTOXIC AGGREGATES/MISFOLDED PROTEINS

Recent studies have demonstrated the role of ER accumulation of misfolded proteins and UPR activation in the pathogenesis of several animal models of CMT associated with point mutations in myelin-related genes, including *PMP22* and *MPZ*. Furthermore, treatment with an agent that relieves ER stress (curcumin) improved the phenotype of both models. Therefore, compounds that either relieve ER stress or reduced UPR activation are promising therapeutic strategies to treat patients with mutations that cause misfolded proteins to accumulate in the ER of Schwann cells.

TARGETING TRANSPORT DEFECTS

Treatment strategies for axonal forms of CMT have not been as easily identified as for demyelinating forms. Recently, histone deacetylase-6 inhibitors have been shown to correct axonal transport defects in a mouse model of CMT2F associated with point mutations in the *HSPB1* gene, rescuing the axonal loss and clinical phenotype of these mice. It remains to be shown whether this same strategy could be useful in other forms of axonal CMT, but correcting axonal transport defects may be a common treatment option for most of these CMT types.

CELLULAR REPROGRAMMING AND HIGH-THROUGHPUT DRUG SCREENING

Two new technologies recently developed hold enormous potential in the search for compounds to treat CMT: cellular reprogramming and high-throughput drug screening. Cellular reprogramming is a technique that allows the generation of specific cell types (including stem cell–like cells, neurons, and glia) by genetically modifying readily available somatic cells such as fibroblasts or lymphocytes. Using this technology, researchers are able to generate unlimited supplies of patient-specific cell lines for use in mechanistic studies and drug development. These patient-specific cell lines will be particularly useful when combined with high-throughput screening of drug libraries containing thousands of compounds. In these highly automated platforms, the process of identifying compounds capable of correcting certain disease-related cell phenotypes is streamlined, allowing for a faster target selection of compounds to be tested in phase 1 animal studies. The use of patient-derived human cells offer the theoretical advantage of a more translational platform, which could facilitate the process of moving from phase 1 studies to human clinical trials. Whether this is actually true remains to be proven.

OUTCOME

Phenotypic variability occurs within given phenotypes, and natural history studies of most forms of CMT are lacking. Nevertheless, most patients remain ambulatory throughout life and life span is not typically shortened. Some patients do not develop symptoms until adult years.

Vital to clinical trials in inherited neuropathy is the establishment of solid outcome measures. With neuropathies that progress slowly over many years, this can be challenging. To this end, a validated scoring system (CMT neuropathy score) based on symptoms, signs, and neurophysiologic data has been developed for adults with excellent inter- and intraobserver correlations and which can detect changes over 1 year. A more sensitive pediatric score exists for those patients between the ages of 3 and 21 years which takes into account growth-related changes and should prove useful in future clinical trials. Sequential yearly magnetic resonance imaging (MRI) of limb muscles looking at progressive replacement of muscle with fatty tissue may also prove to be a valuable outcome measurement and is currently under investigation in a cohort of CMT1A patients.

CONCLUSIONS

Although CMT is a genetically heterogeneous condition, it is often possible to determine the type of CMT a person has by distinguishing characteristics. The prevalence of the various mutations, inheritance pattern, nerve conductions, and age of onset should be taken into account when deciding what genetic testing should be ordered. New genes causing CMT continue to be found, prevalence continues to be studied, and recommendations for testing will continue to evolve over time. Just as the past two decades have witnessed a surge in gene discovery and molecular diagnosis of CMT subtypes, this knowledge will lead to innovative therapeutic directions in the upcoming years. Beyond directing genetic counseling and prognosis in the specific patient, accurate genotyping of individuals with CMT will allow gene/pathway-specific clinical trials and, ultimately, individualization of therapy according to the underlying molecular defect.

SUGGESTED READINGS

Burns J, Ouvrier R, Estilow T, et al. Validation of the Charcot-Marie-Tooth disease pediatric scale as an outcome measure of disability. *Ann Neurol.* 2012;71:642–652.

Harel T, Lupski JR. Charcot-Marie-Tooth disease and pathways to molecular based therapies. *Clin Genet.* 2014;86(5):422–431.

Lewis RA, Sumner AJ, Shy ME. Electrophysiological features of inherited demyelinating neuropathies: a reappraisal in the era of molecular diagnosis. *Muscle Nerve.* 2000;23:1472–1487.

Murphy SM, Herrmann DN, McDermott MP, et al. Reliability of the CMT neuropathy score (second version) in Charcot-Marie-Tooth disease. *J Peripher Nerv Syst.* 2011;16:191–198.

Murphy SM, Laura M, Fawcett K, et al. Charcot-Marie-Tooth disease: frequency of genetic subtypes and guidelines for genetic testing. *J Neurol Neurosurg Psychiatry.* 2012;83:706–710.

Niemann A, Berger P, Suter U. Pathomechanisms of mutant proteins in Charcot-Marie-Tooth disease. *Neuromolecular Med.* 2006;8:217–242.

Pareyson D, Marchesi C, Salsano E. Dominant Charcot-Marie-Tooth syndrome and cognate disorders. *Handb Clin Neurol.* 2013;115:817–845.

Pareyson D, Reilly MM, Schenone A, et al; CMT-TRIAAL; CMT-TRAUK groups. Ascorbic acid in Charcot-Marie-Tooth disease type 1A (CMT-TRIAAL and CMT-TRAUK): a double-blind randomised trial. *Lancet Neurol.* 2011;10:320–328.

Reilly MM, Shy ME. Diagnosis and new treatments in genetic neuropathies. *J Neurol Neurosurg Psychiatry.* 2009;80:1304–1314.

Rossor AM, Kalmar B, Greensmith L, et al. The distal hereditary motor neuropathies. *J Neurol Neurosurg Psychiatry.* 2012;83:6–14.

Rossor AM, Polke JM, Houlden H, et al. Clinical implications of genetic advances in Charcot-Marie-Tooth disease. *Nat Rev Neurol.* 2013;9:562–571.

Rotthier A, Baets J, Timmerman V, et al. Mechanisms of disease in hereditary sensory and autonomic neuropathies. *Nat Rev Neurol.* 2012;8:73–85.

Saporta AS, Sottile SL, Miller LJ, et al. Charcot-Marie-Tooth disease subtypes and genetic testing strategies. *Ann Neurol.* 2011;69:22–33.

Saporta MA, Shy ME. Inherited peripheral neuropathies. *Neurol Clin.* 2013;31:597–619.

Sivera R, Sevilla T, Vilchez JJ, et al. Charcot-Marie-Tooth disease: genetic and clinical spectrum in a Spanish clinical series. *Neurology.* 2013;81:1617–1625.

Christina M. Ulane and Lewis P. Rowland

INTRODUCTION

Pathology at the neuromuscular junction can occur at the presynaptic or postsynaptic membrane. Autoimmune disorders, hereditary diseases, and toxins are the main types of disease which affect the neuromuscular junction.

MYASTHENIA GRAVIS

Myasthenia gravis (MG) is caused by a defect of neuromuscular transmission (NMT) owing to antibody-mediated attack on nicotinic acetylcholine receptors (AChR) or muscle-specific tyrosine kinase (MuSK) at neuromuscular junction. It is characterized by fluctuating weakness that is improved by inhibitors of cholinesterase.

EPIDEMIOLOGY

Greater awareness and improved diagnosis has led to an increased incidence of MG. A systematic review spanning 1980 to 2007 of 31 studies mostly conducted in Europe found incidence rates from 3 to 30 per million per year. The prevalence in the United States is estimated at 20 per 100,000 by Philips in 2003. MG is equally present in men and women older than the age of 40 years; however, it is three times more common in women than men under 40 years of age. MuSK myasthenia is also more common in women.

Systemic autoimmune disorders are found with greater incidence in patients with MG. Thyroid disorders are present in up to 15% of patients with MG. Other autoimmune disorders with increased incidence in patients with MG include rheumatoid arthritis and systemic lupus erythematosus (SLE).

Familial cases are rare; single members of pairs of fraternal twins and several sets of identical twins have been affected. Young women with MG tend to have HLA-B8, HLA-DR3, and HLA-DQB1*0102 haplotypes; in young Japanese women, HLA-A12 is prominent. These observations imply the presence of a linked immune response gene that encodes a protein involved in the autoimmune response. First-degree relatives show an increased incidence of other autoimmune diseases (SLE, rheumatoid arthritis, thyroid disease) and HLA-B8 haplotype.

PATHOBIOLOGY

The purpose of the neuromuscular junction is to transmit the electrical impulse from the motor neuron to the muscle fiber and trigger contraction. The complex synapse is depicted in Figure 89.1. An electrical signal reaching the terminal motor axon results in

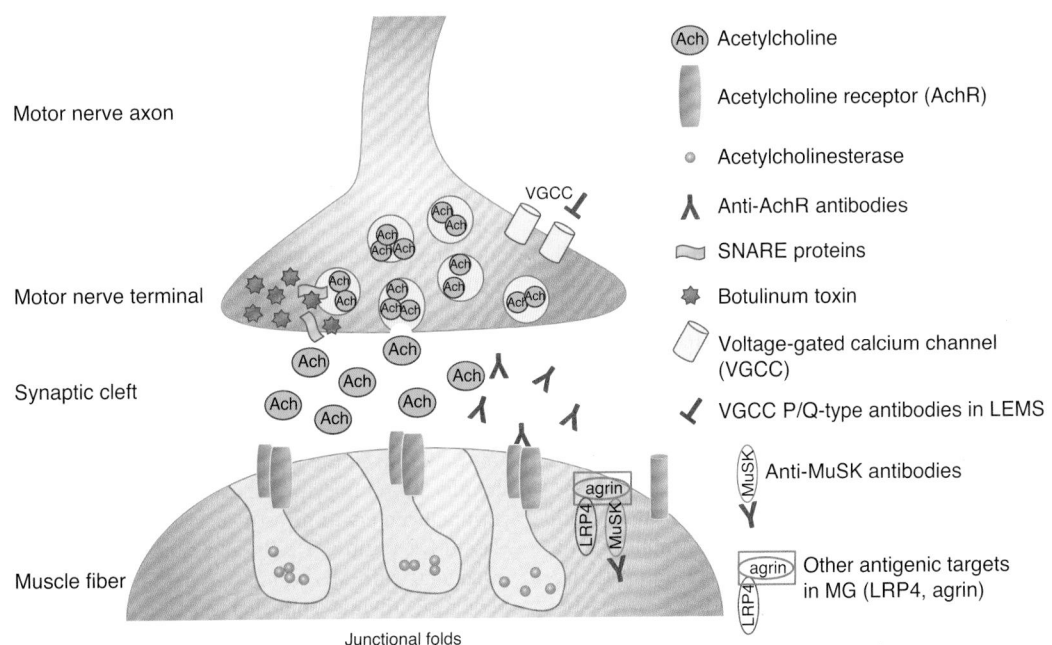

FIGURE 89.1 The neuromuscular junction. Key components of the neuromuscular junction are depicted including the motor axon and muscle endplate, the synaptic cleft, and the muscle fiber. When an action potential reaches the terminal, ACh is released into the synapse and binds to the nicotinic Ach receptors on the sarcolemma, triggering a muscle fiber action potential and contraction. The antigenic targets in myasthenia gravis and LEMS are indicated, as is the site of action of botulinum toxin. LEMS, Lambert–Eaton myasthenic syndrome; MG, myasthenia gravis.

the release of acetylcholine (ACh) quanta into the synaptic cleft through fusion of vesicles with the membrane. The released ACh serves as a chemical signal, which then travels across the synaptic cleft and binds to AChR on the postsynaptic muscle fiber membrane, triggering a muscle fiber action potential and subsequent contraction or twitch.

The neuromuscular junction is susceptible to autoimmune pathology because there is no blood–nerve barrier to protect the neuromuscular junction. The precise mechanisms triggering autoimmunity at the neuromuscular junction are unknown; however, there is considerable knowledge regarding the pathobiology. MG is an antibody-mediated disorder in which the autoantibodies are clearly pathogenic. This is deduced from several lines of evidence:

1. Identification of circulating serum antibodies against the AChR and other components of the neuromuscular junction
2. Immunization of experimental animal models with purified AChR induces high titers of anti-AChR antibodies, weakness, and pathologic and electrophysiologic features of MG.
3. Passive transfer of human immunoglobulin G (IgG) from persons with MG to mice reproduces electrophysiologic features of MG.
4. Plasma exchange reduces anti-AChR antibody titers and ameliorates MG signs and symptoms.

Extensive research has shown the complex autoimmune nature of MG. Antibodies against the AChR are found in 80% to 85% of patients with MG. A majority of these are AChR "binding" antibodies. AChR "modulating" antibodies are found in less than 1% of MG patients without binding antibodies, and "blocking" antibodies are found in approximately 10% of MG patients without binding antibodies. The polyclonal IgG antibodies to AChR are produced by plasma cells in peripheral lymphoid organs, bone marrow, and thymus. These cells are derived from B cells that have been activated by antigen-specific T-helper (CD41) cells. The T cells have also been activated, in this case, by binding to AChR antigenic peptide sequences (epitopes) that rest on the histocompatibility antigens on the surface of antigen-presenting cells.

Most common are anti-AChR binding antibodies, which bind to the AChR on the postsynaptic membrane and cause the complement-mediated destruction of the junctional folds and accelerate internalization and degradation of AChR. Blocking antibodies prevent ACh binding to the AChR. Modulating antibodies distort the neuromuscular junction and folds. The end result in all cases is a loss of functional AChR. The AChR antibodies react with multiple determinants, and enough antibodies circulate to saturate up to 80% of all AChR sites on muscle. A small percentage of the anti-AChR molecules interfere directly with the binding of ACh, but the major damage to endplates seems to result from actual loss of receptors owing to complement-mediated lysis of the membrane and to acceleration of normal degradative processes (internalization, endocytosis, lysosomal hydrolysis) with inadequate replacement by new synthesis. As a consequence of the loss of AChR and the erosion and simplification of the endplates, the amplitude of miniature endplate potentials is about 20% of normal, and patients are abnormally sensitive to the competitive antagonist curare. The characteristic decremental response to repetitive stimulation of the motor nerve reflects failure of endplate potentials to reach threshold so that progressively fewer fibers respond to arrival of a nerve impulse. Most AChR antibodies are directed against antigenic determinants on the extracellular portion of the protein farthest out from the membrane rather than the ACh-binding site. The summed effects of the polyclonal anti-AChR antibodies, especially

those that fix complement, result in destruction of the receptors. Physiologic studies indicate impaired postsynaptic responsiveness to ACh, which accounts for the physiologic abnormalities, clinical symptoms, and beneficial effects of drugs that inhibit acetylcholinesterase (AChE). If binding or blocking antibodies are absent, tests can be done for "modulating" antibodies that enhance degradation of the receptors in cultured cells, bringing the number of positive tests to 90%, according to Howard et al.

The MuSK protein is localized to the inner surface of the muscle membrane and is involved in AChR clustering. Approximately 10% of all patients with MG and 50% of patients without antibodies to the AChR will have antibodies against MuSK. There is prominent atrophy of muscles in anti-MuSK MG. Anti-MuSK antibodies are pathogenic by inhibiting the clustering of the AChR, demonstrated in passive transfer of human IgG from patients with anti-MuSK MG to rodents.

Beginning in 2011, multiple groups of researchers found other antigenic targets in seronegative MG patients. Lipoprotein-related protein 4 (LRP4) is essential for neuromuscular junction formation, serving as an agrin receptor and participating in agrin-activated MuSK and AChR clustering. Antibodies against LRP4 were found in MG patients seronegative for AChR antibodies and MuSK antibodies. Antibodies against agrin were identified in patients both with anti-AChR antibodies and in seronegative patients. There are likely additional autoantibodies to components of the neuromuscular junction which are yet to be discovered and account for the remainder of the "seronegative" MG patients.

How the autoimmune disorder starts is not known. In human disease, in contrast to experimental MG in animals, the thymus gland is almost always abnormal; often multiple lymphoid follicles show germinal centers ("hyperplasia of the thymus"), and in about 15% of patients, there is an encapsulated benign tumor, a thymoma. These abnormalities are impressive because the normal thymus is responsible for the maturation of T cells that mediate immune protection without promoting autoimmune responses. AChR antibodies are synthesized by B cells in cultures of hyperplastic thymus gland. The hyperplastic glands contain all the elements needed for antibody production: class II HLA-positive antigen-presenting cells, T-helper cells, B cells, and AChR antigen; that is, mRNA for subunits of AChR has been detected in thymus, and "myoid cells" are found in both normal and hyperplastic thymus. The myoid cells bear surface AChR and contain other muscle proteins. When human myasthenic thymus was transplanted into severely congenitally immunodeficient mice, the animals produced antibodies to AChR that bound to their own motor endplates, even though weakness was not evident.

T lymphocytes are responsible for initiating and maintaining the autoantibody response, and the thymus gland is the site of overt pathology. About 70% of thymus glands from adult patients with MG are not involuted, weigh more than normal, and demonstrate lymphoid hyperplasia. In contrast, germinal centers in non-myasthenics are numerous in the lymph nodes and spleen but are sparse in the thymus. Immunocytochemical methods indicate that the thymic germinal centers in myasthenics contain B cells, plasma cells, HLA class II DR-positive T cells, and dendritic cells. Approximately 10% of patients with MG will have lymphoepithelial thymomas, and the neoplastic thymic epithelial cells express self-antigens including the AChR and other skeletal muscle proteins such as titin and the ryanodine receptor. The lymphoid cells in these tumors are T cells; the neoplastic elements are epithelial cells. Benign thymomas may nearly replace the gland with only residual glandular material at the edges, or they may rest within a large hyperplastic gland. Thymomas tend to occur in older patients, but in one series, 15% were found in patients between ages 20 and 29 years. They may invade contiguous pleura, pericardium, or blood vessels or seed onto more distant thoracic structures, including the diaphragm; however, they almost never spread to other organs. In older patients without thymoma, the thymus gland appears involuted, often showing hyperplastic foci within fatty tissue on microscopic examination of multiple samples. Excessive and inappropriately prolonged synthesis of thymic hormones that normally promote differentiation of T-helper cells may contribute to the autoimmune response. Still another possible initiating factor is immunogenic alteration of the antigen AChR at endplates; penicillamine therapy in patients with rheumatoid arthritis may initiate a syndrome that is indistinguishable from MG except that it subsides when administration of the drug is stopped.

There are few familial cases of the acquired autoimmune disease, but disproportionate frequency of some HLA haplotypes (B8, DR3, DQB1) in MG patients suggests that genetic predisposition may be important. Other autoimmune diseases also seem to occur with increased frequency in patients with MG, especially hyperthyroidism and other thyroid disorders, SLE, rheumatoid arthritis, pernicious anemia, and pemphigus.

In about 50% of cases, muscles contain lymphorrhages, which are focal clusters of lymphocytes near small necrotic foci without perivascular predilection. In a few cases, especially in patients with thymoma, there is diffuse muscle fiber necrosis with infiltration of inflammatory cells; similar lesions are only rarely encountered in the myocardium. Lymphorrhages are not seen near damaged neuromuscular junctions (although inflammatory cells may be seen in necrotic endplates in rat experimental autoimmune MG), but morphometric studies have shown loss of synaptic folds and widened clefts. Some nerve terminals are smaller than normal, and multiple small terminals are applied to the elongated, simplified postsynaptic membrane; others are absent. Other endplates appear normal. On residual synaptic folds, immunocytochemical methods show Y-shaped antibody-like structures, IgG, complement components 2 and 9, and complement membrane attack complex.

CLINICAL FEATURES

The symptoms of MG have three general characteristics that together provide a diagnostic combination (Table 89.1). Formal diagnosis depends on clinical features, demonstration of the response to cholinergic drugs, electrophysiologic evidence of abnormal neuromuscular transmission, and demonstration of circulating antibodies to AChR or MuSK.

The fluctuating nature of myasthenic weakness is unlike any other disease. The weakness varies in the course of a single day, sometimes within minutes, and it varies from day to day or over longer periods. Major prolonged variations are termed *remissions* or *exacerbations*; when an exacerbation involves respiratory muscles to a degree that intubation and assisted mechanical ventilation, it is called a *crisis*. An "exacerbation" may be ameliorated by noninvasive ventilation or may be a transient worsening without respiratory distress. Variations sometimes seem related to exercise; this and the nature of the physiologic abnormality have long been termed *excessive fatigability*, but there are practical reasons to de-emphasize fatigability as a central characteristic of MG. Patients with the disease less often complain of fatigue or symptoms that might be construed as fatigue except when there is incipient respiratory muscle weakness. Myasthenic symptoms are always owing to weakness and not to rapid tiring. Fatigue is common in MG, and at times can be difficult (especially for patients) to differentiate from true myasthenic exacerbation.

The second characteristic of MG is the distribution of weakness. Ocular muscles are affected first in about 40% of patients and are ultimately involved in about 85%. Ptosis and diplopia are the symptoms

TABLE 89.1	Cardinal Clinical Features of Myasthenia Gravis
• **Fluctuating weakness**	
• Proximal arms or legs	
• Sometimes distal arms/hands	
• Axial: neck flexors > neck extensors	
• **Diplopia**	
• Extraocular muscle weakness	
• May resemble INO	
• **Ptosis**	
• Often asymmetric	
• **Dysarthria**	
• Nasal speech	
• LMN	
• **Dysphagia**	
• **Respiratory insufficiency**	
• Dyspnea	
• Hypoxia is a late finding.	

INO, internuclear ophthalmoplegia; LMN, lower motor neuron.

that result. Other common symptoms affect facial or oropharyngeal muscles, resulting in dysarthria, dysphagia, and limitation of facial movements. Together, oropharyngeal and ocular weakness cause symptoms in virtually all patients with acquired MG. Limb and neck weakness is also common in conjunction with cranial weakness. Almost never are the limbs affected alone. MuSK myasthenia particularly involves ocular, facial, and bulbar muscles and has high risk of respiratory insufficiency. MuSK myasthenia can follow a rapidly progressive and more severe course.

Aside from the fluctuating nature of the weakness, MG is not a steadily progressive disease. The general nature of the disease, however, is usually established within weeks or months after the first symptoms. If myasthenia is restricted to ocular muscles for 2 years, certainly if it is restricted after 3 years, it is likely to remain restricted, and only in rare cases does it then become generalized. Distinguishing solely ocular myasthenia from generalized myasthenia soon after onset is challenging.

Vital signs and findings on general physical examination are usually normal, unless the patient is in crisis. Weakness of the facial and levator palpebrae muscles produces a characteristic expressionless appearance with drooping eyelids, which can be asymmetric (Fig. 89.2A). Weakness of ocular muscles (Fig. 89.2B) may cause paralysis or weakness of isolated ocular muscles, limitation of conjugate gaze, complete ophthalmoplegia in one or both eyes, or a pattern resembling internuclear ophthalmoplegia. Proximal limb weakness is manifest by difficulty in raising the arms above the head (Fig. 89.2C) and difficulty climbing stairs, whereas weakness of the neck flexor and extensor muscles may result in head drop (Fig. 89.2D). Weakness of oropharyngeal or limb muscles, when present, can be shown by appropriate tests. Respiratory muscle weakness can be detected by pulmonary function tests, which should not be limited to measurement of vital capacity but should also include inspiratory and expiratory pressures, the measurement of which may be abnormal even before overt symptoms are evident. Muscular wasting of variable degree is found in about 10% of patients but is not focal and

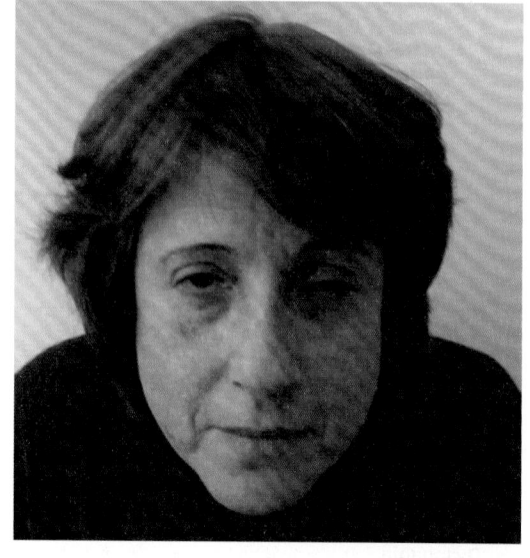
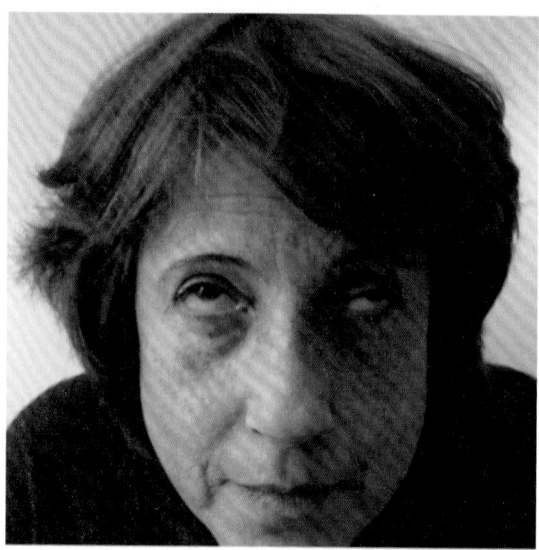
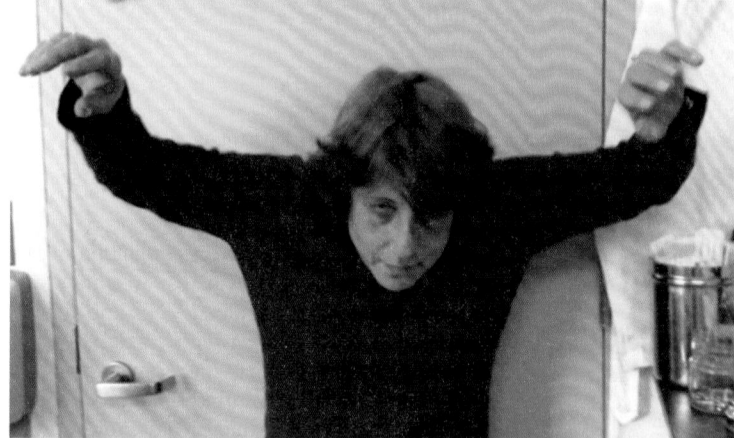
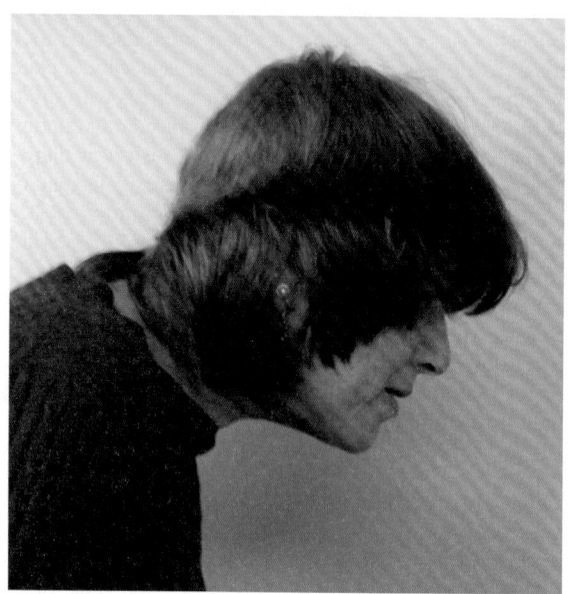

FIGURE 89.2 Clinical features of myasthenia gravis. **A:** Bifacial weakness and asymmetric ptosis. **B:** Weakness of extraocular muscles causing dysconjugate gaze. **C:** Proximal arm weakness. **D:** Neck flexor weakness causing head drop. (Courtesy of C. M. Ulane.)

is usually encountered only in patients with malnutrition caused by severe dysphagia. Fasciculations do not occur, unless the patient has received excessive amounts of cholinergic drugs. Sensation is normal and the reflexes are preserved, even in muscles that are weak.

Crisis is most likely to occur in patients with oropharyngeal or respiratory muscle weakness. It seems to be provoked by respiratory infection in many patients or by surgical procedures, including thymectomy, although it may occur with no apparent provocation. Both emotional stress and systemic illness may aggravate myasthenic weakness for reasons that are not clear; in patients with oropharyngeal weakness, aspiration of secretions may occlude lung passages to cause rather abrupt onset of respiratory difficulty. Major surgery may be followed by respiratory weakness without aspiration, however, so this cannot be the entire explanation.

DIAGNOSIS

Clinical

Clear clinical picture of fluctuating weakness, improved with rest, and ocular symptoms can make diagnosis of MG straightforward. However, ocular MG can at times be challenging to diagnose when clinical signs are minimal during examination, symptoms do not significantly fluctuate, and symptoms are mild. The ice test is performed at bedside on patients with ptosis: A pack of ice is placed over the ptotic eye for 1 to 2 minutes, and resolution or improvement in the ptosis is considered positive and highly specific for MG.

The dramatic improvement that follows the injection of neostigmine bromide (Prostigmin) or edrophonium (Tensilon) makes the administration of these drugs pertinent. The Tensilon test administers the short-acting AChE inhibitor edrophonium; improvement in a subsequent clinical assessment is considered similarly positive and specific for MG. A test dose of 2 mg edrophonium is given intravenously, followed by up to 8 mg intravenously. Muscles weak from MG will respond within 30 to 45 seconds, with a response lasting up to 5 minutes; an objective improvement in muscle strength is considered a positive result. Although risk of serious cardiac complications is low, life-threatening bradyarrhythmias and ventricular fibrillation can occur with the Tensilon test, and it should be carried out with close monitoring and atropine at the bedside. Patients must be monitored for acute decompensation with cholinergic crisis causing increased secretions in patients with oropharyngeal weakness, cholinergic weakness, bradycardia, and gastrointestinal intolerance.

False positives can occur in motor neuron and other diseases, and the sensitivity of the Tensilon test is 60%. Both the ice test and Tensilon test require objectively measurable outcomes and thus are most useful in cases of ptosis and oculomotor abnormalities, rather than limb weakness. The only other conditions in which clinical improvement has been documented after use of edrophonium are other disorders of neuromuscular transmission: botulinum intoxication, snake bite, organophosphate intoxication, or unusual disorders that include features of both MG and the Lambert–Eaton syndrome. Denervating disorders, such as motor neuron disease or peripheral neuropathy, do not show a reproducible or unequivocal clinical response to edrophonium or neostigmine. The response should be unequivocal and reproducible. If a structural lesion of the third cranial nerve seems to respond, the result should be photographed (and published).

Laboratory and Electrodiagnostics

Routine examinations of blood, urine, and cerebrospinal fluid (CSF) are normal. Antibodies to AChR are found in 85% to 90% of patients of all ages with generalized MG if human muscle is used as the test antigen (Table 89.2). Antibodies may not be detected in patients with strictly ocular disease, in some patients in remission (or after thymectomy), or even in some patients with severe symptoms. The titer does not match the severity of symptoms; patients in complete clinical remission may have high titers. For pure ocular MG, AChR antibodies present in serum support the diagnosis; however, the sensitivity is rather low (range 25% to 70%). Antibodies to myofibrillar proteins (titin, myosin, actin, actomyosin) are found in 85% of patients with thymoma and may be the first evidence of thymoma in some cases. In the first report of seronegative myasthenia, there were no clinical differences between patients who had or lacked AChR antibodies. Subsequently, more than half of these seronegative patients were found to have antibodies to MuSK. Patients with anti-MuSK antibodies were found to have a similar clinical picture almost always with generalized MG with predominantly bulbar signs, poor and inconsistent responses to pyridostigmine, immunosuppressants, or thymectomy but excellent response to plasmapheresis. Antibodies to rapsyn-clustered AChR were detected on human embryonic kidney cells by fluorescence-activated cell sorting in 66% (25/38) of sera from patients that had previously tested negative for binding to AChR in solution. Other serologic abnormalities are encountered with varying frequency, and in several studies, antinuclear factor, rheumatoid factor, and thyroid antibodies were encountered more often than in control populations.

The characteristic electrodiagnostic abnormality is progressive decrement in the amplitude of compound muscle action potentials evoked by repetitive nerve stimulation at 3 or 5 Hz (Fig. 89.3). In generalized MG, the decremental response can be demonstrated in about 90% of patients if at least three neuromuscular systems are used (median-thenar, ulnar-hypothenar, accessory-trapezius). Repetitive nerve stimulation testing is often negative in ocular MG (in both distal and proximal muscles). In single-fiber electromyography (EMG), a small electrode measures the interval between evoked potentials of the muscle fibers in the same motor unit.

TABLE 89.2	Diagnostic Testing for Myasthenia Gravis
Laboratory Test	**Comments**
Acetylcholine receptor (AChR) antibodies	
• AChR binding • AChR blocking • AChR modulating	• 80%–85% of all MG • 50% of ocular MG • Binding most common • Blocking positive in ~10% of MG with negative binding • Modulating positive in <1% of MG with negative binding
MusK antibodies	• 10% of all MG • 50% of AchR-negative MG
Other antibodies	
• Striational • (titin, RyR, myosin, actin) • LRP4, agrin	• Present in 75%–85% of thymomatous MG • May be associated with more severe disease (titin, RyR) • Found in other disorders
Electrodiagnostic Test	
Nerve conduction studies	• Repetitive nerve stimulation reveals decrement (≥10%). • Sensitivity 53%–100% in generalized MG • Sensitivity 10%–48% in ocular MG • Not specific
Single-fiber EMG	• Most sensitive test for MG (>95%) but not specific (~70%)
Radiology	
Computed tomography of the chest	• 10% thymoma

MG, myasthenia gravis; EMG, electromyography.

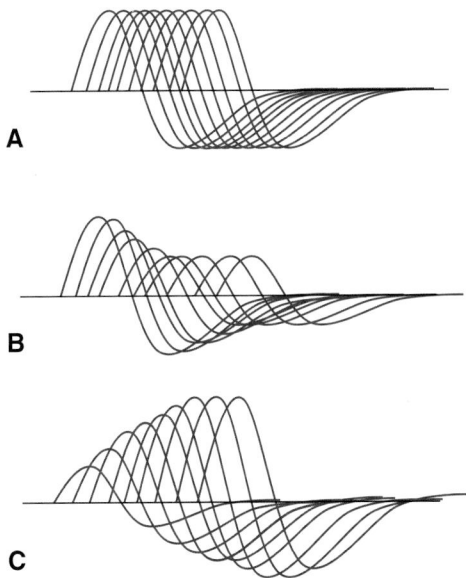

FIGURE 89.3 Repetitive nerve stimulation. Slow (3 Hz) repetitive nerve stimulation (RNS) of the median nerve-abductor pollicis brevis system reveals normal response, decrement and facilitation of the compound muscle action potential. **A:** Normal response to RNS with minimal decrement. **B:** Decremental response in MG. **C:** Facilitation in Lambert–Eaton myasthenic syndrome and botulism.

This interval normally varies, a phenomenon called *jitter*, and the normal temporal limits of jitter have been defined. In MG, the jitter is increased, and an impulse may not appear at the expected time; this is called *blocking*, and the number of blockings is increased in myasthenic muscle. All these electrophysiologic abnormalities are characteristic of MG, but blocking and jitter are also seen in other disorders. Single-fiber EMG is the most sensitive test for MG but is not specific.

The standard-needle EMG is usually normal, occasionally shows a myopathic pattern, and almost never shows signs of denervation unless some other condition supervenes. Similarly, nerve conduction velocities are normal.

All patients diagnosed with MG should be screened for the presence of thymoma. Computed tomography (CT) of the mediastinum demonstrates all but microscopic thymomas. Magnetic resonance imaging (MRI) is not more sensitive than CT.

The differential diagnosis includes all diseases that are accompanied by weakness of oropharyngeal or limb muscles, such as the muscular dystrophies, amyotrophic lateral sclerosis (ALS), progressive bulbar palsy, ophthalmoplegia of other causes, and the asthenia of psychoneurosis or hyperthyroidism. There is usually no difficulty in differentiating these conditions from MG by the findings on examination and by the failure of symptoms in these conditions to improve after parenteral injection of neostigmine or edrophonium. Occasionally, blepharospasm is thought to mimic ocular myasthenia, but the forceful eye closure in that condition involves both the upper and the lower lids; the narrowed palpebral fissure and signs of active muscle activity are distinctive.

TREATMENT

Treatment for MG is tailored to the individual patient. A general algorithm for treatment of MG is presented in Figure 89.4. Clinicians must choose the sequence and combination of therapy: anticholinesterase drug therapy, corticosteroids, immunosuppressives, plasmapheresis, intravenous immunoglobulins (IVIG), and thymectomy (Table 89.3).

Cholinesterase Inhibitors

In 1934, Dr. Mary Walker discovered the beneficial effects of AChE inhibitors in patients with MG. To this day, this remains a mainstay of treatment, yet there are no randomized trials of these agents in MG. A Cochrane review in 2011 reaffirmed the lack of controlled studies but concluded that the results from observational studies were so clear that it would be difficult to justify a trial. It is generally agreed that anticholinesterase drug therapy should be given as soon as the diagnosis is made. Of the three available drugs—neostigmine, pyridostigmine bromide, and ambenonium—pyridostigmine is the most popular but has not been formally assessed in controlled comparison with the other drugs. The muscarinic side effects of abdominal cramps and diarrhea are the same for all three drugs but are least severe with pyridostigmine; none has more beneficial or adverse effects than another and all can be regarded as safe. The usual starting dose of pyridostigmine is 60 mg given orally every 4 hours while the patient is awake. Depending on clinical response, the dosage may be increased, but incremental benefit is not to be expected in amounts greater than 120 mg every 2 hours. If patients have difficulty eating, doses can be taken about 30 minutes before a meal. If patients have special difficulty on waking in the morning, an extended-release 180-mg tablet of pyridostigmine can be taken at bedtime. Muscarinic symptoms can be ameliorated by preparations containing atropine (0.4 mg) with each dose of pyridostigmine. Excessive doses of atropine can cause psychosis, but the amounts taken in this regimen have not had that effect. Other drugs may be taken if diarrhea is prominent. Combinations of two drugs are no better than any single drug alone.

Although cholinergic drug therapy sometimes gives impressive results, there are serious limitations. In ocular myasthenia, ptosis may be helped, but some diplopia almost always persists. In generalized MG, patients may improve remarkably, but some symptoms usually remain. Cholinergic drugs do not return function to normal, and the risk of crisis persists because the disease is not cured. Therefore, one of the other treatments is used promptly to treat

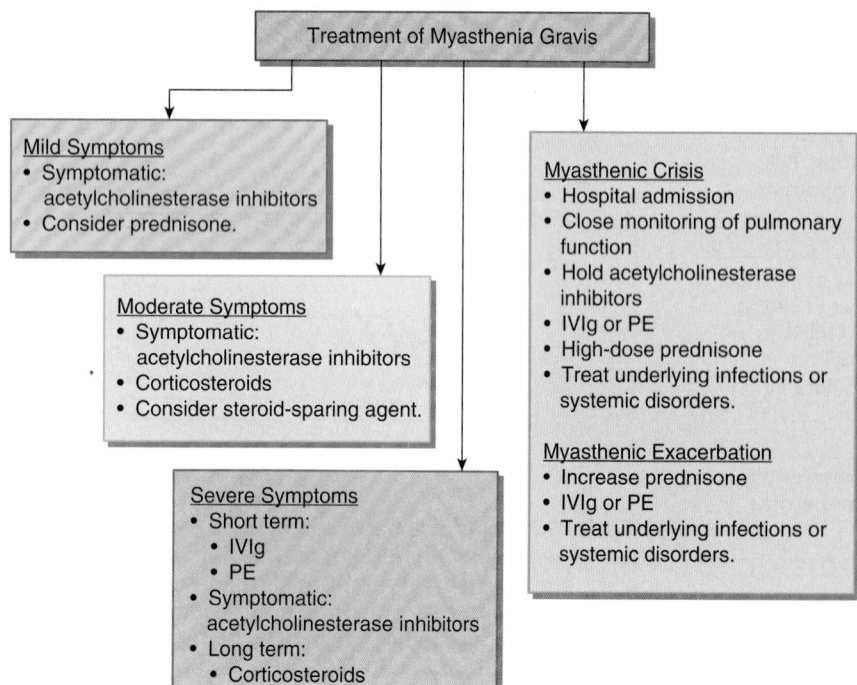

FIGURE 89.4 General treatment guidelines for MG. Treatment of MG is highly individualized and depends on many factors. Shown here are general principles to guide physicians in the treatment of MG based on severity of symptoms. IVIG, intravenous immunoglobulins; PE, plasma exchange.

Treatment of Myasthenia Gravis

Mild Symptoms
• Symptomatic: acetylcholinesterase inhibitors
• Consider prednisone.

Moderate Symptoms
• Symptomatic: acetylcholinesterase inhibitors
• Corticosteroids
• Consider steroid-sparing agent.

Severe Symptoms
• Short term:
  • IVIg
  • PE
• Symptomatic: acetylcholinesterase inhibitors
• Long term:
  • Corticosteroids
  • Steroid-sparing agents

Myasthenic Crisis
• Hospital admission
• Close monitoring of pulmonary function
• Hold acetylcholinesterase inhibitors
• IVIg or PE
• High-dose prednisone
• Treat underlying infections or systemic disorders.

Myasthenic Exacerbation
• Increase prednisone
• IVIg or PE
• Treat underlying infections or systemic disorders.

TABLE 89.3   Medications Used to Treat Myasthenia Gravis

Agent	Dose	Monitoring Parameters	Side Effects
Pyridostigmine	30–90 mg q4–6h Extended release: 180 mg q.h.s	Clinical response	Common: fasciculations, diarrhea Overdose: cholinergic crisis, weakness, dysphagia, respiratory failure Rare: bromism (acute psychosis)
Prednisone	1 mg/kg/day (usually 60–80 mg/day) Alternate-day dosing Taper over months after sustained clinical response Concomitant: PPIs, H2 blockers Calcium, vitamin D	May cause initial worsening Blood pressure Serum glucose Yearly ophthalmologic exam	Hyperglycemia Hypertension Weight gain Fluid retention Cataracts/glaucoma Osteoporosis/avascular necrosis Steroid myopathy Peptic ulcer disease Depression/psychiatric effects
IVIG	2 g/kg over 4–5 days	Heart rate Blood pressure Clinical response (usually within 1 wk)	Common: headache, chills, fever, nausea Rare: acute renal failure (solute-induced), aseptic meningitis, thrombosis (DVT/PE, stroke, MI), leukopenia
Plasma exchange	five to six exchanges	Heart rate Blood pressure Coagulation studies Fibrinogen Ionized calcium	Paresthesias Hypotension Transient arrhythmias Nausea, light-headedness, chills Complications of central lines
Azathioprine	Start at 50 mg/day Titrate up to 2–3 mg/kg/day	Complete blood count Hepatic function	Infections Gastrointestinal upset Hepatoxicity Cytopenias Malignancy
Mycophenolate mofetil	1g b.i.d., up to 3g total daily[a]	Complete blood count Hepatic function	Infections Cytopenias Nausea Diarrhea Abdominal pain If used with other immunosuppressives: PML
Cyclosporine A	5–6 mg/kg b.i.d. Goal trough: 75–150 ng/mL	Blood pressure Renal function	Infections Renal toxicity Hypertension Many medication interactions
Tacrolimus	3–5 mg/day	Blood pressure Renal function Glucose	Infections Hyperglycemia Renal toxicity Hypertension Malignancy
Cyclophosphamide	Monthly pulsed doses 500 mg/m^{2b}	Complete metabolic panel Urine studies Complete blood count	Myelosuppression Hemorrhagic cystitis Hyponatremia Seizures Opportunistic infection Malignancy

[a]Recent randomized controlled trials (RCTs) suggest no benefit.

[b]Usually reserved for severe refractory MG.

PPIs, proton pump inhibitors; IVIG, intravenous immunoglobulin; DVT, deep vein thrombosis; PE, pulmonary embolism; MI, myocardial infarction; PML, progressive multifocal leukoencephalopathy.

generalized MG. MuSK MG patients often do not respond as well to anticholinesterases.

Glucocorticoids

Despite the widespread use and agreed upon efficacy of glucocorticoids in the treatment of MG, there are no randomized controlled

studies, and at this point, it would be unethical to withhold a known beneficial treatment. Several controlled and blinded studies initially suggested the benefit of steroids for MG. Numerous retrospective studies show that steroids can induce remission in 27% to 42% and marked improvement in 29% to 52% of patients with MG. Prednisone, 60 to 100 mg daily, will achieve a response within a few days or weeks. Within the first 2 weeks of starting prednisone, patients may experience worsening of their symptoms, and caution must be taken in those with prominent bulbar or respiratory symptoms. An equally satisfactory response can be seen with a lower dosage, but it takes longer; for instance, if the dose is 25 to 40 mg, benefit may be seen in 2 to 3 months. Once improvement is achieved, the dosage should be gradually tapered to 20 to 35 mg every other day. This has become a popular treatment for disabled patients, but there has been no controlled trial. If the patient does not improve in about 6 months or if there are unacceptable side effects from the steroids, treatment with steroid-sparing agents is pursued.

Prednisone, 15 to 35 mg on alternate days, is also recommended by some clinicians for ocular myasthenia, weighing risks against potential benefit. For some patients in sensitive occupations, the risks of prednisone therapy may be necessary (e.g., actors, police officers, roofers or others who work on heights, or those who require stereoscopic vision). Ocular myasthenia is not a threat to life, and pyridostigmine may alleviate ptosis. An eye patch can end diplopia, and prisms help some patients with stable horizontal diplopia. Currently, the Efficacy of Prednisone in the Treatment of Ocular Myasthenia (EPITOME) trial is ongoing and seeks to study the safety and efficacy of prednisone for ocular MG in a multicenter, randomized controlled trial.

Steroid-Sparing Agents

Azathioprine is one of the most studied in this category. It is a purine antimetabolite, which acts by inhibiting T- and B-cell proliferation. It is often well tolerated but it can take more than 12 months to achieve maximal benefit. Common side effects include gastrointestinal upset and an idiosyncratic flulike reaction. In addition, azathioprine may cause hepatotoxicity and transaminases need to be monitored. Rare but serious adverse effects include leukopenia and pancytopenia, which can occur at any time during treatment. In 1998, a randomized controlled trial demonstrated the benefit of azathioprine in addition to prednisolone. Patients receiving both had fewer exacerbations, longer remission, and lower total daily dose of maintenance prednisolone [**Level 1**].[1] Another study suggests that azathioprine alone may be as effective or more effective than prednisone alone in preventing clinical deterioration after 2 to 4 years of treatment [**Level 1**].[2]

Mycophenolate mofetil inhibits T- and B-cell proliferation by selectively blocking purine synthesis. Initial pilot and retrospective studies showed promising benefit for the treatment of MG. In one report, 73% of 85 patients improved; adverse effects led to discontinuation of treatment in 6% [**Level 1**].[3] However, two randomized controlled trials in 2008 showed no benefit over placebo [**Level 1**].[4,5] Many experts still use mycophenolate and consider it effective, and it has a favorable side effect profile. Critiques of the negative studies suggested that the patients chosen had mild disease, a better than expected response to low-dose prednisone and the overall short duration of the trial may have obscured a positive effect.

Cyclosporine acts as a calcineurin inhibitor, thus reducing the function of effector T cells. It is used less due to renal toxicity; however, it has been shown to be effective in several randomized, controlled trials [**Level 1**].[6,7]

Cyclophosphamide can also be considered in doses up to 2.5 mg/kg daily for an adult [**Level 1**].[8] It is often reserved for refractory cases due to toxicity. Another agent with benefit is tacrolimus [**Level 1**].[9]

Methotrexate may also be considered as a second-line agent for the treatment of MG, but there is no quality data to support its efficacy. Side effects are often mild with mucositis, alopecia, and gastrointestinal intolerance, but serious adverse events such as interstitial pneumonitis, hepatotoxicity, and bone marrow suppression can occur.

The numerous side effects of prednisone must be weighed against the possibilities of marrow suppression, susceptibility to infection, or delayed malignancy in patients who are given immunosuppressive drugs.

Intravenous Immunoglobulins and Plasma Exchange

Plasma exchange (PE) is also used for exacerbations; the resulting improvement, seen in most patients, may be slight or dramatic and may last only a few days or several months. PE is safe but expensive and is not convenient for many patients. Indwelling catheters may lead to bleeding or infection. In general, 5 sessions of PE are given every other day.

IVIG therapy is usually given in five daily doses to a total of 2 g/kg body weight. There is some evidence that 1g/kg may be sufficient for treating exacerbation [**Level 1**].[10] A randomized, double-masked, placebo-controlled trial of IVIG for the treatment of moderate to severe MG exacerbations found benefit that was both statistically significant and clinically meaningful [**Level 1**].[11] Side effects include headache, aseptic meningitis, and a flulike syndrome that can be alarming but subsides in 1 or 2 days. Thromboembolic events, including stroke, can occur. IVIG is easier to administer but is even more expensive. It is preferred over PE in those with poor venous access, including children.

Both IVIG and PE are also available for management of exacerbations. Given the differences in availability at various treatment centers and different side effect profiles, it is important to consider each carefully. A study compared IVIG to PE for moderate to severe exacerbations in a randomized, masked fashion and found both to be equally effective treatments for worsening MG with similar duration of benefits and safety profiles [**Level 1**].[12]

Other Immunomodulatory Agents

There is great interest in new immunosuppressive and modulatory therapies to treat MG. Recently, there is significant focus on the use of rituximab (a monoclonal antibody to CD20 B-cells which acts to deplete B-cell reserves) in MG. Many case reports and series suggest a robust response in patients in particular with MuSK antibody MG. It is also used off-label at times for refractory generalized MG. There is currently an ongoing trial to assess its efficacy in the treatment of MG.

There is interest in eculizumab for the treatment of MG; eculizumab acts to prevents terminal complement activation and therefore could function to preserve AChR and neuromuscular junction transmission in MG. Promising results from a phase II trial have instigated the initiation of a phase III trial regarding its efficacy.

Thymectomy

Thymectomy was originally reserved for patients with serious disability because the operation had a high mortality. With advances in surgery and anesthesia, however, the operative mortality is now negligible in major centers. About 80% of patients without thymoma become asymptomatic or go into complete remission after thymectomy; although there has been no controlled trial of thymectomy, these results seem to diverge from the natural history of the untreated disease. Currently, there is an ongoing randomized trial of thymectomy in MG to address this exact question.

Decisions made for children or patients older than 65 years must be individualized. Although it is safe, thymectomy is a major operation and is not usually recommended for patients with ocular myasthenia unless there is a thymoma. The thymoma should be resected but so should the remaining thymus that may show hyperplasia. The beneficial effects of thymectomy are usually delayed for months or years. It is never an emergency measure, and other forms of therapy are used in the interim. Mantegazza et al. found a remission rate of about 50% at 6 years after surgery with either the standard transsternal operation or a minimally invasive thorascopic operation.

Patients with thymoma are likely to have more severe MG and are less likely to improve after thymectomy; nevertheless, many of these patients also improve if the surrounding thymus gland is excised in addition to the tumor.

Myasthenic Crisis

Myasthenic crisis arises in about 10% of myasthenic patients. It is more likely to occur in patients with dysarthria, dysphagia, and documented respiratory muscle weakness, presumably because they are liable to aspirate oral secretions, but crisis may also occur in other patients after respiratory infection or major surgery (including thymectomy). The principles of treatment are those of respiratory failure in general. Numerous retrospective studies have investigated what clinical and laboratory factors in MG crisis predict the need for mechanical ventilation. See Table 89.4 for clinical and laboratory features of impending respiratory failure in patients with MG. Cholinergic drug therapy is usually discontinued once an endotracheal tube has been placed and positive pressure respiration started; this practice avoids questions about the proper dosage or cholinergic stimulation of pulmonary secretions. Crisis is viewed as a temporary exacerbation that subsides in a few days or weeks. The therapeutic goal is to maintain vital functions and to avoid or treat infection until the patient spontaneously recovers from the crisis. Cholinergic drug therapy need not be restarted unless fever and other signs of infection have subsided, there are no pulmonary complications, and the patient is breathing without assistance. Myasthenic crisis and exacerbations can be triggered by infections, surgery, and medications (Table 89.5).

TABLE 89.4	Signs of Impending Respiratory Failure in Myasthenia Gravis
Clinical features	Significant bulbar dysfunction
	• Dysarthria, dysphagia
	• Impaired gag reflex
	Tachypnea, dyspnea
	Use of accessory muscles
	Paradoxical breathing
	Count out loud in single exhale
	Poor cough
	Impaired secretion clearance
Laboratory signs	**Pulmonary function tests:**
	VC <15–20 mL/kg (or VC <1 L)
	NIF > −20 cm H_2O
	MEP <40 cm H_2O
	Tidal volume <4–5 mL/kg
	Laboratory:
	PCO_2 ≥50 mm Hg[a]

[a]Hypoxia is a late finding.
VC, vital capacity; NIF, negative inspiratory force; MEP, maximal expiratory pressure.

TABLE 89.5	Medications That Exacerbate Myasthenia Gravis
Contraindicated	α-Interferon Penicillamine Telithromycin Botulinum toxin
Use with caution (may worsen MG)	**Cardiac medications** • β-Blockers (propranolol, timolol maleate eye drops) • Calcium channel blockers • Quinine, quinidine, procainamide **Neuromuscular blocking agents** • Succinylcholine • d-Tubocurarine **Antibiotics** • Aminoglycosides (gentamicin, kanamycin, streptomycin, neomycin) • Macrolides (erythromycin, azithromycin) • Quinolones (ciprofloxacin, levofloxacin, norfloxacin, ofloxacin) **Magnesium salts** (laxatives, antacids)

MG, myasthenia gravis.

Outcome

Before the advent of intensive care units (ICUs) and the introduction of positive pressure respirators in the 1960s, crisis was a life-threatening event. In the past 60 to 70 years, advances in pulmonary critical care and in the diagnosis of MG have reduced mortality rates for myasthenic crisis from 33% to 60% to approximately 4%. With improved respiratory care, patients rarely die of MG, except when cardiac, renal, or other disease complicates the picture. Even so, pulmonary intensive care is now so effective that crisis is almost never fatal and many patients go into a remission after recovery from crisis. Because of advances in therapy, MG is still serious but not so grave.

SPECIAL FORMS OF MYASTHENIA GRAVIS

Neonatal Myasthenia

About 12% of infants born to myasthenic mothers have a syndrome characterized by impaired sucking, weak cry, limp limbs, and, exceptionally, respiratory insufficiency. Symptoms begin in the first 48 hours and may last several days or weeks, after which the children are normal. The mothers are usually symptomatic but may be in complete remission; in either case, AChR antibodies are demonstrable in both mother and child. Symptoms disappear as the antibody titer in the infant declines. Severe respiratory insufficiency may be treated by exchange transfusion, but the natural history of the disorder is progressive improvement and total disappearance of all symptoms within days or weeks. Respiratory support and nutrition are the key elements of treatment. Rare instances of arthrogryposis multiplex congenita (a syndrome of multiple joint contractures present at birth) have been attributed to transplacental transfer of antibodies that inhibit fetal AChR.

Congenital Myasthenia

Children with congenital MG, although rarely encountered, show several characteristics. The mothers are asymptomatic and do not have circulating anti-AChR in the blood. Usually, no problem occurs in the neonatal period; instead, ophthalmoplegia is the dominant sign later in infancy. Limb weakness may be evident. The condition is often familial. Antibodies to AChR are not found, but there are decremental responses to repetitive stimulation. Ultrastructural and biochemical examination of motor endplates, microelectrode analysis, and identification of mutations have delineated a series of disorders that include both presynaptic, synaptic, and postsynaptic proteins including not only AChR but also the ColQ part of AChE, choline acetylase, rapsyn, MuSK, the $Na_v1.4$ sodium channel, plectin, and Dok-7. Disorders of the ion channel formed by the AChR molecule include the slow-channel syndrome, in which the response to ACh is enhanced because the opening episodes of the channel are abnormally prolonged. Forearm extensors tend to be selectively weak. More than 11 different mutations have been identified in different AChR subunits. Quinidine shortens the prolonged openings and gives therapeutic benefit. A fast-channel syndrome, with impaired response to ACh, has been reported in rare patients with mutations of the ϵ-subunit. Another mutation in the same subunit leads to abnormal kinetics of AChR activation so that the channel opens more slowly and closes more rapidly than normal. The 38 known mutations in the ϵ-subunit are inherited recessively and result in severe lack of AChR in the endplates. One syndrome results from mutations in the collagen tail subunit of AChE, creating a deficiency of the enzyme. Subsequently, clinical differences were identified between those with mutations in the AChR ϵ-subunit and those with mutations in rapsyn, the endplate AChR clustering protein. The receptor mutations caused congenital ophthalmoplegia, bulbar symptoms, and limb weakness. The rapsyn mutations caused an early-onset syndrome with arthrogryposis and life-threatening crises in childhood or a late-onset syndrome beginning in adolescence or later and resembling seronegative myasthenia. Dok-7 binding impairs MuSK signaling and this myasthenic syndrome is relatively common. It is associated with a proximal (limb-girdle) weakness. Slow-channel syndrome benefits from quinidine; fast-channel syndromes, from 3,4-diaminopyridines. Anticholinesterase drugs may help in some of these disorders, but parents should be warned that sudden apneic spells may be induced by mild infections.

Drug-Induced Myasthenia

The best example of this condition occurs in patients treated with penicillamine for rheumatoid arthritis, scleroderma, or hepatolenticular degeneration (Wilson disease). The clinical manifestations and AChR antibody titers are similar to those of typical adult MG, but both disappear when drug administration is discontinued. Cases attributed to the anticonvulsant trimethadione have been less thoroughly studied.

LAMBERT–EATON MYASTHENIC SYNDROME

The Lambert–Eaton myasthenic syndrome (LEMS) is an autoimmune disease of peripheral cholinergic synapses. Antibodies are directed against voltage-gated calcium channels in peripheral nerve terminals (see Fig. 89.1).

EPIDEMIOLOGY

LEMS is rare and found essentially only in adults. It can be either autoimmune or paraneoplastic. About half of LEMS cases are paraneoplastic, and of these, 80% occur with small cell carcinoma of the lung. The neurologic symptoms almost always precede those of the

tumor; the interval may be as long as 5 years. Other tumors have also been implicated, but about 33% of cases are not associated with a tumor. Tumor-free individuals tend to show the HLA-B8 and HLA-DR3 haplotype, which are not found in those with neoplasms.

PATHOBIOLOGY

Cell lines derived from the lung cancer bear voltage-gated calcium channels displaying the antigenic sites. If tumor cells are grown in the presence of IgG from a patient with LEMS, the number of functional channels declines. Similar antigens are found on voltage-gated calcium channels from neuroendocrine tumors. The cultured carcinoma cells also bear receptors for dihydropyridines.

The abnormality of neurotransmission is attributed to inadequate release of ACh from nerve terminals at both nicotinic and muscarinic sites and is related to P/Q voltage-dependent calcium channels. When IgG from affected patients is injected into mice, the number of ACh quanta released by nerve stimulation is reduced, and there is disarray of the active zone particles that can be detected by freeze-fracture ultrastructural analysis.

Purified calcium channel proteins can be directly radiolabeled. An alternative label can be generated by the use of specific ligand, omega-conotoxin, which is prepared from a marine snail (*Conus magus*) and has been used to identify P/Q-type calcium channels in extracts of small cell carcinoma, neuroblastoma, and other neuroendocrine cell lines. A diagnostic test for the autoantibodies is based on radiolabeled preparations, but it is not fully specific. In one series 92% of 72 patients had a positive reaction. A glial cell nuclear antigen identified in small cell lung carcinoma (SCLC) (a developmental transcription factor) is reactive in 22% of SCLC patients and has been identified in 64% of patients with both LEMS and SCLC but none of those with LEMS alone. This could provide a marker of concurrent SCLC in patients with LEMS. There have been a few positive tests for this antigen in paraneoplastic cerebellar disorders. Some patients have both LEMS and a cerebellar syndrome.

CLINICAL FEATURES

LEMS may be suspected in patients with symptoms of proximal limb weakness who have lost knee and ankle jerks and complain of dry mouth or myalgia. Other less common autonomic symptoms include impotence, constipation, and hypohidrosis. LEMS differs clinically from MG because diplopia, dysarthria, dysphagia, and dyspnea are lacking. Autonomic symptoms are more common in LEMS than in MG.

DIAGNOSIS

The disease is defined, and the diagnosis made, by the characteristic incremental response to repetitive nerve stimulation, a pattern that is the opposite of MG. The first evoked potential has an abnormally low amplitude, which decreases even further at low rates of stimulation. At rates greater than 10 Hz, however, there is a marked increase in the amplitude of evoked response (2 to 20 times the original value) (see Fig. 89.3C). The increment results from facilitation of release of transmitter at high rates of stimulation, which can also be achieved by exercise. At low rates, the number of quanta released per impulse (quantal content) is inadequate to produce endplate potentials that reach threshold. Similar abnormalities are found in preparations exposed to botulinum toxin or to a milieu low in calcium or high in magnesium.

Appropriate search for malignancy should be done in all patients diagnosed with LEMS, including CT chest, and possibly positron emission tomography (PET) scan. If initially negative, screening should be repeated in the ensuing years, as the LEMS may precede the malignancy.

Some patients with LEMS have ptosis with antibodies to AChR. This combined syndrome may be an example of multiple autoimmune diseases in the same individual.

TREATMENT

Treatment is directed to the concomitant tumor. The neuromuscular disorder is treated with drugs that facilitate release of ACh, such as 3,4-diaminopyridine. Two randomized controlled trials showed both clinical and electrophysiologic improvement with 3,4-diaminopyridine in patients with LEMS [**Level 1**].[13,14] A combination of pyridostigmine bromide and 3,4-diaminopyridine improves strength, but other aminopyridines may be hazardous. 4-Aminopyridine causes convulsions. 3,4-Diaminopyridine is not currently approved by the U.S. Food and Drug Administration (FDA) but is available through expanded access studies in the United States. Other drugs that facilitate release of ACh have also had adverse effects. For instance, guanidine hydrochloride (20 to 30 mg/kg/day) may depress bone marrow or cause severe tremor and cerebellar syndrome.

Other treatments that may be helpful include PE, IVIG, steroids, and immunosuppressive agents. A small randomized placebo-controlled crossover trial showed short-term benefit in strength for LEMS patients treated with IVIG, presumably due to the lower levels of circulating antibodies [**Level 1**].[15]

BOTULISM

EPIDEMIOLOGY AND PATHOBIOLOGY

Botulism is a disease in which nearly total paralysis of nicotinic and muscarinic cholinergic transmission is caused by botulinum toxin, which acts on presynaptic mechanisms for release of ACh in response to nerve stimulation. The heavy chain of the toxin mediates binding of the toxin to surface receptors on motor nerve terminals. This allows the toxin molecule to be internalized via endocytosis, and the light chain is then translocated into the cytoplasm. The light chain functions as a zinc-dependent protease that cleaves different components of synaptic vesicles depending on the serotype of the toxin. Toxin types A and E cleave SNAP-25; type B, synaptotagmin, and both B, F, and G, synaptobrevin so that exocytosis of vesicles is blocked (see Fig. 89.1).

The toxins are produced by spores of clostridial agents. *Clostridium botulinum*, which may contaminate foods grown in soil, produces types A, B, F, and G or in fish, type E; *Clostridium butyricum* produces type E and *Clostridium barati* produces type F. Intoxication results if contaminated food is inadequately cooked and the spores are not destroyed or if fish are not eviscerated before drying or salt curing. Toxin can be produced in anaerobic wounds that have been contaminated by organisms and spores. Ingestion or inhalation of spores by infants may cause botulism when toxins type A or B are produced in the gastrointestinal tract during periods of constipation. An analogous syndrome occurs in adults with growth of *C. botulinum* in the intestine after surgery from gastric achlorhydria or from antibiotic therapy. The toxin does not cause cell death, although it disrupts exocytosis. The effects slowly disappear over several months.

CLINICAL FEATURES

Isolated cases in children and adolescents may be thought to be Guillain–Barré syndrome, MG, or even diphtheria. Ptosis has

responded to intravenous edrophonium chloride in a few patients, but response to anticholinesterase drugs is neither sufficiently extensive nor sufficiently prolonged to be therapeutic. Infants with botulism are usually younger than 6 months. They show generalized weakness, which is manifested by reduced spontaneous movements, lethargy, poor sucking, and drooling. Sucking and gag reflexes are decreased or absent. There is facial diplegia, ptosis, and ophthalmoparesis.

DIAGNOSIS

Diagnosis is made by the following characteristics: symmetry of signs, dry mouth or absence of saliva, pupillary paralysis, and the characteristic incremental response to repetitive nerve stimulation (see Fig. 89.3C). The Centers for Disease Control and Prevention (CDC; with a dedicated emergency 24-hour telephone number) or appropriate state laboratories should be notified so that the toxin can be identified in refrigerated samples of serum, stool, or residual food samples. In suspected infantile botulism, feces should be evaluated for the presence of *C. botulinum* as well as toxin.

Electrophysiologic evidence of severely disturbed neuromuscular transmission includes an abnormally small single-muscle action potential evoked in response to a supramaximal nerve stimulus. When the synapse is driven by repetitive stimulation at high rates (20 to 50 Hz), the evoked response is potentiated up to 400% (see Fig. 89.3C). In affected infants, muscle action potentials are unusually brief, of low amplitude, and overly abundant. This is presumably related to involvement of terminal nerve twigs in endings of many motor units. In patients treated for blepharospasm or other movement disorders by intramuscular injections of botulinum toxin, single-fiber EMG shows increased jitter in muscles remote from those injected, and the jitter is maximally increased at low firing rates. These abnormalities are not symptomatic but imply an effect of circulating toxin.

C. botulinum toxin is called the *most poisonous poison* (the lethal dose for a mouse is 10^{-12} g/kg body weight). If a patient survives and reaches a hospital, symptoms include dry, sore mouth and throat; blurred vision; diplopia; nausea; and vomiting. Signs include hypohidrosis; total external ophthalmoplegia; and symmetric descending facial, oropharyngeal, limb, and respiratory paralysis. Pupillary paralysis, however, is not invariable. Not all patients are equally affected, suggesting variable toxin intake or variable individual responses. When cases occur in clusters, the diagnosis is usually suspected immediately.

TREATMENT

Patients should be treated in intensive care facilities for respiratory care. Specific therapy includes antitoxin (a horse serum product that may cause serum sickness or anaphylaxis), available from the CDC, and guanidine hydrochloride, which promotes release of transmitter from residual spared nerve endings but may depress bone marrow. Botulinum immune globulin (BIG) is given in cases of infant botulism to reduce time on ventilator as well as time in the hospital.

ANTIBIOTIC-INDUCED DISORDERS OF THE NEUROMUSCULAR JUNCTION

Aminoglycoside antibiotics (neomycin sulfate, streptomycin sulfate, kanamycin sulfate, gentamicin, and amikacin) and polypeptide antibiotics (colistin sulfate and polymyxin B sulfate) may cause symptomatic block in neuromuscular transmission in patients without any identified neuromuscular disease. Antibiotics occasionally aggravate MG. The problem surfaces when blood levels are excessively high, which usually occurs in patients with renal insufficiency, but levels may be within the therapeutic range. Studies of bath-applied streptomycin in neuromuscular preparations disclosed inadequate release of ACh; the effect was antagonized by an excess of calcium ion. In addition, the sensitivity of the postjunctional membrane to ACh was reduced. Different compounds varied in relative effects on presynaptic and postsynaptic events. Neomycin and colistin produced the most severe derangements. The effects of kanamycin, gentamicin sulfate, streptomycin, tobramycin sulfate, and amikacin sulfate were moderate; tetracycline, erythromycin, vancomycin hydrochloride, penicillin G, and clindamycin had negligible effects. Patients who fail to regain normal ventilatory effort after anesthesia or who show delayed depression of respiration after extubation and are receiving one of the more potent agents should receive ventilatory support until the agent can be discontinued or another antibiotic substituted.

LEVEL 1 EVIDENCE

1. Palace J, Newsom-Davis J, Lecky B. A randomized double-blind trial of prednisolone alone or with azathioprine in myasthenia gravis. Myasthenia Gravis Study Group. *Neurology.* 1998;50(6):1778–1783.

2. A randomised clinical trial comparing prednisone and azathioprine in myasthenia gravis. Results of the second interim analysis. Myasthenia Gravis Clinical Study Group. *J Neurol Neurosurg Psychiatry.* 1993;56(11):1157–1163.

3. Meriggioli MN, Ciafaloni E, Al-Hayk KA, et al. Mycophenolate mofetil for myasthenia gravis: an analysis of efficacy, safety, and tolerability. *Neurology.* 2003;61(10):1438–1440.

4. Sanders DB, Hart IK, Mantegazza R, et al. An international, phase III, randomized trial of mycophenolate mofetil in myasthenia gravis. *Neurology.* 2008;71(6):400–406. doi:10.1212/01.wnl.0000312374.95186.cc.

5. Muscle Study Group. A trial of mycophenolate mofetil with prednisone as initial immunotherapy in myasthenia gravis. *Neurology.* 2008;71(6):394–399. doi:10.1212/01.wnl.0000312373.67493.7f.

6. Tindall RS, Rollins JA, Phillips JT, et al. Preliminary results of a double-blind, randomized, placebo-controlled trial of cyclosporine in myasthenia gravis. *N Engl J Med.* 1987;316(12):719–724. doi:10.1056/NEJM198703193161205.

7. Tindall RS, Phillips JT, Rollins JA, et al. A clinical therapeutic trial of cyclosporine in myasthenia gravis. *Ann N Y Acad Sci.* 1993;681:539–551.

8. De Feo LG, Schottlender J, Martelli NA, et al. Use of intravenous pulsed cyclophosphamide in severe, generalized myasthenia gravis. *Muscle Nerve.* 2002;26(1):31–36. doi:10.1002/mus.10133.

9. Nagane Y, Utsugisawa K, Obara D, et al. Efficacy of low-dose FK506 in the treatment of myasthenia gravis—a randomized pilot study. *Eur Neurol.* 2005;53(3):146–150. doi:10.1159/000085833.

10. Gajdos P, Tranchant C, Clair B, et al. Treatment of myasthenia gravis exacerbation with intravenous immunoglobulin: a randomized double-blind clinical trial. *Arch Neurol.* 2005;62(11):1689–1693. doi:10.1001/archneur.62.11.1689.

11. Zinman L, Ng E, Bril V. IV immunoglobulin in patients with myasthenia gravis: a randomized controlled trial. *Neurology.* 2007;68(11):837–841. doi:10.1212/01.wnl.0000256698.69121.45.

12. Barth D, Nabavi Nouri M, Ng E, et al. Comparison of IVIg and PLEX in patients with myasthenia gravis. *Neurology.* 2011;76(23):2017–2023. doi:10.1212/WNL.0b013e31821e5505.

13. Sanders DB, Massey JM, Sanders LL, et al. A randomized trial of 3,4-diaminopyridine in Lambert-Eaton myasthenic syndrome. *Neurology.* 2000;54(3):603–607.

14. McEvoy KM, Windebank AJ, Daube JR, et al. 3,4-Diaminopyridine in the treatment of Lambert-Eaton myasthenic syndrome. *N Engl J Med.* 1989;321(23):1567–1571. doi: 10.1056/NEJM198912073212303.

15. Bain PG, Motomura M, Newsom-Davis J, et al. Effects of intravenous immunoglobulin on muscle weakness and calcium-channel autoantibodies in the Lambert-Eaton myasthenic syndrome. *Neurology.* 1996;47(3):678–683.

SUGGESTED READINGS

Beeson D, Higuchi O, Palace J, et al. Dok-7 mutations underlie a neuromuscular junction synaptopathy. *Science.* 2006;313:1975–1978.

Benatar M, Rowland LP. The muddle of mycophenolate mofetil in myasthenia. *Neurology.* 2008;71(6):390–391.

Benatar M, Sanders DB, Wolfe GI, et al. Design of the efficacy of prednisone in the treatment of ocular myasthenia (EPITOME) trial. *Ann N Y Acad Sci.* 2012;1275:17–22.

Bever CT Jr, Chang HW, Penn AS, et al. Penicillamine-induced myasthenia gravis: effects of penicillamine on acetylcholine receptor. *Neurology.* 1982;32:1077–1082.

Burke G, Cossins J, Maxwell S, et al. Distinct phenotypes of congenital acetylcholine receptor deficiency. *Neuromuscul Disord.* 2004;14:356–364.

Ciafaloni E, Massey JM. Myasthenia gravis and pregnancy. *Neurol Clin.* 2004;22(4):771–782.

Donaldson JO, Penn AS, Lisak RP, et al. Antiacetylcholine receptor antibody in neonatal myasthenia gravis. *Am J Dis Child.* 1981;135:222–226.

Drachman DB, Adams RN, Hu R, et al. Rebooting the immune system with high-dose cyclophosphamide for treatment of refractory myasthenia gravis. *Ann N Y Acad Sci.* 2008;1132:305–314.

Eaton LM, Lambert EH. Electromyography and electric stimulation of nerves in diseases of motor unit: observations in myasthenic syndrome associated with malignant tumors. *J Am Med Assoc.* 1957;163:1117–1124.

Engel AG, Sine SM. Current understanding of congenital myasthenic syndromes. *Curr Opin Pharmacol.* 2005;5:308–321.

Evoli A, Tonali PA, Padua L, et al. Clinical correlates with anti-MuSK antibodies in generalized seronegative myasthenia gravis. *Brain.* 2003;126:2304–2311.

Gajdos P, Chevret S, Toyka K. Intravenous immunoglobulin for myasthenia gravis. *Cochrane Database Syst Rev.* 2008;(1):CD002277.

Gronseth GS, Barohn RJ. Practice parameter: thymectomy for autoimmune myasthenia gravis (an evidence-based review): report of the Quality Standards Subcommittee of the American Academy of Neurology. *Neurology.* 2000;55(1):7–15.

Guillermo GR, Téllez-Zenteno JF, Weder-Cisneros N, et al. Response of thymectomy: clinical and pathological characteristics among seronegative and seropositive myasthenia gravis patients. *Acta Neurol Scand.* 2004;109:217–221.

Guptill JT, Sanders DB, Evoli A. Anti-MuSK antibody myasthenia gravis: clinical findings and response to treatment in two large cohorts. *Muscle Nerve.* 2011;44:36–40.

Hoff JM, Daltveit AK, Gilhus NE. Myasthenia gravis: consequences for pregnancy, delivery, and the newborn. *Neurology.* 2003;61:1362–1366.

Howard FM Jr, Lennon VA, Finley J, et al. Clinical correlations of antibodies that bind, block, or modulate human acetylcholine receptors in myasthenia gravis. *Ann N Y Acad Sci.* 1987;505:526–538.

Howard JF Jr, Barohn RJ, Cutter GR, et al. A randomized, double-blind, placebo-controlled phase II study of eculizumab in patients with refractory generalized myasthenia gravis. *Muscle Nerve.* 2013;48:76–84.

Illa I, Diaz-Manera J, Rojas-Garcia R, et al. Sustained response to rituximab in anti-AChR and anti-MuSK positive myasthenia gravis patients. *J Neuroimmunol.* 2008;201–202:90–94.

Jaretzki A, Steinglass KM, Sonett JR. Thymectomy in the management of myasthenia gravis. *Semin Neurol.* 2004;24(1):49–62.

Juel V. Evaluation of neuromuscular junction disorders in the electromyography laboratory. *Neurol Clin.* 2012;30:621–639.

Katzberg HD, Barnett C, Merkies ISJ, et al. Minimal clinically important difference in myasthenia gravis: outcomes from a randomized trial. *Muscle Nerve.* 2014;49:661–665.

Kondo K, Monden Y. Thymoma and myasthenia gravis: a clinical study of 1,089 patients from Japan. *Ann Thorac Surg.* 2005;79(1):219–224.

Leite MI, Jacob S, Viegas S, et al. IgG1 antibodies to acetylcholine receptors in "seronegative" myasthenia gravis. *Brain.* 2008;131(pt 7):1940–1952.

Lindstrom J, Seybold M, Lennon VA, et al. Antibody to acetylcholine receptor in myasthenia gravis: prevalence, clinical correlates, and diagnostic value. *Neurology.* 1976;26:1054–1059.

McGrogan A, Sneddon S, de Vries CS. The incidence of myasthenia gravis: a systematic literature review. *Neuroepidemiology.* 2010;34:171–183.

Mehndiratta MM, Pandey S, Kuntzer T. Acetylcholinesterase inhibitor treatment for myasthenia gravis. *The Cochrane Library.* 2011; 2: 1–17.

Padua L, Stalberg E, LoMonaco M, et al. SFEMG in ocular myasthenia gravis diagnosis. *Clin Neurophysiol.* 2000;111:1203–1207.

Pasnoor M, He J, Herbelin L, et al. Phase II trial of methotrexate in myasthenia gravis. *Ann N Y Acad Sci.* 2012;1275:23–28.

Patrick J, Lindstrom J. Autoimmune response to acetylcholine receptor. *Science.* 1973;180:871–872.

Phillips LH II. The epidemiology of myasthenia gravis. *Ann N Y Acad Sci.* 2003;998:407–412.

Pinching AJ, Peters DK. Remission of myasthenia gravis following plasma exchange. *Lancet.* 1976;2(8000):1373–1376.

Prigent H, Orlikowski D, Letilly N, et al. Vital capacity versus maximal inspiratory pressure in patients with Guillain-Barré syndrome and myasthenia gravis. *Neurocrit Care.* 2012;17:236–239.

Rowland LP, Hoefer PFR, Aranow H Jr. Myasthenic syndromes. *Res Publ Assoc Res Nerv Ment Dis.* 1961;38:548–600.

Rowland LP, Hoefer PF, Aranow H Jr, et al. Fatalities in myasthenia gravis: a review of 39 cases with 26 autopsies. *Neurology.* 1956;6:307–326.

Ruff RL, Lennon VA. How myasthenia gravis alters the safety factor for neuromuscular transmission. *J Neuroimmunol.* 2008;201–202:13–20.

Sanders DB, El-Salem K, Massey JM, et al. Clinical aspects of MuSK antibody positive seronegative MG. *Neurology.* 2003;60:1978–1980.

Silvestri NJ, Wolfe GI. Treatment-refractory myasthenia gravis. *J Clin Neuromuscular Dis.* 2014;15(4):167–178.

Sonett JR, Jaretzki A III. Thymectomy for nonthymomatous myasthenia gravis: a critical analysis. *Ann N Y Acad Sci.* 2008;1132:315–328.

Toyka KV, Drachman DB, Pestronk A, et al. Myasthenia gravis: passive transfer from man to mouse. *Science.* 1975;190:397–399.

Vincent A. Autoantibodies in different forms of myasthenia gravis and in the Lambert–Eaton syndrome. *Handb Clin Neurol.* 2008;91:213–227.

Vincent A, McConville J, Farrugia ME, et al. Seronegative myasthenia gravis. *Semin Neurol.* 2004;24(1):125–133.

Wolfe GI, Barohn RJ, Foster BM, et al; Myasthenia Gravis-IVIG Study Group. Randomized, controlled trial of intravenous immunoglobulin in myasthenia gravis. *Muscle Nerve.* 2002;26(4):549–552.

Wu JY, Kuo PH, Fan PC, et al. The role of non-invasive ventilation and factors predicting extubation outcome in myasthenic crisis. *Neurocrit Care.* 2009;10:35–42.

Zhang B, Tzartos JS, Belimezi M, et al. Autoantibodies to lipoprotein-related protein 4 in patients with double-seronegative myasthenia gravis. *Arch Neurol.* 2012;69(4):445–451.

Inflammatory Myopathies 90

Rebecca Traub, Christina M. Ulane, and Kurenai Tanji

INTRODUCTION

Myopathies, or disorders of skeletal muscle, are due to a variety of hereditary and acquired causes. Myopathies with genetic underpinnings are discussed in Chapters 93 and 95 and throughout Section 19. Acquired myopathies due to systemic disorders and toxins is the subject of Chapter 92. This chapter focuses on acquired myopathies due to inflammation. The focus is on prototypical, noninfectious immune-mediated inflammatory myopathies: dermatomyositis, polymyositis, inclusion body myositis, and necrotizing myopathy. Distinguishing these disorders from hereditary or toxic myopathies is essential for appropriate management of patients with muscle diseases which may have similar clinical presentations.

DERMATOMYOSITIS

EPIDEMIOLOGY

Dermatomyositis (DM) is rare and exact epidemiologic data is lacking. A recent systematic review and meta-analysis estimates an incidence of approximately 7.98 cases per million per year and a prevalence of 14 per 100,000 (range 2.4 to 33.8 per 100,000) for all inflammatory myopathies.

DM occurs in all decades of life, with peaks of incidence before puberty and at about age 40 years. In young adults, women are more likely to be affected. Familial cases are rare. Adult cases are associated with an increased risk of malignant neoplasms; most often ovarian, lung, or breast cancer, although others such as nasopharyngeal carcinoma have been reported. Most studies report 15% to 25% of adult DM is associated with malignancy.

Juvenile DM is extremely rare, with estimated incidence of 2 to 5 per 1 million children per year younger than 16 years of age. It much more common in girls than boys (5:1) and essentially never associated with malignancy.

PATHOBIOLOGY

DM is thought to be an autoimmune disease with vasculopathy of muscle and skin. The antigenic target appears to be the endothelium of intramuscular microvessels, activating complement pathways to cause vascular injury. The loss of capillaries is thought to cause muscle ischemia resulting in myofiber injury and loss. Lymphocytic infiltrates are composed of both B and T cells, as contrasted to the T-cell–predominant inflammatory process of polymyositis and inclusion body myositis.

CLINICAL MANIFESTATIONS

The typical clinical presentation of DM is a combination of myopathy with characteristic skin findings. The rash may precede weakness by several weeks, but weakness alone is almost never the first symptom. Sometimes, the rash is so typical that the diagnosis can be made even without evidence of myopathy (amyopathic

DM). In other cases, weakness may not be evident but there is electrophysiologic, pathologic, or serum creatine kinase (CK) evidence of myopathy.

Weakness in DM primarily affects the proximal muscles in the arms and legs and may be accompanied by discomfort (myalgias) and tenderness. Patients often describe difficulty going up stairs, standing from a seated position, and lifting their arms above the head. Cranial muscles may be involved, causing facial weakness, dysphagia, and esophageal involvement. Neck weakness may occur, causing head drop. Sensation is preserved and reflexes are lost only when the myopathy is severe.

The typical rash is on the face, often on the upper eyelids as a purplish discoloration with edema (heliotrope rash). An erythematous macular rash may be found on the face, neck and chest (V-sign), and upper back (shawl sign). The initial redness may be replaced later by brownish pigmentation. Gottron sign is denoted by red-purple scaly macules on the extensor surfaces of finger joints. Dusky discoloration of the knuckles has been called *mechanic's hands* and is associated with the antisynthetase syndrome of arthritis, Raynaud phenomenon, and interstitial lung disease.

Subcutaneous calcifications can occur, more often in chronic cases and in pediatric DM. These calcifications may erode through the skin and cause ulceration and secondary infection.

Interstitial lung disease may accompany DM and is more common in the setting of anti–Jo-1 antibodies or antisynthetase syndrome, and patients should be questioned about respiratory symptoms and referred for pulmonary evaluation when appropriate. Cardiac involvement can occur, so clinical history should include questions of chest pain, palpitations, and syncope, and cardiac screening is advised.

Juvenile DM presents with a similar rash and proximal weakness.

DIAGNOSIS

DM is a clinical diagnosis (Table 90.1) aided by muscle biopsy (see the "Muscle Pathology" section later in this chapter). There should be elevations in muscle enzymes, including CK and aldolase. Other lab testing should include antinuclear antibodies (ANA), antibodies for other nuclear antigens, and myositis-specific antibodies (Table 90.2). Anti–Jo-1, which is the most common antisynthetase antibody, is associated with interstitial lung disease, arthritis, and Raynaud phenomenon. Nonsynthetase antibodies to Mi-2 are associated with a more acute onset and better response to therapy and prognosis. The presence of anti-Ro, anti-La, anti-Sm, RNP, anti-PM/Scl, and anti-Ku antibodies, among others, may suggest an overlap syndrome of a systemic rheumatologic disorder with associated myopathy.

Electrodiagnostic testing typically demonstrates normal nerve conduction studies with myopathic findings on electromyogram (EMG) with fibrillations, positive sharp waves, complex repetitive discharges, and sometimes myotonia, suggesting an inflammatory process. Magnetic resonance imaging (MRI) of the muscles can be used to look for evidence of inflammation and direct a target for muscle biopsy.

TABLE 90.1 Bohan and Peter Criteria for Myositis

Criterion	Description
Symmetric proximal weakness (over weeks to months)	Neck flexors, limb-girdle musculature
Consistent muscle biopsy findings	Necrosis, regeneration, phagocytosis, atrophy, mononuclear cell infiltrates
Elevated muscle enzymes	Creatine kinase, aldolase, transaminases, lactate dehydrogenase
Electromyographic evidence for myopathy	Muscle fiber irritability (positive sharp waves, fibrillations), short duration, small amplitude, polyphasic motor unit potentials, with spontaneous bizarre high-frequency discharges
Characteristic skin rash	Gottron sign, Gottron papules, heliotrope

Definite PM: four criteria. Definite DM: three or four criteria plus rash.
Possible PM: two criteria. Possible DM: one criterion plus rash.
PM, polymyositis; DM, dermatomyositis.

TABLE 90.2 Myositis-Specific Antibodies

Antibody	Clinical Features
Antisynthetase Antibodies	
Anti–Jo-1	Seen in polymyositis, dermatomyositis, and interstitial lung disease
Anti–PL-7	
Anti–PL-12	
Anti-EJ	
Anti-OJ	
Anti-KS	
Anti-Zo	
Anti-Ha	
Dermatomyositis-Specific Antibodies	
Anti-Mi-2	Treatment responsive
Anti-MDA5 (CADM-140)	Minimal myopathy; ILD
Anti-155/140	Cancer associated
Anti-140	Juvenile dermatomyositis, calcinosis
Anti-SAE	Amyopathic DM
Antibodies in Immune-mediated Necrotizing Myopathy	
Anti-SRP	Severe, acute presentation, resistant to treatment
Anti-HMGCR	Related to statin use

ILD, interstitial lung disease; DM, dermatomyositis.
Adapted from Albayda J, Mammen AL. Is statin-induced myositis part of the polymyositis disease spectrum? *Curr Rheumatol Rep.* 2014;16:433.

The differential diagnosis for DM includes the other inflammatory myopathies, hereditary muscular dystrophies, and toxic myopathies. Clinical features, electrodiagnostic findings, muscle pathology, and genetic testing can help distinguish these entities (Tables 90.3 and 90.4).

Once the diagnosis of DM is suspected, testing should include evaluation for underlying malignancy and associated pulmonary fibrosis. Computed tomography (CT) of the chest, abdomen, and pelvis is usually sufficient, with the addition of pelvic ultrasound in woman, although positron emission tomography (PET) may be indicated in some cases.

Cancer screening is recommended in all patients diagnosed with DM, including routine mammography and colonoscopy. CT of the chest, abdomen, and pelvis, and sometimes PET scan are indicated depending on the clinical scenario.

TREATMENT

The initial treatment for both DM and polymyositis is prednisone, typically starting with high dose (60 mg daily or higher) and then tapering slowly over months in conjunction with the addition of steroid-sparing therapies.

The usual first-line steroid-sparing agent used in DM and polymyositis is azathioprine [Level 1].[1,2] Azathioprine is started at a low dose (50 mg daily) and slowly increased (goal of 2 to 3 mg/kg/day), with monitoring of cell counts and hepatic function. Methotrexate is another first-line alternative, given orally (start 7.5 mg/wk, titrate up by 2.5 mg weekly to goal of 10 to 20 mg weekly; given with folic acid 1 mg daily) with close monitoring of cell counts, hepatic function, and renal function. In patients with myositis refractory to these agents or with intolerable side effects, second-line options include rituximab (1,000 mg IV on days 1 and 15 may be repeated every 24 weeks) and intravenous immunoglobulin (IVIG) (doses vary, typically 1 to 2 g/kg IV every 2 to 4 weeks). Rituximab, a monoclonal anti-CD20 antibody, when studied for treatment of DM and polymyositis in a randomized controlled trial, failed to meet the primary outcome measure, but clinical improvement and a significant reduction in steroid dose was seen in all patients receiving the treatment [Level 1].[3] A randomized controlled trial of IVIG in treatment-resistant cases of DM showed it to be effective in 9 of 12 cases [Level 1].[4] The American Academy of Neurology 2012 guidelines recommend IVIG as a possibly effective therapy for refractory DM. Other medications occasionally used for refractory cases include cyclosporine (starting 2.5 mg/kg daily divided b.i.d.), tacrolimus (0.075 mg/kg/day divided b.i.d.), mycophenolate mofetil (starting 500 to 1,000 mg daily), and cyclophosphamide (doses starting at 300 mg/m² every 4 weeks). Many of these second- and third-line immunosuppressive medications have significant toxicities and side effects and should be prescribed by specialists familiar with their use.

Treatment must include management of associated systemic manifestations, with close coordination of rheumatology, neurology, pulmonology, cardiology, and oncology when appropriate.

Physical therapy, occupational therapy, and low-intensity exercise are generally recommended for all patients with inflammatory myopathies to prevent deconditioning, help with gait training, and improve muscle strength.

Treatment of juvenile DM is similar and high-dose daily oral prednisone or pulsed intravenous methylprednisolone is considered the gold standard and must be initiated promptly to prevent significant morbidity and mortality. Other steroid-sparing immunosuppressives in those who do not respond to or cannot tolerate steroids including methotrexate and cyclosporine may be used.

TABLE 90.3 Key Features of Inflammatory and Necrotizing Autoimmune Myopathies

	Dermatomyositis	Polymyositis	Inclusion Body Myositis	Necrotizing Autoimmune Myopathy
Autoantibodies	Antisynthetase antibodies (anti–Jo-1 and others)	Antisynthetase antibodies (anti–Jo-1 and others)	Possibly anti-cytosolic 5'-nucleotidase 1A (cN1A)	Anti-SRP Anti-HMGCR
	Dermatomyositis-specific antibodies (anti–Mi-2 and others)	Antibodies of systemic rheumatologic disease		
Muscle enzymes	Up to 50× ULN	Up to 50× ULN	Up to 15× ULN	Often >10× ULN
Associated disorders	Interstitial lung disease (antisynthetase)	Interstitial lung disease (antisynthetase)	None	HMGCR—statin use
	Malignancy (ovarian, lung, others)	Systemic rheumatologic disorders		
Treatment (see dermatomyositis treatment for typical doses)	Prednisone	Prednisone	None	Prednisone
	Azathioprine	Azathioprine		Rituximab
	Methotrexate	Methotrexate		
	Rituximab	Rituximab		
	IVIG	IVIG		
	Others	Others		

SRP, signal recognition particle; HMGCR, 3-hydroxy-3-methylglutaryl-coenzyme A reductase; ULN, upper limit of normal; IVIG, intravenous immunoglobulin.

POLYMYOSITIS

Polymyositis (PM), as a clinical syndrome of myopathic weakness, is similar in presentation and treatment to DM, absent the typical dermatologic findings of the latter. Pathologically, however, it is a distinct entity and associates more closely with systemic autoimmune disorders. Although treated similarly with regard to immunosuppression, distinguishing PM and DM is important to establish risk of underlying malignancy or rheumatologic disease (see Tables 90.3 and 90.4).

EPIDEMIOLOGY

Idiopathic inflammatory myopathies as a whole are reported with a prevalence of approximately 14 in 100,000. The percentage of inflammatory myopathies identified as PM vary widely from 2% to over 50% in different series.

TABLE 90.4 Features Differentiating Dermatomyositis from Polymyositis

Dermatomyositis	Polymyositis
Typical dermatologic manifestations	No rash unless lupus associated
May be associated with malignancy	Not typically associated with malignancy
Not generally associated with systemic rheumatologic disease, except sometimes scleroderma	Often associated with a systemic rheumatologic disease, including lupus, systemic sclerosis, vasculitis
Childhood form exists	Adult disease
Muscle biopsy findings (perimysial and perivascular inflammation)	Muscle biopsy findings (endomysial inflammation)

PATHOBIOLOGY

PM is considered an autoimmune disease of disordered cellular immunity (in contrast to the presumed humoral abnormalities of DM). The antigenic target is not known, however, and the nature of the immunologic aberration is not known. The association with collagen-vascular disease increases the likelihood of autoimmune disorder. Although there is some increased risk of malignancy in association with PM, the association is not as high as that seen in DM.

CLINICAL MANIFESTATIONS

The symptoms of PM are those of a myopathy that primarily affects proximal limb muscles, similar in distribution to DM: difficulty climbing stairs or rising from low seats, lifting packages or dishes, or working with the arms overhead. Weakness of neck muscles may result in head drop. Typically, cranial muscles are spared, although dysphagia can occur when the disease is severe. Respiratory muscles are only rarely affected. Pain, or myalgias, may be present, but sensory symptoms are otherwise absent.

Symptoms of systemic disease may occur in the setting of PM related to a systemic rheumatologic disorder, including arthralgia or Raynaud symptoms. The typical rash of DM is absent, but there may be a rash of lupus in association with PM.

Interstitial lung disease can occur in PM but is more commonly associated with DM and anti–Jo-1 antibodies.

There is a mild increase in cancer risk in PM compared to the general population, but the association is not nearly as strong as that seen in DM.

Cardiac involvement can occur with PM with myocarditis, arrhythmia, and rarely, congestive heart failure. Cardiology evaluation in all patients with inflammatory myopathy is advised.

DIAGNOSIS

The diagnosis of PM is made in the appropriate clinical setting with a combination of electrodiagnostic and muscle biopsy findings

TABLE 90.5	Differential Diagnosis of Polymyositis
Mimic	Differentiating Characteristics
Dermatomyositis	Associated rash, specific pathologic findings on muscle biopsy, myositis-specific antibodies
Necrotizing myopathy	Specific pathologic findings on muscle biopsy, drug/statin exposure, more resistant to immunosuppressant therapy
Inclusion body myositis	Slower progression, older age of onset, distribution of muscle weakness, specific pathologic findings on muscle biopsy, lack of response to immunosuppressants
Overlap syndrome	Associated rheumatologic diagnosis (e.g., lupus, rheumatoid arthritis)
Muscular dystrophy	Age of onset, slower progression, family history, specific pathologic findings on muscle biopsy, genetic testing, lack of response to immunosuppressants
Metabolic myopathy	Age of onset, slower progression, family history, pathology, genetic testing, lack of response to immunosuppressants
Fibromyalgia	Prominent pain, no weakness, normal muscle biopsy
Polymyalgia rheumatica	High ESR/CRP, normal CK, normal EMG

ESR, erythrocyte sedimentation rate; CRP, C-reactive protein; CK, creatine kinase; EMG, electromyogram.

(see "Muscle Pathology" section for the latter). The differential diagnosis includes other inflammatory myopathies, toxic myopathies, and hereditary muscle diseases (Table 90.5). Motor neuron disease (amyotrophic lateral sclerosis[ALS]) may be included in the differential diagnosis because of modestly elevated CK levels, although the clinical and electrodiagnostic findings are distinctive in ALS.

The electrodiagnostic findings of PM are indistinguishable from those in DM. Nerve conduction studies are normal except in the case of severe myopathy, in which case motor CMAP amplitudes may be reduced. Needle EMG shows fibrillations, complex repetitive discharges, and other "inflammatory" findings in combination with myopathic motor unit potentials, which are low amplitude, short duration, polyphasic, and with early recruitment.

Lab testing will demonstrate elevations in serum CK and aldolase as markers of muscle inflammation. Antibody testing in PM may be suggestive of an underlying rheumatologic disorder, including positive ANA or scleroderma antibodies. SRP antibodies have been reported in PM but are more associated with necrotizing myopathy. Although myositis-specific antibodies (see Table 90.2) are less common in PM than DM, it is recommended that they be checked in all patients with inflammatory myopathies, as their presence may suggest association with interstitial lung disease or help guide immunotherapy.

As in DM, muscle MRI is sometimes useful in targeting muscle biopsy.

TREATMENT

Treatment of PM is similar to DM, and many clinical trials include both disorders in their recruitment. First-line and initial treatment is with high-dose steroids, typically prednisone, with the same consideration for steroid sparing and options for refractory disease as elaborated in the dermatomyositis treatment section earlier.

INCLUSION BODY MYOSITIS

Inclusion body myositis (IBM) is considered an inflammatory myopathy distinct in clinical features and treatment response to DM and PM. In addition, IBM exhibits unique pathologic features, suggesting that IBM may have dual aspects of inflammatory and degenerative muscle diseases.

EPIDEMIOLOGY

The prevalence of IBM varies from 4.9 per million in the Netherlands to 71 per million in Olmstead County, Minnesota. Both prevalence and incidence increase if restricted to age older than 50 years. There is a 2:1 to 3:1 male predominance, unlike most autoimmune disorders with female predominance. IBM is rare in African-Americans and nonwhites. Up to 15% will have an associated autoimmune disease such as lupus, Sjögren syndrome, thrombocytopenia, or sarcoidosis. There are inherited forms, the most common called *hereditary inclusion body myositis* (hIBM) or IBM2, which is found in 1 in 1,500 persons of Iranian Jewish descent.

PATHOBIOLOGY

The cause of IBM is unknown, but it is thought to be both autoimmune and neurodegenerative. The inflammatory response in the muscle and acquired nature suggest an immune etiology (see "Muscle Pathology" section). A novel autoantibody has been identified from sera of 50% of patients with IBM that recognized a 43-kDa muscle protein that was not found in other diseases or healthy controls. The protein was identified as the cytosolic 59-nucleotidase 1A (cN1A), and moderate reactivity is 70% sensitive and 92% specific.

Poor responsiveness to immunotherapy may suggest a degenerative component of the disease. Histologically, protein aggregates are found in the vacuolated muscle fibers of IBM that are not typically seen in other inflammatory myopathies. These aggregates, which are thought to be accumulation of misfolded proteins, share similar components to those found in other neurodegenerative diseases.

There are a few genetic mutations causing hIBM. hIBM/IBM2 is an autosomal recessive disorder due to specific mutation in the *GNE* gene, which encodes a dual-function enzyme (epimerase and kinase) which is important in the synthesis of the abundant Neu5Ac sugar moiety. IBM3 is an autosomal dominant disorder related to mutations in the gene encoding myosin heavy chain IIa (MYHC2A), with the initial reports described in a Swedish family. Inclusion body myopathy with early-onset Paget disease with or without frontotemporal dementia 1 (IBMPFD1) is an autosomal dominant disease caused by mutation in the VCP gene with incomplete penetrance for the clinical phenotypes described in its name. In 30% of patients with IBMPFD, the isolated symptoms are neuromuscular.

CLINICAL MANIFESTATIONS

The clinical symptoms of IBM, in its classic form, are distinct from other inflammatory myopathies in the distribution and time course of weakness. The onset of weakness is typically slow, with worsening over the course of years, as compared to PM and DM, which typically have a more subacute presentation. Many patients will have symptoms for years before diagnosis is established. Muscles first affected are usually proximal legs, with predilection for the quadriceps muscle group, as opposed to other myopathies affecting proximal muscles, which typically have more hip flexor involvement. In the arms, distal muscles tend to be first and more severely affected, with prominent involvement of the finger and wrist flexors in the forearm. Atrophy is often greater than is seen in other inflammatory myopathies and is usually symmetric. Pronounced atrophy, and weakness which can be asymmetric distinguishes IBM from PM and DM, and is cause for diagnostic confusion with motor neuron disease. Muscle pain (myalgia) is present in approximately 40% of patients. Neck muscles are often involved and can lead to head drop. Dysphagia occurs in half or more of patients, making it a more common symptom in IBM than in other inflammatory myopathies and may be the initial symptom. Rarely, there is involvement of respiratory muscles. Prognosis is for slow progression over years, typically leading to use of wheelchair. Death may occur as complication of respiratory infection or aspiration, but this may be 10 or more years after symptoms begin.

DIAGNOSIS

The diagnosis of IBM is often suspected based on history and physical exam findings, supported by electrodiagnostic studies, but relying on muscle pathology for confirmation (see "Muscle Pathology" section). Lab testing shows mild elevations in CK, up to 15 times the upper limit of normal but may be normal. There should be no elevation in erythrocyte sedimentation rate (ESR) or other inflammatory markers, although there are reports of an association with ANA and Sjögren antibodies. Testing should include antibodies for systemic rheumatologic disorders and myositis-specific antibodies to look for PM and DM, which are included in the differential diagnosis of IBM (Table 90.6).

Electrodiagnostic studies show primarily a myopathic pattern with inflammatory features, similar to that seen in DM and PM. There are fibrillations and abnormal spontaneous activity consistent with an inflammatory process, with short duration and low-amplitude motor unit potentials and early recruitment. In some patients with IBM, however, there is a mixed electrodiagnostic picture, with both myopathic and neurogenic features. These mixed findings on EMG in combination with normal sensory responses can make the diagnosis more challenging and occasionally leads to the misdiagnosis of motor neuron disease in patients with IBM.

Muscle MRI is increasingly being used for diagnosis in inflammatory myopathies, and in IBM, it will show atrophy and/or fatty replacement of muscle with predominant involvement of the anterior thigh muscles.

There have been a number of diagnostic criteria used to establish the definite or probable diagnosis of IBM for clinical and research use. The most recent of these is the criteria defined in the ENMC workshop in 2011 (Table 90.7).

TREATMENT

IBM is notorious for being refractory to the treatments that are effective for other inflammatory myopathies. In some patients, there is an initial response to corticosteroids; however, all will eventually become refractory. Other immunosuppressive agents have not proven to alter the natural course of IBM. A randomized controlled trial of methotrexate showed improved CK levels but no effect on strength [**Level 1**].[5] Randomized controlled trials of IVIG with and without steroids also have not shown significant benefits for patients with IBM [**Level 1**].[6,7] Two randomized controlled pilot studies by the Muscle Study Group did not show any benefit for IBM patients treated with interferon [**Level 1**].[8] Despite negative trials, some neuromuscular specialists will treat patients with IBM with prednisone, steroid-sparing agents, such as methotrexate or azathioprine, or IVIG on a trial basis based on the observation that a small subset of patients appear to improve or stabilize with regard to muscle strength with treatment, but whether to offer immunotherapy is a controversial topic.

Given the limited, if any, benefit with immunomodulating therapy for IBM, treatment should focus on symptomatic and supportive therapies to improve quality of life. Low-intensity physical therapy can help with strength and mobility. Falls prevention and gait training are important for preventing complications of worsening weakness. Speech therapy can help in managing dysphagia and preventing aspiration.

NECROTIZING AUTOIMMUNE MYOPATHY

Necrotizing autoimmune myopathy (NAM) or immune-mediated necrotizing myopathy (IMNM) is a distinct type of immune-mediated myopathy that show on biopsy various degree of myofiber necrosis associated with little or no inflammatory response except for myophagocytosis. NAM may occur in isolation (with or without anti–signal recognition particle [SRP] antibodies) or in association with statin use (with anti–3-hydroxy-3-methylglutaryl-coenzyme A reductase [HMGCR] antibodies) with certain connective tissue disorders and possibly with malignancies. Originally discovered as novel myositis antibodies, the target was identified as HMGCR.

EPIDEMIOLOGY

Cases of NAM in the context of statin use were reported initially in the 1980s, and subsequent case series describe myopathy that progress after statin cessation, with features on biopsy of NAM and response to immunosuppressant medication. The exact incidence of NAM is unclear. However, 21% of NAM is associated with systemic lupus erythematosus (SLE), and in patients with anti-SRP antibodies, most are female, with an average age of onset of 45 years, 65% have

TABLE 90.6	Differential Diagnosis for Inclusion Body Myositis
Dermatomyositis	Associated skin findings
	Muscle pathology
Polymyositis	Associated autoantibodies
	Muscle pathology
Hereditary distal myopathies	Family history
	Early age of onset
	Genetic testing
Drug-induced (toxic) myopathies	History of toxic or medication exposure
Motor neuron disease	Upper motor neuron findings
	Electrodiagnostic testing
	Muscle biopsy—neurogenic changes
Myasthenia gravis	Ocular and prominent bulbar symptoms
	Acetylcholine receptor or muscle-specific kinase (MuSK) antibodies
	Abnormal repetitive stimulation
	Response to immunotherapy

TABLE 90.7	Diagnostic Criteria for Inclusion Body Myositis from the European Neuromuscular Center Workshop, 2011	
Classification	**Clinical Features**	**Pathologic Features**
Clinicopathologically defined IBM	Duration over 12 mo Age at onset older than 45 yr Quadriceps weakness greater than hip flexor weakness and/or finger flexor weakness greater than shoulder abductor weakness Serum CK not greater than 15× the upper limit of normal	Endomysial inflammation and rimmed vacuoles and protein accumulation (amyloid or other proteins) Or Filaments 15–18 nm
Clinically defined IBM		One or more of the following: Endomysial inflammation Or increased MHC-1 staining Or rimmed vacuoles Or protein accumulation (amyloid Or other proteins) Or filaments 15–18 nm
Probable IBM		One or more of the following: Endomysial exudate Or increased MHC-1 staining Or rimmed vacuoles Or protein accumulation (amyloid Or other proteins) Or filaments 15–18 nm

IBM, inclusion body myositis; CK, creatine kinase. Adapted from Barohn R, Dimachkie M. Inclusion body myositis. *Neurol Clin.* 2014;32:629–646; Machado P, Brady S, Hanna MG. Update in inclusion body myositis. *Curr Opin Rheumatol.* 2013;25(6):763–771.

comorbid hypertension, 23% have diabetes mellitus, and up to 37% will have interstitial lung disease (ILD). One-third of NAM cases do not have any myositis-specific antibodies, and these are most often associated with SLE and systemic scleroderma.

PATHOBIOLOGY

NAM is characterized by muscle biopsies showing necrosis and degeneration but without the typical inflammatory cell infiltrate seen in DM and PM, despite its autoimmune physiology.

In the case of the statins, there is increased expression of HMGCR on regenerating muscle fibers, which likely triggers and immune response and the subsequent development of anti-HMGCR antibodies. This upregulation persists even after statins have been discontinued, presumably why the symptoms continue and even progress after the statin is discontinued. Whether these antibodies are pathogenic or an associated finding is unknown, especially as the target is an intracellular protein. HMGCR is the rate-limiting enzyme in cholesterol synthesis and is the target of statin medications.

Beginning in 1986, antibodies recognizing the SRP on the endoplasmic reticulum membrane were found in association with myopathy. It is also unclear if this antibody is pathogenic, as it too is intracellular. However, titers of anti-SRP antibodies and serum CK are found to correlate with one another during treatment.

CLINICAL MANIFESTATIONS

Similar to PM, patients present with symmetric proximal weakness over the course of weeks to months. However, in patients with anti-SRP antibodies, the onset may be acute and severe, and 66% to 80% of this group will have myalgias. Anti-SRP myopathy patients can have dyspnea (50%) which may be due to either neuromuscular weakness or ILD (21% to 37%). Symptoms in statin-related

cases can occur at any time in treatment (2 months to 3 years) but on average, after 3 years of treatment. Symptoms continue or even worsen with cessation of statin and myalgias are a prominent feature (75%). Rarely, patients can present with HMGCR-positive myopathy in the absence of statin exposure.

DIAGNOSIS

As in other inflammatory myopathies, NAM is diagnosed with a combination of clinical, lab, and electrodiagnostic features but often relying on muscle pathology to confirm diagnosis (see "Muscle Pathology" section).

Serum CK levels are often elevated, usually more than 5,000 U/mL, as in other inflammatory myopathies. Serum can be tested for the presence of anti-SRP and anti-HMGCR antibodies which are extremely helpful in each case. Patients with anti-SRP myopathy typically do not have any other myositis-specific antibodies. Patients with non-NAM statin-induced myotoxicity do not have anti-HMGCR antibodies. Anti-SRP antibodies are found in approximately 16% of NAM.

Electrodiagnostic testing shows findings similar to that seen in PM and DM with normal nerve conduction studies, unless weakness is severe, in which case CMAP amplitudes may be reduced. There is abnormal spontaneous activity, with fibrillations and other irritable features. Motor unit potentials are myopathic, with short duration and low amplitude, and recruitment is early.

Muscle MRI shows findings similar to other inflammatory myopathies, with muscle edema, atrophy, and fatty replacement. MRI is sometimes helpful in targeting muscle biopsy.

TREATMENT

Treatment of NAM relies on both discontinuing any toxic trigger for the disease process (i.e., stopping statins) when implicated.

Although typical statin-induced myopathy will improve after discontinuation of the medication, the course of NAM is of worsening weakness despite stopping the triggering medication. Immunosuppressive treatment is necessary to address the underlying autoimmune pathophysiology in NAM. Most patients respond to steroids. Other steroid-sparing agents which have been used with success include methotrexate, azathioprine, mycophenolate mofetil, rituximab, and intravenous immunoglobulin.

MUSCLE PATHOLOGY

DERMATOMYOSITIS

Muscle pathology in DM shows perimysial, and in particular perivascular, inflammation which is often composed of a mixed population of T lymphocytes (especially helper T cells) and B lymphocytes (Fig. 90.1). Plasmacytoid dendritic cells are also present. The extent and the degree of inflammation, however, greatly vary from case to case. Except for amyopathic cases, necrotic/degenerative or regenerating fibers are present across all sections or in a perifascicular pattern (see Fig. 90.1). The endomysial capillary density may be significantly reduced. Immune complexes containing IgG, IgM, and complement, especially membrane attack complex (MAC), are found deposited in the microvessels, although it remains unclear how the complement pathway is activated. Putative antigen(s) are expressed by the endothelial cells of the microvasculature. Immunohistochemical staining of the fibers, especially in the perifascicular areas, often show the expression of MHC class I and variable expression of MHC class II. Ultrastructurally, endothelial cells of affected microvessels may show necrosis, swelling, or reactive/degenerative changes. Reactive/degenerative endothelial cells may exhibit tubuloreticular structures that appear closely related to endoplasmic reticulum and are thought to reflect type 1 interferon (INF) exposure.

POLYMYOSITIS AND INCLUSION BODY MYOSITIS

PM and IBM share certain pathologic features including muscle fiber necrosis and regeneration and lymphocyte infiltration, mainly in the endomysium (Fig. 90.2A). The infiltrating inflammatory

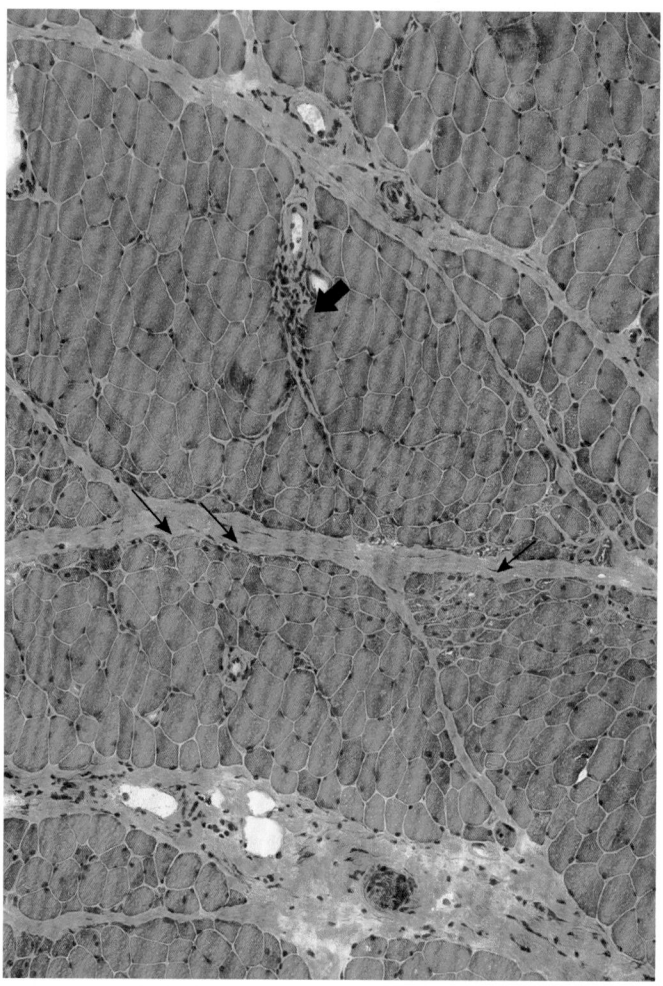

FIGURE 90.1 Muscle pathology in dermatomyositis. Perivascular inflammation (*large arrow*) and perifascicular pattern (*small arrows*) of myocyte injury. (Hematoxylin and eosin stain, ×200 magnification.)

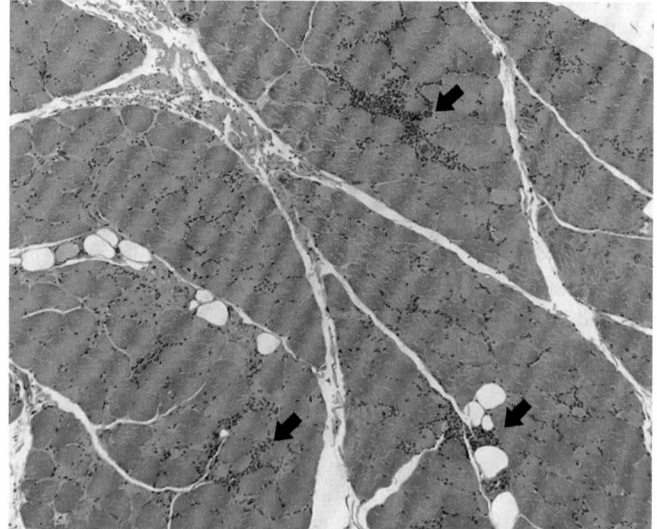

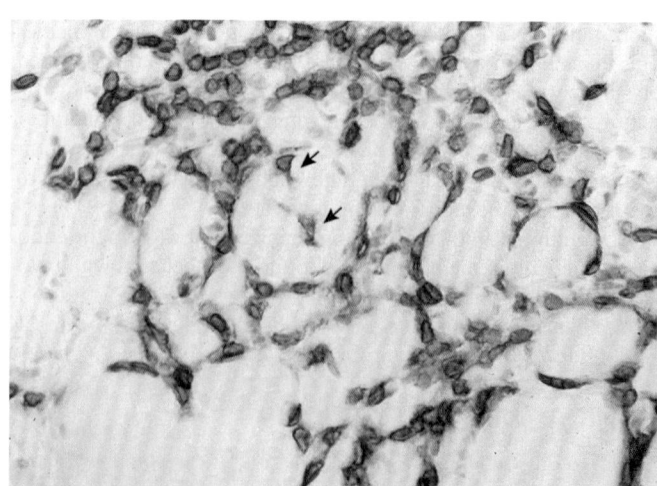

A   B

FIGURE 90.2 Muscle pathology in polymyositis. **A:** Endomysial lymphocytic infiltration (*arrows*) (hematoxylin and eosin stain, ×200 magnification). **B:** Cytotoxic T-cell infiltrate invading myofibers (*arrows*) (immunohistochemical staining for CD8, ×400 magnification).

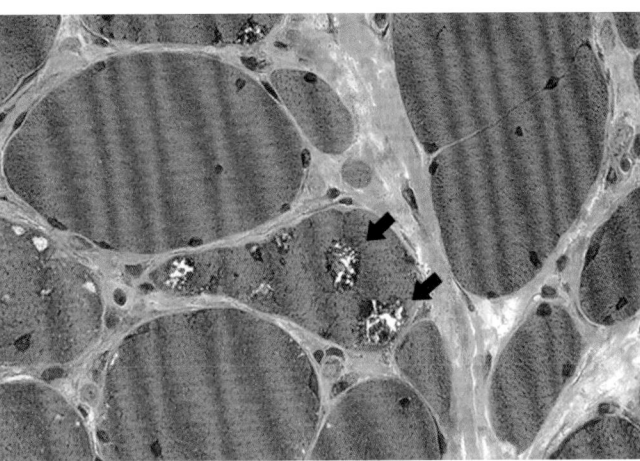

FIGURE 90.3 Muscle pathology in inclusion body myositis. Rimmed vacuoles (*arrows*). (Hematoxylin and eosin stain, ×400 magnification.)

cells are T cells (with a large proportion of cytotoxic T cells), macrophages/histiocytes, and myeloid dendritic cells. Occasionally, cytotoxic T cells invading into non–necrotic-appearing sarcoplasm can be captured on muscle biopsy by using immunohistochemical staining for the CD8 molecule (Fig. 90.2B). Typically, untreated cases of PM and IBM show immunohistochemical expression of MHC class I expression along the surface of myofibers; there is often association with MHC class II expression. In general, muscle biopsy in IBM will display greater chronic myopathic changes than PM; other features of IBM may include rimmed vacuoles (Fig. 90.3) and mitochondrial abnormalities. Congophilic, intracytoplasmic amyloid associated with vacuoles, considered to be a hallmark of IBM, can be visualized in frozen sections stained with Congo red dye under rhodamine optics using a fluorescence microscope. The recognition of insoluble protein aggregates associated with rimmed vacuoles prompted immunohistochemical evaluation for and identified the presence of several proteins including phosphorylated tau, β-amyloid, and TAR DNA binding protein-43 (TDP43). The similarity of these protein aggregates to those found in other neurodegenerative disorders of the central nervous system and the typically poor response of IBM to immunotherapy supports a possible neurodegenerative pathobiology.

IMMUNE-MEDIATED (AUTOIMMUNE) NECROTIZING MYOPATHY

Muscle biopsy in NAM shows scattered necrotic myofibers associated with phagocyte (macrophage) infiltration (Fig. 90.4). There is minimal or absent T-lymphocytic infiltration and inflammation. Microvascular deposition of MAC may be present, but unlike in DM, perivascular inflammation is scant or absent and there are no tuboreticular aggregates in the endothelial cells of the microvasculature. MHC class I and II are reported to be variably upregulated in anti-SRP–associated NAM, paraneoplastic NAM, and statin-associated NAM. MHC class I upregulation is consistently seen in the originally reported cases of statin-associated NAM.

LEVEL 1 EVIDENCE

Dermatomyositis and Polymyositis

1. Bunch TW. Prednisone and azathioprine for polymyositis: long-term followup. *Arthritis Rheum.* 1981;24:45–48.
2. Bunch TW, Worthington JW, Combs JJ, et al. Azathioprine with prednisone for polymyositis. A controlled, clinical trial. *Ann Intern Med.* 1980;92:365–369.
3. Oddis CV, Reed AM, Aggarwal R, et al. Rituximab in the treatment of refractory adult and juvenile dermatomyositis and adult polymyositis: a randomized, placebo-phase trial. *Arthritis Rheum.* 2013;65:314–324.
4. Dalakas MC, Illa I, Dambrosia JM, et al. A controlled trial of high-dose intravenous immune globulin infusions as treatment for dermatomyositis. *N Engl J Med.* 1993;329:1993–2000.

Inclusion Body Myositis

5. Badrising UA, Maat-Schieman ML, Ferrari MD, et al. Comparison of weakness progression in inclusion body myositis during treatment with methotrexate or placebo. *Ann Neurol.* 2002;51:369.
6. Dalakas MC, Koffman B, Fukii M, et al. A controlled study of intravenous immunoglobulin combined with prednisone in the treatment of IBM. *Neurology.* 2001;56:323–327.
7. Dalakas MC, Sonies B, Dambrosia J, et al. Treatment of inclusion-body myositis with IVIg: a double-blind, placebo-controlled study. *Neurology.* 1997;48:712–716.
8. The Muscle Study Group. Randomized pilot trial of high-dose beta-interferon-1a in patients with inclusion body myositis. *Neurology.* 2004;63:718–720.

SUGGESTED READINGS

Inflammatory Myopathies (General)

Amato AA, Barohn RJ. Evaluation and treatment of inflammatory myopathies. *J Neurol Neurosurg Psychiatry.* 2009;80:1060–1068.

Amato AA, Greenberg SA. Inflammatory myopathies. *Continuum (Minneap Minn).* 2013;19:1615–1633.

Dalakas MC. Inflammatory disorders of muscle: progress in polymyositis, dermatomyositis and inclusion body myositis. *Curr Opin Neurol.* 2004; 17:561–567.

Dimachkie MM, Barohn RJ, Amato AA. Idiopathic inflammatory myopathies. *Neurol Clin.* 2014;32:595–628, vii.

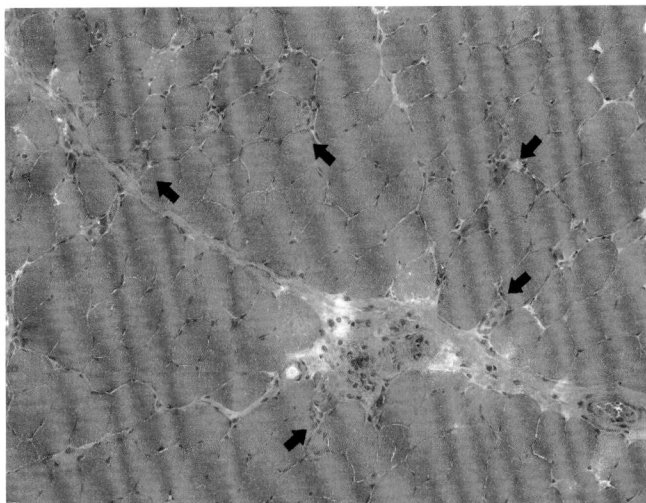

FIGURE 90.4 Muscle pathology in necrotizing autoimmune myopathy. Necrotic myofibers with minimal inflammation (*arrows*). (Hematoxylin and eosin stain, ×200 magnification.)

Joffe MM, Love LA, Leff RL, et al. Drug therapy of the idiopathic inflammatory myopathies: predictors of response to prednisone, azathioprine, and methotrexate and a comparison of their efficacy. *Am J Med.* 1993;94:379–387.

Katzap E, Barilla-LaBarca ML, Marder G. Antisynthetase syndrome. *Curr Rheumatol Rep.* 2011;13:175–181.

Mahler EA, Blom M, Voermans NC, et al. Rituximab treatment in patients with refractory inflammatory myopathies. *Rheumatology (Oxford).* 2011; 50:2206–2213.

Marie I, Josse S, Hatron PY, et al. Interstitial lung disease in anti-Jo-1 patients with antisynthetase syndrome. *Arthritis Care Res (Hoboken).* 2013;65:800–808.

Patwa HS, Chaudry V, Katzberg H, et al. Evidence-based guideline: intravenous immunoglobulin in the treatment of neuromuscular disorders: report of the Therapeutics and Technology Assessment Subcommittee of the American Academy of Neurology. *Neurology.* 2012;78:1009–1015.

Salaroli R, Baldin E, Papa V, et al. Validity of internal expression of the major histocompatibility complex class I in the diagnosis of inflammatory myopathies. *J Clin Pathol.* 2012;65:14–19.

Soueidan SA, Dalakas MC. Treatment of autoimmune neuromuscular diseases with high-dose intravenous immune globulin. *Pediatr Res.* 1993;33: S95–S100.

Dermatomyositis and Polymyositis

Andras C, Ponyi A, Constantin T, et al. Dermatomyositis and polymyositis associated with malignancy: a 21-year retrospective study. *J Rheumatol.* 2008;35:438–444.

Bendewald MJ, Wetter DA, Li X, et al. Incidence of dermatomyositis and clinically amyopathic dermatomyositis: a population-based study in Olmsted County, Minnesota. *Arch Dermatol.* 2010;146:26–30.

Bohan A, Peter JB. Polymyositis and dermatomyositis (first of two parts). *N Engl J Med.* 1975;292:344–347.

Bohan A, Peter JB. Polymyositis and dermatomyositis (second of two parts). *N Engl J Med.* 1975;292:403–407.

Chinoy H, Fertig N, Oddis CV, et al. The diagnostic utility of myositis autoantibody testing for predicting the risk of cancer-associated myositis. *Ann Rheum Dis.* 2007;66:1345–1349.

Emslie-Smith AM, Engel AG. Microvascular changes in early and advanced dermatomyositis: a quantitative study. *Ann Neurol.* 1990;27:343–356.

Engel AG, Hohlfeld R. The polymyositis and dermatomyositis syndromes. In: Engel AG, Franzini-Armstrong C, ed. *Myology.* 3rd ed. New York: McGraw-Hill; 2004:1321–1388.

Feldman BM, Rider LG, Reed AM, et al. Juvenile dermatomyositis and other idiopathic inflammatory myopathies of childhood. *Lancet.* 2008; 371:2201–2212.

Hengstman GJ, Hoogen FH, van Engelen BG. Treatment of dermatomyositis and polymyositis with anti-tumor necrosis factor-alpha: long-term follow-up. *Eur Neurol.* 2004;52:61–63.

Hill CL, Zhang Y, Sigurgeirsson B, et al. Frequency of specific cancer types in dermatomyositis and polymyositis: a population-based study. *Lancet.* 2001;357:96–100.

Hoogendijk JE, Amato AA, Lecky BR, et al. 119th ENMC international workshop: trial design in adult idiopathic inflammatory myopathies, with the exception of inclusion body myositis, 10–12 October 2003, Naarden, The Netherlands. *Neuromuscul Disord.* 2004;14:337–345.

Levine TD. Rituximab in the treatment of dermatomyositis: an open-label pilot study. *Arthritis Rheum.* 2005;52:601–607.

Mendez EP, Lipton R, Ramsey-Goldman R, et al. US incidence of juvenile dermatomyositis, 1995–1998: results from the National Institute of Arthritis and Musculoskeletal and Skin Diseases Registry. *Arthritis Rheum.* 2003;49: 300–305.

Mimori T, Imura Y, Nakashima R, et al. Autoantibodies in idiopathic inflammatory myopathy: an update on clinical and pathophysiological significance. *Curr Opin Rheumatol.* 2007;19:523–529.

Mimori T, Nakashima R, Hosono Y. Interstitial lung disease in myositis: clinical subsets, biomarkers, and treatment. *Curr Rheumatol Rep.* 2012;14:264–274.

Morganroth PA, Kreider ME, Werth VP. Mycophenolate mofetil for interstitial lung disease in dermatomyositis. *Arthritis Care Res (Hoboken).* 2010; 62:1496–501.

Newman ED, Scott DW. The use of low-dose oral methotrexate in the treatment of polymyositis and dermatomyositis. *J Clin Rheumatol.* 1995;1:99–102.

Noss EH, Hausner-Sypek DL, Weinblatt ME. Rituximab as therapy for refractory polymyositis and dermatomyositis. *J Rheumatol.* 2006;33:1021–1026.

Pachman LM, Hayford JR, Chung A, et al. Juvenile dermatomyositis at diagnosis: clinical characteristics of 79 children. *J Rheumatol.* 1998;25:1198–1204.

Quartier P, Gherardi RK. Chapter 149: juvenile dermatomyositis. *Handbook of Clin Neurol.* 2013;113:1457–1463.

Rowin J, Amato AA, Deisher N, et al. Mycophenolate mofetil in dermatomyositis: is it safe? *Neurology.* 2006;66:1245–1247.

Sigurgeirsson B, Lindelof B, Edhag O, et al. Risk of cancer in patients with dermatomyositis or polymyositis. A population-based study. *N Engl J Med.* 1992;326:363–367.

Stone KB, Oddis CV, Fertig N, et al. Anti-Jo-1 antibody levels correlate with disease activity in idiopathic inflammatory myopathy. *Arthritis Rheum.* 2007;56:3125–3131.

Inclusion Body Myositis

Argov Z, Eisenberg I, Grabov-Nardini G, et al. Hereditary inclusion body myopathy: the Middle Eastern genetic cluster. *Neurology.* 2003;60:1519–1523.

Askanas V, Engel WK. Inclusion-body myositis, a multifactorial muscle disease associated with aging: current concepts of pathogenesis. *Curr Opin Rheumatol.* 2007;19:550–559.

Badrising UA, Maat-Schieman M, van Duinen SG, et al. Epidemiology of inclusion body myositis in the Netherlands: a nationwide study. *Neurology.* 2000;55:1385–1387.

Benveniste O, Guiguet M, Freebody J, et al. Long-term observational study of sporadic inclusion body myositis. *Brain.* 2011;134:3176–3184.

Brannagan TH, Hays AP, Lange DJ, et al. The role of quantitative electromyography in inclusion body myositis. *J Neurol Neurosurg Psychiatry.* 1997;63:776–779.

Cox FM, Reijnierse M, van Rijswijk CS, et al. Magnetic resonance imaging of skeletal muscles in sporadic inclusion body myositis. *Rheumatology (Oxford).* 2011;50:1153–1161.

Dabby R, Lange DJ, Trojaborg W, et al. Inclusion body myositis mimicking motor neuron disease. *Arch Neurol.* 2001;58:1253–1256.

Dimachkie MM, Barohn RJ. Inclusion body myositis. *Neurol Clin.* 2014;32: 629–646, vii.

Griggs RC. The current status of treatment for inclusion-body myositis. *Neurology.* 2006;66:S30–S32.

Larman HB, Salajegheh M, Nazareno R, et al. Cytosolic 5'-nucleotidase 1A autoimmunity in sporadic inclusion body myositis. *Ann Neurol.* 2013;73:408–418.

Lotz BP, Engel AG, Nishino H, et al. Inclusion body myositis. Observations in 40 patients. *Brain.* 1989;112(pt 3):727–747.

Machado P, Brady S, Hanna MG. Update in inclusion body myositis. *Curr Opin Rheumatol.* 2013;25:763–771.

Needham M, Mastaglia FL, Garlepp MJ. Genetics of inclusion-body myositis. *Muscle Nerve.* 2007;35:549–561.

Pluk H, van Hoeve BJ, van Dooren SH, et al. Autoantibodies to cytosolic 5'-nucleotidase 1A in inclusion body myositis. *Ann Neurol.* 2013;73:397–407.

Wilson FC, Ytterberg SR, St Sauver JL, et al. Epidemiology of sporadic inclusion body myositis and polymyositis in Olmsted County, Minnesota. *J Rheumatol.* 2008;35:445–447.

Necrotizing Autoimmune Myopathy

Albayda J, Mammen AL. Is statin-induced myositis part of the polymyositis disease spectrum? *Curr Rheumatol Rep.* 2014;16:433.

Allenbach Y, Benveniste O. Acquired necrotizing myopathies. *Curr Opin Neurol.* 2013;26:554–560.

Christopher-Stine L, Casciola-Rosen LA, Hong G, et al. A novel autoantibody recognizing 200-kd and 100-kd proteins is associated with an immune-mediated necrotizing myopathy. *Arthritis Rheum.* 2010;62:2757–2766.

Ellis E, Ann Tan J, Lester S, et al. Necrotizing myopathy: clinicoserologic associations. *Muscle Nerve.* 2012;45:189–194.

Mammen AL, Chung T, Christopher-Stine L, et al. Autoantibodies against 3-hydroxy-3-methylglutaryl-coenzyme A reductase in patients with statin-associated autoimmune myopathy. *Arthritis Rheum.* 2011;63:713–721.

Miller T, Al-Lozi MT, Lopate G, et al. Myopathy with antibodies to the signal recognition particle: clinical and pathological features. *J Neurol Neurosurg Psychiatry.* 2002;73:420–428.

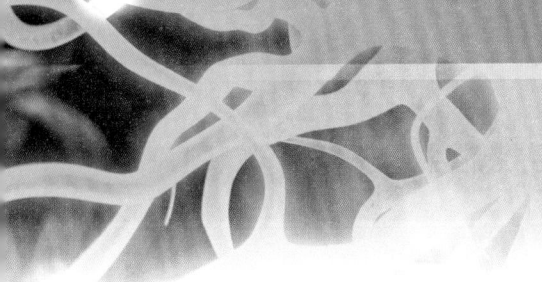

Critical Illness Myopathy and Neuropathy 91

Michio Hirano and Louis H. Weimer

INTRODUCTION

Although critically ill individuals in intensive care units are typically weak due to their severe medical illnesses, a subgroup of patients develops critical illness myopathy (CIM), critical illness polyneuropathy (CIP), or both. The first case of acute quadriplegic myopathy (AQM, later renamed CIM) was reported in 1977 by MacFarlane and Rosenthal in a 24-year-old woman who received high-dose corticosteroids for status asthmaticus. In 1984, Bolton and colleagues described five critically ill patients with sepsis and multiorgan failure who developed severe sensorimotor peripheral neuropathies. Since then, hundreds of patients with CIM and CIP have been reported.

EPIDEMIOLOGY

Although incidence rates of CIM and CIP vary in reported series based on patient populations and detection methods, the disorders appear frequently common in the intensive care unit (ICU) setting. In one report, about 25% of patients in the ICU developed weakness, whereas electrophysiologic studies have detected neuromuscular abnormalities in up to 84% of patients. Among patients with sepsis or systemic inflammatory response syndrome (SIRS), the incidence has been estimated to be 70% and virtually 100% in patients with septic shock or sepsis plus coma. In most case series, the incidence of CIM has been greater than CIP; however, some patients manifest both.

PATHOBIOLOGY

For CIM, corticosteroids, nondepolarizing neuromuscular blocking agents, or both are considered the prime inciting factors, but it has appeared in some individuals who received neither agent. Patients undergoing treatment for status asthmaticus, organ transplantation, and severe trauma seem to be particularly vulnerable. In contrast, for CIP, sepsis, SIRS, and multiorgan failure are risk factors. Other factors that may contribute to CIM and CIP include severity of the illness, duration of ICU stay, duration of organ dysfunction, renal failure, neurologic failure, hyperosmolarity, hyperglycemia, and vasopressor and catecholamine supportive treatment.

Pathophysiologic mechanisms responsible for these conditions are not fully understood. In patients with CIM, direct muscle stimulation has shown a loss of muscle fiber excitability, which has been attributed to voltage-gated sodium channel fast inactivation, based on animal models of steroid-treated denervated muscle as well as biopsied muscle. Enhanced expression of ubiquitin, lysosomal enzymes, and calcium-activated proteases (calpains) has been observed in muscle and could play a pathogenic role. These catabolic pathways may be activated in muscle by induction of transforming growth factor-β/mitogen activated protein kinase pathways. Immune activation by cytokines may also contribute to the myopathy.

Although direct evidence is lacking, CIP has been attributed to microcirculation defects including increased vessel permeability and vasodilation leading to the axonal degeneration. Peripheral nerve biopsies from CIP patients have revealed expression of E-selectin in the vascular endothelium of epineural and endoneurial vessels. Because E-selectin is not normally expressed in vascular endothelium, its presence may increase nerve microvasculature permeability, which would allow circulating neurotoxins to enter the endoneurium and promote endoneural edema.

CLINICAL MANIFESTATIONS

In CIM, severe quadriplegia and muscle atrophy commence 4 to more than 100 days after initiation of intensive care therapy. The weakness may be primarily distal or proximal but is usually diffuse; many patients lose tendon reflexes. Ophthalmoparesis and facial muscle weakness are occasionally present. Persistent respiratory muscle weakness complicates weaning patients from mechanical ventilation. Patients often manifest diffuse muscle atrophy, which can be severe. Improvement is generally evident in 1 to several months in most individuals who survive their critical illness, but protracted recovery or persistent deficits are common.

CIP presents as acute distal limb weakness and sensory loss with diminished or absent tendon reflexes. Involvement of the phrenic and intercostal nerves causes respiratory muscle weakness that often requires prolonged mechanical ventilation therapy (Table 91.1).

DIAGNOSIS

Diagnosis of CIM and CIP is typically suspected when patients have unexplained severe limb weakness, inability to weak patients off mechanical ventilation, or both. Marked muscle atrophy is common in CIM, whereas areflexia and stocking–glove sensory loss (in alert patients) are characteristic of CIP. CIM and CIP must be distinguished from the persistent weakness that may follow administration of nondepolarizing blocking agents to a person with impaired hepatic metabolism, reduced renal excretion, or both.

In patients with CIM, laboratory studies have shown normal or elevated serum creatine kinase levels. Nerve conduction studies (NCS) demonstrate absent or low-amplitude compound motor action potentials with decreased duration. Sensory nerve action potentials are normal, reduced, or absent but frequently hampered by technical constraints in the ICU environment and by limb edema. Electromyography (EMG) variably shows signs of denervation from muscle necrosis and myogenic or normal motor unit action potentials; however, motor unit and recruitment analysis are frequently suboptimal owing to severe weakness, encephalopathy, sedation, or other confounding factors. Direct muscle stimulation has shown a loss of muscle fiber excitability.

Muscle biopsies demonstrate myopathic changes. Three distinct histologic features have been described in skeletal muscle biopsies;

TABLE 91.1	Major Characteristics of Critical Illness Myopathy and Critical Illness Polyneuropathy	
	Critical Illness Myopathy (CIM)	**Critical Illness Polyneuropathy (CIP)**
Clinical features	Weakness, typically diffuse including respiratory muscles. Muscle atrophy is common.	Distal limb weakness and sensory loss with diminished or absent tendon reflexes. Respiratory muscle weakness is common.
Risk factors	Treatment with corticosteroid, nondepolarizing neuromuscular blocking agent, or both	Sepsis, systemic inflammatory response syndrome (SIRS), multiorgan failure
Nerve conduction study and electromyography abnormalities	Myogenic abnormalities	Neurogenic abnormalities with signs of acute denervation
Muscle biopsy findings	Myofiber atrophy predominantly affecting type 2 fibers. Loss of thick (myosin) filaments is characteristic but is not always seen.	Signs of acute denervation
Treatment	Reduce exposure to corticosteroids and nondepolarizing neuromuscular blocking agents.	Intensive insulin treatment to maintain normal blood glucose levels

the abnormalities may be present in isolation or in variable combinations. Muscle fiber atrophy, often more prominent in type 2 fibers, is routinely seen. In patients with markedly elevated creatine kinase levels, necrosis of muscle fibers has been observed. The most striking feature revealed by electron microscopy is loss of thick (myosin) filaments, corroborated by antimyosin-antibody stains and reduced myosin mRNA levels but is not seen in many cases.

In CIP, NCS typically show signs of axonopathy with decreased or absent sensory and compound motor action potentials with mildly reduced conduction velocities; these changes may appear as early as 72 hours after ICU admission and can precede clinical manifestations. Electrophysiologic studies of the peroneal nerve have been proposed as a rapid and sensitive diagnostic test for CIP. EMG shows fibrillations and positive sharp waves due to acute denervation, which can be difficult to distinguish from acute muscle necrosis from CIM.

Muscle biopsies in CIP can show signs of acute denervation. Nerve biopsies are generally not useful in CIP, which typically manifests nonspecific signs of axonal neuropathy; however, if other forms of peripheral neuropathy (e.g., vasculitis or chronic inflammatory demyelinating polyneuropathy) are suspected, then nerve biopsies may be indicated.

TREATMENT

Treatment of patients with CIM and CIP is primarily directed at the underlying acute medical condition(s). Supportive care, particularly mechanical ventilation, is important. Because corticosteroids and neuromuscular blocking agents appear to trigger CIM, reducing exposure to these agents is generally recommended.

Two randomized trials of ICU patients have demonstrated that intensive insulin treatment (IIT) aimed at maintaining normal glucose levels reduces the incidence of CIP by nearly half (relative risk 0.65, 95% confidence interval 0.55–0.77) as well as duration of mechanical ventilation and 180-day mortality compared to conventional insulin treatment [**Level 1**].[1,2] Physical therapy to passively stretch muscles may reduce muscle atrophy and may increase functional independence.

OUTCOME

Both CIM and CIP cause prolonged and often severe disability. The weakness can persist for months to years or even indefinitely. About 28% of patients with CIP, CIM, or both may not recover ability to ambulate independently or weak completely off ventilation. CIP is more likely to cause permanent disability than CIM. The majority of patients with CIM recover in 3 to 6 months.

LEVEL 1 EVIDENCE

1. Van den Berghe G, Schoonheydt K, Becx P, et al. Insulin therapy protects the central and peripheral nervous system of intensive care patients. *Neurology*. 2005;64:1348–1353.

2. Hermans G, Wilmer A, Meersseman W, et al. Impact of intensive insulin therapy on neuromuscular complications and ventilator dependency in the medical intensive care unit. *Am J Respir Crit Care Med*. 2007;175:480–489.

SUGGESTED READINGS

Allen DC, Arunachalam R, Mills KR. Critical illness myopathy: further evidence from muscle-fiber excitability studies of an acquired channelopathy. *Muscle Nerve*. 2008;37:14–22.

Apostolakis E, Papakonstantinou NA, Baikoussis NG, et al. Intensive care unit-related generalized neuromuscular weakness due to critical illness polyneuropathy/myopathy in critically ill patients. *J Anesth*. 2015;29:112–121.

Argov Z, Latronico N. Neuromuscular complications in intensive care patients. *Handb Clin Neurol*. 2014;121:1673–1685.

Bird SJ. Diagnosis and management of critical illness polyneuropathy and critical illness myopathy. *Curr Treat Options Neurol*. 2007;9:85–92.

Bolton CF, Gilbert JJ, Hahn AF, et al. Polyneuropathy in critically ill patients. *J Neurol Neurosurg Psychiatry*. 1984;47:1223–1231.

Coakley JH, Nagendran K, Yarwood GD, et al. Patterns of neurophysiological abnormality in prolonged critical illness. *Intensive Care Med*. 1998;24:801–807.

De Jonghe B, Sharshar T, Lefaucheur JP, et al. Paresis acquired in the intensive care unit: a prospective multicenter study. *JAMA*. 2002;288:2859–2867.

De Letter MA, van Doorn PA, Savelkoul HF, et al. Critical illness polyneuropathy and myopathy (CIPNM): evidence for local immune activation by cytokine-expression in the muscle tissue. *J Neuroimmunol.* 2000;106:206–213.

Di Giovanni S, Molon A, Broccolini A, et al. Constitutive activation of MAPK cascade in acute quadriplegic myopathy. *Ann Neurol.* 2004;55:195–206.

Fenzi F, Latronico N, Refatti N, et al. Enhanced expression of E-selectin on the vascular endothelium of peripheral nerve in critically ill patients with neuromuscular disorders. *Acta Neuropathol.* 2003;106:75–82.

Goodman BP, Harper CM, Boon AJ. Prolonged compound muscle action potential duration in critical illness myopathy. *Muscle Nerve.* 2009;40:1040–1042.

Guarneri B, Bertolini G, Latronico N. Long-term outcome in patients with critical illness myopathy or neuropathy: the Italian multicentre CRIMYNE study. *J Neurol Neurosurg Psychiatry.* 2008;79:838–841.

Helliwell TR, Wilkinson A, Griffiths RD, et al. Muscle fibre atrophy in critically ill patients is associated with the loss of myosin filaments and the presence of lysosomal enzymes and ubiquitin. *Neuropathol Appl Neurobiol.* 1998;24:507–517.

Hermans G, De Jonghe B, Bruyninckx F, et al. Interventions for preventing critical illness polyneuropathy and critical illness myopathy. *Cochrane Database Syst Rev.* 2014;1:CD006832.

Hirano M, Ott BR, Raps EC, et al. Acute quadriplegic myopathy: a complication of treatment with steroids, nondepolarizing blocking agents, or both. *Neurology.* 1992;42:2082–2087.

Koch S, Spuler S, Deja M, et al. Critical illness myopathy is frequent: accompanying neuropathy protracts ICU discharge. *J Neurol Neurosurg Psychiatry.* 2011;82:287–293.

Koch S, Wollersheim T, Bierbrauer J, et al. Long-term recovery in critical illness myopathy is complete, contrary to polyneuropathy. *Muscle Nerve.* 2014;50:431–436.

Kraner SD, Novak KR, Wang Q, et al. Altered sodium channel-protein associations in critical illness myopathy. *Skelet Muscle.* 2012;2:17.

Lacomis D, Petrella JT, Giuliani MJ. Causes of neuromuscular weakness in the intensive care unit: a study of ninety-two patients. *Muscle Nerve.* 1998;21:610–617.

Latronico N, Tomelleri G, Filosto M. Critical illness myopathy. *Curr Opin Rheumatol.* 2012;24:616–622.

MacFarlane IA, Rosenthal FD. Severe myopathy after status asthmaticus. *Lancet.* 1977;2:615.

Matsuda N, Kobayashi S, Tanji Y, et al. Widespread muscle involvement in critical illness myopathy revealed by MRI. *Muscle Nerve.* 2011;44:842–844.

Minetti C, Hirano M, Morreale G, et al. Ubiquitin expression in acute steroid myopathy with loss of myosin thick filaments. *Muscle Nerve.* 1996;19:94–96.

Segredo V, Caldwell JE, Matthay MA, et al. Persistent paralysis in critically ill patients after long-term administration of vecuronium. *N Engl J Med.* 1992;327:524–528.

Tennila A, Salmi T, Pettila V, et al. Early signs of critical illness polyneuropathy in ICU patients with systemic inflammatory response syndrome or sepsis. *Intensive Care Med.* 2000;26:1360–1363.

Trojaborg W, Weimer LH, Hays AP. Electrophysiologic studies in critical illness associated weakness: myopathy or neuropathy—a reappraisal. *Clin Neurophysiol.* 2001;112:1586–1593.

Weber-Carstens S, Deja M, Koch S, et al. Risk factors in critical illness myopathy during the early course of critical illness: a prospective observational study. *Crit Care.* 2010;14:R119.

Weber-Carstens S, Schneider J, Wollersheim T, et al. Critical illness myopathy and GLUT4: significance of insulin and muscle contraction. *Am J Respir Crit Care Med.* 2013;187:387–396.

Witt NJ, Zochodne DW, Bolton CF, et al. Peripheral nerve function in sepsis and multiple organ failure. *Chest.* 1991;99:176–184.

Zink W, Kollmar R, Schwab S. Critical illness polyneuropathy and myopathy in the intensive care unit. *Nat Rev Neurol.* 2009;5:372–379.

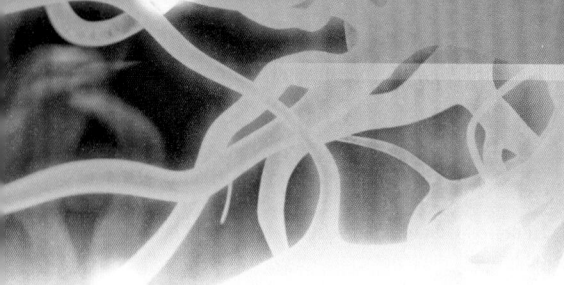

Endocrine and Toxic Myopathies 92

Christina M. Ulane

INTRODUCTION

Muscle comprises a large proportion of all tissues in the body and the energy required for its function renders it susceptible to metabolic abnormalities from endocrine dysfunction and toxic effects of medications and environmental exposures. Muscle tissue is affected by the metabolic and trophic effects of various components of the endocrine system and by direct and indirect effects of toxins. This chapter highlights features of the most common endocrinopathies and toxins affecting muscle, concisely reviews the many others, and emphasizes the fundamental principles in diagnosis and treatment of these disorders.

ENDOCRINE MYOPATHIES

EPIDEMIOLOGY

Myopathy in endocrine disorders is rather common, but the earlier diagnosis and treatment of endocrinopathies has reduced the severity of myopathic symptoms. Thyroid disorders and corticosteroid abnormalities (most often from exogenous sources) are the most common endocrinopathies encountered and thus discussed in most detail. Exogenous corticosteroid administration at doses of 30 mg or more per day of prednisone confers the highest risk.

Historical studies suggest that up to 75% of patients with hyperthyroidism will experience myopathy, but current data regarding incidence of true myopathy in endocrinopathies is not available, likely a result of earlier diagnosis and treatment. Myopathy is also found in association with acromegaly, hypopituitarism, hyperparathyroidism, and hypoparathyroidism.

PATHOBIOLOGY

The exact basis of myopathy in endocrinopathy is unknown and may be multifactorial. Often, weakness and fatigue are out of proportion to muscle wasting, suggesting energy failure as a mechanism. Thyroxine has catabolic effects on muscle, may reduce efficiency of muscle contraction, alter membrane excitability, and lead to reduced potassium in muscle and serum, leading to weakness in hyperthyroidism. Hypothyroidism reduces glycogenolysis (animal studies indicate this occurs via reduced expression of β-adrenergic receptors on muscle cells), which may be responsible for cramps and fatigue. Hypothyroidism can also reduce mitochondrial oxidation, and studies in rats demonstrate changes in myosin from fast-twitch to slow-twitch muscle types. Thyroid-associated ophthalmopathy leads to edema in the extraocular muscles from both glycoprotein accumulation and inflammation. Corticosteroids cause muscle catabolism and stimulate protein degradation.

CLINICAL FEATURES

Myopathy from endocrine disorders causes nonspecific symptoms of myopathy. Proximal limb weakness, fatigue, and cramps are common. In some cases, myalgias are present. In steroid myopathy, symptoms may occur as early as after a few weeks of treatment. See Table 92.1 for clinical features of thyroid-associated myopathies and Table 92.2 for other endocrine-associated myopathies, including that due to exogenous steroid administration.

DIAGNOSIS

Other features related to specific endocrine disorders are usually apparent and suggest the diagnosis. However, if corticosteroids are

TABLE 92.1	Myopathies Associated with Thyroid Disorders		
Disorder	**Clinical**	**Diagnostics**	**Treatment**
Hypothyroidism	• Muscle stiffness, pain, and cramps, especially with cold and exercise • Delayed relaxation (pseudo-myotonia)	• CK elevated, up to 10× normal • EMG: myopathic, +/− fibrillations, positive sharp waves • Biopsy: normal or nonspecific changes	• Thyroxine (T4) supplementation (start 25–50 μg daily, increase to 1.6 μg/kg/day, and monitor TSH)
Hyperthyroidism	• Proximal weakness, wasting (shoulder girdle, scapular winging) • May involve respiratory, bulbar, or distal muscles	• CK is normal (except in thyroid storm) • EMG: myopathic in proximal muscles • Biopsy: nonspecific, type 1 and 2 fiber atrophy	• Correction of thyroxine levels to normal (antithyroid medications, radioactive iodine, thyroidectomy) • Weakness may take months to resolve. • Propranolol (start 10 mg t.i.d. to q.i.d., may increase to 40 mg q.i.d.) may hasten recovery.

(continued)

TABLE 92.1 Myopathies Associated with Thyroid Disorders (continued)

Disorder	Clinical	Diagnostics	Treatment
Thyrotoxic periodic paralysis	• Severe weakness lasting hours to days, precipitated by cold, exercise, or high-carbohydrate intake • More common in men from Japan and China	• Potassium levels low during attacks • +/− low magnesium or phosphorus • Associated HLA haplotypes	• Correction of thyroid abnormality • Propranolol (start 10 mg t.i.d. to q.i.d., may increase to 40 mg q.i.d.) may prevent attacks.
Thyroid ophthalmopathy	• Exophthalmos, pain, diplopia • May have compressive optic neuropathy • Mostly occurs with hyperthyroidism (sometimes with hypothyroidism, euthyroidism)	• Edema of extraocular muscles on MRI	• Correction of thyroid abnormality • Guanethidine eye drops (β-adrenergic) • Local steroid injection • Systemic steroids (prednisone 30–100 mg PO daily for at least 4 wks followed by taper or methylprednisolone 500 mg IV for one dose followed by 250 mg IV weekly) • Selenium 100 mg b.i.d. for 6 mo

CK, creatine kinase; EMG, electromyography; TSH, thyroid-stimulating hormone; HLA, human leukocyte antigen; MRI, magnetic resonance imaging; PO, by mouth; IV, intravenous.

TABLE 92.2 Myopathies Associated with Other Endocrinopathies

Disorder	Clinical	Diagnostics	Treatment
Cushing disease/ exogenous corticosteroid administration	• Painless proximal weakness (legs affected more than arms) • +/− muscle wasting • Fluorinated corticosteroids more likely to cause myopathy (triamcinolone, betamethasone, dexamethasone)	• CK is normal. • EMG: may be normal or show myopathic features • Biopsy: type 2 fiber atrophy, increased glycogen	• Treat underlying Cushing etiology, but recovery may be slow or incomplete • Reduce exogenous steroid dose to minimum possible • Alternate-day steroid dosing • Use of nonfluorinated corticosteroids • Use of steroid-sparing agents
Adrenal insufficiency	• General weakness • Fatigue, cramps	• CK is normal. • EMG: normal • Biopsy: nonspecific	• Glucocorticoid replacement. Hydrocortisone 5 mg/m^2 total daily, given b.i.d. with 2/3 of dose in AM and 1/3 in PM.
Acromegaly	• Slowly progressive proximal weakness and pain • Decreased exercise tolerance • Minimal muscle wasting	• CK is normal or mildly elevated • EMG: +/− myopathy • Biopsy: hypertrophy or atrophy of type 1 and 2 fibers, excess lipofuscin, glycogen	Correction of excess GH: • Bromocriptine: start 1.25–1.5 mg daily, increase to 20–30 mg daily • Pituitary adenoma resection • Irradiation
Hyperparathyroidism	• Generalized weakness, stiffness • Proximal weakness, wasting (especially legs) • Tongue fasciculations • +/− hyperreflexia • Chronic renal failure (secondary hyperparathyroidism)	• CK is normal. • EMG: +/− myopathic • Biopsy: nonspecific	• Parathyroidectomy
Osteomalacia	• Proximal weakness and myalgias	• CK is normal or mildly elevated • EMG: myopathic • Biopsy: nonspecific	• Vitamin D supplementation (50,000 units vitamin D_2 or D_3 weekly for 6 wks then 800 units D_3 daily) • Supplementation as needed: calcium 1,000 mg daily and phosphorus 30–80 mmol total daily given t.i.d. or q.i.d.

CK, creatine kinase; EMG, electromyography; GH, growth hormone.

being used for the treatment of a disease that also causes weakness (such as polymyositis or myasthenia gravis), it can be challenging to determine whether progression of the underlying disorder or the corticosteroid treatment is the cause of weakness. Laboratory testing for serum levels of thyroid function, adrenocorticotrophic hormone, cortisol, metabolic panel, parathormone, and growth hormone can be diagnostic. Serum creatine kinase (CK) levels are helpful in many cases.

Electromyography (EMG) testing will often show myopathic abnormalities and occasionally, signs of irritative myopathy, but may be normal. Muscle biopsy may be required to distinguish other underlying causes, but findings in endocrine myopathies are usually nonspecific. Please see Tables 92.1 and 92.2 for laboratory, EMG, and muscle biopsy findings in various endocrine myopathies.

TREATMENT

Treatment is directed at correcting the underlying endocrine abnormality, through hormone replacement therapy or by reducing circulating hormone levels. In the case of hyperthyroid myopathy, propranolol may improve time to recovery through β-adrenergic blockade. If exogenous corticosteroids are the cause for myopathy, treatment of the disease for which the steroids are indicated must be balanced with reducing the contribution of steroids to the myopathy. Several strategies can be helpful, including alternate-day dosing and the use of steroid-sparing agents when possible (see Tables 92.1 and 92.2).

OUTCOME

Most persons with endocrinopathy causing myopathy will recover completely with correction of the underlying abnormality. Rarely, in Cushing disease, recovery may be incomplete.

TOXIC MYOPATHIES

EPIDEMIOLOGY

Toxic myopathies arise from environmental exposures and increasingly often from medications (Table 92.3). The large number of people prescribed statin medications makes this potentially myotoxic agent a commonly encountered clinical problem. Up to 20% of people taking statins will experience myalgias or cramps. Most of statin myotoxicity is mild and self-limited; however, severe toxic necrotizing myopathy can occur in rare cases. Myotoxicity from statin use is increased in those with obesity, preexisting hepatic disease, hypothyroidism, and advanced age. There is also a dose-dependent myotoxic effect: 1.6% on 80 mg/day versus 0.1% on 20 mg/day of simvastatin. Certain statins pose greater risk (atorvastatin, simvastatin, and pravastatin), whereas others are associated with lower risk (fluvastatin, rosuvastatin). In 2001, cerivastatin was withdrawn from the market in connection with cases of fatal rhabdomyolysis. Rhabdomyolysis due to statins is rare, occurring 0.44 per 10,000 patient-years.

Genome-wide association studies identified *SLCO1B1* gene polymorphisms as a predisposition to statin-induced myopathy. This gene encodes a protein involved in the hepatic uptake of statins, and persons homozygous for the polymorphism (2% of the general population) have increased serum levels of statins and 15% develop self-limited statin myopathy (not the autoimmune necrotizing myopathy). Concomitant use of medications metabolized by the CYP3A4 (such as calcium channel blockers, antibiotics,

TABLE 92.3	Toxic Myopathies
Pathophysiology	**Medications/Toxins**
Necrotizing	Statins (toxic necrotizing or toxic necrotizing autoimmune)
	Other cholesterol-lowering agents (fibrates, red yeast rice)
	Immunophilins (cyclosporine, tacrolimus)
	Ethanol
	Labetalol, propofol (rare)
	Snake venom
Amphiphilic (autophagic lysosomal)	Chloroquine/hydroxychloroquine (may have associated cardiomyopathy, correlates with duration of use and dose)
	Amiodarone (also causes hypothyroidism, neuropathy, tremor, ataxia)
Antimicrotubular	Colchicine
	Vincristine
Hypokalemic	Diuretics
	Laxatives
	Amphotericin
	Toluene
	Licorice
	Steroids
	Ethanol
Mitochondrial	Zidovudine
	Antiretrovirals
Inflammatory	L-tryptophan
	D-penicillamine
	Phenytoin
	Lamotrigine
	Interferon-α
	Hydroxyurea
	Imatinib (20%–50% will have myalgias)
	Cimetidine (rare; with interstitial nephritis)

antidepressants, and antiretrovirals) increases serum levels of statins and thus the risk of myotoxicity. Likewise, simultaneous use of fibric acid derivatives, especially gemfibrozil, increases the probability of statin myopathy.

PATHOBIOLOGY

Toxins cause myopathy either by directly affecting the muscle or indirectly through electrolyte imbalance or triggering immune reactions. Various types of pathophysiology account for toxic myopathies. Toxins may induce necrotizing myopathy, as with alcohol and statins. Autophagic lysosomal pathology is seen with amphiphilic agents such as chloroquine and amiodarone. Colchicine and vincristine induce myopathy through antimicrotubular effects. Many agents can cause an inflammatory myopathy. Antiretroviral agents lead to mitochondrial myopathy, and diuretics and laxatives among others cause hypokalemic myopathy. Self-limited

TABLE 92.4	Myotoxicity Associated with Statins
Syndrome	**Management**
Asymptomatic hyperCKemia	• May continue statin • Monitor CK and for clinical symptoms.
Myalgias, cramps	• Discontinue statin; most symptoms will resolve in 2–3 mo. • Retrial at lower dose or switch to lower risk statin. • If symptoms persist or progress, consider muscle biopsy for underlying neuromuscular disorder or myositis. • Potential role for vitamin D (mainly in those with deficiency), coenzyme Q10
Toxic necrotizing myopathy	• Discontinue statin (improve within 2–3 mo). • Hospital admission • Intravenous hydration • Supportive measures • Hemodialysis if needed • Risk/benefit analysis regarding need for statin
Necrotizing autoimmune myopathy	• Discontinue statin (myopathy persists or progresses despite discontinuation). • Long-term immunosuppressive treatment (see Chapter 90)

CK, creatine kinase.

statin myotoxicity likely is due to muscle membrane destabilization secondary to reduced levels of lipid precursors, affecting mitochondrial electron transport and coenzyme Q10 production. The immune-mediated necrotizing myopathy caused by statins is discussed in detail in Chapter 90.

CLINICAL FEATURES

Symptoms of toxic myopathies are nonspecific. Proximal weakness is common, with or without associated pain. Rarely are the respiratory and bulbar muscles affected.

DIAGNOSIS

History and temporal correlation with medication use are crucial in determining whether a toxin is the cause of myopathy. Resolution of symptoms following withdrawal of the potentially offending agent is helpful in diagnosis.

Laboratory studies including CK, metabolic panel, hepatic function testing, thyroid function testing, and vitamin D can assist in diagnosis but also aid in identifying readily correctable abnormalities that may worsen myopathy. EMG may show myopathic findings. On occasion, a myotoxic medication may identify an underlying metabolic or hereditary myopathy.

TREATMENT

Most often, removal of exposure to the offending agent will reduce or resolve myopathy completely. In the case of statin-associated necrotizing autoimmune myopathy, ongoing immunosuppressive treatment is needed (see Chapter 90). Results are mixed as to whether supplementation with coenzyme Q10 is beneficial for statin-associated myopathy. Vitamin D supplementation is recommended only for those with laboratory evidence of deficiency and it is unclear if it is helpful in the absence of deficiency. The high prevalence of dyslipidemia and ensuing statin use suggests a tiered approach to the treatment of statin-associated myopathy (Table 92.4).

OUTCOME

Prognosis for toxic myopathies depends on the etiology and specific syndrome. In general, withdrawal of the offending agent results in resolution or significant improvement of myopathy.

SUGGESTED READINGS

Harper CR, Jacobson TA. Evidence-based management of statin myopathy. *Curr Atheroscler Rep.* 2010;12:322–330.

Ishii M. Neurologic complications of nondiabetic endocrine disorders. *Continuum (Minneap Minn).* 2014;20(3):560–579.

Kendall-Taylor P, Turnbull DM. Endocrine myopathies. *Br Med J (Clin Res Ed).* 1983;287:705–708.

Mammen AL. Toxic myopathies. *Continuum (Minneap Minn).* 2013;19(6): 1634–1649.

Mastaglia FL, Needham M. Update on toxic myopathies. *Curr Neurol Neurosci Rep.* 2012;12:54–61.

Orrell RW. Endocrine myopathies. *Handb Clin Neurol.* 2007;86:343–355.

Pasnoor M, Barohn RJ, Dimachkie MM. Toxic myopathies. *Neurol Clin.* 2014; 32:647–670.

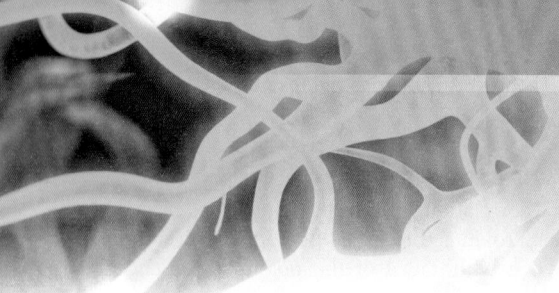

Periodic Paralysis and Other Channelopathies 93

Comana M. Cioroiu and Lewis P. Rowland

INTRODUCTION

Muscle channelopathies comprise a heterogeneous group of diseases of skeletal muscle that include both syndromes of episodic weakness (periodic paralyses) and muscle fiber hyperexcitability (nondystrophic myotonias). The clinical phenotype depends on the particular channel mutation involved, and attacks can vary in severity, duration, and constellation of symptomatic triggers (Table 93.1). Most of these disorders are inherited in an autosomal dominant fashion, although sporadic mutations do exist. Changes in neuronal membrane depolarization secondary to various ion channel mutations can either lead to sustained depolarization and resultant overt muscle weakness or to a more mild constant depolarization (or reduced repolarization) leading to myotonia and stiffness. On occasion, there is overlap between the two, and some patients may have episodes of both myotonia and paralysis. There are three main types of periodic paralysis: hypokalemic periodic paralysis, hyperkalemic periodic paralysis, and Andersen–Tawil syndrome (periodic paralysis with cardiac arrhythmia and dysmorphic features). The nondystrophic myotonic disorders are primarily composed of myotonia congenita, paramyotonia congenita, as well as a subgroup of potassium aggravated myotonic disorders. Electrodiagnostic testing is important in helping to identify particular patterns and make a correct diagnosis. Needle electromyogram (EMG) is needed to detect myotonic discharges or other abnormal spontaneous activity. In addition to routine nerve

| TABLE 93.1 | Clinical Features of Hereditary Periodic Paralysis and Nondystrophic Myotonias |

	Hypokalemic Periodic Paralysis	Hyperkalemic Periodic Paralysis	Andersen–Tawil Syndrome	Paramyotonia Congenita	Myotonia Congenita
Gene	CACN1AS or SCN4A	SCN4A	KCNJ2	SCN4A	CLCN-1 (AD) or SCN4A (AR)
Age of onset	Usually second or latter part of first decade	First decade	First or second decade	First decade	First decade
Sex	Male preponderance	Equal	Equal	Equal	Male preponderance
Frequency of paralytic episodes	Daily to yearly	Hourly to daily	Daily to yearly	May not be present; otherwise, weekly to monthly	Usually not present, variable frequency in AR form
Degrees of paralysis	Tends to be severe	Tends to be mild but can be severe	Variable	Tends to be mild but can be severe	Lasting seconds to minutes in AR form, usually not present in AD form
Effect of cold	May induce an attack	May induce an attack	May induce an attack	Tends to induce an attack	No effect
Oral potassium	Relieves or prevents an attack	Precipitates an attack	May relieve or prevent an attack	May precipitate an attack	No effect
Myotonia	Absent	May be present	Absent	Present	Present
Precipitants	Carbohydrate-rich food, cold	Fasting, stress, rest after exercise, K-rich foods	Carbohydrate-rich food, rest after exercise	Fasting, stress, cold, rest after exercise	Exercise
Exercise testing	Increase in CMAP with gradual decline with long exercise testing; short exercise testing normal (Fournier V)	Increase in amplitudes with gradual decrease in both short and long exercise testing (Fournier IV)	Unknown	Prominent drop in amplitudes with cooling in both long and short exercise testing; PEMPs present (Fournier I)	AD: drop in amplitude on short exercise testing, less drop with repeated testing AR: drop in amplitude with slow recovery (Fournier II)

AD, autosomal dominant; AR, autosomal recessive; K, potassium; CMAP, compound muscle action potential; PEMP, postexercise myotonic potential.
Modified from Hudson AJ. Progressive neurological disorder and myotonia congenita with paramyotonia. *Brain.* 1963;86:811.

conduction studies, short and long exercise tests are uniquely used to help characterize specific patterns. In short exercise testing, the patient is asked to exercise a muscle (typically the abductor digiti minimi), and a compound muscle action potential (CMAP) is recorded every 10 seconds thereafter and compared to a baseline. In the long exercise test, the patient is asked to exercise the muscle for an extended amount of time (usually 5 minutes), and CMAPs are recorded every 2 minutes thereafter for about 1 hour and compared to baseline. Changes in CMAP amplitude in both short and long exercise testing can be used to differentiate between the various channelopathies. For instance, CMAP amplitudes typically increase in the periodic paralyses and decrease in the myotonias. Different electrodiagnostic patterns diagnostic of each particular disease were described in 2004 by Emmanuel Fournier and are still used today and are known as *Fournier patterns*. Targeted confirmatory genetic testing is often done thereafter to confirm the diagnosis. Although patients with these diseases have a normal life expectancy, they may struggle with persistent pain or progressive weakness causing significant functional impairment.

HYPOKALEMIC PERIODIC PARALYSIS

EPIDEMIOLOGY AND PATHOBIOLOGY

Hypokalemic periodic paralysis (hypoKPP) is the most common of the periodic paralyses, yet it is still rare, affecting only about 1.7 per 1,000,000 people in England. Clinical onset is usually within the first 2 years of life (although it may be delayed into the sixth decade) and is more prevalent in men than women in a ratio of about 2:1. Most of these patients have mutations in either the CACN1AS gene (CaV1.1, chromosome 1q31-32) encoding an L-type calcium channel or less commonly, the SCN4A sodium channel gene (NaV1.4, chromosome 17q23). In the presence of these mutations, muscle fibers become depolarized and electrically inexcitable, leading to weakness. Just how these mutations cause persistent depolarization is unknown; however, one mouse model of such a calcium channel mutation proposed a possible explanation via a "gating pore current," described as an anomalous inward current at the resting potential triggered by low extracellular potassium content, leading to depolarization and sodium channel inactivation. At the structural level, mutations in the calcium channel lead to a vacuolar myopathy, whereas sodium channel mutations are associated with the development of transverse tubular aggregates and less vacuolization.

CLINICAL MANIFESTATIONS AND DIAGNOSIS

Patients with hypoKPP typically note transient weakness after a period of rest after exercise. These episodes are often more prominent during sleep or on rising in the morning and are worse after a meal rich in sodium or carbohydrates. The extent of paralysis can be variable and asymmetric and can vary from slight leg weakness to complete flaccid quadriplegia. Bulbar and respiratory muscles are typically spared, but urinary or fecal retention may be seen. The duration of attacks can be variable and last anywhere from a few hours to several days. The interval between attacks may be as long as 1 year, although in some patients, attacks can occur daily. Patients have normal strength in between attacks, but some eventually develop fixed proximal weakness. Attacks may be associated with pain either preceding or following weakness. In a mild attack, tendon reflexes are diminished in proportion to the degree of weakness and are completely absent in a severe attack. Sensation remains normal.

Diagnosis can be made on the basis of the presence of similar attacks of transient weakness in family members. Confirmatory tests include the finding of low potassium content (3.0 mEq/L or less) and high sodium content in the serum during an attack and the ability to induce an attack with an IV infusion of glucose and regular insulin. Serum creatine kinase (CK) levels are typically normal or mildly elevated. Short exercise electrodiagnostic testing is usually normal, but an increase in CMAP amplitude with a delayed decline can be seen with long exercise testing (Fournier pattern V). Needle EMG does not show myotonic discharges. Prior to making a diagnosis of hypoKPP, it is of crucial importance to exclude other conditions than may also lead to periodic paresis and hypokalemia including hyperaldosteronism, diuretic use, gastrointestinal loss, and thyrotoxicosis (Table 93.2). The latter in particular must be considered (particularly in those of Asian ancestry). Also, attacks of hypoKPP have been described in patients with hyperthyroidism linked to the potassium channel β subunit gene *KCNE3*, which responds completely with treatment of the thyroid disorder.

TREATMENT AND OUTCOME

Acute attacks may be treated safely with oral potassium (20 to 100 mEq), and rarely, IV potassium can be used, although it comes with the risk of subsequent hyperkalemia and cardiac arrhythmias. Prophylaxis of recurrent attacks is usually accomplished with the carbonic anhydrase inhibitor acetazolamide (Diamox) in doses of 250 to 1,000 mg daily. About 50% of patients respond to acetazolamide, and there is a greater benefit in patients with the CACNA1S

TABLE 93.2	Potassium and Paralysis: Noninherited Forms

Hypokalemic

- Excessive urinary loss
- Hyperaldosteronism (Conn syndrome)
- Drugs: glycyrrhizae (licorice), thiazide diuretics, furosemide, chlorthalidone, ethacrynic acid, amphotericin B, duogastrone, barium, corticosteroids
- Pyelonephritis, renal tubular acidosis
- Recovery from diabetic acidosis
- Ureterocolostomy
- Excessive gastrointestinal loss (diarrhea, vomiting, fistula)
- Malabsorption syndrome
- Laxative abuse
- Pancreatic tumor, villous adenoma
- Thyrotoxicosis

Hyperkalemic

- Uremia
- Hypoaldosteronism
- Addison disease
- Potassium-sparing diuretics (i.e., spironolactone)
- Excessive intake/supplementation of potassium
- Iatrogenic
- Geophagia

calcium mutation than in those with the SCN4A sodium channel mutation. In fact, on occasion, it may worsen attacks in patients with sodium channel mutations. The mechanism whereby it helps attacks of weakness is uncertain but may be related to induction of a mild metabolic acidosis, improved chloride conductance, or activation of the KCa^{2+} channel. Dichlorphenamide, another carbonic anhydrase inhibitor, has also been shown to be efficacious in reducing attacks in both hyper- and hypoKPP. Other agents that may be beneficial include triamterene or spironolactone, which promote retention of potassium. More recently, bumetanide (an Na-K-2Cl inhibitor) has been effective in preventing recurrent attacks of weakness and restoring force in a mouse model of hypoKPP with either a NaV1.4 sodium channel or CaV1.1 calcium channel mutation. Patients are also encouraged to avoid strenuous exercise and meals rich in carbohydrates. In those cases of hypoKPP secondary to a general medical condition (i.e., thyroid disease), the underlying disorder must be treated.

With time, patients with hypoKPP experience less attacks as they age and attacks may cease altogether after age 40 or 50 years. The disease does not shorten overall survival, and death due to respiratory involvement is rare. A progressive and persistent proximal myopathy may develop with time and cause functional impairment and disability. Finally, it should be mentioned that susceptibility to malignant hyperthermia has been linked to the CACNA1S gene (although it is usually caused by a mutation in the RYR1 gene encoding a ryanodine receptor), and cases of malignant hyperthermia have been described in patients with hypoKPP. However, to date, no conclusive evidence of a clear genetic link has been found.

HYPERKALEMIC PERIODIC PARALYSIS

EPIDEMIOLOGY AND PATHOBIOLOGY

Hyperkalemic periodic paralysis (hyperKPP) was first described by Frank Tyler at the University of Utah in 1951, when he recognized a form of periodic paralysis not accompanied by a decrease in serum potassium. The disease is caused by an autosomal dominant genetic mutation with complete penetrance, affecting the SCN4A sodium channel gene. It is thought to cause defective inactivation of the sodium channel, thereby resulting in a complete loss of membrane excitability and weakness. Mutations involving the SCN4A gene cause three clinical variations of hyperKPP—episodic weakness without myotonia, episodic weakness with myotonia, and episodic weakness associated with paramyotonia congenita triggered by cold (to be discussed in a subsequent section of this chapter). Overall prevalence is estimated to be about 1.3 per 1,000,000 people with onset before the age of 10 years. The pathophysiology of hyperKPP was first studied by Rudel et al. in the 1980s and led to the suspicion that a defective sodium channel protein might be responsible. First, using microelectrode studies of intercostal muscle, they confirmed that muscle isolated from patients with hyperKPP was partially depolarized at rest. The abnormal depolarization was blocked by tetrodotoxin, which specifically affects the α subunit of the sodium channel. Patch clamp experiments showed faulty inactivation, leading to the conclusion that excessive sodium influx causes repetitive firing of action potentials (myotonia) and eventual inactivation of the membrane (weakness). Cloning and analysis of the gene encoding the voltage-gated sodium channel identified more than 20 missense mutations in the SCN4A gene. Some mutations exhibit both interfamilial and intrafamilial phenotypic variability. Muscle biopsy may reveal intracytoplasmic vacuoles.

CLINICAL MANIFESTATIONS AND DIAGNOSIS

As opposed to hypoKPP, attacks in hyperKPP tend to occur more frequently in the daytime and are shorter (less than 2 hours on average) and less severe. Involvement of bulbar or respiratory muscles is rare. The frequency of attacks varies but they tend to occur more often than those in hypoKPP. Attacks may be precipitated by potassium-rich food, rest after exercise, fasting, and cold temperature. Strength is normal in between attacks, and during attacks, patients are areflexic. Fixed proximal weakness may develop over time. Minimal clinical myotonia may be observed, with myotonic lid lag or lingual myotonia.

Serum potassium levels may be normal or elevated during an attack, at times in excess of 5.0 mEq/L. Serum CK can also be normal or mildly elevated. Needle EMG may show fibrillations or myotonic discharges in up to 50% to 75% of patients (indicative of hyperexcitability and muscle irritation), and later in the clinical course, motor units may become myopathic in appearance. Both short and long exercise testing reveal a rise in CMAP amplitude that decreases over time (Fournier pattern IV). Confirmatory genetic testing for the responsible mutation is often done. As with hypoKPP, noninherited causes of hyperkalemia must be excluded, such as uremia, Addison disease, and excessive potassium supplementation.

TREATMENT AND OUTCOME

Attacks may be terminated by administration of calcium gluconate, glucose, and insulin to stabilize cardiac membranes and reduce serum potassium levels. Acetazolamide in doses of 250 mg to 1 g orally may reduce the number of attacks or completely abolish them. Potassium-wasting diuretics such as thiazides can promote urinary excretion of potassium and also be effective clinically. Rarely, β-adrenergic agents can be used as well, although come with a risk of cardiac arrhythmias. In those patients with myotonia, mexiletine may give symptomatic relief but comes with a small risk of cardiovascular effects (including arrhythmias) and an electrocardiogram (ECG) is needed prior to its initiation. Patients are encouraged to avoid fasting, potassium-rich foods, and exposure to cold temperatures. As in hypoKPP, life expectancy is not affected but patients' morbidity may be related to episodic and progressive proximal weakness and myalgia with muscle stiffness may result from myotonia.

ANDERSEN–TAWIL SYNDROME

EPIDEMIOLOGY AND PATHOBIOLOGY

Also known as *Klein–Lisak–Andersen syndrome*, this rare disease is inherited in an autosomal dominant fashion (with some sporadic cases) and is most frequently due to mutations in the KCNJ2 gene encoding an inward-rectifying potassium channel, and several mutations in this gene exist. It accounts for less than 10% of all people with periodic paralysis. The syndrome is characterized by the clinical triad of periodic paralysis, ventricular arrhythmias with a prolonged QT interval, and dysmorphic features, which are usually skeletal abnormalities. Not all patients show the complete triad. The disease typically starts with episodes of periodic paralysis in the first or second decade, and serum levels of potassium vary.

CLINICAL MANIFESTATIONS AND DIAGNOSIS

Attacks are highly variable in frequency, duration, and severity. There is usually no associated myotonia or weakness in between episodes, but some patients demonstrate mild neck flexor or facial weakness. Developmental abnormalities include hypertelorism, clinodactyly, low-set ears, scoliosis, and syndactyly, and patients are usually short statured and may have a cleft or high-arched palate. Some patients may have cognitive abnormalities. The associated cardiac manifestations of Andersen–Tawil syndrome (ATS) are inherent and unique to the diagnosis. Over 50% of patients have a prolonged QT syndrome, and an even larger proportion develops arrhythmias such as bidirectional or polymorphic ventricular tachycardia. Ventricular tachyarrhythmias are less frequent and often asymptomatic, although cardiac arrest may occur in up to 10% of patients. Patients must be questioned about any unexplained syncopal events, which may be indicative of an underlying arrhythmia. An ECG is a crucial component of the diagnostic workup because some patients may benefit from pacing or antiarrhythmic agents. Electrophysiologic testing is often useful, as long as exercise testing shows an immediate increase in CMAP amplitude with a subsequent decline. Genetic testing for the *KCNJ2* gene mutation is confirmatory. As with hyper- and hypoKPP, secondary causes of periodic paralysis must be excluded (including thyroid disease, renal failure, and others).

TREATMENT AND OUTCOME

Management of ATS is aimed at treatment of both the episodic paralysis and the cardiac manifestations, and a multidisciplinary approach is therefore crucial. Carbonic anhydrase inhibitors may decrease the frequency of clinical attacks, as in other forms of periodic paralysis. Cardiac evaluation includes yearly ECG and Holter monitoring, as some patients benefit from a pacemaker or defibrillator. More often, however, pharmacologic agents such as β-blockers and other antiarrhythmics are used to control arrhythmias. Patients must be counseled to avoid medications that may further prolong the QT interval.

NONDYSTROPHIC MYOTONIAS

EPIDEMIOLOGY AND PATHOBIOLOGY

Paramyotonia congenita (PC; sometimes known as *Eulenburg disease*) is also caused by a mutation in the SCN4A sodium channel gene and, given the shared genetic locus, often overlaps with hyperKPP and different phenotypes may exist in the same family. It is typically inherited as an autosomal dominant disorder and symptoms begin early in life. Infants may have difficulty opening their eyes while crying (eyelid-opening myotonia). In PC, poor inactivation of the sodium channel prolongs the neuronal action potential and slows the rate of repolarization, thereby causing a mild state of persistent depolarization leading to clinical myotonia. This phenotype differs from hyperKPP, and there is probably a different kind of functional defect in the SCN4A gene in the two syndromes accounting for this variability. Genetic defects causing persistent sodium currents may lead to paralysis via stable and persistent depolarization (hyperKPP), whereas myotonic discharges result from instability of channel activation that is more variable. Histopathologically, muscle biopsy may show myopathic features with intracytoplasmic vacuolization and tubular aggregates.

Also known as *Thomsen disease*, myotonia congenita (MC) is also autosomal dominant and is caused by mutations in the CLCN1 chloride channel gene. Men are affected more than women. In the autosomal dominant form, changes in chloride channel function lead to a loss of chloride conductance, thereby leading to delayed repolarization and increased neuronal excitability due to

potassium accumulation in T-tubules and resultant membrane depolarization. An autosomal recessive form also exists, also known as *Becker disease*, and involves a mutation in the SCN4A sodium channel gene.

CLINICAL MANIFESTATIONS AND DIAGNOSIS

The first clinical signs of PC are typically seen in the first decade of life. Patients demonstrate "paradoxical" myotonia, which is defined as myotonia or stiffness that worsens with repeated exercise (as opposed to the "warm-up phenomenon" seen in other myotonic syndromes, in which myotonia decreases with exercise.) Cold ambient temperatures worsen clinical myotonia and stiffness, and short and long exercise testing in a cooled limb shows a drop in amplitude with a slow recovery (Fournier pattern I). With more trials, a further drop in amplitude can be seen, which is an electrophysiologic equivalent of the paradoxical myotonia seen clinically. Many patients demonstrate postexercise myotonic potentials (PEMPs), which are after discharges of decreasing amplitude seen after exercise. Needle EMG may show signs of muscle irritability in the form of fibrillations and myotonic discharges, which disappear completely with colder temperatures as the muscle weakens. Given the occasional overlap with periodic paralysis, in some patients, cold temperature or potassium intake can induce a paretic attack. Fixed progressive muscle weakness may develop with time.

Symptoms of Thomsen disease begin in the first decade of life with clinical signs of myotonia—for instance, infants may have trouble opening their eyes after crying and may fall when learning to walk. In MC, myotonia demonstrates the classic warm-up phenomenon, whereby the myotonia improves with exercise and repeated muscle contraction. Both percussion and grip myotonia may be observed. Patients are described as being "herculean" with excessive muscle mass attributed to the nearly constant state of muscle contraction, although they usually do not complain of pain. Episodes of weakness are rare in the autosomal dominant form, but in Becker disease, they may occur at the onset of physical activity, lasting seconds to minutes. Moreover, in these patients, symptoms commence later in life and they may also develop proximal weakness. Serum CK is typically normal, as is serum potassium. Short exercise testing shows a transient drop in amplitude (more pronounced with cooling in autosomal dominant form) with a smaller drop with repeated trials (corresponding to the warm-up phenomenon seen clinically), consistent with a Fournier II pattern. Long exercise testing shows little if any change and PEMPs may be seen. Genetic testing confirms the diagnosis.

TREATMENT AND OUTCOME

Muscle stiffness related to myotonia is often the primary complaint of patients with PC and MC, and strategies aimed at mitigating this pain vary. Mexiletine, a class IB antiarrhythmic medication, has been used for many years for symptomatic relief in both dystrophic and nondystrophic myotonic syndromes. One placebo-controlled trial done by Statland et al. in 2012 demonstrated significant improvement in stiffness after mexiletine treatment for 4 weeks in patients with nondystrophic myotonia. Mexiletine is thought to work via enhancement of fast inactivation of sodium channels, although its efficacy is not restricted to only those patients with myotonia related to SCN4A (sodium channel) mutations. The medication is generally well tolerated and is typically started at a dose of 150 mg daily, then slowly increased to a dose of 300 mg three times per day. Cardiac testing including an ECG is often done prior to initiating the drug trial, particularly in patients with cardiac symptoms or known cardiovascular disease. Some patients may find relief from other medications with different mechanisms of action such as carbamazepine, phenytoin, or diuretics such as acetazolamide or hydrochlorothiazide.

SUGGESTED READINGS

Bendahhou S, Donaldson MR, Plaster NM, et al. Defective potassium channel Kir2.1 trafficking underlies Andersen-Tawil syndrome. *J Biol Chem.* 2003;278(51):51779–51785. doi:10.1074/jbc.M310278200.

Bendheim PE, Reale EO, Berg BO. Beta-adrenergic treatment of hyperkalemic periodic paralysis. *Neurology.* 1985;35(5):746–749.

Benstead TJ, Camfield PR, King DB. Treatment of paramyotonia congenita with acetazolamide. *Can J Neurol Sci.* 1987;14(2):156–158.

Borg K, Hovmoller M, Larsson L, et al. Paramyotonia congenita (Eulenburg): clinical, neurophysiological and muscle biopsy observations in a Swedish family. *Acta Neurol Scand.* 1993;87(1):37–42.

Cannon SC. An expanding view for the molecular basis of familial periodic paralysis. *Neuromuscul Disord.* 2002;12(6):533–543.

Cannon SC. Pathomechanisms in channelopathies of skeletal muscle and brain. *Annu Rev Neurosci.* 2006;29:387–415. doi:10.1146/annurev.neuro.29.051605.112815.

Cavel-Greant D, Lehmann-Horn F, Jurkat-Rott K. The impact of permanent muscle weakness on quality of life in periodic paralysis: a survey of 66 patients. *Acta Myol.* 2012;31(2):126–133.

Comi G, Testa D, Cornelio F, et al. Potassium depletion myopathy: a clinical and morphological study of six cases. *Muscle Nerve.* 1985;8(1):17–21. doi:10.1002/mus.880080104.

Dias Da Silva MR, Cerutti JM, Arnaldi LA, et al. A mutation in the KCNE3 potassium channel gene is associated with susceptibility to thyrotoxic hypokalemic periodic paralysis. *J Clin Endocrinol Metab.* 2002;87(11):4881–4884. doi:10.1210/jc.2002-020698.

Donaldson MR, Yoon G, Fu YH, et al. Andersen-Tawil syndrome: a model of clinical variability, pleiotropy, and genetic heterogeneity. *Ann Med.* 2004;36(suppl 1):92–97.

Evers S, Engelien A, Karsch V, et al. Secondary hyperkalaemic paralysis. *J Neurol Neurosurg Psychiatry.* 1998;64(2):249–252.

Fournier E, Arzel M, Sternberg D, et al. Electromyography guides toward subgroups of mutations in muscle channelopathies. *Ann Neurol.* 2004;56(5):650–661. doi:10.1002/ana.20241.

Griggs RC, Engel WK, Resnick JS. Acetazolamide treatment of hypokalemic periodic paralysis. Prevention of attacks and improvement of persistent weakness. *Ann Intern Med.* 1970;73(1):39–48.

Heatwole CR, Statland JM, Logigian EL. The diagnosis and treatment of myotonic disorders. *Muscle Nerve.* 2013;47(5):632–648. doi:10.1002/mus.23683.

Horga A, Raja Rayan DL, Matthews E, et al. Prevalence study of genetically defined skeletal muscle channelopathies in England. *Neurology.* 2013;80(16):1472–1475. doi:10.1212/WNL.0b013e31828cf8d0.

Jurkat-Rott K, Lehmann-Horn F. Periodic paralysis mutation MiRP2-R83H in controls: interpretations and general recommendation. *Neurology.* 2004;62(6):1012–1015.

Jurkat-Rott K, Lerche H, Lehmann-Horn F. Skeletal muscle channelopathies. *J Neurol.* 2002;249(11):1493–1502. doi:10.1007/s00415-002-0871-5.

Kostera-Pruszczyk A, Potulska-Chromik A, Pruszczyk P, et al. Andersen-Tawil syndrome: report of three novel mutations and high risk of symptomatic cardiac involvement. *Muscle Nerve.* 2015;51(2):192–196. doi:10.1002/mus.24293.

Layzer RB, Lovelace RE, Rowland LP. Hyperkalemic periodic paralysis. *Arch Neurol.* 1967;16(5):455–472.

Lehmann-Horn F, Rudel R, Ricker K, et al. Two cases of adynamia episodica hereditaria: in vitro investigation of muscle cell membrane and contraction parameters. *Muscle Nerve.* 1983;6(2):113–121. doi:10.1002/mus.880060206.

Levitt JO. Practical aspects in the management of hypokalemic periodic paralysis. *J Transl Med.* 2008;6:18. doi:10.1186/1479-5876-6-18.

Lisak RP, Lebeau J, Tucker SH, et al. Hyperkalemic periodic paralysis and cardiac arrhythmia. *Neurology.* 1972;22(8):810–815.

Marchant CL, Ellis FR, Halsall PJ, et al. Mutation analysis of two patients with hypokalemic periodic paralysis and suspected malignant hyperthermia. *Muscle Nerve.* 2004;30(1):114–117. doi:10.1002/mus.20068.

Matthews E, Portaro S, Ke Q, et al. Acetazolamide efficacy in hypokalemic periodic paralysis and the predictive role of genotype. *Neurology.* 2011;77(22):1960–1964. doi:10.1212/WNL.0b013e31823a0cb6.

Minaker KL, Meneilly GS, Flier JS, et al. Insulin-mediated hypokalemia and paralysis in familial hypokalemic periodic paralysis. *Am J Med.* 1988;84(6):1001–1006.

Moxley RT III, Ricker K, Kingston WJ, et al. Potassium uptake in muscle during paramyotonic weakness. *Neurology.* 1989;39(7):952–955.

Ponce SP, Jennings AE, Madias NE, et al. Drug-induced hyperkalemia. *Medicine (Baltimore).* 1985;64(6):357–370.

Ptacek LJ, Trimmer JS, Agnew WS, et al. Paramyotonia congenita and hyperkalemic periodic paralysis map to the same sodium-channel gene locus. *Am J Hum Genet.* 1991;49(4):851–854.

Rajabally YA, El Lahawi M. Hypokalemic periodic paralysis associated with malignant hyperthermia. *Muscle Nerve.* 2002;25(3):453–455.

Rudel R, Ricker K, Lehmann-Horn F. Genotype-phenotype correlations in human skeletal muscle sodium channel diseases. *Arch Neurol.* 1993;50(11):1241–1248.

Sansone V, Griggs RC, Meola G, et al. Andersen's syndrome: a distinct periodic paralysis. *Ann Neurol.* 1997;42(3):305–312. doi:10.1002/ana.410420306.

Sansone V, Tawil R. Management and treatment of Andersen-Tawil syndrome (ATS). *Neurotherapeutics.* 2007;4(2):233–237. doi:10.1016/j.nurt.2007.01.005.

Statland JM, Barohn RJ. Muscle channelopathies: the nondystrophic myotonias and periodic paralyses. *Continuum (Minneap Minn).* 2013;19(6)(Muscle Disease):1598–1614. doi:10.1212/01.CON.0000440661.49298.c8.

Statland JM, Bundy BN, Wang Y, et al; Consortium for Clinical Investigation of Neurologic Channelopathies. Mexiletine for symptoms and signs of myotonia in nondystrophic myotonia: a randomized controlled trial. *JAMA.* 2012;308(13):1357–1365. doi:10.1001/jama.2012.12607.

Striessnig J, Hoda JC, Koschak A, et al. L-type Ca2+ channels in Ca2+ channelopathies. *Biochem Biophys Res Commun.* 2004;322(4):1341–1346. doi:10.1016/j.bbrc.2004.08.039.

Tawil R, McDermott MP, Brown R Jr, et al. Randomized trials of dichlorphenamide in the periodic paralyses. Working Group on Periodic Paralysis. *Ann Neurol.* 2000;47(1):46–53.

Tricarico D, Barbieri M, Camerino DC. Acetazolamide opens the muscular KCa2+ channel: a novel mechanism of action that may explain the therapeutic effect of the drug in hypokalemic periodic paralysis. *Ann Neurol.* 2000;48(3):304–312.

Tricarico D, Servidei S, Tonali P, et al. Impairment of skeletal muscle adenosine triphosphate-sensitive K+ channels in patients with hypokalemic periodic paralysis. *J Clin Invest.* 1999;103(5):675–682. doi:10.1172/JCI4552.

Tristani-Firouzi M, Jensen JL, Donaldson MR, et al. Functional and clinical characterization of KCNJ2 mutations associated with LQT7 (Andersen syndrome). *J Clin Invest.* 2002;110(3):381–388. doi:10.1172/JCI15183.

Venance SL, Cannon SC, Fialho D, et al; CINCH Investigators. The primary periodic paralyses: diagnosis, pathogenesis and treatment. *Brain.* 2006;129 (pt 1):8–17. doi:10.1093/brain/awh639.

Venance SL, Jurkat-Rott K, Lehmann-Horn F, et al. SCN4A-associated hypokalemic periodic paralysis merits a trial of acetazolamide. *Neurology.* 2004;63(10):1977.

Vicart S, Sternberg D, Fournier E, et al. New mutations of SCN4A cause a potassium-sensitive normokalemic periodic paralysis. *Neurology.* 2004;63(11):2120–2127.

Vijayakumar A, Ashwath G, Thimmappa D. Thyrotoxic periodic paralysis: clinical challenges. *J Thyroid Res.* 2014;2014:649502. doi:10.1155/2014/649502.

Vroom FW, Jarrell MA, Maren TH. Acetazolamide treatment of hypokalemic periodic paralysis. Probable mechanism of action. *Arch Neurol.* 1975;32(6):385–392.

Webb J, Cannon SC. Cold-induced defects of sodium channel gating in atypical periodic paralysis plus myotonia. *Neurology.* 2008;70(10):755–761. doi:10.1212/01.wnl.0000265397.70057.d8.

Wu F, Mi W, Cannon SC. Beneficial effects of bumetanide in a CaV1.1-R528H mouse model of hypokalaemic periodic paralysis. *Brain.* 2013;136(12):3766–3774. doi:10.1093/brain/awt280.

Wu F, Mi W, Cannon SC. Bumetanide prevents transient decreases in muscle force in murine hypokalemic periodic paralysis. *Neurology.* 2013;80(12):1110–1116. doi:10.1212/WNL.0b013e3182886a0e.

Wu F, Mi W, Hernandez-Ochoa EO, et al. A calcium channel mutant mouse model of hypokalemic periodic paralysis. *J Clin Invest.* 2012;122(12):4580–4591. doi:10.1172/JCI66091.

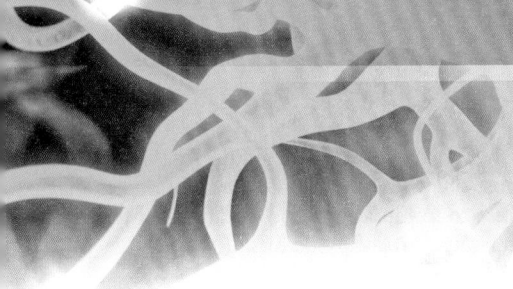

Stiff Person Syndrome and Peripheral Nerve and Muscle Hyperexcitability 94

Jonathan Perk, Christina M. Ulane, and Lewis P. Rowland

INTRODUCTION

The terms *muscle stiffness* and *cramps* are used for commonly experienced symptoms that are often transient and benign. Rarely, they may be harbingers of more serious pathology. Persistent limb muscle stiffness arises from involuntary continuous muscle contraction, whereas cramps and spasms are brief contractions. Lesions throughout the motor system have been implicated in generating muscle stiffness or spasm. Excessive muscular activation may result from dysfunction of inhibitory systems in central nervous system (CNS) pathology or inappropriate activation or hyperexcitability in peripheral nervous system (PNS) pathology. Table 94.1 outlines features of various causes of muscle cramps and stiffness.

STIFF PERSON SYNDROME

In 1956, Moersch and Woltman, senior neurologists at the Mayo Clinic, described patients with a rare clinical syndrome of progressive fluctuating muscular rigidity and painful spasms. This condition is currently known by the gender neutral name *stiff person syndrome* (SPS). A focal variant of the disorder has been called the *stiff limb syndrome*.

EPIDEMIOLOGY

SPS occurs more often in women, but both men and women can be affected (average age of symptom onset is 35 years) and develop progressive symptoms over several months or years. SPS is quite rare and exact epidemiologic data is lacking; the estimated prevalence is one in a million. It is most often an immunologically mediated disorder with the presence of anti–glutamic acid decarboxylase-65 (anti-GAD65) antibodies; it may coexist with other autoimmune disorders including type 1 diabetes mellitus (in at least 35% of patients with SPS), Hashimoto thyroiditis, Graves disease, pernicious anemia, vitiligo, and celiac disease. A paraneoplastic form of SPS accounts for about 5% of cases, most often associated with breast cancer but also reported with thyroid, renal, or colon

TABLE 94.1 Disorders Causing Muscle Stiffness and Hyperexcitability

Localization of Abnormality	Disorder	Principal Manifestations	Treatment
Brain, brain stem, and spinal cord	Stiff person syndrome (SPS)	Rigidity and reflex spasms Anti-GAD65 antibodies	Diazepam, IVIG, treatment of underlying cancer if paraneoplastic
	Progressive encephalomyelitis with rigidity and myoclonus (PERM)	Rigidity and reflex spasms, focal neurologic deficits Anti-GlyRα1 antibodies	Similar to SPS
	Tetanus	Rigidity and reflex spasms	Diazepam, supportive care
Peripheral nerve	Acquired neuromyotonia (Isaac syndrome)	Stiffness, myokymia, delayed relaxation Anti-VGKC antibodies	Immunotherapy, phenytoin, carbamazepine, mexiletine, treatment of underlying cancer if paraneoplastic
	Schwartz–Jampel syndrome	Stiffness and myotonia	Phenytoin, carbamazepine
	Tetany	Carpopedal spasm	Correction of calcium, magnesium, or acid–base derangement
Muscle	Myotonic disorders	Delayed relaxation, percussion myotonia	Mexiletine, phenytoin, carbamazepine (see Chapter 142)
	Metabolic myopathies	Cramps during intense or ischemic exercise	See Chapter 95 and Section 19.
	Neuroleptic malignant syndrome	Rigidity during dopamine block	Supportive care, bromocriptine, dantrolene
	Malignant hyperthermia	Rigidity during anesthesia	Supportive care, dantrolene
Unknown	Ordinary muscle cramps	Cramps during sleep or ordinary activity	Stretching affected muscle to relieve cramp, medications may be used if severe (see text)

IVIG, intravenous immunoglobulin; VGKC, voltage-gated potassium channel.

cancer. The disorder is extremely rare in children (eight cases identified older than 29 years at Mayo Clinic and 12 other case reports).

PATHOBIOLOGY

CNS γ-aminobutyric acid (GABA)–secreting neurons play a major role in the normal inhibition of excessive continuous motor activation. GABA synthesis from glutamic acid is catalyzed by the enzyme glutamic acid decarboxylase (GAD). The discovery of antibodies against the 65-kilodalton GAD protein in most patients suggests immunologically mediated dysfunction of inhibitory synapses. Figure 94.1 illustrates the inhibitory synapse and subcellular localization of antigenic targets of antibodies found in SPS. Reported association of SPS with autoimmune diseases as pernicious anemia, thyroid disease, type 1 diabetes mellitus, and others provides further support for the role of autoimmunity. The presence of anti-GAD65 antibodies with other neurologic disorders, including cerebellar ataxia (with or without coexisting SPS), epilepsy, or progressive encephalitis with rigidity and myoclonus (PERM) suggests a spectrum of pathology associated with neuronal disinhibition in which SPS is one subtype. Although there is often an association of anti-GAD65 antibodies and SPS, the direct pathogenic role of anti-GAD65 antibodies remains uncertain. One major puzzle is that the antigenic GAD65 enzyme is intracellular and therefore supposedly hidden from the offensive antibodies. Furthermore, unlike myasthenia gravis, another antibody-mediated autoimmune disease where antibodies are directed against surface nicotinic acetylcholine receptors, passive transmission of antibodies (e.g., in maternal placental transfer) does not confer the SPS.

It may be that other associated antibodies are the pathologic culprits as, for example, the anti-GABA receptor–associated protein (GABARAP) autoantibody. Dalmau and colleagues found that antibodies directed against the glycine receptor subunit alpha 1 (GlyRα1) IgG antibodies are present in 12% of SPS patients and are found in other hyperexcitable disorders affecting brain stem and spinal cord, most often PERM. Anti-GlyRα1 antibodies may predict good response to immunotherapy. Mutations in the gene encoding the GlyRα1 cause *hyperekplexia* or *startle disease*.

Over the years, a paraneoplastic subgroup form of SPS patients was identified. Many of those patients were positive for autoantibodies directed against other molecules in the inhibitory synapse such as amphiphysin (breast and small cell lung cancer) and gephyrin (mediastinal cancer).

CLINICAL MANIFESTATIONS

Progressive stiffness and intermittent spasms of the axial musculature characterize the classic form of SPS, but distal limb muscles may also be affected. Aching discomfort and stiffness tend to predominate in the axial and proximal limb muscles, causing a hyperlordotic posture, with awkward gait and slowness of movements. Unlike tetanus, trismus does not occur, but facial and oropharyngeal muscles may be affected. In some cases, respiratory muscles are involved. The stiffness diminishes during sleep and under general anesthesia, differentiating it from other motor unit hyperexcitable syndromes such as neuromyotonia. The spasms may lead to joint deformities and are powerful enough to rupture muscles, rip surgical sutures, and fracture bones. Painful reflex spasms and falls occur in response to movement, sensory stimulation, or emotional changes. Fear of attacks elicited by environmental stimulation may lead to a debilitating avoidance of public places. Anxiety and task-specific phobias can be dominant features in SPS and may contribute to the often observed delay in diagnosis or misdiagnosis.

Physical examination shows markedly increased axial and proximal muscle tone. However, strength, coordination, and sensation are preserved. Passive muscle stretch provokes an exaggerated reflex contraction that lasts several seconds. Table 94.2 highlights the dominant features of classic SPS. The startle reactions of SPS are similar to those in hyperekplexia.

DIAGNOSIS

Laboratory Data

The diagnosis of SPS is aided by the presence of serum (or cerebrospinal fluid [CSF]) antibodies against GAD65 in high titers (2,000 U/mL or more) which are found in approximately 80% of cases. Anti-GAD65 antibodies are supportive of the diagnosis of SPS but not specific; they are found in other neurologic disorders (including

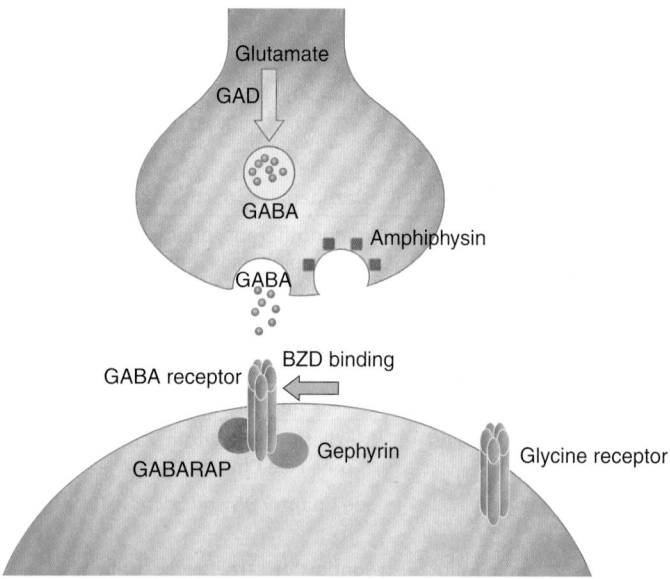

FIGURE 94.1 The neuronal inhibitory synapse. GABA and glycine are primary inhibitory neurotransmitters. Dysfunction of components of the synapse (presynaptic, synaptic, and postsynaptic) can lead to loss of inhibition and clinical stiffness and spasms. GAD, glutamic acid decarboxylase; GABARAP, GABA receptor–associated protein; BZD, benzodiazepine.

TABLE 94.2	**Defining Characteristics of the Stiff Person Syndrome**

- Prodromal stiffness of axial muscles
- Slow progress to proximal limbs, walking awkward
- Fixed deformity of the spine, lordosis, "permanent shrug" (neck drawn down to shoulder girdle)
- Spasms precipitated by startle, jarring, noise, emotional upset
- Otherwise normal findings on motor and sensory examination
- Anxiety and task-specific phobias
- Normal intellect and affect
- Continuous motor activity in affected muscles relieved by intravenous or oral diazepam

Modified from Lorish TR, Thorsteinsson G, Howard FM Jr. Stiff-man syndrome updated. *Mayo Clin Proc.* 1989;64(6):629–636.

cerebellar ataxia, PERM, and Batten disease), and low titers are associated with other autoimmune diseases (up to 22% of persons with type 1 diabetes mellitus). Other autoantibodies present in SPS include anti-GABARAP in 65% of SPS cases, anti-GlyRα1 antibodies in up to 10% of cases, antiamphiphysin in up to 5% of paraneoplastic cases, and antigephyrin (found in one case of paraneoplastic SPS).

Electrophysiology

Electromyography (EMG) reveals continuous firing of normal motor unit action potentials (MUAPs) even at rest. This excessive firing may be inhibited by administration of intravenous diazepam. Another hallmark of the SPS is cocontraction of agonist and antagonist muscles. Normally, contraction of an agonist muscle is associated with inhibition of the activity of the antagonist, but this is not so in SPS (Fig. 94.2).

Imaging

Magnetic resonance (MR) imaging of the brain and spinal cord is normal in SPS and are most useful in ruling out other pathologies. Brain MR spectroscopy, however, shows a marked reduction of the inhibitory GABA neurotransmitter.

TREATMENT AND OUTCOMES

Until the discovery of anti-GAD and other autoantibodies, GABA-enhancing medications were used both for diagnosis and symptomatic treatment. The realization that autoimmunity likely plays a role opened new diagnostic and treatment possibilities. Dalakas showed clear benefit for patients with SPS treated with intravenous immunoglobulin (IVIG) in a randomized, double-blind, placebo-controlled study involving 16 patients with SPS [**Level 1**].[1] Although most patients experience benefit after initial dose of IVIG, many require repeat treatment to sustain response. Steroids, plasmapheresis, and rituximab (antibodies directed against B cells) were all tried with varying success.

Benzodiazepines are the mainstay for rigidity and spasms, and patients often require titration up to high doses; on average 40 mg/day, but some require several hundred milligrams per day. Baclofen may be used as an adjunct and doses of 60 to 100 mg/day may be required. Other medications that may be helpful are gabapentin (300 to 1,200 mg three times daily), pregabalin (50 to 100 mg three times daily), levetiracetam (500 to 1,500 mg twice daily), and in refractory cases, dantrolene sodium (starting at 25 mg daily and titrating up to a maximum of 100 mg four times daily). Dantrolene should be used with caution and monitoring for cardiac side effects and hepatotoxicity. Some may respond to intrathecal baclofen.

OTHER CENTRAL NERVOUS SYSTEM DISORDERS OF MUSCLE STIFFNESS

Common CNS disorders can show increased muscle tone. Stroke, multiple sclerosis, amyotrophic lateral sclerosis, and primary lateral sclerosis are examples where loss of normal inhibition of the motor system occurs. These relatively more common entities are discussed elsewhere in this book.

Although tetanus and tetany share a similar name and also some clinical features, they are entirely distinct. Tetanus is discussed in Chapter 63 and is only briefly mentioned here because of the pathogenic similarities to SPS at the inhibitory synapse. Tetanus is caused by the toxin tetanospasmin released from the bacteria *Clostridium tetani* in contaminated wounds. This toxin reaches nerve terminals and travels by retrograde axonal transport to reach inhibitory interneurons in the spinal cord and brain stem. Tetanospasmin prevents the release of GABA and glycine into the synapse, effectively blocking inhibitory neurotransmission in a similar mechanism to SPS. However, unlike SPS, tetanus has a predilection for the brain stem, possibly due to the shorter length of cranial nerve axons, eliciting distinct features such as trismus and forceful satanic-like smile ("risus sardonicus"). Opisthotonic spasm of axial muscles may cause fractures and respiratory failure. Treatment includes respiratory support, antibiotics, antitoxin treatment, and muscle relaxants. Tetanus is best prevented by immunization, which is unfortunately unavailable in many developing countries. Risus sardonicus is also seen in strychnine intoxication with a similar mechanism of action; however, the clinical setting and toxin exposure set the two syndromes apart.

Tropical spastic paraparesis is caused by the human T-lymphotrophic virus (HTLV-1) retrovirus and is prevalent in the adult population of the Caribbean islands. This infectious myelopathy primarily affects the thoracic spinal cord and is manifest by progressive spasticity and weakness, bladder dysfunction, and minor sensory symptoms. There are no current effective disease-modifying agents, which alter the long-term debilitating course. Corticosteroids, interferon-α and interferon-β, as well as other agents have been tried with limited success. Treatment is largely symptomatic and directed to relieve spasticity, painful muscle spasms, and loss of bladder control.

There are hereditary forms of spastic paraparesis, most notably the hereditary spastic paraplegias (HSPs). These are clinically and genetically heterogeneous. Clinical syndromes may be "pure" if only manifesting as spasticity and weakness in the legs with bladder dysfunction, or "complicated" if additional neurologic and systemic symptoms are present. These can be autosomal dominant, autosomal recessive, or X-linked and may be diagnosed genetically.

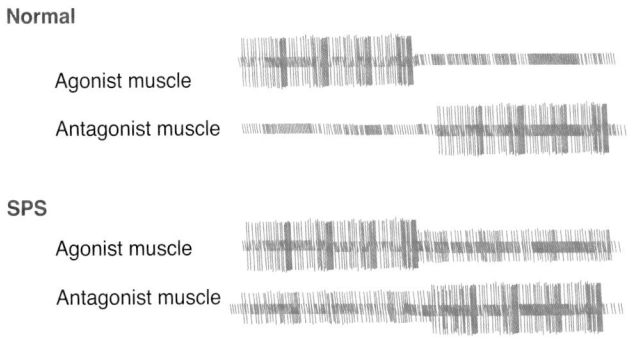

FIGURE 94.2 Schematic depiction of simultaneous agonist/antagonist electromyography recordings in stiff person syndrome. The normal response tracings (*top*) show runs of agonist muscle MUAPs associated with inhibition of MUAPs in the antagonist and vice versa. In contrast, paired tracings recorded in a stiff person patient (*bottom pair*) show uninhibited simultaneous activation of both agonist and antagonist muscles. MUAP, motor unit action potential.

PERIPHERAL NERVE AND MUSCLE HYPEREXCITABILITY

ACQUIRED NEUROMYOTONIA (ISAAC SYNDROME)

Isaac first described this disorder as a state of "continuous muscle fiber activity." The invariable clinical manifestation is myokymia, visibly apparent constant muscle twitching likened to a bag of writhing worms. As a result of the continuous activity, patients may develop muscle cramps or abnormal postures of the limbs, which may be persistent or intermittent and are identical to carpal or pedal spasm.

Epidemiology

Neuromyotonia is a rare disorder; no specific information regarding incidence or prevalence is available. The acquired autoimmune forms can be seen in association with multiple other autoimmune diseases, either neurologic (such as myasthenia gravis) or systemic. Neuromyotonia is at times a paraneoplastic syndrome associated mainly with thymoma or small cell lung cancer but also with breast carcinoma or lymphoma.

Pathobiology

In the autoimmune form, neuromyotonia was first attributed to the presence of antibodies directed against voltage-gated potassium channels (VGKC). Anti-VGKC complex antibodies were also found in some patients with limbic encephalitis and additionally in patients with the syndrome of benign fasciculations with cramps. This wide phenotypic spectrum associated with anti-VGKC was puzzling. However, advances in specific antibody identification have improved our understanding of the hyperexcitability syndromes and aided in clinical classification. More recent studies show that, rather than binding the potassium channel itself, the "anti-VGKC antibodies" bind antigenic neuronal targets of the macromolecular complex associated with the channel. The two main antigens are the leucine-rich glioma-inactivated protein 1 (LGI1) and contactin-associated protein-like 2 (CASPR2). Anti-LGI1 antibodies target CNS structures and are more commonly associated with limbic encephalitis. Anti-CASPR2 antibodies on the other hand, target both central and peripheral nervous tissue. They may be associated with neuromyotonia as well as the cramp-fasciculation syndrome, which may be a mild variant of Isaac syndrome. It is reasonable therefore to consider this spectrum of phenotypes under the umbrella of *autoimmune peripheral nerve hyperexcitability disorders*.

Clinical Manifestations

Isaac syndrome affects children, adolescents, or young adults and begins insidiously, progressing slowly for months or a few years. Symptoms most often begin in the distal arms and legs. Slow movement, clawing of the fingers, and toe walking are later joined by stiffness of proximal and axial muscles; occasionally, oropharyngeal or respiratory muscles are affected. The motor symptoms are often accompanied by the profuse sweating syndrome of hyperhidrosis. The stiffness and myokymia are seen at rest but, unlike SPS, continue in sleep and under general anesthesia. Voluntary contraction may induce a spasm that persists during attempted relaxation.

If patients develop higher cortical dysfunction manifest by sleep disorders, personality changes, and delirium, the condition is named the *Morvan syndrome*. The fixed postures of the limbs in Isaac syndrome can be simulated by the rare genetic Schwartz–Jampel syndrome (SJS). However, SJS is characterized by the additional features of a unique facial appearance (blepharophimosis), short stature, and bony abnormalities. In "ocular neuromyotonia," the limbs and cranial muscles are spared and the disorder is confined to one or more extraocular muscles.

Diagnosis

Antibodies reactive against the VGKC are detected in 30% to 40% of patients with Isaac syndrome and in 80% of those with coexisting thymoma but may also be seen at very low titers in asymptomatic people (2%). They may also be found in patients with painful small-fiber neuropathy. The prevalence of distinct antibodies to CASPR2 and LGI1 in this population is unknown. It is reasonable to perform a malignancy screening, as 20% to 25% of patients with Isaac have an underlying malignancy (although the Isaac may precede malignancy by many years).

EMG shows characteristic findings. The EMG recorded from stiff muscles reveals prolonged myokymic or neuromyotonic discharges. In electrical myokymia, grouped fasciculations fire at rates up to 60 Hz and sound like marching soldiers. Myokymia may be found in the EMG of some individuals without any clinically visible twitching. Furthermore, myokymia is not restricted to Isaac syndrome; it may appear in other clinically distinct entities as postradiation neuropathy, multiple sclerosis, or after exposure to the Timber rattlesnake venom. In electrical *neuromyotonia*, on the other hand, continuous discharges occur at rates of 150 to 300 Hz, tend to start or stop abruptly, and sound like a "NASCAR engine" or a "dive bomber." Voluntary effort triggers more intense discharges that persist during relaxation, accounting for the myotonia-like aftercontraction, but electrical myotonia is not found. In SJS, the more frequent EMG pattern is that of myotonic discharges, but there may be continuous motor activity with both myokymic and neuromyotonic discharges.

Treatment

The treatment of the peripheral nerve hyperexcitability disorders is multitiered. The muscle contraction symptoms are usually controlled with anticonvulsants as carbamazepine (200 to 1,200 mg daily in divided doses) or phenytoin (100 to 300 mg daily). Mexiletine may also be used at doses of 100 to 300 mg three times daily but with caution in patients at risk of cardiac arrhythmias (monitor for QTc prolongation) and can rarely cause hepatotoxicity. Plasmapheresis (three to five sessions every other day) and intravenous immunoglobulin therapy (2 g/kg over 4 to 5 days) are effective in some patients, and in the paraneoplastic group, treatment is directed primarily against the underlying cancer.

TETANY

Tetany is a clinical syndrome characterized by convulsions, paresthesias, prolonged spasms of limb muscles, or laryngospasm; it is accompanied by signs of hyperexcitability of peripheral nerves. Tetany occurs in patients with hypocalcemia, hypomagnesemia, or alkalosis. Hyperventilation may unmask latent hypocalcemic tetany, but respiratory alkalosis itself only rarely causes outright tetany.

Intense circumoral and digital paresthesias generally precede the typical carpopedal spasms, which consist of adduction and extension of the fingers, flexion of the metacarpophalangeal joints, and equinovarus postures of the feet. In severe cases, the spasms spread to the proximal and axial muscles, eventually causing opisthotonus. In all forms of tetany, the nerves are hyperexcitable, as manifested by the reactions to ischemia (Trousseau sign) or percussion (Chvostek sign). The spasms are owing to spontaneous firing of peripheral nerves, starting in the proximal portions of the longest nerves. EMG shows individual motor units discharging independently at a rate of 5 to 25 Hz (at times up to 300 Hz); each discharge consists of a group of two or more identical potentials.

The treatment of tetany consists of correcting the underlying metabolic disorder. In hypomagnesemia, tetany does not respond to correction of the accompanying hypocalcemia unless the magnesium deficit is also corrected.

NEUROLEPTIC MALIGNANT SYNDROME AND MALIGNANT HYPERTHERMIA

Acute diffuse symptoms of muscle stiffness maybe associated with exposure to neuroleptic medications that inhibit dopamine. The neuroleptic malignant syndrome (NMS) may be dramatic and life-threatening if not aggressively treated (see also Chapter 128, Neurotoxicology). The syndrome comprises acute alteration of mental status, fever, autonomic dysfunction, and muscle breakdown with high serum levels of creatine kinase (CK). Muscle necrosis may release intracellular potassium and myoglobin into the serum; the resulting hyperkalemia may lead to cardiac arrhythmias and renal failure. An often overlooked cause of sudden dopamine loss with possible similar consequences may occur with abrupt discontinuation of dopaminergic medications used by patients with Parkinson disease. The mainstay treatment of NMS is supportive with body cooling, intravenous fluids, and respiratory support. Dopamine agonists such as bromocriptine (5 to 10 mg three to four times daily) and the potentially hepatotoxic muscle relaxant dantrolene may be helpful (start 25 mg daily, titrate up to 100 mg three to four times daily).

Another syndrome similar to NMS is seen in patients exposed to anesthetic agents causing the malignant hyperthermia syndrome (MHS). The most common offensive agents are the neuromuscular blocking agent succinylcholine and the inhaled general anesthetics like halothane, sevoflurane, and desflurane. High fever is the hallmark of the syndrome, but muscle stiffness, consequences of muscle breakdown ("rhabdomyolysis" or myoglobinuria), and cardiorespiratory collapse are virtually undistinguishable from NMS. Treatment is similar to that of NMS as well. Patients with the rare inherited myopathy central core disease have mutations in the ryanodine receptor RYR1 and are most susceptible to MHS.

MUSCLE CRAMPS

The common *muscle cramp* is a sudden, forceful, painful muscle contraction that lasts from a few seconds to several minutes. Muscle cramps are most often benign but can also accompany various neuromuscular disorders such as peripheral nerve hyperexcitability syndromes, lower motor neuron disease, medications, and myopathies (metabolic, mitochondrial, or dystrophic).

Epidemiology

Most adults have at least one episode of benign leg cramps during a lifetime, with no significant prevalence difference between men and women. In some populations, such as elderly veterans, up to 50% experience nocturnal leg cramps, as do 30% to 50% of pregnant women, worsening as pregnancy progresses. Most cramps occur only at night (73%), some have both day and night-time cramps, and a few have daytime-only cramps. In up to 40% of those who have cramps, the attacks occur several times per week, and 6% experience daily cramps. Cramps are common (32%) in children with CMT1A. Frequent cramps tend to accompany hypothyroidism, uremia, profuse sweating or diarrhea, hemodialysis, electrolyte abnormalities, hypoglycemia, and anterior horn cell diseases. Statins and diuretics may provoke cramps as well.

Pathobiology

A cramp often starts with fasciculations, after which the muscle becomes intermittently hard and knot-like as the involuntary contraction waxes and wanes, passing from one part of the muscle to another. Normally, when an a-motor neuron fires, acetylcholine is released into the neuromuscular junction, which then binds to and elicits an action potential in the muscle fiber. This action potential is then translated into contraction by release of calcium from the sarcoplasmic reticulum and the interaction of actin and myosin to cause muscle shortening (twitch or contraction). The process ends when calcium concentration decreases; both muscle contraction and relaxation require adenosine triphosphate. If calcium levels remain elevated, relaxation cannot occur. Stretch of the muscle spindle 1a fiber excites the motor neuron and also causes muscle contraction (monosynaptic muscle stretch reflex). Inhibition occurs within the spinal cord by inhibitory interneurons.

The neuroanatomic origin and propagation of cramps is a topic of ongoing debate, and both peripheral and central mechanisms are invoked. Cramps may result from hyperexcitability of the motor neurons (induced by afferent input) resulting in an autonomous positive feedback loop, implicating a spinal contribution. Cramps can be induced distal to a peripheral nerve block with electrical stimulation, and such cramps can be terminated by stretching the muscle, favoring a nerve terminal site of origin.

Clinical Manifestations

Muscle cramps are experienced as abrupt, painful spasms lasting seconds to minutes. Cramps may be provoked by a trivial movement or by voluntary contraction of a shortened muscle. They may occur during vigorous exercise but are more likely to occur after exercise ceases. Benign fasciculations or myokymia may be associated with frequent muscle cramps in apparently healthy people. The legs and in particular the calves are most often affected by cramps. Nocturnal cramps typically cause forceful flexion of the ankle and toes. However, cramps can affect almost any voluntary muscle.

Most people have cramps at some time, but a few people have inordinately frequent cramps, often accompanied by fasciculations. This syndrome of *benign fasciculations* is disproportionately more frequent among physicians and other medical workers because they are more likely to know the ominous implications of fasciculations for the diagnosis of motor neuron disease. In fact, however, motor neuron disease almost never starts with fasciculations alone. If neither weakness nor wasting is seen, motor neuron disease is essentially excluded. The syndrome of benign fasciculation has been reported many times with variations on the name.

True cramps must be distinguished from cramp-like muscle pain unaccompanied by spasm. The cramps of McArdle disease (myophosphorylase deficiency) occur during exercise because of the block of glycogen metabolism. Because no electrical activity is evident in the EMG during the painful shortening of muscle affected by McArdle disease, the term *contracture* is used. The origin of the contracture is not known but depletion of adenosine triphosphate in muscle has long been suspected. Muscle breakdown is associated with myoglobinuria and elevated CK values in serum.

Mild dystrophinopathies, with little or no clinical weakness, may be manifested by exertional muscle pain and myoglobinuria. These symptoms have been referred to as *muscle cramps*, but actual muscle spasm has not been described in such cases; the pain may simply be a measure of muscle injury. The dystrophic and nondystrophic myotonic disorders are discussed elsewhere in this textbook.

Myalgia and cramps are believed to be especially common in *myoadenylate deaminase deficiency*, but because this condition is common in asymptomatic people (found in 1% to 3% of all muscle biopsies), the association is difficult to confirm. Moreover, in affected families, the muscle enzyme deficiency and clinical symptoms are not well linked.

Diagnosis

The diagnosis of the common muscle cramp is essentially based on the clinical history. It is important to exclude underlying medical and neurologic causes for cramps. Routine laboratory testing for electrolytes and other underlying medical disorders can be performed as clinically indicated on a case-by-case basis. Tests may include complete blood cell count, metabolic panel, and CK.

Electrodiagnostic testing is useful in diagnosing an underlying peripheral nerve or muscle disorder, as well as characterizing any abnormal spontaneous muscle activity. EMG of a cramp shows brief, periodic bursts of motor unit potentials discharging at a frequency of 200 to 300 Hz, appearing irregularly, and intermingling with similar discharges from adjacent motor units. Several foci within the same muscle may discharge independently. This electrical activity clearly arises within the lower motor neuron.

Treatment

Passive stretching of the affected muscle usually terminates a cramp. However, a 2010 analysis by the American Academy of Neurology (AAN) found insufficient evidence for nonpharmacologic treatment (such as stretching and hydration) of muscle cramps [**Level 1**].[2]

A Cochrane Review in 2010 found that the administration of quinine derivatives at doses of 200 to 500 mg per day were effective, although modestly, with few serious adverse events [**Level 1**].[3] Rare but serious adverse effects of quinine include thrombocytopenia, bleeding diathesis, cardiac arrhythmias, and acute hypersensitivity reactions, which may occur in 2% to 4% of persons treated. Other serious adverse effects include hypoglycemia, vision loss, psychosis, tinnitus, and esophagitis. Given the adverse effect profile, the U.S. Food and Drug Administration (FDA) has issued multiple warnings and both the FDA and AAN recommend against the use of quinine for the routine treatment of muscle cramps. Use of quinine is recommended only when cramps are disabling, not relieved by other agents, and with full patient education and monitoring for possibly serious side effects [**Level 1**].[1]

Despite the frequency of common cramps, no other agents have been sufficiently studied, but agents that may be effective for cramps include vitamin B complex (thiamine 50 mg, cobalamin 250 μg, pyridoxine 30 mg, riboflavin 5 mg), naftidrofuryl (not available in the United States; 100 mg three times daily), and diltiazem (30 mg daily). Other agents commonly used with variable success include baclofen, benzodiazepines, carbamazepine, oxcarbazepine, verapamil, magnesium citrate, and gabapentin; however, evidence is insufficient regarding these agents. For cramps associated with hemodialysis, vitamin E and C may be effective, and zinc sulfate and branched chain amino acids may be helpful in cramps associated with cirrhosis. For cramps occurring in association with ALS, gabapentin and tetrahydrocannabinol are ineffective.

Outcome

The common muscle cramp has a good prognosis, but pain and discomfort can be troublesome. Nocturnal cramps can interrupt sleep.

LEVEL 1 EVIDENCE

1. Dalakas MC. The role of IVIg in the treatment of patients with stiff person syndrome and other neurological diseases associated with anti-GAD antibodies. *J Neurol.* 2005;252 (suppl 1):I19–I25.

2. Katzberg HD, Khan AH, So YT. Assessment: symptomatic treatment for muscle cramps (an evidence-based review): report of the therapeutics and technology assessment subcommittee of the American Academy of Neurology. *Neurology.* 2010;74(8):691–696.

3. El-Tawil S, Al Musa T, Valli H, et al. Quinine for muscle cramps. *Cochrane Database Syst Rev.* 2010;(12):CD005044.

SUGGESTED READINGS

Stiff Person Syndrome

Alexopoulos H, Dalakas MC. A critical update on the immunopathogenesis of stiff person syndrome. *Eur J Clin Invest.* 2010;40(11):1018–1025.

Barker RA, Revesz T, Thom M, et al. Review of 23 patients affected by the stiff man syndrome: clinical subdivision into stiff trunk (man) syndrome, stiff limb syndrome, and progressive encephalomyelitis with rigidity. *J Neurol Neurosurg Psychiatry.* 1998;65:633–640.

Butler MH, Hayashi A, Ohkoshi N, et al. Autoimmunity to gephyrin in stiff-man syndrome. *Neuron.* 2000;26(2):307–312.

Carvajal-Gonzalez A, Leite MI, Waters P, et al. Glycine receptor antibodies in PERM and related syndromes: characteristics, clinical features and outcomes. *Brain.* 2014;137:2178–2192.

Chang T, Alexopoulos H, McMenamin M, et al. Neuronal surface and glutamic acid decarboxylase autoantibodies in nonparaneoplastic stiff person syndrome. *JAMA Neurol.* 2013;70(9):1140–1149.

De Camilli P, Thomas A, Cofiell R, et al. The synaptic vesicle-associated protein amphiphysin is the 128-kD autoantigen of stiff-man syndrome with breast cancer. *J Exp Med.* 1993;178:2219–2223.

Levy LM, Levy-Reis I, Fujii M, et al. Brain gamma-aminobutyric acid changes in stiff-person syndrome. *Arch Neurol.* 2005;62(6):970–974.

Lorish TR, Thorsteinsson G, Howard FM Jr. Stiff-man syndrome updated. *Mayo Clin Proc.* 1989;64(6):629–636.

McKeon A, Martinez-Hernandez E, Lancaster E, et al. Glycine receptor autoimmune spectrum with stiff-man syndrome phenotype. *JAMA Neurol.* 2013;70(1):44–50.

McKeon A, Robinson MT, McEvoy KM, et al. Stiff-man syndrome and variants: clinical course, treatments, and outcomes. *Arch Neurol.* 2012;69(2):230–238.

Moersch FP, Woltman HW. Progressive fluctuating muscular rigidity and spasm (stiff-man syndrome): report of a case and some observations in 13 other cases. *Proc Staff Meet Mayo Clin.* 1956;31:421–427.

Petzold GC, Marcucci M, Butler MH, et al. Rhabdomyolysis and paraneoplastic stiff-man syndrome with amphiphysin autoimmunity. *Ann Neurol.* 2004;55:286–290.

Rakocevic G, Floeter MK. Autoimmune stiff person syndrome and related myelopathies: understanding of electrophysiological and immunological processes. *Muscle Nerve.* 2012;45(5):623–634.

Cramps and Related Disorders

Alvarez MV, Driver-Dunckley EE, Caviness JN, et al. Case series of painful legs and moving toes: clinical and electrophysiologic observations. *Mov Disord.* 2008;23(14):2062–2066.

Blexrud MD, Windebank AJ, Daube JR. Long-term follow-up of 121 patients with benign fasciculations. *Ann Neurol.* 1993;34:622–625.

Layzer RB. Motor unit hyperactivity states. In: Engel AG, Franzini-Armstrong C, eds. *Myology.* 3rd ed. London, United Kingdom: Churchill Livingstone; 2004.

Layzer RB. The origin of muscle fasciculations and cramps. *Muscle Nerve.* 1994;17:1243–1249.

Minetto MA, Holobar A, Botter A, et al. Origin and development of muscle cramps. *Exerc Sport Sci Rev.* 2013;41(1):3–10.

Rowland LP. Cramps, spasms, and muscle stiffness. *Rev Neurol (Paris).* 1985;4:261–273.

Rowland LP, Trojaborg W, Haller RG. Muscle contracture: physiology and clinical classification. In: Serratrice G, Pouget J, Azulay J-Ph, eds. *Exercise Intolerance and Muscle Contracture.* Paris, France: Springer; 1999:161–170.

Thompson PD. Muscle cramp syndromes. *Handbook of Clin Neurol.* 2007; 86:389–396.

Neuromyotonia

Hart IK, Maddison P, Newsom-Davis J, et al. Phenotypic variants of autoimmune peripheral nerve hyperexcitability. *Brain*. 2002;125:1887–1895.

Irani SR, Alexander S, Waters P, et al. Antibodies to Kv1 potassium channel-complex proteins leucine-rich, glioma inactivated 1 protein and contactin-associated protein-2 in limbic encephalitis, Morvan's syndrome and acquired neuromyotonia. *Brain*. 2010;133(9):2734–2748.

Klein CJ, Lennon VA, Aston PA, et al. Insights from LGI1 and CASPR2 potassium channel complex autoantibody subtyping. *JAMA Neurol*. 2013;70(2):229–234.

Lai M, Huijbers MG, Lancaster E, et al. Investigation of LGI1 as the antigen in limbic encephalitis previously attributed to potassium channels: a case series. *Lancet Neurol*. 2010;9(8):776–785.

Lancaster E, Huijbers MG, Bar V, et al. Investigations of caspr2, an autoantigen of encephalitis and neuromyotonia. *Ann Neurol*. 2011;69(2):303–311.

Maddison P. Neuromyotonia. *Clin Neurophysiol*. 2006;117(10):2118–2127.

Paterson RW, Zandi MS, Armstrong R, et al. Clinical relevance of positive voltage-gated potassium channel (VGKC)-complex antibodies: experience from a tertiary referral centre. *J Neurol Neurosurg Psychiatry*. 2014;85:625–630.

Takahashi H, Mori M, Sekiguchi Y, et al. Development of Isaacs' syndrome following complete recovery of voltage-gated potassium channel antibody-associated limbic encephalitis. *J Neurol Sci*. 2008;275(1–2):185–187.

Taylor RG, Layzer RB, Davis HS, et al. Continuous muscle fiber activity in the Schwartz–Jampel syndrome. *Electroencephalogr Clin Neurophysiol*. 1972;33:497–509.

Vincent A. Autoimmune channelopathies: John Newsom-Davis's work and legacy. A summary of the Newsom-Davis Memorial Lecture 2008. *J Neuroimmunol*. 2008;15:201–202, 245–249.

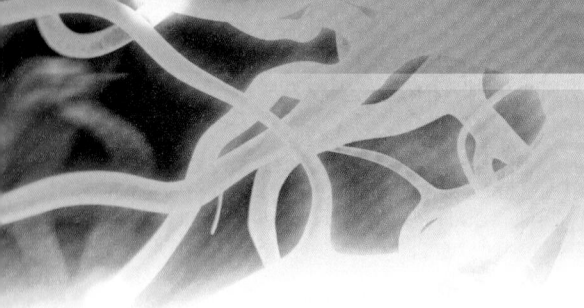

*Michio Hirano, Salvatore DiMauro,
and Lewis P. Rowland*

INTRODUCTION

Metabolic myopathies comprise a clinically and etiologically diverse group of disorders due to defects in cellular energy metabolism, including the breakdown of carbohydrates and fatty acids to generate adenosine triphosphate (ATP), predominantly through mitochondrial respiratory chain oxidative phosphorylation. Accordingly, metabolic myopathies can be etiologically classified into three broad categories: glycogen storage diseases (GSDs), fatty acid oxidation (FAO) disorders, and mitochondrial diseases. These metabolic myopathies present with a clinical spectrum ranging from severe infantile-onset multisystemic diseases to mild adult-onset isolated myopathies. In this chapter, we focus on metabolic myopathies that affect adults.

EPIDEMIOLOGY

Metabolic myopathies are rare diseases. The most common of these disorders is Pompe (acid maltase deficiency) disease with variable ethnic and geographic incidence from 1:14,000 births annually in African-Americans to 1:100,000 in people of European descent. Prevalence of late-onset Pompe disease has been estimated to be 1:60,000. Other frequent metabolic myopathies include McArdle disease (myophosphorylase deficiency) and carnitine palmitoyltransferase II (CPT II) deficiency. The prevalence of McArdle disease has been estimated to be 1:100,000 in the Dallas–Fort Worth, Texas region and a minimum of 1:170,000 in Spain. The prevalence of CPT II deficiency is unknown; however, over 300 patients have been reported. Although individual mitochondrial diseases are rare, collectively, the prevalence of mitochondrial disorders in adults is approximately 1:5,000.

PATHOBIOLOGY

Energy in the form of ATP is required to drive numerous cellular functions including muscle contraction. The main fuels used to generate ATP are glycogen, glucose, and free fatty acids (FFAs). Glycogen is metabolized in the cytoplasm to pyruvate, which enters mitochondria (Fig. 95.1). Short-chain and medium-chain fatty acids cross freely into the mitochondria, whereas long-chain fatty acids require binding to carnitine for transport across the mitochondrial membrane, a process mediated by acyl-carnitine translocase and CPTs I and II (Fig. 95.2). Once in the mitochondria, all these substrates are turned into acetyl-coenzyme A (CoA), which feeds into the Krebs cycle. In this critical cycle, reducing equivalents (electrons) combined with protons are bound to intermediate molecules, nicotinamide adenine dinucleotide (NADH) and flavin adenine dinucleotide, reduced (FADH$_2$), which deliver the electrons to the mitochondrial respiratory chain to produce ATP and water (H$_2$O).

Defects in any of these pathways—glycogen catabolism (glycogenolysis and glycolysis), fatty acid oxidation, Krebs cycle, and mitochondrial respiratory chain and oxidative phosphorylation—cause human disorders that often predominantly affect muscle due to its high energy requirements, particularly during exercise. Because most of the enzyme defects are partial, many of these diseases manifest in adulthood with muscle symptoms either in isolation or with other clinical features.

Abundant glucose is stored in liver and skeletal muscle in the form of a polysaccharide called *glycogen*. The glycogenoses include disorders characterized by genetic mutations in glycogen synthesis (glyconeogenesis), degradation (glycogenolysis), or glucose degradation (glycolysis). To date, 15 glycogenoses have been identified (see Fig. 95.1); most are autosomal recessive except for phosphoglycerate kinase (PGK) and phosphorylase *b* kinase deficiency, which are X-linked.

Fatty acids are the primary energy source for muscle at rest and during periods of prolonged low-intensity exercise. Fatty acids are catabolized by the β-oxidation enzymes, which cleave two-carbon fragments with each cycle. Thus, lipidoses arise due to failure of fatty acid transport into mitochondria secondary to carnitine or CPT I or II deficiencies or to defects of intramitochondrial β-oxidation. These disorders are inherited as autosomal recessive traits. The more severe variants present in infancy or childhood with primary involvement of liver or brain, whereas the milder adult forms are predominantly myopathic and include the myopathic variant of CPT II deficiency, trifunctional protein deficiency (TFP), and very long chain acyl-CoA dehydrogenase deficiency (VLCAD).

In addition to catabolizing lipids, mitochondria perform additional essential functions including Krebs cycle and amino acid metabolism as well as energy production through the respiratory chain and oxidative phosphorylation. The respiratory chain is composed of four multisubunit enzymatic complexes (I, II, III, and IV), which generate a proton gradient across the inner mitochondrial membrane (IMM) that, in turn, drives ATP synthesis by complex V. In addition, CoQ$_{10}$ and cytochrome *c* are critical components of the mitochondrial respiratory chain, serving as "electron shuttles" between the complexes. Originally restricted to primary defects of the respiratory chain and oxidative phosphorylation, mitochondrial diseases have expanded to encompass defects of mitochondrial transcription, translation, protein importation, lipid membranes, and organellar dynamics (fusion, fission, and movement) (see Chapter 139).

CLINICAL FEATURES

From a clinical point of view, metabolic myopathies can be categorized into two different groups: (1) those that show symptoms and signs related to exercise (exercise intolerance, cramps, myalgias, myoglobinuria) with normal interictal examination and (2) those with fixed symptoms such as muscle weakness often associated with systemic involvement (such as encephalopathies or endocrinopathies). When evaluating a patient with

FIGURE 95.1 Scheme of glycogen metabolism and glycolysis. *Roman numerals* denote muscle glycogenoses due to defects in the following enzymes: *0*, glycogen synthase; *II*, acid maltase; *III*, debrancher; *IV*, brancher; *V*, myophosphorylase; *VII*, phosphofructokinase; *VIII*, phosphorylase *b* kinase; *IX*, phosphoglycerate kinase; *X*, phosphoglycerate mutase; *XI*, lactate dehydrogenase; *XII*, aldolase; *XIII*, β-enolase; *XIV*, phosphoglucomutase 1; and *XV*, glycogenin-1. *Red numerals* designate glycogenoses associated with exercise intolerance, cramps, and myoglobinuria. *Blue italic numerals* correspond to glycogenoses causing weakness.

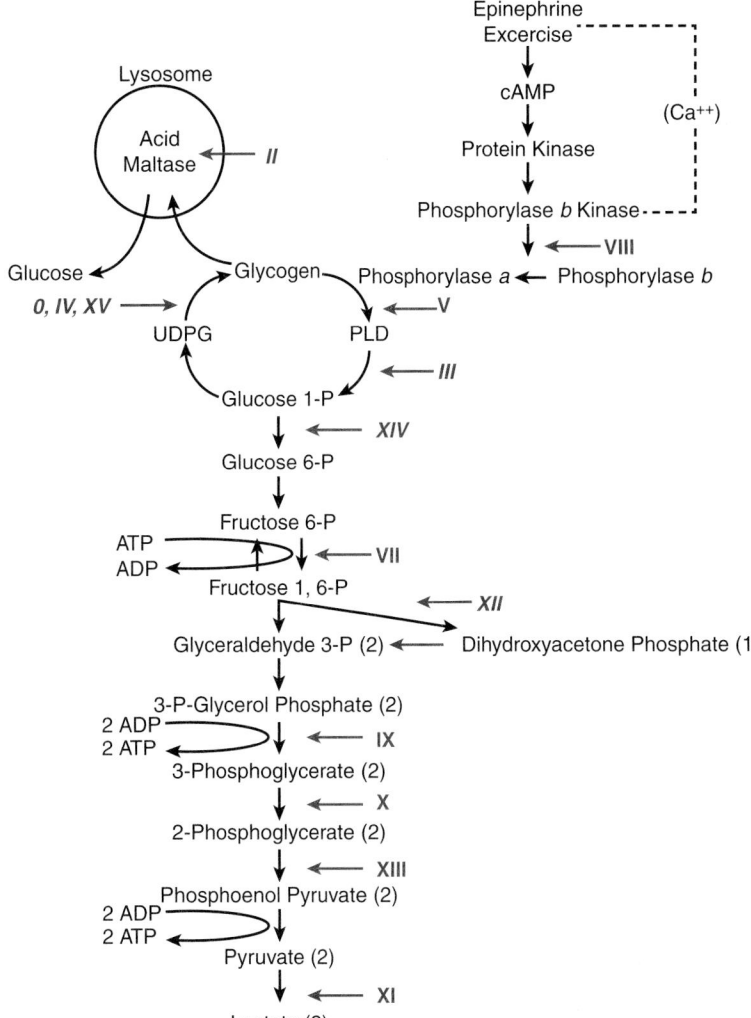

exercise-related symptoms, clinicians should ask two questions: (1) What type of exercise provokes symptoms? (2) Are there associated triggering factors? If short bursts of high-intensity exercise cause muscle cramps or myoglobinuria, the patient may have a defect of glycogen metabolism. Examples of this type of activity include weight lifting or sprinting. In young patients who play baseball or softball, the "home run" sign (Haller sign), inability to sprint around the bases due to exercise-induced muscle spasms, is a typical complaint in patients with glycogenoses, such as McArdle disease. In contrast, if the patient complains that prolonged exercise (such as hiking or playing soccer) triggers myalgias, fatigue, and myoglobinuria without acute contractures, the patient is likely to have a defect of fatty acid oxidation. The symptoms often occur when the patient is fasting or under stress. A prototypical example is a young adult with CPT II deficiency who enlists in military service and has difficulty completing long marches due to fatigue and myalgias followed by myoglobinuria.

In the past, the term *myoglobinuria* was reserved for grossly pigmented urine, but modern techniques can detect amounts of this protein so minute that discoloration may not be evident. (Determination of serum myoglobin content by radioimmunoassay has similar diagnostic significance as measurement of serum creatine kinase [CK] activity.) The clinically important syndromes, however, are associated with gross pigmenturia. Numerous conditions

cause myoglobinuria (Table 95.1). Sometimes, the disorder can be recognized without direct demonstration of myoglobin in the urine: For instance, acute renal failure in a patient with levels of serum CK activity over 1,000 units would suggest myoglobinuric renal failure. Inexplicably, the cumbersome neologism *rhabdomyolysis* was favored for a few years, but a 2015 Medline search found that "myoglobinuria" is holding fast. Myoglobin is the visible pigment in the urine, and it is a toxin that injures the kidney; the syndrome originates with muscle necrosis, which does not need a new name.

Some patients with glycolytic, lipid, or mitochondrial disorders can develop isolated progressive myopathy and persistent weakness. More typically, patients with mitochondrial diseases can show a wide range of extramuscular manifestations. In this section, general clinical aspects of these metabolic myopathies with emphasis on the more common forms are described.

DISORDERS OF GLYCOGEN METABOLISM (GLYCOGENOSES)

Clinical presentations of muscle glycogenoses are protean, ranging from profound multisystem disease in infancy to exercise intolerance or isolated progressive muscle weakness in adults. Here, we focus on the adult patients. Myophosphorylase deficiency (McArdle disease, glycogenosis type V) is a prototypical

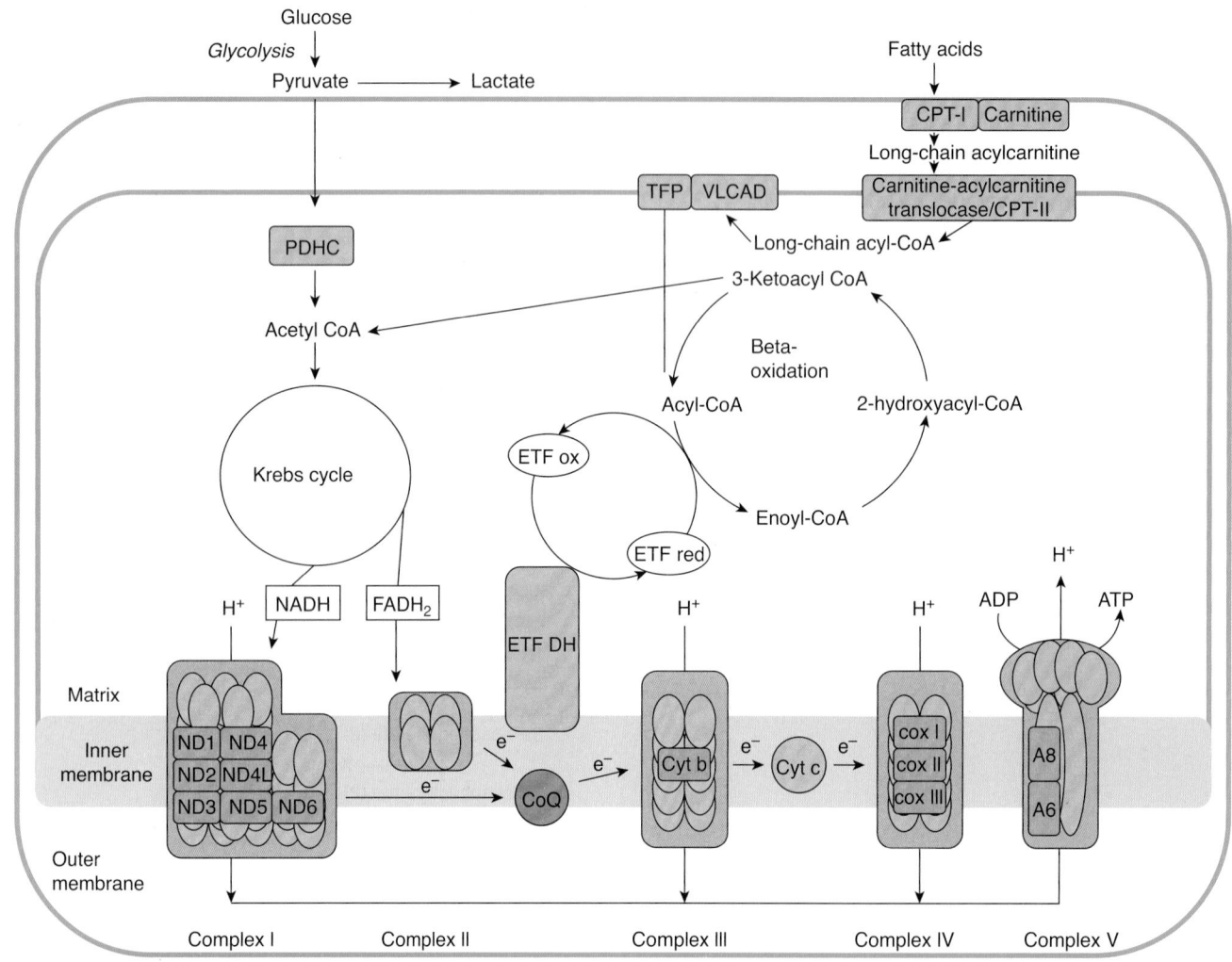

FIGURE 95.2 Schematic representation of mitochondrial metabolism. CPT, carnitine palmitoyltransferase; TFP, trifunctional enzyme; VLCAD, very long chain acyl-CoA dehydrogenase; PDHC, pyruvate dehydrogenase complex; CoA, coenzyme A; ETF ox and red, electron transfer flavoprotein oxidized and reduced; NADH, nicotinamide adenine dinucleotide; FADH₂, flavin adenine dinucleotide, reduced; ETF DH, electron transfer flavoprotein dehydrogenase; CoQ, coenzyme Q; Cyt c, cytochrome c.

glycogenolytic disorder with episodic muscle dysfunction and myoglobinuria. It is the most common disorder of skeletal muscle carbohydrate metabolism and one of most frequent genetic myopathies. Patients with McArdle disease typically exhibit intolerance to static or isometric muscle contractions and also to dynamic exercise that can trigger episodes of reversible "muscle crises." Acute crises manifest mainly in the form of premature fatigue and contractures, frequently accompanied by muscle breakdown (rhabdomyolysis) with elevated serum CK and sometimes by myoglobinuria. In addition to McArdle disease, five other forms of glycogenoses manifest exercise-induced myoglobinuria: type VII (phosphofructokinase [PFK] deficiency, Tarui disease), type VIII (phosphorylase b kinase), type IX (PGK deficiency), type X (phosphoglycerate mutase [PGAM] deficiency), type XI (lactate dehydrogenase deficiency), and type XIV (phosphoglucomutase 1 deficiency).

Another important sign considered pathognomonic is the "second wind," which is a marked improvement in exercise tolerance about 10 minutes into aerobic exercise involving large muscle masses (jogging or cycling). The second wind, as manifested by a marked decrease in early exertional tachycardia (e.g., a decrease from ~140 to 150 beats per minute to ~120 beats per minute)

starting after around 7 minutes of exercise, does not occur in patients with other disorders that are also associated with exercise intolerance, such as PFK deficiency and other glycogenoses, mitochondrial myopathies, or disorders of lipid metabolism. This phenomenon is due to increased uptake of glucose and use of fatty acid.

Hemolytic anemia (elevated indirect bilirubin and reticulocytes) is seen in glycogenosis due to defects in genes partially expressed in erythrocytes such as PFK, PGK, and aldolase A. Cognitive deficits are often associated with the adult polyglucosan body disease (APBD) form of branching enzyme deficiency (type IV) and PGK deficiency.

Acid maltase or acid α–glucosidase (GAA) is an enzyme responsible for the catabolism of glycogen within lysosomes. Infantile-onset acid maltase deficiency (type II, Pompe disease) presents as a myopathy and cardiomyopathy, which, if untreated, is typically fatal in the first year of life. In contrast, in the late-onset form of Pompe disease beginning in childhood through adulthood, patients have slowly progressive fixed proximal muscle weakness and early respiratory insufficiency. Although myopathy is the predominant manifestation, patients with Pompe disease also develop basilar

TABLE 95.1 Classification of Human Myoglobinuria

Hereditary Myoglobinuria

Disorders of Glycogen Metabolism

Myophosphorylase deficiency (McArdle; MIM 232600)

Phosphofructokinase deficiency (Tarui; MIM 171840)

Phosphoglycerate kinase (DiMauro 3; MIM 311800)

Phosphoglycerate mutase (DiMauro 2; MIM 261670)

Lactate dehydrogenase (Kanno; MIM 150000)

Disorders of Lipid Metabolism

Carnitine palmitoyltransferase II deficiency (DiMauro 1; MIM 255110)

LPIN1 mutations (MIM 268200)

VLCAD deficiency (MIM 201375)

Trifunctional protein deficiency (MIM 609015)

Mitochondrial Myopathies

Mitochondrial DNA (MTCYB) mutations

Coenzyme Q_{10} deficiency

Other Genetic Myopathies

RYR1 deficiency (with malignant hyperthermia MIM 145600, without malignant hyperthermia)

Becker/Duchenne muscular dystrophy

Fascioscapulohumeral dystrophy (FSHD)

Limb-girdle muscular dystrophy 1C (Caveolin deficiency)

Limb-girdle muscular dystrophy 2C (SGCG, γ-sarcoglycan deficiency)

Limb-girdle muscular dystrophy 2D (SGCA, α-sarcoglycan deficiency)

Limb-girdle muscular dystrophy 2E (SGCB, β-sarcoglycan deficiency)

Limb-girdle muscular dystrophy 21 (FKRP deficiency)

Limb-girdle muscular dystrophy 2L (ANO5 mutations)

Sporadic Myoglobinuria

Exertion in Untrained Individuals

"Squat-jump" and related syndromes

Anterior tibial syndrome

Convulsions

High-voltage electric shock, lightning stroke

Agitated delirium, restraints

Status asthmaticus

Prolonged myoclonus or acute dystonia

Crush Syndrome

Compression by fallen weights

Compression by body in prolonged coma

Sporadic Myoglobinuria (continued)

Ischemia

Arterial occlusion

Cardioversion

Coagulopathy in sickle cell disease or disseminated intravascular coagulation

Ischemia in compression and anterior tibial syndromes

Laparoscopic nephrectomy

Ligation of vena cava

Surgery on morbidly obese people, including bariatric surgery

Metabolic Depression

Barbiturate, carbon monoxide, narcotic coma

Cold exposure

Diabetic acidosis

General anesthesia

Hyperglycemic, hyperosmolar coma

Hypothermia

Exogenous Toxins and Drugs

Alcohol abuse

Amphotericin B

Carbenoxolone

Clopidogrel (and heart transplant)

Gemfibrozil (plus statin)

Glycyrrhizae

Haff disease

Heatstroke

Heroin

Hypokalemia, chronic, any cause

Interferon α-2B

Isotretinoin

Malayan sea-snake bite poison

Malignant neuroleptic syndrome

Plasmocid

Phenylpropanolamine

Statin drugs

Succinylcholine

Toxic shock syndrome

Viral infection (CMV, influenza, others)

Wasp stings

Progressive Muscle Disease

Alcoholic myopathy

Polymyositis or dermatomyositis

Cause unknown

CMV, cytomegalovirus.

artery and aortic aneurysms, bladder or bowel incontinence, and dysphagia. An autopsy study of a late-onset Pompe patient revealed ultrastructural abnormalities in the smooth muscle of blood vessels, gastrointestinal tract, and bladder, thereby accounting for the extraskeletal muscle manifestations. Hearing loss has also been reported in this disease. It is important to diagnose Pompe disease, as enzyme replacement therapy with recombinant human GAA (rhGAA) dramatically improves the cardiomyopathy in the infantile form and less effectively improves the myopathy in both infantile and late-onset forms.

In other cases such as debrancher deficiency (type III, Cori–Forbes disease), distal muscle weakness can be combined with cardiomyopathy and peripheral neuropathy in patients who had shown in infancy hepatomegaly, hypoglycemia, and failure to thrive, all of which usually improve around puberty. Thus, adult patients with debrancher deficiency can manifest distal muscle weakness and wasting with electromyographic myogenic and neurogenic abnormalities.

Branching enzyme deficiency (type IV) presents with heterogeneous phenotypes ranging from congenital or infantile neuromuscular disorders to late-onset APBD, which manifests as progressive upper and lower motor neuron dysfunction, stocking-glove sensory loss, bladder dysfunction, and dementia. Muscle and nerve biopsies of APBD patients reveal periodic acid–Schiff (PAS)–positive but diastase-resistant polyglucosan bodies. Although reported in various ethnic groups, APBD is particularly frequent in the Ashkenazi Jewish population due to founder mutations. Polyglucosan bodies are also characteristic of a juvenile-onset myopathy often accompanied by cardiomyopathy due to mutations in *RBCK1*, which encodes a ubiquitin ligase.

Striking absence of glycogen is characteristic of two disorders: glycogenosis type 0, glycogen synthase (GS1) deficiency, and glycogenosis type XV, glycogenin-1 deficiency. Both enzymes are required for the synthesis of glycogen. GS1 deficiency has presented as childhood exercise intolerance, cardiomyopathy, sudden death, or cardiomyopathy and myopathy. Glycogenin-1 deficiency has been described in one adult patient with myopathy and cardiac arrhythmias as well as in seven other adult patients with childhood or adult onset myopathy with polyglucosan bodies but without cardiopathy.

DISORDERS OF LIPID METABOLISM

Since DiMauro and DiMauro-Melis described the first patients with CPT II deficiency, this disease has been the most frequently diagnosed disorder of lipid metabolism. The first symptoms most often occur between 6 and 20 years of age, but age at onset may be older than 50 years. The symptomatology usually consists of recurrent attacks of myalgias and muscle stiffness or weakness, often associated with myoglobinuria. The duration of the attacks are usually acute and the consequences may be prolonged up to several weeks. The patients are usually asymptomatic between attacks. The frequency of these attacks is highly variable. The rhabdomyolysis may occasionally be complicated by two types of life-threatening events: more commonly, acute renal failure secondary to myoglobinuria and, much less frequently, respiratory insufficiency secondary to respiratory muscle involvement. Symptoms are usually prompted by prolonged exercise and less commonly by prolonged fasting, high-fat intake, exposure to cold, mild infection (especially in children), fever, emotional stress, general anesthesia, or drugs such as diazepam or ibuprofen. In all cases, the clinical symptomatology is restricted to skeletal muscle without liver or heart involvement.

Defects of most β-oxidation enzymes typically manifest in infancy with severe multisystem disease; however, the clinical presentation of VLCAD deficiency may be indistinguishable from CPT II deficiency. Trifunctional enzyme catalyzes three steps in long-chain fatty acid β-oxidation: enoyl-CoA hydratase, long-chain 3-hydroxyacyl-CoA dehydrogenase (LCHAD), and acylthiolase (see Fig. 95.2). Adults with trifunctional protein (TFP) deficiency present with recurrent rhabdomyolysis triggered by prolonged exercise, fasting, or infections similar to CPT II and VLCAD deficiencies; however, TFP mutations are often associated with peripheral neuropathy and pigmentary retinopathy.

Multiple acyl-CoA dehydrogenation deficiency (MADD), also known as *glutaric aciduria type II* (GA II), is an autosomal recessive disorder due to mutations in genes encoding either one of the two subunits of the electron transferring flavoprotein (*ETFA* and *ETFB*) or to mutations in the gene encoding the electron transfer flavoprotein dehydrogenase (*ETF DH*) and resulting in abnormal fatty acid, amino acid, and choline metabolism. Less severely affected patients might present with progressive muscle weakness and lipid storage myopathies with secondary muscle CoQ$_{10}$ deficiency, mainly in adulthood and are sometimes responsive to riboflavin treatment (riboflavin responsive MADD), CoQ$_{10}$ supplementation, or both.

The myopathic form of coenzyme Q$_{10}$ (CoQ$_{10}$) deficiency is characterized by proximal myopathy with premature fatigue, weakness, and increased serum levels of CK and lactate. Muscle biopsies show excessive numbers of lipid droplets, predominantly in type 1 fibers, combined deficiency of respiratory chain complexes I and III, and CoQ$_{10}$ levels below 50% of normal. Mutations in the *ETF DH* gene, leading to a decrement in complex electron transfer flavoprotein-ubiquinone oxidoreductase (ETF:QO) activity have been identified in adult-onset MADD and some cases of myopathy with CoQ$_{10}$ deficiency indicating that that they can be allelic diseases.

Neutral lipid storage disease (NLSD) present with mild to moderate proximal limb weakness with striking accumulation of lipid in skeletal muscle and other tissues as well as in leukocytes (Jordan anomaly). CK is persistently elevated and has preceded weakness. Mutations in *PNPLA2* encoding adipocyte triglyceride lipase (ATGL) cause neutral lipid storage myopathy, whereas mutations in *ABHD5*, which encodes CGI-58 (activator of ATGL), cause lipid storage myopathy with ichthyosis (Chanarin–Dorfman syndrome).

MITOCHONDRIAL DISEASES

Although mitochondrial diseases frequently present as infantile- or childhood-onset multisystemic diseases, many adult patients have myopathy as the predominant or only manifestation with either fixed weakness, exercise intolerance, or both. Myoglobinuria is less common in respiratory chain oxidative phosphorylation disorders relative to other metabolic myopathies.

Like most myopathies, mitochondrial myopathies cause proximal limb weakness, but extraocular muscles are also frequently affected, leading to ptosis and chronic progressive external ophthalmoplegia (CPEO). CPEO begins in childhood or adulthood and typically manifests with symmetric and slowly progressive impairment of eye movements accompanied by ptosis. Occasionally, the extraocular muscle weakness can be strikingly asymmetric. CPEO is sometimes misdiagnosed as myasthenia gravis; however, fixed weakness with minimal or no fluctuations, absence of acetylcholine receptor and muscle specific tyrosine kinase (MUSK) antibodies, as well as absence of neuromuscular junction dysfunction on electrophysiologic studies should lead clinicians to screen for myopathies such as CPEO.

CPEO often remains a pure myopathy with limb weakness and variable dysphagia and respiratory muscle involvement. In contrast, CPEO can be part of a multisystemic disease such as Kearns–Sayre syndrome (KSS) or sensory ataxic neuropathy dysarthria ophthalmoplegia (SANDO) (see Chapter 139). Some individuals are classified as CPEO-plus because they develop additional neurologic manifestations but lack features to fulfill criteria for KSS, SANDO, or other defined clinical syndromes. CPEO can be due to maternally inherited mitochondrial DNA (mtDNA) point mutations, sporadic single large-scale deletions of mtDNA, or primary autosomal dominant or recessive mutations that cause secondary multiple deletions of mtDNA.

In patients with mitochondrial myopathies, exercise intolerance presents with premature fatigue with activities as mild as walking up a single flight of stairs. After a short rest, patients usually can resume their activity but symptoms recur. Mitochondrial disease patients often report subjective heaviness or burning of muscles with exertion but, in contrast to patients with glycogenoses, do not typically manifest stiffness, cramps, or second wind phenomenon. The exercise intolerance is often disproportionately severe relative to muscle weakness. This symptom can be isolated or associated with muscle weakness and multisystemic involvement. Exercise testing is particularly helpful as an evaluation and screening tool in mitochondrial myopathies. Elevated lactate levels at rest and exaggerated lactate responses after even trivial exercise are useful clues to the diagnosis of mitochondrial disease. One of the hallmarks of mitochondrial myopathies is a reduction in maximal whole body oxygen consumption (VO_2 max) demonstrated by a characteristic deficit in peripheral oxygen extraction (A to V O_2 difference) and an enhanced oxygen delivery (hyperkinetic circulation). Alternatively, in specialized referral centers, ^{31}P nuclear magnetic resonance (NMR) spectroscopy can reveal decreased basal levels of high-energy phosphate compounds (e.g., ATP and phosphocreatine [P-Cr]) at rest or prolonged recovery of ATP and P-Cr after exercise in patients with mitochondrial myopathies.

An unusual group of mitochondrial disease patients present with sporadic isolated myopathies with exercise intolerance variably accompanied by proximal muscle weakness and myoglobinuria. It is important for clinicians to be aware of this condition, which in several cases, was misdiagnosed as chronic fatigue syndrome or fibromyalgia. Resting venous lactic acid is elevated in most patients with this condition; therefore, blood lactate is a useful noninvasive screening test for this syndrome. In most cases, muscle biopsies reveal ragged-red fibers that are cytochrome c oxidase (COX)–positive because the gene defect is often a mutation in the cytochrome b gene, which encodes a subunit of complex III, or in an ND gene, encoding a subunit of complex I. In addition, other mutations in mtDNA have been associated with exercise intolerance, including transfer RNA (tRNA) mutations as well as mutations in protein coding genes for subunits of respiratory chain complex I or IV. Because the mutations are not detectable in blood in most of these patients, muscle biopsy is generally required to make the diagnosis.

A rare clinical form of CoQ_{10} deficiency presents as encephalomyopathy in childhood with the triad of encephalopathy (seizures, mental retardation, or ataxia), muscle weakness often with myoglobinuria, and ragged-red fibers in muscle. Patients have been diagnosed in adolescence or adulthood and have improved with CoQ_{10} supplementation.

A rare childhood-onset mitochondrial myopathy has been identified in Northern Swedish patients who have exercise intolerance.

In these patients, modest exercise triggers fatigue, tachycardia, shortness of breath, and myoglobinuria due to a founder splice site mutation in *ISCU*, which encodes the iron-sulfur (Fe-S) scaffold protein required by Fe-S subunit containing enzymes such as aconitase and complexes I, II, and III of the mitochondrial respiratory chain.

DIAGNOSIS

The diagnosis of glycogenosis should be considered in patients with recurrent myoglobinuria triggered by brief intense exercise. Presence of the "second wind" is indicative of McArdle disease (myophosphorylase deficiency), whereas in adults, signs of hemolytic anemia with elevated uric acid (and occasionally gout) is suggestive of PFK or PGK deficiency in adults. The specific glycolytic defect can be identified by sequencing blood DNA or by measuring biochemical activity of seven glycolytic enzymes (myophosphorylase, PFK, phosphorylase b kinase, phosphoglycerate kinase, PGAM, lactate dehydrogenase, and phosphoglucomutase 1). In patients with limb weakness, early respiratory muscle involvement, and EMG evidence of prominent spontaneous activity of paraspinal muscles, the diagnosis of Pompe disease should be considered. A dried blood spot test can detect acid maltase deficiency. Definitive diagnosis is made by sequencing *GAA* in blood or by a muscle biopsy showing increased membrane-bound glycogen with markedly reduced acid maltase activity. Debrancher enzyme deficiency should be considered in patients with fixed distal greater than proximal limb weakness with EMG myogenic and neurogenic abnormalities and visceral organ involvement. Branching enzyme deficiency is clinically recognizable by the combination of upper and lower motor neuron dysfunction, sensorimotor neuropathy, sphincter dysfunction, and dementia. Both debrancher and branching enzyme deficiencies can be diagnosed by DNA sequencing. In many cases, muscle histology showing excessive free glycogen lead to the diagnosis of debrancher deficiency, whereas detection of polyglucosan bodies is indicative of APBD. Detecting biochemical defects of muscle debrancher or branching enzyme is diagnostic, particularly in cases when DNA sequencing reveals variants of uncertain significance.

In patients with recurrent myoglobinuria triggered by prolonged exercise, fasting, or both, defects of fatty acid oxidation should be considered. Acylcarnitine profile may reveal elevated acylcarnitines (e.g., long-chain acylcarnitines in CPT II and VLCAD deficiencies) particularly after overnight fasting; however, the profiles are often normal. The diagnosis can be made by blood DNA testing. CPT II activity can be measured in skeletal muscle or cultured fibroblasts.

In patients with suspected mitochondrial myopathy, measurement of free-flowing blood lactate and pyruvate can be useful; elevated resting lactate especially when the lactate-to-pyruvate ratio is high (i.e., >20:1) is indicative of a mitochondrial respiratory chain oxidative phosphorylation defect. In patients with evidence of maternal inheritance, whole mtDNA sequencing offers a cost-effective approach to identifying mtDNA point mutations. Individuals with sporadic CPEO, CPEO-plus, or KSS should be screened for single large-scale mtDNA deletions, which are usually undetectable in blood and occasionally identified in urine sediment but most reliably detected in muscle biopsies. In patients with autosomal CPEO, CPEO-plus, and SANDO, sequencing of nuclear genes, particularly *POLG* encoding the mtDNA polymerase catalytic subunit, can reveal the causative mutation(s). If blood and urine DNA screening is negative or ambiguous, muscle biopsy for histology, measurement of mitochondrial respiratory chain activities, and potential molecular genetic testing (e.g., screening for mtDNA deletions or depletion) are often useful.

Although not a metabolic disorder, mutations in *RYR1* encoding the skeletal muscle ryanodine receptor are frequent causes of recurrent exercise-induced myoglobinuria. Heat, and to a lesser degree, viral infections, alcohol, and drugs can trigger episodes of myoglobinuria.

TREATMENT

Treatment of metabolic myopathies is limited. Enzyme replacement therapy for Pompe disease is the only disease-modifying therapy; however, efficacy is limited in adults. There is Level 1 evidence of mild beneficial effects of enzyme replacement therapy on respiratory function and ambulation in patients with late-onset Pompe disease [**Level 1**].[1] Avoidance of precipitating factors (e.g., intense exercise in patients with myoglobinuria due to glycogenesis) is critical.

Glucose or sucrose intake before exercise exacerbates muscle's symptoms (out-of-wind phenomenon) in PFK deficiency where the metabolic block occurs below the entry of glucose into glycolysis, whereas in McArdle disease, sugar intake ameliorates symptoms because the metabolic block is upstream of glucose catabolism. In other cases, such as PGAM or PFK deficiencies, this intervention does not produce changes in the exercise performance.

In patients with FAO disorders, a carbohydrate-rich diet and avoidance of fasting is often beneficial. In patients with CPT II, VLCAD, and TP deficiencies, supplementation with medium-chain triglycerides can be beneficial.

For patients with mitochondrial myopathies, symptomatic therapy is important. Patients with severe ptosis that impairs vision, eyelid crutches, or eyelid slings can be beneficial. Screening for heart block in patients with KSS or CPEO is important, as timely placement of a pacemaker can be lifesaving. Aerobic exercise training improves oxidative capacity in patients with heteroplasmic mtDNA mutations.

OUTCOME

The long-term prognosis of patients with metabolic myopathies due to defects of glycogen or lipid metabolism is generally favorable. In patients with severe myoglobinuria, compartment syndrome and renal failure are serious complications that must be treated aggressively. In patients with recurrent myoglobinuria due to myophosphorylase or PFK deficiency, moderate fixed weakness often develops late in life. In contrast, patients with late-onset Pompe disease can develop severe restrictive lung disease that is amenable to continuous positive airway pressure (CPAP) and bilevel positive airway pressure (BiPAP) support.

The prognosis for patients with mitochondrial myopathies is variable. Patients with CPEO can have a very benign outcome with moderate to severe extraocular weakness as the main problem; however, some patients with CPEO have developed symptomatic dysphagia, restrictive lung disease, and marked limb weakness. Patients with KSS, SANDO, and other multisystemic mitochondrial diseases frequently progress and can develop severe encephalopathies and in the case of KSS, severe cardiomyopathy or visceral organ dysfunction that can be fatal in early to mid-adulthood.

LEVEL 1 EVIDENCE

1. van der Ploeg AT, Clemens PR, Corzo D, et al. A randomized study of alglucosidase alfa in late-onset Pompe's disease. *N Engl J Med.* 2010;362:1396–1406.

SUGGESTED READINGS

Andreu AL, Hanna MG, Reichmann H, et al. Exercise intolerance due to mutations in the cytochrome b gene of mitochondrial DNA. *N Engl J Med.* 1999;341:1037–1044.

Aure K, Ogier de Baulny H, Laforet P, et al. Chronic progressive ophthalmoplegia with large-scale mtDNA rearrangement: can we predict progression? *Brain.* 2007;130:1516–1524.

Bao Y, Kishnani P, Wu JY, et al. Hepatic and neuromuscular forms of glycogen storage disease type IV caused by mutations in the same glycogen-branching enzyme gene. *J Clin Invest.* 1996;97:941–948.

Berardo A, DiMauro S, Hirano M. A diagnostic algorithm for metabolic myopathies. *Curr Neurol Neurosci Rep.* 2010;10:118–126.

Bertrand C, Largiliere C, Zabot MT, et al. Very long-chain acyl-CoA dehydrogenase deficiency: identification of a new inborn error of mitochondrial fatty acid oxidation in fibroblasts. *Biochim Biophys Acta.* 1992;1180:327–329.

Bruno C, Dimauro S. Lipid storage myopathies. *Curr Opin Neurol.* 2008;21:601–606.

DiMauro S. Mitochondrial encephalomyopathies—fifty years on: the Robert Wartenberg Lecture. *Neurology.* 2013;81:281–291.

DiMauro S, DiMauro-Melis PM. Muscle carnitine palmitoyltransferase deficiency and myoglobinuria. *Science.* 1973;182:929–931.

DiMauro S, Schon EA, Carelli V, et al. The clinical maze of mitochondrial neurology. *Nat Rev Neurol.* 2013;9:429–444.

Dlamini N, Voermans NC, Lillis S, et al. Mutations in RYR1 are a common cause of exertional myalgia and rhabdomyolysis. *Neuromuscul Disord.* 2013;23:540–548.

Garone C, Rubio JC, Calvo SE, et al. MPV17 mutations causing adult-onset multisystemic disorder with multiple mitochondrial DNA deletions. *Arch Neurol.* 2012;69:1648–1651.

Haller RG, Vissing J. Spontaneous "second wind" and glucose-induced second "second wind" in McArdle disease: oxidative mechanisms. *Arch Neurol.* 2002;59:1395–1402.

Kanno T, Sudo K, Takeuchi I, et al. Hereditary deficiency of lactate dehydrogenase M-subunit. *Clin Chim Acta.* 1980;108:267–276.

Kaufmann P, El-Schahawi M, DiMauro S. Carnitine palmitoyltransferase II deficiency: diagnosis by molecular analysis of blood. *Mol Cell Biochem.* 1997;174:237–239.

Kearns TP, Sayre GP. Retinitis pigmentosa, external ophthalmoplegia, and complete heart block. *AMA Arch Ophthalmol.* 1958;60:280–289.

Kishnani PS, Steiner RD, Bali D, et al. Pompe disease diagnosis and management guideline. *Genet Med.* 2006;8:267–288.

Kollberg G, Tulinius M, Gilljam T, et al. Cardiomyopathy and exercise intolerance in muscle glycogen storage disease 0. *N Engl J Med.* 2007;357:1507–1514.

Lossos A, Barash V, Soffer D, et al. Hereditary branching enzyme dysfunction in adult polyglucosan body disease: a possible metabolic cause in two patients. *Ann Neurol.* 1991;30:655–662.

Malfatti E, Nilsson J, Hedberg-Olfors C, et al. A new muscle glycogen storage disease associated with glycogenin-1 deficiency. *Ann Neurol.* 2014;76:891-898.

McArdle B. Myopathy due to a defect in muscle glycogen breakdown. *Clin Sci.* 1951;10:13–33.

Mochel F, Knight MA, Tong WH, et al. Splice mutation in the iron-sulfur cluster scaffold protein ISCU causes myopathy with exercise intolerance. *Am J Hum Genet.* 2008;82:652–660.

Moraes CT, DiMauro S, Zeviani M, et al. Mitochondrial DNA deletions in progressive external ophthalmoplegia and Kearns-Sayre syndrome. *N Engl J Med.* 1989;320:1293–1299.

Moslemi AR, Lindberg C, Nilsson J, et al. Glycogenin-1 deficiency and inactivated priming of glycogen synthesis. *N Engl J Med.* 2010;362:1203–1210.

Ogasahara S, Engel AG, Frens D, et al. Muscle coenzyme Q deficiency in familial mitochondrial encephalomyopathy. *Proc Natl Acad Sci U S A*. 1989;86: 2379–2382.

Ogilvie I, Pourfarzam M, Jackson S, et al. Very long-chain acyl coenzyme A dehydrogenase deficiency presenting with exercise-induced myoglobinuria. *Neurology*. 1994;44:467–473.

Oldfors A, DiMauro S. New insights in the field of muscle glycogenoses. *Curr Opin Neurol*. 2013;26:544–553.

Olsson A, Lind L, Thornell LE, et al. Myopathy with lactic acidosis is linked to chromosome 12q23.3-24.11 and caused by an intron mutation in the ISCU gene resulting in a splicing defect. *Hum Mol Genet*. 2008;17: 1666–1672.

Paradas C, Gutierrez Rios P, Rivas E, et al. TK2 mutation presenting as indolent myopathy. *Neurology*. 2013;80:504–506.

Ronchi D, Garone C, Bordoni A, et al. Next-generation sequencing reveals DGUOK mutations in adult patients with mitochondrial DNA multiple deletions. *Brain*. 2012;135:3404–3415.

Rowland LP. Progressive external ophthalmoplegia. In: Vineken PJ, Bruyn GW, Klawans HL, eds. *Handbook of Clinical Neurology*. Amsterdam, The Netherlands: Elsevier Sciences Publishers; 1992:287–329.

Schaefer J, Jackson S, Dick DJ, et al. Trifunctional enzyme deficiency: adult presentation of a usually fatal beta-oxidation defect. *Ann Neurol*. 1996;40:597–602.

Sharp LJ, Haller RG. Metabolic and mitochondrial myopathies. *Neurol Clin*. 2014;32:777–799.

Sobreira C, Hirano M, Shanske S, et al. Mitochondrial encephalomyopathy with coenzyme Q10 deficiency. *Neurology*. 1997;48:1238–1243.

Stojkovic T, Vissing J, Petit F, et al. Muscle glycogenosis due to phosphoglucomutase 1 deficiency. *N Engl J Med*. 2009;361:425–427.

Tarui S, Okuno G, Ikura Y, et al. Phosphofructokinase deficiency in skeletal muscle. A new type of glycogenosis. *Biochem Biophys Res Commun*. 1965;19:517–523.

Tsujino S, Shanske S, DiMauro S. Molecular genetic heterogeneity of myophosphorylase deficiency (McArdle's disease). *N Engl J Med*. 1993;329:241–245.

Tyynismaa H, Sun R, Ahola-Erkkila S, et al. Thymidine kinase 2 mutations in autosomal recessive progressive external ophthalmoplegia with multiple mitochondrial DNA deletions. *Hum Mol Genet*. 2012;21:66–75.

Vissing J, Haller RG. The effect of oral sucrose on exercise tolerance in patients with McArdle's disease. *N Engl J Med*. 2003;349:2503–2509.

Zeviani M, Carelli V. Disorders of mitochondrial DNA maintenance. In: Greenamyre JT, ed. *Medlink Neurology*. San Diego, CA: Medlink Corporation; 2013.

Gliomas 96

Mikael L. Rinne and Patrick Y. Wen

INTRODUCTION

Gliomas are a group of primary central nervous system (CNS) neuroepithelial tumors that appear to arise from glial progenitor cells in the brain or spinal cord. Based on their resemblance to glial lineages, gliomas have been classified into different tumor types, including astrocytomas, oligodendrogliomas, mixed oligoastrocytomas, ependymomas, and several less common types of glioneuronal tumors. Gliomas are the most common type of tumor arising in the brain. Because they rarely metastasize outside of the CNS, gliomas are not staged like systemic malignancies. Instead, gliomas are graded based on histopathologic features that predict aggressiveness; tumors with malignant features are often referred to as *high-grade gliomas* (HGGs), in contrast to "low-grade" gliomas (LGGs), which in spite of their more benign histologic appearance, are not clinically benign. The location and invasiveness of most LGGs that occur in adults often makes them difficult to completely resect, leading to recurrent disease, as well as significant morbidity and mortality. The lowest grade gliomas (such as pilocytic astrocytomas) are an exception and are often surgically curable but they rarely occur in adults.

EPIDEMIOLOGY

Gliomas are relatively rare tumors with an estimated annual incidence of 4.67 to 6.02 per 100,000 persons. HGGs have an increasing incidence with age and are significantly more common than their low-grade counterparts, which appear more frequently in young adults. In general, the incidence of gliomas is higher in men than in women and in non-Hispanic whites than in blacks, Hispanics, Asians, or Native Americans.

There are very few known risk factors for the development of glioma, and no preventative measures or lifestyle changes are known to decrease an individual's risk. Several rare genetic tumor predisposition syndromes are associated with increased glioma incidence, including the neurofibromatoses, tuberous sclerosis, Cowden, Li-Fraumeni, and Turcot syndromes. Exposure to ionizing radiation is the only established environmental risk factor that can lead to glioma development. Frequent concerns about head injury, pesticides, occupational exposures, and foods containing N-nitroso compounds or aspartame appear to be unfounded or at least unproven. Although there has been concern about cell phones and other electromagnetic fields, existing evidence is conflicting and often limited by confounding recall bias and other shortcomings of retrospective study design. To date, there is no convincing evidence that cell phone use increases the risk of brain tumors, although studies continue.

CLINICAL FEATURES

Like patients with brain metastases, patients with gliomas present with diverse nonspecific clinical symptoms and signs that are related to tumor location, size, and growth rate rather than tumor type, except perhaps seizures which may be more common from oligodendrogliomas. Focal symptoms such as hemiparesis, aphasia, ataxia, visual field deficits, or cranial neuropathies result from localized invasion or compression of critical brain structures, whereas generalized symptoms such as headache, vomiting, lethargy, and confusion tend to be the result of increased intracranial pressure from tumor mass, edema, or hydrocephalus. Seizures resulting from an underlying glioma invariably begin focally but may rapidly generalize, making it difficult to recognize their partial onset. Although seizures or symptoms from hemorrhage appear suddenly, most other symptoms produced by gliomas present subacutely over days to weeks. HGGs tend to present with more rapidly progressive focal or generalized symptoms, whereas LGGs frequently precipitate seizures without progressive neurologic deficits. Depending on location, even large tumors can produce surprisingly few symptoms, as in the case of LGGs, to which the brain can gradually adapt. Consequently, an apparently normal neurologic exam cannot rule out an underlying glioma, and a thorough history and physical exam must be coupled with a high degree of clinical suspicion in order to know when to consider the diagnosis and obtain neuroimaging.

DIAGNOSIS

Brain or spinal cord magnetic resonance imaging (MRI) with and without gadolinium contrast is the imaging modality of choice when a CNS tumor is suspected. MRI provides superior resolution and tissue characterization compared to computed tomography (CT) scanning and has become an integral part of tumor diagnosis, treatment planning, surveillance, and therapeutic monitoring. MRI sequences required for adequate tumor characterization include T2/fluid-attenuated inversion recovery (FLAIR) and T1 pre– and post–gadolinium contrast–enhanced images. High-resolution three-dimensional (3D) T1-weighted sequences allow improved visualization in multiple orientations and are often used in presurgical planning and subsequent monitoring. Additional useful imaging includes diffusion-weighted images (DWI) with apparent diffusion coefficient (ADC) maps, as well as susceptibility-weighted images (SWI).

Gliomas generally appear as infiltrating, poorly defined white matter lesions that are hyperintense on T2/FLAIR and hypointense on T1-weighted images. Gliomas predominantly arise in the cerebral hemispheres, although brain stem and cerebellar locations are common in children. Although there are exceptions, most LGGs in adults tend to be infiltrative and nonenhancing with mild to moderate mass effect, whereas HGGs are more often heterogeneously enhancing, frequently with regions of necrosis and marked surrounding T2/FLAIR hyperintense edema contributing to more significant mass effect. Gadolinium enhancement is the result of contrast leakage from abnormal tumor vessels, and although the extent of enhancement does not always correlate with degree of malignancy, the development of new contrast enhancement can signal transformation to higher grade. It is important to remember that the area of enhancement does not define the extent of the tumor, particularly in invasive gliomas. Because of their abnormal vasculature, various tumor types, including HGGs can present with hemorrhage. For this reason, it is important to obtain delayed follow-up imaging in any patient presenting with an unexplained intracerebral hemorrhage. Similarly, although restricted diffusion on MRI is often equated with infarction or abscess, hypercellular gliomas can similarly restrict water diffusion. This finding can lead to some confusion about the diagnosis, although gliomas tend to spare cortical gray matter and do not remain confined to a single vascular territory.

In recent years, advanced imaging techniques have been developed to improve diagnostic capability and surgical planning for glioma patients. Many of these techniques aim to move beyond anatomic characterization in order to gain greater insights into tumor biology. Some of the techniques being studied for their use in glioma include magnetic resonance (MR) diffusion tensor imaging, MR perfusion, MR spectroscopy, and positron emission tomography (PET)/CT.

PATHOBIOLOGY

The diagnosis of a glioma is made based on histopathologic appearance under light microscopy, occasionally aided by immunohistochemistry and specific molecular testing. Morphologic similarity to normal glial cells is used to assign tumors to particular glioma subtypes, including astrocytoma, oligodendroglioma, mixed oligoastrocytoma, ependymoma, and glioneuronal tumors. Within each of these tumor types, the presence or absence of specific anaplastic features is used to infer tumor behavior and growth rate and to assign tumors to pathologic grades, with implications for prognosis and treatment. Some of the features that determine tumor grade include cellular atypia, anaplasia, mitotic activity, endothelial proliferation, and necrosis. Gliomas are graded using the World Health Organization (WHO) classification system that includes grades I to IV. WHO grades I and II are considered low-grade tumors, whereas WHO grades III and IV are considered high-grade, malignant tumors. Based on their pathologic appearance, LGGs have occasionally been referred to as *benign*; however, this term is a misnomer, as the clinical course of LGGs in adults almost always includes recurrence and progression to higher grade malignancy and death (except the lowest grade tumors such as pilocytic astrocytomas described further in the following text).

Glioma grade is determined by the highest grade features identified, even if those features are restricted to a small region within the tumor. Because of the location and marked heterogeneity of many gliomas, there is a risk of sampling error and undergrading, particularly when the diagnosis is made based on a stereotactic biopsy.

A rapidly increasing understanding of the molecular pathogenesis of gliomas has the potential to improve diagnosis and lead to the discovery of more effective treatments. Currently, there are a number of molecular biomarkers used to assist in establishing the diagnosis, estimating prognosis, and predicting treatment responsiveness in several glioma subtypes. Numerous additional molecular features are being studied as markers or potential targets of molecularly directed therapeutics in an attempt to improve glioma treatment.

TREATMENT

There are a number of challenges that clinicians face in the treatment of gliomas, including the location of tumors in the CNS, the tendency of gliomas to infiltrate surrounding brain or spinal cord, the potential for even low-grade tumors to transform to higher grade malignancies with aggressive behavior, the pathologic and molecular heterogeneity of many gliomas, and the ever-present blood–brain barrier that can make it difficult for systemic therapies to reach infiltrating tumor cells. Depending on the individual glioma subtype, treatment can involve any of several approaches, including surgery, radiation, and chemotherapy, in addition to medical management and close clinical and radiographic monitoring.

SURGERY

Surgical options in the management of glioma include stereotactic biopsy, subtotal resection, or more extensive surgery with attempts at gross total resection. Because of the location and invasiveness of many gliomas, complete surgical resection is often unachievable. Unfortunately, in addition, even when all visible tumors can be excised, viable microscopic glioma cells generally remain and eventually regrow. Therefore, except in cases of certain WHO grade I gliomas, where gross total resection can be curative, surgery alone is generally inadequate to serve as definitive therapy in the management of gliomas. Still, determining the extent of resection is an important consideration in the approach to glioma treatment. Because of feasibility, it has been difficult to conduct prospective randomized trials to determine whether there is a survival benefit from more extensive surgical resection. However, existing retrospective evidence and post hoc subset analyses of prospectively conducted studies support maximal safe resection and demonstrate a survival advantage with gross or near-gross total resection over biopsy. Of course, retrospective surgical data can be confounded by selection bias, as there is some evidence that tumors amendable to more extensive resection may have a more favorable prognosis independent of the extent of their resection. Still, in most cases, maximal safe resection is the goal, where the extent of resection is balanced with preservation of neurologic function. Because many gliomas can be difficult to distinguish from surrounding normal brain, intraoperative assessments of resection are often inaccurate, and the extent of resection should be measured by a postoperative MRI within 72 hours of the procedure. Functional magnetic resonance imaging (fMRI), intraoperative mapping, and the emerging use of intraoperative imaging can enable more extensive resection, particularly when tumors occupy eloquent brain regions. Even in the case of partial resection, surgery can often improve neurologic function, reduce symptoms and mass effect, and decrease corticosteroid requirements. In addition, because tissue obtained at surgery is important not only for diagnosis but also for molecular and clinical trial testing, subtotal resection can be a reasonable approach in many cases. In those cases where no significant resection can be achieved because of tumor location, a stereotactic biopsy should be performed in order to establish the diagnosis, although the limited amount of tissue obtained may preclude molecular characterization. In the end, the major objectives of surgery for most gliomas are to obtain adequate tissue for an accurate histologic diagnosis, to reduce mass effect when necessary, and if possible, to remove as much of the tumor as can be safely resected. Following surgery for many glioma subtypes, radiation and chemotherapy can serve as important adjuncts, although the optimal timing and dose may vary.

RADIATION THERAPY

Radiation therapy (RT) induces DNA strand breaks either directly (in the case of particle therapy) or indirectly through the production of reactive oxygen free radicals (in the case of photon therapy). Cells undergoing mitosis are more sensitive to the damaging effects of RT, and cancer cells are targeted by virtue of their rapid division and impaired DNA repair mechanisms. RT is generally delivered in repeated doses known as *fractions* in order to allow normal cells to repair sublethal damage. The radiation tolerance of the CNS is primarily influenced by the dose per fraction, and radiation side effects in the late-reacting CNS tend to appear months to years after RT is completed. Most RT for glioma involves fractionated external beam photon (x-ray) therapy generated by linear accelerators. Treatment involves delivery of radiation beams from several directions converging on the treatment area of interest. Dose varies depending on the tumor type, but fractions of 1.8 to 2 Gy are typically delivered to a total dose of 40 to 60 Gy. RT planning involves targeting the T2/FLAIR-defined glioma volume plus a 1.5- to 2-cm margin for subclinical infiltrative disease and a small volume for uncertainties in planning or treatment delivery.

A number of RT techniques improve the ability to more precisely target tumor while sparing normal surrounding brain tissue with the intent of minimizing toxicity. Intensity-modulated radiation therapy (IMRT), together with 3D conformal planning, allows for delivery of RT that better conforms to the contours of the intended treatment area. Single fraction stereotactic radiosurgery (SRS) or radiotherapy (SRT) given in a few fractions, involves the use of many focused radiation beams to target a small, well-defined area while delivering minimal dose to surrounding structures. Because of its small well-defined target volume, SRS/SRT is not ideal for most infiltrating gliomas and is not used routinely for initial radiotherapy, although it is occasionally used for focal recurrences. Proton beam RT is a particle-based therapy whose advantage is the delivery of ionizing radiation at a defined target depth while sparing tissue both superficial and deep to the target. Because of limited availability and waiting time, proton therapy is generally reserved for pediatric patients with low-grade tumors who are likely to benefit most from decreased risk of long-term side effects following RT to a developing brain. In spite of high-dose focal RT, most gliomas eventually recur at the original site of treatment, suggesting persistence of residual disease. Unfortunately, efforts to increase RT dose and to develop RT sensitizers have been unsuccessful to date. Reirradiation carries an increased risk of neurotoxicity and radiation necrosis, although it can be considered when tumor growth occurs outside of the prior radiation field or when substantial time has elapsed since the prior treatment.

CHEMOTHERAPY

Because of the infiltrative nature of glial neoplasms, microscopic cancer cells extend beyond the area of MRI abnormality. Local therapy with surgery and RT are often not enough to prevent tumor recurrence, and systemic therapy is generally required. Numerous chemotherapeutic agents have been used in the treatment of both LGGs and HGGs, including alkylating agents, antimetabolites, topoisomerase inhibitors, and taxanes, to name a few. Most traditional chemotherapeutics work by inducing DNA damage or blocking DNA replication, with the greatest effect seen in rapidly dividing cells. Unfortunately, very few drugs have been proven to be effective in the treatment of gliomas. Alkylating agents such as the nitrosoureas and temozolomide have been the most successful agents in the treatment of glioma and remain a mainstay of current therapy (Table 96.1).

More recently, molecularly targeted agents have been developed in an attempt to inhibit glioma growth. Bevacizumab is a humanized monoclonal antibody that binds vascular endothelial growth factor (VEGF) preventing activation of VEGF receptors (VEGFRs), one of the major signals used by tumors to recruit new blood vessels. In highly vascular HGGs, bevacizumab has been shown to normalize abnormal tumor vessels and improve enhancement, mass effect, and edema. Bevacizumab is used in the treatment of recurrent HGGs and occasionally newly diagnosed HGGs in select circumstances, although its ultimate benefits and role are still being defined. A large number of other molecularly targeted agents are being tested in clinical trials with gliomas. Significant preclinical research and clinical trial work aimed at identifying effective treatments for glioma are ongoing.

ASTROCYTOMAS

PILOCYTIC ASTROCYTOMA

Definition and Epidemiology

Pilocytic astrocytomas are relatively well-circumscribed World Health Organization (WHO) grade I astrocytic gliomas that primarily occur in children and young adults. Pilocytic astrocytomas make up 5% to 6% of all gliomas and are the most common glioma in children but only rarely appear in older adults. They exhibit slow indolent growth, and unlike most other LGGs, can often be cured with complete resection. Pilocytic astrocytomas are associated with neurofibromatosis type I where they are estimated to occur in 15% to 20% of patients.

Clinical and Imaging Features

Pilocytic astrocytomas can occur anywhere in the neuraxis, although they most frequently arise in the cerebellum. They also have a predilection for the anterior optic pathway, particularly in NF1, where they display an even more indolent course than sporadic tumors. In fact, optic pathway pilocytic astrocytomas are so characteristic of NF1 that any child diagnosed with this tumor should be evaluated for NF1. Pilocytic astrocytomas present insidiously with symptoms related to their location. Infratentorial tumors often present with progressive headache, nausea, and vomiting related to hydrocephalus, whereas optic pathway tumors present with progressive visual loss or proptosis. Seizures are an uncommon presentation, as these tumors rarely involve cerebral cortex. On MRI, pilocytic astrocytomas appear well-circumscribed with bright contrast enhancement and frequent cyst formation. Despite their defined border, pilocytic astrocytomas do not have a true capsule, and although they are considered noninvasive, they often microscopically infiltrate surrounding brain parenchyma.

Pilocytic astrocytomas generally maintain their WHO grade I status for years and only rarely undergo malignant transformation. Approximately 60% to 80% of sporadic non–NF1-associated pilocytic astrocytomas have been shown to contain a novel BRAF-KIAA

TABLE 96.1 Overview of Chemotherapeutic Agents Used Most Frequently in the Treatment of Glioma

Drug	Indication	Dose Regimen	Side Effects	Monitoring

Temozolomide	GBM
	Anaplastic astrocytoma/
	  oligodendroglioma
	Low-grade glioma
		Chemoradiation: 75 mg/m^2/
		  day PO daily for 6 wk
		Adjuvant: 150–200 mg/m^2/day
		  for 5 days every 28 days
			Nausea, vomiting
			Fatigue
			Myelosuppression—
			  especially lymphope-
			  nia, thrombocytopenia
				CBC with differen-
				  tial weekly during
				  chemoradiation,
				  days 21 and 28 dur-
				  ing adjuvant dosing,
				  or more frequently

Lomustine CCNU (PCV)	GBM (recurrent)
	Low-grade glioma
	Anaplastic
	Oligodendroglioma
		90–110 mg/m^2 PO as single
		  dose every 6 wk
			Nausea, vomiting,
			  myelosuppression—
			  especially lymphopenia,
			  thrombocytopenia
			Pulmonary fibrosis
				CBC with differential
				  weekly × 6 wk,
				Hepatic and renal
				  function
				Pulmonary func-
				  tion at baseline
				  and periodically
				  thereafter

Carmustine BCNU	GBM (recurrent)	150–200 mg/m^2 IV as single
		  dose every 6 wk
			Nausea, vomiting,
			  myelosuppression
			Pulmonary fibrosis
			Headache, rare infusion
			  reaction	

Carmustine wafers	GBM	Up to eight wafers (61.6 mg)
		  implanted in the surgical
		  bed at time of resection
			CNS edema/local inflam-
			  mation, infection, CSF
			  leak, seizures
				Clinical monitoring
				  for seizure/CNS
				  infection/edema

Procarbazine (PCV)	Low-grade glioma
	Anaplastic
	Oligodendroglioma
		60–75 mg/m^2 PO days 8–21
		  every 6 wk
			Nausea, vomiting,
			  myelosuppression,
			  encephalopathy
				CBC with differential
				Hepatic and renal
				  function tests

Vincristine (PCV)	Low-grade glioma
	Anaplastic
	Oligodendroglioma
		1.4 mg/m^2 IV days 8 and 29
		  every 6 wk
			Sensorimotor peripheral
			  neuropathy, seizures
				CBC with differential,
				  electrolytes, hepatic
				  function, uric acid
				  levels

Bevacizumab	Recurrent GBM	10 mg/kg IV every 2 wk	Hemorrhage, thrombosis,
			  impaired wound heal-
			  ing, HTN, proteinuria
				CBC with differential,
				  blood pressure,
				  urine protein

GBM, glioblastoma; PO, by mouth; CBC, complete blood count; PCV, procarbazine, lomustine, and vincristine; IV, intravenous; CNS, central nervous system; CSF, cerebrospinal fluid; HTN, hypertension.

fusion that appears to predict improved survival following partial resection and raises the possibility that these tumors could be treated with BRAF inhibition.

Treatment and Outcome

Gross total resection of pilocytic astrocytomas can be curative and should be the primary treatment consideration whenever possible. Even partial resection can lead to long-term survival with up to 87% and 82% of patients surviving at 10 and 20 years, although significant morbidity can result from persistent unresected tumor. Regardless of the extent of resection, patients must be followed long-term to monitor for infrequent progression. Because of their indolent natural history, even partially resected pilocytic astrocytomas can be subsequently monitored without adjuvant therapy until there is evidence of further growth. Documented cases of spontaneous remission following partial resection appear to validate this wait-and-see approach. RT or chemotherapy (temozolomide, bevacizumab, and irinotecan have been used) can be considered in cases with inoperable or progressive tumors, although the long-term benefits of these modalities are uncertain. The prognosis from pilocytic astrocytoma depends on resectability, as those that cannot be completely resected tend to recur. Malignant transformation only occurs in a minority (~5%) of cases, although there is unfortunately no way to predict which tumors will transform.

DIFFUSE ASTROCYTOMA

Definition and Epidemiology

Diffuse astrocytomas are WHO grade II infiltrative astrocytic tumors that typically affect otherwise healthy young adults. They are fairly well-differentiated tumors with a slow, indolent early course, although they have the tendency to eventually undergo malignant transformation to high grade (Fig. 96.1). Diffuse astrocytomas make up 10% to 15% of all astrocytic tumors with an annual incidence of 1.4 per 1 million and a peak incidence in the fourth decade of life.

Clinical and Imaging Features

Diffuse astrocytomas can occur anywhere in the CNS, although they preferentially arise in the cerebral hemispheres in adults. In children, they often occur in the brain stem as diffuse intrinsic pontine gliomas. Diffuse astrocytomas most frequently present with seizures but depending on location can also cause focal symptoms or cognitive and behavioral change. Diffuse astrocytomas generally appear as ill-defined homogeneous regions with T1 hypointense signal and T2/FLAIR hyperintensity, although they tend to infiltrate beyond the T2/FLAIR margins visible on MRI. Diffuse astrocytomas generally have minimal contrast enhancement, and the

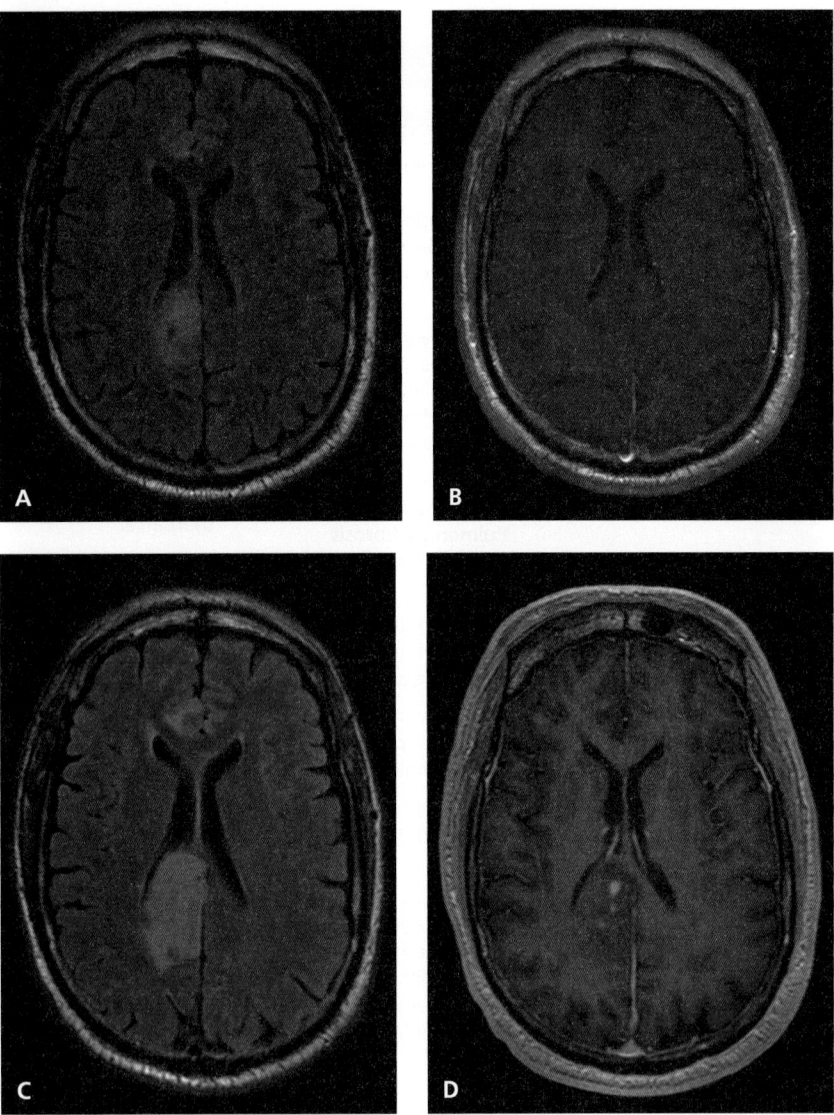

FIGURE 96.1 Diffuse astrocytoma, WHO II with progression to anaplastic astrocytoma WHO III. T2-weighted FLAIR **(A)** and gadolinium contrast–enhanced T1-weighted. **(B)** MRI sequences of a patient with diffuse astrocytoma that despite radiation years gradually progressed over 10 years with more extensive T2/FLAIR signal **(C)** and the development of patchy enhancement **(D)** that was proven by biopsy to represent transformation to anaplastic astrocytoma.

development of new contrast enhancement can signal progression to higher grade (see Fig. 96.1).

Pathologic and Molecular Features

Diffuse astrocytomas are made up of well-differentiated astrocytes with increased cellularity and occasionally demonstrate nuclear atypia but rare mitotic activity, with Ki-67/MIB-1 staining growth fraction typically less than 4%. By definition, diffuse astrocytomas have no necrosis or endovascular proliferation. Although they appear fairly benign histologically, diffuse astrocytomas are not clinically benign, with a high rate of transformation to malignancy over the course of years. Point mutations in the isocitrate dehydrogenase enzyme IDH1 (R132), or rarely IDH2 (R172), are present in the majority (65% to 80%) of grades II and III gliomas, including 75% of diffuse astrocytoma. The presence of an IDH mutation is a favorable prognostic factor regardless of tumor type, and IDH mutation can be detected by immunohistochemistry, polymerase chain reaction (PCR), and MR spectroscopy. Methylation of the O6-methylguanine-DNA methyltransferase (MGMT) promoter, which leads to MGMT gene silencing is also common in diffuse astrocytoma and is associated with improved prognosis and alkylating agent chemosensitivity.

Treatment and Outcome

The approach to diffuse astrocytoma is complex, and a number of questions remain regarding various aspects treatment. Management incorporating observation, surgery, RT, and chemotherapy is individualized based on tumor location, molecular profile, and patient characteristics. Because of the indolent nature of diffuse astrocytoma, the potential benefits of treatment must also be weighed against the risk of long-term side effects, and there may be a role for delayed intervention in minimally symptomatic patients with limited disease. Although diffuse astrocytoma is a low-grade tumor, current therapies do not offer a cure, and the goal of treatment is to ameliorate symptoms and delay or prevent transformation to high grade, balanced against treatment-induced toxicities. The mainstay of initial treatment involves surgery and RT, although uncertainty remains surrounding the timing of these interventions as well as the ultimate role of chemotherapy.

Available evidence increasingly supports surgical resection over observation and appears to suggest a survival benefit from more extensive resection. Immediate surgery is generally recommended for patients with large symptomatic tumors, although the management of small minimally symptomatic tumors is less clear. In this patient population, available studies also appear to show a trend toward improved survival with immediate surgery, although monitoring for clinical or radiographic progression is also an option. Of course, the diffuse infiltrative nature of these tumors makes gross total resection difficult, and subtotal resection or a biopsy is often the only viable option. For patients with significant residual tumor remaining after surgery, adjuvant RT or chemotherapy is often considered.

Although RT is a frequent component of the treatment of diffuse astrocytoma, the optimal timing remains somewhat unclear. Clinical trial evidence has attempted to define the optimal parameters of RT as well as its benefits in diffuse astrocytoma. Two studies addressing RT dose found that lower doses of RT (either 45 or 50.4 Gy) were equivalent to higher dose RT (59.4 or 64.8 Gy) [**Level 1**],[1,2] and as a result, most patients currently receive 50 to 54 Gy. Regarding the timing of RT, one seminal study showed that postoperative RT delayed the time to progression but did not prolong overall survival [**Level 1**].[3] In light of the potential long-term neurocognitive effects of RT, these results have been used to justify delaying RT, although tumor progression may also negatively impact cognitive function. Early treatment may be most justified in patients with significant symptoms or radiographic progression or in patients at high risk for progression (those older than 40 years old, with >5-cm preoperative tumor or incomplete resection, MIB-1 >3%).

The role for chemotherapy in diffuse astrocytoma continues to be defined. Most studies addressing this question do not separate diffuse astrocytoma from other LGGs (such as oligodendrogliomas that are often more responsive to chemotherapy), making it difficult to draw specific conclusions about individual tumor types. A study examining the role of chemotherapy in "high-risk LGGs" (defined as age younger than 40 years with subtotal resection or biopsy or age older than 40 years with any extent of resection), including diffuse astrocytoma, compared RT alone to RT followed by 6 months of chemotherapy with procarbazine, lomustine, and vincristine (PCV) [**Level 1**].[4] Long-term follow-up demonstrated a statistically significant improvement in overall survival (13.3 years vs. 7.8 years) from the addition of PCV chemotherapy to RT versus RT alone. Details have not yet been published, including how much of this effect is explained by the more chemosensitive oligodendrogliomas. The specific type of chemotherapy is also an area of uncertainty; PCV and temozolomide have both been studied, but there have been no trials directly comparing the two. Regardless, temozolomide is often preferred because it has fewer side effects and is easier to administer. Preliminary results of a study comparing chemotherapy to RT in high-risk LGG patients showed no difference in overall survival, although patients with retained 1p19q appeared to have improved outcomes with RT.

The prognosis for patients with diffuse astrocytoma is highly variable, driven largely by the rate of transformation to higher grade. Mean survival is in the range of 6 to 8 years, and prognostic features include age; functional status; neurologic deficits; tumor size and degree of resection; presence of enhancement; and molecular markers such as MIB-1, MGMT methylation, IDH mutation, and 1p19q codeletion. Regardless of treatment, tumors inevitably recur and often transform to anaplastic astrocytoma or glioblastoma.

ANAPLASTIC ASTROCYTOMA AND GLIOBLASTOMA

Definition and Epidemiology

Anaplastic astrocytoma is a diffusely infiltrating WHO grade III glioma with significant proliferative activity and rapid growth (see Fig. 96.1C and D). Anaplastic astrocytomas have a strong tendency to progress to glioblastoma (GBM), a WHO grade IV glioma with highly infiltrative, vascular, necrotic growth (Fig. 96.2). These tumors are characterized as high-grade or malignant gliomas. GBM is the most common primary malignant brain tumor, with an annual incidence of approximately three or four cases per 100,000 persons. GBM accounts for 60% to 80% of malignant gliomas, whereas anaplastic astrocytomas make up 10% to 15%, and the remainder consists of anaplastic oligodendrogliomas, anaplastic oligoastrocytomas, and anaplastic ependymomas (see the following section). These rapidly progressive, uniformly fatal glial neoplasms can either evolve from LGGs or can arise de novo. They primarily affect adults with a mean age at diagnosis around 45 years for anaplastic astrocytoma and 64 years for GBM.

Clinical and Imaging Features

Anaplastic astrocytomas and GBMs preferentially arise in the white matter of the cerebral hemispheres. Symptoms result from tumor location and mass effect and can include headaches, focal neurologic deficits, or seizures. More than half of patients present with headache, and although classic brain tumor headaches occur in the morning and are associated with nausea and vomiting, these symptoms are only seen in a minority of patients; most headaches are indistinguishable from tension headache. Seizures are more common in anaplastic gliomas than GBM. Malignant gliomas are hypointense on T1-weighted MRI sequences and hyperintense on T2/FLAIR with poorly defined margins. They generally have marked heterogeneous enhancement, although some anaplastic astrocytomas do not enhance. Marked central necrosis and surrounding edema are frequent in GBM (see Fig. 96.2) and typically less prominent in anaplastic astrocytoma. Importantly, in up to 40% of patients receiving initial treatment with RT and chemotherapy, early imaging can demonstrate increased enhancement and edema. Although these findings appear consistent with early tumor progression, in up to half of patients, the changes are actually the result of increased vessel permeability from treatment, a phenomenon known as *pseudoprogression*. A role for MR spectroscopy, MR perfusion, and PET is being explored to better diagnose malignant glioma and to distinguish tumor progression from treatment-related pseudoprogression.

Pathologic and Molecular Features

Anaplastic astrocytomas contain diffusely infiltrating astrocytes that have increased cellularity and atypia compared with LGGs, as well as evidence of mitotic activity. GBMs additionally contain either microvascular proliferation or regions of necrosis or both.

Malignant gliomas are thought to arise as a cumulative result of a series of oncogenic alterations, and it is clear that tumors that arise de novo possess distinct molecular alterations from those that evolve from lower grade tumors. GBM was among the first human tumors to undergo comprehensive genomic characterization, and the results defined significantly amplified and deleted and mutated genes that led to an appreciation of the high incidence of p53, Rb, and receptor tyrosine kinase (RTK) pathway dysregulation in GBM. Expression profiling was subsequently used to define GBM subclasses. There are significant ongoing efforts to design and test therapeutics that will specifically target the molecular alterations found in malignant glioma. For the time being, however, and despite all that is known about the genetic alterations and subclasses within HGG, the best available treatment continues to be conventional approaches, including surgery, RT, and chemotherapy.

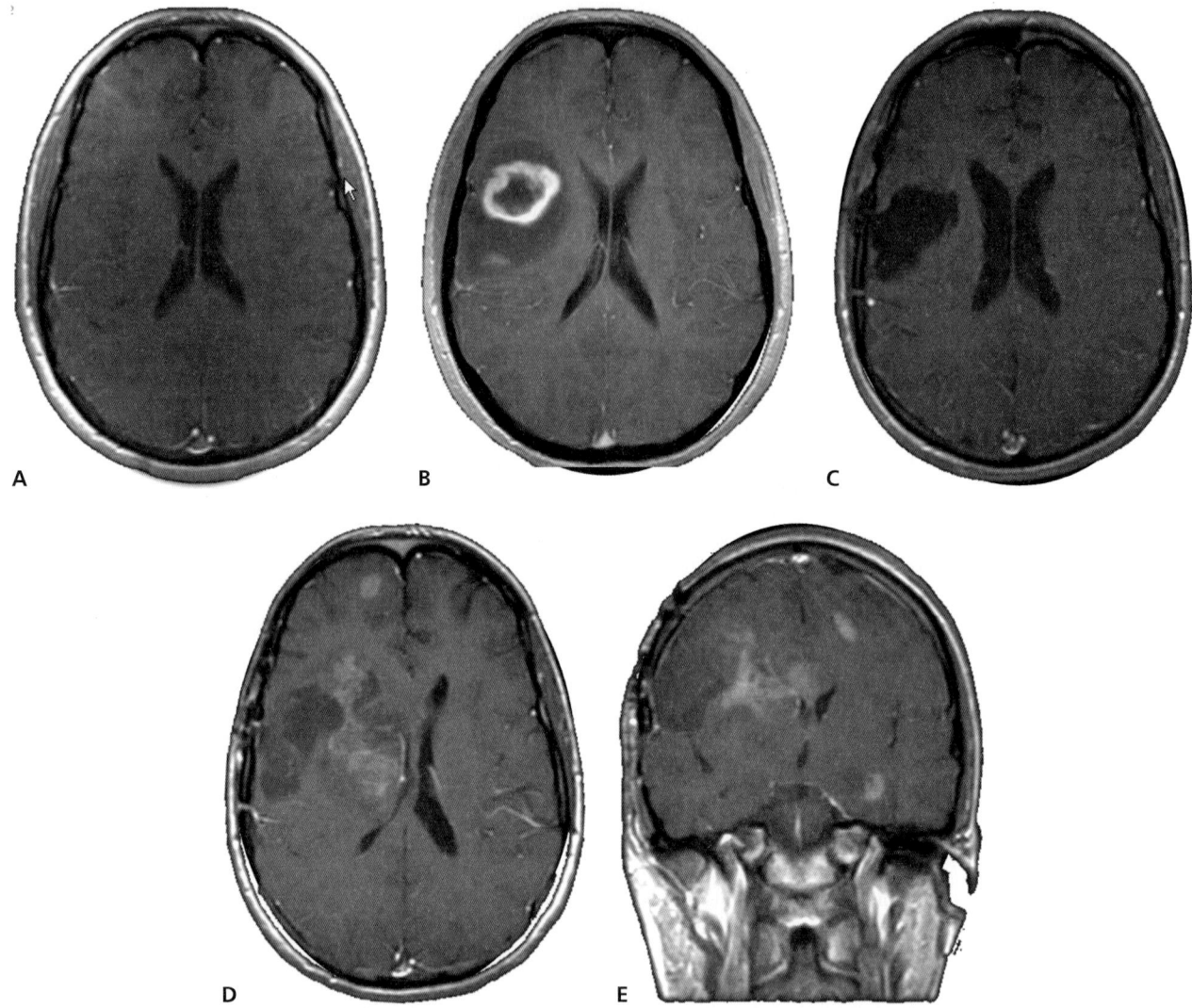

FIGURE 96.2 Glioblastoma. Gadolinium contrast–enhanced T1-weighted MRI images of a patient who initially presented with headaches and had unremarkable imaging **(A)**. The patient developed facial weakness that led to a repeat MRI just 3 months later that revealed a centrally necrotic peripherally enhancing mass **(B)**. Gross total resection led to the diagnosis of glioblastoma **(C)**, but despite chemoradiation, within 6 months, the patient's tumor recurred **(D)** and infiltrated the contralateral hemisphere **(E)**.

Treatment and Outcome

The overall approach to the treatment of HGGs involves maximal safe resection followed by RT and chemotherapy (Fig. 96.3). Because anaplastic astrocytoma is much less common than GBM, the approach for both tumor types is generally based on treatment established in GBM although this approach is controversial.

In spite of the fact that malignant glioma's infiltrative nature precludes a complete resection of all tumor cells, current evidence suggests that there is a survival advantage from more extensive resection. Although the data is largely retrospective, several studies have proposed thresholds for extent of resection (88% to 89% or 95% to 98%), above which there is a significant improvement in overall survival. Resection also enhances diagnostic accuracy and provides tissue for molecular testing that is important for prognostication and some treatment decisions. Still, in spite of attempts to achieve gross total resection in patients with malignant glioma, viable tumor cells inevitably remain and local recurrence is the rule

(see Fig. 96.2), necessitating additional treatment with RT and systemic agents.

RT plays a central role in the treatment of patients with malignant glioma and is important for treating both gross and microscopic infiltrative disease that cannot be resected. Adjuvant RT following surgery has had the greatest impact on the survival of patients with GBM, prolonging overall survival on average from 3 to 4 months to 7 to 12 months. RT should be considered in all patients and typically consists of involved field external beam RT delivered 5 days per week in fractions of 1.8 to 2.0 Gy to a total dose of 60 Gy. Because of the infiltrative character of malignant gliomas, there is no clear role for stereotactic radiosurgery or brachytherapy in the up-front treatment of malignant glioma. In spite of prior attempts to treat microscopic disease with larger fields and higher RT doses, the majority of malignant gliomas recur at the original site, and increasing the field size increases toxicity without improving survival. Further complicating the early picture is the fact that

FIGURE 96.3 Overview of the treatment of glioblastoma.

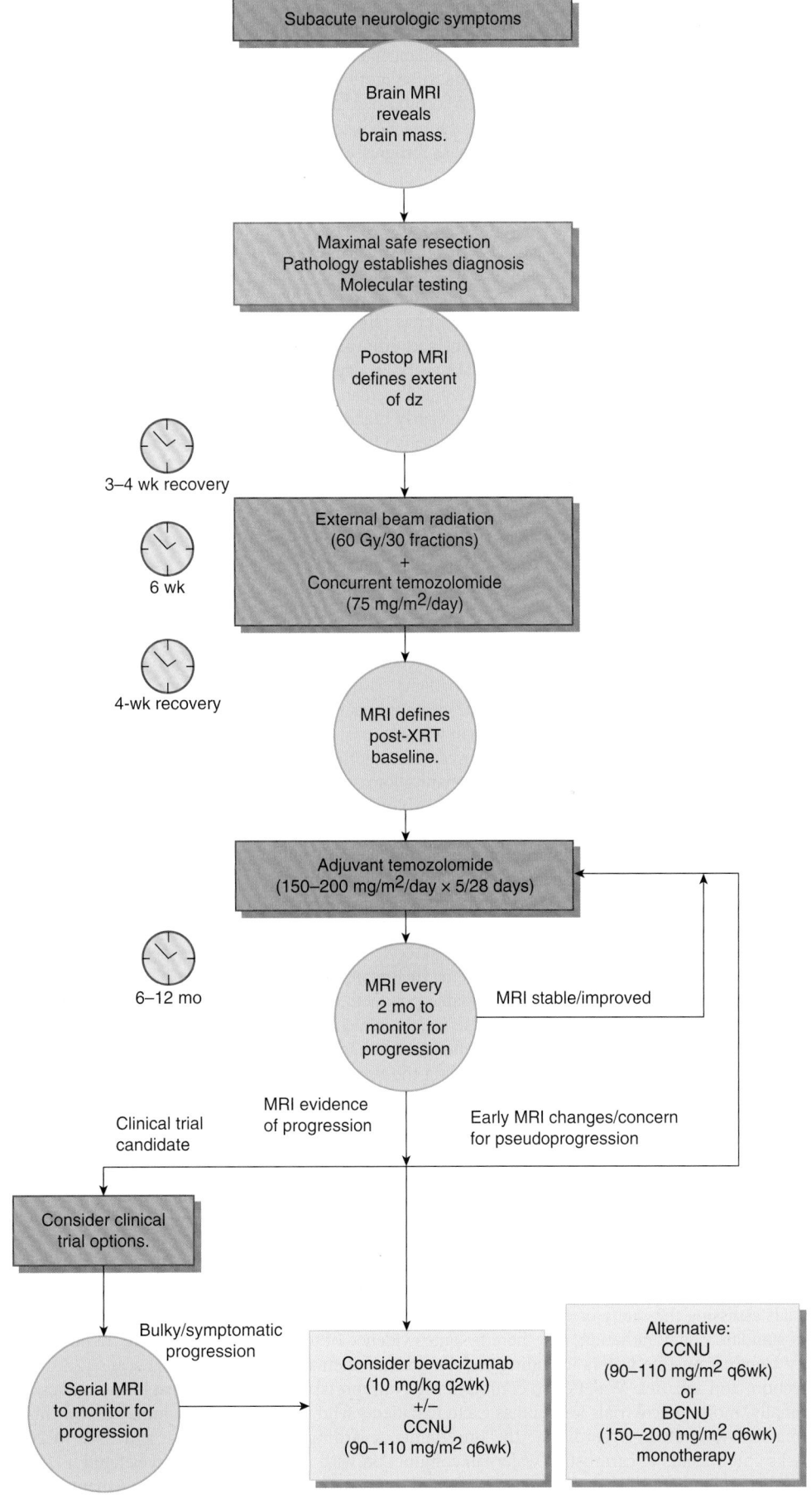

early MRI changes related to RT and chemotherapy can mimic disease progression (pseudoprogression), as either can destabilize the blood–brain barrier, leading to nonspecific enhancement, edema, and mass effect. Pseudoprogression appears to be more common in patients with tumors that harbor MGMT promoter methylation, although MGMT methylation status cannot be relied on to distinguish pseudoprogression from disease progression in an individual patient.

Chemotherapy plays an important role in the management of patients with malignant glioma. Temozolomide is an oral DNA alkylating agent that is administered together with RT, followed by at least six monthly adjuvant cycles as a part of the current standard of care in GBM [**Level 1**].[5,6] Temozolomide was shown to improve overall survival in a randomized phase III study that compared RT alone to RT plus concurrent and adjuvant temozolomide (150 to 200 mg/m^2/day for 5 days every 28 days for six cycles). The addition of temozolomide prolonged median survival from 12.1 to 14.6 months and led to significantly higher rates of survival at 2 years (26.5% vs. 10.4%) and 5 years (10% vs. 2%). A companion study analyzed tumor tissue for epigenetic silencing of MGMT, the DNA repair protein that is responsible in part for reversing the effects of temozolomide. That study found that patients whose tumors had methylation of the MGMT promoter had a greater benefit from temozolomide (21.7-month median survival and 46% 2-year survival) compared with patients without promoter methylation (12.7-month median survival, 13.8% 2-year survival) [**Level 1**].[7] Therefore, MGMT promoter methylation has subsequently been established as a predictor of benefit from temozolomide, especially in elderly patients. However, patients with GBMs that do not harbor MGMT promoter methylation also survive longer with temozolomide than without it. Therefore, in the absence of proven effective alternatives, temozolomide continues to be used in the treatment of malignant glioma regardless of MGMT promoter methylation status. Temozolomide is easily administered and generally well tolerated, with an acceptable side effect profile that consists primarily of nausea, fatigue, and mild myelosuppression, with the greatest effects on platelet number. Perhaps more importantly, MGMT methylation is also a prognostic marker in newly diagnosed GBM, associated with longer survival regardless of treatment administered.

Another chemotherapeutic approach to the treatment of malignant glioma involves the use of biodegradable polymers containing the alkylating agent carmustine. These wafers, which can be implanted into a tumor bed immediately after resection, gradually release carmustine into the tissue surrounding the resection cavity in order to kill residual tumor cells. A phase III trial for newly diagnosed disease suggested a modest survival benefit from wafer implantation at the time of resection, with median survival increasing from 11.6 to 13.9 months, which led to U.S. Food and Drug Administration (FDA) approval for the initial treatment of malignant glioma [**Level 1**].[8] However, the up-front use of carmustine wafers was not compared with standard temozolomide chemotherapy, so data are lacking to indicate whether there is a survival advantage over standard therapy. In addition, there are no trials assessing the safety or efficacy of adding carmustine wafers to standard chemoradiation, and there is some evidence of toxicity from carmustine wafers including increased brain edema, infection, and seizures. Wafers also confound MRI interpretability. Finally, most clinical trials for gliomas exclude patients who were treated with wafers. Accordingly, the uncertainty regarding the risks and benefits of carmustine wafers in conjunction with standard chemoradiation has limited the adoption of this approach in the initial treatment of malignant glioma, and they have fallen out of favor in recent years.

Despite aggressive treatment with surgery, RT, and chemotherapy, malignant gliomas inevitably recur, on average 7 to 10 months after initial diagnosis. As mentioned earlier, progressive disease can be difficult to distinguish from the early radiographic changes caused by concurrent chemoradiation. Tissue sampling can be required to distinguish between progressive disease and pseudoprogression, although even pathology can demonstrate a mixture of both processes. Patients with early imaging changes are typically continued on adjuvant temozolomide with close radiographic follow-up, unless significant symptoms warrant treatment with corticosteroids, surgery, or bevacizumab. If reresection is considered for the treatment of recurrent disease, consideration may also be given to carmustine wafers, which have been shown to prolong survival compared with placebo (31 vs. 23 weeks) in a randomized phase III trial [**Level 1**].[9] Unfortunately, for most patients, surgery cannot be considered because of the location, extent, or multifocality of the recurrent tumor. Alternatively, reirradiation can occasionally be considered if tumor recurrence arises outside of the prior radiation field or if it has been some time since initial radiotherapy. SRS or SRT are occasionally used for focal recurrences, although the role of these treatment modalities is still being defined, as the disease is inherently diffuse.

In most cases of recurrent malignant glioma, where surgery and RT are not viable options, systemic agents are the primary therapeutic consideration. Unfortunately, none of the available salvage therapies has been definitively shown to prolong survival, and therefore, the risks of treatment need to be carefully weighed. In patients with adequate performance status, participation in clinical trials should be seriously considered. There are a large number of clinical trials testing a host of different agents in recurrent GBM, although fewer trial options exist for patients with anaplastic astrocytoma. In patients who are not clinical trial candidates, a number of salvage chemotherapy options exist, including readministration of temozolomide or other alkylating agents including nitrosoureas or carboplatin or treatment with the antiangiogenic agent bevacizumab. Another treatment that has been FDA approved for use in recurrent GBM is a portable device that applies low-intensity alternating electrical fields to the scalp. The NovoTTF-100A was approved based on a phase III trial that showed comparable efficacy but less toxicity than salvage chemotherapy. Unfortunately, the trial did not employ a noninferiority design necessary to make an adequate comparison between treatments, and the role of NovoTTF in the treatment of recurrent GBM therefore remains unclear.

Particularly for those patients with significant symptoms or mass effect, bevacizumab is an important therapeutic option at recurrence, either alone or in combination with cytotoxic chemotherapy. Bevacizumab is a humanized monoclonal antibody directed against VEGF, a key mediator of vascular permeability and angiogenesis. In highly vascular malignant glioma, bevacizumab often results in normalization of tumor blood vessels and a rapid decrease in enhancement, peritumoral edema, and mass effect. A phase II study of bevacizumab with or without concurrent administration of the topoisomerase inhibitor irinotecan in GBM demonstrated radiographic responses in the form of improved brain MRI scans (28% to 39%) with an increase in the percentage of patients experiencing disease control at 6 months (42% to 50%) compared with historical controls (5% to 9% radiographic response and 15% to 20% disease control at 6 months), which led to accelerated FDA approval of bevacizumab for recurrent GBM. Improvements on MRI are often accompanied by symptom improvement and decreased corticosteroid requirements, although the effects on overall survival are less clear. Uncontrolled data suggests marginally prolonged median survival compared to historical controls, and recent evidence suggests that bevacizumab administered in combination with lomustine may lead to improved overall survival compared with either bevacizumab or lomustine alone [**Level 1**].[10] Randomized studies of bevacizumab in the recurrent setting are ongoing.

However, two up-front phase III trials of bevacizumab in combination with temozolomide and RT confirmed an improvement in clinical and radiographic disease control but no overall survival benefit [**Level 1**].[11,12] At this time, bevacizumab appears to be most beneficial for patients with significant symptoms who could benefit from tumor shrinkage or decreased peritumoral edema, either at the time of initial treatment or at recurrence. Bevacizumab is generally very well tolerated, although it does carry a low risk of thromboembolism or hemorrhage. However, even in highly vascular GBM, the risk of intracerebral hemorrhage is fairly low at approximately 2% to 3%, and the benefits of treatment generally outweigh these risks. The duration of optimal therapy is uncertain, and there is some concern that withdrawal of the antiangiogenic effects of bevacizumab, even when there is evidence of progression, may lead to a rebound in the tumor-associated edema and mass effect. In fact, there is some evidence to support a continued role of bevacizumab even after progression on that treatment. However, following progression on bevacizumab, prognosis is extremely poor (3- to 4-month median survival) and no chemotherapeutic agents have proven to prolong either disease control or survival following failure of bevacizumab. Regardless of treatment, malignant glioma carries a dismal prognosis that in spite of significant scientific and technical advances has not significantly changed in the last several decades.

Median survival for patients with anaplastic astrocytoma is approximately 3 years, whereas patients with GBM have a median survival of around 15 months. Of course, prognosis varies significantly between individuals, and a small subset of patients can live a decade or longer with anaplastic astrocytoma or rarely even GBM. Prognosis is influenced by both patient factors, such as age and functional status, as well as tumor-related factors such as grade, location, extent of resection, and molecular determinants such as deletion of chromosome 1p and 19q (most common in oligodendrogliomas), MGMT promoter methylation, and the presence of IDH1/2 mutation. The best prognosis is generally found among young, otherwise healthy patients with a gross total resection and MGMT methylation and IDH1/2 mutation, but even in these cases, treatment may control disease for a time, but tumor growth inevitably recurs. In light of the significant morbidity and mortality from malignant glioma, there is a desperate need for improved treatment in this disease.

OLIGODENDROGLIOMAS

DEFINITION AND EPIDEMIOLOGY

Oligodendroglial tumors are diffusely infiltrating gliomas composed of neoplastic cells that morphologically resemble oligodendrocytes. Although these tumors exist on a continuum from well-differentiated to overtly malignant, they are categorized into two distinct prognostic groups: low-grade (WHO grade II) oligodendrogliomas and anaplastic (WHO grade III) oligodendrogliomas. Together, these tumors make up approximately 5% of all glial neoplasms, but unlike astrocytic tumors, the majority of oligodendroglial tumors are low grade, with 65% to 80% being WHO grade II oligodendrogliomas. These tumors tend to occur in patients in their 30s to 50s, with grade II lesions appearing in younger patients than their grade III counterparts.

CLINICAL AND IMAGING FEATURES

Oligodendrogliomas preferentially arise in the cortex and subcortical white matter of the cerebral hemispheres, most frequently in the frontal lobe. Approximately two-thirds of patients present with seizures, although headache or focal deficits are also common. Anaplastic oligodendrogliomas can arise de novo or as a result of progression from a WHO grade II oligodendroglioma, on average 6 to 7 years after initial diagnosis. Oligodendrogliomas respond better to treatment and have a more favorable prognosis than astrocytomas. In fact, even the presence of an oligodendroglial component, seen in mixed oligoastrocytomas, may confer a better prognosis than pure astrocytic histology. Unlike most other gliomas, oligodendroglial tumors are uniquely chemosensitive, which has led to an increasing role for chemotherapy in this disease. On MRI, oligodendrogliomas are T2/FLAIR hyperintense and infiltrative with indistinct borders (Fig. 96.4). Low-grade oligodendrogliomas

FIGURE 96.4 Low-grade oligodendroglioma, WHO II. Gadolinium contrast–enhanced T1-weighted **(A)** and T2-weighted **(B)** MRI of a patient with a largely nonenhancing infiltrative oligodendroglioma.

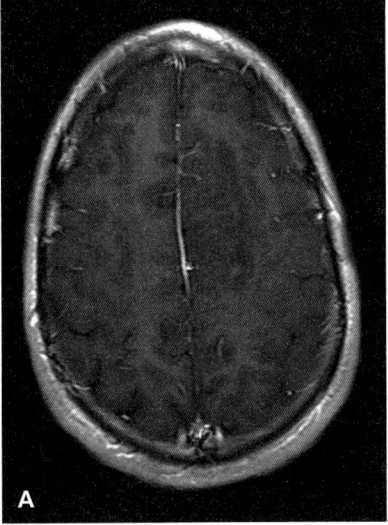
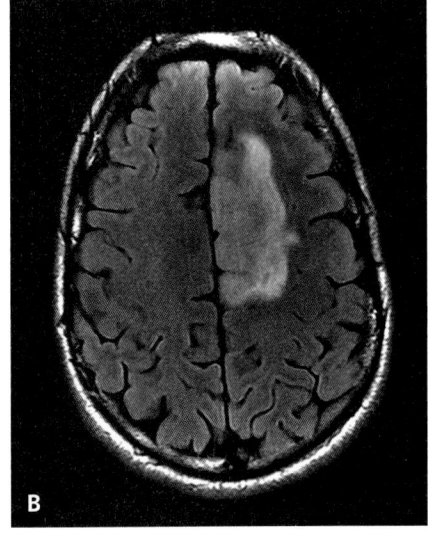

are generally nonenhancing, whereas anaplastic lesions frequently have some degree of enhancement, and calcification is characteristic of oligodendrogliomas, although this finding is not specific.

PATHOLOGIC AND MOLECULAR FEATURES

Oligodendrogliomas are composed of monomorphic cells with round nuclei and characteristic perinuclear halos that are said to look like "fried eggs" in a dense "chicken wire" network of branching capillaries. WHO grade II oligodendrogliomas may have marked cellular atypia and occasional mitoses, but the appearance of significant mitotic activity or microvascular proliferation is consistent with a diagnosis of anaplastic oligodendroglioma. The presence of necrosis warrants a diagnosis of GBM, although GBM with oligodendroglial features may have a somewhat better prognosis than a typical GBM. The majority of oligodendroglial neoplasms have evidence of codeletion of the short arm of chromosome 1 (1p) and the long arm of chromosome 19 (19q) that results from an imbalanced translocation of 1p to 19q. The frequency of 1p19q codeletion is estimated to be 80% to 90% in grade II oligodendrogliomas and 50% to 70% in anaplastic oligodendrogliomas and can be used to support the diagnosis in cases of atypical histology. This codeletion corresponds to a longer natural history and an improved response to chemotherapy and may be used to help guide therapeutic decision making. As a result of its diagnostic, prognostic, and predictive value, testing for 1p19q should be performed on all oligodendroglial tumors. Mutation in IDH1/2 is also very common, occurring in 60% to 80% of grade II and III oligodendrogliomas, where it strongly correlates with 1p19q codeletion and an improved prognosis. Recent data suggests 1p19q deleted tumors are a subset of those with IDH mutation, which also carries independent and favorable prognostic value. Together with MGMT methylation, these three correlating features are highly prognostic for longer survival of patients with oligodendroglial tumors.

TREATMENT

The approach to the management of WHO grade II oligodendrogliomas is complex, and the optimal treatment strategy for these low-grade tumors remains controversial. Because most studies have not distinguished between glioma subtypes, much of the approach to treatment is similar to that of other LGGs, although important differences are emerging. Oligodendrogliomas can be managed with a combination of observation, surgery, RT, and chemotherapy, which unfortunately, despite the indolent nature of these low-grade tumors, do not offer a cure. In light of their long natural history (average survival of approximately 10 years) and the neurotoxicity from both tumor and treatment, the central therapeutic challenge is to balance efforts to extend survival with the preservation of neurocognitive function. Although initial treatment is clearly indicated in patients older than 45 to 50 years of age, those with neurologic deficits, or with large or rapidly growing lesions, observation with close neuroradiologic follow-up can be considered in young asymptomatic patients with small or completely resected tumors.

As with other gliomas, surgery is recommended to obtain pathologic confirmation of the diagnosis, improve neurologic symptoms, and reduce tumor bulk. Gross total resection is the goal if tumor location will allow it, although tumor cells invariably remain and will eventually recur. Particularly given the highly epileptogenic nature of oligodendrogliomas, even a partial resection can improve seizure control and should be considered in cases of refractory seizure. Regardless of the extent of resection, additional therapy beyond surgery is eventually required in all patients.

Both adjuvant RT and chemotherapy are important components of treatment following resection, although optimal timing is somewhat uncertain. Early postoperative treatment is generally considered in patients who had evidence of growth, mass effect, or neurologic deficits prior to surgery but may also be considered in older patients or those with significant residual disease or large initial tumor diameter (>5 cm). Young asymptomatic patients or those with isolated preoperative seizures may be monitored closely after resection with further treatment being reserved until there is evidence of recurrent tumor growth on MRI.

In patients with oligodendroglioma that require adjuvant therapy, the roles of chemotherapy and RT continue to be defined. Early postoperative RT has been shown to improve symptoms and time to progression but not overall survival, potentially justifying delayed RT in this population with the potential for long-term survival. Some early evidence suggests that patients without 1p19q codeletion may have better outcomes with RT than chemotherapy, and adjuvant radiotherapy may be the modality of choice in this subset of patients.

In contrast, because oligodendrogliomas with 1p19q codeletion are known to be particularly chemosensitive, initial postoperative treatment with chemotherapy alone may be considered in order to delay subsequent RT and the risks of long-term neurologic side effects. Of course, the optimal chemotherapeutic regimen remains uncertain; PCV and temozolomide have both been studied, and although no trials directly compare the two, temozolomide is often preferred because of its better side effect profile and ease of administration.

With regard to survival, there is growing evidence supporting the use of both RT and chemotherapy in low-grade glioma, including oligodendroglioma, as discussed earlier with regard to low-grade astrocytoma [**Level 1**].[4] The long-term results of a study examining the addition of chemotherapy to RT have recently been released, in which high-risk low-grade glioma patients (subtotally resected or age older than 40 years) were treated with RT alone or RT followed by 6 months of PCV. Results demonstrated a statistically significant improvement in overall survival with the addition of PCV to RT (13.3 years vs. 7.8 years). Because the details have not yet been published, including whether a particular diagnostic or molecular subgroup accounts for the survival advantage, it is difficult to draw specific conclusions about oligodendrogliomas versus astrocytomas or mixed oligoastrocytomas. However, knowing that oligodendrogliomas with 1p19q codeletion are particularly sensitive to chemotherapy, it seems likely that the benefits of adjuvant chemotherapy would be greatest in this tumor type. As a result, the argument could be made that adjuvant therapy in oligodendroglioma should include both RT and chemotherapy over radiotherapy alone. Whether chemotherapy alone (with radiotherapy at recurrence rather than diagnosis to avoid late neurocognitive toxicity) shortens survival is not clear at this time.

OUTCOME

Regardless of initial treatment, oligodendrogliomas eventually recur, frequently with evidence of transformation to a higher grade. If there is radiographic evidence of new enhancement or rapid growth concerning for a malignant transformation, biopsy or reresection to confirm tumor grade may be considered. At the time of recurrence, either RT or chemotherapy may be considered, particularly if one or the other was not used during initial treatment. Reirradiation after a prior complete course of RT is not usually considered out of concern for neurotoxicity, although it can occasionally be entertained if it's been several years since initial treatment.

A return to a previously effective chemotherapeutic (either PCV or temozolomide) is another option if progression has occurred off of treatment. Other agents with some reported activity include melphalan, platins, and etoposide. Even though oligodendroglioma is a low-grade tumor with marked chemosensitivity, tumor recurrence and progression to high grade significantly shorten life expectancy. There is marked variability between individuals with median survival ranging from 8 to 16 years, and some patients can survive decades without recurrence. Prognostic features include age; functional status; neurologic deficits; original tumor size and extent of resection; as well as molecular features such as 1p19q co-deletion, IDH1 mutation, and MGMT methylation. However, regardless of prognostic features, most patients with oligodendroglioma will eventually undergo malignant transformation to anaplastic oligodendroglioma or GBM.

OLIGODENDROGLIOMA SUBTYPES

Anaplastic Oligodendroglioma

Similar to low-grade oligodendrogliomas, there is no commonly accepted standard approach to the treatment of WHO grade III anaplastic oligodendroglioma. Because of the malignant growth of anaplastic oligodendrogliomas, early treatment with surgery, RT, and/or chemotherapy is necessary. Recognition of the chemosensitivity that corresponds to 1p19q codeletion in these tumors has led to the incorporation of molecular genetic analysis in treatment decision making.

In the surgical approach to these tumors, evidence suggests an association between extent of resection and survival, and although tumor location may only allow biopsy or partial resection, maximal safe resection is preferred whenever possible. Given the high likelihood of recurrence following surgery for anaplastic tumors, adjuvant treatment with RT and/or chemotherapy is recommended. Both RT and chemotherapy are active in anaplastic oligodendroglioma, although the timing and order are less clear. Codeletion of 1p19q is a strong predictive biomarker associated with improved response to chemotherapy and evidence suggests that 1p19q status can be used to guide the choice of adjuvant therapy.

Postoperative RT has been shown to improve disease control and overall survival in HGG, and although its effectiveness has not been specifically demonstrated in anaplastic oligodendroglioma, radiotherapy is considered a central component of the treatment of these tumors.

The further addition of chemotherapy to RT has recently been evaluated in randomized clinical trials of anaplastic oligodendroglioma. The long-term results of two large complementary trials demonstrated that the addition of PCV to radiotherapy was associated with dramatically improved progression-free and overall survival in tumors with 1p19q codeletion. However, for tumors with retained 1p19q, there appeared to be limited benefit from the addition of chemotherapy. Therefore, patients with 1p19q retained anaplastic oligodendroglioma may benefit most from treatment with adjuvant radiotherapy alone, whereas patients with 1p19q codeleted anaplastic oligodendroglioma should be treated with both RT and chemotherapy [Level 1].[13] One study suggests that IDH mutation, in the absence of 1p19q deletion, also predicts benefit from chemotherapy, but this result has not been validated to date. Open questions remain about the order of therapy (RT then chemotherapy or vice versa), although guidelines support the use of chemotherapy after RT because of better tolerability. In addition, the optimal chemotherapy is unclear whether temozolomide, which is better tolerated and easier to administer, can

be substituted for PCV. Although no direct comparison has been made, current evidence suggests that both regimens are similarly active, and studies directly comparing the two are ongoing. Finally, given the chemosensitivity of anaplastic oligodendrogliomas and the concern for delayed neurotoxicity from RT, there is some interest in using adjuvant chemotherapy alone to delay radiotherapy, and this approach is currently being studied in clinical trials.

Regardless of the treatment approach taken, anaplastic oligodendrogliomas invariably recur. Reresection or reirradiation can be considered in select patients depending on the location of the recurrence and the overall clinical picture. In addition, both temozolomide and PCV have been shown to have activity at the time of recurrence, and one strategy is to treat with the regimen not used previously. Other agents with some minor evidence of activity include paclitaxel, irinotecan, carboplatin, and etoposide. Finally, although bevacizumab has beneficial effects and approval in GBM, the evidence is much less clear in anaplastic oligodendroglioma and may carry a higher risk of intratumoral hemorrhage than in GBM. In spite of attempts at salvage, the prognosis from anaplastic oligodendrogliomas is significantly worse than low-grade tumors, with median survival of 4.5 years compared with 9.8 years for oligodendroglioma. Still, some patients survive significantly longer, including younger patients with gross total resection; good functional status; and evidence of 1p19q codeletion, IDH mutation, and MGMT methylation.

Mixed Oligoastrocytomas

Mixed oligoastrocytomas are infiltrating gliomas with morphologic features of both oligodendroglioma and astrocytoma and represent an intermediate category between these two major tumor subtypes. Mixed histology can be present in WHO grade II oligoastrocytomas or in WHO grade III anaplastic oligoastrocytomas, although the proportion of oligodendroglial features required for these diagnoses is not explicitly established. Because the criteria for diagnosis are not clearly defined, the incidence of these tumors is unclear, although they may make up as much as 10% of adult gliomas depending on the pathologist. Clinically, these tumors have similar symptoms, location, and appearance to astrocytomas and oligodendrogliomas. The natural history and treatment responsiveness of mixed oligoastrocytomas likely lies somewhere between that of astrocytomas and oligodendrogliomas, and the molecular genetic alterations present in these mixed tumors reveal that some tumors are genetically similar to oligodendrogliomas and others are more like astrocytomas. Codeletion of 1p19q occurs in approximately 30% to 50% of mixed gliomas; between the frequencies observed in oligodendrogliomas and astrocytomas. Because chemoresponsiveness correlates with 1p19q codeletion, most mixed oligoastrocytomas with 1p19q loss are treated as oligodendrogliomas, whereas those with retained 1p19q are treated as astrocytomas. As with other aspects of these mixed tumors, their prognosis is likely intermediate between that of oligodendrogliomas and astrocytomas.

EPENDYMOMAS

DEFINITION AND EPIDEMIOLOGY

Ependymomas are glial neoplasms that arise from the ependymal cells lining the walls of the ventricles or spinal canal. They are uncommon tumors that primarily affect children and young adults, where the majority are infratentorial, most frequently involving the fourth ventricle. In contrast, the majority of ependymomas in adults arise in the spinal cord, especially the cervical and thoracic spine. Ependymomas account for somewhere between 2% and 9% of all gliomas, including up to 10% of pediatric brain tumors and nearly 50% to 60% of spinal gliomas in adults. Most are well-defined slow-growing WHO grade II ependymomas, although more rapid malignant growth is seen with WHO grade III anaplastic ependymomas. In addition, rare benign WHO grade I ependymal tumors include subependymomas, which are found in the lateral or fourth ventricles and myxopapillary ependymomas, which exclusively involve the conus medullaris and filum terminale.

CLINICAL AND IMAGING FEATURES

Although ependymomas generally appear adjacent to the ventricular system, they may also arise within the parenchyma of the brain without obvious ependymal attachment. Posterior fossa ependymomas often cause cerebrospinal fluid (CSF) outflow obstruction producing headache, nausea, vomiting, and ataxia or increasing head circumference in children younger than the age of 2 years. Spinal cord ependymomas present with sensory dysesthesias or motor deficits, often with difficulty walking. Typical MRI findings in ependymoma include a well-circumscribed T1 hypointense, T2 hyperintense lesions with prominent heterogeneous enhancement. Cysts, hemorrhage, and calcification are also common. Proximity or involvement of the ventricular system, particularly the fourth ventricle, is an important clue to the diagnosis of ependymoma, although supratentorial parenchymal ependymomas can be difficult to distinguish from other types of glioma. Because of a risk of leptomeningeal dissemination, all patients should have CSF cytology and imaging of the entire neuraxis to exclude metastatic disease.

PATHOLOGIC AND MOLECULAR FEATURES

Ependymomas contain histologic features reminiscent of ependymal cells lining the ventricles. Although mitoses are rare or absent in WHO grade II ependymoma, brisk mitotic activity with microvascular proliferation and necrosis are signs of WHO grade III anaplastic ependymoma.

TREATMENT AND OUTCOME

The treatment of ependymal tumors depends on tumor histology, anatomic location, and extent of resection. The most important component of initial therapy involves maximal safe resection. Observational evidence suggests improved survival from gross total resection, which is the goal of surgery when possible. WHO grade I ependymal tumors including subependymoma and myxopapillary ependymoma can be cured with gross total resection. However, in the case of grade II ependymoma or grade III anaplastic ependymoma, tumors often recur following surgery and adjuvant RT is generally used to reduce the risk of recurrence.

In the past, prophylactic craniospinal RT was advocated for all resected ependymomas, but because most tumors recur at the original site, local radiotherapy targeting a margin around the surgical cavity has become the standard of care. More extensive radiation fields are indicated if either neuroimaging or CSF cytology reveal evidence of tumor dissemination. In the case of patients with gross total resection of supratentorial WHO grade II ependymoma, retrospective data suggests there may be a role for observation with postponement of RT until there is evidence of recurrence. This is particularly relevant for young children with ependymoma in whom RT is associated with significant long-term neurocognitive side effects.

The role of chemotherapy in the treatment of ependymoma is still being defined. Cisplatin, carboplatin, and etoposide have all been shown to have activity in ependymoma, with the best responses seen following combination therapy. Chemotherapy has been shown to be effective in patients with partially resected ependymoma, suggesting a potential role for chemotherapy in incompletely resected disease prior to either radiotherapy or a second-look surgery. Chemotherapy has also been used in an attempt to delay or avoid RT altogether, and uncontrolled results suggest that there may be some efficacy in this setting, although further study is necessary. Finally, chemotherapy is being examined as adjuvant therapy following RT, although results to date are mixed. Additional study is necessary to better define the role of chemotherapy in the treatment of ependymoma, although it may be considered in patients with incompletely resected ependymomas prior to RT.

Patients with ependymoma that develop recurrent disease after radiotherapy have a poor long-term prognosis, and most eventually die from progressive disease. Unfortunately, no treatment strategies have been proven to be effective in this setting. Treatment options include reresection, reirradiation, chemotherapy, and bevacizumab. In the end, the overall prognosis from ependymoma depends on the extent of resection, tumor location, and performance status, with the best prognosis seen in patients with gross total resection. The 5-year overall survival of ependymoma ranges from 40% to 80%, with 10-year survival ranging from 47% to 68%.

GLIONEURONAL TUMORS

Glioneuronal tumors are a group of rare neoplasms that have histologic evidence of both glial and neuronal differentiation. For the most part, they are slow-growing WHO grade I and II tumors with rare transformation to malignancy. Each of the tumors in this class has unique features that justify subclassification; however, because they are so uncommon, knowledge about natural history and optimal clinical management is limited. Much of what is known about these tumors is based on small series and case reports. There are a number of glioneuronal tumor subtypes, and although a detailed discussion of each is beyond the scope of this text, we will attempt to highlight the most important features of a couple of the most common tumors.

GANGLIOGLIOMA

Ganglioglioma is a rare WHO grade I tumor composed of neoplastic glial cells together with neoplastic mature ganglion cells. Tumors composed of neoplastic ganglion cells alone are known as *gangliocytomas*. Both are well-differentiated slow-growing tumors that can occur anywhere in the neuraxis, although the majority (>70%) are found in the temporal lobes. Most patients present with seizures, and gangliogliomas are the most frequent tumor found in patients with epilepsy, with a reported incidence of 15% to 25% of patients undergoing epilepsy surgery. They affect individuals across a wide age range and are estimated to make up approximately 1% of all primary brain tumors in adults and 4% of pediatric brain tumors. Gangliogliomas are typically well-circumscribed masses that are T1 hypointense and T2 hyperintense on MRI with frequent homogeneous enhancement, although they are occasionally nonenhancing. Many have large cystic components with an enhancing mural nodule. Gangliogliomas only rarely induce surrounding edema and they generally exhibit little to no mass effect. Although gangliogliomas can infiltrate adjacent normal brain, they generally do not behave aggressively. Rarely, gangliogliomas may undergo anaplastic transformation involving their subpopulation of glial cells, and these anaplastic tumors are considered WHO grade III tumors with behavior similar to other high-grade gliomas. The optimal treatment for gangliogliomas has not been established, although initial treatment typically involves surgical resection. Complete resection can be achieved in most patients and may be curative. Seizures can improve even in cases where only a partial resection is possible. Radiotherapy does not seem to improve outcomes following complete resection, but it may be beneficial following partial resection or in patients with evidence of recurrence after gross total resection. Even patients with anaplastic components may be followed after resection and treated with reresection and RT at recurrence. A role for chemotherapy in ganglioglioma is not well defined, although nitrosoureas, retinoic acid, and cisplatin have all been reported to be active in this disease. In general, the prognosis of ganglioglioma is very good with greater than 90% of patients achieving long-term progression-free survival (7.5-year recurrence-free survival of 94% in one report), although anaplastic features may indicate more aggressive behavior and less favorable outcomes.

DYSEMBRYOPLASTIC NEUROEPITHELIAL TUMOR

Dysembryoplastic neuroepithelial tumors (DNETs) are benign, slow-growing WHO grade I lesions that contain both glial elements and mature neurons. They are cortically based supratentorial tumors believed to have a malformative origin, and up to 80% are associated with cortical dysplasia. They have a predilection for the temporal lobes and nearly all patients develop long-standing drug-resistant epilepsy. They occur most often in children and young adults, with 90% of patients developing seizure prior to the age of 20 years. However, they may not initially be recognized as the cause of seizures, only to be discovered at the time of epilepsy surgery, where they are found in approximately 12% to 13% of surgeries. On MRI, DNETs appear as T1 hypointense, T2 hyperintense regions of cortical expansion with infrequent extension to the subcortical white matter. They may be sharply or poorly demarcated and often appear as multiple nodules or pseudocysts although they have little or no mass effect or surrounding edema. Most have little to no contrast enhancement, and in those that do, the enhancement generally represents ischemia or hemorrhage rather than transformation. As evidence of their benign slow growth, DNETs often demonstrate some deformation of the overlying calvarium. They rarely have nuclear pleomorphism, mitoses, or endothelial proliferation and essentially never undergo malignant transformation. Treatment involves surgery and is indicated in patients with refractory seizures. Gross total resection is curative, although even partial resection can improve seizure control. No additional therapy is required after surgery and even in cases of subtotal resection, patients typically do not have evidence of recurrence in long-term follow-up.

LEVEL 1 EVIDENCE

1. Karim AB, Maat B, Hatlevoll R, et al. A randomized trial on dose-response in radiation therapy of low-grade cerebral glioma: European Organization for Research and Treatment of Cancer (EORTC) Study 22844. *Int J Radiat Oncol Biol Phys*. 1996;36:549–556.

2. Shaw E, Arusell R, Scheithauer B, et al. Prospective randomized trial of low- versus high-dose radiation therapy in adults with supratentorial low-grade glioma: initial report of a North Central Cancer Treatment Group/Radiation Therapy Oncology Group/Eastern Cooperative Oncology Group study. *J Clin Oncol*. 2002;20:2267–2276.

3. van den Bent MJ, Afra D, de Witte O, et al. Long-term efficacy of early versus delayed radiotherapy for low-grade astrocytoma and oligodendroglioma in adults: the EORTC 22845 randomised trial. *Lancet*. 2005;366:985–990.

4. Shaw EG, Wang M, Coons SW, et al. Randomized trial of radiation therapy plus procarbazine, lomustine, and vincristine chemotherapy for supratentorial adult low-grade glioma: initial results of RTOG 9802. *J Clin Oncol*. 2012;30:3065–3070.

5. Stupp R, Hegi ME, Mason WP, et al. Effects of radiotherapy with concomitant and adjuvant temozolomide versus radiotherapy alone on survival in glioblastoma in a randomised phase III study: 5-year analysis of the EORTC-NCIC trial. *Lancet Oncol*. 2009;10:459–466.

6. Stupp R, Mason WP, van den Bent MJ, et al. Radiotherapy plus concomitant and adjuvant temozolomide for glioblastoma. *N Engl J Med*. 2005;352:987–996.

7. Hegi ME, Diserens AC, Gorlia T, et al. MGMT gene silencing and benefit from temozolomide in glioblastoma. *N Engl J Med*. 2005;352:997–1003.

8. Westphal M, Hilt DC, Bortey E, et al. A phase 3 trial of local chemotherapy with biodegradable carmustine (BCNU) wafers (Gliadel wafers) in patients with primary malignant glioma. *Neuro Oncol*. 2003;5:79–88.

9. Brem H, Piantadosi S, Burger PC, et al. Placebo-controlled trial of safety and efficacy of intraoperative controlled delivery by biodegradable polymers of chemotherapy for recurrent gliomas. The Polymer-brain Tumor Treatment Group. *Lancet*. 1995;345:1008–1012.

10. Taal W, Oosterkamp HM, Walenkamp AM, et al. Single-agent bevacizumab or lomustine versus a combination of bevacizumab plus lomustine in patients with recurrent glioblastoma (BELOB trial): a randomised controlled phase 2 trial. *Lancet Oncol*. 2014;15(9):943–953.

11. Gilbert MR, Dignam JJ, Armstrong TS, et al. A randomized trial of bevacizumab for newly diagnosed glioblastoma. *N Engl J Med*. 2014;370:699–708.

12. Chinot OL, Wick W, Mason W, et al. Bevacizumab plus radiotherapy-temozolomide for newly diagnosed glioblastoma. *N Engl J Med*. 2014;370:709–722.

13. Cairncross G, Wang M, Shaw E, et al. Phase III trial of chemoradiotherapy for anaplastic oligodendroglioma: long-term results of RTOG 9402. *J Clin Oncol*. 2013;31:337–343.

SUGGESTED READINGS

General Considerations in Glioma

Andronesi OC, Kim GS, Gerstner E, et al. Detection of 2-hydroxyglutarate in IDH-mutated glioma patients by in vivo spectral-editing and 2D correlation magnetic resonance spectroscopy. *Sci Transl Med*. 2012;4:116ra4.

Bondy ML, Scheurer ME, Malmer B, et al. Brain tumor epidemiology: consensus from the Brain Tumor Epidemiology Consortium. *Cancer*. 2008;113: 1953–1968.

Jansen M, Yip S, Louis DN. Molecular pathology in adult gliomas: diagnostic, prognostic, and predictive markers. *Lancet Neurol*. 2010;9:717–726.

Louis DN, Ohgaki H, Wiestler OD, et al. The 2007 WHO classification of tumours of the central nervous system. *Acta Neuropathol*. 2007;114:97–109.

Omuro A, DeAngelis LM. Glioblastoma and other malignant gliomas: a clinical review. *JAMA*. 2013;310:1842–1850.

Ostrom QT, Gittleman H, Farah P, et al. CBTRUS statistical report: primary brain and central nervous system tumors diagnosed in the United States in 2006–2010. *Neuro Oncol*. 2013;15(suppl 2):ii1–ii56.

Pardo FS, Aronen HJ, Kennedy D, et al. Functional cerebral imaging in the evaluation and radiotherapeutic treatment planning of patients with malignant glioma. *Int J Radiat Oncol Biol Phys*. 1994;30:663–669.

Upadhyay N, Waldman AD. Conventional MRI evaluation of gliomas. *B J Radiol*. 2011;84(2):S107–S111.

Wen PY, Macdonald DR, Reardon DA, et al. Updated response assessment criteria for high-grade gliomas: response assessment in neuro-oncology working group. *J Clin Oncol*. 2010;28:1963–1972.

Principles of Treatment

Batchelor TT, Sorensen AG, di Tomaso E, et al. AZD2171, a pan-VEGF receptor tyrosine kinase inhibitor, normalizes tumor vasculature and alleviates edema in glioblastoma patients. *Cancer Cell*. 2007;11:83–95.

Beiko J, Suki D, Hess KR, et al. IDH1 mutant malignant astrocytomas are more amenable to surgical resection and have a survival benefit associated with maximal surgical resection. *Neuro Oncol*. 2014;16:81–91.

Mayer R, Sminia P. Reirradiation tolerance of the human brain. *Int J Radiat Oncol Biol Phys*. 2008;70:1350–1360.

Senft C, Bink A, Franz K, et al. Intraoperative MRI guidance and extent of resection in glioma surgery: a randomised, controlled trial. *Lancet Oncol*. 2011;12:997–1003.

Stummer W, Pichlmeier U, Meinel T, et al. Fluorescence-guided surgery with 5-aminolevulinic acid for resection of malignant glioma: a randomised controlled multicentre phase III trial. *Lancet Oncol*. 2006;7:392–401.

Wallner KE, Galicich JH, Krol G, et al. Patterns of failure following treatment for glioblastoma multiforme and anaplastic astrocytoma. *Int J Radiat Oncol Biol Phys*. 1989;16:1405–1409.

Astrocytic Tumors

Bikowska-Opalach B, Szlufik SA, Grajkowska WA, et al. Pilocytic astrocytoma: a review of genetic and molecular factors, diagnostic and prognostic markers. *Histol Histopathol*. 2014;29(10):1235–1248.

Brandes AA, Franceschi E, Tosoni A, et al. MGMT promoter methylation status can predict the incidence and outcome of pseudoprogression after concomitant radiochemotherapy in newly diagnosed glioblastoma patients. *J Clin Oncol*. 2008;26:2192–2197.

Brandsma D, Stalpers L, Taal W, et al. Clinical features, mechanisms, and management of pseudoprogression in malignant gliomas. *Lancet Oncol*. 2008;9:453–461.

Brem H, Piantadosi S, Burger PC, et al. Placebo-controlled trial of safety and efficacy of intraoperative controlled delivery by biodegradable polymers of chemotherapy for recurrent gliomas. The Polymer-brain Tumor Treatment Group. *Lancet*. 1995;345:1008–1012.

Chaichana KL, Jusue-Torres I, Navarro-Ramirez R, et al. Establishing percent resection and residual volume thresholds affecting survival and recurrence for patients with newly diagnosed intracranial glioblastoma. *Neuro Oncol*. 2014;16:113–122.

Forsyth PA, Shaw EG, Scheithauer BW, et al. Supratentorial pilocytic astrocytomas. A clinicopathologic, prognostic, and flow cytometric study of 51 patients. *Cancer*. 1993;72:1335–1342.

Friedman HS, Prados MD, Wen PY, et al. Bevacizumab alone and in combination with irinotecan in recurrent glioblastoma. *J Clin Oncol*. 2009;27: 4733–4740.

Hart MG, Garside R, Rogers G, et al. Temozolomide for high grade glioma. *Cochrane Database Syst Rev*. 2013;4:CD007415.

Jones DT, Kocialkowski S, Liu L, et al. Tandem duplication producing a novel oncogenic BRAF fusion gene defines the majority of pilocytic astrocytomas. *Cancer Res*. 2008;68:8673–8677.

Quant EC, Norden AD, Drappatz J, et al. Role of a second chemotherapy in recurrent malignant glioma patients who progress on bevacizumab. *Neuro Oncol*. 2009;11:550–555.

Quinn JA, Reardon DA, Friedman AH, et al. Phase II trial of temozolomide in patients with progressive low-grade glioma. *J Clin Oncol*. 2003;21:646–651.

Sabel M, Giese A. Safety profile of carmustine wafers in malignant glioma: a review of controlled trials and a decade of clinical experience. *Curr Med Res Opin*. 2008;24:3239–3257.

Sanai N, Chang S, Berger MS. Low-grade gliomas in adults. *J Neurosurg*. 2011;115:948–965.

Smith JS, Chang EF, Lamborn KR, et al. Role of extent of resection in the long-term outcome of low-grade hemispheric gliomas. *J Clin Oncol*. 2008;26:1338–1345.

Taal W, Brandsma D, de Bruin HG, et al. Incidence of early pseudo-progression in a cohort of malignant glioma patients treated with chemoirradiation with temozolomide. *Cancer*. 2008;113:405–110.

Whittle IR. What is the place of conservative management for adult supratentorial low-grade glioma? *Adv Tech Stand Neurosurg*. 2010;35:65–79.

Oligodendroglial Tumors

Baumert BG, Mason WP, Ryan G, et al. Temozolomide chemotherapy versus radiotherapy in molecularly characterized (1p loss) low-grade glioma: a randomized phase III intergroup study by the EORTC/NCIC-CTG/TROG/MRC-CTU (EORTC 22033–26033). *J Clin Oncol*. 2013;31(suppl). Abstract 2007.

Buckner JC, Gesme D Jr, O'Fallon JR, et al. Phase II trial of procarbazine, lomustine, and vincristine as initial therapy for patients with low-grade oligodendroglioma or oligoastrocytoma: efficacy and associations with chromosomal abnormalities. *J Clin Oncol*. 2003;21:251–255.

van den Bent MJ, Brandes AA, Taphoorn MJ, et al. Adjuvant procarbazine, lomustine, and vincristine chemotherapy in newly diagnosed anaplastic oligodendroglioma: long-term follow-up of EORTC Brain Tumor Group study 26951. *J Clin Oncol*. 2013;31:344–350.

van den Bent MJ, Taphoorn MJ, Brandes AA, et al. Phase II study of first-line chemotherapy with temozolomide in recurrent oligodendroglial tumors: the European Organization for Research and Treatment of Cancer Brain Tumor Group study 26971. *J Clin Oncol*. 2003;21:2525–2528.

Wick W, Hartmann C, Engel C, et al. NOA-04 randomized phase III trial of sequential radiochemotherapy of anaplastic glioma with procarbazine, lomustine, and vincristine or temozolomide. *J Clin Oncol*. 2009;27:5874–5880.

Ependymal Tumors

Garvin JH Jr, Selch MT, Holmes E, et al. Phase II study of pre-irradiation chemotherapy for childhood intracranial ependymoma. Children's Cancer Group protocol 9942: a report from the Children's Oncology Group. *Pediatr Blood Cancer*. 2012;59:1183–1189.

Grundy RG, Wilne SA, Weston CL, et al. Primary postoperative chemotherapy without radiotherapy for intracranial ependymoma in children: the UKCC-SG/SIOP prospective study. *Lancet Oncol*. 2007;8:696–705.

Guyotat J, Signorelli F, Desme S, et al. Intracranial ependymomas in adult patients: analyses of prognostic factors. *J Neuro Oncol*. 2002;60:255–268.

Reni M, Brandes AA, Vavassori V, et al. A multicenter study of the prognosis and treatment of adult brain ependymal tumors. *Cancer*. 2004;100:1221–1229.

Glioneuronal Tumors

Blumcke I, Wiestler OD. Gangliogliomas: an intriguing tumor entity associated with focal epilepsies. *J Neuropathol Exp Neurol*. 2002;61:575–584.

Luyken C, Blumcke I, Fimmers R, et al. Supratentorial gangliogliomas: histopathologic grading and tumor recurrence in 184 patients with a median follow-up of 8 years. *Cancer*. 2004;101:146–155.

Luyken C, Blumcke I, Fimmers R, et al. The spectrum of long-term epilepsy-associated tumors: long-term seizure and tumor outcome and neurosurgical aspects. *Epilepsia*. 2003;44:822–830.

McLendon RE, Provenzale J. Glioneuronal tumors of the central nervous system. *Brain Tumor Pathol*. 2002;19:51–58.

Metastatic Tumors 97

Enid Choi, Graeme F. Woodworth, and
Minesh P. Mehta

INTRODUCTION

It is estimated that 13.7 million people living in the United States today are alive with a diagnosis of cancer. The American Cancer Society projects that 1,665,540 new cancer diagnoses will be made in 2014. The American Society of Clinical Oncology predicts that cancer will overtake heart disease as the most common cause of death by 2030, and it is already the leading cause of death in England and in Americans younger than 85 years old. Metastatic disease, that is, cancer that has spread from its site of origin (from the Greek *meta*, meaning "next," and *stasis*, meaning "placement"), is the cause of death in the vast majority of cancer patients. This chapter will focus on these tumors, first discussing them in general and then discussing more specific clinical entities, including brain metastasis, epidural spinal column metastasis, and leptomeningeal metastasis (LM).

METASTATIC TUMORS

EPIDEMIOLOGY

Although the number of new cases of metastasis to the central nervous system diagnosed yearly is estimated at over 200,000, the exact incidence remains unknown. The reason for this is that although cancer as a disease is reportable, sites of metastatic disease are not routinely reported to any registry. Autopsy studies have reported the presence of intracranial metastases in 10% to 30% of all cancer patients (15% to the brain, 5% to the leptomeninges, 5% to the dura) as well as occult LM in an average of 20% of all cancer patients. The incidence of brain metastases has risen steadily over the last few decades, a phenomenon which is likely multifactorial: High-resolution imaging allows brain metastases to be detected more readily, and increasingly effective treatments lead to prolonged survival and thus a longer period during which neural metastases may develop. One conjectured reason for the very high incidence of metastatic disease to the brain is the highly selective permeability of the blood–brain barrier, which allows tumor cells sanctuary in the central nervous system (CNS) both from immune surveillance and the cytotoxic effects of chemotherapy, as most of these agents fail to cross the barrier adequately.

Although the brain parenchyma is the location most likely to be involved (80%) with metastatic disease to the nervous system, other common sites include the epidural space and leptomeninges. Less common sites include the dura, intramedullary spinal cord, optic apparatus, and cranial and peripheral nerves. Data regarding these less common sites are generally limited to case reports and small series, and therefore, this discussion will focus on CNS metastases, primarily of the parenchymal brain.

PATHOBIOLOGY

The molecular processes within cancer cells and their microenvironment that ultimately result in the development of metastatic disease are poorly understood and are the focus of much ongoing research. It is known that the shedding of tumor cells into systemic circulation is an early phenomenon in the natural history of malignancy, but these circulating tumor cells do not always lead to metastasis. It is estimated that less than 0.01% of these cells are able to establish a metastatic lesion at a distant anatomic site. This could well be a consequence of immune surveillance mechanisms. It is also known that certain malignancies have a predilection to metastasize to particular organs. This may be due in part to simple anatomy and physiology but may also be dependent on specific molecular characteristics, including the secretion of specific chemotactic factors by the organ or site involved; neurotropic growth factors in the CNS are thought to play such a role. Another possible factor is the expression of specific surface molecules on tumor cells that allow them to home to certain tissues. Melanoma cells are presumed to possess such molecular features, which allow them to have among the highest probabilities of metastasizing to the brain.

Possible pathways for spread of cancer include hematogenous, lymphatic, intrathecal, and perineural. (Fig. 97.1). Although not technically metastatic, tumors may directly extend into neighboring structures, including the CNS; for example, large tumors of the head and neck may invade the brain or spinal cord. The intravasation of the cancer cell requires multiple signals between that cell and its surrounding microenvironment. Some data suggest that transformation of the malignant cell into a mesenchymal, or connective tissue–like, state is crucial for this, a phenomenon referred to as *epithelial-to-mesenchymal transformation*, or EMT.

Once intravasated and in circulation, normal anatomic organs may act as a barrier. Regional lymph nodes may trap tumor cells. The hepatocytes of the liver filter the blood as the venous return from abdominal organs passes through it, and the liver is a frequent site of metastatic disease from gastrointestinal primaries. The blood–brain barrier presents another obstacle for circulating tumor cells. Logically, organs with a large volume of blood flow are more prone to metastatic disease, such as the pulmonary capillary bed with its high flow. The CNS and the bones receive approximately 20% of the cardiac output; it is therefore not surprising that the liver, lung, CNS, and bones are the most common sites of metastatic disease.

When cancer cells arrive at a distant site, they must extravasate from circulation and establish at this location, a complex process that requires multiple interactions with the new microenvironment. The nascent metastasis must also be capable of angiogenesis, the formation of new blood vessels, in order to sustain growth larger than approximately 1 mm. Despite all these required steps for the formation of distant metastases, metastatic disease from cancer is an all too real and common phenomenon, indicating that

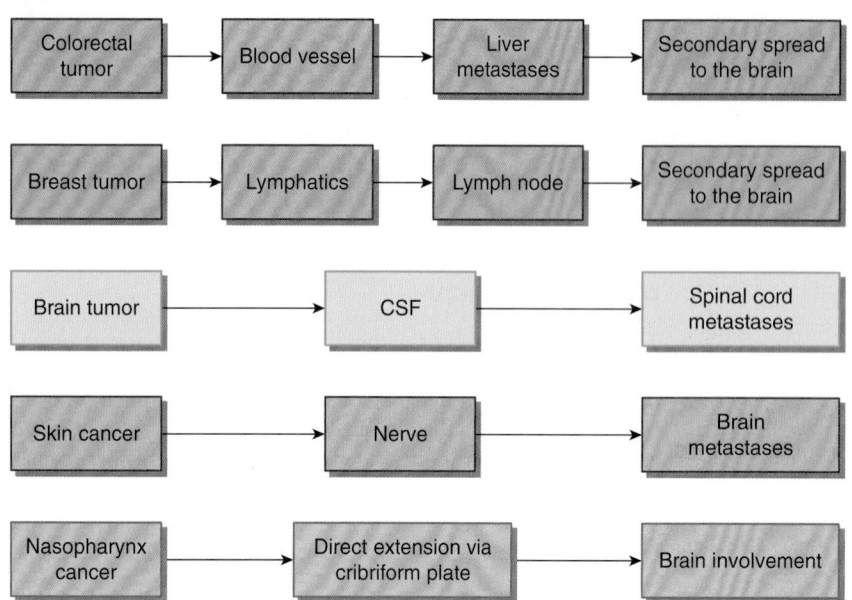

FIGURE 97.1 Routes of metastases. CSF, cerebrospinal fluid.

this orchestrated process of dissociation, intravasation, circulation, avoidance of immune surveillance, extravasation, and metastatic growth is efficiently coordinated by a significant number of malignancies through sophisticated genetic interplay.

CLINICAL FEATURES AND WORKUP

Metastatic disease to the nervous system may present with or without symptoms, and an appropriate clinical workup is indicated to make the diagnosis. In asymptomatic patients, metastatic disease is often found incidentally during their cancer workup and staging process or while concomitant nonmalignant comorbidities are being investigated. CNS metastases are often diagnosed in the context of a known history of malignancy, but symptomatic CNS metastasis may also be the initial clinical presentation of a previously unidentified malignancy. In this situation, biopsy or resection is required in order to pathologically confirm a diagnosis of cancer and to guide treatment. The most common primary malignancy that presents with metastatic disease in the brain is lung cancer. The most common primary malignancies that presents with metastatic disease to the spine are breast and prostate cancer. In some cases, the primary malignancy responsible for the metastatic disease is never identified despite a complete and thorough evaluation.

History and Physical Exam

The clinical presentation of CNS metastasis is highly dependent on the specific neurologic structure involved and the degree to which it has been compromised. Symptoms may be of gradual or abrupt onset, which provides insight not only to the pathologic process but also prognosis and likelihood of recovery. Clinical workup of a new neurologic deficit must begin with a thorough history and physical exam, with particular focus on the elucidation of any neurologic deficits.

Laboratory Studies

Blood work has limited use in the workup of CNS metastatic disease, but one exception is tumor markers: cancer-specific or cancer-associated proteins that are measurable in the blood or cerebrospinal fluid (CSF). If markers are elevated, especially in the CSF, then systemic metastases, including neurologic, are more likely. The converse statement, however, is not true; a tumor marker value within normal limits does not preclude malignancy or metastatic disease. Despite this limited use, any patient with general neurologic symptoms, such as altered mental status, headache, or seizures, should have basic labs drawn in order to rule out other etiologies such as infection, electrolyte imbalance, toxins, and blood gas abnormalities.

Imaging

Magnetic resonance imaging (MRI), with and without gadolinium contrast, is the gold standard imaging test for suspected CNS cancer. Computed tomography (CT) is used in patients who cannot tolerate MRI and occasionally to further evaluate hemorrhage. Magnetic resonance spectroscopy can suggest whether a lesion is neoplastic, inflammatory, or other. At present, positron emission tomography (PET) with ^{18}F-fluorodeoxyglucose (FDG) has limited use in evaluation of brain cancers due to the high background activity of the normal brain. It is important to note that none of these imaging techniques replaces histology for diagnostic accuracy.

Tissue Diagnosis

In many cases, histologic confirmation of a CNS metastasis is unnecessary, as the likelihood of metastatic disease from a known primary, especially in the setting of systemic disease, outweighs the likelihood of a new primary CNS tumor. This is particularly true if the imaging studies have characteristics consistent with metastatic disease. In other cases, however, the diagnosis of CNS metastasis is unclear from the history, physical exam, laboratory values, and radiographic studies. If the diagnosis of metastatic disease is in question, and if the lesion is surgically accessible with reasonable safety, biopsy should be performed to provide histopathologic diagnosis.

Another important possible method of identifying metastasis to the CNS is sampling of the CSF with a lumbar puncture (LP). LP may also rule in or out other etiologies and clarify the diagnosis of LM (also termed *leptomeningeal carcinomatosis*, *neoplastic meningitis*, or *carcinomatous meningitis*). It will not, however, diagnose parenchymal brain metastases in the absence of CSF involvement. LP is contraindicated due to the risk of brain herniation in cases where increased intracranial pressure (ICP) is suspected.

TREATMENT

Both symptomatic and definitive treatments are important. Symptomatic treatment includes corticosteroids, treatment of seizures, and anticonvulsant prophylaxis. Definitive treatment includes surgery, radiation therapy, and chemotherapy.

Corticosteroids and Antiepileptics

Metastatic disease may cause marked edema due to extravasation of plasma from leaky tumor vasculature. Within the narrow anatomic confines of the CNS, this edema may cause increased ICP and significant compression of the normal neural tissue (Fig. 97.2A). Symptoms of increased ICP include headache and blurred vision. Intravenous corticosteroids, most commonly dexamethasone, should be given immediately to symptomatic patients and often result in rapid improvement in symptoms. One widely used dosing of steroids begins with an intravenous bolus of 10 mg of dexamethasone (although the actual value of the intravenous route over oral as well as the larger 10-mg dose in terms of symptom resolution is unclear), followed by 4 mg given every 6 hours.

The dose should be titrated upward or downward as needed. Large doses can cause acute psychiatric symptoms, and chronic administration has myriad toxicities including candidiasis, increased risk of pneumocystis pneumonia, metabolic imbalance, sleep and mood disturbance, muscle atrophy and wasting, weight gain, osteopenia and pathologic fractures, gastrointestinal irritability, and perforation. Steroids should be tapered as rapidly as tolerated once definitive therapy has been initiated.

Symptomatic patients or those with radiographic evidence of significant mass effect should be stabilized with steroids as soon as possible. Steroids have been shown to improve or resolve symptoms in up to two-thirds of patients and may confer a small survival benefit compared to no treatment. Patients who present with seizures should be stabilized with antiepileptic medications, preferably selecting agents that do not induce cytochrome p450 hepatic enzymes, as such induction could interfere with some chemotherapies. Antiepileptics are generally not indicated in patients with no history of seizure, as they have no proven benefit given prophylactically and may have significant adverse effects, including fatigue and decreased cognition; however, studies suggesting

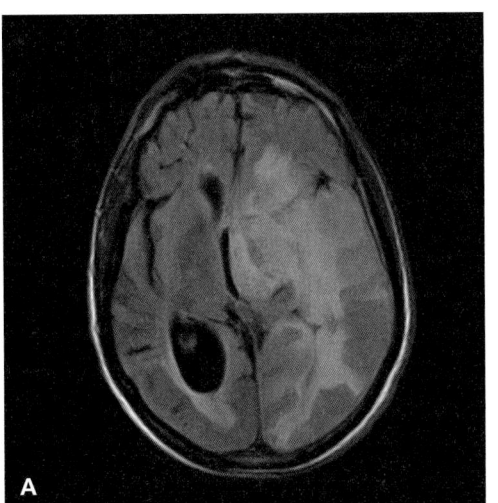
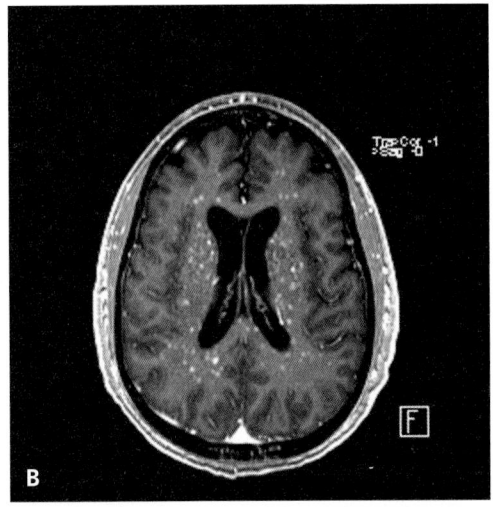
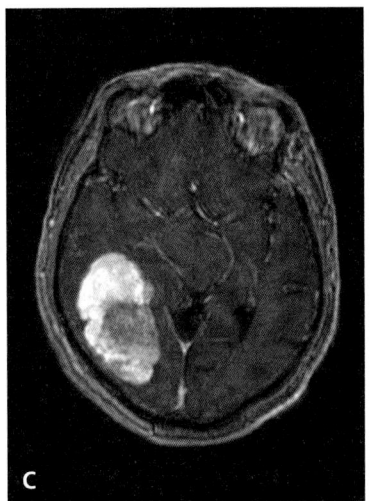
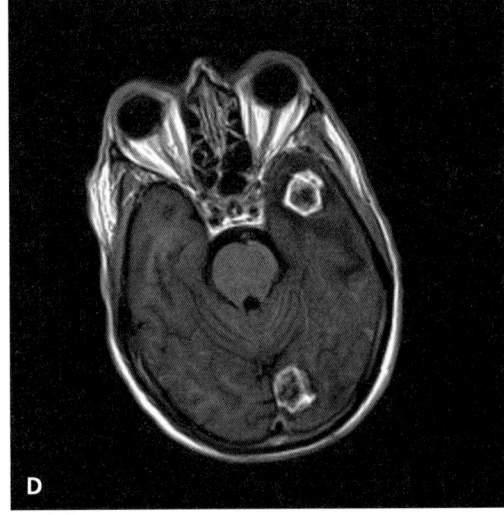
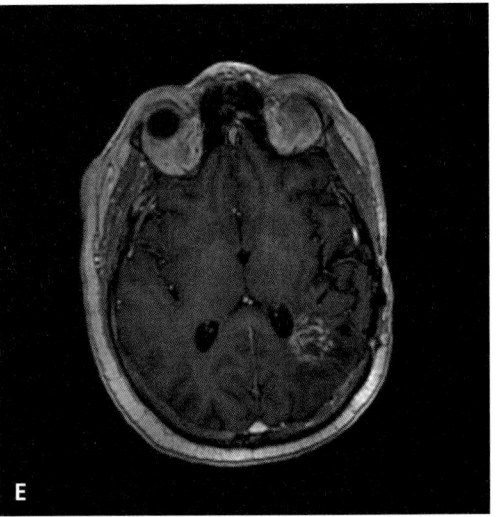

FIGURE 97.2 A: Edema from brain metastases causing significant mass effect and midline shift. **B:** Miliary brain metastases. **C:** Hemorrhagic brain metastasis. **D:** Classic appearance of brain metastases. **E:** Radiation necrosis. These are axial contrast-enhanced MR images **(B-E)** except for **(A)** which is an axial FLAIR MR sequence.

antepileptics have risk outweighing benefit in seizure naive patients were conducted before some of the more modern drugs, such as levetiracetam, were developed, and definitive data are lacking in the modern era [**Level 1**].[1]

Surgery

In general, surgical management is considered for patients who are medically fit, with large tumors (>2 to 3 cm), one or few tumors, and/or a tumor associated with significant brain swelling, mass effect, and neurologic deficits. The benefits of direct tumor removal with surgery include rapid improvement in symptoms and improved local disease control. The decision for or against surgery depends on many factors, including overall clinical performance status; status of systemic disease; and location, size, and number of metastases. Surgery may be followed by radiation or, less commonly, chemotherapy. Risks of surgery include bleeding, infection, CSF leak, and transient or permanent neurologic deficit.

Radiation Therapy

Radiation therapy (RT) may be used in combination with surgery, typically as adjuvant therapy following maximal resection or as primary therapy for unresected disease. Tumor regression following radiation is a gradual process, and the therapeutic effects lack the immediacy of surgical resection, making radiation second-line therapy in situations where immediate decompression is indicated.

For patients with known brain metastases too numerous to target individually, RT is generally delivered to the entire brain (whole brain radiation therapy [WBRT]) with the rationale that the presence of brain metastases indicates that the entire organ has been compromised. The likelihood of other tumor cells with metastatic potential elsewhere within the brain is high, and WBRT not only treats the known lesions but also may prevent the development of macroscopic disease elsewhere in the brain.

WBRT alone may reduce or eliminate symptoms from brain metastases in 60% to 80% of patients and may result in a significant radiographic response in about half of all patients. WBRT is also associated with improved median survival 4 to 6 months as opposed to 1 month without treatment. Side effects include neurocognitive decline, radiation necrosis, and damage related to the specific area of the brain being irradiated.

WBRT is classically given to a total dose of 30 Gy delivered in 10 fractions, although several other fractionation schedules have been shown to have similar efficacy with no significant difference in toxicity (20 Gy in 5 fractions, 30 Gy in 15, 37.5 Gy in 15, 40 Gy in 15, and 40 Gy in 20). Doses higher than this (50 to 54.4 Gy) and hyperfractionation (more and smaller fractions) did not show a survival benefit, and larger fraction sizes were found to be detrimental, with shorter progression-free survival and higher neurologic toxicity [**Level 1**].[2–4] Prophylactic cranial irradiation (PCI) is WBRT in the absence of known macrometastatic disease in the brain in order to decrease the likelihood of developing such brain metastasis. PCI is indicated in small cell lung cancer, which has a very high propensity for brain metastasis. Other tumors, particularly classic pediatric brain tumors such as medulloblastoma, have a high incidence of metastatic disease to not only elsewhere in the brain but also the spinal cord. Prophylactic craniospinal irradiation (CSI) is given to the entire CNS axis in these situations.

Stereotactic radiosurgery (SRS) is a more targeted radiation technique in which a much larger dose of radiation is given in a single treatment. The advantages of SRS include shorter treatment time (1 day vs. 2 to 3 weeks) and decreased radiation dose to the surrounding normal brain tissue. SRS may be used safely to treat multiple brain lesions and may also be given in combination with WBRT. In certain situations, the precision of SRS is combined with the delivery of a few large fractions of radiation, as opposed to a single fraction, an approach referred to as *stereotactic radiotherapy*.

Chemotherapy

Chemotherapy has traditionally had a limited role in the treatment of CNS metastases because the blood–brain and the blood–CSF barriers inhibit the ability of systemic agents to penetrate to the brain and spinal cord. Some agents with good CNS penetration include high-dose intravenous methotrexate and temozolomide. Chemotherapy may also be administered intrathecally, typically via a port placed into the ventricular system, which helps circumvent these natural anatomic barriers, but intrathecal chemotherapy only penetrates into brain parenchyma by a few millimeters at most and is generally ineffective against parenchymal brain metastases. Another limitation to using chemotherapy to treat neurologic metastasis is that the primary malignancy might have previously been treated with the same agent, leading to acquired resistance.

Cancer histologies for which chemotherapy has shown efficacy, albeit modest, in CNS metastases include germ cell tumors (where the effect is dramatic), small cell lung cancer, and breast cancer. Cancers harboring specific driver mutations such as epidermal growth factor receptor (EGFR) mutations in non–small cell lung cancer (NSCLC) may respond well to appropriate targeted therapeutics (e.g., EGFR tyrosine kinase inhibitors), which do at least partially penetrate the blood–brain barrier.

BRAIN METASTASIS

EPIDEMIOLOGY AND CLINICAL MANIFESTATIONS

The most common type of cancer of the brain is metastatic disease; brain metastases outnumber primary brain tumors by a ratio of approximately 9:1. Up to 20% to 40% of all cancer patients will develop lesions in the brain. The brain may be a site of relapse at any time in the clinical course. The median time interval between the development of brain metastasis and the original cancer diagnosis is approximately 1 year, but the range can exceed 10 years. NSCLC is the most common source of brain metastases, likely because it is more common than other cancers. In comparison, a larger proportion of patients with diagnoses such as melanoma, small cell lung cancer, and specific subsets of breast cancer will develop brain metastases, but due to the lower number of patients diagnosed with these diseases, the total incidence from these primary tumors is lower than that from NSCLC.

Symptoms of CNS metastases result from both focal pressure on surrounding tissue, destruction of normal neurons, and global increases in ICP from the metastases or associated peritumoral edema. Presenting symptoms most often include headache (49%), altered mental status (32%), focal weakness (30%), ataxia (21%), and seizures (18%). Diffuse, small, miliary lesions scattered throughout the brain parenchyma are particularly associated with leukemia and small cell lung cancer and may manifest as a generalized encephalopathy (Fig. 97.2B).

Untreated brain metastases generally produce worsening symptoms over days to weeks. In some cases, symptoms are more acute and may mimic ischemic or hemorrhagic stroke. The more abrupt clinical course may particularly be seen with bleeding within the metastasis; hemorrhagic brain metastases are classically associated with certain histologies, including melanoma, renal carcinoma, choriocarcinoma, NSCLC, and thyroid (Fig. 97.2C).

IMAGING

In the setting of a known diagnosis of cancer and new neurologic symptoms, multiple, spheroidal, enhancing brain lesions, mostly at the gray–white junction, with a disproportionate degree of edema on MRI, strongly suggest a diagnosis of brain metastases. Differential diagnosis include primary brain tumor, lymphoma, abscess, other infectious processes, stroke, multifocal demyelination, radiation necrosis, etc. A seminal series of 54 patients with a single brain lesion seen on imaging who underwent resection or biopsy reported pathologic discordance in 11%; in other words, 1 of 10 patients with MRI findings consistent with a single metastatic lesion in the brain might not have a brain metastasis.

Brain metastases may be single or multiple. The classic appearance of metastatic disease in the brain is a round, irregular, ring-enhancing lesion at the gray–white matter interface with associated vasogenic edema (Fig. 97.2D). In comparison, high-grade gliomas may appear more infiltrative and irregularly shaped; gliomas are most commonly single and rarely present as multiple distinct lesions. CNS lymphoma tends to appear as periventricular, homogenously enhancing disease. Intracranial abscesses are high on the list of differentials in the setting of immunosuppression. These appear as well-circumscribed, thick-rimmed, ring-enhancing masses with central hypodensity. Stroke, both hemorrhagic and ischemic, may produce both similar symptoms and imaging findings as brain metastases. Multifocal demyelination has been reported after treatment with certain chemotherapy agents (5-fluorouracil and levamisole) and may also mimic metastases in appearance. Radiation necrosis is a known potential complication from RT, particularly SRS, and may also appear as a contrast-enhancing mass (Fig. 97.2E).

About 80% of brain metastases involve the cerebral hemispheres, 10% the cerebellum, and 5% the brain stem, a rate of incidence that appears consistent with the relative volume and percentage of blood flow. A high proportion of brain metastases are seen in the watershed regions. This is most likely due to smaller blood vessels and slower blood flow in these areas. For reasons that are not fully understood, different histologies may preferentially metastasize to different brain locations; lung cancer tends to metastasize to the cerebrum, whereas gastrointestinal malignancies tend to metastasize to the cerebellum.

TREATMENT

Approximately 30% to 50% of patients with metastatic disease to the brain will die from progressive intracranial disease. Therefore, when considering treatment options, one must consider not only the extent of intracranial disease but also overall disease burden, clinical status, and prognosis. To predict survival in the setting of intracranial metastasis, the Radiation Therapy Oncology Group (RTOG) developed a recursive partitioning analysis (RPA) classifier that stratifies patients based on performance status, age, control of primary tumor, and presence of extracranial metastatic disease. The graded prognostic assessment (GPA) index also takes into account the number of brain metastases and is histology-specific. Based on these categories, predictions may be made regarding overall survival, which may then be used to potentially guide therapy.

Two clinical scenarios merit additional clarification: (1) a single brain lesion, meaning known disease elsewhere with only one lesion in the brain and (2) a solitary brain lesion, meaning the one metastasis to the brain is the only known site of disease. (It should

be noted the literature often uses single and solitary interchangeably.) Single or solitary brain lesions generally warrant aggressive management, as this may have a significant impact on survival. A series by Flannery et al., reported that treatment of single, synchronous brain metastases from NSCLC in addition to definitive thoracic treatment improved survival.

After medical stabilization, definitive treatment with surgery, focused radiation with SRS, WBRT, chemotherapy (including targeted agents in highly selected patients), or different combinations of these modalities are considered. The only clinical trials that have ever demonstrated survival advantage from more aggressive therapy are in patients with single (inclusive of solitary) brain metastasis.

Focal Treatment

Brain metastases may be focally treated with either surgery or SRS. To date, there are no completed prospective clinical trials directly comparing surgery with radiosurgery in the treatment of brain metastases, but in retrospective comparisons, outcomes appear generally similar [**Level 1**].[5]

SURGERY

Resection of a limited number of brain metastases, usually one, results in improved outcomes, both for locoregional recurrence and overall survival. For patients with solitary or single brain metastases with controlled systemic disease, resection followed by WBRT prolongs survival (median 40 to 50 weeks) and functional independence and improved neurologic function versus WBRT alone. Table 97.1 summarizes the key randomized surgical trials [**Level 1**].[6–8] Appropriate patient selection is crucial because resection of single metastases in patients with a greater burden of systemic disease or with poorer performance status generally does not lengthen survival. This is believed to be the reason behind the lack of survival benefit seen in the trial by Mintz et al., as this study included patients with Karnofsky performance status (KPS) of 50, compared to KPS of 70 in the other two trials. The results of this trial were also potentially confounded by a high rate of surgery following disease progression among patients randomized to WBRT alone.

Surgery is preferred to radiation in the setting of extensive edema and increased ICP, as it is the most efficacious therapy for immediate reduction of mass effect. Surgery is also preferred for cases in which a pathologic sample is desired to guide treatment and for lesions larger than 4 cm. Wider application of surgery is limited by the risk of morbidity, particularly for multiple metastases for which multiple craniotomies might be necessary. Retrospective studies of resection of up to two metastases in well-selected patients suggest a possible survival advantage, but level 1 evidence to support this approach is lacking.

TABLE 97.1	Comparison of Overall Survival for Surgery plus Whole-Brain Radiation Therapy versus Whole-Brain Radiation Therapy Alone			
Trial	N	Surgery + WBRT	WBRT Alone	P Value
Patchell et al.	48	40 wk	15 wk	<.01
Noordijk et al.	63	~40 wk	~24 wk	.04
Mintz et al.	84	~22.4 wk	~25.2 wk	NS

WBRT, whole-brain radiation therapy; NS, not significant.

Stereotactic Radiosurgery

SRS is used to deliver a single, high-dose treatment of radiation to a small, circumscribed target and is frequently used for metastatic disease that is not amenable to surgery due to location or to patient comorbidities. Additionally, unlike surgery, SRS may be considered in the treatment of multiple lesions. SRS results in either stability or decrease in tumor size in over 80% of patients and represents an effective means to achieve local control. With submillimetric treatment precision accomplished with increasingly sophisticated immobilization and imaging and extremely sharp dose gradients, SRS is capable of safely delivering high doses of radiation to the target with markedly reduced dose to neighboring structures. This capability for dose escalation means that metastases from radioresistant histologies, such as melanoma and renal cell carcinoma, are more likely to respond. The prescribed dose of radiation delivered by SRS is determined by the size of the lesion, with larger lesions receiving lower doses due to the increased risk of inducing unacceptable edema and necrosis. Also for this reason, the largest lesion that may be safely treated with SRS is on the order of 3 to 4 cm, although lesions up to 5 cm in size have been treated with diminishing local control.

SRS is frequently used in combination with WBRT. A randomized trial compared WBRT plus SRS to one to three brain metastases versus WBRT alone and found an overall survival advantage with the addition of SRS in patients with a single lesion; on post hoc analysis, other subgroups with survival benefit were identified and included patients with lung cancer with up to three lesions and RTOG RPA class I patients [**Level 1**].[9] A recent reanalysis of these data, using the GPA scoring system revealed that patients with high GPA scores irrespective of the number of lesions (up to three) experienced a survival advantage.

An active area of investigation is the use of SRS to prevent local recurrence post resection. Resection bed SRS is more complex than targeting an enhancing tumor due to uncertainties regarding the interpretation of a postoperative MRI. Soltys et al. reported a 1-year local control rate of 94% when a 2-mm margin was added around the defined tumor bed versus 78% when no margin was added. One concern regarding surgical bed SRS is the possibility of leptomeningeal spread secondary to the resection, especially for patients with breast cancer and those with posterior fossa disease. The North Central Cancer Treatment Group (NCCTG), in collaboration with RTOG, is conducting a randomized study comparing postoperative WBRT versus resection bed SRS. Some institutions use preoperative SRS to obviate the tumor bed definition challenges and contend that the leptomeningeal dissemination rate is lower, but no prospective evaluations of pre- versus postoperative SRS have been conducted.

Whole-Brain Radiation Therapy in Addition to Focal Treatment

Although focal therapy such as surgery or SRS can effectively control the treated lesion, the rate of relapse in the rest of the brain is still approximately 30% to 70%. WBRT following resection or radiosurgery of a single (or up to four) brain metastases yields dramatic improvement in intracranial failure and death from neurologic progression and also improves local control. The addition of WBRT to focal treatment unquestionably reduces relapse in the brain, but cognitive decline consequential to the late effects of WBRT may result in a proportion of patients. Neurocognitive effects may be seen within months, and fixed deficits become pronounced years after treatment. Half or more of all patients with brain metastases die from systemic progression rather than from their intracranial disease, but certainly, some patients have prolonged survival and clinicians must therefore consider and discuss the possible late complications of WBRT. Recent data support a protective effect for the drug memantine [**Level 1**].[10] There are also new data suggesting that sparing critical structures within the brain, such as the perihippocampal regenerative subgranular stem cell niche, may reduce the development of neurocognitive deficits from brain radiation.

One crucial question is whether there exists a subgroup of patients with lower risk of intracranial relapse for whom WBRT can be safely withheld altogether. As an example, a retrospective analysis by Sawrie et al. demonstrated that of 100 patients treated with SRS alone, 18 could be identified as "low-risk," with a 1-year freedom from distant brain failure rate of 83% compared to the 26% risk in all other patients. Low-risk patients included those with three or fewer brain metastases, nonmelanoma histology, and controlled extracranial disease. The median time to brain relapse was considerably longer in these "low-risk" patients, implying that brain "seeding" probably occurs at much later times in some subgroups who could therefore be treated with upfront SRS alone. Ayala-Peacock et al. recently reported a nomogram that can be used to predict an individual patient's risk of distant brain failure after SRS, and although not yet independently validated, such a tool could prove useful in selecting appropriate patients for withholding WBRT.

SRS is increasingly used alone, particularly in elderly patients or others with fragile baseline mentation or in those whose overall prognosis is excellent. In one small randomized trial, SRS alone actually produced neurocognitive preservation superior to WBRT plus SRS; however, the small trial size unfortunately cannot exclude selection imbalance [**Level 1**].[11] In a larger Japanese trial, cognitive function, as measured using the Mini-Mental State Examination (MMSE) trended toward superiority for the SRS + WBRT arm, with a longer period to MMSE decline favoring the WBRT arm [**Level 1**].[12] In a European Organisation for Research and Treatment of Cancer (EORTC) trial of either resection or radiosurgery, with or without WBRT, adjuvant WBRT negatively impacted some aspects of health-related quality of life (HRQOL), although these effects were transitory. However, compliance with HRQOL was only 88.3% at baseline and dropped to an abysmal low of 45% at 1 year; in trials with such large components of missing data, imputing superiority is fraught with a lot of inherent biases [**Level 1**].[13] A larger intergroup trial in patients with up to three metastases has recently been completed and included survival as well as cognitive and quality of life end points, but results are not available to date. Another limited institution trial is testing the same concept in patients with up to 10 brain metastases. At the American Society for Therapeutic Radiology and Oncology (ASTRO) 2014 Annual Meeting, Sahgal et al. reported a meta-analysis of three trials (EORTC 22952, JRSOG99-1, NCT 00460395) with an SRS +/− WBRT design, none of which were powered to determine a survival benefit. These trials included patients with brain metastases from various histologies; included varying number of brain lesions (one to four) with significant differences in entry criteria, salvage treatment, systemic therapy, enrollment eras, SRS dose, nonspecified follow-up imaging criteria, and variable follow-up; and also included some patients having undergone resection. The overall conclusion was that overall survival was superior in the subset of approximately 70 patients (roughly 35 patients in each cohort) receiving SRS alone and aged 35 to 50 years; no biologic explanation for this finding was offered. Crucially, none of the trials mandated pre-SRS restaging of their systemic cancer, an element that would be crucially necessary to ensure that the survival benefit was not a spurious finding because of greater systemic disease burden in one cohort. A fundamental limitation of such an analysis was articulated by Patchell et al. wherein they pointed out that to establish whether WBRT could be safely omitted in unselected groups of patients, a noninferiority design for the SRS arm would be necessary, and with an assumed median survival of 8 months, this would require in the order of 2,250 patients.

Therefore, these findings must be interpreted cautiously, especially in the context of other reports in the literature, such as the oft-forgotten study by Pirzkall et al. involving 236 patients, wherein SRS + WBRT, compared to SRS alone (not a randomized trial), yielded better tumor control and reduced intracranial relapse and a trend toward improved survival, especially in patients with no extracranial disease (15.4 vs. 8.3 months, $P = .08$), underscoring the logical expectation that WBRT added to SRS improves brain disease control, and this has the potential to translate to a survival advantage, only in patients who are less likely to succumb to extracranial progression, once again underscoring the need to perform systemic disease restaging in trials attempting to define a survival difference.

The American Society of Radiation Oncology, in 2014, recommended against routine use of WBRT in certain selected patients with limited intracranial disease treated with SRS, but if these patients have limited extracranial disease, they may well be the exact group which might actually experience a survival benefit with WBRT, analogous to the survival benefit that accrues to small cell lung cancer patients when WBRT is used to treat presumed intracranial microscopic disease in the context of well-controlled extracranial disease (the so-called prophylactic cranial irradiation, although there is nothing truly "prophylactic" about this strategy, but in reality it is therapeutic for micrometastatic intracranial disease).

It is important to understand that recurrence of cancer in any organ frequently leads to functional deterioration within that organ, and the brain should not be expected to be an exception to this; therefore, deferring WBRT or additional SRS until relapse may have potential detrimental neurocognitive and overall survival consequences, as relapse in the brain may present with potentially devastating and irreversible symptoms. Very few studies carefully analyze the mode of death; Regine et al., in a single institution experience reported considerably increased intracranial relapses in patients treated with SRS alone but more importantly noticed that these were most often (71%) symptomatic and associated with a neurologic deficit. Patchell et al., in their seminal trial of resection, +/− WBRT tracked cause of death and identified neurologic death as occurring far more frequently in patients not receiving WBRT, a logical outcome of increased intracranial failure [**Level 1**].[14] One option around this is frequent monitoring with screening MRI scans after initial SRS and salvage with repeat SRS at presymptomatic recurrence. However, such an option, even if it were shown to be effective in a randomized trial, would likely be associated with increased societal costs consequential to the intense MRI and salvage with repeat SRS, usually on more than one occasion. All of these factors must be weighed for each individual patient in order to optimize treatment.

Reirradiation

Despite good initial responses, most patients will eventually experience disease progression in the brain, and so the role of reirradiation

must also be considered. SRS may be used to treat recurrence after WBRT and vice versa. In some cases, WBRT may be repeated and has been reported to improve symptoms in 40% to 70% of patients. To date, there is no level 1 evidence regarding the role or reirradiation for brain metastases, and clinical decisions must be made on a case-by-case basis [**Level 1**].[15]

Chemotherapy and Targeted Agents

The role of chemotherapy, targeted therapy, or immunotherapy is not well defined. There is no level 1 evidence favoring the use of systemic therapy, and therefore no standard cytotoxic chemotherapy is routinely used for the treatment of brain metastases. In patients with brain metastases that have failed local therapy, the same chemotherapeutic agents employed for the treatment of extracranial disease are often used. Alternatively, drugs with good CNS penetration, such as temozolomide, topotecan, irinotecan, and high-dose methotrexate may be employed, even in patients in whom the chemotherapy might have at most minor efficacy against the primary tumor.

Improved understanding of tumor biology has led to the identification of specific molecular drivers of cancer development and progression. Alterations involving the *EGFR* gene and *EML4–ALK* chromosomal translocation in lung cancer, HER2 protein overexpression in breast cancer, and *BRAF* mutation in melanoma are examples of distinct subsets of cancer amenable to unique treatment approaches. There have been several prospective studies in the last 3 to 5 years particularly focusing on targeted therapies or immunotherapy.

EGFR INHIBITORS IN NON–SMALL CELL LUNG CANCER

The RTOG 0320 trial did not show any additional benefit of temozolomide or erlotinib when added to WBRT and SRS in unselected patients with NSCLC with one to three brain metastases [**Level 1**].[16] One of the limitations of this study was that patients were not stratified according to *EGFR* mutational status. In a phase II study of 40 NSCLC patients with brain metastases, WBRT and erlotinib was safe and the median survival time was 11.8 months. In the 17 patients with known *EGFR* status, the benefit of erlotinib was more pronounced in the mutant *EGFR* patients (overall survival [OS] of 19.1 months) as compared to the wild-type *EGFR* patients (OS of 9.3 months). In a large cohort of 110 patients with *EGFR* mutant lung cancer with newly diagnosed brain metastases, patients treated with WBRT (32 patients) had longer median time to intracranial progression compared to 63 patients who received erlotinib therapy upfront (24 vs. 16 months).

In a phase II study of gefitinib in 41 NSCLC patients unselected for *EGFR* mutation, an objective response rate of 10% in the brain was seen. Higher response rates were reported in studies of EGFR inhibitors in enriched with patients with known *EGFR* mutations. Recently, Gerber et al., reported that the survival of *EGFR*-mutated NSCLC patients with brain metastases is notably long, with a median of 33 months; those receiving radiosurgery had a dramatic median survival of 64 months.

ALK INHIBITORS IN NON–SMALL CELL LUNG CANCER

Although crizotinib has limited blood–brain barrier penetrability, initial results of the novel Alk inhibitors such as alectinib, ceritinib, AP26113, etc., show better control of intracranial metastases and are in early evaluation phases regarding their activity against established brain metastases in patients with Alk-rearrangement tument NSCLC with brain metastases.

HER2 INHIBITORS FOR BREAST CANCER

Several prospective clinical trials have evaluated the role of lapatinib-based therapy in *HER2*-positive breast cancer patients with active brain metastases. In one phase II study of lapatinib in patients with *HER2*-positive breast cancer with progressive brain metastases after WBRT and/or SRS, a CNS response rate of only 6% was seen. In a single-arm, phase 2 study, 29 of the 45 patients with newly diagnosed, previously untreated brain metastases from *HER2*-positive breast cancer achieved an objective CNS response (66%) with the combination of lapatinib and capecitabine [**Level 1**].[17] Newer agents such as trastuzumab emtansine are demonstrating intracranial activity in anecdotal reports.

INHIBITORS TARGETING BRAF IN MELANOMA

Activating *BRAF* mutations that result in constitutive activation of the mitogen-activated protein kinase (MAPK) pathway affect approximately half of melanoma patients and more than 95% of these are the V600E mutations (substitution of valine by glutamic acid at the 600th amino acid position). In an open-label phase II study, 172 patients with V600E or V600K mutation–positive melanoma metastatic to the brain were treated with dabrafenib. Patients in cohort A had not received any prior local therapy and cohort B had disease progression in the brain following local therapy (surgery, WBRT, SRS). Twenty-nine of 74 patients (39%) with V600E *BRAF*-mutant melanoma in cohort A and 20 of 65 patients in cohort B achieved an overall intracranial response. This study provided initial evidence that dabrafenib has activity in patients with V600E *BRAF*-mutant melanoma brain metastases irrespective of prior local therapy.

In a prospective study, 24 patients with V600E *BRAF* mutation–positive melanoma brain metastases were treated with vemurafenib. Of 19 patients with measurable intracranial disease, 7 (37%) achieved greater than 30% intracranial tumor regression, and 3 (16%) achieved a confirmed partial response (PR), whereas 13/21 patients (62%) had extracranial responses. A phase II study of vemurafenib in 146 patients with V600 *BRAF* mutation–positive melanoma brain metastases (NCT01378975) with or without prior treatment for their brain metastases has completed accrual, and results are pending.

IMMUNE-MODULATING APPROACHES

The development of immune-modulating agents, specifically immune checkpoint inhibitors, offers an exciting opportunity for treating patients with brain metastases. Recent research has demonstrated that activated T cells can be effective in brain metastases and other intracranial tumors. In a phase II study, 72 melanoma patients with brain metastases (51 asymptomatic [cohort A], 21 symptomatic and on steroids [cohort B]) were treated with ipilimumab, a monoclonal antibody against CTLA-4. Twelve of 51 patients (24%) in cohort A and 2 of 21 patients (10%) in cohort B achieved CNS disease control. Median OS was 7.0 months in cohort A and 3.7 months in cohort B. This study demonstrated that ipilimumab could have some activity in recurrent brain metastases, and further evaluation especially in a combinatorial manner is proceeding.

In the expanded access programme (EAP) in Italy, the feasibility of ipilimumab (3 mg/kg every 3 weeks for four doses) in patients with stage III (unresectable) or IV melanoma and asymptomatic brain metastases who had failed or did not tolerate previous treatments was investigated. Of 855 patients, 146 had asymptomatic brain metastases. With a median follow-up of 4 months, the overall disease control rate was 27%, including 4 patients with a complete response and 13 with a partial response. Median progression-free survival and overall survival were 2.8 and 4.3 months, respectively, and approximately one-fifth of patients were alive 1 year after starting ipilimumab.

There is considerable interest in combining these immune checkpoint inhibitors with radiation. A retrospective analysis of 13 patients treated with WBRT within 30 days of ipilimumab showed that 4/9 patients (44 %) experienced partial response or stable disease. There was a high rate of intratumoral hemorrhage, with 10 of 10 patients with posttreatment imaging demonstrating new or increased intratumoral bleeding after WBRT. In another retrospective review, the median survival of patients with melanoma with brain metastases treated with ipilimumab and brain SRS was comparable to patients without brain metastases.

EPIDURAL SPINAL COLUMN METASTASIS

EPIDEMIOLOGY AND CLINICAL MANIFESTATIONS

Metastatic disease to the spine can be leptomeningeal (discussed in the following section) or intramedullary, but by far, the most common site is epidural. Epidural spinal metastases can cause severe neurologic compromise by compressing the thecal sac and ultimately the spinal cord. The cancers that most often are responsible for epidural metastatic disease of the spine include breast, prostate, and lung cancers. This is in part due to the relatively high incidence of these malignancies but also for their predilection for metastatic spread to bones; the spinal column is the most common site of bone metastasis.

Epidural spinal cord compression can be a surgical emergency that occurs in up to 15% of patients with a history of cancer. This complication typically occurs in the setting of known bone metastases but, as with brain lesions, may be the presenting symptom for a new diagnosis of primary malignancy or for new diagnosis of metastatic disease. The most common level of cord compression is thoracic (59% to 78%), followed by lumbar (16% to 33%) and cervical (4% to 15%) (Fig. 97.3). In up to 50% of patients, disease may involve multiple levels of the vertebral column. As with bone metastases, pain is the most common presenting symptom of spinal cord compression (96%). This may be not only from the bone itself but also from spinal cord or nerve root involvement. As compression worsens, patients may also develop other signs and symptoms of spinal cord compression including gait ataxia, focal weakness (76% to 86%), sensory disturbances (51% to 80%), and autonomic dysfunction (40% to 64%). In most cases, epidural spinal cord compression occurs due to extension of disease from the bony vertebrae, but it sometimes may be due to infiltration of the neural foramina or paravertebral spaces or from pathologic vertebral fracture. Compression of the spinal cord and blood vessels causes mechanical nerve damage and ultimately ischemia and infarction. The longer the cord is compromised, the more likely that the damage is irreversible; it is well established that long-standing, gradually worsening neurologic symptoms are unlikely to be markedly improved due to the chronic nature of the damage.

The diagnostic test of choice for spine metastasis of any kind is a contrast-enhanced MRI scan, but if the patient's condition is rapidly deteriorating, or if the patient is unable to tolerate the length of this study, a noncontrast MRI may be adequate. If, however,

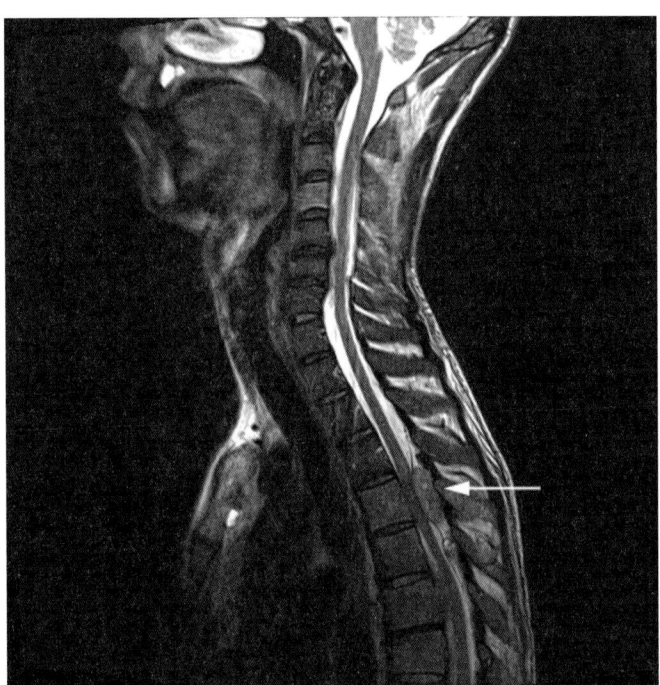

FIGURE 97.3 Spinal cord compression from metastatic disease, sagittal, T2 MRI.

there is clinical suspicion for either intramedullary or leptomeningeal disease, then intravenous contrast is absolutely indicated. The entire spine should be studied in order to evaluate for multilevel involvement. Patients who are unable to undergo MRI should have a CT myelogram.

TREATMENT

Initial palliation of pain from spinal metastasis is often with nonsteroidal anti-inflammatory drugs (NSAIDs), narcotics, agents to ameliorate neuropathic pain, and steroids.

For spinal cord compression, the goals of care are to preserve neurologic function and to relieve pain. The early recognition and initiation of treatment, even prior to definitive diagnosis, are critical due to the time-sensitive chance of recovery from a neurologic deficit. As soon as clinical suspicion for cord compression is raised, treatment should begin with early administration of high-dose corticosteroids to decrease swelling, as this has been shown to improve outcomes in acute spinal cord injury [**Level 1**].[18]

Surgery is the primary modality for relieving spinal cord compression, particularly in the setting of limited disease, as it can result in immediate decompression. The seminal prospective study comparing the addition of surgery to radiation in the setting of spinal cord compression showed not only improved neurologic and functional outcomes with surgery, including ambulation, continence, and decreased steroid and narcotic requirements, but also an overall survival benefit (126 vs. 100 days, $P = .033$) [**Level 1**].[19] Even in the absence of cord compression, surgical management should be considered in the setting of an unknown primary malignancy or new metastatic disease in order to confirm the diagnoses. For patients with vertebral fracture or spinal instability, stabilization of the spine through surgical means should be considered. Anterior epidural metastases are more challenging to access and may require thoracotomy, whereas posterior lesions are likely to be amenable to laminectomy.

Given the grave consequences of progressive disease in the spine, RT, which is a highly effective palliative treatment with up to 90% of patients experiencing a significant reduction of pain, should be considered at an early stage. This is important because pain from a compression fracture and compressive symptoms from retropulsed bony fragments are almost never adequately relieved by any modality except surgery. RT can reduce the likelihood of a pathologic fracture, as may vertebroplasty. Should a fracture occur, surgical repair is the best option when possible, and postoperative radiation is the standard of care. RT in this setting decreases the likelihood of local recurrence, which may compromise the integrity of the surgical repair. The typical timeframe is 1 to 2 weeks after surgery in order to allow adequate wound healing. In selected patients, percutaneous vertebroplasty or kyphoplasty may be effective in relieving symptoms. None of these treatments will prolong survival but may have a significant positive impact on quality of life.

RT is also a common palliative treatment for epidural spinal cord metastases, particularly for cases in which surgery is not feasible (i.e., multilevel cord involvement, multiple medical comorbidities) and in the postoperative setting. As with brain metastases, the effect from radiation is gradual and lacks the immediate decompression of surgery. RT is therefore suboptimal in the setting of spinal cord compression. The classic regimen for palliative RT is 30 Gy in 10 fractions, but other equivalent fractionation schedules exist. The target volume typically includes one whole vertebral body above and below the area involved with disease. For primary malignancies involving the bone, such as multiple myeloma or sarcoma, the prescribed dose may be lower or higher and the target volume more conservative to avoid overtreating neighboring structures, particularly the spinal cord.

RT may be contraindicated in patients who have received previous RT to the same site or for relatively radioresistant tumors such as renal cell carcinoma. Reirradiation may be considered using a highly focused, intensity-modulated technique, as this has been shown to stabilize or improve neurologic status in the majority of patients with minimal risk of radiation myelopathy. Stereotactic body radiation therapy (SBRT), highly focal fractionated radiation with sharp dose gradients similar to SRS, may also be employed in this setting in order to minimize unnecessary dose to the spinal cord. Sahgal et al. report that normalized biologically effective doses less than a point maximum of 20 to 25 Gy carry a low risk for myelopathy so long as the total effective dose does not exceed approximately 70 Gy, and the SBRT maximum dose is less than half the total normalized dose. A prospective series of 59 patients from MD Anderson who underwent reirradiation of spinal metastases demonstrated 92% freedom from neurologic deterioration from any cause at 1 year. An ongoing RTOG phase II/III trial exploring SRS in the up-front treatment of spine metastases may ultimately provide insight regarding the use of this approach [**Level 1**].[20] The phase II trial supported the feasibility of single fraction SRS for spinal metastases with no serious treatment-related toxicities. Phase III compares SRS versus classic fractionated external beam treatments with regard to pain relief and quality of life.

By far, the strongest prognostic factor for neurologic outcome is the patient's neurologic status prior to treatment. The best odds for regain of function are with surgery. With radiation, 80% of ambulatory patients remained ambulatory, but only 50% of patients with paresis and less than 10% of those with paralysis will regain the ability to walk. Pain may be relieved in over 90% of patients treated with corticosteroids and radiation. Overall survival is most strongly determined by systemic disease burden.

LEPTOMENINGEAL METASTASIS

EPIDEMIOLOGY AND CLINICAL PRESENTATION

LM refers to metastasis to the pia and arachnoid. The disease may be focal or disseminated, but any involvement of the meninges with cancer indicates that the entire CSF compartment is compromised. This devastating complication occurs in up to 5% to 10% of cancer patients, with acute lymphocytic leukemia and other hematologic malignancies representing the most common sources. The most common solid tumors that spread to the leptomeninges are breast cancer, NSCLC, melanoma, and gastrointestinal cancers. Over half (50% to 80%) of patients with known brain metastases also have LM. Surgical resection of brain lesions, particularly of the posterior fossa, has been reported as a risk factor for the development of LM. Most cases of LM are diagnosed in the setting of known metastatic disease, but LM may be an isolated phenomenon, particularly for hematologic cancers.

The median survival without treatment is 4 to 6 weeks. Appropriate treatment may prolong survival to several months, particularly for lymphoma, leukemia, and to a lesser extent breast cancer. Treatment may also potentially reverse or prevent further neurologic symptoms. The presence of systemic disease, obstruction of the CSF, gross CNS metastases, and poor performance status are negative prognostic factors.

Headache is a common presenting symptom (30% to 50%), as are altered mental status and signs of focal neuropathy. Patients most commonly present with multifocal neurologic symptoms from spinal cord (60%), cerebral (50%), or cranial nerve involvement (40%). Increased ICP or hydrocephalus may develop due to obstruction of CSF flow or from disruption of the blood–brain barrier. Seizures occur in up to 25% of patients.

In the workup of LM, MRI of the entire CNS should be performed. Even though the sensitivity and specificity of imaging are relatively low (76% and 77%), obvious LM on imaging obviates the need for CSF sampling by lumbar or other puncture. If LM is visualized, it appears as enhancement of the leptomeninges, cranial nerves, or nerve roots or as gross tumor nodules. Visible LM is most commonly seen at the base of brain, sylvian fissures, and cauda equina, perhaps due to slower CSF flow in these regions.

LP should be performed for CSF analysis, particularly if the clinical suspicion for LM is high and MRI is negative. LP may show a combination of malignant cells, elevated opening pressure, low glucose, high protein, and leukocytosis, typically of lymphocytes. Assessing the CSF for tumor marker levels, although not standard, may aid in diagnosis. The false-negative rate for initial LP in the diagnosis of LM is relatively high at 50%, and therefore, this procedure may need to be repeated multiple times to increase diagnostic yield if clinically indicated. In as many as 20% of patients with clinical or radiographic LM, the CSF may be nondiagnostic despite multiple samples. LP is contraindicated if there is a risk for brain herniation and should therefore follow MRI to make this assessment.

TREATMENT

LM is generally an incurable condition with a poor prognosis, and a careful balance of risks and benefits must be individualized. The focus of treatment is primarily palliation of symptoms. Treatment must address the entire CSF compartment, and therefore, focal therapy with surgery and radiation has limited use. Nevertheless, neurosurgical evaluation should be considered for CSF shunting, typically to the peritoneum, or for placement of an intrathecal reservoir. CSF shunting carries a theoretical risk of spread of tumor cells into the destination space, but this risk is generally not clinically significant in the context of such limited survival.

Symptomatic or bulky focal lesions may be treated with radiation in a similar fashion to epidural metastases. CSI is not routinely indicated, as it does not improve outcomes and can cause significant morbidity, especially in adults (nausea, dysphagia, fatigue, myelosuppression).

Intrathecal chemotherapy (ITC) is the mainstay of treatment of LM as it allows circulation to the entire CSF volume; specific agents include methotrexate, cytarabine (in both standard and depot formulations), and thiotepa. Cytarabine, especially the depot form, should be preceded and followed by 2 to 3 days of corticosteroid prophylaxis, as a severe chemical meningitis can otherwise result. Combination chemotherapy may be considered, although data showing increased efficacy are sparse. ITC is less effective in patients with obstruction of the CSF and contraindicated in the setting of increased ICP. Occasionally, a combination ventruloperitoneal shunt/Ommaya reservoir device is implanted to both reduce ICP and serve as a method for ITC delivery; however, this requires careful coordination of valve positioning and all too often becomes obstructed with CSF cells. ITC is typically administered intraventricularly using an implanted Ommaya reservoir. Administration via LP is also possible, but this method is more cumbersome and painful and less reliable. ITC carries a risk of meningitis, myelosuppression, and encephalopathy.

Disruption in the normal flow of CSF is a common phenomenon with LM. This has important implications in the administration of ITC, as it can both decrease efficacy and increase toxicity. Assessment of the CSF flow with radionuclide cisternogram prior to ITC is beneficial but not universally available. MRI-based flow studies are emerging but the level of resolution is limited in this context. Identification of sites of obstruction may allow focal treatment with radiation prior to ITC, which may improve flow even in the absence of a discrete lesion. WBRT may be considered, as it is well tolerated and may improve CSF flow.

Systemic chemotherapy has limited use in the treatment of LM due to the blood–brain barrier, but this is an area of ongoing investigation. Additional palliative care with analgesics, steroids, antiseizure medications, and CSF shunting should be initiated as indicated.

CONCLUSIONS

Metastatic disease to the neurologic system, particularly the CNS, is a widespread and clinically important scenario. The diagnosis is generally made with a combination of history, physical exam, and imaging. In some cases, blood work, biopsy, or CSF sampling may also aid in diagnosis. Management of CNS metastases is accomplished with corticosteroids, surgery, radiation, chemotherapy, or a combination of these modalities. The treatment plan and clinical outcome depend on the specific factors of that individual patient, including the location and extent of metastatic lesions, duration of symptoms, and the patient's ability to tolerate treatment.

LEVEL 1 EVIDENCE

1. Glantz MJ, Cole BF, Forsyth PA, et al. Practice parameter: anticonvulsant prophylaxis in patients with newly diagnosed brain tumors. Report of the Quality Standards Subcommittee of the American Academy of Neurology. *Neurology.* 2000;54(10):1886–1893.

2. Borgelt B, Gelber R, Larson M, et al. Ultra-rapid high dose irradiation schedules for the palliation of brain metastases: final results of the first two studies by the Radiation Therapy Oncology Group. *Int J Radiat Oncol Biol Phys.* 1981;7(12):1633–1638.

3. Kurtz JM, Gelber R, Brady LW, et al. The palliation of brain metastases in a favorable patient population: a randomized clinical trial by the Radiation Therapy Oncology Group. *Int J Radiat Oncol Biol Phys.* 1981;7(7):891–895.

4. Murray KJ, Scott C, Greenberg HM, et al. A randomized phase III study of accelerated hyperfractionation versus standard in patients with unresected brain metastases: a report of the Radiation Therapy Oncology Group (RTOG) 9104. *Int J Radiat Oncol Biol Phys.* 1997;39(3):571–574.

5. Muacevic A, Wowra B, Siefert A, et al. Microsurgery plus whole brain irradiation versus Gamma Knife surgery alone for treatment of single metastases to the brain: a randomized controlled multicentre phase III trial. *J Neurooncol.* 2008;87(3):299–307.

6. Patchell RA, Tibbs PA, Walsh JW, et al. A randomized trial of surgery in the treatment of single metastases to the brain. *N Engl J Med.* 1990;322(8):494–500.

7. Noordijk EM, Vecht CJ, Haaxma-Reiche H, et al. The choice of treatment of single brain metastasis should be based on extracranial tumor activity and age. *Int J Radiat Oncol Biol Phys.* 1994;29(4):711–717.

8. Mintz AH, Kestle J, Rathbone MP, et al. A randomized trial to assess the efficacy of surgery in addition to radiotherapy in patients with a single cerebral metastasis. *Cancer.* 1996;78(7):1470–1476.

9. Andrews DW, Scott CB, Sperduto PW, et al. Whole brain radiation therapy with or without stereotactic radiosurgery boost for patients with one to three brain metastases: phase III results of the RTOG 9508 randomised trial. *Lancet.* 2004;363(9422):1665–1672.

10. Brown PD, Pugh S, Laack NN, et al. Memantine for the prevention of cognitive dysfunction in patients receiving whole-brain radiotherapy: a randomized, double-blind, placebo-controlled trial. *Neuro Oncol.* 2013;15(10):1429–1437.

11. Chang EL, Wefel JS, Hess KR, et al. Neurocognition in patients with brain metastases treated with radiosurgery or radiosurgery plus whole-brain irradiation: a randomised controlled trial. *Lancet Oncol.* 2009;10(11):1037–1044.

12. Aoyama H, Shirato H, Tago M, et al. Stereotactic radiosurgery plus whole-brain radiation therapy vs stereotactic radiosurgery alone for treatment of brain metastases: a randomized controlled trial. *JAMA.* 2006;295(21):2483–2491.

13. Kocher M, Soffietti R, Abacioglu U, et al. Adjuvant whole-brain radiotherapy versus observation after radiosurgery or surgical resection of one to three cerebral metastases: results of the EORTC 22952-26001 study. *J Clin Oncol.* 2011;29(2):134–141.

14. Patchell RA, Tibbs PA, Regine WF, et al. Postoperative radiotherapy in the treatment of single metastases to the brain: a randomized trial. *JAMA.* 1998;280(17):1485–1489.

15. Ammirati M, Cobbs CS, Linskey ME, et al. The role of retreatment in the management of recurrent/progressive brain metastases: a systematic review and evidence-based clinical practice guideline. *J Neurooncol.* 2010;96(1):85–96.

16. Sperduto PW, Wang M, Robins HI, et al. A phase 3 trial of whole brain radiation therapy and stereotactic radiosurgery alone versus WBRT and SRS with temozolomide or erlotinib for non-small cell lung cancer and 1 to 3 brain metastases: Radiation Therapy Oncology Group 0320. *Int J Radiat Oncol Biol Phys.* 2013;85(5):1312–1318.

17. Bachelot T, Romieu G, Campone M, et al. Lapatinib plus capecitabine in patients with previously untreated brain metastases from HER2-positive metastatic breast cancer (LANDSCAPE): a single-group phase 2 study. *Lancet Oncol.* 2013;14(1):64–71.

18. Sørensen S, Helweg-Larsen S, Mouridsen H, et al. Effect of high-dose dexamethasone in carcinomatous metastatic spinal cord compression treated with radiotherapy: a randomised trial. *Eur J Cancer.* 1994;30A(1):22–27.

19. Patchell RA, Tibbs PA, Regine WF, et al. Direct decompressive surgical resection in the treatment of spinal cord compression caused by metastatic cancer: a randomised trial. *Lancet.* 2005;366(9486):643–648.

20. Ryu S, Pugh SL, Gerszten PC, et al. RTOG 0631 phase 2/3 study of image guided stereotactic radiosurgery for localized (1-3) spine metastases: phase 2 results. *Pract Radiat Oncol.* 2014;4(2):76–81.

SUGGESTED READINGS

Abu Hejleh T, Clamon G. Advances in the systemic treatment of leptomeningeal cancer. *Clin Adv Hematol Oncol.* 2012;10(3):166–170.

American Cancer Society. Cancer facts and figures 2014. American Cancer Society Web site. http://www.cancer.org/research/cancerfactsstatistics/cancerfactsfigures2014/index. Accessed February 15, 2015.

American Society of Clinical Oncology. The state of cancer care in America, 2014: a report by the American Society of Clinical Oncology. *J Oncol Pract.* 2014;10(2):119–142.

Auchter RM, Lamond JP, Alexander E, et al. A multiinstitutional outcome and prognostic factor analysis of radiosurgery for resectable single brain metastasis. *Int J Radiat Oncol Biol Phys.* 1996;35(1):27–35.

Barajas RF Jr, Cha S. Imaging diagnosis of brain metastasis. *Prog Neurol Surg.* 2012;25:55–73.

Bindal RK, Sawaya R, Leavens ME, et al. Surgical treatment of multiple brain metastases. *J Neurosurg.* 1993;79(2):210–216.

Ceresoli GL, Cappuzzo F, Gregorc V, et al. Gefitinib in patients with brain metastases from non-small-cell lung cancer: a prospective trial. *Ann Oncol.* 2004;15(7):1042–1047.

Chamberlain MC, Kormanik P. Carcinoma meningitis secondary to non-small cell lung cancer: combined modality therapy. *Arch Neurol.* 1998;55(4):506–512.

Chin LS, Regine WF. *Principles and Practice of Stereotactic Radiosurgery.* New York: Springer; 2008.

Coleman RE. Skeletal complications of malignancy. *Cancer.* 1997;80(8 suppl):1588–1594.

Cooper JS, Steinfeld AD, Lerch IA. Cerebral metastases: value of reirradiation in selected patients. *Radiology.* 1990;174(3, pt 1):883–885.

Davies H, Bignell GR, Cox C, et al. Mutations of the BRAF gene in human cancer. *Nature.* 2002;417(6892):949–954.

Davis PC, Hudgins PA, Peterman SB, et al. Diagnosis of cerebral metastases: double-dose delayed CT vs contrast-enhanced MR imaging. *AJNR Am J Neuroradiol.* 1991;12(2):293–300.

Delattre JY, Krol G, Thaler HT, et al. Distribution of brain metastases. *Arch Neurol.* 1988;45(7):741–744.

Dummer R, Goldinger SM, Turtschi CP, et al. Vemurafenib in patients with BRAF(V600) mutation-positive melanoma with symptomatic brain metastases: final results of an open-label pilot study. *Eur J Cancer.* 2014;50(3):611–621.

Fink KR, Fink JR. Imaging of brain metastases. *Surg Neurol Int.* 2013;4(suppl 4):S209–S219.

Flannery TW, Suntharalingam M, Regine WF, et al. Long-term survival in patients with synchronous, solitary brain metastasis from non-small-cell lung cancer treated with radiosurgery. *Int J Radiat Oncol Biol Phys.* 2008;72(1):19–23.

Fuller BG, Heiss J, Oldfield EH. Spinal cord compression. In: DeVita VT Jr, Lawrence TS, Rosenburg SA, eds. *Cancer: Principles and Practice of Oncology.* Philadelphia: Lippincott Williams & Wilkins; 2001:2617–2633.

Garg AK, Wang XS, Shiu AS, et al. Prospective evaluation of spinal reirradiation by using stereotactic body radiation therapy: the University of Texas MD Anderson Cancer Center experience. *Cancer.* 2011;117(15):3509–3516.

Gaspar L, Scott C, Rotman M, et al. Recursive partitioning analysis (RPA) of prognostic factors in three Radiation Therapy Oncology Group (RTOG) brain metastases trials. *Int J Radiat Oncol Biol Phys.* 1997;37(4):745–751.

Gerber NK, Yamada Y, Rimner A, et al. Erlotinib versus radiation therapy for brain metastases in patients with EGFR-mutant lung adenocarcinoma. *Int J Radiat Oncol Biol Phys.* 2014;89(2):322–329.

Gleissner B, Chamberlain MC. Neoplastic meningitis. *Lancet Neurol.* 2006; 5(5):443–452.

Goblirsch MJ, Zwolak PP, Clohisy DR. Biology of bone cancer pain. *Clin Cancer Res.* 2006;12(20, pt 2):6231s–6235s.

Gondi V, Tomé WA, Mehta MP. Why avoid the hippocampus? A comprehensive review. *Radiother Oncol.* 2010;97(3):370–376.

Gutiérrez AN, Westerly DC, Tomé WA, et al. Whole brain radiotherapy with hippocampal avoidance and simultaneously integrated brain metastases boost: a planning study. *Int J Radiat Oncol Biol Phys.* 2007;69(2):589–597.

Halperin EP, Wazer DE, Perez CA. The discipline of radiation oncology. In: Halperin EP, Wazer DE, Perez CA, et al, eds. *Perez and Brady's Principles and Practice of Radiation Oncology.* Philadelphia: Lippincott Williams & Wilkins; 2013.

Kim DY, Lee KW, Yun T, et al. Comparison of intrathecal chemotherapy for leptomeningeal carcinomatosis of a solid tumor: methotrexate alone versus methotrexate in combination with cytosine arabinoside and hydrocortisone. *Jpn J Clin Oncol.* 2003;33(12):608–612.

Kurup P, Reddy S, Hendrickson FR. Results of re-irradiation for cerebral metastases. *Cancer.* 1980;46(12):2587–2589.

Le Rhun E, Taillibert S, Chamberlain MC. Carcinomatous meningitis: leptomeningeal metastases in solid tumors. *Surg Neurol Int.* 2013;4(suppl 4):S265–S288.

Lin NU, Diéras V, Paul D, et al. Multicenter phase II study of lapatinib in patients with brain metastases from HER2-positive breast cancer. *Clin Cancer Res.* 2009;15(4):1452–1459.

Long GV, Trefzer U, Davies MA, et al. Dabrafenib in patients with Val600Glu or Val600Lys BRAF-mutant melanoma metastatic to the brain (BREAK-MB): a multicentre, open-label, phase 2 trial. *Lancet Oncol.* 2012;13(11):1087–1095.

Margolin K, Ernstoff MS, Hamid O, et al. Ipilimumab in patients with melanoma and brain metastases: an open-label, phase 2 trial. *Lancet Oncol.* 2012;13(5):459–465.

Mehta MP, Vogelbaum MA, Chang S, et al. Neoplasms of the central nervous system. In: DeVita VT Jr, Lawrence TS, Rosenberg SA, eds. *Cancer: Principles and Practice of Oncology.* Philadelphia: Lippincott Williams & Wilkins; 2011:1700–1749.

Nichols EM, Patchell RA, Regine WF, et al. Palliation of brain and spinal cord metastases. In: Halperin EP, Wazer DE, Perez CA, et al, eds. *Perez and Brady's Principles and Practices of Radiation Oncology.* Philadelphia: Lippincott Williams & Wilkins; 2013:1766.

O'Neill BP, Iturria NJ, Link MJ, et al. A comparison of surgical resection and stereotactic radiosurgery in the treatment of solitary brain metastases. *Int J Radiat Oncol Biol Phys.* 2003;55(5):1169–1176.

Park SJ, Kim HT, Lee DH, et al. Efficacy of epidermal growth factor receptor tyrosine kinase inhibitors for brain metastasis in non-small cell lung cancer patients harboring either exon 19 or 21 mutation. *Lung Cancer.* 2012; 77(3):556–560.

Rades D, Stalpers LJ, Veninga T, et al. Effectiveness and toxicity of reirradiation (Re-RT) for metastatic spinal cord compression (MSCC) [in German]. *Strahlenther Onkol.* 2005;181(9):595–600.

Rades D, Stalpers LJ, Veninga T, et al. Evaluation of five radiation schedules and prognostic factors for metastatic spinal cord compression. *J Clin Oncol.* 2005;23(15):3366–3375.

Ruderman NB, Hall TC. Use of glucocorticoids in the palliative treatment of metastatic brain tumors. *Cancer.* 1965;18:298–306.

Sahgal A, Ma L, Weinberg V, et al. Reirradiation human spinal cord tolerance for stereotactic body radiotherapy. *Int J Radiat Oncol Biol Phys.* 2012; 82(1):107–116.

Sawrie SM, Guthrie BL, Spencer SA, et al. Predictors of distant brain recurrence for patients with newly diagnosed brain metastases treated with stereotactic radiosurgery alone. *Int J Radiat Oncol Biol Phys.* 2008;70(1):181–186.

Schiff D, Shaw EG, Cascino TL, et al. Outcome after spinal reirradiation for malignant epidural spinal cord compression. *Ann Neurol.* 1995;37(5):583–589.

Schöggl A, Kitz K, Reddy M, et al. Defining the role of stereotactic radiosurgery versus microsurgery in the treatment of single brain metastases. *Acta Neurochir (Wien).* 2000;142(6):621–626.

Shaw E, Scott C, Souhami L, et al. Single dose radiosurgical treatment of recurrent previously irradiated primary brain tumors and brain metastases: final report of RTOG protocol 90-05. *Int J Radiat Oncol Biol Phys.* 2000;47(2):291–298.

Soltys SG, Adler JR, Lipani JD, et al. Stereotactic radiosurgery of the postoperative resection cavity for brain metastases. *Int J Radiat Oncol Biol Phys.* 2008; 70(1):187–193.

Son CH, Jimenez R, Niemierko A, et al. Outcomes after whole brain reirradiation in patients with brain metastases. *Int J Radiat Oncol Biol Phys.* 2012; 82(2):e167–e172.

Sperduto CM, Watanabe Y, Mullan J, et al. A validation study of a new prognostic index for patients with brain metastases: the Graded Prognostic Assessment. *J Neurosurg.* 2008;109(suppl):87–89.

Townsend PW, Rosenthal HG, Smalley SR, et al. Impact of postoperative radiation therapy and other perioperative factors on outcome after orthopedic stabilization of impending or pathologic fractures due to metastatic disease. *J Clin Oncol.* 1994;12(11):2345–2350.

Twombly R. Cancer surpasses heart disease as leading cause of death for all but the very elderly. *J Natl Cancer Inst.* 2005;97(5):330–331.

Welsh JW, Komaki R, Amini A, et al. Phase II trial of erlotinib plus concurrent whole-brain radiation therapy for patients with brain metastases from non-small-cell lung cancer. *J Clin Oncol.* 2013;31(7):895–902.

Wen PY, Black PM, Loeffler JS. Treatment of metastatic cancer. In: DeVita VT, Heilman S, Rosenberg SA, eds. *Cancer: Principles and Practice of Oncology.* Philadelphia: Lippincott Williams & Wilkins; 2001:2655–2670.

Wilson EH, Weninger W, Hunter CA, et al. Trafficking of immune cells in the central nervous system. *J Clin Invest.* 2010;120(5):1368–1379.

Wong WW, Schild SE, Sawyer TE, et al. Analysis of outcome in patients reirradiated for brain metastases. *Int J Radiat Oncol Biol Phys.* 1996;34(3):585–590.

Wu YL, Zhou C, Cheng Y, et al. Erlotinib as second-line treatment in patients with advanced non-small-cell lung cancer and asymptomatic brain metastases: a phase II study (CTONG-0803). *Ann Oncol.* 2013;24(4):993–999.

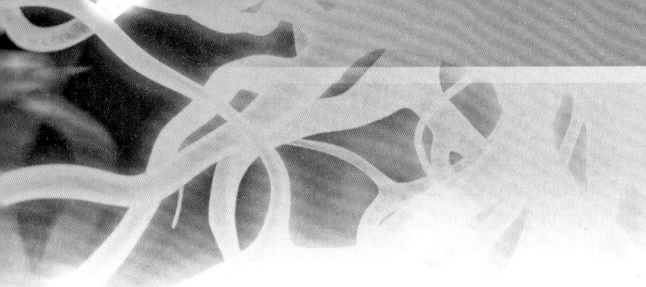

INTRODUCTION

Diseases of the dura are rather uncommon, except for meningiomas. Not just the most common dural disease, meningiomas are the most common intracranial primary tumor in adults. Especially in the current environment of neuroimaging with computed tomography (CT) or magnetic resonance imaging (MRI) being performed for any and every possible neurologic symptom, both symptomatic and more frequently asymptomatic meningiomas will be found. Accordingly, meningiomas may become the most common intracranial tumor neurologists, and most physicians, will encounter. Although they are usually benign, they may enlarge and/or cause neurologic dysfunction depending on the location and because the cranium has only a limited capacity to accommodate an expanding mass. Surgery remains the treatment of choice, but not all meningiomas are amenable to complete resection, and some will recur and require further therapy. This chapter will outline the major dural diseases with the majority devoted to meningiomas.

MENINGIOMAS

EPIDEMIOLOGY

Meningiomas are the most common primary "brain" tumor in adults, although technically, they are tumors of the brain covering rather than brain parenchyma. The Central Brain Tumor Registry of the United States estimates an incidence of approximately 20,000 new meningioma cases diagnosed per year. This represents 36% of all primary brain tumors (World Health Organization [WHO]). These tumors have a clear female predominance with an almost 2:1 female-to-male ratio. These tumors are quite rare in children except within a predisposing neurogenetic syndrome. They are substantially more common in adults and tend to increase in incidence with age, particularly older than the age of 65 years. Autopsy series suggest a prevalence of 2%, typically asymptomatic and discovered incidentally during life or postmortem.

The only clear risk factors for meningiomas are prior radiotherapy involving the head and neck region as well as predisposing neurogenetic syndromes, such as neurofibromatosis type 2 (NF2). Ionizing radiation has also been demonstrated to be clear risk factor for future meningioma development. Prior radiation therapy for an extracranial malignancy such as head and neck cancer or childhood leukemia is the most common. These meningiomas that develop as a result of prior radiotherapy tend to be more aggressive in their clinical course. The latency for meningioma development is inversely proportional to the dose of radiation delivered.

Although no longer performed, scalp radiation for tinea capitis, a fungal infection, has been linked to meningioma development. Similarly, older less refined dental x-rays have been inconclusively linked to meningiomas. Currently, however, radiotherapy is no longer performed for scalp infections and newer dental x-rays probably do not have significant risk, different from the older less refined variant. Probably the most controversial potential link to

meningiomas in the recent media and scientific literature has been the use of cellular phones and potential radiation exposure. To date, there has been no proven definitive link between cellular phones and the development of a meningioma.

PATHOBIOLOGY

Meningiomas are tumors that arise from the arachnoid coverings of the brain. Histologically, these tumors have various appearances depending on the subtype of meningioma, although most physicians frequently recall the whorling pattern of tumor cells which is most common and calcium collections known as *psammoma bodies*. The WHO classifies meningiomas into three grades (in the following text).

The most common neurogenetic syndrome predisposing the patient to meningiomas is NF2, the less common form of neurofibromatosis. NF2 is an autosomal dominant disorder with full penetrance caused by alteration of the *NF2* gene (also known as *chromosome 22*, which encodes for the tumor suppressor protein merlin (moesin-ezrin-radixin-like protein), also called *neurofibromin*. Approximately 80% of sporadic meningiomas also harbor *NF2* alterations. However, there is no clear selective therapy to target merlin alterations.

Recent research efforts have focused on understanding the biology of cancer as a whole and using targeted therapies that disrupt a specific biologic pathway, typically a growth factor ligand/receptor-mediated pathway. Meningiomas are highly vascular tumors with elevated expression of the vascular endothelial growth factor (VEGF) receptor and its ligand, VEGF. Other growth factor pathways such as platelet-derived growth factor (PDGF), epidermal growth factor (EGF), insulin-like growth factor (IGF), and somatostatin are also expressed in meningiomas. Efforts at targeting these pathways are discussed in the following text.

A major thrust of cancer investigation over the last decade has been whole genome sequencing to identify drugable oncogenic driver mutations. Mutations in two pathways recently were identified in approximately 20% of meningiomas: AKT and SMO. AKT mutations disrupt the homeostasis that normally regulates cancer cell survival, proliferation, angiogenesis, and metabolism. SMO mutations alter a key pathway responsible for controlling cancer cell self-renewal.

In the Clark et al. paper, genomic analysis revealed oncogenic mutations in *AKT1* and *SMO* in 13% and 4% of specimens, respectively. These mutated tumors tend to occur more frequently in skull base locations, which also tend to be the most surgically challenging or inaccessible areas. Patients with *AKT* mutations harbored the E17K mutation, a well-characterized oncogenic mutation present in several other cancer types. The E17K mutation can be found in breast cancer, colorectal cancer, and lung cancer and results in constitutive AKT activation, which in turn stimulates downstream mTOR activity, resulting in overactivity of the PI3K pathway. PI3K pathway activation in turn stimulates multiple oncogenic processes including cell proliferation and angiogenesis. The *SMO* mutations included the L412F seen in a subset of medulloblastomas and the

W535L alteration seen in basal cell carcinoma and predictive of sensitivity to U.S. Food and Drug Administration (FDA)–approved therapy with vismodegib, a hedgehog inhibitor. When the SMO protein is activated, it results in ligand-independent downstream activation of the hedgehog pathway resulting in cell proliferation and cancer stem cell self-renewal.

In the Brastianos et al. paper, 65 meningioma specimens underwent analysis and revealed similar results identifying *AKT* and *SMO* mutations in a subset of patients. Five patients (8%) demonstrated AKT mutations, all E17K. Three patients (5%) demonstrated *SMO* mutations, two of which were the W535L mutation seen in basal cell carcinoma and one L412F alteration previously described in desmoplastic medulloblastoma. They then studied an additional 46 grade I tumors and 49 grade II and III tumors and found 6 AKT1 E17K mutated tumors (1 grade III, 5 grade I), and 2 SMO L412F mutated tumors (both grade I).

In summary, these two studies demonstrated that PI3K pathway activation and hedgehog pathway activation occurs in a subset of meningioma patients. The mutations seen are well characterized in other cancer types and in the case of basal cell cancer, predict therapeutic response to inhibition with an available agent. Future studies hope to define the role, if any, of these agents in the treatment of these particular molecular subtypes of meningioma.

CLINICAL MANIFESTATIONS

As with most other brain tumors, the clinical presentation of meningiomas is highly variable, depending on tumor location, size, and shape. Tumors may manifest as visual disturbances, speech dysfunction, weakness, sensory dysfunction, neurocognitive dysfunction, personality changes, or seizures. Because meningiomas are typically slow-growing neoplasms, they rarely cause acute increases in intracranial pressure, resulting in symptoms such as headache, nausea, vomiting, or alteration of consciousness. In fact, because they are such slow-growing tumors, they can often become surprisingly large without causing any clinical neurologic dysfunction. However, even a "benign" meningioma can result in disabling neurologic dysfunction if it grows beyond the capacity of the skull to accommodate the increase in volume. Rarely, these tumors may metastasize outside the central nervous system (CNS), usually to bone. This is an exceptionally rare event and typically only with malignant meningiomas.

DIAGNOSIS

Meningiomas are best visualized on an MRI with contrast, which demonstrates a brightly enhancing mass arising off of the dura which typically has a linear continuation with the dura known as *a dural tail* (Fig. 98.1). CT with contrast may demonstrate the same pattern of enhancement, but MRI provides a better visualization of the underlying brain. CT may be superior for demonstrating any changes in the neighboring bone, as meningiomas can trigger a reactive hyperostosis in the bone adjacent to the meningioma itself, seen in approximately 25% of patients. Without contrast, meningiomas appear on both CT and MRI as either hypodense or hypointense, or isodense or isointense.

As with most tumors, neuroimaging alone cannot definitively diagnose a meningioma, which depends on tissue analysis

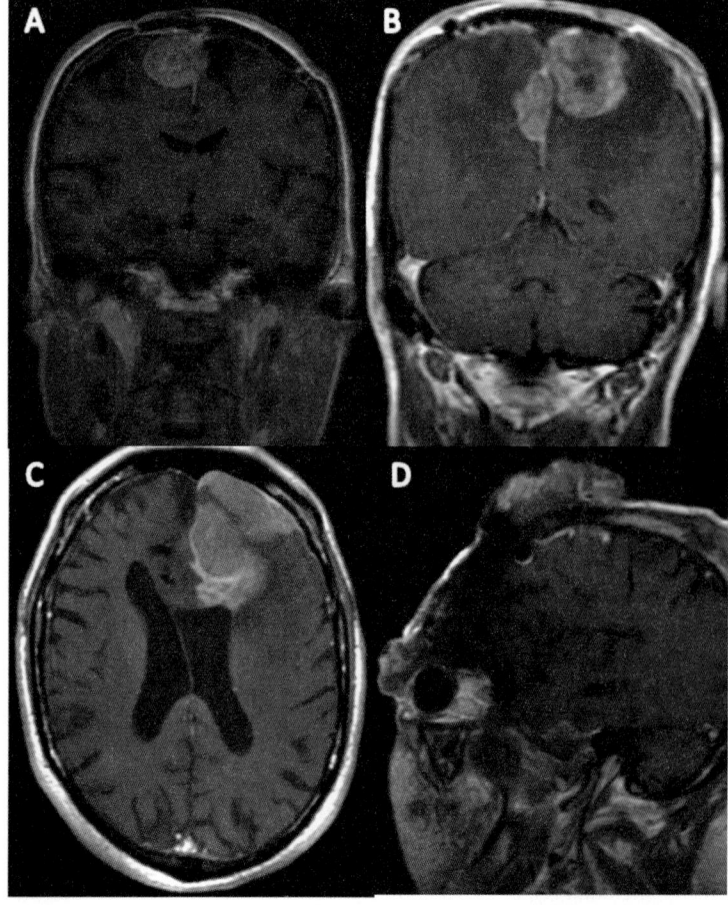

FIGURE 98.1 MRI appearance of meningiomas. **A:** Coronal T1 postcontrast image demonstrating a recurrent grade I meningioma. **B:** Coronal T1 postcontrast image demonstrating an atypical meningioma noting significant peritumoral edema. **C:** Axial T1 postcontrast image demonstrating an anaplastic meningioma noting brain invasion. **D:** Sagittal T1 postcontrast image demonstrating extracranial growth of a recurrent surgery and radiation refractory meningioma.

TABLE 98.1	World Health Organization Grading Criteria for Meningiomas

WHO Grade I Meningioma

Angiomatous
Fibrous
Lymphoplasmacyte-rich
Meningothelial
Metaplastic
Microcystic
Psammomatous
Secretory
Transitional

WHO Grade II Meningioma

Clear cell
Chordoid
Atypical: greater than four mitoses per 10 high-power fields or at least three of the following features:
- Increased cellularity
- Small cells with a high nuclear-to-cytoplasmic ratio
- Prominent nucleoli
- Patternless or sheetlike growth
- Necrosis

WHO Grade III Meningioma

Rhabdoid
Papillary
Anaplastic (malignant): ≥20 mitoses per 10 high-power fields and/or malignant characteristics including the following:
- Loss of typical growth patterns
- Brain invasion
- Abundant mitoses with atypical forms
- Multifocal necrosis

acquired by biopsy or resection. The WHO classifies meningiomas in three grades (Table 98.1). WHO grade I meningiomas are classified as "benign" meningiomas and makeup approximately 80% of meningiomas. They are typically slow-growing tumors that basically fail to demonstrate any of the characteristics of higher grade meningiomas. Grade I meningiomas include most of the histologic subtypes: angiomatous, fibrous, lymphoplasmacyte-rich, meningothelial, metaplastic, microcystic, psammomatous, secretory, and transitional meningiomas. WHO grade II meningiomas include the clear cell and chordoid histologic variants, as well as atypical tumors that harbor increased mitotic activity as evidenced by four or more mitoses per 10 high-power fields or at least three of the following features: increased cellularity, small cells with a high nuclear-to-cytoplasmic ratio, prominent nucleoli, patternless or sheet-like growth, or necrosis. Importantly, brain invasion is associated with increased rates of recurrence and is sufficient to diagnose a WHO grade II tumor, regardless of the presence of other atypical features. WHO grade III meningiomas include rhabdoid, papillary, and anaplastic (malignant). The criteria for anaplastic meningiomas include increased mitotic activity as evidenced by 20 or more mitoses per 10 high-power fields and/or malignant characteristics resembling carcinoma, sarcoma, or melanoma, such as the loss of usual meningioma growth patterns, infiltration of underlying brain, abundant mitoses with atypical forms, and multifocal necrosis. Anaplasia is sufficient to diagnose a WHO grade III regardless of the presence of brain invasion.

TREATMENT

Despite advances in cancer therapy, the treatment of meningioma remains primarily surgical with the goal of maximum safe surgical resection. In patients in whom a meningioma is unresectable due to location yet needs treatment, or in patients whose tumor is only amenable to a subtotal resection with persistent neurologic symptoms or dysfunction, radiation therapy is typically offered. Oftentimes, the biggest clinical question revolves around the timing of each of these therapies, which we will discuss further within the individual grades of meningioma and is outlined in Figure 98.2.

Surgery

The goal of surgical resection is always maximum resection balanced against minimal neurologic surgical morbidity. The degree of surgical resection is graded on the Simpson grading scale, ranging from grade I which includes complete removal of not only the meningioma but also any involved dura or bone through grade 5 which only includes decompression, with or without biopsy of the tumor. However, in clinical practice, the most commonly used terminology is *gross total resection* (removal of all visible tumor), *subtotal resection* (partial resection), or *biopsy* (only a small piece of tissue was removed for histologic diagnosis).

Radiotherapy

The two forms of radiotherapy used most often are external beam radiation therapy and stereotactic radiosurgery. External beam radiation therapy (EBRT) uses standard radiation techniques of delivering a lower dose of radiation per day over a longer course of treatment. Stereotactic radiosurgery (SRS) delivers a very high dose of radiation, typically within one session. SRS goes by many different names depending on the machine that is used, the energy source, and planning platform. Some centers use Gamma Knife machines, CyberKnife machines, or LINAC systems. EBRT and SRS have never been compared against one another in a randomized prospective fashion. However, both forms of radiation demonstrated efficacy in treating meningiomas in multiple retrospective series. Similarly, the different forms of SRS have never been compared against one another in a randomized fashion, but they are likely all comparable. The decision of whether to use EBRT or SRS is typically determined by the location of the tumor, potential complications of radiation, and expertise of the physician administering the treatment.

Chemotherapy

Unlike surgery and radiation, chemotherapy has yet to demonstrate a benefit in the treatment of meningioma. However, there is a need for effective medical or chemotherapy for certain subsets of patients with meningiomas, especially those with meningiomas refractory to surgery and radiation. In this subset, no medical therapy has yet proven effective. The other subset for which a viable chemotherapy approach is needed is that subset of tumors in whom surgery and/or radiation is either technically not feasible or not advisable due to other circumstances.

Many chemotherapies have been studied in the treatment of meningioma; unfortunately, no therapy has demonstrated clear efficacy in a randomized phase III trial (Table 98.2), and no FDA-approved therapies exist. Studies investigating traditional cytotoxic chemotherapies (temozolomide, hydroxyurea, irinotecan, and triple therapy with cyclophosphamide + doxorubicin + vincristine), hormonal therapies (progesterone and estrogen modulators), interferon α-2b, somatostatin analogues, and molecularly targeted therapies including inhibitors of PDGF (imatinib) and epidermal

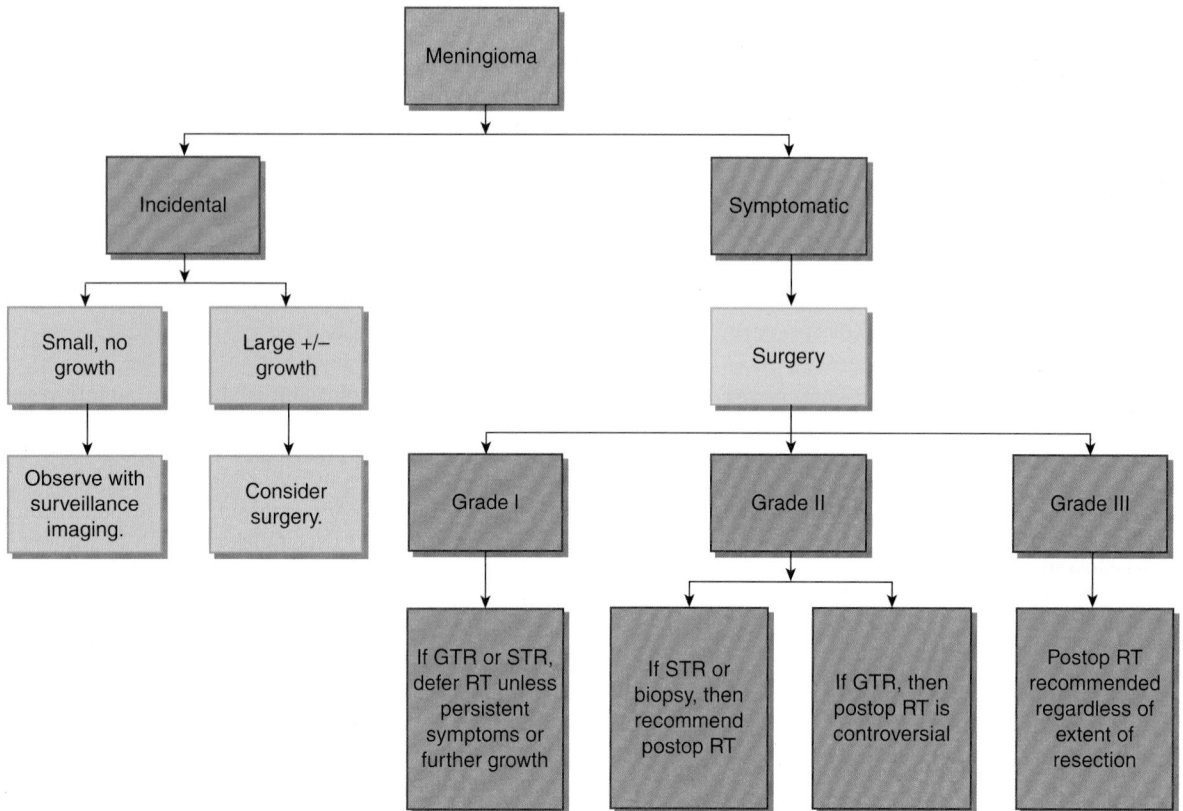

FIGURE 98.2 Algorithm for the treatment of meningiomas. GTR, gross total resection; STR, subtotal resection; RT, radiation therapy.

growth factor receptor (EGFR; gefitinib and erlotinib) have all been disappointing. The 6-month progression-free survival rates are less than 20%, similar to those for the most common and aggressive parenchymal brain tumor, glioblastomas.

Meningiomas are highly vascular and targeting tumor vasculature may be a potentially effective strategy. Targeted therapy to disrupt tumor angiogenesis (the development of new blood vessels) such as vascular endothelial growth factor receptor (VEGFR) with the tyrosine kinase inhibitor sunitinib and targeting the VEGF ligand with the monoclonal antibody bevacizumab have shown some possible benefit and may represent a viable future treatment strategy.

The recent discovery of oncogenic driver mutations in either AKT in the PI3K pathway or SMO in the hedgehog pathway may provide potential therapeutic targets in a subset of patients. Inhibitors of AKT and SMO are currently in clinical trial development. However, *AKT* and *SMO* mutant tumors are a minority, additional discoveries are desperately needed.

OUTCOMES

World Health Organization Grade I Meningioma

The preferred treatment of WHO grade I meningiomas remains surgical resection whenever feasible. With gross total resection, the 5-year recurrence rate is approximately 10% to 25% (Rogers et al.). With subtotal resection, it is approximately 25% to 50%. With either gross total resection or subtotal resection, postoperatively, these patients are managed with observation and surveillance imaging. Radiation is typically reserved for when patients have persistent neurologic dysfunction due to a tumor that cannot be completely resected or for patients who suffer a recurrence or progressive growth of their tumor.

World Health Organization Grade II Meningioma

As with grade I tumors, the initial and preferred management of WHO grade II meningiomas is also maximum safe surgical resection. If gross total resection is not achieved, postoperative radiotherapy is standard absent a contraindication. However, there is substantial controversy whether the benefits of immediate postoperative radiotherapy outweigh the risks for completely resected tumors. The 5-year recurrence rate after surgery alone is approximately 50%, and numerous retrospective series have demonstrated an increase in progression-free survival with the addition of postoperative radiotherapy. However, immediate postoperative radiotherapy (as opposed to radiotherapy at the time of recurrence) has yet to demonstrate an overall survival advantage and has risks. Fortunately, a randomized trial is ongoing.

World Health Organization Grade III Meningioma

After surgery alone, the chance of recurrence at 5 years is 70% to 80% after gross total resection and 100% after subtotal resection. Therefore, postoperative radiation is nearly always offered to these patients in an attempt to increase the time before inevitable recurrence. Regardless, however, nearly all patients recur.

Incidental Meningioma

The incidental meningioma is a common yet often puzzling clinical situation. With imaging alone, there is uncertainty as to the histology, grade, and pace of growth (if any) of the incidentally found lesion. Often, the meningioma itself is asymptomatic and unrelated to the initial complaint that led to the neuroimaging. In the case of a

TABLE 98.2	Medical Therapies Investigated for Meningioma
Drug	**Mechanism of Action**
Hydroxyurea	Ribonucleotide reductase inhibitor
Temozolomide	Alkylating chemotherapy
Irinotecan	Topoisomerase 1 inhibitor
Cyclophosphamide + Adriamycin + vincristine	Combination cytotoxic chemotherapy
Interferon-α	Immunomodulation
Mifepristone (RU-486)	Antiprogesterone
Megestrol acetate	Progesterone receptor agonist
Medroxyprogesterone acetate	Synthetic progesterone
Tamoxifen	Antiestrogen
Octreotide	Somatostatin analogue
Sandostatin LAR	Somatostatin analogue
Pasireotide LAR (SOM230C)	Somatostatin analogue
Imatinib	PDGFR TKI
Erlotinib	EGFR TKI
Gefitinib	EGFR TKI
Vatalanib	VEGFR + PDGFR TKI
Sunitinib	VEGFR + PDGFR TKI
Bevacizumab	Anti-VEGF antibody
NovoTTF-100A (*external device, trial ongoing*)	Microtubule inhibition

PDGFR, platelet-derived growth factor receptor; TKI, tyrosine kinase inhibitor; EGFR, epidermal growth factor receptor; VEGFR, vascular endothelial growth factor receptor; VEGF, vascular endothelial growth factor.

small asymptomatic incidentally found meningioma, the preferred treatment is one of observation. If repeat imaging demonstrates further stability, then these tumors can be followed expectantly with periodic imaging and clinical evaluations. If there is growth, then typically, a surgical intervention is offered to these patients.

OTHER DURAL DISEASES

HEMANGIOPERICYTOMAS

Hemangiopericytomas (HPC) are tumors that also may arise off the dura and appear radiographically similar to meningiomas. However, they usually behave more like sarcomas with a more aggressive course, multiple recurrences, and metastases to extracranial organs (particularly bone, liver, and lung). Surgery and postoperative radiation are standard, although recurrence is nearly universal.

DURAL METASTASES

The radiographic appearance of metastases to the dura from extracranial malignancies (such as breast cancer) is usually very similar to that of meningiomas. However, dural metastases are more often multiple, may appear as diffuse dural thickening (in the following text), and usually have a faster growth rate on subsequent images. These are more common in lymphoma and possibly breast cancer

but should really be suspected in any patient with a systemic malignancy. The breast cancer patient is a particular challenge, as these patients also have an increased incidence of meningioma. Short-interval imaging and reassessment can usually differentiate between dural metastasis and meningioma on the basis of the growth rate (faster with metastases, slower with benign meningiomas). Occasionally, these entities are mixed ("collision" tumor). Treatment is similar to metastatic disease elsewhere in the brain, considering radiation and chemotherapy, and occasionally surgery (especially if histology is in question). Dural metastases do differ from parenchymal metastases in that dural metastases are not protected by a blood–brain barrier such as parenchymal disease.

HYPERTROPHIC PACHYMENINGITIS

Hypertrophic pachymeningitis refers to a thickening of the dura, either focally or diffusely, that may be caused by a variety of different etiologies. In general, this is a rather rare disorder, although the differential is broad including infections (tuberculosis, fungal, syphilis), autoimmune (rheumatoid arthritis, Sjögren disease), vasculitic (Wegener, giant cell arteritis, Behçet disease), sarcoid, histiocytosis, and metastases from systemic malignancies, as well as "idiopathic" hypertrophic pachymeningitis (IHP) where no underlying etiology is identified.

The most common symptoms are headache, followed by visual dysfunction, then other cranial nerve dysfunction, and cerebellar dysfunction. Seizures may occur due to local irritation of underlying brain. Imaging features on MRI are typically diffuse dural enhancement, which may be either nodular or smooth. Evaluation for underlying causes should be sought and lumbar puncture is typically necessary. In the idiopathic variety, there is typically a pleocytosis (usually lymphocytic) and elevated protein. Treatment is directed at the underlying cause or in the case of IHP with immunosuppressive therapy, often starting with corticosteroids.

SUGGESTED READINGS

Black PM, Morokoff AP, Zauberman J. Surgery for extra-axial tumors of the cerebral convexity and midline. *Neurosurgery*. 2008;62(6)(suppl 3):1115–1121.

Bondy M, Ligon BL. Epidemiology and etiology of intracranial meningiomas: a review. *J Neurooncol*. 1996;29:197–205.

Brastianos PK, Horowitz PM, Santagata S, et al. Genomic sequencing of meningiomas identifies oncogenic SMO and AKT1 mutations. *Nat Genet*. 2013;45:285–289.

Clark VE, Erson-Omay EZ, Serin A, et al. Genomic analysis of non-NF2 meningiomas reveals mutations in TRAF7, KLF4, AKT1, and SMO. *Science*. 2013;339:1077–1080.

Custer BS, Koepsell TD, Mueller BA. The association between breast carcinoma and meningioma in women. *Cancer*. 2002;94:1626–1635.

Grunberg SM, Rankin C, Townsend J, et al. Phase III double-blind randomized placebo-controlled study of mifepristone (RU) for the treatment of unresectable meningioma. *Proc Am Soc Clinical Oncol*. 2001;20:56a.

Hatano N, Behari S, Nagatani T, et al. Idiopathic hypertrophic cranial pachymeningitis: clinicoradiological spectrum and therapeutic options. *Neurosurgery*. 1999;45:1336–1344.

Hosler MR, Turbin RE, Cho E-S, et al. Idiopathic hypertrophic pachymeningitis mimicking lymphoplasmacyte-rich meningioma. *J Neuroophthalmol*. 2007;27:95–98.

Kaley T, Barani I, Chamberlain M, et al. Historical benchmarks for medical therapy trials in surgery- and radiation-refractory meningioma: a RANO review. *Neuro Oncol*. 2014;16:829–840.

Kaley TJ, Wen P, Schiff D, et al. Phase II trial of sunitinib for recurrent and progressive atypical and anaplastic meningioma. *Neuro Oncol*. 2015; 17:116–121.

Kupersmith MJ, Martin V, Heller G, et al. Idiopathic hypertrophic pachymeningitis. *Neurology*. 2004;62:686–694.

Longstreth WT Jr, Phillips LE, Drangsholt M, et al. Dental X-rays and the risk of intracranial meningioma. *Cancer*. 2004;100:1026–1034.

Louis DN, Ohgaki H, Wiestler OD, et al. *WHO Classification of Tumours of the Central Nervous System*. 4th ed. Lyon, France: International Agency for Research and Cancer; 2007.

Nakamura M, Roser F, Michel J, et al. The natural history of incidental meningiomas. *Neurosurgery*. 2003;53:62–70; discussion 70–71.

Nayak L, Iwamoto FM, Rudnick JD, et al. Atypical and anaplastic meningiomas treated with bevacizumab. *J Neurooncol*. 2012;109(1):187–193.

Norden AD, Drappatz J, Wen PY. Advances in meningioma therapy. *Curr Neurol Neurosci Rep*. 2009;9(3):231–240.

Ostrom QT, Gittleman H, Farah P, et al. CBTRUS statistical report: primary brain and central nervous system tumors diagnosed in the United States in 2006-2010. *Neuro Oncol*. 2013;15(suppl 2):ii1–ii56.

Quant EC, Wen PY. Response assessment in neuro-oncology. *Curr Oncol Rep*. 2011;13:50–56.

Rogers L, Barani I, Chamberlain M, et al. Knowledge base, treatment outcomes, and uncertainties. A RANO review. *J Neurosurg*. 2015;122:4–23.

Rudnik A, Larysz D, Gamrot J, et al. Idiopathic hypertrophic pachymeningitis—case report and literature review. *Folia Neuropathol*. 2007;45: 36–42.

Sadetzki S, Flint-Richter P, Ben-Tal T, et al. Radiation-induced meningioma: a descriptive study of 253 cases. *J Neurosurg*. 2002;97:1078–1082.

Voller B, Vass K, Wanschitz J, et al. Hypertrophic chronic pachymeningitis as a localized immune process in the craniocervical region. *Neurology*. 2001;56:107–109.

Wen PY, Lee EQ, Reardon DA, et al. Current clinical development of PI3K pathway inhibitors in glioblastoma. *Neuro Oncol*. 2012;14(7):819–829.

Wen PY, Quant E, Drappatz J, et al. Medical therapies for meningiomas. *J Neurooncol*. 2010;99:365–378.

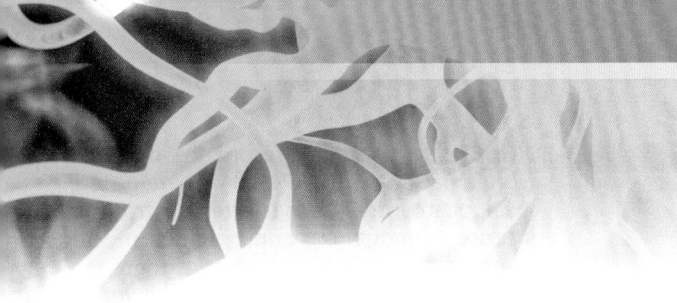

Primary Central Nervous System Lymphoma 99

Tracy T. Batchelor

INTRODUCTION

Primary central nervous system lymphoma (PCNSL) is an extranodal non-Hodgkin lymphoma confined to the brain, leptomeninges, eyes, or spinal cord. The prognosis of PCNSL is inferior to that of other non-Hodgkin lymphoma subtypes. The diagnosis and management of PCNSL differs from that of other primary brain cancers and non-Hodgkin lymphoma in other parts of the body.

EPIDEMIOLOGY

PCNSL is a rare brain tumor and subtype of non-Hodgkin lymphoma. An estimated 3,855 cases of PCNSL were diagnosed in the United States from 2004 to 2006, and the number of cases is expected to increase further with the aging of the U.S. population. The median age at diagnosis is 65 years and PCNSL is slightly more common among men. PCNSL accounts for approximately 3% of all the primary central nervous system (CNS) tumors diagnosed each year in the United States. Between 1970 and 2000, the incidence of PCNSL increased, largely due to the HIV pandemic. The annual incidence rate is 0.47 cases per 100,000 person-years. Since 2000, there has been a further increase in the incidence of PCNSL, especially in the elderly. Congenital or acquired immunodeficiency is the only established risk factor for PCNSL and individuals infected with the HIV are at greater risk of developing this tumor. However, the incidence of HIV-related PCNSL has declined dramatically, and this chapter focuses on PCNSL in the immunocompetent host.

PATHOBIOLOGY

Approximately 90% of PCNSL cases are diffuse large B-cell lymphomas (DLBCL), with the remainder consisting of T-cell lymphomas, poorly characterized low-grade lymphomas, or Burkitt lymphomas. Primary CNS DLBCL is composed of centroblasts or immunoblasts clustered in the perivascular space, with reactive lymphocytes, macrophages, and activated microglial cells intermixed with the tumor cells. Most tumors express pan–B-cell markers including CD19, CD20, CD22, and CD79a. The molecular mechanisms underlying transformation and localization to the CNS are poorly understood. Limitations in molecular studies of PCNSL include the rarity of the disease and the limited availability of tissue because the diagnosis is most often made with stereotactic needle biopsy. Like systemic DLBCL, PCNSL harbors chromosomal translocations of the *BCL6* gene, deletions in 6q, and aberrant somatic hypermutation in protooncogenes including *MYC* and *PAX5*. Inactivation of *CDKN2A* is also commonly observed in both entities. Also like DLBCL, PCNSL can be classified into the three molecular subclasses by gene expression profiling: type 3 large B-cell lymphoma, germinal center B-cell (GCB) lymphoma, and activated B-cell lymphoma (ABC). In all DLBCL cases, the ABC gene expression profile is associated with an inferior prognosis versus the GCB profile. The ABC subclass accounts for a higher proportion of primary CNS DLBCL cases versus other types of DLBCL. This higher prevalence of the ABC gene expression profile subtype in PCNSL may partially account for the relatively inferior prognosis of this lymphoma versus other forms of DLBCL. Moreover, certain molecular features distinguish primary CNS DLBCL from systemic DLBCL. Gene expression profiles demonstrate that PCNSL is characterized by differential expression of genes related to adhesion and the extracellular matrix pathways, including *MUM1*, *CXCL13*, and *CHI3L1*. The ongoing somatic hypermutation with biased use of V_H gene segments that has been observed in PCNSL is suggestive of an antigen-dependent proliferation. These observations are consistent with the hypothesis that PCNSL is secondary to antigen-dependent activation of circulating B cells, which subsequently localize to the CNS by expression of various adhesion and extracellular matrix–related genes. However, further molecular studies to investigate the transforming events and the subsequent events responsible for CNS tropism in PCNSL are needed. Insights into the molecular pathogenesis of PCNSL may allow the development of targeted therapeutic approaches for this tumor.

CLINICAL MANIFESTATIONS

The median age of immunocompetent patients diagnosed with PCNSL is 60 years. The presenting symptoms and signs are variable. In 248 immunocompetent patients, 43% had neuropsychiatric signs, 33% had symptoms of increased intracranial pressure, 14% had seizures, and 4% had ocular symptoms. Seizures are less common than with other types of brain tumors probably because PCNSL involves predominantly subcortical white matter rather than epileptogenic gray matter. Unlike patients with systemic non-Hodgkin lymphoma, PCNSL patients rarely manifest B symptoms.

DIAGNOSIS

The International PCNSL Collaborative Group (IPCG) has developed guidelines to determine extent of disease. A gadolinium-enhanced brain magnetic resonance imaging (MRI) scan is the most sensitive radiographic study for the detection of PCNSL (Fig. 99.1). Most PCNSL patients present with a single brain mass. The mass is typically isointense to hyperintense on T2-weighted MRI sequences and homogeneously enhancing on postcontrast images. The diagnosis of PCNSL is typically made by stereotactic brain biopsy, by cerebrospinal fluid (CSF) analysis, or by analysis of vitreous aspirate in patients with ocular involvement. Given the possible delay in diagnosis and treatment with the latter two methods, prompt stereotactic biopsy is advised in almost all cases that are surgically accessible. Secondary CSF and ocular involvement occurs in approximately 15% to 20% and 5% to 20% of PCNSL patients, respectively. Presenting symptoms of

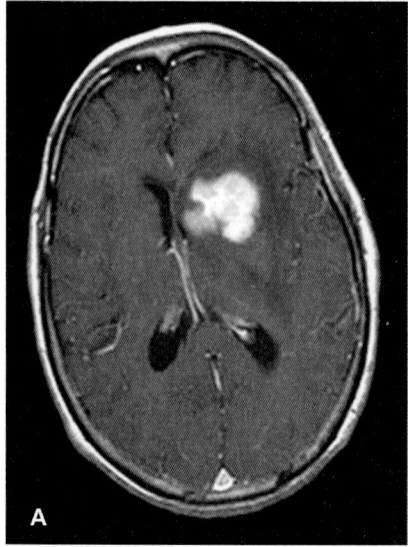 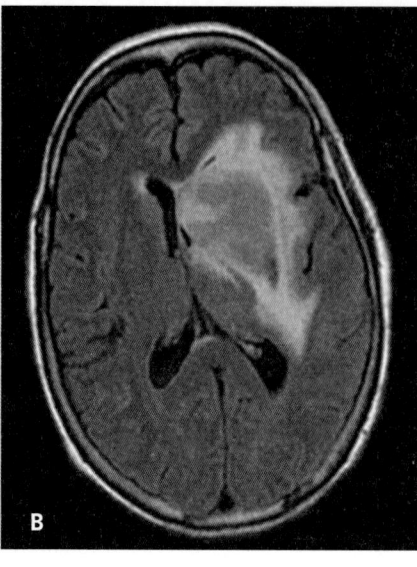

FIGURE 99.1 Magnetic resonance images from a patient with PCNSL. A T1-weighted, axial, postcontrast scan **(A)** demonstrates intense, homogenous enhancement of the tumor in the region of the left caudate nucleus. An axial T2/fluid-attenuated inversion recovery (FLAIR) scan at the same anatomic level **(B)** demonstrates hyperintense signal surrounding the tumor, reflecting vasogenic cerebral edema. (Courtesy of Priscilla K. Brastianos, MD.)

ocular involvement include eye pain, blurred vision, and floaters. B symptoms such as weight loss, fevers, and night sweats are infrequent in PCNSL. A thorough diagnostic evaluation is needed to establish the extent of the lymphoma and to confirm localization to the CNS. Physical examination should consist of a lymph node examination, a testicular examination in men, and a comprehensive neurologic examination. A lumbar puncture should be performed if not contraindicated, and CSF should be assessed by flow cytometry, cytology, and immunoglobulin heavy-chain gene rearrangement. Because extraneural disease must be excluded to establish a diagnosis of PCNSL, computed tomography (CT) or CT/positron emission tomography (PET) scans of the chest, abdomen, and pelvis and a bone marrow biopsy and aspirate should be performed to exclude occult systemic disease. Involvement of the optic nerve, retina, or vitreous humor should be excluded with a comprehensive eye evaluation by an ophthalmologist that includes a slit lamp examination. Blood tests should include a complete blood count, a basic metabolic panel, serum lactate dehydrogenase, and HIV serology.

Two prognostic scoring systems have been developed specifically for PCNSL. In a retrospective review of 105 PCNSL patients, the International Extranodal Lymphoma Study Group (IELSG) identified age older than 60 years, Eastern Cooperative Oncology Group (ECOG) performance status greater than 1, elevated serum lactate dehydrogenase (LDH) level, elevated CSF protein concentration, and involvement of deep regions of the brain as independent predictors of poor prognosis. In patients with zero or one factor, two or three factors, and four or five factors, the 2-year survival proportions were 80%, 48%, and 15%, respectively. In another prognostic model, PCNSL patients were divided into three groups based on age and performance status: (1) younger than 50 years old, (2) 50 years or older with a Karnofsky performance status (KPS) greater than or equal to 70, and (3) 50 years or older with a KPS less than 70. Based on these three divisions, significant differences in overall and failure-free survival were observed. There is no staging system that correlates with prognosis or response to treatment in PCNSL. However, because PCNSL is a multicompartmental disease potentially involving the brain, spinal cord, eye, and CSF, the IPCG recommends an extent of disease evaluation, as noted earlier, that will enable clinicians to follow the response to therapy.

TREATMENT

NEWLY DIAGNOSED PRIMARY CENTRAL NERVOUS SYSTEM LYMPHOMA

Treatment for newly diagnosed PCNSL consists of remission-induction (induction) and remission-consolidation (consolidation) phases. Typically, induction consists of chemotherapy with the objective of achieving a complete response/remission. Once this response/remission is achieved, a different chemotherapy regimen or whole brain radiation therapy (WBRT) is administered to "consolidate" the response/remission. Defining response to treatment in PCNSL requires assessment of all sites (brain, CSF, eye) potentially involved by disease. The IPCG has established response criteria that have been adopted into most prospective clinical trials of PCNSL (Table 99.1).

Corticosteroids decrease tumor-associated edema and may result in partial radiographic regression of PCNSL. An initial response to corticosteroids is associated with a favorable outcome in PCNSL. However, after an initial response to corticosteroids, almost all patients quickly relapse. Corticosteroids should be avoided if possible prior to a biopsy, given the risk of disrupting cellular morphology, resulting in a nondiagnostic pathologic specimen.

Surgical resection is not part of the standard treatment approach for PCNSL given the multifocal nature of this tumor and has not been shown to prolong survival because most patients also receive additional treatment. Accordingly, the role of neurosurgery in PCNSL is to establish a diagnosis via stereotactic biopsy. However, it can be considered as a lifesaving intervention in extreme cases with large lesions and impending herniation.

Standardized induction and consolidation treatment for PCNSL has yet to be defined. Historically, PCNSL was treated only with WBRT at doses ranging from 36 to 45 Gy, which resulted in a high proportion of radiographic responses but also rapid relapse. In a multicenter phase 2 trial, 41 patients were treated with WBRT to 40 Gy plus a 20 Gy tumor boost and achieved a median overall survival (OS) of only 12 months. Given the lack of durable responses to radiation and the risk of neurotoxicity associated with this modality of therapy, WBRT alone is no longer a recommended treatment for most patients with PCNSL. Moreover, because PCNSL is an infiltrative, multifocal disease, focal radiation or

TABLE 99.1 International Primary Central Nervous System Lymphoma Collaborative Group Consensus Guidelines for the Assessment of Response in Primary Central Nervous System Lymphoma

Response	Brain Imaging	Steroid Dose	Ophthalmologic Examination	CSF Cytology
Complete response	No contrast-enhancing disease	None	Normal	Negative
Unconfirmed complete response	No contrast-enhancing disease	Any	Normal	Negative
	Minimal enhancing disease	Any	Minor RPE abnormality	Negative
Partial response	50% decrease in enhancement[a]	NA	Normal or minor RPE abnormality	Negative
	No contrast-enhancing disease	NA	Decrease in vitreous cells or retinal infiltrate	Persistent or suspicious
Progressive disease	25% increase in enhancing disease	NA	Recurrent or new disease	Recurrent or positive
	Any new site of disease[a]			
Stable disease	All scenarios not covered by responses above	—	—	—

[a]Based on longest single dimension of lesion.
CSF, cerebrospinal fluid; NA, not applicable; RPE, retinal pigment epithelium.

radiosurgery is not recommended. The most effective treatment for PCNSL is intravenous, high-dose methotrexate (HD-MTX) at variable doses (1 to 8 g/m^2), typically used in combination with other chemotherapeutic agents and/or WBRT. However, there is no consensus on the optimal dose of HD-MTX or on the role of radiation in combination with methotrexate in the management of PCNSL. A number of randomized trials are ongoing to address these issues. Doses of methotrexate 3 g/m^2 or higher result in therapeutic concentrations in the brain parenchyma and CSF and when combined with WBRT lead to more durable treatment responses. In a phase 2 trial, 79 PCNSL patients were randomized to receive either (1) HD-MTX (3.5 g/m^2, day 1) *versus* (2) HD-MTX (3.5 g/m^2, day 1) + cytarabine (2 g/m^2 b.i.d., days 2 and 3) [**Level 1**].[1] Each chemotherapy cycle was 21 days. All patients underwent consolidative WBRT after induction chemotherapy. The HD-MTX + cytarabine arm had a higher proportion of complete radiographic responses and a superior 3-year OS. However, it is now widely recognized that there is a high incidence of neurotoxicity with combined modality treatment that includes WBRT. The latter observation prompted studies using *lower doses* of WBRT. In a multicenter phase 2 study, no significant neurocognitive decline was observed after consolidative reduced-dose WBRT (23.4 Gy) and cytarabine in patients who had achieved a complete response to induction chemotherapy including HD-MTX. However, further study and longer neuropsychological follow-up of these patients is necessary to definitively assess the safety of this regimen because numerous studies have demonstrated the delayed neurotoxic effects of WBRT in the PCNSL population and the reduced risk of neurotoxicity in regimens consisting of chemotherapy alone. Given the risk of clinical neurotoxicity, other studies have assessed whether WBRT can be *eliminated* from the initial management of PCNSL. In a multicenter phase 3 trial, patients were randomized to receive HD-MTX–based chemotherapy with or without WBRT [**Level 1**].[2] Five hundred fifty-one patients were enrolled, of whom 318 were treated per protocol. Intent to treat analysis revealed that patients treated in the combined modality arm (chemotherapy + WBRT) achieved prolonged progression-free survival (PFS) but no improvement in OS, demonstrating that the elimination of WBRT from the treatment regimen did not compromise OS. This has led to deferral of WBRT

and the application of chemotherapy alone approaches for newly diagnosed PCNSL patients. These approaches are based on a foundation of HD-MTX. Variable doses and schedules of HD-MTX have been used, but in general, dose 3 g/m^2 or higher delivered as an initial bolus followed by an infusion over 3 hours administered every 10 to 21 days is recommended for optimal outcomes and adequate CSF concentrations. Multiple phase 2 studies have demonstrated the safety, efficacy, and relatively preserved cognition of HD-MTX–based chemotherapy regimens. Moreover, longer duration of induction chemotherapy with HD-MTX (>6 cycles) results in higher complete response proportions.

Several first-generation chemotherapy regimens for PCNSL included intrathecal chemotherapy. However, a number of nonrandomized studies that included intrathecal chemotherapy did not improve outcomes in PCNSL relative to regimens that did not include intrathecal injections of chemotherapy. Moreover, the ability to consistently achieve micromolar concentrations of methotrexate in the CSF at a dose of 8 g/m^2 has led to the elimination of intrathecal chemotherapy from most of the induction chemotherapy regimens currently in use. However, the question regarding the role of intrathecal chemotherapy in the management of PCNSL should ultimately be addressed in a randomized trial.

Rituximab, a chimeric monoclonal antibody targeting the CD20 antigen on B lymphocytes, is being incorporated in combination regimens for PCNSL. When rituximab is administered intravenously at doses of 375 to 800 mg/m^2, CSF levels from 0.1% to 4.4% of serum levels are achieved. Despite limited CSF penetration, radiographic responses have been observed in relapsed PCNSL patients treated with rituximab monotherapy and this antibody has been incorporated into contemporary regimens for PCNSL. Moreover, in historical comparisons, the complete radiographic response rates are higher with induction regimens that include rituximab versus those in which there is no rituximab. In a cooperative group phase 2 study, 44 PCNSL patients were treated with induction chemotherapy consisting of HD-MTX at 8 g/m^2 (day 1), rituximab at 375 mg/m^2 (day 3), and temozolomide at 150 mg/m^2 (days 7 to 11), all drugs with demonstrated efficacy as monotherapy in PCNSL. This induction chemotherapy was followed by consolidation chemotherapy consisting of intravenous etoposide 5 mg/kg as a continuous infusion over 96 hours and cytarabine at 2 g/m^2 every 12 hours for eight doses. Sixty-six percent of these patients achieved complete response (CR); median PFS of the entire group was 2.4 years and median OS was not reached at the time of publication. These results are comparable to any regimen that *includes* WBRT. It is noteworthy that PFS was shorter in PCNSL patients in whom chemotherapy was delayed longer than 1 month after diagnosis compared to those patients who promptly initiated chemotherapy (3-year PFS of 20% vs. 59%, $P = .05$). This observation highlights the importance of early diagnosis and prompt initiation of chemotherapy in PCNSL patients.

Given the limited durability of responses observed in many studies of PCNSL, there is interest in high-dose chemotherapy (HDT) followed by autologous stem cell transplantation (ASCT) as consolidative therapy for newly diagnosed PCNSL. Conditioning regimens including thiotepa have demonstrated the most encouraging results. In a multicenter phase 2 study, 79 patients were treated with induction HD-MTX, cytarabine, rituximab, and thiotepa, followed by carmustine and thiotepa conditioning prior to ASCT. The overall radiographic response (ORR) was 91%, 2-year OS was 87%, and treatment-related deaths occurred in less than 10% of enrolled patients. The toxicities, mostly cytopenias, were manageable. There are three ongoing, multicenter, randomized trials comparing the efficacy of consolidative HDT/ASCT versus chemotherapy or WBRT for newly diagnosed PCNSL (Table 99.2).

TREATMENT OF PRIMARY CENTRAL NERVOUS SYSTEM LYMPHOMA IN ELDERLY PATIENTS

Elderly patients account for more than half of all the subjects diagnosed with PCNSL. The risk of neurotoxicity is highest in this population, and in general, chemotherapy alone is the preferred option for this subgroup. The majority of PCNSL patients older than 60 years of age develop clinical neurotoxicity after treatment

---

TABLE 99.2 Randomized Trials in Primary Central Nervous System Lymphoma

Induction	Consolidation
Completed Trials	
Medical Research Council Phase 2, $n = 53$ (stopped early) CHOP vs. WBRT followed by CHOP	**G-PCNSL-SG-1—NCT00153530** Phase 3, $n = 551$, age 18 yr or older *Arm 1: methotrexate ± ifosfamide => WBRT* *Arm 2: methotrexate ± ifosfamide*
IELSG 20—NCT00210314 Phase 2, $n = 79$, ages 18–75 yr *Induction arm 1: methotrexate + cytarabine => WBRT* *Induction arm 2: methotrexate => WBRT*	
ANOCEF-GOELAMS—NCT00503594 Phase 2, $n = 95$, age 60 yr or older *Arm 1: methotrexate, procarbazine, vincristine, cytarabine* *Arm 2: methotrexate, temozolomide*	
Ongoing Trials	
IESLG 32—NCT01011920 Phase 2, $n = 200$, ages 18–70 yr *Induction arm 1: methotrexate, cytarabine* *Induction arm 2: methotrexate, cytarabine, rituximab* *Induction arm 3: methotrexate, cytarabine, rituximab, thiotepa*	**IESLG 32—NCT01011920** Phase 2, $n = 104$, ages 18–70 yr *Consolidation arm 1: WBRT* *Consolidation arm 1: HDT/ASCT*
ALLG/HOVON—EudraCT 2009-014722-42 Phase 3, $n = 200$, ages 18–70 yr *Arm 1: R-MBVP* *Arm 2: MBVP*	**ANOCEF-GOELAMS—NCT00863460** Phase 2, $n = 100$, ages 18–60 yr *R-MBVP =>* *Consolidation arm 1: HDT/ASCT* *Consolidation arm 2: WBRT*
—	**RTOG 1114—NCT01399372** Phase 2, $n = 84$, age 18 yr or older Methotrexate, procarbazine, vincristine, rituximab => *Consolidation arm 1: WBRT (lower dose) => cytarabine* *Consolidation arm 2: cytarabine*
	Alliance 51101—NCT01511562 Phase 2, $n = 160$, ages 18–75 yr Methotrexate, temozolomide, rituximab, cytarabine => *Consolidation arm 1: HDT/ASCT* *Consolidation arm 2: etoposide, cytarabine*

CHOP, Cytoxan, hydroxyrubicin (Adriamycin), Oncovin (vincristine), prednisone (chemotherapy regimen); WBRT, whole brain radiation therapy; ANOCEF, Association des Neuro-Oncologue d'Expression Française; GOELAMS, Groupe Ouest Est d'Etude des Leucémies et Autres Maladies du Sang; G-PCNSL-SG, German Primary CNS Lymphoma Study Group; NCT, National Clinical Trial; IELSG, International Extranodal Lymphoma Study Group; HDT/ASCT, high-dose chemotherapy and autologous stem cell transplantation; ALLG, Australasian Leukaemia and Lymphoma Group; HOVON, Stichting Hemato-Oncologie voor Volwassenen Nederland (Dutch-Belgian Cooperative Trial Group for Hematology Oncology); BCNU, 1,3-bis(2-chloroethyl)-1-nitrosourea; R-MBVP, rituximab, methotrexate, BCNU, teniposide, prednisone; RTOG, Radiation Therapy Oncology Group.

with a WBRT-containing regimen and some of these patients die of treatment-related complications, rather than recurrent disease. Several studies have indicated that HD-MTX at doses of 3.5 to 8 g/m^2 is well tolerated in elderly patients with manageable grade 3 or 4 renal and hematologic toxicity. In a multicenter, randomized, phase 2 trial of chemotherapy alone in elderly patients with PCNSL, 98 patients were randomized to receive three 28-day cycles of either MPV-A (methotrexate 3.5 g/m^2, days 1 and 15; procarbazine 100 mg/m^2, days 1 to 7; vincristine 1.4 mg/m^2, days 1 and 15) or MT (methotrexate 3.5 g/m^2, days 1 and 15; temozolomide 100 to 150 mg/m^2, days 1 to 5 and 15 to 19) with one additional cycle of cytarabine (3 g/m^2/day for 2 consecutive days) in the MPV arm only [**Level 1**].[3] Although trends favored the MPV-A regimen over the simpler, less toxic MT regimen with respect to complete response rate, PFS, and OS, none of these differences reached statistical difference. Subsequent studies suggest that the addition of rituximab to both MPV and MT could increase the radiographic response rate. Both of these chemotherapy regimens are options in elderly PCNSL patients.

RELAPSED AND REFRACTORY PRIMARY CENTRAL NERVOUS SYSTEM LYMPHOMA

Despite high initial response rates with HD-MTX–based induction therapy, most patients with PCNSL relapse. Moreover, there is a small subset of patients who have HD-MTX–refractory disease. Prognosis of relapsed or refractory PCNSL is poor with a limited number of prospective, phase 2 studies for guidance on management. Rechallenge with HD-MTX is effective in patients who had previously responded to this agent. In a multicenter, retrospective study of 22 relapsed PCNSL patients with a history of prior response to HD-MTX, 91% had a radiographic response to the first salvage treatment with HD-MTX and 100% to second salvage. The median OS from the first salvage was 61.9 months. In patients who have not previously been treated with HDT/ASCT, this is also an option at the time of relapse. In a phase 2 trial of 43 patients with relapsed or refractory PCNSL, salvage therapy with high-dose cytarabine and etoposide was followed by HDT/ASCT with a conditioning regimen consisting of thiotepa, busulfan, and cyclophosphamide. Twenty-seven patients ultimately proceeded to transplantation. Twenty-six of 27 patients had a CR and the median PFS and OS in this group were 41.1 and 58.6 months, respectively. It is noteworthy that in a small series of patients with relapsed PCNSL after initial HDT/ASCT, a second autotransplantation was successful as salvage treatment. Finally, WBRT in patients who have not received it as a part of their initial treatment is an effective option in the relapsed PCNSL setting, although the risk of neurotoxicity remains high. Many clinicians reserve WBRT for those patients with chemotherapy-refractory disease or at the time of relapse. In a series of 27 relapsed or refractory PCNSL patients treated with WBRT (median dose 36 Gy), 74% achieved an overall radiographic response and the median OS was 10.6 months. Delayed neurotoxicity rates of 15% were noted at doses greater than 36 Gy even in the setting of short survival. Novel therapeutics currently under study for systemic DLBCL have entered early-phase clinical trials in primary CNS DLBCL and include bendamustine, lenalidomide, pomalidomide, everolimus, and pemetrexed.

NEUROTOXICITY

The most frequent complication in long-term PCNSL survivors is delayed neurotoxicity. Although this risk is high, the exact incidence of delayed neurotoxicity is unclear, as most studies did not systematically assess neurocognitive function with serial neuropsychological testing. The elderly are at highest risk for this complication, with nearly all patients older than the age of 60 years developing clinical neurotoxicity following combined modality therapy. Treatment with WBRT has been identified as the major risk factor for the development of late neurotoxicity. Common symptoms and signs include deficits in attention, memory, executive function, gait ataxia, and incontinence. These deficits have a detrimental impact on quality of life. Radiographic findings include periventricular white matter changes, ventricular enlargement, and cortical atrophy. Pathologic studies reveal demyelination, hippocampal neuronal loss, and large-vessel atherosclerosis. Although the pathophysiology is unclear and likely multifactorial, damage to neural progenitor cells has been implicated to play an important role in radiation-related neurotoxicity. Currently, there are no treatments to reverse these delayed neurotoxic effects. Neuropsychological function was maintained in one long-term follow-up study of PCNSL patients treated with chemotherapy alone. It is critical that serial neuropsychological assessments are incorporated into the management of patients with PCNSL, as cognitive outcome is a critical end point. The IPCG has developed an instrument for this purpose, which is composed of quality of life questionnaires and standardized neuropsychological tests that include assessment of executive function, attention, memory, and psychomotor speed.

OUTCOME

As treatment improves for PCNSL, more patients are living longer, emphasizing the need to optimize neurocognitive function and quality of life. The IPCG recommends a schedule of follow-up neuroimaging studies and cognitive assessment in PCNSL survivors.

LEVEL 1 EVIDENCE

1. Ferreri AJ, Reni M, Foppoli M, et al. High-dose cytarabine plus high-dose methotrexate versus high-dose methotrexate alone in patients with primary CNS lymphoma: a randomised phase 2 trial. *Lancet*. 2009;374:1512–1520.
2. Thiel E, Korfel A, Martus P, et al. High-dose methotrexate with or without whole brain radiotherapy for primary CNS lymphoma (G-PCNSL-SG-1): a phase 3, randomised, noninferiority trial. *Lancet Oncol*. 2010;11:1036–1047.
3. Omuro A, Chinot O, Taillandier L, et al. Multicenter randomized phase II trial of methotrexate (MTX) and temozolomide (TMZ) versus MTX, procarbazine, vincristine, and cytarabine for primary CNS lymphoma (PCNSL) in the elderly: an Anocef and Goelams Intergroup study. Paper presented at: 49th Annual Meeting of the American Society of Clinical Oncology; May 31–June 4, 2013; Chicago, IL.

SUGGESTED READINGS

Abrey LE, Batchelor TT, Ferreri AJ, et al. Report of an international workshop to standardize baseline evaluation and response criteria for primary CNS lymphoma. *J Clin Oncol*. 2005;23:5034–5043.

Abrey LE, Ben-Porat L, Panageas KS, et al. Primary central nervous system lymphoma: the Memorial Sloan-Kettering Cancer Center prognostic model. *J Clin Oncol*. 2006;24:5711–5715.

Bataille B, Delwail V, Menet E, et al. Primary intracerebral malignant lymphoma: report of 248 cases. *J Neurosurg*. 2000;92:261–266.

Batchelor T, Carson K, O'Neill A, et al. Treatment of primary CNS lymphoma with methotrexate and deferred radiotherapy: a report of NABTT 96-07. *J Clin Oncol.* 2003;21:1044–1049.

Batchelor TT, DeAngelis LM, eds. *Lymphoma and Leukemia of the Nervous System.* 2nd ed. New York: Springer; 2013.

Batchelor TT, Grossman SA, Mikkelsen T, et al. Rituximab monotherapy for patients with recurrent primary CNS lymphoma. *Neurology.* 2011;76:929–930.

Bellinzona M, Roser F, Ostertag H, et al. Surgical removal of primary central nervous system lymphomas (PCNSL) presenting as space occupying lesions: a series of 33 cases. *Eur J Surg Oncol.* 2005;31:100–105.

Chan CC, Rubenstein JL, Coupland SE, et al. Primary vitreoretinal lymphoma: a report from an International Primary Central Nervous System Lymphoma Collaborative Group symposium. *Oncologist.* 2011;16:1589–1599.

Correa DD, Maron L, Harder H, et al. Cognitive functions in primary central nervous system lymphoma: literature review and assessment guidelines. *Ann Oncol.* 2007;18:1145–1151.

DeAngelis LM, Seiferheld W, Schold SC, et al. Combination chemotherapy and radiotherapy for primary central nervous system lymphoma: Radiation Therapy Oncology Group Study 93-10. *J Clin Oncol.* 2002;20:4643–4648.

Dolecek TA, Propp JM, Stroup NE, et al. CBTRUS statistical report: primary brain and central nervous system tumors diagnosed in the United States in 2005-2009. *Neuro Oncol.* 2012;14(suppl 5):v1–v49.

Doolittle ND, Korfel A, Lubow MA, et al. Long-term cognitive function, neuroimaging and quality of life in primary CNS lymphoma. *Neurology.* 2013;81:84–92.

Ferreri AJ, Blay JY, Reni M, et al. Prognostic scoring system for primary CNS lymphomas: the International Extranodal Lymphoma Study Group experience. *J Clin Oncol.* 2003;21:266–272.

Ferreri AJ, Guerra E, Regazzi M, et al. Area under the curve of methotrexate and creatinine clearance are outcome-determining factors in primary CNS lymphomas. *Br J Cancer.* 2004;90:353–358.

Glantz MJ, Cole BF, Recht L, et al. High-dose intravenous methotrexate for patients with nonleukemic leptomeningeal cancer: is intrathecal chemotherapy necessary? *J Clin Oncol.* 1998;16:1561–1567.

Holdhoff M, Ambady P, Abdelaziz A, et al. High-dose methotrexate with or without rituximab in newly diagnosed primary CNS lymphoma. *Neurology.* 2014;83:235–239.

Hottinger AF, DeAngelis LM, Yahalom J, et al. Salvage whole brain radiotherapy for recurrent or refractory primary CNS lymphoma. *Neurology.* 2007;69:1178–1182.

Illerhaus G, Fritsch K, Egerer G, et al. Sequential high dose immuno-chemotherapy followed by autologous peripheral blood stem cell transplantation for patients with untreated primary central nervous system lymphoma—a multicentre study by the Collaborative PCNSL Study Group Freiburg. Paper presented at: 54th Annual Meeting of the American Society of Hematology; December 8–11, 2012; Atlanta, GA.

Jahnke K, Korfel A, Martus P, et al. High-dose methotrexate toxicity in elderly patients with primary central nervous system lymphoma. *Ann Oncol.* 2005;16:445–449.

Juergens A, Pels H, Rogowski S, et al. Long-term survival with favorable cognitive outcome after chemotherapy in primary central nervous system lymphoma. *Ann Neurol.* 2010;67:182–189.

Kasenda B, Schorb E, Fritsch K, et al. Primary CNS lymphoma—radiation-free salvage therapy by second autologous stem cell transplantation. *Biol Blood Marrow Transplant.* 2011;17:281–283.

Khan RB, Shi W, Thaler HT, et al. Is intrathecal methotrexate necessary in the treatment of primary CNS lymphoma? *J Neurooncol.* 2002;58:175–178.

Lai R, Abrey LE, Rosenblum MK, et al. Treatment-induced leukoencephalopathy in primary CNS lymphoma: a clinical and autopsy study. *Neurology.* 2004;62:451–456.

Mathew BS, Carson KA, Grossman SA. Initial response to glucocorticoids. *Cancer.* 2006;15:383–387.

Mead GM, Bleehen NM, Gregor A, et al. A medical research council randomized trial in patients with primary cerebral non-Hodgkin lymphoma: cerebral radiotherapy with and without cyclophosphamide, doxorubicin, vincristine, and prednisone chemotherapy. *Cancer.* 2000;89:1359–1370.

Monje ML, Vogel H, Masek M, et al. Impaired hippocampal neurogenesis after treatment for central nervous system malignancies. *Ann Neurol.* 2007;62:515–520.

Morris PG, Correa DD, Yahalom J, et al. Rituximab, methotrexate, procarbazine and vincristine followed by consolidation reduced-dose whole-brain radiotherapy and cytarabine in newly diagnosed primary CNS lymphoma: final results and long-term outcome. *J Clin Oncol.* 2013;31:3971–3979.

Nayak L, Batchelor TT. Recent advances in treatment of primary central nervous system lymphoma. *Curr Treat Options Oncol.* 2013;14:539–552.

Nelson DF, Martz KL, Bonner H, et al. Non-Hodgkin's lymphoma of the brain: can high dose, large volume radiation therapy improve survival? Report on a prospective trial by the Radiation Therapy Oncology Group (RTOG): RTOG 8315. *Int J Radiat Oncol Biol Phys.* 1992;23:9–17.

Nguyen PL, Chakravarti A, Finkelstein DM, et al. Results of whole-brain radiation as salvage of methotrexate failure for immunocompetent patients with primary CNS lymphoma. *J Clin Oncol.* 2005;23:1507–1513.

Ostrom QT, Gittleman H, Farah P, et al. CBTRUS statistical report: primary brain and central nervous system tumors diagnosed in the United States 2006-2010. *Neuro Oncol.* 2013;14(suppl 2):ii1–ii56.

Plotkin SR, Betensky RA, Hochberg FH, et al. Treatment of relapsed central nervous system lymphoma with high-dose methotrexate. *Clin Cancer Res.* 2004;10:5643–5646.

Ponzoni M, Issa S, Batchelor TT, et al. Beyond high-dose methotrexate and brain radiotherapy: novel targets and agents for primary CNS lymphoma. *Ann Oncol.* 2014;25:316–322.

Rubenstein JL, Hsi ED, Johnson JL, et al. Intensive chemotherapy and immunotherapy in patients with newly diagnosed primary CNS lymphoma: CALGB 50202 (Alliance 50202). *J Clin Oncol.* 2013;31:3061–3068.

Sierra Del Rio M, Ricard D, Houillier C, et al. Prophylactic intrathecal chemotherapy in primary CNS lymphoma. *J Neurooncol.* 2012;106:143–146.

Soussain C, Hoang-Xuan K, Taillandier L, et al. Intensive chemotherapy followed by hematopoietic stem-cell rescue for refractory and recurrent primary CNS and intraocular lymphoma: Societe Francaise de Greffe de Moelle Osseuse-Therapie Cellulaire. *J Clin Oncol.* 2008;26:2512–2518.

Swerdlow SH, Campo E, Harris NL, et al, eds. *WHO Classification of Tumours of the Haematopoietic and Lymphoid Tissues.* Lyon, France: IARC Press; 2008.

Villano JL, Koshy M, Shaikh H, et al. Age, gender, and racial differences in incidence and survival in primary CNS lymphoma. *Br J Cancer.* 2011;105:1414–1418.

Zhu JJ, Gerstner ER, Engler DA, et al. High-dose methotrexate for elderly patients with primary CNS lymphoma. *Neuro Oncol.* 2009;11:211–215.

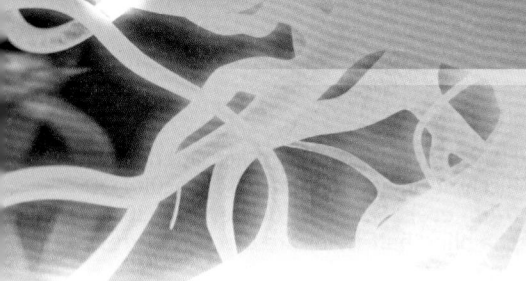

Tumors of the Pituitary Gland 100

John Ausiello, Pamela U. Freda,
and Jeffrey N. Bruce

INTRODUCTION

Pituitary tumors are a common medical problem often found incidentally on routine magnetic resonance imaging (MRI) scans. These tumors are overwhelmingly benign but may cause symptoms due to mass effect, compression of the optic chiasm, excess hormonal secretion, or hypopituitarism. As such, the diagnosis and management of these tumors involves the coordinated efforts of neurosurgeons, endocrinologist, and ophthalmologists.

EPIDEMIOLOGY

The true prevalence of pituitary adenomas is difficult to ascertain because most are asymptomatic; autopsy estimates of prevalence range from 1.7% to 24%. No sexual predilection exists, but the tumors are most common in adults, peaking in the third and fourth decades. Children and adolescents account for approximately 10% of cases. Pituitary tumors are not hereditary except for rare families with multiple endocrine neoplasia I (MEN-I), an autosomal dominant condition manifested by a high incidence of pituitary adenomas and tumors of other endocrine glands.

PATHOBIOLOGY

Pituitary tumors can be classified in four ways: by size, endocrine function, clinical findings, or histology. The first two remain the most common, as the majority of tumors are histologically benign and the clinical findings usually reflect the size or endocrinologic function of the tumor. With regard to size, microadenomas are less than 1 cm in diameter and macroadenomas are greater than 1 cm. Typically, when microadenomas cause symptoms, it is due to excess hormone secretion, whereas with macroadenomas, it is via compression of normal glandular or neural structures. Macroadenomas may invade the dura or bone and may infiltrate surrounding structures such as the cavernous sinus, cranial nerves, blood vessels, sphenoid bone, and sinus or brain. These locally invasive pituitary adenomas are nearly always histologically benign. In some studies, but not all, the proliferation index correlates with growth velocity and recurrence. However, their invasive character may be independent of their growth rate.

A second manner by which tumors can be classified is by the presence (or absence) of endocrine function, dividing tumors into secreting or nonsecreting tumors. Secreting tumors are less common and produce one or more anterior pituitary hormones, including prolactin (the most common secreting tumor), growth hormone (GH), adrenocorticotropic hormone (ACTH) (causing Cushing disease), follicle-stimulating hormone (FSH), or luteinizing hormone (LH). Mixed secretory tumors account for 10% of adenomas; interestingly, these adenomas still have a monoclonal origin. Secretion of more than one hormone has implications for medical therapy, as all excess hormone secretion must be treated. *Null cells*, or nonsecreting adenomas, demonstrate no clinical or immunohistochemical evidence of hormone secretion.

In general, adenomas grow more slowly in older patients than younger patients. *Pituitary carcinomas* are rare but highly invasive, rapidly growing, and anaplastic. Unequivocal diagnosis relies on the presence of distant metastases, as certain histologic findings including pleomorphism and mitotic figures may be seen in benign adenomas.

The posterior pituitary, which contains the terminal processes of hypothalamic neurons and supporting glial cells, is a rare site of neoplasia. *Infundibulomas* are rare tumors of the neurohypophysis; they are variants of pilocytic astrocytomas. *Granular cell tumors* (e.g., *myoblastomas* or *choristomas*), also rare tumors of the neurohypophysis, are of uncertain origin.

CLINICAL MANIFESTATIONS

Clinical manifestations arise either from endocrine dysfunction or mass effect with invasion or compression of surrounding neural and vascular structures. The manifestations and management of hormonally active tumors are discussed in Chapter 117. Here, discussion is primarily limited to nonsecretory tumors, most of which are macroadenomas by the time they come to clinical attention. Macroadenomas may present with panhypopituitarism if the normal pituitary gland is destroyed. Headaches result from stretching of the diaphragma sellae and adjacent dural structures that transmit sensation through the first branch of the trigeminal nerve. Visual field abnormalities are caused by compression of the crossing fibers in the optic chiasm, first affecting the superior temporal quadrants and then the inferior temporal quadrants, leading to a bitemporal hemianopia. Further expansion compromises the noncrossing fibers and affects the lower nasal quadrants and finally the upper nasal quadrants (Fig. 100.1).

Visual loss may be accompanied by optic disc pallor and loss of central visual acuity although papilledema is rare. Patients usually complain of blurring or dimming of vision but often are unaware of peripheral visual loss. Formal visual field testing is important because some tumors affect only the macular fibers, causing central hemianopic scotomas that may be missed on routine screening. Bitemporal hemianopia is most common, but any pattern of visual loss is possible, including unilateral or homonymous hemianopia.

Lateral extension of the tumor with compression or invasion of the cavernous sinus may compromise third, fourth, or sixth cranial nerve functions, manifesting as diplopia. The third cranial nerve is most commonly affected. Numbness may occur in the V1 or V2 distribution. Overall, however, cranial nerve dysfunction is not a common feature of adenomas and may be more suggestive of other neoplasms of the cavernous sinus.

Adenomas can become quite large before causing symptoms. Suprasellar extension may compress the foramen of Monro, causing hydrocephalus and symptoms of increased intracranial pressure (ICP). Hypothalamic dysfunction could lead to diabetes insipidus but this condition is relatively rare. If diabetes insipidus is present, it is more suggestive of inflammation or possible tumor invasion of the pituitary stalk. Extensive subfrontal extension with compression of both

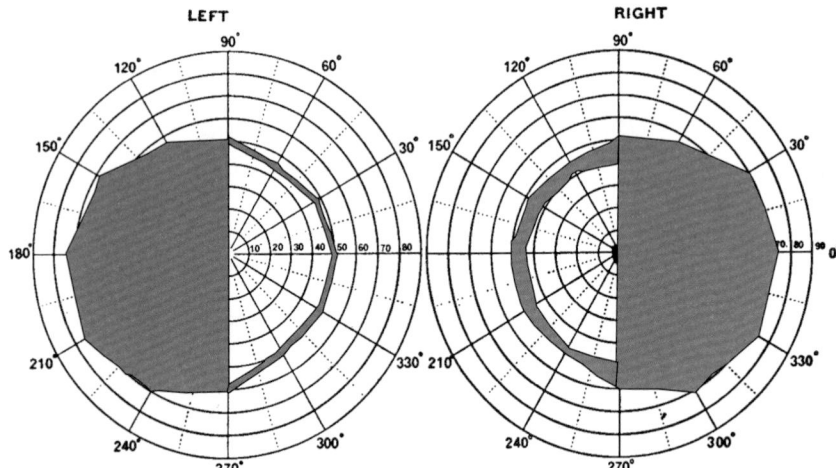

FIGURE 100.1 Pituitary macroadenoma. Bitemporal hemianopia; visual acuity OD (*right eye*) 15/200, OS (*left eye*) 15/30. The blind half-fields are black. (Courtesy of Dr. Max Chamlin.)

frontal lobes may cause personality changes or dementia. There may be seizures or motor and sensory dysfunction. Erosion of the skull base is a risk factor for the development of cerebrospinal fluid (CSF) rhinorrhea.

In about 5% of pituitary tumors, the first symptoms are those of pituitary apoplexy caused by hemorrhage or infarction of the adenoma. Symptoms include sudden onset of severe headache, oculomotor palsies, nausea, vomiting, altered mental state, diplopia, and rapidly progressive visual loss. Apoplexy is diagnosed by computed tomography (CT) or MRI and occasionally is an indication for emergency surgery (Fig. 100.2). Histologically, the adenoma shows massive necrosis and hemorrhage. Apoplexy is almost always caused

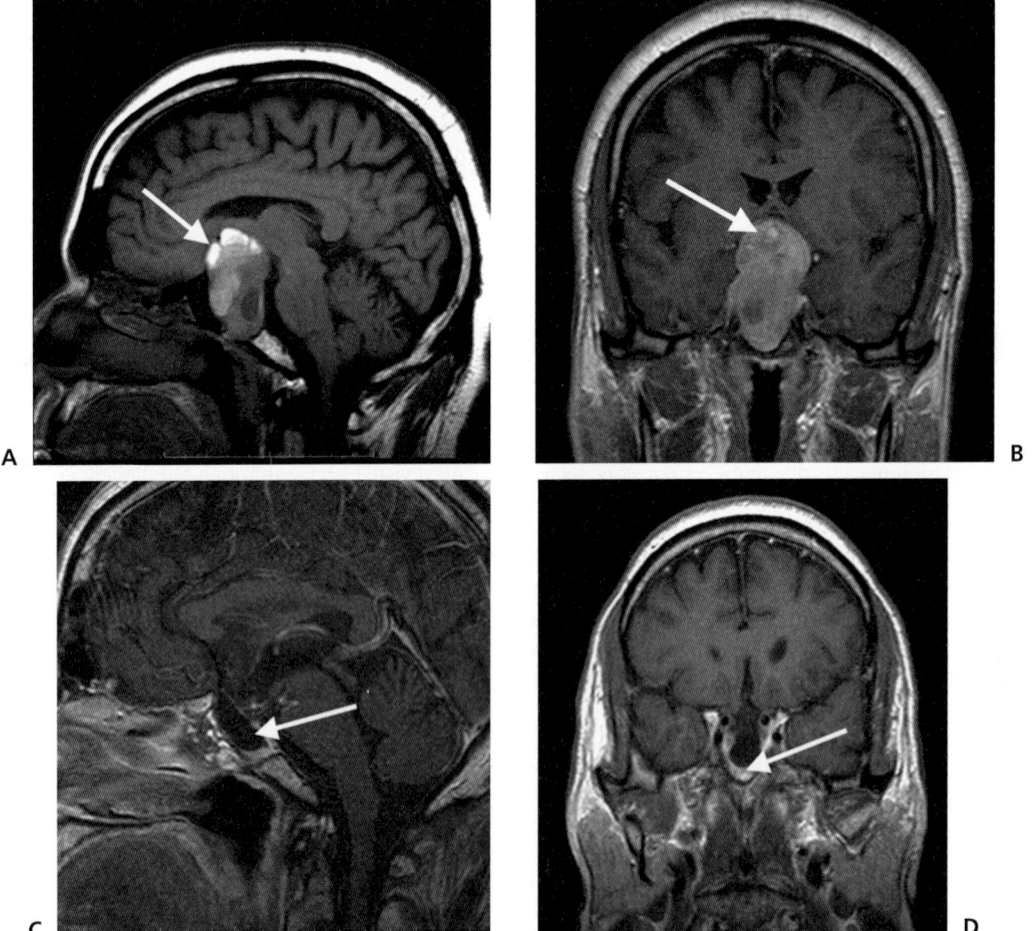

FIGURE 100.2 Pituitary apoplexy. **A:** T1-weighted sagittal and **(B)** coronal MRI demonstrating a pituitary mass that turned out to be partially hemorrhagic in a patient with apoplexy. Hyperintensity (*arrows*) corresponds to the hemorrhagic component. **C:** Postoperative sagittal MRI following successful tumor resection through a standard transsphenoidal approach shows CSF within the enlarged sella (*arrow*). **D:** Coronal MRI shows normal gland (*arrow*) along the floor of the sella with no residual tumor.

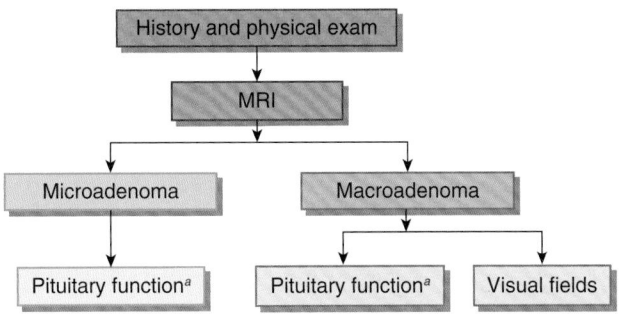

*a*Initial tests include prolactin, TSH, FT4, LH/FSH, E2, testosterone, ACTH, cortisol, GH, and IGF-1. Additional tests including dynamic studies may be needed to assess functional status.

FIGURE 100.3 Initial assessment of pituitary tumors. TSH, thyroid-stimulating hormone; FT4, free thyroxine; LH, luteinizing hormone; FSH, follicle-stimulating hormone; E2, estradiol; ACTH, adrenocorticotropic hormone; GH, growth hormone; IGF-1, insulin-like growth factor 1.

by a pituitary tumor, but it has been reported in other conditions, such as lymphocytic hypophysitis. Pituitary adenomas may enlarge during pregnancy, causing acute symptoms or even apoplexy.

DIAGNOSIS

An algorithm for the initial assessment of a pituitary mass is shown in Figure 100.3.

RADIOGRAPHIC FEATURES

MRI is the best way to evaluate pituitary pathology because soft tissue is seen clearly without interference from the bony surroundings of the sella. MRI also produces images in any plane, which helps define the relationship of the tumor to the surrounding structures. Vascular structures such as the adjacent carotid artery are easily visualized by signal void. Normally, the anterior lobe of the pituitary gland has the same signal as white matter on T1-weighted imaging. With gadolinium, the normal gland enhances homogeneously. Small punctate areas of heterogeneity may be the result of local variations in vascularity, microcyst formation, or granularity within the gland. The posterior lobe shows increased signal on T1-weighted images, probably representing neurosecretory granules in the antidiuretic hormone (ADH)–containing axons.

Microadenomas are sometimes difficult to see directly on MRI but may be inferred by glandular asymmetry, focal sellar erosion, asymmetric convexity of the upper margin of the gland, or displacement of the infundibulum (Fig. 100.4).

The normal gland usually shows more enhancement than a microadenoma (Fig. 100.5). In the presence of a macroadenoma, the normal gland may not be visualized and the bright signal of the posterior lobe may be absent. Areas of increased signal on the T1-weighted image may stem from hemorrhage; areas of low signal may represent cystic degeneration. MRI alone is usually sufficient, but CT may show the bony anatomy in better detail. MRI typically excludes an aneurysm, but magnetic resonance angiography (MRA) or an angiogram is indicated if aneurysm is a serious diagnostic concern.

ACTH-secreting tumors may be too small to visualize on MRI. Diagnosis is suggested by the clinical features of Cushing disease, elevated 24-hour urinary free-cortisol levels, loss of ACTH suppression by high-dose as opposed to low-dose glucocorticoids, and elevated ACTH levels. However, the specific differentiation of an ACTH-secreting pituitary tumor from ectopic sources of ACTH may require measurement of ACTH peripherally and in each inferior petrosal sinus which drains the pituitary gland.

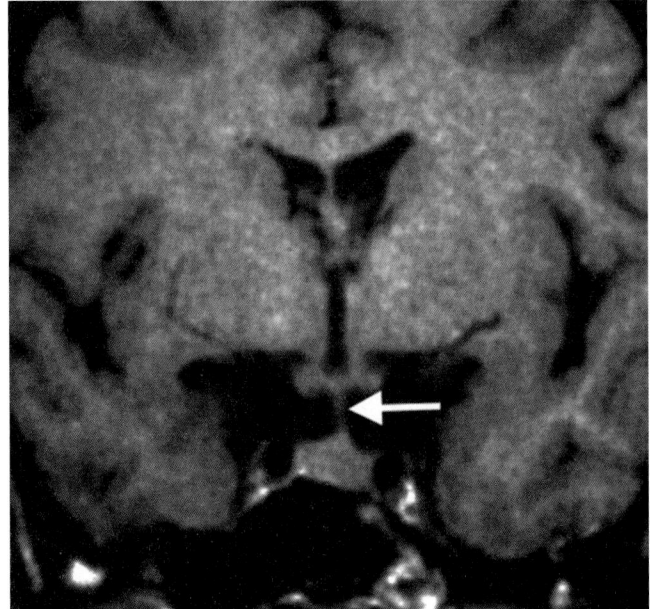
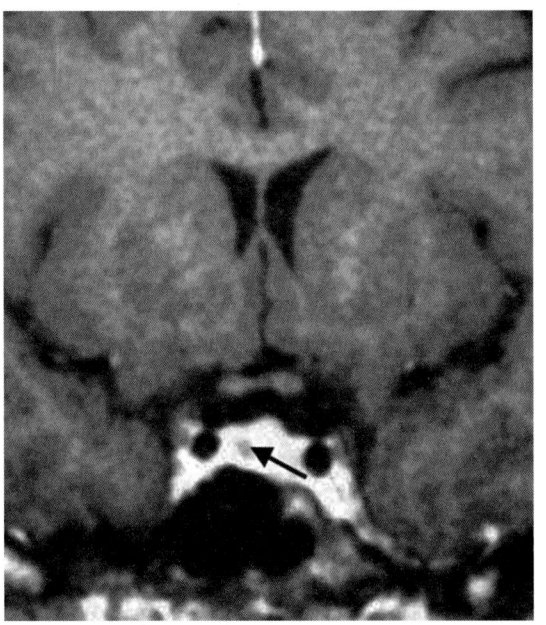

A   B

FIGURE 100.4 Pituitary microadenoma. **A:** T1-weighted coronal MRI shows slight tilting of the pituitary stalk to the left (*arrow*), with questionable fullness of the right pituitary gland. These are secondary signs of pituitary microadenoma but are not sufficient to establish the diagnosis radiographically. **B:** T1-weighted coronal scan after gadolinium enhancement demonstrates a tiny focus of relative hypointensity within the right pituitary gland (*arrow*) consistent with a microadenoma. (Courtesy of Dr. S. Chan.)

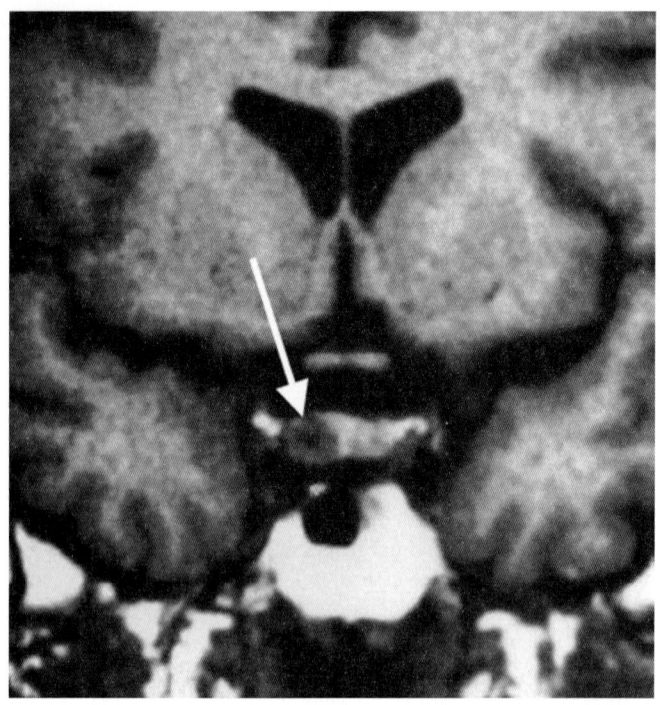

FIGURE 100.5 Pituitary adenoma. T1-weighted coronal MRI after gadolinium enhancement demonstrates a discrete focus of hypointensity (*arrow*) in the right pituitary gland, most consistent with pituitary adenoma. (Courtesy of Dr. S. Chan.)

ENDOCRINE EVALUATION

Complete endocrine evaluation is necessary for all patients with pituitary tumors, not only to establish the diagnosis of a secreting adenoma but also to determine the presence of hypopituitarism (Tables 100.1 and 100.2), which may result from compression of the normal pituitary gland.

Serum hormone levels should be obtained in all patients with adequate hormone replacement administered for any deficiencies identified. Long-term follow-up monitoring is essential because hypopituitarism may develop years after diagnosis and treatment. Nonsecreting tumors may cause slight elevations of serum prolactin levels (typically <100 ng/mL) via compression of the pituitary stalk leading to interruption of dopaminergic fibers that inhibit prolactin release. Mild elevations are common and must be distinguished from prolactin-secreting macroadenomas that are more likely when prolactin levels are more than 200 ng/mL. This distinction is important therapeutically because nonsecreting tumors do not respond to dopamine agonists (e.g., cabergoline or bromocriptine).

DIFFERENTIAL DIAGNOSIS

Most lesions in the differential diagnosis have characteristic radiographic or clinical syndromes that distinguish them from

TABLE 100.1	Symptoms of Pituitary Failure

1. Gonadotroph failure
   Sexual dysfunction
   Amenorrhea
   Infertility

2. Thyrotroph failure
   Fatigue
   Malaise
   Apathy
   Constipation
   Weight gain

3. Somatotroph failure
   Weight gain
   Reduced bone mass
   Hypercholesterolemia
   Muscle weakness

4. Corticotroph failure
   Fatigue
   Weight loss
   Decreased appetite
   Hypoglycemia

TABLE 100.2	Symptoms of Pituitary Hypersecretion

1. Gonadotroph excess
   Typically asymptomatic
   Ovarian hyperstimulation

2. Thyrotroph excess
   Weight loss
   Heat intolerance
   Palpitations
   Tremors
   Loose stools

3. Somatotroph excess
   Enlargement of hands, feet, jaw bone, forehead
   Arthralgias, myalgias, carpal tunnel
   Cardiac disease
   Colonic polyps

4. Corticotroph excess
   Increase appetite and weight gain
   Hypertension
   Hyperglycemia
   Myopathy
   Osteoporosis

pituitary adenomas. Craniopharyngiomas have a predilection for children, are calcified, and usually include cystic areas that contain highly proteinaceous fluid with cholesterol crystals. Rathke cleft cysts are similar to craniopharyngiomas but have a cystic appearance without any solid component. Meningiomas are commonly found in the diaphragma sellae, planum sphenoidale, and tuberculum sellae and may be difficult to distinguish from a macroadenoma. Distinguishing characteristics of meningiomas include enhancement, visualization of a cleavage plane between the mass and the sellar contents, normally sized sella, and the presence of a dural tail of enhancement. Optic glioma, hypothalamic glioma, germinoma, dermoid tumor, metastasis, and nasopharyngeal carcinoma are less commonly seen entities that should be considered. Chordomas characteristically show extensive bony destruction of the clivus. Mucoceles of the sphenoid sinus may simulate pituitary adenoma. Visual symptoms and sellar enlargement may also result from chronic, increased ICP of any origin. Characteristic signal voids on MRI usually distinguish an aneurysm. The differential diagnosis also includes sarcoidosis, lymphoma, lymphocytic hypophysitis, and other granulomatous diseases.

Herniation of the subarachnoid space into the sella through an incompetent diaphragma sellae may produce the empty sella syndrome, with enlargement of the sella and flattening of the pituitary gland on its floor (Fig. 100.6). This syndrome may be associated with pseudotumor cerebri or CSF rhinorrhea. Although most are not symptomatic, an empty sella may be associated with headaches and occasionally with mild hypopituitarism, but the visual fields are usually normal. The condition is readily seen on MRI and may be a complication of previous transsphenoidal surgery.

TREATMENT

Pituitary tumors are histologically benign tumors but can be associated with a significant decrease in a patient's quality of life and

functional capacity. Early intervention may minimize disability and must address both endocrinologic and neurologic function.

Treatment of pituitary adenomas begins with replacement of any deficient pituitary hormone; replacement of thyroid and adrenal hormones remains the most important. Steroid replacement must be adequate for stressful situations, including surgery on the pituitary lesion. Typically, in patients with normal adrenal function prior to surgery, dexamethasone 4 mg is administered preoperatively and tapered off by postoperative day 2 (in patients requiring a craniotomy, the starting dose may be dexamethasone 10 mg perioperatively with a more prolonged taper). A morning cortisol level can be evaluated prior to discharge. Patients with known secondary adrenal insufficiency preoperatively should be continued on replacement doses after surgery.

The goals of treatment differ according to the functional activity of the tumor. For endocrinologically active tumors, an aggressive approach toward reversing hypersecretion is essential while preserving normal pituitary function. This may often be achieved by surgical excision, although prolactinomas are generally better controlled by giving dopamine agonists, such as cabergoline, that achieve tumor shrinkage and normalization of prolactin levels in almost all microadenomas and a majority of macroadenomas (Fig. 100.7). In a subset of patients with hormonally active tumors (typically ACTH-secreting) refractory to standard therapy, chemotherapy has been used but further discussion of this treatment modality is beyond the scope of this chapter.

Candidates for surgical treatment include patients with prolactinomas who fail to respond medically or those who do not tolerate the side effects of medication. The treatment strategies for secretory adenomas are covered in detail in Chapter 117.

Nonsecreting tumors are best treated by surgical reduction of the mass while maintaining pituitary function. Resection also offers the advantage of establishing the correct diagnosis. Incidentally discovered asymptomatic adenomas require no intervention but should be followed with periodic visual field examination and

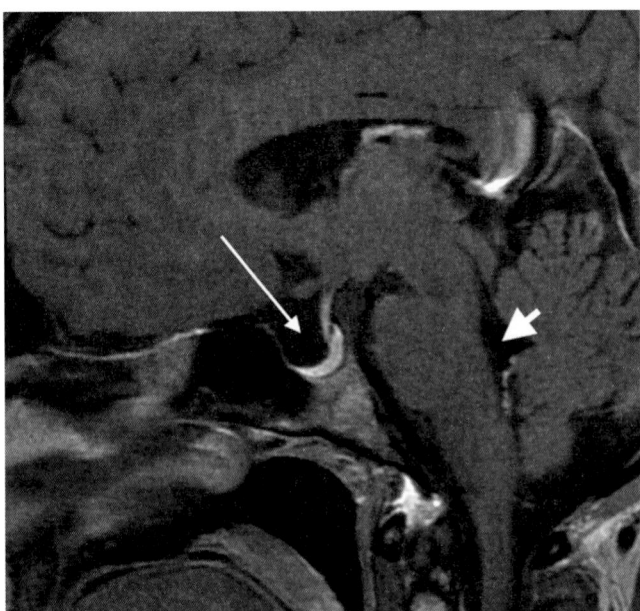
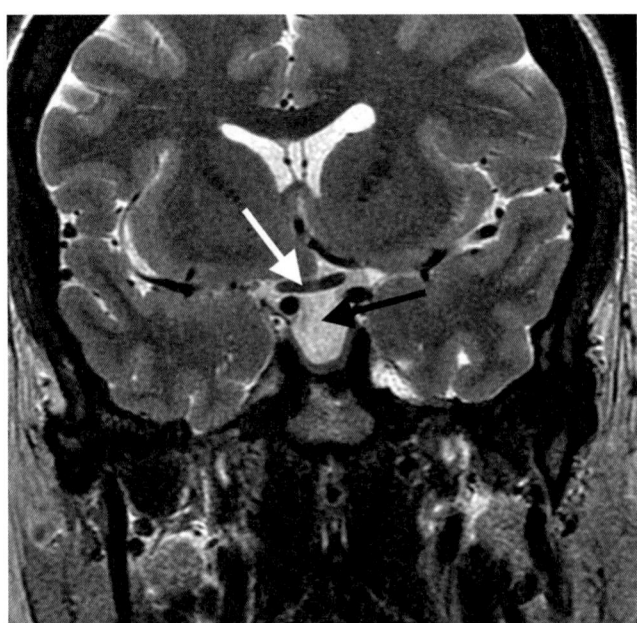

A   B

FIGURE 100.6 Empty sella. **A:** Sagittal T1-weighted MRI demonstrates low-intensity intrasellar signal (*long arrow*) representing CSF (compare with same signal within the fourth ventricle—*short arrow*). **B:** Coronal T2-weighted MRI increased signal within the sella (*black arrow*) representing CSF and normal optic chiasm (*white arrow*). (Courtesy of Dr. Alex Khandji.)

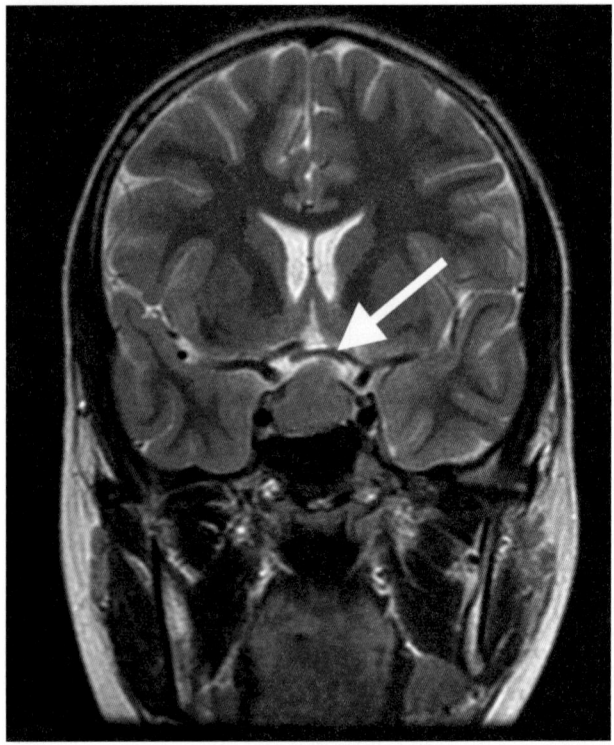
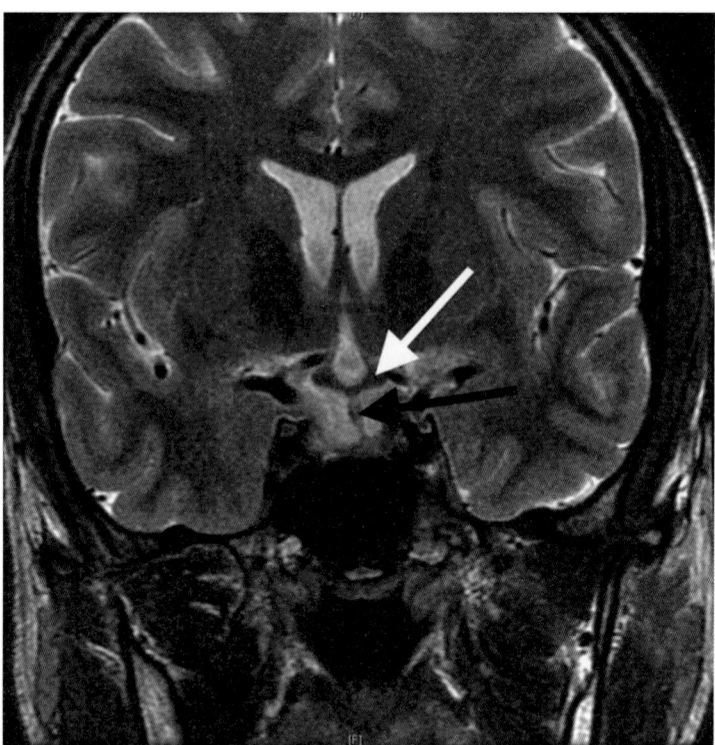

A **B**

FIGURE 100.7 Prolactinoma. **A:** T2-weighted coronal MRI of a 19-year-old man with a markedly elevated serum prolactin level. The tumor is partially compressing the optic chiasm (*arrow*). **B:** Coronal MRI after treatment with a dopamine agonist shows marked decrease in the tumor size such that the infundibulum (*black arrow*) and optic chiasm (*white arrow*) are decompressed.

MRI. Onset of symptoms or MRI documentation of growth is an indication for treatment.

SURGERY

The efficacy and safety of the transsphenoidal approach make it the procedure of choice for the removal of adenomas. Endoscopic approaches have become increasingly popular and seem to produce equivalent results. Most tumors are soft and friable; transsphenoidal access, although limited, permits complete removal even if there is suprasellar extension or the sella is not enlarged. Transsphenoidal surgery was originally developed by Cushing but refinements in microsurgery and the availability of steroid replacement and antibiotics have dramatically improved the results.

A transcranial approach may be preferred for resection of exceptionally large tumors or those extending into the middle fossa or the suprasellar space through an intact diaphragma sellae with a waistband constriction of the tumor (Fig. 100.8). A transcranial approach may be necessary to decompress the optic structures before radiation when a transsphenoidal approach fails to adequately debulk the tumor or there is persistent major visual loss.

RADIATION THERAPY

Radiation therapy is complementary to surgery in preventing progression or recurrence. Standard radiation now uses conformal treatment planning to avoid unnecessary dosage to the temporal lobes. Doses of 4,500 to 5,000 cGy, delivered in 180 cGy

fractions, are recommended. Radiation may be the only treatment for patients who are poor operative risks, but histologic confirmation is generally desired. Radiation therapy is usually not the initial treatment for hormonally active tumors because full normalization of hormone levels often does not occur for years afterwards.

Radiation therapy is indicated for patients with recurrent, medically refractory, hypersecreting tumors or administered postoperatively to patients with invasive or large, incompletely removed adenomas. It is not routinely administered after gross total resection; these patients are followed with serial MRI and visual field examination, and radiation is reserved for documented tumor regrowth.

Early complications of radiation therapy are transient and involve minor inconveniences such as epilation, dry mouth, and altered taste or smell. The most common and important delayed complication is hypopituitarism which may occur any time from 6 months to 10 years after treatment. Annual endocrine evaluation is necessary to treat this appropriately. Other rare complications include visual loss, radiation necrosis of the temporal lobes, and radiation-induced tumors. To minimize risk of visual loss, optic structures should be decompressed before radiation therapy.

New techniques, such as radiosurgery using proton beam, Gamma Knife, or the linear accelerator, are being investigated. In these methods, a single high-dose fraction is directed to a limited volume, giving a high biologic effect. These methods may produce more rapid clinical and hormonal responses, potentially with less toxicity. However, there is concern about damage to the optic chiasm

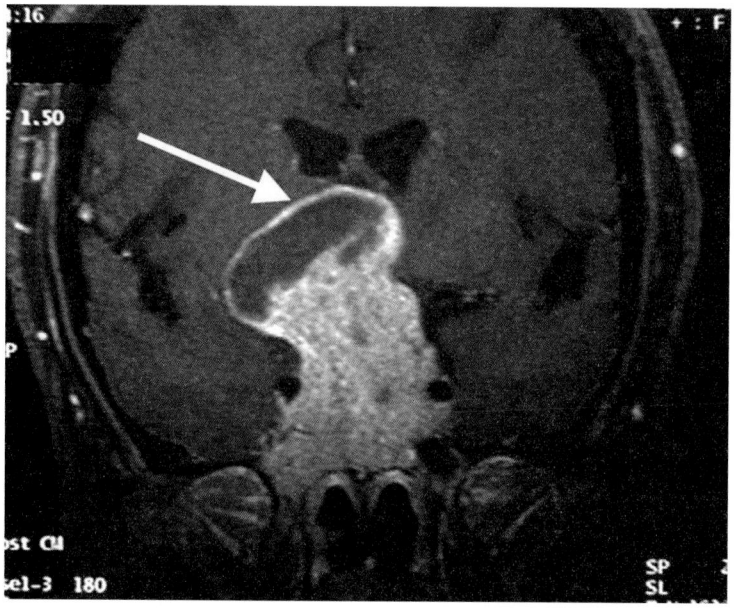
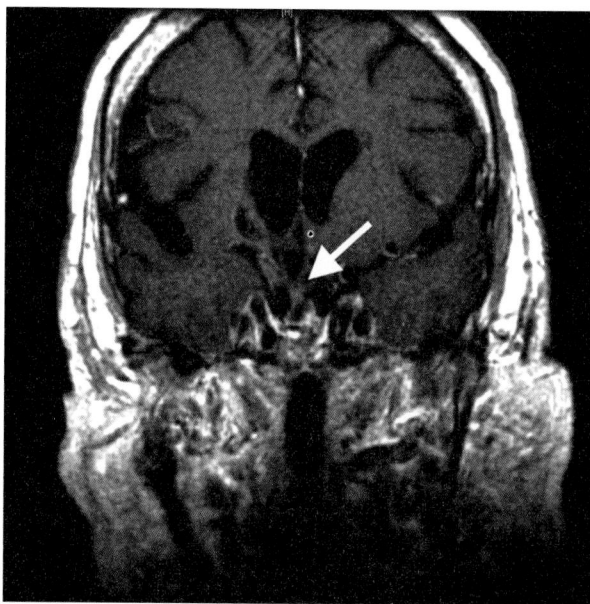

FIGURE 100.8 Large pituitary adenoma. **A:** T1-weighted coronal MRI with gadolinium showing a contrast-enhancing giant pituitary adenoma reaching up to the floor of the third ventricle with extension laterally to the right (*arrow*). A large tumor such as this often requires a craniotomy to decompress the optic structures adequately. **B:** Coronal MRI after a gross total resection of the pituitary adenoma through a craniotomy. There is no residual tumor, and the optic chiasm and a portion of the infundibulum may be seen clearly (*arrow*).

or cranial nerves. Radiosurgery is not used for large tumors or those less than 3 mm distance from the optic apparatus; this therapy may also be associated with a higher incidence of hypopituitarism.

RECURRENT TUMORS

Patients with recurrent tumors are difficult to manage, and treatment must be individualized. If the patient has not had prior radiation, then radiation would be the treatment of choice. Otherwise, repeat transsphenoidal surgery is usually indicated. Other treatment options include stereotactic radiosurgery, which may be effective and safe even in the patient who has had standard external beam radiotherapy.

OUTCOMES

Given the diverse clinical spectrum seen with pituitary masses, outcomes are variable and dependent on the size and characteristics of the tumor, the therapeutic modality being assessed, and the preexisting comorbidities of the patient at time of diagnosis.

SURGERY

Transsphenoidal surgery is safe with mortality rates less than 1% and major morbidity rates less than 3.5%. Morbidity includes stroke, visual loss, meningitis, CSF leak, or cranial nerve palsy; diabetes insipidus may also develop but is usually transient.

Assessing long-term clinical outcomes in patients with nonsecreting adenomas is challenging due to the scarcity of definitive data. Total resection at time of surgery is dependent on the size of tumor and the experience of the surgeon; in selected centers, it may be as high as 75%. Rates of recurrence vary from different surgical series but have been estimated to be 20%. They are

dependent on a host of clinical and nonclinical factors including tumor size, presence of symptoms on presentation, nature of the tumor (solid vs. cystic), and the skill of the surgeon. The presence of a residual adenoma on postoperative MRI has been shown to correlate with increased risk of recurrence. Some improvement in visual function is estimated to occur in 80% of patients. Restoration of normal endocrine function is dependent on preoperative status in addition to the aforementioned factors. Patients with preexisting hormonal deficiencies typically will not have restoration of full pituitary function.

Regarding functional tumors, outcomes are dependent on tumor type and a full discussion is beyond the scope of this chapter. For patients with Cushing or acromegaly, cure is possible if the tumor is small and symptoms are mild on presentation but risk of recurrent or residual disease increases with larger tumors or more advanced symptoms at time of diagnosis.

RADIATION THERAPY

Radiation therapy is highly effective in controlling tumor growth (80% or higher depending on length of follow up). Gamma Knife therapy may be more effective in patients who are candidates for this modality. Some degree of hypopituitarism occurs in 30% to 50% of patients across all radiation modalities.

MEDICAL THERAPY

Dopamine agonists (cabergoline is most commonly used with starting dose of 0.25 mg once or twice a week that may be titrated based on prolactin levels and radiographic response) are highly effective in treating prolactinomas and reducing prolactin levels and tumor size in greater than 90% of cases. Tumor size does impact outcomes, as macroprolactinomas have lower response rates than microprolactinomas but nonetheless, a majority will still respond to dopamine agonists.

SUGGESTED READINGS

Ausiello JC, Bruce JN, Freda PU. Postoperative assessment of the patient after transsphenoidal pituitary surgery. *Pituitary*. 2008;11(4):391–401.

Jho DH, Biller BM, Agarwalla PK, et al. Pituitary apoplexy: large surgical series with grading system. *World Neurosurg*. 2014;82(5):781–790. doi:10.1016/j.wneu.2014.06.005.

Camara Gomez R. Non-functioning pituitary tumors: 2012 update. *Endocrinol Nutr*. 2014;61(3):160–170.

Cappabianca P, de Divitiis E. Endoscopy and transsphenoidal surgery. *Neurosurgery*. 2004;54(5):1043–1048; discussions 1048–1050.

Chandler WF, Barkan AL. Treatment of pituitary tumors: a surgical perspective. *Endocrinol Metab Clin North Am*. 2008;37(1):51–66,viii.

Chen Y, Wang CD, Su ZP, et al. Natural history of postoperative nonfunctioning pituitary adenomas: a systematic review and meta-analysis. *Neuroendocrinology*. 2012;96(4):333–342.

Dekkers OM, Pereira AM, Roelfsema F, et al. Observation alone after transsphenoidal surgery for nonfunctioning pituitary macroadenoma. *J Clin Endocrinol Metab*. 2006;91(5):1796–1801.

Fernandez A, Karavitaki N, Wass JA. Prevalence of pituitary adenomas: a community-based, cross-sectional study in Banbury (Oxfordshire, UK). *Clin Endocrinol (Oxf)*. 2010;72(3):377–382.

Fernandez-Balsells MM, Murad MH, Barwise A, et al. Natural history of nonfunctioning pituitary adenomas and incidentalomas: a systemic review and metaanalysis. *J Clin Endocrinol Metab*. 2011;96(4):905–912.

Frank G, Pasquini E, Farneti G, et al. The endoscopic versus the traditional approach in pituitary surgery. *Neuroendocrinology*. 2006;83(3–4):240–248.

Freda PU, Beckers AM, Katznelson L, et al. Pituitary incidentaloma: an endocrine society clinical practice guideline. *J Clin Endocrinol Metab*. 2011;96(4):894–904.

Gertner ME, Kebebew E. Multiple endocrine neoplasia type 2. *Curr Treat Options Oncol*. 2004;5(4):315–325.

Goel A, Nadkarni T, Muzumdar D, et al. Giant pituitary tumors: a study based on surgical treatment of 118 cases. *Surg Neurol*. 2004;61(5):436–445; discussion 445–456.

Heaney AP. Clinical review: pituitary carcinoma: difficult diagnosis and treatment. *J Clin Endocrinol Metab*. 2011;96(12):3649–3660.

Honegger J, Prettin C, Feuerhake F, et al. Expression of Ki-67 antigen in nonfunctioning pituitary adenomas: correlation with growth velocity and invasiveness. *J Neurosurg*. 2003;99(4):674–679.

Ibrahim AE, Pickering RM, Gawne-Cain ML, et al. Indices of apoptosis and proliferation as potential prognostic markers in non-functioning pituitary adenomas. *Clin Neuropathol*. 2004;23(1):8–15.

Jane JA Jr, Laws ER Jr. The surgical management of pituitary adenomas in a series of 3,093 patients. *J Am Coll Surg*. 2001;193(6):651–659.

Johnson MD, Woodburn CJ, Vance ML. Quality of life in patients with a pituitary adenoma. *Pituitary*. 2003;6(2):81–87.

Joshi SM, Cudlip S. Transsphenoidal surgery. *Pituitary*. 2008;11(4):353–360.

Komninos J, Vlassopoulou V, Protopapa D, et al. Tumors metastatic to the pituitary gland: case report and literature review. *J Clin Endocrinol Metab*. 2004;89(2):574–580.

Kreutzer J, Fahlbusch R. Diagnosis and treatment of pituitary tumors. *Curr Opin Neurol*. 2004;17(6):693–703.

Laws ER, Sheehan JP, Sheehan JM, et al. Stereotactic radiosurgery for pituitary adenomas: a review of the literature. *J Neurooncol*. 2004;69(1–3):257–272.

Lee MS, Pless M. Apoplectic lymphocytic hypophysitis. Case report. *J Neurosurg*. 2003;98(1):183–185.

Loeffler JS, Shih HA. Radiation therapy in the management of pituitary adenomas. *J Clin Endocrinol Metab*. 2011;96(7):1992–2003.

Losa M, Valle M, Mortini P, et al. Gamma knife surgery for treatment of residual nonfunctioning pituitary adenomas after surgical debulking. *J Neurosurg*. 2004;100(3):438–444.

Ma W, Ikeda H, Yoshimoto T. Clinicopathologic study of 123 cases of prolactin-secreting pituitary adenomas with special reference to multihormone production and clonality of the adenomas. *Cancer*. 2002;95(2):258–266.

Mejico LJ, Miller NR, Dong LM. Clinical features associated with lesions other than pituitary adenoma in patients with an optic chiasmal syndrome. *Am J Ophthalmol*. 2004;137(5):908–913.

Melmed S. Update in pituitary disease. *J Clin Endocrinol Metab*. 2008;93(2):331–338.

Molitch ME. Management of incidentally found nonfunctional pituitary tumors. *Neurosurg Clin N Am*. 2012;23(4):543–553.

Mortini P, Losa M, Barzaghi R, et al. Results of transsphenoidal surgery in a large series of patients with pituitary adenoma. *Neurosurgery*. 2005;56(6):1222–1233; discussion 1233.

Park KJ, Kano H, Parry PV, et al. Long-term outcomes after gamma knife stereotactic radiosurgery for nonfunctional pituitary adenomas. *Neurosurgery*. 2011;69(6):1188–1199.

Pollock BE, Carpenter PC. Stereotactic radiosurgery as an alternative to fractionated radiotherapy for patients with recurrent or residual nonfunctioning pituitary adenomas. *Neurosurgery*. 2003;53(5):1086–1091; discussion 1091–1094.

Rajaratnam S, Seshadri MS, Chandy MJ, et al. Hydrocortisone dose and postoperative diabetes insipidus in patients undergoing transsphenoidal pituitary surgery: a prospective randomized controlled study. *Br J Neurosurg*. 2003;17(5):437–442.

Scheithauer BW, Kovacs KT, Laws ER Jr, et al. Pathology of invasive pituitary tumors with special reference to functional classification. *J Neurosurg*. 1986;65(6):733–744.

Sheehan JP, Starke RM, Mathieu D et al. Gamma Knife radiosurgery for the management of nonfunctioning pituitary adenomas: a multicenter study. *J Neurosurg*. 2013;119(2):446–456.

Swearingen B. Update on pituitary surgery. *J Clin Endocrinol Metab*. 2012;97(4):1073–1081.

Tanaka Y, Hongo K, Tada T, et al. Growth pattern and rate in residual nonfunctioning pituitary adenomas: correlations among tumor volume doubling time, patient age, and MIB-1 index. *J Neurosurg*. 2003;98(2):359–365.

Pineal Region Tumors 101

Jeffrey N. Bruce

INTRODUCTION

The pineal gland is composed of glandular tissue, glia, endothelial cells, and sympathetic nerve terminals. The numerous cell types that make up the normal gland and surrounding periventricular region may lead to a diverse group of tumors ranging from benign to malignant (Table 101.1), all of which may have a similar clinical presentation. Despite the common presentation, the specific histology has important implications for treatment and outcome. Optimal management of pineal region tumors therefore necessitates establishment of an accurate histologic diagnosis.

EPIDEMIOLOGY

Pineal tumors account for about 1% of all intracranial tumors in the United States. In Asia, where germ cell tumors (GCTs) are common, pineal cell tumors constitute 4% to 7% of all intracranial tumors. GCTs are found almost exclusively during the first three decades of life, whereas pineal cell tumors have a mean age of diagnosis around 30 years of age. Although intracranial germ cell tumors are overwhelmingly more common in men, there seems to be no strong gender preference among other pineal tumor types.

PATHOBIOLOGY

The pineal gland is an encapsulated structure situated between the velum interpositum of the posterior and the tectum of the midbrain. The gland produces melatonin in response to light–dark cycles and may play an ill-defined role in circadian rhythms. Pineocytomas and pineoblastomas arise from pineal glandular elements, astrocytomas and oligodendrogliomas from glial cells, hemangioblastomas from endothelial cells, and chemodectomas from sympathetic nerve cells. Arachnoid cells in the reflections of the tela choroidea, adjacent to the pineal gland, give rise to meningiomas. Ependymomas arise from ependymal cells that line the third ventricle. GCTs derive from primitive germ cell rests that are retained in the pineal and other midline structures after embryologic migration.

GERM CELL TUMORS

GCTs account for approximately one-third of all pineal tumors and are histologically identical to gonadal GCTs. They predominate in men and usually occur in children and adolescents. Pineal GCTs occur almost exclusively in boys, but suprasellar tumors occur equally in boys and girls. GCTs fall into two major categories: germinomas and nongerminomatous (NGGCT) that include choriocarcinomas, embryonal cell carcinomas, teratocarcinomas, and endodermal sinus tumors. Benign, mature teratomas may also be seen.

Germinomas arise in the midline, usually in the pineal area and suprasellar cistern and occasionally in both areas simultaneously. Rarely do they develop in the cerebral hemispheres. Germinomas account for about half of all intracranial GCTs. They are histologically identical to the testicular seminoma and ovarian dysgerminoma. Germinomas are highly malignant; pathologically, they are frequently infiltrated by lymphocytes, which may occasionally confuse the diagnosis. Germinomas label with placental alkaline phosphatase; some contain syncytiotrophoblastic elements that produce β-human chorionic gonadotropin (β-hCG), which confers a slightly worse prognosis in some studies (Table 101.2). Germinomas may occasionally seed the cerebrospinal fluid (CSF).

NGGCTs are highly malignant and more aggressive than germinomas; they metastasize to the CSF more frequently than germinomas. Choriocarcinoma contains cyto- and syncytiotrophoblastic cells that produce β-hCG. Endodermal sinus tumors contain yolk sac elements that produce α-fetoprotein (AFP). High levels

TABLE 101.1	Summary of Pathologically Verified Pineal Tumors at the New York Neurological Institute (1990–2013)			
Type	Benign	Malignant	Male-to-Female Ratio	Average Age (yr)
Germ cell	3	29	15:1	22
Pineal cell	16	29	1:1	41
Glial cell	18	20	1:1.5	38
Meningioma	9	2	1:2.7	46
Pineal cyst	14	0	1:2.5	36
Miscellaneous (including metastases)	3	15	1:1	40
Total	63	95	1.1:1	36

TABLE 101.2	Biologic Markers in Germ Cell Tumors		
Tumors		β-hCG	AFP
Immature teratoma		?	+
Germinoma		−	−
Germinoma with syncytiotrophoblastic cells		+	−
Embryonal cell carcinoma		+	+
Choriocarcinoma		++	−
Endodermal sinus tumor		−	++

β-hCG, β-human chorionic gonadotropin; AFP, α-fetoprotein.

of β-hCG or AFP in the CSF or serum indicate the presence of malignant germ cell elements. When markers are elevated, a tissue diagnosis is not necessary and patients are treated with radiation and chemotherapy.

All patients with histologically confirmed GCTs, regardless of subtype, should have serum and CSF tested for markers (if not done preoperatively), a complete spine magnetic resonance imaging (MRI) with gadolinium, and cytologic examination of CSF to complete staging prior to treatment.

Treatment first involves surgical resection to establish the diagnosis and debulk the tumor; if possible, gross total excision is the surgical goal. Patients with pure germinomas should be treated with radiotherapy, usually to 50.4 Gy; the port must include the whole ventricular system, and some radiotherapists treat the whole brain. If the tumor is disseminated in the CSF, craniospinal radiation is required. Chemotherapy may be useful at recurrence but is not recommended at diagnosis because most germinoma patients are cured with radiotherapy alone. NGGCTs require craniospinal radiotherapy and adjuvant chemotherapy in all cases after maximal resection. Benign GCTs such as teratomas, dermoids, and epidermoids are generally curable with surgery alone.

PINEAL CELL TUMORS

Primary pineal cell tumors are classified as low-grade pineocytomas (World Health Organization [WHO] grade I), pineal parenchymal tumors of intermediate differentiation (PPTID, WHO grade II or III), or the highly malignant pineoblastoma (WHO grade IV). Pineoblastomas are the same entity as primitive neuroectodermal tumors (PNET) of the pineal region. The higher grade tumors tend to occur in children and young adults, whereas pineocytomas usually occur in adults. Pineal tumors of all histologic grades may seed the leptomeninges, but pineocytomas do so only rarely. Complete resection of a pineocytoma does not require additional therapy, but incomplete resection should be followed by radiation. Intermediate-grade pineocytomas require radiotherapy, and pineoblastomas require neuraxis radiation and chemotherapy.

GLIOMAS

Gliomas account for one-third of pineal tumors. Most are invasive and have a prognosis comparable to astrocytomas of the upper brain stem. Some gliomas are low-grade, cystic, and may be surgically curable. Anaplastic astrocytomas and glioblastomas are less common. Oligodendrogliomas and ependymomas may also occur. Treatment of these tumors is identical to the treatment of gliomas in other areas of the central nervous system.

MENINGIOMAS

Meningiomas may arise from the velum interpositum or from the tentorial edge. They occur predominantly in middle-aged patients and in the elderly. They are amenable to surgical resection.

METASTASIS AND OTHER MISCELLANEOUS TUMORS

The pineal gland does not have a blood–brain barrier and, like the pituitary gland, may be underrecognized as a site of brain metastasis from systemic tumors. Miscellaneous tumors include sarcoma, hemangioblastoma, choroid plexus papilloma, lymphoma, and chemodectoma.

PINEAL CYSTS

Benign cysts of the pineal gland are often found incidentally on imaging studies, and it is important to distinguish them from cystic tumors. They are normal variants of the pineal gland and consist of a cystic structure surrounded by normal pineal parenchymal tissue (Fig. 101.1). Radiographically, they are up to 2 cm in diameter and often have some degree of peripheral enhancement as a result of the compressed normal pineal gland. Pineal cysts may be found in 4% of all MRI scans. These cysts are static, anatomic variants and need no treatment unless they become symptomatic. The most common symptoms are headaches, followed by visual symptoms. The cysts may be sufficiently large to cause obstructive hydrocephalus. Decompression can occasionally be accomplished by third-ventricular endoscopic resection of the cyst.

CLINICAL FEATURES

Pineal region tumors may become symptomatic from one of three mechanisms: increased intracranial pressure (ICP) from hydrocephalus, direct compression of brain stem and cerebellum, or endocrine dysfunction. Headache, associated with hydrocephalus, is the most common symptom at onset and is caused by obstruction of third-ventricular outflow at the aqueduct of Sylvius (Table 101.3). Leptomeningeal dissemination can produce a multitude of symptoms depending on the area affected, analogous to leptomeningeal metastases from other cancers. Hydrocephalus must be surgically addressed in most patients, preferably by an endoscopic third ventriculostomy. A ventriculoperitoneal shunt is an acceptable alternative but carries greater long-term risks including peritoneal seeding of malignant tumors.

More advanced hydrocephalus may result in papilledema, gait disorder, nausea, vomiting, lethargy, and memory disturbance.

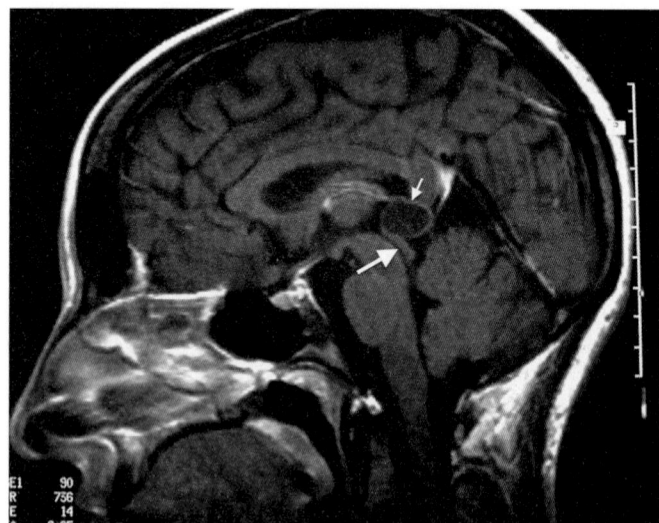

FIGURE 101.1 Sagittal T1-weighted gadolinium-enhanced MRI of a pineal cyst. These cysts may have rim enhancement (*small arrow*) and may be up to 2 cm in diameter. They rarely cause compression of the sylvian aqueduct (*larger arrow* on patent aqueduct) and are rarely symptomatic. Histologically, they are normal variants of the pineal gland and require no treatment; they must be distinguished from cystic tumors. Growth of the cyst on serial MRIs or the development of hydrocephalus is sufficient cause to doubt the diagnosis, and surgical resection should be considered.

TABLE 101.3	Presenting Symptoms and Signs in 100 Consecutive Patients with Pineal Region Tumors at the New York Neurological Institute		
Symptoms	Number	Signs	Number
Headache	87	Parinaud syndrome	75
Nausea/vomiting	32	Ataxia	39
Gait unsteadiness	32	Papilledema	36
Diplopia	31	Normal exam	12
Blurred vision	19	Fourth nerve palsy	5
Memory impairment	16	Obtundation	4
Lethargy	11	Sixth nerve palsy	3
Altered consciousness	9	Spasticity	3
Personality change	9	Visual field deficit	1
Visual obscurations	4	Psychomotor retardation	1
Syncope	3		
Polyuria/polydipsia	3		
Seizures	3		
Tremor	3		
Neck stiffness	2		
Numbness	2		
Developmental delay	2		
Incontinence	2		
Precocious puberty	1		
Rigidity	1		
Amenorrhea	1		
Subarachnoid hemorrhage	1		

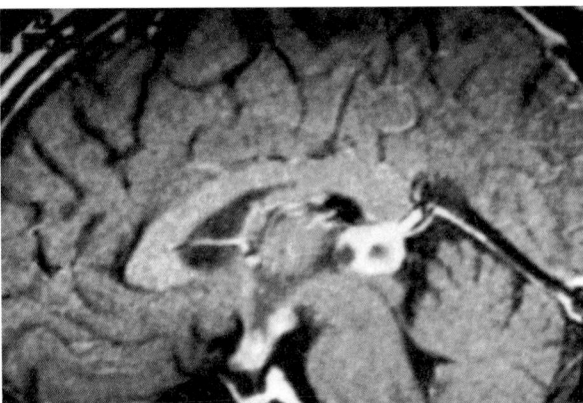

FIGURE 101.2 Sagittal MRI with gadolinium showing multi-centric germinoma involving the pineal region and infiltrating the mammillary bodies, optic chiasm, and pituitary stalk. This patient presented with diminished visual fields and diabetes insipidus.

cells and ectopic secretion of β-hCG. In boys, the luteinizing hormone–like effects of β-hCG may stimulate Leydig cells to produce androgens that induce development of secondary sexual characteristics and pseudopuberty. This phenomenon does not occur in girls with pineal region tumors because GCTs are rare in females, and both luteinizing hormone and follicle-stimulating hormone (FSH) are necessary to trigger ovarian estrogen production.

DIAGNOSIS

MRI with gadolinium is mandatory for all pineal tumors to determine the presence of hydrocephalus and evaluate tumor size, vascularity, and homogeneity. In particular, sagittal MRI reveals the relationship of the tumor to surrounding structures and also evaluates possible ventricular seeding. Angiography is not performed unless a vascular anomaly is suspected. Measurement of AFP and β-hCG in serum and CSF is required in the preoperative workup. If β-hCG or AFP levels are elevated, malignant germ cell elements must be present so a tissue diagnosis is not necessary and treatment with radiation and chemotherapy can commence. Despite improved imaging and CSF markers, a definite histologic diagnosis requires pathologic examination of tumor tissue, and all patients should undergo surgery.

TREATMENT

Given the rarity of pineal region tumors, studies establishing level 1 standards do not exist. Owing to the wide variety of pineal region tumor subtypes, the general approach to these tumors is to first establish a histologic diagnosis by obtaining tumor tissue through an open surgical approach or a stereotactic-guided needle biopsy (Fig. 101.3). Subsequent management is dependent on the tumor type (Fig. 101.4).

SURGERY

The pineal region may be reached surgically from one of several approaches, above or below the tentorium, depending on tumor size and coexistent hydrocephalus (Fig. 101.5). Complete excision

Direct midbrain compression may cause disorders of ocular movements, such as Parinaud syndrome (paralysis of upgaze, convergence or retraction nystagmus, and light-near pupillary dissociation) or the sylvian aqueduct syndrome (paralysis of downgaze or horizontal gaze superimposed upon a Parinaud syndrome). Either lid retraction (Collier sign) or ptosis may follow dorsal midbrain compression or infiltration. Fourth nerve palsy with diplopia and head tilt may be seen. Ataxia and dysmetria may result from direct cerebellar compression.

Endocrine dysfunction is rare, usually arising from secondary effects of hydrocephalus or tumor spread to the hypothalamic region (Fig. 101.2). The symptoms may occur early, before any radiographic documentation of hypothalamic seeding.

Although precocious puberty has been linked with pineal masses, documented cases are rare. Precocious puberty is actually precocious pseudopuberty because the hypothalamic–gonadal axis is not mature. It occurs in boys with choriocarcinomas or germinomas with syncytiotrophoblastic

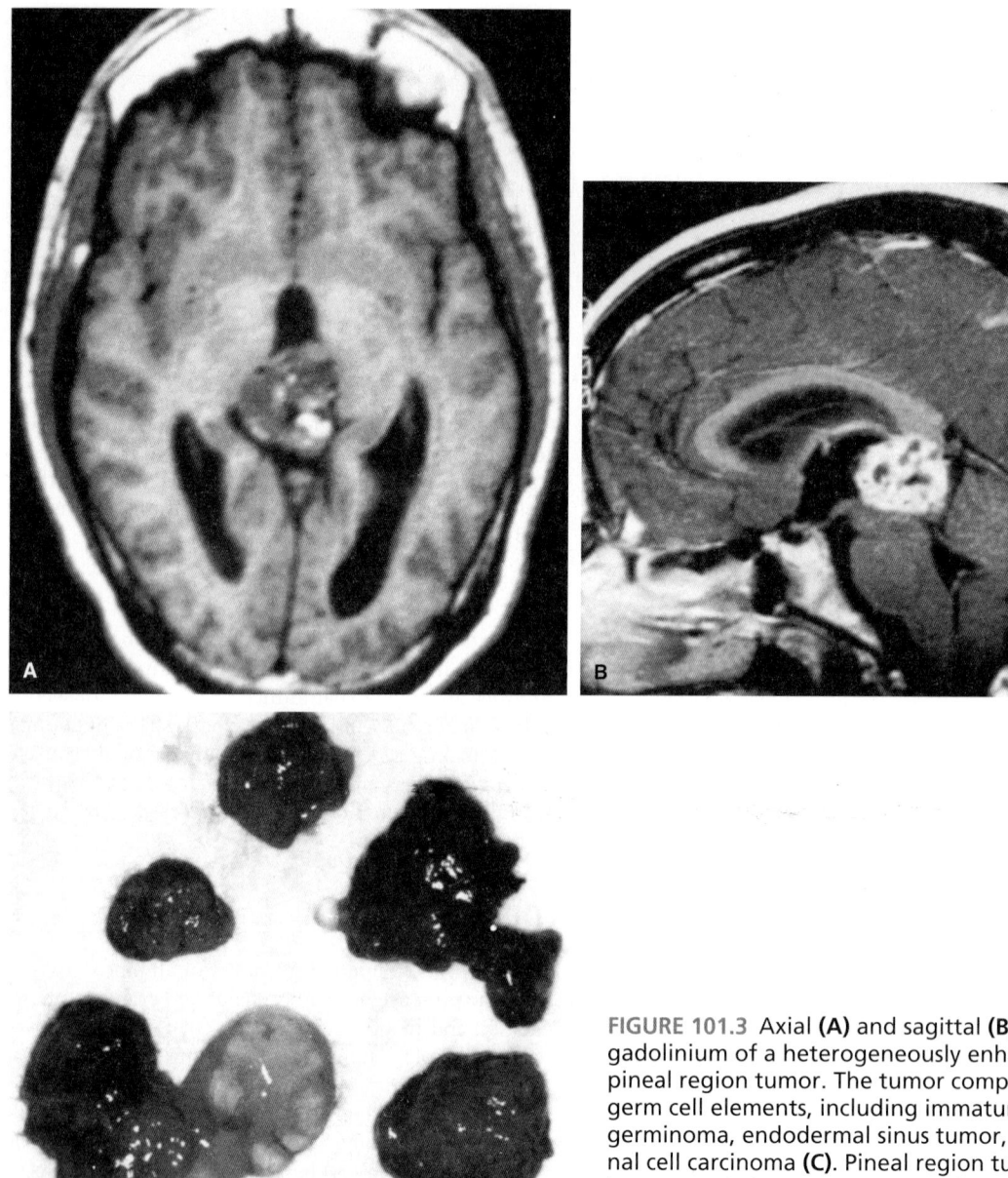

FIGURE 101.3 Axial **(A)** and sagittal **(B)** MRIs with gadolinium of a heterogeneously enhancing pineal region tumor. The tumor comprised several germ cell elements, including immature teratoma, germinoma, endodermal sinus tumor, and embryonal cell carcinoma **(C)**. Pineal region tumors may be extremely heterogeneous, and extensive tumor sampling is necessary to avoid diagnostic errors.

is the goal for any pineal tumor. Nearly one-third of pineal tumors are benign and curable with complete resection alone. With malignant tumors, aggressive tumor resection provides the best opportunity for accurate histologic diagnosis and may increase the effectiveness of adjuvant radiotherapy or chemotherapy. The overall operative mortality is about 4%, with an additional 3% permanent major morbidity. The most serious complication of surgery is hemorrhage into a partially resected malignant tumor. The most common postoperative complications are ocular palsies, altered mental status, and ataxia, which are usually transient. For patients with obviously disseminated tumor or those with medical problems that pose excessive surgical risks, biopsy via a stereotactic or endoscopic approach is a reasonable alternative for obtaining diagnostic tissue. Although gaining in popularity, stereotactic biopsy is not performed routinely because of possible sampling error through insufficient tissue analysis, increased

risk of hemorrhage from the adjacent deep venous system and highly vascular pineal tumors, and a better prognosis that follows aggressive resection.

POSTOPERATIVE STAGING

All patients with pineal cell tumors and GCTs are evaluated for CSF seeding (Fig. 101.6). High-resolution gadolinium-enhanced MRI of the complete spine should be performed. Even if the spine MRI is negative, CSF analysis for cytology and markers is still required in all patients.

RADIOTHERAPY

Germinomas and pineal parenchymal tumors of intermediate differentiation require radiation to a dose of 50 to 60 Gy with coverage of the ventricles. All patients with pineoblastomas, NGGCT,

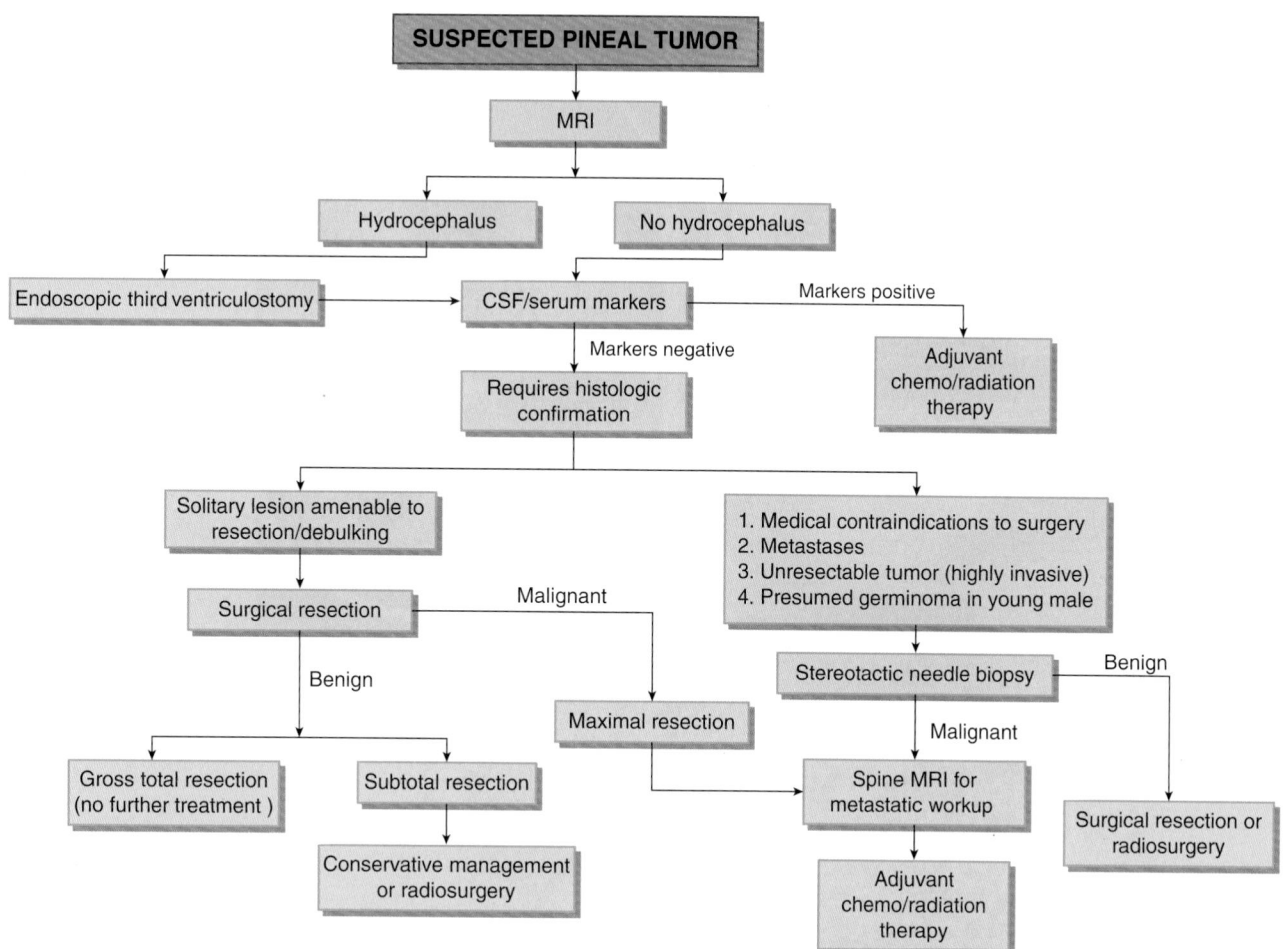

FIGURE 101.4 Algorithm for management of pineal region tumors.

and disseminated germinomas require neuraxis radiotherapy, usually to a total dose of about 36 Gy, with a boost to the primary site to achieve a dose of at least 54 Gy. Gliomas are treated according to histologic subtype.

Experience with stereotactic radiosurgery is limited because pineal tumors are rare. There are reports of tumor control using radiosurgery as the sole treatment for some low-grade tumors such as pineocytoma, but it rarely produces complete tumor regression and is probably not optimal initial therapy. The main problem with radiosurgery is not the response of the targeted mass but the potential for recurrence outside of the treatment volume. It has been used with some success for tumors less than 3 cm in diameter at recurrence, provided there is no evidence of CSF dissemination.

CHEMOTHERAPY

Chemotherapy has been of most benefit with NGGCTs and pineoblastomas. The most commonly used regimens are combinations of cisplatin, vinblastine, and bleomycin or cisplatin and VP-16 (e.g., etoposide). Chemotherapy is usually given after completion of neuraxis radiation, except in young children in whom radiotherapy is avoided because of the risk of severe, long-term effects on growth and cognition. Young children are treated with chemotherapy alone, and radiotherapy is deferred until they are at least 3 years or older.

Initial attempts to avoid radiation in all patients by using aggressive chemotherapy resulted in an unacceptably high incidence (50%) of recurrence at 2 years, including patients with germinoma, which is curable with radiation alone. Therefore, chemotherapy is not used as part of the initial treatment of localized germinomas.

OUTCOME

Generally, benign pineal tumors and pineal cysts are curable with surgery alone. For malignant tumors, meta-analysis of small clinical series suggests that maximal surgical resection provides survival benefits; however, class I or II evidence is lacking. Prognosis is highly dependent on tumor histology. Germinomas have a 90% 10-year survival rate following surgery and radiotherapy. Patients with NGGCT have 5-year survival rates in the range of 50%, but some may be salvaged with additional chemotherapy. Greater than 80% of patients with pineocytomas survive 5 years particularly following aggressive surgical resection. Median survival for patients with pineoblastomas is much more variable ranging from 1 to 5 years, with prognosis influenced by extent of resection, age, and disseminated disease. The outcome for patients with glial tumors is similar to gliomas found in other regions of the brain.

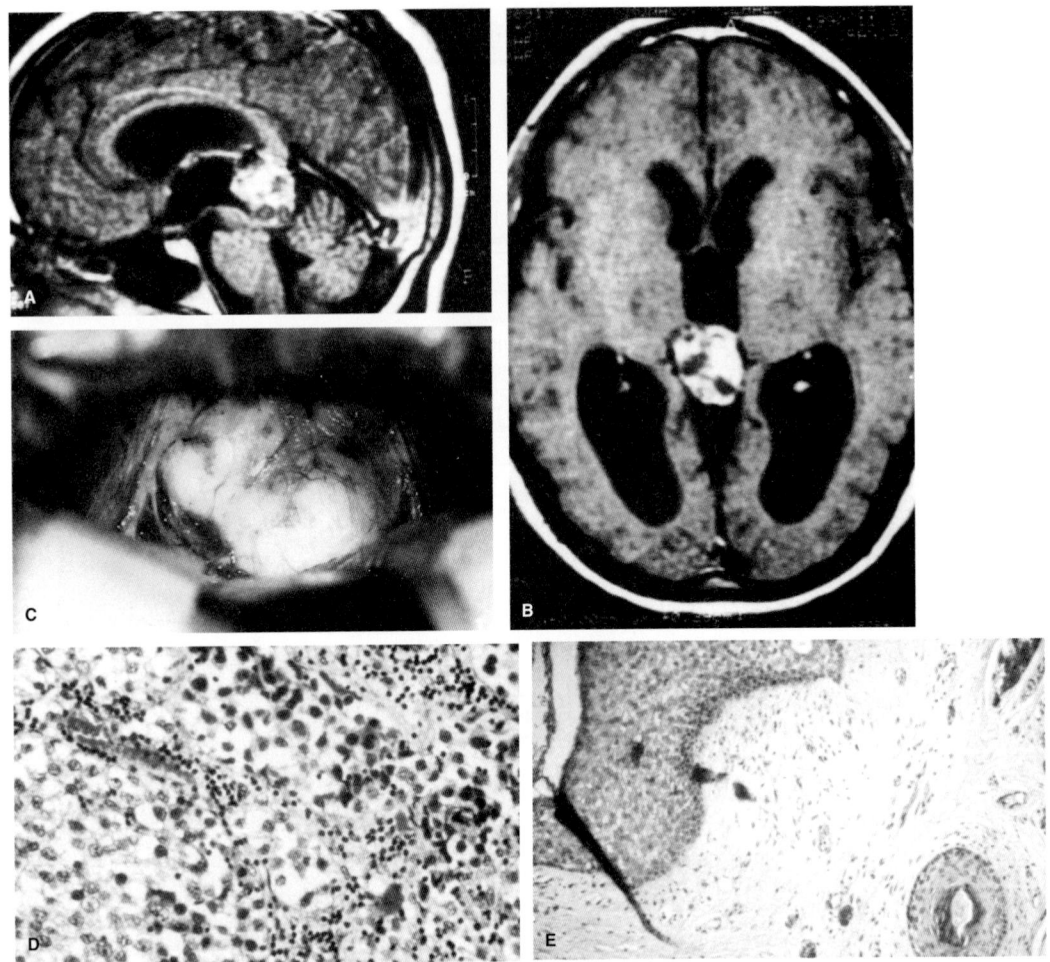

FIGURE 101.5 Sagittal **(A)** and axial **(B)** MRIs with gadolinium of a mixed dermoid/germinoma causing hydrocephalus. **C:** Intraoperative photograph shows the tumor, which was completely resected through a supracerebellar–infratentorial approach without neurologic deficits (cerebellum is at the bottom of the photograph covered by a retractor). **D and E:** Histologic analysis revealed a mixed dermoid/germinoma.

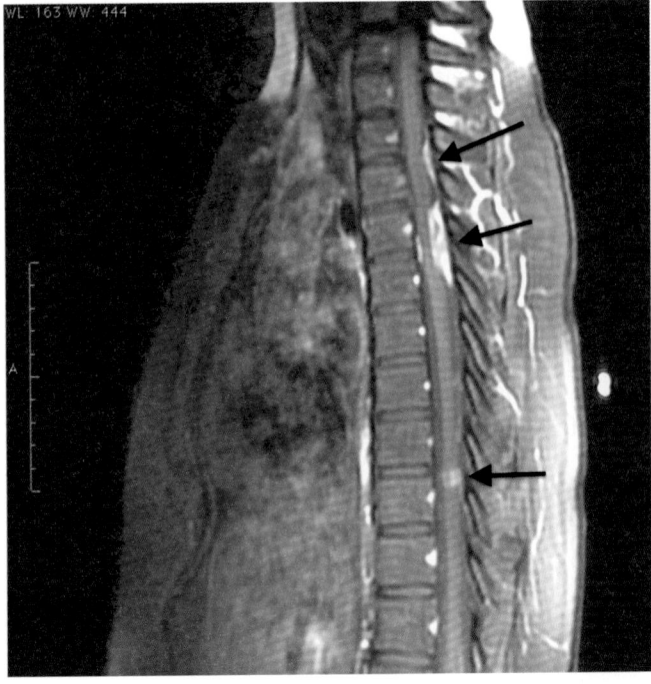

FIGURE 101.6 Intradural seeding from a pineoblastoma. Thoracic MRI showing enhancing drop metastases (*arrows*) in thoracic spinal canal.

SUGGESTED READINGS

Anan M, Ishii K, Nakamura T, et al. Postoperative adjuvant treatment for pineal parenchymal tumour of intermediate differentiation. *J Clin Neurosci.* 2006;13(9):965–968.

Baehring J, Vives K, Duncan C, et al. Tumors of the posterior third ventricle and pineal region: ependymoma and germinoma. *J Neurooncol.* 2004;70(2):273–274.

Balmaceda C, Finlay J. Current advances in the diagnosis and management of intracranial germ cell tumors. *Curr Neurol Neurosci Rep.* 2004;4(3):253–262.

Balossier A, Blond S, Touzet G, et al. Role of radiosurgery in the management of pineal region tumours: indications, method, outcome [published online ahead of print]. *Neurochirurgie.* 2014.

Bruce JN. Pineal tumors. In: Winn H, ed. *Youmans Neurological Surgery.* Vol. 2. 6th ed. Philadelphia: Elsevier; 2011:1359–1372.

Bruce JN, Ogden AT. Surgical strategies for treating patients with pineal region tumors. *J Neurooncol.* 2004;69(1–3):221–236.

Calaminus G, Bamberg M, Jurgens H, et al. Impact of surgery, chemotherapy and irradiation on long term outcome of intracranial malignant nongerminomatous germ cell tumors: results of the German cooperative trial MAKEI 89. *Klin Padiatr.* 2004;216(3):141–149.

Chernov MF, Kamikawa S, Yamane F, et al. Neurofiberscopic biopsy of tumors of the pineal region and posterior third ventricle: indications, technique, complications, and results. *Neurosurgery.* 2006;59(2):267–277; discussion 267–277.

Choy W, Kim W, Spasic M, et al. Pineal cyst: a review of clinical and radiological features. *Neurosurg Clin N Am.* 2011;22(3):341–351, vii.

Clark AJ, Sughrue ME, Ivan ME, et al. Factors influencing overall survival rates for patients with pineocytoma. *J Neurooncol.* 2010;100(2):255–260.

Constantini S, Mohanty A, Zymberg S, et al. Safety and diagnostic accuracy of neuroendoscopic biopsies: an international multicenter study. *J Neurosurg Pediatr.* 2013;11(6):704–709.

Deshmukh VR, Smith KA, Rekate HL, et al. Diagnosis and management of pineocytomas. *Neurosurgery.* 2004;55(2):349–355; discussion 355–357.

Fetell MR, Bruce JN, Burke AM, et al. Non-neoplastic pineal cysts. *Neurology.* 1991;41:1034–1040.

Fevre-Montange M, Champier J, Szathmari A, et al. Microarray analysis reveals differential gene expression patterns in tumors of the pineal region. *J Neuropathol Exp Neurol.* 2006;65(7):675–684.

Fevre-Montange M, Hasselblatt M, Figarella-Branger D, et al. Prognosis and histopathologic features in papillary tumors of the pineal region: a retrospective multicenter study of 31 cases. *J Neuropathol Exp Neurol.* 2006;65(10):1004–1011.

Hanft SJ, Isaacson SR, Bruce JN. Stereotactic radiosurgery for pineal region tumors. *Neurosurg Clin N Am.* 2011;22(3):413–420, ix.

Hasegawa T, Kondziolka D, Hadjipanayis CG, et al. The role of radiosurgery for the treatment of pineal parenchymal tumors. *Neurosurgery.* 2002;51(4):880–889.

Jackson C, Jallo G, Lim M. Clinical outcomes after treatment of germ cell tumors. *Neurosurg Clin N Am.* 2011;22(3):385–394, viii.

Kellie SJ, Boyce H, Dunkel IJ, et al. Primary chemotherapy for intracranial nongerminomatous germ cell tumors: results of the second International CNS Germ Cell Study Group protocol. *J Clin Oncol.* 2004;22(5):846–853.

Kennedy BC, Bruce JN. Surgical approaches to the pineal region. *Neurosurg Clin N Am.* 2011;22(3):367–380, viii.

Knierim DS, Yamada S. Pineal tumors and associated lesions: the effect of ethnicity on tumor type and treatment. *Pediatr Neurosurg.* 2003;38(6):307–323.

Kochi M, Itoyama Y, Shiraishi S, et al. Successful treatment of intracranial nongerminomatous malignant germ cell tumors by administering neoadjuvant chemotherapy and radiotherapy before excision of residual tumors. *J Neurosurg.* 2003;99(1):106–114.

Konovalov AN, Pitskhelauri DI. Principles of treatment of the pineal region tumors. *Surg Neurol.* 2003;59(4):250–268.

Korogi Y, Takahashi M, Ushio Y. MRI of pineal region tumors. *J Neurooncol.* 2001;54(3):251–261.

Lassman AB, Bruce JN, Fetell MR. Metastases to the pineal gland. *Neurology.* 2006;67(7):1303–1304.

Lutterbach J, Fauchon F, Schild SE, et al. Malignant pineal parenchymal tumors in adult patients: patterns of care and prognostic factors. *Neurosurgery.* 2002;51(1):44–55; discussion 55–56.

Mandera M, Marcol W, Bierzynska-Macyszyn G, et al. Pineal cysts in childhood. *Childs Nerv Syst.* 2003;19(10–11):750–755.

Matsutani M. Clinical management of primary central nervous system germ cell tumors. *Semin Oncol.* 2004;31(5):676–683.

Matsutani M, Sano K, Takakura K, et al. Primary intracranial germ cell tumors: a clinical analysis of 153 histologically verified cases. *J Neurosurg.* 1997;86:446–455.

Michielsen G, Benoit Y, Baert E, et al. Symptomatic pineal cysts: clinical manifestations and management. *Acta Neurochir (Wien).* 2002;144(3):233–242; discussion 42.

Ogawa K, Toita T, Nakamura K, et al. Treatment and prognosis of patients with intracranial nongerminomatous malignant germ cell tumors: a multiinstitutional retrospective analysis of 41 patients. *Cancer.* 2003;98(2):369–376.

Parwani AV, Baisden BL, Erozan YS, et al. Pineal gland lesions: a cytopathologic study of 20 specimens. *Cancer.* 2005;105(2):80–86.

Regis J, Bouillot P, Rouby-Volot F, et al. Pineal region tumors and the role of stereotactic biopsy: review of the mortality, morbidity, and diagnostic rates in 370 cases. *Neurosurgery.* 1996;39:907–914.

Schild SE, Scheithauer BW, Haddock MG, et al. Histologically confirmed pineal tumors and other germ cell tumors of the brain. *Cancer.* 1996;78(12):2564–2571.

Silvani A, Eoli M, Salmaggi A, et al. Combined chemotherapy and radiotherapy for intracranial germinomas in adult patients: a single-institution study. *J Neurooncol.* 2005;71(3):271–276.

Smith AA, Weng E, Handler M, et al. Intracranial germ cell tumors: a single institution experience and review of the literature. *J Neurooncol.* 2004;68(2):153–159.

Spunt SL, Walsh MF, Krasin MJ, et al. Brain metastases of malignant germ cell tumors in children and adolescents. *Cancer.* 2004;101(3):620–626.

Villano JL, Propp JM, Porter KR, et al. Malignant pineal germ-cell tumors: an analysis of cases from three tumor registries. *Neuro Oncol.* 2008;10(2):121–130.

Yamini B, Refai D, Rubin CM, et al. Initial endoscopic management of pineal region tumors and associated hydrocephalus: clinical series and literature review. *J Neurosurg.* 2004;100(5)(suppl Pediatrics):437–441.

Yianni J, Rowe J, Khandanpour N, et al. Stereotactic radiosurgery for pineal tumours. *Br J Neurosurg.* 2012;26(3):361–366.

Zacharia BE, Bruce JN. Stereotactic biopsy considerations for pineal tumors. *Neurosurg Clin N Am.* 2011;22(3):359–366, viii.

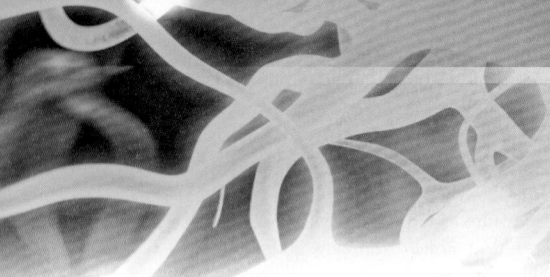

VESTIBULAR SCHWANNOMA (ACOUSTIC NEUROMA)

EPIDEMIOLOGY

Vestibular schwannomas (e.g., acoustic neuroma, acoustic neurofibroma) are slow-growing, benign extra-axial tumors that arise commonly from the superior vestibular portion of the eighth cranial nerve (CN VIII). Vestibular schwannomas comprise 8% to 10% of intracranial tumors. Tumors may arise either sporadically (95%) or in association with neurofibromatosis type 2 (NF2). The incidence of sporadic cases is believed to be 1 per 100,000 person-years, with a median age of 50 years. As a result of the prevalence of magnetic resonance imaging (MRI), the incidence of vestibular schwannomas has increased recently, whereas the typical size at diagnosis has decreased.

PATHOBIOLOGY

Vestibular schwannomas are histopathologically benign tumors that grow slowly from the Schwann cell sheath surrounding the vestibular branch of CN VIII. Tumors are composed of Antoni A (narrow elongated bipolar cells) and Antoni B fibers (loose reticulated pattern of cells). Verocay bodies are frequently seen and consist of acellular eosinophilic areas surrounded by parallel arrangements of spindle-shaped Schwann cells.

Vestibular schwannomas are typically unilateral lesions. Bilateral vestibular schwannomas occur in less than 5% of patients and are a defining characteristic of NF2, an autosomal dominant disorder involving the *NF2* gene located on chromosome 22 band q11-13.1. This gene normally encodes the protein merlin (schwannomin), which is thought to play a role in membrane stability through interactions with cytoskeletal and integral membrane proteins. Loss of function of merlin in Schwann cells has been associated with both sporadic and NF2-related vestibular schwannomas, and the gene is often considered a classic tumor suppressor. Cytologically, vestibular schwannomas that arise in NF2 are identical to sporadic cases but with a greater tendency to infiltrate the nerve rather than displace it. In addition to patients with bilateral lesions, any patient younger than 40 years of age with a unilateral vestibular schwannoma should also undergo evaluation for NF2.

Tumors often originate within the internal acoustic meatus (intracanalicular; Fig. 102.1) and may extend into the cerebellopontine angle (extracanalicular). Mass effect from extracanalicular tumor may compromise function of cranial nerves, brain stem nuclei, and the cerebellum. Tumors typically follow three growth patterns: (1) no or

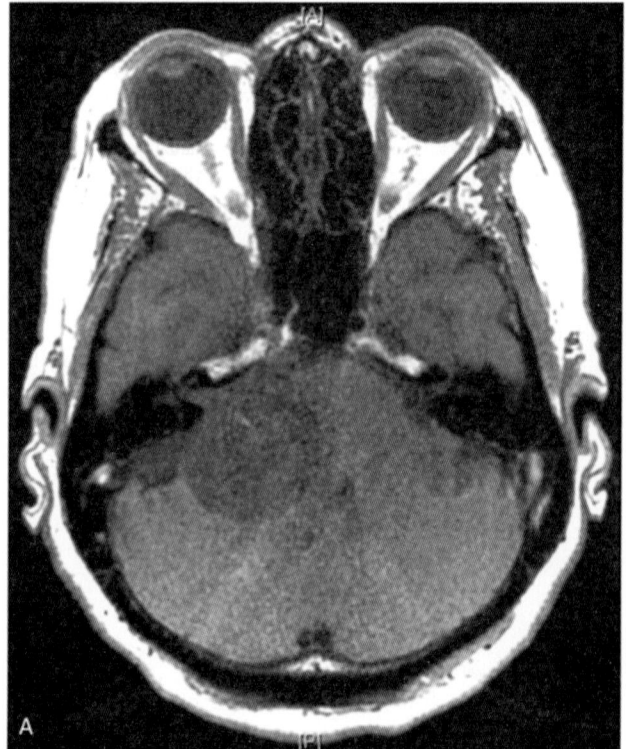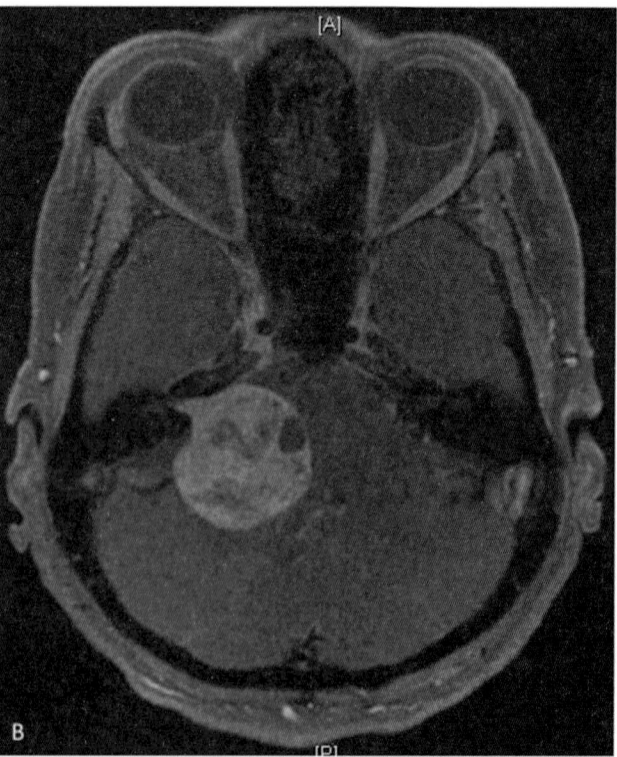

FIGURE 102.1 Vestibular Schwannoma. **A:** T1-weighted axial MRI before contrast shows large hypo intense mass within the CPA angle exerting mass effect on the brainstem. **B:** T1-weighted axial MRI post-contrast shows a vestibular schwannoma with expansion of the internal auditory meatus.

TABLE 102.1	Symptoms in Vestibular Schwannoma (1,000 Patients)
Symptoms	**%**
Hearing loss	95
Tinnitus	63
Dysequilibrium/vertigo	61
Headache	12
Trigeminal nerve disturbance	9
Facial paresis	5.2
Caudal cranial nerve disturbances	2.7
Change of taste	2
Diplopia	1.8

From Matthies C, Samii M. Management of 1000 vestibular schwannomas (acoustic neuromas): clinical presentation. *Neurosurgery.* 1997;40(1):1–9; discussion 9–10.

very slow growth; (2) slow growth (2 mm/yr linear growth on imaging studies); or (3) fast growth (>8 mm/yr) as a result of the enlargement of cystic components or rarely, intratumoral hemorrhage.

CLINICAL FEATURES

Vestibular schwannomas most commonly present with progressive unilateral hearing loss, characterized by difficulty with speech discrimination, especially when talking on the telephone. The next most common symptoms include tinnitus, followed by balance difficulties (Table 102.1). This triad of symptoms is related to pressure on the eighth nerve complex in the internal auditory canal. Other presenting symptoms include facial paralysis, trigeminal neuralgia, and rarely, hydrocephalus and brain stem compression in the setting of larger tumors. Although this constellation of symptoms may occur with any mass in the cerebellopontine angle, including meningioma, cholesteatoma, or trigeminal neuroma, only rarely will these other lesions cause tinnitus or hearing dysfunction.

DIAGNOSIS

Patients with hearing loss often undergo audiometric evaluation with pure tone audiogram and speech discrimination evaluation. Those with vestibular disturbances may undergo vestibular test-

ing. Hearing loss is typically insidious and progressive, with 70% of patients demonstrating a high-frequency loss pattern and impaired word discrimination (especially noticeable in telephone conversation). Tinnitus is usually high-pitched. Weber test lateralizes to the uninvolved side, and Rinne test will be positive on both sides if there is enough preserved hearing.

Asymmetric sensorineural hearing loss, or defects in other cranial nerves, indicates the need for imaging. Gadolinium-enhanced MRI is the gold standard for diagnosing vestibular schwannomas. Tumors enhance brightly, and an origin within the internal auditory canal suggests vestibular schwannoma rather than meningioma. Contrast-enhanced computed tomography (CT) can also be used to diagnose vestibular schwannomas greater than 15 mm in diameter for patients who cannot undergo MRI.

TREATMENT

The goal of treatment is to cure the tumor while preserving intact neurologic function. Following diagnosis, patients with vestibular schwannomas have several options for managing their tumor including observation with serial imaging, stereotactic radiosurgery (SRS), fractionated radiotherapy (RT), and microsurgery. Selection of treatment modality depends on tumor size, symptoms, patient age, patient health, and patient preference. Figure 102.2 represents a decision tree following initial diagnosis of vestibular schwannoma. In general, noncystic, non-NF2 intracanalicular tumors or cerebellopontine angle (CPA) tumors 20 mm or smaller may be followed with serial imaging and hearing tests. Tumors larger than 15 to 20 mm should be treated. NF2 patients present a challenge and should be evaluated on a case-by-case basis.

Observation/Expectant Management

Observation with serial clinical assessment and follow-up MRI to monitor for signs of tumor growth is an option in the management of vestibular schwannoma. Patients using this approach are monitored using MRI until progression of symptoms or tumor growth warrants more invasive treatment. Imaging is performed every 6 months for 2 years after diagnosis. If stable, imaging occurs annually until year 5 after diagnosis and then occurs at year 7, 9, and 14 after diagnosis. However, observation is not without risk, as tumor growth rates and progression of symptoms are not predictable. By 10 years, most clinical experience demonstrates that the majority of patients will have tumor growth and progression of symptoms. Therefore, the "wait and scan" approach should mainly

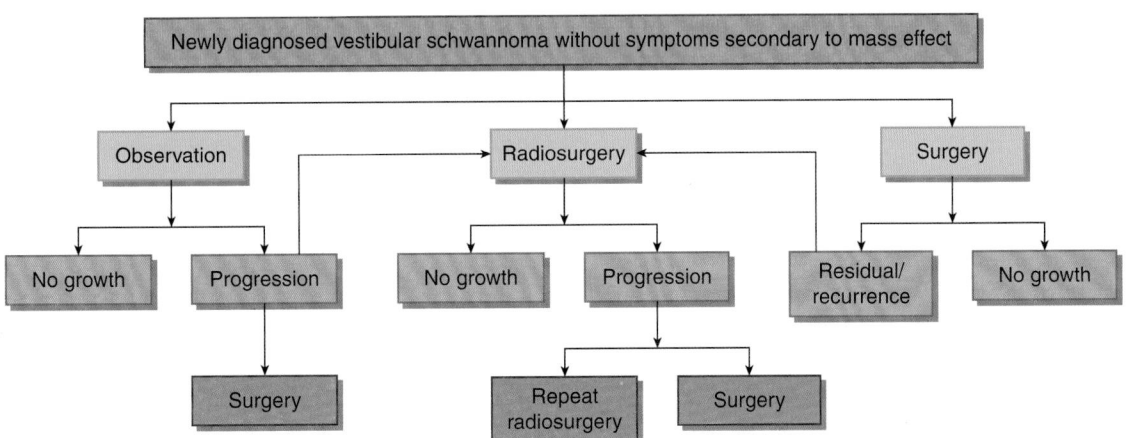

FIGURE 102.2 Treatment algorithm for vestibular schwannoma management.

be used in older patients and those whose medical comorbidities preclude other treatment options.

Stereotactic Radiosurgery

Radiosurgery is a therapeutic option that improves tumor control and hearing preservation compared with observation in patients presenting with small tumors (<30-mm diameter), serviceable hearing, or in those who wish to avoid surgery due to preference or anxiety. A dose of 12 to 13 Gy is prescribed typically and associated with improved hearing preservation. Long-term tumor control rates ranging from 91% to 98% have been reported in large series after radiosurgery, with 1.6% to 4.2% ultimately requiring resection for progressive enlargement. When applied early after diagnosis, long-term hearing preservation is achieved in greater than 60% of patients with doses of 13 Gy or lower, with higher rates achievable with intracanalicular tumors. Minimizing the radiation exposure to nearby structures (i.e., the cochlea, semicircular canals, and brain stem in larger tumors) minimizes morbidity rates associated with radiosurgery without sacrificing efficacy. Preservation of facial and trigeminal nerve function is also possible in the majority of patients.

For smaller tumors, hearing preservation and tumor control rates are equivalent following radiosurgery or surgical resection. However, radiosurgery is more effective than surgical resection in preserving postoperative facial function and is associated with lower rates of trigeminal neuropathy and other treatment-associated morbidity. In addition, hospital lengths of stay and management costs are less after radiosurgery and in general, hospital postoperative functional outcomes and patient satisfaction have been found to be greater after radiosurgery when compared with microsurgery.

Surgical Resection

Microsurgical resection remains the best cytoreductive therapy for vestibular schwannomas and is generally indicated in the setting of tumor progression after previous interventions and for those with large tumors (>30 mm diameter). In particular, microsurgery remains the preferred treatment for large lesions causing mass effect and obstructive hydrocephalus. Additional treatment is necessary in less than 2% of cases after microsurgical treatment. Facial nerve function may be preserved in more than 95% of patients with small tumors less than 20 mm, with rates of preservation dropping in the setting of tumors larger than 30 mm. Serviceable hearing, otherwise known as *useful hearing*, is assessed using the combined results of pure tone audiogram that evaluates the functionality of hearing and speech discrimination tests. Serviceable hearing is maintained in 32% to 44% of cases, with rates closer to 50% in the setting of tumors less than 30 mm. Recent data suggest that planned near-total or extensive subtotal resections, followed by radiosurgery for residual tumor, may be appropriate for large tumors, with excellent rates of facial nerve preservation and functional outcomes and no decrease in tumor control.

Chemotherapy

Patients with progressive acoustic neuromas in the setting of NF2 may derive benefit from treatment with bevacizumab, an anti–vascular endothelial growth factor (VEGF) monoclonal antibody with imaging response rates reported as high as 60% and minimal associated morbidity.

MALIGNANT TUMORS OF THE SKULL AND SKULL BASE

METASTASIS TO THE SKULL BASE

The skull is a common site of metastases from systemic cancers, with skull metastases occurring in 4% of cancer patients. The most common metastatic tumors to the skull base include breast, lung, and prostate cancers. Not surprisingly, prostate carcinoma is the most frequent cause of skull metastases (although it almost never metastasizes to the brain parenchyma) in men, whereas breast carcinoma is the most common in women (which also frequently metastasizes to the brain). Colon, renal, and thyroid cancers, as well as lymphoma, melanoma, and neuroblastoma may also metastasize to the skull base.

The clinical manifestation of metastases to the skull base depends on the location of the lesion (Table 102.2). Cranial nerves are vulnerable to compression by osseous metastases as they exit through the bony foramina of the skull. In addition, although metastases to the skull base are often painless, craniofacial pain in a patient with known cancer may be an initial symptom.

Contrast-enhanced MRI is the gold standard for detection of metastases to the skull base. CT scan is less effective than MRI for detecting contrast-enhancing soft-tissue masses but is the best method to demonstrate lytic bone lesions. Radionuclide bone scans have great sensitivity in detecting bone metastases. Although biopsy may be difficult and hazardous, it may be necessary to establish a diagnosis. Examination of cerebrospinal fluid (CSF) may be important to evaluate meningeal carcinomatosis in select patients.

The prognosis of skull base metastases depends on the extent of the primary disease, the location and associated extension of the tumor, and the surgical accessibility of the metastasis itself. In addition to symptomatic treatments with steroids and analgesia, specific treatments include radiotherapy, chemotherapy, and surgery. Treatment depends on the nature of the underlying tumor. Palliative radiotherapy is generally the standard treatment with a

TABLE 102.2	Clinical Syndromes Associated with Metastases to the Skull Base	
Syndrome	Symptoms	Cranial Nerves Affected
Orbital	Proptosis, diplopia, facial numbness, pain	II, V_1
Parasellar	Unilateral frontal headache, diplopia, facial numbness	II, IV, VI, V_1
Petrous apex	Facial pain, diplopia	V, VI
Middle fossa or gasserian ganglion	Facial pain, facial numbness, diplopia	V_2, V_3, VI
Jugular foramen	Hoarseness, dysphagia, pharyngeal pain	IX, X, XI
Occipital condyle or hypoglossal canal	Occipital pain, unilateral tongue weakness	XII

total dose of at least 30 Gy given in 3 Gy fractions with excellent symptomatic relief. Some patients benefit from chemotherapy or hormonal therapy for appropriately sensitive tumors. Gamma Knife radiosurgery is useful for small tumors or tumors previously irradiated. Select patients may benefit from surgical resection. In general, the overall prognosis is poor with median survival less than 3 years for most tumors. Note that metastases to the skull are not synonymous with metastases to the brain and are not protected by the blood–brain barrier, an important consideration when choosing chemotherapeutics.

EXTENSION OF MALIGNANT TUMORS TO THE SKULL BASE

Several malignant tumors involve the skull base by direct extension (Fig. 102.3). These include squamous cell carcinoma (nasal sinuses and temporal bone), adenoid cystic carcinoma (salivary glands), esthesioneuroblastoma (olfactory mucosa), and nasopharyngeal carcinoma. Involvement of the skull base by these tumors may result in pain and cranial neuropathies. Erosion of the skull base and the presence of a contrast-enhancing soft-tissue mass are generally identified on CT or MRI. Biopsy of accessible lesions is diagnostic and small tumors may be cured by wide excision prior to invasion of sensitive neural structures. However, most tumors are extensive at the time of diagnosis, and prognosis is poor despite radical excision and radiation therapy.

PRIMARY MALIGNANT TUMORS OF THE SKULL AND SKULL BASE

Chondrosarcoma

Chondrosarcoma is a malignant cartilage tumor originating in the enchondral bones of the skull base that most commonly affects men in the fourth decade. Tumors arise in the paranasal sinuses,

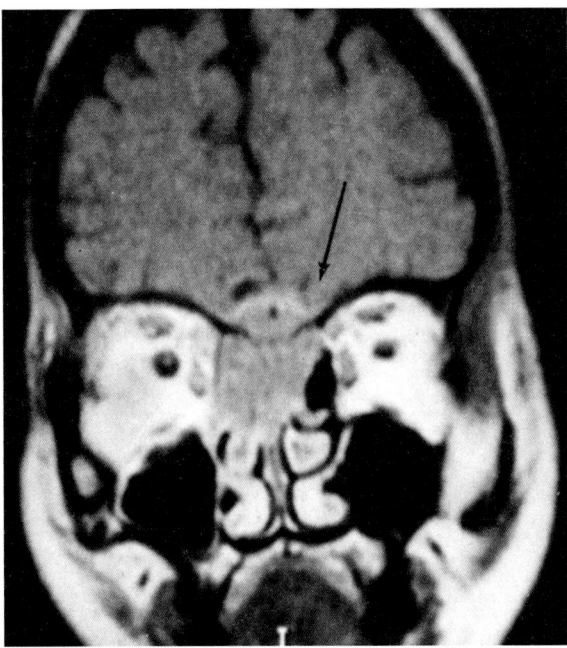

FIGURE 102.3 Esthesioneuroblastoma. Coronal MRI demonstrates an esthesioneuroblastoma in the ethmoid sinus with intradural extension (*arrow*). This tumor arises from olfactory mucosa.

the parasellar areas, or the cerebellopontine angle, with variable symptoms depending on location. CT and MRI are the preferred imaging modalities. Maximal safe debulking followed by adjuvant radiotherapy or observation is the treatment of choice.

Chordoma

Chordoma is a rare, histologically benign, locally aggressive bone tumor associated with destruction of surrounding tissues. Derived from remnants of notochord within the axial skeleton, tumors distribute equally between the skull base, mobile spine, and sacrum with predominance in men between 50 and 60 years of age. Chordomas of the skull base often arise in the clivus and cause cranial nerve palsies. Histologically, tumors are distinguished by the presence of physaliferous cells. Treatment involves maximal safe aggressive resection with an emphasis on preservation of neurologic function, followed by advanced radiotherapy such as proton beam radiation. High rates of recurrence make their prognosis similar to malignant tumors.

Osteogenic Sarcoma

Osteogenic sarcoma (osteosarcoma) is the most common primary bone malignancy. Osteosarcoma primarily affects long bones with rare involvement of the skull or skull base. Lesions are the result of osteoid or immature bone production by malignant spindle cells and are associated with destruction of normal bone (Fig. 102.4). Patients may report history of prior radiation, chemotherapy, Paget disease, fibrous dysplasia, or chronic osteomyelitis. Symptoms are variable by location. Treatment is maximal safe surgical resection with an emphasis on preserving neurologic function and avoiding cosmetic defects. Tumors are relatively radioresistant and chemotherapy with cisplatin, doxorubicin, and high-dose methotrexate may offer benefits.

Soft-Tissue Sarcoma

Soft-tissue sarcomas of the skull base are rare. Malignant fibrous histiocytoma, fibrosarcoma, angiosarcoma, and malignant peripheral nerve sheath tumors are the most frequently encountered lesions. CT and MRI are essential for assessing tumor size and location. Treatment is aggressive safe resection. However, because anatomic constraints of the skull base often limit wide excision, patients will often receive adjuvant radiotherapy and chemotherapy.

GLOMUS JUGULARE TUMORS

Jugular paragangliomas ("glomus jugulare") are the most common tumor arising within the jugular foramen. These rare, slow-growing, locally invasive tumors arise from chromaffin cells in the region of the jugular bulb and course along the glossopharyngeal nerve, the tympanic branch of the glossopharyngeal nerve (Jacobsen nerve), or the auricular branch of the vagus nerve (Arnold nerve). Tumors are highly vascularized and symptoms are the result of both compression and infiltration of adjacent temporal and occipital bone and involvement of nearby cranial nerves. In addition, tumors may extend into the middle ear and cause conductive hearing loss, pulsatile tinnitus, and audible bruits or may be discovered as a small vascular mass within the middle ear cavity. MRI with contrast best visualizes tumors, and magnetic resonance angiography (MRA) reveals their extensive vascularity. CT with contrast may also be considered in patients who cannot undergo MRI. Digital subtraction angiography (DSA) is performed for diagnosis and preoperative embolization is essential to decrease tumor vascularity and

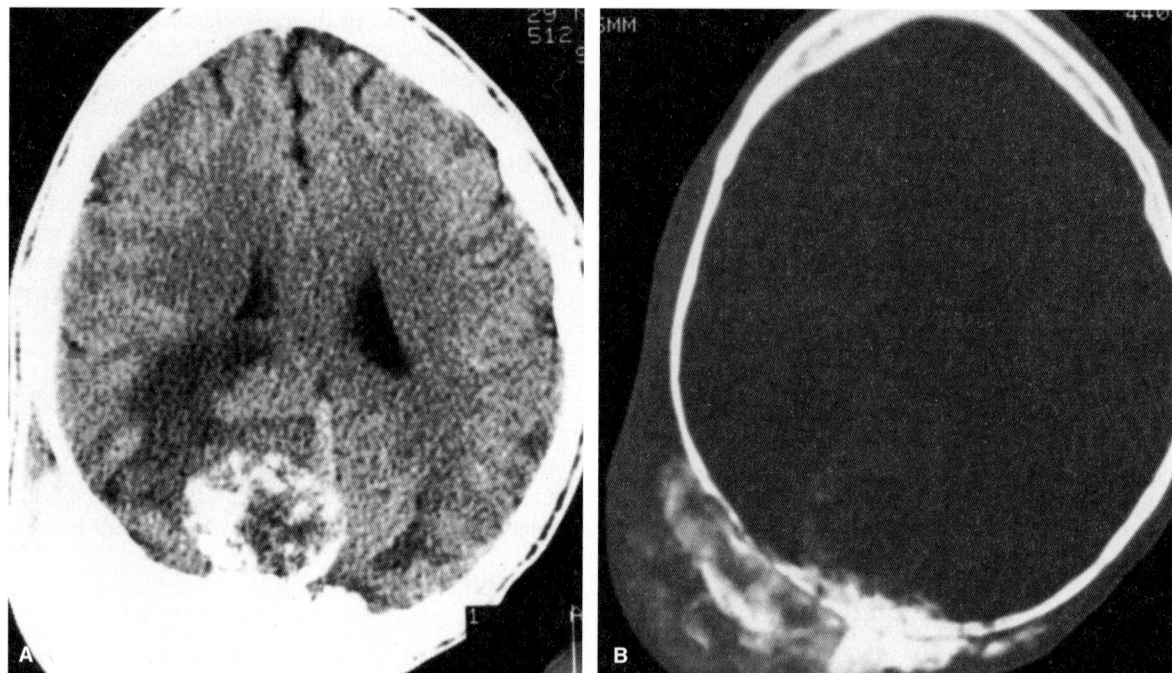

FIGURE 102.4 Osteogenic sarcoma (osteosarcoma). **A:** Noncontrast axial CT shows a calcified mass within the medial right parietooccipital lobes with massive extracranial soft-tissue swelling. **B:** Corresponding bone window shows thinning and eroded calvarium with several large areas of calcification and ossification noted within the extracranial soft tissues in the right parietooccipital region. These findings are classic for osteosarcoma.

facilitate resection. Interestingly, some paragangliomas secrete catecholamines, which may be ascertained by a 24-hour urine assay and must be blocked prior to surgery. Malignant transformation of these lesions is rare.

Surgery offers the best chance of cure for glomus jugulare tumors and results in cessation of cardiovascular symptoms and normalization of catecholamine levels in patients symptomatic from secreting tumors. However, total removal is difficult and accompanied by significant morbidity due to the vascularity and invasiveness of the lesions. Observation may be appropriate until patients become symptomatic or tumors demonstrate growth on imaging. Gamma Knife radiosurgery may offer improved rates of tumor control with lower risks of morbidity compared with surgery for patients with nonsecreting tumors.

BENIGN TUMORS OF THE SKULL

OSTEOMA

Osteomas are rare, benign slow-growing tumors of the skull. Histologically, tumors are composed of well-differentiated mature, compact, or cancellous bone arising from either the inner table or the outer table of the skull. Lesions frequently occur in the paranasal sinuses but may arise within the frontoethmoidal region, the petrous bone (mastoid sinuses), the cranial vault, and the mandible. Tumors are generally asymptomatic but may be associated with headache, recurrent sinusitis, and proptosis and orbital deformities secondary to orbital invasion. Rarely, tumors may present with pneumocephalus, rhinorrhea, meningitis, dural erosion, and abscess formation. Calvarial lesions are hard, painless localized masses with minimal intracranial extension. Diagnosis is based on the characteristic appearance of a circumscribed homogenous

hyperdensity involving the skull that is best seen with CT scan (Fig. 102.5). Symptomatic lesions are treated surgically, and reconstruction may be necessary for extensive lesions.

CHONDROMA

Chondromas are rare, slow-growing benign tumors arising from cartilage rests at the basilar synchondroses of the skull base. Lesions have a predilection for the sphenoethmoidal, sphenopetrosal, spheno-occipital, or petro-occipital regions. However, rare dural, intraparenchymal, and intraventricular lesions have been described. Clinical presentation varies by anatomic location and slow-growing tumors may remain asymptomatic for prolonged periods of time. Radiographically, tumors appear as lytic lesions, with sharp margins and erosion of surrounding bone. Stippled calcification within the lesion may be apparent and helps distinguish chondroma from metastasis or chordoma. Chondromas typically display high intensity on T2-MRI and low to intermediate intensity on T1-MRI, with a heterogeneous ring-and-arc enhancement pattern after administration of gadolinium. Treatment involves radical resection for symptomatic lesions with extension to normal bone margins to prevent recurrence. Progression to malignant chondrosarcoma is rare.

HEMANGIOMA

Hemangiomas are benign, vascular bone tumors representing 0.2% of bony neoplasms of the skull. Lesions may involve the calvaria or the skull base (or vertebral bodies of the spine), with a predilection for the cavernous sinus. Commonly discovered incidentally after CT or MRI performed for other reasons, hemangiomas may present as a slowly enlarging lump associated with headaches that worsen with lesion expansion. However, neurologic findings are uncom-

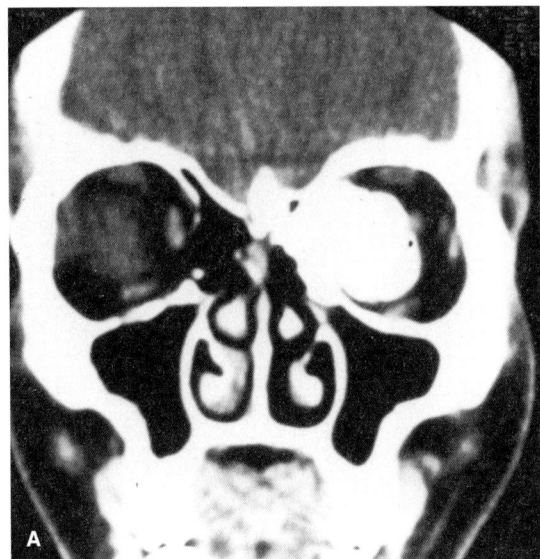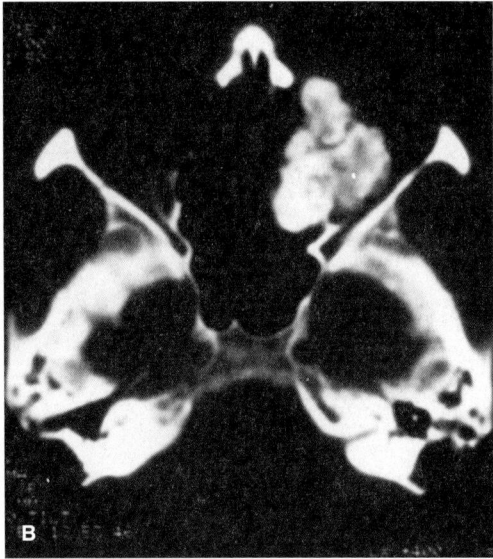

FIGURE 102.5 Orbital osteoma. Coronal **(A)** and axial **(B)** CT with bone windows show an osteoma involving the orbit.

mon, as hemangiomas rarely extend intracranially. Radiographically, tumors appear as well-circumscribed, expansive hypodense regions with a honeycomb or polka-dotted pattern on CT. MRI demonstrates heterogeneous signal on both T1- and T2-weighted sequences and may demonstrate flow voids suggestive of a vascular lesion. However, the radiographic appearance of skull base hemangiomas is variable and pathologic examination is often required for diagnosis. Resection is indicated for neurologic compromise, unremitting headache, mass effect, cosmetic deformity, or tissue diagnosis. Treatment is by safe maximal resection and the use of preoperative embolization may be beneficial. The use of radiation for incompletely resected, or multiple tumors, remains controversial.

DERMOID AND EPIDERMOID TUMORS

Dermoid and epidermoid cysts are benign, extra-axial developmental lesions arising from trapped ectodermal tissue during closure of the neural tube. Cysts are lined with stratified squamous epithelium and contain keratin, cellular debris, cholesterol (epidermoids), and elements of the dermis, including hair and sebaceous glands (dermoids). Epidermoids most commonly arise in the cerebellopontine angle and the parasellar region but may occur in the middle cranial fossa and spinal canal. Dermoids are predominantly midline lesions, arising commonly in the diploe of the fontanel extradurally and in the parasellar region intradurally.

Cysts may remain asymptomatic for years due to slow growth, with rare acute presentations due to hemorrhage or trauma. Cyst rupture is a rare complication that can cause severe chemical or aseptic meningitis. Epidermoids and dermoids typically appear as hypodense areas on CT. On MRI, epidermoids present as polycystic irregular lesions with extensive growth in the CSF spaces. Epidermoids have slightly higher signal intensity than CSF on T1- and T2-weighted images and heterogeneous features on fluid-attenuated inversion recovery (FLAIR) sequences. Diffusion-weighted imaging (DWI) facilitates identification of epidermoids. Dermoids are usually hyperintense on both T1- and T2-weighted images. Radical surgical excision is the preferred treatment when possible and can be curative. Malignant degeneration is rare.

NEOPLASTIC-LIKE LESIONS OF THE SKULL

HYPEROSTOSIS

Hyperostosis of nonneoplastic etiology may involve either the inner or the outer table of the skull. Outer table hyperostosis is clinically insignificant aside from cosmetic concerns. Hyperostosis of the inner table may rarely become large enough to compress intracranial contents. Hyperostosis frontalis interna (HFI) is a condition occurring in postmenopausal women, characterized by increased bone deposition along the inner table of the frontal bone. HFI is usually an incidental finding on CT or MRI, although excessive growth can cause compression of brain tissue.

FIBROUS DYSPLASIA

Fibrous dysplasia is a benign condition in which normal bone is replaced by poorly organized woven bone. Progressive growth of lesions may result in swelling, cosmetic deformities, and pain. Fibrous dysplasia is most commonly monostotic with involvement of a single bone. However, 25% of cases are polyostotic involving more than 50% of the skeleton and can be associated with fractures and skeletal deformities. Fibrous dysplasia may also occur as part of McCune–Albright syndrome. Lesions mostly occur in the ribs or craniofacial bones, particularly the maxilla. Localized involvement of the skull base and sphenoid wing, particularly by the sclerotic variety, may cause symptoms secondary to cranial nerve entrapment. X-rays and CT classically demonstrate a ground-glass appearance due to thin spicules of woven bone (Fig. 102.6). Chemotherapy and radiation are not effective treatments and radiation may predispose to higher rates of malignant transformation. Neurosurgical involvement may be required for skull lesions producing refractory pain or neurologic symptoms.

PAGET DISEASE (OSTEITIS DEFORMANS)

Paget disease is a disorder of osteoclasts causing rapid remodeling of bone. Increased bone resorption is followed by reactive osteoblastic overproduction of sclerotic, brittle woven bone that

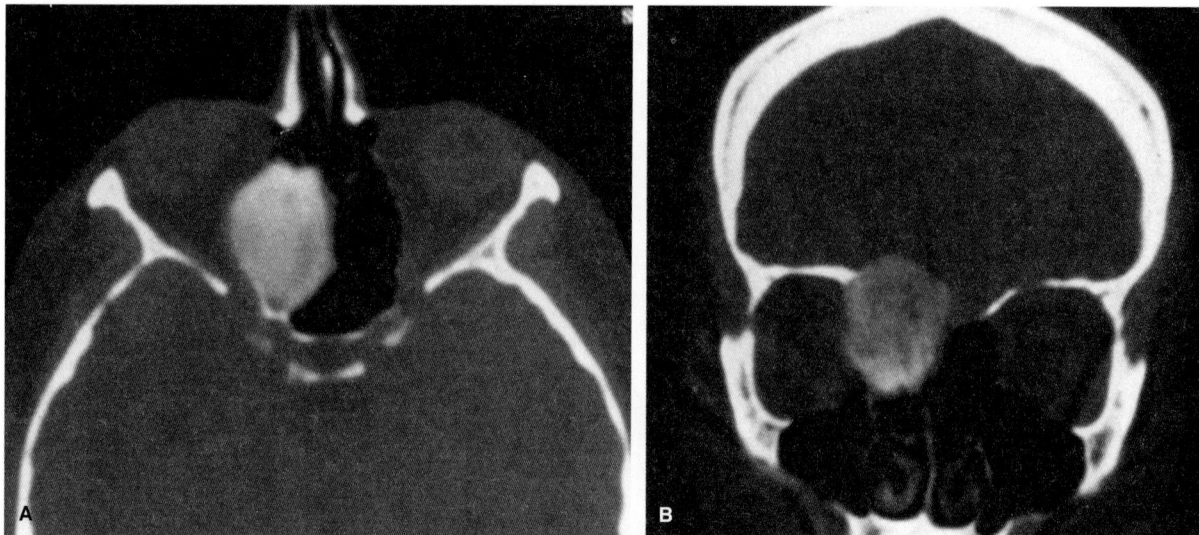

FIGURE 102.6 Fibrous dysplasia. Axial **(A)** and coronal **(B)** CT with bone windows demonstrate classic ground-glass appearance of fibrous dysplasia of the orbit and ethmoid sinus.

produces a characteristic mosaic pattern on x-ray. Family history is present in 15% to 30% of discovered cases and about 1% degenerate into sarcoma with the possibility of systemic metastases. Lesions commonly involve the axial skeleton, long bones, and the skull. Mostly asymptomatic or incidentally discovered, facial and skull base remodeling may result in localized pain, cranial nerve compression with deafness being the most prominent finding in most cases, or basilar invagination. Markedly elevated serum alkaline phosphatase is a constant feature. Surgical intervention should be reserved for diagnosis or relief of symptoms.

MUCOCELE

Occlusion of a nasal air sinus may result in an encapsulated collection of mucus or pus, known as a *mucocele*. Progressive expansion of mucoceles may result in erosion through the skull base with subsequent compression of intracranial contents. Lesions frequently enhance with intravenous contrast on MRI and CT (Fig. 102.7). Surgery with reconstruction is the treatment of choice.

MISCELLANEOUS

A variety of systemic disease may additionally involve the skull. These include histiocytosis X (eosinophilic granuloma is the mildest form), multiple myeloma, plasmacytoma, brown tumor of hyperparathyroidism, Wegener granulomatosis, and lethal midline granuloma. Infectious lesions such as tuberculosis, syphilis, leprosy, and fungal infections (especially aspergillosis and mucormycosis) may also occur within the skull base. In addition, lesions within the nose may communicate with the intracranial cavity such as nasopharyngeal carcinoma, esthesioneuroblastoma, encephalocele, and nasal gliomas.

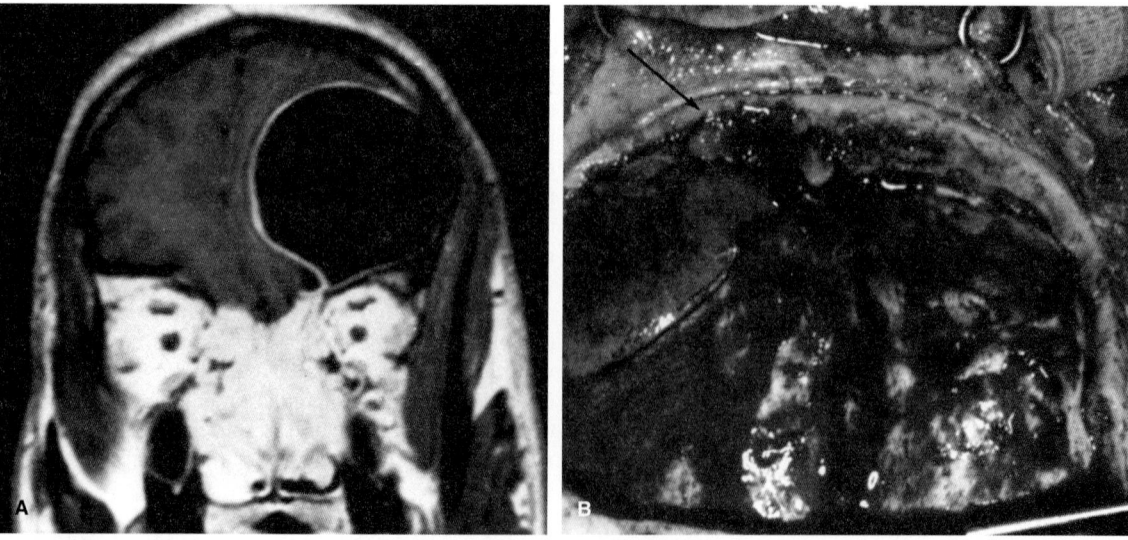

FIGURE 102.7 Mucocele. **A:** Coronal contrast-enhanced MRI shows a large mucocele compressing the frontal lobe, with chronic inflammation of the nasal mucosa obstructing the nasal sinuses. **B:** Intraoperative photograph shows the mucocele before its resection and subsequent skull base reconstruction. The frontal sinus contains inflammatory tissue (*arrow*) that had caused obstruction of the sinus.

SUGGESTED READINGS

Arthurs BJ, Fairbanks RK, Demakas JJ, et al. A review of treatment modalities for vestibular schwannoma. *Neurosurg Rev.* 2011;34(3):265–277; discussion 277–279.

Bakkouri WE, Kania RE, Guichard JP, et al. Conservative management of 386 cases of unilateral vestibular schwannoma: tumor growth and consequences for treatment. *J Neurosurg.* 2009;110(4):662–669.

Bowers CA, Taussky P, Couldwell WT. Surgical treatment of craniofacial fibrous dysplasia in adults. *Neurosurg Rev.* 2014;37(1):47–53.

Chennupati SK, Norris R, Dunham B, et al. Osteosarcoma of the skull base: case report and review of literature. *Int J Pediatr Otorhinolaryngol.* 2008;72(1):115–119.

Combs SE, Welzel T, Schulz-Ertner D, et al. Differences in clinical results after LINAC-based single-dose radiosurgery versus fractionated stereotactic radiotherapy for patients with vestibular schwannomas. *Int J Radiat Oncol Biol Phys.* 2010;76(1):193–200.

de Bree R, van der Waal I, de Bree E, et al. Management of adult soft tissue sarcomas of the head and neck. *Oral Oncol.* 2010;46(11):786–790.

Eversole R, Su L, ElMofty S. Benign fibro-osseous lesions of the craniofacial complex. A review. *Head Neck Pathol.* 2008;2(3):177–202.

Fayad JN, Keles B, Brackmann DE. Jugular foramen tumors: clinical characteristics and treatment outcomes. *Otol Neurotol.* 2010;31(2):299–305.

Flickinger JC, Kondziolka D, Niranjan A, et al. Acoustic neuroma radiosurgery with marginal tumor doses of 12 to 13 Gy. *Int J Radiat Oncol Biol Phys.* 2004;60(1):225–230.

Fong B, Barkhoudarian G, Pezeshkian P, et al. The molecular biology and novel treatments of vestibular schwannomas. *J Neurosurg.* 2011;115(5):906–914.

Fountas KN, Stamatiou S, Barbanis S, et al. Intracranial falx chondroma: literature review and a case report. *Clin Neurol Neurosurg.* 2008;110(1):8–13.

Gologorsky Y, Shrivastava RK, Panov F, et al. Primary intraosseous cavernous hemangioma of the clivus: case report and review of the literature. *J Neurol Surg Rep.* 2013;74(1):17–22.

Gormley WB, Tomecek FJ, Qureshi N, et al. Craniocerebral epidermoid and dermoid tumours: a review of 32 cases. *Acta Neurochir (Wien).* 1994;128(1–4):115–121.

Haddad FS, Haddad GF, Zaatari G. Cranial osteomas: their classification and management. Report on a giant osteoma and review of the literature. *Surg Neurol.* 1997;48(2):143–147.

Hall FT, Perez-Ordonez B, Mackenzie RG, et al. Does catecholamine secretion from head and neck paragangliomas respond to radiotherapy? Case report and literature review. *Skull Base.* 2003;13(4):229–234.

Haque R, Wojtasiewicz TJ, Gigante PR, et al. Efficacy of facial nerve-sparing approach in patients with vestibular schwannomas. *J Neurosurg.* 2011;115(5):917–923.

Harner SG, Laws ER Jr. Clinical findings in patients with acoustic neurinoma. *Mayo Clin Proc.* 1983;58(11):721–728.

Karpinos M, The BS, Zeck O, et al. Treatment of acoustic neuroma: stereotactic radiosurgery vs. microsurgery. *Int J Radiat Oncol Biol Phys.* 2002;54(5):1410–1421.

Kondziolka D, Lunsford LD, McLaughlin MR, et al. Long-term outcomes after radiosurgery for acoustic neuromas. *N Engl J Med.* 1998;339(20):1426–1433.

Kondziolka D, Mousavi SH, Kano H, et al. The newly diagnosed vestibular schwannoma: radiosurgery, resection, or observation? *Neurosurg Focus.* 2012;33(3):E8.

Kondziolka D, Nathoo N, Flickinger JC, et al. Long-term results after radiosurgery for benign intracranial tumors. *Neurosurgery.* 2003;53(4):815–821; discussion 821–822.

Laigle-Donadey F, Taillibert S, Martin-Duverneuil N, et al. Skull-base metastases. *J Neurooncol.* 2005;75(1):63–69.

Matthies C, Samii M. Management of 1000 vestibular schwannomas (acoustic neuromas): clinical presentation. *Neurosurgery.* 1997;40(1):1–9; discussion 9–10.

Myrseth E, Møller P, Pedersen PH, et al. Vestibular schwannomas: clinical results and quality of life after microsurgery or gamma knife radiosurgery. *Neurosurgery.* 2005;56(5):927–935; discussion 927–935.

Neff BA, Welling DB, Akhmametyeva E, et al. The molecular biology of vestibular schwannomas: dissecting the pathogenic process at the molecular level. *Otol Neurotol.* 2006;27(2):197–208.

Ostrom QT, Gittleman H, Farah P, et al. CBTRUS statistical report: primary brain and central nervous system tumors diagnosed in the United States in 2006–2010. *Neuro Oncol.* 2013;15(suppl 2):ii1–ii56.

Plotkin SR, Stemmer-Rachamimov AO, Barker FG II, et al. Hearing improvement after bevacizumab in patients with neurofibromatosis type 2. *N Engl J Med.* 2009;361(4):358–367.

Pollock BE, Driscoll CL, Foote RL, et al. Patient outcomes after vestibular schwannoma management: a prospective comparison of microsurgical resection and stereotactic radiosurgery. *Neurosurgery.* 2006;59(1):77–85; discussion 77–85.

Pollock BE, Lunsford LD, Kondziolka D, et al. Outcome analysis of acoustic neuroma management: a comparison of microsurgery and stereotactic radiosurgery. *Neurosurgery.* 1995;36(1):215–224; discussion 224–229.

Régis J, Carron R, Park MC, et al. Wait-and-see strategy compared with proactive Gamma Knife surgery in patients with intracanalicular vestibular schwannomas. *J Neurosurg.* 2010;113(suppl):105–111.

Régis J, Pellet W, Delsanti C, et al. Functional outcome after gamma knife surgery or microsurgery for vestibular schwannomas. *J Neurosurg.* 2002;97(5):1091–1100.

Schiefer TK, Link MJ. Epidermoids of the cerebellopontine angle: a 20-year experience. *Surg Neurol.* 2008;70(6):584–590; discussion 590.

Schmidinger A, Rosahl SK, Vorkapic P, et al. Natural history of chondroid skull base lesions—case report and review. *Neuroradiology.* 2002;44(3):268–271.

She R, Szakacs J. Hyperostosis frontalis interna: case report and review of literature. *Ann Clin Lab Sci.* 2004;34(2):206–208.

Suárez C, Rodrigo JP, Bödeker CC, et al. Jugular and vagal paragangliomas: systematic study of management with surgery and radiotherapy. *Head Neck.* 2013;35(8):1195–1204.

Sughrue ME, Yang I, Aranda D, et al. The natural history of untreated sporadic vestibular schwannomas: a comprehensive review of hearing outcomes. *J Neurosurg.* 2010;112(1):163–167.

Walcott BP, Nahed BV, Mohyeldin A, et al. Chordoma: current concepts, management, and future directions. *Lancet Oncol.* 2012;13(2):e69–e76.

Yang I, Sughrue ME, Han SJ, et al. A comprehensive analysis of hearing preservation after radiosurgery for vestibular schwannoma. *J Neurosurg.* 2010;112(4):851–859.

Yang I, Sughrue ME, Han SJ, et al. Facial nerve preservation after vestibular schwannoma Gamma Knife radiosurgery. *J Neurooncol.* 2009;93(1):41–48.

David Cachia, Claudio E. Tatsui, and Mark R. Gilbert

INTRODUCTION

Tumors of the spinal cord or nerve roots are similar to intracranial tumors in cellular type. They may arise from the parenchyma of the cord, nerve roots, meninges, intraspinal blood vessels, sympathetic nerves, or vertebrae. Metastases may arise from remote tumors.

Spinal tumors are divided by location into three groups: intramedullary, extramedullary intradural, or extradural (or epidural) (Fig. 103.1). Occasionally, an extradural tumor extends through an intervertebral foramen to be partially within and partially outside the spinal canal (e.g., dumbbell or hourglass tumors; Fig. 103.2).

EPIDEMIOLOGY

Spinal cord tumors are much less prevalent than intracranial tumors, in a ratio of 1:4, but this varies by histology. The intracranial-to-spinal ratio of astrocytoma is 10:1, and the ratio for ependymomas varies from 3:1 to 20:1, although spinal tumors are the most prevalent location of ependymoma in adults. Men and women are affected equally often, except that meningiomas are more common in women and ependymomas are more common in men. Spinal tumors occur predominantly in young or middle-aged adults and are less common in childhood or after age 60 years.

Spinal tumors appear most often in the thoracic region, but if the relative lengths of the divisions of the spinal cord are considered, the distribution is comparatively equal.

PATHOBIOLOGY

The histologic characteristics of primary and secondary tumors are similar to those of intracranial tumors. An analyses of data from the Surveillance, Epidemiology, and End Results (SEER) and National Program of Cancer Registries that included 11,712 cases of primary spinal tumors identified over a 4-year period showed that of these, 78% were benign and 22% malignant. Histologically, the three most common tumors were meningioma, nerve sheath tumors, and ependymoma.

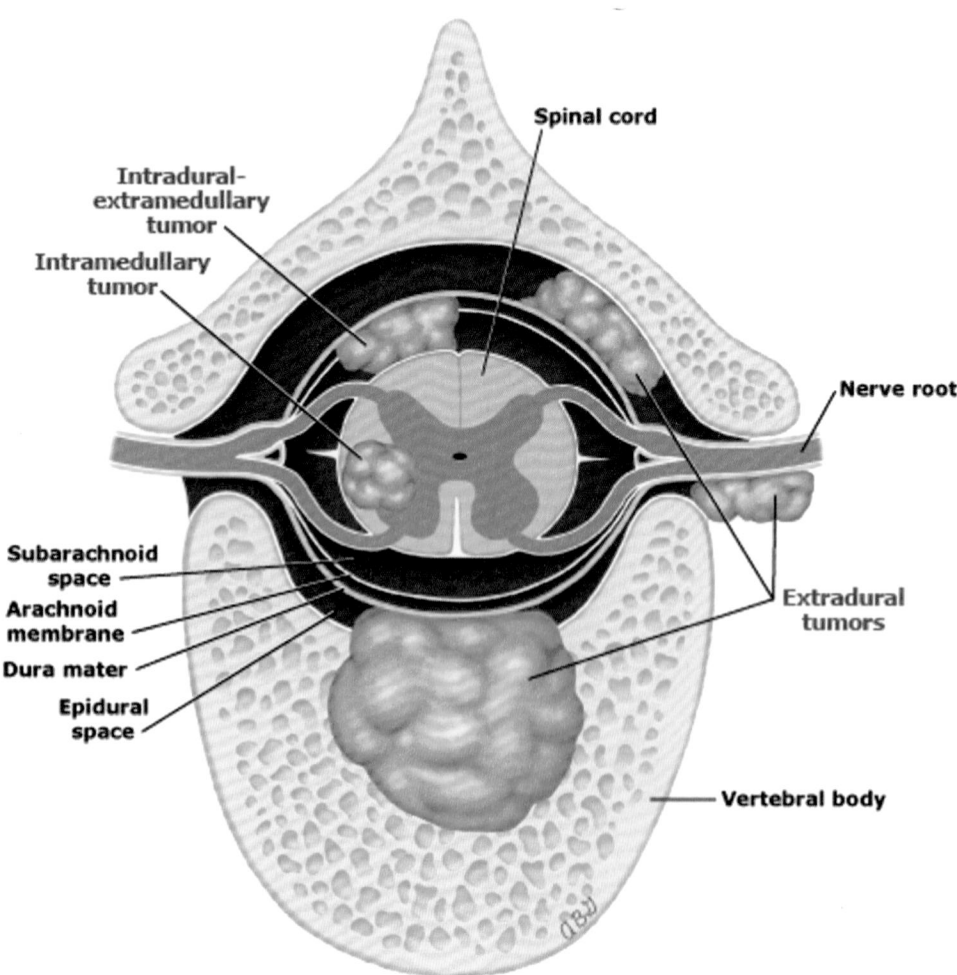

Spinal cord

Intradural-extramedullary tumor

Intramedullary tumor

Nerve root

Subarachnoid space

Arachnoid membrane

Dura mater

Epidural space

Extradural tumors

Vertebral body

FIGURE 103.1 Location of spinal tumors in relationship to spinal anatomy. (Reproduced with permission from Welch WC, Schiff D, Gerszten PC. Spinal cord tumors. UpToDate Web site. http://www.uptodate.com/contents/spinal-cord-tumors. Accessed April 9, 2015.)

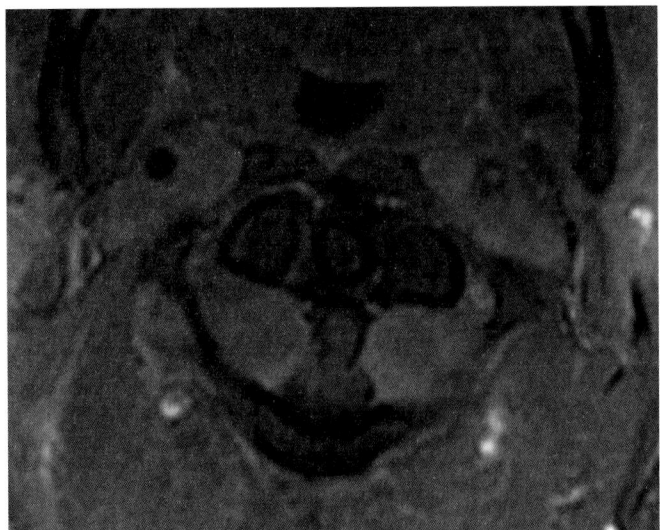
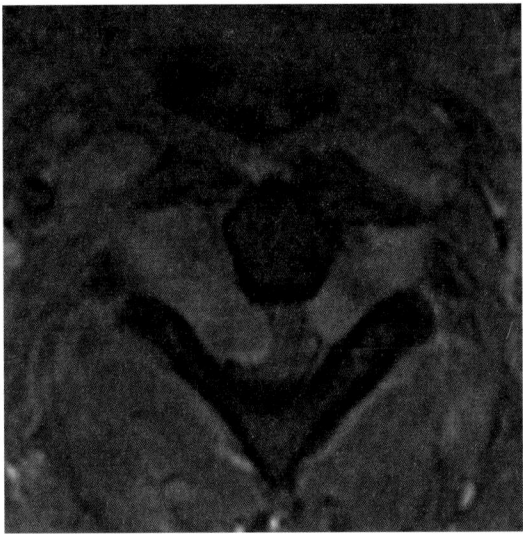

A   B

FIGURE 103.2 Neurofibromatosis. **A:** Gadolinium-enhanced T1-weighted axial MRI demonstrates bilateral neurofibromas seen at C1–C2, causing severe central spinal canal stenosis. **B:** Axial contrast-enhancing MRI at C2–C3 shows a large foraminal neurofibroma extending into the canal on the right and causes moderate central spinal canal stenosis.

The most recent Central Brain Tumor Registry of the United States (CBTRUS) data on primary brain and CNS tumors showed that in the age group 0 to 19 years, the most common histology were ependymal tumors followed by other neuroepithelial tumors, whereas in the 20 years and older age group, tumors of the meninges predominate (Fig. 103.3).

The most frequent extradural or epidural tumors are metastasis with the most common primary sites of metastatic tumors to the spine being, in order of frequency—lung, breast, and prostate. Other common metastatic malignancies include tumors of the gastrointestinal tract, lymphomas, melanomas, kidney, sarcomas, thyroid, multiple myeloma, and plasmocytomas.

CLINICAL MANIFESTATIONS

Extramedullary tumors cause symptoms by compressing nerve roots or spinal cord or by occluding the spinal blood vessels resulting in regional ischemia and infarct. The symptoms of intramedullary tumors result from direct interference with the intrinsic structures of the spinal cord from mass effect, edema, or development of syringomyelia. Descriptions of special syndromes follow.

EXTRAMEDULLARY TUMORS

These tumors may be either intradural or extradural (epidural). They usually involve a few spinal cord levels and cause focal signs by compressing nerve roots, particularly the dorsal roots. Extramedullary tumors may ultimately affect the spinal cord, potentially progressing to complete loss of function below the level of the lesion. The first symptoms are typically focal pain and paresthesias, arising from pressure on the dorsal nerve roots. This symptom pattern is soon followed by sensory loss, weakness, and muscular wasting in the distribution of the affected roots. Compression of the spinal cord first interrupts the functions of the pathways that lie at the periphery of the spinal cord. The early signs of cord compression usually include those referable to upper motor neurons such as spastic weakness below the lesion, overactive tendon reflexes, Babinski signs; impairment of cutaneous and proprioceptive sen-

sation below the lesion; impaired control of the bladder and, less often, the rectum; and loss of superficial abdominal reflexes. Occasionally, symptoms may be those of lower motor neurons, such as underactive or absent reflexes with flaccid weakness, especially if the compression occurs abruptly as in spinal "shock" from trauma. If untreated, this syndrome may lead to signs and symptoms of complete transection of spinal cord, with wasting and atrophy of muscles at the level of the root lesion and, below the lesion, paraplegia or quadriplegia. The earliest and only sign can be pain, and the absence of other signs or symptoms may give the misleading impression that the cord is not compressed.

The severity and distribution of weakness and sensory loss varies, depending in part on the location of the tumor in relation to the anterior, lateral, or posterior portion of the spinal cord. Eccentrically placed tumors may cause a typical Brown-Séquard syndrome, namely, ipsilateral signs of posterior column and pyramidal tract dysfunction, with contralateral loss of pain and temperature due to involvement of the lateral spinothalamic tract. Usually, however, because of the external compression, the Brown-Séquard features are incomplete.

Spinal vessels may be occluded by extradural tumors, particularly metastatic carcinoma, lymphoma, or abscess. When the arteries destined for the spinal cord are occluded, the resulting myelomalacia causes signs and symptoms similar to those of a severe intradural process leading to necrosis of the spinal cord. Occlusion of major components of the anterior spinal artery, however, results in segmental lower motor neuron signs at the appropriate level, bilateral loss of pain and temperature sensation, and upper motor neuron signs below the lesion with preservation of dorsal column function (proprioception, discriminative tactile function, and vibration).

Extradural (Epidural) Tumors

Extradural lesions constitute the most frequent group of spinal tumors. Metastatic spinal disease accounts for 95% of those lesions, whereas primary bone tumors account for the remaining 5% of spinal lesions. In general, benign lesions within the vertebral bones are usually asymptomatic and found incidentally, whereas malignant

A

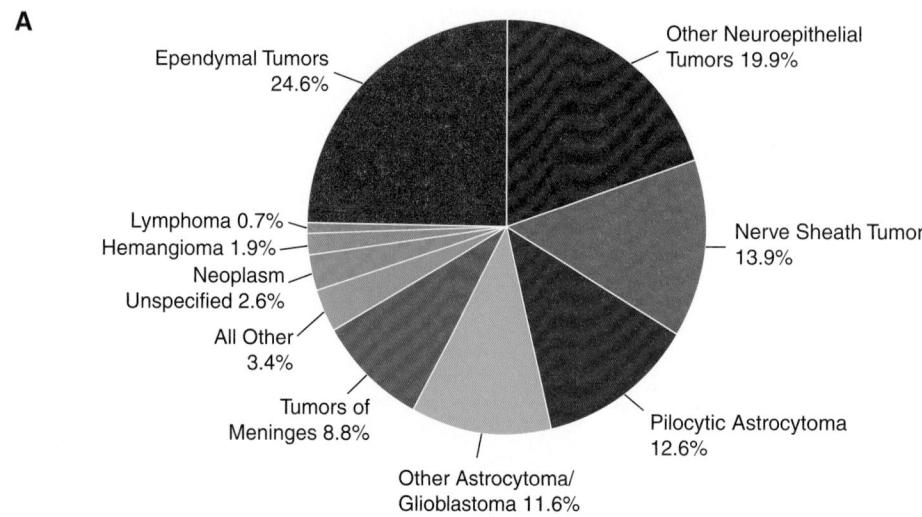

B

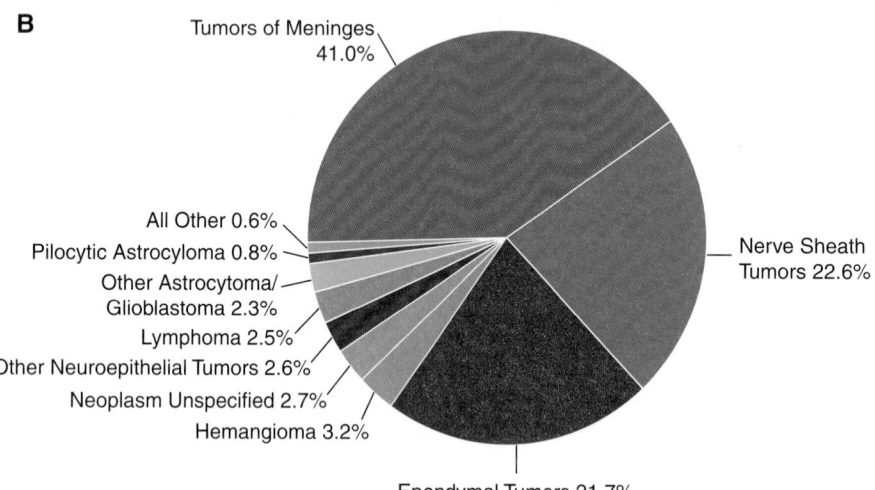

FIGURE 103.3 Distribution of spinal cord, spinal meninges, and cauda equina tumors by age group and histology. **A:** Ages 0 to 19 years (*N* = 1,067). **B:** Ages 20 years and older (*N* = 14,013). Central Brain Tumor Registry (CB-TRUS) Statistical Report: National Program of Cancer Registries (NPCR) and the National Cancer Institute, Surveillance, Epidemiology, and End Results (SEER Program, 2006–2010). (From Ostrom QT, Gittleman H, Farah P, et al. CBTRUS statistical report: primary brain and central nervous system tumors diagnosed in the United States in 2006–2010. *Neuro Oncol.* 2013;15[suppl 2]:ii1–ii56.)

vertebral tumors cause back pain, mechanical instability, pathologic fractures, and sometimes neurologic symptoms due to spinal cord compression. In addition to metastatic cancers, other malignant extradural tumors include multiple myeloma (Fig. 103.4), chordoma, Ewing sarcoma, and chondrosarcoma.

The most frequent benign bone lesions are hemangioma, enostosis, osteoid osteoma–osteoblastoma, aneurismal bone cyst, eosinophilic granuloma (histiocytosis), giant cell tumor, and osteochondroma. Although considered benign, these lesions can be locally aggressive associated with pain, spinal deformity, pathologic fractures, and neural elements compression. Spinal cord metastases will be discussed in greater detail in the following section.

Epidural Spinal Cord Metastasis

Epidural spinal metastasis may be considered a disorder of the vertebral column; the neurologic consequences result from extension of tumor into the spinal canal. Although currently estimated to occur in about 5% to 10% of all cancer patients, as the survival of patients with systemic cancers improves, the incidence of epidural spinal cord compression has increased. Most studies have demonstrated that treatment of cord compression does not prolong survival, but prompt treatment may have an important palliative role, alleviating pain and preventing neurologic disability.

Signs and symptoms of epidural spinal cord compression can be overlooked in a patient with disseminated cancer because of the presence of diffuse pain and asthenia. However, persistent neck and back pain which typically gets worse at night or at rest should prompt an investigation, not waiting for neurologic dysfunction to ensue. Limb weakness or paresthesias in the distribution of a nerve root and bowel or bladder dysfunction make this a neurooncologic emergency that commands prompt evaluation and treatment. Rarely, aside from pain, the only manifestation of cord compression may be a gait disorder, often due to sensory ataxia, without overt evidence of weakness or cutaneous sensory loss. In this situation, it may even be difficult to demonstrate impaired proprioception. The ataxia may be caused by compression of spinocerebellar pathways. The primary malignancy in more than 50% of cases of epidural cord compression is lung (Fig. 103.5) or breast cancer. Overall, more than 80% of cases arise from primary tumors in lung, breast, prostate, gastrointestinal system, melanoma, or lymphoma.

The mechanism of spread of these tumors to the epidural space includes a direct extension from a paravertebral focus through a nerve root foramen; hematogenous metastasis to the vertebrae with extension from bone into the epidural space; or retrograde spread along the venous plexus of Batson. Hematogenous spread to bone is the most common form, and computed tomography (CT) typically shows lytic

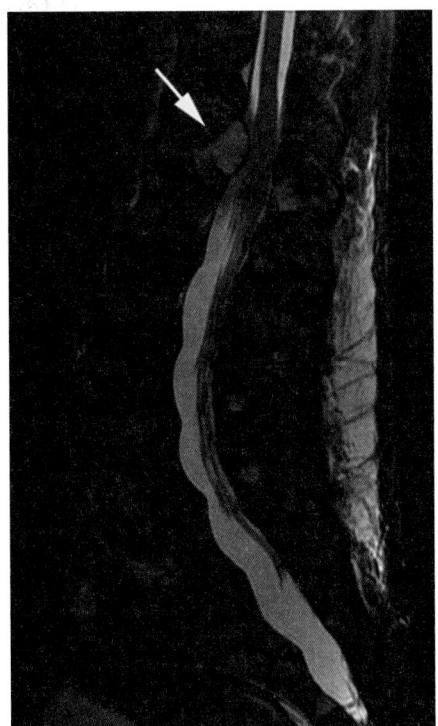
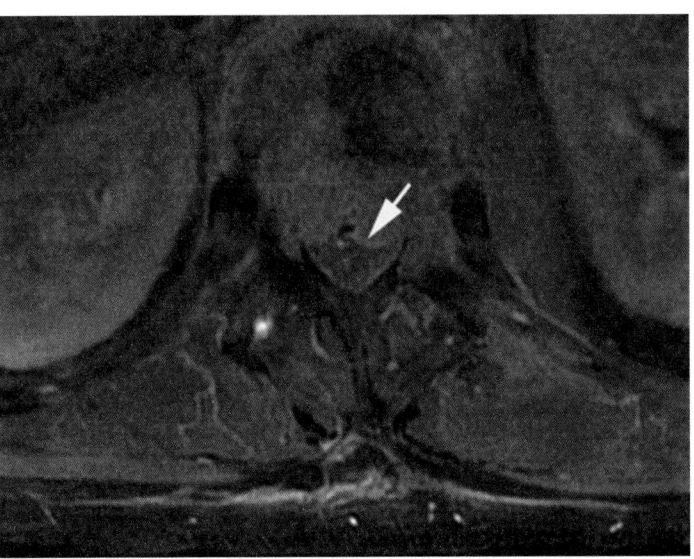

A   B

FIGURE 103.4 Epidural spinal metastases. **A:** T2-weighted sagittal MRI demonstrates destruction and mild collapse of the T12 vertebra (*arrow*) in a patient with multiple myeloma. Note the hyperintense marrow signal at multiple levels in the spine indicating additional metastatic deposits. **B:** Axial T1 with contrast MRI at T12 level shows moderate canal stenosis (*arrow*).

or blastic changes in the vertebral bodies in 85% of those patients. Osteoblastic changes are common with prostate carcinoma and are occasionally seen with breast cancer, whereas osteolytic changes are typically seen in multiple myeloma. CT and magnetic resonance imaging (MRI) are sensitive techniques for the detection of spinal osseous metastases. Importantly, involvement of paraspinal lymph nodes with spread to the spinal canal is common with lymphoma. In this

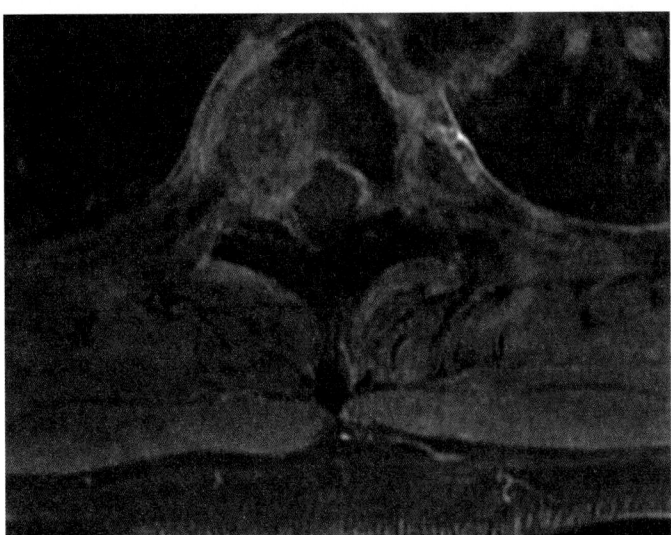

FIGURE 103.5 Epidural spinal metastases. Axial T1-weighted contrast-enhanced sequence at T5 demonstrates epidural extension of metastatic lung non–small cell carcinoma with bone destruction at this level.

situation, the vertebral bone may be normal on imaging studies and use of screening spinal x-rays will be misleading.

Intradural, Extramedullary Tumors

Neurofibromas, schwannomas, and meningiomas are the most commonly occurring primary intradural tumors of the spinal cord. On MRI with gadolinium, the lesions enhance brightly. Meningiomas may be identified by the presence of a dural tail, where the tumor attaches to the dura (Figs. 103.6 and 103.7). Symptoms may occur slowly and some may be asymptomatic despite large size, presumably because of slow growth allowing the spinal cord an opportunity to adapt to the mass effect.

Leptomeningeal metastasis and drop metastases of intracranial tumors also involve the intradural space, but typically, they appear as small nodules attached to the surface of the cord or cauda equina nerve roots (Fig. 103.8), although many (approximately 70%) or not visible on imaging of brain or spine and are detected only by cerebrospinal fluid (CSF) analyses.

INTRAMEDULLARY TUMORS

Primary Intramedullary Tumors

The most common intramedullary tumors are ependymomas and astrocytomas. A diagnosis of von Hippel–Lindau syndrome, an autosomal dominant disorder, should be considered when a spinal hemangioblastoma is present (most commonly involving the thoracic cord) because this association occurs in one-third of the cases. However, rarely, hemangioblastoma can also occur in the intradural extramedullary and extradural locations. Although a single lesion is the most common presentation, multiple lesions occur in one-fifth of cases.

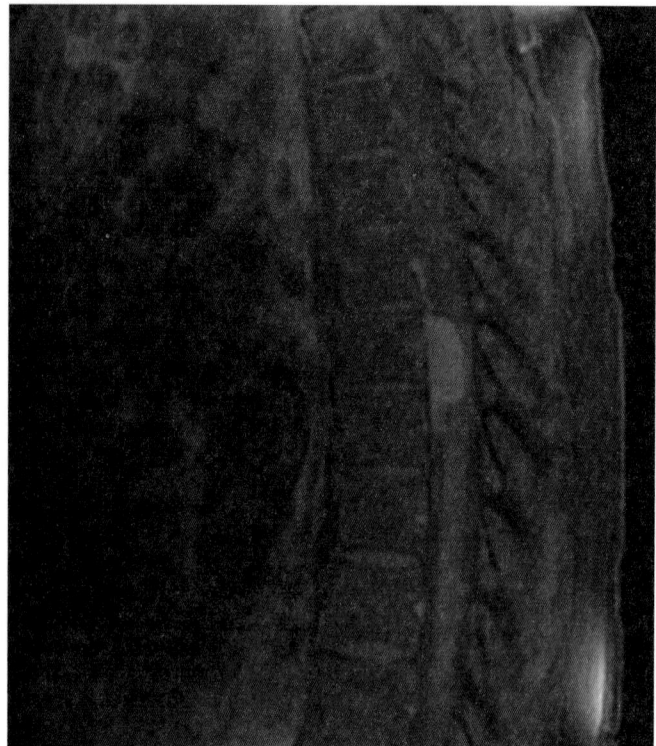

A

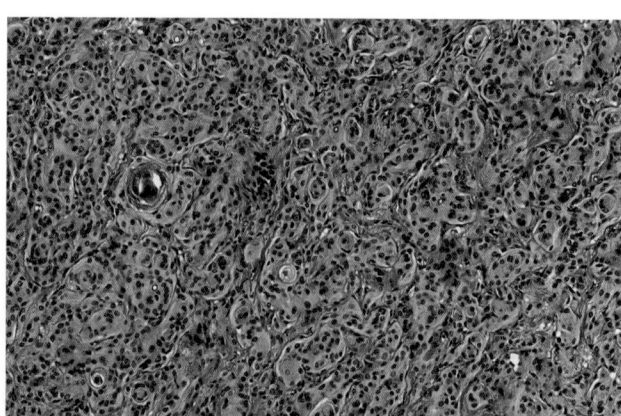

FIGURE 103.7 Meningothelial meningioma of the spinal cord. The classic variant of meningioma is composed of lobules of meningothelial cells separated by fine collagen fibers. The intercellular borders are ill-defined characteristic of a syncytial pattern. Nuclear clearing and whorl formation are frequent. Calcifications (psammoma bodies) might be present. (Courtesy of Dr. Adriana Olar, Department of Pathology, MD Anderson Cancer Center.)

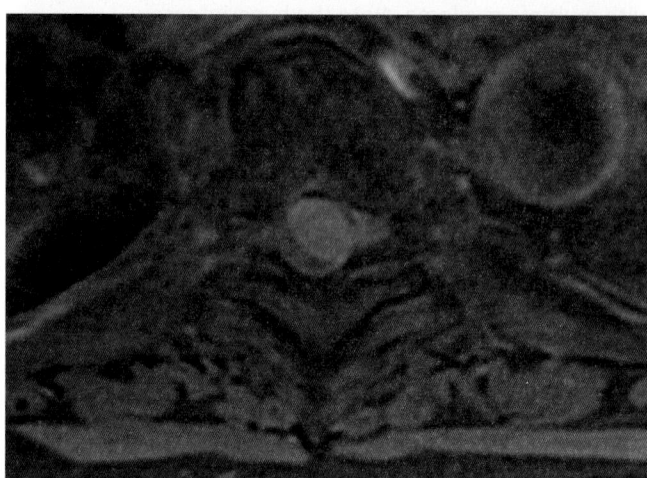

B

FIGURE 103.6 Thoracic meningioma. **A:** T1-weighted contrast-enhanced sagittal MRI demonstrates a large intradural mass at T6–T7 with dural tail sign. **B:** Axial MRI demonstrates the large size of this lesion, probably a meningioma. Despite marked spinal cord compression, the patient had no abnormality on neurologic examination and only complained of left-sided thoracic pain.

Primary intramedullary tumors usually extend over many segments, causing dilatation of the spinal cord and sometimes causing syringomyelia, which can involve the whole length of the spinal cord. For this reason, the signs and symptoms of intramedullary tumors are more variable than those of extramedullary tumors (Figs. 103.9 and 103.10).

If the tumor is restricted to one or two segments, the clinical presentation can be similar to that of an extramedullary tumor. Pain may be an early manifestation if the dorsal root entry zone is affected. Compression of the crossing pain fibers in the central

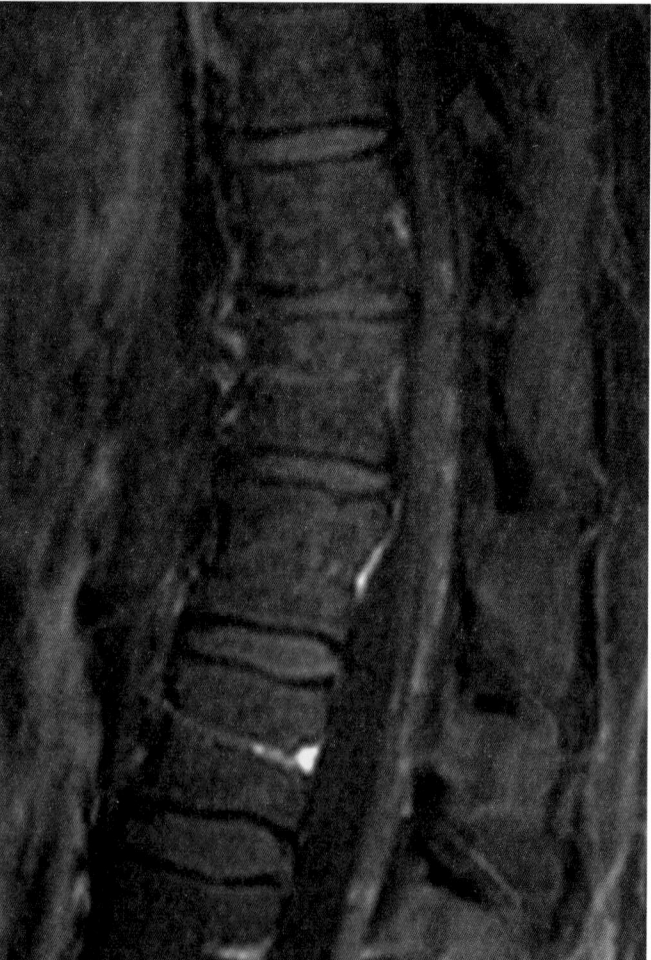

FIGURE 103.8 Leptomeningeal disease. Sagittal T1-weighted contrast-enhanced MRI shows tumor deposits along the surface of the distal thoracic cord and the nerve roots of the cauda equine in a patient with breast carcinoma.

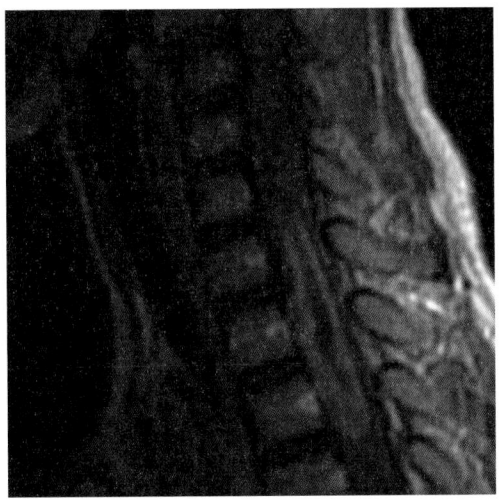
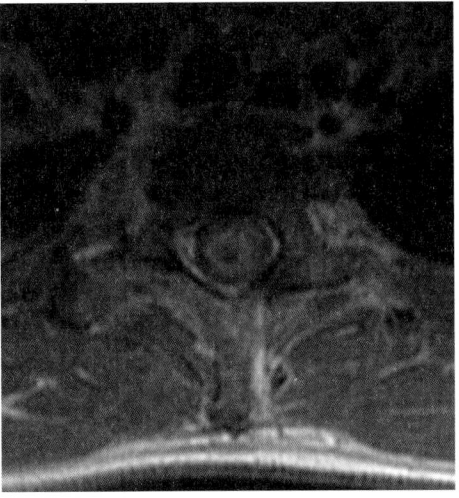

FIGURE 103.9 Intramedullary glioblastoma. **A:** Sagittal T1-weighted contrast-enhanced MRI demonstrates T1–T4 intramedullary lesion with peripheral enhancement and hypointense center that expands the cord. **B:** T1-weighted MRI shows a contrast-enhancing intramedullary tumor at the T1–T2 level. At operation, a spinal glioblastoma with necrotic center was removed.

cord may cause loss of pain and temperature only in the affected segments. As the tumor spreads peripherally, the spinothalamic tracts may be affected; in the thoracic and cervical areas, pain and temperature fibers from the sacral area lie near the external surface of the cord and may be spared (e.g., sacral sparing). Involvement of the central gray matter destroys the anterior horn cells, with local weakness and atrophy resulting. However, pyramidal fibers may be spared. The clinical picture may be identical to that of syringomyelia with a "suspended" sensory level.

Intramedullary Metastases

Although rare, the most common tumors that cause intramedullary metastases are lung cancer or breast cancer. Intramedullary metastases typically occur with advanced metastatic disease, and at autopsy, 61% of patients with intramedullary metastases are found to have had multiple sites of cerebral or spinal lesions.

Contrast-enhanced MRI is the preferred method for detection of intramedullary metastases. Reversal or stabilization of neurologic signs depends on early diagnosis, but survival is poor; 80% of patients in one series died within 3 months of diagnosis, likely a manifestation of the extent of systemic disease at the time of the spinal cord involvement.

REGIONAL SYNDROMES

Foramen Magnum Tumors

Tumors in the region of the foramen magnum may extend up into the posterior fossa or down into the cervical region. The syndrome from tumor in the foramen magnum typically shows signs and symptoms of dysfunction of the lower cranial nerves, primarily those pertaining to the eleventh, twelfth, and rarely, the ninth and tenth. The most characteristic foramen magnum tumor, the

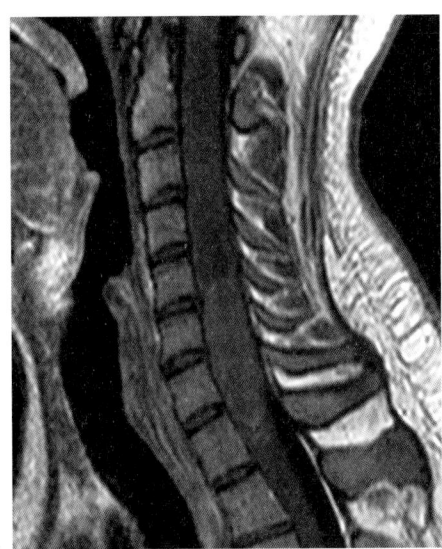
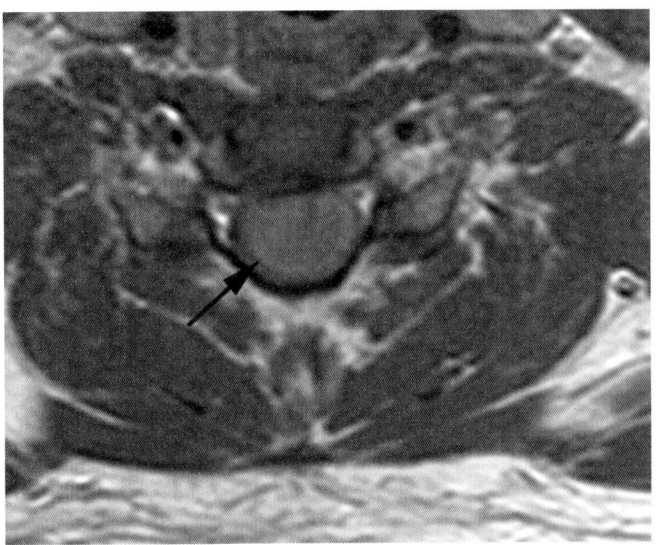

FIGURE 103.10 Intramedullary ependymoma. **A:** Sagittal T1-weighted MRI shows an intramedullary enhancing mass at C5–T1. **B:** Axial T1-weighted image with contrast shows expansion and significant displacement of the cord by the tumor at C6 (*arrow*).

ventrolateral meningioma, compresses the spinal cord at the cervicomedullary junction to cause long tract signs: loss of position, vibratory, and light touch perception, with more prominent symptoms in the arms than the legs. Upper motor neuron signs are seen in all four limbs. There may be cutaneous sensory loss in distribution of C2 or the occiput, with posterior cranial headaches and high cervical pain. Progression of sensory and motor symptoms may involve the limbs asymmetrically.

Cervical Tumors

Tumors of the upper cervical segments cause pain or paresthesias in the occipital or cervical region, with stiff neck, weakness, and wasting of neck muscles. Below the lesion, there may be a spastic tetraplegia or hemiplegia. Cutaneous sensation may be affected below the lesion, and the descending trigeminal nucleus may be involved. Characteristic findings make it possible to localize the upper level of spinal tumors in the middle and lower cervical segments or T1 as shown in Table 103.1.

Other signs of cervical tumors include nystagmus, which is attributed to involvement of the descending portion of the median longitudinal fasciculus. A Horner syndrome may be found with intramedullary lesions in any portion of the cervical cord if the descending sympathetic pathways are affected.

Thoracic Tumors

Clinical localization of tumors in the thoracic region of the cord is best made by the sensory level. It is not possible to determine the location of a lesion in the upper half of the thoracic cord by testing the strength of intercostal muscles. Lesions that affect the abdominal muscles below T10 but spare the upper ones may be localized by the Beevor sign (i.e., the umbilicus moves upward when the patient, lying in the supine position, attempts to flex the neck against resistance). Abdominal skin reflexes are absent below the lesion.

Lumbar Tumors

Lesions in the lumbar region may be localized by the level of the sensory loss and motor weakness typically following a dermatome or myotome distribution. Tumors that compress only the L1 and L2 nerve roots cause loss of the cremasteric reflexes and weakness in the iliopsoas muscle. The abdominal reflexes are preserved, as are the knee and ankle jerks. Lesions affecting the L3 and L4 nerve roots may present with weakness in the quadriceps muscle, loss of patellar reflex, and pain in the anteromedial portion of the lower extremity.

The typical involvement of the L5 nerve root causes weakness of eversion, inversion, and dorsiflexion of the foot and hallux. Decreased sensation over the anterolateral calf and dorsum of the foot, with pain radiating down the leg to the hallux which can be exacerbated by the straight leg testing (Lasègue sign) is also characteristic. The presence of weakness of foot inversion in an L5 radiculopathy is an important distinguishing factor from a peroneal palsy where foot inversion strength is typically normal.

A tumor affecting the S1 root may present with weakness of the gastrocnemius and hamstring, with absent ankle jerk and decreased sensation over the lateral calf and lateral foot including the sole.

The involvement of multiple nerve roots can occur at any lumbar level and it is usually described as cauda equina syndrome, which typically presents as flaccid paralysis of the legs with loss of knee and ankle reflexes associated with urinary retention and bowel incontinence. If both the spinal cord and cauda equina are asymmetrically affected, there may be spastic paralysis of one leg with an overactive ankle reflex on that side and flaccid paralysis with loss of reflexes on the other side.

Finally, tumors affecting the sacrum at the level of S2–S4 can cause perineal or saddle anesthesia and loss of bowel and bladder control without motor deficits observable in the lower extremities because the motor roots (L1–S1) are not affected.

Tumors of the Conus and Cauda Equina

Although a conus lesion is intramedullary involving the parenchyma of the terminal spinal cord, a cauda equina lesion is extramedullary affecting multiple exiting nerve roots. Distinguishing between the two entities is not always possible as many of the clinical features are similar. Moreover, in neoplastic processes, there is frequent involvement of both.

The first symptom of a tumor that involves the conus or cauda equina is pain in the back, rectal area, or both lower legs, often leading to the preliminary diagnosis of sciatica. Loss of bladder function and impotence are seen early especially with conus involvement. As the tumor grows, there may be flaccid paralysis of the legs, with atrophy of leg muscles, and foot drop. Fasciculation may be evident. Sensory loss may affect the perianal or saddle area and the remaining sacral and lumbar dermatomes. This loss may

TABLE 103.1	Localization in the Cervical and T1 Region Based on Symptomatology
C4	Paralysis of the diaphragm
C5	Atrophy and paralysis of the deltoid, biceps, supinator longus, rhomboid, and spinati muscles. The upper arms hang limp at the side. The sensory level extends to the outer surface of the arm. The biceps and supinator reflexes are lost.
C6	Paralysis of triceps and wrist extensors. The forearm is held semiflexed and there is a partial wristdrop. The triceps reflex is lost. Sensory impairment extends to a line running down the middle of the arm slightly to the radial side.
C7	Paralysis of the flexors of the wrist and of the flexors and extensors of the fingers. Efforts to close the hands result in extension of the wrist and slight flexion of the fingers (e.g., preacher's hand). The sensory level is similar to that of the sixth cervical segment but slightly more to the ulnar side of the arm.
C8	Atrophy and paralysis of the small muscles of the hand with resulting clawhand (main-en-griffe). Horner syndrome, unilateral or bilateral, results from lesions at this level and is characterized by the triad of ptosis, small pupil (i.e., miosis), and loss of sweating on the face. Sensory loss extends to the inner aspect of the arm and involves the fourth and fifth fingers and the ulnar aspect of the middle finger.
T1	Lesions rarely cause motor symptoms because the T1 nerve root normally provides little functional innervation of the small hand muscles.

be slight or so severe that a trophic ulcer develops over the lumbosacral region, buttocks, hips, or heels.

DIAGNOSIS

Tumors compressing the spinal cord or the cauda equina typically cause radicular pain. The slow evolution of signs of an incomplete transverse lesion of the cord or signs of compression of the conus medullaris or cauda equina usually bring patients to medical attention. In addition to cord compression, extradural tumors may obstruct the blood supply to the cord; if this occurs, the symptoms are often of sudden onset. In a patient with neurofibromatosis 1 (von Recklinghausen disease), the skin lesions may focus the differential diagnosis to neurofibroma, glioma, or ependymoma.

The diagnosis of an intraspinal tumor may be established before the operative procedure, with visualization by CT, MRI, or myelography. Vascular malformations or vascular tumors may be best visualized by spinal angiography. CSF examination with cytologic studies may also be helpful if positive, but negative cytology does not exclude a neoplastic process.

RADIOGRAPHY

CT and MRI have replaced standard radiographic studies (plain x-rays). However, when conventional x-ray imaging is performed, the abnormalities (listed in the following text) are seen in about 15% of spinal neoplasms:

1. Localized destruction of the vertebrae is manifest by scalloping of the posterior margin of the vertebral body or lucency of a portion of the vertebra or pedicle.
2. Changes occur in the contour or separation of the pedicles (e.g., the interpediculate distance may be measured and compared with normal values). Localized enlargement of foramina is seen with dumbbell neurofibromas. Localized enlargement of the spinal canal is usually diagnostic of an intraspinal tumor but enlargement of many segments may be a developmental anomaly.
3. Paraspinal tissues are distorted by tumors, frequently neurofibromas that extend through the intervertebral foramen or by tumors that originate in the paraspinal structures.
4. Proliferation of bone, which is rare except in osteomas and sarcomas, is also occasionally seen in hemangiomas of bone and meninges.
5. Calcium deposits are occasionally present in meningiomas or congenital tumors.

MRI has largely supplanted myelography for imaging both intramedullary and extramedullary processes. MRI is the most useful test for evaluating spinal tumors. The vertebral bodies, spinal canal, and spinal cord, itself, are clearly delineated. Most spinal neoplasms display contrast enhancement. When a metastatic tumor is suspected or demonstrated, it is advisable to image the entire cord because more than one lesion may be present.

CT is the modality of choice for imaging of the bony structures but is more limited than MRI in demonstrating the soft tissues. Injection of contrast in the lumbar cistern is used for a CT myelogram, which is an alternative in cases of contraindication for MRI (i.e., pacemakers or ferromagnetic implants). A CT myelogram may demonstrate the soft-tissue changes of intraspinal tumors and is particularly useful in the diagnosis of cystic lesions in the subarachnoid space, where the contrast material may accumulate around and create a negative contrast of the cyst. It is also useful to evaluate if there is communication between the subarachnoid space and intradural cystic lesions (i.e., arachnoid cysts, syringomyelia, or cystic tumors).

CEREBROSPINAL FLUID

When there is a complete subarachnoid block, the CSF is xanthochromic as a result of the high protein content (Froin's syndrome). It may be only slightly yellow or even colorless if the subarachnoid block is incomplete. The cell count is usually normal, but a slight pleocytosis is found in about 30% of patients. Cell counts of between 25 and 100 per cubic millimeter are found in about 15% of patients. The protein content is increased in more than 95%. Values of over 100 mg/dL are present in 60% of the patients and values of over 1,000 mg/dL are present in 5% and may, in rare cases, lead to communicating hydrocephalus. The glucose content is normal unless there is meningeal spread. Cytologic evaluation of the CSF is useful when malignant tumors are suspected, although as mentioned previously, negative cytology does not exclude leptomeningeal cancer. More than one CSF sampling procedure may be required (some advocate up to five), although the remainder of the CSF profile (cells, protein, tumor markers) is usually abnormal in the setting of leptomeningeal metastases, notwithstanding the absence of malignant cells on cytologic analysis.

DIFFERENTIAL DIAGNOSIS

Spinal tumors must be differentiated from other disorders of the spinal cord, including transverse myelitis, multiple sclerosis (MS), syringomyelia, combined system disease, syphilis, amyotrophic lateral sclerosis, anomalies of the cervical spine and base of the skull, spondylosis, adhesive arachnoiditis, radiculitis of the cauda equina, hypertrophic arthritis, ruptured intervertebral disks, diastematomyelia, and vascular anomalies.

MS, with a complete or incomplete transverse lesion of the cord, may usually be differentiated from spinal cord tumors by the remitting course, signs and symptoms of more than one lesion, evoked potential studies, cranial MRI, and the presence of CSF oligoclonal bands. Acute transverse myelitis may occasionally enlarge the cord to simulate an intramedullary tumor.

Determining the differential diagnosis between spontaneous syringomyelia and intramedullary tumor-related syrinx is complicated because intramedullary cysts mimicking a syrinx are commonly associated with these tumors. Extramedullary tumors in the cervical region may give rise to localized pain and muscular atrophy in conjunction with a Brown-Séquard syndrome, producing a clinical picture similar to that of syringomyelia. The differential diagnosis may often be made by contrast-enhanced MRI that reveals a tumor nodule.

The combination of atrophy of hand muscles and spastic weakness in the legs in amyotrophic lateral sclerosis may suggest the diagnosis of a cervical cord tumor. Tumor is excluded by the lack of paresthesias, and normal sensation on examination, and by the presence of fasciculation or atrophy in leg muscles or tongue, and by imaging.

Cervical spondylosis may cause stenosis of the spinal canal and cause symptoms and signs of root irritation and/or compression of the spinal cord. Degenerative changes are extremely common and the modality of choice for diagnosis is MRI. Clinical correlation with image findings is critical for the treatment decision because most changes on imaging studies are incidental findings or do not have a clinical correlation.

Anomalies in the cervical region or at the base of the skull, such as platybasia or Klippel–Feil syndrome, are diagnosed by CT or MRI. Occasionally, arachnoiditis may interfere with the circulation of CSF causing signs and symptoms of a transverse lesion. The CSF protein content is usually elevated. Diagnosis is made by complete or partial arrest of the contrast column on myelography or by fragmentation of the material at the site of the lesion. Slowed CSF flow will be seen using magnetic resonance flow techniques.

Epidural lipomatosis is a complication of prolonged steroid therapy but sometimes occurs without apparent cause; the fat accumulations act as an extradural mass lesion, causing low back pain and compression of the spinal cord or cauda equina.

TREATMENT

INTRADURAL EXTRAMEDULLARY TUMORS

Once the diagnosis of an intraspinal tumor has been made, the treatment is surgical removal of the tumor whenever possible. When the neurologic disorder is severe or rapidly progressing, emergency surgery is indicated. The best results are obtained when the signs and symptoms are due solely to compression by a benign encapsulated extramedullary tumor. Some of these tumors, especially meningiomas, may lie anterior to the spinal cord and a complete resection of the involved dura is not possible or carries a significant risk of morbidity. In these cases, a gross total resection of the mass with cauterization of the dural insertion of tumor is performed. In cases of recurrence, another surgical resection may be necessary. The functional outcome of patients harboring extramedullary tumors is predicated by the severity of the preoperative neurologic disability. Overall, surgery aiming at a gross total resection is the modality of choice for the intradural extramedullary tumors (Video 103.1) and ideally should be performed before installment of neurologic dysfunction because when this occurs, it might represent evidence of irreversible damage to the spinal cord due to compression or ischemia. Radiotherapy is typically not indicated for benign intradural extramedullary tumors. In fact, most of these lesions are low-grade tumors with no tissue separation between the lesion and the spinal cord. This increases the risk of radiation-induced myelopathy, especially in cases where preexisting damage is suspected (i.e., evidence of myelomalacia or ischemia due to long-dated compression). In cases of recurrence, a second surgical procedure is usually considered a better alternative than radiation, which in general is reserved for cases where a high surgical comorbidity precludes surgery.

INTRAMEDULLARY TUMORS

In almost all World Health Organization (WHO) grade I (myxopapillary) and WHO grade II ependymomas, complete microsurgical resection of the tumor is the treatment of choice (Video 103.2). There is no consensus on the use of radiotherapy for WHO grade I and WHO grade II spinal cord tumors and overall radiation is reserved for cases with incomplete resection, with bulky residual disease or symptomatic tumor recurrence when the patient is considered not to be a good surgical candidate. Radiation treatment is indicated after initial surgery for all patients with WHO grade III ependymoma. Astrocytomas are typically infiltrating and often lack a plane of cleavage. In this case, an attempt at complete resection or extensive debulking is associated with significant risk of neurologic decline. Although radiotherapy should be given for spinal cord astrocytomas, the results particularly for WHO grade III and IV tumors are discouraging. For other less common intramedullary tumors, such as hemangioblastomas, teratomas, or dermoids, if complete removal has been achieved, typically, no further treatment is recommended aside from surveillance.

Intramedullary tumors are typically approached with multilevel laminectomies, which create disruption in the posterior tension band of the ligaments stabilizing the spine. As a result, spinal deformities that may have been present preoperatively may worsen and other deformities may develop, eventually requiring surgical correction with spinal instrumentation and fusion. If allowed to progress, these deformities may create additional functional impairment, especially in skeletally immature patients. Some surgeons have advocated replacement of the lamina after definitive surgery, rather than the standard laminectomy. However, the occurrence of postoperative kyphosis is common and the natural history of this deformity is uncertain. The additional use of radiotherapy for intraspinal tumors in younger patients may affect the growth of the spine and in adults may increase the muscle atrophy and degenerative changes leading to the development or worsening of preexisting deformities of the spine.

EPIDURAL DISEASE FROM METASTATIC CANCER

Treatment of epidural metastasis is palliative in nearly all patients. Prognostic scoring systems based on patient age, performance status, extent of spinal and extraspinal disease, tumor histology, and availability of systemic treatments are useful to predict the expected survival of patients harboring spinal metastasis. However, management has to be individualized in order to achieve the best balance between morbidity and palliation. A randomized trial [**Level 1**][1] has demonstrated that surgery for spinal decompression and spinal stabilization followed by radiation is superior to conventional radiation alone in maintenance and recovery of ambulation, duration of ambulation, and maintenance of sphincter continence. Loss of bowel or bladder function is an ominous prognostic sign and is usually irreversible. Among patients diagnosed and treated early, 94% remain ambulatory until they die.

Conventional radiation therapy is the mainstay of treatment for most patients with spinal metastases, even those who had surgical decompression, with the typical treatment plan comprising 3,000 cGy divided in 10 fractions of 300 cGy each. More recently, high-dose hypofractionated radiotherapy using image-guided techniques (spinal stereotactic radiotherapy) has emerged as an effective modality overcoming the relative radioresistance of some tumors to conventional radiation. However, in cases of symptomatic or high-degree spinal cord compression, a judicious combination of surgery to separate the tumor from the spinal cord prior to stereotactic radiation has been shown to achieve a high degree of local control with relative low morbidity.

In general, surgery provides spinal stabilization and spinal cord and nerve roots decompression, whereas radiation therapy provides local tumor control. Usually, radiation treatment is well tolerated even by patients who are seriously ill, and in most cases, palliation is often achieved with relief of pain. In general, indications for surgery include spinal cord compression due to radioresistant tumors (renal cell carcinoma, sarcomas, melanomas, etc.), spinal instability, unknown tissue diagnosis, or rapid progression of neurologic dysfunction. Judicious use of surgery is critical to achieve a meaningful clinical improvement in patients with advanced systemic disease because the anticipated recovery time has to be weighed against the expected duration of survival.

OUTCOME

Epidural spinal cord compression is an emergency because without treatment, irreversible loss of neurologic function will lead to significant morbidity and mortality. It is estimated that patients who were ambulatory preoperatively were 2.3 times more likely to be able to walk postoperatively. Treatment should be initiated early, as neurologic status at presentation is predictive of functional outcome. Critical to this is the education of patients, patient families, and health care providers to recognize warning signs of cord compression early on. Recent studies do support the notion that patients with cord compression are presenting earlier. In fact, although a study published in 1998 showed that only 33% were ambulatory and 53% were catheter free at the time of initiation of therapy, in another study published in 2010, 62% of patients were ambulatory at presentation. It has also been shown that nonambulatory patients if treated surgically require more extensive surgery with consequent higher complication rates and morbidity. It is therefore of paramount importance that a careful patient selection process is pursued, always taking into consideration the patient's overall prognosis and presumed benefits balanced against the treatment-related morbidity.

For intramedullary tumors, the prognosis and outcome from surgery is strongly related to tumor histology and the occurrence of a plane of surgical dissection between the lesion and the surrounding spinal cord and nerve roots. When a plane of cleavage exists, such as in ependymomas, a complete surgical resection is potentially curative. With more diffusely infiltrating tumors such as spinal cord astrocytic tumors, the goal of surgery in most cases is diagnostic and especially in high-grade tumors, treatment is palliative with a dismal outcome irrespective of treatment.

Overall, intradural extramedullary tumors have slow progression and usually, treatment is recommended when symptomatic or when there is a significant degree of spinal cord compression. With improved imaging, neurophysiologic monitoring, and sound microsurgical techniques, the goals of treatment for these lesions is gross total resection with curative intent. Good functional outcomes are generally observed and overall recurrence rates range between 0% and 13%.

This is in contrast to the prognosis of patients with leptomeningeal metastasis from systemic cancer where the prognosis, irrespective of the cancer of origin, is typically around 2 to 3 months, although there are exceptions, most often patients with lymphoma and occasionally breast cancer.

Videos can be found in the companion e-book edition. For a full list of video legends, please see the front matter.

LEVEL 1 EVIDENCE

1. Patchell RA, Tibbs PA, Regine WF, et al. Direct decompressive surgical resection in the treatment of spinal cord compression caused by metastatic cancer: a randomised trial. *Lancet.* 2005;366(9486):643–648.

SUGGESTED READINGS

Aghakhani N, David P, Parker F, et al. Intramedullary spinal ependymomas: analysis of a consecutive series of 82 adult cases with particular attention to patients with no preoperative neurological deficit. *Neurosurgery.* 2008;62: 1279–1286.

Aghayev K, Vrionis F, Chamberlain MC. Adult intradural primary spinal cord tumors. *J Natl Compr Canc Netw.* 2011;9(4):434–447.

Al-Khawaja D, Seex K, Eslick GD. Spinal epidural lipomatosis—a brief review. *J Clin Neurosci.* 2008;15:1323–1326.

Aryan HE, Farin A, Nakaji P, et al. Intramedullary spinal cord metastasis of lung adenocarcinoma presenting as Brown-Sequard syndrome. *Surg Neurol.* 2004;61:72–76.

Borba LA, de Oliveira JG, Giudicissi-Filho M, et al. Surgical management of foramen magnum meningiomas. *Neurosurg Rev.* 2009;32:49–58.

Chamberlain MC, Tredway TL. Adult primary intradural spinal cord tumors: a review. *Curr Neurol Neurosci Rep.* 2011;11:320–328.

Chaichana KL, Woodworth GF, Sciubba DM, et al. Predictors of ambulatory function after decompressive surgery for metastatic epidural spinal cord compression. *Neurosurgery.* 2008;62:683–692.

Cheshire WP, Santos CC, Massey EW, et al. Spinal cord infarction: etiology and outcome. *Neurology.* 1996;47:321–330.

Clarke JL. Leptomeningeal metastasis from systemic cancer. *Continuum.* 2012;18:328–342.

Dam-Hieu P, Seizeur R, Mineo JF, et al. Retrospective study of 19 patients with intramedullary spinal cord metastasis. *Clin Neurol Neurosurg.* 2009;11: 10–17.

Duong LM, McCarthy BJ, McLendon RE, et al. Descriptive epidemiology of malignant and nonmalignant primary spinal cord, spinal meninges, and cauda equina tumors, United States, 2004–2007. *Cancer.* 2012;118:4220–4227.

Ebner FH, Roser F, Acioly MA, et al. Intramedullary lesions of the conus medullaris: differential diagnosis and surgical management. *Neurosurg Rev.* 2009;32:287–300.

Elsberg CA. *Surgical Diseases of the Spinal Cord, Membranes and Nerve Roots.* New York: Paul B. Hoeber; 1941.

Eule JM, Erickson MA, O'Brien MF, et al. Chiari I malformation associated with syringomyelia and scoliosis: a twenty-year review of surgical and nonsurgical treatment in a pediatric population. *Spine (Phila Pa 1976).* 2002;27:1451–1455.

Gerszten PC, Burton SA, Ozhasoglu C, et al. Radiosurgery for spinal metastases: clinical experience in 500 cases from a single institution. *Spine (Phila Pa 1976).* 2007;32:193–199.

Hanbali F, Fourney DR, Marmor E, et al. Spinal cord ependymoma: radical surgical resection and outcome. *Neurosurgery.* 2002;51:1162–1174.

Husband DJ. Malignant spinal cord compression: prospective study of delays in referral and treatment. *BMJ.* 1998;317(7150):18–21.

Jallo GI, Danish S, Velasquez L, et al. Intramedullary low-grade astrocytomas: long-term outcome following radical surgery. *J Neurooncol.* 2001;53:61–66.

Jallo GI, Freed D, Epstein F. Intramedullary spinal cord tumors in children. *Childs Nerv Syst.* 2003;19:641–649.

Jankowski R, Nowak S, Zukiel R, et al. Application of internal stabilisation in the surgical treatment of spinal metastases. *Neurol Neurochir Pol.* 2008;42:323–331.

King AT, Sharr MM, Gullan RW, et al. Spinal meningiomas: a 20-year review. *Br J Neurosurg.* 1998;12:521–526.

Laufer I, Iorgulescu JB, Chapman T, et al. Local disease control for spinal metastases following "separation surgery" and adjuvant hypofractionated or high-dose single-fraction stereotactic radiosurgery: outcome analysis in 186 patients. *J Neurosurg Spine.* 2013;18:207–214.

Lonser RR, Weil RJ, Wanebo JE, et al. Surgical management of spinal cord hemangioblastomas in patients with von Hippel-Lindau disease. *J Neurosurg.* 2003;98:106–116.

Manzano G, Green BA, Vanni S, et al. Contemporary management of adult intramedullary spinal tumors-pathology and neurological outcomes related to surgical resection. *Spinal Cord.* 2008;46:540–546.

Maranzano E, Trippa F, Chirico L, et al. Management of metastatic spinal cord compression. *Tumori.* 2003;89:469–475.

Mathew P, Todd NV. Intradural conus and cauda equina tumours: a retrospective review of presentation, diagnosis and early outcome. *J Neurol Neurosurg Psychiatry.* 1993;56:69–74.

Matson DD. *Neurosurgery of Infancy and Childhood.* 2nd ed. Springfield, IL: Charles C Thomas; 1969.

McCormick PC, Stein BM. Intramedullary tumors in adults. *Neurosurg Clin North Am.* 1990;1:609–630.

McGirt MJ, Goldstein IM, Chaichana KL, et al. Extent of surgical resection of malignant astrocytomas of the spinal cord: outcome analysis of 35 patients. *Neurosurgery.* 2008;63:55–60; discussion 60–61.

Mechtler LL, Nandigam K. Spinal cord tumors: new views and future directions. *Neurol Clin.* 2013;31:241–268.

Nakamura M, Ishii K, Watanabe K, et al. Surgical treatment of intramedullary spinal cord tumors: prognosis and complications. *Spinal Cord.* 2008;46:282–286.

Ogden AT, Feldstein NA, McCormick PC. Anterior approach to cervical intramedullary pilocytic astrocytoma. Case report. *J Neurosurg Spine*. 2008;9: 253–257.

Ostrom QT, Gittleman H, Farah P, et al. CBTRUS statistical report: primary brain and central nervous system tumors diagnosed in the United States in 2006–2010. *Neuro Oncol*. 2013;15(suppl 2):ii1–ii56.

O'Toole JE, McCormick PC. Midline ventral intradural schwannoma of the cervical spinal cord resected via anterior corpectomy with reconstruction: technical case report and review of the literature. *Neurosurgery*. 2003;52:1482–1485.

Parsa AT, Chi JH, Acosta FL Jr, et al. Intramedullary spinal cord tumors: molecular insights and surgical innovation. *Clin Neurosurg*. 2005;52:76–84.

Putz C, Wiedenhöfer B, Gerner HJ, et al. Tokuhashi prognosis score: an important tool in prediction of the neurological outcome in metastatic spinal cord compression?: a retrospective clinical study. *Spine*. 2008;15;33: 2669–2674.

Rades D, Huttenlocher S, Dunst J, et al. Matched pair analysis comparing surgery followed by radiotherapy and radiotherapy alone for metastatic spinal cord compression. *J Clin Oncol*. 2010;28:3597.

Ribas ES, Schiff D. Spinal cord compression. *Curr Treat Options Neurol*. 2012; 14:391–401.

Robertson SC, Traynelis VC, Follett KA, et al. Idiopathic spinal epidural lipomatosis. *Neurosurgery*. 1997;41:68–74.

Sandalcioglu IE, Hunold A, Müller O, et al. Spinal meningiomas: critical review of 131 surgically treated patients. *Eur Spine J*. 2008;17:1035–1041.

Santi M, Mena H, Wong K, et al. Malignant astrocytomas. Clinicopathologic features in 36 cases. *Cancer*. 2003;98(3):554–561.

Schild SE, Nisi K, Scheithauer BW, et al. The results of radiotherapy for ependymomas: the Mayo Clinic experience. *Int J Radiat Oncol*. 1998;42:953–958.

Smoker WR, Khanna G. Imaging the craniocervical junction. *Childs Nerv Syst*. 2008;24:1123–1145.

Tokuhashi Y, Matsuzaki H, Oda H, et al. A revised scoring system for preoperative evaluation of metastatic spine tumor prognosis. *Spine (Phila Pa 1976)*. 2005;30:2186–2191.

Tomita K, Kawahara N, Kobayashi T, et al. Surgical strategy for spinal metastases. *Spine (Phila Pa 1976)*. 2001;26:298–306.

Van Goethem JW, van den Hauwe L, Ozsarlak O, et al. Spinal tumors. *Eur J Radiol*. 2004;50:159–176.

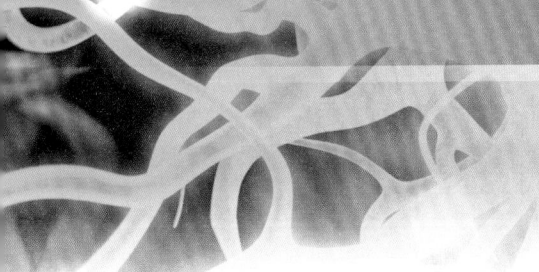

Paraneoplastic Syndromes 104

Lauren R. Schaff and Lewis P. Rowland

INTRODUCTION

Neurologic paraneoplastic disorders are caused by indirect damage to central or peripheral nervous system structures from a systemic cancer, resulting in a wide spectrum of neurologic signs and symptoms. The cause is thought to be immune-mediated as opposed to the direct effects of tumor invasion, metastases, toxicity from treatment, malnutrition, or coincidental infection.

EPIDEMIOLOGY

Paraneoplastic syndromes are quite rare, affecting less than 0.1% of all patients with malignancy. However, other studies suggest up to 7% of patients with malignancy are afflicted. They are associated with a broad range of symptoms that are typically subacute in onset, evolving over weeks to months. Most patients develop neurologic symptoms before a cancer is identified. After onset of symptoms, the cancer may still be small enough to elude detection and may not be identified for many months or years, sometimes discovered only postmortem.

Any cancer may be associated with a paraneoplastic syndrome but some syndromes are associated with a specific cancer or a particular group of neoplasms. Small cell lung cancer (SCLC) is one of the most common tumors associated with paraneoplastic syndromes. Other tumors that are associated with these syndromes are those that express neuroendocrine proteins, those that affect organs with immunoregulatory functions, or those derived from cells that produce immunoglobulins.

PATHOBIOLOGY

The pathogenesis of paraneoplastic syndromes is thought to be immune-mediated. It is generally accepted that malignancies causing these syndromes express proteins normally restricted to the nervous system. The host mounts an immune attack against those antigens in the tumor but the response is directed against central or peripheral neural antigens, resulting in neurologic deficits. In many paraneoplastic syndromes, the detection of characteristic antibodies has served as a useful diagnostic tool but the pathogenesis of these antibodies is not clearly understood.

In general, antibodies associated with paraneoplastic syndromes are classified based on location of their targeted antigen, either intracellular or on the neuronal surface. This distinction has further implications on the understanding of the pathogenic role of the antibody and the diagnostic value of its detection. Antibodies targeted against intracellular antigens, or onconeural antibodies, may predict with high frequency the presence of an underlying tumor and may be used to establish a neurologic symptom as paraneoplastic. The pathogenic role of these antibodies is not clearly understood and they may be present (often at lower levels) in a patient with an underlying cancer but without neurologic symptoms. There is evidence to suggest that the mechanism for

neuronal damage is sometimes mediated by cytotoxic T cells, and these syndromes are typically poorly responsive to immunomodulatory therapy. Conversely, antibodies against surface antigens are thought to be pathogenic—interfering with neuronal cell signaling or synaptic transmission. These antibodies are often associated with well-characterized central nervous system (CNS) syndromes, although their presence does not necessarily denote a malignancy. Some syndromes are responsive to immunomodulatory therapy, often with a correlation between antibody titers and outcome. Notably, there are many cases where a neurologic syndrome exists that is suspected to be paraneoplastic without the detection of any associated antibodies.

CLINICAL MANIFESTATIONS

Paraneoplastic syndromes encompass a broad range of clinical manifestations. Onset is typically acute (as in paraneoplastic cerebellar degeneration) or subacute. There are some symptoms that are almost always associated with a malignancy (Lambert–Eaton myasthenic syndrome, cerebellar degeneration, and opsoclonus–myoclonus as examples) and others that may occur without malignancy (encephalitides, sensory neuropathies). Discussed in the following text are some of the most well-recognized symptoms of paraneoplastic syndromes (Table 104.1).

ENCEPHALITIS/MYELITIS

Encephalitis and *myelitis* are terms used to describe inflammation of the CNS, ranging from the cerebrum to the spinal cord. When limbic structures are affected, there is a characteristic set of manifestations referred to as *limbic encephalitis*. Brain stem encephalitis may also occur resulting in bulbar symptoms. Myelitis may cause focal neurologic deficits localizable to the spinal cord. When more than one area is affected in the setting of likely malignancy, this is referred to as *paraneoplastic encephalomyelitis*.

Paraneoplastic Encephalomyelitis

Paraneoplastic encephalomyelitis (PEM) is a multifocal inflammatory disorder that can result in a variety of syndromes, which can occur in isolation or in various combinations. The cause is disseminated neuronal loss and inflammatory lesions of the nervous system. Common features are limbic encephalitis, myelitis, cerebellar ataxia, sensory neuropathies, and autonomic failure. Symptoms can be associated with almost any cancer but the majority are in patients with SCLC. The most common antibodies are anti-Hu, anti-CV2/CRMP5, and antiamphiphysin. The syndrome is poorly responsive to treatment although can stabilize or sometimes improve with tumor therapy.

Limbic Encephalitis

Limbic encephalitis manifests as rapidly progressive personality and mood changes and within weeks is dominated by delirium and dementia with severe memory loss, often accompanied by seizures. The psychiatric symptoms may be confused with a primary

TABLE 104.1 Paraneoplastic Syndromes, Associated Cancers, and Antibodies

Syndrome	Frequent Associated Tumors	Frequent Associated Antibodies
PEM	SCLC, thymoma, breast	Anti-Hu (ANNA-1), anti-CV2/CRMP5, antiamphiphysin
Limbic encephalitis	SCLC, testicular cancer, teratoma, thymoma, breast	Anti-Hu (ANNA-1), anti-CV2/CRMP5, antiamphiphysin, **anti-VGKC**, anti-Ma2 (Ta), **anti-NMDAR, anti-AMPAR, anti-GABABR**
Paraneoplastic cerebellar degeneration	Ovarian, breast, SCLC, Hodgkin lymphoma	Anti-Yo (PCA-1), anti-Ri (ANNA-2), anti-Hu (ANNA-1), anti-CV2/CRMP5, anti-Tr
Sensory neuronopathy	SCLC, breast	Anti-Hu (ANNA-1), anti-CV2/CRMP5
Opsoclonus–myoclonus	Neuroblastoma, SCLC, breast cancer, ovarian cancer	Anti-Ri (ANNA-2)
Retinopathies	SCLC, melanoma	Antirecoverin, antiretinal bipolar cell, anti-CV2/CRMP5
LEMS	Thymoma, SCLC	**Anti-VGCC**, anti-SOX-1
Stiff person syndrome	SCLC, breast cancer, thymoma, Hodgkin lymphoma, adenocarcinoma	Anti-GAD, antiamphiphysin, anti-Ri (ANNA-2)

Bold antibodies are directed against cell surface antigens.

PEM, paraneoplastic encephalomyelitis; SCLC, small cell lung cancer; LEMS, Lambert–Eaton myasthenic syndrome.

psychiatric syndrome. Symptoms may be part of PEM and can be associated with brain stem findings or sensory neuropathy. Cerebrospinal fluid (CSF) often reveals pleocytosis with elevated protein. Limbic encephalitis is one of the only paraneoplastic diseases in which imaging may be useful in establishing the diagnosis because increased T2 signal or mild enhancement of the medial temporal lobes on magnetic resonance imaging (MRI) is often seen. Tissue evaluation frequently reveals neuronal loss, perivascular infiltration by leukocytes, and microglial proliferation.

The most common associated cancers are SCLC (associated with anti-Hu), testicular germ cell tumors (associated with anti-Ma2), and teratomas (anti–N-methyl-D-aspartate [NMDA] receptor). Antibodies in limbic encephalitis may be targeted against intracellular antigens (anti-Hu, anti-Ma2, anti-CV2/CRMP5), in which case immune response is mediated by cytotoxic T-cell mechanisms and response to treatment is often poor. If an associated malignancy is discovered, the most effective treatment tends to be cancer-directed therapy. Encephalitides associated with antibodies against cell surface antigens tend to be reversible and responsive to immunomodulatory therapy (anti-NMDA receptor, anti–voltage-gated potassium channel [VGKC]). In some cases, there is no associated malignancy and these cases are often particularly responsive to treatment.

Brain stem Encephalitis

Symptoms of brain stem encephalitis are usually part of a more widespread encephalomyelitis in the anti-Hu syndrome, but bulbar symptoms with cranial nerve dysfunction may be the first manifestation. It can also occur as an isolated syndrome in lung and other cancers associated with the anti-Ma antibody. Common findings are oculomotor disorders including nystagmus and supranuclear vertical gaze palsy, as well as hearing loss, dysarthria, dysphagia, and abnormal respiration. Movement disorders may be prominent.

Myelitis

Spinal cord symptoms evolve over days or weeks with clinical evidence of a focal lesion. Symptoms may be monophasic or relapsing and are often associated with other neurologic symptoms of encephalomyelitis. Some patients have severe isolated myelopathy

with T2 changes on MRI and faint enhancement. Antiamphiphysin and anti-CV2/CRMP5 antibodies have been described, typically in the setting of SCLC or breast cancer. CSF may show pleocytosis with high protein content and normal sugar; oligoclonal bands may be present.

PARANEOPLASTIC CEREBELLAR DEGENERATION

Paraneoplastic cerebellar degeneration (PCD) is almost always associated with malignancy. Symptoms manifest as a pancerebellar syndrome with ataxia of gait and limbs, dysarthria, nystagmus, and oscillopsia. PCD can be the presenting symptom of PEM and as such can be associated with bulbar symptoms, corticospinal tract signs, dementia, and peripheral neuropathy. Differential diagnosis may include viral encephalitis, multiple sclerosis, Creutzfeldt–Jakob disease, alcoholic cerebellar degeneration, and hereditary spinocerebellar atrophy. CSF may reveal a modest pleocytosis with high protein content with elevated immunoglobulin G (IgG) and oligoclonal bands. Computer tomography (CT) and MRI are usually normal but occasionally, diffuse hyperintensity of the cerebellum on T2-weighted images or contrast enhancement of the folia can be seen. Over time, diffuse cerebellar atrophy can occur. On autopsy, there is a loss of Purkinje cells and the dentate nucleus may also be affected. PCD is most often associated with anti-Yo antibodies in gynecologic cancers, anti-Hu antibodies with SCLC, anti-Tr with Hodgkin disease, or anti-Ri with breast cancers. Cases in which cerebellar symptoms progress to PEM are typically associated with anti-Hu or anti-CV2/CRMP5 antibodies in SCLC. Often, there may be no antibody detected. Prognosis of PCD is poor and most patients do not improve due to early and irreversible neuronal destruction. If a patient is diagnosed while symptoms are still progressing, immunosuppression may stabilize the course. Onset is typically rapid.

SENSORY NEURONOPATHY

Sensory neuronopathy is generally subacute in onset and results in the progressive loss of all sensory modalities as a result of inflammatory or autoimmune-mediated destruction of the dorsal root ganglia. The first symptom is often a painful neuropathy that frequently progresses to result in a severe sensory ataxia. Motor function is spared or minimally affected. The pattern is often asymmetric and may affect cranial nerves, unlike more common peripheral neuropathies. Symptoms may be associated with a number of cancers but SCLC with anti-Hu antibodies in the context of PEM is the most common. Patients may experience partial improvement with steroids. Tumors responsive to treatment have been associated with improvement in symptoms.

OPSOCLONUS–MYOCLONUS

The term *opsoclonus–myoclonus* implies chaotic motion of the eyes—arrhythmic, irregular in direction, or tempo, with associated myoclonic muscle movements. The disordered physiology is not clear. In children, findings are associated with neuroblastoma and may portend a better oncologic prognosis. Symptoms respond to treatment of the tumor and directed immunotherapy although long term; these children are noted to struggle with speech and motor delays, cognitive deficits, and behavioral problems. In adults, symptoms range across a broad spectrum from opsoclonus with mild truncal ataxia to severe symptoms of opsoclonus, myoclonus, and ataxia that can progress to encephalopathy and death. Opsoclonus may be associated with tumors of the breast or gynecologic malignancies with anti-Ri antibodies although in many cases, antibodies are not well classified. In both children and adults, opsoclonus–myoclonus is due to a paraneoplastic process in only a minority of patients and other etiologies should be considered. Paraneoplastic opsoclonus–myoclonus is among the paraneoplastic syndromes that are most responsive to treatment.

VISUAL SYMPTOMS

The most common causes of visual symptoms in patients with malignancy are metastatic infiltration of the optic nerves or neurotoxicity from chemotherapy and radiation. Paraneoplastic causes include cancer-associated retinopathy (CAR) and melanoma-associated retinopathy (MAR). CAR can occur with any solid tumor but is most commonly associated with SCLC. More than 20 antibodies have been described but the most common is an antibody to recoverin (a calcium-binding photoreceptor protein). MAR is associated with antibodies that react with the bipolar cells of the retina. Onset of symptoms typically occurs months to years after diagnosis. Diagnosis is made with an electroretinogram and supported by antibody studies. CAR and MAR are difficult to treat and have poor response to immunotherapy although there are case reports of improvement with intravenous immunoglobulin (IVIG), plasmapheresis, and tumor treatment.

Paraneoplastic optic neuropathy causes subacute, painless, and bilateral visual loss. Examination may reveal papilledema or optic atrophy. Symptoms may occur in the context of PEM. Bilateral diffuse uveal melanocytic proliferation (BDUMP) is the result of diffuse proliferation of melanocytes in the uveal tract and causes bilateral vision loss. Symptoms typically precede a cancer diagnosis and have been described in carcinomas of the reproductive tract (in women) or of the lung and pancreas (in men). Corticosteroids are typically ineffective, and radiation may worsen symptoms.

MOTOR NEURON DISEASE

When cancer and motor neuron disease occur together, it is usually a coincidence of two common illnesses in the elderly. Epidemiologic studies have not definitively shown increased incidence of cancer in amyotrophic lateral sclerosis (ALS) patients. However, some patients have neurologic symptoms that disappear with treatment

of the tumor. Also, there have been more than 60 reports of patients with motor neuron and lymphoproliferative disease. Lower motor neuron signs (amyotrophy) including fasciculations are also sometimes seen in combination with PEM and anti-Hu antibodies. A purely upper motor neuron syndrome (primary lateral sclerosis) has been reported in women with breast cancer, but several of those patients later developed lower motor neuron signs and the disorder became typical ALS.

SENSORIMOTOR PERIPHERAL NEUROPATHY

Sensorimotor peripheral neuropathy with or without slow conduction velocity is common after age 50 years. In cancer patients in particular, treatment with neurotoxic chemotherapies can result in distal and symmetric symptoms. Paraneoplastic syndromes rarely can result in a similar presentation. Prominent features may include stocking-glove paresthesias and sensory loss, distal limb weakness, or both. Autonomic failure may be prominent with disorders of gastrointestinal motility, especially diarrhea or pseudo-obstruction. Cranial symptoms are lacking. The syndrome is typically slow in evolution and may respond to immunotherapy. Among the diverse causes are anti–myelin-associated glycoprotein (MAG) paraproteinemic peripheral neuropathy associated with Waldenström macroglobulinemia and paraneoplastic neuropathy. Vasculitis is found in some acute neuropathies and can result in proximal muscle weakness.

Sensory symptoms that are asymmetric or affect cranial nerves should raise the question of leptomeningeal spread, although sensory neuronopathy in PEM can present similarly. Mononeuropathies or plexopathies raise the possibility of metastatic infiltration of the nerves or plexuses.

NEUROMUSCULAR DISORDERS

The association of myasthenia gravis with thymoma is described in another chapter; myasthenia is not known to be associated with other malignancies. Lambert–Eaton myasthenic syndrome (LEMS) is associated with SCLC approximately two-thirds of the time, with malignancy frequently diagnosed 2 years after diagnosis of LEMS. Voltage-gated calcium channel (VGCC) antibodies are present in nearly all cases but do not differentiate between paraneoplastic and nonparaneoplastic cases. Sox1 antibody is also a marker of paraneoplastic LEMS. Treatment often involves a combination of treatment of cancer and immunosuppression. A 3,4-diaminopyrine increases the release of acetylcholine and results in neurologic improvement in many patients. Paraneoplastic neuromyotonia is associated most often with thymoma but also with SCLC or other tumors. Stiff person syndrome is manifest by limb muscle stiffness, rigidity, and muscle aches and spasms, developing over months. Approximately 80% of cases are paraneoplastic and the most common malignancies are breast cancer, SCLC, thymoma, and Hodgkin lymphoma. Associated antibodies are anti–glutamic acid decarboxylase (GAD) and antiamphiphysin.

MYOPATHIES

About 20% of patients with dermatomyositis starting after age 40 years have an associated tumor, which can be of almost any type. Whether there is a higher than expected association of tumor with polymyositis has not been proven.

DIAGNOSIS

Diagnosis of a paraneoplastic syndrome is not always simple and often requires a high level of suspicion based on a clinical history

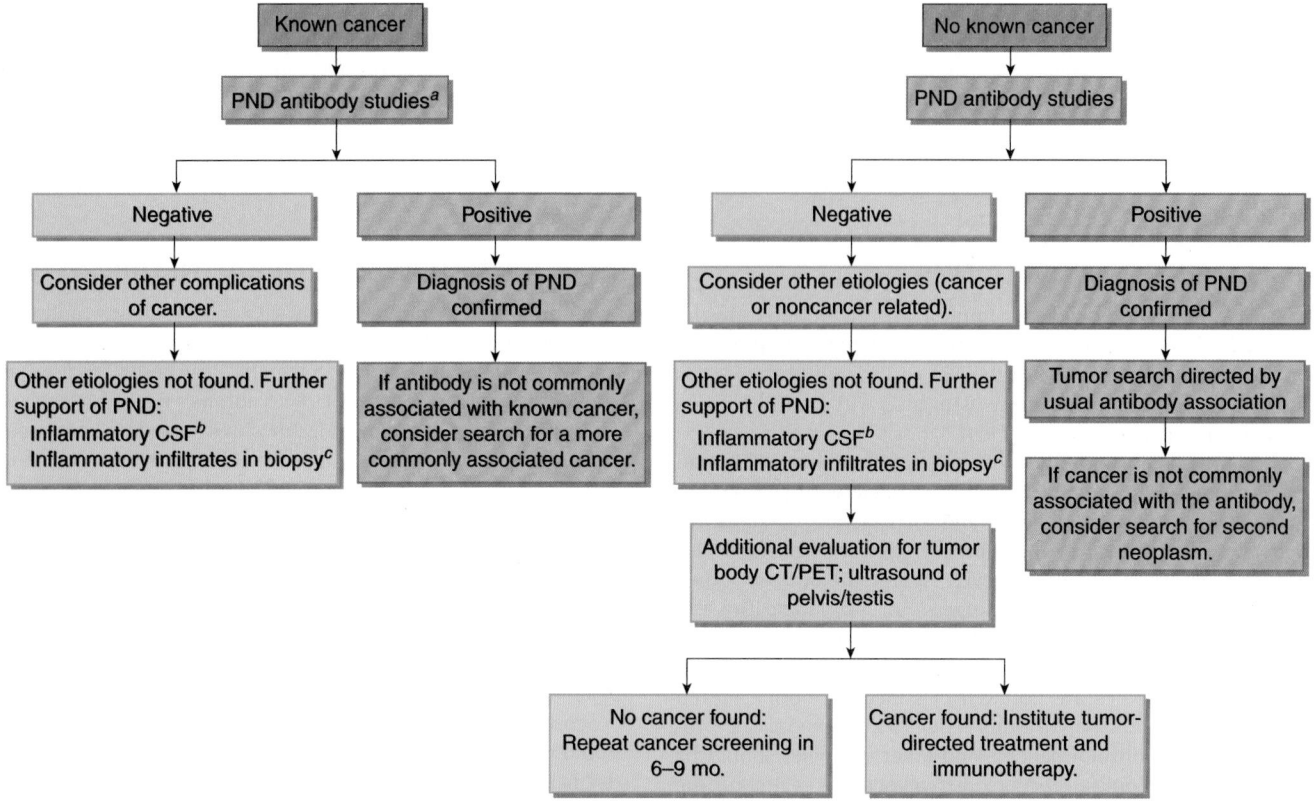

FIGURE 104.1 Diagnostic approach in a patient with a suspected paraneoplastic neurologic disorder. [a]PND antibody studies refer to well-characterized paraneoplastic antibodies. [b]CSF inflammatory changes include lymphocytic pleocytosis, elevated IgG index, and oligoclonal band with or without elevated protein concentration. [c]Biopsy should be directed to symptomatic area of the nervous system (clinical or by MRI). PND, paraneoplastic neurologic disorder; CSF, cerebrospinal fluid; CT, computed tomography; PET, positron emission tomography. (Adapted from Dalmau J. Rosenfeld MR. Paraneoplastic syndromes of the CNS. *Lancet Neurol.* 2008;7:327–340.)

of subacute neurologic dysfunction. In some cases, the diagnosis of malignancy has already been made but frequently, symptoms of paraneoplastic syndromes antedate the diagnosis of a cancer. CSF may be normal or may demonstrate elevated protein or pleocytosis. CSF sugar content is almost always normal; hypoglycorrhachia (low sugar) in a patient with malignancy suggests meningeal spread of tumor cells. MRI is usually normal and may or may not show subtle abnormalities of white or gray mater. The diagnosis of peripheral neuropathy depends in part on the demonstration of conduction abnormalities, and LEMS is virtually defined by the demonstration of an incrementing response to repetitive nerve stimulation. Ideally, the diagnosis of a paraneoplastic syndrome is established by demonstrating a specific antibody in a patient with a characteristic syndrome. Commercial tests for paraneoplastic panels are testable in serum and CSF. If the CNS is affected, tests performed on CSF may be more sensitive because high antibody titers result from intrathecal synthesis. The presence of an antibody is not always confirmed—if a paraneoplastic syndrome is suspected, the lack of a diagnostic antibody should not preclude diagnosis and malignancy workup may still need to be pursued (Fig. 104.1).

DETECTION OF CANCER

If a paraneoplastic syndrome is highly suspected or confirmed with an antibody screen in the absence of a known malignancy,

patients should undergo thorough cancer screening. Identification of a particular antibody may guide workup based on the associated cancer. If there is no identified antibody, a thorough cancer screen should be performed with whole body positron emission tomography (PET), mammography, pelvic ultrasound, testicular ultrasound, body CT, or MRI. If an underlying malignancy is not found, it is recommended that patients undergo regular cancer screening, as malignancy can be found months or even years later.

TREATMENT

The mainstay of treatment in paraneoplastic syndromes is cancer-targeted therapy. If no underlying malignancy is discovered but there is an identified antibody that has a strong association with a particular cancer type, surgical exploration or removal of the likely affected organ can be considered (e.g., orchiectomy in a patient with anti-Yo antibodies or oophorectomy with anti-NMDA). In cases in which an identified antibody is pathogenic, syndromes may be responsive to immunomodulatory therapies such as high-dose steroids, IVIG, and plasmapheresis. Peripheral disorders such as sensorimotor polyneuropathy, LEMS, and myasthenia gravis are particularly sensitive to this treatment. When these therapies fail, rituximab, cyclophosphamide, azathioprine, tacrolimus, or cyclosporine may be appropriate.

Concerns that immunosuppression in malignancy could favor tumor growth have remained unfounded and immunomodulatory therapy is typically well tolerated in patients receiving chemotherapy. Paraneoplastic syndromes that are likely mediated by T-cell mechanisms or have no identified pathogenic antibody tend to be poorly responsive to therapy of any type. In general, the best chance for optimal neurologic outcome is administration of treatment while the syndrome is progressing, as this may lead to stabilization of symptoms.

OUTCOME

Outcome in paraneoplastic syndromes is variable and depends on identification and treatment of the underlying malignancy and pathogenesis of the neurologic disorder. In some cases, such as PCD, neuronal damage is permanent and irreversible. Syndromes in which the identified antibody is known to be pathogenic are frequently responsive to immunomodulatory therapies.

SUGGESTED READINGS

Bataller L, Gaus F, Saiz A, et al. Clinical outcome in adult onset idiopathic or paraneoplastic opsoclonus-myoclonus. *Brian.* 2001;124:437–443.

Boronat A, Sabater L, Saiz A, et al. GABA(B) receptor antibodies in limbic encephalitis and anti-GAD associated neurologic disorders. *Neurology.* 2011;76: 795–800.

Cooper R, Khakoo Y, Matthay KK, et al. Opsoclonus-myoclonus-ataxia syndrome in neuroblastoma: histopathologic features—a report from the Children's Cancer Group. *Med Pediatr Oncol.* 2001;36:623–629.

Dalmau J, Gleichman AJ, Huges EG, et al. Anti-NMDA-receptor encephalitis: case series and analysis of the effects of antibodies. *Lancet Neurol.* 2008;7(12): 1091–1098.

Dalmau J, Rosenfeld MR. Paraneoplastic syndromes of the CNS. *Lancet Neurol.* 2008;7:327–340.

Dalmau J, Rosenfeld MR. Update on paraneoplastic neurologic disorders. *Oncologist.* 2010;15(6):603–617.

Darnell JC, Albert ML, Darnell RB. Cdr2, a target antigen of naturally occurring human tumor immunity, is widely expressed in gynecological tumors. *Cancer Res.* 2000;60:2136–2139.

Darnell RB. Paraneoplastic neurologic disorders: windows into neuronal function and tumor immunity. *Arch Neurol.* 2004;61:30–32.

Darnell RB, Posner JB. *Paraneoplastic Syndromes.* New York: Oxford University Press; 2011.

Darnell RB, Posner JB. Paraneoplastic syndromes involving the nervous system. *N Engl J Med.* 2003;349:1543–1554.

Didelot A, Honnorat J. Update on paraneoplastic neurological syndromes. *Curr Opin Neurol.* 2009;21:566–572.

Flanagan EP, McKeon A, Lennon VA, et al. Paraneoplastic isolated myelopathy: clinical course and neuroimaging clues. *Neurology.* 2011;76:2089–2095.

Giometto B, Grisold W, Vitaliani R, et al. Paraneoplastic neurologic syndrome in the PNS Euronetwork database: a European study from 20 centers. *Arch Neurol.* 2010;67(3):330–335.

Gordon PH, Rowland LP, Younger DS, et al. Lymphoproliferative disorders and motor neuron disease. *Ann Neurol.* 1997;48:1671–1678.

Graus F, Dalmau J. Paraneoplastic neurological syndromes. *Curr Opin Neurol.* 2012;25(6):795–801.

Graus F, Keime-Guibert F, Rene R, et al. Anti-Hu associated paraneoplastic encephalomyelitis: analysis of 200 patients. *Brain.* 2001;124:1138–1148.

Graus F, Saiz A, Dalmau J. Antibodies and neuronal autoimmune disorders of the CNS. *J Neurol.* 2010;257:509–517.

Gultekin SH, Rosenfeld MR, Voltz R, et al. Paraneoplastic limbic encephalitis: neurological symptoms, immunological findings and tumour association in 50 patients. *Brain.* 2000;123:1481–1494.

Hart IK, Maddison P, Newsom-Davis J, et al. Phenotypic variants of autoimmune peripheral nerve hyperexcitability. *Brain.* 2002;125(pt 8):1887–1895.

Hayward K, Jeremy RJ, Jenkins S, et al. Long-term neurobehavioral outcomes in children with neuroblastoma and opsoclonus-myoclonus-ataxia syndrome: relationship to MRI findings and anti-neuronal antibodies. *J Pediatr.* 2001;139: 552–559.

Hoffmann LA, Jarius S, Pellkofer HL, et al. Anti-Ma and anti-Ta associated paraneoplastic neurological syndromes: 22 newly diagnosed patients and review of previous cases. *J Neurol Neurosurg Psychiatry.* 2008;79(7): 767–773.

Jarius S, Hoffmann LA, Stich O, et al. Relative frequency of VGKC and "classical" paraneoplastic antibodies in patients with limbic encephalitis. *J Neurol.* 2008;255(7):1100–1101.

Ko MW, Dalmau J, Galetta SL. Neuro-ophthalmologic manifestations of paraneoplastic syndromes. *J Neuroophthalmol.* 2008;28(1):58–68.

Koike H, Tanaka F, Sobue G. Paraneoplastic neuropathy: wide-ranging clinicopathological manifestations. *Curr Opin Neurol.* 2011;24:504–551.

Lahrmann H, Albrecht G, Drlicek M, et al. Acquired neuromyotonia and peripheral neuropathy in a patient with Hodgkin's disease. *Muscle Nerve.* 2001;24: 834–838.

Lawn ND, Westmoreland BF, Kiely MJ, et al. Clinical, magnetic resonance imaging, and electroencephalographic findings in paraneoplastic limbic encephalitis. *Mayo Clinic Proc.* 2003;78:1363–1368.

McCabe DJ, Turner NC, Chao D, et al. Paraneoplastic "stiff person syndrome" with metastatic adenocarcinoma and anti-Ri antibodies. *Neurology.* 2004;62(8): 1402–1404.

Nagashima T, Mizutani Y, Kawahara H, et al. Anti-Hu paraneoplastic syndrome presenting with brainstem-cerebellar symptoms and Lambert-Eaton myasthenic syndrome. *Neuropathology.* 2003;23:230–238.

Posner JB, ed. *Neurologic Complications of Cancer.* Philadelphia: FA Davis; 1995: 353–385.

Rosenfeld MR, Dalmau J. Update on paraneoplastic neurologic disorders. *Oncologist.* 2010;15(6):603–617.

Rosenfeld MR, Eichen JG, Wade DF, et al. Molecular and clinical diversity in paraneoplastic immunity to Ma proteins. *Ann Neurol.* 2001;50:339–348.

Russo C, Cohn SL, Petruzzi MJ, et al. Long-term neurologic outcome in children with opsoclonus-myoclonus associated with neuroblastoma: a report from the Pediatric Oncology Group. *Med Pediatri Oncol.* 1997;28: 284–288.

Stockton D, Doherty VR, Brewster DH. Risk of cancer in patients with dermatomyositis or polymyositis, and follow-up implications: a Scottish population-based cohort study. *Br J Cancer.* 2001;85:41–45.

Thomas L, Kwok Y, Edelman MJ. Management of paraneoplastic syndromes in lung cancer. *Curr Treat Options Oncol.* 2004;5:51–62.

Titulaer MJ, Lang B, Verschuuren JJ. Lambert-Eaton myasthenic syndrome: from clinical characteristics to therapeutic strategies. *Lance Neurol.* 2011;10: 1098–1107.

Titulaer MJ, Soffietti R, Dalmau J, et al. Screening for tumours in paraneoplastic neurological syndromes: report of an EFNS Task Force. *Eur J Neurol.* 2011;18(1):19–e3.

Toothaker T, Rubin M. Paraneoplastic neurological syndromes. *Neurologist.* 2009;15:21–33.

Vernino S, Lennon VA. Ion channel and striational antibodies define a continuum of autoimmune neuromuscular hyperexcitability. *Muscle Nerve.* 2002;26: 702–707.

Vincent A, Bien CG. Anti-NMDA-receptor encephalitis: a cause of psychiatric, seizure, and movement disorders in young adults. *Lancet Neurol.* 2008;12: 1074–1075.

Wakabayashi K, Horikawa Y, Oyake M, et al. Sporadic motor neuron disease with severe sensory neuronopathy. *Acta Neuropathol.* 1998;95:426–430.

Jasmin Jo and David Schiff

INTRODUCTION

Neurologic complications of cancer therapy are relatively common and may be disabling. Understanding these complications may mitigate or halt progression of injury to the nervous system through early recognition and prompt management. In this chapter, we will discuss neurotoxicities associated with the various agents used in the treatment of cancer.

NEUROLOGIC COMPLICATIONS OF RADIOTHERAPY

Cranial and spinal radiation used to treat primary or secondary central nervous system (CNS) tumors as well as for prophylaxis in certain systemic malignancies is a recognized cause of neurologic complications. The cranial and peripheral nerves are also vulnerable to adverse effects when included in the radiation field for CNS or non-CNS tumors. The risk for radiation injury increases with higher total dose and fractions, larger treatment volume, and coadministration of chemotherapy. Patients younger than 10 and older than 70 years old are more susceptible to complications of radiotherapy (RT).

PATHOBIOLOGY

Tissue injury from RT is categorized in sequential stages: acute (<1 month), early-delayed (1 to 6 months), and late-delayed reactions (>6 months). The timing is helpful in predicting reversibility of tissue damage. Capillary injury and leakiness leading to edema is the mechanism during acute injury. Late injury is generally associated with permanent tissue damage. In the brain and spinal cord, the proposed mechanism for late effects is a combination of vascular injury involving the small- and medium-sized vessels,

demyelination with loss of oligodendrocytes, and immunologic response to antigens released from damaged glial cells. The pathologic end state is radiation necrosis, involving coagulation necrosis and gross demyelination. Tissue atrophy is seen upon long-term follow-up. Table 105.1 summarizes RT injuries and their corresponding manifestations based on location.

CLINICAL MANIFESTATIONS AND DIAGNOSIS

Brain

Acute encephalopathy, consisting of somnolence, headache, nausea, vomiting, and exacerbation of preexisting deficits, usually develops days after initiation of RT and generally responds to corticosteroids. No specific neuroimaging findings are associated with acute injury. Early-delayed complications include the somnolence syndrome, characterized by drowsiness, fatigue, anorexia, irritability, and transitory cognitive disturbances primarily affecting attention and short-term memory. Neuroimaging at this time may be unchanged or show increased edema and contrast enhancement within the tumor bed that mimics tumor progression, termed *pseudoprogression* (Fig. 105.1). The exact frequency with which this phenomenon occurs is difficult to estimate because of varying criteria defined in different reports. However, it occurs in at least 10% to 20% of patients with glioblastoma receiving concurrent RT and temozolomide; it manifests most commonly 1 to 3 months posttreatment (although may occur later) and usually improves within a few months. Late injury is associated with focal radionecrosis (causing seizures, focal neurologic symptoms, and signs of increased intracranial pressure) and leukoencephalopathy (leading to cognitive dysfunction and severe dementia). Diffuse white matter changes and atrophy are seen in the neuroimaging in nearly all cases. Magnetic resonance imaging (MRI) does not distinguish between radiation necrosis and tumor progression. Metabolic and

---

TABLE 105.1 Neurologic Complications of Radiotherapy

| Type | Onset | Pathology | Symptoms according to Sites | | | |
			Brain	Spinal Cord	Cranial Nerves	Peripheral Nerves
Acute	<1 mo	BBB disruption Edema	Acute encephalopathy Pseudoprogression	—	—	Paresthesia
Early-delayed	1–6 mo	Edema Demyelination	Somnolence syndrome Transient cognitive impairment Pseudoprogression	Lhermitte sign	Painless visual loss Tongue weakness Hearing loss Anosmia	Transient plexopathy Pain
Late-delayed	>6 mo	Vascular injury Demyelination Necrosis Cellular loss	Focal radionecrosis Leukoencephalopathy Cognitive impairment Dementia	Brown-Séquard syndrome Spastic paraplegia	Hearing loss Visual loss Lower CN palsies	Irreversible plexopathy Myokymia on EMG

BBB, blood–brain barrier; CN, cranial nerves; EMG, electromyography.

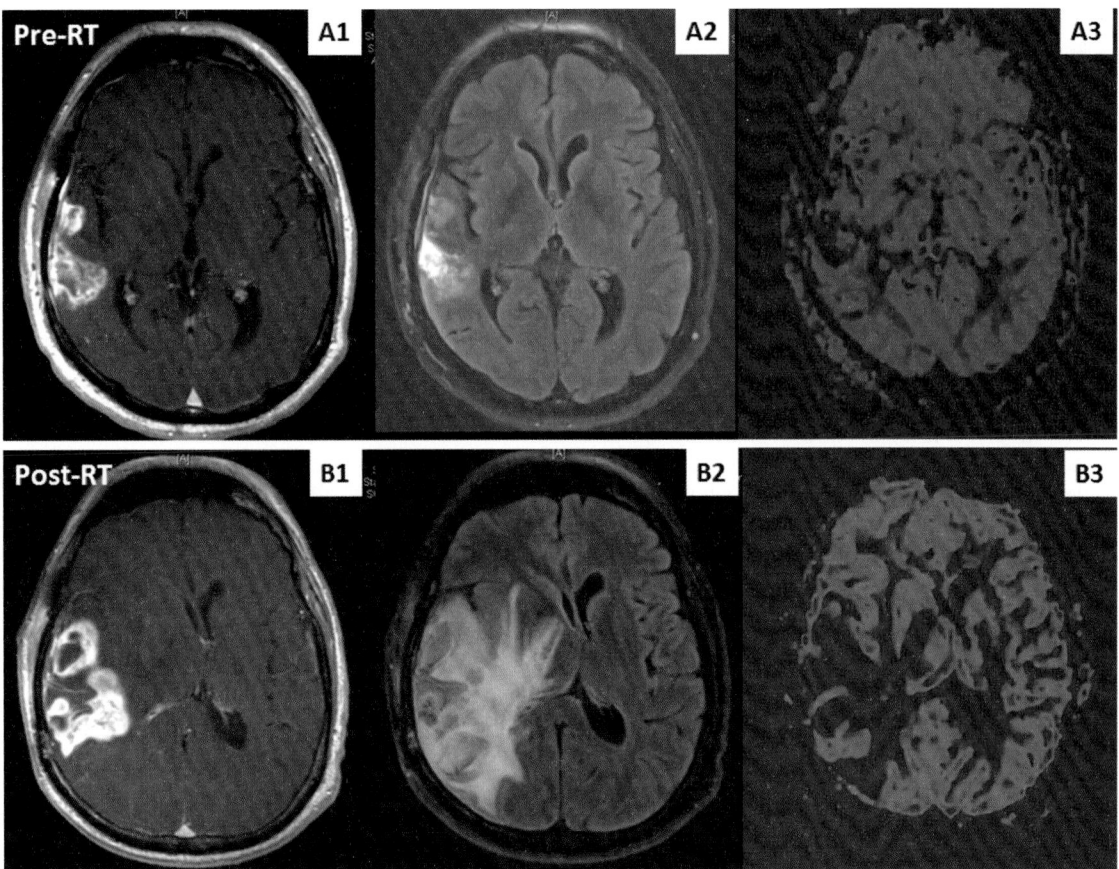

FIGURE 105.1 Pseudoprogression in a 52-year-old man with right temporal glioblastoma, methylguanine-DNA methyltransferase (MGMT) methylated. **A:** Pretreatment MRI showed nodular enhancement along the surgical cavity **(A1)** in the right temporal lobe with minimal surrounding fluid-attenuated inversion recovery (FLAIR) signal abnormality **(A2)**. No elevated cerebral blood volume noted in the perfusion study **(A3)**. **B:** Repeat MRI 4 weeks after concurrent radiotherapy and temozolomide demonstrated significant increase in the size of the irregularly enhancing mass **(B1)** associated with increase in surrounding FLAIR signal abnormality with mass effect **(B2)** without evidence of elevated cerebral blood volume **(B3)**. The patient underwent second resection and pathology revealed reactive changes, scattered atypical cells, and thickened vessels consistent with radiation treatment effects.

perfusion imaging studies may help discriminate the two entities, but surgery remains the gold standard to confirm the diagnosis.

Spinal Cord

Radiation-induced damage to the spinal cord is categorized into early-delayed (6 weeks to 6 months) and late-delayed (>6 months) myelopathy. Acute worsening should prompt investigation for intratumoral hemorrhage or tumor progression. Early-delayed RT myelopathy is characterized clinically by Lhermitte sign that typically resolves spontaneously, with no distinctive imaging finding. Patients with late-delayed radiation myelopathy often presents with Brown-Séquard syndrome, spastic paraplegia with impaired sensory and autonomic functions. The condition may begin abruptly or insidiously and is most often irreversible. MRI demonstrates increase T2 hyperintensity and enhancement in the affected spinal cord levels.

Peripheral Nervous System

Any cranial nerves may be involved if included in the radiation field. The hypoglossal nerve is the most vulnerable followed by the vagus nerve and the recurrent laryngeal nerve, believed to be due to absorption of higher amount of energy from RT to the neck region.

Optic neuropathy results in painless and progressive visual loss or visual field constriction. The oculomotor, trochlear, trigeminal, abducens, and facial nerves are less vulnerable and can be affected from focal RT for skull base tumors. Trigeminal neuropathy is quite rare and may result from radiosurgery for vestibular schwannoma and trigeminal neuralgia. Radiation-induced injury to vestibulocochlear nerve is rare, except in RT for acoustic neuroma. Hearing impairment, especially at high frequency, may be due to changes in the cochlea and/or retrocochlear auditory pathway. Permanent damage to cranial nerves is rare and usually occurs due to delayed effect.

RT-induced brachial and lumbosacral plexopathies may result from treatment of breast, lung, and pelvic cancers. The usual presentation includes paresthesia and hypesthesia, followed by weakness and amyotrophy. Pain is usually relatively mild and occurs late in the course, as opposed to severe pain in patients with malignant plexopathy. Myokymia seen on electromyography and hypointensity in T1- and T2-weighted sequences and absence of mass on MRI suggest RT plexopathy.

Indirect Complications to Nervous System

RT can indirectly cause endocrine dysfunction such as hypothalamic–pituitary impairment resulting in hypothyroidism, hypogonadism, hyperprolactinemia, and panhypopituitarism; vascular damage leading to stroke, hemorrhage, vascular malformations, and rarely, SMART syndrome (stroke-like migraine attacks after radiation therapy); and secondary tumors such as meningioma, glioma, and sarcoma.

TREATMENT AND PREVENTION

Corticosteroid (dexamethasone, intravenous [IV] or oral, initially at 16 mg/day) generally reverses symptoms from acute and early-delayed injuries but has variable benefit in radiation necrosis. Anti–vascular endothelial growth factor (VEGF) agents such as bevacizumab (10 mg/kg every 2 weeks or 7.5 mg/kg every 3 weeks IV) have demonstrated beneficial effects in patients with cerebral radiation necrosis. In rare occasions, surgical resection of cerebral radiation necrosis is indicated, providing both therapeutic and diagnostic benefits. The use of memantine at 20 mg/day within 3 days of initiating RT for 24 weeks results in delayed time to cognitive decline and reduced rate of decline in memory, executive function, and processing speed in patients with brain metastases receiving whole brain RT [**Level 1**].[1] Hippocampal sparing during brain RT may also reduce the incidence of neurocognitive injury. Pain management and physical therapy are important aspects in the management of RT-induced plexopathy. Hyperbaric oxygen and anticoagulation may ameliorate the effects of radiation necrosis, but their efficacy is limited.

OUTCOME

Recovery of symptoms is typically expected in acute and early-delayed RT injuries. However, delayed complications of RT are progressive and irreversible, leading to poor outcome and quality of life for long-term survivors.

NEUROLOGIC COMPLICATIONS OF CHEMOTHERAPY

Cytotoxic chemotherapeutic agents may cause toxic effects to the peripheral and central nervous system, often leading to reduction or cessation of treatment. The severity depends on the treatment dose, duration, route, existing comorbidities, and coadministration of other neurotoxic agents.

PATHOBIOLOGY

The mechanism of chemotherapy-induced peripheral neuropathy (CIPN) depends on the cytotoxic agents used. Antimitotic agents, such as vinca alkaloids and taxanes, disrupt microtubule-based axonal transport leading to length-dependent axonal injury. Platinum agents such as cisplatin cause neuropathy by apoptosis of sensory neurons in dorsal root ganglion, whereas oxaliplatin additionally causes transient Na-gated channel dysfunction resulting in altered nerve excitability, particularly refractoriness. Despite the presence of the blood–brain barrier (BBB), the CNS remains susceptible to neurotoxicity effects if the protective barrier is breached by direct effects of tumor through endothelium damage or by RT, if the agent crosses the intact BBB, or if the agents are administered directly to the cerebrospinal fluid (CSF) or into the cerebral vasculature. Chemotherapy can also cause damage to neural progenitor cells responsible for neurogenesis and maintenance of white matter integrity.

CLINICAL MANIFESTATIONS

Central Nervous System

Chemotherapy agents such as ifosfamide, high-dose methotrexate, and procarbazine can cause acute toxicities occurring during or few days after treatment, characterized by confusion, hallucination,

seizures, and drowsiness. A cerebellar syndrome may develop from high-dose cytarabine. Intrathecal (IT) methotrexate and cytarabine can cause aseptic meningitis and myelopathy. IT vincristine causes severe neurotoxicity that is nearly always fatal and must be avoided. Posterior reversible encephalopathy syndrome (PRES), manifesting as acute or subacute onset of headache, seizures, confusion, and visual changes, has been reported from cisplatin, cyclophosphamide, high-dose corticosteroids, and gemcitabine. Chronic leukoencephalopathy, characterized by progressive personality change, dementia, ataxia, and incontinence, may occur months to years following methotrexate, especially when given during or soon after whole brain RT. Therefore, whole brain RT should be administered after systemic or IT methotrexate.

Peripheral Nervous System

CIPN typically presents with symmetric distal paresthesia, loss of proprioception and vibratory sense, and loss of ankle reflexes. Distal motor weakness and autonomic dysfunction including atonic bladder, impotence, and orthostatic hypotension may also occur with certain agents (Table 105.2). Vestibulocochlear toxicity, with hearing loss, vertigo, and ataxia, is associated with cisplatin. Acute cold-induced dysesthesia involving the distal extremities, throat, mouth, or face occur commonly with oxaliplatin.

DIAGNOSIS

In acute CNS syndromes, the brain MRI may be unremarkable or demonstrate edema. Diffuse white matter disease, cortical–subcortical atrophy, and ventricular dilation are typical imaging findings in chronic leukoencephalopathy. Nerve conduction studies in CIPN may demonstrate decreased sensory nerve action potential, prolonged latencies, and delayed conduction velocities. For classic presentations of CIPN, diagnostic testing is not usually required. Identification and treatment of coexisting conditions that cause peripheral neuropathy, such as diabetes, alcohol abuse, and vitamin B_{12} deficiency, is imperative in the management of CIPN. Paraneoplastic neuropathy should be distinguished from CIPN, as treatment involves further cancer-directed treatment. Patients with small cell lung cancer may develop a subacute sensory paraneoplastic neuropathy associated with anti-Hu antibodies.

TABLE 105.2	Peripheral Nervous System Toxicities from Cytotoxic and Targeted Agents
Neuropathic Syndromes	**Agents**
Acute sensory dysesthesia	Oxaliplatin, ifosfamide, cytarabine (rare)
Chronic pure sensory neuropathy	Cisplatin, oxaliplatin, carboplatin, docetaxel, procarbazine, etoposide, bortezomib, thalidomide
Chronic sensorimotor neuropathy	Vincristine, vinorelbine, nelarabine, paclitaxel, ixabepilone, etoposide, fludarabine, 5-fluorouracil, procarbazine, bortezomib, thalidomide (rare)
Chronic autonomic neuropathy	Vincristine, thalidomide, ixabepilone (rare)
Vestibulocochlear toxicity	Cisplatin

TREATMENT AND PREVENTION

Most patients who develop acute CNS syndromes recover within a few days with supportive treatment. Methylene blue may be effective in treatment (50 mg IV 6× per day) or prophylaxis (50 mg, IV or oral, 4× per day) of ifosfamide-induced encephalopathy. Discontinuation of the offending agent is indicated if a patient experience acute myelopathy or cerebellar syndromes. There are no effective treatments for neurocognitive toxicities. Erythropoietin (40,000 units weekly), methylphenidate (10 mg twice daily), modafinil (200 to 400 mg/day), and cholinesterase inhibitors such as donepezil (5 to 10 mg/day), nonsteroidal anti-inflammatory agents (i.e., aspirin 100 mg daily), as well as cognitive rehabilitation have been studied but no definite recommendations can be made.

Dose-reduction or discontinuation of chemotherapeutic agents causing CIPN usually improves the symptoms. Antiepileptic agents, tricyclic antidepressants, serotonin–norepinephrine reuptake inhibitors (SNRI), opioids, and topical local anesthetics may provide symptomatic relief of CIPN (Table 105.3) [**Level 1**].[2] Neuroprotective agents have been used to prevent or limit neurotoxicity. However, calcium and magnesium infusion (1 g of each given immediately before and after each dose of oxaliplatin) did not substantially decrease oxaliplatin-induced sensory neurotoxicity in a recent phase III randomized controlled trial [**Level 1**].[3] Some nutritional supplements may worsen rather than improve CIPN [**Level 1**].[4]

OUTCOMES

Acute CNS toxicities usually resolve within few days with supportive treatments. Chronic leukoencephalopathy are often progressive and irreversible. CIPN most often resolves on appropriate dose reduction or discontinuation of the offending agents. However, worsening of peripheral neuropathy ("coasting") may occur for a few months after cessation of treatment (e.g., cisplatin, thalidomide), preventing timely discontinuation of treatment.

NEUROLOGIC COMPLICATIONS OF BIOLOGIC AGENTS

MONOCLONAL ANTIBODIES

Bevacizumab, a humanized antibody against VEGF, increases the risk of thromboembolic stroke and intracranial hemorrhage and may cause PRES and rarely, optic neuropathy. Discontinuation

of the drug, management of hypertension, and appropriate supportive care are recommended. Rituximab, a chimeric monoclonal antibody (MAb) against CD20 antigen found on the surface of normal and malignant B lymphocytes, may cause headache, myalgia, paresthesia, dizziness, and rarely, progressive multifocal leukoencephalopathy and PRES.

TARGETED MOLECULAR AGENTS

Small molecule protein kinase inhibitors target both membrane-bound and intracellular molecules and interfere with corresponding enzymatic activities. Most agents have minimal neurotoxicity such as headache and dizziness. Mild visual disturbance is seen in 45% of patients receiving crizotinib (ALK and c-MET inhibitor). Bortezomib (proteasome inhibitor) causes a length-dependent, painful, small-fiber sensory axonal neuropathy, which occurs in about 35% of patients and can be dose limiting. Nerve conduction study is consistent with small-fiber sensory neuropathy but may also be normal. Symptoms improve with discontinuation or dose reduction of the offending agent. Lower rates of neuropathy are observed with newer proteasome inhibitor such as carfilzomib.

IMMUNOTHERAPY

Immunomodulatory agents stimulate the immune system by administration of proinflammatory cytokines such as interferon and interleukin to boost the immune system to attack cancer cells. Neurotoxicity associated with these agents tends to be dose-related. Neurologic adverse effects from ipilimumab, a human MAb that blocks cytotoxic T-lymphocytes antigen-4 used to treat melanoma, includes inflammatory myopathy, aseptic meningitis, severe meningoradiculoneuritis, temporal arteritis, and Guillain–Barré syndrome. Pituitary failure can also lead to metabolic encephalopathy associated with various endocrinopathies. Chronic inflammatory demyelinating polyneuropathy, transverse myelitis and concurrent myositis, and myasthenia gravis–type syndrome have also been reported with ipilimumab. Discontinuation of the drug and administration of high-dose IV steroids (methylprednisolone 125 mg IV for 3 days) or plasmapheresis (three to five sessions) are recommended, which generally improve neurologic symptoms within 2 weeks. Neuropsychiatric symptoms, most commonly depression, encephalopathy, hallucination, and seizures, are frequently reported with interferon-α (IFN-α). These symptoms usually improve after discontinuation of therapy, although permanent dementia and persistent vegetative state have been reported. Interleukin-2 (IL-2) crosses the BBB, causing direct toxicity to the neurons and glial cells. Transient encephalopathy and neurocognitive symptoms may develop toward the end of therapy and resolve within hours to days after discontinuation of treatment.

NEUROLOGIC COMPLICATIONS OF HEMATOPOIETIC STEM CELL TRANSPLANTATION

HSCT is commonly used for treatment of leukemias and lymphomas. The myeloablative doses of chemotherapy sometimes result in neurotoxicity not encountered with conventional doses, including seizures with busulfan; encephalopathy with ifosfamide, melphalan, etoposide, and thiotepa; and neuropathy with carboplatin, cyclophosphamide, and etoposide. Intracerebral hemorrhage due to thrombocytopenia from bone marrow suppression can also be encountered. Immunosuppressant agents such as calcineurin inhibitors cyclosporine and tacrolimus and muromonab-3 (OKT3)

TABLE 105.3	Therapeutic Agents Commonly Used for Chemotherapy-Induced Peripheral Neuropathy	
Agents	**Dose**
Carbamazepine	200 mg/day; target plasma level 4–6 mg/L
Gabapentin	100–2,700 mg/day
Pregabalin	75–150 mg/day
Lamotrigine	25–300 mg/day
Duloxetine	30–60 mg/day
Amitriptyline	50 mg/day
Morphine	10–15 mg every 4–6 h
Topical gel	Twice daily

are typically used to prevent graft-versus-host disease (GVHD). Major CNS complications from calcineurin inhibitors include headache, altered mental status, seizures, cortical blindness, visual and auditory hallucinations, spasticity, paresis, and ataxia. PRES is also reported, perhaps due to direct toxicity to vascular endothelium. Neurologic symptoms eventually resolve after reducing or stopping the treatment. As a result of immunosuppression, 5% to 8% of patients develop opportunistic CNS infection including toxoplasmosis; herpesvirus, cytomegalovirus, and JC virus reactivation; nocardia; and aspergillosis. Treatment is directed toward the inciting pathogen.

NEUROLOGIC COMPLICATIONS OF BRAIN TUMOR TREATMENTS

Treatment for brain tumors, including surgery, radiation therapy, and/or chemotherapy, can cause neurotoxicity. Surgical complications are typically acute, consisting of hemorrhage, vascular damage, infarcts, coagulopathies, cerebral edema with herniation syndromes, and postoperative infections. Major neurologic morbidity from parenchymal tumor resection occurs in 8.5% of patients; usually in patients with tumor in eloquent or near-eloquent brain regions. Risk factors for chronic neurotoxicity from RT and chemotherapy include age, therapeutic modality and dosage, combination therapy, genetic background, and idiosyncratic patient predilections. Leukoencephalopathy may result from treatment with high-dose methotrexate in patients with primary central nervous system lymphoma (PCNSL), especially when given concurrently with or soon after RT. Neurocognitive dysfunction is a well-recognized long-term toxicity from RT. Several strategies have been studied to reduce or delay neurotoxicity from RT, such as use of 3D conformal RT in patients with gliomas, deferring whole brain radiotherapy (WBRT) in subsets of patients with brain metastases, reducing dose in patients with PCNSL who achieved complete remission after high-dose methotrexate therapy, modification of radiation delivery such as stereotactic radiosurgery or proton therapy, and sparing of hippocampus and neural stem cell during WBRT. Secondary tumors can develop years to decades after irradiation, including meningiomas, nerve sheath tumors, pituitary adenomas, gliomas, sarcomas, and embryonal neoplasm.

CONCLUSION

Neurologic complications of cancer treatment can result from direct toxicity to the nervous system, indirectly through toxic–metabolic effects, or from immunosuppressant effects resulting in opportunistic infection. Early recognition and differentiation from metastatic disease or paraneoplastic syndromes are imperative for proper management, as well as avoidance of inappropriate discontinuation or dose reduction of therapeutic agents.

LEVEL 1 EVIDENCE

1. Brown PD, Pugh S, Laack NN, et al. Memantine for the prevention of cognitive dysfunction in patients receiving whole-brain radiotherapy: a randomized, double-blind, placebo-controlled trial. *Neuro Oncol.* 2013;15:1429–1437.
2. Hershman DL, Lacchetti C, Dworkin RH, et al. Prevention and management of chemotherapy-induced peripheral neuropathy in survivors of adult cancers: American Society of Clinical Oncology clinical practice guideline. *J Clin Oncol.* 2014;32:1941–1967.

3. Loprinzi CL, Qin R, Dakhil SR, et al. Phase III randomized, placebo-controlled, double-blind study of intravenous calcium and magnesium to prevent oxaliplatin-induced sensory neurotoxicity (N08CB/Alliance). *J Clin Oncol.* 2014;32:997–1005.
4. Hershman DL, Unger JM, Crew KD, et al. Randomized double-blind placebo-controlled trial of acetyl-L-carnitine for the prevention of taxane-induced neuropathy in women undergoing adjuvant breast cancer therapy. *J Clin Oncol.* 2013;31: 2627–2633.

SUGGESTED READINGS

Neurologic Complications of Radiotherapy

Arlt W, Hove U, Muller B, et al. Frequent and frequently overlooked: treatment-induced endocrine dysfunction in adult long-term survivors of primary brain tumors. *Neurology.* 1997;49:498–506.

Brandsma D, Stalpers L, Taal W, et al. Clinical features, mechanisms, and management of pseudoprogression in malignant gliomas. *Lancet Oncol.* 2008;9:453–461.

Brown PD, Pugh S, Laack NN, et al. Memantine for the prevention of cognitive dysfunction in patients receiving whole-brain radiotherapy: a randomized, double-blind, placebo-controlled trial. *Neuro Oncol.* 2013;15:1429–1437.

Chi D, Behin A, Delattre JY. Neurologic complications of radiation therapy. In: Schiff D, Kesari S, Wen P, eds. *Cancer Neurology in Clinical Practice Neurologic Complications of Cancer and Its Treatment.* 2nd ed. Totowa, NJ: Springer; 2008:259–286.

Crossen JR, Garwood D, Glatstein E, et al. Neurobehavioral sequelae of cranial irradiation in adults: a review of radiation-induced encephalopathy. *J Clin Oncol.* 1994;12:627–642.

Esik O, Csere T, Stefanits K, et al. A review on radiogenic Lhermitte's sign. *Pathol Oncol Res.* 2003;9:115–120.

Gondi V, Tome WA, Mehta MP. Why avoid the hippocampus? A comprehensive review. *Radiother Oncol.* 2010;97:370–376.

Jaeckle KA. Neurologic manifestations of neoplastic and radiation-induced plexopathies. *Semin Neurol.* 2010;30:254–262.

Kargiotis O, Kyritsis AP. Radiation-induced peripheral nerve disorder. In: Wen P, Schiff D, Lee EQ, eds. *Neurologic Complications of Cancer Therapy.* New York: Demos Medical Publishing; 2012:355–368.

Kerklaan JP, Lycklama a Nijeholt GJ, Wiggenraad RG, et al. SMART syndrome: a late reversible complication after radiation therapy for brain tumours. *J Neurol.* 2011;258:1098–1104.

Levin VA, Bidaut L, Hou P, et al. Randomized double-blind placebo-controlled trial of bevacizumab therapy for radiation necrosis of the CNS. *Int J Radiat Oncol Biol Phys.* 2011;79:1487–1495.

Li JJ, Guo YK, Tang QL, et al. Prospective study of sensorineural hearing loss following radiotherapy for nasopharyngeal carcinoma. *J Laryngol Otol.* 2010;124:32–36.

Lin YS, Jen YM, Lin JC. Radiation-related cranial nerve palsy in patients with nasopharyngeal carcinoma. *Cancer.* 2002;95:404–409.

Pettorini BL, Park YS, Caldarelli M, et al. Radiation-induced brain tumours after central nervous system irradiation in childhood: a review. *Childs Nerv Syst.* 2008;24:793–805.

Posner J. Side effects of radiation therapy. In: Posner J, ed. *Neurologic Complications of Cancer.* Philadelphia: F.A. Davis Company; 1995:311–337.

Qayyum A, MacVicar AD, Padhani AR, et al. Symptomatic brachial plexopathy following treatment for breast cancer: utility of MR imaging with surface-coil techniques. *Radiology.* 2000;214:837–842.

Ricard D, Psimaras D, Soussain C, et al. Central nervous system complications of radiation therapy. In: Wen P, Schiff D, Lee EQ, eds. *Neurologic Complications of Cancer Therapy.* New York: Demos Medical Publishing; 2012: 301–313.

Rogers LR. Neurologic complications of radiation. *Continuum (Minneap Minn).* 2012;18:343–354.

Torcuator R, Zuniga R, Mohan YS, et al. Initial experience with bevacizumab treatment for biopsy confirmed cerebral radiation necrosis. *J Neurooncol.* 2009;94:63–68.

Neurologic Complications of Chemotherapy

Arrillaga-Romany IC, Dietrich J. Imaging findings in cancer therapy-associated neurotoxicity. *Semin Neurol.* 2012;32:476–486.

Chi D, Behin A, Delattre JY. Neurologic complications of radiation therapy. In: Schiff D, Kesari S, Wen P, eds. *Cancer Neurology in Clinical Practice: Neurologic Complications of Cancer and Its Treatment.* 2nd ed. Totowa, NJ: Springer; 2008:259–286.

Davis J, Ahlberg FM, Berk M, et al. Emerging pharmacotherapy for cancer patients with cognitive dysfunction. *BMC Neurol.* 2013;13:153.

Dietrich J, Wen PY. Neurologic complications of chemotherapy. In: Schiff D, Kesari S, Wen PY, eds. *Cancer Neurology in Clinical Practice: Neurologic Complications of Cancer and Its Treatment.* 2nd ed. Totowa, NJ: Humana Press; 2008:287–326.

Gill JS, Windebank AJ. Cisplatin-induced apoptosis in rat dorsal root ganglion neurons is associated with attempted entry into the cell cycle. *J Clin Invest.* 1998;101:2842–2850.

Grisold W, Cavaletti G, Windebank AJ. Peripheral neuropathies from chemotherapeutics and targeted agents: diagnosis, treatment, and prevention. *Neuro Oncol.* 2012;14(suppl 4):iv45–iv54.

Joseph EK, Chen X, Bogen O, et al. Oxaliplatin acts on IB4-positive nociceptors to induce an oxidative stress-dependent acute painful peripheral neuropathy. *J Pain.* 2008;9:463–472.

Krishan AV, Goldstein D, Friedlander M, et al. Oxaliplatin-induced neurotoxicity and the development of neuropathy. *Muscle Nerve.* 2005;32:51–60.

Kwong YL, Yeung DY, Chan JC. Intrathecal chemotherapy for hematologic malignancies: drugs and toxicities. *Ann Hematol.* 2009;88:193–201.

Lee EQ, Arrillaga-Romany IC, Wen PY. Neurologic complications of cancer drug therapies. *Continuum (Minneap Minn).* 2012;18:355–365.

Loprinzi CL, Qin R, Dakhil SR, et al. Phase III randomized, placebo-controlled, double-blind study of intravenous calcium and magnesium to prevent oxaliplatin-induced sensory neurotoxicity (N08CB/Alliance). *J Clin Oncol.* 2014;32:997–1005.

Monje M, Dietrich J. Cognitive side effects of cancer therapy demonstrate a functional role for adult neurogenesis. *Behav Brain Res.* 2012;227: 376–379.

Omuro AM, Ben-Porat LS, Panageas KS, et al. Delayed neurotoxicity in primary central nervous system lymphoma. *Arch Neurol.* 2005;62:1595–1600.

Pelgrims J, De Vos F, Ven den Brande J, et al. Methylene blue in the treatment and prevention of ifosfamide-induced encephalopathy: report of 12 cases and a review of the literature. *Br J Cancer.* 2000;82:291–294.

Rowinsky EK. Antimitotic drugs. In: Chabner BA, Longo DL, eds. Cancer Chemotherapy and Biotherapy: Principles and Practice. Philadelphia: Lippincott Williams & Wilkins; 2011:216–266.

Schiff D, Wen PY, van den Bent MJ. Neurological adverse effects caused by cytotoxic and targeted therapies. *Nat Rev Clin Oncol.* 2009;6:596–603.

Sioka C, Kyritsis AP. Central and peripheral nervous system toxicity of common chemotherapeutic agents. *Cancer Chemother Pharmacol.* 2009;63:761–767.

Vaughn C, Zhang L, Schiff D. Reversible posterior leukoencephalopathy syndrome in cancer. *Curr Oncol Rep.* 2008;10:86–91.

Neurologic Complications of Biologic Agents

Armstrong T, Wen P, Gilbert M, et al. Management of treatment-associated toxicities of anti-angiogenic therapy in patients with brain tumors. *Neuro Oncol.* 2012;14:1203–1214.

Lee EQ, Wen P. Neurologic complications of cancer treatment with biologic agents. UpToDate Web site. http://www.uptodate.com/contents/neurologic-complications-of-cancer-treatment-with-biologic-agents. Accessed December 30, 2013.

Sherman JH, Aregawi DG, Lai A, et al. Optic neuropathy in patients with glioblastoma receiving bevacizumab. *Neurology.* 2009;73:1924–1926.

Targeted Molecular Agents

Bang YJ. The potential for crizotinib in non-small cell lung cancer: a perspective review. *Ther Adv Med Oncol.* 2011;3:279–291.

Lee EQ, Norden A, Schiff D, et al. Neurologic complications of targeted therapy. In: Wen P, Schiff D, Lee EQ, eds. *Neurologic Complications of Cancer Therapy.* New York: Demos Medical Publishing; 2012:149–165.

Richardson PG, Briemberg H, Jagannath S, et al. Frequency, characteristics, and reversibility of peripheral neuropathy during treatment of advance multiple myeloma with bortezomib. *J Clin Oncol.* 2006;24:3113–3120.

Immunotherapy

Apfel SC. Neurologic complications of immunomodulatory agents. In: Wen P, Schiff D, Lee EQ, eds. *Neurologic Complications of Cancer Therapy.* New York: Demos Medical Publishing; 2012:93–106.

Liao B, Shroff S, Kamiya-Matsuoka C, et al. Atypical neurological complications of ipilimumab therapy in patients with metastatic melanoma. *Neuro Oncol.* 2014;16:589–593.

Meyers CA, Scheibel RS, Forman AD. Persistent neurotoxicity of systemically administered interferon-alpha. *Neurology.* 1991;41:672–676.

Rohatiner AZ, Prior PF, Burton AC, et al. Central nervous system toxicity of interferon. *Br J Cancer.* 1983;47:419–422.

Tarhini A. Immune-mediated adverse events associated with ipilimumab CTLA-4 blockade therapy: the underlying mechanisms and clinical management. *Scientifica (Cairo).* 2012;2013:857519.

Neurologic Complications of Hematopoietic Stem Cell Transplantation

Giglio P, Gilbert MR. Neurologic complications of cancer and its treatment. *Curr Oncol Rep.* 2010;12:50–59.

Hinchey J, Chaves C, Appignani B, et al. A reversible posterior leukoencephalopathy syndrome. *N Engl J Med.* 1996;334:494–500.

Quant EC, Wen P. Neurological complications of hematopoietic stem cell transplantation. In: Schiff D, Kesari S, Wen P, eds. *Cancer Neurology in Clinical Practice: Neurologic Complications of Cancer and Its Treatment.* Totowa, NJ: Humana Press; 2008:327–352.

Sklar EM. Post-transplant neurotoxicity: what role do calcineurin inhibitors actually play? *AJNR Am J Neuroradiol.* 2006;27:1602–1603.

Neurologic Complications of Brain Tumor Treatments

Cahan WG, Woodard HQ, Higinbotham NL, et al. Sarcoma arising in irradiated bone: report of eleven cases. 1948. *Cancer.* 1998;82:8–34.

Kleinschmidt-DeMasters BK, Kang JS, Lillehei KO. The burden of radiation-induced central nervous system tumors: a single institution's experience. *J Neuropathol Exp Neurol.* 2006;65:204–216.

Marsh JC, Godbole RH, Herskovic AM, et al. Sparing of the neural stem cell compartment during whole-brain radiation therapy: a dosimetric study using helical tomotherapy. *Int J Radiat Oncol Biol Phys.* 2010;78:946–954.

Perry A, Schmidt RE. Cancer therapy-associated CNS neuropathology: an update and review of the literature. *Acta Neuropathol.* 2006;111:197–212.

Sawaya R, Hammoud M, Schoppa D, et al. Neurosurgical outcomes in a modern series of 400 craniotomies for treatment of parenchymal tumors. *Neurosurgery.* 1998;42:1044–1055; discussion 1055–1056.

Scoccianti S, Detti B, Cipressi S, et al. Changes in neurocognitive functioning and quality of life in adult patients with brain tumors treated with radiotherapy. *J Neurooncol.* 2010;108:291–308.

Hydrocephalus 106

Michelle L. Ghobrial, Leon D. Prockop, and Fred Rincon

INTRODUCTION

Hydrocephalus is characterized by an imbalance in the production, drainage, and reabsorption of cerebrospinal fluid (CSF) resulting in a dilation of the cerebral ventricles. The choroid plexus produces about 500 mL of CSF daily. The CSF circulates from the lateral ventricles to the third ventricle through the foramen of Monro. It then flows to the fourth ventricle via the cerebral aqueduct and exits into the subarachnoid space via the foramina of Magendie and Luschka. The arachnoid villi granulations reabsorb the CSF into the venous system.

CLASSIFICATION

Although various classifications of hydrocephalus have evolved historically, the several types are recognized (Table 106.1). Although all types of hydrocephalus are obstructive to some degree, the anatomic localization and severity of resistance to normal anterograde CSF flow can vary. *Obstructive hydrocephalus* is used to describe conditions that result near complete blockage of CSF flow within the ventricular system. *Communicating hydrocephalus* describes conditions in which the ventricles are enlarged despite an open flow system from within the ventricles into the basal cisterns and over the convexities. Walter Dandy first described communicating hydrocephalus in 1914. He injected a tracer dye into one of the lateral ventricles. If the dye appeared in lumbar CSF, the hydrocephalus was termed *communicating*; if the dye did not appear in lumbar CSF, the hydrocephalus was termed *noncommunicating*. Because it proved useful in surgical-shunt placement, this functional classification was widely accepted; however, by this definition, noncommunicating hydrocephalus refers only to that caused by obstruction within the ventricular system. Communicating hydrocephalus infers CSF obstruction due to damage to the absorptive system after exiting the ventricles. Normal pressure hydrocephalus (NPH) is a form of communicating hydrocephalus.

Hydrocephalus can be *acute* or *chronic*. Acute hydrocephalus can be an immediate threat to life when it develops rapidly over several hours and leads to intracranial hypertension and downward central herniation of the brain. By contrast, even massive ventriculomegaly can be minimally symptomatic if it develops gradually over weeks, months, or years and does not represent a threat to life.

Another classification of hydrocephalus is congenital versus acquired. Congenital hydrocephalus is present at birth. Acquired hydrocephalus can develop any time after birth. These forms of hydrocephalus are distinguished from *hydrocephalus ex vacuo* in which CSF volume increases without change in CSF pressure because of cerebral atrophy.

EPIDEMIOLOGY

Population-based statistics for hydrocephalus are difficult to provide given the scope of varying ages of onset and causes. Congenital hydrocephalus occurs with an incidence of 0.5 to 1.8 per 1,000 births per year and may result from either genetic or nongenetic causes. Posthemorrhagic hydrocephalus occurs with an incidence of 25% to 70%, depending on the severity of the hemorrhage. Approximately 10% of infants with intraventricular hemorrhage (IVH) will require a shunt. The incidence of acute acquired hydrocephalus is unknown. Recent population-based studies have estimated the prevalence of NPH to be about 0.5% in those older than 65 years, with an incidence of about 5.5 patients per 100,000 per year. This is in accordance with comparable findings stating that although NPH occurs in both men and women of any age, it is found more often in the elderly population, with a peak onset generally in the sixth to seventh decades. Low-pressure hydrocephalus is reported in the literature as case series but no population statistics are known due to its uncommon occurrence.

PATHOBIOLOGY

OBSTRUCTIVE HYDROCEPHALUS

In intraventricular obstructive hydrocephalus, the obstruction causes proximal dilation of the ventricles with preservation of

---

TABLE 106.1 Classification of Hydrocephalus

Obstructive hydrocephalus

- Congenital malformations (i.e., aqueductal stenosis)
- Mass lesions causing ventricular obstruction (i.e., acute intraventricular hemorrhage, third ventricular colloid cyst)

Communicating hydrocephalus (CH)

- Defective reabsorption of CSF (i.e., postinflammatory or posthemorrhagic)
- Normal pressure hydrocephalus (NPH)
- Venous insufficiency
- Overproduction of CSF (i.e., colloid plexus tumor)
- External hydrocephalus (i.e., preponderance of excess CSF over the convexities)

Hydrocephalus ex vacuo

CSF, cerebrospinal fluid.

normal ventricular size distally. Obstruction may occur at the foramen of Monro, the third ventricle, the aqueduct of Sylvius, the fourth ventricle, or the fourth ventricular outflow foramina of Luschka and Magendie. Obstructive hydrocephalus can be caused by congenital malformations, developmental lesions, mass lesions, or posthemorrhagic ventricular obstructions.

Congenital Malformations and Developmental Lesions

Common nongenetic causes include intracranial hemorrhage (ICH) secondary to birth trauma or prematurity and meningitis as a cause for congenital hydrocephalus. Genetically, at least 43 mutants/loci linked to hereditary hydrocephalus have been identified in animal models and humans. In some, aqueductal stenosis has been documented by magnetic resonance imaging (MRI) or at postmortem examination. It is not clear whether aqueductal lesions (e.g., gliosis or fibrosis) occur developmentally or are the residue of prior viral inflammatory disease contracted in utero or in early life (Fig. 106.1). In some families, the occurrence of aqueductal stenosis, hydrocephalus of undetermined anatomic type, and the Dandy–Walker syndrome in siblings of both sexes suggests other modes of inheritance. In the Dandy–Walker syndrome, there is expansion of the fourth ventricle and the posterior fossa with obstruction of the foramina of Luschka and Magendie (Fig. 106.2). The Arnold–Chiari malformation may be associated with hydrocephalus at birth or it may develop later.

Mass Lesions

Intracranial neoplasms may cause obstructive hydrocephalus (Fig. 106.3). Tumors clustered about the third or fourth ventricles or the sylvian aqueduct, including pineal tumors, colloid cysts, gliomas, ependymoma, and metastases, are commonly implicated in intraventricular obstructive hydrocephalus. Prognosis, after shunting, is largely related to the type of tissue in the tumor. Other mass-like lesions, such as intraparenchymal cerebral hemorrhage, cerebellar infarction, or cerebellar hemorrhage, which assert local pressure on the ventricles may lead to acute hydrocephalus. Basilar artery ectasia and other vascular abnormalities (e.g., vein of Galen malformation) have also been associated with hydrocephalus.

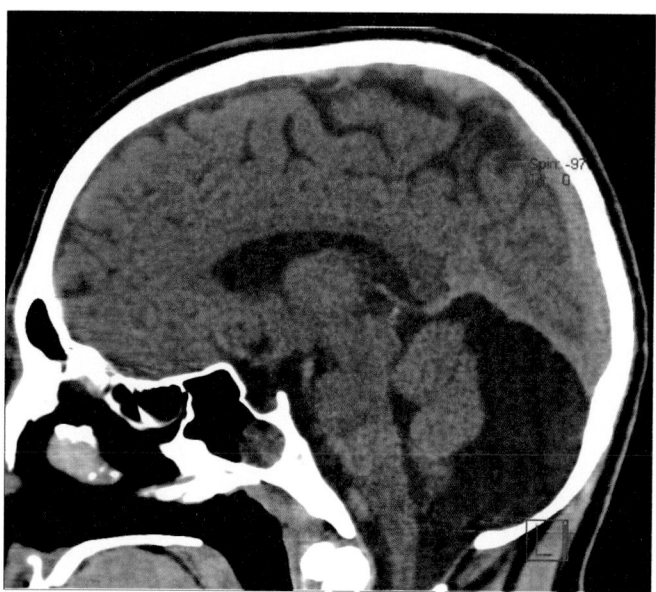

FIGURE 106.2 Sagittal CT scan showing a Dandy–Walker malformation.

Posthemorrhagic Ventricular Obstruction

Intracerebral hemorrhage complicated by IVH in adults also causes hydrocephalus (Fig. 106.4). In some patients, CSF flow obstruction is transient; therefore, intracranial pressure (ICP) increases and hydrocephalus appears but then disappears spontaneously. Other patients exhibit progressive hydrocephalus.

COMMUNICATING HYDROCEPHALUS

When neither an intraventricular nor an extraventricular obstruction is documented, three other mechanisms may cause hydrocephalus: oversecretion of CSF, venous insufficiency, or impaired absorption of CSF by arachnoid villi. The absorptive capacity of the subarachnoid space is about three times the normal CSF formation rate of 0.35 mL/min (20 mL/h or 500 mL/day). Formation rates greater than 1.0 mL/min may produce hydrocephalus. Clinically, choroid plexus papilloma is the only known cause of oversecretion hydrocephalus.

Posthemorrhagic Hydrocephalus

Posthemorrhagic hydrocephalus is a major complication of cerebral IVH in low birth weight infants. Hydrocephalus results when a clot within the ventricular system obstructs CSF flow by a process of obliterative basilar arachnoiditis or by cortical arachnoiditis. Hydrocephalus also occurs in adults after subarachnoid bleeding caused by head trauma or ruptured aneurysm (see Fig. 106.4). After subarachnoid hemorrhage, distension of the arachnoid villi by packed red cells suggests an absorptive defect as a pathogenic mechanism for hydrocephalus. Consequently, fibrotic impairment of extraventricular CSF pathways after ICH may be complicated by dysfunction of arachnoid villi. In preterm infants, there is a predisposition to germinal matrix (GM) hemorrhage leading to periventricular hemorrhagic infarction (PHI) and IVH causing hydrocephalus. GM hemorrhage is graded by severity, as I through IV, whereby grades III and IV usually develop progressive hydrocephalus that requires shunting.

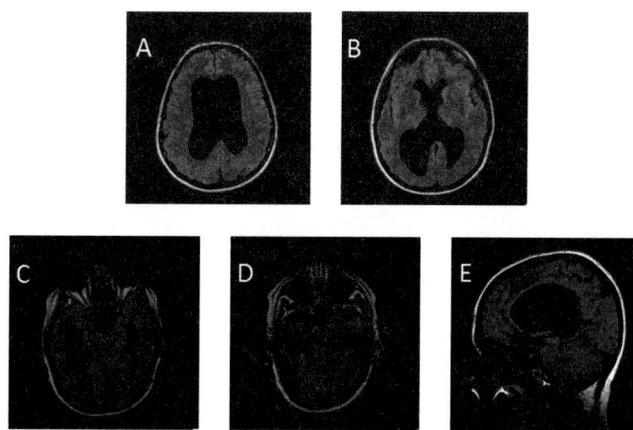

FIGURE 106.1 A 76-year-old man presented with 1-month history of gait dysfunction, memory loss, and urinary incontinence. **A, B, C,** and **D** are axial FLAIR MRI images and **E** is a sagittal T1 MRI image of chronic hydrocephalus secondary to aqueductal stenosis.

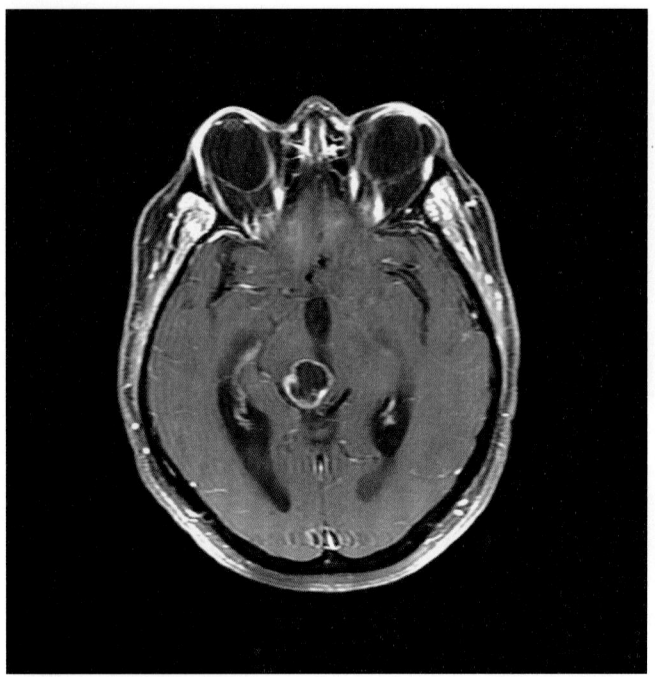
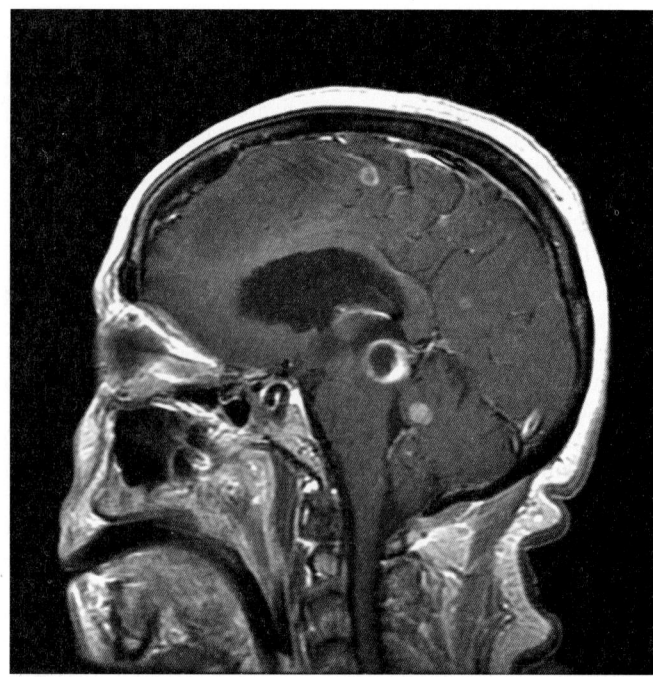

A

B

FIGURE 106.3 A and B: A 61-year-old female with a history of breast cancer presented with nausea and vomiting. She was found to have hydrocephalus secondary to brain metastasis as seen here in this T1 post-contrast MRI.

Postinfectious Hydrocephalus

Among infectious diseases, bacterial, fungal, tubercular, or syphilitic meningitis may cause chronic hydrocephalus secondary to basal arachnoiditis (Fig. 106.5). Among parasitic infections, neurocysticercosis may produce both communicating and noncommunicating hydrocephalus.

Otitic Hydrocephalus

Otitic hydrocephalus occurs in children after chronic otitis media or mastoiditis with lateral sinus thrombosis. Otherwise, impaired cerebral venous drainage, for example, thrombosis of cortical veins or intracranial venous sinuses, rarely causes hydrocephalus. Rarely, hydrocephalus due to impairment of extracranial venous

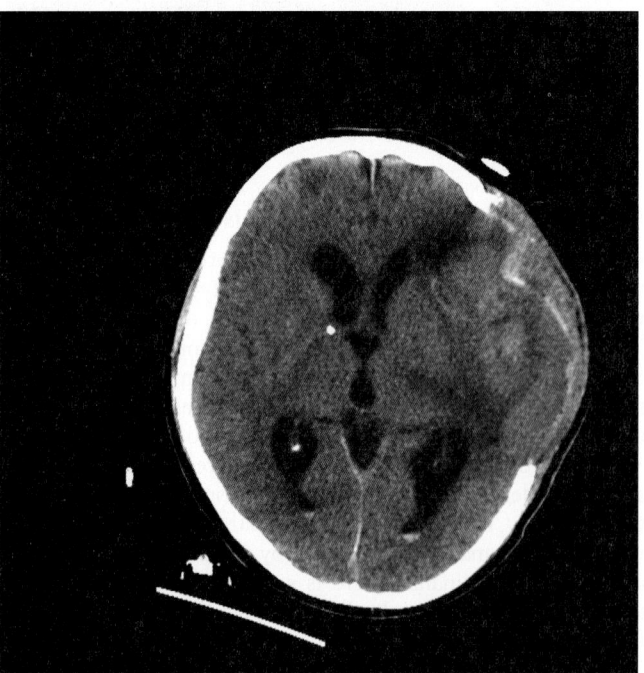
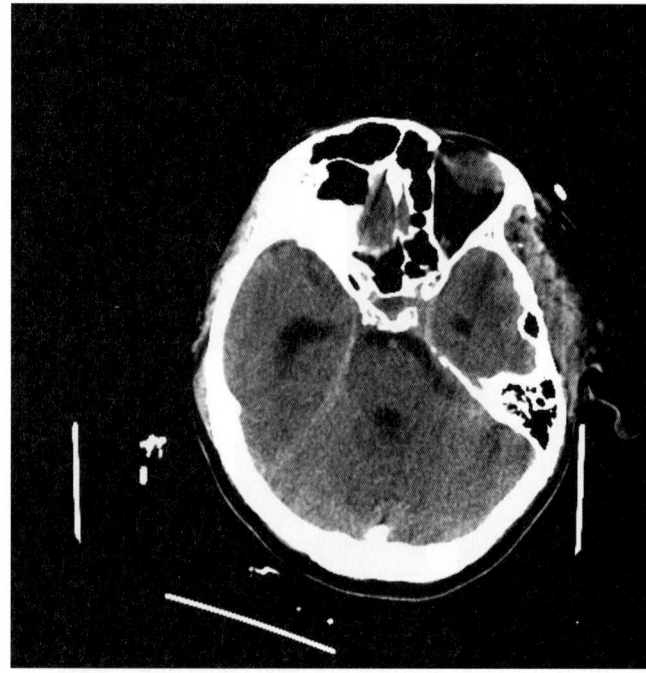

A

B

FIGURE 106.4 A 54-year-old man found unresponsive. He underwent endovascular coiling of a large left middle cerebral artery (MCA) aneurysm and decompressive hemicraniectomy **(A)**. The hydrocephalus persisted and he required a ventriculoperitoneal shunt after a restorative cranioplasty **(B)**.

FIGURE 106.5 A 47-year-old man with ventriculitis and secondary communicating hydrocephalus. **A** and **B** are post-contrast T1 MRI images. **C** and **D** are FLAIR MRI images.

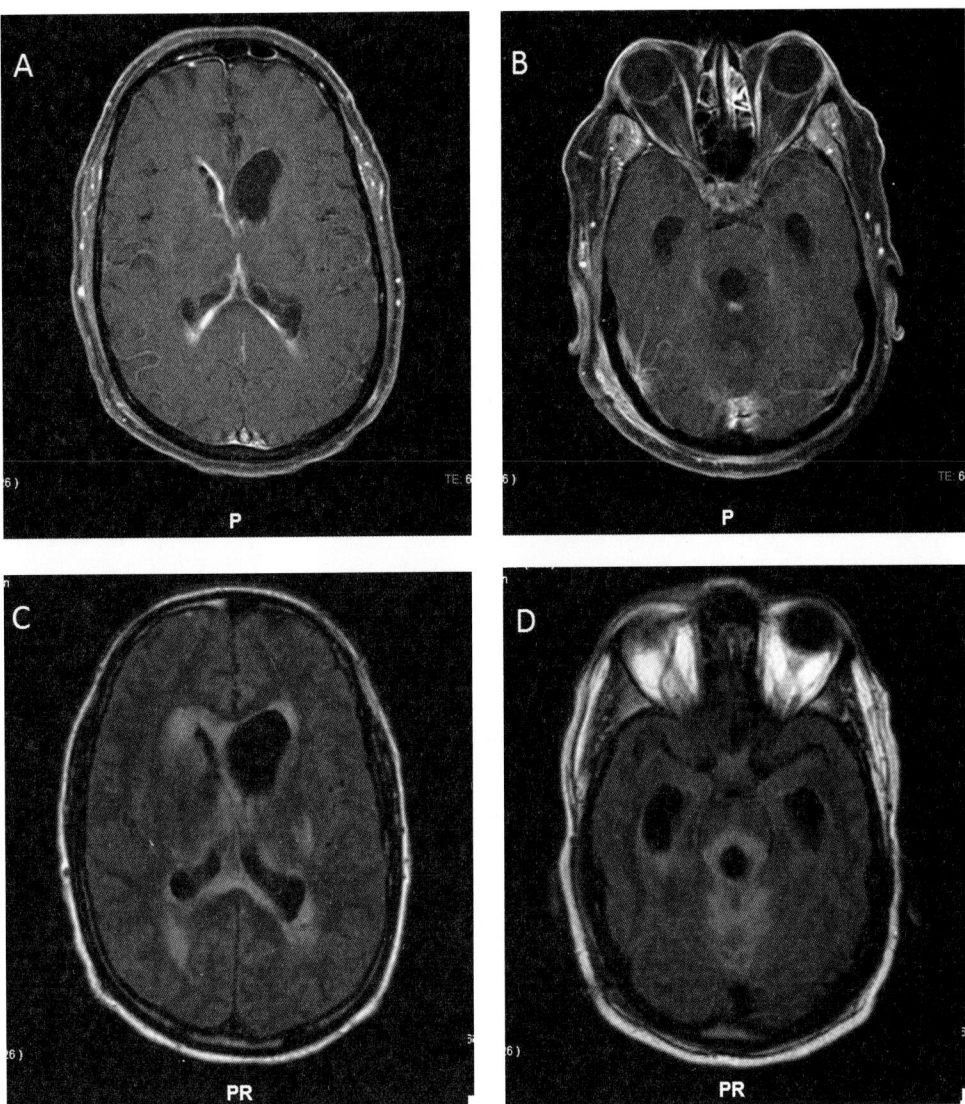

drainage follows radical neck dissection or obstruction of the superior vena cava.

Congenital Agenesis of the Arachnoid Villi

Communicating hydrocephalus has been attributed to congenital agenesis of the arachnoid villi with consequent impairment of CSF absorption. Because detailed pathologic study of the number of villi and their structural characteristics is difficult and rarely performed, this defect may be more common than statistics indicate. Likewise, dysfunction of arachnoid villi without obstruction of basilar or transcortical CSF pathways is not easy to assess.

Hyperproteinorraquia

Hydrocephalus has also been described when lumbar CSF protein content exceeds 500 mg/dL, as in polyneuritis or spinal cord tumor. The protein may interfere with CSF absorption. Ependymoma, the most common spinal cord tumor associated with hydrocephalus, may cause tumor seeding of the arachnoid villi.

Normal Pressure Hydrocephalus

NPH is a form of chronic communicating hydrocephalus with incomplete obstruction of the normal pathway of CSF flow. NPH most likely results from a serial pattern of increased resistance to normal CSF flow at the foramen of Monro, sylvian aqueduct, fourth ventricular outflow tracts, and the arachnoid granulations. The result is a relative increase in the volume of the lateral and third ventricles, with normal ICP. Symptoms are produced by stretching and secondary dysfunction and degeneration of white matter pathways in the corona radiata, which encase the lateral ventricles, and to a lesser extent white matter tracts in the internal capsule and below.

NPH is often "idiopathic" and may relate simply to an abnormal brain aging process, whereas in some cases, it may follow subarachnoid hemorrhage from trauma or aneurysm, meningitis, tumor, or surgery. Irrespective of the underlying etiology, the ventricles expand at the expense of brain volume, causing both brain compression and periventricular white matter changes. These changes are thought to arise from brain edema caused by transependymal flow of fluid (Fig. 106.6) or to ischemic demyelination caused by compression of brain tissue. There may also be neuronal dysfunction from the compression. However, the overall effect is sufficiently chronic, or compensated, so that the CSF pressure is normal.

Low-Pressure Hydrocephalus

A clinical state has been described with low CSF pressures and acute symptomatic hydrocephalus in the setting of medium pressure

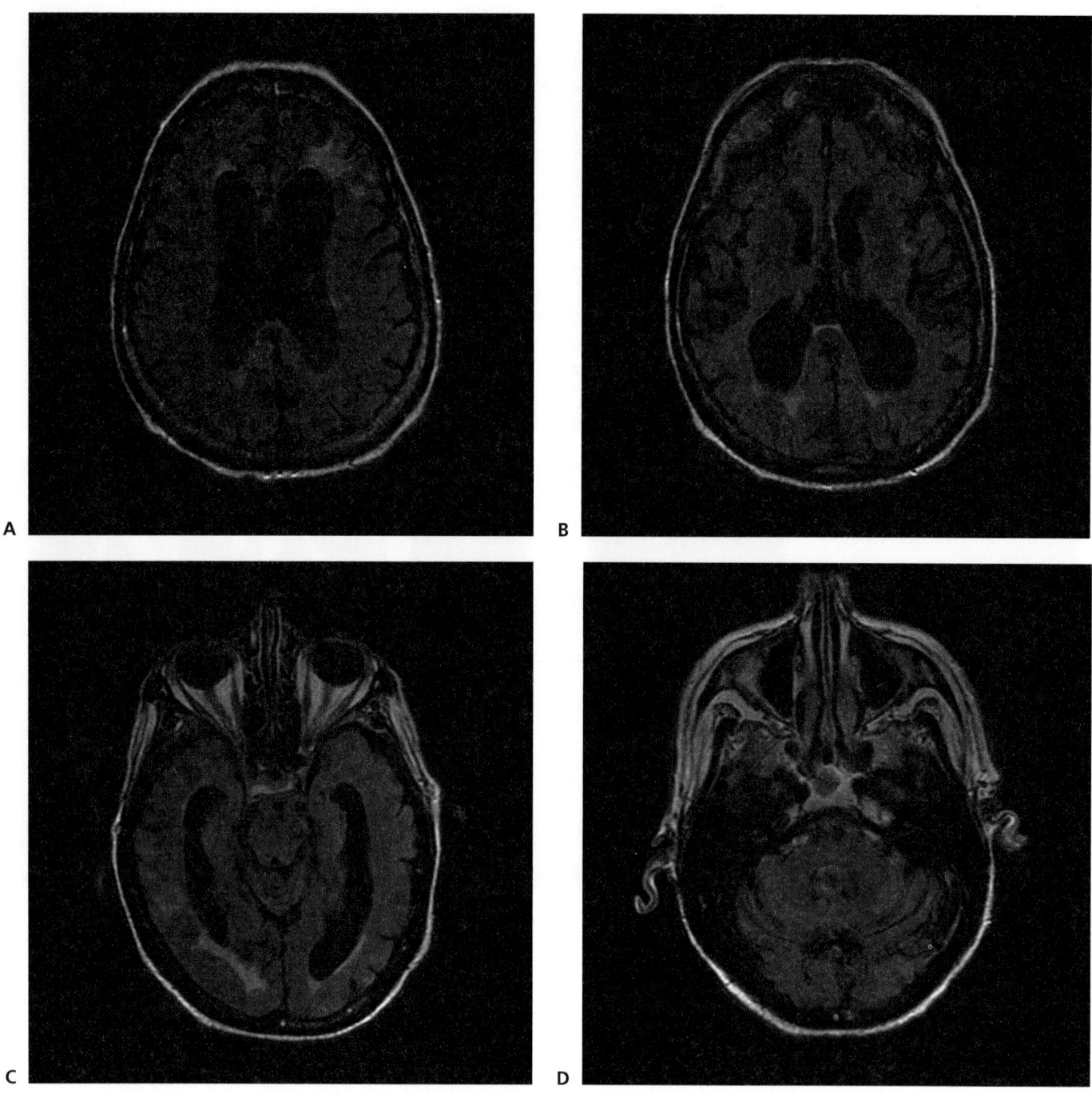

FIGURE 106.6 A to D: An 85-year-old man presented with gait dysfunction and urinary incontinence for 3 months. His symptoms improved after a large-volume LP. Axial FLAIR MRI images of a patient with NPH. Note periventricular transependymal interstitial edema.

CSF diversion and ventriculomegaly. Chronic shunting, subarachnoid hemorrhage, IVH, and tumors have been associated with low-pressure hydrocephalus. It has been postulated that a decrease in cerebral elasticity coupled with the ventricular enlargement produces this syndrome. There are different viscoelastic theories that have been applied in attempts to delineate this physiologic occurrence. Ultimately, this condition improves with subzero CSF drainage.

External Hydrocephalus

External hydrocephalus presents as collections of subarachnoid fluid over the convexities, with or without coexisting ventriculomegaly.

It can occur in both children and adults. In some cases, it can be difficult to determine whether the collection of fluid is truly in the subarachnoid or subdural space, and in some cases, both may exist. The criteria for diagnosis of benign external hydrocephalus in children is a rapidly enlarging head circumference along with a computed tomography (CT) scan showing enlarged subarachnoid spaces, particularly in the frontal regions, and normal ventricular size. The etiology in most cases is idiopathic, but it has been reported in many different conditions such as prematurity with IVH, subarachnoid hemorrhage, meningitis, steroid therapy, chemotherapy, neurosurgery, and trauma. Children with external hydrocephalus also have at least one close relative with macrocephaly in 40% of cases. An autosomal dominant mode of transmission is suspected. The most common theory of etiology in these children is immaturity of arachnoid villi. In adults, external hydrocephalus may be seen after trauma or subarachnoid hemorrhage. Another cause is after surgical hemicraniectomy if the bone has not been replaced. It is important to differentiate adult external hydrocephalus from subdural hygromas, as the latter will worsen if ventricular shunting is attempted.

CLINICAL MANIFESTATIONS

CONGENITAL OR INFANTILE HYDROCEPHALUS

The manifestation of hydrocephalus is influenced by the patient's age. Infants will experience tension hydrocephalus if the insult occurs before the cranial sutures fuse at the end of the third year. This will cause skull enlargement and wide fontanels. If the hydrocephalus occurs recently after suture closure, they may be separated by the pressure (suture diastasis). The face will appear relatively small and with stretching of the skin of the scalp, prominent veins appear. Upon percussion of the skull, a "cracked pot" sound is noted, known as *Macewen sign*. Scalp necrosis in these children can lead to CSF leakage and infections. If left untreated, there is failure to thrive due to poor feeding and frequent vomiting. Parinaud syndrome is caused by damage to midbrain tegmentum. The symptoms include paralysis or spasm of convergence, convergence–retraction nystagmus, visual loss and eventual optic atrophy, pseudo-Argyll Robertson pupils, eyelid retraction (Collier sign), and impaired upgaze or forced downgaze (setting-sun sign). Signs of corticospinal tract dysfunction include spasticity, increased deep tendon reflexes, positive Babinski sign, and wasting of trunk and limb muscles. The child will be developmentally delayed in motor and cognitive function.

In otitic hydrocephalus, the child may be febrile and listless. Eardrum perforation and purulent otic discharge usually occur. Often, ipsilateral sixth nerve paralysis and papilledema are noted.

ACUTE HYDROCEPHALUS

In acute hydrocephalus, there will first be headache and nausea/vomiting. This is followed by decreased mental status and may lead to coma. Corticospinal manifestations include lower extremity spasticity, increased deep tendon reflexes, and bilateral Babinski signs. It can progress to extensor posturing. The pupils are normal early in the process. Parinaud syndrome symptoms may appear as well. If untreated, pupillary mydriasis will develop. Depending on the speed of evolution, papilledema can be seen.

NORMAL PRESSURE HYDROCEPHALUS

A different symptom complex is seen with NPH, as the hydrocephalus in this disease process is slow and insidious. Patients present with a triad of gait ataxia, dementia, and urinary incontinence. Gait change is usually the first symptom, as well as the most frequent symptom, of NPH. This change may be subacute, fluctuating, or more chronic but most often worsens over weeks or months. The gait disturbance is often inconsistent and variable but has parkinsonian features, with shuffling, shortened stride length, imbalance, and often initial slowness. Frequently, the gait is wide-based (not commonly a feature of Parkinson disease), often with external rotation of the legs. The gait is classically described as "magnetic,"

with inability to lift the feet off the floor. It is also described as a gait "apraxia" because it appears that motor program involved in starting to move the legs is impaired, without evident impairment of strength. In addition to difficulty with the initiation of gait, there may also be difficulty maintaining gait, and there may be "freezing," with problems reinitiating movement. Tremor is uncommon, but falls are common.

Urinary symptoms are also frequent in NPH and may go unrecognized, consisting only of urinary urgency or frequency. Urinary incontinence itself is common, presumably due to loss of descending control mechanisms, with consequent unsuppressed bladder contractions, together with decreased voluntary ability to control the bladder outlet. A characteristic feature is said to be incontinence in which there is little evident concern regarding the problem.

Impaired cognition, ranging from subtle to severe, occurs in NPH, usually following after the onset of gait and urinary dysfunction. The characteristics of dementia associated with hydrocephalus include "subcortical" features. Symptoms may include not only forgetfulness but also slowness in mental processing, inertia, apathy, and impaired executive function, including decision making and task switching. Memory impairment in hydrocephalus may differ from that seen in cortical dementias such as Alzheimer disease (AD). As in AD, preservation of long-term knowledge can be seen, although the memory deficits more clearly involves poor learning. Impairment in delayed recall of learned material could relate to deficits in learning but may also involve initiation and speed of retrieval. For example, recall with simple cues may be much better than free recall, indicating a dominant deficit in retrieval rather than defective encoding of learned material. Advanced hydrocephalus results in severe slowing of mentation and possibly an akinetic mute state.

DIAGNOSIS

In infants, hydrocephalus must be distinguished from other forms of macrocephaly such as subdural hematoma. Sonography, described in Chapter 23, is useful in evaluating subependymal hemorrhage and IVH in high-risk premature infants and in following the infants for possible later development of progressive hydrocephalus (Fig. 106.7). Results correlate well with CT. As a bedside procedure, sonography requires minimal manipulation of critically ill infants. Plain-skull radiographs and skull measurements are useful to follow the course of hydrocephalus in infants and children. Skull x-ray may also demonstrate erosion of the sella turcica or thinning of the inner table, "beaten silver cranium." Overall, CT and MRI are the best diagnostic aids for all forms of hydrocephalus. In X-linked hydrocephalus, laboratory testing for genetic analysis and counseling can be useful.

In adults, the first test to be performed in suspected hydrocephalus is CT or MRI. Although CT can essentially exclude hydrocephalus, MRI is required for accurate assessment of subtle findings such as transependymal edema. The characteristic feature of hydrocephalus is ventricular enlargement out of proportion to sulcal enlargement. In general, brain atrophy due to degenerative disease or aging involves both "central" (ventricular) and "peripheral" (sulcal) spaces. But judging whether the ventricular enlargement is disproportionate can be difficult and is often fraught with interobserver disagreement. Thus, auxiliary features can be useful in assessing the likelihood of hydrocephalus. Abnormal periventricular white matter, with low attenuation by CT or increased

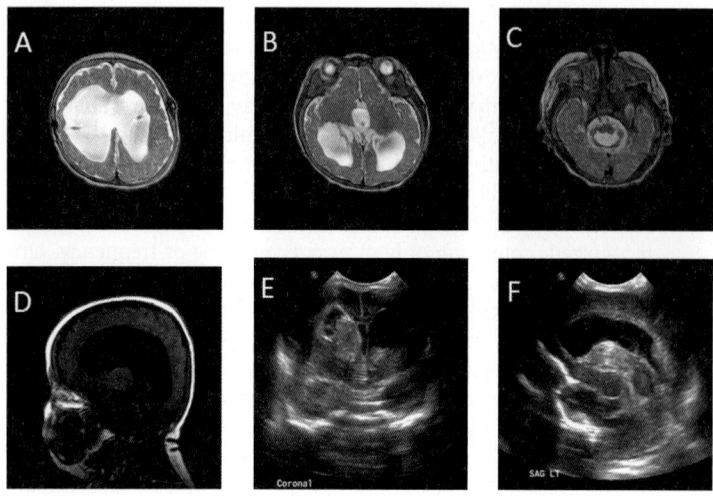

FIGURE 106.7 This former 24-week premature infant suffered grade IV IVH and subsequent posthemorrhagic hydrocephalus. **A, B,** and **C** are axial T2-weighted MRI images and **D** is a sagittal T1 MRI image 3 months after hemorrhage. **E** and **F** are transcranial ultrasound (US) images (coronal and sagittal, respectively) 1 week after birth.

T2-weighted or fluid-attenuated inversion recovery (FLAIR) signal by MRI, suggests transependymal fluid flow, consistent with hydrocephalus, but periventricular white matter signal change is nonspecific and may arise from microvascular ischemic disease. Other allied structural changes suggesting hydrocephalus may include "ballooning" of the frontal horns of the ventricles, markedly dilated temporal horns, and bowing and thinning of the corpus callosum. Rapid longitudinal change can be diagnostically useful, but multiple CT or MRI studies over several years may not be available.

Confirmatory tests are often sought in hydrocephalus because of these uncertainties in clinical diagnosis and neuroimaging. When NPH is suspected, additional tests may be useful for diagnosis and to determine the likelihood of response to CSF shunting. Lumbar puncture (LP) is indicated to measure CSF pressure and to determine whether it contains blood or signs of chronic inflammatory or infectious disease. The opening pressure on LP in NPH may be in the upper range of normal (14 to 20 cm H_2O), and such relatively higher "normal" pressures may also be indicative of a greater likelihood of benefit from CSF shunting. Continuous monitoring of intraventricular pressure (IVP) may reveal higher pressures than lumbar CSF pressures. Either lumbar or intraventricular monitoring may reveal the presence of Lundberg B waves, mild transient ICP elevations (<10 minutes in duration and generally <20 mm Hg in amplitude).

The response of the patient with suspected NPH to CSF diversion via a ventriculoperitoneal shunt (VPS) is best evaluated with a 48-hour trial of lumbar drainage. This test, which requires hospital admission, essentially mimics the effect of a VPS, with the caveat that the CSF is drained out of the lumbar space (10 mL every 2 hours) rather than the ventricular space. The main outcome measure of the test is subjective and objective observation of gait before, during, and after the procedure. Objective measurement is best made by videotaped recording of the patient prior to and at 24-hour intervals after the tap. In responders, gait typically improves during the first few days, with gradual loss of benefit over the next week after the lumbar drain has been removed. Cognition or urination may also improve, although this is usually less evident and more difficult to assess objectively. Lack of benefit from the tap points to likely lack of likelihood of benefit from CSF shunting. Response of symptoms to a single or repeated large-volume (30 to 40 mL) LPs (the CSF "tap test") can also be attempted, but this test is not sensitive and may not detect improvement that can result from more sustained CSF diversion.

Radionuclide cisternogram to assess CSF flow in NPH, with a positive finding being delayed appearance of radiotracer in the lateral ventricles, does not appear to be prognostically useful for assessing the likely clinical response to VPS. MRI evidence of an increased aqueductal CSF flow void, or an increased volume of CSF pulsing back and forth in the aqueduct ("aqueductal CSF stroke volume"), are similarly inconsistent and problematic as predictors of shunt-responsive NPH.

TREATMENT

The goal of treatment in hydrocephalic patients is to normalize CSF hydrodynamics. Treatment for every patient with hydrocephalus must be individualized. If the obstruction to flow is between the third and fourth ventricle, an endoscopic fenestration procedure can be attempted. In the case of a tumor obstructing CSF circulation, a surgical resection can be curative. If the cause of the alteration in CSF hydrodynamics is transient, the hydrocephalus may resolve during initial treatment, and temporary external ventricular drainage or serial LPs may be the only intervention needed. However, LP should only be employed in communicating hydrocephalus. In all forms of hydrocephalus, pharmacologic therapy is of limited value; however, there have been favorable reports of acetazolamide 500 mg orally (PO) three times a day (t.i.d.) as an adjunctive therapy to serial LP. Despite all this, most patients with symptomatic hydrocephalus will require CSF diversion through shunt insertion.

Shunt systems establish a connection between a CSF space (ventricular or lumbar) and a drainage cavity (peritoneum, pleural space, right atrium). The components of a CSF shunt include a proximal catheter, reservoir, valve, and distal catheter (Fig. 106.8). The proximal catheter is positioned intraventricularly, ideally away from choroid plexus, and exits through a burr hole to connect with a reservoir in the subcutaneous tissue. CSF may be sampled via this reservoir. A one-way valve regulates CSF flow into the distal catheter, which is subcutaneously tunneled to drain into a body cavity capable of reabsorbing fluid. All ventricular catheters are

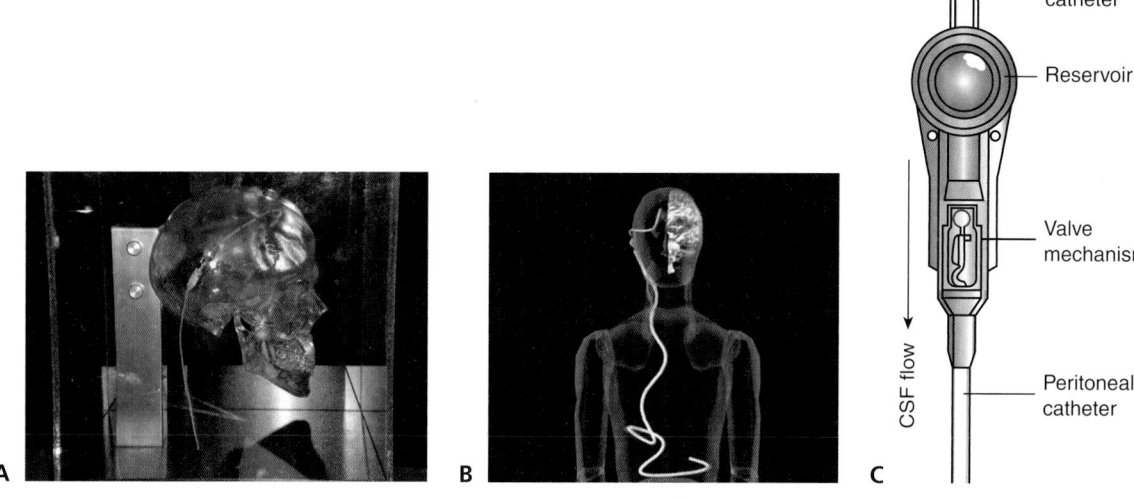

FIGURE 106.8 CSF shunt system. **A:** Cranial segment with reservoir located behind the ear. **B:** Path of shunt tubing in the subcutaneous anterior which ends in the peritoneal space. **C:** Cut-away view of shunt reservoir with one-way valve. Valve pictured is a Codman valve.

composed of silicone rubber and may vary in terms of length, internal/external diameter, shape, tip configuration, stiffness, and radiopaque markings. The valves now used include differential pressure regulators (static and programmable), flow regulators, siphon-resistive devices, and gravity-activated valves. The valves open or close based on a differential pressure, which is the pressure at the outlet (drainage cavity) minus the pressure at the inlet (intraventricular).

There are currently three different valve designs: slit, diaphragm, and spring-loaded ball-in-cone. The slit valve is an older design with a slit in the wall of the distal catheter, which opens with sufficient fluid pressure in the lumen of the catheter. The mechanical properties of the slit (silicone stiffness, wall thickness, length of slit) determine its operating pressure. Diaphragm valves have a flexible membrane, which moves in response to pressure differentials allowing CSF to flow around it. Finally, spring-loaded ball-in-cone valves contain a metallic coiled or flat spring, which applies force to a ball located in a cone-shaped housing. When CSF pressure is high enough, the ball is pressed against the spring, which opens the valve. CSF pressures change with posture (lying, sitting, or standing) and blood flow, which can alter shunt function. There are devices, which help prevent CSF siphoning during posture changes (standing up) by reacting to hydrostatic pressure across the two ends of the catheter and closing the valve. Gravitational devices use metal balls that fall into a cone-shaped seat upon standing, adding resistance to the flow in the shunt pathway equal to the height of a hydrostatic column. When the patient returns to a horizontal position, the balls move away from the fluid pathway, creating little resistance to the flow of CSF. Overdrainage regulatory devices control CSF shunting during postural and vasogenic effects. Flow regulatory devices help maintain a continual flow through the valve at different pressures by varying the size of the valve opening and thus resistance to flow. Another treatment option for hydrocephalus is endoscopic fenestration.

Endoscopic treatment of CSF pathway obstructions can effectively treat obstructive hydrocephalus, especially with aqueductal stenosis, and be used as an adjunct in treating loculated hydrocephalus. In endoscopic third ventriculostomy (ETV), a frontal region burr hole is made after a trajectory is chosen to provide a straight line linking the foramen of Monro and the tuber cinereum, the space between the mammillary bodies posteriorly and the infundibulum of the pituitary gland anteriorly (Fig. 106.9). Stereotactic neuronavigation is commonly used for this. The endoscope is inserted and the foramen of Monro is first visualized in the lateral ventricle. The scope is advanced into the third ventricle and the tuber cinereum is identified. A probe is used to make a fenestration in the floor of the third ventricle and a balloon enlarges this hole. Endoscopic fenestration can also be performed prior to shunt insertion in cases where both foramen of Monro are obstructed. The procedure creates a connection through the septum pellucidum in these cases.

The decision which procedure is best for a patient should be individualized. In particular, treatment for NPH is neurosurgical and involves CSF diversion. ETV is less likely to be a definitive management option for these patients. Shunting is most likely to be efficacious in those patients whose symptoms initially involved only gait and in those with milder cognitive dysfunction. It may also be more effective in those with a history of meningitis, subarachnoid hemorrhage, or other identifiable "secondary" cause of hydrocephalus. More successful outcomes are obtained in patients with positive spinal tap test and if the measured ICP is higher. Patients with severe dementia, marked sulcal atrophy, or those whose first symptom is dementia, with subsequent gait and urinary involvement, are less likely to respond favorably to CSF shunting. This may relate to irreversibility of symptoms or perhaps a greater likelihood of underlying AD.

OUTCOME

Before CSF shunts were available 50 years ago, acute obstructive hydrocephalus used to be a lethal or severely disabling disease. If untreated, progressive infantile hydrocephalus carries a mortality rate as high as 50% at age 1 year and 75% at age 10 years. Treatment greatly improves these figures. For example, with shunting, the survival rate is at least 50% after age 15 years but with a 15% incidence of mental retardation. If ICH leads to hydrocephalus in

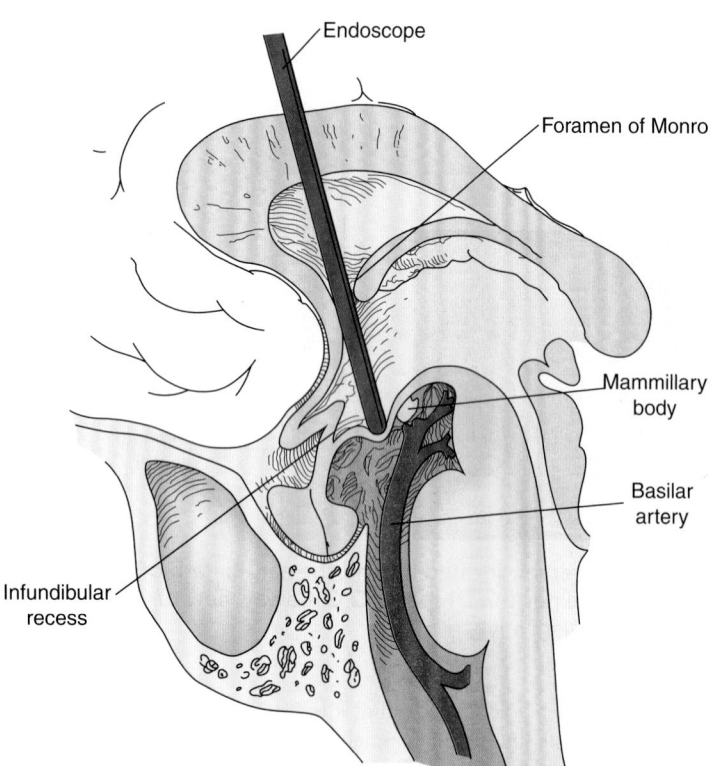

Endoscope

Foramen of Monro

Mammillary body

Basilar artery

Infundibular recess

FIGURE 106.9 Endoscopic third ventriculostomy surgical approach.

high-risk premature infants, the outcome is usually related to factors (e.g., asphyxia) other than shunt responsiveness.

Prognosis is sometimes related to an underlying disease (e.g., cerebral neoplasm). In such cases, treatment of hydrocephalus may be only palliative. However, because management of eventually terminal conditions prolongs life with quality, relief of obstructive hydrocephalus by a shunting procedure is often indicated to prevent acute brain herniation and death. Likewise, in nonneoplastic but serious conditions, such as the Dandy–Walker syndrome or postbasal arachnoiditis, shunting is indicated but eventual outcome depends on the underlying disease.

In adult-onset obstructive (noncommunicating) hydrocephalus, ETV is an established treatment, with success rates of 60% to 80%. Its role in posthemorrhagic and postinflammatory hydrocephalus is debated. Common complications of this procedure include bleeding from injury to the basilar artery, intraventricular vessels, or brain parenchyma; infection; CSF leak; and hypothalamic injury. A large series published a mortality rate of 1% and permanent morbidity rate of 1.6% for ETV. Complications are more common with shunt procedures.

A shunt complication is any problem that requires repeat surgical intervention. This may occur due to mechanical failure causing improper device function, functional failure secondary to inadequate flow rate despite a working shunt system, or infection. The risk of shunt failure is highest in the first few months postoperatively, with a 25% to 40% failure rate at 1 year. The mean survival time for a shunt system is 5 years.

Complications can arise from any component of the shunt system. Shunt obstruction is the most frequent cause of mechanical failure in patients, with fracture of shunt tubing coming in second (Fig. 106.10). Occlusion can occur proximally at the ventricular catheter entry point, at the level of the valve, or at the end of the distal catheter. Proximal occlusions can be caused by CSF debris,

a collapsed ventricle, or choroid plexus ingrowth. Valve obstruction can be the consequence of debris accumulation, bacterial proliferation, or the development of an immune reaction. Distal occlusion is most common in distal slit catheters due to accumulation of granulomatous nodules. Disconnection or fracture can occur at any fixation point, which causes tension along the catheter course or as a host reaction to foreign material causing degradation and calcification of the catheter. The functional complication of overdrainage occurs more frequently in the older adult population. Overdrainage may cause subdural collections or slit ventricle syndrome, a state of high ICP thought to be secondary to the CSF compartment decrease removing the buffer for volume change in blood or brain tissue. Problems such as migration, misplacement, skin problems, subcutaneous CSF effusions, pediatric craniostenosis, and ventricular loculation occur less frequently. Arachnoiditis and acquired tonsillar herniation are complications unique to lumboperitoneal shunts.

Infection remains an important and potentially devastating cause of shunt failure. In large databases, the infection rate is reported as 5% to 10%. It can be divided by site of infection: meningitis, wound infection, peritonitis, or shunt equipment infection. Symptoms correlate to the site of infection. Most shunt infections occur within 2 months of surgery. In early postoperative infections, *Staphylococcus epidermidis* and *Staphylococcus aureus* are the most common organisms, but other bacteria related to skin flora such as *Propionibacterium acnes* also occur. Gram-negative bacteria are associated with late shunt infections. Treatment requires intravenous antibiotics; ceftriaxone plus vancomycin is an acceptable empiric treatment regimen. The infected hardware must be removed and external ventricular drainage performed until infection clear. Ventriculoatrial shunts may cause bacterial endocarditis as an infectious complication.

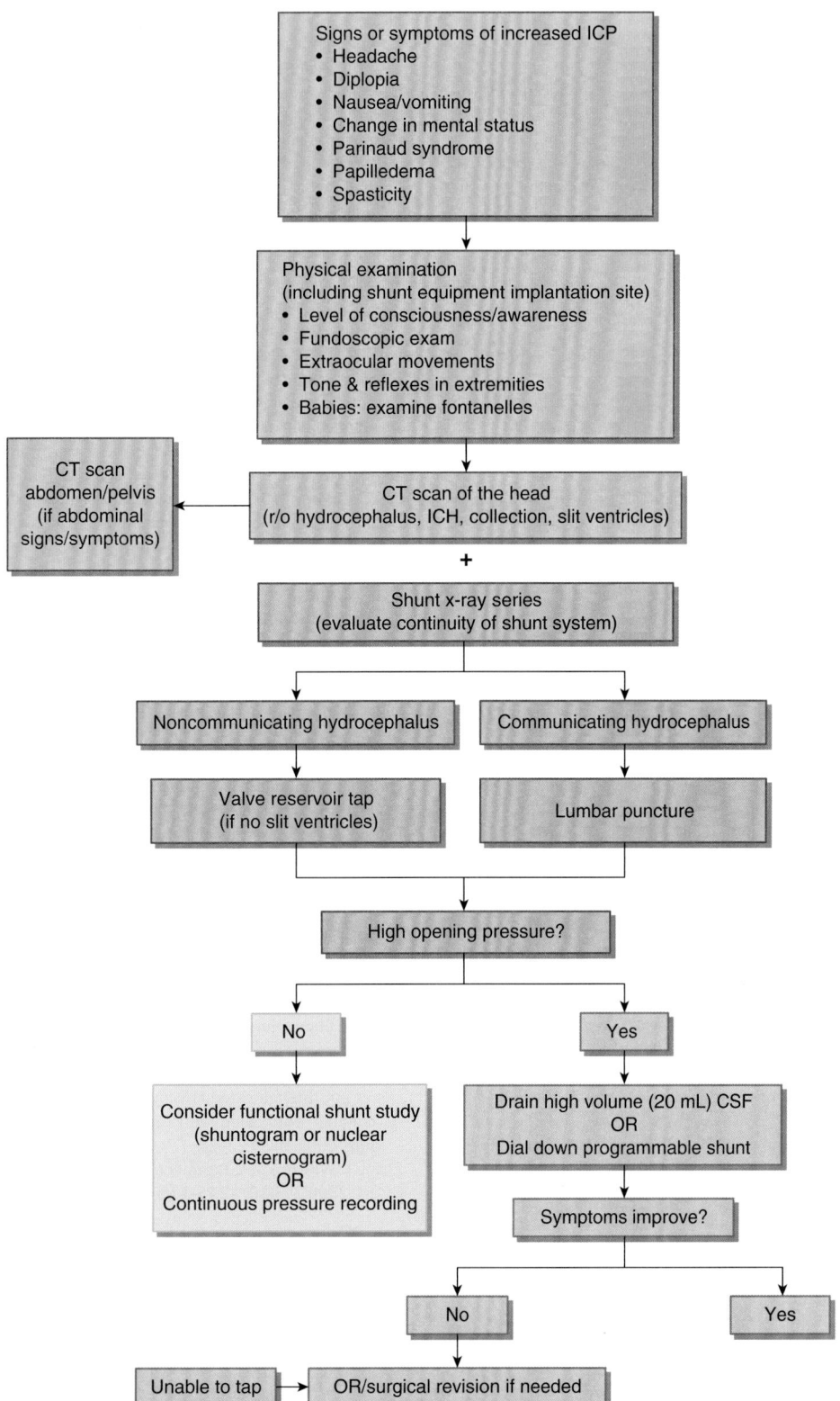

FIGURE 106.10 Approach to suspected shunt malfunction. ICP, intracranial pressure; CT, computed tomography; ICH, intracranial hemorrhage; OR, operating room.

SUGGESTED READINGS

Adams RD, Fisher CM, Hakim S, et al. Symptomatic occult hydrocephalus with "normal" cerebrospinal fluid pressure: a treatable syndrome. *N Engl J Med.* 1965;273:117–126.

Arthur AS, Whitehead WE, Kestle JRW. Duration of antibiotic therapy for the treatment of shunt infection: a surgeon and patient survey. *Pediatr Neurosurg.* 2002;36(5):256–259.

Atkins PT, Guppy KH, Axelrod YV, et al. The genesis of low pressure hydrocephalus. *Neurocrit Care.* 2011;15:561–468.

Boschert J, Dieter H, Krauss J. Endoscopic third ventriculostomy for shunt dysfunction in occlusive hydrocephalus: long-term follow-up and review. *J Neurosurg.* 2003;98:1032–1039.

Brockmeyer D. Techniques of endoscopic third ventriculostomy. *Neurosurg Clin N Am.* 2004;15:51–59.

Brodbelt A, Stoodley M. CSF pathways: a review. *Br J Neurosurg.* 2007;21(5):510–520.

Buckle C, Smith JK. Choroid plexus papilloma of the third ventricle. *Pediatr Radiol.* 2007;37(7):725.

Callen PW, Hashimoto BE, Newton TH. Sonographic evaluation of cerebral cortical mantle thickness in the fetus and neonate with hydrocephalus. *J Ultrasound Med.* 1986;5:251–255.

Carrion E, Hertzog JH, Medlock MD, et al. Use of acetazolamide to decrease cerebrospinal fluid production in chronically ventilated patients with ventriculopleural shunts. *Arch Dis Child.* 2001;84:68–71.

Chang S, Agarwal S, Williams MA, et al. Demographic factors influence cognitive recovery after shunt for normal-pressure hydrocephalus. *Neurologist.* 2006;12:39–42.

Dalen K, Bruarøy S, Wentzel-Larsen T, et al. Intelligence in children with hydrocephalus, aged 4–15 years: a population-based, controlled study. *Neuropediatrics.* 2008;39(3):146–150.

Devito EE, Pickard JD, Salmond CH, et al. The neuropsychology of normal pressure hydrocephalus (NPH). *Br J Neurosurg.* 2005;19:217–224.

Edwards RJ, Dombrowski SM, Luciano MG, et al. Chronic hydrocephalus in adults. *Brain Pathol.* 2004;14(3):325–336.

Gallia GL, Rigamonti D, Williams MA. The diagnosis and treatment of idiopathic normal pressure hydrocephalus. *Nat Clin Pract Neurol.* 2006;2:375–381.

Ginsberg HJ. Physiology of cerebrospinal fluid shunt devices. In: Winn HR, ed. *Youmans Neurological Surgery.* 5th ed. Philadelphia: WB Saunders; 2004:3374–3385.

Gnanalingham KK, Lafuente J, Thompson D, et al. The natural history of ventriculomegaly and tonsillar herniation in children with posterior fossa tumors—an MRI study. *Pediatr Neurosurg.* 2003;39(5):246–253.

Graff-Radford NR. Normal pressure hydrocephalus. *Neurol Clin.* 2007;25:809–832.

Greitz D. Radiological assessment of hydrocephalus: new theories and implications for therapy. *Neurosurg Rev.* 2004;27(3):l45–165; discussion 166–167.

Jack CR, Mokri B, Laws ER, et al. MR findings in normal-pressure hydrocephalus: significance and comparison with other forms of dementia. *J Comput Assist Tomogr.* 1987;11:923–931.

Johnston I, Teo C. Disorders of CSF hydrodynamics. *Childs Nerv Syst.* 2000;16:776–799.

Joseph VB, Rahuram L, Korah P, et al. MR ventriculography for the study of CSF flow. *AJNR Am J Neuroradiol.* 2003;24(3):373–381.

Khan A, Jabbar A, Banerjee A, et al. Cerebrospinal shunt malfunction: recognition and emergency management. *Br J Hosp Med.* 2007;68(12):651–655.

Khoromi S, Prockop LD. Disturbances of cerebrospinal fluid circulation, including hydrocephalus and meningeal reactions. In: Greenburg JO, ed. *Neuroimaging.* 2nd ed. New York: McGraw-Hill; l999:335–374.

Klinge P, Fischer J, Heissler HE, et al. PET and CBF studies of chronic hydrocephalus: a contribution to surgical indication and prognosis. *J Neuroimaging.* 1998;8:205–209.

Klinge P, Marmarou A, Bergsneider M, et al. Outcome of shunting in idiopathic normal-pressure hydrocephalus and the value of outcome assessment in shunted patients. *Neurosurgery.* 2005;57(suppl 3):S40–S52.

Kuczkowski J, Narozny W, Mikaszewski B. Diagnosis and management of otitic hydrocephalus. *Am J Otolaryngol.* 2009;30(1):69.

Lan CC, Wong TT, Chen SJ, et al. Early diagnosis of ventriculoperitoneal shunt infections and malfunctions in children with hydrocephalus. *J Microbiol Immunol Infect.* 2003;36(1):47–50.

Luetmer PH, Huston J, Friedman JA, et al. Measurement of cerebrospinal fluid flow at the cerebral aqueduct by use of phase-contrast magnetic resonance imaging: technique validation and utility in diagnosing idiopathic normal pressure hydrocephalus. *Neurosurgery.* 2002;50(3):534–542.

Meier U, Konig A, Miethke C. Predictors of outcome in patients with normal-pressure hydrocephalus. *Eur Neurol.* 2004;51(2):59–67.

Našel C, Gentzsch S, Heimberger K. Diffusion-weighted magnetic resonance imaging of cerebrospinal fluid in patients with and without communicating hydrocephalus. *ACTA Radiologica.* 2008;14(54):768–773.

Poca MA, Sahuquillo J. Short-term medical management of hydrocephalus. *Expert Opin Pharmacother.* 2005;6(9):1525–1538.

Pratt R, Mayer SA. Normal pressure "herniation." *Neurocrit Care* 2005;2:172–175.

Ratilal B, Costa J, Sampaio C. Antibiotic prophylaxis for surgical introduction of intracranial ventricular shunts: a systematic review. *J Neurosurg Pediatrics.* 2008;1:48–56.

Rekate HL. Hydrocephalus in children. In: Winn HR, ed. *Youmans Neurological Surgery.* 5th ed. Philadelphia: WB Saunders; 2004:3387–3404.

Sgouros S, John P, Walsh AR, et al. The value of colour Doppler imaging in assessing flow through ventriculo-peritoneal shunts. *Childs Nerv Syst.* 1996;12:454–459.

Volpe JJ. Brain injury in the premature infant: neuropathology, clinical aspects, pathogenesis, and prevention. *Clin Perinatol.* l997;24(3):567–587.

Yasuda T, Tomita T, McLone DG, et al. Measurement of cerebrospinal fluid output through external ventricular drainage in one hundred infants and children: correlation with cerebrospinal fluid production. *Pediatr Neurosurg.* 2002;36(1):22–28.

Zhang J, Williams MA, Rigamonti D. Genetics of human hydrocephalus. *J Neurol.* 2006;253(10):1255–1266.

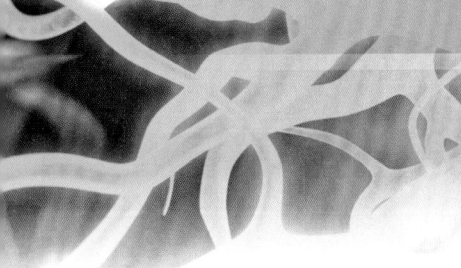

Stephan A. Mayer

INTRODUCTION

Brain edema accompanies a wide variety of pathologic processes. It plays a major role in head injury, stroke, brain tumor, and cerebral infections such as brain abscess, encephalitis, and meningitis. Less common but equally devastating causes of brain edema include fulminant hepatic encephalopathy, hypertensive encephalopathy and posterior reversible encephalopathy syndrome (PRES), hydrocephalus, hypoxic–ischemic injury, hyponatremia, and other disorders associated with acute hypo-osmolality (Table 107.1). Brain edema occurs in many different forms; clearly, it is not a single pathologic or clinical entity.

BRAIN EDEMA

Brain edema is defined as an increase in brain volume caused by an increase in water and sodium content. When well localized or mild in degree, brain edema is associated with little or no clinical evidence of brain dysfunction; however, when severe, it can cause massive intracranial mass effect and potentially fatal brain stem herniation. Because the brain is encased in a rigid cranial vault, focal or generalized brain edema results in intracranial hypertension when it is severe enough to exceed the compensatory mechanisms that modulate intracranial pressure (ICP).

Brain tissue shifting or *herniation* results from the generation of compartmentalized mass effect and ICP gradients within the skull. The major forms of herniation are central, transtentorial (or uncal), subfalcine (or cingulate), and cerebellar (see Fig. 18.5).

Brain edema and vascular engorgement are different processes. *Brain engorgement* is an increase in the blood volume of the brain caused by obstruction of the cerebral veins and venous sinuses or by arterial vasodilatation, such as that caused by hypercapnia. Hypertension severe enough to overwhelm the brain's capacity to autoregulate and maintain a constant level of cerebral blood flow (CBF) is another common cause of brain engorgement. Brain engorgement is also known as *hyperemia* or *luxury perfusion*.

PATHOBIOLOGY

Brain edema has conventionally been classified into three major categories: *vasogenic*, *cytotoxic*, and *interstitial*. The basic features of these three forms of cerebral edema are summarized in Table 107.2 with regard to pathogenesis, location and composition of the edema

---

TABLE 107.1   Conditions Characterized by Brain Edema

Intracellular Edema	Vasogenic (continued)
Cytotoxic	• Lead encephalopathy
• Cerebral infarction	• Immunosuppressants (tacrolimus/FK-506, cyclosporine A, interferon alpha [IFN-α]), intravenous immunoglobulin (IVIG)
• Hypoxic–ischemic injury	
• Reye syndrome	• Chemotherapeutic agents (cisplatin, cytarabine)
Osmotic	• Erythropoietin
• Acute hyponatremia	• End-stage renal disease
• Diabetic ketoacidosis	*Interstitial*
• Dialysis dysequilibrium syndrome	• Hydrocephalus
Extracellular Edema	**Combined Intracellular and Extracellular Edema**
Vasogenic	*Vasogenic and cytotoxic*
• Brain tumor	• Intracerebral hemorrhage
• Abscess	• Subarachnoid hemorrhage
• Postendarterectomy hyperperfusion syndrome	• Dural sinus thrombosis
• High-altitude cerebral edema	• Traumatic brain injury
• Acute intermittent porphyria	• Encephalitis
• MS	• Meningitis
• Posterior reversible encephalopathy syndrome	• Hepatic encephalopathy
• Hypertensive encephalopathy	
• Eclampsia	

MS, multiple sclerosis.

TABLE 107.2 Classification of Brain Edema

	Vasogenic	Cellular	Interstitial
Pathogenesis	Increased capillary permeability	Cellular swelling caused by energy failure or osmotic forces	Increased brain fluid due to block of CSF absorption
Location of edema	Primarily white matter	Gray and white matter	Periventricular white matter
Edema fluid composition	Plasma filtrate including plasma proteins	Increased intracellular water and sodium	CSF
Extracellular fluid volume	Increased	Decreased	Increased
Capillary permeability to large molecules	Increased	Normal	Normal
Clinical disorders	Brain tumor, abscess, infarction (late), trauma, intracerebral hemorrhage, hepatic encephalopathy, high-altitude cerebral edema	Hypoxia–ischemia (early), hypo-osmolality (e.g., hyponatremia), dialysis dysequilibrium syndrome	Obstructive hydrocephalus, idiopathic intracranial hypertension
Therapeutic effects			
Steroids	Beneficial in brain tumor, abscess	Not effective	Not effective
Osmotherapy	Effectiveness limited by blood–brain barrier disruption	Effective	Rarely useful

CSF, cerebrospinal fluid.
Modified from Fishman RA. Brain edema. In: Fishman RA, ed. *Cerebrospinal Fluid in Diseases of the Nervous System.* 2nd ed. Philadelphia: WB Saunders, 1992:116–137.

fluid, and changes in capillary permeability. A newer classification scheme focuses on the primary location of the edema fluid as *intracellular* or *extracellular*. In this scheme, the two main forms of intracellular edema are *cytotoxic* and *osmotic*, and the two main forms of extracellular edema are *vasogenic* and *interstitial* (hydrocephalic). Many causes of brain edema, including hemorrhagic stroke, venous infarction, and trauma, lead to a combination of these different forms of brain edema, and the varying contributions of each form of edema may change over time.

Vasogenic Edema

Vasogenic edema is a form of extracellular edema characterized by increased permeability of the blood–brain barrier to fluid, solutes, and macromolecules such as the plasma proteins, whose entry is normally limited by tight junctions between the capillary endothelial cells. The increase in permeability is visualized when contrast enhancement is observed with computed tomography (CT) or magnetic resonance imaging (MRI). Increased cerebrospinal fluid (CSF) protein levels are also indicative of increased endothelial permeability. MRI fluid-attenuated inversion recovery (FLAIR) sequences are more sensitive than CT for demonstrating the increases in brain tissue water content and extracellular volume that characterize vasogenic edema.

The biochemical basis of the changes in membrane integrity that underlie vasogenic edema involves the effects of free radicals (i.e., superoxide ions, hydroxyl radicals, singlet oxygen, and nitric oxide) and polyunsaturated fatty acids, most notably arachidonic acid, in the peroxidation of membrane phospholipids. The ability of glucocorticoids to inhibit the release of arachidonic acid from cell membranes may explain their beneficial effects in vasogenic edema. By contrast, steroids such as dexamethasone have not been shown to be therapeutically useful in the treatment of cytotoxic edema or vasogenic brain edema associated with stroke or trauma.

Vasogenic edema is characteristic of clinical disorders in which a local tissue inflammatory response occurs when angiogenesis is stimulated by neoplasm or when severe hypertension overwhelms the brain's capacity to autoregulate CBF. These disorders include brain tumor, abscess, hemorrhage, infarction with reperfusion, hypertensive encephalopathy, and traumatic contusion. Vasogenic edema related to varying degrees of vasodilation and blood–brain barrier disruption is also seen with acute demyelinating lesions in multiple sclerosis, hepatic or lead encephalopathy, Reye syndrome, and meningitis or encephalitis. Functional manifestations of vasogenic edema include focal neurologic deficits, focal electroencephalogram (EEG) slowing, disturbances of consciousness, and severe intracranial hypertension. In patients with brain tumor, whether primary or metastatic, the clinical signs are often caused more by the surrounding edema than by the tumor mass itself.

Cytotoxic (Osmotic) Edema

Cytotoxic edema is characterized by swelling of all the cellular elements of the brain (neurons, glia, and endothelial cells) with a concomitant reduction in the volume of the extracellular fluid space of the brain. Capillary permeability is usually not affected by osmotic edema (i.e., hyponatremia) or in the early phase of a hypoxic–ischemic insult. The biologic basis of cytotoxic or osmotic brain edema involves astrocytic calcium signaling and activation of aquaporin-4 channels, which are the major influx route for water into the cell. Patients with pure cytotoxic edema have a normal CSF protein, and CT and MRI do not reveal contrast enhancement. MRI diffusion-weighted imaging (DWI) reflects the restricted diffusion of water within swollen cells and is by far the most sensitive method for imaging cytotoxic edema (see also Chapter 21).

There are several causes of cytotoxic or osmotic edema, the most important being hypoxia–ischemia, acute hypo-osmolality of the plasma relative to the intracellular compartment, and the osmotic dysequilibrium syndromes. *Hypoxia* after cardiac arrest or asphyxia results in cerebral energy depletion. The cellular swelling is determined by the appearance of increased intracellular osmoles (especially sodium, lactate, and hydrogen ions) that induce the rapid entry of water into cells. Cytotoxic edema also plays a large role in the tissue swelling that occurs after cerebral infarction. *Acute hypo-osmolality of the plasma* and extracellular fluid is caused by acute dilutional hyponatremia, syndrome of inappropriate secretion of antidiuretic hormone (SIADH), or severe sodium depletion (see also Chapter 12). *Osmotic dysequilibrium syndromes* occur with hemodialysis or diabetic ketoacidosis, in which excessive brain intracellular solutes result in excessive cellular hydration when the plasma osmolality is rapidly normalized with therapy. In the case of renal failure, the intracellular solutes presumably include a number of organic acids recovered in the dialysis bath. In diabetic ketoacidosis, the intracellular solutes include glucose and ketone bodies; however, there are also unidentified, osmotically active, intracellular solutes termed *idiogenic osmoles* that favor cellular swelling.

Major changes in cerebral function can result from processes that result in cytotoxic edema, including encephalopathy, stupor or coma, ICP elevation, brain stem herniation, asterixis, myoclonus, and focal or generalized seizures. As a general rule, intracellular edema caused by osmotic derangements is much more treatable than cytotoxic edema resulting from hypoxic–ischemic injury because cellular function remains viable. The extent of cellular swelling and neurologic dysfunction resulting from acute hypo-osmolality is directly related with how quickly it develops; chronic states of extreme hypo-osmolality that are reached gradually lead to minimal symptomatology. Hypoxic–ischemic injury causes cytotoxic edema and selective cellular necrosis. If the process progresses to frank tissue infarction, vasogenic edema follows. The delay in visualizing contrast enhancement with CT following an ischemic stroke illustrates that time is needed for defects in endothelial cell permeability to develop.

Interstitial (Hydrocephalic) Edema

Interstitial edema is the third type of edema best characterized in obstructive hydrocephalus, in which the water and sodium content of the periventricular white matter is increased because of the movement of CSF across the ventricular ependymal surface. Obstruction of the CSF outflow results in the transependymal movement of CSF and thereby an absolute increase in the volume of the extracellular fluid of the brain. Interstitial edema thus is strictly periventricular on CT and MRI, with predominance at the anterior and posterior aspects of the lateral ventricles. The composition of interstitial edema is similar to CSF. The clinical manifestations of interstitial edema (dementia, psychomotor slowing, and gait disorder) are often difficult to separate from those seen with normal pressure hydrocephalus in which there is physical traction on the periventricular white matter fiber tracts.

SELECTED CAUSES OF BRAIN EDEMA

Cerebral Infarction

Most patients with arterial occlusion initially have cytotoxic edema followed by vasogenic edema, which are together termed *ischemic brain edema*. The cytotoxic phase takes place over minutes to hours and may be reversible. At this point, DWI may show dramatic changes well before evidence of completed tissue infarction can be demonstrated on MRI FLAIR sequences or by CT. Although osmotic or vasogenic edema can also be DWI positive, a phenomenon called *T2 shine through*, cytotoxic edema can be further differentiated from these causes on MRI because it is always associated with a reduction

(low signal) in the apparent diffusion coefficient (ADC) of water. The vasogenic phase of infarction takes place over hours to days as the tissue swells; in many cases, spontaneous vessel recanalization may occur and accelerate this process. A patchy and heterogenous pattern of contrast enhancement on CT or MRI at this point is characteristic. Despite the theoretical concern that osmotic therapy with mannitol or hypertonic saline may aggravate tissue edema because these osmotically active substances may leak through disrupted endothelial cells into the infarcted brain tissue, clinical experience indicates that these treatments can effectively reverse the early stages of brain stem herniation. *Hemicraniectomy* is the definitive treatment of choice for younger patients (younger than 60 years) who are at risk for brain stem herniation due to complete infarction of the middle cerebral artery territory (see also Chapter 35).

Intracerebral Hemorrhage

Perihematomal brain edema is a form of vasogenic edema that progressively increases over the first week after intracerebral hemorrhage (ICH, see also Chapter 38). Symptomatic mass effect related to edema formation is the major cause of delayed neurologic deterioration after ICH. Perihematomal edema is caused by the local infiltration of plasma rich in thrombin and other coagulation proteins into the surrounding brain tissue. The thrombin then triggers a unique form of *neuro-hemo-inflammation*, stimulating the surrounding tissue to produce prostaglandins, complement, leukotrienes, and other inflammatory mediators that promote apoptotic cell death and blood–brain barrier disruption. Dexamethasone is not effective for treating perihematomal edema [**Level 1**].[1] By contrast, large doses of 20% mannitol (1.4 g/kg) have been shown to effectively reduce ICP and reverse clinical brain stem herniation in uncontrolled cohort studies.

Subarachnoid Hemorrhage

Subarachnoid hemorrhage (SAH, see also Chapter 39) can cause global cerebral edema that typically occurs at onset in poor-grade patients, as well as a variety of forms of focal edema related to focal hematoma formation, cerebral infarction, brain retraction injury, and other causes. The global brain edema is mostly vasogenic in nature (Fig. 107.1). The pathophysiology is thought to reflect

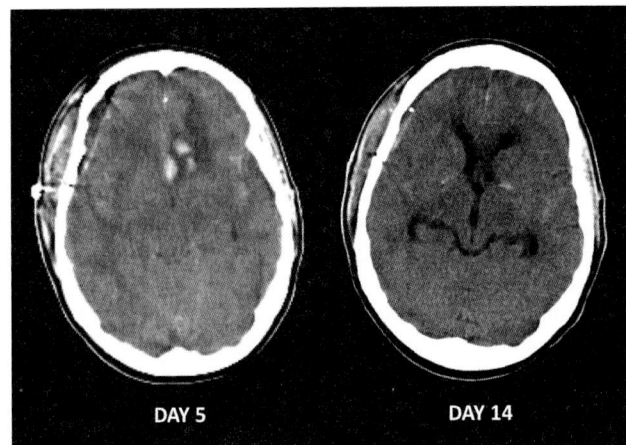

FIGURE 107.1 Global cerebral edema in a patient with subarachnoid hemorrhage. Day 5: CT shows global swelling of the brain with effacement of the quadrigeminal cisterns. A focus of hemorrhage with surrounding edema is also evident in the left inferior frontal lobe. The patient was undergoing induced hypertension, which later was felt to be exacerbating brain edema. Day 14: Resolution of global cerebral edema is evident.

transient hypoperfusion as a brief period of intracranial circulatory arrest associated with a massive surge in ICP, followed by reperfusion injury of the brain, with reflex hypertension in the setting of impaired autoregulation causing vascular engorgement. Global cerebral edema on CT affects 20% of patients and is associated with increased mortality and poor functional and cognitive outcome after SAH. Placement of an external ventricular drain is the first step in attaining ICP control; hypertonic saline and hypothermia are promising but untested potential interventions for mitigating further tissue damage.

Venous Infarction

Venous infarction results from occlusion of the cerebral venous and dural sinuses usually in the setting of dural sinus thrombosis (Chapter 40) or as a complication of a neurosurgical procedure. The result is tissue hypoperfusion with congestion and engorgement of the microcirculation, which results in a combination of cytotoxic and prominent vasogenic edema. Imaging shows extensive mass effect, patchy enhancement, and secondary hemorrhagic transformation of the infarct in most cases. In addition to standard measures to control ICP, treatment is directed at preventing clot propagation within the venous system with heparin anticoagulation. Interventional approaches to restore venous flow with local thrombolytic therapy can also be attempted as a heroic measure.

Cardiac Arrest

After cardiac arrest (Chapter 37), massive swelling of the brain that develops over the next several days is an ominous sign. Patients are usually in deep coma, and recovery is rare. Standard measures to treat brain edema at that point are usually pointless because the extent of cellular necrosis throughout the brain is very severe.

Traumatic Brain Injury

Traumatic brain injury (TBI) can result in both focal and global brain edema (see also Chapter 46). The global form of edema is largely vasogenic in nature and is felt to reflect neurogenic vascular engorgement and hyperemia in the setting of autoregulatory failure and dysfunction of vasomotor centers in the brain stem. In some cases, the patients present with a lucid interval after experiencing a concussion, followed an hour later by rapid progression to coma, as the brain massively swells. *Second impact syndrome* refers to rapid and catastrophic swelling of the brain that occurs when a person experiences a second concussion before symptoms of an earlier one have resolved. Standard measures to control ICP, with emphasis on hyperventilation and blood pressure (BP) control to reduce cerebral blood volume, are effective. Focal brain edema can result from contusional injury, brain compression from epidural or subdural hematoma, thrombin-mediated perihematomal edema, or cerebral infarction when brain herniation results in compression of the anterior or posterior cerebral arteries (see also Chapter 46). Steroids are not effective, and in one study, high-dose intravenous (IV) methylprednisolone (Solu-Medrol) was shown to increase mortality, which was presumably due to immunosuppression, hyperglycemia, increased muscle catabolism, and impaired wound healing [**Level 1**].[2]

Brain Tumors

Brain neoplasms (see also Section 13 and Chapter 145) cause a pure form of vasogenic brain edema, which is caused by the local release of cytokines, angiogenic factors, and other proinflammatory proteins that result in blood–brain barrier disruption. Malignant and highly vascular tumors as a rule cause much more local edema of the surrounding brain tissue than do benign neoplasms such as meningiomas, although exceptions can occur. The edema characteristically tracks along the white matter pathways on MRI or CT. Vasogenic edema associated with brain neoplasm is highly responsive to glucocorticoid therapy. In addition to standard measures to control ICP, *dexamethasone* is the treatment of choice; a typical starting dose is 4 to 10 mg every 6 hours.

Fulminant Hepatic Encephalopathy

Acute fulminant liver failure from any cause can result in hepatic encephalopathy producing clouding of consciousness with prominent asterixis (see also Chapter 119). As the severity of neurologic dysfunction progresses from lethargy to stupor to coma, massive swelling of the brain can occur resulting in dangerous elevations of ICP and brain stem herniation. The cause of the brain edema is poorly understood, and its onset can be unpredictable. Initially, the edema is primarily vasogenic with a large component of vascular engorgement. Ammonia (NH_3) and other substances normally metabolized by the liver cross the blood–brain barrier where they cause astrocytes to swell and disrupt endothelial tight junctions. Treatment relies on standard measures to control ICP; lactulose does not control brain edema when it is present. Optimal management requires placement of an ICP monitor after meticulous correction of the coagulopathy that usually is present. Transcranial Doppler sonography and jugular venous oxygen saturation monitoring demonstrate findings consistent with excessive hyperemia and can be used as end points to ensure that hyperventilation and BP control are not excessive. Mild to moderate hypothermia (33°C) has been shown to be effective in addition to more standard measures for controlling ICP, but liver transplantation is the only known definitive treatment. If the process is uncontrolled, herniation and brain death are a common outcome.

Reye Syndrome

Reye syndrome is a form of acute hepatitis with prominent fatty changes resulting from viral infection and exposure to aspirin that can occur in children. It is often accompanied by an encephalopathy characterized by progressive stupor and coma and a combination of cytotoxic and, to a lesser extent, vasogenic brain edema. Uncontrolled intracranial hypertension can lead to fatal brain stem herniation, and the pathogenesis is obscure. The disease is rarely seen today because of restrictions of the use of aspirin in pediatric patients.

Brain Abscess

Brain abscesses (Chapter 62) caused by localized infection with bacteria, toxoplasmosis, cysticercosis, fungal infection, or other causes result in a pure form of vasogenic edema very similar to that produced by brain tumors. Local release of various inflammatory mediators results in increased vascular permeability. As is the case with neoplasms, the edema is highly responsive to dexamethasone 6 mg every 6 hours.

Viral Encephalitis

MRI DWI sequences in patients with viral encephalitis (Chapter 66) reveal cytotoxic edema in the limbic cortex, including the medial temporal and inferior frontal lobes, insula, and cingulate gyrus without mass effect. In milder cases, FLAIR and CT may be negative and the lesions are only apparent on DWI. In rare cases, viral encephalitis can result in a more fulminant pattern of generalized cytotoxic and vasogenic edema that requires ICP monitoring and treatment.

Meningitis

Severe generalized brain edema can occur with acute purulent bacterial or tuberculous meningitis (see also Chapter 61). Such edema is caused by the inflammatory response generated by infiltrating polymorphonuclear white blood cells (WBCs) and has been termed *granulocytic brain edema*. Vasogenic edema predominates, but interstitial edema may also occur as the result of communicating hydrocephalus. Dexamethasone 10 mg every 6 hours for 4 days diminishes the inflammatory response and has been shown to improve survival and reduce cranial nerve injury in adults and children with bacterial meningitis regardless of whether brain edema is evident on imaging [**Level 1**].[3] A similar steroid regimen is also commonly used to reduce the inflammatory response in patients with tuberculous meningitis. Placement of an external ventricular drain may be required in cases with a significant component of hydrocephalus and is usually sufficient to control ICP.

Posterior Reversible Encephalopathy Syndrome

PRES is a clinical syndrome characterized by neurologic dysfunction and a characteristic pattern of brain edema that predominates in the white matter of the parietal and occipital lobes (Fig. 107.2). The edema is primarily vasogenic with cerebral perfusion pressure (CPP) breakthrough and disruption of the blood–brain barrier playing a large role in the pathogenesis of the disorder (see also Chapter 43). FLAIR imaging is highly sensitive and often reveals scattered microbleeds on gradient echo (T2*) sequences. A wide variety of very different pathologic entities can cause PRES, including hypertensive encephalopathy resulting from poorly controlled essential hypertension, eclampsia, a variety of immunosuppressive agents, and end-stage renal disease (see also Chapter 43). Clinical manifestations start with headache, confusion, visual disturbances (including cortical blindness in some cases), and seizures and can progress to stupor or coma. Massive swelling of the brain that requires ICP monitoring and therapy is unusual but can occur. Treatment is directed at removing any possible triggering agent and BP control with treatment for seizures and elevated ICP as needed. Continuous infusion antihypertensive agents that allow precise BP control, such as labetalol and nicardipine, are preferred. Magnesium sulfate 4-g bolus followed by 10 to 12 g/h has been shown to improve outcome in women with eclampsia [**Level 1**].[4]

High-Altitude Cerebral Edema

This condition is a form of global and purely vasogenic cerebral edema caused by excessive cerebral vasodilation triggered by hypoxia in high altitudes. In addition to vascular engorgement,

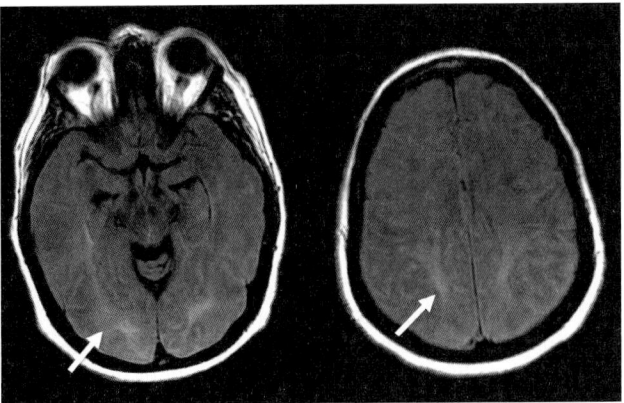

FIGURE 107.2 PRES. FLAIR images show abnormally increased signal (*arrows*) in the occipital and parietal white matter.

endothelial disruption results in fluid leakage into the brain. The condition can be rapidly fatal. MRI shows posterior white matter edema with a predilection for the splenium of the corpus callosum. Immediate descent (600 to 1,200 m), acetazolamide 500 mg every 6 hours, and delivery of supplemental oxygen are the treatments of choice.

Postendarterectomy Hyperperfusion Syndrome

This unusual complication of carotid endarterectomy or stenting occurs in patients who have long-standing high-grade carotid stenosis. Immediately after revascularization, the cerebral circulation remains maximally dilated and is unable to recover the capacity to autoregulate. The result is a pulsatile headache; more severe cases involve focal neurologic defects related to vasogenic edema in the downstream anterior circulation. In some cases, hemorrhagic conversion occurs. Meticulous BP control can minimize the extent of injury, and the syndrome typically resolves over several days.

INTRACRANIAL PRESSURE MANAGEMENT

General Approach

As outlined earlier, the optimal therapy of brain edema depends on the cause. A patent airway, maintenance of an adequate BP, and the avoidance of hypoxia are fundamental requirements in the care of these patients. The administration of appropriate parenteral fluids to meet the needs of patients is also essential. Administration of salt-free hypotonic fluids to patients with cerebral edema should be strictly avoided because serum hypo-osmolality increases brain swelling. As a general rule, inflammatory processes that predominantly involve vasogenic edema respond to dexamethasone (with the exception of vasogenic edema in patients with stroke or trauma) and measures to minimize brain engorgement and cerebral blood volume, including tight BP control and hyperventilation. By contrast, cytotoxic or cellular edema resulting from fluid and solute overload on the intracellular compartment responds best to osmotic therapy.

Neurosurgical decompression of the cranial vault can be life-saving and should always be the *first and last* consideration when patients are at risk for secondary deterioration due to compartmentalized intracranial mass effect. Surgical options include placement of an external ventricular or lumbar drain for drainage, craniotomy to remove an intracranial mass lesion, or as a last resort, hemicraniectomy with duraplasty to definitively decompress the cranial vault (Fig. 107.3). In all comatose patients where (1) intracranial hypertension elevation is suspected, (2) imaging shows mass effect due to brain edema, and (3) aggressive intensive care unit (ICU) care is indicated, placement of an ICP monitor is essential. Empiric treatment of suspected ICP should be performed in the short term but only when ICP and CPP are actually being measured can the problem be optimally treated.

In a monitored patient for whom all current neurosurgical options have been exhausted, medical management of elevated ICP is best performed according to an algorithm that emphasizes the logical stepwise application of various interventions (Table 107.3). In addition to the avoidance of hypotension and hypoxia, fluid resuscitation with isotonic crystalloids, seizure prophylaxis and fever control, and head elevation to 30 degrees lowers ICP by reducing jugular venous pressure and should be performed as a general measure in all patients (Table 107.4). Subsequent first-line pharmacologic treatment of brain edema resulting in increased ICP should then progress through the steps outlined in Table 107.3. In this

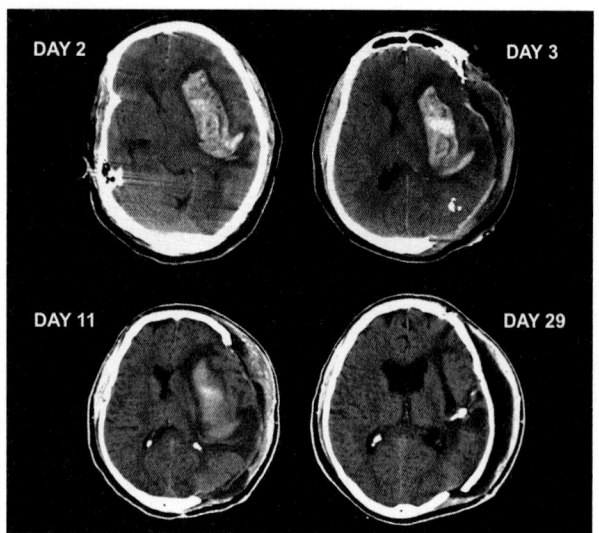

FIGURE 107.3 Decompressive hemicraniectomy in a 58-year-old man with left putamen ICH. On day 3, he experienced brain stem herniation with bilateral motor posturing and a fixed and dilated left pupil despite aggressive medical intervention. He underwent urgent hemicraniectomy and duraplasty with restoration of midline positioning of the brain evident on day 11. The day 29 image shows normalization of brain morphology after replacement of the bone flap. The patient made a near-complete recovery.

algorithm, sedation is the fundamental first step to controlling ICP after rescue neurosurgical intervention has been performed. Sedation lowers thoracic and jugular venous pressure and can calm arterial hypertension and autonomic instability. CPP, calculated as mean arterial pressure minus ICP, can aggravate intracranial hypertension when it is either extremely low or extremely high (Fig. 107.4). Osmotherapy in the form of 20% mannitol or 23.4% hypertonic saline solution is the mainstay intervention for reducing ICP in critical "brain code" situations. Mannitol should be hung wide open, and 30 mL of 23.4% saline should be pushed through a central venous line over 5 minutes. Doses can be repeated as often

TABLE 107.3	Initial Stepwise Management Protocol for Intracranial Pressure Crisis (>20 mm Hg for >10 Minutes) in a Monitored Patient

1. **Neurosurgical intervention** including ventricular drainage or craniotomy

2. **Sedate** to attain a motionless, quiet state with fentanyl and propofol

3. **Optimize cerebral perfusion pressure** (generally 70–100 mm Hg) to minimize excessive vasodilation from low hypotension or perfusion pressure breakthrough

4. **Bolus osmotherapy** with mannitol 0.5–1.51 g/kg IV or 30 mL 23.4% hypertonic saline repeated up to every 30 min as needed

5. **Hyperventilation** to PCO$_2$ levels of 30–34 mm Hg

6. **Hypothermia** with external or catheter-based cooling to 35°C

See text for details.
IV, intravenous.

TABLE 107.4	Baseline Treatment Measures for Patients at Risk for Intracranial Pressure

• Avoid hypotension and hypoxia.

• Administer only isotonic fluids (avoid all sources of free water).

• Head elevation to 30 degrees

• Control fever.

• Consider seizure prophylaxis.

as every 30 minutes as needed. Hyperventilation often does not have a sustained effect and should be administered in bursts, typically in tandem with bolus osmotherapy in response to ICP crisis.

In patients with ICP refractory to the aforementioned measures, consideration should be given to proceeding with decompressive hemicraniectomy. If this is not feasible or desired, the final step in first-line ICP intervention is to induce mild hypothermia to a target temperature of 35°C.

As outlined in Figure 107.5, escalation beyond the first line of medical intervention for refractory ICP becomes more nuanced and should be tailored to the specific clinical situation and available resources and expertise. These second-tier interventions for super-refractory ICP crisis are extensions of each step of first-line intervention. Decompressive hemicraniectomy should be reconsidered. CPP can be further optimized with invasive brain multimodality monitoring with the intention of normalizing CBF or brain tissue oxygen tension (PbtO2) (see Chapter 33). After a patient is sedated with conventional agents such as propofol, paralysis or barbiturate anesthesia with pentobarbital can be considered. Bolus osmotherapy can be escalated with continued good effect on ICP to serum osmolality levels far above 320 mOsm/L. When brain hyperemia is considered an important contributing factor, aggressive hyperventilation to PCO$_2$ levels far below 30 mm Hg can be safely attained with concurrent monitoring of PbtO2, CBF, or jugular venous oxygen saturation (normally 70% to 90%). Finally, hypothermia can be pushed to 33°C. Temperature levels below 30°C are thought to cause an unacceptable risk of arrhythmia and other cardiac complications.

SPECIFIC TREATMENTS FOR BRAIN EDEMA

Glucocorticoids

Glucocorticoids dramatically and rapidly (in hours) begin to reduce the focal and general signs of brain edema around tumors and abscesses but are not effective for treating the edema that results from cerebral infarction, ICH, SAH, or TBI. The major mechanism explaining the usefulness in vasogenic brain edema is a direct normalizing effect on endothelial cell function and permeability when the process is triggered by local release of cytokines, angiogenic factors, vascular adhesion molecules, and other inflammatory mediators.

Long-acting, high-potency glucocorticoids are most widely used for the treatment of vasogenic edema related to tumor or infection. The usual dosage of dexamethasone is a starting dose of 10 mg followed by 4 to 6 mg administered four times a day thereafter—a dose equivalent in potency to more than 400 mg of cortisol daily. These large doses are about 20 times the normal rate of human endogenous cortisol production. There are no convincing data, clinical or experimental, that glucocorticoids have beneficial effects for the treatment of cytotoxic or osmotic cellular edema regardless of cause.

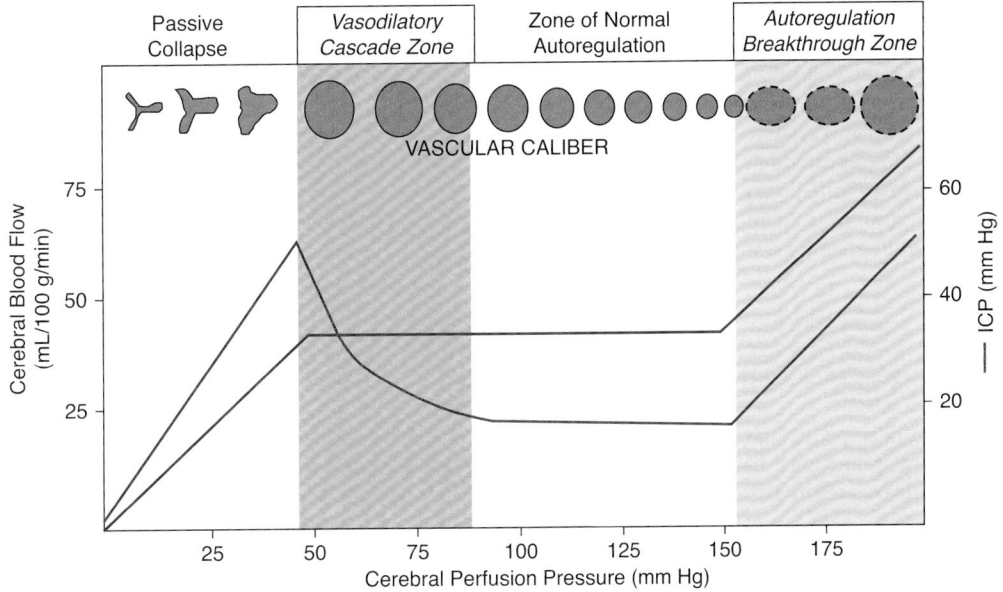

FIGURE 107.4 Cerebral autoregulation curve (*blue line*) and relationship between CPP and ICP in states of abnormal intracranial compliance (*red line*). Under normal circumstances, CBF is held constant across a wide range of CPP (50 to 150 mm Hg), and changes in vessel caliber have no effect on ICP. In disease states with reduced intracranial compliance, ICP can become elevated when CPP is low due to autoregulatory vasodilation and increased CBV (vasodilatory cascade physiology) or when CPP is too high due to passive increases in CBV due to increased hydrostatic pressure and hyperemia (autoregulation breakthrough physiology).

Steroids are also commonly used by neurosurgeons to enhance brain compliance and relaxation during craniotomy despite little evidence of its effectiveness. Steroids may be useful in the management of less common conditions characterized by an inflammatory CSF and brain edema, such as postinfectious acute disseminated encephalomyelitis (ADEM), CNS vasculitis, and meningeal sarcoidosis.

Mannitol

IV mannitol is the most widely used solute for the treatment of intracranial hypertension associated with brain edema. Given in a 20% solution at a dose of 0.25 to 1.5 g/kg, mannitol dehydrates brain tissue and mediates an ICP-lowering effect through several mechanisms. First, it is an osmotic diuretic that creates a concentration gradient across the blood–brain barrier and pulls free water from the brain. This decreases volume of the brain parenchyma and lowers ICP. Second, mannitol increases CPP through plasma expansion and promotes vasoconstriction and cerebral blood volume reduction by decreasing blood viscosity and improving CBF. Finally, mannitol is excreted in the urine resulting in a net clearance of free water and increased serum osmolality.

When given as a bolus infusion, mannitol can lower ICP within as little as 10 to 30 minutes. Dosing may be repeated as frequently

FIGURE 107.5 Stepwise ICP management protocol. Escalation of ICP therapy should advance through first-line interventions to ensure that vital steps are not skipped. The need for repeated bolus osmotherapy, burst hyperventilation, or induction of hypothermia defines ICP crisis. At the level of super-refractory ICP crisis, second-line interventions can be added based on the clinical situation and available resources and expertise. RASS, Richmond Agitation Sedation Scale; MMM, multimodality monitoring.

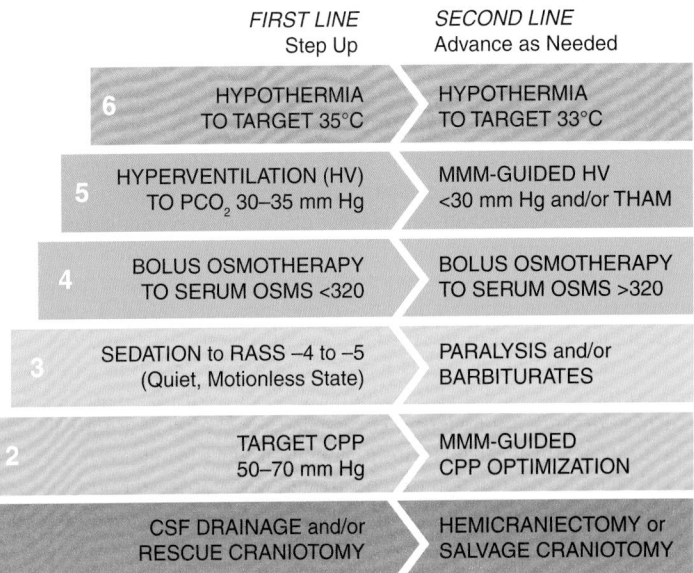

	FIRST LINE Step Up	SECOND LINE Advance as Needed
6	HYPOTHERMIA TO TARGET 35°C	HYPOTHERMIA TO TARGET 33°C
5	HYPERVENTILATION (HV) TO PCO₂ 30–35 mm Hg	MMM-GUIDED HV <30 mm Hg and/or THAM
4	BOLUS OSMOTHERAPY TO SERUM OSMS <320	BOLUS OSMOTHERAPY TO SERUM OSMS >320
3	SEDATION to RASS −4 to −5 (Quiet, Motionless State)	PARALYSIS and/or BARBITURATES
2	TARGET CPP 50–70 mm Hg	MMM-GUIDED CPP OPTIMIZATION
1	CSF DRAINAGE and/or RESCUE CRANIOTOMY	HEMICRANIECTOMY or SALVAGE CRANIOTOMY

as once an hour when ICP is elevated. Complications of mannitol therapy include dehydration, electrolyte depletion, and osmotically mediated renal failure. A widened gap of more than 10 mOsm/L between the measured and calculated osmolality may indicate incomplete mannitol clearance by the kidneys and an increased risk of renal tubular necrosis. With repeated bolus, dosing a "rebound effect" with successive increases in ICP may occur. Although it is sometimes stated that mannitol loses its efficacy when serum osmolality exceeds 320 mOsm/L, there is scant evidence to support this contention.

Hypertonic Saline

Hypertonic saline has an osmotic effect on the brain because of its high tonicity and ability to effectively remain outside the blood–brain barrier. Numerous animal studies have suggested that fluid resuscitation with hypertonic saline after hemorrhagic shock prevents the ICP increase that follows resuscitation with isotonic fluids. Hypertonic saline solutions may have favorable effects on CBF by producing a boost in CPP and via local effects on the cerebral microvasculature. A clinical trial comparing hypertonic saline with isotonic crystalloid for TBI patients, however, failed to show any benefit. Infusion of a bolus dose of 3%, 7%, 10%, or 23% hypertonic saline solution results in maximal ICP reduction between 30 and 120 minutes accompanied by a surge in CPP. In the United States, use of 30-mL "bullets" of 23.4% saline has become the most popular form of hypertonic saline bolus osmotherapy. Common complications of hypertonic saline administration include volume overload, pulmonary edema, and electrolyte depletion.

IDIOPATHIC INTRACRANIAL HYPERTENSION

Idiopathic intracranial hypertension (IIH) describes a heterogeneous group of disorders characterized by increased ICP when intracranial mass lesions, obstructive hydrocephalus, intracranial infection, and hypertensive encephalopathy have been excluded. IIH is also termed *pseudotumor cerebri*. The best documented risk factors for IIH are obesity, hypervitaminosis A, steroid withdrawal, and female gender. The term *benign* has been used because spontaneous recovery is characteristic, but the condition is far from harmless: Serious threats to vision make accurate diagnosis and therapeutic intervention a necessity.

CAUSES OF IDIOPATHIC INTRACRANIAL HYPERTENSION

Endocrine and Metabolic Disorders

IIH is most commonly seen in healthy women with a history of menstrual dysfunction. Frequently, the women are moderately or markedly overweight (without evidence of alveolar hypoventilation). Menstrual irregularity or amenorrhea is common; galactorrhea is an unusual symptom. The histories often emphasize excessive premenstrual weight gain. Endocrine studies have not revealed specific abnormalities of urinary gonadotropins or estrogens, and the pathogenesis is unknown. IIH has a complex relationship to adrenal hormones. Rarely, IIH is a complication of Addison disease or Cushing disease. Improvement occurs after restoration of a normal adrenal state; the mechanism in either circumstance is unknown.

IIH has also occurred in patients treated with corticosteroids for prolonged periods. Many of the patients had allergic skin disorders or asthma during childhood; IIH generally occurs when the steroid dosage is reduced but evidence of hyperadrenalism persisted.

Hypoparathyroidism may also present with increased ICP; hypocalcemic seizures or cerebral calcifications may further complicate the clinical picture. IIH has also been reported in women taking oral progestational drugs.

Drugs and Toxins

IIH has been reported in otherwise healthy adolescents who are taking large doses of vitamin A for the treatment of acne. Oral doses as low as 25,000 IU daily may cause headache and papilledema with rapid improvement after cessation of the therapy. The syndrome is said to have occurred in Arctic explorers who consumed polar bear liver, a great source of vitamin A. Some cases of IIH that are manifested by bulging fontanel and papilledema have been reported in children given tetracycline. The mechanisms involved are obscure. Spontaneous, rapid recovery occurs when the drugs are stopped. Amiodarone and lithium carbonate, as well as the insecticide chlordecone, have also been reported to cause IIH.

Hematologic and Connective Tissue Disorders

Papilledema and increased ICP have been attributed to severe iron deficiency anemia with striking improvement after treatment of the anemia. Presumably, the mechanism partly reflects the marked increase in CBF that accompanies profound anemia. IIH has also been observed as a manifestation of systemic lupus erythematosus.

Pulmonary Encephalopathy

IIH may be a major complication of chronic, hypoxic hypercapnia caused by paralytic states such as muscular dystrophy and cervical myelopathy; it may also be a complication of obstructive pulmonary disease and obstructive sleep apnea. There is a chronic increase of CBF because of hypoxia and carbon dioxide retention. Patients usually appear mentally dull and encephalopathic and thus differ from most patients with IIH.

Spinal Cord Diseases

IIH rarely occurs with tumors of the spinal cord or cauda equina or with polyneuritis. Papilledema and headache disappear with treatment of the spinal lesion or regression of the polyneuropathy. The mechanism may involve the effects of an elevated CSF protein on CSF absorption at the arachnoid villi in both cranial and spinal subarachnoid spaces. Occurrence of this syndrome, however, does not correlate with the degree of protein elevation.

PATHOBIOLOGY

Several mechanisms have been considered as possible explanations for the pathophysiology of IIH. These include an increased rate of CSF formation, a sustained increase in intracranial venous pressure, a decreased rate of CSF absorption by arachnoid villi apart from venous occlusive disease, and an increase in brain volume caused by an increase in blood volume or extravascular fluid volume simulating a form of brain edema.

No data are available regarding the rate of CSF formation, and the only condition in which increased CSF formation has been demonstrated is choroid plexus papilloma. Increased CSF production might explain the pathophysiology in some of the diverse conditions associated with IIH, but this mechanism remains unproven. A sustained increase in intracranial venous pressure associated with decreased CSF absorption has similarly not been documented in IIH. The currently most favored explanation for IIH is decreased CSF absorption (in the absence of venous occlusion) resulting from altered function of the arachnoid villi. For reasons that are unclear, however, hydrocephalus does not occur in IIH. On the contrary, very often, the brain appears swollen and the ventricles are smaller than normal. It has been hypothesized that IIH might have caused by an increase in brain volume secondary to an increase in extracellular fluid volume. An increase in brain volume would be expected if the extracellular space of the brain were expanded; this might occur if there was a defect in the ability to absorb brain interstitial fluid.

Any theory of the pathogenesis of IIH must be consonant with the rapid therapeutic response of IIH to shunting of CSF by an implanted lumbar peritoneal shunt. Impaired CSF absorption or increased CSF formation would explain the occurrence of IIH in most cases; however, the limited data available, currently, do not allow any firm conclusions.

One of the more common forms of IIH appears in otherwise healthy persons in the absence of any of the aforementioned etiologic factors. Both genders are affected, women more than men, and occurrence is most often in patients between 10 and 50 years of age.

CLINICAL FEATURES

Typically, the first symptoms are headache and impaired vision. The headache may be worse on awakening and aggravated by coughing and straining. It is often mild or may be entirely absent. In some cases, pulse-synchronous tinnitus occurs. The most common ocular complaint is visual blurring, a manifestation of papilledema. Some patients complain of brief, fleeting moments of dimming or complete loss of vision occurring many times during the day, at times accentuated or precipitated by coughing and straining. This ominous symptom indicates that vision is in jeopardy. Visual loss may be minimal despite severe chronic papilledema, including retinal hemorrhages; however, blindness occasionally develops rapidly (i.e., <24 hours). Visual field testing characteristically shows enlargement of the blind spots and may show constriction of the peripheral fields and central or paracentral scotoma. Diplopia caused by unilateral or bilateral sixth nerve palsy may develop as a result of increased ICP. The neurologic examination is otherwise normal. A major clinical point is that patients with IIH usually look well; their apparent well-being belies the ominous appearance of the papilledema. Although the disorder most often lasts for months, it may persist for years without serious sequelae. Remissions may be followed by one or more recurrences in 5% to 10% of cases. In some patients, IIH may be responsible for development of the *empty sella syndrome*, in which radiographic image showing enlargement of the sella turcica simulates the appearance of a pituitary tumor. CT reveals that the enlarged sella is filled with CSF flowing from a defect of its diaphragm.

DIAGNOSIS

The patient with headache and papilledema without other neurologic signs suggest the diagnosis of IIH. Although the diagnosis of IIH may be suspected by the appearance of well-being and a history of some of the associated etiologic features listed previously, the diagnosis is essentially one of exclusion and depends on ruling out the more common structural causes of increased ICP. Brain tumor, particularly when located in relatively "silent" areas such as the frontal lobes or right temporal lobe or when obstructing the ventricular system, may be manifested only by headache and papilledema. Patients with chronic subdural hematoma, without a history of significant trauma, may have the same symptoms. Other important conditions to exclude include viral meningitis and other CNS infections and dural sinus thrombosis.

Diagnostic evaluation depends on MRI with venography and lumbar puncture. Lumbar puncture should be deferred until imaging indicates that the perimesencephalic cisterns are open. Diagnostic lumbar puncture is mandatory to establish the diagnosis of IIH. In obesity, the normal upper limit of CSF pressure is 250 mm Hg. In IIH, the CSF pressure is elevated, usually between 250 and 600 mm Hg, but the fluid is otherwise normal. The protein content is often in the lower range of normal, and lumbar CSF protein levels of 10 to 20 mg/dL are common. CSF protein content greater than 50 mg/dL, decreased CSF glucose, or increased cell count throws doubt on the diagnosis of IIH and suggests other disease conditions.

Pseudopapilledema may be a source of diagnostic confusion. In this developmental anomaly of the fundus, the ophthalmic appearance may be indistinguishable from true papilledema; there is elevation of the optic disc, although exudates and hemorrhages are absent. Visual acuity is normal, but visual fields may show enlargement of the blind spots. The unchanging appearance of the fundus in subsequent examinations favors the diagnosis of pseudopapilledema, as does the finding of normal CSF pressure on lumbar puncture. Optic neuritis is differentiated from IIH by visual loss and normal CSF pressure.

TREATMENT

The common form of IIH in patients with menstrual disorders and obesity requires individualized management. This syndrome is self-limited in most cases, and after some weeks or months, spontaneous remissions occur, making evaluation of therapy outcomes difficult. Recurrent episodes have been noted in about 5% to 10% of patients, and the illness seldom lasts for years. In the extremely obese patient, weight reduction is recommended. Daily lumbar puncture was used in the past to lower CSF pressure to normal levels by removing sufficient fluid; 15 to 30 mL of fluid may be removed, but the value of this procedure is dubious. A CSF shunt procedure, such as a lumboperitoneal shunt, is useful in patients with intractable headache and progressive visual impairment. It may dramatically relieve symptoms. Optic nerve decompression has its advocates as the procedure of choice to preserve vision.

Acetazolamide 500 mg two to four times a day has been used because this carbonic anhydrase inhibitor reduces CSF formation. The Neuro-Ophthalmology Research Disease Investigator Consortium (NORDIC) trial has demonstrated that acetazolamide 1,000 mg titrated upward, along with a weight reduction diet, results in modest improvement in visual field function for patients with mild pseudotumor cerebri [**Level 1**].[5] Hypertonic IV solutions (20% mannitol) to lower ICP may be used in acute situations when there is rapidly failing vision and surgical intervention is awaited. When the pseudotumor syndrome is a manifestation of hypoadrenalism or hypoparathyroidism, replacement therapy is indicated. Vitamin A intoxication disappears when administration of the vitamin is stopped.

SPONTANEOUS INTRACRANIAL HYPOTENSION

Spontaneous intracranial hypotension (SIH) was first described in 1938. The cardinal symptom is postural headache, which is markedly exacerbated when upright and relieved by lying down. In more severe cases, downward traction on the cranial nerves can cause diplopia, visual field defects, tinnitus, and hearing loss. The symptoms are often self-limited, resolving spontaneously within several weeks to months. The peak age at onset is 40 years, and women are affected more than men.

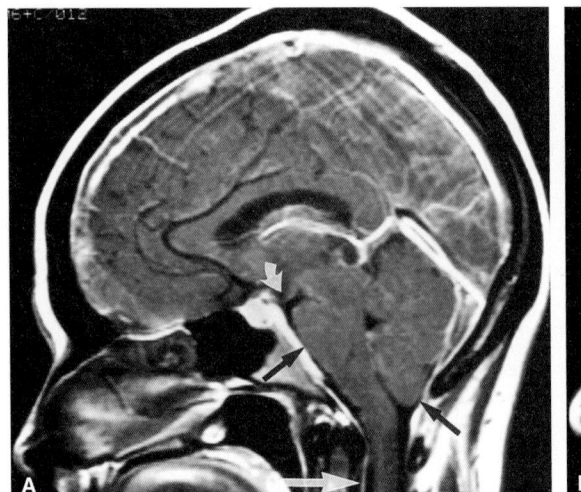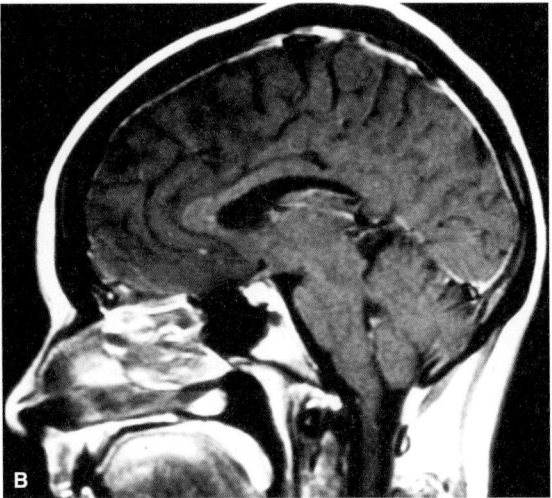

FIGURE 107.6 Sagging brain in spontaneous intracranial hypotension. **A:** Gadolinium-enhanced T1-weighted sagittal MRI prior to lumbar epidural blood patch demonstrates enhancement of the dura, venous engorgement, displacement of the pons and cerebellum below the level of the prepontine cistern (*black solid arrows*), and inferior displacement of the optic chiasm and third ventricle (*curved white arrow*). Enhancement of the ventral cervical dura is also present (*long white arrow*). **B:** Gadolinium-enhanced T1-weighted images 5 days after large-volume (20 mL) lumbar epidural blood patch showing resolution of dural enhancement and restoration of the cisterns with elevation of the pons, tonsils, and optic chiasm. (From Fishman RA, Dillon WP. Dural enhancement and cerebral displacement secondary to intracranial hypotension. *Neurology*. 1993;43:609–610, with permission.)

SIH is most often caused by the formation of CSF leak via dural fistulas along a thoracic spinal nerve root. Such defects commonly reflect rupture of arachnoid (Tarlov) cyst that occurs without trauma. These lesions can be identified on contrast CT myelography. Cervical subarachnoid injection (C2 or C3 level) is often preferred over lumbar injection because it is usually more proximate to the CSF fistulae, which may be intracranial, cervical, or thoracic and less likely lumbosacral. Delayed CT myelography can often pinpoint the site of contrast leak and CSF leakage.

Lumbar puncture typically reveals normal CSF with a low opening pressure (<10 cm H$_2$O). Brain MRI in SIH commonly reveals striking, diffuse dural enhancement, which reflects meningeal venous engorgement due to a compensatory increase in cerebral venous blood volume in response to a reduction in CSF volume. MRI may also reveal subdural fluid collections, pituitary engorgement, and sagging of the brain, which manifests as effacement of the quadrigeminal cisterns, flattening of the optic chiasm, and displacement of the pons against the clivus and cerebellar tonsils below the foramen magnum. These changes resolve rapidly after closure of the CSF fistula. Figure 107.6 shows the characteristic MRI findings in the sagging brain together with their resolution 5 days after a successful, large-volume, epidural lumbar blood patch.

SIH usually resolves with bed rest and IV hydration analogous to post–lumbar puncture headache. For intractable cases, treatment with a large-volume lumbar epidural blood patch is usually preferred, with the head and spine then tilted downward (30 degrees for 10 minutes) to facilitate the movement of blood, extradurally, to the thoracic and cervical regions. In persistent cases, surgical closure of the fistula may be necessary. This requires CT myelography to identify the precise location of the fistula.

Although postural headaches in the erect position are typical of SIH, some patients are headache free despite characteristic radiologic changes. The occurrence of somnolence and stupor caused by a sagging brain has been observed. Head-down Trendelenburg positioning is the initial treatment of choice. Restoration of CSF volume and pressure to normal by the intrathecal injection of normal saline or preferably Elliotts B solution (a pH-adjusted buffered saline) dramatically and rapidly restores consciousness and a normal mental state.

LEVEL 1 EVIDENCE

1. Poungvarin N, Bhoopat W, Viriyavejakul A, et al. Effects of dexamethasone in primary supratentorial intracerebral hemorrhage. *N Engl J Med*. 1987;316(20):1229–1233.
2. Roberts I, Yates D, Sandercock P, et al. Effect of intravenous corticosteroids on death within 14 days in 10,008 adults with clinically significant head injury (MRC CRASH trial): randomised placebo-controlled trial. *Lancet*. 2004;364:1321–1328.
3. van de Beek D, de Gans J, McIntyre P, et al. Steroids in adults with acute bacterial meningitis: a systematic review. *Lancet Infect Dis*. 2004;3:139–143.
4. Magpie Trial Collaborative Group. Do women with preeclampsia, and their babies, benefit from magnesium sulfate? The Magpie Trial: a randomised placebo-controlled trial. *Lancet*. 2002;359:1877–1890.
5. The NORDIC Idiopathic Intracranial Hypertension Study Group Writing Committee, Wall M, McDermott MP, et al. Effect of acetazolamide on visual function in patients with idiopathic intracranial hypertension and mild visual loss: the Idiopathic Intracranial Hypertension Treatment Trial. *JAMA*. 2014;311(16):1641–1651. doi:10.1001/jama.2014.3312

SUGGESTED READINGS

Brain Edema

Claassen J, Carhuapoma JR, Kreiter KT, et al. Global cerebral edema after subarachnoid hemorrhage: frequency, predictors, and impact on outcome. *Stroke*. 2002;33:1225–1232.

Fishman RA. Brain edema. In: *Cerebrospinal Fluid in Diseases of the Nervous System*. 2nd ed. Philadelphia: WB Saunders; 1992:116–137.

Hackett PH, Yarnell PR, Hill R, et al. High-altitude cerebral edema evaluated with magnetic resonance imaging. *JAMA*. 1998;280:1920–1925.

Ho ML, Rojas R, Eisenberg RL. Cerebral edema. *AJR Am J Roentgenol*. 2012;199(3):W258–W273.

Jha SK. Cerebral edema and its management. *MJAFI*. 2003;59:326–331.

Lee KR, Colon KP, Betz AL, et al. Edema from intracerebral hemorrhage: the role of thrombi. *J Neurosurg*. 1996;84:91–96.

Qureshi AI, Suarez JI. Use of hypertonic saline solutions in treatment of cerebral edema and intracranial hypertension. *Crit Care Med*. 2000;28:3301–3313.

Schilling L, Wahl M. Mediators of cerebral edema. *Adv Exp Med Biol*. 1999;474:123–141.

Walcott BP, Kahle KT, Simard JM. Novel treatment targets for cerebral edema. *Neurotherapeutics*. 2012;9:65–72.

Idiopathic Intracranial Hypertension

Ball A, Clarke C. Idiopathic intracranial hypotension. *Lancet Neurol*. 2006;5:433–442.

Bastin ME, Sinha S, Farrall AJ, et al. Diffuse brain edema in idiopathic intracranial hypertension: a quantitative magnetic resonance study. *J Neurol Neurosurg Psychiatry*. 2003;74:1693–1696.

Binder DK, Horton JC, Lawton MT, et al. Idiopathic intracranial hypertension. *Neurosurgery*. 2004;54:538–552.

Fishman RA. Pseudotumor cerebri. In: *Cerebrospinal Fluid in Diseases of the Nervous System*. 2nd ed. Philadelphia: WB Saunders; 1992:138–151.

Ridsdale L, Moseley I. Thoracolumbar intraspinal tumors presenting features of raised intracranial pressure. *J Neurol Neurosurg Psychiatry*. 1978;41:737–745.

Sinclair AJ, Woolley R, Mollan SP. Idiopathic intracranial hypertension. *JAMA*. 2014;312(10):1059–1060.

Wakerley BR, Tan MH, Ting EY. Idiopathic intracranial hypertension. *Cephalalgia*. 2015;35(3):248–261. doi:10.1177/0333102414534329.

Spontaneous Intracranial Hypotension

Fishman RA, Dillon WP. Dural enhancement and cerebral displacement secondary to intracranial hypotension. *Neurology*. 1993;43:609–610.

Horton JC, Fishman RA. Neurovisual findings in the syndrome of spontaneous intracranial hypotension from dural cerebrospinal fluid leak. *Ophthalmology*. 1994;101:244–251.

Mokri B, Piepgras DG, Miller GM. Syndrome of orthostatic headaches and diffuse pachymeningeal gadolinium enhancement. *Mayo Clin Proc*. 1997;72:400–413.

Pleasure SJ, Abosch A, Friedman J, et al. Spontaneous intracranial hypotension resulting in stupor caused by diencephalic compression. *Neurology*. 1998;50:1854–1857.

Renowden SA, Gregory R, Hyman N, et al. Spontaneous intracranial hypotension. *J Neurol Neurosurg Psychiatry*. 1995;59(5):511–515.

Schievink, Wouter I. Stroke and death due to spontaneous intracranial hypotension. *Neurocrit Care*. 2013;18(2):248–251.

Tarlov IM. Spinal perineural and meningeal cysts. *J Neurol Neurosurg Psychiatry*. 1970;33:833–843.

Emitseilu K. Iluonakhamhe, Tiffany R. Chang,
and Kiwon Lee

INTRODUCTION

In 1825, Magendie described a patient with symptoms of unsteadiness and vertigo resulting from hypotension of spinal fluid and ventricular collapse. A century later in 1938, Georg Schaltenbrand described a condition, which he termed *spontaneous or essential aliquorrhea*, that was marked by postural headache and low cerebrospinal fluid (CSF) pressure. Intracranial hypotension occurs when there is loss of CSF volume. The loss of CSF can occur at different location of the neural axis depending on the underlying etiology. For example, CSF leaks can occur at a skull base fracture from trauma and post–dural puncture CSF leaks can occur at the spinal level of needle insertion. A similar syndrome of intracranial hypotension can be seen in patients with excessive CSF drainage by ventriculoperitoneal shunts and post craniotomy (i.e., brain sagging). An increasingly recognized etiology of intracranial hypotension is spontaneous intracranial hypotension (SIH).

SPONTANEOUS INTRACRANIAL HYPOTENSION

SIH is the result of an idiopathic CSF leak. Most spontaneous CSF leaks occur at the cervicothoracic junction or thoracic spine. Some of the proposed mechanisms include spontaneous rupture of an arachnoid membrane and a variety of dura abnormalities such as meningeal diverticula, perineural (Tarlov) cyst, localized absence of dura, as well as spontaneous dura tears occurring where the spinal roots leave the subarachnoid space. Some spontaneous leaks have been attributed to underlying connective tissue disorders such as Marfan syndrome and Ehlers–Danlos syndrome (type II). Other predisposing etiologies include autosomal dominant polycystic kidney disease, Lehman syndrome, and neurofibromatosis type 1.

The true incidence of SIH is unknown, but the estimated annual incidence is 5 per 100,000 and a prevalence of 1 case per 50,000. It occurs more in women than men in a 2:1 ratio. Symptoms typically begin in the fourth to fifth decade of life; however, it has been reported in all age groups.

CLINICAL FEATURES

The most common initial presentation is a new onset of headache, typically orthostatic in nature. Additional symptoms include visual changes, diplopia, hearing changes, neck pain and/or stiffness, convulsions, nausea, and vomiting. Atypical presentations include parkinsonism, dementia, hypopituitarism, seizures, and coma. Symptoms are typically reversible with normalization of CSF pressure. Spinal symptoms including radicular symptoms and quadriparesis are rare. The onset and exacerbation of symptoms can be associated with coughing, laughing, Valsalva maneuver, and post coitus.

The diagnostic criteria for SIH as defined in *International Classification of Headache Disorders*, 3rd edition (ICHD-3), is noted in Table 108.1. A diagnosis of SIH cannot be made if patient had a dural puncture within a month of onset of headache. The headache quality resembles post–dural puncture headache, but the postural component may not be as dramatic. The onset of headache in SIH is minutes to hours compared to seconds as in postdural headaches. The location is often holocephalic but may be localized to the frontal or occipital region. It is usually described as a throbbing or pressure-like headache but can also be dull in quality. The headache is alleviated by lying flat for about 15 to 30 minutes, but resolution can be delayed or incomplete. The headache is thought to be the result of loss of CSF buoyancy resulting in downward displacement of the brain, causing traction on pain-sensitive structures such as the dura or compensatory engorgement of pain-sensitive intracranial venous structures. If unmanaged, SIH can lead to a chronic daily headache that may not be orthostatic or relieved by recumbency. It is important to elicit the orthostatic nature of the headache at the initial onset, as this feature may become less obvious to the patient as the headache becomes chronic.

Important complications of spontaneous CSF leaks include subdural hematoma, bibrachial amyotrophy, cerebral venous thrombosis (CVT), and, rarely, superficial siderosis.

DIAGNOSIS

In addition to history and physical examination, use of magnetic resonance imaging (MRI) of the brain, particularly T1-weighted

TABLE 108.1	Diagnostic Criteria for Spontaneous Intracranial Hypotension as Defined in *International Classification of Headache Disorders*, 3rd Edition	
A	Any new-onset headache with at least two of the following:	
	• Headache develops exclusively during upright posture.	
	• Headache spontaneously improves in horizontal posture.	
	• Headache is mostly in the back of the neck, sometimes spreading upwards to the occipital region ("coat hanger distribution").	
B	Low CSF opening pressure (<6 cm H$_2$O) and/or evidence of CSF leakage on imaging	
C	Headache has developed in temporal relation to the low CSF leakage or has led to its discovery	
D	Not better accounted for by another *ICHD-3* diagnosis	

CSF, cerebrospinal fluid; *ICHD-3, International Classification of Headache Disorders*, 3rd edition.

images post gadolinium injection, is useful in making the diagnosis (Fig. 108.1). Five characteristic features seen on post–gadolinium-enhanced MRI of the brain are subdural fluid collections, diffuse enhancement of pachymeninges, engorgement of venous structures, pituitary hyperemia, and sagging of the brain, which make up the mnemonic SEEPS (Table 108.2). Most observed MRI of the brain findings are a result of a compensatory change due to the loss of CSF volume. Based on the Monroe–Kellie principle, a decrease in CSF volume will result in brain sag and compensatory venous engorgement. There are several case reports that demonstrate improvement in MRI findings after successful treatment of CSF leak. It is important to note that in about 20% of patients diagnosed with SIH, the MRI findings will be normal; therefore, a normal MRI does not exclude the diagnosis of SIH.

Opening CSF pressure can be obtained by performing lumbar puncture (LP). It is typically employed if there is a high suspicion of SIH although MRI findings are normal. LP should be performed after MRI of the brain is obtained to avoid post-LP MRI pachymeningeal enhancement, which can confound the diagnosis. A CSF opening pressure of less than 6 cm H_2O is a diagnostic criterion for SIH but not a requirement. In approximately 25% of patients with SIH, the CSF opening pressure is normal. In addition to low CSF opening pressure, lymphocytic pleocytosis as well as elevated protein concentration and xanthochromia have been reported.

If the MRI and CSF findings are inconclusive despite having high suspicion of SIH, computed tomographic (CT) myelography with iodinated contrast or magnetic resonance (MR) myelography with gadolinium of the spine as well as radionucleotide cisternography is advocated. Likewise, if initial treatment is ineffective and localization of the CSF leaks is desired for direct surgical intervention, these imaging modalities can accurately define the location and extent of CSF leak. CT myelography is the most accurate study for localization of CSF leak. It can also reveal the underlying

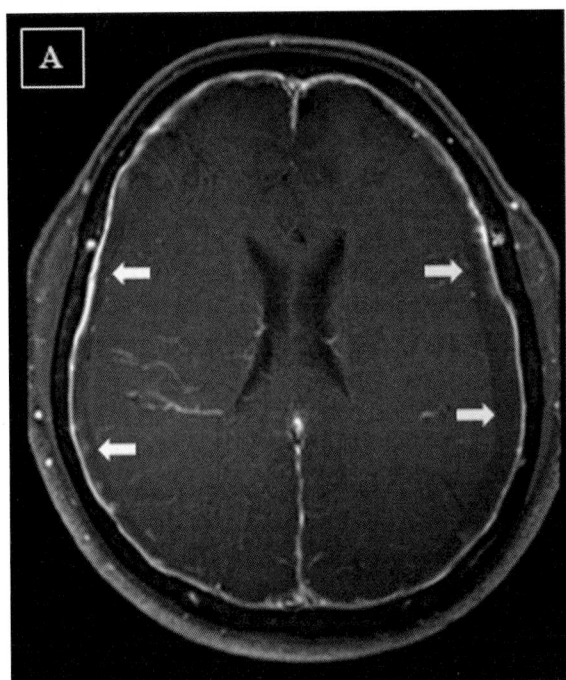

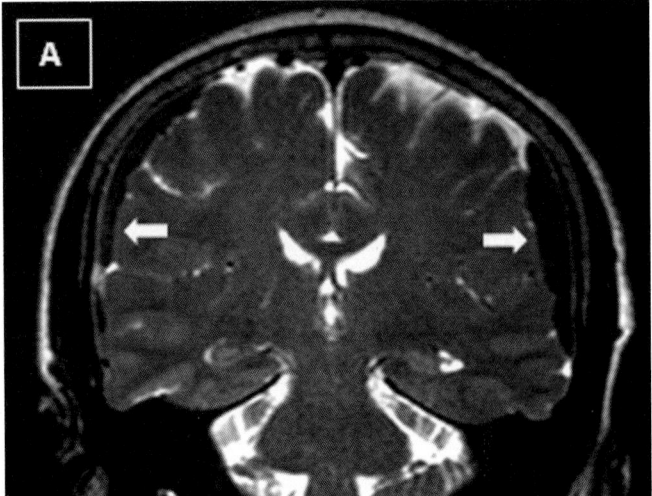

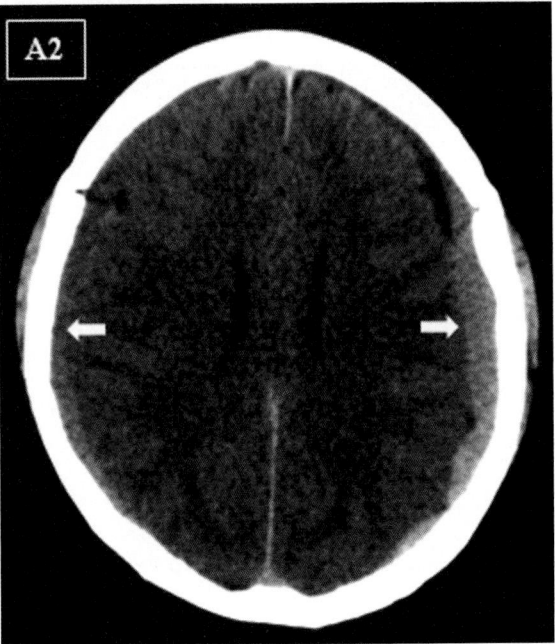

FIGURE 108.1 Cardinal MRI findings of spontaneous intracranial hypotension (mnemonic, SEEPS). **A:** Axial postcontrast T1 **(left)** and coronal T2 **(right)** MRI of the brain showing subdural fluid collections (*arrows*), noncontrasted axial CT of the head **(bottom)** showing bilateral subdural hemorrhage. (*continued*)

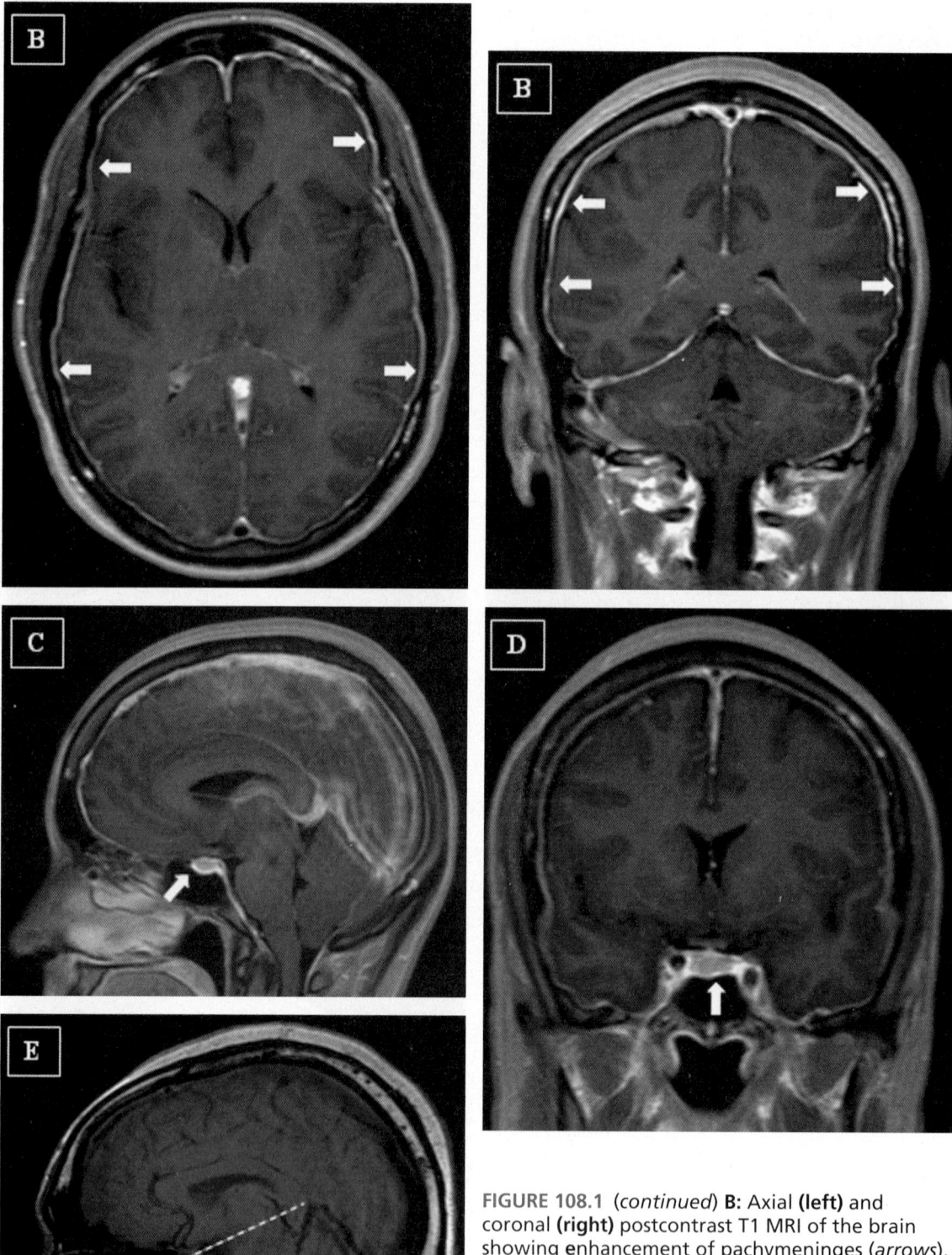

FIGURE 108.1 (*continued*) **B:** Axial **(left)** and coronal **(right)** postcontrast T1 MRI of the brain showing enhancement of pachymeninges (*arrows*). **C:** Sagittal view of postcontrast T1 MRI of the brain showing engorgement of venous structures as well as pituitary hyperemia (*arrow*). **D:** Coronal view of postcontrast T1 MRI of the brain showing pituitary hyperemia (*arrow*). **E:** Sagittal view of T1 MRI of the brain showing sagging of the brain, descent of cerebellar tonsils (*arrow*), and descent of the iter below incisural line (*dashed line*).

TABLE 108.2	Magnetic Resonance Imaging Features of Spontaneous Intracranial Hypotension (SEEPS)
Subdural fluid collections	
Enhancement of pachymeninges	
Engorgement of venous structures	
Pituitary hyperemia	
Sagging of the brain	

etiology of the leak, such as meningeal diverticula. It is recommended that early and delayed cuts are obtained at each spinal level to detect both fast and slow CSF leaks. MR myelography with intrathecal gadolinium and noninvasive MR myelography have been used increasingly as a reasonable alternative. Although historically, radionucleotide cisternography has been used as an indirect indicator of CSF leak, it is seldom employed when CT or MR myelography is available, as it is less sensitive. However, simultaneous use of CT and single-photon emission computed tomography (SPECT) has improved the sensitivity of radionucleotide cisternography detecting the exact location of CSF leak.

Although findings from CT of the brain are not as conclusive as MRI findings, it is useful when MRI is unavailable. Nontraumatic subdural fluid collections, ventricular collapse, obliteration of subarachnoid cisterns, and displacement of pons and cerebellar tonsils below the foramen magnum all contribute to making the diagnosis (see Fig. 108.1A).

MRI of the spine may demonstrate spinal manifestations of intracranial hypotension; however, it is not always useful in localizing the site of the CSF leak. Some imaging findings on MRI of the spine include dural enhancement, meningeal diverticula, dilated epidural or intradural veins, syringomyelia, retrospinal C1–C2 fluid, and extrathecal CSF collections. Use of MRI of the spine may be indicated if patient has neuropathic or myelopathic symptoms.

TREATMENT

Many cases of SIH are self-limited, although the time course for resolution is variable. Thus, the initial treatment is usually conservative medical management with bed rest, oral hydration, oral or intravenous caffeine, and abdominal binders. Epidural and/or intrathecal infusion of saline has been used to improve symptoms by temporarily increasing CSF volume. Caffeine has been used to serve as a vasoconstrictor to mitigate symptoms that are attributable to compensatory venous engorgement.

For patients who do not benefit from conservative medical management and continue to have persistent and debilitating symptoms, the mainstay reported treatment is the use of epidural blood patch (EBP). It involves injection of about 10 to 20 mL of autologous blood into the spinal epidural space. It can be injected directly at the level of CSF leak if known or can be placed in the safer lower lumbar region (Fig. 108.2). The patient is usually placed in Trendelenburg for up to 60 minutes after injection. The proposed mechanism is twofold; first to replace the lost CSF volume with blood volume in the spinal canal and second to serve as a sealant for any dural defect. Although there are no randomized controlled trials to evaluate the effectiveness of EBP use, it is reported to improve symptoms in 30% to 70% of patients after the first injection. Symptomatic relief is almost immediate but may not provide complete or permanent resolution of symptoms. Two or

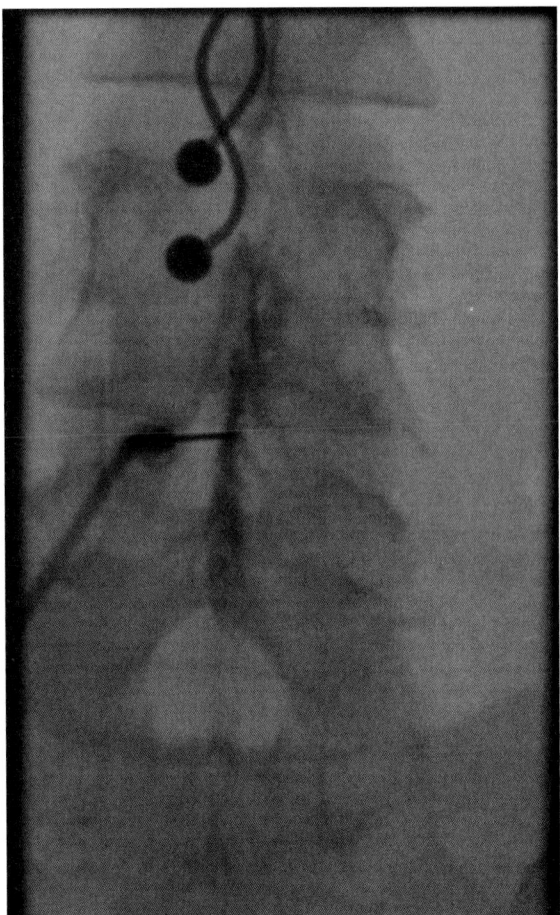

FIGURE 108.2 EBP placement in L4/L5 level under fluoroscopy.

more EBP may be required to achieve sustained relief. Thirty percent to 50% of patients may benefit from multiple administrations of EBP. After the initial one, subsequent EBP may be done with much larger volume of blood (up to 100 to 150 mL). It is expected that symptomatic relief should be sustained for at least a few days. Complications from EBP are rare, but they include neck and back pain, worsening of headache due to dural puncture, meningeal irritation, and rebound intracranial hypertension.

If the exact site of CSF leak is known from imaging studies and EBP does not provide sustained relief, use of percutaneous placement of fibrin sealant or directed EBP is advised. In refractory cases where the symptoms are debilitating and the site of leak is known, surgical repair using suture, aneurysm clip, muscle pledget with fibrin sealant, and Gelfoam may be considered.

POSTCRANIOTOMY BRAIN SAGGING

CLINICAL FEATURES

"Brain sagging" or "sinking brain syndrome" is a serious postoperative complication. It should be part of the differential diagnosis for any patient who clinically declines after craniotomy. Brain sagging may be diagnosed with three classic criteria: (1) clinical signs of transtentorial herniation, (2) excessive intracranial air with effacement of the basal cisterns (often with an oblong brain stem), and (3) improvement of symptoms when patient is placed in Trendelenburg position (Table 108.3). The syndrome typically develops as

TABLE 108.3	Criteria for Postcraniotomy "Brain Sagging" Syndrome

- Clinical signs of transtentorial herniation (e.g., reduced level of consciousness, motor posturing, pupillary and oculomotor abnormalities)
- Radiographic signs of excess intracranial air and effacement of the basal cisterns
- Improvement of symptoms in Trendelenburg (head down) position

an immediate postoperative finding, or within 48 hours of surgery, often once sedation is stopped. The hallmark presentation is anisocoria with acute mental status decline. Early recognition is paramount to avoid irreversible transtentorial herniation leading to permanent damage. Reported risk factors include presurgical presence of global cerebral edema, intraoperative lumbar drain, ventriculostomy, and prolonged surgery.

DIAGNOSIS

Neuroimaging, CT or MRI of the brain, may reveal crowding of the posterior fossa as well as flattening of the optic chiasm and anterior pons, descent of the brain stem and cerebellar tonsils, and reduction of subarachnoid cisternal spaces. On imaging, patients may have a significant amount of pneumocephalus and demonstrate Mount Fuji sign, peaking of the frontal lobes with excessive intracranial air (Fig. 108. 3). Remote hemorrhage, most often cerebellar in location, may also be seen on brain imaging following cranial or spinal surgery. This is attributed to venous bleeding secondary to intraoperative CSF loss. Remote cerebellar hemorrhage may give the appearance of a "zebra sign" on neuroimaging and can be associated with local edema and mass effect (Fig. 108.4).

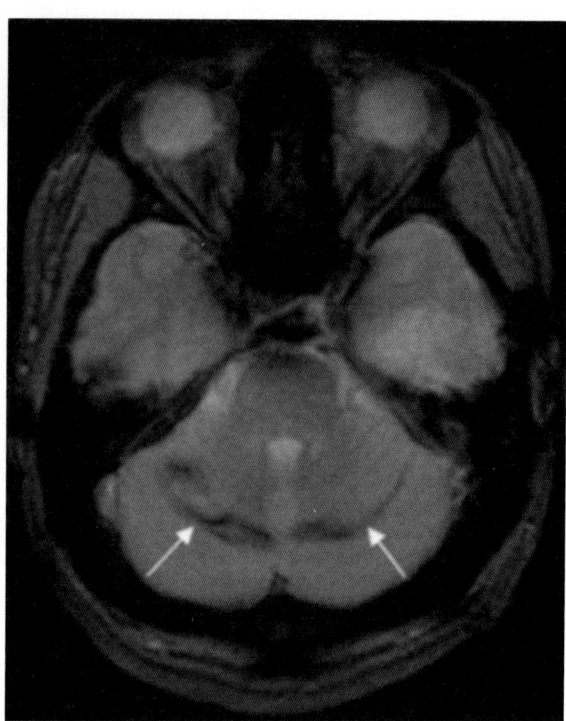

FIGURE 108.4 Gradient echo MRI of brain showing bilateral low intensity (*white arrows*) within the cerebellar sulci consistent with chronic hemosiderin staining due to remote cerebellar hemorrhage. This pattern of irregular stripes are alternating blood and cerebellum that is sometimes referred to as the *zebra sign*. (From Paul J, Jhaveri MD, Lewis SL. Teaching neuroimages: remote cerebellar hemorrhage following resection of a supratentorial tumor. *Neurology.* 2011;77[14]:e82–e83.)

TREATMENT

Most patients with brain sagging respond quickly when placed in Trendelenburg position. If after hours of Trendelenburg position does not improve neurologic condition, one should question the diagnosis and search for other causes of mental status deterioration. An injection of 10 to 15 mL of autologous blood (blood patch) into the lumbar space can resolve persistent symptoms of postural headache and neurologic symptoms (e.g., dizziness, lethargy, dysarthria) once the herniation syndrome has been reversed. In extreme cases of brain stem herniation from CSF hypovolemia, controlled infusion of isotonic crystalloid solution via a lumbar catheter has been reported to reverse the syndrome. Conservative management with bed rest, caffeine, oral hydration, and use of an abdominal binder has also been reported as effective in less severe cases.

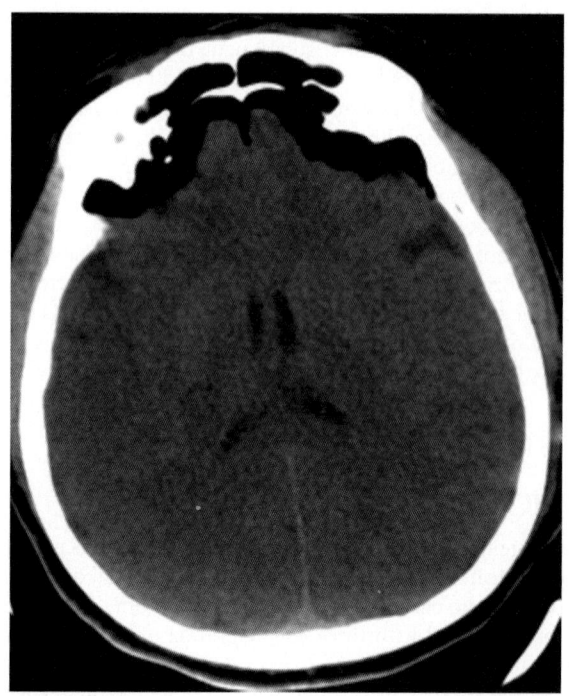

FIGURE 108.3 Pneumocephalus (*Mount Fuji sign*) after craniotomy for evacuation of subdural hemorrhage.

SUGGESTED READINGS

Albayram S, Kara B, Ipek H, et al. Isolated cortical venous thrombosis associated with intracranial hypotension syndrome. *Headache.* 2009;49(6):916–919.

Amoozegar F, Guglielmin D, Hu W, et al. Spontaneous intracranial hypotension: recommendations for management. *Can J Neurol Sci.* 2013;40(2):144–157.

Brockmann MA, Groden C. Remote cerebellar hemorrhage: a review. *Cerebellum.* 2006;5(1):64–68.

Chalela JA, Monroe T, Kelley M, et al. Cerebellar hemorrhage caused by remote neurological surgery. *Neurocrit Care.* 2006;5(1):30–34.

Chazen JL, Talbott JF, Lantos JE, et al. MR myelography for identification of spinal CSF leak in spontaneous intracranial hypotension. *AJNR Am J Neuroradiol.* 2014;35(10):2007–2012.

Chiapparini L, Ciceri E, Nappini S, et al. Headaches and intracranial hypotension: neuroradiological findings. *Neurol Sci.* 2004;25(suppl 3):S138–S141.

Davenport RJ, Chataway SJ, Warlow CP. Spontaneous intracranial hypotension from a CSF leak in a patient with Marfan's syndrome. *J Neurol Neurosurg Psychiatry.* 1995;59(5):516–519.

Hadizadeh DR, Kovacs A, Tschampa H, et al. Postsurgical intracranial hypotension: diagnostic and prognostic imaging findings. *AJNR Am J Neuroradiol.* 2010;31(1):100–105.

Headache Classification Committee of the International Headache Society. The International Classification of Headache Disorders, 3rd edition (beta version). *Cephalalgia.* 2013;33(9):629–808.

Kelley GR, Johnson PL. Sinking brain syndrome: craniotomy can precipitate brainstem herniation in CSF hypovolemia. *Neurology.* 2004;62(1):157.

Komotar RJ, Mocco J, Ransom ER, et al. Herniation secondary to critical postcraniotomy cerebrospinal fluid hypovolemia. *Neurosurgery.* 2005;57(20):286–292.

Komotar RJ, Ransom ER, Mocco J, et al. Critical postcraniotomy cerebrospinal fluid hypovolemia; risk factors and outcome analysis. *Neurosurgery.* 2006;59(2):284–290.

Lin WC, Lirng JF, Fuh JL, et al. MR findings of spontaneous intracranial hypotension. *Acta Radiol.* 2002;43(3):249–255.

Mathew L, Komotar R. Epidural blood patch for severe postoperative intracranial hypotension. *J Neurosurg Anesthesiol.* 2008;20(1):49–52.

Mokri B. Spontaneous CSF leaks low CSF volume syndromes. *Neurol Clin.* 2014;32:397–422.

Mokri B, Maher CO, Sencakova D. Spontaneous CSF leaks: underlying disorder of connective tissue. *Neurology.* 2002;58(5):814–816.

Mokri B, Posner JB. Spontaneous intracranial hypotension: the broadening clinical and imaging spectrum of CSF leaks. *Neurology.* 2000;55(12):1771–1772.

Schaltenbrand G. Normal and pathological physiology of the cerebrospinal fluid circulation. *Lancet.* 1953;1(6765):805–808.

Schievink WI. Novel neuroimaging modalities in the evaluation of spontaneous cerebrospinal fluid leaks. *Curr Neurol Neurosci Rep.* 2013;13(7):358.

Schievink WI. Spontaneous spinal cerebrospinal fluid Leaks and intracranial hypotension. *JAMA.* 2006;295(19):2286–2296.

Schievink WI, Maya MM, Louy C, et al. Diagnostic criteria for spontaneous spinal CSF leaks and intracranial hypotension. *AJNR Am J Neuroradiol.* 2008;29(5):853–856.

Schievink WI, Torres VE. Spinal meningeal diverticula in autosomal dominant polycystic kidney disease. *Lancet.* 1997;349(9060):1223–1224.

Intervertebral Disk Disease and Radiculopathy 109

Peter D. Angevine, Hani R. Malone, and Paul C. McCormick

INTRODUCTION

Intervertebral disk disease is responsible for a range of pain syndromes that have been recognized since the time of Hippocrates. The first reported treatment of intervertebral disk pathology occurred in 1909, when Krause operated on a patient who had been diagnosed by Oppenheimer as suffering from a lesion localized to the L4 root. In surgery, Krause found an extradural mass that was described pathologically as a chondroma and the operation to remove it apparently affected a cure. In 1934, Mixter and Barr were the first to point out that these lesions were actually fragments of intervertebral disks and that they were responsible for radicular pain. They further proved the efficacy of surgical treatment in their series of 58 patients treated with laminectomy and diskectomy for lumbar disk herniation.

EPIDEMIOLOGY

Symptoms related to intervertebral disk disease, particularly low back pain, are common. Pathologic studies have demonstrated that almost all individuals older than the age of 30 years have some evidence of disk degeneration. As individuals age, spondylosis and osteochondrosis, the long-term sequelae of degenerative disk disease, become more and more prominent. Intervertebral disk rupture is most common in the fourth to sixth decades of life. It is relatively rare before age 25 years and less common after age 60 years.

Importantly, pathologic or radiographic findings consistent with disk disease are often asymptomatic and clinically insignificant. Although some maintain that degenerative disk disease is a by-product of the modern human environment, there is no conclusive evidence that back pain has significantly increased over the past 50 years. Fortunately, the efficacy and morbidity associated with treating intervertebral disk disease has improved considerably.

PATHOPHYSIOLOGY

INTERVERTEBRAL DISK DISEASE

Displaced disk material may cause signs and symptoms by bulging or protruding beneath an attenuated annulus fibrosus, or the material may extrude through a tear in the annulus and project directly into the spinal canal (Fig. 109.1). In either case, the encroaching disk material may irritate or compress nerve roots as they approach their exit through the neural foramina. In cervical and thoracic regions, the problem is more neurologically complex because the spinal cord itself, as well as the adjacent nerve roots, may be involved. At cervical and thoracic levels, signs and symptoms are caused either by cord compression or a combination of cord and nerve root compression. In the lumbar region, signs and symptoms solely relate to the compression of nerve roots or to compression of the cauda equina if the disk is large enough to crowd the entire spinal canal.

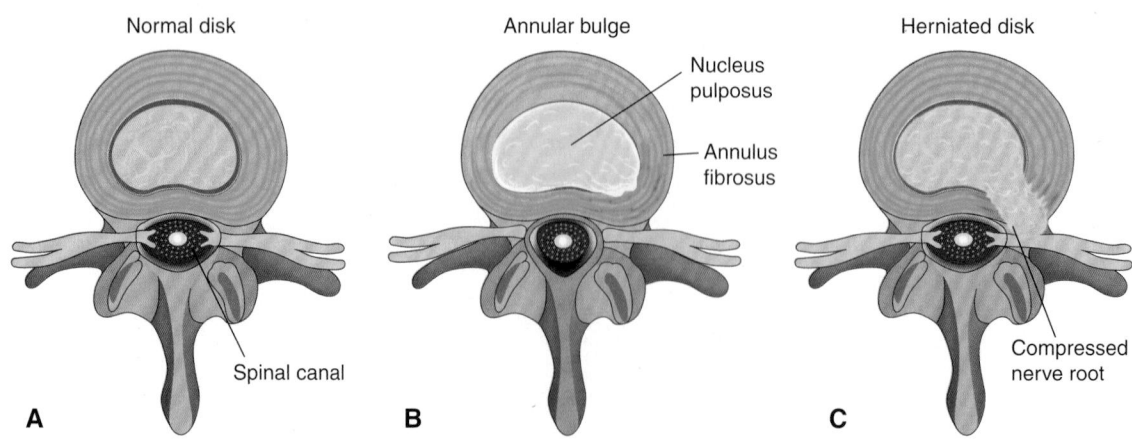

FIGURE 109.1 Anatomic illustration of the spinal canal and intervertebral disk. **A:** Demonstrating normal anatomy of the lumbar spine. **B:** An annular "disk bulge." **C:** An annular tear with herniation of the nucleus pulposus causing nerve root impingement.

There are eight spinal nerve roots in the cervical spine (C1–C8), which are numbered according to the caudal vertebra of the corresponding disk space. For example, the C4 nerve root exits through the neural foramen at the C3–C4 level and the C5 nerve root exits via the C4–C5 foramen. The C8 nerve root courses through the C7–T1 intervertebral foramen, as there is no C8 vertebra. Conversely, nerve roots in the thoracic and lumbar spine are numbered according to the vertebrae rostral to their exit through the intervertebral foramen. For example, the L5 nerve root exits the spinal canal at the level of L5–S1.

Importantly, paramedian lumbar disk herniations generally impinge on nerve roots that exit the spinal canal, a level below the site of disk herniation. For example, a paramedian herniated disk at the L4–L5 level compresses the L5 nerve root, which exits the spinal canal through the L5–S1 intervertebral foramen. This is not the case for *far lateral* disk herniations, which extend laterally to compress the rostral lumbar nerve root at the affected level. A far lateral L3–L4 lumbar disk herniation, for example, may compress the L3 nerve root either within the foramen or more distally as the root passes over the disk space (Fig. 109.2). Far lateral disk herniations account for 10% of all lumbar disk herniations, affect higher lumbar levels, and are likely to cause objective neurologic deficit. A far lateral disk herniation should be suspected with acute onset of an isolated upper lumbar radiculopathy that affects L2, L3, or L4.

In the cervical spine, degenerative disk disease most commonly affects the C5–C6 and C6–C7 levels. In the lumbar spine, most disk degeneration occurs at the L4–L5 and L5–S1 levels. This pattern suggests that the dynamics of pathologic change are partly related to wear and tear and to the trauma of motion.

Thoracic disk protrusions, except at the lower thoracic levels, differ from cervical and lumbar disorders in both genesis and histopathology. Motion does not play a significant role, as thoracic vertebrae are designed for stability rather than motion, and the heavy rib cage contributes to the rigidity of this region. Ruptured thoracic disks are markedly different on gross and microscopic examination and their consistency seldom resembles that of cervical and lumbar ruptured disks. These pathologic differences suggest a separate mechanism of injury in thoracic disk disease. Trauma has been accepted as a prime cause of thoracic disk herniation, but genetic predisposition also likely plays a role. Trauma may aggravate this susceptibility and ultimately catalyze rupture. Intervertebral disk disease is far less common in the thoracic spine compared to lumbar and cervical segments.

The signs and symptoms of herniated disks relate not only to the size and strategic location of the disk fragments but also to the size and configuration of the spinal canal. Congenital spinal stenosis, which is an abnormally narrow spinal canal, is an example of an inherited anomaly that influences the clinical impact of disk disease. Degenerative spondylosis leads to spinal stenosis and narrowing of the neural foramina through osteophyte formation and hypertrophy of the ligamentum flavum and facet joints. Degenerative spondylosis and congenital spinal stenosis are major contributors to compression syndromes of the spinal cord and cauda equina, as even small disk protrusions in these patients can further compromise an already limited canal. In a canal of normal dimensions, the severity of neural compression and the clinical impact of a protruded disk fragment depends more on the site of rupture and the volume of the extruded material.

CLINICAL FEATURES

CHRONIC LOW BACK PAIN

In the United States, back pain is the most common reason for limiting physical activity in people younger than 45 years; it is the second most frequent cause of visits to a physician, the fifth cause of hospital admissions, and the third leading cause of surgery. In many countries, it is the most common cause of absenteeism from work, accounting for more than 12% of sick days. The aggregate economic cost in the Netherlands in 1991 was estimated to be 1.7% of gross national product. This figure likely represents the typical cost incurred by developed nations. In the United States, the aggregate cost of lower back pain is estimated to exceed $100 billion per year.

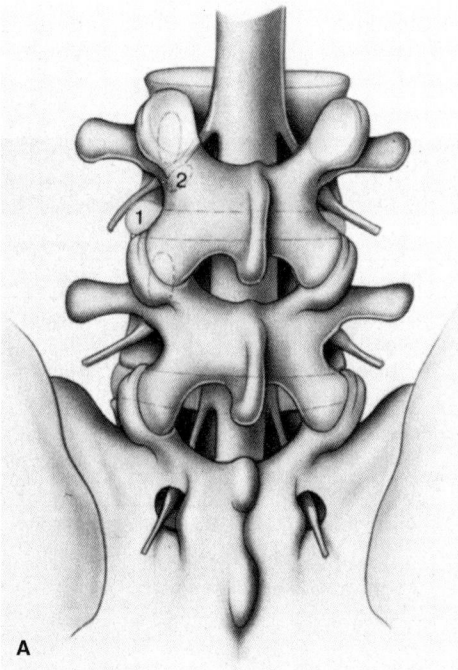 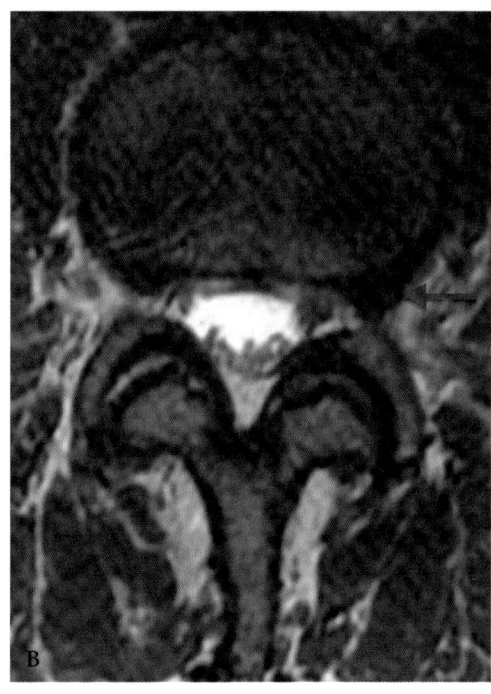

FIGURE 109.2 Far lateral disk herniation. A: Two sites of possible upper nerve root compression from a far lateral disk herniation. Root compression may occur at the level of the disk space (*1*) or from a rostrally migrated fragment into the foramen of the upper nerve root (*2*). **B:** MRI demonstrates a left far lateral disk herniation at the L3–L4 level (*arrow*).

According to Andersson, "Chronic low back pain has become a diagnosis of convenience for many people who are actually disabled for socioeconomic, work-related, or psychological reasons." The complexity of the problem is measured in a lengthy literature and a long list of approaches to therapy. Medications and other therapies include nonsteroidal anti-inflammatory drugs, opiates, and antidepressants; extradural injection of steroids; decompressive surgery; physical therapy, including massage and exercise; chiropractic treatment; and acupuncture. In Finland, a third of the direct costs were spent on complementary therapies. Multidisciplinary spine centers and pain centers may be sources of the most effective approach to management.

RADICULAR PAIN AND LUMBAR DISK DISEASE

Root syndromes of intervertebral disk disease are often episodic, so remissions are characteristic. The pain may be restricted to the back or follow a radicular distribution in one or both legs. Lumbar pain may increase after heavy lifting or twisting of the spine. No matter how severe the pain is when the patient is erect, characteristically, it is relieved when the patient lies down. Some patients, however, are more comfortable sitting and many find no comfortable position.

Physical examination often reveals loss of lumbar lordosis or flattening of the lumbar spine with splinting and asymmetric prominence of the long erector muscles. Range of motion of the lumbar spine is reduced by the protective splinting of paraspinal muscles, and attempted movement in some planes induces severe back pain. There may be tenderness of the adjacent vertebrae. When the patient is erect, one gluteal fold may hang down and show added skin creases because the gluteus is wasted—evidence of involvement of the S1 root. Passive straight leg raise is reduced in range and increases back and leg pain. Muscle atrophy and weakness or sciatic tenderness and discomfort may occur on direct pressure at some point along the nerve from the sciatic notch to the calf. This is particularly true in older patients.

The typical syndromes of root compression at lumbar levels are described in Table 109.1. Importantly, clinical signs may not be as distinct in actual practice as the table implies. More than 80% of syndromes affect the L5 or S1 nerve roots (Table 109.2). Compression of the nerve root at these levels results in "sciatica," a sharp and burning pain that radiates down the posterior/lateral aspect of the leg to the foot or ankle (Fig. 109.3). When the lesion affects L4 or higher roots, straight leg raise does not stretch the roots above L5. The affected roots may be tensed, however, by extension of the limb with the knee flexed when the patient is prone, thus reproducing the typical radicular spread of pain. Nerve root compression is often associated with numbness and tingling. Radicular pain resulting from disk disease classically intensifies with Valsalva (coughing, defecating, sneezing).

THORACIC DISK RUPTURE

The thoracic spine is designed for rigidity rather than excursion, thus wear and tear from motion and stress may not cause thoracic disk protrusion, and clinical disorders are rare. Thoracic disk disease may result from chronic vertebral changes incident to Scheuermann disease or juvenile osteochondritis with later trauma. The radiographic changes of Scheuermann disease, when seen with thoracic cord compression, should raise the possibility of disk protrusion (Fig. 109.4). The small capacity of the thoracic spinal canal makes this region vulnerable to cord compression from disk herniation. By the same token, decompressive operations are more precarious and require meticulous care to avoid damaging the spinal cord. Calcific changes are common in pathologic thoracic intervertebral disks, which pose additional challenges when performing diskectomy. The lower thoracic levels, however, are more capacious, and although the conus medullaris or cauda equina may be damaged by disk protrusions, surgical approaches are less hazardous compared to higher levels.

CERVICAL DISK DISEASE

Cervical disk herniation may involve both the nerve root and spinal cord depending on the volume of the canal and the size of the lesion. Spinal cord compression is uncommon, except with spinal stenosis or massive rupture of a disk. The sites of the most frequent disk herniations are C5–C6 and C6–C7; C4–C5 and C7–T1 are less frequently affected (Table 109.3). Movement of the cervical spine is normally incremental and any process contributing to focal stress at individual levels adds to progressive pathologic changes in the disk and to deficits in joint mechanics (Fig. 109.5). Development of a new fulcrum of motion above

TABLE 109.1 Common Root Syndromes of Intervertebral Disk Disease

Disk Space	L3–L4	L4–L5	L5–S1	C4–C5	C5–C6	C6–C7	C7–T1
Root affected	L4	L5	S1	C5	C6	C7	C8
Muscles affected	Quadriceps	Peroneals, anterior tibial, extensor hallucis longus	Gluteus maximus, gastrocnemius, plantar flexors of toes	Deltoid, biceps	Biceps	Triceps, wrist extensors	Intrinsic hand muscles
Area of pain and sensory loss	Anterior thigh, medial shin	Great toe, dorsum of foot	Lateral foot, small toe	Shoulder, anterior arm	Radial forearm	Thumb, middle fingers	Index, fourth, and fifth fingers
Reflex affected	Knee jerk	Posterior tibial	Ankle jerk	Biceps	Biceps	Triceps	Triceps
Straight leg raising	Many do not increase pain	Aggravates root pain	Aggravates root pain	—	—	—	—

TABLE 109.2	*Signs of Lumbar Disk Herniation in 97 Patients*			
Disk Space	L2–L3	L3–L4	L4–L5	L5–S1
Patients (*n*)	1	9	45	42
Weak muscles				
Anterior tibial, extensor hallucis	0	3	13	3
Gastrocnemius, plantar responses of foot	0	0	2	3
Quadriceps	0	3	0	0
Reflex affected				
Knee jerk	1	6	4	0
Ankle jerk	0	1	12	23

Data are numbers of patients. From Hardy RW Jr, Plank NM. Clinical diagnosis of herniated lumbar disc. In: Hardy RW, ed. *Lumbar Disc Disease.* New York: Raven Press; 1982:17–28.

a fusion or congenital block vertebrae increases susceptibility to these changes.

The signs and symptoms of cervical disk disease usually begin with stiff neck, reactive splinting of the erector capital muscles, and discomfort at the medial border of the scapula. Radicular paresthesias and pain supervene when the root is more severely compromised. These symptoms are worsened by movements of the head and neck as well as by stretching of the dependent arm. For relief, the patient often adopts a position with the arm elevated and flexed behind the head, unlike the patient with shoulder disease who maintains the arm in a dependent position avoiding elevation or abduction at the shoulder joint.

As compression proceeds, discrete root syndromes appear (see Table 109.1). C5 lesions cause pain in the shoulder and dermatomic sensory diminution with weakness and atrophy of the deltoid. C6 lesions cause paresthesias of the thumb and depression of the biceps reflex with weakness and atrophy of that muscle. In C7 lesions, paresthesias may involve the index and middle fingers, and even the thumb with atrophy and weakness in the triceps muscles, wrist extensors, and pectoral muscles, as well as a parallel reflex depression. C8 subserves important intrinsic muscle functions in the hand and sensation in the fourth and fifth fingers. Because these are important in discriminatory and fine finger maneuvers, C8 damage may be disabling.

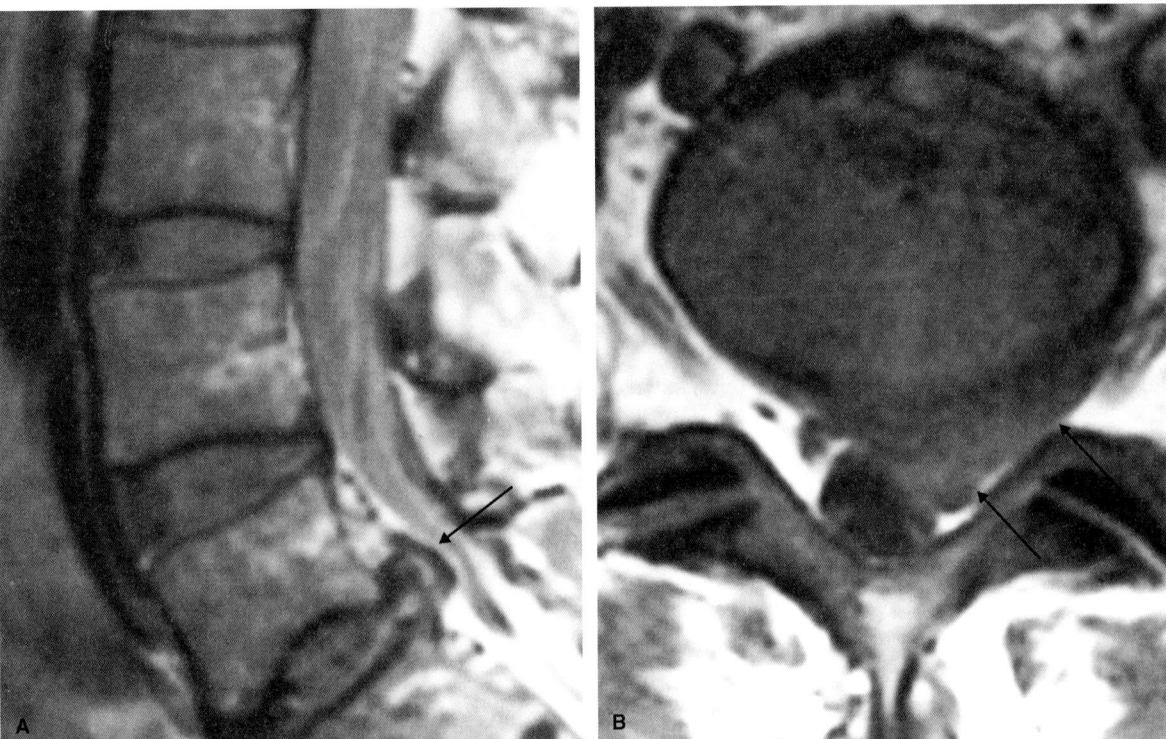

FIGURE 109.3 MRI of lumbosacral disk herniation. Sagittal proton-density **(A)** and axial T1-weighted **(B)** MRI demonstrate a large L5–S1 disk herniation on the left side. Clinically, this patient had an S1 radiculopathy that did not respond to conservative therapy. Complete relief of symptoms followed lumbar diskectomy.

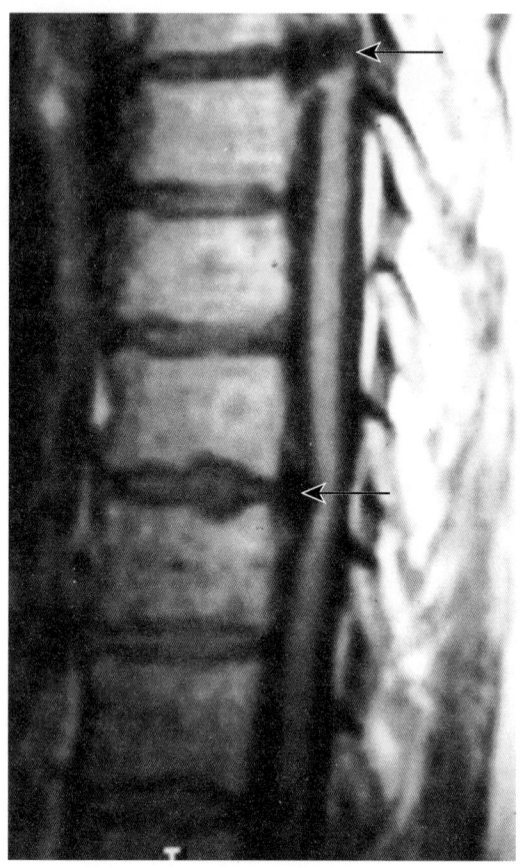

FIGURE 109.4 Thoracic disk herniation. Sagittal T1-weighted MRI demonstrates two large thoracic disks (*arrows*) in a patient with a subacute myelopathy.

TABLE 109.3	Frequency of Compression of the Cervical Roots by Ruptured Intervertebral Disk
Root	**Percent**
C5	2
C6	19
C7	69
C8	10

MYELOPATHY

Large disk protrusions in the thoracic and cervical spine, particularly with concurrent spinal stenosis, may compress the spinal cord resulting in myelopathic signs on clinical exam. Clinical signs of myelopathy reflect injury to upper motor neurons. Reflexes and tone are increased, whereas coordination and balance are diminished. Patients with cervical myelopathy often have difficulty using their hands for fine motor tasks and adopt a broad-based gait to improve balance while upright. Other signs of myelopathy on routine physical exam include Hoffman and Babinski signs, a positive Romberg test, and sustained clonus. Myelopathy is often combined with lower motor neuron weakness and may be subtle if compression of the cord is mild.

DIAGNOSIS

INITIAL MANAGEMENT AND EVALUATION

Radiculopathy is a clinical diagnosis based on careful history and physical examination. Immediate diagnostic testing with magnetic resonance imaging (MRI) is not necessary in patients with new-onset radicular pain that have not failed conservative measures.

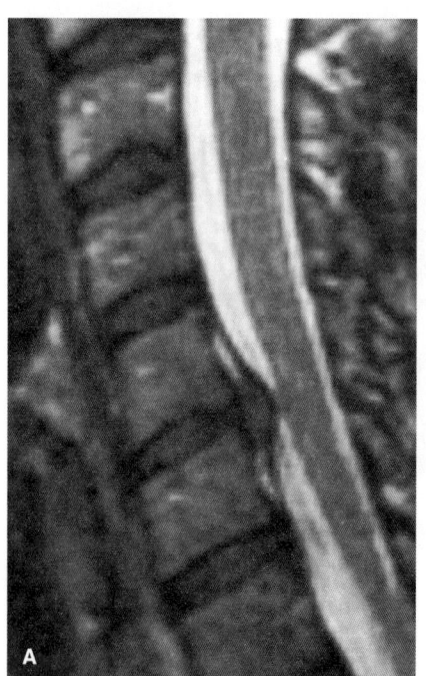
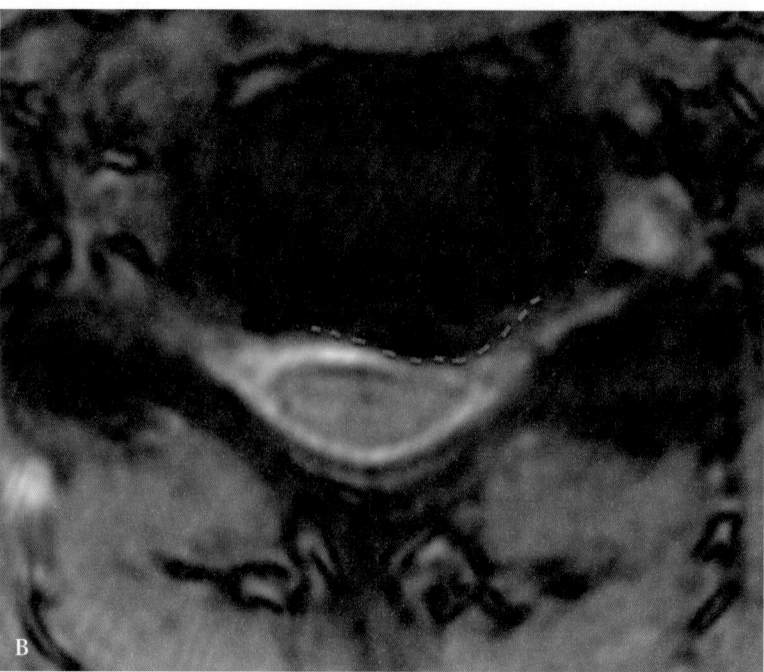

FIGURE 109.5 Cervical disk herniation. T2-weighted MRI shows C5–C6 disk herniation (*dashed line* in **B**) in a patient with radiculopathy in **(A)** sagittal and **(B)** axial planes.

Patients with low back and/or radicular pain should undergo at least 6 weeks of pain control, rest, and physical therapy.

Immediate imaging should be obtained in those patients with acute and/or progressive neurologic deficits. Diagnostic imaging is particularly urgent in patients with urinary retention and or saddle anesthesia, signs of cauda equina syndrome. MRI should also not be delayed in cases with a high clinical suspicion of neoplastic or infectious systemic disease, as symptoms in these patients may be secondary to spinal metastases or epidural abscesses.

In those patients who fail conservative management, MRI should be used to confirm a diagnosis of disk disease before considering invasive treatment. When no correlation exists between radiographic and clinical findings, electromyography (EMG) and nerve conduction studies (NCS) can help elucidate the etiology of presenting symptoms.

Considerations in the Cervical Spine

Lesions such as supraspinatus tendinitis, arthritic changes in the acromioclavicular joint, and rotator cuff tears may be difficult to differentiate from cervical root compression, especially because prolonged pain and lack of range of motion lead to atrophy and frozen shoulder in these syndromes. C8 and T1 lesions commonly cause a partial Horner syndrome. A diagnostic workup for syndromes of these levels must include apical lordotic views of the chest, and special care must be taken to rule out pulmonary neoplasms and abnormal cervical ribs.

Other Diagnostic Considerations

Because many disk syndromes are genetic, abnormal skeletal features throughout the spine may be sought on radiographs. These include spinal stenosis, spondylolisthesis, widespread disk disease, or Marfan syndrome. Acquired disorders, such as osteochondritis juvenilis, and metabolic states such as osteoporosis, may contribute to pathologic changes in the disk and adjacent joints, as do several forms of arthritis. Importantly, disk syndromes may be duplicated by tumors (e.g., primary or metastatic), infections (e.g., epidural abscess), and arachnoiditis. Epidural lipomatosis, a rare cause of low back syndromes, is a complication of steroid therapy.

IMAGING AND ELECTRODIAGNOSTIC STUDIES

Magnetic Resonance Imaging

MRI is the imaging procedure of choice for disk disorders (see also Chapter 21). MRI identifies spinal cord or root compression and also shows the degree of degenerative change within the disk. It clearly delineates both intra- and extradural structures and is the ideal screening procedure for a differential diagnosis that includes structural disorders affecting the spinal cord and nerve roots.

Importantly, evidence of degenerative disk disease and even disk rupture on MRI may not correlate with clinically significant pathology that requires intervention. In studies of asymptomatic individuals, bulging and herniated disks have been identified in 50% and 27% of adults, respectively. Abnormal findings on MRI of the lumbar spine in asymptomatic adults do not appear to predict future development of low back pain. In the absence of progressive neurologic deficit or suspicion of systemic illness, such as cancer or infection, MRI should be reserved for those individuals with at least 6 weeks of persistent low back/radicular pain despite conservative therapy (see "Initial Management and Evaluation").

Myelography and X-ray

Computed tomography (CT) myelography is more invasive than MRI, exposing patients to the intrathecal administration of contrast as well as ionizing radiation. Accordingly, CT myelography is rarely indicated. It does effectively visualize spinal nerve roots and their trajectory though the neural foramina, particularly the anatomy of the nerve root sleeve. However, myelography is unrevealing in the evaluation of far lateral disk herniations, which occur lateral to the spinal canal and root sleeve. Myelography is useful for patients with intolerance of, or contraindications to, MRI, such as cardiac pacemakers and other implanted electrical devices. In addition, CT myelography may be preferred for patients who have surgically placed spinal hardware that produces magnetic artifacts. Plain radiographs effectively depict bony anatomy but not herniated disks. Radiographs do provide valuable information related to spinal alignment and segmental stability prior to surgical intervention.

Electromyography and Nerve Conduction Studies

The primary electrodiagnostic studies used in the evaluation of radiculopathy are EMG and NCS. These studies can be used to accurately identify radiculopathy that has been accompanied by weakness for 3 weeks or more, but they are seldom essential. Electrodiagnostic studies are most useful when radiographic findings do not correlate with clinical presentation (see also Chapter 26).

TREATMENT

Most acute attacks of back pain improve in days or weeks, and only a small minority of patients require surgery. In one meta-analysis, 82% of patients with acute low back pain returned to work within a month of onset. In the absence of neurologic deficit, conservative treatment should be pursued so long as the patient continues to improve with analgesics and bedrest for lumbar disk disorders and immobilization of the neck by a collar for cervical disk disorders. Some clinicians use epidural steroid injections, which decrease edematous swelling and thereby relieve pressure on the affected nerve root.

EXPERT REFERRAL

In the acute phase, indications for referral to a treatment specialist are similar to indications for urgent MRI. Patients who present with signs/symptoms of acute or progressive neurologic deficit, including motor weakness, myelopathy, or signs of cauda equina syndrome, should be urgently evaluated by a neurosurgeon or orthopedic surgeon with experience in spine surgery. This referral should not delay MRI, which is an essential component of any potential surgical decision making. Of note, there is no evidence that early referral to a spine surgeon, in the absence of the aforementioned criteria, improves outcome. For those patients who lack acute or progressive neurologic deficit but have persistent symptoms impairing quality of life, surgery can be scheduled on an elective basis. Importantly, no randomized trial demonstrating the benefits of surgery has enrolled patients with less than 6 weeks of conservative therapy.

LUMBAR DISKECTOMY

Lumbar diskectomy is indicated in patients with evidence of nerve root compression on neuroimaging and either corresponding radicular pain refractory to conservative therapy or corresponding acute/progressive weakness. Surgery represents an effective treatment option in properly selected patients, as diskectomy of a herniated lumbar disk fragment almost always results in long-term satisfactory relief of symptoms. Lumbar fusion is rarely required for treatment of radiculopathy from a herniated lumbar disk. Excessively prolonged physiotherapy and bed rest may cause emotional exhaustion, muscle loss, or drug dependence.

Evidence from an early randomized controlled trial by Weber and colleagues comparing prolonged conservative management to diskectomy suggests that surgery offers greater relief from radiculopathy caused by herniated lumbar disks in the short term [**Level 1**].[1] However, patients randomized to both surgical and nonsurgical groups experienced considerable symptomatic improvement over time and the difference between groups was not statistically significant at long-term follow up. This may be partially explained by unintended crossover between groups, as approximately one-quarter of patients randomized to nonsurgical therapy elected to have a diskectomy presumably due to persistent symptoms with conservative management.

In a large multicenter, prospective, randomized, controlled trial, researchers with The Spine Patient Outcomes Research Trial (SPORT) demonstrated substantial improvement with both surgical and nonsurgical treatment of lumbar disk disease with radiculopathy. Although short-term results were consistently in favor of surgery, differences in primary outcomes were not statistically different [**Level 1**].[2] At long-term follow up (4 and 8 years), patients treated with surgery demonstrated greater improvement in secondary outcomes, including "sciatica bothersomeness," self-rated improvement, and patient satisfaction with symptoms [**Level 1**].[3] Primary outcomes (bodily pain, physical function, and disability index) also favored surgery, but these differences were not significant between groups. The results of the SPORT research effort were widely touted by the lay press, and some in the medical community, as evidence for the equivalence between modern surgical and nonsurgical treatment techniques. However, as the study authors rightly conclude, "conclusions about the superiority or equivalence of the treatments under study are not warranted based on the intent-to-treat analysis." Crossover between groups again served as a major confounder that may underestimate the relative benefit of surgery, as approximately half (49%) of patients assigned to nonoperative management ultimately elected to have surgery after a trial of conservative therapy.

Surgical techniques for lumbar diskectomy can be broadly segregated into three categories: open diskectomy, microdiskectomy, and minimally invasive diskectomy. Traditional open diskectomy involves a standard laminectomy and is performed with eyepiece magnification. Microdiskectomy is the most commonly performed procedure and typically involves a smaller incision with less bone removal in the form of a hemilaminotomy and use of the operative microscope to remove the offending disk fragment.

Minimally invasive techniques have become extremely common in modern practice. Typically, minimally invasive lumbar diskectomy includes the use of a tubular retractor system inserted through small incisions over a guidewire with fluoroscopic guidance. This technique uses muscle spitting, as opposed to the muscle cutting/detachment inherent to other methods, which its advocates purport reduces postoperative pain and recovery time. Currently, this position is not supported by data from randomized controlled trials. Arts and colleagues randomized 328 patients to minimally invasive versus conventional microdiskectomy for lumbar radiculopathy. At 2-year follow-up, similar functional and clinical outcomes were reported between groups [**Level 1**].[4] Of note, recovery time was not shorter among patients treated with minimally invasive tubular diskectomy. A recently published meta-analysis of randomized controlled trials comparing tubular diskectomy to conventional microdiskectomy found that both methods lead to a substantial and equivalent long-term improvement in leg pain. Incidental durotomies occurred significantly more frequently during minimally invasive surgery, but total complications did not differ between study arms [**Level 1**].[5]

CERVICAL DISKECTOMY

Indications for surgery to relieve radiculopathy from disk disease in the cervical spine are similar to the indications for lumbar diskectomy. Good surgical candidates have persistent radicular pain despite at least 6 weeks of conservative treatment or acute/progressive motor weakness. Clinical evidence of myelopathy with radiographic evidence of cord compression from a herniated disk represents an additional indication for diskectomy.

Generally, spinal cord compression requires consideration of decompressive measures as soon as it is recognized. Root syndromes of the cervical spine may be separated into those that require careful supervision and early operation and those that tolerate and may respond to conservative care. The muscles served by C5 may rapidly atrophy, leaving abduction paresis, poor prognosis for restoration of function, and a painful frozen shoulder. C8 is also vulnerable, and unrelieved compression may lead to irreversible atrophy with complex shoulder–arm–hand disorders that include circulatory and sweating abnormalities. C6 and C7 innervate large muscles and tolerate pressure more benignly even for long periods and may have good functional return. Cervical root syndromes are less likely to recur than lumbar disorders, and conservative therapy is worthwhile within the outlines described.

Removal of a cervical herniated disk may be performed either through a posterior laminotomy or through an anterior approach. In most case, particularly in patients with cervical kyphosis, an anterior approach is preferred. Anterior cervical diskectomy with fusion (ACDF) is one of the most successful and widely practiced procedures in spine surgery. By combining anterior decompression with a strut graft (usually allograft) to promote fusion across the vacated intervertebral disk space, lordosis can be restored across the segment. Excellent results may be anticipated in appropriately selected patients.

Persson and colleagues conducted a randomized controlled trial comparing anterior cervical diskectomy to nonoperative therapy in 81 patients with clinical and radiologic signs of cervical nerve root compression lasting 12 weeks or more. Patients in the nonoperative arm were prescribed physical therapy and immobilization with a hard cervical collar. Individuals with clinical signs of myelopathy or radiographic evidence of cord compression were excluded. Patients treated with surgery demonstrated greater improvement in both pain and motor strength at 4 months follow up. At 1 year, no significant difference in pain remained, but patients in the surgical arm maintained a small advantage in muscle strength [**Level 1**].[6]

Prospective observational studies by Heckmann and Sampath provide further support for the efficacy of anterior cervical diskectomy in the treatment of cervical radiculopathy without myelopathy. At 2-year follow-up, patients who underwent surgery showed greater improvements in both pain and weakness compared to conservatively treated patients. Overall, approximately 75% of patients experienced significant relief from symptoms after surgery.

SUMMARY

Radiculopathy resulting from intervertebral disk disease is self-limited in the majority of patients. Symptoms generally improve with rest, pain control, physical therapy, and time. If symptoms persist after at least 6 weeks of conservative therapy, patients should be referred for MRI. If intervertebral disk disease identified on neuroimaging correlates with clinical presentation, patients should be referred to a spine surgeon. More urgent referral should be initiated in the presence of symptoms of cauda equina syndrome, myelopathy, or acute/progressive motor weakness. Randomized controlled trials comparing diskectomy to conservative therapy in the lumbar and cervical spine demonstrate similar long-term outcomes between groups that modestly favor surgery in appropriately selected patients. The short-term benefits of surgery have been more consistently realized across studies. Crossover between randomized arms may contribute to an underestimation of the benefit of surgery, as patients frustrated by the severity of their symptoms and the slow pace of recovery with conservative therapy commonly opt to have surgery.

LEVEL 1 EVIDENCE

1. Weber H. Lumbar disc herniation. A controlled, prospective study with ten years of observation. *Spine.* 1983;8(2):131–140.
2. Weinstein JN, Tosteson TD, Lurie JD, et al. Surgical vs nonoperative treatment for lumbar disk herniation: the Spine Patient Outcomes Research Trial (SPORT): a randomized trial. *JAMA.* 2006;296(20):2441–2450.
3. Lurie JD, Tosteson TD, Tosteson ANA, et al. Surgical versus nonoperative treatment for lumbar disc herniation: eight-year results for the spine patient outcomes research trial. *Spine.* 2014;39(1):3–16.
4. Arts MP, Brand R, van den Akker ME, et al. Tubular diskectomy vs conventional microdiskectomy for the treatment of lumbar disk herniation: 2-year results of a double-blind randomized controlled trial. *Neurosurgery.* 2011;69(1):135–144.
5. Dasenbrock HH, Juraschek SP, Schultz LR, et al. The efficacy of minimally invasive discectomy compared with open discectomy: a meta-analysis of prospective randomized controlled trials. *J Neurosurg Spine.* 2012;16(5):452–462.

6. Persson LC, Moritz U, Brandt L, et al. Cervical radiculopathy: pain, muscle weakness and sensory loss in patients with cervical radiculopathy treated with surgery, physiotherapy or cervical collar. A prospective, controlled study. *Eur Spine J.* 1997;6(4):256–266.

SUGGESTED READINGS

Andersson GB. Epidemiological features of chronic low-back pain. *Lancet.* 1999;354(9178):581–585.

Atlas SJ, Nardin RA. Evaluation and treatment of low back pain: an evidence-based approach to clinical care. *Muscle Nerve.* 2003;27(3):265–284.

Butterman GR. Treatment of lumbar disc herniation: epidural steroid injection compared with discectomy. A prospective, randomized study. *J Bone Joint Surg Am.* 2004;86A(4):670–679.

Chou R, Fu R, Carrino JA, et al. Imaging strategies for low-back pain: systematic review and meta-analysis. *Lancet.* 2009;373:463–472.

Hansen FR, Bendix T, Skov P, et al. Intensive, dynamic back muscle exercises, conventional physiotherapy, or placebo-control treatment of low back pain: a randomized, observer-blind trial. *Spine.* 1993;18:98–108.

Heckmann JG, Lang CJ, Zöbelein I, et al. Herniated cervical intervertebral discs with radiculopathy: an outcome study of conservatively or surgically treated patients. *J Spinal Disord.* 1999;12(5):396–401.

Hemmila HM. Quality of life and cost of care of back pain patients in Finnish general practice. *Spine.* 2002;27(6):647–653.

Katz JN. Lumbar disc disorders and low-back pain: socioeconomic factors and consequences. *J Bone Joint Surg Am.* 2006;88(suppl 2):21–24.

Kraemer J. History and terminology. In: Kraemer J, ed. *Intervertebral Disk Diseases: Causes, Diagnosis, Treatment, and Prophylaxis.* 3rd ed. Stuttgart, Germany: Georg Thieme Verlag; 2009:3–9.

McCormick PC. The Spine Patient Outcomes Research Trial results for lumbar disc herniation: a critical review. *J Neurosurg Spine.* 2007;6(6):513–520.

Mixter WJ, Barr JS. Rupture of the intervertebral disc with involvement of the spinal canal. *N Engl J Med.* 1934;211:210.

Peul WC, van Houwelingen HC, van den Hout WB, et al. Surgery versus prolonged conservative treatment for sciatica. *N Engl J Med.* 2007;356(22):2245–2256.

Sampath P, Bendebba M, Davis JD, et al. Outcome in patients with cervical radiculopathy. Prospective, multicenter study with independent clinical review. *Spine.* 1999;24(6):591–597.

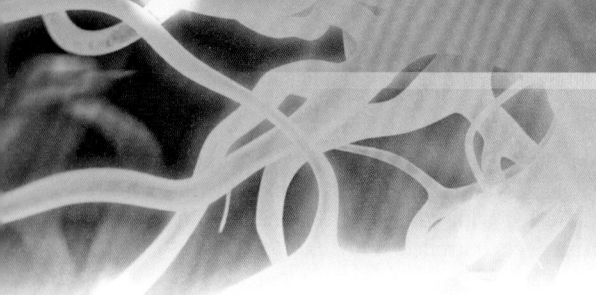

Lewis P. Rowland and Paul C. McCormick

INTRODUCTION

Cervical and lumbar spinal stenosis are the most common causes of neck and back pain and spinal cord and cauda equina or nerve root dysfunction and represent the most frequent indications for spinal surgery in adults older than the age of 55 years.

PATHOBIOLOGY

The term *spinal stenosis* describes an acquired condition of progressive narrowing of the spinal canal usually due to age-related progressive arthritic degeneration of the intervertebral disks and facet joints. This process results in disk bulging, facet overgrowth, synovial cyst development, and bone spur formation, as well as ligamentum flavum and facet joint capsule hypertrophy. These proliferative, so-called spondylotic, changes that occur in response to accumulated mechanical stress in the spine lead to progressive narrowing of the spinal canal and/or foramina. In some patients, these degenerative changes may compromise the mechanical integrity of the spine leading to deformity (e.g., degenerative scoliosis, kyphosis) or spondylolisthesis that may further exacerbate the clinical condition produced by spinal stenosis. In a smaller subset of patients, narrowing of the spinal canal may be due to degenerative and/or destructive changes to the articulating joints from systemic conditions such as rheumatoid arthritis, or enthesopathies such as ossification of the posterior longitudinal ligament (OPLL), ankylosing spondylitis, or diffuse idiopathic skeletal hyperostosis (DISH). OPLL may be focal or diffuse and seems to be most common in people of Asian heritage. These conditions much more commonly affect the cervical spine.

Progressive stenosis of the cervical, or rarely thoracic, spinal canal from these conditions may damage the spinal cord producing a condition known as *cervical spondylotic myelopathy* (CSM). Such myelopathy is attributed to one or more of three possible mechanisms: (1) direct compression of the spinal cord by bony or fibrous tissue overgrowth, (2) ischemia caused by compromise of the vascular supply to the cord, and (3) repeated trauma in the course of normal neck movement. Similarly, ongoing progressive or intermittent narrowing of the nerve root foramen may cause injury to the cervical nerve roots. Although the cauda equina seems less susceptible than the spinal cord to permanent injury from lumbar spinal stenosis, advanced, nontreated severe stenosis may result in irreversible injury to these nerve roots similar to cervical myelopathy.

In the cervical spine, spondylotic bars may leave deep indentations (e.g., visible at autopsy) on the ventral surface of the spinal cord. At what may be several levels of lesions, there is degeneration of the gray matter, sometimes with necrosis and cavitation. Above the compression, there is degeneration of the posterior columns; below the compression, corticospinal tracts are demyelinated. A similar process occurs in the lumbar spine where the proliferative changes due to the normal aging process produces progressive narrowing of the lumbar spinal canal and compression of the cauda equina.

CAUSES OF CERVICAL AND LUMBAR STENOSIS

Normal, albeit accentuated, wear and tear degenerative changes in the spine is the most common cause of spinal stenosis both in the cervical and lumbar spine. The water content of the intervertebral disk and annulus fibrosus declines progressively with advancing age. Concomitantly, there are degenerative changes in the disk. The intervertebral space narrows and may be obliterated, and the annulus fibrosus protrudes into the spinal canal. Osteophytes form at the margins of the vertebral body, converge on the protruded annulus, and may convert it into a bony ridge or bar. The bar may extend laterally into the intervertebral foramen; there is also fibrosis of the dural sleeves of the nerve roots. All these changes narrow the canal, a process that may be aggravated by fibrosis and hypertrophy of the ligamenta flava. In some cases, this narrowing may be exacerbated by acute or chronic disk herniation, synovial cyst development from the facet joint, or degenerative spondylolisthesis. These last two conditions are much more common in the lumbar spine of women, especially at the L4–L5 level. The likelihood of spinal cord or cauda equina compression or vascular compromise increases in direct relation to the decrease in the original diameter of the spinal canal.

Most cases of degenerative cervical or lumbar stenosis are sporadic in occurrence, although there may be a family history in some patients. The term *congenital spinal stenosis* is a bit of a misnomer because stenosis connotes an acquired narrowing. A *developmentally small spinal canal* is a more accurate term than congenital stenosis. Patients with a developmentally small canal, a familial characteristic, may be more susceptible to develop symptomatic stenosis simply because they have less capacity to accommodate the proliferative degenerative changes associated with the progressive arthritic process of the spine. Spinal stenosis tends to develop at the most mobile and mechanically stressed spinal levels. The C5–C6 and C6–C7 levels are most commonly involved in the cervical spine, whereas L4–L5 and L3–L4 are the most commonly affected lumbar levels. Both C4–C5 and L5–S1 are slightly less commonly involved. Concomitant symptomatic cervical and lumbar stenosis can be seen in up to 15% of patients. Patients who have either congenital (i.e., Klippel–Feil syndrome) or previously performed surgical spinal fusion may be prone to develop spinal stenosis at levels adjacent to the fused level.

Systemic conditions such as rheumatoid arthritis may cause destructive changes of synovial joints, especially in the upper cervical spine leading to cervical instability and stenosis with spinal cord compression. The term *enthesis* describes the site where ligaments or tendons attach to bone. In the spine, a number of different enthesopathies may involve the spine to produce spinal stenosis. The most common of these is OPLL, where calcification of the posterior longitudinal ligament can produce progressive spinal stenosis, particularly in the cervical spine, and myelopathy. Less commonly, diffuse idiopathic skeletal hyperostosis or ankylosing spondylitis may result in excessive ossification of either the posterior or anterior longitudinal spinal ligaments leading to spinal rigidity, fragility, and spinal stenosis.

CLINICAL MANIFESTATIONS

CERVICAL STENOSIS

Neck pain may be prominent and chronic in nature. Root pain is common in patients with predominant or concomitant foraminal stenosis, but most patients present with either myelopathy or radiculopathy. A combined "myeloradicular" presentation is unusual. The most common symptom of myelopathy is spastic gait disorder (Table 110.1). Clumsiness of the hands and loss of dexterity and fine motor control with such tasks as writing, typing, and buttoning are common early complaints in patients with CSM. Weakness and wasting of the hands may be seen but only as the condition becomes more advanced. Predominate proximal arm weakness with difficulty lifting the arm over the head is the presenting complaint in a small number of patients. Bowel bladder complaints are usually not common in the early stages of CSM. Fasciculations are rarely noted in the early stages of CSM. Overt sensory loss is uncommon, but the patient may note that the hands feel numb and clumsy.

The course of the disorder is slowly progressive, but the natural history is not well delineated. In some patients, the condition may wax and wane with periods of relative quiescence or even improvement followed by progressive worsening. Acute worsening precipitated by a fall or other traumatic event may exacerbate existing symptoms or a central cord syndrome that is characterized by a sudden onset of predominant, often distal, upper extremity numbness/weakness with relative preservation of lower extremity function. These injuries most likely occur from sudden hyperextension of the cervical spine with infolding of the ligamentum flavum causing a pincer-type impingement of the spinal cord. Spontaneous substantial recovery from acute central cord syndromes commonly occurs.

LUMBAR STENOSIS

The classic presentation of patients with lumbar spinal stenosis is neurogenic claudication. Patients typically present with symptoms of lower extremity pain, weakness, and/or numbness with standing or walking that are reliably relieved with sitting or leaning forward. The reason for this is that upright postures and positions tend to exacerbate the degree of lumbar stenosis by infolding of the ligamentum flavum into the spinal canal. Sitting and leaning forward straightens the ligamentum flavum to increase lumbar spinal canal dimensions. Symptoms can vary from patient to patient in terms of quality (pain or numbness), distribution (bilateral or unilateral, multiroot or single root), severity, and duration. Most patients do not have a fixed neurologic deficit by the time of clinical presentation. Fixed deficits (e.g., footdrop) or cauda equina syndrome is now rare, although they can be seen in long-standing untreated patients or acute presentations from a large central disk herniation.

TABLE 110.1	Clinical Manifestations of Cervical Spondylotic Myelopathy
Symptoms or Signs	**% of Patients**
Reflexes	
Hyperreflexia	87
Babinski sign	51
Hoffmann sign	13
Spastic gait disorder	49
Bladder symptoms	49
Sensation	
Vague sensory level	41
Proprioceptive sensory loss	39
Cervical dermatome sensory loss	33
Motor functions	
Arm weakness	31
Paraparesis	21
Hemiparesis	18
Quadriparesis	10
Brown-Séquard syndrome	18
Hand atrophy	13
Fasciculation	13
Pain	
Radicular arm	41
Radicular leg	13
Neck	8

Data from Lunsford LD, Bissonette DJ, Zorub DS. Anterior surgery for cervical disc disease. Part 2: treatment of cervical spondylotic myelopathy in 32 cases. *J Neurosurg.* 1980;53:12–19.

DIAGNOSIS

The diagnosis of cervical or lumbar stenosis is confirmed with imaging of the spinal canal. It is important to appreciate that spinal stenosis is a clinical, rather than radiologic, diagnosis because many individuals may have a narrow, or stenotic, spinal canal but no neurologic signs or symptoms. With few exceptions, these asymptomatic patients are not in need of treatment.

Formerly, the most important diagnostic tests were plain radiographs of the cervical spine and myelography. Plain radiographs show narrowing of the disk spaces and the presence of osteophytes, especially at C5–C6 and C6–C7. Posterior osteophytes tend to be smaller than anterior projections and may not be seen without computerized tomography (CT). The disk bodies may be normal or may show sclerosis. Changes in the zygapophyseal joints account for the designation of osteoarthritis and may encroach on the intervertebral foramen; the changes may cause subluxation of the articular surfaces or compression of vertebral arteries. These invasive studies have largely been supplanted by noninvasive imaging.

Magnetic resonance imaging (MRI) is the imaging procedure of choice for the evaluation of both cervical and lumbar stenosis. It is noninvasive and provides exquisite resolution of spinal cord, exiting nerve roots, and cauda equina (Figs. 110.1–110.3). MRI allows evaluation of spondylosis and the alternative possibilities: Chiari malformation, arteriovenous malformation, extramedullary or intramedullary tumor, syringomyelia, or demyelinating conditions such as multiple sclerosis. MRI may also identify physical changes within the spinal cord such as increase T2 signal abnormalities reflecting edema, ischemia, cyst formation, and spinal cord injury.

CT complements MRI and provides additional detail regarding bone and calcified disks. It is particularly important in patients suspected of having calcified spurs, often in association with OPLL or DISH.

Somatosensory-evoked responses add little to aid in diagnosis of either cervical or lumbar stenosis, although they may help in

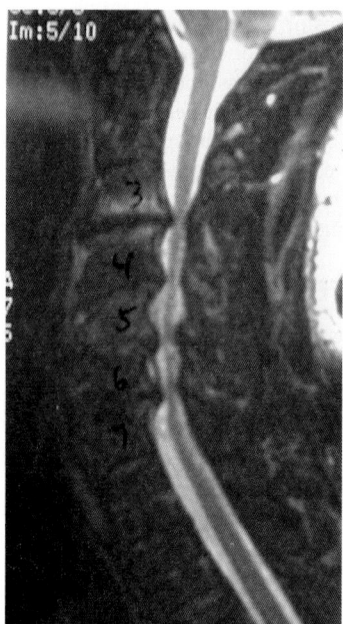

FIGURE 110.1 Sagittal proton-density MRI demonstrates extensive spinal cord compression caused by a combination of ventral bone spurs and preexisting (i.e., congenital) canal stenosis.

the differential diagnosis of anterior horn cell disease (amyotrophic lateral sclerosis) or peripheral neuropathy. The cerebrospinal fluid (CSF) is usually normal or the protein concentration may be 50 to 100 mg/dL. Higher protein levels or CSF pleocytosis should raise the question of multiple sclerosis or tumor, including meningeal carcinomatosis. The role of transcranial magnetic stimulation in diagnosis remains to be ascertained, but motor-evoked potentials may be more contributory than sensory potentials.

DIFFERENTIAL DIAGNOSIS

Two types of problems arise in the differential diagnosis. In one group, there is compression of the cervical spinal cord but not by spondylosis or not by spondylosis alone. Spinal tumors are the best example of this kind of problem. These lesions are revealed by MRI. In other compressive lesions, the primary bony changes are congenital (e.g., anomalies of the craniocervical junction) or acquired (e.g., rheumatoid arthritis or basilar impression) and may be further complicated by spondylosis. These disorders are recognized by CT or MRI. Arteriovenous malformations may also be found.

Another group of myelopathies presents more of a diagnostic problem. Cervical spondylosis is so common in the general population that it may be present by chance and may be harmless in a person with another disease of the spinal cord. The ultimate test of the pathogenic significance of spondylosis would be complete relief of symptoms after decompressive surgery, but this is rarely seen. Among the other diseases that may cause clinical syndromes similar to those attributed to spondylosis are multiple sclerosis (MS), amyotrophic lateral sclerosis (ALS), neurosyphilis, and possibly subacute combined system disease with vitamin B_{12} deficiency (see also Chapter 111). In one series, 12% of patients diagnosed with spondylotic myelopathy proved to have some other condition.

MS is probably the most common cause of spastic paraplegia in middle life and is probably the actual cause of the disorder in some people who have had a cervical laminectomy. These conditions can generally be distinguished based on clinical presentation and imaging but for equivocal cases, it is important to test for MS by use of visual, somatosensory, and brain stem–evoked responses; examine CSF for γ-globulin content and oligoclonal bands; and carry out an MRI examination of the cerebral white matter, foramen magnum, brain stem, and cervical spinal cord. Proper use and interpretation of these test results often remove diagnostic uncertainty.

ALS must be considered whenever wasting and fasciculations are seen in arm and hand muscles and especially when there are

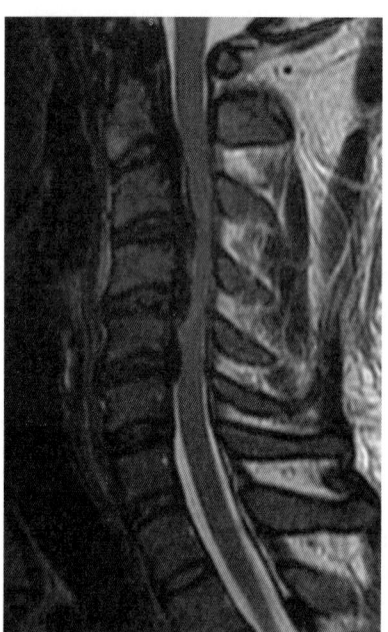
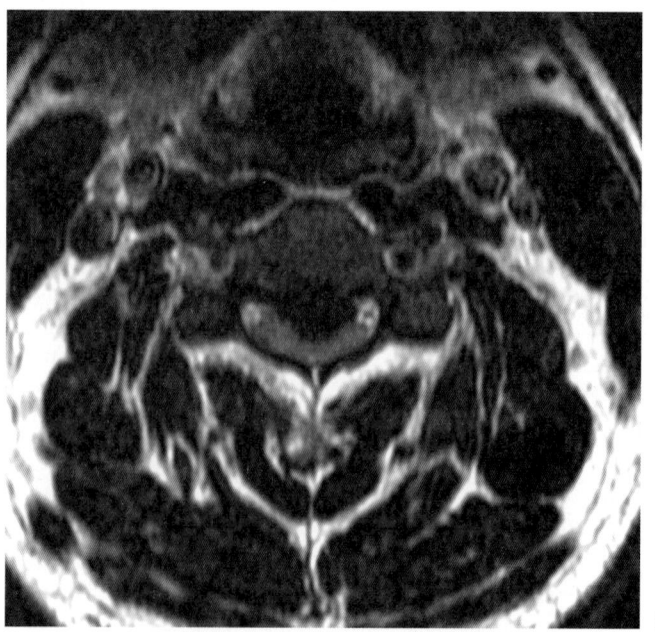

FIGURE 110.2 A: Sagittal T1-weighted MRI shows severe upper spinal cord compression from OPLL, which appears as dark bulges anterior to the cord along the posterior aspects of the C 3/4, C 4/5, and C 5/6 discs. This dense calcification is typical of OPLL. **B:** Axial MRI in same patient.

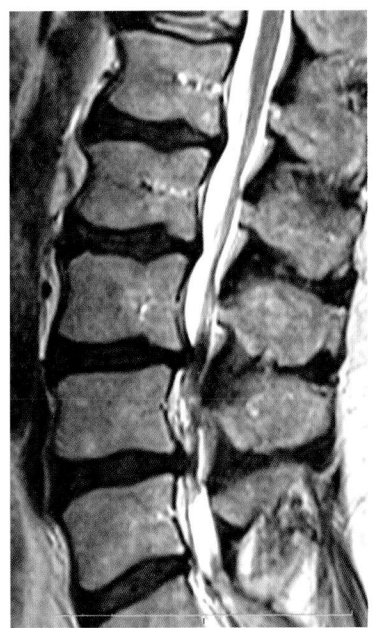
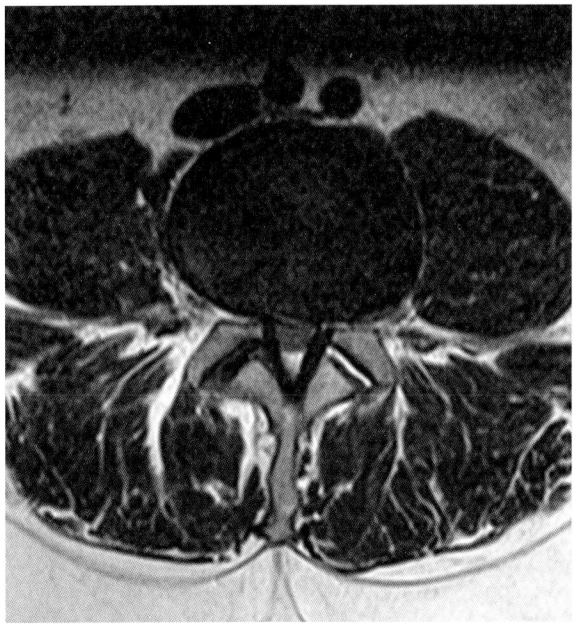

FIGURE 110.3 A: T2-weighted sagittal MRI of lumbar spine demonstrates severe lumbar spinal stenosis at the L3–L4 and L4–L5 spinal levels. **B:** T2-weighted axial MRI shows severe stenosis at the L4–L5 level in same patient.

fasciculations in the legs. The presence of overt fasciculation makes it unlikely that spondylotic myelopathy is the cause of symptoms; when fasciculation is visible, caution is warranted when laminectomy is being considered. There is no diagnostic test for ALS, however, and the distinction may be difficult.

Rare causes of spastic paraplegia in middle life are the myelopathy caused by human T-cell lymphotropic virus type I or adult-onset adrenoleukodystrophy. The diagnosis of exclusion, when no other cause is identified, is primary lateral sclerosis, which is almost as common a cause of spastic paraparesis as MS.

In northern England, a prospective survey of 585 patients with nontraumatic spastic paraparesis gave the following order of frequency of diagnosis: CSM, 24%; tumor, 16%; MS, 18%; diagnosis uncertain, 19%; and ALS, 4%. The absence of primary lateral sclerosis from this list suggests regional differences in making a diagnosis. Of course, the real problem is ascertaining the diagnosis of spondylotic myelopathy.

TREATMENT

CERVICAL STENOSIS

The treatment of cervical stenosis depends on many factors. As previously noted, radiographic stenosis in the absence of signs or symptoms of neurologic symptoms rarely necessitates intervention. Occasionally, a patient with severe stenosis (<7-mm canal diameter) and an intramedullary signal abnormality within the spinal cord may present with little or no neurologic symptoms. In these patients, preemptive surgical decompression may be offered but it is not clear if the benefit of surgery outweighs the risks in this patient population. Often, patients with minimal or no neurologic signs/symptoms are followed both clinically and with imaging over time. Surgical decompression is usually recommended if clinical progression is documented. Patients with radicular symptoms from nerve root compression from foraminal stenosis are initially managed with conservative measures such as activity modulation, physical therapy, judicious use of anti-inflammatory medications, and/or steroidal spinal injections. Surgery for decompression of the nerve root either through a posterior foraminotomy or anterior diskectomy is an option for patients with persistent radiculopathy that is not responsive to conservative management.

The natural history of CSM varies greatly and is unpredictable in individual patients. The Cochrane Library listed a single, controlled trial for spondylotic myelopathy, that of Bednarik et al.; in 1999, they reported early benefit for surgery over conservative therapy but did not find differences after 1 year. However, they studied only 49 patients. Therefore, there have still been no adequately controlled trials of surgical therapy. Additionally, several different operations have been advocated (e.g., ventral vs. dorsal, with or without fusion, and with or without different kinds of stabilizing hardware). Therefore, uniform recommendations for treatment have been difficult to establish but is usually recommended for patients with progressive neurologic dysfunction. Decompressive operations include posterior laminectomy or laminoplasty, anterior diskectomy, or vertebrectomy with spinal fusion.

Conservative treatment with physical therapy for gait training and with neck immobilization with a firm collar may be appropriate for some patients with mild myelopathy. Surgery should be considered if the myelopathy progresses despite conservative treatment.

LUMBAR STENOSIS

Unlike cervical stenosis, most patients with lumbar stenosis do not have neurologic deficit. Thus, treatment options are more variable. For patients with mild symptoms, conservative management with activity modification, physical therapy, and/or periodic epidural steroidal injections may provide durable stability or even improvement from the symptoms of spinal stenosis of lumbar spinal stenosis. However, if symptoms become increasingly problematic to the patient in terms of symptoms, function, or quality of life, then surgical intervention for decompression may be offered.

SURGICAL EFFICACY

The outcome following surgical treatment for cervical stenosis is variable and difficult to predict on an individual basis. Although contemporary surgical series report a 70% to 80% rate of improvement, only about 50% of patients show satisfactory functional improvement or complete reversal of symptoms that is maintained over time and up to one-third of patients show no improvement following decompressive surgery for CSM. In some patients, their condition may even become worse as a result of surgery. In these cases, irreversible injury from spinal stenosis may have already occurred or surgery did not optimally achieve the operative objective. Surgical decompression for nerve root compression in the foramina provides more reliably achieved improvement in neurologic symptoms than does surgical treatment for cord compression.

At this point, it is unlikely that any randomized trial comparing surgery to nonoperative management or no treatment for CSM will be forthcoming due to the lack of clinical equipoise. Randomized controlled trials are underway, however, to evaluate both the comparative efficacy as well as the cost-effectiveness of various surgical techniques that are commonly used to treat these patients. In the absence of clear guidelines, management should be tailored to the specific circumstances of individual patients and to the experiences of the treating physicians and surgeons.

The results of surgery for lumbar spinal stenosis in patients who have failed to respond to nonoperative treatments is much more favorable and predictable than for cervical stenosis. The Spine Patient Outcomes Research Trial (SPORT) provides level 1 evidence of both the efficacy and durability of spinal decompression through lumbar laminectomy to relieve the symptoms of spinal stenosis in appropriately selected patients who have failed to improve with standard nonoperative measures [**Level 1**].[1,2] Additionally, level 1 evidence provided by the SPORT also demonstrated the efficacy and durability of lumbar decompression and fusion for patients with lumbar stenosis and degenerative spondylolisthesis [**Level 1**].[3,4]

LEVEL 1 EVIDENCE

1. Weinstein JN, Lurie JD, Tosteson TD, et al. Surgical versus nonsurgical therapy for lumbar spinal stenosis. *N Engl J Med.* 2008;358(8):794–810.
2. Weinstein JN, Lurie JD, Tosteson TD, et al. Surgical versus nonsurgical treatment for lumbar degenerative spondylolisthesis. *N Engl J Med.* 2007;356(22):2257–2270.
3. Weinstein JN, Tosteson TD, Lurie JD, et al. Surgical versus nonoperative treatment for lumbar spinal stenosis: four-year results of the spine patients outcomes research trial. *Spine.* 2010;35(14):1329–1338.
4. Weinstein JN, Lurie JD, Tosteson TD, et al. Surgical compared with nonoperative treatment for lumbar degenerative spondylolisthesis: four-year results of the spine patient outcomes research trial. *J Bone Joint Surg Am.* 2009;91:1295–1304.

SUGGESTED READINGS

Aliabadi H, Biglari D, Gonzalez LF, et al. Diffuse idiopathic skeletal hyperostosis versus ankylosing spondylitis: brief case review. *Barrow Quarterly.* 2006;22(4):10–14.

Azuma S, Seichi A, Ohnishi I, et al. Long-term results of operative treatment for cervical spondylotic myelopathy in patients with athetoid cerebral palsy: an over 10-year follow-up study. *Spine.* 2002;27(9):943–948.

Baptiste DC, Fehlings MG. Pathophysiology of cervical myelopathy. *Spine J.* 2006;6:190S–197S.

Bednarik J, Kadanka Z, Dusek L, et al. Presymptomatic spondylotic cervical myelopathy: an updated predictive model. *Eur Spine J.* 2008;17(3):421–431.

Bednarik J, Kadanka Z, Vohanka S, et al. The value of somatosensory- and motor-evoked potentials in predicting and monitoring the effect of therapy in spondylotic cervical myelopathy. Prospective randomized study. *Spine.* 1999;24(15):1593–1598.

Behrbalk E, Salame K, Regev GJ, et al. Delayed diagnosis of cervical spondylotic myelopathy by primary care physicians. *Neurosurg Focus.* 2013;35(1):1–6.

Chen J, Song D, Wang X, et al. Is ossification of posterior longitudinal ligament an enthesopathy? *Int Orthopedics.* 2011;(35):1511–1516.

Chin KR, Eiszner JR, Huang JL, et al. Myelographic evaluation of cervical spondylosis: patient tolerance and complications. *J Spinal Disord Tech.* 2008;21(5):334–337.

Ebara S, Yonenobu K, Fujiwara K, et al. Myelopathy hand characterized by muscle wasting: a different type of myelopathy hand in patients with cervical spondylosis. *Spine.* 1988;13:785–791.

Emery SE, Bohlman HH, Bolesta MJ, et al. Anterior cervical decompression and arthrodesis for the treatment of cervical spondylotic myelopathy. Two- to seventeen-year follow-up. *J Bone Joint Surg Am.* 1998;80:941–951.

Fessler RG, Steck JC, Giovanni MA. Anterior cervical corpectomy for cervical spondylotic myelopathy. *Neurosurgery.* 1998;43:257–265.

Fouyas IP, Sandercock PA, Statham PF, et al. Surgery for cervical radiculomyelopathy. *Cochrane Database Syst Rev.* 2007;(2):CD001466.

Ghogawala Z, Benzel EC, Heary RF, et al. Cervical spondylotic myelopathy surgical (CSM-C) trial: randomized controlled trial design and rationale. *Neurosurgery.* 2014;75(4):334–346.

Ghogawala Z, Coumans J-V, Benzel EC, et al. Ventral versus decompression for cervical spondylotic myelopathy: surgeons' assessment of eligibility for randomization in a proposed randomized controlled trial: results of a survey of the Cervical Spine Research Society. *Spine.* 2007;32:429–436.

Ghogawala Z, Martin B, Benzel EC, et al. Comparative effectiveness of ventral vs dorsal surgery for cervical spondylotic myelopathy. *Neurosurgery.* 2011;68:622–631.

Lo YL, Chan LL, Lim W, et al. Systematic correlation of transcranial magnetic stimulation and magnetic resonance imaging in cervical spondylotic myelopathy. *Spine.* 2004;29:1137–1145.

Lunsford LD, Bissonette DJ, Zorub DS. Anterior surgery for cervical disc disease. Part 2: treatment of cervical spondylotic myelopathy in 32 cases. *J Neurosurg.* 1980;53:12–19.

Lyu RK, Tang LM, Chen CJ, et al. The use of evoked potentials for clinical correlation and surgical outcome in cervical spondylotic myelopathy with intramedullary high signal intensity on MRI. *J Neurol Neurosurg Psychiatry.* 2004;75:256–261.

Matz PG. Does nonoperative management play a role in the treatment of cervical spondylotic myelopathy? *Spine J.* 2006;6(6)(suppl):175S–181S.

Moore AP, Blumhardt LD. A prospective survey of the causes of non-traumatic spastic paraparesis and tetraparesis in 585 patients. *Spinal Cord.* 1997;5:361–367.

Nakamura K, Kurokawa T, Hoshino Y, et al. Conservative treatment for cervical spondylotic myelopathy: achievement and sustainability of a level of "no disability." *J Spinal Disord.* 1998;11:175–179.

Nguyen HV, Ludwig SC, Silber J, et al. Rheumatoid arthritis of the cervical spine. *Spine J.* 2004;(4):329–334.

Nurick S. The natural history and results of surgical treatment of the spinal cord disorder associated with cervical spondylosis. *Brain.* 1972;95:101–108.

Nurick S. The pathogenesis of the spinal cord disorder associated with cervical spondylosis. *Brain.* 1972;95:87–100.

Persson LCG, Carlsson C-A, Carlsson JY. Long-lasting cervical radicular pain managed with surgery, physiotherapy, or a cervical collar. A prospective, randomized study. *Spine.* 1997;22(7):751–758.

Resnick DK, ed. Special issue on cervical myelopathy. *Spine J.* 2006;6(6)(suppl 1):S175–S322.

Rowland LP. Surgical treatment of cervical spondylotic myelopathy: time for a controlled trial. *Neurology.* 1992;42:5–13.

Sampath P, Bendebba M, Davis JD. Outcome of patients treated for cervical myelopathy. A prospective multicenter study with independent clinical review. *Spine.* 2000;25:670–676.

Shimomura T, Sumi M, Nishida K, et al. Prognostic factors for deterioration of patients with cervical spondylotic myelopathy after nonsurgical treatment. *Spine.* 2007;32(22):2474–2479.

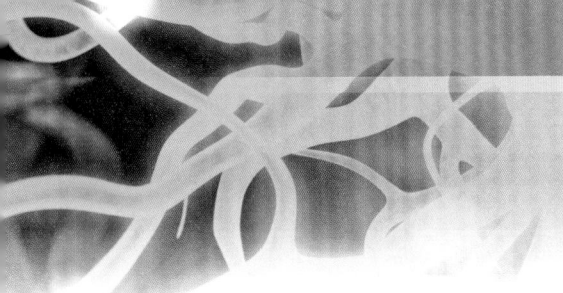

Acquired and Hereditary Myelopathies 111

Acquired and Hereditary Myelopathies 111

Natalie R. Weathered and Noam Y. Harel

INTRODUCTION

Myelopathy indicates pathology of the spinal cord leading to dysfunction of central motor and sensory circuits, as opposed to radiculopathy (pathology of spinal roots), which affects solely peripheral circuits. A large number of conditions may cause myelopathy (Table 111.1). This chapter expands on key inflammatory, infectious, vascular, metabolic, genetic, and toxic insults.

SYRINGOMYELIA

A syrinx is an intramedullary fluid-filled cavity typically found within the cervical to midthoracic spinal cord (Fig. 111.1), but extension down to the conus medullaris is also possible as is upward extension to the brain stem in which case it is called *syringobulbia*. The cavity is most commonly filled with cerebrospinal fluid (CSF). However, syringomyelia should be regarded as distinct from simple cystic expansion of the central canal for which the term *hydromyelia* applies.

EPIDEMIOLOGY

The prevalence of syringomyelia in Western countries is approximately 8.4 cases per 100,000. It typically presents in the third to fourth decade of life, and men are more frequently affected than women. It is uncommon in childhood or late-adult years.

PATHOBIOLOGY

Generally speaking, primary syringomyelia arises from an impairment of normal CSF flow dynamics. Although congenital cases of primary syringomyelia do exist, syringomyelia more often arises secondary to Arnold–Chiari type 1 malformation. There has long been debate about exactly how this posterior malformation leads to syringomyelia, with no definite consensus on a single theory.

Spinal cord tumors may also cause secondary syringomyelia by altering local CSF flow dynamics. Additionally, syringomyelia may be seen in the chronic phase after trauma, either as an ex vacuo lesion that persists after absorption of an intramedullary hematoma or due to local inflammation of the pia–arachnoid resulting in adhesions between the meninges and spinal cord. In animal models, these adhesions lead to ischemia, demyelination, and ultimately, cavitation.

CLINICAL FEATURES

The classic presentation of cervicothoracic syringomyelia is a cape-like distribution of decreased pain and temperature sensation in the back, arms, and hands, which occurs due to disruption of the crossing spinothalamic tracts. There may be varying degrees of weakness in the arms (lower motor neuron type due to involvement of cervical anterior horn cells) and legs (upper motor neuron type due to involvement of lateral corticospinal fibers). A Horner syndrome may be present if a cervicothoracic syrinx affects the intermediolateral columns. Bowel and bladder function are generally preserved unless the syrinx extends toward the sacral cord segments.

DIAGNOSIS

Magnetic resonance imaging (MRI) allows visualization not only of the syrinx but also of any associated abnormalities such as Arnold–Chiari malformation, neoplasm, or arachnoid granulations. Full cord imaging should be strongly considered. MRI CSF flow studies may also be useful in guiding treatment. There are no biomarkers associated with syringomyelia. CSF is often normal or may have a nonspecific, mild elevation in protein.

TREATMENT

Conservative observation is warranted in cases with no or only minor symptoms and in cases of Arnold–Chiari malformation with tonsillar herniation less than 5 mm below the foramen magnum in the setting of normal CSF flow studies. In more severe cases of Arnold–Chiari, however, posterior fossa decompression and cervical laminectomy with or without duraplasty is frequently pursued in hopes of restoring normal CSF flow dynamics.

In cases of syringomyelia secondary to neoplasm, if resection is not possible, then fenestration or marsupialization of the syrinx may be attempted. Lysis of adhesions and/or shunting of the syrinx to the pleural or peritoneal cavities is also performed, although the benefits have not been proven and are very difficult to predict in individual patients.

OUTCOME

A recent study by Alfieri and Pinna found that surgical decompression for Arnold–Chiari type 1 malformation associated with syringomyelia tends to be well tolerated with few complications. Additionally, 93.4% of patients experienced some degree of clinical improvement.

In contrast, a study of surgical treatment for posttraumatic syringomyelia showed much lower clinical success rates, with only 51% of patients reporting clinical improvement. Forty-one percent of patients experienced no clinical change, and 8% had further clinical deterioration. Notably, among those patients in whom surgery was not recommended based on lack of significant neurologic symptoms, 84% remained stable at 10 years. The high progression-free rate and the unsure evidence for surgical efficacy both argue for the clinician to take a conservative, watchful approach to posttraumatic syringomyelia if at all possible.

METASTATIC CORD COMPRESSION

Neoplasm should be high on the differential anytime someone presents with a previously undiagnosed myelopathy. Metastatic disease is much more common than a primary central nervous system (CNS) tumor. In fact, an estimated 12% to 20% of patients

TABLE 111.1 Differential Diagnosis of Myelopathy

Acute Myelopathy

Compressive/mechanical
- Trauma
- Disk herniation/subluxation
- Epidural abscess
- Epidural hematoma
- Epidural neoplasm/metastasis
- Vertebral compression fracture

Vascular
- Stroke
- Dural arteriovenous fistula
- Arteriovenous malformation
- Cavernous malformation

Infectious
- Viral gray matter/acute flaccid paralysis
  - Poliovirus
  - Enterovirus
  - Coxsackieviruses A and B
  - West Nile virus (WNV)
  - Japanese encephalitis (JE)
  - Tick-borne encephalitis
- Viral white matter/longitudinal myelitis
  - Herpes simplex virus (HSV)
  - Varicella-zoster virus (VZV)
  - Cytomegalovirus (CMV)
  - Epstein–Barr virus (EBV)
  - Influenza
- Bacterial
  - *Mycoplasma pneumoniae*
  - Syphilis
  - Tuberculosis
  - Lyme
- Fungal
  - *Cryptococcus neoformans*
  - *Coccidioides immitis*
  - *Blastomyces dermatitidis*
  - *Histoplasma capsulatum*
  - *Candida* species
  - *Aspergillus* species
  - Zygomycetes
- Parasitic
  - *Schistosoma* species
  - *Toxoplasma gondii*
  - *Taenia solium* (cysticercosis)

Inflammatory
- Multiple sclerosis
- Neuromyelitis optica
- Transverse myelitis
- Acute disseminated encephalomyelitis (ADEM)
- Sarcoidosis
- Paraneoplastic
- Systemic lupus erythematosus (SLE)
- Antiphospholipid antibody syndrome (APS)
- Sjögren syndrome
- Mixed connective tissue disease (MCTD)
- Behçet disease

Acute Myelopathy *(continued)*

Toxic/metabolic
- Heroin
- Konzo
- Arachnoiditis after angiographic/myelographic contrast agents
- Methotrexate toxicity
- Cytarabine toxicity
- Amphotericin B toxicity

Neoplasm

Subacute Myelopathy

Inflammatory
- Multiple sclerosis
- Neuromyelitis optica
- Transverse myelitis
- ADEM
- Sarcoidosis
- Paraneoplastic
- SLE
- APS
- Sjögren syndrome
- MCTD
- Behçet disease

Vascular
- Dural arteriovenous fistula
- Arteriovenous malformation
- Cavernous malformation

Neoplasm

Postinfectious myelitis

Chronic Myelopathy

Compressive/mechanical
- Disk herniation/subluxation
- Arachnoid cyst
- Spinal stenosis
- Ligamentous ossification
- Paget disease
- Syringomyelia

Neoplasm
- Ependymoma
- Glioma (astrocytoma > oligodendroglioma)
- Hemangioblastoma
- Lymphoma
- Leukemia
- Meningioma
- Neurofibroma

Infection
- HIV
- Human T-lymphotropic virus (HTLV)
- Syphilis
- Tuberculosis

TABLE 111.1 Differential Diagnosis of Myelopathy *(continued)*

Chronic Myelopathy *(continued)*

Toxic/metabolic
- Nutritional deficiency
  - Cyanocobalamin (B_{12})
  - Thiamine (B_1)
  - Folate (B_9)
  - Vitamin E
  - Copper
- Cyanide poisoning (cassava plant ingestion)
- Hexacarbon toxicity (glue sniffing)
- Nitrous oxide toxicity
- Organophosphate toxicity
- 1-Bromopropane toxicity (aerosol exposure, dry cleaning)
- Fluorosis
- Lathyrism
- Hepatic myelopathy

Chronic Myelopathy *(continued)*

Genetic
- Distal motor–sensory axonopathy
  - Hereditary spastic paraplegia
- Motor neuron disease
  - Amyotrophic lateral sclerosis (ALS)
  - Primary lateral sclerosis (PLS)
  - Spinobulbar muscular atrophy (Kennedy syndrome)
- Disorders of metabolism
  - Adrenomyeloneuropathy
  - Krabbe disease
  - Metachromatic leukodystrophy
  - Methylene tetrahydrofolate reductase deficiency
  - Cobalamin C disease
  - Arginase deficiency
  - Hyperornithinemia–hyperammonemia–homocitrullinuria
  - Abetalipoproteinemia (Bassen–Kornzweig syndrome)
- Spinocerebellar degeneration
  - Friedreich ataxia
  - Spinocerebellar ataxia types 1–28
- Spinal muscular atrophy

with cancer present with spinal metastasis as the initial symptom. Primary spinal cord tumors are much rarer, with an estimated incidence of 0.74 cases per 100,000—these neoplasms are discussed elsewhere in this volume. Further information on metastatic neoplasm may also be reviewed in Chapter 97.

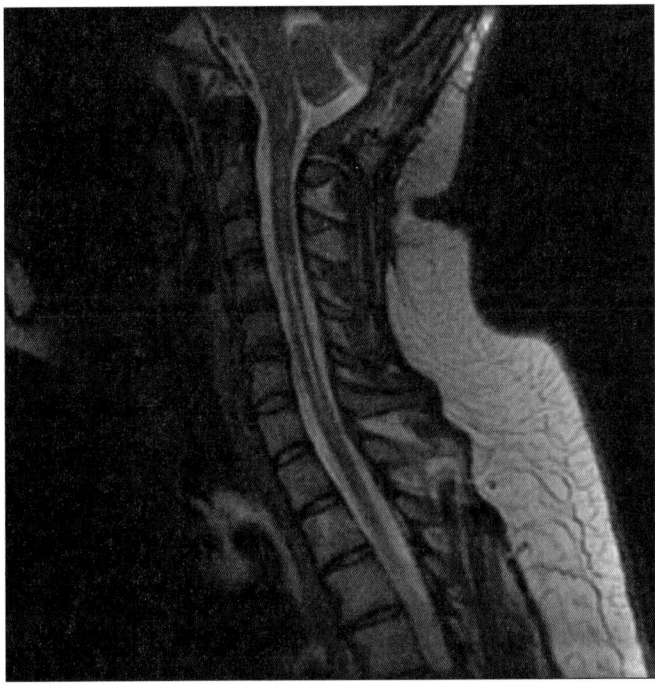

FIGURE 111.1 Syringomyelia on a T2-weighted MRI. The syrinx, which appears as a high-intensity linear lesion in the central cord, extends from C4 to C7. (From Peleggi AF, Lovely TJ. Treatment of delayed Chiari malformation and syringomyelia after lumboperitoneal shunt placement: case report and treatment recommendations. *Surg Neurol Int.* 2012;3:101, with permission.)

It is important to bear in mind that not all myelopathy in the setting of neoplasm is a direct consequence of the neoplasm itself but rather may be secondary to radiation injury, chemotherapy toxicity, or a paraneoplastic disorder.

EPIDEMIOLOGY

The cancers that most frequently metastasize to the spinal column are lung, breast, renal, hematopoietic, melanoma, prostate, and gastrointestinal. At least 95% of spinal metastases are extradural, usually to the vertebrae, and may remain asymptomatic. Autopsy studies suggest that over 30% of patients with advanced systemic cancer have pathologic evidence of vertebral metastases at the time of death. In the rostrocaudal axis, the majority of spinal metastases localize to the lumbar spine. However, due to the narrower diameter of the spinal canal within the thoracic segments, most symptomatic metastases are within the thoracic spine.

PATHOBIOLOGY

Most spinal metastases travel hematologically either through the arterial system or retrogradely through Batson venous plexus. As the vertebral column comprises a large proportion of the body's bone marrow rich in growth factors, the vertebrae may provide a particularly hospitable environment for metastatic cells. Leptomeningeal metastases can also result from either extension from nearby bone or spread through the CSF.

CLINICAL FEATURES

In addition to the usual myelopathic symptoms of weakness, sensory loss, and urogenital dysfunction, spinal neoplasms are often marked by pain. The pain may be local or radicular. It may accompany myelopathic symptoms acutely, or it may precede myelopathic symptoms by weeks to months. Although nonspecific, red flags of concern for a cancerous cause of back pain include age older than 60 years, associated weight loss, worse at night, thoracic rather than lumbar pain, and tenderness to palpation. The rate of symptom progression may range from slowly progressive (as a result of compressive tumor growth) to an acute onset (such as a pathologic vertebral fracture secondary to intravertebral tumor). In addition, metastases may alter arterial perfusion and/or venous drainage, resulting in acute ischemia, hemorrhage, or venous compression.

DIAGNOSIS

Although a computed tomography scan performs well at detecting bony metastases, MRI with contrast remains the test of choice, as it visualizes the extent of cord and soft-tissue involvement, as well as vasogenic and cytotoxic edema. If a neoplasm is identified, full neuraxis imaging should be completed to evaluate for additional lesions, as these may alter treatment and prognosis. Additionally, if the patient is not otherwise known to have cancer, then a full assessment for the primary tumor should be initiated. If the spinal lesion is intradural, a high-volume lumbar puncture should be sent for cytology and flow cytometry although the sensitivity of these studies is not high. Ultimately, biopsy of either the spinal lesion or a suspected primary tumor source if easier to access remains the diagnostic gold standard.

TREATMENT

The mainstay of treatment has traditionally been glucocorticoid and radiation therapy. Radiation tends to be well tolerated, and 65% to 80% of patients report improvement of symptoms. High-dose corticosteroids such as dexamethasone 100 mg intravenous push (IVP), followed by 10 mg every 6 hours with a rapid taper over the next few days, is often used concurrently for symptom management. A randomized trial has shown that decompressive surgical resection plus radiation therapy for acute paraplegia results in greater ability to walk (84% vs. 57%), and a better chance of regaining the ability to walk (62% vs. 19%), compared to radiation therapy alone [**Level 1**].[1]

OUTCOME

As mentioned, the prognosis after diagnosis of a spinal metastasis is poor, with an average life expectancy of 4 to 15 months. The emphasis in management, therefore, is typically in maintaining the highest quality of life possible.

INFECTIOUS MYELOPATHY

Numerous infectious causes of myelopathy may induce symptoms through direct neuroinvasion, compression, or as an inflammatory response. Symptoms may occur at the time of the acute infection, as in the case of viral myelitis, meningoencephalitis, or abscess, or they may be delayed by days to weeks as in the case of postinfectious or postvaccination myelitis or even years in the case of neurosyphilis or HIV.

This chapter expands on viral myelitis and human T-cell lymphotropic virus (HTLV)–associated myelitis. Many other infectious syndromes are detailed elsewhere in this book. Additional reference may be made to Chapters 61 to 67.

VIRAL MYELITIS

Epidemiology

The true incidence of viral myelitis is unknown. Worldwide, the viral syndrome of acute flaccid paralysis, one form of viral myelitis, occurs in approximately 40 per 1,000,000 individuals per year. Prior to widespread vaccination, polio accounted for the vast majority of cases of acute flaccid paralysis. In recent times, West Nile virus (WNV) and Japanese encephalitis are the more likely culprits. Cases of transverse myelitis number approximately 1 to 4 cases per 1,000,000 individuals per year. Viral myelitis tends to be more common in the summer and early fall with a bimodal incidence peak in adolescence and the fourth decade of life.

Pathobiology

Viral myelitis may occur through direct cellular toxicity or through parainfectious inflammation. In particular, gray matter and anterior horn cells are often targeted by enteroviruses (including poliovirus, coxsackieviruses A and B, echovirus) and flaviviruses (WNV, Japanese encephalitis, tick-borne encephalitis). In contrast, herpesviruses, including herpes simplex virus (HSV), varicella-zoster virus (VZV), cytomegalovirus (CMV), and Epstein–Barr virus, have a higher predilection for glial cells of the white matter and sensory neurons in the dorsal horn.

Clinical Features

Acute flaccid paralysis typically presents with fever and headache followed a few days later by the onset of flaccid paralysis of at least one extremity. Alterations in cognition may be seen, reflecting a common association between flaccid paralysis and meningitis and encephalitis. Sensory symptoms and alterations in bowel and bladder control are notably absent. In comparison, transverse myelitis often has prominent sensory (usually symmetric) and bowel/bladder abnormalities in addition to weakness with or without cognitive symptoms that evolves over the period of hours to days.

Diagnosis

MRI with and without contrast may show evidence of edema, demyelination, meningeal enhancement, or necrosis. In addition to cord imaging, brain MRI is warranted to evaluate for intracranial involvement—abnormalities of the deep gray matter indicate viral encephalitis, whereas white matter findings would redirect the diagnosis toward an autoimmune etiology such as postviral or parainfectious inflammation, multiple sclerosis, or neuromyelitis optica.

All patients with suspected viral myelitis should undergo lumbar puncture. Typical CSF findings include pleocytosis with a lymphocytic or mononuclear predominance, normal glucose, but elevated total protein. Additionally, most pathogenic viruses may be directly detected within CSF using either polymerase chain reaction amplification of viral nucleic acid or specific antibody titers.

Treatment

In the setting of suspected viral myelitis, supportive care is fundamental. Specific antiviral medications include intravenous (IV) acyclovir, which is typically started upon presentation and may be discontinued if testing for HSV and VZV are negative. If CMV is suspected in the setting of HIV or other type of immunosuppression, then it would be reasonable to start ganciclovir and foscarnet. If the pathogen is WNV, there is mixed data supporting the use of intravenous immunoglobulin (IVIG) and interferon-α-2b. Finally, to combat parainfectious inflammation, IV methylprednisolone is often used in parallel with these other treatments.

Outcome

Prognosis depends in no small part on whether the damage involves gray matter or white matter, with better recovery in the latter. Age, severity of abnormalities, and timing of initiation of specific treatment also affect recovery.

HUMAN T-CELL LYMPHOTROPIC VIRUS–ASSOCIATED MYELOPATHY/TROPICAL SPASTIC PARAPARESIS

Epidemiology

HTLV types 1 and 2 cause insidious, progressive myelopathy in approximately 20 million people worldwide, with the highest infection rates in Japan, South America, the Caribbean, and equatorial Africa. Similar to HIV, HTLV transmission generally occurs as a result of unprotected sex, mother-to-child via breastfeeding, sharing of needles, or blood transfusions. Roughly 3% to 5% of infected individuals develop an aggressive T-cell leukemia, whereas an additional 0.25% to 3% develops a spastic paraparesis. Women are 1.5 to 3.5 times more likely to develop human T-cell lymphotropic virus–associated myelopathy/tropical spastic paraparesis (HAM/TSP) than men and may experience a faster progression of disease.

Pathobiology

Like HIV, HTLV predominantly infects CD4+ T lymphocytes. As a retrovirus, it reverse transcribes its RNA genome into DNA that then integrates into the host genome as a provirus. How HTLV infection leads to chronic, inflammatory/demyelinating myelopathy is not well understood. Autopsy studies show perivascular infiltrates containing HTLV-infected lymphocytes as well as multiple inflammatory cytokines resulting in breakdown of the blood–brain barrier (BBB).

Clinical Features

HAM/TSP is an insidious disease that begins initially with subtle weakness or stiffness of the lower extremities, followed by progression—without remissions—toward spastic paraparesis and spastic bladder. Paresthesias in the lower extremities are also common, although sensory levels are not usually seen.

Diagnosis

In the early stages of the disease, MRI is often unremarkable. With progression, nonspecific subcortical and periventricular white matter demyelinating lesions appear in the brain followed eventually by spinal cord atrophy.

Lumbar puncture typically shows mild pleocytosis with elevated total protein and normal glucose. HTLV-1 antibodies and a proviral load can be detected in the CSF. Oligoclonal bands and evidence of intrathecal immunoglobulin G (IgG) synthesis are often present.

Treatment

Several antiretroviral drugs used against HIV have been trialed against HTLV, so far without success. In the cancer literature, there are some reports of decreased HTLV-1 expression with interferon-α treatment. Other immune-modulating medications such as corticosteroids and cyclosporine may improve HAM/TSP symptoms, but these are far from proven therapies. As such, the mainstays of treatment are symptomatic.

Outcome

HAM/TSP remains a chronic, progressive, untreatable disease. Patients almost invariably become wheelchair bound with significant bladder and bowel dysfunction.

INFLAMMATORY MYELOPATHY

The noninfectious inflammatory causes of myelopathy include transverse myelitis, multiple sclerosis (MS; see Chapter 69), systemic lupus erythematosus (SLE), antiphospholipid antibody syndrome, Sjögren syndrome, mixed connective tissue disease, sarcoidosis, Behçet disease, neuromyelitis optica (NMO), acute disseminated encephalomyelitis (ADEM), paraneoplastic syndromes (see Chapter 104), and others that remain to be identified. It is important to note that the cause remains unidentified in up to 30% of cases of spinal cord inflammation resulting in the diagnosis of idiopathic transverse myelitis.

CLINICAL FEATURES

As with any other cause of myelopathy, symptoms of inflammatory myelopathy depend on the location of the lesion. Most classically, patients present with sensory symptoms in a bandlike distribution associated with bladder dysfunction. Symptoms often progress to include motor deficits over the course of hours to days.

DIAGNOSIS

MRI with contrast usually reveals T2-hyperintense white matter lesions, often with contrast enhancement (Fig. 111.2). The pattern of cord and brain MRI involvement may help narrow the differential—for example, longitudinally extensive cord lesions suggest NMO, whereas deep brain gray matter lesions suggest ADEM. However, as many as 40% of cases may not show any MRI abnormality. CSF studies must include testing for oligoclonal bands (OCB) and IgG synthesis rate. Although not highly specific,

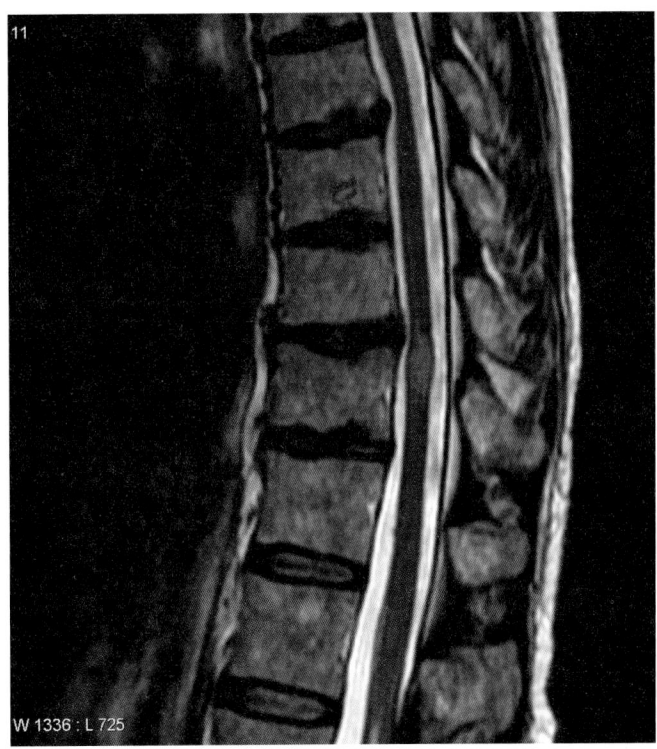

FIGURE 111.2 An MRI showing a transverse myelitis lesion (the lesion is the lighter, oval shape at center right). This MRI was taken 3 months after patient recovered. (From Gaillard F. Transverse myelitis. Radiopaedia.org Web site. http://radiopaedia.org/cases/transversemyelitis. Accessed April 25, 2015.)

several of the most common inflammatory myelopathies are associated with characteristic CSF profiles. For example, MS tends to feature normal protein, lack of pleocytosis, and positive OCB/IgG synthesis; in contrast, NMO usually demonstrates increased protein and cell count and a lower rate of positive OCB/IgG synthesis. Specific serum and CSF biomarkers include aquaporin-4 antibody (NMO), angiotensin-converting enzyme (ACE) (sarcoidosis), antinuclear and anti–double-stranded DNA antibodies (SLE), anti-Ro/SSA antibodies, anti-La/SSB antibodies (Sjögren), anti–scl-70 antibodies (scleroderma), and paraneoplastic antibodies. Visual-evoked potentials and somatosensory-evoked potentials may be useful ancillary tests if MRI and CSF are unrevealing. In up to 30% of cases, none of these studies are abnormal. These cases earn the diagnostic label of idiopathic transverse myelitis, a label that has steadily become less frequent due to improved diagnostic understanding.

TREATMENT

Once infection is ruled out, most cases of paraparesis related to acute transverse myelitis are treated with a 3- to 5-day course of IV corticosteroids, most commonly IV methylprednisolone 1,000 mg daily. More aggressive diseases such as NMO, SLE, Sjögren scleroderma, and others are treated with plasmapheresis or chronic immunosuppressive therapy.

OUTCOME

Prognosis varies widely depending on the disease, the extent of the lesion, the rate of symptom progression, and the patient's age. Disease course may be monophasic or relapsing, with complete remission or permanent disability.

VASCULAR MYELOPATHY

SPINAL CORD INFARCTION

Epidemiology

Compared to cerebrovascular ischemia, spinal cord infarction is quite rare, accounting for only 1% to 2% of vascular neurologic deficits and 5% to 8% of all acute myelopathies. In one small study by Cheshire and colleagues, men were almost twice as likely to experience an infarction of the spinal cord as women, but to our knowledge, this has not been studied in a larger context.

Pathobiology

The spinal cord is perfused mainly by direct branches of the aorta. The most common causes of spinal cord ischemia are secondary to aortic pathology and injury, such as dissection, traumatic rupture, and surgical procedures. Additionally, traditional causes of stroke in the cerebral vasculature can also cause stroke in the spinal cord vasculature—therefore, etiologies such as cardioembolism, hypercoagulable state, atherosclerosis, and vasculitis should be considered. The vast majority of spinal infarcts occur in the territory supplied by the anterior spinal artery (see Chapter 16, Fig 16.2). Due to a relative paucity of collateral perfusion, the thoracic cord is especially susceptible to systemic hypotension.

Clinical Features

Symptom onset typically occurs acutely over minutes to hours, although some patients experience a slower progression of symptoms in the setting of arterial insufficiency. Back pain frequently accompanies other typical myelopathic symptoms. On acute exam, flaccid paralysis and a sensory level to pinprick and temperature below the level of the ischemic lesion will usually be present. Vibration and proprioception are typically preserved, as the dorsal columns are supplied by the posterior spinal arteries. Reflexes are initially reduced or absent but transition to hyperreflexia over subsequent days to weeks.

Diagnosis

When cord ischemia is suspected, MRI and magnetic resonance (MR) angiography should be performed, with special attention to diffusion-weighted and apparent diffusion coefficient sequences. However, due to difficulties with resolution in the spinal canal, a negative scan does not rule out the diagnosis of ischemia, especially in the first few hours after presentation. There are no specific laboratory abnormalities to confirm the diagnosis. However, as part of the diagnostic workup and to guide secondary prevention, an echocardiogram, telemetry, a lipid panel, and hemoglobin A1c are typically ordered, along with a hypercoagulable disease workup if the patient is younger than 50 years or has a concerning family history.

Treatment

No randomized trials have looked at treatment of acute spinal cord infarction as a unique entity.

Induced hypertension with phenylephrine (20 to 100 μg/min) in association with spinal drainage to reduce CSF pressure (<5 cm H_2O) and increase spinal cord perfusion pressure has been described, in particular when spinal cord infarction occurs as a complication of aortic aneurysm surgery.

There are no reports of use of tissue plasminogen activator for the treatment of acute spinal cord infarction. This is most likely a result of the broad differential diagnosis of acute paraplegia (see Table 111.1).

Outcome

The classic teaching is that prognosis for recovery of motor or sphincter function after a spinal infarct is quite poor. However, Robertson and colleagues recently showed in a study of 115 patients that functional recovery of both ambulation and bladder control is possible in over one-third of survivors, especially if there is even a small degree of residual motor function within the first 6 months.

SPINAL ARTERIOVENOUS MALFORMATIONS

Epidemiology

Arteriovenous malformations (AVM) are inappropriate arteriovenous connections involving arteries that normally supply neural tissue. In contrast, dural arteriovenous fistulas (DAVF) are improper connections that involve the radiculomeningeal arteries. The vast majority, approximately 70%, of all spinal vascular malformations are DAVF. DAVF occur most frequently after the fourth decade of life and are more common in men than women. Intradural AVF are most common within the lower thoracic and lumbar spine. Extradural AVF are most common within the cervical cord. In comparison, spinal AVMs have no gender predominance and tend to present between the ages of 20 and 60 years old. Just over half of spinal AVMs are found within the thoracic cord, almost a third are cervical and the remaining are in the lumbar spine.

Pathobiology

Frank hemorrhage is not necessary to cause many of the symptoms of spinal vascular malformations. In both DAVF and AVM, the abnormal direct arterial flow into the venous system may result in myelopathy via cord compression as well as via the development of venous hypertension which leads to intramedullary edema. Additionally, in the setting of large arteriovenous lesions, vascular steal may occur, resulting in cord ischemia. Finally, symptoms may occur when arterial pressure overwhelms the accommodation of the venous wall, leading to hemorrhage; this is more common in AVM than DAVF.

Clinical Features

Chronically progressive motor deficits, especially paraparesis, are the most common presenting symptom. The weakness may worsen with exercise. Almost half of patients will have pain, often radicular, referable to the lesion. The diagnosis often eludes detection for years, although one clinical key may be the stepwise pattern of progression. Notably, in the case of AVMs, approximately half of patients present acutely with sudden onset of myelopathic symptoms due to hemorrhage.

Diagnosis

On standard MRI sequences, signs of AVM and DAVF include cord edema and enhancement. Gradient echo–based MRI sequences may detect characteristic abnormal flow voids. Conventional digital subtraction angiography remains the gold standard over MR angiography for diagnosis. It also has the added benefit of allowing for therapeutic intervention if the diagnosis is confirmed.

Treatment

Treatment options for AVM and DAVF include embolization of the feeding arteries, surgical clipping or resection, and gamma knife radiosurgery. Frequently, a combination of these treatment modalities is necessary. The treatment of asymptomatic and unruptured cranial lesions, especially AVM, is quite controversial. The A Randomized Multicenter Clinical Trial of Unruptured Brain AVMs (ARUBA) was stopped prematurely due to an increased rate of adverse events in the intervention arm—including all of these options—as compared to conservative medical therapy. Although this trial excluded spinal AVMs, these results should be considered.

Outcome

Prognosis can be difficult to predict; as may be expected, the patient's age, duration, and severity of myelopathic symptoms are critical variables that influence response to treatment. Overall, complete obliteration of the vascular lesion may be difficult to attain—especially with AVMs—however, in most cases, even partial treatment can result in significant clinical improvement.

TOXIC/METABOLIC CAUSES OF MYELOPATHY

Numerous causes of toxic or metabolic myelopathy may present with similar progressive myelopathic symptoms. The specific diagnosis derives from a combination of history of past exposures, systemic manifestations, and laboratory testing. Nutritional deficiencies, especially those of cyanocobalamin, thiamine, folate, vitamin E, and copper, are discussed extensively in Chapter 123.

MYELOPATHY DUE TO RADIATION OR CHEMOTHERAPY

Radiation therapy and a number of medications, especially chemotherapeutics, have been reported to cause myelopathy. The risk of myelopathy as a consequence of radiation therapy increases nonlinearly with the dose of radiation, with a reported prevalence of approximately 5% of patients who receive 60 cGy to the spinal cord as compared to only 1% of patients who were treated with 50 cGy. Radiation-induced myelopathy typically onsets months to years after treatment. Of the chemotherapeutics, methotrexate and cytarabine are the most frequent offenders and are most likely to lead to a myelopathy in those treated intrathecally or with systemic doses that are high enough to penetrate the BBB. If chemotherapy-related myelopathy occurs, it generally does so within hours to weeks after treatment and usually after the patient has received multiple doses. A number of other chemotherapeutics have been reported to cause myelopathy including fludarabine, cladribine, thiotepa, doxorubicin, and daunorubicin. In addition, amphotericin B has been reported to contribute to development of myelopathy.

NITROUS OXIDE TOXICITY

Nitrous oxide (NO) is an inhaled anesthetic that is used primarily for dental procedures. Therefore, occupational exposure is a risk, although NO toxicity more frequently results from recreational abuse in the form of "whippets," derived from whipped cream canisters. NO-induced myelopathy typically results relatively rapidly after abuse and is associated with functional B_{12} deficiency due to interference with B_{12} metabolism. Accordingly, the clinical picture is identical to subacute combined degeneration, with prominent proprioceptive loss in addition to spastic paraparesis. If a patient is expected to undergo a procedure with NO anesthesia and has moderately low B_{12} levels, supplementation with cyanocobalamin for a few weeks prior to the procedure can prevent this complication.

HEPATIC MYELOPATHY

Hepatic myelopathy is an uncommon and overlooked consequence of advanced cirrhosis. It is characterized by a spastic paraparesis that almost always spares the arms and which progresses slowly over years. Sensory and autonomic symptoms are typically absent. The myelopathy is often preceded by hepatic encephalopathy and most frequently occurs in the setting of a portosystemic shunt. MRI is often normal, especially early in the disease; however, motor-evoked potentials may confirm an abnormality. The pathobiology is unknown. There is mixed literature on improvement after liver transplantation, with some suggesting that transplantation before symptoms become too severe may allow for some degree of recovery.

GENETIC CAUSES OF MYELOPATHY

The genetic causes of myelopathy include hereditary spastic paraplegia, motor neuron disease, disorders of metabolism, and spinocerebellar degeneration. Within this section, we focus primarily on hereditary spastic paraplegia. Additional chapters expanding on these etiologies include Chapters 79, 85, 133, 134, and 137.

HEREDITARY SPASTIC PARAPLEGIA

Epidemiology

Hereditary spastic paraplegia (HSP) is a heterogeneous group of neurodegenerative disorders associated with mutations in any of over 50 genes that may have either autosomal dominant (AD) or autosomal recessive (AR) inheritance. HSP has a prevalence of 5.5 cases per 100,000. Among families with AD inheritance, the most frequent culprit mutations occur in SPG4 followed by SPG3A. Among families with AR inheritance, mutations within SPG11 are the most common, with SPG15 and SPG5 mutations as the second and third most common anomalies. X-linked and mitochondrial causes also exist, but the epidemiology of these is not as well studied. In addition, de novo mutations can occur in the absence of family history.

Pathobiology

HSP is classically associated with axonal degeneration at the distal ends of the lateral corticospinal tracts, often accompanied by distal degeneration within the fasciculus gracilis as well. The molecular basis for these abnormalities varies widely depending on the particular causal gene, with abnormalities involving axonal and endosomal trafficking, endoplasmic reticulum morphogenesis, lipid metabolism, and mitochondrial regulation. Further information can be found in recent reviews by Fink as well as Noreau and colleagues.

Clinical Features

HSP can present at any age. It typically begins as a gait abnormality due to impaired dorsiflexion secondary to extensor spasticity. Especially early in the disease, spasticity is a more prominent finding than actual weakness and may be mildly asymmetric. As the disease progresses, more proximal leg muscles become involved leading to a scissoring gait (adductor spasticity). Abnormalities of vibratory and position sense as well as bowel and bladder control may also be seen. The arms are generally spared except for possible hyperreflexia. "Complicated" HSP refers to cases with additional symptoms such as cognitive impairment, epilepsy, parkinsonism, ataxia, peripheral neuropathy, amyotrophy, or vision or hearing loss.

Diagnosis

A presumptive diagnosis of HSP is usually made based on a combination of personal and family history and physical exam. Genetic testing finds the causative gene in only 33% to 55% of autosomal dominantly inherited cases and 18% to 29% of autosomal recessively inherited cases. MRI is often normal but may show distal spinal cord atrophy, especially later in disease course. Sensory-evoked potentials are often abnormal, even in patients without clinical evidence of sensory abnormalities.

Treatment

Treatment is symptomatic. Muscle relaxants such as baclofen, tizanidine, or diazepam may aid with spasticity. Botulinum toxin injection may prove helpful in more resistant cases. Physical therapy is recommended to help maintain range of motion and mobility. Symptoms of spastic bladder can be treated with anticholinergic medications such as oxybutynin.

Outcome

HSP does not typically shorten life expectancy, and many patients will experience a plateau in neurologic decline after which the degree of disability seems to stabilize. At what point this plateau will occur, however, will vary with the patient and is difficult to predict.

LEVEL 1 EVIDENCE

1. Patchell RA, Tibbs PA, Regine WF, et al. Direct decompressive surgical resection in the treatment of spinal cord compression caused by metastatic cancer: a randomised trial. *Lancet.* 2005;366:643–648.

SUGGESTED READINGS

Alfieri A, Pinna G. Long-term results after posterior fossa decompression in syringomyelia with adult Chiari Type 1 malformation. *J Neurosurg Spine.* 2012;17:381–387.

Cachat A, Chevalier SA, Alais S, et al. Alpha interferon restricts human T-lymphocytic virus type 1 and 2 de novo infection through PRK activation. *J Virol.* 2013;87:13386–13396.

Caldwell C, Werdiger N, Jakab S, et al. Use of model for end-stage liver disease exception points for early liver transplantation and successful reversal of hepatic myelopathy with a review of the literature. *Liver Transpl.* 2010;16:818–826.

Cheshire WP, Santos CC, Massey EW, et al. Spinal cord infarction: etiology and outcome. *Neurology.* 1996;47:321–330.

Cheung AT, Weiss SJ, McGarvey ML, et al. Interventions for reversing delayed-onset postoperative paraplegia after thoracic aortic reconstruction. *Ann Thorac Surg.* 2002;74:413–419.

Cho W-S, Kim K-J, Kwon O-K, et al. Clinical features and treatment outcomes of the spinal arteriovenous fistulas and malformations. *J Neurosurg Spine.* 2013;19:207–216.

Cree BAC. Acute inflammatory myelopathies. *Handb Clin Neurol.* 2014;122: 613–667.

Fink JK. Hereditary spastic paraplegia: clinico-pathologic features and emerging molecular mechanisms. *Acta Neuropathol.* 2013;126:307–328.

Fuzii HT, da Silva Dias GA, de Barros RJS, et al. Immunopathogenesis of HTLV-1-associated myelopathy/tropical spastic paraparesis (HAM/TSP). *Life Sci.* 2014;104:9–14.

Goncalves DU, Proietti FA, Ribas JGR, et al. Epidemiology, treatment, and prevention of human T-cell leukemia virus type-1-associated diseases. *Clin Microbiol Rev.* 2010;23:577–589.

Hathout L, El-Saden S. Nitrous oxide-induced B_{12} deficiency myelopathy: perspectives on the clinical biochemistry of vitamin B_{12}. *J Neurol Sci.* 2011;301:1–8.

Heldner MR, Arnold M, Nedeltchev K, et al. Vascular diseases of the spinal cord: a review. *Curr Treat Options Neurol.* 2012;14:509–520.

Hrabalek L. Intramedullary spinal cord metastases: review of the literature. *Biomed Pap Med Fac Univ Palacky Olomouc Czech Repub.* 2010;154:117–122.

Irani DN. Aseptic meningitis and viral myelitis. *Neurol Clin.* 2008;26:635–655.

Jacobs WB, Perrin RG. Evaluation and treatment of spinal metastases: an overview. *Neurosurg Focus.* 2001;11:e10.

Kim J, Losina E, Bono C, et al. Clinical outcome of metastatic spinal cord compression treated with surgical excision ± radiation versus radiation therapy alone: a systematic review of literature. *Spine (Phila Pa 1976).* 2012;37:78–84.

Kincaid O, Lipton HL. Viral myelitis: an update. *Curr Neurol Neurosci Rep.* 2006;6:469–474.

Klekamp J. Treatment of posttraumatic syringomyelia. *J Neurosurg Spine.* 2012;17:199–211.

Koyanagi I, Houkin K. Pathogenesis of syringomyelia associated with Chiari type 1 malformation: review of evidences and proposal of a new hypothesis. *Neurosurg Rev.* 2010;33:271–285.

Krings T, Geibprasert S. Spinal dural arteriovenous fistulas. *AJNR Am J Neuroradiol.* 2009;30:639–648.

Kumar N. Metabolic and toxic myelopathies. *Semin Neurol.* 2012;32:123–136.

Lad SP, Santarelli JG, Patil CG, et al. National trends in spinal malformations: a review. *Neurosurg Focus.* 2009;26:1–5.

Lima M, Bica R, Araujo A. Gender influence on the progression of HTLV-1 associated myelopathy/tropical spastic paraparesis. *J Neurol Neurosurg Psychiatry.* 2005;76:294–296.

Loher TJ, Bassetti CL, Lovblad KO, et al. Diffusion-weighted MRI in acute spinal cord ischaemia. *Neuroradiology.* 2003;45:557–561.

Marcus J, Schwarz J, Singh IP, et al. Spinal dural arteriovenous fistulas: a review. *Curr Atheroscler Rep*. 2013;15:335.

Martin F, Castro H, Gabriel C, et al. Ciclosporin A proof of concept study in patients with active, progressive HTLV-1 associated myelopathy/tropical spastic paraparesis. *PLoS Negl Trop Dis*. 2012;6:e1675.

Mihai C, Jubelt B. Infectious myelitis. *Curr Neurol Neurosci Rep*. 2012;12:633–641.

Nagpal S, Clarke JL. Neoplastic myelopathy. *Semin Neurol*. 2012;32:137–145.

Nardone R, Holler Y, Storti M, et al. Spinal cord involvement in patients with cirrhosis. *World J Gastroenterol*. 2014;20:2578–2585.

Newton HB. Neurological complications of chemotherapy to the central nervous system. *Handb Clin Neurol*. 2012;105:903–916.

Noreau A, Dion PA, Rouleau GA. Molecular aspects of hereditary spastic paraplegia. *Exp Cell Res*. 2014;325:18–26.

Robertson CE, Brown RD, Wijdicks EF, et al. Recovery after spinal cord infarcts: long-term outcome in 115 patients. *Neurology*. 2012;78:114–121.

Roy AK, Slimack NP, Ganju A. Idiopathic syringomyelia: retrospective case series, comprehensive review, and update on management. *Neurosurg Focus*. 2011;31:E15.

Ruano L, Melo C, Silva MC, et al. The global epidemiology of hereditary ataxia and spastic paraplegia: a systematic review of prevalence studies. *Neuroepidemiology*. 2014;42:174–183.

Satran R. Spinal cord infarction. *Stroke*. 1988;19:529–532.

Scotti G, Gerevini S. Diagnosis and differential diagnosis of acute transverse myelopathy: the role of neuroradiological investigations and review of the literature. *Neurol Sci*. 2001;22:S69–S73.

Transverse Myelitis Consortium Working Group. Proposed diagnostic criteria and nosology of acute transverse myelitis. *Neurology*. 2002;59:499–505.

Vandertop WP. Syringomyelia. *Neuropediatrics*. 2014;45:3–9.

West TW, Hess C, Cree BAC. Acute transverse myelitis: demyelinating, inflammatory, and infectious myelopathies. *Semin Neurol*. 2012;32:97–113.

Neurogenic Orthostatic Hypotension, Autonomic Failure, and Acquired and Familial Autonomic Neuropathy

112

Louis H. Weimer

INTRODUCTION

Autonomic disorders are generally considered to be uncommon conditions, but in fact, autonomic dysfunction is ubiquitous in neurologic disease, including highly prevalent processes such as seizures, strokes, mass lesions, infections, multiple sclerosis (MS) plaques, and others, but dysautonomia is often a secondary concern. A limited number of disorders produce severe or isolated dysautonomia or autonomic failure (AF). Because autonomic systems affect virtually all organ systems, symptoms produced are multiple and varied, often affecting functions not considered by most neurologists. Problems can arise from any site of autonomic control including the central cortical and subcortical autonomic network, brain stem, spinal cord, autonomic ganglia, or peripheral autonomic nerves. The range of pathogenic mechanisms is highly varied, including degenerative, hereditary, immune-mediated, paraneoplastic, aberrant reflex, and metabolic, among others. Suspicion of autonomic dysfunction rests with the clinician and can be missed if symptoms that can appear to be nonspecific are considered in isolation (Table 112.1). Early symptoms of the most characteristic finding, orthostatic hypotension (OH), may appear as postural fatigue, cognitive change, anxiety, or vertigo. This lack of certainty in many cases makes more objective assessment desirable in these instances (see Chapter 27). Postural hypotension (OH) is a prevalent clinical sign seen in numerous and diverse neurologic and nonneurologic conditions. Shibao et al. estimated over 80,000 U.S. OH-related hospitalizations in 2004; OH was the primary diagnosis in 35%. One consensus agreement defines OH as a fall in systolic blood pressure (SBP) of 20 or 10 mm Hg diastolic within 3 minutes of standing or similar orthostatic challenge, such as upright tilt, although some require a 30 mm Hg decline. OH, however, may be asymptomatic, especially in the elderly, and varies according to underlying conditions or confounding factors (Table 112.2). The sign is one marker of advanced AF caused by either diseases of central autonomic pathways or autonomic neuropathy. Some severe and important causes are discussed; a more comprehensive list is provided in Table 112.3. Acute and subacute processes are generally considered separately from more chronic conditions.

ACUTE AND SUBACUTE AUTONOMIC DISORDERS

Acute or subacute autonomic neuropathy (AAN) or acute pandysautonomia is an unusual but distinct entity, which primarily affects peripheral autonomic nerves. Roughly, half are preceded by a viral prodrome similar to Guillain–Barré syndrome (GBS). Patients typically develop generalized AF including OH, anhidrosis, parasympathetic failure, and gastrointestinal dysfunction, although predominantly adrenergic

and cholinergic variants are seen. The illness is monophasic with acute or subacute onset over several weeks. Recovery generally occurs but is often slow and incomplete. Acute signs such as ileus may develop into lesser degrees of gastrointestinal dysmotility including bloating, early satiety, nausea, vomiting, and alternating diarrhea and constipation. Antecedent viruses include herpes simplex, mononucleosis, rubella, and nondescript febrile illnesses. Roughly 25% have a restricted cholinergic form (acute cholinergic neuropathy) characterized by dry eyes and mouth, gastrointestinal dysmotility, bladder dysfunction, hypohidrosis, unreactive pupils, fixed heart rate, and sexual dysfunction but without significant OH. Abnormalities on formal autonomic testing are prominent in the involved systems. Nerve conduction studies are typically normal or show minor sensory abnormalities. The lack of OH in cholinergic cases complicates the diagnosis.

Demonstration of high-titer antibodies to nicotinic ganglionic AChR α-3 subunits, which are similar but distinct from those at the neuromuscular junction (α-1 subunits), supports an immune-mediated basis. A paraneoplastic form, which develops in a similar time course and is indistinguishable on clinical or laboratory

---

TABLE 112.1   Autonomic Review of Symptoms

- Secretomotor: dry eyes and mouth, often required natural tears or frequent sips of water. Excessive saliva can also occur.
- Orthostatic: dizziness, weakness, fatigue, cognitive changes, visual disturbance, vertigo, anxiety, palpitations, pallor, nausea, syncope
- Postprandial: bloating, fullness, nausea, dizziness, sweating, orthostatic hypotension
- GI: constipation, nocturnal or intermittent diarrhea
- Genitourinary (GU): urinary retention, difficulty with initiation, incomplete emptying, incontinence
- Sexual: erectile failure, ejaculatory dysfunction, retrograde ejaculation into bladder
- Visual: blurred vision, sensitivity to light/glare, reduced night vision
- Sudomotor: reduced loss of sweating ability (distally in polyneuropathies); excessive, paroxysmal, or inappropriate sweating; mixed pattern of loss and excessive areas, heat intolerance
- Vasomotor: distal color changes, change in skin appearance, persistently cold extremities, Raynaud phenomenon, loss of skin wrinkling in water, heat intolerance
- Other: unexplained syncope

GI, gastrointestinal

TABLE 112.2	Factors Affecting Orthostatic Hypotension
Aggravating Factors	

- Warm environment, hot bath
- Post exercise
- Prolonged motionless standing
- Large meals (carbohydrate load)
- Early morning
- Valsalva maneuver, isometric exercise
- Volume depletion
- Rising after prolonged bed rest
- Rapid postural change
- Space flight
- Alcohol
- Medications
- Beneficial maneuvers
- Squatting, leg crossing
- Abdominal and leg compression
- Nighttime slight upright tilt
- Isotonic exercise

grounds, may appear prior to tumor discovery, most commonly thymoma. In screening patients with autonomic disorders and controls, Vernino et al. found that 41% of patients with idiopathic autonomic neuropathy had high antibody titers; paraneoplastic neuropathy patients were frequently positive as well. Rarely, patients with chronic OH and AF have high antibody titers and respond to immunotherapy, such as intravenous immunoglobulin (IVIG) or plasma exchange. Some patients with orthostatic intolerance, discussed later, and idiopathic gastrointestinal dysmotility, but none with chronic degenerative autonomic processes, also had positive assays at lower titers. Knockout mouse models of the α-3 subunit gene, rabbits immunized against the subunit, and passive antibody transfer to other animals all induce signs of AF supporting the assertion that the antibodies are causative. Antibody titers also correlate with disease severity. Of note, low-level titers may occur in patients with other disorders or nonspecific symptoms. One-third of AAN patients recover, one-third have a partial recovery with substantial deficits, and the remainder do not improve. Gastrointestinal dysfunction and OH are usually the most debilitating manifestations. Supportive care and management of the OH and system-specific problems are the mainstays of treatment. Rare cases with AAN and myasthenia gravis have both types of AChR antibodies. Autonomic involvement is common in typical GBS, discussed in Chapter 87, especially in more severe cases, and is a prominent cause of morbidity and mortality.

PARANEOPLASTIC AUTONOMIC NEUROPATHY

Subacute autonomic neuropathy or predominantly enteric neuropathy is also seen in isolation or with somatic sensory neuropathy and other underlying antibodies, especially type 1 antineuronal nuclear antibodies (ANNA-1, anti-Hu) usually in patients with small cell lung cancer. Paraneoplastic neuropathy is also associated with other paraneoplastic antibodies including Purkinje cell cytoplasmic anti-

body type 2 (PCA-2) and collapsing response mediator protein-5 (CRMP-5). Botulism (cholinergic), acute intermittent porphyria, and toxic neuropathy are other diagnostic considerations. A rare chronic form associated with high titers to ganglionic antibodies is known that can mimic degenerative AF. Autonomic manifestations are also common in patients with Lambert–Eaton myasthenic syndrome, especially cholinergic complaints and manifestations (see Chapter 89).

ORTHOSTATIC INTOLERANCE

Exaggerated orthostatic tachycardia may be evident in some cases without significant cardiac denervation. This led to the proposal that some patients with the common syndrome of idiopathic orthostatic intolerance without OH (postural orthostatic tachycardia syndrome), also known as orthostatic intolerance, may have an attenuated form of acute autonomic neuropathy. Orthostatic intolerance symptoms include postural lightheadedness, fatigue, cognitive changes, and presyncope despite minimal changes in blood pressure (BP). Potential mechanisms are multiple, including excessive venous pooling, idiopathic hypovolemia, adrenergic hypersensitivity, and altered cerebrovascular autoregulation. Some may have an attenuated form of AAN supported by abnormalities of sudomotor and other autonomic systems in one-third of cases and an overrepresentation of antecedent viral infection in these patients. The common physiologic thread is presumed bouts of cerebral hypoperfusion, despite a seemingly adequate systemic BP. This syndrome is the most common cause of consultation in most autonomic centers. The condition is much more common in women, roughly 5:1 and commonly initially develops between ages 15 and 25 years, often after an acute illness, such as a viral syndrome. An association with joint hypermobility and presumed or documented Ehlers–Danlos syndrome type III is increasingly recognized. Patients with grade I Chiari malformations also typically have multiple autonomic symptoms, including orthostatic intolerance. Roughly, 40% of patients have additional vasovagal syncopal episodes. The condition must be distinguished from depression, vestibular disorders, chronic fatigue, fibromyalgia, and panic disorders but many overlap cases exist; many patients have coincident chronic and not postural fatigue, insomnia, and chronic pain. Uncommon symptomatic causes must be considered, such as adrenal insufficiency, pheochromocytoma, and Sjögren syndrome. The syndrome often leads to secondary deconditioning, which complicates recovery. An indistinguishable hereditary form resulting from a mutation in a norepinephrine transporter gene is known but is exceedingly rare. Similar symptoms can be seen in patients with predominantly painful small fiber neuropathy due to additional involvement of distal autonomic nerves. Treatment must be individualized based on the most prominent symptoms but is generally based on improving standing BP, increasing blood volume, minimizing anemia, and increasing activity levels. Beta blockade is helpful in patients with bothersome palpitations and hyperadrenergic forms but is counterproductive in other subtypes.

CHRONIC NEUROGENIC ORTHOSTATIC HYPOTENSION AND AUTONOMIC NEUROPATHY

PARKINSONIAN SYNDROMES AND PURE AUTONOMIC FAILURE

Marked AF in patients with multiple system atrophy (MSA), especially the former Shy–Drager syndrome, is frequent. Other autonomic

TABLE 112.3 Selected Disorders of Autonomic Function

Isolated Degenerative Autonomic	**Hereditary**
Pure autonomic failure (PAF), "Bradbury–Eggleston syndrome"	Familial amyloidosis, hereditary sensory and autonomic neuropathies (see Chapter 88), dopamine β-hydroxylase deficiency, porphyria, Fabry disease, norepinephrine transporter deficiency, fragile X premutation–associated tremor/ataxia syndrome, CANVAS syndrome, Hirschsprung megacolon, Ehlers–Danlos type III, myopathy, external ophthalmoplegia, neuropathy, gastrointestinal encephalopathy (MNGIE), Machado–Joseph disease, prion-induced diarrhea, and autonomic neuropathy
Multisystem Degenerative Disorders	
MSA	
Parkinson disease with autonomic failure	
Central	**Toxins and Medications**
Brain tumors (posterior fossa, third ventricle, hypothalamus), syringobulbia, MS, tetanus, Wernicke–Korsakoff syndrome, fatal familial insomnia	Botulism, vincristine, cisplatin, taxoids, amiodarone, pyriminil (Vacor), hexacarbon, carbon disulfide, heavy metals, podophyllin, alcohol
Spinal Cord	**Drug and Medication Effects**
MS, syringomyelia, transverse myelitis, trauma, mass lesion	Anticholinergics: tricyclic antidepressants, atropine, oxybutynin
Peripheral	β-Adrenergic blockers: propranolol and others
Immune mediated	α2-Agonists: clonidine, prazosin, α-methyl dopa, terazosin, doxazosin
Guillain–Barré syndrome (see Chapter 87), acute and subacute autonomic neuropathy, acute cholinergic neuropathy, Sjögren disease, SLE, rheumatoid arthritis, Holmes–Adie syndrome, Ross syndrome, Harlequin syndrome, acute anhidrosis	α1-Antagonists: phentolamine, phenoxybenzamine, guanabenz
	Ganglionic blockers: guanethidine, hexamethonium, mecamylamine
Metabolic	Others: hydralazine, nitrates, diuretics, calcium channel blockers, ACE inhibitors, antihistamines, antipsychotics, Sinemet, narcotics, sildenafil, tadalafil
Diabetes, vitamin B_{12} and thiamine deficiency, uremia	Reduced orthostatic tolerance
Paraneoplastic	Neurocardiogenic syncope, POTS, mitral valve prolapse syndrome, prolonged bed rest or weightlessness, Chiari malformation
Paraneoplastic autonomic neuropathy and paraneoplastic syndromes with autonomic neuropathy (ANNA-1, α3-AchR ganglionic, CRMP-5, PCA-2 antibodies), enteric neuropathy, Lambert–Eaton myasthenic syndrome (cholinergic)	**Others**
Infectious	Acquired amyloidosis, chronic idiopathic autonomic neuropathies, small-fiber neuropathy, idiopathic hyperhidrosis, idiopathic anhidrosis, Horner syndrome
Chagas disease (cholinergic), syphilis, leprosy, HIV, Lyme disease, diphtheria	

MSA, multiple system atrophy; MS, multiple sclerosis; SLE, systemic lupus erythematosus; CRMP-5, collapsing response mediator protein-5; PCA-2, Purkinje cell cytoplasmic antibody type 2; CANVAS, cerebellar ataxia, neuropathy, vestibular areflexia syndrome; MNGIE, mitochondrial neurogastrointestinal encephalomyopathy; ACE, angiotensin-converting enzyme; POTS, postural orthostatic tachycardia syndrome.

symptoms often predate OH, including impotence, decreased sweating, and urinary incontinence. MSA is a group of disorders with overlapping neuropathology and may have autonomic, parkinsonian, or cerebellar symptoms at onset or later, as discussed in Chapter 84. Other common manifestations include sleep apnea, incontinence, impotence, dystonia, inspiratory stridor, hoarseness, lack of rest tremor, and ineffective or transient L-dopa response. Virtually all MSA patients eventually show autonomic signs or symptoms, regardless of initial manifestations. Demonstration of argyrophilic glial cytoplasmic inclusions (GCIs) in oligodendroglia is a characteristic but not a pathognomonic MSA hallmark. GCIs are prominent in sites of central autonomic control and correlate better with clinical findings than do areas of neuronal loss. Consensus diagnostic criteria first published in 1996 were simplified and refined in 2008. Increased risk of MSA has been found in families and some sporadic cases from various mutations in the gene COQ2, which is essential for the biosynthesis of coenzyme Q10. Median survival from symptom onset

is approximately 10 years based on the most recent natural history studies; parkinsonism at onset and incomplete bladder emptying were the most predictive factors for faster progression.

Many patients with idiopathic Parkinson disease (IPD) also have autonomically mediated complaints, most commonly constipation and urinary dysfunction, but measurable OH is often asymptomatic. However, the prevalence of autonomic symptoms in IPD patients is increasingly recognized. Exacerbation or inducement of OH from medications such as L-dopa is recognized and variably clinically significant.

Some patients with otherwise typical IPD have more severe AF including symptomatic OH and are designated Parkinson disease (PD) with AF. A separate disorder known as *pure autonomic failure* (PAF) or idiopathic OH, first described by Bradbury and Eggleston in 1925, is a profound, slowly progressive disorder with disabling OH, usually starting after age 50 years. By definition, no other neurologic impairment is seen, and the ultimate diagnosis is often delayed 3 to 5 years to ensure that MSA or parkinsonism does not emerge. Autopsies show a similar pattern of classic Lewy bodies in peripheral autonomic and enteric ganglia in both PD with AF and PAF. Similarities between these Lewy body disorders are further supported by cardiac fluorodopamine positron emission tomography (PET) studies demonstrating loss of cardiac sympathetic innervation in both conditions but not in MSA patients. The shared neurodegenerative mechanisms between IPD, diffuse Lewy body dementia, and PAF is increasingly recognized.

Dopamine β-hydroxylase deficiency is a very rare but treatable entity with severe OH, syncope, and nearly undetectable norepinephrine and epinephrine leading to a failure of BP maintenance while standing. The norepinephrine precursor L-threo-dihydroxyphenylserine (L-DOPS; droxidopa), which can be beneficial for these patients and in patients with other forms of AF, was U.S. Food and Drug Administration (FDA) approved in 2014, commonly titrated to a target dose of 100 mg three times a day.

Cerebellar ataxia, neuropathy, and vestibular areflexia syndrome (CANVAS) is a recently recognized neurodegenerative ganglionopathy that commonly includes OH; in one series, 83% had evidence of autonomic dysfunction.

Numerous other common and uncommon disorders affecting the brain and spinal cord affect autonomic function but less commonly cause symptomatic OH (see Table 112.3). Additionally, some processes may be pathway or organ specific such as predominantly cholinergic, adrenergic, regional, or organ-specific disorders. Anhidrosis or hypohidrosis occurs with a variety of process, notably in length-dependent neuropathy. Regional and segmental hypohidrosis can occur; when associated with Adie pupils and hyporeflexia, the condition is known as *Ross syndrome*; some cases occur following viral infection and are presumed to be immune-mediated. Acute or subacute generalized anhidrosis also occurs. Patients, however, more commonly note increased sweating. Compensatory proximal sweating is common in patients with large areas of reduced sweating from any cause. Essential hyperhidrosis is diffuse tendency for excessive sweating and is often hereditary. Treatments directed at reducing sweating include traumatizing sweat glands with water iontophoresis, chemodenervation, or strong antiperspirants; simple anticholinergic medications are typically ineffective at tolerable dosage. Surgical endoscopic sympathectomy is an option for severe cases.

CHRONIC AUTONOMIC NEUROPATHIES

Many of the scores of different peripheral neuropathies induce autonomic dysfunction, often limited to distal sweating and vasomotor control, especially those disproportionately affecting small-diameter fibers. The consequence is dry, cool distal extremities common in many neuropathy patients. Dysfunction is generally insufficient to impair peripheral vasoconstriction or postural reflexes enough to produce symptomatic OH. A few entities, however, lead to severe or targeted autonomic dysfunction, which can produce frank AF and symptomatic OH. Particularly noteworthy causes include diabetes, familial and acquired amyloidosis, paraneoplastic neuropathies, and selected hereditary, infectious, and toxic neuropathies. Some of the more prominent examples are listed in Table 112.3.

Diabetic autonomic neuropathy (DAN) is the most common and important cause of autonomic neuropathy and the most extensively examined. Somatic peripheral neuropathy is usually concurrent. Much attention has focused on the impact of diabetic autonomic dysfunction on long-term survival. Ewing et al. found 56% of 73 patients with DAN died within 5 years, many owing to nonautonomic complications such as renal failure. Later studies showed an increased but less ominous DAN mortality rate in diabetics without other initial complications (23% at 8 years) compared with diabetics without DAN and similar disease duration (3% at 8 years). The added autonomic dysfunction risk is independent of coronary perfusion deficits. Upper gastrointestinal dysmotility, bladder complaints, impotence, sudomotor loss, constipation, episodic diarrhea, and gustatory sweating are a few common manifestations that aid in diagnosis and may require symptomatic treatment.

Amyloidosis, including both hereditary and acquired forms, is another important consideration in patients with severe AF. Certain mutations in transthyretin (TTR) are associated with more severe autonomic neuropathy than mutations in apolipoprotein A1 or gelsolin. Some forms commonly cause neuropathy, whereas others rarely do. Hepatic, bone marrow, and stem cell transplantation are evolving treatments; several other modalities of treatments such as an oligonucleotide antisense drug are in late-stage clinical trials.

Immune-mediated and paraneoplastic neuropathy are potentially treatable and often begin subacutely. A chronic form is also seen in isolation or in association with other autoimmune disorders, notably Sjögren disease. A notable report in 2005 complicated diagnosis by demonstrating a patient with presumed, very long-standing, stable AF, who demonstrated high AChR ganglionic antibodies, typically reserved for acute and subacute neuropathy, and responded markedly and repeatedly to recurrent IVIG infusions.

Idiopathic painful, small-fiber neuropathy often affects distal autonomic function but rarely causes symptomatic OH or symptomatic AF. Other forms of autonomic neuropathy are listed in Table 112.3.

HEREDITARY SENSORY AND AUTONOMIC NEUROPATHY AND FAMILIAL DYSAUTONOMIA

The onset of some autonomic disorders occurs much earlier than those already discussed, including some congenital and infantile hereditary conditions. The most common and important entities are discussed.

FAMILIAL DYSAUTONOMIA (RILEY–DAY SYNDROME)

Hereditary sensory and autonomic neuropathy type III, also known as *familial dysautonomia* (FD) and was first described by Riley et al. in 1949, is a rare autosomal recessive disease with complete penetrance but variable expression. Virtually all patients are of eastern European (Ashkenazi) Jewish descent. The carrier rate may be as high as 1 in 25 and the disease prevalence was 1 in 4,100 live births. However, following the availability of genetic testing, subsequent to the gene discovery in 2001, the incidence sharply dropped. In 2009, only five new FD cases were diagnosed worldwide. There is no sex predilection in either affected individuals or carriers. The condition affects the survival and development of sensory, sympathetic, and some parasympathetic neurons. Autonomic symptoms are prominent, and general somatic growth is affected.

The causative gene is IKBKAP (I kappa B kinase complex–associated protein) on chromosome 9q31-q33. Two mutations in the gene IKBKAP are implicated. The major FD mutation is a splice defect that displays tissue-specific expression and causes aberrant mRNA splicing. The second more infrequent mutation is a missense mutation. The end result is a nonfunctional IKAB protein and a congenital sensory and autonomic neuropathy. Specific assay for mutations of IKBKAP have facilitated carrier screening for FD in the Ashkenazi Jewish population. Prenatal diagnosis is available, and preimplantation genetic diagnosis is also available for at-risk couples.

The condition can be identified in the neonatal period; clinical manifestations tend to increase with age. FD is currently classified as hereditary, sensory, and autonomic neuropathy type III (HSAN III).

Clinical Manifestations

Neurologic abnormalities detected in the neonatal period include decreased muscle tone, diminished or absent deep tendon reflexes, absent corneal responses, reduced Moro reflex, and weak cry and suck. The tongue tip lacks fungiform papillae and appears smooth. Uncoordinated swallowing with resultant regurgitation may cause aspiration and pneumonia. Some infants require tube feeding, gastrostomy, and fundoplication because of gastroesophageal reflux. Absence of overflow tears, which can be normal for the first 3 months, persists and becomes a consistent feature. Corneal ulceration can occur.

During the first 3 years of life, affected children show delayed physical and developmental milestones, episodic vomiting, excessive sweating, excessive drooling, blotchy erythema, and breath-holding spells. Up to one-third of patients have seizures during early life, usually associated with fever or hypoxia. Less than 10% of patients have subsequent epilepsy. Dysautonomic crises occur usually after age 3 years characterized by irritability, self-mutilation, negativistic behavior, diaphoresis, tachycardia, hypertension, and thermal instability; however, episodes share many characteristics of autonomic seizures and typically respond to anticonvulsants. Episodic vomiting is frequent and can be cyclic, requiring hospitalization for stabilization with parenteral hydration and sedation.

School-aged patients tend to have short stature, awkward gait, and nasal speech. School performance may be poor, frequently 20 or more intelligence points below unaffected siblings. Scoliosis is frequent and can begin in childhood and progress during preadolescence. The prevalence of spinal deformity is high in FD patients older than 20 years. Vomiting and dysautonomic crises tend to decrease during adolescence when more frequent symptoms center on decreased exercise tolerance, poor general coordination, emotional difficulties, and postural hypotension. Vasovagal syncope may occur randomly, after micturition, or during laryngeal intubation for anesthesia.

There is a high incidence of sudden death in FD. There is also an incidence of syncope, electrocardiographic abnormalities including asystole, bradycardia, atrioventricular (AV) block, and prolonged QT interval. Pacemaker placement to protect FD patients has not been found to be protective against fatal bradyarrhythmias but may decrease the incidence of syncope.

Diagnosis

The diagnosis should be suspected because of the specific clinical symptoms and findings and the familial Ashkenazi Jewish background. The FD gene test provides definitive confirmation. DNA diagnoses and genetic screening of the Ashkenazi Jewish population is available. If both parents are carriers, prenatal diagnosis can be done by chorionic villus sampling (10th to 11th gestational week) or by amniocentesis (14th to 17th gestational week). Preimplantation diagnosis is available for at risk couples who would not consider pregnancy termination.

The intradermal histamine phosphate test can provide additional diagnostic confirmation. An intradermal injection of 1:1,000 histamine phosphate (0.03 to 0.05 mL) normally produces pain and erythema. A central wheel forms within minutes and is surrounded by an axon flare that is a zone of erythema measuring 2 to 6 cm in diameter. The flare lasts for several minutes. In dysautonomic patients, the pain is greatly reduced and there is no axon flare. In infants, a saline solution of 1:10,000 histamine should be substituted.

Biochemical and Pathologic Data

The protein product is part of a six-protein elongator complex that plays a key role in transcription of products that affect the cytoskeleton and cell motility. How this disruption of function leads to FD is not currently understood. Plasma levels of both norepinephrine and dopamine are markedly elevated during dysautonomic crises.

Pathologic data reveal hypoplastic cervical sympathetic ganglia with diminished volume and neuronal counts. Sympathetic preganglionic spinal cord neurons seem reduced in number and size. Patients are deficient in nonmyelinated and small-fiber neurons. Lingual submucosal neurons and sensory axons are reduced. Taste buds are scant; circumvallate papillae are hypoplastic.

Treatment

Preventative treatment and supportive therapies include maintaining eye moisture to control absence of tearing, fundoplication with gastrostomy to control vomiting and reflux, and the use of benzodiazepine and clonidine for dysautonomic crises.

The use of epidural or deep conscious sedation forms of anesthesia have been advocated for surgical procedures to avoid intubation and the sometimes fatal complications of general anesthesia.

OH is treated similarly to adult forms. Symptomatic treatment is indicated for dysautonomic crises with parenteral fluids, diazepam, sedation, and antiemetic therapy. GH treatment in selected patients with FD may have the potential to increase growth.

Tocotrienols may elevate IKBKAP gene expression and cause increased functional cellular levels of IKAP protein and increased levels of monoamine oxidase A in cells and tissues. Other agents such as kinetin are under investigation for their possible therapeutic potential to improve gene splicing and increase functional protein levels.

Outcome

Long-term survival is documented; more than 40% of surviving patients are older than 20 years. Some women with FD have had pregnancies and delivered normal infants. Infant and childhood fatalities may be a result of aspiration pneumonia, gastric hemorrhage, or dehydration. A second cluster of fatalities between the ages of 14 and 24 years has been secondary to pulmonary complications, sleep deaths, and cardiopulmonary arrests. The few oldest patients are now in their fifth and sixth decades.

OTHER HEREDITARY AUTONOMIC DISORDERS

A novel prion disease associated with diarrhea and hereditary sensory and autonomic neuropathy associated with a defect in the PRNP gene was described late in 2013. Other types of hereditary sensory and autonomic neuropathy (HSAN) typically cause more severe sensory ganglionopathy or sensory neuropathy and are often considered as a separate congenital category.

DIAGNOSIS AND TREATMENT OF AUTONOMIC DISORDERS

Nonautonomic conditions can cause OH and mimic AF; most important are adrenal failure and pheochromocytoma. Asymptomatic OH is a prevalent sign in the elderly, and causes are often multifactorial. Formal laboratory evaluation of autonomic disorders is discussed in Chapter 27. Treatment of AF is directed at symptomatic relief and improved quality of life, especially for generally the most disabling symptom—OH. Numerous pharmacologic and nonpharmacologic interventions are available to lessen OH and improve orthostatic tolerance. Asymptomatic hypotension on standing usually requires no treatment; reasonable precautions and avoidance of precipitating factors may be adequate. An exercise reflex, which immediately but transiently lowers BP on standing may become symptomatic requiring standing slowly and in stages. However, lesser indicators of hypoperfusion such as postural "coat hanger" pattern shoulder fatigue and headache (local muscle ischemia), pure postural vertigo, postprandial fatigue, and cognitive slowing are possible indicators of OH. Supplemental water and salt intake (0.5 to 2 g/day) have been independently shown to be beneficial and lessen the need for medications. Raising the head of the bed 4 inches stimulates baroreceptors and decreases nocturnal diuresis. Useful postural and physical measures to attempt and others to avoid are listed in Table 112.2. Cumbersome compressive garments with abdominal compression are mildly effective in reducing venous pooling but are problematic for many with neurologic disorders; abdominal binders alone may help to a lesser degree. Small, frequent meals low in carbohydrates lessen postprandial hypotension. Reevaluation of the need for prescribed BP lowering and autonomically active agents should be considered.

If these measures are insufficient, first-line medications include fludrocortisone (starting at 0.1 mg/day) or the α-adrenergic agonist midodrine or both. Midodrine is shorter acting, and the dosage must cover vulnerable periods, especially early morning, and is not given after 6 PM; generally 2.5 to 10 mg doses three times a day. Droxidopa was FDA approved in 2014 and may become an additional treatment option commonly titrated to a target dose of 100 mg three times a day. Excessive fluid retention and heart failure are concerns, especially in the elderly. Relative anemia exacerbates OH. Pyridostigmine, which enhances autonomic ganglionic neural transmission, increases standing greater than supine BP and is a common off-label option, especially in patients with supine hypertension, which is a perennial and unresolved controversial concern with fludrocortisone, midodrine, and droxidopa. Typically, 30 or 60 mg doses are given every 6 to 8 hours. Clinical judgment is required to balance the need for adequate standing and reasonable supine pressures; this balance is challenging in severe cases. Second-line agents are numerous and are sometimes effective if earlier agents have failed. Concomitant treatment of urinary dysfunction, gastric and intestinal dysmotility, impotence, and secretomotor dysfunction is often necessary. In MSA, inspiratory stridor may lead to tracheostomy, and nocturnal positive pressure ventilation may be needed for sleep apnea.

Exacerbating factors are important considerations for both patient and physician to take appropriate precautions or avoid certain situations (see Table 112.2). Patients with delayed OH (3 to 15 minutes after standing) or situational triggers must anticipate potential problems. Patients with chronic, symptomatic OH may learn to recognize these conditions but often need physician instruction. Chronic OH also results in optimized cerebral autoregulation and relative tolerance of low BP but provides a narrow window between an asymptomatic state and syncope.

ACKNOWLEDGMENT

The author acknowledges Dr. Alan M. Aron for contributions to an earlier version of the hereditary autonomic disorder section of this chapter.

SUGGESTED READINGS

Acute and Subacute Autonomic Neuropathy

Camdessanche JP, Antoine JC, Honnorat J, et al. Paraneoplastic peripheral neuropathy associated with anti-Hu antibodies. A clinical and electrophysiological study of 20 patients. *Brain.* 2002;125:166–175.

Etienne M, Weimer LH. Immune-mediated autonomic neuropathies. *Curr Neurol Neurosci Rep.* 2006;6(1):57–64.

Gibbons CH, Vernino SA, Freeman R. Combined immunomodulatory therapy in autoimmune autonomic ganglionopathy. *Arch. Neurol.* 2008;65:213–217.

Koike H, Atsuta N, Adachi H, et al. Clinicopathological features of acute autonomic and sensory neuropathy. *Brain.* 2010;133:2881–2896.

Lennon VA, Ermilov LG, Szurszewski JH, et al. Immunization with neuronal nicotinic acetylcholine receptor induces neurological autoimmune disease. *J Clin Invest.* 2003;111:64–65.

Sandroni P, Vernino S, Klein CM, et al. Idiopathic autonomic neuropathy: comparison of cases seropositive and seronegative for ganglionic acetylcholine receptor antibody. *Arch Neurol.* 2004;61:44–48.

Shannon JR, Flattem NL, Jordan J, et al. Orthostatic intolerance and tachycardia associated with norepinephrine-transporter deficiency. *N Engl J Med.* 2000;342:541–549.

Suarez GA, Fealey RD, Camilleri M, et al. Idiopathic autonomic neuropathy: clinical, neurophysiologic and follow-up studies on 27 patients. *Neurology.* 1994;44:1675–1682.

Vernino S, Low PA, Fealey RD, et al. Autoantibodies to ganglionic acetylcholine receptors in autoimmune autonomic neuropathies. *N Engl J Med.* 2000;343:847–855.

Wallman D, Weinberg J, Hohler AD. Ehlers-Danlos syndrome and postural tachycardia syndrome: a relationship study. *J Neurol Sci.* 2014;340(1–2):99–102.

Young RR, Asbury AK, Corbett JL, et al. Pure pandysautonomia with recovery. *Brain.* 1975;98:613–636.

Zochodne DW. Autonomic involvement in Guillain–Barré syndrome: a review. *Muscle Nerve.* 1994;17:1145–1155.

Chronic Autonomic Neuropathy, Central Autonomic Failure, and Neurogenic Orthostatic Hypotension

Benarroch EE. Postural tachycardia syndrome: a heterogeneous and multifactorial disorder. *Mayo Clin Proc.* 2012;87(12):1214–1225.

Benarroch EE, Schmeichel AM, Sandroni P, et al. Involvement of vagal autonomic nuclei in multiple system atrophy and Lewy body disease. *Neurology.* 2006;66(3):378–383.

Cersosimo MG, Benarroch EE. Autonomic involvement in Parkinson's disease: pathology, pathophysiology, clinical features, and possible peripheral biomarkers. *J Neurol Sci.* 2012;313:57–63.

Cheshire WP, Freeman R. Disorders of sweating. *Semin Neurol.* 2003;23:399–406.

Ewing DJ, Campbell IW, Clarke BF. The natural history of diabetic autonomic neuropathy. *Q J Med.* 1980;49:95–108.

Freeman R. Clinical practice. Neurogenic orthostatic hypotension. *N Engl J Med.* 2008;358:615–624.

Freeman R, Wieling W, Axelrod FB, et al. Consensus statement on the definition of orthostatic hypotension, neurally mediated syncope and the postural tachycardia syndrome. *Auton Neurosci.* 2011;161:46–48.

Furness JB. The enteric nervous system and neurogastroenterology. *Nat Rev Gastroenterol Hepatol.* 2012;9:286–294.

Gerritsen J, Dekker JM, TenVoorde BJ, et al. Impaired autonomic function is associated with increased mortality, especially in subjects with diabetes, hypertension, or a history of cardiovascular disease: the Hoorn study. *Diabetes Care.* 2001;24:1793–1798.

Gilman S, Wenning GK, Low PA, et al. Second consensus statement on the diagnosis of multiple system atrophy. *Neurology.* 2008;71(9):670–676.

Goldstein DS, Holmes CS, Dendi R, et al. Orthostatic hypotension from sympathetic denervation in Parkinson's disease. *Neurology*. 2002;58:1247–1255.

Hague K, Lento P, Morgello S, et al. The distribution of Lewy bodies in pure autonomic failure: autopsy findings and review of the literature. *Acta Neuropathol (Berl)*. 1997;94:192–196.

Kaufmann H, Freeman R, Biaggioni I, et al. Droxidopa for neurogenic orthostatic hypotension: a randomized, placebo-controlled, phase 3 trial. *Neurology*. 2014;83(4):328–335.

Klein CM, Vernino S, Lennon VA, et al. The spectrum of autoimmune autonomic neuropathies. *Ann Neurol*. 2003;53:752–758.

Magalhães M, Wenning GK, Daniel SE, et al. Autonomic dysfunction in pathologically confirmed multiple system atrophy and idiopathic Parkinson's disease—a retrospective comparison. *Acta Neurol Scand*. 1995;91:98–102.

Multiple-System Atrophy Research Collaboration. Mutations in COQ2 in familial and sporadic multiple-system atrophy. *N Engl J Med*. 2013;369:233–244.

Muppidi S, Vernino S. Autoimmune autonomic failure. *Handb Clin Neurol*. 2013;117:321–327.

Schroeder C, Vernino S, Birkenfeld AL, et al. Plasma exchange for primary autoimmune autonomic failure. *N Engl J Med*. 2005;353(15):1585–1590.

Shibao C, Grijalva CG, Raj SR, et al. Orthostatic hypotension-related hospitalizations in the United States. *Am J Med*. 2007;120:975–980.

Shy GM, Drager GA. A neurological syndrome associated with orthostatic hypotension: a clinical-pathologic study. *Arch Neurol*. 1960;2:511–527.

Singer W, Paola Sandroni P, Opfer-Gehrking TL, et al. Pyridostigmine treatment trial in neurogenic orthostatic hypotension. *Arch Neurol*. 2006;63:513–518.

Stefanova N, Bucke P, Duerr S, et al. Multiple system atrophy: an update. *Lancet Neurol*. 2009;8:1172–1178.

The Consensus Committee of the American Autonomic Society and the American Academy of Neurology. Consensus statement on the definition of orthostatic hypotension, pure autonomic failure, and multiple system atrophy. *Neurology*. 1996;46:1470.

Vagaonescu TD, Saadia D, Tuhrim S, et al. Hypertensive cardiovascular damage in patients with primary autonomic failure. *Lancet*. 2000;355:725–726.

Verbaan D, Marinus J, Visser M, et al. Patient-reported autonomic symptoms in Parkinson disease. *Neurology*. 2007;69(4):333–341.

Vernino S, Sandroni P, Singer W, et al. Autonomic ganglia: target and novel therapeutic tool. *Neurology*. 2008;70(20):1926–1932.

Weimer LH, Zadeh P. Syncope and orthostatic intolerance. *Med Clin N Am*. 2009;93(2):427–449.

Wenning GK, Geser F, Krismer F, et al. The natural history of multiple system atrophy: a prospective European cohort study. *Lancet Neurol*. 2013;12:264–274.

Wu TY, Taylor JM, Kilfoyle DH, et al. Autonomic dysfunction is a major feature of cerebellar ataxia, neuropathy, vestibular areflexia "CANVAS" syndrome. *Brain*. 2014;137(pt 10):2649–2656.

Hereditary Autonomic Neuropathies

Anderson SL, Coli R, Daly IW, et al. Familial dysautonomia is caused by mutations of the IKAP gene. *Am J Hum Genet*. 2001;3:753–758.

Anderson SL, Rubin BY. Tocotrienols reverse IKAP and monamine oxidase deficiencies in familial dysautonomia. *Biochem Biophys Res Commun*. 2005;336(1):150–156.

Axelrod FB. Familial dysautonomia. *Muscle Nerve*. 2004;3:352–363.

Axelrod FB. Familial dysautonomia: a review of the current pharmacological treatments. *Expert Opin Pharmacother*. 2005;6(4):561–567.

Axelrod FB, Gold-von Simson G. Hereditary sensory and autonomic neuropathies: types II, III, and IV. *Orphanet J Rare Dis*. 2007;3:2–39.

Axelrod FB, Rolnitzky L, Gold von Simson G, et al. A rating scale for the functional assessment of patients with familial dysautonomia (Riley Day syndrome). *J Pediatr*. 2012;161(6):1160–1165.

Blumenfeld A, Slaugenhaupt SA, Axelrod FB. Localization of the gene for familial dysautonomia on chromosome 9 and definition of DNA markers for genetic diagnosis. *Nat Genet*. 1993;4:160–164.

Couzin-Frankel J. Chasing a disease to the vanishing point. *Science*. 2010;328(5976):298–300.

Hims MM, Ibrahim EC, Leyne M, et al. Therapeutic potential and mechanism of kinetin as a treatment for the human splicing disease familial dysautonomia. *J Mol Med*. 2007;85(2):149–161.

Mead S, Gandhi S, Beck J, et al. A novel prion disease associated with diarrhea and autonomic neuropathy. *N Engl J Med*. 2013;369:1904–1914.

Rechitsky S, Verlinsky O, Kuliev A, et al. Preimplantation genetic diagnosis for familial dysautonomia. *Reprod Biomed Online*. 2003;6(4):488–493.

Riley CM, Day RL, Greely DM, et al. Central autonomic dysfunction with defective lacrimation; report of five cases. *Pediatrics*. 1949;3:468–478.

Smith AA, Dancis J. Responses to intradermal histamine in familial dysautonomia—a diagnostic test. *J Pediatr*. 1963;63:889–894.

Szald A, Udassin R, Maayan C, et al. Laparoscopic-modified Nissen fundoplication in children with familial dysautonomia. *J Pediatr Surg*. 1996;31:1560–1562.

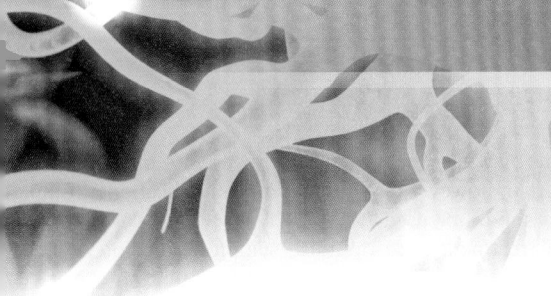

Paroxysmal Sympathetic Hyperactivity after Acute Brain Injury

113

*Huimahn Alex Choi, Sophie Samuel, and
Teresa A. Allison*

INTRODUCTION

After surviving acute brain injury, patients can develop paroxysmal sympathetic hyperactivity (PSH), a syndrome of episodic physiologic hyperactivation manifesting in fevers, diaphoresis, tachycardia, tachypnea, hypertension, and dystonic posturing. Since the first description in 1929 by Wilder Penfield, numerous terms have been used to describe this syndrome: episodic autonomic instability, dysautonomia, autonomic dysregulation, central autonomic dysfunction, paroxysmal autonomic instability with dystonia (PAID), sympathetic storming, autonomic storming, dysautonomic crises, and diencephalic fits. First believed to be epileptic in nature and now believed to be a syndrome caused by a disconnection of inhibitory pathways, the etiology of PSH is still not well understood. The unifying principle describing this syndrome is the episodic nature of the dysregulation of the autonomic nervous system, manifesting as episodic sympathetic hyperactivity.

PSH can develop abruptly and last a short time period but can also be prolonged and a main driver of complications after acute brain injury. Delayed recognition leading to unnecessary workup and medications can further prolong hospitalization with potentially harmful results to patients. Additionally, uncontrolled symptoms can lead to secondary brain injury from hypertension, hyperthermia, cardiac damage, and even death.

EPIDEMIOLOGY

The absence of a unified diagnostic criterion, the unclear etiology, and the multiple different causes of PSH has hindered the study of the syndrome. There are widely differing estimates of prevalence of PSH from 8% to 33% of patients admitted to the intensive care unit (ICU), reflecting the differences in population of patients.

The cause of brain injury is an important risk factor for the development of PSH. Most reported cases of PSH result from traumatic brain injury (TBI) (80%), followed by hypoxic brain injury (10%) and stroke (5.4%). The main risk factor for developing PSH after acute brain injury is the severity of the initial brain injury, younger age, and male gender. Although TBI may be the etiology for most cases of PSH, patients with other diseases may actually be at a higher risk for PSH. For instance, N-methyl-D-aspartate (NMDA) receptor–associated encephalitis is characterized by an aggressive and difficult to treat PSH-like syndrome.

PATHOBIOLOGY

Most believe PSH is caused by a functional disconnection leading to unbalanced activation of brain stem systems controlling the autonomic nervous system. Brain regions implicated range from the cerebral cortex to the anterior hypothalamus to the medulla and the connections in between. Regardless of the lesion location, the final common pathway is an imbalance of adrenergic outflow.

The Excitatory-to-Inhibitory Ratio (EIR) Model has been used to explain the pathophysiology of PSH and it takes into account the hypersensitive, overreactive nature of the responses to normal stimuli. Autonomic efferents at the level of the spinal cord are modulated centrally by a balance of sympathetic and parasympathetic inputs from higher brain stem nuclei. Afferents from the spinal cord can modulate this balance in response to stimuli from the environment. The EIR model proposes that the afferent stimuli from the spine have an allodynic tendency, which is normally controlled by tonic inhibitory drive from diencephalic centers. Damage to these inhibitory centers or their inhibitory processes down to the mesencephalon releases the inhibition of the allodynic tendency. Once the tonically inhibitory cycle is broken, there is a positive feedback loop that produces sympathetic overactivity to any afferent stimuli. This model explains how a normally nonnoxious stimulus can become a very noxious stimulus associated with an uncontrolled sympathetic response.

Imaging studies have shown that injury to the deep brain structures, periventricular white matter, corpus callosum, diencephalon, or brain stem may be associated with the development of PSH. PSH is associated with an increased number of lesions in the midbrain and upper pons compared with number of lesions in cerebral cortex, subcortex, corpus callosum, and diencephalon. Bilateral diencephalic lesions have also been attributed to PSH in hypoxic–ischemic encephalopathy. The evidence from imaging studies showing damage to brain stem structures emphasizes the importance of the diencephalic and mesencephalic regions to the pathophysiology of PSH.

CLINICAL MANIFESTATIONS

PSH usually occurs, or at least is noticed, once patients are being weaned off of continuous intravenous sedation and they begin to awaken. Usually, it occurs in patients with a depressed mental status and episodes are associated with worsening mental status. The clinical manifestation of PSH define the syndrome: Episodic increases in heart rate, blood pressure, respiratory rate, temperature, diaphoresis, at times with pupillary dilatation, and motor hyperactivity manifested in abnormal posturing and dystonic movements. Episodes of exacerbation may last from minutes to hours and can occur several times a day or in refractory cases nearly continuously. PSH can be difficult to differentiate from opiate withdrawal or agitation from mechanical ventilation. It may persist into the rehabilitation phase and last weeks to months after the injury. In severe cases, it may persist for a year.

DIAGNOSIS

The overlapping symptoms of PSH with other neurologic sequelae of acute brain injury make the diagnosis difficult and only made after excluding other causes for symptoms. Clinical suspicion and careful examination are of paramount importance in the detection of PSH. Infections, sepsis, pain, opiate withdrawal, and seizures are all diagnoses that have overlapping clinical presentations that need to be excluded in order to diagnose PSH.

There are at least nine unique diagnostic criteria describing this syndrome. Most include increased heart rate, diaphoresis, motor hyperactivity, tachypnea, hyperthermia, and hypertension. Some diagnostic criteria have included pupillary dilatation and decreased level of consciousness. Although multiple proposed diagnostic criteria overlap significantly in descriptive ways, consensus regarding specifics of timing, severity, and number of episodes does not exist. Characteristically, PSH tends to be triggered by minimal external stimuli, such as touching, passive movement (turning, moving limbs, and bathing), or endotracheal tube suctioning. This feature of overreactivity, allodynic response, may be a helpful characteristic for diagnostic purposes.

TREATMENT

Effective clinical management of PSH requires a combination of pharmacologic as well as nonpharmacologic treatment modalities. There are few large-scale prospective studies and no level 1 evidence is available. Management is guided predominantly by case reports, case series, and personal experience using different medications and treatment strategies. Therapy is focused on control of symptoms. Medical treatments for PSH include opioids, β-blockers, dopamine agonists, α2-agonists, GABAergic agents, benzodiazepines, gabapentin, and muscle relaxants (Table 113.1).

The mechanisms by which these agents improve symptoms of PSH remain speculative; however, a combination of medications from different classes should be used.

The goal of treatment is to optimize symptom control while minimizing side effects, mainly sedation and hypotension. Treatment should focus on nonpharmacologic management first. Potential stimuli which can trigger acute episodes of exacerbation should be identified and minimized. Because patients usually are unable to communicate, this process can be difficult but an important first step. Pharmacologic management of PSH focuses on three treatment approaches: maintenance, symptom abortion, and refractory treatment. A suggested treatment algorithm is presented on Figure 113.1.

When a paroxysm of hyperactivity occurs, abortive medications are indicated to control discrete breakthrough episodes. These medications have a rapid onset of action with a short half-life. The targets of the abortive medications usually depend on the predominant symptoms: treating hyperthermia with antipyretics, agitation with sedation, and hypertension with antihypertensive agents. Morphine, other opiates, and short-acting benzodiazepines are first-line treatment options for this indication. Dose of medication should be titrated to symptom relief and is limited by the potential side effects, mainly sedation, respiratory depression, and hypotension. Medications with a short half-life should be used for abortive treatment to minimize undesired effects. If frequency bouts of hyperactivity occur, maintenance medication should be adjusted accordingly. Importantly, once the frequency of episodes of exacerbation is controlled, maintenance medications should be aggressively tapered to maximize the alertness of patients.

First-line maintenance pharmacologic agents include medications which are less sedating and reduce the frequency and intensity of exacerbations. These medications include nonselective β-blockers, α2-agonists, bromocriptine, baclofen, gabapentin, opiates, and long-acting benzodiazepines such as clonazepam.

TABLE 113.1 Medications Used for Treatment of Paroxysmal Sympathetic Hyperactivity

Medication	Location of Action	Proposed Mechanism	Symptoms Treated
Baclofen	Centrally	GABA$_B$ agonist	Pain, clonus, rigidity
Benzodiazepines	Centrally	GABA$_A$ agonist	Agitation, hypertension, tachycardia, posturing
Bromocriptine	Centrally; at hypothalamus	Dopamine agonist	Dystonia, fever, posturing
Clonidine	Centrally; decreased sympathetic outflow	α_2-Receptor agonist	Agitation, hypertension, tachycardia
Dantrolene	Peripherally	Direct-acting skeletal muscle relaxant	Muscle rigidity, posturing
Dexmedetomidine	Centrally; decreased sympathetic outflow	α_2-Receptor agonist	Agitation, hypertension, tachycardia
Gabapentin	Centrally	GABA agonist	Spasticity, allodynic response
Opioids	Centrally; medullary vagal nuclei and peripherally	μ-Opioid receptor agonist	Hypertension, tachycardia, allodynic response
Propofol	Centrally	GABA$_A$ agonist	Agitation, hypertension, tachycardia
Propranolol	Peripherally; decreasing effect of catecholamines	Nonselective β-blocker	Hypertension, tachycardia, fever

GABA, γ-aminobutyric acid.

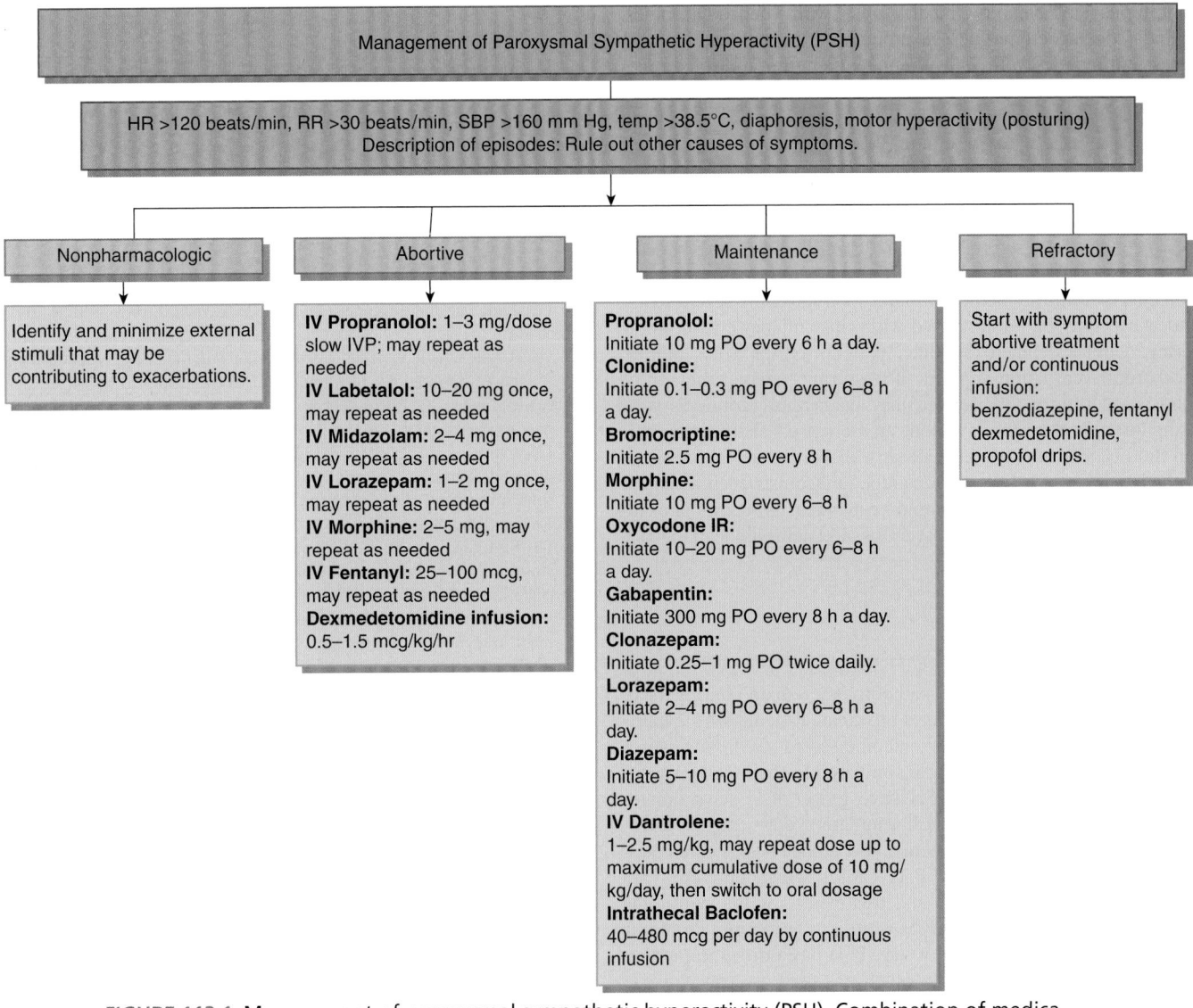

FIGURE 113.1 Management of paroxysmal sympathetic hyperactivity (PSH). Combination of medications from different doses likely results in the most effective approach in managing PSH.

Propranolol, a competitive nonselective β-blocker, is an ideal drug for controlling symptoms of PSH due to its mechanism of action and broad control of symptoms with minimum sedation. In addition to its cardiovascular effects, propranolol decreases the hyperthermic response to brain injury. Clonidine, a presynaptic α2-receptor agonist, is a useful agent to manage hypertension and tachycardia. Because increased blood pressure due to excitation of the sympathetic nervous system is one of the major features of PSH, clonidine is often an effective medication. Its use as monotherapy usually does not work in resolution of other symptoms. Morphine is a potent μ-opioid receptor agonist. In addition to morphine's analgesic properties, its cholinergic effects and histamine-releasing actions make it a good agent for the management of tachycardia and hypertension. Morphine is the most commonly used medication and can be used as maintenance as well as abortive treatment for breakthrough episodes. Bromocriptine is a synthetic dopamine agonist, the mechanism by which resolution of symptoms including hyperpyrexia and dysautonomia are achieved is unclear. Baclofen, a γ-aminobutyric acid (GABA)$_B$ receptor agonist, is indicated for treatment of spasticity associated with PSH and to

improve mobility. The benefit is to decrease the number and severity of spasms, thus relieving associated pain, clonus, and muscle rigidity. Benzodiazepines, GABA$_A$ receptor agonists, are useful for symptoms of motor activity, tachycardia, and hypertension. The concern with benzodiazepines is the possibility of worsening neurologic functioning in newly injured brain. A long-acting benzodiazepine, clonazepam, is helpful as a maintenance medication to reduce episodes. Gabapentin, an analog of GABA, was originally developed as an anticonvulsant. However, it may be more useful in the management of painful neuropathies, spasticity, and tremor. It is most useful as an adjunct medication, which is less sedating than benzodiazepines. Dantrolene acts directly on skeletal muscle, decreasing the force of contraction by interfering with release of calcium ion from sacroplasmic reticulum and can be used in cases when severe dystonia or posturing continues to persist. Dantrolene can possibly be effective for the amelioration of dystonic posturing, but the risk of causing hepatotoxicity can limit its use.

Finally, in some cases, patients develop refractory PSH when symptoms do not respond to isolated intermittent treatment modalities and symptoms become life threatening. In these cases, continuous intravenous medications with benzodiazepines, opioids, dexmedetomidine, or propofol drips are required. At times, antipyretics with or without temperature control devices is necessitated for aggressive temperature modulation. In addition to continuous infusions of opiates (morphine, fentanyl) and benzodiazepines, dexmedetomidine, an α2-receptor agonist, can be administered as a continuous intravenous infusion predominantly for sedation. Given its favorable effects on heart rate, blood pressure, and agitation, dexmedetomidine is a useful intravenous treatment choice. If symptoms are not controlled with other medications, propofol, a general anesthetic, can be used. However, the side effects from the medication limit its use to only severe cases, and it can only be administered with close intensive care monitoring. Unlike dexmedetomidine, patients on propofol require mechanical ventilation support. If posturing persists, the use of intrathecal infusion of baclofen may be helpful. Concerns with using intrathecal infusions include an increased risk in cerebrospinal fluid (CSF) leak and infection as well as mechanical problems with the catheter or pump. Dopamine antagonists such as chlorpromazine and haloperidol should be avoided, as reports of exacerbation of cognitive deficits, psychosis, and neuroleptic malignant syndrome have been reported.

OUTCOME

Although the risk factors and pathobiology remain controversial, the impacts on clinical outcomes are clear. Patients who experience PSH have worse Glasgow outcome scores (GOS) and worse functional independent measures compared to their counterparts. Additionally, patients with PSH have longer ICU stays, longer hospital stay, longer mechanical ventilation days, higher infectious episodes, more tracheostomy, and higher health care costs. The mechanisms as to how PSH causes worse outcomes are multifactorial. The symptoms and treatments for the symptoms cause longer period of days on the ventilator, leading to more tracheostomy and longer length of stay. PSH has a direct impact on fever burden after brain injury, which has been associated worse outcome after brain injury. In addition, the influence of the autonomic nervous system and its effects on inflammation has been studied in other disease states and may be very active in the acutely brain-injured population. The dysregulated autonomic nervous system may have an influence in causing unopposed inflammation and leading to secondary brain injury.

SUGGESTED READINGS

Baguley IJ. The excitatory:inhibitory ratio model (EIR model): an integrative explanation of acute autonomic overactivity syndromes. *Med Hypotheses.* 2008;70:26–35.

Baguley IJ, Heriseanu RE, Gurka JA, et al. Gabapentin in the management of dysautonomia following severe traumatic brain injury: a case series. *J Neurol Neurosurg Psychiatry.* 2007;78:539–541.

Baguley IJ, Nott MT, Slewa-Younan S, et al. Diagnosing dysautonomia after acute traumatic brain injury: evidence for overresponsiveness to afferent stimuli. *Arch Phys Med Rehabil.* 2009;90:580–586.

Chioléro RL, Breitenstein E, Thorin D, et al. Effects of propranolol on resting metabolic rate after severe head injury. *Crit Care Med.* 1989;17:328–334.

Fernandez-Ortega JF, Prieto-Palomino MA, Garcia-Caballero M, et al. Paroxysmal sympathetic hyperactivity after traumatic brain injury: clinical and prognostic implications. *J Neurotrauma.* 2012;29:1364–1370.

Fernández-Ortega JF, Prieto-Palomino MA, Quesada-García G, et al. Findings in the magnetic resonance of paroxysmal sympathetic hyperactivity. *J Neurotrauma.* 2011;28:1327–1328.

Hinderer SR, Lehmann JF, Price R, et al. Spasticity in spinal cord injured persons: quantitative effects of baclofen and placebo treatments. *Am J Phys Med Rehabil.* 1990;69:311–317.

Ko SB, Kim CK, Lee SH, et al. Morphine-sensitive paroxysmal sympathetic storm in pontine intracerebral hemorrhage. *Neurologist.* 2010;16:384–385.

Lv LQ, Hou LJ, Yu MK, et al. Prognostic influence and magnetic resonance imaging findings in paroxysmal sympathetic hyperactivity after severe traumatic brain injury. *J Neurotrauma.* 2010;27:1945–1950.

Lv LQ, Hou LJ, Yu MK, et al. Risk factors related to dysautonomia after severe traumatic brain injury. *J Trauma.* 2011;71:538–542.

Payen D, Quintin L, Plaisance P, et al. Head injury: clonidine decreases plasma catecholamines. *Crit Care Med.* 1990;18:392–395.

Penfield W. Diencephalic autonomic epilepsy. *Arch Neurol Psychiatry.* 1929;22:358–374.

Perkes I, Baguley IJ, Nott MT, et al. A review of paroxysmal sympathetic hyperactivity after acquired brain injury. *Ann Neurol.* 2010;68:126–135.

Perkes IE, Menon DK, Nott MT, et al. Paroxysmal sympathetic hyperactivity after acquired brain injury: a review of diagnostic criteria. *Brain Inj.* 2011;25:925–932.

Pranzatelli MR, Pavlakis SG, Gould RJ, et al. Hypothalamic-midbrain dysregulation syndrome: hypertension, hyperthermia, hyperventilation, and decerebration. *J Child Neurol.* 1991;6:115–122.

Rossitch E Jr, Bullard DE. The autonomic dysfunction syndrome: aetiology and treatment. *Br J Neurosurg.* 1988;2:471–478.

Russo RN, O'Flaherty S. Bromocriptine for the management of autonomic dysfunction after severe traumatic brain injury. *J Paediatr Child Health.* 2000;36:283–285.

Srinivasan S, Lim CCT, Thirugnanam U. Paroxysmal autonomic instability with dystonia. *Clin Auton Res.* 2007;17:378–381.

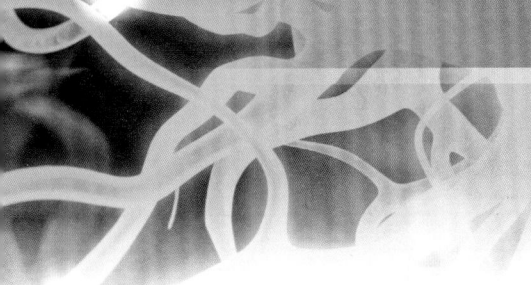

Carl W. Bazil and Andrew J. Westwood

INTRODUCTION

Sleep and sleep disorders are frequently overlooked as a cause or exacerbating factor in neurologic dysfunction. Neuronal activity and the networks involved are different in each state of sleep (non–rapid eye movement [NREM] and rapid eye movement [REM] sleep) compared with the normal waking brain. Sleep and sleep disorders therefore offer unique opportunities to understand the physiology of the brain and its impact on daily functioning. Sleep is involved in the regulation of endocrine and autonomic output and is integral to learning and memory, areas whose complexity and relationship to sleep are only beginning to be understood.

This chapter begins with a brief description of normal sleep and its impact on functioning. Diagnostic testing in sleep is discussed in Chapter 29. An overview of sleep disorders follows with particular relation to their impact on neurologic diseases.

PHYSIOLOGY OF NORMAL SLEEP

Sleep is an active process that involves numerous distinct neuronal networks, which are ultimately expressed as altered physiologic functions. Heart rate, blood pressure, gas exchange, gastrointestinal function, hormonal secretion, and even kidney function are altered during sleep. The exact purpose of sleep remains unclear, but there is considerable evidence of essential associations with immune function, memory, learning, energy conservation, and toxin clearance.

Sleep is classified into stages based on three parameters: electroencephalography (EEG), eye movement or electro-oculography (EOG), and muscle tone as assessed by electromyography (EMG) of the mentalis muscle. Arbitrary classification of 30 second recordings, or epochs, divide the process into wakefulness, three stages of NREM sleep (stages N1, N2, and N3), and one stage of REM sleep (stage R).

Wakefulness (stage W) is identified by a low-voltage fast-frequency EEG, high muscle tone, and REMs. *Stage N1* sleep is characterized by a low-voltage, mixed-frequency EEG and slow, rolling eye movements. Reactivity to outside stimuli is decreased, and mentation may proceed but is slowed. *Stage N2* consists of a moderate low-voltage background EEG with sleep spindles (bursts of 12- to 16-Hz activity lasting 0.5 to 2 seconds) and K complexes (brief high-voltage discharges with an initial negative deflection followed by a positive component). *Slow-wave sleep (stage N3)* consists of high-amplitude delta (0 to 2 Hz) frequencies occupying 20% or more of the epoch. During this deeper sleep, heart and respiratory rates are slowed and regular. In NREM sleep, the tonic chin EMG is of moderately high amplitude but less than that of quiet wakefulness (Fig. 114.1).

The EEG pattern during REM sleep (stage R) consists of low-voltage, mixed-frequency activity and is similar to that of stage N1 sleep. Moderately high-amplitude, 3- to 6-Hz triangular waveforms referred to as *sawtooth waves* are intermittently present and are unique to REM sleep. Intermittent bursts of rapid conjugate eye movements occur. Tonic chin EMG activity is absent or markedly reduced, and phasic muscle discharges occur in irregular bursts. The decreased EMG activity is a reflection of muscle paralysis resulting from active inhibition of muscle activity. During REM sleep, surges of parasympathetic and sympathetic activity are denoted by greater variability in heart and respiratory rates. This stage is also associated with complex vivid imagery, but visual imagery can occur in all sleep stages. When occurring in deep NREM sleep, dream images are typically fragmented and may be associated with actions such as the sensation of falling.

During a normal night, sleep comprises recurring cycles. Within each cycle of 90 to 120 minutes, NREM sleep alternates with REM sleep. The normal healthy adult typically falls asleep within 10 minutes and goes through the sequence of stages N1 through N3, followed by reversion to stage N2 sleep. Afterward, the first REM sleep period occurs 70 to 100 minutes into sleep. The first REM period is usually the shortest, about 10 minutes. This pattern of NREM and REM sleep is repeated three to five times during a normal night's sleep. Typically, most stage N3 sleep is seen in the first two sleep cycles, and REM sleep periods increase in duration and intensity of REM activity as the night progresses. Stage N2 sleep, however, is the most common sleep stage, typically making up half of a normal adult's night. In the normal adult, wakefulness accounts for approximately 5% of the night. N3 and REM sleep typically account for 25% each of total sleep and N1 approximately 5% (Fig. 114.2).

NEUROANATOMY AND NEUROCHEMISTRY OF SLEEP

Anatomically, NREM sleep is expressed when a network of neurons in the anterior hypothalamus suppresses the reticular activating system and monoaminergic neuronal activity. This network causes a functional disconnection of sensory input to the cortex and decreases the metabolic rate of most of the cortex. During stage N3, cortical neuronal synchrony is promoted, and this may be related to synaptic pruning. REM sleep, however, is an activation of cholinergic neurons in the pontine dorsal tegmentum that subsequently excite neurons responsible for REM-associated atonia, REMs, increase in cortical metabolic rate, loss of thermoregulation, and other features. REM sleep is inhibited by activation of the dorsal raphe and locus ceruleus. A network of neurons in the hypothalamus midbrain and thalamus seems to regulate REM sleep cycling.

Hypocretin—named so because it structurally resembles secretin in the gut—appears to stabilize the ability to remain awake. It is also referred to as *orexin* codiscovered by another group—named so because of its ability to stimulate food intake (from the Greek *orexis* meaning appetite).

Throughout the 24-hour day, the human body has a symphony of endocrinologic and metabolic variations that are timed to maximize performance during wakefulness and promote quality rejuvenation during sleep. Because we evolved on a planet that

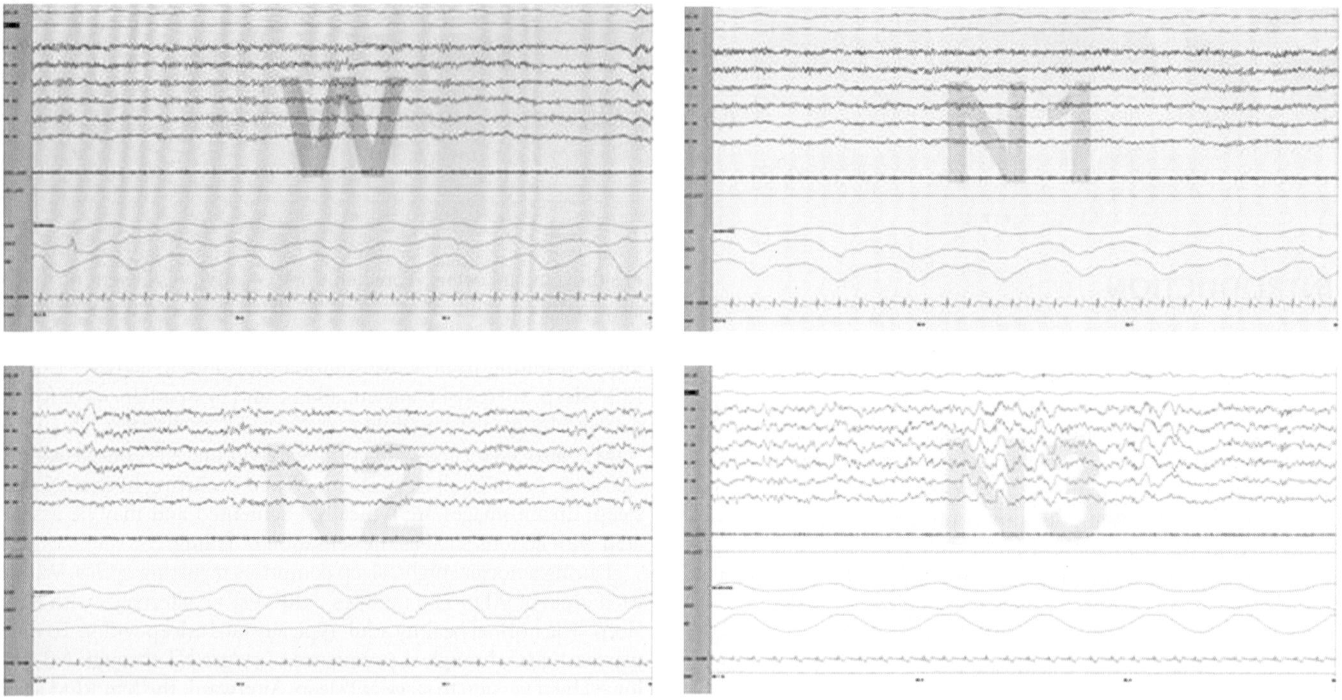

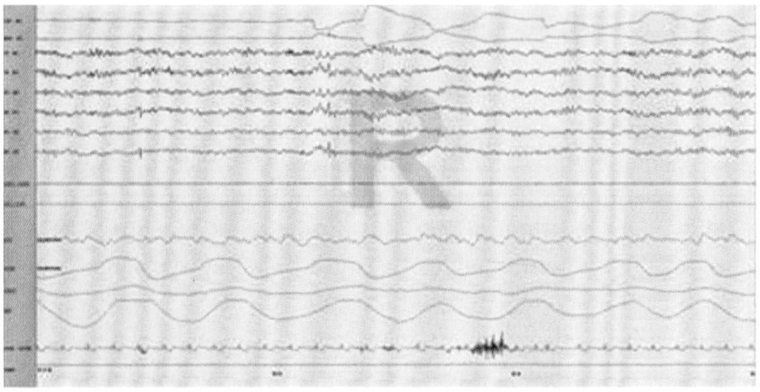

FIGURE 114.1 Stages of sleep. Each 30-second recording represents a different stage of sleep. Wake (*W*), NREM is divided into three stages (*N1, N2, N3*) and REM (*R*). For each recording, the top two channels are electro-oculogram (LOC-A2 and ROC-A1); the following six are EEG, followed by chin EMG and leg EMG (LAT1-LAT2), airflow, chest and abdominal movements, ECG, and oxygen saturation.

rotates every 24 hours, we developed a delicate neurochemistry anticipatory cycle that prepares the body for the upcoming sleep–wake state. This circadian cycle is approximately 1 day as captured in the Greek meaning of *circadian*. Many body functions, including body temperature, plasma and urine hormones, renal functions,

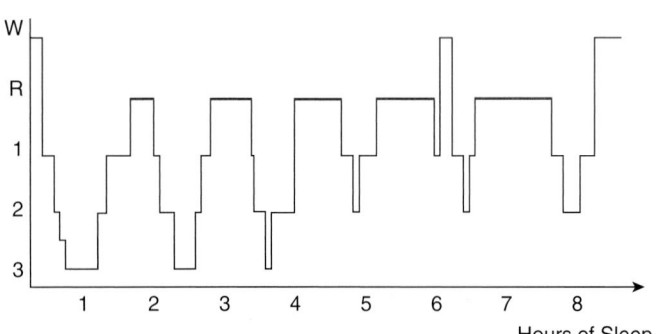

FIGURE 114.2 Hypnogram. Graphical representation of sleep stages as a function of time. This hypnogram shows normal sleep architecture with the majority of slow-wave sleep in the first third of the night, REM sleep majority in the last third of the night, and progressive longer durations of REM.

psychological performance measures, and internal sleep-stage organization, participate in this circadian rhythm. Humans have a circadian rhythm that is approximately 24.3 hours and is driven by the suprachiasmatic nucleus. This nucleus is influenced by external time clues to synchronize the body clock with the outside world, including bright light, activity, meals, and social interactions. Evidence for the importance of circadian rhythms comes from studies of acute phase shifts, such as those that occur after jet lag or shift work. Because our internal clock is longer than 24 hours, adaptation is slower after an eastward flight (phase advance) than after a westward flight (phase delay).

SPECIFIC DISORDERS OF SLEEP

Diagnostic procedures are discussed in Chapter 29.

Nearly all patients with disorders of the central nervous system (CNS) are at high risk for sleep dysfunction, which may be a direct result or a secondary effect of the neurologic condition. Sleep disorders may exacerbate the symptoms of the underlying neurologic disorder and impair quality of life. In this chapter, we describe selected disorders. *Fatal familial insomnia*, a prion disease, is discussed in Chapter 68. Sleep-associated headache disorders and epilepsy syndromes are also discussed in their respective chapters.

INSOMNIA

Insomnia can consist of difficulty falling asleep (sleep-onset insomnia), difficulty staying asleep (sleep maintenance insomnia), both, or sleep that is nonrefreshing or nonrestorative. The daytime symptoms include excessive fatigue, impaired performance, or emotional change. Most people have an occasional night fraught with difficulty falling asleep or trouble maintaining sleep, usually caused by an alerting response to short-term stress; this is a normal property of the brain and is not considered insomnia if it resolves quickly. In the past, insomnia has been categorized into primary or secondary types but these were difficult to reliably ascertain. Insomnia is now considered as *short-term, chronic,* or *other* [**Level 1**].[1]

Short-term insomnia lasting less than 3 months duration might be closely linked to the surrounding events, psychological disturbances, or sudden changes in a medical condition. Typically, there is an identifiable precipitant that an individual is able to recall. Individuals may complain of disturbances fewer than three times per week but this results in a general dissatisfaction in their quality of sleep. It may also result in the individual catastrophizing that they may never sleep again. The 1-year prevalence of short-term insomnia is around 20% in the general adult population. Circadian rhythm disorders should be considered as mimickers of insomnia. In delayed sleep phase syndrome, individuals typically complain that they cannot fall asleep until later in the night and due to morning commitments have to curtail their sleep, and this results in sleep deprivation. Early morning arousal raises the possibility of advanced sleep phase if the patient falls asleep early in the evening.

Chronic insomnia, lasting greater than 3 months on 3 or more days per week, is usually attributed to multiple factors. The factors may be divided into predisposing, precipitating, and perpetuating, which outline the formation of insomnia as an ongoing process. Characteristics that predispose an individual for insomnia are female gender, older age, psychiatric or chronic medical illness, lower socioeconomic status, poor education, obsessive–compulsive nature, poor coping strategies, and hyperalertness (Table 114.1).

Insomnia may be precipitated by sudden changes in environment or challenges to the body or mind. These challenges may come in the form of acute medical illness, psychological or psychiatric events, shift in schedule, or changes in medications or supplements. After the start of the insomnia, patients adopt behaviors or

rituals that perpetuate the insomnia. Patients may use maladaptive habits that occur during the day or night and include heavy caffeine or alcohol use; watching television, working, or playing video games while in bed; or even eating or exercising during the usual sleep period. They may become dependent on certain somnogenic substances. Some patients develop associations of not sleeping with the bedroom and may fear going to bed. These poor associations and expectations of poor sleep promote the apprehension toward sleep. The insomnia symptom complex may indicate an underlying disorder related to primary failure of the sleep mechanism or one in which sleep disruption is a result of another disorder. Patients with obstructive sleep apnea, restless legs syndrome, and even narcolepsy may complain of insomnia. Sleep diaries, accounting bedtime and wake time, can be useful in determining potential links to schedule or circadian rhythm issues. Perception of good sleep is an important factor in evaluating the complaint of insomnia.

Some patients exaggerate their symptoms, whereas other patients may not perceive they are asleep. These individuals display the normal physiologic parameters of sleep but do not recognize that they have slept. This is referred to as *sleep-state misperception* or *paradoxical insomnia.*

Insomnia may also be produced by medical or neurologic disorders. Derangement of almost any system in the body can disrupt sleep. Patients with diseases affecting the nervous system, heart, liver, kidneys, gastrointestinal tract, or lungs commonly complain of insomnia. Musculoskeletal discomfort such as in arthritis or other rheumatologic disorders may become worse with periods of rest. Pain from entrapment neuropathies such as carpal tunnel are typically worse at night, and headaches such as cluster headache or pain related to increased intracranial pressure or brain mass lesions can become more intense during sleep. Nearly all of the psychiatric illnesses have some link to poor sleep. Patients with depression or anxiety disorders may have insomnia years prior to the presentation of the affective component. Although a causal relationship is still in debate, the association is clear. Insomnia may also herald the onset of psychosis or mania.

Treatment of insomnia should be directed toward symptom improvement and avoidance of maladaptive behaviors. Therapy for neurologic and psychiatric disorders should be optimized, and a multipronged approach addressing the patient's behaviors, psychological attitudes, and the potential underlying neurochemistry should be constructed. Cognitive behavioral therapy for insomnia (CBT-i) consisting of sleep restriction therapy, relaxation therapy, stimulus control, and sleep hygiene (see Table 114.1) provides a solid therapeutic foundation. CBT-i is the most effective long-term therapy for insomnia. The use of acupuncture for insomnia remains equivocal due to the lack of methodologic consistency in the trials [**Level 1**].[2]

There are also a number of safe, effective hypnotic substances that may be used particularly in short-term insomnia to help restore normal sleep patterns and reverse negative associations with sleep time and the bedroom environment. These differ mainly in half-life, with zaleplon (5 to 20 mg) very short acting, zolpidem (5 to 10 mg) short, and eszopiclone (1 to 3 mg) the longest (therefore most useful in sleep maintenance insomnias). Ramelteon (8 mg) is a melatonin agonist that is also a mild hypnotic. Suvorexant (5 to 20 mg), a nonselective orexin antagonist was approved in 2014 for insomnia. When these agents fail, benzodiazepines and sedating antidepressant drugs are alternatives. Short-acting benzodiazepines are usually preferable to avoid daytime sedation, although if anxiety is also present, longer acting compounds can be useful. Many medications are used off-label for insomnia particularly if there are concomitant symptoms

TABLE 114.1	Principles of Good Sleep Hygiene Are the Basis for a Sound Night of Sleep
Principles of Sleep Hygiene	

- Establish regular bedtimes.
- Wake regularly at a fixed time.
- Regulate the amount of sleep obtained each night.
- Exercise daily and regularly (particularly aerobic) but not in the late evening.
- Sleep in a quiet, cool, comfortable environment.
- Avoid caffeinated beverages and other stimulants (including tobacco) especially close to bedtime.
- Avoid alcohol within 3 h of bedtime.
- Avoid hypnotic drugs.
- Do something relaxing before bedtime.

TABLE 114.2 A List of Current Medications Approved by the U.S. Food and Drug Administration for Insomnia

Class	FDA-Approved Pharmaceutical Treatment of Insomnia			
	Agent	Dosage (mg)	Half-life (h)	Comments
Nonbenzodiazepine-benzodiazepine receptor agonists (NBZRAs)	Zaleplon	5–20	1	—
	Zolpidem	5 (women) 5–10 (men)	1.4–3.6	Available as oral, oral spray, and sublingual forms
	Zolpidem ER	6.25–12.5	1.4–3.6	Women metabolize zolpidem at a lower rate than men.
	Eszopiclone	1–3	5–7	—
Orexin antagonist	Suvorexant	5–20	8–14	—
Benzodiazepines	Estazolam	0.5–2	10–24	—
	Flurazepam	15–30	47–100	—
	Quazepam	7.5–15	47–100	—
	Temazepam	7.5–30	8–20	—
	Triazolam	0.0625–0.125	1.5–5.5	—
Tricyclic antidepressants	Doxepin	3–6	8–24	Approved in low-dose 3- and 6-mg formulations only
Selective melatonin receptor agonist	Ramelteon	8	8	—

Many others are used off-label.

FDA, U.S. Food and Drug Administration.

that could be effectively treated at the same time, such as headaches or depression. Many medications typically used for insomnia have not received formal approval by the U.S. Food and Drug Administration (FDA) because they have not applied for insomnia as a specific indication. Substances that promote alertness should be minimized when possible, and additional medicinal therapy should be directed toward a specific disease process. The goal of treatment with any hypnotic should be to help restore normal sleeping patterns, followed by slow elimination of the drug (Table 114.2).

When an individual has less sleep than what is generally considered normal, concern may arise from those around them. Some individuals are *short sleepers* requiring less than 6 hours of sleep but do not complain of sleep/wake disturbances and therefore are not insomniacs per se. Others may spend excessive amounts of time in bed. This pattern may occur, for example, from parents allocating too much time for their children to sleep, but the child functions normally. Some adult individuals are *long sleepers*, requiring 10 or more hours of sleep to function without signs of sleep deprivation. Although frustrating to patients, this condition is best treated with longer sleep times so long as no other source of ineffective sleep is found.

THE HYPERSOMNIAS

Sleepiness is defined as the propensity to enter sleep. This is a normal feeling as one approaches a typical sleep period, but excessive sleepiness occurs when one enters sleep at an inappropriate time or setting. Excessive sleepiness can occur in degrees. In mild sleepiness, one might have only limited impairment, such as falling asleep while reading a book. Greater degrees of sleepiness, however, may be associated with bouts of irresistible sleep or sleep attacks that intrude on such activities as driving, having a conversation, or eating meals. This degree of sleepiness places the

patient at significant risk for accidents and has a major impact on the person's well-being. It must occur for at least 3 months prior to diagnosis.

Clinicians should always question their hypersomnic patients for clues of potential sleep debt, sleep disorders, or other medical or psychiatric causes. Sleep deprivation is the most common cause of sleepiness. Information regarding sleep habits, schedule during the week and weekends, and environment often discloses other important contributing factors. Excessive sleepiness may result from a wide range of medical disorders and medications. Patients with heart, kidney, or liver failure or rheumatologic or endocrinologic disorders such as hypothyroidism and diabetes may note sleepiness and fatigue. Neurologic disorders such as strokes, tumors, demyelinating diseases, epilepsy, and head trauma can evoke excessive sleepiness. Sleepiness is frequently the cardinal symptom of many sleep disorders (Table 114.3). Patients with sleep apnea, narcolepsy, restless legs syndrome–periodic limb movements, or even parasomnias may note excessive daytime sleepiness as their main complaint. Thus, the clinician should question the patient further to elucidate potential etiologies.

About 2% of men and 1.5% of women report sleeping at least 10 hours per night and are regarded as *long sleepers* (in children, it is 2 hours more than the age-specific normative data). The additional sleep time is spent in REM and N2 compared to other individuals. Providing that these individuals obtain sufficient sleep prior to testing, the multiple sleep latency test (MSLT) is normal.

Narcolepsy

Narcolepsy is an incurable lifelong neurologic disorder characterized by the tetrad of (1) excessive daytime sleepiness, (2) cataplexy, (3) sleep paralysis, and (4) hypnagogic hallucinations. Patients with narcolepsy also typically have fragmentation of nocturnal sleep. Estimates of prevalence range between 2 and 10

TABLE 114.3	Differential Diagnosis of Excessive Daytime Sleepiness

- Insufficient sleep syndrome
- Sleep apnea syndromes
- Narcolepsy
- Idiopathic hypersomnia
- Demyelinating disease
- Infections
- Sarcoidosis
- Neurodegenerative diseases
- Tumors of the hypothalamus or rostral midbrain
- Metabolic disorders, e.g., hypothyroidism, pancreatic insufficiency, renal insufficiency, hepatic encephalopathy
- Drugs, e.g., antidepressants, hypnotics, and antihistamines
- Withdrawal of stimulants
- Periodic limb movement disorder
- Circadian rhythm disorders
- Depression

per 10,000 individuals in North America and Europe. It is about five times more prevalent in Japan, and the incidence is only 1 per 500,000 in Israel. The symptoms of narcolepsy typically present between ages 10 and 30 years, although cases have been reported with onset as early as age 2 years and as late as 76 years. Men and women are equally affected. There appears to be a bimodal distribution occurring in teenage years and later around age 35 years. Symptoms gradually develop over several years but once it has fully developed, there is usually only a minor fluctuation in the severity. Sleepiness is often minimized or thought to be related to other causes, and diagnosis can be delayed for years or even decades. As weight gain and depression are common other causes for excessive daytime sleepiness in a previously well-rested individual should be considered.

Narcolepsy is a prototype disorder of loss of control of sleep–wake determination. Patients have bouts of irresistible sleep and frequent arousals during nocturnal sleep, with episodes of partial intrusion of REM sleep into wakefulness. Intrusion of fragments of REM sleep into wakefulness is most evident in the presence of the symptoms of cataplexy, sleep paralysis, and hypnagogic hallucinations.

Daytime sleepiness is usually the first and most prominent symptom to appear, but hyperactivity may be seen in children as they attempt to fight off sleep. Patients often complain of attacks of irresistible sleep that occur at inappropriate times, such as during conversation, driving, and eating. Brief naps for some are refreshing. The symptom of excessive daytime sleepiness is disabling and often leads to personal, social, and economic problems.

Cataplexy is the abrupt onset of paralysis or weakness of voluntary muscles without change in consciousness; it is typically precipitated by strong emotions. Events can be triggered by a joke, surprise, anger, fear, or athletic endeavors. These events last seconds to minutes, and patients have clear memory for the complete event with no postictal confusion or deficits. Longer events may proceed to the patient entering sleep. The severity of cataplexy is variable. Some patients may have as few as two or three

episodes in a lifetime, whereas others may have several episodes every day. A full range of severity exists between these extremes. Cataplexy may be partial and affect only certain muscles; common examples include dysarthria; drooping of the head, face, and eyelids; and slight buckling of the knees. Severe global attacks affect all skeletal muscles except muscles of respiration and cause collapse. Onset of the attack usually takes seconds with brief moments of partial regaining of muscle tone at the beginning. Examination of the patient during the cataplectic attack will demonstrate paralysis with diffuse hypotonia, absence of deep tendon reflexes, diminished corneal reflexes, preserved pupillary responses, and phasic muscle twitching with preserved consciousness. Phasic muscle twitching can occur as single jerks or repetitive muscle twitching and is most frequently seen in the face. Most episodes last only seconds to 1 minute, but severe attacks can last minutes. Sudden withdrawal of antidepressants can result in status cataplecticus. Cataplexy typically follows onset of excessive daytime somnolence, usually beginning within 5 years if present.

The combination of excessive daytime sleepiness and cataplexy is nearly always related to narcolepsy. Cataplexy can rarely be seen as an isolated symptom, suggesting an underlying neurologic disorder. Cataplexy has been reported in cases of demyelinating disease, stroke, and Niemann–Pick type C. The historical feature of clear emotional triggers differentiates cataplexy from hypotension, vertebral basilar insufficiency, and the group of neuromuscular disorders known to produce periodic paralysis. Autoimmune or paraneoplastic disorders associated with the aquaporin-4 or anti-Ma2 as well as myotonic dystrophy, parkinsonism, and severe head trauma can also present with narcolepsy.

The presence of cataplexy was previously diagnostic of narcolepsy; however, narcolepsy type 1 now requires an abnormal MSLT (as described in Chapter 29) and/or cerebrospinal fluid (CSF) hypocretin-1 concentration, measured by immunoreactivity to be less than 110 pg/mL. Cataplexy does not need to be present if hypocretin-1 levels are below 110 pg/mL. Ten percent of individuals with cataplexy will not have hypocretin-1 levels below this cutoff and are now considered to be narcolepsy type 2. Narcolepsy type 2 is diagnosed if the patient has an abnormal MSLT but cataplexy is absent or CSF measurements are greater than 110 pm/mL (or not measured). In the *Diagnostic and Statistical Manual of Mental Disorders*, 5th edition (*DSM-5*), narcolepsy with the absence of cataplexy is considered *primary hypersomnia*.

Sleep paralysis is a global paralysis of voluntary muscles that occurs at the entry into or emergence from sleep. These events may include the feeling of being chased or impending danger. The terror associated with the events can be recounted by the patient years later. The events are aborted with a tactile stimulation. The paralysis associated with the event is thought to result from the same motor inhibition that occurs in REM sleep. Sleep paralysis without narcolepsy can occur in an isolated form in sleep-deprived healthy individuals but is also frequently seen in patients with depression. Prevalence of a single episode of sleep paralysis is estimated to be between 15% and 40% of the general population. Differential diagnoses for sleep paralysis should include cataplexy, atonic seizures, and familial periodic paralysis syndromes.

Hypnic hallucinations are vivid dreamlike images that occur during sleep onset (hypnogogic) or at sleep offset (hypnopompic). They may include simple to complex visual, auditory, or somatosensory hallucinations. Patients are usually aware of their surroundings and may have difficulty in discerning the hallucinations from reality. The hallucinations can be relatively pleasant or terrifying. Patients may note a feeling of weightlessness, falling, or flying or have out of body–like experiences that may sometimes terminate with a sudden jerk (hypnic jerk). Hypnic hallucinations are most likely the result of dissociated CNS processes involved in dreaming during REM sleep. They can be precipitated by sleep deprivation, medications, and alcohol in normal individuals. Hallucinations typically accompany sleep paralysis in 25% to 75% of cases.

Narcolepsy has been associated with several of the human leukocyte antigen (HLA) subtypes. *DQB1*0602* is found in isolation in blacks and together with *DR2/DRB1*1501* in Caucasians and Asians. Most with narcolepsy type 1 will have the DQB1*0602 but it is also found in 12% to 38% of the general population. The risk of narcolepsy type 1 in first-degree relatives is approximately 1% to 2%.

Identification of the hypocretin-orexin gene and receptors in mouse models and humans revealed that narcolepsy type 1 is associated with loss of hypocretin-orexin–producing neurons in the lateral hypothalamus. Hypocretin-orexin in the CSF is found low in patients with cataplexy. Brains from narcolepsy patients show a loss of hypocretin-orexin–producing neurons. This loss of hypocretin-orexin–producing neurons is thought to permit the rapid switching between sleep and wake states.

Narcolepsy symptoms produce major social, familial, educational, and economic consequences for both the patient and the family. Patients often do not achieve their intellectual potential and suffer frequent failures of occupation, education, and marriage. Family members, friends, and even patients often interpret the symptoms as indicating laziness, lack of ambition, delayed maturation, or psychological defects. Because these symptoms begin during the crucial period of maturation from puberty to adulthood, misinterpretation and lack of diagnosis can greatly affect a patient's personality and feelings of self-esteem (Table 114.4).

The current treatment for the sleepiness of narcolepsy is the use of stimulant drugs, behavioral modifications, and/or γ-hydroxybutyrate (6 to 9 g). The stimulants can be categorized into the amphetamine and nonamphetamines types. Modafinil (100 to 200 mg) and armodafinil (the R-enantiomer of modafinil, [150 to 250 mg]) are wake-promoting agents chemically and pharmacologically distinct from the amphetamine stimulants [**Level 1**].[3] Use of stimulant drugs should be carefully monitored; patients and physicians should cooperate in adjusting the amount

and timing of doses to meet functional daytime needs and scheduling of patients' activities. Cataplexy, when present to a significant degree, is usually well controlled with the selective serotonin reuptake inhibitors (paroxetine hydrochloride [20 to 60 mg] or fluoxetine hydrochloride [20 to 60 mg]) and tricyclic compounds (imipramine hydrochloride [10 to 100 mg], protriptyline hydrochloride [5 to 60 mg], or clomipramine [10 to 150 mg]); however, impotence may be an undesirable side effect in men. These medications are thought to treat cataplexy effectively because they suppress REM sleep. γ-Hydroxybutyrate (6 to 9 g) is given at bedtime and again during the night to improve sleep and reduce the frequency and severity of both sleepiness and cataplexy. Due to its potential for abuse, it is highly regulated and only available from a single central pharmacy.

An important adjunctive treatment for narcolepsy is the rational scheduling of daytime naps, two 20-minute naps for example, and the maintenance of proper sleep hygiene. The physician's role in providing the patient with a clear understanding of the nature of the symptoms and with emotional support in coping with the many adaptive difficulties cannot be overemphasized.

Kleine–Levin Syndrome

Kleine–Levin syndrome (recurrent hypersomnia) consists of recurrent episodes of hypersomnia and binge eating lasting from 2 days to 5 weeks (rarely to 80 days), with intervals less than 18 months between episodes. Neurobehavioral and psychological changes, such as disorientation, automatic behavior, forgetfulness, depression, depersonalization, hallucinations, irritability, aggression, and sexual hyperactivity, often accompany the episodes of hypersomnia. During the episodes, the EEG shows general slowing with 0.5- to 2-second bursts of bisynchronous generalized moderate- to high-voltage 5- to 7-Hz waves. This resolves in between episodes. Onset is typically in early adolescent boys and is less common in girls. Prevalence is estimated to be around one or two cases per million. Episodes decrease in frequency and severity with age and are rarely present after the fourth decade. Differential diagnosis for this condition includes encephalitis, hyperammonemic encephalopathy, demyelinating disease, head trauma, porphyria, basilar migraine, and complex partial status epilepticus as well as psychiatric conditions such as

TABLE 114.4	Comparison between the *International Classification of Sleep Disorders-3* and the *Diagnostic and Statistical Manual of Mental Disorders-5* for the Criteria of Narcolepsy Variants		
DSM-5 Criteria	Narcolepsy-Hypocretin Deficiency	Primary Hypersomnia	
ICSD-3 Criteria	Narcolepsy Type 1	Narcolepsy Type 2	Idiopathic Hypersomnia
Findings on MSLT	<8 min with two or more SOREMPs	<8 min with two or more SOREMPs	<8 min and fewer than two SOREMPs[a]
Cataplexy	Present	Rarely present	Absent
CSF hypocretin	<110 pg/mL	>110 pg/mL	>110 pg/mL
Description of naps	Short and refreshing	Short and refreshing	Long and unrefreshing
Sleep efficiency	Low	Low	High (>90%)

[a]If longer than 8 minutes, the individual must have 11 hours of sleep in a 24-hour polysomnogram or averaged from 7-day wrist actigraphy.

DSM, Diagnostic and Statistical Manual of Mental Disorders; ICSD, International Classification of Sleep Disorders; MSLT, multiple sleep latency test; SOREMPs, sleep onset rapid eye movement periods; CSF, cerebrospinal fluid.

depression, seasonal affective disorder, or somatoform disorder. A menstrual variant of this condition has been reported in 18 women worldwide.

A definitive treatment for Kleine–Levin syndrome is not known, but there are reports of limited success with stimulants (especially amantadine [100 to 200 mg]), sodium valproate [250 to 60 mg/kg], and antidepressant therapy (including lithium [300 to 1,800 mg]).

SLEEP-RELATED BREATHING DISORDERS

Control of respiration during sleep is an excellent model of state-dependent neuronal regulation. Respiratory patterns vary with sleep stage. Near sleep onset, occasionally, individuals will have normal pauses in breathing. Mild periodicity to breathing can be noted in light sleep, but on entrance into slow-wave sleep, breathing is very regular and response to high CO_2 and low oxygen levels is blunted. During REM sleep, chest musculature is paralyzed and ventilation occurs only via diaphragmatic movement. REM sleep is also characterized by significant variation in respiratory pattern and the least response to high CO_2 levels and low oxygen. Each of these stages allows for the expression of dysfunction in the regulation of breathing during sleep. Some individuals with brain or cardiac pathology may express dramatic periodic breathing or Cheyne–Stokes respiration in NREM sleep, whereas others who have impairment of ventilation owing to diaphragmatic impairment or impediment will demonstrate hypoventilation during REM sleep. More commonly, individuals may have obstruction of the upper airway during sleep.

Snoring

Snoring is created by turbulent airflow vibrating upper airway soft tissue and is more prominent during inspiration and loudest during N3 and REM sleep (the periods of greatest muscle relaxation). Snoring occurs in approximately two-thirds of adults, more commonly in men and over 10% of children. Persistent loud snoring is a classic symptom of obstructive sleep apnea syndrome (OSAS), but the absence of snoring does not exclude the diagnosis. Some patients' airways do not resonate to produce snoring. This is especially true in patients who have had upper airway surgical procedures that tightened tissue. Other individuals may not generate enough inspiratory force, such as those with neuromuscular disorders.

Catathrenia

Catathrenia is the term associated with sleep-related groaning typically associated with a prolonged expiration that disturbs the bed partner or family members. It is more common in men although remains rare. There are no known long-term consequences of it and it can be treated effectively with positive airway pressure.

Sleep Apnea

Apnea refers to a pause in breathing, and on overnight sleep studies, the pause must persist for at least 10 seconds to be considered apnea. *Hypopneas* are defined as the partial reduction in airflow for a similar time. These respiratory events are accompanied by oxygen desaturation and/or arousals. Apneas and hypopneas are typically more prevalent during light NREM sleep and REM sleep.

Historically, bed partners may describe these events as though the breathing has stopped or the patient is holding his or her breath during sleep. These events may be aborted with a loud gasp, snort, body jerks, or the quiet resumption of breathing. Some patients

have hundreds of events per night and are unable to obtain quality sleep. These individuals are typically unaware of any sleep disruption but feel unrefreshed in the morning. Patients with neurologic disorders are also at higher risk for sleep apnea. Sleep apnea is more commonly seen in individuals with CNS disease such as epilepsy, strokes, and head trauma and "classical" peripheral disease such as muscular dystrophy and myotonic dystrophy. Sleep apnea is classified into two major forms: obstructive and central.

Obstructive apnea is the most common form of sleep apnea. These apneas occur due to obstruction or collapse of the upper airway. The OSAS is the cluster of features including snoring, witnessed apneas, excessive daytime sleepiness, insomnia, morning headache, and impairment of daytime performance caused by the repetitive apneas. However, up to half of patients with documented obstructive sleep apnea on overnight polysomnography have no complaints of daytime symptoms. OSAS is frequently seen in individuals with hypertension, diabetes mellitus, and vascular disease. In adults, OSAS occurs predominantly between the fourth and sixth decades and is more common in men. The prevalence of OSAS increases with age and is higher in individuals with habitual snoring and obesity. Many patients are obese, yet some have normal body habitus. Common structural abnormalities such as narrow nasal passage, long soft palate, large tonsils, or retroflexed mandible leading to a small airway contribute to airway obstruction. Individuals with CNS disease are found to have a higher prevalence of sleep apnea than the general population.

OSAS is an independent risk for hypertension and the development of vascular disease. Recognized systemic complications of OSAS are systemic hypertension, pulmonary hypertension, diabetes mellitus, cardiac enlargement, myocardial infarction, stroke, elevated hematocrit, and an increased risk of sudden death during sleep.

Sleep apnea also occurs in infants and children. In infants, sleep apnea is associated with familial, congenital, and acquired dysautonomia syndromes and craniofacial disorders. Distinguishing apnea from normal periodic breathing is critical in infants, as some of these disorders are associated with either central or obstructive apneas. In children, obstructive sleep apnea is often associated with adenotonsillar hypertrophy, and daytime sequelae of hyperactivity, poor school performance, behavior problems, and limited growth have been associated.

Central apnea is the absence of ventilation owing to an absence of generation of respiratory effort. Central apneas can cause complaints of frequent awakenings and restless unrefreshing sleep. These respiratory events can be caused by neurologic abnormalities involving respiratory regulatory neuronal networks. Apneas may also follow neurologic events such as nocturnal seizures or acute strokes. One form of periodic breathing, Cheyne–Stokes breathing, can be seen in individuals with heart/renal failure, neurologic lesions, and metabolic or toxic encephalopathies. Patients with central apnea need a complete cardiac and neurologic examination. Certain medications such as opiates may also result in central sleep apnea.

When a single event is a combination of the two, the term *mixed apnea* is used. The term *complex sleep apnea* has no standard definition and should be avoided. Some may use it to describe an individual who has both central and obstructive events on diagnostic testing; others use it to describe the emergence of central events when obstructive events are treated.

Treatment for sleep apnea consists primarily of methods of promoting airway patency for obstructive apnea and stimulation of breathing in central apnea. Continuous positive airway pressure

(CPAP) is the most common and effective treatment. Constant air pressure is generated by a small pump and delivered via tubing to a mask covering the nose and/or mouth. Patients may be given this treatment during polysomnography to determine the pressure required to alleviate airway obstruction during sleep. Autotitrating devices alter the pressure required depending on the level of resistance; these can be prescribed for most individuals without in-laboratory titrations. In some circumstances, the positive airway pressure may need to be altered in both inspiration and expiration to maximize each breath. A bilevel-CPAP device is then used. In some cases of central sleep apnea, adaptive servoventilation may be required. These devices provide variable support to overcome the oscillations between hyperpneas and hypoventilation seen in this condition and may reduce mortality in certain individuals. It is unclear whether treatment is needed for individuals where central sleep apnea is related to opioid use. This breathing pattern resolves with cessation of the offending medications [**Level 1**].[4]

In those with neuromuscular disorders, volume-assured pressure support (VAPS) may be indicated although there is no clear benefit compared to bilevel CPAP. It can, however, adapt as the disease progresses. Typically, those with progressive neuromuscular disorders are monitored with nocturnal oximetry for evidence of sleep-related hypoventilation.

In individuals unable to tolerate any devices but have desaturations during sleep, oxygen may be prescribed. However, there is limited evidence whether sleep-related desaturations (with the absence of wake-related desaturations) are deleterious to health.

Key elements for compliance with positive airway pressure therapy include patient education of the importance of therapy, close follow-up, and addressing patient problems with the therapy. Oral appliances advancing the mandible are reasonable alternative therapies for patient with mild sleep apnea particularly if unable to tolerate positive airway pressure.

The level of obstruction in obstructive sleep apnea may be found at various levels of the airway. In some patients, especially children and young adults, the removal of enlarged tonsils and adenoids relieves the obstruction. Stimulation devices of the airway have recently been developed to reduce the risk of airway collapse during sleep. The surgical procedure, uvulopalatopharyngoplasty, has been an inconsistently beneficial treatment, and selection criteria are not well established. Genioglossal and maxillary–mandibular advancements have successfully treated patients with structural abnormalities causing hypopharyngeal obstruction. Other treatments for less severe cases have been sustained weight loss and (for those with significant sleep apnea only when supine) sleeping in the lateral position.

Hypoventilatory and Hypoxemic Disorders

Several causes of hypoventilation during sleep are known and require detection of hypercarbia (sleep-related hypoxemia requires a diagnosis of hypoxia). *Obesity hypoventilation syndrome* result in sleep as well as daytime hypercarbia and requires a body mass index (BMI) of 30 or to be greater than the 95th percentile for age and sex in children. *Congenital central alveolar hypoventilation syndrome*, previously Ondine's curse, is a syndrome of the automatic central control of breathing due to the PHOX2B gene. It must be distinguished from mimickers such as Chiari malformation, obesity hypoventilation syndrome, Leigh disease, or congenital heart disease when cor pulmonale coexists. *Late-onset central hypoventilation with hypothalamic dysfunction* presents after the first few years of life with hyperphagia and respiratory failure from

minor provocation. Temperature dysregulation, precocious puberty, thyroid disease, and other endocrinologic disorders may occur from inappropriately elevated or reduced levels of hypothalamic hormones.

SLEEP-RELATED MOVEMENT DISORDERS

RESTLESS LEGS SYNDROME AND PERIODIC LIMB MOVEMENT DISORDER

Periodic limb movements in sleep (PLMS) are found in most patients with restless legs syndrome who are studied with polysomnography but are more commonly associated without symptoms of restless legs syndrome. Although most patients do not complain of symptoms related to the PLMS, patients or their bed partner may notice leg or arm movements during sleep. These movements may occur as periodic events or appear random. PLMS are repetitive stereotyped movements of any of the extremities. These most commonly occur in NREM sleep and activate the lower extremities as extension of the great toe with dorsiflexion of the ankle and flexion of the knee and hip. Movements can also occur in the arms and axial muscles. The individual movements are relatively brief, lasting 0.5 to 5.0 seconds, occur at 20- to 90-second intervals, and may continue for minutes to hours. Limb movements may be accompanied by an arousal or awakening. In contrast to most movement disorders, which are diminished by sleep (e.g., cerebellar and extrapyramidal tremors, chorea, dystonia, hemiballism), PLMS are initiated by sleep or drowsiness. They are also different from *hypnic jerks* (sleep starts), which are normal, nonperiodic, isolated myoclonic movements. Similar to restless legs syndrome, periodic limb movements are provoked by uremia, anemia, peripheral neuropathy, antiemetics, antidepressants, and caffeine use.

In individuals with restless legs syndrome, limb movements can be seen on the polysomnography. Periodic limb movements of sleep, however, are not necessary and are not correlative with restless legs syndrome. Eighty percent of sufferers have periodic limb movements of sleep. Periodic limb movements during wakefulness have also been noted and have been proposed as a better marker.

Restless legs syndrome is discussed in detail in Chapter 75. It is important to note that restless legs syndrome is a clinical diagnosis based on questioning the individual. It does not require a sleep study to diagnose.

In a case of hypersomnia where all medical causes, psychiatric diseases, and other sleep disorders have been excluded and the only abnormality is periodic limb movements, then *periodic limb movement disorder* is diagnosed. Periodic limb movement disorder is mutually exclusive of restless legs syndrome and the two disorders cannot be codiagnosed. There is limited literature on the treatment but is empirically treated with similar therapeutic approaches as restless legs syndrome.

Sleep-Onset Movements

Some movements occur at the transition between wake and sleep. *Sleep-related rhythmic movement disorder* involves large muscle groups moving in a stereotyped repetitive fashion that is not a tremor. It may involve the head, torso, or limbs in isolation. Sleep-related movement disorder is common in children and typically does not require treatment except protection from injury if movements are violent. It rarely persists into adulthood, in which case it can be disruptive to bed partners and treated with low-dose clonazepam (0.25 to 1 mg). When smaller muscle groups are involved, other diagnoses such as bruxism, thumb sucking, or hypnagogic foot tremor, excessive fragmentary myoclonus should be considered. *Propriospinal myoclonus* results in difficulty initiating sleep and affects mainly the abdomen, trunk, and neck. When it is persistent into the daytime, a structural cause is found in 15% to 20% of cases. It typically spreads slow to rostral and caudal muscles from the axial muscles. *Sleep starts* or *hypnic jerks* involve one or more body segments in a single contraction and often asymmetrically. These may occur in association with a sensory component such as loud noise or a sensation of falling. Sleep deprivation, excessive stimulants, prior intense exercise, and emotional stress can increase frequency and severity of sleep starts. They are also prominent in heredity hyperekplexia [**Level 1**].[5]

Sleep-Related Movements

Body movements may occur during sleep such as the presentation of parasomnias or sleep-related leg cramps. *Benign sleep myoclonus of infancy* occurs only in sleep, whereas myoclonic seizures and myoclonic encephalopathy will also occur in wakefulness.

CIRCADIAN RHYTHM DISORDERS

Disorders of the circadian sleep–wake cycle are divided into two major categories, transient and persistent. The *transient disorders* include the temporary sleep disturbance following an acute work shift change and a rapid time zone change (jet lag). Both sleep deprivation and the circadian phase shift produce symptoms including insomnia, disrupted sleep, and excessive sleepiness. These disorders usually resolve as external and internal cycles become aligned. The *DSM-5* removed jet lag disorder from its list of conditions; however, the *International Classification of Sleep Disorders* still recognizes its existence.

Other disorders are more persistent. Sleep–wake cycle disorders that persist are divided into several major clinical categories. Persons who voluntarily and frequently change their sleep–wake schedule (e.g., shift workers) have a mixed pattern of excessive sleepiness alternating with arousal at inappropriate times of the day or have minimal circadian pattern. Sleep is typically short and disrupted. Waking is associated with a decrease in performance and vigilance. This syndrome often disrupts social and family life.

The *delayed sleep phase type* is a specific chronobiologic sleep disorder characterized by going to bed late and waking up late in the morning. Patients are typically unable to fall asleep earlier and go to sleep between 1 and 6 AM. On weekends and vacation days, they sleep until late morning or early afternoon and feel refreshed but have great difficulty awakening at the required 7 or 8 AM for work or school. These patients have a normal sleep length and internal organization of sleep when clock time of sleep onset and sleep offset coincides with the circadian timing that controls daily sleep.

Successful treatment has been a phase shift of the time of the daily sleep episode by progressive phase delay of the sleep time. By delaying the time of going to sleep and awakening by 2 or 3 hours each day (i.e., a 26- or 27-hour sleep–wake cycle), the patient's sleep timing can be successfully reset to the preferred clock time. Additionally, treatment with bright light in the morning and melatonin (0.2 to 0.5 mg) or a melatonin agonist in the evening may help shift and lock the circadian rhythm to a desired schedule [**Level 1**].[6]

The *advanced sleep phase type* is a condition in which individuals go to bed early in the evening and wake early in the morning. Typical sleep onset is between 6 and 8 PM, with wake times between 1

and 3 AM despite efforts to delay sleep time. This pattern is more likely to occur in elderly persons. Treatment of bright light in the evening and extended-release melatonin may help the sleep–wake schedule.

The rare individual with the free running type or *nonentrained type* maintains a 25- to 27-hour biologic day that does not entrain to the world's 24-hour cycle. This is more common in individuals who have prechiasmatic blindness, as light stimulus (a primary zeitgeber) does not reach the suprachiasmatic nucleus. This is in contrast to a person with an *irregular sleep–wake type* consisting of considerable irregularity without an identifiable persistent sleep–wake rhythm. There are frequent daytime naps at irregular times and a disturbed nocturnal sleep pattern. This disorder indicates dysfunction of the pacemaker, and most patients with this syndrome have congenital, developmental, or degenerative brain dysfunction, although it does occur rarely in cognitively intact patients. Treatment is difficult but should include regularly scheduled activities and time in bed based on sleep hygiene principles.

NOCTURNAL BEHAVIORS

Parasomnias

Parasomnias are undesirable physical or behavioral phenomena that occur predominantly during sleep. They include disorders of arousals, such as sleepwalking or night terrors; sleep–wake transition disorders, such as sleep talking; and REM parasomnias, such as REM sleep behavior disorder (RBD). These behavioral events may mimic epileptic seizures or other psychiatric events. Key features of age of onset, time of night of the events, stereotypic behavior, memory for the events, and family history are important in historically distinguishing the etiologies. Although RBD is the only disorder requiring polysomnography for diagnosis, most patients require polysomnographic recording (with complete EEG if epilepsy is in the differential) to delineate the cause or other potential sleep disorders provoking the parasomnia.

Non–Rapid Eye Movement Parasomnias

The classic disorders of arousal occur out of slow-wave sleep and include *sleepwalking, sleep terrors*, and *confusional arousals*. These behaviors are more common in children and adolescents and are characterized as events occurring as partial arousals from the deeper stages of NREM sleep. These patients are caught in a transition of part of the brain in NREM sleep and another portion in wake. These nonstereotypic events are more common in the first half of the night (when N3 is more prevalent), and typically, patients have little to no memory for the events; recall may increase with age. Sleepwalking usually involves a series of simple motor behaviors, such as sitting up in bed, walking, opening and closing doors, or climbing stairs, however, can rarely result in jumping out of bed as well as violent behaviors. Higher cognitive functions are significantly impaired, and there is reduced vigilance although motor behavior is intact. Self-injury and injury to those around them can occur.

Sleep terrors, however, start with a piercing scream or fright with significant sympathetic nervous system output. Patients have tachycardia, pupillary dilation, and sweating and appear wide eyed and inconsolable. A subgroup of patients may be harmful to themselves or others, such as fighting, throwing objects, and climbing out or walking through a window.

Confusional arousals occur following sudden awakening and may be accompanied with disorientation and the patient striking out. Other variations include sleep-related eating disorder, which is hallmarked by patients eating in a messy, haphazard manner with little or no recall. Sleep-related abnormal sexual behaviors can involve masturbatory behavior and sexual vocalizations and may have criminal consequences due to the initiation of sexual intercourse, molestation, or assault.

A small nightly dose of a benzodiazepine, such as clonazepam (0.25 to 4 mg) or temazepam (7.5 to 30 mg), is useful, especially when potential exists for the patient or bed partner to be injured. Medication such as zolpidem, phenothiazines, anticholinergics, and lithium may provoke these episodes. Hypnosis has also been used. Generally, treatment is not required but safety is a priority especially when the individual has a tendency to leave the bed.

Rapid Eye Movement Parasomnias

RBD, a REM sleep–related parasomnia, is characterized by intermittent loss of REM sleep atonia with dream enactment. Patients usually have clear recall of the dream, and witnesses can relate the activity to the dream mentation. Events are more likely to occur in the latter half of the night (when REM is more prevalent) and do not have stereotypic behavior. Injury to self or bed partner is common. It appears that as many as 80% of those with idiopathic RBD progress to a synucleinopathic neurodegenerative condition within a decade; this association is less clear when idiopathic RBD begins at a younger age. The prevalence of RBD is unknown but appears to be more common in older men. Some patients may develop RBD due to structural lesions interrupting the REM atonia pathway. Medications such as serotonin reuptake blockers and norepinephrine reuptake blockers have been cited to result in RBD-like behavior, although there is no evidence currently that these predispose to the condition.

The diagnosis is usually suggested by history and is required to be confirmed by polysomnography. Recordings show persistent muscle tone and complex behaviors during REM sleep. Most patients respond to clonazepam (0.25 to 4 mg) at bedtime, but success has been reported with melatonin (2 to 12 mg) and donepezil (10 to 15 mg) [**Level 1**].[7] Restraints to the individual during the night are sometimes required to avoid self-injury and to those around them, such as bedrails or placing the individual in a sleeping bag (Table 114.5).

Other REM parasomnias include painful erections, nightmares, and REM sleep–related sinus arrest, which are beyond the scope of this chapter.

TABLE 114.5	Differential Diagnosis of Dream Enactment Behavior

- REM behavior disorder
- Severe obstructive sleep apnea
- Periodic limb movement disorder
- Frontal lobe epilepsy
- Disorders of arousal
- Oneiric stupor
- Hallucinations in dementia
- Confusional awakenings in dementia
- Dissociative disorder

REM, rapid eye movement.

CONCLUSION

Nearly every CNS process has been associated with disruption of sleep. The ubiquity of sleep and the brain makes this dynamic relationship even more important. Sleep may be abnormal because of involvement of brain structures that control and regulate sleep and wakefulness or because of abnormal movements or behaviors that occur during sleep. Additionally, the loss of sleep provokes further dysfunction of the brain. For example, patients with epilepsy have fewer seizures once treated for their previously unrecognized obstructive sleep apnea. Other small studies have shown patients with neuromuscular disorders improve their daytime function when their sleep-related respiratory disturbances are treated. As neurologists, we must be keenly aware that sleep provides another dimension of diagnostic and therapeutic avenues for diseases of the nervous system. More importantly perhaps, we need to be vigilant for sleep disorders contributing to morbidity in our patients, particularly as nearly all are treatable, potentially resulting in increased quality of life.

LEVEL 1 EVIDENCE

1. American Academy of Sleep Medicine. *International Classification of Sleep Disorders*. 3rd ed. Darien, IL: American Academy of Sleep Medicine; 2014.
2. Morgenthaler T, Kramer M, Alessi C, et al; American Academy of Sleep Medicine. Practice parameters for the psychological and behavioral treatment of insomnia: an update. *Sleep*. 2006;29(11):1415–1419.
3. Morgenthaler TI, Kapur VK, Brown TM, et al. Practice parameters for the treatment of narcolepsy and other hypersomnias of central origin. *Sleep*. 2007;30:1705–1711.
4. Aurora N, Chowdhuri S, Ramar K, et al. The treatment of central sleep apnea syndromes in adults: practice parameters with an evidence-based literature review and meta-analyses. *Sleep*. 2012;35(1):17–40.
5. Chesson AL Jr, Wise M, Davila D, et al. Practice parameters for the treatment of restless legs syndrome and periodic limb movement disorder. An American Academy of Sleep Medicine report. Standards of Practice Committee of the American Academy of Sleep Medicine. *Sleep*. 1999;22:961–968.
6. Morgenthaler TI, Lee-Chiong T, Alessi C, et al. Practice parameters for the clinical evaluation and treatment of circadian rhythm sleep disorders sleep. 2007;30(11):1445–1459.
7. Aurora RN, Zak RS, Maganti RK, et al; Standards of Practice Committee; American Academy of Sleep Medicine. Best practice guide for the treatment of REM sleep behavior disorder (RBD). *J Clin Sleep Med*. 2010;6(1):85–95.

SUGGESTED READINGS

Ackermann S, Rasch B. Differential effects of non-REM and REM sleep on memory consolidation? *Curr Neurol Neurosci Rep*. 2014;14:430.

Berry RB, Brooks R, Gamaldo CE, et al; for the American Academy of Sleep Medicine. *The AASM Manual for the Scoring of Sleep and Associated Events: Rules, Terminology and Technical Specifications*. Version 2.1. Westchester, IL: American Academy of Sleep Medicine; 2014.

Billiard M. Idiopathic hypersomnia. *Neurol Clin*. 1996;14:573–582.

Black J, Houghton WC. Sodium oxybate improves excessive daytime sleepiness in narcolepsy. *Sleep*. 2006;29(7):939–946.

Boeve BF. Idiopathic REM sleep behaviour disorder in the development of Parkinson's disease. *Lancet Neurol*. 2013;12(5):469–482. doi:10.1016/S1474-4422(13)70054-1.

Claassen DO, Josephs KA, Ahlskog JE, et al. REM sleep behavior disorder preceding other aspects of synucleinopathies by up to half a century. *Neurology*. 2010;75:494–499.

de Lecea L, Kilduff TS, Peyron C, et al. The hypocretins: hypothalamus-specific peptides with neuroexcitatory activity. *Proc Natl Acad Sci U S A*. 1998;95:322–327.

Drummond SP, Walker M, Almklov E, et al. Neural correlates of working memory performance in primary insomnia. *Sleep*. 2013;36(9):1307–1316.

Feber R. Childhood sleep disorders. *Neurol Clin*. 1996;14:493–511.

Giles TL, Lasserson TJ, Smith BH, et al. Continuous positive airways pressure for obstructive sleep apnoea in adults. *Cochrane Database Syst Rev*. 2006;(3):CD001106.

Greenstone M, Hack M. Obstructive sleep apnoea. *BMJ*. 2014;348:g3745.

Harris SF, Monderer RS, Thorpy M. Hypersomnias of central origin. *Neurol Clin*. 2012;30(4):1027–1044.

Iliff JJ, Wang M, Liao Y, et al. A paravascular pathway facilitates CSF flow through the brain parenchyma and the clearance of interstitial solutes, including amyloid β. *Sci Transl Med*. 2012;4(147):147ra111.

Kang JE, Lim MM, Bateman RJ, et al. Amyloid-beta dynamics are regulated by orexin and the sleep-wake cycle. *Science*. 2009;326(5955):1005–1007.

Kryger MH, Roth T, Dement WC, eds. *Principles and Practice of Sleep Medicine*. 5th ed. Philadelphia: WB Saunders; 2010.

Lopez R, Dauvilliers Y. Pharmacotherapy options for cataplexy. *Expert Opin Pharmacother*. 2013;14(7):895–903.

Mahowald MW, Schenck CH. NREM sleep parasomnias. *Neurol Clin*. 1996;14:675–696.

Malhotra RK, Avidan AY. Parasomnias and their mimics. *Neurol Clin*. 2012;30(4):1067–1094.

Martin TJ, Sanders MH. Chronic alveolar hypoventilation: a review for the clinician. *Sleep*. 1995;18:617–634.

Mason M, Welsh EJ, Smith I. Drug therapy for obstructive sleep apnoea in adults. *Cochrane Database Syst Rev*. 2013;5:CD003002.

Menaker M, Murphy ZC, Sellix MT. Central control of peripheral circadian oscillators. *Curr Opin Neurobiol*. 2013;23(5):741–746.

Mignot E, Lammers GJ, Ripley B, et al. The role of cerebrospinal fluid hypocretin measurement in the diagnosis of narcolepsy and other hypersomnias. *Arch Neurol*. 2002;59(10):1553–1562.

Mignot E, Nishino S. Emerging therapies in narcolepsy–cataplexy. *Sleep*. 2005;28(6):754–763.

Newman AB, Nieto FJ, Guidry U, et al; Sleep Heart Health Study Research Group. Relation of sleep-disordered breathing to cardiovascular disease risk factors: the Sleep Heart Health Study. *Am J Epidemiol*. 2001;154(1):50–59.

Obermeyer WH, Benca RM. Effects of drugs on sleep. *Neurol Clin*. 1996;14:827–840.

Oliveira MM, Conti C, Prado GF. Pharmacological treatment for Kleine-Levin syndrome. *Cochrane Database Syst Rev*. 2013;8:CD006685.

Postuma RB, Gagnon JF, Tuineaig M, et al. Antidepressants and REM sleep behavior disorder: isolated side effect or neurodegenerative signal? *Sleep*. 2013;36(11):1579–1585.

Prinz PN. Sleep and sleep disorders in older adults. *J Clin Neurophysiol*. 1995;12:139–145.

Rasch B, Born J. About sleep's role in memory. *Physiol Rev*. 2013;93(2):681–766.

Richardson GS, Malin HV. Circadian rhythm sleep disorders: pathophysiology and treatment. *J Clin Neurophysiol*. 1996;13:17–31.

Riemann D, Spiegelhalder K, Feige B, et al. The hyperarousal model of insomnia: a review of the concept and its evidence. *Sleep Med Rev*. 2010;14(1):19–31.

Roth T, Dauvilliers Y, Mignot E, et al. Disrupted nighttime sleep in narcolepsy. *J Clin Sleep Med*. 2013;9(9):955–965.

Sabater L, Gaig C, Gelpi E, et al. A novel non-rapid-eye movement and rapid-eye-movement parasomnia with sleep breathing disorder associated with antibodies to IgLON5: a case series, characterisation of the antigen, and post-mortem study. *Lancet Neurol*. 2014;13(6):575–586.

Sack RL, Auckley D, Auger RR, et al; American Academy of Sleep Medicine. Circadian rhythm sleep disorders. An American Academy of Sleep Medicine review. *Sleep*. 2007;30(11):1460–1501.

Sakurai T, Amemiya A, Ishii M, et al. Orexins and orexin receptors: a family of hypothalamic neuropeptides and G-protein coupled receptors that regulate feeding behaviour. *Cell*. 1998;92:573–585.

Saper CB. The central circadian timing system. *Curr Opin Neurobiol*. 2013;23(5):747–751.

Saper CB, Scammell TE, Lu J. Hypothalamic regulation of sleep and circadian rhythms. *Nature*. 2005;437(7063):1257–1263.

Schenck CH, Mahowald MW. REM sleep parasomnias. *Neurol Clin*. 1996;14:697–720.

Schmidt-Nowara W, Lowe A, Wiegand L, et al. Oral applications for the treatment of snoring and obstructive sleep apnea: a review. *Sleep*. 1995;18:501–510.

Silber MH. Sleep-related movement disorders. *Continuum (Minneap Minn)*. 2013;19(1 Sleep Disorders):170–184.

Thorpy MJ. The clinical use of the multiple sleep latency test. *Sleep*. 1992;15:268–276.

Tononi G, Cirelli C. Sleep and the price of plasticity: from synaptic and cellular homeostasis to memory consolidation and integration. *Neuron*. 2014;81(1):12–34.

Vignatelli L, Billiard M, Clarenback P, et al. EFNS guidelines on management of restless legs syndrome and periodic limb movement disorder in sleep. *Eur J Neurol*. 2006;13:1049–1065.

Wise MS. Narcolepsy and other disorders of excessive sleepiness. *Med Clin North Am*. 2004;88:597–610.

Wozniak DR, Lasserson TJ, Smith I. Educational, supportive and behavioural interventions to improve usage of continuous positive airway pressure machines in adults with obstructive sleep apnoea. *Cochrane Database Syst Rev*. 2014;1:CD007736.

Yaggi HK, Concato J, Kernan WN, et al. Obstructive sleep apnea as a risk factor for stroke and death. *N Engl J Med*. 2005;353(19):2034–2041.

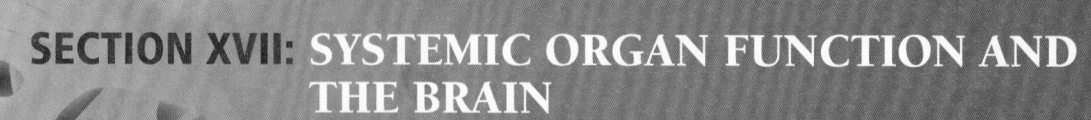

Heart–Brain Interactions 115

Shouri Lahiri and Stephan A. Mayer

INTRODUCTION

The heart–brain interaction is a vital physiologic circuit often implicated in neurologic and cardiovascular injury. Cerebral complications of cardiac procedures and stroke due to atrial arrhythmias represent important causes of neurologic disability. Recent advances and complications of cardiopulmonary support with left ventricular assist device and extracorporeal membrane oxygenation have opened the door to new neurologic diagnostic and therapeutic challenges. Conversely, severe acute brain injury is being increasingly recognized as a cause of catecholamine-mediated myocardial dysfunction, an entity that is known by many names (Table 115.1) but is most accurately described as *neurogenic stunned myocardium*.

Autonomic storming is similarly caused by exaggerated sympathetic effect after brain injury and is characterized by cardiovascular abnormalities including coexistent hypertension and tachycardia. Neurogenic hypotension in the absence of cardiac dysfunction usually results from abnormal vasomotor tone and is discussed in Chapter 112.

CEREBRAL COMPLICATIONS OF CARDIAC PROCEDURES

EPIDEMIOLOGY

Cerebrovascular injury is one of the most feared complications of cardiac surgery. Ischemic strokes occur in 0.8% to 5.2% of coronary artery bypass graft (CABG) surgeries, although the incidence may be decreasing with more recent publications from 2011 reporting incidence closer to 1.6%. One single-center study of more than 45,000 patients found that 40% of the strokes occurred intraoperatively with the postoperative risk for stroke peaking at 40 hours following surgery. The risk for stroke is greater for patients undergoing CABG with aortic atherosclerosis and concomitant carotid artery disease and the risk is directly proportional to the degree of stenosis. Other risk factors for perioperative stroke with CABG include atrial fibrillation, prior stroke or transient ischemic attack

TABLE 115.1	Synonyms for Neurogenic Stunned Myocardium
Takotsubo cardiomyopathy	
Apical ballooning syndrome	
Broken heart syndrome	
Stress-induced cardiomyopathy	
Contraction band necrosis	

(TIA), and female gender. Cognitive disability in the absence of acute infarct occurs in up to 70% of patients following CABG. The reported incidences of postoperative cognitive decline are widely variable and likely reflect variability of the cardiac procedure itself to differing neuropsychiatric testing methods and control groups.

Atrial fibrillation occurs in up to 40% of patients within a few days following CABG. It occurs in up to 50% of patients after valve surgery and up to 60% of patients following valve replacement plus CABG. Eleven percent of patients develop atrial fibrillation as a late complication of CABG. In the general population, the most common causes of atrial fibrillation are hypertension, coronary heart disease, and rheumatic heart disease, with the latter being uncommon in developed countries. The risk of ischemic stroke due to atrial fibrillation may be stratified using scoring systems such as CHADS$_2$, which incorporate additional risk factors for stroke including heart failure, advanced age, diabetes, prior stroke, female gender, etc. Refer to Chapter 44 for detailed discussion of stroke risk due to atrial fibrillation.

Left ventricular assist device (LVAD) and extracorporeal membrane oxygenation (ECMO) have dramatically changed the therapeutic landscape of severe, medically refractory cardiopulmonary failure. Neurologic complications are, however, common and occur in 8% to 25% of patients with LVADs. In a series from the University of Pittsburgh Medical Center, 61% of LVAD-related neurologic complications were due to embolic strokes and 25% were intracerebral hemorrhages. In another single center study from Columbia University, 14% of patients with LVADs developed neurologic complications of which 81% were either due to ischemic or hemorrhagic stroke. A recent review on LVAD-related bleeding and thrombosis from 2012 found that the incidence of ischemic strokes was 0.04 to 0.13 per patient-year and 0.05 to 0.8 per patient-year and for hemorrhagic strokes. Relatively, little has been reported on the neurologic complications of adult patients on ECMO. In one series, 50% of patients receiving ECMO suffered neurologic injury of which 17% were strokes defined as either ischemic stroke, hemorrhagic stroke, or subarachnoid hemorrhage. The frequency of neurologic events was likely underestimated in this study, as less than one-third of the patients underwent cerebral imaging.

PATHOBIOLOGY

The majority of strokes after cardiac surgery are ischemic, although hemorrhagic conversion of ischemic infarcts is possible. Intraoperative strokes occur due to arterial emboli arising from atherosclerosis of major vessels such as the aorta or carotid arteries or due to cerebral hypoperfusion resulting from intraoperative hypotension or diminished cardiac output. Fat and air emboli may also occur. Transcranial Doppler (TCD) ultrasonography monitoring of the middle cerebral artery has been used to quantify microemboli during coronary bypass surgery, which in some cases exceed 60 per operation. High-risk periods for embolization include manipulation of the heart and aorta, particularly during aortic clamping and cannulation. No causal relationship has been confirmed between number of microemboli and cognitive decline, although increased burden of new ischemic lesions has been associated with postoperative cognitive decline.

Postoperative strokes are generally cardioembolic and related to postoperative arrhythmias such as atrial or ventricular fibrillation. Cerebral complications of atrial fibrillation occur due to embolization of thrombus from the left atrium or atrial appendage. Strokes due to atrial fibrillation are more likely to cause large-vessel occlusion and hemispheric injury than embolic sources arising from the carotid arteries. This was demonstrated in a study that showed that cardioembolic etiologies of stroke were 25 times likely to cause hemispheric events than retinal events. The presumed mechanism for this difference is the larger size of cardioembolic particles compared to emboli arising from the carotid arteries.

LVADs pose extraordinary challenges related to coagulopathy. Although anticoagulation is required to decrease risk of device thrombosis and thromboembolism, this comes at the cost of increased hemorrhagic complications. Furthermore, high-shear stress conditions related to LVADs are thought to induce an acquired von Willebrand syndrome by mechanical destruction of von Willebrand multimers. As a result, LVAD patients are at higher risk for both hemorrhagic and ischemic strokes. Hemorrhagic strokes in patients with mechanical circulatory devices should raise suspicion for endocarditis. The role of infections and inflammatory milieu on neurologic complications is an ongoing debate in patients both with and without mechanical circulatory devices. In one study of LVAD patients, 42% of cerebrovascular accidents occurred in patients with infections. An elevated white blood cell count was noted in patients with neurologic complications regardless of the presence or absence of infection, although it is unclear whether this represented a stress reaction from acute brain injury. The same study found thromboelastogram abnormalities in periods with infection than without infection suggesting that infection may activate platelet function and contribute to the risk of neurologic injury.

Similar to the LVAD, anticoagulation is required to decrease the risk of ECMO-related thrombosis and thromboembolism. Also analogous to the LVAD, increased platelet activation and consumption due to exposure to foreign surface area is common, further contributing to a bleeding diathesis. The net result is a significantly increased risk of bleeding in up to 40% of patients receiving ECMO. Thromboembolic complications are more common in venoarterial compared to venovenous ECMO, as blood is infused directly to the systemic circulation with the former. Greater risk of retrograde aortic blood flow and stasis of the blood due to worsening left ventricular output also increase the risk of thrombus formation.

CLINICAL FEATURES

The clinical manifestations of post-CABG strokes (or strokes due to atrial fibrillation) reflect the dysfunction of the affected neuro-anatomic structures. Approximately 20% of strokes involve the posterior circulation. Symptoms attributable to the posterior circulation such as eye movement abnormalities, behavioral abnormalities, and cortical blindness should raise suspicion for a "top of the basilar" syndrome. Hemiparesis is not an invariable finding of post-CABG strokes, as isolated aphasia syndromes or cortical blindness is also encountered. When hemiparesis is present, it may be limited to hand or fine finger movements and mistaken for a compression neuropathy.

The clinical manifestations of LVAD- or ECMO-related stroke are similar to post-CABG stroke patients. Intracranial hemorrhagic complications related to these devices are more likely to have a more fulminant presentation with impairment in consciousness and rapid progression of symptoms.

DIAGNOSIS

Initial diagnosis of stroke is suggested by history and physical examination and then corroborated by cerebral imaging. The National Institute of Health Stroke Scale is a reliable 15-item scale that is validated as a measure of stroke impairment (see Chapter 15). Computed tomography (CT) of the brain is often used as an initial diagnostic test for intracranial hemorrhage because hyperacute ischemic changes may not be evident. Magnetic resonance imaging of the brain with diffusion-weighted imaging may detect ischemic abnormalities as early as within 3 minutes of symptom onset, however, may be contraindicated in patients with metallic devices such as LVADs and certain pacemakers. Blood cultures, fungal cultures, and transesophageal echocardiograms should be obtained when there is a suspicion for endocarditis and septic emboli and particularly in patients with mechanical circulatory devices. Cerebral angiography may be indicated to diagnose mycotic aneurysms.

TREATMENT

Prevention

It is critical to employ measures to prevent neurologic complications during cardiac surgery. Preoperative evaluation involves assessment of risk factors including carotid stenosis. The risk of stroke during cardiac surgery may be lowered by performing simultaneous carotid endarterectomy. Avoiding relative hypotension during cardiac surgery may improve outcomes. This was shown in a randomized trial of 248 patients where maintaining higher pressures (mean artery pressures 80 to 100 mm Hg vs. 50 to 60 mm Hg) during cardiopulmonary bypass was significantly associated with lower rates of neurologic and cardiac complications or death at 6 months [**Level 1**].[1] Systemic hypothermia at 32°C for closed chamber and 28°C for open chamber procedures during cardiopulmonary bypass may reduce cerebral metabolic rate and prevent ischemia. Transesophageal echocardiogram reduces the risk of intraoperative strokes by enhanced detection of aortic atheroma enabling the surgeon to alter technique to reduce risk of embolization. Electroencephalography can also be used to detect cerebral ischemia during cardiac surgery, although the use of this is debated.

Acute Ischemic Stroke

Thrombolytic therapy is often contraindicated for acute ischemic stroke during the postoperative period and in patients being treated with therapeutic levels of anticoagulation. Strokes occurring due to septic emboli from infected hardware also increase the risk of hemorrhage due to thrombolysis. Alternative reperfusion techniques including endovascular therapies may be considered in the appropriate circumstances. In patients with LVADs or patients receiving ECMO, the benefits of anticoagulation for thromboembolism need to be balanced with the risks of hemorrhagic conversion of ischemic infarct for a given patient based on stroke severity and size. There are currently limited data on the optimal time frame for restarting antithrombotics; however, significant delays in restarting these medications further increase the considerable risk of thromboembolism. Other management strategies of acute ischemic stroke are discussed in Chapter 15.

Intracranial Hemorrhage

Intracranial hemorrhage is primarily a risk of LVAD and ECMO support due to the need for anticoagulation and concurrent risk of brain embolism. Initial management should involve discontinuation of all antiplatelet medications and anticoagulation. Anticoagulation reversal should be strongly considered for life-threatening hemorrhages with the understanding that these interventions may increase the risk of device thrombosis in patients with cardiopulmonary devices. Hemostatic therapy should be tailored to the specific anticoagulant exposure (see Table 38.2). For example, protamine sulfate may be used for heparin-related intracerebral hemorrhage and vitamin K with prothrombin complex concentrate/fresh frozen plasma may be used for warfarin-related intracerebral hemorrhage. Antifibrinolytics and recombinant factor VIIa may also be considered in the appropriate clinical setting. Patients undergoing treatment with LVAD or ECMO should receive platelet transfusions and DDAVP. Blood pressure should be managed as per current guidelines (see Table 38.2). Endocarditis should be treated with antibiotics and surgical evaluation (see also Chapter 63). There is currently limited data on when to restart antithrombotics after intracerebral hemorrhage. A rational approach that balances the risk of hemorrhage expansion with the considerable benefits of thromboembolic prophylaxis based on the individual clinical circumstance is appropriate until further research is available.

OUTCOME

Perioperative stroke increases hospital mortality by up to 10-fold and long-term survival is worse among stroke survivors. A study by Tarakji et al. found that perioperative stroke decreased the likelihood of survival at 1, 10, and 20 years by 25%, 41%, and 23%, respectively.

In The Randomized Evaluation of Mechanical Assistance in Treatment of Chronic Heart Failure trial, cerebrovascular complications were the third leading cause of death (9.8%). This finding was supported by two other publications; 1 of over 1,000 LVADs where a central nervous system event was the third leading cause of mortality accounting for 14% of deaths. Little has been reported on neurologic complications of adult ECMO patients. This may be in part due to the difficulty in knowing whether the neurologic consequences are the result of the pathology prompting ECMO or related to the ECMO process itself. In one series, 63% of subjects who underwent cerebral imaging had pathologically abnormal findings, and 90% of patients who underwent brain autopsy had evidence of intracranial pathology ranging from ischemic/hemorrhagic lesions to diffuse cerebral edema. In one study of infants receiving ECMO, major intracranial hemorrhage accounted for 55% of deaths.

CARDIOVASCULAR COMPLICATIONS OF NEUROLOGIC INJURY

NEUROGENIC STUNNED MYOCARDIUM

Epidemiology

Neurogenic stunned myocardium may be defined as an acute, reversible cardiac injury commonly associated with various forms of acute brain injury including subarachnoid hemorrhage, intracerebral hemorrhage, ischemic stroke, and seizures. Electrocardiographic abnormalities are seen in up to 70% of patients with subarachnoid hemorrhage and in up to 40% of patients with intracerebral hemorrhage and ischemic stroke. Left ventricular systolic dysfunction has been found in 10% to 28% of patients with subarachnoid hemorrhage, and diastolic dysfunction is seen in up 71% of patients.

Pathobiology

Neurogenic stunned myocardium (NSM) is presumed to occur due to dysregulation of autonomic control, primarily of the sympathetic system. A proposed instigating mechanism is injury to the insular cortex or hypothalamus, which are important areas for autonomic control. Right cerebral hemispheric injury is more likely to be associated with sympathetic dysautonomia, whereas the left cerebral hemisphere predominantly causes parasympathetic responses. Similar neuroanatomic specialization was demonstrated in cats where lateral hypothalamic stimulation caused sympathetic responses such as tachycardia and ST-segment depressions, whereas anterior hypothalamic stimulation caused parasympathetic responses such as bradycardia. There is evidence that primary brain stem injury in the setting of transtentorial herniation can also produce a massive sympathetic discharge. All of these states are characterized by abnormal hyperactivity of the locus coeruleus, a nucleus in the pons that mediates sympathetic tone.

Catecholamine release and overload, primarily released by the cardiac sympathetic nerves, produces a state of overstimulation of myocardial cells with a characteristic histopathology termed *contraction band necrosis*. Affected myocardial cells are overloaded with calcium, remain hypercontracted, and no longer respond to β1-receptor agonists due to uncoupling of the adenyl cyclase secondary messenger system. For this reason, attempts to improve left ventricular contractility with exogenous catecholamines such as norepinephrine in patients with cardiogenic shock tend to be ineffective.

Clinical Features

NSM tends to occur in the setting of acute severe brain injury. Subarachnoid hemorrhage is the best known and most common cause of NSM, but the condition can develop in response to any cause of massive sympathetic outflow, including intracerebral hemorrhage, cerebral infarction with herniation; Guillain–Barré syndrome; acute hydrocephalus; traumatic brain injury; or status epilepticus, acute emotional stress, and pheochromocytoma. Mild to moderate elevations in cardiac enzymes may accompany characteristic electrocardiographic features, which include long QT intervals, widespread symmetric inverted T waves, and U waves. Left ventricular dysfunction manifests as diastolic dysfunction in mild cases. More severely affected patients develop regional left ventricular wall motion abnormalities that do not respect typical vascular territories in association with mild to moderate reduction of the left ventricular (LV) ejection fraction (20% to 40%). In fulminant cases, patient can develop acute cardiogenic shock with ejection fractions of 20% or less. The level of cardiac enzyme elevation is typically low in relation to the extent of LV dysfunction. A retrospective study to differentiate between acute coronary syndrome and NSM found troponin levels were 10-fold higher with infarcted heart (based on historic controls) compared to stunned myocardium (2.8 ng/mL vs. 0.22 ng/mL). A troponin level of less than 2.8 ng/mL and ejection fraction less than 40% in the setting of acute aneurysmal were consistent with stunned myocardium rather than acute coronary syndrome.

Acute neurogenic pulmonary edema (NPE) can occur in isolation, or in addition to, NSM. In its purest sense, NPE is thought to represent a neurally mediated noncardiogenic form of pulmonary edema characterized by disruption of the integrity of the pulmonary

FIGURE 115.1 Diagram explaining how neurogenic stunned myocardium and pulmonary edema characterized by increased pulmonary vascular permeability can coexist after subarachnoid hemorrhage and other forms of catastrophic brain injury. The unifying inciting event is a massive catecholamine discharge (*b*), which leads to concomitant decreased left ventricular contractility and leaky lung pulmonary edema after the initial phase of injury (*c*). RA, right atrium; RV, right ventricle; LA, left atrium; LV, left ventricle. (Adapted from Mayer SA, Swarup R. Neurogenic cardiac injury after subarachnoid hemorrhage. *Current Opinion Anaesth.* 1996;9:356–361.)

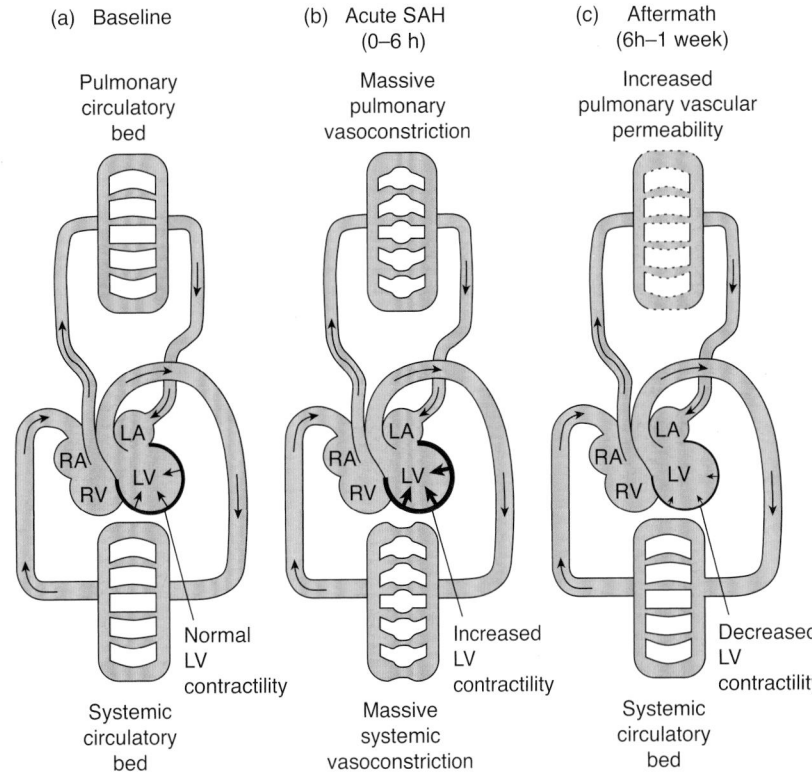

microvasculature (i.e., "leaky lung" pulmonary edema). Acute peripheral vasoconstriction has been shown to cause a massive increase in intrathoracic blood volume, which causes a "blast effect" which then leads to increased pulmonary vascular permeability (Fig. 115.1).

Diagnosis

The takotsubo variant of NSM features characteristic echocardiographic findings of apical akinesis and ballooning with left ventricular diastolic and systolic dysfunction (Video 115.1). It is important to appreciate that NSM occurs on a spectrum of variants that includes a "reverse takotsubo" pattern where the apex of the heart is normal and the base is hypokinetic (Video 115.2). If clinical suspicion is high for acute coronary syndrome, coronary angiography may be required to definitively exclude underlying coronary artery disease. Serial echocardiography by definition shows progressive improvement and eventual normalization of LV function over days to weeks.

Treatment and Outcome

Patients with severe acute intracranial pathology should have continuous electrocardiographic monitoring for at least 72 hours and cardiac enzymes should be obtained. Management should be focused on treating the underlying cause of the neurogenic stunning such as securing the ruptured aneurysm. Euvolemia should be maintained using isotonic intravenous fluids as needed. There is evidence from cohort studies that NSM is less common among subarachnoid hemorrhage patients previously on β-blockers; for this reason, there may be some rationale for use of the β1-blocker esmolol (starting at 50 μg/kg/min, titrated to attain heart rate below 100 beats per minute). When cardiac function is significantly diminished, inotropic vasopressors or inotropes such as norepinephrine, dobutamine, and milrinone may be required to augment cardiac output. There is

evidence that milrinone, a phosphodiesterase inhibitor, is a more effective inotrope than norepinephrine because it bypasses β1 receptors, which are prone to receptor desensitization. NPE tends to be fragile and often responds to gentle diuresis with furosemide. Reversibility is a hallmark feature of NSM and echocardiographic abnormalities usually improve within days.

PAROXYSMAL SYMPATHETIC STORMING

Synonyms for paroxysmal sympathetic storming include autonomic storming, paroxysmal dysautonomia (PDA), autonomic dysfunction syndrome, hypothalamic–midbrain dysregulation syndrome, paroxysmal autonomic instability with dystonia (PAID), and neurostorming. The condition is characterized by irregular, recurrent violent sympathetic discharges in the acute or subacute phase of severe brain injury in the intensive care unit.

Epidemiology

Paroxysmal sympathetic storming occurs in up to 33% of patients with severe traumatic brain injury and severe diffuse axonal shearing injury and is also relatively common in patients with anoxic brain injury. It is less frequently seen in poor-grade subarachnoid hemorrhage, coma resulting from intracerebral hemorrhage, malignant middle cerebral artery infarction syndrome, and in patients with brain stem pathology. It seems to be more common in younger patients.

Clinical Features

Autonomic storming presents with paroxysmal episodes of hypertension and tachycardia, fever, hyperventilation, diaphoresis, extensor posturing, and severe dystonia. The onset typically occurs days to weeks after the original brain injury event. The posturing and dystonia may at times resemble generalized seizures consistent with prior descriptions of autonomic storming as "diencephalic seizures."

TABLE 115.2	Diagnostic Criteria for Paroxysmal Sympathetic Storming

Four of the following, occurring in episodic surges at intervals of 30 min to 4 h:

- Fever (>38.3°C)
- Tachycardia (120 beats/min or 100 beats/min if on β-blockers)
- Tachypnea (respiratory rate >30 breaths/min)[a]
- Hypertension (systolic blood pressure >160 mm Hg or pulse pressure >80 mm Hg)
- Diaphoresis
- Extensor posturing or motor dystonia
- Severe dystonia

[a]In the absence of sepsis or airway obstruction.

Diagnosis

Autonomic storming is a clinical diagnosis. A diagnostic algorithm is summarized in Table 115.2. One of the easiest ways to make the diagnosis is to establish the presence of episodic parallel urges in blood pressure and heart rate when reviewing vital signs over 24 hours on a bedside monitor. Seizures may need to be excluded using continuous video electroencephalography because the episodes are often paroxysmal. Autonomic storming may need to be differentiated from the typical pressor response to elevated intracranial pressure or cerebral ischemia, which is a common compensatory sequel of acute brain injury and likely reflects efforts to maintain adequate cerebral perfusion pressure in the face of elevated intracranial pressure.

Management

Management of sympathetic storming is focused on brain sedation, analgesics that blunt nociceptive inputs that trigger storms, agents that specifically suppress the locus coeruleus, and blunting of the peripheral manifestations of hypertension and tachycardia with β-blockers. Acute control of severe symptoms can be quickly attained with infusion of propofol (50 to 200 μg/kg/min), fentanyl (50 to 100 mg/h), or dexmedetomidine (0.7 to 1.4 μg/kg/h) alone or in combination (Fig. 115.2).

Pharmacotherapeutic options to control symptoms and allow weaning of analgosedative infusions in the intensive care unit (ICU) are summarized in Table 115.3. These agents should be started sequentially and evaluated during daily interruptions of continuous intravenous (IV) analgosedation. Concurrent use of IV antihypertensive agents such as nicardipine or labetalol is rarely needed after IV sedative agents have been administered. It is important to realize that neurogenic autohypertension is fragile and can be easily overtreated and result in impaired cerebral perfusion pressure. As such, antihypertensive medications may need to be started at lower doses and titrated up while monitoring response.

Outcome

Paroxysmal sympathetic storming typically persists for weeks to months before it resolves. Storming treated with prolonged IV infusions of analgosedatives such as propofol and fentanyl leads to increased ICU length of stay and a concomitant increase in the risk of hospital-acquired infections and complications. Outcome can be improved by aggressively advancing the agents used for subacute to chronic control of symptoms in Table 115.3, which allows discontinuation of IV sedation, liberation from the ventilator, and advancement to rehabilitation.

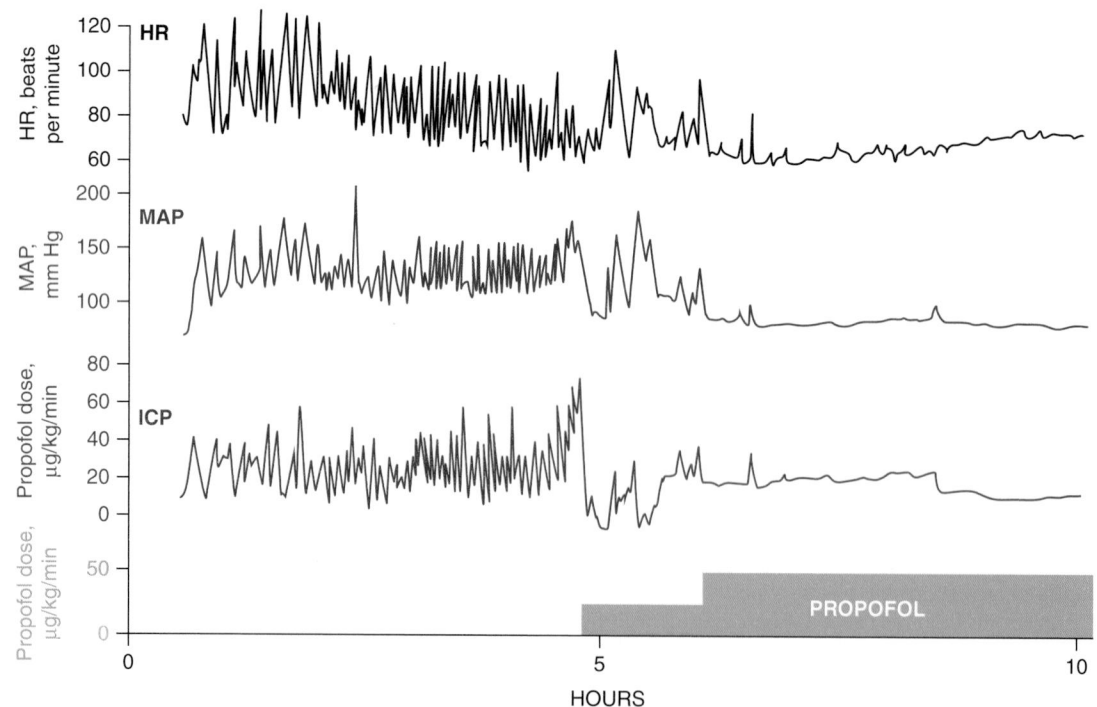

FIGURE 115.2 Suppression and stabilization of sympathetic storming with propofol infusion in a patient with paroxysmal sympathetic storming. Note the immediate stabilizing effect on intracranial pressure, which fell from levels as high as 70 mm Hg to normal at the start of the infusion. HR, heart rate; MAP, mean arterial pressure; ICP, intracranial pressure.

TABLE 115.3	Pharmacotherapy for Paroxysmal Sympathetic Storming during the Subacute to Chronic Phase
Analgosedatives	• Fentanyl patch 25–300 μg/h
	• Morphine (Roxanol, MS Contin) 5–20 mg q4h
	• Lorazepam 2–24 mg/day
	• Klonopin 1–8 mg/day
β-Blockers	• Propranolol 160–640 mg/day
	• Labetalol 400–3,600 mg/day
Central antiadrenergic agonists	• Clonidine PATCH 0.1–0.9 mg/day
	• Bromocriptine 10–40 mg/day
Muscle relaxants	• Baclofen 10 mg t.i.d.
	• Dantrolene PO 25–100 mg q.i.d.
Anticonvulsants	• Gabapentin 900–3,600 mg/day

Videos can be found in the companion e-book edition. For a full list of video legends, please see the front matter.

LEVEL 1 EVIDENCE

1. Gold JP, Charlson ME, Williams-Russo P, et al. Improvement of outcomes after coronary artery bypass. A randomized trial comparing intraoperative high versus low mean arterial pressure. *J Thorac Cardiovasc Surg.* 1995;110(5):1302–1311.

SUGGESTED READINGS

Neurologic Complications of Cardiac Interventions

Barber PA, Hach S, Tippett LJ, et al. Cerebral ischemic lesions on diffusion-weighted imaging are associated with neurocognitive decline after cardiac surgery. *Stroke.* 2008;39(5):1427–1433.

Biswas AK, Lewis L, Sommerauer JF. Aprotinin in the management of life-threatening bleeding during extracorporeal life support. *Perfusion.* 2000;15(3):211–216.

Eckman PM, John R. Bleeding and thrombosis in patients with continuous-flow ventricular assist devices. *Circulation.* 2012;19;125(24):3038–3047.

Filsoufi F, Rahmanian PB, Castillo JG, et al. Incidence, topography, predictors and long-term survival after stroke in patients undergoing coronary artery bypass grafting. *Ann Thorac Surg.* 2008;85(3):862–870.

Kato TS, Schulze PC, Yang J, et al. Pre-operative and post-operative risk factors associated with neurologic complications in patients with advanced heart failure supported by a left ventricular assist device. *J Heart Lung Transplant.* 2012;31(1):1–8.

Maisel WH, Rawn JD, Stevenson WG. Atrial fibrillation after cardiac surgery. *Ann Intern Med.* 2001;135(12):1061–1073.

Mateen FJ, Muralidharan R, Shinohara RT, et al. Neurological injury in adults treated with extracorporeal membrane oxygenation. *Arch Neurol.* 2011;68(12):1543–1549.

McKhann GM, Grega MA, Borowicz LM Jr, et al. Stroke and encephalopathy after cardiac surgery: an update. *Stroke.* 2006;37(2):562–571.

Selnes OA, Gottesman RF, Grega MA, et al. Cognitive and neurologic outcomes after coronary-artery bypass surgery. *N Engl J Med.* 2012;366(3):250–257.

Selnes OA, McKhann GM. Neurocognitive complications after coronary artery bypass surgery. *Ann Neurol.* 2005;57(5):615–621.

Tarakji KG, Sabik JF III, Bhudia SK, et al. Temporal onset, risk factors, and outcomes associated with stroke after coronary artery bypass grafting. *JAMA.* 2011;305(4):381–390.

Tsukui H, Abla A, Teuteberg JJ, et al. Cerebrovascular accidents in patients with a ventricular assist device. *J Thorac Cardiovasc Surg.* 2007;134(1):114–123.

Wittenstein B, Ng C, Ravn H, et al. Recombinant factor VII for severe bleeding during extracorporeal membrane oxygenation following open heart surgery. *Pediatr Crit Care Med.* 2005;6(4):473–476.

Neurogenic Stunned Myocardium

Guglin M, Novotorova I. Neurogenic stunned myocardium and takotsubo cardiomyopathy are the same syndrome: a pooled analysis. *Congest Heart Fail.* 2011;17(3):127–132.

Mayer SA, Fink ME, Homma S, et al. Cardiac injury associated with neurogenic pulmonary edema following subarachnoid hemorrhage. *Neurology.* 1994;44:815–820.

Melville KI, Blum B, Shister HE, et al. Cardiac ischemic changes and arrhythmias induced by hypothalamic stimulation. *Am J Cardiol.* 1963;12:781–791.

Murthy SB, Shah S, Rao CP, et al. Neurogenic stunned myocardium following acute subarachnoid hemorrhage pathophysiology and practical considerations [published online ahead of print November 7, 2013]. *J Intensive Care Med.*

Nguyen H, Zaroff JG. Neurogenic stunned myocardium. *Curr Neurol Neurosci Rep.* 2009;9(6):486–491.

Oppenheimer SM, Gelb A, Girvin JP, et al. Cardiovascular effects of human insular cortex stimulation. *Neurology.* 1992;42(9):1727–1732.

Samuels MA. The brain-heart connection. *Circulation.* 2007;116(1):77–84.

Wittstein IS, Thiemann DR, Lima JA, et al. Neurohumoral features of myocardial stunning due to sudden emotional stress. *N Engl J Med.* 2005;352:539–548.

Sympathetic Storming

Blackman JA, Patrick PD, Buck ML, et al. Paroxysmal autonomic instability with dystonia after brain injury. *Archives of Neurology.* 2004;61(3):321–328.

Boeve BF, Wijdicks EF, Benarroch EE, et al. Paroxysmal sympathetic storms ("diencephalic seizures") after severe diffuse axonal head injury. *Mayo Clin Proc.* 1998;73(2):148–152.

Perkes I, Baguley IJ, Nott MT, et al. A review of paroxysmal sympathetic hyperactivity after acquired brain injury. *Ann Neurol.* 2010;68(2):126–135.

Rabinstein AA. Paroxysmal sympathetic hyperactivity in the neurological intensive care unit. *Neurol Res.* 2007;29(7):680–682.

Rossitch E Jr, Bullard DE. The autonomic dysfunction syndrome: aetiology and treatment. *Br J Neurosurg.* 1988;2(4):471–478.

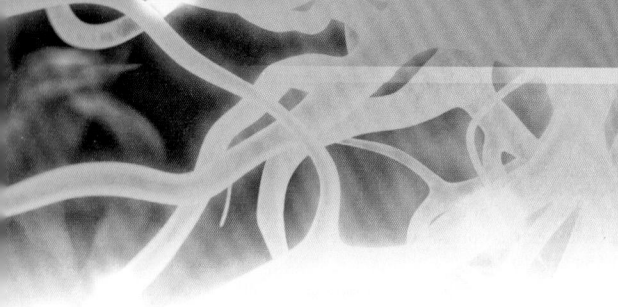

INTRODUCTION

Much of the high morbidity and mortality from acute neurologic disorders results from abnormalities of breathing. Respiratory abnormalities can themselves worsen neurologic injury, whereas neurologic abnormalities conversely predispose to aspiration, impaired airway clearance, atelectasis, and pneumonia. In stroke, traumatic brain injury, status epilepticus, Guillain–Barré syndrome, myasthenia gravis, and many other neurologic disorders, oropharyngeal and respiratory muscle weakness predispose to aspiration of secretions into the airways, mucus plugging, hypoventilation, atelectasis, and pneumonia. Accordingly, respiratory monitoring and support are among the most common indications for the admission of neurologic patients to an intensive care unit (ICU).

RESPIRATORY PHYSIOLOGY AND PATHOPHYSIOLOGY

PULMONARY GAS EXCHANGE

Hypoxemia is characterized by reduced oxygen content of the bloodstream. Hypoxemia is caused by five conditions: (1) a low inspired oxygen concentration, (2) alveolar hypoventilation, or impaired gas exchange within the lungs due to (3) ventilation–perfusion (V/Q) mismatching, (4) transpulmonary or intracardiac right-to-left shunting, or (5) impaired diffusion of gases between the alveoli and the capillaries. It can also be caused by low mixed venous oxygen saturation.

Impaired gas exchange can be quantified by measuring the gradient between the partial pressure of oxygen in the alveoli and the arterial blood (the A/a gradient, which is normally <20 mm Hg) or the P/F ratio, which is the partial pressure of oxygen in the arterial blood (PaO_2, normally 90 to 100 mm Hg) divided by the fraction of inspired oxygen (FiO_2, normally 21% in room air). Alveolar oxygen tension (PaO_2) can be calculated from the equation $PaO_2 = (FiO_2 \times 713) - (PaCO_2/0.8)$, where $PaCO_2$ is the arterial carbon dioxide tension.

The cause of impaired gas exchange leading to hypoxemia can be differentiated according to the response to supplemental oxygen. *Shunting*, defined as hypoxia unresponsive to oxygen supplementation, results from the direct transfer of deoxygenated venous blood into the arterial circulation through an intracardiac atrial septal defect, pulmonary arteriovenous malformation, or perfused but nonventilated lung parenchyma (i.e., dense airspace consolidation due to pneumonia). With V/Q mismatching, ventilation and perfusion relationships are heterogeneously deranged, but systemic oxygenation improves in response to a higher FiO_2. Diffusion abnormalities are characterized by abnormalities of the intra-alveolar septae, which may be fibrotic (i.e., interstitial lung disease), reduced in number and surface area (i.e., emphysema), and inflamed or edematous (i.e., acute respiratory distress syndrome, congestive heart failure). Low inhaled FiO_2 is typical of extreme altitude but can also result from equipment malfunction such as rebreathing of exhaled gases.

Hypercarbia results from impaired alveolar ventilation and is caused by some combination of inadequate "bellows function" of the lung (characterized by reduced minute ventilation, the product of the respiratory rate and tidal volume), increased carbon dioxide production, and impaired gas exchange. Hypoventilation can only be mechanism of hypoxia when concomitant hypercarbia is present.

RESPIRATORY FAILURE

The diagnosis of *respiratory failure* depends on arterial blood gas analysis and on the chronicity of the event. Three separate processes can contribute to the development of respiratory failure: (1) hypoxia, which results from impaired gas exchange in the lung; (2) ventilatory failure, which results from inadequate ability to move air into and out of the lungs; and (3) failure to protect the upper airway, which can result in airflow obstruction or aspiration of secretions, food, or gastric contents.

Chronic respiratory failure is said to be present when a patient cannot maintain adequate oxygenation (PaO_2 >59 mm Hg) or ventilation (PCO_2 <50 mm Hg) without supplemental oxygen or ventilatory assistance. In contrast, *acute hypoxemic respiratory failure* describes a state in which adequate oxygenation cannot be maintained despite supplemental oxygen delivery. In these patients, positive pressure ventilation and supplemental oxygen administered through an endotracheal tube or by noninvasive positive pressure ventilation are required to maintain normal oxygenation of arterial blood. In the hospital, hypoxemia can be easily and noninvasively diagnosed and monitored by measuring the percent oxygen saturation of hemoglobin in the blood (SpO_2). The clinical hallmark of hypoxemic respiratory failure is cyanosis.

Hypercarbic respiratory failure may be clinically obvious, as seen when the accessory muscles of respiration are activated and the patient appears "working hard to breathe" or can be subtle, manifest only by decreased mental acuity, myoclonus, confusion, agitation, or lethargy. Acute hypercapnia leads to acidosis and cerebral vasodilatation, which in turn can cause depressed level of consciousness ("CO_2 narcosis"), aggravation of elevated intracranial pressure (ICP), and blunted respiratory drive, leading to further hypoventilation. Arterial blood gas analysis is the most reliable method for diagnosing hypercarbic respiratory failure, but end-tidal carbon dioxide monitoring has gained popularity as a noninvasive method to monitor changes in alveolar carbon dioxide tension.

Failure of airway protection is diagnosed clinically when patients appear to be aspirating oral secretions, cannot maintain the upper airway open for gas exchange, have a rapid neurologic decline with a diminished gag and cough reflexes, or are experiencing repeated oxyhemoglobin desaturation due to intermittent plugging of the airways by secretions. Under unstable conditions, such as during a period of acute neurologic instability or during patient transport between hospitals or departments, it is advisable to intubate these patients and start mechanical ventilation to prevent sudden respiratory decompensation. Conversely, it may be safe to extubate such patients later in their hospital course under controlled

TABLE 116.1   Pulmonary Function Tests in Neuromuscular Respiratory Failure

	Normal	Criteria for Intubation and Weaning	Criteria for Extubation
Vital capacity (mL/kg)	40–70	15	25
Maximal inspiratory pressure (cm H2O)	>80	20	40
Maximal expiratory pressure (cm H2O)	>140	40	50

Adapted from Mayer SA. Intensive care of the myasthenic patient. *Neurology.* 1997;48(suppl 5):S70–S75.

circumstances, despite significantly decreased mental status. There is no absolute measure of adequate upper airway protection, and unfortunately, such determinations remain for most part subjective.

The pathophysiology of neuromuscular respiratory failure resembles a vicious cycle. Increased mucus production and/or weak cough leads to mucus plugging and atelectasis, which in turn cause decreased efficiency of ventilation. Hypoxemia usually precedes hypercapnia because atelectasis and V/Q mismatching are an early development. As fever and infection develop, carbon dioxide production increases, and ventilatory needs rise. The downward spiral of increasing carbon dioxide production, decreasing efficiency of ventilation, and progressive mucus plugging and atelectasis ultimately results in hypercarbia and respiratory failure. As ventilation fails, rapid shallow breathing and hypercapnia develop. At this stage, ventilatory reserves are exhausted, and there is the danger of sudden life-threatening hypoxemia, respiratory acidosis, or respiratory arrest.

EFFECTS OF RESPIRATORY COMPROMISE ON NEUROLOGIC INJURY

Many types of neurologic injury are exacerbated by respiratory compromise. Carbon dioxide and pH are powerful determinants of cerebral vascular tone, and the intended or unintended effects of hyperventilation (decreased cerebral blood flow, decreased intracranial blood volume, and decreased ICP) should be anticipated and monitored by clinicians. Conversely, hypoventilation and hypercapnia cause cerebral vasodilation and increased ICP. Hyperoxia is a potent exacerbant of reperfusion injury, whereas hypoxia is strongly associated with worse outcome in stroke, hypoxic–ischemic encephalopathy, and traumatic brain injury. Finally, when work of breathing is markedly increased, up to 50% of the cardiac output may be diverted to the respiratory muscles, driving metabolic stress, and potentially "stealing" blood flow from the ischemic brain or spinal cord. This metabolic stressor can be effectively managed by sedation, intubation, and initiation of full mechanical ventilatory support.

PULMONARY FUNCTION TESTING

Pulmonary function testing should be routinely used to monitor respiratory function in patients with neuromuscular respiratory compromise (Table 116.1). Arterial blood gases and end-tidal carbon dioxide monitoring are helpful, but abnormalities of gas exchange usually develop later in the cycle of respiratory decompensation and are therefore insensitive for early detection of ventilatory decline. Forced vital capacity (FVC), the volume of air exhaled after maximal inspiration and exhalation, normally ranges from 40 to 70 mL/kg. Reduction in vital capacity to 30 mL/kg is associated with a weak cough, accumulation of oropharyngeal secretions,

atelectasis, and nocturnal hypoxemia. FVC below 15 mL/kg (1 L in a 70-kg person) is the level at which invasive or noninvasive ventilatory support should be considered (Table 116.2). Maximal inspiratory pressure (MIP), normally more than 80 cm H$_2$O, measures the strength of the diaphragm and other muscles of inspiration and generally reflects the ability to maintain normal lung expansion and avoid atelectasis, whereas maximal expiratory pressure (MEP), normally more than 140 cm H$_2$O, measures the strength of the muscles of expiration and correlates with cough and the ability to clear secretions from the airway.

MANAGEMENT OF RESPIRATORY FAILURE

EXAMINATION

The initial management of the patient with impending respiratory failure is directed toward assessing the adequacy of oxygenation and ventilation, workload and stability of breathing, and assessment of the airway. In patients with fulminant respiratory failure, intubation can be lifesaving and is preferentially performed under safe, controlled circumstances well before the threat of impending cardiopulmonary arrest.

The patient's overall comfort and anxiety levels and the rate of progression of respiratory compromise should be assessed. Hypoxia is usually easy to diagnose with pulse oximetry and arterial blood gas analysis. Hypoventilation and hypercarbia may be present without distress or increased work of breathing if central respiratory drive is compromised, whereas increased respiratory

TABLE 116.2   Criteria for Intubation and Mechanical Ventilation

- PaO$_2$ <70 mm Hg with maximal oxygen delivery by face mask
- PaCO$_2$ >50 mm Hg associated with acidosis (pH <7.35), which cannot be rapidly and durably reversed
- Severe oropharyngeal paresis or decreased level of arousal with inability to protect or maintain the airway
- Need for deep sedation or general anesthesia to control seizures or elevated ICP
- Maximal inspiratory pressure <25 cm H$_2$O or FVC <15 mL/kg
- Respiratory rate >35 breaths/min or visibly excessive work of breathing

These physiologic criteria are intended to serve only as guidelines; treatment decisions must be individualized. As a general rule, intubation in neurologic patients with impending respiratory failure should be performed *before* significant blood gas abnormalities develop.

PaO$_2$, partial pressure of oxygen; PaCO$_2$, partial pressure of carbon dioxide; pH, potential of hydrogen; ICP, intracranial pressure; FVC, forced vital capacity.

effort with intact respiratory drive manifests as respiratory alkalosis. Sidestream end-tidal carbon dioxide monitoring, less well established than oximetry but effective, is increasingly used to provide early warning of hypoventilation in patients at risk. Rapid, shallow breathing, the use of accessory muscles of the neck and the shoulder, and visible gulping or gasping with inability to generate adequate tidal volumes are signs of respiratory muscle fatigue and impending collapse, although such signs may be absent when central respiratory drive is impaired. Diaphragmatic strength can be estimated by palpating for normal outward movement of the abdomen with inspiration; with severe diaphragmatic paralysis, inspiration is associated with spontaneous inward movement of the diaphragm (abdominal paradox). Activation of respiratory muscles during the expiratory phase often indicates airflow obstruction.

When neuromuscular weakness is present, ventilatory reserves can be assessed by checking the patient's ability to count from 1 to 20 in a single breath. The strength of the patient's cough should be noted. A wet gurgled voice and pooled oropharyngeal secretions are clinical signs of dysphagia and ongoing aspiration. When severe, weakness of the glottic and oropharyngeal muscles can lead to stridor, which indicates possibly life-threatening obstruction of the upper airway.

Dysphagia is assessed by asking the patient to sip 3 ounces of water; coughing is diagnostic of aspiration, and if present, oral feeding should be avoided until swallowing can be formally assessed. Patients with decreased cough and gag reflexes, however, may have aspiration without obvious clinical signs. Clinicians should have a low threshold to arrange for formal swallowing evaluation in patients with bulbar dysfunction.

NONINVASIVE POSITIVE PRESSURE VENTILATION

Mechanical ventilatory support is the primary treatment of respiratory failure. If airway protection is adequate and the patient is relatively cooperative, noninvasive positive pressure ventilation (NPPV) administered via a snug-fitting face mask should be considered. In medical patients with an acute exacerbation or chronic obstructive pulmonary disease or congestive heart failure, NPPV has fewer complications than invasive mechanical ventilation. In neurologic patients, the use of NPPV is becoming increasingly common as an initial intervention for early neuromuscular respiratory failure from myasthenic exacerbation and in others with chronic neuromuscular weakness and acute respiratory disease. Its

use in Guillain–Barré syndrome is suspected, however, with mixed results and some concerns about safety due to the potential for respiratory arrest.

Among patients with neuromuscular weakness, early use of NPPV maintains lung expansion, reduces the work of breathing, and minimizes the risk of severe respiratory failure requiring intubation. Only patients with adequate airway protective reflexes should be treated, and NPPV should *not* be used as a substitute for endotracheal intubation when acute respiratory failure is severe or complete elimination of the work of breathing is desirable. NPPV requires close observation in a monitored setting and the availability of rapid intubation in the event of respiratory decompensation. Many clinicians prefer the security of invasive mechanical ventilation with an endotracheal tube (ETT) or tracheostomy, but neurologists should be aware that in ICUs where high-quality, safe NPPV can be provided; it is often strongly preferred by patients and reduces the incidence of hospital-acquired infections, the need for sedation and analgesia, and the length of ICU stay. NPPV should be used in conjunction with mechanical cough assist devices to aid in airway clearance—a combination that effectively treats mucus plugging and atelectasis and keeps many patients off the ventilator.

ENDOTRACHEAL INTUBATION AND MECHANICAL VENTILATION

Indications for endotracheal intubation due to respiratory failure may include compromised ventilation or oxygenation, the need for airway protection, or both. For patients needing endotracheal intubation, clinicians should consider the patient's comfort level, as well as intracranial and arterial pressures. IV access should be obtained prior to intubation and infusion because sedation and positive pressure ventilation may cause a precipitous drop in BP. All patients should be preoxygenated with an FiO_2 of 100% prior to intubation, and in patients with elevated ICP, mild hyperventilation should be considered before lowering the head of the bed, and extra efforts made to avoid hypoventilation.

Special concerns related to the intubation of neurologic patients are described in Table 116.3.

The administration of 50 to 100 mg of IV lidocaine immediately before intubation blunts the anticipated rise in ICP. *Rapid sequence intubation* involves administration of a combination of IV sedatives (i.e., etomidate or fentanyl), amnestics (i.e., midazolam), and muscle relaxants (i.e., vecuronium); depolarizing muscle relaxants

TABLE 116.3	Intubation and Respiratory Concerns Specific to Patients with Neurologic Disease	
Problem	Assessment	Management
Elevated ICP	Mass lesion, cerebral edema, hydrocephalus	Preadministration of mannitol or hypertonic saline solution, minimize head-flat positioning, adequate analgesia and sedation, avoidance of hypoventilation
Brain ischemia	Acute stroke with penumbra	Administration of fluids and/or vasopressors, avoidance of vasodilators, end-tidal CO_2 monitoring, avoidance of hyperventilation
Cervical spine injury or instability	Mechanism of injury suggesting cervical spine injury or radiographic injury	In-line spinal stabilization Intubation techniques to minimize anteroposterior cord displacement
Ischemia-reperfusion injury	Minimize biochemical harm	Normalize oxygenation (keep PaO_2 60–300 mm Hg) and ventilation (keep $PaCO_2$ 30–50 mm Hg or $ETCO_2$ 30–45 mm Hg)

ICP, intracranial pressure; CO_2, carbon dioxide; PaO_2, partial pressure of oxygen; $PaCO_2$, partial pressure of carbon dioxide; $ETCO_2$, end-tidal carbon dioxide.

TABLE 116.4	Ventilator Modes and Functions
Abbreviation	**Stands for Description**
SIMV	Synchronized intermittent mandatory ventilation
CMV	Continuous mandatory ventilation
PS	Pressure support
CPAP	Continuous positive airway pressure
PEEP	Positive end-expiratory pressure

such as succinylcholine should be avoided in patients suffering from immobility or paresis because of a possibly abrupt rise in serum potassium level after drug-induced muscle depolarization. The trachea may be intubated orally or nasally; a high-volume, low-pressure cuff is then inflated in the trachea to prevent leakage of air and secretions around the tube.

Modes of mechanical ventilatory support include volume- and pressure-cycled ventilation, pressure support with continuous positive airway pressure (CPAP), and many others (Table 116.4). Although no ventilatory mode is intrinsically superior to the others, in general, patients should be ventilated according to the basic principles of lung-protective ventilation to avoid ventilator-induced lung injury (VILI). Lung-protective ventilation endeavors to minimize barotrauma and volutrauma due to overdistention of aerated lung segments, trauma from atelectasis due to repetitive opening and closing of collapsed alveoli, and biotrauma due to inflammation. This is accomplished by minimizing peak and plateau airway pressures (goal <30 cm H_2O), providing positive end-expiratory pressure (PEEP) to prevent alveolar collapse at end-expiration and to recruit collapsed lung units, limiting exposure to toxic levels of oxygen and using small tidal volumes (4 to 6 mL/kg of *ideal* body weight) to prevent overdistention of vulnerable alveolar units. In general, "permissive" hypercapnia and hypoxia—part of most "lung protective ventilation" protocols—should be employed cautiously and after consideration of the effects of dysventilation on neurophysiology. Unless required for control of elevated intracranial pressure, prolonged uninterrupted "deep" sedation and paralysis are discouraged because spontaneous respiratory efforts by the patient prevent dependent atelectasis and respiratory muscle atrophy.

MANIPULATION OF VENTILATION: EFFECTS ON INTRACRANIAL PRESSURE AND CEREBRAL BLOOD FLOW

Hyperventilation results in acute hypocarbia and respiratory alkalosis. This causes arteriolar constriction in the brain, leading immediately to decreased cerebral blood flow and lower intracranial pressure (ICP). Conversely, hypoventilation results in hypercarbia and cerebral arteriolar dilation, causing increased cerebral blood flow and intracranial pressure. These physiologic responses are frequently manipulated to treat elevations of intracranial pressure and because of the potential for harm should be carefully monitored in patients with impaired cerebral perfusion or elevated ICP.

Hyperventilation is a powerful tool to reverse critical increases in ICP and is a standard measure to reverse uncal or transtentorial herniation syndromes. The negative effects of hyperventilation on cerebral blood flow prohibit prolonged and excessive usage unless

brain oxygenation is concurrently monitored (see Chapter 33). Hyperventilation should not be used at all when active brain ischemia is present, such as in acute large vessel stroke or cerebral vasospasm. In addition to the danger of precipitating brain ischemia, prolonged hyperventilation is rarely effective as a treatment for elevated ICP, as compensatory mechanisms in the central nervous system rapidly buffer the pH changes in peripheral pH, and CBF is restored. Hyperventilation below a PCO_2 of 20 mm Hg causes progressive hemodynamic deterioration but does not result in additional arterial constriction or reduction in ICP. It is not known whether spontaneous hyperventilation puts the brain at risk of ischemia or whether it simply reflects a physiologic compensatory mechanism at work.

End-tidal carbon dioxide ($ETCO_2$) tension correlates modestly well with the partial pressure of alveolar carbon dioxide, and inline $ETCO_2$ can be monitored as a continuous vital sign in mechanically ventilated patients, whereas sidestream $ETCO_2$ is used to monitor alveolar carbon dioxide tension in nonintubated patients. $ETCO_2$ tends to run slightly lower than arterial PCO_2; differences between the two measurements reflect not only dead space ventilation but also increasing age, chronic obstructive pulmonary disease (COPD), and circumstances in which alveolar dead space increases such as hypovolemia, pulmonary embolism, and a low cardiac output state.

PREVENTION OF VENTILATOR-ASSOCIATED PNEUMONIA

Ventilator-associated pneumonia (VAP) is the most common and serious complication of endotracheal intubation. The endotracheal tube serves as a conduit for bacterial invasion of the airway and deep lung segments and compromises natural defenses against infection. About 20% of patients who are intubated for more than 1 week develop VAP, which adds an average of 1 week to the ICU length of stay, $40,000 to the cost of care, and carries an attributable mortality exceeding 30%. The clinical diagnosis is established by the appearance of a new pulmonary infiltrate on chest radiography more than 48 hours after intubation and the new onset of fever, leukocytosis, or purulent secretions. Neurologic patients are at particularly high risk for VAP because they are immobile and tend to aspirate.

A standardized protocol of measures that minimize bacterial colonization of the upper airway and digestive tract and the risk of aspiration can reduce the risk of VAP. These measures include 30-degree head elevation to minimize gastric regurgitation, mouth care with chlorhexidine-based solutions, avoidance of unnecessary antibiotics, and removal of the ETT as soon as possible by combining daily interruption of sedation with spontaneous breathing trials (SBTs). Some ICUs employ selective gut decontamination or prophylactic antibiotics in patients with neurologic disease to decrease the incidence of respiratory infections, but these measures are not widely recommended and require further study.

WEANING FROM MECHANICAL VENTILATION

Weaning from mechanical ventilation is a continuous process that should begin as soon as a moderate level of medical and respiratory stability is achieved. Although excessive work of breathing should be avoided as a stressor in patients with neurologic or cardiac ischemia, respiratory work is necessary to prevent muscle atrophy, and the duration of mechanical ventilation is strongly correlated with the development of VAP and other medical complications.

TABLE 116.5 Contraindications to a Daily Spontaneous Breathing Trial

- FiO_2 >80%, PEEP >10 cm H_2O, or high risk of lung derecruitment in severe ARDS
- Deep sedation or paralysis for control of seizures, ICP, or shivering
- Active and clinically important brain or myocardial ischemia
- Severe and unstable cerebral vasospasm

FiO_2, fraction of inspired oxygen; PEEP, positive end-expiratory pressure; ARDS, acute respiratory distress syndrome; ICP, intracranial pressure.

Ventilator weaning should be delayed in only dire circumstances (Table 116.5).

Weaning of mechanical ventilation begins with the downward titration of FiO_2 and mean airway pressure to levels consistent with spontaneous ventilation and face mask oxygen delivery. This is typically consistent with an FiO_2 of 40% and PEEP of 5 cm H_2O. Compared to gradually reducing the respiratory rate using synchronized mandatory ventilation or the level of pressure support triggered by each breath, the best results are obtained through the use of daily SBTs. SBTs vary widely in design but reflect a measured period of breathing in which most or all of the work of breathing is performed by the patient and after which a protocolized assessment is performed to determine suitability for the discontinuation of mechanical ventilation. The most common types of SBTs involve placing the patient on CPAP with a low-level pressure support (usually 5 cm H_2O) sufficient to overcome ETT resistance and T-piece trials, in which the patient breathes spontaneously for a predetermined duration through an open tubing system with oxygen flow-by.

The ability of the patient to tolerate a T-piece or CPAP trial for 2 hours, while maintaining a ratio of respiratory rate (breaths/minute) to tidal volume (liters) less than 100, is a useful predictor of successful extubation. In patients with depressed level of consciousness or neuromuscular respiratory weakness, the ability to tolerate a T-piece or CPAP ventilation overnight offers additional reassurance that the patient has adequate stamina to tolerate breathing off the ventilator indefinitely. Indications of tiring during an SBT include an increasing respiratory rate with decreasing tidal volumes, a drop in arterial oxygen saturation, diaphoresis, the progressive use of accessory muscles of respiration, or hemodynamic instability. Failure of a weaning trial is a physiologic stressor, and patients with these signs should be returned to mechanical ventilation.

In patients with tracheostomy or receiving NPPV, detachment from and reconnection to the ventilator is uneventful and easy to perform. Extubation and reintubation, however, always entail risk. Before a planned extubation, the patient's volume status, airway reactivity, secretions, and cardiac function should be optimized (Table 116.6). Despite the best predictors of successful extubation, it is not possible to evaluate the airway itself prior to extubation. Even with careful patient selection and medical optimization, as many as 20% of extubated patients are reintubated within 48 hours, and patients with neurologic diseases are among the most difficult to predict.

TRACHEOSTOMY

Clinicians have traditionally performed tracheostomy when mechanical ventilation has been used for more than 14 days. Tracheostomy has several advantages over prolonged endotracheal intubation, including increased comfort, reduced risk of permanent

TABLE 116.6 General Criteria for Extubation

- Successful completion of a spontaneous breathing trial
- Neurologic and medical condition is stable or improving
- Cough and gag reflexes present, minimal pooling of secretions
- PaO_2 >70 mm Hg with 40% oxygen and PEEP ≤8 cm H_2O
- Minute ventilation <12 L/min at rest
- Vital capacity >15 mL/kg and maximal inspiratory pressure >25 mm Hg
- No pending procedures, operations, or radiographic studies requiring airway protection
- Minimal secretions or moderate secretions with strong cough
- Volume status optimized, airway reactivity assessed and treated, feeds held
- Equipment, medications, and personnel necessary for reintubation readily available

PaO_2, partial pressure of oxygen; PEEP, positive end-expiratory pressure.

tracheolaryngeal injury, increased ease of weaning from the ventilator (reduced dead space and less resistance to flow from the ETT), and improved ability to manage and suction secretions. In comatose patients or in those with profound neuromuscular weakness for whom a prolonged period of ventilator dependence is anticipated, early tracheostomy within 3 to 5 days of intubation extends these benefits and has been associated with reduced ICU length of stay and mortality. Most patients with significant bulbar dysfunction following an acute brain injury will require tracheostomy for secretions management, although they can often be weaned rapidly from mechanical ventilation, and many will ultimately be decannulated when cough strength and airway protective reflexes have partially recovered.

Percutaneous tracheostomy creates a temporary stoma that is easily and rapidly reversible upon decannulation, whereas surgical tracheostomy creates a more durable and permanent stoma that typically requires surgical closure. In some patients with severe persistent oropharyngeal muscle weakness, a tracheostomy is necessary to manage secretions and prevent aspiration, even though respiratory muscle function is adequate.

LONG-TERM VENTILATION

In chronic respiratory failure (CRF), patients and clinicians should work together to determine the best interface for mechanical ventilatory support. Patients with good bulbar function and normal level of consciousness can often tolerate intermittent daytime and continuous nocturnal NPPV by nasal or face mask, whereas those at high risk of aspiration, or with a low or waxing and waning level of arousal, are more safely ventilated by tracheostomy. Patients with CRF often describe improved quality of life with NPPV and may be at lower risk of developing respiratory infections than patients with permanent tracheostomy—this has been dramatically demonstrated in patients with respiratory failure due to progressive Duchenne muscular dystrophy. Yet patients with a tracheostomy can sometimes speak and eat; an experienced speech therapist can determine the safety of and capacity for these activities. Adjustments in tidal volume and tracheostomy size may be important in facilitating speech, and cuff deflation dramatically improves the ability to speak and swallow but leaves the airway open to aspiration.

Some patients need ventilatory support for months or years. Small suitcase- or laptop-sized ventilators are available for use at home, and battery-powered portable ventilators can allow wheelchair-bound patients to travel out of the home. For patients with respiratory failure after brain stem or high cervical cord lesions, an implantable phrenic nerve pacemaker can be used to stimulate diaphragmatic contraction, liberating the patient from connection to a machine.

SUGGESTED READINGS

Aboussouan LS, Khan SU, Meeker DP, et al. Effect of noninvasive positive-pressure ventilation on survival in amyotrophic lateral sclerosis. *Ann Intern Med.* 1997;127:450–453.

Bach JR. Continuous noninvasive ventilation for patients with neuromuscular disease and spinal cord injury. *Semin Respir Crit Care Med.* 2002;23(3):283–292.

Bach JR, Saporito LR, Shah HR, et al. Decanulation of patients with severe respiratory muscle insufficiency: efficacy of mechanical insufflation-exsufflation. *J Rehabil Med.* 2014;46(10):1037–1041.

Benditt JO. Management of pulmonary complications in neuromuscular disease. *Phys Med Rehabil Clin N Am.* 1998;9:116–185.

Bolton CF. Assessment of respiratory function in the intensive care unit. *Can J Neurol Sci.* 1994;21:S28–S34.

Bösel J, Schiller P, Hook Y, et al. Stroke-related Early Tracheostomy versus Prolonged Orotracheal Intubation in Neurocritical Care Trial (SETPOINT): a randomized pilot trial. *Stroke.* 2013;44(1):21–28.

British Thoracic Society Standards of Care Committee. Non-invasive ventilation in acute respiratory failure. *Thorax.* 2002;57:192–211.

Carrera E, Schmidt JM, Fernandez L, et al. Spontaneous hyperventilation and brain tissue hypoxia in patients with severe brain injury. *J Neurol Neurosurg Psychiatry.* 2010;81(7):793–797.

Chalela JA. Pearls and pitfalls in the intensive care management of Guillain-Barré syndrome. *Semin Neurol.* 2001;21:399–405.

Coplin WM, Pierson DJ, Cooley KD, et al. Implications of extubation delay in brain-injured patients meeting standard weaning criteria. *Am J Respir Crit Care Med.* 2000;161:1530–1536.

Curley G, Kavanagh BP, Laffey JG. Hypocapnia and the injured brain: more harm than benefit. *Crit Care Med.* 2010;38(5):1348–1359.

Diringer MN, Videen TO, Yundt K, et al. Regional cerebrovascular and metabolic effects of hyperventilation after severe traumatic brain injury. *J Neurosurg.* 2002;96(1):103–108.

Esteban A, Frutos F, Tobin MJ, et al. A comparison of four methods of weaning patients from mechanical ventilation. Spanish Lung Failure Collaborative Group. *N Engl J Med.* 1995;332:345.

Farrero E, Prats E, Povedano M, et al. Survival in amyotrophic lateral sclerosis with home mechanical ventilation. *Chest.* 2005;127:2132–2138.

Howard RS, Wiles CM, Hirsch NP, et al. Respiratory involvement in primary muscle disorders: assessment and management. *Q J Med.* 1993;86:175–189.

Koh WY, Lew TWK, Chin NM, et al. Tracheostomy in a neuro-intensive care setting: indications and timing. *Anaesth Intensive Care.* 1997;25:365–368.

Kress JP, Pohlman AS, O'Connor MF, et al. Daily interruption of sedative infusions in critically ill patients undergoing mechanical ventilation. *N Engl J Med.* 2000;342:1471–1477.

Laghi F, Tobin MJ. Disorders of the respiratory muscles. *Am J Respir Crit Care Med.* 2003;168:10–48.

Levine S, Nguyen T, Taylor N, et al. Rapid disuse atrophy of diaphragm fibers in mechanically ventilated humans. *N Engl J Med.* 2008;358:1327–1335.

MacDuff A, Grant IS. Critical care management of neuromuscular disease, including long-term ventilation. *Curr Opin Crit Care.* 2003;9:106–112.

Nieszkowska A, Combes A, Luyt CE, et al. Impact of tracheotomy on sedative administration, sedation level, and comfort of mechanically ventilated ICU patients. *Crit Care Med.* 2005;33:2527–2533.

Perrin C, Unterborn JN, Ambrosio CD, et al. Pulmonary complications of chronic neuromuscular diseases and their management. *Muscle Nerve.* 2004;29:5–27.

Qureshi AI, Suarez JI, Parekh PD, et al. Prediction and timing of tracheostomy in patients with infratentorial lesions requiring mechanical ventilatory support. *Crit Care Med.* 2000;28:1383–1387.

Rabinstein A, Wijdicks EF. BiPAP in acute respiratory failure due to myasthenic crisis may prevent intubation. *Neurology.* 2002;59:1647–1649.

Rabinstein AA, Wijdicks EF. Warning signs of imminent respiratory failure in neurological patients. *Semin Neurol.* 2003;23:97–104.

Seder DB, Riker RR, Jagoda A, et al. Emergency neurological life support: airway, ventilation, and sedation. *Neurocrit Care.* 2012;17(suppl 1):4–20.

Seneviratne J, Mandrekar J, Wijdicks EFM, et al. Noninvasive ventilation in myasthenic crisis. *Arch Neurol.* 2008;65:54–58.

Seneviratne J, Mandrekar J, Wijdicks EFM, et al. Predictors of extubation failure in myasthenic crisis. *Arch Neurol.* 2008;65:929–933.

Thomas CE, Mayer SA, Gungor Y, et al. Myasthenic crisis: clinical features, mortality, complications, and risk factors for prolonged intubation. *Neurology.* 1997;48:1253–1260.

Tobin MJ. Mechanical ventilation. *N Engl J Med.* 1994;330:1056–1061.

Varelas PN, Chua HC, Natterman J, et al. Ventilatory care in myasthenia gravis crisis: assessing the baseline adverse event rate. *Crit Care Med.* 2002;30:2663–2668.

Wijdicks EFM, Borel CO. Respiratory management in acute neurologic illness. *Neurology.* 1998;50:11–20.

Yang KL, Tobin MJ. A prospective study of indexes predicting the outcome of trials of weaning from mechanical ventilation. *N Engl J Med.* 1991;324:1445–1450.

Yavagal DL, Mayer SA. Respiratory complications of rapidly progressive neuromuscular syndromes: Guillain-Barré syndrome and myasthenia gravis. *Semin Respir Crit Care Med.* 2002;23:221–229.

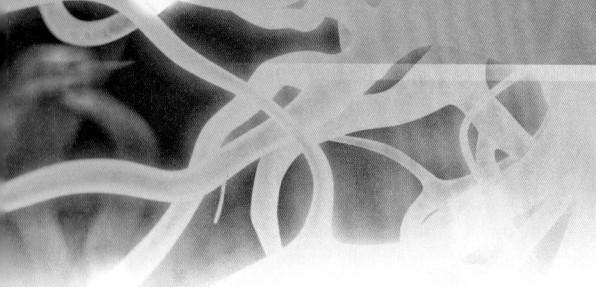

INTRODUCTION

Endocrine secretions and disorders of metabolism have a profound influence on the nervous system. Disturbances of consciousness and cognition along with a variety of other neurologic symptoms may accompany primary endocrine diseases. In addition, endocrine secretions may influence the expression of neurologic disorders such as migraine, epilepsy, or movement disorders. This chapter considers common endocrine conditions that may cause important neurologic symptoms.

PARATHYROID DISEASE

HYPERPARATHYROIDISM

Epidemiology

Primary hyperparathyroidism is the most common cause of hypercalcemia. The most recent estimated incidence was approximately 22 cases per 100,000 per year. The incidence peaks in the seventh decade and there is a fivefold excess of women in those older than 75 years. The incidence is similar in men and women before 45 years of age. A single-gland adenoma secreting excess parathyroid hormone (PTH) is the most common cause (75% to 85%).

Pathobiology

PTH regulates calcium by direct effects on kidney and bone and indirect effects on the gastrointestinal tract. PTH secretion, in turn, is regulated by ionized calcium concentration in extracellular fluid. Thyrocalcitonin and vitamin D also play important roles in calcium metabolism. The principle effects of PTH on the nervous system are via calcium regulation. However, PTH receptors occur in the brain and an endogenous neuropeptide is the natural ligand. Their exact function is uncertain.

Clinical Features

The classic syndrome of hyperparathyroidism is hypercalcemia with a combination of renal lithiasis, osteitis, and peptic ulcer disease ("stones, bones, and abdominal groans"). However, with the ease of determining serum calcium concentration by routine automated blood chemistry tests, the diagnosis is frequently made with minimal clinical symptoms and the classic triad is rarely seen today. Currently, it is estimated that 70% to 80% of individuals have no symptoms or signs of disease at the time of diagnosis.

Common symptoms include fatigue and subjective weakness. Mental status changes include impaired memory, personality changes, affective disorders, delirium, and psychosis. Elderly patients may be particularly susceptible to the effects of hypercalcemia. Parkinsonism and a syndrome resembling motor neuron disease reversing with parathyroid surgery have been described. "Brown tumors" seen in osteitis fibrosa cystica may cause myelopathy. Neuromuscular symptoms include proximal weakness, muscle pain and stiffness, and paresthesias. Tendon reflexes may be normal or hyperactive.

Diagnosis

The initial diagnosis typically occurs by finding hypercalcemia with hypophosphatemia on routine laboratory screening. This will be followed by an elevated PTH level. Differential diagnosis includes other causes of hypercalcemia, including drugs or conditions causing secondary hyperparathyroidism (e.g., renal failure) or familial hypocalciuric hypercalcemia. Hypercalcemia with low or undetectable PTH levels may suggest cancer-associated hypercalcemia mediated by PTH-related protein, or alternatively, ectopic production of PTH. Electromyography (EMG) and muscle biopsy can show evidence of myopathic or neuropathic disease. Brown tumors show variable intensities on T2-weighted images with intense enhancement on T1-weighted contrast studies. Fluid-filled cysts may be detected.

Treatment

Parathyroidectomy normalizes serum calcium and is the treatment of choice for patients with symptomatic primary hyperparathyroidism. Localization of a parathyroid adenoma with a variety of imaging techniques or by an experienced surgeon occurs in 95% of cases. In patients with mild disease or who are not surgical candidates, bisphosphonates are an option. The calcimimetic drug cinacalcet often normalizes serum calcium concentration and modestly decreases PTH levels.

Outcome

Although the degree of hypercalcemia does not always correlate with clinical severity, most neurologic and neuromuscular manifestations typically improve with treatment. It remains controversial as to whether symptoms such as fatigue, subjective weakness, or neuropsychiatric symptoms remit with parathyroidectomy.

HYPOPARATHYROIDISM

Epidemiology

Hypoparathyroidism occurs most commonly after thyroidectomy (~1% to 2 % with experienced endocrine surgeons) or other neck surgery. Autoimmune hypoparathyroidism is the next most common cause. Hypoparathyroidism may also be a feature of inherited disorders (e.g., Kearns–Sayre syndrome or DiGeorge syndrome) or glandular destruction from infiltrative processes or radiation. An estimated 60,000 individuals may have chronic hypoparathyroidism in the United States.

Pathobiology

Hypoparathyroidism is due to deficiency of PTH or lack of peripheral response to PTH (pseudohypoparathyroidism). The latter results from abnormal PTH receptors, defects in receptor-linked enzyme activity, or circulating antagonists. Chronic PTH deficiency has profound effects on the skeleton, and hypoparathyroidism disrupts normal calcium and phosphorus metabolism. Intracranial calcifications occur in vascular and perivascular locations. The action of PTH in brain is unknown but is hypothesized to be a cause of behavioral deficits seen in some forms of hypoparathyroidism.

Clinical Features

Tetany is the most distinctive sign that may be manifested by carpopedal spasm. Latent tetany can be demonstrated by contracture of the facial muscles on tapping the facial nerve in front of the ear (Chvostek sign) or by evoking carpal spasm by inducing ischemia in the arm with an inflated blood pressure cuff (Trousseau sign). Patients may also present with paresthesias and cramps, and if hypocalcemia is acute, may manifest with seizures, bronchospasm, laryngospasm, or cardiac arrhythmias. Seizures are usually generalized, tend to be frequent, and respond poorly to anticonvulsant drugs.

Intracranial calcifications are common in hypoparathyroidism. The basal ganglia are the predominant site for calcium deposition, but other regions such as the cerebellum may be affected. The calcifications are usually not associated with symptoms, but cognitive impairment and a variety of hypokinetic (parkinsonism) and hyperkinetic (choreoathetosis, hemiballismus, torticollis) movement disorders have been reported. Increased intracranial pressure may complicate hypoparathyroidism. The mechanism is unexplained. Sensorineural hearing loss and myopathy occur rarely.

Diagnosis

Hypocalcemia with an inappropriate low intact PTH level should lead to the suspicion of hypoparathyroidism. Hypomagnesemia can lower calcium and PTH. Hypocalcemia with low PTH essentially rules out other causes of hypocalcemia, such as vitamin D deficiency, malabsorption syndrome, or renal disease. In pseudohypoparathyroidism, PTH levels will be elevated and there are a variety of associated physical abnormalities. In most cases, there may be a relevant prior surgery or history of some destructive process (e.g., radiotherapy) involving the parathyroid. Autoimmune hypoparathyroidism may present with vitiligo or hypoadrenalism. Other forms of hypoparathyroidism may be associated with developmental anomalies (e.g., DiGeorge syndrome or Kearns–Sayre syndrome).

Treatment

There are no formal guidelines for management of chronic hypoparathyroidism. Treatment options include the use of calcium, vitamin D metabolites and analogues, and thiazide diuretics to enhance renal calcium reabsorption. Various forms of PTH are also being explored for treatment. Antiepileptic drugs that increase metabolism of vitamin D (e.g., phenytoin) should be avoided so as not to potentially interfere with calcium absorption from the gut or calcium mobilization from bone.

Outcome

Neuromuscular symptoms and seizures resolve with restoration of calcium to normal levels. Movement disorders may also be reversible with appropriate treatment. However, the response of cognitive–behavioral symptoms is variable. A study of women with postsurgical hypoparathyroidism treated to maintain calcium in a therapeutic range did not improve elevated levels of anxiety and sense of well-being.

ADRENAL DISEASE

HYPERADRENALISM

Epidemiology

Excessive secretion of glucocorticoids from the adrenal glands produces *Cushing syndrome*. However, the most common cause of Cushing syndrome is exposure to exogenous, often supraphysiologic doses of glucocorticoids. The incidence of endogenous Cushing syndrome is 0.7 to 2.4 per million population per year. There are two main forms, corticotropin (adrenocorticotropic hormone [ACTH])-dependent (80%) and ACTH-independent (20%). ACTH-dependent Cushing syndrome (Cushing disease) is primarily due to pituitary tumors hypersecreting ACTH and is addressed in Chapter 115. Approximately 20% of ACTH-dependent Cushing syndrome is due to ectopic production of ACTH, usually from carcinoid tumors or small cell carcinoma of the lung. ACTH-independent Cushing syndrome is usually due to an adrenal tumor.

Pathobiology

Hippocampus, amygdala, and cerebral cortex are rich in glucocorticoid receptors. Global cerebral atrophy occurs with Cushing syndrome. Hippocampal atrophy occurs and hippocampal formation volume is positively associated with performance on cognitive testing. Glucocorticoids decrease protein synthesis and increase protein degradation in muscles.

Clinical Features

The physical examination in Cushing syndrome may demonstrate hypertension, plethoric facies, hirsutism, centripetal obesity, a posterior neck fat pad (buffalo hump), purple abdominal striae, and bruising. Diabetes mellitus (DM), gonadal dysfunction, and osteoporosis are prominent features. Cognitive changes (impaired memory, visual–spatial processing, verbal learning, and language performance) with mood disorders (particularly major depression), myopathic weakness, and headache are the most common neurologic features. Myelopathy or radiculopathy may result from epidural lipomatosis.

Diagnosis

The diagnosis of Cushing syndrome is very challenging and despite the classical clinical manifestations, the presentation can be quite nonspecific. The initial step is distinguishing Cushing syndrome from individuals with Cushing-like states where hypercortisolism is a common feature. These include obesity, depression, or alcoholism. There is no test that has absolute diagnostic accuracy, with first-line screening being a 24-hour urinary free cortisol and overnight dexamethasone suppression test or late night salivary cortisol. After Cushing syndrome has been established, plasma ACTH is measured. If ACTH is elevated, then ACTH-dependent causes should be investigated. If ACTH is suppressed, then adrenal-dependent Cushing is suspected. There are many potential pitfalls, thus consultation with an experienced endocrinologist is essential. Adrenal tumors or tumors as a source of ectopic ACTH will require imaging for localization.

Treatment

Treatment depends on the etiology. In cases where there is an adrenal tumor secreting cortisol or an ACTH-secreting tumor, surgical removal of the tumor is the first-line treatment. Medical therapy includes various drugs that interfere with synthesis and secretion of cortisol. Ketoconazole (200 to 400 mg twice a day to three times a day), an antifungal compound that inhibits steroidogenesis, is the most widely used medication in the United States for this purpose.

Outcome

Evidence suggests that resolution of hypercortisolism does not completely resolve symptoms. After successful surgery, hippocampal volume increased and correlated with the magnitude of decrease in cortisol levels. Caudate volume increase has also been described with improvements in depression, anxiety, and obsessive–compulsive behavior. However, reduced brain volume and cognitive behavioral symptoms may only be partially reversible. Cognitive problems and psychopathology may persist even after long-term serum cortisol normalization.

HYPERALDOSTERONISM

Epidemiology

Hyperaldosteronism is the most common disorder of the adrenal zona glomerulosa with a prevalence of 5% to 20% of patients with resistant hypertension. It is the most common form of secondary hypertension.

Pathobiology

Aldosterone, typically produced by an adrenal adenoma or bilateral adrenal hyperplasia, is inappropriately elevated. The resulting volume expansion causes hypokalemic alkalosis and hypertension, although hypokalemia and hypertension are not generally correlated with aldosterone levels. Activity-dependent conduction block responsive to potassium replacement has been reported with neurophysiologic studies obtained in a patient with primary aldosteronism, weakness, and severe hypokalemia.

Clinical Features

The principle clinical feature is hypertension. There appears to be an excess incidence of stroke in patients with hypertension from primary aldosteronism versus essential hypertension. Hypokalemic alkalosis can lead to muscle weakness, paresthesias, tetany, or paralysis. Recurrent attacks of muscle weakness may simulate periodic paralysis. Paresthesias may occur as a result of the alkalosis. Vertigo may be caused by abrupt fluid and electrolyte shifts. Idiopathic intracranial hypertension has been reported. Many patients may suffer from an anxiety disorder and diminished sense of well-being.

Diagnosis

Endocrine Society clinical practice guidelines recommend case detection for a variety of types of individuals with hypertension including individuals with a family history of early-onset hypertension or stroke at a young age (younger than 40 years). The aldosterone-to-renin ratio is a widely used screening test, but many antihypertensive medications, oral contraceptives, or selective serotonin reuptake inhibitors can compromise sensitivity or specificity.

Treatment

Normalization of blood pressure should be a goal, but some adverse effects of primary aldosteronism seem to be partially independent of the hypertension. Surgical removal of adrenal tissue/

tumor is recommended where appropriate. Medical therapy with spironolactone can be effective, with several other agents now available.

Outcome

Surgery is essentially curative and corrects the hypokalemia. Antihypertensives may need to be withdrawn gradually.

HYPOADRENALISM

Epidemiology

Primary adrenal insufficiency, also known as *Addison disease*, has a prevalence of approximately 100 per million and an incidence of 5 per million in white populations. Age of diagnosis peaks in the fourth decade with women more frequently affected than men. In developed countries, 80% to 90% is due to autoimmune adrenalitis, occasionally in association with other autoimmune disorders, such as thyroid disease, hypoparathyroidism, or DM. Secondary adrenal insufficiency due to reduced pituitary ACTH has an estimated prevalence of 150 to 280 per million and is also more frequent in women. The peak age is in the sixth decade and is related to therapeutic administration of glucocorticoids.

Pathobiology

Destruction of the adrenal gland results in both corticosteroid and mineralocorticoid deficiency. It also results in dehydroepiandrosterone deficiency, which leads to androgen deficiency in women. In secondary adrenal insufficiency, mineralocorticoid production is preserved. These hormones are critical for sustaining the function of multiple physiologic systems. Glucocorticoids have pleiotropic effects on the nervous system, working at both the genomic level to alter gene expression and protein synthesis and at cell membranes to affect cell permeability and neurotransmitter release. They have effects on brain microstructure and influence production of nerve growth factors. The absence of adrenal hormones has widespread cognitive and behavioral consequences.

Adrenocortical insufficiency due to mutations in the ABCD1 gene results in abnormal metabolism of long-chain fatty acids that characterizes X-linked adrenoleukodystrophy. It may be the only clinical expression in about 10% of cases. In one study, one-third of young boys or men diagnosed with primary adrenal failure (Addison disease) were found to have adrenoleukodystrophy after measurement of long-chain fatty acids (see also Chapter 134).

Clinical Features

In primary adrenal insufficiency, typical systemic features are fatigue, anorexia, weight loss, hypotension, changes in skin, and hair loss. Headache is a common complaint. Mineralocorticoid deficiency produces hyponatremia with salt craving. Cortisol deficiency leads to increased production of melanocyte-stimulating hormone derived from pituitary proopiomelanocortin, which stimulates melanocytes to produce hyperpigmentation. These characteristics distinguish primary from secondary adrenal insufficiency. Cerebral symptoms include apathy, depression, confusion, and rarely, psychosis. Muscle pain and cramping may occur and hyperkalemic periodic paralysis has been observed.

In adrenoleukodystrophy, there is progressive central demyelination with impairment of cognition, vision, hearing, and motor function in children. In a second phenotype with onset in the late 20s, adrenomyeloneuropathy, there is spastic paraparesis and sphincter disturbances.

Diagnosis

Measurement of early morning serum cortisol and plasma ACTH generally separates patients with primary adrenal insufficiency from healthy individuals and those with secondary adrenal insufficiency. The standard short corticotropin test, in which serum cortisol is measured after intravenous ACTH, demonstrates the impairment of the adrenal cortex response to ACTH. In secondary adrenal insufficiency, there may be little difference in baseline hormone measurements from healthy individuals. The insulin tolerance test, which is a powerful activator of the hypothalamic–pituitary axis, remains the gold standard for assessment of secondary pituitary insufficiency. However, this test poses a significant burden on both the patient and the physician and tests such as the short corticotropin test, which capitalizes on the relative adrenal unresponsiveness to ACTH in secondary disease, are used. Because hypoadrenalism may antedate neurologic symptoms in adrenoleukodystrophy or adrenomyeloneuropathy, this diagnosis should be considered in young men with adrenal insufficiency.

Treatment

Hydrocortisone 15 to 25 mg/day is given in two or three divided doses daily, with a larger dose administered in the morning to mimic the pattern of physiologic cortisol secretion. Mineralocorticoid replacement (fludrocortisone (50 to 200 μg/day) is required only for primary adrenal insufficiency. Dehydroepiandrosterone (50 mg daily) can be replaced in a single morning dose.

Outcome

Glucocorticoids are lifesaving in acute adrenal insufficiency. However, despite adequate adrenal hormone replacement to meet basic physiologic requirements, health-related quality of life is reduced in adrenal insufficiency. Chronic complaints include fatigue, lack of energy, depression, and anxiety. Dehydroepiandrosterone replacement may improve well-being and libido in women.

PHEOCHROMOCYTOMA

Epidemiology

Pheochromocytomas are rare neuroendocrine tumors with approximately 80% arising from the chromaffin cells of the adrenal medulla. They secrete catecholamines and cause an estimated 0.1% to 0.6% of cases of secondary hypertension.

Pathobiology

Pheochromocytomas may occur sporadically or as part of a hereditary syndrome. Pheochromocytoma may be seen with neurofibromatosis, von Hippel–Lindau disease, ataxia-telangiectasia, Sturge–Weber syndrome, or multiple endocrine neoplasia type 2 consistent with the neuroectodermal origin of the adrenal medulla. It is estimated that 25% are associated with known genetic mutations.

Clinical Features

Hypertension of a moderate or severe degree is characteristic. The hypertension may be paroxysmal or sustained and is associated with palpitations, episodic hyperhidrosis, headaches, and other nonspecific systemic symptoms, such as nausea, emesis, or diarrhea. Anxiety attacks are common. Death may result from cerebral hemorrhage, pulmonary edema, or cardiac failure complicating an acute attack or as a result of sustained hypertension.

Diagnosis

Diagnosis is made by demonstrating increased excretion of catecholamine metabolites in urine and localization of the tumor. Measurement of fractionated plasma or urine metanephrines (or both) is recommended. Food, caffeinated beverages, strenuous physical activity, or smoking are not permitted for at least 8 to 12 hours prior to testing. A greater than fourfold elevation of plasma metanephrines is highly suggestive of the presence of the tumor. Tumors may occur in sites other than the adrenal (e.g., organs of Zuckerkandl). Computed tomography (CT), magnetic resonance imaging (MRI), or functional imaging techniques are helpful in localization.

Treatment

Surgical removal of the pheochromocytoma is the treatment of choice. Preoperative blockade of catecholamines, most commonly with phenoxybenzamine (10 mg once or twice a day), for 2 weeks prior to surgery is required. Volume contraction is associated with chronic vasoconstriction; thus, volume expansion is recommended to reduce postoperative hypotension.

Outcome

Surgery is curative for local disease and surgical debulking for more advanced disease will facilitate radiotherapy or chemotherapy. Essential hypertension may persist in up to 20% of cases. Long-term follow-up with yearly measurement of catecholamines is recommended and is especially important for patients identified with mutations associated with pheochromocytoma.

THYROID DISEASE

HYPOTHYROIDISM

Epidemiology

Hypothyroidism is a common disorder with an estimated prevalence of 0.4% to 1.2% in the United States. Approximately 40% of cases are overt, with 60% being subclinical. Congenital hypothyroidism due to maternal iodine deficiency or dysgenesis of the thyroid occurs in 1:3,000 to 1:4,000 births.

Pathobiology

The most common causes of hypothyroidism are autoimmune destruction and thyroidectomy or radioablation of the gland. Thyroid hormone is important in early growth and development, and the neurologic consequences of hypothyroidism depend on the age when the deficiency begins. Severe thyroid deficiency *in utero* or early life results in delayed physical and mental development (cretinism) or myxedema in adults. Thyroid hormone affects neurofilament gene expression, mitochondrial protein synthesis, and the appearance and distribution of laminin, which provides guidance to migrating neurons. Hypothyroidism is associated with pathologic changes in muscle, including accumulation of glycogen and lipids, abnormal and increased mitochondria, dilated sarcoplasmic reticulum, and focal myofibrillar degeneration. The biochemical changes produced in the brain or muscle induced by hypothyroidism are still not well correlated with clinical symptomatology.

Clinical Features

CONGENITAL HYPOTHYROIDISM

In congenital hypothyroidism, subcutaneous tissue thickens; the cry becomes hoarse; the tongue enlarges; and the infant has widely spaced eyes, a potbelly, and an umbilical hernia. Neurologically, there is mental retardation with pyramidal and extrapyramidal signs in a proximal and truncal distribution. Strabismus, deafness, and primitive reflexes are common. The severity of physical and mental retardation in juvenile hypothyroidism is usually less than in infantile myxedema. Precocious puberty may occur. Idiopathic intracranial hypertension has been reported in hypothyroid children receiving thyroid replacement therapy.

NEUROLOGIC MANIFESTATIONS

The neurologic complications of hypothyroidism include headache, disorders of the cranial and peripheral nerves, sensorimotor abnormalities, and changes in cognition and level of consciousness. Mental status changes may be prominent, with decreased attentiveness, poor concentration, lethargy, and dementia. Psychiatric symptoms—delirium, depression, or frank psychosis (myxedema madness)—may appear, depending on the severity and duration of thyroid deficiency. Cranial nerve abnormalities, other than visual and acoustic nerve problems, are unusual. Decreased vision from chiasmal compression may occur secondary to pituitary hypertrophy. Hearing loss, vertigo, and tinnitus may be present.

MYXEDEMA

Adult myxedema is primarily associated with primary thyroid failure as opposed to secondary hypothyroidism due to hypothalamic–pituitary disease. It is characterized by lethargy, somnolence, or impairment of attention and concentration; weakness; slowness of speech; nonpitting edema of the subcutaneous tissues; coarse, pale skin; dry, brittle hair; thick lips; macroglossia; and increased sensitivity to cold. In severe cases, myxedema coma may occur, accompanied by hypothermia, hypotension, and respiratory and metabolic disturbances. If untreated, myxedema coma has a high mortality rate.

NEUROMUSCULAR MANIFESTATIONS

Neuromuscular findings include slowing of voluntary movements and slow relaxation of tendon reflexes, particularly the ankle jerks. Electrically silent mounding of muscles on direct percussion is called *myoedema*. There may be exercise intolerance or myopathic weakness. In hypothyroid infants, a remarkable generalized enlargement or hypertrophy of muscles ("infant Hercules";

Fig. 117.1) constitutes the Kocher–Debré–Sémélaigne syndrome. Enlargement of muscles with pain and stiffness in adults produces the Hoffmann syndrome.

A mild, primarily sensory neuropathy is characterized mainly by paresthesias in the hands and feet. Entrapment neuropathy of the median nerve (carpal tunnel syndrome) is attributed to the accumulation of acid mucopolysaccharides in the nerve and surrounding tissues. Cerebellar ataxia (myxedema staggers) may occur in adults, manifesting as incoordination with a slow or stiff, unstable gait. Sleep apnea may result from myxedematous changes in the upper airway and hypertrophy of the tongue.

Diagnosis

The characteristic findings are low circulating thyroxine (T4) and triiodothyronine (T3), elevated thyrotropin (thyroid-stimulating hormone [TSH]), and low radioiodine uptake by the thyroid. Hypothyroidism due to hypothalamic–pituitary disease will have reduced circulating thyroid hormones with low TSH. Cerebrospinal fluid (CSF) protein content is increased; values greater than 100 mg/mL are not exceptional. Electroencephalogram (EEG) abnormalities include slowing and generalized decrease in amplitude. Serum creatine kinase levels are elevated with myopathy.

Treatment

The treatment of hypothyroidism depends on the severity of the deficiency. Myxedema coma should be treated rapidly with intravenous administration of T4 (200 to 400 μg), although the optimal approach to rapid thyroid hormone replacement is still uncertain. In other patients, gradually increasing doses of oral levothyroxine (to 1.6 μg/kg/day) are recommended. Older patient should be started on lower doses (25 to 50 μg daily). Angina pectoris or heart failure can be precipitated by too rapid replacement in adults. In secondary hypothyroidism, thyroid replacement should not be started without concomitant corticosteroid replacement, so as not to precipitate cortisol insufficiency. Prophylactic treatment of cretinism is important in goiter districts, where iodine should be given to all pregnant women.

Treatment of subclinical thyroid disease (i.e., normal thyroid hormone levels with elevated or depressed TSH levels) is controversial. Subclinical hypothyroidism has been reported to be associated with deficits in working memory that were reversible with T4 replacement.

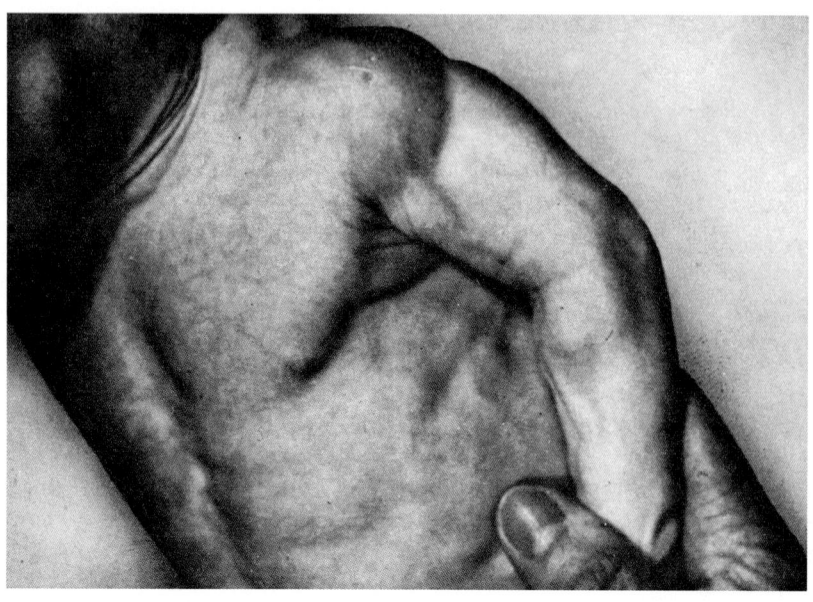

FIGURE 117.1 Enlargement of muscles in the Kocher–Debré–Sémélaigne syndrome. (Courtesy of Dr. Arnold Gold.)

Outcome

In many patients, thyroid hormone therapy administered within the first 2 months of life results in nearly complete restoration of normal physical and mental function. Treatment should begin during the first 2 weeks of life for optimal intellectual development. Despite early treatment, mild hearing and vestibular dysfunction may persist. Mortality for myxedema coma may be as high as 20%. In general, neuromuscular signs and symptoms resolve with treatment.

HYPERTHYROIDISM

Epidemiology

Hyperthyroidism or thyrotoxicosis has several causes, the most common being Graves disease. It affects an estimated 1% of the U.S. population, with 40% of cases being overt and 60% being subclinical. It affects women more commonly than men.

Pathobiology

In Graves disease, which is characterized by diffuse goiter, ophthalmopathy, and dermopathy, immunologic mechanisms play an important role in the thyroid, eye, and skin manifestations. In Graves ophthalmopathy, there is an increase in the orbital contents with edema, hypertrophy, infiltration, and fibrosis of the extraocular muscles (Fig. 117.2). Other common causes of hyperthyroidism are thyroid nodules, thyroiditis, or ingestion of thyroid hormone.

Clinical Features

Hyperthyroidism typically presents with an increased metabolic rate, abnormal cardiovascular and autonomic functions, tremor,

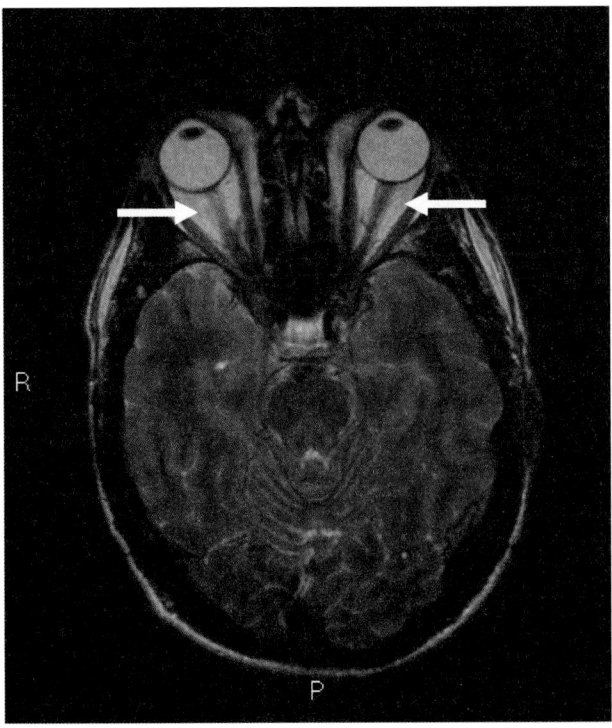

FIGURE 117.2 Magnetic resonance imaging of the orbits, showing congestion of the retroorbital space and enlargement of the extraocular muscles (*arrows*) consistent with the diagnosis of Graves ophthalmopathy.

and nervousness. Hyperthyroidism may be subtle in older patients, with apathy, myopathy, and cardiovascular disease as the most prominent symptoms. It is associated with atrial fibrillation and cardioembolic stroke. Mental disturbances range from mild irritability to psychosis.

THYROID STORM

Thyroid "storm" or "crisis" is usually precipitated by infection, surgery, or trauma in individuals with unrecognized hyperthyroidism. The cardinal symptom is fever greater than 102°F accompanied by cardiac symptoms and central nervous system (CNS) dysfunction. Nausea, vomiting, and abdominal discomfort are common. Affected individuals are confused or agitated and may present with psychosis. If untreated, level of consciousness may deteriorate to coma with seizures. Neurologic signs such as bulbar weakness and corticospinal tract dysfunction have been observed.

OCULAR SYMPTOMS

Ocular symptoms are common. These may be seen as infrequent blinking, lid lag, or weakness of convergence and are distinct from the infiltrative ophthalmopathy known as *Graves ophthalmopathy*. The relationship of the eye disorder to thyroid status is not entirely clear. Onset of symptoms is gradual; exophthalmos is often accompanied by diplopia secondary to paresis of one or more ocular muscles. Clinically, eyelid retraction (Dalrymple sign) is the first evidence in 75% of cases, and pain is the most common symptom. Both eyes may be involved simultaneously, or exophthalmos in one eye may precede the other by several months. Papilledema sometimes occurs, and ulcerations of the cornea may develop secondary to failure of the lid to protect the eye. The symptoms progress rapidly for a few months and may lead to complete ophthalmoplegia.

NEUROMUSCULAR MANIFESTATIONS

Thyrotoxic myopathy is characterized by painless weakness and wasting of proximal muscles of the arms and legs. Tendon reflexes are normal or hyperactive, and sensation is normal. The occurrence of hyperthyroidism and periodic paralysis (see Chapter 93) is more common in people of Asian ancestry and is similar to hypokalemic periodic paralysis in terms of precipitants and treatment. There is an association between hyperthyroidism and myasthenia gravis (see Chapter 89). About 5% of patients with myasthenia gravis have hyperthyroidism.

Diagnosis

A low TSH is the best test for diagnosis. This should be followed by obtaining a free T4. If the free T4 is not elevated, a free T3 measurement may be elevated, indicative of T3 toxicosis. The radioiodine uptake by the thyroid is the next test, which will be most helpful in distinguishing the different causes of hyperthyroidism. Other tests are available if the use of radioisotope studies is contraindicated. Orbital imaging will be abnormal in thyroid ophthalmopathy.

Treatment

β-Adrenergic blockade (e.g., propranolol 10 to 40 mg four times a day [q.i.d.]) is appropriate for symptomatic treatment of tremor or myopathy. Methimazole (5 to 120 mg daily, depending on severity) and propylthiouracil (50 to 300 mg t.i.d. to q.i.d.) are antithyroid medications that inhibit thyroid hormone synthesis. Ablation with radioactive iodine (^{131}I) or thyroidectomy is useful in treating various etiologies of hyperthyroidism that cannot be managed with medical therapies. Thyroid storm is a medical emergency with a mortality of around 20%. Immediate goals of treatment are to inhibit thyroid hormone synthesis and release, control cardiac symptoms, and support systemic circulation. Treatment of thyroid ophthalmopathy is controversial and may include immune suppression with corticosteroids, radiotherapy, or surgical decompression of the orbit.

Outcome

Successful treatment of hyperthyroidism results in improvement of most symptoms. Patients will need to be followed at varying intervals depending on the type of treatment that is selected.

PANCREATIC DISEASE

HYPOGLYCEMIA

Epidemiology

Hypoglycemia is uncommon in the general population but accounts for approximately 3% of deaths in patients with type 1 DM. The average patient with type 1 DM experiences two episodes of symptomatic hypoglycemia per week with one episode of temporarily disabling hypoglycemia each year.

Pathobiology

Hypoglycemia is most commonly associated with an overdose of insulin in the treatment of DM. Spontaneous hypoglycemia is usually the result of pancreatic hyperinsulinism. Hypersecretion of insulin by the pancreas may be due to a tumor of the islet cells or functional overactivity of these cells. Hypoglycemia may also occur when liver function is impaired or when there is severe damage to the pituitary or adrenal glands. The CNS depends almost entirely on glucose for its metabolism; dysfunction develops rapidly when the amount of glucose in the blood falls below critical levels. Hypoglycemia may cause cerebral ischemic damage, possibly by inducing endothelial dysfunction.

Clinical Features

The symptoms of hypoglycemia and hyperinsulinism are paroxysmal, tending to occur when the blood glucose could be expected to be low (in the morning before breakfast, after a fast, or after heavy exercise). Occasionally, symptoms follow a meal. The duration of symptoms varies from minutes to hours. The severity also varies. There may be only nervousness, anxiety, or tremulousness, which is relieved by the ingestion of food. Severe attacks last for hours, during which the patient may perform automatic activity with complete amnesia for the entire period or seizures followed by coma. The frequency of attacks varies from several per day to infrequent episodes.

Spontaneous hypoglycemia is occasionally seen in infants. Risk factors include immaturity, low birth weight, or severe illness. Infants of diabetic mothers may exhibit hyperinsulinism. A host of genetic or metabolic defects may cause hypoglycemia, including galactosemia, fructose intolerance, or leucine sensitivity. The symptoms of infantile hypoglycemia are muscular twitching, myoclonic jerks, and seizures. Mental retardation results if the condition is not recognized and adequately treated.

Hypoglycemic symptoms can be divided into two groups: autonomic and cerebral. Sympathetic symptoms are present in most patients at the onset of hypoglycemia, usually preceding the more serious cerebral manifestations. Autonomic symptoms include light-headedness, sweating, nausea, vomiting, pallor, palpitations, precordial pressure, headache, abdominal pain, and hunger. In DM, hypoglycemia-associated autonomic failure may occur due to repeated episodes of hypoglycemia with attenuation of the physiologic and, subsequently, symptomatic responses to hypoglycemia.

Cerebral symptoms usually occur with the sympathetic phenomena but may be the only manifestations. The most common manifestations are paresthesias, diplopia, and blurred vision, which may be followed by tremor, focal neurologic abnormalities, abnormal behavior, or convulsions. After prolonged severe hypoglycemia, coma may ensue. Confusion and abnormal behavior from episodic hypoglycemia may simulate complex partial seizures, although hyperinsulinism only rarely causes epilepsy. Chronic or repeated hypoglycemia may produce dementia or other behavioral abnormalities. Distal axonal neuropathy has also been observed.

Diagnosis

Findings on neurologic examination are usually normal, except during attacks of hypoglycemia. The diagnosis is established by documentation of hypoglycemia during a symptomatic episode, but the timing of the specimen is important because homeostatic mechanisms may return the blood glucose level to normal. The level of blood glucose at which symptoms appear varies from person to person but is generally less than 30 to 40 mg/dL. The EEG shows focal or widespread dysrhythmia during an attack of hypoglycemia and, in some patients, even in the interval between attacks.

The diagnosis of hyperinsulinism is made by the paroxysmal appearance of signs of autonomic and cerebral dysfunction in association with a low blood glucose level and an inappropriately high circulating insulin level. Factitious hypoglycemia may be caused by self-administration of insulin or inappropriate use of oral hypoglycemic agents. If it is not possible to obtain a blood specimen during an attack, a diagnostic fast should be considered. After 12 to 14 hours, 80% of patients with islet cell tumors have low glucose and high insulin levels. Longer fasts may be needed. The diagnosis of islet cell adenoma can be difficult; additional endocrine tests and imaging studies may be required. Hypoglycemia associated with diseases of the liver, adrenal, or pituitary can usually be distinguished by other signs and symptoms of disease in these organs.

Treatment

Ingestion of glucose or carbohydrate-containing foods can correct insulin-induced hypoglycemia. Administration of 10 g of oral glucose can raise blood glucose levels by approximately 40 mg/dL over 30 minutes and 20 g of oral glucose can raise blood glucose levels by 60 mg/dL over 45 minutes. Administration of glucagon is the treatment of choice for severe hypoglycemia. Comatose patients should be given glucose intravenously. Long-term management of hyperinsulinism is directed at optimizing diabetic control and/or identification and correction of the underlying cause.

Outcome

Early intensive treatment of acute hypoglycemia is important to prevent CNS damage. Long-term effects include adverse cardiovascular events and cognitive impairment.

DIABETES MELLITUS

Epidemiology

DM is a systemic metabolic disorder characterized by hypoinsulinism or peripheral resistance to the action of insulin that affects an estimated 250 million people worldwide. The primary neurologic complication of DM is peripheral neuropathy, which is the most frequent type of neuropathy in Western countries. DM neuropathy affects up to 60% of individuals with diabetes. It increases with duration of DM and with poor glycemic control.

Pathobiology

Abnormalities reported in diabetic neuropathy include axonal degeneration in nerve fibers, primary demyelination resulting from Schwann cell dysfunction, secondary segmental demyelination related to impairment of the axonal control of myelination, onion bulb formations, and hypertrophy of the basal lamina. Endoneurial capillaries often show signs of diabetic microangiopathy with marked thickening of the basal lamina. Metabolic and ischemic mechanisms have a role in diabetic neuropathies. Mononeuropathies are attributed to inflammatory and/or vascular lesions of peripheral nerves, whereas metabolic abnormalities are likely to predominate in length-dependent diabetic polyneuropathy. Genetic factors might explain why some individuals develop a more severe polyneuropathy than others with similar diabetic status.

Clinical Features

The neuropathies include mononeuropathies (peripheral and cranial nerves), polyneuropathy, autonomic neuropathy, radiculopathies, and entrapment neuropathy (median, ulnar, and peroneal; see Chapter 87). Common cranial neuropathies involve the oculomotor and abducens nerves. Pupillary sparing is common but not invariable and is related to the pattern of presumed vascular damage within the oculomotor nerve. The prognosis for recovery from mononeuropathy or radiculopathy is good.

Diagnosis

Onset of symptoms is rapid, and pain is common in both mononeuropathies and radiculopathies caused by DM. In the more common distal symmetric polyneuropathies, there is typically a gradual onset of symptoms, the character of which depending on the type(s) of peripheral nerve fiber affected. Numbness and burning are common complaints. In symptomatic diabetic neuropathy, there is slowing of nerve conduction velocity owing to demyelination and loss of large myelinated fibers and a decrease in nerve action potentials owing to loss of axons. However, if the neuropathy primarily affects small myelinated or unmyelinated fibers, nerve conduction studies may be normal.

Treatment

Optimal glycemic control diminishes the risk of developing a disabling peripheral neuropathy. Attention should be paid to protection of hyposensitive areas, notably the foot. Treatment of neuropathic pain is addressed in Chapter 57. Treatment of autonomic dysfunction is addressed in Chapter 130. Painful diabetic polyradiculopathies often respond to antineuralgia medications, such as carbamazepine, gabapentin, and pregabalin.

Outcome

Spontaneous improvement in focal diabetic neuropathies typically occurs. Good glycemic control is the only way to minimize occurrence and/or progression of neuropathy.

PITUITARY DISEASE

HYPOPITUITARISM

Epidemiology

In one population-based study, the prevalence of hypopituitarism was 45.5 cases per 100,000 with an incidence of 4.2 cases per 100,000 per year. Tumors were the most common cause. In recent years, there has been increased recognition that hypopituitarism is frequently associated with traumatic brain injury, subarachnoid hemorrhage, and cranial irradiation.

Pathobiology

Pituitary dysfunction can be caused by mechanical vascular or neural disconnection from the hypothalamus as is seen with various mass lesions of the sellar region, such as pituitary adenomas or craniopharyngiomas. Direct damage to the hypothalamus or altered neurotransmitter input is the likely cause of neuroendocrine dysfunction leading to hypopituitarism associated with cranial irradiation, traumatic brain injury, or subarachnoid hemorrhage. Hypotension or shock from obstetric hemorrhage or infection causes occlusive spasm of pituitary arteries with anoxic–ischemic necrosis (apoplexy) of a pituitary gland that has hypertrophied under estrogen stimulation from pregnancy (Sheehan syndrome).

Clinical Features

The skin is often thin, smooth, and dry; the peculiar pallor (alabaster skin) and inability to tan have been related to loss of melanocyte-stimulating hormone or ACTH. Axillary and pubic hair may be sparse, with relatively infrequent facial shaving. Depending on the severity of the decrease in ACTH and TSH, patients may note lethargy, weakness, fatigability, cold intolerance, and constipation. There may be an acute adrenal crisis with nausea, vomiting, hypoglycemia, hypotension, and circulatory collapse, particularly in response to stress. Loss of vasopressin will lead to diabetes insipidus with polyuria and polydipsia, which is potentially life threatening in patients with obtundation or coma. In children, loss of growth hormone (GH) will result in reduced growth velocity. In adults, the clinical manifestation of GH deficiency is less clear, but emerging data suggest that GH therapy may improve cognitive function. Loss of prolactin inhibitory factor (dopamine) from the hypothalamus can lead to raised prolactin concentrations which may cause galactorrhea and breast tenderness. Both hyperprolactinemia and loss of gonadotropins may manifest with symptoms of hypogonadism. The presentation of hypopituitarism may often be accompanied by signs and symptoms of the underlying disease responsible for pituitary dysfunction.

Diagnosis

Evaluation of patients with pituitary insufficiency depends on measurement of pituitary hormone levels in the peripheral blood, coupled with functional assessment of the target organs. The basic endocrine evaluation includes thyroid function tests (T4, T3, and TSH), prolactin determination, and assessment of adrenal reserve, such as ACTH stimulation for cortisol responsiveness. Pituitary hormone levels must be interpreted in the context of clinical findings. For example, normal gonadotropin levels (follicle-stimulating hormone, luteinizing hormone) may indicate pituitary insufficiency after menopause when elevated levels would be expected. Elevated levels of gonadotropins or TSH suggest primary gonadal or thyroid failure but, rarely, may be secreted by pituitary tumors. Dynamic tests of pituitary reserve or stimulation tests with synthetic hypothalamic releasing factors are sometimes needed to detect mild hypopituitarism or to distinguish between pituitary and hypothalamic causes of hypopituitarism.

Treatment

Treatment is initially determined by cause. Medical or surgical treatment of a pituitary tumor or other mass lesion may restore pituitary function (see Chapter 100). Hormone replacement is essential to restore normal adrenal and thyroid status, with replacement therapy of corticosteroids preceding thyroid replacement. Treatment of hypogonadism in both women and men can restore libido and sense of well-being and protect bone mass and in men, restore sexual function and increase muscle mass. There are oral, intranasal, and intravenous options for vasopressin replacement to treat diabetes insipidus.

Outcome

Replacement of pituitary hormones can greatly reduce morbidity and mortality and enhance quality of life. Hormonal needs may change with time and patients should be monitored regularly, especially during the first year after diagnosis. In many situations, such as traumatic brain injury, the issue of optimal hormone replacement remains uncertain and will depend on clinical judgment.

SEX HORMONE DYSFUNCTION

The brain–pituitary–ovarian axis provides an excellent example of the rich interplay between the brain and endocrine organs (Fig. 117.3). Hormonal changes linked to specific phases of the menstrual cycle, pregnancy, and menopause may impact the release and metabolism of neurotransmitters and neuromodulators and give rise to or modify a host of neurologic and neuropsychiatric conditions. Migraine is about three times as common in adult women as in men. Meningeal tumors are more prevalent in women than men. Early menopause has been touted as a risk factor for the development of Parkinson disease.

Pathobiology

MIGRAINE

The decline in plasma estradiol in the late luteal phase plays an important role in the expression of catamenial migraine. Estrogens may influence migraine by acting directly on vascular smooth muscle or by modulating the activity of vasoactive substances at the neurovascular junction. Perimenstrual fluctuations in circulating estrogens may also stimulate vasoregulatory elements in the hypothalamus or brain stem resulting in symptomatic alterations in cerebrovascular tone.

CEREBROVASCULAR DISEASE

Estrogen induces hypercoagulability by increasing plasma levels of fibrinogen and clotting factors VII, VIII, IX, X, and XII; enhancement of platelet aggregation; and suppression of antithrombin III activity and fibrinolysis. Fluctuating sex hormone levels may compromise the integrity of cerebral arterial walls akin to their effects on endometrial spiral arteries. Sex hormones may also exert direct trophic influences on arteriovenous malformations analogous to their effects on other highly vascularized lesions such as gingival epulis, spider angiomas, and meningiomas.

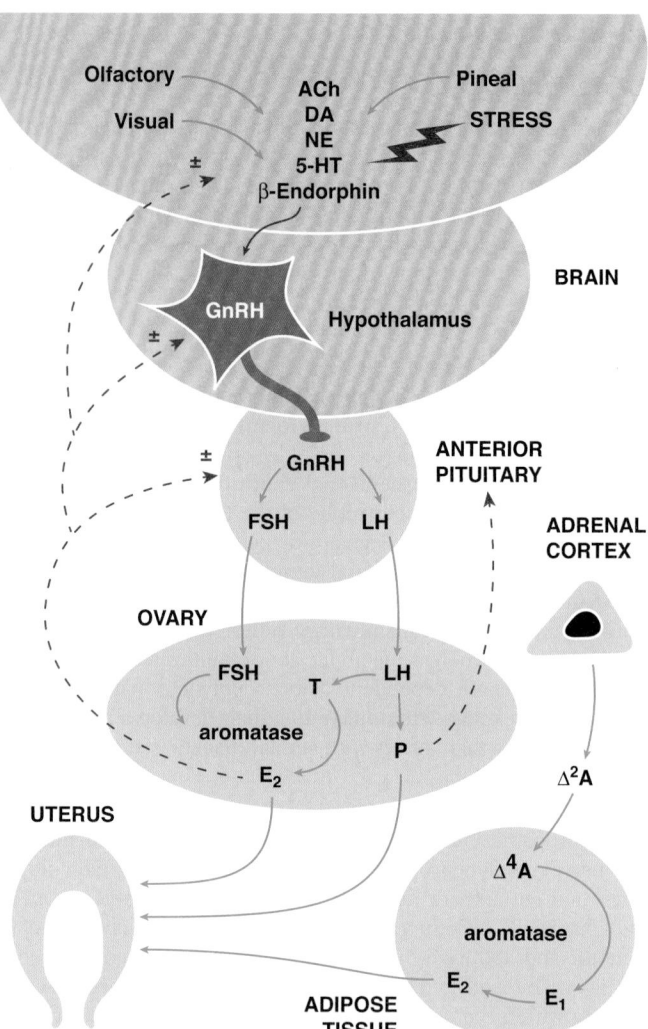

FIGURE 117.3 The brain–pituitary–ovarian axis. Δ4A, delta-4-androstenedione; ACh, acetylcholine; DA, dopamine; NE, norepinephrine; 5-HT, 5-hydroxytryptamine (serotonin); GnRH, gonadotropin-releasing hormone; FSH, follicle-stimulating hormone; LH, luteinizing hormone; T, testosterone; E2, estradiol; P, progesterone. (Modified from Schipper HM, Jay CA, Abrams GM. Sex hormone, pituitary, parathyroid, and adrenal disorders and the nervous system. In: Aminoff MJ, Josephson SA, eds. *Aminoff's Neurology and General Medicine.* 5th ed. San Diego, CA: Academic Press; 2014:369–397.)

MOVEMENT DISORDERS

Pregnancy may unmask latent chorea by facilitating dopaminergic neurotransmission in basal ganglia previously injured by hypoxic or rheumatic encephalopathy. Estrogens may influence motor manifestations of parkinsonism by modulating dopaminergic tone within the nigrostriatum.

BRAIN TUMORS

Perimenstrual and gestational changes in tumor size may be due to direct trophic effects of gonadal hormones on meningioma cells, steroid-induced fluid retention by the tumor, or increased vascular engorgement of the lesion. Gonadal steroid receptors or biologic responsiveness to sex hormones has been described in cases of pituitary adenomas, acoustic neuromas, ependymomas, and other neuraxial tumors. Astrocytomas may selectively bind estrogens, progestins, or androgens. In astroglial neoplasms, expression levels of estrogen receptor–beta may vary inversely with the degree of histopathologic dedifferentiation.

PORPHYRIA

Estradiol and other steroid hormones may trigger porphyric crises by inducing the heme biosynthetic enzyme, δ-aminolevulinic acid synthase. In women with acute intermittent porphyria, cyclical attacks may occur during the late luteal phase or at ovulation.

EPILEPSY

Estrogens and progestins have epileptogenic and anticonvulsant properties, respectively. Perimenstrual seizure activity may be precipitated by rising estrogen-to-progesterone ratios during the late luteal phase.

Clinical Features

Perimenstrual worsening of headaches (catamenial migraine) occurs in approximately 60% of female migraineurs (see also Chapter 54). The severity or frequency of migraine attacks often diminishes with pregnancy, particularly in individuals whose headaches are associated with the menstrual cycle. Menstruation, pregnancy, and menopause may also influence cluster headache, other autonomic cephalalgias, and hemicrania continua.

Pregnancy may be complicated by the appearance of choreiform movements, which are more prevalent in individuals with prior rheumatic fever and Sydenham chorea. Women with gestational chorea may additionally exhibit fever, neuropsychiatric symptoms, dysarthria, pendular reflexes, or limb hypotonia. Fluctuating sex hormone levels have also been reported to influence symptoms in other movement disorders including Parkinson disease, Tourette syndrome, tardive dyskinesia, and posthypoxic myoclonus.

Various seizure disorders may worsen premenstrually (catamenial epilepsy), at ovulation, or during pregnancy. Women may experience exacerbations of symptoms related to meningiomas in the luteal phase of the menstrual cycle. There is clinical and radiologic evidence for the rapid growth of meningiomas during pregnancy, followed by their spontaneous regression postpartum. Astrocytomas have been reported to expand during pregnancy and regress in the puerperium.

Endometriosis may cause back or pelvic pain by invading lumbar vertebrae, the lumbosacral plexus, or the sciatic nerve sheath (catamenial sciatica). Pain usually begins several days before the onset of menses and may continue until cessation of flow. Leg weakness, numbness, and loss of ankle reflexes may accompany the pain. Rarely, subarachnoid hemorrhage may be cyclic in women with hormone-sensitive ectopic endometriomas of the spinal canal.

Diagnosis

In patients with suspected chorea gravidarum, appropriate clinical and laboratory investigations may be indicated to exclude other etiologies, such as hyperthyroidism, rheumatic fever, Wilson disease, or systemic lupus erythematosus. Neuroimaging in endometriotic sciatica is generally unremarkable. Surgical exploration of the sciatic nerve may be required for diagnosis. Characteristic glandular elements are observed at histopathology.

Treatment

Perimenstrual migraine can usually be managed with standard dietary, psychological, and pharmacologic modalities employed in the general migraine population. Treatment with estrogen implants and the antiestrogen tamoxifen have yielded contradictory results. There are reports of significant symptom alleviation in women with menstrual migraine following treatment with the testosterone derivative danazol or the dopamine agonist bromocriptine. Late luteal phase therapy with prostaglandin inhibitors and mild diuretics may be helpful in refractory cases of severe catamenial migraine.

Approaches to the management of catamenial epilepsy include (1) premenstrual or periovulatory supplementation of anticonvulsant doses or addition of an adjunctive antiepileptic drug, (2) cyclic administration of a mild diuretic such as acetazolamide (which has weak anticonvulsant activity), and (3) progesterone supplementation by mouth or suppository.

Chorea gravidarum and oral contraceptive–related dyskinesias usually resolve by parturition or after discontinuation of the medication, respectively. In severe cases, neuroleptics may afford symptomatic relief. Individuals with a history of chorea gravidarum or contraceptive-induced dyskinesias should probably avoid further exposure to estrogen-containing medications.

In porphyria, chronic administration of GnRH agonists, such as leuprolide or D-His, downregulates gonadotrope GnRH receptors, resulting in long-term suppression of the pituitary–ovarian axis. In one report, complete remission of catamenial acute intermittent porphyria was observed during 6 months of D-His treatment. Subsequent cases of perimenstrual acute intermittent porphyria and hereditary coproporphyria also exhibited beneficial responses to GnRH agonist therapy.

Symptoms of endometriotic sciatica and periodic subarachnoid hemorrhage due to spinal canal endometriosis may improve dramatically with standard therapy for endometriosis, including progestins, danazol, GnRH agonist, or (in refractory cases) oophorectomy.

SUGGESTED READINGS

Parathyroid Disease

Arit W, Fremerey C, Callies F, et al. Well-being, mood and calcium homeostasis in patients with hypoparathyroidism receiving standard treatment with calcium and vitamin D. *Eur J Endocrinol.* 2002;146:215–222.

Bhadada SK, Bhansali A, Upreti V, et al. Spectrum of neurological manifestations of idiopathic hypoparathyroidism and pseudohypoparathyroidism. *Neurol India.* 2011;59:596–589.

Bilezekian JP, Khan A, Potts JT, et al. Hypoparathyroidism in the adult: epidemiology, diagnosis, pathophysiology, target organ involvement, treatment, and challenges for future research. *J Bone Miner Res.* 2011;26:2317–2337.

Dai CL, Sun ZJ, Zhang X, et al. Elevated muscle enzymes and muscle biopsy in idiopathic hypoparathyroidism patients. *J Endocrinol Invest.* 2012;35:286–289.

De Sanctis V, Soliman A, Fiscina B. Hypoparathyroidism: from diagnosis to treatment. *Curr Opin Endocrinol Diabetes Obes.* 2012;19:435–442.

Douglas M. Neurology of endocrine disease. *Clin Med.* 2010;10:387–390.

Fraser WD. Hyperparathyroidism. *Lancet.* 2009;374:145–158.

Marcocci C, Cetani F. Primary hyperparathyroidism. *N Engl J Med.* 2011;365:2389–2397.

Powers J, Joy K, Ruscia A, et al. Prevalence and incidence of hypoparathyroidism in the United States using a large claims database. *J Bone Miner Res.* 2013;28:2570–2576.

Wen HY, Schumacher HR, Zhang LY. Parathyroid disease. *Rheum Dis Clin North Am.* 2010;36:647–664.

Adrenal Disease

Anderson NE, Chung K, Willoughby, et al. Neurological manifestations of phaeochromocytomas and secretory paragangliomas: a reappraisal. *J Neurol Neurosurg Psychiatry.* 2013;84:452–457.

Bertorini T, Perez A. Neurologic complications of disorders of the adrenal glands. *Hand Clin Neurol.* 2014;120:749–771.

Bleicken B, Hahner S, Ventz M, et al. Delayed diagnosis of adrenal insufficiency is common: a cross-sectional study of 216 patients. *Am J Med Sci.* 2010;339:525–531.

Bourdeau I, Bard C, Noel B, et al. Loss of brain volume in endogenous Cushing's syndrome and its reversibility after correction of hypercortisolism. *J Clin Endocrinol Metab.* 2002;87:1949–1954.

Carey RM. Primary aldosteronism. *J Surg Oncol.* 2012;106:575.

Catena C, Colussi G, Nadalini E, et al. Cardiovascular outcomes in patients with primary aldosteronism after treatment. *Arch Int Med.* 2008;168:80–85.

Chakera AJ, Vaidya B. Addison disease in adults: diagnosis and management. *Am J Med.* 2010;123:409–413.

Chen H, Sippel RS, O'Dorisio MS, et al. The North American Neuroendocrine Tumor Society consensus guideline for the diagnosis and management of neuroendocrine tumors: pheochromocytoma, paraganglioma, and medullary thyroid cancer. *Pancreas.* 2010;39: 775–783.

Funder JW, Carey RM, Fardella C, et al. Case detection, diagnosis, and treatment of patients with primary aldosteronism: an Endocrine Society clinical practice guideline. *J Clin Endocrinol Metab.* 2008;93:3266–3281.

Hsieh S, White PC. Presentation of primary adrenal insufficiency in childhood. *J Clin Endocrinol Metab.* 2011;96:E925–E928.

Kiehna EN, Keil M, Lodish M, et al. Pseudotumor cerebri after surgical remission of Cushing's disease. *J Clin Endocrinol Metab.* 2010;95:1528–1532.

Krishnan AV, Colebatch JG, Kiernan MC. Hypokalemic weakness in hyperaldosteronism: activity dependent conduction block. *Neurology.* 2005;65:1309–1312.

Moser HW, Raymond GV, Dubey P. Adrenoleukodystrophy. *JAMA.* 2005; 294:3131–3134.

Neiman LK, Biller BMK, Findling JW, et al. The diagnosis of Cushing's syndrome: an Endocrine Society clinical practice guideline. *J Clin Endocrinol Metab.* 2008 93;1526–1540.

Pivonello R, De Martino MC, De Leo M, et al. Cushing's syndrome. *Endocrinol Metab Clin North Am.* 2008;37:135–149.

Sathi N, Makkuni D, Mitchell WS, et al. Musculoskeletal aspects of hypoadrenalism: just a load of aches and pains? *Clin Rheumatol.* 2009;28:631–638.

Starkman MN. Neuropsychiatric findings in Cushing syndrome and exogenous glucocorticoid administration. *Endocrinol Metab Clin North Am.* 2013;42:477–488.

Sukor N. Primary aldosteronism: from bench to bedside. *Endocrine.* 2012;41:31–39.

Tritos NA, Biller BMK. Advances in medical therapies for Cushing's syndrome. *Discovery Med.* 2012;13:171–179.

Tsirlin A, Oo Y, Sharma R, et al. Pheochromocytoma: a review. *Maturitas.* 2014; 77:229–238.

Valassi E, Crespo I, Santos A, et al. Clinical consequences of Cushing's syndrome. *Pituitary.* 2012;15:319–329.

Thyroid Disease

Alix JJP, Shaw PJ. Thyroid disease and the nervous system. In: Aminoff MJ, Josephson SA, eds. *Aminoff's Neurology and General Medicine.* 5th ed. San Diego, CA: Academic Press; 2014:369–397.

Bahn RS. Grave's ophthalmopathy. *N Eng J Med.* 2010;362:726–738.

Feldman AZ, Shrestha RT, Hennessey JV. Neuropsychiatric manifestations of thyroid disease. *Endocrinol Metab Clin North Am.* 2013;42:453–475.

Gaitonde DY, Rowley KD, Sweeney LB. Hypothyroidism: an update. *Am Fam Phys.* 2012;86:244–251.

Halpern JF, Boyages SC, Maberly GF, et al. The neurology of endemic cretinism. A study of two endemias. *Brain.* 1991;114:825–841.

Kwaku MP, Burman KD. Myxedema coma. *J Intensive Care Med.* 2007;22:224–231.

McDermott MT. Hyperthyroidism. *Ann Int Med.* 2012;157:1–16.

Pavlu J, Carey MP, Winer JB. Hypothyroidism and nemaline myopathy in an adult. *J Neurol Neurosurg Psychiatry.* 2006;77:708–709.

Squizzato A, Gerdes VE, Brandjes DPM, et al. Thyroid diseases and cerebrovascular disease. *Stroke.* 2005;36:2302–2310.

Tashko V, Davachi F, Baboci R, et al. Kocher-Debrâe-Sâemâelaigne syndrome. *Clin Pediatr.* 1999;38:113–115.

Pancreatic Disease

Awoniyi O, Rehman R, Dagogo-Jack S. Hypoglycemia in patients with type 1 diabetes: epidemiology, pathogenesis, and prevention. *Curr Diab Rep.* 2013;13:660–678.

Cryer PE. Mechanisms of hypoglycemia-associated autonomic failure in diabetes. *N Engl J Med.* 2013;369:367–372.

Martin CL, Albers JW, Pop-Busui R; DCCT/EDIC Research Group. Neuropathy and related findings in the diabetes control and complications trial/epidemiology of diabetes interventions and complications study. *Diabetes Care.* 2014;37:31–38.

Mohseni S. Hypoglycemic neuropathy. *Acta Neuropathol (Berl).* 2001;102:413–421.

Said G. Diabetic neuropathy—a review. *Nat Clin Pract Neurol.* 2007;36: 331–340.

Singleton JR, Smith AG. The diabetic neuropathies: practical and rational therapy. *Sem Neurol.* 2012;32:196–203.

Strachan MWJ, Reynolds RM, Marioni RE, et al. Cognitive function, dementia and type 2 diabetes mellitus in the elderly. *Nat Rev Endocrinol.* 2011;7: 108–114.

Pituitary Disease

Appleman Dykstra NM, Kokshoorn NE, Dekkers OM, et al. Pituitary dysfunction in adult patients after cranial radiotherapy: systemic review and meta-analysis. *J Clin Endocrinol Metab.* 2011;96(8):2330–2340.

Nyberg F, Halberg M. Growth hormone and cognitive function. *Nat Rev Endocrinol.* 2013;9:357–365.

Randva HS, Schoebel J, Byrne J, et al. Classical pituitary apoplexy: clinical features, management and outcome. *Clin Endocrinol (Oxf).* 1999;51:181–188.

Schneider HJ, Aimaretti G, Kreitschmann-Andermahr I, et al. Hypopituitarism. *Lancet.* 2007;369:1461–1470.

Schneider HJ, Kreitschmann-Andermahr I, Ghigo E, et al. Hypothalamo-pituitary dysfunction following traumatic brain injury and aneurysmal subarachnoid hemorrhage. *JAMA.* 2007;298:1429–1438.

Tesnow AH, Wilson JD. The changing face of Sheehan's syndrome. *Am J Med Sci.* 2010;340:402–406.

Wiebke F, Allolio B. Current state and future perspectives in the diagnosis of diabetes insipidus: a clinical review. *J Clin Endocrinol Metab.* 2012;97:3426–3437.

Sex Hormone Dysfunction

Dworetzky BA, Townsend MK, Pennell PB, et al. Female reproductive factors and risk of seizure or epilepsy: data from the Nurses' Health Study II. *Epilepsia.* 2012;53(1):e1–e4.

Floyd JR, Keeler ER, Euscher ED, et al. Cyclic sciatica from extrapelvic endometriosis affecting the sciatic nerve. *J Neurosurg Spine.* 2011;14:281–289.

Frantzen C, Kruizinga RC, van Asselt SJ, et al. Pregnancy-related hemangioblastoma progression and complications in von Hippel-Lindau disease. *Neurology.* 2012;79:793–796.

Loder E. Rizzoli P. Golub J. Hormonal management of migraine associated with menses and the menopause: a clinical review. *Headache.* 2007;47(2): 329–340.

Maia DP, Fonseca PG, Camargos ST, et al. Pregnancy in patients with Sydenham's chorea. *Parkinsonism Relat Disord.* 2012;18:458–461.

Nicoletti A, Nicoletti G, Arabia G, et al. Reproductive factors and Parkinson's disease: a multicenter case-control study. *Mov Disord.* 2011;26:2563–2566.

Pines A. Hormone therapy and brain tumors. *Climacteric.* 2011;14:215–216.

Schipper HM, Jay CA, Abrams GM. Sex hormone, pituitary, parathyroid, and adrenal disorders and the nervous system. In: Aminoff MJ, Josephson SA, eds. *Aminoff's Neurology and General Medicine.* 5th ed. San Diego, CA: Academic Press; 2014:369–397.

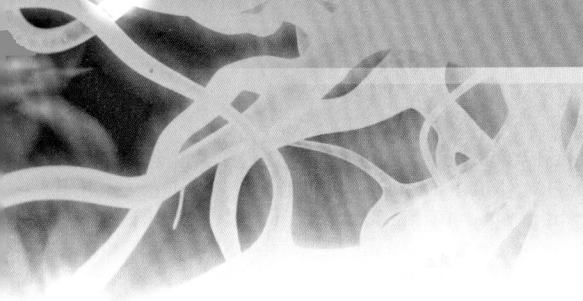

RED BLOOD CELL DISORDERS

Anemia is a common complication of acute, severe neurologic illnesses such as stroke and traumatic brain injury. Maturation of hematopoietic stem cells into red blood cells (RBCs) in bone marrow is regulated by the glycoprotein hormone erythropoietin (EPO), which is released by peritubular cells in the kidneys in response to reductions in oxygen (O_2) delivery. Production of RBCs is also dependent on sufficient quantities of bone marrow substrate, including iron, folate, and vitamin B_{12}. RBCs normally have a life span of 100 to 120 days before being removed by the spleen.

ANEMIA

Anemia is defined as a hemoglobin (HB) concentration of less than 12 g/dL in women and 13 g/dL in men. There are numerous possible etiologies for anemia, which are presented in Figure 118.1. Measurement of the reticulocyte count helps determine whether the bone marrow is responding "appropriately" to anemia—if so, it implies that the cause is hemorrhage or hemolysis; if not, there is a problem with RBC production. RBC indices, especially the mean cell volume (MCV), provide further information concerning the differential diagnosis. Microcytosis (MCV <80) implies that there is a cytoplasmic problem with the production of HB and the maturation of RBCs. Specific causes of microcytic anemia include iron deficiency and various hemoglobinopathies. Macrocytosis (MCV >100) implies that there is a nuclear defect in developing RBCs, which may be due to vitamin B_{12} and folate deficiency or drug toxicity. Normocytic anemia suggests that there is a pathologic bone marrow process or that there is reduced stimulation for RBC production.

This section will focus on the neurologic implications of anemia and on sickle cell disease, which is a major cause of stroke in children and young adults.

Anemia and Transfusion in Hospitalized and Critically Ill Neurologic Patients

Anemia is one of the most common medical complications to be encountered among hospitalized patients, especially in the intensive care unit. The development of an HB concentration less than 10 g/dL has been reported in about 40% to 50% of neurocritical care patients with traumatic brain injury (TBI) or subarachnoid hemorrhage (SAH). The etiology of anemia in hospitalized patients is multifactorial. RBC production is impaired during systemic inflammation, as cytokines blunt the production of EPO and prevent progenitor cells from incorporating iron. RBC loss is accelerated by the need for frequent phlebotomy, reduced RBC survival, and (in some cases) hemorrhage. Hemodilution produced by administration of large volumes of intravenous fluids or phlebotomy may also contribute.

Optimal care of patients with acute brain injury and various forms of stroke involves the protection of salvageable brain tissue and the prevention of secondary injury. Reduced O_2 delivery to ischemic penumbra may produce increasing neurologic damage. The amount of O_2 reaching tissues is the product of local blood flow and arterial O_2 content, which in turn is dependent on the HB concentration and the degree to which it is saturated with O_2.

Anemia is initially well tolerated by most patients for several reasons: systemic O_2 delivery exceeds O_2 consumption by a large amount, tissues have the capacity to increase O_2 extraction in the

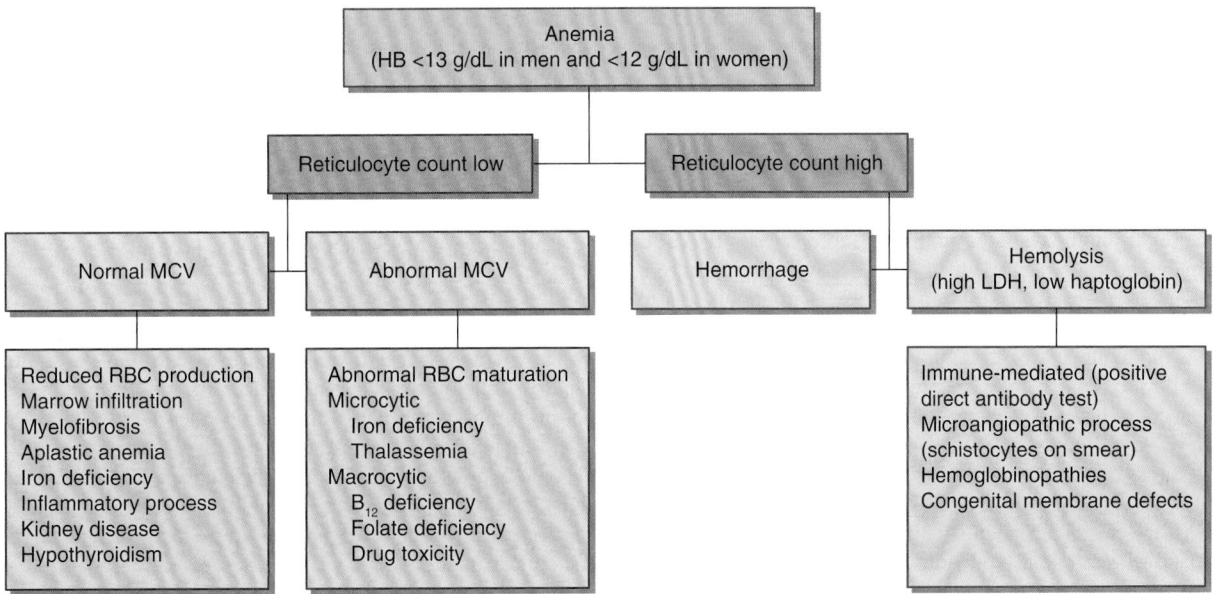

FIGURE 118.1 Approach to determining the etiology of anemia. MVC, mean cell volume; LDH, lactate dehydrogenase; RBC, red blood cell.

setting of reduced delivery, and sympathetic stimulation results in increased cardiac output. In the brain, the normal response to anemia is cerebral vasodilation, with a resulting increment in cerebral blood flow (CBF). Experiments in healthy volunteers demonstrate that neurocognitive impairment begins at an HB concentration below approximately 7 g/dL. It is likely that the HB threshold for neurologic deterioration is higher in brain-injured patients, in whom autoregulatory mechanisms may be impaired.

The development of anemia is associated with worsened outcomes in patients with TBI, SAH, and intracerebral hemorrhage (ICH). Studies using invasive multimodal neurologic monitoring have found that anemia is associated with lower brain tissue O_2 tension and high cerebral lactate concentrations. Patients with SAH, in particular, are vulnerable to delayed cerebral ischemia. Administration of RBC transfusions improves O_2 delivery to the brain and increases physiologic "reserve" in regions of the brain with a high O_2 extraction fraction.

Historically, clinicians would give RBC transfusions to maintain HB concentrations greater than 9 to 10 g/dL in brain-injured patients. However, allogeneic RBC transfusions have potential adverse effects, including transfusion-related acute lung injury (TRALI) and immunosuppression with an increased risk of nosocomial infections. Randomized trials in general critical care patients have found no advantage, and possible harm, when RBC transfusions are used to maintain HB concentrations above 10 g/dL compared with a transfusion threshold of 7 g/dL [**Level 1**].[1,2] However, there were few brain-injured patients in these studies and HB concentrations of 7 to 9 g/dL may be too low in some brain-injured patients. There is substantial variability of practice, which will continue until clinical trials are performed specifically in brain-injured patients. Consensus guidelines in the setting of SAH recommend maintaining HB levels greater than 8 to 10 g/dL.

Sickle Cell Disease

Sickle cell disease (SCD) is a group of genetic disorders characterized by the presence of "sickle hemoglobin" (HBS) caused by a mutation in the β-globin gene, whereby the sixth amino acid changes from glutamic acid to valine. The most common and severe form is sickle cell anemia, which occurs in patients homozygous for the HBS allele. There are other SCD variants where HBS is inherited form one parent and another abnormal HB from the other. Stroke is the most common neurologic complication of SCD.

EPIDEMIOLOGY

The global burden of SCD is increasing, especially in Africa and India. About 8% of African-Americans are heterozygous for HBS and 1 in 600 are homozygous. Another 2% to 3% carry the HBC allele, which is attributable to a glutamic acid to lysine substitution. The incidence of stroke in children with SCD is about 300 to 400 times higher than the rate of stroke in other children, such that the chance of having a stroke by 20, 30, and 45 years of age is estimated to be about 11%, 15%, and 24%, respectively. The highest incidence occurs between the ages of 2 and 9 years. Intracranial hemorrhage is less common but increases in incidence between 20 and 30 years of age. Stroke is a major cause of premature death and disability in patients with SCD. Untreated, stroke may recur in as many as two-thirds of patients within 2 years. By far the strongest risk factor for stroke is a previous stroke or transient ischemic attack (TIA). Other risk factors include the degree to which HB is reduced, hypertension, frequent episodes of acute chest pain syndrome, leukocytosis, and lower pulse oximetry values.

Even in patients who have not developed overt stroke, magnetic resonance imaging (MRI) studies demonstrate that silent cerebral infarcts are common, occurring in more than a third of patients. Previous infarcts are seen especially in watershed regions and are associated with cognitive impairment and a higher subsequent risk of overt stroke. Areas of restricted diffusion, suggestive of recent cerebral ischemia, can be detected even when patients are asymptomatic, suggesting that patients are at constant risk. Identified risk factors for silent cerebral infarcts include lower baseline HB concentration, higher systolic blood pressure, and male gender.

PATHOBIOLOGY

O_2 is normally transported by adult hemoglobin (HBA) consisting of two α and β polypeptide chains that encircle a heme moiety. Unlike HBA, HBS has a tendency to polymerize when it is deoxygenated, which in turn disrupts the normal architecture and flexibility of RBCs, causing them to take on sickle-shaped morphology. Sickling of RBCs interferes with their transit through capillaries and venules, causes them to adhere to endothelium, and increases blood viscosity, all of which may produce microvascular occlusion and tissue ischemia. Increased hemolysis occurs in the spleen. Most of the clinical manifestations of sickle cell anemia are attributable either to vaso-occlusion or hemolysis.

Multiple factors other than just stasis and sluggish microvascular flow are implicated in causing cerebral ischemia. Adherence of sickled RBCs to vascular endothelium induces a cascade of events that produce leukocyte recruitment, inflammation, intimal hyperplasia, fibrosis, and thrombosis. Intravascular hemolysis and release of free HB scavenges nitric oxide, the production of which may also be impaired by endothelial damage, thereby interfering with maintenance of normal vascular tone. These factors contribute to impaired CBF autoregulation, making the brain vulnerable both to hyperemia and ischemia.

Imaging studies with digital subtraction or magnetic resonance (MR) angiography demonstrate that many patients have various forms of vasculopathy. By far the most common cerebrovascular abnormality is stenosis of proximal intracranial vessels, especially in the anterior circulation, which may be accompanied by relative hypoperfusion if perfusion imaging is performed. Involvement of extracranial vessels is less common but does occur and may lead to cervical artery dissection and/or embolic strokes. Over time, with persistent severe intracranial stenosis, there may be development of collateral vessels resembling those of Moyamoya disease. The presence of such collaterals is a marker of a greater degree of vasculopathy and has been identified as a major risk factor for future stroke. These friable vessels are also vulnerable to bleeding. Intracranial aneurysms may develop in unusual locations with a possible predilection for the posterior circulation.

CLINICAL MANIFESTATIONS

SCD patients with cerebrovascular disease present most often with TIA or ischemic stroke. Among those with hemorrhage, SAH is more common than ICH or intraventricular hemorrhage. Repeated silent infarcts cause progressive neurologic deterioration. Children in whom previous infarcts are detected on a MRI scan have, on average, lower performance on neurocognitive testing and worse school performance. They are also more likely to have psychological concerns, such as anxiety and depression. Similar observations have been made in adults with sickle cell anemia, in whom the degree of anemia is associated with more severely impaired cognitive function. Neuroimaging reveals that patients with SCD have a greater degree of thinning of the frontal lobe cortex, as well as reduced basal ganglia and thalamus volumes.

SCD may rarely cause complications in the spinal cord and peripheral nervous system. There have been numerous case reports of spinal cord infarction, most often involving the cervical cord and causing quadriparesis. Ischemic injury of peripheral nerves presents as mononeuritis multiplex. Functional asplenia is a well-recognized complication of SCD. The resulting immunosuppression predisposes to bacterial infections, including meningitis, with the risk being high enough to justify prophylactic penicillin usage until at least the age of 5 years. Fever should therefore be considered a medical emergency.

DIAGNOSIS

The diagnosis of SCD is confirmed by HB electrophoresis. Quantification of the percentage of HBS, determined by high-performance light chromatography, is important for therapeutic decision making. Ischemic strokes are rare in the absence of detectable abnormalities in the cerebral vasculature. When vasculopathy is present, the risk of stroke can be significantly ameliorated with appropriate therapy. Thus, screening of patients for cerebrovascular disease is important. Cerebral vasculature is best imaged with digital subtraction angiography (DSA), but noninvasive imaging is preferred. Both computed tomography (CT) and MR angiography can be used, although published experience is larger with the latter. Previous concerns that intravenous contrast could precipitate sickling crisis have likely been exaggerated.

In experienced hands, transcranial Doppler (TCD) ultrasonography correlates well with angiography. Increased TCD velocities in the anterior circulation are highly predictive of the risk of subsequent stroke [Level 1].[3] In one prospective single-center study, the sensitivity and specificity for subsequent overt stroke exceeded 85% when TCD velocity exceeded 170 cm/s. In children, when TCD velocities in either middle cerebral or intracranial internal carotid artery consistently exceed 200 cm/s, a randomized controlled trial demonstrated that a stroke prevention strategy using RBC transfusions decreased the risk of stroke over the ensuing 2 years from 16% to 2% [Level 1].[4] The risk of stroke is even higher if there are elevated velocities in more than one vessel. Annual screening with TCD is recommended for children with SCD beginning at 2 years of age. Implementation of screening has been temporally associated with a reduction in the incidence of stroke in some jurisdictions. Most studies assessing the use of TCD in SCD have been in children. TCD velocities that are associated with vascular stenosis seem to be somewhat lower in adults, and it is unclear whether TCD is as predictive of subsequent stroke risk.

Apart from imaging of the intra- and extracranial cerebral vasculature, patients with SCD who develop ischemic strokes should undergo a similar diagnostic evaluation to that of other patients, including an echocardiogram, lipid panel, and assessment for diabetes mellitus. In patients with SAH or ICH, if CT or MR angiography does not demonstrate a cause, a DSA should be considered to ensure that a small aneurysm or vascular abnormality is not being missed.

TREATMENT

SCD is a multisystem condition, and the management of neurologic complications occurs in the context of other concomitant treatment considerations. In the management of cerebrovascular complications, therapeutic goals are the primary and secondary prevention of strokes, including those that are silent and may contribute to cognitive decline as well as minimization of brain injury when strokes do occur.

Transfusion Strategies and Stroke Prevention

The Stroke Prevention Trial in Sickle Cell Anemia (STOP) demonstrated that using RBC transfusions to keep the fraction of HBS less than 30% (Table 118.1) significantly reduces the risk of stroke [Level 1].[4] Apart from diluting HBS with the addition of HBA, transfusions also temporarily reduce EPO production, thereby reducing the production of new HBS. O_2 binds more efficiently to HBA than HBS, such that the O_2 saturation is temporarily increased. Although the STOP trial was a primary prevention study, chronic transfusion therapy has also been widely adopted as a secondary prevention strategy. The target HB concentration is generally greater than 9 g/dL. Simple transfusions can be performed when patients are very anemic. Exchange transfusions refer to the transfusion of RBCs together with the removal of the patient's blood, which is more effective at reducing the concentration of HBS and at lowering stroke incidence.

The need for regular transfusions also has risks, most notably the development of iron overload. Over time, excess iron overwhelms the capacity of reticuloendothelial system to sequester it, and iron begins to accumulate in organs, especially the liver. The consequence of unchecked iron accumulation is hepatic fibrosis and eventually cirrhosis. Rather than performing repeated biopsies, liver iron burden can be accurately monitored noninvasively with annual quantitative MRI scans. Increasing liver iron concentration or serum ferritin (>1,500 µg/L) is an indication to initiate treatment with an iron chelator, most often deferasirox, which has similar efficacy to deferoxamine but is orally available. In an attempt to avoid long-term dependence on blood transfusions, the STOP 2 trial assessed the safety of discontinuing prophylactic transfusions in children whose TCD results had normalized over time. Unfortunately, cessation of transfusions was associated with a clear increment in TCD velocities over time as well as an increased risk of recurrent stroke [Level 1].[5]

Post hoc analyses of the STOP trials indicated that new silent infarcts were reduced by the use of transfusions and that discontinuation of transfusions led to an increment in the occurrence of new infarcts. However, patients treated with chronic transfusion still commonly develop progressive cerebral vasculopathy. Increased TCD velocities are not necessarily predictive of the development of

TABLE 118.1	Indications for Chronic Transfusion Program for the Prevention of Stroke in Patients with Sickle Cell Disease

Primary prevention (screen annually with TCDs of MCA and distal ICA between 2 and 16 yr)

- If >220 cm/s, initiate transfusion program
- If 200–220 cm/s, repeat TCDs in 1–2 wk and initiate transfusion program if confirmed >200 cm/s
- If 170–200 cm/s, repeat TCDs in 3–6 mo; consider MRI scan to assess for SCI.
- If <170 cm/s, repeat TCDs annually; consider MRI scan to assess for SCI.

Secondary prevention (if patient has had symptomatic stroke)

MRI evidence of silent cerebral infarction (Note: Optimal frequency of MRI screening has not yet been defined.)

TCD, transcranial Doppler; MCA, middle cerebral artery; ICA, internal carotid artery; MRI, magnetic resonance imaging; SCI, silent cerebral infarction.

silent infarcts. MR angiography may be more predictive, but the relationship between burden of vasculopathy and risk of infarction is imperfect. Until recently, it was unclear whether performing serial MRI scans to document silent infarcts is helpful and should modify the therapeutic approach. However, the Silent Cerebral Infarct trial has demonstrated that regular transfusions to maintain HBS less than 30% and HB greater than 9 g/dL reduces the incidence of subsequent overt or silent infarcts [**Level 1**].[6] Patients should be periodically screened for silent infarcts (the optimal interval has not been defined) and enrolled in a transfusion program if they are present.

Management of Acute Stroke

There have been no randomized trials of thrombolysis in the treatment of pediatric stroke. The pathophysiology of acute stroke in the setting of SCD may not be the same as in other settings. Nevertheless, although the risk of iatrogenic hemorrhage may be higher, the presence of SCD is not necessarily a contraindication for the use of thrombolytics, especially if the stroke mechanism involves acute thrombotic or embolic vascular occlusion. CT angiography, performed immediately after an initial noncontrast CT scan, can help clarify the mechanism while concomitantly identifying vascular abnormalities that may constitute a relative contraindication. Urgent transfusion to lower the HBS concentration and raise the total HB concentration to about 10 g/dL is appropriate to maximize O_2 delivery to the affected penumbra. Adequate hydration and avoidance of hypotension, hyperglycemia, and fever are other standard measures. Antiplatelet therapy is indicated in adults sustaining acute strokes in other settings but there is no data specifically in patients with SCD. The very high risk of recurrent stroke with SCD justifies the use of chronic transfusion for secondary prevention.

Hydroxyurea as an Alternative to Chronic Transfusion

Fetal hemoglobin (HBF) consists of two gamma, rather than beta, globulins. For this reason, an increased concentration of HBF in the circulation prevents the sickling of RBCs. Hydroxyurea is thought to exert its beneficial effects in SCD by increasing the formation of HBF. A large randomized trial found hydroxyurea to reduce painful vaso-occlusive crises. Long-term follow-up demonstrated a possible mortality benefit [**Level 1**].[7] Hydroxyurea is currently recommended in patients older than 24 months with frequent pain crises, acute chest syndrome, or severe symptomatic anemia. There has been interest in using hydroxyurea as an alternative to chronic transfusion in the prevention of cerebrovascular disease.

Early data suggested that hydroxyurea might be efficacious. However, the recent Stroke with Transfusions Changing to Hydroxyurea (SWiTCH) trial demonstrated that discontinuing regular transfusions and instead treating patients with hydroxyurea resulted in an increased stroke risk [**Level 1**].[8]

Intracranial Hemorrhage and Moyamoya Syndrome

Supportive care of SAH and ICH is not different compared with patients who do not have SCD. Immediate priorities with SAH are cardiopulmonary stabilization and treatment of hydrocephalus. Cerebral angiography (invasive or noninvasive) is required to identify the source of bleeding. Most aneurysms with SCD appear to be saccular and are amenable to clip ligation or coil embolization. Some aneurysms are fusiform and can be treated with endovascular stenting. Nimodipine should be used for prevention of delayed cerebral ischemia.

Moyamoya syndrome, a syndrome of progressive intracranial large-vessel occlusion, is a recognized and relatively common complication of sickle cell vasculopathy that is associated with an increased risk of stroke and cognitive decline (see also Chapter 43). There are no controlled studies assessing the optimal management of moyamoya syndrome in the context of SCD. In the setting of an acute ischemic stroke, physiologic targets (blood pressure, partial pressure of carbon dioxide and O_2, core body temperature) should be directed at optimizing cerebral perfusion and protecting vulnerable ischemic penumbra. Surgical revascularization is generally preferred for secondary prevention. Small case series have suggested a reduced risk of ischemic stroke with surgery. In adults, direct revascularization with a superficial temporal artery to middle cerebral artery bypass procedure may be possible. In children or in adults without a suitable target vessel, indirect revascularization procedures (e.g., pial synangiosis) are more often performed.

POLYCYTHEMIA

Polycythemia is present when the HB concentration is greater than 16.5 g/dL in women and 18.5 g/dL in men (or the hematocrit is >48% and 52%, respectively). True polycythemia should not be attributable solely to a reduction in plasma volume (hemoconcentration). "Primary" polycythemia refers to increased production of RBCs without increased release of EPO and occurs as a result of congenital or acquired mutations in RBC progenitors. "Secondary" polycythemia is an appropriate response to increased EPO production (Fig. 118.2). Management of secondary polycythemia should be directed at the underlying cause.

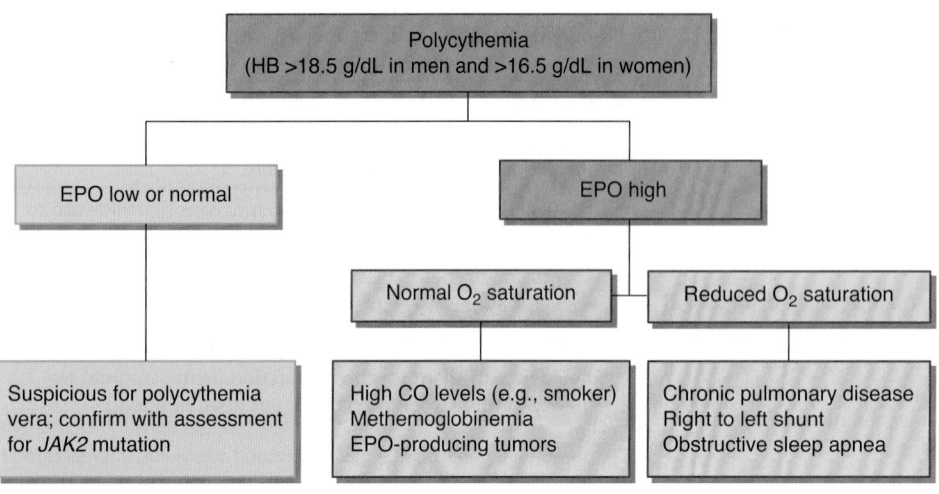

FIGURE 118.2 Approach to determining the etiology of polycythemia. EPO, erythropoietin; O_2, oxygen; CO, carbon monoxide.

Polycythemia Vera

Polycythemia vera (PV) is of interest to neurologists primarily as a cause of stroke. The median age of diagnosis is about 60 years, but PV can occur across all age categories. In almost all cases, PV is associated with a mutation involving JAK2, a gene located on chromosome 9 that codes for the production of tyrosine kinase, a family of proteins that participate in the regulation of hematopoietic cell proliferation. The same mutation is present in about 50% of patients with essential thrombocythemia (ET) and primary myelofibrosis.

PATHOBIOLOGY

PV is a myeloproliferative neoplasm characterized by the clonal proliferation of RBC progenitors resulting in an elevated RBC mass. A small proportion of patients with PV will develop leukemic transformation usually after many years. A major concern with PV and other myeloproliferative disorders is a predisposition to thrombosis. It is thought that persistently elevated viscosity produces high shear stress in blood vessels, which in turn is complicated by endothelial dysfunction, as well as platelet and leukocyte activation. Increased levels of thromboxane and other markers of platelet activation can be detected in the blood of patients with PV. High viscosity may reduce CBF to a degree that overall O_2 delivery is impaired despite the higher O_2-carrying capacity produced by a higher HB concentration. However, other factors must be at play because there is no clear evidence that secondary polycythemia increases the risk of thrombosis.

CLINICAL MANIFESTATIONS

PV is sometimes detected incidentally on routine blood work. However, a sizable proportion of patients have already had thrombotic events by the time they come to medical attention. Arterial thrombosis is more common than venous thrombosis. Patients may also present with transient visual disturbances, headaches, and dizziness attributable to hyperviscosity and sluggish blood flow. Other common complaints include pruritus that is exacerbated by contact with water and erythromelalgia (burning sensation in extremities with erythema or pallor). Physical examination commonly demonstrates hepato- and splenomegaly as well as facial plethora. Apart from an elevated HB concentration, other laboratory findings include thrombocytosis, leukocytosis, high lactate dehydrogenase (LDH), and low EPO levels. Major diagnostic criteria for PV include an elevated HB concentration and the presence of the JAK2 mutation. Minor criteria include characteristic findings on a bone marrow aspirate or biopsy and reduced serum EPO.

TREATMENT

The goal of treatment is to reduce symptoms and the risk of thrombosis while also minimizing long-term complications, especially leukemia. In a multicenter randomized trial involving patients with JAK2-positive PV, treatment with phlebotomy or hydroxyurea to achieve a hematocrit of less than 45% was associated with a significant reduction in thrombotic events. This target hematocrit should therefore be maintained with phlebotomy in essentially all patients [**Level 1**].[9] For patients at especially high risk of thrombosis (those older than the age of 60 years or having had previous thrombotic events), treatment with hydroxyurea is recommended, as it appears to further reduce the risk of thrombosis with a smaller increase in the risk of leukemia over time compared with other myelosuppressive drugs. The addition of low-dose aspirin (80 mg/day) can further reduce thrombotic risk [**Level 1**].[10]

WHITE BLOOD CELL DISORDERS

MALIGNANCIES OF LYMPHOID CELLS

Lymphoma and Lymphoblastic Leukemia

Lymphoid malignancies present primarily as mass lesions, which are referred to as *lymphoma*, or with cancer cells in the blood, referred to as *leukemia*. They are most often categorized using the World Health Organization classification system. Lymphoma is divided broadly as Hodgkin (HL) and non-Hodgkin (NHL). NHL encompasses a heterogeneous group of malignancies, arising from B lymphocytes in about 85% to 90% of cases, and T lymphocytes in about 10% to 15% of cases. B- and T-cell lymphomas are further subdivided based on whether the malignancy involves proliferation of immature precursor cells or mature cells. Neurologic involvement is rare with HL. However, with NHL and acute lymphoblastic leukemia (ALL), neurologic complications may occur because of direct infiltration of cancer cells into the central nervous system (CNS) (Table 118.2).

EPIDEMIOLOGY

The distribution of NHL subtypes varies by region. In western countries, diffuse large B-cell lymphoma and follicular lymphoma account for more than 50% of cases. CNS involvement is most common with very high-grade lymphomas, especially Burkitt lymphoma and acute lymphoblastic lymphoma, where it may be present at the time of diagnosis in as many as a third. However, CNS involvement also occurs with intermediate- and high-grade

TABLE 118.2 Classification of Most Common Subtypes of Non-Hodgkin Lymphoma and Approximate Prevalence of Central Nervous System Involvement	
Type of Lymphoma	**Prevalence of CNS Involvement**
Indolent lymphomas	1%–3%
• Follicular lymphoma (grades I and II)	
• Marginal zone B-cell lymphoma	
• Small lymphocytic lymphoma/ B-cell CLL	
Aggressive lymphomas	3%–5%
• Diffuse large B-cell lymphoma	Note: prevalence higher with certain risk factors (e.g., involvement of testes, orbits, nasopharynx, breasts, multiple extranodal sites, high serum LDH)
• Follicular lymphoma (grade III)	
• Mantle cell lymphoma	
• Peripheral T-cell lymphoma	
• Anaplastic large cell lymphoma	
Highly aggressive lymphomas	25%–50%
• Burkitt lymphoma	
• Precursor T and B lymphoblastic lymphoma	
• Adult T-cell lymphoma	

CNS, central nervous system; CLL, chronic lymphocytic leukemia; LDH, lactate dehydrogenase.

lymphoma subtypes (e.g., diffuse B-cell lymphoma, the most common subtype in North America), especially when there is lymphoma spread to testes, orbits, or the nasopharynx and when there is a high serum LDH concentration. Most cases with neurologic involvement manifest as disease relapses during or after initial treatment, even when there has been a favorable systemic response to treatment, suggesting that subclinical disease was present at the time of diagnosis. The proportion of patients developing CNS relapses may have decreased over time with the addition of rituximab to standard CHOP therapy.

More than half of cases of ALL occur in children, with a peak incidence between the ages of 2 and 5 years. CNS infiltration is detected at diagnosis in about 5% to 10% of patients. This is likely to be an underestimate, given that identification of CNS involvement may be challenging and is not routinely pursued. Before routine use of prophylactic therapy, CNS relapses occurred in as many as 80% of cases. CNS involvement was sometimes identified at autopsy in patients previously thought to have had more limited disease. Risk factors for CNS leukemia include younger age, high white blood cell (WBC) count, positive Philadelphia chromosome, and T-cell ALL.

CLINICAL MANIFESTATIONS

The usual location of CNS involvement is the leptomeninges and subarachnoid space. Brain parenchyma involvement is less common. The predilection of certain tumor subtypes for CNS penetration may relate to expression of various surface adhesion molecules. The most frequent manifestations of leptomeningeal involvement include headache, neck pain, and various cranial neuropathies. If there is spread to the lumbar cistern, patients may develop low back pain and radiculopathies. The degree of subarachnoid involvement may occasionally be severe enough to interfere with CSF flow and cause hydrocephalus. With brain parenchymal involvement, there is a risk of developing seizures and focal deficits. Intramedullary spinal cord involvement is rare. In contrast, NHL and multiple myeloma are among the most common malignancies to cause epidural spinal cord compression (see Chapter 16).

DIAGNOSIS

Gadolinium-enhanced MRI can identify leptomeningeal or brain parenchymal spread. There may be enhancement and thickening of the meninges or individual cranial nerves or nerve roots. There are no characteristic MRI features that definitively identify cerebral mass lesions as lymphoma rather than other tumors; surgical biopsy may be required. CSF findings include lymphocytic pleocytosis, elevated protein, reduced glucose, and high opening pressure, although most patients do not have all of these findings. CSF cytology and flow cytometry should both be performed, as they provide complementary information. Sampling CSF more than once may reduce false-negative rate. CNS leukemia is defined by the presence of leukemic blasts in CSF. Blasts may occur regardless of whether or not the CSF WBC count is increased. The presence of CSF blasts predicts a worse prognosis.

TREATMENT

Lymphoma

When NHL is complicated by secondary CNS involvement, the usual treatment approach must be modified. Options include intensification of the chemotherapeutic regimen, with inclusion of higher doses of drugs that cross the blood–brain barrier or delivering chemotherapy directly into the CNS using either an Ommaya reservoir or repeated lumbar puncture. It is unclear which of these approaches is preferred, as they have not been compared in large clinical trials.

When systemic chemotherapy is used, the regimen usually includes high-dose methotrexate. Combining high-dose chemotherapy with autologous stem cell transplantation appears to be a particularly promising approach. Intrathecal therapy consists of methotrexate in combination with cytarabine. Preliminary data suggest that cytarabine is more efficacious when administered as a slow-release liposomal formulation, which has the additional advantage of requiring less frequent administration. Systemic corticosteroids are effective in some patients at temporarily ameliorating neurologic symptoms and providing analgesia. Radiation therapy may be helpful in selected cases where there are radiographically visible lesions that are causing symptoms.

Because the prognosis of NHL is much worse with relapses that involve the CNS, some experts favor administration of prophylactic CNS therapy as a component of the initial chemotherapeutic regimen in patients deemed to be at high risk. The risk of CNS involvement, even if not documented at diagnosis, is sufficiently high with Burkitt lymphoma and lymphoblastic lymphoma to justify CNS prophylaxis. This may also be appropriate other forms of NHL if risk factors for CNS involvement are present.

Acute Lymphoblastic Leukemia

Phases of treatment for ALL include induction, consolidation, and maintenance. Induction therapy includes glucocorticoids, vincristine, asparaginase, and possibly an anthracycline. Philadelphia chromosome–positive patients have a worse prognosis and are also treated with tyrosine kinase inhibitors. Essentially all treatment protocols include CNS prophylaxis, which is administered during the induction phase. Consolidation and maintenance therapy involves the administration of further chemotherapy or, in some high-risk cases, hematopoietic cell transplantation.

Cranial radiotherapy used to be a standard component of CNS prophylaxis but induces CNS toxicity in a substantial proportion of patients. Radiation has been largely replaced by use of intrathecal chemotherapy [**Level 1**].[10] A variety of regimens have been used but most often include intrathecal methotrexate, cytarabine, and hydrocortisone. Neurotoxicity, with MRI evidence of leukoencephalopathy, has been described with high doses of intrathecal methotrexate.

Established CNS leukemia at the time of diagnosis is still commonly treated with the combination of whole-brain irradiation and intrathecal methotrexate. Given that the prognosis of adults with CNS leukemia is guarded, there may be a role for allogeneic hematopoietic cell transplantation, but further research is required.

Plasma Cell Malignancies

MULTIPLE MYELOMA

Multiple myeloma (MM) is a malignancy of marrow plasma cells characterized by the production of monoclonal immunoglobulins. It is the most prevalent hematologic malignancy after NHL and is particularly common in the elderly with a median onset age in the early 60s. MM has a higher incidence in African-Americans and in men.

Plasma cell proliferation in the marrow interferes with the production of other hematopoietic cells, resulting in anemia and thrombocytopenia. Lytic bone lesions cause pain and make patients vulnerable to pathologic fractures. Increased bone metabolism precipitates hypercalcemia. Production of immunoglobulins by other plasma cells is impaired, resulting in hypogammaglobulinemia and impaired humeral immunity with increased vulnerability to bacterial infections. Renal failure may occur for a variety of reasons, including acute tubular necrosis from light-chain casts, glomerulonephropathy from amyloidosis, and the effects of hypercalcemia.

The various complications of MM (e.g., hypercalcemia, infections, or uremia) may produce neurologic symptoms (e.g., altered level of consciousness). Vertebral body fractures or plasmacytomas can cause spinal cord compression. Brain involvement is less common and may be due to plasmacytoma extension from the skull or the development of leptomeningeal myelomatosis with resultant cranial nerve palsies or spinal radiculopathies. CNS involvement can generally be diagnosed with MRI scans and assessment of CSF. There have been no prospective studies assessing optimal therapy of CNS involvement, but preliminary experience with adjunctive intrathecal chemotherapy and selective use of cranial irradiation has been favorable.

MM is the second most common cause of hyperviscosity syndrome (discussed in the following text). There have been an increasing number of case reports of hyperammonemic encephalopathy complicating MM. Although myeloma cells appear to produce significant quantities of ammonia, the pathogenesis remains unclear. As with other causes of hyperammonemia, patients develop lethargy, confusion, and seizures. In severe cases, there may be diffuse cerebral edema and coma. The relationship between serum ammonia concentration and clinical manifestations is imperfect, although most reported cases had markedly elevated levels. Clinical improvement has been reported with the initiation of chemotherapy. In several reports, hemodialysis was used successfully to lower ammonia levels more rapidly.

WALDENSTRÖM MACROGLOBULINEMIA

Waldenström macroglobulinemia (WM) is a form of lymphoplasmacytic lymphoma associated with production of circulating immunoglobulin (Ig) M monoclonal antibodies. Other lymphoid malignancies (e.g., chronic lymphocytic leukemia), as well as monoclonal gammopathy of undetermined significance and primary amyloidosis, may also result in increased production of IgM antibodies. WM is a rare condition with an incidence of only 3 per million population per year.

As with MM, patients may develop clinical manifestations related to tumor infiltration in hematopoietic tissues. However, most neurologic complications are related to the effects of circulating IgM. WM is the most common cause of the hyperviscosity syndrome, which is present in as many as one-third of patients at the time of diagnosis. Serum viscosity is generally expressed in centipoises (cP), where 1 cP is the viscosity of water. Serum usually has a viscosity of 1.4 to 1.8 cP. Clinical manifestations typically occur when viscosity exceeds 4 cP and are almost always present above 6 cP. High viscosity results in sluggish blood flow and relative hypoperfusion. Consequently, patients develop blurry vision, altered mental status, and focal neurologic deficits. In severe cases, cerebral venous thrombosis or ischemic strokes may occur. Circulating proteins also interfere with platelet aggregation, leading to prolonged bleeding time and a tendency toward mucosal hemorrhage. Funduscopy classically demonstrates segmental dilatation of retinal veins, as well as retinal hemorrhages or exudates. A significant proportion of patients with WM also develop a progressive sensorimotor peripheral neuropathy. The neuropathy is usually demyelinating, affects sensation to a greater degree than motor function, and targets primarily the lower extremities. Monoclonal IgM antibodies are detected by serum protein electrophoresis and direct measurement of IgM levels. Bone marrow biopsy reveals infiltration of lymphocytes with plasma cell differentiation (>10% of cells).

Hyperviscosity syndrome is a medical emergency. The need for treatment is based primarily on the presence of clinical manifestations rather than the specific serum viscosity. Apart from fluid resuscitation, patients should undergo urgent plasmapheresis using albumin rather than plasma for fluid replacement. Each treatment reduces serum viscosity by about 20% to 30% and repeated plasmapheresis is performed until symptoms have resolved. Further therapy consists of appropriate chemotherapy administered together with rituximab [**Level 1**].[11]

ACUTE MYELOID LEUKEMIA

Acute myeloid leukemia (AML) is a group of hematologic malignancies involving clonal proliferation of myeloid precursor cells (destined to become granulocytes, monocytes, RBCs, or platelets). AML may occur because of defined genetic abnormalities as part of the natural history of myelodysplastic syndrome or as a complication of exposure to cytotoxic drugs. AML "not otherwise specified" is most often categorized according to the French, American, and British classification system based on the specific cell type that is implicated.

Patients with AML usually come to medical attention with manifestations attributable to pancytopenia, such as fatigue, weakness, infections, or bleeding. Leukemic infiltration of various tissues can produce additional symptoms. If the WBC is high enough, manifestations of hyperviscosity ("leukostasis") may develop, which may be severe enough to cause stupor and coma. There appears to be an increased risk of ICH for several days after the high WBC has been corrected, possibly because of reperfusion injury.

CNS leukemic involvement is uncommon at presentation and is less of a concern for AML than with ALL. It is more common with acute monocytic and myelomonocytic leukemia, as well as with relapses of acute promyelocytic leukemia. In studies where lumbar puncture is routinely performed, the incidence of CNS disease approaches 20%. Additional risk factors include African-American ethnicity, younger age, and a high serum LDH. Cytarabine is commonly used as part of combination chemotherapy in AML and is thought to be relatively effective at treating CNS leukemia even when clinicians are unaware that it is present. CNS disease with AML may manifest especially with meningeal involvement and cranial neuropathies. Although the pathogenesis is not always clear, some patients have evidence of raised intracranial pressure with headaches, visual impairment, and papilledema. Patients may present with extramedullary granulocytic sarcomas, which sometimes develop in the brain. Other manifestations may include intracranial hemorrhage and spinal cord compression.

CNS leukemia is most often detected by lumbar puncture. There is, however, a concern that traumatic lumbar puncture could introduce leukemic cells into CSF. Traumatic lumbar puncture is more common in the presence of thrombocytopenia, such that some experts recommend only performing the procedure once the platelet count has been corrected to more than 40,000 to 50,000. Apart from the presence of blast cells, CSF protein counts are usually moderately elevated and glucose levels may be low. MRI scans may be helpful in occasional patients who have intracranial mass lesions.

There have been no clinical trials to specifically direct therapy of AML involving the CNS, such that treatment strategies are largely extrapolated from experience with other malignancies. Initial intrathecal treatment usually consists of either intrathecal methotrexate or cytarabine. As with lymphoid malignancies, intrathecal therapy can be administered either by repeated lumbar puncture or an Ommaya reservoir. The dosage is reduced by about 20% when drug is delivered directly into cerebral ventricles. Treatment is usually given two or three times per week until leukemic cells have cleared and then approximately every week for 1 year. Liposomal cytarabine has the advantage that it only needs to be administered every 2 weeks initially and then monthly. Radiation therapy is reserved for refractory cases or when patients have intracranial mass lesions or cranial neuropathies.

HEMATOPOIETIC CELL TRANSPLANTATION

Hematopoietic cell transplantation (HCT) refers to the use of high-dose preparative chemotherapy followed by the intravenous infusion of autologous or allogeneic progenitor cells. The source of transplanted cells can be bone marrow, peripheral blood, or umbilical cord blood. HCT is used primarily to treat hematologic and lymphoid cancers but occasionally also nonmalignant marrow disorders. Pretransplant preparative regimens may be myeloablative or nonmyeloablative with the goal of eradicating malignant cells. In the case of allogeneic transplantation, conditioning regimens also provide immunosuppression to prevent graft rejection. Nonmyeloablative "reduced-intensity conditioning" (RIC) regimens are used in patients who may not tolerate more intensive induction therapy. The efficacy of RIC depends in part on a graft-versus-tumor effect. Frequently used myeloablative drugs include busulfan, cyclophosphamide, and melphalan. In the treatment of lymphoma, the most common myeloablative regimen consists of combination chemotherapy with carmustine, etoposide, cytosine arabinoside, and melphalan ("BEAM"). Fludarabine is used in RIC regimens and may also be combined with lower doses of the same drugs used for myeloablation. Coadministration of total body irradiation targets sites that may not otherwise be affected by chemotherapy. Monoclonal antibodies directed at specific antigens on bone marrow cells can be radiolabeled and used to provide directed radiation therapy, which helps avoid the adverse systemic effects of total body irradiation. Conditioning regimens are invariably complicated by the development of pancytopenia within a few days.

One of the major complications of allogeneic HCT is *graft-versus-host disease* (GVHD), which becomes more common with a greater degree of disparity in HLA matching. Calcineurin inhibitors (cyclosporine and tacrolimus), in combination with either mycophenolate or methotrexate, are used in the prevention of GVHD. T-lymphocyte depletion with antithymocyte globulin is performed in high-risk cases.

In the setting of autologous HCT, peripheral blood progenitor cells are preferred over bone marrow because this approach leads to more rapid engraftment and fewer complications. With allogeneic HCT, there seems to be little difference in survival between use of peripheral progenitor cells and bone marrow. Peripheral cells are associated with more rapid engraftment but a somewhat higher rate of GVHD. Umbilical cord blood is another widely available source of progenitor cells that is increasingly used, but it is associated with a higher rate of graft failure and delayed immune reconstitution. Engraftment typically requires between 10 days and 4 weeks, during which patients are at especially high risk of bacterial infections and require repeated RBC and platelet transfusions.

Epidemiology

Neurologic complications occur in about 15% to 20% of patients within the first 3 to 4 months after HCT. If carefully sought, delirium may develop at some point in as many half of patients. The risk of CNS complications is higher with allogeneic compared with autologous HCT, especially when donors are unrelated and there is a greater degree of HLA mismatch. The most common causes of CNS complications are drug toxicity and infections. Ischemic stroke and intracranial hemorrhage are relatively unusual. Some late CNS complications may be due to disease relapse.

Pathobiology

During the initial 2 to 4 weeks after HCT, before engraftment, patients are neutropenic, resulting in a relative loss of phagocytic defenses. Chemotherapy-induced mucositis enables pathogens to translocate from the gut. Patients are therefore especially vulnerable to bacterial and fungal infections and sepsis is a common cause of nonfocal encephalopathy. Common respiratory virus (e.g., influenza) and herpes simplex virus (HSV) infections may occur throughout the post-HCT course but do not usually involve the CNS. Opportunistic viruses that reactivate in the setting of impaired cell-mediated immunity, including cytomegalovirus (CMV) and varicella-zoster virus (VZV), become a concern in the postengraftment period. Patients remain vulnerable to such infections for months. Toxoplasmosis and mycobacteria are nonviral pathogens that may reactivate. During the late postengraftment period, months to years after HCT, reactivation of Epstein–Barr virus (EBV) may induce polyclonal B-cell proliferation, which causes posttransplant lymphoproliferative disorder, a syndrome that resembles lymphoma and may involve the CNS. Because of the concerns about infection, many HCT protocols use prophylactic antimicrobials. Fluoroquinolones (e.g., levofloxacin) are typically used as prophylaxis against bacteria. Acyclovir and fluconazole are the most common regimens used for prophylaxis and against HSV and fungal infections. Surveillance for CMV and *Aspergillus* sp. enables preemptive therapy if infection is considered to be imminent.

Clinical Manifestations, Diagnosis, and Treatment

COMPLICATIONS OF CONDITIONING DRUGS

Potential neurologic complications of drugs used in HCT conditioning are summarized in Table 118.3. Several drugs, especially busulfan, have been associated with development of seizures. Some centers give prophylaxis to patients who receive busulfan. Although data to support this practice is limited, the incidence of seizures appears to be very low with prophylaxis. Because of concerns about drug interactions, clonazepam or levetiracetam are preferred over phenytoin by some clinicians. Although less common, there have also been case reports of neurotoxicity with cyclophosphamide, melphalan, fludarabine, and cytarabine, all of which may present with encephalopathy.

COMPLICATIONS OF CALCINEURIN INHIBITORS

Cyclosporine and tacrolimus are widely used in the prevention of GVHD (see Table 118.3). Posterior reversible leukoencephalopathy syndrome (PRES) is the most common serious neurologic complication of calcineurin inhibitors (see also Chapter 43). This condition is characterized by vasogenic edema that preferentially (but not exclusively) involves the posterior regions of the brain. Typical manifestations of PRES include seizures, an altered or depressed level of consciousness, and visual disturbances. The diagnosis is

TABLE 118.3	Neurologic Complications of Chemotherapeutic Drugs Used in Hematopoietic Cell Transplantation	
Drug	**Indication**	**Associated Complications**
Busulfan	Conditioning	Seizures
Carboplatin	Conditioning	PRES, peripheral neuropathy, ototoxicity
Carmustine	Conditioning	Delayed encephalopathy
Cyclophosphamide	Conditioning	Transient encephalopathy
Cyclosporine	GVHD prophylaxis	PRES, seizures, movement disorders, optic neuropathy, mutism, pseudotumor cerebri, polyneuropathy
Cytarabine	Systemic: conditioning Intrathecal: CNS prophylaxis	Seizures, cerebellar dysfunction, lymphocytic meningitis, cauda equine syndrome
Etoposide	Conditioning	PRES, peripheral neuropathy, acute dystonia
Fludarabine	Reduced intensity conditioning	Toxic leukoencephalopathy, PRES, retinal toxicity
Ifosfamide	Refractory lymphoma	Encephalopathy, seizures, movement disorders
Melphalan	Conditioning	Encephalopathy
Methotrexate	Systemic: conditioning Intrathecal: CNS prophylaxis, GVHD prophylaxis	PRES, necrotizing leukoencephalopathy, transient stroke-like syndrome (may have restricted diffusion), seizures, movement disorders, optic neuropathy
Sirolimus	GVHD prophylaxis	PRES, polyneuropathy
Tacrolimus	GVHD prophylaxis	PRES, seizures, movement disorders, optic neuropathy, mutism, polyneuropathy, hearing loss, demyelinating lesions

PRES, posterior reversible leukoencephalopathy syndrome; GVHD, graft-versus-host disease; CNS, central nervous system.

established with MRI. Substitution with another immunosuppressive drug is generally required. Other complications that have been reported include tremors and other movement disorders, optic neuropathy, pseudotumor cerebri, akinetic mutism, plexopathy, and demyelinating lesions.

BACTERIAL INFECTIONS

Encephalopathy attributable to sepsis is a common neurologic complication in the early post-HCT period. However, bacterial infections specifically involving the CNS are unusual. Initial antibiotic coverage with sufficient dosing to reach the CNS needs to be broadly directed at both gram-positive and gram-negative organisms. *Listeria monocytogenes* is a pathogen that occurs particularly in immunosuppressed patients and requires additional coverage with high-dose ampicillin or, in penicillin-allergic patients, trimethoprim-sulfamethoxazole.

FUNGAL INFECTIONS

Candida does not have a particular predilection for the CNS, but involvement may occur in the context of disseminated disease. *Candida tropicalis* is the most likely species to be implicated. It most often causes meningitis but may also produce microabscesses. The CSF WBC count is usually elevated with either a predominance of neutrophils or leukocytes. Liposomal amphotericin B is the preferred drug because it achieves relatively high CNS concentrations and has a higher rate of success compared with other agents. It can be transitioned to fluconazole after the initial 2 weeks of therapy, but a total duration of several weeks is required, depending on the clinical and radiographic course.

Severe and prolonged neutropenia, as well as GVHD, predisposes patients to invasive *Aspergillus* infections, which most often appear early in the postengraftment period. CNS involvement may occur in the context of disseminated disease or because of local spread from sinuses and has a particular predilection for the corpus callosum. Patients usually present with seizures or focal neurologic deficits. Imaging may demonstrate multiple ring-enhancing mass lesions, sometimes with concomitant infarction. The diagnosis of invasive *Aspergillus* infections can be challenging because cultures of sputum and CSF are not always positive. A positive serum galactomannan assay has a sensitivity of about 60% to 70% and specificity for invasive disease of about 90%. The sensitivity is further increased if galactomannan can be detected in a bronchoscopy sample. When feasible, histologic assessment of biopsy material can be diagnostic. The mortality associated with CNS *Aspergillus* infections is high. Voriconazole in combination with an echinocandin, as well as surgical abscess drainage when feasible, is the preferred treatment [**Level 1**].[12]

VIRAL INFECTIONS

Although rare, several viruses have been reported to cause encephalitis after HCT. Human herpesvirus 6 (HHV-6) infections have been reported to occur in as many as 3% to 4% of patients undergoing allogeneic HCT, with a median posttransplant time interval of about 3 weeks. A major risk factor is the use of umbilical cord hematopoietic cells. MRI findings, if present, are most likely to involve the temporal lobes. Other viruses tend to occur later in the course. VZV reactivation is common after HCT but usually does not involve the CNS. Cases used to occur in the immediate postengraftment period. However, with use of antiviral prophylaxis, infections more often develop weeks to months later. Cases of encephalitis due to CMV, EBV, HSV, and West Nile virus have also been primarily described well after engraftment. Diagnosis of viral infections is supported by MRI findings and relevant cerebrospinal fluid polymerase chain reaction (PCR) analysis.

Progressive multifocal leukoencephalopathy (PML) is a demyelinating condition attributable to John Cunningham (JC) virus. PML may complicate various conditions characterized by significant immune suppression. PML has been described after both allogeneic and autologous HCT with a median lag of about 11 months. Clinical manifestations include seizures and subacute onset of focal neurologic deficits, ataxia, and visual disturbances. MRI shows white matter lesions, which may show contrast enhancement. The diagnosis can be made in most cases with PCR of CSF for JC virus, which has a sensitivity of about 75% to 85% and a specificity of more than 90%. Falsely negative cases can only be diagnosed definitively with brain biopsy. There is no specific therapy for JC virus. Apart from cessation of immunosuppressive agents, drugs with theoretical action against JC virus include cidofovir and mefloquine. Mirtazapine has also been administered based on the observation that JC virus uses serotonin receptors to infect cells.

PROTOZOAL INFECTIONS

The protozoan *Toxoplasma gondii* exists in a quiescent form in some recipients of HCT and may reactivate in the postengraftment period because of impaired cell-mediated immunity. Most patients who develop invasive disease are seropositive before undergoing transplantation. The presence of moderate to severe GVHD is a risk factor. Onset of symptoms typically occurs after about 2 to 3 months. Toxoplasmosis may present with isolated CNS involvement or as part of a disseminated infection. Clinical manifestations include fever, seizures, and a depressed level of consciousness. Extracerebral manifestations may include pneumonitis or chorioretinitis. Neuroimaging usually reveals ring-enhancing lesions. A presumptive diagnosis can be based on characteristic clinical findings in patients who have positive *Toxoplasma* serology and did not receive prophylaxis. The diagnosis can be made with CSF PCR with a high specificity but variable sensitivity. Biopsy of affected brain is usually diagnostic in patients that can safely undergo the procedure. Initial therapy consists of pyrimethamine, sulfadiazine, and leucovorin for about 6 weeks. Corticosteroids should be considered for patients with evidence of significant vasogenic edema and mass effect.

GRAFT-VERSUS-HOST DISEASE

Acute GVHD affects primarily the gastrointestinal tract, skin, liver, eyes, and lungs; neurologic involvement is uncommon. Chronic GVHD (occurring after >100 days) involves the peripheral nervous system more often than the CNS. Conditions that have been associated with GVHD include polymyositis, immune-mediated polyneuropathy comparable to Guillain–Barré syndrome and myasthenia gravis. CNS conditions that have been associated with GVHD include vasculitis, acute demyelinating encephalomyelitis, and aseptic meningitis. In most cases, it is unclear to what degree the GVHD is causative, and treatment does not differ from idiopathic cases.

PLATELET DISORDERS

THROMBOCYTOPENIA

After formation in the bone marrow from megakaryocytes, platelets circulate for 7 to 10 days. Thrombocytopenia is defined as a platelet count less than 150,000/μL. The risk of spontaneous hemorrhage, including intracranial hemorrhage, increases especially below 10,000 to 20,000/μL. A review of reported cases of ICH among children in the United States with immune thrombocytopenic purpura (ITP) found that 90% had counts less than 20,000/μL and

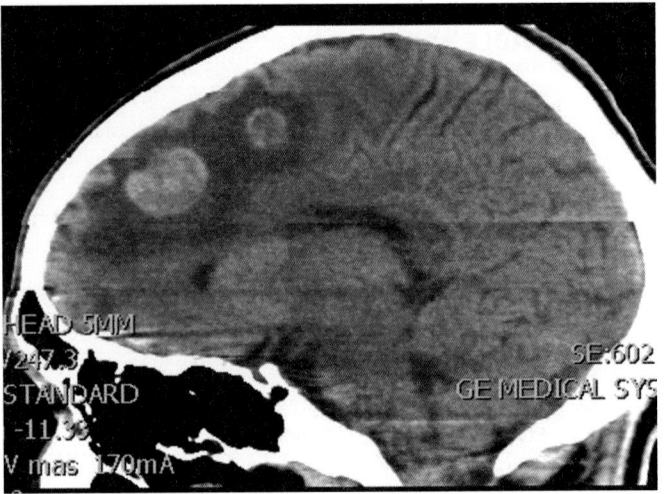

FIGURE 118.3 CT scan of a 19-year-old man who presented with acute promyelocytic leukemia, complicated by disseminated intravascular coagulation and severe thrombocytopenia, demonstrating multiple areas of hyperdensity consistent with intracerebral hemorrhage.

75% had counts less than 10,000/μL. Excessive bleeding during surgery may be encountered below 50,000/μL. Thrombocytopenia may occur because of reduced production, increased destruction or consumption, and splenic sequestration (Figs. 118.3 and 118.4).

Prophylactic platelet transfusions are generally not recommended unless the platelet count reaches 10,000/μL. Transfusion strategies that are even more restrictive than this have been associated with a higher risk of spontaneous bleeding [**Level 1**].[13,14] The minimum platelet count required before performing lumbar puncture is not well defined but is recommended to be greater than 40,000 to 50,000/μL, particularly because the consequences of iatrogenic hemorrhage could be catastrophic. For neurosurgical procedures, counts greater than 80,000 to 100,000/μL have been suggested. A similar target seems reasonable when spontaneous ICH occurs in thrombocytopenic patients, especially in the first few hours. The expected increment in the platelet concentration per unit transfused is about 10,000/μL. More frequent administration of lower doses may be a more efficient approach, with less overall need for allogeneic platelets than less frequent higher doses [**Level 1**].[15] Certain causes of thrombocytopenia have other important neurologic effects and merit further discussion.

Thrombotic Thrombocytopenic Purpura and Hemolytic Uremic Syndrome

Thrombotic thrombocytopenic purpura (TTP) is a clinical syndrome characterized by the presence of microangiopathic hemolytic anemia, thrombocytopenia, and various degrees of organ failure in the absence of another recognized cause (e.g., malignant hypertension or scleroderma). TTP and hemolytic uremic syndrome (HUS) are likely to represent different spectrums of the same disease, with the former classically having neurologic manifestations and the latter presenting with renal involvement. The comprehensive term *thrombotic thrombocytopenic purpura-hemolytic uremic syndrome* (TTP-HUS) is increasingly used. The classic "pentad" consisting of hemolysis, thrombocytopenia, fever, neurologic manifestations, and kidney failure is not required for a diagnosis of TTP-HUS and is actually not present in the majority of cases. It is possible that, over time, TTP-HUS has been recognized and treated earlier, such that

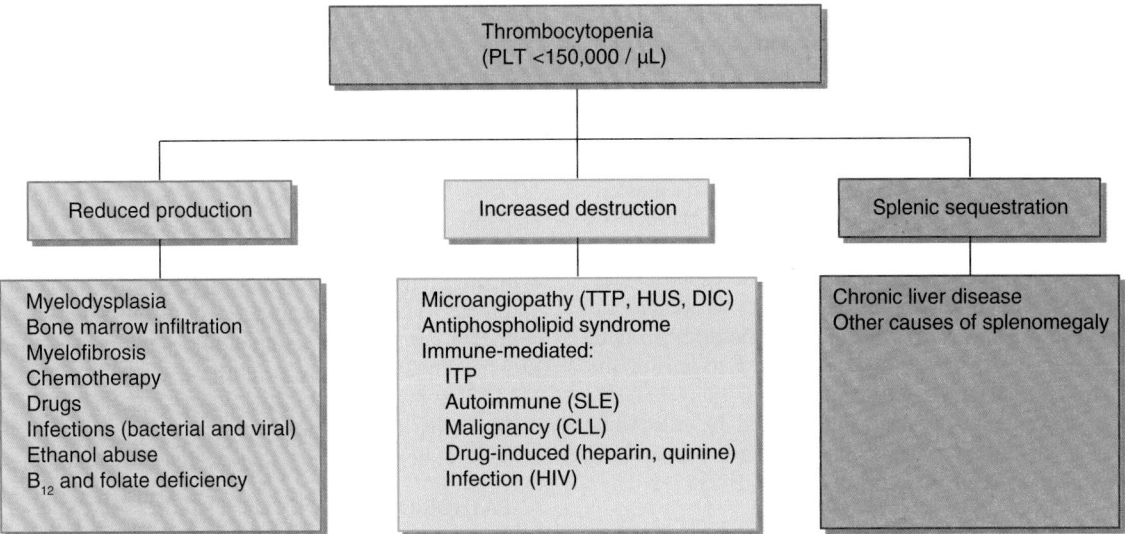

FIGURE 118.4 Causes of thrombocytopenia. PLT, platelet; TTP, thrombotic thrombocytopenic purpura; HUS, hemolytic uremic syndrome; DIC, disseminated intravascular coagulation; ITP, immune thrombocytopenic purpura; SLE, systemic lupus erythematosus; CLL, chronic lymphocytic leukemia.

progression to fulminant disease has become less common. Some patients with TTP-HUS have reduced activity of ADAMTS13, a metalloprotease responsible for cleaving von Willebrand factor (vWF). About half of patients with TTP-HUS have neurologic involvement.

EPIDEMIOLOGY

The incidence of TTP-HUS is about 4 to 11 cases per million population per year. About 40% of cases are idiopathic; about a third occur in the setting of various autoimmune, infectious, or malignant disorders; and the remainder is associated with various drugs, HCT, or pregnancy. A form of TTP-HUS that is particularly common in children follows diarrheal illness caused by toxin-producing enterohemorrhagic *Escherichia coli* (EHEC).

PATHOBIOLOGY

TTP is characterized pathologically by the formation of platelet-rich thrombi in arterioles and capillaries. There is also thickening of the intima, hypertrophy of underlying smooth muscle, and deposition of fibrin. Many idiopathic cases of TTP-HUS are associated with severe deficiency of ADAMTS13 activity (<10% of normal). Reduced activity is commonly related to an inhibitory antibody. The consequent accumulation vWF multimer promotes platelet activation and aggregation. Other mechanisms that have been implicated include relative deficiency of vascular endothelial growth factor, increased amounts of plasminogen activator inhibitor type 1, and dysregulation of complement. In patients with TTP-HUS complicating EHEC diarrheal illness, toxins penetrate into the circulation bound to neutrophils and then target endothelial cells. Although kidney involvement is common with this disorder, it is not universal and some patients present with neurologic manifestations.

Some chemotherapeutic agents (e.g., cisplatin) and immunosuppressive drugs (e.g., cyclosporine) produce direct endothelial toxicity that resembles TTP-HUS. The most common drug to be implicated in causing TTP-HUS is quinine; in this case, the pathogenesis appears to be antibody-mediated. The mechanism of TTP-HUS that is occasionally associated with use of the antiplatelet agent clopidogrel is not well understood. Although the pathogenesis of TTP-HUS occurring in pregnancy is not clear, it has been noted that ADAMTS13 levels decline progressively beginning in the second trimester, which may increase vulnerability.

Autopsy specimens show similar changes in cerebral microvasculature as in other organs. Some patients develop acute ischemic strokes but these do not usually involve large vascular territories. In a series of patients with TTP who had neurologic manifestations and underwent brain MRI scans, about a third had small ischemic strokes. When angiography is performed, large-vessel occlusion is rarely observed. By far the most common radiographic findings are those of PRES, which was present in almost half of cases. As with other causes of PRES, the mechanism likely involves vasogenic edema induced by endothelial damage and disruption of the blood–brain barrier. When clinicians observe hypodensities on CT scans, they should not necessarily conclude that they are infarcts or that they are irreversible.

CLINICAL MANIFESTATIONS

TTP-HUS is invariably characterized by the presence hemolysis and thrombocytopenia. Hemolysis results in increased concentrations of serum indirect bilirubin and LDH and reductions in serum haptoglobin. Levels of LDH are often very high and can be used as a surrogate for response to therapy. RBCs become fragmented by fibrin in the microcirculation, resulting in the formation of schistocytes, which can be visualized on peripheral blood smears. Thrombocytopenia ranges from profound to relatively mild. In patients with renal involvement, there may be some hematuria and proteinuria, although it is usually not as severe as in patients with glomerulonephritis. A minority of patients requires renal replacement therapy. The most common neurologic manifestation is altered mental status occurring in about one-third of all patients. Seizures occur in about 15% to 20%, whereas coma and strokes occur in about 10%. When PRES occurs in its most characteristic location, cortical blindness may ensue.

DIAGNOSIS

In patients who are anemic and thrombocytopenic, crucial diagnostic tests to assess for TTP-HUS are a peripheral blood smear, serum LDH, and bilirubin. Sepsis with disseminated intravascular coagulation (DIC) produces some of the same findings as TTP-HUS but usually also causes prolongation of the prothrombin time (PT) and partial thromboplastin time (PTT) and a reduction in serum fibrinogen levels. Measurement of ADAMTS13 is recommended. A low level of ADAMTS13 activity (<10%) is a specific finding that essentially confirms the diagnosis of TTP-HUS. On the other hand, patients with TTP-HUS may not have low ADAMTS13 activity, and intermediate (10% to 50%) or normal (>50%) values should not be used as criteria to stop therapy. Patients who present with higher ADAMTS13 activity do, however, appear less likely to relapse after initial therapy.

If patients have acute kidney injury that does not response readily to fluid resuscitation, a kidney biopsy can be considered and may be diagnostic. Potential causes of TTP-HUS should be sought. If there is a history of diarrhea, stool should be assessed for the presence of toxin-producing bacteria, especially *E. coli* O157:H7. In women of appropriate age, pregnancy should be ruled out. Clinicians should determine whether patients have been taking various drugs that have been associated with TTP-HUS.

TREATMENT

In original descriptions of TTP-HUS, mortality was very high. Outcomes have improved markedly with use of plasma exchange (PLEX), which has been demonstrated to be efficacious in randomized controlled trials [**Level 1**].[16] It is thought that one of the main mechanisms of PLEX is the removal of inhibitory antibodies targeting ADAMTS13 and concomitant replacement with plasma. However, the efficacy of PLEX is not necessarily limited to patients who are shown to be ADAMTS13 deficient. It is therefore reasonable to initiate PLEX even before the diagnosis is entirely certain. The benefit of PLEX is less clear in TTP-HUS associated with other conditions compared with idiopathic cases. PLEX is usually performed daily until platelet counts have normalized and evidence of hemolysis (high LDH and presence of schistocytes) is abating. Because of the presumed autoimmune etiology of idiopathic TTP-HUS, some experts recommend treatment with corticosteroids. Preliminary data suggest rituximab may be beneficial in refractory cases. When TTP-HUS occurs in pregnancy, it may be difficult to distinguish from other obstetrical syndromes, including preeclampsia and HELLP syndrome, such that early delivery should be considered. PLEX is safe during pregnancy and should not be withheld.

Treatment of neurologic complications is largely supportive. Usual measures aimed at preventing and treating cerebral edema should be implemented. Neurologic involvement in TTP-HUS is a clear risk factor for failure to respond to therapy and worse outcomes. Longer term follow-up of patients who survived TTP-HUS reveals that many have persistent neurocognitive deficits. Future research should investigate whether modifications in the care of patients with TTP-HUS might prevent such deficits.

Heparin-Induced Thrombocytopenia

Heparin is one of the most common medications known to induce thrombocytopenia. Immune-mediated heparin-induced thrombocytopenia (HIT) occurs after at least 5 days of heparin exposure and is associated with a high risk of thrombotic (rather than hemorrhagic) complications, including stroke. The incidence is approximately 2% to 3% with more than 5 days of heparin exposure. The risk is higher with unfractionated rather than low molecular weight heparin in surgical patients and in women. Onset beyond 2 weeks of heparin exposure is relatively uncommon.

PATHOBIOLOGY AND CLINICAL FEATURES

HIT is due to the formation of antibodies targeting the heparin-platelet factor 4 (PF4) complex. When antibodies bind to this complex on platelet surfaces, they induce platelet activation and aggregation, which in turn promotes thrombin generation. Consumption and clearance of activated platelets causes the platelet concentration to fall. The risk of thrombosis over the 4 weeks following the diagnosis of HIT is greater than 50%. Most patients with HIT have relatively mild thrombocytopenia (rarely <20,000/μL). The development of lower extremity deep venous thrombosis (DVT) is the most common complication of HIT, but arterial thrombosis can occur. Neurologic complications, primarily arterial ischemic strokes and to a lesser degree cerebral venous thrombosis, have been reported to occur in 3% to 9% of patients with established HIT.

DIAGNOSIS

A clinical scoring system, the 4T score, can be used to assess the pretest probability that a patient could have HIT (Table 118.4). Patients are assigned 0 to 2 points for each of four variables: the degree of thrombocytopenia, the timing of the drop in platelets, the development of thrombosis, and the presence of alternative causes of thrombocytopenia. A score of 0 to 3 indicates a low risk of HIT and is justification to not pursue additional testing. A score of 4 to 5 suggests an intermediate risk and 6 to 8 indicates a

---

TABLE 118.4 The 4T Score in the Diagnosis of Heparin-Induced Thrombocytopenia

Variable	2 Points	1 Point	0 Point
Thrombocytopenia severity	Platelet fall >50% and platelet nadir ≥20	Platelet fall 30%–50% or platelet nadir 10–19	Platelet fall <30% or platelet nadir <10
Timing of platelet count reduction	Clear onset day 5–10 or ≤1 day with prior heparin exposure past 30 days	Consistent with day 5–10 fall but not clear; onset after day 10; or fall ≤1 day with prior heparin 30–100 days ago	Platelet fall <4 days without recent exposure
Thrombosis	New thrombosis, skin necrosis	Progressive or recurrent thrombosis	None
Thrombocytopenia alternative causes	None apparent	Possible	Definite

Score of 0 to 3: <1% chance of HIT; score of 4 to 5: 10% to 15% chance of HIT; score of 6 to 8: >50% chance of HIT.

Data from Cuker A, Gimotty PA, Crowther MA, et al. Predictive value of the 4Ts scoring system for heparin-induced thrombocytopenia: a systematic review and meta-analysis. *Blood*. 2012;120:4160–4167.

high risk. Heparin-PF4 complexes can be detected with enzyme-linked immunosorbent assay (ELISA) with a high sensitivity but somewhat lower specificity. The gold standard test, with sensitivity and specificity greater than 95%, is the C^{14}-serotonin release assay, which is only performed at specialized centers.

TREATMENT

When HIT is suspected, all heparin must be discontinued, including that used for DVT prophylaxis or to flush venous or arterial catheters. If the suspicion for HIT is at least moderate, the risk of thrombosis is sufficiently high to justify therapeutic anticoagulation with an alternative drug that does not cross-react with heparin. Appropriate alternatives include the direct thrombin inhibitors argatroban, bivalirudin, or danaparoid. Successful use of the pentasaccharide fondaparinux has been described in a few patients, but this drug has also been reported to induce HIT and is therefore currently not preferred. Treatment with warfarin is recommended after the platelet count has risen to more than 150,000/μL. Warfarin should overlap with the thrombin-specific inhibitor for at least 5 days and should then be continued with a target international normalized ratio (INR) of 2 to 3 for 3 months in the setting of thrombosis and 4 to 6 weeks for HIT without thrombosis.

IMPAIRED PLATELET FUNCTION

Platelet function may be impaired by numerous genetic disorders and acquired medical conditions, including uremia, plasma cell dyscrasias, advanced liver disease, and myeloproliferative disorders. More often, platelet dysfunction is iatrogenic from antiplatelet drugs used in the prevention and treatment of cardiovascular disease.

Many patients that develop spontaneous ICH or subdural hematomas are receiving antiplatelet drugs. The degree of hematoma expansion over the initial few hours after intracranial hemorrhage is a crucial predictor of outcome. Although literature is conflicting, numerous studies have suggested that the degree of hematoma expansion and the chance of poor outcomes are greater among patients receiving antiplatelet drugs. Aspirin (ASA) is the most common agent and works by inhibiting the effects of cyclooxygenase-1 (COX-1) in converting arachidonic acid to prostaglandin H_2, thereby reducing levels of thromboxane A_2, an inducer of platelet aggregation. The antiplatelet effects of ASA are irreversible and last for the life span of the platelet. Clopidogrel is a thienopyridine drug, which works by permanently modifying platelet ADP receptors, thereby inhibiting platelet aggregation. The addition of clopidogrel to ASA is particularly important for patients who have undergone percutaneous coronary interventions (PCI). Prasugrel and ticagrelor are newer antiplatelet drugs that work on the same receptor as clopidogrel and may have a greater degree of antiplatelet effect and in turn a slightly higher risk of bleeding.

Newer assays enable point-of-care assessment of platelet function, thereby allowing the effects of antiplatelet drugs to be rapidly measured. This information could potentially be used in therapeutic decision making. Platelet transfusions can improve platelet activity and may reduce hematoma expansion. Similarly, desmopressin improves platelet activity by promoting the release of vWF from endothelium. However, whether platelet transfusions or desmopressin improve outcomes in acute ICH requires further study.

THROMBOCYTOSIS

Thrombocytosis refers to an elevation in the concentration of platelets and is usually defined using a threshold of 450,000/μL. Thrombocytosis may be "reactive" in response to a systemic condition or may be a manifestation of ET or another myeloproliferative disorder ("autonomous thrombocytosis"). A reactive etiology (e.g., inflammation, tissue damage, anemia) is much more common, even when thrombocytosis is extreme (>1,000,000/μL). Clinical manifestations, including vasomotor symptoms (e.g., headache and visual disturbances) as well as thrombotic or hemorrhagic complications, occur with autonomous thrombocytosis and are uncommon with reactive thrombocytosis.

Essential Thrombocythemia

ET is a clonal myeloproliferative disorder characterized by an elevated platelet count. There is no specific diagnostic test for ET and excluding reactive thrombocytosis and other myeloproliferative disorders makes the diagnosis. ET is associated with an increased risk of thrombosis, including stroke. The median age of patients diagnosed with ET is about 60 years and it is more common in women.

PATHOBIOLOGY

Numerous factors contribute an increased risk of thrombosis, including activation of platelets, resistance to the effects of endogenous coagulation inhibitors (protein C and S), increased levels of thrombomodulin, and activation of leukocytes. Risk factors for thrombosis include a previous history of thrombotic events, the presence of the JAK2 mutation, leukocytosis, and other cardiovascular risk factors.

CLINICAL MANIFESTATIONS

Many patients are asymptomatic at the time of diagnosis. The most common complaints are vasomotor symptoms and erythromelalgia. The risk of thrombosis is not directly related to the degree of platelet elevation. The risk of thrombotic events over 15 years is about 20% and stroke develops in about 10% to 15% of patients. A small proportion of patients eventually develop AML or myelofibrosis.

DIAGNOSIS

Bone marrow aspirates and biopsies demonstrate hyperplasia of megakaryocytes. Cytogenetic studies reveal absence of the Philadelphia chromosome (characteristic of chronic myelogenous leukemia). About half of patients with ET will have the JAK2 mutation. To be diagnosed with ET, there should be no evidence of myelofibrosis and a normal RBC mass.

TREATMENT

Patients at low risk of thrombosis include those younger than 60 years, with no previous events and a platelet count less than 1,000,000/μL. These patients do not necessarily require treatment. Vasomotor symptoms and erythromelalgia often respond to treatment with low-dose ASA. Patients with previous thrombosis and those who are older than 60 years are generally treated with a combination of ASA and hydroxyurea, with an initial dose of 15 mg/kg/day, adjusted to achieve a target platelet count less than 600,000/μL [**Level 1**].[17] Achieving counts less than 400,000/μL may further reduce the risk of subsequent thrombosis.

COAGULATION DISTURBANCES

Coagulation disturbances develop when there is insufficient production, increased consumption, or inhibition of clotting factors. Apart from rare congenital deficiencies of specific clotting factors (e.g., factor VIII with hemophilia A), reduced production of clotting factors occurs because of liver disease, vitamin K deficiency, or the use of the vitamin K antagonist warfarin. Other anticoagulants work primarily by inhibiting thrombin. Consumption of clotting factors occurs with DIC and massive hemorrhage. Coagulation disturbances are of interest to neurologists and neurosurgeons because of their association with intracranial hemorrhage.

NORMAL COAGULATION

When endothelium is damaged, there is immediate activation and aggregation of platelets. Apart from forming an initial barrier to bleeding, the platelet plug also provides the phospholipid template upon which coagulation can proceed. Tissue factor is a membrane protein that is expressed by subendothelial cells and interacts with circulating factor VII, which in turn activates factor X. This process is further amplified by factors VIII and IX. Activated factor X, together with factor V, converts prothrombin to thrombin, which in turn promotes conversion of fibrinogen to fibrin. Thrombin also has a positive feedback effect, whereby it further activates platelets, factor VIII, and factor XI (Fig. 118.5).

To avoid unregulated clotting, there exist a number of natural anticoagulant mechanisms. Antithrombin is a protease inhibitor that blocks the activity of factor X. Thrombomodulin is protein on the surface of endothelial cells that inhibits thrombin and activates protein C, which together with protein S inactivates factors V and VIII. The endothelial enzyme tissue plasminogen activator (tPA) stimulates the conversion of plasminogen to plasmin, which is responsible for cleaving cross-lined fibrin.

IMPAIRED COAGULATION

Warfarin-Induced Intracranial Hemorrhage

Warfarin is widely used to reduce the risk of thromboembolic complications in patients with atrial fibrillation, to prevent valve thrombosis in patients with mechanical heart valves, and as treatment of venous thromboembolism. Warfarin antagonizes the formation of vitamin K–dependent clotting factors (II, VII, IX, and X) in the liver. Its effect on clotting is measured by the PT and the measurement is standardized using the INR. For most conditions,

the target INR is 2 to 3. The risk of intracranial hemorrhage with warfarin has been in the range of 1% in clinical trials, but it is somewhat higher in usual practice, where patients may not be as carefully selected and the INR not as carefully monitored. Warfarin use has traditionally accounted for as many as a quarter of spontaneous ICH cases at some centers, although this proportion will decrease with increasing use of new oral anticoagulants.

Hematoma expansion is more pronounced and outcomes worse among patients with warfarin-induced ICH. Although fresh frozen plasma (FFP) reverses the effects of warfarin, the time required for cross-matching, thawing, and administering 20 to 40 mL/kg of fluid results in major delays. The INR can be corrected more rapidly with the use of four-factor prothrombin complex concentrate (PCC), which contains vitamin K–dependent clotting factors in a relatively small volume of fluid that can be administered over a few minutes [**Level 1**].[18] Several commercially available three-factor PCC products lack factor VII and do not appear to be as effective in normalizing the INR. The 2010 iteration of American Heart Association guidelines recommends the use of either FFP or PCC, whereas the 2012 American College of Chest Physicians guidelines recommend the use of four-factor PCC. The optimal dose of PCC remains unclear but is generally recommended to include 25 to 50 IU/kg of factor IX activity. Vitamin K should also be administered either enterally or intravenously.

Reversal of Novel Oral Anticoagulants

Several novel oral anticoagulants (NOACs) have been demonstrated to be equally or more efficacious than warfarin in the prevention of stroke among patients with atrial fibrillation, with a comparable or lower risk of intracranial hemorrhage. Dabigatran is a direct thrombin inhibitor, whereas rivaroxaban, apixaban, and edoxaban are all factor X_a inhibitors. The PTT and INR do not measure the effects of these agents. Measurement of the thrombin time (TT) or ecarin clotting time (ECT), if available, provides a better reflection of the anticoagulant effect of dabigatran. Anti–factor X_a activity can be measured to assess the effects of X_a inhibitors.

There are currently no specific reversing agents available when use of newer oral anticoagulants is complicated by intracranial hemorrhage. Because these drugs do not reduce levels of clotting

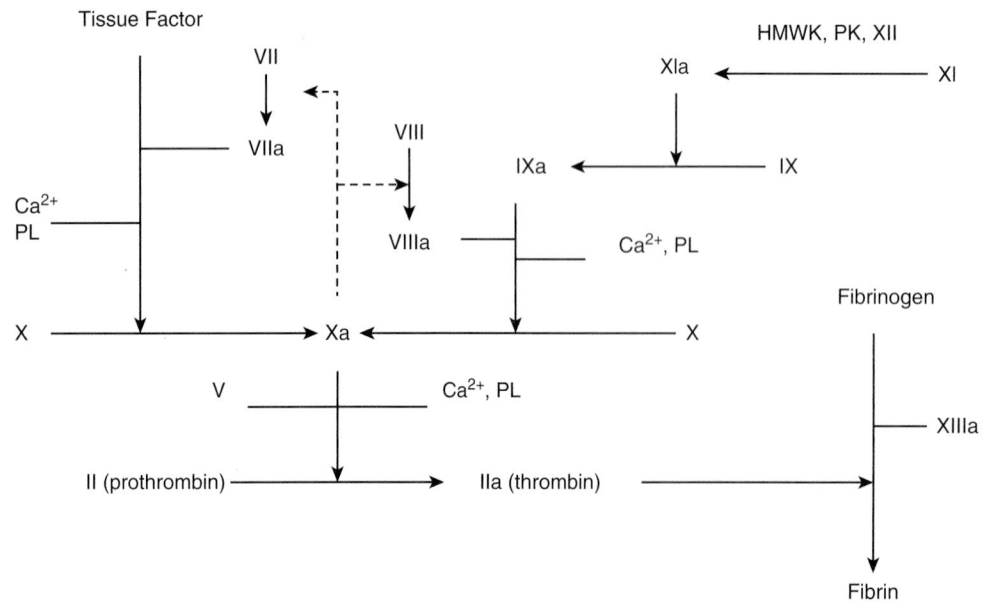

FIGURE 118.5 Traditional model of the coagulation cascade with extrinsic (*left*) and intrinsic (*right*) pathways. Although this laboratory model is useful to understand the factors which may influence coagulation times (PT, *left*; PTT, *right*), it is not a physiologic model that describes exactly how coagulation functions in vivo. HMWK, high molecular weight kininogen; PK, prekallikrein; PL, phospholipid.

factors, FFP is ineffective at reversing the coagulopathy. In contrast, standard PCC, activated PCC (factor VIII inhibitor bypassing activity), and recombinant factor VIIa may all have some limited efficacy. Despite the inability to reverse newer oral anticoagulants, outcomes do not appear to be worse than with warfarin-induced ICH. Hemodialysis can be used to rapidly reduce levels of dabigatran, but it is unlikely that this can be accomplished in a time frame that would have a major impact in preventing hematoma expansion in ICH.

Bleeding Associated with Thrombolytic Therapy

When tPA is administered to treat acute ischemic stroke, the risk of intracranial hemorrhage is in the range of 3% to 7%. This rate is 1% to 2% when tPA is used for other conditions, such as myocardial infarction or pulmonary embolism. Apart from discontinuation of the infusion, patients should receive 10 units of cryoprecipitate to increase fibrinogen levels because there is some evidence that hemorrhagic infarction after tPA is associated with a systemic consumption coagulopathy and fibrinogen depletion.

HYPERCOAGULABLE STATES

Familial Thrombophilia

The possibility of thrombophilia should be considered, especially when stroke occurs in children and young adults. It should also be pursued when there are recurrent thromboembolic events or when there is a strong family history. Several familial conditions cause deficiencies or dysfunction of naturally occurring anticoagulants, including protein S, protein C, antithrombin III, and factor V. A mutation of prothrombin (factor II) has been identified as a risk factor for both ischemic strokes and cerebral venous thrombosis, especially with concomitant use of oral contraceptives.

Antiphospholipid Antibody Syndrome

The antiphospholipid syndrome (APLS) is a condition characterized by arterial or venous thrombosis and/or pregnancy morbidity, occurring in combination with persistently detectable antiphospholipid (APL) antibodies. It is of interest to neurologists primarily because it predisposes patients to ischemic stroke and cerebral venous thrombosis and is also associated with neuropsychiatric manifestations and cognitive decline.

EPIDEMIOLOGY

Approximately half of patients have "primary" APLS, whereas the remainder has either systemic lupus erythematosus (SLE) or another connective tissue disorder. APLS is more common in women and has a mean age at diagnosis of 40 to 45 years. Ischemic strokes occur in 10% to 20% and TIAs in about 5% to 15% of patients meeting established criteria for APLS.

PATHOBIOLOGY

There are several mechanisms whereby APL antibodies may contribute to an increased risk of thrombosis, including interference with natural anticoagulant mechanisms (e.g., inhibition of protein C and antithrombin III activity), activation of platelets and endothelial cells, and triggering of the complement cascade. Some cases of ischemic stroke in APLS develop because of in situ thrombosis, whereas others are cardioembolic. Valvular cardiac abnormalities that can be detected by transesophageal echocardiography range from thickening of valve leaflets to the development of frank vegetations (nonbacterial endocarditis). The mitral valve is affected more often than the aortic valve. Spontaneous echo contrast is also sometimes found in the left atrium, but a definitive association with stroke risk has not been established.

CLINICAL MANIFESTATIONS

Prospective studies have shown that APL antibodies can be detected in a sizable proportion of patients diagnosed with ischemic strokes. However, in some cases, the antibodies are only transiently and slightly elevated and therefore not consistent with true APLS. Studies are somewhat conflicting regarding the question of whether the presence of detectable APL antibodies purports an increased risk of subsequent stroke. The association with stroke appears to be strongest and most definitive in young women and when more than one type of APL antibody is elevated.

Venous thrombosis is more common than arterial thrombosis with APLS. The possibility of APLS should always be considered in patients presenting with idiopathic cerebral venous thrombosis. A significant proportion of patients with APLS develop cognitive deficits even without previously diagnosed strokes. The specific mechanism is not well understood, although MRI scans commonly reveal white matter disease. Apart from pregnancy loss and thrombosis, APLS can also present in some cases with microangiopathy, similar to TTP-HUS. Catastrophic APLS refers to a small subset of patients who develop multiorgan failure as a result of widespread thrombosis; this occurs in less than 1% of patients.

DIAGNOSIS

APLS should be considered in the setting of idiopathic episodes of thrombosis, recurrent pregnancy loss, unexplained thrombocytopenia or abnormal PTT, and thrombotic microangiopathy. APL antibody titers should not be routinely assessed in all patients with ischemic strokes. Diagnostic workup for APLS consists of ELISA testing for IgG and IgM anticardiolipin and anti–β2-glycoprotein antibodies, as well as testing for a lupus anticoagulant. If positive, these assays should be repeated after at least 12 weeks for confirmation. Criteria for catastrophic APS have been proposed and include a history of APLS, thrombosis in three or more organ systems within a week, biopsy confirmation of microthrombosis, and exclusion of other causes of thrombosis. Patients are considered to have definite catastrophic APLS if all four criteria are met. Patients have probable APLS if there are only two organs involved, if the only missing criterion is histopathology, or if the time frame of recurrent thrombosis exceeds 1 week but is less than 1 month.

TREATMENT

Optimal treatment of stroke in the context of APLS is somewhat controversial. American Stroke Association guidelines state that antiplatelet drugs remain appropriate treatment for patients with cryptogenic ischemic stroke or TIA in whom APL antibodies are detected (class 2b, level of evidence B). The rationale for this recommendation is that the largest prospective series have not demonstrated a difference in the rate of subsequent thrombotic events based on whether or not APL antibodies are present. On the other hand, the guidelines also state that oral anticoagulation is appropriate therapy for patients in whom a diagnosis of APLS is confirmed, which would be the case for any patient with stroke in whom repeat antibody testing after 12 weeks is confirmatory. In several retrospective series of confirmed APLS, treatment with aspirin had limited efficacy.

Despite availability of newer oral anticoagulants, most experience treating APLS has been with warfarin. The goal INR is 2 to 3. Although some older literature advocated for more intensive anticoagulation (INR 3 to 4), subsequent clinical trials did not demonstrate any advantage to justify the higher risk of hemorrhage [**Level 1**].[19,20] For patients with thrombosis in the setting of APS, indefinite anticoagulation is recommended. For patients with other reasons for a thrombotic event, in whom the elevation in APL antibody titers is mild or transient, cessation of therapy after a few months can be considered.

For patients with APL antibodies and risk factors for stroke, it is reasonable to administer antiplatelet drugs as primary prophylaxis. Antiplatelet therapy is also recommended for patients with APL antibodies and neuropsychiatric manifestations but no clear evidence of a stroke. There are no randomized trials specifically in patients meeting criteria for catastrophic APLS. Retrospective series suggest that mortality may be lower when patients are treated not only with anticoagulation but also with corticosteroids and PLEX.

LEVEL 1 EVIDENCE

1. Hebert PC, Wells G, Blajchman MA, et al. A multi-center randomized, controlled clinical trial of transfusion requirements in critical care. *N Engl J Med.* 1999;340:409–417.

2. Lacroix J, Hebert PC, Hutchison JS, et al. Transfusion strategies for patients in pediatric intensive care units. *N Engl J Med.* 2007;356:1609–1619.

3. Adams R, McView V, Nichols F, et al. The use of transcranial ultrasonography to predict stroke in sickle cell disease. *N Engl J Med.* 1992;326:605–610.

4. Adams RJ, McKie VC, Hsu L, et al. Prevention of a first stroke by transfusions in children with sickle cell anemia and abnormal results on transcranial Doppler ultrasonography. *N Engl J Med.* 1998;339:5–11.

5. Adams RJ, Brambilla D; Optimizing Primary Stroke Prevention in Sickle Cell Anemia (STOP 2) Trial Investigators. Discontinuing prophylactic transfusions used to prevent stroke in sickle cell disease. *N Engl J Med.* 2005;353:2769–2778.

6. DeBaun MR, Gordon M, McKinstry RC, et al. Controlled trial of transfusions for silent cerebral infarcts in sickle cell anemia. *N Engl J Med.* 2014;371:699.

7. Steinberg MH, Barton F, Castro O, et al. Effect of hydroxyurea on mortality and morbidity in adult sickle cell anemia: risks and benefits up to 9 year of treatment. *JAMA.* 2003;289:1645.

8. National Institutes of Health. Stroke prevention study in children with sickle cell anemia, iron overload stopped early. National Institutes of Health Web site. http://www.nih.gov/news/health/jun2010/nhlbi-03.htm. Accessed May 15, 2014.

9. Marchioli R, Finazzi G, Specchia G, et al. Cardiovascular events and intensity of treatment in polycythemia vera. *N Engl J Med.* 2013;368:22.

10. Pui CH, Campana D, Pei D, et al. Treating childhood acute lymphoblastic leukemia without cranial irradiation. *N Engl J Med.* 2009;360:2730.

11. Buske C, Hoster E, Dreyling M, et al. The addition of rituximab to front-line therapy with CHOP (R-CHOP) results in a higher response rate and longer time to treatment failure in patients with lymphoplasmacytic lymphoma: results of a randomized trial of the German Low-grade Lymphoma Study Group (GLSG). *Leukemia.* 2009;23:153.

12. Herbrecht R, Denning DW, Patterson TF, et al. Voriconazole versus amphotericin B for primary therapy of invasive aspergillosis. *N Engl J Med.* 2002;347:408.

13. Rebulla P, Finazzi G, Marangoni F, et al. The threshold for prophylactic platelet transfusions in adults with acute myeloid leukemia. *N Engl J Med.* 1997;337:1870–1875.

14. Stanworth SJ, Estcourt LJ, Powter G, et al. A no-prophylaxis platelet-transfusion strategy for hematologic cancers. *N Engl J Med.* 2013;368:1771–1780.

15. Slichter SJ, Kaufman RM, Assmann SF, et al. Dose of prophylactic platelet transfusions and prevention of hemorrhage. *N Engl J Med.* 2010;362:600–613.

16. Michael M, Elliott EJ, Ridley GF. Interventions for haemolytic uremic syndrome and thrombotic thrombocytopenic purpura. *Cochrane Database Syst Rev.* 2009;(1):CD003595.

17. Cortelazzo S, Finazzi G, Ruggeri M, et al. Hydroxyurea for patients with essential thrombocythemia and a high risk of thrombosis. *N Engl J Med.* 1995;332:1132.

18. Sarode R, Milling TJ Jr, Refaai MA, et al. Efficacy and safety of a 4-factor prothrombin complex concentrate in patients on vitamin K antagonists presenting with major bleeding: a randomized, plasma-controlled, phase IIIb study. *Circulation.* 2013;128:1234–1243.

19. Crowther MA, Ginsberg JS, Denburg JJ, et al. A comparison of two intensities of warfarin for the prevention of recurrent thrombosis in patients with the antiphospholipid antibody syndrome. *N Engl J Med.* 2003;349:1133.

20. Finazzi G, Marchioli R, Brancaccio V, et al. A randomized clinical trial of high-intensity warfarin vs. conventional antithrombotic therapy for the prevention of recurrent thrombosis in patients with the antiphospholipid syndrome (WAPS). *J Thromb Haemost.* 2005;3:848.

SUGGESTED READINGS

Baehring JM, Hochberg EP, Raje N, et al. Neurological manifestations of Waldenstrom macroglobulinemia. *Nat Clin Pract Neurol.* 2008;4:547.

Burrus T, Wijdicks E, Rabinstein A. Brain lesions are most often reversible in acute thrombotic thrombocytopenic purpura. *Neurology.* 2009;73:66–70.

Cuker A, Gimotty PA, Crowther MA, et al. Predictive value of the 4Ts scoring system for heparin-induced thrombocytopenia: a systematic review and meta-analysis. *Blood.* 2012;120:4160–4167.

Denier C, Bourhis JH, Lacroix C, et al. Spectrum and prognosis of neurologic complications after hematopoietic transplantation. *Neurology.* 2006;67:1990–1997.

Dhar R, Zazulia AR, Videen TO, et al. Red blood cell transfusion increases cerebral oxygen delivery in anemic patients with subarachnoid hemorrhage. *Stroke.* 2009;40:3039–3044.

Erkan D, Espinosa G, Cervera R. Catastrophic antiphospholipid syndrome: updated diagnostic algorithms. *Autoimmune Rev.* 2010;10:74.

Flaherty ML, Tao H, Haverbusch M, et al. Warfarin use leads to larger intracerebral hematomas. *Neurology.* 2008;71:1084.

Gruppo Italiano Studio Policitemia. Polycythemia vera: the natural history of 1213 patients followed for 20 years. *Ann Intern Med* 1995;123:656.

Kramer AH, Zygun DA. Anemia and red blood cell transfusion in neurocritical care. *Crit Care.* 2009;13:R89.

Lamonte MP, Brown PM, Hursting MJ. Stroke in patients with heparin-induced thrombocytopenia and the effect of argatroban therapy. *Crit Care Med.* 2004;32:976–980.

LeRoux PD; Participants in the International Multi-disciplinary Consensus Conference on the Critical Care Management of Subarachnoid Hemorrhage. Anemia and transfusion after subarachnoid hemorrhage. *Neurocrit Care.* 2011;15:342–353.

Mackins RS, Insel P, Truran D, et al. Neuroimaging abnormalities in adults with sickle cell anemia: associations with cognition. *Neurology.* 2014;82:835–841.

Meloni G, Proia A, Antonini G, et al. Thrombotic thrombocytopenic purpura: prospective neurologic, neuroimaging and neurophysiologic evaluation. *Haematologica.* 2011;86:1194–1199.

Ohene-Frempong K, Weiner SJ, Sleeper LA, et al. Cerebrovascular accidents in sickle cell disease: rates and risk factors. *Blood*. 1998;91:288–294.

Pohl C, Harbrecht U, Greinacher A, et al. Neurologic complications of immune-mediate heparin induced thrombocytopenia. *Neurology*. 2000;54:1240–1245.

Posfai E, Marton I, Szoke A, et al. Stroke in essential thrombocythemia. *J Neurol Sci*. 2014;336:260–262.

Psaila B, Petrovic A, Page LK, et al. Intracranial hemorrhage (ICH) in children with immune thrombocytopenia (ITP): study of 40 cases. *Blood*. 2009;114:4777–4783.

Pruitt AA, Graus F, Rosenfeld MF. Neurologic complications of transplantation: part I: hematopoietic cell transplantation. *Neurohospitalist*. 2013;3:24–38.

Quinn CT, McKinstry RC, Dowling MM, et al. Acute silent cerebral ischemic events in children with sickle cell anemia. *JAMA Neurol*. 2013;70:58–65.

Rozovski U, Ohanian M, Ravandi F, et al. Incidence of and risk factors for acute myeloid leukemia involvement of the central nervous system. *Leuk Lymphoma*. 2014;11:1–19.

Saloheimo P, Ahonen M, Juvela S, et al. Regular aspirin-use preceding the onset of primary intracerebral hemorrhage is an independent predictor for death. *Stroke*. 2006;37:129–133.

Tefferi A, Rumi E, Finazzi G, et al. Survival and prognosis among 1545 patients with contemporary polycythemia vera: an international study. *Leukemia*. 2013;27:1874.

Tektonidou MG, Varsou N, Kotoulas G, et al. Cognitive deficits in patients with antiphospholipid syndrome: association with clinical, laboratory, and magnetic resonance imaging findings. *Arch Intern Med*. 2006;166:2278.

Thomas X, Le QH. Central nervous system involvement in adult acute lymphoblastic leukemia. *Hematology*. 2008;13:293.

Urbanus RT, Siegerink B, Roest M, et al. Antiphospholipid antibodies and risk of myocardial infarction and ischemic stroke in young women in the RATIO study: a case control study. *Lancet Neurol*. 2009;8:998–1005.

Vichinsky EP, Neumayr LD, Gold JI, et al. Neuropsychological dysfunction and neuroimaging abnormalities in neurologically intact adults with sickle cell anemia. *JAMA*. 2010;303:1823–1831.

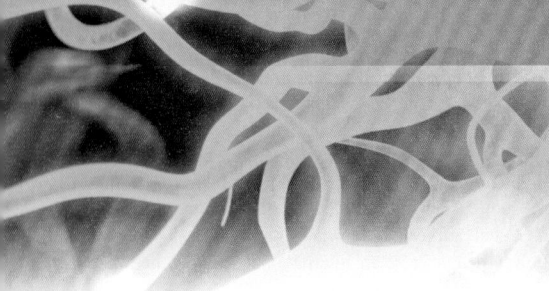

Hepatic Disease and the Brain 119

Charles L. Francoeur and Stephan A. Mayer

INTRODUCTION

Neurologic manifestations of liver disease have been recognized for centuries. The liver is indispensable in its functions of synthesis, metabolism, and detoxification, and its dysfunction can cause symptoms ranging from subtle neuropsychiatric finding to rapid death. Tremendous advances in our understanding of the pathophysiology and in available treatments now allow for better outcomes. In this chapter, we will focus on two distinct clinical presentations of hepatic disease: hepatic encephalopathy (HE) associated with chronic cirrhotic liver disease (CLD) and the syndrome of encephalopathy and brain edema caused by fulminant acute liver failure (ALF).

HE associated with cirrhosis is a neuropsychiatric syndrome ranging from barely detectable changes to profound coma. It often presents in an episodic and recurrent fashion, can be precipitated by extrinsic factors, and is graded according to the West Haven Scale (Table 119.1). As a general rule, the severity of the encephalopathy is proportional to the underlying severity of liver disease. ALF, on the other hand, is a less common but highly lethal entity. Core components include the acute onset of hepatocellular dysfunction, which triggers a different set of complications dominated by cerebral edema with intracranial hypertension, unregulated systemic inflammation, and multisystem organ failure.

CIRRHOSIS AND HEPATIC ENCEPHALOPATHY

EPIDEMIOLOGY

In 2013, chronic liver disease was the 12th leading cause of death in the United States accounting for more than 36,000 deaths and over 100,000 hospitalizations. Those figures are probably an underestimate and the prevalence is steadily increasing. Hepatitis C patients, typically born between 1945 and 1965, are contributing to a large number of new cases and the obesity epidemic accounts for an increase in nonalcoholic fatty liver disease.

The less severe form of neurologic impairment, minimal hepatic encephalopathy (MHE), afflicts between 60% and 80% of cirrhotic patients. Often qualified of "subclinical," MHE is nonetheless a tremendous social burden with the majority of patients being unfit to drive and half of them unable to keep a permanent job.

Overt hepatic encephalopathy occurs in 30% to 45% of cirrhotic patients. It is responsible for the bulk of hospitalization days attributed to cirrhosis and its complications. Depending on the time course, it is subdivided into episodic, recurrent (6 months or less between episodes), or persistent (behavioral alterations that are always present).

PATHOBIOLOGY

Causes of chronic liver damage are numerous (Table 119.2), and the final common pathway is cirrhosis defined by parenchymal fibrosis with hepatic architecture distortion and the formation of regenerative nodules. The numerous associated complications are related to a loss of synthetic and metabolic functions, relative immunosuppression, and portal hypertension often associated to portosystemic shunting.

TABLE 119.1 West Haven Hepatic Encephalopathy Grading Scale

Grade	Description
Minimal	• Psychometric or neuropsychological alterations of tests exploring psychomotor speed/executive functions or neurophysiologic alterations without clinical evidence of mental change
1	• Trivial lack of awareness • Shortened attention span • Impaired performance of addition • Euphoria or anxiety
2	• Lethargy or apathy • Minimal disorientation for time or place • Subtle personality change • Inappropriate behavior • Impaired performance of subtraction
3	• Somnolence to semistupor, responsive to verbal stimuli • Confusion • Gross disorientation, bizarre behavior
4	• Coma (unresponsive to verbal or noxious stimuli)

TABLE 119.2 Causes of Cirrhosis

• Alcoholic Liver Disease	• Wilson Disease
• Chronic viral hepatitis (hepatitis B and C)	• α_1-Antitrypsin deficiency
• Hemochromatosis	• Polycystic liver disease
• Nonalcoholic fatty liver disease	• Veno-occlusive disease (including Budd–Chiari syndrome)
• Autoimmune hepatitis	• Infections (e.g., brucellosis, syphilis, echinococcosis, schistosomiasis)
• Primary and secondary biliary cirrhosis	• Medication (e.g., isoniazid, methotrexate)
• Primary sclerosing cholangitis	• Celiac disease

Most of the existing evidence points to ammonia (NH_3) as the main culprit behind HE. It is generated from glutamine by the enterocytes and from catabolism of nitrogenous products (proteins and urea) by colonic bacteria. Detoxification normally takes place in the liver through the conversion of NH_3 to urea and glutamine basically reversing what took place in the digestive tract. Cirrhosis and portosystemic shunting bypasses this process, allowing systemic levels of NH_3 to rise, which easily crosses the blood–brain barrier by diffusion and ion channels. Once in the brain, NH_3 is taken up by astrocytes, where it triggers oxidative stress, increases intracellular calcium, induces mitochondrial dysfunction, and activates NF-kB and an inflammatory response. Some data suggest that severity of HE correlates more with inflammatory indices than with NH_3 levels. Many other molecules have been implicated in the pathobiology of HE, such as neurosteroids. Synthetized by astrocytes and microglia, they appear to upmodulate the γ-aminobutyric acid (GABA)–A receptors leading to the clinically obvious increased GABA-ergic tone (depression of central nervous system [CNS] function) seen in HE.

CLINICAL FEATURES

Cirrhosis

Compensated cirrhotic patients may be asymptomatic, but eventually, most will develop one of the myriad of possible clinical manifestations as the disease progresses (Fig. 119.1). They may report nonspecific symptoms like anorexia, weight loss, fatigue, and weakness. They often have a low blood pressure, and they may present jaundice, pruritus, severe muscle cramps, or abdominal distention from ascites.

Classically, cirrhotic patients are classified according to the Child–Turcotte–Pugh score. Designed 30 years ago to predict outcome after surgery for portal hypertension (Table 119.3) (http://www.mdcalc.com/child-pugh-score-for-cirrhosis-mortality), it is now used to grade clinical severity and follow the evolution of most patients. Alternatively, the Model for End-Stage Liver Disease (MELD) score evaluates serum creatinine, bilirubin, and international normalized ratio (INR) to predict 3-month mortality following transjugular intrahepatic portosystemic shunt (TIPS) procedures (http://www.mdcalc.com/meld-score-model-for-end-stage-liver-disease-12-and-older/). The MELD score is currently used to prioritize candidates for liver transplantation scaled from 6 (less ill) to 40 (gravely ill).

Minimal Hepatic Encephalopathy

Patients with MHE, by definition, have no clinically detectable abnormalities at the bedside but manifest clear deficits on psychometric testing. They usually reveal impairment of vigilance, alertness and orientation, executive functions, working memory, learning processes, visuospatial coordination, and reaction time. When looked at closely, daily functioning is usually impaired in all spheres. They have a higher risk of car accidents with less than 20% of them fit to drive. Verbal ability is characteristically unimpaired.

Overt Hepatic Encephalopathy

Overt hepatic encephalopathy (OHE) can manifest itself from subtle clinical signs to profound coma. As it sets in, one of the earliest manifestations is usually a change in the sleep pattern (usually hypersomnia). Once it progresses, behavioral changes such as apathy, anxiety, and irritability appear. Attention span diminishes and short-term memory becomes impaired. Patients sometimes suffer from visual perception disturbances, both as a result of cortical and retinal dysfunction, with visual agnosia, macropsia, spatial disorientation, and problems with visuospatial construction. Visual hallucinations can occur. Neuromuscular impairments include ataxia, dysarthria, hyperreflexia, and extensor plantar responses. Asterixis, although not pathognomonic, was first described in HE patients. This "flapping tremor" is a negative myoclonus characterized by brief interruptions of sustained voluntary muscle contractions causing loss of postural tone. It is usually bilateral, nonrhythmic, and with a frequency of 3 to 5 Hz. It can be elicited by hyperextension of the wrists but is also seen in the feet, tongue, or eyelids. Parkinsonian features are at times prominent with tremor, rigidity, bradykinesia, hypomimia, slowness of speech, and monotony. Focal deficits have been described but are rare. As patients deteriorate, the most striking feature is the mental status change from lethargy to stupor and coma. At the point of coma, most patients are hyperventilating and have loss of deep tendon reflexes. Seizures are unusual. Mental status and motor changes do not always progress in a synchronized fashion.

Hepatic Myelopathy

Another well-described long-term neurologic complication of cirrhosis is hepatic myelopathy (HM). It is characterized by severe spastic paraparesis with minimal sensory involvement. Spasticity

FIGURE 119.1 Common complications of cirrhosis. GI, gastrointestinal.

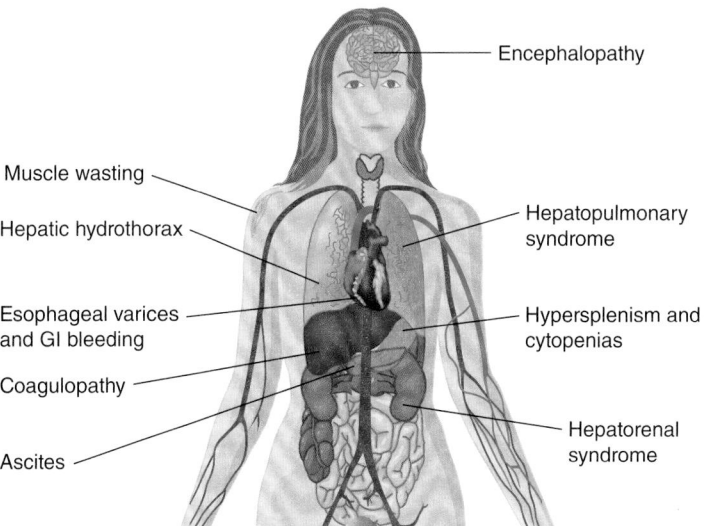

Encephalopathy

Muscle wasting

Hepatic hydrothorax

Esophageal varices and GI bleeding

Coagulopathy

Ascites

Hepatopulmonary syndrome

Hypersplenism and cytopenias

Hepatorenal syndrome

TABLE 119.3 Child–Turcotte–Pugh Score

	1	2	3
Bilirubin	<2 mg/L	2–3 mg/L	>3 mg/L
Albumin	>3.5 g/L	2.8–3.5 g/L	<2.8 g/L
INR	<1.7	1.7–2.2	>2.2
Ascites	No ascites	Ascites, medically controlled	Ascites, poorly controlled
Encephalopathy	No encephalopathy	Encephalopathy, medically controlled	Encephalopathy, poorly controlled

Interpretation: 5 to 6 points, child class A; 7 to 9 points, child class B; 10 to 15 points, child class C.

INR, international normalized ratio.

and weakness usually affect the lower limbs more severely and are progressive. It is caused by symmetric demyelination of the lateral pyramidal tracts. It does not respond to NH_3-lowering therapy, although some improvement might follow liver transplantation.

Persistent Hepatic Encephalopathy

Often preceded by multiple episodes of OHE, a chronic and largely irreversible syndrome characterized by dementia, dysarthria, gait ataxia, intention tremor, and choreoathetosis might appear. This persistent form of HE, previously referred to as *acquired hepatolenticular degeneration*, afflicts 4% of cirrhotic patients. The associated neuropathologic findings are neuronal necrosis in basal ganglia, cerebellum, and cerebral cortex in addition to Alzheimer type II astrocytosis. It does not respond to standard therapies.

DIAGNOSIS

Minimal Hepatic Encephalopathy

MHE diagnosis cannot be made at the bedside with usual examination techniques and requires neuropsychometric or neurophysiologic testing. Numerous tests have been designed and, although sensitive enough, they are usually not very specific. Most importantly, many are time-consuming or require specialized personnel, and the lack of standardized testing is a hindrance to routine testing implementation. The reader is referred to the suggested readings for a comprehensive description and critical analysis of available tests.

Overt Hepatic Encephalopathy

The diagnosis of OHE is made with the compatible clinical picture in the context of cirrhosis after exclusion of plausible alternative explanations. It is graded according to the West Haven criteria (see Table 119.1). The majority of OHE episodes are not spontaneous and precipitated by an event, and the absence of such cause in the setting of altered mental status should alert the clinician for other organ failures. Although blood NH_3 level per se does not allow staging or prognostication in chronic liver disease, a normal level puts the diagnosis of OHE in question. Brain imaging does not help in diagnosis but is used to rule out other pathologies, such as intracerebral hemorrhage, which is five times more prevalent in this population.

TREATMENT

Minimal Hepatic Encephalopathy

MHE rarely presents in clinical practice as a medical complaint and has not been widely evaluated in clinical trials. Several lines of evidence suggest a benefit on cognitive function and quality of life when patients are treated with lactulose, rifaximin, or probiotics, as discussed in the following text. Whether the benefits outweigh the costs is unknown at present.

Overt Hepatic Encephalopathy

OHE management focuses on identification and correction of the precipitating factor, exclusion of alternative causes for mental status changes, and measures to lower blood levels of NH_3 (Table 119.4), all the while supporting the patient appropriately.

Identification of the precipitating factor is paramount because its specific treatment is central to recovery. Precipitants are not always obvious and a careful history, physical examination, and appropriate laboratory tests are required. The most common causes are infection (especially spontaneous bacterial peritonitis and urinary tract infection), alcohol abuse, gastrointestinal (GI) bleeding, and iatrogenic insults such as dehydration from diuretics or lactulose or oversedation from benzodiazepines or opiates.

The mainstay of NH_3-lowering therapy is the use of nonabsorbable disaccharides such as lactulose, although efficacy in clinical trials has been variable. The putative mechanisms of action are multiple. The cathartic effect due to the osmolar load is thought to reduce time allowed for NH_3 absorption, as well as to increase fecal nitrogen excretion. Lactulose catabolism generates lactic acid, thereby acidifying colonic contents, which causes protonation of NH_3 into ammonium (NH_4^+), which is poorly absorbed, remains trapped in the lumen, and is excreted. Lactulose is titrated to achieve two to three bowel movements per day.

Sodium benzoate also lowers NH_3 levels by combining with glycine to form hippurate, which is water-soluble and allows greater elimination of NH_3 through renal excretion. It has been shown to improve symptoms of HE improvement just as well as lactulose.

A concomitant approach is through modulation of fecal flora with antibiotics. The most promising treatment by far is rifaximin, a minimally absorbed antibiotic with broad-spectrum activity against gram-positive, gram-negative, and anaerobic bacteria. Its preferential site of action is the small bowel, where it lowers the bacterial load up to 1,000-fold. Recent data demonstrated that it is more effective for improvement of OHE as an add-on therapy than lactulose alone and, most importantly, showed a significant reduction in mortality [**Level 1**].[1]

General care measures include appropriate hydration and nutritional support with protein intake of 1.2 to 1.5 g/kg/day and correction of electrolyte abnormalities. Treatment of chronic hyponatremia must be done carefully, as cirrhotic patients are at higher risk

TABLE 119.4 Ammonia-Reducing Pharmacologic Therapies

Agent	Dose
Lactulose	15–45 mL PO b.i.d. to q.i.d.
Sodium benzoate	5 mg PO b.i.d.
Rifaximin	400 mg PO t.i.d.

PO, by mouth.

of osmotic demyelination syndrome. Correction of hyponatremia should be performed no faster than 12 mmol/L per 24 hours. Correction of hypokalemia is also an essential component of therapy because it increases renal NH₃ production. After a first episode of OHE, secondary prophylaxis is recommended with lactulose and rifaximin to prevent recurrence. This therapy should be continued indefinitely.

OUTCOME

Even without obvious clinical manifestations, MHE patients do not fare well. After diagnosis, 50% of patients will be hospitalized within a year and 75% will die within the next 4 years. The future is even grimmer after a first episode of OHE: 40% will have a recurrent episode by the end of the year. The cumulative survival at 1 year is 42% and at 3 years, it is a mere 23%.

ACUTE LIVER FAILURE AND CEREBRAL EDEMA

EPIDEMIOLOGY

ALF is rare in developed countries, with an incidence ranging from 1 to 8 cases per million per year representing approximately 2,000 cases annually in the United States. It is seen most commonly in previously healthy adults in their 30s, and the most prominent cause is drug-induced liver injury dominated by acetaminophen-induced hepatotoxicity (Fig. 119.2). It is of interest to the neurologist to know that causes of ALF include carbamazepine, phenytoin, and valproic acid.

PATHOBIOLOGY

Multiple Organ Failure

Acute liver dysfunction results in a shutdown of its synthetic, metabolic, detoxification, and immunologic functions. Loss of coagulation factor synthesis leads to coagulopathy, and necrotic hepatocytes trigger an intense systemic inflammatory syndrome. This inflammatory state produces vasoparesis and is often complicated by acute renal failure and acute lung injury. Loss of neoglucogenesis may lead to hypoglycemia and reduced lactate clearance. Immunoparesis puts patients at high risk of sepsis, and bone marrow suppression manifests as cytopenia.

Encephalopathy and Cerebral Edema

Acute NH₃ accumulation produces different consequences than the chronic hyperammonemia seen in cirrhotic patients. The rapid transformation of NH₃ to glutamine inside the astrocytes does not

allow for compensatory mechanisms such as the release of taurine or myoinositol. The osmotic effect causes astrocytes to take in water and swell, creating cytotoxic brain edema. This is why arterial NH₃ levels in ALF are highly correlated with prognosis and the extent of cerebral edema. Patients with NH₃ levels less than 75 μmol/L usually do not develop encephalopathy at all, and those with NH₃ greater than 200 μmol/L have a 55% risk of developing cerebral edema with concomitant intracranial hypertension. The rapid buildup of glutamine is partially transformed to glutamate, which may explain the aggressive and agitated delirium seen in some patients and their propensity for seizures. Numerous other causal pathways explaining cerebral dysfunction are being studied, including loss of autoregulation, elevated cerebral lactate concentrations, and inflammatory cytokines.

CLINICAL FEATURES

The clinical picture of ALF is dominated by acute hepatic dysfunction, unregulated systemic inflammation with multiorgan dysfunction, and cerebral edema with intracranial hypertension, which is the most feared complication (Fig. 119.3).

The characteristic sleepiness and asterixis of cirrhotic patients are not reliable indicators of early encephalopathy in ALF. Instead, forewarning signs of impending cerebral edema are usually onset of aggressive behavior and agitated delirium associated with hyperreflexia and ankle clonus. Mental status changes can quickly follow with the patient lapsing into coma in just a few hours. Multifocal myoclonus and excessive startle response are well described and later stages may reveal spasticity and extensor posturing, as well extensor plantar responses. Pupillary responses are impaired only when intracranial pressure (ICP) is frankly elevated and brain herniation has occurred. Oculomotor dysfunction is uncommon but dysconjugate gaze and periodic alternating gaze deviation are reported. Cushing response is a late and unreliable finding. Seizures, albeit generally nonconvulsive, are also a frequent occurrence in ALF. Up to 30% of patients monitored with continuous electroencephalogram (cEEG) have evidence of electrographic seizures.

DIAGNOSIS

ALF is defined as the onset of coagulopathy (INR >1.5) and encephalopathy (any degree of altered mentation) secondary to liver injury in a patient without preexisting liver disease. The time from the start of illness to encephalopathy is variable from hyperacute (less than a week) to subacute (up to 26 weeks). Patients with Wilson disease, vertically transmitted hepatitis B virus, or autoimmune hepatitis may be included if the disease has only been recognized for less than 6 months.

When ALF is suspected, the history must be very thorough, with a focus on drug and medication ingestion, including over-the-counter medications or supplements, as well a possible viral exposure, including travel history. Although the cause of ALF remains unknown in close to 20% of cases, it is the single most important prognostic factor and might call for specific treatment, so it must be sought aggressively. In addition to laboratory testing and imaging, serial biochemical testing should be done, including NH₃, glucose, and lactate levels; liver and renal function; electrolytes; and coagulation panels.

TREATMENT

General Management

Patients with a diagnosis of ALF must be hospitalized, and those developing encephalopathy should be transferred to a critical care unit, as they can deteriorate in a matter of hours. Frequent neurologic assessments are mandatory in ALF patients. Special attention should

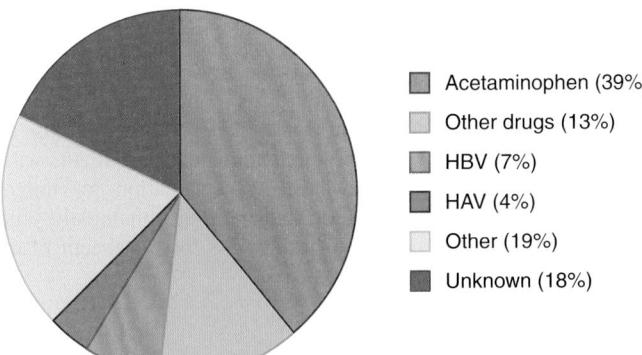

Acetaminophen (39%)
Other drugs (13%)
HBV (7%)
HAV (4%)
Other (19%)
Unknown (18%)

FIGURE 119.2 Common causes of acute liver failure in the United States. HAV, hepatitis A virus; HBV, hepatitis B virus.

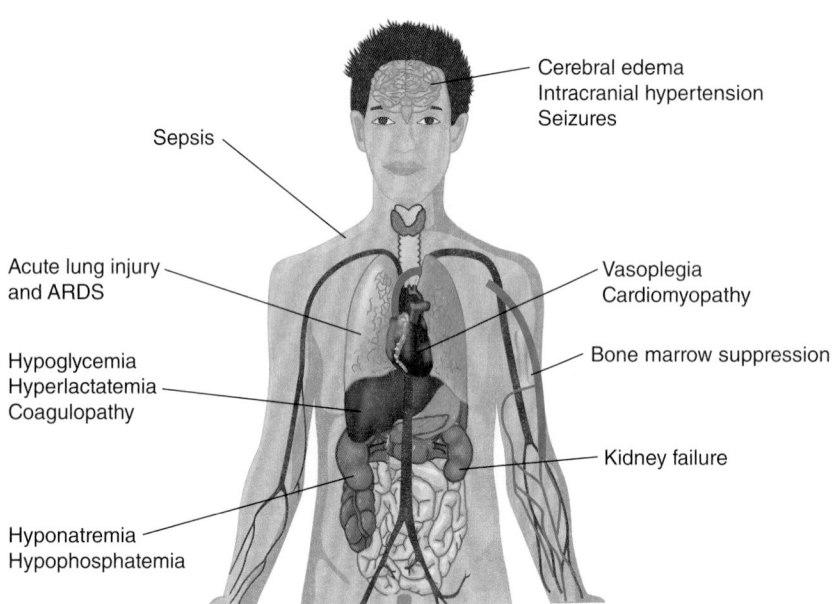

FIGURE 119.3 Multiorgan dysfunctions associated with acute liver failure. ARDS, acute respiratory distress syndrome.

be dedicated to development of delirium, mental status changes, abnormal motor tone and deep tendon reflexes, and myoclonus. Those progressing to West Haven stage III or IV (see Table 119.1), which usually corresponds to a Glasgow Coma Scale score of 8 and less (see Table 18.1), should be intubated and strong consideration should be given to invasive ICP monitoring. Communication with a transplant center is essential and transfer criteria have to be determined very early in the evaluation process. Depending on the etiology of ALF, specific treatment should be instituted promptly, especially in the case of acetaminophen poisoning (Table 119.5). Hypoglycemia and hyponatremia are common, can exacerbate the severity of neurologic insult, and must be carefully prevented.

Intracranial Pressure and Transcranial Doppler Monitoring

Patients with grade III encephalopathy (see Table 119.1) have a risk of experiencing elevated ICP of 30%, whereas in grade IV

patients, it climbs to 70%. Noncontrast head computed tomography (CT) is often done to rule out other concomitant pathologies, such as bleeding, but the usual finding that implies a high risk of intracranial hypertension is global cerebral edema with convexity sulcal effacement, effacement of the basal cisterns and small ventricles, and loss of gray–white matter differentiation.

Transcranial Doppler (TCD) is a noninvasive technique allowing indirect evaluation of both cerebral blood flow (CBF) and ICP (see Chapter 23). In ALF, because the global cerebral edema is primarily vasogenic and caused by hyperemia and vasodilation, the rise in ICP is usually preceded by an increase in CBF and hence in TCD flow velocities. Early on, TCD flow velocities are elevated above normal values (60 cm/s in a healthy young person), and the pulsatility index (peak systolic minus diastolic flow velocity divided by mean flow velocity) is reduced below the normal value of 1.0 due to downstream vasodilation. Brain injury is highly reversible at this stage, and for this reason, the triad of coma, global cerebral edema on CT, and elevated flow velocities on TCD is the ideal time for an ICP monitor to be inserted.

After ICP has been massively elevated for a sustained period of time, the brain remains engorged but hypoperfused, CBF falls, metabolic changes in the brain cause cellular swelling, and cytotoxic brain edema ensues. At this late stage, TCD evolves toward a picture consistent with brain death: Mean flow velocities drop, the pulsatility index increases, and eventually, readings evolve to isolated systolic flow velocity spikes with diastolic flow arrest diagnostic of brain death (see Chapter 19).

As for other neurocritical care patients, invasive ICP monitoring (see Chapter 33) is the gold standard for monitoring when intracranial hypertension is the main threat to life. Although its use in ALF is still contentious, it is now recommended in patients with high-grade encephalopathy awaiting transplantation in centers with appropriate expertise. Associated with encephalopathy, the following factors are considered indications for placement of an ICP monitor.

- Global cerebral edema on CT
- Arterial NH_3 greater than 150 mmol/L
- Age younger than 40 years
- TCD indices of high CBF
- Concurrent renal or cardiovascular organ failure

TABLE 119.5	Acute Liver Failure Etiologies and Specific Treatments
Etiology	**Specific Treatment**
Acetaminophen poisoning	IV NAC[a]
Nonacetaminophen ALF	IV NAC[a]
Drug-induced liver injury	IV NAC[a]
Mushroom poisoning (*Amanita phalloides*)	Penicillin G (1 million U/kg/day) and IV NAC[a]
HBV	Lamivudine
Herpesvirus or varicella-zoster virus	Acyclovir (10 mg/kg IV every 8 h)
Autoimmune	Prednisone (40–60 mg/day)
ALF of pregnancy or HELLP	Delivery

[a]Loading dose is 150 mg/kg in 5% dextrose over 15 minutes; maintenance dose is 50 mg/kg given over 4 hours followed by 100 mg/kg administered over 16 hours (or 6 mg/kg/h).

IV, intravenous; NAC, *N*-acetylcysteine; ALF, acute liver failure; HBV, hepatitis B virus; HELLP, hemolysis, elevated liver enzymes, low platelets.

The main concern of placing an invasive ICP monitor is bleeding because most patients with ALF are coagulopathic. Recent series report clinically significant bleeding in ALF patients after standard reversal procedures at the same order of magnitude as for other intracranial pathologies. Reversal of coagulopathy when placing an intracranial monitoring device should be taken seriously. Off-label usage of recombinant factor VIIa (40 µg/kg given 30 minutes before the procedure) is used at many liver transplant centers throughout the world to correct the coagulopathy prior to ICP monitor placement. Recombinant factor VIIa has been associated with a 5% risk of thrombotic complications, including brain and myocardial infarction.

We also recommend keeping platelets over 50,000 and to correct hypofibrinogenemia (fibrinogen <100 mg/dL) with cryoprecipitate prior to insertion. Elevated prothrombin time (PT)/INR can also be corrected with fresh frozen plasma (15 mL/kg).

Intracranial Pressure Management

Usual ICP management principles (see Chapter 107) apply to ALF patients but with some particularities. Hypertonic saline (30%) given prophylactically (at a rate of 5 to 20 mL/h) with a sodium target of 145 to 155 mEq/L has been shown to reduce the incidence and severity of ICP crisis. Prophylactic induction of hypernatremia is thus recommended [**Level 1**][2] in high-risk patients (encephalopathy grade III or IV, N H_3 >150 µmol/L, acute renal failure or requiring vasopressors). In the event of a herniation event, mannitol boluses (20% solution at a dose of 0.5 to 1 g/kg) are successful in resolving ICP crisis in ALF patients and it improves survival compared to placebo. Corticosteroids are useless in cerebral edema caused by ALF and are probably harmful and should not be used [**Level 1**].[2]

The role of therapeutic hypothermia is debated. Case series show great improvement in ICP control and impressive survival rates, but a randomized controlled trial (RCT) and retrospective cohort studies have failed to show better outcomes with cooling, albeit showing no higher rates of bleeding or infection. Induction of hypothermia to 33°C may be considered as a rescue intervention in patients with refractory ICP crisis, refractory to sedation and paralysis, bolus osmotherapy, and hyperventilation as a bridge to liver transplantation. Indomethacin (25 mg intravenously [IV]) has been shown in a few ALF patients with ICP refractory to mannitol to dramatically reduce ICP without documented adverse effects.

Seizures

With a reported frequency of nonconvulsive seizures in up to 30% of patients, grade III or IV encephalopathy should be monitored with cEEG. Prophylactic phenytoin failed to improve outcomes in one RCT and is thus not recommended.

Ammonia Clearance

Therapies used for HE, such as lactulose, have not been proven useful in acutely reducing blood level of NH_3 in ALF patients. Recent clinical data shows that hemofiltration with continuous renal replacement therapy (CRRT) might be the best way to control arterial NH_3 levels. Clearance is closely correlated with ultrafiltration rate up to 90 mL/kg/h, and glutamine is also likely to be cleared in the process. CRRT also allows for tighter control of serum sodium levels, intravascular volume, pH, and temperature.

Artificial Liver Support Systems

Numerous extracorporeal liver support systems have been developed; currently, the only U.S. Food and Drug Administration (FDA)–approved device is the Molecular Adsorbent Recirculating System (MARS). This nonbiologic artificial liver support system is based on a dialysis technique using an albumin-coated membrane. It allows detoxification by removal of water-soluble toxins but also, in contrast to CRRT, albumin-bound substances. Among proven benefits in ALF patients, there is improvement in hemodynamic stability, reduction in ICP, and improvement of HE. The only large RCT did not show a survival benefit, although it was highly underpowered. At present, MARS should only be considered as a "bridge to transplant."

Transplantation

Orthotopic liver transplantation is the only definitive therapy for those whose liver function does not recover. Given the usually rapid evolution toward cerebral edema, candidacy must be assessed promptly. Numerous prognostic scores have been developed trying to predict who has a poor prognosis with medical management alone and hence who will benefit most from emergent liver transplantation. None of them is universally accepted, but the most widely used are the King's College criteria (Table 119.6). Adult patients with sudden acute- and severe-onset ALF according to the King's College criteria have a life expectancy less than 7 days without transplant and are granted 1A status, making them the highest priority, but up to 25% will die while on the waiting list. As of 2012, more than 12,000 patients were on the liver transplant waiting list in the United States with about 10% of livers usually allocated to ALF patients.

TABLE 119.6	King's College Criteria for Acute Liver Failure
Acetaminophen-Induced ALF	
Strongly consider OLT listing	• Arterial lactate >3.5 mmol/L after early fluid resuscitation
List for OLT	• pH <7.3 *or* • Arterial lactate >3.0 mmol/L after adequate fluid resuscitation
List for OLT if all three occur within a 24-h period	• Presence of grade 3 or 4 hepatic encephalopathy • INR >6.5 • Creatinine >3.4 mg/dL
Non–Acetaminophen-Induced ALF	
List for OLT	• INR >6.5 *and* • Encephalopathy present (irrespective of grade)
List for OLT if any three of the following (and any grade of encephalopathy present)	• Age younger than 10 yr or older than 40 yr • Jaundice for >7 days before development of encephalopathy • INR ≥3.5 • Serum bilirubin ≥17 mg/dL • Unfavorable etiology, such as Wilson disease, idiosyncratic drug reaction, seronegative hepatitis

ALF, acute liver failure; OLT, orthotopic liver transplantation; INR, international normalized ratio.

OUTCOME

With optimization of medical management and improved organ allocation system, the overall mortality of ALF is now between 30% and 40%. The etiology of ALF is one of the most important predictors of outcome. For example, transplant-free survival is largely over 50% for acetaminophen poisoning, hepatitis A, or pregnancy-related disease. On the contrary, survival without transplantation is less than 25% in Wilson disease, Budd–Chiari syndrome, or autoimmune hepatitis. With emergent transplantation, although the survival at 1 year is less than for elective transplantation (mainly due to infection in the first 3 months), ALF patients have a better long-term survival.

LEVEL 1 EVIDENCE

1. Sharma BC, Sharma P, Lunia MK, et al. A randomized, double-blind, controlled trial comparing rifaximin plus lactulose with lactulose alone in treatment of overt hepatic encephalopathy. *Am J Gastroenterol*. 2013;108:1458–1463.
2. Lee WM, Larson AM, Stravitz RT. *AASLD Position Paper: The Management of Acute Liver Failure: Update 2011*. Baltimore: American Association for the Study of Liver Diseases; 2011.

SUGGESTED READINGS

Cirrhosis and Hepatic Encephalopathy

Frederick RT. Current concepts in the pathophysiology and management of hepatic encephalopathy. *Gastroenterol Hepatol (N Y)*. 2011;7(4):222–233.

Prakash RK, Sowjanya K, Mullen KD. Evolving concepts: the negative effect of minimal hepatic encephalopathy and role for prophylaxis in patients with cirrhosis. *J Clin Therapeutics*. 2013;35(9):1458–1473.

Sharma BC, Sharma P, Lunia MK, et al. A randomized, double-blind, controlled trial comparing rifaximin plus lactulose with lactulose alone in treatment of overt hepatic encephalopathy. *Am J Gastroenterol*. 2013;108:1458–1463.

Vilstrup H, Amodio P, Bajaj J, et al. Hepatic encephalopathy in chronic liver disease: 2014 practice guideline by the American Association for the Study of Liver Diseases and the European Association for the Study of the Liver. *Hepatology*. 2014;60(2):715–735.

Acute Liver Failure and Cerebral Edema

Bernal W, Wendon J. Acute liver failure. *N Engl J Med*. 2013;369:2525–2534.

DellaVolpe JD, Garavaglia JM, Huang DT. Management of complications of end-stage liver disease in the intensive care unit. *J Intensive Care Med*. 2014;1–10.

Karvellas CJ, Stravitz RT, Battenhouse H, et al; US Acute Liver Failure Study Group. Therapeutic hypothermia in acute liver failure: a multicenter retrospective cohort analysis. *Liver Transpl*. 2015;21.

Krisl JC, Meadows HE, Greenberg CS, et al. Clinical usefulness of recombinant activated factor VII in patients with liver failure undergoing invasive procedures. *Ann Pharmacother*. 2011;45:1433–1438.

Lee WM, Larson AM, Stravitz RT. *AASLD Position Paper: The Management of Acute Liver Failure: Update 2011*. Baltimore: American Association for the Study of Liver Diseases; 2011.

Mohsenin V. Assessment and management of cerebral edema and intracranial hypertension in acute liver failure. *J Crit Care*. 2013;28:783–791.

Murphy N, Auzinger G, Bernel W, et al. The effect of hypertonic sodium chloride on intracranial pressure in patients with acute liver failure. *Hepatology*. 2004;39:464–470.

Nevens F, Laleman W. Artificial liver support devices as treatment option for liver failure. *Best Pract Res Clin Gastroenterol*. 2012;26:17–26.

Rabadán AT, Spaho N, Hernández D, et al. Intraparenchymal intracranial pressure monitoring in patients with acute liver failure. *Arq Neuropsiquiatr*. 2008;66(2-B):374–377.

Shawcross DL, Wendon JA. The neurological manifestations of acute liver failure. *Neurochem Int*. 2012;60:662–671.

Slack AJ, Auzinger G, Willars C, et al. Ammonia clearance with haemofiltration in adults with liver disease. *Liver Int*. 2014;34:42–48.

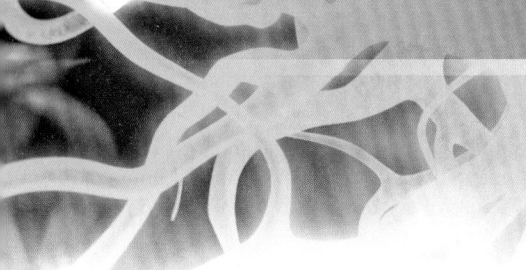

Renal Disease and the Brain

J. Kirk Roberts and Stephan A. Mayer

INTRODUCTION

Renal disease is most commonly associated with neurologic disease when both are related to an underlying condition (e.g., diabetes mellitus, hypertension) that damages both systems. However, renal disease and resultant azotemia (blood urea nitrogen elevation or uremia) can injure both the central nervous system (CNS) and the peripheral nervous system. With the increase in aggressive kidney dialysis and transplantation, the incidence of many neurologic conditions associated with chronic renal failure has declined, but a new constellation of neurologic complications associated with dialysis and transplantation has become more important.

UREMIC ENCEPHALOPATHY

The differential diagnosis of encephalopathy in a patient with renal failure is wide and includes metabolic, infectious, structural, and other causes. Fluid and electrolyte disturbances are common. Drugs that are excreted in the urine may accumulate and dosing must be adjusted.

PATHOBIOLOGY

Uremia itself can cause encephalopathy. The symptoms of *uremic encephalopathy* are usually more severe in patients with more severe azotemia; they are often evident earlier and more severely in patients with acute as opposed to chronic renal failure. The specific factors that cause encephalopathy are still not identified. The earliest indicator is sensorial clouding, which progresses to delirium, obtundation, and even coma. In addition to cognitive changes, patients are usually weak, uncoordinated, and unsteady. Focal symptoms or signs may wrongly suggest a focal process. Asterixis is a dramatic problem, with jerking movements arising from lapses of posture holding, as of the outstretched hands. Multifocal myoclonus, involuntary twitches occurring randomly throughout the body, may become apparent, usually after stupor or coma has supervened. Tetany may be overt, with spontaneous carpopedal spasm, or latent as manifest by a Trousseau sign (sustained muscle contraction and cupping of the hand, induced by arterial occlusion). Seizures are a manifestation of uremic encephalopathy. Fluctuation of clinical symptoms and signs from day to day is characteristic.

DIAGNOSIS

No laboratory value, including specific evaluations of renal function, correlates well with clinical symptoms and signs of uremia. Lumbar puncture may reveal elevated cerebrospinal fluid (CSF) protein, sometimes exceeding 100 mg/dL, and occasionally a mild pleocytosis but is primarily performed to exclude an infectious cause of encephalopathy. Computed tomography (CT) or magnetic resonance imaging (MRI) findings are usually nonspecific but may help to exclude ischemic stroke, intracerebral hemorrhage, subdural hematoma, or hydrocephalus. Electroencephalogram (EEG),

like the clinical state, is usually more strikingly abnormal in acute renal failure than in chronic renal failure. The background activity is slow with theta and delta waves more prominent in the frontal regions. Triphasic waves may appear. Nonconvulsive status epilepticus is an important treatable cause of encephalopathy that can be identified only by EEG with dramatic improvement when appropriately managed.

TREATMENT

Uremic encephalopathy usually responds dramatically to dialysis, suggesting that one or more dialyzable substances are responsible. Sometimes, response is delayed for 1 to 2 days. A variety of metabolites acting toxically when accumulating have been postulated as the etiology of uremic encephalopathy, but no single substance has been identified as the sole or major cause. Hormonal changes, electrolyte abnormalities, altered calcium homeostasis, and imbalance of excitatory and inhibitory neurotransmission are all thought to play a role.

DIALYSIS DISEQUILIBRIUM SYNDROME

Dialysis disequilibrium syndrome is usually seen with rapid correction of uremia at the start of a dialysis program. It is more common in those with more severe azotemia. Symptoms vary from mild headache, nausea, and muscle cramps to, rarely, delirium, obtundation, and convulsions. The syndrome is usually self-limited, subsiding in hours, but delirium may persist for several days. Although the pathogenesis is controversial, shift of water into brain is probably the cause of syndrome. The rapid reduction in blood osmoles cannot be paralleled as rapidly by a reduction in brain osmoles, resulting in an osmotic gradient between blood and brain, causing movement of water into brain and cerebral edema and encephalopathy. With improvements in dialysis, this syndrome is much less frequent now. Gradual initiation of dialysis may help prevent. Before diagnosing dialysis disequilibrium, other causes of cerebral symptoms should be excluded. If it seems likely, dialysis should be stopped and supportive care provided. Some have suggested hypertonic saline or mannitol for severe cases but this is not routine.

DIALYSIS DEMENTIA

A subacute, progressive, usually fatal encephalopathy rarely occurs in patients who are chronically dialyzed. The first symptom is usually a stammering, hesitancy of speech and at times, speech arrest. The speech disorder is intensified during and immediately after dialysis and at first may be seen only during these periods. As the disorder progresses, speech becomes more dysarthric and aphasic along with personality change, psychosis, myoclonus, seizures, and occasionally focal neurologic abnormalities. Brain imaging and CSF findings are usually unremarkable and, again, are most helpful in excluding other causes of encephalopathy. Increased dialysis time and renal transplantation do not seem to alter the course of the disease. Aluminum content is consistently elevated in the cerebral gray matter of patients who die from this condition. Municipal water supplies heavily contaminated with aluminum have been linked to the syndrome in epidemiologic studies. The frequency of the disease markedly diminished when aluminum was removed from the water used during dialysis but did not disappear completely. Another possible source is absorption of aluminum from orally administered phosphate-binding agents that are given to uremic patients.

CEREBROVASCULAR DISEASE

Stroke is prevalent in patients with renal failure, mostly because of shared risk factors. However, renal failure may additionally promote atherogenesis through several mechanisms. Hypotension during dialysis may result in watershed infarction. Renal failure is associated with platelet dysfunction, and anticoagulants used during hemodialysis may contribute to intracerebral hemorrhage or subdural hematoma. Chronic subdural hematoma may present with an encephalopathic picture without focal motor or sensory symptoms and signs. Autosomal dominant polycystic kidney disease is associated with an increased risk of saccular aneurysm and subarachnoid hemorrhage (SAH).

RESTLESS LEGS SYNDROME

At least 20% of patients with chronic renal failure suffer from creeping, crawling, prickling, and pruritic sensations deep within the legs particularly when at rest and improving with movement (see Chapter 75). Periodic limb movements of sleep may coexist. Dialysis often does not lead to significant improvement, and treatment is similar to that in patients without renal failure.

BENIGN INTRACRANIAL HYPERTENSION

Benign intracranial hypertension or pseudotumor cerebri is thought to occur more frequently in patients with chronic renal failure (see also Chapter 107). Symptoms typically include headache, visual obscurations, and possibly sixth nerve palsies. Focal mass lesions and CSF infections must be excluded. Treatment consists of managing renal failure, weight loss, low-salt diet, and often diuretics, in particular, acetazolamide 500 mg orally (PO) three times a day (t.i.d.).

PERIPHERAL NEUROPATHY

The most common neurologic consequence of chronic renal failure is a distal, symmetric, predominantly axonal, mixed sensorimotor neuropathy affecting the legs more than the arms. Cranial nerves, particularly vision and hearing, and the autonomic nervous system may be affected. The rate of progression, severity, prominence of motor or sensory symptoms and signs, and degree of pain varies. Decreased vibratory and temperature sense in the feet are the earliest signs and sensory symptoms and signs usually predate motor. In general, the neuropathy evolves over several months but may be fulminant.

PATHOBIOLOGY

Pathologically, uremic neuropathy is usually a primary axonal degeneration with secondary segmental demyelination; there is also a predominantly demyelinating type. Because uremic neuropathy improves with hemodialysis, it seems likely that the neuropathy re-

sults from the accumulation of dialyzable metabolites. The control of neuropathy in some patients depends on increased hours of dialysis each week. The use of erythropoietin has also been reported to improve uremic neuropathy.

DIAGNOSIS

Other causes must always be considered given the coexistence of renal diseases and conditions that predispose to peripheral neuropathy (e.g., diabetes mellitus, amyloidosis). Mononeuropathies, such as carpal tunnel syndrome caused by damage to the median nerve at the wrist or ulnar neuropathy, may occur, perhaps owing to an increased susceptibility of at-risk nerves to injury or as a vascular steal phenomenon after arteriovenous fistula. Electrophysiologic studies are often abnormal, even in those with no symptoms, with both decreased amplitudes and slowing. Among most patients who enter chronic dialysis programs, the neuropathy stabilizes or improves slowly. Patients with mild neuropathy often recover completely, but those who begin dialysis with severe neuropathy rarely recover even after several years, and some may continue to progress. However, lack of improvement or progression of symptoms while on dialysis should suggest an evaluation for an alternative diagnosis.

TREATMENT

Successful renal transplantation often leads to a significant beneficial effect on uremic neuropathy. Motor nerve conduction velocities can increase within days of transplantation along with continued improvement for several months, sometimes with complete recovery, unless there was severe axonal degeneration before transplantation.

The symptomatic treatment of painful uremic neuropathy is similar to the treatment of any painful peripheral neuropathy (see Chapter 87) but with careful attention to medication dosing, given the presence of renal failure.

MYOPATHY

In patients with renal failure, myopathy with proximal limb weakness, fatigability, and atrophy is a poorly understood condition. Muscle enzymes and electromyogram (EMG) are usually normal. Muscle biopsy may reveal nonspecific alterations and sometimes type II fiber atrophy. Electrolyte abnormalities, in particular potassium, calcium, and magnesium, must be considered. If the patient has been treated with a kidney transplant and is taking steroids, a steroid myopathy may be considered.

NEUROLOGIC COMPLICATIONS OF RENAL TRANSPLANTATION

Renal transplantation is the preferred treatment of end-stage renal disease, and with advances in transplantation medicine, these patients live longer and are more at risk for the adverse consequences of long-term immunosuppression.

A femoral neuropathy may complicate renal transplant surgery caused by perioperative compression or traction. It can usually be managed expectantly.

Transplant patients suffering systemic features of rejection may also present with encephalopathic symptoms including confusion and even seizures. Symptoms usually begin within a few months of transplant, but some occur later. Treatment of rejection usually leads to improvement.

POSTERIOR REVERSIBLE ENCEPHALOPATHY SYNDROME

Several drugs are used to prevent transplant rejection, and each has adverse effects. Of particular interest to the neurologist is the *posterior reversible encephalopathy syndrome* (PRES) usually seen in those patients treated with cyclosporine or tacrolimus (see also Chapter 43). PRES may also be seen in nontransplanted patients with renal disease and hypertension. Symptoms include headache, visual disturbance, encephalopathy, and seizures. Blood pressure is usually elevated. MRI reveals changes in the white matter, most extensive in the occipital and parietal regions, that suggest vasogenic edema. Treatment involves lowering blood pressure and, whenever possible, discontinuing immunosuppressive agents. Obviously, patients with transplanted organs require immunosuppression; if medications are substituted, the patient will need continued monitoring for PRES. Patients with seizures should be treated with anticonvulsants. Late recurrence of seizures after successful treatment is low and the anticonvulsant can usually be discontinued in the uncomplicated patient once symptoms and imaging have resolved, although some advocate continuing for 1 to 3 months.

PRIMARY CENTRAL NERVOUS SYSTEM LYMPHOMA

The risk that a lymphoma will develop after a transplant is about 35 times more than in normal people; the increased risk depends almost entirely on the increased incidence of primary CNS lymphoma. These are almost always B-cell lymphomas developing from immunosuppression-related Epstein–Barr virus (EBV) infection causing lymphocyte proliferation. The tumor typically appears between 5 and 45 months after transplantation. The resulting clinical syndromes include increased ICP, rapidly evolving focal neurologic signs, or combinations of these. Convulsions are rare. The lymphoma may be multicentric and may involve the meninges. Treatment may include immunosuppression withdrawal, chemotherapy, and radiation.

OPPORTUNISTIC INFECTIONS

Infections occur often in transplant patients, and a high index of suspicion must be maintained because the usual inflammatory response may be impaired diminishing the severity of symptoms. New headache or mental changes should lead the clinician to consider brain imaging and lumbar puncture. Viral infections with cytomegalovirus (CMV), herpes zoster virus (HZV), varicella-zoster virus (VZV), human herpes virus (HHV)-6, EBV, and John Cunningham (JC) virus can often be diagnosed on CSF with culture or polymerase chain reaction (PCR). Bacterial and tuberculous meningitis are also considerations. Systemic fungal infections are common and secondary brain abscess formation may occur. In almost all cases, the primary source of infection is in the lung. Chest radiographs and the presence of fever aid in differentiating fungal brain abscess from brain tumor in recipients of transplants. *Aspergillus* has a unique predilection for dissemination to brain and accounts for most fungal brain abscesses; *Candida*, *Nocardia*, and *Histoplasma* are found in the others. The clinical syndrome resulting from these infections is usually delirium accompanied by seizures. Headache, stiff neck, and focal signs also occur but not commonly. The CSF is often remarkably bland, and brain biopsy may be the only reliable way to establish a diagnosis. The distinction of fungal brain abscess from possibly radiosensitive brain tumor makes it important to consider this procedure.

HYPONATREMIA

Sodium and fluid homeostasis is under the control of the brain and kidneys. The neurologist, particularly in the neurologic intensive care unit (ICU), is frequently confronted by hyponatremia (serum sodium <135 mEq/L). In this setting, the most common causes of hyponatremia are volume depletion, the syndrome of inappropriate antidiuretic hormone secretion (SIADH), and cerebral salt wasting (CSW).

CLINICAL FEATURES

Hyponatremia can not only be caused by brain injury but can also further impair neurologic function and cause a vast array of clinical manifestations, ranging from mild confusion to death. The severity of symptomatology is primarily related to the speed of sodium reduction, rather than the absolute sodium level itself. Sodium is the principle osmotically active solute in the extracellular fluid compartment. If the sodium concentration falls quickly (>1 mEq/h), free water moves into the intracellular compartment, leading to cellular swelling and edema. Unlike other organs, the CNS tolerates this process extremely poorly. Acute hyponatremia can lead to global cerebral edema and dramatic clinical manifestations, including seizures, coma, or death from brain stem herniation.

When sodium levels drop gradually, cells compensate by reducing the intrinsic osmolality of the intracellular compartment. This process, which involves release of intracellular electrolytes such as potassium and elimination of organic osmolytes, takes hours to days. As a result, normal cellular volume is maintained in chronic hyponatremia, but subtle neurologic dysfunction in the form of neurocognitive dysfunction, impaired reaction times, and gait instability results from these intrinsic changes in neuronal intracellular composition. Hospitalized patients with chronic hyponatremia have an increased risk of mortality and a two- to fourfold increased fall risk compared to normonatremic patients.

DIAGNOSIS

The medical history is an important first step in the evaluation of hyponatremia and in particular includes information about fluid loss (or excess intake), low protein intake, medications, history of heart failure, cirrhosis, kidney failure, hypothyroidism, adrenal insufficiency, lung cancer, and, of course, CNS disease.

In addition to the history, physical examination should start with an assessment of *volume status* by evaluating blood pressure and heart rate, skin turgor, the mucous membranes, and jugular venous pressure. Measurement of fluid inputs and outputs (Is and Os) typically demonstrate positive net fluid balance in patients who are hypovolemic, as the kidneys appropriately retain fluid to correct the problem. A spot urine sodium concentration is typically low in hypovolemic states (<25 mEq/L), representing avid renal sodium retention. A low central venous pressure (CVP) is fairly specific for hypovolemia; otherwise, CVP is a poor indicator of volume status. Advanced diagnostic methods in the ICU for evaluating volume status include use of bedside ultrasound to diagnose collapsibility of the inferior vena cava (IVC) with spontaneous respirations and cardiac output monitors that can measure the global end-diastolic volume index (GEDI) of the heart.

Essential laboratory testing in hyponatremia includes serum osmolality, urine osmolality, and urine electrolytes, in addition to standard serum chemistries. If serum osmolality is low, then

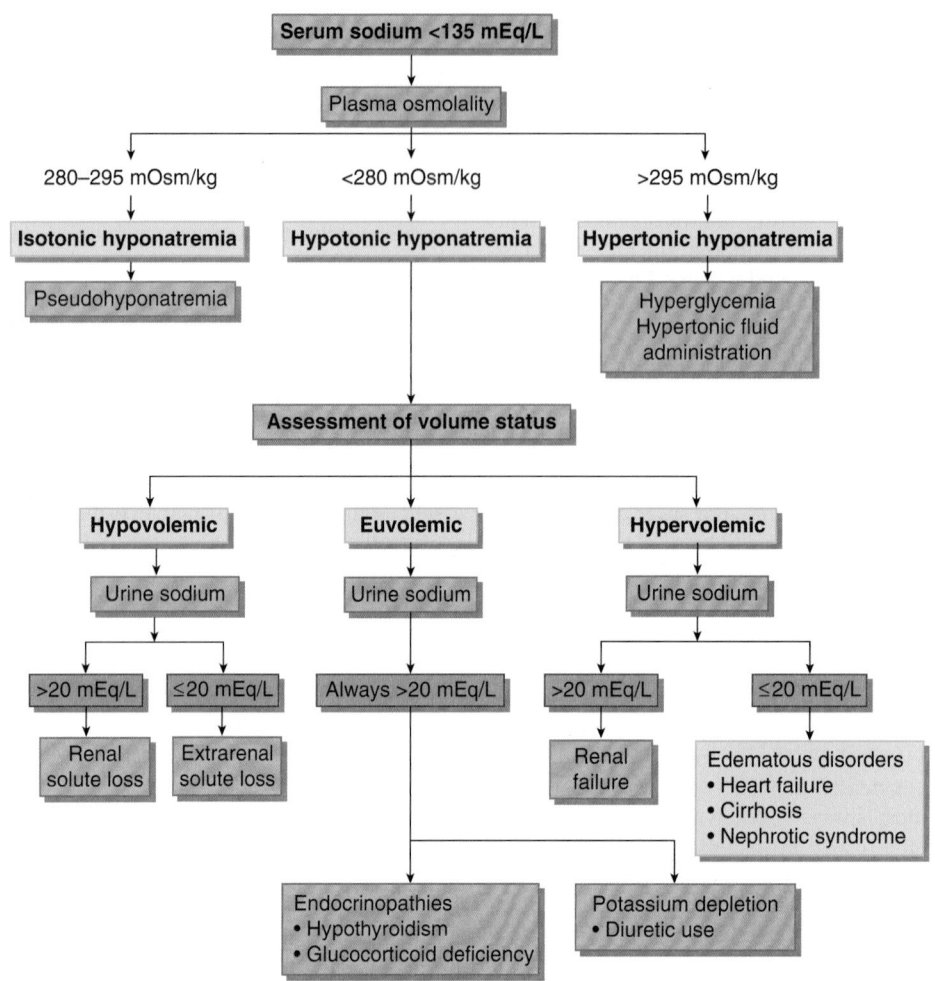

FIGURE 120.1 Diagnostic algorithm for identifying the cause of hyponatremia. Step 1 is to confirm the presence of hypotonic hyponatremia by checking serum osmolality. Step 2 is to evaluate volume status. Euvolemic hyponatremia is usually due to SIADH. Hypovolemia hyponatremia may be due to extrarenal sodium losses such as vomiting or diarrhea, or inappropriate renal losses, as occurs with cerebral salt wasting.

true hypotonic hyponatremia is confirmed (Fig. 120.1). If serum sodium is low but serum osmolality is normal, elevated lipids or proteins may account for a measured pseudohyponatremia. If sodium is low and osmolality is elevated, then another substance is contributing to osmoles such as glucose, urea, alcohol, or mannitol.

When hypotonic hyponatremia is confirmed, classification of volume status as hypovolemic, euvolemic, or hypervolemic is key for identifying the cause (see Fig. 120.1). Analysis of urine sodium is a key ancillary test. Calculation of the fractional excretion of sodium (FENa; Table 120.1) is less than 1% in patients who are hypovolemic or have reduced effective circulating blood volume and normal renal function, reflecting a corrective pattern of avid sodium retention. An important exception is when fluid losses and hypovolemia are caused by excessive and inappropriate sodium excretion, as occurs with untreated CSW (Table 120.2).

In this setting of SIADH, patients are euvolemic, spot urine sodium is greater than 40 mEq/L, and the FENa is greater than 1%. Because antidiuretic hormone (ADH) is inappropriately elevated, urine osmolality is more than a maximally dilute urine of 100 mOsm/kg and usually more than 300 mOsm/kg.

SIADH from enhanced ADH release may occur in the setting of almost any CNS disease, including stroke, trauma, brain tumor, or encephalitis, and with acute peripheral neuropathies such as Guillain–Barré syndrome.

CSW is typically encountered in patients with SAH but can occur with other forms of acute CNS injury as well. In this condition, sympathetic nervous system activation release of circulating factors such as brain natriuretic factor drive excessive sodium excretion while suppressing the normal renin-angiotensin system response to hypovolemia. CSW as a cause of hyponatremia is about one-tenth as common as SIADH. In some cases, most often SAH, hyponatremia can be the result of dual physiologic processes that favor the combination of excessive sodium losses and inappropriate ADH elevation.

TREATMENT

Acute Symptomatic Hyponatremia

Treatment of hyponatremia in neurologic patients, whether acute or chronic, is important. Symptomatic acute hyponatremia leading to brain edema is a medical emergency and should be treated

TABLE 120.1 Syndrome of Inappropriate Antidiuretic Secretion versus Cerebral Salt Wasting

	SIADH	CSW
Serum sodium (mEq/L)	<135	<135
Serum osmolality (mOsm/kg)	<275	<275
Urine osmolality (mOsm/kg)	>100 (usually >300)	>100 (usually >300)
Urine sodium (mEq/L)	>40	>40
Volume status	Euvolemic to hypervolemic	Hypovolemic
Response to isotonic saline	No effect	Improved hyponatremia

SIADH, syndrome of inappropriate antidiuretic secretion; CSW, cerebral salt wasting.

with hypertonic saline. The mainstay of therapy is a 3% sodium chloride–acetate solution, infused at a rate of 0.25 to 1.0 mL/kg/h, depending on the severity of symptoms and sodium level. Serum sodium level should be monitored every 4 hours, with the rate of the infusion adjusted to attain a rate of correction of no more than 12 mEq/L over 24 hours (0.5 mEq/L/h). More rapid aggressive correction of hyponatremia must be avoided because of the possibility of osmotic demyelination or central pontine myelinolysis (CPM; see Chapter 70).

Chronic Hyponatremia

The mainstay of treating *hypovolemic hyponatremia*, whatever the cause, is isotonic fluid resuscitation in the form of normal (0.9%) saline. In most cases, correction of the volume deficit results in normalization of the sodium concentration.

The conventional first-line treatment for SIADH commonly involves fluid restriction, but this should more correctly be termed *free water restriction*. All sources of free water, whether oral or in the form of hypotonic intravenous (IV) fluids or enteral feeds, should be restricted in SIADH, but isotonic crystalloids can still be given to maintain intravascular volume, particularly in SAH patients who require volume expansion.

In most cases of SIADH, the usual treatment of oral free water restriction is slow; this treatment prevents more free water from being retained but does not eliminate the free water excess that currently exists. Addition of sodium tablets also does little to correct the problem because 2 g of sodium chloride is the equivalent of only 34 mEq of NaCl, an amount not nearly sufficient to correct the problem.

Recently, a novel therapy of vasopressin receptor blockade has been introduced, which targets the V2 receptor in the distal collecting tubule. By causing a conformational change, aquaporin-2 allows more free water to exit ("aquaresis") leading to a significant free water clearance. *Tolvaptan* 15 mg PO daily leads to an average increase in serum sodium of 3 mEq/L over 24 hours, whereas *conivaptan* 20 mg IV over 1 hour, followed by a 20 mg infusion over 24 hours, results in an mean increase in sodium 6 mEq/L over 24 hours. By blocking the ADH receptor, so-called vaptan therapy targets the underlying pathophysiologic abnormality that underlies SIADH. Both agents have a U.S. Food and Drug Administration (FDA) indication for patients with euvolemic or hypervolemic hyponatremia due to SIADH.

SUGGESTED READINGS

Benna P, Lacquaniti F, Triolo G, et al. Acute neurologic complications of hemodialysis. Study of 14,000 hemodialyses in 103 patients with chronic renal failure. *Ital J Neurol Sci.* 1981;2:53–57.

Brouns R, De Deyn PP. Neurological complications in renal failure: a review. *Clin Neurol Neurosurg.* 2004;107:1–16.

Burns DJ, Bates D. Neurology and the kidney. *J Neurol Neurosurg Psychiatry.* 1998;65:810–821.

Campistol JM. Uremic myopathy. *Kidney Int.* 2002;62:1901–1913.

Chang D, Nagamoto G, Smith WE. Benign intracranial hypertension and chronic renal failure. *Cleve Clin J Med.* 1992;59:419–422.

Cheung AK, Sarnak MJ, Yan G, et al. Atherosclerotic cardiovascular disease risks in chronic hemodialysis patients. *Kidney Int.* 2000;58:353–362.

Cohen JA, Raps EC. Critical neurologic illness in the immunocompromised patient. *Neurol Clin.* 1995;13:659–677.

TABLE 120.2 Interpretation of Fractional Excretion of Sodium (FENa) and Urinary Sodium Concentration

	Prerenal	Intrinsic Renal Disease	Postrenal Obstruction
FENa	<1%	>1%	>4%
U_{Na} (mmol/L)	<20	>40	>40
Examples	Hypovolemia	Acute tubular necrosis	Bladder obstruction
	Heart failure	Glomerulonephritis	Ureteral obstruction
	Renal artery stenosis	Acute nephritis	

U_{Na}, urine sodium.

FENa is calculated as $[(P_{Cr} \times U_{Na}) / (P_{Na} \times U_{Cr})] \times 100$

Dunea G. Dialysis dementia: an epidemic that came and went. *ASAIO J.* 2001;47:192–194.

Ellison DH, Berl T. Clinical practice. The syndrome of inappropriate antidiuresis. *N Engl J Med.* 2007;356:2064–2072.

Galassi G, Ferrari S, Cobelli M, et al. Neuromuscular complications of kidney disease. *Nephrol Dial Transplant.* 1998;13(suppl 7):41–47.

Gross ML, Sweny P, Pearson RM, et al. Rejection encephalopathy. An acute neurological syndrome complicating renal transplantation. *J Neurol Sci.* 1982;56:23–34.

Lederman RJ, Henry CF. Progressive dialysis encephalopathy. *Ann Neurol.* 1978;4:199–204.

Lee JJ, Kilonzo K, Nistico A, et al. Management of hyponatremia. *CMAJ.* 2014;186(8):E281–E286.

Lehrich RW, Ortiz-Melo DI, Patel MB, et al. Role of vaptans in the management of hyponatremia. *Am J Kidney Dis.* 2013;62(2):364–376.

Pastan S, Bailey J. Dialysis therapy. *N Engl J Med.* 1998;338:1428–1437.

Patchell RA. Neurological complications of organ transplantation. *Ann Neurol.* 1994;36:688–703.

Raskin NH, Fishman RA. Neurologic disorders in renal failure. *N Engl J Med.* 1976;294:143–148, 204–210.

Renneboog B, Musch W, Vandemergel X, et al. Mild chronic hyponatremia is associated with falls, unsteadiness, and attention deficits. *Am J Med.* 2006;119(1):71.e1–71.e8.

Ropper AH. Accelerated neuropathy of renal failure. *Arch Neurol.* 1993;50:536–539.

Singh S, Bohn, Carlottti AP, et al. Cerebral salt wasting: truths, fallacies, theories, and challenges. *Crit Care Med.* 2002;30:2575–2579.

Sterns RH, Hix JK, Silver SM. Management of hyponatremia in the ICU. *Chest.* 2013;144(2):672–679.

Sterns RH, Silver SM. Cerebral salt wasting versus SIADH: what difference? *J Am Soc Nephrol.* 2008;19:194–196.

Winkelman JW, Chertow GM, Lazarus JM. Restless legs syndrome in end-stage renal disease. *Am J Kidney Dis.* 1996;28:372–378.

Yeakes KE, Singer M, Morton AR. Salt and water: a simple approach to hyponatremia. *CMAJ.* 2004;170:365–369.

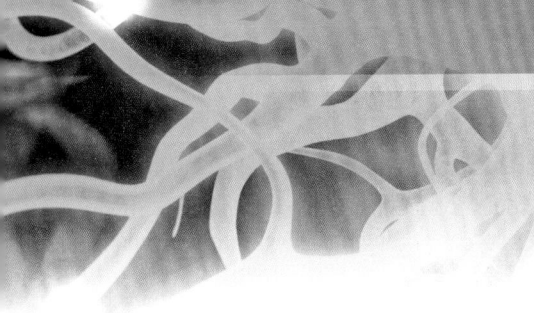

Gastric and Genitourinary Function and the Brain 121

Alden Doerner Rinaldi and Charles C. Esenwa

INTRODUCTION

The brain shares intricate connections with the gastrointestinal (GI) and genitourinary (GU) organ systems. Injury to the nervous system at any anatomic level and by a number of mechanisms—ischemia, trauma, inflammation, infection, toxic–metabolic insult, developmental anomaly, or degeneration—can provoke GI or GU symptoms. Inversely, primary GI disorders may have deleterious effects on neurologic function. In both cases, the human consequences, in terms of quality of life, morbidity, and mortality can be enormous. Here we describe (1) the general neurologic mechanisms that lead to disruption of the healthy physiologic function of the GI and GU systems, (2) specific neurologic disorders that have comorbid GI or GU manifestations, and (3) GI disorders that are associated with neurologic complications.

NEUROANATOMY

The autonomic nervous system is central in the regulation of the GI and GU systems. Autonomic impulses are mediated by the cortex and hypothalamus and affect nuclei in the brain stem, thoracolumbar, and sacral spinal cord. Parasympathetic cholinergic outflow from the dorsal nucleus of the vagus nerve in the medulla promotes the vegetative functions of secretion, digestion, absorption, and gut motility, whereas sacral parasympathetics stimulate voiding, defecation, and tumescence.

Sympathetic adrenergic outflow from the thoracolumbar cord directly opposes parasympathetic function by decreasing secretions, gut motility, and splanchnic blood flow while also increasing sphincter tone to promote urinary and fecal continence. Somatic motor neurons arising from Onuf's nucleus at the S2–S4 segments of the sacral cord pass via the pudendal nerve to innervate muscles of the pelvic floor and sphincters at the anus and urethra maintaining volitional control over continence (Fig. 121.1).

GASTROINTESTINAL MANIFESTATIONS OF NEUROLOGIC DISEASE

The enteric nervous system (ENS) is a quasi-independent branch of the autonomic nervous system with an estimated 400,000 to 600,000 neurons, nearly equal to that of the entire spinal cord.

FIGURE 121.1 Peripheral neuroanatomy of the GI and GU systems. Somatic innervation predominantly by cranial nerves V, VII, IX, and XI as well as the pudendal nerves appear in *yellow*. Parasympathetic innervation, depicted in *red*, is carried rostrally from the brain stem to the oropharynx and proximal enteric nervous system by the vagus nerve (cranial nerve X). Caudal parasympathetic innervation arising from the sacral cord, instead, travels by way of the pelvic nerves. Sympathetic output, on the other hand, reaches the enteric nervous system by way of three principle ganglia—the celiac, superior, and inferior mesenteric. The pelvic organs receive their sympathetic innervation via the hypogastric nerve, which complexes with sacral parasympathetic outputs at the pelvic to richly innervate the distal colon, rectum, and GU organs.

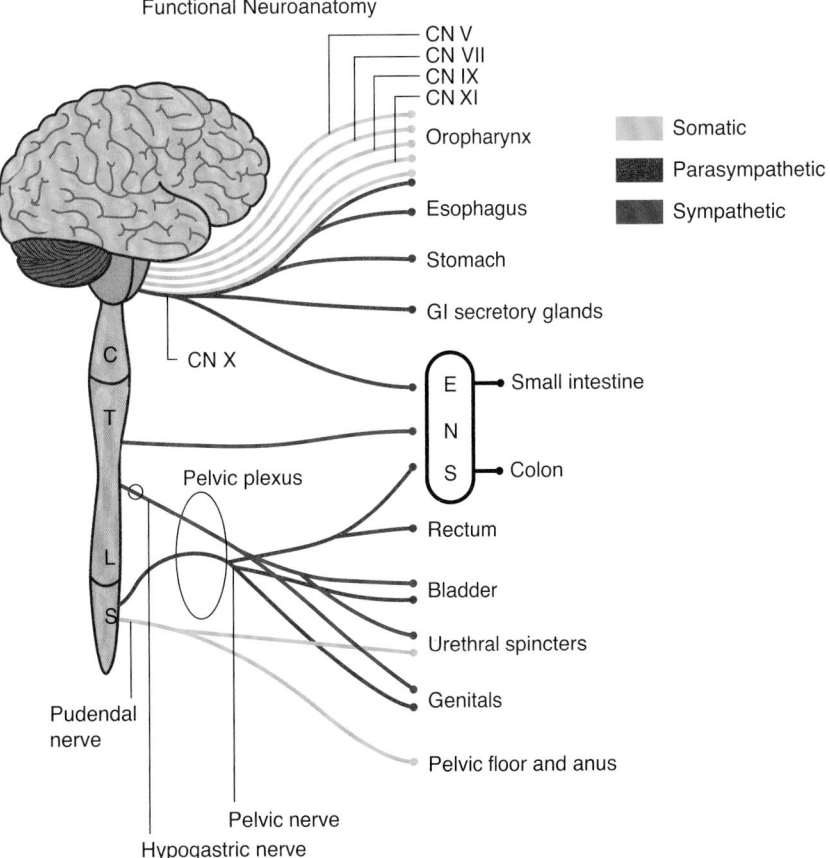

Its function is to (1) orchestrate gut motility, (2) control secretomotor function, (3) regulate local blood flow, (4) control fluid and nutrient absorption, and finally, (5) interact with and modulate the enteric immune system. It has two anatomically distinct subdivisions. The submucosal plexus, which includes Meissner plexus, is located in the gut wall and monitors the local epithelial environment exerting secretomotor control in response to parasympathetic stimuli, whereas the myenteric, or Auerbach, plexus located superficially in the muscular layer of the gut, mediates motility through both sympathetic and parasympathetic inputs. The most proximal and distal parts of the GI tract are somatically innervated, making these areas particularly susceptible to neurologic injury.

DYSPHAGIA

The process of deglutition is initiated in the cerebral cortex and overseen by the nucleus ambiguus in the medulla. Chewing, bolusing, and initiation of the swallow reflex occur in the oropharynx through a coordinated effort involving multiple cranial nerves. The swallow reflex and esophageal peristalsis are the involuntary phases and are overseen by glossopharyngeal and vagal inputs. Difficulty with swallowing, or dysphagia, can manifest as drooling, inability to effectively maneuver the food bolus, a sensation of esophageal fullness, and choking or coughing when attempting to ingest food.

A disease process affecting the primary motor cortex or supplementary motor areas, such as stroke or neurodegenerative dementia, can disrupt the preparatory and oral phases of swallowing. Direct injury to the brain stem or corticobulbar tracts by ischemia, the Parkinson-plus syndromes, or multiple sclerosis (MS) can disrupt inputs to the nucleus ambiguus, affecting the involuntary phase of swallowing. Motor neuron disorders such as amyotrophic lateral sclerosis (Lou Gehrig disease) or spinal and bulbar muscular atrophy (Kennedy disease) cause prominent dysphagia by affecting the motor neurons that supply the muscles of mastication, the oropharynx, and upper esophagus. Peripherally, disorders of the neuromuscular junction, such as myasthenia gravis and botulism, and disorders of muscle, including the muscular dystrophies and inflammatory myopathies, can also have significant effects on all phases of deglutition.

Videofluoroscopy has been the gold standard in the evaluation of dysphagia and direct visualization using videoendoscopy is now being used more commonly. In stroke, where deglutition is expected to recover, percutaneous endoscopic gastrostomy (PEG) is sometimes used as a bridge to independent swallowing. Dysphagia due to a degenerative disorder, although mitigated by swallow therapy, will naturally progress to malnutrition, dehydration, and ultimately carries a high risk of aspiration pneumonia.

ESOPHAGEAL DYSMOTILITY

The lower esophageal sphincter (LES) is controlled by the dorsal motor nucleus of the vagus nerve and is meant to serve as a one-way valve for food contents passing from the esophagus to the stomach. Achalasia is characterized by loss of esophageal peristalsis with sustained contraction of LES leading to megaesophagus and a classic "bird's beak" appearance on videofluoroscopy. Although typically a primary idiopathic disorder, there is evidence implicating an underlying inflammatory or autoimmune process affecting the ganglion cells of the myenteric plexus. Similarly, in the chronic stages of Chagas disease, achalasia can occur by infectious destruction of the myenteric plexus by the protozoa *Trypanosoma cruzi*.

GASTROPARESIS

Peristalsis in the stomach is controlled by independent rhythmic contractile waves paced by the interstitial cells of Cajal and overseen by vagal inputs. Gastroparesis is delayed gastric emptying from impaired antral motility and usually presents as postprandial bloating, pain, nausea, and vomiting. Diabetic vagal neuropathy and diabetic autonomic neuropathy are common causes that can similarly affect bowel motility, causing alternating diarrhea and constipation. Prokinetic agents such as metoclopramide, cisapride, and erythromycin are used to treat acute exacerbations, whereas severe cases may require venting gastrostomy with feeding enterostomy.

STRESS GASTRIC ULCER

Neurologic dysfunction from traumatic brain injury, spinal cord injury, or neurologic surgery predisposes to stress-related mucosal injury and hemorrhage. Stress ulcers are particularly exacerbated by injury involving brain stem and diencephalon. Dysregulation of hypothalamic function with simultaneous overactivation of parasympathetic and sympathetic efferents both increase gastric acid production and compromise mucosal protection. Stress ulcer prophylaxis is recommended in patients with coagulopathy or those requiring mechanical ventilation but should also be considered in patients with traumatic brain or spinal cord injury. Proton pump inhibitors serve as first-line therapy.

BOWEL DYSMOTILITY

Motility of the small and large intestines is coordinated exclusively by reflex loops made up of motor neurons, interneurons, and intrinsic sensory neurons. Primary Hirschsprung disease is a condition in which this neuronal network fails to form. Failure of neural crest cells to migrate during development leaves a section of colon or rectum without functional enteric plexus. Newborns can have delay in passage of meconium and in severe instances will have massive secondary dilation of the bowel termed *megacolon*. In less severe cases, diagnosis can be delayed to late childhood and even adulthood. Patients in this subgroup come to medical attention because of chronic symptoms of constipation. Diagnosis is suggested by videofluoroscopy and is made by rectal biopsy. Surgical resection of the affected bowel is the mainstay in treatment. Destruction of the enteric plexus by *T. cruzi* infection in Chagas disease is a secondary form of megacolon that has a similar diagnostic and therapeutic approach.

INCONTINENCE

Much like the esophagus, autonomic and somatic nerves innervate the anorectum. Reflex muscle contractions and paired inhibitions drive fecal movements through the rectum and into the anal vault. Motor neurons arising from Onuf's nucleus at the sacral level traverse the lower sacral plexus and pudendal nerves, ultimately exerting their effect on the external anal sphincter and muscles of the pelvic floor. Lower motor neuron injuries at this level cause sphincter dysfunction with loss of formed stool and fecal incontinence. Anorectal manometry and anal sphincter electromyography can help in such cases.

URINARY MANIFESTATIONS OF NEUROLOGIC DISEASE

The lower urinary tract (LUT) serves as both reservoir and outlet by the reciprocal action of detrusor and urethral sphincter muscles.

Anatomically, the periaqueductal gray (PAG), located in the pons, integrates rostral input from the midbrain, limbic system, and cortex to promote bladder compliance and storage through a direct tonic inhibition of the pontine micturition center (PMC). This inhibition results in a *storage reflex* by which suppression of parasympathetic and activation of sympathetic pathways causes synergistic detrusor relaxation and urethral smooth muscle contraction to close the urethral outlet. A *voiding reflex* is similarly directed by the PAG, whereby release of the PMC activates parasympathetically driven circuits throughout the thoracosacral spinal cord. Cholinergic stimulation contracts the bladder, whereas nitric oxide (NO) released from nonadrenergic noncholinergic parasympathetic (NANC) fibers relaxes the internal urethral sphincter. This action is facilitated by volitional control of somatically innervated striated muscle of the external urethral sphincter to open the urethral outlet and permit micturition. These distinct reflexes may be disrupted by neurologic injury leading to symptoms that are broadly classifiable as (1) *voiding dysfunction* with hesitancy, intermittency, slow stream, straining, terminal dribble, and retention or (2) *storage dysfunction* with urgency, frequency, nocturia, incontinence, and altered bladder sensation (Fig. 121.2).

VOIDING DYSFUNCTION

Lower motor neuron lesions of the sacral roots, plexus, or peripheral nerves cause parasympathetic denervation of the detrusor muscle resulting in a large, areflexic, and underactive bladder. When occurring alone, functional voiding symptoms may be difficult to differentiate from urinary outlet obstruction, but decreased rectal tone and impaired defecation often accompany. In the extreme form, the patient will have acute urinary retention, which is a urologic emergency. Causes include spinal cord shock from traumatic injury, Guillain–Barré syndrome, conus medullaris syndrome, and cauda equina syndrome; however, additional neurologic symptoms such as sensory loss, weakness, and areflexia will typically predominate in all of these. Less commonly, acute infection of the sacral roots by varicella or herpesviruses can also cause

urinary retention accompanied by unilateral sacral pain, sensory loss, and classic zoster or herpetic rash. Opiates, anticholinergic medications, α-adrenoreceptor agonists, benzodiazepines, nonsteroidal anti-inflammatory agents, and calcium channel blockers can all cause reversible voiding dysfunction.

Upper motor neuron lesions of the spinal cord can functionally uncouple the reciprocal action of the pathways responsible for bladder control. Although typically associated with storage dysfunction, it can cause detrusor–sphincter dyssynergia (DSD) with intermittent and simultaneous contraction of the detrusor and urethral sphincter muscles and resultant urinary retention accompanied by hesitancy and interrupted stream.

Bladder scan, postvoid residuals (PVR), urinalysis, and voiding diary will help assess degree of dysfunction, whereas spinal magnetic resonance imaging (MRI), clinical neurophysiology, and lumbar puncture can help to determine the underlying etiology. Patients with either acute or chronic voiding dysfunction are at high risk of developing urinary tract infections and bladder stones and may require intermittent urethral catheterization or a continuous suprapubic catheter. Less definitive symptomatic management may include reflex voiding by suprapubic pressure (Credé maneuver), vibratory stimulation, or cold water applied to the genitals. Detrusor areflexia has a variable response to muscarinic receptor agonists or a parasympathomimetic agent such as bethanechol. Relaxation of the urethral sphincter by α-adrenergic blockade or botulinum toxin injection can provide additional benefit.

STORAGE DYSFUNCTION

Upper motor neuron injury, either above or below the level of the pons, can result in detrusor overactivity (DO). Typically, the bladder is small and hyperreflexic. The patient will suffer from increased urinary frequency, urgency, and incontinence, a symptomatic triad commonly referred to as *overactive bladder (OAB) syndrome.* A chronic elevation of intravesicular pressures results and over time can lead to detrusor hypertrophy, vesicoureteric reflux, hydronephrosis, renal impairment, and even end-stage renal disease.

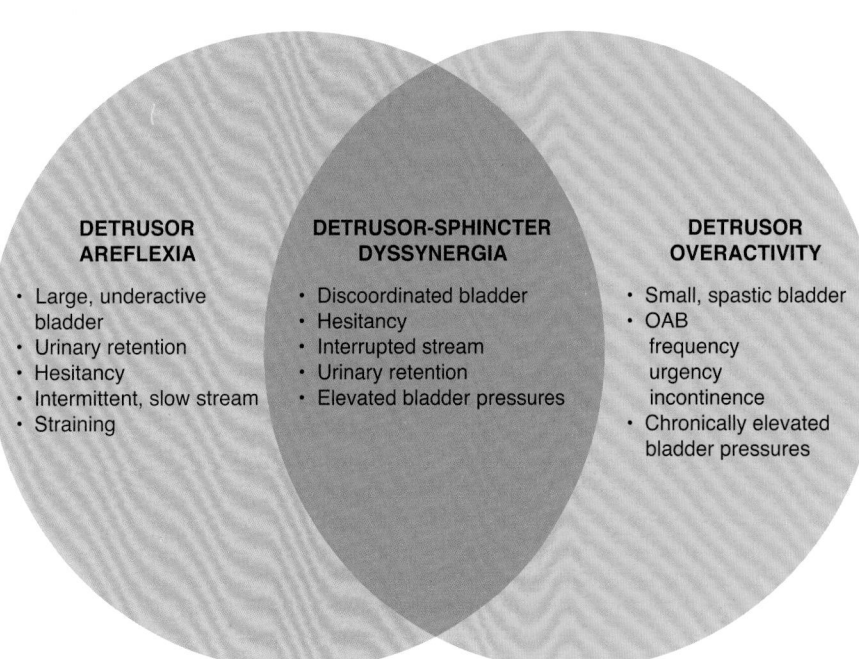

FIGURE 121.2 Symptoms of neurogenic bladder dysfunction. Particular bladder symptoms may be classified as relating to voiding dysfunction, storage dysfunction, or a mixed picture in which both occur simultaneously. Pure voiding (*purple area*) and storage (*coral area*) dysfunction are synonymous with detrusor areflexia and detrusor overactivity, respectively, whereas a combination of voiding and storage dysfunction (*area of overlap*) will lead to detrusor–sphincter dyssynergia. Each condition leads to its own unique pattern of symptomology as listed. OAB, overactive bladder.

VOIDING DYSFUNCTION **STORAGE DYSFUNCTION**

DETRUSOR AREFLEXIA
- Large, underactive bladder
- Urinary retention
- Hesitancy
- Intermittent, slow stream
- Straining

DETRUSOR-SPHINCTER DYSSYNERGIA
- Discoordinated bladder
- Hesitancy
- Interrupted stream
- Urinary retention
- Elevated bladder pressures

DETRUSOR OVERACTIVITY
- Small, spastic bladder
- OAB
  frequency
  urgency
  incontinence
- Chronically elevated bladder pressures

Here too, urodynamic testing should be pursued to better assess the pathology and help plan more invasive management of refractory symptoms.

Therapeutic approaches to storage dysfunction address OAB symptoms while mitigating the long-term consequences of persistently elevated bladder pressure. Nonpharmacologic interventions such as avoiding caffeine, pelvic floor exercises, and bladder training may be efficacious for mild symptoms. Antimuscarinic agents improve bladder compliance and are considered the mainstay of pharmacotherapy. Their use is sometimes limited by adverse central nervous system (CNS) effects, constipation, and urinary retention, in which case muscarinic acetylcholine receptor M_3 specific or blood–brain barrier impermeable agents, such as darifenacin and trospium, can be employed. Desmopressin can also reduce symptoms of urinary frequency but does so by decreasing urine production. When OAB symptoms persist despite optimal pharmacotherapy, therapeutic options include detrusor botulinum toxin injection, sacral neuromodulation, and posterior tibial nerve stimulation. As an option of last resort, surgical augmentation by cystoplasty, urinary diversion, or sphincterotomy can be done to definitively reduce bladder pressures.

SEXUAL MANIFESTATIONS OF NEUROLOGIC DISEASE

The medial preoptic area (MPOA) of the hypothalamus mediates sexual stimuli and initiates the sexual response. Caudal projections to midbrain and brain stem nuclei—including the paraventricular nucleus of the hypothalamus, the ventral tegmental area, the raphe, and gigantocellular nuclei—drive spinal reflexes that initiate tumescence, emission, and ejaculation. Tumescence may occur by both psychogenic and reflexogenic mechanisms driven by cerebrum and spinal cord, respectively. A preponderance of parasympathetic tone transmitted via the pelvic plexus and cavernous nerves to the genital soft tissue relaxes the smooth muscle of the corpora cavernosa and helicine penile arteries. NO released from NANC fibers further increases blood flow and intracavernosal pressure. Subsequent venous compression against the tunic albuginea restricts the outflow of blood to enhance and maintain erection. In women, tumescence occurs with increased vaginal blood flow and lubrication. Afferent signals carried by the pudendal and hypogastric nerves are distributed rostrally throughout the CNS. As sexual stimulation increases, sympathetic tone builds with glandular emission of the various components of sperm and the formation of semen. At sexual climax, sympathetic surge through the hypogastric nerves results in a coordinated autonomic and somatic reflex. In the male, this results is simultaneous closure of the bladder neck and expulsion of semen by rhythmic contractions of striated muscle.

MALE SEXUAL DYSFUNCTION

Injury rostral to the thoracolumbar cord preserves reflexogenic erection and ejaculation but blocks the psychogenic facilitation of the human sexual response resulting in difficulty maintaining erection. Disconnecting sympathetic pathways by injury to either the thoracolumbar cord or hypogastric nerves, often by lymph node dissection or sigmoidectomy, similarly spares reflexogenic erection but frequently inhibits ejaculation. Sacral spinal cord and root injury, on the other hand, interrupts parasympathetic outflow and reflexogenic sexual response. Plasticity of thoracolumbar outputs to the pelvic plexus provides an alternative pathway by which psychogenic erection and ejaculation may reemerge.

Phosphodiesterase-5 inhibitors improve erectile function, but their use must be weighed against the cardiovascular side effects, to which neurologic patients with autonomic dysfunction are particularly prone. Apomorphine, a dopamine agonist, acts centrally to initiate erection but requires intact efferent spinal pathways to be of benefit. Intracavernous injections of prostaglandin E1, papaverine, and phentolamine, as well as intraurethral alprostadil are effective second-line therapies. Ejaculatory dysfunction and sexual function in general may be treated with yohimbine, a mild monoamine oxidase (MAO) inhibitor, whereas midodrine, an $\alpha 1$ agonist, has been shown effective in facilitating ejaculation in men with spinal cord injury. In addition, an array of mechanical and electrostimulatory techniques for men may enable sexual function, reproduction, and improve quality of life.

FEMALE SEXUAL DYSFUNCTION

Female sexual dysfunction (FSD) is a frequent, although poorly explored, comorbidity of neurologic disease, which may be categorized as disorder of sexual desire, arousal, orgasm, or sexual pain. FSD negatively impacts quality of life, both directly and by compromising sexual relationships and, thereby, psychosocial health. The prevalence of FSD in MS is double that of the general population with more than 80% of female MS patients reporting symptoms of low desire, decreased arousal, and difficulty achieving orgasm. In MS, these symptoms of sexual dysfunction typically correlate with impaired cognitive function, depressive symptoms, bladder and bowel incontinence, Expanded Disability Status scores, and MS subtype but not time since diagnosis. Similarly, FSD is overrepresented among women with epilepsy, most commonly as a lack of sexual desire and orgasmic dysfunction. Both dysregulated hypothalamic function due to ictal and interictal discharges and effects of enzyme-inducing drugs on circulating testosterone levels may contribute. Given the clear importance of sexual health on overall quality of life, a detailed sexual history should be included in any comprehensive neurologic assessment exploring any impediment to healthy sexual function, satisfaction, and relationship.

NEUROLOGIC DISORDERS AND THE GASTROINTESTINAL AND GENITOURINARY SYSTEMS

PERIPHERAL NEUROPATHY

Peripheral autonomic fibers are particularly susceptible to neuropathy with resultant and often concurrent cardiovascular, GI, and GU dysfunction. Acute cholinergic neuropathies are the exception, causing isolated GI and GU manifestations. GI symptomology includes postprandial fullness, nausea, paralytic ileus, constipation, intermittent diarrhea, and bowel incontinence. GU symptoms are also varied, but urinary retention and erectile dysfunction, a sensitive indicator of early autonomic dysfunction, predominate. Diabetes mellitus is the most common cause of autonomic neuropathy. LUT symptoms, gastroparesis, and constipation are present in over half of diabetic patients. Pudendal compressive injury, known as *Alcock syndrome*, is classically associated with bicycle riding or labor and results in genital sensory loss, erectile dysfunction, and fecal and urinary incontinence.

SPINAL CORD INJURY

Spina bifida is one of the most common birth defects worldwide with an incidence of 1 or 2 per 1,000 births. In addition to lower extremity weakness and orthopedic problems, decreased bladder sensation and storage dysfunction commonly occur. This developmental anomaly or its surgical correction is also associated with tethered cord syndrome with traction of the filum terminale and displacement of the conus medullaris below the L1–L2 disk space. As a consequence, flexion or extension of the spine may provoke pain, sphincter dysfunction, and incontinence.

In the acute phase of traumatic spinal cord injury, autonomic and reflex activities may be lost below the level of injury with paralytic ileus and voiding dysfunction. In the chronic phase, these disabled reflexes reemerge with exaggerated function. Hyperreflexia and loss of voluntary control increases bladder and colon wall tone and tightens the external anal sphincter leading to OAB with simultaneous constipation and mild incontinence. Chronic constipation requires attentive bowel care to help prevent stercoral rectal ulcers. With spinal cord transection at or above the level of T6, potentially fatal autonomic dysreflexia can occur after an uninhibited sympathetic surge is triggered by a noxious stimulus, such as bladder or bowel distention.

MULTIPLE SCLEROSIS

Bladder dysfunction is common in MS, affecting 80% to 100% of patients over the course of their disease. Given that there are often incomplete and multilevel spinal cord lesions, patients usually give a mixed picture of urinary tract dysfunction, although storage dysfunction with OAB is most frequently encountered. In addition to conventional approaches, cannabis and the cannabinoid-derived nabiximol have shown modest results in increasing bladder control and improving quality of life. Sexual dysfunction affects more than half of men and women with MS. Decreased libido and arousal; dyspareunia; and inability to achieve erection, orgasm, and ejaculation may be further compounded by associated fatigue, immobility, and allodynia.

PARKINSONISM

Patients with Parkinson disease (PD) have been shown to develop Lewy body pathology in the ENS early in the course of the disease. Moreover, involvement of the dorsal motor nucleus of the vagus nerve causes parasympathetic dysfunction and prominent gastric symptoms. Dysphagia with pooling of saliva and drooling, postprandial fullness from delayed gastric emptying, bowel dysmotility, and constipation frequently occur. Loss of libido and erectile and ejaculatory dysfunction are also common. Pathologic hypersexuality, however, may be seen in the setting of dopamine dysregulation syndrome. Late in the disease course, there can be loss in dopamine-mediated inhibition of the PMC leading to urinary storage dysfunction and OAB.

Multiple system atrophy (MSA) is characterized by ubiquitin and α-synuclein inclusion bodies and cell loss in the brain stem, basal ganglia, cerebellum, motor cortex, and central autonomic system with subsequent autonomic failure, parkinsonism, cerebellar ataxia, and pyramidal signs. Compared to PD, urogenital dysfunction is a relatively early feature. Erectile dysfunction is the initial symptom in an estimated 41% of male patients and eventually affects almost all men with MSA. Symptoms of voiding dysfunction and urinary retention develop early in the course of the disease. As a consequence, more than half of patients with MSA suffer from recurrent urinary tract infections.

CORTICAL AND SUBCORTICAL WHITE MATTER DISEASE

Urodynamic testing in patients with cortical neurodegenerative disorders such as Lewy body dementia and Alzheimer disease frequently demonstrates subclinical storage dysfunction. In normal pressure hydrocephalus (NPH), incontinence is usually the presenting symptom in the triad of gait disturbance and cognitive impairment. DO is the most common form of incontinence after stroke and has a significant impact on poststroke quality of life. Even subclinical leukoaraiosis is thought to contribute to storage dysfunction. The shared mechanism across these disparate conditions is thought to be disruption of frontal white matter tracts.

NEUROLOGIC CONSEQUENCES OF PRIMARY GASTROINTESTINAL DISEASE

Irritable bowel syndrome (IBS) is a common GI syndrome that affects up to 20% of adults. It is defined by cramping abdominal pain, altered bowel habits, and changes in stool form and frequency. The underlying cause, although largely unknown, has been related to abnormally low threshold for neurogenic gut simulation by inflammatory mediators such as serotonin, histamine, and corticotropin-releasing factor resulting in dysregulated postprandial gut motility and visceral hyperalgesia.

Gluten sensitivity and celiac disease cause small bowel inflammation with dietary exposure to gluten. Diverse neurologic manifestations can occur, often before the GI symptoms are apparent. Gluten ataxia typically presents insidiously in the fifth decade of life as pure cerebellar ataxia. It can be accompanied by myoclonus, opsoclonus, palatal tremor, or chorea. A majority will have cerebellar atrophy on imaging. Nearly a quarter of patients with established celiac disease on a gluten-free diet will have electrophysiologic evidence of peripheral nerve damage. Although most commonly a sensorimotor axonal neuropathy, sensory ganglionopathy, small-fiber neuropathy, and pure motor neuropathy have been reported. Rarely, encephalopathy with headaches, diffuse or focal CNS white matter abnormalities, and cognitive deficits can be seen in association. Gradually progressive white matter disease can also occur and may be difficult to distinguish from MS. Other neurologic disorders reported in association with gluten sensitivity include stiff person syndrome, myopathy, and myelopathy. The common mechanism for these varied clinical manifestations is thought to involve perivascular inflammation, breakdown of the blood–brain barrier, and loss of the CNS immunoprivilege.

Inflammatory bowel disease (IBD) is made up of two entities: ulcerative colitis (UC) and Crohn disease (CD). Similar to gluten sensitivity, neurologic presentations of IBD occasionally precede GI symptoms and involve both the central and peripheral nervous systems. Peripheral neuropathies, including chronic-demyelinating or large- and small-fiber axonal types, are the most common neurologic complications affecting approximately one-third of patients and are typically unresponsive to the treatment of underlying IBD.

IBD is a hypercoagulable state with increased levels of factors V and VII, fibrinogen, and von Willebrand factor; decreased levels of protein S and antithrombin; and thrombocytosis and platelet dysfunction. Cerebral venous thrombosis is a common neurologic manifestation of UC. IBD-related arterial ischemic stroke can also occur and can have multiple underlying etiologies including small-vessel disease, artery-to-artery embolism, cardioembolism with or without endocarditis, paradoxical embolism, or vasculitis. Melkersson–Rosenthal syndrome has been described in patients with IBD and is characterized by a triad of recurrent orofacial swelling, relapsing facial paralysis, and fissured tongue.

SUGGESTED READINGS

Beach TG, Adler CH, Sue LI, et al. Multi-organ distribution of phosphorylated alpha-synuclein histopathology in subjects with Lewy body disorders. *Acta Neuropathol.* 2010;119(6):689–702.

Beckel JM, Holstege G. Neuroanatomy of the lower urinary tract. In: Anderson KE, Michel MC, eds. *Urinary Tract.* Berlin, Germany: Springer-Verlag; 2011:99–116.

Beckel JM, Holstege G. Neurophysiology of the lower urinary tract. In: Anderson KE, Michel MC, eds. *Urinary Tract.* Berlin, Germany: Springer-Verlag; 2011:149–170.

Birder L, De Groat W. Autonomic control of the urinary tract. In: Robertson D, Biaggioni I, Burnstock G, et al, eds. *Primer on the Autonomic Nervous System.* 3rd ed. London, United Kingdom: Elsevier; 2012:225–228.

Bresalier RS. The clinical significance and pathophysiology of stress-related gastric mucosal hemorrhage. *J Clin Gastroenterol.* 1991;13(suppl 2):S35–S43.

Camillieri M. Gastrointestinal function. In: Robertson D, Biaggioni I, Burnstock G, et al, eds. *Primer on the Autonomic Nervous System.* 3rd ed. London, United Kingdom: Elsevier; 2012:205–209.

Chadwick VS, Chen W, Shu D, et al. Activation of the mucosal immune system in irritable bowel syndrome. *Gastroenterology.* 2002;122(7):1778–1783.

Chancellor MB, Patel V, Leng WW, et al. OnabotulinumtoxinA improves quality of life in patients with neurogenic detrusor overactivity. *Neurology.* 2013;81:841–848.

Chapple C. Overview of the lower urinary tract. In: Anderson KE, Michel MC, eds. *Urinary Tract.* Berlin, Germany: Springer-Verlag; 2011:1–14.

Cook DJ, Fuller HD, Guyatt GH, et al. Risk factors for gastrointestinal bleeding in critically ill patients. Canadian Critical Care Trials Group. *N Engl J Med.* 1994;330(6):377–381.

De Ridder D, Van Der Aa F, Debruyne J, et al. Consensus guidelines on the neurologist's role in the management of neurogenic lower urinary tract dysfunction in multiple sclerosis. *Clin Neurol Neurosurg.* 2013;115:2033–2040.

Drake M, Parsons B. Bladder function in health and disease. In: Robertson D, Biaggioni I, Burnstock G, eds. *Primer on the Autonomic Nervous System.* 3rd ed. London, United Kingdom: Elsevier; 2012:229–232.

Everaert K, de Waard WIQ, Van Hoof T, et al. Neuroanatomy and neurophysiology related to sexual dysfunction in male neurogenic patients with lesions to the spinal cord or peripheral nerves. *Spinal Cord.* 2010;48:182–191.

Faaborg PM, Christensen P, Krassioukov A, et al. Autonomic dysreflexia during bowel evacuation procedures and bladder filling in subjects with spinal cord injury. *Spinal Cord.* 2014;52(6):1–5.

Furness JB. The enteric nervous system and neurogastroenterology. *Nat Rev Gastroenterol Hepatol.* 2012;9(5):286–294.

Griffiths DJ. Use of functional imaging to monitor central control of voiding in humans. In: Anderson KE, Michel MC, eds. *Urinary Tract.* Berlin, Germany: Springer-Verlag; 2011:81–98.

Grundy D, Al-Chaer ED, Aziz Q, et al. Fundamentals of neurogastroenterology: basic science. *Gastroenterology.* 2006;130(5):1391–1411.

Hadjivassiliou M, Sanders DS, Grunewald RA, et al. Gluten sensitivity: from gut to brain. *Lancet Neurol.* 2010;9:318–330.

Hertzler II DA, DePowell J, Stevenson CB, et al. Tethered cord syndrome: a review of the literature from embryology to adult presentation. *Neurosurg Focus.* 2010;29:1–9.

Hilz M. Physiology and pathophysiology of female sexual function. In: Robertson D, Biaggioni I, Burnstock G, ed. *Primer on the Autonomic Nervous System.* 3rd ed. London, United Kingdom: Elsevier; 2012:235–238.

Kanai AJ. Afferent mechanism in the urinary tract. In: Anderson KE, Michel MC, ed. *Urinary Tract.* Berlin, Germany: Springer-Verlag; 2011:171–206.

Koppel BS, Brust JCM, Fife T, et al. Systematic review: efficacy and safety of medical marijuana in selected neurologic disorders. *Neurology.* 2014;82: 1556–1563.

Linsenmeyer TA. Post-CVA voiding dysfunctions: clinical insights and literature review. *NeuroRehabilitation.* 2012;30:1–7.

McKeown SJ, Stamp L, Hao MM, et al. Hirschsprung disease: a developmental disorder of the enteric nervous system. *Wiley Interdiscip Rev Dev Biol.* 2013;2:113–129.

Panicker JN, Fowler CJ. The bare essentials: uro-neurology. *Pract Neurol.* 2010;10:178–185.

Papatsoris AG, Papapetropoulos S, Singer C, et al. Urinary and erectile dysfunction in multiple system atrophy (MSA). *Neurourol Urodyn.* 2008;27:22–27.

Perkin GD, Murray-Lyon I. Neurology and the gastrointestinal system. *J Neurol Neurosurg Psychiatry.* 1998;65(3):291–300.

Peters KM, Kandagatia P, Killinger KA, et al. Clinical outcomes of sacral neuromodulation in patients with neurologic conditions. *Urology.* 2013;81(4): 738–744.

Pfeiffer RF. Gastrointestinal, urological, and sexual dysfunction in Parkinson's disease. *Mov Disord.* 2010;25:S94–S97.

Ransmayr GN, Holliger S, Schletterer K, et al. Lower urinary tract symptoms in demential with Lewy bodies, Parkinson disease, and Alzheimer disease. *Neurology.* 2008;70:299–302.

Rossiter CD, Norman WP, Jain M, et al. Control of lower esophageal sphincter pressure by two sites in dorsal motor nucleus of the vagus. *Am J Physiol.* 1990;259(6, pt 1):G899.

Ruffion A, Castro-Diaz D, Patel H, et al. Systematic review of the epidemiology of urinary incontinence and detrusor overactivity among patients with neurogenic overactive bladder. *Neuroepidemiology.* 2013;41:146–155.

Sakakibara R, Kanda T, Sekido T, et al. Mechanism of bladder dysfunction in idiopathic normal pressure hydrocephalus. *Neurourol Urodyn.* 2008;27:507–510.

Schirmer CM, Kornbluth J, Heilman CB, et al. Gastrointestinal prophylaxis in neurocritical care. *Neurocrit Care.* 2012;16:184–193.

Siaud P, Puech R, Assenmacher I, et al. Adrenergic innervation of the dorsal vagal motor nucleus: possible involvement in inhibitory control of gastric acid and pancreatic insulin secretion. *Cell Tissue Res.* 1990;259(3):535–542.

Utomo E, Groen J, Blok BFM. Surgical management of functional bladder outlet obstruction in adults with neurogenic bladder dysfunction. *Cochrane Database Syst Rev.* 2014;5:CD004927.

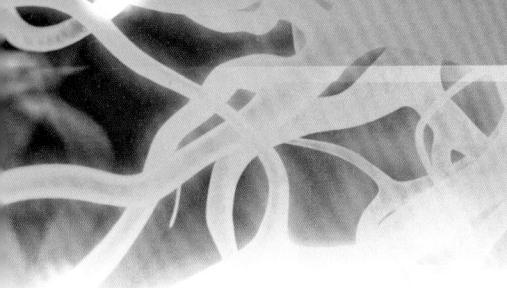

Bone Diseases and the Central Nervous System 122

Roger N. Rosenberg and Alison M. Pack

PAGET DISEASE

This chronic disease of the adult skeleton, formerly known as *osteitis deformans*, is characterized by bowing and irregular flattening of the bones. Any or all skeletal bones may be affected, but the tibia, skull, and pelvis are the most frequent sites. Usually, multiple bones are affected, but in 15%, only one is involved. The disease is symptomatic in 15% to 20% of affected individuals. Pain is the most common symptom. Except for the skeletal deformities and pain, the disease causes disability only when the skull or spine is involved.

EPIDEMIOLOGY

There is a postmortem incidence of 3% in patients older than 40 years of age. Men and women are equally affected. The most common age at onset is in the fourth to sixth decades; it is rare before age 30 years. Genetic and environmental factors such as paramyxovirus infection and dietary deficiency of calcium may influence the presentation.

PATHOBIOLOGY

In affected bones, there is an imbalance between the formation and the resorption of bone. In most cases, there is a mixture of excessive bone formation and bone destruction. The areas of bone destruction are filled with hyperplastic vascular connective tissue. New bone formation may occur in the destroyed areas in an irregular disorganized manner. The metabolic disturbance is unknown.

CLINICAL FEATURES

Two types of neurologic symptoms appear: those owing to the abnormalities in bone and those owing to arteriosclerosis, a common accompaniment. The cerebral manifestations that occur with arteriosclerosis are identical to those seen in patients with arteriosclerosis in the absence of Paget disease.

The neurologic defects of osteitis deformans are usually related to pressure on the central nervous system (CNS) or nerve roots by the overgrowth of bone. Convulsive seizures, generalized or neuralgic head pain, cranial nerve palsies, and paraplegia occur in a few cases. Deafness caused by pressure on the auditory nerves is the most common symptom; unilateral facial palsy is the next most common. Loss of vision in one eye, visual field defects, or exophthalmos may occur when the sphenoid bone is affected. Compression of the spinal cord is more common than compression of the brain, which is extremely rare except when there is sarcomatous degeneration of the lesions. Platybasia may occur in advanced cases. Paget disease has also been described in a patient with basilar impression and Arnold–Chiari type I malformation.

DIAGNOSIS

The diagnosis of Paget disease is made from the patient's appearance and the characteristic radiographic changes. Involvement of the skull in advanced cases is manifested by a generalized enlargement of the calvarium, anteroflexion of the head, and depression of the chin on the chest. When the spine is involved, the patient's stature is shortened, the spine is flexed forward, and spinal mobility is greatly reduced.

Radiographically, the skull shows areas of increased bone density with loss of normal architecture, mingled with areas in which the density of the bone is decreased (Fig. 122.1). The margins of the bones are fuzzy and indistinct. The general appearance is that of an enormous skull with the bones of the vault covered with cotton wool. In advanced cases, there may be a flattening of the base of the skull on the cervical vertebrae (*platybasia*) with signs of damage to the lower cranial nerves, medulla, or cerebellum. Both computed tomography (CT) and magnetic resonance imaging (MRI) aid diagnosis.

The serum calcium content is normal, and the serum phosphorus is normal or only slightly increased. Serum alkaline phosphatase activity is increased; the level varies with the extent and activity of the process. It may be only slightly elevated when the disease is localized to one or two bones.

Diagnosis may be difficult if the clinical symptoms are mainly neurologic. In these instances, radiographs of the pelvis and legs or a general survey of the entire skeleton may establish the diagnosis. Rarely, it may be impossible to distinguish monophasic Paget disease of the skull from osteoblastic metastases. Search for a primary neoplasm, particularly in the prostate, or biopsy of one of the lesions in the skull may be necessary in those cases.

TREATMENT

Bisphosphonates such as pamidronate, alendronate, risedronate, and zoledronic acid are considered the treatment of choice. These agents inhibit osteoblastic bone resorption. They have been shown to heal radiologic lesions and restore normal histology. The long-term effects of these drugs on disease progression have not been adequately studied. The most common indication is for pain. Less potent second-line choices include etidronate and tiludronate. Calcium and vitamin D repletion is necessary to avoid hypocalcemia secondary to bisphosphonates. The value of these medical therapies can be evaluated by reduction of serum levels of alkaline phosphatase measured at 4-month intervals and annual radiographs of specific lesions. Decompression of the spinal cord may be indicated for myelopathy secondary to stenosis created by the enlarged vertebrae. Similarly, platybasia may require to decompression of the posterior fossa to relieve cranial nerve dysfunction.

Calcitonin may also be given to inhibit the osteolytic process. Salmon calcitonin is given in subcutaneous injections of 50 to 100 units daily. Improvement of osteolytic lesions and reversal of neurologic manifestations have been noted with long-term therapy. About 25% of the patients develop serum antibodies to salmon calcitonin, sometimes in titers high enough to make the person resistant to the hormonal action of calcitonin; under these circumstances, human calcitonin may be effective.

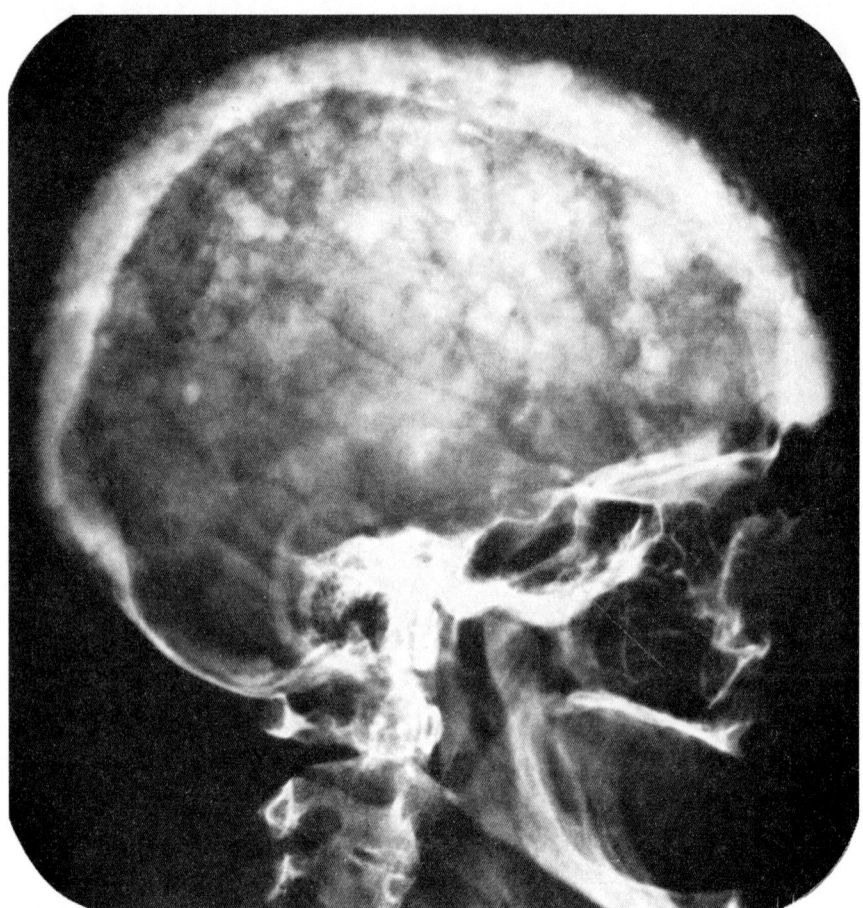

FIGURE 122.1 Osteitis deformans (Paget disease) of the skull. (Courtesy of Dr. Juan Taveras.)

OUTCOME

The course is variable but usually extends for decades. The neurologic lesions seldom lead to serious disability other than deafness, convulsive seizures, or compression of the spinal cord.

FIBROUS DYSPLASIA

The skull and the bones in other parts of the body are occasionally involved by a process characterized by small areas of bone destruction or massive sclerotic overgrowth. The clinical picture of fibrous dysplasia is related to the site and extent of the bone overgrowth. Fibrous dysplasia can involve one (monostotic form) or multiple (polyostotic form) bones. Both types may be associated with hyperfunctional endocrinopathies and café au lait lesions referred to as the *McCune–Albright syndrome*. Fibrous dysplasia and McCune–Albright syndrome are caused by a sporadic postzygotic missense mutation in the somatic cells of the GNAS complex locus located on chromosome 20q13. Overall, this leads to defects in osteoblast differentiation and proliferation of osteoblast progenitors leading to abnormal bone. The bones of the skull most often affected are the frontal (56%) and sphenoid (48%) bones. A recent Danish case series of 26 subjects revealed that 80% had involvement of craniofacial bones. Diffuse involvement of the entire skull produces leontiasis ossea, with exophthalmos, optic atrophy, and cranial nerve palsies (Fig. 122.2).

In addition to the disfiguration of the skull in the polyostotic form, symptoms of the monostotic form of the disease include headache, convulsions, exophthalmos, optic atrophy, and deafness. Most patients are, however, asymptomatic. Symptoms may begin at any age, but onset usually occurs in early adult life. The family history is negative, and there is no racial or sexual predominance.

Treatment is limited. Surgical intervention can be used to treat fracture and bony deformities. Although not well studied, bisphosphonates have been used to treat bone pain. Results are mixed and no randomized clinical trial has been done.

ACHONDROPLASIA

Achondroplasia (*chondrodystrophy*) is the most frequent form of skeletal dysplasia causing dwarfism. It is characterized by short arms and legs, lumbar lordosis, and enlargement of the head caused by mutations in the fibroblast growth factor receptor 3 gene (FGFR3). The gene product is expressed in cartilage. A frequent FGFR3 mutation is a Gl 138A codon mutation with GGG to AGG or CGG substitutions, resulting in an exchange of glycine at position 380 in the FGFR3 protein to arginine. This mutation results in a gain of negative function, producing an inactive FGFR and resultant dwarfism. The disease is rare and is estimated to occur in 15 of 1 million births in the United States. It is inherited as an autosomal dominant trait, although 80% of cases are sporadic.

Symptoms of involvement of the nervous system sometimes develop as a result of hydrocephalus, compression of the medulla and cervical cord at the level of the foramen magnum, compression of the spinal cord by ruptured intervertebral disk, and bone compression of the lower thoracic or lumbar cord. Seizures, ataxia, and paraplegia are the most common symptoms. Mental development is usually normal. Mortality rates are significantly elevated secondary to accidental, neurologic, and heart disease–related causes.

The diagnosis is made from the characteristic body configuration of short arms and legs, normal-sized trunk, enlargement of the head, and changes in the radiographs of the skeleton. Previously, CT was used to evaluate neurologic complications of achondroplasia. Currently, MRI of the brain and spine best define the presence of hydrocephalus and degree of ventricular compensation as well as whether cord compression is present. Somatosensory-evoked potential may be useful for detecting cervical myelopathy. Many affected infants die in the perinatal period, although a normal life span is possible for patients with less severe involvement of the bones.

Shunting procedures may be needed for hydrocephalus caused by involvement of the bones at the base of the skull. Laminectomy is indicated for signs of cord compression. The mutations in the FGFR3 gene at 4p are usually new mutations and result in autosomal dominant inheritance.

ANKYLOSING SPONDYLITIS

Ankylosing spondylitis is considered the prototype of the spondyloarthropathies. It typically occurs in younger persons and men are affected two to three times more commonly than women. Its etiology is likely secondary to multiple genetic and environmental factors including a strong association with the gene for human leukocyte antigen (HLA)-B27. The condition is common, affecting an estimated 1.4% of the general population. Neurologic symptoms have been considered to be uncommon but have only received limited study. A recent study investigated this question further among 24 patients recruited from an Egyptian outpatient rheumatologic clinic compared to age and sex matched controls.

Neurologic manifestations occurred in 25% of the patients; 8.3% had myelopathy and 16.7% had radiculopathy. Subclinical neurologic complications as evident by neurophysiologic test abnormalities were common, as over 70% had at least one abnormal finding.

This inflammatory disorder affects ligamentous insertions into bones; at first, it usually affects the sacroiliac joints and lumbar spine. In some patients, the entire spine is involved, with ossification of the ligaments and fusion of the vertebra. The spine becomes rigid and susceptible to a variety of disorders that may affect the spinal cord, including fractures and dislocations, atlanto-occipital dislocation, and spinal stenosis.

A cauda equina syndrome may appear in patients with long-standing spondylitis. Signs and symptoms are symmetric, with weakness, wasting, and sensory loss in lumbosacral myotomes. Autonomic dysfunction and more specifically parasympathetic dysfunction may occur. Bladder and bowel are commonly affected, and pain may be severe. The mechanism is not clear. Although concomitant arachnoiditis has been suspected as the cause, the syndrome appears late, when there is little evidence that the underlying spondylitis is active. Moreover, there is little inflammation at postmortem examination, which is likely to show chronic fibrosis. There is erosion of posterior bone elements, and, in earlier days, myelography showed enlargement of the caudal sac and prominent diverticulae of the arachnoid. CT shows similar pathology, but MRI is more illuminating, showing nerve root thickening and sometimes enhancement of dura and nerve roots; that pattern suggests inflammation of the arachnoid structures, supporting the earlier theory. Surgery is generally ineffective and has sometimes been deleterious, although there have been rare reports of some relief. Steroid therapy has been similarly without benefit. Physical therapy may be useful. Studies suggest the use of nonsteroidal anti-inflammatory drugs (NSAIDs) or selective cyclo-oxygenase-2 inhibitors for symptomatic patients. Tumor necrosis factor (TNF) inhibitors are useful for patients whose symptoms persist despite treatment with NSAIDs.

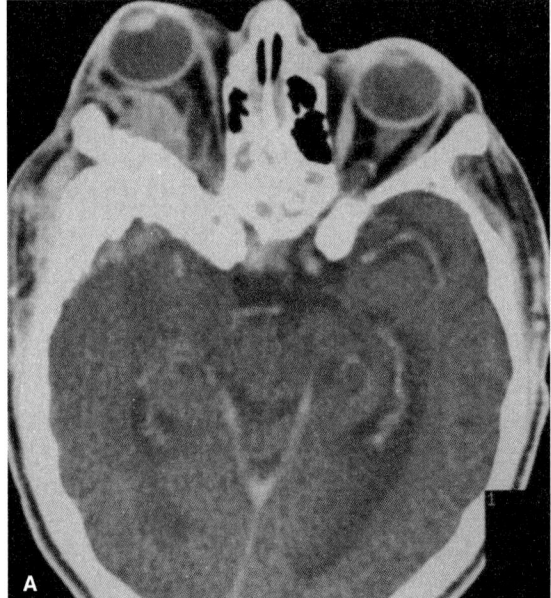
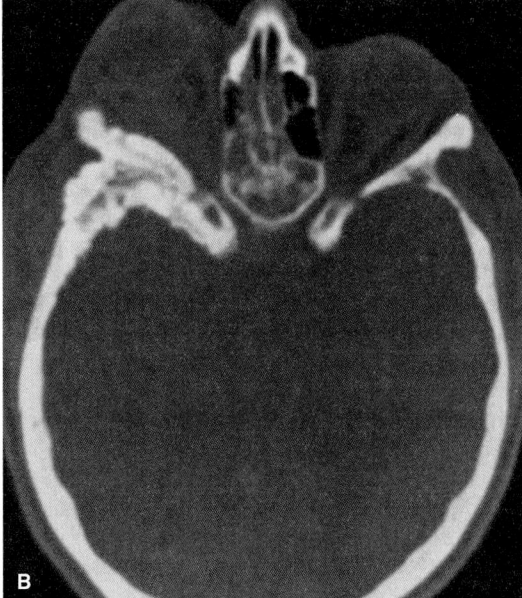

FIGURE 122.2 Fibrous dysplasia. CT. **A:** Axial contrast-enhanced scan shows proptosis on *right* with abnormal soft-tissue enhancement within orbit and middle cranial fossa. **B:** Bone window depicts pronounced thickening of sphenoid bone. (Courtesy of Dr. T. L. Chi.)

ATLANTOAXIAL DISLOCATION

Subluxation of C1 on C2 occurs in many conditions that render the odontoid process of C2 ineffective as a stabilizing post. This occurs most often as a complication of cervical trauma but also as a congenital malformation (alone or in combination with other anomalies of the cervical spine or cranium) and is seen with disproportionate frequency with Down syndrome, ankylosing spondylitis, and rheumatoid arthritis. It can be demonstrated with plain spine films, CT, or MRI. There is risk of cervical myelopathy or medullary compression and sudden death has been reported. For symptomatic cases, surgical stabilization is indicated. For asymptomatic cases, there has to be consideration of the risks of surgery against uncertain risks of no surgery. A general recommendation is to consider stabilization or decompression if imaging shows deformation of the neuraxis, symptomatic or not. A closed reduction and brace immobilization was successfully applied to a patient with traumatic bilateral rotatory dislocation of the atlantoaxial joints.

FRACTURES AND SECONDARY OSTEOPOROSIS: NEUROLOGIC CAUSES

Epilepsy, stroke, multiple sclerosis (MS), and Parkinson disease are all neurologic diseases associated with secondary osteoporosis resulting in increased risk of fracture. In addition, certain treatments of neurologic diseases including glucocorticosteroids, antiepileptic drugs (AEDs), and unfractionated heparin have an independent negative effect on bone. Steroid-induced osteoporosis is the most common cause of secondary osteoporosis. Enzyme-inducing AEDs such as phenytoin, phenobarbital, and carbamazepine are independently associated with lower bone mineral density (BMD). Vitamin D insufficiency is reported in all of these neurologic conditions contributing to reduced BMD and increased fracture risk.

Fracture rates are increased approximately twofold in persons with epilepsy. Falls secondary to seizure activity, gait imbalance because of AED treatment, and potential direct effects of AED therapy on bone including secondary osteoporosis all contribute. Similarly, fractures occur two to seven times more commonly in patients with stroke than in patients without stroke. The fractures usually occur relatively late after stroke onset and more commonly affect the paretic side of the body. The tendency to fall as a result of poststroke hemiplegia and disuse osteoporosis increase the fracture risk. Fracture rates are also higher in patients with MS because of reduced BMD secondary to immobility, prolonged corticosteroid use, and vitamin D insufficiency. Finally, fracture risk is increased in persons with Parkinson disease. In Parkinson disease, the femur is the most commonly fractured bone, whereas in the community, it is the radius. Higher percentages of osteoporosis are found in persons with Parkinson disease.

Clinically, it is important to recognize that persons with neurologic diseases are at increased risk for secondary osteoporosis and fracture. Screening of patients at risk includes serologic 25-hydroxyvitamin D testing and BMD assessment using dual-energy x-ray absorptiometry. When necessary, vitamin D supplementation should be encouraged. For those taking enzyme-inducing AEDs, higher doses of vitamin D supplementation will be needed. Bisphosphonates are commonly used to slow progression of osteoporosis and reduce fracture risk. Randomized controlled trials have found an increase in BMD, a reduction in fracture when bisphosphonates were given to patients with epilepsy [Level 1][1] or Parkinson disease [Level 1],[2] and an open-label study found similar benefits amongst stroke survivors [Level 1].[3] No study has assessed their impact among MS patients.

Some reports suggest that bisphosphonates are associated with an increased risk of atrial fibrillation and may increase the risk of ischemic stroke. A Danish case-control population-based study did not find an association between oral bisphosphonates and risk of ischemic stroke. A nonsignificant increased risk was found in association with an intravenous formulation (zoledronic acid) in an international multicenter randomized study. Interestingly, animal models suggest that bisphosphonates have an antiatherosclerotic effect, and in one population study, persons who received bisphosphonates had a lower risk of stroke when followed for a 2-year period. These results need to be followed up with a randomized clinical trial.

LEVEL 1 EVIDENCE

1. Lazzarri AA, Dussault PM, Thakore-James M, et al. Prevention of bone loss and vertebral fractures in patients with chronic epilepsy—antiepileptic drug and osteoporosis prevention trial. *Epilepsia*. 2013;54(11):1997–2004.
2. Sato Y, Iwamoto J, Honda Y. Once-weekly risedronate for prevention of hip fracture in women with Parkinson's disease: a randomized controlled trial. *J Neurol Neurosurg Psychiatry*. 2011;82:1390–1393.
3. Sato Y, Honda Y, Iwamoto J, et al. Effect of folate and mecobalamin on hip fractures in patients with stroke: a randomized controlled trial. *JAMA*. 2005;293(9):1082–1088.

SUGGESTED READINGS

Paget Disease
Chen JR, Rhee RS, Wallach S, et al. Neurologic disturbances in Paget disease of bone: response to calcitonin. *Neurology*. 1979;29:448–457.
Colina M, La Corte R, De Leonardis F, et al. Paget's disease of bone: a review. *Rheumatol Int*. 2008;28(11):1069–1075.
Corey JM. Genetic disorders producing compressive radiculopathy. *Semin Neurol*. 2006;26(5):515–522.
Douglas DL, Kanis JA, Duckworth T, et al. Paget's disease: improvement of spinal cord dysfunction with diphosphonates and calcitonin. *Metab Bone Dis Relat Res*. 1981;3:327–335.
Gruener G, Camacho P. Paget's disease of bone. *Handb Clin Neurol*. 2014;119:529–540.
Hadjipavlou A, Lander P. Paget disease of the spine. *J Bone Joint Surg Am*. 1991;73:1376–1381.
Hosking D, Lyles K, Brown JP, et al. Long-term control of bone turnover in Paget's disease with zoledronic acid and risedronate. *J Bone Miner Res*. 2007;22:142–148.
Hullar TE, Lustig LR. Paget's disease and fibrous dysplasia. *Otolaryngol Clin North Am*. 2003;36:707–732.
Iglesias-Osma C, Gómez Sánchez JC, Suquia Múgica B, et al. Paget's disease of bone and basilar impression with an Arnold–Chiari type-I malformation [in Spanish]. *An Med Intern*. 1997;14:519–522.
Langston AL, Campbell MK, Fraser WD, et al. Randomized trial of intensive bisphosphonate treatment versus symptomatic management in Paget's disease of bone. *J Bone Miner Res*. 2010;25:20–31.
Moiyadi AV, Praharaj SS, Pillai VS, et al. Hydrocephalus in Paget's disease. *Acta Neurochir (Wien)*. 2006;148(12):1297–1300.

Ralston SH, Langston AL, Reid IR. Pathogenesis and management of Paget's disease of bone. *Lancet.* 2008;372(9633):155–163.

Wallach S. Treatment of Paget's disease. *Adv Neurol.* 1982;27:1–43.

Watts GD, Wymer J, Kovach MJ, et al. Inclusion body myopathy associated with Paget disease of bone and frontotemporal dementia is caused by mutant valosin-containing protein. *Nat Genet.* 2004;36:377–381.

Fibrous Dysplasia

Albright F. Polyostotic fibrous dysplasia: a defense of the entity. *J Clin Endocrinol Metab.* 1947;7:307–324.

Bhansali A, Sharma BS, Sreenivasulu P, et al. Acromegaly with fibrous dysplasia: McCune–Albright Syndrome—clinical studies in 3 cases and brief review of literature. *Endocr J.* 2003;50:793–799.

Candeliere GA, Roughley PJ, Glorieux FH. Polymerase chain reaction-based technique for the selective enrichment and analysis of mosaic Arg201 mutations in G alpha S from patients with fibrous dysplasia of bone. *Bone.* 1997;21:201–206.

Chao K, Katznelson L. Use of high-dose oral bisphosphonate therapy for symptomatic fibrous dysplasia of the skull. *J Neurosurg.* 2008;109(5):889–892.

Chapurlat RD, Orcel P. Fibrous dysplasia of bone and McCune–Albright syndrome. *Best Pract Res Clin Rheumatol.* 2008;22(1):55–69.

Fitzpatrick KA, Taljanovic MS, Speer DP, et al. Imaging findings of fibrous dysplasia with histopathologic and intraoperative correlation. *AJR Am J Roentgenol.* 2004;182:1389–1398.

Leet AI, Magur E, Lee JS, et al. Fibrous dysplasia in the spine: prevalence of lesions and association with scoliosis. *J Bone Joint Surg Am.* 2004;86-A:531–537.

Lisle DA, Monsour PA, Maskiell CD. Imaging of craniofacial fibrous dysplasia. *J Med Imaging Radiat Oncol.* 2008;52(4):325–332.

Sassin JF, Rosenberg RN. Neurologic complications of fibrous dysplasia of the skull. *Arch Neurol.* 1968;18:363–376.

Selmani Z, Aitasalo K, Ashammakhi N. Fibrous dysplasia of the sphenoid sinus and skull base presents in an adult with localized temporal headache. *J Craniofac Surg.* 2004;15:261–263.

Thomsen MD, Rejnmark L. Clinical and radiological observations in a case series of 26 patients with fibrous dysplasia. *Calcif Tissue Int.* 2014;94:384–395.

Achondroplasia

Dandy WF. Hydrocephalus in chondrodystrophy. *Bull Johns Hopkins Hosp.* 1921;32:5–10.

Dennis JP, Rosenberg HS, Alvord EC Jr. Megalocephaly, hydrocephalus and other neurological aspects of achondroplasia. *Brain.* 1961;84:427–445.

Gollust SE, Thompson RE, Gooding HC, et al. Living with achondroplasia: attitudes toward population screening and correlation with quality of life. *Prenat Diagn.* 2003;23:1003–1008.

Haga N. Management of disabilities associated with achondroplasia. *J Orthop Sci.* 2004;9:103–107.

Hecht JT, Bodensteiner JB, Butler IJ. Neurologic manifestations of achondroplasia. *Handb Clin Neurol.* 2014;119:551–563.

Horton WA, Lunstrum GP. Fibroblast growth factor receptor 3 mutations in achondroplasia and related forms of dwarfism. *Rev Endocr Metab Disord.* 2002;3:381–385.

McKusick VA. 1997 Albert Lasker Award for special achievement in medical science. Observations over 50 years concerning intestinal polyposis, Marfan syndrome and achondroplasia. *Nat Med.* 1997;3:1065–1068.

Richette P, Bardin T, Stheneur C. Achondroplasia: from genotype to phenotype. *Joint Bone Spine.* 2008;75(2):125–130.

Shiang R, Thompson LM, Zhu YZ, et al. Mutations in the transmembrane domain of FGFR3 cause the most common genetic form of dwarfism, achondroplasia. *Cell.* 1994;78:335–342.

Smoker WR, Khanna G. Imaging the craniocervical junction. *Childs Nerv Syst.* 2008;24(10):1123–1145.

Thompson NM, Hecht JT, Bohan TP, et al. Neuroanatomic and neuropsychological outcome in school-age children with achondroplasia. *Am J Med Genet.* 1999;88:145–153.

Wynn J, King TM, Gambello MJ, et al. Mortality in achondroplasia study: a 42-year follow-up. *Am J Med Genet A.* 2007;143A(21):2502–2511.

Yamanaka Y, Ueda K, Seino Y, et al. Molecular basis for the treatment of achondroplasia. *Horm Res.* 2003;60(suppl 3):60–64.

Ankylosing Spondylitis

Borman P, Gokoglu F, Kocaoglu S, et al. The autonomic dysfunction in patients with ankylosing spondylitis: a clinical and electrophysiological study. *Clin Rheumatol.* 2008;27:1267–1273.

Braun J, Sieper J. Biological therapies in the spondyloarthritides—the current state. *Rheumatology (Oxford).* 2004;43:1072–1084.

Fox MW, Onofrio BM, Kilgore JE. Neurological complications of ankylosing spondylitis. *J Neurosurg.* 1993;78:871–878.

Haywood KL, Garratt AM, Jordan K, et al. Spinal mobility in ankylosing spondylitis: reliability, validity and responsiveness. *Rheumatology (Oxford).* 2004;43:750–757.

Khedr EM, Rashad SM, Hamed SA, et al. Neurological complications of ankylosing spondyltitis: neurophysiological assessment. *Rheumatol Int.* 2009;29:1031–1040.

Ostrowski RA, Takagishi T, Robinson J. Rheumatoid arthritis, spondyloarthropathies, and relapsing polychondritis. *Handb Clin Neurol.* 2014;119:449–461.

Sangala JR, Dakwar E, Uribe J, et al. Nonsurgical management of ankylosing spondylitis. *Neurosurg Focus.* 2008;24(1):E5.

Zhou H, Buckwalter M, Boni J, et al. Population-based pharmacokinetics of the soluble TNFr etanercept: a clinical study in 43 patients with ankylosing spondylitis compared with post hoc data from patients with rheumatoid arthritis. *Int J Clin Pharmacol Ther.* 2004;42:267–276.

Atlantoaxial Dislocation

Braganza SF. Atlantoaxial dislocation. *Pediatr Rev.* 2003;24(3):106–107.

Crossman JE, Thompson D, Hayward RD, et al. Recurrent atlantoaxial rotatory fixation in children: a rare complication of a rare condition. Report of four cases. *J Neurosurg.* 2004;100(3 suppl Spine):307–311.

Ostrowski RA, Takagishi T, Robinson J. Rheumatoid arthritis, spondyloarthropathies, and relapsing polychondritis. *Handb Clin Neurol.* 2014;119:449–461.

Stevens JM, Chong WK, Barber C, et al. A new appraisal of abnormalities of the odontoid process associated with atlantoaxial subluxation and neurological disability. *Brain.* 1994;117:133–l48.

Yamashita Y, Takahashi M, Sakamoto Y, et al. Atlantoaxial subluxation. Radiography and MRI correlated to myelopathy. *Acta Radiol.* 1989;10:135–140.

Fractures and Secondary Osteoporosis: Neurologic Causes

Black DM, Reid IR, Boonen SR, et al. The effect of 3 versus 6 years of zoledronic acid treatment of osteoporosis: a randomized extension to the HORIZON-Pivotal Fracture Trial (PFT). *J Bone Miner Res.* 2012;27(2):243–254.

Blalock SJ, Norton LL, Patel RA, et al. Patient knowledge, beliefs, and behavior concerning the prevention and treatment of glucocorticoid-induced osteoporosis. *Arthritis Rheum.* 2005;53(5):732–739.

Christensen S, Mehnert F, Chapurlat RD, et al. Oral bisphosphonates and risk of ischemic stroke: a case–control study. *Osteoporos Int.* 2011;22:1773–1779.

Cosman F, Nieves J, Komar L, et al. Fracture history and bone loss in patients with MS. *Neurology.* 1998;51(4):1161–1165.

Jørgensen L, Engstad T, Jacobsen BK. Higher incidence of falls in long-term stroke survivors than in population controls: depressive symptoms predict falls after stroke. *Stroke.* 2002;33(2):542–547.

Kang JH, Keller JJ, Lin HC. A population-based 2-year follow-up study on the relationship between bisphosphonates and the risk of stroke. *Osteoporos Int.* 2012;23:2551–2557.

Komoroski M, Azad N, Camacho P. Disorders of bone and bone mineral metabolism. *Handb Clin Neurol.* 2014;119:865–887.

Mazziotti G, Angeli A, Bilezikian JP, et al. Glucocorticoid-induced osteoporosis: an update. *Trends Endocrinol Metab.* 2006;17(4):144–149.

Ozgocmen S, Bulut S, Ilhan N, et al. Vitamin D deficiency and reduced bone mineral density in multiple sclerosis: effect of ambulatory status and functional capacity. *J Bone Miner Metab.* 2005;23(4):309–313.

Pack AM, Morrell MJ, Marcus R, et al. Bone mass and turnover in women with epilepsy on antiepileptic drug monotherapy. *Ann Neurol.* 2005;57(2):252–257.

Pack AM, Morrell MJ, Randall A, et al. Bone health in young women with epilepsy after one year of antiepileptic drug monotherapy. *Neurology.* 2008;70(18):1586–1593.

Sato Y, Honda Y, Iwamoto J. Risedronate and ergocalciferol prevent hip fracture in elderly men with Parkinson disease. *Neurology.* 2007;68(12):911–915.

Sato Y, Iwamoto J, Honda Y. An open-label trial comparing alendronate and alphacalcidol in reducing falls and hip fractures in disabled stroke patients. *J Stroke Cerebrovasc Dis.* 2011;20:41–46.

Sato Y, Iwamoto J, Kanoko T, et al. Risedronate sodium therapy for prevention of hip fracture in men 65 years or older after stroke. *Arch Intern Med.* 2005;165(15):1743–1748.

Souverein PC, Webb DJ, Petri H, et al. Incidence of fractures among epilepsy patients: a population-based retrospective cohort study in the General Practice Research Database. *Epilepsia.* 2005;46(2):304–310.

Souverein PC, Webb DJ, Weil JG, et al. Use of antiepileptic drugs and risk of fractures: case-control study among patients with epilepsy. *Neurology.* 2006;66(9):1318–1324.

Vaserman N. Parkinson's disease and osteoporosis. *Joint Bone Spine.* 2005;72(6):484–488.

Weinstock-Guttman B, Gallagher E, Baier M, et al. Risk of bone loss in men with multiple sclerosis. *Mult Scler.* 2004;10(2):170–175.

Wood B, Walker R. Osteoporosis in Parkinson's disease. *Mov Disord.* 2005;20(12):1636–1640.

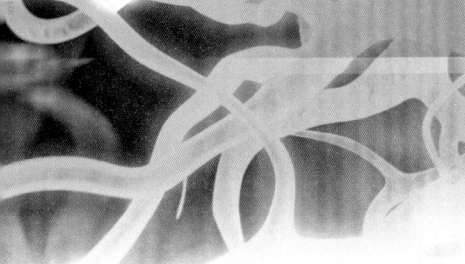

Malnutrition, Malabsorption, and B₁₂ and Other Vitamin Deficiencies 123

Rebecca Traub and Laura Lennihan

INTRODUCTION

Malnutrition and malabsorption lead to isolated and multiple nutritional deficiencies with neurologic manifestations that are ascribed to lack of vitamins or other essential nutrients. An excess of certain vitamins or minerals may also cause neurologic syndromes. Obesity and caloric excess also contribute directly and indirectly to neurologic health status. The wide range of neurologic complications of obesity and dietary excess including ischemic stroke, diabetic neuropathy, and degenerative disease of the spine are covered elsewhere in this text. Treatments for the epidemic of obesity have also led to nutritional disorders and neurologic disease.

Although this chapter describes typical syndromes associated with specific vitamin deficiencies, it should be noted that in clinical practice, vitamin deficiency and malnutrition are often multifactorial with multiple deficiencies occurring together to lead to clinical symptoms and signs.

CAUSES OF NUTRITIONAL DEFICIENCIES

Nutritional deficiency may occur due to inadequate dietary intake or impaired absorption related to intrinsic or iatrogenic gastrointestinal disorders. In developing countries, inadequate nutritional intake is often due to inadequate access to food and natural sources of vitamin and minerals. In developed or industrialized countries, causes of impaired intake may include alcoholism, eating disorders, or other causes of severely restricted dietary intake. Alcohol abuse is a major cause of malnutrition and is associated with numerous neurologic syndromes, the pathophysiology of which may be direct toxicity of ethanol, single or multiple vitamin deficiencies, or a combination. Another common cause of malnutrition is *anorexia nervosa*. Severely reduced caloric intake related to eating disorders often causes neuropathy, myopathy, and other syndromes related to multiple vitamin deficiencies.

Malabsorption may arise for any of several reasons, both intrinsic and iatrogenic. Bowel diseases causing malabsorption include inflammatory bowel disease, celiac disease, and disorders of pancreatic enzyme function. In patients with these disorders, neurologic abnormalities seem to be disproportionately frequent. Alone or in combination, there may be evidence of myopathy, sensorimotor peripheral neuropathy, and degeneration of corticospinal tracts and posterior columns and cerebellum. Optic neuritis, atypical pigmentary degeneration of the retina, and dementia are less common signs of malabsorption. Bariatric surgery to treat obesity and its associated complications typically involves restricting gastric volume. Neurologic complications are uncommon but typically are attributed to a combination of malabsorption and hyperemesis resulting in multivitamin deficiency state. Vitamin and mineral supplementation is routinely instituted after bariatric surgery to prevent such complications.

VITAMIN DEFICIENCY AND EXCESS SYNDROMES

Although many presentations of neurologic disorders related to malnutrition are attributed to deficiencies of multiple vitamins and minerals occurring together, there are particular syndromes and neurologic disorders that are typically described with specific deficiencies (Tables 123.1 and 123.2). Oversupplementation of some vitamins or minerals may also lead to neurologic disorders. In the following sections are descriptions of some of these more commonly seen syndromes.

VITAMIN B₁₂ (COBALAMIN) DEFICIENCY

Pernicious anemia, caused by vitamin B₁₂ deficiency, includes the triad of anemia, neurologic symptoms, and atrophy of the epithelial surface of the tongue. The term *combined degeneration of the spinal cord* to describe the nervous system consequences of B₁₂ deficiency was introduced around 1900. Replacement therapy began in the 1920s with dietary liver and parenteral liver extract in 1948, the year that vitamin B₁₂ was identified. B₁₂ deficiency continues to be common, with increased risk with older age related to atrophic gastritis, decreased dietary intake, and use of medications that interfere with acid secretion.

Physiology of B₁₂ Metabolism

Cobalamin is synthesized only in specific microorganisms, and animal products are the sole dietary source. Gastric acid is needed for peptic digestion to release the vitamin from proteins. The freed B₁₂ is bound by R proteins and then by gastric intrinsic factor, a

TABLE 123.1	Neurologic Syndromes Attributed to Vitamin or Mineral Deficiency
Vitamin or Mineral	**Neurologic Symptoms or Signs in Deficiency**
B₁ (thiamine)	Seizures (infants), Wernicke encephalopathy, Korsakoff dementia, subacute peripheral neuropathy
B₆ (pyridoxine)	Peripheral neuropathy, ataxia, altered mental status, seizures
B₉ (folate)	Neural tube defects (prenatal deficiency)
B₁₂ (cobalamin)	Myeloneuropathy
A	Xerophthalmia
D	Myopathy
E	Neuropathy, myopathy, ataxia
Copper	Myeloneuropathy
Iron	Restless legs syndrome

TABLE 123.2	Neurologic Syndromes Attributed to Vitamin or Mineral Excess
Vitamin or Mineral	**Neurologic Symptoms and Signs in Excess States**
B₆ (pyridoxine)	Neuropathy/ganglionopathy
A	Intracranial hypertension
Manganese	Parkinsonism
Selenium	Neuropathy
Zinc	Myeloneuropathy (through copper deficiency)

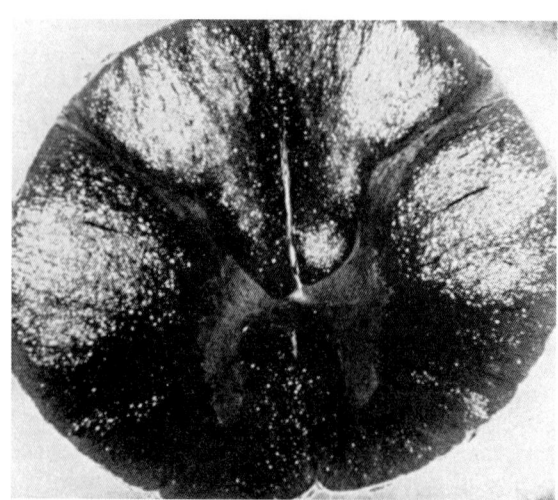

FIGURE 123.2 Subacute combined degeneration. Destruction of myelin predominating in the posterior and lateral columns. Swelling of affected myelin sheaths causes spongy appearance.

glycoprotein produced by gastric parietal cells, which is needed for transport of B₁₂ and which is absent in people with pernicious anemia. The combined intrinsic factor–cobalamin complex is transported across the terminal ileum and binds to transcobalamin, which then enters cells for use in metabolic processes.

Pathobiology of B₁₂ Deficiency

About 80% of adult-onset pernicious anemia is caused by lack of gastric intrinsic factor secondary to atrophic gastritis. The disorder is thought to be autoimmune in origin because antibodies to gastric parietal cells are found in 90% and antibodies to intrinsic factor occur in up to 76% of people with pernicious anemia. Pernicious anemia also coexists with other autoimmune diseases. In those with normal intrinsic factor, the vitamin is not absorbed because of jejunal diverticulosis, tropical or celiac sprue, or loss of the stomach or ileum by surgical resection. Proton pump inhibitors and H2-blocker medications to treat gastroesophageal reflux or peptic ulcer disease also can cause B₁₂ deficiency. Chronic recreational or occupational exposure to nitrous oxide can interfere with cobalamin metabolism and cause neuropathy or combined system disease. Long-term metformin therapy for diabetes mellitus can also lead to B₁₂ deficiency through interference with calcium-dependent ileal membrane function.

Pathology of B₁₂ Deficiency

In the spinal cord, white matter is affected more than gray. Symmetric loss of myelin sheaths occurs more often than axonal loss; changes are most prominent in the posterior and lateral columns (*combined system disease*; Figs. 123.1 and 123.2). The thoracic

cord is affected first and then the process extends into the cervical or lumbar spinal cord. Patchy demyelination may be seen in the frontal white matter, correlating with cognitive clinical symptoms.

Clinical Features

Today, most people with B₁₂ deficiency are probably asymptomatic. If the deficiency persists, symptoms may be those of anemia, neurologic disorder, or other problems such as vitiligo, sore tongue, or prematurely gray hair. About 40% of all patients with B₁₂ deficiency have some neurologic symptoms or signs, and these are often the first or most prominent manifestations of the disease. Usually, there are features of both myelopathy and peripheral neuropathy. The most common symptom is acroparesthesia—burning and painful sensations that affect the hands and feet. There may be sensory ataxia due to loss of proprioception. Memory loss, visual loss (owing to optic neuropathy), orthostatic hypotension, anosmia, impaired taste (dysgeusia), sphincter symptoms, and impotence are other symptoms and signs that have been described. B₁₂ levels should be checked in all people undergoing evaluation of cognitive impairment, as it is a treatable cause of memory loss.

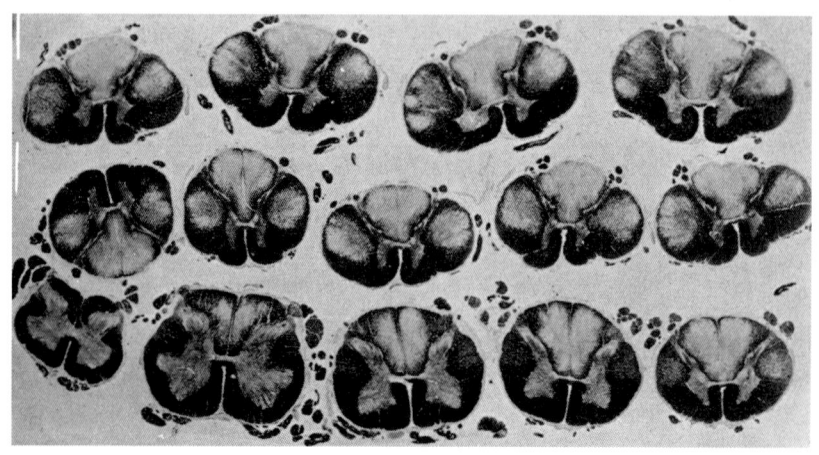

FIGURE 123.1 Subacute combined degeneration. Sections of spinal cord at various levels showing segmental loss of myelin, which is most intense in the dorsal and lateral columns.

Diagnosis

The diagnosis rests on demonstration of serum levels of vitamin B_{12} under 200 pg/mL, but low-normal values (200 to 350 pg/mL) may be found in people who respond to therapy. Some people with low values are not deficient, and additional tests may be useful. Both methylmalonic acid and homocysteine accumulate when there is impairment of cobalamin-dependent reactions; both metabolites are abnormally increased in serum in more than 99% of patients with true cobalamin deficiency. There are limitations to these tests in certain populations, with elevated homocysteine in hereditary homocysteinemia and elevated methylmalonic acid in patients with renal failure. Pernicious anemia, which often underlies B_{12} deficiency, is best assessed with intrinsic factor antibodies. Sensitivity of these antibodies is only 50% to 70% but specificity is nearly 100%. Antiparietal cell antibodies are more sensitive but less specific.

In patients with neurologic signs, only about 20% have severe anemia. Both the hematocrit and mean corpuscular volume may be normal, although anemia and macrocytosis are the classic abnormalities. Bone marrow biopsy reliably shows megaloblastic abnormalities.

Other testing in B_{12} deficiency may include magnetic resonance imaging (MRI) or electrodiagnostic testing. MRI may show increased T2-weighted signal and contrast enhancement of the posterior and lateral columns of the spinal cord (Fig. 123.3), with return to normal on treatment. Nerve conduction tests show an axonal sensorimotor neuropathy, although may be normal. B_{12} deficiency must be considered in any sensorimotor neuropathy, myelopathy, autonomic neuropathy, dementia, or optic neuropathy.

Treatment

B_{12} replacement is given intramuscularly in a dosage of 1,000 µg daily for the first week, followed by weekly injections for the first month, and then monthly injections for at least a number of months. Although some patients require lifelong B_{12} injections,

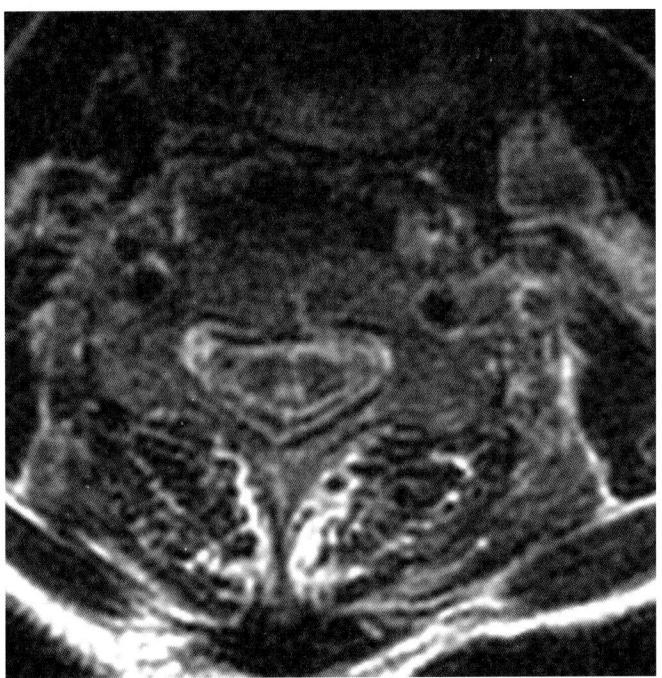

FIGURE 123.3 Increased T2 signal in the posterior columns on spine MRI in vitamin B₁₂ deficiency. (Courtesy of Dr. Gul Moonis, Associate Professor of Radiology, Columbia University.)

particularly those with pernicious anemia or surgical procedures affecting the terminal ileum, others may be transitioned to oral or sublingual formulations for maintenance therapy. There are some studies suggesting that high-dose oral vitamin B_{12} (1,000 to 2,000 µg daily) may even be a sufficient treatment in place of intramuscular therapy as initial treatment of deficiency.

After injection of B_{12}, hematologic improvement may be evident within 48 hours, as well as a subjective sense of general improvement. Paresthesias are often the first neurologic symptoms to improve and do so within 2 weeks; corticospinal and cognitive abnormalities are slower to respond, typically within 3 months but sometimes with continued improvement up to a year. If there is no response in 3 months, the condition is probably not from B_{12} deficiency. About half of the patients are left with some neurologic abnormality on examination; the residual disability, both related to the myelopathy or cognitive injury, depends on the duration and severity of symptoms at the time that treatment is started.

VITAMIN B₁ (THIAMINE) DEFICIENCY

Thiamine is an important cofactor in the metabolism of amino acids and carbohydrates. Thiamine also plays a role in the neuromuscular junction and neurotransmission. Thiamine deficiency most often occurs as a complication of severe caloric restriction, as in alcoholism, eating disorders, or after gastric surgery. The elderly may be at particular risk of thiamine deficiency due to poor absorption of the vitamin.

Clinical Features

The typical manifestations of thiamine deficiency include beriberi, both infantile and adult, and Wernicke–Korsakoff syndrome. Infantile beriberi typically occurs in the first few months of life, with primarily a cardiopulmonary picture, although a neurologic syndrome of vomiting, nystagmus, and seizures may occur. Infants fed with formula deficient in thiamine have developed beriberi, with a cluster of cases seen in Israel in 2003. Adult beriberi has traditionally been divided into two subtypes. Dry beriberi refers to a sensorimotor neuropathy, which usually occurs with a subacute presentation. The neuropathy can be severe, causing near quadriplegia. Wet beriberi refers to the high-output heart failure sometimes accompanying the neuropathy of adult thiamine deficiency.

Wernicke–Korsakoff syndrome is a central nervous system (CNS) manifestation of thiamine deficiency. Wernicke encephalopathy refers to the acute presentation of altered mental status, ataxia, and ophthalmoplegia. This syndrome has traditionally been described in alcoholics although can be seen in anyone with malnutrition or malabsorption. Many do not have the full clinical triad and rather have isolated ataxia or ophthalmoplegia. *Korsakoff syndrome* refers to the more chronic manifestations of CNS injury due to thiamine deficiency: dementia with prominent or isolated memory deficits and confabulation.

Diagnosis

Thiamine can be measured in a number of ways, most often as a blood level. Supplementation, often given intravenously in the emergency department or ambulance, will usually invalidate tests for B_1 deficiency. The diagnosis is usually made based on historical and clinical grounds, unless a B_1 level is measured before supplementation. In Wernicke–Korsakoff syndrome, MRI of the brain may demonstrate typical abnormalities, including T2-hyperintense signal and restricted diffusion in the mamillary bodies and thalami (Fig. 123.4). These MRI findings are often reversible with treatment.

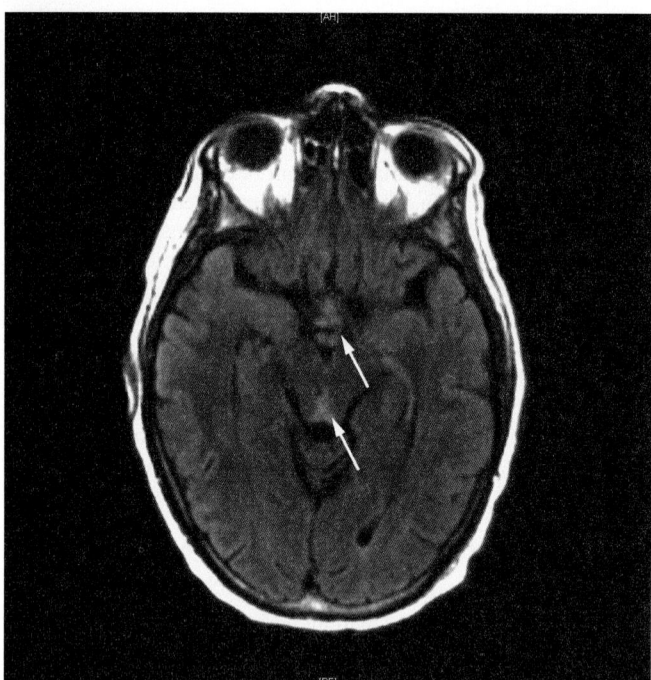

FIGURE 123.4 Increased T2 signal in the mamillary bodies and midbrain tectum in Wernicke encephalopathy due to thiamine deficiency.

Treatment

Thiamine can be given intravenously or intramuscularly for deficiency conditions, typically 100 mg daily for 7 to 14 days, followed by oral supplementation. Acute Wernicke encephalopathy is treated with even higher doses, 500 mg intravenously three times daily for 3 days, then once daily for an additional 5 days. In any patient at risk for thiamine deficiency (e.g., history of alcoholism or other risk factors for malnutrition), thiamine should be given in the emergency setting prior to glucose administration to avoid precipitation of acute Wernicke encephalopathy, as glucose metabolism increases demand for thiamine. Some advise prophylactic oral thiamine supplementation in alcoholics, elderly, or others at risk for deficiency.

VITAMIN B_6 (PYRIDOXINE) DEFICIENCY OR EXCESS

Vitamin B_6 has a number of critical cofactor roles, including metabolism of amino acids, lipids, and carbohydrates. It also serves in neurotransmitter formation, plays a role in endocrine function through effects on steroid hormones, and plays a role in both the humoral and cell-mediated immune system. B_6 deficiency occurs typically in combination with other vitamin deficiencies and is seen in any medical condition that causes malnutrition or malabsorption. Uremia and dialysis are specific risk factors for B_6 deficiency.

Clinical Features of B_6 Deficiency

Low B_6 levels have been associated with peripheral neuropathy, although isolated B_6 deficiency causing neuropathy is probably rare. Ataxia and altered mental status have also been reported with low levels of this vitamin. Severe B_6 deficiency leads to seizures, rarely seen from dietary deficiency. The genetic condition of pyridoxine-dependent seizures is a treatable cause of refractory epilepsy in neonates.

Clinical Features of B_6 Toxicity

Excessive supplementation with B_6 can cause sensory neuropathy and in severe cases, sensory ganglionopathy. Most cases are at doses of B_6 over 250 mg daily, although some have occurred at doses as low as 100 mg daily.

Diagnosis of B_6 Deficiency or Excess

Pyridoxine levels can be measured in plasma. A fasting specimen is the most accurate measure of B_6 tissue stores. In an individual person with neuropathy, it may be difficult to interpret a modestly elevated or reduced B_6 level and know whether it is responsible for clinical symptoms. The lab testing must be combined with clinical history and symptomatology to interpret values.

Treatment

Vitamin B_6 is orally supplemented in cases of deficiency at a dose of 50 to 100 mg daily.

VITAMIN B_9 (FOLIC ACID) DEFICIENCY

Folate is found in many vegetables, legumes, and animal products and in many fortified grains and foods. The primary neurologic role of folate supplementation is in women during pregnancy (or chance of pregnancy), where it plays a critical role in neural tube formation. Prenatal folic acid supplementation reduces the risk of neural tube defects by 50% to 70%. Supplements are recommended at least a month before conception, given the development of the neural tube occurs during the first weeks of embryonic development. In women at low risk for neural tube defects, 0.4 to 0.8 mg daily is recommended. In those on antiepileptics that interfere with folate absorption or use or with a prior history of pregnancy with neural tube defect, 4 mg daily is recommended.

In adults, folate deficiency has primarily hematologic manifestations, with rare, if any, neurologic symptoms. There is limited benefit to checking folate levels in patients presenting with dementia, neuropathy, or other neurologic syndromes. It should be noted that folic acid supplementation may mask vitamin B_{12} deficiency by correcting some of the associated anemia and allowing the associated neurologic syndrome to go undiagnosed. Therefore, B_{12} levels should be assessed before initiating folate replacement.

VITAMIN A DEFICIENCY OR TOXICITY

Vitamin A is a fat-soluble vitamin found in plants (beta-carotene or provitamin A) and animal sources, particularly fish, dairy, and meat, especially liver (retinol, preformed vitamin A). Retinoids are compounds related to retinol, many with actions similar to vitamin A. Physiologically, vitamin A has critical roles in fetal eye development and maintenance of retinal photoreceptor cells. Vitamin A deficiency is uncommon in developed countries but remains one of the most common nutritional deficiencies worldwide. In developed countries, vitamin A deficiency may occur in disorders of fat absorption, as in cystic fibrosis, pancreatic disorders, and celiac disease.

Vitamin A deficiency causes *xerophthalmia*, a term used to describe the spectrum of eye diseases related to deficiency, from night blindness to complete blindness and dryness or ulceration of the conjunctiva and cornea. Diagnosis of vitamin A deficiency is typically made on clinical grounds, although serum retinol levels may be measured.

Vitamin A toxicity (hypervitaminosis A) may also cause neurologic disease, with a clinical presentation of increased cerebrospinal fluid pressure (pseudotumor cerebri). Most cases occur with ingestion of excessive amounts of supplements, although it has also been described in people consuming large amounts of dietary liver. Isotretinoin, a retinoic acid derivative used for the treatment of acne, can similarly cause pseudotumor cerebri, presumably through similar mechanism of action.

VITAMIN D DEFICIENCY

Vitamin D is a fat-soluble vitamin obtained through diet or skin exposure to ultraviolet rays in sunlight. Deficiency may occur due to inadequate dietary intake, disorders of fat absorption, and inadequate exposure to sunlight. The primary manifestations of vitamin D deficiency are related to bone development and maintenance, with rickets in children and osteomalacia in adults. However, vitamin D is implicated in a number of neurologic conditions. Severe vitamin D deficiency has been described causing myopathy but only at very low serum levels, typically in cases of malabsorption. Patients with epilepsy are at increased risk for low bone density and fracture. This increased risk is multifactorial and complex, partially related to cytochrome P450 enzyme inducing antiepileptics, which increase vitamin D metabolism. Because of this risk of bone loss in many epilepsy patients, vitamin D and calcium supplementation is generally advised. Vitamin D has effects on multiple cellular functions of the immune system, and studies have demonstrated an association between vitamin D deficiency and a number of autoimmune disorders, including multiple sclerosis (MS). Whether supplementing vitamin D in patients already diagnosed with MS is beneficial from a clinical standpoint has yet to be established.

Diagnosis of vitamin D deficiency is made by measuring 25-hydroxyvitamin D (25[OH]D) levels to assess vitamin D status. There is some variation in goal levels, with most recommending 30 to 40 ng/mL.

VITAMIN E

Vitamin E is a fat-soluble vitamin found in many foods, including meat, oil, eggs, and vegetables. It is an antioxidant and a component of cell membranes. Risk factors for vitamin E deficiency are disorders that impair fat absorption, including cholestasis and pancreatic deficiencies. There are genetic diseases causing deficient vitamin E absorption and frequent neurologic impairments. The typical neurologic manifestations of vitamin E deficiency include neuropathy, myopathy, and ataxia.

MINERAL DEFICIENCY AND EXCESS SYNDROMES

COPPER DEFICIENCY AND TOXICITY

Copper, a trace mineral present in many foods, is absorbed in the stomach and proximal small intestine. In the liver, it becomes part of ceruloplasmin, which is transported through the body. Deficiency has multisystemic effects on skin and hair, liver, bone, and the nervous system. Risk factors for copper deficiency are malabsorption, including gastric surgery and celiac disease, and excessive zinc ingestion through supplements or zinc-containing denture creams.

Symptoms of Copper Deficiency

The neurologic syndrome of copper deficiency is typically myelopathy or myeloneuropathy, often mimicking vitamin B₁₂ deficiency. There is gait ataxia, sensory loss, and spasticity, with physical exam demonstrating prominent loss of vibration and joint position sense, hyperreflexia, and extensor plantar responses.

Diagnosis of Copper Deficiency

Lab testing in copper deficiency will show a low serum copper and/or ceruloplasmin level. When excessive zinc ingestion is suspected as a cause of copper deficiency, serum zinc and 24-hour urinary zinc can be measured. Given the similar clinical features, vitamin B₁₂ levels should always be checked in patients with suspected copper deficiency myeloneuropathy, and imaging of the spinal cord is often indicated, showing abnormal signal in the posterior columns.

Treatment of Copper Deficiency

Copper is supplemented at a dose of 2 mg daily. Some recommend higher doses for initial treatment in the symptomatic patient. Usually, oral supplementation suffices; however, intravenous and intramuscular forms can be used if there is concern for severe impaired absorption.

Wilson Disease

Wilson disease, which is described in more detail in Chapter 134, is a hereditary, autosomal recessive disorder of excessive copper accumulation, which leads to liver disease and a characteristic neurologic syndrome of ataxia, dysarthria, dystonia, tremor, and parkinsonism.

OTHER MINERAL DEFICIENCIES AND TOXICITIES

- *Iron:* Iron deficiency in childhood is associated with developmental delays. In adults, iron deficiency is a treatable cause of restless legs syndrome.
- *Manganese:* Manganese toxicity, primarily occurring through occupational exposure, although also reported in patients receiving parenteral nutrition, can cause symptoms similar to those seen in Parkinson disease.
- *Selenium:* Selenium toxicity, typically occurring in excessive supplementation, causes neuropathy in association with dermatologic symptoms.
- *Zinc:* Excessive zinc ingestion, as described earlier, causes a secondary copper deficiency and associated myeloneuropathy.

SUGGESTED READINGS

Allen RP, Auerbach S, Bahrain H, et al. The prevalence and impact of restless legs syndrome on patients with iron deficiency anemia. *Am J Hematol.* 2013;88:261–264.

Bloomberg RD, Fleishman A, Nalle JE, et al. Nutritional deficiencies following bariatric surgery: what have we learned? *Obes Surg.* 2005;15:145–154.

Butler CC, Vidal-Alaball J, Cannings-John R, et al. Oral vitamin B₁₂ versus intramuscular vitamin B₁₂ for vitamin B₁₂ deficiency: a systematic review of randomized controlled trials. *Fam Pract.* 2006;23:279–285.

Butterworth RF. Thiamin deficiency and brain disorders. *Nutr Res Rev.* 2003;16:277–284.

Castelli MC, Friedman K, Sherry J, et al. Comparing the efficacy and tolerability of a new daily oral vitamin B₁₂ formulation and intermittent intramuscular vitamin B₁₂ in normalizing low cobalamin levels: a randomized, open-label, parallel-group study. *Clin Ther.* 2011;33:358.e2–371.e2.

Chang CG, Adams-Huet B, Provost DA. Acute post-gastric reduction surgery (APGARS) neuropathy. *Obes Surg.* 2004;14:182–189.

Chin RL, Sander HW, Brannagan TH, et al. Celiac neuropathy. *Neurology.* 2003;60:1581–1585.

Czeizel AE, Dudas I. Prevention of the first occurrence of neural-tube defects by periconceptional vitamin supplementation. *N Engl J Med.* 1992;327:1832–1835.

de Jager J, Kooy A, Lehert P, et al. Long term treatment with metformin in patients with type 2 diabetes and risk of vitamin B-12 deficiency: randomised placebo controlled trial. *BMJ*. 2010;340:c2181.

De-Regil LM, Fernandez-Gaxiola AC, Dowswell T, et al. Effects and safety of periconceptional folate supplementation for preventing birth defects. *Cochrane Database Syst Rev*. 2010;(10):CD007950.

Goodman BP, Bosch EP, Ross MA, et al. Clinical and electrodiagnostic findings in copper deficiency myeloneuropathy. *J Neurol Neurosurg Psychiatry*. 2009;80:524–527.

Green PH, Alaedini A, Sander HW, et al. Mechanisms underlying celiac disease and its neurologic manifestations. *Cell Mol Life Sci*. 2005;62:791–799.

Green R, Kinsella LJ. Current concepts in the diagnosis of cobalamin deficiency. *Neurology*. 1995;45:1435–1440.

Hack JB, Hoffman RS. Thiamine before glucose to prevent Wernicke encephalopathy: examining the conventional wisdom. *JAMA*. 1998;279:583–584.

Healton EB, Savage DG, Brust JC, et al. Neurologic aspects of cobalamin deficiency. *Medicine (Baltimore)*. 1991;70:229–245.

Imdad A, Herzer K, Mayo-Wilson E, et al. Vitamin A supplementation for preventing morbidity and mortality in children from 6 months to 5 years of age. *Cochrane Database Syst Rev*. 2010;(12):CD008524.

Jaiser SR, Winston GP. Copper deficiency myelopathy. *J Neurol*. 2010;257:869–881.

Juhasz-Pocsine K, Rudnicki SA, Archer RL, et al. Neurologic complications of gastric bypass surgery for morbid obesity. *Neurology*. 2007;68:1843–1850.

Kinsella LJ, Green R. "Anesthesia paresthetica": nitrous oxide-induced cobalamin deficiency. *Neurology*. 1995;45:1608–1610.

Koffman BM, Greenfield LJ, Ali II, et al. Neurologic complications after surgery for obesity. *Muscle Nerve*. 2006;33:166–176.

Kopelman MD, Thomson AD, Guerrini I, et al. The Korsakoff syndrome: clinical aspects, psychology and treatment. *Alcohol Alcohol*. 2009;44:148–154.

Kumar N. Nutritional neuropathies. *Neurol Clin*. 2007;25:209–255.

Kumar N, Gross JB Jr, Ahlskog JE. Copper deficiency myelopathy produces a clinical picture like subacute combined degeneration. *Neurology*. 2004;63:33–39.

MacFarquhar JK, Broussard DL, Melstrom P, et al. Acute selenium toxicity associated with a dietary supplement. *Arch Intern Med*. 2010;170:256–261.

Mayo-Smith MF. Pharmacological management of alcohol withdrawal. A meta-analysis and evidence-based practice guideline. American Society of Addiction Medicine Working Group on Pharmacological Management of Alcohol Withdrawal. *JAMA*. 1997;278:144–151.

Mayo-Wilson E, Imdad A, Herzer K, et al. Vitamin A supplements for preventing mortality, illness, and blindness in children aged under 5: systematic review and meta-analysis. *BMJ*. 2011;343:d5094.

Mechanick JI, Youdim A, Jones DB, et al. Clinical practice guidelines for the perioperative nutritional, metabolic, and nonsurgical support of the bariatric surgery patient—2013 update: cosponsored by American Association of Clinical Endocrinologists, the Obesity Society, and American Society for Metabolic & Bariatric Surgery. *Endocr Pract*. 2013;19:337–372.

Mikati MA, Dib L, Yamout B, et al. Two randomized vitamin D trials in ambulatory patients on anticonvulsants: impact on bone. *Neurology*. 2006;67:2005–2014.

Nations SP, Boyer PJ, Love LA, et al. Denture cream: an unusual source of excess zinc, leading to hypocupremia and neurologic disease. *Neurology*. 2008;71:639–643.

Pack AM. Bone disease in epilepsy. *Curr Neurol Neurosci Rep*. 2004;4:329–334.

Patchell RA, Fellows HA, Humphries LL. Neurologic complications of anorexia nervosa. *Acta Neurol Scand*. 1994;89:111–116.

Penniston KL, Tanumihardjo SA. The acute and chronic toxic effects of vitamin A. *Am J Clin Nutr*. 2006;83:191–201.

Russell JSR, Batten FE, Collier J. Subacute combined degeneration of the spinal cord. *Brain*. 1900;23:39–110.

Savage DG, Lindenbaum J, Stabler SP, et al. Sensitivity of serum methylmalonic acid and total homocysteine determinations for diagnosing cobalamin and folate deficiencies. *Am J Med*. 1994;96:239–246.

Stabler SP. Clinical practice. Vitamin B$_{12}$ deficiency. *N Engl J Med*. 2013;368:149–160.

Victor M, Lear AA. Subacute combined degeneration of the spinal cord. *Am J Med*. 1956;20:896–911.

Wald NJ. Folic acid and the prevention of neural-tube defects. *N Engl J Med*. 2004;350:101–103.

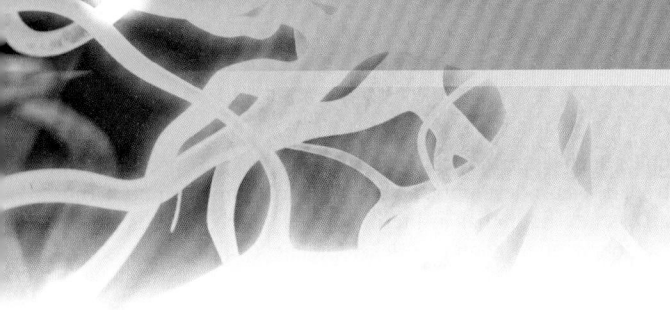

Alison M. Pack

INTRODUCTION

Pregnancy and the postpartum period are times of major biologic and social changes. Pregnancy may be associated with alterations in preexisting neurologic conditions, such as epilepsy or migraine, or herald the emergence of neurologic disorders such as peripheral nerve entrapment or a movement disorder. This chapter addresses the diagnosis, management, and treatment of neurologic disorders arising in or altered by pregnancy.

BIOLOGY OF PREGNANCY

Physiologic changes during pregnancy may influence the expression of neurologic disease and complicate management. Alterations in neuroactive steroid hormones may influence the phenotypic appearance of the disease. Changes in pharmacokinetics, medication compliance, and sleep patterns may make disease management more challenging.

The concentration and type of circulating steroid hormones change during pregnancy. Estrogen production increases. In the nonpregnant state, the main circulating estrogens are estradiol, which is synthesized by ovarian thecal cells, and estrone, which is produced by the extraglandular conversion of androstenedione. Estriol is a peripheral metabolite of estrone and estradiol. In pregnancy, the concentrations of all these estrogens, particularly estriol, increase. As pregnancy progresses, maternal steroids and dihydroisoandrostene from developing fetal adrenal glands are converted principally to estriol. Progesterone production also increases dramatically. These hormonal changes may affect neurologic conditions that are hormone responsive, including migraine, epilepsy, and multiple sclerosis (MS).

Drug pharmacokinetics is affected by the physiologic changes of pregnancy (Table 124.1). Renal blood flow and glomerular filtration increase as a function of increased cardiac output. Plasma volume, extravascular fluid, and adipose tissue increase to create

TABLE 124.1	Physiologic Changes during Pregnancy
Variable	Change
Extracellular volume	Increases 4–6 L
Plasma volume	Increases 40%
Renal blood flow	Increases 30%–50%
Glomerular filtration rate	Increases 30%–50%
Cardiac output	Increases 30%–50%
Serum albumin	Decreases 20%–30%

Data from Silberstein SD. Drug treatment and trials in women. In: Kaplan PW, ed. *Neurologic Disease in Women*. New York: Demos Medical Publishing; 1998:25–44.

a larger volume of distribution. Serum albumin decreases, which reduces drug binding, increases the free fraction, and increases drug clearance. These pharmacokinetic alterations may affect drug concentrations and are most important for drugs that are highly protein bound, hepatically metabolized, or renally cleared.

Other events of pregnancy that may compromise management are hyperemesis gravidarum, sleep deprivation, and poor compliance. Hyperemesis gravidarum can make it difficult to maintain adequate concentrations of oral medications. Sleep deprivation aggravates many neurologic conditions and can be a particular problem in the third trimester. Compliance may deteriorate because of a woman's concern that taking medication might harm her baby. Women are often advised by friends, relatives, and even medical personnel to minimize fetal drug exposure. This may lead to skipped doses, reduced doses, or even self-discontinuation of an indicated medication.

EPILEPSY

Each year, 20,000 women with epilepsy become pregnant. This number has grown as marriage rates have increased for women with epilepsy, as parenting has become more socially supported, and as the medical management of pregnancy in women with epilepsy has improved.

Although most women do maintain good seizure control throughout pregnancy, particularly if they have been seizure free for the 9 months preceding conception, seizure frequency may change. Changes responsible for this include changes in sex hormones, antiepileptic drug (AED) metabolism, sleep schedules, and medication compliance. AED concentrations may change. The total AED concentration falls because of an increase in volume of distribution, decreased drug absorption, and increased drug clearance. Lamotrigine (Lamictal) concentrations decrease throughout pregnancy because of markedly increased clearance. Monitoring of this medication should be performed at least monthly and appropriate adjustments made. Concentrations of levetiracetam (Keppra), oxcarbazepine (Trileptal), and topiramate (Topamax) also decrease in pregnancy and doses need to be adjusted. For some AEDs that are highly protein bound, although the total concentration decreases, the proportion of unbound or free drug increases because albumin levels and protein binding decline. Therefore, it is necessary to follow the non–protein-bound drug concentrations for AEDs that are highly protein bound, including carbamazepine (Tegretol), phenytoin sodium (Dilantin), and sodium valproate (Depakene). Dose adjustments should maintain a stable non–protein-bound fraction.

TERATOGENICITY

The incidence of major congenital malformations (MCMs) in association with in utero AED exposure is increased at least two- or threefold when compared to the general population. Current published risks are derived from data gathered from international prospective registries. A prospective U.S.-based North American registry continues to gather information about pregnancy and fetal outcome in women using AEDs. This registry should be contacted regarding any woman who becomes pregnant while taking AEDs (1-888-233-2334). A European registry includes countries throughout Europe, Asia, and the continent of Australia and prospectively records information about the effects of AEDs as monotherapy on the developing fetus. The Australian group has independently published their findings. A U.K. register is also actively following pregnant women with epilepsy. MCMs related to AED exposure include cleft lip and palate, cardiac defects (atrial septal defect, tetralogy of Fallot, ventricular septal defect, coarctation of the aorta, patent ductus arteriosus, and pulmonary stenosis), and urogenital defects.

Data is available for many of the commonly used AEDs. Among the currently available AEDs, valproate is consistently associated with the highest rate of MCMs including a higher risk of neural tube defects. When compared to other AEDs, the relative risk is threefold and the absolute risk is 6% to 9% of exposed pregnancies. Results from the European Surveillance of Congenital Anomalies (EUROCAT) found that in utero valproate exposure resulted in a 12.7-fold increase (odds ratio [OR] 12.7, 95% confidence interval [CI] 7.7 to 20.7) of spina bifida when compared to those with no exposure. Findings suggest the risk of valproate-associated MCMs increases at doses above 700 mg/day. Phenobarbital, which is used throughout the world, particularly in developing countries, results in a significantly increased risk of MCMs, notably cardiac malformations. First-trimester topiramate exposure is associated with an increased risk of oral clefts. The rate of oral clefts in the North American Registry was 1.4% (approximately 10-fold higher than control prevalence of 0.11%) and the U.K. Register was 2.2% (U.K. population prevalence is 0.2%). Although carbamazepine has a lower total risk of MCMs (2.6% to 3.8%) than valproate, results from EUROCAT found a 2.6-fold increased risk of spina bifida (OR 2.6, 95% CI 1.2 to 5.3) when compared to those with no exposure. The range of MCMs for lamotrigine in different studies is between 2.0% and 4.6%. Emerging data are encouraging for levetiracetam (Keppra) with published rates of MCMs between 0.7% and 2.4%. Data is limited for other commonly used AEDs including gabapentin, lacosamide, oxcarbazepine, pregabalin, and zonisamide.

Polytherapy is an independent risk factor for teratogenicity. Rates of major malformations are elevated in children exposed to multiple AEDs. Studies find that the children of pregnant women who took multiple AEDs have a higher rate of teratogenicity.

Several mechanisms have been postulated to explain the teratogenicity of AEDs. Some AEDs may be teratogenic because of free radical intermediates that bind with RNA and disrupt DNA synthesis and organogenesis. Higher concentrations of oxide metabolites increase the risk of fetal malformations. Some AEDs cause folic acid deficiency, which is associated with higher occurrence and recurrence rates of neural tube defects. The American Academy of Neurology (AAN) and American Epilepsy Society (AES) recommend that all women with epilepsy of childbearing age receive at least 0.4 mg of folic acid per day. There is currently insufficient evidence to know if higher doses of folic acid offer greater benefit.

EFFECTS OF ANTIEPILEPTIC DRUGS ON COGNITION

In addition to the teratogenicity of AEDs, AEDs may also affect cognitive outcomes of exposed infants. Retrospective and prospective studies suggest a negative effect of valproate; children whose mothers took valproate have lower scores on neuropsychological tests and have more special needs. Early studies were limited by retrospective design, size, and inability to control for confounding variables such as maternal IQ. Data from the prospective well-controlled Neurodevelopmental Effects of Antiepileptic Drugs (NEAD) study finds that in utero valproate exposure was associated with impaired cognitive development. Children exposed to valproate had significantly lower IQ scores at age 6 years (analyses controlled for maternal IQ, AED dose, gestational age, and folic acid use) when compared to children whose mothers took carbamazepine, lamotrigine, or phenytoin. In addition, findings from NEAD suggest that verbal abilities may specifically be at risk from valproate as well as the other studied AEDs (carbamazepine, lamotrigine, and phenytoin). Periconceptional folic acid use resulted in improved cognitive outcomes. The mean IQs were higher in children exposed to periconceptional folic acid (mean 108, 95% CI 106 to 111) when compared to unexposed children for all AEDs (mean 101, 95% CI 98 to 104; $P = .0009$). Valproate exposure has also been reported to increase the risk of autism and autism disorders among in utero exposed children. Cognitive outcome data is limited for other commonly used AEDs.

MANAGEMENT OF EPILEPSY DURING PREGNANCY

Management of epilepsy in women of reproductive age should focus on maintaining effective control of seizures while minimizing fetal exposure to AEDs. This applies to dosage and number of AEDs. Medication reduction or substitution should be considered prior to conception. Altering medication during pregnancy increases the risk of breakthrough seizures and exposes the fetus to an additional AED. The recommended AED management in pregnancy is monotherapy at the lowest effective dose. Higher AED doses are associated with higher risks of MCMs as well as poorer cognitive outcomes. If there is a family history of neural tube defects, an agent other than valproate and carbamazepine should be considered.

Seizures in pregnancy may result in miscarriage, preterm labor, fetal bradycardia, and injury to the mother and child. Seizures do not appear to increase the risk of MCMs. Frequent generalized tonic–clonic seizures increase risk of impaired cognitive development.

Once a woman is pregnant, prenatal diagnostic testing includes a maternal serum α-fetoprotein (AFP) and an anatomic ultrasound at 14 to 18 weeks. This combination will identify more than 95% of infants with neural tube defects. In some instances, amniocentesis may be indicated.

Enzyme-inducing AEDs may result in AED-related vitamin K deficiency, which increase the risk of early fetal hemorrhage. Although earlier AAN guidelines recommended that women taking enzyme-inducing AEDs be given supplemental vitamin K (vitamin K_1, 10 mg/day) for the last month of gestation, a recent review concluded that there was insufficient evidence to determine if prenatal vitamin K supplementation reduces neonatal hemorrhagic complications. Importantly, all neonates receive vitamin K at delivery.

For pregnant women with new-onset seizures, the diagnostic strategy is similar to that for any patient with a first-time seizure. The neurologic history and examination can be directed to signs of a specific cause, such as acute intracranial hemorrhage or central nervous system (CNS) infection. Evaluation should include screening for hypertension, proteinuria, and edema to exclude eclampsia. Follow-up studies include serologic tests for syphilis and HIV, electroencephalogram (EEG), and magnetic resonance imaging (MRI), which is the preferred imaging technique for pregnant women. As in nonpregnant women with a first-time seizure, treatment depends on seizure type and cause.

PREECLAMPSIA AND ECLAMPSIA

Preeclampsia and eclampsia are most often seen in young primigravida women and in multiparous women with a change in partner. Preeclampsia is a multisystem disorder that is diagnosed clinically by hypertension, proteinuria, and edema. Modern consensus definitions define preeclampsia as pregnancy-induced hypertension beginning after 20th week with proteinuria. Women are also defined as having *preeclampsia* if they have pregnancy-induced hypertension without proteinuria if they have other common symptoms including cerebral symptoms, epigastric or right upper quadrant pain with nausea or vomiting, or thrombocytopenia and abnormal liver enzymes. Preeclampsia is associated with hepatic and coagulation abnormalities, hypoalbuminemia, increased urate levels, and hemoconcentration. Studies suggest that secreted antiangiogenic factors such as fms-like tyrosine kinase 1 contribute to the acute symptomatology and potential long-term effects. Women who develop preeclampsia/eclampsia should be screened for glomerular and cardiovascular disease throughout life.

EPIDEMIOLOGY

Preeclampsia can progress to eclampsia, a syndrome of diffuse multifocal brain edema that can result in posterior reversible encephalopathy syndrome (PRES; see also Chapter 43). Fewer than 5% of women with preeclampsia progress to eclampsia. The incidence in Europe and other developed countries is 1 per 2,000. In developing countries, the incidence varies from 1 in 100 to 1 in 1,700. Worldwide, eclampsia probably accounts for 50,000 deaths annually. The main cause of death is pulmonary edema.

CLINICAL FEATURES

Neurologic abnormalities associated with *eclampsia* may include headaches, confusion or lethargy, seizures, cortical blindness or visual field defects, coma, brain hemorrhage, or death due to herniation from massive global cerebral edema. Seizures are most often generalized but may be partial. Common neurologic findings on exam include memory deficits, increased deep tendon reflexes, visual perception deficits, visual information–processing deficits, altered mental status, and cranial nerve deficits. Cortical blindness and visual field defects may occur because occipital lobes are preferentially involved.

DIAGNOSIS

The differential diagnosis of eclampsia includes subarachnoid hemorrhage and cerebral venous thrombosis. The diagnosis is established by appropriate clinical features in the presence of increased blood pressure plus proteinuria, edema, or both. A significant increase in blood pressure is defined as an increase of more than 15 mm Hg diastolic or 30 mm Hg systolic above baseline measurements obtained before or early in pregnancy. If no early reading is available, a blood pressure of 140/90 mm Hg or higher in late pregnancy is significant.

Neuroimaging, EEG, cerebrospinal fluid (CSF) analysis, and angiography may help in diagnosis. Computed tomography (CT) is usually normal in eclampsia but may show hypodense regions in areas of cerebral edema. MRI provides better detection of edema in the cortical mantle and is the mainstay for confirming the diagnosis. MRI characteristically shows sulcal hyperintensity and small multifocal microinfarcts and hemorrhages, with a predilection for the occipital lobes (Fig. 124.1). EEG may show spike-and-wave

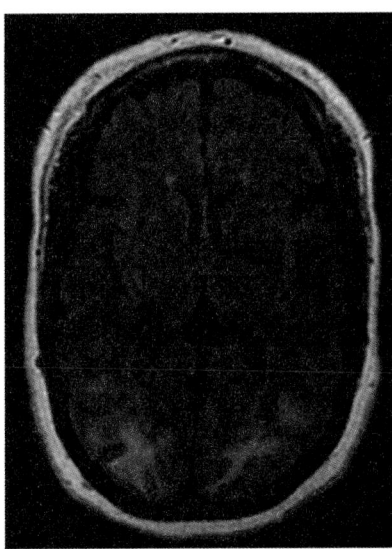

FIGURE 124.1 Symmetric posterior edema on MRI T2 fluid-attenuated inversion recovery (FLAIR) images characteristic of PRES in a hypertensive pregnant woman who presented with visual changes (patches in her vision). (From Hosley CM, McCullough LD. Acute neurologic issues in pregnancy and the peripartum. *Neurohospitalist.* 2011;1:104–116.)

discharges. The CSF is usually normal in preeclampsia but the protein content may be moderately elevated, and the pressure may be increased. In some patients, angiography shows arterial spasm. A subset of patients with severe eclampsia also develop HELLP syndrome.

Pathologic examination of eclamptic brains reveals petechial hemorrhages in cortical and subcortical patches. Microscopically, these petechial hemorrhages are ring hemorrhages about capillaries and precapillaries occluded by fibrinoid material. Areas that are predisposed include the parietooccipital and occipital regions.

TREATMENT

The most accepted treatment of eclampsia is delivery of the fetus, if possible. Hypertension should be treated with continuous infusion antihypertensive agents, initially directed toward attaining the patient's baseline premorbid blood pressure levels or a 20% reduction in systolic blood pressure, whichever is higher. Presently, magnesium sulfate (a 4- to 6-g loading dose, followed by an infusion of 1 to 2 g an hour, with a target serum magnesium level of 2.0 to 3.5 mmol/L) is the first-line treatment for the prevention and treatment of eclamptic seizures and other symptoms of eclampsia. Randomized trials have compared magnesium sulfate and other agents including phenytoin and diazepam, and the results suggest that magnesium sulfate is the agent of choice. An international randomized placebo-controlled trial (MAGPIE trial) compared the use of magnesium sulfate and placebo for preeclampsia; magnesium sulfate halved the risk of eclampsia and reduced the risk of maternal death from 1.9% to 0.8% [**Level 1**].[1] Hypertension refractory to magnesium alone can be treated with intravenous nicardipine, clevidipine, or labetalol. There were no substantive harmful effects to mother or baby in the short term. For women at high risk for preeclampsia, the U.S. Preventive Services Task Force recommends low-dose aspirin as preventive medication after 12 weeks of gestation [**Level 1**].[2]

STROKE

EPIDEMIOLOGY

Pregnancy is a risk factor for stroke, and the postpartum period is the most vulnerable time. The reported incidence of stroke secondary to pregnancy varies between 4 and 34 deliveries per 100,000. Data from the National Inpatient Sample of the Healthcare Cost and Utilization Project suggest that the incidence of pregnancy-associated stroke has risen since the 1990s. The analysis, which included all types of pregnancy-associated strokes found a 47% when comparing the time periods 1994–1995 to 2006–2007. Concurrent hypertensive disorders and heart disease explain most of the increase. Mortality is approximately 10% to 13% and is higher in black women, older women, and those with no prenatal care. Factors that increase the risk for stroke include pregnancy-related hypertension and cesarean delivery. Certain medical conditions may also increase the risk (Table 124.2). Presumptive mechanisms include changes in the coagulation and fibrinolytic systems leading to a hypercoagulable state and an increase in viscosity and stasis, which can promote thrombosis. In the postpartum period, the large decrease in blood volume at childbirth, rapid changes in hormone status that alter hemodynamics and coagulation, and the strain of delivery may predispose to a stroke. The risk of thrombosis in the postpartum period persists until at least 12 weeks after delivery.

ISCHEMIC STROKE

Arterial occlusion resulting in cerebral infarction (see also Chapter 35) approximately one-half strokes in pregnant women. Arterial occlusion occurs primarily in the second and third trimesters. Arterial strokes are generally a consequence of identifiable risk factors, including premature atherosclerosis, moyamoya disease, Takayasu arteritis, fibromuscular dysplasia, and primary CNS vasculitis.

CEREBRAL VENOUS THROMBOSIS

Cerebral venous thrombosis (see also Chapter 40) is the second most common cause of stroke in pregnant women, causing approximately one-third of strokes in pregnant women. Cerebral venous thrombosis usually occurs late in pregnancy or in the postpartum period.

TABLE 124.2	Medical Conditions that Increase the Risk of Stroke in Pregnancy
Hypertension	
Diabetes	

Hematologic disorders:
  Sickle cell disease
  Antiphospholipid syndrome
  Thrombotic thrombocytopenic purpura
  Hyperhomocysteinemia
  Mutations in prothrombin gene
  Deficiencies in antithrombin III, protein C, protein S, and factor V Leiden	

Cardiac disease	
Systemic lupus erythematosus	
Smoking	
Alcohol use	
Recreational drug use (particularly cocaine)	

The pathophysiology of venous infarctions differs from strokes associated with arterial occlusion, as they occur in the setting of venous thrombosis secondary to venous congestion and rise in pressure. Contributing factors include the underlying hypercoagulable state in pregnancy, alterations in platelet function, prothrombotic and antithrombotic proteins, as well as iron deficiency anemia and adaptive response to hemorrhage of labor and delivery. Testing for free protein S deficiency, an acquired hypercoagulable state, is positive in many patients. The clinical presentation is variable, as the woman can present with headaches (the most common presenting symptom), focal neurologic deficits, depressed mental status, or seizures. Hematologic disorders can play an etiologic role in arterial and venous strokes (see Table 124.2). Other causes are cardiogenic and paradoxic emboli.

DIAGNOSIS

The key to early diagnosis of stroke in pregnancy is prompt neuroimaging. As with nonpregnant patients, CT and MRI should be done to identify areas of stroke as well as study cerebral vasculature. Angiography including magnetic resonance (MR), CT, or transfemoral catheter angiography may be needed to assess stroke etiology. The current gold standard for diagnosing cerebral venous thrombosis is magnetic resonance venography (MRV) in combination with MRI. Imaging of cerebral venous thrombosis reveals thrombus within cerebral vein or venous sinus either without parenchymal changes or with evidence of cerebral edema, apparent ischemic stroke, or hemorrhage. Hemorrhage occurs in almost half of those with cerebral venous thrombosis (see hemorrhage section for further discussion). Further evaluation such as cardiac ultrasound and serologic studies to evaluate for conditions associated with an increased stroke risk should be pursued. With the exception of protein C, protein S, and antithrombin III deficiency, other hypercoagulable studies can be performed. Evaluation of protein C, protein S, and antithrombin III factors should occur at least 6 weeks after delivery, as they are directly affected by pregnancy itself.

TREATMENT

Treatment of strokes in pregnancy is directed to the specific cause.

Tissue Plasminogen Activator

Intravenous (IV) recombinant tissue plasminogen activator (tPA) is the only U.S. Food and Drug Administration (FDA)–approved thrombolytic drug available for acute ischemic stroke. As pregnant women were excluded from the trials, no controlled studies are available. IV tPA has a short half-life and does not cross the placenta. Potential concern therefore relates to maternal hemorrhage, placental hemorrhage and abruption, fetal loss, and preterm and not increased teratogenicity. In the literature, there are reports of six pregnant women with stroke who received IV tPA. Of those six women, three had no hemorrhagic complications, one had minor hemorrhagic transformation of the stroke, and one had an intrauterine hematoma. No fetal complications occurred in three, and in two cases, the pregnancy was terminated allowing no further analysis. The sixth patient and fetus died as a result not of a direct effect of the systemic tPA but from arterial dissection complicating angioplasty.

Unfractionated and Low Molecular Weight Heparin

Anticoagulation is a treatment option for prevention of recurrent stroke in patients with stroke due to arterial dissection (see also Chapter 43). Unfractionated heparin does not cross the placenta.

However, long-term use (>1 month) is associated with osteoporosis and thrombocytopenia. Use of low molecular weight heparin (LMWH) is thus considered to be a more preferable choice than unfractionated heparin, as the development of osteoporosis, thrombocytopenia as well as allergies is less likely. Indeed, LMWH is the drug of choice for treatment of venous thromboembolism from deep vein thrombosis, one of the leading causes of maternal mortality and morbidity in the developed world. Warfarin (Coumadin) crosses the placenta and is a known teratogen. It is therefore recommended only for women who cannot tolerate heparin or who have recurrent thromboembolic events. Aspirin complications in pregnancy include teratogenic effects and bleeding in the neonate. However, low-dose aspirin (<150 mg) is safe in the second and third trimesters, with no increase in maternal or neonatal adverse effects.

Anticoagulation is also the treatment of choice for cerebral venous thrombosis including those with cerebral hemorrhage. Acutely, early anticoagulation with either unfractionated heparin or LMWH is recommended. Studies find that among nonpregnant patients, patients who received heparin had lower mortality when compared to those who did not. In one study, no worsening with anticoagulation occurred in those with hemorrhage (see Chapter 40). Prolonged anticoagulation is also recommended, typically for 3 to 6 months. Warfarin can be used in the postpartum period. In those cases of cerebral venous thrombosis during pregnancy, LMWH is used and is held during labor and delivery.

CEREBRAL HEMORRHAGE

The risk of cerebral hemorrhage increases in pregnancy. Cerebral hemorrhage occurs in 1 to 5 pregnancies per 10,000, with an associated mortality of 30% to 40%. Factors that predispose to hemorrhage include physiologic changes of pregnancy such as hypertension, high concentrations of estrogens causing arterial dilation, and increases in cardiac output, blood volume, and venous pressure. Pregnancy-related conditions also increase the risk of hemorrhage. These include eclampsia, metastatic choriocarcinoma, cerebral emboli, and coagulopathies.

Subarachnoid hemorrhage accounts for 50% of all intracranial bleeding in pregnancy and carries a high mortality. Cerebral aneurysms and arteriovenous malformations cause most subarachnoid hemorrhages in pregnancy. Other causes include eclampsia, cocaine use, coagulopathies, ectopic endometriosis, moyamoya disease, and choriocarcinoma. Aneurysmal bleeding usually occurs in older patients in the second and third trimesters. In contrast, hemorrhages from arteriovenous malformations (see Chapter 41) occur in younger women throughout gestation, with the highest risk during labor and the puerperium. A recent large study from China did not, however, find an increased risk of hemorrhage in patients with cerebral arteriovenous malformation during pregnancy and the puerperium.

As discussed previously, cerebral venous thrombosis may also result in cerebral bleeding as a complication of venous infarction. Stasis of flow leads to infarction and secondary hemorrhage. The hemorrhage can extend to multiple areas of the brain including subarachnoid, subdural, and intraventricular spaces.

The diagnosis and treatment of subarachnoid hemorrhage (see Chapter 39) and intracerebral hemorrhage (see Chapter 38) in pregnant women are similar to those in nonpregnant patients. Subarachnoid hemorrhage is diagnosed by clinical manifestations and CT. If brain CT is normal and the clinical signs are consistent with intracranial hemorrhage, lumbar puncture should be performed.

Once intracranial hemorrhage is detected, follow-up studies include MRI and four-vessel angiography. Noncontrast CT is also the most sensitive means of diagnosing intracerebral hemorrhage. As previously discussed, cerebral venous thrombosis is best initially diagnosed using MRV in combination with MRI. Digital subtraction angiography with careful venography may be necessary in equivocal cases but is less preferable due to fetal exposure to radiation. Treatment of these conditions is directed to supporting the mother and fetus and preventing complications. Blood pressure should be carefully monitored, and fetal monitoring is indicated. The specific treatment depends on the etiology of the hemorrhage and may require emergent surgery, especially in setting of aneurysmal subarachnoid hemorrhage, when the risk of early rebleeding is high. As in nonpregnant patients, management of intracranial pressure (ICP) is important. Current practice suggests that monitoring ICP and cerebral perfusion pressure (CPP) plays a role in guiding therapy in cerebral hemorrhage, particularly for patients at high risk for developing hydrocephalus (see also Chapter 107).

MULTIPLE SCLEROSIS

MS affects 1 in 10,000 people in Western countries, primarily women in the childbearing years. MS is classified as either relapsing remitting or chronic progressive with the majority having the relapsing remitting subtype. Pregnancy is common among women with MS, as 20% to 33% of women with MS will have children after being diagnosed. Approximately 97% of these women have the relapsing remitting subtype. Initial presentation of MS during pregnancy is unusual. In contrast, pregnancy may prevent MS. An Australian case-control study of 282 women with a clinically isolated MS attack and 542 controls found that a higher number of pregnancies/births decreased the likelihood of experiencing a first attack. Prospective studies and other surveys find that the relapse rate decreases in pregnancy, especially in the third trimester, and increases in the first 3 months postpartum. A high relapse rate or disability before pregnancy is associated with an increased risk of postpartum attacks. Although prior reports suggested that long-term disability was not affected by pregnancy, studies now suggest that pregnancy may have a protective effect. A recent cross-sectional study of 973 women with relapsing, remitting MS who had two or more pregnancies were less likely to reach a standardized disability marker. A similar outcome was not seen for women with the progressive subtype. The outcome of the pregnancy itself is not affected by MS.

The mechanisms responsible for the change in the rate of relapses include humoral and immunologic changes, as seen also in pregnant women with other autoimmune diseases such as rheumatoid arthritis or systemic lupus erythematosus. There is no correlation of relapse rate with the physical stress of childbirth and caring for the newborn, sleep deprivation, type and dose of anesthesia, breastfeeding, or socioeconomic factors.

Some reports suggest that women with MS are more likely to have inductions and operative interventions during delivery when compared to control groups of women without MS and that MS is associated with lower birth weight. A recent meta-analysis, however, reports that women with MS are not at significant risk for obstetric or neonatal complications.

Treatment of MS is divided into three categories: disease-modulating, acute, and symptomatic therapies. Data regarding pregnancy outcomes and disease-modulating therapies is limited. Among the disease-modulating therapies, glatiramer acetate is currently considered the safest, as it is safe in animal models at doses above those used to treat MS. In a review that included 97 cases, there was no association with low birth weight, congenital anomaly, pre-term labor, or spontaneous abortion. The interferon βs are commonly used modulating therapies. They have abortifacient effects in primate models at higher doses than used in humans. Multiple international registry studies have not found an increased risk of birth defects or spontaneous abortions. A systematic review of over 750 pregnancies did find an association with interferon β exposure and lower mean birth weight, shorter mean birth length, and preterm labor. Natalizumab use in animal studies resulted in decreased survival and hematologic abnormalities. Both a prospective early pregnancy study ($n = 362$) and review of 35 cases found no adverse outcomes. In contrast, eight of nine children born to women with rapidly progressive disease who were treated through-out pregnancy had hematologic abnormalities. Fingolimod and BG-12 are also associated with adverse outcomes in animal studies but human data is lacking. Teriflunomide is FDA category X, as it is teratogenic in animal models. The use of disease-modulating thera-pies during pregnancy should be limited to cases whereby potential benefits outweigh the risks. If a severe relapse does occur with preg-nancy, a short course of corticosteroid therapy is recommended. Use in early pregnancy should be avoided if possible, as it may increase the risk of oral clefts and lower birth weight. In addition, neonatal adrenal suppression may follow maternal corticosteroid use, and large prenatal doses in animals caused growth retardation and compromised development of the CNS. Symptomatic thera-pies should be minimized in pregnancy. Intrathecal baclofen may be safe for the treatment of severe spasticity due to MS.

MIGRAINE

Migraine is diagnosed in 18% of women of childbearing years, and 60% to 70% of migraine headaches improve during pregnancy, especially for migraines without aura. Women who had migraine onset at menarche or who have had menstrual migraines are more likely to experience improvement, especially in the first or second trimester. Higher levels of estrogen are probably responsible for this improvement during pregnancy. The subsequent fall in es-trogen levels may cause postpartum headaches. Postpartum head-aches are common, occurring in approximately 30% of women typically during 3 to 6 days postpartum. They are associated with both personal and family histories of migraine headaches.

Migraines may also arise during pregnancy. Studies suggest these headaches are more likely to be with aura. If migraine arises in preg-nancy, the differential diagnosis must be considered. A new-onset migraine with aura can be a symptom of vasculitis, brain tumor, or occipital arteriovenous malformation. Subarachnoid hemorrhage can cause headache any time during pregnancy or delivery. Other disorders with headache include stroke, cerebral venous thrombo-sis, eclampsia, pituitary tumor, and choriocarcinoma.

Medication use during pregnancy should be limited. Acetamino-phen is the analgesic of choice, as studies confirm that it is safe at therapeutic doses of 4 g or less per day. If necessary, codeine or other narcotics may be used. Chronic use though can result in neona-tal withdrawal. Low-dose aspirin may also be given but should be avoided toward the end of pregnancy because of increased risk of prolonged labor, postpartum hemorrhage, and neonatal bleeding. Ibuprofen is the nonsteroidal anti-inflammatory drug (NSAID) of choice during pregnancy and can be given in the first and second trimesters. Both aspirin and NSAIDs are associated with prema-ture closure of the fetal ductus arteriosus. NSAIDs are also associ-ated with an increased risk of oligohydramnios. Antiemetics such as

metoclopramide or prochlorperazine may relieve the headache and associated nausea and vomiting. These agents are generally safe and effective. Ergotamine and dihydroergotamine mesylate (DHE 45) should be avoided. The triptans are effective and widely used for the treatment of headache. Current evidence does not support adverse outcomes associated with their use in pregnancy. However, as lim-ited information is available, their use in pregnancy is not recom-mended. Sumatriptan has been available the longest and is the most widely used particularly in the first trimester. Current data suggest that first-trimester exposure of sumatriptan is not associated with any significant increase in congenital malformations or poor pregnancy outcomes. For someone with recurrent headaches, a β-adrenergic blocker, such as propranolol, may be used prophylactically. How-ever, adverse effects including intrauterine growth retardation have been reported with β-adrenergic blockers. In addition, treatment should be stopped 2 to 3 days before delivery to reduce risk of fetal bradycardia and reduction in uterine contraction. Other agents used to prophylactically treat migraine headaches include valproate and topiramate. These agents should be discontinued prior to conception, as they are both associated with higher than expected rates of MCMs. In conclusion, the choice of medication for migraine in pregnant women should balance the mother's comfort with the least fetal risk.

NEOPLASMS

Brain tumors rarely become symptomatic during pregnancy. The types of tumors arising in pregnancy differ from those in non-pregnant women. Glioma is the most common, followed by me-ningioma, acoustic neuroma, and then a variety of other tumors, including pituitary tumors. Tumor growth may be exacerbated by pregnancy, especially meningioma. Possible mechanisms include increased blood volume, fluid retention, and stimulation of tumor growth by hormones.

Systemic cancer is unusual in young women and rarely begins during pregnancy. Choriocarcinoma is the only systemic tumor specifically associated with pregnancy. Brain metastases are com-mon in choriocarcinoma; among patients diagnosed with chorio-carcinoma, 3% to 20% have brain disease at diagnosis.

Cerebral neoplasms cause headaches, seizures, focal signs, or symptoms of increased ICP. The seizures may be partial or gen-eralized. Nausea and vomiting in the first trimester can be con-fused with morning sickness. All women suspected of having a brain tumor should be examined with MRI. Studies suggest that pregnancy is not a contraindication to biopsy and/or resection. Radiation therapy should be avoided. Chemotherapy is definitely contraindicated. Caesarian section is preferable to vaginal delivery to avoid increased intracranial pressure secondary to Valsalva.

NEUROPATHIES

Women are at an increased risk for peripheral neuropathy dur-ing pregnancy and the puerperium. Backache and poorly localized paresthesias are common. At least 50% of pregnant women have back pain. Among the specific rare neuropathies that occur with a higher incidence during pregnancy are carpal tunnel syndrome, facial nerve palsy, meralgia paresthetica, and chronic inflammatory demyelinating polyneuropathy (CIDP).

Carpal tunnel syndrome is the most frequent neuropathy of pregnancy. Estimated incidence ranges from 1% to 60% with approximately 17% described in prospective studies. It usually begins in the third trimester and disappears after delivery. It is attributed to generalized edema. Other potential hypotheses include the effect of hormones such as relaxin on ligamentous laxity, changes in sleep position, and increased adipose tissue. A prospective study found that 30% of women noted resolution of symptoms soon after delivery, 11% during lactation, and 5% after interruption of lactation. Prognosis was better for those who developed symptoms later in pregnancy. *Bell palsy* appears with a slightly higher frequency during pregnancy, mostly in the third trimester. Prognosis for recovery is excellent and is similar to that in nonpregnant women. Corticosteroid use within 3 to 7 days of presentation is the current treatment recommendations for the general population. Steroids are FDA category C and are probably safe in pregnancy. The potential risks in pregnancy particularly if the woman has poorly controlled hypertension or hyperglycemia need to be considered. The AAN guidelines do not find conclusive evidence to support use of antiviral agents; they are, however, safe in pregnancy. As studies suggest that women who develop Bell palsy have an increased incidence of hypertension and preeclampsia, these women should be monitored closely. *Meralgia paresthetica*, a sensory neuropathy of the lateral femoral cutaneous nerve of the thigh, is attributed to compression of the nerve under the lateral part of the inguinal ligament. Swelling during pregnancy, increased body weight, and increased lordosis during pregnancy are possible causes. Numbness, burning, tingling, or pain in the lateral thigh suggests the diagnosis. A local anesthetic with or without steroids is usually all that is necessary. Most women improve in the postpartum period. The incidence of CIDP is slightly higher during pregnancy. As in nonpregnant women, treatment includes plasmapheresis, intravenous immunoglobulin (IVIG), or steroids.

MYASTHENIA GRAVIS

Symptoms of myasthenia gravis (MG) improve in approximately 30% to 40% of patients, remains unchanged in 30% to 40% of patients, and worsen in 20% to 30% of patients. Exacerbations occur more likely in the first trimester, in the final 4 weeks of gestation, or puerperium. The total rate of pregnancy complications particularly preterm rupture of the amniotic membranes is higher among women with MG than in the general population. An association between MG and preeclampsia has been described. Pregnancy does not affect the long-term outcome of MG.

Treatment of myasthenia during pregnancy includes immunosuppressant drugs, plasmapheresis, and IVIG. Use of prednisone in the first trimester is associated with a small increase in cleft palate, and high doses may lead to premature rupture of membrane. Use of cyclosporine is not recommended because of reported increased risk of spontaneous abortions, prematurity, and low birth weight. Azathioprine and mycophenolate mofetil should not be used, as they can result in significant risk to the fetus and are designated by the FDA as category X. Anticholinesterase drugs are reportedly safe. Thymectomy is deferred until long after delivery. The long-term outcome of MG is not affected by pregnancy. (Myasthenia is also discussed in Chapter 89.)

Neonatal MG affects 12% to 20% of infants born to mothers with MG. The occurrence of neonatal MG does not correlate with maternal disease severity or titer of maternal anticholinesterase receptor antibodies. The symptoms clear within a few weeks.

MOVEMENT DISORDERS

Movement disorders are unusual in young women, but those that specifically occur during pregnancy include the restless legs syndrome, chorea, and drug-induced movement disorders.

The *restless legs syndrome* is the most common movement disorder of pregnancy. It is a chronic condition that has an autosomal dominant pattern of inheritance and is characterized by a crawling, burning, or aching sensation in the calves with an irresistible urge to move the legs. It occurs in 10% to 20% of pregnant women and can occur for the first time in pregnancy, usually in the second and third trimesters. For women with preexisting restless legs syndrome, there can be a worsening of symptoms. In a study of 606 pregnant women, 59 had preexisting restless legs syndrome and among those women, 36 reported worsening of symptoms. Iron deficiency has been found in patients with restless legs syndrome, and treatment of iron deficiency in pregnant women has been advocated but therapeutic trials have yet not been performed. Also, lower folate levels are associated with the restless legs syndrome and treatment recommendations include folate supplementation. Other treatments include massage, flexion and extension, walking, benzodiazepines, opiates, or levodopa.

Chorea gravidarum occurs in pregnancy (see Chapter 81). Treatment is reserved for those with violent and disabling chorea and includes haloperidol or benzodiazepines.

Drugs that block dopamine receptors are often used to treat the nausea and vomiting of pregnancy. These drugs can cause new-onset chorea, tremor, dystonia, or parkinsonism. *Idiopathic Parkinson disease* is uncommon in women younger than 40 years. More common is secondary parkinsonism caused by medication or toxins. There is no definite evidence that Parkinson disease worsens during pregnancy, and there is little information about the toxicity of antiparkinson medications. Successful pregnancies have been reported in women taking levodopa.

LEVEL 1 EVIDENCE

1. Magpie Trial Collaborative Group. Do women with pre-eclampsia, and their babies, benefit from magnesium sulfate? The Magpie Trial: a randomised placebo-controlled trial. *Lancet.* 2002;359:1877–1890.
2. LeFevre ML. Low-dose aspirin use for the prevention of morbidity and mortality from preeclampsia: U.S. Preventive Services Task Force recommendation statement. *Ann Intern Med.* 2014;161(11):819–826.

SUGGESTED READINGS

Biology of Pregnancy

Neuroendocrinology. In: Speroff L, Fritz M, eds. *Clinical Gynecologic Endocrinology and Fertility.* 7th ed. Baltimore: Lippincott Williams & Wilkins; 2004:145–186.

Silberstein SD. Drug treatment and trials in women. In: Kaplan PW, ed. *Neurologic Disease in Women.* 2nd ed. New York: Demos Medical Publishing; 2006.

Epilepsy

Artama M, Gissler M, Malm H, et al; Drug and Pregnancy Group. Effects of maternal epilepsy and antiepileptic drug use during pregnancy on perinatal health in offspring: nationwide, retrospective cohort study in Finland. *Drug Saf.* 2013;36(5):359–369.

Baxter P. Valproate and folic acid in pregnancy: associations with autism. *Dev Med Child Neurol.* 2014;56(7):604.

Bech BH, Kjaersgaard MI, Pedersen HS, et al. Use of antiepileptic drugs during pregnancy and risk of spontaneous abortion and stillbirth: population based cohort study. *BMJ.* 2014;349:g5159.

Bromley R, Weston J, Adab N, et al. Treatment for epilepsy in pregnancy: neurodevelopmental outcomes in the child. *Cochrane Database Syst Rev.* 2014;10:CD010236.

Christensen J, Grønborg TK, Sørensen MJ, et al. Prenatal valproate exposure and risk of autism spectrum disorders and childhood autism. *JAMA.* 2013;309(16):1696–1703.

Cohen MJ, Meador KJ, Browning N, et al. Fetal antiepileptic drug exposure: motor, adaptive, and emotional/behavioral functioning at age 3 years. *Epilepsy Behav.* 2011;22(2):240–246.

Harden CL. Pregnancy and epilepsy. *Continuum (Minneap Minn).* 2014;20(1):60–79.

Hernandez-Díaz S, Smith CR, Shen A, et al; North American AED Pregnancy Registry. Comparative safety of antiepileptic drugs during pregnancy. *Neurology.* 2012;78(21):1692–1699.

Jentink J, Loane MA, Dolk H, et al; EUROCAT Antiepileptic Study Working Group. Valproic acid monotherapy in pregnancy and major congenital malformations. *N Engl J Med.* 2010;362(23):2185–2193.

Johnson EL, Stowe ZN, Ritchie JC, et al. Carbamazepine clearance and seizure stability during pregnancy. *Epilepsy Behav.* 2014;33:49–53.

Kilic D, Pedersen H, Kjaersgaard MI, et al. Birth outcomes after prenatal exposure to antiepileptic drugs—a population-based study. *Epilepsia.* 2014;55(11):1714–1721.

Margulis AV, Mitchell AA, Gilboa SM, et al; National Birth Defects Prevention Study. Use of topiramate in pregnancy and risk of oral clefts. *Am J Obstet Gynecol.* 2012;207(5):405.e1–e7.

Mawhinney E, Craig J, Morrow J, et al. Levetiracetam in pregnancy: results from the UK and Ireland epilepsy and pregnancy registers. *Neurology.* 2013;80(4):400–405.

Meador KJ. Epilepsy: pregnancy in women with epilepsy-risks and management. *Nat Rev Neurol.* 2014;10(11):614–616.

Meador KJ, Baker GA, Browning N, et al; NEAD Study Group. Fetal antiepileptic drug exposure and cognitive outcomes at age 6 years (NEAD study): a prospective observational study. *Lancet Neurol.* 2013;12(3):244–252.

Pennell PB, Klein AM, Browning N, et al; NEAD Study Group. Differential effects of antiepileptic drugs on neonatal outcomes. *Epilepsy Behav.* 2012;24(4):449–456.

Thomas SV, Syam U, Devi JS. Predictors of seizures during pregnancy in women with epilepsy. *Epilepsia.* 2012;53(5):e85–e88.

Tomson T, Battino D, Bonizzoni E, et al; EURAP study group. Dose-dependent risk of malformations with antiepileptic drugs: an analysis of data from the EURAP epilepsy and pregnancy registry. *Lancet Neurol.* 2011;10(7):609–617.

Tomson T, Landmark CJ, Battino D. Antiepileptic drug treatment in pregnancy: changes in drug disposition and their clinical implications. *Epilepsia.* 2013;54(3):405–414.

Vajda FJ, Graham J, Roten A, et al. Teratogenicity of the newer antiepileptic drugs—the Australian experience. *J Clin Neurosci.* 2012;19(1):57–59.

Vajda FJ, O'Brien TJ, Lander CM, et al. Teratogenesis in repeated pregnancies in antiepileptic drug-treated women. *Epilepsia.* 2013;54(1):181–186.

Vajda FJ, O'Brien T, Lander C, et al. The efficacy of the newer antiepileptic drugs in controlling seizures in pregnancy. *Epilepsia.* 2014;55(8):1229–1234.

Vajda FJ, O'Brien TJ, Lander CM, et al. The teratogenicity of the newer antiepileptic drugs—an update. *Acta Neurol Scand.* 2014;130(4):234–238.

Werler MM, Ahrens KA, Bosco JL, et al; National Birth Defects Prevention Study. Use of antiepileptic medications in pregnancy in relation to risks of birth defects. *Ann Epidemiol.* 2011;21(11):842–850.

Preeclampsia and Eclampsia

Burrows RF, Burrows EA. The feasibility of a control population for a randomized control trial of seizure prophylaxis in the hypertensive disorders of pregnancy. *Am J Obstet Gynecol.* 1995;173:929–935.

Feske SK, Singhal AB. Cerebrovascular disorders complicating pregnancy. *Continuum (Minneap Minn).* 2014;20(1):80–99.

Lucas MJ, Leveno KJ, Cunningham FG. A comparison of magnesium sulfate with phenytoin for the prevention of eclampsia. *N Engl J Med.* 1995;333:201–205.

Paternoster DM, Fantinato S, Manganelli F, et al. Recent progress in the therapeutic management of pre-eclampsia. *Expert Opin Pharmacother.* 2004;5(11):2233–2239.

Postma IR, Slager S, Kremer HP, et al. Long-term consequences of the posterior reversible encephalopathy syndrome in eclampsia and preeclampsia: a review of the obstetric and nonobstetric literature. *Obstet Gynecol Surv.* 2014;69(5):287–300.

Sibai BM. Etiology and management of postpartum hypertension-preeclampsia. *Am J Obstet Gynecol* 2012;206(6):470–475.

Thadhani R, Mutter WP, Wolf M, et al. First trimester placental growth factor and soluble fms-like tyrosine kinase 1 and risk for preeclampsia. *J Clin Endocrinol Metab.* 2004;89(2):770–775.

Stroke

Del Zotto E, Giossi A, Volonghi I, et al. Ischemic stroke during pregnancy and puerperium. *Stroke Res Treat.* 2011;2011:606–780.

Feske SK, Singhal AB. Cerebrovascular disorders complicating pregnancy. *Continuum (Minneap Minn).* 2014;20(1):80–99.

Grear KE, Bushnell CD. Stroke and pregnancy: clinical presentation, evaluation, treatment, and epidemiology. *Clin Obstet Gynecol.* 2013;56(2):350–359.

Guimicheva B, Czuprynska J, Arya R. The prevention of pregnancy-related venous thromboembolism. *Br J Haematol.* 2015;168(2):163–174.

Gulati D, Strbian D, Sundararajan S. Cerebral venous thrombosis: diagnosis and management. *Stroke.* 2014;45(2):e16–e18.

Hovsepian DA, Sriram N, Kamel H, et al. Acute cerebrovascular disease occurring after hospital; discharge for labor and delivery. *Stroke.* 2014;45(7):1947–1950.

Johnson DM, Kramer DC, Cohen E, et al. Thrombolytic therapy for acute stroke in late pregnancy with intra-arterial recombinant tissue plasminogen activator. *Stroke.* 2005;36(6):e53–e55.

Kamel H, Navi BB, Sriram N, et al. Risk of a thrombotic event after the 6-week postpartum period. *N Engl J Med.* 2014;370(14):1307–1315.

Kuklina EV, Tong X, Bansil P, et al. Trends in pregnancy hospitalizations that included a stroke in the United States from 1994 to 2007: reasons for concern? *Stroke.* 2011;42(9):2564–2570.

Liang CC, Chang SD, Lai SL, et al. Stroke complicating pregnancy and the puerperium. *Eur J Neurol.* 2006;13(11):1256–1260.

Leonhardt G, Gaul C, Nietsch HH, et al. Thrombotic therapy in pregnancy. *J Thromb Thrombolysis.* 2006;21(3):271–276.

Mantoan Ritter L, Schüler A, Gangopadhyay R, et al. Successful thrombolysis of stroke with intravenous alteplase in the third trimester of pregnancy. *J Neurol.* 2014;261(3):632–634.

Murugappan A, Coplin WM, Al-Sadat AN, et al. Thrombolytic therapy of acute ischemic stroke during pregnancy. *Neurology.* 2006;66(5):768–770.

Singhal AB, Kimberly WT, Schaefer PW, et al. Case records of the Massachusetts General Hospital. Case 8-2009. A 36-year-old woman with headache, hypertension, and seizure 2 weeks post partum. *N Engl J Med.* 2009;360(11):1126–1137.

Star M, Flaster M. Advances and controversies in the management of cerebral venous thrombosis. *Neurol Clin.* 2013;31(3):765–783.

Starke RM, Komoter RJ, Hickman ZL, et al. Clinical features, surgical treatment, and long-term outcome of adult moyamoya patients. *J Neurosurg.* 2009;111(5):936–942.

Wabnitz A, Bushnell C. Migraine, cardiovascular disease, and stroke during pregnancy: systematic review of the literature. *Cephalalgia.* 2015;35(2):132–139.

Wiese KM, Talkad A, Mathews M, et al. Intravenous recombinant tissue plasminogen activator in a pregnant woman with cardioembolic stroke. *Stroke.* 2006;37(8):2168–2169.

Headache

Banhidy F, Acs N, Horvath-Puho E, et al. Pregnancy complications and delivery outcomes in pregnant women with severe migraine. *Eur J Obstet Gynecol Reprod Biol.* 2007;134(2):157–163.

Browne ML, Van Zutphen AR, Botto LD, et al. Maternal butalbital use and selected defects in the national birth defects prevention study. *Headache.* 2014;54(1):54–66.

Cripe SM, Frederick IO, Qiu C, et al. Risk of preterm delivery and hypertensive disorders of pregnancy in relation to maternal co-morbid mood and migraine disorders during pregnancy. *Paediatr Perinat Epidemiol.* 2011;25(2):116–123.

David PS, Kling JM, Starling AJ. Migraine in pregnancy and lactation. *Curr Neurol Neurosci Rep.* 2014;14(4):439.

Frederick IO, Qiu C, Enquobahrie DA, et al. Lifetime prevalence and correlates of migraine among women in a pacific northwest pregnancy cohort study. *Headache.* 2014;54(4):675–685.

MacGregor EA. Headache in pregnancy. *Continuum (Minneap Minn)*. 2014;20(1): 128–147.

Nezvalová-Henriksen K, Spigset O, Nordeng H. Triptan exposure during pregnancy and the risk of major congenital malformations and adverse pregnancy outcomes: results from the Norwegian Mother and Child Cohort Study. *Headache*. 2010;50(4):563–575.

Nezvalová-Henriksen K, Spigset O, Nordeng H. Triptan safety during pregnancy: a Norwegian population registry study. *Eur J Epidemiol*. 2013;28(9):759–769.

Wabnitz A, Bushnell C. Migraine, cardiovascular disease, and stroke during pregnancy: systematic review of the literature. *Cephalalgia*. 2015;35(2):132–139.

Cerebral Hemorrhage

Feske SK, Singhal AB. Cerebrovascular disorders complicating pregnancy. *Continuum (Minneap Minn)*. 2014;20(1):80–99.

Helbok R, Olson DM, Le Roux PD, et al; Participants in the International Multidisciplinary Consensus Conference on Multimodality Monitoring. Intracranial pressure and cerebral perfusion pressure monitoring in non-TBI patients: special considerations. *Neurocrit Care*. 2014;21(suppl 2): 85–94.

Liu XJ, Wang S, Zhao YL, et al. Risk of cerebral arteriovenous malformation rupture during pregnancy and puerperium. *Neurology*. 2014;82(20): 1798–1803.

Nasr DM, Brinjikji W, Cloft HJ, et al. Mortality in cerebral venous thrombosis: results from the national inpatient sample database. *Cerebrovasc Dis*. 2013;35(1):40–44.

Star M, Flaster M. Advances and controversies in the management of cerebral venous thrombosis. *Neurol Clin*. 2013;31(3):765–783.

Wang J, Wang R, Zhao J. Ruptured cerebral aneurysm from choriocarcinoma. *J Clin Neurosci*. 2013;20(9):1324–1326.

Multiple Sclerosis

Coyle PK. Multiple sclerosis pregnancy. *Continuum (Minneap Minn)*. 2014;20(1): 42–59.

Coyle PK, Sinclair SM, Scheuerle AE, et al. Final results from the Betaseron (interferon β-1b) Pregnancy Registry: a prospective observational study of birth defects and pregnancy-related adverse events. *BMJ Open*. 2014;4(5):1–8.

D'hooghe MB, Haentjens P, Nagels G, et al. Menarche, oral contraceptives, pregnancy and progression of disability in relapsing onset and progressive onset multiple sclerosis. *J Neurol*. 2012;259(5):855–861.

Ebrahimi N, Herbstritt S, Gold R, et al. Pregnancy and fetal outcomes following natalizumab exposure in pregnancy. A prospective, controlled observational study. *Mult Scler*. 2014;21(2):198–205.

Fagius J, Burman J. Normal outcome of pregnancy with ongoing treatment with natalizumab. *Acta Neurol Scand*. 2014;129(6):e27–e29.

Finkelsztejn A, Brooks JB, Paschoal FM Jr, et al. What can we really tell women with multiple sclerosis regarding pregnancy? A systematic review and meta-analysis of the literature. *BJOG*. 2011;118(7):790–797.

Fragoso YD. Glatiramer acetate to treat multiple sclerosis during pregnancy and lactation: a safety evaluation. *Expert Opin Drug Saf*. 2014;13(12):1743–1748.

Fragoso YD, Finkelsztejn A, Kaimen-Maciel DR, et al. Long-term use of glatiramer acetate by 11 pregnant women with multiple sclerosis: a retrospective, multicenter case series. *CNS Drugs*. 2010;24(11):969–976.

Haghikia A, Langer-Gould A, Rellensmann G, et al. Natalizumab use during the third trimester of pregnancy. *JAMA Neurol*. 2014;71(7):891–895.

Hellwig K, Haghikia A, Rockhoff M, et al. Multiple sclerosis and pregnancy: experience from a nationwide database in Germany. *Ther Adv Neurol Disord*. 2012;5(5):247–253.

Karp I, Manganas A, Sylvestre MP, et al. Does pregnancy alter the long-term course of multiple sclerosis? *Ann Epidemiol*. 2014;24(7):504–508.

Lu E, Wang BW, Guimond C, et al. Disease modifying drugs for multiple sclerosis in pregnancy. *Neurology*. 2012;79(11):1130–1135.

Ponsonby AL, Lucas RM, van der Mei IA, et al. Offspring number, pregnancy, and risk of a first clinical demyelinating event. The AusImmune Study. *Neurology*. 2012;78(12):867–874.

Portaccio E, Ghezzi A, Hakiki B, et al. Breastfeeding is not related to postpartum relapse in multiple sclerosis. *Neurology*. 2011;77(2):145–150.

Ramagopalan S, Yee I, Byrnes J, et al. Term pregnancies and the clinical characteristics of multiple sclerosis: a population based study. *J Neurol Neurosurg Psychiatry*. 2012;83(8):793–795.

Romero RS, Lünzmann C, Bugge JP. Pregnancy outcomes in patients exposed to interferon beta-1b. *J Neurol Neurosurg Psychiatry*. 2015;86(5):587–589.

Sandberg-Wollheim M, Alteri E, Moraga MS, et al. Pregnancy outcomes in multiple sclerosis following subcutaneous interferon beta-1a therapy. *Mult Scler*. 2011;17(4):423–430.

van der Kop ML, Pearce MS, Dahlgren L, et al. Neonatal and delivery outcomes in women with multiple sclerosis. *Ann Neurol*. 2011;70(1):41–50.

Vukusic S, Durand-Dubief F, Benoit A, et al. Natalizumab for the prevention of post-partum relapses in women with multiple sclerosis [published online ahead of print October 10, 2014]. *Mult Scler*.

Neoplasms

Bonfield CM, Engh JA. Pregnancy and brain tumors. *Neurol Clin*. 2012;30(3): 937–946.

Daras M, Cone C, Peters KB. Tumor progression and transformation of low-grade glial tumors associated with pregnancy. *J Neurooncol*. 2014;116(1): 113–117.

Scarrott LJ, Raina A, Madej T, et al. Recurrent glioblastoma multiforme in pregnancy. *J Obstet Gynaecol*. 2012;32(7):704–705.

Verheecke M, Halaska MJ, Lok CA, et al; ESGO Task Force "Cancer in Pregnancy." Primary brain tumours, meningiomas and brain metastases in pregnancy: report on 27 cases and review of literature. *Eur J Cancer*. 2014;50(8):1462–1471.

Zwinkels H, Dörr J, Kloet F, et al. Pregnancy in women with gliomas: a case-series and review of the literature. *J Neurooncol*. 2013;115(2):293–301.

Peripheral Nerve Disorders

Guidon AC, Massey EW. Neuromuscular disorders in pregnancy. *Neurol Clin*. 2012;30(3):889–911.

Massey EW, Guidon AC. Peripheral neuropathies in pregnancy. *Continuum (Minneap Minn)*. 2014;20(1):100–114.

Mondelli M, Rossi S, Monti E, et al. Prospective study of positive factors for improvement of carpal tunnel syndrome in pregnant women. *Muscle Nerve*. 2007;36(6):778–783.

Myasthenia Gravis

Guidon AC, Massey EW. Neuromuscular disorders in pregnancy. *Neurol Clin*. 2012;30(3):889–911.

Hoff JM, Daltveit AK, Gilhus NE. Myasthenia gravis in pregnancy and birth: identifying risk factors, optimising care. *Eur J Neurol*. 2007;14(1):38–43.

Massey JM, DeJusus-Acosta CD. Pregnancy and myasthenia gravis. *Continuum (Minneap Minn)*. 2014;20(1):115–127.

Niks EH, Verrips A, Semmekrot BA, et al. A transient neonatal myasthenic syndrome with anti-MUSK antibodies. *Neurology*. 2008;70(14):1215–1216.

O'Carroll P, Bertorini TE, Jacob G, et al. Transient neonatal myasthenia gravis in a baby born to a mother with new-onset anti-MuSK-mediated myasthenia gravis. *J Clin Neuromuscul Dis*. 2009;11(2):69–71.

Oskoui M, Jacobson L, Chung WK, et al. Fetal acetylcholine receptor inactivation syndrome and maternal myasthenia gravis. *Neurology*. 2008;71(24):2010–2012.

Wen JC, Liu TC, Chen YH, et al. No increased risk of adverse pregnancy outcomes for women with myasthenia gravis: a nationwide population-based study. *Eur J Neurol*. 2009;16(8):889–894.

Movement Disorders

Bordelon YM, Smith M. Movement disorders in pregnancy. *Semin Neurol*. 2007;27(5):467–475.

Earley CJ. Restless legs syndrome. *N Engl J Med*. 2003;348:2103–2109.

Golbe LI. Pregnancy and movement disorders. *Neurol Clin*. 1994;12:497–508.

Kranick S, Mowry E, Colcher A, et al. Movement disorders and pregnancy: a review of the literature. *Mov Disord*. 2010;25(6):665–671.

Manconi M, Govoni V, De Vito A, et al. Restless legs syndrome and pregnancy. *Neurology*. 2004;63(6):1065–1069.

Miyasaki JM, AlDakheel A. Movement disorders in pregnancy. *Continuum (Minneap Minn)*. 2014;20(1):148–161.

Rogers JD, Fahn S. Movement disorders and pregnancy. In: Devinsky O, Feldmann E, Hainline B, eds. *Neurological Complications of Pregnancy*. New York: Raven; 1994:163–178.

Scott M, Chowdhury M. Pregnancy in Parkinson's disease: unique case report and review of the literature. *Mov Disord*. 2005;20(8):1078–1079.

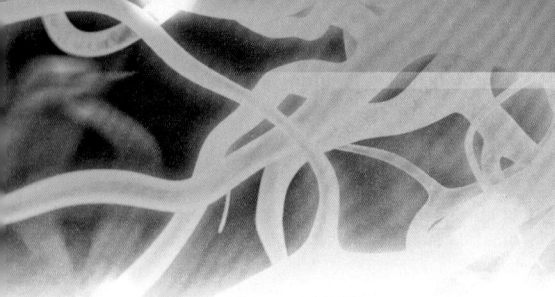

Neurologic Complications of Organ Transplantation 125

Eelco F. M. Wijdicks

INTRODUCTION

Organ transplantation has been associated with a distinct spectrum of neurologic complications. Complications can emerge during pretransplant preparation (e.g., hematopoietic stem cell transplantation and chemotherapy), perioperative support (e.g., cardiac transplantation with cardiopulmonary bypass), and postoperative management (e.g., newly introduced immunosuppression). Some neurologic complications, particularly peripheral nerve injury, are related to the surgical procedure and are less specific.

When large series are reported, neurologic complications from organ transplantation occur in approximately 5% to 10% of patients. Of course, the prevalence depends on the motivation of transplant teams to consult a neurologist and thus is a reflection of how relevant a neurologic complication is when seen in the whole of the clinical picture. Prospective incidence studies may not capture all the postoperative neurologic events if they are not carefully examined by neurologists. Moreover, over the years, there has been a continuous decline in neurologic complications in some types of organ transplantation (e.g., renal, liver).

Neurologic complications are major when they involve recurrent seizures, postoperative failure to awaken, immunosuppression neurotoxicity, or acute disabling neuromuscular disease. Familiarity with the administration and dosing of the main intravenous immunosuppressive drugs has reduced the risk of major neurotoxicity, and extreme cases with coma and seizures and neuroimaging showing diffuse white matter edema are now rarely seen.

This chapter does not attempt to fully discuss all neurologic complications described over the years but will concentrate on the most common considerations (Table 125.1).

TABLE 125.1	Neurologic Syndromes in Transplant Recipients and Causes
Failure to awaken or acute coma	Hypoxic–ischemic brain injury, brain edema, oversedation, acute graft failure, calcineurin neurotoxicity, intracranial hemorrhage, fulminant CNS infection
Seizures	Calcineurin neurotoxicity, intracranial hemorrhage, new mass (abscess, tumor), posterior reversible encephalopathy syndrome
Aphasia, dysarthria	Calcineurin neurotoxicity, ischemic stroke
Hemiparesis	Brachial plexopathy, ischemic or hemorrhagic stroke, brain tumor, brain abscess
Tremors	Calcineurin neurotoxicity
Myoclonus, asterixis	Acute liver, renal, or pulmonary disease; drug toxicity

CNS, central nervous system.

GENERAL CONSIDERATIONS

Generally speaking, and not surprisingly, a patient with more elaborate surgery has a higher risk of an early neurologic complication. For instance, liver transplantation carries a much higher risk of early neurologic complications than renal transplantation. Once the patient goes successfully through the first critical weeks, a later phase includes a proclivity for central nervous system (CNS) infections, and much later—although it may be only a few months—serious malignancies may appear. Dramatic is the appearance of posttransplant lymphoproliferative disease (PTLD) and likely explained from introducing genetic material of an Epstein–Barr virus (EBV)–seropositive donor into an EBV-seronegative recipient. It may involve the CNS.

The threshold for cerebral fluid examination should be low even if meningitis is not suspected. Because an infectious mass lesion may be present, a computed tomography (CT) scan may need to be performed to exclude such a lesion. An acutely febrile patient with an abnormal level of consciousness should prompt an aggressive search for a CNS infection. Immunosuppressed transplant recipients have a proclivity for infections with *Listeria monocytogenes*, *Nocardia*, or *Aspergillus*. Infections with *Cryptococcus neoformans* or *Toxoplasma gondii* are rarely seen within 6 months after transplantation. All of these infections present often with meningeal enhancement on a CT or magnetic resonance imaging scan, solitary or multiple abscesses, or ring lesions. None of them are specific and can only be documented by biopsy.

Neurologic complications may result in an increased risk of early demise. Most instructively—when reviewed in more detail—the majority of patients with a lung transplantation were found to have a neurologic manifestation or complication with a third seriously affecting quality of life or resulting in a fatal outcome. That leaves the question of whether neurologic complications are sufficiently recognized.

There are several other considerations. First, neurologic complications may be specific to the type of transplantation. Neurologic complications associated with bone marrow transplantation are quite different than those from organ transplants such as a kidney or liver. Second, seizures are often drug related and less commonly due to a permanent structural lesion. It is a difficult task to implicate certain drugs, but several drugs lower the seizure threshold (i.e., calcineurin inhibitors and antibiotics such as imipenem). Third, any structural lesion in the brain, whether it has the appearance of a cerebritis or ring enhancing, is most often due to an infectious cause and requires immediate treatment. Fourth, major sodium abnormalities and osmotic shifts can be seen after liver transplantation causing osmotic demyelination.

ENCEPHALOPATHY AND DELIRIUM

In actuality, there are particular syndromes that most often present to the neurologist. The most commonly encountered reason for a consultation has to do with assessment of an "altered state of consciousness." The appearance of a new encephalopathy may be due to rejection causing dysfunction of the graft or may have other causes.

Acute confusional state remains difficult to define in transplant recipients and can be considered if it lasts more than 2 to 3 consecutive days. Postoperative hyperactive delirium associated with hallucinations is common post transplantation, and some circumstances should be recognized. If patients are seen in the immediate postoperative period, both hyperactive and hypoactive delirium after liver transplantation occurs in about a third of the patients. This is more often in patients who had a pretransplant encephalopathy and is more often seen in alcoholic liver disease.

In evaluating patients with impaired consciousness, some guidance can be provided. All potential sedative drugs should be carefully scrutinized, and the time remaining to clearance should be calculated. Physicians should consider administration of flumazenil or naloxone to eliminate the remaining effects. Neurotoxicity of immunosuppressive drugs is frequently implicated, and it continues to be a concern to be dealt with. None of these drugs do cause other structural disease other than a leukoencephalopathy, which cannot be clinically or radiographically distinguished from posterior reversible encephalopathy syndrome (PRES) (see also Chapter 43).

DRUG TOXICITY

There are many drugs and medications that need to be considered in acute confusion. This includes the use of calcineurin inhibitors, opioid antagonists, β-adrenergic blockers, and high-dose corticosteroids. All of these drugs can be implicated. Other commonly used drugs, such as midazolam and propofol, may impact level of consciousness, particularly because they have different pharmacokinetics in transplant patients. Midazolam, for example, although relatively short acting in comparison with other sedative agents, has a prolonged activity if the liver graft is not functioning fully. It is also highly protein bound, and preexisting low protein levels may increase its sedative effects. Clearance of propofol is dependent on hepatic blood flow and cardiac output; and if both are disturbed, awakening from propofol may be markedly delayed, and the patient may not characteristically awaken as usually anticipated 10 to 15 minutes after discontinuation of infusion. Opioids may continue to linger after cardiac transplantation; typically, very large doses are used during the procedure.

Neurotoxicity associated with cyclosporine or tacrolimus is often considered but less often diagnosed. Breakdown of the blood–brain barrier is needed for cyclosporine to enter because no lipoprotein transport system exists. Cyclosporine is very lipophilic from aliphatic groups but cannot cross the blood–brain barrier because of tight junctions. How crossing occurs remains unknown and perhaps impairment of the blood–brain barrier is facilitated by surgery-associated ischemic insults due to hypotension. The predilection of the posterior areas of the brain may also be related to a less-developed blood–brain barrier that quickly opens when challenged. Oligodendroglia is more susceptible than astrocytes. This characteristic fits nicely with the largely white matter lesions on magnetic resonance imaging.

The pathway of neurotoxicity associated with cyclosporine or tacrolimus has not been resolved at a molecular level. Both immunosuppressive drugs bind to an immunophilin, a protein with an affinity for both drugs, and consequently trigger a cascade of actions that include blockade of calcineurin. Calcineurin is involved in cell signaling and maintenance of cytoskeletal protein function,

particularly in oligodendrocytes. Inhibition of calcineurin activity, therefore, may lead to neuronal death or apoptosis. It remains very likely, however, that extremely high doses in the earlier days of transplantation due to unfamiliarity with the drugs has been the major driving factor. This possibility is also supported by the very low incidence of cyclosporine neurotoxicity using oral preparations, resulting in stable blood levels and avoidance of extreme blood levels during intravenous loading. The earliest abnormality seems to be neurotoxicity from fluid extravasation (vasogenic edema) and not cell destruction (cytotoxic edema). Very limited pathology studies are available, and some have suggested demyelination.

One should obtain serum levels of cyclosporine or tacrolimus and trend the values. A marked increase in levels may indicate development of neurotoxicity but such an association is only plausible if it is seen outside of the usual intravenous loading period that is within the first week of treatment. Many transplant surgeons titrate toward increasing plasma levels, and these levels should not be misinterpreted as indicative of neurotoxicity. Recent laboratory values should be obtained and should include electrolyte panel, liver and renal function tests, serum ammonia, arterial blood gas, and where indicated, antiepileptic drug levels.

Finally, a mistake is to label postoperative encephalopathy as multifactorial and it often does nothing to find the possible triggers. For example, a liver transplant recipient may have severe hyponatremia and rising creatinine and blood urea nitrogen (BUN) and show signs of early rejection. Cefepime toxicity may be the cause of decline in consciousness, and new myoclonus and improvement can be expected when the drug is discontinued.

ORGAN-SPECIFIC COMPLICATIONS

LUNG TRANSPLANTATION

Lung transplant patients, due to significant challenges in oxygenation, may have severe neurologic complications in a third of the patients. Most severe complications are perioperative stroke and encephalopathy, and when neurologic complications occur, there is a higher mortality. Acute hyperammonemia—an unexpected and not completely explained metabolic derangement in lung transplant recipients—has also been described causing seizures and profound encephalopathy. Cyclosporin neurotoxicity is not a major cause of complications in lung transplant recipients.

CARDIAC TRANSPLANTATION

Cardiac transplantations are obviously at risk of ischemic injury as a result of embolization from aortic atheroembolism but also perioperative cardiogenic shock requiring extreme measures such as intra-aortic balloon pump support or extracorporeal membrane oxygenation (ECMO). Intracerebral hemorrhage is rarely seen after cardiac transplantation, but poorly controlled hypertension may cause a lobar or basal ganglia hemorrhage.

LIVER TRANSPLANTATION

One relatively uncommon but dramatic clinical scenario is a patient with acute fulminant hepatic failure (FHF) followed by rapid listing for liver transplantation. This condition is very unique with many clinical uncertainties and neurologists and neurosurgeons are often asked to be part of rapidly changing clinical decisions making. There are three immediate concerns. First, the transition of hepatic encephalopathy (basically a metabolic injury) to brain edema (now a structural injury) must be recognized. Second, intracranial pressure may rise steeply and requires prompt treatment. Third, some patients may have already progressed to brain death, which would preclude transplantation.

The mechanism of brain edema in an FHF (see also Chapter 119) is influenced by multiple factors. Hyperosmolarity due to increased ammonia and also the development of oxidative stress may contribute. Brain edema is mostly vasogenic and is usually first confirmed by the appearance of severe brain swelling on CT. A useful method to identify the development of vasogenic brain edema in encephalopathic patients with FHF is to identify increased cerebral blood flow velocity associated with reduced waveform pulsatility on transcranial Doppler (see Chapter 23).

Once identified, brain edema requires aggressive treatment to prevent transtentorial herniation and is best guided by an intracranial pressure (ICP) monitor (see Chapter 107). However, patients who have an ICP monitoring device placed and are treated aggressively do not have a better outcome or higher percentage of liver transplantation and that could question the role of ICP-based management. Most centers place an intraparenchymal ICP in comatose patients with evidence of cerebral edema on CT, but the situation is further complicated by the presence of coagulopathy, which invariably complicated FHF. Use of recombinant factor VII (4 mg intravenous push [IVP]) or prothrombin complex concentrate (25 to 50 U/kg, depending on baseline international normalized ratio [INR]) is an important new development in countering coagulopathy in FHF. Their use has significantly decreased the frequency of bleeding complications, particularly related to ICP monitor insertion.

INTESTINAL TRANSPLANTATION

Intestinal transplantation for a short bowel syndrome due to thrombosis, inflammatory bowel disease, and radiation enteritis has become another "organ" that can be transplanted but experience is only in a few hundred patients. The initial experience is not sufficient to potentially identify specific complications and most reported are in the known categories such as encephalopathy, CNS infection, seizures, stroke, and neuromuscular complications. Early assessment suggests rate of neurologic complications is much higher than solid organ transplants. One possible explanation is the higher immunosuppression as a result of relative lower resistance to rejection of the intestine.

LONG-TERM EFFECTS OF IMMUNOSUPPRESSION

Any transplant recipient is at risk of developing B-cell lymphomas or glioblastoma multiforme or progressive multifocal leukoencephalopathy (PML). These disorders are extremely uncommon but can present within months after transplantation. Most notorious is the occurrence of CNS lymphoma several weeks after transplantation (may vary from a few weeks to more than two decades after transplantation). Most posttransplantation lymphomas are monoclonal B-cell lymphomas, but multiclonal B-cell lymphomas or T-cell lymphomas have been reported. EBV infection has been linked to B-cell lymphoma. CNS lymphoma debuts with both brain and spinal cord involvement, but presentation is nonspecific with new behavioral changes, visual hallucinations, or focal signs such as hemiparesis. In most patients, a change in personality may be the only key sign. Meningeal involvement may produce headache. The diagnosis can only be considered if the CT scan shows a new mass lesion in the periventricular region and with proportionally large amount of perilesional edema. A biopsy might be necessary to find the lesion followed by aggressive treatment with radiation. Outcome, however, remains very poor with ultimate demise in all patients.

PML is caused by JC virus (see also Chapter 66), and the disorder is usually relentless (Fig. 125.1). Withdrawal of immunotherapy or highly active antiretroviral treatment is considered with some good outcomes reported.

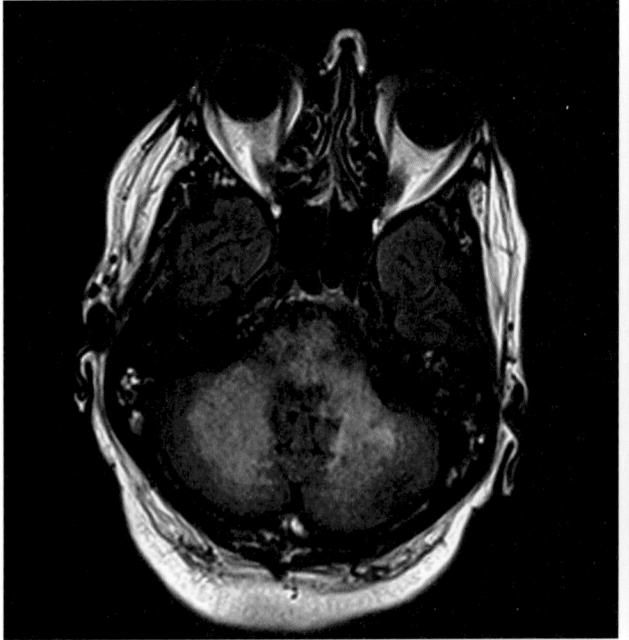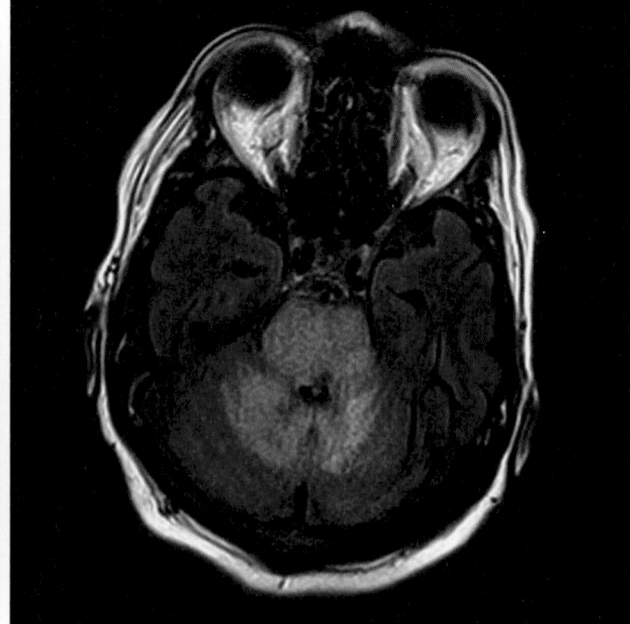

FIGURE 125.1 Magnetic resonance image of PML after liver transplantation.

CONCLUSIONS

There are early and late neurologic complications after organ transplantation. The nature of neurologic complications may change with new treatment protocols and new drug approaches. Neurotoxicity from immunosuppressive drugs remains commonly implicated but is not common except if the dosing is high. Other complications relate to common operative stressors (hypotension) or perioperative concerns (infections, hemorrhage). This field—neurology of organ transplantation—requires special expertise and frequent reassessment of the spectrum of complications.

SUGGESTED READINGS

Amodio P, Biancardi A, Montagnese S, et al. Neurological complications after orthotopic liver transplantation. *Dig Liver Dis*. 2007;39(8):740–747.

Buis CI, Wiesner RH, Krom RA, et al. Acute confusional state following liver transplantation for alcoholic liver disease. *Neurology*. 2002;59(4):601–605.

Cui R, Fayek S, Rand EB, et al. Central pontine myelinolysis: a case report and clinical-pathological review. *Pediatr Transplant*. 2012;16(6):E251–E256.

Fugate JE, Kalimullah EA, Hocker SE, et al. Cefepime neurotoxicity in the intensive care unit: a cause of severe, underappreciated encephalopathy. *Crit Care*. 2013;17(6):R264.

Ghaus N, Bohlega S, Rezeig M. Neurological complications in liver transplantation. *J Neurol*. 2001;248(12):1042–1048.

Goldstein LS, Haug MT III, Perl J II, et al. Central nervous system complications after lung transplantation. *J Heart Lung Transplant*. 1998;17(2):185–191.

Guarino M, Benito-Leon J, Decruyenaere J, et al. EFNS guidelines on management of neurological problems in liver transplantation. *Eur J Neurol*. 2006;13(1):2–9.

Hocker S, Rabinstein AA, Wijdicks EF. Pearls & oy-sters: status epilepticus from hyperammonemia after lung transplant. *Neurology*. 2011;77(10):e54–e56.

Knight JS, Tsodikov A, Cibrik DM, et al. Lymphoma after solid organ transplantation: risk, response to therapy, and survival at a transplantation center. *J Clin Oncol*. 2009;27(20):3354–3362.

Lewis MB, Howdle PD. Neurologic complications of liver transplantation in adults. *Neurology*. 2003;61(9):1174–1178.

Mateen FJ, Dierkhising RA, Rabinstein AA, et al. Neurological complications following adult lung transplantation. *Am J Transplant*. 2010;10(4):908–914.

Mateen FJ, Muralidharan R, Carone M, et al. Progressive multifocal leukoencephalopathy in transplant recipients. *Ann Neurol*. 2011;70(2):305–322.

Munoz P, Valerio M, Palomo J, et al. Infectious and non-infectious neurologic complications in heart transplant recipients. *Medicine (Baltimore)*. 2010;89(3):166–175.

Ohara H, Kataoka H, Nakamichi K, et al. Favorable outcome after withdrawal of immunosuppressant therapy in progressive multifocal leukoencephalopathy after renal transplantation: case report and literature review. *J Neurol Sci*. 2014;341(1–2):144–146.

Pittock SJ, Rabinstein AA, Edwards BS, et al. OKT3 neurotoxicity presenting as akinetic mutism. *Transplantation*. 2003;75(7):1058–1060.

Pruitt AA, Graus F, Rosenfeld MR. Neurological complications of solid organ transplantation. *Neurohospitalist*. 2013;3(3):152–166.

Schiff D, O'Neill B, Wijdicks E, et al. Gliomas arising in organ transplant recipients: an unrecognized complication of transplantation? *Neurology*. 2001;57(8):1486–1488.

Silveira FP, Husain S, Kwak EJ, et al. Cryptococcosis in liver and kidney transplant recipients receiving anti-thymocyte globulin or alemtuzumab. *Transpl Infect Dis*. 2007;9(1):22–27.

Singh N. How I treat cryptococcosis in organ transplant recipients. *Transplantation*. 2012;93(1):17–21.

Uchida H, Sakamoto S, Sasaki K, et al. Central pontine myelinolysis following pediatric living donor liver transplantation: a case report and review of literature. *Pediatr Transplant*. 2014;18(4):E120–E123.

van de Beek D, Patel R, Daly RC, et al. Central nervous system infections in heart transplant recipients. *Arch Neurol*. 2007;64(12):1715–1720.

Weber SC, Uhlenberg B, Raile K, et al. Polyoma virus-associated progressive multifocal leukoencephalopathy after renal transplantation: regression following withdrawal of mycophenolate mofetil. *Pediatr Transplant*. 2011;15(2):E19–E24.

Wijdicks EFM. *Neurologic Complications in Organ Transplant Recipients*. Boston, MA: Butterworth-Heinemann; 1999.

Wijdicks EFM, Hocker SE. Neurologic complications of liver transplantation. *Handb Clin Neurol*. 2014;121:1257–1266.

Wijdicks EFM, Wiesner RH, Krom RA. Neurotoxicity in liver transplant recipients with cyclosporine immunosuppression. *Neurology*. 1995;45(11):1962–1964.

Zhao CZ, Erickson J, Dalmau J. Clinical reasoning: agitation and psychosis in a patient after renal transplantation. *Neurology*. 2012;79(5):e41–e44.

Zivkovic SA, Eidelman BH, Bond G, et al. The clinical spectrum of neurologic disorders after intestinal and multivisceral transplantation. *Clin Transplant*. 2010;24(2):164–168.

Alcoholism 126

John C. M. Brust

INTRODUCTION

In the United States, 7% of all adults and 19% of adolescents are "problem drinkers": psychically or physically dependent on ethanol or, even if abstinent most of the time, likely to get into trouble when they drink. Ethanol-related deaths exceed 100,000 each year, accounting for 5% of all deaths in the United States. The devastation is direct (from intoxication, addiction, and withdrawal) or indirect (from nutritional deficiency or other ethanol-related diseases).

ACUTE ETHANOL SYNDROMES

INTOXICATION

Ethanol acts at many levels of the neuraxis. Although specific ethanol receptors comparable to opioid receptors do not appear to exist, ethanol interacts directly with membrane proteins of a number of neurotransmitter systems, and much of its actions depend on facilitation at inhibitory γ-aminobutyric acid (GABA) receptors and inhibition at excitatory glutamate receptors.

To obtain a mildly intoxicating blood ethanol concentration (BEC) of 100 mg/dL, a 70-kg person must drink about 50 g (2 oz) of 100% ethanol. Following zero-order kinetics, ethanol is metabolized at about 70 to 150 mg/kg of body weight per hour, with a fall in BEC of 10 to 25 mg/dL/h. Thus, most adults require 6 hours to metabolize a 50-g dose, and the ingestion of only 8 g of additional ethanol per hour would maintain the BEC at 100 mg/dL.

Symptoms and signs of acute ethanol intoxication are a result of cerebral depression, possibly at first of the reticular formation with cerebral disinhibition and later of the cerebral cortex itself. Manifestations depend not only on the BEC but also on the rate of climb and the person's tolerance, which is related less to increased metabolism than to poorly understood adaptive changes in the brain. At any BEC, intoxication is more severe when the level is rising than when it is falling, when the level is reached rapidly, and when the level has only recently been achieved. A single BEC determination therefore is not a reliable indicator of drunkenness, and the correlations of Table 126.1 are broad generalizations. Death from respiratory paralysis may occur with a BEC of 400 mg/dL, and survival may occur at 700 mg/dL; a level of 500 mg/dL would be fatal in 50% of individuals.

Low to moderate BECs cause slow saccadic eye movements and interrupted jerky pursuit movements that may impair visual acuity. Esophoria and exophoria cause diplopia. With a BEC of 150 to 250 mg/dL, there is increased electroencephalography (EEG) beta activity ("beta buzz"); higher BECs cause EEG slowing. During sleep, suppression of the REM stage is followed by REM rebound after a few hours.

TABLE 126.1	Correlation of Symptoms with Blood Ethanol Concentration
BEC	**Symptoms**
50–150 mg/dL	• Euphoria or dysphoria, shyness or expansiveness, friendliness or argumentativeness • Impaired concentration, judgment, and sexual inhibitions
150–250 mg/dL	• Slurred speech and ataxic gait, diplopia, nausea, tachycardia, drowsiness, or labile mood with sudden bursts of anger or antisocial acts
300 mg/dL	• Stupor alternating with combativeness or incoherent speech, heavy breathing, vomiting
400 mg/dL	• Coma
500 mg/dL	• Respiratory paralysis

BEC, blood ethanol concentration.

The term *pathologic intoxication* refers to sudden extreme excitement with irrational or violent behavior after even small doses of ethanol. Episodes are said to last for minutes or hours, followed by sleep and, on awakening, amnesia for the events that took place. Delusions, hallucinations, and homicide may occur during bouts of pathologic intoxication. Some cases might be psychological dissociative reactions; others may be owing to the kind of paradoxic excitation that sometimes follows barbiturate administration. These syndromes are more likely to occur in younger people that have had little prior exposure to alcohol.

The term *alcoholic blackout* refers to amnesia for periods of intoxication, sometimes lasting several hours, even though consciousness at the time did not seem to be disturbed. Although sometimes considered a sign of physiologic dependence, blackouts also occur in occasional drinkers. The amnesia is a direct effect of ethanol on memory encoding.

Acute ethanol poisoning causes more than 1,000 deaths each year in the United States. In stuporous alcoholic patients, subdural hematoma, meningitis, and hypoglycemia are important diagnostic considerations, but it is equally important to remember that ethanol intoxication alone can be fatal.

Blood ethanol causes a rise of blood osmolality, about 22 mOsm/L for every 100 mg/dL of ethanol; however, there are no transmembrane shifts of water, and the hyperosmolarity does not cause symptoms.

TABLE 126.2 Treatment of Acute Ethanol Intoxication

For Obstreperous or Violent Patients

- Isolation, calming environment, and reassurance—avoid sedatives.
- Close observation

For Stuporous or Comatose Patients

- If hypoventilation, artificial respiration in an ICU
- If serum glucose in doubt, intravenous 50% glucose with parenteral thiamine 100 mg
- Careful monitoring of blood pressure; correction of hypovolemia or acid–base imbalance
- Consider hemodialysis if patient is severely acidotic, deeply comatose, or apneic.
- Avoid emetics or gastric lavage.
- Avoid analeptics.
- Do not forget other possible causes of coma in an alcoholic.

ICU, intensive care unit.

Ethanol overdose should be considered in any comatose patient whose serum osmolarity is higher than predicted by calculation of the sum of serum sodium, glucose, and urea.

Patients stuporous or comatose from ethanol intoxication are generally managed similarly to those poisoned by other depressant drugs (Table 126.2). Death comes from respiratory depression, and mechanical ventilation in an intensive care unit is the mainstay of treatment. Hypovolemia, acid–base or electrolyte imbalance, and abnormal temperature require attention, and if there is any uncertainty about the blood glucose level, 50% glucose is given intravenously, along with parenteral thiamine. Because ethanol is rapidly absorbed, gastric lavage does not help unless other drugs have been ingested. In obstreperous or violent patients, sedatives (including benzodiazepines and dopamine-blocking agents) should be used with caution because they may push patients into stupor and respiratory depression. Patients being addressed may appear alert but then lapse into stupor or coma when stimuli are decreased.

In a nonhabitual drinker, a BEC of 400 mg/dL can take 20 hours to return to zero. The only practical agent that might accelerate ethanol metabolism and elimination is fructose, but this causes gastrointestinal upset, lactic acidosis, and osmotic diuresis. Hemodialysis or peritoneal dialysis can be used for BECs greater than 600 mg/dL; for severe acidosis; for concurrent ingestion of methanol, ethylene glycol, or other dialyzable drugs; or for severely intoxicated children. Analeptic agents such as ethamivan, caffeine, or amphetamine have no useful role and can cause seizures and cardiac arrhythmia. Although patients are often depleted of magnesium, administration of magnesium sulfate may further depress the sensorium in intoxicated patients. Anecdotal reports describe temporary reversal of ethanol intoxication with the mu-opioid antagonist naloxone.

ETHANOL–DRUG INTERACTIONS

The combination of ethanol with other drugs, often in suicide attempts, causes 2,500 deaths annually or 13% of all drug-related fatalities. Ethanol is often taken with marijuana, barbiturates, opioids, cocaine, hallucinogens, and inhalants—with varying interactions. Alcoholics often abuse barbiturates, and although ethanol

and barbiturates are cross-tolerant, each lowers the lethal dose of the other when they are taken in combination. Ethanol with chloral hydrate ("Mickey Finn") may be especially dangerous.

Impaired judgment and respiratory depression are also hazards when ethanol is combined with hypnotics, such as methaqualone (Quaalude), sedating antihistamines, antipsychotic agents, and benzodiazepines. Hypnotic drugs with long half-lives may cause potentially dangerous incoordination when ethanol is consumed the following day.

The cross-tolerance of ethanol with general anesthetics raises the threshold to sleep induction, but synergistic interaction then increases the depth and length of the anesthetic stage reached. Tricyclic antidepressants do not have a consistent effect; desipramine antagonizes the effects of ethanol and amitriptyline potentiates them. Ethanol and morphine, repeatedly used, can increase each other's potency, and methadone addicts not only frequently become alcoholic but also then develop a characteristic encephalopathy. Death has followed ethanol taken with propoxyphene. A mild reaction resembling that caused by disulfiram occurs when patients combine ethanol with sulfonylureas such as tolbutamide or with some antibiotics, including chloramphenicol, griseofulvin, isoniazid, metronidazole, and quinacrine.

ETHANOL WITHDRAWAL

The term *hangover* refers to the headache, nausea, vomiting, malaise, nervousness, tremulousness, and sweating that can occur in anyone after brief but excessive drinking. Hangover does not imply ethanol dependence, but *ethanol withdrawal* does imply dependence and encompasses several disorders (Table 126.3), which may occur alone or in combination after reduction or cessation of drinking. Severity depends on the length and degree of a particular binge. Withdrawal syndromes are particularly common during hospitalization and can be exacerbated by concurrent illness.

Tremulousness, the most common ethanol withdrawal symptom, usually appears in the morning after several days of drinking. It is usually promptly relieved by ethanol, but if drinking cannot continue, tremor becomes more intense, with insomnia, easy startling, agitation, facial and conjunctival flushing, sweating, anorexia, nausea, retching, weakness, tachypnea, tachycardia, and systolic hypertension. Except for inattentiveness and inability to fully recall the events that occurred during the binge, mentation is usually intact. In some patients, tremulousness can persist for weeks or longer.

Perceptual disturbances, with variable insight, occur in about 25% of ethanol-dependent patients and include nightmares, illusions, and hallucinations, which are most often visual but may be auditory, tactile, olfactory, or a combination of these. Imagery includes insects, animals, or people. Hallucinations are usually fragmentary,

TABLE 126.3 Ethanol Withdrawal Syndromes

Early (<48 hours after last drink)

Tremulousness

Hallucinosis

Seizures

Late (>48 hours after last drink)

Delirium tremens

lasting minutes at a time for several days. Sometimes, however, auditory hallucinations of threatening content last much longer and may even progress to a persistent state of auditory hallucinosis with paranoid delusions requiring care in a mental hospital. Repeated bouts of acute auditory hallucinosis may predispose to the chronic form.

Ethanol can precipitate *seizures* in any epileptic; seizures usually occur the morning after weekend or even single-day drinking rather than during inebriation. Alcohol-related seizures affecting alcoholics not otherwise epileptic have traditionally been considered a withdrawal phenomenon, usually occurring within 48 hours of the last drink in persons who have abused ethanol chronically or in binges for months or years. The minimal duration of drinking sufficient to cause seizures is uncertain, but the risk is dose-related, beginning at only 50-g absolute ethanol daily. (In the United States, a "standard drink" usually means 12 ounces of beer, 5 ounces of wine, or 1.5 ounces of 80 proof spirits, each containing 14 g of absolute ethanol.) Seizures usually occur singly or in a brief cluster; status epilepticus is infrequent. Focal features are present in 25% and do not consistently correlate with evidence of previous head injury or other structural cerebral pathology. Alcohol seizures sometimes accompany tremulousness or hallucinosis, but they may occur in otherwise asymptomatic individuals. Their frequent appearance during active drinking or after more than 1 week of abstinence is consistent with mechanisms other than withdrawal per se.

The diagnosis of alcohol-related seizures depends on an accurate history and exclusion of other cerebral lesions. Workup should include brain computed tomography (CT) or magnetic resonance imaging (MRI) and consideration of lumbar puncture. Alcohol withdrawal can trigger new-onset seizures in patients with intracranial hemorrhage, central nervous system (CNS) infection, or brain neoplasm. Fewer than 10% of patients with alcohol-related seizures have spontaneous EEG abnormalities, compared with 50% of those with idiopathic epilepsy.

Transient *parkinsonism* during alcohol withdrawal is described in older patients. Transient chorea and dystonia are described in younger patients.

In contrast to tremor, hallucinosis, or seizures, which usually occur early and within 48 hours of abstinence, *delirium tremens* usually begins from 48 to 72 hours after the last drink. Patients with delirium tremens are often hospitalized for other reasons. Delirium tremens may follow withdrawal seizures either before the postictal period has cleared or after 1 or 2 asymptomatic days, but when seizures occur during a bout of delirium tremens, some other diagnosis (e.g., meningitis) should be considered.

Symptoms of delirium tremens typically begin and end abruptly, lasting from hours to a few days. There may be alternating periods of confusion and lucidity. Infrequently, relapses may prolong the disorder for a few weeks. Patients are typically agitated, inattentive, and grossly tremulous, with fever, tachycardia, and profuse sweating. They pick at the bed clothes or stare wildly about and intermittently shout at or try to fend off hallucinated people or objects. "Quiet" delirium is infrequent. Mortality is as high as 15%; death is usually owing to other diseases (e.g., pneumonia or cirrhosis), but it may be attributed to unexplained shock or lack of response to therapy or have no apparent cause.

The pathophysiologic basis of ethanol withdrawal in its several forms is probably a combination of glutamate receptor upregulation and GABA receptor downregulation. Neuronal excitotoxicity during withdrawal could then set the stage for a kindling pattern of repeated withdrawal episodes, further excitotoxicity, a permanently lowered seizure threshold, and the occurrence of seizures temporally independent of withdrawal.

Treatment of ethanol withdrawal includes prevention or reduction of early symptoms, prevention of delirium tremens, and management of delirium tremens after it starts (Table 126.4). Benzodiazepines, which have cross-tolerance with ethanol, are appropriately given to recently abstinent alcoholics or those with mild early withdrawal symptoms. Lorazepam (Ativan) 2 to 4 mg every 4 hours is a reasonable starting agent and dose. It is important to adjust the dose to symptom response, level of consciousness, and respiratory status after initiating therapy. A loading dose may cause symptoms of mild intoxication (calming, dysarthria, ataxia, fine nystagmus); dosage can then be adjusted to avoid both intoxication and tremulousness, and after 1 or 2 days, it can be gradually tapered, with reinstitution should withdrawal symptoms reappear.

Compared to fixed dose schedules, symptom-triggered pharmacotherapy more effectively decreases the likelihood of progression to delirium tremens and is less likely to result in sedative accumulation. Among standard protocols for symptom-triggered therapy, the Clinical Institute for Withdrawal Assessment for Alcohol (CIWA-Ar) scale assesses at regular intervals vital signs, nausea/vomiting, tremor, paroxysmal sweating, anxiety, agitation, tactile, visual or auditory disturbances, headache, and orientation/clouding of consciousness.

β-Adrenergic blockers such as propranolol and α-2 agonists such as clonidine or dexmedetomidine are helpful as adjunctive therapy to help control symptoms of sympathetic overdrive, but they are not cross-tolerant with alcohol and have reportedly triggered hallucinosis. Phenobarbital, which has a different GABAergic mechanism of action than benzodiazepines, has also been used as add-on treatment.

TABLE 126.4 **Treatment of Ethanol Withdrawal**

Prevention or Reduction of Early Symptoms

- Lorazepam 1–4 mg PO or IV; diazepam 5–20 mg; or chlordiazepoxide 25–100 mg repeated hourly until sedation or mild intoxication; successive daily doses tapered with resumption of higher dose if withdrawal symptoms recur
- Thiamine 100 mg and multivitamins IM or IV
- Magnesium, potassium, and calcium replacement as needed

Delirium Tremens

- Lorazepam 2–4 mg IV or IM or diazepam 10 mg IV, repeated every 5–15 min until calming; maintenance dose every 1–4 h p.r.n.
- If refractory to benzodiazepines, phenobarbital 260 mg IV repeated in 30 min p.r.n.
- If refractory to phenobarbital, propofol 25–100 μg/kg/min, with endotracheal intubation and repeated doses to produce general anesthesia
- Careful attention to fluid and electrolyte balance; several liters of saline per day, or even pressors, may be needed.
- Cooling blanket for high fever
- Prevent or correct hypoglycemia.
- Thiamine and multivitamin replacement
- Consider coexisting illness (e.g., liver failure, pancreatitis, meningitis, subdural hematoma).

PO, by mouth; IV, intravenous; IM, intramuscular; p.r.n., as needed.

Numerous anticonvulsants, especially those with GABAergic actions, have been subjected to randomized trials comparing them to benzodiazepine or placebo. A Cochrane review of 56 such trials concluded that evidence was insufficient to recommend their use. Similar conclusions were reached in Cochrane reviews of baclofen or γ-hydroxybutyric acid compared to benzodiazepines in the treatment of alcohol withdrawal.

Intravenous parenteral ethanol solutions have been used to treat delirium tremens. Treating with parenteral ethanol has the disadvantage of a low therapeutic index, and because ethanol is directly toxic to many organs, it should be avoided during hospitalization, even though most patients resume drinking on discharge. Haloperidol and phenothiazines are less likely to prevent hallucinosis or delirium tremens than drugs cross-tolerant with ethanol, and they can lower seizure threshold, prolong the QT interval, cause hypotension, and impair thermoregulation. They are appropriately considered in patients whose only symptoms are hallucinations or in whom hallucinations have outlasted other withdrawal symptoms.

Parenteral lorazepam given to patients following an ethanol withdrawal seizure reduces the likelihood of recurrence. Status epilepticus during ethanol withdrawal is treated as in other situations. Long-term anticonvulsants are not indicated in patients whose seizures occur only during withdrawal; abstainers do not need them, and drinkers do not take them. Alcoholics whose seizures occur independent of withdrawal and epileptics whose seizures are exacerbated by ethanol unfortunately do need anticonvulsant prophylaxis even though compliance is unlikely.

Hypomagnesemia is common during early ethanol withdrawal, and although it may not be the primary cause of symptoms, magnesium sulfate should be given to hypomagnesemic patients. Hypokalemia and hypocalcemia may also be present, and the latter may respond to treatment only when hypomagnesemia is corrected. Parenteral thiamine and multivitamins are given even if there are no clinical signs of depletion.

Delirium tremens, once it appears, cannot be abruptly reversed by any agent, and the mainstay of treatment is a parenteral benzodiazepine in dosage sufficient to produce adequate sedation. The required doses might be fatal in a normal person (see Table 126.4), but one cannot predict in any individual patient how high the tolerable dose is. Liver disease decreases the metabolism of benzodiazepines, and patients with cirrhosis are more vulnerable to the depressant effects of sedatives; as delirium tremens clears, hepatic encephalopathy can take its place.

General medical management in delirium tremens is intensive. Although dehydration may be severe enough to cause shock, patients with liver damage may retain sodium and water. Hypokalemia can cause cardiac arrhythmias. Hypoglycemia may be masked, as may other serious coexisting illnesses, such as alcoholic hepatitis, pancreatitis, meningitis, or subdural hematoma.

CHRONIC ETHANOL SYNDROMES

WERNICKE–KORSAKOFF SYNDROME

Although they share the same pathology, Wernicke and Korsakoff syndromes are clinically distinct. Wernicke syndrome, when full-blown, consists of mental, eye movement, and gait abnormalities. Korsakoff syndrome is a mental disorder that differs qualitatively from Wernicke syndrome (Table 126.5). Both are the result of thiamine deficiency.

In acute Wernicke syndrome, mental symptoms most often consist of a global confusional state that appears over days or

TABLE 126.5	Major Nutritional Disturbances in Alcoholics	
Disorder	Clinical Disorder	Deficiency
Wernicke syndrome	Dementia with lethargy, inattentiveness, apathy, and amnesia; Ophthalmoparesis; Gait ataxia	Thiamine
Korsakoff syndrome	Dementia, mainly amnesia, with or without confabulation	Thiamine
Cerebellar degeneration	Gait ataxia; limb coordination relatively preserved	Probably thiamine plus other vitamins plus ethanol neurotoxicity
Polyneuropathy	Distal limb sensory loss and weakness; less often autonomic dysfunction	Probably thiamine plus other vitamins plus ethanol neurotoxicity
Amblyopia	Optic atrophy, decreased visual acuity, central scotomas; total blindness rare	Probably thiamine plus other vitamins plus ethanol neurotoxicity

weeks; there is inattentiveness, indifference, decreased spontaneous speech, disorientation, impaired memory, and lethargy. Selective amnesia is unusual. Disordered perception is common; a patient might identify the hospital room as his or her apartment or a bar. In fewer than 10%, mentation is normal.

Abnormal eye movements include nystagmus (horizontal with or without vertical or rotatory components), lateral rectus palsy (bilateral but usually asymmetric), and conjugate gaze palsy (horizontal with or without vertical), progressing to complete external ophthalmoplegia. Although sluggishness of pupillary reaction is common, total loss of reactivity to light and ptosis are rare. Mental symptoms, including progression to coma, can occur without evident abnormal eye movements in patients with pathologically verified acute Wernicke syndrome.

Truncal ataxia, present in more than 80% of patients, may prevent standing or walking. Dysarthria and limb ataxia, especially in the arms, are infrequent. Peripheral neuropathy, which occurs to some degree in most patients, may cause weakness sufficient to mask the ataxia. Abnormalities of vestibular caloric testing are common, with gradual improvement, often incomplete, over several months.

Patients with the Wernicke syndrome frequently have signs of nutritional deficiency (e.g., skin changes, tongue redness, cheilosis) or liver disease. Autonomic signs are common. Although beriberi heart disease is rare, acute tachycardia, dyspnea on exertion, and postural hypotension unexplained by hypovolemia are common, and sudden circulatory collapse may follow mild exertion. Hypothermia is less frequent; fever usually indicates infection.

In acute Wernicke syndrome, the EEG may show diffuse slowing or it may be normal. Cerebrospinal fluid (CSF) is normal except for occasional mild protein elevation. Elevated blood pyruvate, falling with treatment, is not specific. Decreased blood transketolase (which requires thiamine pyrophosphate as cofactor) and serum thiamine level may be depressed, but in most centers, the diagnosis depends on history and examination (and thiamine and multivitamins should be given to any alcoholic patient, symptomatic or not).

In most patients, the more purely amnestic syndrome of Korsakoff emerges as the other mental symptoms of Wernicke syndrome respond to treatment. How often Korsakoff syndrome occurs without a background of Wernicke syndrome is disputed and bound up with the question of "alcoholic dementia" (see later in the text). Pathologic changes of Wernicke–Korsakoff are sometimes encountered unexpectedly at autopsy, suggesting the presence of subclinical or atypical forms, including unexplained coma.

The amnesia of Korsakoff syndrome is both anterograde, with inability to retain new information, and retrograde, with rather randomly lost recall for events months or years old. Alertness, attentiveness, and behavior are relatively preserved, but there tends to be a lack of spontaneous speech or activity. Confabulation is not invariable and, if initially present, tends gradually to disappear. Insight is usually impaired, and there may be flagrant anosognosia for the mental disturbance.

The histopathologic lesions of Wernicke–Korsakoff syndrome consist of variable degrees of neuronal, axonal, and myelin loss; prominent blood vessels; reactive microglia, macrophages, and astrocytes; and, infrequently, small hemorrhages. Nerve cells may be relatively preserved in the presence of extensive myelin destruction and gliosis, and astrocytosis may predominate chronically.

Lesions affect the thalamus (especially the anterior and dorsomedial nuclei and the medial pulvinar), the hypothalamus (especially the mammillary bodies), the midbrain (especially the oculomotor and periaqueductal areas), and the pons and medulla (especially the abducens and medial vestibular nuclei). Such lesions sometimes produce abnormal signals on MRI, including diffusion-weighted imaging (DWI). Diffusion tensor imaging reveals disruption of the fornix. In the anterior–superior vermis of the cerebellum, severe Purkinje cell loss and astrocytosis accompany lesser degrees of neuronal loss and gliosis in the molecular and granular layers.

Memory impairment in Korsakoff syndrome correlates best with lesions involving the anterior nuclei of the thalamus; other components of the so-called Papez circuit (e.g., the mammillary bodies) probably contribute. The global confusion of Wernicke syndrome can occur without visible thalamic lesions and may be a biochemical disorder. Periaqueductal, oculomotor, or abducens nucleus lesions probably explain ophthalmoparesis. Both cerebellar and vestibular lesions likely contribute to ataxia.

Experimental and clinical evidence ascribes a specific role to thiamine in the Wernicke–Korsakoff syndrome. A genetic influence is implied because only a few alcoholic or otherwise malnourished people are affected, and whites seem more susceptible than blacks.

Untreated Wernicke–Korsakoff syndrome can be fatal, and the mortality rate is 10% among treated patients. Concomitant liver failure, infection, or delirium tremens often makes the cause of death unclear. Postural hypotension and tachycardia call for strict bed rest; associated medical problems may require intensive care. The cornerstone of treatment is thiamine, 1,000 mg daily, until a normal diet can be taken; intramuscular or intravenous administration is preferred because thiamine absorption is impaired in chronic alcoholics. Hypomagnesemia may retard improvement after thiamine treatment; magnesium is therefore replaced, along with other vitamins. Protein intake may have to be titrated against the patient's liver status.

With thiamine treatment, the ocular abnormalities (especially abducens and gaze palsies) improve within a few hours and usually resolve within 1 week; in about 35% of patients, horizontal nystagmus persists indefinitely. Global confusion may improve in hours or days and usually resolves within 1 month, leaving Korsakoff amnesia in more than 80%. In less than 25% of these patients, there is eventual clearing of the memory deficit. Ataxia may improve in a few days, but recovery is complete in less than 50% of patients, and nearly 35% do not show improvement at all.

Nonalcoholics who develop Wernicke encephalopathy (e.g., as a result of starvation or hyperemesis gravidarum) are less likely to have Korsakoff amnesia following treatment, consistent with a contributory role for alcohol itself in the pathogenesis of Wernicke–Korsakoff syndrome.

ALCOHOLIC CEREBELLAR DEGENERATION

Cerebellar cortical degeneration may occur in nutritionally deficient alcoholics without Wernicke–Korsakoff syndrome (see Table 126.5). Instability of the trunk is the major symptom, often with incoordination of leg movements. Arm ataxia is less prominent; nystagmus and dysarthria are rare. Symptoms evolve in weeks or months and eventually stabilize, sometimes even with continued drinking and poor nutrition. Ataxia without Wernicke disease is less likely to appear abruptly or to improve.

Pathologically, the superior vermis is invariably involved, with nerve cell loss and gliosis in the molecular, granular, and especially the Purkinje cell layers. There may be secondary degeneration of the olives and of the fastigial, emboliform, globose, and vestibular nuclei. Involvement of the cerebellar hemispheric cortex is exceptional and limited to the anterior lobes. Pathologic evidence of Wernicke disease may coexist, even though it is unsuspected clinically. CT and autopsies, moreover, have revealed cerebellar atrophy in alcoholics who were not clinically ataxic.

Although similar cerebellar lesions occur in malnourished nonalcoholics, most patients with alcoholic cerebellar degeneration do not have clinical or pathologic evidence of Wernicke disease. The disorder is probably the result of both nutritional deficiency and ethanol toxicity, perhaps involving glutamate.

ALCOHOLIC POLYNEUROPATHY

Alcoholic polyneuropathy is a sensorimotor disorder that stabilizes or improves with abstinence and an adequate diet (see Table 126.5). Neuropathy is found in most patients with Wernicke–Korsakoff syndrome but more often occurs alone. Paresthesia is usually the first symptom; there may be burning or lancinating pain and exquisite tenderness of the calves or soles. Impaired vibratory sense is usually the earliest sign; proprioception tends to be preserved until other sensory loss is substantial. Loss of ankle jerks is another early sign; eventually, there is diffuse areflexia. Weakness appears at any time and may be severe. Distal leg muscles are affected first, although proximal weakness may be marked. Radiologically demonstrable neuropathic arthropathy of the feet is common, as are skin changes (e.g., thinning, glossiness, reddening, cyanosis, hyperhidrosis). Peripheral autonomic abnormalities are usually less prominent than in diabetic neuropathy but may cause urinary and fecal incontinence, hypotension, hypothermia, cardiac arrhythmia, dysphagia, dysphonia, impaired esophageal peristalsis, altered sweat patterns, or abnormal Valsalva ratio. Pupillary parasympathetic denervation is rare. The CSF is usually normal except for occasional mild elevation of protein content.

Pathologically, the neuropathy is axonal, and clinical and experimental evidence suggests that it is both toxic and nutritional in origin. A clinical and pathologic study found that pure thiamine deficiency neuropathy (TDN) differs from pure alcoholic neuropathy (ALN); ALN is sensory dominant, slowly progressive, and painful and causes predominantly small-fiber axonal loss, whereas TDN is motor dominant and acutely progressive and causes predominantly large-fiber axonal loss.

Peripheral nerve pressure palsies, especially radial and peroneal, are common in alcoholics. Nutritional polyneuropathy may increase the vulnerability of peripheral nerves to compression injury in intoxicated individuals, who tend to sleep deeply in unusual locations and positions. Recovery usually takes days or weeks; splints during this period can prevent contractures.

ALCOHOLIC AMBLYOPIA

Alcoholic amblyopia is a visual impairment that progresses over days or weeks, with development of central or centrocecal scotomas and temporal disc pallor (see Table 126.5). Demyelination affects the optic nerves, chiasm, and tracts, with predilection for the maculopapular bundle. Retinal ganglion cell loss is secondary. Although amblyopia improves in patients who receive dietary supplements but continue to smoke and drink ethanol, direct toxicity from ethanol and from compounds in tobacco smoke (perhaps cyanide) could be contributory. Alcoholic amblyopia does not progress to total blindness; it may remain stable without change in drinking or eating habits. Improvement, which is often incomplete, nearly always follows abstinence and nutritional replacement.

PELLAGRA

Nicotinic acid deficiency in alcoholics causes pellagra, with dermatologic, gastrointestinal, and neurologic symptoms. Altered mentation progresses over hours, days, or weeks to amnesia, delusions, hallucinations, or delirium. Nicotinic acid therapy (plus other vitamins, deficiency of which can be contributory) usually results in prompt improvement.

ALCOHOLIC LIVER DISEASE

Alcoholic liver disease, progressing from reversible steatosis through steatohepatitis to cirrhosis, is a major cause of death among alcoholics. Altered mentation in an alcoholic always raises the possibility of hepatic encephalopathy, which may accompany intoxication, withdrawal, Wernicke syndrome, meningitis, subdural hematoma, hypoglycemia, or other alcohol states. Hepatic encephalopathy is discussed in detail in Chapter 119. Other neurologic disorders encountered in alcoholic cirrhotics include a poorly understood syndrome of altered mentation, myoclonus, and progressive myelopathy following portacaval shunting, as well as acquired chronic hepatocerebral degeneration, a characteristic syndrome of dementia, dysarthria, ataxia, intention tremor, choreoathetosis, muscular rigidity, and asterixis, which usually occurs in patients who have had repeated bouts of hepatic coma. Heavy ethanol use greatly increases the risk for acetaminophen hepatotoxicity and for cirrhosis and hepatocellular carcinoma in patients with hepatitis C infection.

HYPOGLYCEMIA

Metabolism of ethanol by alcohol dehydrogenase and of acetaldehyde by mitochondrial aldehyde dehydrogenase uses nicotinamide adenine dinucleotide (NAD). The resulting elevated NADH-to-NAD ratio impairs gluconeogenesis, and if food is not being eaten and liver glycogen is depleted, there may be severe hypoglycemia with altered behavior, seizures, coma, or focal neurologic deficit. Residual symptoms are common, including dementia. Even after appropriate treatment with intravenous 50% dextrose, these patients require close observation; blood glucose may fall again, with the return of symptoms and possibly permanent brain damage. Ethanol stimulates intestinal release of secretin, which aggravates reactive hypoglycemia, especially in children, by enhancing glucose-stimulated insulin release.

ALCOHOLIC KETOACIDOSIS

In alcoholic ketoacidosis, β-hydroxybutyric acid and lactic acid accumulate in association with heavy drinking. The mechanism relates to starvation, increased lipolysis, and impaired fatty acid oxidation. Typical patients are young binge drinkers who stop drinking when they are overcome by anorexia. Vomiting, dehydration, confusion, obtundation, and hyperventilation ensue. Blood glucose may be normal, low, or moderately elevated, with little or no glycosuria. A large anion gap is accounted for by β-hydroxybutyrate, lactate, and lesser amounts of pyruvate and acetoacetate. Serum insulin levels are low, and serum levels of growth hormone, epinephrine, glucagon, and cortisol are high, but glucose intolerance usually clears without insulin and is not demonstrable on recovery. It is not unusual for patients to have repeated attacks of alcoholic ketoacidosis.

Alcoholics may have other reasons for metabolic acidosis with a large anion gap (e.g., methanol or ethylene glycol poisoning). When β-hydroxybutyrate is the major ketone present, the nitroprusside test (Acetest) may be negative. Treatment includes infusion of glucose (and thiamine), correction of dehydration or hypotension, and replacement of electrolytes such as potassium, magnesium, and phosphate. Small amounts of bicarbonate may be given. Insulin is usually not needed.

INFECTION IN ALCOHOLICS

Alteration of white blood cell (WBC) function contributes to the alcoholic's predisposition to infection (e.g., bacterial and tuberculous meningitis). Infectious meningitis must always be considered in alcoholics with seizures or altered mental status, even when the clinical picture seems to be that of intoxication, withdrawal, thiamine deficiency, hepatic encephalopathy, hypoglycemia, or other alcoholic disturbances. Alcoholic intoxication is a risk factor for HIV infection.

TRAUMA IN ALCOHOLICS

Thrombocytopenia, a direct effect of ethanol and a consequence of cirrhosis, increases the likelihood of intracranial hematomas after head injury. Abnormalities of clotting factors also increase the possibility of intracranial hematomas. Experimentally, moreover, acute ethanol enhances blood–brain barrier leakage around areas of cerebral trauma. Close observation is essential after even mild head injury in intoxicated patients; an abnormal sensorium must not be dismissed as drunkenness.

ALCOHOL AND CANCER

Independently of tobacco, ethanol in moderate amounts increases the risk of carcinoma of the mouth, esophagus, pharynx, larynx, liver, and, probably, large bowel and breast.

ALCOHOL AND STROKE

As with coronary artery disease, epidemiologic studies suggest that low to moderate amounts of ethanol decrease ischemic stroke risk, whereas higher amounts increase it. Although reports have been inconsistent, meta-analysis of rigorously designed cohort and case-control studies found a J-shaped association between ethanol consumption and the risk of ischemic stroke and a linear association between ethanol consumption and the risk of hemorrhagic stroke. In the United States, the relationship holds for men and women; for blacks, whites, and Hispanics; and for spirits, beer, and wine. Whether extra risk is temporally associated with binge drinking and whether special benefit is conferred by wine (especially red wine) is less clear. In asymptomatic subjects, moderate ethanol consumption reduces the risk of both carotid atherosclerosis and leukoaraiosis. Ethanol could either prevent or cause stroke by several mechanisms. Acutely and chronically, ethanol causes hypertension. It reportedly lowers blood levels of low-density lipoproteins, raises levels of high-density lipoproteins, decreases fibrinolytic activity, increases or inhibits platelet reactivity, increases or decreases C-reactive protein, dilates or constricts cerebral vessels, and indirectly reduces cerebral blood flow through dehydration. The antioxidant properties of flavonoids in red wine might confer special protection. Alcoholic cardiomyopathy predisposes to embolic stroke.

ALCOHOLIC MYOPATHY

Alcoholic myopathy is of two types. Chronic myopathy produces painless proximal weakness; serum creatine kinase (CK) can be elevated or normal, and pathologically, there is atrophy affecting especially type 2 fibers (a nonspecific finding also seen with disuse or glucocorticoid toxicity). Cardiomyopathy may be present. Acute alcoholic myopathy consists of rhabdomyolysis, painful swelling, and myoglobinuria with renal injury. Both types of myopathy are attributed to direct effects of ethanol on muscle independent of malnutrition. Acute rhabdomyolysis often occurs hours or days after binge drinking. Workup includes checking for potassium or phosphate depletion, which are common in alcoholics. Treatment is supportive, and symptoms improve with abstinence.

CENTRAL PONTINE MYELINOLYSIS AND MARCHIAFAVA–BIGNAMI DISEASE

Central pontine myelinolysis occurs in both alcoholics and nondrinkers and is a consequence of overvigorous correction of hyponatremia. Marchiafava–Bignami disease is nearly always associated with alcoholism (including wine, beer, and whiskey). It is of unknown origin and causes symptoms, including death, that are scarcely explained by the characteristic callosal lesions. Marchiafava–Bignami disease and central pontine myelinolysis are discussed in detail in Chapter 70.

ALCOHOLIC DEMENTIA

Whether ethanol, as a direct neurotoxin, can cause progressive mental decline in the absence of nutritional deficiency, brain trauma, or other indirect mechanisms has been controversial for decades. Properly controlled animal studies reveal dose-related impaired learning and neuropathologic changes in hippocampus and other brain regions. Brains of alcoholics without evident nutritional deficiency have reduced volume especially affecting white matter; reports of cortical or hippocampal neuronal loss are less consistent, but neuropathologic changes appear to correlate with memory and other cognitive impairment. A plausible mechanism is inhibition of glutamate neurotransmission with receptor upregulation and rebound excitotoxicity. It is possible that ethanol neurotoxicity and thiamine deficiency are synergistic in this regard.

Numerous cohort and case-control studies addressing dose-related effects of ethanol on cognition have found that compared to nondrinking, low to moderate alcohol intake actually reduces the risk of dementia. As with ischemic stroke, a J-shaped curve reflects ethanol's long-term effects on cognition: Compared to nondrinking, moderate intake reduces the risk of dementia and heavy intake increases it. Ethanol's protective effect is independent of its benefit on cerebrovascular disease. Wine, beer, and spirits are each protective, with some studies finding special benefit in red wine (perhaps related to antioxidant polyphenols such as resveratrol). The mechanism of ethanol's protective effects against nonvascular dementia is otherwise unclear.

FETAL ALCOHOL SPECTRUM DISORDERS

Ethanol ingestion during pregnancy causes congenital malformations and delayed psychomotor development. Major clinical features of the *fetal alcohol syndrome* (FAS) include cerebral dysfunction, growth deficiency, and distinctive facies (Table 126.6); less often, there are abnormalities of the heart, skeleton, urogenital organs, skin, and muscles. Neuropathologic abnormalities include absence or displacement of the corpus callosum, hydrocephalus, cerebellar dysplasia, abnormal neuronal migration, heterotopic cell clusters, and microcephaly. These changes occur independently of other potentially incriminating factors, such as maternal malnutrition, smoking, other drug use, or age. Binge drinking, which may produce high ethanol levels at a critical fetal period, may be more important than chronic ethanol exposure, and early gestation appears to be the most vulnerable period.

The face of a typical patient with FAS is distinctive and as easily recognized at birth as that of an infant with Down syndrome. Irritability and tremulousness with poor suck reflex and hyperacusis are usually present at birth and last weeks or months. Of these children, 85% perform more than two standard deviations below the mean on tests of mental performance; those who are not grossly retarded rarely have even average mental ability. Older children are often hyperactive and clumsy, and there may be hypotonia or hypertonia. Except for neonatal seizures, epilepsy is not a component of the syndrome.

Some children of alcoholic mothers have milder cognitive or behavioral features—for example, depression, anxiety, or hyperactivity. The broad continuum of ethanol's fetal effects is referred to as *fetal alcohol spectrum disorders* (FASDs), comprising mental, emotional, craniofacial, physiologic, and immunologic abnormalities that occur alone or in combination. Dysregulation of the hypothalamic–pituitary–adrenal (HPA) axis, with hyperstress responses, is a major feature in many subjects.

Ethanol is directly teratogenic to many animals. Proposed mechanisms include apoptosis secondary to blockade of N-methyl-D-aspartate (NMDA) glutamate receptors during a critical period of synaptogenesis, toxicity to adhesion molecules essential for neuronal migration, and fetal vasospasm and CNS ischemia. Twin studies show genetic vulnerability to FASD (100% concordance in monozygotes, 63% in dizygotes), and ethanol has epigenetic effects which in animals are transgenerational. Epigenetics might explain observations that paternal drinking also carries risk for FASD.

In humans, the risk of alcohol-induced birth defects is established with more than 3 oz of absolute alcohol daily. Below that, the risk is uncertain; a threshold of safety has not been defined. As rates of ethanol use in the United States rose during the 1990s, so did the incidence of FAS. On the basis of data from the United States and France, it was estimated that the incidence of FASD is nearly 1% of all live births. FASD may affect 1% of infants born to women who drink 1 oz of ethanol daily early in pregnancy. More than 30% of the offspring of heavy drinkers are affected by FAS,

TABLE 126.6 Clinical Features of Fetal Alcohol Syndrome

Feature	Majority	Minority
CNS	Mental retardation	—
	Microcephaly	
	Hypotonia	
	Poor coordination	
	Hyperactivity	
Impaired growth	Prenatal for length and weight	—
	Postnatal for length and weight	
	Diminished adipose tissue	
Abnormal face	Short palpebral fissures	Ptosis
Eyes	—	Strabismus
		Epicanthal folds
		Myopia
		Microphthalmia
		Blepharophimosis
		Cataracts
		Retinal pigmentary abnormalities
Nose	Short, upturned	—
	Hypoplastic philtrum	
Mouth	Thin vermilion lip borders	Prominent lateral palatine ridges
	Retrognathia in infancy	Cleft lip or palate
	Micrognathia or prognathia in adolescence	Small teeth with faulty enamel
Maxilla	Hypoplastic	—
Ears	—	Posteriorly rotated
		Poorly formed concha
Skeletal	—	Pectus excavatum or carinatum
		Syndactyly, clinodactyly, or camptodactyly
		Limited joint movements
		Nail hypoplasia
		Radioulnar synostosis
		Bifid xiphoid
		Scoliosis
		Klippel–Feil anomaly
Cardiac	—	Septal defects
		Great vessel anomalies
Cutaneous	—	Abnormal palmar creases
		Hemangiomas
		Infantile hirsutism
Muscular	—	Diaphragmatic, inguinal, or umbilical hernias
		Diastasis recti
Urogenital	—	Labial hypoplasia
		Hypospadias
		Small rotated kidneys
		Hydronephrosis

CNS, central nervous system.

which thus may be the leading teratogenic cause of mental retardation in the Western world.

TREATMENT OF CHRONIC ALCOHOLISM

The literature on the treatment of alcoholism is voluminous, and strong opinions outweigh scientific data. Not all problem drinkers consume physically addicting quantities of ethanol, no personality type defines an alcoholic, and the relative roles of genetics and social deprivation vary from patient to patient. (Animal and human studies indicate polygenetic influences in alcoholism.) Of course, such variability of alcoholic populations means that no treatment modality (e.g., psychotherapy, group psychotherapy, family or social network therapy, drug therapy, behavioral [aversion] therapy) or no single therapeutic setting (e.g., general hospital, halfway house, vocational rehabilitation clinic, Alcoholics Anonymous) is appropriate for all. For example, the success rate of Alcoholics Anonymous has been estimated to be 34%.

Use of tranquilizing and sedating drugs is especially controversial because they may lead to switching of dependency or to drug–ethanol interactions. Some clinicians espouse short-term use of these drugs in doses high enough to reduce the psychological tensions that lead to ethanol use but low enough not to block symptoms of ethanol withdrawal.

Disulfiram inhibits aldehyde dehydrogenase and reduces the rate of oxidation of acetaldehyde, accumulation of which accounts for the symptoms that appear soon after someone taking disulfiram drinks ethanol. Within 5 to 10 minutes, there is throbbing headache, dyspnea, nausea, vomiting, sweating, chest pain, palpitations, hypotension, anxiety, and confusion. The severity and duration of these symptoms depend on the amount of ethanol drunk; severe reactions can last hours or be fatal and require hospital admission, with careful management of hypotension and cardiac arrhythmia.

Taken in the morning, when the urge to drink is least, disulfiram, 0.25 to 0.5 g daily, does not alter the taste for ethanol and helps only patients who strongly desire to abstain. Side effects of disulfiram that are unrelated to ethanol ingestion include drowsiness, psychiatric symptoms, and cardiovascular problems. Paranoia, impaired memory, ataxia, dysarthria, and even major motor seizures may be difficult to distinguish from ethanol effects. So may peripheral neuropathy, which can be fulminant. Hypersensitivity hepatitis also occurs.

Naltrexone and acamprosate are both U.S. Food and Drug Administration (FDA) approved for treatment of alcoholism. Naltrexone might work by decreasing dopaminergic activity in reward circuits. Acamprosate might work by modulating glutamate neurotransmission and resetting a disrupted balance between GABA and glutamate systems. Placebo-controlled trials suggest that acamprosate (1,332 to 3,000 mg/day) is more effective than naltrexone in maintaining abstinence, whereas naltrexone (50 to 100 mg/day) is more effective in reducing heavy drinking and craving should drinking be resumed.

Topiramate affects both dopaminergic and glutamatergic pathways, and placebo-controlled trials demonstrate benefit (at doses ranging from 50 to 300 mg/day) both for maintaining abstinence and for reducing heavy drinking.

SUGGESTED READINGS

Amato L, Minozzi S, Davoli M. Efficacy and safety of pharmacological interventions for the treatment of the alcohol withdrawal syndrome. *Cochrane Database Syst Rev.* 2011;(6):CD008537.

Bijjal S, Subodh BN, Narayanaswamy JC, et al. Dystonia as a presenting feature of alcohol withdrawal. *J Neuropsychiatry Clin Neurosci.* 2012;24:E15–E16.

Blodgett JC, Del Re AC, Maisel NC, et al. A meta-analysis of topiramate's effects for individuals with alcohol use disorders. *Alcohol Clin Exp Res.* 2014;38:1481–1488.

Brathen G, Ben-Manachem E, Brodtkarb E, et al. EFNS guideline on the diagnosis and management of alcohol-related seizures: report of an EFNS task force. *Eur J Neurol.* 2005;12:575–581.

Brust JCM. A 74-year-old man with memory loss and neuropathy who enjoys alcoholic beverages. *JAMA.* 2008;299:1046–1054.

Brust JCM. Alcohol withdrawal: diagnosis and treatment. *Handb Clin Neurol.* 2014;125:123–131.

Brust JCM. Ethanol and cognition: indirect effects, neurotoxicity and neuroprotection: a review. *Int J Environ Res Public Health.* 2010;7:1540–1557.

Brust JCM. *Neurological Aspects of Substance Abuse.* 2nd ed. Boston, MA: Butterworth-Heinemann; 2004:317–425.

Brust JCM. Stroke and substance abuse. In: Mohr JP, Choi D, Grotta J, et al, eds. *Stroke: Pathophysiology, Diagnosis, and Management.* 5th ed. Philadelphia: Elsevier/Saunders; 2011;362–383.

Brust JCM. Wine, flavonoids, and the "water of life." *Neurology.* 2002;59:1300–1301.

Carlson RW, Kumar NN, Wong-Mckinstry E, et al. Alcohol withdrawal syndrome. *Crit Care Clin.* 2012;28:549–585.

Cassidy EM, O'Sullivan I, Bradshaw P, et al. Symptom-triggered benzodiazepine therapy for alcohol withdrawal syndrome in the emergency department: a comparison with the standard fixed dose benzodiazepine regimen. *Emerg Med J.* 2012;29:802–804.

De la Monte SM, Kril JJ. Human alcohol-related neuropathology. *Acta Neuropathol.* 2014;127:71–90.

Frazee EN, Personett HA, Leung JG, et al. Influence of dexmedetomidine therapy on the management of severe alcohol withdrawal syndrome in critically ill patients. *J Crit Care.* 2014;29:298–302.

Harding A, Halliday G, Caine D, et al. Degeneration of anterior thalamic nuclei differentiates alcoholics with amnesia. *Brain.* 2000;123:141–154.

Hillbom M, Saloheimo P, Fujioka S, et al. Diagnosis and management of Marchiafava-Bignami disease: a review of CT/MRI confirmed cases. *J Neurol Neurosurg Psychiatry.* 2014;85:168–173.

Hughes JC, Cook CC. The efficacy of disulfiram: a review of outcome studies. *Addiction.* 1997;92:381–395.

Jung MK, Callaci JJ, Lauing KL, et al. Alcohol exposure and mechanisms of tissue injury and repair. *Alcohol Clin Exp Res.* 2011;35:392–399.

Koike H, Iijima M, Sugiura M, et al. Alcoholic neuropathy is clinicopathologically distinct from thiamine-deficiency neuropathy. *Ann Neurol.* 2003;54:19–29.

Kril JJ, Harper CG. Neuroanatomy and neuropathology associated with Korsakoff's syndrome. *Neuropsychol Rev.* 2012;22:72–80.

Lee H, Roh S, Kim DJ. Alcohol-induced blackout. *Int J Environ Res Public Health.* 2009;6:2783–2792.

Leone MA, Vigna-Taglianti F, Avanzi G, et al. Gamma-hydroxybutyrate (GHB) for treatment of alcohol withdrawal and prevention of relapses. *Cochrane Database Syst Rev.* 2010;17(2):CD0006266.

Liu J, Wang L. Baclofen for alcohol withdrawal. *Cochrane Database Syst Rev.* 2011;19(1):CD008502.

Maisel NC, Bloodgett JC, Wilbourne PL, et al. Meta-analysis of naltrexone and acamprosate for treating alcohol use disorders: when are these medications most helpful? *Addiction.* 2013;108:275–293.

Manzo G, De Gennaro A, Cozzolino A, et al. MR imaging findings in alcoholic and nonalcoholic acute Wernicke's encephalopathy: a review. *Biomed Res Int.* 2014;2014:503596. doi:10.1155/2014/503596.

Mead EA, Sarkar AK. Fetal alcohol spectrum disorders and their transmission through genetic and epigenetic mechanisms. *Front Genet.* 2014;5:1–10.

Mellion M, Gilchrist JM, de la Monte S. Alcohol-related peripheral neuropathy: nutritional, toxic, or both? *Muscle Nerve.* 2011;43:309–316.

Minozzi S, Amato L, Vecchi S, et al. Anticonvulsants for alcohol withdrawal. *Cochrane Database Syst Rev.* 2011;17(3):CD005064.

Mukamal KJ, Ascherio A, Mittleman MA, et al. Alcohol and risk for ischemic stroke in men: the role of drinking patterns and usual beverage. *Ann Intern Med.* 2005;142:11–19.

Mukamal KJ, Kuller LH, Fitzpatrick AL, et al. Prospective study of alcohol consumption and the risk of dementia in older adults. *JAMA*. 2003;289:1405–1413.

Muzyk AJ, Fowler JA, Norwood DK, et al. Role of alpha-2 agonists in the treatment of acute alcohol withdrawal. *Ann Pharmacother*. 2011;45:649–657.

Nahum L, Pignat J-M, Bouzerda-Wahlen A, et al. Neural correlate of anterograde amnesia in Wernicke-Korsakoff syndrome [published online ahead of print August 23, 2014]. *Brain Topogr*. doi:10.1007/s10548-014-00391-5.

Noble JM, Weimer LH. Neurologic complications of alcoholism. *Continuum (Minneap Minn)*. 2014;20:624–641.

Ntais C, Pakos E, Kyzas P, et al. Benzodiazepines for alcohol withdrawal. *Cochrane Database Syst Rev*. 2005;(3):CD005063.

Pitel AL, Segobin SH, Ritz L, et al. Thalamic abnormalities are a cardinal feature of alcohol-related brain dysfunction [published online ahead of print August 6, 2014]. *Neurosci Biobehav Rev*. doi:10.1016/j.neubiorev.2014.07.023.

Reynolds K, Lewis LB, Nolan JDL, et al. Alcohol consumption and risk of stroke. A meta-analysis. *JAMA*. 2003;289:579–588.

Rosenbloom MJ, Pfefferbaum AMD. Magnetic resonance imaging of the living brain: evidence for brain degeneration among alcoholics and recovery with abstinence. *Alcohol Res Health*. 2008;31:362–376.

Rosenson J, Clements C, Simon B, et al. Phenobarbital for acute alcohol withdrawal: a prospective randomized double-blind placebo-controlled study. *J Emerg Med*. 2013;44(3):592–598.

Sabia S, Elbaz A, Britton A, et al. Alcohol consumption and cognitive decline in early old age. *Neurology*. 2014;82:332–339.

Sacco RL, Elkind M, Baden-Albala B, et al. The protective effect of moderate alcohol consumption on ischemic stroke. *JAMA*. 1999;281:53–60.

Samokhvalov AV, Irving H, Mohapatra S, et al. Alcohol consumption, unprovoked seizures, and epilepsy: a systematic review and meta-analysis. *Epilepsia*. 2010;51:1177–1184.

Solfrizzi V, D'Introno A, Colacicco AM, et al. Alcohol consumption, mild cognitive impairment, and progression to dementia. *Neurology*. 2007;68:1790–1799.

Victor M, Adams RD, Collins GH. *The Wernicke–Korsakoff Syndrome*. 2nd ed. Philadelphia: FA Davis; 1989.

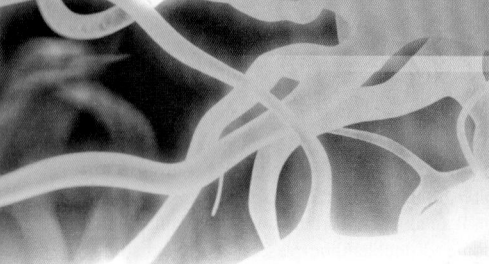

Drug Intoxication and Withdrawal 127

John C. M. Brust

INTRODUCTION

There are two kinds of drug dependence. *Psychic dependence* leads to craving and drug-seeking behavior. *Physical dependence* produces somatic withdrawal symptoms and signs. Depending on the particular drug and the circumstances of its administration, psychic and physical dependence can coexist or occur alone. *Addiction* is psychic dependence.

In the United States, dependence of one or both types is encountered with a variety of agents, licit and illicit (Table 127.1). Different classes of drugs produce diverse symptoms of intoxication and withdrawal as well as medical and neurologic complications.

DRUGS OF DEPENDENCE

OPIOIDS

Opioids include agonists, antagonists, and mixed agonist–antagonists (Table 127.2). Heroin, the opioid most often abused, is illegal in the United States. During the past decade, however, escalation in the use of prescription opioids for noncancer pain resulted in an epidemic of prescription opioid recreational use, especially oxycodone, hydrocodone, methadone, morphine, fentanyl, and hydromorphone. During the same period, heroin use also increased sharply, in many cases representing escalation from prescription opioid use.

Desomorphine, a reduction of codeine that is more potent but also often contains more impurities, is termed *crocodile* for the green-black skin lesions found on parenteral users.

At desired levels of intoxication, agonist opioids produce drowsy euphoria; analgesia; cough suppression; miosis; and often nausea, vomiting, sweating, pruritus, hypothermia, postural hypotension, constipation, and decreased libido. Taken parenterally or smoked (often in combination with alkaloidal crack cocaine), heroin produces a "rush," a brief ecstatic feeling followed by euphoria and either relaxed "nodding" or garrulous hyperactivity. Overdose causes coma, respiratory depression, and pinpoint (but reactive) pupils. For adults with respiratory depression, treatment consists of respiratory support and naloxone, 2 mg intravenously, repeated as needed up to 20 mg; for those with normal respirations, smaller doses (0.4 to 0.8 mg) are given to avoid precipitation of withdrawal signs. Naloxone is short acting, and so patients receiving it require admission and close observation.

Opioid agonist withdrawal symptoms include irritability, lacrimation, rhinorrhea, sweating, yawning, mydriasis, myalgia, muscle spasms, piloerection, nausea, vomiting, abdominal cramps, fever, hot flashes, tachycardia, hypertension, and orgasm. In adults, seizures and delirium are not features of opioid withdrawal, which is rarely life threatening and can usually be prevented or treated with 20 mg of methadone taken once or twice daily. By contrast, untreated opioid withdrawal in newborns is severe and protracted, probably causes seizures, and is often fatal. Treatment is with titrated doses of methadone or paregoric; a barbiturate can be added if additional drug withdrawal is suspected or if seizures require treatment.

Effective pharmacotherapy for opioid dependence consists of substitution with oral methadone or buprenorphine. Treatment failure is usually attributable to inadequate dosage. Antagonist therapy with naltrexone proved disappointing.

TABLE 127.1 Drugs of Dependence

Opioids
Psychostimulants
Sedatives/hypnotics
Marijuana
Hallucinogens
Inhalants
Phencyclidine
Anticholinergics
Ethanol
Tobacco

TABLE 127.2 Commonly Used Opioids

Agonist
• Camphorated tincture of opium (paregoric)
• Morphine
• Meperidine
• Methadone
• Fentanyl
• Hydromorphone
• Oxycodone
• Hydrocodone
• Propoxyphene
• Heroin

Antagonist
• Naloxone
• Naltrexone

Mixed Agonist–Antagonist
• Pentazocine
• Butorphanol
• Buprenorphine

TABLE 127.3 Commonly Used Psychostimulants
Dextroamphetamine
Methamphetamine
Ephedrine
Pseudoephedrine
Methylphenidate
Pemoline
Phenmetrazine
Phentermine
Phenylpropanolamine (no longer produced in the United States)
Methylenedioxymethamphetamine (MDMA; ecstasy)
Cocaine
Cathinone, methcathinone

PSYCHOSTIMULANTS

Psychostimulants include amphetamine-like agents and cocaine (Table 127.3). 3,4-methylenedioxymethamphetamine (MDMA; "ecstasy") appears to combine the psychostimulant properties of amphetamine with the hallucinogenic properties of lysergic acid diethylamide (LSD). An East African–Arabian shrub, khat (*Catha edulis*), is chewed for the effects of its psychoactive ingredient cathinone. A related and easily manufactured compound, methcathinone, as well as numerous designer analogs, are marketed as "bath salts" in Europe and North America. Also available are designer psychostimulants chemically characterized as aminoindanes, piperazines, and pipradol.

Desired effects of psychostimulants include alert euphoria with increased motor activity and physical endurance. Taken parenterally or smoked as alkaloidal cocaine ("crack") or methamphetamine ("ice"), psychostimulants produce a rush clearly distinguishable from that of opioids. With repeated use, there is stereotypic activity progressing to bruxism or other dyskinesias and paranoia progressing to frank hallucinatory psychosis. Overdose causes headache, chest pain, tachycardia, hypertension, flushing, sweating, fever, and excitement. There may be delirium, cardiac arrhythmia, myoclonus, seizures, myoglobinuria, shock, coma, and death. Malignant hyperthermia and disseminated intravascular coagulation are described. Treatment includes benzodiazepine sedation, oxygen, bicarbonate for acidosis, anticonvulsants, cooling, an antihypertensive (preferably an α-blocker such as phenoxybenzamine or a direct vasodilator such as sodium nitroprusside), respiratory and blood pressure (BP) support, and cardiac monitoring.

Psychostimulant withdrawal produces fatigue, depression, and increased hunger and sleep. Objective signs are few, but depression or somnolence can require treatment or even hospitalization.

An effective pharmacotherapy for psychostimulant dependence does not exist.

SEDATIVES

Sedative agents include barbiturates, benzodiazepines, and miscellaneous products (Table 127.4). Desired effects and overdose both resemble ethanol intoxication, although respiratory depression is much milder with benzodiazepines. Treatment is supportive; for severe benzodiazepine poisoning, there is a specific antagonist, flumazenil. Withdrawal causes tremor and seizures, which can be prevented or treated with titrated doses of a benzodiazepine such as lorazepam 5 mg every 4 hours. Delirium tremens is a medical emergency requiring intensive care.

γ-Hydroxybutyric acid (GHB) and two of its precursors, γ-butyrolactone and 1,4-butanediol, are notorious as "date rape" drugs. Often taken with ethanol, they cause sedation and respiratory depression. Treatment is supportive. Dependence occurs and withdrawal signs resemble those of other sedatives and ethanol, including seizures and delirium tremens.

MARIJUANA

Marijuana, from the hemp plant *Cannabis sativa*, contains many cannabinoid compounds, of which the principal psychoactive

TABLE 127.4 Sedative/Hypnotic Drugs
Barbiturates
• Phenobarbital
• Primidone
• Amobarbital
• Butalbital (only in mixtures, e.g., Fioricet)
• Pentobarbital
• Secobarbital
• Methohexital
• Thiopental
Benzodiazepines
• Alprazolam
• Clorazepate
• Chlordiazepoxide
• Diazepam
• Lorazepam
• Oxazepam
• Flurazepam
• Temazepam
• Triazolam
• Clonazepam
• Midazolam
Miscellaneous Agents
• Buspirone
• Chloral hydrate
• Paraldehyde
• Diphenhydramine
• Ethchlorvynol
• Glutethimide
• Hydroxyzine
• Meprobamate
• Methaqualone (no longer produced in the United States)
• Zolpidem
• Zaleplon
• γ-Hydroxybutyric acid

agent is δ-9-tetrahydrocannabinol (THC). Hashish refers to preparations made from the plant resin, which contains high concentrations of psychoactive cannabinoids. δ-9-THC acts at cannabinoid receptors in the brain, and the pharmaceutical development of synthetic receptor agonists was soon followed by their availability as recreational agents. Marketed as "Spice" or "K2," they are often many times more potent than δ-9-THC.

Usually smoked, marijuana produces a relaxed dreamy euphoria, often with jocularity, disinhibition, depersonalization, subjective slowing of time, conjunctival injection, tachycardia, and postural hypotension. High doses cause auditory or visual hallucinations, confusion, and psychosis, but fatal overdose has not been documented. Withdrawal symptoms, other than craving, are minimal; there may be jitteriness, anorexia, and headache. Psychic dependence is common, however.

HALLUCINOGENS

Hallucinogenic plants are used ritualistically or recreationally around the world. In the United States, the most popular agents are the indolealkylamines psilocybin and psilocin (from several mushroom species), the phenylalkylamine mescaline (from the peyote cactus), and the synthetic ergot compound LSD. Increasingly popular is the herb *Salvia divinorum*, which contains the kappa-opioid receptor agonist salviorum A. Other synthetic hallucinogens carry such street names as "fly" and "dragonfly."

The acute effects of hallucinogens are perceptual (distortions or hallucinations, usually visual and elaborately formed), psychologic (depersonalization or altered mood), and somatic (dizziness, tremor, and paresthesia). Some users experience paranoia or panic and some, days to months after use, have flashbacks, the spontaneous recurrence of drug symptoms without taking the drug. High doses of LSD cause hypertension, obtundation, and seizures, but fatalities are usually the result of accidents or suicide. Treatment of overdose consists of a calm environment, reassurance, and, if necessary, a benzodiazepine. Withdrawal symptoms do not occur.

INHALANTS

Recreational inhalant use is especially popular among children and adolescents, who sniff a wide variety of products, including aerosols, spot removers, glues, lighter fluid, fire-extinguishing agents, bottled fuel gas, marker pens, paints, and gasoline. Compounds include aliphatic hydrocarbons such as *n*-hexane, aromatic hydrocarbons such as toluene, and halogenated hydrocarbons such as trichloroethylene; in addition, nitrous oxide is sniffed from whipped-cream dispensers and butyl or amyl nitrite from room odorizers. Despite such chemical diversity, desired subjective effects are similar to those of ethanol intoxication. Overdose can cause hallucinations, seizures, and coma; death has resulted from cardiac arrhythmia, accidents, and aspiration of vomitus. Symptoms tend to clear within a few hours, and treatment consists of respiratory and cardiac monitoring. There is no predictable abstinence syndrome other than craving.

PHENCYCLIDINE

Developed as an anesthetic, phencyclidine hydrochloride (PCP or "angel dust") was withdrawn because it caused psychosis. As a recreational drug, it is usually smoked. The related agents ketamine, dextromethorphan, and methoxetamine are also used recreationally. Low doses of PCP cause euphoria or dysphoria and a feeling of numbness; with increasing intoxication, there is agitation, nystagmus, tachycardia, hypertension, fever, sweating, ataxia, paranoid

or catatonic psychosis, hallucinations, myoclonus, rhabdomyolysis, seizures, coma, respiratory depression, and death. Treatment includes a calm environment with benzodiazepine sedation and restraints as needed, gastric suctioning, activated charcoal, forced diuresis, cooling, antihypertensives, anticonvulsants, and monitoring of cardiorespiratory and renal function. Neuroleptics, which can aggravate seizures, hypotension, and myoglobinuria, are best avoided. Symptoms can persist for hours or days. Psychic dependence to PCP occurs, but withdrawal signs are infrequent, usually consisting of nervousness, tremor, and upset stomach.

ANTICHOLINERGICS

The recreational use of anticholinergics includes ingestion of the plant *Datura stramonium*, popular among American adolescents, as well as use of antiparkinson drugs and the tricyclic antidepressant amitriptyline. Intoxication produces decreased sweating, fever, tachycardia, dry mouth, dilated unreactive pupils, and delirium with hallucinations. Severe poisoning causes myoclonus, seizures, coma, and death. Treatment includes intravenous (IV) physostigmine, 0.5 to 3 mg, repeated as needed every 30 minutes to 2 hours, plus gastric lavage, cooling, bladder catheterization, respiratory and cardiovascular monitoring, and, if necessary, anticonvulsants. Neuroleptics, which have anticholinergic activity, are contraindicated. There is no withdrawal syndrome.

COMPLICATIONS OF DRUG TOXIDROMES

TRAUMA

Trauma may be a consequence of a drug's acute effects, for example, automobile and other accidents during marijuana, inhalant, or anticholinergic intoxication; violence in psychostimulant or PCP users; and self-mutilation during hallucinogen psychosis. Trauma among users of illicit drugs, however, is most often the result of the illegal activities necessary to distribute and procure them. Overprescribing of sedatives is a major contributor to falls in the elderly.

INFECTION

Parenteral users of any drug are subject to an array of local and systemic infections, which in turn can affect the nervous system. Hepatitis leads to encephalopathy or hemorrhagic stroke. Cellulitis and pyogenic myositis produce more distant infection, including vertebral osteomyelitis with myelopathy or radiculopathy. Endocarditis, bacterial or fungal, leads to meningitis, cerebral infarction or abscess, and septic ("mycotic") aneurysm. Tetanus, often severe, affects drug injectors, and botulism occurs either at injection sites or, among cocaine snorters, in the nasal sinuses. Malaria affects heroin users in endemic areas. Anthrax has affected users of contaminated heroin.

Parenteral drug use is a major risk factor for HIV infection. Users are subject to the same neurologic complications that affect nondrug users, especially syphilis and tuberculosis, including drug-resistant forms. Because of promiscuity and associated sexually transmitted diseases, nonparenteral cocaine users are also at increased risk for AIDS. Heroin and cocaine are themselves immunosuppressants (heroin users were vulnerable to unusual fungal infections before the AIDS epidemic), yet their use in HIV-seropositive individuals does not seem to accelerate the development of AIDS.

Progressive myelopathy occurs in parenteral drug users infected with either human T-lymphotropic virus (HTLV)-I or HTLV-II.

SEIZURES

Seizures are a feature of withdrawal from sedatives, including, infrequently, benzodiazepines. Methaqualone (no longer legally available in the United States) and glutethimide have reportedly caused seizures during intoxication. Opioids lower seizure threshold, but seizures are seldom encountered during heroin overdose. Myoclonus and seizures more often occur in meperidine users, a consequence of the active metabolite normeperidine. Seizures may occur in cocaine users without other evidence of overdose. In animals, repeated cocaine administration produces seizures in a pattern suggestive of kindling. Amphetamine and other psychostimulants are less epileptogenic than cocaine, but seizures did affect users of the no longer legal over-the-counter anorectic phenylpropanolamine. A case-control study found that marijuana was protective against the development of new-onset seizures. In animal studies, the nonpsychoactive cannabinoid compound cannabidiol is anticonvulsant.

STROKE

Illicit drug users frequently abuse ethanol and tobacco, increasing their risk for ischemic and hemorrhagic stroke. Parenteral drug users are subject to stroke through systemic complications such as hepatitis, endocarditis, and AIDS. Heroin users develop nephropathy with secondary hypertension, uremia, and bleeding. Heroin has also caused stroke in the absence of other evident risk factors, perhaps through immunologic mechanisms.

Amphetamine users are prone to intracerebral hemorrhage following acute hypertension and fever. They are also at risk for occlusive stroke secondary to cerebral vasculitis affecting either medium-sized arteries (resembling polyarteritis nodosa) or smaller arteries and veins (resembling hypersensitivity angiitis). Ischemic and hemorrhagic stroke is also a frequent consequence of cocaine use, regardless of route of administration. Over 600 cases have been reported, roughly half hemorrhagic and half ischemic. Most hemorrhagic strokes are probably consequent to acute surges of hypertension; most ischemic strokes are probably secondary to cocaine's vasoconstrictive actions on cervical and intracranial circulation. Cerebral saccular aneurysms and vascular malformations are often found in patients undergoing angiography for cocaine-related intracranial hemorrhage.

Because of their association with stroke, diet pills and decongestants containing phenylpropanolamine were banned by the U.S. Food and Drug Administration (FDA). Similar association led to a number of states banning dietary supplements containing ephedra. Intracerebral and subarachnoid hemorrhages are described in MDMA users.

Anecdotal and epidemiologic reports describe marijuana use as a risk factor for ischemic stroke. A proposed mechanism is reversible cerebral vasoconstriction. Ischemic stroke was reported in young smokers of the synthetic cannabinoid Spice.

LSD and PCP are vasoconstrictive, and occlusive and hemorrhagic strokes have followed their use.

ALTERED MENTATION

Dementia in illicit drug users may be the result of concomitant ethanol abuse, malnutrition, head trauma, or infection. Parenteral drug users are at risk for HIV encephalopathy. Whether the drugs themselves cause lasting cognitive or behavioral change is more difficult to establish, for predrug mental status is nearly always uncertain and many drug users are probably self-medicating preexisting psychiatric conditions (e.g., cocaine for depression).

Clinical studies describe significant impairments in working memory, verbal fluency, and "cognitive impulsivity" among users of opioids, including prescription opioids and methadone maintenance therapy. Functional imaging studies demonstrate reduced cerebral gray matter density, decreased white matter fractional anisotropy, and abnormal connectivity patterns.

Controversy exists over whether psychostimulants predispose to lasting depression or if PCP predisposes to schizophrenia. In animals and humans, methamphetamine damages both dopaminergic and serotonergic nerve terminals and MDMA destroys serotonin nerve terminals. Impaired memory is described in abstinent methamphetamine users, and among MDMA users followed prospectively, only a few years of use was associated with cognitive decline and abnormal fractional anisotropy in multiple brain areas.

Cocaine is not neurotoxic to axon terminals, but impaired cognition is described as well as morphologic abnormalities in hippocampus, frontostriatal and limbic systems, and cerebral white matter.

Clinical, imaging, and animal studies convincingly demonstrate that marijuana use, especially during adolescence, causes lasting behavioral and cognitive alteration. Long-term marijuana users demonstrate axonal microstructural alterations and volume reductions in brain regions rich in cannabinoid receptors. Epidemiologic studies provide persuasive evidence that marijuana is a significant risk factor for schizophrenia.

Sedatives can cause reversible dementia in the elderly and delayed learning in small children.

Lead encephalopathy is described in gasoline sniffers, and cerebral white matter lesions with dementia are described in toluene sniffers.

FETAL EFFECTS

The effects of illicit drugs on intrauterine development are also difficult to separate from damage secondary to ethanol, tobacco, malnutrition, and inadequate prenatal care or home environment. Infants exposed in utero to heroin have reportedly been small for gestational age, at risk for respiratory distress, and cognitively impaired later in life.

Prenatal methamphetamine exposure is an independent risk factor for fetal growth restriction. Studies of cocaine's fetal effects, including cognitive, are conflicting. Studies have described impaired memory and language and brain morphologic abnormalities. A 10-year prospective study controlling for such confounders as additional drugs and environmental influences concluded that first-trimester cocaine exposure confers risk for reduced height, weight, and head circumference and for abnormal behavior. Animal studies demonstrate that in utero cocaine exposure detrimentally affects learning.

Long-term cohort studies of in utero marijuana exposure have demonstrated impaired attention and memory and smaller head size. Animal studies show abnormal axonal connectivity. Organic solvents are teratogenic in animals.

MISCELLANEOUS EFFECTS

Guillain–Barré-type neuropathy and *brachial* or *lumbosacral plexopathy*, probably immunologic in origin, have been associated with heroin use. (Brachial plexopathy has also resulted from septic aneurysm of the subclavian artery.) Severe sensorimotor polyneuropathy occurs in sniffers of glue containing *n*-hexane. *Myoglobinuria* and renal failure have followed use of heroin, amphetamine, cocaine, and PCP.

Myeloneuropathy indistinguishable from cobalamin deficiency occurs in nitrous oxide sniffers. Anemia is absent, and serum vitamin B$_{12}$ levels are usually normal. The mechanism is inactivation of the cobalamin-dependent enzyme methionine synthetase.

Possibly vascular in origin, acute myelopathy occurs in parenteral heroin users.

Severe irreversible parkinsonism developed in Californians exposed to a meperidine analog contaminated with 1-methyl-4-phenyl-1,2,3,6-tetrahydropyridine (MPTP), a metabolite of which is toxic to neurons in the substantia nigra. Symptoms responded to levodopa.

Dementia, ataxia, quadriparesis, blindness, and *death* occur in smokers of heroin pyrolysate ("chasing the dragon"). Autopsies show spongiform changes in the central nervous system (CNS) white matter. The responsible toxin has not been identified.

Parenteral methcathinone users are subject to *extrapyramidal gait disturbance* and *hypophonia*, a consequence of hypermagnesemia following the use of potassium permanganate in the preparation of the drug.

Blindness developed in a heroin user whose mixture contained large quantities of quinine.

Chronic cocaine users experience *dystonia* and *chorea*, and cocaine can precipitate symptoms in patients with *Tourette syndrome*.

Marijuana inhibits luteinizing and follicle-stimulating hormones, causing *reversible impotence* and *sterility* in men and *menstrual irregularity* in women.

Ataxia and *cerebellar white matter* changes have occurred in toluene sniffers.

Hallucinogen users not only experience flashbacks but, in some cases, visual phenomena persist for years (*hallucinogen-persisting perception disorder*).

U.S. cocaine is frequently adulterated with the immunomodulatory drug levamisole, complications of which include leukopenia, vasculitis, and leukoencephalopathy.

SUGGESTED READINGS

Baldacchino A, Balfour DJK, Passetti F, et al. Neuropsychological consequences of chronic opioid use: a quantitative review and meta-analysis. *Neurosci Biobehav Rev.* 2012;36:2056–2068.

Battistella G, Fornari E, Annoni JM, et al. Long-term effects of cannabis on brain structure. *Neuropsychopharmacology.* 2014;39(9):2041–2048. doi:10.1038/nnp.2014.67.

Bolla KI, Brown K, Eldreth D, et al. Dose-related neurocognitive effects of marijuana use. *Neurology.* 2002;59:1337–1343.

Broussard CS, Rasmussen SA, Reefhuis J, et al. Maternal treatment with opioid analgesics and risk for birth defects. *Am J Obstet Gynecol.* 2011;204:314.e1–e11.

Brust JCM. Cognition and cannabis: from anecdote to advanced technology. *Brain.* 2012;135:2004–2005.

Brust JCM, ed. *Neurological Aspects of Substance Abuse.* 2nd ed. Boston, MA: Butterworth-Heinemann; 2004.

Brust JCM. Seizures, illicit drugs, and ethanol. *Curr Neurol Neurosci Rep.* 2008;8:333–338.

Brust JCM. Spice, pot, and stroke. *Neurology.* 2013;81:2064–2065.

Brust JCM. Stroke and substance abuse. In: Mohr JP, Wolf PA, Grotta JC, et al, eds. *Stroke: Pathophysiology, Diagnosis, and Management.* 5th ed. Philadelphia: Elsevier/Saunders; 2011:790–813.

Brust JCM. Substance abuse and movement disorders. *Mov Disord.* 2010;25:2010–2020.

Buckingham-Howes S, Berger SS, Scaletti LA, et al. Systematic review of prenatal cocaine exposure and adolescent development. *Pediatrics.* 2013;131:e1917–e1937.

Corazza O, Schifano F, Simonato P, et al. Phenomenon of new drugs on the internet: the case of ketamine derivative methoxetamine. *Hum Psychopharmacol.* 2012;27:145–149.

deWin MM, Jager G, Booij J, et al. Sustained effects of ecstasy on the human brain: a prospective imaging study in novel users. *Brain.* 2008;131:2936–2945.

Freeman MJ, Rose DZ, Myers MA, et al. Ischemic stroke after use of the synthetic marijuana "spice." *Neurology.* 2013;81:2090–2093.

Fried PA, Smith AM. A literature review of the consequences of prenatal marijuana exposure. An emerging theme of a deficiency in aspects of executive function. *Neurotoxicol Teratol.* 2001;23:1–11.

Grund JP, Latypov A, Harris M. Breaking worse: the emergence of krokodil and excessive injuries among people who inject drugs in Eurasia. *Int J Drug Policy.* 2013;24:265–274.

Gwira Baumblatt JA, Weideman C, Dunn R, et al. High risk use by patients prescribed opioids for pain and its role in overdose deaths. *JAMA Intern Med.* 2014;174(5):796–801.

Hanczaruk M, Reischi U, Grass G, et al. Injectional anthrax in heroin users. Europe, 2000–2012. *Emerg Infect Dis.* 2014;20(2):322–323.

Hermle L, Simon M, Ruchsow M, et al. Hallucinogen-persisting perception disorder. *Ther Adv.* 2012;2:199–205.

Iverson L, White M, Treble R. Designer psychostimulants: pharmacology and differences. *Neuropharmacology.* 2014;87:59–65. doi:10.1016/j.neuropharm.2014.01.015.

Johanson CE, Frey KA, Lundahl LH, et al. Cognitive function and nigrostriatal markers in abstinent methamphetamine abusers. *Psychopharmacology.* 2006;185:327–338.

Kaufman MJ, Levin JM, Ross MH, et al. Cocaine-induced cerebral vasoconstriction detected in humans with magnetic resonance angiography. *JAMA.* 1998;279:376–380.

Khattak S, K-Moghtader G, McMartin K, et al. Pregnancy outcome following gestational exposure to organic solvents. A prospective controlled study. *JAMA.* 1999;281:1106–1109.

Kosten TR, O'Connor PG. Management of drug and alcohol withdrawal. *N Engl J Med.* 2003;348:1786–1795.

Kriegstein AR, Shungu DC, Millar WS, et al. Leukoencephalopathy and raised brain lactate from heroin vapor inhalation ("chasing the dragon"). *Neurology.* 1999;53:1765–1773.

LaRocque A, Hoffman RS. Levamisole in cocaine: unexpected news from an old acquaintance. *Clin Toxicol.* 2012;50:231–241.

Levine SR, Brust JCM, Futrell N, et al. Cerebrovascular complications of the use of the "crack" form of alkaloidal cocaine. *N Engl J Med.* 1990;323:699–704.

Lineberry TW, Bostwick JM. Methamphetamine abuse: a perfect storm of complications. *Mayo Clin Proc.* 2006;81:77–84.

Mattick RP, Breen C, Kimber J, et al. Buprenorphine maintenance versus placebo or methadone maintenance for opioid dependence. *Cochrane Database Syst Rev.* 2014;2:CD002207.

Meier MH, Caspi A, Ambler A, et al. Persistent cannabis users show neuropsychological decline from childhood to midlife. *Proc Natl Acad U S A.* 2012;109(40):E2657–E2664.

Murphy PN, Wareing M, Fisk JE, et al. Executive working memory deficits in abstinent ecstasy/MDMA users: a critical review. *Neuropsychobiology.* 2009;60:159–175.

Ng SKC, Brust JCM, Hauser WA. Illicit drug use and the risk of new onset seizures. *Am J Epidemiol.* 1990;132:47–57.

Pujol J, Blanco-Hinojo L, Batalla A, et al. Functional connectivity alterations in brain networks relevant to self-awareness in chronic cannabis users. *J Psychiatric Res.* 2014;51:68–78.

Qiu Y, Jiang G, Su H, et al. Progressive white matter microstructure damage in male chronic heroin dependent individuals: a DTI and TBSS study. *PLoS One.* 2013;8(5):e63212. doi:10.137/journal.pone.0663212.

Richardson GA, Goldschmidt L, Larkby C, et al. Effects of prenatal cocaine exposure on child behavior and growth at 10 years of age. *Neurotoxicol Teratol.* 2013;40:1–8. doi:10.1016/j.ntt.2013.08.001.

Rosenbaum CD, Carreiro SP, Babu KM. Here today, gone tomorrow . . . and back again? A review of herbal marijuana alternatives (K2, Spice), synthetic cathinones (bath salts), Kratom, Salvia divinorum, methoxetamine, and piperazines. *J Med Toxicol.* 2012;8:15–32.

Smith LM, LaGrasse LL, Derauf C, et al. The infant development, environment, and lifestyle study: effects of prenatal methamphetamine exposure, polydrug exposure, and poverty on intrauterine growth. *Pediatrics.* 2006;118:1149–1156.

Stephens A, Logina I, Liguts V, et al. A parkinsonian syndrome in methcathinone users and the role of manganese. *N Engl J Med.* 2008;358:1009–1017.

Tarabar AF, Nelson LS. The gamma-hydroxybutyrate withdrawal syndrome. *Toxicol Rev.* 2004;23:45–49.

Tortoriello G, Morris CV, Alpar A. Miswiring the brain: delta-9-tetrahydrocannabinol disrupts cortical development by inducing an SCG10/stathmin-2 degradation pathway. *EMBO J.* 2014;33:668–685.

Van Winkel R, Kuepper R. Epidemiological, neurobiological, and genetic clues to the mechanisms linking cannabis use to risk for nonaffective psychosis. *Annu Rev Clin Psychol.* 2014;10:767–791.

Volkow ND, Baler RD, Compton WM, et al. Adverse health effects of marijuana use. *N Engl J Med.* 2014;370:2219–2227.

Wang Y, Zhu J, Li Q, et al. Altered fronto-striatal and fronto-cerebellar circuits in heroin-dependent individuals: a resting-state FMRI study. *PLoS One.* 2013;8(3):e58098. doi:10.1371/journal.pone.0058098.

Weiner WJ, Rubinstein A, Lewin B, et al. Cocaine-induced persistent dyskinesias. *Neurology.* 2001;56:964–965.

Westover AN, McBride S, Haley RW. Stroke in young adults who abuse amphetamines and cocaine. A population-based study of hospitalized patients. *Arch Gen Psychiatry.* 2007;64:495–502.

Wolff V, Armspach JP, Lauer V, et al. Cannabis-associated stroke: myth or reality? *Stroke.* 2013;44:558–563.

Zvosec D, Smith SW, McCutcheon Jr, et al. Adverse events, including death, associated with the use of 1,4-butanediol. *N Engl J Med.* 2001;344:87–94.

INTRODUCTION

Xenobiotics are substances within an organism that are not normally found in or produced by that organism. *Neurotoxicology* refers to the adverse effects of xenobiotics, or poisons, on the nervous system. This is a massive field with well over 350 documented neurotoxic xenobiotics. To facilitate digestibility and clinical use of the topic, this chapter will focus on acute neurotoxicology. Chronic neurotoxic associations and syndromes will be listed and briefly described. Neurotoxicology with reference to neurodevelopment, withdrawal syndromes, and psychiatric disorders, such as psychosis and mood disorders, will be minimally discussed.

Xenobiotics can include medications; industrial chemicals such as heavy metals, air pollution, solvents, and vapors; substances produced by other organisms (e.g., marine toxins, snake venom); food additives; herbal products and botanicals; recreational drugs; and insecticides, herbicides, rodenticides, and other household products. Acute neurotoxic events have been better described and causational links are more convincing. Neurotoxic effects from chronic exposures are more challenging to prove, as the clinical symptoms may be temporally distant from the exposure or the concentration of the xenobiotic in the organism is so low that it may be difficult to detect.

EPIDEMIOLOGY

The specific incidence, prevalence, and demographics of specific neurotoxins, where available, will be mentioned individually in the following sections. Age, gender, and certain comorbidities have been associated with the occurrence and severity of various toxicity syndromes.

Clinical toxicity is more commonly seen in older patients for several reasons. Age-related decrements in renal and hepatic function impair the ability to clear and eliminate xenobiotics. Reductions in neuronal quantity increase the sensitivity to the presence of xenobiotics. Finally, changes in mitochondrial function are known to occur with advanced age, increasing the possibility of excitotoxicity.

Gender has been associated with certain clinical manifestations in the setting of xenobiotics. Bruxism and dystonia are more prevalent in males, whereas tardive dyskinesia and parkinsonism are more frequently observed in females.

Comorbidities can increase the risk of neurotoxicity if they impair elimination of the xenobiotic (e.g., renal insufficiency or cirrhosis) or facilitate its entry into the central nervous system (CNS) via disturbance of the blood–brain barrier (e.g., meningitis, encephalitis). The presence of or prior exposure to other nonneurotoxic xenobiotics (e.g., prescription medications) can influence the relative neurotoxicity of a xenobiotic by impairing its metabolism or elimination; hastening its conversion to a neurotoxic metabolite; and altering gene expression, neurotransmitter production, release, breakdown, and neurotransmitter receptor density

or function. Efflux transporters on the blood–brain barrier, such as P-glycoproteins and organic acid transport proteins, are typically responsible for shuttling xenobiotics out of the CNS. Some medications and conditions are known to inhibit the function of P-glycoproteins (Table 128.1), increasing the concentration of the neurotoxic xenobiotics in the CNS. Some nutrition inadequacies, such as heavy metal deficiencies, can enhance the uptake of neurotoxic xenobiotics. Lastly, some neurologic disorders can be unmasked with the introduction of a xenobiotic (Table 128.2).

PATHOBIOLOGY

For neurotoxicity to occur, a xenobiotic must come into contact with the nervous system. CNS toxicity occurs when certain xenobiotics cross the blood–brain barrier via endocytosis, transport proteins, or diffusion. Lipophilic xenobiotics gain entry via diffusion, whereas hydrophilic ones must engage with one of the two other mechanisms.

Neurotoxicity occurs through a variety of mechanisms that are summarized in Table 128.3. The most elusive mechanism to associate with a xenobiotic are those that alter gene expression, as the appearance of clinical toxicity may not occur until the xenobiotic has been eliminated from the system. *Excitotoxicity* is a common end point for several of the neurotoxic xenobiotics whether it is through activation of excitatory pathways or via retarded energy production, which leads to metabolic failure in the setting of neuroexcitation.

Neurotoxicity can manifest pathophysiologically as central or peripheral demyelination, neuronal death, clinical syndromes

TABLE 128.1	Selected P-glycoprotein Inhibitors and Inducers	
Inhibitors	**Inducers**
• Amiodarone	• Avasimibe
• Ceftriaxone	• Carbamazepine
• Clarithromycin, erythromycin	• Clotrimazole
• Cyclosporine	• Phenytoin
• Diltiazem	• Phenobarbital
• Hydrocortisone	• Rifampin
• Ketoconazole, itraconazole	• St. John's wort
• Nicardipine	• Tipranavir/ritonavir
• Propranolol	• Prazosin
• Ritonavir, saquinavir, nelfinavir	• Progesterone
• Tamoxifen	
• Tacrolimus	
• Verapamil	

TABLE 128.2	Neurologic Disorders Unmasked by Xenobiotics
Xenobiotic	**Neurologic Disorder**
Aminoglycosides	Myasthenia gravis
Vincristine	Charcot–Marie–tooth
Antiretrovirals	HIV-related peripheral neuropathy

related to the activation or inhibition of neurotransmitter pathways, or impaired function due to disrupted neuronal or glial processes.

CLINICAL FEATURES

Neurotoxic presentations are protean and may include seizures or status epilepticus, ataxia, tremor, encephalopathy, movement disorders, peripheral neuropathies, lethargy, stupor, coma, cognitive impairment, neuropsychiatric behavioral disturbances, or diffuse weakness. Lateralization of neurologic deficits is uncommon unless the toxicity is unmasking a prior neurologic insult.

Seizures are a not uncommon neurotoxic presentation. Table 128.4 lists some xenobiotics known to cause seizures. A variety of movement disorders have been reported to be caused by xenobiotics, including dyskinesias, akathisia, chorea, parkinsonism, dystonias, myoclonus, and asterixis (Table 128.5). Tremors associated with xenobiotics, which can be resting, sustention, or kinetic, are summarized in Table 128.6. Medications and toxins known to cause ataxia are listed in Table 128.7. Cranial and/or peripheral neuropathies can be the result of demyelination, axonal injury, or failed transmission at the neuromuscular junction (NMJ) or of the action potential and present with diffuse weakness, autonomic dysfunction, and/or sensory disturbances. Tables 128.8 and 128.9 summarize xenobiotics associated with each of these mechanisms. Lastly, Table 128.10 lists xenobiotics associated with myopathies, which present with diffuse myalgias and weakness.

TABLE 128.3	Mechanisms of Neurotoxicity	
Cellular	**Membrane**	**Cellular Signaling**
• Oxidative injury/ neuroexcitation	• Disrupted ion homeostasis	• Altered neurotransmitter production, release, metabolism, or uptake
• Disturbed energy production	• Antagonism/ agonism of ion channels	• Blunted or exaggerated neurotransmitter receptor activation
• Altered gene expression or transcription		• Mimics neurotransmitter, stimulating receptor
• Altered protein function or structure		

DIAGNOSIS

Many of the neurotoxic xenobiotics or their metabolites can be detected in the serum, urine, or other body tissues or fluids. Of note, the detection of a neurotoxic xenobiotic should not universally lead the clinician to conclude that it is the culprit for the clinical complaint or ailment. The clinical symptoms should be consistent with a well-documented neurotoxicity or syndrome in a patient with a known exposure to the toxin. Otherwise, a neurotoxin can be suspected to be the cause of the clinical symptoms, but other etiologies should be excluded. Improving symptoms in the setting of neurotoxin elimination serves to increase confidence in the diagnosis of neurotoxicity. Additional diagnostic clues can be obtained when certain odors are perceived that are suggestive of a particular xenobiotic (Table 128.11).

TREATMENT

In any acute neurotoxic presentation, the first steps are to rule out hypoglycemia and remove the victim from the exposure. If the toxin is on the patient's clothing or skin, they should be promptly decontaminated. Health care workers should employ universal precautions when approaching such patients to prevent self-exposure. Entry into an enclosed environment should be delayed until decontamination can be performed so as to not poison other patients or health care providers. If providing glucose, *thiamine 100 mg* intravenous (IV) should be considered prior to doing so as to not induce Korsakoff syndrome in those with a (relative) thiamine deficiency. In hypopneic or apneic patients with miotic pupils, *naloxone 0.4 to 2.0 mg IV* can be administered to reverse a potential opiate overdose.

The core components of treating any neurotoxic presentation include reducing absorption of the toxin, enhancing its elimination, provision of an antidote, and supportive care. Performing gastric lavage, administering activated charcoal, and/or providing whole bowel irrigation (WBI) has the potential to reduce the absorption of an ingested xenobiotic.

Gastric lavage has largely become antiquated, as it is resource intensive, often requires endotracheal intubation, and has not been objectively shown to be beneficial. However, it still has a role in the hyperacute ingestions (within 1 hour) of highly toxic substances that are not effectively absorbed by activated charcoal and do not have an effective antidote. Due to the risk for inadvertent aspiration, hydrocarbons and alkaline caustics should not be lavaged.

Similarly, the use of activated charcoal has decreased over the years, as published evidence has failed to demonstrate appreciable efficacy. It is not to be used in those with a depressed level of consciousness, at risk for aspiration, and after some ingestions (Table 128.12). WBI can be considered in those with an ingestion of a highly toxic sustained-release medication or xenobiotics that are not absorbed by activated charcoal.

Options for enhanced elimination include the provision of hemodialysis, hemoperfusion, urinary alkalinization, and rarely, exchange transfusion. The elimination of protein-bound xenobiotics is not appreciably enhanced with dialysis.

Table 128.13 summarizes some neurotoxins and their antidotes. Benzodiazepines are the preferred treatment for neurotoxin-induced seizures. Ion channel dysfunction is a not uncommon mechanism for several of the seizure-inducing neurotoxins, which may be made worse with the administration of many of the commonly used antiepileptics (e.g., phenytoin or valproic acid).

TABLE 128.4   Xenobiotics Known to Induce Seizures

Xenobiotic Category	Specific Agents	Xenobiotic Category	Specific Agents
Antihistamines	**Diphenhydramine**, doxylamine	Methylxanthines	Caffeine, **theophylline**
Anticholinergics	Benztropine mesylate, scopolamine	Other medications	Levodopa, baclofen, levothyroxine, allopurinol, bromocriptine, colchicine, corticosteroids
Antibiotics	**Isoniazid**, beta-lactams (penicillins, cephalosporins, carbapenems), ciprofloxacin	Alcohols	Ethylene glycol, methanol
Antivirals	Acyclovir, valacyclovir, amantadine	Recreational drugs	Cocaine, MDMA (ecstasy or molly), amphetamines, phencyclidine, nicotine
Antimalarials	**Chloroquine**, mefloquine, pyrimethamine	Rodenticides	**Tetramethylenedisulfotetramine (TETS)**, thallium, zinc phosphide, arsenic
Nonsteroidal anti-inflammatories	Mefenamic acid, phenylbutazone (veterinary NSAID), ibuprofen, naproxen, salicylates	Pesticides/insecticides	Pyrethrins (insecticides), organochlorines (e.g., Lindane), organic phosphorus compounds (e.g., Malathion)
Opioids	*Meperidine*, propoxyphene, tramadol	Botanicals	**Cicutoxin** (water hemlock), picrotoxin (*Anamirta cocculus*, plant and performance enhancers), ackee fruit, daphne, rhododendrons
Local anesthetics	Bupivacaine, lidocaine, procaine, tetracaine	Heavy metals	Thallium, arsenic, copper, lead, nickel, manganese
Antiepileptics	Phenytoin, carbamazepine, valproic acid, ethosuximide	Household and industrial toxins	Carbon monoxide, **camphor**, cyanide, fluoride, phenols (e.g., paint strippers), 1,4-dichlorobenzene (e.g., mothballs), **monomethylhydrazine (rocket fuel)**, carbon disulfide, hydrogen sulfide, methyl bromide, triazine, various hydrocarbons, chlorophenoxy herbicides
Antineoplastics	Bleomycin, busulphan, carmustine, chlorambucil, cisplatin, cytarabine, mechlorethamine, methotrexate, vinblastine, vincristine		
Antidepressants	***Bupropion***, fluoxetine, maprotiline, mianserin, trazodone		
Tricyclic antidepressants	All of them	Ingestion	Domoic acid (amnestic shellfish poisoning), **ciguatera** (moray eels, barracuda, red snapper) tetrodotoxin (puffer fish species, blue-ringed octopus, horseshoe crab), **gyromitrin (*Gyromitra* fungus species)**, herbals (lobelia, passion flower, periwinkle, wormwood, *Galega*, mandrake, jimson weed).
Antipsychotics, mood stabilizers	All antipsychotics, especially *chlorpromazine, clozapine*, and *phenothiazines*, lithium		
Stimulants	Methylphenidates, pemoline		
Antiemetics	*Prochlorperazine*, metoclopramide, *promethazine*, droperidol		
Cardiovascular drugs	Propranolol, flecainide, digoxin		
Ergotamines	Dihydroergotamine, ergotamine	Envenomations	Pit viper, tick bite, scorpion

The **xenobiotics** in **bold** are reported to have caused status epilepticus, and those in *italics* frequently cause seizures. **Strychnine poisoning** causes nonepileptic convulsions and is intentionally excluded from these lists.
MDMA, 3,4-methylenedioxymethamphetamine.

OUTCOME

Outcomes following a neurotoxin exposure are dependent on the pathophysiology of the neurotoxic insult. Mechanisms that lead to neuronal injury or death are more likely to produce permanent deficits than mechanisms that interfere with the functioning of neurotransmitters or cell signaling. In some circumstances, toxins that alter cell signaling or action potential propagation can lead to permanent changes in the structure, function, or density of neurotransmitter receptors or ion channels, increasing the possibility of lasting effects. Many of the toxicities are dependent on the peak concentration of the toxin in the patient and its concentration over time. Clinical outcomes can be worsened with delays in toxic elimination or the provision of an antidote. Reexposure tends to produce exponentially severe clinical symptoms, which are more likely to be permanent.

COMMON NEUROTOXIDROMES

Neurotoxins with similar mechanisms of action typically produce distinct syndromes that allow for their clinical recognition and commonalities in their treatment. This section will summarize several syndromes, provide lists of known culprit neurotoxins, outline treatment options, and describe their expected clinical outcomes.

ANTICHOLINERGIC TOXICITY

Approximately 20,000 patients are exposed to anticholinergic xenobiotics per year. This is likely an underestimate, as this only accounts for the recognized and reported cases. To be specific, these substances have antimuscarinic properties that produce their characteristic clinical symptoms. Xenobiotics with antinicotinic actions are separate and distinct from those mentioned here. Hundreds of medications have anticholinergic properties, which

TABLE 128.5 Movement Disorders Associated with Xenobiotics

Chorea	Dystonia	Reversible Parkinsonism	Irreversible Parkinsonism
• Anticholinergics	• Anticholinergics	• Carbon disulfide	• Calcium channel blockers
• Antiepileptics	• Dopamine antagonists	• Carbon monoxide	• Chemotherapeutics (several)
• Levodopa	• Levodopa	• Copper	• Cyclosporine
• Amantadine		• Cyanide	• Antipsychotics
• Bromocriptine		• Heroin	• Antiemetics
• Carbon monoxide		• Manganese	• Sertraline
• Corticosteroids		• MPTP	• Valproate
• Dopamine antagonists			• Trazodone
• Toluene			• Progesterone
• Sympathomimetics			• Kava-kava
• Oral contraceptives			
• Lithium			

Dyskinesia	Akathisia	Myoclonus
• Antidopaminergics	• Antidepressants	• Anticholinergics
• Calcium channel blockers	• Antidopaminergics	• Antiepileptics
	• Calcium channel blockers	• Sedatives/hypnotics
	• Tetrabenazine	• Bismuth
	• AMPT	• Ethanol
		• Lead
		• Levodopa
		• Mercury
		• Tricyclic antidepressants

MPTP, 1-methyl-4-phenyl-1,2,3,6-tetrahydropyridine; AMPT, alpha-methyl-p-tyrosine.

places many patients at risk for subtle toxicities that may manifest in mild behavioral or cognitive disturbances.

Clinical Features

Clinical symptoms of anticholinergic toxicity are summarized in Table 128.14 and are secondary to antimuscarinic actions. Patients rarely have all of the associated symptoms; tachycardia and dry mucous membranes are the most commonly seen. The most severe exposures produce hyperthermia, coma, and/or seizures. Xenobiotics with antimuscarinic activity are summarized in Table 128.15. Note that ophthalmic drops are absorbed systemically and therefore can produce anticholinergic symptoms in the setting of liberal administration. Additionally, recreational drugs have been contaminated with anticholinergic adulterants on more than one occasion (e.g., heroin tainted with scopolamine).

Treatment

Treatment is largely supportive. Hyperthermia should be rapidly corrected with conductive and evaporative measures. Agitation and seizures should be controlled with benzodiazepines such as *lorazepam* 2–4 mg IV repeated as needed. Antipsychotics should be avoided, as they lower the seizure threshold and nearly all of them have antimuscarinic actions as well (see Table 128.15). Antiepileptics are typically not effective in the treatment of anticholinergic-induced seizures and their action on ion channels may increase the

risk for cardiac arrhythmias. Status epilepticus is rarely the result of antimuscarinic toxicity; if present, other etiologies should be considered.

Physostigmine is an acetylcholinesterase inhibitor that has been used to treat anticholinergic toxicity and is the only acetylcholinesterase inhibitor that crosses the blood–brain barrier. A dose of 0.02 mg/kg can be given over 5 minutes and repeated every 10 to 15 minutes. It has a rapid onset and short duration of action (~1 hour). Extreme caution must be exercised when using physostigmine, as it may produce symptoms of cholinergic toxicity, severe bradycardia, and even asystole. Anticholinergic toxicity is quite rarely fatal with supportive therapy; therefore, the use of physostigmine is rarely justified, given its associated risks. It is contraindicated in atrioventricular and intraventricular conduction delays and in tricyclic antidepressant toxicity.

SYMPATHOMIMETIC TOXICITY AND ACUTE EXCITED STATE

The clinical presentation of patients with a toxin-induced excited delirium and those with sympathomimetic toxicity is largely indistinguishable. The risk factors, patient characteristics, and management are largely the same as well, so they will be discussed together. Some pertinent idiosyncrasies of some of the xenobiotics will be mentioned. Table 128.16 summarizes the various agents known to cause excited delirium.

TABLE 128.6 **Xenobiotics Associated with Tremors**

Resting Tremor	Sustention Tremor	Kinetic Tremor
• Hypoglycemics	• Amiodarone	• Amiodarone
• Calcium channel blockers	• Hypoglycemics	• Hypoglycemics
• Antidopaminergics	• Methylxanthines	• Sedative/hypnotics
• Carbon disulfide	• Carbon disulfide	• Carbamazepine
• Carbon monoxide	• Carbon monoxide	• Colistin
• Captopril	• Antidopaminergics	• Lithium
• Lithium	• Sympathomimetics	• Phenytoin
• Manganese	• MAOIs	• Valproic acid
• Methanol	• TCAs	
• MPTP	• Ethanol	
• Phenytoin	• Sedative/hypnotics	
• Tetrabenazine	• Phenytoin	
	• Valproic acid	
	• Phencyclidine	
	• Corticosteroids	
	• Arsenic, lead	
	• Lithium	
	• Levodopa	

MAOIs, monoamine oxidase inhibitors; TCAs, tricyclic antidepressants; MPTP, 1-methyl-4-phenyl-1,2,3,6-tetrahydropyridine .

Widespread use of prescription, botanical, and recreational stimulants and hallucinogens has brought the neurotoxic effects of these substances into daily clinical conversation. There are well over 100,000 presentations to emergency departments each year in the United States related to these xenobiotics. Their neurotoxic effects are exerted through manipulation of the mechanisms carried out by the central monoamine neurotransmitters (serotonin, norepinephrine, and dopamine). This includes increased neurotransmitter release, exaggerated effects at its postsynaptic receptor, decreased neurotransmitter breakdown, and receptor agonism or antagonism, among other mechanisms. In several cases, the culprit xenobiotic's effects are not isolated to one neurotransmitter or receptor, making their clinical manifestations less predictable and reliable.

Clinical Features

Clinically, these patients will present with hypervigilance, agitation, paranoia, hallucinations, stereotyping, dyskinesias, choreoathetoid movements, tachycardia, hypertension, mydriasis, and/or diaphoresis. More severe toxicity can cause delirium, combativeness, severe hyperthermia (>40°C), and seizures. Wide complex tachycardia can be seen in the setting of cocaine- (due to its sodium channel blockade) or rhabdomyolysis-induced hyperkalemia. The patient may have a depressed level of consciousness due to other co-ingested intoxicants. Diaphoresis is absent in anticholinergic toxicity, making this finding suggestive of excited delirium. However, it can be absent in sympathomimetic toxicity if the patient is volume depleted.

Diagnosis

Diagnosis is largely based on the clinical presentation and history. When the circumstances are unknown, the provider must exclude life-threatening, treatable etiologies, such as an intracranial hemorrhage, status epilepticus, or CNS infection. Urine drug screens are frequently performed, but they are fraught with false positives and negatives. Furthermore, a positive finding on a urine drug screen may be the result of a prior exposure and is not the cause of the patient's current

TABLE 128.7 **Medications and Toxins Associated with Ataxia**

- **Antiepileptics:** phenytoin, carbamazepine, oxcarbazepine, gabapentin, levetiracetam, lamotrigine, valproate sodium
- **Antineoplastic agents:** cytarabine, methotrexate, 5-fluorouracil, asparaginase
- **Heavy metals:** methylmercury, arsenic, lead, thallium, manganese
- **Lithium**
- **Hydrocarbons:** toluene, benzene, *n*-hexane, carbon tetrachloride
- **Sedatives/hypnotics:** benzodiazepines, barbiturates, ethanol
- **Amiodarone**
- **Carbon disulfide**
- **Cyclosporine**
- **Tacrolimus**
- **Metronidazole**
- **Bismuth**
- **High-dose corticosteroids**

TABLE 128.8 Neuropathies Associated with Xenobiotics

Xenobiotic	Acute			Subacute/Chronic			Cranial Nerve
	Sens	Motor	Aut	Sens	Motor	Aut	
5-Flurouracil				My	My	My	
Acrylamide				Ax	Ax		
Allyl chloride				Ax	Ax		
Amiodarone				My	My		II, III
Ammonia							II
Amphotericin B				My	My	My	
Arsenic	My	My		Ax	Ax		
Buckthorn				My	Ax, My	My	
Carbon disulfide				Ax	Ax		
Cisplatin							II
Clioquinol							II
Colchicine				Ax			
Cyclosporine				My	My	My	
Dapsone					Ax		
Deferoxamine							II
Diethylene glycol				My	My	My	II, III, VI, VII, VIII
Dimethyl mercury							II
Disulfiram				Ax	Ax		
Ethambutol				Ax			
Ethanol					Ax		
Ethionamide				Ax			
Ethylene glycol							V, VII, VIII, IX, X
Ethylene oxide				Ax	Ax		
Fludarabine				My	My	My	
Glutethimide				Ax			
Gold				Ax, My	Ax, My		
Hexacarbons	Ax	Ax	Ax	Ax	Ax		
Hydralazine				Ax	Ax		
Hydrogen sulfide							I
Hydroxychloroquine				Ax	Ax	Ax	
Interferon-α				Ax, My	Ax, My	Ax, My	II, III
Isoniazid				Ax	Ax		
L-Tryptophan				My	My	My	
Levamisole				My	My	My	
Linezolid				Ax	Ax	Ax	
Lithium							VI
MDMA							VI
Mercury					Ax		
Methanol				Ax	Ax	Ax	II
Methotrexate				My	My	My	II
Methyl bromide				Ax	Ax		
Methyl iodide							II, III
Metronidazole				Ax	Ax		

(continued)

TABLE 128.8 Neuropathies Associated with Xenobiotics *(continued)*

Xenobiotic	Acute Sens	Acute Motor	Acute Aut	Subacute/Chronic Sens	Subacute/Chronic Motor	Subacute/Chronic Aut	Cranial Nerve
Misonidazole				Ax	Ax		
Nitrofurantoin				Ax	Ax		
Nitroglycerin							VI
Nitrous oxide				Ax, My	My	My	
Nucleoside analogs				Ax	Ax	Ax	
OPCs				Ax	Ax		
Oxaliplatin				Ax	Ax	Ax	II, V, VI
Phenytoin				Ax	Ax		
Polychlorinated biphenyls				Ax	Ax		
Procainamide				My	My	My	
Pyridoxine	Ax						
Quinine							II, VIII
Salicylates							VIII
Solvents							II, VIII
Tacrolimus				My	My	My	
Taxol				Ax			
Thallium	Ax	Ax		Ax	Ax		III, IV, VI
TNF-α inhibitors				My	My	My	
Triorthocresyl phosphate	Ax	Ax					
Vacor	Ax		Ax	My	My	My	
Vincristine				Ax, My	Ax, My	My	V
Zinc				My	My	My	

Sens, sensory; Aut, autonomic; Ax, axonopathy; My, myelinopathy; MDMA, 3,4-methylenedioxy-methamphetamine; OPCs, organic phosphorus compounds.

symptoms. A basic metabolic panel should be obtained. Hyponatremia has been known to occur in 3,4-methylenedioxymethamphetamine (MDMA) ingestions causing status epilepticus.

Treatment

Treatment is largely supportive. Agitation should be treated with liberal *benzodiazepine* administration with the goal of minimizing muscle activity to prevent hyperthermia. Antipsychotics are not typically used so as to avoid administering drugs with anticholinergic actions that may increase the risk for seizures, delirium, and hyperthermia. If they are used, the *butyrophenones* (haloperidol, droperidol) are the best option, so long as the patient's QTc interval is normal. Antiepileptics are best avoided, as these patients frequently have electrolyte abnormalities and are at higher risk for complications when they are given. Benzodiazepines, propofol, or barbiturates are preferred for seizure management. Hyperthermia must be avoided or rapidly corrected. IV hydration should be provided to prevent rhabdomyolysis-induced kidney injury and hyperkalemia. Cocaine-induced wide complex tachycardia may be treated with sodium bicarbonate. Persistent hypertension despite adequate sedation can be treated with *phentolamine* 5 mg IV repeated as needed or nitroglycerine IV 5 to 20 μg/min. β-Blockers are best avoided given the potential for worsened vasospasm due

to unopposed α-agonist activity. With optimal acute management, outcomes are typically outstanding.

CHOLINERGIC TOXICITY: ORGANOPHOSPHATES AND CARBAMATES

Organophosphates (OPs) and carbamates are acetylcholinesterase (AChE) inhibitors that have been recognized and used since the mid-19th century. OPs are used as weapons of war (e.g., sarin gas), insecticides, and for medicinal purposes. Carbamates have medical applications (e.g., physostigmine) and are used as insecticides. Some xenobiotics that are carbamates do not inhibit AChE.

Epidemiology

Exposure to OPs and carbamates has been on the decline in the United States, falling to less than 10,000 reports per year in the mid-2000s. This is in contrast to the hundreds of thousands of deaths that occur each year in rural Asia. Chronic and delayed sequelae are subject to underreporting, as the association between the exposure and clinical event may go unrecognized.

Pathobiology

OPs and carbamates are highly lipophilic xenobiotics that penetrate tissues with ease. Systemic toxicity occurs following dermal

TABLE 128.9 Neuromuscular Junction and Peripheral Nerve Action Potential Propagation Dysfunction Related to Xenobiotics

Xenobiotic	Presynaptic	Postsynaptic	Axonal Transmission
Aminoglycosides	X	X	
Azathioprine	X		
β-Adrenergic agonists	X	X	
Chloroquine	X	X	
Ciguatera toxin			X
Clindamycin	X	X	
Corticosteroids			
Crotaline venom	X		
D-Penicillamine		X	
Elapid snake venom	X		X
Gymnothoratoxin			X
Holocyclotoxin (tick paralysis)	X		X
Latrodectus mactans venom (black widow)	X		X
Lithium	X	X	
Magnesium	X		
Nicotine alkaloids		X	X
OPCs, carbamates		X	
Phenothiazines		X	
Phenytoin	X	X	
Polymyxins	X	X	
Procainamide	X	X	
Quinidine	X	X	
Saxitoxin			X
Scorpion venom			X
Tetrodotoxin			X
Trimethaphan		X	
Verapamil	X		

OPCs, organic phosphorus compounds.

exposure via cutaneous absorption, inhalation, or less commonly, ingestion. The initial binding of AChE by OPs is reversible and then becomes irreversible, a process termed *aging*. The time to "aging" varies by OP and ranges from a few hours to a couple of days, with the weapons of war having the shortest time to aging. Once the bond is "aged," the antidote *pralidoxime* (2-PAM) is not effective. Carbamates, on the other hand, do not age, and their effects dissipate upon their clearance.

Clinical Features

The clinical manifestations of OP or carbamate exposure are the result of increased acetylcholine (ACh) in all neuronal junctions (i.e., parasympathetic and sympathetic postganglionic muscarinic, parasympathetic and sympathetic preganglionic nicotinic, CNS, and NMJ nicotinic; Fig. 128.1). Symptom onset ranges from a few minutes to several hours. The high lipophilicity of the compounds causes them to be absorbed in adipose tissues; delayed effects can be seen when they diffuse into the circulation. A syndrome of OP-induced delayed axonal neuropathy is the result of inhibition of a neuronal lysophospholipase neuropathy target esterase (NTE).

Clinical full range of manifestations of OP or carbamate exposure are summarized in Table 128.15. The most common presentation includes miosis, diaphoresis, and dyspnea due to bronchorrhea. CNS manifestations range from restlessness and confusion to stupor, coma, and seizure activity. The increased ACh at the NMJ leads to muscle fasciculations, weakness, and finally, paralysis. A syndrome of delayed NMJ dysfunction seen in 25% of patients 1 to 4 days after OP exposures, characterized by muscle weakness without fasciculations and respiratory insufficiency, has been called *intermediate syndrome*. Some patients experience an OP-induced delayed polyneuropathy (OPIDN) that involves the upper and lower motor neurons days to weeks after exposure.

Diagnosis

The diagnosis of OP/carbamate toxicity is best made based on known exposure and subsequent symptoms. In cases of uncertain exposure or atypical or subtle presentations, measurement of plasma and red blood cell (RBC) *cholinesterase levels* can assist in the diagnosis. There are several caveats to their interpretation that are beyond the scope of this text. Spontaneous repetitive potentials

TABLE 128.10	Xenobiotics Associated with Myopathy
Xenobiotic Category	**Specific Agents**
Antiretrovirals	Azidothymidine, zidovudine
Antibiotics	Penicillin, D-penicillamine, rifampin, sulfonamides
Antimalarials	Chloroquine, hydroxychloroquine
Lipids-lowering medications	Clofibrate, HMG-CoA reductase inhibitors (statins), niacin
Immunosuppressives and antineoplastics	Cyclosporine, vincristine, glucocorticoids (especially when combined with a neuromuscular blocker)
Other medications	Amiodarone, cimetidine, colchicine, doxylamine, ε-aminocaproic acid, ipecac, procainamide, propylthiouracil, suxamethonium (succinylcholine)
Recreational drugs	Ethanol, heroin, phencyclidine
Envenomations	Snakes: *Bothrops asper* (pit viper), *Agkistrodon* (pit viper), *Acanthophis* (elapid snakes), other crotaline snakes
	Spider: *Loxosceles* sp. (recluse spider)

HMG-CoA, hydroxymethylglutaryl-coenzyme A.

on single-nerve electromyography (EMG) are a sensitive finding of AChE inhibition.

Treatment

Patients with OP exposure must be rapidly decontaminated by removing all clothing and liberally irrigating the skin. The initial treatment begins with liberal amounts of *atropine* (starting dose 1 to 2 mg IV doubled every 5 minutes until respiratory secretions are ceased). It is not uncommon for patients to require nearly 500 mg of atropine during the initial hour of care. Additionally, an oxime, typically *pralidoxime* (2-PAM), should be administered as soon as the syndrome is suspected (1 to 2 mg IV every 4 hours for at least 24 hours) to prevent aging and ir-

TABLE 128.11	Smells and Odors Suggestive of Neurotoxic Xenobiotics
Odor or Smell	**Xenobiotic**
Mothballs	Camphor
Garlic	Organophosphates, arsenic, thallium
Peanuts	Vacor
Carrots	Cicutoxin (water hemlock)
Wintergreen	Methyl salicylates
Fruity	Chlorinated hydrocarbons
Glue	Solvents, toluene
Rotten eggs	DMSA, hydrogen sulfide
Shoe polish	Nitrobenzene

DMSA, dimercaptosuccinic acid.

TABLE 128.12	Xenobiotic Ingestions that Should Not Be Treated with Activated Charcoal

- Heavy metals (e.g., lead, arsenic, etc.)
- Acids
- Alkalis
- Hydrocarbons
- Alcohols
- Inorganic ions (e.g., lithium, fluoride, calcium, etc.)
- Oils

reversible inhibition of AChE. Of note, the evidence supporting oxime use is conflicting. Benzodiazepines, particularly *diazepam* 5 to 10 mg IV every 4 to 6 hours, have been observed to decrease cerebral injury resulting from OP-induced seizures and mitigate OP-induced respiratory depression. *Ketamine* (1 to 4 mg/kg loading dose followed by 0.1 to 0.5 mg/min IV infusion) and other

TABLE 128.13	Neurotoxins and Their Antidotes/Specific Treatments
Neurotoxin/Toxidrome	**Antidote/Treatment**
Arsenic, lead, mercury	BAL
TCAs	Bicarbonate
Rattlesnake envenomation	CroFab antivenin
Serotonin syndrome	Cyproheptadine
Arsenic, lead, mercury	D-Penicillamine
NMS, sympathomimetic hyperpyrexia	Dantrolene
Iron	Cefuroxime
Digoxin	Digoxin-specific Fab
Lead	DMSA
Lead	EDTA
Methanol, ethylene glycol	Ethanol
Benzodiazepines	Flumazenil
Methanol, methotrexate	Folate/folinic acid
Ethylene glycol, methanol	Fomepizole
Cyanide, hydrogen sulfide	Hydroxycobalamin, sodium thiosulfate, sodium nitrite
Local anesthetics, TCAs	Intralipid 20%
Valproic acid	l-Carnitine
Black widow spider envenomation	Lactrodectus antivenin
Opioids	Naloxone
Anticholinergics	Physostigmine
Organophosphates, carbamates	Pralidoxime (2-PAM)
Isoniazid, monomethylhydrazine, ethylene glycol	Pyridoxine

BAL, dimercaprol; TCAs, tricyclic antidepressants; NMS, neuroleptic malignant syndrome; DMSA, dimercaptosuccinic acid; EDTA, ethylenediaminetetraacetic acid.

TABLE 128.14 Clinical Findings of Neurotoxic Syndromes

Anticholinergic	• Flushed skin • Anhidrosis • Dry mucus membranes • Urinary retention • Constipation/ileus/decreased bowel sounds • Hyperthermia • Mydriasis • Blurred vision (impaired accommodation) • Agitation, confusion, delirium, psychosis • Visual hallucinations • Myoclonus, choreoathetosis, picking behavior • Stupor/coma (higher doses) • Seizures (very rarely status epilepticus)	**Organophosphate and carbamate toxicity (*continued*)**	• Muscle fasciculations • Seizures/convulsions • Confusion to stupor/coma • Blurred vision/miosis[a] • Bronchospasm[a] • Bradycardia[a] • Hypotension[a]
Sympathomimetic	• Diaphoretic • Hypertensive • Tachycardic • Hyperthermia • Agitation, combativeness, psychosis • Hallucinations • Mydriasis • Seizures	**Neuroleptic malignant syndrome**	• Confusion/delirium • Catatonia/mutism • Stupor/coma • Lead pipe rigidity • Hyperthermia • Tachycardia • Hypertension • Tachypnea
Organophosphate and carbamate toxicity	• Restlessness • Diarrhea • Lacrimation • Salivation • Urination • Bronchorrhea • Diaphoresis	**Serotonin syndrome**	• Agitation, hypervigilance • Confusion, delirium • Hyperthermia • Tachycardia • Hypertension • Diaphoresis • Diarrhea • Ocular clonus • Mydriasis • Akathisia • Tremor • Rigidity • Hyperreflexia[b] • Clonus[b]

[a]Cholinergic activity at the preganglionic sympathetic fibers leads to increased release of norepinephrine at the postganglionic nerve terminals in the target organs. Clinically, this results in activation of the sympathetic and parasympathetic pathways, which may lead to normocardia, tachycardia, normotension, bronchodilation, or mydriasis.

[b]More pronounced in the lower extremities.

TABLE 128.15 Xenobiotics with Anticholinergic Properties

Category	Specific Agents
Antihistamines	Cetirizine, chlorpheniramine, cimetidine, diphenhydramine, doxylamine, hydroxyzine, loratadine, ranitidine
Antipsychotics	Chlorpromazine, clozapine, olanzapine, quetiapine, risperidone, ziprasidone
Antiemetics	Doxylamine, metoclopramide, promethazine, scopolamine
Antivertigo	Meclizine, scopolamine
Tricyclic antidepressants	Amitriptyline, desipramine, doxepin, imipramine, nortriptyline
Antidepressants	Mirtazapine, paroxetine
Antiparkinsonian	Benztropine, biperiden, carbidopa/levodopa, procyclidine, selegiline, trihexyphenidyl
Ophthalmic	Atropine, cyclopentolate, homatropine, tropicamide
Bronchodilators	Ipratropium, tiotropium
Antispasmodics	Dicyclomine, hyoscyamine, loperamide, oxybutynin[a], propantheline
Muscle relaxants	Baclofen, carisoprodol, cyclobenzaprine, methocarbamol
Others	Amantadine, glycopyrrolate[a], trazodone
Botanicals	Deadly nightshade (atropine, *Atropa belladonna*), henbane (*Hyoscyamus niger*), jimson weed (scopolamine, *Datura stramonium*), mandrake (*Mandragora officinarum*)

[a]Does not cross blood–brain barrier.

TABLE 128.16   Xenobiotics Causing Sympathomimetic Toxicity/Acute Excited State

Category	Source	Specific Agents	Comments
Cocaine	Coca plant (*Erythroxylum coca*)	Cocaine hydrochloride, methy-lecgonidine, and ecgonidine ("crack")	WCT/arrhythmias and local anesthetic due to Na channel blockage
Methamphetamines	Synthetic	"crank," "crystal," "chalk," "ice," etc.	Lead toxicity can be seen due to contamination.
Designer (recreational) amphetamines	Synthetic	MDMA ("ecstasy," "XTC," or "Adam"), MDA, MDEA ("Eve"), PMA ("death"), DOM ("STP"), DOI, DOB, others	Hyponatremia not uncommonly seen that may be due to ADH-like action with MDMA; irreversible damage to serotoninergic neurons seen on MRI
Prescription amphetamines	Synthetic	Dextroamphetamine, lisdexamfetamine	
Prescription piperazine compounds	Synthetic	Methylphenidate	
NMDA receptor antagonists	Synthetic	PCP, ketamine, dextromethorphan	
Synthetic cannabinoid	Synthetic	HU-210, JWH-018, JWH-073, JWH-200, CP-47, and cannabicyclohexanol (all largely referred to as *K2* or *spice*)	New compounds rapidly cycled in as DEA adds them to controlled substances lists.
Ephedrine	Ephedra (*ma-huang*)	Various recreation, herbal, and weight loss compounds	
Cathinone	Khat (*Catha edulis*)	Consumed by chewing or in teas	Manganese toxicity from contamination has produced EPS.
Cathinone derivatives	Synthetic	Mephedrone, methylone, ethylone, butylone, pyrovalerone, MDPV, methcathinone, ethcathinone, others ("bath salts" marketed under many names)	
Methylxanthines	*Coffea arabica*, many other botanicals	Caffeine	
N-substituted piperazine compounds	Synthetic	"Legal E," "legal X," BZP ("A2"), TFMPP ("Molly"), CPP, 25I-NBOMe ("N-bomb")	
Mescaline	Cacti (*Lophophora williamsii, Lophophora diffusa, Trichocereus pachanoi*)	"Peyote"	
LSD	Synthetic		
LSD-like substances	Hawaiian baby woodrose (*Argyreia nervosa*), Hawaiian woodrose (*Merremia tuberosa*), morning glory (*Ipomoea violocea*), oliliuqui (*Rivea corymbosa*)		
Hallucinogen: tryptamines (indole alkaloids)	*Psilocybe, Panaeolus,* and *Conocybe* mushrooms Various plants and organisms Synthetics	Psilocybin and psilocin "magic mushrooms" DMT, 5-MeO-DMT AMT, DiPT, 5-MeO-DiPT ("foxy" or "foxy-methoxy")	Drank as *ayahuasca*
Hallucinogens: botanicals	*Salvia divinorum* *Mitragyna speciosa* Korth tree African rain forest shrub (*Tabernanthe iboga*) Wormwood tree extract (*Artemisia absinthium*) Isoxazole mushrooms (*Amanita muscaria, Amanita pantherina, Amanita gemmata,* and *Amanita cothurnata*)	Salvinorin A or divinorin A Kratom, specific compound uncertain, suspect mitragynine Iboga (ibogaine) Thujone ("absinthe") Ibotenic acid and muscimol	Ion channel effects, 11 deaths reported from cardiac arrest Inhibitor of GABA-A receptor→ seizures

WCT, wide complex tachycardia; MDMA, 3,4-methylenedioxymethamphetamine; MDA, 3,4-methylenedioxyamphetamine; MDEA, 3,4-methylenedioxyethamphetamine; PMA, paramethoxyamphetamine; DOM, 4-methyl-2,5-dimethoxyamphetamine; DOI, 2,5-dimethoxy-4-iodoamphetamine; DOB, 2,5-dimethoxy-4-bromoamphetamine; STP, serenity, tranquility, and peace; PCP, phencyclidine; EPS, extrapyramidal symptoms; MDPV, methylenedioxypyrovalerone; BZP, 1-benzylpiperazine; TFMPP, 1-(trifluoromethylphenyl)piperazine; CPP, 1-(chlorophenyl)piperazine; 25I-NBOMe, 2-(4-iodo-2,5-dimethoxyphenyl)-*N*-[(2-methoxyphenyl)methyl]ethanamine; LSD, lysergic acid diethylamide; DMT, dimethyltryptamine; 5-MeO-DMT, 5-methoxy-dimethyltryptamine, diisopropyl; 5-MeO-DiPT, 5-methoxy-tryptamine; DiPT, diisopropyltryptamine; AMT, alpha-methyltryptamine.

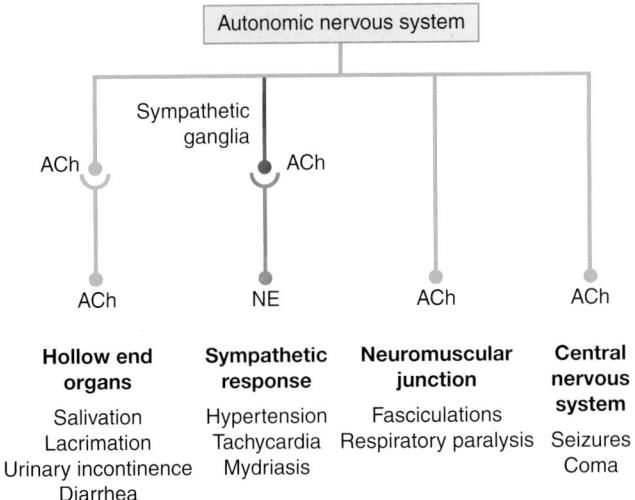

FIGURE 128.1 Sites of action of organophosphates and carbamates. ACh, acetylcholine; NE, norepinephrine.

N-methyl-D-aspartate (NMDA) receptor antagonists have been shown to reduce OP-induced seizures and enhance survival in mice. When endotracheal intubation is being performed, succinylcholine is best avoided.

Outcome

The case fatality rate ranges from 10% to 40%. Evidence is lacking that describes neurologic outcomes with precision following acute and chronic poisoning. Residual deficits with an incomplete recovery are common in those with OPIDN. Cognitive deficits have been observed after acute OP exposure.

NEUROLEPTIC MALIGNANT SYNDROME

Neuroleptic malignant syndrome (NMS) is an idiosyncratic life-threatening neurologic emergency seen in those on neuroleptic (antidopaminergic) agents or after withdrawal of dopaminergic medications (Table 128.17). Precise estimates of its incidence are lacking. It can occur at any age of life and is seen more often in

TABLE 128.17	Examples of Medications that Cause Neuroleptic Malignant Syndrome	
Dopaminergic Agents (Discontinuation)	**Antipsychotics**	**Antiemetics**
Bromocriptine	Aripiprazole	Droperidol
Amantadine	Chlorpromazine	Metoclopramide
Rimantadine	Clozapine	Prochlorperazine
Memantine	Haloperidol	Promethazine
Levodopa	Olanzapine	
Cabergoline	Quetiapine	
Dihydroergocryptine (DHEC)	Risperidone	
Pergolide	Thioridazine	
	Ziprasidone	

men, but this is proportional to the increased use of neuroleptics in the male gender. NMS is frequently seen within the first 2 weeks of treatment with a neuroleptic, but it may occur at any time even in those on antipsychotics for years. The risk of NMS is higher with rapid dose escalation, parenteral administration, switching of agents, and when higher doses are used. The precise pathophysiology is not known, but it is believed to be the result of a relative dopamine deficit in the CNS. Genetic studies have identified a specific allele of the D2 receptor that results in a decreased amount and function of dopamine receptors to be a risk factor.

Clinical Features

Clinical features include mental status changes, muscular rigidity, hyperthermia, and autonomic dysfunction; symptoms typically present in this sequence. Mental status changes may precede the other symptoms by 24 hours or more. Mental status changes range from confusion and delirium to catatonia, mutism, stupor, and coma. Cogwheeling, dystonia, and other dyskinesias can be seen in addition to the lead pipe rigidity. The majority of patients will have a temperature higher than 38°C, with nearly half exceeding 40°C. Autonomic dysfunction manifests as tachycardia, hypertension, and tachypnea. Laboratory abnormalities may include an elevated creatine kinase (>4× normal), transaminitis, and leukocytosis.

Diagnosis

The diagnosis is clinical. A scoring system has been proposed, but it has not been validated. The evaluation is typically targeted toward identifying metabolic derangements that require correction and the exclusion of other differential diagnoses. Cerebral edema has been observed on magnetic resonance imaging (MRI). Seizures are not typically seen in NMS. Cerebral spinal fluid evaluation may reveal a mild protein elevation without pleocytosis or hypoglycorrhachia.

Treatment

Treatment includes aggressive supportive therapy, temperature correction, and cessation of any possible offending agent (or resumption of a discontinued one). *Dantrolene* (1 to 2.5 mg/kg IV), a skeletal muscle relaxant that works by inhibiting calcium release from the sarcoplasmic reticulum, maybe used to reduce rigidity and help to correct hyperthermia and rhabdomyolysis. It should not be used if there is a significant transaminitis. *Amantadine* (100 mg orally [PO] every 12 hours) and *bromocriptine* (2.5 mg PO every 6 hours) are dopamine agonists that may be considered in the treatment of NMS. Summated evidence from retrospective observations and cases suggests that they may hasten recovery and reduce mortality, but this is far from conclusive. There are reports of electroconvulsive therapy (ECT) being used, but its true efficacy is far from clear. In fact, several patients are reported to have gone into cardiac arrest during ECT.

OUTCOME

Recovery typically occurs within 2 weeks of stopping the neuroleptic (or resuming the dopamine agonist), with some exceptions being reported. The mortality ranges from 5% to 20%. Relapse upon resumption of neuroleptics is very difficult to predict. If they must be resumed, lower potency agents should be selected at the lowest possible dose. Weak evidence suggests lithium therapy may increase the risk of developing NMS; therefore, it is best avoided if possible.

TABLE 128.18	Xenobiotics Known to Potentially Cause Serotonin Syndrome
Category	**Specific Examples**
SSRIs	Citalopram, escitalopram, fluoxetine, paroxetine, sertraline
SNRIs	Desvenlafaxine, duloxetine, milnacipran, venlafaxine
TCAs	Amitriptyline, clomipramine, desipramine, doxepin, imipramine, nortriptyline, protriptyline, trimipramine
MAOIs	Isocarboxazid, moclobemide, phenelzine, tranylcypromine
DNRIs	Bupropion
SARIs	Nefazodone, trazodone, and vilazodone
Recreational drugs	Cocaine, methamphetamine, designer amphetamines (e.g., MDMA ["ecstasy"], see Table 128.16), LSD
AEDs	Carbamazepine, valproate
Triptans	Almotriptan, eletriptan, frovatriptan, rizatriptan, sumatriptan, zolmitriptan
Ergots	Ergotamine, methylergonovine
Amphetamines	Dextroamphetamine, lisdexamfetamine
Opioids	Meperidine, tramadol, pentazocine, fentanyl
Appetite suppressants	Fenfluramine, phentermine, dexfenfluramine, sibutramine
Parkinson medications	Levodopa, carbidopa/levodopa, rasagiline, selegiline
5-HT$_3$ receptor antagonists	Dolasetron, granisetron, ondansetron, palonosetron
Antibiotics	Linezolid, tedizolid
Others	Tryptophan, St. John's wort, cyclobenzaprine, dextromethorphan, buspirone, lithium, methylene blue, procarbazine

SSRIs, selective serotonin reuptake inhibitors; SNRIs, serotonin–norepinephrine reuptake inhibitors; TCAs, tricyclic antidepressants; MAOIs, monoamine oxidase inhibitors; DNRIs, dopamine–norepinephrine uptake inhibitors; SARIs, serotonin antagonist and reuptake inhibitors; AEDs, antiepileptic drugs; MDMA, 3,4-methylenedioxymethamphetamine; LSD, lysergic acid diethylamide.

SEROTONIN SYNDROME

Serotonin syndrome is a life-threatening neurologic emergency resulting from a relative serotonin excess. The death of Libby Zion at New York Hospital in 1984, which was reported in the mainstream media and eventually led to the creation of the contemporary laws that limit resident work hours, was suspected to be the result of serotonin syndrome. The syndrome can be precipitated when two or more serotonergic medications are coadministered but can occur with monotherapy as well (see Table 128.18 for a list of serotonergic xenobiotics). There are over 25,000 reported cases of potential toxic exposure to serotonergic agents annually in the United States, with nearly 10,000 of them suspected to cause serotonin syndrome resulting in nearly 100 deaths. Serotonin syndrome occurs on a spectrum. Mild symptoms are likely to go unrecognized and are underreported.

TABLE 128.19	Hunter Serotonin Toxicity Criteria

Any of the following are present after a serotonergic agent is introduced:

- Spontaneous clonus
- Inducible or ocular clonus with agitation or diaphoresis
- Inducible or ocular clonus with hypertonicity and fever
- Tremor with hyperreflexia

Pathobiology

Serotonin receptors are primarily found in the CNS in the brain stem (midline raphe nuclei) and peripherally in the gastrointestinal tract, vasculature, and platelets. Rapid increases in serotonin concentration at these sites produce the symptoms of serotonin syndrome. Mild symptoms include tremor, diarrhea, and restlessness or hypervigilance. More severe symptoms result in further autonomic dysfunction, hyperthermia (>40°C), and more significant deficits in mental status (see Table 128.14). Clonus (ocular, spontaneous, and induced) and hyperreflexia are specific for serotonin syndrome and are more pronounced in the lower extremities. The onset is typically within minutes to hours of exposure to the serotonergic agent.

Diagnosis

Table 128.19 outlines the Hunter Serotonin Toxicity Criteria, which have a sensitivity of 84% and specificity of 97% for diagnosing serotonin syndrome. The diagnosis is completely clinical. Laboratory and imaging investigations are done to evaluate for metabolic derangements and to exclude alternative diagnoses.

Management

Symptoms resolve promptly upon the cessation of all serotonergic agents, making this the cornerstone of treatment. Unfortunately, some selective serotonin reuptake inhibitors (SSRIs) have long half-lives (e.g., fluoxetine's half-life is 1 week). In such cases, prolonged supportive therapy is necessary. Agitation should be treated with benzodiazepines. If agitation persists or if autonomic dysfunction persists despite control of agitation, *cyproheptadine*, a histamine and serotonin antagonist, maybe used. It is only available for oral administration. The initial dose is 12 mg followed by 2 mg every 2 hours. There is little evidence beyond case reports to confirm that it has any therapeutic benefit. Outcomes can be expected to be excellent with optimal supportive care and prompt withdrawal of the serotonergic agent(s).

CARBON MONOXIDE POISONING

Carbon monoxide (CO) intoxication is a common cause of neurotoxic damage and death. Deaths averaged 5,600 annually over a 10-year period in the United States and split between accidental and intentional. Statistics on nonfatal CO encephalopathy and the delayed CO-induced neuropsychiatric syndrome are imprecise. CO competes with oxygen for binding to hemoglobin, myoglobin, and cytochrome *c* oxidase resulting in tissue hypoxia and disordered cellular energy generation.

Clinical Features

Clinical presentations range from mild, viral syndrome–like symptoms, such as headache, malaise, dizziness, nausea, difficulty concentrating, and dyspnea, to coma, particularly in the setting of smoke inhalation. In survivors, neurologic symptoms include dementia, cerebellar dysfunction, and parkinsonism. A delayed neuropsychiatric syndrome may follow acute exposure by 3 to 240 days with cognitive and personality changes and psychotic behavior. This syndrome occurs in 10% to 30% of CO poisonings. Although up to 10% of victims show gross neurologic or psychiatric impairment, more frequently there is only a subtle, persistent neuropsychiatric deficit. Computed tomography (CT), MRI, magnetic resonance spectroscopy (MRS), and isotopic imaging can disclose the brain damage. Postmortem findings include multifocal necrosis and myelinopathy with discrete lesions in the globus pallidus, cortex, and white matter.

Diagnosis

The diagnosis is made by measuring the serum carboxyhemoglobin (COHb) level. Normal levels are less than 5% in nonsmokers and can be as high as 12% in two-pack-per-day smokers. Although serious toxicity is often associated with levels greater than 25%, neurologic damage is not always directly related to the COHb level. Furthermore, serum levels may have fallen by the time the patient reaches the emergency department such that a normal COHb level does not rule out CO poisoning. Blood taken at the scene by emergency technicians can be used. Measurement of CO in expired air and in the exposure area's ambient air can also be useful. The U.S. government standard for CO prohibits exposure to more than 35 ppm, averaged over an 8-hour workday.

Treatment

Initial treatment is 100% oxygen by a nonrebreather face mask, which will reduce the elimination half-life of COHb from 4 to 5 hours to 1 to 2 hours. Treatment continues until the COHb levels are below 10%. Most experts advocate hyperbaric oxygen (HBO) for treatment of symptomatic CO poisoning. It enhances elimination of COHb with an average half-life of 20 minutes at three atmospheres, but randomized trials have not clarified whether it hastens recovery or reduces the rate of late sequelae. Coma, ischemic symptoms, acidosis, levels over 25%, and pregnancy with levels over 20% are indications for HBO.

MALIGNANT HYPERTHERMIA

Malignant hyperthermia (MH) is a life-threatening reaction that occurs in approximately 1/100,000 exposures to volatile anesthetics or succinylcholine. It results from the improper opening of the ryanodine receptors on the sarcoplasmic reticulum in skeletal muscle. Its presentation is on a spectrum, with the most pronounced episodes being characterized by diffuse muscle rigidity despite neuromuscular blockade. The first signs are an elevation of the end-tidal CO_2 and tachycardia. Fever develops later, with the temperature being prone to rapid elevations. Untreated, rhabdomyolysis and hyperthermia and their associated complications lead to death. Rapid treatment with *dantrolene* (2.5 mg/kg IV followed by 1 mg/kg IV until symptoms resolve) is the cornerstone of treatment.

Epidemiologically, MH is most commonly the result of a mutation of the ryanodine receptor or dihydropyridine receptor. Additional cases are seen in those with several hereditary myopathies. Population-based screening is not justifiable. Genetic testing is specific but not sensitive. Contracture testing is much more sensitive, but it is invasive and only available at select centers. Additionally, contracture testing has a 20% false-positive rate.

STRYCHNINE POISONING

Strychnine, a competitive antagonist of glycine, causes involuntary tonic–clonic activity in otherwise awake individuals. It is derived from the seeds of the tree *Strychnos* nux vomica. Contemporary poisonings are usually the result of the adulteration of recreational drugs and less commonly in herbal medications. It is absorbed through all routes, including dermal, with an onset of 10 to 20 minutes. It is largely eliminated by the liver with a half-life of approximately 12 hours. The diagnosis is clinical. Rhabdomyolysis and its associated complications are a significant threat as well as respiratory arrest from an inability to properly ventilate. Treatment is supportive with benzodiazepine or propofol use.

METHANOL (METHYL ALCOHOL)

Methanol ingestion occurs when it is substituted for ethanol or in suicide attempts. Poisoning is related to the conversion of methanol to formaldehyde and formic acid, which results in a severe metabolic acidosis. The initial clinical presentation is similar to acute ethanol intoxication with gastrointestinal symptoms, drunkenness, and coma. The mortality rate is approximately 35%. Visual loss is common and attributed to retinal metabolism of methanol to formic acid. Cerebral imaging has demonstrated petechial hemorrhages and edema. Inhibitors of aldehyde dehydrogenase (ethanol and fomepizole) block the conversion of methanol to formaldehyde, allowing it to be excreted in the urine.

VOLATILE ORGANIC COMPOUNDS

Neurologic syndromes caused by volatile organic compounds (VOC) (*solvents*) occur after either occupational or deliberate exposure by inhalation abuse. The agents include aromatic and aliphatic hydrocarbons, alcohols, esters, ketones, aliphatic nitrates, anesthetic agents, halogenated solvents, and propellants. Aromatic hydrocarbons, especially *toluene*, produce cerebral and cerebellar damage. Aliphatic hydrocarbons caused outbreaks of peripheral neuropathy in industrial or recreational exposures to *n*-hexane or methyl-*n*-butyl ketone, which begin in the lower extremities and ascend, resembling Guillain–Barré syndrome. Pathophysiologically, neurofilamentous axonal swelling and distal axonal degeneration are seen.

Other organic compounds that induce axonal neuropathy by industrial exposure are acrylamide, carbon disulfide, methyl bromide, and triorthocresyl phosphate. Halogenated hydrocarbons are toxic for the CNS by damaging nerve cell membranes and altering neurotransmission; an excitatory phase is rapidly followed by CNS depression. The compounds include chloroform, methylene chloride, and tetrachloroethane. The neurotoxic potential of one substance is sometimes facilitated by others in the same commercial product.

NITROUS OXIDE MYELOPATHY

Nitrous oxide (NO), commonly known as *laughing gas*, is used as an inhaled anesthetic. Chronic exposure to NO, also known as *Layzer syndrome*, was described in the last 1970s in a series of dentists with occupational exposure or chronic NO abuse. It has also been described in those with a vitamin B_{12} deficiency that are exposed to NO. Because NO interferes with the action of vitamin B_{12}, symptoms mimic its deficiency and include paresthesias, Lhermitte symptoms, ataxia, leg weakness, impotence, and sphincter disturbances. Examination showed signs of sensorimotor polyneuropathy, often implicating the posterior and lateral columns of the spinal cord, which can be confirmed on MRI. Electrodiagnostic tests showed axonal polyneuropathy. Animal studies have suggested that methionine has a protective role. Improvement has been reported to occur over weeks to months after exposure ceased.

HEAVY METALS

Lead

Acute lead encephalopathy in children is typically attributed to pica or ingestion of flaking lead-containing paint. Children with blood levels above 80 μg/dL are more susceptible than adults to overt lead encephalopathy with delirium, ataxia, seizure, stupor, or coma with associated cerebral edema. Adults with chronic lead exposure yielding blood lead levels of 25 to 60 μg/dL may experience irritability, headache, myalgias, anorexia, nausea, crampy abdominal pain, and depression with signs of impaired visual–motor dexterity and reaction times. Objective neuropathies that manifest in muscle weakness and atrophy occur with long-term levels of 60 μg/dL or more. Because of links between lead and cognitive dysfunction, behavioral problems, as well as stunted growth in children, the Centers for Disease Control and Prevention has declared levels exceeding blood concentration of 5 μg/dL to be abnormal and requiring case management. Periodic screening of children aged 9 to 36 months is advocated, especially because the symptoms are nonspecific, including lethargy, anorexia, intermittent abdominal pain with vomiting, or constipation. Testing blood lead levels is recommended for children with presumed autism, attention deficit disorder (ADD), pervasive development disorder, mental retardation, or language problems.

A diagnosis of lead intoxication is supported if blood zinc protoporphyrin exceeds 100 μg/dL or if urinary aminolevulinic acid excretion is more than 15 mg/L. With blood lead levels of 10 μg/dL, the activity of aminolevulinic acid dehydratase is low. At higher lead levels, the activities of coproporphyrinogen oxidase and ferrochelatase are also low. Anemia and basophilic stippling of erythrocytes are characteristic. Nerve conduction velocities are nonspecifically slow in lead and other neuropathies.

Treatment combines decontamination, supportive care, and the judicious use of chelating agents. In affected people, chelation therapy commences with levels of 40 to 45 μg/dL. Supportive care may include treatment of increased ICP by standard use of IV mannitol and glucocorticoids, the latter because the pathophysiology of lead encephalopathy involves capillary leak. In patients with lead encephalopathy, calcium disodium edetate or calcium ethylenediaminetetraacetic acid (EDTA) should be administered at 30 mg/kg every 24 hours. Some advocate initiating chelation with a single dose of dimercaprol (British anti-Lewisite [BAL]) 4 to 5 mg/kg deep intramuscularly. Alternatively, meso-2,3-dimercaptosuccinic acid (DMSA or succimer) is advocated for treatment of moderately severe chronic lead intoxication. Childhood lead exposure carries a risk of long-lasting health impairment, especially with neurocognitive and neurobehavioral sequelae, emphasizing the need for primary prevention and for obtaining occupational and environmental information.

Mercury

The relations between elemental, inorganic, and organic forms of mercury involve transformations from one form to another. Modern epidemics include Minamata disease from fish contaminated by methyl mercury (MeHg), which affected 2,500 people in Japan, and erethism (abnormal sensitivity to stimulation of any type)—also known as the *mad hatter syndrome*—from mercuric nitrate used in the hatting industry. Acute toxicity from elemental mercury may include encephalopathy and seizures, whereas its chronic toxicity includes peripheral sensorimotor neuropathy, dysarthria, and parkinsonism. Subclinical nerve conduction and neuropsychiatric abnormalities have been documented in the modern workplace.

Organic mercury includes MeHg, the cause of Minamata disease, and ethyl mercury. Excessive MeHg intake has been reported in fish-eating communities in Greenland, the Faroe Islands, the Seychelles, the Madeira Basin of the Amazon River, and New Zealand. Symptoms of organic mercury toxicity include tremor; ataxia; dysarthria; paresthesias of the hands, feet, and mouth; visual field constriction; erethism; and spasticity. Prenatal exposure to MeHg can cause severe congenital abnormalities such as micrognathia, microcephaly, mental retardation, blindness, and motor deficits. Minamata disease produces neuropathologic abnormalities in the cerebral cortex, cerebellum, and peripheral nerves.

The 24-hour urine mercury concentration may assess both recent exposure and elimination of tissue burden. The normal blood concentration is less than 10 to 20 μg/L, and the urinary level is less than 20 μg/L. Treatment consists of decontamination and chelation with established guidelines. If the person is symptomatic, dimercaprol is given intramuscularly 3 to 5 mg/kg every 4 hours on day 1, every 12 hours on day 2, and then once a day for the next 3 days followed by a 2-day interruption. Other agents are DMSA and 2,3-dimercapto-propane-1-sulfonate, a water-soluble form of BAL. All agents are somewhat effective for organic and inorganic mercury poisoning.

Arsenic

Arsenic toxicity is a global health problem. It is estimated that tens of millions of people, for example, in Bangladesh, are at risk of excessive arsenic levels from natural geologic sources leaching into aquifers, contaminated drinking water, mining, and other industrial processes. Arsenicosis can result in cancer at various sites, encephalopathy, and axonal peripheral neuropathy. The chronic version is "blackfoot disease" with vascular changes, gangrene, and a less severe peripheral neuropathy. The use of arsenic trioxide to treat leukemia may cause arsenic neuropathy.

Vomiting, bloody diarrhea, myoglobinuria, renal failure, arrhythmias, hypotension, seizures, coma, and death characterize acute arsenic poisoning. In survivors, *Mees lines* on the fingernails and sensorimotor neuropathy appear in 7 to 14 days. Slow and incomplete recovery takes years. Cognition may be impaired in some survivors depending on the severity of the acute encephalopathy.

The diagnosis of arsenic intoxication is confirmed by urinary levels more than 75 μg/dL. Hair analysis has been used but is not reliable. BAL therapy is also used for acute arsenic poisoning. It is most effective before symptoms of neuropathy appear. BAL is considered more effective than penicillamine in treating the chronic neuropathy. Hemodialysis is another treatment for an acute episode.

Thallium

Despite the ban on manufacture of thallium rodenticides in the United States, accidental and suicidal exposures still occur because the poisons are available in other countries. After an acute exposure, gastrointestinal symptoms occur first with paresthesias occurring a few weeks later with the onset of a neuropathy. The encephalopathy presents with cognitive impairment and choreoathetosis, myoclonus, or other involuntary movements. Alopecia, which is unique to thallium toxicity, begins 1 to 3 weeks after exposure.

After acute exposure, blood tests are not useful for detecting thallium because it is rapidly taken up by the cells. Normal urinary thallium values are 0.3 to 0.8 μg/L. Levels of 200 to 300 μg/L are seen in overt poisoning. A provocative test uses potassium chloride (KCl), which is given orally in a dose of 45 mEq. Potassium displaces thallium from tissue stores, blood levels rise, and urinary content can be followed serially.

Treatment of acute poisoning depends in part on enhancing urinary and fecal excretion of thallium by giving laxatives and using Prussian blue or activated charcoal to retard absorption. Urinary excretion is enhanced by forced diuresis and administration of KCl. Hemodialysis may be effective.

Manganese

Manganese intoxication, still a threat in industrial settings, reproduces the essential motor features of parkinsonism but with sufficient clinical and pathologic differences to indicate the conditions are not identical; for instance, exaggerated tendon reflexes and behavioral features occur early in manganese toxicity. The outlook is gloomy, including severe cognitive loss. Responses to levodopa and to chelation therapy are limited.

Aluminum

Dialysis dementia (see also Chapter 120) has been attributed to aluminum in the dialysis water and also in ingested phosphate binders used to control blood phosphorus levels. Treatment of the water and avoidance of the binders have decreased the incidence. Encephalopathy, however, has also occurred in uremic patients dialyzed with deionized water and also in those that ingest the phosphate binders without dialysis. Paresthesias and weakness were part of "potroom palsy," a complex syndrome in workers in a smelter who were exposed to pots that had not been vented properly. Other manifestations included ataxia, tremor, and memory loss.

PLANT, ANIMAL, AND MARINE NEUROTOXINS

Ciguatera poisoning or the *marine neurotoxic syndrome* is the most common nonbacterial form of food poisoning in the United States and is endemic in subtropical regions. Toxins are found in tropical reef fish, which acquire them when they consume dinoflagellates. Initial symptoms are gastrointestinal followed by sensory symptoms, paresthesias, and pruritus. *Sensory inversion*, manifested as cold feeling hot and vice versa, dysuria, and dyspareunia are particular to this poisoning. Myalgia, fasciculations, areflexia, trismus, and carpopedal spasm are also reported. Respiratory failure is uncommon. There is no formal laboratory or clinical criteria for diagnosis. Mechanistically, most associated toxins open sodium channels. Treatment is symptomatic, with a randomized trial of mannitol showing no advantage.

Shellfish poisoning can result from contamination of mollusks by saxitoxin, which blocks sodium channels. The symptoms are similar to ciguatera but more severe, and respiratory depression is a greater risk. Cerebellar ataxia was the dominant finding and hypertension is common. Binding assays and liquid chromatography identify the toxin in serum and urine. In Japan, the agent of puffer fish poisoning is tetrodotoxin. Treatment of these conditions is symptomatic.

Amnesic shellfish poison is due to consuming domoic acid, a glutamate receptor agonist, in mussels, which can result in a transient encephalopathy. There is no specific treatment.

Many plants contain pharmacologically active substances that cross the blood–brain barrier with resulting delirium, hallucinations, seizures, and sedation. *Cicutoxin*, from *water hemlock*, produces a clinical state of agitation and confusion followed by sedation. *Andromedotoxin* from *rhododendron* is a depressant. Over 100,000 potential toxic exposures to botanicals are reported per year.

Neurolathyrism presents with spastic paraparesis in impoverished countries and is seen during times of drought when the *Lathyrus* plant is consumed. *Konzo* is a disease due to prolonged consumption of the bitter cassava *Manihot esculenta* prevalent in sub-Saharan Africa with a similar presentation. Cassava contains a cyanoglucoside linamarin, which is enzymatically converted to cyanide, which then damages neural calls. The clinical picture is a sudden, symmetric, and permanent spastic paraplegia. Males are predominately affected in both conditions. Hearing loss, visual impairment, and dysarthria may be seen in cassavaism but not neurolathyrism.

ACKNOWLEDGMENTS

Leon D. Prockop, Louis H. Weimer, and Lewis P. Rowland contributed to the content in this chapter in previous editions. Edward (Mel) J. Otten is to be thanked for his mentorship and advisement on the content of this Chapter.

SUGGESTED READINGS

Aaron CK. Organophosphate poisoning-induced intermediate syndrome: can electrophysiological changes help predict outcome? *PLoS Med.* 2008;5(7):e154.

Anderson HR, Nielsen JB, Grandjean P. Toxicologic evidence of developmental neurotoxicity of environmental chemicals. *Toxicology.* 2000;144(1–3): 121–127.

Arora A, Neema M, Stankiewicz J, et al. Neuroimaging of toxic and metabolic disorders. *Semin Neurol.* 2008;28:495–510.

Awada A, Kojan S. Neurological disorders and travel. *Int J Antimicrob Agents.* 2003;21(2):189–192.

Bellinger DC, Trachtenberg F, Barregard L, et al. Neuropsychological and renal effects of dental amalgam in children: a randomized clinical trial. *JAMA.* 2006;295(15):1775–1783.

Bouchard M, Mergler D, Baldwin ME, et al. Manganese cumulative exposure and symptoms: a follow-up study of alloy workers. *Neurotoxicology.* 2008;29(4):577–583.

Buckley NA, Eddleston M, Li Y, et al. Oximes for acute organophosphate pesticide poisoning. *Cochrane Database Syst Rev.* 2011;(2):CD005085.

Buckley NA, Juurlink DN, Isbister G, et al. Hyperbaric oxygen for carbon monoxide poisoning. *Cochrane Database Syst Rev.* 2011;(4):CD002041.

Chateau-Degat ML, Beuter A, Vauterin G, et al. Neurologic signs of ciguatera disease: evidence of their persistence. *Am J Trop Med Hyg.* 2007;77(6):1170–1175.

Chiang WK. Mercury. In: Ford MD, Delaney KA, Ling LJ, et al, eds. *Clinical Toxicology.* Philadelphia: WB Saunders; 2001:737–743.

Clancy C, Klein Schwarz W. Plants: central nervous system toxicity. In: Ford MD, Delaney KA, Ling LJ, et al, eds. *Clinical Toxicology.* Philadelphia: WB Saunders; 2001:909–921.

DeCarvalho M, Jacinto J, Ramos N, et al. Paralytic shellfish poisoning. Clinical and electrophysiological observations. *J Neurol.* 1998;2245:551–554.

Feldman RG. *Occupational and Environmental Neurology.* Philadelphia: Lippincott-Raven; 1999.

Ford MD, Delaney KA, Ling LS, et al. *Clinical Toxicology.* Philadelphia: WB Saunders; 2001.

Goldfrank LR, Flomenbaum NE, Hoffman RS, et al. *Goldfrank's Toxicologic Emergencies.* 10th ed. New York: McGraw-Hill; 2015.

Greenburg MI, Hamilton R, Phillips SD, et al. *Occupational, Industrial, and Environmental Toxicology.* Philadelphia: Mosby; 2003.

Hadzic A, Glab K, Sanborn KV, et al. Severe neurologic deficit after nitrous oxide anesthesia. *Anesthesiology*. 1995;83:863–866.

Hampson NB, Hauff NM. Risk factors for short-term mortality from carbon monoxide poisoning treated with hyperbaric oxygen. *Crit Care Med*. 2008;36(9):2523–2527.

Jeffery B, Barlow T, Moizer K, et al. Amnesic shellfish poison. *Food Chem Toxicol*. 2004;42(4):545–557.

Juntunen J, Matikainen E, Antti-Poika M, et al. Nervous system effects of long-term occupational exposure to toluene. *Acta Neurol Scand*. 1985;72: 512–517.

Kim JH, Chang KH, Song IC, et al. Delayed encephalopathy of acute carbon monoxide intoxication: diffusivity of cerebral white matter lesions. *AJNR*. 2003;24:1592–1597.

Layzer RB. Myeloneuropathy after prolonged exposure to nitrous oxide. *Lancet*. 1978;2:1227–1230.

Lidsky TI, Schneider JS. Lead neurotoxicity in children: basic mechanisms and clinical correlates. *Brain*. 2003;126(pt 1):5–19.

Meyer-Baron M, Schäper M, Knapp G, et al. Occupational aluminum exposure: evidence in support of its neurobehavioral impact. *Neurotoxicology*. 2007;28(6):1068–1078.

Moretto A, Lotti M. Poisoning by organophosphorus insecticides and sensory neuropathy. *J Neurol Neurosurg Psychiatry*. 1998;64:463–468.

Myers JE, teWaterNaude J, Fourie M, et al. Nervous system effects of occupational manganese exposure on South African manganese mine workers. *Neurotoxicology*. 2003;24:649–656.

Nayak P. Aluminum: impacts and disease. *Eviron Res*. 2002;89(2):101–115.

Perkins RA, Morgan SS. Poisoning, envenomation, and trauma from marine creatures. *Am Fam Physician*. 2004;69:885–890.

Prockop LD. Carbon monoxide. In: Dobbs MR, ed. *Clinical Toxic and Environmental Neurology*. New York: Elsevier; 2008.

Prockop LD, Alt M, Tison J. Huffer's neuropathy. *JAMA*. 1974;229:1083–1084.

Prockop LD, Brock C, Spencer PS. Neurotoxic disorders. In: Rosenberg R, ed. *Atlas of Clinical Neurology*. Philadelphia: Current Medicine LLC; 2008.

Rutchik JS, Wittman RI. Neurologic issues with solvents. *Clin Occup Environ Med*. 2004;4(4):621–656.

Schaumberg H, Albers JW. Identification of neurotoxic disease. *Continuum: Lifelong Learn Neurol*. 2008;14(5):11–34.

Sethi NK, Mullin P, Torgovnick J, et al. Nitrous oxide "whippit" abuse presenting with cobalamin responsive psychosis. *J Med Toxicol*. 2006;2(2): 71–74.

Shrot S, Ramaty E, Biala Y, et al. Prevention of organophosphate-induced chronic epilepsy by early benzodiazepine treatment. *Toxicology*. 2014;323: 19–25.

Spencer PS, Schaumburg HH, Ludolph A. *Experimental and Clinical Neurotoxicology*. 2nd ed. New York: Oxford University Press; 1999.

Steenland K, Jenkins B, Ames RG, et al. Chronic neurologic sequelae to organophosphate pesticide poisoning. *Am J Public Health*. 1994;84:731–736.

Stepens A, Logina I, Liguts V, et al. A parkinsonian syndrome in methcathinone users and the role of manganese. *N Engl J Med*. 2008;358(10): 1009–1017.

Struwe G. Psychiatric and neurological symptoms in workers occupationally exposed to organic solvents—results of a differential epidemiological study. *Acta Psychiatr Scand Suppl*. 1983;303(suppl):100–104.

Vahidnia A, van der Voet GB, de Wolff FA. Arsenic neurotoxicity–a review. *Hum Exp Toxicol*. 2007;26(10):823–832.

Wang DZ. Neurotoxins from marine dinoflagellates: a brief review. *Mar Drugs*. 2008;6(2):349–371.

Weaver LK. Clinical practice. Carbon monoxide poisoning. *N Engl J Med*. 2009;360(12):1217–1225.

Weaver LK, Hopkins RO, Chan KJ, et al. Hyperbaric oxygen for acute carbon monoxide poisoning. *N Engl J Med*. 2002;347(14):1057–1067.

Weissman BA, Raveh L. Therapy against organophosphate poisoning: the importance of anticholinergic drugs with antiglutamatergic properties. *Toxicol Appl Pharmacol*. 2008;232(2):351–358.

Zhao G, Ding M, Zhang B, et al. Clinical manifestations and management of acute thallium poisoning. *Eur Neurol*. 2008;60(6):292–297.

INTRODUCTION

The first known description of nervous system injury by radiation was in 1930 by Fischer and Holfelder. Contemporary medicine's use of radiotherapy to treat malignancies has brought radiation injury into daily clinical discussion. The expansion of nuclear energy programs during the 1970s increased the risk for widespread radiation injury in the event of nuclear plant failure. The Three Mile Island accident in 1979 and disasters at the Chernobyl Nuclear Power Station in 1986 and the Fukushima Nuclear Power Plant following a tsunami in 2011 have provided real reminders of the ongoing risk.

Radiation injury is the result of exposure to ionizing radiation. Nonionizing radiation does not cause neurologic injury; its biologic injury is limited to thermal surface injury. Nervous system injury results from x-rays or gamma rays; alpha and beta particles also produce ionizing radiation, but they do not penetrate tissue by more than 8 mm and therefore do not reach the central or peripheral nervous system. Internal injury can result when alpha or beta particles are ingested, but even in such cases, their proximity to central neurologic structures limits their ability to produce significant neurologic injury.

The amount of radiation absorbed is described in terms of *gray* (Gy), where one Gy is equal to one joule of radiation absorbed per kilogram of tissue. A *radiation-absorbed dose* (rad) is equal to 100th of a Gy (i.e., 100 rad = 1 Gy). One rad is also equal to one *roentgen equivalent man* (rem), that is, 1 rad = 1 rem. In contrast, the dose of radiation delivered is described in sieverts (Sv), where 1 Sv is equal to 100 rem. To provide context, we are exposed to approximately 3 millisieverts (mSv) per year from natural radioactive material and cosmic radiation. Furthermore, one head computed tomography (CT) delivers 2 mSv of radiation.

Radiation effects on the nervous system and other organ systems (Table 129.1) can be difficult to predict, as the amount of radiation delivered is not necessarily equal to the amount absorbed, particularly when considering occupational or environmental exposures. The clinical effects of radiation are related to the individual susceptibility, dose rate, dose absorbed, and distribution of the dose.

EPIDEMIOLOGY

As mentioned earlier, the incidence of radiation injury is related to individual patient characteristics, the dose amount, dose rate, and distribution of the exposure. Hypertension and diabetes mellitus increase the risk of radiation injury. Radiation injury may occur after scalp radiation for tinea capitis, radiotherapy to the head or neck for malignancy, whole-brain radiation for acute lymphoblastic leukemia (ALL) or small cell carcinoma, brachytherapy, or radiotherapy for intracranial malignancies.

Acute cerebral edema may occur days to weeks after radiation. It rarely occurs at doses below 2 Gy and is seen in about half of the time after doses over 7.5 Gy. Delayed leukoencephalopathy and/or demyelination typically occur between 1 and 6 months after exposure. Radiation necrosis is seen between 6 months and 7.5 years after radiotherapy, with a median onset of 14 months, and 75% of patients experience symptoms within 3 years. The cumulative dosing threshold for necrosis is reported as being 50 to 60 Gy, with a 5% incidence in those receiving a total of 50 Gy in daily doses of 2 Gy.

Myelopathy occurs 1 to 3 years after radiation, with peaks in incidence at 12 to 14 months and 24 to 28 months. Similar to radiation necrosis, 5% of patients receiving total doses of approximately 60 Gy to the spinal cord have been reported to develop myelopathy, but this is not consistent.

Intracranial and extracranial vasculopathy have been seen over 20 years after radiation exposure. Stroke-like migraine attacks after radiation therapy (*SMART*) syndrome has been reported many years after whole-brain radiation. It is rare with an incidence and risk factors that are not well described.

Plexopathy and neuropathy (including cranial and optic neuropathy) are typically seen after radiation directed at the affected region. Brachial plexopathy after radiation for breast cancer has a median onset of 4.5 months. Transient symptoms are seen in 1% to 2% of those receiving doses of 50 Gy. Lumbosacral plexopathy is rarely seen, even at doses of up to 70 to 80 Gy. Neuropathy is rarely seen at doses under 60 Gy. Optic neuropathy is seen within 3 years of exposure when it occurs.

The radiation dose threshold associated with neuroendocrine disorders in children is less than that for the previously mentioned injuries. Growth hormone (GH) deficiency is seen in fractionated doses of less than 20 Gy. Sixty-five percent of children undergoing prophylactic cranial radiation for ALL in a total dose of 20 to 30 Gy are observed to have a GH deficit. Other neuroendocrine disorders occur at total doses over 40 to 50 Gy, including gonadotropin deficiency, thyrotropin deficiency, adrenocorticotropic hormone deficiency, and hyperprolactinemia.

TABLE 129.1	Radiation Effects

- Acute cerebral edema
- Early-delayed leukoencephalopathy or demyelination
- Late-delayed radiation necrosis
- Myelopathy
- Vasculopathy
- Plexopathy
- Neuropathy (including cranial and optic neuropathy)
- Neuroendocrine disorders
- Radiation-induced tumors
- Neuropsychiatric, behavioral, and cognitive disturbances

Cognitive and neuropsychiatric disturbances are all too common in children receiving radiation for malignancies, with some series reporting rates of 100%. Radiotherapy that traverses the hippocampus or frontostriatal brain circuitry is felt to increase the risk of occurrence.

Radiation-induced tumors include meningiomas, sarcomas, gliomas, and peripheral nerve tumors. Meningiomas have a latency of up to 37 years at doses of 8.5 Gy and as short as 18 months after 20 Gy. Sarcomas are seen about 10 years after doses of 50 Gy with an unclear frequency. The relationship between glioma occurrence and radiation therapy is not agreed upon. However, high-volume cell phone use has been associated with the occurrence of gliomas (and meningiomas) and the risk appears to be related to the "dose" of cell phone use. Peripheral nerve tumors are seen in about 10% of patients receiving radiation therapy directed through a peripheral nerve.

PATHOBIOLOGY

Ionizing radiation causes biologic injury by damaging the most basic elements that make up cellular structures and conduct cellular processes. The x-rays and/or gamma rays collide with electrons, causing elements to become ionized that were not otherwise, altering their ability to conduct cellular functions. This will damage DNA, leading to mutations that contribute to the increased malignancy risk. Cells that have high rates of turnover are the most vulnerable to this damage (e.g., hematopoietic, mucosal, endothelial, and gastrointestinal cells).

The early cerebral edema is suspected to be secondary to vascular endothelial dysfunction, causing vasogenic edema (hence its clinical response to corticosteroids). The latently observed leukoencephalopathy is thought to be the result of a transient demyelination due to oligodendrocyte dysfunction, as the time frame corresponds with expected myelin turnover.

Radiation necrosis is predominately a white matter process that may occur by one or more of the following mechanisms: glial dysfunction, vasculopathy, or immunologic. Glial dysfunction is supported by histologic changes including white matter necrosis, cystic cavitation with gliosis, and patchy demyelination suspected to be the result of oligodendrocytes injury. Alternatively, vascular injury has been observed histologically as perivascular lymphocytic infiltration, endothelial proliferation, fibrinoid degeneration, capillary occlusion, and intraluminal thrombosis of medium- and small-sized arteries. Endothelial cell injury then causes vasogenic edema.

A *mineralizing microangiopathy* is seen in nearly 20% of patients at autopsy and can be appreciated clinically as calcifications at the gray–white junction on head CT. Lastly, an *immunologic mechanism* is suspected to occur when irradiated glial cells release antigens that induce an autoimmune reaction.

In myelopathy, white matter necrosis is seen after higher radiation doses, whereas lower doses are observed to cause vascular damage, with a more delayed presentation. Asymptomatic animals are found to have a spongy vacuolation of the spinal cord white matter. In contrast, the animals with paralysis were found to have tissue destruction and vascular changes, predominantly in the posterior and lateral columns.

Plexopathies and neuropathies can be the result of an occlusion of an artery (e.g., subclavian artery stenosis causing a brachial plexopathy) or radiation fibrosis, producing external compression around the nerve. Peripheral nerve ischemia due to radiation injury to the vasa nervorum is also suspected. Autopsies of those with radiation vasculopathy reveal myointimal proliferation, hyalinization, and occlusion.

CLINICAL FEATURES

Acutely radiated victims of an occupational or environmental event or accident typically do not know the dose of radiation they were exposed to. Symptoms of acute radiation sickness (ARS) on presentation include nausea, vomiting, diarrhea, or headache. The onset, persistence, and severity of symptoms are used to gage the dose and therefore prognosis of the victim. If neurologic symptoms are present acutely and are not the result of an injury sustained from a blast or other traumatic force, such as a decreased level of consciousness, ataxia, and seizures, the estimated radiation exposure is greater than 10 Gy and mortality is 100%. Those with a moderate radiation dose (2 to 6 Gy) may develop some mild transient cognitive impairment. Those with a higher dose (~6 to 10 Gy) will have more significant disturbances in cognition and consciousness that persist beyond 24 hours and have an expected survival of less than 5%. If the radiation dose remains uncertain due to confounders or an ambivalent presentation, the absolute lymphocyte count at 48 hours can provide further insight into the estimated radiation dose absorbed (Table 129.2).

Symptoms of cerebral edema from radiation injury following therapeutic radiotherapy with high daily dose fractions appear within a few days to weeks and include headache, nausea, and vomiting. Alopecia and scalp erythema may also be seen. Injury to

TABLE 129.2	Acute Radiation Syndrome Prognosis Based on Acute Symptoms and 48-Hour Absolute Lymphocyte Count			
Radiation Dose (Gy)	Acute Symptoms	24-hour CNS Symptoms	48-hour Absolute Lymphocyte Count	Prognosis/ Mortality
0–0.4	None to very mild, onset ~6 h	None to very mild headache	1,400–3,000 (normal)	Excellent, <5%
0.5–2	None to mild, onset 2–6 h	None to headache	1,000–1,399	Good, <5%
2–4	Mild to moderate, onset 1–2 h	Brief cognitive impairments	500–999	Fair, 5–50%
4–8	Moderate to severe, onset 10–60 min	Drowsy to confused	100–499	Poor, 50–100%
>8	Severe, onset within 10 min	Immediate lethargy, coma, seizures	100	Dismal, 100%

CNS, central nervous system.

the pharyngeal mucosa may cause pharyngitis and eustachian tube dysfunction leading to otitis media. A delayed leukoencephalopathy can present 4 to 10 weeks after radiation with somnolence and headache. A posterior fossa syndrome of ataxia, dysarthria, and nystagmus may follow radiation to the middle ear area for glomus jugulare tumors.

Radiation necrosis is a delayed-late consequence of radiation that presents between 6 months and 7.5 years after radiotherapy with clinical manifestations that may mimic the original tumor. Other presentations may include seizures, headaches, or increased intracranial pressure (ICP). Focal or lateralizing neurologic deficits can be neuroanatomically linked to the site of the treated malignancy or distant from it.

Early-delayed radiation myelopathy is transient and presents within 6 months of radiotherapy. Lhermitte sign (i.e., flexion of the neck causes an electric shock sensation down the spine) is reported in up to 15% of those receiving radiation for Hodgkin lymphoma. Delayed radiation myelopathy presents 1 to 3 years following radiotherapy and presents with painless numbness and paresthesias, which then progress to include a spastic gait, sphincter symptoms, and limb weakness. Less commonly, acute paraplegia occurs acutely over a few hours and in this instance is thought to be the result of vascular injury causing infarction. Also worth mentioning is a syndrome that simulates motor neuron disease, which progress over 1 to 2 years and then plateaus.

Radiation-induced vasculopathy typically presents as a transient ischemic attack and/or ischemic stroke. Cerebrovascular malformations have been reported in the field of irradiated tissue as well. This time course to onset can be short or several decades after radiotherapy. SMART syndrome presents many years after whole-brain radiation and presents with seizures, headaches, and stroke-like symptoms.

Radiation plexopathy is observed in three distinct clinical syndromes. A transient plexus injury presents 3 to 6 months following radiotherapy with paresthesias, pain, or weakness. Acute ischemic brachial neuropathy has an acute presentation that does not progress and is painless. Radiation fibrosis presents with painless paresthesias involving the upper (brachial) plexus +/− swelling of the arm about 4 years after radiotherapy. Tumor recurrence can also present in a delayed fashion with paresthesias, but there is typically no swelling, it is painful, and it affects the lower plexus.

Optic neuropathy presents with painless visual loss, decreased visual acuity, and/ or abnormal visual fields within 3 years of radiotherapy. Exam demonstrates papilledema followed by optic atrophy and hemorrhagic exudates.

Endocrine dysfunction presents with growth arrest in children, a decrease in muscle mass, and an increase in adipose tissue in adults. Gonadotropin deficiency manifests as a failure to enter puberty in children and with amenorrhea, infertility, sexual dysfunction, and decreased libido in adults. Thyrotropin deficiency presentations may include weight gain and lethargy. Adrenocorticotropic hormone deficiency is uncommon and presents with lethargy, fatigue, fasting hypoglycemia, and hyponatremia. Hyperprolactinemia is featured by delayed puberty, galactorrhea, and amenorrhea in women and decreased libido and impotence in men.

Neuropsychological sequela of radiation is most conspicuous when it manifests with a delayed IQ decline, learning disability, or academic failure. Detailed neuropsychiatric testing can reveal deficits in memory, executive function, processing speed, and verbal selective reminding. A syndrome of ataxia, cognitive disturbance, and urinary incontinence has been described that resolves with ventriculoperitoneal shunting.

DIAGNOSIS

The diagnosis for many of the aforementioned clinical sequela rests on the identification of their clinical features, time frame between radiation exposure and onset of symptoms, and exclusion of other conditions or inflictions that can produce the same symptoms. The early onset of cerebral edema after radiotherapy can be appreciated on head CT and brain magnetic resonance imaging (MRI) (T2 or fluid-attenuated inversion recovery [FLAIR]), but the clinical diagnosis is often assumed if there is improvement in symptoms after the administration of corticosteroids. Early-delayed leukoencephalopathy is suspected by the time between radiation exposure and symptom onset. T2 and FLAIR sequences on MRI may demonstrate hyperintensities, which are not specific for the condition. Confidence in the diagnosis of early-delayed leukoencephalopathy is strengthened by the gradual improvement in symptoms without treatment or intervention.

Radiation necrosis is suspected when symptoms begin more than 6 months after radiotherapy. Neuroradiologic abnormalities range from focal mass lesions to diffuse white matter changes. Mass lesions are typically at the site of the original tumor/malignancy or in the path of delivered radiotherapy. CT and/or MRI may demonstrate ringlike or heterogeneous enhancement mimicking the original neoplasm. Angiography will demonstrate that the lesion is avascular. Initially, changes are typically seen in the white matter but may progress to involve the gray matter over a period of 6 months to 2 years. Diffuse white matter changes are seen as areas of hypodensity on CT or increased signal intensity on T2/FLAIR on MRI (with MRI being more sensitive), do not necessarily correlate with clinical symptoms, and are typically not reversible. Mild or early changes are seen adjacent to the frontal and occipital horns of the lateral ventricles. More extensive or progressive changes extend to include the centrum semiovale. The most advanced show diffuse lesions with a characteristic scalloped configuration. Accompanying changes include cortical atrophy or ventricular dilatation. In all stages, mass effect is rare, and if seen an alternative process or focal necrosis should be considered.

Distinguishing tumor recurrence from radiation necrosis may be difficult. Single-photon emission computed tomography (SPECT) and positron emission tomography (PET) may be helpful. Hypometabolic areas on PET are suggestive of radiation necrosis. A reduction in choline levels on *magnetic resonance* (MR) *spectroscopy* suggests tumor necrosis (and therefore radiation necrosis), whereas an increase could suggest tumor recurrence. Lactate elevations are suggestive (but not diagnostic) of necrosis due to vasculopathy. The clinicians should avoid anchoring themselves to a diagnosis based on neuroimaging alone and should have a low threshold for performing a biopsy to increase their diagnostic certainty.

Radiation myelopathy is diagnosed via exclusion of other processes and its time of onset in relation to the radiation administration (~1 to 3 years after radiotherapy). MRI may demonstrate cord swelling, atrophy, or complete subarachnoid block, but it also maybe normal. Signal changes on TI (low intensity) or T2 (high intensity) and contrast enhancement may appear 1 month after the onset of clinical symptoms. Beginning about 1 year after onset of symptoms, cord atrophy is seen and there is no further contrast enhancement. The diagnostic approach should seek to exclude other possible etiologies of the patient's myelopathy, such as extra- or intramedullary tumors, leptomeningeal metastases, or cord compression due to vertebral body abnormalities.

Unilateral gyriform enhancement on MRI many years after whole brain radiation in a patient with headaches, seizures, and/or focal neurologic findings is suggestive of SMART syndrome. Radiation vasculopathy is suspected based history, location of the vasculopathy, and region of prior radiotherapy. Radiation plexopathy due to fibrosis is favored with electromyography (EMG) demonstrates myokymia. CT and MRI changes consistent with fibrosis increase the likelihood of a causational link but are not conclusive. Endocrinopathies and pituitary dysfunction are diagnosed as described elsewhere in this text. Cognitive and neurobehavioral disturbances are detected through neuropsychiatric assessment.

TREATMENT

The nervous system effects from ARS do not have specific therapies. The treatment of ARS is described in other texts and largely includes supportive care and granulocyte-stimulating drugs when significant lymphopenia is seen. Corticosteroids do not have a role in ARS, as immunosuppression is one of the most feared and deadly consequences of high-dose ionizing radiation exposures.

Cerebral edema, early-delayed leukoencephalopathy, late-delayed radiation necrosis, myelopathy, plexopathies, and neuropathies are often treated with corticosteroids. Among these inflictions, only cerebral edema seems to have an appreciable clinical response. Not uncommonly, there is a transient improvement with corticosteroids in radiation necrosis and myelopathies, but they are not expected to alter the ultimate course of the disease. Surgical resection should be considered when focal radiation necrosis produced marked mass effect, as it can be lifesaving and mitigate further neurologic injury from herniation syndromes.

There are no known effective treatments for radiation myelopathy. Large artery vasculopathy has been treated successfully with stenting. Treatments for plexopathy include the prevention of shoulder subluxation, treating lymphedema, and providing analgesia.

SMART syndrome does not have any proven or specific treatments; patients often receive a course of corticosteroids and antiepileptics. Some authors advocate for antiplatelet agents and/or statins.

OUTCOME

Outcomes after acute radiation syndromes are displayed in Table 129.2. Early cerebral edema and early delayed leukoencephalopathy/demyelination are nearly always self-limited and reversible. Radiation necrosis can be progressive and fatal and is typically not reversible. Symptoms of radiation myelopathy are also not expected to improve. Outcomes after vasculopathy are related to the efficacy and timing of revascularization efforts. Outcomes after SMART syndrome have only been described in case series, but up to 50% appear to have residual neurologic deficits. Radiation plexopathy, neuropathy, and optic neuropathy are usually irreversible. Cognitive deficits are typically not reversible and not uncommonly progressive, resulting in death or permanent disability and dependence.

SUGGESTED READINGS

Ballesteros-Zebadúa P, Chavarria A, Celis MA, et al. Radiation-induced neuroinflammation and radiation somnolence syndrome. *CNS Neurol Disord Drug Targets*. 2012;11(7):937–949.

Ben Arush MW, Elhasid R. Effects of radiotherapy on the growth of children with leukemia. *Pediatr Endocrinol Rev*. 2008;5(3):785–788.

Diaz AZ, Choi M. Radiation-associated toxicities in the treatment of high-grade gliomas. *Semin Oncol*. 2014;41(4):532–540.

Doyle DM, Einhorn LH. Delayed effects of whole brain radiotherapy in germ cell tumor patients with central nervous system metastases. *Int J Radiat Oncol Biol Phys*. 2008;70(5):1361–1364.

Genc M, Genc E, Genc BO, et al. Significant response of radiation induced CNS toxicity to high dose steroid administration. *Br J Radiol*. 2006;79(948): e196–e199.

Greene-Schloesser D, Robbins ME, Peiffer AM, et al. Radiation-induced brain injury: a review. *Front Oncol*. 2012;2:73.

Hopewell JW, Millar WT, Ang KK. Toward improving the therapeutic ratio in stereotactic radiosurgery: selective modulation of the radiation responses of both normal tissues and tumor. *J Neurosurg*. 2007;107(1):84–93.

Hottinger AF, DeAngelis LM, Yahalom J, et al. Salvage whole brain radiotherapy for recurrent or refractory primary CNS lymphoma. *Neurology*. 2007;69(11): 1178–1182.

Jahnke K, Kraemer DF, Knight KR, et al. Intraarterial chemotherapy and osmotic blood-brain barrier disruption for patients with embryonal and germ cell tumors of the central nervous system. *Cancer*. 2008;112(3):581–588.

Kim JH, Brown SL, Jenrow KA, et al. Mechanisms of radiation-induced brain toxicity and implications for future clinical trials. *J Neurooncol*. 2008;87(3): 279–286.

Knab B, Connell PP. Radiotherapy for pediatric brain tumors: when and how. *Expert Rev Anticancer Ther*. 2007;7(12)(suppl):S69–S77.

Kramer K, Humm JL, Souweidane MM, et al. Phase I study of targeted radioimmunotherapy for leptomeningeal cancers using intra-Ommaya 131-I-3F8. *J Clin Oncol*. 2007;25(34):5465–5470.

Lampert PW, Devis RL. Delayed effects of radiation on the human CNS— "early" and "late" delayed reactions. *Neurology*. 1964;14:912–917.

Lo SS, Chang EL, Yamada Y, et al. Stereotactic radiosurgery and radiation therapy for spinal tumors. *Expert Rev Neurother*. 2007;7(1):85–93.

Mettler FA, Voelz G. Major radiation exposure: what to expect and how to respond. *N Engl J Med*. 2002;346(20):1554–1561.

Mody R, Li S, Dover DC, et al. Twenty-five-year follow-up among survivors of childhood acute lymphoblastic leukemia: a report from the Childhood Cancer Survivor Study. *Blood*. 2008;111(12):5515–5523.

Rogers LR. Neurologic complications of radiation. *Continuum (Minneap Minn)*. 2012;18(2):343–354.

Schiff D, Wen P. Central nervous system toxicity from cancer therapies. *Hematol Oncol Clin North Am*. 2006;20(6):1377–1398.

Siegal D, Keller A, Xu W, et al. Central nervous system complications after allogeneic hematopoietic stem cell transplantation: incidence, manifestations, and clinical significance. *Biol Blood Marrow Transplant*. 2007;13(11):1369–1379.

Verma N, Cowperthwaite MC, Burnett MG, et al. Differentiating tumor recurrence from treatment necrosis: a review of neuro-oncologic imaging strategies. *Neuro Oncol*. 2013;15(5):515–534.

Warrington JP, Ashpole N, Csiszar A, et al. Whole brain radiation-induced vascular cognitive impairment: mechanisms and implications. *J Vasc Res*. 2013;50(6):445–457.

Radiation: Central Nervous System Effects

Al-Mefty O, Kersh JE, Routh A, et al. The long-term side effects of radiation therapy for benign brain tumors in adults. *J Neurosurg*. 1990;73:502–512.

Archibald Y, Lunn D, Ruttan L, et al. Cognitive functioning in long-term survivors of high-grade gliomas. *J Neurosurg*. 1994;80:247–253.

Black DF, Morris JM, Lindell EP, et al. Stroke-like migraine attacks after radiation therapy (SMART) syndrome is not always completely reversible: a case series. *AJNR Am J Neuroradiol*. 2013;34(12):2298–2303.

Buchpiguel CA, Alavi JB, Alavi A, et al. PET versus SPECT in distinguishing radiation necrosis from tumor in the brain. *J Nucl Med*. 1995;36:159–164.

Chernov MF, Ono Y, Abe K, et al. Differentiation of tumor progression and radiation-induced effects after intracranial radiosurgery. *Acta Neurochir Suppl*. 2013;116:193–210.

Coderre JA, Morris GM, Micca PL, et al. Late effects of radiation on the central nervous system: role of vascular endothelial damage and glial stem cell survival. *Radiat Res*. 2006;166:495–503.

DeAngelis LM, Delattre JY, Posner JB. Radiation-induced dementia in patients cured of brain metastases. *Neurology*. 1989;39:789–796.

Donahue B. Short- and long-term complications of radiation therapy for pediatric brain tumors. *Pediatr Neurosurg*. 1992;18:207–217.

Doyle WK, Budinger TF, Valk PE, et al. Differentiation of cerebral radiation necrosis from tumor recurrence by [¹⁸F]FDG and ⁸²RB positron emission tomography. *J Comput Assist Tomogr*. 1987;11:563–570.

Fischer AW, Holfeder H. Lokales Amyloid im Gehirn. *Dtsch Z Chir*. 1930;227: 475–483.

Harris J, Levene M. Visual complications following irradiation for pituitary adenomas and craniopharyngiomas. *Radiology*. 1976;120:167–171.

Landau K, Killer HE. Radiation damage [letter]. *Neurology*. 1996;46:889.

Loeffler JS, Siddon RL, Wen PY, et al. Stereotactic radiosurgery of the brain using a standard linear accelerator: a study of early and late effects. *Radiother Oncol*. 1990;17:311–321.

Macdonald D, Rottenberg D, Schutz J, et al. Radiation-induced optic neuropathy. In: Rottenberg D, ed. *Neurological Complications of Cancer Treatment*. Boston, MA: Butterworth-Heinemann; 1991:37–61.

Marks JE, Baglan RJ, Prassad SC, et al. Cerebral radionecrosis: incidence and risk in relation to dose, time, fractionation and volume. *Int J Radiat Oncol Biol Phys*. 1981;7:243–252.

Mayer R, Sminia P. Reirradiation tolerance of the human brain. *Int J Radiat Oncol Biol Phys*. 2008;70:1350–1360.

Meadows A, Gordon J, Massari DJ, et al. Declines in IQ scores and cognitive dysfunctions in children with acute lymphocytic leukemia treated with cranial irradiation. *Lancet*. 1981;2:1015–1018.

Minniti G, Clarke E, Lanzetta G, et al. Stereotactic radiosurgery for brain metastases: analysis of outcome and risk of brain radionecrosis. *Radiat Oncol*. 2011;6:48.

Mitomo M, Kawai R, Miura T, et al. Radiation necrosis of the brain and radiation-induced cerebrovasculopathy. *Acta Radiol Suppl*. 1986;369:227–230.

Moss H, Nannis E, Poplack DG. The effects of prophylactic treatment of the central nervous system on the intellectual functioning of children with acute lymphocytic leukemia. *Am J Med*. 1981;71:47–52.

Mostow EN, Byrne J, Connelly RR, et al. Quality of life in long-term survivors of CNS tumors of childhood and adolescence. *J Clin Oncol*. 1991;9:592–599.

Mulhern RK, Kovnar E, Langston J, et al. Long-term survivors of leukemia treated in infancy: factors associated with neuropsychologic status. *J Clin Oncol*. 1992;10:1095–1102.

Nightingale S, Dawes PJDK, Cartlidge NEF. Early-delayed radiation rhombencephalopathy. *J Neurol Neurosurg Psychiatry*. 1982;45:267–270.

Norris AM, Carrington BM, Slevin NJ. Late radiation change in the CNS: MR imaging following gadolinium enhancement. *Clin Radiol*. 1997;52:356–362.

Packer RJ, Meadows AT, Rorke LB, et al. Long-term sequelae of cancer treatment on the central nervous system in childhood. *Med Pediatr Oncol*. 1987;15:241–253.

Parsons J, Fitzgerald C, Hood C, et al. The effects of irradiation on the eye and the optic nerve. *Int J Radiat Oncol Biol Phys*. 1983;9:609–622.

Phuphanich S, Jacobs M, Murtagh FR, et al. MRI of spinal cord radiation necrosis simulating recurrent cervical cord astrocytoma and syringomyelia. *Surg Neurol*. 1996;45:362–365.

Plowman PN. Haematologic toxicity during craniospinal irradiation—the impact of prior chemotherapy. *Med Pediatr Oncol*. 1997;28:238–239.

Pomeranz HD, Henson JW, Lessell S. Radiation-associated cerebral blindness. *Am J Ophthalmol*. 1998;126:609–611.

Ruben JD, Dally M, Bailey M, et al. Cerebral radiation necrosis: incidence, outcomes, and risk factors with emphasis on radiation parameters and chemotherapy. *Int J Radiat Oncol Biol Phys*. 2006;65:499–508.

Schultheiss TE, Kun LE, Ang KK, et al. Radiation response of the central nervous system. *Int J Radiat Oncol Biol Phys*. 1995;31:1093–1112.

Schüttrumpf LH, Niyazi M, Nachbichler SB, et al. Prognostic factors for survival and radiation necrosis after stereotactic radiosurgery alone or in combination with whole brain radiation therapy for 1-3 cerebral metastases. *Radiat Oncol*. 2014;9:105.

Sheline GE, Wara WM, Smith V. Therapeutic irradiation and brain therapy. *Int J Radiat Oncol Biol Phys*. 1980;6:1215–1228.

Sonoda Y, Kumabe T, Takahashi T, et al. Clinical usefulness of ¹¹C-MET PET and ²⁰¹Tl SPECT for differentiation of recurrent glioma from radiation necrosis. *Neurol Med Chir (Tokyo)*. 1998;38:342–347.

Tada E, Matsumoto K, Nakagawa M, et al. Serial magnetic resonance imaging of delayed radiation necrosis treated with dexamethasone: case illustration. *J Neurosurg*. 1997;86:1067.

Telera S, Fabi A, Pace A, et al. Radionecrosis induced by stereotactic radiosurgery of brain metastases: results of surgery and outcome of disease. *J Neurooncol*. 2013;113(2):313–325.

Twijnstra A, Boon PJ, Lormans ACM, et al. Neurotoxicity of prophylactic cranial irradiation in patients with small cell carcinoma of the lung. *Eur J Cancer Clin Oncol*. 1987;23:983–986.

Valk PE, Budinger TF, Levin VA, et al. PET of malignant cerebral tumors after interstitial brachytherapy. *J Neurosurg*. 1988;69:830–838.

Wald LL, Nelson SJ, Day MR, et al. Serial proton magnetic resonance spectroscopy imaging of glioblastoma multiforme after brachytherapy. *J Neurosurg*. 1997;87:525–534.

Radiation Myelopathy

Alfonso ED, De Gregorio MA, Mateo P, et al. Radiation myelopathy in over-irradiated patients: MR imaging findings. *Eur Radiol*. 1997;7:400–404.

Delattre JY, Rosenblum MK, Thaler HT, et al. A model of radiation myelopathy in the rat: pathology, regional capillary permeability changes and treatment with dexamethasone. *Brain*. 1988;111:1319–1336.

Goldwein JW. Radiation myelopathy: a review. *Med Pediatr Oncol*. 1987;15:89–95.

Grunewald R, Chroni E, Panayiotopoulos C, et al. Late onset radiation-induced motor neuron syndrome. *J Neurol Neurosurg Psychiatry*. 1992;55:741–742.

Hopewell JW. Radiation injury to the central nervous system. *Med Pediatr Oncol*. 1998;(suppl 1):1–9.

Jeremic B, Djuric L, Mijatovic L. Incidence of radiation myelitis of the cervical spinal cord at doses of 5,500 cGy or greater. *Cancer*. 1991;68:2138–2141.

Koehler PJ, Verbiest H, Jager J, et al. Delayed radiation myelopathy: serial MR imaging and pathology. *Clin Neurol Neurosurg*. 1996;98:197–201.

Komachi H, Tsuchiya K, Ikeda M, et al. Radiation myelopathy: a clinicopathological study with special reference to correlation between MRI findings and neuropathology. *J Neurol Sci*. 1995;132:228–232.

Melki PS, Halimi P, Wibault P, et al. MRI in chronic progressive radiation myelopathy. *J Comput Assist Tomogr*. 1994;18:1–6.

Phuphanich S, Jacobs M, Murtagh FR, et al. MRI of spinal cord recognition necrosis stimulating recurrent cervical cord astrocytoma and syringomyelia. *Surg Neurol*. 1996;45:362–365.

Schultheiss TE, Higgins EM, El-Mahdi AM. The latent period in clinical radiation myelopathy. *Int J Radiat Oncol Biol Phys*. 1984;10:1109–1115.

Tashima T, Morioka T, Nishio S, et al. Delayed cerebral radionecrosis with a high uptake of ¹¹C-methionine on positron emission tomography and ²⁰¹Tl-chloride on single-photon emission computed tomography. *Neuroradiology*. 1998;40:435–438.

Thornton AF, Zimberg SH, Greenberg HS, et al. Protracted Lhermitte's sign following head and neck irradiation. *Arch Otolaryngol Head Neck Surg*. 1991;117:1300–1303.

Van der Kogel AJ. Radiation tolerance of the rat spinal cord: time-dose relationships. *Radiology*. 1977;122:505–509.

Wang PY, Shen WC, Jan JS. Serial MRI changes in radiation myelopathy. *Neuroradiology*. 1995;37:374–377.

Wara W, Phillips T, Sheline G, et al. Radiation tolerance of the spinal cord. *Cancer*. 1975;35:1558–1562.

Radiation: Vascular Complications

Benson PJ, Sung JH. Cerebral aneurysms following radiotherapy for medulloblastoma. *J Neurosurg*. 1989;70:545–550.

Chang SD, Vanefsky MA, Havton LA, et al. Bilateral cavernous malformations resulting from cranial irradiation of a choroid plexus papilloma. *Neurol Res*. 1998;20:529–532.

Hirata Y, Matsukado Y, Mihara Y, et al. Occlusion of the internal carotid artery after radiation therapy for the chiasmal lesion. *Acta Neurochir (Wien)*. 1985;74:141–147.

Houdart E, Mounayer C, Chapot R, et al. Carotid stenting for radiation-induced stenosis. *Stroke*. 2001;32:118–121.

Kreisl TN, Toothaker T, Karimi S, et al. Ischemic stroke in patients with primary brain tumors. *Neurology*. 2008;70(24):2314–2320.

McGuirt WF, Feehs RS, Strickland JL, et al. Irradiation-induced atherosclerosis: a factor in therapeutic planning. *Ann Otol Rhinol Laryngol*. 1992;101:222–228.

Murros KE, Toole JF. The effect of radiation of carotid arteries: a review article. *Arch Neurol.* 1989;46:449–455.

Pozzati E, Giangaspero F, Marliani F, et al. Occult cerebrovascular malformations after irradiation. *Neurosurgery.* 1996;39:677–682.

Werner MH, Burger PC, Heinz ER, et al. Intracranial atherosclerosis following radiotherapy. *Neurology.* 1988;38:1158–1160.

Stroke-like Migraine Attacks after Radiation Therapy (SMART) Syndrome

Armstrong AE, Gillan E, DiMario FJ Jr. SMART syndrome (stroke-like migraine attacks after radiation therapy) in adult and pediatric patients. *J Child Neurol.* 2014;29(3):336–341.

Black DF, Morris JM, Lindell EP, et al. Stroke-like migraine attacks after radiation therapy (SMART) syndrome is not always completely reversible: a case series. *AJNR Am J Neuroradiol.* 2013;34(12):2298–2303.

Radiation-Induced Plexopathy

Bowen BC, Verma A, Brandon AH, et al. Radiation-induced brachial plexopathy: MR and clinical findings. *AJNR Am J Neuroradiol.* 1996;17:1932–1936.

Georgion A, Grigsby PW, Perez CA. Radiation induced lumbosacral plexopathy in gynecologic tumors: clinical findings and dosimetric analysis. *Int J Radiat Oncol Biol Phys.* 1993;26:479–482.

Harper CM, Thomas J, Cascino T, et al. Distinction between neoplastic and radiation-induced brachial plexopathy, with emphasis on the role of EMG. *Neurology.* 1989;39:502–506.

Jaeckle KA, Young DF, Foley KM. The natural history of lumbosacral plexopathy in cancer. *Neurology.* 1985;35:8–15.

Kori SH, Foley KM, Posner JB. Brachial plexus lesions in patients with cancer: 100 cases. *Neurology.* 1981;31:45–50.

Olsen NK, Pfeiffer P, Johannsen L, et al. Radiation-induced brachial plexopathy: neurological follow-up in 161 recurrence-free breast cancer patients. *Int J Radiat Oncol Biology Phys.* 1993;26:43–49.

Thomas JE, Cascino TL, Earle JD. Differential diagnosis between radiation and tumor plexopathy of the pelvis. *Neurology.* 1985;35:1–7.

Wouter van Es H, Engelen AM, Witkamp TD, et al. Radiation-induced brachial plexopathy: MR imaging. *Skeletal Radiol.* 1997;26:284–288.

Endocrine Dysfunction

Burstein S. Poor growth after cranial irradiation. *Pediatr Rev.* 1997;18:442–444.

Constine LS, Woolf PD, Cann D, et al. Hypothalamic-pituitary dysfunction after radiation for brain tumors. *N Engl J Med.* 1993;328:87–94.

Duffner PK, Cohen ME, Voorhess ML, et al. Long-term effects of cranial irradiation on endocrine function in children with brain tumors: a prospective study. *Cancer.* 1985;56:2189–2193.

Mechanik JI, Hochberg FH, LaRocque A. Hypothalamic dysfunction following whole-brain irradiation. *J Neurosurg.* 1986;65:490–494.

Rappaport R, Brauner R. Growth and endocrine disorders secondary to cranial irradiation. *Pediatr Res.* 1989;25:561–567.

Shalet SM. Radiation and pituitary dysfunction. *N Engl J Med.* 1993;238:131–133.

Woo E, Lam K, Yu YL, et al. Temporal lobe and hypothalamic-pituitary dysfunctions after radiotherapy for nasopharyngeal carcinoma: a distinct clinical syndrome. *J Neurol Neurosurg Psychiatry.* 1988;51:1302–1307.

Radiation: Neuropsychological Effects

Anderson V, Godber T, Smibert E, et al. Neurobehavioural sequelae following cranial irradiation and chemotherapy in children: an analysis of risk factors. *Pediatr Rehabil.* 1997;1:63–76.

Armstrong C, Ruffer J, Corn B, et al. Biphasic patterns of memory deficits following moderate-dose partial-brain irradiation: neuropsychologic outcome and proposed mechanisms. *J Clin Oncol.* 1995;13:2263–2271.

Crossen JR, Garwood D, Glatstein E, et al. Neurobehavioral sequelae of cranial irradiation in adults: a review of radiation-induced encephalopathy. *J Clin Oncol.* 1994;12:627–642.

Duffey P, Chari G, Cartlidge NEF, et al. Progressive deterioration of intellect and motor function occurring several decades after cranial irradiation. *Arch Neurol.* 1996;53:814–818.

Edelmann MN, Krull KR, Liu W, et al. Diffusion tensor imaging and neuro-cognition in survivors of childhood acute lymphoblastic leukaemia. *Brain.* 2014;137(pt 11):2973–2983.

Glauser TA, Packer RJ. Cognitive deficits in long-term survivors of childhood brain tumors. *Childs Nerv Syst.* 1991;7:2–12.

Kazda T, Jancalek R, Pospisil P, et al. Why and how to spare the hippocampus during brain radiotherapy: the developing role of hippocampal avoidance in cranial radiotherapy. *Radiat Oncol.* 2014;9:139.

Krull KR, Minoshima S, Edelmann M, et al. Regional brain glucose metabolism and neurocognitive function in adult survivors of childhood cancer treated with cranial radiation. *J Nucl Med.* 2014;55(11):1805–1810.

Roman DD, Sperduto PW. Neuropsychological effects of cranial radiation: current knowledge and future directions. *Int J Radiat Oncol Biol Phys.* 1998;31:983–998.

Sklar CA, Copstine LS. Chronic neuropsychological sequela of radiation therapy. *Int J Radiat Oncol Biol Phys.* 1995;31:1113–1121.

Radiation Damage to Peripheral Nerves

Giese WL, Kinsella TJ. Radiation injury to peripheral and cranial nerves. In: Gutin PH, Leibel SA, Sheline GE, eds. *Radiation Injury to the Nervous System.* New York: Raven Press; 1991:383–403.

Gillette EL, Mahler PA, Powers BE, et al. Late radiation injury to muscle and peripheral nerves. *Int J Radiat Oncol Biol Phys.* 1995;31:1309–1318.

Radiation-Induced Tumors

Coureau G, Bouvier G, Lebailly P, et al. Mobile phone use and brain tumours in the CERENAT case-control study. *Occup Environ Med.* 2014;71(7):514–522.

Dweik A, Maheut-Lourmiere J, Lioret E, et al. Radiation-induced meningioma. *Childs Nerv Syst.* 1995;11:661–663.

Ecemis GC, Atmaca A, Meydan D. Radiation-associated secondary brain tumors after conventional radiotherapy and radiosurgery. *Expert Rev Neurother.* 2013;13(5):557–565.

Foley KM. Radiation-induced malignant and atypical peripheral nerve sheath tumors. *Ann Neurol.* 1980;7:311–318.

Harrison MJ, Wolfe DE, Lau TS, et al. Radiation-induced meningiomas: experience at the Mount Sinai Hospital and review of the literature. *J Neurosurg.* 1991;75:564–574.

Kumar PP, Good RR, Skultety FM, et al. Radiation-induced neoplasms of the brain. *Cancer.* 1987;59:1274–1282.

Nadeem SQ, Feun LG, Bruce-Gregorios JH, et al. Post radiation sarcoma (malignant fibrous histiocytoma) of the cervical spine following ependymoma (a case report). *J Neurooncol.* 1991;11:263–268.

Ron E, Modan B, Boice JD Jr, et al. Tumors of the brain and nervous system after radiotherapy in childhood. *N Engl J Med.* 1988;319:1033–1039.

Shapiro S, Mealey J, Sartorius C. Radiation-induced intracranial malignant gliomas. *J Neurosurg.* 1989;71:77–82.

Radiation Optic Neuropathy

Danish-Meyers HV. Radiation-induced optic neuropathy. *J Clin Neurosci.* 2008;15:95–100.

McClellan RL, el Gammal T, Kline LB. Early bilateral radiation-induced optic neuropathy with follow-up MRI. *Neuroradiology.* 1995;37:131–133.

Piquemal R, Cottier JP, Arsene S, et al. Radiation-induced optic neuropathy 4 years after radiation: report of a case followed up with MRI. *Neuroradiology.* 1998;40:439–441.

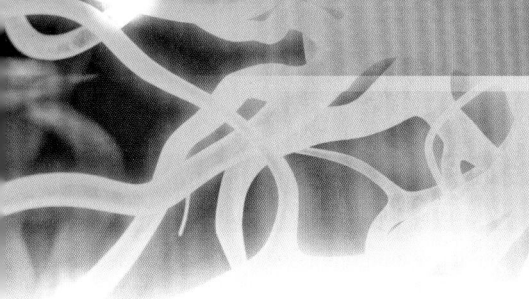

Electrical and Lightning Injury 130

Christopher Zammit and Edward (Mel) J. Otten

INTRODUCTION

Electrical injuries (EI) and lightning strikes (LS) have been reported to cause a variety of neurologic injuries. Interestingly, although some of the associated neurologic sequelae are seen acutely, others develop in a delayed fashion. Although both EI and LS produce injury via the creation of an electrical current, the neurologic complications of each can be quite different.

Low-voltage electrical injuries (LVEI) are defined as resulting from exposures of less than 1,000 V, whereas greater exposures are termed *high-voltage electrical injuries* (HVEI). They are to be further distinguished as being the result of a direct current (DC) or alternating current (AC), with the latter producing approximately three times as much injury as the former. LS are exceptionally brief, with voltages on the order of the millions, and produce a unique constellation of immediate and delayed injuries.

EPIDEMIOLOGY

The first death in the United States related to an artificial electrical source occurred in front of a crowd in Buffalo, New York in 1881 when an intoxicated man came into contact with a generator. His death was seen as being quite painless, leading to the use of electrocution as a humane method of capital punishment. Formal reporting of electrical and lightning injuries is not required, limiting the accuracy of existing epidemiologic data.

There are an estimated 3,000 EI per year in the United States, including 1,000 deaths. Children are more likely to suffer LVEI, whereas adolescents and adults more commonly experience HVEI, which are frequently occupationally related.

Over 15,000 police departments across the United States use conducted energy weapons (CEW), such as stun guns and TASER devices to restrain suspects. Cardiac arrests have occurred after the uses of CEW, but a causational link has been proposed in only a minority of cases. In the majority of circumstances, excited delirium and/or intoxicates ingested by the victim are blamed for causing the arrest.

Three hundred to 1,000 lightning injuries occur per year in the United States, with an estimated mortality rate of 10%. Many victims either do not seek care at the time of the injury, and half of the immediate deaths are transported directly to the coroner and never reported. Victims are usually men (4.5:1 male-to-female ratio) in their second to third decade of life and are performing outdoor recreational or occupational activities.

PATHOBIOLOGY

ELECTRICAL INJURIES

The severity of LVEI is subject to the pathway of the current and proportional to the duration of exposure and amount of current (milliamperes [mA]). Low-voltage AC, in contrast to low-voltage DC, can produce continuous involuntary muscle contractions. If the victim grips an AC electrical source with their hand, tetany of the flexors of the upper extremity prove stronger than the extensors, causing the victim's grasp of the source to be strengthened. Currents of 6 to 9 mA or greater, which can be achieved via exposure to a standard 110-V household outlet, exceed the "let-go threshold," rendering the victim incapable of dissociating himself/herself from the source. If the current flows through the thorax, tetany of the muscles of respiration can occur, causing the victim to suffocate. Currents of approximately 50 to 100 mA can cause ventricular fibrillation; the current threshold is inversely proportional to the duration of exposure.

Direct contact with a high-voltage electrical source more commonly produces diffuse, sudden, and violent muscle contractions that thrust the victim away from the source, causing traumatic insults in addition to the EI. Even with brief exposures, the high voltages convey a tremendous amount of energy, which is released via electrothermal heating at points of high resistance (e.g., the skin, where full-thickness burns are seen). Internally, the current is carried along tissues of low resistance, such as the nerves, muscles, and blood vessels. Immediate effects include muscle necrosis and small-vessel thrombosis, resulting in threats to extremity viability and peripheral nerve integrity through compartment syndromes and limb ischemia.

In contrast to a direct contact injury, a spark can jump from a highly charged source to a ground source, forming an electrical arc, where temperatures can reach 2,500°C. When a victim is caught in the path of the arc, he or she suffers cutaneous thermal burns and blast injuries when the suddenly heated air rapidly cools, in addition to a HVEI by becoming part of the conduction pathway of the current.

CEWs are reported to be high voltage (with an initial charge of ~50,000 V). However, the victim does not experience this voltage. Instead, it allows for an arc to be created if the barbs do not make contact with the skin, which happens about 30% of the time. Once contact is made, the voltage immediately decreases to provide a current of approximately 2 mA in brief pulses at a rate of 20 times per second, producing involuntary muscle clonus (much like an AC circuit), preventing the suspect from resisting. Because of the low current, EI is rare with CEWs, and most injuries, when they do occur, are traumatic and related to when the victim falls to the ground.

LIGHTNING STRIKES

Lightning victims can be directly struck with the discharge, receive current via an adjacent object that was directly struck (side flash), become part of the ground current when their feet are apart (step voltage), be the conduit for currents that originate from the ground and discharge toward the clouds (upward stream), and/or experience a concussive or blast injury from the rapid heating and cooling of the air (thunder). Curiously, some of the injuries typically seen with direct contact HVEI are not found in lightning injuries and entry and exit wounds are only seen in a minority of cases, suggesting that most, if not all, of the current flows external to the victim. This is thought to result in a powerful magnetic field being created over the victim, causing electrical currents to flow internally through low-resistance tissues (i.e., nerves, muscles, blood vessels), resulting in powerful muscle contractions and medullary dysfunction leading to apnea, asystole, and a tremendous catecholamine surge.

Ball lightning (BL) is a poorly understood, spherical, mobile electrical field observed floating along power lines, down aisles of airplanes, or through the air during lightning storms. Neurologic sequela has been reported in those that have come into contact with BL.

The pathophysiology of neuronal injury after EI and LS is not clear and several plausible mechanisms have been reported. The low resistance of nerves makes them a conduit for the electrical current, causing tremendous excitatory discharges, which result in microglia activation, electroporation, and chromatolysis. Electroporation is the destabilization of neuronal cell membranes from electrical current–induced changes in cellular proteins, resulting in their dysfunction and perhaps ultimate death. Microglia activation produces an inflammatory response suspected to result in injury to neurons and oligodendrocytes. Upregulation of postsynaptic cortical γ-aminobutyric acid (GABA)-B receptors is also a suggested consequence of the excitatory impulse based on the results of experiments using transcranial magnetic stimulation in patients with HVEI. Axonal injury and demyelination have been observed in EI and LS victims on MRI, nerve conduction studies, and autopsy.

Blood vessels similarly conduct electrical current, which has been observed to cause microvascular thrombosis and large vessel vasospasm, with some case reports of cerebral thrombosis. Endothelial cell dysfunction at the capillary level resulting in tissue ischemia is a proposed etiology for some of the delayed clinical consequences.

Muscles are also low resistance and therefore conduct a great deal of electrical current. Sarcolemmal injury is a proposed cause of the protracted fatigue reported by many victims of HVEI.

CLINICAL FEATURES

The immediately clinical presentation of EI and LS can range from a minor contact burn to a victim in cardiac arrest. In EI due to direct contact, particularly HVEI, there are often significant cutaneous burns with much more extensive internal burn injuries, particularly involving muscles, small vessels, and tendons. Limb amputation is not uncommonly required and rhabdomyolysis is frequent in HVEI. Traumatic injuries to the head and spinal cord are also common. Vasospasm and cerebral arterial thrombosis, both immediate and delayed, have been reported. Myelopathy is frequently reported and occurs at a spinal level consistent with the path of the electrical current. Contact injuries to the head and LS may cause a multiple-level myelopathy when the current exits through the foot. Myelopathy is not uncommonly delayed in presentation, with a time period that is inversely proportional to the patient's age. Curiously, peripheral neuropathy is not commonly seen, but when it does occur, it tends to affect motor nerves more than sensory and recently has been described to be axonal.

Neuropsychiatric symptoms, cognitive and memory impairment, autonomic dysfunction, fatigue, chronic headaches, and sleep disturbances are quite common among survivors. The constellation of symptoms is quite similar to those seen after a traumatic brain injury.

Cherington has divided the neurologic complications of lightning injury into four categories. Category I are temporary and benign, category II are prolonged and permanent, category III

TABLE 130.1	Neurologic Complication in Victims of Lightning Strikes
Category I	Headache, numbness, weakness, depressed level of consciousness, keraunoparalysis (Charcot paralysis)
Category II	Hypoxic encephalopathy; cognitive deficits; memory and attention impairment; mood, behavioral, and sleep disturbances; fatigue; autonomic dysfunction; cold insensitivity; acute ischemic stroke; intracerebral hemorrhage (basal ganglia or brain stem); myelopathy
Category III	Parkinsonism, progressive motor disease, focal dystonia, and tics
Category IV	Traumatic intracranial hemorrhage, spinal cord injury due to fractures, or hemorrhages

includes delayed symptoms, and category IV are traumatic neurologic injuries that occur secondary to falls, sudden violent muscle contractions, or blast effects. Table 130.1 summarizes these injuries.

Keraunoparalysis, or Charcot paralysis, is an immediate, transient paralysis seen in some LS victims. It involves the lower extremities more than the upper, lasts for less than an hour, and is characterized by pale limbs with diminished or absent pulses, sensory symptoms, and hypertension. A catecholamine surge has been suspected, but not proven, to be the cause.

Several case reports have attempted to suggest a link between EI/LS and amyotrophic lateral sclerosis; however, several recent reviews have summarized the available data and reports and concluded that any link is quite unlikely.

DIAGNOSIS

Victims of EI or LS with an altered level of consciousness, focal deficit, or paralysis on presentation should have emergent diagnostic imaging of the head and/or spine performed to evaluate for traumatic injuries or acute ischemia, which may warrant prompt interventions. Acute cerebral ischemia many be secondary to thrombosis or vasospasm; emergent computed tomography (CT) or conventional angiography should be considered.

TREATMENT

Specific treatments for the neurologic sequela of electrical and lighting injuries have not been described. Intravenous thrombolytics and/or endovascular therapy (clot retrieval if thrombosis or angioplasty/intra-arterial therapy if vasospasm) should be considered in patients presenting with a sudden onset of focal neurologic deficits after an EI or LS. Victims who are resuscitated after a cardiac arrest and not following commands should be considered candidates for targeted temperature management, barring other contraindications. Similarly, if the victim remains comatose for longer than 2 hours without an alternate explanation, it may suggest he or she was transiently asystolic and/or apneic, particularly in the setting of an LS. Cardiac automaticity and ventilation may have spontaneously resumed but not without suffering a hypoxic–ischemic cerebral injury. The astute clinician should consider targeted temperature management in this setting as well because the event is the equivalent of return of spontaneous circulation in a cardiac arrest patient who received an active resuscitation. Traumatic injuries should be treated accordingly. Survivors of EI and LS may be referred to an international support group, Lightning Strike and Electric Shock Survivors International, Inc. (http://www.lightning-strike.org).

OUTCOME

The neuropsychiatric complications, cognitive deficits, and autonomic disturbances seen after EI and LS are most commonly permanent and at times progressive. Myelopathy may improve, and recovery has been seen in some victims, but most are left with persistent symptoms. Cardiopulmonary resuscitation (CPR) success rates have been higher in victims of electrical and lightning injuries than from other causes even when the interval from injury has been prolonged. Outcomes after EI or LS complicated by a cerebral infarction or hypoxic–ischemic injury are only found in case reports or case series, making accurate estimations impossible.

SUGGESTED READINGS

Abhinav K, Al-Chalabi A, Hortobagyi T, et al. Electrical injury and amyotrophic lateral sclerosis: a systematic review of the literature. *J Neurol Neurosurg Psychiatry*. 2007;78:450–453.

Cherington M. Neurologic manifestations of lightning strikes. *Neurology*. 2003;60:182–185.

Cherington M. Spectrum of neurologic complications of lightning injuries. *NeuroRehabilitation*. 2005;20:3–8.

Cherington M, Yarnell PR, Lane J, et al. Lightning-induced injury on an airplane: coronal discharge and ball lightning. *J Trauma*. 2002;52(3):579.

Critchley M. Neurological effects of lightning and electricity. *Lancet*. 1934;1:68–72.

Davidson GS, Deck JH. Delayed myelopathy following lightning strike: a demyelinating process. *Acta Neuropathol*. 1988;77:104–108.

Jain RS, Gupta P, Handa R, et al. Vertebrobasilar territory ischemic stroke and electrical injury: delayed sequelae. *J Stroke Cerebrovasc Dis*. 2014;23(6):1721–1723.

Jost W, Schonrock L, Cherington M. Autonomic nervous system dysfunction in lightning and electrical injuries. *NeuroRehabilitation*. 2005;20:19–23.

Kashigar A, Udupa K, Fish J, et al. Neurophysiological assessment of fatigue in electrical injury patients. *Exp Brain Res*. 2014;232:1013–1023.

Kleinschmidt-DeMasters DK. Neuropathology of lightning-strike injuries. *Semin Neurol*. 1995;15:323–328.

Kwon KH, Kim SH, Minn WK. Electrodiagnostic study of peripheral nerves in high-voltage electrical injury. *J Burn Care Res*. 2014;35:e230–e233.

Primeau M. Neurorehabilitation of behavioral disorders following lightning and electrical trauma. *NeuroRehabilitation*. 2005;20:25–33.

Reisner A. Possible mechanisms for delayed neurological damage in lightning and electrical injury. *Brain Injury*. 2013;27(5):565–569.

Roshanzamir S, Dabbaghmanesh A, Ashraf A. Predicting post-electrical injury autonomic dysfunction symptom occurrence by a simple test. *Burns*. 2013;40:624–629.

Vilke GM, Bozeman WP, Chan TC. Emergency department evaluation after conducted energy weapon use: review of the literature. *J Emerg Med*. 2011;40:598–604.

Decompression Illness 131

Christopher Zammit and Edward (Mel) J. Otten

INTRODUCTION

The symptoms of decompression illness (DCI) have been observed in underwater and caisson workers since the early 1800s, when it was coined "caisson disease." Today, DCI refers to the sequela that result from arterial gas embolism (AGE) and decompression sickness (DCS). Both conditions are the result of rapid changes in ambient pressure that cause dissolved inert gases to emerge in the circulation as bubbles. The rapid growth in popularity of underwater diving with a self-contained underwater breathing apparatus (SCUBA), particularly by travelers, has made DCS a diagnostic possibility even in land-locked areas. Although this chapter focuses on DCI, other dysbaric conditions with neurologic inflictions or complaints are also briefly discussed, which include middle ear barotrauma (MEBT), inner ear barotrauma (IEBT), alternobaric vertigo (ABV), carbon monoxide poisoning, nitrogen narcosis, oxygen toxicity, and swallow water blackouts.

EPIDEMIOLOGY

DCS has been observed in those who perform submersion activities (e.g., SCUBA, saturation, or breath-hold diving), high-altitude aviation (e.g., U-2 pilots), and simulated altitude ascents. AGE can occur after resurfacing from depths of only 1 to 1.5 m, whereas DCS is never seen after surfacing from depths of less than 6 m and very rarely occurs after dives less than 10 m in depth. AGE can occur if the diver rapidly ascends to the surface, holds his or her breath during ascent, or has intrinsic lung disease, particularly those with blebs and asthmatics. DCS risk factors include longer submersion times, deeper submersions, high exertion and warm temperatures during the dive, cold temperatures after the dive, older age, obesity, dehydration, and male gender. Divers with a patent foramen ovale (PFO) appear to be at increased risk (odds ratios of 2.6 to 5.6) for neurologic DCI when compared with divers without a PFO. Dive computers and tables are available to advise whether "decompression stops" are required during ascent to mitigate the DCS risk.

DCI is estimated to occur in 3 out of every 10,000 dives, with higher rates in U.S. Navy and commercial divers and the lower rates in recreational divers. The Divers Alert Network produces an annual report, which profiles diving-related complications. Data from the most recent report are outlined in Table 131.1.

DCS is less commonly seen in high-altitude flying, when compared with submersion activities, and when observed, the symptoms are typically less severe and rarely include neurologic manifestations. A notable recent exception are Air Force U-2 pilots who fly at altitudes of up to 70,000 ft in suits that are pressurized to approximately 30,000 feet above sea level.

PATHOBIOLOGY

DCI is believed to result from bubbles of inert gas, particularly nitrogen, being formed in the circulation during decompression. In the case of submersion, at increasing pressures, inert gases, mostly nitrogen, become intensely dissolved in the blood and tissues of the body. The amount dissolved will increase if the temperature rises. Upon ascent (whether that is resurfacing from a dive or ascending in elevation, as in aviation), these inert gases come out of solution. Ideally, the gas is delivered to the alveoli, where it is expired. In reality, gas bubbles can be observed in the blood of all divers via ultrasound upon emergence from a dive. Typically, the pulmonary circulation filters the bubbles and the diver does not experience any symptoms. However, if the quantity of bubbles is too great, they will buildup and occlude small veins and lymphatic vessels. At high bubble loads, the pulmonary vasculature also develops occlusions, increasing right heart pressures and raising the possibility of opening an otherwise closed PFO through which bubbles can pass into the arterial circulation.

In addition to vessel occlusion, intravascular bubbles are known to irritate the endothelium, causing capillary leakage, and platelet, complement, and cytokine activation, leading to third spacing, hemoconcentration, small-vessel thrombosis, and eventually hypotension. The occlusive action in the venules combined with small-vessel thrombosis is hypothesized to be the cause of the cerebral, vestibular, and spinal cord injuries and dysfunction in neurologic DCS. Inert gases preferentially dissolve in tissue with a high lipid content, such as the central nervous system (CNS), where the emergence of nitrogenous bubbles are suspected to contribute to neurologic dysfunction and injury.

AGE has a slightly different pathophysiology. Alveolar gas that abruptly expands on decompression (Boyle law) and is not ventilated appropriately will force itself through the alveolar–capillary membrane and directly enter the arterial circulation, where it produces mechanical obstructions. The most notable clinical sequela occur when the cerebral or coronary vessels are occluded, producing ischemic strokes and myocardial infarctions.

TABLE 131.1 2008 Diving-Related Deaths and Morbidity in the United States		
Condition	**Confirmed**	**Suspected**
Fatalities	144[a]	—
Decompression sickness (DCS)	122	209
Cerebral DCS	16	10
Spinal DCS	28	15
Arterial gas embolism	—	11
Middle ear barotrauma	—	344
Inner ear barotrauma	—	26
Alternobaric vertigo	—	6

[a]83 U.S./Canadian residents.

Data from the Divers Alert Network annual report.

MEBT and IEBT occur during compression when the eustachian tube collapses and the middle ear cannot equalize its pressure with the ambient pressure. In MEBT, the tympanic membrane ruptures, exposing the middle ear to the water, causing vertigo and, at times, a seventh cranial nerve palsy. IEBT is the result of a sudden equalization of pressure in the inner ear, causing injury to the cochleo-vestibular system. In contrast, ABV occurs during ascent when gases expand in the middle ear but cannot escape to allow equalization.

Nitrogen narcosis is a result of high concentrations of dissolved nitrogen that can occur at depth of greater than 100 ft. CNS oxygen toxicity can occur when the partial pressure of oxygen exceeds 1.4 atm. Compressed air tanks can be contaminated with carbon monoxide or carbon dioxide if the compressor's exhaust is too close to the air intake, causing carbon monoxide poisoning. Symptoms would be expected to occur during decent or at depth, in contrast to DCI that occurs with ascent or after surfacing. Swallow water blackouts occur in divers who hyperventilate ambient air prior to a dive, driving their arterial carbon dioxide levels very low without increasing their arterial oxygen content. During the dive, carbon dioxide levels do not increase sufficiently to increase respiratory drive, whereas oxygen levels fall, causing a loss of consciousness.

CLINICAL FEATURES

DCS has been divided into two clinical categories, type 1 (DCS1) and type 2 (DCS2). The majority of the time, DCS presents within 24 hours of decompression, but delayed presentation have been seen, particularly in those that have flown or ascended in altitude shortly after decompression. DCS1 includes signs and symptoms related to the integumentary, lymphatic, or musculoskeletal system. The patient will describe joint aches and pains, itching, or extremity edema, and a lenticular skin rash believed to be due to venous status, known as *cutis marmorata*, can be observed.

DCS2 can include features of DCS1 with additional symptoms related to the CNS, lungs, or vestibular system. The pulmonary symptoms, which include a cough, dyspnea, or chest pain, have been called *the chokes*. Vestibular symptoms, also known as the *staggers*, manifest as vertigo, nystagmus, nausea, or vomiting and can be difficult to differentiate from ABV because both can occur on ascent. The symptoms of cerebral DCS can include headache, diplopia, dysarthria, personality changes, disorientation, fatigue, ataxia, drowsiness, and even lethargy. Visual disturbances include optic neuropathy, homonymous hemianopsia, and central retinal artery occlusion. Spinal cord DCS presents with limb weakness, numbness, paresthesias, incontinence, priapism, urinary retention, or back/pelvic pain.

AGE has a dramatic and abrupt presentation, occurring during ascent or within 10 minutes of surfacing, and is commonly found to be the cause of death in diving fatalities. The presentation can include a variety of neurologic changes, including stroke syndromes, and may include pulmonary symptoms in about half of the cases. It can be difficult to distinguish AGE from DCS2. Alas, their treatment is the same, so sorting out the diagnosis is of academic interest only.

MEBT, IEBT, and ABV all have similar symptoms. MEBT will often include a ruptured tympanic membrane. IEBT should be distinguished, as the symptoms will be persistent and often require referral to an otolaryngologist. IEBT and vestibular DCS may be difficult to distinguish as well. A history of a sudden symptom onset upon equalization of pressures suggests IEBT. Cerebellar infarcts have been seen as a result of DCS and should be treated the same as vestibular DCS.

DIAGNOSIS

The diagnosis of DCS is clinical. Any symptoms upon decompression consistent with DCS should be treated as such. There are sporadic reports of carotid artery dissection and one report of an epidural spinal hematoma in a breath-hold diver, but these cases are the exception, and recompression should not be delayed. Magnetic resonance imaging (MRI) lesions have been seen in cerebral and spinal DCS, but they lack sensitivity, as even those with incomplete recovery have been observed to have normal serial imaging. Spinal cord MRI lesions have been observed in the white and gray matter. Cerebral MRI findings include foci of ischemia and T2 hyperintensities, which have been found in the anterior and posterior circulations and in the subcortical white and cortical gray matter. Divers without a history of neurologic DCS have rarely been reported to have abnormal MRIs, but there are only a handful of controlled studies to fully describe the specificity of neuroimaging. Spinal canal stenosis has been associated with the occurrence of spinal DCS and MRI lesions, but it is not associated with clinical outcomes.

TREATMENT

DCI is a medical emergency that calls for the immediately administration of 100% oxygen and recompression. Large-scale observational evidence suggests that timely recompression optimizes outcomes and hastens recovery. More recent publications challenge whether time to recompression impacts the rates of recovery in those with neurologic DCS, but the datasets are small and limited to observations. Therefore, expeditious recompression remains the standard of care, and DCS must be considered a medical emergency.

Hyperbaric therapy (HBT) can be provided in monoplace or multiplace chambers, with the later allowing for hands-on treatment of the patient, if needed. HBT recommendations for DCS and AGE can be found in the U.S. Navy Diving Manual (see "Suggested Readings"). Serial HBT dives are performed until benefit is not seen with consecutive treatments. Patients requiring air transport to HBT should be flown at the lowest safe altitude (recent recommendations are <500 ft above surface level) or in a pressurized aircraft. Portable chambers that allow for partial recompression are available. For chamber locations and emergency information, U.S. physicians should contact the Divers Alert Network, at 919-681-4326, a 24-hour hotline.

Isotonic, non–dextrose-containing intravenous fluids should be administered, as many of these patients are hemoconcentrated. If AGE is suspected, intravenous lidocaine is commonly provided, as randomized evidence from the cardiac surgery literature, where AGE and cerebral injury are commonly seen, suggests it has neuroprotective benefits. Aspirin is considered by many, without evidence to support its use. An randomized controlled trial (RCT) of tenoxicam for DCS demonstrated that is hastened recovery and reduce the number of required recompressions from 3 to 2, but clinical outcomes were no different [**Level 1**].[1] Preliminary evidence is promising for perfluorocarbons, but clinical trials are needed. A small study from the 1990s suggested that a helium-oxygen mixture might be superior to an air-oxygen mixture during recompression, but the results have not been reproduced. A recent study of PFO closure in divers suggests it reduces the incidence of DCS and the quantity of ischemic brain lesions on MRI.

OUTCOME

Cerebral DCS outcomes are similar to ischemic stroke survivors, as one series found the National Institutes of Health Stroke Scale (NIHSS) to have a similar ability to predict outcomes in both conditions. Spine DCS outcomes have been found to be worse in those older than 42 years of age, with bladder symptoms, with progressive symptoms upon decompression, with initial severe symptoms, and with MRI abnormalities. One-quarter to one-third of spinal cord DCS victims will make an incomplete recovery.

LEVEL 1 EVIDENCE

1. Bennett M, Mitchell S, Dominguez A. Adjunctive treatment of decompression illness with a non-steroidal anti-inflammatory drug (tenoxicam) reduces compression requirement. *Undersea Hyperb Med.* 2003;30(3):195–205.

SUGGESTED READINGS

Bennett MH, Lehm JP, Mitchell SJ, et al. Recompression and adjunctive therapy for decompression illness. *Cochrane Database Syst Rev.* 2012;5:CD005277.

Billinger M, Zbinden R, Mordasini R, et al. Patent foramen ovale closure in recreational divers: effect on decompression illness and ischaemic brain lesions during long-term follow-up. *Heart.* 2011;97(23):1932–1937.

Blatteau JE, Gempp E, Constantin P, et al. Risk factors and clinical outcome in military divers with neurological decompression sickness: influence of time to recompression. *Diving Hyperb Med.* 2011;41(3):129–134.

Blatteau JE, Gempp E, Simon O, et al. Prognostic factors of spinal cord decompression sickness in recreational diving: retrospective and multicentric analysis of 279 cases. *Neurocrit Care.* 2011;15(1):120–127.

Byyny RL, Shockley LW. Scuba diving and dysbarism. In: Marx J, Hockberger R, Walls R, et al, eds. *Rosen's Emergency Medicine.* 7th ed. Philadelphia: Elsevier/Saunders; 2014.

Diagnosis and treatment of decompression sickness and arterial gas embolism. In: *U.S. Navy Diving Manual.* Vol 5. Revision 6.Washington, DC: Naval Sea Systems Command; 2008. http://www.supsalv.org/pdf/Dive%20Manual%20Chapter%2020%20with%20Change%20A.pdf.

Dutka AJ. Long term effects on the central nervous system. In: Brubakk AO, Neumann TS, eds. *Bennett and Elliott's Physiology and Medicine of Diving.* 6th ed. New York: W.B. Saunders; 2003.

Gao GK, Wu D, Yang Y, et al. Cerebral magnetic resonance imaging of compressed air divers in diving accidents. *Undersea Hyperb Med.* 2009;36(1):33–41.

Gempp E, Blatteau JE. Risk factors and treatment outcome in scuba divers with spinal cord decompression sickness. *J Crit Care.* 2010;25(2):236–242.

Gempp E, Blatteau JE, Stephant E, et al. MRI findings and clinical outcome in 45 divers with spinal cord decompression sickness. *Aviat Space Environ Med.* 2008;79(12):1112–1116.

Gempp E, Louge P, Lafolie T, et al. Relation between cervical and thoracic spinal canal stenosis and the development of spinal cord decompression sickness in recreational scuba divers. *Spinal Cord.* 2014;52(3):236–240.

Germobpre P. Patent foramen ovale and diving. *Cardiol Clin.* 2005;23:97–104.

Holck P, Hunter RW. NIHSS applied to cerebral neurological dive injuries as a tool for dive injury severity stratification. *Undersea Hyperb Med.* 2006;33(4):271–280.

Kizer KW, Van Hoesen. Diving medicine. In: Auerbach PS, ed. *Wilderness Medicine.* 6th ed. Philadelphia: Elsevier/Mosby; 2012.

Kohshi K, Tamaki H, Lemaître F, et al. Brain damage in commercial breath-hold divers. *PLoS One.* 2014;9(8):e105006.

MacDonald RD, O'Donnell C, Allan GM, et al. Interfacility transport of patients with decompression illness: literature review and consensus statement. *Prehosp Emerg Care.* 2006;10(4):482–487.

McGuire S, Sherman P, Profenna L, et al. White matter hyperintensities on MRI in high-altitude U-2 pilots. *Neurology.* 2013;81(8):729–735.

Moon RE. Adjunctive therapy for decompression illness: a review and update. *Diving Hyperb Med.* 2009;39(2):81–87.

Ryles MT, Pilmanis AA. The initial signs and symptoms of altitude decompression sickness. *Aviat Space Environ Med.* 1996;67:983–989.

Shupak A, Melamed Y, Ramon Y, et al. Helium and oxygen treatment of severe air-diving-induced neurologic decompression sickness. *Arch Neurol.* 1997;54(3):305–311.

Vann RD, Butler FK, Mitchell SJ, et al. Decompression illness. *Lancet.* 2010;377:153–164.

Neonatal Neurology 132

Arthur M. Mandel

INTRODUCTION

Pediatric neurologists treat many children with brain injuries that originate in the perinatal period and cause mental retardation, cerebral palsy, and/or seizures. This chapter will focus on some of the most common disease processes affecting neonates.

PERIVENTRICULAR-INTRAVENTRICULAR HEMORRHAGE

EPIDEMIOLOGY

Premature, low birth weight neonates are especially at risk for periventricular-intraventricular hemorrhage, and the incidence and severity of intraventricular hemorrhage (IVH) increases with earlier prematurity and lower birth weight. The prevalence of periventricular IVH in newborns weighing less than 1,500 g has declined, falling from approximately 40% in 1980 to 20% since the late 1990s. Corticosteroid therapy prenatally and surfactant use after birth have contributed to the decline of IVH. However, with the increased survival rate of extremely low birth weight infants, there are more infants at highest risk, with a risk of 45% in infants less than 1,000 g. In a population-based study in Switzerland, IVH decreased by 3.5% with each added week of gestation.

Additionally, severe IVH increases with decreasing gestational age. In a large, multicenter registry of infants of very low gestational age (22 to 28 weeks) and birth weight (401 to 1,500 g), born between 2003 and 2007 in the United States, 16% overall had severe IVH, and the prevalence increased with decreasing gestational age, from 38% at 22 weeks to 7% at 28 weeks.

PATHOBIOLOGY

In premature neonates, the vascular germinal plate near the foramen of Monro, in the region of the caudate, is friable and susceptible to hemorrhage. The risk for hemorrhage is further exacerbated by disturbances in cerebral blood flow, either through hypotension and lower cerebral perfusion, possibly lowered further by positive pressure ventilation through endotracheal intubation, and/or through hypoperfusion-reperfusion coupled with immaturity of intrinsic cerebral vasoreactivity and autoregulatory mechanisms. Other factors potentially increasing risk of IVH during prematurity are metabolic (hypoglycemia, hypernatremia), hematologic (anemia, thrombocytopenia), and immunologic (chorioamnionitis, immaturity of antioxidant responses, or other immune responses).

The Papile grading system, with some modification, is the most commonly used scale to describe the severity of the IVH (Fig. 132.1). The IVH may remain in the matrix area (grade I), but 50% can rupture into the lateral ventricles (grade II), which can result in ventricular enlargement or distension (grade III). Grade IV, now termed *periventricular hemorrhagic infarction* (PVHI), refers to extensive IVH with parenchymal involvement, likely due to terminal venous occlusion, venous infarction, and subsequent secondary hemorrhage.

Late in the course after IVH (1 to 3 weeks after the initial hemorrhage), especially with more severe IVH, there can be posthemorrhagic hydrocephalus (PHH), or progressive ventricular dilatation (PVD), thought to result from impaired reabsorption of cerebrospinal fluid (CSF) because of inflammation of the subarachnoid villi. Usually, impaired reabsorption results in a communicating hydrocephalus, although there can also be a noncommunicating hydrocephalus due to localized obstruction or scarring.

CLINICAL MANIFESTATIONS

Most IVH in premature infants occurs within the first 5 postnatal days. Late IVH is associated with low cerebral blood flow, usually from systemic processes.

The clinical presentation of IVH varies depending on severity. Grade I IVH is usually asymptomatic. Many grade II and some III hemorrhages are clinically silent, but there may be a saltatory course evolving over hours to days, characterized by nonspecific findings of altered level of consciousness, hypotonia, eye movement changes, subtle changes in movement, decreased spontaneous movements, and disturbed respiratory function. Some grade III hemorrhages produce hydrocephalic symptoms of varying severity, and if seen in combination with PVHI, there may be signs of severe apnea, bradycardia, extensor posturing, and opisthotonus. There also may be flaccid weakness, cranial nerve abnormalities including fixed pupils to light, most likely leading to unresponsiveness and death within hours. There may be clonic limb movements, which some clinicians have labeled as seizures, although there is usually little electroencephalogram (EEG) correlation. Most infants who die have other lesions, such as periventricular leukomalacia (see the section "Periventricular Leukomalacia"), brain stem necrosis, or cerebellar necrosis.

DIAGNOSIS

Cranial ultrasonography is the preferred imaging modality because of its portability, its ability to delineate blood in the parenchyma and ventricles as well as ventricular size, and its lack of ionizing radiation. Routine ultrasound screening should be performed in all infants with a gestational age younger than 30 weeks and should be strongly considered in infants with abnormal clinical signs such as changes in neurologic or respiratory status or with systemic conditions which can predispose to IVH.

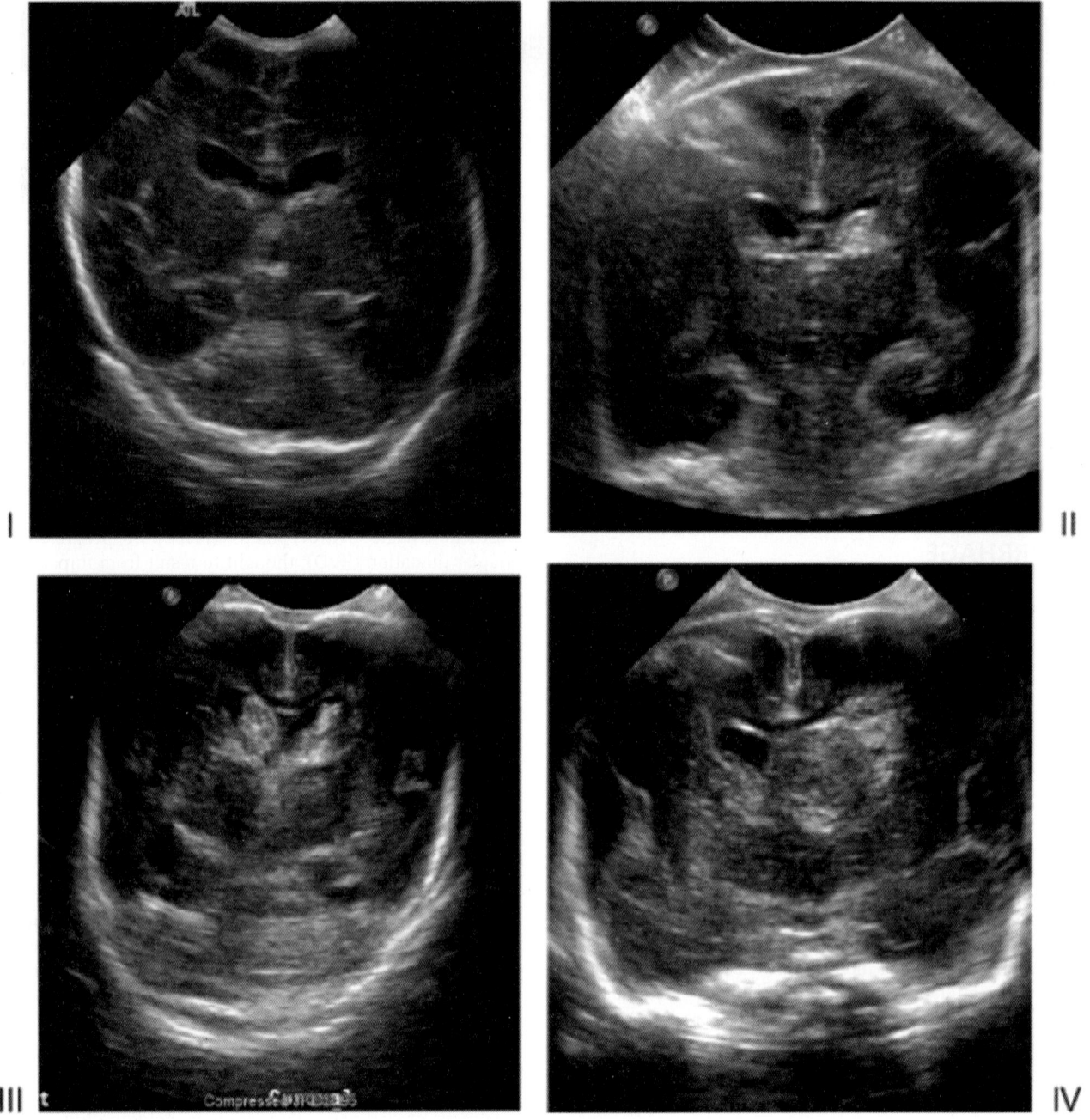

FIGURE 132.1 Papile grading system for neonatal IVH, shown by head ultrasonography. Echodensities are seen in periventricular region (**I**, grade I), with rupture into the lateral ventricles (**II**, grade II) and with ventricular enlargement (**III**, grade III). PVHI (**IV**) has parenchymal involvement. (From El-Dib M, Massaro AN, Bulas D, et al. Neuroimaging and neurodevelopmental outcome of premature infants. *Am J Perinatol.* 2010;27[10]:803–818.)

Computed tomography (CT) or magnetic resonance imaging (MRI) have limited usefulness as routine screening tools because of their lack of portability, exposure to ionizing radiation (CT), and a longer examination time (MRI). However, these modalities may be helpful in documenting other lesions, such as parenchymal abnormalities or subdural or posterior fossa hemorrhages. CT scanning is generally avoided because of the exposure to ionizing radiation, if MRI is available.

Lumbar puncture may be helpful if ultrasonography is unavailable. The red blood cell count is typically high, with a protein concentration of 250 to 1,200 mg/dL. Later, the CSF becomes xanthochromic, and glucose concentration frequently decreases.

TREATMENT

Prevention

The most effective prevention strategy is avoidance of premature birth. When preterm birth is inevitable, there are some prenatal and delivery room practices associated with a lowered risk of IVH. Corticosteroids given antenatally, at a dose of two 12-mg intramuscular injections of betamethasone at 24-hour intervals, reduce risk of IVH. Delayed clamping of the umbilical cord (30 to 60 seconds) has been associated with a reduction in the relative risk of IVH, although it is not clear whether there is a correlative decrease in severe IVH. Maternal transport to a perinatal center before delivery reduces risk of IVH in very low birth weight infants as compared with infant transport after delivery.

General measures of neonatal care are widely accepted to reduce risk of IVH in the postnatal period. Resuscitation should be prompt and hemodynamic instability, hypoxia, hypercarbia, hyperoxia, and hypocarbia should be avoided. Hypotension and hypertension should be avoided and corrected (in a gradual fashion to avoid large acute changes in blood pressure). Coagulopathies and metabolic abnormalities should be corrected. Bicarbonate therapy is associated with an increased risk of IVH and should be avoided.

Medical Therapies

There are no medical interventions that have been shown to safely reduce the long-term effects of IVH. Indomethacin, usually administered as three 0.1 or 0.2 mg/kg doses beginning 6 or 12 hours after birth, with a dosing interval of 12 or 24 hours, may reduce the rate of severe IVH but has not been shown to affect long-term outcomes such as death or severe neurologic impairment.

Procedural or Surgical Intervention

In general, no treatment is needed for grade I and II hemorrhages, although they should be followed for progression by regular cranial ultrasonography. For grade III hemorrhage or PVHI, ongoing monitoring should be performed, with weekly head ultrasounds with daily head circumference measurement and frequent clinical assessment for increased intracranial pressure (ICP). If there is evidence of significant lateral ventricular dilatation or increased ICP, intervention may be needed. Serial lumbar punctures can be done, although they should be coupled with cranial ultrasonography to ensure that there is a resultant decrease in ventricular size. As a temporizing measure, ventricular drainage with a direct extraventricular drain or with a subcutaneous drain to a subcutaneous reservoir or a ventriculosubgaleal shunt may be helpful. Usually, if a drain is needed, eventually, a permanent ventricular shunt, usually a ventriculoperitoneal shunt, will be needed, although a

third ventriculostomy may be effective as well in some cases. Every attempt should be made to delay shunting until the newborn attains as much somatic growth as possible.

OUTCOME

Grades I and II IVH usually has a good short-term outcome, with an 80% to 90% survival rate without an obvious neurologic abnormality (Table 132.1). However, there may be long-term disorders of learning and behavior, especially with extremely low birth weight neonates (<1,000 g).

The mortality rate of grade III IVH and PVHI is approximately 20%, with 75% of the surviving infants developing PHH. Long-term prognosis worsens with decreasing gestational age and increasing severity of IVH, with higher rates of developmental delay, cerebral palsy, bilateral deafness, and bilateral blindness associated with more severe bleeds and extreme prematurity. Some infants with PVHI survive without disability, especially when the infarctions are small.

HYPOXIC–ISCHEMIC ENCEPHALOPATHY

EPIDEMIOLOGY

In developed countries, birth asphyxia affects 3 to 5 newborns per 1,000 live births and causes moderate to severe hypoxic–ischemic encephalopathy (HIE) in 0.5 to 1 per 1,000 live births. Globally, 10% to 60% of neonates with HIE die, and 25% have long-term neurodevelopmental difficulties.

PATHOBIOLOGY

HIE is most commonly associated with severe maternal hypotension, uterine rupture, placental abruption, and placental or umbilical cord dysfunction. In addition, there may be associated hypoxic cardiopulmonary, hepatic, or renal injury.

Brain pathology depends on the level of maturity at the time of the insult, as well as the duration and location of the insult. In infants injured younger than 32 weeks' gestation, periventricular leukomalacia (PVL) is commonly seen because of the vulnerability of late oligodendroglial precursors. After 36 weeks' gestation, hypoxic lesions are frequently located in the cerebral gray matter, deep gray nuclei, brain stem, and Purkinje cells of the cerebellum.

TABLE 132.1 **Intraventricular Hemorrhage Clinical Features, Treatment, and Outcome**

IVH Grade	Clinical Syndrome	Treatment	Outcome
I	Usually asymptomatic	Follow clinically and with cranial ultrasound.	Usually normal; may have long-term behavioral/learning problems if low birth weight
II	Frequently asymptomatic, may display subtle neurologic signs affecting mental status, tone, eye or muscle movements, or respiration		
III	May show signs of hydrocephalus; may show other neurologic signs similar to grade II	If signs of increased intracranial pressure, may require intervention: serial lumbar punctures, ventricular drainage, ventricular shunt, or third ventriculostomy	20% mortality; 75% show PHH. May progress to developmental delay, cerebral palsy, bilateral deafness, especially with bilateral blindness associated with more severe bleeds and extreme prematurity. May be normal if small hemorrhage.
PVHI	May show more severe neurologic signs including apnea, bradycardia, opisthotonus, posturing		

IVH, intraventricular hemorrhage; PHH, posthemorrhagic hydrocephalus; PVHI, periventricular hemorrhagic infarction.

On a cellular and molecular level, hypoxia–ischemia acutely causes neuronal loss in the cerebral sulci, often with edema and infarction. Chronically, there is neuronal loss and astrocytosis, with possible atrophy, cystic encephalomalacia, ulegyria, status marmoratus, and cerebellar atrophy. Energy failure from hypoxia stems from loss of mitochondrial function, which can be confirmed by measuring increased lactic acid levels in the CSF or by magnetic resonance spectroscopy (MRS). There is accompanying membrane depolarization and an increase in neurotransmitter release, as well as excessive activation of glutamate receptors. Resultant is excitotoxic cellular injury, leading to an increase in intracellular calcium that leads to a cascade of pathologic pathways leading to secondary cell death. In addition, there is oxidative stress, which produces reactive oxygen species and subsequent reactive nitrogen radicals, also contributing to cell toxicity. After the anoxic insult, many cells undergo reoxygenation and reperfusion. Reperfusion contributes further to oxidative stress by producing more reactive oxygen species and further cellular injury.

CLINICAL MANIFESTATIONS

HIE initially presents with low Apgar scores, which translate into bradycardia, depressed respiration, diminished responsiveness, and decreased muscle tone (Table 132.2). One of three clinical patterns then evolves: (1) mild: awake, irritable, hyperalert, with jitteriness, dilated pupils, increased deep tendon reflexes, and normal muscle tone; (2) moderate: lethargy with depressed deep tendon reflexes, frequently with seizures; and (3) severe: apathy, with severe hypotonia, poorly reactive pupils, an absent Moro reflex, depression or coma, and seizures. There is usually clinical improvement with the mild and moderate cases as the newborns become more alert, improve their tone, and are able to feed. Seizures or therapy for seizures may delay recovery. Newborns with severe encephalopathy will usually become stuporous; develop frequent seizures, respiratory depression, or brain stem abnormalities; and may show signs of decerebration. They become unresponsive and lose sucking reflexes and the Moro response, and even with vigorous supportive and anticonvulsant therapy, 20% to 30% of these newborns die. If the neonate survives, seizures usually stop after 48 to 72 hours, and there is usually some recovery.

DIAGNOSIS

HIE should be distinguished from other causes of encephalopathy in the newborn period. Strict diagnostic criteria for HIE includes the presence of a sentinel obstetric event in the immediate prenatal or perinatal period, nonreassuring fetal heart rate tracing in the prenatal or perinatal period, fetal umbilical artery acidemia with a pH less than 7.0 and/or a base deficit greater than or equal to 12 mmol/L, Apgar scores of 0 to 3 for 5 minutes or longer, and imaging evidence of acute multifocal or diffuse cerebral injury. There may be multisystem organ failure consistent with HIE, such as renal, hepatic, or cardiac dysfunction; hematologic abnormalities; metabolic derangements such as low serum glucose or sodium or elevated CSF lactate; and/or gastrointestinal injury. All of these criteria lie on a continuum, so, for example, more severe acidemia increases the likelihood of an intrapartum hypoxic injury.

Certain patterns of brain injury seen in neuroimaging of late preterm or term infants are commonly seen in HIE, including parasagittal injury in an arterial watershed distribution and/or injury to the deep gray nuclei (Figs. 132.2 and 132.3). Neuroimaging, alternatively, may reveal another cause of encephalopathy, such as a developmental brain malformation or a focal area of infarction. Brain MRI is the most sensitive imaging modality for most lesions and usually yields the most useful information, although it requires transport, monitoring, and support. MRS, if available, can be useful for diagnosis of HIE if a lactate peak is seen. Head CT is useful for detecting intracranial hemorrhage and brain calcifications but is less sensitive for detecting mild brain edema or white matter injury, which is somewhat obscured because of the high water content of the newborn white matter. The posterior fossa is not adequately imaged with CT because of bony artifact. Cranial ultrasonography can be done at the bedside but is not very sensitive for detection of white matter abnormalities or lesions in the outer cerebral cortex.

Along with revealing seizure activity that may be inapparent clinically, EEG can be helpful to indicate the degree of HIE: Indications of severity include a burst-suppression pattern and/or a relatively inactive background. Amplitude-integrated EEG, although not as sensitive as standard EEG, may show low voltage in the setting of severe HIE and is able to detect some but not all seizure activity.

TREATMENT

Because multiple organ systems are involved in addition to the brain, management and therapeutic measures include maintenance of physiologic homeostasis, including providing adequate ventilation, maintenance of perfusion and metabolism, avoidance of brain edema, and seizure control. Therapeutic hypothermia has been shown in multiple randomized controlled trials to lower mortality and major neurodevelopmental disability in term

TABLE 132.2	Apgar Scores		
	Score of 0	Score of 1	Score of 2
Color	Blue or pale, entire body	Blue at extremities, body pink	No cyanosis
Heart rate	Absent	<100	>100
Reflex irritability	No response to stimulation	Feeble cry or grimace when stimulated	Cry or pull away when stimulated
Muscle tone	None	Some flexion	Flexed arms and legs
Respiratory effort	Absent	Weak, gasping, irregular	Strong, lusty cry

Adapted from Apgar V. A proposal for a new method of evaluation of the newborn infant. *Curr Res Anesth Analg.* 1953;32(4):260–267.

FIGURE 132.2 MRI of full-term infant with birth asphyxia (from ruptured uterus). **A:** Inversion recovery sequence shows increased intensity within thalami and basal ganglia. Diffusion-weighted imaging **(B–D)** shows restricted diffusion in the ventrolateral thalami, lentiform nuclei, cerebral peduncles, and perirolandic cortex. (From de Vries LS, Groenendaal F. Patterns of neonatal hypoxic-ischaemic brain injury. *Neuroradiology.* 2010;52[6]:555–566.)

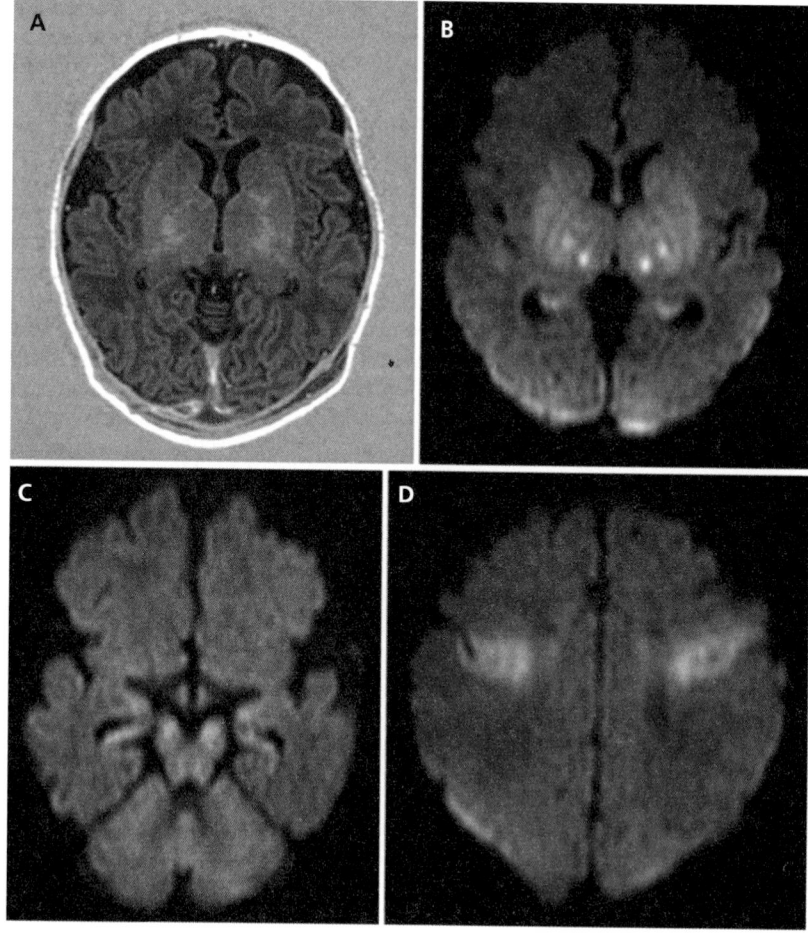

and late preterm infants with moderate or severe HIE [**Level 1**].[1] There are some adverse effects of hypothermia, including an increase in sinus bradycardia and in thrombocytopenia, but the benefits of cooling outweigh these short-term adverse effects. Questions still remaining are the optimal timing of the cooling after birth (research protocols have started cooling before 6 hours of age), the duration of cooling needed (most research protocols have cooled for 72 hours), the level of hypothermia required, and the method (selective head cooling vs. whole body cooling).

OUTCOME

Long-term prognosis of HIE remains a challenge for the neonatal neurologist, especially with the relatively recent introduction of therapeutic hypothermia. Most infants with mild HIE have a normal outcome. Children with severe HIE who survive the neonatal period usually have low cognitive ability and scholastic achievement, serious motor disability, and epilepsy. Children with moderate HIE form a heterogenous group, depending on how the outcomes are measured and how the degree of encephalopathy is defined.

FIGURE 132.3 MRI of full-term infant born with severe anemia, showing watershed pattern of injury. **A:** T2-weighted sequence shows loss of cortical ribbon, with increased signal intensity in corpus callosum. **B:** Apparent diffusion coefficient (ADC) map shows decreased signal intensity in posterior watershed areas, splenium of corpus callosum, and optic radiation. (From de Vries LS, Groenendaal F. Patterns of neonatal hypoxic-ischaemic brain injury. *Neuroradiology.* 2010;52[6]:555–566.)

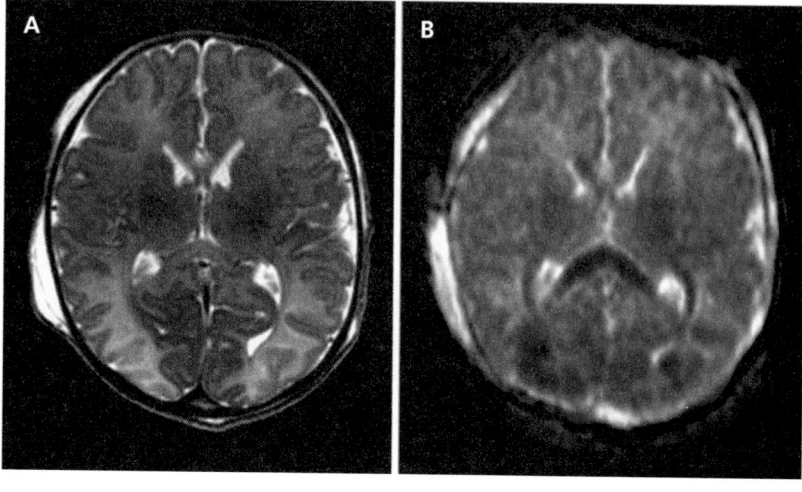

NEONATAL SEIZURES

EPIDEMIOLOGY

Neonatal brains are particularly susceptible to seizures because of a relative abundance of excitatory neurotransmitters and the relative underdevelopment of inhibitory systems. Seizures occur in 1 to 3.8 per 1,000 newborns and are often an urgent clinical problem requiring prompt diagnosis and treatment.

PATHOBIOLOGY

The vast majority of neonatal seizures are due to specific etiologic causes rather than epileptic syndromes (Table 132.3). The most common causes are encephalopathy (often HIE) in term infants and IVH in premature babies. Other important causes include other hemorrhage (intracerebral, subdural, subarachnoid), infection (meningitis, encephalitis, or intrauterine), infarction, metabolic (hypoglycemia, hypocalcemia, hypomagnesemia), chromosomal anomalies, cerebral malformations, neurodegenerative disorders, inborn errors of metabolism (nonketotic hyperglycinemia, urea cycle defects, phenylketonuria, maple sugar urine disease, lactic or organic acidurias), and maternal drug withdrawal or intoxication. Some seizures are responsive to vitamin treatment, including B_6, pyridoxal phosphate, and folinic acid. There has been a decrease in seizure frequency from transient metabolic causes or infection, most likely because of the advances in neonatal care over the past few decades.

There are three well-recognized neonatal epilepsy syndromes as classified by the International League Against Epilepsy: benign neonatal familial convulsions (BFNS), early myoclonic encephalopathy (EME), and early infantile epileptic encephalopathy (EIEE or Ohtahara syndrome). (The formerly recognized syndrome of benign idiopathic neonatal convulsions has been eliminated because of its diminished occurrence since the 1970s, when it was first described.) BFNS is a dominantly inherited condition, and diagnosis depends on a family history of neonatal seizures. There are two identified genes: *KCNQ2* and *KCNQ3*, which are voltage-gated potassium channel genes. EME and EIEE may be secondary to multiple etiologies, usually a severe metabolic cause for EME or a structural lesion for EIEE.

On a molecular level and cellular level, both animal models and human studies indicate that the developmental regulation of excitatory and inhibitory synaptic networks play a crucial role in the greater susceptibility of neonates to seizures. In particular, both AMPA and N-methyl-D-aspartate (NMDA) subtypes of glutamate receptors, which are excitatory, have high expression and are expressed with subunit composition enhancing excitability of neuronal networks in the period around birth in humans and in animal models. Additionally, the inhibitory class of γ-aminobutyric acid (GABA) receptors is underexpressed during this time period.

CLINICAL MANIFESTATIONS

Seizure semiology and EEG features of neonatal seizures differ from those of older children and adults. Consequently, classification schemes for seizures in older children and adults are not appropriate for neonates. Neonatal seizure classification schemes most often rely on dominant clinical features. Focal clonic, focal tonic, and some myoclonic seizures have associated ictal EEG discharges. Other paroxysmal movements, such as generalized tonic posturing, and motor automatisms (mouthing, pedaling, and rotatory arm movements) have unreliable or inconsistent EEG equivalents and may reflect etiologies other than seizures such as HIE. Generalized tonic–clonic seizures do not occur in newborns because of the immaturity of the cerebral white matter.

DIAGNOSIS

As with older patients with seizures, history is essential, especially details about the pregnancy, delivery, and family history. Head circumference, the presence of congenital anomalies, neurocutaneous markings, and organomegaly are all relevant findings. The neurologic exam should also note any abnormal posturing or unusual movements.

Laboratory evaluation should focus first on common metabolic or infectious disorders that are treatable—serum should be studied for levels of glucose, calcium, magnesium, sodium, and acid–base levels, as well as culture. CSF should be evaluated for meningitis and hemorrhage. EEG should be done promptly if there are abnormal movements or unexplained behavioral changes. Continuous EEG should be done if available, as there can be seizures without clinical manifestations. Ultrasound may identify hemorrhage and hydrocephalus. Amplitude-integrated EEG may be able to detect seizures, although localization is limited and some seizures may be missed. CT also shows hemorrhage and hydrocephalus and, in addition, demonstrates parenchymal calcifications and major cerebral malformations. MRI is usually necessary to detect more subtle developmental abnormalities, such as partial lissencephaly, polymicrogyria, or cortical dysplasia.

Timing of the first seizure may aid in the diagnosis. Seizures due to severe brain malformations, intracerebral hemorrhage, and hypoxic–ischemic injury occur within 24 to 48 hours. Seizures caused by infection and inborn errors of metabolism typically begin later in the first week of life. Seizures due to drug withdrawal usually occur in the first 3 days (e.g., alcohol or short-acting barbiturates) but may not appear for 2 to 3 weeks (e.g., methadone).

TABLE 132.3	Etiology of Neonatal Seizures
Cause	**Examples**
Encephalopathy	HIE
Hemorrhage	IVH, also intracerebral, subdural, subarachnoid
Infarction	Embolic stroke
Infection	Meningitis, encephalitis, intra-uterine
Metabolic	Hypoglycemia, hypocalcemia, hypomagnesemia
Genetic	Chromosomal anomaly, neonatal epilepsy syndrome (EME, EIEE, BFNS)
Structural	Heterotopia or other migrational anomaly
Inborn error of metabolism	Nonketotic hyperglycinemia, urea cycle defect, maple syrup urine disease, lactic aciduria, organic aciduria
Maternal	Drug withdrawal, intoxication
Vitamin dependency	B_6, pyridoxal phosphate, folinic acid

HIE, hypoxic–ischemic encephalopathy; IVH, intraventricular hemorrhage; EME, early myoclonic encephalopathy; EIEE, early infantile epileptic encephalopathy; BFNS, benign neonatal familial convulsions.

TABLE 132.4 Treatments for Metabolic Causes of Seizures

Cause	Treatment	Maintenance
Hypoglycemia	10% glucose IV 2 mL/kg	8 mg/kg/min
Hypocalcemia	10% calcium gluconate (100 mg/kg or 1 mL/kg IV) infused over 5–10 min, checking HR and infusion site, repeated in 10 min if no response *OR* Calcium chloride (20 mg/kg or 0.2 mL/kg)	Add calcium gluconate to IV solution.
Hypomagnesemia (may be associated with hypocalcemia)	50% solution IM 0.25 mL/kg or 125 mg/kg, repeat every 12 h until normalized	
Pyridoxine-responsive seizures	Pyridoxine 100 mg IV or pyridoxal phosphate 30 mg/kg/day divided t.i.d.	Pyridoxine 15–18 mg/kg/day and folinic acid 3–5 mg/kg/day
Pyridoxal phosphate–responsive seizures	Pyridoxal phosphate 30 mg/kg/day divided t.i.d. or q.i.d. for 3–5 days and folinic acid 3–5 mg/kg/day	Pyridoxal phosphate 30 mg/kg/day divided q.i.d.

IV, intravenous; HR, heart rate; IM, intramuscular.

Seizures must be distinguished from other paroxysmal phenomena that occur in newborns, including jitteriness, which can be triggered or stopped by manipulation of a limb, benign sleep myoclonus, dyskinesias (e.g., seen commonly with severe bronchopulmonary dysplasia), and the movements that occur during rapid eye movement (REM) sleep. Brief, generalized, tonic postures that occur with poor cerebral perfusion or with resolving encephalopathies are usually not epileptic seizures, and they respond poorly or not at all to antiepileptic drugs.

TREATMENT

Etiology of seizures is a crucial determinant for choosing an appropriate treatment protocol. If there is a metabolic or infectious cause, for example, there may be specific therapies to address the seizures. Treatment of metabolic causes of neonatal seizures is presented in Table 132.4.

First-line anticonvulsant therapy for seizures in most nurseries is phenobarbital, and other agents are fosphenytoin (preferred over phenytoin because of fewer cardiac side effects) and benzodiazepines such as lorazepam and midazolam. There are some initial indications of the use of other agents such as levetiracetam, lidocaine, topiramate, and bumetanide. Recommendations are to start with one anticonvulsant and increase levels to maximum tolerance if needed, before starting with another anticonvulsant. Treatment of acute symptomatic neonatal seizures is presented in Table 132.5.

Goals of treatment remain an open question for certain clinical scenarios. Certainly, electroclinical seizures should be treated

TABLE 132.5 Treatment of Acute Symptomatic Neonatal Seizures

Medication	Dosage	Notes
Phenobarbital	Load: 20 mg/kg IV, repeated once as needed. Daily dosing: 5 mg/kg/day (target serum level 40–60 μg/mL)	Side effects: respiratory depression, depressed level of consciousness, hypotension, hypotonia, hepatotoxicity, blood dyscrasia, skin rash
Fosphenytoin (and phenytoin)	Load: 20 mg/kg IV. Daily dosing 5 mg/kg/day (target level 10–20 μg/mL)	Cardiovascular, CNS, cutaneous side effects, which are less often seen with fosphenytoin compared with phenytoin. Variability in pharmacokinetics may result in inconsistent serum levels.
Levetiracetam	Load: 40–60 mg/kg IV. Daily dosing 30 mg/kg/day	Optimal dosing regimen not known
Lorazepam	Load: 0.05–0.1 mg/kg IV	Side effects: respiratory depression, depressed consciousness, hypotension
Midazolam	Load: 0.2 mg/kg IV, then continuous infusion (1 μg/kg/min), increasing by 0.5–1 μg/kg/min every 2 min to 2–5 μg/kg/min	Side effects: respiratory depression, depressed consciousness, hypotension
Lidocaine	Load: 2 mg/kg over 10 min, then continuous infusion 6 mg/kg/h during first 12 h, then 4 mg/kg/h for next 4 h, then 2 mg/kg/h. Lower doses when infant is being treated with therapeutic hypothermia.	Side effect: arrhythmia. Should only be given in ICU setting with continuous cardiac monitoring. Avoid concurrent treatment with proarrhythmic drugs such as phenytoin. Avoid in patient with congenital heart disease.

IV, intravenous; CNS, central nervous system; ICU, intensive care unit.
Adapted from Glass HC. Neonatal seizures: advances in mechanisms and management. *Clin Perinatol.* 2014;41(1):177–190.

as long as there are no compromises in respiratory or circulatory function. Subclinical seizures may result in long-term behavioral or cognitive effects.

OUTCOME

Prognosis usually depends on etiology, and, as discussed earlier, it is essential to address and remedy the underlying cause of the seizures if possible. HIE, severe IVH, and cerebral malformations are particularly associated with poor outcomes. An interictal EEG showing a suppression-burst pattern, a low-voltage background, and/or continuous multifocal epileptiform discharges frequently correlates with disabling brain damage.

Approximately 15% to 30% of neonates with seizures will develop epilepsy. There has been a decrease in overall mortality during the past few decades from neonatal seizures, from approximately 40% to 20%, although the prevalence of long-term neurodevelopmental sequelae has been unchanged at approximately 30%, perhaps because sicker infants are surviving the acute illness but then developing chronic manifestations. There is also some question about whether seizures directly cause brain injury, in particular when there is already an underlying defect in energy metabolism such as in HIE.

STROKE AND SINUS VENOUS THROMBOSIS

EPIDEMIOLOGY

Acute symptomatic perinatal stroke can be classified into three clinical groups (with incidence): arterial–ischemic stroke (70%), sinus venous thrombosis (20%), and hemorrhagic stroke (10%). The incidence is approximately 10-fold higher than in childhood stroke in general. In retrospective studies, the prevalence of perinatal ischemic stroke has been found to be approximately 1 per 3,500, but this prevalence is undoubtedly an underestimate because it is based in part on database searches, which may not account for all cases.

PATHOBIOLOGY

Pathophysiologic mechanisms leading to neonatal ischemic stroke include embolism, arteriopathy, or thrombosis. Most commonly, there is an infarction in the distribution of the middle cerebral artery (MCA), usually on the left. Neonates are at particular risk for thromboembolism because of multiple factors, including placental pathology or the normal thrombosis of placental vessels seen at birth; right-to-left shunts that may result from a patent foramen ovale or another congenital heart lesion; or indwelling umbilical vessel catheters, commonly used in neonatal intensive care units. Prothrombotic states, either from a systemic condition such as infection or from an inherited coagulation disorder may also play a contributory role.

Sinus venous thrombosis may also result from placental conditions resulting in a prothrombotic state or from a prothrombotic disorder. Most occur in the superior sagittal or transverse sinus, and there is frequently infarction, which may be hemorrhagic.

CLINICAL MANIFESTATIONS

In arterial ischemic stroke, seizures are frequently seen, with contralateral focal seizures if there is unilateral cerebral infarction. There may also be hemiparesis, which may appear as a subtle asymmetry of spontaneous movements. There may be a normal neonatal course, however, with hemiparesis presenting only after

many months. Sinus venous thrombosis usually presents with seizures and/or alteration of consciousness.

DIAGNOSIS

CT or, preferably, MRI/magnetic resonance angiography (MRA) will show complete or branch infarcts, usually in the MCA distribution. An infarct may be detected early with diffusion-weighted imaging. MRA can also be helpful if there are congenital vascular anomalies or carotid artery dissection. In sinus venous thrombosis, MRI/magnetic resonance venography (MRV) or CT may show the "empty delta" sign and/or associated stroke or hemorrhage (Fig. 132.4).

If the infant presents with seizures, a thorough evaluation for systemic causes, such as infection, inborn errors of metabolism, or toxicity should be performed. EEG may show focal attenuation, slowing, and/or epileptiform discharges. An echocardiogram should be done to evaluate for a congenital anomaly or a thrombus.

Hypercoagulability should be evaluated in the setting of ischemic stroke (Table 132.6). The workup includes maternal studies for lupus anticoagulant, anticardiolipin antibody, and antinuclear antibodies. The placenta should be examined for infarcts or clots. Protein S, protein C, and antithrombin III are usually tested at 3 to 4 months of age because newborns normally have low values of these proteins. Genetic analysis can be performed for factor V

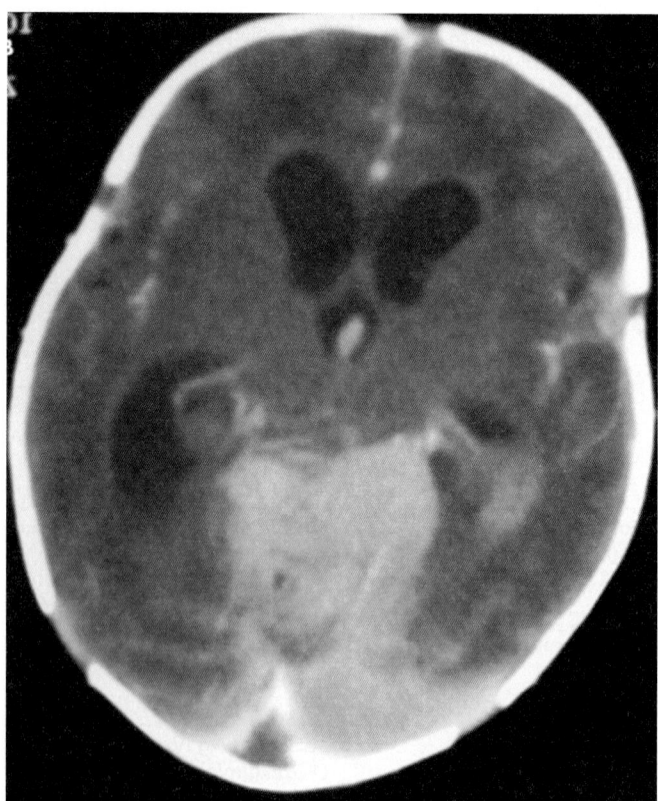

FIGURE 132.4 Sagittal venous sinus thrombosis in a near-term neonate, as shown by head computed tomography. "Empty delta sign" of the torcular herophili and associated posterior fossa hemorrhage, ventriculomegaly. (From Fumagalli M, Ramenghi LA, Mosca F. Palpebral ecchymosis and cerebral venous thrombosis in a near term infant. *Arch Dis Child Fetal Neonatal Ed*. 2004;89:F530.)

TABLE 132.6	Hypercoagulability Workup for Ischemic Stroke
Test	**Comment**
Lupus anticoagulant	
Anticardiolipin antibody	
Antinuclear antibodies	
Protein S, protein C, antithrombin III	Examine at age 3–4 mo.
Factor V Leiden	
Prothrombin G20210A	
Homocystinuria	Test for maternal homocysteine concentration or methylene tetrahydrofolate reductase mutations.
Placenta	Examine for infarct or clot.

Leiden and prothrombin G20210A mutations. Homocystinuria, if not part of regular newborn screening, can be assessed with the maternal homocysteine concentration or methylene tetrahydrofolate reductase mutations.

TREATMENT

Supportive care for stroke includes maintenance of adequate oxygenation; treatment of acidosis, electrolyte disturbances, dehydration, and anemia; and antibiotic or anticonvulsant treatment if needed. For arterial ischemic stroke, treatment with anticoagulants or antiplatelet agents is restricted to patients with a documented cardioembolic source or recurrent arterial ischemic stroke or patients who are at risk for recurrent stroke because of severe thrombophilic disorders.

Historically, there has been some controversy regarding anticoagulation therapy for sinus venous thrombosis, although there is now growing evidence supporting its safety, and there is some evidence that treatment reduces the occurrence of clot propagation. Current recommended guidelines suggest anticoagulation for 6 weeks if there is no significant intracerebral hemorrhage, to continue for 6 more weeks unless there is complete recanalization, and to consider anticoagulation in the setting of significant hemorrhage, beginning anticoagulation if there is thrombus propagation at 5 to 7 days.

OUTCOME

Long-term prognosis for ischemic stroke depends on the location and extent of the ischemic injury. Hemiparesis occurs in 25% to 30% of infants with unilateral infarction and is more often seen when there is infarction of the entire MCA territory. Milder neuromotor dysfunction occurs in another 30% with unilateral damage. Epilepsy occurs in 10% to 30% of patients with acute perinatal stroke. Cognitive impairment occurs in 20% to 25% of patients with unilateral infarction, with a worse risk if there is bilateral infarction or a large injury. The involvement of deep gray nuclei worsens cognitive outcome.

Outcome of sinus venous thrombosis varies. Most neonates (80% to 97%) survive the immediate neonatal period. Motor deficit occurs in approximately 60% of survivors, with cognitive impairment in approximately 25% to 50% and epilepsy in 20% to 40%.

PERIVENTRICULAR LEUKOMALACIA

EPIDEMIOLOGY

PVL is a focal injury, usually from infection or ischemia, to the cerebral white matter, in the periventricular region, occasionally with more diffuse injury. It is more commonly seen in premature infants, especially in infants younger than 32 weeks' gestational age, although it can be seen in term infants as well. Prevalence based on ultrasound diagnosis ranges from 5% to 15% of very low birth weight infants, but the prevalence is higher when MRI, which is a more sensitive imaging modality, is used.

PATHOBIOLOGY

The cerebral white matter of premature neonates is particularly vulnerable to injury because of a number of factors: (1) diminished vascularization and subsequent reduced blood flow in the periventricular area; (2) inadequate cerebral vascular autoregulation (with reduced cerebral perfusion in the setting of hypotension); and (3) the susceptibility of preoligodendrocytes (the predominant cell in white matter at early gestational ages and the precursor to normal myelin-producing cells) to injury and cell death from glutamate toxicity, which stems from hypoxia. Maternal infection, which is a risk factor for premature birth itself and lead to umbilical cord funisitis, or neonatal sepsis, is associated with PVL because of cytokines such as interleukin-1 beta, interleukin-6, and tumor necrosis factor-α producing free radicals which then activate astrocytes and microglia, which in turn release reactive oxygen species, toxic to the susceptible preoligodendrocytes.

CLINICAL MANIFESTATIONS

Hypomyelination is seen in periventricular fibers descending from the frontal lobes to the peripheral neurons in the legs. Consequently, the classical presentation is spastic diplegia and cerebral palsy, which may not be present in the newborn period. The involvement of the visual radiations in the posterior white matter can result in visual impairment. There may also be ex vacuo ventriculomegaly, with associated decreased gray matter volume, which may cause behavioral abnormalities and subnormal IQ scores.

DIAGNOSIS

Ultrasonography typically reveals echodensities adjacent to the lateral ventricles, throughout the periventricular region, and usually evolve over time, with potential development of echolucent cysts within weeks and then ventriculomegaly over months. More sensitive is MRI, which can detect more subtle diffuse white matter injuries or noncystic lesions. Diffusion-weighted imaging may allow for earlier detection of PVL or white matter injuries.

TREATMENT

Infants with PVL need to be closely monitored for development of neurologic sequelae, with the appropriate therapy provided for spasticity, cognitive, and visual complications.

OUTCOME

Infants with more extensive injury and ventriculomegaly are more likely to experience more severe motor and cognitive difficulties. Cyst formation is more likely to result in cerebral palsy. White matter injuries are a risk factor for cortical abnormalities and reduction in gray matter volume.

LEVEL 1 EVIDENCE

1. Jacobs SE, Berg M, Hunt R, et al. Cooling for newborns with hypoxic ischaemic encephalopathy. *Cochrane Database Syst Rev.* 2013;1:1–112.

SUGGESTED READINGS

Periventricular-Intraventricular Hemorrhage

Aly H, Hammad TA, Essers J, et al. Is mechanical ventilation associated with intraventricular hemorrhage in preterm infants? *Brain Dev.* 2012;34(3):201–205.

Aschner JL, Poland RL. Sodium bicarbonate: basically useless therapy. *Pediatrics.* 2008;122(4):831–835.

Bajwa NM, Berner M, Worley S, et al. Population based age stratified morbidities of premature infants in Switzerland. *Swiss Med Wkly.* 2011;24:141–146.

Ballabh P. Intraventricular hemorrhage in premature infants: mechanism of disease. *Pediatr Res.* 2010;67(1):1–8.

Bolisetty S, Dhawan A, Abdel-Latif M, et al. New South Wales and Australian Capital Territory Neonatal Intensive Care Units' Data Collection. Intraventricular hemorrhage and neurodevelopmental outcomes in extreme preterm infants. *Pediatrics.* 2014;133(1):55–62.

El-Dib M, Massaro AN, Bulas D, et al. Neuroimaging and neurodevelopmental outcome of premature infants. *Am J Perinatol.* 2010;27(10):803–818.

Fowlie PW, Davis PG. Prophylactic indomethacin for preterm infants: a systematic review and meta-analysis. *Arch Dis Child Fetal Neonatal Ed.* 2003;88(6):F464–F466.

Kluckow M, Evans N. Low superior vena cava flow and intraventricular haemorrhage in preterm infants. *Arch Dis Child Fetal Neonatal Ed.* 2000;82(3):F188–F194.

Kuint J, Barak M, Morag I, et al. Early treated hypotension and outcome in very low birth weight infants. *Neonatology.* 2009;95(4):311–316.

Levene MI, Wigglesworth JS, Dubowitz V. Hemorrhagic periventricular leukomalacia in the neonate: a real-time ultrasound study. *Pediatrics.* 1983;71(5):794–797.

McCrea HJ, Ment LR. The diagnosis, management, and postnatal prevention of intraventricular hemorrhage in the preterm neonate. *Clin Perinatol.* 2008;35(4):777–792.

Mohamed MA, Aly H. Transport of premature infants is associated with increased risk for intraventricular haemorrhage. *Arch Dis Child Fetal Neonatal Ed.* 2010;95(6):F403–F407.

Rabe H, Diaz-Rossello JL, et al. Effect of timing of umbilical cord clamping and other strategies to influence placental transfusion at preterm birth on maternal and infant outcomes. *Cochrane Database Syst Rev.* 2012;8:1–84.

Robinson S. Neonatal posthemorrhagic hydrocephalus from prematurity: pathophysiology and current treatment concepts. *J Neurosurg Pediatr.* 2012;9(3):242–258.

Stoll BJ, Hansen NI, Bell EF, et al. Neonatal outcomes of extremely preterm infants from the NICHD Neonatal Research Network. *Pediatrics.* 2010;126(3):443–456.

Tarby TJ, Volpe JJ. Intraventricular hemorrhage in the premature infant. *Pediatr Clin North Am.* 1982;29(5):1077–1104.

Volpe J. *Neurology of the Newborn.* 5th ed. Philadelphia: Saunders; 2008.

Wilson-Costello D, Friedman H, Minich N, et al. Improved survival rates with increased neurodevelopmental disability for extremely low birth weight infants in the 1990s. *Pediatrics.* 2005;115(4):997–1003.

Whitelaw A. Periventricular hemorrhage: a problem still today. 2012;88(12):965–969.

Hypoxic–Ischemic Encephalopathy

American Academy of Pediatrics. Neonatal encephalopathy and neurologic outcome, second edition. Report of the American College of Obstetricians and Gynecologists' Task Force on Neonatal Encephalopathy. *Obstet Gynecol.* 2014;123(4):896–901.

Armstrong-Wells J, Bernard TJ, Boada R, et al. Neurocognitive outcomes following neonatal encephalopathy. *NeuroRehabilitation.* 2010;26(1):27–33.

Azzopardi D. Clinical management of the baby with hypoxic ischaemic encephalopathy. *Early Hum Dev.* 2010;86(6):345–350.

Azzopardi D, Strohm B, Marlow N, et al. Effects of hypothermia for perinatal asphyxia on childhood outcomes. *N Engl J Med.* 2014;371(2):140–149.

Back SA, Luo NL, Borenstein NS, et al. Late oligodendrocyte progenitors coincide with the developmental window of vulnerability for human perinatal white matter injury. *J Neurosci.* 2001;21(4):1302–1312.

de Vries LS, Groenendaal F. Patterns of neonatal hypoxic-ischaemic brain injury. *Neuroradiology.* 2010;52(6):555–566.

Ferriero DM. Neonatal brain injury. *N Engl J Med.* 2004;351(19):1985–1995.

Kurinczuk JJ, White-Koning M, Badawi N. Epidemiology of neonatal encephalopathy and hypoxic-ischaemic encephalopathy. *Early Hum Dev.* 2010;86(6):329–338.

Martinez-Biarge M, Diez-Sebastian J, Wusthoff CJ, et al. Antepartum and intrapartum factors preceding neonatal hypoxic-ischemic encephalopathy. *Pediatrics.* 2013;132(4):e952–e959.

van Handel M, Swaab H, de Vries LS, et al. Behavioral outcome in children with a history of neonatal encephalopathy following perinatal asphyxia. *J Pediatr Psychol.* 2010;35(3):286–295.

van Laerhoven H, de Haan TR, Offringa M, et al. Prognostic tests in term neonates with hypoxic-ischemic encephalopathy: a systematic review. *Pediatrics.* 2013;131(1):88–98.

Volpe JJ. Neonatal encephalopathy: an inadequate term for hypoxic-ischemic encephalopathy. *Ann Neurol.* 2012;72(2):156–166.

Yager JY, Armstrong EA, Black AM. Treatment of the term newborn with brain injury: simplicity as the mother of invention. *Pediatr Neurol.* 2009;40(3):237–243.

Neonatal Seizures

Boylan GB, Stevenson NJ, Vanhatalo S. Monitoring neonatal seizures. *Semin Fetal Neonatal Med.* 2013;18(4):202–208.

Cobo NH, Sankar R, Murata KK, et al. The ketogenic diet as broad-spectrum treatment for super-refractory pediatric status epilepticus: challenges in implementation in the pediatric and neonatal intensive care units. *J Child Neurol.* 2014;50(1):101–103.

Cowan LD. The epidemiology of the epilepsies in children. *Ment Retard Dev Disabil Res Rev.* 2002;8(3):171–181.

Gillam-Krakauer M, Carter BS. Neonatal hypoxia and seizures. *Pediatr Rev.* 2012;33(9):387–396.

Glass HC. Neonatal seizures: advances in mechanisms and management. *Clin Perinatol.* 2014;41(1):177–190.

Lundqvist M, Ågren J, Hellström-Westas L, et al. Efficacy and safety of lidocaine for treatment of neonatal seizures. *Acta Paediatr.* 2013;102(9):863–867.

Shellhaas RA, Chang T, Tsuchida T, et al. The American Clinical Neurophysiology Society's guideline on continuous EEG monitoring in neonates. *J Clin Neurophysiol.* 2011;28:611–617.

Silverstein FS, Jensen FE. Neonatal seizures. *Ann Neurol.* 2007;62(2):112–120.

Stockler S, Plecko B, Gospe SM Jr, et al. Pyridoxine dependent epilepsy and antiquitin deficiency: clinical and molecular characteristics and recommendations for diagnosis, treatment and follow-up. *Mol Genet Metab.* 2011;104(1–2):48–60.

Tekgul H, Gauvreau K, Soul J, et al. The current etiologic profile and neurodevelopmental outcome of seizures in term newborn infants. *Pediatrics.* 2006;117(4):1270–1280.

Stroke and Sinus Venous Thrombosis

Agrawal N, Johnston SC, Wu YW, et al. Imaging data reveal a higher pediatric stroke incidence than prior US estimates. *Stroke.* 2009;40:3415.

Armstrong-Wells J, Johnston SC, Wu YW, et al. Prevalence and predictors of perinatal hemorrhagic stroke: results from the Kaiser pediatric stroke study. *Pediatrics.* 2009;123:823.

deVeber G, Andrew M, Adams C, et al. Cerebral sinovenous thrombosis in children. *N Engl J Med.* 2001;345(6):417–423.

Govaert P, Ramenghi L, Taal R, et al. Diagnosis of perinatal stroke I: definitions, differential diagnosis and registration. *Acta Paediatr.* 2009;98:1556.

Moharir MD, Shroff M, Stephens D, et al. Anticoagulants in pediatric cerebral sinovenous thrombosis: a safety and outcome study. *Ann Neurol.* 2010;67:590–599.

Monagle P, Chan AK, Goldenberg NA, et al. American College of Chest Physicians. Antithrombotic therapy in neonates and children: Antithrombotic Therapy and Prevention of Thrombosis, 9th ed: American College of Chest Physicians Evidence-Based Clinical Practice Guidelines. *Chest.* 2012;141(2)(suppl):e737S-e801S.

Raju TN, Nelson KB, Ferriero D, et al. Ischemic perinatal stroke: summary of a workshop sponsored by the National Institute of Child Health and Human Development and the National Institute of Neurological Disorders and Stroke. *Pediatrics.* 2007;120:609.

Roach ES, Golomb MR, Adams R, et al. Management of stroke in infants and children: a scientific statement from a Special Writing Group of the American Heart Association Stroke Council and the Council on Cardiovascular Disease in the Young. *Stroke.* 2008;39(9):2644–2691.

Rutherford MA, Ramenghi LA, Cowan FM. Neonatal stroke. *Arch Dis Child Fetal Neonatal Ed.* 2012;97:F377–F384.

Periventricular Leukomalacia

Folkerth RD. Periventricular leukomalacia: overview and recent findings. *Pediatr Dev Pathol.* 2006;9(1):3–13.

Kinney HC. The near-term (late preterm) human brain and risk for periventricular leukomalacia: a review. *Semin Perinatol.* 2006;30(2):81–88.

Krägeloh-Mann I, Horber V. The role of magnetic resonance imaging in elucidating the pathogenesis of cerebral palsy: a systematic review. *Dev Med Child Neurol.* 2007;49(2):144–151.

Kwon SH, Vasung L, Ment LR, et al. The role of neuroimaging in predicting neurodevelopmental outcomes of preterm neonates. *Clin Perinatol.* 2014;41(1):257–283.

Volpe JJ. Brain injury in premature infants: a complex amalgam of destructive and developmental disturbances. *Lancet Neurol.* 2009;8(1):110–124.

Woodward LJ, Anderson PJ, Austin NC, et al. Neonatal MRI to predict neurodevelopmental outcomes in preterm infants. *N Engl J Med.* 2006;355(7):685–694.

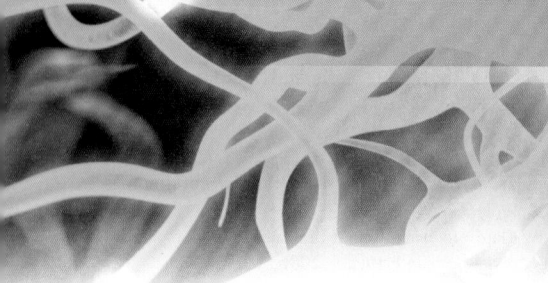

INTRODUCTION

Induced by underlying mesodermal structures, such as the notochord, and inhibited by surrounding ectodermal tissue, the nervous system begins as a thickened layer of poorly differentiated cells in the developing ectoderm of a 14-day human embryo. By 21 days, ridge-like structures have formed in the lateral most aspects of the neuroectoderm and begin to appose and to close in multiple closure sites, with the first in the cervical region. This forms a tube-like structure termed the *neural tube*, and this closure is normally complete by 26 days before most women know that they are pregnant. Errors in this process lead to myelomeningoceles (L5 and more rostral) and encephaloceles.

At the most caudal end of this tube is a mixed cell mass of ectoderm and mesoderm termed the *caudal cell mass*, which is induced by the presence of the neural tube to form the sacrum, the filum terminale, the conus medullaris, and the cauda equina. Errors in these processes lead to tethered spinal cords, caudal regression, fatty filum terminale, sacral pits and tracks, and other sacral defects.

The neural crest cells form from the extreme lateral aspects of the neuroectoderm and give rise to many of the sensory ganglia of cranial and spinal nerves in addition to the sympathetic chain and other structures.

Once the neural tube is completely formed, patterning or segmentation of this tube leads to the beginning of the well-described vesicles of the developing nervous system (prosencephalon, mesencephalon, and rhombencephalon). The prosencephalon divides in the midline to two telencephalic vesicles that will become the cerebral hemispheres. Precursors lining the ventricles of the developing nervous systems become postmitotic and migrate radially to populate developing structures such as the cortex. Axons sprout and cross the midline to form the corpus callosum and thereby connect the two developing hemispheres. Neurons extend axons to connect in a very deliberate and use-dependent fashion to the appropriate targets. This is basic nervous system development. To understand nervous system malformations, some additional genetic, molecular, and basic neurobiology insight is needed.

This chapter will summarize normal and abnormal human central nervous system (CNS) formation and describe the genetic aberrations that cause congenital malformations of the CNS. Much of human CNS development is inferred from animal studies and from abnormal developmental processes. Without being exhaustive, the proteins believed to be involved in the individual components of CNS development and those involved in pathologic alterations of normal development will be listed. The functions of some of the genes responsible for abnormal development can be surmised by examining the pathologic consequences. Hence, one is able to correlate genetic abnormalities with developmental neuropathology. Other genes and molecules involved in abnormal human CNS formation have well-studied counterparts in animals that provide insight into their function in humans.

The study of the genetics of human development is rapidly changing, and important new genetic mechanisms are being described often. Although the information regarding human genes involved in normal and abnormal brain formation was as up-to-date as possible at the time that this chapter was written, important new insights into the genetics of human CNS development have likely been made since this was written. Therefore, please visit Online Mendelian Inheritance in Man (OMIM) for more current information (http://www.ncbi.nlm.nih.gov/omim). As is the convention for the time that this chapter is written, terms such as *pathogenic variant* for those previously termed *mutation* will be used herein.

Emphasis is placed on important information for the clinician in this chapter, but there is plenty of knowledge of human nervous system development that could be covered herein. However, the space limitations and lack of current applicability to clinical neurology limit the amount of information that can be communicated here. Instead, the covered pathologic entities are presented in the context of the developmental processes that are believed to have gone awry, disorders previously categorized as migration abnormalities might, on the basis of new genetic insights, be found in the discussion of cellular differentiation or segmentation for example. As further insights are made into human brain developmental disorders leading to neurologic disorders, the following categorization scheme will probably have to be altered.

FORMATION OF NEUROECTODERM

The human brain is formed from the *neuroectoderm*, a placode of cells that are induced by the underlying notochord to differentiate from the ectoderm beginning at 14 days of gestation. The nature of the inducible factor(s) (actually inhibiting factors—bone morphogenic protein 4) involved in this process remain largely unknown. The molecular action of these molecules probably is similar to that of the retinoids that likely bind to a nuclear receptor to promote or suppress specific genes (Fig. 133.1).

NEURAL TUBE CLOSURE

PRIMARY NEURULATION

The neuroectoderm placode develops ridges (folds) laterally and begins to approximate in the region of the future medulla at 22 days of gestation before most women are aware they are pregnant. This closure, a process known as *neurulation*, results in a tube that continues to extend by the process of approximation of the neural folds in multiple locations rostrally and caudally until a complete neural tube is formed at 28 days of gestation, with the latter period marking the end of caudal neural tube closure (future spinal cord). The rostral neural tube, which closes at approximately 24 days of gestation, serves as the foundation for further brain development; the caudal end of the tube forms the spinal cord.

A

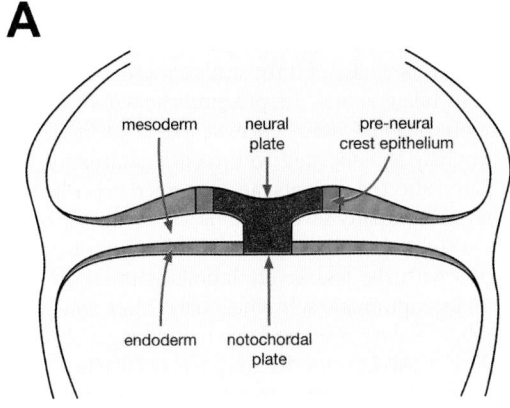

B

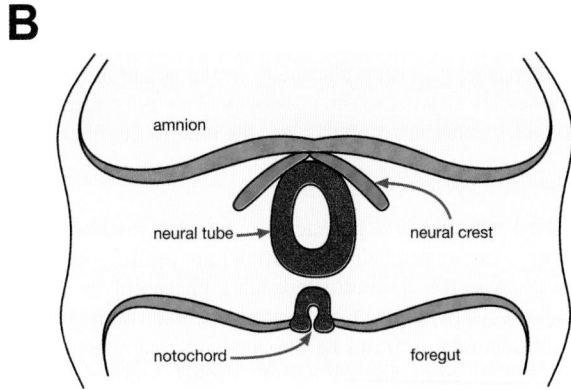

C

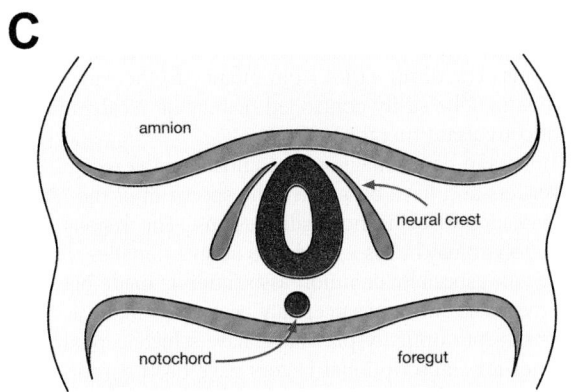

D

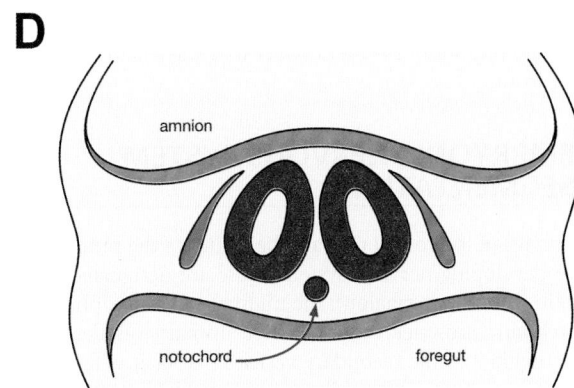

FIGURE 133.1 **A:** Notochord plate induces the neuroepithelium to differentiate from surrounding ectoderm. At the periphery of the neuroepithelium, neural crest forms. **B:** Neural tube closes. **C and D:** Rostral neural tube is induced by ventral notochord (Sonic Hedgehog and other factors) to split into two telencephalic vesicles that will become the cerebral hemispheres. (Drawings by Nathan Lucy, http://www.nathanlucy.com/.)

Although the specific molecules and genes involved in the processes of neural tube closure in humans are largely unknown, clearly a combination of genetic and environmental factors leads to disorders of these processes. Studies in mice suggest that a codeletion of *Paxl*, a gene for a *transcriptional factor* that mediates notochord signaling, and *Pdgfra*, the platelet-derived growth factor alpha gene, may lead to a spina bifida–like phenotype.

Certain ethnic groups experience a higher incidence of neural tube closure defects than do others, and genetic disorders with an apparent autosomal recessive inheritance that include neural tube defects have been described. In addition, teratogens are involved in neural tube pathology. The most notable teratogens for the neurologist are the anticonvulsants valproate and carbamazepine, each of which imposes a risk of 1% to 6% for a neural tube defect in offspring exposed in utero to these common drugs. Whereas folate supplementation appears to prevent neural tube defects in large population studies, this vitamin may or may not be protective when these disorders are associated with the aforementioned anticonvulsants. Given that short-term treatment with folate is probably benign, it seems prudent to offer this vitamin (400 to 4,000 μg daily, depending on risk factors) to women of childbearing age who are on anticonvulsants.

SPECIFIC NEURAL TUBE DEFECTS

In humans, multiple genes and factors probably are involved in the pathogenesis of disorders of neural tube formation and closure. The human disorders of neural tube closure include craniorachischisis (a complete failure of neural tube closure along the entire neuraxis), anencephaly (a failure of anterior neural tube closure), myeloschisis (a failure of posterior neural tube closure), spina bifida (myelomeningocele, a failure of closure of a portion of posterior neural tube), and encephalocele (a partial defect in anterior neural tube closure). Fetal recognition of myelomeningocele with correction in utero prior to 26 weeks' gestation can dramatically alter the need for subsequent ventriculoperitoneal shunting (reduced by 42%) and reduces the incidence of intellectual disability. The risk is to the mother.

Encephaloceles

Encephaloceles (brain substance outside of the skull) and meningoceles (meninges and cerebrospinal fluid [CSF] only) vary in location, in the amount of brain involved, and therefore in the clinical manifestations of the lesions. In most cases, the neural tube is closed, and the gyral pattern of the protruding brain appears normal. In the western hemisphere, most encephaloceles are occipital and midline. In the eastern hemisphere, anterior encephaloceles (nasal and frontal) surpasses that of posterior lesions. One should avoid nasogastric tube placement in the situation of a nasal mass in a newborn owing to the possibility of a nasal encephalocele; it is possible in this situation to place the tube in the brain substance.

Meckel Syndrome

Meckel syndrome, a genetic disorder that involves an occipital encephalocele, cerebellar malformations (molar tooth anomaly—see discussion in Joubert syndrome), microcephaly, renal dysplasia (polycystic kidneys), polydactyly, retinal dystrophy, and other malformations, appears to be caused by pathogenic variants in genes involved in ciliary function. Meckel syndrome is allelic with Joubert syndrome and the same genetic aberrations are present in both disorders. Most of these disorders are inherited in an autosomal recessive fashion, although some are inherited in a dominant fashion and others X-linked dominant or recessive. The genes involved are part of a ciliary complex that determines cell polarity and are important for the migration of early neurons in the posterior fossa.

EMBRYONIC NERVOUS SYSTEM SEGMENTATION

Flexures of the rostral neural tube delineate the primary vesicles of the developing nervous system; these are designated as the hindbrain (rhombencephalon), the midbrain (mesencephalon), and the forebrain (prosencephalon). These primary vesicles then further subdivide into the secondary vesicles that later will form the adult brain structures. The hindbrain consists of the metencephalon and myelencephalon; these structures will become the pons, the cerebellum, and the medulla oblongata of the adult. Rostrally, the mesencephalon will become the midbrain of the adult. The forebrain is further divided into the telencephalon and the diencephalon. The telencephalon will become the cerebral hemispheres, and the diencephalon will become the thalamus and hypothalamus of the adult.

TRANSCRIPTIONAL FACTORS AND HOMEOBOX GENES

Regional specification of the developing nervous system is an important step in human CNS development and is likely under the control of a number of genes that encode transcriptional factors and of a number of molecules that influence these genes. These genes were first described in *Drosophila* and are involved in the regional specification of the fly embryo. Not surprisingly, the function of the proteins encoded by the comparable genes in mammals differs considerably from that in fruit flies, but the general role of these proteins appears to be that of regional specification of clones of cells destined to form structures in the fully developed nervous system.

Transcriptional factors are proteins with distinct sequences that participate in DNA binding and thus influence DNA. In *Drosophila*, transcriptional factors encoding homeobox genes, empty spiracles, *ems* have been shown to specify head structures. For example, the rudimentary structures of mutant flies that are devoid of *ems* seem to be a result of failure of regional specification of a clone of cells that are destined to form those structures. In humans, pathogenic variants in the comparable gene *EMX2* may result in schizencephaly, cleft in the cortical mantle. The clefts in this disorder extend from the pia to the ventricle and are lined with a polymicrogyric gray matter (see the discussion in "Polymicrogyria").

The pia and ependyma are usually in apposition, especially in severe cases. The defect is termed *open lipped* if the cleft walls are separated by CSF and *closed lipped* if the walls appose. These clefts may be unilateral or bilateral and the prognosis appears to be dependent on location, bilateral occurrence, or extent of the lesion. Bilateral schizencephaly is associated with mental retardation and spastic cerebral palsy; affected patients often are microcephalic. Seizures almost always accompany severe lesions, especially the open-lipped and bilateral schizencephalic clefts. The exact frequency of seizures in patients with the less severe lesions is uncertain, nor is the incidence of asymptomatic schizencephaly. Most patients in whom schizencephaly is diagnosed undergo neuroimaging because of seizure. Therefore, a bias in favor of a universal occurrence of seizure in this disorder is noted. Hence, patients with schizencephaly who do not have epilepsy might exist, but the malformation remains undetected because no imaging is done. With fetal imaging, asymptomatic schizencephaly has been noted (Fig. 133.2).

Seizure type and onset may vary in this disorder. Patients may experience focal or generalized seizures. Some will present with infantile spasms. The onset varies from infancy to the early adult years. Seizures may be easily controlled or may be recalcitrant to standard anticonvulsant therapy.

Improvements in neuroimaging have enhanced the recognition of these disorders and have broadened the spectrum of the radiographic appearance of schizencephalic lesions. The lesions may occur in isolation or may be associated with other anomalies of brain development. An especially common association is made between septo-optic dysplasia and schizencephaly because as many as 50% of patients with septo-optic dysplasia also have schizencephaly.

Other genes for transcriptional factors have been described in the mouse. *Pax3*, *PaxS*, *Pax6*, *Dlxl*, *Dlx2*, *Dbx*, and the *Hox* genes are found in specific brain regions. In general, the *Pax* genes tend to be expressed in midbrain and the *Dlx* genes tend to be expressed in the ventral forebrain, ventral telencephalon, and dorsal telencephalon; *Dlx2* is important for the genesis of GABAergic interneurons from the median ganglionic eminence. The *Hox* genes seem to specify the neuromeres and rhombomeres of the hindbrain.

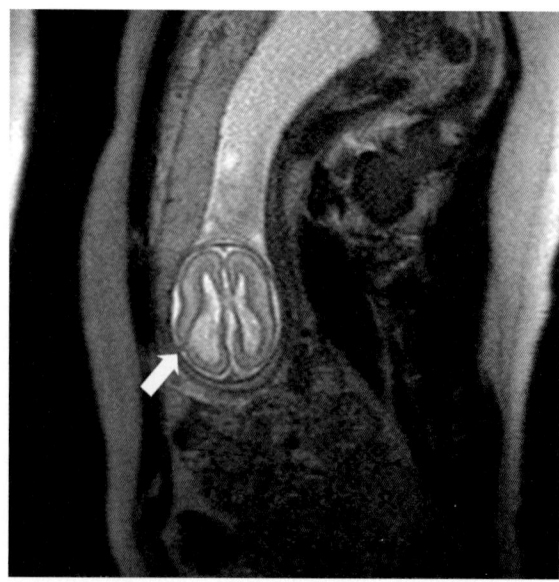

FIGURE 133.2 Segmentation or patterning defect—schizencephalic cleft in a developing fetus at 21 weeks' gestation. *Arrow* points to the cleft in the developing cortex.

Furthermore, in an interesting link to the ventral inductive events described later, when applied to proliferating cells at critical times in development, the protein sonic hedgehog can alter the expression of the homeobox genes. This ties the inductive proteins to the expression of homeobox genes and gives a hint as to the mechanisms involved in inductive processes. Further, a gradient of retinoic acid in a rostral (less) to caudal (more) fashion seems to be important for *Hox* and other patterning gene expression patterns in the hindbrain, neck, and other structures of the head. Retinoic acid activity also decreases the sonic hedgehog signaling (see "Ventral Induction [Prosencephalon Cleavage]"). It is for this reason that retinoids are highly regulated and should not be given to women who may become pregnant.

SEPTO-OPTIC DYSPLASIA

Septo-optic dysplasia (de Morsier syndrome) is a disorder characterized by absence of the septum pellucidum, optic nerve hypoplasia, agenesis of the corpus callosum, and hypothalamic dysfunction. This disorder should be considered in any patient who exhibits at least two of these, and all such patients should have hypothalamic function screening. Fifty percent of patients with septo-optic dysplasia have schizencephaly. Although this is a rare disorder, genetic syndromes with this phenotype and with some risk of recurrence have been described. For instance, pathogenic variants in homeobox gene expressed in ES cells, *HESX1*, have caused a dominantly inherited disorder in siblings. This disorder can be suspected in utero but magnetic resonance imaging (MRI) of the fetus may be necessary to assure a proper diagnosis. The prognosis for development is highly variable, with learning, intellectual, and motor impairments often described. Asymptomatic patients probably only come to medical attention if there are needs for neuroimaging. Pathogenic variants in *COL11A2* and *PAX6* have also been described. Because most of the genes related to this phenotype are undiscovered and no genetic panels exist, it is recommended that clinicians consider exome sequencing in order to delineate the recurrence risk in a family.

VENTRAL INDUCTION (PROSENCEPHALON CLEAVAGE)

NORMAL PROSENCEPHALON DIVISION

The telencephalon is formed by medial division of a rostral single tube-like structure (prosencephalon); the two vesicles (telencephalon) formed in this division become the two cerebral hemispheres. The ventral and anterior portion of this division is induced by midline facial structures and the notochord via soluble factors. Abnormalities of this induction and division lead to midline abnormalities of the brain such as holoprosencephaly. These disruptions of normal development occur before 42 days of gestation.

Sonic hedgehog, which was described first in *Drosophila* as a soluble factor (protein) that influences dorsoventral patterning of the developing embryo, is probably the most important of the soluble factors influencing ventral induction. Sonic hedgehog is expressed in the notochord (also in ventral forebrain and floor plate— future facial structures), interacts through a well-defined signaling pathway that includes *PTCH*, a human homolog of *patched*, and alters the expression of transcriptional factors (homeobox and other related gene products).

Other molecules of interest in this inductive process are the retinoids (discussed previously in segmentation), which are lipids capable of crossing membranes and have been shown to exist in gradients across embryos. Retinoic acid can alter the pattern of transcriptional factors in neuroepithelial cells, and it can also downregulate sonic hedgehog, perhaps explaining some of the midfacial defects and holoprosencephaly seen in retinoid embryopathy. Also, cholesterol and cholesterol-derived lipids serve as a cofactor for sonic hedgehog, thus perhaps explaining telencephalic cleavage issues (holoprosencephaly) in Smith–Lemli–Opitz syndrome (7-dehydrocholesterol reductase deficiency).

DISORDERS OF VENTRAL INDUCTION: HOLOPROSENCEPHALY

The holoprosencephaly syndromes are heterogeneous disorders of ventral induction and telencephalic cleavage that result from a failure of the prosencephalic vesicle to medially cleave normally. At least three forms of this disorder have been described: alobar, semilobar, and lobar. In the alobar form, the telencephalic vesicle completely fails to divide, producing a single horseshoe-shaped ventricle, sometimes with a dorsal cyst, fused thalami, and a malformed cortex (Fig. 133.3). In the semilobar form, the interhemispheric fissure is present posteriorly, but the frontal and, sometimes, parietal lobes continue across the midline. In the lobar form, only minor changes may be seen: The anterior falx is absent, the frontal lobes and horns are hypoplastic, there may be partial fusion of the thalami, and the genu of the corpus callosum may be abnormal. Holoprosencephaly is a common human malformation leading to spontaneous abortion.

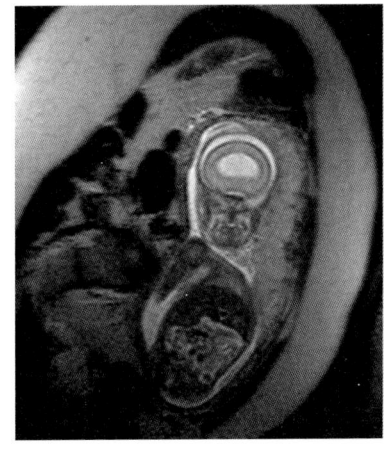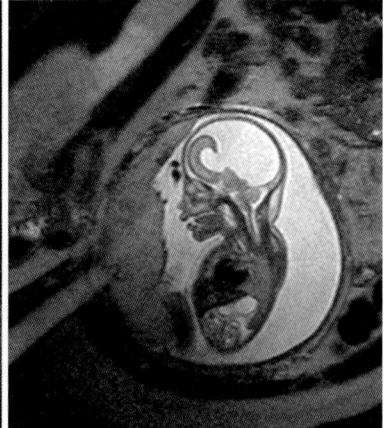

FIGURE 133.3 Failure of telencephalic cleavage— holoprosencephaly in a fetus at 32 weeks' gestation. Note the single ventricle with no division of the cerebrum into hemispheres on a coronal view **(left panel)**. On a sagittal view **(right panel)**, a dorsal cyst is noted that is typical for the alobar holoprosencephaly.

Because sonic hedgehog and patched are expressed in the developing face, it is not surprising that holoprosencephaly is associated with a spectrum of midline facial defects. These include cyclopia, in which there is a single central eye and a supraorbital proboscis; ethmocephali, in which the nose is replaced by a proboscis located above the hypoteloric eyes; cebocephaly, in which hypotelorism and a nose with a single nostril are seen; and premaxillary agenesis, with hypotelorism, a flat nose, a single frontal incisor, and a midline cleft lip.

Only children who have the semilobar and lobar forms are known to survive for more than a few months. An infant affected with the severe form is microcephalic (unless aqueduct stenosis and hydrocephalus are present), hypotonic, and visually inattentive. In infants with the less severe forms of holoprosencephaly, myoclonic seizures frequently develop and, if the infant survives, autonomic dysfunction, failure to thrive, psychomotor retardation, and atonic or spastic cerebral palsy often are present. Some infants with the lobar form may be only mildly affected. Pituitary defects may be associated with these malformations and may result in neuroendocrine dysfunction.

Holoprosencephaly has been reported to be associated with maternal diabetes, retinoic acid exposure, cytomegalovirus, and rubella. Chromosomal abnormalities associated with this disorder include trisomies 13 and 18; duplications in 3p, 13q, and 18q; and deletions in 2p, 7q, 13q, and 18q. Autosomal dominant forms exist in which the pathogenic variant is in *sonic hedgehog* or in *ZIC2*. In this form, the clinical features vary. In their mildest form, presence of a single central incisor, attention deficit disorder, or a choroid fissure coloboma may be the only clinical manifestation of an autosomal dominant disorder.

NEURONAL AND GLIAL PROLIFERATION

NORMAL CELL PROLIFERATION

Lining the interior of the newly developed telencephalic vesicles is a proliferative, primitive neuroepithelium. Neuroepithelial processes extend from the ventricular surface to the pial surface, and the nuclei of the primitive neuroepithelial cells move from the cortical surface in a premitotic phase to a mitotic phase near the ventricle. Cells divide at the most ventricular aspects of the developing telencephalon and, after division, move back toward the pial surface. The pial processes of neuroepithelial cells near the ventricle often will detach from the cortical surface before a new cycle begins.

Neuroepithelial cells divide in so-called proliferative units such that each unit will undergo a specific number of divisions resulting in the appropriate number of cells for the future cortex. Abnormalities in the number of proliferative units or in the total number of divisions can lead to disorders of brain manifested by abnormal brain size and, therefore, an unusually small (microcephaly) or large head (macrocephaly). Disorders in which too many cells are generated in the proliferative phase result in megalencephaly (large brain) or, if proliferative events go awry on only one side of the developing cortex, hemimegalencephaly. Once the appropriate complement of cells is generated in the proliferative phase, the cells that will become the neurons of the cerebral cortex become postmitotic and are referred to as *neuroblasts*. Others undergo a programmed cell death—apoptosis. The genetics of apoptosis are best characterized in the simple nematode *Caenorhabditis elegans*. Approximately 10% of the cells generated during development of this worm will undergo apoptotic or programmed cell death. Pathogenic variants leading to smaller or larger numbers of surviving cells result in smaller or larger nematodes, respectively. The molecular characterization of these pathogenic variants has led to identification of a number of "death" genes and of genes that prevent apoptosis. The mammalian counterparts of the nematode death genes encode enzymes that are cysteine aspartate–specific proteases, also known as *caspases*. At least one function of such enzymes is that of an interleukin-converting enzyme common in the inflammatory response of the body. These enzymes have been shown to promote neuronal death; in addition, when an animal is produced without caspase 3, a larger than normal brain results.

DISORDERS OF NEURONAL AND GLIAL PROLIFERATION

Microcephaly

Although primary familial microcephaly may be a normal variant, in the classic symptomatic form, clinical and radiologic examinations reveal a receding forehead, flat occiput, early closure of fontanelles, and hair anomalies such as multiple hair whirls and an anterior cowlick. Neuroimaging may show small frontal and occipital lobes, open opercula, and an uncovered cerebellum. The cortex may appear malformed (polymicrogyria, pachygyria, diminished white matter).

Neurologic findings also vary. Only mild psychomotor retardation may be noted, sometimes associated with pyramidal signs, or more severe intellectual disability, seizures, and an atonic cerebral palsy might be present. Primary microcephaly is seen in many genetic syndromes and, in its isolated form, may be autosomal recessive. Autosomal dominant and X-linked transmission has also been reported. *Microcephaly vera* is the term applied to this genetic form of microcephaly. Affected children present with a head circumference that is usually more than two standard deviations below the mean, hypotonia, and intellectual disability. They later show intellectual disability, dyspraxias, motor incoordination, and sometimes seizures.

Destructive lesions of the forming brain, such as those caused by teratogens and by infectious agents, also may result in microcephaly. Teratogens of note are alcohol, cocaine, and hyperphenylalaninemia (maternal phenylketonuria). Intense radiation exposure (such as in a nuclear explosion) in the first trimester can cause microcephaly. Microcephaly and intracranial calcifications are likely due to well-recognized in utero infections caused by cytomegalovirus, toxoplasmosis, or the HIV, among others.

Although now usually recognized in utero, patients with pathologic microcephaly or pathologic macrocephaly have been, in the past, identified by their pediatricians. Neuroimaging may reveal an etiology in such patients. Because multiple genetic or teratogenic etiologies must be considered, one must use neuroimaging as a clue to possible etiologies (presence of malformations, calcifications, etc.). The prognosis varies greatly and depends on the etiology. Familial microcephaly and familial macrocephaly with benign outcomes have been described.

Megalencephaly and Hemimegalencephaly

The terms *megalencephaly* and *hemimegalencephaly* refer to disorders in which the brain volume is greater than normal (not owing to the abnormal storage of material); usually, the enlarged brain is accompanied by macrocephaly or a large head. Although considered by some to be a migration disorder, the increase in brain size in these disorders appears to be attributable to errors in neuroepithelial proliferation, as the microscopic appearance of the brain is that of an increase in number of cells (both neurons and glia) and in cell size.

Typically, patients are noted to have large heads at birth and may manifest an accelerated head growth in the first few months of life. Children with megalencephaly or hemimegalencephaly may come to medical attention when presenting with seizures, a developmental disorder (intellectual disability), hemihypertrophy, or a hemiparesis (opposite the affected hemisphere). Seizures vary both in onset and in type and usually are the most problematic symptom, sometimes necessitating hemispherectomy or callosotomy.

Approximately 50% of patients with linear sebaceous nevus syndrome have hemimegalencephaly associated with *HRAS* or *KRAS* somatic-mosaic pathogenic variants. Many patients with hypomelanosis of Ito also have hemimegalencephaly. The neuropathologic and clinical pictures in these conditions appear to be identical to the isolated hemimegalencephalies. Interestingly, the genetic aberrations suggest an upregulation of the mammalian target of rapamycin (mTOR) pathway via a downregulation of phosphoinositol kinase 3 (PI3 kinase).

Microscopic examination of the affected brain usually reveals an increase in cellularity, large bizarre neurons, enlarged glia, cortical lamination defects, and heterotopias. The cortex usually is thickened, and malformed neurons are disturbed in polarity. Interestingly, the cytologic basis for the increase in brain size may be the abundant cytoplasm of individual cells.

NEURONAL DIFFERENTIATION

At the time of neuronal differentiation, the neural tube consists of four contiguous layers: (1) the ventricular zone, which gives rise to neurons and all the glia of the CNS; (2) the subventricular zone, which is the more superficial layer and is the staging area from which postmitotic neurons begin to differentiate and to migrate; (3) the intermediate zone, which is the contiguous, more superficial zone and which is destined to become the cortical plate and the future cerebral cortex; and (4) the marginal zone, which is the outermost zone and is composed of the cytoplasmic extensions of ventricular neuroblasts, corticopetal fibers, and the terminal processes of radial glia (which, at this time, are completely spanning the neural tube).

Differentiation of neuroepithelial cells begins in the subventricular layer at approximately gestational day 26. Neuroepithelial cells were destined to become neurons at the time of the final mitotic division of the neuroepithelial cell precursor before moving to the subventricular zone, the staging area for neuronal migration. At this point, these neuroblasts lack electrically polarized membranes as would commonly be seen in neurons. The fate of the neuroblast probably is determined before this final mitosis has occurred, as the postmitotic neuroblast has the properties of many neuron types. The older, larger pyramidal cells are the first cells to be born and probably differentiate early in order to act as targets or barriers in the migration of the nervous system.

No disorders of solely neuronal differentiation have yet been identified, although some disorders may be found to fit into this category. For instance, premature neuroblast differentiation could result in an inability of these cells to migrate and thus could be manifest as a migration abnormality. The megalencephaly and hemimegalencephaly syndromes may yet be found to be the results

of disturbances in differentiation, as discussed earlier. Disorders such as tuberous sclerosis, in which both tumor development and areas of migration abnormalities are seen, seem to be a differentiation disorder due to upregulation of mTOR. The brain manifestations of this disorder include hamartomas of the subependymal layer (tubers), areas of cortical migration abnormalities (cortical dysgenesis), and the development of giant cell astrocytomas in upwards of 5% of patients. Two genes for tuberous sclerosis have been identified: TSC1 (encodes for hamartin) has been localized to 9q34 and TSC2 (encodes for tuberin) has been localized to 16p13.3. Both proteins suppress mTOR and when lost or dysfunctional lead to overactivation of this important protein in development. The frequency of gene abnormalities in tuberous sclerosis patients has been estimated to be almost equally distributed between TSC1 and TSC2. Interestingly, recently type IIB cortical dysplasias were found to harbor human papilloma virus 16 and its oncogenic protein E6, which exerts its effect by upregulating mTOR by, in part, depressing TSC2.

NEURONAL MIGRATION

NORMAL MIGRATION

At the most rostral end of the neural tube in the 40-day-old fetus, the first mature neuron arrives at the developing cortical surface. These first neurons are the *Cajal–Retzius cells*, which are the major neurons of the cortex by day 43. Cajal–Retzius cells, along with corticopetal nerve fibers, form a so-called preplate. These cells will be the major cell type of the most superficial layer of the cerebral cortex, layer I. At the same time that the Cajal–Retzius cells are arriving at the most superficial layer of cortex, other pioneering neurons differentiate and form a so-called subplate. The pioneering neurons of the subplate and the preplate act as the police officers of the developing nervous system and define the limits of the developing cortical plate, which will become the six-layered cortex of the adult brain. Most of the cells of the subplate will die postnatally in a programmed cell death (see earlier discussion of apoptosis).

Near the end of the proliferative phase of neurodevelopment, billions of postmitotic neurons are poised to begin the trip to the cortical surface and to form the cortical plate. This tremendous number of neurons accomplishes this task, for the most part, by attaching to and migrating along radial glia (radially spanning from ventricle to pial surface) in a process known as *radial migration* (Fig. 133.4). In the process of migration, the deepest layer of the cortical plate forms before the other layers. Therefore, the first neurons to arrive at the future cortical plate are layer VI neurons. More superficial layers of cortex then are formed such that the neurons of layer V migrate and pass the neurons of layer VI; the same process occurs for layers IV, III, and II. The cortex therefore is formed in an inside-out fashion (see Fig. 133.4).

The molecules and the interactions between neurons and glia are extremely important in this process of neuronal migration. Reelin, the protein involved in the migration mouse mutant, reeler, appears to be one such important molecule. Reelin appears to promote an attachment of neurons to glia and, when abnormal, as in the mouse mutant reeler, it leads to an inverted cortex such that the most superficial neurons are the first to arrive and the later-arriving neurons are deeper. This mouse mutant cortex appears to be due to an abnormally adhesive interaction between neurons and glia. Additional molecules that appear to act in an adhesive manner are laminin, astrotactin, L1 antigen, fibronectin, neural cell adhesion molecules (NCAM), and adhesion molecule on glia (AMOG).

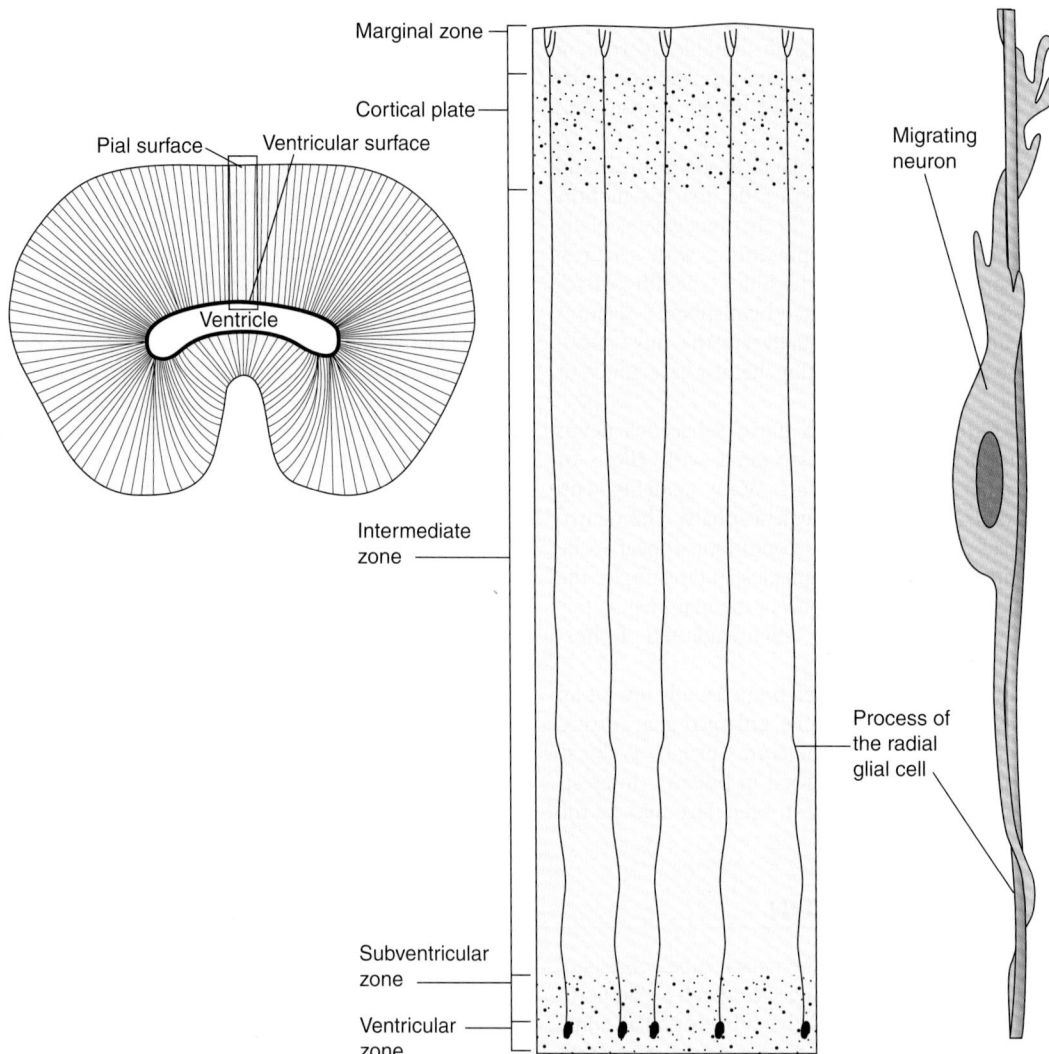

Marginal zone

Cortical plate

Pial surface Ventricular surface

Ventricle

Intermediate zone

Subventricular zone

Ventricular zone

Migrating neuron

Process of the radial glial cell

FIGURE 133.4 Neuronal radial migration in cortical development—*upper left* depicts a single cortical vesicle stained for glia. Glia radially project from the ventricle to the cortical surface. The *right figure* depicts the apposition of the migrating neuron to a radial glial cell. Cells migrate past their predecessor to deposit in an inside out fashion.

Neuroblast movement on radial glia involves an extension of a leading process, a neural outgrowth having an orderly arrangement of microtubules. *Microtubules* are cytoskeletal elements with a polymerizing (positive) end and a depolymerizing (negative) end. They serve as the major structural element that gives shape to long neural processes. When microtubules depolymerize, or slide, long neural processes are shortened. Shortening of the leading process of migrating neurons has been associated with forward movement of the soma of migrating neurons in vitro. Cytoskeletal changes in leading processes have been purported to be responsible for this shortening and somal movement.

A possible mode of movement in neuronal migration on glia would be the attachment of the neuron to a matrix secreted by either the glia or the neurons. This matrix is likely to consist of the aforementioned adhesion molecules. The attachment of the neuron would be through *integrin* receptors, cytoskeletal-linking membrane-bound recognition sites for adhesion molecules. That attachment serves as a stronghold for the leading process and soma of the migrating neuron. Shortening of the leading process owing

to depolymerization or shifts of microtubules results in movement of the soma relative to the attachment points. This theory of movement of neurons also must include a phase of detachment from the matrix at certain integrin receptors so that the neuroblast can navigate successfully along as much as 6 cm of developing cortex (the maximum estimated distance of radial migration of a neuroblast in humans). Finally, the movement of cells must stop at the appropriate location, the boundary between layer I and the forming cortical plate. Therefore, some stop signal must be given in order for the migrating neuroblast to detach from the radial glia and begin to differentiate into a cortical neuron. This is obviously deficient in such disorders as cobblestone lissencephalies (discussed in the following section).

Other forms of neuronal migration occur in brain development. Some evidence exists for a tangential migration of neurons in the cortex and in the early granule cell migration in the cerebellum. A so-called chain migration of neurons on other neurons occurs in the formation of the olfactory bulbs. In this chain migration, neuroblasts from the subventricular zone of the lateral ventricle migrate to the olfactory bulb through a sheath of glial cells, but the actual migration occurs on other neurons.

CORTICAL NEURONAL MIGRATION DISORDERS

Many clinical entities are associated with neuronal migration disorders. In some, abnormalities are limited to the nervous system but, in others, malformations involving other organs also are present. The responsible genetic mechanism has been identified in some of these disorders, and new genetic mechanisms are being identified regularly. Although the role of the gene product in producing many of these migration disorders may not yet be entirely clear, the disorders provide important clues to mechanisms that are responsible for normal brain development.

Modern neuroimaging techniques, particularly MRI, have allowed the recognition of major migration disorders. Some of these disorders are associated with typical clinical features that might alert the clinician to the presence of such abnormalities even before imaging is obtained. In other disorders, the clinical features are so varied that a strong correlation between imaging and clinical presentation does not exist. High-field MRI and other research techniques may further refine the clinician's ability to refine diagnoses.

Lissencephaly

Although the term *lissencephaly* (smooth brain) refers to the external appearance of the cerebral cortex in those disorders in which a neuronal migration aberration leads to improper number of neurons at the surface of the cortex (Fig. 133.5), the most important observation in such cases is the thickened cortex with neurons in what should be white matter. In such deficits of migration, gyri and sulci do not form properly because the cortical–cortical attractive forces that result from strong associations are decreased, owing to improper axon pathways (i.e., the targets for synapses are malpositioned). It is important to note that the term *lissencephaly* is applied to cortical disorders in which there is a thickened cortex (migration deficit) and a cortical surface abnormality; rarely, there is a completely smooth brain. At least two types of lissencephaly have been identified: type I, or classic, lissencephaly and type II, or cobblestone, lissencephaly. This classification is based on both the external appearance of the brain and the underlying histology.

TYPE I (CLASSIC) LISSENCEPHALY

Type I lissencephaly most often accompanies the *Miller–Dieker syndrome*. In this disorder, an inadequate radial migration of neurons appears to have taken place. The cortex is described as being composed of a four-layered abnormal sequence consisting of an outer molecular layer (layer 1), which is similar to normal layer I; a disorganized cellular layer of neurons near the normal location for the outer cortex (layer 2) (cells that should be in layers II to VI of the normal cortical plate); a cell-sparse zone (layer 3); and a heterotopic zone of neurons that have been arrested in neuronal migration (layer 4). The most extensive layer in this lissencephalic sequence is layer 4, the heterotopic zone. The neurons and cells of this zone have the appearance of cells that would normally be in layers II to IV of the normal cortical plate; however, these neurons are highly disorganized. Therefore, the later waves of neuronal migration that form the outer cortical plate appear to be those most affected by the migration abnormality in this disorder.

Hallmarks on imaging are a lack of opercularization (covering of the sylvian fissure), large ventricles with colpocephaly (fetal-like configuration of the occipital horns), and agyria or pachygyria

(see Fig. 133.5). The corpus callosum is almost never absent, and the posterior fossa has a normal appearance on neuroimaging (except in lissencephaly with ambiguous genitalia). Head size typically is in the low-normal range at birth, but most patients develop microcephaly owing to a decreased rate of brain growth over the first year of life. Nearly all patients with this disorder will develop seizures within this first year, and more than 80% of them will have infantile spasms. This seizure frequency is far greater than that seen in other neuronal migration disorders.

In the Miller–Dieker syndrome, facial dysmorphism, cardiac abnormalities (40%), sacral abnormalities (70%), deep palmar creases and, in male patients, genital abnormalities (70%) may be seen. The sacral abnormalities include deep sacral dimples, sacral pits, and sacral tracks. Facial abnormalities include upturned nares; a short nose; a thin, "pouty" upper lip; a long philtrum; micrognathia; and bitemporal hollowing. Although the bitemporal hollowing may be the result of the underlying brain abnormality, the other facial features would be difficult to explain on the basis of the brain abnormality alone. Therefore, these abnormalities are believed to result from deficits of genes near the lissencephaly gene on the 17th chromosome. Larger deletions of the distal short arm of chromosome 17 appear to result in the full Miller–Dieker phenotype, whereas microdeletions of just the lissencephaly gene *LIS1* result in isolated lissencephaly. Therefore, a deletion in the lissencephaly gene appears to be sufficient for the brain abnormalities, but other genes (14-3-3) must be deleted for the full phenotypic manifestations of the Miller–Dieker syndrome to be seen.

Miller–Dieker lissencephaly is one of the migration disorders of brain in which the responsible genetic defect has been identified. By both molecular and cytogenetic techniques, deletions in the terminal portion of one arm of chromosome 17 can be found in approximately 90% of Miller–Dieker lissencephaly cases. These patients typically have dysmorphic features and other congenital anomalies (see earlier discussion). The deletions of the terminal part of chromosome 17 in these cases have included microdeletions, ring 17 chromosome, pericentric inversions, and a partial monosomy of 17p13.3. These genetic abnormalities can be the result of an inherited unbalanced translocation from a parent with a balanced translocation involving this region of chromosome 17; multiple mechanisms of inheritance similar to this have been described for this disorder. Of course, a parent with a balanced translocation of chromosome 17p is at a greatly increased risk of having another child with Miller–Dieker lissencephaly. In families that are affected in this manner, screening with amniocentesis can be performed in subsequent pregnancies.

Current chromosomal microarray testing will detect deletions of *LIS1* and of the neighboring 14-3-3 gene, thus genetically distinguishing Miller–Dieker syndrome from isolated lissencephaly. Some patients with isolated lissencephaly (no facial, skeletal, or cardiac abnormalities) also have deletions (often submicroscopical) of the terminal portion of the short arm of chromosome 17. Therefore, some researchers suspected that within one deleted region of chromosome 17 was a gene that, when deleted, was sufficient to result in the lissencephaly phenotype. In 1993, the human gene for this form of lissencephaly was identified as *LIS1*.

The protein encoded by *LIS1* has 99% homology to a 45-kD subunit of a bovine brain platelet-activating factor acetylhydrolase (in humans PAFAH1B1). Subsequently, depletion of this protein has been demonstrated in the brains of patients with Miller–Dieker syndrome and with isolated lissencephaly. Interestingly, whereas the message for *LIS1* in mice is expressed ubiquitously, the *LIS1* protein product has been localized to the neuropile, Cajal–Retzius cells, and

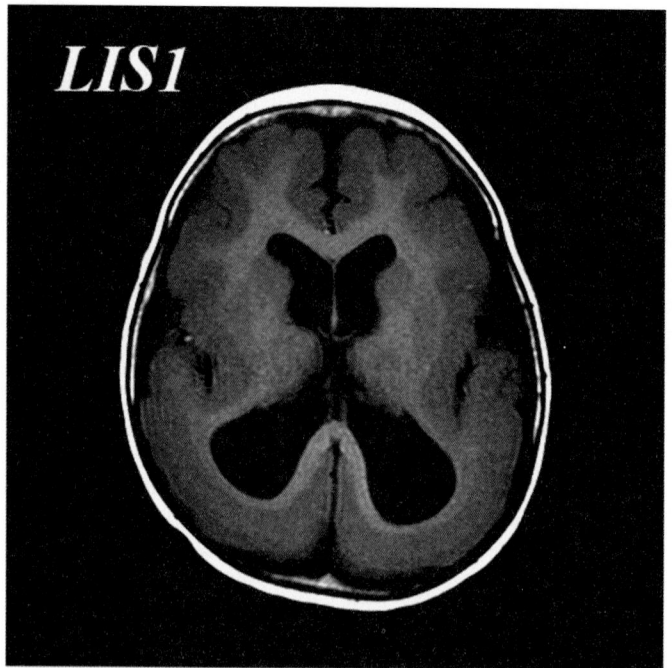
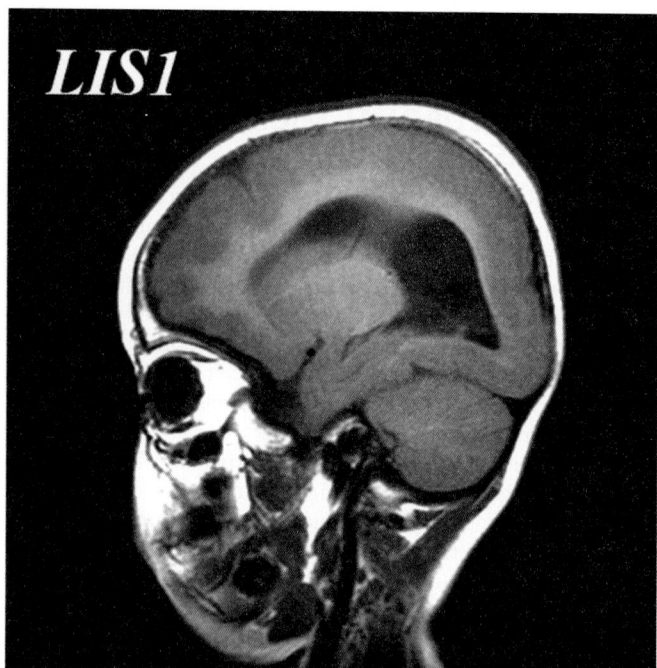
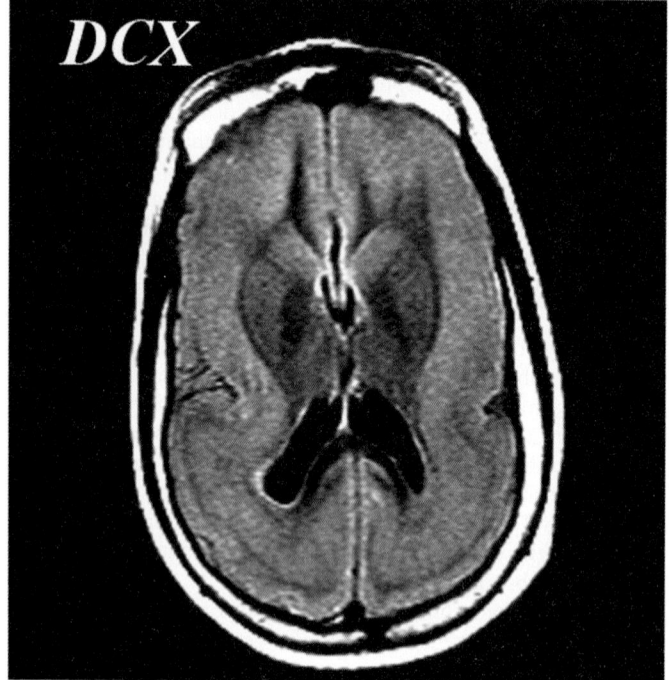
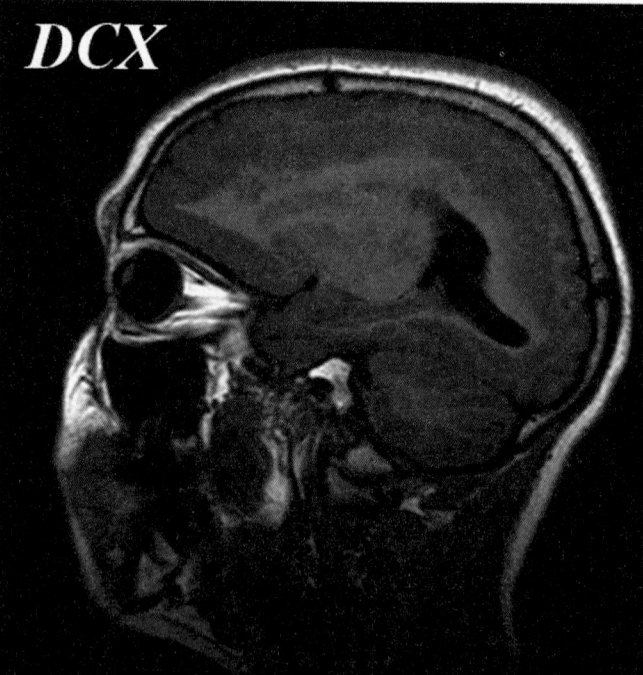

FIGURE 133.5 Lissencephaly spectrum—**top panels** are from a patient harboring an *LIS1* deletion. To the **left** is an axial T1 magnetic resonance image demonstrating agyria posteriorly and pachygyria anteriorly. To the **right** is a lateral sagittal T1 magnetic resonance image from the same patient demonstrating the same gradient of posterior worse than anterior malformation. **Bottom panels** are from a female with a *doublecortin* (*DCX*) mutation demonstrating the so-called double cortex (subcortical band heterotopia).

ventricular neuroepithelium at the time of human neuronal migration. However, it is not the lack of enzyme activity that leads to the brain malformation; rather, it appears that the catalytic units of this enzyme complex regulate the available level of LIS1 protein.

The brain malformations in LIS1 deficiencies are usually worse posteriorly as compared with X-linked lissencephaly, which is worse anteriorly as discussed in the following text (see Fig. 133.5). However, in Miller–Dieker syndrome the malformation may be equally severe anteriorly and posteriorly, thus making a distinction phenotypically difficult. This lesion can be detected in utero but late and beyond time for termination of a pregnancy. The life expectancy is dependent on the severity of the neurologic impairment.

X-linked lissencephaly looks nearly identical to the LIS1 deletion form of this disorder: Patients have classic lissencephaly, and the neurologic presentation is the same. However, the malformation is usually worse anteriorly, and the skeletal and other anomalies seen in the Miller–Dieker syndrome are not noted in this form of lissencephaly. In addition, X-linked lissencephaly occurs mostly in boys. Females who are heterozygous for the same gene have band heterotopia. Women with band heterotopia have been noted to give birth to boys with lissencephaly (see Fig. 133.5).

The *X-linked lissencephaly–band heterotopia syndrome* has been linked to Xq22.3. In female patients, the less severe phenotype probably is attributable to random X inactivation, such that in a variable percentage of cells, normal gene expression is seen and, in the remaining cells, the gene for X-linked lissencephaly, doublecortin, is expressed. This protein doublecortin is a microtubule-associated protein that appears to stabilize the cytoskeletal structure. It appears that this is a cell autonomous disorder, in other words, the cell expressing the abnormal X chromosome manifests aberrant migration or disturbed substrate on which cells can migrate.

The band heterotopia or double-cortex syndrome is a unique form of a neuronal migration defect that almost exclusively occurs in girls and is allelic with X-linked lissencephaly in boys. In this disorder, a circumferential, thick band of tissue is isointense with cerebral gray matter located within what should be the white matter of the hemispheres (see Fig. 133.5). This band is most obvious in the frontocentroparietal regions in keeping with the anterior worse than posterior gradient in disorders associated with *doublecortin* pathogenic variants. The inner and outer margins at its interface with the adjacent white matter usually are smooth. The overlying gyral appearance may vary from normal cortex to a one with abnormal sulcation. This anomaly represents incomplete neuronal migration. The exact mechanism is unclear, but possibilities include a lack of separation of the migrating neuron from the radial fiber or an arrest on the path to a normal cortical location.

Patients with band heterotopia typically present with seizures and a developmental disorder. The seizure type is variable, and the onset of epilepsy usually is between 2 months and 11 years of age. Patients may present with infantile spasms or, even though the migration abnormality is diffuse, some patients may present with focal seizures. Control of the epilepsy varies, some patients being controlled with monotherapy and others being entirely refractory to all agents.

Most patients with the X-linked lissencephaly–band heterotopia syndrome (double cortex) have impaired intellectual development that ranges from severe retardation to low-normal IQs; one girl had an IQ of 91. Generally, individuals with this syndrome are less impaired than are patients with other diffuse neuronal migration defects such as lissencephaly. Patients in whom seizures are of later onset generally have less developmental impairment. Neurologic findings include mild dysarthria and mild bilateral pyramidal syndromes.

Heterozygous pathogenic variants in *TUBA1A* can cause isolated lissencephaly but may cause other malformations such as polymicrogyria. The lissencephaly with cerebellar hypoplasia phenotype may be caused by pathogenic variants in *TUBA1A*.

Lissencephaly with ambiguous genitalia is associated with pathogenic variants leading to loss of function in the X chromosome gene *ARX*. The brain is small in this disorder and there is usually no corpus callosum. The basal ganglia are small or may have cysts. Interestingly, *ARX* poly A expansions may lead to West syndrome (infantile spasms) and ARX is responsible for the formation of

TABLE 133.1	**Type I (Classic) Lissencephaly Disorders**	
Gene	Inheritance/ Mechanism	Phenotype(s)
LIS1	Hemizygous, de novo deletion 17p13.3, pathogenic variants	Agyria, pachygyria worse posteriorly
LIS1 and *14-3-3ε*	Hemizygous, de novo deletion 17p13.3	Agyria, pachygyria worse posteriorly
Doublecortin (DCX)	X-linked dominant (hemizygous), usually de novo, but germ line inheritance described	Males: lissencephaly, worse anteriorly Females: band heterotopia (double cortex) worse anteriorly
TUBA1A	De novo pathogenic variants	Lissencephaly or lissencephaly with cerebellar hypoplasia
REELN	Recessive pathogenic variants (compound heterozygote or homozygote [with consanguinity])	Lissencephaly with cerebellar hypoplasia
ARX	X-linked de novo pathogenic variants	Lissencephaly, microcephaly, agenesis of the corpus callosum, cysts in basal ganglia, ambiguous genitalia

inhibitory neurons of the cortex. It is important to remember that repeats are not detected well with exome sequencing (Table 133.1).

TYPE II (COBBLESTONE) LISSENCEPHALY

In type II lissencephaly, the brain may have a smooth appearance or may exhibit polymicrogyria and pachygyria. The underlying cortical histology is that of a bizarre arrangement of neurons. Typically, in the most affected areas, normal cortical plate formation is not evident. Rather, bizarre whirls of cells are found. In addition, cells seem to penetrate the molecular layer and may spill into the subarachnoid space as if part of a volcanic eruption. This deposition of neurons in the subarachnoid space imparts a cobblestone street–like appearance to the brain surface; thus, the term *cobblestone lissencephaly* has been used to describe the cortex in these disorders. The Walker–Warburg, muscle–eye–brain, and Fukuyama muscular dystrophy syndromes appear to be genetically distinct. Abnormalities that may or may not be seen in these disorders include muscular dystrophy, ocular anterior chamber abnormalities, retinal dysplasias (abnormal electroretinogram and visual-evoked responses), hydrocephalus (usually of an obstructive type, requiring shunting), and encephaloceles. The Walker–Warburg syndrome or muscle–eye–brain disorder might be diagnosed even if the ocular examination and muscle biopsies are normal. On MRI, an abnormal white matter signal, hypoplastic brain stem and cerebellum, and a thickened falx suggest the Walker–Warburg diagnosis. Neuroimaging of the muscle–eye–brain disorders might reveal focal white matter abnormalities. This disorder and other cobblestone lissencephalies have been diagnosed in utero.

In the cobblestone lissencephaly spectrum, despite the widespread cortical abnormalities, only one-third of patients develop seizures. The typical presentation is that of a child with marked hypotonia, macrocephaly (obstructive hydrocephalus), and eye abnormalities. Depending on the degree of brain and of muscle involvement, this disorder may not be compatible with life. Long-term survival is rare. Syndromes accompanying type II lissencephaly include the Walker–Warburg syndrome, HARD-1-E (hydrocephalus, agyria, retinal dysplasia, with or without eye [anterior chamber] abnormalities) syndrome, muscle–eye–brain disease, and Fukuyama muscular dystrophy. These are all the result of recessive inheritance of pathogenic variants in extracellular matrix proteins or in the cell receptors for the extracellular matrix.

Fukuyama muscular dystrophy is distinguished from the Walker–Warburg–like syndromes by the severity of the muscular dystrophy, by the cortical malformation that includes polymicrogyria, and by Japanese inheritance. This disorder is seen more often in Japan than in the Western hemisphere, probably because it is the result of a founder pathogenic variant (a viral transposon insertion) in a gene termed *fukutin*. Patients typically present with evidence of a neuronal migration defect (cobblestone lissencephaly with polymicrogyria, hypotonia, and depressed reflexes).

Not surprisingly, patients with other pathogenic variants of *fukutin* have been described to have muscle, eye, brain, and even cardiac abnormal phenotypes. The protein fukutin interacts with laminin, an extracellular protein expressed in brain, muscle, and eyes, and with α-dystroglycans on muscle membranes. There is further interaction with fukutin-related protein (FKRP), which seems to promote glycosylation of α-dystroglycans in coordination with fukutin; FKRP pathogenic variants may cause Walker–Warburg, muscle–eye–brain, HARD-1-E, muscular dystrophy, or may be asymptomatic. Table 133.2 lists known genes involved in cobblestone lissencephalies; only about 50% of patients have genetic aberrations identified. This makes the case for exome sequencing in these disorders.

TABLE 133.2		**Cobblestone Lissencephaly Disorders**
Gene	Inheritance	Phenotype(s)
POMT1	AR	Cobblestone lissencephaly, muscular dystrophy
POMT2	AR	Intellectual disability, "mild brain malformations," muscular dystrophy
Fukutin	AR	Fukuyama muscular dystrophy, cobblestone lissencephaly, Walker–Warburg, limb-girdle muscular dystrophy
FKRP	AR	Walker–Warburg, muscle–eye–brain, cardiomyopathy, limb-girdle muscular dystrophy
LARGE	AR	Brain malformations, congenital muscular dystrophy
ISPD	AR	Cobblestone lissencephaly, limb-girdle muscular dystrophy

AR, autosomal recessive.

All these syndromes probably are accompanied by muscle abnormalities; the most extreme muscle involvement is in the Fukuyama muscular dystrophy patients. In the Walker–Warburg syndrome, the muscle abnormalities may or may not be clinically apparent (normal creatinine kinase [CK], no apparent myopathy on clinical exam).

Kallmann Syndrome

The Kallmann syndrome is an X-linked disorder characterized by anosmia and a defect in gonad development. Patients with this disorder may have other neurologic signs and symptoms, including cerebellar dysfunction and eye movement abnormalities. Therefore, abnormalities in other areas of brain, especially cerebellum, have been suspected in this disorder. Gonadal dysfunction is thought to result from a deficiency in gonadotropin-releasing hormone. Because the neurons that produce gonadotropin-releasing hormone are derived from the olfactory plate and actually migrate back into the forebrain via the olfactory nerve, the abnormality of this hormone is likely due to an arrest in migration of the gonadotropin-releasing hormone neurons.

The gene for Kallmann syndrome has been localized to the X chromosome and appears to encode a fibronectin type III–like molecule. Because fibronectin type III has been proposed to be a neural adhesion molecule, the gene for Kallmann syndrome probably also encodes a neural adhesion molecule involved in olfactory and hypothalamic neuron migration.

Zellweger Syndrome

Zellweger syndrome is an autosomal recessive peroxisomal disorder characterized by neuronal migration abnormalities, hepatomegaly, renal cysts, and stippled calcification of the patella. The neuronal migration defects include pachygyria and polymicrogyria, with underlying abnormalities best characterized as a nonlayered appearance of the cortex. Migration abnormalities are also noted in the cerebellum and in the brain stem in this disorder. Children with Zellweger syndrome present in the neonatal period with severe hypotonia, characteristic facies, hepatomegaly, and seizures. A mouse model of Zellweger syndrome has been produced; migration abnormalities were noted in the cerebellum and cortex despite normal-appearing radial glia. Disturbed maturation of neurons and apoptotic neurons also are noted in this mouse model; perhaps similar mechanisms are operative in the comparable Human disorder. More than 12 PEX genes have been implicated in Zellweger or Zellweger-like disorders; all are inherited in an autosomal recessive pattern.

Zellweger syndrome results from the body's inability to make peroxisomes owing to a deficiency of one of the 12 proteins encoded by the *PEX* genes. A number of peroxisomal enzymes are abnormal and lead to the accumulation of very long chain fatty acids. Therefore, testing for this disorder includes an assay of very long chain fatty acids.

Polymicrogyria

Polymicrogyria (many small gyri) is a disorder often considered to be a neuronal migration disorder; it is important to recognize that this malformation may result from both genetic and destructive processes. The microscopic appearance of the lesion is that of too many small abnormal gyri. The gyri may be shallow and separated by shallow sulci, which may be associated with an apparent increased cortical thickness on neuroimaging. The multiple small convolutions may not have intervening sulci, or the sulci may be bridged by fusion of overlying molecular layer, which may give a smooth appearance to the brain's surface; alternatively, the brain may appear to have pachygyria.

Polymicrogyria takes two distinct histologic forms: four-layered and unlayered. The four-layered form consists of an outer layer, a neuronal layer, a cell-sparse layer, and a deeper neuronal layer. One theory is that the lower cell-sparse layer of the four-layered types represents a glial scar from a laminar necrosis. On the basis of examination of fetuses in which the occurrence of the insult causing the malformation has been accurately timed, this pattern is believed to occur as a result of insults late in the first or early in the second trimester. Others believe that this is a postmigration insult resulting from distorted migration of cells through an injured area, the outcome of which is the cell-sparse layer. A cell-sparse layer between the upper and lower neuronal layers is absent from the unlayered form. Insults that occur early in the second trimester before migration is completed are believed to be the origin of unlayered polymicrogyria. Identical twin pregnancies discordant for polymicrogyria have been described; the theory being that global insults can lead to polymicrogyria. The common association of congenital cytomegalovirus infection with polymicrogyria supports the hypothesis that a destructive process can be involved in these disorders.

Polymicrogyria has also been associated with genetic and chromosomal disorders. It is found in disorders of peroxisomal metabolism such as Zellweger syndrome (see earlier discussion) and neonatal adrenal leukodystrophy. It has also been associated with the Bloch–Sulzberger syndrome, Meckel–Gruber syndrome, thanatophoric dysplasia, and Fukuyama congenital muscular dystrophy. Familial bilateral frontal polymicrogyria and bilateral perisylvian polymicrogyria have been reported. Therefore, if no identifiable cause of the polymicrogyric malformation is found, the recurrence risk may be that of an autosomal recessive disorder (25%) or an X-linked disorder in boys. A bilateral parasagittal parietooccipital polymicrogyria has also been described. Multiple chromosomal deletions and duplications including X-linked potential inheritance have been described. Multiple recessively inherited disorders have also been identified, including GPR56 and WDR62 pathogenic variants in families with recurrences of polymicrogyria with variable phenotypes.

The clinical picture varies depending on the location, extent, and etiology of the abnormality. Microcephaly with severe developmental delay and hypertonia may result when polymicrogyria is diffuse. When polymicrogyria is unilateral, focal deficits might be seen. Epilepsy often is present, characterized by partial complex seizures or partial seizures that secondarily generalize. The age at presentation and severity of seizures depends on the extent of the associated pathology.

The lesions are most clearly recognized by MRI and are best noted on sagittal views. They often are recognized by the rough appearance of the surface of the cortex on a thin-cut T2-weighted image. If MRI cuts are thick, these lesions may be confused with pachygyria. Because the genetic implications of pachygyria and polymicrogyria differ considerably, distinguishing between these two conditions is important.

Congenital Bilateral Perisylvian Syndrome

Advances in neuroimaging have led to the recognition of the congenital bilateral perisylvian syndrome, also known as the *Foix–Chavany–Marie syndrome*. MRI demonstrates bilateral abnormalities in the opercular and perisylvian regions. The cortex is irregular, and the sylvian fissure may be noted to extend to the top of the convexity.

Striking clinical features include a pseudobulbar palsy with abnormal tongue movements, dysarthria, dysphasia, mental retardation, absent or hyperactive gag reflex, drooling, and pyramidal signs in more than 70% of the reported cases. These patients may be intellectually disabled, and nearly all have severe language disorders. Dysphagia can impair proper nutrition. Seizures are present in most of the affected patients. Several patients have had infantile spasms during the first year of life. Seventy percent of the patients experience seizures before the age of 10 years. The etiology of this syndrome is similar to other forms of polymicrogyria (deletions, duplications, insults [cytomegalovirus, twin pregnancies], Aicardi syndrome [see later discussion], and recessively inherited pathogenic variants in genes).

Heterotopias

Heterotopias are collections of normal-appearing neurons in an abnormal location probably secondary to a disturbance in radial migration. The exact mechanism of the migration aberration has not been established. Various hypotheses include damage to the radial glial fibers, premature transformation of radial glial cells into astrocytes, or a deficiency of specific molecules on the surface of neuroblasts or of the radial glial cells (or the receptors for those molecules) that results in disruption of the normal migration process. Heterotopias often occur as isolated defects that may result in only epilepsy. However, when they are multiple, heterotopias might also be associated with a developmental disorder and cerebral palsy (usually spastic). In addition, if other migration defects such as gyral abnormalities are present, the clinical syndrome may be more profound. Usually, no cause is apparent. Occasionally, heterotopias may be found in a variety of syndromes, including neonatal adrenal leukodystrophy, glutaric aciduria type II, GM_2 gangliosidosis, neurocutaneous syndromes, multiple congenital anomaly syndromes, chromosomal abnormalities, and fetal toxic exposures.

Heterotopias may be classified by their location: subpial, within the cerebral white matter, and in the subependymal region. Leptomeningeal heterotopias often contain astrocytes mixed with ectopic neurons and may resemble a gliotic scar. They may be related to discontinuities in the external limiting membrane and often are associated with type II lissencephaly. These *subarachnoid heterotopias* are responsible for the pebbled appearance of the surface of the brain (therefore the name cobblestone lissencephaly). *White matter heterotopias* may be focal, subcortical, or diffuse. They may cause distortion of the ventricles and may be associated with diminished white matter in the surrounding area. When diffuse, they may take the form of a circumferential subcortical layer of heterotopic gray matter, which has been called *band heterotopia* or the *double-cortex syndrome* (see previous discussion in "Type I [Classic] Lissencephaly"). Laminar heterotopia may consist of sheets of ectopic gray matter that may be split into elongated islands. A central ovoid mass of white matter may be present within the band. Patients with this form of subcortical heterotopia have a high prevalence of developmental delay, hemiplegia, and seizures. Nodular subcortical heterotopias may be seen in association with subependymal heterotopias.

Subependymal heterotopias often are associated only with epilepsy. Most patients will have normal intelligence and no motor deficits. These heterotopias are located just beneath and about the ependymal lining of the lateral ventricles. They may be either bilateral or unilateral and are located most often adjacent to the occipital horns and trigones and, less commonly, within the temporal horns and frontal horns. Seizure onset in patients with subependymal heterotopias is relatively late, often in the second decade, and more often affects women. The seizures may be partial complex, tonic–clonic, or focal motor. Subependymal heterotopias have been identified as an X-linked dominant syndrome linked to markers in the distal Xq28 locus and pathogenic variants in *filamin A* have been found to be causative. Filamin A, a cytoskeletal protein, must be important for the initiation of migration because cells are arrested in the ventricular zone. An increased incidence of spontaneous abortions, patent ductus arteriosus, spontaneous hemorrhage, and a much higher than expected incidence of female offspring are noted in affected women, suggesting that inheritance of *filamin A* pathogenic variants may be lethal for male embryos. Some variants in this gene may result in male phenotypes. A syndrome marked by periventricular heterotopia, mental retardation, and syndactyly has recently been described in male patients.

Patients with diffuse gray matter heterotopias, whether subependymal or in the white matter, usually are candidates for medical treatment of the epilepsies present. Occasionally, patients who are refractory to medical management may be considered for hemispherectomies or focal cortical resections. In the case of bilateral temporal lobe periventricular heterotopias, the prognosis for a surgical cure may be poor.

Cortical Dysgenesis

Cortical dysgenesis refers to disorders of cortical formation. In general, many of the disorders just discussed are considered to be within the spectrum of this entity. In this section, an emphasis on those focal macroscopic and microscopic lesions that do not fit into the preceding classifications will be discussed.

The terms *cortical dysplasia* and *cortical dysgenesis* often are used synonymously for the same disorders. Included in these terms are not only the obvious malformations such as smooth gyri and clefts but also lesions classified as focal cortical dysplasias and microdysgenesis. Focal cortical dysplasia may involve a major part of a lobe and may be characterized by the congregation of large, bizarre neurons and abnormal glial cells in the subadjacent white matter. *Microdysgenesis*, by definition, can be detected only histologically and is beyond the imaging capability of current MRI scans. It consists of unipolar and bipolar neurons under the pia, increased neurons in the first layer of the cortex, indistinct boundaries between the first and second layers of the cortex, neuronal glial heterotopias in the pia, persistence of columnar architecture of the cortex, and an increased number of neurons in the white matter. Patients with microdysgenesis are reported only in series of patients undergoing epilepsy surgery. Microdysgenesis is not detected in patients with controlled epilepsy and thus the incidences of migration disorders and of microdysgenesis responsible for epilepsy are unknown.

Microdysgenesis was the most common migration disorder noted in a series of pathologic examinations of brain tissue removed from epileptic patients. Malformations of this type were found in 14% of epileptic brains; the frequency of other abnormalities in epileptic brains was microgyria, 4.7%; heterotopia, 15%; and pachygyria, 8%. In patients with microdysgenesis, seizure onset occurs between 2 and 20 years of age.

A surprisingly high incidence of microdysgenesis has been reported in brain tissue removed from adults to treat recalcitrant seizures. The lesions noted included ectopic neurons within the subcortical white matter in 42% of the specimens and neuronal clustering in 28%; in addition, bare areas were present within layers II to VI. Similar findings have been reported in epilepsy surgical specimens from children. Thus, microscopic abnormalities have been found in 20% to 40% of specimens from patients

undergoing surgical therapy for intractable epilepsy, the most common lesions being microdysgenesis and cortical dysplasias.

As mentioned earlier, MRI has been useful in detecting migration abnormalities and generally has been found to be more sensitive than computed tomography (CT) scanning. MRI-apparent migration abnormalities have been detected in as many as 50% of patients who underwent epilepsy surgery. Of those patients with epilepsy alone, 6.7% had migration abnormalities; in those who had both mental retardation and epilepsy, such abnormalities were found in 13.7%. The abnormalities included pachygyria or polymicrogyria or both, schizencephaly, heterotopias, and hemimegalencephaly. Of 222 adults with temporal lobe epilepsy studied by MRI, 7.2% were found to have malformations of the temporal lobe. These malformations consisted of heterotopias, focal neocortical dysgenesis, hippocampal malformations, or a combination of various lesions.

Cortical dysgenesis has also been associated with hippocampal sclerosis, leading some to believe that hippocampal sclerosis is a disorder of brain formation. Raymond and colleagues studied 100 patients with hippocampal sclerosis diagnosed by histologic examination or MRI and found that 15 of the patients also had cortical dysgenesis. The most common abnormality was subependymal heterotopia. The cortical dysplasia was, at times, contralateral to the hippocampal sclerosis.

Clearly, migration aberrations need not be manifested by abnormal motor function; rather, epilepsy and mental retardation might be the only clinical symptoms in these disorders.

The severity of the migration disorder correlates with clinical symptoms. Patients with milder forms of neuronal migration defects (i.e., focal cortical dysplasias, heterotopias, microdysgenesis) may appear normal. Most often, migration disorders are diagnosed in patients with epilepsy, as neuroimaging is performed for seizure. These patients generally have partial seizures and normal life expectancies. Some patients with these disorders will have developmental delays, mild intellectual deficits, or spastic or atonic cerebral palsy. Profound defects are associated with more severe symptoms.

Children presenting with intractable epilepsy, significant intellectual disability, and neurologic signs more often have diffuse migration abnormalities on MRI scanning. Therefore, not surprisingly, the degree of abnormality on MRI scans correlates well with the degree of neurologic involvement. The age of onset of seizures varies from early childhood to young adult life. Generally, the severity of the seizures and the severity of the pathology correlate positively. Severe abnormalities are associated with seizures in the first year of life, whereas microdysgenesis may be associated with adult onset of seizures. Later onset seizures also tend to correlate with subependymal heterotopias.

Although the pathogenic mechanisms involved in focal dysgenesis remain poorly understood, mechanisms similar to those involved in global or more extensive migration disorders probably are operative. Therefore, definition of the pathogenic mechanisms causing these disorders is important. An important insight into the pathogenesis of focal developmental lesions may have come from the observation that the human papilloma virus (HPV) 16 RNA, and its oncogenic protein E6 are present in focal cortical dysplasia type IIB resected for epilepsy. This fascinating observation potentially ties HPV with tuberous sclerosis because the E6 protein encoded by HPV exerts its oncogenic effect via depression of TSC2, thereby upregulating mTOR as occurs in tuberous sclerosis. In support of this hypothesis is the fact that cortical dysplasia type IIB also occurs in tuberous sclerosis. Indeed, other viruses could have similar effects on the developing nervous system and could explain microdysgenesis and other lesions of the nervous system described earlier.

POSTERIOR FOSSA FORMATION AND MALFORMATION

Posterior fossa malformations are best understood in terms of the normal developmental processes that have gone awry. At 4 weeks of human gestation, the hindbrain and/or rhombencephalon bends and divided into two vesicles, the metencephalon and the myelencephalon; the pons develops in the floor of the metencephalon and the lateral walls of the myelencephalon form the medulla oblongata. The cerebellum develops from the dorsal hindbrain (neuromere 1, rhombic lip) with contributions from the lower mesencephalon, which forms the vermis and the metencephalon, which forms the cerebellar hemispheres. As this development progresses, mesenchymal tissue from the forming skull and meninges invade to form the choroid plexus. This invasion of mesenchymal tissue is caudal to the developing rhombic lip and this invasion penetrates the developing fourth ventricle. The roof of the developing fourth ventricle is divided by this invading mesenchymal tissue into two areas, the anterior membranous area and the posterior membranous area. The rhombic lip, the developing cerebellum, grows over the structures as it enlarges to form the cerebellum. As the cerebellum develops, the anterior membranous area involutes and the posterior membranous area protrudes outward from the developing nervous system. This performs the so-called Blake pouch cyst, which may persist normally until 4 months gestation. Eventually, the foramen of Magendie form in this Blake pouch cyst and the protrusion normally involutes. The foramen of Luschka also developed around this time.

A proliferative zone of cells in the ventricular region of the rhombic lip give rise to future Purkinje cells which migrate radially toward the surface of the developing cerebellum. At the tip of the rhombic lip, cerebellar granule cells are born that migrate over the surface of the rhombic lip and then, in a reverse radial migration, penetrate the developing cerebellum, pass Purkinje cells, and deposit in the developing internal granule cell layer. Amazingly, this process of cerebellar granule cell formation is occurring in the first year of human life. Prior to this, other neurons are born in interventricular zone and migrate to the various nuclei of the brain stem.

For the purposes of this chapter, I will divide posterior fossa malformations into predominantly neuronal structural malformations and malformations of the foramina and ventricular and transient cyst structures of the developing brain. This division is in all likelihood further defined by the genetic abnormalities that are involved in neuronal genesis, migration, and patterning (predominantly neuronal structural malformations) and those of mesenchymal support structures that are important in the formation of the transient cyst of the developing posterior fossa.

JOUBERT, MECKEL–GRUBER, AND OTHER CILIOPATHIES

In the classic form, Joubert syndrome is a recessively inherited disorder with clinical features of variable intellectual impairment, respiratory rate dysregulation, oculomotor movement abnormalities (classically oculomotor apraxia), hypotonia, and ataxia. Kidney, liver, renal, and retinal abnormalities may accompany these symptoms and signs. Radiologically, Joubert syndrome is recognized by the molar tooth anomaly and accompanying vermian hypoplasia or aplasia. The molar tooth malformation results from thin cerebellar peduncles that extend dorsally at right angles to the brain stem and absence or hypoplasia of the vermis giving the appearance of roots of a molar tooth. Absence of the cerebellar peduncle decussation and disturbance of the cortical spinal tract decussation combined with brain stem nuclei abnormalities result in a thinning of the brain stem with a prominent isthmus giving the ventral brain stem the appearance of the crown of a molar tooth. Cerebellar foliation defects may be noted along with other brain stem abnormalities.

The Meckel–Gruber syndrome may include the aforementioned brain stem and cerebellar abnormalities but is distinguished by the presence of an occipital encephalocele that is usually located near the level of the torcula and may contain supratentorial contents or infratentorial contents or both. This may be accompanied by syndactyly and renal, liver, retinal, or kidney problems and the developmental outcomes are more severe than those of Joubert syndrome.

Genetically, Joubert and Meckel–Gruber are caused by recessive loss of function pathogenic variants in primary ciliary genes. The primary cilia are the polarity antenna of many cells, are not motile, nor have motility functions other than to determine directionality in development.

RHOMBENCEPHALOSYNAPSIS

Rhombencephalosynapsis is fusion of the cerebellar hemispheres with absence of the vermis. The development of this lesion is unknown but apparently results from a dorsal lack of division of the developing cerebellum. Clinical manifestations may be developmental or this lesion may be noted in asymptomatic patients. To date, the genetics of this lesion is undetermined with the exception of an implication of ZIC2 in a combination of holoprosencephaly and rhombencephalosynapsis noted in two half sisters concordant for a pathogenic variant in this gene.

DANDY–WALKER

Possibly failure to form the foramen of Magendie or failure to involute the anterior membranous area results in an enlargement of the fourth ventricle, thereby lifting, externally rotating, and compressing the vermis. The cerebellar hemispheres are splayed outward and the torcula may be elevated. The posterior fossa is enlarged and in 80% of cases, there is obstructive hydrocephalus requiring postnatal shunting from either failure to form the foramina and therefore outflow from the fourth ventricle or from compression of the aqueduct of Sylvius (Fig. 133.6). Surprisingly, this lesion is associated with good neurologic outcomes if there are no accompanying distinct malformations of the brain or if not accompanying trisomy 9, 13, 18, 21, or other chromosomal aberrations. Some of the genes associated with this disorder are expressed in meninges and developing skull (FOXC1) and others in the dorsal cerebellum during development (ZIC1, ZIC4). The single gene defects thus far associated with this brain lesion are heterozygote deletions or loss of function mutations.

Unfortunately, a rather loose use of the terms *Dandy–Walker* and *Dandy–Walker variant* have made the literature regarding these malformations very difficult to interpret and to the impression that these lesions carry poor prognoses; for the most part, they do not. It is my opinion that the terms *Dandy–Walker* and *Dandy–Walker variant* should be reserved for those malformations that solely involve enlargement of the fourth ventricle with its consequences such that in the case of Dandy–Walker variant, the lesion should include at least upward rotation of the vermis.

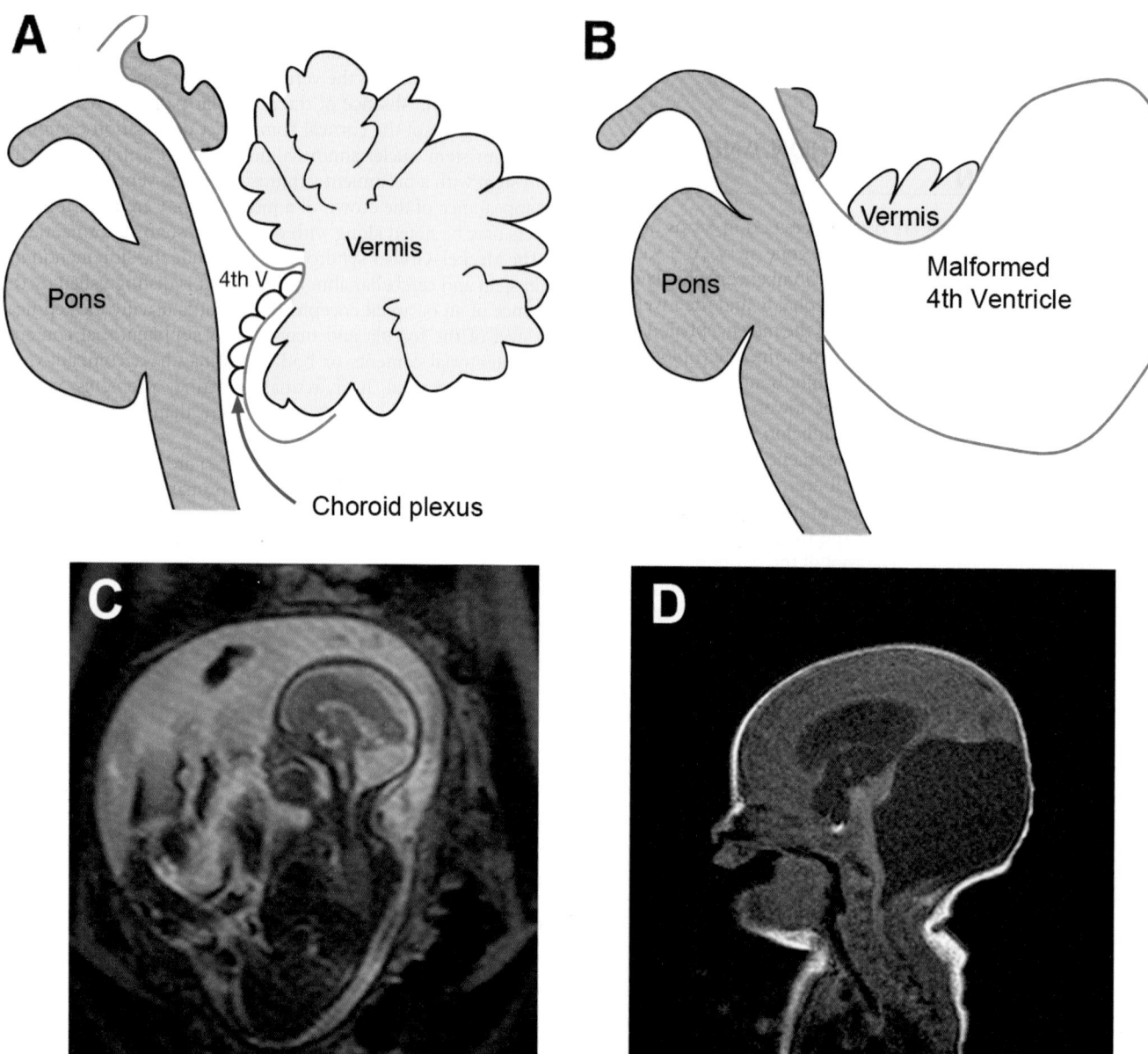

FIGURE 133.6 Dandy–Walker malformation. **A:** Midsagittal drawing of the posterior fossa with normal fourth ventricle. **B:** Midsagittal drawing of the posterior fossa in Dandy–Walker malformation. The foramen of Magendie has not opened resulting in large fourth ventricle that rotates, compresses, and elevates the vermis and the torcula. **C:** A 21-week-old fetus with Dandy–Walker malformation **D:** Dandy–Walker malformation with obstructive hydrocephalus in a newborn. (A and B by Nathan Lucy, http://www.nathanlucy.com/.)

An enlarged cisterna magna forms embryologically in a different fashion, although *FOXC1* is implicated in both enlarged cisterna magna and in Dandy–Walker. Further, arachnoid cysts may form in the posterior fossa resulting in enlargement of the posterior fossa and even compression of developing structures, but because these form distinctly from the dilatation of the fourth ventricle in Dandy–Walker, the term *Dandy–Walker* should be applied to these lesions nor should the expectations be the same. Similarly, in the earlier described lesions of the posterior fossa that do not expand it, there may be hypoplasia of the brain stem, malformations of the cerebellum, or other malformations that disturb the posterior fossa. The developmental consequences of these lesions are usually dire and to use the term *Dandy–Walker* in any form

to describe these is not accurate embryologically and lowers the developmental expectations for true Dandy–Walker patients.

PROCESS OUTGROWTH AND SYNAPSE FORMATION

CORPUS CALLOSUM

Callosal formation begins surprisingly early in human development; the first axons crossing from one developing hemisphere to the other side is apparent at 6 weeks' gestation. By 11 to 12 weeks, there is an identifiable corpus callosum and by 18 to 20 weeks, all of the structures of the corpus callosum are present (rostrum, body, splenium). Errant formation of this structure can result in complete agenesis, so-called partial agenesis or dysgenesis. The corpus callosum continues to form and differences in appearance may be seen through adolescence owing to myelination and pruning of crossing fibers.

The outcome depends on the genetic disorder and outcome data is heavily biased toward poor outcomes. There is an ascertainment bias in many brain developmental disorders, but perhaps none more than in callosal disorders. Most patients with callosal agenesis/dysgenesis have neuroimaging because they have presented to a neurologist owing to developmental or neurologic issues. Asymptomatic people with callosal agenesis or dysgenesis are therefore not recognized. However, with commonplace fetal imaging, it is possible that more accurate data regarding outcomes in these disorders may be noted. In fact, in a French cohort of 20 patients with agenesis or dysgenesis of the corpus callosum identified in utero (without prejudice), 80% have had normal outcomes up to 10 years later.

Multiple etiologies of agenesis/dysgenesis of the corpus callosum have been described and the potential etiologies are legion and could deserve a chapter. For the clinician, the division into accompanying other brain malformations, isolated and symptomatic seems the most useful. Examples of accompanying other brain malformations include Walker–Warburg and other muscle–eye–brain disorders, ciliopathies (see "Posterior Fossa Formation and Malformation"), X-linked lissencephaly with ambiguous genitalia (*ARX* pathogenic variants), and Aicardi syndrome.

Aicardi syndrome occurs mostly in females (in XXY males), is accompanied by other brain anomalies (polymicrogyria, intracranial cysts, nodular heterotopia), and is defined by chorioretinal lacunae; the genetic basis of this disorder is unknown. The prognosis is poor and epilepsy is nearly a certainty.

It is important for the clinician to recognize that structural brain disease can result from metabolic disorders. Nonketotic hyperglycinemia may result in agenesis/dysgenesis of the corpus callosum. With the structural brain disease and lack of acidosis, the neurologist and neonatologist may easily assume that the seizures, hypotonia, and depressed mental status at birth are the result of the brain malformation. Similarly, pyruvate dehydrogenase complex deficiency may result in callosal agenesis/dysgenesis with or without lactic acidosis.

An important review of the genetics of callosal dysgenesis was published as an editorial by Dobyns and nicely catalogs observations with and without other CNS malformations associated with duplications, deletions, trisomies, and point pathogenic variants (recessive, X-linked, and dominant). A reasonable evaluation of a patient symptomatic from a callosal dysgenesis would include an ophthalmologic exam if female to rule out Aicardi, metabolic studies to include CSF glycine to serum glycine ratios, urine organic acids, and chromosomal microarray and if these are negative, consideration for whole exome sequencing should be made.

Fetal recognition of isolated agenesis of the corpus callosum may carry a different prognosis as discussed earlier. Eighty percent of the fetuses so identified will be normal in follow-up. When evaluating the fetus with a corpus callosum malformation, it is important to recognize that Aicardi syndrome, with its poor prognosis, needs to be considered as a possibility for females.

NORMAL SYNAPSE FORMATION

Even as neurons are arriving in the cortical plate, important neural outgrowths and synapses are forming. The process by which neurons sprout new extensions (neurites) that grow impressive distances to make precise synaptic connections is remarkable and has been well studied, although it is still being elucidated. During development, many more synapses are made than are needed; these subsequently are pruned to improve precision of synaptic connections. Such pruning occurs while other synapses are strengthened. Pruning may be a phenomenon peculiar to the developing nervous system, but synapse strengthening probably continues throughout life.

Most early neurites will form axons. The distance and the terrain that a forming axon must negotiate to reach its target are often formidable, yet this process occurs with little error. Neurites consist of a long shaft of dynamic cytoskeletal elements that terminate in a growth cone, a highly motile structure capable of responding to chemical cues.

The nature of the chemical cues that guide growth cones and, thus, developing axons are threefold: adhesive, chemoattractive, and chemorepulsive. Adhesive molecules, such as those in the NCAM family, line projection pathways; integrin receptors on growth cones and neurites link the internal cytoskeleton of these structures with the extracellular adhesive molecules. These adhesive molecules provide a substrate on which the motile growth cone and neurite can respond to the chemical cues that determine the final synaptic target.

Diffusible cues appear to provide a trophic influence on developing axons through a chemoaffinity mechanism. One hypothesis is that gradients of chemotactic substances, emitted at the targets for synapse formation, interact with receptors on the growth cone that steer the growth cone toward the target.

Although it appears not to play a role in the early stages of synapse formation, synaptic activity is critical for subsequent remodeling. Pathways apparently are overrepresented often in early postnatal life, and "exuberant" projections of axons must be appropriately pruned. This occurs in a use-dependent fashion such that pathways used for neural activity are retained and those not used are eliminated. The classic studies of Hubel and Wiese have demonstrated that this process is critical in the formation of the proper synaptic connections of the visual cortex. In their studies, the eyelid of one kitten eye was closed temporarily, and the eye deprived of light was underrepresented, whereas the eye that remained open was overrepresented in the visual cortex. This phenomenon is noted in children who have significant amblyopia (so-called lazy eye). If this amblyopia is not recognized during a critical period of synapse remodeling, these children can be cortically blind in the affected eye.

Throughout life, significant synaptic plasticity persists. Memory is believed to result from a strengthening of heavily used synapses, a phenomenon known as *long-term potentiation*. Considering the lessons learned about the role neuronal activity plays in the remodeling of connectivity in sensory systems, one wonders whether early life experiences, such as seizures, could also alter local circuit remodeling for the recurrent axon collaterals of hippocampal pyramidal cells. Hence, during hippocampal development, if repeated seizures occurred, the synchronous discharging of pyramidal cells might prevent axonal remodeling that normally takes place, and so an excess in axonal branching present in early life could be maintained into adulthood. In turn, this consolidation could result in an imbalance between recurrent excitation and inhibition and lead to the production of a chronic epileptic focus in hippocampus.

DISORDERS OF PROCESS OUTGROWTH

The disorders of process outgrowth probably are poorly recognized, given the current limitations of neuroimaging. Many children with cerebral palsy and normal neuroimaging scans likely have disorders involving dendritic branching and axonal growth. Although there are likely many synapse disorders, a number have been well characterized.

Down syndrome (trisomy 21) includes a static encephalopathy characterized by mental retardation and hypotonia. The major neuropathologic changes in Down syndrome are a reduction in both the dendritic spines and the number of synapses.

Rett syndrome is a progressive disorder that affects girls and is due to a loss of function of MECP2. After a normal gestation, normal birth, and normal first 6 months of development, regression in intellect and motor function is seen. Girls affected with this disorder develop a gait and a truncal apraxia, loss of purposeful hand movements, stereotypic hand movements, progressive spasticity, autism-like social withdrawal, and intellectual disability. Accompanying this decline is a deceleration in head growth, which occurs during a time that brain development mainly involves glial proliferation and neuronal process outgrowth. Although patients typically have normal head sizes at birth, they become microcephalic during the time of their decline in function.

Pathologic examinations of the brains of patients with Rett syndrome support a disturbance in neuronal process outgrowth. The size of individual neurons is reduced, which is accompanied by an increase in packing density in the cerebral cortex, thalami, and basal ganglia. Abnormal dendritic branching has been noted in affected brain; this is especially prominent in layers III and V neurons of the frontal, motor, and temporal cortices. Because dendritic branching is believed to occur in response to axonal innervation, an examination of Rett syndrome brains for axonal aberrations was undertaken. This examination revealed significantly lower numbers of axons entering cortex as compared to normal.

Fragile X syndrome is the most common nonchromosomal, genetic form of mental retardation seen in boys and men. The disorder results from the disturbance of the FMR1 gene on the long arm of the X chromosome by a triplicate repeat. The brain in this disorder appears normal but, on microscopic examination, dendritic spine abnormalities are apparent.

Autistic spectrum disorders may turn out to be disorders of synapses. Male patients with autism may have an abnormal acceleration in head growth before age of 2 years. Neuroligins and other synapse-specific targeting proteins are on the X chromosome, perhaps explaining, in part, the increased incidence of autism in boys.

CONCLUSIONS

Exciting, new genetic and molecular insights regarding nervous system development and disturbances in that development have led to this attempt to give the clinician the framework to understand malformations of the human CNS and to evaluate patients afflicted by these disorders. Obtaining an etiology in such situations is of value to the patient, the family, and potentially to society. With new technologies such as exome sequencing, the potential for obtaining an etiology is vastly enhanced.

SUGGESTED READINGS

Ackroyd MR, Whitmore C, Prior S, et al. Fukutin-related protein alters the deposition of laminin in the eye and brain. *J Neurosci.* 2011;31:12927.

Adzick NS, Thom EA, Spong C, et al. A randomized trial of prenatal versus postnatal repair of myelomeningocele. *N Engl J Med.* 2011;364:993.

Aicardi J. Aicardi syndrome. *Brain Dev.* 2005;27:164.

Aldinger KA, Lehmann OJ, Hudgins L, et al. FOXC1 is required for normal cerebellar development and is a major contributor to chromosome 6p25.3 Dandy-Walker malformation. *Nat Genet.* 2009;41:1037.

Allendoerfer K, Shatz CJ. The subplate, a transient neocortical structure: its role in the development of connections between thalamus and cortex. *Ann Rev Neurosci.* 1994;17:185.

American Academy of Pediatrics, Committee on Genetics. Folic acid for the prevention of neural tube defects. *Pediatrics.* 1999;104:325.

Amir RE, Van den Veyver IB, Wan M, et al. Rett syndrome is caused by mutations in X-linked MECP2, encoding methyl-CpG-binding protein. *Nat Genet.* 1999;23:185.

Angevine JBJ, Sidman RL. Autoradiographic study of cell migration during histogenesis of cerebral cortex in the mouse. *Nature.* 1961;192:766.

Aravind L, Koonin EV. The fukutin protein family—predicted enzymes modifying cell-surface molecules. *Curr Biol.* 1999;9:R836.

Arimura T, Hayashi YK, Murakami T, et al. Mutational analysis of fukutin gene in dilated cardiomyopathy and hypertrophic cardiomyopathy. *Circ J.* 2009;73:158.

Armstrong DD. Review of Rett syndrome. *J Neuropathol Exp Neurol.* 1997;56:843.

Armstrong DD. The neuropathology of temporal lobe epilepsy. *J Neuropathol Exp Neurol.* 1993;52:433.

Armstrong DD, Antalffy B, Dunn JK. Quantitative golgi studies of dendrites in Rett syndrome and trisomy 21. *J Neuropathol Exp Neurol.* 1996;55:630.

Armstrong D, Dunn JK, Antalffy B, et al. Selective dendritic alterations in the cortex of Rett syndrome. *J Neuropathol Exp Neurol.* 1995;54:195.

Baes M, Gressens P, Baumgart E, et al. A mouse model for Zellweger syndrome. *Nat Gen.* 1997;17:49.

Bahi-Buisson N, Poirier K, Boddaert N, et al. GPR56-related bilateral frontoparietal polymicrogyria: further evidence for an overlap with the cobblestone complex. *Brain.* 2010;133:3194.

Baker EM, Khorasgani MG, Gardner-Medwin D, et al. Arthrogryposis multiplex congenita and bilateral parietal polymicrogyria in association with the intrauterine death of a twin. *Neuropediatrics.* 1996;27:54.

Balci B, Uyanik G, Dincer P, et al. An autosomal recessive limb girdle muscular dystrophy (LGMD) with mild mental retardation is allelic to Walker-Warburg syndrome (WWS) caused by a mutation in POMT1 gene. *Neuromuscul Disord.* 2005;15:271.

Barkovich AJ, Chuang SH. Unilateral megalencephaly: correlation of MR imaging and pathologic characteristics. *Am J Neuroradiol.* 1990;11:523.

Barkovich AJ, Gressens P, Evrard P. Formation, maturation, and disorders of brain neocortex. *Am J Neuroradiol.* 1992;13:423.

Barkovich AJ, Kjos BO. Gray matter heterotopias: MR characteristics and correlation with developmental and neurologic manifestations. *Radiology.* 1992;182:493.

Barkovich AJ, Kjos BO. Nonlissencephalic cortical dysplasias: correlation of imaging findings with clinical deficits. *AJNR Am J Neuroradiol.* 1992;13:95.

Beedle AM, Nienaber PM, Campbell KP. Fukutin-related protein associates with the sarcolemmal dystrophin-glycoprotein complex. *J Biol Chem.* 2007;282:16713.

Belichenko PV, Hagberg B, Dahlström A. Morphological study of neocortical areas in Rett syndrome. *Acta Neuropathol.* 1997;93:50.

Belichenko PV, Oldfors A, Hagberg B, et al. Rett syndrome: 3-D confocal microscopy of cortical pyramidal dendrites and afferents. *Neuroreport.* 1994;5:1509.

Beltran-Valero de Bernabé D, Voit T, Longman C, et al. Mutations in the FKRP gene can cause muscle-eye-brain disease and Walker-Warburg syndrome. *J Med Genet.* 2004;41:e61.

Blank MC, Grinberg I, Aryee E, et al. Multiple developmental programs are altered by loss of Zic1 and Zic4 to cause Dandy-Walker malformation cerebellar pathogenesis. *Development.* 2011;138:1207.

Brickman JM, Clements M, Tyrell R, et al. Molecular effects of novel mutations in Hesx1/HESX1 associated with human pituitary disorders. *Development.* 2001;128:5189.

Brockington M, Blake DJ, Prandini P, et al. Mutations in the fukutin-related protein gene (FKRP) cause a form of congenital muscular dystrophy with secondary laminin alpha2 deficiency and abnormal glycosylation of alpha-dystroglycan. *Am J Hum Genet.* 2001;69:1198.

Brockington M, Yuva Y, Prandini P, et al. Mutations in the fukutin-related protein gene (FKRP) identify limb girdle muscular dystrophy 2I as a milder allelic variant of congenital muscular dystrophy MDC1C. *Hum Mol Genet.* 2001;10:2851.

Brown SA, Warburton D, Brown LY, et al. Holoprosencephaly due to mutations in ZIC2, a homologue of Drosophila odd-paired. *Nat Genet.* 1998;20:180.

Brunelli S, Faiella A, Capra V, et al. Germline mutations in the homeobox gene EMX2 in patients with severe schizencephaly. *Nat Gen.* 1996;12:94.

Caviness VS, Takahashi T. Proliferative events in the cerebral ventricular zone. *Brain Dev.* 1995;17:159.

Chang W, Winder TL, LeDuc CA, et al. Founder Fukutin mutation causes Walker-Warburg syndrome in four Ashkenazi Jewish families. *Prenat Diagn.* 2009;29:560.

Chen J, Tsai V, Parker WE, et al. Detection of human papillomavirus in focal cortical dysplasia type IIB. *Ann Neurol.* 2012;72:881.

Chong SS, Pack SD, Roschke AV, et al. A revision of the lissencephaly and Miller-Dieker syndrome critical chromosome 17p13.3. *Hum Mol Genet.* 1997;6:147–155.

Cirak S, Foley AR, Herrmann R, et al. ISPD gene mutations are a common cause of congenital and limb-girdle muscular dystrophies. *Brain.* 2013;136:269.

Clark GD. Brain development and the genetics of brain development. *Neurol Clin.* 2002;20:917.

Clark GD, Mizuguchi M, Antalffy B, et al. Predominant localization of the LIS family of gene products to Cajal-Retzius cells and ventricular neuroepithelium in the developing human cortex. *J Neuropathol Exp Neurol.* 1997;56:1044.

Clarke NF, Maugenre S, Vandebrouck A, et al. Congenital muscular dystrophy type 1D (MDC1D) due to a large intragenic insertion/deletion, involving intron 10 of the LARGE gene. *Eur J Hum Genet.* 2011;19:452.

Cotarelo RP, Valero MC, Prados B, et al. Two new patients bearing mutations in the fukutin gene confirm the relevance of this gene in Walker-Warburg syndrome. *Clin Genet.* 2008;73:139.

Courchesne E, Karns CM, Davis HR, et al. Unusual brain growth patterns in early life in patients with autistic disorder: an MRI study. *Neurology.* 2001;57:245.

Dalton D, Chadwick R, McGinnis W. Expression and embryonic function of empty spiracles: a Drosophila homeo box gene with two patterning functions on the anterior-posterior axis of the embryo. *Genes Dev.* 1989;3:1940.

Darling DL, Yingling J, Wynshaw-Boris A. Role of 14-3-3 proteins in eukaryote signaling and development. *Curr Top Dev Biol.* 2005;68:281.

Dattani MT, Martinez-Barbera JP, Thomas PQ, et al. Mutations in the homeobox gene HESX1/Hesx1 associated with septo-optic dysplasia in human and mouse. *Nat Genet.* 1998;19:125.

Daube JR, Chou SM. Lissencephaly: two cases. *Neurology.* 1966;16:179.

Davis EE, Zhang Q, Liu Q, et al. TTC21B contributes both causal and modifying alleles across. *Nat Genet.* 2011;43:189.

de Bernabé DB, van Bokhoven H, van Beusekom E, et al. A homozygous nonsense mutation in the fukutin gene causes a Walker-Warburg syndrome phenotype. *J Med Genet.* 2003;40:845.

De Ciantis A, Barkovich AJ, Cosottini M, et al. Ultra-High-Field MR imaging in polymicrogyria and epilepsy. *AJNR Am J Neuroradiol.* 2015;36:309–316.

de Paula F, Vieira N, Starling A, et al. Asymptomatic carriers for homozygous novel mutations in the PKRP gene: the other end of the spectrum. *Eur J Hum Genet.* 2003;11:923.

De Rosa MJ, Secor DL, Barsom M, et al. Neuropathologic findings in surgically treated hemimegalencephaly: immunohistochemical, morphometric, and ultrastructural study. *Acta Neuropathol.* 1992;84:250.

Dieker H, Edwards RH, Zu Rhein G. The lissencephaly syndrome. *Birth Defects.* 1969;5:53.

Dobyns WB. Absence makes the search grow longer. *Am J Hum Genet.* 1996;58:7.

Dobyns WB. Agenesis of the corpus callosum and gyral malformations are frequent manifestations of nonketotic hyperglycinemia. *Neurology.* 1989;39:817.

Dobyns WB. Cerebral dysgenesis: causes and consequences. In Miller G, Ramer JC, eds. *Static Encephalopathies of Infancies and Childhood.* New York: Raven Press; 1992:235.

Dobyns WB, Andermann E, Andermann F, et al. X-linked malformations of neuronal migration. *Neurology.* 1996;47:331.

Dobyns WB, Guerrini R, Czapansky-Beilman DK, et al. Bilateral periventricular nodular heterotopia with mental retardation and syndactyly in boys: a new X-linked mental retardation syndrome. *Neurology.* 1997;49:1042.

Dobyns WB, Mirzaa G, Christian SL, et al. Consistent chromosome abnormalities identify novel polymicrogyria loci in 1p36.3, 2p16.1-p23.1, 4q21.21-q22.1, 6q26-q27, and 21q2. *Am J Med Genet A.* 2008;146A:1637.

Dobyns WB, Patton MA, Stratton RF, et al. Cobblestone lissencephaly with normal eyes and muscle. *Neuropediatrics.* 1996;27:70.

Dobyns WB, Truwit CL. Lissencephaly and other malformations of cortical development: 1995 update. *Neuropediatrics.* 1995;26:132.

Faust PL, Hatten ME. Targeted deletion of the PEX2 peroxisome assembly gene in mice provides a model for Zellweger syndrome, a human neuronal migration disorder. *J Cell Biol.* 1997;139:1293.

Fox JW, Lamperti ED, Eksioglu YZ, et al. Mutations in filamin 1 prevent migration of cerebral cortical neurons in human periventricular heterotopia. *Neuron.* 1998;21:1315.

Frosk P, Greenberg CR, Tennese AA, et. The most common mutation in FKRP causing limb girdle muscular dystrophy type 2I may have occurred only once and is present in Hutterites and other populations. *Hum Mutat.* 2005;25:38.

Geranmayeh F, Clement E, Feng LH, et al. Genotype-phenotype correlation in a large population of muscular dystrophy patients with LAMA2 mutations. *Neuromuscul Disord.* 2010;20:241.

Gleeson JG, Allen KM, Fox JW, et al. Doublecortin, a brain-specific gene mutated in human X-linked lissencephaly and double cortex syndrome, encodes a putative signaling protein. *Cell.* 1998;92:63.

Gleeson JG, Lin PT, Flanagan LA, et al. Doublecortin is a microtubule-associated protein and is expressed widely by migrating neurons. *Neuron.* 1999;23:257.

Gleeson JG, Luo RF, Grant PE, et al. Genetic and neuroradiological heterogeneity of double cortex syndrome. *Ann Neurol.* 2000;47:265.

Godfrey C, Clement E, Mein R. Refining genotype phenotype correlations in muscular dystrophies with defective glycosylation of dystroglycan. *Brain.* 2007;130:2725.

Goodman CS, Shatz CJ. Developmental mechanisms that generate precise patterns of neuronal connectivity. *Cell.* 1993;72:77.

Greenberg F, Stratton R, Lockhart L, et al. Familial Miller-Dieker syndrome associated with pericentric inversion of chromosome 17. *Am J Med Genet.* 1986;23:853.

Grinberg I, Northrup H, Ardinger H, et al. Heterozygous deletion of the linked genes ZIC1 and ZIC4 is involved in Dandy-Walker malformation. *Nat Genet.* 2004;36:1053.

Guerrini R, Dubeau F, Dulac O, et al. Bilateral parasagittal parietooccipital polymicrogyria and epilepsy. *Ann Neurol.* 1997;41:65.

Harel T, Goldberg Y, Shalev SA, et al. Limb-girdle muscular dystrophy 2I: phenotypic variability within a large consanguineous Bedouin family associated with a novel FKRP mutation. *Eur J Hum Genet.* 2004;12:38.

Haslam R, Smith DW. Autosomal dominant microcephaly. *J Pediatr.* 1979;95:701.

Hattori M, Adachi H, Tsujimoto M, et al. Miller-Dieker lissencephaly gene encodes a subunit of brain platelet-activating factor acetylhydrolase [corrected]. *Nature.* 1994;370:216.

Hehr U, Gross C, Diebold U, et al. Wide phenotypic variability in families with holoprosencephaly and a sonic hedgehog mutation. *Eur J Pediatr.* 2004;163:347.

Helms JA, Kim CH, Hu D, et al. Sonic hedgehog participates in craniofacial morphogenesis and is down-regulated by teratogenic doses of retinoic acid. *Dev Biol.* 1997;187:25.

Helwig U, Imai K, Schmahl W, et al. Interaction between undulated and Patch leads to an extreme form of spina bifida in double-mutant mice. *Nat Genet.* 1995;11:60.

Hinton VJ, Brown WT, Wisniewski K, et al. Analysis of neocortex in three males with the fragile X syndrome. *Am J Med Genet.* 1991;41:289.

Hopkins B, Sutton VR, Lewis RA, et al. Neuroimaging aspects of Aicardi syndrome. *Am J Med Genet.* 2008;146A:2871.

Hopkins IJ, Humphrey I, Keith CG, et al. The Aicardi syndrome in a 47, XXY male. *Austr Paedtr J.* 1979;15:278.

Horesh D, Sapir T, Francis F, et al. Doublecortin, a stabilizer of microtubules. *Hum Mol Genet.* 1999;8:1599.

Hubel DH, Wiesel TN. The period of susceptibility to the physiological effects of unilateral eye closure in kittens. *J Physiol.* 1970;206:419.

Ismail S, Schaffer AE, Rosti RO, et al. Novel mutation in the fukutin gene in an Egyptian family with Fukuyama congenital muscular dystrophy and microcephaly. *Gene.* 2014;539:279.

Jamain S, Quach H, Betancur C, et al; Paris Autism Research International Sibpair Study. Mutations of the X-linked genes encoding neuroligins NLGN3 and NLGN4 are associated with autism. *Nat Genet.* 2003;34:27.

Jansen AC, Oostra A, Desprechins B, et al. TUBA1A mutations: from isolated lissencephaly to familial polymicrogyria. *Neurology.* 2011;76:988.

Jones KL, Gilbert EF, Kaveggia EG. The MIller-Dieker syndrome. *Pediatrics*. 1980;66:277.

Kallmann FJ, Schoenfeld WA, Barrera SE. The genetic aspects of primary eunuchoidism. *Am J Ment Defic*. 1944;48:203.

Kava M, Chitayat D, Blaser S, et al. Eye and brain abnormalities in congenital muscular dystrophies caused by fukutin-related protein gene (FKRP) mutations. *Pediatr Neurol*. 2013;49:374.

Ke N, Ma H, Diedrich G, et al. Biochemical characterization of genetic mutations of GPR56 in patients with bilateral frontoparietal polymicrogyria (BFPP). *Biochem Biophys Res Commun*. 2008;366:314.

Keynes R, Krumlauf R. Hox genes and regionalization of the nervous system. *Ann Rev Neurosci*. 1994;17:109.

Kim MH, Cierpicki T, Derewenda U, et al. The DCX-domain tandems of doublecortin and doublecortin-like kinase. *Nat Struct Biol*. 2003;10:324.

Kitamura K, Yanazawa M, Sugiyama N, et al. Mutation of ARX causes abnormal development of forebrain and testes in mice and X-linked lissencephaly with abnormal genitalia in humans. *Nat Genet*. 2002;32:359.

Kobayashi K, Nakahori Y, Miyake M, et al. An ancient retrotransposal insertion causes Fukuyama-type congenital muscular dystrophy. *Nature*. 1998;394:388.

Kumar RA, Pilz DT, Babatz TD, et al. TUBA1A mutations cause wide spectrum lissencephaly (smooth brain) and suggest that multiple neuronal migration pathways converge on alpha tubulins. *Hum Mol Genet*. 2010;19:2817.

Kuzniecky R. Magnetic resonance imaging in developmental disorders of the cerebral cortex. *Epilepsia*. 1994;35(suppl 6):S44.

Kuzniecky R, Andermann F. The congenital bilateral perisylvian syndrome: imaging findings in a multicenter study. CBPS Study Group. *AJNR Am J Neuroradiol*. 1994;15:139.

Kuzniecky R, Andermann F, Guerrini R. Congenital bilateral perisylvian syndrome: study of 31 patients. The CBPS Multicenter Collaborative Study. *Lancet*. 1993;341:608.

Kuzniecky R, Garcia JH, Faught E, et al. Cortical dysplasia in temporal lobe epilepsy: magnetic resonance imaging correlations. *Ann Neurol*. 1991;29:293.

Ledbetter SA, Kuwano A, Dobyns WB, et al. Microdeletions of chromosome 17p13 as a cause of isolated lissencephaly. *Am J Hum Genet*. 1992;50:182.

Lee JE, Gleeson JG. A systems-biology approach to understanding the ciliopathy disorders. *Genome Med*. 2011;3:59.

Lee JH, Silhavy JL, Lee JE, et al. Evolutionarily assembled cis-regulatory module at a human ciliopathy locus. *Science*. 2012;335:966.

Lehéricy S, Dormont D, Semah F, et al. Developmental abnormalities of the medial temporal lobe in patients with temporal lobe epilepsy. *AJNR Am J Neuroradiol*. 1995;16:617.

Liesi P, Seppälä I, Trenkner E. Neuronal migration in cerebellar microcultures is inhibited by antibodies against a neurite outgrowth domain of laminin. *J Neurosci Res*. 1992;33(1):170.

Lin YC, Murakami T, Hayashi YK, et al. A novel FKRP gene mutation in a Taiwanese patient with limb-girdle muscular dystrophy 2I. *Brain Dev*. 2007;29:234.

Lindhout D, Omtzigt JG, Cornel MC. Spectrum of neural-tube defects in 34 infants prenatally exposed to antiepileptic drugs. *Neurology*. 1992;42:111.

Longman C, Brockington M, Torelli S, et al. Mutations in the human LARGE gene cause MDC1D, a novel form of congenital muscular dystrophy with severe mental retardation and abnormal glycosylation of alpha-dystroglycan. *Hum Mol Genet*. 2003;12:2853.

Louhichi N, Triki C, Quijano-Roy S, et al. New FKRP mutations causing congenital muscular dystrophy associated with mental retardation and central nervous system abnormalities. Identification of a founder mutation in Tunisian families. *Neurogenetics*. 2004;5:27.

MacLeod H, Pytel P, Wollmann R, et al. A novel FKRP mutation in congenital muscular dystrophy disrupts the dystrophin glycoprotein complex. *Neuromusc Disord*. 2007;17:285.

Matsuo N, Kawamoto S, Matsubara K, et al. Cloning and developmental expression of the murine homolog of doublecortin. *Biochem Biophys Res Commun*. 1998;252:571.

McConnell S. The control of neuronal identity in the developing cerebral cortex. *Curr Opin Neurobiol*. 1992;2(1):23.

Meencke HJ, Veith G. Migration disturbances in epilepsy. In: Angel J, Wasterlain C, Cavalhiero EA, et al, eds. *Molecular Neurobiology of Epilepsy*. Amsterdam, The Netherlands: Elsevier; 1992:31.

Mercuri E, Topaloglu H, Brockington M, et al. Spectrum of brain changes in patients with congenital muscular dystrophy and FKRP gene mutations. *Arch Neurol*. 2006;63:251.

Mizuguchi M, Takashima S, Kakita A, et al. Lissencephaly gene product. Localization in the central nervous system and loss of immunoreactivity in Miller-Dieker syndrome. *Am J Pathol*. 1995;147:1142.

Morris-Rosendahl DJ, Najm J, Lachmeijer AM, et al. Refining the phenotype of alpha-1a tubulin (TUBA1A) mutation in patients with classical lissencephaly. *Clin Genet*. 2008;74:425.

Moutard ML, Kieffer V, Feingold J, et al. Agenesis of corpus callosum: prenatal diagnosis and prognosis. *Childs Nerv Syst*. 2003;19:471.

Moutard ML, Kieffer V, Feingold J, et al. Isolated corpus callosum agenesis: a ten-year follow-up after prenatal diagnosis (how are the children without corpus callosum at 10 years of age?). *Prenat Diagn*. 2012;32:277.

Muntoni F, Brockington M, Godfrey C, et al. Muscular dystrophies due to defective glycosylation of dystroglycan. *Acta Myol*. 2007;26:129.

Murdock DR, Clark GD, Bainbridge MN, et al. Whole-exome sequencing identifies compound heterozygous mutations in WDR62 in siblings with recurrent polymicrogyria. *Am J Med Genet A*. 2011;155A:2071.

Nakagawa Y, Kaneko T, Ogura T, et al. Roles of cell-autonomous mechanisms for differential expression of region-specific transcription factors in neuroepithelial cells. *Development*. 1996;122:2449.

Nakano KK. Anencephaly: a review. *Dev Med Child Neurol*. 1973;15:383.

Novarino G, Akizu N, Gleeson JG. Modeling human disease in humans: the ciliopathies. *Cell*. 2011;147:70.

Nyberg DA, Mack LA, Bronstein A, et al. Holoprosencephaly: prenatal sonographic diagnosis. *AJR Am J Radiol*. 1987;149:1051.

Ogawa M, Miyata T, Nakajima K, et al. The reeler gene-associated antigen on Cajal-Retzius neurons is a crucial molecule for laminar organization of cortical neurons. *Neuron*. 1995;14:899.

Optiz JM, Holt MC. Microcephaly: general considerations and aids to nosology. *J Craniofac Genet Dev Biol*. 1990;10:175.

Pinard JM, Motte J, Chiron C, et al. Subcortical laminar heterotopia and lissencephaly in two families: a single X linked dominant gene. *J Neurol Neurosurg Psychiatry*. 1994;57:914.

Poirier K, Keays DA, Francis F, et al. Large spectrum of lissencephaly and pachygyria phenotypes resulting from de novo missense mutations in tubulin alpha 1A (TUBA1A). *Hum Mutat*. 2007;28:1055.

Poussaint TY, Fox JW, Dobyns WB, et al. Periventricular nodular heterotopia in patients with filamin-1 gene mutations: neuroimaging findings. *Pediatr Radiol*. 2000;30:748.

Powers JM. The pathology of peroxisomal disorders with pathogenetic considerations. *J Neuropathol Exp Neurol*. 1995;54:710.

Puckett RL, Moore SA, Winder TL, et al. Further evidence of Fukutin mutations as a cause of childhood onset limb-girdle muscular dystrophy without mental retardation. *Neuromusc Disord*. 2009;19:352.

Ramocki MB, Scaglia F, Stankiewicz P, et al. Recurrent partial rhombencephalosynapsis and holoprosencephaly in siblings with a mutation of ZIC2. *Am J Med Genet A*. 2011;155A:1574.

Raymond AA, Fish D, Sisodiya S, et al. Abnormalities of gyration, heterotopias, tuberous sclerosis, focal cortical dysplasia, microdysgenesis, dysembryoplastic neuroepithelial tumour and dysgenesis of the archicortex in epilepsy. Clinical, EEG and neuroimaging features in 100 adult patients. *Brain*. 1995;118:629.

Raymond AA, Fish DR, Stevens JM, et al. Association of hippocampal sclerosis with cortical dysgenesis in patients with epilepsy. *Neurology*. 1994;44:1841.

Reiner O, Carrozzo R, Shen Y, et al. Isolation of a Miller-Dieker lissencephaly gene containing G protein beta-subunit-like repeats. *Nature*. 1993;364:717.

Renier WO, Gabreëls FJM, Jasper TWJ, et al. An X-linked syndrome with microcephaly, severe mental retardation, spasticity, epilepsy and deafness. *J Ment Defic Res*. 1982;26:27.

Renowden S, Squier M. Unusual magnetic resonance and neuropathological findings in hemimegalencephaly: report of a case following hemispherectomy. *Dev Med Child Neurol*. 1994;36:357.

Rett A. On a unusual brain atrophy syndrome in hyperammonemia in childhood [in German]. *Wien Med Wochenschr*. 1966;116:723.

Rijntjes-Jacobs EG, Lopriore E, Steggerda SJ, et al. Discordance for Schimmelpenning-Feuerstein-Mims syndrome in monochorionic twins supports the concept of a postzygotic mutation. *Am J Med Genet A*. 2010;152A:2816.

Roessler E, Belloni E, Gaudenz K, et al. Mutations in the human Sonic Hedgehog gene cause holoprosencephaly. *Nat Genet.* 1996;14:357.

Rugarli EI, Ballabio A. Kallmann syndrome. From genetics to neurobiology. *JAMA.* 1993;270:2713.

Rugarli EI, Lutz B, Kuratani SC, et al. Expression pattern of the Kallmann syndrome gene in the olfactory system suggests a role in neuronal targeting. *Nat Genet.* 1993;4:19.

Saredi S, Ruggieri A, Mottarelli E, et al. Fukutin gene mutations in an Italian patient with early onset muscular dystrophy but no central nervous system involvement. *Muscle Nerve.* 2009;39:845.

Sattar S, Gleeson JG. The ciliopathies in neuronal development: a clinical approach to investigation of Joubert syndrome and Joubert syndrome-related disorders. *Dev Med Child Neurol.* 2011;53:793.

Sharief N, Craze J, Summers D, et al. Miller-Dieker syndrome with ring chromosome 17. *Arch Dis Child.* 1991;66:710.

Sheen VL, Dixon PH, Fox JW, et al. Mutations in the X-linked filamin 1 gene cause periventricular nodular heterotopia in males as well as in females. *Hum Mol Genet.* 2001;10:1775.

Shevell MI, Matthews PM, Scriver CR, et al. Cerebral dysgenesis and lactic acidemia: an MRI/MRS phenotype associated with pyruvate dehydrogenase deficiency. *Pediatr Neurol.* 1994;11:224.

Sidman R, Rakic P. Neuronal migration, with special reference to developing human brain: a review. *Brain Res.* 1973;62:1.

Stone DM, Hynes M, Armanini M, et al. Lissencephaly and pachygyria: an architectonic and topographical analysis. *Nature.* 1996;384:129.

Sugama S, Kusano K. Monozygous twin with polymicrogyria and normal co-twin. *Pediatr Neurol.* 1994;11:62.

Sunohara N, Sakuragawa N, Satoyoshi E, et al. A new syndrome of anosmia, ichthyosis, hypogonadism, and various neurological manifestations with deficiency of steroid sulfatase and arylsulfatase C. *Ann Neurol.* 1986;19:174.

Swann JW, Hablitz JJ. Cellular abnormalities and synaptic plasticity in seizure disorders of the immature nervous system. *Ment Retard Dev Disabil Res Rev.* 2000;6:258.

Takada K, Becker LE, Chan F. Aberrant dendritic development in the human agyric cortex: a quantitative and qualitative Golgi study of two cases. *Clin Neuropathol.* 1988;7:111.

Toda T, Chiyonobu T, Xiong H, et al. Fukutin and alpha-dystroglycanopathies. *Acta Myol.* 2005;24:60.

Tohyama J, Kato M, Kawasaki S, et al. Dandy-Walker malformation associated with heterozygous ZIC1 and ZIC4 deletion: Report of a new patient. *Am J Med Genet.* 2011;155A:130.

Topaloglu H, Brockington M, Yuva Y, et al. FKRP gene mutations cause congenital muscular dystrophy, mental retardation, and cerebellar cysts. *Neurology.* 2003;60:988.

Trovato R, Astrea G, Bartalena L, et al. Elevated serum creatine kinase and small cerebellum prompt diagnosis of congenital muscular dystrophy due to FKRP mutations. *J Child Neurol.* 2014;29:394.

Turner D, Cepko C. A common progenitor for neurons and glia persists in rat retina late in development. *Nature.* 1987;328:131.

van den Bosch H, Schrakamp G, Hardeman D, et al. Ether lipid synthesis and its deficiency in peroxisomal disorders. *Biochimie.* 1993;75:183.

Volpe J, Adams R. *Acta Neuropathol.* 1972;20:175.

Walter MC, Petersen JA, Stucka R, et al. FKRP (826C>A) frequently causes limb-girdle muscular dystrophy in German patients. *J Med Genet.* 2004;41:e50.

Wan M, Lee SS, Zhang X, Houwink-Manville I, et al. Rett syndrome and beyond: recurrent spontaneous and familial MECP2 mutations at CpG hotspots. *Am J Hum Genet.* 1999;65:1520.

Willer T, Lee H, Lommel M, et al. ISPD loss-of-function mutations disrupt dystroglycan O-mannosylation and cause Walker-Warburg syndrome. *Nat Genet.* 2012;44:575.

Yamamoto LU, Velloso FJ, Lima BL, et al. Muscle protein alterations in LGMD2I patients with different mutations in the Fukutin-related protein gene. *J Histochem Cytochem.* 2008;56:995.

Yamamoto T, Kato Y, Karita M, et al. Fukutin expression in glial cells and neurons: implication in the brain lesions of Fukuyama congenital muscular dystrophy. *Acta Neuropathol.* 2002;104:217.

Yan W, Assadi AH, Wynshaw-Boris A, et al. Previously uncharacterized roles of platelet-activating factor acetylhydrolase 1b complex in mouse spermatogenesis. *Proc Natl Acad Sci U S A.* 2003;100:7189.

Zutt M, Strutz F, Happle R, et al. Schimmelpenning-Feuerstein-Mims syndrome with hypophosphatemic rickets. *Dermatology.* 2003;207:72.

Inborn Errors of Metabolism 134

Marc C. Patterson

INTRODUCTION

There are hundreds of inborn errors of metabolism, each individually rare, but collectively sufficiently common to constitute a significant public health burden. Most severe inborn errors of metabolism involve the nervous system, either directly, or by producing neurologic dysfunction through intoxication with toxic substrates, energy deficiency (to which the brain is especially prone), deficiency of essential substrates or neurotransmitters, or combinations thereof. Although the complexity of these disorders defies easy classification, they may be conveniently divided into small and large molecule disorders for clinical purposes. The former group includes amino and organic acidopathies and urea cycle disorders, among others. Most result from enzyme deficiencies that impair the body's ability to cope with substrate loads. In severe forms, they present in neonates exposed to normal substrates for the first time without their mother's metabolic machinery to compensate. Lesser degrees of impairment may present later and intermittently under conditions of unusual stress.

In contrast, large molecule disorders, which include the lysosomal, peroxisomal, and glycogen storage diseases, have a slowly but inexorably progressive course, paralleling the accumulation of macromolecules within cells. The most severe phenotypes exhibit specific patterns of neurodegeneration, reflecting the loci of storage in the nervous system. Thus, predominantly neuronal storage, as seen in the neuronal ceroid lipofuscinoses and neuroaxonal dystrophies, presents as poliodystrophies. Disorders in which white matter bears the major burden of disease are designated as leukodystrophies.

This chapter surveys some of the more prominent of these disorders but cannot be comprehensive. Indeed, the major text of inherited metabolic disease (*Metabolic and Molecular Bases of Inherited Disease* [*MMBID*]) was last published in print form in 2001 when it was felt that its 4,600 pages spread over four volumes had reached the limits of print publishing. The *MMBID* is now only available as an electronic text (*Online Metabolic and Molecular Bases of Inherited Disease* [*OMMBID*]), and the interested reader is referred to it and the recommended reading lists in each of the following sections for more comprehensive data on disorders of interest.

SMALL MOLECULE DISORDERS

GLUCOSE TRANSPORTER TYPE 1 DEFICIENCY SYNDROME

Clinical Syndrome

In 1991, De Vivo et al. described two children with infantile seizures, delayed motor and behavioral development, acquired microcephaly, and ataxia. Lumbar puncture revealed low cerebrospinal fluid (CSF) glucose concentrations (hypoglycorrhachia) and low-normal to low CSF lactate concentrations.

Seizures begin in early infancy, and the seizure types vary with the age of the patient. In infancy, the dominant seizure types include behavioral arrest, pallor and cyanosis, eye deviation

simulating opsoclonus, and apnea. The electroencephalogram (EEG) at this stage may be normal or show focal spikes and evolves to a generalized spike-wave pattern in childhood. In childhood, the seizures typically include astatic seizures, atypical absence seizures, and generalized tonic–clonic seizures. The seizures are refractory to antiepileptic drugs but respond to a ketogenic diet. Other paroxysmal events, including abnormal eye movements, ataxia, paralysis (with or without migraine), and dyskinesias are frequent. Many patients exhibit static defects, of which intellectual disability, ataxia, dystonia, and spasticity are prominent.

Laboratory Data

Diagnosis requires awareness of the clinical manifestations and documentation of hypoglycorrhachia. A low or low-normal CSF lactate concentration strengthens the presumptive diagnosis.

Molecular Genetics and Pathogenesis

D-Glucose is the obligate fuel for brain metabolism under virtually all circumstances. With fasting, the brain adapts to use ketone bodies (β-hydroxybutyrate and acetoacetate) in partial lieu of glucose. The transport of D-glucose across the blood–brain barrier and into brain cells is selectively mediated by glucose transporter 1 (GLUT1), a member of a multigene family of protein transporters that facilitate the diffusion of sugar molecules across tissue barriers. GLUT1 is encoded by SLC2A1 on chromosome 1p34.1 and is present in high abundance in brain capillaries, astroglial cells, and erythrocyte membranes.

The molecular basis of the syndrome is GLUT1 haploinsufficiency; a few patients are hemizygous, but most are heterozygous with a variety of mutations. This syndrome is the first genetically determined abnormality of the blood–brain barrier; it may be familial and transmitted as an autosomal dominant trait.

Diagnosis

Lumbar puncture for measurement of glucose and lactate (with simultaneous serum assays of both) is critical in establishing the diagnosis. Confirmatory evidence is provided by sequencing of the SLC2A1 gene; mutations are found in more than 90% of cases; severe phenotypes have been associated with microdeletions in the SLC2A1 region.

Treatment

Standard treatment is the ketogenic diet, which controls the seizures, at least early in the course, but is less effective in improving cognition and behavior. More recently, anaplerotic therapy with triheptanoin has been studied, with evidence of benefit. Antiepileptic drugs have been uniformly ineffective.

HYPERAMMONEMIA

Introduction

Hyperammonemia has many genetic and acquired causes. The hepatic urea cycle is the major mammalian system for the detoxification of ammonia and defects have been described in all six urea cycle enzymes. The prevalence of these disorders is 1:35,000; two-thirds present after the newborn period. The mortality is 24% in neonates and 11% in older individuals. An additional pathway from arginine to citrulline generates the putative second messenger and neurotransmitter, nitric oxide, catalyzed by nitric oxide synthetase. The enzyme is found in many tissues, including brain. Animal studies suggest that derangement of this pathway, cerebral energy metabolism, amino acid and neurotransmitter pathways, mitochondrial permeability, signal transduction, and oxidative stress all contribute to the brain injury associated with exposure to high levels of ammonia.

Neonatal Hyperammonemia

Transient hyperammonemia is occasionally seen in otherwise well premature infants and rarely requires treatment. Hyperammonemia may reflect liver damage associated with birth asphyxia or congenital hepatic disease; the birth history usually establishes the diagnosis.

The ill neonate with hyperammonemia without other explanation often has an inborn error of metabolism that, directly or indirectly, affects the urea cycle. Marked hyperammonemia causes progressive lethargy, vomiting, poor feeding, apneic episodes, and seizures. These nonspecific symptoms occur in many disorders, such as sepsis, that can also precipitate hyperammonemia. The age at onset of these symptoms is a useful differential diagnostic point. Infants with hyperammonemia owing to urea cycle enzymopathies or organic acidurias typically are well until they have received 1 to 3 days of protein feeding. In contrast, infants with hyperammonemia secondary to impaired pyruvate metabolism are symptomatic within the first 24 hours. Pyruvate dehydrogenase and (type B) pyruvate carboxylase deficiencies feature lactic acidosis, and these diagnoses can be confirmed by an assay of enzyme activities in fibroblasts.

Organic acidurias lead to ketoacidosis (but maple syrup urine disease does not), which distinguishes them from urea cycle enzymopathies. Severe deficiency of urea cycle enzymes, other than arginase, causes similar clinical syndromes. The affected child is well for the first 24 hours but signs of hyperammonemia appear as protein feedings continue. Respiratory alkalosis with hyperventilation is classic but not always present, and infants with sepsis or vomiting may have metabolic acidosis or alkalosis. Plasma amino acid and orotic acid assays help to distinguish different urea cycle defects (Table 134.1). Direct sequencing of urea cycle genes will make the diagnosis in more than 80% of cases; tissue enzyme analysis is required in the remainder. All of the urea cycle genes are autosomal recessive, except for ornithine carbamyl transferase deficiency, which is X-linked. Prenatal screening is available.

Long exposure to high levels of ammonia damages the brain. Thus, acute hyperammonemic coma in the newborn is a medical emergency, and rapid reduction in ammonia levels is necessary. Peritoneal dialysis is more effective than exchange transfusion; hemodialysis may also be effective. Useful adjuncts include intravenous administration of sodium benzoate and sodium phenylbutyrate. A block in the urea cycle (other than at arginase) renders arginine an essential amino acid, which must be supplemented. Protein catabolism should be minimized by temporarily eliminating protein from the diet and by ensuring adequate caloric intake, principally as glucose. Long-term management depends on the specific enzyme defect.

Hyperammonemia in Older Children and Adults

Primary metabolic disease is much less likely a cause of hyperammonemia in an older child or adult than in neonates. Partial urea cycle defects (as seen in ornithine transcarbamylase [OTC] heterozygotes—i.e., women) may cause episodic hyperammonemia during periods of metabolic stress and should be considered, especially if there are affected relatives. Allopurinol loading, popular historically, has been supplanted by sequencing of urea cycle genes. Heterozygotes for OTC deficiency have impaired neuropsychological function compared to controls; impeccable metabolic control is critical in preserving neurologic function. The older child or adult with hyperammonemia usually has severe liver disease or drug-induced hyperammonemia.

Valproate-Associated Hyperammonemia

Valproate therapy is one of the most common causes of hyperammonemia in clinical neurologic practice. Malnourished patients with carnitine deficiency and those with unrecognized urea cycle and fatty acid oxidation defects seem to be at higher risk of this complication. This dose-related laboratory finding may occur without clinical symptoms. The pathogenesis is disputed but may result from inhibition of hepatic N-acetylglutamate synthase activity by valproyl-coenzyme A (CoA). It is unclear whether patients become symptomatic from the increased ammonia under these circumstances.

L-Carnitine supplementation can prevent the development of hyperammonemia in animals and humans receiving valproate; the clinical significance of this reduction is unclear. Some authors routinely supplement L-carnitine in patients with reduced serum carnitine levels. In severe acute valproate hepatotoxicity with hyperammonemia, a disorder with high mortality, intravenous L-carnitine has been shown to improve survival compared to oral therapy with the same agent.

TABLE 134.1   **Plasma Amino Acid and Urinary Orotic Acid Findings in Urea Cycle Defects**

Enzymatic Deficiency	Citrulline	Argininosuccinic Acid	Orotic Acid	Arginine
Carbamyl phosphate synthetase (CPS deficiency)	0 to trace	0	↓	↓
Ornithine transcarbamylase (OTC deficiencies)	0 to trace	0	↑↑	↓
Argininosuccinate synthetase (citrullinuria)	↑↑	0	↑	↓
Argininosuccinase (argininosuccinic aciduria)	↑	↑↓	nl	↓
Arginase	nl	0	↑	↑↑
Transient hyperammonemia of newborn	nl or slightly ↑	0	nl	nl

↓, decreased; ↑, increased; nl, normal.

DISORDERS OF AMINO ACID METABOLISM

Introduction

Mass screening for disorders of amino acid metabolism has resulted in early biochemical diagnosis of phenylketonuria (PKU) and other aminoacidopathies. In one screening program in New South Wales, Australia, the incidence of PKU was 1:10,000 live births per year, the incidence of defects of amino acid transport was about 2:10,000 live births per year, and the combined incidence of all other aminoacidopathies was less than 8:100,000 live births per year. Although these conditions are rare, they are important because neurologic damage is potentially preventable with early treatment and because they provide information about the development and functions of the brain. PKU is described in some detail as a model for this family of disorders.

Phenylketonuria

INTRODUCTION

Phenylalanine hydroxylase deficiency is an autosomal recessive inborn error of metabolism manifested by impaired hepatic hydroxylation of phenylalanine to tyrosine. Untreated, the disorder causes a clinical picture highlighted by intellectual disability, seizures, and imperfect hair pigmentation.

The disease has been found in all parts of the world. The prevalence in the general population of the United States, as determined by screening programs, is about 1:11,700.

PATHOGENESIS AND PATHOLOGY

The hydroxylation of phenylalanine to tyrosine is an irreversible and complex reaction that requires phenylalanine hydroxylase and five other enzymes, in addition to several nonprotein components. Phenylalanine hydroxylase is normally found in liver, kidney, and pancreas but not in brain or skin fibroblasts.

In classic PKU, enzyme activity is generally less than 5% of normal. More than 40% of PKU subjects and more than 80% of those with mild PKU are tetrahydrobiopterin (BH_4) responsive when challenged with 20 mg/kg BH_4.

In some 1% to 3% of subjects, hyperphenylalaninemia results from a deficiency of BH_4. The BH_4-deficient hyperphenylalaninemias comprise a genetically heterogeneous group of disorders caused by mutations in the genes encoding enzymes involved in the synthesis or regeneration of the coenzyme BH_4. Three genetic defects in the synthesis of BH_4 have been described. These involve guanosine-5′-triphosphate (GTP) cyclohydrolase, I,6-pyruvoyltetrahydropterin synthase and sepiapterin reductase. In addition, there are two disorders in the regeneration of the aromatic amino acid–hydroxylating system: dihydropteridine reductase and pterin-4a-carbinolamine dehydratase. All these conditions lead to hyperphenylalaninemia associated with progressive neurologic deterioration, along with a variety of dyskinesias.

Children with classic PKU are born with only slightly elevated phenylalanine blood levels, but these rise rapidly on an unrestricted diet. Phenylalanine is converted to phenylpyruvic acid, phenylacetic acid, and phenylacetylglutamine, which impart a characteristic odor to the urine.

Brain changes are nonspecific and diffuse and involve both gray and white matter; they include interference with normal maturation of the brain, defective myelination, and diminished or absent pigmentation of the substantia nigra and locus ceruleus.

SYMPTOMS AND SIGNS

PKU exhibits a wide range of clinical and biochemical severity. In the classic form, untreated infants appear normal at birth. Vomiting and irritability in the first few months is followed by cognitive delay; ultimate intellectual disability may be severe. Seizures, including epileptic spasms, usually present in the first 18 months.

Untreated children are fairer with lighter irides than unaffected sibs and may have eczema and a peculiar musty ("mousey") odor. Focal neurologic abnormalities are rare, but microcephaly, mild spastic paraparesis, and tremor may occur.

Magnetic resonance imaging (MRI) usually shows white matter signal hyperintensity on T2-weighted sequences, mainly in the posterior watershed regions.

DIAGNOSIS

Most PKU patients are identified through newborn screening. If the diagnosis of a case of classic PKU is missed, the most likely reason is laboratory error, rather than insufficient protein intake or too early testing of the infant.

Mutation analysis facilitates carrier detection and the prenatal diagnosis of PKU in families with at least one previously affected child. Newborn screening programs have also detected conditions other than PKU with neonatal hyperphenylalaninemia. Patients with moderate and mild PKU and mild hyperphenylalaninemia, as these entities are termed, have phenylalanine levels that tend to be lower than those seen in classic PKU.

TREATMENT

All infants whose blood phenylalanine concentration is greater than 10 mg/dL (600 μM/L) and whose tyrosine concentration is low or normal (i.e., 1 to 4 mg/dL) should be started on a low-phenylalanine diet immediately. Infants whose blood phenylalanine concentrations remain in the range of 6.6 to 10.0 mg/dL (400 to 600 μM/L) on an unrestricted diet are generally not treated, and on follow-up evaluations, children of this group have normal intelligence and a normal MRI.

Therapy for classic PKU is restriction of the dietary phenylalanine using one of several low-phenylalanine formulas. Milk is added to the diet in amounts sufficient to maintain blood levels of the amino acid between 2 and 6 mg/dL (120 to 360 μM/L). Generally, patients tolerate this diet quite well, and within 1 to 2 weeks, the serum concentration of phenylalanine becomes normal.

Weekly serum phenylalanine determinations are essential to monitor dietary adherence for life. Strict dietary control should be maintained for life, and most centers strive to keep levels below 6 mg/dL (360 μM/L) in all patients with PKU. Dietary lapses are frequently accompanied by progressive white matter abnormalities on MRI. The addition of sapropterin (5 to 20 mg/kg/day), an orally active synthetic form of BH_4, permits a less restrictive diet for those patients who respond to a BH_4 challenge.

Phenylalaninemia caused by BH_4 deficiency requires diet, administration of BH_4 or a synthetic pterin, and replacement of neurotransmitter precursors (L-dopa/carbidopa and 5-hydroxytryptophan), whose synthesis is also impaired.

Early detection and dietary control of PKU has increased the number of homozygous PKU women achieving pregnancy. Maternal hyperphenylalaninemia causes intellectual disability, microcephaly, seizures, and congenital heart defects in affected children. During pregnancy, phenylalanine levels must be monitored as closely as during infancy because the fetus is exposed to even higher phenylalanine concentrations than the mother.

OUTCOME

When a child with classic PKU is maintained on a low-phenylalanine diet, seizures disappear and the EEG normalizes. Abnormally blond hair regains natural color, and head growth resumes.

Cognitive effects are less clear cut. In most studies, some deficit in intellectual development has been found, even in infants who had been diagnosed and treated as neonates. This could be a consequence of prenatal brain damage induced by high phenylalanine levels in the fetus.

Although the measured IQ is normal in most, deficits have been noted in executive functioning, attention, verbal memory, verbal fluency, and expressive naming. There is no threshold below which phenylalanine has no effect on cognition. Neurologic deterioration during adult life is generally the consequence of dietary lapses.

Other Amino Acid Disorders

Several other aminoacidopathies have distinguishing features that enable the clinician to suspect the diagnosis. Maple syrup urine disease, a disorder of branched-chain amino acid metabolism, produces a characteristic odor (detectable in cerumen as well as urine) and classically presents in the first week of life with acute encephalopathy and opisthotonic posturing. Isoleucine, leucine, and valine are present in excess in the urine. Emergent diagnosis and management is necessary to preserve life and neurologic function; a few patients are thiamine-responsive. Later onset forms may also occur.

Homocystinuria is manifest as tall stature, dislocated lenses, and varying degrees of intellectual impairment; a subgroup of patients responds to therapy with cobalamin. Thromboembolic episodes may begin in infancy. Disorders of sulfur amino acids are summarized in Table 134.2.

Hartnup disease is a disorder of renal tubular transport of tryptophan and other neutral amino acids; it causes intermittent ataxia with a pellagra-like rash. The disorders of amino acid transport are summarized in Table 134.3.

ORGANIC ACIDURIAS

Progress in diagnostic techniques in the 1950s enabled the identification of a family of disorders of distal steps in intermediary metabolism marked by the accumulation of nonamino organic acids, not detectable in bodily fluids by older methods, that are preferentially excreted in the urine. These compounds are mono-, di- and tricarboxylic acids derived from the breakdown of amino acids through the intramitochondrial degradation of CoA-activated carbonic acids. They are separated from the amino acid disorders only because of the analytical methods employed in their diagnosis, not because of any fundamental biologic difference. The classic organic acidurias have a number of common clinical features, including precipitation of acute encephalopathy, acidosis and hyperammonemia, and other multisystem manifestations by an excess substrate load or metabolic stress in the form of fever or other illness. Profound brain and systemic injury follows unless rapid and effective intervention is undertaken. This usually involves substrate restriction; suppression of aberrant pathways by providing alternate energy sources; and removal of offending metabolites by dialysis, hemofiltration, or by activating alternate pathways. The classical organic acidurias include propionic aciduria, methylmalonic aciduria, and isovaleric aciduria. The first named is associated with a poor long-term neurologic outcome, as assessed by cognitive measures and the presence of basal ganglia lesions; isovaleric aciduria with excellent outcome and methylmalonic aciduria is associated with intermediate impairment of neurologic function. Early diagnosis and tight metabolic control are necessary, but not always sufficient, to achieve the best outcome in these disorders.

Most of these diseases result from deficient activity of enzymes or their cofactors and present as neonatal encephalopathies in their most severe forms; less profound defects may present intermittently in older children. Slowly progressive disorders with predominant or exclusive neurologic manifestations are designated as cerebral organic

---

TABLE 134.2   Disorders of Sulfur Amino Acids

Disorder	Enzyme Deficiency	Neurologic Picture
Homocystinuria	Cystathionine-β-synthase	Multiple thromboembolic episodes starting in first year of life, mental retardation, ectopia lentis
Homocystinuria and mild homocysteinemia	$N^{5,10}$-methylenetetrahydrofolate reductase	Seizures, microcephaly, spastic paraparesis, ataxia
Cystathioninuria	γ-Cystathionase	Asymptomatic
Homocystinuria with megaloblastic anemia	—	—
Cbl E	Methionine synthase reductase	Severe developmental delay, lethargy, staring spells, hypotonia
Cbl G	Methionine synthase	Failure to thrive, mental retardation, cerebral atrophy
Cbl C	Synthesis of methyl and adenosyl cobalamin	Marfanoid habitus, mental retardation, acute psychosis, subacute spinal cord degeneration
Cbl D	Synthesis of methyl and adenosyl cobalamin	Acute psychosis, mental retardation, subacute spinal cord degeneration, Marfanoid habitus
Cbl F	Cobalamin lysosomal release	Developmental delay, sudden death in infancy
Sulfite oxidase deficiency	Sulfite oxidase	Seizures starting in neonatal period, profound mental retardation, subluxation of lens
Molybdenum cofactor deficiency	Molybdenum cofactor deficiency	As for sulfite oxidase deficiency

Cbl, cobalamin.

TABLE 134.3 Defects in Amino Acid Transport

Transport System	Condition	Biochemical Features	Clinical Features
Basic amino acids	Cystinuria (three types)	Impaired renal clearance, defective intestinal transport of lysine, arginine, ornithine, and cystine	Renal stones, no neurologic disease
	Lowe syndrome	Impaired intestinal transport of lysine and arginine, impaired tubular transport of lysine	Severe mental retardation, congenital glaucoma, cataracts, myopathy
Acidic amino acids	Dicarboxylic aminoaciduria	Increased excretion of glutamic, aspartic acids	Severe mental retardation glaucoma, cataracts, myopathy, sex-linked transmission
Neutral amino acids	Hartnup disease	Defective intestinal and renal tubular transport of tryptophan and other neutral amino acids	Intermittent cerebellar ataxia, photosensitive rash
Proline, hydroxyproline, glycine	Iminoglycinuria	Impaired tubular transport of proline, hydroxyproline, and glycine	Harmless variant
β-Amino acids	None known	Excretion of β-aminoisobutyric acid and taurine in β-alaninemia is increased due to competition at the tubular level	Harmless variant

acidopathies and include glutaric aciduria, type 1, L-2-hydroxyglutaric aciduria, D-2-hydroxyglutaric aciduria, and succinic semialdehyde dehydrogenase deficiency (SSADH) and Canavan disease.

Glutaric aciduria, type 1, results from glutaryl-CoA dehydrogenase deficiency and manifests as macrocephaly, hypotonia, and mild motor delay; affected children can decompensate suddenly in the face of metabolic stress and exhibit a hyperkinetic movement disorder that is refractory to most therapy. MRI shows enlarged extra-axial spaces over the frontal and temporal convexities, with widened sylvian fissures. Signal hyperintensity and eventual necrosis occurs in the striatum in untreated cases and corresponds to the presence of movement disorder. Glutaric acid and 3-methylglutaric acid are excreted in excess in the urine, as is glutaryl carnitine. Carnitine supplementation is of proven benefit in preventing neurologic progression but must be introduced before the onset of basal ganglia injury.

L-2-Hydroxyglutaric aciduria is associated with mutations in the L2HGDH gene and presents with progressive ataxia and intellectual disability in children; adult onset with similar, more slowly progressive symptoms also occurs on occasion. MRI shows a characteristic pattern that involves the basal ganglia and dentate nuclei and the subcortical, but not cerebellar, white matter. Patients with this disorder have an increased risk of primary brain tumors, attributed to the putative "oncometabolite" 2-hydroxyglutarate.

D-2-Hydroxyglutaric aciduria (D-2-HGA) is genetically and clinically heterogenous. Some patients who excrete D-hydroxyglutaric acid in the urine are asymptomatic; others exhibit facial dysmorphism, seizures, hypotonia, and developmental delay. About half of the patients have recessive mutations in D2HGDH, designated type 1 D-2-HGA. The remainder, designated type 2 D-2-HGA, harbor dominant mutations in IDH2, a gene which is mutated in some cases of acute myeloid leukemia and gliomas. A few patients have

been described with combined D- and L-2-hydroxyglutaric aciduria resulting from mutations in the SLC25A1 gene. The phenotype is severe, with hypotonia, delay, and intractable seizures; it is important to recognize, as it may respond to therapy with citrate.

SSADH deficiency is a disorder of γ-aminobutyric acid (GABA) metabolism that results from mutations in ALDH5A1 and presents with hypotonia, developmental delay, and ataxia. Epilepsy, which may be difficult to control, occurs in more than half of affected children, along with movement disorders and behavioral disturbances. MRI may show hyperintensities in the basal ganglia, specifically the globus pallidus, and less frequently in the dentate nuclei, brain stem, and subcortical white matter. 4-Hydroxybutyric acid is increased in urine and CSF and may be detected by magnetic resonance (MR) spectroscopy. Treatment is symptomatic; vigabatrin (50 mg/kg/day; 500 to 1,500 mg twice daily), which inhibits the production of succinic semialdehyde, is a logical choice as an antiepileptic drug but is not always effective. Valproate (10 to 60 mg/kg/day) is relatively contraindicated but can be cautiously employed if seizures are refractory to other agents. A trial of taurine is currently in progress.

Canavan disease is a spongiform leukodystrophy in which deficient activity of aspartoacylase leads to accumulation of N-acetylaspartic acid (NAA) in bodily fluids and the brain. It is commonly manifest as hypotonia and progressive macrocephaly in infants, followed by loss of milestones, spasticity, seizures, and premature death. MRI shows diffuse white matter hyperintensity, and MR spectroscopy demonstrates marked elevation of NAA. The diagnosis is made by demonstrating defective aspartoacylase activity in leucocytes and corresponding mutations in the ASPA gene. Antenatal diagnosis is possible using gene sequencing. Gene therapy using an AAV2 vector has shown reduced NAA levels and evidence of clinical stabilization in an open-label study in humans with Canavan disease.

DISORDERS OF PURINE AND PYRIMIDINE METABOLISM

Introduction

Purines and pyrimidines are heterocyclic compounds that participate in nucleotide synthesis, generation of energy compounds (i.e., adenosine diphosphate [ADP] and adenosine triphosphate [ATP]), and in signaling pathways (i.e., cyclic adenosine monophosphate [AMP]). Several disorders of purine and pyrimidine metabolism have been recognized; see Table 134.4. Findings include anemia, immunodeficiency, hypo- or hyperuricemia (i.e., with nephrolithiasis and renal failure in severe cases), and a variety of neurologic phenotypes. The latter range through sensorineural hearing loss, developmental delays, intellectual disability, autism, seizures, and movement disorders. The archetype and most frequently recognized of these disorders is the Lesch–Nyhan syndrome, described in more detail in the following paragraphs.

Lesch–Nyhan Syndrome

In 1964, Lesch and Nyhan described two brothers with hyperuricemia, intellectual disability, choreoathetosis, and self-destructive biting of the lips and fingers. Most cases are boys, but at least one symptomatic female with skewed X-inactivation has been described. The trait is X-linked recessive. The basic defect is the lack of hypoxanthine-guanine phosphoribosyltransferase (HPRT).

The enzyme deficiency increases the rate of purine biosynthesis, and uric acid reaches high levels in blood, urine, and CSF. Urate is deposited in the kidneys and joints and may result in nephropathy and gout.

The neurologic manifestations include severe intellectual disability, spasticity, and choreoathetosis that start in the first year. The characteristic self-mutilating behavior appears in the second year. Death is usually caused by renal failure and may occur in the second or third decade of life. Sudden death may occur at any time because of acute respiratory failure, often related to the motor disorder. Milder variants are recognized, in which self-mutilation may be absent and manifestations may be restricted to cognitive impairment with mild motor symptoms or progressive spastic paraparesis. The pathogenesis of the cerebral symptoms is not known.

Diagnosis depends on recognition of the clinical manifestations and may be made precisely by biochemical assay of the enzyme in erythrocyte hemolysates or cultured fibroblasts. DNA analysis confirms the diagnosis and may be used for prenatal diagnosis and carrier detection; mutations can be detected in most affected individuals. More than 400 mutations have been described.

Gout is treated effectively with allopurinol, but the neurologic disorder is daunting. Restraints may be needed to prevent the child from damaging himself or herself or others; dental extraction is often required to prevent facial mutilation. Diazepam (1 to 2.5 mg by mouth three or four times daily), carbamazepine (10 to 35 mg/kg/day), gabapentin (10 to 40 mg/kg/day), and botulinum

TABLE 134.4 Disorders of Purine and Pyrimidine Metabolism

Enzyme	Anemia	ID	Uric Acid	MR	SNHL	Seizures	Ataxia	MD	Other
NT	+	+	−	+		+	+	+	Symptoms improve with uridine
Purine Pathway									
PRPS	−	−	+	+	+	−	+	−	Autism
ADSL	−	−	0	+	−	+	−	−	Autism
AMPD1	−	−	0	−	−	−	−	−	Muscle cramps, increased CK
ADA	−	+	0	+	−	−	−	+	Spasticity
NP	+	+	−	+	−	−	−	+	Spasticity
XDH	−	−	−	−	−	−	−	−	Myopathy, arthropathy
HPRT	−	−	+	+	−	+	−	+	Self-mutilation, spasticity, 6-thioguanine resistance
APRT	−	−	+	−	−	−	−	−	
Pyrimidine Pathway									
UMPS	+	−	0	+	−	−	−	−	
UMPH	+	−	0	−	−	−	−	−	
DPYD	−	−	0	+	−	+	−	−	Microcephaly, 5-fluorouracil sensitivity, autism
DPYS	−	−	0	+	−	+	−	−	
UP	−	−	0	+	−	+	−	+	

+, present (or increased for uric acid); −, absent (or decreased for uric acid); 0, unchanged; ID, immunodeficiency; MR, developmental delay, mental retardation; SNHL, sensorineural hearing loss; MD, movement disorder; NT, 5′-nucleotidase; PRPS, phosphoribosyl pyrophosphate synthetase superactivity; ADSL, adenylosuccinate lyase deficiency; AMPD1, adenosine monophosphate deaminase 1; CK, creatine kinase; ADA, adenosine deaminase deficiency; NP, nucleoside phosphorylase deficiency; XDH, xanthine dehydrogenase (= xanthine oxidase) deficiency (xanthinuria; secondary impairment in molybdenum cofactor deficiency); HPRT, hypoxanthine-guanine phosphoribosyltransferase deficiency (Lesch–Nyhan syndrome); APRT, adenosine phosphoribosyltransferase deficiency; UMPS, uridine monophosphate synthase deficiency (hereditary orotic aciduria); UMPH, uridine monophosphate hydrolase (= pyrimidine 5′-nucleotidase) deficiency; DPYD, dihydropyrimidine dehydrogenase deficiency; DPYS, dihydropyrimidinase deficiency; UP, ureidopropionase deficiency.

toxin are sometimes helpful, but physical restraint is often required in classic cases. Deep brain stimulation surgery, targeted to the globus pallidus, has improved or abolished self-mutilation in some cases. Neither enzyme replacement nor gene therapy is available for Lesch–Nyhan syndrome.

Other Purine Disorders

Neurologic abnormalities are also seen in patients who are without other enzymes of purine-nucleoside metabolism. Adenosine deaminase deficiency causes severe, combined immunodeficiency in infants; some patients have extrapyramidal or pyramidal signs and psychomotor development and may be retarded. Partial exchange transfusion may be clinically beneficial. Also, a few patients lacking purine-nucleoside phosphorylase with impaired cellular immunity have shown a form of spastic paraparesis in childhood. 5'-Nucleotidase superactivity produces a complex phenotype with all of the features of purine and pyrimidine disorders that responds to oral uridine therapy. These patients may have autistic features that may also be prominent in phosphoribosyl pyrophosphate synthetase (PRPS), adenylosuccinate lyase (ADSL), and dihydropyrimidine dehydrogenase (DPYD) deficiencies.

PORPHYRIA

The porphyrias are a family of disorders in which the synthesis of heme and its precursors are impaired. They are traditionally divided into hepatic and erythropoietic subgroups according to the major sites of gene expression. Acute intermittent porphyria (AIP) is the most frequent of these disorders and the most likely to present to a neurologist.

AIP is an autosomal dominant disorder with low penetrance caused by deficiency of hydroxymethylbilane synthase (HMBS, also known as *porphobilinogen deaminase*), most frequently observed in Sweden and South Africa, which typically presents as an acute encephalopathy with pronounced behavioral changes (including frank psychosis) that may be accompanied by seizures, autonomic neuropathy causing abdominal pain, tachycardia and hypertension, or a painful motor neuropathy that may progress to quadriplegia with respiratory failure in severe cases. Patients may have hyponatremia as a consequence of inappropriate antidiuretic hormone (ADH) secretion. Decompensation may be provoked by fasting or by exposure to alcohol or any one of a number of drugs that interact with this pathway, including older anesthetic agents, barbiturates, and oral contraceptives; pregnancy may also precipitate an attack. Drugs appear to precipitate attacks of AIP by inducing delta-amino levulinic acid synthase, thereby leading to hepatic heme depletion, or by inhibiting the P-450 cytochrome system. Understanding these mechanisms facilitates prediction of the likely toxicity of drugs in affected individuals.

The diagnosis of AIP requires timely assay of urine porphobilinogen, with subsequent confirmation by sequencing of the HMBS gene. Acute management, which must not be delayed for definitive diagnosis, requires the removal of precipitants, careful attention to fluid and electrolyte balance, the administration of intravenous Panhematin or heme arginate to shut down the synthetic pathway, appropriate analgesia with agents such as gabapentin (10 to 40 mg/kg/day), and management of seizures with safe agents such as benzodiazepines that do not exacerbate the metabolic block.

A number of atypical presentations have been reported in AIP, including posterior reversible encephalopathy syndrome, acute cortical blindness, and progressive muscular atrophy.

Long-term management hinges on education of the patients and their medical providers to recognize and avoid situations and agents that provoke decompensation. In rare cases, liver transplantation may be indicated to manage hepatic failure or recurrent attacks when conservative management is ineffective.

Acute variegate porphyria (AVP), a dominant disorder associated with decreased activity of the mitochondrial enzyme protoporphyrinogen oxidase (PPOX), can present in a clinically indistinguishable fashion from AIP because the typical blistering rash may be absent in as many as half of affected individuals in acute crises. It is managed in the same fashion as AIP.

DISORDERS OF METAL METABOLISM

Several inherited neurologic diseases are associated with abnormal handling of metals in the brain. These may be conveniently divided into disorders of copper and iron metabolism.

Disorders of Copper Metabolism

WILSON DISEASE

Kinnier Wilson described his eponymous disease in 1912 as hepatolenticular degeneration, a disorder characterized by progressive dystonia, tremor, and psychiatric disturbances, usually beginning in adolescence, and accompanied by cirrhosis. A decade earlier, Kayser and Fleischer had reported the brown corneal rings now known to represent the accumulation of copper in Descemet's membrane. These have proven to be an excellent gauge of excess copper stores, which regress in the face of effective copper removal, only to reappear if treatment is discontinued.

Wilson disease is caused by mutations in the transporter, encoded by the ATP7B gene that transports copper from hepatocytes to the bile and blood; its dysfunction leads to accumulation of copper in the liver, where it provokes fibrosis and eventually cirrhosis. When this store is exhausted, copper begins to deposit in the lenticular nuclei, causing extrapyramidal dysfunction and if untreated, destruction of the nuclei.

Neurologic presentations are rare in the first decade of life; Wilson disease is more likely to present in young children with acute or chronic liver failure, hemolytic anemia, or renal tubular dysfunction, reflecting the tissues in which copper is toxic. Affected adolescents have a typical appearance, in which the upper lip is drawn back to expose the teeth, accompanied by a wing-beating tremor and dystonic posturing. Spasticity, dysphagia, and dysarthria are commonly seen, and parkinsonian features are most prominent in some cases. Psychiatric manifestations are frequent and may dominate the clinical picture.

Laboratory tests may show elevated transaminases, low serum uric acid, and elevated urine copper, amino acids, and urate secondary to tubular dysfunction. Serum copper and ceruloplasmin are low. Apart from the demonstration of two mutations in trans in the ATP7B gene, no single test is diagnostic for Wilson disease. A diagnostic scoring system has been developed to assist the clinician; this includes presence or absence of Kayser–Fleischer rings or neurologic symptoms, serum ceruloplasmin, liver copper content, urinary copper excretion, and mutation analysis of the ATP7B gene.

Penicillamine (750 to 1,500 mg/day administered in two or three divided doses daily for adults; dosing in children is 20 mg/kg/day rounded off to the nearest 250 mg, given in two or three divided doses) is the traditional chelating agent used in Wilson disease, but its adverse effect profile has led to the employment of zinc (which impairs copper absorption) (150-mg elemental zinc/day for adults; for children ,50 kg in body weight, 75 mg/day, administered in three divided doses, 30 minutes before meals) and trientine (which increases urinary copper excretion) (900 to 2,700 mg/day in two or three divided doses, with 900 to 1,500 mg/day used for maintenance therapy; in children, the weight-based dose is not established, but the dose generally used is 20 mg/kg/day rounded off to the nearest 250 mg, given in two or three divided doses) as preferred treatments today. Vitamin E may have a role as an antioxidant, but no dosage regimen has been widely accepted. If copper stores can be removed before permanent tissue damage has occurred, the prognosis is excellent, provided that treatment is continued lifelong. Liver transplantation is an option in those with irreversible hepatic failure or who cannot tolerate other treatments.

MENKES DISEASE

In contrast to Wilson disease, the manifestations of Menkes disease reflect the effects of copper deficiency on the brain and other tissues. Menkes disease is caused by mutations in the X-linked ATP7A gene that encodes the protein that facilitates transport of copper from the gut to the circulation. The resultant systemic deficiency of copper leads to dysfunction of multiple enzyme systems, including cytochrome *c* oxidase, lysyl oxidase, and dopamine b-hydroxylase. The disease manifests in boys in the first 2 months with developmental regression; hypotonia; seizures; twisted, sparse, fair hair (often absent through easy breakage); hypothermia; and hypoglycemia. They have a cherubic appearance secondary to abnormal collagen formation, which is also responsible for the bony anomalies (metaphyseal flaring) and dilatation of the urinary collecting system and blood vessels. The latter may rupture spontaneously, leading to intracranial hemorrhage, sometimes mistakenly attributed to child abuse. Without treatment, most boys die by 3 years, although survival into the fourth decade has been reported in one treated patient with a mild phenotype.

The diagnosis is suspected clinically and confirmed by ATP7A mutation analysis. Bypassing the impaired gut absorption by administering subcutaneous copper histidine has shown benefit in morbidity and mortality, provided that treatment is instituted before permanent damage has occurred.

Females with ATP7A mutations can present when X-autosome translocation has occurred or in theory, in cases of Turner syndrome. Their clinical manifestations resemble those in boys.

Two allelic variants have been recognized in patients with ATP7A mutations. The occipital horn syndrome manifests as calcification of the insertions of the trapezius muscles, associated with joint laxity, a dilated urinary collecting system, and tortuous blood vessels, with only mild, if any, cognitive impairment. A distal motor neuropathy resembling Charcot–Marie–Tooth syndrome has also been described in adult males; it lacks any other findings in common with Menkes disease.

Disorders of Iron Metabolism

A family of rare diseases, embraced by the acronym NBIA (neurodegeneration with brain iron accumulation) has been delineated in recent years. All feature varying combinations of basal ganglia dysfunction associated with neuropsychiatric symptoms. Eight of the 10 known subtypes are autosomal recessive disorders; BPAN is X-linked dominant and neuroferritinopathy is autosomal dominant. The core disorders in this family are pantothenate kinase–associated neurodegeneration (PKAN; NBIA 1), formerly known as *Hallervorden–Spatz disease* and *PLA2G6-associated neurodegeneration* (PLAN), or NBIA 2.

PKAN or NBIA 1 is a childhood-onset neurodegenerative disorder that most often presents in the first decade with intellectual delay and progressive gait and oromandibular dystonia; more subtle disturbances of cognitive function and gait may occur with later onset forms of the disease. Saccadic eye movement disorders including vertical supranuclear gaze palsy have been described. The classic phenotype also includes retinal pigmentation, acanthocytes, and deposition of iron in the globus pallidus. This causes signal hypointensity in the globus pallidus on MRI early in the course of the disease; with progression, a central area of hyperintensity appears in the medial globus pallidus, producing the "eye of the tiger" sign. Although highly suggestive of the diagnosis, the absence of this finding does not rule out the diagnosis of PKAN, which is established by sequencing of the PANK2 gene. Although there is no definitive therapy for PKAN, small studies suggest a stabilizing effect of iron chelation using deferiprone.

NBIA 2, PARK14, or PLAN, first recognized as infantile neuroaxonal dystrophy, is associated with mutations in PLA2G6, which encodes calcium-independent phospholipase A2. The key features are the combination of ataxia, truncal hypotonia, spasticity, nystagmus, and optic atrophy with peripheral neuropathy. MRI shows cerebellar atrophy and iron deposition in the globus pallidus—without hyperintensity. Later onset forms may have a dystonia–Parkinson phenotype. Axonal spheroids are the pathologic hallmark of the disease, and their demonstration in biopsies was critical to the diagnosis before mutation analysis was available. Only symptomatic therapy is available.

DISORDERS ASSOCIATED WITH ACANTHOCYTOSIS

Acanthocytes are irregularly shaped red cells with spiny projections whose appearance reflects abnormal membrane structure. They are found in PKAN (see the following text) and in Huntington-like disorder 2 (HDL2), a triplet repeat disease affecting the gene encoding junctophilin-3, a protein involved in sarcoplasmic and plasma membranes.

Chorea-acanthocytosis is an autosomal recessive disorder in which patents experience the onset of a hyperkinetic movement disorder in early adulthood, which eventually evolves into parkinsonism. The movements are often drug resistant but may respond to deep brain stimulation. A neuropsychiatric syndrome, beginning with features of obsessive–compulsive disorder may evolve into dementia; some patients also have an axonal neuropathy and seizures. Death usually occurs within 15 years; there is no disease-modifying therapy. Patients have mutations in CHAC, the human analog of the yeast vacuolar protein sorting 13 (VPS13). The gene product, chorein, interacts with β-adducin and β-actin, membrane cytoskeletal proteins expressed at synapses and red cell membranes.

Two related disorders of lipid metabolism are also associated with acanthocytosis. Abetalipoproteinemia (Bassen–Kornzweig syndrome) is caused by mutations in the gene encoding the microsomal triglyceride transfer protein. This leads to severe diarrhea and almost complete absence of apolipoprotein B (apoB)–containing proteins in the blood, with very low levels of cholesterol (often <40 mg/dL) and other blood lipids. Fat-soluble vitamins are correspondingly low; perhaps the most significant is vitamin E, whose deficiency causes a spinocerebellar syndrome progressive ophthalmoplegia and pigmentary retinopathy. Vitamin K deficiency may cause serious bleeding. The presence of very low serum cholesterol and acanthocytes should suggest the diagnosis, which can be confirmed by mutation analysis. Treatment with vitamin E and vitamin K is effective if begun early. Hypobetalipoproteinemia results from mutations in the apoB gene itself; the phenotype is indistinguishable from abetalipoproteinemia; the treatment is the same.

McLeod syndrome is an X-linked disorder, originally recognized in asymptomatic individuals donating blood. They have abnormal expression of Kell blood group antigens secondary to mutations in the XK gene. A subgroup of people with this finding has a symptomatic neuromyopathy associated with elevated creatine kinase levels, hemolysis, and involuntary movements. Some also have seizures. MRI shows caudate atrophy and increased signal in the putamen. Cardiomyopathy may occur and lead to premature death. Electromyography (EMG) shows axonal degeneration and muscle biopsy may show myopathy and denervation. Complex phenotypes likely result from contiguous gene syndromes; XK is adjacent to CYBB (causing X-linked chronic granulomatous disease), DMD (Duchenne muscular dystrophy), and RPGR (X-linked retinitis pigmentosa) on the X chromosome.

LARGE MOLECULE DISORDERS

LYSOSOMAL AND ASSOCIATED LARGE MOLECULE DISORDERS

Introduction

Lysosomal diseases are characterized by the accumulation of macromolecules within lysosomes because of genetically determined deficiency of a catabolic enzyme or related gene product. The stored materials comprise complex lipids, saccharides, or proteins, and the central nervous system (CNS) is usually affected. Both autosomal and X-linked inheritance occur. Carrier detection and prenatal diagnosis are available for most of these disorders. Specific treatment in the form of enzyme replacement therapy (ERT) for mucopolysaccharidosis (MPS) I, II, and VI; Gaucher, Fabry, and Pompe disease; substrate reduction therapy for Gaucher disease; and hemopoietic stem cell transplantation for several lysosomal storage diseases has now entered practice, albeit with varying evidence of efficacy.

Lipidoses

Lipid storage diseases involve all three major lipid classes: neutral lipids (i.e., cholesterol ester, fatty acid, and triglycerides), polar lipids (i.e., glycolipids and phospholipids), and very polar lipids (i.e., gangliosides).

GM2-GANGLIOSIDOSES

Hexosaminidase-deficiency diseases result from a genetically determined deficiency of the enzyme hexosaminidase, which causes accumulation in cells (especially in neurons) of GM2-ganglioside and other glycosphingolipids.

For full activity, hexosaminidase requires two different subunits: the α-subunit, coded for by the hexosaminidase A locus on chromosome 15, and the β-subunit, coded for by the hexosaminidase B locus on chromosome 5. Three isozymes of hexosaminidase have a defined subunit structure: hexosaminidase A ($\alpha\beta$), hexosaminidase B ($\beta\beta$), and hexosaminidase S ($\alpha\alpha$). Hexosaminidase A is required for cleavage of GM2-ganglioside, but the true substrate is the ganglioside bound to a protein activator whose deficiency also causes a GM2-gangliosidosis (the so-called AB variant). The GM2-gangliosidoses are classified according to the phenotype, the genetic locus, and the allele involved.

Progressive infantile encephalopathy was the most common clinical pattern in the past. The success of carrier screening in the Ashkenazi Jewish community dramatically reduced its incidence,

and later onset variants are now seen more commonly. Hexosaminidase deficiencies show diverse phenotypes from infancy to adulthood. This diagnosis can be suspected with nearly any degenerative neurologic disorder, except demyelinating neuropathy or myopathy. Sensory dysfunction, ocular palsies, neurogenic bladder, and extraneural involvement are not prominent features.

The diagnosis is made by assaying hexosaminidase activity in blood serum and leukocytes and by sequencing the hexosaminidase genes.

Infantile Encephalopathy with Cherry-red Spots

Three disorders in this group are well known: classic infantile Tay–Sachs disease (α-locus), infantile Sandhoff disease (β-locus), and the so-called AB variant (activator locus). Heterozygosity for α-locus mutations occurs in 1 in 30 Ashkenazi Jews (compared with 1 in 300 for the general population), accounting for the ethnic concentration of classic Tay–Sachs disease and genetic compounds containing α-locus mutations.

In all three conditions, the infants appear normal until 4 to 6 months of age. They learn to smile and reach for objects but do not sit or crawl. A myoclonic jerk reaction to sound (traditionally, but misleadingly, termed *hyperacusis*) and the macular cherry-red spot are constant findings. The cherry-red macular spot is a funduscopic finding reflecting a combination of foveal atrophy and perifoveal lipid accumulation. The former improves visualization of the underlying choroid (whose color may range from bright red to brown in different individuals), which is contrasted with the more opaque surrounding lipid-laden retinal tissue. Cherry-red spots may be seen in GM2 and GM1 gangliosidoses, Niemann–Pick disease types A and B (but not in C), and sialidosis type 1 (cherry-red spot myoclonus syndrome) and has been occasionally reported in Krabbe disease.

Affected infants become floppy and weak but have hyperactive reflexes, clonus, and extensor plantar responses. Visual deterioration, apathy, and loss of developmental milestones lead to a vegetative state by the second year. Seizures and myoclonus are prominent for the first 2 years. The infants eventually become decorticate. They need tube feeding, have difficulty with secretions, and are blind. Head circumference enlarges progressively to about the 90th percentile, from ages 1 to 3 years, and then stabilizes. Death is due to intercurrent infection, usually pneumonia. The disease is confined to the nervous system, apart from variable hepatosplenomegaly in Sandhoff disease.

By light microscopy, grossly ballooned neurons are found throughout the brain, cerebellum, and spinal cord. By electron microscopy, membranous cytoplasmic bodies (i.e., distended lysosomes) are seen, with regularly spaced, concentric, dark, and pale lamellae.

GM2-ganglioside content is markedly increased in the brain and to a much lesser degree, in the viscera. Other glycosphingolipids such as asialo-GM2 and globoside accumulate to a lesser degree.

The storage results from the deficiency of hexosaminidase. In classic Tay–Sachs disease, hexosaminidase A is absent, and hexosaminidase B increased. Heterozygous carriers have a partial decrease of hexosaminidase A.

In infantile Sandhoff disease, hexosaminidases A and B are deficient. Carriers have partially decreased hexosaminidases A and B. In one form of the AB variant, a hexosaminidase A–activating protein is missing. Although levels of hexosaminidases A and B are increased, GM2-ganglioside cannot be cleaved. Diagnosis requires the use of the natural substrate, GM2-ganglioside, or direct testing for the activator or activator mutations. In a second form of the

AB variant, the residual hexosaminidase A cleaves artificial but not sulfated-artificial or natural substrate. Although this is detected as an AB variant, it is an α-locus disorder.

Late-Infantile, Juvenile, and Adult GM2-Gangliosidoses

These present with dementia and ataxia with or without macular cherry-red spots. Spasticity, muscle wasting stemming from anterior horn cell disease, and seizures are frequently seen. Hexosaminidase A deficiency or hexosaminidases A and B deficiency are found on biochemical study of serum, leukocytes, and cultured skin fibroblasts.

Other late-onset forms of GM2-gangliosidosis present as cerebellar ataxia or spinocerebellar ataxia. Hexosaminidase A or hexosaminidases A and B deficiency are found on biochemical study.

Motor neuron disease resembling spinal muscular atrophy type III may be the first evidence of late-onset GM2-gangliosidoses. Upper motor neuron findings may also be present, giving an amyotrophic lateral sclerosis–like phenotype.

Many, perhaps most, of these late-onset cases are compound heterozygotes. Diagnosis requires both enzyme assay and DNA sequencing.

GM1-GANGLIOSIDOSIS

This group of disorders is characterized by the deficiency of GM1-ganglioside β-galactosidase and storage of GM1-ganglioside, asialo-GM1, keratan sulfate–like oligosaccharides, and glycoproteins. Other β-galactosidases such as those that cleave galactosylceramide and lactosylceramide are not deficient, and these compounds do not accumulate. There are at least three forms of deficiency of this enzyme: primary deficiency of β-galactosidase, causing infantile and late-infantile GM1-gangliosidosis and an adult form; combined neuraminidase and β-galactosidase deficiency, galactosialidosis; and combined deficiency of β-galactosidase and several other lysosomal enzymes in I cell disease, mucolipidosis II (ML I). The latter two types are discussed under MLs.

Infantile GM1-Gangliosidosis

Infantile GM1-gangliosidosis is earlier in onset, more severe, and more rapidly progressive than infantile Tay–Sachs disease. Soon after birth, these infants become hypotonic, with poor sucking ability and slow weight gain. They have frontal bossing, coarsened features, large low-set ears, and an elongated philtrum. Gum hypertrophy, macroglossia, peripheral edema, and often faint corneal haze are noted. Strabismus and nystagmus may be seen. About half the patients develop macular cherry-red spots. Development is slow, and they do not sit or crawl. By the age of 6 months, liver and spleen are enlarged; joint stiffness and claw-hand deformities may be seen, and the skin is thickened. Seizures may develop. Infants typically die before age 2 years of pneumonia or cardiac arrhythmias.

MRI of the brain may be normal initially, but as the head grows rapidly, diffuse signal hyperintensity appears throughout the white matter (Fig. 134.1). X-rays show changes similar to those of Hurler syndrome after 6 to 12 months, with anterior beaking of vertebral bodies and a J-shaped sella turcica. Peripheral blood smears show vacuolated lymphocytes, and foamy histiocytes are found in the bone marrow.

Diagnosis is suggested by the characteristic oligosaccharide pattern in urine and confirmed by assay of GM1-ganglioside β-galactosidase in blood leukocytes or cultured skin fibroblasts and mutation analysis.

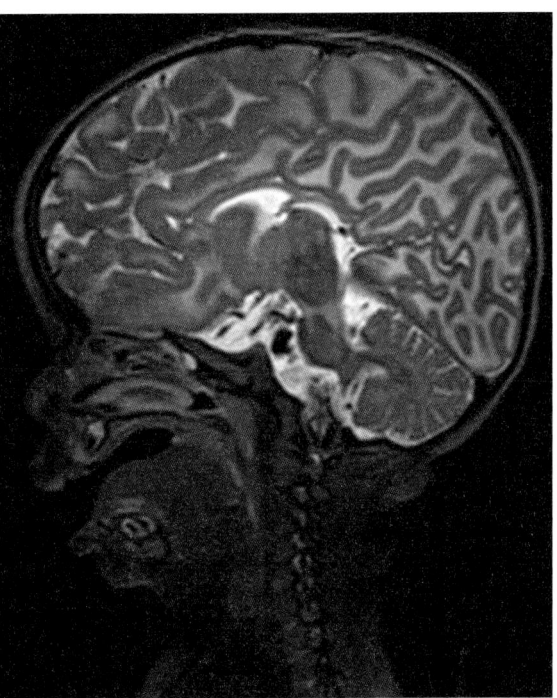

FIGURE 134.1 Sagittal T2-weighted MRI of an infant with GM1-gangliosidosis showing macrocephaly and signal hyperintensity throughout the white matter.

Late-Infantile GM1-Gangliosidosis

Symptoms begin between ages 1 and 3 years, with gait ataxia, hypotonia, hyperreflexia, dysarthria, and speech regression. Seizures, dementia, and spastic quadriplegia lead to death, usually by pneumonia. Optic atrophy and evidence of anterior horn cell disease may be found. Corneas are clear, organomegaly is absent, and bone changes are scanty.

FABRY DISEASE

Fabry disease is an X-linked disorder in which the skin, kidney, peripheral and autonomic nervous systems, and blood vessels store trihexosylceramide, a breakdown product of globoside. Trihexosylceramide accumulates because of a deficiency of β-galactosidase A. Recent studies have found that female heterozygotes are frequently clinically affected, albeit less severely and later than hemizygotes.

Symptoms usually commence in childhood or adolescence, with lancinating pains in the limbs, especially the feet and hands, often brought on by temperature changes and accompanied by paresthesia or abdominal crises. Anhydrosis and unexplained fever are common.

Angiokeratomas, which become more numerous with age, are purple; macular and maculopapular; hyperkeratotic; 1 to 3 mm in size; and with a predilection for the groin, buttocks, scrotum, and umbilicus. Glycolipid storage in the renal glomeruli and tubules begins with asymptomatic proteinuria in children; it progresses to renal failure and hypertension in the third or fourth decade. Glycolipid storage in blood vessel walls may cause stroke. Edema of the limbs, whorled corneal clouding (cornea verticillata) visible by slit lamp, and myocardial involvement may occur. ERT has been demonstrated to reverse lipid storage in the kidney, heart, and blood vessels and to produce corresponding improvement or reversal of renal impairment, pain, cardiac function, and cerebral blood flow. In some cases, renal transplant may still be required when renal failure supervenes. The lancinating pains may respond to phenytoin (5 to 8 mg/kg/day), carbamazepine (10 to 35 mg/kg/day), or gabapentin (10 to 40 mg/kg/day).

Heterozygous women may also be affected, but manifestations are less marked. Skin lesions are few or absent. Corneal opacity is more common. If renal or cardiac involvement occurs, they are later in onset and less severe. Fabry disease is diagnosed by finding decreased β-galactosidase activity in plasma and leukocytes and a mutation in the β-galactosidase gene.

GAUCHER DISEASE

Gaucher disease is an autosomal recessive sphingolipidosis in which glucocerebroside is stored as a result of deficiency of glucocerebroside β-glucosidase (or glucocerebrosidase). At least four forms have been described: the infantile neuronopathic form, the juvenile neuronopathic form, the adult neuronopathic form, and the adult nonneuronopathic form.

These distinctions seem to be artificial, with overlapping manifestations occurring across a broad spectrum of phenotypes. The adult (nonneuronopathic) form (type I) is more common in Ashkenazi Jews than in the general population. Diagnosis of all forms is made by demonstrating reduced glucocerebroside β-glucosidase activity in cultured skin fibroblasts or blood leukocytes and is further refined by demonstrating mutations in the β-glucosidase gene.

Type II (Infantile Neuronopathic) Gaucher Disease

This disease occurs in the first year of life, often in the first 3 months. The course is rapid, with developmental regression and death before age 2 years. Affected infants lose weight, reflecting the mechanical compression of the gut and the hypercatabolic state associated with pronounced hepatosplenomegaly. The neurologic signs reflect severe brain stem dysfunction and include stridor, difficulty in sucking and swallowing, strabismus, retrocollis, spasticity, and hyperreflexia. Bilateral esotropia is typical. Later, they enter a vegetative state, becoming flaccid and weak. Seizures may occur. Macular cherry-red spots and optic atrophy do not occur.

Type III (Juvenile Neuronopathic) Gaucher Disease

The manifestations range from a severe form, presenting in infancy as pulmonary infiltrates, splenomegaly, and cardiorespiratory failure, to a progressive myoclonic dementia in adolescents or adults (common in the northern provinces of Norrbotten and Västerbotten in Sweden). Horizontal supranuclear gaze palsy, with characteristic looping movements, in which the inability to generate horizontal saccades is partially compensated by generating vertical saccades accompanied by a horizontal head thrust, is an important clue to the diagnosis.

Type I (Adult) Gaucher Disease

These patients have visceral (e.g., liver, lymph nodes, lung) and skeletal manifestations without primary neurologic disease. Multiple myeloma may be a late complication. It is most common in Ashkenazi Jews. Type 1 Gaucher disease presents at any age from infancy to the seventh decade. Splenectomy should be avoided unless ERT is not possible or the mechanical and hematologic manifestations are not otherwise controlled. Lesions of long bones, pelvis, or vertebral bodies may be painful. Severe cases may require surgical intervention, including joint replacement. ERT, with purified modified β-glucosidase (i.e., alglucerase) or recombinant β-glucosidase (i.e., imiglucerase), reverses all of the manifestations

of type 1 Gaucher disease, provided that treatment begins before severe tissue damage has occurred.

Adult Neuronopathic Gaucher Disease

Parkinsonism has been found to be more frequent in several studies of adults with Gaucher disease and in heterozygotes for glucocerebrosidase mutations. The relation now appears well established; the mechanism remains uncertain, and nonspecific lysosomal dysfunction may play a role in several neurodegenerative diseases, including parkinsonism.

NIEMANN–PICK DISEASE

This group of disorders includes several diseases that were grouped together in 1958 by Crocker and Farber on the basis of the overlapping pathology (i.e., visceral foam cells) and biochemistry (i.e., lysosomal storage of the glycosphingolipid sphingomyelin). Crocker subsequently proposed four groups. It is now recognized that his groups A and B are primary sphingomyelinase deficiencies, whereas groups C and D are allelic disorders, whose primary defect is not deficiency of a lysosomal hydrolase but in intracellular lipid trafficking. Patients with types A and B Niemann–Pick disease have deficient activity of the sphingomyelin-cleaving enzyme acid, sphingomyelinase. The diagnosis should be suspected in patients with progressive hepatosplenomegaly, with or without cerebral symptoms. The bone marrow contains characteristic mulberry storage cells (i.e., distinct from Gaucher cells). Decreased sphingomyelinase activity may be shown in cultured skin fibroblasts, leukocytes, or tissue.

Infantile Niemann–Pick Disease, Type A

This is the most severe form of Niemann–Pick disease and occurs more commonly in Ashkenazi Jews than in the general population. Transient neonatal jaundice is followed by progressive hepatosplenomegaly; developmental regression and weight loss lead to dementia, hypotonia, and death by age 2 years. About one-half of patients develop macular cherry-red spots. Seizures are uncommon. Bone involvement is mild. Skin often has a brownish-yellow tinge. Most patients have diffuse haziness or patchy infiltrates in the lungs.

Diagnosis is made by the characteristic clinical picture, by demonstration of near-total deficiency of sphingomyelinase in leukocytes or cultured skin fibroblasts, and/or by demonstrating mutations in the acid sphingomyelinase gene.

Juvenile Nonneuronopathic, Type B

This form presents with asymptomatic splenomegaly or hepatosplenomegaly without neurologic disorder in infants, children, or adults, although cherry-red spots may be found. These patients have more residual sphingomyelinase (i.e., 15% to 20% of normal) than those with type A (i.e., up to 10%). ERT is currently in clinical trials for Niemann–Pick disease, type B.

Niemann–Pick Disease, Type C

Niemann–Pick disease, type C (NPC), may arise at any age from fetal life (i.e., with ascites) to the fifth or sixth decades. Early-onset disease is dominated by hepatic and pulmonary failure, which are usually lethal in infancy. Classic childhood-onset disease more often presents insidiously with school failure and clumsiness that evolve into a progressive syndrome of ataxia, dystonia, and dementia. Vertical supranuclear gaze palsy is characteristic and almost invariably presents early, although often unrecognized. About 50%

of patients have seizures, and 20% experience gelastic cataplexy. Hepatosplenomegaly is variable, and its absence does not rule out NPC. Genetic isolates have been described in Nova Scotia (i.e., formerly Niemann–Pick disease, type D) and in Hispanics in Colorado and New Mexico.

Most patients with NPC are compound heterozygotes for mutations in NPC1; the gene product is a large transmembrane protein localized to the late endosomal–lysosomal pathway. Dysfunction of this protein is associated with impaired trafficking of large molecules in this pathway, with accumulation of glycolipids, sphingomyelin, and cholesterol in lysosomes. The diagnosis rests on demonstration of this defect. Direct DNA analysis can be used as a first-line diagnostic test, but false negatives occur owing to the size of the gene and the large number of mutations (more than 300 recognized to date). The standard biochemical test requires demonstration of accumulation of free cholesterol in lysosomes, which is identified by filipin staining. This is an indirect index of the functional defect, with a significant number of variant cases with results that may be difficult to distinguish from heterozygotes. Assay of 3-β, 5-α, 6-β-cholestane triol in blood is a sensitive and specific marker of NPC and is likely to enter clinical practice as a first-line diagnostic test within the lifetime of this text. There is no approved therapy for NPC in the United Sates, although miglustat has been approved for management of its neurologic manifestations in the European Union and several other countries. Clinical trials are planned or underway for intrathecal cyclodextrin, oral vorinostat, and oral arimoclomol in NPC.

A small number of cases of NPC are associated with mutations in a second gene, *NPC2*, whose gene product is a soluble, lysosomal protein. Recent studies suggest that NPC2 interacts with NPC1 either through transfer of unesterified cholesterol, responding to oxysterol signals, or some combination of both. Hematopoietic stem cell transplantation may be helpful in this disorder.

FARBER DISEASE

Farber disease is caused by deficiency of acid ceramidase. Infants with this disease have profound reduction of enzyme activity and present with painful swollen joints, hoarseness, vomiting, respiratory difficulty, or limb edema in the first few months of life, sometimes as early as 2 weeks of age. Most patients die of pulmonary disease before age 2 years, but some survive into adolescence. Hematopoietic stem cell transplantation has produced improvement in several findings. Children with higher residual acid ceramidase activity (>10%) may present with a spinal muscular atrophy–progressive myoclonic epilepsy phenotype, distinct from that associated with SMN1 mutations.

CEREBROTENDINOUS XANTHOMATOSIS (CHOLESTANOL STORAGE DISEASE)

Patients with cerebrotendinous xanthomatosis (CTX) often have early cognitive impairment, but cataracts, tendon xanthomas, and progressive spasticity, usually associated with ataxia, commonly do not begin before adolescence or young adulthood. The spasticity and ataxia are severe and progressive. Speech is affected. Neuropathy may appear with distal muscle wasting. Sensory deficits and Babinski signs are seen. Pseudobulbar palsy develops terminally. Death from neurologic disease or myocardial infarction usually occurs in the fourth to sixth decade. Some patients have apparently normal mental function.

Tendon xanthomas are almost always seen on the Achilles tendon and may occur elsewhere. The cerebellar hemispheres contain large (i.e., up to 1.5 cm) granulomatous xanthomas with extensive demyelination. The brain stem and spinal cord may be involved.

Diagnosis is based on demonstration of elevated blood cholestanol levels and mutations in the sterol 27-hydroxylase gene (CYP27). Treatment with chenodeoxycholic acid may be beneficial.

Mucopolysaccharidoses

The MPS are defined by a characteristic phenotype and by the tissue storage and urinary excretion of acid mucopolysaccharide. They were originally considered a single disease, but eight clinical types, and numerous subtypes, are now known. Each is caused by deficiency of a lysosomal hydrolase required for degradation of one or more of three sulfated mucopolysaccharides: dermatan sulfate, heparan sulfate, and keratan sulfate.

Diagnosis is suspected based on the clinical picture, the presence of excessive amounts of one or more acid mucopolysaccharides in urine, and is confirmed by demonstrating a specific enzyme defect. Urine screening tests for excess mucopolysaccharides are useful but are subject to false-positive and false-negative results. Positive screening tests require confirmation by quantitative and qualitative determination of urinary mucopolysaccharides and demonstration of the enzyme defect. False negatives are relatively frequent in Sanfilippo and Morquio syndromes. If clinical suspicion for an MPS is high, diagnostic evaluation should be pursued, despite a negative urine screening test. Prenatal diagnosis of these disorders is available.

HURLER SYNDROME (MUCOPOLYSACCHARIDOSIS I)

This is the most severe of the MPS and is characterized by onset in infancy, progressive disability, and death usually occurring before 10 years of age. Nearly all the features found in other types are present in Hurler syndrome. Corneal clouding and lumbar gibbus occur in the first year of life, followed by stiff joints with periarticular swelling; short, stubby hands and feet; claw hands; lumbar lordosis; chest deformity; and dwarfing by 2 or 3 years of age. The facies are characteristic, with thickened eyelids and lips; frontal bossing; bushy eyebrows; a depressed nasal bridge; ocular hypertelorism; enlarged tongue; noisy breathing; rhinorrhea; and widely spaced, peg-like teeth. Psychomotor slowing is followed by dementia, but seizures are not typical. Deafness is frequent, and few patients develop speech. Leptomeningeal thickening, arachnoid cysts, and hydrocephalus may occur. Cardiac murmurs resulting from valvular heart disease, coronary occlusion, and cardiac enlargement may occur and cause death. Abdominal distention is common, with inguinal and umbilical hernias and hepatomegaly. Corneal clouding progresses and with retinal degeneration impairs vision. Cervical cord compression with quadriplegia may occur.

Radiographic changes support the diagnosis of MPS but do not reliably distinguish the various types. Findings include ovoid or beaked lumbar vertebrae, peg-shaped metacarpals, a J-shaped sella turcica, and spatulate ribs. Peripheral leukocytes and bone marrow cells contain metachromatic granules. Clear vacuoles are seen in hepatocytes and other cells. Zebra bodies containing lipids occur in the brain. Both dermatan sulfate and heparan sulfate are stored. The diagnosis is made by demonstrating severe deficiency of α-L-iduronidase in cultured skin fibroblasts and leukocytes. Mutation analysis of the α-L-iduronidase gene confirms the diagnosis and permits prenatal diagnosis.

Scheie syndrome (MPS IS), a milder allelic variant of Hurler syndrome, is characterized by juvenile onset of joint stiffness with the development of claw hands and deformed feet. A phenotype intermediate between that of the Hurler and Scheie syndromes is referred to as the *Hurler–Scheie compound* (MPS I HS).

HUNTER SYNDROME (MUCOPOLYSACCHARIDOSIS II)

Hunter syndrome includes mild and severe forms. Both are X-linked recessive and show iduronate-2-sulfatase deficiency. A Hunter-like phenocopy in girls with iduronate-2-sulfatase deficiency occurs in the context of total sulfatase deficiency (metachromatic leukodystrophy [MLD], Austin type).

Boys with the severe form experience juvenile-onset joint stiffness, typical facial features (Fig. 134.2), dysostosis multiplex, hepatosplenomegaly, diarrhea, dwarfing, and mental deterioration. Progressive deafness is prominent. Pigmentary retinal deterioration, papilledema, and hydrocephalus may be seen. Nodular or pebbled-skin change over the scapulae and absence of corneal clouding are important features distinguishing Hunter syndrome from Hurler syndrome. Patients usually die as teenagers.

Patients with the mild form of Hunter syndrome may be asymptomatic or have only mild systemic findings

SANFILIPPO SYNDROME (MUCOPOLYSACCHARIDOSIS III)

Patients with this syndrome outnumber all other forms of MPS combined. They exhibit progressive cognitive impairment, mild somatic involvement, and urinary excretion of heparan sulfate alone. Four biochemically distinct forms reflect four metabolic steps required for the degradation of heparan sulfate but not dermatan sulfate or keratan sulfate. Sanfilippo patients have juvenile-onset dementia, with delay or deterioration of speech or school performance. Children presenting with psychiatric disorder, intellectual disability, or dementia should be carefully examined for mild coarsening of facial features, hepatosplenomegaly, hirsutism, joint stiffness, and radiographic changes of dysostosis multiplex. These patients deteriorate neurologically, with progressive dementia, spastic quadriparesis, tetraballism, athetosis, incontinence, and seizures. Cardiac involvement may occur. Corneal clouding is absent. Bone changes, dwarfing, and organ enlargement are slight. Patients may die in adolescence or survive into the third decade of life.

The diagnosis is made by the characteristic clinical picture, excess heparan sulfaturia, demonstration of the specific enzyme defect, and mutations analysis. Screening tests for mucopolysacchariduria may be negative in Sanfilippo syndrome.

Mucolipidoses

The MLs resemble the Hurler phenotype but lack excess urinary mucopolysaccharide, having instead, excess urinary oligosaccharides or glycopeptides, most of which are fragments of more complex structures. Urinary thin-layer chromatography for oligosaccharides is a useful screening test.

SIALIDOSIS (MUCOLIPIDOSIS I)

Patients with sialidoses have deficiency of α-L-neuraminidase, also known as *sialidase*. In most forms, sialic acid–containing glycoproteins, oligosaccharides, and glycolipids accumulate in tissue, and sialyloligosaccharides are excreted in urine.

The diagnosis is based on clinical findings, the presence of abnormal sialyloligosaccharides in the urine, and deficiency of the appropriate sialidase in cultured skin fibroblasts, tissue, or leukocytes. There are at least two distinct lysosomal sialidases.

In addition to the isolated sialidase deficiencies, two other groups of MLs have sialidase deficiency. In one, galactosialidosis, both sialidase and β-galactosidase are deficient because a stabilizing protein they share is defective. In the second group, ML II and ML III, sialidase and several other lysosomal hydrolases are deficient owing to deficient activity of the phosphotransferase that

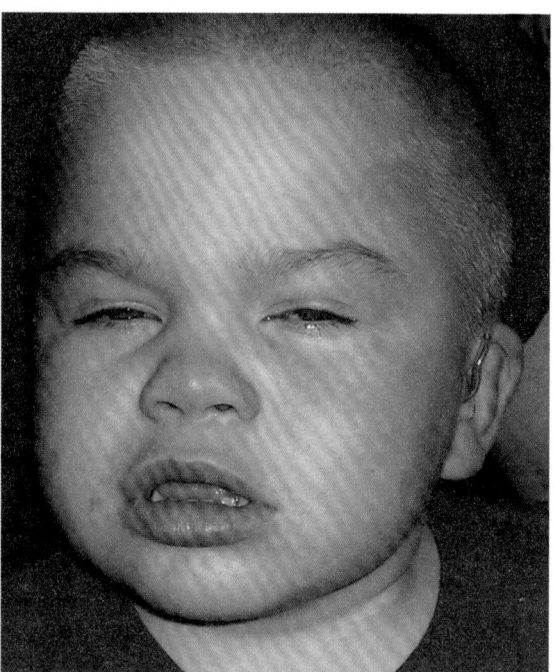

FIGURE 134.2 Mucopolysaccharidosis type II (Hunter syndrome); note periorbital fullness, increased tissue thickness of the lips and cheeks, and hearing aid.

is responsible for creating the mannose-6-phosphate motif that targets enzymes to the lysosome.

Sialidoses with isolated sialidase deficiency have a highly variable clinical picture. Neonates with congenital sialidoses have hydrops fetalis, hepatosplenomegaly, and short survival times. Infants with nephrosialidosis resemble the Hurler phenotype and develop macular cherry-red spots and renal disease. Children with ML I (i.e., lipomucopolysaccharidosis), a milder disorder, are similarly affected but develop ataxia, myoclonic jerks, and seizures. The mildest form is the cherry-red spot myoclonus disorder, in which adolescents, who are usually mentally normal, develop macular cherry-red spots, myoclonus, and myoclonic seizures. There is a predilection for individuals of Italian descent.

MUCOLIPIDOSES II AND III

ML II, or I cell disease, and ML III, or pseudo-Hurler polydystrophy, are allelic disorders associated with deficiency of the enzyme, glycoprotein *N*-acetylglucosaminyl phosphotransferase, whose activity is required for mannose-6-phosphate targeting of glycoproteins, including many lysosomal hydrolases, to the lysosome.

ML II is a severe disorder that resembles Hurler syndrome without corneal clouding. Cultured fibroblasts contain coarse inclusions (I cells). Diagnosis is made by finding excess sialo-oligosaccharides in the urine and deficiencies of multiple lysosomal enzymes in cultured skin fibroblasts, with elevated levels of these enzymes in plasma. In brain and viscera, only β-galactosidase is consistently deficient.

ML III is a milder clinical disorder than ML II that may present with joint stiffness, carpal tunnel syndrome, or mild intellectual impairment.

MUCOLIPIDOSIS IV

Patients with ML IV present with corneal clouding as early as 6 weeks of age. Mild retardation progresses to severe mental and motor defect. The disease occurs almost exclusively in Ashkenazi Jews. Achlorhydria is universal, and measurement of elevated serum gastrin levels is a convenient and reliable screening test for ML IV. Diagnosis may now be made by mutation analysis of the MCOLN 1 gene, which codes for mucolipin, a protein that may function in cation channels and in membrane trafficking in the endosomal–lysosomal system.

Neuronal Ceroid Lipofuscinoses

The neuronal ceroid lipofuscinoses (NCLs) are a family of lysosomal diseases characterized by varying degrees of progressive dementia, epilepsy, and visual impairment associated with retinal pigmentation and profound cortical atrophy. They were previously defined by histologic and ultrastructural features and a plethora of confusing and inconsistently applied eponyms, but are now classified according to genotypes. The common pathologic features include neurons engorged with periodic acid–Schiff (PAS)–positive and autofluorescent material on light microscopy and typical profiles, including granular osmiophilic deposits, curvilinear and fingerprint bodies (or combinations of these), on electron microscopy. Although the signs and symptoms are confined to the nervous system, the abnormal cytosomes are widely distributed in skin, muscle, peripheral nerves, leukocytes, urine sediment, and viscera.

Thirteen genes have been associated with 14 NCL loci; the gene associated with one locus (CLN9) has not yet been identified. All are autosomal recessive, except for the Parry form of adult NCL, which is associated with dominant mutations in DNAJC5. Some phenotypes may be associated with mutations in several genes (such as adult NCL, associated with mutations in CTSD, PPT1, CLN3, CLN5, CLN6, CTSF, and GRN) and some genes may cause several different phenotypes, such as PPTI, which is associated with infantile, late-infantile, and juvenile NCL.

The diagnosis of PPT1-, TPP1-, and CTSD-deficient forms of NCL may be made by enzyme assay and confirmed by mutational analysis. A database listing NCL mutations is available online at http://www.ucl.ac.uk/ncl/mutation.shtml.

Supporting investigations include an abnormal electroretinogram in the infantile, late-infantile, and juvenile forms and electron microscopic examination of tissue (i.e., skin, nerve, muscle, or rectal biopsy for autonomic neurons). Abnormal autofluorescence is seen on examination of frozen section of biopsied muscle, enabling rapid diagnosis.

The most frequent phenotypes are late infantile (NCL2) and juvenile (NCL3). The former presents between 2 and 4 years with seizures, associated with developmental regression, ataxia, myoclonus, and spasticity. Retinal degeneration occurs later in the course and eventually leads to blindness.

Juvenile NCL begins in the latter half of the first decade with progressive loss of vision and later onset of epilepsy. Patients may survive into the fourth decade.

Leukodystrophies

The leukodystrophies are progressive, genetic metabolic disorders causing dysmyelination, in contrast to leukoencephalopathies that are often acquired.

Disorders such as Krabbe disease, MLD, adrenoleukodystrophy (ALD) (discussed with other peroxisomal disorders), Alexander disease, and classic Pelizaeus–Merzbacher disease were defined by traditional clinical and pathologic investigations. Careful clinical and MR phenotyping combined with molecular biology have led to the identification of a variety of additional leukodystrophies, including childhood ataxia with central hypomyelination or CACH (also known as *vanishing white matter disease*), and megalencephalic leukoencephalopathy with subcortical cysts (MLC), hypomyelination of the basal ganglia and cerebellum (H-ABC), oculodentodigital dysplasia (ODDD), and leukoencephalopathy involving the brain stem and spinal cord with lactate elevation (LBSL). This leaves a heterogeneous, but shrinking group, of unclassified leukodystrophies, sometimes called *orthochromatic* or *sudanophilic leukodystrophies*. Diffuse sclerosis (Schilder disease) is included in this chapter, although it resembles multiple sclerosis more than traditional leukodystrophies.

METACHROMATIC LEUKODYSTROPHY

MLD is a group of autosomal recessive disorders with degeneration of central and peripheral myelin, striking metachromasia of the stored substances, primarily sulfatides, and deficiency of the sulfatide-cleaving enzyme, sulfatase A, also called *arylsulfatase A*. Late-infantile–onset disease is most common.

The diagnosis of MLD is complicated by the existence of sulfatase A pseudodeficiency, an autosomal recessive condition in which sulfatase A activity is greatly diminished by the usual enzyme assays, but there is no neurologic disease. An additional complication is the requirement of sulfatase A for the sulfatide-activator protein. Patients with genetic deficiency of sulfatide-activator protein may have MLD, but the commonly used enzyme assays may fail to diagnose normal.

Late-Infantile Metachromatic Leukodystrophy

Affected infants have onset of difficulty in walking after the first year of life, usually between ages 12 and 30 months. Flaccid paresis and diminished, or absent, tendon reflexes are typical, but occasionally, spastic paresis develops. Genu recurvatum, hyperextension of the knee, may be noted. Progressive dementia and dysarthria follow.

Peripheral neuropathy leads to loss of tendon reflexes and may be accompanied by limb pain. Later, patients become bedridden and quadriplegic, with feeding difficulties, bulbar and pseudobulbar palsies, and optic atrophy. Children so affected usually die in the first decade of life, blind and in a vegetative state. Investigations show increased CSF protein content, impaired gallbladder function, metachromatic lipids on sural nerve biopsy, and increased urinary-sulfatide excretion.

Sulfatide accumulates in brain, peripheral nerves, and some extraneural tissues (e.g., kidney). Sulfatide causes brown metachromasia, with acetic acid-cresyl violet staining in glial cells, Schwann cells, myelin lamellae, and neurons. Characteristic "tuffstone" bodies are seen by electron microscopy.

The diagnosis is based primarily on enzyme analysis, supported by ARSA gene sequencing.

Late-onset Metachromatic Leukodystrophy

Juvenile MLD patients resemble those with late-infantile MLD but for the later onset of symptoms (i.e., usually ages 3 to 10 years) and slower progression of the disease. Emotional disturbance and dementia are more common presentations, although gait disorder may be the initial symptom. Nystagmus and tremor may be noted. Nerve conduction velocities are slowed and CSF protein concentrations are elevated. The diagnosis can usually be suspected from MRI of the brain, which shows diffuse, confluent

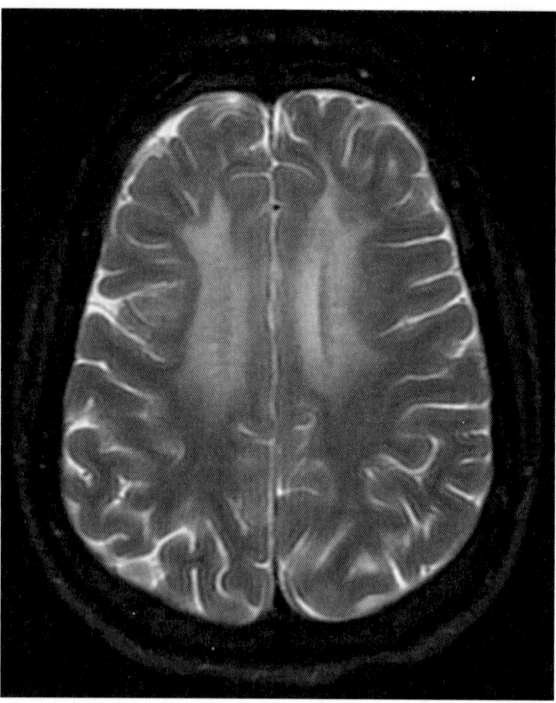

FIGURE 134.3 Axial T2-weighted MRI of an 18-year-old with metachromatic leukodystrophy, illustrating the characteristic "tigroid" appearance of the white matter.

signal hyperintensity in the white matter of the centra semiovale, with a striated "tigroid" appearance (Fig. 134.3).

MLD commonly starts in adults in the third or fourth decade as a psychiatric disorder (mimicking schizophrenia) or progressive dementia. Other findings may include truncal ataxia, hyperactive reflexes, and seizures. Both psychiatric and motor manifestations may coexist in association with certain mutations. CSF protein concentration is usually not elevated. The illness runs a protracted course, averaging 15 years.

KRABBE (GLOBOID CELL) LEUKODYSTROPHY

Patients are normal at birth but may have subtle findings such as fisting in the first few weeks. At 3 to 6 months, irritability, inexplicable crying, fevers, rigidity, seizures, feeding difficulty, vomiting, and slowing of mental and motor development occur. Later, psychomotor regression occurs, accompanied by increasing tone and extensor posturing. Reflexes may be increased before being lost. Optic atrophy is frequent. Patients may develop flaccidity or flexor postures before death, at about 2 years of age.

CSF protein is increased and nerve conduction velocities are slowed. Galactocerebrosidase activity is deficient in serum, leukocytes, and cultured skin fibroblasts. Psychosine, a substrate for this enzyme, is increased at least 200-fold over levels in the normal brain. Psychosine toxicity is probably the cause of the disease, based on studies showing its ability to produce characteristic lesions in animal models.

A few patients with juvenile-onset and slower progression of dementia, optic atrophy, and pyramidal tract signs, without neuropathy, have had galactocerebrosidase deficiency. An adult-onset disorder with a similar but more slowly progressive course has been described.

Hematopoietic stem cell transplantation in the first 3 weeks of life is effective in prolonging life in infants with early infantile

Krabbe disease, although many such children have significant neurologic disabilities. The availability of this therapy has led to the implementation of newborn screening for Krabbe disease in New York and other states.

ALEXANDER DISEASE

Alexander disease is an autosomal dominant progressive leukodystrophy associated with mutations in the GFAP gene that encodes glial fibrillary acidic protein. As such, it is a primary disorder of astrocytes, in contrast to other leukodystrophies, in which the major affected cell type is the oligodendrocyte. The classic presentation occurs in infants, who manifest macrocephaly, developmental regression, seizures, and progressive spasticity. MRI shows a pattern of frontal predominant white matter hyperintensity, sometimes with cavitation, with periventricular hyperintensity with or without enhancement and "garlands" and increased signal in the medulla, middle cerebellar peduncles, and long tracts, with or without atrophy (particularly in later onset cases) (Figs. 134.4 and 134.5). Some patients develop hydrocephalus secondary to compression of the aqueduct of Sylvius by swollen midbrain astrocytes. The affected areas show accumulation of Rosenthal fibers.

In adolescents and adults, Alexander disease is much less likely to be associated with macrocephaly and may be manifest as cognitive and emotional disturbance, with relatively mild long tract signs or ataxia; persistent vomiting may be prominent. Oculopalatal myoclonus has been described as a classical finding in such patients but is often absent. The anatomic and clinical patterns overlap with neuromyelitis optica (NMO), which is an acquired disorder of astrocytes, in which antibodies are directed at aquaporin, expressed in water channels in astrocytes.

There is no disease-modifying therapy available for Alexander disease, but given its prolonged course, particularly in later onset forms, vigorous supportive treatment is strongly encouraged.

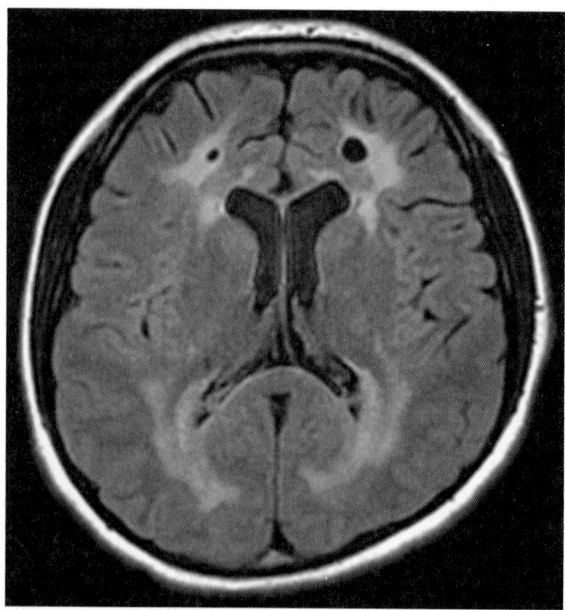

FIGURE 134.4 Axial T2 fluid-attenuated inversion recovery (FLAIR) MRI of a 12-year-old with Alexander disease showing frontal predominant white matter hyperintensity with cavitation and periventricular hyperintensity.

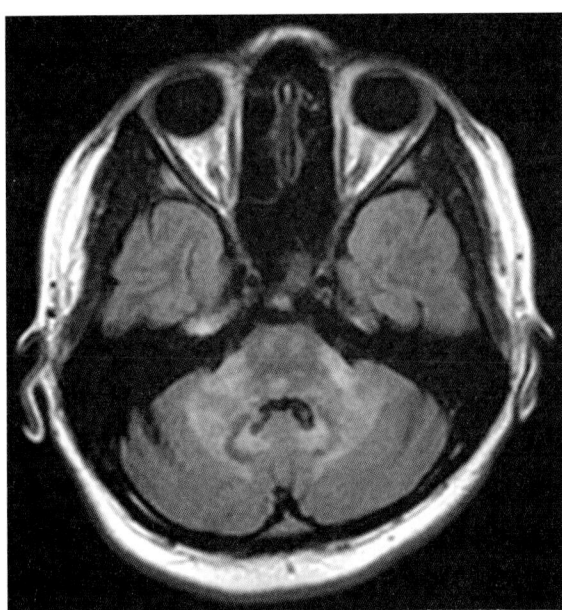

FIGURE 134.5 Axial T2 FLAIR MRI of a 12-year-old with Alexander disease showing increased signal in the medulla, middle cerebellar peduncles, and long tracts.

PELIZAEUS–MERZBACHER DISEASE

Pelizaeus–Merzbacher disease (PMD) is an X-linked hypomyelinating disorder associated with duplications, deletions, and point mutations in the gene encoding central proteolipid protein (PLP1). Infantile forms of the disease present with profound hypotonia and unusual pendular nystagmus with gray optic discs. The most severely affected infants do not develop further and succumb to their illness in the first few years of life, but some boys make developmental gains and survive into the second decade, although they rarely walk or talk. In those who survive into childhood, intellectual disability, progressive ataxia, spasticity, and choreoathetosis are often observed. The MRI in PMD shows profound hypomyelination with reduced white matter volume. Some patients with mild mutations in PLP1 have a slowly progressive spastic paraplegia classified as SPG2. There is no established therapy for PMD, but a trial of human CNS stem cells implanted into the cerebral hemispheres is currently in progress.

A number of families, who lack mutations in PLP1, have been recognized with a PMD-like illness. Recessive mutations in GJA12/GJC2, which encodes a protein essential in gap junction formation in myelin, have been identified in some such families; TUBB4A mutations have been identified in another case mimicking PMD.

VANISHING WHITE MATTER DISEASE

In 1994, Schiffmann and colleagues described four girls with progressive ataxic diplegia, whose imaging studies showed confluent white matter disease early in the course of the illness; the peripheral nerves and intellect were spared, and extensive investigation for previously described leukodystrophies was uninformative. Biopsy specimens showed hypomyelination, demyelination, and gliosis and reduced quantities but qualitatively normal lipids. MR spectroscopy showed reduced NAA, choline, and creatine restricted to the white matter. They named this disorder *childhood ataxia with central hypomyelination*. A year earlier, Hanefeld et al. had described three children with identical features, whose disease they named *myelinopathia centralis diffusa* (MCD).

In 1997, van der Knaap's group described nine more patients with this phenotype. They emphasized the unusual combination of slowly progressive ataxia with episodic decompensation in the face of minor trauma (motor change) or intercurrent infection (coma). They also recognized that the white matter signal eventually disappeared to be replaced by CSF intensity signal. The latter was found to correspond to extensive cystic degeneration of the cerebral white matter with preserved cortex in an autopsied case. Subsequent studies have emphasized the relative preservation of oligodendrocytes with abundant foamy cytoplasm and scarcity of astrocytes as the specific neuropathologic hallmark of the disease.

van der Knaap's descriptive term, *vanishing white matter disease* (VWM), which emphasizes the most dramatic aspect of this illness, has subsequently dominated the literature. MCD was never widely accepted, but CACH is still encountered, most often in tandem with VWM.

VWM is caused by mutations in any one of the genes coding for the subunits of the eukaryotic translation initiation factor 2 b (eIF2B); VWM is the first disease recognized that is associated with mutations in a translation factor. eIF2B is the major regulator of protein synthesis under conditions of mild stress, such as temperatures up to 41°C. The gene is expressed in all tissues, yet VWM is restricted to the cranial white matter. In vitro studies of VWM brain have shown that all three pathways of the unfolded protein response are inappropriately activated but only in white matter. This remarkable specificity remains unexplained, as is the case for other disorders involving mutations of DNA housekeeping machinery that are expressed in specific regions of the nervous systems, such as spinal muscular atrophy.

As has proven to be the case in other inborn errors of metabolism, the appearance and use of a diagnostic test for VWM has been followed by the recognition of a broader range of phenotypes than those originally described. Thus, Cree leukoencephalopathy and ovarioleukodystrophy have both been shown to be associated with mutations in eIF2B. The former is an autosomal recessive leukodystrophy, lethal in the first 2 years, that is observed in the native North American Cree and Chippewayan population where high rates of consanguinity prevail. Death in the context of a common viral infection may be the presenting feature. The latter phenotype can be associated with either primary or secondary amenorrhea and a more indolent neurologic course, with variable dementia, gait ataxia, sphincter dysfunction, optic atrophy, and episodic decompensation. Other unusual features have been reported, including marked macrocephaly in a child with survival into the third decade, adult presentation with psychosis, and precipitation of symptoms after being frightened by a horse.

Despite the availability of DNA diagnostic testing, confirmation of the diagnosis may be technically difficult because VWM can result from mutations in any of the five genes coding for subunits of eIF2B and because there is a high frequency of private and low-frequency mutations in the cases described to date.

There is, as yet, no specific treatment for VWM. Avoidance of the precipitating factors is obviously advisable but difficult to accomplish in practice, given the propensity of children to bump their heads and catch colds.

DIFFUSE SCLEROSIS

Schilder described new syndromes of diffuse demyelination of the brain in 1912, 1913, and 1924. Later advances identified the 1913 description as one of ALD, and the 1924 patient had subacute sclerosing panencephalitis. Nevertheless, the 1912 case delineated a clinical and pathologic syndrome that is still seen, even though cases of uncomplicated diffuse sclerosis are so few that each encounter results in a case report. In 1994, Afifi and colleagues counted 12 cases since 1912; Yilmaz and others added 16 more between 1998 and 2008.

Schilder disease was and is regarded as a variant of multiple sclerosis, but the etiology and pathogenesis are not known.

At autopsy, there are large areas of demyelination in the centrum ovale, with relative preservation of axons. Subcortical U-fibers are often spared. In acute lesions, there is perivascular infiltration by CD45-positive lymphocytes and giant cells; there may be necrosis. The lesions are similar to those of multiple sclerosis. In fact, in most cases that include large areas of demyelination, there are also smaller, more typical lesions of multiple sclerosis. For these cases, the term *transitional sclerosis* has been used. It is assumed that the small lesions coalesce to form the large ones. The demyelinating lesions contain CD68-positive macrophages and GFAP-positive astrocytes with long processes.

The clinical syndrome is a leukoencephalopathy, with progressive dementia, psychosis, corticospinal signs, and loss of vision caused by either optic neuritis with papilledema or cerebral blindness. Brain stem signs may include nystagmus and internuclear ophthalmoplegia. The disease is relentlessly progressive, with average survival of about 6 years but sometimes as long as 45 years.

Diagnosis depends on imaging; MRI shows gadolinium enhancement of large white matter lesions. There may be CSF pleocytosis with evidence of intrathecal synthesis of gamma globulin and oligoclonal bands. Brain biopsy may be needed to identify the few cases that simulate mass lesions.

Steroid therapy was followed by complete resolution of lesions or only minor sequelae in 10 of 16 cases reported in the decade up to 2008 (Yilmaz et al.); 9 cases subsequently recurred. Intravenous immunoglobulin has been used successfully; surgical resection is occasionally required to manage herniation complicating a large lesion.

DISORDERS OF CARBOHYDRATE METABOLISM

Glycogen Storage Diseases

Abnormal metabolism of glycogen and glucose may occur in a series of genetically determined disorders, each representing a specific enzyme deficiency (Table 134.5). The signs and symptoms of each disease are largely determined by the tissues in which the enzyme defect is expressed. Virtually all enzymes of glycogen metabolism, including tissue-specific isoforms or subunits, have been assigned to chromosomal loci and the corresponding genes have been cloned and sequenced. Numerous mutations have been identified and genotype–phenotype correlation is taking shape.

Severe fasting hypoglycemia may result in periodic episodes of lethargy, coma, convulsions, and anoxic brain damage in *glucose-6-phosphatase deficiency (glycogenosis type I)* or in *glycogen synthetase deficiency*. The liver is enlarged in both diseases. Clinical manifestations tend to become milder in patients who survive the first few years of life.

The CNS is directly affected by the enzyme defect in generalized glycogen storage diseases, even though neurologic symptoms are lacking in some disorders and in others, it may be ascribed to liver rather than to brain dysfunction. The following enzyme defects seem to be generalized: acid maltase (type II), debrancher (type III), brancher (type IV), and phosphoglycerate kinase (type IX).

Acid maltase (acid α-1,4 and α-1,6 glucosidase) deficiency is a lysosomal disorder due to mutations in the *GAA* gene on chromosome 17. In the infantile form of acid maltase deficiency (Pompe disease), pathologic involvement of the CNS has been documented, with accumulation of both free and intralysosomal glycogen in all cells, especially spinal motor neurons and neurons of the brain stem nuclei. Peripheral nerve biopsy specimens show accumulation of glycogen in Schwann cells. The profound generalized weakness of infants with Pompe disease is probably due to combined effects of glycogen storage in muscle, anterior horn cells, and peripheral nerves. In four patients with the childhood form of acid maltase deficiency, increased glycogen deposition in neurons of the brain stem was related to fatal intractable hyperpyrexia. No morphologic changes were seen in the CNS of a patient with adult-onset acid maltase deficiency despite marked decrease of enzyme activity. However, the enzyme defect predisposes to dilative arteriopathy and cerebral aneurysm formation, sometimes leading to stroke.

Patients with debrancher deficiency (glycogenosis type III, due to mutations in the *AGL* gene on chromosome 1) have hepatomegaly, fasting hypoglycemia, and seizures in infancy and childhood, which usually remit around puberty. Although overt signs of peripheral neuropathy are rare, abnormal deposits of glycogen have been documented both in axons and in Schwann cells and may explain, in part at least, the distal wasting and mixed EMG pattern observed in adult patients with neuromuscular involvement.

In branching enzyme deficiency (glycogenosis type IV, due to mutations in the *GBE1* gene on chromosome 3), the clinical picture is typically dominated by liver disease, with progressive cirrhosis and chronic hepatic failure causing death in childhood. However, the neuromuscular system is involved more often than it was previously realized, with congenital, juvenile, or adult presentations. The severe congenital myopathy, sometime associated with cardiomyopathy, may simulate spinal muscular atrophy type I (Werdnig–Hoffmann disease). Deposits of a basophilic, intensely PAS-positive material that is partially resistant to β-amylase digestion (polyglucosan) have been found in all tissues; in the CNS, spheroids composed of branched filaments were present in astrocytic processes, particularly in the spinal cord and medulla. Ultrastructurally, the storage material was composed of aggregates of branched osmiophilic filaments, 6 nm in diameter often surrounded by normal glycogen particles.

In phosphoglycerate kinase deficiency (glycogenosis type IX, due to mutations in the *PGK1* on the X chromosome), the type and severity of clinical manifestations vary in different genetic variants of the disease and are probably related to the severity of the enzyme defect in different tissues. In several families, the clinical picture was characterized by the association of severe hemolytic anemia, with intellectual disability and seizures.

LAFORA DISEASE AND OTHER POLYGLUCOSAN STORAGE DISEASES

Myoclonus epilepsy with Lafora bodies (Lafora disease) is an autosomal recessive disease that is characterized by the triad of epilepsy, myoclonus, and dementia. Inconstant other neurologic manifestations include ataxia, dysarthria, spasticity, and rigidity. Onset is in adolescence, and the course progresses rapidly to death, which occurs between 17 and 24 years in 90% of patients. Negative criteria or manifestations that imply some other disease include onset before 6 or after age 20 years, optic atrophy, macular degeneration, prolonged course, or normal intelligence. Epilepsy, with predominantly occipital seizures, is the first manifestation in

TABLE 134.5 Classification of Glycogen Storage Disease

Type	Affected Tissues	Clinical Presentation	Glycogen Structure	Enzyme Defect	Mode of Transmission
I	Liver and kidney	Severe hypoglycemia; hepatomegaly	Normal	Glucose-6-phosphatase	AR
II	—	—	—	—	—
Infancy	Generalized	Cardiomegaly; weakness; hypotonia; death younger than age 1 yr	Normal	—	AR
Childhood	Generalized	Myopathy-simulating Duchenne dystrophy; respiratory insufficiency	Normal	Acid maltase	AR
Adult	Generalized	Myopathy-simulating limb-girdle dystrophy or polymyositis; respiratory insufficiency	Normal	—	AR
III	Generalized	Hepatomegaly; fasting hypoglycemia; progressive weakness	PLD	Debrancher	AR
IV	Generalized	Hepatosplenomegaly; cirrhosis of liver; neuromuscular disease; APBD	Polyglucosan	Brancher	AR
V	Skeletal muscle	Intolerance to intense exercise; cramps; myoglobinuria	Normal	Muscle phosphorylase	AR
VI	Liver; RBC	Mild hypoglycemia; hepatomegaly	Normal	Liver phosphorylase	AR
VII	Skeletal muscle; RBC	Intolerance to intense exercise; cramps; myoglobinuria	Normal (± polyglucosan)	PFK-M	AR
VIII	Liver	Asymptomatic hepatomegaly	Normal	Phosphorylase kinase	XR
—	Liver and skeletal muscle	Hepatomegaly; growth retardation; hypotonia	Normal	Phosphorylase kinase	AR
—	Skeletal muscle	Exercise intolerance; myoglobinuria	Normal	Phosphorylase kinase	XR; AR (?)
—	Heart	Fatal infantile cardiomyopathy	Normal	Phosphorylase kinase	AR
IX	Generalized	Hemolytic anemia; seizures; mental retardation	Normal (?)	PKG	XR
—	—	Intolerance to intense exercise; myoglobinuria	—		
X	Skeletal muscle	Intolerance to intense exercise; myoglobinuria	Normal (?)	PGAM-M	AR
XI	Skeletal muscle	Intolerance to intense exercise; myoglobinuria	Normal (?)	LDH-M	AR
XII	Skeletal muscle RBC	Exercise intolerance	Normal (?)	Aldolase A	AR
XIII	Skeletal muscle	Exercise intolerance	Normal (?)	β-Enolase	AR
—	Generalized	Myoclonus epilepsy (Lafora disease)	Polyglucosan	Laforin	AR
0	Muscle	Cardiomyopathy; exercise intolerance	Glycogen deficiency	Glycogen synthetase	AR

?, not yet definitively documented; AR, autosomal recessive; PLD, phosphorylase-limit dextrin; APBD, adult polyglucosan body disease; RBC, red blood cell; PFK-M, muscle phosphofructokinase; XR, X-linked recessive; PKG, phosphoglycerate kinase; PGAM-M, muscle phosphoglycerate mutase; LDH-M, muscle lactate dehydrogenase.

most patients; status epilepticus is common in terminal stages. Myoclonus usually appears 2 or 3 years after the onset of epilepsy, may affect any area of the body, is sensitive to startle, and is absent during sleep. Intellectual deterioration generally follows the appearance of seizures by 2 or 3 years and progresses rapidly to severe dementia. Therapy is symptomatic and is designed to suppress seizures and reduce the severity of myoclonus; some control of myoclonus is achieved with benzodiazepines.

Laboratory findings are normal except for EEG changes; bilaterally synchronous discharges of wave-and-spike formations are commonly seen in association with myoclonic jerks. EEG abnormalities may be found in asymptomatic relatives. The pathologic hallmark of the disease is the presence in the CNS of the bodies first described by Lafora in 1911: round, basophilic, strongly PAS-positive intracellular inclusions that vary in size from dust-like bodies less than 3 nm in diameter to large bodies up to

30 nm in diameter. The medium and large bodies often show a dense core and a lighter periphery. Lafora bodies are seen only in neuronal perikarya and processes and are most numerous in cerebral cortex, substantia nigra, thalamus, globus pallidus, and dentate nucleus.

Ultrastructurally, Lafora bodies are not membrane bound. They consist of two components in various proportions: amorphous, electron-dense granules and irregular filaments. The filaments, which are about 6 nm in diameter, are often branched and frequently continuous with the granular material.

Irregular accumulations of a material similar to that of the Lafora bodies are found in liver, heart, skeletal muscle, skin, and retina, suggesting that Lafora disease is a generalized storage disease. Both histochemical and biochemical criteria indicate that the storage material is a branched polysaccharide composed of glucose (polyglucosan) similar to the amylopectin-like polysaccharide that accumulates in branching enzyme deficiency. The activity of branching enzyme, however, was normal in several tissues, including brain, of patients with Lafora disease. About half of the cases of Lafora disease are due to mutations in the *EPM2A* gene, which encodes laforin, a member of the dual-specificity protein phosphatase family that additionally contains a glycogen-binding domain. Lafora disease is genetically heterogeneous, and pathogenic mutations have been identified in a second gene, *EPM2B*, which encodes an E3 ubiquitin ligase called *malin*. Laforin and malin act cooperatively to mediate polyglucosan degradation; the laforin–malin complex also protects against endoplasmic reticulum stress-induced apoptosis. Although over 100 mutations have been identified in these two genes, not all patients have mutations in either one, and there is good evidence for involvement of yet a third gene.

A clinically distinct form of polyglucosan body disease (*adult polyglucosan body disease* or *APBD*) occurs in patients with a complex but stereotyped chronic neurologic disorder characterized by progressive upper and lower motor neuron involvement, sensory loss, sphincter problems, neurogenic bladder, and in about half of the cases, dementia; there is no myoclonus or epilepsy. Onset is in the fifth or sixth decade of life, and the course ranges from 3 to 20 years. Electrophysiologic studies show axonal neuropathy. In some cases, the clinical picture simulates amyotrophic lateral sclerosis. Throughout the CNS, polyglucosan bodies are present in processes of neurons and astrocytes but not in perikarya. There are also polyglucosan accumulations in peripheral nerve and in other tissues, including liver, heart, and skeletal and smooth muscle. As in debranching enzyme deficiency and Lafora disease, the abnormal polysaccharide in APBD seems to have longer peripheral chains than normal glycogen. Branching enzyme activity was significantly decreased in leukocytes from Israeli patients, and this finding was confirmed in both leukocytes and peripheral nerve specimens from American Ashkenazi Jewish patients. Mutations in the gene encoding the branching enzyme (*GBE1*) have been found in both Ashkenazi Jewish families with APBD and in non-Jewish patients, confirming that APBD is a clinical variant of branching deficiency. The observation that APBD is often associated with "mild" *GBE1* mutations or even heterozygous mutations may explain the late onset of symptoms.

Another form of polyglucosan is in *corpora amylacea*, which accumulate progressively and nonspecifically with age. They are more commonly seen within astrocytic processes in the hippocampus and in subpial and subependymal regions; however, they also occur in intramuscular nerves in patients older than 40 years.

PEROXISOMAL DISEASES: ADRENOLEUKODYSTROPHY, ZELLWEGER SYNDROME, AND REFSUM DISEASE

Peroxisomes are ubiquitous cellular organelles that participate in a variety of essential biochemical functions. Peroxisomes are enclosed by a single membrane and contain no DNA, implying that all peroxisomal-associated proteins are encoded by nuclear genes. A complex shuttle system transports peroxisomal enzymes and structural proteins from the cytosolic polyribosomes (where they are made) to the peroxisome. This system involves at least two recognition sequences (peroxisomal targeting sequences) that are embedded in the protein products themselves and several receptors or transporters; the system is ATP dependent.

Peroxisomes participate in both anabolic and catabolic cellular functions, especially in the metabolism of lipids. For example, peroxisomes contain a complete series of enzymes for the β-oxidation of fatty acids. These enzymes are distinct from the mitochondrial enzymes of β-oxidation in both genetic coding and substrate specificity. Because mitochondrial enzymes of β-oxidation cannot metabolize carbon chain lengths greater than 24, the peroxisomal system is required for the degradation of endogenous and exogenous very long-chain fatty acids (VLCFA). The peroxisome is also the site of the initial and rate-limiting steps of the synthesis of plasmalogens, ether-linked lipids that constitute the major portion of the myelin sheath. Other key functions include cholesterol and bile acid biosynthesis, degradation of pipecolic and phytanic acids, and transamination of glyoxylate.

Human diseases caused by disruption of peroxisome function are divided into two broad categories (Table 134.6). The first category is characterized by abnormalities in more than one metabolic pathway, often accompanied by morphologic changes of the peroxisome. The prototype of this class is the Zellweger syndrome, discussed in the following paragraphs. Milder phenotypes in the Zellweger spectrum include neonatal ALD, infantile Refsum disease, and hyperpipecolic acidemia. A second phenotype, distinct from the Zellweger spectrum and termed *rhizomelic*

TABLE 134.6	Human Genetic Diseases due to Peroxisomal Dysfunction
Peroxisomal Biogenesis Disorders	**Single Peroxisomal Enzyme Disorders**
Zellweger syndrome	X-linked adrenoleukodystrophy
Neonatal adrenoleukodystrophy	Oxidase deficiency (pseudoneonatal adrenoleukodystrophy)
Infantile Refsum disease	Bifunctional enzyme deficiency
Hyperpipecolic acidemia	Thiolase deficiency (pseudo-Zellweger)
Rhizomelic chondrodysplasia punctate	DHAP acyl transferase deficiency
	Alky1 DHAP synthase deficiency
	Glutaric aciduria type III (one case only)
	Refsum disease
	Hyperoxaluria type 1
	Acatalasia

DHAP, dihydroxyacetone phosphate.

chondrodysplasia punctata (RCDP), is associated with severe growth failure, profound developmental delay, cataracts, rhizomelia (disproportionate length of proximal limbs, such as short limbs of achondroplasia), epiphyseal calcifications, and ichthyosis. Patients with RCDP have decreased plasmalogen levels and elevated phytanic acid, but unlike the Zellweger spectrum, the β-oxidation pathway and VLCFA levels are normal. In recognition of the similar cellular pathophysiology in these phenotypes, *peroxisome biogenesis disorder* (PBD) is now the preferred term for all Zellweger spectrum and RCDP conditions.

The second class of human peroxisomal diseases shows the genetic and biochemical features of single enzyme defects. In addition to X-linked ALD and Refsum disease discussed later in this chapter, this category includes defects in the β-oxidation pathway of VLCFA, which cause a Zellweger-like phenotype, and defects in plasmalogen synthesis, which result in an RCDP-like phenotype.

Zellweger Syndrome

The Zellweger syndrome (*cerebrohepatorenal syndrome*) is an autosomal recessive disease with no ethnic or racial predilection. It results from mutations in any one of a large number of genes named *pexins*, whose gene products are required for normal peroxisome assembly. Affected newborns are strikingly floppy and inactive and lack neonatal reflexes. The characteristic facies includes a high narrow forehead, round cheeks, flat root of the nose, wide-set eyes with shallow orbits, puffy eyelids, pursed lips, narrow high-arched palate, and small chin. The head circumference is normal, but the fontanels and sutures are wide open. Eye findings include pigmentary retinopathy, retinal arteriolar attenuation, and optic atrophy. The pinnas may be abnormal and posteriorly rotated. Affected infants suck and swallow poorly and often require tube feeding. Some have congenital heart disease, notably patent ductus arteriosus or septal defects. The liver is cirrhotic and either enlarged or shrunken; some children are jaundiced, and some develop splenomegaly and a bleeding diathesis. Cystic dysplasia of the kidneys may be palpable and may cause mild renal failure. Genital anomalies include an enlarged clitoris, hypospadias, and cryptorchidism. Minor skeletal anomalies include contractures of large and small joints, polydactyly, low-set rotated thumbs, and clubfeet; there are also stippled calcifications of the patella and epiphyseal cartilage. The children are apathetic, poorly responsive to environmental stimuli, and limp. Tendon reflexes are absent or hypoactive. Many children have seizures and fail to thrive or develop; most succumb within the first few months of life.

Typical but nonspecific laboratory findings include elevated bilirubin levels, abnormal liver enzymes, elevated serum iron, saturated iron-binding capacity, and transferrin. The CSF protein content may be elevated. The EEG is abnormal, and MRI shows poor myelination, brain atrophy, pachygyria, polymicrogyria, and neuronal heterotopias. Diffusion-weighted and tensor-diffusion MRI identify regions of injury in patients with PBD that are not apparent with conventional MRI.

The hallmark of Zellweger syndrome is dysfunction in multiple enzymatic pathways, including the following:

1. Levels of VLCFA—those with 24 or more carbons—are increased in plasma, fibroblasts, and chorionic villus;
2. In plasma and urine, increased content of intermediates of bile acid metabolism includes trihydroxycholestanoic acid and dihydroxycholestanoic acid;
3. Levels of pipecolic and phytanic acids increase;
4. Plasmalogen levels decrease.

Pathologically, the absence of functional peroxisomes in hepatocytes is a pathognomonic feature of Zellweger syndrome and one that helps distinguish it from other PBDs and from single enzyme disorders such as pseudo-Zellweger disease. Membrane proteins may assemble with membrane lipids to form rudimentary "ghosts" of peroxisomes that seem unable to import enzymes. Secondary abnormalities are also seen in mitochondria that show an abnormally dense matrix and distorted cristae.

Therapy for Zellweger syndrome is primarily supportive and limited because of the multisystem impairment already present at birth. Reliable prenatal diagnosis is available by mutation analysis when the genotype has been established in the proband.

Adrenoleukodystrophy

ALD is an X-linked incompletely recessive disorder with variable expressivity; it is well defined genetically, clinically, and pathologically. The ALD gene has been cloned and encodes a member of the ATP-binding cassette transporter class of proteins (ABCD1). The most common phenotype is the childhood cerebral form, which appears in boys who have normal early development. Behavioral change is the most common initial feature, with abnormal withdrawal, aggression, poor memory, or difficulties in school, ultimately evolving into progressive dementia. Visual loss with optic atrophy reflects demyelination along the entire visual pathway. The outer retina is notably spared. Progressive gait disturbance with pyramidal tract signs is an important feature. Dysphagia and deafness may occur. Seizures are common late in the disease but are occasionally the first manifestation. Some patients have overt signs of adrenal failure, including fatigue, vomiting, salt craving, and hyperpigmentation that is most prominent in skin folds. The course is relentlessly progressive. Patients enter a vegetative state and die from adrenal crisis or other causes 1 to 10 years after onset.

Several other clinical phenotypes have been described. Adrenomyeloneuropathy (AMN) is the most common of the variant phenotypes. Typical features are spastic paraparesis, peripheral neuropathy, and adrenal insufficiency, beginning in the second decade. Hypogonadism, impotence, and sphincter disturbance are also seen. Cerebellar dysfunction and dementia have been reported. A similar syndrome is found in about 15% of women who are heterozygous for mutation at the *ALD* gene. MRI frequently reveals cortical demyelinating lesions in AMN patients, even in those without signs or symptoms of cortical involvement. Pathologic findings in AMN include demyelination and dying-back changes in the cord and lamellar cytoplasmic inclusions in brain, adrenal gland, and testis; the findings are similar to those of ALD.

An adolescent cerebral form of ALD is similar to the childhood form but for its onset. In adults, X-linked ALD may present as dementia, schizophrenia, or focal cerebral syndromes such as aphasia, Klüver–Bucy syndrome, or hemianopia; adrenal insufficiency is usually present. Adult ALD includes spastic paraparesis, frontal lobe syndromes, cerebellar dysfunction, or olivopontocerebellar atrophy. Female heterozygotes may be symptomatic with adult ALD. Adrenal insufficiency can be seen without neurologic disorder; ALD should be considered in any boy with unexplained Addison disease. Finally, children and adults with the biochemical defect may be asymptomatic or presymptomatic. Phenotypic heterogeneity is the rule within families with multiple affected individuals; the disparate manifestations are probably the result of modifying genetic loci or environmental factors.

Laboratory evaluation of the patient with ALD reveals elevated CSF protein and posteriorly predominant white matter signal hyperintensity with marginal enhancement. Occasionally, the onset is frontal or cerebellar. The corticotropin stimulation test usually shows adrenal insufficiency, even in the absence of clinical signs. Characteristic inclusions, accumulations of lamellar lipid profiles, may be seen in the brain, adrenal glands, sural nerve biopsy, or testis. The primary finding in the brain is extensive diffuse demyelination, sparing U-fibers in the centrum semiovale and elsewhere. In involved areas of white matter, perivascular infiltration of lymphocytes and plasma cells is prominent.

Diagnosis is suggested by the characteristic clinical findings of neurologic deterioration, demonstration of adrenal hypofunction, and MRI abnormalities. The demonstration of elevated VLCFA levels in plasma and cultured skin fibroblasts without disruption of other peroxisomal functions should be followed by ABCD1 mutation analysis.

Several approaches have been taken to treat ALD. Ideally, cases would be detected at birth, which would allow immediate treatment and genetic counseling for parents. A method for newborn screening is under investigation.

Steroid replacement therapy is given during stressful periods, such as intercurrent illness, or if there is evidence of adrenal insufficiency. Dietary avoidance of VLCFA alone does not lead to biochemical change because of endogenous synthesis. Efforts to lower endogenous synthesis using glycerol trierucate oil and glycerol trioleate oil (Lorenzo oil) in conjunction with dietary restriction do produce a fall in VLCFA levels in both affected individuals and female carriers. Unfortunately, this striking biochemical change does not have an equally striking clinical correlate; its use is most likely limited to presymptomatic boys. Bone marrow transplantation cures the biochemical defect in ALD, but the morbidity and mortality are high, and neither neurologic defects nor radiologic abnormalities revert, although favorable outcomes have been reported in boys who are transplanted when few neurologic signs are present. In all cases, radiologic abnormalities and progression almost invariably precede neurologic progression; it is therefore imperative that every child whose family might consider bone marrow transplantation is closely followed radiographically. Immunotherapy has been considered in X-ALD because of the inflammatory component of the central lesions, but β-interferon and thalidomide have not been effective. Finally, the cloning and characterization of the ALD locus may lead to a gene or protein product replacement therapy.

Refsum Disease

This autosomal recessive disease (also known as *heredopathia atactica polyneuritiformis*) is unique among the lipidoses because the stored lipid (phytanic acid) is not synthesized in the body, but is exclusively dietary in origin. This has enabled successful therapy by dietary management. Symptoms begin in early childhood in some patients but may be delayed until the fifth decade in others. Progressive night blindness usually appears in the first or second decade, followed by limb weakness and gait ataxia. Symptoms are progressive, but abrupt exacerbations and gradual remissions may occur with intercurrent illness or pregnancy. There are no seizures, but some patients have psychiatric symptoms. Peripheral neuropathy is manifest by loss of tendon reflexes, weakness and wasting, and distal sensory loss. Ataxia may be seen. A granular pigmentary retinopathy is universally present. Other findings include ichthyosis; nerve deafness (often severe); cataracts; miosis and pupillary asymmetry; pes cavus; and bone deformities with shortening of the metatarsal bones, epiphyseal dysplasia, and, in some, kyphoscoliosis. CSF protein content is elevated. Nerve conduction velocities are slowed. ECG changes include conduction abnormalities. Peripheral nerves may feel thickened and, on histologic study, may

show hypertrophic interstitial changes and onion-bulb formation. The course is generally progressive with exacerbations and remissions. Peripheral visual fields may ultimately be lost, with resulting telescopic vision. Sudden death may result from cardiac arrhythmia.

The biochemical defect in Refsum disease has been identified as phytanoyl-CoA hydroxylase (PHYH) deficiency; the responsible gene in most cases is *PAHX*. Several kindreds with typical Refsum disease have lacked *PAHX* mutations or linkage to chromosome 10; they proved to be heterozygous for mutations in *PEX 7*. That gene encodes the receptor for the type 2 peroxisomal targeting signal (PTS2), whose normal function is essential for PHYH import to peroxisomes. Diagnosis is made by the characteristic clinical picture and elevation of phytanic acid levels in the plasma. Studies in rat brain suggest that phytanic acid exerts direct neurotoxic effects by binding to the inner mitochondrial membrane, impairing mitochondrial ATP supply and membrane permeability.

Therapy limits dietary phytanic acid and its precursor, phytol, a branched chain fatty alcohol, which is abundantly present in nature as part of the chlorophyll molecule. When dairy products, ruminant fat, and chlorophyll-containing foods are eliminated, plasma phytanic acid levels are reduced and tissue stores are mobilized, with improvement of symptoms. Paradoxically, symptoms may worsen and plasma phytanic acid levels may rise shortly after institution of dietary therapy, especially if patients reduce caloric intake and lose weight. Increased plasma phytanic acid causes anorexia, increased weight loss, and still more severe symptoms. Adequate caloric intake helps prevent weight loss and abrupt fat mobilization. Plasmapheresis helps to prevent or treat exacerbations. Induction of phytanic acid ω-oxidation might be helpful.

Another rare peroxisomal phenotype can be confused with Refsum disease. Patients with α-methylacyl-CoA racemase (AMACR) deficiency may have retinopathy, peripheral neuropathy plus a variety of cerebral findings, including seizures, progressive cognitive decline, and relapsing encephalopathy.

SUGGESTED READINGS

Glucose Transporter Type 1 Deficiency Syndrome

Bertoli S, Trentani C, Ferraris C, et al. Long-term effects of a ketogenic diet on body composition and bone mineralization in GLUT-1 deficiency syndrome: a case series. *Nutrition*. 2014;30:726–728.

De Vivo DC, Trifiletti RR, Jacobson RI, et al. Defective glucose transport across the blood–brain barrier as a cause of persistent hypoglycorrhachia, seizures, and developmental delay. *N Engl J Med*. 1991;325:703–709.

Ito Y, Takahashi S, Kagitani-Shimono K, et al. Nationwide survey of glucose transporter-1 deficiency syndrome (GLUT-1DS) in Japan [published online ahead of print December 5, 2014]. *Brain Dev*.

Levy B, Wang D, Ullner PM, et al. Uncovering microdeletions in patients with severe Glut-1 deficiency syndrome using SNP oligonucleotide microarray analysis. *Mol Genet Metab*. 2010;100:129–135.

Pascual JM, Liu P, Mao D, et al. Triheptanoin for glucose transporter type I deficiency (G1D): modulation of human ictogenesis, cerebral metabolic rate, and cognitive indices by a food supplement. *JAMA Neurol*. 2014;71:1255–1265.

Pearson TS, Akman C, Hinton VJ, et al. Phenotypic spectrum of glucose transporter type 1 deficiency syndrome (Glut1 DS). *Curr Neurol Neurosci Rep*. 2013;13:342.

Hyperammonemia

Aires CC, van Cruchten A, Ijlst L, et al. New insights on the mechanisms of valproate-induced hyperammonemia: inhibition of hepatic N-acetylglutamate synthase activity by valproyl-CoA. *J Hepatol*. 2011;55:426–434.

Batshaw ML, Tuchman M, Summar M, et al. A longitudinal study of urea cycle disorders. *Mol Genet Metab.* 2014;113:127–130.

Haberle J. Clinical practice: the management of hyperammonemia. *Eur J Pediatr.* 2011;170:21–34.

Hadjihambi A, Khetan V, Jalan R. Pharmacotherapy for hyperammonemia. *Expert Opin Pharmacother.* 2014;15:1685–1695.

Schousboe A, Waagepetersen HS, Leke R, et al. Effects of hyperammonemia on brain energy metabolism: controversial findings in vivo and in vitro. *Metab Brain Dis.* 2014;29:913–917.

Sprouse C, King J, Helman G, et al. Investigating neurological deficits in carriers and affected patients with ornithine transcarbamylase deficiency. *Mol Genet Metab.* 2014;113:136–141.

Vazquez M, Fagiolino P, Maldonado C, et al. Hyperammonemia associated with valproic acid concentrations. *Biomed Res Int.* 2014;2014:217269.

Yamamoto Y, Takahashi Y, Imai K, et al. Risk factors for hyperammonemia in pediatric patients with epilepsy. *Epilepsia.* 2013;54:983–989.

Disorders of Amino Acid Metabolism

Alkufri F, Harrower T, Rahman Y, et al. Molybdenum cofactor deficiency presenting with a parkinsonism-dystonia syndrome. *Mov Disord.* 2013;28:399–401.

Allmendinger AM, Desai NS, Burke AT, et al. Neuroimaging and renal ultrasound manifestations of oculocerebrorenal syndrome of Lowe. *J Radiol Case Rep.* 2014;8:1–7.

Azmanov DN, Rodgers H, Auray-Blais C, et al. Persistence of the common Hartnup disease D173N allele in populations of European origin. *Ann Hum Genet.* 2007;71:755–761.

Bailey CG, Ryan RM, Thoeng AD, et al. Loss-of-function mutations in the glutamate transporter SLC1A1 cause human dicarboxylic aminoaciduria. *J Clin Invest.* 2011;121:446–453.

Belaidi AA, Schwarz G. Molybdenum cofactor deficiency: metabolic link between taurine and S-sulfocysteine. *Adv Exp Med Biol.* 2013;776:13–19.

Burrage LC, Nagamani SC, Campeau PM, et al. Branched-chain amino acid metabolism: from rare Mendelian diseases to more common disorders. *Hum Mol Genet.* 2014;23:R1–R8.

Christ SE, Moffitt AJ, Peck D, et al. Decreased functional brain connectivity in individuals with early-treated phenylketonuria: evidence from resting state fMRI. *J Inherit Metab Dis.* 2012;35:807–816.

Diaz VM, Camarena C, de la Vega A, et al. Liver transplantation for classical maple syrup urine disease: long-term follow-up. *J Pediatr Gastroenterol Nutr.* 2014;59:636–639.

Groselj U, Tansek MZ, Battelino T. Fifty years of phenylketonuria newborn screening—a great success for many, but what about the rest? *Mol Genet Metab.* 2014;113:8–10.

Hichri H, Rendu J, Monnier N, et al. From Lowe syndrome to Dent disease: correlations between mutations of the OCRL1 gene and clinical and biochemical phenotypes. *Hum Mutat.* 2011;32:379–388.

Higuchi R, Sugimoto T, Tamura A, et al. Early features in neuroimaging of two siblings with molybdenum cofactor deficiency. *Pediatrics.* 2014;133:e267–e271.

Jaeken J, Creemers J, Regal L. Evaluation of the pediatric patient with hypotonia: don't forget the hypotonia-cystinuria syndrome! *Dev Med Child Neurol.* 2012;54:288.

Klee D, Thimm E, Wittsack HJ, et al. Structural white matter changes in adolescents and young adults with maple syrup urine disease. *J Inherit Metab Dis.* 2013;36:945–953.

Leuzzi V, Mannarelli D, Manti F, et al. Age-related psychophysiological vulnerability to phenylalanine in phenylketonuria. *Front Pediatr.* 2014;2:57.

Lewis RA, Nussbaum RL, Brewer ED. Lowe syndrome. GeneReviews Web site. http://www.ncbi.nlm.nih.gov/books/NBK1480/. Accessed January 12, 2015.

Lindegren ML, Krishnaswami S, Reimschisel T, et al. A systematic review of BH4 (sapropterin) for the adjuvant treatment of phenylketonuria. *JIMD Rep.* 2013;8:109–119.

Manara R, Del Rizzo M, Burlina AP, et al. Wernicke-like encephalopathy during classic maple syrup urine disease decompensation. *J Inherit Metab Dis.* 2012;35:413–417.

Mendel RR. The molybdenum cofactor. *J Biol Chem.* 2013;288:13165–13172.

Picker JD, Levy HL. Homocystinuria caused by cystathionine beta-synthase deficiency. GeneReviews Web site. http://www.ncbi.nlm.nih.gov/books/NBK1524/. Accessed January 12, 2015.

Rosini F, Rufa A, Monti L, et al. Adult-onset phenylketonuria revealed by acute reversible dementia, prosopagnosia and parkinsonism. *J Neurol.* 2014;261:2446–2448.

Skovby F, Gaustadnes M, Mudd SH. A revisit to the natural history of homocystinuria due to cystathionine beta-synthase deficiency. *Mol Genet Metab.* 2010;99:1–3.

Strauss KA, Puffenberger EG, Morton DH. Maple syrup urine disease. GeneReviews Web site. http://www.ncbi.nlm.nih.gov/books/NBK1319/. Accessed January 12, 2015.

Strisciuglio P, Concolino D. New strategies for the treatment of phenylketonuria (PKU). *Metabolites.* 2014;4:1007–1017.

Weisfeld-Adams JD, Bender HA, Miley-Akerstedt A, et al. Neurologic and neurodevelopmental phenotypes in young children with early-treated combined methylmalonic acidemia and homocystinuria, cobalamin C type. *Mol Genet Metab.* 2013;110:241–247.

Organic Acidurias

Hoshino H, Kubota M. Canavan disease: clinical features and recent advances in research. *Pediatr Int.* 2014;56:477–483.

Kolker S, Burgard P, Sauer SW, et al. Current concepts in organic acidurias: understanding intra- and extracerebral disease manifestation. *J Inherit Metab Dis.* 2013;36:635–644.

Kranendijk M, Struys EA, van Schaftingen E, et al. IDH2 mutations in patients with D-2-hydroxyglutaric aciduria. *Science.* 2010;330:336.

Leone P, Shera D, McPhee SW, et al. Long-term follow-up after gene therapy for canavan disease. *Sci Transl Med.* 2012;4:165ra163.

Matalon R, Michals-Matalon K. Canavan disease. GeneReviews Web site. http://www.ncbi.nlm.nih.gov/books/NBK1234/. Accessed January 12, 2015.

Muhlhausen C, Salomons GS, Lukacs Z, et al. Combined D2-/L2-hydroxyglutaric aciduria (SLC25A1 deficiency): clinical course and effects of citrate treatment. *J Inherit Metab Dis.* 2014;37:775–781.

Nizon M, Ottolenghi C, Valayannopoulos V, et al. Long-term neurological outcome of a cohort of 80 patients with classical organic acidurias. *Orphanet J Rare Dis.* 2013;8:148.

Nunes J, Loureiro S, Carvalho S, et al. Brain MRI findings as an important diagnostic clue in glutaric aciduria type 1. *Neuroradiol J.* 2013;26:155–161.

Pearl PL, Dorsey AM, Barrios ES, et al. Succinic semialdehyde dehydrogenase deficiency. GeneReviews Web site. http://www.ncbi.nlm.nih.gov/books/NBK1195/. Accessed January 12, 2015.

Steenweg ME, Salomons GS, Yapici Z, et al. L-2-Hydroxyglutaric aciduria: pattern of MR imaging abnormalities in 56 patients. *Radiology.* 2009;251:856–865.

Testai FD, Gorelick PB. Inherited metabolic disorders and stroke part 2: homocystinuria, organic acidurias, and urea cycle disorders. *Arch Neurol.* 2010;67:148–153.

Vogel KR, Pearl PL, Theodore WH, et al. Thirty years beyond discovery—clinical trials in succinic semialdehyde dehydrogenase deficiency, a disorder of GABA metabolism. *J Inherit Metab Dis.* 2013;36:401–410.

Weimar C, Schlamann M, Krageloh-Mann I, et al. L-2 hydroxyglutaric aciduria as a rare cause of leukencephalopathy in adults. *Clin Neurol Neurosurg.* 2013;115:765–766.

Zinnanti WJ, Lazovic J, Housman C, et al. Mechanism of metabolic stroke and spontaneous cerebral hemorrhage in glutaric aciduria type I. *Acta Neuropathol Commun.* 2014;2:13.

Purine and Pyrimidine Disorders

Abel TJ, Dalm BD, Grossbach AJ, et al. Lateralized effect of pallidal stimulation on self-mutilation in Lesch-Nyhan disease. *J Neurosurg Pediatr.* 2014;14:594–597.

Goodman EM, Torres RJ, Puig JG, et al. Consequences of delayed dental extraction in Lesch-Nyhan disease. *Mov Disord Clin Pract (Hoboken).* 2014;1:225–229.

Gottle M, Prudente CN, Fu R, et al. Loss of dopamine phenotype among midbrain neurons in Lesch-Nyhan disease. *Ann Neurol.* 2014;76:95–107.

Guibinga GH, Barron N, Pandori W. Striatal neurodevelopment is dysregulated in purine metabolism deficiency and impacts DARPP-32, BDNF/TrkB expression and signaling: new insights on the molecular and cellular basis of Lesch-Nyhan syndrome. *PLoS One.* 2014;9:e96575.

Jinnah HA, Sabina RL, Van Den Berghe G. Metabolic disorders of purine metabolism affecting the nervous system. *Handb Clin Neurol.* 2013;113:1827–1836.

Micheli V, Camici M, Tozzi MG, et al. Neurological disorders of purine and pyrimidine metabolism. *Curr Top Med Chem.* 2011;11:923–947.

Nyhan WL, O'Neill JP, Jinnah HA, et al. Lesch-Nyhan syndrome. GeneReviews Web site. http://www.ncbi.nlm.nih.gov/books/NBK1149/. Accessed January 12, 2015.

Schretlen DJ, Varvaris M, Vannorsdall TD, et al. Brain white matter volume abnormalities in Lesch-Nyhan disease and its variants. *Neurology.* 2015; 84(2):190–196.

Torres RJ, Peters GJ, Puig JG. Novel developments in metabolic disorders of purine and pyrimidine metabolism and therapeutic applications of their analogs. *Nucleosides Nucleotides Nucleic Acids.* 2014;33:165–173.

Porphyria

Hift RJ, Thunell S, Brun A. Drugs in porphyria: from observation to a modern algorithm-based system for the prediction of porphyrogenicity. *Pharmacol Ther.* 2011;132:158–169.

Kuo HC, Huang CC, Chu CC, et al. Neurological complications of acute intermittent porphyria. *Eur Neurol.* 2011;66:247–252.

Singal AK, Parker C, Bowden C, et al. Liver transplantation in the management of porphyria. *Hepatology.* 2014;60:1082–1089.

Stein P, Badminton M, Barth J, et al. Best practice guidelines on clinical management of acute attacks of porphyria and their complications. *Ann Clin Biochem.* 2013;50:217–223.

Stein PE, Badminton MN, Barth JH, et al. Acute intermittent porphyria: fatal complications of treatment. *Clin Med.* 2012;12:293–294.

Whatley SD, Badminton MN. Acute intermittent porphyria. GeneReviews Web site. http://www.ncbi.nlm.nih.gov/books/NBK1193/. Accessed. January 12, 2015.

Zhao B, Wei Q, Wang Y, et al. Posterior reversible encephalopathy syndrome in acute intermittent porphyria. *Pediatr Neurol.* 2014;51:457–460.

Disorders of Metal Metabolism

Cossu G, Abbruzzese G, Matta G, et al. Efficacy and safety of deferiprone for the treatment of pantothenate kinase-associated neurodegeneration (PKAN) and neurodegeneration with brain iron accumulation (NBIA): results from a four years follow-up. *Parkinsonism Relat Disord.* 2014;20: 651–654.

Dusek P, Litwin T, Czlonkowska A. Wilson disease and other neurodegenerations with metal accumulations. *Neurol Clin.* 2015;33:175–204.

Ferenci P. Whom and how to screen for Wilson disease. *Expert Rev Gastroenterol Hepatol.* 2014;8:513–520.

Gregory A, Hayflick S. Neurodegeneration with brain iron accumulation disorders overview. GeneReviews Web site. http://www.ncbi.nlm.nih.gov/books/NBK121988/. Accessed January 12, 2015.

Kaler SG. ATP7A-related copper transport diseases-emerging concepts and future trends. *Nat Rev Neurol.* 2011;7:15–29.

Kaler SG. ATP7A-related copper transport disorders. GeneReviews Web site. http://www.ncbi.nlm.nih.gov/books/NBK1413/. Accessed January 12, 2015.

Kaler SG. Neurodevelopment and brain growth in classic Menkes disease is influenced by age and symptomatology at initiation of copper treatment. *J Trace Elem Med Biol.* 2014;28:427–430.

Kurian MA, Hayflick SJ. Pantothenate kinase-associated neurodegeneration (PKAN) and PLA2G6-associated neurodegeneration (PLAN): review of two major neurodegeneration with brain iron accumulation (NBIA) phenotypes. *Int Rev Neurobiol.* 2013;110:49–71.

Schilsky ML. A century for progress in the diagnosis of Wilson disease. *J Trace Elem Med Biol.* 2014;28:492–494.

Schneider SA, Dusek P, Hardy J, et al. Genetics and pathophysiology of neurodegeneration with brain iron accumulation (NBIA). *Curr Neuropharmacol.* 2013;11:59–79.

Smpokou P, Samanta M, Berry GT, et al. Menkes disease in affected females: the clinical disease spectrum. *Am J Med Genet A.* 2015;167(2):417–420.

Tchan MC, Wilcken B, Christodoulou J. The mild form of Menkes disease: a 34 year progress report on the original case. *JIMD Rep.* 2013;9:81–84.

Weiss KH. Wilson disease. GeneReviews Web site. http://www.ncbi.nlm.nih.gov/books/NBK1512/. Accessed January 12, 2015.

Disorders Associated with Acanthocytosis

Connolly BS, Hazrati LN, Lang AE. Neuropathological findings in chorea-acanthocytosis: new insights into mechanisms underlying parkinsonism and seizures. *Acta Neuropathol.* 2014;127:613–615.

Jung HH, Danek A, Walker RH, et al. McLeod neuroacanthocytosis syndrome. GeneReviews Web site. http://www.ncbi.nlm.nih.gov/books/NBK1354/. Accessed January 12, 2015.

Lee J, Hegele RA. Abetalipoproteinemia and homozygous hypobetalipoproteinemia: a framework for diagnosis and management. *J Inherit Metab Dis.* 2014;37:333–339.

Miquel M, Spampinato U, Latxague C, et al. Short and long term outcome of bilateral pallidal stimulation in chorea-acanthocytosis. *PLoS One.* 2013;8:e79241.

Miranda M, Jung HH, Danek A, et al. The chorea of McLeod syndrome: progression to hypokinesia. *Mov Disord.* 2012;27:1701–1702.

Shiokawa N, Nakamura M, Sameshima M, et al. Chorein, the protein responsible for chorea-acanthocytosis, interacts with beta-adducin and beta-actin. *Biochem Biophys Res Commun.* 2013;441:96–101.

Lysosomal and Associated Large Molecule Disorders

Afifi AK, Bell WE, Menezes AH, et al. Myelinoclastic diffuse sclerosis (Schilder's disease): report of a case and review of the literature. *J Child Neurol.* 1994; 9:398–403.

Alcalay RN, Dinur T, Quinn T, et al. Comparison of Parkinson risk in Ashkenazi Jewish patients with Gaucher disease and GBA heterozygotes. *JAMA Neurol.* 2014;71:752–757.

Alqahtani E, Huisman TA, Boltshauser E, et al. Mucopolysaccharidoses type I and II: new neuroimaging findings in the cerebellum. *Eur J Paediatr Neurol.* 2014;18:211–217.

Bacigaluppi S, Polonara G, Zavanone ML, et al. Schilder's disease: non-invasive diagnosis? A case report and review. *Neurol Sci.* 2009;30:421–430.

Barczykowski AL, Foss AH, Duffner PK, et al. Death rates in the U.S. due to Krabbe disease and related leukodystrophy and lysosomal storage diseases. *Am J Med Genet A.* 2012;158A:2835–2842.

Boustany RM. Lysosomal storage diseases—the horizon expands. *Nat Rev Neurol.* 2013;9:583–598.

Ding XQ, Bley A, Ohlenbusch A, et al. Imaging evidence of early brain tissue degeneration in patients with vanishing white matter disease: a multimodal MR study. *J Magn Reson Imaging.* 2012;35:926–932.

Ganesh A, Bruwer Z, Al-Thihli K. An update on ocular involvement in mucopolysaccharidoses. *Curr Opin Ophthalmol.* 2013;24:379–388.

Gotoh L, Inoue K, Helman G, et al. GJC2 promoter mutations causing Pelizaeus-Merzbacher-like disease. *Mol Genet Metab.* 2014;111:393–398.

Graff-Radford J, Schwartz K, Gavrilova RH, et al. Neuroimaging and clinical features in type II (late-onset) Alexander disease. *Neurology.* 2014;82:49–56.

Hanefeld F, Holzbach U, Kruse B, et al. Diffuse white matter disease in three children: an encephalopathy with unique features on magnetic resonance imaging and proton magnetic resonance spectroscopy. *Neuropediatrics.* 1993;24(5):244–248.

Herwerth M, Schwaiger BJ, Kreiser K, et al. Adult-onset vanishing white matter disease as differential diagnosis of primary progressive multiple sclerosis: a case report. *Mult Scler.* 2015;21(5):666–668.

Irun P, Mallen M, Dominguez C, et al. Identification of seven novel SMPD1 mutations causing Niemann-Pick disease types A and B. *Clin Genet.* 2013;84: 356–361.

Kraus D, Konen O, Straussberg R. Schilder's disease: non-invasive diagnosis and successful treatment with human immunoglobulins. *Eur J Paediatr Neurol.* 2012;16:206–208.

Laukka JJ, Stanley JA, Garbern JY, et al. Neuroradiologic correlates of clinical disability and progression in the X-linked leukodystrophy Pelizaeus-Merzbacher disease. *J Neurol Sci.* 2013;335:75–81.

Lee NC, Chien YH, Wong SL, et al. Outcome of early-treated type III Gaucher disease patients. *Blood Cells Mol Dis.* 2014;53:105–109.

Lin Y, Pang X, Huang G, et al. Impaired eukaryotic translation initiation factor 2B activity specifically in oligodendrocytes reproduces the pathology of vanishing white matter disease in mice. *J Neurosci.* 2014;34:12182–12191.

Lopez G, Sidransky E. Predicting parkinsonism: new opportunities from Gaucher disease. *Mol Genet Metab.* 2013;109:235–236.

Lyseng-Williamson KA. Miglustat: a review of its use in Niemann-Pick disease type C. *Drugs.* 2014;74:61–74.

Messing A, Brenner M, Feany MB, et al. Alexander disease. *J Neurosci.* 2012; 32:5017–5023.

Mole SE, Williams RE. Neuronal ceroid-lipofuscinoses. GeneReviews Web site. http://www.ncbi.nlm.nih.gov/books/NBK1428/. Accessed January 12, 2015.

Motta M, Camerini S, Tatti M, et al. Gaucher disease due to saposin C deficiency is an inherited lysosomal disease caused by rapidly degraded mutant proteins. *Hum Mol Genet.* 2014;23:5814–5826.

Patterson M. Niemann-Pick disease type C. GeneReviews Web site. http://www.ncbi.nlm.nih.gov/books/NBK1296/. Accessed January 12, 2015.

Patterson MC, Hendriksz CJ, Walterfang M, et al. Recommendations for the diagnosis and management of Niemann-Pick disease type C: an update. *Mol Genet Metab.* 2012;106:330–344.

Prada CE, Grabowski GA. Neuronopathic lysosomal storage diseases: clinical and pathologic findings. *Dev Disabil Res Rev.* 2013;17:226–246.

Schiffmann R, Moller JR, Trapp BD, et al. Childhood ataxia with diffuse central nervous system hypomyelination. *Ann Neurol.* 1994;35(3):331–340.

Schulz A, Kohlschutter A, Mink J, et al. NCL diseases—clinical perspectives. *Biochim Biophys Acta.* 2013;1832:1801–1806.

Shayman JA, Larsen SD. The development and use of small molecule inhibitors of glycosphingolipid metabolism for lysosomal storage diseases. *J Lipid Res.* 2014;55:1215–1225.

Shimojima K, Okumura A, Ikeno M, et al. A de novo TUBB4A mutation in a patient with hypomyelination mimicking Pelizaeus-Merzbacher disease. *Brain Dev.* 2015;37(3):281–285.

Simonati A, Pezzini F, Moro F, et al. Neuronal ceroid lipofuscinosis: the increasing spectrum of an old disease [published online ahead of print October 10, 2014]. *Curr Mol Med.*

Stevenson DA, Steiner RD. Skeletal abnormalities in lysosomal storage diseases. *Pediatr Endocrinol Rev.* 2013;10(suppl 2):406–416.

van der Knaap MS, Barth PG, GabreëlsGabreels FJ, et al. A new leukoencephalopathy with vanishing white matter. *Neurology.* 1997;48(4):845–855.

van der Lei HD, van Berkel CG, van Wieringen WN, et al. Genotype-phenotype correlation in vanishing white matter disease. *Neurology.* 2010;75:1555–1559.

Vanier MT. Complex lipid trafficking in Niemann-Pick disease type C. *J Inherit Metab Dis.* 2015;38(1):187–199.

van Karnebeek CD, Mohammadi T, Tsao N, et al. Health economic evaluation of plasma oxysterol screening in the diagnosis of Niemann-Pick Type C disease among intellectually disabled using discrete event simulation. *Mol Genet Metab.* 2015;114(2):226–232.

Vitner EB, Futerman AH. Neuronal forms of Gaucher disease. *Handb Exp Pharmacol.* 2013;(216):405–419.

Weiss K, Gonzalez AN, Lopez G, et al. The clinical management of type 2 Gaucher disease. *Mol Genet Metab.* 2015;114:110–122.

Winchester B. Lysosomal diseases: diagnostic update. *J Inherit Metab Dis.* 2014;37:599–608.

Wraith JE. Mucopolysaccharidoses and mucolipidoses. *Handb Clin Neurol.* 2013;113:1723–1729.

Yilmaz Y, Kocaman C, Karabagli H, et al. Is the brain biopsy obligatory or not for the diagnosis of Schilder's disease? Review of the literature. *Childs Nerv Syst.* 2008;24:3–6.

Zafeiriou DI, Batzios SP. Brain and spinal MR imaging findings in mucopolysaccharidoses: a review. *AJNR Am J Neuroradiol.* 2013;34:5–13.

Disorders of Carbohydrate Metabolism

Boentert M, Karabul N, Wenninger S, et al. Sleep-related symptoms and sleep-disordered breathing in adult Pompe disease. *Eur J Neurol.* 2015;22(2):369–376.

Falk DJ, Todd AG, Lee S, et al. Peripheral nerve and neuromuscular junction pathology in Pompe disease. *Hum Mol Genet.* 2015;24(3):625–636.

Hobson-Webb LD, Austin SL, Bali DS, et al. The electrodiagnostic characteristics of glycogen storage disease type III. *Genet Med.* 2010;12:440–445.

Kishnani PS, Beckemeyer AA. New therapeutic approaches for Pompe disease: enzyme replacement therapy and beyond. *Pediatr Endocrinol Rev.* 2014;12(suppl 1):114–124.

Magoulas PL, El-Hattab AW. Glycogen storage disease type IV. GeneReviews Web site. http://www.ncbi.nlm.nih.gov/books/NBK115333/. Accessed January 12, 2015.

Malfatti E, Nilsson J, Hedberg-Oldfors C, et al. A new muscle glycogen storage disease associated with glycogenin-1 deficiency. *Ann Neurol.* 2014;76:891–898.

Mochel F, Schiffmann R, Steenweg ME, et al. Adult polyglucosan body disease: natural history and key magnetic resonance imaging findings. *Ann Neurol.* 2012;72:433–441.

Quinlivan R, Martinuzzi A, Schoser B. Pharmacological and nutritional treatment for McArdle disease (glycogen storage disease type V). *Cochrane Database Syst Rev.* 2014;11:CD003458.

Sun B, Fredrickson K, Austin S, et al. Alglucosidase alfa enzyme replacement therapy as a therapeutic approach for glycogen storage disease type III. *Mol Genet Metab.* 2013;108:145–147.

van der Meijden JC, Gungor D, Kruijshaar ME, et al. Ten years of the international Pompe survey: patient reported outcomes as a reliable tool for studying treated and untreated children and adults with non-classic Pompe disease [published online ahead of print August 12, 2014]. *J Inherit Metab Dis.*

Wang Y, Ma K, Wang P, et al. Laforin prevents stress-induced polyglucosan body formation and Lafora disease progression in neurons. *Mol Neurobiol.* 2013;48:49–61.

Peroxisomal Diseases: Adrenoleukodystrophy, Zellweger Syndrome, and Refsum Disease

Baldwin EJ, Gibberd FB, Harley C, et al. The effectiveness of long-term dietary therapy in the treatment of adult Refsum disease. *J Neurol Neurosurg Psychiatry.* 2010;81:954–957.

Crane DI. Revisiting the neuropathogenesis of Zellweger syndrome. *Neurochem Int.* 2014;69:1–8.

Engelen M, Barbier M, Dijkstra IM, et al. X-linked adrenoleukodystrophy in women: a cross-sectional cohort study. *Brain.* 2014;137:693–706.

Engelen M, Kemp S, Poll-The BT. X-linked adrenoleukodystrophy: pathogenesis and treatment. *Curr Neurol Neurosci Rep.* 2014;14:486.

Menon GK, Orso E, Aslanidis C, et al. Ultrastructure of skin from Refsum disease with emphasis on epidermal lamellar bodies and stratum corneum barrier lipid organization. *Arch Dermatol Res.* 2014;306:731–737.

Rosewich H, Waterham H, Poll-The BT, et al. Clinical utility gene card for: Zellweger syndrome spectrum [published online ahead of print November 19, 2014]. *Eur J Hum Genet.* doi:10.1038/ejhg.2014.250.

Steinberg SJ, Moser AB, Raymond GV. X-linked adrenoleukodystrophy. GeneReviews Web site. http://www.ncbi.nlm.nih.gov/books/NBK1315/. Accessed January 12, 2015.

Theda C, Gibbons K, Defor TE, et al. Newborn screening for X-linked adrenoleukodystrophy: further evidence high throughput screening is feasible. *Mol Genet Metab.* 2014;111:55–57.

van Geel BM, Poll-The BT, Verrips A, et al. Hematopoietic cell transplantation does not prevent myelopathy in X-linked adrenoleukodystrophy: a retrospective study. *J Inherit Metab Dis.* 2015;38(2):359–361. doi:10.1007/s10545-014-9797-1.

Wanders RJA, Waterham HR, Leroy BP. Refsum disease. GeneReviews Web site. http://www.ncbi.nlm.nih.gov/books/NBK1353/. Accessed January 12, 2015.

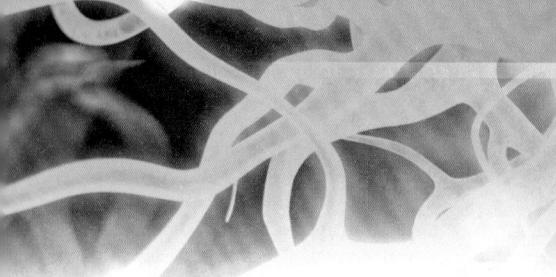

Marc C. Patterson

INTRODUCTION

Rearrangements of the human genome, ranging from grossly disordered chromosome number to submicroscopic variations in copy numbers can profoundly affect development and function of the nervous system. Likewise, defects in the machinery that maintain the integrity and duplication fidelity of DNA lead to a family of rare disorders characterized by varying combinations of neurodegeneration, premature aging, immunodeficiency, and susceptibility to malignancy.

CHROMOSOMAL DISORDERS

Human chromosomal anomalies are manifested as change in the total number of chromosomes, structural rearrangements, imprinting abnormalities, or variations in copy number. Examples of abnormal chromosome number (i.e., aneuploidy) are sex-chromosomal aneuploidy, such as 45,X (Turner syndrome), and autosomal aneuploidy, such as 47,XX +21 (trisomy 21, Down syndrome). Structural abnormalities include regional deletions or insertions, segmental translocations (i.e., reciprocal or Robertsonian) or inversions (i.e., pericentric or paracentric), duplications, and ring chromosomes. There are many chromosomal syndromes, which result primarily from these numeric or segmental anomalies, producing a functional change of gene dosage; gene imprinting is also recognized as a critical modifier of expression. The most common manifestation of chromosomal anomalies is intellectual disability. Congenital malformations occur with variable frequency and differences in severity. In the sex-chromosome disorders, infertility is the most common feature. Table 135.1 summarizes the features of several classic chromosome disorders as examples: trisomy 21 syndrome, Prader–Willi syndrome (PWS), Angelman syndrome (AS), and a common idiopathic intellectual disability syndrome caused by subtelomeric anomalies of chromosomes. A variety of mechanisms underlie these disorders. Trisomy 21 results from chromosomal nondisjunction (maternal 80%, paternal 20%), an age-related phenomenon in most cases, and unbalanced translocation in the remainder. PWS and AS result from loss of paternally or maternally imprinted alleles in the same chromosomal region (15 q11-13); such loss may reflect abnormal imprinting (methylation—see the following section), chromosomal deletion, translocation or inversion, or point mutations in a specific gene (UBE3A for AS). CATCH-22 is a deletion syndrome—the manifestations are at least in part a reflection of the amount of genetic material that is lost.

GENOMIC IMPRINTING

Genomic imprinting is an epigenetic phenomenon that permits nonmendelian inheritance in the mammalian genome. Several autosomal genes are inherited, in a silent state, on one parental allele and in an active state on the other parental allele. This parent-of-origin–specific gene expression is called *genomic imprinting*.

The diseases that arise from these genes are mostly caused by mutation of the active allele, duplication of the nonactive allele, or imprinting errors resulting in silencing of the active allele. Over 20 imprinted genes have now been identified in the mouse genome; many of them have human homologs. For example, the *IGF-2* gene is paternally active, and only when the gene defect is inherited from the father do the offspring express the dwarfing phenotype. In PWS and AS, deletions in the PWS critical region on the paternal chromosome, or maternal uniparental disomy, result in silencing the paternally active allele and the PWS phenotype, whereas deletion of the AS critical region on the maternal chromosome, or paternal uniparental disomy, results in the silencing of the maternal allele and the AS phenotype.

The molecular mechanism of genomic imprinting is incompletely understood. The isolation of a *cis*-acting imprinting center, located upstream to the promotor region of the *SNRPN* gene, has helped us understand the molecular basis of genomic imprinting. Deletions or mutations in this imprinting center have been shown to associate with PWS or AS, depending on the origin of parental germ lines. It is postulated that the imprinting center confers a male or female imprint by use of an imprinting switch during gametogenesis. In the female germ line, the imprinting switch is needed to reset the male chromosome from the maternal grandfather to confer the characteristics of a female chromosome. In the male germ line, the same process is needed to reset the female chromosome from the paternal grandmother to confer the characteristics of a male chromosome. This epigenetic mark is thought to be achieved by DNA methylation. In the case of PWS, the inactive allele on the maternal chromosome is hypermethylated, which suppresses gene transcription. The hypermethylated cytosine residues on the DNA sequences may repel the transcription factors needed for the activation of gene transcription. In other imprinted genes such as the IGF-2 receptor, DNA methylation is associated with the active allele on the maternal chromosome. Therefore, other factors in addition to DNA methylation may be involved in genomic imprinting.

AUTISM SPECTRUM DISORDER AND GENOMIC IMPRINTING

Autism is a neurodevelopmental disorder characterized by language and social impairments and prominent repetitive, stereotypic behaviors (see also Chapter 138). Interstitial duplication of maternal chromosome 15q11–13 region is one of the more common chromosomal anomalies in autism. Clinically, there are some phenotypic overlaps between autism spectrum disorders (ASDs) and PWS. Interestingly, among the children with PWS, those who express two maternally imprinted alleles are twice more likely to have ASD than those with PWS caused by deletion of paternally imprinted alleles. The identification of mutations in the methyl CpG-binding protein 2 (*MeCP2*) gene as the major cause of Rett syndrome suggested that DNA methylation (and hence genomic imprinting) may play important roles in other neurodevelopmental disorders.

TABLE 135.1 Common Chromosomal Disorders

Genetic Abnormality/Eponym	Key Clinical Features	Diagnosis
Trisomy 21; chromosome 14/21 translocation; Down syndrome	Intellectual disability, hypotonia, atlantoaxial instability, short stature. Characteristic round facies with epicanthal folds. Early-onset dementia. Congenital heart disease, increased risk of leukemia.	Chromosome analysis
Prader–Willi syndrome; 15q11-13 deletion	Neonatal hypotonia and failure to thrive followed by uncontrolled appetite with obesity (hypothalamic dysfunction); characteristic facial features, intellectual disability and behavior (obsessiveness, mood swings, skin picking)	DNA methylation analysis (loss of paternal allele at *SNRPN* locus: includes 15q11-13 deletion, uniparental disomy, and imprinting defects—detects 99% of cases)
Angelman syndrome; 15q11-13 deletion	Characteristic facies, microbrachy cephaly, protruding tongue, jerky limb movements (features may not be apparent until after 1 yr); developmental delays; and intellectual disability	DNA methylation analysis (loss of maternal allele: includes 15q11-13 deletion, uniparental disomy, and imprinting defects—78% of cases); UBE3A mutation analysis 11% of cases; chromosome analysis (translocations, inversions—1% of cases); no diagnostic test findings—10% of cases
22q11 deletion syndrome (CATCH-22; DiGeorge; velocardiofacial syndrome)	Cardiac malformations, facial clefts, other cranial and brachial arch anomalies, dysmorphism, intellectual disability, and psychiatric disorders (schizophrenia, OCD, PDD, and ADHD)	FISH, MLPA, chromosomal microarray (detects 95+% of cases)

OCD, obsessive–compulsive disorder; PDD, pervasive developmental disorder; ADHD, attention deficit hyperactivity disorder; FISH, fluorescent in situ hybridization; MLPA, multiplex ligation-dependent probe amplification.

Subtle chromosomal anomalies such as subtelomeric and submicroscopic deletion or duplication frequently give rise to neurologic phenotypes, without necessarily causing somatic manifestations. Techniques using subtelomeric probes led the way in improving cytogenetic diagnosis but have been largely supplanted by array comparative genomic hybridization (CGH) in the investigation of idiopathic intellectual disability and cancers.

INTELLECTUAL DISABILITY ASSOCIATED WITH SUBTELOMERIC CHROMOSOMAL DELETION

Telomeres are the chromosome ends that contain complex DNA protein structures. The DNA sequence is a repetitive-hexanucleotide motif, TTAGGG, ranging from 2 to 15 kb in length. This repetitive sequence and its specific DNA-binding proteins form a cap structure at the chromosome ends. This cap structure enables cells to distinguish chromosome ends, prevents fusion or degradation of chromosomes, and facilitates chromosomal segregations during cellular divisions. A reverse transcriptase named *telomerase* recognizes this terminal repetitive DNA sequence and works to maintain the chromosomal integrity by adding telomeric DNA onto chromosome ends, when a lagging strand is created during replication. Anomalies of these DNA protein structures

change the chromosomal length. Shortening of telomeric length is seen in normal aging of somatic cells, whereas unchecked telomerase activation results in chromosomal fusion, as is often seen in cancer cells. Intellectual disability is a common developmental disorder. The etiology of about 30% to 40% of moderate to severe intellectual disability (IQ <50) remains unknown, despite extensive diagnostic testing. These patients have a normal karyotype using routine- or high-resolution chromosomal-banding techniques.

Since the early 1990s, researchers have developed DNA probes to detect subtle subtelomeric chromosomal anomalies in humans. At least 5% of children with idiopathic intellectual disability harbor subtelomeric chromosomal rearrangements, detected by a set of subtelomeric probes in different fluorescent in situ hybridization (FISH) studies. These rearrangements include subtelomeric deletions, duplications, or derivative chromosomes resulting in partial monosomy–trisomy states. The positive detection rate increases when screening criteria include severe intellectual disability, positive family history of intellectual disability, and at least one physical dysmorphism. These results suggest that subtelomeric FISH study remains a useful tool for identifying the etiology of the disorders of patients with idiopathic intellectual disability. More recently, single nucleotide polymorphism (SNP) arrays have been recommended as an efficient screening test in populations with intellectual disability, with a diagnostic yield greater than 10% in one study.

IDENTIFICATION OF DNA COPY NUMBER VARIATIONS BY ARRAY COMPARATIVE GENOMIC HYBRIDIZATION

Chromosomal disorders arising from segmental deletion or duplication contribute to variations of copy numbers of DNA fragments. These fragments are often not visualized by current high-resolution chromosomal banding. This submicroscopic genomic copy number variation is thought to be the most common cause of idiopathic developmental delay, including intellectual disability. Recent advances in high-throughput microarray technology, coupled with sophisticated data analysis, have allowed rapid and accurate detection of these submicroscopic genomic copy number variations. In CGH, the patient's DNA is hybridized to arrayed genomic DNA targets (genomic clones or oligonucleotides) on a glass slide or gene chip. The signal intensities of each hybridized genomic target are compared with those of the control standards (or the parents). Variation of copy numbers can be readily detected. This new genetic diagnostic tool has led to the identification of an ever-growing family of novel microdeletion syndromes. The repetitive observation of microscopic chromosomal anomalies and their correlation with certain clinical phenotypes is likely to identify the genetic causes of many idiopathic neurodevelopmental disorders whose cause is currently unknown. Investigators have reported relatively high yields of CGH in cohorts with intellectual disability and autism in both children and adults.

DISORDERS OF DNA MAINTENANCE, TRANSCRIPTION, AND TRANSLATION

Except for components of the respiratory chain encoded by DNA, the DNA of the nucleus is responsible for the production of the molecules essential to the cellular economy. Disorders that impair the maintenance of the integrity of DNA, or its timely and accurate transcription and translation, frequently lead to neurodegeneration, impaired growth, premature aging, and a propensity to develop malignancies. The brain is particularly vulnerable to these disorders because cerebral neurons are, for practical purposes, irreplaceable and their high metabolic rate mandates high levels of oxygen consumption; both of these factors render the CNS more susceptible to damage by reactive oxygen species and other metabolites than less richly endowed tissues.

This section provides an introduction to the processes involved and the rare diseases resulting from derangement of these controls. It is likely that the number of these disorders will continue to grow in parallel with the relevant basic science. Neurologists in the 21st century must have a firm grasp of the essential principles to diagnose and manage people with these diseases.

DNA MAINTENANCE AND TRANSCRIPTION

DNA is subject to errors in its duplication during cell division and during the process of repair following exposure to a variety of mutagens (environmental, toxic, and therapeutic). The elaborate machinery includes helicases that unwind the strands of DNA in preparation for transcription into RNA, RNA polymerase, which directs the formation of mRNA on the DNA template, and DNA polymerase, which catalyses the duplication of DNA. The process is fine-tuned by a large family of transcription factors; investigators are constantly adding to their number. This process is highly dependent on sites of replication origin, which change during development and in the face of disease.

A complex system has evolved to correct errors in nucleic acid duplication. When single bases are incorrectly inserted into the new DNA molecules, they are removed by the process of base excision repair, mediated by specific DNA glycosylases and endonucleases and DNA polymerases and ligases. Longer segments of 25 to 32 bases are frequently damaged by exposure to ultraviolet radiation and are removed by nucleotide excision repair, which requires its own family of proteins. Breaks of double-stranded DNA activate a mechanism that requires the participation of DNA protein kinase and recombination proteins. The processes are even more complex than is implied by this brief overview, because many of the involved proteins play multiple, mutually modifying roles in repair and transcription.

Precursor-mRNA (pre-mRNA) is transcribed from the genomic DNA template and includes the sequences of both expressed sequences (exons) and intervening sequences (introns). Introns are removed from pre-mRNA by RNA splicing to produce the mRNA used in translation of the message into protein. This process requires the participation of five additional RNA molecules (small nuclear RNAs or snRNAs) and more than 50 proteins. The snRNAs are added to multiprotein complexes known as *spliceosomes*. The steps involved in pre-mRNA processing into mRNA occur in the nucleus and conclude with export of the mRNA to the cytoplasm via the nuclear pore complex.

DNA TRANSLATION AND MODIFICATION

Translation of mRNA requires intact ribosomal function, factors to control the initiation and duration of translation, and machinery to modify the nascent polypeptide chains by the addition of smaller molecules, particularly oligosaccharides. This modification amplifies the ability of the organism to respond to changing needs at different stages of development (such as differing proportions of enzyme or structural protein isoforms) or in response to external stimuli (as in the modification of T-cell receptor populations and other elements of the immune system to target invading microorganisms). The most important of such processes are *N*- and *O*-linked glycosylation.

CELL CYCLE CONTROL

The activity of the systems responsible for DNA transcription, maintenance, and translation is related to the phase of the cell cycle, which is regulated by a highly conserved family of protein kinases known as *cyclin-dependent kinases* (CDKs). CDKs are themselves regulated by inhibitory phosphorylation (Wee 1), dephosphorylation (Cdc25), the binding of inhibitor proteins (CKIs), and through cyclical proteolysis (ubiquitin ligases and activators—SCF, APC, Cdc20, Hct 1) and gene regulatory proteins (E2F, p53).

SPECIFIC DISORDERS

Table 135.2 summarizes selected monogenic DNA disorders. The categorization of specific disorders in one category is an arbitrary oversimplification because the gene products have multiple actions in many cases.

TABLE 135.2 Selected Disorders of DNA Synthesis, Maintenance, Transcription, and Translation

Disorder	Inheritance	Gene and Protein	Mechanism (Known or Putative)	Specific Features
DNA Maintenance and Transcription				
Cockayne syndrome, type 1 (CSA)	Autosomal recessive (AR)	*CSA (ERCC8)* Excision repair cross-complementing rodent repair deficiency 8 protein	CSA/ERCC8 interacts with p44, CSB, and TFIIH. Mutations thus lead to RNA polymerase II dysfunction and impaired nucleotide excision repair.	Intellectual disability, accelerated aging, pigmentary retinal degeneration, optic atrophy, deafness, marble epiphyses, photosensitivity, and basal ganglia/cerebellar calcification
COFS	AR	*CSB (ERCC6)* Excision repair cross-complementing rodent repair deficiency 6 protein	Abnormal nucleotide excision repair resulting from disturbed RNA polymerase I–TFIIH interaction within the CSBIP/150 complex, of which CSB/ERCC6 is a component	Microcephaly, microphthalmia, cataracts, dysmorphism, failure to thrive, recurrent pneumonias, axial hypotonia, appendicular hypertonia, hyperreflexia, and progressive contractures. Calcifications in the periventricular frontal white matter and basal ganglia.
Progeria	AR	*LMNA* Lamin A	Lamins are structural components of the nuclear membrane. Mutations in LMNA are associated with both defective nuclear mechanics and impaired transcriptional activation.	Postnatal onset of short stature, failure to thrive and accelerated aging, loss of scalp hair and subcutaneous fat, joint stiffness, and early atherosclerosis leading to strokes and myocardial infarcts and premature death. Elevated prothrombin time, platelets, and phosphorous; conductive hearing loss is also reported. Cognition is spared.
Xeroderma pigmentosum (XP) (de Sanctis-Cacchione syndrome—most commonly complementation group D-XPD)	AR	*ERCC2* Excision repair cross-complementing rodent repair deficiency 2 protein	Abnormal nucleotide excision repair: XPD (ERCC2) interacts with the p44 subunit of TFIIH stimulating 5-prime-to-3-prime helicase activity. Mutations in XPD prevent the interaction with p44, leading to decreased XPD helicase activity.	Intellectual disability, short stature, facial freckling, spasticity, hypogonadism, and olivopontocerebellar atrophy
Trichothiodystrophy (TTD 1)	AR	*ERCC2* Excision repair cross-complementing rodent repair deficiency 2 protein	As for XP, TFIIH also stabilizes thyroid hormone receptors in TTD mouse brain.	Intellectual disability, hair shaft abnormalities, ichthyosis, immature sexual development, short stature, and facial dysmorphism
Rett syndrome	X-linked	*MECP2* Methyl CpG-binding protein 2	Regulation of gene expression, chromatin composition, and chromosomal architecture through binding to methylated DNA. MeCP2 is expressed ubiquitously by neurons; levels of MeCP2 expression increase during neuronal differentiation and remain at high levels in the adult brain.	Classic phenotype restricted to females. Normal development for first 6 mo, followed by acquired microcephaly, loss of hand skills and replacement by stereotypies, regression of skills, seizures, spasticity, and scoliosis.
Spinal muscular atrophy 1, 2, and 3	AR	*SMN1* Survival motor neuron protein	SMN1 is a key component of the spliceosome complex; selective vulnerability of anterior horn cells is not yet understood.	Loss of anterior horn cells (and neurons of brain stem and thalami in severe cases)

(table continues on page 1178)

TABLE 135.2   Selected Disorders of DNA Synthesis, Maintenance, Transcription, and Translation *(continued)*

Disorder	Inheritance	Gene and Protein	Mechanism (Known or Putative)	Specific Features
DNA Translation and Translational Modification				
CACH, Cree leuko-encephalopathy, ovarioleukodystrophy	AR	*eIF2B* Eukaryotic translation initiation factor 2B	Translation initiation factor 2B catalyzes exchange of GDP for GTP, an essential stage in recycling of translation initiation factor 2 (eIF2); guanine nucleotide exchange factor (GEF) activity. Mutations in any of the five genes coding for subunits of eIF2B cause loss of normal downregulation of protein translation under stress, resulting in protein denaturation and accumulation of aggregates producing cellular toxicity.	Slowly progressive ataxia with diffuse loss of white matter. Episodes of coma with fever and motor impairment with minor trauma.
Congenital disorder of glycosylation 1a (CDG 1a)	AR	*PMM2* Phosphomannomutase 2	PMM2 is one of a family of enzymes catalyzing the assembly of the lipid-linked oligosaccharide (LLO) precursor that is attached to the nascent polypeptide chain during cotranslational modification by *N*-linked glycosylation.	Intellectual disability, short stature, progressive ataxia, peripheral neuropathy, stroke-like episodes, seizures, immune dysfunction, intermittent hepatic failure, coagulopathies
Cell Cycle Regulation				
Angelman syndrome	Multiple mechanisms, including maternal deletion of 15q11-13, paternal uniparental disomy, imprinting defects, and point mutations or small UBE3A intragenic deletions. Some patients have MECP2 mutations.	*UBE3A* Ubiquitin-protein ligase E3A	The Ube3a gene encodes sense and antisense RNA transcripts in the brain with neuron-specific imprinting of Ube3a in primary brain cell cultures. The maternal UBE3A allele is preferentially expressed in the neuronal nucleus and at synapses; absence of this allele is associated with abnormal dendritic spine morphology.	Psychomotor retardation, ataxia, hypotonia, epilepsy, absence of speech, large mandible, and tongue thrusting. Optic atrophy and albinism in some.
Ataxia-telangiectasia	AR	*ATM* Ataxia-telangiectasia mutated (ATM) protein	The ATM protein is a phosphatidylinositol-3 kinase that phosphorylates key substrates involved in DNA repair and/or cell cycle control	Progressive ataxia, choreoathetosis, anterior horn cell loss, immune deficiency, scleral telangiectasia
Seckel syndrome 1	AR	*Ataxia-telangiectasia and Rad3-related (ATR) protein; CEP152* Centrosomal protein 152	ATR is a phosphatidylinositol kinase (PIK) involved in cell cycle progression, DNA recombination, and the detection of DNA damage; CEP152 regulates genomic integrity and cellular response to DNA damage.	Short stature, dysmorphism ("bird-headed dwarf"), congenital microcephaly, intellectual disability. No immune deficiency or cancers.

CSB, Cockayne syndrome group B; TFIIH, transcription factor II H; COFS, cerebro-oculo-facio-skeletal syndrome; CACH, childhood ataxia with central nervous system hypomyelination.

SUGGESTED READINGS

Chromosomal Disorders

Aypar U, Brodersen PR, Lundquist PA, et al. Does parent of origin matter? Methylation studies should be performed on patients with multiple copies of the Prader-Willi/Angelman syndrome critical region. *Am J Med Genet.* 2014;164:2514–2520.

Barlow DP, Bartolomei MS. Genomic imprinting in mammals. *Cold Spring Harb Perspect Biol.* 2014;6(2).

Bird LM. Angelman syndrome: review of clinical and molecular aspects. *Appl Clin Genet.* 2014;7:93–104.

Butler MG. Prader-Willi syndrome: obesity due to genomic imprinting. *Curr Genomics.* 2011;12:204–215.

Cassidy SB, Schwartz S, Miller JL, et al. Prader-Willi syndrome. *Genet Med.* 2012;14:10–26.

Cho SC, Yim SH, Yoo HK, et al. Copy number variations associated with idiopathic autism identified by whole-genome microarray-based comparative genomic hybridization. *Psychiatr Genet.* 2009;19:177–185.

Dagli A, Buiting K, Williams CA. Molecular and clinical aspects of Angelman syndrome. *Mol Syndromol.* 2012;2:100–112.

Dykens EM, Lee E, Roof E. Prader-Willi syndrome and autism spectrum disorders: an evolving story. *J Neurodev Disorder.* 2011;3:225–237.

Fan YS, Jayakar P, Zhu H, et al. Detection of pathogenic gene copy number variations in patients with mental retardation by genomewide oligonucleotide array comparative genomic hybridization. *Hum Mutat.* 2007;28:1124–1132.

Jonas RK, Montojo CA, Bearden CE. The 22q11.2 deletion syndrome as a window into complex neuropsychiatric disorders over the lifespan. *Biol Psychiatry.* 2014;75:351–360.

Knight SJ, Flint J. Perfect endings: a review of subtelomeric probes and their use in clinical diagnosis. *J Med Genet.* 2000;37:401–409.

LaSalle JM, Yasui DH. Evolving role of MeCP2 in Rett syndrome and autism. *Epigenomics.* 2009;1:119–130.

Liyanage VR, Rastegar M. Rett syndrome and MeCP2. *Neuromolecular Med.* 2014;16:231–264.

Lott IT. Neurological phenotypes for Down syndrome across the life span. *Prog Brain Res.* 2012;197:101–121.

Mabb AM, Judson MC, Zylka MJ, et al. Angelman syndrome: insights into genomic imprinting and neurodevelopmental phenotypes. *Trends Neurosci.* 2011;34:293–303.

Mezei G, Sudan M, Izraeli S, et al. Epidemiology of childhood leukemia in the presence and absence of Down syndrome. *Cancer Epidemiol.* 2014;38:479–489.

Millan Sanchez M, Heyn SN, Das D, et al. Neurobiological elements of cognitive dysfunction in Down syndrome: exploring the role of APP. *Biol Psychiatry.* 2012;71:403–409.

Monteiro FP, Vieira TP, Sgardioli IC, et al. Defining new guidelines for screening the 22q11.2 deletion based on a clinical and dysmorphologic evaluation of 194 individuals and review of the literature. *Eur J Pediatr.* 2013;172:927–945.

Murrell A. Cross-talk between imprinted loci in Prader-Willi syndrome. *Nat Genet.* 2014;46:528–530.

Navon D, Shwed U. The chromosome 22q11.2 deletion: from the unification of biomedical fields to a new kind of genetic condition. *Soc Sci Med.* 2012;75:1633–1641.

Peters J. The role of genomic imprinting in biology and disease: an expanding view. *Nat Rev Genet.* 2014;15:517–530.

Rabinovitz S, Kaufman Y, Ludwig G, et al. Mechanisms of activation of the paternally expressed genes by the Prader-Willi imprinting center in the Prader-Willi/Angelman syndromes domains. *Proc Natl Acad Sci U S A.* 2012;109:7403–7408.

Sadikovic B, Fernandes P, Zhang VW, et al. Mutation update for UBE3A variants in Angelman syndrome. *Hum Mutat.* 2014;35(12):1407–1417.

Schaefer GB, Starr L, Pickering D, et al. Array comparative genomic hybridization findings in a cohort referred for an autism evaluation. *J Child Neurol.* 2010;25:1498–1503.

Squarcione C, Torti MC, Di Fabio F, et al. 22q11 deletion syndrome: a review of the neuropsychiatric features and their neurobiological basis. *Neuropsychiatr Dis Treat.* 2013;9:1873–1884.

Stobbe G, Liu Y, Wu R, et al. Diagnostic yield of array comparative genomic hybridization in adults with autism spectrum disorders. *Genet Med.* 2014;16:70–77.

Thibert RL, Larson AM, Hsieh DT, et al. Neurologic manifestations of Angelman syndrome. *Pediatr Neurol.* 2013;48:271–279.

Ueno M. Roles of DNA repair proteins in telomere maintenance. *Biosci Biotechnol Biochem.* 2010;74:1–6.

Utine GE, Haliloglu G, Volkan-Salanci B, et al. Etiological yield of SNP microarrays in idiopathic intellectual disability. *Eur J Paedtr Neurol.* 2014;18:327–337.

Valente KD, Varela MC, Koiffmann CP, et al. Angelman syndrome caused by deletion: a genotype-phenotype correlation determined by breakpoint. *Epilepsy Res.* 2013;105:234–239.

Weaver JR, Bartolomei MS. Chromatin regulators of genomic imprinting. *Biochim Biophys Acta.* 2014;1839:169–177.

Webb CJ, Wu Y, Zakian VA. DNA repair at telomeres: keeping the ends intact. *Cold Spring Harb Persperct Biol.* 2013;5(6).

Whittington J, Holland A. Neurobehavioral phenotype in Prader-Willi syndrome. *Am J Genet C Semin Med Genet.* 2010;154C:438–447.

Disorders of DNA Maintenance, Transcription, and Translation

Aamann MD, Muftuoglu M, Bohr VA, et al. Multiple interaction partners for Cockayne syndrome proteins: implications for genome and transcriptome maintenance. *Mech Ageing Dev.* 2013;134:212–224.

Agirrezabala X, Frank J. From DNA to proteins via the ribosome: structural insights into the workings of the translation machinery. *Hum Genomics.* 2010;4:226–237.

Arancio W, Pizzolanti G, Genovese SI, et al. Epigenetic involvement in Hutchinson-Gilford progeria syndrome: a mini-review. *Gerontology.* 2014;60:197–203.

Arnold WD, Kassar D, Kissel JT. Spinal muscular atrophy: diagnosis and management in a new therapeutic era. *Muscle Nerve.* 2015;51(2):157–167.

Bahi-Buisson N. Genetically determined encephalopathy: Rett syndrome. *Handb Clin Neurol.* 2013;111:281–286.

Breitling J, Aebi M. N-linked protein glycosylation in the endoplasmic reticulum. *Cold Spring Harb Persperct Biol.* 2013;5:a013359.

Bugiani M, Boor I, Powers JM, et al. Leukoencephalopathy with vanishing white matter: a review. *J Neuropathol Exp Neurol.* 2010;69:987–996.

Chaudhary MW, Al-Baradie RS. Ataxia-telangiectasia: future prospects. *Appl Clin Genet.* 2014;7:159–167.

Cleaver JE, Bezrookove V, Revet I, et al. Conceptual developments in the causes of Cockayne syndrome. *Mech Ageing Dev.* 2013;134:284–290.

Del Bigio MR, Greenberg CR, Rorke LB, et al. Neuropathological findings in eight children with cerebro-oculo-facio-skeletal (COFS) syndrome. *J Neuropathol Exp Neurol.* 1997;56:1147–1157.

Edens BM, Ajroud-Driss S, Ma L, et al. Molecular mechanisms and animal models of spinal muscular atrophy. *Biochim Biophys Acta.* 2015;1852(4):685–692.

Farooqi AA, Attar R, Arslan BA, et al. Recently emerging signaling landscape of ataxia-telangiectasia mutated (ATM) kinase. *Asian Pac J Cancer Prev.* 2014;15:6485–6488.

Ghosh S, Zhou Z. Genetics of aging, progeria and lamin disorders. *Curr Opin Genet Dev.* 2014;26C:41–46.

Gómez-Escoda B, Wu PY. The programme of DNA replication: beyond genome duplication. *Biochem Soc Trans.* 2013;41:1720–1725.

Hoskins AA, Moore MJ. The spliceosome: a flexible, reversible macromolecular machine. *Trends Biochem Sci.* 2012;37:179–188.

Jaeken J. Congenital disorders of glycosylation. *Handb Clin Neurol.* 2013;113:1737–1743.

Kalay E, Yigit G, Aslan Y, et al. CEP152 is a genome maintenance protein disrupted in Seckel syndrome. *Nat Genet.* 2011;43:23–26.

Kralund HH, Ousager L, Jaspers NG, et al. Xeroderma pigmentosum-trichothiodystrophy overlap patient with novel XPD/ERCC2 mutation. *Rare Dis.* 2013;1:e24932.

Lambert WC, Gagna CE, Lambert MW. Trichothiodystrophy: photosensitive, TTD-P, TTD, Tay syndrome. *Adv Exp Med Biol.* 2010;685:106–110.

Laugel V. Cockayne syndrome: the expanding clinical and mutational spectrum. *Mech Ageing Dev.* 2013;134:161–170.

Lehmann AR, McGibbon D, Stefanini M. Xeroderma pigmentosum. *Orphanet J Rare Dis*. 2011;6:70.

Maher RL, Branagan AM, Morrical SW. Coordination of DNA replication and recombination activities in the maintenance of genome stability. *J Cell Bio*. 2011;112:2672–2682.

Mantha AK, Sarkar B, Tell G. A short review on the implications of base excision repair pathway for neurons: relevance to neurodegenerative diseases. *Mitochondrion*. 2014;16:38–49.

Marteijn JA, Lans H, Vermeulen W, et al. Understanding nucleotide excision repair and its roles in cancer and ageing. *Nat Rev Mol Cell Biol*. 2014;15:465–481.

Naegeli H, Sugasawa K. The xeroderma pigmentosum pathway: decision tree analysis of DNA quality. *DNA Repair (Amst)*. 2011;10:673–683.

O'Driscoll M, Ruiz-Perez VL, Woods CG, et al. A splicing mutation affecting expression of ataxia-telangiectasia and Rad3-related protein (ATR) results in Seckel syndrome. *Nat Genet*. 2003;33:497–501.

Parsons JL, Dianov GL. Co-ordination of base excision repair and genome stability. *DNA Repair (Amst)*. 2013;12:326–333.

Rulten SL, Caldecott KW. DNA strand break repair and neurodegeneration. *DNA Repair (Amst)*. 2013;12:558–567.

Saijo M. The role of Cockayne syndrome group A (CSA) protein in transcription-coupled nucleotide excision repair. *Mech Ageing Dev*. 2013;134:196–201.

Shababi M, Lorson CL, Rudnik-Schöneborn SS. Spinal muscular atrophy: a motor neuron disorder or a multi-organ disease? *J Anat*. 2014;224:15–28.

Trovesi C, Manfrini N, Falcettoni M, et al. Regulation of the DNA damage response by cyclin-dependent kinases. *J Mol Biol*. 2013;425:4756–4766.

Velez-Cruz R, Egly JM. Cockayne syndrome group B (CSB) protein: at the crossroads of transcriptional networks. *Mech Ageing Dev*. 2013;134:234–242.

Weidenheim KM, Dickson DW, Rapin I. Neuropathology of Cockayne syndrome: evidence for impaired development, premature aging, and neurodegeneration. *Mech Ageing Dev*. 2009;130:619–636.

Darryl C. De Vivo and Jahannaz Dastgir

INTRODUCTION

Tone opposes gravity and maintains postural attitude. The term *hypotonia* refers to a state of low muscle tone. Infants who are hypotonic are often referred to as *floppy* because their limbs and head hang limply rather than firmly extended when held by an examiner in the prone position. These infants also may show a diminished resistance to passive limb movement when examined. The floppy infant seems to be weak, but the examiner may find it difficult to distinguish between true weakness and apparent weakness due to hypotonia and/or hyperlaxity.

Causes for hypotonia in infants are many, and it is the responsibility of the clinician to create a relevant differential diagnosis for the clinical presentation (Fig. 136.1). The clinician should first focus on the presenting history, noting weeks of gestation, intrauterine drug exposure, perinatal ultrasound abnormalities (e.g., cerebral dysgenesis, reduced fetal movements, oligohydramnios, or polyhydramnios), intrauterine infections (herpes simplex, cytomegalovirus, toxoplasmosis, rubella), and perinatal drug exposure or trauma (global or focal). A notation also should be made on whether the infant had low tone, limb contractures, difficulty breathing, or a weak cry at birth. This information helps determine whether the condition began before, at, or after birth. Hypotonia, emerging days after birth suggests an inborn error of metabolism. Additional history, when evaluating an infant in the first month of life, should include the strength of the infant's suck and whether the infant chokes with feeds. Potential exposures to *Clostridium botulinum* (via honey or corn syrup consumption or dirt) are important. Family history may reveal an inherited risk for hypercoagulability (including prior maternal spontaneous abortions), immune-mediated conditions, genetic syndromes (premature death may suggest a metabolic syndrome), neuropathies, myasthenia gravis, or myopathies/muscular dystrophies (developmental delay and weakness).

The aforementioned history will complement a careful neurologic exam that identifies (1) unique dysmorphic features; (2) a highly arched palate or tenting of the mouth (suggestive of congenital tongue weakness); (3) respiratory distress; (4) heart, abdominal, genitourinary, skin (birthmarks, doughy quality), or musculoskeletal abnormalities (congenital scoliosis, kyphosis, contractures, hip dysplasia, torticollis, hyperextensibility of joints); (5) level of alertness; (6) quality of cry; (7) cranial nerve dysfunction (facial weakness, ptosis, limited extraocular movements, tongue fasciculations, tongue atrophy, strength of suck); (8) focal or diffuse weakness; (9) evidence of hypertonicity (increased jitteriness and rigidity of the limbs) or hypotonicity (frog-legged posture while supine, lack of spontaneous movement, scarf sign, tendency to keep the trunk flexed while held in horizontal suspension, slip through); and (10) tendon reflex responses. The pertinent findings on examination, in conjunction with a thorough history, will guide the clinician to whether the infant's presentation is related to a nonneurologic (structural, toxic, or genetic syndrome) or neurologic etiology that may be central (brain and spinal cord) or peripheral (peripheral nerves, neuromuscular junction, or muscle).

If the clinician believes that the hypotonia is neurologic and central in nature, additional workup would include brain imaging (magnetic resonance imaging [MRI] or computed tomography [CT] scan), electroencephalography (EEG), and cerebrospinal fluid (CSF) studies. If the hypotonia is neurologic and peripheral, confirmatory studies may include electromyography (EMG), nerve conduction studies (NCS), serum creatine kinase (CK) levels, muscle ultrasound or MRI, and muscle and/or nerve biopsy. If the findings from these tests raise concerns for a dystrophy or myopathy, additional processing of the muscle for electron microscopy (to identify distinctive ultrastructural abnormalities), immune staining, or biochemical assays for specific enzyme deficiencies should be performed.

If the clinician finds that the hypotonia is nonneurologic, confirmatory diagnostic workup should address a particular genetic syndrome (chromosomal microarray, whole exome sequencing, or targeted gene sequencing), inborn error of metabolism (blood studies—e.g., glucose, electrolytes, blood gas, ammonium, lactate and pyruvate, carnitine profile, liver function testing, very long-chain fatty acids, plasma amino acids, 7-dehydrocholesterol, isoimmune electrophoresis for transferrin; urine studies—e.g., urinalysis, urine amino acids, urine organic acids; CSF studies—e.g., amino acids, lactate, pyruvate, neurotransmitters, pterins, and 5-methyltetrahydrofolate), or structural abnormality (bone films, spinal MRI). These studies complement the newborn screening.

CAUSES OF CENTRAL HYPOTONIA

Central hypotonia refers to decreased tone due to lesions above the anterior horn cells of the spinal cord. Such hypotonia is often symmetric and affects the upper and lower limbs equally. It may also present with additional features of developmental delay (speech, motor, or global), seizures, and/or brisk reflexes.

HYPOXIC–ISCHEMIC ENCEPHALOPATHY

Hypoxic–ischemic encephalopathy (HIE) develops in the setting of perinatal hypoxia. The initial presentation of HIE in the newborn period may be hypotonia in addition to seizures, decreased level of alertness, and/or irritability. Over time, the initial presentation of hypotonia may evolve into increased tone and spasticity.

NEURONAL MIGRATION DISORDERS

Neuronal migration disorders include holoprosencephaly, anencephaly, lissencephaly, pachygyria, polymicrogyria, and/or heterotopias. It should be noted that neuronal migration disorders might be part of a larger syndrome, and some of these syndromes also present with peripheral hypotonia either in the form of myopathy, muscular dystrophy, or neuropathy (e.g., merosin-deficient congenital muscular dystrophy, Fukuyama congenital muscular dystrophy, Walker–Warburg syndrome, or muscle–eye–brain disease).

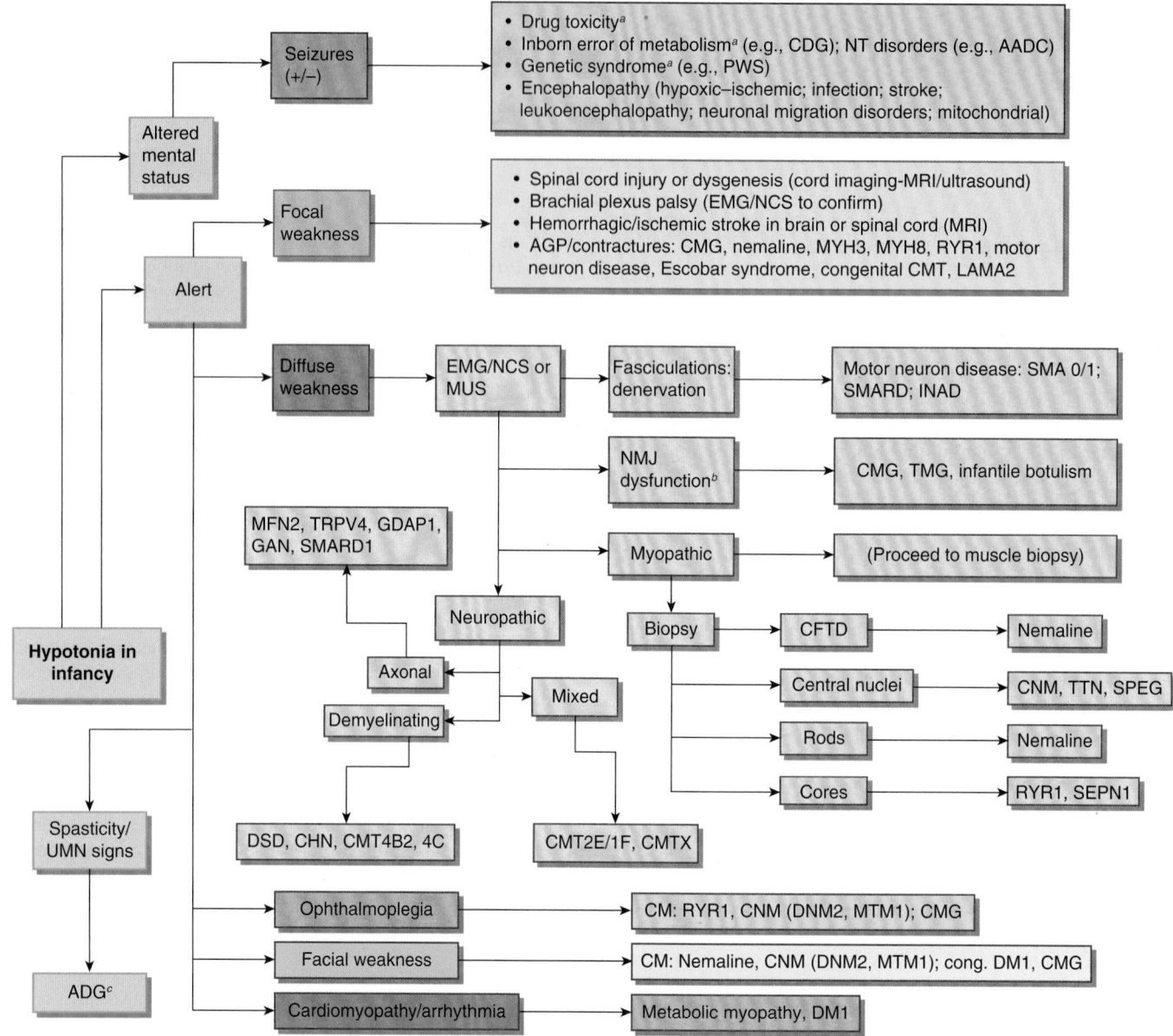

FIGURE 136.1 Differential diagnosis for hypotonia in infants. [a]May be associated with pathognomonic dysmorphic features. [b]Muscle ultrasound (MUS) is not diagnostic for neuromuscular junction dysfunction but can visualize fasciculations and fibrofatty replacement in muscle either due to myopathy, neuropathy, or motor neuron disease. [c]May also present with seizures.

AADC, aromatic l-amino acid decarboxylase deficiency; ADG, α-dystroglycanopathy; AGP, arthrogryposis; CDG, congenital disorder of glycosylation; CFTD, congenital fiber-type disproportion; CHN, congenital hypomyelinating neuropathy; CM, congenital myopathy; CMG, congenital myasthenia gravis; CMT, Charcot–Marie–Tooth; CNM, centronuclear myopathy; DM1, myotonic dystrophy; DNM2, dynamin 2 gene; DSD, Dejerine–Sottas disease; EMG, electromyography; GAN, giant axonal neuropathy; GDAP1, ganglioside induced differentiation associated protein 1; INAD, infantile neuroaxonal dystrophy; LAMA2, laminin α-2 gene; MFN2, mitofusin 2 gene; MRI, magnetic resonance imaging; MTM1, myotubularin 1 gene; MUS, muscle ultrasound; MYH, myosin heavy chain; MYH3, myosin heavy chain 3 gene; MYH8, myosin heavy chain 8 gene; NCS, nerve conduction studies; NMJ, neuromuscular junction; NT, neurotransmitter; PWS, Prader–Willi syndrome; RYR, ryanodine receptor 1 gene; SEPN1, selenoprotein 1 gene; SMA, spinal muscular atrophy; SMARD1, spinal muscular atrophy and respiratory distress type 1; SPEG, striated muscle preferentially expressed protein kinase; TMG, transient myasthenia gravis; TRPV4, transient receptor potential cation channel, subfamily V, member 4; TTN, titin gene; UMN, upper motor neuron.

LEUKODYSTROPHIES

Leukodystrophies may also present with a concomitant demyelinating neuropathy (see "Peripheral Neuropathy" section).

Leukodystrophies are disorders of central nervous system (CNS) myelin development and maintenance (divided into disorders of dysmyelination, hypomyelination, or demyelination). They are genetically determined and may present in infancy with hypotonia, encephalopathy, and/or developmental delays.

VASCULOPATHIES: ISCHEMIC OR HEMORRHAGIC

Neonatal stroke may initially present as hypotonia and later evolve into hypertonia with spasticity.

CONGENITAL INFECTIONS

Congenital infections include toxoplasmosis, *Treponema pallidum*, rubella, cytomegalovirus, herpesvirus, hepatitis B and C viruses, HIV, varicella, and parvovirus B19. These may present with hypotonia in addition to other features of intracranial calcifications or cysts, abnormal liver function, skin rash, hearing loss, encephalopathy, seizures, and/or retinitis or optic nerve atrophy.

INBORN ERRORS OF METABOLISM

Refer to Chapters 134 and 139. Some inborn errors of metabolism may also cause peripheral neuropathy.

GENETIC SYNDROME

Genetic syndromes that most commonly present with hypotonia include Down syndrome, Prader–Willi syndrome, fragile X syndrome, trisomy 18, 1p36 deletion, 22q13 deletion syndrome, 22q11.2 deletion syndrome, DiGeorge/velocardiofacial syndrome, Williams syndrome, trisomy 13, Smith–Magenis syndrome, Sotos syndrome, Lowe syndrome, Smith–Lemli–Opitz syndrome, Wolf–Hirschhorn syndrome, Kabuki syndrome, Cri-du-chat syndrome.

TOXICITY

Intrauterine exposure to drugs such as lamotrigine, lithium, and benzodiazepines have been associated with hypotonia. Antepartum or peripartum maternal exposure to high levels of magnesium sulfate for the treatment of eclampsia and prevention of cerebral palsy has also been associated with congenital hypotonia.

NERVE/CORD INJURY OR STRUCTURAL ABNORMALITY

For discussion of spinal dysraphism/spina bifida, refer to Chapter 133.

Spinal cord injury may be secondary to intrauterine malpositioning or trauma/severe asphyxia during birth (via hypoperfusion between the anterior spinal artery and paired spinal arteries) that subsequently damages the lower motor neurons of the spinal cord. Autopsy studies of fatally asphyxiated neonates demonstrate prominent, ischemic necrosis of anterior spinal cord gray matter. Infants with spinal cord injury often present with hypotonia, weakness, and absent tendon reflexes only in the regions distal to the site of injury. Ultrasound/MRI of the spine also may be used to identify cord ischemia or spinal dysraphism.

CAUSES OF PERIPHERAL HYPOTONIA

Peripheral hypotonia refers to disorders of the motor unit/anterior horn cell, peripheral nerve, neuromuscular junction, and/or muscle.

Identifying whether or not there is focality to the weakness often helps with diagnosing its etiology.

FOCAL WEAKNESS: BRACHIAL PLEXUS INJURY

Epidemiology

Brachial plexus injury is variable and ranges from 0.38 to 3 per 1,000 live births in industrialized countries. Birth incidence depends on the type of obstetric care and the average birth weight (strongest predictor) of infants in different geographic regions.

Pathobiology

Shoulder dystocia is a strong predictor for brachial plexus palsy. Vaginal deliveries associated with vacuum extraction or direct compression of the fetal neck during delivery by forceps can cause stretching of the cervical nerve roots (via misdirected traction or hyperextension of the arms) and eventually, brachial plexus injury. A prolonged second stage of labor may also increase the risk.

Clinical Features

Brachial plexus palsies are divided into four categories based on location of injury: (1) upper (Erb palsy, C5–C7, most common palsy presenting with adducted arm that is internally rotated at the shoulder; wrist is flexed and fingers are extended in a "waiter's tip" posture), (2) intermediate (C7 and sometimes C8 and T1), (3) lower (Klumpke paralysis—C8, T1—poor hand grasp with more intact proximal muscles), and (4) total plexus palsy (C5–C8 and sometimes T1—second most common and the most devastating—claw hand and flaccid arm with no sensation). Additional finding that may be associated with a poor prognosis is Horner syndrome.

Diagnosis

X-rays of the chest, spine, and upper limbs are most important for brachial plexus palsies because they reveal associated injuries (fracture of ribs, transverse process, clavicle, humerus, or phrenic nerve injury). MRI of the upper limb/shoulder and spinal MRI also should be performed to rule out nerve root evulsion. CT myelography may be used if MRI is not possible. EMG/NCS may identify the severity of the neural lesion and detect signs of reinnervation. Serial EMG/NCSs within the first 48 hours after birth will distinguish between prenatal and obstetric causes of brachial plexus palsy. Sensory-evoked potentials can be used to assess the integrity of sensory conduction.

Treatment

For brachial plexus palsy, supportive therapy to maintain passive range of motion and muscle strength is recommended. The optimal timing of surgical exploration remains controversial but most recommend intervention in the first 6 months of life if there is no evidence of clinical recovery.

Outcome

The majority (70% to 95%) of patients with brachial plexus palsy make complete spontaneous recovery, but both the extent (upper, lower, total) and the severity (avulsion, rupture) of the injury influence the prognosis (lower plexopathies tend to be more severe). A small proportion of infants, managed conservatively, have severe permanent disability.

DIFFUSE WEAKNESS

For motor neuron disease, refer to Chapter 141. For congenital myopathies and muscular dystrophies, refer to Chapter 142. For metabolic myopathies, refer to Chapter 134.

Peripheral Neuropathy

Peripheral neuropathies in infancy are rare and can present with hypotonia, weakness, sensory alteration, areflexia, ataxia, contractures, congenital hip dysplasia, and predominantly distal muscle wasting. They may be described according to neurophysiologic findings (via EMG/NCS) and/or findings on nerve biopsy. Inherited neuropathies of the demyelinating or axonal type are described in the following text. Acquired causes are less common in infants and include Guillain–Barré syndrome, nutritional deficiencies (B_{12}, thiamine, or vitamin E), and toxic or infectious (e.g., diphtheria) causes. These will not be discussed in this section (see Chapter 88).

DEMYELINATING NEUROPATHIES

Dejerine–Sottas Disease (Also Known as CMT3 or HMSN Type III)

Pathobiology: Dejerine–Sottas disease (DSD) may be due to PMP22 point mutations, duplications, or deletions. Mutations in myelin protein zero (MPZ), EGR2, NEFL, periaxin, frabin (FGD4 gene/ also referred to as *CMT4H*), and FIG4 (also referred to as *CMT4J*) have also been noted. PMP22 is a glycoprotein with four putative transmembrane domains and accounts for 2% to 5% of compact myelin of the peripheral nervous system. It may play a role in the proliferation and differentiation of Schwann cells. MPZ is a member of the immunoglobulin gene superfamily that functions as a hemophilic adhesion molecule playing an important role in myelin adhesion and compaction. EGR2 is a zinc finger transcription factor, which binds regulatory domains of target genes, including those critical for myelin formation and maintenance. Periaxin is a cytoskeleton-associated protein expressed exclusively in myelinating Schwann cells. It is important for the elongation of Schwann cells and myelination during development. FGD4 is a Rho GDP/GTP nucleotide exchange factor expressed in the peripheral nerve. FGD4 induces changes in Schwann cell shape.

Clinical Features: DSD presents around 6 months with motor delays, hypotonia, and areflexia. Weakness is more distal than proximal. Most patients acquire the skill of walking. Cases associated with PMP22 point mutations may also have sensorineural hearing loss, facial weakness, rarely nystagmus, vestibular dysfunction, ptosis, limited extraocular movements, and bladder symptoms. Adie pupil may be associated with MPZ mutations. EGR2-related neuropathies have a high frequency of cranial nerve involvement. FIG4-related neuropathies have the unusual features of asymmetric involvement and sometimes rapid progression of muscle weakness precipitated by trauma.

Diagnosis: Profound slowing of motor conduction velocities (<10 to 12 m/s) supports the diagnosis. Nerve biopsies show significant reduction in density of myelinated fibers with hypomyelination and/or demyelination and extensive onion bulb formations. In periaxin mutation–related cases, immunohistochemistry demonstrates absent C-terminal L-periaxin staining.

Congenital Hypomyelinating Neuropathy

Pathobiology: Congenital hypomyelinating neuropathy (CHN) is due to PMP22 point mutations (autosomal dominant [AD] or autosomal recessive [AR]), MPZ (AD, AR), or EGR2 (AD, AR) mutations. It is thought to reflect a defect in myelin synthesis.

Clinical Features: Severe cases of CHN present at birth with profound weakness, hypotonia, arthrogryposis, and respiratory insufficiency. Tongue fasciculations may be present. Less severe cases may present in infancy with hypotonia and motor delay.

Diagnosis: NCSs demonstrate very slow or absent responses. Nerve biopsies show complete absence of peripheral nerve myelin without classic onion bulb formations, although some may have unusual "basal lamina onion bulbs" consisting of concentric whorls of double-layered Schwann cell basement membrane. Evidence of myelin degeneration is absent on pathology.

CMT4B2

Pathobiology: CMT4B2 is due to mutations in the myotubularin-related protein (MTMR13) gene (also known as *SET binding factor 2* [SBF2]).

Clinical Features: Some children present with early-onset glaucoma that precedes the onset of neuropathy and delayed motor milestones.

Diagnosis: NCSs show slowing of motor nerve conduction velocities.

CMT4C

Pathobiology: CMT4C is due to mutations in SH3TC2 or KIAA1985 gene. SH3TC is expressed exclusively in Schwann cells and is thought to play a role in endosomal recycling and membrane trafficking processes that are required for normal myelin formation.

Clinical Features: Early-onset severe spinal deformities are often the presenting symptom. Hypotonia is noted in the first few months of life with delayed motor development. Most children achieve walking. Foot deformity is common and may precede weakness. Hearing loss is the most common form of cranial nerve involvement, although facial weakness, nystagmus, and tongue atrophy/fasciculations are also reported. Respiratory insufficiency or hypoventilation may also occur.

Diagnosis: NCSs confirm a demyelinating neuropathy. Nerve biopsy shows loss of myelinated fibers, thinly myelinated fibers, basal lamina onion bulbs, and large cytoplasmic Schwann cell processes surrounding multiple unmyelinated axons.

Infantile Demyelinating Neuropathies with Central Nervous System Involvement

- CNS hypomyelination
  - Hypomyelination with congenital cataracts/DRCTNNBIA gene
  - Peripheral demyelinating neuropathy, central dysmyelinating leukodystrophy, Waardenburg syndrome, and Hirschsprung disease (PCWH)/SOX10 gene
  - Pelizaeus–Merzbacher disease/PLP1
  - Pelizaeus–Merzbacher–like disease/GJA12
  - Cockayne syndrome/ERCC6 and ERCC8 genes
- CNS white matter changes
  - Metachromatic leukodystrophy/ARSA gene
  - Krabbe disease/GALC gene
  - Niemann–Pick disease, type C/NPC1 and NPC2 genes
  - Merosin-deficient congenital muscular dystrophy/LAMA2 gene
  - Navajo neurohepatopathy/MPV17 gene
- Other CNS involvement
  - Congenital disorders of glycosylation/multiple genes
  - Congenital cataracts, facial dysmorphism, and neuropathy (CCFDN)/CTP1 gene
  - POLG-related hepatocerebral mtDNA deletion syndromes/POLG1 gene
  - Leigh syndrome/multiple genes

AXONAL NEUROPATHIES

CMT2A/Mitofusin 2 Mutations

Pathobiology: Mitofusin 2 (MFN2) is a transmembrane GTPase located in the outer mitochondrial membrane. It is important for mitochondrial fusion, axonal mitochondrial transport, and tethering of the mitochondria to the endoplasmic reticulum. Most mutations are dominant (30% to 40% de novo), and some are compound heterozygous and homozygous.

Clinical Features: CMT2A may start in early childhood with distal weakness. Most children reach ambulation, but progression is rapid and usually leads to wheelchair dependence by the end of the second decade. Children may have complete distal paralysis and claw hands. Planus foot is universal in all cases. Early proximal weakness of the lower limbs is also noted and may produce a waddling gait with foot drop. Optic atrophy is noted in 10% to 20% of cases.

Diagnosis: NCSs show axonal and sensory neuropathy with normal velocities. Motor and sensory responses may be unrecordable. Nerve biopsy shows severe loss of large, myelinated fibers and abnormal aggregations of small round mitochondria on electron microscopy.

CMT2C/TRPV4 Mutations

Pathobiology: TRPV4 is a Ca2+ permeable nonselective cationic channel widely expressed in a number of tissues (cartilage, motor neurons, and dorsal root ganglia). Mutations result in neurotoxic gain of function effect from increased Ca2+ influx. How this translates to a neuromuscular disorder is unknown.

Clinical Features: Those who present in infancy usually have a congenital distal spinal muscular atrophy phenotype presenting with congenital foot deformities (often talipes equinovarus) and contractures of the hips, knees, and Achilles tendons. Congenital hip dysplasia and scoliosis are also common. CMT2C may be associated with vocal cord paresis presenting as stridor or respiratory distress due to diaphragmatic involvement. Additional features include hearing loss, mild sensory loss, hand tremor, and bladder dysfunction.

Diagnosis: NCSs show motor and sensory axonal neuropathy. Findings on biopsy include moderate loss of myelinated fibers and clusters of regenerating axons.

CMT4A/GDAP1 Mutations

Pathobiology: The GDAP1 protein is expressed in axons localized to the outer mitochondrial membrane and involved in mitochondrial fission and regulation of the mitochondrial network.

Clinical Features: CMT4A presents in the first year of life with prominent foot deformities, gait difficulties, and distal weakness. Some children are hypotonic at birth, but many have normal early motor development and walk by 2 years. Hand weakness develops in the first decade and rapidly evolves to "claw hands." Progressive proximal weakness renders patients wheelchair dependent by the second decade. Vocal cord paresis or hoarseness is a frequent feature. Diaphragmatic dysfunction and restrictive lung disease is also very common. Optic atrophy has been noted.

Diagnosis: Both axonal and demyelinating features are present on NCSs. On nerve biopsy, the most common finding is axonal degeneration, regeneration, and pseudo–onion bulbs. Some patients have a predominantly demyelinating process with a decrease in the number of myelinated fibers and segmental demyelination.

Giant Axonal Neuropathy

Pathobiology: Giant axonal neuropathy is due to recessive mutations in the gigaxonin (GAN) gene, which is ubiquitously expressed and involved in the maintenance of microtubule networks. Mutations are thought to cause defective ubiquitin-mediated degradation of microtubule-related proteins leading to neuronal toxicity and impaired retrograde axonal transport.

Clinical Features: Children with GAN have severe, early-onset motor and sensory neuropathy with CNS involvement and characteristic "kinky" hair. Most present with delayed development and gait difficulties. Additional CNS involvement (cerebellar signs and/or spasticity) may or may not present early or throughout the course of the disease. The clinical course is progressive with most kids being wheelchair dependent in the second decade.

Diagnosis: NCSs show an axonal sensorimotor neuropathy sometimes with mild slowing of nerve conduction. Visual, somatosensory, and auditory brain stem–evoked potentials are abnormal. EEG may show diffuse slowing with occasional sharp waves. MRI may show periventricular and cerebellar white matter signal abnormalities and/or cerebral, cerebellar, and brain stem atrophy. Biopsy shows characteristic giant axons (large axonal swellings in thinly myelinated/unmyelinated nerve fibers) with densely packed structurally normal bundles of neurofilaments.

Spinal Muscular Atrophy with Respiratory Distress Type I

This is also known as *SMARD1* or *infantile axonal neuropathy with respiratory failure.*

Pathobiology: SMARD1 is due to mutation in the IGHMBP2 gene.

Clinical Features: Children with SMARD1 present with respiratory failure and progressive distal weakness.

Diagnosis: NCSs show absent responses in most cases. Nerve biopsy demonstrates decreased myelinated fibers, active axonal degeneration or active evidence of regeneration, and no onion bulb formations.

Infantile Neuroaxonal Dystrophy/Neuronal Brain Iron Accumulation Syndrome

Pathobiology: Infantile neuroaxonal dystrophy (INAD) is due to recessive mutations in the PLA2G6 gene.

Clinical Features: INAD present with early-onset hypotonia and psychomotor regression. Onset is between 6 months and 3 years after a period of normal development. Children evolve from hypotonia to a spastic tetraparesis, although some children have obvious features of a neuropathy with amyotrophy and areflexia. Gait ataxia, ophthalmologic abnormalities (optic atrophy, nystagmus, and strabismus), and dystonia are frequent. Seizures are rare. Mean age of death is 9 years.

Diagnosis: NCSs shows a sensorimotor axonal neuropathy and EMG evidence of denervation. Abnormal visual-evoked potentials may also be noted. Muscle ultrasound may show fasciculations. Almost all children have cerebellar atrophy on MRI along with T2/fluid-attenuated inversion recovery (FLAIR) hyperintensities in the cerebellum. Around 50% have abnormal iron accumulation in the globus pallidus. Nerve biopsy electron microscopy shows dystrophic axons.

MIXED AXONAL AND DEMYELINATING NEUROPATHY

CMT2E/1F

Pathobiology: CMT2E is due to NEFL mutations (also seen in DSD). Severe, early-onset cases can be caused by dominant or recessive mutations. NEFL assembles into heteropolymers with heavy and medium neurofilaments forming the major intermediate filament in axons. Neurofilaments determine axonal diameter and thus conduction velocity. NEFL mutations disrupt neurofilaments assembly and axonal transport resulting in decreased axonal diameter and contributing to slowed conduction.

Clinical Features: CMT2E presents in infants with hypotonia, delayed motor development, and/or foot deformity (e.g., pes cavus). Distal weakness and wasting may be severe, and proximal weakness may be present. Additional features include intellectual disability, pyramidal signs, hearing loss, ataxia, and tremor.

Diagnosis: NCSs show mixed axonal and demyelinating features. Compound motor action potentials (CMAPs) are usually moderately to severely reduced and distal motor latencies may be significantly prolonged. Nerve biopsy shows loss of large myelinated fibers with regenerating clusters. Some individuals have giant axons containing accumulations of irregularly oriented neurofilaments.

CMTX

Pathobiology: CMTX is due to mutations in the gap junction protein beta-1 (GJB1 or connexin 32). This is an X-linked CMT. CMTX2 is associated with cognitive impairment. CMTX4 is associated with hearing loss and cognitive deficits.

Clinical Features: CMTX presents with delayed motor development in infancy. Neuropathy is slowly progressive and most patients remain ambulant. Sensorineural hearing loss may occur.

Diagnosis: NCS velocities are in the intermediate range and CMAP amplitudes are usually low. Demyelinating and axonal features are present on nerve biopsies with reduced myelinated fiber density, thinned myelin sheaths, and onion bulb formations. Paranodal abnormalities are also described.

Disorders of the Neuromuscular Junction

For congenital myasthenia, please refer to Chapter 89.

BOTULISM

Epidemiology

As of 2006, infant botulism was reported in at least 26 different countries around the world, with the largest number of cases in the United States (mainly California, Utah, and Eastern Pennsylvania).

Pathobiology

Infant botulism results from the ingestion of *C. botulinum* spores. This bacterium is a gram-positive spore that produces seven different toxins (A→ G), and only types A, B, E, and F are known to cause disease in humans. Upon ingestion of *C. botulinum* spores, colonization occurs in the infant's intestinal tract, which lacks the competitive microbial flora that normally inhibits growth of ingested spores. The spores then produce neurotoxins that are absorbed into the blood and eventually bind to the presynaptic nerve terminals. This prevents the binding, fusion, and release of acetylcholine and causes a symmetric, descending motor weakness and flaccid paralysis with autonomic dysfunction.

Clinical Features

Botulinum toxicity often presents with rather acute manifestations of feeding difficulties, decreased gag, ileus, constipation, hypotonia, weakness, pupillary dilation and paralysis, ophthalmoplegia, decreased tendon reflexes, bulbar palsy, and apneic spells.

Diagnosis

Botulism diagnosis may be confirmed by the recovery of the bacterium and the exotoxin in the feces.

Treatment

Treatment for infant botulism is highly dependent on early clinical diagnosis (examination and EMG/NCS) confirmed with identification of the *C. botulinum* organism in the patient's stool. Stool samples should be collected carefully, as the botulinum toxin is poisonous. Baby botulism immune globulin is available only to infants who are diagnosed with suspected botulism within 7 days of hospital admission and after consultation with an Infant Botulism Treatment and Prevention Program (IBTPP) physician.

Outcome

Patients diagnosed with infant botulism are expected to make a complete recovery if spared any secondary complications. Botulism immune globulin intravenous (BIG-IV) shortens hospital stays.

SUGGESTED READINGS

Abbassi-Ghanavati M, Alexander JM, McIntire DD, et al. Neonatal effects of magnesium sulfate given to the mother. *Am J Perinatol.* 2012;29:795–800.

Baets J, Deconinck T, De Vriendt E, et al. Genetic spectrum of hereditary neuropathies with onset in the first year of life. *Brain.* 2011;134:2664–2676.

Bönnemann CG, Wang CH, Quijano-Roy S, et al. Diagnostic approach to the congenital muscular dystrophies. *Neuromuscul Disord.* 2014;24:289–311.

Brun L, Ngu LH, Keng WT, et al. Clinical and biochemical features of aromatic L-amino acid decarboxylase deficiency. *Neurology.* 2010;75(1):64–71.

Chien YH, Hwu WL, Lee NC. Pompe disease: early diagnosis and early treatment make a difference. *Pediatr Neonatol.* 2013;54:219–227.

Dubowitz V. *The Floppy Infant.* Cambridge, United Kingdom: Cambridge University Press; 1993.

Gordon HB, Letsou A, Bonkowsky JL. The leukodystrophies. *Semin Neurol.* 2014;34(03):312–320.

Hantaï D, Nicole S, Eymard B. Congenital myasthenic syndromes: an update. *Curr Opin Neurol.* 2013;26:561–568.

Hirano M, DiMauro S. Metabolic myopathies. *Adv Neurol.* 2002;88:217–234.

Jones HR, De Vivo DC, Darras BT, eds. *Neuromuscular Diseases of Infancy, Childhood, and Adolescence.* Philadelphia: Butterworth-Heinemann; 2003.

Kamboj M. Clinical approach to the diagnoses of inborn errors of metabolism. *Pediatr Clin North Am.* 2008;55(5):1113–1127.

Kang PB, Gooch CL, McDermott MP, et al. The motor neuron response to SMN1 deficiency in spinal muscular atrophy. *Muscle Nerve.* 2014; 49: 636–644.

Kinali M, Beeson D, Pitt MC, et al. Congenital myasthenic syndromes in childhood: diagnostic and management challenges. *J Neuroimmunol.* 2008;201–202:6–12.

Kozma C. Neonatal toxicity and transient neurodevelopmental deficits following prenatal exposure to lithium: another clinical report and a review of the literature. *Am J Med Genet A.* 2005;132A:441–444.

Lehman LL, Rivkin MJ. Perinatal arterial ischemic stroke: presentation, risk factors, evaluation, and outcome. *Pediatr Neurol.* 2014;51:760–768.

Leyenaar J, Camfield P, Camfield C. A schematic approach to hypotonia in infancy. *Paediatr Child Health.* 2005;10(7):397–400.

Lott IT. Neurological phenotypes for Down syndrome across the life span. *Prog Brain Res.* 2012;197:101–121.

Menezes MP, North K. Inherited neuromuscular disorders: pathway to diagnosis. *J Paediatr Child Health.* 2012;48:458–465.

Monani UR, De Vivo DC. Neurodegeneration in spinal muscular atrophy: from disease phenotype and animal models to therapeutic strategies and beyond. *Future Neurol.* 2014;9(1):49–65.

Neu N, Duchon J, Zachariah P. TORCH infections. *Clin Perinatol.* 2015;42(1): 77–103, viii. doi:10.1016/j.clp.2014.11.001.

North KN, Wang CH, Clarke N, et al. Approach to the diagnosis of congenital myopathies *Neuromuscul Disord.* 2014;24:97–116.

Pearl PL, Taylor JL, Trzcinski S, et al. The pediatric neurotransmitter disorders. *J Child Neurol.* 2007;22(5):606–616.

Pifko E, Price A, Sterner S. Infant botulism and indications for administration of botulism immune globulin. *Pediatr Emerg Care.* 2014;30:120–127.

Prasad AN, Prasad C. Genetic evaluation of the floppy infant. *Semin Fetal Neonatal Med.* 2011;16:99–108.

Prendergast P, Magalhaes S, Campbell C. Congenital myotonic dystrophy in a national registry. *Paediatr Child Health.* 2010;15(8):514–518.

Scott K, Gadomski T, Kozicz T, et al. Congenital disorders of glycosylation: new defects and still counting. *J Inherit Metab Dis.* 2014;37(4):609–617.

Takcı Ş, Bayhan C, Çelik T, et al. Hypotonia and poor feeding in an infant exposed to lamotrigine and valproic acid in utero. *Turk J Pediatr.* 2013;55:546–548.

Tuysuz B, Kartal N, Erener-Ercan T, et al. Prevalence of Prader–Willi syndrome among infants with hypotonia. *J Pediatr.* 2014;164:1064–1067.

Uzun S, Kozumplik O, Jakovljevic M, et al. Side effects of treatment with benzodiazepines. *Psychiatr Danub.* 2010;22(1):90–93.

Wilmshurst JM, Ouvrier R. Hereditary peripheral neuropathies of childhood: an overview for clinicians. *Neuromuscul Disord.* 2011;21:763–775.

Wilmshurst JM, Pollard JD, Nicholson G, et al. Peripheral neuropathies of infancy. *Dev Med Child Neurol.* 2003;45:408–411.

Yiu EM, Ryan MM. Demyelinating prenatal and infantile developmental neuropathies. *J Peripher Nerv Syst.* 2012;17:32–52.

Yiu EM, Ryan MM. Genetic axonal neuropathies and neuronopathies of prenatal and infantile onset. *J Peripher Nerv Syst.* 2012;17:285–300.

Zafeiriou DI, Psychogiou K. Obstetrical brachial plexus palsy. *Pediatr Neurol.* 2008;38:235–242.

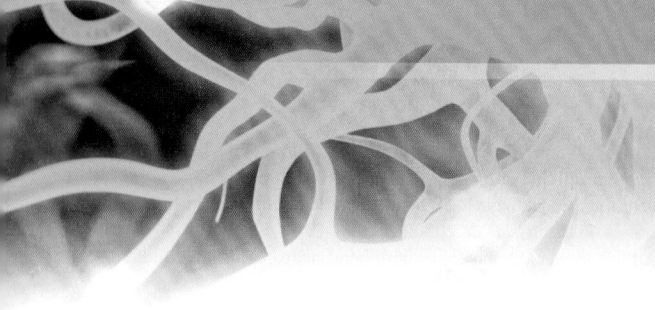

INTRODUCTION

Infancy and early childhood are marked by rapid brain growth and development. A wide variety of genetic and nongenetic factors may affect the immature brain during this period and manifest as a delay in the acquisition of milestones in one or more developmental domains: motor (gross and fine), speech/language, social, and cognitive. The delay may be isolated to one domain. When development in more than one domain is significantly delayed in children younger than the age of 5 years, the term *global developmental delay* applies.

Developmental delay is a common reason for referral to a child neurologist. The aims of the initial neurologic evaluation of a child with developmental delay are, first, to confirm the nature and severity of the suspected delay and second, to characterize any specific findings that may provide a clue to the underlying diagnosis. A detailed history is the key starting point. Items of particular importance include the family history (presence of neurologic or developmental disorders in the siblings, parents, grandparents, aunts, or uncles), perinatal history (complications during pregnancy, birth, or the neonatal period, including prematurity), and history of any coexisting medical problems. With regard to the presenting problem (e.g., motor delay), important items include the age at which the initial concern arose, the child's developmental progress over time, and whether or not there has been developmental regression. On general examination, the child's head circumference, height and weight, and the presence of any dysmorphic features should be noted. The eyes and optic fundi should be thoroughly examined, and skin should be checked for stigmata of neurocutaneous syndromes. Specific features of interest in the neurologic examination will be outlined in the relevant sections below.

DISORDERS OF MOTOR DEVELOPMENT

The acquisition of motor skills features prominently in the first year of life (Table 137.1). As a result, conditions that affect the motor system often present during infancy with motor developmental delay. Motor delay may also be the first manifestation of a condition that affects development globally because impaired motor function becomes apparent earlier than impairments in other domains such as cognition and language. Motor delay may be accompanied by specific motor symptoms such as stiffness, floppiness, and involuntary movements.

APPROACH TO THE CHILD WITH MOTOR DELAY

The neurologic examination begins with observation, particularly in the infant or toddler. Observe the child's spontaneous posture and movements for asymmetry, paucity of movement that may hint at weakness, abnormal postures, and excessive or involuntary movements. On cranial nerve examination, look for eye movement abnormalities including restricted range of movement and nystagmus. If the child can speak, note whether speech is clear or dysarthric. Turning attention to the body, assess muscle tone

in the trunk and limbs. Low truncal tone is common to many disorders that present with motor delay in infancy. Are the limbs hypotonic or spastic? Check whether tendon reflexes are abnormally brisk, suggesting an upper motor neuron lesion, or reduced, suggesting a neuromuscular abnormality. Assess coordination on targeted reaching movements (looking for dysmetria) and, in an older child, rapid alternating movements such as repetitive hand tapping. If the child is able, ask them to rise to standing from the floor (looking for a Gowers sign, which indicates proximal lower limb weakness). Note whether the gait is narrow or wide based and steady or unsteady. If involuntary movements are present, note their body distribution, their quality (e.g., sustained, writhing, or jerky), whether they are random or repetitive and stereotyped, and in what contexts they appear (e.g., at rest, during movement).

Following the clinical evaluation, brain imaging may be considered. Magnetic resonance imaging of the brain is indicated if there is a history of developmental regression, marked micro- or

TABLE 137.1	Motor Developmental Milestones in the First 5 Years
Gross Motor	**Age Range**
Hold head steady	2–4 mo
Roll over	2–5 mo
Sit without support	5½–7 mo
Pull to stand	8–10 mo
Walk	11–15 mo
Run	14–20 mo
Jump	21–28 mo
Hop	3–4 yr
Balance on one foot for 4 s	3½–5 yr
Fine Motor	**Age Range**
Grasp rattle	3–4 mo
Reach	4–6 mo
Transfer objects	5–8 mo
Pincer grasp	7–10 mo
Scribble	12–17 mo
Feed self with spoon	13–18 mo
Stack two blocks	13–21 mo
Hold crayon using fingers (not fist)	2–3 yr
Copy a circle	3–4 yr
Refined tripod pencil grip, print own name, copy a square	4–5 yr

Age range indicates approximately the 25th to 90th percentile for each milestone according to the Denver II Developmental Screening Tool.

TABLE 137.2	Features that Should Prompt Evaluation for a Possible Genetic or Metabolic Disorder in a Child Presenting with Symptoms of Cerebral Palsy

- Parent or sibling with a neurologic disorder
- Absent history of perinatal complications
- Normal brain imaging
- Developmental regression
- Progressive neurologic symptoms
- Ataxia or involuntary movements
- Signs of peripheral neuromuscular disease (reduced or absent reflexes, sensory loss)
- Fluctuating motor symptoms, for example, diurnal variation, worsening during fasting or exercise (may be symptoms of a treatable condition, e.g., a neurotransmitter disorder or Glut1 deficiency syndrome)

macrocephaly (>2 standard deviations from the mean), abnormal rate of head growth, or any abnormalities on neurologic examination including cranial nerve dysfunction, focal weakness, spasticity, abnormally brisk reflexes, or involuntary movements. Other investigations, such as genetic testing, may be indicated by the clinical syndrome or brain imaging results. In all cases, the aim is to determine a specific etiologic diagnosis whenever possible in order to guide the most appropriate management strategy. If the clinical syndrome and brain imaging findings are compatible with a developmental malformation or static brain lesion, then symptomatic management will be the most important consideration (see "Cerebral Palsy" below). On the other hand, several individually rare genetic and metabolic disorders may present with motor delay and mimic cerebral palsy. It is vital that the child neurologist be alert to signs that may indicate one of these conditions (Table 137.2). Making the correct diagnosis in these selected cases has important implications for management. In some cases, there is a disease-specific treatment that may dramatically improve the clinical course. Even if no disease-specific treatment yet exists, accurate diagnosis makes it possible to provide prognostic information and genetic counseling regarding recurrence risk in future pregnancies to the family.

CEREBRAL PALSY

Cerebral palsy (CP) is an umbrella term that describes a group of disorders characterized by motor impairment due to a developmental anomaly or nonprogressive lesion that arose in the developing fetal or infant brain. CP is not a specific disease and does not imply any one specific etiology. The term remains useful if considered not as a diagnosis in itself, but rather as a descriptive term which has widespread familiarity and conveys a recognized set of clinical characteristics and physical needs.

CP is common, with a birth prevalence of 2 or 3 per 1,000 live births in developed countries. Risk factors include a perinatal history of prematurity, intrauterine growth retardation, multiple gestation, and antepartum hemorrhage. One common misconception is that CP is usually caused by birth asphyxia, but in fact, fewer than 20% of patients with CP have documented perinatal asphyxia in many studies, and the actual proportion may be less than 10%. Other causes of CP include periventricular leukomalacia (the most

common form of ischemic brain injury in very preterm infants), cerebral malformations, stroke, and infection. The etiology is usually, but not always, evident on brain imaging.

CP may be classified according to the predominant motor abnormality: spasticity, dyskinesia (involuntary movements including dystonia, chorea, or athetosis), or ataxia. In some cases, there is a mixture of more than one motor feature, such as spasticity and dystonia. Spastic CP may be further classified according to the affected body regions: diplegia (both legs), quadriplegia (all four limbs), and hemiplegia (one side of the body). An accurate characterization of the motor syndrome is important for two reasons. First, it assists the interpretation of the clinical history and brain imaging findings in establishing the etiology of a child's CP. Second, it guides management decisions.

Spastic Diplegia

Approximately one-third of children with CP have spastic diplegia (or diparesis), in which spasticity is predominantly found in the legs. The arms may be mildly affected or unaffected. Parents may notice leg stiffness and a tendency for the legs to cross ("scissoring") due to increased tone in the hip adductor muscles. The increased lower limb tone may lead an infant to roll over or bear weight through the legs at an atypically early age. An older child with mild to moderate symptoms may have a narrow-based, scissoring gait and toe walking. On examination, there is increased tone in the lower limb muscle groups, particularly hip adductors, hamstrings, and calves. Tendon reflexes are brisk and plantar responses are extensor. The most commonly associated brain imaging abnormality is bilateral periventricular white matter lesions, particularly in children with a history of prematurity. The white matter lesions may be periventricular leukomalacia, consequences of intraventricular hemorrhage, or both.

Spastic Quadriplegia

Spastic quadriplegia (found in 20% to 25% of children with CP) is the most severe form. It is frequently associated with diffuse brain injury or dysgenesis. Brain imaging may demonstrate abnormalities in both gray and white matter, such as cystic encephalomalacia resulting from diffuse hypoxic injury. Severe limb hypertonia is often associated with hypotonia in the neck and trunk. A subset of patients has lesions in the deep gray nuclei (basal ganglia or thalamus) and may have a coexisting movement disorder. Most children with spastic quadriplegia are unable to walk and are dependent on a wheelchair for mobility and on support from caregivers for routine daily activities. Due to the diffuse nature of the cerebral insult, a number of comorbidities are often present, including seizures, cognitive impairment, and swallowing and speech difficulties. If swallowing is impaired, a feeding gastrostomy is often required to ensure adequate nutrition. For children who have both the inability to speak and limited voluntary control of hand movements, communication can be very challenging. Effective use of a communication device such as a board or tablet to which the child can point, or devices with eye tracking capability, may vastly improve the quality of life for both the child and their caregivers.

Spastic Hemiparesis

Spastic hemiplegia is found in about one-third of children with CP and results from a unilateral corticospinal tract lesion, such as a cerebral infarct (often in the territory of the middle cerebral artery), focal malformation (e.g., schizencephaly, cortical dysplasia), or posthemorrhagic porencephalic lesion in the white matter.

Such lesions may have been acquired prenatally or perinatally, but symptoms tend to manifest around age 6 months, when parents notice that the child exhibits a strong preference to use one hand over the other. Handedness normally develops at age 2 to 3 years, and so an obvious hand preference younger than 12 months of age should prompt clinical evaluation for a hemiparesis.

The hemiparesis usually affects the arm and hand more than the leg. Children with spastic hemiplegic CP are able to walk, although walking may be delayed, and an asymmetric gait pattern with toe walking and circumduction of the affected leg on the affected side is observed. In mild cases, upper limb weakness may only be evident as a subtle loss of hand dexterity or abnormal arm posturing during running. On the other hand, large lesions that involve both the white matter and the cortex can be associated with pronounced weakness as well as cortical sensory loss, leading to little or no functional hand use. Speech and language development is often delayed in the setting of a unilateral lesion of either hemisphere, but most children develop age-appropriate spoken language by the time they enter school. Longitudinal follow-up studies describe the emergence of subtle cognitive weaknesses in school-aged children with a history of perinatal stroke. Seizures are an additional factor that may adversely impact long-term cognitive outcome.

Dyskinetic Cerebral Palsy

Involuntary movements are the predominant motor finding in 5% to 10% of children with CP. The majority of children with dyskinetic CP have a history of term birth. Several types of involuntary movements may occur either alone or in combination. *Dystonia* describes stereotyped, abnormal twisting postures that may be fixed or intermittent. When severe dystonia causes fixed postures that make the limb appear hypertonic, it may be difficult to distinguish from severe spasticity. *Athetosis* refers to continuous writhing or wriggly movements, whereas *chorea* appears as discrete, random-appearing, jerky movements. Children with dyskinetic CP often have a history of hypotonia during early infancy, and their underlying muscle tone also tends to be low. A key feature of the involuntary movements is their tendency to worsen with increased activity or attempts to initiate voluntary movement. Often, muscles of the face and neck are involved in addition to the trunk and limbs.

Basal ganglia lesions are the most common abnormality seen on brain imaging in children with dyskinetic CP. These lesions may result from hypoxic–ischemic injury (in which cortical injury is also often seen) or neonatal hyperbilirubinemia (*kernicterus*, usually caused by maternal–fetal blood group incompatibility and now rare in developed countries). In instances where the cortex is spared, children may have good cognitive function despite severe motor disability and speech impairment.

Ataxic Cerebral Palsy

Ataxic CP is the least common form of CP (<5%) and is characterized by hypotonia, trunk and gait ataxia, and limb ataxia (intention tremor, dysmetria). If speech is affected, dysarthria with a slow and scanning quality is typical. Brain imaging may demonstrate a cerebellar malformation or lesion, although it is often normal. Both dyskinetic and ataxic CP are associated with normal brain imaging in a significant proportion of children (approximately one-third and one-half, respectively). In these cases, it is important to consider further investigation for an underlying treatable or neurodegenerative condition (Table 137.3).

Management of Cerebral Palsy

Children with CP should be referred to a multidisciplinary specialty center and to an early intervention program for therapy services as soon as they are identified. Hearing and vision should both be assessed early. Interventions are directed toward: (1) spasticity management; (2) management of involuntary movements; and (3) improvement of strength, motor abilities, function, and self-care. Effective management requires ongoing regular follow-up as the child grows and develops so that realistic expectations and achievable goals can be set and periodically reevaluated.

TABLE 137.3 Selected Genetic Conditions that May Mimic Dyskinetic and Ataxic Cerebral Palsy

Condition	Features
Neurotransmitter disorders	Hypotonia, dystonia with diurnal variation (better in morning and after sleep), oculogyric crises. Diagnosed by CSF neurotransmitter metabolite assay, genetic testing. Many forms respond to levodopa treatment.
Glut1 deficiency syndrome	Seizures, acquired microcephaly, ataxia, spasticity, dystonia, paroxysmal dyskinesia (may be triggered by exercise, fasting); treatment: ketogenic diet
Creatine deficiency	Intellectual disability, seizures, autism, progressive dystonia in guanidinoacetate methyltransferase (GAMT) deficiency. Treated with creatine monohydrate supplementation.
Benign hereditary chorea	Hypotonia, chorea, dystonia, myoclonus; may be associated with hypothyroidism, neonatal respiratory distress, or asthma.
Lesch–Nyhan syndrome	Hypotonia, dystonia, self-injurious behavior, elevated plasma urate
Ataxia-telangiectasia	Slowly progressive ataxia; chorea; dystonia (involuntary movements may preceed onset of ataxia); oculocutaneous telangiectasia; immunodeficiency; elevated serum α-fetoprotein; reduced levels of serum IgA, IgE, IgG$_2$
Pelizaeus–Merzbacher disease	Initial hypotonia then spastic quadriparesis, ataxia, ± dystonia and chorea, nystagmus (in classic form)
Niemann–Pick disease type C	Initial hypotonia followed by vertical supranuclear gaze palsy, slowly progressive ataxia, dystonia; ± hepatosplenomegaly

CSF, cerebrospinal fluid; Ig, immunoglobulin.

Spasticity management aims to reduce hypertonia in order to maximize the child's ability to gain muscle strength and range of movement through physical therapy, and to prevent long-term complications such as joint contractures and deformity. Functional goals depend on the severity of the child's impairment. For example, the goal for a child with moderate spastic diparesis may be to achieve independent ambulation. In a child with severe spastic quadriplegia, seizures, and intellectual disability, the goal may be to improve comfort and ease the caregivers' burden of care during daily activities such as dressing and bathing. The effect of spasticity on a child's posture and motor function can change over time, often increasing noticeably during periods of rapid growth.

Botulinum toxin injections are an effective tool for reducing spasticity, particularly when targeted toward a limited number of muscle groups. The toxin's effect lasts approximately 3 to 4 months, so injections typically need to be repeated up to three times per year. Sometimes, injections may be combined with serial casting to treat mild contractures. Oral medications such as baclofen (starting dose: 2.5 to 5 mg/day) and diazepam (starting dose: 1 to 5 mg/day depending on age and size) are useful when symptoms are generalized and offer modest benefit, but side effects such as sedation often limit the dose and efficacy.

Neurosurgical options for the management of spasticity include placement of an intrathecal baclofen pump and selective dorsal rhizotomy. Compared to oral baclofen, intrathecal baclofen may achieve a greater reduction in spasticity, particularly in the lower limbs, with fewer side effects. However, this potential benefit must be weighed against the long-term effort needed to maintain the pump and risk of complications. Rhizotomy aims to produce a permanent reduction in tone and is a good treatment option for some patients. Traditionally, the "ideal" rhizotomy candidate has been an ambulating child aged 3 to 8 years with spastic diparesis, in whom the goal of surgery is to optimize gait and independent function. Rhizotomy may also be appropriate in selected patients with spastic quadriparesis in order to ease caregivers' burden of care and reduce the need for future botulinum toxin injections and orthopedic procedures. If musculoskeletal complications such as joint contractures develop despite medical and surgical attempts to control spasticity, orthopedic surgery (such as tendon release procedures) may be indicated.

Children with dyskinetic CP often benefit from symptomatic treatment of their involuntary movements. For dystonia, trihexyphenidyl, starting at a low dose (1 to 2 mg/day) and titrated gradually to the point of tolerance (with common side effects being sedation, constipation, and urinary retention), may reduce abnormal posturing. Levodopa (starting dose: 25 to 50 mg/day) is beneficial in some children with dystonic CP. Hyperkinetic movements, such as chorea or athetosis, may respond to tetrabenazine (starting dose: 6.25 to 12.5 mg/day). Deep brain stimulation, with electrodes placed in the globus pallidus pars interna, may be a surgical option in severe, treatment-refractory cases of dyskinetic CP, although experience regarding efficacy and long-term outcome remains limited.

The rehabilitation team, composed of a physiatrist; orthotist; and physical, occupational, and speech/language therapists, plays an essential role in the care of a child with CP. Physical therapy aims to improve strength and range of movement, train ambulation, and stretch muscles to prevent joint deformity. Occupational therapy focuses on upper limb function and gaining independence with practical skills. Speech and language therapy focuses on communication. It is important to assess the child's home and school environments and determine equipment to facilitate mobility and daily activities.

Although diagnosed during childhood, CP is a lifelong condition, and all interventions made early in life are performed with an eye to the child's future as an adult. Children with severe motor and intellectual disability will require lifelong care, either from a parent or relative or in a nursing home setting. Less affected children need a school and therapy program targeted to their abilities, aiming to maximize their potential for future independence and well-being.

DEVELOPMENTAL COORDINATION DISORDER

Developmental coordination disorder (DCD) affects about 5% to 6% of children and is characterized by subtle impairments in gross and fine motor skills that typically manifest as difficulties in daily activities such as dressing, writing, or learning to ride a bike. Affected children are often described as "clumsy." In contrast to CP, the neurologic examination in DCD is normal apart from subtle signs such as mild hypotonia and dysdiadochokinesia. The underlying neurophysiologic basis remains poorly understood. DCD often co-occurs with other developmental disorders including attention deficit hyperactivity disorder, learning disabilities, and speech/language impairment.

DISORDERS OF HIGHER CEREBRAL FUNCTIONS

Assessment of speech and language, cognitive, academic, and reciprocal social abilities is an essential component of the evaluation of a child with developmental delay. The disorders that affect these domains of development are all defined behaviorally, lacking a single biologic marker or gold standard diagnostic instrument. Consequently, thorough assessment is crucial for proper diagnosis and effective management. The groups of developmental disorders of higher cerebral development under consideration are listed in Table 137.4.

APPROACH TO THE CHILD WITH LANGUAGE, COGNITIVE, OR ACADEMIC DELAYS

The age and manner in which children acquire speech and language varies considerably. Knowledge of normal developmental language milestones is essential in order to properly assess a child (Table 137.5). Speech and/or language delays are one of the most common presenting complaints to a child neurologist, especially in toddlers and preschool children. Hearing impairment must be excluded in all children with speech and language delays. The main diagnostic considerations in toddlers/preschoolers are developmental language disorders, autism spectrum disorders, intellectual disability, and attention deficit hyperactivity disorder (ADHD), although a definitive diagnosis of the latter may be postponed until a child is older if symptoms are not severe.

The mental status examination is the most informative part of the neurologic examination in the evaluation of a developmental disability involving higher cerebral function. The mental status exam in the toddler/preschooler relies heavily on observation. Watch the child play with representational toys (e.g., tiny dolls in a dollhouse, cars and trucks at a fire station, people and animals at a farm), assess his or her ability to talk to and play with the examiner or parent, and observe his or her interest and ability to focus on an activity introduced by another person (playing ball, looking at pictures, drawing). Particular attention should be paid to

TABLE 137.4 Developmental Disorders of Higher Cerebral Functions

Disorder	Function Affected	Location of Brain Dysfunction
Intellectual disability	Cognition	Diffuse or multifocal
Dysphasia (developmental language disorder)	Oral language	Language systems
Dyslexia (reading disability)	Written language (phonologic processing)	Language systems (left perisylvian)
Dyscalculia (math disability)	Math (spatial cognition)	Posterior right hemisphere
Nonverbal learning disability (NVLD)	Visuospatial, math, social cognition	Right parietal
Attention deficit hyperactivity disorder (ADHD)	Focused attention (executive functioning)	Prefrontal
Autism spectrum disorders (ASDs)	Social cognition	Connectivity

the child's ability to engage in creative/imaginative play, imitation, behavioral flexibility (ability to switch activities), attention span, and joint attention (the ability to draw another person's attention to an object of interest through the use of eye gaze and gestures, such as pointing).

Speech and/or language disorders can be subdivided based on the area of deficit: expressive or receptive. Expressive disorders can exist in isolation, but receptive disorders always coexist with expressive deficits. Speech and language skills should be assessed in the following areas: (1) production: amount of speech and its intelligibility, fluency, length and syntactic complexity of sentences, and richness of vocabulary; (2) pragmatics: knowing how to engage another person in conversation, turn taking, topic maintenance, appropriate eye gaze, awareness of tone of voice, facial expression, gestures, and body postures; (3) comprehension: following commands, answering simple questions (e.g., what's that? where is_?), answering complex, open-ended questions (e.g., why? when? how?); and (4) abnormal features: immediate echolalia, delayed echolalia (overlearned scripts), perseveration, abnormal prosody, and narrow range of topics.

In school-age children, school failure or underachievement is a common presenting complaint. In this age group, the differential diagnosis includes those disorders under consideration in the toddler/preschool years but expands to include disorders affecting academic achievement, for example, learning disabilities. Thus, the evaluation of the older child must include an assessment of academics in the areas of reading, writing, spelling, and mathematics. An assessment of cognitive ability is the first step, as the diagnosis of learning disability implies at least average intelligence. Attention should also be evaluated, as attention deficit hyperactivity disorder can now be diagnosed more reliably than in the toddler/preschooler. Language screening in the office is best done through a combination of informal assessment (as described for the preschooler) and standardized measures to assess vocabulary, word retrieval, word fluency, and automaticity of retrieval. General fund of knowledge, reading, spelling, writing, arithmetic, drawing (visuospatial skills), attention, and social reciprocity should also be evaluated. These skills can be assessed qualitatively; however, standardized screening tests are advisable to increase reliability.

Many children will come to the office with a detailed quantitative report generated by a psychologist or neuropsychologist detailing the strengths and weaknesses in cognitive, linguistic, and academic domains. It is important to be knowledgeable in the interpretation of these tests, and their scores as parents rely on neurologists to synthesize the findings for diagnostic clarification and developing an effective management plan. If a child has not had a formal assessment, it is advisable to have a comprehensive evaluation by a psychologist (preferably a neuropsychologist) and speech language pathologist to assess the child's cognitive and linguistic strengths and weaknesses. This should include a report of school achievement tests when learning disabilities are suspected. Attention disorders (with or without hyperactivity) frequently co-occur with learning disability; therefore, it is essential to diagnose these conditions accurately, as management strategies are quite different (i.e., educational vs. pharmacologic).

DEVELOPMENTAL LANGUAGE DISORDERS

Developmental language disorders (DLD), often lumped under the umbrella term *specific language impairment* (SLI) or *developmental dysphasias*, are a heterogeneous group of disorders characterized by inadequate language acquisition at the expected age despite otherwise normal development. The diagnostic criteria remain controversial, but DLD is usually ascribed when there is evidence that expressive and/or receptive language deficit is not attributable to inadequate hearing, intellectual disability, extreme and prolonged social deprivation (not simply social impoverishment), or a known brain lesion. Dysphasias can affect phonology (speech sounds) and syntax (word order, grammar) or higher order language processing skills, for example, semantic (word meaning) and pragmatics (communicative and conversational use of language). Genetics is the major cause of the developmental dysphasias, which occur more frequently in boys than girls.

Autism spectrum disorder (ASD) is an important diagnostic consideration in any child with a speech and/or language delays. Children with ASDs differ from children with DLD in their lack of drive to communicate. Unlike ASD, children with DLD use gestures, such as pointing and head nodding, which are usually well coordinated with eye gaze and facial expressions. Children with ASD have abnormal features such as echolalia, overlearned scripts, and perseverative language, in addition to the hallmark of impaired social reciprocity (see Chapter 138).

The occurrence of language regression in a child raises alarm in most families and sets off a cascade of neurodiagnostic testing that usually involves performing an electroencephalography (EEG). The exceptionally rare acquired epileptic aphasia or *Landau–Kleffner syndrome* (LKS) refers to previously normal children who lose their language skills, usually due to word deafness (i.e., auditory verbal agnosia), in the setting of clinical seizures or an epileptiform EEG, activated in sleep. Electrical status epilepticus during slow-wave sleep (ESES) is the electroencephalographic pattern seen in LKS. Similarly, approximately one-third of children with ASDs experience regression during

TABLE 137.5 Language and Social/Emotional Milestones

Age	Receptive Skills	Expressive Skills	Social/Emotional
0–2 mo	Startle, eye widening to sound	Range of cries (from hunger to pain)	Smiles spontaneously
2–4 mo	Quiets to voice, eye blinking to sound	Coos in response to voice	Smiles responsively
4–9 mo	Head turns to sound, responds with raised arms when mom says "up" and reaches for child, responds appropriately to friendly or angry voices	Babbling, repeats self-initiated sounds	Laughs to social attentions
9–12 mo	Listens selectively to familiar words, begins to respond to "no" and to one-step commands (usually accompanied by gesture), understands 10 words	Repeats parent-initiated sounds, symbolic gestures, jargoning, says "mama/dada" nonspecifically	Responds and plays social games: pat-a-cake, peek-a-boo. Joint attention emerges.
12–18 mo	Points to three body parts, understands up to 50 words, recognizes common objects by name, follows one-step commands accompanied by gestures	Uses words to express needs, 10 words by 18 mo, word usage may be inconsistent and mixed with jargon	Responds to name, joint attention established, functional play
18 mo–2 yr	Points to pictures when asked "show me," begins to distinguish "you" from "me"	Telegraphic two-word phrases "go bye-bye," "mama up," "baby go," 2 yr: vocab of at least 50 words and 50% intelligible by strangers	Symbolic play (feed baby, mix food in bowls)
2 ½ yr	Follows two-step commands, can identify actions in pictures and objects by use	2–3-word sentences develop, adjectives and adverbs appear, begins to ask questions	Imaginative play
3 yr	Knows several colors, knows what to do when we are hungry, thirsty, or sleepy; aware of past and future, understands "today" and "not today"	Uses pronouns and plurals, sentence length increases to 3–5 words, can tell stories that begin to be understood; uses negatives "I can't" and "I won't"; verbalizes toileting needs; tells full name, age, and gender	Starts to join in play with other children, begins dramatic play
3 ½ yr	Answers questions as "do you have a doll?" and "what toys do you have?"	Can relate experiences in sequential order, asks for permission	More independent in play with other children, shares toys and takes turns with assistance
4 yr	Understands same versus different, can follow three-step commands, understands why we have houses, umbrellas . . .	Can tell a story, uses past tense, names primary colors, asks many questions, nearly all speech understood by strangers	Fully plays and interacts with other children, improving in turn taking and cooperation, very imaginative with self and others
5 yr	Understands what we do with eyes and ears; understands "if," "because," "when," "why"; understands differences and comparisons; begins to understand left and right	Asks definition of specific words, makes serious inquiries ("how does this work?" "what does it mean?"), language is now complete in structure and form, all parts of speech are used as well as all types of sentences and clauses	Respects reasonable authority, wants to do what is expected, plays games with rules

the first 1 to 3 years of life, commonly referred to as *autistic regression*. EEGs in these children can be epileptiform. Children with autistic regression, however, undergo a more global loss of skills involving language, nonverbal communication, and sociability, unlike those with LKS who tend to maintain nonverbal communication skills and reciprocal social capabilities. The degree of overlap between LKS, ESES, and autistic regression with epileptiform EEG is currently poorly understood, although it is known that ESES is rarely seen in children with a more global autistic regression.

INTELLECTUAL DISABILITY

Intellectual disability (ID), also known as *intellectual developmental disorder*, requires limitations in both intellectual ability and deficits in adaptive skills relative to the child's age, experience, and environment. The onset of both deficits must occur during the developmental period. Deficits in intellectual functioning must be confirmed through clinical evaluation and standardized IQ testing. The IQ definition of ID uses 100 as the mean and 15 as the standard deviation. An IQ score of 65 to 75 (approximately 2 standard deviations below the mean, with a variation of +/− 5 points) is the demarcation point. The level and severity of ID (mild, moderate, severe, and profound) is defined on the basis of adaptive skills rather than the IQ score. The definition links the severity of ID to the degree of community support required to achieve optimal independence. Mild ID indicates the need for intermittent support, moderate ID for limited support, severe ID for extensive support, and profound ID for pervasive support. Although both intellectual and adaptive functioning are pertinent in defining ID, impairment of adaptive function is more likely to be the presenting feature than low IQ; however, it is expected that there is an association between intellectual functioning and adaptive skills.

The term *global developmental delay* (GDD) is used to describe children younger than the age of 5 years with significant delays in developmental milestones in several areas of functioning. GDD can be diagnosed using a standardized test, which shows performance at least two standard deviations below the mean in at least two developmental domains: motor, speech and language, cognition, personal–social, and/or adaptive (daily living). The diagnosis of ID is not used for children younger than 5 years old because IQ scores are not reliable until after 5 years and because some children with GDD will not meet criteria for ID as they get older.

The prevalence of ID varies due to differences in diagnostic approach, population characteristics, and study design but is generally considered to be 1%. Mild ID represents the majority (85%) and severe ID the minority (0.5% to 1%). Those with severe ID are more likely to have a definable etiology, whereas those with mild ID tend to come from socially disadvantaged backgrounds, often with a family history of mild ID or borderline intellectual function. The prevalence of GDD (in children younger than 5 years) is estimated at 1% to 3%.

The yield of diagnostic testing in determining a cause for GDD/ID is quite variable. The diagnostic evaluation should focus on clues for a genetic versus acquired etiology for ID. Recent years have seen important progress in identifying the genes involved in ID and currently, genetic defects are found in approximately 25% to 50%. A history of consanguinity, pregnancy losses/stillbirths, postnatal deaths of prior offspring, or birth defects should raise suspicion for a genetic etiology. If there is a family member known to have GDD/ID, testing specific to the known disorder should be performed, and if not known, a comprehensive genetics evaluation should be initiated. Observed dysmorphic features may prompt specific testing (e.g., Down syndrome, fragile X syndrome).

Other neurodiagnostic investigations should be undertaken based on the clinical picture. Inherited metabolic diseases are responsible for 1% to 5% of unspecified ID, and testing should be undertaken if clinical indicators are present. An EEG is appropriate if an underlying epilepsy syndrome is suspected or when there are paroxysmal behaviors concerning for seizures. Neuroimaging is recommended as part of the diagnostic evaluation of a child with GDD. Magnetic resonance imaging is more sensitive than computed tomography (CT), with abnormalities found in approximately one-half to one-third of children with global delay. The chance of detecting an abnormality increases if physical abnormalities, particularly CP, are present.

The management of children with ID focuses on finding the appropriate educational setting for children with mild ID, vocational training for those with moderate ID, and determining home or institutional placement for those with severe and profound ID. Available evidence demonstrates the benefits of early intervention through a variety of programs, at least with respect to short-term outcomes, and suggests that early diagnosis of a child with global delay may improve long-term outcome.

LEARNING DISABILITIES

Learning disabilities (LDs) occur in approximately 10% to 15% of school-aged children and can affect one or more academic skills. LDs involve reading (dyslexia), spelling (dysorthographia), writing (dysgraphia), mathematics (dyscalculia), and visuospatial skills (nonverbal learning disability [NVLD]). Executive functioning deficits are seen in LDs and also in disorders of attention, for example, attention deficit hyperactivity disorder. Specific learning disabilities do not refer to those children whose learning problems result from visual, hearing, or motor handicaps or are a consequence of emotional disturbance, environmental, cultural, or economic disadvantage. The term *learning disability* implies at least average intelligence.

DYSLEXIA

Developmental dyslexia is the most widely recognized and most common LD. It occurs in as many as 10% of school-aged children and comprises 80% of LDs. Boys are more often affected than girls. Dyslexia is characterized by an unexpected difficulty learning to read despite at least average intelligence, adequate instruction, and sociocultural opportunity. Major sensory functions must be normal. Dyslexia has a significant genetic component with heritability estimated at 54% to 84%. Dyslexia-susceptibility-1-candidate-1 (DYX1C1) was the first gene reported to be associated with dyslexia. Numerous candidate dyslexia susceptibility genes have subsequently been identified including several that affect neuronal migration.

There are different subtypes of dyslexia but the most common involves impaired phonologic processing. Children with dyslexia have difficulties with accurate and/or fluent word recognition, poor spelling, and decoding abilities. They have problems segmenting and sequencing speech into phonemes (e.g., speech sounds). Measures that assess phonologic functioning (e.g., segmenting words [say *cowboy* without the *boy*, say *smack* without the *m*], word and nonword blending, sound matching of first and last syllables) best differentiate dyslexic from normal readers.

A history of language delay and/or a family history of reading disabilities are often found in those with dyslexia. The elemental neurologic examination is normal. Routine imaging is normal and unnecessary, except perhaps in children with abnormalities on neurologic examination, seizures, or large discrepancies between verbal and spatial skills. All children with dyslexia should have a formal neuropsychological evaluation to determine their cognitive abilities (strengths and weaknesses) and to determine if there are co-occurring conditions that might affect treatment (e.g., ADHD).

Dyslexia is a lifelong disorder; however, most children with early reading problems learn to read at average to above-average levels if they are diagnosed by age 8 to 9 years (i.e., third or fourth grade) and evidence-based reading instruction is provided. Early diagnosis is essential, as children diagnosed late are likely to continue to have reading problems, even if remediated. Large population studies suggest that some degree of reading disability persists into adulthood in most, and occupational attainment may be lower in some.

NONVERBAL LEARNING DISABILITIES

Mycklebust and Johnson coined the term *nonverbal learning disabilities* in 1967. It described a predominantly social emotional disorder that in many ways resembled the current concepts of the ASDs but included some spatial difficulties as well. The distinction between NVLDs and high-functioning ASD is widely debated. Some differentiate NVLD from ASD based on the lack of restrictive behaviors and the presence of greater verbal than performance IQ in the former. Subtypes of NVLD were subsequently described that involved varying degrees of social cognitive impairments, visuoperceptual skills, math difficulties, attention, and executive functioning relative to average or above-average reading (decoding) and spelling. NVLD does not appear in the *Diagnostic and Statistical Manual of Mental Disorders*, 5th edition (*DSM-5*), but is referred to by various other names, including *right hemisphere syndrome* and *visuospatial learning disability*. The exact prevalence is unknown largely due to varying definitions but it is generally thought to account for approximately 10% of all LDs.

The basis for the identification of children with NVLDs is usually their higher verbal as compared with performance IQ scores on neuropsychological assessment batteries. This is an indicator of their visuospatial and visuomotor difficulties, which are a core feature of the disorder. A complete neuropsychological evaluation is required for diagnosis. Suggested management for NVLDs often trades on developing verbal strengths to compensate for the nonverbal deficits.

DYSCALCULIA

Developmental dyscalculia involves any or all aspects of mathematics from difficulties representing and manipulating numeric information to learning and remembering arithmetic facts to executing arithmetic procedures. The prevalence of dyscalculia is approximately 3% to 6%, affecting both genders equally. A developmental Gerstmann syndrome (right/left disorientation, finger agnosia, dysgraphia, dyscalculia, and sometimes constructional apraxia) occurs in as many as 2% of school-aged children. ADHD co-occurs in one-fourth of individuals and approximately one-fifth have dyslexia.

Comprehensive neuropsychological evaluations are recommended in individuals suspected of having dyscalculia. Children with neuropsychological signs of both left and right hemisphere dysfunction can have dyscalculia. Both groups have similar problems on arithmetic batteries, but those with left hemisphere dysfunction seem to perform significantly worse in addition, subtraction, complex multiplication, and division and also make more visuospatial errors. Math remediation is appropriate for the child with isolated difficulties or with mathematics difficulties in combination with other learning difficulties.

ATTENTION DEFICIT HYPERACTIVITY DISORDER

Attention deficit hyperactivity disorder begins in childhood with symptoms of hyperactivity, impulsivity, and/or inattention. For children younger than 17 years of age, the *DSM-5* diagnosis requires six or more symptoms of hyperactivity and impulsivity and six or more symptoms of inattention. For individuals 17 years and older, five or more symptoms per category are required. Depending on the predominance of symptoms, ADHD is divided into three subtypes: predominantly inattentive, predominantly hyperactive-impulsive, and combined type. Symptoms of hyperactivity/

impulsivity and inattention must occur often; be present in more than one setting, such as school or work and home; persist for at least 6 months; be present before age 12 years; impair academic, social, or occupational functioning; and be excessive for the developmental level of the child.

The reported prevalence of ADHD in school-aged children ranges from 1% to 20%. The *DSM-5* conservatively estimates the prevalence of ADHD as about 5% of children and 2.5% of adults in most cultures. The variation in prevalence is secondary to differing techniques of ascertainment and invariably reflects the lack of a biologic marker for the disorder. ADHD occurs approximately twice as often in males. Affected females are more likely to present primarily with inattentive features.

ADHD occurs and can be diagnosed in the toddler (although the false-positive rate is relatively high). The diagnosis is more reliably made when a child reaches 4 years old. Hyperactive and impulsive symptoms typically increase during the next 3 to 4 years, peaking at age 7 to 8 years. By adolescence, hyperactivity symptoms diminish, although symptoms of impulsivity and feelings of restlessness persist. Symptoms of inattention usually are not obvious until the child is 8 to 9 years old. ADHD persists into adulthood in two-thirds to three-fourths of people diagnosed with ADHD in childhood.

Attention disorders (with or without hyperactivity) are diagnosed based on history obtained from parents, observations of the child, questionnaires from parents and teachers, and in some instances, computerized tests of attention. As the disorder must affect functioning in at least two settings (i.e., school and home), it is advisable to obtain some written or verbal report from the child's teacher or school personnel. Given the high rate of psychiatric comorbidities in ADHD (e.g., anxiety and mood disorders, oppositional defiant disorder, conduct disorder), both narrow-band questionnaires that specifically assess for ADHD and broad-band questionnaires that assess for ADHD as well as other psychiatric comorbidities should be used. The elemental neurologic examination is generally normal, although minor findings are common (e.g., synkinesis during repetitive finger tapping and sequencing tasks). Neuropsychological testing is not absolutely necessary unless comorbid learning disabilities are suspected. The neuropsychological profile usually reveals average intelligence, but low scores are common on the Wechsler IQ subtests that demand attention or rapid processing (e.g., digit span, coding, arithmetic, symbol search) and intratest scatter often is found, reflecting variability in attention. Executive frontal lobe functioning, the ability to initiate, inhibit, sustain, and shift attention, working memory, and organizational skills, is often impaired.

ADHD has a substantial genetic component. Reported heritability of ADHD ranges from 0.70 to 0.88 in twins. ADHD frequently co-occurs with other neurobehavioral disorders such as Tourette syndrome, obsessive–compulsive disorder, anxiety, and learning disabilities, raising the question of possible shared susceptibility genes.

Dopamine appears to be the primary neurotransmitter involved in ADHD. Medications that increase levels of dopamine, in particular psychostimulants, are the mainstay of treatment. The National Institutes of Health (NIH)–sponsored Multimodal Treatment Study of ADHD (MTA) has shown both behaviorally and by neuropsychological testing that stimulants work and that they work better than behavioral modification [**Level 1**].[1] Approximately 75% of children respond to stimulants initially. Side effects may limit treatment (e.g., weight loss, rebound depression or irritability, flat affect) in 5% to 10%. Many different formulations of the stimulants exist, with different durations of action. Tics are not a contraindication to stimulant use in ADHD, although they may affect medication choices. Comorbid mood or anxiety disorders also influence medication choice. Medications other than stimulants can be used to treat ADHD. Atomoxetine (starting dose: 0.5 mg/kg q.d.) and α-agonists clonidine (starting dose: 0.05 to 0.1 mg q.d.), guanfacine (starting dose: 0.5 to 1 mg q.d.), Intuniv (starting dose: 1 mg q.d.), and Kapvay (starting dose: 0.1 mg q.h.s.) are accepted nonstimulant medication choices. Tricyclic antidepressants, selective serotonin reuptake inhibitors, serotonin–norepinephrine reuptake inhibitors, bupropion, and modafinil have all been used generally in those who failed to respond to stimulants. In addition to medication, treatment should focus on parent skills training, educational accommodations (preferential seating, extended time/separate testing site for testing, organizational supports), and behavioral modification.

LEVEL 1 EVIDENCE

1. The Multimodal Treatment Study of Children with Attention-Deficit/Hyperactivity Disorder Cooperative Group. A 14-month randomized clinical trial of treatment strategies for attention-deficit/hyperactivity disorder. *Arch Gen Psychiatry.* 1999;56(12):1073–1086.

SUGGESTED READINGS

Disorders of Motor Development

Bax M, Tydeman C, Flodmark O. Clinical and MRI correlates of cerebral palsy: the European Cerebral Palsy Study. *JAMA.* 2006;296(13):1602–1608.

Ellenberg JH, Nelson KB. The association of cerebral palsy with birth asphyxia: a definitional quagmire. *Dev Med Child Neurol.* 2013;55(3):210–216.

Gupta R, Appleton RE. Cerebral palsy: not always what it seems. *Arch Dis Child.* 2001;85(5):356–360.

Himmelmann K, McManus V, Hagberg G, et al. Dyskinetic cerebral palsy in Europe: trends in prevalence and severity. *Arch Dis Child.* 2009;94(12):921–926.

Kan P, Gooch J, Amini A, et al. Surgical treatment of spasticity in children: comparison of selective dorsal rhizotomy and intrathecal baclofen pump implantation. *Childs Nerv Syst.* 2008;24(2):239–243.

Krageloh-Mann I, Cans C. Cerebral palsy update. *Brain Dev.* 2009;31(7):537–544.

Krageloh-Mann I, Horber V. The role of magnetic resonance imaging in elucidating the pathogenesis of cerebral palsy: a systematic review. *Dev Med Child Neurol.* 2007;49(2):144–151.

McIntyre S, Morgan C, Walker K, et al. Cerebral palsy—don't delay. *Dev Disabil Res Rev.* 2011;17(2):114–129.

Nelson KB. Causative factors in cerebral palsy. *Clin Obstet Gynecol.* 2008;51(4):749–762.

Olaya JE, Christian E, Ferman D, et al. Deep brain stimulation in children and young adults with secondary dystonia: the Children's Hospital Los Angeles experience. *Neurosurg Focus.* 2013;35(5):E7.

Quality Standards Subcommittee of the American Academy of Neurology and the Practice Committee of the Child Neurology Society; Delgado MR, Hirtz D, et al. Practice parameter: pharmacologic treatment of spasticity in children and adolescents with cerebral palsy (an evidence-based review): report of the Quality Standards Subcommittee of the American Academy of Neurology and the Practice Committee of the Child Neurology Society. *Neurology.* 2010;74(4):336–343.

Schaefer GB. Genetics considerations in cerebral palsy. *Semin Pediatr Neurol.* 2008;15(1):21–26.

Steinbok P. Selective dorsal rhizotomy for spastic cerebral palsy: a review. *Childs Nerv Syst.* 2007;23(9):981–990.

Tilton A. Management of spasticity in children with cerebral palsy. *Semin Pediatr Neurol.* 2009;16(2):82–89.

Vidailhet M, Yelnik J, Lagrange C, et al. Bilateral pallidal deep brain stimulation for the treatment of patients with dystonia-choreoathetosis cerebral palsy: a prospective pilot study. *Lancet Neurol.* 2009;8(8):709–717.

Westmacott R, MacGregor D, Askalan R, et al. Late emergence of cognitive deficits after unilateral neonatal stroke. *Stroke.* 2009;40(6):2012–2019.

Zwicker JG, Missiuna C, Harris SR, et al. Developmental coordination disorder: a review and update. *Eur J Paediatr Neurol.* 2012;16(6):573–581.

Disorders of Higher Cerebral Functions

Baron IS. *Neuropsychological Evaluation of the Child.* New York: Oxford University Press; 2004.

Bates E, Thal D, Finlay B, et al. Early language development and its neural correlates. In: Segalowitz SJ, Rapin I, eds. *Handbook of Neuropsychology. Child Neuropsychology.* Part II. Vol 8. 2nd ed. Amsterdam, The Netherlands: Elsevier Science; 2003.

Cortese S. The neurobiology and genetics of attention-deficit/hyperactivity disorder (ADHD): what every clinician should know. *J Europ Paed Neurol Soc.* 2012;16:422–433.

Cortese S, Holtmann M, Banaschewski T. Practitioner review: current best practice in the management of adverse events during treatment with ADHD medications in children and adolescents. *J Child Psychol Psychiatry.* 2013;54(3):227–246.

Flore LA, Milunsky JM. Updates in the genetic evaluation of the child with global developmental delay or intellectual disability. *Semin Pediatr Neurol.* 2012;19:173–180.

Gibson CJ, Gruen JR. The human lexinome: genes of language and reading. *J Commun Disord.* 2008;41(5):409–420.

Kaminsky EB, Kaul V, Paschall J, et al. An evidence-based approach to establish the functional and clinical significance of copy number variants in intellectual and developmental disabilities. *Genet Med.* 2011;13(9):777–784.

Michelson DJ, Shevell MI, Sherr EH, et al. Evidence report: genetic and metabolic testing on children with global developmental delay. *Neurology.* 2011;77:1629–1635.

Miller DT, Adam MP, Aradhya S. Consensus statement: chromosomal microarray is a first-tier clinical diagnostic test for individuals with developmental disabilities or congenital anomalies. *Amer J Human Gen.* 2010;86:759–764.

Peterson RL, Pennington BF. Developmental dyslexia. *Lancet.* 2012;379:1997–2007.

Rapin I, Dunn M, Allen DA. Developmental language disorders. In: Segalowitz SJ, Rapin I, eds. *Handbook of Neuropsychology. Clinical Neuropsychology.* Part II. Vol 8. 2nd ed. Amsterdam, The Netherlands: Elsevier Science; 2003:593–630.

Rudel RG, Holmes J, Pardes J. *Assessment of Developmental Learning Disorders: A Neuropsychological Approach.* New York: Basic Books; 1988.

Scerri TS, Schulte-Korne G. Genetics of developmental dyslexia. *Eur Child Adolesc Psychiatry.* 2010;19:179–197.

Schubiner H, Katragadda S. Overview of epidemiology, clinical features, genetics, neurobiology, and prognosis of adolescent attention-deficit/hyperactivity disorder. *Adolesc Med State Art Rev.* 2008;19(2):209–215.

Shalev RS. Developmental dyscalculia. In: Segalowitz SJ, Rapin I, eds. *Handbook of Neuropsychology. Child Neuropsychology.* Part II. Vol 8. 2nd ed. Amsterdam, The Netherlands: Elsevier Science; 2003.

Sharp SI, McQuillin A, Gurling H. Genetics of attention-deficit hyperactivity disorder (ADHD). *Neuropharmacology.* 2009;57:590–600.

Shaywitz SE, Shaywitz BA. Paying attention to reading: the neurobiology of reading and dyslexia. *Dev Psychopathol.* 2008;20(4):1329–1349.

Shevell M. Global developmental delay and mental retardation or intellectual disability: conceptualization, evaluation, and etiology. *Pediatr Clin North Am.* 2008;55(5):1071–1084.

Shevell M, Ashwal S, Donley D, et al. Practice parameter: evaluation of the child with global developmental delay. *Neurology.* 2003;60:367–380.

Spencer TJ, Brown A, Seidman LJ, et al. Effect of psychostimulants on brain structure and function in ADHD: a qualitative literature review of magnetic resonance imaging-based neuroimaging studies. *J Clin Psychiatry.* 2013;74(9):902–917.

Whitmore K, Hart H, Willems G, eds. *A Neurodevelopmental Approach to Specific Learning Disorders.* London, United Kingdom: Mac Keith Press; 1999.

Autism Spectrum Disorders 138

Reet K. Sidhu

INTRODUCTION

Autism spectrum disorders (ASD) are a heterogeneous group of biologically based neurodevelopmental disorders of brain function. They are a behaviorally defined group of disorders that are characterized by impairments in two areas: (1) deficits in social communication and social interactions and (2) restricted and repetitive patterns of behavior, interests, and activities. The term *autism* (originating from the Greek word *autos* meaning *self*) was adopted by Leo Kanner in 1943 to describe children whose behavior was "governed rigidly and consistently by the powerful desire for aloneness and sameness."

The ASDs have been defined in the *Diagnostic and Statistical Manual of Mental Disorders* (*DSM*) of the American Psychiatric Association under many different names including the umbrella term *pervasive developmental disorder* or PDD, causing much confusion for both families and professionals. With the most recent 2013 revision, *Diagnostic and Statistical Manual of Mental Disorders*, 5th edition (*DSM-5*), ASD now subsumes what were previously separate diagnostic categories of autistic disorder (also referred to as *classic autism* or *early infantile autism*), pervasive developmental disorder–not otherwise specified (PDD-NOS), and Asperger syndrome. These changes are based on research results which have failed to document these categories as separate biologic entities.

Under the *DSM-5*, a diagnosis of ASD requires an individual to exhibit three deficits in social communication and at least two symptoms in the category of restricted range of activities/repetitive behaviors. The prior version of the diagnostic manual also included deficits in language expression as a separate criterion, but this is no longer the case, as not all children with ASD have specific language disorders. Pragmatic language skills, however, are incorporated into the social domain, as all individuals with ASD have deficits in this domain of language. Within the second category, a new symptom is included: hyper- or hyporeactivity to sensory input or unusual interests in sensory aspects of the environment. Deficits in social communication and interactions include those in social reciprocity; nonverbal communication; and skills in developing, maintaining, and understanding relationships. Symptoms must be present in early development but need not be shown until social demands exceed the individual's capacity. Furthermore, *DSM-5* specifies three levels of severity (mild, moderate, severe) rated separately for social communication and restricted, repetitive behaviors based on what level of support the individual requires. In addition to the diagnosis, individuals are also described in terms of any known genetic cause (e.g., fragile X syndrome, Rett syndrome), level of language and intellectual disability, and presence of medical conditions such as seizures, psychiatric disorders (e.g., anxiety, depression), and/or gastrointestinal disorders. The variability in severity and range of disabilities seen in children with ASD cannot be overemphasized. A full description of the *DSM-5* criteria for ASD can be found in the American Psychiatric Association, *Diagnostic and Statistical Manual of Mental Disorders*, 5th edition.

EPIDEMIOLOGY

There has been a significant increase in the prevalence of ASD in the United States, particularly since the late 1990s when the estimated frequency was about 1 per 1,000 for autism and 2.8 per 1,000 for all ASD subtypes (autistic disorder, Asperger syndrome, and PDD-NOS). The estimated prevalence is much higher now. The Autism and Developmental Disabilities Monitoring Network (2010, 2014) that identifies ASD through screening and review of health and education records that document behaviors associated with ASD in 11 sites in the United States most recently reported a prevalence rate of 14.7 per 1,000 (1 in 68) among 8-year-olds, with prevalence estimates varying from 5.7 to 21.9 per 1,000 in the different sites. Non-Hispanic white children were approximately 30% more likely to be identified with ASD than non-Hispanic black children and almost 50% more than Hispanic children. ASDs are four times more likely in males than in females.

Factors such as increased awareness among parents and professionals, broadening of the diagnosis with emphasis on the spectrum aspect of the disorder, including mildly affected individuals, change in referral patterns, and using the diagnosis as a basis for intervention services may account for increased prevalence rates. The theory that vaccines, in particular the measles, mumps, rubella (MMR) vaccine, play any role in the increased prevalence of autism has been completely discredited.

PATHOBIOLOGY

NEUROPATHOLOGY

ASDs are characterized as neurodevelopmental disorders because their signs and symptoms have been demonstrated to be the result of alterations in brain structure and function. Although much remains to be discovered, a great deal is now known about the fundamental alterations in the brain in ASD. ASDs are now considered disorders of the development of connectivity of neurons of cerebral cortex, which results in disturbances in the highly specialized connections that provide for uniquely human abilities. Studies of brain structure have implicated multiple events in prenatal and postnatal brain development, particularly neuronal organizational events. The generalized enlargement of the brain resulting from premature overgrowth attests to the broadness of the involvement of the brain, precluding focal brain theories and single primary deficit theories. The occurrence of mutations in genes that act on molecular signaling pathways involved in the development and maintenance of neuronal and synaptic connections have reinforced the centrality of disruption of cortical connectivity in ASD.

The most consistent abnormality seen on neuroimaging studies and in postmortem examination is an increase in brain weight and volume in children with ASDs compared to controls. Very young children with ASD (18 months to 4 years) have a 5% to 10% increase in brain volume, especially in the frontal lobe, which parallels the increasing head circumference during this period. By adolescence and adulthood, however, brain volumes seem to be lower than in controls, suggesting brain overgrowth within the first few years of life followed by volume loss. Increased brain volume in childhood is attributed primarily to enlargement of white matter, specifically the corona radiata and U-fibers, whereas the size of the corpus callosum is reduced, perhaps resulting in decreased interhemispheric communication. The white matter abnormalities result in abnormality of connectivity. At the cytoarchitectonic level, minicolumns that determine connectivity are abnormal, especially in the dorsolateral prefrontal cortex. As a result, and well delineated on diffusion tensor (DT) imaging, short-range connectivity is increased, and long-range connectivity is decreased. The hyperconnected local networks may become partially isolated and acquire novel functional properties. By contrast, the decrease in long-range connections could explain the problems with top-down control and integration.

Imaging studies also highlight the dissociation between white matter tract overgrowth and gray matter dendritic and synaptic underdevelopment. Also found is an enlargement of the cerebellum and caudate nuclei. Larger caudate volumes are associated with more severe stereotyped motor mannerisms. Volumes of the amygdala and hippocampus have been more variable. In addition to showing an increase in short-range connectivity and decrease in long-range connectivity, DT imaging also demonstrates an alteration of white matter tracts in brain regions implicated in social cognition, including the fusiform gyrus, superior temporal gyrus, ventromedial prefrontal cortex, anterior cingulate, and temporoparietal junction. Magnetic resonance (MR) spectroscopy studies suggest that gray matter is abnormal and dendritic arborization and synaptosome density reduced with lower levels of neuronal N-acetylaspartate and alterations in choline and creatinine metabolism.

Positron emission tomography (PET) and single-photon emission computed tomography (SPECT) suggest reduced brain perfusion and abnormalities of serotonin synthesis. Functional imaging studies (functional magnetic resonance imaging [fMRI]) have shown atypical patterns of brain activation during tasks of face processing, language, and emotional understanding. Activation of the mirror neuron system—a network within the inferior frontal gyrus and posterior parietal lobe that is thought to subserve imitation and understanding of intentions of other people—is reduced in individuals with ASDs, suggesting a role for this network in the pathogenesis of autism.

Neuropathologic studies have generally consisted of few subjects, but postmortem abnormalities include inflammatory changes and reduced width and increased number of cortical minicolumns compared with controls. A recent postmortem study supports a prenatal onset of ASD occurring during the second and third trimester of pregnancy. Focal patches of abnormal laminar cytoarchitecture and cortical disorganization of neurons, but not glia, were found in the prefrontal and temporal cortical tissue from 10 of 11 children with autism and from 1 of 11 unaffected children, supporting a probable dysregulation of layer formation and layer-specific neuronal differentiation prenatally.

GENETICS

ASDs are clinically and etiologically heterogeneous. Twin and family studies provide evidence for ASD as a highly genetic disorder with heritability estimates of 85% to 92%. Genetic heterogeneity is suspected. Using currently available technology, a genetic cause can be identified in 30% to 40% of children with ASD. This number has increased with the use of chromosomal microarrays (CMAs).

Known genetic causes of ASD include cytogenetically visible chromosomal abnormalities (5%), copy number variants (CNVs) (e.g., submicroscopic deletions and duplications) (10% to 20%), and single gene disorders in which neurologic findings are associated with ASD (5%). CMA is rapidly replacing high-resolution chromosomes as the initial test of choice to evaluate children with ASD. CMA has identified clinically relevant de novo genetic imbalances in up to 20% of individuals with autism of unknown cause. The most common autism-related CNVs are the 15q11.2-11.3 duplications, reciprocal 16p11.2 microdeletions and duplications, and the 7q11.23 duplication. Taken together, these CNVs seem to confer susceptibility to ASD in up to 1% of individuals. A number of other CNVs have been described in a few autism families, and although none seems to be particularly common, they highlight the potential of array-based techniques to point autism researchers toward specific autism genes within the CNVs.

The microarray technology is evolving with more advanced types of arrays, including those used in research studies, picking up more and smaller CNVs. Unfortunately, it is often not possible to know whether many of the small CNVs are pathologic or benign. In some cases, a variant might be reported that has no known phenotypic consequence or that the consequence is not known to be related to the ASD. Parental testing is frequently performed to assist in interpretation of abnormal findings. Informed genetic counseling is very important in this context. Children identified with CNVs of unclear significance should be followed periodically by the geneticist so new information can be shared with the family as it becomes available. It should be noted that CMA will not detect balanced translocations or low-level mosaicism; a karyotype should be done when there is a family history of multiple miscarriages or there is high suspicion of mosaic aneuploidy.

For individuals with ASD in whom the etiology is known, genetic counseling and risk assessment are based on the genetics of that specific disorder. For ASD of unknown cause, the empiric aggregate risk to siblings is 5% to 10% for autism and 10% to 15% for milder conditions including language, social, and psychiatric disorders. For families with two or more affected children, the recurrence risk approaches 35%. Recurrence risk may be up to 20% for families who have one autistic child plus another child or relative with mild autistic symptoms. The amount of weight to place on mild autistic symptoms in siblings, parents, and other relatives when estimating recurrence risk for families is unknown. Families contemplating additional pregnancies should be offered genetics evaluation and counseling by a medical geneticist.

In addition to clinically identifying known genetic disorders which may predispose to ASD, intense efforts have been directed to identifying genes that specifically cause or increase the risk of developing ASD. Methods used include both large genome-wide association studies and investigation of candidate genes. A number of genes of interest, including neuroligin 3 and 4, neurexin 1, contactin 4, contactin-associated protein-like 2, and SHANK 3, play a role in synapse formation and function. Other genes have a role in serotonin, glutamate, or γ-aminobutyric acid (GABA) neurotransmission. This is an area of tremendous interest in the scientific community and is rapidly evolving.

CLINICAL FEATURES

Social communication dysfunction is the hallmark of ASDs. Deficits in sociability are variable but an essential and defining feature. Early signs include failure to respond to name, abnormal eye gaze (gaze aversion), paucity of gestures, and impairment of joint attention (the ability to draw another person's attention to an object of interest through the use of eye gaze and gestures, such as pointing). Children appear aloof with a lack of interest in others and mainly interact with others when they need something rather than to share their interests, enjoyment, and achievements. As children age, a lack of empathy becomes apparent along with difficulty interpreting and reciprocating the social and emotional behaviors of others. Pragmatic language skills are always impaired, that is, the social rules for communicating are not well understood. These individuals have a hard time taking turns in conversations, talk only about topics of their interest or knowledge, talk *at* people without checking to see if anyone is listening or interested, fail to maintain appropriate interpersonal distance, and are inappropriately intrusive or persistent. There is an impaired ability to read facial expressions, body language, and tone of voice of others, which contributes to these deficits. They are often described as "odd" or "annoying," as their social approaches are peculiar.

Another cardinal feature of ASD is a restricted range of behaviors, interests, and activities that are often repetitive or stereotyped. These include motor stereotypies such as hand flapping or licking, finger flicking, spinning, and body rocking. They may have unusual preoccupations and interests and play skills are impaired. These children can watch the same video for hours, play with unusual objects (e.g., a piece of string), or line up toys instead of playing with them imaginatively. Some children have routines or rituals that need to be followed and many such children have difficulty making transitions. Overall, there is a tolerance for monotony and a resistance to change.

Although no longer a criterion for a diagnosis of ASD, verbal communication disturbances are commonly found. The most common presenting complaint is a delay in language development. Despite this delay, there is a lack of compensation through nonverbal modes of communication, such as gesture and imitation. Spoken language is often echolalic with repetitive and stereotyped phrases. Some children will recite scripts from television or videos. Some children fail to process language and despite normal hearing, appear deaf (verbal auditory agnosia). Abnormalities in syntax (word order), semantics (word meaning), and most prominently pragmatics are present in higher functioning individuals. These children are often extremely literal and concrete and have difficulties understanding jokes, humor, or sarcasm. Speech prosody (melody of language) is impaired, as evidenced by mechanical, monotonous, excessively rapid, high-pitched, and high-volume speech. There can be a fascination with letters and numbers in the early toddler years and some children may learn to read without instruction, e.g. hyperlexia, although comprehension is limited.

Intelligence is not a defining feature but strongly influences prognosis. Intellectual disability (IQ <70) occurs in approximately 55% of individuals with ASD, although many have average or even superior intellectual ability. Prodigious or savant skills can be seen in visuospatial ability, memory, calculation, or music ability. IQ is a key predictor of long-term outcome in autism, especially for those with an IQ of less than 50 who generally fare poorly. Average to superior IQ is a positive prognostic sign. Having a higher verbal IQ at 2 to 3 years of age appears to predict better outcome, particularly if intervention is delivered early.

Developmental regression or loss of previously established skills during the first 1 to 3 years of life has been estimated as occurring in approximately one-third of children with ASD. There is debate as to whether children with ASD and regression develop better, worse, or the same on IQ, language, and social functioning than those with no regression, but good recovery in children with regressive symptoms is rare.

MEDICAL COMORBIDITIES

Medical comorbidities frequently occur in ASD. Among them include epilepsy, gastrointestinal dysfunction, sleep disorders, and psychiatric conditions (e.g., anxiety, depression, obsessive–compulsive disorder [OCD]). It is important to consider medical causes for any change in behavior, especially in those individuals who are nonverbal or with limited language capability. Examples of such medical conditions include, but are not limited to, the following: pain (due to migraine headaches, ear infection, fractures, etc.), gastrointestinal disorders (e.g., gastroesophageal reflux disease [GERD], constipation), genitourinary conditions (e.g., urinary tract infection [UTI]), hormonal imbalance/endocrine dysfunction (e.g., menstruation), and sleep disturbance (e.g., sleep apnea).

EPILEPSY

The association of epilepsy with autism provided one of the first clues to suggest that autism was a neurodevelopmental disorder of brain function. It is now well established that individuals with ASD have a higher risk of epilepsy as compared with the general population. Epilepsy is commonly reported to occur in approximately one-third of individuals with ASD but the exact prevalence is unknown with reports in the literature ranging from 5% to 50%. Variation in estimates is likely related to multiple factors such as sample ascertainment, degree of intellectual disability, age, gender, and type of ASD (idiopathic vs. complex). Intellectual disability and motor impairments (e.g., cerebral palsy) have been identified most commonly as significant risk factors for epilepsy in ASD, with higher rates in those with more severe cognitive impairments. A community-based study of ASD in children with epilepsy has found that only 5% to 15% of children with epilepsy have autism.

Age of onset of epilepsy in ASD has generally been thought to occur in two peaks, one in early childhood (0 to 5 years) and the other in adolescence (10 to 15 years). The peak before age 5 years, however, includes those children with ASD secondary to infantile spasms (frequently as part of tuberous sclerosis) and other epileptic encephalopathies.

Given the prevalence of epilepsy in autism, it is important to consider the possibility of seizures when evaluating an individual with autism but currently, there is inadequate evidence to recommend electroencephalogram (EEG) in all individuals with autism. Although all seizure types are present in ASD, the most commonly observed are complex partial seizures (85%) and generalized tonic–clonic seizures (7%). Absence and myoclonic seizures occur less commonly (1% to 4%).

ASD can occur in the context of other comorbid medical conditions. Some of the most widely recognized syndromes associated with ASD and epilepsy include tuberous sclerosis, fragile X syndrome, Rett syndrome, Angelman syndrome, and 15q duplication syndrome. A targeted physical examination should consider other risk factors for epilepsy including head circumference (microcephaly), dysmorphism, skin lesions (tuberous sclerosis, neurofibromatosis type 1 [NF-1]), and focal neurologic findings. It is crucial to assess for medical comorbidities, which may mimic seizures including sleep disorders, gastroesophageal reflux and other gastrointestinal disorders, and psychiatric disorders including attention deficit hyperactivity disorder (ADHD).

Epileptiform EEG abnormalities are frequently seen in children with ASD, with or without epilepsy. Because these background or epileptiform EEG abnormalities can occur in ASD individuals without a clinical history of seizures, they are not to be considered evidence for epilepsy. The significance of these abnormalities, especially in the absence of clinical seizures, is quite unclear. At the present time, there are no data to support the use of antiepileptic drugs or epilepsy surgery in the treatment of these abnormalities in the absence of clinical seizures.

The relationship of autistic regression to epilepsy and epileptiform EEG abnormalities is unclear. Findings in the literature are inconsistent with some studies reporting higher rates of epilepsy in children with ASD and regression and others showing no relationship. However, language regression is a hallmark of Landau–Kleffner syndrome (LKS), a rare childhood-onset epileptic encephalopathy in which loss of previously acquired language skills occurs in the context of an epileptiform EEG, activated in sleep. Electrical status epilepticus during slow-wave sleep (ESES) is the electroencephalographic pattern seen in LKS. The degree of overlap between LKS, ESES, and autistic regression with epileptiform EEG is currently poorly understood, although it is known that this ESES is rarely seen in children with a more global autistic regression. At the current time, there are no data to support the use of LKS- or ESES-specific treatment regimens in those with more classic autistic regression and epileptiform EEG without clinical seizures.

DIAGNOSIS

EVALUATION

ASDs are diagnosed based on clinical history and observations of the child. Research indicates that ASDs may be identified as young as 18 months of age or younger. By age 2 years, it is expected that a qualified professional can reliably make the diagnosis. The American Academy of Pediatrics recommends screening all children at well-child visits at 18 months and at 24 months of age. A number of questionnaires and observation measures are available to screen for ASDs. Probably the most commonly used is the Modified Checklist for Autism in Toddlers-Revised (M-CHAT-R), which is a parent-completed questionnaire designed to identify children at risk for autism in the general population. The Social Communication Questionnaire (SCQ) is another commonly used screening questionnaire that has established validity against the Autism Diagnostic Interview-Revised (see ADI-R in the following text) in children 4 years or older. It is a parent questionnaire that can be completed and scored easily.

There are a number of tools used to assess ASDs, but experts believe that no single tool should be used to make a diagnosis. The Autism Diagnostic Observation Schedule-2 (ADOS-2) is considered the "gold standard" in diagnosing ASD. It consists of a semistructured, standardized assessment of social interaction, play, and imaginative use of material for individuals suspected of having ASDs from toddlers through adults. A recent toddler module was designed to assess children who are 18 months of age onwards. The ADOS often is used in conjunction with the ADI-R, a clinical diagnostic interview for diagnosing autism in children and adults with mental ages of 18 months and older that focuses on assessing reciprocal social interactions, communication, and language and restricted and repetitive, stereotyped interests and behaviors. Both the ADOS and ADI-R are time consuming and require special training to administer and score, making them less practical for the average office setting. Other well-known assessments include the Childhood Autism Rating Scale-2nd edition (CARS-2) that is appropriate for children older than age 2 years and draws from observations on different areas of behavior associated with ASDs and can be helpful to quantify office observations in addition to the Gilliam Autism Rating Scale-3rd edition (GARS-3), which helps teachers, parents, and clinicians in diagnosis of the disorder.

NEUROLOGIC EXAMINATION

Observations of the child are the key aspect of the neurologic examination. The remainder of the examination is fairly unremarkable. Motor findings include mild hypotonia with incoordination and motor apraxia. Toe walking and motor stereotypies are very common. Many children have a constellation of symptoms that are referred to as *sensory deficits*; however, the neurologic basis for this is unclear. These include a preoccupation with sensory features of objects, over- or underresponsiveness to environmental stimuli, or paradoxical responses to sensory stimuli (e.g., excessive sniffing or licking, oral aversions, intolerant to loud noises, or tactile contact). Macrocephaly (occipitofrontal circumference [OFC] >2 standard deviations [SD] above mean) occurs in approximately 30% of children with autism and usually becomes apparent between the age of 2 and 4 years, reflecting an increase in brain volume. Macrocephaly in adults with autism is less common than in children with ASD, suggesting volume loss. Microcephaly is not a common finding and should prompt neuroimaging. The skin examination requires careful attention, especially given the high co-occurrence with tuberous sclerosis. Examination for dysmorphology is important for making genetic diagnoses (e.g., fragile X, velocardiofacial syndrome, and Smith–Magenis syndrome).

NEURODIAGNOSTIC TESTING

There are many different causes of ASD. The purpose of performing neurodiagnostic testing is to potentially identify any diagnosable or treatable condition. A clinical rationale for performing diagnostic testing is advisable. There are clinical practice guidelines for performing genetic testing but other diagnostic investigations, such as neuroimaging, EEGs, or metabolic laboratory investigations follow "best practice" recommendations, as evidenced-based guidelines are not available.

All children with ASD should have a comprehensive medical history and examination to assess for symptoms or signs of an underlying genetic disorder. Having an etiologic diagnosis offers clinicians the opportunity to provide better guidance regarding recurrence risks as well as prognostic information and obviates the need for additional testing. Furthermore, a specific diagnosis can alert clinicians to be aware of other comorbidities associated with certain genetic syndromes. CMA and fragile X are considered first tier testing in the diagnostic workup of ASD. MECP2 sequencing for Rett syndrome and phosphatase and tensin homolog [PTEN] testing for those with head circumferences greater than 2.5 SD above the mean are recommended second-tier testing. See Table 138.1 for genetic disorders associated with an ASD phenotype.

The clinical rationale for neuroimaging in children with ASD is an attempt to determine a specific etiopathologic diagnosis for an individual. In a minority of cases, the detection of an abnormality of the brain may lead to determination of a specific cause for the child's ASD. This is true especially if the lesion is pathognomonic for a given disorder, for example, a neurocutaneous syndrome. However, it should be noted that abnormalities on neuroimaging are not necessarily causally related to the ASD. In many cases, the etiology of the brain abnormality is still unknown and the relationship to the ASD unclear. Nonetheless, the MRI may help guide more focused etiologic investigations that could further lead to specific diagnoses in a limited number of cases. For these reasons, imaging is not a routine part of the evaluation of individuals with ASD. See Table 138.2 for clinical indicators to consider neuroimaging in ASD.

TABLE 138.1 Genetic Disorders Associated with Autism Spectrum Disorders

Single Gene Disorders

Fragile X

PTEN macrocephaly syndrome

Rett syndrome

Tuberous sclerosis complex (TSC)

Angelman syndrome

Sotos syndrome

Timothy syndrome

Joubert syndrome

Williams syndrome

Sanfilippo syndrome

Cohen syndrome

Cornelia de Lange syndrome

22q11.1 deletion syndrome

Duchenne muscular dystrophy

Neurofibromatosis, type 1

Cytogenetically Visible Chromosomal Abnormalities

15q duplication syndrome

Trisomy 21

Turner syndrome (45,X)

Copy Number Variants (CNVs)

15q11.2-11.3 duplications

Reciprocal 16p11.2 microdeletions and duplications

7q11.23 duplication

PTEN, phosphatase and tensin homolog.

Hearing impairment should be excluded by a formal audiology assessment. EEG, including a sleep record or overnight video-EEG monitoring, is appropriate when seizures occur or if developmental regression has occurred (see "Epilepsy" section).

There are multiple metabolic causes of ASD, many of which are not usually associated with any dysmorphology. The diagnosis of a primary inborn error of metabolism in simple autism is a rare occurrence. On careful history taking and examination, usually

TABLE 138.2 Clinical Indicators that Might Prompt Neuroimaging with Brain Magnetic Resonance Imaging

- Seizures or history of focal EEG
- Microcephaly
- Extreme (>3 SD above mean) or progressive macrocephaly
- Neurocutaneous lesions
- Suspicion of CNS structural abnormality
- Focal motor findings or a change in motor examination
- Active or recurrent regression

EEG, electroencephalogram; CNS, central nervous system.

TABLE 138.3 Red Flags that Might Indicate a Metabolic Etiology for Autism Spectrum Disorders

History or *symptoms* of any of the following:

- Active or recurrent regression
- Profound intellectual disability or global developmental delay
- Severe growth retardation
- Deafness
- Unexplained intractable seizures
- Fatigue with daily activities or exercise
- Recurrent or relapsing history of decompensation with illness
- Family history suggestive of metabolic disease

Any of the following *physical* or *laboratory* findings:

- Objective neurologic abnormalities (e.g., significant hypotonia with gross motor delay, muscle weakness, microcephaly, macrocephaly, dystonia/chorea)
- Multiple organ system involvement
- Unrelated signs suggesting an inborn error of metabolism (e.g., hypoglycemia, metabolic acidemia)
- MRI abnormality suggestive of metabolic disease

List is not meant to be exhaustive.
MRI, magnetic resonance imaging.

one or more "red flags" is identified in children whose ASD is part of a presentation of an inborn error of metabolism (Table 138.3). Treatable conditions include phenylketonuria (PKU), hyperammonemia/urea cycle defects, and creatine synthesis/creatine transporter defects. Other conditions include purine and pyrimidine abnormalities, Smith–Lemli–Opitz syndrome, and lysosomal storage disorders. Primary mitochondrial disease and ASD is a subject of much debate. Some investigators report a significant incidence of mitochondrial DNA changes or functional disturbances in children with ASD but whether these are the primary cause of ASD remains to be defined. The extent of the evaluation for an underlying metabolic disorder depends on clinical suspicions and the relevance to family counseling. Table 138.4 lists metabolic disorders that can be associated with an ASD phenotype.

TREATMENT

There are no known cures for ASDs; however, early and intensive behavioral and educational interventions are highly effective in most individuals and provide the best chance for a favorable outcome. Both behavioral and educational interventions target the core symptoms of ASDs. Usually, children with ASD require a combination of therapies and interventions to address their individual groups of symptoms. It is recommended that children receive educational intervention as soon as they are suspected of having ASD, with services being provided a minimum of 20 to 25 hours a week on a yearly basis.

Intensive behavioral interventions, such as applied behavior analysis (ABA), based on the work of Lovaas, uses multiple prompting paradigms, reinforcement schedules, and imitation and modeling. Another type of intervention, the Treatment and Education of Autistic and Related Communication-Handicapped Children (TEACCH) method uses structured teaching to help improve skills, with the therapist functioning as a generalist in treating the whole child.

TABLE 138.4	Metabolic Disorders Associated with Autism Spectrum Disorders
Phenylketonuria	
Mitochondrial disorders	
Mucopolysaccharidosis, including Sanfilippo	
Smith–Lemli–Opitz syndrome	
Urea cycle disorders	
Adenylosuccinate lyase deficiency	
Cerebral folate deficiency	
Disorders of creatine transport or metabolism	
Succinic semialdehyde dehydrogenase deficiency	
Dihydropyrimidinase deficiency	
Cystathionine β-synthase deficiency	
Homocysteine	
Biotinidase deficiency	

Developmental and relationship-based models, such as the Developmental Individual Difference Relationship approach (DIR or Floortime) focus on teaching skills, such as social communication and interpersonal skills. The Early Start Denver Model (ESDM) is considered an integrative approach as it uses a combination of intensive ABA and developmental and relationship-based intervention and includes parents as therapists. A randomized controlled trial that compared the ESDM program with interventions commonly available in the community demonstrated significant gains in language, cognitive, and adaptive functioning in toddlers over a 2-year period [**Level 1**].[1]

Parental involvement is considered an important part of the treatment program. Social skills training programs are very helpful, especially in higher functioning individuals. Maladaptive behaviors can develop and become extremely challenging to manage. It is very important to evaluate and treat problem behaviors appropriately. Medical causes need to be excluded (see "Medical Comorbidities" section). Functional behavioral analysis is important to identify the antecedents, consequences, and functions of behaviors. A combined approach of pharmacotherapy and behavioral modification therapy is often necessary. Medications are used to treat comorbid symptoms/conditions such as irritability, aggression, self-injury, inattention, hyperactivity/impulsivity, OCD, anxiety, depression, sleep disturbance, and seizures.

OUTCOME

The symptoms of ASD, like other developmental disorders, often change with age. Outcome studies of children diagnosed with ASD suggest that although 40% show overall improvement during adolescence, as many as a third may deteriorate. The onset of seizures can contribute to this decline. In addition, psychiatric comorbidities commonly develop in adolescence and adulthood: depression, anxiety, and even catatonia. A minority of patients, usually the higher functioning group, improve significantly during adolescence. Approximately two-thirds of adults with autism show poor social adjustment (limited independence in social relations), and half require institutionalization. Autistic adults who are not intellectually impaired tend to improve more than those who are intellectually impaired. Even though higher functioning individuals with ASD (including those previously diagnosed as Asperger syndrome) have the best outcome, only 15% to 30% have fair to good outcomes, and only 5% to 15% become competitively employed, lead independent lives, marry, and raise families. Probably, some "odd" adults go undiagnosed in childhood and adolescence, thus increasing the proportion of those with ASD who ultimately function in the mainstream.

LEVEL 1 EVIDENCE

1. Dawson G, Rogers S, Munson J, et al. Randomized controlled trial of an intervention for toddlers with autism: the early Denver model. *Pediatrics.* 2010;125:e17–e23.

SUGGESTED READINGS

American Psychiatric Association. *Diagnostic and Statistical Manual of Mental Disorders.* 5th ed. Washington, DC: American Psychiatric Association; 2013.

Aylward EH, Minshew NJ, Field K, et al. Effects of age on brain volume and head circumference in autism. *Neurology.* 2002;59:175–183.

Ballaban-Gil K, Tuchman R. Epilepsy and epileptiform EEG: association with autism and language disorders. *Ment Retard Dev Disabil Res Rev.* 2000;6:300–308.

Baribeau DA, Anagnostou E. An update on medication management of behavioral disorders in autism. *Curr Psychiatry Rep.* 2014;16:437.

Barnea-Goraly N, Kwon H, Menon V, et al. White matter structure in autism: preliminary evidence from diffusion tensor imaging. *Biol Psychiatry.* 2004;55:323–326.

Baron-Cohen S. The extreme male brain theory of autism. *Trends Cogn Sci.* 2002;6(6):248–254.

Baron-Cohen S, Tager-Flusberg H, Cohen D. *Understanding Other Minds II: Perspectives from Autism and Cognitive Neuroscience.* Oxford, United Kingdom: Oxford University Press; 2000.

Bauman ML, Kemper TL. Neuroanatomic observations of the brain in autism. In: Bauman ML, Kemper TL, eds. *The Neurobiology of Autism.* Baltimore: Johns Hopkins University Press; 1994:119–145.

Casanova MF, Buxhoeveden DP, Switala AE, et al. Minicolumnar pathology in autism. *Neurology.* 2002;58:428–432.

Chugani DC, Muzik O, Behen M, et al. Developmental changes in brain serotonin synthesis capacity in autistic and nonautistic children. *Ann Neurol.* 1999;45:287–295.

Courchesne E, Carper R, Akshoomoff N. Evidence of brain overgrowth in the first year of life in autism. *JAMA.* 2003;290:337–344.

Courchesne E, Karns CM, Davis HR, et al. Unusual brain growth patterns in early life in patients with autistic disorder: an MRI study. *Neurology.* 2001;57:245–254.

Critchley HD, Daly EM, Bullmore ET, et al. The functional neuroanatomy of social behaviour: changes in cerebral blood flow when people with autistic disorder process facial expressions. *Brain.* 2000;123:2203–2212.

Dapretto M, Davies MS, Pfeifer JH, et al. Understanding emotions in others: mirror neuron dysfunction in children with autism spectrum disorders. *Nat Neurosci.* 2006;9(1):29–30.

Dementieva YA, Vance DD, Donnelly SL, et al. Accelerated head growth in early development in individuals with autism. *Pediatr Neurol.* 2005;32:102–108.

Filipek PA, Accardo PJ, Ashwal S, et al. Practice parameter: screening and diagnosis of autism. Report of the Quality Standards Subcommittee of the American Academy of Neurology and the Child Neurology Society. *Neurology.* 2000;55:468–479.

Fombonne E. Epidemiological surveys of autism and other pervasive developmental disorders: an update. *J Autism Dev Disord.* 2003;33(4):365–382.

Fombonne E. Epidemiology of autistic disorder and other pervasive developmental disorders. *J Clin Psychiatry.* 2005;66:3–8.

Friedman SD, Shaw DW, Artru AA, et al. Regional brain chemical alterations in young children with autism spectrum disorder. *Neurology.* 2003;60:100–107.

Gaugler T, Klei L, Sanders S, et al. Most genetic risk for autism resides with common variation. *Nat Genet.* 2014;46:881–885.

Groen WB, Zwiers MP, van der Gaag RJ, et al. The phenotype and neural correlates of language in autism: an integrative review. *Neurosci Biobehav Rev.* 2008;32(8):1416–1425.

Haas RH. Autism and mitochondrial disease. *Dev Disabil Res Rev.* 2010;16:144–153.

Herbert MR, Ziegler DA, Deutsch CK, et al. Dissociations of cerebral cortex, subcortical and cerebral white matter volumes in autistic boys. *Brain.* 2003;126:1182–1192.

Herbert MR, Ziegler DA, Makris N, et al. Localization of white matter volume increase in autism and developmental language disorder. *Ann Neurol.* 2004;55:530–540.

Hollander E, Anagnostou E, Chaplin W, et al. Striatal volume on magnetic resonance imaging and repetitive behaviors in autism. *Biol Psychiatry.* 2005;58:226–232.

Howlin P, Goode S, Hutton J, et al. Adult outcome in children with autism. *J Child Psychol Psychiatry.* 2004;45:212–229.

Jamain S, Quach H, Betancur C, et al. Mutations of the X-linked genes encoding neuroligins NLGN3 and NLGN4 are associated with autism. *Nat Genet.* 2003;34:27–29.

Kagan-Kushnir T, Roberts SW, Snea OC III. Screening electroencephalograms in autism spectrum disorders: evidence-based guideline. *J Child Neurol.* 2005;20:197–206.

Kanner L. Autistic disturbances of affective contact. *Nerv Child.* 1943;2:217–250.

Kim HG, Kishikawa S, Higgins AW, et al. Disruption of neurexin 1 associated with autism spectrum disorder. *Am J Hum Genet.* 2008;82:199–207.

Knaus TA, Silver AM, Lindgren KA, et al. fMRI activation during a language task in adolescents with ASD. *J Int Neuropsychol Soc.* 2008;14(6):967–979.

Lee JE, Bigler ED, Alexander AL, et al. Diffusion tensor imaging of white matter in the superior temporal gyrus and temporal stem in autism. *Neurosci Lett.* 2007;424(2):127–132.

Levitt JG, O'Neill J, Blanton RE, et al. Proton magnetic resonance spectroscopic imaging of the brain in childhood autism. *Biol Psychiatry.* 2003;54:1355–1366.

Lovaas OI, Smith T. A comprehensive behavioral theory of autistic children: paradigm for research and treatment. *J Behav Ther Exp Psychiatry.* 1989;20(1):17–29.

MacDonald R, Parry-Cruwys D, Dupere S, et al. Assessing progress and outcome of early intensive behavioral intervention for toddlers with autism. *Res Dev Dis.* 2014;35(12):3632–3644.

McDougle CJ, Naylor ST, Cohen DJ, et al. A double-blind, placebo-controlled study of fluvoxamine in adults with autistic disorder. *Arch Gen Psychiatry.* 1996;53:1001–1008.

Moessner R, Marshall CR, Sutcliffe JS, et al. Contribution of SHANK3 mutations to autism spectrum disorder. *Am J Hum Genet.* 2007;81(6):1289–1297.

O'Roak BJ, State MW. Autism genetics: strategies, challenges, and opportunities. *Autism Res.* 2008;1:4–17.

Pierce K, Muller RA, Ambrose J, et al. Face processing occurs outside the fusiform "face area" in autism: evidence from functional MRI. *Brain.* 2001;124:2059–2073.

Polimeni MA, Richdale AL, Francis AJ. A survey of sleep problems in autism, Asperger's disorder and typically developing children. *J Intellect Disabil Res.* 2005;49:260–268.

Ramocki MB, Zoghbi HY. Failure of neuronal homeostasis results in common neuropsychiatric phenotypes. *Nature.* 2008;455:912–918.

Rapin I, Tuchman RF. Autism: definition, neurobiology, screening, diagnosis. *Pediatr Clin North Am.* 2008;55(5):1129–1146.

Redcay E, Courchesne E. When is the brain enlarged in autism? A meta-analysis of all brain size reports. *Biol Psychiatry.* 2005;58:1–9.

Schaefer GB, Mendelsohn NJ. Clinical genetics evaluation in identifying the etiology of autism spectrum disorders: 2013 guideline revisions. *Genet Med.* 2013;15(5):399–407.

Schultz RT, Gauthier I, Klin A, et al. Abnormal ventral temporal cortical activity during face discrimination among individuals with autism and Asperger syndrome. *Arch Gen Psychiatry.* 2000;57:331–340.

Sebat J, Lakshmi B, Malhotra D, et al. Strong association of de novo copy number mutations with autism. *Science.* 2007;316(5823):445–449.

Seltzer MM, Shattuck P, Abbebuto L, et al. Trajectory of development in adolescents and adults with autism. *Ment Retard Dev Disabil Res Rev.* 2004;10:234–247.

Silani G, Bird G, Brindley R, et al. Levels of emotional awareness and autism: an fMRI study. *Soc Neurosci.* 2008;3(2):97–112.

Stoner R, Chow ML, Boyle MP, et al. Patches of disorganization in the neocortex of children with autism. *New Engl J Med.* 2014;370:1209–1219.

Tang O, Gudsnuk K, Kuo S, et al. Loss of mTOR-dependent macroautophagy causes autistic-like synaptic pruning deficits. *Neuron.* 2014;83(5): 1131–1143.

Tuchman RF, Rapin I, Shinnar S. Autistic and dysphasic children II. Epilepsy. *Pediatrics.* 1991;88:1219–1225.

Vargas DL, Nascimbene C, Krishnan C, et al. Neuroglial activation and neuroinflammation in the brain of patients with autism. *Ann Neurol.* 2005;57: 67–81.

Volkmar FR, Siegel M, Woodbury-Smith M, et al. Practice parameter for the assessment and treatment of children and adolescents with autism spectrum disorder. *J Am Acad Child Adolesc Psychiatry.* 2014;53(2):237–257.

Wilcox J, Tsuang MT, Ledger E, et al. Brain perfusion in autism varies with age. *Neuropsychobiology.* 2002;46:13–16.

Mitochondrial Encephalomyopathies 139

Salvatore DiMauro and Michio Hirano

INTRODUCTION

Mitochondria are uniquely intriguing organelles, not only for the variety of biologic functions that they perform but also because of their regulation by two genomes—their own DNA (mtDNA) and that of the nucleus (nDNA). Accordingly, mitochondrial diseases can be due to mutations in either genome (Table 139.1). The main function of mitochondria is aerobic production of adenosine triphosphate (ATP) energy through oxidative phosphorylation. Because brain and muscle have high-energy requirements, mitochondrial disorders frequently manifest as encephalomyopathies. Advances in this rapidly expanding field have been covered extensively in recent reviews, but here we provide general overview of the genetically and clinically heterogeneous mitochondrial diseases.

TABLE 139.1	Genetic Classification of Mitochondrial Diseases with Representative Clinical Syndromes

1. Defects of mitochondrial DNA

A. Single deletions (usually sporadic)

  a. Kearns–Sayre syndrome (KSS)

  b. Chronic progressive external ophthalmoplegia (CPEO) and CPEO-plus

  c. Pearson syndrome

B. Point mutations (maternal transmission)

  a. Mitochondrial encephalomyopathy, lactic acidosis, and stroke-like episodes (MELAS);

  b. Myoclonus epilepsy with ragged red fibers (MERRF);

  c. Leber hereditary optic neuropathy (LHON);

  d. Neuropathy, ataxia, and retinitis pigmentosa (NARP)

2. Defects of nuclear DNA (mendelian or X-linked transmission)

A. "Direct hits": mutations in genes encoding subunits of the respiratory chain enzyme complexes with biochemical defects of complex I, II, III, or IV presenting as Leigh syndrome or a multisystemic disorder

B. "Indirect hits": defects of respiratory chain enzyme complex assembly factors with biochemical defects of complex I, II, III, or IV presenting as Leigh syndrome or a multisystemic disorder

C. Defects of mitochondrial transcription

D. Defects of mitochondrial translation

E. Defects of mitochondrial lipid composition

F. Defects of mitochondrial dynamics (fusion, fission, movement)

G. Defects of mitochondrial DNA maintenance

H. Defects of mitochondrial importation

I. Defects of mitochondrial metal metabolism

HISTORY

In 1962, the first human disease attributed to mitochondrial dysfunction was described as a hypermetabolic state in a patient with normal thyroid function and excessive number of abnormally large mitochondria in skeletal muscle. Biochemical studies showed "loose coupling" of oxidative phosphorylation. This syndrome was named after the endocrinologist Rolf Luft. Since then, however, there has been only one other known case of Luft syndrome and its etiology remains unknown.

Later in the 1960s, mitochondrial diseases were brought to prominence by Milton Shy and Nicholas Gonatas, who defined this new organellar disorder by the electron microscopic appearance of overabundant or enlarged mitochondria with paracrystalline inclusions. Soon thereafter, W. King Engel noted that abnormal proliferation of mitochondria could be identified under the light microscope as *ragged red fibers* (RRF) with a modified Gomori trichrome stain. For the next two decades, this histologic hallmark was the basis for recognition of mitochondrial diseases based on an initial biochemical classification.

The molecular era of mitochondrial disease began in 1988 when the first two pathogenic mutations in mtDNA were described: a point mutation in Leber hereditary optic neuropathy patients and single large deletions causing mitochondrial myopathy.

EPIDEMIOLOGY

Although mitochondrial diseases have been detected worldwide, epidemiologic data are limited. The prevalence of mitochondrial diseases has been estimated to be 7.6 per 100,000 births per year in Southern Australia whereas the prevalence in the working age adult population has been assessed to be 9.6 per 100,000 in the northeast of England.

PATHOBIOLOGY

We will consider separately the pathobiology associated with mtDNA mutations and with nDNA mutations.

PATHOBIOLOGY OF mtDNA MUTATIONS: MITOCHONDRIAL GENETICS VERSUS MENDELIAN INHERITANCE

Human mtDNA is a small (16.6 kb) circle of double-stranded DNA (Fig. 139.1) comprising only 37 genes. Of these, 13 encode polypeptides, all subunits of the respiratory chain: 7 subunits of complex I (NADH-ubiquinone oxidoreductase), 1 subunit of complex III (ubiquinone–cytochrome *c* oxidoreductase), 3 subunits of complex IV (cytochrome *c* oxidase [COX]), and 2 subunits of complex V (ATP synthase). The other 24 genes encode 22 transfer RNAs (tRNAs) and 2 ribosomal RNAs (rRNAs) that are required for translation of messenger RNAs on mitochondrial ribosomes

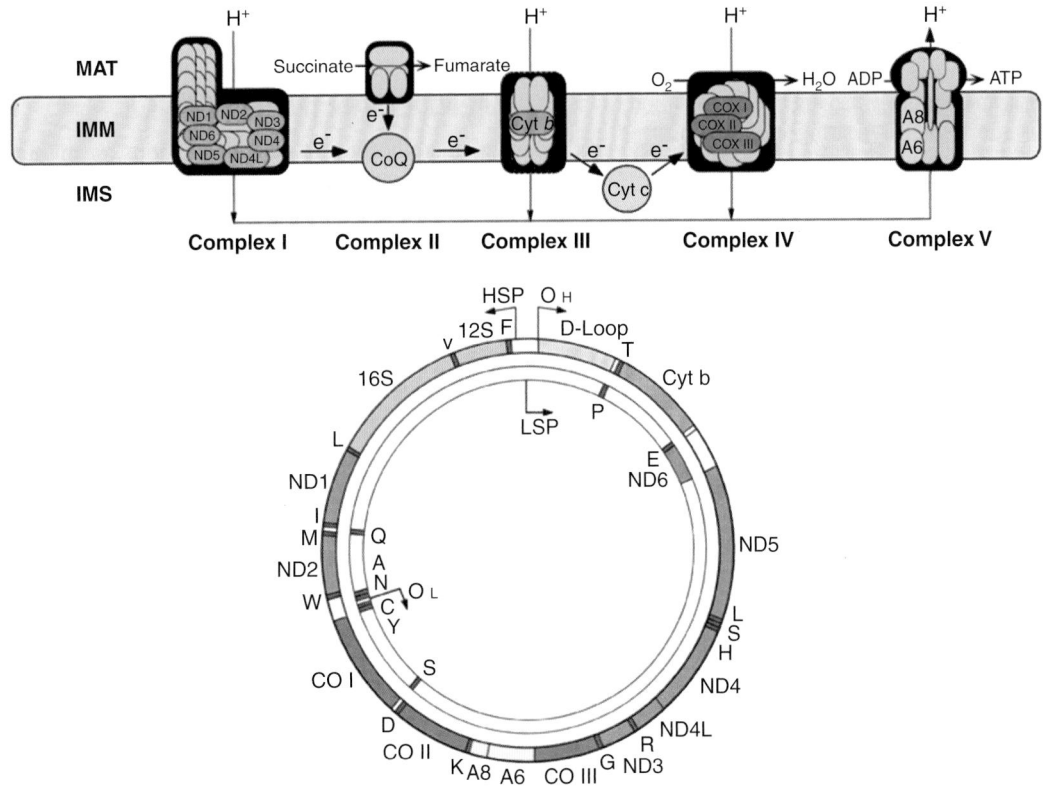

FIGURE 139.1 The respiratory chain **(top)** and mitochondrial DNA (mtDNA; **bottom**). Genes and corresponding gene products are similarly color-coded. ND denotes the subunits of NADH-coenzyme Q oxidoreductase (complex I); cyt *b*, cytochrome *b*; subunits of cytochrome *c* oxidase are labeled CO in the mtDNA scheme and COX in the respiratory chain rendition; *A6* and *A8* indicate subunits 6 and 8 of ATP synthase. The 22 tRNA genes are denoted by one-letter amino acid nomenclature, whereas *12S* and *16S* denote ribosomal RNAs (rRNAs). O_H and O_L are the origin of heavy- and light-strand replication; HSP and LSP are the promoters of heavy- and light-strand transcription.

(mitoribosomes). The subunits of complex II (succinate dehydrogenase [SDH]–ubiquinone oxidoreductase) and the enzymes required for synthesis of small electron carriers (coenzyme Q_{10} [ubiquinone] and cytochrome *c*) are encoded exclusively by nDNA.

The following main principles distinguish mitochondrial genetics from mendelian genetics and help explain many of the clinical peculiarities of mtDNA-related disorders.

1. *Polyplasmy.* Most cells contain multiple mitochondria and each mitochondrion contains multiple copies of mtDNA so that there are thousands of mitochondrial genomes in each cell.
2. *Heteroplasmy.* When an mtDNA pathogenic mutation affects some but not all genomes, a cell, a tissue, indeed a whole individual will harbor two populations of mtDNA, normal (or wild-type) and mutant, a condition known as *heteroplasmy*; in normal tissues, all mtDNA were considered identical, a situation called *homoplasmy*. However, highly sensitive next-generation sequencing has revealed the coexistence of mutated mtDNA variants (0.2% to 2.0% heteroplasmy) and wild-type mtDNA within a cell in blood and skeletal muscle of clinically unaffected individuals (a phenomenon termed *universal heteroplasmy*).
3. *Threshold effect.* The functional impairment associated with a pathogenic mtDNA mutation is largely determined by the degree of heteroplasmy, and a minimal critical number of mutant genomes (the mutation load) is required before tissue dysfunction becomes evident (and related clinical signs become manifest), a concept aptly termed *threshold effect*. This is, however, a relative concept: Tissues with high metabolic demands, such as brain, heart, and muscle, tend to have lower tolerance for mtDNA mutations than do metabolically less active tissues.
4. *Mitotic segregation.* Both organellar division and mtDNA replication are apparently stochastic events unrelated to cell division: Thus, the number of mitochondria (and mtDNA) can vary not only in space (i.e., among cells and tissues) but also in time (i.e., during development or aging). Moreover, at cell division, the proportion of mutant mtDNAs in daughter cells may drift, allowing for relatively rapid changes in genotype; therefore, if and when the threshold is exceeded, a clinical phenotype may manifest.
5. *Maternal inheritance.* At fertilization, all mitochondria (and all mtDNA) in the zygote are derived from the oocyte. Therefore, a mother carrying an mtDNA pathogenic mutation will pass it on to all her children, males and females, but only her daughters will transmit to their progeny, in a vertical matrilineal line. When maternal inheritance is evident in a clinical setting, it provides strong evidence that an mtDNA mutation must underlie the disease in question. However, the other features of mitochondrial genetics (e.g., heteroplasmy degree and

the threshold effect) often mask maternal inheritance by causing striking intrafamilial clinical heterogeneity. Thus, when suspecting an mtDNA-related disorder, it is crucial to collect the family history meticulously, paying special attention to "soft signs" (such as short stature, hearing loss, or migraine headache) in potentially oligosymptomatic maternal relatives.

More than 250 point mutations of mtDNA have been identified (Fig. 139.2). Ten pathogenic mutations in mtDNA have been observed frequently in neonatal cord blood of over 3,000 well babies, and a surprisingly high frequency, 1 in 200, harbored a pathogenic mtDNA mutation. The frequent occurrence of mtDNA mutations leads to a correspondingly high prevalence of mtDNA-related diseases: In the northeast of England, for example, 1 in

10,000 people are clinically affected by mtDNA-related disorders, and 1 in 6,000 individuals are considered at risk.

MENDELIAN INHERITANCE

The identification of nDNA mutations for mitochondrial diseases has accelerated rapidly since the discovery in 1995 of the first "direct hit" mutation in an nDNA-encoded gene for one of four subunits of complex II, exclusively controlled by nuclear genetics. These advances have been made possible by rapidly evolving technologies, from linkage analysis, homozygosity mapping, sequencing of candidate genes, and—ultimately—to next-generation genome-wide (whole-exome) sequencing (WES) or to screening of the portion of the genome that encodes the approximately 1,700 mitochondrial

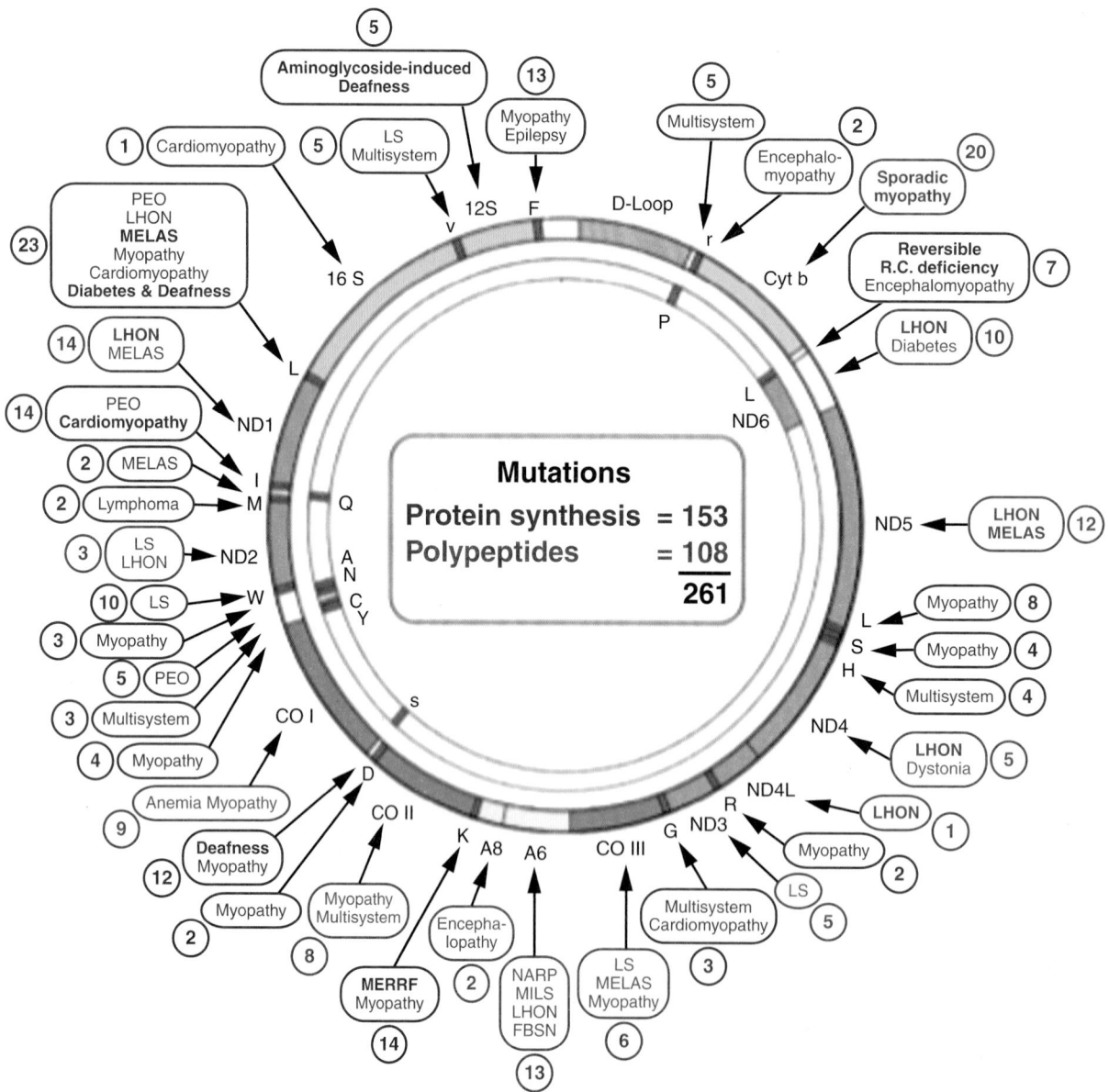

FIGURE 139.2 Morbidity map of the human mtDNA. Disorders caused by mutations in protein-coding genes are shown in *red*. Disorders caused by mutations in gene controlling protein synthesis are shown in *blue*. FBSN, familial bilateral striatal necrosis; LHON, Leber hereditary optic neuropathy; LS, Leigh syndrome; MELAS, mitochondrial encephalomyopathy, lactic acidosis, and stroke-like episodes; MERRF, myoclonus epilepsy with ragged red fibers; MILS, maternally inherited Leigh syndrome; NARP, neuropathy, ataxia, and retinitis pigmentosa; PEO, progressive external ophthalmoplegia.

proteins in a process known as *mito-exome sequencing*. The advantages of high-throughput DNA sequencing are eminently practical, enabling rapid diagnosis of puzzling cases and informing genetic counseling.

Direct Hits Mutations

"Direct hits" refer to pathogenic mutations that directly affect nDNA-encoded respiratory chain subunits in all five complexes but most commonly affecting the 16 of the 45 structural subunits of the gigantic complex I. In contrast, only a few direct hits affect complex II (affecting any of the four subunits), complex III (2 of the 11 subunits harbor damaging mutations, UQCRB and UQCRQ), complex IV (COX), of which only COX subunits 6B1 and 7B harbor deleterious mutations, and complex V (ATP synthase, containing a direct hit in a single gene, *ATP5E*). In keeping with the all-or-none effect of mostly recessive mendelian mutations, as opposed to the variegated effect of heteroplasmic mtDNA mutations, disorders to direct hits to the mitochondrial respiratory chain generally manifest at or soon after birth and are severe, often being lethal in infancy, most often associated with Leigh syndrome.

Indirect Hits Mutations

Even when all nDNA-encoded subunits of the various complexes are expressed correctly, they must be translated, imported into mitochondria, and directed to the inner mitochondrial membrane (IMM). At this site, they assemble with their mtDNA-encoded counterparts, acquire prosthetic groups, if necessary multimerize, and further assemble into supercomplexes (respirasomes). Mutations in these pathways are referred to as *indirect hits*, as they indirectly affect the mitochondrial respiratory chain.

In 1998, the search for the molecular basis of COX-deficient Leigh syndrome led to simultaneous discovery by two groups of the first mutant mitochondrial assembly gene, *SURF1*. Mutations in SURF1 are among the most common causes of Leigh syndrome. Mutations in at least seven more COX assembly factors (SCO1, SCO2, COX10, COX14, COX15, COA5, FAM36A, and TACO1) have been associated with various human diseases, predominantly encephalopathy, but cardiopathy often occurs with some mutations (*SCO2, COX10, COX15,* and *COA5*), whereas hepatopathy is associated with the *SCO1* mutations.

In patients with complex I deficiencies that are difficult to define molecularly, mutant assembly factors have been identified through next-generation sequencing of DNA. The clinical manifestations of these indirect hits tend to be more clinically heterogeneous than those associated with direct hits; all described patients have had encephalopathy resembling Leigh syndrome, but many have had leukodystrophy rather than gray matter involvement. Cardiomyopathy is often the dominating feature, presenting in infancy or in early childhood and early death.

The first assembly defect in complex III was identified in 2002 in Finnish infants with an extremely severe syndrome named GRACILE, an acronym aptly summarizing the symptoms and signs: growth *r*etardation, *a*minoaciduria, *c*holestasis, *i*ron overload, and early death. The mutated protein was the mitochondrial chaperone BCSL1, needed for insertion of the iron–sulfur (Fe-S) subunit into complex III.

A new group of disorders attributed to deficiency of coenzyme Q_{10} (CoQ$_{10}$) can be related to indirect hits that consist of mutations in a cascade of biosynthetic enzymes. They result in deficiency of this relatively simple component, CoQ$_{10}$, which is an integral part of the respirosome, where it shuttles electrons from complex I and complex II to complex III, acts as an antioxidant and modulates apoptosis. Molecular defects in genes encoding CoQ$_{10}$ biosynthetic enzymes (*PDSS2* and *COQ2*) were initially discovered in 2006, but mutations in other biosynthetic genes (*PDSS1*, *COQ6*, *ADCK3*, and *COQ9*) followed. Five clinical syndromes are attributed to CoQ$_{10}$ deficiency and they will be considered in the following section.

Defects of mtRNA Translation

The mitochondrial genome is transcribed into 13 mRNAs, which are translated by mitoribosomes into the 13 mtDNA-encoded respiratory chain subunits. As described in a comprehensive review, this process can be divided into two phases: a posttranscriptional phase (involving tRNA modifications, aminoacyl-tRNA synthetases, and processing of ribosomal proteins) and mtRNA translation (initiation, elongation, termination, and recycling). Representative examples of defects of each step of the mitochondrial translation process are briefly highlighted.

ABNORMAL tRNA MODIFICATIONS

Pseudouridylation modification is thought to promote stability and conformation of mitochondrial and nuclear tRNAs. Mutations in pseudouridine synthase 1 (*PUS1*) differentially impair nuclear and mitochondrial tRNA maturation causing mitochondrial myopathy, lactic acidosis, and sideroblastic anemia (*MLASA*); in addition, psychiatric symptoms and facial dysmorphism are likely due to abnormal cytosolic protein synthesis.

The conundrum of spontaneous improvement in *infantile reversible COX-deficient myopathy* (more accurately designated reversible infantile respiratory chain deficiency [RIRCD]) was resolved by elucidation of the tRNA modification processes in this disorder. RIRCD is due to homoplasmic mutations in *MT-TE*, which encodes mt-tRNA^{Glu}. Pathogenesis of the disease became more complex when patients in two families were found to harbor mutations in the *TRMU* gene, which modifies a wobble uridine base in mt-tRNA-^{Glu}. Skeletal muscle from infants in the initial symptomatic phase showed significantly decreased 2-thiouridylation due to defective TRMU activity, which exacerbated the effect of the mtRNA^{Glu} mutation and triggered the mitochondrial translation defect, thus demonstrating an nDNA-modifying effect on the mtDNA mutation.

Mutations in nine highly specialized aminoacyl-tRNA synthetases (ARs), which covalently link an amino acid to its cognate tRNA (tRNA charging), are associated with multiple specific clinical syndromes. Mitoribosomes consist of two mRNA components (12S and 16S rRNAS) and of novel about 30 and 50 nDNA-encoded proteins. Of the roughly 80 ribosomal proteins, 3 have been firmly linked to mitochondrial diseases: MRPS16, MRPS22, and MRPL3. Patients with defects of mitochondrial elongation factor genes (*GFM1* encoding EFG1; *TUFM*, EF-Tu$_{mt}$; and *TSFM*, EF-TS$_{mt}$) typically present with infantile-onset multisystemic diseases. Of the three known mitochondrial translation termination factors, which catalyze release of fully synthesized polypeptides, mutations have only been identified in a poorly characterized ribosome-recycling factor encoded by *C12orf65* in two unrelated families with LS, optic atrophy, and ophthalmoplegia. Mutations in two mitochondrial translation activators, both required for COX, have been linked to human diseases. Mutations in the gene *TACO1* (encoding translational activator for COX I), cause late-onset Leigh syndrome and COX deficiency, whereas mutations in *LRPPRC* (which encodes a leucine-rich pentatricopeptide repeat–containing protein) have been identified as the cause of a distinctive Leigh syndrome prevalent in French Canadians. Mutations of *RMND1* cause mitochondrial translational defects affecting multiple organs; however, the function of the encoded protein, which contains a domain of unknown function (DUF 155), remains a mystery.

Defects of the Inner Mitochondrial Membrane Lipid Milieu

The respiratory chain resides in the phospholipid component of the IMM and alterations in the lipid milieu are increasingly associated with mitochondrial encephalomyopathy. Cardiolipin, a dimeric molecule composed of two phosphatidylglycerol moieties connected by a glycerol group, is the signature mitochondrial phospholipid and a major component of the IMM, where it is synthesized. Cardiolipin deficiency was first documented—together with mutations in the gene encoding tafazzin (*TAZ*)—in patients with Barth syndrome, an X-linked mitochondrial myopathy and cardiomyopathy, with neutropenia and stunted growth.

Similar to Barth syndrome, Sengers syndrome affects primarily heart and muscle, with the distinctive additional clinical feature of congenital cataracts. Whole exome sequencing revealed mutations in the acylglycerol kinase (*AGK*) gene. Notably, lack of phosphatidic acid is a precursor of cardiolipin, thus providing a point of convergence in Sengers syndrome and Barth syndrome, which could account for the clinical similarities between the two disorders.

The mitochondrial-associated endoplasmic reticulum (ER) membrane (MAM) is the close physical and functional association between ER and mitochondria. MAMs are involved in multiple functions, including lipid transport, cholesterol metabolism, calcium signaling, energy metabolism, apoptosis, and mitochondrial dynamics.

New diseases have been associated with MAM dysfunction, including the MEGDEL syndrome (3-methylglutaconic aciduria type IV, deafness, and Leigh syndrome), in which the SERAC protein is located in the MAM and controls exchange of phospholipids between the ER and mitochondria. Interestingly, a central role of MAM in the pathogenesis of Alzheimer disease has been well documented.

Defects of Mitochondrial Dynamics

Mitochondria are highly dynamic organelles that move around the cell on microtubular tracks and, similar to their bacterial precursors, they fuse and divide, thus forming tubular networks that favor a balanced distribution of energy throughout the cell. Impairment of mitochondrial motility, fusion, or fission causes the nervous system particularly susceptible, as it is highly dependent on oxidative energy, and mitochondria must travel long distances along central axons and peripheral nerves.

Mitochondrial fusion requires coordinated action of multiple guanosine triphosphatases (GTPases) in the outer mitochondrial membrane (OMM), namely mitofusins MFN1 and MFN2, and in the IMM, namely OPA1.

Mitochondrial fission requires cytosolic dynamin-related protein 1 (DRP1; also a GTPase), which is recruited to the OMM together with two partners, mitochondrial fission (FIS1) and mitochondrial fission factor (MFF). Once recruited to the OMM, DRP1 forms a spiral that wraps around the mitochondrion like a noose and severs the mitochondrial membrane using guanosine triphosphate (GTP) hydrolysis.

DEFECTS OF MITOCHONDRIAL MAINTENANCE

These disorders have been traditionally subdivided into two groups: (1) mtDNA depletion syndromes manifesting early in life

and presenting as myopathy, hepatocerebral disease, or encephalomyopathy and (2) multiple mtDNA deletions, usually associated with chronic progressive external ophthalmoplegia with other manifestations that are predominantly neurologic (progressive external ophthalmoplegia [PEO]–plus).

The disorders of intergenomic communication are usually caused either by defects of mtDNA replication that are catalyzed by polymerase γ (genes *POLG* and *POLG2*) and by the helicase Twinkle (*PEO1*) or by altered homeostasis of the intramitochondrial deoxynucleoside triphosphates (dNTPs) pool that is controlled by multiple genes including *TK2* (encoding thymidine kinase 2), *DGUOK* (encoding deoxyguanosine kinase), and *TYMP* (encoding thymidine phosphorylase). In addition, the gene encoding adenine nucleotide translocase 1 (*ANT1*) causes autosomal dominant progressive external ophthalmoplegia (adPEO). Another mutant gene (*OPA1*), which is required mitochondrial fusion, has curiously been associated with autosomal dominant PEO-plus.

It is evident that mtDNA depletion and multiple mtDNA deletions often coexist in the same patient and are often caused by the same genes that cause either isolated depletion or multiple deletions of mtDNA (Table 139.2). A peculiarity of these disorders is that—although they are unequivocally mendelian—they share many features of mitochondrial genetics, including heteroplasmy and the threshold effect.

DISORDERS OF MITOCHONDRIAL PROTEIN IMPORTATION

A prerequisite for the assembly of any respiratory chain complex is the import of nDNA-encoded subunits from the cytoplasm into mitochondria, thus adding one more category to the indirect hits, namely defects in the mitochondrial importation machinery.

CLINICAL FEATURES

mtDNA-RELATED DISEASES

Mitochondria and mtDNA are ubiquitous, which explains why every tissue in the body can be affected by mtDNA mutations. This is illustrated in Figure 139.2 depicting mtDNA as a veritable Pandora box (abbreviated morbidity map). Table 139.2 is a compilation of symptoms and signs reported in patients with three different types of mtDNA mutations, including single deletions, point mutations in two distinct tRNA genes, and point mutations in a protein-coding gene. As shown by the boxes, certain constellations of symptoms and signs are sufficiently characteristic to make the diagnosis relatively easy in typical patients. On the other hand, because of the peculiar rules of mitochondrial genetics, different tissues harboring the same mtDNA mutation may be affected to different degrees or not at all, which explains the sometimes puzzling variety of syndromes associated with carriers of mtDNA mutations, even within a single pedigree.

Among the maternally inherited encephalomyopathies, four syndromes are more frequent. The first is *MELAS* (*mitochondrial encephalomyopathy, lactic acidosis, and stroke-like episodes*), which usually presents in children or young adults after normal early development. Symptoms include seizures, migraine-like headache, and stroke-like episodes causing cortical blindness, hemiparesis, or hemianopia. Magnetic resonance imaging (MRI) of the brain shows "infarcts" that do not correspond to the distribution of major vessels, raising the question of whether the strokes are vascular due to

TABLE 139.2 Paradigms of mtDNA-mutation Disorders

Tissue	Symptom/Sign	mtDNA Single Deletions		tRNA		ATPase6	
		KSS	Pearson	MERRF	MELAS	NARP	MILS
CNS	Seizures	−	−	+	+	−	+
	Ataxia	+	−	+	+	+	±
	Myoclonus	−	−	+	±	−	−
	Psychomotor retardation	−	−	−	−	−	+
	Psychomotor regression	+	−	±	+	−	−
	Hemiparesis/hemianopia	−	−	−	+	−	−
	Cortical blindness	−	−	−	+	−	−
	Migraine-like headaches	−	−	−	+	−	−
	Dystonia	−	−	−	+	−	+
PNS	Peripheral neuropathy	±	−	±	±	+	−
Muscle	Weakness	+	−	+	+	+	+
	Ophthalmoplegia	+	±	−	−	−	−
	Ptosis	+	−	−	−	−	−
Eye	Pigmentary retinopathy	+	−	−	−	+	±
	Optic atrophy	−	−	−	−	±	±
	Cataracts	−	−	−	−	−	−
Blood	Sideroblastic anemia	±	+	−	−	−	−
Endocrine	Diabetes mellitus	±	−	−	±	−	−
	Short stature	+	−	+	+	−	−
	Hypoparathyroidism	±	−	−	−	−	−
Heart	Conduction block	+	−	−	±	−	−
	Cardiomyopathy	±	−	−	±	−	±
GI	Exocrine pancreas dysfunction	±	+	−	−	−	−
	Intestinal pseudo-obstruction	−	−	−	−	−	−

Typical features are highlighted in red for each disorder except MILS, which is diagnosed neuropathologically.

KSS, Kearns–Sayre syndrome; MERRF, myoclonus epilepsy with ragged red fibers; MELAS, mitochondrial encephalomyopathy, lactic acidosis, and stroke-like episodes; NARP, neuropathy, ataxia, and retinitis pigmentosa; MILS, maternally inherited Leigh syndrome; CNS, central nervous system; PNS, peripheral nervous system; GI, gastrointestinal.

mitochondrial microangiopathy (Fig. 139.3). The most common cause of MELAS is *m3243A>G* in the *tRNA^Leu(UUR)* gene, but more than 20 other mutations have been associated with this disorder.

The second syndrome is *MERRF (myoclonus epilepsy with ragged red fibers)*, characterized by myoclonus, seizures, myopathy, and cerebellar ataxia. Less common signs include dementia, hearing loss, peripheral neuropathy, and multiple lipomas. The typical mtDNA mutation in MERRF is the m.8344A>G in the *tRNA^Lys* gene, but other mutations in the same gene have been reported.

The third syndrome has two clinical presentations. The first is *NARP (neuropathy, ataxia, and retinitis pigmentosa)*, which usually affects young adults and causes retinitis pigmentosa, dementia, seizures, ataxia, proximal weakness, and sensory neuropathy. The second is maternally inherited Leigh syndrome (*MILS*), a more severe infantile encephalopathy with characteristic symmetric lesions in the basal ganglia and the brain stem (see Fig. 139.3). As noted by the late Anita Harding in her original description of this syndrome, the two major causative mutations (m.8993G>T or m.8993C>T,

both affecting the same gene *MTATP6*) affect maternal relatives in the same family with those afflicted with MILS having higher mutation loads than individuals with NARP.

The fourth syndrome, *Leber hereditary optic neuropathy* (LHON), is characterized by acute or subacute loss of vision in young adults, more frequently males, due to bilateral optic atrophy. Mutations in three genes of complex I (ND genes) have been associated with LHON, *m.11778G>A* in *ND4, m.3460G>A* in *ND1*, and *m.14484T>C* in *ND6*. Epidemiologic studies have shown that LHON is the most common mtDNA-related disorder in adults. Epigenetic factors contribute to disease expression in homoplasmic patients by virtue of increased penetrance due to the European mtDNA haplogroup J and a protective effect of estrogens in women who are less frequently affected than men.

Three sporadic conditions are associated with mtDNA single deletions, *Kearns–Sayre syndrome* (KSS), *chronic progressive external ophthalmoplegia* (CPEO), and *Pearson syndrome* (PS). All three conditions are typically sporadic; however, a few cases of maternal

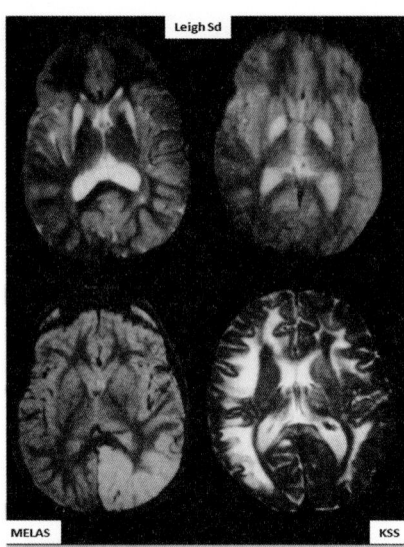

FIGURE 139.3 Characteristic brain MRI abnormalities in mitochondrial encephalomyopathies. These T2-weighted images show bilateral putaminal hyperintensities in a child with cytochrome *c* oxidase (COX)–associated Leigh syndrome **(top left panel)**, bilateral globus pallidus hyperintensities in a child with a familial Leigh syndrome phenotype **(top right)**, a left posterior cerebral hyperintense stroke-like lesion in a child with MELAS **(bottom left)**, and bilateral white matter hyperintensities in a child with Kearns–Sayre syndrome (KSS) **(bottom right)**.

transmission have been reported. A multicenter retrospective study of 226 families has confirmed that women carrying single mtDNA deletions have a low risk of having affected children (1 in 24).

KSS is a multisystem disorder with the obligate triad of onset before age 20 years of impaired eye movements (PEO and ptosis), pigmentary retinopathy plus heart block (requiring installment of a pacemaker), ataxia, or markedly elevated cerebrospinal fluid (CSF) protein (>100 mg/dL). Frequent additional signs include dementia, endocrinopathies (diabetes mellitus, growth hormone deficiency, and hypoparathyroidism), and lactic acidosis.

CPEO is a relatively benign disorder characterized by ptosis, PEO, and proximal myopathy. In addition, patients often develop dysphagia and ataxia.

PS, characterized by sideroblastic anemia and exocrine pancreatic dysfunction, is usually a fatal disorder of infancy. Due to *mitotic segregation* of deleted mtDNAs resulting in loss of the mutant mtDNA from blood cells but increased mutation burden in muscle and other postmitotic cells, the phenotype often evolves into CPEO or KSS in some surviving babies.

It is often stated that any patient having multiple organ involvement and evidence of maternal inheritance should be suspected of harboring a pathogenic mtDNA point mutation until proven otherwise. Although this "rule of thumb" has some practical value, it is also important to keep in mind that patients with involvement of a single tissue can still have pathogenic point mutations of mtDNA. This is especially true for skeletal muscle. As described earlier, isolated myopathy with PEO can be due to single large-scale mtDNA deletions, but isolated myopathy without PEO has been associated with point mutations in several tRNA genes, which can be due to generalized but skewed heteroplasmy in muscle. However, a simple nonmaternal inherited rule can be applied to pure mitochondrial myopathies due to somatic mutations in protein-coding mtDNA

genes, including subunits of complex I, complex III (including cytochrome *b*, *MTCYB*), or complex IV, accompanied by severe exercise intolerance, myalgia, and myoglobinuria.

MENDELIAN INHERITANCE

Leigh syndrome (LS) is the most important mitochondrial disease affecting infants and children, and reflecting the ravages of energy shortage on the developing nervous system, LS is a defined neuropathologically or neuroradiologically entity by bilateral symmetric lesions all along the neuraxis but especially in the basal ganglia, thalamus, brain stem, and cerebellar roof nuclei. Microscopically, there is neuronal loss, proportionate loss of myelin, reactive astrocytosis, and proliferation of cerebral microvessels. Clinically, these children have psychomotor retardation or regression, respiratory abnormalities, hypotonia, failure to thrive, seizures, and optic atrophy. Although we have highlighted mtDNA mutations in complex V genes causing LS (NARP/MILS), several other defects in mtDNA-encoded complex I (ND) genes as well as mutations in nuclear encoded subunits of complexes I, II, and IV frequently cause LS.

Besides LS, four distinct presentations have been attributed to direct hits in complex I deficiency: fatal infantile lactic acidosis (FILA), neonatal cardiomyopathy with lactic acidosis, leukodystrophy with macrocephaly, and hepatopathy with renal tubulopathy. Likely, these disorders represent variations of the common LS theme rather than separate clinical entities: Usually, these children are fine at birth or early in life, but disease progression is rapid and relentless, leading to death often before 1 year of age.

It has long been known that complex IV deficiency is a common cause of LS, but years went by before a mutated gene (*SURF1*) was associated with LS, the first example of an "indirect hit." Mutations in the COX assembly gene *SCO2* cause a severe combination of neonatal cardiomyopathy with encephalopathy, which is fatal in the first weeks or months of life. Importantly, *SCO2* mutations can simulate spinal muscular atrophy (SMA); therefore, it is important to consider *SCO2* mutations in patients with the clinical picture of SMA but without mutations in the SMN gene and with cardiomyopathy and COX-deficiency in muscle histology. Mutations in several other genes encoding COX assembly proteins have been associated with encephalopathy resembling LS together with involvement of other tissues. However, mutations in *SCO1* cause encephalohepatopathy, mutations in *COX10* cause encephalonephropathy, and mutations in *COX15* cause encephalocardiopathy as do mutations in *C2orf64*. Additional disorders due to indirect hits and resulting in generalized COX deficiency, including an unusual "toxic" mechanism of COX inhibition, have been reported. Indirect hits in complex V are rather frequently associated with mutations in the gene *TMEM70*, resulting in defective assembly of ATP synthase. Most patients harboring *TMEM70* mutations were severely affected with neonatal hypotonia, apneic spells, psychomotor delay, hypertrophic cardiomyopathy, and profound lactic acidosis, whereas a minority presented with additional infantile-onset cataracts, early-onset gastrointestinal dysfunction, and multiple joint contractures.

Indirect hits include those encompassing five major phenotypes due to CoQ_{10} deficiency. These disorders are important to diagnose, as they often respond to CoQ_{10} supplementation. The first patients reported in 1989 were a pair of sisters, ages 12- and 14-year-old with a mitochondrial disorder characterized by encephalopathy (mental retardation, seizures, and mild ataxia) and myopathy with recurrent myoglobinuria. The triad of mitochondrial myopathy, myoglobinuria, and encephalopathy has been reported in a few other patients. The second syndrome is childhood-onset cerebellar atrophy and ataxia, with variable additional symptoms, including neuropathy, seizures, mental retardation, and muscle weakness. The molecular basis of this phenotype was identified in some but not all patients, and the mutated gene was *ADCK3/CABC1*. The third syndrome was an infantile multisystemic disease, which typically manifests as encephalopathy and nephropathy (particularly steroid-resistant nephrotic syndrome). This syndrome was initially associated with mutations in COQ2 and PDSS and subsequently in additional genes required for CoQ$_{10}$ biosynthesis including *PDSS1*, *PDSS2*, and *COQ9*. The fourth syndrome, dominated by severe nephropathy and typically leading to end-stage renal disease, was originally attributed to *COQ2* gene mutations, whereas steroid-resistant nephrosis and end-stage renal failure associated with sensorineural deafness was linked to *COQ6* mutations. The fifth syndrome is isolated myopathy and, in a few cases, has been due to multiple acyl-CoA dehydrogenases deficiency causing secondary CoQ$_{10}$ deficiency.

Defects of the Inner Mitochondrial Membrane Lipid Milieu

Phospholipid metabolism and the lipid composition of the IMM were relatively neglected in the study of mitochondrial diseases, but there was a recent awakening of this subject and several new disorders were discovered, thanks in part to whole exome sequencing.

Barth syndrome is an X-linked disorder characterized by mitochondrial cardiac and skeletal myopathy, cyclic neutropenia, and growth retardation and, as previously noted, is due to *TAZ* mutations that alter cardiolipin, the most abundant phospholipid component of the IMM.

Sengers syndrome, an autosomal recessive disorder, was described in 1975 and consisted of congenital cataracts, hypertrophic cardiomyopathy, skeletal myopathy, exercise intolerance, and lactic acidosis. This syndrome was ultimately attributed through exome sequencing to mutations in the gene (*AGK*) encoding acylglycerol kinase.

A third disorder of the mitochondrial lipid milieu was identified in 15 patients with a *congenital myopathy* characterized by early-onset muscle weakness and mental retardation with protracted course (most patients were alive at the time of publication and only four had died between the ages of 2½ and 28 years). The hallmark of the disease was the presence in muscle of greatly enlarged mitochondria (megaconial disease) displaced at the periphery of the fibers and the genetic cause was due to mutations in the gene (*CHKB*) encoding choline kinase beta.

A genetic alteration of phospholipid metabolism explained a syndrome characterized by 3-methylglutaconic aciduria (3-methlylglutagonic aciduria type IV, deafness, and Leigh-like encephalopathy, which was dubbed *MEGDEL*). This syndrome was caused by mutations in the phospholipid remodeling gene *SERAC1*, a key player in intracellular cholesterol trafficking and a member of the MAMs.

Defects of Mitochondrial Translation

Mitochondrial translational defects typically present with diverse clinical phenotypes with multisystemic disease and LS being the most prevalent; however, a few distinct phenotypes have emerged in this group of heterogeneous disorders. As previously noted, MLASA can be caused not only by *PUS1* mutations but also *YARS* mutations. RIRCD to a homoplasmic tRNA^{Glu} is particularly important to diagnose because, with proper supportive care, children typically improve spontaneously and eventually become clinically normal.

Pathogenic mutations in the gene *DARS* (encoding aspartyl-tRNA synthethase) cause brain stem and spinal cord involvement and lactate elevation (*LBSL*) in affected children with cerebellar ataxia, spasticity, dorsal column dysfunction, and mild cognitive decline. Equally severe mutations in the gene *RARS2* (encoding arginyl-tRNA synthetase) have been identified in three patients with severe infantile encephalopathy with *pontocerebellar hypoplasia*. Mutations in *EARS2*, encoding glutamyl-tRNA synthetase, were identified by whole exome sequencing in a cohort of 11 unrelated cases with symmetric cerebral white matter abnormalities and signal abnormalities of the thalami, midbrain, pons, medulla oblongata, and cerebellar white matter. All patients share an infantile-onset and rapidly progressive disease with severe lactic acidosis. Mutations in *MARS2*, encoding the methionyl-tRNA synthetase, were found to be responsible for *autosomal recessive spastic ataxia with leukoencephalopathy* (*ARSAL*).

Defects of mitoribosomes have been associated with complex multisystemic disorders; however, in one family with *MPRL3* mutations, four siblings manifested fatal infantile-onset hypertrophic cardiomyopathy and psychomotor retardation. Similarly, patients with abnormal mitochondrial translational elongation factors typically present with fatal infantile diseases with early hepatoencephalopathy with *GFM1* (EFG1) mutations and macrocystic leukodystrophy and micropolygyria due to *TUFM* (EF-Tu$_{mt}$) defects.

Defects of Mitochondrial Dynamics

There is a group of disorders due to numerous mutations in mitochondrial fusion proteins and, less commonly, in fission proteins. Mutations in fusion proteins, such as OPA1, result in a dominantly inherited optic atrophy (DOA or Kjer disease), the nDNA blindness corresponding to the mtDNA disorder LHON. Other mutations in fusion proteins, such as MFN2 or GADP1, result in Charcot–Marie–Tooth neuropathies (types 2A and 4A).

Two infants with distinct mutations in fission genes (*DRP1* and *MFF*) showed both mitochondrial and peroxisomal abnormalities, and they were severely affected with rapidly fatal encephalopathy and lactic acidosis.

DEFECTS OF mtDNA MAINTENANCE

Here, we consider the main clinical phenotypes associated with mtDNA depletion syndromes (MDS), with multiple mtDNA syndromes (PEO-plus), and, finally, with combined appearance of mtDNA depletion and of multiple mtDNA deletions.

mtDNA Depletion Syndromes

MYOPATHIC mtDNA DEPLETION SYNDROMES

Patients usually present in the first year of life with failure to thrive, hypotonia, weakness, and sometimes PEO. They usually die in childhood from pulmonary insufficiency but severity of weakness and survival vary considerably. The myopathic MDS is most commonly due to mutations in the gene (*TK2*) encoding mitochondrial thymidine kinase 2. About 20 mutations have been reported in as many patients. Notably, mutations in *TK2* can also cause a phenocopy of SMA; therefore, it is of practical importance to screen for *TK2* mutations in patients with SMA but without mutations in the *SMN1* gene.

ENCEPHALOMYOPATHIC mtDNA DEPLETION SYNDROMES

Two variants of this condition are both due to a defect of succinyl-CoA lyase activity in the Krebs cycle. Mutations in the gene (*SUCLA2*) encoding the ATP-dependent succinyl-CoA lyase SUCLA2 cause severe psychomotor retardation, muscle hypotonia, hearing loss, generalized seizures, knee and hip contractures, mild ptosis, lactic acidosis, and methylmalonic aciduria. There is only moderate mtDNA depletion (about 30%) in muscle, whereas MRI of the brain is suggestive of LS. Mutations in the gene (SUCLG1) encoding the GTP-dependent isoform SUCLG1 cause a much more severe and rapidly fatal phenotype with mtDNA depletion in both muscle and liver, characterized clinically by dysmorphic features, congenital lactic acidosis, and methylmalonic aciduria. A less dismal course, more like the SUCLA2 phenotype, is correlated to the degree of residual activity.

Patients with mtDNA depletion are due to mutations in RRM2B (encoding the small subunit, p53R2, of the p53-inducible ribonucleotide reductase protein). Infants are hypotonic and children are weak but may also manifest nephropathy and central nervous system involvement with microcephaly, seizures, and developmental delay.

HEPATOCEREBRAL mtDNA DEPLETION SYNDROMES

Mutations in three other genes, DGUOK, MPV17, and POLG also cause liver and brain involvement. Mutations in DGUOK, encoding the mitochondrial deoxyguanosine kinase (dGK), were first reported in 2001. Severe mutations cause fatal infantile hepatopathy and brain involvement, whereas milder mutations cause isolated liver disease and are compatible with longer survival.

Mutations in MPV17, which encodes a small mitochondrial membrane protein of unknown function, cause a rather typical hepatocerebral syndrome in Caucasian children but is associated with a peculiar neurohepatopathy that is prevalent in the Navajo population due to a founder MPV17 mutation. The clinical features of NNH include peripheral and central nervous system involvement, acral mutilation, corneal scarring or ulceration, liver failure, and immunologic derangement.

Alpers–Huttenlocher syndrome (AHS) is the most important form of hepatocerebral MDS and it has been attributed to mutations in POLG. AHS is defined as a disorder of childhood by the tetrad of refractory seizures, episodic psychomotor regression, cortical blindness, and hepatopathy with micronodular cirrhosis. It is crucially important not to expose these children to valproate, which often precipitates fulminant hepatic failure.

Syndromes due to Multiple mtDNA Deletions

MUTATIONS IN ANT1

Mutations in the gene for one isoform of the adenine nucleotide translocator (ANT1) have been identified in patients with autosomal dominant PEO, sometime associated with psychiatric disorders. In a seminal paper, multiple mtDNA deletions were most abundant in brain, followed by cardiac and skeletal muscle. Sporadic PEO may also infrequently be due to mutations in ANT1 and the association of mitochondrial myopathy and cardiomyopathy, even in patients with recessive inheritance and without PEO, should raise the question of ANT1 mutations.

MUTATIONS IN PEO1

In 2001, autosomal dominant PEO with multiple mtDNA deletions was associated with mutations in the gene (PEO1), encoding a mitochondrial helicase called Twinkle, an essential factor for mtDNA maintenance and for the regulation of mtDNA copy number. A review of 33 patients from 26 families showed that the most common symptoms were ptosis (97%) and ophthalmoparesis (94%), followed by exercise intolerance (52%) and mild proximal weakness. (33%). Central nervous system involvement was infrequent and included visual impairment, migraine, lethargy, hearing loss, and epilepsy. Cardiac problems were noted in 24% of the patients. A relatively benign long-term progression was noted in a large family with autosomal dominant isolated PEO.

MUTATIONS IN POLG

Mutations in the gene encoding the only mitochondrial polymerase, polymerase γ (POLG) have emerged as major causes of a vast array of mitochondrial disorders. Over 150 mutations have been described in all three domains of the gene, exonuclease, linker, and polymerase and may cause either autosomal dominant or autosomal recessive PEO, a syndrome comprising autosomal recessive sensory ataxic neuropathy, dysarthria, and ophthalmoparesis (SANDO), mitochondrial recessive ataxia syndrome (MIRAS), or parkinsonism with or without PEO.

MUTATIONS IN OPA1

One unexpected gene was recently added to those described earlier and associated with myopathy and PEO, OPA1. This was unexpected because mutations in OPA1 had been initially associated with a purely ophthalmologic condition, dominant optic atrophy (DOA) or Kjer disease, and because the gene product is a mechanoenzyme associated with mitochondrial fusion rather than with mitochondrial maintenance.

However, a syndromic disorder, often dubbed DOA-plus, has emerged, which is characterized more or less sequentially by optic atrophy with visual failure, sensorineural deafness, ataxia, myopathy, axonal sensory motor polyneuropathy, and PEO. Muscle biopsy in these patients shows scattered ragged blue, COX-negative fibers and multiple mtDNA deletions. The relationship between this defect of mitochondrial dynamics and altered mitochondrial maintenance is intriguing. Two explanations have been proposed: decreased ability by the organelles to repair stress-induced mtDNA damage or accelerated accumulation of preexisting age-associated somatic mtDNA mutations.

Coexistence of mtDNA Depletion and mtDNA Multiple Deletions

MITOCHONDRIAL NEUROGASTROINTESTINAL ENCEPHALOMYOPATHY

One of the disorders in which the coexistence of multiple mtDNA deletions and mtDNA depletion was first recognized is mitochondrial neurogastrointestinal encephalomyopathy (MNGIE). This autosomal recessive multisystemic syndrome is characterized by mitochondrial myopathy with ptosis and PEO, peripheral neuropathy, gastrointestinal dysmotility causing severe cachexia, and leukoencephalopathy without cognitive impairment. MNGIE is due to mutations in the gene (TYMP) encoding thymidine phosphorylase (TP), resulting in elevated levels of thymidine and deoxyuridine in plasma and tissues. The disease starts in young adults and is relentlessly progressive, with an average age of death at 37 years. Molecular analysis has shown over 50 TYMP mutations resulting in mtDNA multiple deletions, depletion, and site-specific somatic mtDNA point mutations in multiple tissues. A mouse model has demonstrated that increased levels of thymidine and deoxyuridine imbalance mitochondrial deoxynucleotide triphosphate pools, resulting in mtDNA instability.

Infantile-onset spinocerebellar ataxia (IOSCA) was described in the 1970s in Finland. Between 9 and 18 months, children develop acutely or subacutely ataxia, hypotonia, athetosis, and areflexia, and by teenage years, they lose independent ambulation. Additional symptoms include PEO, optic atrophy, sensorineural hearing loss, cognitive impairment, sensory neuropathy, and autonomic nervous system dysfunction. In 2005, this autosomal recessive disorder was attributed to mutations in *PEO1*. Both brain and liver showed mtDNA depletion.

In addition to causing early childhood-onset myopathic mtDNA depletion, mutations in *TK2* can also cause adult-onset myopathy with mtDNA depletion and even late-onset PEO with multiple mtDNA deletions rather than mtDNA depletion.

Mutations in *RRM2B* can also be associated with autosomal dominant or recessive PEO and multiple mtDNA deletions.

Exome sequencing revealed *DGUOK* mutations in five adult patients with PEO and mitochondrial myopathy with multiple mtDNA deletions: Only one of these patients had had liver problems in childhood. Mutations in *MPV17*, in addition to causing juvenile-onset mtDNA depletion, can also cause adult-onset PEO-plus with multiple mtDNA deletions in muscle.

DIAGNOSIS

LABORATORY

Lactic acidosis is a common finding in defects of the respiratory chain, and the lactate-to-pyruvate ratio is usually elevated (>20:1). Information about CSF lactate and pyruvate is important because CSF values can be increased in children with encephalopathy and normal blood lactate. However, lack of lactic acidosis does not exclude the diagnosis. For example, in patients with NARP or MILS, blood lactate and pyruvate can be normal or only mildly elevated. Serum creatine kinase (CK) levels are usually normal or modestly increased except, of course, in patients with myopathy during episodes of myoglobinuria. As another exception to this rule, and a useful diagnostic clue, serum CK values can be markedly elevated in children with the myopathic form of mtDNA depletion, such as those with mutations in the gene (*TK2*) encoding mitochondrial thymidine kinase. Another important laboratory test is plasma thymidine, which is greatly increased in patients with MNGIE, an autosomal recessive disease due to mutations in *TYMP* encoding thymidine phosphorylase.

NEURORADIOLOGY

Bilateral MRI T2 signal hyperintensities in basal ganglia and brain stem are indicative of LS. Stroke-like lesions predominantly affecting the cortex, often in the posterior cerebral hemispheres, are typically seen in patients with MELAS. Increased MRI T2 signal abnormality of the central white matter is sometimes observed in KSS, whereas basal ganglia calcifications are common in both MELAS and KSS syndrome (see Fig. 139.3). White matter signal abnormalities are distinctively seen in patients with complex I deficiency or in children with mtDNA translation defects or in several patients with problems of mtDNA maintenance. Proton magnetic resonance spectroscopy reveals lactate accumulation in the CSF and in specific areas of the brain, where lactate concentration can be compared to the concentration of *N*-acetylaspartate (NAA), an indicator of cell viability.

EXERCISE PHYSIOLOGY

Impaired oxygen extraction by exercising muscle can be detected by near-infrared spectroscopy, which measures the degree of deoxygenation of hemoglobin. A simpler test is based on the measurement of the partial pressure of oxygen (PO_2) in cubital venous blood after forearm aerobic exercise. PO_2 rises paradoxically in patients with mitochondrial myopathy or PEO, and the degree of rise reflects the severity of oxidative impairment. By ^{31}P-magnetic resonance spectroscopy, the ratio of phosphocreatine to inorganic phosphate (PCr to Pi) can be measured in muscle at rest, during exercise, and during recovery. In patients with mitochondrial dysfunction, PCr to Pi ratios are lower than normal at rest, decrease excessively during exercise, and return to baseline more slowly than normal.

PATHOLOGY

SKELETAL MUSCLE

Muscle biopsy has a central role in the diagnosis of primary mtDNA-related disorders but is equally important in diagnosing patients with defects of mtDNA maintenance, who have strictly mendelian inheritance and secondary mtDNA alterations. In both types of disorders, abnormal mitochondrial proliferation, a hallmark of mitochondrial dysfunction, can be revealed with the modified Gomori trichrome stain (RRF) or better with the SDH reaction (ragged blue fibers) (Fig. 139.4). RRF are present in muscle biopsies from patients with most disorders due to mtDNA mutations although rare exceptions include NARP/MILS and LHON. Most cases of mendelian inheritance rarely are diagnosable by the presence of RRF or ragged blue fibers, but these types of fibers are exceptionally detectable in patients with either mtDNA depletion or mtDNA multiple deletions.

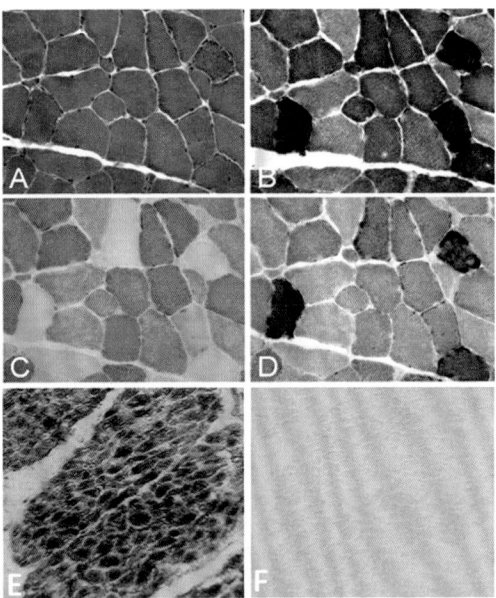

FIGURE 139.4 Serial sections from the muscle biopsy of a patient with MERRF syndrome. With the modified Gomori trichrome stain **(A)**, two ragged red fibers are evident. The same fibers appear *ragged-blue* with the succinate dehydrogenase (SDH) stain **(B)**, are pale with the cytochrome *c* oxidase (COX) stain **(C)**, and appear more or less intensely blue with the combined COX/SDH stain **(D)**. In contrast to the checkerboard appearance of the muscle biopsy in an mtDNA-related disease, the biopsy from a patient with mutations in *SCO2*, an nDNA assembly gene of COX, shows normal fiber type–related variability in SDH staining intensity **(E)** but uniform lack of COX activity **(F)**.

The COX histochemical reaction typically reveals scattered COX-negative and COX-deficient fibers, which usually correspond to—but are not confined to—RRF. RRF are COX-positive in two main conditions: (1) typical MELAS syndrome and (2) mutations in mtDNA genes encoding cytochrome *b* or complex I subunits. To confirm the pathogenicity of an mtDNA mutation, single fibers can be dissected out of thick cross-sections of muscle and used to determine the levels of a given mutation by polymerase chain reaction (PCR). Finding higher levels of the mutation in affected (ragged red or COX-negative fibers) than in unaffected (non–ragged red, COX-positive fibers) is strong evidence that the mutation in question is pathogenic.

Electron microscopy has lost much of its historical diagnostic value but it can reveal focal accumulations of mitochondria or mitochondria with paracrystalline inclusions in cases in which histochemical results are equivocal.

NEUROPATHOLOGY

The major neuropathologic findings in mitochondrial encephalomyopathies consist of four histologic lesions: spongy degeneration, neuronal loss, gliosis, and demyelination. Although these lesions are nonspecific, their distribution patterns vary in patients with different mtDNA-related disorders. Thus, the neuropathology of KSS is characterized by spongiform degeneration, which is usually generalized and affects both gray and white matter. In MELAS, multifocal necrosis predominates, affecting not only the cerebral cortex or the subcortical white matter but also the cerebellum, thalamus, and basal ganglia. Calcification of basal ganglia is also common. In MERRF, neuronal degeneration, astrocytosis, and demyelination affect preferentially the cerebellum (especially the dentate nucleus), the brain stem (especially the olivary nucleus), and the spinal cord. In LS, due to either mtDNA-related diseases or to mendelian conditions, there are symmetric, bilateral foci of necrosis in the basal ganglia, thalamus, midbrain, and pons. Microscopically, the lesions show vascular proliferation, gliosis, neuronal loss, demyelination, and cystic cavitation.

BIOCHEMICAL FINDINGS

All 13 proteins encoded by mtDNA are components of the mitochondrial respiratory chain. Seven (ND1 to ND5, ND4L, ND6) are subunits of complex I, one (cytochrome *b*) is part of complex III, three (COX I, COX II, and COX III) are subunits of complex IV, and two (adenosine triphosphatase [ATPase] 6 and ATPase 8) are subunits of complex V (see Fig. 139.1). Therefore, disorders owing to mutations of mtDNA are usually associated with biochemical defects of oxidative phosphorylation. Skeletal muscle is the preferred tissue for biochemical analysis because it is rich in mitochondria, it is invariably affected in multisystem disorders (mitochondrial encephalomyopathies), and it is the most common tissue affected in isolation (mitochondrial myopathies). There is some controversy about whether fresh muscle tissue is needed or frozen tissue suffices. It is our view that—except for the rare cases in which freshly isolated mitochondria for polarographic analyses are required—frozen specimens provide adequate biochemical information. Because mitochondrial proliferation in muscle (RRF) is a common occurrence, activities of respiratory chain complexes should be referred to the activity of citrate synthase, a nuclear-encoded enzyme of the mitochondrial matrix that is a good marker of mitochondrial abundance.

Biochemical studies in muscle extract from patients with mtDNA-related disorders yield two main types of results. The first pattern consists of partial defects in the activities of multiple complexes containing mtDNA-encoded subunits (I, III, and IV) contrasting with normal or increased activities of SDH (complex II) and citrate synthase. The second pattern is a severe deficiency in the activity of one specific respiratory complex. As a rule, the first pattern is found in patients with single mtDNA deletions (e.g., KSS) or mutations in tRNA genes (e.g., MELAS, MERRF) because these genetic errors impair mitochondrial protein synthesis *in toto*. The second pattern is typical of mutations in mtDNA protein-coding genes. For example, mutations in the cytochrome *b* gene cause isolated complex III deficiency. However, mutations in ND genes, which are encountered with increasing frequency in patients with MELAS, LS, LHON, or overlap syndromes, cause inconsistent and often modest impairment of complex I activity.

Specific enzyme defects are documentable in mendelian conditions, especially clear in "direct" and "indirect" hits of complex I and complex IV. However, universal decrease of all respiratory chain enzymes (except for complex II) typically appears in conditions of mtDNA depletion syndromes and—equally devastating—it typically also characterizes most disorders due to mtDNA translation syndromes. Occasionally, defects in Fe-S assembly proteins show biochemical decreases of three specific respiratory chain enzymes (complex I, complex II, complex III) and of one specific enzyme of the Krebs cycle (aconitase) of which Fe-S are components.

TREATMENT

No panacea for respiratory chain dysfunction and no universal therapy for mitochondrial disorders currently exist. Nevertheless, symptomatic pharmacologic treatments (e.g., antiepileptic drugs) and surgical remedies (such as blepharoplasty) are useful in prolonging and improving the lives of patients with mitochondrial disease. Exercise therapy has been demonstrated to improve exercise tolerance and quality of life in patients with mitochondrial diseases. Several strategies aimed at curing (or even preventing) mitochondrial diseases have shown promise *in vitro* or in animals or have produced encouraging preliminary results in humans and are briefly reviewed in the following sections.

MITOCHONDRIAL TRANSFER

For mtDNA-related diseases, many of which are devastating and undiagnosable prenatally, the ultimate goal is to prevent their occurrence altogether via mitochondrial replacement. In this approach, the nucleus of an *in vitro*–fertilized oocyte from an mtDNA mutation carrier is transferred to an enucleated oocyte from a normal donor: The embryo will have the nDNA of the biologic parents but the mtDNA of a normal mitochondrial donor. In nonhuman primate experiments using oocyte spindle-chromosomal complex transfer, the infants were healthy and devoid of original maternal mtDNA. The same technique was applied to fertilized and unfertilized but parthenogenically activated human oocytes, and the cells were found to develop into normal blastocysts and contain virtually exclusively donor mtDNA. Moreover, only donor mtDNA was detected after stem cell lines from blastocysts were differentiated into neurons, cardiomyocytes and *β* cells. Similar results were obtained in the United Kingdom after pronuclear transfer in abnormally fertilized human oocytes developed to the blastocyst stage. Despite some concerns, the stage seems set for approval of this technique for therapeutic application both in the United Kingdom and the United States.

SHIFTING HETEROPLASMY

For mtDNA-related disorders, an obvious but challenging goal is to shift heteroplasmy in patients, thereby lowering the mutation load to subthreshold levels. When deprived of glucose and exposed to ketogenic media, cybrids harboring single mtDNA deletions shifted their heteroplasmy level and recovered mitochondrial function, probably through selective mitochondrial autophagy (mitophagy). A genetic approach to heteroplasmic shifting involves use of restriction endonucleases to eliminate specific pathogenic mutations.

ENHANCEMENT OF RESPIRATORY CHAIN FUNCTION

The most obvious therapeutic approach to mitochondrial disorders is to enhance respiratory chain function, thereby mitigating both energy crisis (ATP deficit) and oxidative stress (toxic buildup of reactive oxygen species [ROS]). The compound used almost universally in patients with mitochondrial disease is CoQ_{10}, given the pivotal role of this molecule in electron transport, its antioxidant properties, and its safety even at high doses. Two synthetic analogs of CoQ_{10}—idebenone and parabenzoquinone—seem more promising. Idebenone, a short-chain benzoquinone, has shown positive results at 900 mg daily in two studies of patients with LHON. The second compound, a parabenzoquinone labelled EPI-743, has so far been tested only in open studies: This compound at 100 to 400 mg three times daily reversed vision loss in four of five patients with LHON, produced clinical improvement in 12 children with various mitochondrial disorders, and arrested or reversed disease progression in 13 children with genetically proven LS.

ELIMINATION OF NOXIOUS COMPOUNDS

The second logical therapeutic approach to mitochondrial disease is to eliminate the noxious compounds that accumulate in these disorders. To decrease brain lactate in patients with MELAS, we used dichloroacetate (DCA), which keeps pyruvate dehydrogenase in the active form and favors lactate oxidation. Unfortunately, this agent had unacceptable neurotoxicity and treatment had to be discontinued. A more promising "detoxifying therapy" seems to be allogeneic hematopoietic stem cell transplantation (AHSCT) aimed at restoring sufficient thymidine phosphorylase activity in patients with MNGIE to normalize the circulating toxic levels of thymidine and deoxyuridine. As of 2012, 9 of 24 patients with MNGIE who had undergone AHSCT were alive and had normal blood thymidine phosphorylase activity, virtually undetectable levels of thymidine and deoxyuridine, and mild clinical improvements. A safety study of AHSCT in patients with MNGIE is under way to assess if transplants can be performed with low morbidity in mildly to moderately affected individuals.

ALTERATION OF MITOCHONDRIAL DYNAMICS

Mitochondrial dynamics could be exploited therapeutically in two opposing ways. We could enhance mitochondrial fission and favor mitophagy, a natural "quality control" function that sequesters and eliminates dysfunctional mitochondria, perhaps sensing their abnormally low membrane potential. Alternatively, enhancement of mitochondrial fusion and "networking" would allow complementation of "bad" and "good" mitochondria and normalization of overall mitochondrial function.

Although natural mitochondrial proliferation (e.g., RRF) is a futile compensatory mechanism, preliminary studies indicate

it may be possible to improve on nature's strategy by enhancing mitochondrial biogenesis through activation of the transcriptional coactivator PGC-1α AMPK pathway or Sirtuin1. The advantage over disease-induced mitochondrial proliferation, which appears to favor mutated mtDNAs, is that upregulation of mitochondrial biosynthesis increases numbers of all mtDNAs, allowing wild-type genomes to compensate for mutated ones. Encouraging results have been obtained in four mouse models of COX deficiency.

SUGGESTED READINGS

General Reviews

DiMauro S. Mitochondrial encephalomyopathies—fifty years on: the Robert Wartenberg Lecture. *Neurology.* 2013;81:281–291.

DiMauro S, Bonilla E. Mitochondrial disorders due to mutations in the mitochondrial genome. In: Rosenberg RN, DiMauro S, Paulson HL, et al, eds. *The Molecular and Genetic Basis of Neurological and Psychiatric Disease.* 4th ed. Boston, MA: Butterworth-Heinemann; 2008:169–176.

DiMauro S, Schon EA, Carelli V, et al. The clinical maze of mitochondrial neurology. *Nat Rev Neurol.* 2013;9:429–444.

Koopman WJ, Willems PH, Smeitink JA. Monogenic mitochondrial disorders. *N Engl J Med.* 2012;366:1132–1141.

History

DiMauro S, Bonilla E, Lee CP, et al. Luft's disease. Further biochemical and ultrastructural studies of skeletal muscle in the second case. *J Neurol Sci.* 1976;27:217–232.

Engel WK, Cunningham CG. Rapid examination of muscle tissue: an improved trichrome stain method for fresh-frozen biopsy sections. *Neurology.* 1963; 13:919–923.

Holt IJ, Harding AE, Morgan-Hughes JA. Deletions of muscle mitochondrial DNA in patients with mitochondrial myopathies. *Nature.* 1988;331:717–719.

Luft R, Ikkos D, Palmieri G, et al. A case of severe hypermetabolism of nonthyroid origin with a defect in the maintenance of mitochondrial respiratory control: a correlated clinical, biochemical, and morphological study. *J Clin Invest.* 1962;41:1776–1804.

Shy GM, Gonatas NK, Perez M. Childhood myopathies with abnormal mitochondria. I. Megaconial myopathy-pleoconial myopathy. *Brain.* 1966;89:133–158.

Wallace DC, Singh G, Lott MT, et al. Mitochondrial DNA mutation associated with Leber's hereditary optic neuropathy. *Science.* 1988;242:1427–1430.

Pathobiology

Alexander C, Votruba M, Pesch UE, et al. OPA1, encoding a dynamin-related GTPase, is mutated in autosomal dominant optic atrophy linked to chromosome 3q28. *Nat Genet.* 2000;26:211–215.

Area-Gomez E, Del Carmen Lara Castillo M, Tambini MD, et al. Upregulated function of mitochondria-associated ER membranes in Alzheimer disease. *EMBO J.* 2012;31:4106–4123.

Bione S, D'Adamo P, Maestrini E, et al. A novel X-linked gene, G4.5. is responsible for Barth syndrome. *Nat Genet.* 1996;12:385–389.

Boczonadi V, Smith PM, Pyle A, et al. Altered 2-thiouridylation impairs mitochondrial translation in reversible infantile respiratory chain deficiency. *Hum Mol Genet.* 2013;22:4602–4615.

Bourdon A, Minai L, Serre V, et al. Mutation of RRM2B, encoding p53-controlled ribonucleotide reductase (p53R2), causes severe mitochondrial DNA depletion. *Nat Genet.* 2007;39:776–780.

Bourgeron T, Rustin P, Chretien D, et al. Mutation of a nuclear succinate dehydrogenase gene results in mitochondrial respiratory chain deficiency. *Nature Genet.* 1995;11:144–149.

Bykhovskaya Y, Casas K, Mengesha E, et al. Missense mutation in pseudouridine synthase 1 (PUS1) causes mitochondrial myopathy and sideroblastic anemia (MLASA). *Am J Hum Genet.* 2004;74:1303–1308.

Calvo SE, Compton AG, Hershman SG, et al. Molecular diagnosis of infantile mitochondrial disease with targeted next-generation sequencing. *Sci Transl Med.* 2012;4:118ra110.

Calvo SE, Tucker EJ, Compton AG, et al. High-throughput, pooled sequencing identifies mutations in NUBPL and FOXRED1 in human complex I deficiency. *Nat Genet.* 2010;42:851–858.

Chen H, Chan DC. Mitochondrial dynamics—fusion, fission, movement, and mitophagy—in neurodegenerative diseases. *Hum Mol Genet.* 2009;18:R169–176.

Cuesta A, Pedrola L, Sevilla T, et al. The gene encoding ganglioside-induced differentiation-associated protein 1 is mutated in axonal Charcot-Marie-Tooth type 4A disease. *Nat Genet.* 2002;30:22–25.

Delettre C, Lenaers G, Griffoin JM, et al. Nuclear gene OPA1, encoding a mitochondrial dynamin-related protein, is mutated in dominant optic atrophy. *Nat Genet.* 2000;26:207–210.

DiMauro S, Tanji K, Schon EA. The many clinical faces of cytochrome c oxidase deficiency. *Adv Exp Med Biol.* 2012;748:341–357.

Elpeleg O, Miller C, Hershkovitz E, et al. Deficiency of the ADP-forming succinyl-CoA synthase activity is associated with encephalomyopathy and mitochondrial DNA depletion. *Am J Hum Genet.* 2005;76:1081–1086.

Fernandez-Vizarra E, Berardinelli A, Valente L, et al. Nonsense mutation in pseudouridylate synthase 1 (PUS1) in two brothers affected by myopathy, lactic acidosis and sideroblastic anaemia (MLASA). *J Med Genet.* 2007;44:173–180.

Garcia-Diaz B, Barros MH, Sanna-Cherchi S, et al. Infantile encephaloneuromyopathy and defective mitochondrial translation are due to a homozygous RMND1 mutation. *Am J Hum Genet.* 2012;91:729–736.

Gempel K, Topaloglu H, Talim B, et al. The myopathic form of coenzyme Q10 deficiency is caused by mutations in the electron-transferring-flavoprotein dehydrogenase (ETFDH) gene. *Brain.* 2007;130:2037–2044.

Gorman GS, Schaefer AM, Ng Y, et al. Prevalence of nuclear and mitochondrial DNA mutations related to adult mitochondrial disease. *Ann Neurol.* 2015;77:753–759.

Hakonen AH, Goffart S, Marjavaara S, et al. Infantile-onset spinocerebellar ataxia and mitochondrial recessive ataxia syndrome are associated with neuronal complex I defect and mtDNA depletion. *Hum Mol Genet.* 2008;17:3822–3835.

Heeringa SF, Chernin G, Chaki M, et al. COQ6 mutations in human patients produce nephrotic syndrome with sensorineural deafness. *J Clin Invest.* 2011;121:2013–2024.

Holt IJ, Harding AE, Petty RK, et al. A new mitochondrial disease associated with mitochondrial DNA heteroplasmy. *Am J Hum Genet.* 1990;46:428–433.

Horvath R, Kemp JP, Tuppen HA, et al. Molecular basis of infantile reversible cytochrome c oxidase deficiency myopathy. *Brain.* 2009;132:3165–3174.

Indrieri A, van Rahden VA, Tiranti V, et al. Mutations in COX7B cause microphthalmia with linear skin lesions, an unconventional mitochondrial disease. *Am J Hum Genet.* 2012;91:942–949.

Janer A, Antonicka H, Lalonde E, et al. An RMND1 mutation causes encephalopathy associated with multiple oxidative phosphorylation complex deficiencies and a mitochondrial translation defect. *Am J Hum Genet.* 2012;91:737–743.

Lagier-Tourenne C, Tazir M, Lopez LC, et al. ADCK3, an ancestral kinase, is mutated in a form of recessive ataxia associated with coenzyme Q10 deficiency. *Am J Hum Genet.* 2008;82:661–672.

López LC, Schuelke M, Quinzii C, et al. Leigh syndrome with nephropathy and CoQ10 deficiency due to *decaprenyl diphosphate synthase subunit 2 (PDSS2)* mutations. *Am J Hum Genet.* 2006;79:1125–1129.

Mandel H, Szargel R, Labay V, et al. The deoxyguanosine kinase gene is mutated in individuals with depleted hepatocerebral mitochondrial DNA. *Nat Genet.* 2001;29:337–341.

Massa V, Fernandez-Vizarra E, Alshahwan S, et al. Severe infantile encephalomyopathy caused by a mutation in COX6B1, a nucleus-encoded subunit of cytochrome c oxidase. *Am J Hum Genet.* 2008;82:1281–1288.

McShane MA, Hammans SR, Sweeney M, et al. Pearson syndrome and mitochondrial encephalopathy in a patient with a deletion of mtDNA. *Am J Hum Genet.* 1991;48:39–42.

Mimaki M, Hatakeyama H, Komaki H, et al. Reversible infantile respiratory chain deficiency: a clinical and molecular study. *Ann Neurol.* 2010;68:845–854.

Mitsuhashi S, Ohkuma A, Talim B, et al. A congenital muscular dystrophy with mitochondrial structural abnormalities caused by defective de novo phosphatidylcholine biosynthesis. *Am J Hum Genet.* 2011;88:845–851.

Mollet J, Giurgea I, Schlemmer D, et al. Prenyldiphosphate synthase, subunit 1 (PDSS1) and OH-benzoate polyprenyltransferase (COQ2) mutations in ubiquinone deficiency and oxidative phosphorylation disorders. *J Clin Invest.* 2007;117:765–772.

Mootha VK, Lepage P, Miller K, et al. Identification of a gene causing human cytochrome c oxidase deficiency by integrative genomics. *Proc Natl Acad Sci U S A.* 2003;100:605–610.

Naviaux RK, Nguyen KV. POLG mutations associated with Alpers' syndrome and mitochondrial DNA depletion. *Ann Neurol.* 2004;55:706–712.

Ogasahara S, Engel AG, Frens D, et al. Muscle coenzyme Q deficiency in familial mitochondrial encephalomyopathy. *Proc Nat Acad Sci U S A.* 1989;86:2379–2382.

Ostergaard E, Christensen E, Kristensen E, et al. Deficiency of the alpha subunit of succinate-coenzyme A ligase causes fatal infantile lactic acidosis with mitochondrial DNA depletion. *Am J Hum Genet.* 2007;81:383–387.

Ostergaard E, Schwartz M, Batbayli M, et al. A novel missense mutation in SUCLG1 associated with mitochondrial DNA depletion, encephalomyopathic form, with methylmalonic aciduria. *Eur J Pediatr.* 2010;169:201–205.

Payne BA, Wilson IJ, Yu-Wai-Man P, et al. Universal heteroplasmy of human mitochondrial DNA. *Hum Mol Genet.* 2013;22:384–390.

Quinzii C, Naini A, Salviati L, et al. A mutation in para-hydroxybenzoate-polyprenyl transferase (COQ2) causes primary coenzyme Q10 deficiency. *Am J Hum Genet.* 2006;78:345–349.

Scheper GC, van der Klok T, van Andel RJ, et al. Mitochondrial aspartyl-tRNA synthetase deficiency causes leukoencephalopathy with brain stem and spinal cord involvement and lactate elevation. *Nat Genet.* 2007;39:534–539.

Schlame M, Towbin JA, Heerdt PM, et al. Deficiency of tetralinoleoyl-cardiolipin in Barth syndrome. *Ann Neurol.* 2002;51:634–637.

Schon EA, Area-Gomez E. Mitochondria-associated ER membranes in Alzheimer disease. *Mol Cell Neurosci.* 2013;55:26–36.

Spelbrink JN, Li FY, Tiranti V, et al. Human mitochondrial DNA deletions associated with mutations in the gene encoding Twinkle, a phage T7 gene 4-like protein localized in mitochondria. *Nat Genet.* 2001;28:223–231.

Spinazzola A, Viscomi C, Fernandez-Vizarra E, et al. MPV17 encodes an inner mitochondrial membrane protein and is mutated in infantile hepatic mitochondrial DNA depletion. *Nat Genet.* 2006;38(5):570–575.

Steenweg ME, Ghezzi D, Haack T, et al. Leukoencephalopathy with thalamus and brainstem involvement and high lactate "LTBL" caused by EARS2 mutations. *Brain.* 2012;135:1387–1394.

Tatuch Y, Christodoulou J, Feigenbaum A, et al. Heteroplasmic mtDNA mutation (T->G) at 8993 can cause Leigh disease when the percentage of abnormal mtDNA is high. *Am J Hum Genet.* 1992;50:852–858.

Tiranti V, Hoertnagel K, Carrozzo R, et al. Mutations of SURF-1 in Leigh disease associated with cytochrome c oxidase deficiency. *Am J Hum Genet.* 1998;63:1609–1621.

Tiranti V, Viscomi C, Hildebrandt T, et al. Loss of ETHE1, a mitochondrial dioxygenase, causes fatal sulfide toxicity in ethylmalonic encephalopathy. *Nat Med.* 2009;15:200–205.

Visapaa I, Fellman V, Vesa J, et al. GRACILE syndrome, a lethal metabolic disorder with iron overload, is caused by a point mutation in BCS1L. *Am J Hum Genet.* 2002;71:863–876.

Waterham HR, Koster J, van Roermund CW, et al. A lethal defect of mitochondrial and peroxisomal fission. *N Engl J Med.* 2007;356:1736–1741.

Wortmann SB, Vaz FM, Gardeitchik T, et al. Mutations in the phospholipid remodeling gene SERAC1 impair mitochondrial function and intracellular cholesterol trafficking and cause dystonia and deafness. *Nat Genet.* 2012;44:797–802.

Zhu Z, Yao J, Johns T, et al. SURF1, encoding a factor involved in the biogenesis of cytochrome c oxidase, is mutated in Leigh syndrome. *Nat Genet.* 1998;20:337–343.

Zuchner S, Mersiyanova IV, Muglia M, et al. Mutations in the mitochondrial GTPase mitofusin 2 cause Charcot-Marie-Tooth neuropathy type 2A. *Nat Genet.* 2004;36:449–451.

Clinical Features

Amati-Bonneau P, Valentino ML, Reynier P, et al. OPA1 mutations induce mitochondrial DNA instability and optic atrophy "plus" phenotypes. *Brain.* 2008;131:338–351.

Andreu AL, Hanna MG, Reichmann H, et al. Exercise intolerance due to mutations in the cytochrome *b* gene of mitochondrial DNA. *New Engl J Med.* 1999;341:1037–1044.

Behin A, Jardel C, Claeys KG, et al. Adult cases of mitochondrial DNA depletion due to TK2 defect: an expanding spectrum. *Neurology.* 2012;78:644–648.

Carelli V, Barboni P, Sadun AA. Mitochondrial ophthalmology. In: DiMauro S, Hirano M, Schon EA, eds. *Mitochondrial Medicine.* Oxon, United Kingdom: Informa Healthcare; 2006:105–142.

Carrozzo R, Dionisi-Vici C, Steuerwald U, et al. SUCLA2 mutations are associated with mild methylmalonic aciduria, Leigh-like encephalomyopathy, dystonia and deafness. *Brain.* 2007;130:862–874.

Chinnery PF, DiMauro S, Shanske S, et al. Risk of developing a mitochondrial DNA deletion disorder. *Lancet.* 2004;364:592–596.

DiMauro S, Nicholson JF, Hays AP, et al. Benign infantile mitochondrial myopathy due to reversible cytochrome c oxidase deficiency. *Ann Neurol.* 1983;14:226–234.

Elliott HR, Samuels DC, Eden JA, et al. Pathogenic mitochondrial DNA mutations are common in the general population. *Am J Hum Genet.* 2008;83:254–260.

Emmanuele V, Lopez LC, Berardo A, et al. Heterogeneity of coenzyme Q10 deficiency: patient study and literature review. *Arch Neurol.* 2012;69:978–983.

Fratter C, Gorman GS, Stewart JD, et al. The clinical, histochemical, and molecular spectrum of PEO (Twinkle)-linked adPEO. *Neurology.* 2010;74:1619–1626.

Fratter C, Raman P, Alston CL, et al. RRM2B mutations are frequent in familial PEO with multiple mtDNA deletions. *Neurology.* 2011;76:2032–2034.

Garone C, Rubio JC, Calvo SE, et al. MPV17 mutations causing adult-onset multisystemic disorder with multiple mitochondrial DNA deletions. *Arch Neurol.* 2012;69:1648–1651.

Hirano M, Kaufmann P, De Vivo DC, et al. Mitochondrial neurology I: encephalopathies. In: DiMauro S, Hirano M, Schon EA, eds. *Mitochondrial Medicine.* London: Informa Healthcare; 2006:27–44.

Hudson G, Amati-Bonneau P, Blakely EL, et al. Mutation of OPA1 causes dominant optic atrophy with external ophthalmoplegia, ataxia, deafness and multiple mitochondrial DNA deletions: a novel disorder of mtDNA maintenance. *Brain.* 2008;131:329–337.

Hudson G, Schaefer AM, Taylor RW, et al. Mutation of the linker region of the polymerase gamma-1 (POLG1) gene associated with progressive external ophthalmoplegia and Parkinsonism. *Arch Neurol.* 2007;64:553–557.

Karadimas CL, Vu TH, Holve SA, et al. Navajo neurohepatopathy is caused by a mutation in the MPV17 gene. *Am J Hum Genet.* 2006;79:544–548.

Koene S, Rodenburg RJ, van der Knaap MS, et al. Natural disease course and genotype-phenotype correlations in complex I deficiency caused by nuclear gene defects: what we learned from 130 cases. *J Inherit Metab Dis.* 2012;35:737–747.

Luoma P, Melberg A, Rinne JO, et al. Parkinsonism, premature menopause, and mitochondrial DNA polymerase gamma mutations: clinical and molecular genetic study. *Lancet.* 2004;364:875–882.

Mancuso M, Orsucci D, Angelini C, et al. Phenotypic heterogeneity of the 8344A>G mtDNA "MERRF" mutation. *Neurology.* 2013;80:2049–2054.

Paradas C, Gutierrez Rios P, Rivas E, et al. TK2 mutation presenting as indolent myopathy. *Neurology.* 2013;80:504–506.

Ronchi D, Garone C, Bordoni A, et al. Next-generation sequencing reveals DGUOK mutations in adult patients with mitochondrial DNA multiple deletions. *Brain.* 2012;135:3404–3415.

Rotig A, Appelkvist EL, Geromel V, et al. Quinone-responsive multiple respiratory-chain dysfunction due to widespread coenzyme Q10 deficiency. *Lancet.* 2000;356:391–395.

Saneto RP, Naviaux RK. Polymerase gamma disease through the ages. *Dev Disabil Res Rev.* 2010;16:163–174.

Sengers RC, Trijbels JM, Willems JL, et al. Congenital cataract and mitochondrial myopathy of skeletal and heart muscle associated with lactic acidosis after exercise. *J Pediatr.* 1975;86:873–880.

Tyynismaa H, Sun R, Ahola-Erkkila S, et al. Thymidine kinase 2 mutations in autosomal recessive progressive external ophthalmoplegia with multiple mitochondrial DNA deletions. *Hum Mol Genet.* 2012;21:66–75.

Tyynismaa H, Ylikallio E, Patel M, et al. A heterozygous truncating mutation in RRM2B causes autosomal-dominant progressive external ophthalmoplegia with multiple mtDNA deletions. *Am J Hum Genet.* 2009;85:290–295.

Yu-Wai-Man P, Chinnery PF. Dysfunctional mitochondrial maintenance: what breaks the circle of life? *Brain.* 2012;135:9–11.

Yu-Wai-Man P, Griffiths PG, Gorman GS, et al. Multi-system neurological disease is common in patients with OPA1 mutations. *Brain.* 2010;133:771–786.

Pathology

Hays AP, Oskoui M, Tanji K, et al. Mitochondrial neurology II: myopathies and peripheral neuropathies. In: DiMauro S, Hirano M, Schon EA, eds. *Mitochondrial Medicine.* Oxon, United Kingdom: Informa Healthcare; 2006:27–44.

Tanji K, Kunimatsu T, Vu TH, et al. Neuropathological features of mitochondrial disorders. *Semin Cell Dev Biol.* 2001;12:429–439.

Therapy

Cerutti R, Pirinen E, Lamperti C, et al. NAD(+)-dependent activation of Sirt1 corrects the phenotype in a mouse model of mitochondrial disease. *Cell Metab.* 2014;19:1042–1049.

Craven L, Elson JL, Irving L, et al. Mitochondrial DNA disease: new options for prevention. *Hum Mol Genet.* 2011;20:R168–R174.

Craven L, Tuppen HA, Greggains GD, et al. Pronuclear transfer in human embryos to prevent transmission of mitochondrial DNA disease. *Nature.* 2010;465:82–85.

Enns GM, Kinsman SL, Perlman SL, et al. Initial experience in the treatment of inherited mitochondrial disease with EPI-743. *Mol Genet Metab.* 2012;105:91–102.

Gilkerson RW, De Vries RL, Lebot P, et al. Mitochondrial autophagy in cells with mtDNA mutations results from synergistic loss of transmembrane potential and mTORC1 inhibition. *Hum Mol Genet.* 2012;21:978–990.

Hirano M, Garone C, Quinzii CM. CoQ(10) deficiencies and MNGIE: two treatable mitochondrial disorders. *Biochim Biophys Acta.* 2012;1820:625–631.

Kaufmann P, Engelstad K, Wei Y, et al. Dichloroacetate causes toxic neuropathy in MELAS: a randomized, controlled clinical trial. *Neurology.* 2006;66:324–330.

Klopstock T, Yu-Wai-Man P, Dimitriadis K, et al. A randomized placebo-controlled trial of idebenone in Leber's hereditary optic neuropathy. *Brain.* 2011;134:2677–2686.

Martinelli D, Catteruccia M, Piemonte F, et al. EPI-743 reverses the progression of the pediatric mitochondrial disease—genetically defined Leigh syndrome. *Mol Genet Metab.* 2012;107:383–388.

Paull D, Emmanuele V, Weiss KA, et al. Nuclear genome transfer in human oocytes eliminates mitochondrial DNA variants. *Nature.* 2013;493:632–637.

Sadun AA, Chicani CF, Ross-Cisneros FN, et al. Effect of EPI-743 on the clinical course of the mitochondrial disease Leber hereditary optic neuropathy. *Arch Neurol.* 2012;69:331–338.

Tachibana M, Amato P, Sparman M, et al. Towards germline gene therapy of inherited mitochondrial diseases. *Nature.* 2013;493:627–631.

Tachibana M, Sparman M, Sritanaudomchai H, et al. Mitochondrial gene replacement in primate offspring and embryonic stem cells. *Nature.* 2009;461:367–372.

Taivassalo T, Haller RG. Exercise and training in mitochondrial myopathies. *Med Sci Sports Exerc.* 2005;37:2094–2101.

Tanaka M, Borgeld HJ, Zhang J, et al. Gene therapy for mitochondrial disease by delivering restriction endonuclease SmaI into mitochondria. *J Biomed Sci.* 2002;9:534–541.

Viscomi C, Bottani E, Civiletto G, et al. In vivo correction of COX deficiency by activation of the AMPK/PGC1α axis. *Cell Metab.* 2011;14:80–90.

Wenz T, Diaz F, Spiegelman BM, et al. Activation of the PPAR/PGC-1alpha pathway prevents a bioenergetic deficit and effectively improves a mitochondrial myopathy phenotype. *Cell Metab.* 2008;8:249–256.

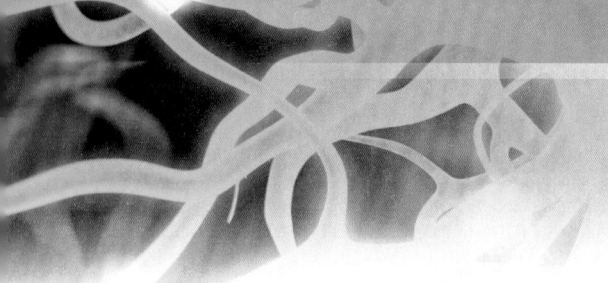
INTRODUCTION

Several genetic diseases involve both the skin and nervous system. These are called *neurocutaneous disorders* or *neuroectodermatoses*. In the past, they were referred to as the *phakomatoses* (*phakos* is the Greek word for lentil, flat plate, or spot).

Any part of the central nervous system (CNS) or peripheral nervous system can be affected by these hereditary diseases; their expressivity is quite variable both between and within kindreds.

NEUROFIBROMATOSIS

INTRODUCTION

Although neurofibromatosis (NF) was first described at least as early as the 17th century and a comprehensive clinical review was published in 1849, the clinical and pathologic phenotypes were first linked by von Recklinghausen in 1882. NF is one of the most common single-gene disorders of the CNS. Cardinal features include multiple cutaneous hyperpigmented marks (*café au lait spots*); multiple neurofibromas; and lesions in bone, CNS, peripheral nervous system, or other organs. The best characterized forms are neurofibromatosis type 1 (NF-1; *von Recklinghausen disease* or *peripheral NF* [MIM 162200]), neurofibromatosis type 2 (NF-2; *central NF* or the *bilateral acoustic neuroma syndrome* [MIM 101000]) and schwannomatosis, a phenotype characterized by the presence of multiple schwannomas, associated with intractable pain, without vestibular involvement. The three conditions differ in genetics, pathogenesis, and clinically.

EPIDEMIOLOGY

Both sexes are affected equally, and the condition is found worldwide in all racial and ethnic groups. Incidence figures must be a minimal estimate, because mild cases are often unrecognized.

MOLECULAR GENETICS AND PATHOBIOLOGY

NF-1, NF-2, and schwannomatosis are autosomal dominant conditions; penetrance of NF-1 is almost 100%, but expressivity varies. Mutations account for 50% of new cases. The *NF-1* gene has been mapped to chromosome 17q11.2. The gene product is called *neurofibromin*, a tumor suppressor gene that acts through the RAS/MAPK pathway. Translocations, large megabase deletions, large internal deletions, small rearrangements, and point mutations all occur in the *NF-1* gene. Although the genotypes differ, the phenotypes are indistinguishable. The marked clinical variability within families having an identical *NF-1* gene mutation equals the variability among families with different *NF-1* gene mutations. The exception occurs with large megabase deletions associated with cognitive dysfunction and more severe clinical manifestations generally. Mutation inactivates the gene, and, by analogy with other oncogenes, loss of the allelic gene later in life could result in tumor formation. It is not known how the other manifestations of the

disease arise. Several potential genetic modifiers in associated signalling pathways have been identified in screening studies.

The *NF-2* gene maps to chromosome 22q12. The gene product is similar to that of the moezin-ezrin-radixin-like protein gene; for this reason, it is called *merlin*. Deletions of the gene have been found in schwannoma and meningioma cells, the major tumors in NF-2 patients. NF-2 inhibits the Rac/CDC42-dependent Ser/Thr kinase PAK1, which activates both Ras transformation and NF-1 through two separate domains. Specific inhibitors of PAK1 selectively inhibit the growth of NF-2–deficient cancer cells, suggesting that PAK1 is essential for the malignant growth of NF-2–deficient cells. Inhibitors of PAK1 might have a future role as therapies for these tumors.

Schwannomatosis has been linked to mutations in three genes: SMARCB1, LZTR1, and COQ6. The SMARCB1 gene product is a subunit of the SWI/hSHNF chromatin remodeling complex. Mutations in this gene account for about half of familial schwannomatosis but only about 10% of sporadic cases. LZTR1 encodes a protein that acts as a tumor suppressor; COQ6 mutations impair the synthesis of coenzyme Q10.

NEUROPATHOLOGY

Dysplasia, hyperplasia, and neoplasia of neural-supporting tissues involves the central, peripheral, and autonomic nervous systems. Visceral manifestations result from hyperplasia of the autonomic ganglia and nerves within the organ. Dysplastic and neoplastic changes also affect skin, bone, endocrine glands, and blood vessels. Developmental anomalies include thoracic meningocele and syringomyelia. Patients affected by NF-1 are more likely than others to have neoplastic disorders, including neuroblastoma, Wilms tumor, leukemia, pheochromocytoma, and sarcomas.

Neoplasms involving the peripheral nervous system and spinal nerve roots include schwannomas and neurofibromas. Intramedullary spinal cord tumors include ependymomas (especially of the conus medullaris and filum terminale) and astrocytomas (although some of these may actually be ependymomas when electron microscopy is used); gangliomas are rare. The most common intracranial tumors are hemispheric astrocytomas of any histologic grade from benign to highly malignant; posterior fossa tumors are rare. Pilocytic astrocytic gliomas of the optic nerve and optic chiasm are also characteristic and generally progress very slowly. Bilateral acoustic neuromas and solitary or multicentric meningiomas occur in adults with NF-2.

CLINICAL MANIFESTATIONS

There are at least four forms of NF. *Peripheral NF* (NF-1) as described by von Recklinghausen is most common. *Central NF* (NF-2) is manifested by bilateral acoustic neuromas with mild cutaneous changes. *Segmental NF* arises from mosaic-type microdeletions in NF-1; it is characterized by café au lait spots and neurofibromas that are limited, usually affecting an upper body segment. The lesions extend to the midline and include the ipsilateral arm but spare the head and neck. *Cutaneous NF* is limited to pigmentary changes; there are numerous café au lait spots but no other clinical manifestations. One percent to 4% of patients with a mild NF phenotype (café au lait spots only) have a related disorder, Legius syndrome, which is associated with mutations in the SPRED1 gene.

NF-1–Noonan syndrome has the clinical manifestations of NF-1 coupled with a Noonan syndrome phenotype. The clinical features of the Noonan syndrome include ocular hypertelorism, downward-slanting palpebral fissures, webbed neck, low-set ears, and pulmonic stenosis.

NF-1 has protean and progressive manifestations. Families and physicians often anticipate a fate like that of Joseph Merrick (the Elephant Man, who almost certainly had the Proteus syndrome, not NF-1). In reality, many patients with the disease are functionally indistinguishable from normal. Often, they have only cutaneous lesions and are not diagnosed until they see a physician because of a learning disability, scoliosis, or another problem.

Cutaneous Manifestations

The café au lait macule is the pathognomonic lesion, being present in almost all patients (Figs. 140.1 and 140.2). Six or more café au lait spots larger than 5 mm in diameter before puberty and greater than 15 mm in diameter after puberty are diagnostic. The spots are usually present at birth but may not appear until age 1 or 2 years. Increasing in both size and number during the first decade of life, the macules tend to be less evident after the second decade because they blend into the surrounding hyperpigmented skin. These discrete, tan macules involve the trunk and limbs in a random fashion but tend to spare the face.

Other cutaneous manifestations may include freckles over the entire body, but freckles usually involve the axilla and other intertriginous areas. Larger, darker hyperpigmented lesions are often associated with an underlying plexiform neurofibroma; if this involves the midline, it may indicate the presence of a spinal cord tumor.

Ocular Findings

Pigmented iris hamartomas (Lisch nodules) (Fig. 140.3) are pathognomonic and consist of small translucent yellow or brown elevations on slit lamp examination. The nodules increase in number with age and are present in almost all patients older than 20 years.

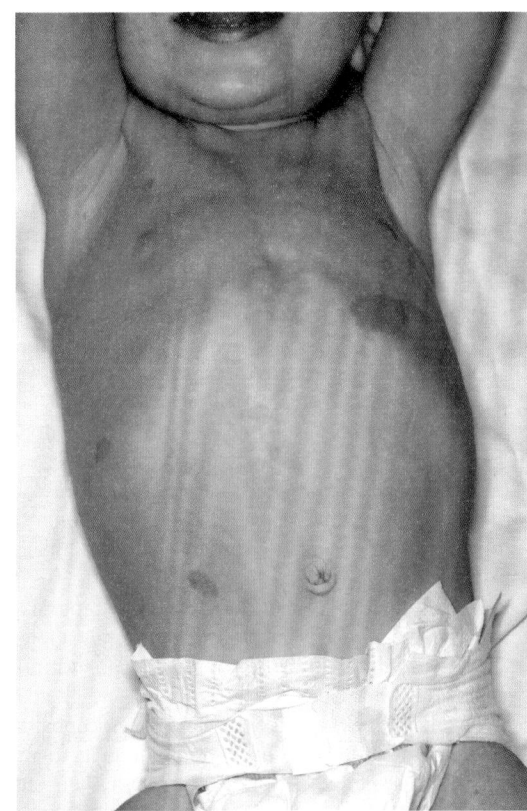

FIGURE 140.2 Cafe-au-lait patches on the abdomen. (Courtesy of Marc C. Patterson, MD.)

Neurologic Symptoms

Neurofibromas are highly characteristic lesions and usually become clinically evident at age 10 to 15 years. They always involve the skin, ultimately developing into sessile, pedunculated lesions. The nodules are found on deep peripheral nerves or nerve roots and on the autonomic nerves that innervate the viscera and blood vessels. The lesions increase in size and number during the second and third decades. There may be a few or many thousands. These benign tumors consist of neurons, Schwann cells, fibroblasts, blood vessels, and mast cells. They rarely give rise to any symptoms other

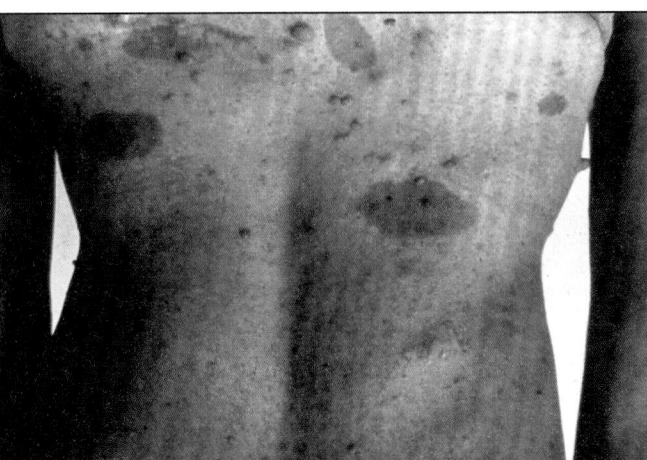

FIGURE 140.1 Café au lait patches and neurofibromas on the back. (Courtesy of Suresh Kotagal, MD.)

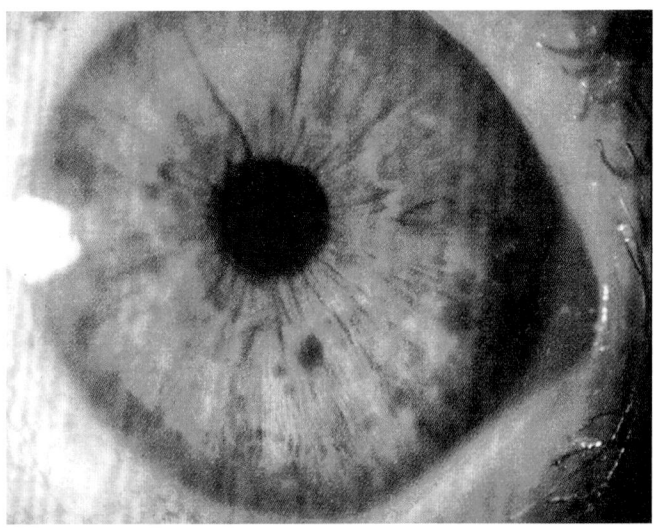

FIGURE 140.3 Lisch nodules.

than pain as a result of pressure on nerves or nerve roots; however, they may undergo sarcomatous degeneration in the third and fourth decades of life. Neurofibromas involving the terminal distribution of peripheral nerves form vascular plexiform neurofibromas that result in localized overgrowth of tissues or segmental hypertrophy of a limb. Spinal root or cauda equina neurofibromas are often asymptomatic when they are small, but large tumors may cause myelopathy. The number and size of neurofibromas may increase during pregnancy.

Optic gliomas, astrocytomas, acoustic neuromas, neurilemmomas, and meningiomas have a combined frequency of 5% to 10% in all patients with NF. Optic nerve gliomas and other intracranial neoplasms are often evident before age 10 years; acoustic neuromas become symptomatic at about age 20 years. When optic glioma is associated with NF, it commonly involves the optic nerve or is multicentric; less frequently, it involves the chiasm. Optic nerve glioma must be distinguished from the commonly observed nonneoplastic optic nerve hyperplasia. The optic glioma of NF is slowly progressive and has a better prognosis than similar tumors without this association.

NF-2 is clinically evident at about age 20 years; symptoms include hearing loss, tinnitus, imbalance, and headache. Only a few café au lait spots and neurofibromas are seen. Intracranial and intraspinal neoplasms include meningiomas, schwannomas, and gliomas.

CNS involvement in NF is highly variable. Macrocephaly, a common clinical manifestation of postnatal origin, is an incidental finding not related to academic performance, seizures, or neurologic function. Specific learning disabilities or attention deficit disorder, with or without impaired speech, are the most common neurologic complications of NF. Intellectual disability or convulsive disorders each occur in about 5% of the patients. Brain stem tumors associated with NF-1 have a more indolent course than those without NF.

Occlusive cerebrovascular disease is rare but is sometimes seen in children, resulting in acute hemiplegia and convulsions. Magnetic resonance angiography (MRA) or conventional angiography may demonstrate tapering occlusion of the supraclinoid portion of the internal carotid artery at the origin of the anterior and middle cerebral arteries with associated collaterals in the adjacent basal ganglia (moyamoya disease).

A more severe form of NF-1, often clinically apparent in young children, is due to a contiguous gene deletion on chromosome 17q11 that includes neurofibromin. In addition to the clinical features of NF-1, there are dysmorphic features, major malformations, and intellectual disability.

Skeletal and Limb Manifestations

Skeletal anomalies characteristic of NF include (1) unilateral defects in the posterosuperior wall of the orbit, with pulsating exophthalmos, usually associated with dural ectasia; (2) a defect in the lambdoid with underdevelopment of the ipsilateral mastoid; (3) dural ectasia with enlargement of the spinal canal and scalloping of the posterior portions of the vertebral bodies (also seen in connective tissue disorders such as Marfan and Ehlers–Danlos syndromes); (4) scoliosis, affecting between 21% and 49% of patients with NF-1; (5) pseudarthrosis, especially involving the tibia (5% of cases) and radius; (6) "twisted ribbon" rib deformities; and (7) enlargement of long bones.

Miscellaneous Features

Pheochromocytomas occur in 0.1% to 5.7% of patients with NF-1; they are rare in children. Hypertension may be due to a pheochromocytoma (20% to 50% of cases) or a neurofibroma of

a renal artery. Malignant tumors occurring less frequently in NF include sarcoma, leukemia, Wilms tumor, ganglioglioma, and neuroblastoma. Medullary thyroid carcinoma and hyperparathyroidism are rare. Precocious puberty and, less commonly, sexual infantilism result from involvement of the hypothalamus by glioma or hamartoma. Cystic lesions, malignancy, and interstitial pneumonia are pulmonary complications.

DIAGNOSIS

Diagnosis of NF-1 or NF-2 is based on clinical, radiologic, and pathologic findings, as well as the family history. Diagnostic criteria were established by a National Institutes of Health consensus conference (Table 140.1). Some investigators have suggested updating the criteria to account for new knowledge regarding "anaemic nevi, unidentified bright objects, choroidal hamartomas, and a typical neuropsychological phenotype" in NF-1.

Laboratory Data

Diagnosis is usually made by clinical presentation and family history. Molecular genetic studies are available, but many subjects who meet consensus diagnostic criteria do not have detectable mutations in the NF-1 gene. Most affected individual have de novo mutations.

All patients and those at risk should receive a tailored evaluation to confirm the diagnosis and assess the extent of disease. A comprehensive evaluation may include psychoeducational and psychometric testing; electroencephalogram (EEG); ophthalmologic and audiologic testing; cranial computed tomography (CT), including orbital views; CT of the spine and internal auditory foramina; magnetic resonance imaging (MRI) of brain and spine; and quantitative measurement of 24-hour urinary catecholamines.

TABLE 140.1	Diagnostic Criteria for Neurofibromatosis

Neurofibromatosis 1 (Any Two or More)
Six or more café au lait macules
Before puberty >5-mm diameter
After puberty >15-mm diameter
Freckling in the axillary or inguinal areas
Two or more neurofibromas or one plexiform neurofibroma
A first-degree relative with NF-1
Two or more Lisch nodules (iris hamartomas)
Bone lesion
Sphenoid dysplasia
Thinning of the cortex of long bones with or without pseudarthrosis
Neurofibromatosis 2
Bilateral eighth nerve tumor (MRI, CT, or histologic confirmation)
A first-degree relative with NF-2 and a unilateral eighth nerve tumor
A first-degree relative with NF-2 and any two of the following: neurofibroma, meningioma, schwannoma, glioma, or juvenile posterior subcapsular lenticular opacity

NF-1, neurofibromatosis type 1; MRI, magnetic resonance imaging; CT, computed tomography; NF-2, neurofibromatosis type 2.

TREATMENT

There is no specific treatment for NF, but its manifestations may be ameliorated with early recognition and prompt therapeutic intervention. Learning disabilities should be considered in all children with NF-1 and may be complicated by comorbid conditions (such as attention deficit hyperactivity disorder) that warrant educational therapy or behavioral modification, psychotherapy, and pharmacotherapy. Speech problems require a language evaluation and formal speech therapy, and seizures should be managed with appropriate antiepileptic drugs. Progressive kyphoscoliosis usually requires surgical intervention. Surgery may be necessary for removal of pheochromocytomas and intracranial or spinal neoplasms; cutaneous neurofibromas require extirpation when they compromise function or are disfiguring. Preliminary data suggest that thalidomide might have a role in treating neurofibromas. Radiation therapy is reserved for some CNS neoplasms, including optic glioma. Genetic counseling by a qualified geneticist or genetic counselor is essential, and psychotherapy with family counseling is often indicated.

TUBEROUS SCLEROSIS COMPLEX

INTRODUCTION

Tuberous sclerosis complex (TSC) was first described by von Recklinghausen in 1863. In 1880, Bourneville coined the term *sclérose tubéreuse* for the potato-like lesions in the brain. In 1890, Pringle described the facial nevi or *adenoma sebaceum*. Vogt later emphasized the classic triad of seizures, intellectual disability, and adenoma sebaceum. TSC (MIM 191400) is a progressive genetic disorder characterized by the development in early life of hamartomas, malformations, and congenital tumors of the CNS, skin, and viscera.

EPIDEMIOLOGY

Incidence figures are considered minimal because milder varieties are often unrecognized. Clinical surveys suggest a prevalence between 1 in 10,000 and 1 in 170,000. Pulmonary lymphangioleiomyomatosis, progressive and often fatal, occurs almost exclusively in young women.

GENETICS

Tuberous sclerosis is an autosomal dominant trait, with a high incidence of sporadic cases and protean clinical expression. This variability is attributed to modifier genes. The defective genes map to chromosome 9q34 (TSC1) and chromosome 16p13.3 (TSC2). TSC1 or TSC2 is mutated in 75% to 85% of TSC patients; no mutation is found in 15%. *Hamartin* is the gene product for TSC1, and *tuberin* is the gene product for TSC2. Hamartin and tuberin form heterodimers that inhibit the mammalian target of rapamycin (mTOR); phosphorylation is an important aspect of this complex process, which involves over 50 interacting proteins.

PATHOLOGY AND PATHOBIOLOGY

The pathologic changes are widespread and include lesions in the nervous system, skin, bones, retina, kidney, lungs, and other viscera. Multiple small nodules often line the ventricles.

TSC is characterized by the presence of hamartias and hamartomas. Hamartias (from the Greek for "flaw") are malformations in which cells native to a tissue display abnormal architecture and morphology. These lesions do not grow disproportionately for the tissue or organ in which they are found. Hamartomas have the same characteristics but grow excessively for their site of origin. This old concept is valuable in recognizing the proliferative potential of lesions found in TSC. Thus, cortical tubers are hamartias and do not grow excessively, whereas angiomyolipomas are hamartomas that grow disproportionately and may produce symptoms as a consequence.

The brain is usually normal in size, but variable numbers of hard nodules occur on the surface of the cortex. These nodules are smooth, round, or polygonal and project slightly above the surface of the neighboring cortex. They are white, firm to the touch, and of various sizes. Some involve only a small portion of one convolution; others encompass the convolutions of one whole lobe or a major portion of a hemisphere. In addition, there may be developmental anomalies of the cortical convolutions in the form of pachygyria or microgyria. On sectioning of the hemispheres, sclerotic nodules may be found in the subcortical gray matter, the white matter, and the basal ganglia. The lining of the lateral ventricles is frequently the site of numerous small nodules that project into the ventricular cavity. Sclerotic nodules are less frequently found in the cerebellum. The brain stem and spinal cord are rarely involved.

Histologically, the nodules are characterized by a cluster of atypical glial cells in the center and giant cells in the periphery. Calcifications are relatively frequent. Other features include heterotopia, vascular hyperplasia (sometimes with actual angiomatous malformations), disturbances in the cortical architecture, and, occasionally, development of subependymal giant cell astrocytomas (SEGAs). Intracranial giant aneurysm and arterial ectasia are uncommon findings.

The skin lesions are multiform and include the characteristic facial angiofibromas and fibrous plaques, typically localized to the frontal area. The facial lesions are not adenomas of the sebaceous glands but small hamartomas arising from nerve elements of the skin combined with hyperplasia of connective tissue and blood vessels (angiofibromas) (Fig. 140.4). In late childhood, lesions similar to those on the face are found around or underneath the nails (*periungual* or *subungual fibromas*). Circumscribed areas of

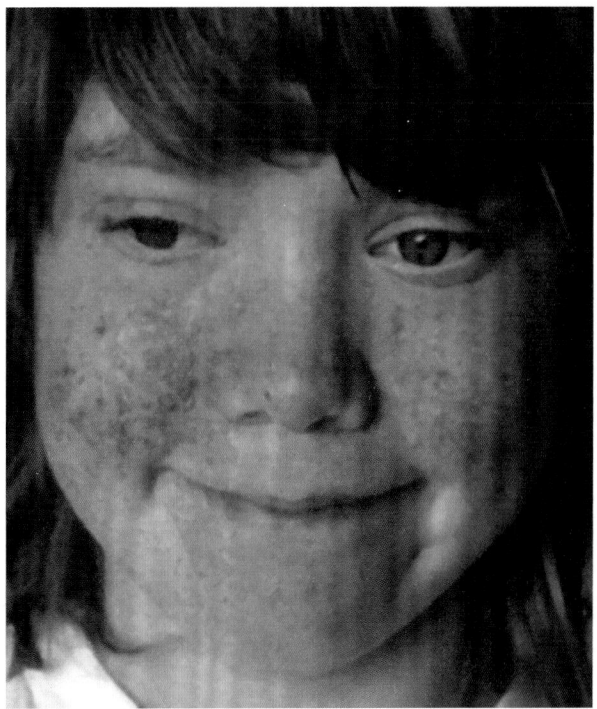

FIGURE 140.4 Facial angiofibromas.

hypomelanosis or depigmented nevi are common in tuberous sclerosis and are often found in infants. Although these depigmented nevi are less specific than the angiofibromas, they are important signals of the diagnosis in infants with seizures. Histologically, the skin appears normal except for the loss of melanin, but ultrastructural studies show that melanosomes are small and have reduced content of melanin. The retinal lesions are small congenital tumors composed of glia, ganglion cells, or fibroblasts. Glioma of the optic nerve has been reported.

Other lesions include cardiac rhabdomyoma; renal angiomyolipoma, renal cysts, and, rarely, renal carcinoma; cystic disease of the lungs and pulmonary lymphangioleiomyomatosis; hepatic angiomas and hamartomas; skeletal abnormalities with localized areas of osteosclerosis in the calvarium, spine, pelvis, and limbs; cystic defects involving the phalanges; and periosteal new bone formation confined to the metacarpals and metatarsals.

CLINICAL MANIFESTATIONS

The cardinal features of tuberous sclerosis are skin lesions, convulsive seizures, and intellectual disability. The disease is characterized by variable expressivity of the clinical manifestations and is often age related: the symptomatic neonate with cardiac rhabdomyoma and heart failure; the infant with hypomelanotic macules and infantile spasms; preschool and school-age children with angiofibromas, developmental delay, learning disability or intellectual disability, and seizures; and adults with dermatologic lesions, subungual fibromas, seizures, and often intellectual disability.

Cutaneous Findings

Depigmented or hypomelanotic macules are the earliest skin lesion (Fig. 140.5). They are present at birth, persist through life, and may be found only with a Wood lamp examination. The diagnosis is suggested if there are three or more macules measuring 1 cm or more in length. Numerous small macules sometimes resemble confetti or depigmented freckles. Most macules are leaf shaped, resembling the leaf of the European mountain ash tree and sometimes following a dermatomal distribution. Facial angiofibromas never present at birth but are clinically evident in more than 90% of affected children by age 4 years. At first, the facial lesion is the size of a pinhead and red because of the angiomatous component. It is distributed symmetrically on the nose and cheeks in a butterfly distribution. The lesions may involve the forehead and chin but rarely involve the upper lip. They gradually increase in size and

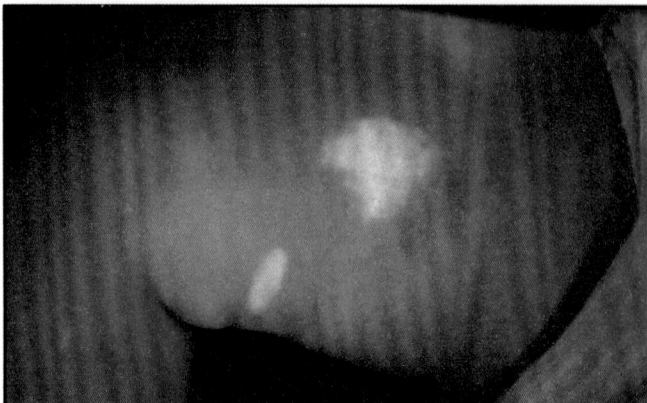

FIGURE 140.5 Hypomelanotic or ash leaf macules under UV light. (Courtesy of Suresh Kotagal, MD.)

become yellowish and glistening. *Shagreen patches*, connective tissue hamartomas, are also characteristic. Rarely present in infancy, the patches become evident after age 10 years. Usually found in the lumbosacral region, shagreen patches are yellowish-brown elevated plaques that have the texture of pigskin (from which the name originated in French). Other skin lesions include café au lait spots, small fibromas that may be tiny and resemble coarse gooseflesh, and ungual fibromas that appear after puberty.

Neurologic Findings

Infantile spasms are the characteristic seizures in young infants and, when associated with hypopigmented macules, are diagnostic of tuberous sclerosis. The older child or adult has generalized tonic–clonic or focal seizures. There is a close relationship between the onset of seizures at a young age and intellectual disability. Intellectual disability rarely occurs without clinical seizures, but intellect may be normal despite seizures. Other than delayed acquisition of developmental milestones, intellectual impairment, or nonspecific language or coordinative deficiencies, the formal neurologic examination is typically nonfocal. TSC is a major cause of autism.

Ophthalmic Findings

Hamartomas of the retina or optic nerve are observed in about 50% of patients. Two types of retinal lesions are seen on funduscopy: first, the easily recognized calcified hamartoma near or at the disc with an elevated multinodular lesion that resembles mulberries, grains of tapioca, or salmon eggs and second, the less distinct, relatively flat, smooth-surfaced, white or salmon-colored, circular or oval lesion located peripherally in the retina. Nonretinal lesions may range from the specific depigmented lesion of the iris to nonspecific, nonparalytic strabismus; optic atrophy; visual field defects; or cataracts.

Visceral and Skeletal Findings

Renal lesions include hamartomas (angiomyolipomas) and hamartias (renal cysts). Typically, both are multiple, bilateral, and usually innocuous and silent. Renal angiomyolipomas grow and occasionally bleed, but most can simply be followed with annual CT scans. Renal cell carcinoma is a rare complication in the older child or adult. In one series, 50% of patients with cardiac rhabdomyoma had tuberous sclerosis. Often asymptomatic, this cardiac tumor may be symptomatic at any age and in infancy can (rarely) result in death.

Pulmonary hamartomas consisting of multifocal alveolar hyperplasia associated with cystic lymphangioleiomyomatosis occur in fewer than 1% of patients. These become symptomatic (often with a spontaneous pneumothorax) in women in the third or fourth decade and are progressive and often lethal. Hamartomatous hemangiomas of the spleen and racemose angiomas of the liver are rare and usually asymptomatic. Sclerotic lesions of the calvarium and cystic lesions of the metacarpals and phalanges are asymptomatic. Enamel pitting of the deciduous teeth and gingival fibromas may aid in diagnosis.

DIAGNOSIS

Clinical diagnosis is possible at most ages. In infancy, three or more characteristic depigmented cutaneous lesions suggest the diagnosis, and this is reinforced by the presence of infantile myoclonic spasms. In the older child or adults, the diagnosis is made by the triad of tuberous sclerosis: facial adenoma sebaceum, epilepsy, and intellectual disability. Retinal or visceral lesions may be diagnostic. The disease, however, is noted for its protean manifestations, and the family history may be invaluable in establishing the diagnosis, which is often reinforced by CT or MRI lesions. Antenatal diagnosis of TSC by fetal ultrasound and MRI is suggested by the presence of a cardiac rhabdomyoma and cortical tubers. Prenatal molecular diagnosis is available for both TSC1 and TSC2.

The differential diagnosis includes other neurocutaneous syndromes that are differentiated by their characteristic skin lesions. Multisystem involvement may complicate the diagnosis of tuberous sclerosis. The Tuberous Sclerosis Complex Consensus Conference has published updated diagnostic criteria (Table 140.2).

Laboratory Data

MRI of the brain is the cornerstone of diagnosis of TSC. Cortical tubers may be hypo- or isointense on T1-weighted images and show varying patterns of hyperintensity on T2 and fluid-attenuated inversion recovery (FLAIR) sequences; calcification may occur over time. Subependymal nodules are common and most calcify over time; radial bands of hyperintense signal from the ventricles to the cortex are characteristic of TSC. SEGAs arise from the caudothalamic groove and may obstruct the ipsilateral foramen of Monro; these tumors most often present in the second decade. Positron emission tomography (PET) often reveals hypometabolic regions that are not obviously abnormal on MRI, indicating a more extensive disturbance of cerebral function.

Visceral lesions are best assessed with imaging studies. Cardiac rhabdomyomas, easily visualized on echocardiography, are frequent in neonates and typically regress over time, whereas renal angiomyolipomas may gradually enlarge and produce symptoms by obstructing the collecting system or bleeding. They are best monitored with ultrasound or CT. Pulmonary lymphangioleiomyomatosis may be detected on routine chest x-rays, but chest CT is more sensitive.

The EEG is often abnormal, especially in patients with clinical seizures. Abnormalities include slow-wave activity and epileptiform discharges such as hypsarrhythmia, focal or multifocal spike or sharp-wave discharges, and generalized spike-and-wave discharges.

Routine laboratory tests of blood and urine are usually normal, except if there is renal dysfunction, including bleeding from angiolipomas.

TREATMENT

Everolimus, a derivative of rapamycin, has been approved for the treatment of SEGAs that are not suitable for surgery. The drug is also being used for off-label indications including topical application for angiofibromas and for adjunctive treatment of intractable epilepsy. The efficacy of the agent for these purposes has not yet been established in clinical trials. Everolimus has a number of adverse effects related to its immunosuppressive actions and so should be administered with careful monitoring. The cutaneous lesions do not compromise function, but cosmetic surgery may be indicated for facial adenoma sebaceum or large shagreen patches. Infantile spasms respond to corticosteroid or corticotropin therapy; currently, vigabatrin is the drug of choice. Focal and generalized seizures are treated with antiepileptic drugs. Patients with focal seizures and minimal developmental delay may experience long-term seizure control following surgical resection of epileptogenic tubers. Progressive cystic renal disease often responds to surgical decompression, but with renal failure, dialysis or renal transplantation may be necessary. Cardiac rhabdomyomas are rarely symptomatic but may be managed medically with standard therapy for arrhythmias or cardiac failure. Surgery is rarely required. Progressive pulmonary involvement is an indication for respiratory therapy, but response is poor and most patients die a few years after the onset of this complication without lung transplantation.

TABLE 140.2	Diagnostic Criteria for Tuberous Sclerosis Complex

A. Genetic Diagnostic Criteria

The identification of either a TSC1 or TSC2 pathogenic mutation in DNA from normal tissue is sufficient to make a definite diagnosis of tuberous sclerosis complex (TSC). A pathogenic mutation is defined as a mutation that clearly inactivates the function of the TSC1 or TSC2 proteins (e.g., out-of-frame indel or nonsense mutation), prevents protein synthesis (e.g., large genomic deletion), or is a missense mutation whose effect on protein function has been established by functional assessment (www.chromium.liacs.nl/LOVD2/TSC/home.php?select_db=TSC1; www.chromium.liacs.nl/LOVD2/TSC/home.php?select_db=TSC2). Other TSC1 or TSC2 variants whose effect on function is less certain do not meet these criteria and are not sufficient to make a definite diagnosis of TSC. Note that 10%–25% of TSC patients have no mutation identified by conventional genetic testing, and a normal result does not exclude TSC or have any effect on the use of clinical diagnostic criteria to diagnose TSC.

B. Clinical Diagnostic Criteria

Major features

1. Hypomelanotic macules (three or more, at least 5-mm diameter)
2. Angiofibromas (three or more) or fibrous cephalic plaque
3. Ungual fibromas (two or more)
4. Shagreen patch
5. Multiple retinal hamartomas
6. Cortical dysplasias[a]
7. Subependymal nodules
8. Subependymal giant cell astrocytoma
9. Cardiac rhabdomyoma
10. Lymphangioleiomyomatosis (LAM)[b]
11. Angiomyolipomas (two or more)[b]

Minor features

1. "Confetti" skin lesions
2. Dental enamel pits (more than three)
3. Intraoral fibromas
4. Retinal achromic patch
5. Multiple renal cysts
6. Nonrenal hamartomas

Definite diagnosis: two major features or one major feature with two or more minor features

Possible diagnosis: either one major feature or two or more minor features

[a]Includes tubers and cerebral white matter radial migration lines.

[b]A combination of the two major clinical features (LAM and angiomyolipomas) without other features does not meet criteria for a definite diagnosis.

OUTCOME

Mild or solely cutaneous involvement often follows a static course, whereas patients with the full-blown syndrome have a progressive course with increasing seizures and cognitive impairment. The child with infantile spasms that are not promptly controlled is at great risk of intellectual disability. Brain tumor, status epilepticus, renal insufficiency, cardiac failure, or progressive pulmonary impairment can lead to death.

ENCEPHALOTRIGEMINAL ANGIOMATOSIS

INTRODUCTION

Encephalotrigeminal angiomatosis (*Sturge–Weber–Dimitri syndrome*; MIM 185300) is manifested by a cutaneous vascular port-wine nevus of the face, contralateral hemiparesis and hemiatrophy, glaucoma, seizures, and intellectual disability. The condition is attributed to partial persistence of a primitive embryonic vascular plexus that develops around the cephalic portion of the neural tube 6 weeks after conception and under the ectoderm in the region destined to become facial skin. In encephalotrigeminal angiomatosis, the vascular plexus persists beyond the ninth week, when it normally regresses. Variability in this process accounts for unilateral or bilateral involvement and also for an incomplete syndrome characterized by leptomeningeal angiomatosis without facial involvement.

EPIDEMIOLOGY

The syndrome occurs in 1:20,000 to 1:50,000 live births.

GENETICS

Almost all patients with encephalotrigeminal angiomatosis, and with nonsyndromic port-wine stains, carry somatic mosaic activating mutations in the GNAQ gene. Mutations in this gene lead to abnormal signaling between G-protein–coupled receptors and downstream effectors. Similar mechanisms have been described in the Proteus and McCune-Albright syndromes.

NEUROPATHOLOGY

The occipital lobe is most often affected, but lesions may involve the temporal and parietal lobes or the entire cerebral hemisphere. Atrophy is characteristically unilateral and ipsilateral to the facial nevus. Leptomeningeal angiomatosis with small venules fills the subarachnoid space. Calcification of the arteries on the surface of the brain and intracerebral calcifications of small vessels are seen. Recent studies have associated focal cortical dysplasia with medically intractable epilepsy in encephalotrigeminal angiomatosis, with important implications for early surgical intervention.

CLNICAL MANIFESTATIONS

Facial nevus and a neurologic syndrome of seizures, hemiplegia, intellectual disability, and glaucoma are characteristic. Typically, other than the facial nevus, the child has normal function for months or years. The subsequent clinical course is highly variable.

Cutaneous Manifestations

The port-wine facial stain, or nevus flammeus, involves variable portions of the face and neck (Fig. 140.6). Most commonly involving the forehead, the nevus may involve one-half of the face and may extend to the neck. The nevus may cross or fall short of the midline. Bilateral facial lesions are seen in about 15% of cases. Recent studies have suggested that the distribution of the nevus flammeus conforms more closely to the embryonic circulation than the divisions of the trigeminal nerve; a nevus involving any part of the forehead is the best clinical indicator of adverse outcome, including glaucoma, seizures, and abnormal development.

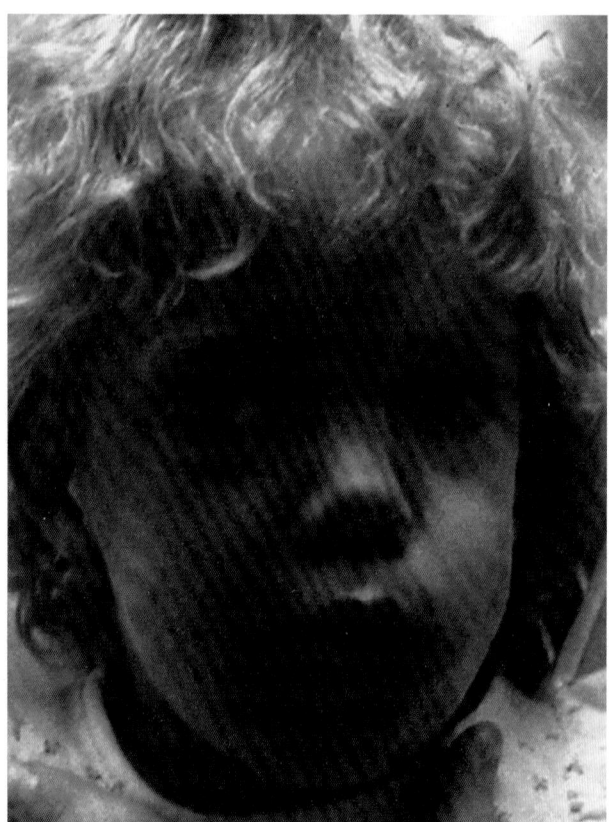

FIGURE 140.6 Facial nevus flammeus. (Courtesy of Suresh Kotagal, MD.)

Neurologic Manifestations

Epilepsy is the most common neurologic manifestation, usually starting in the first year of life with focal or generalized motor or focal dyscognitive seizures. Often refractory to anticonvulsants, the focal motor seizures, hemiparesis, and hemiatrophy are contralateral to the facial nevus. Onset of seizures before age 2 years and refractory epilepsy has prognostic significance; these patients are more likely to be intellectually impaired. Intellectual disability often becomes more marked over time.

Ophthalmologic Manifestations

Raised intraocular pressure with glaucoma and buphthalmos occurs in approximately 30% of patients. Buphthalmos, congenital enlargement of the eye, is more common than glaucoma and results from antenatal intraocular hypertension. Homonymous hemianopia, a common visual field complication, is invariable when the occipital lobe is affected. Other congenital anomalies include coloboma of the iris and deformity of the lens.

DIAGNOSIS

The diagnosis is based on the facial vascular port-wine nevus flammeus and one or more of the following: seizures, contralateral hemiparesis and hemiatrophy, intellectual disability, and ocular findings of glaucoma or buphthalmos. Meningeal involvement is usually obvious on MRI. Rarely, Sturge–Weber–Dimitri syndrome may occur with the neurologic syndrome and the typical meningeal involvement, absent the facial nevus. Encephalotrigeminal angiomatosis must be distinguished from other vascular malformation syndromes, including Klippel–Trenaunay and Parkes Weber syndromes, both of which feature combined vascular malformations, in contrast to the pure capillary lesions of encephalotrigeminal angiomatosis. The identification of GNAQ mutations provides a means of molecular confirmation in biopsies of affected tissue.

Laboratory Data

MRI with contrast-enhanced FLAIR sequences is the most sensitive noninvasive technique to identify leptomeningeal involvement and cortical atrophy. ^{18}F-fluorodeoxyglucose positron emission tomography (FDG-PET) may be helpful in predicting seizure control and cognitive outcome. In a study of 13 children, patients with mild asymmetry of glucose uptake had worse cognitive function than those with marked asymmetry, suggesting that functional reorganization of the cortex is more effective in the latter situation. The capillaries over the affected hemisphere are homogeneously increased, the superficial cortical veins are markedly decreased, and the superior sagittal sinus may be diminished or not seen.

EEG shows low amplitude over the affected areas, and this electrical suppression correlates with the degree of intracranial calcification. The remainder of the hemisphere may show epileptiform activity. The EEG evolves over time, with increasing epileptiform activity, but these electrical changes do not correlate with clinical or seizure severity.

TREATMENT

The facial nevus rarely requires early cosmetic therapy. Later, this blemish can be covered with cosmetics or permanently treated with laser therapy. Seizures may be difficult to control with anticonvulsants. Children with medically intractable seizures often respond to hemispherectomy, even when surgery is delayed. Physical and occupational therapies are indicated for the hemiparesis. Educational therapy and placement in a special school are important for learning-disabled or intellectually impaired patients; vocational training is essential in affected older children and young adults. Behavioral problems are common and include mood disorder, disruptive behavior disorder, and adjustment disorder in children and substance-related disorder in adults. Prophylactic daily low-dose aspirin to prevent venous thrombosis is controversial but can be considered if there are recurrent transient ischemic attacks (TIAs). Yearly monitoring for glaucoma is recommended for all patients and, if present, should be treated aggressively.

INCONTINENTIA PIGMENTI

INTRODUCTION

Incontinentia pigmenti (IP; MIM 308300), described by Bloch and Sulzberger, is a genetic disorder affecting the skin in a characteristic manner and also involving the brain, eyes, nails, and hair.

GENETICS

IP is an X-linked dominant condition that is lethal in males. Mutations in the *NEMO/IKKγ* gene at Xq28 cause the disease. *NEMO/IKKγ* is an essential component of the newly discovered nuclear factor kappa B (NF-κB) signaling pathway. When activated, NF-κB controls the expression of multiple genes, including cytokines and chemokines, and protects cells against apoptosis. *NEMO/IKKγ* deficiency causes the phenotypic expression of the disease via the NF-κB pathway.

Sporadic disease has also appeared in girls with no family history of the disease. In these cases, there is a translocation with a breakpoint at Xp11.21. Some patients and some families do not map to either site, implying *locus heterogeneity*, with still more gene loci to be discovered.

Incontinentia pigmenti achromians (IPA or hypomelanosis of Ito; MIM 146150) resembles IP in that the pigmentary changes respect the lines of Blaschko, but it is otherwise an unrelated syndrome. Blaschko lines are not ordinarily visible, but several cutaneous disorders follow parallel linear streaks. A pregnant woman with IP runs a 25% risk of a spontaneous miscarriage (the affected son); 50% of her infant daughters will be affected and will have the disease. Daughters are likely to be more severely affected than their mothers.

NEUROPATHOLOGY

The neuropathologic findings are nonspecific and include cerebral atrophy with microgyria, focal necrosis with formation of small cavities in the central white matter, and focal areas of neuronal loss in the cerebellar cortex.

CLNICAL MANIFESTATIONS

One-half of affected infants have the initial linear vesicobullous lesions at birth, and most of the remaining children show the lesions in the first 2 weeks of life. About 10% are delayed, appearing as late as age 1 year. The skin lesions can recur and ultimately may undergo a characteristic change to linear verrucous and dyskeratotic growth, usually between the second and sixth weeks of life; pigmentary changes appear between 12 and 26 weeks. Some infants may show the pigmentary lesions at birth without further cutaneous progression. The pigmentation involves the trunk and limbs, is slate gray-blue or brown, and is distributed in irregular marbled or wavy lines (Fig. 140.7). With age, the pigmentary lesions fade and become depigmented with atrophic skin changes.

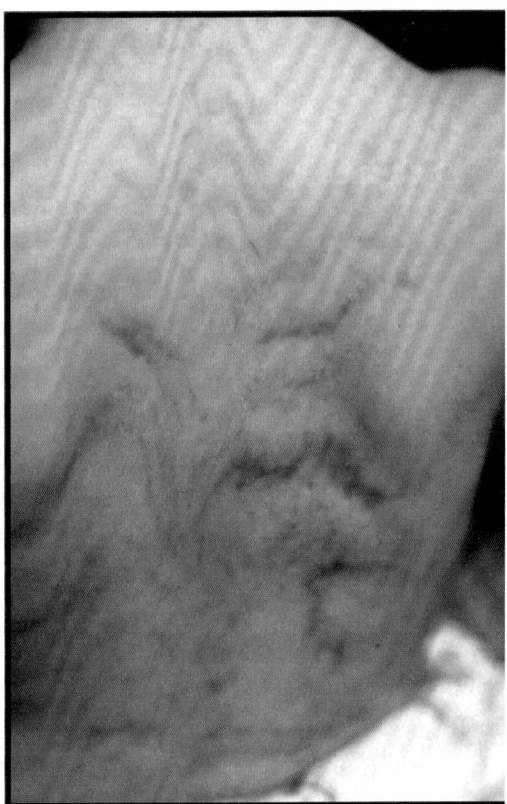

FIGURE 140.7 Incontinentia pigmenti. (Courtesy of Suresh Kotagal, MD.)

Neurologic, Ophthalmic, and Other Symptoms

About 20% of affected children have a neurologic syndrome that may include slow motor development; pyramidal tract dysfunction with spastic hemiparesis, quadriparesis, or diplegia; intellectual disability; and convulsive disorders.

Strabismus, cataracts, and severe visual loss occur in about 20% of affected children. Retinal vascular changes may result in blindness with ectasia, microhemorrhages, avascularity, and later, retinal pigmentation and atrophy.

Partial or total anodontia and peg-shaped teeth are characteristic of IP. Partial or complete diffuse alopecia with scarring and nail dystrophy may also occur.

LABORATORY DATA

Eosinophilia as high as 65% is often seen in infants younger than 1 year, together with an associated leukocytosis. Eosinophils are also found in the vesicobullous lesions and in affected dermis.

TREATMENT

There is no specific treatment for IP, and management is directed at complicating problems, such as anticonvulsants for seizures. Awareness of the ocular manifestations is essential because laser coagulation in retinal ectasia prevents blindness.

INCONTINENTIA PIGMENTI ACHROMIANS (HYPOMELANOSIS OF ITO)

INTRODUCTION

IPA is a syndrome of regions of cutaneous hypopigmentation that conform to the lines of Blaschko, first described by the German dermatologist in 1901, which define the cutaneous distribution of many hereditary dermatoses and acquired inflammatory disorders. The pattern is believed to result from functional autosomal mosaicism transmittable through the action of retrotransposons. IPA is associated with variable involvement of other body systems, particularly the nervous system.

EPIDEMIOLOGY AND GENETICS

IPA is found in all races and sexes and is a syndrome with multiple etiologies. Mutations in the inhibitor of kappa light polypeptide gene enhancer in B-cells gamma kinase (IKBKG), which is also called *NEMO*, gene are the most common single cause of IP in infant girls and anhydrotic ectodermal dysplasia with immunodeficiency (EDA-ID) in infant boys.

Most cases of IPA with an identifiable cause are associated with somatic mosaicism for chromosomal trisomies. Families with IPA have been reported linked to Xp11, but most cases are sporadic.

PATHOBIOLOGY

The pathogenesis of this disease is similar to that of other neurocutaneous disorders. Migration of neural cells to the brain and melanoblasts to the skin from the neural crest occurs between 3 and 6 months' gestational age. A disturbance of this migration results in both brain and cutaneous pigmentary disease.

The hypopigmented skin lesions are characterized by a decrease in the number of dopa-positive melanocytes and decreased pigment production in the basal layer of the epidermis.

CLINICAL MANIFESTATIONS

In infancy, hypopigmented skin lesions appear as whorls or streaks that follow the lines of Blaschko. This lesion is the negative image of IP. In later childhood, affected areas tend to return to normal skin color. The cutaneous lesion is often associated with developmental and neurologic abnormalities with hypotonia, pyramidal tract dysfunction, intellectual disability (approximately 80%), and seizures. Ophthalmologic disorders, including strabismus, optic atrophy, microphthalmia, tessellated fundus (a normal fundus with a pigmented choroid that creates the appearance of dark polygonal areas between choroidal blood vessels), eyelid ptosis, and heterochromia iridis, are also present. Hair, teeth, and the musculoskeletal system may also be affected.

DIAGNOSIS AND LABORATORY DATA

Because there is no pathognomonic laboratory test, diagnosis is clinical. Investigation for chromosomal mosaicism, with karyotyping of blood, fibroblasts, and hair bulbs, should be considered in all cases.

TREATMENT

The whorled, marble-cake hypopigmented skin lesions do not require any treatment. Therapy is directed toward the associated complications, such as anticonvulsants for seizures and specialized educational facilities for the learning-disabled or retarded child.

SUGGESTED READINGS

Neurofibromatosis

Abramowicz A, Gos M. Neurofibromin in neurofibromatosis type 1—mutations in NF1gene as a cause of disease. *Dev Period Med.* 2014;18:297–306.

Arrington DK, Danehy AR, Peleggi A, et al. Calvarial defects and skeletal dysplasia in patients with neurofibromatosis type 1. *J Neurosurg Pediatr.* 2013;11:410–416.

Delucia TA, Yohay K, Widmann RF. Orthopaedic aspects of neurofibromatosis: update. *Curr Opin Pediatr.* 2011;23:46–52.

Duong TA, Bastuji-Garin S, Valeyrie-Allanore L, et al. Evolving pattern with age of cutaneous signs in neurofibromatosis type 1: a cross-sectional study of 728 patients. *Dermatology.* 2011;222:269–273.

Ekvall S, Sjors K, Jonzon A, et al. Novel association of neurofibromatosis type 1-causing mutations in families with neurofibromatosis-Noonan syndrome. *Am J Med Genet A.* 2014;164A:579–587.

Friedman JM. Neurofibromatosis 1: clinical manifestations and diagnostic criteria. *J Child Neurol.* 2002;17:548–554; discussion 571–572, 646–651.

Gupta A, Cohen BH, Ruggieri P, et al. Phase I study of thalidomide for the treatment of plexiform neurofibroma in neurofibromatosis 1. *Neurology.* 2003;60:130–132.

Hagel C, Stemmer-Rachamimov AO, Bornemann A, et al. Clinical presentation, immunohistochemistry and electron microscopy indicate neurofibromatosis type 2-associated gliomas to be spinal ependymomas. *Neuropathology.* 2012;32:611–616.

Hilton DA, Hanemann CO. Schwannomas and their pathogenesis. *Brain pathology.* 2014;24:205–220.

Hulsebos TJ, Plomp AS, Wolterman RA, et al. Germline mutation of INI1/SMARCB1 in familial schwannomatosis. *Am J Hum Genet.* 2007;80:805–810.

Jett K, Friedman JM. Clinical and genetic aspects of neurofibromatosis 1. *Genet Med.* 2010;12:1–11.

Licciulli S, Maksimoska J, Zhou C, et al. FRAX597, a small molecule inhibitor of the p21-activated kinases, inhibits tumorigenesis of neurofibromatosis type 2 (NF2)-associated schwannomas. *J Biol Chem.* 2013;288:29105–29114.

MacCollin M, Chiocca EA, Evans DG, et al. Diagnostic criteria for schwannomatosis. *Neurology.* 2005;64:1838–1845.

Messiaen L, Vogt J, Bengesser K, et al. Mosaic type-1 NF1 microdeletions as a cause of both generalized and segmental neurofibromatosis type-1 (NF1). *Hum Mutat.* 2011;32:213–219.

Neurofibromatosis. *Natl Inst Health Consens Dev Conf Consens Statement.* 1987;6(12):1–7.

Nguyen R, Dombi E, Akshintala S, et al. Characterization of spinal findings in children and adults with neurofibromatosis type 1 enrolled in a natural history study using magnetic resonance imaging. *J Neurooncol.* 2015;121(1):209–215.

Orraca M, Morejon G, Cabrera N, et al. Neurofibromatosis 1 prevalence in children aged 9-11 years, Pinar del Rio Province, Cuba. *MEDICC Rev.* 2014;16:22–26.

Piotrowski A, Xie J, Liu YF, et al. Germline loss-of-function mutations in LZTR1 predispose to an inherited disorder of multiple schwannomas. *Nat Genet.* 2014;46:182–187.

Plotkin SR, Merker VL, Muzikansky A, et al. Natural history of vestibular schwannoma growth and hearing decline in newly diagnosed neurofibromatosis type 2 patients. *Otol Neurotol.* 2014;35:e50–e56.

Rodriguez FJ, Perry A, Gutmann DH, et al. Gliomas in neurofibromatosis type 1: a clinicopathologic study of 100 patients. *J Neuropathol Exp Neurol.* 2008;67:240–249.

Sabbagh A, Pasmant E, Laurendeau I, et al. Unravelling the genetic basis of variable clinical expression in neurofibromatosis 1. *Hum Mol Genet.* 2009;18:2768–2778.

Schroeder RD, Angelo LS, Kurzrock R. NF2/merlin in hereditary neurofibromatosis 2 versus cancer: biologic mechanisms and clinical associations. *Oncotarget.* 2014;5:67–77.

Smith MJ, Higgs JE, Bowers NL, et al. Cranial meningiomas in 411 neurofibromatosis type 2 (NF2) patients with proven gene mutations: clear positional effect of mutations, but absence of female severity effect on age at onset. *J Med Genet.* 2011;48:261–265.

Smith MJ, Wallace AJ, Bowers NL, et al. SMARCB1 mutations in schwannomatosis and genotype correlations with rhabdoid tumors. *Cancer Genet.* 2014;207(9):373–378.

Stowe IB, Mercado EL, Stowe TR, et al. A shared molecular mechanism underlies the human rasopathies Legius syndrome and neurofibromatosis-1. *Genes Dev.* 2012;26:1421–1426.

Tadini G, Milani D, Menni F, et al. Is it time to change the neurofibromatosis 1 diagnostic criteria? *Eur J Intern Med.* 2014;25:506–510.

Zhang K, Lin JW, Wang J, et al. A germline missense mutation in COQ6 is associated with susceptibility to familial schwannomatosis. *Genet Med.* 2014;16:787–792.

Tuberous Sclerosis Complex

Arya R, Tenney JR, Horn PS, et al. Long-term outcomes of resective epilepsy surgery after invasive presurgical evaluation in children with tuberous sclerosis complex and bilateral multiple lesions. *J Neurosurg Pediatr.* 2014;15(1):1–8.

Fallah A, Guyatt GH, Snead OC III, et al. Predictors of seizure outcomes in children with tuberous sclerosis complex and intractable epilepsy undergoing resective epilepsy surgery: an individual participant data meta-analysis. *PloS One.* 2013;8:e53565.

Gallagher A, Tanaka N, Suzuki N, et al. Diffuse cerebral language representation in tuberous sclerosis complex. *Epilepsy Res.* 2013;104:125–133.

Julich K, Sahin M. Mechanism-based treatment in tuberous sclerosis complex. *Pediatr Neurol.* 2014;50:290–296.

Miller JW. Treating epilepsy in tuberous sclerosis with everolimus: getting closer. *Epilepsy Curr.* 2014;14:143–144.

Roth J, Roach ES, Bartels U, et al. Subependymal giant cell astrocytoma: diagnosis, screening, and treatment. Recommendations from the International Tuberous Sclerosis Complex Consensus Conference 2012. *Pediatr Neurol.* 2013;49:439–444.

Thiele EA, Granata T, Matricardi S, et al. Transition into adulthood: tuberous sclerosis complex, Sturge-Weber syndrome, and Rasmussen encephalitis. *Epilepsia.* 2014;55(suppl 3):29–33.

Tillema JM, Leach JL, Krueger DA, et al. Everolimus alters white matter diffusion in tuberous sclerosis complex. *Neurology.* 2012;78:526–531.

van Eeghen AM, Ortiz-Teran L, Johnson J, et al. The neuroanatomical phenotype of tuberous sclerosis complex: focus on radial migration lines. *Neuroradiology.* 2013;55:1007–1014.

Wang S, Fallah A. Optimal management of seizures associated with tuberous sclerosis complex: current and emerging options. *Neuropsychiatr Dis Treat.* 2014;10:2021–2030.

Wiegand G, May TW, Ostertag P, et al. Everolimus in tuberous sclerosis patients with intractable epilepsy: a treatment option? *Eur J Paediatr Neurol.* 2013;17:631–638.

Wu WE, Kirov II, Tal A, et al. Brain MR spectroscopic abnormalities in "MRI-negative" tuberous sclerosis complex patients. *Epilepsy Behav.* 2013;27:319–325.

Zhang BL, Wang LJ, Sun L, et al. Identifying significant crosstalk of pathways in tuberous sclerosis complex. *Eur Rev Med Pharmacol Sci.* 2014;18:2482–2490.

Encephalotrigeminal Angiomatosis

Alkonyi B, Chugani HT, Karia S, et al. Clinical outcomes in bilateral Sturge-Weber syndrome. *Pediatr Neurol.* 2011;44:443–449.

Arulrajah S, Ertan G, M Comi A, et al. MRI with diffusion-weighted imaging in children and young adults with simultaneous supra- and infratentorial manifestations of Sturge-Weber syndrome. *J Neuroradiol.* 2010;37:51–59.

Behen ME, Juhasz C, Wolfe-Christensen C, et al. Brain damage and IQ in unilateral Sturge-Weber syndrome: support for a "fresh start" hypothesis. *Epilepsy Behav.* 2011;22:352–357.

Comi AM. Presentation, diagnosis, pathophysiology, and treatment of the neurological features of Sturge-Weber syndrome. *Neurologist.* 2011;17:179–184.

Comi AM, Marchuk DA, Pevsner J. A needle in a haystack: Sturge-Weber syndrome gene discovery. *Pediatr Neurol.* 2013;49:391–392.

Kossoff EH, Bachur CD, Quain AM, et al. EEG evolution in Sturge-Weber syndrome. *Epilepsy Res.* 2014;108:816–819.

Lance EI, Sreenivasan AK, Zabel TA, et al. Aspirin use in Sturge-Weber syndrome: side effects and clinical outcomes. *J Child Neurol.* 2013;28:213–218.

Lo W, Marchuk DA, Ball KL, et al. Updates and future horizons on the understanding, diagnosis, and treatment of Sturge-Weber syndrome brain involvement. *Dev Med Child Neurol.* 2012;54:214–223.

Maton B, Krsek P, Jayakar P, et al. Medically intractable epilepsy in Sturge-Weber syndrome is associated with cortical malformation: implications for surgical therapy. *Epilepsia.* 2010;51:257–267.

Nakashima M, Miyajima M, Sugano H, et al. The somatic GNAQ mutation c.548G>A (p.R183Q) is consistently found in Sturge-Weber syndrome. *J Hum Genet.* 2014;59(1):691–693.

Parsa CF. Focal venous hypertension as a pathophysiologic mechanism for tissue hypertrophy, port-wine stains, the Sturge-Weber syndrome, and related disorders: proof of concept with novel hypothesis for underlying etiological cause (an American Ophthalmological Society thesis). *Trans Am Opthalmol Soc.* 2013;111:180–215.

Shirley MD, Tang H, Gallione CJ, et al. Sturge-Weber syndrome and port-wine stains caused by somatic mutation in GNAQ. *N Eng J Med.* 2013;368:1971–1979.

Sudarsanam A, Ardern-Holmes SL. Sturge-Weber syndrome: from the past to the present. *Eur J Paedtr Neurol.* 2014;18:257–266.

Turin E, Grados MA, Tierney E, et al. Behavioral and psychiatric features of Sturge-Weber syndrome. *J Nerv Ment Dis.* 2010;198:905–913.

Waelchli R, Aylett SE, Robinson K, et al. New vascular classification of port-wine stains: improving prediction of Sturge-Weber risk. *Br J Dermatol.* 2014;171:861–867.

Wang DD, Blumcke I, Coras R, et al. Sturge-Weber syndrome is associated with cortical dysplasia ilae type IIIc and excessive hypertrophic pyramidal neurons in brain resections for intractable epilepsy [published online ahead of print July 18, 2014]. *Brain Pathol.*

Incontinentia Pigmenti

Conte MI, Pescatore A, Paciolla M, et al. Insight into IKBKG/NEMO locus: report of new mutations and complex genomic rearrangements leading to incontinentia pigmenti disease. *Hum Mutat.* 2014;35:165–177.

Fusco F, Paciolla M, Conte MI, et al. Incontinentia pigmenti: report on data from 2000 to 2013. *Orphanet J Rare Dis.* 2014;9:93.

Hadj-Rabia S, Rimella A, Smahi A, et al. Clinical and histologic features of incontinentia pigmenti in adults with nuclear factor-kappaB essential modulator gene mutations. *J Am Acad Dermatol.* 2011;64:508–515.

Meuwissen ME, Mancini GM. Neurological findings in incontinentia pigmenti; a review. *Eur J Med Genet.* 2012;55:323–331.

Minić S, Trpinac D, Obradović M. Incontinentia pigmenti diagnostic criteria update. *Clin Genet.* 2014;85:536–542.

Minić S, Trpinac D, Obradović M. Systematic review of central nervous system anomalies in incontinentia pigmenti. *Orphanet J Rare Dis.* 2013;8:25.

Pizzamiglio MR, Piccardi L, Bianchini F, et al. Incontinentia pigmenti: learning disabilities are a fundamental hallmark of the disease. *PloS One.* 2014;9:e87771.

Incontinentia Pigmenti Achromians

Assogba K, Ferlazzo E, Striano P, et al. Heterogeneous seizure manifestations in hypomelanosis of Ito: report of four new cases and review of the literature. *Neurol Sci.* 2010;31:9–16.

Bodemer C. Incontinentia pigmenti and hypomelanosis of Ito. *Handb Clin Neurol.* 2013;111:341–347.

Devillers C, Quatresooz P, Hermanns-Le T, et al. Hypomelanosis of Ito: pigmentary mosaicism with immature melanosome in keratinocytes. *Int Dermatol.* 2011;50:1234–1239.

Khaku AS, Hedna VS, Nayak A. Teaching neuroimages: hypomelanosis of Ito. *Neurology.* 2013;80:e130.

Manjila S, Miller BR, Goodman A, et al. Pharmacoresistant epilepsy in hypomelanosis of Ito: palliative surgical treatment with modified anatomic posterior quadrantic resection. *Clin Neurol Neurosurg.* 2014;123: 15–17.

Oiso N, Kawada A. Pigmentary mosaicism of the hypopigmented type (hypomelanosis of Ito): hypopigmented lesions with serrated and irregular borders. *Eur J Dermatol.* 2014;24(6):690–691.

Taibjee SM, Bennett DC, Moss C. Abnormal pigmentation in hypomelanosis of Ito and pigmentary mosaicism: the role of pigmentary genes. *Br J Dermatol.* 2004;151:269–282.

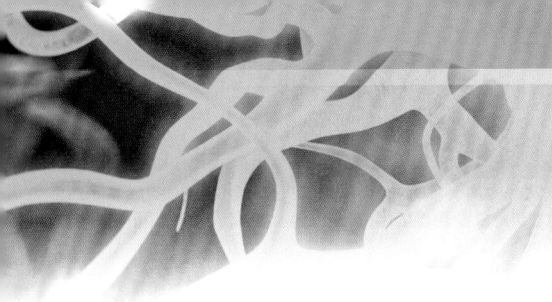

Petra Kaufmann and Darryl C. De Vivo

SPINAL MUSCULAR ATROPHY RELATED TO CHROMOSOME 5 MUTATIONS

GENETIC ETIOLOGY

Spinal muscular atrophy is a motor neuron disease that manifests with muscle atrophy and weakness. Although there are several genetic etiologies, more than 95% of spinal muscular atrophy (SMA) patients carry a homozygous deletion in the *survival motor neurons* (SMN) gene on chromosome 5q11–q13. Based on age at onset and severity of symptoms, three SMA types have historically been described; all are autosomal recessive. The three SMA types are allelic and clinically on a continuous spectrum with SMA1 being the most severe, and SMA3 the milder phenotype. The SMN gene has two almost identical forms on chromosome 5, one telomeric (SMN1) and one centromeric (SMN2). The phenotypic severity of SMA is associated with the SMN2 copy number. SMN1 gene mutation is embryonic lethal in the absence of SMN2 gene. A quantitative study of SMN2 copy number in 375 patients with SMA types 1, 2, and 3 showed that 80% of SMA1 patients had one or two SMN2 copies, 82% of SMA2 patients had three SMN2 copies, and 96% of SMA3 patients had three or four SMN2 copies. In theory, SMA carriers have approximately 50% SMN protein. A mouse model for SMA was made by knocking out the SMN1 gene and introducing the human SMN2 transgene. The murine SMA phenotype is mitigated by increasing the SMN2 copy number, confirming the observation in humans. These findings have become the basis for attempted treatment to increase SMN2 expression in children with SMA.

Direct deletion analysis has high sensitivity and specificity and can be used for diagnosis without muscle biopsy in suspected cases; it is also effective in antenatal diagnosis in an at-risk fetus.

Point mutations are found in the few who lack a deletion. The SMN protein is depleted in the spinal cords of patients. How absence of SMN leads to the disease, however, still has to be elucidated.

CLINICAL MANIFESTATIONS

Infantile SMA type I (*Werdnig–Hoffmann syndrome*; MIM 253300) is evident at birth or soon thereafter, always before age 6 months (Table 14.1). Mothers may notice that intrauterine movements are decreased. In the neonatal period, nursing problems may occur and limb movements are feeble and decreased; this is one of the most common causes of the *floppy infant syndrome* (see also Chapter 136). Proximal muscles are affected before distal muscles, but ultimately, flaccid quadriplegia results. The tongue is often seen to fasciculate, but twitching is seen only rarely in limb muscles, presumably because of the ample subcutaneous fat. Sooner or later, respiration is compromised and paradoxical movements of the chest wall are seen. Tendon reflexes are absent. Without ventilatory and nutritional support, most infants die before age 2 years. The others may survive but never sit; their condition may remain stable for many years.

SMA type II (MIM 253550) patients have clinical onset from 6 months to 1 year and learn to sit but never walk. Respiratory insufficiency and scoliosis are dreaded complications. With proactive pulmonary and rehabilitation management, most patients can lead productive lives and have a normal life expectancy.

Kugelberg–Welander syndrome or SMA type III (MIM 253400) patients learn to walk but have varying degrees of weakness. Symptoms begin with a slowly progressive gait disorder in late childhood or adolescence. The onset is followed by proximal arm weakness and wasting; tendon reflexes are lost. Fasciculations of

---

TABLE 141.1   Spectrum of Phenotypic Severity in Spinal Muscular Atrophy

	SMA 1	SMA 2	SMA 3
Type	Infantile	Intermediate	Mild
Eponym	Werdnig–Hoffmann disease	Dubowitz disease	Kugelberg–Welander disease
Age at onset	0–6 mo	6–18 mo	older than 18 mo
Highest motor milestone achieved	Never able to maintain a sitting position	Sitting	Walking
Life expectancy	Without respiratory and nutritional support typically younger than 2 yr	Normal or slightly reduced	Normal
Typical number of SMN2 copies	2	3	3–4
Notes			Onset may be in adulthood, when it is sometimes referred to as *SMA type 4*.

SMA, spinal muscular atrophy; SMN, centromeric survival motor neurons.

limb muscles, as well as of the tongue, and a tremor of the outstretched limb may be visible. This condition is relatively benign and associated with a normal life span. Others may be handicapped with scoliosis, but serious dysphagia or respiratory compromise is rare. Sensation is spared, and no other organ systems are affected.

DIAGNOSIS

Diagnosis now depends on DNA analysis. Muscle biopsy and electromyography (EMG) are not necessary if a deletion or mutation of SMN is found.

When performed, electrodiagnostic studies show evidence of denervation with normal nerve conductions. Muscle biopsy similarly shows a neurogenic picture. The CSF shows no characteristic changes. Serum levels of sarcoplasmic enzymes, such as creatine kinase, may be increased; in the Kugelberg–Welander type, the increase may be 20 times normal in the range of many myopathies.

TREATMENT

There are promising leads for specific therapy, and clinical trials are underway. Classical gene therapy experiments now can target the SMN1 and SMN2 genes; splice-site enhancers can focus on SMN2 trying to increase the percentage of full-length transcript, and pharmacologic strategies may upregulate the SMN2 transcripts. Histone deacetylase inhibitors are a promising class of compounds that increase full-length SMN protein in vitro. Current treatment is analogous to that described for children with muscular dystrophy using rehabilitative measures, bracing, attention to scoliosis, and assistance in education and social adaptation. Some authorities believe that children with SMA are characteristically of high intelligence; academic programs are important. There is no level 1 evidence to date for an effective treatment of SMA.

OTHER SPINAL MUSCULAR ATROPHIES (NOT RELATED TO CHROMOSOME 5)

SYNDROMES

These syndromes do not map to 5q11 and differ in the focal distribution of symptoms and signs. Most are autosomal recessive, but some families show dominant inheritance.

Fazio–Londe Syndrome

In contrast to the sparing of cranial nerve functions in most juvenile SMA, selective dysarthria and dysphagia in Fazio–Londe syndrome (MIM 211500) begin in late childhood or adolescence. Wasting of the tongue with visible fasciculation occurs. Symptoms may be restricted for years, but weakness of the arms and legs may occur later, and respiration may be affected. It is caused by homozygous or compound heterozygous mutation in the SLC52A3 gene on chromosome 20p13 and may respond to riboflavin.

Scapuloperoneal and Facioscapulohumeral Forms of Spinal Muscular Atrophy

Scapuloperoneal (MIM 271220, 181400) and facioscapulohumeral (FSH; MIM 182970) forms of SMA have been reported. Some may actually have had FSH muscular dystrophy with ambiguous results on EMG and biopsy that led to incorrect classification as a neurogenic disorder. The distinction now depends on DNA analysis.

Childhood Spinal Muscular Atrophy with Known Biochemical Abnormality

Hexosaminidase deficiency (MIM 272800) may cause a syndrome of SMA starting in childhood or adolescence. The pattern of inheritance is autosomal recessive. Some patients also have upper motor neuron signs, as in ALS. Associated psychosis, dementia, or cerebellar signs may appear. Other rare biochemical abnormalities seen with SMA are lysosomal diseases, phenylketonuria, hydroxyisovaleric aciduria, mutations of mtDNA, peroxisomal disease, and ceroid lipofuscinosis.

DIAGNOSIS

Most of the childhood SMAs can be identified by the history and clinical examination. They must be differentiated from muscular dystrophies by DNA analysis, EMG, or muscle biopsy; the family history aids in classification. Hexosaminidase deficiency is suspected in families of Ashkenazi Jewish background, especially if there are known cases of Tay–Sachs disease in the family or if some family members are known to be carriers of the gene. Kennedy syndrome is recognized by onset after age 40 years, distribution of weakness, and gynecomastia.

TREATMENT

For most forms of SMAs, there is no specific treatment. Support and comfort are therefore the goals of treatment, which may include nutritional support, respiratory support, physical and occupational therapy, rehabilitation devices, and other measures as needed.

SUGGESTED READINGS

Awano T, Kim JK, Monani UR. Spinal muscular atrophy: journeying from bench to bedside. *Neurotherapeutics.* 2014;11(4):786–795.

Bosch AM, Abeling NG, Ijlst L, et al. Brown-Vialetto-Van Laere and Fazio-Londe syndrome is associated with a riboflavin transporter defect mimicking mild MADD: a new inborn error of metabolism with potential treatment. *J Inherit Metab Dis.* 2011;34:159–164.

Brzustowicz LM, Lehner T, Castilla LH, et al. Genetic mapping of chronic childhood-onset spinal muscular atrophy to chromosome 5q11.2-13.3. *Nature.* 1990;344:540–541.

Darras BT, Jones HR Jr, Ryan MM, et al. *Neuromuscular Disorders of Infancy, Childhood and Adolescence: A Clinician's Approach.* 2nd ed. Amsterdam, The Netherlands: Academic Press; 2015.

Feldkotter M, Schwarzer V, Wirth R, et al. Quantitative analyses of SMN1 and SMN2 based on real-time lightCyscler PCR: fast and highly reliable carrier testing and prediction of severity of spinal muscular atrophy. *Am J Hum Genet.* 2002;70:358–368.

Gilliam TC, Brzustowicz LM, Castilla LH, et al. Genetic homogeneity between acute and chronic forms of spinal muscular atrophy. *Nature.* 1990; 345:823–825.

Oskoui M, Levy G, De Vivo DC, et al. The natural history of SMA 1. *Neurology.* 2007;69:1931–1936.

Progressive Muscular Dystrophies 142

Mathula Thangarajh, Petra Kaufmann, Louis H. Weimer, Michio Hirano, and Lewis P. Rowland

DEFINITION

A muscular dystrophy has five essential characteristics:

1. It is a myopathy, as defined by clinical, histologic, and electromyographic (EMG) criteria. No signs of denervation or sensory loss are apparent unless there is a concomitant and separate disease.
2. All symptoms are effects of limb or cranial muscle weakness. (The heart and visceral muscles may also be involved.)
3. Symptoms become progressively worse.
4. Histologic changes imply degeneration and regeneration of muscle, but no abnormal storage of a metabolic product is evident.
5. The condition is recognized as heritable, even if there are no other cases in a particular family.

Although not part of the definition, there are two further characterics, which we hope will be reversed in the future:

1. It is incompletely understood why muscles are weak in any of these conditions, even when the affected gene product is known.
2. There is no curative therapy for any of the dystrophies yet, and gene therapy has not yet been successful.

Improvements in medical care and modern rehabilitation measures have improved the life expectancy and opportunities for children with muscular dystrophy. Furthermore, prednisone has been established as a disease-modifying agent for Duchenne muscular dystrophy (DMD) because it delays the loss of ambulation. Newer treatment strategies are currently entering clinical trials. Prevention is another important strategy because genetic counseling and prenatal testing allow parents to make informed choices.

The definition of muscular dystrophies requires qualifications. For instance, some familial myopathies manifest by symptoms other than limb weakness, but those conditions are not called dystrophies. Familial recurrent myoglobinuria, for example, is considered a metabolic myopathy. The several forms of familial periodic paralysis do not qualify as dystrophies even if there is progressive limb weakness because the attacks of weakness are the dominant manifestations in most patients. Syndromes that include myotonia incorporate that word in the name of the disease, as in myotonia congenita, but are called *muscular dystrophy* only when there is progressive limb weakness, as in myotonic muscular dystrophy (MMD). In addition, static conditions, such as congenital myopathies, are not called dystrophies because the weakness does not become progressively more severe. This distinction allows some exceptions: A slowly progressive dystrophy may seem static, and some congenital myopathies slowly become more severe. Another exception is the term *congenital muscular dystrophy* (CMD), which may be severe and static from birth.

CLASSIFICATION

The classification of muscular dystrophies is based on both clinical and genetic characteristics, starting with three main types: DMD, facioscapulohumeral muscular dystrophy (FSHD), and MMD. Each type differs from others in age at onset, distribution of weakness, rate of progression, presence or absence of calf hypertrophy, or high serum levels of creatine kinase (CK), and pattern of inheritance (Table 142.1).

Early investigators recognized that these three types did not include all of the common muscular dystrophies, so they included a fourth subtype of muscular dystrophy, namely, limb-girdle muscular dystrophy (LGMD). Patients with LGMD often have weakness of the shoulder and pelvic girdle muscles. In some forms of LGMD, cardiac and respiratory involvement can be prominent. The identification of several genes associated with LGMD-like phenotype has resulted in a newer classification of LGMD based on whether the disease is inherited in an autosomal dominant or recessive pattern.

Progressive muscular dystrophies result from diverse defects in muscle proteins associated with the extracellular matrix (collagen type VI, merosin); cell membrane and associated proteins (dystrophin, sarcoglycans, caveolin-3, dysferlin, integrins); cellular enzymes (calpain-3), organelle, or sarcomere function (telethonin, myotilin, titin); and nuclear envelope (lamins, emerin) (Fig. 142.1).

LABORATORY DIAGNOSIS

DNA analysis in leukocytes now often obviates the need for EMG and muscle biopsy. Commercially available genetic testing is available for Duchenne, Becker, facioscapulohumeral, scapuloperoneal, myotonic dystrophies, and LGMDs.

The identification of a genetic cause of dystrophinopathy has revolutionized our diagnostic approach to this disorder. In a young boy with gross motor delay and elevated CK and clinical examination suggestive of proximal muscle weakness, the initial testing should focus on large deletions and duplication mutations in the dystrophin gene. Sequencing of the dystrophin gene may be necessary in select cases to confirm diagnosis. Should gene testing in a patient with presumed dystrophinopathy be negative or ambiguous, a muscle biopsy may be performed to establish the diagnosis. Immunocytochemistry and/or Western blot to quantify dystrophin protein may be required. For patients in whom there is mismatch between the clinical phenotype of dystrophinopathy and genetic phenotype, sequencing mRNA from muscle can be performed.

A muscle biopsy can be useful in identifying the appropriate gene for testing in LGMD patients. Histochemical analysis and electrophoretic studies of dystrophin, the associated dystrophin glycoproteins, and other possibly abnormal proteins may be needed for final diagnosis. If unique features are encountered in the biopsy, a regional research center can be consulted. Muscle biopsy is needed to characterize most congenital and metabolic myopathies. Measuring serum CK level and electrocardiogram (ECG) should be included in the workup of all patients with suspected myopathy.

Muscle ultrasound and magnetic resonance imaging (MRI) of skeletal muscle are increasingly used in the diagnostic evaluation.

TABLE 142.1 Features of the Most Common Muscular Dystrophies

	Duchenne (DMD)	Facioscapulohumeral (FSHD)	Myotonic Dystrophy (DM 1) and Proximal Myotonic Myopathy (PROMM, DM 2)
MIM number	310200	158900	DM 1: 16090; DM 2: 60268
Incidence estimates	1 in 3,500 live male births	1 in 20,000 births	1 in 8,000 births
Mode of inheritance	X-linked recessive	Autosomal dominant	Autosomal dominant
Gene defect	Deletion or point mutation in dystrophin gene	FSHD 1: reduced number of tandem repeats in D4Z4: 1–8 repeats (normal 10 to >100 repeats) FSHD 2: mutations in chromatin modifier SMCHD1 causing chromatin relaxation at D4Z4	DM 1: CTG expansion in protein kinase gene; 50 to >2,000 repeats (normal 5–37 repeats) DM 2: CCTG repeat expansion in zinc finger protein 9 gene
Gene location	Xp21.2	4q35	DM 1: 19q13; DM 2: 3q21
Expressivity	Complete	Variable	Variable
Age of onset	Childhood	Adolescence, rarely childhood	DM 1: broad range (infancy to adult life) DM 2: adolescence to adult life
Site of onset	Pelvic girdle	Shoulder girdle	DM 1: face and distal limbs; congenital form: hypotonia, clubfeet, dysphagia, dysmorphism, respiratory distress, mental retardation DM 2: pelvic girdle, neck flexors DM 1 compared to PROMM patients usually have more: facial weakness, dysphagia, and distal weakness and wasting
Calf hypertrophy	Common	Never	DM 1: never DM 2: some
Rate of progression	Relatively rapid	Slow	Variable
Facial weakness	Rare and mild	Common	Common
Contractures	Common	Rare	Rare
Cardiac disease	Usually late (cardiomyopathy)	None	Common (conduction defect)
Other clinical features	Respiratory insufficiency; scoliosis; cognitive function variably impaired (sometimes high function)	High-frequency hearing loss and retinal vasculopathy (rare)	Cataracts, endocrine dysfunction
Genetic heterogeneity	Duchenne and Becker allelic; Becker resembles Duchenne but onset later and less severe	Not all FSHD phenotypes linked to 4q35	Some PROMM patients not linked to 3q21

Muscle ultrasound is painless, less expensive compared to MRI, and offers dynamic images. Muscle imaging can show the selective pattern of muscle involvement associated with some of the muscular dystrophies. For example, there is selective involvement of sartorius and adductor longus in selenoprotein N1 (SEPN1) myopathy with sparing of the gracilis. MRI also offers good delineation between fatty infiltration and skeletal muscle and may guide the choice of the muscle to biopsy.

X-LINKED MUSCULAR DYSTROPHIES

DEFINITIONS

Duchenne and Becker muscular dystrophies (MIM 310200) are dystrophinopathies and are due to mutations in the dystrophin gene located at Xp21. Out-of-frame large deletion or duplication mutations result in the absence of dystrophin protein leading to the severe clinical phenotype (Duchenne), whereas in-frame deletion or duplication mutations in which some dystrophin protein occurs result in the milder clinical phenotype (Becker) (see Table 142.1). Point mutations can cause either Duchenne or Becker muscular dystrophy. There is often overlap in the clinical phenotype, and these children can be classified as having an "intermediate" phenotype. Boys are affected and females are carriers of the mutations. Nondystrophin diseases that map to the same position are called *Xp21 myopathies*.

PREVALENCE AND INCIDENCE

The incidence of DMD is about 1 in 3,500 male births, with no geographic or ethnic variation. Approximately one-third of the

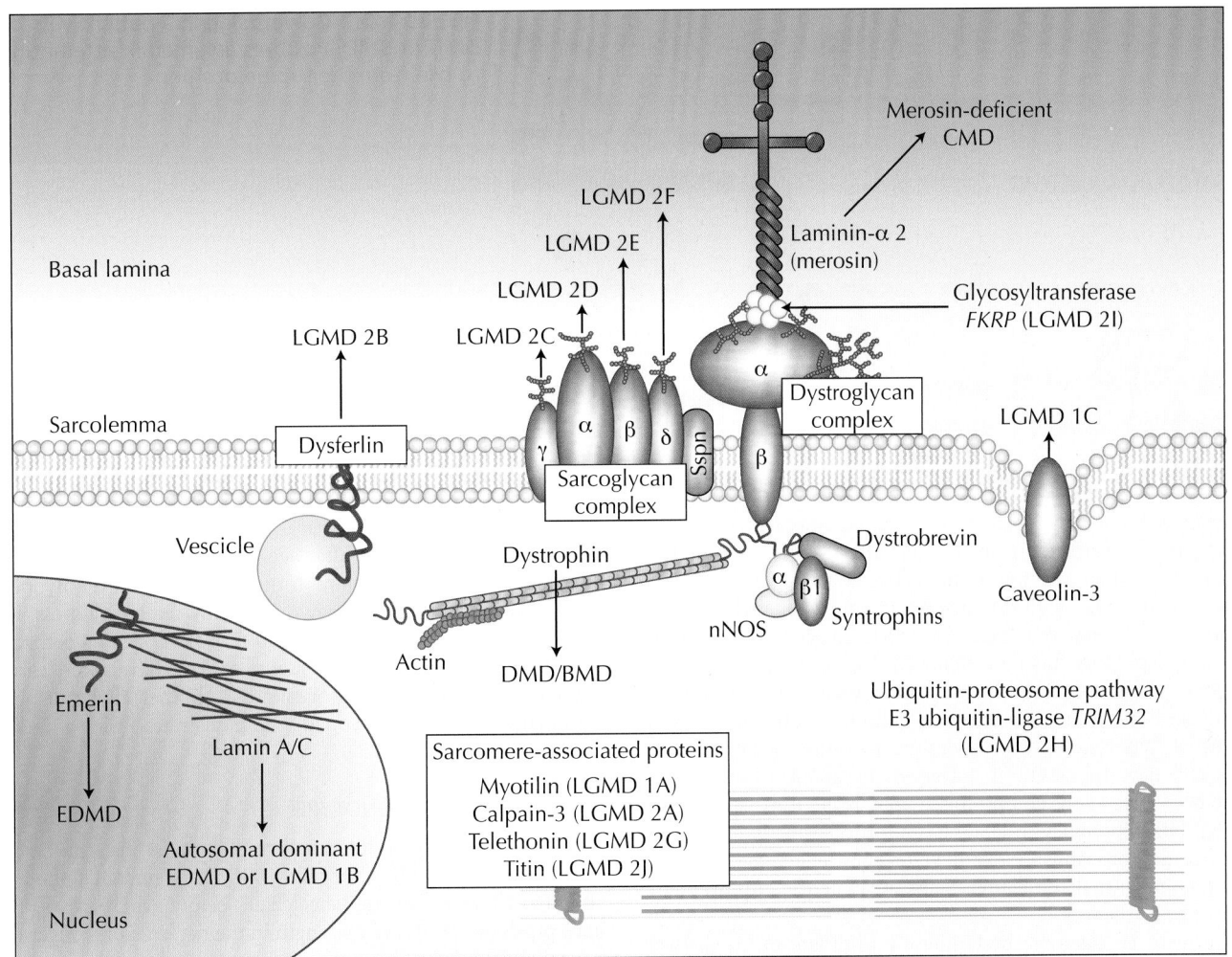

FIGURE 142.1 Skeletal muscle proteins and muscular dystrophies. The dystrophin–glycoprotein complex (DGC) comprises dystrophin, the dystroglycans (α, β), the sarcoglycans (α, β, γ, δ), sarcospan, the syntrophins (α, β_1), and dystrobrevin (α). The complex stabilizes the sarcolemma and protects surface membranes in muscle contraction. Nitric oxide synthetase (nNOS) interacts with the syntrophin complex and laminin-α 2, one of many extracellular ligands of α-dystroglycan. Disease-causing mutations are cited in the text and Table 142.3. LGMD, limb-girdle muscular dystrophy; CMD, congenital muscular dystrophy; DMD, Duchenne muscular dystrophy; BMD, Becker muscular dystrophy; EDMD, Emery–Dreifuss muscular dystrophy. (From Mathews KD, Moore SA. Limb-girdle muscular dystrophy. *Curr Neurol Neurosci Rep*. 2003;3:78–85, with permission.)

cases are caused by de novo mutations; the others are more clearly familial. Because the life span of patients with DMD is shortened, the prevalence is less—about 1 in 18,000 males. Becker muscular dystrophy (BMD) is much less common, with a frequency of about 1 in 20,000.

Duchenne and Becker Muscular Dystrophies

DUCHENNE MUSCULAR DYSTROPHY

The condition may become evident in infancy if serum enzymes are coincidentally measured, for example, for an incidental respiratory infection. A positive family history may also alert an astute physician to the early recognition of motor delay. Authorities often state that symptoms do not begin until age 3 to 5 years but that view may be a measure of the crudeness of muscle evaluation in infants. Infants with DMD score less on scales that evaluate gross motor function. Many boys have hypertrophied calf muscles. Walking is often delayed, and the boys probably never run normally; toe walking and waddling gait are evident. Then, the condition progresses to overt difficulty in walking, climbing stairs, and rising from chairs. An exaggerated lordosis is assumed to maintain balance. The boys tend to fall easily if jostled and then they have difficulty rising from the ground. In doing so, they use a characteristic maneuver called the *Gowers sign* (Fig. 142.2). They roll over to kneel, push down on the ground with extended forearms to raise the rump and straighten the legs, then move the hands to the knees and push up to a standing position. The process has been called *climbing up himself*. It is also seen in other conditions that include proximal limb and trunk weakness, such as spinal muscular atrophy. At this stage, the knee jerks may be lost, whereas ankle jerks are still present; this discrepancy is a measure of the proximal accentuation of weakness.

As the disease progresses, the arms and hands are affected. Slight facial weakness may be seen, but speech, swallowing, and

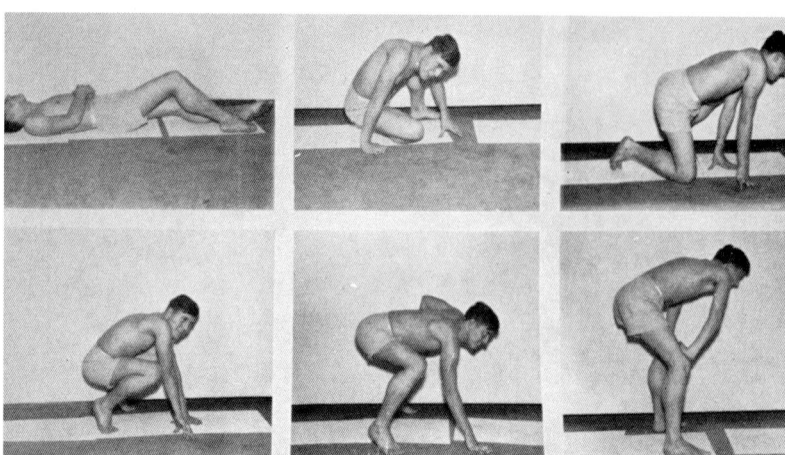

FIGURE 142.2 Gowers sign in a patient with DMD or BMD. Postures assumed in attempting to rise from the supine position.

ocular movements are spared. Iliotibial contractures limit hip extension; heel cord contractures are partly responsible for toe walking. Loss of ambulation occurs between ages 9 and 12 years or later when treated with steroids. Boys then become wheelchair-bound. Scoliosis may then become serious and may compromise limb and respiratory function. Elbow and knee contractures contribute to disability. Respiratory muscle weakness causes progressive decline in lung capacity beginning at about age 8 years. Nocturnal hypoventilation may occur and cause morning headaches and daytime fatigue if untreated. By about age 20 years, respiration is severely compromised that respiratory support is needed. Life expectancy in DMD has improved greatly in the last three decades, probably because of better coordinated medical care and home nocturnal ventilation. Some attribute the improvement to prednisone therapy.

The heart is usually spared clinically until late in the disease when congestive heart failure (CHF) and arrhythmias may develop. The ECG is abnormal in most patients, with increased QRS amplitude in lead V_1 and deep, narrow Q waves in left precordial leads. Echocardiography shows progressively diminished contractility. Signs of cardiomyopathy may not be apparent because of the inability to exercise but may supervene in a few cases. The gastrointestinal system is usually spared, but intestinal hypomotility and acute gastric dilatation are uncommon complications probably related to dystrophin deficiency in smooth muscle. Osteoporosis begins in the ambulatory years, is more severe in the legs, and may contribute to fractures. Intellectual impairment with predominantly verbal difficulties is seen in one-third of boys with DMD, and the average IQ is shifted approximately 1 standard deviation below normal. Therefore, some boys with DMD have average or below average intelligence.

Anesthetic catastrophes may occur with hyperkalemia, extremely high CK levels (even more than 20 times the normal maximum), acidosis, cardiac failure, hyperthermia, and rigidity. The risk can be decreased by avoiding inhaled general anesthetics and depolarizing muscle relaxants, especially succinylcholine. This vulnerability can be considered a form of malignant hyperthermia.

BECKER MUSCULAR DYSTROPHY

This condition is defined by milder skeletal muscle weakness compared to DMD. Calf hypertrophy is present, weakness is greatest proximally, and serum CK levels are high. EMG is myopathic and muscle biopsy reveals some staining of dystrophin. The two clinical features that distinguish it from DMD are differences in age at onset (typically after age 10 years) and rate of progression (still walking after age 16 years, often later). Cognitive impairment is less common than in DMD. Cardiomyopathy usually develops later but may overshadow limb weakness. Cardiac complications contribute to 50% of BMD deaths compared with 20% with DMD. However, some patients have severe cardiomyopathy and mild muscle weakness. Another allelic disorder, X-linked dilated cardiomyopathy, demonstrates little to no skeletal muscle weakness.

INTERMEDIATE PHENOTYPE

Some patients show an intermediate phenotype that can be considered either severe BMD or mild DMD. They remain ambulatory after age 12 years but use wheelchairs before age 16 years. They have preserved antigravity strength in the neck flexors longer than typical DMD patients.

MANIFESTING CARRIERS

DMD is an X-linked recessive condition. Female mutation carriers are usually asymptomatic, but "manifesting carriers" can have limb weakness, calf hypertrophy, cardiomyopathy, or high serum CK levels.

DIAGNOSIS

The diagnosis of Duchenne dystrophy is usually evident from clinical features. In sporadic and atypical cases, spinal muscular atrophy might be mistaken for DMD. Fasciculations and EMG evidence of denervation, however, identify the neurogenic disorder. High CK values are sometimes encountered in screening blood chemistry analysis done for some other purpose; regardless of the clinical findings, this may lead to the erroneous diagnosis of Duchenne dystrophy. However, typical DMD or BMD CK values are at least 20 times normal; few other conditions attain these values, not even interictal phosphorylase deficiency or acid maltase deficiency. Similarly, when a child with an incidental infection has routine blood tests, increased serum liver enzyme values may lead to diagnosis of suspected hepatitis; serum CK should then be assayed, and if it is elevated, a myopathy should be suspected, not a liver disease. In DMD, serum CK levels are highest in the presymptomatic years and then gradually decrease with age.

Increased CK levels are also seen in girls and women who carry the dystrophin mutations, in some patients with spinal muscular atrophy, and, for unknown reasons, in some otherwise asymptomatic individuals (idiopathic or asymptomatic hyperCK-emia). Even before myopathic symptoms begin, high CK values are seen in the dysferlinopathies (LGMD2B or Miyoshi myopathy), which are discussed later in the chapter. Similarly, caveolin-3 mutations (LGMD 1C) may cause hyperCKemia before symptoms of limb-girdle dystrophy become evident.

MOLECULAR GENETICS

The dystrophin gene is involved in both Duchenne and Becker dystrophies, which are allelic diseases. Dystrophin is a cytoskeletal protein located at the plasma membrane. Brain and other organs contain slightly different isoforms. In muscle, dystrophin is associated with membrane glycoproteins that link the cytoskeleton with membrane proteins and then to laminin and the extracellular matrix (see Fig. 142.1). The protein probably plays an essential role in maintaining muscle fiber integrity. If dystrophin is absent, as in Duchenne dystrophy, or is abnormal, as in Becker dystrophy, the sarcolemma becomes unstable in contraction and relaxation, and the damage results in excessive calcium influx, thereby leading to muscle cell necrosis. If specific glycoproteins are abnormal or missing, the same problems arise, as in some LGMDs (described later in the chapter).

These findings have been put to practical use in the diagnosis of Duchenne and Becker dystrophies and in genetic counseling. DNA analysis demonstrates a deletion or duplication at Xp21 in about 65% of DMD and 85% of BMD patients. Patients with DMD typically have "frameshift" mutations that alter the DNA reading frame and consequently change amino acids downstream of the mutation, whereas individuals with BMD have milder "in-frame" rearrangements that maintain the sequence of amino acids flanking the mutation. Point mutations or small rearrangements account for the remainder and can be detected by gene sequencing. The presence of a deletion or point mutation in a patient with compatible clinical findings is diagnostic. Carriers can be similarly identified, and the test can also be used for prenatal diagnosis (Fig. 142.3).

The initial evaluation of a boy suspected to have dystrophinopathy includes a serum CK followed by genetic screening for dystrophin mutations performed on peripheral blood leukocytes. Mutations that interfere with the expression of dystrophin cause DMD and those that leads to abnormal quality or quantity of dystrophin cause BMD. Muscle biopsy is sometimes performed in sporadic cases of unclear phenotype, even when a deletion has been identified, because immunocytochemistry for dystrophin and Western blot for quantitative dystrophin analysis can confirm and refine the diagnosis in these questionable cases. If no deletion is found and if dystrophin sequencing is not available, muscle biopsy is needed.

In Duchenne dystrophy, dystrophin staining is absent by both immunocytochemistry and Western blot. In Becker dystrophy, immunocytochemistry shows an interrupted pattern of staining on the surface membrane, and the Western blot shows decreased dystrophin levels or abnormal protein size. Carriers show a mosaic pattern; some fibers contain normal dystrophin staining and others show no dystrophin staining. The most widely used animal model of DMD is the *mdx-23* mouse, which has a spontaneous mutation in the exon 23 of the murine dystrophin gene.

TREATMENT

Oral corticosteroids are standard of care in DMD. Prednisone (0.75 mg/kg/day) or deflazacort (0.9 to 1.2 mg/kg/day) can be used in DMD. Prednisone therapy improved function and strength in placebo-controlled trials, but the side effects of chronic administration—in particular, weight gain, growth retardation, and behavioral changes—may limit the use of steroids. If not prohibited by side effects, prednisone is usually offered to ambulatory patients older than 5 years of age and may be continued until the patient enters the wheelchair stage. Data on the use of prednisone before age 5 years or during the wheelchair years are insufficient.

Experimental attempts at gene replacement through implanted myoblasts were unsuccessful to date. Drugs encouraging "reading through" nonsense mutations are under investigation as possible treatment for the minority of DMD patients with a point mutation resulting in a premature stop codon. Other treatment approaches currently under investigation include exon skip–mediated correction and gene therapy.

Supportive management is aimed at maintaining function and independence, avoiding complications, and improving quality of life.

Orthopedic and rehabilitation measures include stretching exercises and ankle–foot orthoses during sleep to prevent contractures. Later, standing and walking can be maintained with ankle–foot

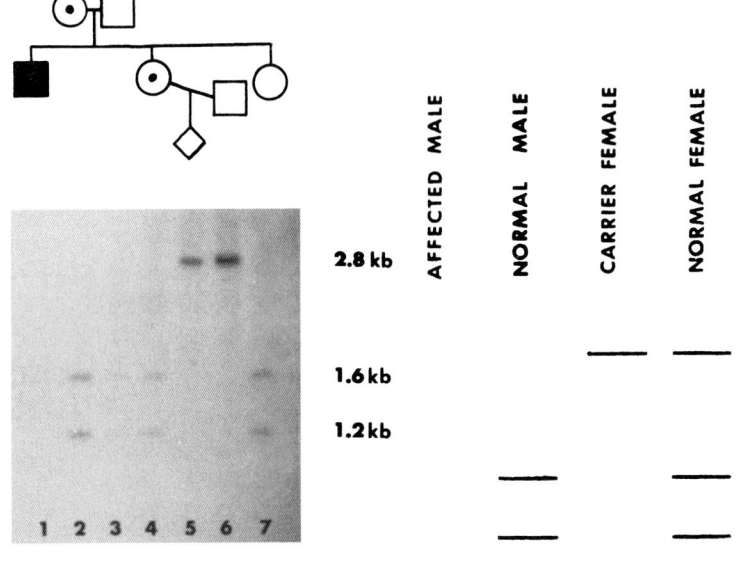

FIGURE 142.3 Prenatal diagnosis in DMD. **A:** Autoradiograph of Southern blot of 1% agarose gel with DNA samples from each individual digested with the restriction enzyme XmnI and probed with pERT87-15. The affected male is deleted (no signal). His sister who was pregnant has a deleted X and an X chromosome with the 1.6/1.2 allele. Her husband's X chromosome contains the 2.8 allele. The fetus contains the husband's X and the deleted X. **B:** Diagram of the four possible outcomes of the prenatal diagnosis. The fetus is a carrier female. (Courtesy of A. D. Roses.)

orthoses or knee–ankle–foot orthoses combined with standing devices or walkers. Surgical release of contractures is only occasionally used for functional reasons, such as maintaining standing or ambulation. During the wheelchair years, surgical scoliosis stabilization can help maintain a comfortable sitting position and may reduce the risk of atelectasis and pneumonia.

Pulmonary function should be monitored regularly in patients with respiratory symptoms and in those who are nonambulatory to detect declines in respiratory muscle strength or ability to cough. Reduced cough strength increases the risk of atelectasis and respiratory infections. Therefore, chest physical therapy and mechanical insufflators/exsufflators are useful. When symptoms of sleep-disordered breathing are suspected, overnight in-home oximetry or laboratory-based sleep studies can confirm nocturnal hypoventilation. Noninvasive nighttime mechanical ventilation should then be considered. Later in the disease when respiratory muscle weakness progresses, continuous noninvasive ventilation is often needed, and sometimes the difficult decision whether to do a tracheostomy arises.

Cardiac function should be assessed prior to any major surgery in those with respiratory insufficiency or cardiac symptoms and, at least annually, in the later stages of the disease. Perindopril (2 to 4 mg/day) is thought to slow the progression of cardiac disease in DMD. Cardiac transplantation has been performed in select BMD patients.

Other measures include precautions with general anesthesia, influenza and pneumococcal vaccinations, weight control, neuropsychological evaluation to guide in educational issues, and social support to aid emotionally and financially. Genetic counseling for families is crucial.

OTHER XP21 MYOPATHIES

Dystrophinopathies

A deletion in a neighboring gene can extend into the dystrophin gene and produce myopathy. The resulting syndrome may be dominated by other neighboring gene changes, including congenital adrenal insufficiency or glycerol kinase deficiency, as well as a myopathy, which may range from mild to severe. These syndromes are customarily called *Becker variants* if appropriate dystrophin abnormalities are found. That nomenclature may be confusing, however, because the original definition of Becker dystrophy was based on clinical criteria, and these syndromes are clinically different. Among them are myopathies that affect girls or women, not only manifesting carriers but also girls with Turner syndrome or balanced translocations that involve Xp21, as well as syndromes of atypical distributions of weakness, such as distal myopathy or quadriceps myopathy. Some syndromes lack limb weakness but are manifested by other symptoms, such as recurrent myoglobinuria or X-linked cramps without weakness. Each of these atypical syndromes warrants studies of dystrophin.

Nondystrophin-Related Xp21 Myopathies

McLeod syndrome (MIM 300842) is a multisystemic disorder first discovered in blood banks because the donors lacked a red cell antigen, the Kell antigen. These individuals were found to have abnormally shaped red blood cells (acanthocytes), and serum CK values were often 29 times normal or even higher. In addition, some had myopathic limb weakness, and the condition mapped to Xp21. Dystrophin is normal in these patients. Deletions in the XK gene cause McLeod syndrome and a chromosomal microarray analysis may be helpful. It is also described in Chapter 134 (acanthocytes).

EMERY–DREIFUSS MUSCULAR DYSTROPHY

Emery–Dreifuss muscular dystrophy (EDMD) is a muscular dystrophy with several distinct manifestations:

1. The characteristic humeroperoneal distribution of weakness is unusual. That is, the biceps and triceps are affected rather than shoulder girdle muscles, and distal muscles are affected more than proximal muscles in the legs. The limb weakness may be mild or severe.
2. Contractures are disproportionately severe and are evident before much weakness is noted. The contractures affect the elbows, knees, ankles, fingers, and spine. A rigid spine develops, and neck flexion is limited.
3. Heart block, atrial paralysis, and atrial fibrillation are found in 95% of patients by age 30 years and lead to placement of a pacemaker. Dilated cardiomyopathy occurs in about 35% of all cases.

EDMD has been associated with six genes. It is characteristically an X-linked recessive disease (MIM 310300) and is linked to mutations in the *EMD* or *emerin* gene on Xq28. Emerin is localized to the nuclear membrane in muscle and other organs. Alternatively, the phenotype is inherited in an autosomal dominant (MIM 181350) or recessive pattern (MIM 604929) linked to the *LMNA* gene on 1q21, encoding lamin A/C. Lamin A/C is located in the inner nuclear lamina and has also been linked to several allelic disorders, as discussed later in the chapter. Mutations in *FHL1* encoding four-and-a-half LIM protein 1 also cause X-linked EDMD. Autosomal dominant EDMD can also be caused by the following genes: *SYNE1*, *SYNE2*, and *TMEM43*.

Symptoms of EDMD often start before age 5 years with difficulty walking. Examination typically shows symmetric contractures and weakness without pseudohypertrophy. Tendon reflexes are hypoactive or absent, and there may be mild facial weakness. Serum CK activity can be mildly elevated to levels less than 10 times normal. The diagnosis is usually confirmed by DNA testing. Absence of emerin can be demonstrated by immunocytochemical study of a muscle biopsy. Emerin staining is absent not only in muscle nuclei but also in circulating white blood cells (WBCs) and skin. As a result, skin biopsy, leukocytes, or inner cheek swabs for exfoliated mucosal cells can be examined diagnostically instead of muscle biopsy. However, DNA or gene product analysis is preferred to establish accurate diagnosis. Cardiac surveillance (including 24-hour ECG and echocardiography) is crucial.

EDMD must be distinguished from other conditions. The rigid spine syndrome includes vertebral and limb contractures but not cardiomyopathy or muscle wasting. Because the cardiac abnormality may not be evident in childhood, some patients with a rigid spine might be expected to have EDMD. Collagen type VI–related disorders (Bethlem myopathy/Ullrich CMD—MIM 158810/254090) include contractures and myopathy but not cardiomyopathy, as discussed later in the chapter.

Management is symptomatic and may include physical therapy and surgical tendon release for contractures. Pacemaker implantation and treatment of cardiomyopathy is often crucial. Female carriers are at risk of arrhythmias and should have regular cardiac evaluations.

FACIOSCAPULOHUMERAL MUSCULAR DYSTROPHY

DEFINITION

FSHD (MIM 158900) is defined by clinical and genetic features that differ from those of DMD. Inheritance is autosomal dominant.

The name designates the characteristic distribution of weakness, which causes symptoms that differ from those of DMD. The face is almost always affected. Severity varies, and some of those affected are asymptomatic but show diagnostic signs. Progression is slow. Symptoms usually begin in adolescence, but signs may be evident in children. Serum CK levels are normal or minimally elevated.

MOLECULAR GENETICS

The disease is autosomal dominant with nearly complete penetrance. Almost all FSHD patients have deletion of the subtelomeric array of 3.3-kilobase repeat elements, termed *D4Z4*, on chromosome 4q35. Normal individuals have 11 to 150 repeats; FSHD patients usually have fewer than 11. The deletion results in inappropriate expression of the double homeobox–containing gene *DUX4* in muscle cells. This common form is referred to as *FSHD1*. About 5% of FSHD patients have chromatin relaxation at D4Z4 without D4Z4 contraction and are due to mutations in the chromatin modifier gene *SMCHD1*. This rare form is referred to as *FSHD2*.

CLINICAL MANIFESTATIONS

The following features are characteristics of FSHD:

1. Facial weakness is evident not only by limitation of lip movements but also in the slightly everted lips and wide palpebral fissures. Patients may state that they have never been able to whistle or blow up a balloon. Some are said by relatives to sleep with eyes open.
2. Scapular winging is prominent. Protrusion of the scapulae is more evident when the patient tries to push against a wall with elbows extended and hands at shoulder level. The winging becomes more evident when the patient tries to raise the arms laterally. The patient cannot raise the arms to shoulder level even though there is no weakness of the deltoids on manual testing. This limitation is caused by inadequate fixation of the scapulae to the chest wall.
3. The shoulder girdle has a characteristic appearance. Viewed from the front, the clavicles seem to sag and the tips of the scapulae project above the supraclavicular fossa. This abnormality becomes more marked when the subject tries to raise the arms laterally to shoulder level. Smallness of the pectoral muscles affects the anterior axillary fold, which is ordinarily diagonal but assumes a vertical position. Abdominal muscle weakness may cause abdominal protrusion and exaggerated lumbar lordosis. The lower abdominal muscles are weaker than the upper causing a positive "Beevor" sign with the navel moving toward the head upon neck flexion in a supine position. The limb muscle weakness is often asymmetric.
4. Leg weakness may affect proximal muscles or, more often, the tibialis anterior and peroneals, resulting in footdrop.

In family studies, asymptomatic individuals can be identified by mild versions of these signs. Within a single family, the condition may vary markedly. Progression is slow, however, and the condition may not shorten longevity. About 20% of patients eventually use a wheelchair. Respiratory insufficiency is rare. Men may be more severely affected than women.

ASSOCIATED DISORDERS

Mild sensorineural hearing loss and vascular retinopathy as well as oropharyngeal symptoms, Coats disease (exudative telangiectasia of the retina), and, possibly, mental retardation are occasionally seen in children with FSHD. However, these findings are not consistent, and it is not known how they relate to the genetic abnormality. Cardiac arrhythmias are rarely seen in FSHD.

LABORATORY STUDIES

In most cases, the diagnosis can be confirmed by leukocyte DNA testing for a contraction of the subtelomeric repeat array on 4q35. Presymptomatic diagnosis is possible in families with more than one affected member, but testing should be done only with appropriate counseling. EMG and muscle biopsy, by definition, should show a myopathic pattern. The histologic changes are mild and nonspecific. Inflammatory cells are found in some patients, raising the question of polymyositis, but immunosuppressive therapy has always failed in these patients. DNA diagnosis resolves this possible confusion and may obviate muscle biopsy. Some patients with typical manifestations do not show the characteristic mutation, which may imply locus heterogeneity (mutation at some other locus) or could exceed the limits of sensitivity of current tests for the mutation.

DIFFERENTIAL DIAGNOSIS

The differential diagnosis includes uncommon myogenic and neurogenic scapuloperoneal syndromes, especially when facial weakness is absent. Additionally, EDMD is sometimes confused with FSHD, but the essential clinical features are different. The increasing availability of genetic testing for FSHD, LGMD, and EDMD is likely to clarify these diagnostic problems. Infantile onset of FSHD is rare, but facial weakness may be severe enough to simulate the Möbius syndrome of congenital facial diplegia.

MANAGEMENT

Albuterol, a β2-agonist sympathomimetic drug, was evaluated in an open-label pilot study followed by a randomized clinical trial of 90 FSHD patients for 12 months comparing two dose levels (8 and 16 mg of albuterol twice daily) to placebo. The primary end point, a difference in global strength, was not reached, but albuterol increased two of the secondary end points: grip strength and muscle mass.

Supportive treatment includes physical therapy, analgesics for joint pain, and ankle–foot orthoses for footdrop. Wiring the scapulae to the chest wall has been used to facilitate use of the arms, but the data seem insufficient to warrant widespread use.

MYOTONIC MUSCULAR DYSTROPHY AND PROXIMAL MYOTONIC MYOPATHY

DEFINITION

Myotonic dystrophy (DM 1, MIM 160900) is an autosomal dominant, multisystem disease of unique distribution that includes muscular dystrophy, myotonia, cardiomyopathy, cataracts, and endocrinopathy. Proximal myotonic myopathy (PROMM, DM 2; MIM 602668) shares many characteristics with DM 1 but differs genetically.

EPIDEMIOLOGY

DM 1 is compatible with long life, and gene penetrance is almost 100%. Because of these characteristics, DM 1 is a disease of high prevalence, about 5 per 100,000 throughout the world, with no specific geographic or ethnic variation. It is probably the most common form of muscular dystrophy. The incidence is about 13.5 per 100,000 live births.

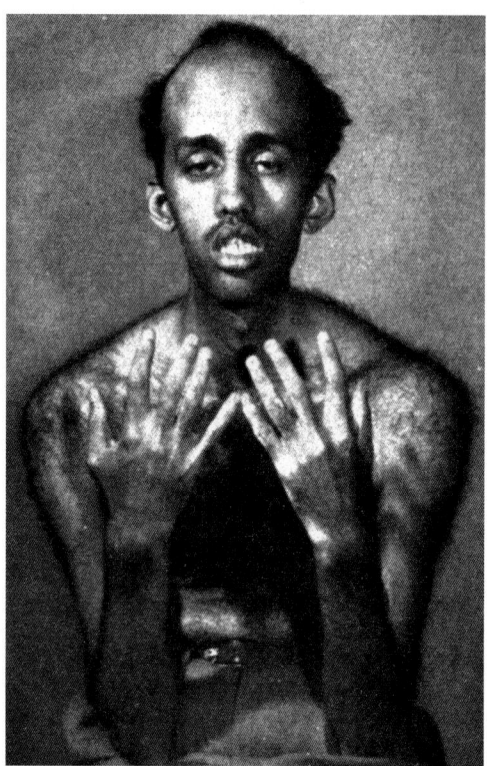

FIGURE 142.4 Myotonic dystrophy. Atrophy of facial, temporal, neck, and hand muscles.

CLINICAL MANIFESTATIONS

In DM 1, as in many other autosomal dominant diseases, variation in age at onset and severity are characteristic. Some affected people are asymptomatic but show signs of the disease on examination. The myopathy is distinctive in distribution (Fig. 142.4). Unlike any of the other major forms of muscular dystrophy, it affects several cranial muscles. Ptosis is common; eye movements may be impaired; and dysarthria and dysphagia may be problems. The temporal muscles are small, and the resulting appearance is distinctive, with a long lean face and ptosis. In men, frontal baldness contributes to the impression. Insensitive clinicians perpetuate unkind words to describe this facial appearance. The sternomastoid muscles are characteristically small and weak. Limb weakness is most pronounced distally and affects the hands and feet equally. This dystrophy is one of the few neuromuscular disorders in which weakness of the finger flexors is prominent. Distal leg weakness may cause a footdrop or steppage gait. Most patients are generally thin, and focal wasting is not prominent. The tendon jerks are lost in proportion to the weakness.

Muscles of respiration may be affected even before there is much limb weakness; this symptom may contribute to the hypersomnia seen in MMD. Sensitivity to general anesthesia may be increased, with prolonged hypoventilation in the postoperative period. MMD, however, is not a muscle disease likely to cause alveolar hypoventilation. The rate of progression is slow and longevity may not be affected, but variation is evident; some people are almost asymptomatic and some become disabled.

Myotonia has a dual definition. First, clinically, it is a phenomenon of impaired relaxation. Second, the EMG shows a distinctive pattern of waxing and waning high-frequency discharges that continue after relaxation begins, thus prolonging and impeding the effort. The EMG pattern is essential to the definition because there are other forms of impaired relaxation (see Chapter 94). Myotonia is most evident in the hands. Symptomatically, it may impair skilled movements or may embarrass the patient by complicating the attempt to shake hands or turn a doorknob because it is difficult to let go. As a sign on examination, the slow relaxation can be elicited by tapping the thenar eminence or, in the forearm, the bellies of the extensors of the fingers. Eliciting percussion myotonia in other limb muscles may be difficult for reasons unknown, but lingual myotonia may be present. Myotonia can also be evoked by asking the patient to grasp forcefully and then relax, which a normal person can do rapidly. In someone with myotonia, however, the grasp is followed by slow relaxation. The abnormal activity arises in the muscle because the response to percussion persists in curarized muscle of these patients; that is, the activity persists after neuromuscular transmission has been blocked.

Cataracts are almost universal but take years to appear. Early findings include characteristic iridescent opacities and posterior opacities.

Endocrinopathy is most readily seen in men. Frontal baldness is almost universal, and testicular atrophy is common; fertility is little diminished, however, so that the disease continues to be propagated in the family. Menstrual irregularities and ovarian failure are not nearly so frequent, and fertility is little decreased in women. Diabetes mellitus may be more common than in the general population, and therefore, annual measurements of glucose and glycosylated hemoglobin should be considered. Hypothyroidism is rare but should be considered so that untreated hypothyroidism does not contribute to muscle weakness.

The *cardiac disorder* is manifested by conduction disturbances, atrial fibrillation and flutter, and ventricular tachyarrhythmias. More than half of the adult patients have abnormalities in the ECG. However, these are often asymptomatic, and pacemakers are needed in only about 5% of patients. CHF and syncope or sudden death may be more common in affected individuals.

Gastrointestinal disorders include impaired swallowing, pseudo-obstruction, or megacolon. *Cognitive impairment* is common in the congenital form of DM 1, but many patients with adult-onset DM 1 are socially well-adjusted. However, mild cognitive and neuropsychiatric impairment may be evident. *Excessive daytime somnolence* is attributed to nocturnal hypoventilation and may be helped by treatment with modafinil or methylphenidate. *Respiratory difficulties* may occur owing to diaphragmatic and intercostal muscle weakness as well as impaired respiratory drive. *Pilomatrixomata* and *epitheliomas* have been associated with DM 1.

Congenital Myotonic Dystrophy

About 5% of children born to a person with DM 1 have symptoms at birth, a condition termed *congenital myotonic dystrophy*. It affects children of either sex who are born to a woman with the usual adult form of the disease, which is often so mild that the woman may be asymptomatic but shows signs of the condition; the mother is the affected parent in almost all cases, but paternal transmission has been reported. The infants have difficulty feeding and breathing in the newborn period, develop slowly, are often mentally retarded, and show developmental anomalies of the face and jaws, as well as severe limb weakness and clubfeet. The genetic basis for the syndrome is discussed later in the text. The clinical syndrome can be confused with other congenital anomalies, and identification of the disease in the mother is therefore essential; this may be difficult because the mother may be asymptomatic or mildly affected. The child may not show EMG evidence of myotonia, but the mother does.

Proximal Myotonic Myopathy

When the mutation causing DM 1 was discovered in 1992, it became evident that some patients did not carry the mutation. Their symptoms and signs are similar to those of DM 1 in many respects, including autosomal dominant myopathy, myotonia, cataracts, and weakness of the sternocleidomastoids. It differs in the distribution of limb weakness because DM 1 is primarily a distal myopathy, and in DM 2, weakness of pelvic girdle muscles is more pronounced than the distal leg weakness. Other differences are less conspicuous. For instance, myotonia is more difficult to elicit, symptoms are less severe, and there may be calf hypertrophy. Congenital DM 1 has not been reported in DM 2 families. Most important, the syndrome does not map to chromosome 19 but maps to chromosome 3q.

LABORATORY STUDIES

EMG shows evidence of myopathy and the characteristic myotonic discharges. Muscle biopsy shows mild and nonspecific changes. Serum CK level may be normal or slightly increased. DNA analysis is now obligatory for precise diagnosis but may raise sensitive questions in a family, and individuals at risk may not wish to be tested. When tested, they should be offered adequate genetic counseling and psychosocial support.

MOLECULAR GENETICS AND PATHOPHYSIOLOGY

The gene for *DM 1* maps to 19q13.2. The mutation is an expansion of a CTG triplet repeat within the DMPK gene. Unaffected people have 5 to 30 CTG repeats; affected individuals have more than 50. Infants with congenital DM 1 have more than 800 repeats, but there is otherwise no strict relation between the number of repeats and clinical severity. Two patients with the same number of repeats may differ in severity. However, the larger the number of repeats, the younger the age at onset, a phenomenon referred to as *anticipation*, and the more severe the syndrome is likely to be (potentiation).

It is not known how the repeat expansion causes the disease. There is no deficiency of the DMPK gene, but mutant mRNA may be retained in the nucleus in structures called *ribonuclear inclusions*. This may reduce the expression of DMPK, but knockout mice do not show a myopathy or myotonia. It has therefore been suggested that the mutant mRNA itself may be toxic, a suspicion confirmed by transgenic mice that show expanded CUG repeats and ribonuclear inclusions and myotonia. The mutant mRNA may bind and sequester essential proteins, such as "muscleblind," which is found in the inclusions of patient's cells. The knockout mouse lacking that gene shows muscle, eye, and RNA splicing abnormalities characteristic of DM.

Locus heterogeneity indicates that a different gene must be involved in *DM 2*, which maps to chromosome 3q21. An expanded CCTG repeat has been found in the gene encoding a zinc finger protein, ZNF9, which is an RNA-binding protein.

Whatever the fundamental fault in these diseases, it must explain how the mutation could cause such a *pleiotropic* disorder, with manifestations in so many different organs.

DIAGNOSIS

The clinical features of DM 1 are so characteristic that the diagnosis is often evident at a glance by noting the long lean face, baldness in men, small sternocleidomastoids, distal myopathy, and myotonia. Early footdrop may lead to confusion with Charcot–Marie–Tooth disease but EMG patterns distinguish the two. Noting an autosomal dominant familial pattern is helpful in general, and diagnosing the mother is especially important in congenital DM 1, which can be mistaken for other causes of mental retardation or chromosome abnormalities. DNA analysis can confirm the diagnosis in most cases.

"Nondystrophic myotonias" are described in other chapters: hyperkalemic periodic paralysis and paramyotonia congenita in Chapter 93 and myotonia congenita and the Schwartz–Jampel syndrome in Chapter 94. "Pseudomyotonia," or impaired relaxation without true myotonic discharges, is seen in the Isaac syndrome or neuromyotonia (see Chapter 94). Myotonic-like discharges, but not clinical myotonia, are seen in patients with acid maltase deficiency. Inclusion body myopathy with both Paget disease and frontotemporal dementia can be associated with myotonia. However, none of these other myotonic syndromes has the characteristic myopathy and multisystem involvement of DM 1 and therefore rarely cause diagnostic confusion.

MANAGEMENT AND GENETIC COUNSELING

Myotonia can be ameliorated with mexiletine (150 to 1,000 mg/day), phenytoin sodium (Dilantin) (300 to 400 mg/day), or other anticonvulsant drugs. However, myotonia is only rarely a bothersome symptom in contrast to other myotonic syndromes; it is the weakness that is disabling. Rehabilitation measures are helpful in keeping the muscles functioning as best as they can and in assisting the patient in the activities of daily living. Orthoses help the footdrop. Ocular and cardiac symptoms are treated as they would be in any patient. An ECG should be recorded annually for adults, and slit lamp examination is also carried out periodically. Glucose metabolism, thyroid function, and, in symptomatic males, testosterone levels should be periodically monitored and when abnormal, treated. Fatigue is common and often responds to pharmacologic treatment such as modafinil (200 to 400 mg/day). Pain is a frequent symptom and should be managed with pharmacologic and other approaches. General anesthesia should be avoided if possible because of increased postoperative pulmonary complications. In congenital DM 1, respiratory support and feeding tubes are often needed. Early intervention with physical, occupational, and speech therapy and special education are indicated to address the problems associated with global developmental delay. The families are educated about the nature of the disease, inheritance, and the availability of DNA diagnosis for adults and for prenatal testing.

LIMB-GIRDLE MUSCULAR DYSTROPHY

HISTORY AND DEFINITION

Limb-girdle muscular dystrophy is a term originally conceived to separate progressive muscular dystrophies that were not X-linked (Duchenne/Becker) or otherwise clinically distinct dystrophies, such as FSHD or DM 1. The group comprises a heterogeneous collection of other progressive muscular dystrophies primarily involving shoulder and pelvic girdle muscles, autosomal dominant or recessive inheritance, and a normal dystrophin gene product. Metabolic myopathies have been separated, especially acid maltase and debrancher enzyme deficiencies; other limb-girdle syndromes proved to be Becker dystrophy, mitochondrial myopathies, polymyositis, inclusion body myositis, or other diseases (Table 142.2). The remaining group was expected to have diverse genetic causes, and in the last 15 years, specific gene defects or chromosomal locations have been discovered for most of the remaining entities; the count currently stands at 27. The disorders are usually not

TABLE 142.2	Conditions Simulating Limb-Girdle Muscular Dystrophy

Acquired Diseases
Inflammatory
Polymyositis, dermatomyositis, inclusion body myositis, sarcoidosis
Toxic myopathies
Chloroquine, steroid myopathy, vincristine, lovastatin, ethanol abuse, phenytoin
Endocrinopathies
Hyperthyroidism, hypothyroidism, hyperadrenocorticism (Cushing syndrome), hyperparathyroidism, hyperaldosteronism
Vitamin deficiency
Vitamin D and vitamin E malabsorption
Paraneoplastic
Lambert–Eaton syndrome, carcinomatous myopathy
Heritable Diseases
Becker muscular dystrophy
Manifesting carrier of Duchenne or Becker gene
Emery–Dreifuss muscular dystrophy
Facioscapulohumeral or scapulohumeral dystrophy
Myotonic muscular dystrophy
Congenital myopathies (centronuclear, central core, nemaline, tubular aggregates, cytoplasmic body, collagen VI–related muscular dystrophy)
Metabolic myopathies: glycogen storage diseases (phosphorylase deficiency, acid maltase deficiency, debrancher deficiency), lipid storage diseases (carnitine deficiencies), mitochondrial myopathies
Myopathy of periodic paralysis

Modified from Jerusalem F, Sieb JP. The limb girdle syndromes. In: Vinken PJ, Bruyn GW, Klawans HL, eds., *Handbook of Clinical Neurology*, Vol. 62. Amsterdam: Elsevier, 1992:179–195.

clinically distinguishable because of marked variability in severity and age onset, even in a single family. However, some characteristic features are seen with specific defects (Table 142.3). The identification of new gene defects has led not only to refinement of this category but has also advanced the understanding of basic muscle cellular biology. The newly identified proteins include many not previously known to play a role in normal muscle function.

CLINICAL MANIFESTATIONS

The diseases are separated into autosomal dominant (type 1) and autosomal recessive (type 2) groups. Individual protein defects are given an additional letter designation in order of discovery. In general, recessive forms are more common, more severe, and of earlier onset. Some have characteristic manifestations but none can be conclusively diagnosed on clinical grounds alone. All of the disorders are characterized by proximal weakness of the pelvic or shoulder girdle muscles and dystrophic signs on muscle biopsy; some include cardiomyopathy. Disorders with primarily distal myopathic weakness are grouped separately as *distal myopathies*. Severity may vary between and within families. Proximal muscle weakness manifesting as difficulty climbing stairs or arising from

a deep-seated chair are common early symptoms. A waddling gait then develops. Difficulty raising the arms and scapular winging may be seen. Knee jerks tend to be lost before ankle jerks. Cranial muscles are usually spared. Serum CK levels are almost always high in recessive types and are often elevated in dominant forms. The progression of disease is slow. Needle examination shows myopathic changes, and muscle biopsy is remarkable for inflammation and dystrophic changes.

MOLECULAR GENETICS

Availability of specific protein antibody markers for muscle biopsy immunohistochemistry and molecular genetic analysis varies for each LGMD, but some are commercially available. A nonprofit federally supported database for both current commercial and research testing can be found at the Web site http://www.genetests.org. Many of the entities, especially dominant ones, have one or more allelic disorders, in some cases with identical gene defects with multiple manifestations (see Table 142.3). Allelic disorders include several with isolated hyperCKemia without muscular weakness (caveolin-3, calpain-3, dysferlin, *ANO5*), some with neurogenic weakness (lamin A/C), and others with other muscle disorders such as rippling muscle disease (CAV3), autosomal dominant EDMD (lamin A/C), and distal myopathy (dysferlin, *ANO5*). The functions of the altered proteins span far wider than maintenance of the sarcolemma as initially postulated. Correlation of genetic defects and clinical manifestations is still in progress.

Autosomal Recessive Limb-Girdle Muscular Dystrophy

Now that specific proteins are recognized with varying manifestations, disorders based on the proteins rather than phenotype may emerge, as in the dystrophinopathies. Currently, the following LGMD classification is still in use (see Table 142.3).

LIMB-GIRDLE MUSCULAR DYSTROPHY 2A

Mutations in the calpain-3 (*CAPN3*) gene on chromosome 15q are among the most common causes of LGMD, and over 130 distinct mutations spanning numerous countries are known. In some populations, these mutations account for 28% to 50% of LGMD cases if sarcoglycanopathies and dystrophinopathies are excluded. The protein is a calcium-sensitive protease that is activated through autolysis. Calpain-3 is a muscle cytoskeletal regulator through cleavage of titin and filamin C. Disease severity varies from asymptomatic hyperCKemia to severe weakness. Onset ranges from 2 to 45 years; some have predominantly distal myopathy. Pelvic weakness initially sparing hip adductors and extensors, scapular winging, abdominal laxity, and contractures are characteristic. CK is moderately elevated. At present, immunostaining of calpain-3 on muscle biopsy is not reliable, and therefore, immunoblotting or Western blot is needed for a definitive diagnosis. Sequencing of the coding region is available for a genetic diagnosis.

LIMB-GIRDLE MUSCULAR DYSTROPHY 2B

Dysferlin mutations are seen in LGMD2B and this disorder is allelic with distal Miyoshi myopathy. Both forms prominently affect the gastrocnemius muscles, but the LGMD2B form progresses proximally. Onset is later than most recessive LGMDs, usually after age 15 years and occasionally much later. CK is elevated more than most LGMDs, likely because dysferlin appears to play an important role in muscle membrane repair. Muscle cell injury induces membrane patches enriched in dysferlin. Muscle immunostaining

TABLE 142.3 Limb-Girdle Muscular Dystrophies

MIM No.	Name	Map Position	Gene Product	Clinical Features	Allelic Disorders	Comment/Diagnosis Method
Autosomal Dominant						
159000	LGMD1A	5q31	Myotilin	Nasal speech, proximal weakness	Myofibrillar myopathy	Rare
159001	LGMD1B	1q11-q21	Lamin A/C	Proximal weakness, cardiac arrhythmias, and dilated cardiomyopathy	AD–EDMD; CMT2B familial lipodystrophy; cardiomyopathy; mandibuloacral dysplasia; Hutchinson–Gilford progeria	Uncommon; DNA analysis
607801	LGMD1C	3p25	Caveolin-3	HyperCKemia, calf hypertrophy, proximal weakness, muscle cramps, childhood onset	Rippling muscle disease; distal myopathy	Muscle
603511	LGMD1D	7q	Unknown	Pelvic girdle greater than shoulder girdle weakness, onset second to sixth decade	—	—
602067	LGMD1E	6q23	Unknown	Proximal weakness, dilated cardiomyopathy	—	—
608423	LGMD1F	7q32.1-q32.2	Unknown	Spanish, pelvic girdle affected before shoulder girdle, juvenile (15 yr) or adult (third or fourth decade), rimmed vacuoles	—	—
609115	LGMD1G	4q21	Unknown	Brazilian, mild proximal weakness, limited toe and finger flexion, onset 30–47 yr	—	—
613530	LGMD1H	3p25.1-p23	Unknown	Proximal arm and leg weakness, calf hypertrophy or proximal muscle atrophy, absent tendon reflexes; onset 15–50 yr	—	—
Autosomal Recessive						
253600	LGMD2A	15q15	Calpain-3	HyperCKemia, proximal weakness, scapular winging, onset 20–40 yr	—	Common DNA[a], muscle
253601	LGMD2B	2p13	Dysferlin	HyperCKemia, distal and/or pelvic girdle weakness, rare calf hypertrophy, onset 17–23 yr	Miyoshi myopathy; distal myopathy	DNA[a], muscle
253700	LGMD2C	13q12	γ-Sarcoglycan	Proximal weakness, calf hypertrophy, onset 3–15 yr	—	DNA[a], muscle
608099	LGMD2D	17q12-21	α-Sarcoglycan (adhalin)	—	—	DNA[a], muscle
604286	LGMD2E	4q12	β-Sarcoglycan	—	—	DNA[a], muscle
601287	LGMD2F	5q33-34	δ-Sarcoglycan	—	—	DNA[a], muscle
601954	LGMD2G	17q11-12	Telethonin	Proximal and distal leg weakness, proximal arm weakness, onset 9–15 yr, rimmed vacuoles	—	Rare
254110	LGMD2H	9q31-34	TRIM32	Manitoba Hutterites, facial weakness possible, proximal leg and neck weakness, onset 1–9 yr	—	Rare

(table continues on page 1242)

TABLE 142.3 Limb-Girdle Muscular Dystrophies *(continued)*

MIM No.	Name	Map Position	Gene Product	Clinical Features	Allelic Disorders	Comment/Diagnosis Method
Autosomal Recessive						
607155	LGMD2I	19q13.3	Fukutin-related protein	Proximal arm greater than leg weakness, onset 1.5–27 yr	CMD1C	Blood[a]
608807	LGMD2J	2q24.3	Titin	Finnish, proximal weakness, tibial muscular dystrophy	—	—
609308	LGMD2K	9q34.1	Protein O-mannosyl-transferase	Turkish, mild proximal greater than distal weakness, hypertrophy, cognitive and language delay, onset 1–3 yr	—	—
611307	LGMD2L	11p13-p12	Anoctamin 5	French Canadian, proximal weakness, quadriceps atrophy, muscle pain, onset 11–50 yr	—	—
611588	LGMD2M	9q31	Fukutin	Hypotonia, proximal weakness, normal cognitive development, onset in infancy	Fukuyama CMD, Walker–Warburg syndrome, dilated cardiomyopathy 1×	—
613158	LGMD2N	14q24	O-mannosyltransferase 2 (POMT2)	Hypotonia, delayed motor milestones, scapular winging	CMD-dystroglycanopathy with mental retardation B2 (MDDGB2)	—
613157	LGMD2O	1p32	Protein O-linked mannose beta 1,2-N-acetylglucosaminyl transferase (POMGnT1)	Onset by age 12 yr; scapular winging; proximal greater than distal weakness; ankle contractures	CMD (MDDGB3)	—
613818	LGMD2P	3p21	α-Dystroglycan (DAG1)	Childhood onset; cognitive delay; ankle contractures; proximal greater than distal weakness	—	—
613723	LGMD2Q	8q24	Plectin	Motor delay, especially ambulation	CMD with familial junctional epidermolysis bullosa	—
615325	LGMD2 R	2q35	Desmin	Facial, proximal muscle weakness; respiratory involvement; cardiomyopathy	—	—
615356	LGMD2 S	4q35.1	Transport protein particle complex 11 (TRAPPC11)	Facial, proximal muscle weakness; cognitive delay	—	—

[a]Commercially available. Muscle, diagnostic muscle biopsy immunostaining; DNA, genetic screening needed; blood, lymphocyte immunoblot analysis.

LGMD, limb-girdle muscular dystrophy; AD–EDMD, autosomal dominant Emery–Dreifuss muscular dystrophy; CMT2B, Charcot–Marie–Tooth type 2B; hyperCKemia, asymptomatic increased creatine kinase; TRIM32, tripartite motif protein 32 (E3–ubiquitin ligase); CMD, congenital muscular dystrophy.

or blood immunoblot for dysferlin as well as DNA sequencing of the coding region are available.

LIMB-GIRDLE MUSCULAR DYSTROPHY 2C THROUGH LIMB-GIRDLE MUSCULAR DYSTROPHY 2F (SARCOGLYCANOPATHIES)

Sarcoglycans are dystrophin-associated glycoproteins (DAGs) integral to sarcolemmal stability. The four primary protein subunits (α, β, γ, and δ) form a complex that provides support and signaling functions for the muscle membrane. These four DAGs have been implicated in specific forms of LGMD. A distinct ϵ subunit replaces α-sarcoglycan in smooth muscle and in some striated muscle cells; ϵ mutations lead to a myoclonus–dystonia syndrome, not LGMD. A mutation in any of the four main subunits typically disrupts the complex as a whole, leading to decreased function and typically loss of muscle immunostaining. α-Sarcoglycan (adhalin) is most commonly screened on muscle biopsy, but DNA analysis is needed to confirm the mutant subunit. Sequencing is commercially available for all four subunits associated with LGMD. Cases with complete complex loss manifest from 3 to 15 years of age and are typically wheelchair users by age 15 years. Partial loss delays onset until the teens or early adulthood. γ-Subunit defects are more severe, often with congenital onset. Duchenne dystrophy can result in secondary DAG deficiency, and dystrophin must be proved normal before a sarcoglycanopathy can be diagnosed by muscle biopsy. Combined mutations in these four subunits represent roughly only 10% of teen- or adult-onset cases; LGMD2D (α-sarcoglycanopathy) is most common. Associated cardiomyopathy is seen more in β and γ and less in α forms, perhaps due to vascular smooth muscle disease that causes vascular constrictions and ischemia. The LGMD, however, appears to be a primary myopathy and not a vasculopathy.

LIMB-GIRDLE MUSCULAR DYSTROPHY 2G THROUGH LIMB-GIRDLE MUSCULAR DYSTROPHY 2Q

The remaining known recessive forms are considerably rarer. LGMD2G is a very rare disorder linked to defects in *telethonin*, which is a muscle-specific protein localized to the Z-disc, associated with *titin*, and likely affects sarcomere structure. LGMD2H is a relatively mild LGMD seen in Canadian Hutterites owing to a defect in *TRIM32*, which is likely involved in targeting proteins for proteasome degradation. LGMD2I is one of a growing number of dystrophies caused by abnormal α-dystroglycan glycosylation and disruption of the link between dystroglycan and laminin. This form is a result of a defect in the fukutin-related protein (FKRP), which also causes CMD 2C, discussed later, but can cause LGMD of variable severity and age of onset. Accurate prevalence data are not yet known, but this form is relatively common in some populations. Muscle hypertrophy and cardiomyopathy may be present. LGMD2J is a rare form of LGMD also known as *tibial muscular dystrophy*; it is caused by defects in the very large *titin* gene. This sarcomeric protein has multiple proposed roles and directly interacts with numerous other proteins discussed in this section. Distal myopathy and familial dilated cardiomyopathy are other titinopathies. Few cases of LGMD2K have been described to date. This condition is associated with mutations in the *POMT1* gene encoding protein O-mannosyl-transferase. Affected individuals have early childhood onset of muscle weakness and global developmental delay with CK levels 20 to 40 times above normal. LGMD2L is due to *ANO5* mutations, which presents with late-onset leg weakness, with mean age of onset being approximately 35 years. Patients with LGMD2L have markedly elevated CK levels, typically 10 to 50 times the upper limit of normal. In the U.K. population, about 25% of LGMD cases

are due to *ANO5* mutations. LGMD2M, 2N, and 2O have defects of dystroglycan glycosylation due to mutations in *FKTN*, *POMT2*, and *POMGNT1*, respectively. In the Turkish population, an ancestral founder mutation in *PLEC* causes LGMD2Q, which presents in early childhood as muscle weakness. Other *PLEC* mutations, however, cause epidermal bullosa simplex with late-onset muscular dystrophy or myasthenic syndrome with late-onset myopathy. *PLEC* encodes a scaffold protein critical for myofiber structure.

Autosomal Dominant Limb-Girdle Muscular Dystrophy

Dominant forms are less common (10% of LGMD) but are associated with greater clinical heterogeneity.

LIMB-GIRDLE MUSCULAR DYSTROPHY 1A

LGMD1A is rare and linked to defects in *myotilin*, localized to the Z-disc near *telethonin*. Affected members are described as having a distinctive, dysarthric speech pattern. Myofibrillar myopathy also occurs with myotilin defects; overexpression in a mouse model causes both pathologies.

LIMB-GIRDLE MUSCULAR DYSTROPHY 1B

LGMD1B is a result of mutations in the LMNA gene that encodes both lamin A and lamin C, which are alternative splice forms. Mutations in this gene lead to multiple distinct phenotypes, including autosomal dominant EDMD, hypertrophic cardiomyopathy, familial partial lipodystrophy, mandibuloacral dysplasia, Hutchinson–Gilford progeria, as well as LGMD. Lamins A and C are found on the inner nuclear membrane and interact with integral nuclear membrane proteins, including *emerin*, as discussed earlier. The LGMD phenotype is relatively mild but often has significant cardiomyopathy and cardiac conduction disease similar to X-linked EDMD; some also have contractures but less severely than EDMD. To add to the heterogeneity and confusion, this gene is also mutated in a form of axonal Charcot–Marie–Tooth disease (2C).

LIMB-GIRDLE MUSCULAR DYSTROPHY 1C

Caveolins are plasma membrane vesicular invaginations important in cellular trafficking and signaling. Caveolin-3 (CAV3) is a muscle-specific caveolin-related protein in skeletal, smooth, and cardiac muscles. In addition to LGMD, mutations of this gene can produce nondystrophic rippling muscle disease, idiopathic and familial asymptomatic hyperCKemia, and a form of distal myopathy. LGMD often begins around age 5 years with cramping, mild weakness, and calf hypertrophy, but mild cases without clinical weakness are also seen. Caveolin-3 appears to interact with dysferlin, and in some patients with LGMD 2B (dysferlin), there is a secondary reduction in CAV3 levels.

LIMB-GIRDLE MUSCULAR DYSTROPHY 1D

LGMD1D (or 1E) (6q) was previously named *familial dilated cardiomyopathy with conduction disease and myopathy* and is due to mutations in the *DES* gene encoding the desmin protein. *DES* mutations more typically cause myofibrillar myopathy or dilated cardiomyopathy.

LIMB-GIRDLE MUSCULAR DYSTROPHY 1E

In two families with autosomal dominant LGMD and vacuoles in skeletal muscles, mutations have been identified in *DNAJB6*, which encodes a molecular cochaperone involved in protecting proteins from irreversible aggregation.

LIMB–GIRDLE MUSCULAR DYSTROPHY 1F

In a large Spanish family with variable juvenile to adult-onset muscular dystrophy and a sporadic LGMD patient, mutations in *TNPO3* were identified. Transportin 3 is a nuclear protein that is a member of the importin-beta/transportin family. Muscle biopsies in the Spanish patients showed abnormally enlarged nuclei.

LIMB–GIRDLE MUSCULAR DYSTROPHY 1G THROUGH LIMB–GIRDLE MUSCULAR DYSTROPHY 1H

These disorders are chromosomally mapped forms awaiting gene identification.

Oculopharyngeal muscular dystrophy (OPMD) is a late-onset autosomal dominant disorder with progressive ptosis, dysphagia, and late-onset proximal limb weakness. Autosomal recessive forms are known. Although originally recognized in French Canadian families, cases have been recognized worldwide. The bulbar onset, however, is usually confused more often with myasthenia gravis than other myopathies. Muscle filamentous intranuclear inclusions are a pathologic hallmark, but rimmed vacuoles are also prominent. The CK is normal or mildly elevated. The disease maps to 14q11.2-q13 and is caused by an expanded GCG repeat in the polyadenylation-binding protein 2 (PABP2). The disease-producing repeat number is unusually short. The normal repeat length is 6, and disease results from lengths of 7 to 13, with 9 and 10 repeats being most common. A more severe autosomal recessive phenotype with earlier onset is described in homozygous patients. *Oculodistal muscular dystrophy* is even less common than OPMD and differs in the distribution of limb weakness but has not yet been mapped.

Collagen type VI–related disorders include a phenotypic spectrum ranging from Bethlem myopathy (MIM 158810) to Ullrich CMD (MIM 254090). *Bethlem myopathy* is an autosomal dominant, progressive muscular dystrophy with onset in infancy or childhood. Contractures are prominent, but CK is only mildly elevated and, in contrast to EDMD, cardiomyopathy is not seen. *Ullrich CMD* is an autosomal recessive collagen type VI–related disorder. It is characterized by congenital hypotonia, proximal weakness and joint contractures, and hyperlaxity of distal joints. Skin biopsy analysis for collagen type VI may be diagnostic.

OTHER RARE DYSTROPHIES

Several forms of scapuloperoneal weakness with dystrophic muscle pathology are not linked to the FSHD site. Some show hyaline bodies. Autosomal dominant and recessive and X-linked–dominant inheritance patterns are described. A similar phenotype is neurogenic (scapuloperoneal muscular atrophy). Mutations in the *FHL1* gene cause X-linked dominant scapuloperoneal myopathy; desmin and myosin heavy-chain 7 gene mutations have been identified in autosomal dominant cases. Other rare discrete entities include epidermolysis bullosa simplex with late-onset muscular dystrophy linked to plectin gene mutations and desmin-related myopathy, one with a defect in the α-β crystalline gene on 11q as well as dominant and recessive forms linked to the desmin gene on 2q. Despite all of the identified genetic defects, additional forms of LGMD will be linked to yet unidentified chromosomal loci and novel pathogenic genes.

DISTAL MYOPATHIES (DISTAL MUSCULAR DYSTROPHIES)

Distal myopathies (distal muscular dystrophies) are defined by clinical manifestations in the feet and hands before proximal limb muscles are affected. As heritable diseases with features of myopathy and slow progression, they are properly considered muscular dystrophies. The distinction from hereditary neuropathies is supported by spared sensation and histologic and electrodiagnostic features of myopathy. Most distal myopathies have been assigned to different map positions, confirming the clinical differences in patterns of inheritance, onset in leg or hands, predominant leg weakness in anterior or posterior compartments, presence or absence of vacuoles, and rise in serum CK (Table 142.4).

TABLE 142.4 **Distal Myopathies**

Type	Heritance	Map/Gene Site	Phenotype	CK	Vacuoles	MIM No.
Onset after Age 40 Yr						
Welander	AD	2p13, TIA1	Hands	Normal	Sometimes	604454
Markesberry–Griggs–Udd	AD	2q31, titin	AC	Normal	Yes	600334
Onset before Age 40 Yr						
Nonaka	AR	9p1-q1, GNE	AC	Normal to 5× normal	Yes	605820
Miyoshi	AR	2p13, dysferlin	PC	Elevated 10 to 150×	No	254130
Nebulin	AR	2q23, nebulin	Toe and finger extensors	Normal	No	—
Gowers-Laing	AD	14q11.2, MYH7	AC	Normal to 3× normal	No	160500
Myopathy with anterior leg sparing	AD	7q32, filamin	Hands and legs	Normal to mild elevation	No	609524
HIBM1	AD	2q35, desmin	Legs, quadriceps	Normal to mild elevation	Yes	—

CK, creatine kinase; MIM, mendelian inheritance in man (McKusick); AD, autosomal dominant; AC, anterior compartment of legs; AR, autosomal recessive; GNE, UDP-*N*-acetylglucosamine-2-epimerase/*N*-acetylmannosamine kinase; PC, posterior compartment.

The most common form is *Welander distal myopathy* (MIM 604454), which was first described in Sweden; inheritance is autosomal dominant. Symptoms begin in adolescence or adult years and progress slowly. The legs are affected before the hands. Histologic changes are mild, but filamentous inclusions may resemble those seen in oculopharyngeal dystrophy or inclusion body myositis. Serum CK is only slightly elevated. The gene maps to chromosome 2p13 but may not be owing to the nearby dysferlin gene.

In the autosomal recessive *Nonaka* variant (MIM 605820), a vacuolar myopathy is seen, the gastrocnemius muscles are spared, and serum enzyme values are only slightly increased. Nonaka distal myopathy and hereditary inclusion body myopathy share clinical and morphologic similarities; both conditions are a result of defects in the UDP-N-acetylglucosamine 2-epimerase/N-acetylmannosamine kinase (GNE) gene. *Miyoshi* (MIM 254130) distal myopathy is also autosomal recessive but differs from Nonaka in that the histologic changes are nonspecific (without vacuoles), the gastrocnemius muscles are affected first, and serum CK values are notably high; hyperCKemia may be noted before symptomatic weakness. Miyoshi myopathy and LGMD type 2B (proximal limb weakness) are allelic, map to 2p17, and are associated with mutations in dysferlin (see Fig. 142.1). Miyoshi type 3 is due to *ANO5* mutations. Some Miyoshi families do not have mutations in either gene, which implies further locus heterogeneity. Other variants of distal myopathies have been described and more are likely to be identified.

SUGGESTED READINGS

Bachinski LL, Udd B, Meola G, et al. Confirmation of the type 2 myotonic dystrophy (CCTG)n expansion mutation in patients with proximal myotonic myopathy/proximal myotonic dystrophy of different European origins: a single shared haplotype indicates an ancestral founder effect. *Am J Hum Genet.* 2003;73:835–848.

Baker NL, Mörgelin M, Pace RA, et al. Molecular consequences of dominant Bethlem myopathy collagen VI mutations. *Ann Neurol.* 2007;62(4):390–405.

Beltran-Valero de Bernabe D, Currier S, Steinbrecher A, et al. Mutations in the O-mannosyltransferase gene POMT1 give rise to the severe neuronal migration disorder Walker–Warburg syndrome. *Am J Hum Genet.* 2002;71:1033–1043.

Betz RC, Schoser BGH, Kasper D, et al. Mutations in CAV3 cause mechanical hyperirritability of skeletal muscle in rippling muscle disease. *Nat Genet.* 2001;28:218–219.

Bolduc V, Marlow G, Boycott KM, et al. Recessive mutations in the putative calcium-activated chloride channel anoctamin 5 cause proximal LGMD2L and distal MMD3 muscular dystrophies. *Am J Hum Genet.* 2010;86(2):213–221.

Bonne G, Di Barletta MR, Varnous S, et al. Mutations in the gene encoding lamin A/C cause autosomal dominant Emery-Dreifuss muscular dystrophy. *Nat Genet.* 1999;21:285–288.

Bönnemann CG, Wang CH, Quijano-Roy S, et al. Diagnostic approach to the congenital muscular dystrophies. *Neuromuscul Disord.* 2014;24(4):289–311.

Brais B. Oculopharyngeal muscular dystrophy. *Handb Clin Neurol.* 2011;101:181–192.

Brockington M, Yuva Y, Prandini P, et al. Mutations in fukutin-related protein gene (FKRP) identify limb-girdle muscular dystrophy 2I as a milder allelic variant of congenital muscular dystrophy MDC1C. *Hum Mol Genet.* 2001;10:2851–2859.

Brown SC, Torelli S, Brockington M, et al. Abnormalities in alpha-dystroglycan expression in MDC1C and LGMD2I muscular dystrophies. *Am J Pathol.* 2004;164:727–737.

Bushby K, Muntoni F, Bourke JP. 107th ENMC international workshop: the management of cardiac involvement in muscular dystrophy and myotonic dystrophy. 7th–9th June 2002, Naarden, the Netherlands. *Neuromuscul Disord.* 2003;13:166–172.

Campbell C, Sherlock R, Jacob P, et al. Congenital myotonic dystrophy; assisted ventilation duration and outcome. *Pediatrics.* 2004;113:811–816.

Campbell KP. Adhalin gene mutations and autosomal recessive limb-girdle muscular dystrophy. *Ann Neurol.* 1995;38:353–354.

Carbone I, Bruno C, Sotgia F, et al. Mutation in the CAV3 gene causes partial caveolin-3 deficiency and hyperCKemia. *Neurology.* 2000;54:1373–1376.

Chaouch M, Allal Y, De Sandre-Giovannoli A, et al. The phenotypic manifestations of autosomal recessive axonal Charcot-Marie-Tooth due to a mutation in lamin A/C gene. *Neuromuscul Disord.* 2003;13:60–67.

Chou FL, Angelini C, Daentl D, et al. Calpain III mutation analysis of a heterogeneous limb girdle muscular dystrophy population. *Neurology.* 1999;52:1015–1020.

Connolly AM, Florence JM, Cradock MM, et al. One year outcome of boys with Duchenne muscular dystrophy using the Bayley-III scales of infant and toddler development. *Pediatr Neurol.* 2014;50(6):557–563.

Danek A, Witt TN, Stockmann HB, et al. Normal dystrophin in McLeod myopathy. *Ann Neurol.* 1990;28(5):720–722.

Day JW, Ranum LP. RNA pathogenesis of the myotonic dystrophies. *Neuromuscul Disord.* 2005;15:5–16.

De Sandre-Giovannoli A, Chaouch M, Kozlov S, et al. Homozygous defects in LMNA, encoding lamin A/C nuclear-envelope proteins, cause autosomal recessive axonal neuropathy in human (Charcot-Marie-Tooth disorder type 2) and mouse. *Am J Hum Genet.* 2002;70:726–736.

Eagle M, Baudouin SV, Chandler C, et al. Survival in Duchenne muscular dystrophy: improvements in life expectancy since 1967 and the impact of home nocturnal ventilation. *Neuromuscul Disord.* 2002;12:926–929.

Fairclough RJ, Wood MJ, Davies KE. Therapy for Duchenne muscular dystrophy: renewed optimism from genetic approaches. *Nat Rev Genet.* 2013;14:373–387.

Fanin M, Pegoraro E, Matsuda-Asada C, et al. Calpain-3 and dysferlin protein screening in patients with limb-girdle dystrophy and myopathy. *Neurology.* 2001;56:660–665.

Fatkin D, MacRae C, Sasaki T, et al. Missense mutations in the rod domain of the lamin A/C gene as causes of dilated cardiomyopathy and conduction-system disease. *N Engl J Med.* 1999;341:1715–1724.

Fischer D, Aurino S, Nigro V, et al. On symptomatic heterozygous alpha-sarcoglycan gene mutation carriers. *Ann Neurol.* 2003;54:674–678.

Flanigan KM. Duchenne and Becker muscular dystrophies. *Neurol Clin.* 2014;32:671–688.

Frosk P, Weiler T, Nylen E, et al. Limb-girdle muscular dystrophy type 2H associated with mutation in TRIM32, a putative E3-ubiquitin-ligase gene. *Am J Hum Genet.* 2002;70:663–672.

Gamez J, Navarro C, Andreu AL, et al. Autosomal dominant limb-girdle muscular dystrophy. A large kindred with evidence for anticipation. *Neurology.* 2001;56:450–454.

Gueneau L, Bertrand AT, Jais JP, et al. Mutations of the FHL1 gene cause Emery-Dreifuss muscular dystrophy. *Am J Hum Genet.* 2009;85(3):338–353.

Gussoni E, Blau HM, Kunkel LM. The fate of individual myoblasts after transplantation into muscles of DMD patients. *Nat Med.* 1997;3:970–977.

Hackman P, Sarparanta J, Lehtinen S, et al. Welander distal myopathy is caused by a mutation in the RNA-binding protein TIA1. *Ann Neurol.* 2013;73(4):500–509.

Harper PS. *Myotonic Dystrophy.* 3rd ed. London, United Kingdom: WB Saunders; 2001.

Hayashi YK. Membrane-repair machinery and muscular dystrophy. *Lancet.* 2003;362:843–844.

Ho M, Chelly J, Carter N, et al. Isolation of the gene for McLeod syndrome that encodes a novel membrane transport protein. *Cell.* 1994;77(6):869–880.

Hoffman EP, McNally EM. Exon-skipping therapy: a roadblock, detour, or bump in the road? *Sci Transl Med.* 2014;6:230.

Jobsis GJ, Boers JM, Barth PG, et al. Bethlem myopathy: a slowly progressive congenital muscular dystrophy with contractures. *Brain.* 1999;122:649–655.

Kanadia RN, Johnstone KA, Mankodi A, et al. A muscleblind knockout model for myotonic dystrophy. *Science.* 2003;302:1978–1980.

Katz JS, Rando TA, Barohn RJ, et al. Late-onset distal muscular dystrophy affecting the posterior calves. *Muscle Nerve.* 2003;28:443–448.

Kissel JT, McDermott MP, Mendell JR, et al. FSH-DY Group. Randomized, double-blind, placebo-controlled trial of albuterol in facioscapulohumeral dystrophy. *Neurology.* 2001;57:1434–1440.

Liang WC, Mitsuhashi H, Keduka E, et al. TMEM43 mutations in Emery-Dreifuss muscular dystrophy-related myopathy. *Ann Neurol.* 2011;69(6):1005–1013.

Lemmers RJ, van der Wielen MJ, Bakker E, et al. Somatic mosaicism in FSHD often goes undetected. *Ann Neurol.* 2004;55:845–850.

Logigian EL, Moxley RT IV, Blood CL, et al. Leukocyte CTG repeat length correlates with severity of myotonia in myotonic dystrophy type 1. *Neurology.* 2004;62:1081–1089.

Mankodi A, Teng-Umnuay P, Krym M, et al. Ribonuclear inclusions in skeletal muscle in myotonic dystrophy types 1 and 2. *Ann Neurol.* 2003;54:760–768.

Mankodi A, Thornton CA. Myotonic syndromes. *Curr Opin Neurol.* 2002;15:545–552.

Maselli RA, Arredondo J, Cagney O, et al. Congenital myasthenic syndrome associated with epidermolysis bullosa caused by homozygous mutations in PLEC1 and CHRNE. *Clin Genet.* 2011;80(5):444–451.

Masny PS, Bengtsson U, Chung SA, et al. Localization of 4q35.2 to the nuclear periphery: is FSHD a nuclear envelope disease? *Hum Mol Genet.* 2004;13:1857–1871.

Melia MJ, Kubota A, Ortolano S, et al. Limb-girdle muscular dystrophy 1F is caused by a microdeletion in the transportin 3 gene. *Brain.* 2013;136:1508–1517.

Meola G, Sansone V, Marinou K, et al. Proximal myotonic myopathy: a syndrome with a favourable prognosis? *J Neurol Sci.* 2002;193:89–96.

Meola G, Sansone V, Perani D, et al. Executive dysfunction and avoidant personality trait in myotonic dystrophy type 1 (DM-1) and in proximal myotonic myopathy (PROMM/DM-2). *Neuromuscul Disord.* 2003;13:813–821.

Mercuri E, Poppe M, Quinlivan R, et al. Extreme variability of phenotype in patients with an identical missense mutation in the lamin A/C gene: from congenital onset with severe phenotype to milder classic Emery-Dreifuss variant. *Arch Neurol.* 2004;61:690–694.

Minetti C, Sotgia F, Bruno C, et al. Mutations in the caveolin-3 gene cause autosomal dominant limb-girdle muscular dystrophy. *Nat Genet.* 1998;18:365–368.

Miske LJ, Hickey EM, Kolb SM, et al. Use of the mechanical in-exsufflator in pediatric patients with neuromuscular disease and impaired cough. *Chest.* 2004;125:1406–1412.

Moreira ES, Wiltshire TJ, Faulkner G, et al. Limb-girdle muscular dystrophy type 2G is caused by mutations in the gene encoding the sarcomeric protein telethonin. *Nat Genet.* 2000;24:163–166.

Muchir A, Bonne G, van der Kooi AJ, et al. Identification of mutations in the gene encoding lamins A/C in autosomal dominant limb girdle muscular dystrophy with atrioventricular conduction disturbances (LGMD1B). *Hum Mol Genet.* 2000;9:1453–1459.

Muntoni F, Fisher I, Morgan JE, et al. Steroids in Duchenne muscular dystrophy: from clinical trials to genomic research. *Neuromuscul Disord.* 2002;12(suppl 1):S162–S165.

Nigro V, Savarese M. Genetic basis of limb-girdle muscular dystrophies: the 2014 update. *Acta Myol.* 2014;33:1–12.

Nonaka I, Noguchi S, Nishino I. Distal myopathy with rimmed vacuoles and hereditary inclusion body myopathy. *Curr Neurol Neurosci Rep.* 2005;5(1):61–65.

Quinzii C, Vu TH, Min C, et al. X-linked dominant scapuloperoneal myopathy is due to a mutation in the gene encoding four-and-a-half LIM protein 1. *Am J Hum Genet.* 2008;82:208–213.

Rafael-Fortney JA, Chimanji NS, Schill KE, et al. Early treatment with lisinopril and spironolactone preserves cardiac and skeletal muscle in Duchenne muscular dystrophy mice. *Circulation.* 2011;124(5):582–588.

Rando TA. The dystrophin-glycoprotein complex, cellular signaling, and the regulation of cell survival in the muscular dystrophies. *Muscle Nerve.* 2001;24:1575–1594.

Sarkozy A, Hicks D, Hudson J, et al. ANO5 gene analysis in a large cohort of patients with anoctaminopathy: confirmation of male prevalence and high occurrence of the common exon 5 gene mutation. *Hum Mutat.* 2013;34(8):1111–1118.

Statlan J, Tawil R. Facioscapulohumeral muscular dystrophy. *Neurol Clin.* 2014;32:721–728.

Takahashi T, Aoki M, Tateyama M, et al. Dysferlin mutations in Japanese Miyoshi myopathy: relationship to phenotype. *Neurology.* 2003;60:1799–1804.

Takeda S, Kondo M, Sasaki J, et al. Fukutin is required for maintenance of muscle integrity, cortical histiogenesis and normal eye development. *Hum Mol Genet.* 2003;12:1449–1459.

Talbot K, Stradling J, Crosby J, et al. Reduction in excess daytime sleepiness by modafinil in patients with myotonic dystrophy. *Neuromuscul Disord.* 2003;13:357–364.

Tawil R, Van Der Maarel SM, Tapscott SJ. Facioscapulohumeral muscular dystrophy. The path to consensus on pathophysiology. *Skelet Muscle.* 2014;4:12.

Tonini MM, Passos-Bueno MR, Cerqueira A, et al. Asymptomatic carriers and gender differences in facioscapulohumeral muscular dystrophy (FSHD). *Neuromuscul Disord.* 2004;14:33–38.

Trip J, Drost G, van Engelen BG, Faber CG. Drug treatment for myotonia. *Cochrane Database Syst Rev.* 2006;1:CD004762.

Tupler R, Gabellini D. Molecular basis of facioscapulohumeral muscular dystrophy. *Cell Mol Life Sci.* 2004;61:557–566.

Udd B. Molecular biology of distal muscular dystrophies—sarcomeric proteins on top. *Biochim Biophys Acta.* 2007;1772:145–158.

Udd B, Meola G, Krahe R, et al. 140th ENMC International Workshop: myotonic dystrophy DM2/PROMM and other myotonic dystrophies with guidelines on management. *Neuromuscul Disord.* 2006;16:403–413.

von Tell D, Bruder CE, Anderson LV, et al. Refined mapping of the Welander distal myopathy region on chromosome 2p13 positions the new candidate region telomeric of the DYSF locus. *Neurogenetics.* 2003;4:173–177.

Wallgren-Pettersson C, Bushby K, Mellies U, et al; ENMC. 117th ENMC workshop: ventilatory support in congenital neuromuscular disorders—congenital myopathies, congenital muscular dystrophies, congenital myotonic dystrophy and SMA (II) 4–6 April 2003, Naarden, The Netherlands. *Neuromuscul Disord.* 2004;14:56–69.

Wheeler TM, Thornton CA. Myotonic dystrophy: RNA-mediated muscle disease. *Curr Opin Neurol.* 2007;20:572–576.

Wohlgemuth M, van der Kooi EL, van Kesteren RG, et al. Ventilatory support in facioscapulohumeral muscular dystrophy. *Neurology.* 2004;63:176–178.

Woodman SE, Sotgia F, Galbiati F, et al. Caveolinopathies: mutations in caveolin-3 cause four distinct autosomal dominant muscular diseases. *Neurology.* 2004;62:538–543.

Yan J, Feng J, Buzin CH, et al. Three-tiered noninvasive diagnosis in 96% of patients with Duchenne muscular dystrophy (DMD). *Hum Mutat.* 2004;23:203–204.

Zhang Q, Bethmann C, Worth NF, et al. Nesprin-1 and -2 are involved in the pathogenesis of Emery Dreifuss muscular dystrophy and are critical for nuclear envelope integrity. *Hum Mol Genet.* 2007;16(23):2816–2833.

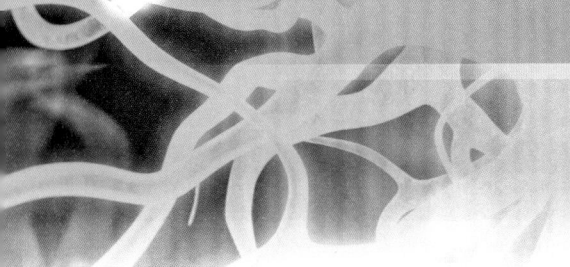

Seizures in Children 143

James J. Riviello Jr and Douglas R. Nordli Jr

INTRODUCTION

A seizure is a paroxysmal neurologic event resulting from excessive central nervous system (CNS) excitation, the hypersynchronous neuronal discharge. Management begins with evaluating the event, formulating a differential diagnosis, selecting appropriate diagnostic studies, and determining treatment, including the need for anticonvulsant medications. Seizures may be precipitated by an acute CNS insult, such as infection, stroke, intracranial hemorrhage, or traumatic brain injury; may result from a primary systemic disorder with secondary effects on the CNS, such as hypoglycemia; or occur with epilepsy, a condition in which recurrent, unprovoked seizures occur. However, many paroxysmal disorders in children are also referred to as *seizures* but are more properly called *nonepileptic paroxysmal events* (NEPE). It is important to consider the differential diagnosis of a seizure because NEPE are not treated with anticonvulsant medications. Seizures and epilepsy are similar in adults and children but certain seizure types and epilepsy syndromes are either peculiar to or more common in children.

The evaluation must determine if the seizure results from an acute CNS insult or if it is the initial presentation of epilepsy. A specific treatment may be needed if the seizure occurs during an intercurrent illness. Benign febrile seizures are frequently encountered in children (see the following text), but a seizure with fever (fever lowers seizure threshold) may occur at any age. In discussing seizures and epilepsy, several terms require definition: seizure, epilepsy, epilepsy syndrome, focal onset, generalized onset, status epilepticus, and refractory status epilepticus (Table 143.1).

EPIDEMIOLOGY

The incidence of unprovoked seizures varies from 42.3 to 61.0 per 100,000 population per year and the incidence of acute symptomatic seizures varies from 20 to 39.0 per 100,000 population per year. In the developed world, the annual incidence of epilepsy is about 46 per 100,000 population per year.

For specific childhood epilepsy syndromes, childhood absence epilepsy is the most common syndrome, occurring in 12% overall in several series, followed by benign rolandic epilepsy, 11.5%, and childhood epilepsy with occipital discharges, 9% (now Panayiotopoulos syndrome). In this series, myoclonic atonic epilepsy occurred in 6%; infantile spasms, 4.1%; and the epileptic encephalopathies, electrical status epilepticus of sleep, 1.1%; and Landau–Kleffner syndrome or epileptic aphasia, 0.5%.

CLASSIFICATION

The classification of the seizure and the actual epilepsy syndrome guides management. The first step is to consider the differential diagnosis because not all events referred to as seizures are epileptic events, such as the NEPE (Table 143.2). The seizure refers to

TABLE 143.1 Terms from International League Against Epilepsy Task Force on Classification and Terminology

Seizure: sudden clinical event with outward change in neurologic function; etiology from the Greek, "to take hold"

Ictus: a neurologic event, including stroke, epileptic seizure, or an anoxic event

Convulsion: excessive, abnormal muscle contractions, usually bilateral, which may be sustained or interrupted

Epileptic seizure: refers to the clinical manifestations of an epileptic pathophysiology (transient hypersynchronous neuronal discharge), usually self-limited, neuronal activity. Adding the descriptor epileptic to seizure clearly signifies an epileptic etiology separating an epileptic from a nonepileptic seizure.

Epilepsy refers to (1) an **epileptic disorder:** a chronic neurologic condition characterized by recurrent epileptic seizures, and (2) **epilepsies:** conditions involving chronic recurrent epileptic seizures.

Epileptic syndromes: a complex of signs and symptoms that define a unique epilepsy condition

Focal: indicates a seizure in which the initial clinical manifestations suggest activation of only one part of a cerebral hemisphere

Febrile seizures: refers to a seizure that occurs in association of a febrile illness
   Simple febrile seizures are isolated, brief generalized convulsions.
   Complex febrile seizures are those that are focal or followed by a postictal deficit (Todd paresis), last >10–15 min, or occur more than once within 24 h.

Generalized: indicates a seizure whose initial clinical manifestations are consistent with more than minimal involvement of both cerebral hemispheres

Status epilepticus: The operational definition of status epilepticus, used for treatment, is a seizure or recurrent seizure without return of consciousness lasting >5 min.

Refractory status epilepticus is now defined as failure to respond to the first two antiepileptic drugs used.

the actual clinical manifestations and the epilepsy syndrome is the constellation of signs and symptoms that cluster around the seizure type. Three major classification systems are used: (1) the location of the seizure onset in the brain, either focal or generalized; (2) the seizure duration; and (3) seizure etiology.

The International League Against Epilepsy (ILAE) developed the International Classification of Epileptic Seizures (ICES), last revised in 2010. The ICES classifies the seizure type, referred to as the *semiology*, the *signs*, and the *epilepsy syndrome*. Seizures are divided into the location of the cortical onset: either focal or

TABLE 143.2	Differential Diagnosis of Seizures

Syncope, convulsive syncope, pallid infantile syncope, breath-holding attacks

Cardiac arrhythmias (prolonged QT syndrome)

Narcolepsy, cataplexy, hypersomnia

Hyperekplexia (startle disease)

Rage attacks, episodic dyscontrol, panic attacks

Migraines, especially benign paroxysmal vertigo, acute confusional state, basilar artery migraine

Movement disorders, paroxysmal dystonia, paroxysmal choreoathetosis, tics (especially ocular tics)

Munchausen syndrome, Munchausen by proxy

Night terrors, somnambulism, parasomnias

Sandifer syndrome, gastroesophageal reflux, esophageal spasm

Ocular movements (nystagmus, spasms, spasmus nutans, ocular tics)

Infantile self-gratification

Nonepileptic seizures (pseudoseizures)

Transient ischemic events

generalized. A focal seizure is defined as one whose initial clinical manifestations indicate activation of only a focal area, or one part of the cortex, or in other words, the initial activation of a focal group of neurons. A generalized seizure is one with "more than minimal involvement of both cerebral hemispheres" or in other words, the initial activation of neurons throughout both hemispheres. A generalized seizure may not simultaneously involve every neuron. This is an important dichotomy because the clinical manifestations of the seizure depend on where the seizure starts and where it spreads and the antiepileptic drugs (AEDs) used to prevent seizure recurrence typically have efficacy for either focal or generalized seizures. The definitions of focal or generalized were revised to emphasize the concept of epileptic networks.

Seizure duration is important because aggressive treatment is needed for longer seizures. Status epilepticus, defined as a prolonged seizure lasting greater than 30 minutes or serial seizures without return of consciousness for 30 minutes, is a medical emergency that requires immediate termination. Five minutes of a continuous seizure or serial seizures without return of consciousness is the operational definition of status epilepticus for the purpose of treatment. Most seizures usually have a short duration, lasting less than several minutes, but status epilepticus is more likely to occur in the critically ill. The staging of status epilepticus has been used to guide treatment (Table 143.3), although the recent guideline from the Neurocritical Care Society defines refractory status epilepticus as failure to respond to the first two AEDs given rather than a stage of status epilepticus.

The third system classifies seizures and epilepsy by etiology, dividing them into symptomatic, cryptogenic, and idiopathic (Table 143.4). A symptomatic seizure is one for which the exact cause is identified. A cryptogenic seizure is one in which an underlying specific etiology is presumed because the neurologic state is abnormal (abnormal development or examination) but is not yet identified. The idiopathic seizure is one in which the etiology is not known, meaning that it arises spontaneously or from an obscure

TABLE 143.3	Stages of Status Epilepticus

Incipient stage (0–5 min)

Early stage (5–30 min)
Special circumstances of the early stage: situations that need immediate seizure control

Transition stage (from early to late; time is variable, depends on underlying condition; e.g., a patient with a brain tumor and increased intracranial pressure may have no remaining compensatory mechanisms)

Late stage (established) (30–60 min)

Refractory stage (>60 min)

Postictal stage

unknown cause. Many of the seizures identified as idiopathic are now identified as being associated with an abnormal gene or a channelopathy. A patient presenting with a new-onset seizure or status epilepticus from a specific cause would have an acute symptomatic seizure (review paper). If a past known CNS insult has caused the seizure, this is called a *remote symptomatic seizure*. However, a patient with epilepsy may have a seizure precipitated by an acute illness, referred to as a *remote symptomatic seizure with an acute precipitant* or an *acute on chronic seizure*.

The 2010 classification revision replaces the categories symptomatic; cryptogenic; and idiopathic with genetic, structural/metabolic, and unknown. The distinction between complex partial and simple partial seizures is also eliminated. However, it is important to be familiar with both systems because the terms symptomatic, cryptogenic, and idiopathic are still in common clinical use.

SPECIFIC PEDIATRIC SEIZURES AND EPILEPSY SYNDROMES

Space limitations preclude an all-inclusive review of pediatric seizures and pediatric epilepsy syndromes. We shall therefore summarize the seizure types and epilepsy syndromes that are peculiar

TABLE 143.4	Classification of Seizure Etiology

Symptomatic seizure: The exact cause of the seizure has been identified.

Cryptogenic seizure: A specific etiology is presumed because the neurologic state is abnormal (abnormal development or examination) but has not yet identified.

Idiopathic seizure: There is no identifiable cause other than a possible hereditary predisposition.

Genetic cause: The concept of genetic epilepsy is that as best understood, the epilepsy is the result of a known genetic defect.

Structural/metabolic cause: There is a distinct structural or metabolic condition or disease that has been demonstrated to be associated with a substantially increased risk of developing epilepsy: stroke, trauma, infection.

Unknown cause: The nature of the underlying cause is not known.

to the younger child. These include febrile seizures, both benign and complex, the most common seizure type and syndrome in childhood, and the severe childhood epilepsy syndromes including infantile spasms and the epileptic encephalopathies. These benign and severe syndromes are distinct from the seizures and epilepsy syndromes that occur in the adult.

FEBRILE SEIZURES

The ILAE defines a febrile seizure as "a seizure in association with a febrile illness in the absence of a CNS infection or acute electrolyte imbalance in children older than 1 month of age without prior afebrile seizures." Febrile seizures are the most common cause of convulsions in children: Between 2% and 4% of all children in the United States and Europe and 9% to 10% of children in Japan have at least one febrile seizure before age 5 years. Hauser (1994) estimated that in 1990, there were 100,000 cases of newly diagnosed febrile seizures in the United States. Genetic predisposition is an important factor. Overall, siblings and offspring of affected probands have a two- to threefold increased risk of seizures with fever. Based on studies of large families with simple febrile seizures, various genetic loci have been mapped. The literature on the genetics of febrile seizures is substantial and it continues to grow. Linkage analysis has implicated many different chromosomes including 1q, 2q, 2p, 5q, 6q, 8q, 12q, 19p, and 19q. An important linkage has been with genes residing on 2q, which is the location of sodium channel genes, including SCN1A. Recently, another gene, SEZ-6, located on chromosome 17q, has been implicated. Some families have a susceptibility to febrile seizures that persists to an unusually late age, and some of these family members later develop epilepsy. These traits are inherited in an autosomal dominant fashion, and the condition has been termed *genetic epilepsy febrile seizures plus* (GEFS+). Mutations in the voltage-gated sodium channel genes SCN1A, SCN1B, and SCN2A are involved as well as the GABRG2 gene.

About two-thirds of febrile seizures occur in the first 24 hours of illness. Indeed, in some children, the seizure is the first indication of illness. Febrile seizures are subdivided into simple and complex types. Simple febrile seizures are most common, representing 80% to 90% of all febrile seizures. Simple febrile seizures are isolated, brief generalized convulsions. Parents commonly report diffuse stiffening followed by rhythmic jerking of all limbs lasting less than 1 to 2 minutes. Complex febrile seizures are those that are focal or followed by a postictal deficit (Todd paresis), last more than 10 to 15 minutes, or occur more than once within 24 hours. Factors predisposing to febrile status epilepticus include a younger age (mean age 15 months vs. 19 months for benign febrile seizures), a lower temperature (102.3°F vs. 103.6°F), female gender, first-degree family history of febrile seizures, and structural temporal lobe abnormalities.

About one-third of children with febrile seizures have more than one attack. Independent risk factors for recurrence are first febrile seizure before the age of 18 months, a family history of febrile seizures, a low peak temperature, and a short duration of fever before the seizure. Febrile seizures represent acute symptomatic seizures, also referred to as *reactive seizures*, and even when recurrent, do not warrant the designation of epilepsy. However, they do have an epileptic pathophysiology.

Children who have an isolated febrile seizure have a risk of developing epilepsy that is similar to that of the general population. This risk increases if simple febrile seizures recur (2% to 3%), if the febrile seizures are complex, there is a family history of afebrile seizures, or neurologic abnormalities were detected before the first febrile convulsion (10% to 13%). When all three features of complex febrile seizures are present (prolonged, focal, repeated), the risk of subsequent epilepsy may be as high as 49%. Mortality is not increased in children with febrile seizures who are neurologically normal.

Simple febrile seizures have not been associated with, nor do they lead to, mental retardation, low IQ, poor school achievement, or behavioral problems. Most studies have also failed to demonstrate any cognitive or behavioral consequences of complex febrile seizures, although some differences have been reported. In children with prolonged febrile convulsions, nonverbal intelligence measures may be slightly lower compared with children with simple febrile seizures and normal controls. Children with complex febrile seizures are also more likely to require special schooling than those with simple febrile seizures.

Whether prolonged febrile seizures cause mesial temporal sclerosis and refractory partial seizures is controversial. Large prospective studies have failed to find an association, but experience in adult epilepsy surgical centers suggests otherwise because many adults with mesial temporal sclerosis have had a prolonged febrile convulsion as a child. Furthermore, magnetic resonance imaging (MRI) in some children with prolonged febrile seizures has shown acute changes in the mesial temporal region that progress over time to mesial temporal sclerosis. There is accumulating evidence that febrile status epilepticus may have long-term consequences. This issue is currently being studied in the United States in a prospective multicenter research effort. The first phase consists of identifying the patients and biomarkers and the next phase will identify who ultimately develops mesial temporal sclerosis.

There are several epilepsy syndromes in pediatric epileptology, besides benign febrile seizures, that must be included: infantile spasms, now called *epileptic spasms*, and epileptic encephalopathy and electrical status epilepticus of sleep with its two major epilepsy syndromes: Landau–Kleffner syndrome and the continuous spikes and waves of sleep. Genetics is very important in many of the epileptic encephalopathies.

INFANTILE SPASMS, WEST SYNDROME

Infantile spasms are an age-dependent epileptic syndrome characterized by the triad myoclonic or tonic seizures, hypsarrhythmia, and mental retardation, referred to as *West syndrome*. The peak onset is between 4 and 7 months and always before 12 months of age. The current classification system now uses the term *epileptic spasms* because spasms may continue or develop after infancy.

Epileptic spasms are divided into symptomatic, cryptogenic, and idiopathic forms. Symptomatic epileptic spasms are secondary to a known neurologic disorder, such as tuberous sclerosis; cryptogenic refers to a suspected but not definitely identified neurologic disorder; idiopathic refers to a case in which no specific disorder has been identified. The etiology must be identified because there are treatable causes and prognosis is worse when the spasms are either symptomatic as opposed to cryptogenic or idiopathic.

The spasms themselves consist of sudden tonic and myoclonic phenomena, including brief head nods, with quick extension and flexion movements of the trunk, arms, and legs, occurring in clusters and especially during transitions from sleeping to awaking. These are also described as flexor, extensor, or mixed. The actual spasms may resolve, but other seizure types occur later.

The classic interictal electroencephalogram (EEG) finding is the hypsarrhythmia pattern, which refers to the high-voltage, disorganized EEG background with multifocal spike and sharp waves. The ictal pattern typically consists of a high-amplitude vertex slow wave, the electrodecremental event (sudden EEG suppression lasting for several seconds), or fast activity and high-voltage spikes or polyspikes and slow waves.

Treatment for epileptic spasms has typically been with steroids or vigabatrin. The American Academy of Neurology (AAN) and Child Neurology Society practice parameter from 2004 concluded that ACTH is probably effective and that vigabatrin was possibly effective for infantile spasms associated with tuberous sclerosis [**Level 1**].[1] A United Kingdom study showed that oral prednisolone was possibly effective.

EPILEPTIC ENCEPHALOPATHY

The ILAE defines an epileptic encephalopathy as a condition in which:

> *The epileptic activity itself may contribute to severe cognitive and behavioral impairments above and beyond what might be expected from the underlying pathology alone (such as a cortical malformation), and that these may worsen over time. Certain syndromes may be referred to as epileptic encephalopathies, but the encephalopathic effects of seizures and epilepsy may potentially occur in association with any form of epilepsy (Berg et al., 2010).*

Electrical status epilepticus of sleep is the term used to describe the extreme form of sleep-activated EEG activity: a spike-wave index (SWI), the number of seconds of non–rapid eye movement (NREM) sleep with spikes/the number of seconds of NREM sleep. The Landau–Kleffner syndrome (LKS) and epileptic encephalopathy with continuous spike and wave during sleep (CSWS) are two of these epileptic encephalopathies that may have electrical status epilepticus of sleep (Fig. 143.1). LKS consists of an acquired epileptic aphasia, typically starting with a receptive aphasia in which the patient first doesn't understand language and then loses expressive language. Children with CSWS typically have seizures, but the hallmark is regression in cognitive functioning and behavior, but not primarily language, as occurs in LKS.

INITIAL MANAGEMENT

Evaluation depends in part on the setting. Is the seizure an acute, new-onset seizure, with the child admitted to the emergency department or is the family reporting the seizure later in an outpatient visit? With an acute presentation, management starts with initial patient stabilization, starting with the airway, breathing, and circulation (ABCs), and then assessing whether the child is acutely ill. Persistent altered awareness could indicate the postictal state or nonconvulsive status epilepticus, with emergent EEG needed to differentiate these.

The specific treatable causes for seizures must always be considered in the first-time seizure, especially in infants and younger children who have a greater incidence of symptomatic seizures. Meningitis and encephalitis must always be excluded, especially in the febrile infant, in whom the classic signs of meningitis may not occur. Fever itself may reduce the seizure threshold in infants and young children, as in the benign febrile seizures.

DIAGNOSTIC EVALUATION

The history and physical examination are important [**Level 1**].[2] Has there been fever, vomiting, diarrhea, or recent trauma? The physical examination includes both a general and neurologic examination, paying particular attention to signs of increased intracranial pressure, such as papilledema, herniation, or focality. For febrile seizures, the diagnosis is made by excluding other possible causes of convulsions, such as meningitis, metabolic abnormalities, or structural brain lesions. Depending on the clinical appearance of the child and the clinician's experience, laboratory tests are not always necessary. Usually, a clinically identifiable illness such as otitis media, upper respiratory infection, or gastroenteritis is present. Fever after immunization may also trigger a febrile seizure. Any suspicion of meningitis, however, mandates lumbar puncture. The typical indicators of meningeal irritation, such as nuchal rigidity and the Brudzinski sign, are not reliable in young infants. Practice guidelines of the American Academy of Pediatrics (1996, 2011) recommend that lumbar puncture be strongly considered if the child is younger than 12 months or if aged between 12 and 18 months, especially if the child has not been immunized or has been pretreated with antibiotics [**Level 1**].[3,4] Although a pleocytosis may occur with a seizure, especially status epilepticus, in 200 children with pure febrile status epilepticus, the cerebrospinal fluid (CSF) cell count was less than 3 in 85%.

ELECTROENCEPHALOGRAPHY

If the seizure has focal features, or if the examination elicits focal neurologic abnormalities, brain imaging is necessary. EEG is not useful in children with simple febrile seizures because it does not provide information regarding either the risk for recurrence of febrile seizures or later development of epilepsy. The role of EEG in the evaluation of children with complex febrile seizures, including febrile status epilepticus, is not yet fully determined.

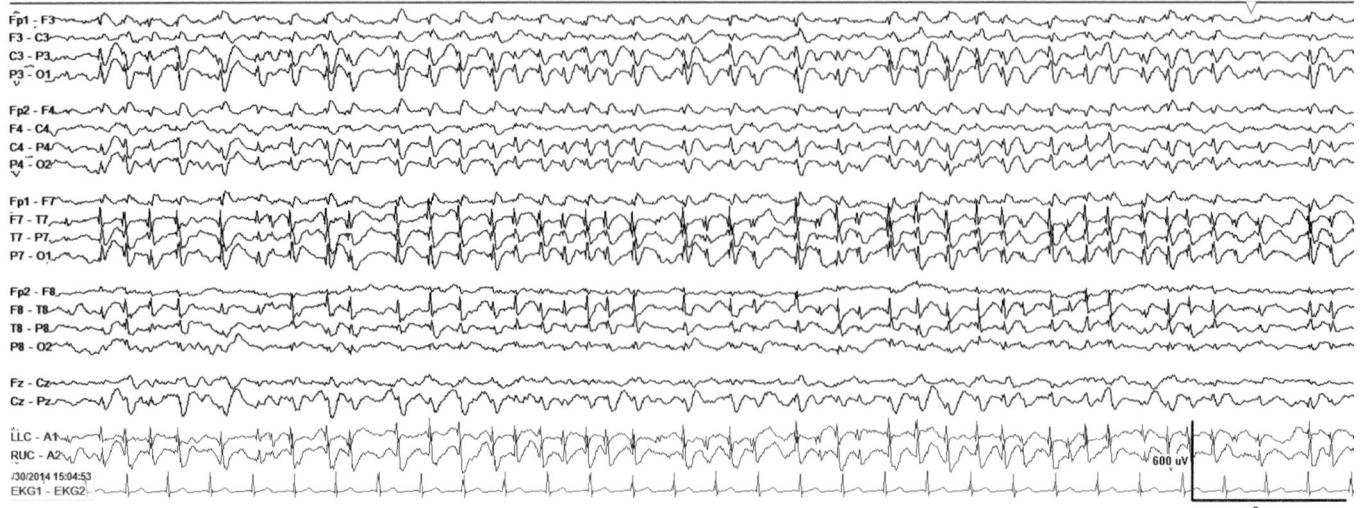

FIGURE 143.1 EEG of electrical status epilepticus of sleep.

The EEG is especially useful in the evaluation and management of seizures and epilepsy syndromes. The AAN practice parameter in 2000 for evaluating a first nonfebrile seizure in children does recommend a routine EEG [**Level 1**].[2] There is controversy regarding the need for EEG after a first afebrile seizure, but EEG findings may help differentiate an epileptic from a nonepileptic event. Syncope can be associated with myoclonus and various motor movements that are thought to be seizures, and cardiac disorders such as the prolonged QT syndrome may present with a "seizure." However, a normal EEG does not exclude the diagnosis of epilepsy, and an abnormal EEG does not, in itself, establish a diagnosis of epilepsy. In a longitudinal study of 3,726 normal children aged 6 to 13 years, 3.5% had epileptiform patterns. The EEG is "diagnostic" of a seizure only when actual clinical manifestations occur at the time of the electrographic discharge.

NEUROIMAGING

Neuroimaging is not mandatory in every child with a seizure. The practice parameter from the AAN in 2000 on the first afebrile seizure recommended that neuroimaging be done based on the specific circumstances. In general, children with focal seizures should have neuroimaging done. Proper classification of the seizure type and epilepsy syndrome is important in determining this. Regarding specific epilepsy syndromes, the generalized syndrome, childhood absence epilepsy, and the focal syndrome "benign rolandic epilepsy" are extremely unlikely to have abnormal neuroimaging and MRI is not recommended. Neuroimaging should be done in every patient with an abnormal neurologic examination, particularly if it is focal or if there is evidence for increased intracranial pressure, with a change in type or severity of seizures, or when seizures are intractable or associated with headaches [**Level 1**].[5]

MRI is now the preferred neuroimaging study for seizures because it is more sensitive than cranial computerized axial tomography (CAT) scan, especially for disorders of neuronal migration. The AAN has produced a practice parameter in 2007 on the use of emergent neuroimaging for seizures [**Level 1**].[6] A study on emergent neuroimaging (cranial CAT scan) in children with new-onset afebrile seizures found that an abnormal CAT scan was more likely in those with underlying disorders or age younger than 33 months with a focal seizure.

GENETIC TESTING

Genetic disorders are a very important cause of seizures in children, both febrile and nonfebrile. These may cause specific genetic syndromes with seizures, such as Rett syndrome or Angelman syndrome, or genetic variants causing seizures. Many of the epilepsies classified previously as idiopathic are now known to result from these variants. Genetic testing includes karyotyping, chromosomal microarray, single gene testing, gene panel testing, whole exome sequencing, and whole genome sequencing. Genetic testing is not typically done for new-onset seizures but can be useful in identifying the etiology of recurrent seizures and the epileptic encephalopathies.

TREATMENT

An important management point is the identification of the child with benign febrile seizures versus the child with epilepsy.

Because most children with simple febrile seizures have no long-term consequences, prophylactic treatment using AEDs should be avoided, even after two or three isolated convulsions. Although both phenobarbital and valproate are effective in reducing recurrence, evidence does not show that treatment alters the risk of later epilepsy. In addition, adverse drug effects occur in as many as 40% of infants and children treated with phenobarbital, and valproate carries a risk of idiosyncratic fatal hepatotoxicity and pancreatitis. Phenytoin and carbamazepine are ineffective.

If treatment is considered at all, it should be reserved for children with a high risk of developing epilepsy or a history of prolonged febrile seizures. A reasonable alternative to chronic drug therapy is abortive treatment using rectal diazepam or intranasal midazolam in children with prolonged seizures. Several studies have shown that administration of diazepam during febrile illnesses is safe and as effective in reducing seizure recurrence as chronic phenobarbital. Although intermittent oral diazepam during acute illnesses has also been shown to be effective, as many as 30% of children experience adverse effects, including ataxia, lethargy, or irritability. Antipyretics may improve the child's comfort during the febrile illness, but they have been shown to be only slightly effective in preventing the recurrence of febrile convulsions.

Watching their child have a convulsion is a frightening experience for parents. The physician therefore must provide reassurance to dispel any myths the family may have, emphasizing in particular that simple febrile seizures are neither life threatening nor damaging to the brain. The American Academy of Pediatrics offers copies of its guidelines and an information sheet for parents through its Web site (www.aap.org), and the Epilepsy Foundation Website (www.epilepsyfoundation.org) provides information about febrile seizures.

RECURRENT SEIZURES

Recurrent seizures raise different questions. Recurrent seizures in infancy require an evaluation to exclude a specific cause. If the child has not been treated with an AED, this decision may need reconsideration. The first step in the treatment of seizures is to establish the diagnosis of epilepsy. Again, there are many nonepileptic disorders that resemble epileptic seizures. If the diagnosis is uncertain, it is better to withhold the diagnosis of epilepsy and not treat with AEDs. Because the overall risk of recurrence of a first seizure varies, these are not usually treated. Although there is agreement that recurrent seizures need treatment with AEDs, after how many seizures should treatment be started remains in question. The decision to treat must be made taking into account the risk-to-benefit ratio: the risk of a recurrent seizure versus the risk of an adverse effect from chronic AED treatment [**Level 1**].[7]

Once the diagnosis of epilepsy has been established and the need for treatment established, the next decision is which AED to use. The choice of an AED is based on the seizure type, the epilepsy syndrome, and the efficacy and toxicity profile of various AEDs (Table 143.5). In general, treatment starts with a single AED; the initial dosing is based on weight, aiming for a specific target dose, and doses increased in increments over several weeks until either complete seizure control is achieved or side effects occur. At this point, another AED is considered. If the first AED does not work, another AED is introduced and the first AED is slowly tapered. AEDs should never be abruptly stopped due to concern for withdrawal seizures unless a major adverse effect occurs. The treatment goal should be monotherapy initially, which results in higher blood levels, fewer side effects, and ultimately, better seizure control. However, polytherapy is frequently used when seizures are hard to control (medically resistant or medically refractory).

If the child is on an AED, management questions include the following: Is the AED dose appropriate, should the AED level be checked, and is it the appropriate AED?

TABLE 143.5 **Choice of Antiepileptic Drugs for Seizure Prophylaxis**

Drug (Generic)	Brand Name	Dose Range (mg/kg/day)	Target Drug Level
Carbamazepine	Tegretol/Carbatrol	10–30	4–12 µg/mL
Clobazam	Onfi	Up to 40	Not done
Ethosuximide	Zarontin	15–40	40–100 µg/mL
Felbamate	Felbatol	15–45	30–100 µg/mL
Gabapentin	Neurontin	30–45	4–20 µg/mL
Lacosamide	Vimpat	5	5–10 µg/mL
Lamotrigine	Lamictal	2–8	2–20 µg/mL
Levetiracetam	Keppra	20–60	10–60 µg/mL
Oxcarbazepine	Trileptal	20–40	10–40 µg/mL
Phenobarbital	Luminal	5	10–45 µg/mL
Phenytoin	Dilantin, fosphenytoin	5	10–20 µg/mL
Primidone	Mysoline		5–10 mg/mL
Rufinamide	Banzel	10–45	3–30 µg/mL
Tiagabine	Gabitril	1–2	20–200 ng/mL
Topiramate	Topamax	5–10	2–25 µg/mL
Valproate	Depakene/Depakote	10–45	50–100 µg/mL
Vigabatrin	Sabril	100–200	Not done
Zonisamide	Zonegran	5–20	10–40 µg/mL

Therapeutic ranges are just guidelines for dosing. Seizures may respond to a low level and toxicity may occur at low levels. Levels above "normal" may be needed to control seizures and can be used if tolerated. It is important to treat the patient and not the "level."

LEVEL 1 EVIDENCE

1. Mackay MT, Weiss SK, Adams-Webber T, et al. Practice parameter: medical treatment of infantile spasms. Report of the American Academy of Neurology and the Child Neurology Society. *Neurology*. 2004;62:1668–1681.
2. Hirtz D, Ashwal S, Berg A, et al. Practice parameter: evaluating a first non-febrile seizure in children. Report of the Quality Standards Subcommittee of the American Academy of Neurology, the Child Neurology Society, and the American Epilepsy Society. *Neurology*. 2000;55:616–623.
3. American Academy of Pediatrics. Committee on Quality Improvement, Subcommittee on Febrile Seizures. Practice parameter: long-term treatment of the child with simple febrile seizures. *Pediatrics*. 1999;103:1307–1309.
4. Subcommittee on Febrile Seizures. Febrile seizures: guideline for the neurodiagnostic evaluation of a child with a simple febrile seizure. *Pediatrics*. 2011;127:389–394.
5. Practice parameter: neuroimaging in the emergency patient presenting with seizure (summary statement). *Ann Emerg Med*. 1996;27:114–118.
6. Harden CL, Huff JS, Schwartz TH, et al. Reassessment: neuroimaging in the emergency patient presenting with seizure (an evidence-based review): report of the Therapeutics and Technology Assessment Subcommittee of the American Academy of Neurology. *Neurology*. 2007;69:1772–1780.
7. Hirtz D, Berg A, Bettis D, et al. Practice parameter: treatment of the child with a first unprovoked seizure. Report of the Quality Standards Subcommittee of the American Academy of Neurology and the Child Neurology Society. *Neurology*. 2003;60:166–175.

SUGGESTED READINGS

American Academy of Pediatrics, Committee on Quality Improvement, Subcommittee on Febrile Seizures. Practice parameter: long-term treatment of the child with simple febrile seizures. *Pediatrics*. 1999;103:1307–1309.

Annegers JF, Hauser WA, Shirts SB, et al. Factors prognostic of unprovoked seizures after febrile convulsions. *N Engl J Med*. 1987;316:493–498.

Baram TZ, Shinnar S, eds. *Febrile Seizures*. San Diego, CA: Academic Press; 2002.

Berg AT, Berkovic SF, Brodie MJ, et al. Revised terminology and concepts for organization of seizures and epilepsies: report of the ILAE commission on classification and terminology, 2005–2009. *Epilepsia*. 2010;51:676–685.

Berg AT, Darefsky AS, Holford TR, et al. Seizures with fever after unprovoked seizures: an analysis in children followed from the time of a first febrile seizure. *Epilepsia*. 1998;39:77–80.

Berg AT, Shinnar S, Darefsky AS, et al. Predictors of recurrent febrile seizures. A prospective cohort study. *Arch Pediatr Adolesc Med*. 1997;151:371–378.

Berg AT, Shinnar S, Shapiro ED, et al. Risk factors for a first febrile seizure: a matched case-control study. *Epilepsia*. 1995;36:334–341.

Blume WT, Luders HO, Mizrahi E. Glossary of descriptive terminology for ictal semiology: report of the ILAE Task Force on Classification and Terminology. *Epilepsia*. 2001;42:1212–1218.

Brophy GB, Bell R, Alldredge A, et al; Neurocritical Care Society Status Epilepticus Guideline Writing Committee. Guidelines for the evaluation and management of status epilepticus. *Neurocrit Care*. 2012;17:3–23.

Camfield C, Camfield P, Gordon K, et al. Does the number of seizures before treatment influence ease of control or remission of childhood epilepsy? Not if the number is 10 or less. *Neurology*. 1996;46:41–44.

Cavazutti GB, Cappella L, Nalin A. Longitudinal study of epileptiform EEG patterns in normal children. *Epilepsia*. 1980;21:43–55.

Chin RFM, Neville BGR, Peckham C, et al. Incidence, cause, and short-term outcome of convulsive status epilepticus in children: prospective, population-based study. *Lancet*. 2006;368:222–229.

Crompton DE, Berkovic SF. The borderland of epilepsy: clinical and molecular features of phenomena that mimic epileptic seizures. *Lancet Neurol.* 2009;8:370–381.

Dura-Trave T, Yoldi-Petri ME, Gallinas-Victoriano F. Incidence of epilepsies and epileptic syndromes in children in Navarre, Spain: 2002–2005. *J Child Neuro.* 2008;23:878–882.

Epi4K Consortium; Epilepsy Phenome/Genome Project. De novo mutations in epileptic encephalopathies. *Nature.* 2013;501:217–222.

Frank LM, Shinnar S, Hesdorffer DC, et al. Cerebrospinal fluid findings in children with fever-associated status epilepticus: results of the consequences of prolonged febrile seizures (FEBSTAT) study. *J Pediatr.* 2012;161:1169–1171.

Gilbert DL, Buncher CR. An EEG should not be obtained routinely after first unprovoked seizure in childhood. *Neurology.* 2000;54:635–641.

Goldstein J, Slomski J. Epileptic spasms: a variety of etiologies and associated syndromes. *J Child Neuro.* 2008;23:407–414.

Goodkin HP, Riviello JJ Jr. Status epilepticus. In: Wyllie E, ed. *The Treatment of Epilepsy: Principles and Practice.* 5th ed. Philadelphia: Lippincott Williams and Wilkins; 2011:469–485.

Greenberg MK, Barsan WG, Starkman S. Neuroimaging in the emergency patient presenting with seizure. *Neurology.* 1996;47:26–32.

Guidelines for epidemiologic studies in epilepsy. Commission on Epidemiology and Prognosis, International League Against Epilepsy. *Epilepsia.* 1993;34:592–596.

Hauser WA. The prevalence and incidence of convulsive disorders in children. *Epilepsia.* 1994;35(suppl 2):S1–S6.

Hauser WA, Beghi E. First seizure definitions and worldwide incidence and mortality. *Epilepsia.* 2008;49(suppl 1):8–12.

Hesdorffer DC, Shinnar S, Lewis DV, et al. Risk factors for febrile status epilepticus: a case-control study. *J Pediatr.* 2013;163:1147–1151.

Hirose S, Mohney RP, Okada M, et al. The genetics of febrile seizures and related epilepsy syndromes. *Brain Dev.* 2003;25:304–312.

Hirtz D, Thurman DJ, Gwinn-Hardy K, et al. How common are the common neurologic disorders? *Neurology.* 2007;68:326–337.

Kotagal P, Costa M, Wyllie E, et al. Paroxysmal nonepileptic events in children and adolescents. *Pediatrics.* 2002;110:e46.

Kramer U, Nevo Y, Neufield MY, et al. Epidemiology of epilepsy in childhood: a cohort of 440 consecutive patients. *Pediatr Neurol.* 1998;18:46–50.

Lempert T, Bauer M, Schmidt M. Syncope: a videometric analysis of 56 episodes of transient cerebral hypoxia. *Ann Neuro.* 1994;36:233–237.

Lothman E. The biochemical basis and pathophysiology of status epilepticus. *Neurology.* 1990;40(suppl 2):13–23.

Lowenstein DH, Bleck T, Macdonald RL. It's time to revise the definition of status epilepticus. *Epilepsia.* 1999;40:120–122.

Lux AL, Edwards SW, Hancock E, et al. The United Kingdom Infantile Spams Study (UKISS) comparing hormonal treatment with vigabatrin on developmental and epilepsy outcomes at 14 months: a multicenter randomized trial. *Lancet Neurol.* 2005;4:712–717.

Lux AL, Edwards SW, Hancock E, et al. The United Kingdom Infantile Spasms study comparing vigabatrin with prednisolone or tetracosactide at 14 days: a multicenter randomized controlled trial. *Lancet.* 2004;364:1773–1778.

MacDonald BK, Johnson AL, Sander JWAS, et al. Febrile convulsions in 220 children—neurological sequelae at 12 years follow-up. *Eur Neurol.* 1999;41:179–186.

Michelucci R, Pasini E, Riguzzi P, et al. Genetics of epilepsy and relevance to current practice. *Curr Neurol Neurosci Rep.* 2012;12:445–455.

Nelson KB, Ellenberg JH. Prognosis in children with febrile seizures. *Pediatrics.* 1978;61:720–727.

Obeid M, Mikati MA. Expanding spectrum of paroxysmal events in children: potential mimickers of epilepsy. *Pediatr Neurol.* 2007;37:309–316.

Olson HE, Poduri A, Pearl PL. Genetic forms of epilepsy and other paroxysmal disorders. *Semin Neurol.* 2014;34:266–279.

Olson H, Shen Y, Avallone J, et al. Copy number variation plays an important role in clinical epilepsy. *Ann Neurol.* 2014;75:943–958.

Pellock JM, Hrachovy R, Shinnar S, et al. Infantile spasms: a U.S. consensus report. *Epilepsia.* 2010;51:2175–2185.

Poduri A, Sheidley BR, Shostak S, et al. Genetic testing in the epilepsies-developments and dilemmas. *Nat Rev Neurol.* 2014;10:293–299.

Riviello JJ. Classification of seizures and epilepsy. *Curr Neurol Neurosci Rep.* 2003;3:325–331.

Riviello JJ. General concepts in seizure management. In: Burg FD, Ingelfinger JR, Polin RA, et al, eds. *Current Pediatric Therapy.* 18th ed. Philadelphia: Elsevier-Mosby; 2006:367–371.

Riviello JJ Jr, Ashwal S, Hirtz D, et al. Practice parameter: diagnostic assessment of the child with status epilepticus (an evidence-based review): report of the Quality Standards Subcommittee of the American Academy of Neurology and the Practice Committee of the Child Neurology Society. *Neurology.* 2006;67(9):1542–1550.

Riviello JJ Jr, Holmes GL. The treatment of status epilepticus. *Semin Pediatri Neurol.* 2004;11:129–138.

Riviello JJ Jr, Scott RC. Seizures. In: Sejersen T, Wang CH, eds. *Acute Pediatric Neurology.* London, United Kingdom: Springer; 2014:23–35.

Rosman NP, Colton T, Labazzo RNC, et al. A controlled trial of diazepam administered during febrile illnesses to prevent recurrence of febrile seizures. *N Engl J Med.* 1993;329:79–84.

Sharma S, Riviello JJ, Harper MB, et al. The role of emergent neuroimaging in children with new-onset afebrile seizures. *Pediatrics.* 2003;111:1–5.

Shinnar S, Hesdorffer DC, Nordli DR, et al. Phenomenology of prolonged febrile seizures: results of the FEBSTAT study. *Neurology.* 2008;71:170–176.

Shorvon SD. The etiologic classification of epilepsy. *Epilepsia.* 2011;52(6):1052–1057.

Tarkka R, Rantala H, Huhari M, et al. Risk of recurrence and outcome after the first febrile seizure. *Pediatr Neurol.* 1998;18:218–220.

VanLandingham KE, Heinz ER, Cavazos JE, et al. MRI evidence of hippocampal injury following prolonged, focal febrile convulsions. *Ann Neurol.* 1998;43:413–426.

Verity CM, Greenwood R, Golding J. Long-term intellectual and behavioral outcomes of children with febrile convulsions. *N Engl J Med.* 1998;338:1723–1728.

Yu ZL, Jiang JM, Wu DH, et al. Febrile seizures are associated with mutation of seizure-related (SEZ) 6, a brain-specific gene. *J Neurosci Res.* 2007;85:166–172.

INTRODUCTION

There are two classifications for pediatric stroke: by age and by stroke subtype. By age, a perinatal stroke occurs during gestation through 28 days of life. Often, a child is discovered to have a chronic infarct in infancy that is presumed to have occurred during the perinatal period. These are referred to as *presumed perinatal strokes*. A stroke that occurs after 28 days through 18 years is a *childhood stroke*. Childhood stroke can be further subdivided into *infancy* (older than 28 days to younger than 2 years), *childhood* (2 to 11 years), and *adolescence* (12 to 18 years). By subtype, pediatric stroke is subdivided as arterial ischemic stroke (AIS), cerebral venous thrombosis (CVT), and hemorrhagic stroke. Hemorrhagic stroke includes intracranial hemorrhage (ICH), intraventricular hemorrhage (IVH), and subarachnoid hemorrhage (SAH). This chapter will begin with a discussion of stroke subtypes, will continue by looking at the unique features of stroke related to sickle cell anemia (SCA) and perinatal and presumed perinatal stroke, and will conclude with a brief review of genetics of pediatric stroke.

ARTERIAL ISCHEMIC STROKE

EPIDEMIOLOGY

Annual incidence for childhood AIS is 1.2 to 7.9 per 100,000 children. After the neonatal period, pediatric AIS peak among school-aged children. From the first 676 patients in the International Pediatric Stroke Study (IPSS) registry, the largest registry of all pediatric stroke, the median age at first AIS presentation was 5.7 years (interquartile range, 1.7 to 11.6 years).

For all childhood stroke, there is a predominance of affected males. In the California discharge database, the relative risk (RR) for ischemic and hemorrhagic stroke was higher among boys than girls: for AIS, RR 1.25 (confidence interval [CI] 1.11 to 1.40); SAH, RR 1.24 (CI 1.00 to 1.53); and ICH, RR 1.34 (CI 1.16 to 1.56). Mortality after AIS was also higher among boys (17% vs. 12%). The ratio of boys-to-girls is generally estimated to be 6:4. IPSS found that 59% of children with AIS are male.

Recent studies in the United States are reporting racial and ethnic disparities in childhood stroke where black children are at higher risk for ischemic and hemorrhagic stroke than white children. Pediatric stroke mortality was found to be higher in stroke belt states (southeastern United States), compared with other U.S. states.

PATHOBIOLOGY

Arteriopathy (50% of Arterial Ischemic Stroke)

Arteriopathy in pediatric stroke is presumed to be nonatheromatous and instead due to inflammation, infection, and inherited disorders of tissue stability and repair. Arteriopathy is found in approximately 50% of childhood AIS, and discrete radiographic and clinical subtypes have begun to be described. Two reported predictors of arteriopathy are a recent upper respiratory infection and SCA. The traditional nomenclature for AIS arteriopathy subtypes are *focal cerebral arteriopathy* (FCA), *moyamoya, intracranial and extracranial arterial dissection, vasculitis, sickle cell arteriopathy, postvaricella arteriopathy*, and other unspecified forms of arteriopathy (Fig. 144.1). (Frequencies of arteriopathy subtypes are as reported in the IPSS registry.)

1. **FCA** (25% of arteriopathy). FCA is typically characterized by unilateral mainstem arterial disease with lenticulostriate infarction. An East Asian study found that FCA was reversible in 68%, progressive in 20%, and stable in 12%. Of the patients with reversible arteriopathy, 53% had early worsening. In European cohorts, the course of unilateral arteriopathy was progressive in only 6%, stabilized in 32%, improved in 45%, and completely normalized in 23%. Among patients with a nonprogressive arteriopathy, 44% had an antecedent varicella infection, and 18% had a recurrent stroke or transient ischemic attack (TIA).

2. **Moyamoya** (22% of arteriopathy). Moyamoya arteriopathy is the progressive development of bilateral occlusive disease of the terminal internal carotid arteries (ICAs) with basal collaterals (see also Chapter 43). There may also be involvement of the mainstem branches of the terminal ICA. Moyamoya syndrome is used when there is an accompanying condition known to be associated with moyamoya arteriopathy and moyamoya disease when the disease is idiopathic. Moyamoya arteriopathy is commonly progressive. In a single-center series, progression developed in 45% over 5.4 ± 3.8 years. Stroke recurrence is also high from 20% over 4 years to 38% over 10 years.

3. **Craniocervical arterial dissection** (CCAD) (20% of arteriopathy). CCAD in childhood includes intracranial and extracranial dissections. In a meta-analysis of arterial dissection in children younger than 18 years, males were affected considerably more than females: 74% male in anterior circulation dissections and 87% male in posterior circulation dissections. This predominance persisted even for nontraumatic dissections. Of dissection involving the anterior circulation, 40% were extracranial and of dissections involving the posterior circulation, 79% were extracranial. One-third of dissections are spontaneous, but less than a fifth are associated with significant trauma. The mean age of presentation is older than all AIS at 8 to 10 years. Common presenting symptoms are hemiparesis and headache. Neck pain was less common in children. Follow-up after an average of 5.2 years showed moderate or severe deficits in 14%, recurrent strokes in 9%, and recurrent dissections only after anterior circulation dissection and in 10% of those patients.

4. **Vasculitis** (12% of arteriopathy). Cerebral vasculitis is rare and can be difficult to diagnose in children (see also Chapter 42). Vasculitis due to systemic inflammatory conditions, viral, fungal, mycobacterial, and even parasitic infections is more likely than primary central nervous system (CNS) angiitis.

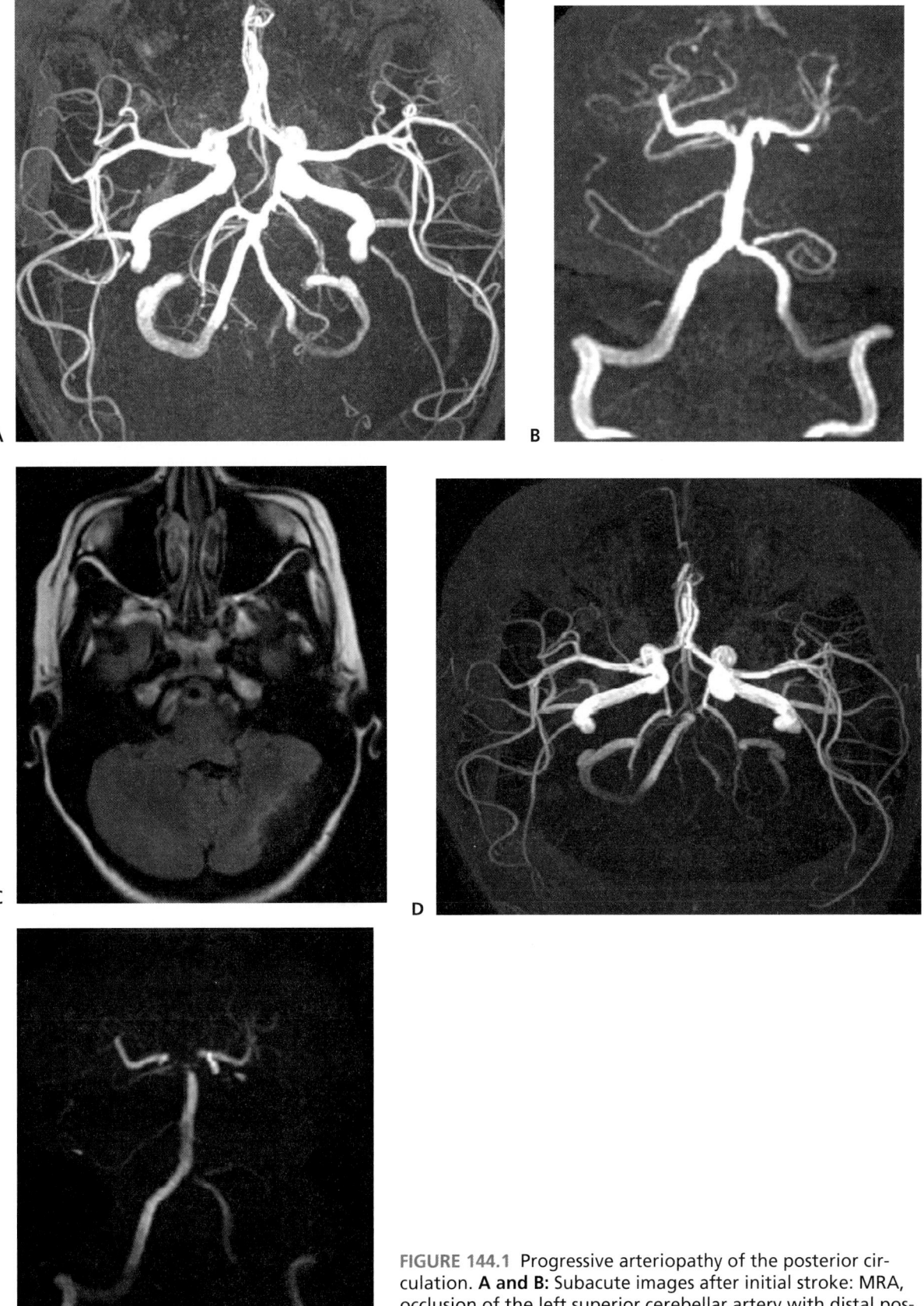

FIGURE 144.1 Progressive arteriopathy of the posterior circulation. **A and B:** Subacute images after initial stroke: MRA, occlusion of the left superior cerebellar artery with distal posterior cerebral artery (PCA) stenosis. **C:** MRI T2, left cerebellar encephalomalacia. **D and E:** Six months later, postural lightheadedness, nausea, fatigue, and left-sided paresthesia: MRA, tip of the basilar and left vertebral stenosis.

Consider vasculitis where there are infarcts in multiple vascular territories with microhemorrhages.

5. **Sickle cell arteriopathy** (8% of arteriopathy). (See later discussion on SCA, and Chapter 118)
6. **Post–varicella angiopathy** (7% of arteriopathy) traditionally stenosis of the distal internal carotid and mainstem branches with lenticulostriate infarction. (See later discussion on "Risk Factors, Infection.")

Cardiogenic (30% of Arterial Ischemic Stroke)

Cardiogenic causes of stroke include congenital heart disease, valvular heart disease, arrhythmias, cardiomyopathy, cardiac surgery and catheterization, extracorporeal membrane oxygenation, and Kawasaki disease.

Congenital heart disease is the most common cardiac risk factor, reported in 59% of those with a cardiogenic stroke. An isolated patent foramen ovale (PFO) was reported in 15% and cardiac catheterization in 8%.

Thromboembolic (15% of Arterial Ischemic Stroke)

Thromboembolic stroke may be due to an indwelling catheter, infection, or a hypercoagulable state that is inherited or acquired. (See "Risk Factors, Thrombophilia Traits.")

Cryptogenic Stroke

Cryptogenic stroke is reported in approximately one-fifth of children.

RISK FACTORS FOR ARTERIAL ISCHEMIC STROKE

Infection (25% of Arterial Ischemic Stroke)

The earliest reports suggesting an association between infection and stroke are in children. Stroke as a complication of bacterial meningitis was thought to be due to inflammation of the vessels traversing infected meninges involving perforating and pial arteries. Subsequently, large-artery involvement and recovery-phase large-artery stenosis was recognized.

Varicella-zoster virus (VZV) was the first viral infection associated with cerebral vasculopathy and ischemia after it was described in a 5-year-old boy following a primary VZV infection. Among young children with AIS, a VZV infection in the preceding year was at least three times more frequent compared with published population rates and controls. On imaging, vascular stenosis in the proximal portion of major arteries was seen in 20 of 22 children with AIS and VZV in the preceding year.

Recently, minor infection is found in association with AIS. In the northern Californian Kaiser Pediatric Stroke Study (1993 to 2003), a minor infection (acute fever, upper respiratory tract infection, pneumonia, acute otitis media, pharyngitis, urinary tract infection, or acute gastroenteritis) independently predicted stroke risk in the month that followed the infection. Similarly, chronic inflammatory conditions such as autoimmune disease were highly associated with stroke risk.

Acute Head and Neck Disorders (25% of Arterial Ischemic Stroke)

Acute head and neck disorders include head trauma, pharyngitis, meningitis, intracranial surgery, otitis media, sinusitis, and mastoiditis.

Acute Systemic Conditions (20% of Arterial Ischemic Stroke)

Acute systemic conditions includes fever longer than 48 hours, sepsis, shock, dehydration, acidosis, and anoxia.

Chronic Systemic Conditions (20% of Arterial Ischemic Stroke)

Chronic systemic conditions include SCA, indwelling catheter, genetic disorders, malignancy, and connective tissue disorders.

Chronic Head and Neck Disorders (10% of Arterial Ischemic Stroke)

Chronic head and neck disorders most commonly refer to migraine, brain tumor, and ventriculoperitoneal (VP) shunt.

Thrombophilia Traits

Most thrombophilic states contribute only a small component to an individual's risk for stroke, but these tendencies are prevalent in the population and may be more important with other risk factors in children with stroke. The largest systematic review to date of thrombophilia risk factors in childhood, AIS and CVT found that in children with first AIS compared with healthy children, there was a significantly greater odds of having an MTHFR C677T, factor V G1691A, or factor II G20210A mutation; antithrombin deficiency; protein C deficiency; protein S deficiency; elevated lipoprotein(a); and antiphospholipid antibodies. The American Heart Association Stroke Council suggests that it is reasonable to test for the more common prothrombotic states even when another stroke risk factor has been identified (Class IIa, Level of Evidence C).

CLINICAL FEATURES

The most common symptoms of an AIS in children is hemiparesis and a speech disturbance. In a single-center pediatric stroke registry, 22% of children with acute AIS presented with seizures. Similarly, an inpatient database in Taiwan found that early symptomatic seizures occurred in 26% of children with AIS.

DIAGNOSIS

Imaging

Patients who present with new focal neurologic deficits should undergo an urgent computed tomography (CT) scan of the head to rule out acute hemorrhage. Early ischemic stroke may not be seen on head CT and should be confirmed with magnetic resonance imaging (MRI). In children with moyamoya disease, transcranial Doppler (TCD) may be useful to follow for stability or progression of vascular disease. (Class IIb, Level of Evidence C).

Stroke Classifications

A new classification system for childhood AIS was recently proposed, the Childhood AIS Standardized Classification and Diagnostic Evaluation (CASCADE) criteria. The system is divided into acute classifications with arteriopathy subdivided by location: small-vessel arteriopathy of childhood, unilateral FCA of childhood, bilateral cerebral arteriopathy of childhood, aortic/cervical arteriopathy, cardioembolic, other, and multifactorial and chronic classifications: progressive, stable, reversible, and indeterminate arteriopathy. These classifications are not yet evidence-based.

TREATMENT

Acute care after AIS begins with maintenance of normal oxygenation, normothermia, normoglycemia, and control of systemic hypertension (Class I, Level of Evidence C). It is reasonable to treat dehydration and anemia (Class IIa, Level of Evidence C). There is no evidence that in children with normal oxygenation, supplemental oxygen provides benefit, and in children without clinical or electrographic seizures, prophylactic administration of antiepileptic medications is not necessary (Class III, Level of Evidence C). There is no data confirming the safety and efficacy of hypothermia as an acute treatment for stroke (Class III, Level of Evidence C). The use of thrombolysis (tissue plasminogen activator [tPA]) is not recommended outside research protocols (Grade 1B). When treatable stroke risk factors are discovered, those conditions should be treated (Class I, Level of Evidence C).

Initial therapy in children without SCA should be unfractionated heparin (UFH) or low molecular weight heparin (LMWH) or aspirin (1 to 5 mg/kg/day) until dissection and embolic causes have been excluded. Once excluded, daily aspirin prophylaxis (1 to 5 mg/kg/day) for a minimum of 2 years should be continued (Grade 1B). In children receiving aspirin who have recurrent AIS or TIAs, consider changing to clopidogrel or an anticoagulant (Grade 2C).

Craniocervical Arterial Dissection

The American Heart Association Stroke Council recommends beginning treatment of an extracranial CCAD with UFH or LMWH and to continue subcutaneous LMWH or bridge to warfarin for 3 to 6 months of treatment (Class IIa, Level of Evidence C). The American College of Chest Physicians recommends anticoagulant therapy for at least 6 weeks, with ongoing treatment dependent on radiologic assessment (Grade 2C). One can also consider using an antiplatelet agent instead of LMWH or warfarin. Beyond 6 months, for recurrent symptoms, it is reasonable to continue anticoagulation or an antiplatelet agent. If symptoms have resolved but there is residual abnormality of the dissected artery on imaging, it is also reasonable to continue an antiplatelet agent beyond 6 months (Class IIa, Level of Evidence C). Surgical procedures may be considered for symptoms due to CCAD despite optimal medical therapy (Class IIb, Level of Evidence C). For an intracranial dissection and for SAH resulting from CCAD, anticoagulation is not recommended (Class III, Level of Evidence C).

Moyamoya Arteriopathy

With moyamoya disease, surgical revascularization can effectively reduce the risk of stroke (Class I, Level of Evidence B). Children with moyamoya should be referred to an appropriate center for consideration of revascularization (Grade 1B). There is less literature to recommend one surgical procedure over another, but indirect revascularization may be preferred in younger children whose small-caliber vessels make direct anastomosis difficult, and direct bypass techniques may be preferable in older individuals (Class I, Level of Evidence C). Indications for revascularization surgery include progressive ischemic symptoms, evidence of inadequate perfusion, or collateral reserve (Class I, Level of Evidence B). After revascularization surgery or in asymptomatic individuals with moyamoya disease, aspirin may be considered (Class IIb, Level of Evidence C). In general, anticoagulants are not recommended with moyamoya disease because of the risk of hemorrhage and the difficulty of maintaining therapeutic levels in children (Class III, Level of Evidence C). Supportive care in children with moyamoya disease includes techniques to reduce anxiety and pain that could lead to

hyperventilation-induced vasoconstriction (Class IIb, Level of Evidence C). Perioperative and intraoperative avoidance of hypotension, hypovolemia, hyperthermia, and hypocarbia may reduce the risk of perioperative stroke (Class IIb, Level of Evidence C).

Cardiogenic Stroke

Treatment for congestive heart failure and congenital heart lesions is recommended and may reduce the likelihood of cardiogenic embolism. This includes resection of an atrial myxoma and does not yet apply to PFOs (Class I, Level of Evidence C). It is reasonable to begin anticoagulation following a cardiac embolism in children who are judged to have a high risk for recurrence. UFH or LMWH can be introduced as a bridge to warfarin (Class IIa, Level of Evidence B). LMWH can be continued instead of warfarin, and it is reasonable to continue either LMWH or warfarin for at least 1 year or until the lesion responsible for the risk has been corrected (Class IIa, Level of Evidence C). For a suspected cardiac embolism with an unknown or lower risk of stroke and that is unrelated to a PFO, it is reasonable to treat with aspirin for at least 1 year (Class IIa, Level of Evidence C). It is reasonable to close large atrial septal defects (excludes PFOs) to prevent stroke (Class IIa, Level of Evidence C).

In patients with endocarditis of a prosthetic valve, it may be reasonable to continue long-term anticoagulation (Class IIb, Level of Evidence C). Anticoagulation should not be used for native valve endocarditis, and it is not necessary to remove a cardiac rhabdomyoma in an individual who has been asymptomatic (Class III, Level of Evidence C).

Inherited Thrombophilic State

In children with AIS or CVT, it is reasonable to measure the serum homocysteine level and to introduce therapies such as diet and supplementation of folate, vitamin B_6, or vitamin B_{12} to lower elevated homocysteine values (Class IIa, Level of Evidence B). In an adolescent with AIS or CVT, it is reasonable to discontinue oral contraceptives (Class IIa, Level of Evidence C).

Other Causes

Children with Fabry disease should receive α-galactosidase replacement therapy (Class I, Level of `Evidence B).

REHABILITATION

A child who has suffered a stroke should be enrolled in age-appropriate rehabilitation and therapy program (Class I, Level of Evidence C). Cognitive and behavioral performance is especially important in school-aged children. The pediatric stroke outcome measure (PSOM) is based on a detailed age-appropriate, neurologic exam and scored for four domains: sensorimotor deficit, language deficit—production (excludes dysarthria), language deficit—comprehension, and cognitive or behavioral deficit. The weight of language and cognitive and behavioral deficits is considerably greater and motor deficits are less weighty compared with similar adult stroke outcome measures. Neuropsychological assessment is useful for planning therapy and educational programs and monitoring cognitive, behavioral, and language deficits after a stroke (Class I, Level of Evidence C).

OUTCOME

Neurologic Deficits

In one single-center series of 90 children followed for a mean of 2.1 years after an AIS, 49% were either normal or mildly impaired by PSOM.

Recurrence

In northern California, the 5-year cumulative recurrence rate was 19% after childhood AIS. All of the recurrences occurred among children with a vascular abnormality. In a large single-center series, 37% of children had a recurrent AIS or TIA at a median of 267 days (range 1 day to 11.5 years). Of the 84% of patients who had reimaging, 11% had clinically silent recurrent ischemia. Among children with arteriopathy in northern California, the 5-year cumulative recurrence rate was 66%. Factors associated with silent reinfarction and clinical recurrences were moyamoya, low birth weight, genetic thrombophilia, previous TIA, bilateral infarction, preexisting condition, and leukocytosis.

Epilepsy

Poststroke seizures and epilepsy is considerable in children. A population-based retrospective study of children with AIS found an average annual incidence rate of first unprovoked seizure of 4.4% (95% CI, 3.3 to 5.8), 16% (95% CI, 12 to 21) at 5 years, and 33% (95% CI, 23 to 46) at 10 years. The risk of epilepsy was 13% (95% CI, 9 to 18) at 5 years and 30% (95% CI, 20 to 44) at 10 years. An inpatient database in Taiwan found epilepsy in 17% of children after AIS.

CEREBRAL VENOUS THROMBOSIS

EPIDEMIOLOGY

Population-based incidence studies report that less than 1 per 100,000 children per year are diagnosed with CVT (see also Chapter 40). Many stroke providers believe true incidence is significantly higher and diagnoses are missed. Among patients with a presumed diagnosis of idiopathic intracranial hypertension (IIH), routine imaging discloses CVT in as many as 26%. CVT also peaks in school-aged children. The mean age of children at the time of diagnosis is 5 to 9 years.

PATHOBIOLOGY

The cerebral veins and sinuses are thin-walled and without valves. Cerebral veins drain into the sinuses that form from dural pockets around the brain. Unlike arterial vascular territories, thrombosis of particular veins does not present with well-defined clinical syndromes. The venous system has considerable anatomic variability, flow can be reversed, and there may be collateral drainage pathways such as through occipital sinuses.

The cerebral veins and sinuses are positioned for thrombotic complications. Venous drainage is slow; it follows a tortuous route and the walls easily distend. A combination of local inflammation in the vessel wall, systemic thrombophilia, hyperosmolality, reduced blood flow, and injury to the vessel wall all work to tip the balance toward cerebral thrombosis. When a thrombus obstructs venous outflow, the pressure becomes high in the venous system. Edema and hemorrhage can develop from high pressure in the capillaries with plasma and red blood cell diapedesis or frank rupture, and the high pressure can exceed arterial perfusion pressure resulting in ischemic infarction. Hydrocephalus with intracranial hypertension will occur when cerebrospinal fluid reabsorption through arachnoid villi and pacchionian body granulations in the dural sinuses becomes impaired. A large thrombus in the superior sagittal sinus, the sinus where most of the reabsorption occurs, will generally lead to a communicating hydrocephalus.

In children, the superior sagittal and lateral sinuses are most often affected, and two or more sinuses or veins are involved. Sinus occlusion may present with intracranial hypertension, whereas an isolated cerebral vein thrombosis may present with focal neurologic signs.

CVT is a complication of many chronic inflammatory, infectious, and prothrombotic states. Inflammatory states and conditions that are recognized to be associated with increased risk for CVT include inflammatory bowel disease, systemic lupus erythematosus, Behçet disease, celiac disease, multiple sclerosis, head injury, brain neoplasm, and a hematologic malignancy. Infectious conditions include mastoiditis, otitis, sinusitis, meningitis, the postoperative period, and postcatheterization. Prothrombotic inherited tendencies and states may be due to nephrotic syndrome, homocystinuria, oral contraceptive use, pregnancy, or exposure to asparaginase. Other conditions associated with CVT are anemia, hydrocephalus, dehydration, and hypoxia.

Prothrombotic tendencies may be present in half of children tested, and more than one abnormality is not uncommon. The meta-analysis of prothrombotic traits in childhood stroke also found a positive association for all of the thrombophilia traits studied with CVT: antithrombin deficiency, protein C deficiency, protein S deficiency, factor V G1691A mutation, and prothrombin G20210A mutation. An antithrombin deficiency was 18-fold higher in children with CVT compared to a control population and protein C or S were six and five times higher in a cohort of children with CVT.

CLINICAL FEATURES

Presenting symptoms are often diffuse and nonspecific. In series of children with CVT, the most common presenting symptoms are headache, vomiting, and visual symptoms. Presenting symptoms may overlap with traditional symptoms of IIH. Other presenting symptoms are lethargy, malaise, irritability, poor appetite, limb weakness, unsteady gait, and seizures.

Common clinical signs on presentation are papilledema, seizure, fever, sixth nerve palsy, and hemiparesis. Other signs include a decreased level of consciousness, visual field defects, cranial nerve palsies, ataxia, speech impairment, and hemisensory loss.

DIAGNOSIS AND IMAGING

The diagnosis is often delayed. A retrospective chart review of 21 children treated from 1997 to 2005 found that there was a mean of 6.3 (range 0 to 26) days from onset of symptoms to hospital presentation, and from hospital presentation to diagnosis, there was a mean of 2.9 (0 to 12) days.

There are pathognomonic imaging signs for CVT. The cord sign is due to dense cortical veins or thrombosed sinuses. The dense-triangle sign due to acutely congealed blood is a very early and transient sign. The delta- or empty-triangle sign is a late finding and is the result of venous flow in the collateral veins in the walls of the sinus compared with absent flow within the sinus.

CT scan is widely available and can be obtained rapidly. At many centers, good quality images can now be obtained with low radiation. In one study, unenhanced CT scan was 73% sensitive for CVT, and there were no false-positive results. CT venogram increases the sensitivity of the study to detect thrombus in the vein and may be superior to magnetic resonance venogram (MRV) in visualization of cerebral veins but requires skilled technicians for appropriate timing of the contrast bolus to avoid arterial contamination. It is also affected by poor cardiac output and conditions associated with increased circulation time.

MRI is superior for the evaluation of parenchymal abnormalities. MRI and MRV do not require contrast but contrast can be helpful to distinguish between a hypoplastic sinus and thrombosis in the lumen. Flow voids can be mistaken for thrombosis where there is slow cerebral flow.

In children with CVT, approximately one-quarter have no parenchymal involvement, one-third have ischemic infarcts, and one-third have ICH. Intraventricular and SAHs are seen in less than 10%.

TREATMENT

Recommendations on anticoagulant use are based on retrospective analysis. While we await a prospective study on anticoagulant use in neonates, a large single-center retrospective analysis of 162 neonates and children from 1992 to 2005 suggests benefit for anticoagulant use even with preexisting hemorrhage. The study was conducted at an institution where a protocol was initiated in 1995 and was practiced. All neonates and children without significant ICH received anticoagulation. If anticoagulation was not started because of significant ICH, a follow-up study was done at 5 to 7 days for clot stability. If the follow-up imaging showed clot propagation, these patients were treated with anticoagulation despite significant ICH. Within 2 weeks of diagnosis, the thrombus propagated in 7% of treated children and 37% of untreated children. Propagation was symptomatic in 60% of children and associated with more severe deficits at discharge. Anticoagulant-related ICH occurred in 5% of treated children and 98% of ICH with anticoagulation occurred in patients with pretreatment ICH. ICH as a complication of anticoagulation was most commonly a subdural hemorrhage and almost all bleeds occurred with additional factors such as supratherapeutic anticoagulation, hypertension, thrombocytopenia, VP shunt surgery, and cerebral atrophy.

The acute management of children with CVT should include hydration, control of clinical and subclinical seizures, and treatment of elevated intracranial pressure (Class I, Level of Evidence C). With severe or long-standing increased intracranial pressure, there is a risk for vision loss. Visual fields and visual acuity should be periodically assessed and appropriate measures to control elevated intracranial pressure should be instituted (Class I, Level of Evidence C). Monitoring the intracranial pressure may be considered during the acute phase of CVT (Class IIb, Level of Evidence C).

Bacterial infection and anemia are treatable causes of CVT, so children with a suspected bacterial infection should receive appropriate antibiotics and a complete blood count should be performed (Class I, Level of Evidence C). There may be benefit to diagnostic testing for underlying infections with blood cultures and sinus radiographs (Class IIb, Level of Evidence B). Performing a thorough thrombophilic screen may be beneficial, and its results could affect the risk of rethrombosis and influence therapeutic decisions (Class IIb, Level of Evidence B). In children who have an impaired mental status and are paralyzed or sedated, subclinical seizures are not uncommon. Continuous electroencephalography monitoring may be considered for these patients (Class IIb, Level of Evidence C).

The American Heart Association Stroke Council suggests that it is reasonable to institute either UFH or LMWH whether or not there is secondary hemorrhage, followed by warfarin therapy for 3 to 6 months. Follow-up neuroimaging studies in children with CVT to confirm vessel recanalization or recurrence of the thrombus may be beneficial (Class IIa, Level of Evidence C). The American College of Chest Physicians recommends initial anticoagulation with UFH or LMWH only in children without significant ICH, followed by LMWH or a vitamin K antagonist for a minimum of 3 months (Grade 1B). If after 3 months of therapy there is incomplete radiologic recanalization of CVT or ongoing symptoms,

anticoagulation should be continued for an additional 3 months (Grade 2C). In children with significant hemorrhage, there is a suggestion to repeat the radiologic evaluation at 5 to 7 days and if there is propagation of thrombus, institute anticoagulation (Grade 2C).

There are case series describing local cerebral thrombolysis for CVT. Reported cases suggest that there may be benefit in the hands of experienced interventionalists but there may also be a considerable risk for hemorrhagic complications. The American Heart Association Stroke Council suggests that in selected children, administration of a thrombolytic agent can be considered (Class IIb, Level of Evidence C). The American College of Chest Physicians suggests thrombolysis, thrombectomy, or surgical decompression only in children with severe CVT in whom there is no improvement with initial UFH therapy (Grade 2C). In children with CVT and ongoing risk factors for thrombosis, such as nephrotic syndrome, or l-asparaginase therapy, prophylactic anticoagulation is suggested (Grade 2C).

OUTCOME

In large-center series, anticoagulation is not associated with increased mortality and severe neurologic outcomes.

Recanalization

At 3 months, more than half of children have recanalization of thrombosed vein. A prothrombotic disorder is associated with nonrecanalization.

Recurrence

Recurrence occurs in 5% to 17% of children. This may depend on the course of the underlying risk factors and residual patency of the cerebral venous system.

Neurologic Deficits

Poor neurologic outcomes after CVT include chronic intracranial hypertension, frequent headaches, cognitive difficulties, hemiparesis, reduced visual acuity, isolated sixth nerve palsy, and epilepsy in 5% to 8%. Predictors for good outcome are anticoagulation, older age, no parenchymal abnormality on imaging, and lateral sinus involvement.

In a small cohort of children followed for a mean of 2.1 years after a CVT, 79% were either normal or mildly impaired by PSOM. In a larger series of children, outcome was unfavorable in 37%.

Mortality

Mortality is reported between 5% and 12%. In one series of children, 88% of whom were not treated with anticoagulation, early mortality was 18%.

HEMORRHAGIC STROKE

ICH, IVH, and SAH (excludes traumatic hemorrhage and germinal matrix hemorrhages)

EPIDEMIOLOGY

In children, approximately half of all strokes are hemorrhagic. The annual incidence rate ranges from 0.63 to 5.11 per 100,000 children without SCA. ICH affects school-aged children. The median age of affected children is 7 to 10 years.

PATHOBIOLOGY

ICH in children is most often intraparenchymal hemorrhage or intraparenchymal hemorrhage with IVH extension. Isolated IVH is rare. Hematoma expansion may occur in one-third of children and the expansion may be significant, requiring urgent evacuation.

Causes of ICH from three pediatric tertiary care centers in the United States are arteriovenous malformations (37%), unknown (17%), cavernous malformations (13%), coagulopathy (11%), anticoagulation (9%), aneurysm (9%), developmental venous anomaly (2%), and moyamoya (2%). In the Baltimore–Washington Cooperative Young Stroke Study, ICH was due to arteriovenous malformations (29%), hematologic causes (23%), vasculopathy (18%), surgical complications (12%), coagulopathy (6%), and indeterminate causes (12%).

CLINICAL FEATURES

Presenting symptoms are headache, focal deficits, altered mental status, and seizures in approximately one-third of children.

DIAGNOSIS AND IMAGING

Children with nontraumatic brain hemorrhage should undergo a thorough risk factor evaluation. When noninvasive imaging does not demonstrate a nidus, conventional cerebral angiography should be performed (Class I, Level of Evidence C). For a patient who presents with symptoms that could be explained by an aneurysm, computed tomography angiography (CTA) or conventional angiography (CA) may be considered even if the patient's magnetic resonance angiography (MRA) fails to show evidence of an aneurysm (Class IIb, Level of Evidence C).

TREATMENT

Children with a severe coagulation factor deficiency should receive appropriate factor replacement therapy, and children with less severe factor deficiency should receive factor replacement after trauma (Class I, Level of Evidence A). There is a recommendation to identify and correct, where clinically feasible, congenital vascular anomalies (Class I, Level of Evidence C). Recently, A Randomised trial of Unruptured Brain Arteriovenous malformations (ARUBA) in adults found that medical management alone was superior to medical management with interventional therapy. This study is changing treatment practice for unruptured arteriovenous malformations.

The child with an acute brain hemorrhage requires urgent care. Attention should be toward assessment of respiratory effort, control of systemic hypertension, control of clinical and subclinical seizures, and managing increased intracranial pressure (Class I, Level of Evidence C). In general, surgical evacuation of a supratentorial intracerebral hematoma is not recommended (Class III, Level of Evidence C). Surgery is reasonable in selected patients at risk for cerebral herniation or who have extremely elevated intracranial pressure; however, it is not clear whether this improves the outcome (Class IIa, Level of Evidence C). Acute hydrocephalus with an ICH requires ventricular drainage. If hydrocephalus persists beyond the acute period, shunting may be indicated (Class I, Level of Evidence B). Low platelet counts should be corrected, and vitamin K should be administered for vitamin K–dependent coagulation disorders (Class I, Level of Evidence B). In the ongoing acute care of patients with SAH, measures to control cerebral vasospasm may be beneficial (Class IIb, Level of Evidence C).

It is reasonable to follow up asymptomatic individuals who have a condition that predisposes them to intracranial aneurysms with a cranial MRA every 1 to 5 years, depending on the perceived level of risk posed by an underlying condition (Class IIa, Level of Evidence C). Given the possible need for repeated studies over a period of years, CTA may be preferable to conventional angiogram for screening individuals at risk for aneurysm (Class IIb, Level of Evidence C).

OUTCOME

Neurologic Deficits

Disability is more prevalent after childhood ICH than other forms of stroke. In a single-center prospective cohort study at a median follow-up of 3.5 months, 71% of survivors had neurologic deficits and 55% had clinically significant disability. A prospective cohort from three centers found severe disability in 12%, moderate disability in one-half, and good recovery in only one-third.

Recurrence

In a population-based study from northern California, the 5-year cumulative recurrence rate was 10%. Sixty-four percent of recurrences were within the first 6 months. Children with idiopathic hemorrhage had no recurrences, compared with children with a structural lesion such as a vascular malformation or tumor who had a 5-year cumulative recurrence rate of 13%.

Epilepsy

In one study, at 2 years, epilepsy developed in less than 15%. A risk factor for late seizures and epilepsy was elevated intracranial pressure requiring acute intervention.

Mortality

Childhood ICH confers mortality in approximately 5%.

SICKLE CELL ANEMIA

The process of neurologic injury that confers long-term cognitive and focal impairment in SCA begins in childhood. Neurologic complications of sickle cell disease include cognitive deficit, ischemic and hemorrhagic stroke due to arterial and venous thrombus, sickle cell arteriopathy, and white matter T2 hyperintensity on brain imaging (see also Chapter 118).

EPIDEMIOLOGY

The Cooperative Study of Sickle Cell Disease, the largest series of stroke in SCA, showed that by the age of 20 years, the risk of stroke was 11% and peak incidence was from 2 to 5 years. There were no gender differences in stroke incidence. In SCA, the annual incidence of stroke is orders of magnitude greater than other childhood stroke. The Baltimore–Washington Cooperative Young Stroke Study found an annual incidence of 285 per 100,000. Ischemic stroke is more common than hemorrhagic stroke in older than 20 years, but in young adults, this trend reverses.

PATHOBIOLOGY

At low oxygen tension, sickle cell hemoglobin (HgbS) polymerizes to form an elongated and rigid sickle shape. This translates to high blood viscosity and the potential for endothelial damage. Sickle cell arteriopathy may be the most important determinant of stroke risk. Over time, arteriopathy tends to progress. Children with a history of stroke were more likely to have progressive vasculopathy than children with abnormal TCDs but no history of stroke. Silent ischemia is twice as common as clinical strokes and confers a high risk for recurrent stroke. Sickle-related arteriopathy more often takes the form of moyamoya arteriopathy with high-grade internal carotid and proximal circle of Willis artery occlusive disease and collateral formation. Older children and adults are at risk for aneurysms, dolichoectasia, and SAH.

RISK FACTORS

The combination of risk factors that result in vascular disease and stroke are still not fully understood. Risk factors such as infection, elevated leukocyte count, acute chest syndrome, inflammation, low hemoglobin concentration, and nocturnal desaturations may all contribute to the risk for stroke in SCA.

Single-nucleotide polymorphisms in genes for a tumor necrosis factor (TNF) promoter, interleukin 4 receptor, adrenoceptor beta 2, leukotriene C4 synthase, vascular cell adhesion molecule 1, and low-density lipoprotein receptor are all reported in association with stroke in children with SCA. These genes are involved in inflammatory pathways.

DIAGNOSIS AND IMAGING

The American Heart Association/American Stroke Association (AHA/ASA) guidelines (2011) recommend TCD for selection of children for primary stroke prevention. MRI and MRA are not similarly established (Class III; Level of Evidence B).

TREATMENT

The only class I recommendations for primary pediatric stroke prevention is in SCA. The recommendations largely derive from the STOP I and II randomized controlled trials. The STOP I trial enrolled children with SCA, mean TCD velocity in the ICA or middle cerebral artery of 200 cm/s or greater, and no history of stroke. Patients were randomized to periodic blood transfusions versus standard of care. The study was terminated early at 130 subjects. In the standard of care arm, there were 10 ischemic and 1 hemorrhagic strokes, compared with the transfusion arm where there was 1 ischemic stroke. Periodic transfusions reduced the risk of stroke by 92%. There is a recommendation to begin TCD screening at 2 years (Class I; Level of Evidence B) TCD should be performed annually and abnormal studies should be repeated in 1 month (Class IIa, Level of Evidence B). Borderline and mildly abnormal TCD studies may be repeated in 3 to 6 months. For TCD velocity greater than 200 cm/s, even in children without a clinical stroke, regular transfusions to reduce the percentage of sickle hemoglobin is recommended to reduce the risk of stroke in children 2 to 16 years of age (Class I, Level of Evidence A) (Grade 1B) (Class I; Level of Evidence B). Children with a confirmed infarction should also receive regular red cell transfusion in conjunction with measures to prevent iron overload (Class I, Level of Evidence B). Prior to undergoing a cerebral angiogram, all children with SCA should be treated with a red blood cell transfusion to reduce sickling precipitated by the procedure (Class I, Level of Evidence C).

When routine transfusions became accepted clinical practice for abnormal TCDs or history of a stroke, the question of when one could safely stop transfusions became widely relevant. Seven years after STOP I, STOP II published its findings. Patients with greater than 30 months on transfusion therapy, no history of a clinical stroke, and reversion to a low-risk TCD (<170 cm/s) were randomly assigned to continuation or discontinuation of transfusions. Again, the trial was stopped early. Of 41 patients in the discontinuation group, 14 developed a high-risk TCD over a mean of 4.5 months and 2 had a stroke. Neither outcome occurred in the continuation group. A long-term transfusion program is currently recommended (Grade 1B) (Class IIa; Level of Evidence B).

There is ongoing research on hydroxyurea as an alternative to routine transfusions. Hydroxyurea increases fetal hemoglobin (HgbF) and mean corpuscular volume (MCV) and it decreases reticulocytes, white blood cells, and platelets. Trials on transition from transfusion to hydroxyurea therapy have not found similar efficacy but are ongoing. Myeloablative stem cell transplantation if successful could reverse high TCD velocities and almost eliminate the risk of stroke in children. Transplantation requires a matched donor, and even if one is identified, rejection and morbidity are considerable. The AHA/ASA guidelines suggests that in children at high risk for stroke, who are not candidates for transfusion, it might be reasonable to consider hydroxyurea or bone marrow transplantation (Class IIb; Level of Evidence C).

In children without SCA and moyamoya arteriopathy, revascularization is an effective treatment for prevention of recurrent stroke. The data in children with SCA and moyamoya arteriopathy is more limited but suggests benefit. The AHA/ASA recommendation is to consider surgical revascularization as a last resort in cases where there is cerebrovascular dysfunction despite optimal medical management (Class IIb, Level of Evidence C).

Acute management of ischemic stroke should include hydration, correction of hypoxemia, and correction of systemic hypotension (Class I, Level of Evidence C). An exchange transfusion to reduce sickle hemoglobin to less than 30% of the total hemoglobin is reasonable (Class IIa, Level of Evidence C) (Grade 1B). A vascular lesion should be considered when there is an ICH (Class IIa, Level of Evidence B). There are no data to indicate that periodic transfusions reduce the risk of ICH caused by SCD (Class III, Level of Evidence B).

OUTCOME

Neurologic Deficits

Compared with healthy children, children with SCA have deficits in working memory and processing speed on neurocognitive testing.

Recurrence

Untreated, the risk of recurrent stroke may be 50%.

Mortality

Overall stroke-related mortality is approximately 10%, and in the 2 weeks after a hemorrhagic stroke, mortality is as high as one-quarter.

PERINATAL AND PRESUMED PERINATAL STROKE: ARTERIAL ISCHEMIC STROKE AND HEMORRHAGIC STROKE

Perinatal stroke is defined as signs and symptoms referable to a vascular event with radiologic or pathologic confirmation of the vascular event. A presumed perinatal stroke is diagnosed when neuroimaging shows a chronic stroke with or without delayed focal neurologic signs referable to the vascular lesion. Perinatal stroke most often affects term infants but it includes strokes that occur from 20 weeks of gestation through 28 postnatal days.

EPIDEMIOLOGY

In the National Hospital Discharge Survey (1980 to 1998), the rate of neonatal ischemic stroke was 17.8/100,000, and hemorrhagic stroke was 6.7/100,000. The overall incidence of neonatal stroke incidence was 26.4/100,000, or 1/4,000 live births, per year. This does not account for infants who present after the first few days of life, children who are diagnosed with a presumed perinatal stroke and undiagnosed hemiplegic cerebral palsy. In northern California, the population prevalence of perinatal AIS was 20 per 100,000 live births. A population-based study from Estonia accounted for neonates diagnosed acutely and retrospectively. Incidence was higher at 63 per 100,000 live births.

PATHOBIOLOGY

The majority of perinatal strokes likely occur in the few days before and after delivery. A nationwide Swedish cohort study showed that the risk of maternal embolism and hemorrhage increased more than 10 times in the 2 days before and 1 day after delivery compared with women in their third trimester. AIS is most common in the anterior circulation and on the left, specifically involving a middle cerebral artery distribution. Bilateral AIS is seen in approximately one-quarter.

Peripartum Factors

Pregnancy and delivery complications have been loosely associated with perinatal stroke. In the Kaiser Permanente Medical Care Program (1997 to 2002), a nested case-control study found that primiparity, history of infertility, preeclampsia, intrauterine growth restriction, oligohydramnios, prolonged rupture of membranes, chorioamnionitis, fetal heart rate abnormality, emergency cesarean delivery, prolonged second stage of labor, vacuum extraction, cord abnormality, 5-minute Apgar less than 7, and resuscitation at birth were more likely in infants with perinatal stroke. In an international series, maternal conditions were uncommon except for gestational hypertension or preeclampsia seen in 10%. Perinatal factors included maternal fever, prolonged rupture of membranes, presence of meconium, a prolonged second stage of labor, and emergent cesarean section seen in 26%. Among neonates, 30% required resuscitation.

Prothrombotic Factors

The meta-analysis on thrombophilia in pediatric stroke showed that neonates with a stroke were more likely to have a factor V Leiden (FVL) mutation (odds ratio [OR] 3.56; 95% CI, 2.29 to 5.53) and a prothrombin 20210 gene mutation (OR, 2.02; 95% CI, 1.02 to 3.99) compared with controls. In a study of mother–infant pairs, 64% of infants and 68% of mothers had evidence of thrombophilia. Compared with controls, infants were more likely to have FVL mutation, protein C deficiency, and antiphospholipid antibodies, and mothers were more likely to have FVL and antiphospholipid antibodies. Most mother–infant pairs were mismatched in their thrombophilia trait.

Infection

Sepsis and meningitis have long been associated with large-artery ischemic strokes and CVT. In an international series of neonates, 23% had a systemic illness around the time of stroke.

Congenital Heart Disease

Intracardiac thrombi due to congenital heart disease are a source of embolic stroke in the newborn. Approximately one-fifth of neonates have a cardiac risk factor most often in the form of congenital heart disease. At one institution, over almost a decade, the risk for AIS or CVT in children with congenital heart disease was 5.4 strokes per 1,000 children undergoing a cardiac surgery. In the Canadian Pediatric Ischemic Stroke Registry, 27% of patients with congenital heart disease had a recurrent stroke within 10 years of the original stroke, and 50% of patients with recurrence were on anticoagulation at the time of recurrence. Aside from inherited heart disease, there is limited data on other cardiac causes of perinatal stroke. In two series of neonates without known congenital heart disease, echocardiography was not informative.

Despite a recent expansion of research in this field, there are no strong predictors of perinatal stroke. Placental abnormality is suspected to be a source of systemic emboli. Research is sparse but ongoing to address this question. Little is known about pathophysiologic mechanisms of perinatal stroke.

CLINICAL FEATURES

Neonatal seizures are the most common presenting sign of a stroke. In one international series on ischemic stroke, 72% of neonates presented with seizures. Other common presenting signs are changes in tone and level of consciousness. More than 50% of neonates with ICH also present with seizures. Neonates are more likely than children to present with diffuse sign of encephalopathy such as lethargy, hypotonia, feeding difficulties, and apnea. In the same series, 63% presented with nonfocal neurologic signs most commonly respiratory and feeding difficulties. An infant with a presumed perinatal stroke may present with delayed milestones, an early hand preference, focal seizures, and hemiparesis.

DIAGNOSIS AND IMAGING

Ultrasound is safe, widely available, and does not require transport of the neonate to an imaging suite. It is sensitive for intraventricular and periventricular blood and chronic infarction, but sensitivity is low for AIS. In one study, only 30% of perinatal AIS was detected on ultrasound. CT scan is often avoided in the neonate because of the availability of ultrasound and in order to avoid exposure to radiation, but where indicated, CT will accurately show superficial ischemic and hemorrhagic lesions. MRI is safe, more sensitive for early ischemic strokes and superficial lesions, and can often be done without anesthesia in newborns.

TREATMENT

Where there is no cardiac indication for aspirin or anticoagulation, there is a recommendation against its use after a first neonatal AIS (Grade 1B). For recurrent AIS, aspirin or anticoagulation are suggested (Grade 2C). Neonates with ICH resulting from coagulation factor deficiency require replacement of the deficient coagulation factors (Class I, Level of Evidence B). Neonates born to mothers exposed to warfarin, phenytoin, or barbiturates may require higher doses of vitamin K. Supportive measures such as treatment of dehydration and anemia should be considered (Class IIa, Level of Evidence C). After a stroke, if there is delayed acquisition of milestones, hypotonia, spasticity, or focal deficits, it is reasonable to institute multispecialty therapy (Class IIa, Level of Evidence B). If an MTHFR mutation with elevated homocysteine levels is discovered, it is reasonable to give folate and B vitamins to normalize homocysteine levels for secondary stroke prevention (Class IIa, Level of Evidence C). Anticoagulation with LMWH and UFH can be considered in selected neonates with severe thrombophilic disorders and multiple cerebral or systemic emboli (Class IIb,

Level of Evidence C). Thrombolytic agents are not recommended in neonates until more information about safety and effectiveness is known (Class III, Level of Evidence C).

OUTCOME

Neurologic Deficits

A review of studies over 30 years on perinatal stroke outcome found that 57% of survivors were neurologically abnormal. In an international series, approximately half of newborns had neurologic deficits at discharge. A small cohort, followed for a mean of 2.1 years, found that by PSOM, children were normal or had only a mild impairment after AIS in 61% and after CVT in 84%. Perinatal stroke is presumed to be the most common cause of hemiplegic cerebral palsy.

Cognitive and Behavioral Deficits

After a unilateral infarction, IQ is generally preserved. Among 46 survivors of a perinatal ischemic stroke, followed for a mean of 42.1 (range 18 to 164) months, neurodevelopmental outcome was abnormal in 67%; multiple disabilities were present in 50%, cerebral palsy in 48%, and cognitive impairment in 41%.

Seizures and Epilepsy

In a single-center prospective stroke registry, at a mean follow-up of 31.3 (SD 16.1) months, 24% of patients with perinatal AIS had at least one seizure and 13% had epilepsy. In a single-center retrospective review, at a median follow-up age of 43 (range, 9 to 197) months, 67% of perinatal stroke survivors had epilepsy.

Recurrence

In northern California, the 5-year cumulative recurrence rate was only 1.2% after perinatal stroke. In another large study from Germany, among 215 neonates followed for median of 3.5 (range, 1 to 8) years, 3.3% experienced a second thromboembolic event including 1.8% who experienced a recurrent AIS.

PERINATAL CEREBRAL VENOUS THROMBOSIS

EPIDEMIOLOGY

Incidence of CVT in neonates is 2 to 3 per 100,000. CVT typically occurs in term or near-term infants. In one study, the mean gestational age was 37 weeks (SD 4 weeks, range 25 to 41 weeks), and 19% of the neonates were preterm. The mean birth weight was 2,720 g (range 770 to 3,960 g).

PATHOBIOLOGY

The deep venous system is more prone to thrombosis in the neonatal period compared with childhood. In one study, involvement of the straight sinus, vein of Galen, or internal cerebral veins was seen in more than two-thirds of neonates.

In neonates, hemorrhagic infarcts are seen in 35% to 50%. IVH is more prevalent than in children and is found in 19% to 38% of neonates. AIS has been reported in 10% and SAH in 5%.

CLINICAL FEATURES

Neonates are more likely to present with seizures and generalized encephalopathy compared with children. Typical neonatal diffuse signs are depressed level of consciousness, jitteriness, irritability, apnea, poor feeding, and low tone.

DIAGNOSIS

Symptoms may begin around the time of birth but diagnosis may be delayed. In one study, the mean age at diagnosis was 9 days.

Doppler ultrasound is portable and well tolerated, but in one neonatal study, only 48% of CVT was detected.

TREATMENT

In the large single-center retrospective analysis, 25% of the neonates were anticoagulated only after thrombus propagation. Within 2 weeks of diagnosis, thrombus propagation occurred in 4% of treated neonates and 28% of untreated neonates. Propagation was asymptomatic but was associated with new venous infarcts in 10%. Anticoagulant-related ICH occurred in 8% and only occurred when there was pretreatment ICH.

Anticoagulation can be considered in neonates with clinical or radiologic evidence of propagating CVT despite supportive therapy (Class IIb, Level of Evidence C). There is insufficient evidence to recommend the initial routine use of anticoagulation in neonates with CVT. Despite this recommendation, at many stroke centers, anticoagulation is started with initial CVT diagnosis when there is not significant hemorrhage.

OUTCOME

Anticoagulation may be safe even in neonates. In the large single-center review, there were no deaths related to anticoagulation in neonates. Recurrence is seen in 8% of neonates. Recanalization may be better in neonates than in older children. In one study at 3 months, 85% of neonates had complete recanalization.

Outcome is more likely to be normal in neonates without parenchymal involvement due to CVT. In neonates with infarction, outcome was normal in only 41% to 43%, and 29% had severe disability at follow-up. The risk of an unfavorable outcome was similar even among neonates with major anticoagulant-related hemorrhage.

Poor outcome includes epilepsy (38% in one series), spastic hemiplegia or tetraplegia, and intellectual disability or developmental delay. A predictor of poor neonatal outcome was absence of anticoagulant treatment.

GENETICS OF STROKE

Study of the genetic association in pediatric stroke may reveal important contributors to stroke mechanism. An excellent review of monogenic disorders associated with childhood AIS and arteriopathy was recently published (Munot et al.). Numerous genetic disorders are associated with an increased risk for stroke. Some of these to consider in patients with additional signs are the hereditary dyslipoproteinemia and hypercholesterolemias, inherited disorders of connective tissue such as Ehlers–Danlos syndrome (type IV) and Marfan syndrome, metabolic disorders such as Menkes syndrome and organic acidemias including glutaric aciduria type II, and disorders of energy metabolism such as mitochondrial encephalomyopathies and Leigh disease.

SUGGESTED READINGS

Adams RJ, Brambilla D; Optimizing Primary Stroke Prevention in Sickle Cell Anemia (STOP 2) Trial Investigators. Discontinuing prophylactic transfusions used to prevent stroke in sickle cell disease. *N Engl J Med.* 2005;353:2769–2778.

Adams RJ, McKie VC, Hsu L, et al. Prevention of a first stroke by transfusions in children with sickle cell anemia and abnormal results on transcranial Doppler ultrasonography. *N Engl J Med.* 1998;339:5–11.

Amlie-Lefond C, Bernard TJ, Sebire G, et al. Predictors of cerebral arteriopathy in children with arterial ischemic stroke: results of the International Pediatric Stroke Study. *Circulation.* 2009;119:1417–1423.

Aygun B, Wruck LM, Schultz WH, et al. Chronic transfusion practices for prevention of primary stroke in children with sickle cell anemia and abnormal TCD velocities. *Am J Hematol.* 2012;87:428–430.

Benders MJ, Groenendaal F, Uiterwaal CS, et al. Maternal and infant characteristics associated with perinatal arterial stroke in the preterm infant. *Stroke.* 2007;38:1759–1765.

Bernard TJ, Manco-Johnson MJ, Lo W, et al. Towards a consensus-based classification of childhood arterial ischemic stroke. *Stroke.* 2012;43:371–377.

Bernaudin F, Socie G, Kuentz M, et al. Long-term results of related myeloablative stem-cell transplantation to cure sickle cell disease. *Blood.* 2007;110:2749–2756.

Beslow LA, Abend NS, Gindville MC, et al. Pediatric intracerebral hemorrhage: acute symptomatic seizures and epilepsy. *JAMA Neurol.* 2013;70:448–454.

Beslow LA, Licht DJ, Smith SE, et al. Predictors of outcome in childhood intracerebral hemorrhage: a prospective consecutive cohort study. *Stroke.* 2010;41:313–318.

Bishop S, Matheus MG, Abboud MR, et al. Effect of chronic transfusion therapy on progression of neurovascular pathology in pediatric patients with sickle cell anemia. *Blood Cells Mol Dis.* 2011;47:125–128.

Braun KP, Bulder MM, Chabrier S, et al. The course and outcome of unilateral intracranial arteriopathy in 79 children with ischaemic stroke. *Brain.* 2009;132:544–557.

deVeber G, Andrew M, Adams C, et al. Cerebral venous thrombosis in children. *N Engl J Med.* 2001;345:417–423.

deVeber GA, MacGregor D, Curtis R, et al. Neurologic outcome in survivors of childhood arterial ischemic stroke and sinovenous thrombosis. *J Child Neurol.* 2000;15:316–324.

Earley CJ, Kittner SJ, Feeser BR, et al. Stroke in children and sickle-cell disease: Baltimore-Washington Cooperative Young Stroke Study. *Neurology.* 1998;51:169–176.

Fox CK, Glass HC, Sidney S, et al. Acute seizures predict epilepsy after childhood stroke. *Ann Neurol.* 2013;74:249–256.

Fullerton HJ, Elkins JS, Johnston SC. Pediatric stroke belt: geographic variation in stroke mortality in US children. *Stroke.* 2004;35:1570–1573.

Fullerton HJ, Wu YW, Sidney S, et al. Recurrent hemorrhagic stroke in children: a population-based cohort study. *Stroke.* 2007;38:2658–2662.

Fullerton HJ, Wu YW, Sidney S, et al. Risk of recurrent childhood arterial ischemic stroke in a population-based cohort: the importance of cerebrovascular imaging. *Pediatrics.* 2007;119:495–501.

Fullerton HJ, Wu YW, Zhao S, et al. Risk of stroke in children: ethnic and gender disparities. *Neurology.* 2003;61:189–194.

Ganesan V, Prengler M, Wade A, et al. Clinical and radiological recurrence after childhood arterial ischemic stroke. *Circulation.* 2006;114:2170–2177.

Goldstein LB, Bushnell CD, Adams RJ, et al. Guidelines for the primary prevention of stroke: a guideline for healthcare professionals from the American Heart Association/American Stroke Association. *Stroke.* 2011;42:517–584.

Golomb MR, MacGregor DL, Domi T, et al. Presumed pre- or perinatal arterial ischemic stroke: risk factors and outcomes. *Ann Neurol.* 2001;50:163–168.

Hankinson TC, Bohman LE, Heyer G, et al. Surgical treatment of moyamoya syndrome in patients with sickle cell anemia: outcome following encephaloduroarteriosynangiosis. *J Neurosurg Pediatr.* 2008;1:211–216.

Hills NK, Johnston SC, Sidney S, et al. Recent trauma and acute infection as risk factors for childhood arterial ischemic stroke. *Ann Neurol.* 2012;72:850–858.

Kenet G, Lutkhoff LK, Albisetti M, et al. Impact of thrombophilia on risk of arterial ischemic stroke or cerebral venous thrombosis in neonates and children: a systematic review and meta-analysis of observational studies. *Circulation.* 2010;121:1838–1847.

Kirton A, Armstrong-Wells J, Chang T, et al. Symptomatic neonatal arterial ischemic stroke: the International Pediatric Stroke Study. *Pediatrics.* 2011;128:e1402–e1410.

Kurnik K, Kosch A, Strater R, et al. Recurrent thromboembolism in infants and children suffering from symptomatic neonatal arterial stroke: a prospective follow-up study. *Stroke.* 2003;34:2887–2892.

Laugesaar R, Kolk A, Tomberg T, et al. Acutely and retrospectively diagnosed perinatal stroke: a population-based study. *Stroke.* 2007;38:2234–2240.

Lee J, Croen LA, Backstrand KH, et al. Maternal and infant characteristics associated with perinatal arterial stroke in the infant. *JAMA.* 2005;293:723–729.

Lynch JK. Epidemiology and classification of perinatal stroke. *Semin Fetal Neonatal Med.* 2009;14:245–249.

Lynch JK, Hirtz DG, DeVeber G, et al. Report of the National Institute of Neurological Disorders and Stroke workshop on perinatal and childhood stroke. *Pediatrics.* 2002;109:116–123.

Mackay MT, Wiznitzer M, Benedict SL, et al. Arterial ischemic stroke risk factors: the International Pediatric Stroke Study. *Ann Neurol.* 2011;69:130–140.

Ment LR, Ehrenkranz RA, Duncan CC. Bacterial meningitis as an etiology of perinatal cerebral infarction. *Pediatr Neurol.* 1986;2:276–279.

Miller ST, Macklin EA, Pegelow CH, et al. Silent infarction as a risk factor for overt stroke in children with sickle cell anemia: a report from the Cooperative Study of Sickle Cell Disease. *J Pediatr.* 2001;139:385–390.

Moharir MD, Shroff M, Stephens D, et al. Anticoagulants in pediatric cerebral venous thrombosis: a safety and outcome study. *Ann Neurol.* 2010;67:590–599.

Monagle P, Chalmers E, Chan A, et al. Antithrombotic therapy in neonates and children: American College of Chest Physicians Evidence-Based Clinical Practice Guidelines (8th Edition). *Chest.* 2008;133:887S–968S.

Munot P, Crow YJ, Ganesan V. Paediatric stroke: genetic insights into disease mechanisms and treatment targets. *Lancet Neurol.* 2011;10:264–274.

Ohene-Frempong K, Weiner SJ, Sleeper LA, et al. Cerebrovascular accidents in sickle cell disease: rates and risk factors. *Blood.* 1998;91:288–294.

Pegelow CH, Macklin EA, Moser FG, et al. Longitudinal changes in brain magnetic resonance imaging findings in children with sickle cell disease. *Blood.* 2002;99:3014–3018.

Powars D, Wilson B, Imbus C, et al. The natural history of stroke in sickle cell disease. *Am J Med.* 1978;65:461–471.

Ricci D, Mercuri E, Barnett A, et al. Cognitive outcome at early school age in term-born children with perinatally acquired middle cerebral artery territory infarction. *Stroke.* 2008;39:403–410.

Roach ES, Golomb MR, Adams R, et al. Management of stroke in infants and children: a scientific statement from a Special Writing Group of the American Heart Association Stroke Council and the Council on Cardiovascular Disease in the Young. *Stroke.* 2008;39:2644–2691.

Rodan L, McCrindle BW, Manlhiot C, et al. Stroke recurrence in children with congenital heart disease. *Ann Neurol.* 2012;72:103–111.

Schoenberg BS, Mellinger JF, Schoenberg DG. Cerebrovascular disease in infants and children: a study of incidence, clinical features, and survival. *Neurology.* 1978;28:763–768.

Sebire G, Meyer L, Chabrier S. Varicella as a risk factor for cerebral infarction in childhood: a case-control study. *Ann Neurol.* 1999;45:679–680.

Sebire G, Tabarki B, Saunders DE, et al. Cerebral venous thrombosis in children: risk factors, presentation, diagnosis and outcome. *Brain.* 2005;128:477–489.

Simchen MJ, Goldstein G, Lubetsky A, et al. Factor v Leiden and antiphospholipid antibodies in either mothers or infants increase the risk for perinatal arterial ischemic stroke. *Stroke.* 2009;40:65–70.

Wu YW, March WM, Croen LA, et al. Perinatal stroke in children with motor impairment: a population-based study. *Pediatrics.* 2004;114:612–619.

Wusthoff CJ, Kessler SK, Vossough A, et al. Risk of later seizure after perinatal arterial ischemic stroke: a prospective cohort study. *Pediatrics.* 2011;127:e1550–e1557.

Zimmerman SA, Schultz WH, Burgett S, et al. Hydroxyurea therapy lowers transcranial Doppler flow velocities in children with sickle cell anemia. *Blood.* 2007;110:1043–1047.

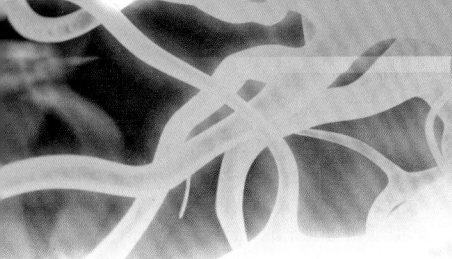

James H. Garvin Jr

INTRODUCTION

Childhood brain tumors range from benign congenital lesions to aggressive, infiltrative cancers. Cure rates for malignant brain tumors are lower than those of most other common childhood cancers, and treatment sequelae may seriously compromise quality of survival. Nonetheless, research advances and refinement of treatment techniques continue to give a sense of cautious optimism. Current research focuses on validating experimental models and identifying molecular targets for novel therapies. An emerging concept is that malignant brain tumors are propagated from stem-like progenitor cells, which may be intrinsically resistant to standard radiation and chemotherapy but could be eliminated by targeted therapy with agents, which disrupt critical signaling pathways or induce differentiation.

EPIDEMIOLOGY

Malignant and benign central nervous system (CNS) tumors may arise at any time in infancy and childhood. Categorization as malignant or benign does not always reflect clinical behavior. Certain benign lesions such as craniopharyngioma can cause extensive damage, whereas low-grade astrocytomas, although classified as malignant, are rarely life-threatening. The peak age for malignant brain tumors is 3 to 4 years. Location is predominantly cerebral or ventricular in infants, cerebellar or brain stem in young children, and midbrain or cerebral in older children and adolescents. Astrocytomas are the largest group, mostly of low-grade histology; pilocytic astrocytomas (World Health Organization [WHO] grade I) account for 24% of all childhood brain tumors. Next in frequency are medulloblastomas, the most common high-grade malignant tumor (16%). After these are a diverse group of congenital and acquired lesions, including high-grade astrocytomas (14%), ependymomas (10%), craniopharyngiomas (5.6%), germ cell tumors (2.5%), and choroid plexus tumors (0.9%). Neuronal tumors (gangliocytoma) and mixed glioneuronal tumors (ganglioglioma, dysembryoplastic neuroepithelial tumor) are relatively uncommon. The principal primary brain tumors of adults (glioblastoma multiforme, meningioma, oligodendroglioma, pituitary adenoma) are rarely seen in children. Moreover, tumorigenesis of high-grade astrocytomas in children differs from that in adults, as deduced from comparative genomic hybridization studies. CNS metastases from solid tumors are also uncommon in children compared to adults. Cerebral metastases are occasionally seen in pediatric germ cell tumors (13.5% incidence), osteosarcoma (6.5%), neuroblastoma (4.4%), melanoma (3.6%), Ewing sarcoma (3.3%), rhabdomyosarcoma (1.9%), and Wilms tumor (1.3%).

Primary CNS malignancies account for about 20% of all childhood cancers, second only to leukemia. Approximately 2,200 cases are diagnosed annually in the United States in children and adolescents age 0 to 19 years, an incidence of 2.9 per 100,000 population in this age group. When nonmalignant lesions are added, the total annual incidence is about 3,750 cases. The reported annual incidence of childhood brain tumors in the United States increased by 35% between 1973 and 1994, led mainly by supratentorial low-grade gliomas and brain stem tumors diagnosed by magnetic resonance imaging (MRI), which became widely available in the mid-1980s. The reported incidence of brain tumors in infants below 12 months of age increased between 1973 and 1986 but has remained stable since then; leading histologies in infants are gliomas, medulloblastoma/primitive neuroectodermal tumor (PNET), and ependymoma.

The causes of congenital and childhood CNS tumors remain unknown. A meta-analysis from 16 international surveys revealed a male-to-female ratio of 1.29. Increased head circumference at birth is positively associated with brain cancer in childhood, with a relative risk of 1.27 per 1-cm increase after adjustment for birth weight, gestational age, and gender, suggesting brain pathology may originate in fetal development. The most common CNS tumors diagnosed in the first year of life are low-grade glioma, medulloblastoma, ependymoma, and choroid plexus tumors.

Most CNS tumors are sporadic, but some are seen in inherited disorders, especially neurocutaneous syndromes. Individuals with *neurofibromatosis type 1* (NF-1) have a 10% chance of developing an intracranial tumor, including optic pathway gliomas and astrocytomas elsewhere in the brain and spinal cord. The NF-1 gene maps to chromosome 17q11.2, and loss of one NF-1 allele is evident in nearly all NF-1–associated pilocytic astrocytomas but only rarely in sporadic pilocytic astrocytomas, suggesting different mechanisms of tumor formation. In the less common *neurofibromatosis type 2* (NF-2), there is a predisposition to bilateral vestibular schwannomas, with chromosome 22q deletions and NF-2 gene mutations in at least half of cases. NF-2 also predisposes to ependymomas, which commonly show a chromosome 22q deletion, but analysis of the NF-2 gene in ependymomas has revealed only a single mutation in a tumor that had lost the remaining wild-type allele.

Children with *tuberous sclerosis* may have a subependymal giant cell astrocytoma or ependymoma. Tuberous sclerosis genes map to chromosomes 9q and 16p, and allelic loss at these loci has been found in some subependymal giant cell astrocytomas, suggesting a tumor suppressor function. Hemangioblastomas of the cerebellum, medulla, and spinal cord are associated with *von Hippel–Lindau disease*, and choroid plexus tumors have occasionally been reported. Loss of chromosome 3p sequences has been described in one choroid plexus tumor, suggesting involvement of the VHL gene. There is an increased risk of brain tumors, particularly choroid plexus carcinoma, in the *Li-Fraumeni syndrome*, involving germ line mutations in *p53* on chromosome 17. *Gorlin syndrome* (*nevoid basal cell carcinoma syndrome*), resulting from *PTCH1* gene mutation, predisposes to medulloblastoma, specifically sonic hedgehog (Shh) subtype (see the following discussion).

Combined cytogenetic and molecular studies of the common sporadic childhood brain tumors have identified genomic alterations that may lead to the identification of genes contributing to tumorigenesis. Isochromosome 17q is found in half of all medulloblastomas implicating a tumor suppressor gene. Clinical outcome is now predictable by gene expression profiles. For example, overexpression of *p53* in malignant gliomas of childhood is associated with adverse outcome. In medulloblastoma, low *MYC* oncogene mRNA expression and high *TrkC* neurotrophin receptor mRNA expression identify a good outcome; the desmoplastic subtype of medulloblastoma is specifically associated with the *basal cell nevus syndrome* (BCNS) (Gorlin syndrome), in which the molecular defect is thought to be a mutation in the human homologue of the Drosophila patched gene. Identification of a novel polymorphism in this gene allows direct detection of allelic loss in BCNS. Desmoplastic medulloblastoma in infants from affected families is reported to have a good prognosis. Conversely, the large cell, anaplastic variant of medulloblastoma and the atypical teratoid/rhabdoid tumor (ATRT) have an unfavorable prognosis. Diagnosis of these variants is based on light microscopic and immunohistochemical findings, and ATRT is further distinguished by chromosome 22q11 deletion with inactivation of the hSNF5/INI1 gene.

Environmental risk factors for CNS tumors include ionizing radiation, which in the distant past was given even for benign conditions such as tinea capitis. In children treated for acute lymphoblastic leukemia, there is a 1.39% cumulative incidence of secondary brain tumors (gliomas and meningiomas) at 20 years, and cranial irradiation is a dose-dependent predisposing factor. Cerebral PNETs may also follow cranial irradiation. Another study with 30-year follow-up found a 3.0% cumulative incidence of brain tumors (excluding meningioma) following *all* treatment. There is no conclusive evidence of risk from prenatal x-ray exposure, prenatal ultrasound, or from electromagnetic fields (from electric blankets or other residential exposure).

Studies have shown an association between farm and animal exposures and childhood brain tumors and a weak association with toxic exposures occurring in the household. Although not implicated in retrospective studies, maternal smoking during pregnancy was associated with slightly increased risk of brain tumors in offspring in a prospective study linking birth and cancer registries. The incidence of medulloblastoma in England declined after 1984 when multivitamin supplementation in pregnancy became widespread following reports that folate reduced the risk of neural tube defects. Maternal intake of folic acid in pregnancy was reported to be protective against PNETs, but this association could not be confirmed in a subsequent study. A seasonal variation has been noted in the incidence of medulloblastoma (but not other brain tumors) in the United States between 1995 and 2001, peaking in October. Possibly related is an observation of increased risk of medulloblastoma/PNET associated with paternal exposure to any heat source, such as electric blanket, in the 3 months prior to the index pregnancy.

PATHOBIOLOGY

Current research on CNS tumorigenesis is based on the molecular genetics of tumor-associated syndromes, rodent models of pediatric brain tumors, and technologic advances in efforts to identify genes that regulate normal and neoplastic cells in the developing CNS. Although the names of brain tumors imply that they originate from normal brain cells (e.g., astrocytoma from astrocytes), the primitive embryonal tumors of childhood that arise during brain development more likely result from aberrant regulation of neurodevelopmental genes. Recently, it has been postulated that brain tumors, like hematologic malignancies, contain small numbers of stem cells (identified as CD133-positive), which have

marked capacity for proliferation and self-renewal. These stem cells can differentiate to phenotypically recognizable brain tumor cells but also maintain clonal proliferation and may be highly resistant to conventional anticancer treatment such as radiation and cytotoxic chemotherapy. Candidate stem cells have been proposed for medulloblastoma, ependymoma, and malignant gliomas. Further characterization of brain tumor stem cells may offer new insights into mechanisms of tumorigenesis and lead to novel treatment strategies based on preferential targeting of tumor stem cells.

SONIC HEDGEHOG, WNT SIGNALING, CEREBELLAR DEVELOPMENT, AND MEDULLOBLASTOMA

In the 19th century, Obersteiner described the cells of the external granular layer (EGL) in the developing cerebellum. Based on morphologic similarity, granule cell precursors (GCPs) were considered the cells of origin in medulloblastoma. Now, gene chip analysis and mouse models have linked medulloblastoma to molecular markers of GCPs. Only medulloblastomas carry these molecular markers of developing cells, whereas supratentorial PNETs do not.

The cerebellum matures through a complex interplay of genes of general CNS development and specifically cerebellar genes. For instance, *Shh* is a glycoprotein involved in the development of the CNS. In cerebellar development, Purkinje cells secrete Shh to activate genes in GCPs and stimulate proliferation of these cells. Activating mutations of the Shh pathway account for desmoplastic medulloblastoma in the nevoid basal cell carcinoma syndrome (Gorlin syndrome), 10% to 20% of sporadic medulloblastomas, and histologically similar tumors in mice that are heterozygous for the equivalent genes. Genome sequencing of Shh-driven medulloblastomas reveals pathway mutations involving PTCH1 (across all age groups), SUFU (infants, including cases of germ line mutation), and SMO (in adults). Functional assays in different Shh-driven medulloblastoma xenografts demonstrated that tumors harboring PTCH mutation were responsive to SMO inhibition, whereas tumors with SUFU mutation or MYCN amplification were resistant.

Wnt proteins also play a role in CNS development and have been linked to medulloblastoma. Patients with Turcot syndrome, which involves defects in the *APC* (*a*denomatous *p*olyposis *c*omplex) gene, are susceptible to colorectal and brain tumors, notably medulloblastoma. *APC* is an element of the *Wnt* signaling pathway, and up to 30% of spontaneous medulloblastomas show mutations in *APC* and other components of this neurodevelopmental signaling cascade. Cell nuclear accumulation of β-catenin protein is also associated with activation of *Wnt/Wg* signaling, and positive immunostain for β-catenin in medulloblastoma has been associated with favorable treatment outcome even with metastatic disease at presentation.

Wnt proteins bind to receptors and modulate *C-myc*, a transcription factor that promotes cell cycle progression. Activation of *C-myc* and *N-myc* leads to proliferation, cell growth, and maintenance of an undifferentiated cellular phenotype; these genes are amplified in some medulloblastomas and are associated with a poor clinical outcome. The same genes are amplified by the *Shh* pathway. *Wnt1* is required for mesencephalon/metencephalon patterning early in development. Cerebellar primordia fail to develop in mice lacking *Wnt1*, and mutations in other *Wnt* pathway components have been implicated not only in medulloblastoma but also in colon cancer, hepatocellular carcinoma, and prostate and ovarian cancers.

Deletion of chromosome 17p, the most frequently detected genetic lesion in medulloblastoma, has been identified as a cause of unrestrained hedgehog signaling. This deletion results in loss of REN(KCTD11), a novel hedgehog antagonist, thus removing a checkpoint of hedgehog-dependent events during cerebellar development and tumorigenesis. Inactivation of the tumor suppressor *p53*, also a resident of chromosome 17, may contribute to the growth of tumors resembling medulloblastoma in mice, but there is neither an increased incidence of medulloblastoma in humans lacking *p53* nor a change in *p53* within the medulloblastoma cells.

The gene *Bmi1*, which induces leukemia through repression of tumor suppressors, is overexpressed in many medulloblastomas and promotes cerebellar GCP proliferation. Linked overexpression of *Bmi1* and patched (*PTCH*) in primary human medulloblastomas, together with rapid induction of Bmi1 expression on addition of *Shh* or overexpression of the *Shh* target Gli1 in cerebellar granule cell culture, implicates *Bmi1* overexpression as an alternative or additive mechanism in medulloblastoma pathogenesis.

ASTROCYTES, GROWTH FACTORS, TUMOR SUPPRESSORS, AND ASTROCYTOMA

Astrocytes develop later than neurons and continue to do so long after neurogenesis stops. Astrocytes retain the capacity for division throughout life and are more susceptible to transformation. Control over astrocyte proliferation and differentiation may be divided into two main categories: cell signaling and cell cycle arrest pathways. During glial development, precursor cells respond to growth factors such as epidermal growth factor (EGF) or platelet-derived growth factor (PDGF). Their receptors (epidermal growth factor receptor [EGFR] and platelet-derived growth factor receptor [PDGFR]) are activated to stimulate tyrosine kinase activity and intracellular pathways that control proliferation and differentiation, programmed cell death, migration, cellular shape, and metabolism.

Amplification and mutation of EGFR are among the most common genetic abnormalities found in adult glioblastomas, particularly those arising de novo (as opposed to lesions progressing from fibrillary astrocytomas). These tumors contain ligands that may activate the receptor, stimulating a pathway that results in tumor progression. In addition, the receptor may be mutated to a constitutively activated form, unable to bind ligand but generating unregulated tyrosine kinase activity. Mice lacking *EGFR* have fewer glial fibrillary acidic protein (GFAP)–positive cells, and massive neuronal degeneration is attributed to a lack of trophic support from the missing glial cells. Amplification of EGFR is uncommon in pediatric high-grade astrocytomas, but significant differential expression of the *EGFR/FKBP12/HIF-2α* growth– and angiogenesis-promoting pathway has been demonstrated. High PDGFR protein expression is associated with malignant histology in pediatric glioma but is not an independent prognostic factor. Attempts to block glioma progression through disruption of the EGFR pathway have led to development of drugs targeting EGFR or PDGFR.

Ras is a downstream effector of several growth factor receptors, signaling through both mitogenic and antiapoptotic pathways. It is under control of the NF-1 gene neurofibromin, and loss of function mutations in neurofibromin underlie the NF-1 syndrome, with predisposition to optic nerve glioma, astrocytoma, and glioblastoma. Neurofibromin functions as a Ras-guanosine triphosphatase-activating protein, but it had been unclear how Ras deregulation was involved in NF-1 pathogenesis. It has now been demonstrated that neurofibromin tightly regulates the mTOR (mammalian target of rapamycin) pathway. mTOR is a highly conserved serine/threonine protein kinase that regulates many steps in cell growth and proliferation, including ribosome biogenesis and protein translation. mTOR

is constitutively activated in NF1-deficient cells and tumors; aberrant mTOR activation depends on Ras and is mediated by the phosphorylation and inactivation of the tuberous sclerosis complex-2 (TSC2)–encoded protein tuberin. Tumor cell lines from NF-1 patients are highly sensitive to the mTOR inhibitor rapamycin, which has therapeutic implications.

Molecular profiling of pediatric glioblastomas identifies at least two subsets. One group is associated with *Ras* and *Akt* pathway activation and exhibits increased expression of genes related to proliferation and a neural stem cell phenotype; this subset has very poor prognosis. A second group with better prognosis is not associated with activation of *Ras* and *Akt* pathways and may originate from astroglial progenitors. Both subsets show overexpression of Y-box protein-1, which may promote oncogenesis.

The tumor suppressor phosphatase with homology to tensin (*PTEN*) is mutated or lost in some pediatric high-grade astrocytomas, as in primary adult glioblastoma. *PTEN* is expressed throughout the embryo and is critical in CNS development. *PTEN* mutations are thought to cause Lhermitte–Duclos disease (dysplastic gangliocytoma of the cerebellum) characterized by enlarged cerebellar foliae, distorted cerebellar cortex, abnormally myelinated axon bundles, and dysplastic neurons. Conditional inactivation of the gene in the cerebellum of developing mice has generated a mammalian model of that disease. Loss of *PTEN* promotes astrocytic growth and survival because it would otherwise act as a repressor of antiapoptotic signaling pathways. *PTEN* is also thought to regulate astrocyte migration and invasion by effects on cell shape and movement. When *PTEN* is overexpressed, it inhibits tumor cell movement; conversely, reduction of *PTEN* activity promotes cell movement, invasiveness, and perhaps metastasis. Loss of *PTEN* has been associated with inferior survival in childhood gliomas. *PTEN* is a component gene in the mTOR pathway; immunohistochemical analysis of Lhermitte–Duclos disease lesions showed high levels of phospho-AKT and phospho-S6 in the large ganglionic cells, indicating activation of the PTEN/AKT/mTOR pathway and suggesting a central role for mTOR in LDD pathogenesis, as well as potential therapeutic intervention through pharmacologic inhibition of mTOR.

The tumor suppressors *retinoblastoma (Rb) protein* and *p53* are also regulators of cell survival and programmed cell death and are intimately involved with astrocytoma. *Rb* mutations in children lead to tumors in the retina, whereas mice null for *Rb* do not survive because of lethally abnormal patterns of neuronal development with pronounced CNS programmed cell death. *Rb* encodes a phosphoprotein important in cell cycle regulation, blocking transcription factors that promote proliferation. In the developing CNS, *Rb* is found in the ventricular zone where neuroblasts proliferate.

Rb is also involved in the regulation of apoptosis through interactions with the tumor suppressor *p53*, a transcription factor upregulated in response to cellular stress to facilitate arrest of the cell cycle for either DNA repair or cell death. Humans with the Li–Fraumeni syndrome lack *p53* and show marked susceptibility to gliomas. *p53* mutant mice develop tumors early in life.

Under conditions of *Rb* inactivation, many cells enter the cell cycle inappropriately and subsequently undergo apoptosis. However, *Rb* loss may synergize with the loss of apoptotic regulators, such as *p53* to promote tumor formation. With the loss of *Rb*, transcription factors go unchecked, which then promotes cell proliferation. Loss of *Rb* might normally lead to apoptosis, but if *p53* is also missing, apoptosis is impaired and tumorigenesis is enhanced. In fact, approximately 75% of adult glioblastomas show impaired apoptotic mechanisms and *p53* pathway defects. Mutations in *p53* were detected in one-third of childhood high-grade astrocytomas, and nearly half over-expressed the p53 protein. This finding was strongly associated with adverse outcome.

Mutations in histone and chromatin remodeling genes appear to be uniquely important in pediatric glioblastoma multiforme. Exome sequencing revealed somatic mutations in the H3.3-ATRX-DAXX chromatin remodeling pathway in nearly half of cases and recurrent mutations in H3F3A (which encodes H3.3) in one-third. H3F3A mutations were specific to GBM, highly prevalent in children and young adults, and tended to be associated with somatic TP53 mutations and alternative telomere lengthening. Increased TERC (telomerase RNA template) and hTERT mRNA (encoding telomerase catalytic component) have been associated with worse overall survival in children with non–brain stem high-grade glioma after controlling for tumor grade and extent of resection.

BRAF alterations (in particular tandem duplication and fusion *BRAF–KIAA1549* on chromosome 7q34) are now widely accepted as molecular markers for pilocytic astrocytoma, in particular for the differential diagnosis of supratentorial pediatric gliomas. Besides their diagnostic use, the evidence of MAPK pathway–activating *BRAF* fusions and mutations in brain tumors has moreover drawn the attention of neurooncologists to the potential use of MEK1/2 and RAF inhibitors in the therapy of high- and low-grade gliomas.

Investigation of molecular aberrations in the most devastating tumor, diffuse intrinsic pontine glioma (DIPG), has lagged because most cases are diagnosed clinically without pathologic confirmation. However, high-resolution single-nucleotide polymorphism–based DNA analysis of a series of DIPGs using postmortem samples revealed recurrent changes distinct from supratentorial high-grade astrocytomas, specifically expression (and gains) of platelet-derived growth factor receptor alpha (PDGFRA) and occasional low-level gains in poly (ADP-ribose) polymerase (PARP)-1. Mutations in

H3F3A (encoding histone H3.3) or HIST1H3B (encoding histone H3.1) appear to be common in DIPG. Whole-genome sequencing has identified three molecular subgroups of DIPG (H3-K27M, silent, and MYCN) and recurrent activating mutations involving the activin receptor gene ACVR1 in some cases.

CLINICAL FEATURES

Children with brain tumors often present with symptoms and signs of increased intracranial pressure (ICP). The ventricular or periventricular location of many tumors, and associated mass effect, results in obstruction of normal cerebrospinal fluid (CSF) pathways and ventriculomegaly. Characteristic signs are headache, vomiting, and diplopia, but the onset may be gradual and nonfocal. Fatigue, personality change, or worsening school performance may be described. Symptoms in infants are nonspecific and include irritability, anorexia, persistent vomiting, and developmental delay or regression, with macrocephaly and seemingly forced-downward deviation of the eyes ("sunset sign"). The median duration of symptoms before diagnosis was 2 months in two series; only one-third of the patients were diagnosed in the first month after onset of symptoms, but diagnostic delay is less important than tumor aggressiveness in determining survival outcome. Persistent vomiting, recurrent headache (awakening the child from sleep), neurologic findings (ataxia, head tilt, weakness, vision loss, papilledema), endocrine disturbance (growth deceleration, diabetes insipidus, precocious puberty), and stigmata of neurofibromatosis should all prompt immediate evaluation for the presence of a CNS tumor.

Symptoms and signs reflect tumor location, and in children (unlike adults), CNS tumors are divided about equally between supratentorial and infratentorial sites (Table 145.1). In a

TABLE 145.1 Location of Central Nervous System Tumors in Infants, Children, and Adolescents

Location	Infant	Child	Adolescent
Cerebral	PNET	Low-grade astrocytoma High-grade astrocytoma PNET Ganglioglioma PXA	High-grade astrocytoma Oligodendroglioma Meningioma Lymphoma
Suprasellar and optic pathway	Low-grade astrocytoma Craniopharyngioma	Low-grade astrocytoma Craniopharyngioma Germ cell tumor	Craniopharyngioma Epidermoid
Ventricular	Choroid plexus tumor Ependymoma Colloid cyst	Ependymoma Low-grade astrocytoma	Colloid cyst Central neurocytoma
Midbrain	Low-grade astrocytoma Dermoid	Low-grade astrocytoma High-grade astrocytoma	High-grade astrocytoma
Pineal	Teratoma Pineocytoma	PNET Germ cell tumor	Germ cell tumor
Posterior fossa	Medulloblastoma Ependymoma Low-grade astrocytoma Gangliocytoma	Medulloblastoma Brain stem glioma Ependymoma Low-grade astrocytoma	Low-grade astrocytoma Medulloblastoma Ependymoma Epidermoid
Spinal cord	Low-grade astrocytoma	Low-grade astrocytoma	Low-grade astrocytoma High-grade astrocytoma

PNET, primitive neuroectodermal tumor; PXA, pleomorphic xanthoastrocytoma.

meta-analysis, the ratio of supra- to infratentorial tumors was 0.92, and infratentorial location was more common between the ages of 3 and 11 years (Table 145.2).

Supratentorial tumors, which predominate in infants and toddlers and also occur in older children, cause headache; limb weakness; sensory loss; and, occasionally, seizures, deteriorating school performance, or personality change. Seizures are a presenting symptom in 10% to 15% of children with brain tumors and may be generalized, focal motor, or psychomotor; electroencephalogram (EEG) is almost always abnormal. Most seizure-associated tumors are in the temporal lobe; frontal lobe tumors more often affect personality and movement, although seizures have been reported with frontal–parietal tumors. The incidence of underlying neoplasm in children with intractable epilepsy approaches 20%, and the increased risk of having a brain tumor is noted even 10 or more years after a diagnosis of epilepsy.

Parietal lobe tumors affect reading ability and awareness of contralateral extremities (hemineglect). Occipital lobe tumors cause visual field disturbance and occasionally, hallucinations. Suprasellar lesions may cause both visual field defects and endocrine dysfunction. The Parinaud syndrome (upgaze paresis and mild pupil dilatation with better reaction to accommodation than light, retraction or convergence nystagmus, and lid retraction) is found in pineal region tumors.

Infratentorial tumors, which predominate from ages 4 to 11 years, typically cause headache, vomiting, diplopia, and imbalance. Bilateral sixth cranial nerve palsy is a frequent sign of increased ICP.

Brain stem tumors cause facial and extraocular muscle palsies, ataxia, and hemiparesis. Leptomeningeal spread occurs at diagnosis or recurrence in up to 15% of children with CNS tumors (more often in medulloblastoma/PNET) and may be asymptomatic or may cause pain, irritability, weakness, or bowel and bladder dysfunction.

DIAGNOSIS

MRI is the preferred imaging modality for evaluation of children with symptoms suggestive of brain tumor (e.g., persistent headache of recent onset, morning vomiting) and abnormal signs on neurologic examination (head tilt, ataxia) or other clinical predictors of brain tumor (diabetes insipidus). Computed tomography (CT) may be the initial evaluation (especially if hydrocephalus or intracranial hemorrhage is suspected), but compared with CT, MRI is more sensitive (especially for nonenhancing, infiltrative tumors and leptomeningeal involvement), may generate images in any plane (e.g., axial, coronal, sagittal), and is not compromised in the posterior fossa by bone artifact. Brain tumors are typically hypo- or isointense on T1-weighted imaging and hyperintense on T2-weighted imaging. Contrast enhancement is a feature of malignant tumors, reflecting blood–brain barrier disruption. Perfusion and diffusion sequences may also be useful in assessing tumor aggressiveness. Magnetic resonance spectroscopy (MRS) can provide additional information; for example, compared to benign

TABLE 145.2	Childhood Central Nervous System Tumors Diagnosed in the United States in 2005 to 2009 by Histology and Age at Diagnosis				
Histology	0–4	5–9	10–14	15–19	Total
Astrocytoma, low grade	1,220	1,084	1,108	890	3,412
Astrocytoma, high grade	207	431	385	407	1,342
Glioma, malignant, NOS	875	789	427	254	2,345
Oligodendroglioma, anaplastic, oligo, oligoastrocytic tumors	58	61	89	187	419
Ependymoma	402	226	211	273	1,112
Choroid plexus tumors	265	40	38	51	394
Neuronal, mixed neuronal–glial, and other neuroepithelial tumors	248	297	429	482	1,486
Pineal region tumors	53	38	32	42	165
Embryonal tumors (medulloblastoma, sPNET, ATRT)	1,232	737	387	261	2,617
Nerve sheath tumors	272	207	252	369	1,100
Meningioma, other meningeal	70	60	176	369	688
Mesenchymal tumors	56	28	31	35	150
Primary melanocytic lesions	—	—	—	—	19
Lymphoma, other hematologic	—	22	20	35	90
Germ cell tumors	129	133	262	299	823
Pituitary tumors	33	107	392	1,362	1,894
Craniopharyngioma	141	251	216	158	766
Hemangioma	49	38	74	132	293
Neoplasm, NOS	173	136	176	242	727
TOTAL	**5,517**	**4,589**	**4,740**	**5,863**	**20,709**

NOS, not otherwise specified; sPNET, supratentorial primitive neuroectodermal tumor; ATRT, atypical teratoid/rhabdoid tumor.

Data from Dolecek TA, Propp JM, Stroup NE, et al. CBTRUS statistical report: primary brain and central nervous system tumors diagnosed in the United States in 2005-2009. *Neuro Oncol.* 2012;14(suppl 5):v1–v49.

tumors or normal brain, malignant tumors have increased choline peaks (reflecting increased membrane turnover) and decreased *N*-acetylaspartate (absence of functional neurons). MRI is repeated postoperatively to confirm extent of tumor resection, although it may be difficult to distinguish tumor from surrounding edema or residual tumor from postoperative changes; for these reasons, postoperative studies should be obtained within 48 hours of surgery.

MRI of the spine has replaced myelography as the standard procedure for evaluation of spinal cord tumors, drop metastases, and leptomeningeal disease. Spine MRI is required in cases of medulloblastoma, ependymoma, choroid plexus carcinoma, ATRT, and pineal region tumors and should be obtained preoperatively if one of these diagnoses is suspected. Lumbar puncture for CSF cytology and tumor markers should also be done in children with these diagnoses. Recommended baseline and surveillance studies, based on tumor aggressiveness and patterns of recurrence, are shown in Table 145.3.

Treatment responses are determined by change in tumor size on MRI based on the most reproducible measurements from T2/fluid-attenuated inversion recovery (FLAIR)–weighted or post-contrast T1-weighted images, whichever gives the best estimate of tumor size. Measurements of the longest tumor dimension and its perpendicular should be recorded for all target lesions (up to 5) and any new lesions. In assessing response, lesions less than twice the combined thickness of the image slice and interslice gap are discounted, and cystic/necrotic elements and/or leptomeningeal disease are generally not measured. Enlargement or reduction of existing lesions should correlate with increase or decrease in two-dimensional measurement, but increased enhancement on T1 without increase in disease bulk on T2/FLAIR is not considered tumor progression, and decreased enhancement without decreased bulk on T2/FLAIR may represent altered contrast permeability rather than regression. Thus, complete or partial response (CR, PR) requires disappearance or greater than 50% reduction of all target lesions, respectively, whereas 25% increase or the appearance of new lesions or newly positive CSF cytology indicates progressive disease (PD). Imaging may be supplemented by positron emission tomography (PET), which characterizes metabolic abnormalities that distinguish high grade from low grade and residual or recurrent tumor from cerebral necrosis. *Thallium-201* single-photon emission computed tomography (SPECT) is sensitive for recurrent tumors, although MRS offers similar capability and is more widely available.

TREATMENT

SURGERY

The mainstay of therapy is *surgery*, which may be curative by itself in resectable congenital and benign tumors. Gross total resection is generally attempted in malignant tumors and contributes to the cure rates of high-grade astrocytoma, medulloblastoma, or ependymoma. Adoption of intraoperative MRI can improve the rate of tumor resection and may alter surgical strategy. Gross total resection (no visible tumor at completion of surgery) or radical subtotal resection (95% to 99% removal of tumor) should be confirmed by postoperative MRI. Radical resection is generally not attempted for lesions deep in the thalamus or for diffuse, intrinsic brain stem tumors; surgery is typically limited to open or closed biopsy (<1% resection) or partial or subtotal resection (10% to 49% and 50% to 95% tumor removal, respectively). Multiple biopsies may be useful in lesions appearing heterogeneous on MRI when major resection is not attempted. The introduction of the operating microscope and ultrasonic aspirator has improved both the safety and effectiveness of surgery. Stereotactic (e.g., CT or MRI guided) techniques are used for biopsy or subtotal resection in difficult-to-reach areas such as the basal ganglia. However, even a 99% resection of a lesion that is 10 cm^3 in size will leave 10^8 tumor cells behind, and

TABLE 145.3 Staging and Surveillance of Children with Central Nervous System Tumors

Diagnosis	Baseline Evaluation	Surveillance (Months from End of Treatment)
Medulloblastoma/PNET Posterior fossa ependymoma Germ cell tumor Atypical teratoid rhabdoid tumor Choroid plexus carcinoma	Brain/spine MRI Lumbar CSF	Brain MRI 3, 6, 9, 12, 16, 20, 24, 30, 36, 48, 60, and annually Spine MRI 12, 24[a], 36, 48[a]
Brain stem glioma Supratentorial ependymoma	Brain/spine MRI Lumbar CSF (for ependymoma)	Brain MRI 4, 8, 12, 16, 20, 24, 30, 36, 48, 60, and annually Spine MRI 18,[a] 48[a]
Cerebellar low-grade astrocytoma Hypothalamic/optic glioma Cerebral low-grade glioma Oligodendroglioma Craniopharyngioma Choroid plexus papilloma	Brain MRI	Brain MRI 6, 12, 18, 24, 36, 48, 60, and annually
Cerebellar or cerebral high-grade astrocytoma	Brain MRI Spine MRI[b] Lumbar CSF[b]	Brain MRI 3, 6, 9, 12, 18, 24, 30, 36, 42, 48, 60, and annually Spine MRI 12,[a] 24,[a] 36,[a] 48[a]

[a]If residual or dissemination.

[b]If symptoms.

PNET, primitive neuroectodermal tumor; MRI, magnetic resonance imaging; CSF, cerebrospinal fluid.

Data from Kramer ED, Vezine LG, Packer RJ, et al. Staging and surveillance of children with central nervous system neoplasms: recommendations of the Neurology and Tumor Imaging Committees of the Children's Cancer Group. *Pediatr Neurosurg.* 1994;20:254–263.

additional postoperative treatment will be necessary to prevent the lesion from regrowing. Surgery is important for establishing a tissue diagnosis and relieving obstructive hydrocephalus. With temporary placement of an external drain or endoscopic third ventriculostomy, followed by tumor resection, it may be possible to avoid the need for a permanent ventriculoperitoneal shunt, in most patients.

Operative mortality is generally not more than 1%, but morbidity varies according to the site and extent of surgery and the condition of the child. A unique and increasingly recognized complication of midline posterior fossa tumor resection is the *cerebellar mutism syndrome*, consisting of diminished speech progressing to mutism, emotional lability, hypotonia, and ataxia. In two prospective trials for standard and high-risk medulloblastoma, cerebellar mutism was reported in 24% of children. In both cohorts, brain stem invasion by tumor was the only predictive feature. At 1 year from diagnosis, nonmotor speech/language deficits, neurocognitive deficits, and/or ataxia persisted in a substantial proportion of patients.

Surgery may be facilitated by intraoperative monitoring of sensory and other evoked potentials. Adjunctive measures include the use of corticosteroids, which counteract tumor edema and are often used in the perioperative period but should be tapered within 1 to 2 weeks, if possible. Patients undergoing surgery for supratentorial tumors are placed on anticonvulsants if they have had seizures or if the surgical approach is likely to cause seizures. Prophylactic anticonvulsants are generally continued for 1 week to 12 months.

RADIATION THERAPY

Radiation therapy is used for nearly all malignant CNS tumors and for some benign lesions. Based on standard x-ray (photon) therapy, doses typically administered to achieve local control range from 45 to 55 Gy, in divided fractions of 150 to 200 cGy, to the tumor as localized on MRI plus 1- to 2-cm margin. Higher doses may be given, often in smaller twice-daily doses (e.g., hyperfractionated technique), but with high total doses, there is increased risk of injuring normal brain tissue. The volume irradiated depends on tumor histology and may include an involved field or whole brain and spine. Presymptomatic craniospinal irradiation is almost always given for medulloblastoma because of its propensity to disseminate throughout the neuraxis. Doses of 36 Gy have been used conventionally, but lower doses (23.4 Gy and possibly 18 Gy) are adequate in standard-risk patients if supplemented with adjuvant chemotherapy.

Newer radiotherapy techniques may increase the effective tumor dose and limit toxicity to the surrounding brain. *Three-dimensional conformal radiation therapy* allows tailoring of treatment to the actual tumor volume rather than arbitrary compartments such as the whole posterior fossa. *Stereotactic irradiation* techniques with arc photons, in conjunction with rigid head fixation systems, permit single high-dose delivery (e.g., radiosurgery), which may be useful for management of recurrent lesions in previously irradiated patients. *Intensity-modulated radiation therapy* (IMRT) uses combinations of variable intensity fields from different beam directions to maximize tumor dose while minimizing dose to adjacent normal tissues. *Proton therapy* takes advantage of the superior physical properties of protons compared to photons, with limited penetration of particles beyond the tumor target, less tissue scatter, and little lateral dispersion. Early applications of proton therapy included ocular melanoma and skull base tumors, but the possibility of comparable tumor control with substantially decreased dose to adjacent normal tissues makes the technique potentially

advantageous for many pediatric indications. *Interstitial radioactive implants* (brachytherapy) may be appropriate in some cases. Use of *radiation sensitizers*, including chemotherapy agents (carboplatin, capecitabine, tipifarnib) and gadolinium derivatives, is currently under study.

Acute side effects of radiation therapy include headache, nausea, alopecia, skin hyperpigmentation and desquamation, and a transient "somnolence syndrome," occurring 4 to 8 weeks after treatment. Radiation therapy to large volumes is problematic in infants and toddlers because of increased neurocognitive sequelae. Dose-intensive chemotherapy may be used to defer irradiation, or involved field treatment with supplemental chemotherapy may be substituted for whole-brain irradiation (as in medulloblastoma).

CHEMOTHERAPY

Chemotherapy is used as an adjunct to radiotherapy, as primary postsurgical treatment in infants, as neoadjuvant therapy in chemotherapy-sensitive tumors (e.g., germ cell tumors), and in recurrent tumors. Effective agents include the nitrosoureas (e.g., carmustine, lomustine), vincristine, cisplatin, carboplatin, etoposide, and cyclophosphamide. Temozolomide appears promising, although response rates in phase II trials have been relatively low. Chemotherapy is generally given systemically and in combination because of complementary mechanisms of action of different agents and to subvert potential tumor resistance. The effectiveness of systemically administered chemotherapy is limited by the blood–brain barrier. Regional delivery of drugs (e.g., intra-arterial, intrathecal, intratumor) potentially circumvents this problem, and responses to intra-arterial carboplatin- or methotrexate-based chemotherapy with osmotic blood–brain barrier disruption are reported for germ cell tumors and primary CNS lymphoma. The dose intensity of conventional, systemic chemotherapy may be increased with the use of hematopoietic growth factors, which shorten the period of myelosuppression and permit the use of higher doses or shorter intervals between treatments. A related approach is the use of extremely high doses of chemotherapy, supported by autologous hematopoietic stem cell rescue, and this approach has been used for chemotherapy-sensitive recurrent tumors or as an intensive consolidation therapy for infants.

The role of adjuvant cisplatin-based chemotherapy following radiation is well established for childhood medulloblastoma, pineoblastoma, and supratentorial PNET. For standard-risk medulloblastoma, use of chemotherapy permits reduction in the dose of radiotherapy. Dose-intensive cyclophosphamide-based chemotherapy has been used following radiation therapy for standard- and high-risk medulloblastoma with the goal of reducing exposure to cisplatin. For high-grade astrocytomas, temozolomide is used routinely with and following radiation therapy, as in adults. Preirradiation chemotherapy is being tested in CNS germ cell tumors and ependymoma but has been generally ineffective in medulloblastoma/PNET and malignant gliomas, including brain stem tumors, presumably because of delaying definitive radiation therapy.

In very young patients (infants and toddlers younger than age 3 to 4 years) with malignant brain tumors, dose-intensive chemotherapy is commonly used postoperatively with the goal of deferring or avoiding radiation therapy. This approach appears effective in medulloblastoma and possibly ependymoma. Intrathecal therapy (intraventricular and intralumbar methotrexate) has also been advocated for medulloblastoma in a protocol designed to avoid radiation therapy.

Chemotherapy is commonly used for recurrent CNS tumors, and patients may receive additional irradiation as well. High-dose chemotherapy with stem cell rescue may offer effective salvage therapy for recurrent medulloblastoma at least when combined with radiation therapy in younger previously unirradiated patients. Established and newer chemotherapy agents can be tested against panels of childhood brain tumor xenografts. Doses of certain chemotherapy agents such as irinotecan may require adjustment if patients are also receiving hepatic enzyme–inducing anticonvulsant drugs such as phenytoin, phenobarbital, carbamazepine, and Mysoline.

Biologic agents in clinical trials for recurrent CNS tumors include differentiation agents (retinoic acid), agents targeting tumor growth factor receptors (erlotinib, gefitinib, imatinib, lapatinib), farnesyltransferase inhibitors (tipifarnib), agents interfering with angiogenesis (bevacizumab, cilengitide, lenalidomide), histone deacetylase inhibitors (suberoylanilide hydroxamic acid, valproic acid), heat shock protein inhibitors (17-allylaminogeldanamycin), and DNA repair enzyme inhibitors (O6-benzylguanine).

Immunotherapy would be an attractive option for treatment of pediatric CNS tumors but remains an elusive goal. Convection-enhanced delivery of immunotoxin conjugates is being evaluated in adult patients. Certain glioma-associated antigens are overexpressed on pediatric brain stem and non–brain stem gliomas and could be suitable candidates for vaccine strategies.

SPECIFIC TYPES OF PEDIATRIC BRAIN TUMORS

Pathologic diagnosis is based on the revised WHO classification published in 2007. This classification distinguishes astrocytic tumors, oligodendroglial tumors and mixed gliomas, ependymal tumors, choroid plexus tumors, and neuronal and mixed neuronal–glial tumors. Among entities newly incorporated in the revised classification are angiocentric glioma, papillary glioneuronal tumor, rosette-forming glioneuronal tumor of the fourth ventricle, papillary tumor of the pineal region, pituicytoma, and spindle cell oncocytoma of the adenohypophysis. Newly described histologic variants of pediatric tumors are pilomyxoid astrocytoma, anaplastic medulloblastoma, and medulloblastoma with extensive nodularity. In addition, the rhabdoid tumor predisposition syndrome was added to the list of familial cancer syndromes.

Some childhood brain tumors, such as supratentorial astrocytomas, are difficult to characterize in the WHO classification. A proposed pediatric classification divides tumors into glial, mixed glial–neuronal, neural, embryonal, and pineal categories. Glial tumors include astrocytoma, ependymoma, oligodendroglioma, and choroid plexus tumor. Mixed glial–neuronal tumors include ganglioglioma and subependymal giant cell tumor. Neural tumors include gangliocytoma. Embryonal tumors are PNET, ATRT, and medulloepithelioma. Pineal tumors are represented by pineocytoma.

Pathologic diagnosis is greatly facilitated by immunostaining for specific markers such as GFAP in glial tumors and neurofilament or synaptophysin in PNETs and gangliogliomas. Other markers have been useful for different tumors: epithelial membrane antigen for ependymoma, α-fetoprotein (AFP) and human chorionic gonadotropin (HCG) for germ cell tumors, S100 for neural tumors, smooth muscle actin (SMA) for ATRT, and cytokeratin for choroid plexus carcinoma (Table 145.4). An important trend in tumor pathology is the application of cytogenetic and DNA approaches. Examples are isochromosome 17q in medulloblastoma, chromosome

1p and 19q deletions in oligodendroglioma, and monosomy or deletion of chromosome 22 (hSNF/INI-1 locus) in ATRT.

CONGENITAL TUMORS

Craniopharyngiomas

Craniopharyngiomas originate from rests of embryonic tissue located in the Rathke pouch, which later form the anterior pituitary gland. They may appear clinically at any age, even later adulthood, and constitute 6% to 10% of intracranial tumors in children. They vary from small, well-circumscribed, solid nodules to huge, multilocular cysts invading the sella turcica. The cysts are filled with turbid fluid that may contain cholesterin crystals. Craniopharyngiomas are histologically benign and may be categorized as mucoid epithelial cysts, squamous epitheliomas, or adamantinomas. Total surgical removal may be difficult because the tumor may invade the hypothalamus or third ventricle and adhere to optic nerves or blood vessels. Manifestations include short stature, hypothyroidism, and diabetes insipidus, with vision loss and signs of increased ICP. Although CT is useful for demonstrating calcification and bony expansion of the sella, MRI is preferred for better definition of the relationship of the tumor to neighboring vessels, optic chiasm and nerves, and the hypothalamus (Fig. 145.1).

A conservative approach is to drain the cyst and resect nonadherent tumor and then administer radiation therapy to the involved area. Alternatively, gross total resection may be attempted, avoiding irradiation. In addition to the standard transsphenoidal approach, there is renewed interest in the endonasal approach. Recurrence rates are similar (20% to 40%), and radical surgery is likely to be accompanied by panhypopituitarism necessitating lifelong hormonal replacement therapy, whereas irradiation has lesser hormonal sequelae but causes cognitive deficits, especially in younger children. Focused treatment by stereotactic radiosurgery (e.g., Gamma Knife) may be advantageous in this regard. Interferon α-2a and pegylated interferon α-2b have been used in recurrent craniopharyngiomas.

Epidermoid Cysts

Epidermoid cysts (cholesteatomas) account for about 2% of all intracranial tumors. They arise within skull tables or adjacent to the dura usually in the suprasellar region, skull base, brain stem or cerebellopontine angle, or within a ventricle. They arise from epithelial cells retained during neural tube closure, have a pearly appearance, and may contain cyst fluid with cholesterol crystals. Clinical onset is usually in young adulthood, with hearing loss, hemifacial spasm, or trigeminal neuralgia. MRI demonstrates a lesion with low T1- and high T2-weighted signal intensity (Fig. 145.2); involvement of multiple cranial nerves and the internal carotid artery is common. Treatment is surgical resection with radical removal of the tumor capsule. *Dermoid tumors* are also cystic, and sebaceous gland secretions impart a dark yellow color to the cyst fluid. Intracranial dermoids are associated with Goldenhar syndrome (i.e., oculo–auriculo–vertebral dysplasia). Treatment is surgical resection. Epidermoid and dermoid cysts occasionally undergo malignant transformation into squamous cell carcinoma. *Arachnoid cysts* are CSF collections within arachnoid membranes, often in the sylvian fissure, presenting with headache and occasionally seizures. Diffusion-weighted imaging can be helpful in distinguishing arachnoid cysts from epidermoid cysts. Surgery is indicated for arachnoid cysts, which are symptomatic (obstructive hydrocephalus, seizures); options include cystectomy, fenestration, or cyst-peritoneal shunting.

TABLE 145.4 Immunohistochemical, Cytogenetic, and Molecular Characteristics of Childhood Brain Tumors

Tumor	Immunohistochemistry	Cytogenetics	Molecular Pathology
Pilocytic astrocytoma	GFAP	+7q34	*BRAF* fusion *NF1* mutation *KRAS* mutation MAP kinase activation
High-grade astrocytoma	GFAP	+1q 10q23 LOH	*TP53* mutation MAP kinase activation *IDH1/2* mutation *EGFR* mutation
Medulloblastoma	Synaptophysin NSE β-Catenin (nuclear)	Iso(17) −6	*PTCH* mutation *TP53* mutation *APC* mutation *MYC* amplification *MYCN* amplification *FOXG1* upregulation
sPNET	Synaptophysin S100 NSE	−9p21 −14q	p16 downregulation
Ependymoma	GFAP EMA	+1q25 −6q25.3	*CDKN2A/B* mutation *EGFR* amplification
ATRT	SMA EMA Vimentin INI-1 negative	del(22q11)	*SMARCB1* mutation
Choroid plexus Ca	Pancytokeratin Vimentin E-cadherin		*TP53* mutation (germ line)
Germ cell tumors	AFP β-HCG	Iso(12p) XXY	*P14* mutation *c-kit* mutation
Oligodendroglioma	S-100	Del(1p/19q)	*IDH1/2* mutation *FUBP1* mutation
Meningioma	Vimentin EMA	−22q	*NF2* mutation PDGFR-β activation

GFAP, glial fibrillary acidic protein; LOH, loss of heterozygosity; NSE, neuron-specific enolase; sPNET, supratentorial primitive neuroectodermal tumor; EMA, epithelial membrane antigen; ATRT, atypical teratoid/rhabdoid tumor; SMA, smooth muscle actin; Ca, carcinoma; AFP, α-fetoprotein; β-HCG, β-human chorionic gonadotropin.

Data from Pfister S, Hartmann C, Korshunov A. Histology and molecular pathology of pediatric brain tumors. *J Child Neurol.* 2009;24(11):1375–1386.

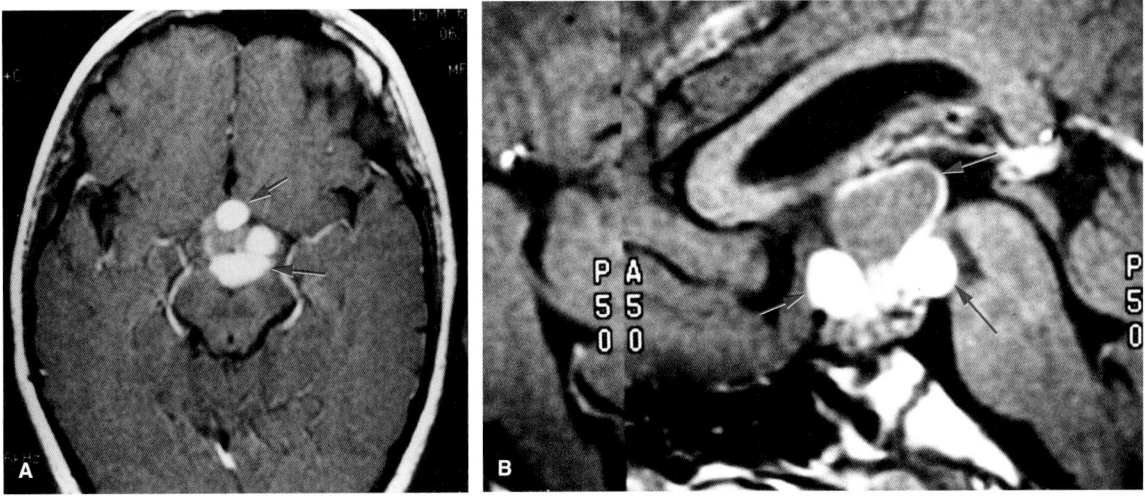

FIGURE 145.1 Axial **(A)** and sagittal **(B)** MRIs of a craniopharyngioma.

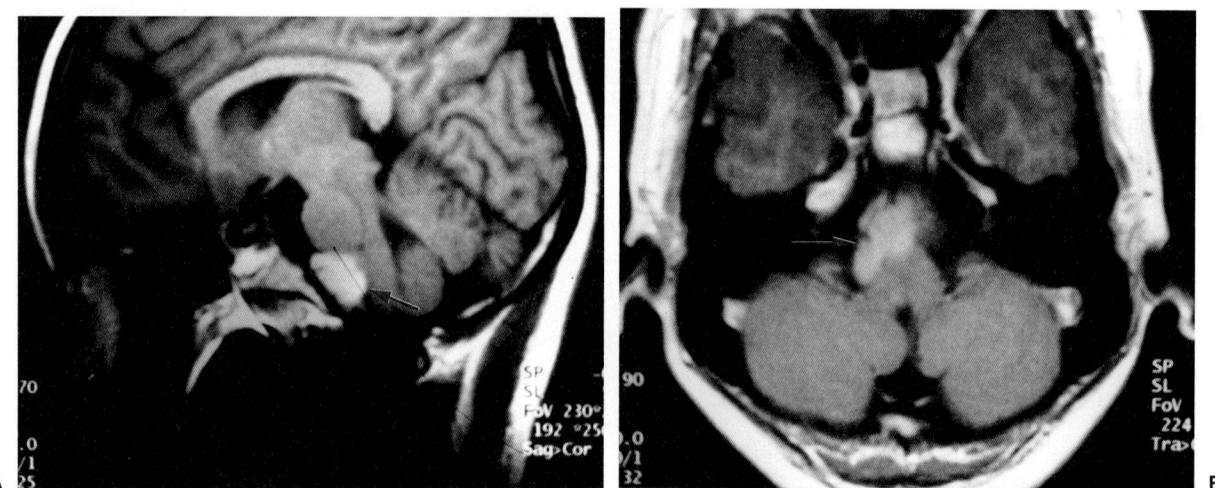

FIGURE 145.2 Sagittal **(A)** and axial **(B)** MRIs of a pontomedullary epidermoid cyst.

Teratomas

Teratomas occur in infants and young children. Prenatal diagnosis of an intracranial teratoma has been reported. Mature teratomas are generally lobulated and cystic, often containing differentiated tissues such as bone, cartilage, teeth, hair, or intestine. Immature and malignant teratomas are less common; posterior fossa immature teratoma in an infant with trisomy 21 has been reported. Teratomas tend to occur in the pineal region, presenting with Parinaud syndrome and hydrocephalus. They comprise about 4% of childhood intracranial tumors and also occur in the spine. Treatment is surgical resection.

Chordomas

Chordomas develop from remnants of the embryonic notochord. Half are in the sacrococcygeal region, one-third at the sphenoid–occipital junction, and the remainder elsewhere along the spinal column. They are rare, accounting for less than 1% of CNS tumors, and usually remain asymptomatic until adulthood. These tumors are locally invasive and cause vision loss or cranial nerve dysfunction. They may invade the nasopharynx or intracranial sinuses and may extend into the neck causing torticollis.

Chordomas have a smooth, nodular surface that resembles cartilage; the characteristic histologic feature is the presence of large masses of physaliferous cells, round or polygonal cells arranged in cords and having large cytoplasmic vacuoles containing mucin. Chordomas grow slowly but may recur after excision. A malignant variant is distinguished by mitotic spindle cells and may metastasize to the lung. Chordoma should be suspected in a patient presenting with multiple cranial nerve palsies or erosion of the skull base. Treatment is surgical resection, although gross total resection is rarely achieved, occasionally with postoperative irradiation. Radiation therapy may be used postoperatively or at recurrence. Proton radiotherapy is advocated because it may confer effective local control and possibly better cosmetic outcome than with conventional irradiation.

Choroid Plexus Tumors

Choroid plexus tumors are rare congenital tumors arising in the choroid plexus of the lateral or fourth ventricles. They may cause symptoms shortly after birth, and most are diagnosed before age 2 years. The first manifestation is likely to be macrocephaly resulting from hydrocephalus, with bulging fontanelle and split sutures

noted in infants. Excess CSF production arising from the tumor may approach 2,000 mL/day. The majority are papillomas (WHO grade I), hamartomatous lesions which grow into the ventricle and tend not to be invasive. Papillomas are often calcified on CT scan and enhance with contrast; they must be distinguished in the infant age group from ependymomas, which lack calcification. *Atypical papillomas* (WHO grade II) have a higher growth fraction (mitotic rate by MIB-1 >2%). Total excision of localized lesions may be curative and stops the excessive CSF production, but malignant transformation of incompletely resected papillomas has been reported.

Choroid plexus carcinomas (WHO grade III) typically invade the brain parenchyma and cause hydrocephalus (Fig. 145.3). Carcinomas are more heterogeneous than papillomas on imaging due to focal necrosis and surrounding vasogenic edema; in nearly half of cases, there is disseminate in the leptomeninges. Choroid plexus carcinomas may be a manifestation of Li–Fraumeni syndrome, and evidence should be sought for germ line mutation in *p53*. Adjuvant chemotherapy or irradiation has been advocated for carcinomas, even following apparent gross total resection, owing to their invasiveness and guarded prognosis (median survival 6 months in one series). For patients undergoing subtotal resection of carcinomas, both chemotherapy and craniospinal irradiation are recommended.

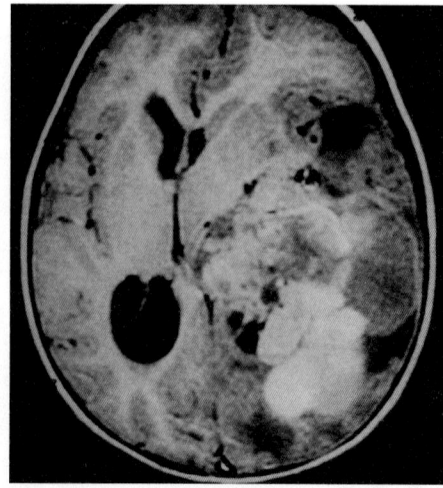

FIGURE 145.3 MRI of a choroid plexus carcinoma of the lateral ventricle with parenchymal invasion.

Colloid Cysts

Colloid cysts presumably arise from the anlage of the paraphysis. These lesions grow in the anterior superior portion of the third ventricle as small, white cysts filled with homogeneous, gelatinous material. They do not usually cause symptoms until adulthood when there may be intermittent hydrocephalus. Disturbance of the limbic system may cause emotional and behavioral changes in some instances. Colloid cysts are T2 hyperintense on MRI without enhancement. Treatment is surgical excision. Endoscopic procedures are gaining acceptance as an alternative to microsurgical resection.

Gangliogliomas

Gangliogliomas are rare, glioneural tumors that account for 2.5% of pediatric brain tumors. The peak age incidence is 10 to 20 years. They arise mainly in the temporal lobe but also in other lobes or spinal cord. The usual syndrome is a long history of refractory epilepsy. Imaging reveals a solid to cystic lesion with calcification on CT and hypometabolic activity on PET. Total surgical resection is recommended, and prognosis for long-term seizure control is excellent. Malignant transformation to glioblastoma may follow incomplete resection. Radiation therapy and chemotherapy are of uncertain benefit.

Desmoplastic infantile ganglioglioma (DIG) is a rare cerebral glioneural tumor of early childhood. DIGs are large hemispheric tumors that are generally benign, but deep lesions may be aggressive. Treatment is resection. Related glioneural tumors include *desmoplastic astrocytoma of infancy* (DACI) and *pleomorphic xanthoastrocytoma* (PXA), which usually cause seizures and headache.

Dysplastic gangliocytoma of the cerebellum (Lhermitte–Duclos *disease*) is a rare, benign entity characterized by loss of normal cerebellar cortical architecture and may be associated with macrocephaly and mental retardation. MRI appearance is a well-circumscribed lesion with characteristic laminar pattern of alternating high and low T2 signal. The disorder has been linked with Cowden disease, with increased risk of breast, uterine, and thyroid cancer and harbors abnormalities in the PTEN/AKT pathway, consistent with germ line mutation in the PTEN tumor suppressor gene in Cowden disease.

Dysembryoplastic Neuroepithelial Tumor

Dysembryoplastic neuroepithelial tumor (DNT) is a rare, low-grade (WHO grade I) mixed neuronal and glial tumor often associated with intractable seizures in children and young adults. DNTs comprise up to 17% of underlying diagnoses in epilepsy surgery series. Cortical dysplasia is found in 30% of cases. Enhancement on MRI is patchy and multifocal; perfusion-weighted MRI and MRS may aid in diagnosis. Unlike other epilepsy-associated glioneuronal tumors, where seizures arise within the lesion, seizures associated with DNT are considered to arise from the surrounding dysplastic brain; thus, extended resection is preferred over lesionectomy alone. Risk factors for recurrent seizures include age older than 10 years and epilepsy duration more than 2 years prior to diagnosis.

ASTROCYTOMAS

Low-Grade Astrocytomas

Low-grade astrocytomas (WHO grades I and II) include superficial lesions in the cerebral or cerebellar cortex and deeper infiltrative lesions of the optic pathways and midbrain. *Cerebellar astrocytomas* constitute about one-third of posterior fossa tumors. The peak

incidence is early in the second decade. These tumors arise most often in the lateral cerebellar hemispheres rather than in the vermis. Symptoms of clumsiness and unsteadiness may be present for months and eventually are accompanied by intermittent morning headache and vomiting. Midline lesions have a shorter symptom interval. Truncal ataxia, dysmetria, and papilledema are usually present at diagnosis. Head tilt may be present, but other cranial nerve palsies or long-tract signs are infrequent and suggest brain stem invasion. Cerebellar astrocytomas may be primarily cystic or solid, and cystic lesions may have a nodule (Fig. 145.4). The typical juvenile pilocytic astrocytoma (WHO grade I) contains areas of compact fibrillated cells with microcysts and eosinophilic structures called *Rosenthal fibers*. These lesions have greater than 90% survival with surgery alone. The tumor and associated cyst should be removed completely, and if residual tumor is identified postoperatively, reresection should be considered, as irradiation will not delay tumor progression. Diffuse astrocytomas (WHO grade II) may infiltrate the brain stem and be more difficult to resect entirely, with more guarded prognosis for survival.

Cerebral hemisphere low-grade gliomas have a peak incidence between ages 2 and 4 years and again in early adolescence. In toddlers, there may be symptoms of increased ICP, developmental delay, and growth retardation and specific signs such as weakness, sensory loss, or vision deficit. These slow-growing pediatric tumors are far less likely than adult gliomas to undergo malignant degeneration. They are infiltrating, however, and may cause seizures, either generalized or focal, the latter particularly suggestive of an occult brain tumor such as a ganglioglioma.

CT often reveals a relatively homogeneous, low-density, variably enhancing lesion with indistinct margins. MRI is more sensitive, showing decreased T1- and increased T2-weighted signal and providing better resolution of tumor and edema. Fibrillary astrocytomas (WHO grade II) are the most frequent histologic variant; protoplasmic and gemistocytic variants are less common. Gross total resection often affords long-term disease control but may not be curative. Five-year survival rates are 75% to 85%. Radiation therapy at doses of 50 to 55 Gy may be given postoperatively following incomplete resection or at progression at least in older children but reoperation should also be considered. For younger children with residual or recurrent tumor, chemotherapy (e.g., vincristine and

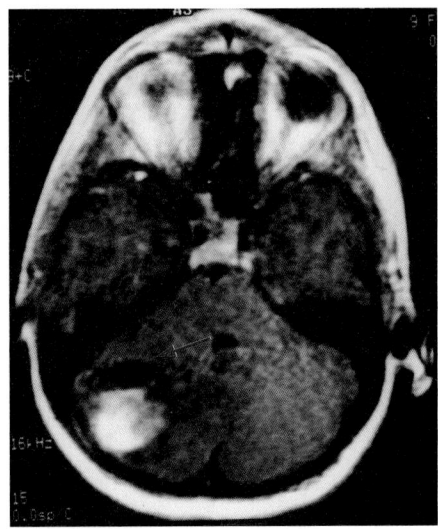

FIGURE 145.4 MRI showing lateral location of a partly cystic, partly solid cerebellar astrocytoma.

carboplatin) has been used in an attempt to defer radiotherapy, and prospective trials evaluating this approach are in progress.

Diencephalic and optic pathway gliomas constitute up to 5% of childhood CNS tumors. Unilateral optic nerve tumors are generally diagnosed in the first decade of life, and optic chiasm tumors tend to present either in infancy or the second decade. An association with NF-1 is present in 50% to 70% of patients with isolated optic nerve tumors and 10% to 20% of patients with optic chiasm tumors. Adolescents are more likely to complain of slowly progressive vision loss. Infants are more likely to be evaluated because of strabismus, nystagmus, or developmental delay. Patients with contiguous optic nerve involvement usually present with proptosis and optic pallor or atrophy. Intraorbital lesions usually cause decrease in central vision, whereas chiasmatic tumors produce bitemporal hemianopic field cuts. Nystagmus may be present in the more involved eye, and amblyopia is common. With routine MRI of NF-1 patients, lesions may be detected before onset of symptoms. There may be endocrine disturbances, such as growth deceleration, precocious puberty, and diencephalic emaciation.

Thalamic lesions may cause acute hemiparesis or hemisensory loss, signs of increased ICP, seizures, or involuntary movements. Infants tend to have macrocephaly, psychomotor delay, and vision deficits. Hypothalamic tumors have insidious onset and may be associated with altered mental status, endocrine dysfunction, and focal neurologic deficits.

On CT or MRI, diencephalic gliomas are hypo- or isodense lesions with variable contrast enhancement. Larger lesions may be cystic (Fig. 145.5A and B). Visual pathway tumors may be confined to the optic chiasm (Fig. 145.6A and B) or may show abnormal enhancement along the optic tracts and radiations. This streaking phenomenon is best appreciated on MRI, particularly with FLAIR sequence. Most diencephalic tumors are low-grade pilocytic astrocytomas.

An increasingly recognized variant in infants and young children is pilomyxoid astrocytoma (WHO grade II), which is locally aggressive. Thalamic tumors are often fibrillary astrocytomas, which can also be locally aggressive. The natural history of these lesions is unpredictable. Spontaneous regression has been noted. An increased MIB-1 labeling index identifies the more aggressive pilocytic astrocytomas. Visual pathway tumors have a particular tendency to spread to contiguous structures. The role of surgery is unclear.

Low-grade astrocytomas of the optic pathway, thalamus, and hypothalamus are generally unresectable. In patients with diffusely infiltrating lesions, especially with NF-1, diagnosis may be confirmed with near certainty on neuroimaging alone, and surgery may be deemed of little benefit. In patients with unilateral blindness, surgery may be recommended for treatment of a severely proptotic eye. However, if some vision persists, local radiotherapy may be recommended. Radiotherapy at doses of 45 to 55 Gy generally reverses tumor progression in nearly all patients and stabilizes or improves vision in most. There may be apparent tumor enlargement at 6 to 12 weeks as a transient effect of the radiation. Patients with very large lesions may benefit from preliminary surgical debulking.

The major disadvantages of radiotherapy are adverse endocrine and neurocognitive effects, especially in younger children. Chemotherapy (based on vincristine and carboplatin) has been beneficial as initial treatment in younger children who have progressive optic pathway and hypothalamic/chiasmatic gliomas, delaying the need for radiotherapy by a median of 4 years; most eventually relapse, however, except for NF-1 patients who tend to have indolent disease. The same chemotherapy regimen has been advocated as initial treatment for infants with tumor-associated diencephalic syndrome of emaciation. Overall survival for optic pathway gliomas exceeds 85% at 10 years but is less than 50% for thalamic low-grade gliomas and considerably worse for high-grade (especially bithalamic) astrocytomas.

Several chemotherapy regimens are active in pediatric low-grade astrocytomas. Two regimens were compared in a Children's Oncology Group study for recurrent/progressive or symptomatic tumors: carboplatin + vincristine (CV) and thioguanine + procarbazine + lomustine (CCNU) + vincristine (TPCV). Five-year event-free and overall survival rates across all tumor locations were 45% and 86%, respectively, with slightly better event-free survival (EFS) with TPCV and inferior survival with tumor location in the thalamus. A regimen of weekly vinblastine shows comparable activity, even in patient previously treated with CV or TPCV. A regimen of cisplatin and etoposide is also widely used.

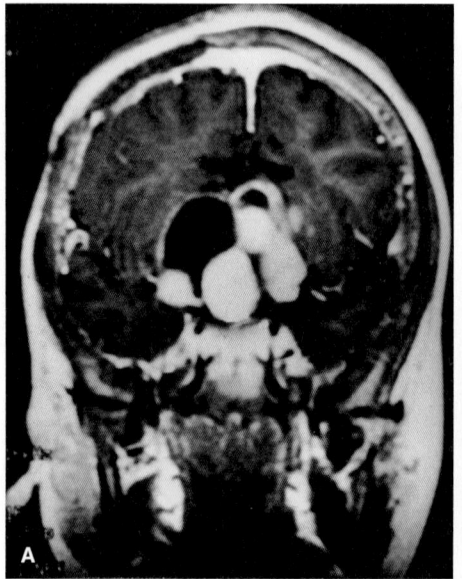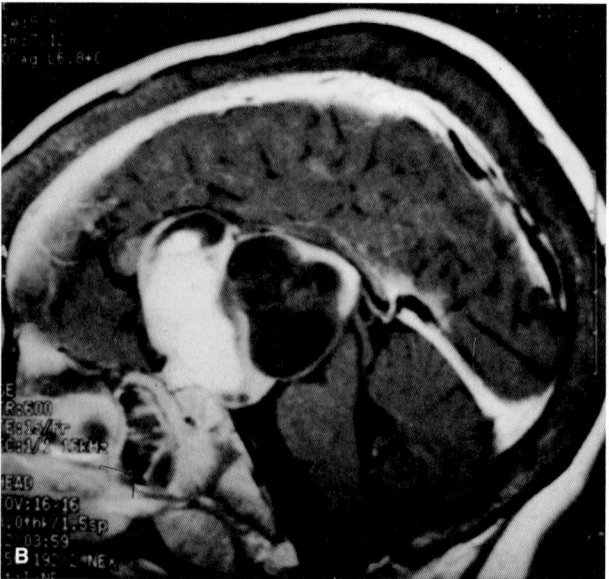

FIGURE 145.5 Coronal **(A)** and sagittal **(B)** MRIs of a large hypothalamic glioma.

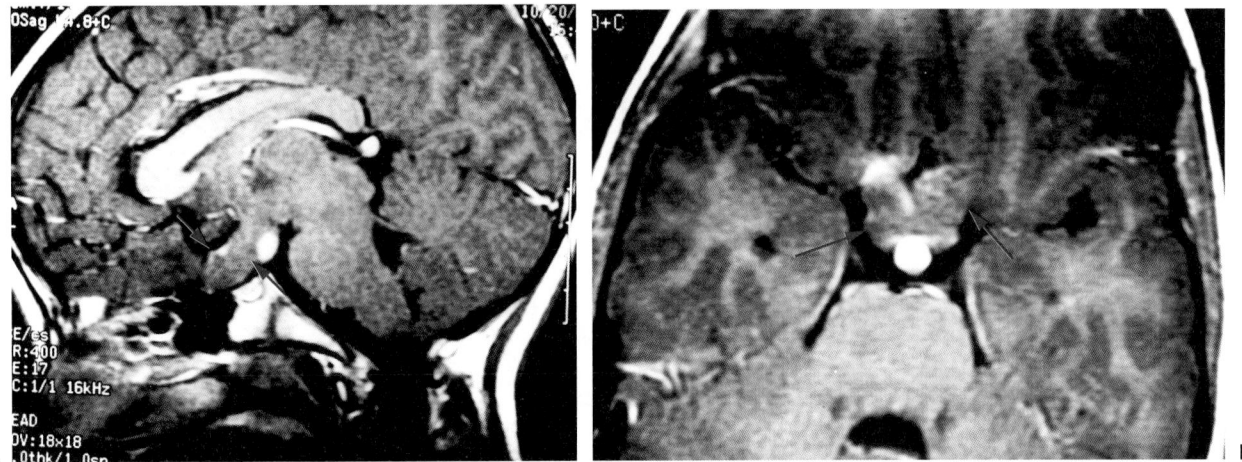

FIGURE 145.6 Sagittal **(A)** and coronal **(B)** MRIs of an optic pathway tumor.

Based on frequent occurrence of *BRAF* mutations in pilocytic astrocytomas, BRAF inhibitors are being tested in children with tumor progression. Because of histologic evidence of vascular proliferation in recurrent low-grade astrocytomas, treatment with antiangiogenic agents such as bevacizumab and lenalidomide has also been explored. Of interest, treatment of children with optic pathway gliomas with bevacizumab produced marked recovery of vision in addition to response on MRI. Experience with sorafenib, a multikinase inhibitor of BRAF, VEGFR, PDGFR, and c-kit, provides a cautionary note, however, as treatment with sorafenib produced unexpected acceleration of tumor growth, perhaps by paradoxical ERK activation. The best example of successful targeted therapy is *subependymal giant cell astrocytoma* (SEGA), a low-grade glioma typically arising in individuals with tuberous sclerosis. SEGAs bear mutations in *TSC1* and *TSC2* genes and have dysregulated activation of mTOR signaling. An mTOR inhibitor, everolimus, showed substantial activity in patients with unresectable SEGAs.

High-grade Astrocytomas

High-grade astrocytomas account for about 10% of brain tumors in children and include anaplastic astrocytoma, oligodendroglioma, and oligoastrocytoma (WHO grade III) and glioblastoma multiforme and gliosarcoma (WHO grade IV). The WHO classification emphasizes degree of cellularity, nuclear and cellular pleomorphism, mitosis, endothelial proliferation, and necrosis. In general, *anaplastic astrocytomas* are composed of astrocytes with increased cellularity, pleomorphism, and numbers of mitoses. There may be focal necrosis, but it may not be so extensive as to form pseudopalisades. In contrast to low-grade pilocytic tumors, anaplastic astrocytomas have an unstable vasculature, with a predominance of immature vessels distinguished by negative immunostaining for α-SMA. Vascular endothelial growth factor and anti-*flt-1/VEGF receptor-1* immunoreactivity was detected in anaplastic astrocytomas but not pilocytic astrocytomas. *Glioblastoma multiforme* has prominent vascular proliferation and a pseudopalisading pattern of necrosis. Cytogenetic analyses developed mainly of tumors from adults has shown consistent chromosomal abnormalities in all tumor grades; however, one aberration—the loss of part or all of chromosome 10—has been specifically associated with glioblastoma multiforme, and amplification and rearrangement of the EGFR gene have also been associated with malignant histology. Gene profiling shows overexpression of hypoxia-inducible transcription factor (HIF)-2α and FK506-binding protein (FKBP)

12–associated genes, including EGFR and insulin-like growth factor–binding protein 2.

Prognosis in high-grade astrocytomas is quite guarded compared to low-grade astrocytomas. Common symptoms of cerebral cortical high-grade astrocytomas include headache, vomiting, seizures, motor weakness, and behavioral abnormalities. Cerebellar lesions may present with ataxia. Symptom duration is generally less than 3 months. Diagnosis is made by CT or MRI. Surgery is important for diagnosis and for removing tumor; major resection improves survival. However, these infiltrative tumors may disseminate in the CSF and will almost certainly recur without further therapy. Postoperative involved-field irradiation (59 to 60 Gy) and adjuvant chemotherapy both increase survival. Adjuvant vincristine plus lomustine was somewhat effective in CCG-943 and CCG-945, but survival rates remained below 35%. Chemotherapy prior to or with radiation therapy may contribute to survival in patients undergoing complete tumor resection. Temozolomide with and following radiation therapy has become standard treatment for adult GBM, yielding 26% 2-year survival, and this regimen appears to have comparable efficacy in children (ACNS0126). Survival is influenced by extent of tumor resection and by histology (e.g., anaplastic astrocytoma vs. glioblastoma multiforme).

Bevacizumab/irinotecan has been the first-line salvage therapy as in adults. High-dose chemotherapy with autologous stem cell rescue afforded occasional long-term survival in recurrent patients with minimal residual tumor following surgical debulking.

Brain Stem Gliomas

Brain stem gliomas are a heterogeneous group. The diffuse, intrinsic pontine lesions carry the worst prognosis of any childhood brain tumor. In contrast, small, intrinsic, tectal gliomas are indolent and may be managed conservatively. Brain stem tumors constitute 10% to 20% of posterior fossa tumors, with a peak incidence at ages 5 to 8 years. Most arise in the pons, and there may be contiguous spread to the medulla or midbrain. Despite the clinical aggressiveness of these tumors, the histologic appearance at initial diagnosis is quite variable, but at autopsy, most show anaplastic features. This may reflect sampling error at initial biopsy or subsequent malignant transformation. These tumors infiltrate the brain stem and compress normal structures while extending superiorly and inferiorly to produce diffuse enlargement of the brain stem. DIPGs are nearly uniformly fatal within 18 to 24 months. Some tumors extend ventrally, laterally, or posteriorly, and the primarily exophytic

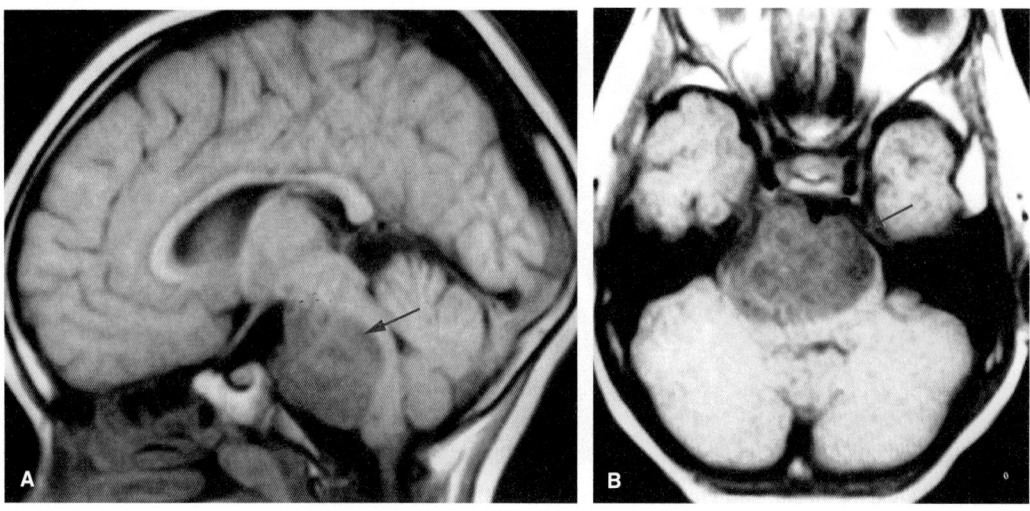

FIGURE 145.7 A: Sagittal MRI of a diffuse brain stem glioma. **B:** Axial image showing infiltration of the medulla.

tumors tend to be more accessible to surgical resection and carry a better prognosis as do focal midbrain lesions.

The course is insidious with slowly progressive cranial neuropathy, motor symptoms and disturbance of gait, swallowing, and speech. Vomiting and headache indicate the presence of hydrocephalus, which is generally a late finding. Children with dorsal exophytic lesions may have more unsteadiness and less evidence of cranial nerve dysfunction. CT shows a low-density lesion in the brain stem, with compression and obliteration of surrounding cisterns but little if any contrast enhancement. Uncommonly, brain stem tumors may be isodense or hyperdense with cystic areas. MRI is preferred because of the detail appreciated on sagittal images typically revealing more extensive disease than appreciated on CT. The magnetic resonance (MR) appearance is of decreased signal intensity on T1-weighted images (Fig. 145.7A) and increased T2-weighted signal. Ring enhancement with contrast administration is prognostically unfavorable. MRI may also demonstrate infiltration of the medulla (Fig. 145.7B) or thalamus.

Given the accuracy of MR diagnosis, the morbidity of surgery, and the variable prognostic impact of biopsy, it has been accepted that surgery is not warranted for most patients with diffuse intrinsic pontine lesions, in whom major resection when attempted has not improved survival. Biopsy may be offered in the context of research protocols accruing tissue samples for molecular studies. Patients with exophytic, cervicomedullary tumors are more likely to benefit from surgery as are patients with atypical clinical courses or MR findings (e.g., symptom duration exceeding 6 months, absence of cranial nerve findings primarily exophytic or focal ring-enhancing lesions). Children younger than age 3 years may fare better. Standard treatment is field-radiation therapy except for completely resected focal lesions. Most children with brain stem gliomas benefit at least transiently from radiation therapy to a dose of 54 to 56 Gy. Although leptomeningeal dissemination may occur, the main risk is for local recurrence. Median survival is only 9 to 12 months with 3-year survival of 13%. Chemotherapy (including temozolomide and topotecan) and immunotherapy (such as β-interferon) have been unsuccessful in this condition, although new agents continue to be studied. Novel approaches include use of the histone deacetylase inhibitor vorinostat or the prodrug capecitabine with and following radiation therapy or regional tumor treatment by convection-enhanced delivery of drugs

and immunotoxins. Determination of responses is complicated by interobserver variability in tumor measurement; the most consistent results are derived from FLAIR images. It has been suggested that clinical trials should incorporate other objective end points, such as survival, rather than radiologic response alone. Children with brain stem tumors should be monitored for signs of hydrocephalus because CSF diversion by shunting or third ventriculostomy can improve quality of life.

Spinal Cord Astrocytomas

Spinal cord astrocytomas account for about 4% of childhood CNS neoplasms. Other primary spinal cord tumors in children include gangliogliomas and ependymomas. Spinal high-grade astrocytomas and PNETs are uncommon. Astrocytomas may occur in any part of the cord but are seen most often in the cervical region, with the solid component extending an average of five spinal segments. Most have benign histologic appearance and grow slowly. Symptoms and signs may include pain (i.e., localized or radicular), weakness or spasticity, gait disturbance, and bowel or bladder dysfunction. Gadolinium-enhanced MRI is preferred for demonstrating the location of the solid tumor, associated cysts, and edema. Treatment may be attempted gross-total or near-total resection or partial resection with decompression of cysts with postoperative radiotherapy.

The degree of neurologic recovery depends on the preoperative condition of the patient. A potential complication is spinal deformity, resulting from laminectomy, radiotherapy, or both. About one-third of patients require a spine stabilization procedure. For children with low-grade tumors, survival rates of 55% at 10 years have been reported after partial resection and radiotherapy. Chemotherapy has been substituted for radiotherapy in very young children. The prognosis for children with high-grade tumors is worse, although 5-year progression-free survival (PFS) of 46% was reported in a study using combined radiation therapy and chemotherapy.

EMBRYONAL TUMORS

Medulloblastomas and Primitive Neuroectodermal Tumors

Medulloblastoma and supratentorial (PNETs) collectively are the most common malignant CNS tumors of childhood. Most PNETs arise in the posterior fossa and are specifically called *medulloblastomas*. Posterior fossa and supratentorial PNETs are histologically identical (WHO grade IV) and have similar epidemiologic profiles but distinct biologic properties. The incidence of medulloblastoma/PNET before age 20 years rose by 23% from 1973 to 1977 to 1993 to 1998.

As described earlier, the presumed cell of origin of *medulloblastoma* is derived from fetal external granular cells of the cerebellum or rests in the posterior medullary velum. These tumors account for about 30% of infratentorial tumors in children but are uncommon in adults. Medulloblastomas typically involve the cerebellar vermis, grow to fill the fourth ventricle, and may infiltrate the floor of the ventricle and adjacent structures. The tumor may arise more laterally, especially in older patients.

Supratentorial PNETs generally arise in the cerebral cortex or pineal region. These lesions appear to originate from the germinal matrix of the primitive neural tube. Most are diagnosed before age 10 years.

"Classic" medulloblastoma has the histologic appearance of a small, round, blue cell tumor with a diffuse pattern of poorly differentiated cells. Neuroblastic ("Homer-Wright") rosettes may be present but are not required for diagnosis. Immunohistochemical staining is typically positive for synaptophysin and occasionally for neurofilament protein or GFAP, although the latter usually represents reactive intratumoral astrocytes. Desmoplastic/nodular (D/N) medulloblastoma typically arises in cerebellar hemispheres and is characterized by nodular islands of differentiating neuroblasts; an "extensively nodular" variant is recognized in infants. Large cell/anaplastic (LCA) medulloblastoma vaguely resembles large cell lymphoma, with large neoplastic cells having vesicular nuclei and prominent nucleoli. Most medulloblastomas fall between these histologic extremes, but one-quarter exhibit at least moderate anaplasia and an associated, aggressive clinical behavior. In infants, medulloblastoma must be distinguished from ATRT, which has a small cell component resembling medulloblastoma but also cords of cells in a mucinous background that resemble chordoma, with a rhabdoid appearance of the cytoplasm of the larger cells.

A specific chromosome abnormality, isochromosome 17q (i.e., duplication of the long arm or deletion of the short arm of chromosome 17), is seen in one-third of cases of medulloblastoma. This could result in inactivation of a tumor suppressor gene, which is located on chromosome 17 but is distinct from *p53*. It is unclear whether chromosome 17p deletions impart poor prognosis, but diploid tumors have worse outcome than aneuploid or hyperdiploid tumors.

It is now apparent that medulloblastomas comprise at least four distinct subtypes based on aberrant activation of signaling pathways regulating cerebellar development or oncogene amplification: (1) WNT tumors (named for drosophila wingless) with classic histology and very good prognosis; (2) Shh tumors (named for sonic hedgehog), relatively more common in infants and adults, with D/N histology and intermediate prognosis (good in infants); (3) "group 3" tumors with overrepresentation of LC/A histology, MYC amplification, very frequent metastasis, and poor prognosis; and (4) "group 4" tumors with classic histology but tendency for metastasis, occasional MYCN amplification, and intermediate prognosis. Immunohistochemical correlations are nuclear positivity for β-catenin in WNT tumors, GAB1 positivity in Shh tumors, and filamin A and YAP1 positivity in both. Correlation with cytogenetic findings shows isochromosome 17q to be typical of group 3 and 4 tumors, monosomy 6 associated with WNT tumors, and 9q and 10q deletion in Shh tumors. Profiling six FISH biomarkers (GLI2; MYC; and chromosomes 11, 14, 17p, and 17q) reliably identifies

very low-risk and very high-risk patients within Shh, group 3, and group 4 medulloblastomas.

Exome sequencing has revealed subtype-specific somatic mutations in known medulloblastoma-related genes (CTNNB1, PTCH1, MLL2, SMARCA4) and genes not previously considered medulloblastoma-related (DDX3X, CTDNEP1, KDM6A, TBR1). In particular, mutant DDX3X potentiates transactivation of a TCF promoter and enhances cell viability in combination with mutant β-catenin. Growth factor–independent 1 family protooncogenes GFI1 and GFI1B have been identified as oncogenic drivers for group 3 and 4 tumors, an example of "enhancer hijacking" wherein coding sequences are juxtaposed proximal to active enhancer elements. Epigenetic alterations also contribute to medulloblastoma tumorigenesis, including highly prevalent regions of hypomethylation correlating with increased gene expression.

Relatively less is known about the cytogenetic and molecular features of supratentorial PNETs, but gene expression analysis shows distinct patterns of gene activation that differ from those of medulloblastoma. Three molecular subgroups have been proposed based on differential expression of cell lineage markers LIN28 and OLIG2: (1) primitive neural (younger females with poorest survival), (2) oligoneural (older males with best survival), and (3) mesenchymal (older males with highest incidence of metastatic disease and intermediate survival). A high-level amplicon involving the chr19q13.41 microRNA cluster (C19MC) identifies an aggressive subgroup of CNS PNET with distinct gene expression profiles and poor survival. ATRTs have monosomy or deletion of chromosome 22, and inactivating mutations of the hSNF5/INI-1 gene at 22q11.2 are considered fundamental to pathogenesis. Loss of chromosome 19 has been reported in ATRT.

Children with medulloblastoma typically have symptoms of increased ICP (e.g., vomiting, lethargy, morning headache), unsteadiness, and diplopia. The median age is 5 years. Symptom duration is generally of less than 3 months. There may be recent onset of head tilt resulting from ophthalmoparesis or incipient cerebellar herniation. Laterally situated lesions present slightly differently with symptoms of cerebellopontine angle disturbance or limb ataxia. These tumors appear isodense or hyperdense on CT and usually enhance homogeneously. Hydrocephalus is seen in more than 80% of patients. Other CT features include small cysts, calcification, and hemorrhage. Children with supratentorial PNET present with headache and vomiting due to increased ICP; infants may have lethargy, irritability, and an enlarging head circumference.

MRI may give better indication of tumor extent (Fig. 145.8A) and possible leptomeningeal dissemination (Fig. 145.8B and C). MRI is also preferred to facilitate evaluation of disseminated spinal tumor, which is found in up to one-third of patients with medulloblastomas. Aggressive surgical resection is recommended for medulloblastoma/PNET. Surgery achieves complete or near-complete resection of medulloblastomas in most cases, limited mainly by tumor infiltration of the fourth ventricle, the brain stem, or one of the cerebellar peduncles. Morbidity may include the posterior fossa syndrome of aseptic meningitis or, less commonly, of mutism, pharyngeal dysfunction, and ataxia. Preoperative ventriculoperitoneal shunting is not done routinely owing to the risk of upward herniation and because hydrocephalus will be relieved by tumor removal in most patients. About 30% to 40% of patients require permanent shunting.

Postoperative CT or MRI is indicated to confirm the extent of resection, and this study should be done within 48 hours when there is less edema than later. Patients with medulloblastoma may be stratified clinically as *average risk* (i.e., localized posterior fossa

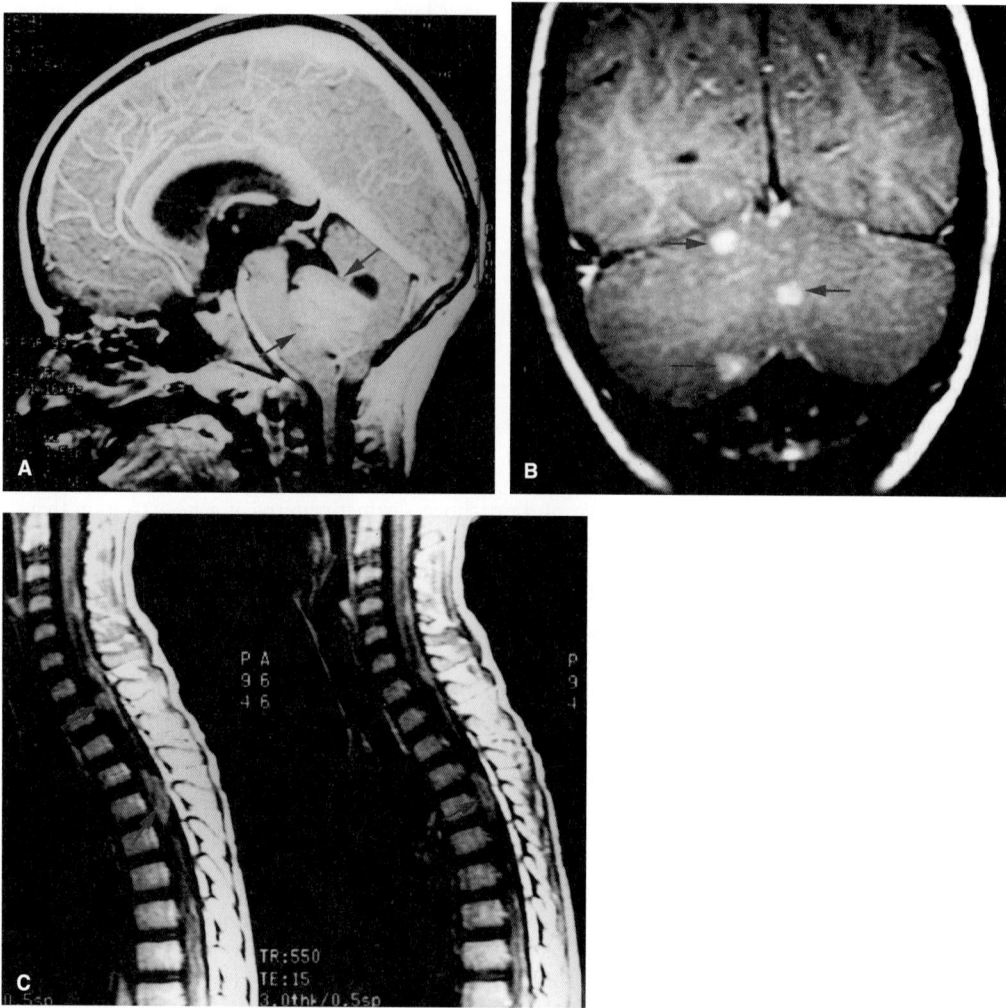

FIGURE 145.8 Sagittal MRI of a medulloblastoma in the posterior fossa **(A)** with **(B)** coronal image showing parenchymal nodules and **(C)** spine images showing seeding of the cord.

medulloblastoma with no more than 1.5 cm² postoperative residual tumor) and *high risk* (i.e., more than 1.5 cm² residual or dissemination outside the posterior fossa, including positive CSF cytology). LC/A medulloblastomas are also categorized as high risk, even if localized and completely resected, because of more aggressive behavior. Average-risk children have 80% 5-year disease-free survival. High-risk children have approximately 65% 5-year survival. Infants younger than age 3 years have inferior outcome and are considered high-risk patients even with localized tumors; an exception appears to be Shh tumors in infants for whom de-escalation of therapy may be considered.

Radiation therapy is the standard postoperative treatment for medulloblastoma/PNET, and craniospinal irradiation is given because the entire neuraxis is at risk for tumor recurrence. Conventional doses are 36 Gy to the brain and spine, with an 18- to 20-Gy boost to the local tumor site. Adjuvant (postirradiation) chemotherapy with vincristine and lomustine was shown to improve survival in advanced stages of medulloblastoma; the addition of cisplatin afforded a remarkable 5-year PFS rate of 85% in one series. Pre-irradiation chemotherapy did not improve survival. Accordingly, adjuvant chemotherapy was introduced for average-risk patients, and the combination of reduced neuraxis irradiation, followed by vincristine, lomustine, and cisplatin chemotherapy (COG A9961), resulted in a 5-year PFS rate of 79%. Even better outcomes have

been reported with dose-intensive adjuvant cyclophosphamide-based adjuvant chemotherapy with hematopoietic stem cell support in both average- and high-risk patients. With recognition of the four subtypes of medulloblastoma, it may be possible through preclinical testing to identify chemotherapeutic agents with selective effectiveness against particular subtypes. For example, screening murine group 3 medulloblastomas against a library of 7,000 compounds in a high-throughput cell-based assay revealed synergistic antitumor activity of pemetrexed and gemcitabine as combination therapy in group 3 tumors overexpressing MYC.

Chemotherapy has also been used preoperatively (following control of hydrocephalus and diagnostic biopsy), and in particular as primary postoperative treatment in infants, to avoid radiotherapy. Current protocols for infants up to age 3 years use this approach, with increasingly intensive regimens (some requiring autologous hematopoietic stem cell support) to enhance the response rate to chemotherapy and to improve the control of leptomeningeal disease. Based on favorable results, the upper age for this approach has been extended to 5 to 6 years. Early tumor progression on chemotherapy has remained a major problem. Addition of high-dose methotrexate to cisplatin-based chemotherapy for young children with newly diagnosed disseminated medulloblastoma (including autotransplant consolidation) resulted in a high response rate and 49% 3-year event-free survival. Some protocols for older infants combine local tumor irradiation (i.e., using confocal techniques) and chemotherapy, either conventional or high dose (with autologous stem cell rescue). Another strategy has been to incorporate intraventricular methotrexate with systemic chemotherapy, avoiding irradiation.

The combination of temozolomide and irinotecan appears active in recurrent medulloblastoma, as does oral etoposide, although overall prognosis after recurrence remains guarded. Recurrence tends to be local in Shh medulloblastoma and metastatic in group 3 and 4 tumors. Targeted therapy with agents such as Shh inhibitors is under investigation. High-dose chemotherapy with hematopoietic stem cell rescue has been used for selected patients with recurrent medulloblastoma who remain chemotherapy sensitive. Increasing pursuit of targeted therapy may be anticipated following successful treatment of a young adult with Shh-driven medulloblastoma with the hedgehog pathway inhibitor GDC-0449 and demonstration of antitumor activity of vismodegib in a child with Shh medulloblastoma.

Supratentorial PNETs are histologically equivalent to medulloblastoma and have been treated with the same approach of resection, craniospinal irradiation, and chemotherapy. Prognosis is worse for these patients, however, with only 40% 5-year survival. A primary postoperative chemotherapy approach in infants and young children resulted in similar outcome without radiotherapy in the majority of patients. As with medulloblastoma, preirradiation chemotherapy seems to compromise survival. Hyperfractionated radiotherapy with cisplatin-based maintenance chemotherapy (HIT 2000) afforded 58% 5-year survival. Pineal region PNETs (i.e., pineoblastomas) have a better outcome than nonpineal supratentorial PNET, approximately 70% 5-year event-free survival, although very young children may do worse. Pineoblastomas must be distinguished from pineal germ cell tumors (see later discussion) and pineocytomas (benign pineal parenchymal tumors treated by surgery alone or with radiotherapy).

Embryonal tumor with multilayered rosettes (ETMR) include three histologic variants with uniform molecular signatures (LIN28A positive, C19MC mRNA amplification, and trisomy 2). *Ependymoblastoma* is an aggressive (WHO grade IV) PNET variant of infants and young children arising in cerebral cortical and paraventricular sites and associated with hydrocephalus and poor outcome. Radical resection, craniospinal irradiation, and/or high-dose chemotherapy with autologous stem cell rescue may offer prolonged survival. *Embryonal tumor with abundant neuropil and true rosettes* (ETANTR) also occurs in young children presenting as a supratentorial mass with increased ICP; prognosis is poor despite multimodality therapy. *Medulloepithelioma* is an aggressive cerebral hemispheric tumor of infants and young children showing a range of differentiation from embryonal primitive neuroepithelioma to mature cells. Outcome is generally poor, although medulloepithelioma arising in the eye or orbit may be cured by gross total resection.

Central neurocytoma is a WHO grade II neuroepithelial intraventricular tumor typically presenting in older children or young adults with hydrocephalus and occasionally seizures. Variants include cerebral (extraventricular) neurocytoma and ganglioneurocytoma (with ganglion cell differentiation. Histologic appearance may resemble oligodendroglioma. Surgical resection is curative.

Atypical Teratoid/Rhabdoid Tumors

CNS ATRT is a rare, highly aggressive embryonal tumor of infants and young children accounting for up to 20% of cases in some infant series. ATRT is associated with somatic mutations of the tumor suppressor gene INI1/hSNF5 on chromosome 22q11, part of the SWI/SNF chromatin remodeling complex. This gene is also mutated in renal rhabdoid tumors, and germ line mutations have been reported in patients with multifocal tumors. Outcome with conventional chemotherapy has been poor (median survival <12 months), but 2-year PFS of 53% was achieved with surgery, radiation therapy, and parenteral and intrathecal chemotherapy based on the Intergroup Rhabdomyosarcoma Study III. Better outcome has been associated with older age, localized presentation, and gross total resection. Addition of myeloablative chemotherapy with autologous stem cell rescue resulted in inferior outcome but demonstrated the possibility of long-term survival without irradiation.

EPENDYMOMAS

Ependymomas are glial neoplasms typically arising within or adjacent to the ependymal lining of the ventricular system, most often in the posterior fossa. Ependymomas constitute 5% to 10% of all primary childhood brain tumors. Most appear to be histologically mature (WHO grade II). Variants include anaplastic ependymoma (WHO grade III), which carries a worse outcome in some series, and the clinically indolent subependymoma and myxopapillary ependymoma (WHO grade I).

Simian virus 40–related DNA sequences have been demonstrated in ependymomas and choroid plexus carcinomas suggesting a viral etiology. Cytogenetic and molecular studies of childhood ependymomas have revealed isochromosome 1q as an early genetic event, as well as rearrangements or deletions of chromosomes 6, 17, and 22. Human telomere reverse transcriptase (hTERT) expression predicts tumor progression. Tumor-derived stem cells show a radial glia phenotype with gene expression patterns corresponding to radial glia cells from anatomically distinct compartments of the CNS. Posterior fossa ependymomas exhibit a CpG island methylator phenotype (CIMP); transcriptional silencing of differentiation genes is driven by CpG methylation. Transcriptional profiling of posterior fossa ependymoma reveals two demographically, genetically, and clinically distinct groups: (1) younger patients (median age 2.5 years) with laterally located tumors with balanced genome, tendency for metastatic recurrence, and poor PFS (18% at 5 years) versus (2) older patients (median age 20 years) with higher degree of tumor genomic instability and cytogenetic aberrations but much better EFS (91% at 5 years).

Clinical symptoms depend on tumor location. Children with ependymomas filling or compressing the fourth ventricle have obstructive hydrocephalus with nausea, vomiting, and morning headaches. Tumors arising low in the fourth ventricle and extending into the lower medulla may cause neck pain, whereas cranial nerve palsies may result from brain stem invasion or compression of cranial nerves. In patients with supratentorial lesions, seizures and focal deficits are seen. Features on CT include calcification and variable enhancement. MRI will better demonstrate invasion by posterior fossa lesions into the brain stem (Fig. 145.9) or upper cervical spinal cord.

The most important predictor of outcome in these cases is the extent of surgical resection as confirmed by postoperative imaging. Successive clinical trials for ependymoma show that the rate of complete resection has increased from 50% to 75%. Resectability of posterior fossa lesions may be limited by brain stem infiltration, extension into the cerebellar pontine angle, or involvement of cranial nerve nuclei. Supratentorial lesions may also be infiltrative and difficult to remove. Gross total resection of ependymomas followed by involved-field irradiation (tumor bed with 1-cm margin)

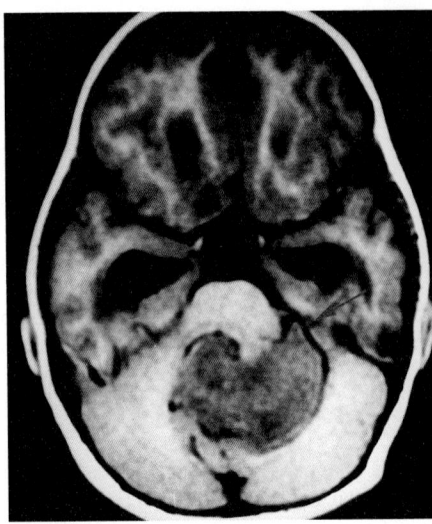

FIGURE 145.9 MR appearance of an ependymoma showing tumor extension through the foramen of Luschka (*arrow*) and invasion of the brain stem.

affords up to 75% survival, whereas local recurrence is the rule following subtotal resection, and survival rates drop below 30%. Patients with tumor dissemination at diagnosis (fewer than 10% of cases) also do poorly.

Postoperative radiation therapy increases survival rates for patients with localized ependymoma, and treatment to an involved field (at a dose of 55 Gy) is generally considered sufficient because relapses are overwhelmingly local. Completely resected supratentorial nonanaplastic ependymomas may be observed without radiation therapy.

Adjuvant chemotherapy may improve outcome based on the responses of recurrent ependymomas to cisplatin and other agents and responses in infants. Preirradiation cisplatin-based chemotherapy for patients with postoperative residual tumor (CCG-9942) produced objective responses in 57% of patients, and 5-year event-free survival of patients receiving chemotherapy for incompletely resected tumors equaled that of patients with complete resection and no chemotherapy (55% vs. 58%). A successor study (ACNS-0831) randomizes all patients to postradiation chemotherapy versus radiation alone.

Primary postoperative chemotherapy with irradiation at progression has been reported in children younger than age 5 years with 59% 4-year survival (23% without irradiation). A similar study in children younger than age 3 years found 61% survival at 3 years leading to a larger study (POG-9233/34) demonstrating that with prolonged dose-intensive chemotherapy, 40% of infants with ependymoma could be cured without radiotherapy. Recurrent ependymomas are managed by reresection and chemotherapy or by stereotactic radiosurgery.

Prospects for targeted therapy focus on histone deacetylase inhibitors, gamma secretase inhibitors (blocking notch signaling pathway activation), telomerase inhibitors (in hTERT-positive ependymoma), and lapatinib (a dual EGFR antagonist). Potential predictive biomarkers were analyzed prospectively in an Italian cooperative group trial; better outcome was associated with lower hTERT mRNA expression and nucleolin protein expression; mRNA expression levels of EGFR and prominin 1 (PROM1)/CD133 were not significant on multivariate analysis, although the PROM/CD133 cancer stem cell marker was strongly expressed in

a substantial fraction of cases and appeared to be associated with more indolent disease.

GERM CELL TUMORS

Germ cell tumors tend to arise in the pineal and suprasellar regions. They account for about half of all pineal tumors and 5% to 10% of parasellar lesions. Pineal germ cell tumors have a male preponderance and usually present in adolescence, whereas suprasellar germ cell tumors predominate in younger females. About 50% to 65% of germ cell tumors are germinomas, histologically primitive lesions resembling gonadal germ cell tumors and presumably derived from embryonic migration of totipotent germ cells. Teratomas and mixed germ cell tumors are variously composed of mature, immature, and malignant elements. Choriocarcinomas are rare but highly malignant. Chromosomal comparative genomic hybridization analysis of CNS germ cell tumors suggests that genomic alterations are essentially indistinguishable from those found in extracranial germ cell tumors.

Symptoms and signs of pineal region germ cell tumors most often include headaches and Parinaud syndrome of upgaze paresis. With extension to the overlying thalamus, there may be hemiparesis, incoordination, vision disturbances, or movement disorders. Suprasellar germ cell tumors produce pituitary and hypothalamic dysfunctions but usually not vision loss. CT appearance is of an irregular lesion of mixed density, occasionally with calcification and with variable enhancement.

MRI is more sensitive for purposes of follow-up evaluation. MRI may reveal a pineal cyst in otherwise healthy children being evaluated for headache; lack of hydrocephalus and Parinaud syndrome should lead one away from the diagnosis of a pineal tumor. Diagnosis may be aided by measurement of AFP and β-subunit of HCG, which are secreted by germ cell tumors but not pineal parenchymal cell tumors or cysts and are detectable in serum and CSF. AFP is elevated in endodermal sinus tumors and some immature teratomas; HCG is elevated in choriocarcinoma and embryonal carcinomas. Elevations associated with both indicate the presence of mixed malignant elements. Even with tumor marker elevation, however, histologic confirmation is recommended.

Surgery for pineal region tumors is technically difficult, but major resections may be achieved with acceptable morbidity rates by the use of supratentorial suboccipital or infratentorial supracerebellar approaches. Most patients require CSF shunting. There may be transient visual migraines caused by occipital lobe contusions. Teratomas may be encapsulated and are therefore easier to remove. Germ cell tumors may disseminate throughout the neuraxis in up to 10% of cases. Radiotherapy is the standard treatment for pure germinomas given typically as 35 to 45 Gy to the brain and spine with a 10- to 15-Gy boost to the area of the tumor affording 90% survival at 5 years. Chemotherapy may allow reductions in the extent of irradiation potentially lessening the considerable endocrine, neuroophthalmologic, and neuropsychological sequelae of treatment.

Survival rates for mixed malignant germ cell tumors are considerably lower, especially with radiotherapy alone, but have improved with the addition of chemotherapy. Current protocols are based on cisplatin- or carboplatin-containing regimens active in gonadal germ cell tumors; patients achieving a complete response to intensive chemotherapy may receive no further treatment, whereas those with incomplete response undergo second-look surgery or irradiation. Five-year overall survival rates are about 75% and the event-free survival rate is 36%. High-dose chemotherapy with autologous stem cell rescue, an effective strategy in recurrent germinomas, is being tested in refractory mixed malignant germ cell tumors.

LYMPHOMAS

Primary CNS lymphomas are rare, constituting fewer than 1% of intracranial tumors. They may occur at any age and are generally of B-lymphocyte origin, including Burkitt type, often seen with congenital or acquired immunodeficiency. The tumor location most commonly seen is the cerebral cortex. CNS lymphomas appear isodense or hyperdense on CT with enhancement. MRI shows an iso- to hypointense lesion on T1-weighted images and iso-, hypo-, or slightly hyperintense lesion on T2-weighted images with variable enhancement. Whole-body ^{18}F-fluorodeoxyglucose positron emission tomography (FDG PET) may reveal extracranial sites of disease not seen on other imaging such as CT scan. Whole-brain irradiation has produced survival rates of 20% to 30%. A prospective trial in immunocompetent adults with primary CNS lymphoma showed that preirradiation, high-dose methotrexate chemotherapy improved survival rates over whole-brain irradiation alone. In addition, there was a 94% objective-response rate to preirradiation chemotherapy, but there was also a 15% incidence of life-threatening, delayed neurologic toxicity. For these reasons, methotrexate- and cytarabine-based chemotherapy without irradiation is now the preferred treatment.

MENINGIOMAS AND MESENCHYMAL TUMORS

Meningiomas are rare in childhood, accounting for 2.5% of pediatric brain tumors. There is an association with NF-2, and this diagnosis should be sought in any child with meningioma. These tumors usually arise on the meningeal surface but (in contrast to adults) may grow as parenchymal lesions presumably from meningeal cell rests. CT and MRI show an isointense or hyperintense lesion enhancing with contrast (Fig. 145.10).

Most lesions are clinically benign, although 10% of pediatric or NF-2–associated tumors show anaplasia and 50% have atypical features. Overall prognosis is worse than in adults. High mitotic index, MIB-1 labeling index, and variant histology (e.g., papillary, clear cell) are associated with invasiveness and adverse outcome. Deletions of NF2, DAL-1, and chromosome 1p and 14q are common. Surgery is the primary treatment. Radiotherapy is of uncertain value but has been used for recurrent tumors, especially

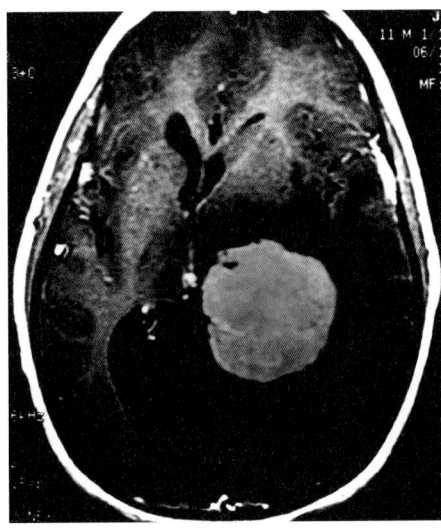

FIGURE 145.10 Axial MRI of a meningioma.

after unsuccessful reresection. Meningiomas may occasionally involve the leptomeninges, primarily, and these tumors (i.e., meningeal sarcomas) tend to behave aggressively. Treatment has been combined radiation and chemotherapy.

Meningeal sarcomas may extend intracranially from the skull or arise directly from the dura or develop within meningiomas. Treatment includes surgery, radiotherapy, and chemotherapy guided by the particular histologic subtype. *Fibrous histiocytomas* arise from the dura or grow in brain parenchyma. Benign variants are curable by surgical resection, but malignant fibrous histiocytoma has guarded prognosis despite multimodality therapy. *Solitary fibrous tumors* arise from the dura and grow slowly; they are distinguished from fibrous meningioma by immunohistochemical positivity for CD34, vimentin, and Bcl-2. Surgical resection is curative. *Hemangiopericytomas* occur mainly in adults, grow rapidly, and may present with seizures. Local recurrence is a problem, as well as neuraxis spread and extracranial metastasis; radiotherapy and chemotherapy (including antiangiogenic agents) may be useful.

Primary malignant melanomas arise in children as well as adults, usually associated with the meninges (whereas metastatic lesions more commonly involve the brain parenchyma), with gadolinium enhancement on MRI and possible leptomeningeal spread. Most lesions contain melanosomes, and electron microscopy can confirm the diagnosis. Prognosis is poor, and tumors are radioresistant, although newer targeted therapies may supplement surgery. *Meningeal melanocytomas* occur mainly in adults and arise in the posterior fossa or spinal cord. Without complete resection, these lesions may transform to malignant melanoma.

LATE EFFECTS OF TREATMENT AND QUALITY OF LIFE

The health of children surviving brain tumors is generally worse than that of survivors of other childhood cancers. Children with supratentorial astrocytomas or craniopharyngioma have a lower health status index than children with other types of brain tumors. A survey of health-related quality of life in childhood brain tumor survivors found cognitive impairment in two-thirds of the children and pain in almost one-third. Global health status was lowest in children given radiation therapy before age 5 years and in those with residual disease. Even among survivors of pediatric low-grade glioma who continue to have excellent long-term survival into adulthood, the greatest risk of death in multivariate analysis was administration of radiation.

Another survey of residual physical handicap in survivors found motor impairment in 56% of patients, cognitive impairment (i.e., IQ score <80) in 30%, visual impairment in 24%, and epilepsy in 21%.

A study of psychological outcomes in long-term survivors found that the prevalence of psychological distress (11%) exceeded that in siblings (5%) and was not a direct result of cancer treatment but rather was associated with diminished social functioning and vocational skills. Another report found increased risk of hospital admission was the focus for psychiatric disorders among patients with brain tumors who had survived at least 3 years from diagnosis compared to other childhood cancer survivors, in whom there was no increased risk.

RADIATION EFFECTS

Radiation effects include a transient somnolence syndrome of sleepiness, irritability, anorexia, and headaches lasting about a week. Radiation necrosis develops in 0.1% to 5.0% of patients after conventional treatment at 50 to 60 Gy in daily fractions of 180 to 200 cGy. The onset may be within 3 months and is usually seen by 3 years, although occasionally not until much later; the symptoms and signs are those of a recurrent intracranial mass with possible seizures and progressive neuropsychological impairment. Surgical resection should be attempted; unresectable lesions may be treated with corticosteroids, but it may be difficult to reduce the dose later. Cavernous hemangiomas (cavernomas) developed in 3.4% of children at a median of 37 months following radiotherapy for brain tumors. Median age at treatment was 7 years. These benign vascular malformations may cause seizures or hemorrhage. Large-vessel thrombosis is a rare complication of radiation therapy occurring between 2 and 30 years after cranial irradiation. The relative risk of stroke for 5-year survivors of brain tumors was 29.0 compared to sibling controls with dose-dependent increased risk following cranial irradiation exceeding 30 Gy. Treatment is symptomatic.

ENDOCRINE DYSFUNCTION

Endocrine dysfunction may follow irradiation to the hypothalamus and pituitary. Doses as low as 18 Gy may produce growth hormone deficiency, and doses above 36 Gy may cause hypothyroidism and gonadal dysfunction in more than half of patients. Nearly 40% of brain cancer survivors in the Childhood Cancer Survivor Study were below the 10th percentile for height. Risk factors included age younger than 5 years at diagnosis and radiation therapy to the hypothalamic–pituitary axis. Growth hormone deficiency in the absence of other anterior pituitary hormone deficiencies in children receiving cranial irradiation for posterior fossa tumors suggests growth hormone is the hormone most sensitive to radiation injury. Hypothalamic obesity, a syndrome of intractable weight gain, is an uncommon but serious complication of hypothalamic irradiation at doses exceeding 50 Gy.

Brain tumor survivors are at risk for hypothyroidism as a collateral effect of cranial or craniospinal irradiation. The incidence of hypothyroidism appears to be considerably lower in children receiving hyperfractionated irradiation compared to those receiving conventional once-daily dosing. Precocious puberty has been noted in nearly one-quarter of girls treated with irradiation. Frank adrenal insufficiency is uncommon, but subtle abnormalities in adrenal function may be present particularly in survivors of craniopharyngioma, other sellar tumors, and medulloblastoma. There is also an increased incidence of osteoporosis.

Children should be followed for measurement of linear growth, periodic thyroid function studies, and additional endocrine evaluation if there is precocious or delayed-onset puberty. Growth hormone treatment improves final height in children with growth hormone deficiency after brain tumor therapy. Growth hormone response depends on adequate thyroid function, and thyroid supplementation may be required. In the subset of patients in whom growth was further limited by early puberty, the combination of gonadotrophin-releasing hormone analogs and growth hormone is reported to improve prospects for attainment of target height. A survey of growth hormone replacement therapy in patients with medulloblastoma suggests a trend toward underutilization, despite ample evidence that there is no increased risk of brain tumor recurrence associated with growth hormone therapy. There is, however, evidence of an increase in the already existing risk for second malignant neoplasms in patients previously treated with radiation therapy. This increased risk of second neoplasms in growth hormone (GH)–treated childhood cancer survivors is now listed in the United States labeling for recombinant human growth hormone (rhGH) products.

CARDIOVASCULAR EFFECTS

Cardiovascular late effects in children treated for brain tumors include increased risk of stroke, blood clots, and angina-like symptoms. Late effects are common in those treated with surgery and radiation and higher still in those treated with surgery, radiation, and chemotherapy. Cardiovascular problems may be compounded by restrictive lung disease and cardiotoxicity in recipients of craniospinal irradiation or intensive chemotherapy. Among survivors of childhood brain cancer whose mean age was 26 years and mean posttreatment interval was 16 years, systolic blood pressures and waist-to-hip ratios were higher than controls, as were blood lipid abnormalities. These findings identify dyslipidemia, central obesity, and hypertension as controllable risk factors for cardiovascular disease.

NEUROLOGIC AND OTHER SEQUELAE

Neurologic and neurosensory sequelae in adult survivors of childhood brain tumors include hearing loss, blindness, cataracts, and diplopia. Nearly half of the survivors have coordination problems, and one-quarter have motor control problems after radiation doses of 50 Gy to frontal brain regions. Seizures are reported in one-quarter of patients, especially after radiation doses of 30 Gy or more. Atonic seizures in particular are difficult to control and are associated with pervasive cognitive impairments. Patients treated with surgery alone generally have no more than minor neurologic impairment that does not interfere with activities of daily living, but one-third have severe ataxia, spastic paresis, visual impairment, or epilepsy.

Radiation therapy is a principal cause of *neurocognitive disorders* in children with CNS tumors. Other factors include acute or chronic increased ICP, tumor mass effect, poorly controlled seizure disorders, hormonal deficits, and complications of surgery and chemotherapy. A neurologic predictor scale has been developed to quantify the influence of the various tumor- and treatment-related risks for neurocognitive problems. Radiologic evaluation of patients treated for medulloblastoma with craniospinal irradiation, with or without chemotherapy, showed reduced volumes of normal white matter, which correlated with full-scale IQ. Neurocognitive problems are more likely in children treated at a young age or with high doses of radiation, especially when applied to cerebral–cortical areas associated with higher functions. The effects may be progressive for years and may include attention deficit, impaired memory, and lowering IQ. In one series, mean observed full-scale IQ was 97.1 for nonirradiated patients and 78.8 for irradiated patients. For children with standard-risk medulloblastoma, hyperfractionated radiotherapy was associated with better executive function than standard radiotherapy without any difference in behavior or quality of life. These children generally require psychological intervention and special education programs.

Chronic neurotoxicity of chemotherapy used in treating CNS tumors includes hearing loss (e.g., especially after cisplatin therapy) and peripheral neuropathy (e.g., with vincristine or occasionally cisplatin and etoposide). Renal impairment and hypertension are associated with cisplatin therapy. Osteopenia is found in half of the children surviving brain tumors, and bone pain may limit physical activity. Chemotherapy may potentiate the deleterious effect of craniospinal irradiation on growth. There is an increased risk (3% to 5%) of second tumors, including meningiomas and sarcomas arising 10 to 20 years after cranial irradiation treatment. Secondary leukemia has been reported after chemotherapy with alkylating agents and etoposide. In a cohort of patients surviving

5 years from diagnosis of a CNS tumor, survival estimates were 91% at 10 years and 86% at 15 years; causes of late mortality were PD (58%), second malignant tumor (21%), and medical complications (18%). Among 5-year survivors treated between 1973 and 1998, the risk of second malignant neoplasms is higher for patients treated after 1985, even controlling for radiotherapy, consistent with increased use of intensive chemotherapy in recent years.

SUGGESTED READINGS

Epidemiology

Amlashi SF, Riffaud L, Brassier G, et al. Nevoid basal cell carcinoma syndrome: relation with desmoplastic medulloblastoma in infancy. A population-based study and review of the literature. *Cancer.* 2003;98:618–624.

Bergsagel DJ, Finegold MJ, Butel JS, et al. DNA sequences similar to those of simian virus 40 in ependymomas and choroid plexus tumors of childhood. *N Engl J Med.* 1992;326:988–993.

Bishop AJ, McDonald MW, Chang AL, et al. Infant brain tumors: incidence, survival, and the role of radiation based on Surveillance, Epidemiology, and End Results (SEER) data. *Int J Radiat Oncol Biol Phys.* 2012;82:341–347.

Blamires TL, Maher ER. Choroid plexus papilloma. A new presentation of von Hippel-Lindau (VHL) disease. *Eye (Lond).* 1992;6:90–92.

Bunin GR, Buckley JD, Boesel CP, et al. Risk factors for astrocytic glioma and primitive neuroectodermal tumor of the brain in young children: a report from the Children's Cancer Group. *Cancer Epidemiol Biomarkers Prev.* 1994;3:197–204.

Bunin GR, Kuijten RR, Buckley JD, et al. Relation between maternal diet and subsequent primitive neuroectodermal brain tumors in young children. *N Engl J Med.* 1993;329:536–541.

Curless RG, Toledano SR, Ragheb J, et al. Hematogenous brain metastasis in children. *Pediatr Neurol.* 2002;26:219–221.

Dolecek TA, Propp JM, Stroup NE, et al. CBTRUS statistical report: primary brain and central nervous system tumors diagnosed in the United States in 2005-2009. *Neuro Oncol.* 2012;14(suppl 5):v1–v49.

Dubuc AM, Northcott PA, Mack S, et al. The genetics of pediatric brain tumors. *Curr Neurol Neurosci Rep.* 2010;10:215–223.

Gold DR, Cohen BH. Brain tumors in neurofibromatosis. *Curr Treat Options Neurol.* 2003;5:199–206.

Green AJ, Smith M, Yates JR. Loss of heterozygosity on chromosome 16p13.3 in hamartomas from tuberous sclerosis patients. *Nat Genet.* 1994;6:193–196.

Gurney JG, Mueller BA, Preston-Martin S, et al. A study of pediatric brain tumors and their association with epilepsy and anticonvulsant use. *Neuroepidemiology.* 1997;16:248–255.

Hader WJ, Drovini-Zis K, Maguire JA. Primitive neuroectodermal tumors in the central nervous system following cranial irradiation: a report of four cases. *Cancer.* 2003;97:1072–1076.

Holly EA, Bracci PM, Mueller BA, et al. Farm and animal exposures and pediatric brain tumors: results from the United States West Coast Childhood Brain Tumor Study. *Cancer Epidemiol Biomark Prev.* 1998;7:797–802.

Kheifets LI, Sussman SS, Preston-Martin S. Childhood brain tumors and residential electromagnetic fields (EMF). *Rev Environ Contam Toxicol.* 1999;159:111–129.

Kluwe L, Hagel C, Tatagiba M, et al. Loss of NF1 alleles distinguish sporadic from NF1-associated pilocytic astrocytomas. *J Neuropathol Exp Neurol.* 2001;60:917–920.

Larouche V, Huang A, Bartels U, et al. Tumors of the central nervous system in the first year of life. *Pediatr Blood Cancer.* 2007;49:1074–1082.

Louis DN, Ohgaki H, Wiestler OD, et al, eds. *WHO Classification of Tumours of the Central Nervous System.* 4th ed. Lyon, France: IARC Press; 2007.

Louis DN, Ramesh V, Gusella JF. Neuropathology and molecular genetics of neurofibromatosis 2 and related tumors. *Brain Pathol.* 1995;5:163–172.

McCarthy BJ, Surawicz T, Bruner JM, et al. Consensus conference on brain tumor definition for registration. *Neuro Oncol.* 2002;4:134–145.

Nabbout R, Santos M, Rolland Y, et al. Early diagnosis of subependymal giant cell astrocytoma in children with tuberous sclerosis. *J Neurol Neurosurg Psychiatry.* 1999;66:370–375.

Ostrom QT, Gittleman H, Farah P, et al. Primary brain and central nervous system tumors diagnosed in the United States in 2006-2010. *Neuro Oncol.* 2013;15(suppl 2):ii1–ii56.

Rickert CH, Paulus W. Epidemiology of central nervous system tumors in childhood and adolescence based on the new WHO classification. *Childs Nerv Syst.* 2001;17:503–511.

Rickert CH, Sträter R, Kaatsch P. Pediatric high-grade astrocytomas show chromosomal imbalances distinct from adult cases. *Am J Pathol.* 2001;158:1525–1532.

Ries LAG, Melbert D, Krapcho M, et al. *SEER Cancer Statistics Review, 1975-2004.* Bethesda, MD: National Cancer Institute; 2007.

Rosso AL, Hovinga ME, Rorke-Adams LB, et al. A case-control study of childhood brain tumors and fathers' hobbies: a Children's Oncology Group study. *Cancer Causes Control.* 2008;19:1201–1207.

Rubio MP, Correa KM, Ramesh V, et al. Analysis of the neurofibromatosis 2 gene in human ependymomas and astrocytomas. *Cancer Res.* 1994;54:45–47.

Shore RE, Moseson M, Harley N, et al. Tumors and other diseases following childhood x-ray treatment for ringworm of the scalp (tinea capitis). *Health Phys.* 2003;85:404–408.

Smith MA, Freidlin B, Ries LA, et al. Trends in reported incidence of primary malignant brain tumors in children in the United States. *J Natl Cancer Inst.* 1998;90:1269–1277.

Stålberg K, Haglund B, Axelsson O, et al. Prenatal ultrasound and the risk of childhood brain tumour and its subtypes. *Br J Cancer.* 2008;98:1285–1287.

Van Wijngaarden E, Stewart PA, Olshan AF, et al. Parental occupational exposure to pesticides and childhood brain cancer. *Am J Epidemiol.* 2003;157:989–997.

Walter AW, Hancock ML, Pui CH, et al. Secondary brain tumors in children treated for acute lymphoblastic leukemia at St Jude Children's Research Hospital. *J Clin Oncol.* 1998;16:3761–3767.

Developmental Biology

Bao S, Wu Q, McLendon R, et al. Glioma stem cells promote radioresistance by preferential activation of the DNA damage response. *Nature.* 2006;444:756–760.

Biegel JA, Tan L, Zhang F, et al. Alterations of the hSNF5/INI1 gene in central nervous system atypical teratoid/rhabdoid tumors and renal and extrarenal rhabdoid tumors. *Clin Cancer Res.* 2002;8:3461–3467.

Buczkowicz P, Hoeman C, Rakopoulos P, et al. Genomic analysis of diffuse intrinsic pontine gliomas identifies three molecular subgroups and recurrent activating ACVR1 mutations. *Nat Genet.* 2014;46:451–456.

Ding H, Roncari L, Shannon P, et al. Astrocyte-specific expression of activated p21-RAS results in malignant astrocytoma formation in a transgenic mouse model of human gliomas. *Cancer Res.* 2001;61:3826–3836.

Dorris K, Sobo M, Onar-Thomas A, et al. Prognostic significance of telomere maintenance mechanisms in pediatric high-grade gliomas. *J Neurooncol.* 2014;117:67–76.

Faury D, Nantel A, Dunn SE, et al. Molecular profiling identifies prognostic subgroups of pediatric glioblastoma and shows increased YB-1 expression in tumors. *J Clin Oncol.* 2007;25:1196–1208.

Hesselager G, Holland EC. Using mice to decipher the molecular genetics of brain tumors. *Neurosurgery.* 2003;53:685–694.

Holland EC, Celestino J, Dai C, et al. Combined activation of RAS and AKT in neural progenitors induces glioblastoma formation in mice. *Nat Genet.* 2000;25:55–57.

Horbinski C. To BRAF or not to BRAF: is that even a question anymore? *Neuropathol Exp Neurol.* 2013;72:2–7.

Judkins AR, Mauger J, Rorke LB, et al. Immunohistochemical analysis of hSNF5/INI1 in pediatric CNS neoplasms. *Am J Surg Pathol.* 2004;28:644–650.

Khatua S, Peterson KM, Brown KM, et al. Prognostic value of epidermal growth factor receptor in patients with glioblastoma multiforme. *Cancer Res.* 2003;63:1865–1870.

Kool M, Jones DT, Jäger N, et al. Genome sequencing of SHH medulloblastoma predicts genotype-related response to smoothened inhibition. *Cancer Cell.* 2014;25:393–405.

Leung C, Lingbeek M, Shakhova O, et al. Bmi1 is essential for cerebellar development and is overexpressed in human medulloblastomas. *Nature.* 2004;428:337–341.

Li J, Yen C, Liaw D, et al. PTEN, a putative protein tyrosine phosphatase gene mutated in human brain, breast, and prostate cancer. *Science.* 1997;275:1943–1947.

Merlo A. Genes and pathways driving glioblastomas in humans and murine disease models. *Neurosurg Rev.* 2003;26:145–158.

Pollack IF, Finkelstein SD, Woods J, et al. Expression of p53 and prognosis in children with malignant gliomas. *N Engl J Med.* 2002;346:420–427.

Pomeroy SL, Tamayo P, Gaasenbeek M, et al. Prediction of central nervous system embryonal tumour outcome based on gene expression. *Nature.* 2002;415:436–442.

Rodriguez FJ, Lim KS, Bowers D, et al. Pathological and molecular advances in pediatric low-grade astrocytoma. *Annu Rev Pathol.* 2013;8:361–379.

Rossi A, Caracciolo V, Russo G, et al. Medulloblastoma: from molecular pathology to therapy. *Clin Cancer Res.* 2008;14:971–976.

Rubin JB, Rowitch DH. Medulloblastoma: a problem of developmental biology. *Cancer Cell.* 2002;2:7–8.

Schwartzentruber J, Korshunov A, Liu XY, et al. Driver mutations in histone H3.3 and chromatin remodeling genes in paediatric glioblastoma. *Nature.* 2012;482:226–231.

Stupp R, Hegi ME. Targeting brain-tumor stem cells. *Nat Biotechnol.* 2007;25:193–194.

Taylor MD, Poppleton H, Fuller C, et al. Radial glia cells are candidate stem cells of ependymoma. *Cancer Cell.* 2005;8:323–335.

Vescovi AL, Galli R, Reynolds B. Brain tumor stem cells. *Nat Rev Cancer.* 2006;6:425–436.

Wang VY, Zoghbi HY. Genetic regulation of cerebellar development. *Nat Rev Neurosci.* 2001;2:484–491.

Wechsler-Reya RJ. Analysis of gene expression in the normal and malignant cerebellum. *Recent Prog Horm Res.* 2003;58:227–248.

Wechsler-Reya R, Scott MP. The developmental biology of brain tumors. *Ann Rev Neurosci.* 2001;24:385–428.

Wu G, Broniscer A, McEachron TA, et al. Somatic histone H3 alterations in pediatric diffuse intrinsic pontine gliomas and non-brainstem glioblastomas. *Nat Genet.* 2012;44:251–253.

Zarghooni M, Bartels U, Lee E, et al. Whole-genome profiling of pediatric diffuse intrinsic pontine gliomas highlights platelet-derived growth factor receptor alpha and poly (ADP-ribose) polymerase as potential therapeutic targets. *J Clin Oncol.* 2010;28:1337–1344.

Zedan W, Robinson PA, High AS. A novel polymorphism in the PTC gene allows easy identification of allelic loss in basal cell nevus syndrome lesions. *Diagn Mol Pathol.* 2001;10:41–45.

Symptoms, Diagnosis, and Management

Borgwardt L, Hojgaard L, Carstensen H, et al. Increased fluorine-18 2-fluoro-2-deoxy-D-glucose (FDG) uptake in childhood CNS tumors is correlated with malignancy grade: a study with FDG positron emission tomography/magnetic resonance imaging coregistration and image fusion. *J Clin Oncol.* 2005;23:3030–3037.

Caruso DA, Orme LM, Neale AM, et al. Results of a phase 1 study utilizing monocyte-derived dendritic cells pulsed with tumor RNA in children and young adults with brain cancer. *Neuro Oncol.* 2004;6:236–246.

Cochrane DD, Gustavsson B, Poskitt KP, et al. The surgical and natural morbidity of aggressive resection for posterior fossa tumors in childhood. *Pediatr Neurosurg.* 1994;20:19–29.

Dahlborg SA, Petrillo A, Crossen JR, et al. The potential for complete and durable response in nonglial primary brain tumors in children and young adults with enhanced chemotherapy delivery. *Cancer J Sci Am.* 1998;4:110–124.

De Vleeschouwer S, Fieuws S, Rutkowski S, et al. Postoperative adjuvant dendritic cell-based immunotherapy in patients with relapsed glioblastoma multiforme. *Clin Cancer Res.* 2008;14:3098–3104.

Dobrovoljac M, Hengartner H, Boltshauser E, et al. Delay in the diagnosis of paediatric brain tumours. *Eur J Pediatr.* 2002;161:663–667.

Duffner PK, Horowitz ME, Krischer JP, et al. Postoperative chemotherapy and delayed radiation in children less than three years of age with malignant brain tumors. *N Engl J Med.* 1993;328:1725–1731.

Duffner PK, Horowitz ME, Krischer JP, et al. The treatment of malignant brain tumors in infants and very young children: an update of the Pediatric Oncology Group experience. *Neuro Oncol.* 1999;1:152–161.

Finlay JF, Goldman S, Wong MC, et al. Pilot study of high-dose thiotepa and etoposide with autologous bone marrow rescue in children and young adults with recurrent CNS tumors. *J Clin Oncol.* 1996;14:2495–2503.

Furchert SE, Lanyers-Kaminsky C, Juurgens H, et al. Inhibitors of histone deacetylases as potential therapeutic tools for high-risk embryonal tumors of the nervous system of childhood. *Int J Cancer.* 2007;120:1787–1794.

Gajjar A, Packer RJ, Foreman NK, et al. Children's Oncology Group's 2013 blueprint for research: central nervous system tumors. *Pediatr Blood Cancer.* 2013;60:1022–1026.

Geoerger B, Gaspar N, Opolon P, et al. EGFR tyrosine kinase inhibition radiosensitizes and induces apoptosis in malignant glioma and childhood ependymoma xenografts. *Int J Cancer.* 2008;123:209–216.

Gilles FH, Brown WD, Leviton A, et al. Limitations of the World Health Organization classification of childhood supratentorial astrocytic tumors. Childhood Brain Tumor Consortium. *Cancer.* 2000;88:1477–1483.

Gilles FH, Leviton A, Tavare CJ, et al. Clinical and survival covariates of eight classes of childhood supratentorial neuroglial tumors. *Cancer.* 2002;95:1302–1310.

Haas-Kogan DA, Banerjee A, Kocak M, et al. Phase I trial of tipifarnib in children with newly diagnosed intrinsic diffuse brainstem glioma. *Neuro Oncol.* 2008;10(3):341–347.

Habrand JL, De Crevoisier R. Radiation therapy in the management of childhood brain tumors. *Childs Nerv Syst.* 2001;17:121–133.

Hug EB, Sweeney RA, Nurre PM, et al. Proton radiotherapy in management of pediatric base of skull tumors. *Int J Radiat Oncol Biol.* 2002;52:1017–1024.

Jacobs JFM, Grauer OM, Brasseur F, et al. Selective cancer-germline gene expression in pediatric brain tumors. *J Neurooncol.* 2008;88:273–280.

Kalifa C, Valtreau D, Pizer B, et al. High-dose chemotherapy in childhood brain tumours. *Childs Nerv Syst.* 1999;15:498–505.

Kellie SJ. Chemotherapy of central nervous system tumours in infants. *Childs Nerv Syst.* 1999;15:592–612.

Kestle JR. Pediatric hydrocephalus: current management. *Neurol Clin.* 2003;21:883–895.

Kirsch DG, Tarbell NJ. New technologies in radiation therapy for pediatric brain tumors: the rationale for proton radiation therapy. *Pediatr Blood Cancer.* 2004;42:461–464.

Kortmann RD, Timmermann B, Becker G, et al. Advances in treatment techniques and time/dose schedules in external radiation therapy of brain tumors in childhood. *Klin Padiatr.* 1998;210:220–226.

Kramer ED, Vezine LG, Packer RJ, et al. Staging and surveillance of children with central nervous system neoplasms: recommendations of the Neurology and Tumor Imaging Committees of the Children's Cancer Group. *Pediatr Neurosurg.* 1994;20:254–263.

Kremer P, Tronnier V, Steiner HH, et al. Intraoperative MRI for interventional neurosurgical procedures and tumor resection control in children. *Childs Nerv Syst.* 2006;22:674–678.

Kukal K, Dobrovoljac M, Boltshauser E, et al. Does diagnostic delay result in decreased survival in paediatric brain tumours? *Eur J Pediatr.* 2009;168(3):303–310.

Lashford LS, Campbell RH, Gattamaneni HR, et al. An intensive multiagent chemotherapy regimen for brain tumours occurring in very young children. *Arch Dis Child.* 1996;74:219–223.

Levisohn L, Cronin-Golomb A, Schmahmann JD. Neuropsychological consequences of cerebellar tumour resection in children: cerebellar cognitive affective syndrome in a paediatric population. *Brain.* 2000;123(pt 5):1041–1050.

Louis DN, Ohgaki H, Wiestler OD, et al. The 2007 WHO classification of tumours of the central nervous system. *Acta Neuropathol.* 2007;114:97–109.

Maria BL, Drane WE, Mastin ST, et al. Comparative value of thallium and glucose SPECT imaging in childhood brain tumors. *Pediatr Neurol.* 1998;19:351–357.

Mason WP, Grovas A, Halpern S, et al. Intensive chemotherapy and bone marrow rescue for young children with newly diagnosed malignant brain tumors. *J Clin Oncol.* 1998;16:210–221.

Medina LS, Kuntz KM, Pomeroy S. Children with headache suspected of having a brain tumor: a cost-effectiveness analysis of diagnostic strategies. *Pediatrics.* 2001;108:255–263.

Merchant TE, Hua C-H, Shukla H, et al. Proton versus photon radiotherapy for common pediatric brain tumors: comparison of models of dose characteristics and their relationship to cognitive function. *Pediatr Blood Cancer*. 2008;51:110–117.

Minn AY, Pollock BH, Garzarella L, et al. Surveillance neuroimaging to detect relapse in childhood brain tumors: a Pediatric Oncology Group study. *J Clin Oncol*. 2001;19:4135–4140.

Nicholson HS, Kretschmar CS, Krailo M, et al. Phase 2 study of temozolomide in children and adolescents with recurrent central nervous system tumors; a report from the Children's Oncology Group. *Cancer*. 2007;110:1542–1550.

Noel G, Habrand JL, Helfre S, et al. Proton beam therapy in the management of central nervous system tumors in childhood: the preliminary experience of the Centre de Protontherapie d'Orsay. *Med Pediatr Oncol*. 2003;40: 309–315.

Okada H, Low KL, Kohanbash G, et al. Expression of glioma-associated antigens in pediatric brain stem and non-brain stem gliomas. *J Neurooncol*. 2008;88:245–250.

Pfister S, Hartmann C, Korshunov A. Histology and molecular pathology of pediatric brain tumors. *J Child Neurol*. 2009;24:1375–1386.

Pollack IF, Keating R. New delivery approaches for pediatric brain tumors. *J Neurooncol*. 2005;75:315–326.

Raffanghello L, Nozza P, Morandi F, et al. Expression and functional analysis of human leukocyte antigen class I antigen-processing machinery in medulloblastoma. *Cancer Res*. 2007;67:5471–5478.

Sandberg DI. Endoscopic management of hydrocephalus in pediatric patients: a review of indications, techniques, and outcomes. *J Child Neurol*. 2008;23:550–560.

Shih C-S, Hale GA, Gronewold L, et al. High-dose chemotherapy with autologous stem cell rescue for children with recurrent malignant brain tumors. *Cancer*. 2008;112:1345–1353.

Steinbok P, Cochrane DD, Perrin R, et al. Mutism after posterior fossa tumour resection in children: incomplete recovery on long-term follow-up. *Pediatr Neurosurg*. 2003;39:179–183.

Tajbakhsh M, Houghton PJ, Morton CL, et al. Initial testing of cisplatin by the pediatric preclinical testing program. *Pediatr Blood Cancer*. 2007;50: 992–1000.

Taylor JS, Langston JW, Reddick WE, et al. Clinical value of proton magnetic resonance spectroscopy for differentiating recurrent or residual brain tumor from delayed cerebral necrosis. *Int J Radiat Oncol Biol Phys*. 1996;36: 1251–1261.

Tzika AA, Vajapeyam S, Barnes PD. Multivoxel proton MR spectroscopy and hemodynamic MR imaging of childhood brain tumors: preliminary observations. *Am J Neuroradiol*. 1997;18:203–218.

Utriainen M, Metsahonkala L, Salmi TT, et al. Metabolic characterization of childhood brain tumors: comparison of 18F-fluorodeoxyglucose and ^{11}C-methionine positron emission tomography. *Cancer*. 2002;95:1376–1386.

Warren KE. NMR spectroscopy and pediatric brain tumors. *Oncologist*. 2004;9:312–318.

Warren KE, Patronas N, Aikin AA, et al. Comparison of one-, two-, and three-dimensional measurements of childhood brain tumors. *J Natl Cancer Inst*. 2001;93:1401–1405.

Wilne S, Collier J, Kennedy C, et al. Presentation of childhood CNS tumours: a systematic review and meta-analysis. *Lancet Oncology*. 2007;8:685–695.

Yousaf J, Avula S, Abernethy LJ, et al. Importance of intraoperative magnetic resonance imaging for pediatric brain tumor surgery. *Surg Neurol Int*. 2012;3(suppl 2):S65–S72.

Congenital Tumors

Abel TW, Baker SJ, Fraser MM, et al. Lhermitte-Duclos disease: a report of 31 cases with immunohistochemical analysis of the PTEN/AKT/mTOR pathway. *J Neuropathol Exp Neurol*. 2005;64(4):341–349.

Allen J, Wissof J, Helson L, et al. Choroid plexus carcinoma: responses to chemotherapy alone in newly diagnosed young children. *J Neurooncol*. 1992;12:69–74.

Bachli H, Avoledo P, Gratzl O, et al. Therapeutic strategies and management of desmoplastic infantile ganglioglioma: two case reports and literature review. *Childs Nerv Syst*. 2003;19:359–366.

Bakhtiar Y, Yonezawa H, Bohara M, et al. Posterior fossa immature teratoma in an infant with trisomy 21: a case report and review of the literature. *Surg Neurol Int*. 2012;3:100.

Chow E, Reardon DA, Shah AB, et al. Pediatric choroid plexus neoplasma. *Int J Radiat Oncol Biol Phys*. 1999;44:249–254.

Dash RC, Provenzale JM, McComb RD, et al. Malignant supratentorial ganglioglioma (ganglion cell–giant cell glioblastoma): a case report and review of the literature. *Arch Pathol Lab Med*. 1999;123:342–345.

Elliott RE, Hsieh K, Hochm T, et al. Efficacy and safety of radical resection of primary and recurrent craniopharyngiomas in 86 children. Clinical article. *J Neurosurg Pediatr*. 2010;5:30–48.

Ferreira J, Eviatar L, Schneider S, et al. Prenatal diagnosis of intracranial teratoma. Prolonged survival after resection of a malignant teratoma diagnosed prenatally by ultrasound: a case report and literature review. *Pediatr Neurosurg*. 1993;19:84–88.

Fornari M, Solero C, Lasio G, et al. Surgical treatment of intracranial dermoid and epidermoid cysts in children. *Childs Nerv Syst*. 1990;6:66–70.

Fouladi M, Jenkins J, Burger P, et al. Pleomorphic xanthoastrocytoma: favorable outcome after complete surgical resection. *Neuro Oncol*. 2001;3:184–192.

Gardner PA, Prevedello DM, Kassam AB, et al. The evolution of the endonasal approach for craniopharyngioma. *J Neurosurg*. 2008;108:1043–1047.

Hamlat A, Hua ZF, Saikali S, et al. Malignant transformation of intra-cranial epithelial cysts: systematic article review. *J Neurooncol*. 2005;74:187–194.

Hellwig D, Bauer BL, Schulte M, et al. Neuroendoscopic treatment for colloid cysts of the third ventricle: the experience of a decade. *Neurosurgery*. 2003;52:525–533.

Im SH, Chung CK, Cho BK, et al. Intracranial ganglioglioma: preoperative characteristics and oncologic outcome after surgery. *J Neurooncol*. 2002;59: 173–183.

Kaylie DM, Warren FM III, Haynes DS, et al. Neurotologic management of intracranial epidermoid tumors. *Laryngoscope*. 2005;115:1082–1086.

Mallucci C, Lellouch-Tubiana A, Salazar C, et al. The management of desmoplastic neuroepithelial tumours in childhood. *Childs Nerv Syst*. 2000;16:8–14.

McEvoy AW, Harding BN, Phipps KP, et al. Management of choroid plexus tumours in children: 20 years experience at a single neurosurgical center. *Pediatr Neurosurg*. 2000;32:192–199.

Meyers SP, Khademian ZP, Chuang SH, et al. Choroid plexus carcinomas in children: MRI features and patient outcomes. *Neuroradiology*. 2004;46:770–780.

Muller HL. Childhood craniopharyngioma. *Hormone Res*. 2008;69:193–202.

Nolan MA, Sakuta R, Chuang N, et al. Dysembryoplastic neuroepithelial tumors in childhood: long-term outcome and prognostic features. *Neurology*. 2004;62:2270–2276.

O'Brien DF, Farrell M, Delanty N, et al. The Children's Cancer and Leukaemia Group guidelines for the diagnosis and management of dysembryoplastic neuroepithelial tumours. *Br J Neurosurg*. 2007;21:539–549.

Rades D, Zwick L, Leppert J, et al. The role of postoperative radiotherapy for the treatment of gangliogliomas. *Cancer*. 2010;116:432–442.

Sarkar C, Sharma MC, Gaikwad S, et al. Choroid plexus papilloma: a clinicopathological study of 23 cases. *Surg Neurol*. 1999;52:37–39.

Stripp DC, Maity A, Janss AJ, et al. Surgery with or without radiation therapy in the management of craniopharyngiomas in children and young adults. *Int J Radiat Oncol Biol Phys*. 2004;58:714–720.

Tabori U, Shlien A, Baskin B, et al. TP53 alterations determine clinical subgroups and survival of patients with choroid plexus tumors. *J Clin Oncol*. 2010;28:1995–2001.

Tamburrini G, Colosimo C Jr, Giangaspero F, et al. Desmoplastic infantile ganglioglioma. *Childs Nerv Syst*. 2003;19:292–297.

Uliel-Sibony S, Kramer U, Fried I, et al. Pediatric temporal low-grade glial tumors: epilepsy outcome following resection in 48 children. *Childs Nerv Syst*. 2011;27:1413–1418.

Vinchon M, Dhellemmes P. Craniopharyngiomas in children: recurrence, reoperation and outcome. *Childs Nerv Syst*. 2008;24:211–217.

Wolff JE, Sajedi M, Brant R, et al. Choroid plexus tumours. *Br J Cancer*. 2002;87:1086–1091.

Wrede B, Liu P, Wolff JEA. Chemotherapy improves the survival of patients with choroid plexus carcinoma: a meta-analysis of individual cases with choroid plexus tumors. *J Neurooncol*. 2007;85:345–351.

Yasuda M, Bressor D, Chibbaro S, et al. Chordomas of the skull base and cervical spine: clinical outcomes associated with a multimodal surgical resection combined with proton-beam radiation in 40 patients. *Neurosurg Rev*. 2012;35:171–182.

Yeung JT, Pollack IF, Panigrahy A, et al. Pegylated interferon-α-2b for children with recurrent craniopharyngioma. *J Neurosurg Pediat.* 2012;10:498–503.

Zacharia BE, Bruce SS, Goldstein H, et al. Incidence, treatment and survival of patients with craniopharyngioma in the surveillance, epidemiology and end results program. *Neuro Oncol.* 2012;14:1070–1078.

Zentner J, Wolf HK, Ostertun B, et al. Gangliogliomas: clinical, radiological, and histopathological findings in 51 patients. *J Neurol Neurosurg Psychiatry.* 1994;57:1497–1502.

Astrocytomas

Albright AL, Packer RJ, Zimmerman R, et al. Magnetic resonance scans should replace biopsies for the diagnosis of diffuse brain stem gliomas: a report from the Children's Cancer Group. *Neurosurgery.* 1993;33:1026–1029.

Amano T, Inamura T, Nakamizo A, et al. Case management of hydrocephalus associated with the progression of childhood brain stem gliomas. *Childs Nerv Syst.* 2002;18:599–604.

Ater JL, Zhou T, Holmes E, et al. Randomized study of two chemotherapy regimens for treatment of low-grade gliomas in young children: a report from the Children's Oncology Group. *J Clin Oncol.* 2012;30:2641–2647.

Avery RA, Hwang EI, Jakacki RI, et al. Marked recovery of vision in children with optic pathway gliomas treated with bevacizumab. *JAMA Ophthalmol.* 2014;132:111–114.

Benesch M, Eder HG, Sovinz P, et al. Residual or recurrent low-grade glioma in children after tumor resection: is re-treatment needed? A single center experience from 1983 to 2003. *Pediatr Neurosurg.* 2006;42:159–164.

Bouffet E, Jakacki R, Goldman S, et al. Phase II study of weekly vinblastine in recurrent or refractory pediatric low-grade glioma. *J Clin Oncol.* 2012;30:1358–1363.

Bowers DC, Gargan L, Kapur P, et al. Study of the MIB-1 labeling index as a predictor of tumor progression in pilocytic astrocytomas in children and adolescents. *J Clin Oncol.* 2003;21:2968–2973.

Bowers DC, Krause TP, Aronson LJ, et al. Second surgery for recurrent pilocytic astrocytoma in children. *Pediatr Neurosurg.* 2001;34:229–234.

Bredel M, Pollack IF, Hamilton RL, et al. Epidermal growth factor receptor expression and gene amplification in high-grade non-brainstem gliomas of childhood. *Clin Cancer Res.* 1999;5:1786–1792.

Bronisder A, Laningham FH, Sanders RP, et al. Young age may predict a better outcome for children with diffuse pontine glioma. *Cancer.* 2008;113(3):566–572.

Cohen KJ, Pollack IF, Zhou T, et al. Temozolomide in the treatment of high-grade gliomas in children: a report from the Children's Oncology Group. *Neuro Oncol.* 2011;13:317–323.

Daglioglu E, Cataltepe O, Akalan N. Tectal gliomas in children: the implications for natural history and management strategy. *Pediatr Neurosurg.* 2003;38:223–231.

Finlay JL, Boyett JM, Yates AJ, et al. Randomized phase III trial in childhood high-grade astrocytoma comparing vincristine, lomustine, and prednisone with the eight-drugs-in-1-day regimen. *J Clin Oncol.* 1995;13:112–123.

Finlay JL, Dhall G, Boyett JM, et al. Myeloablative chemotherapy with autologous bone marrow rescue in children and adolescents with recurrent malignant astrocytoma: outcome compared with conventional chemotherapy: a report from the Children's Oncology Group. *Pediatr Blood Cancer.* 2008;51:806–811.

Fisher PG, Tihan T, Goldthwaite PT, et al. Outcome analysis of childhood low-grade astrocytomas. *Pediatr Blood Cancer.* 2008;51:245–250.

Gajjar A, Heideman RL, Kovnar EH, et al. Response of pediatric low-grade gliomas to chemotherapy. *Pediatr Neurosurg.* 1993;19:113–120.

Gesundheit B, Klement G, Senger C, et al. Differences in vasculature between pilocytic and anaplastic astrocytomas of childhood. *Med Pediatr Oncol.* 2003;41:516–526.

Gnekow AK, Kortmann RD, Pietsch T, et al. Low grade chiasmatic-hypothalamic glioma—carboplatin and vincristine chemotherapy effectively defers radiotherapy within a comprehensive treatment strategy—report from the multicenter treatment study for children and adolescents with a low grade glioma—HIT-LGG 1996—of the Society of Pediatric Oncology and Hematology (GPOH). *Klin Padiatr.* 2004;216:331–342.

Gropman AL, Packer RJ, Nicholson HS, et al. Treatment of diencephalic syndrome with chemotherapy: growth, tumor response, and long term control. *Cancer.* 1998;83:166–172.

Gururangan S, Fangusaro J, Poussaint TY, et al. Efficacy of bevacizumab plus irinotecan in children with recurrent low-grade gliomas—a Pediatric Brain Tumor Consortium study. *Neuro Oncol.* 2014;16:310–317.

Hargrave D, Bartels U, Bouffet E. Diffuse brainstem glioma in children: critical review of clinical trials. *Lancet Oncology.* 2006;7:241–248.

Hayward RM, Patronas N, Baker EH, et al. Inter-observer variability in the measurement of diffuse intrinsic pontine gliomas. *J Neurooncol.* 2008;90(1):57–61.

Heidemen RL, Kuttesch J Jr, Gajjar AJ, et al. Supratentorial malignant gliomas in childhood. A single institution perspective. *Cancer.* 1997;80:497–504.

Huang EI, Jakacki RI, Fisher MJ, et al. Long-term efficacy and toxicity of bevacizumab-based therapy in children with recurrent low-grade glioma. *Pediatr Blood Cancer.* 2013;60:776–781.

Jallo GI, Biser-Rohrbaugh A, Freed D. Brainstem gliomas. *Childs Nerv Syst.* 2004;20:143–153.

Jallo GI, Freed D, Epstein F. Intramedullary spinal cord tumors in children. *Childs Nerv Syst.* 2003;19:641–649.

Jansen MH, Veidhuijzen van Zanter SE, Sanchez Aliaga E, et al. Survival prediction model of children with diffuse intrinsic pontine glioma based on clinical and radiological criteria. *Neuro Oncol.* 2014;17(1):160–166.

Janss AJ, Grundy R, Cnaan A, et al. Optic pathway and hypothalamic/chiasmatic gliomas in children younger than age 5 years with a 6-year follow-up. *Cancer.* 1995;75:1051–1059.

Jennings MT, Sposto R, Boyett JM, et al. Preradiation chemotherapy in primary high-risk brainstem tumors: phase II study CCG-9941 of the Children's Cancer Group. *J Clin Oncol.* 2002;20:3431–3437.

Karajannis MA, Legault G, Fisher MJ, et al. Phase II study of sorafenib in children with recurrent or progressive low-grade astrocytomas. *Neuro Oncol.* 2014;16(10):1408–1416.

Khatua S, Peterson KM, Brown KM, et al. Overexpression of the EGFR/FKBP12/ HIF-2alpha pathway identified in childhood astrocytomas by angiogenesis gene profiling. *Cancer Res.* 2003;63:1865–1870.

Komotar RJ, Burger PC, Carson BS, et al. Pilocytic and pilomyxoid hypothalamic/ chiasmatic astrocytomas. *Neurosurgery.* 2004;54:72–79.

Krueger DA, Care MM, Holland K, et al. Everolimus for subependymal giant-cell astrocytomas in tuberous sclerosis. *N Engl J Med.* 2010;363:1801–1811.

Laithier V, Grill J, Le Deley M-C, et al. Progression-free survival in children with optic pathway tumors: dependence on age and the quality of the response to chemotherapy—results of the first French prospective study for the French Society of Pediatric Oncology. *J Clin Oncol.* 2003;21: 4572–4578.

Lashford LS, Thiesse P, Jouvet A, et al. Temozolomide in malignant gliomas of childhood: a United Kingdom Children's Cancer Study Group and French Society for Pediatric Oncology Intergroup Study. *J Clin Oncol.* 2002;20:4684–4691.

Lewis J, Lucraft H, Gholkar A. UKCCSG study of accelerated radiotherapy for pediatric brain stem gliomas. United Kingdom Childhood Cancer Study Group. *Int J Radiat Oncol Biol Phys.* 1997;38:925–929.

Listernick R, Louis DN, Packer RJ, et al. Optic pathway gliomas in children with neurofibromatosis 1: consensus statement from the NF1 Optic Pathway Glioma Task Force. *Ann Neuro.* 1997;41:143–149.

Lowis SP, Pizer BL, Coakham H, et al. Chemotherapy for spinal cord astrocytoma: can natural history be modified? *Childs Nerv Syst.* 1998;14:317–321.

Martinez-Lage JF, Perez-Espejo MA, Esteban JA, et al. Thalamic tumors: clinical presentation. *Childs Nerv Syst.* 2002;18:405–411.

Massimino M, Spreafico F, Cefalo G, et al. High response rate to cisplatin/ etoposide regimen in childhood low-grade glioma. *J Clin Oncol.* 2002;20:4209–4216.

Packer RJ, Boyett JM, Zimmerman RA, et al. Hyperfractionated radiation therapy (72 Gy) for children with brain stem gliomas: a Children's Cancer Group phase I/II trial. *Cancer.* 1993;72:1414–1421.

Packer RJ, Prados M, Phillips P, et al. Treatment of children with newly diagnosed brain stem gliomas with intravenous recombinant beta-interferon and hyperfractionated radiation therapy: a Children's Cancer Group phase I/II study. *Cancer.* 1996;77:2150–2152.

Pencalat P, Maixner W, Sainte-Rose C, et al. Benign cerebellar astrocytomas in children. *J Neurosurg.* 1999;90:265–273.

Pollack IF, Finkelstein SD, Woods J, et al. Expression of p53 and prognosis in children with malignant gliomas. *N Engl J Med.* 2002;346:420–427.

Pollack IF, Hamilton RL, Burnham J, et al. Impact of proliferation index on outcome in childhood malignant gliomas: results in a multi-institutional cohort. *Neurosurgery*. 2002;50:1238–1244.

Pollack IF, Hamilton RL, Sobol RW, et al. O⁶-methylguanine-DNA methyltransferase expression strongly correlates with outcome in childhood malignant gliomas: results from the CCG-945 cohort. *J Clin Oncol*. 2006;24: 3431–3437.

Reardon DA, Gajjar A, Sanford RA, et al. Bithalamic involvement predicts poor outcome among children with thalamic glial tumors. *Pediatr Neurosurg*. 1998;29:29–35.

Sanghavi SN, Needle MN, Krailo MD, et al. A phase I study of topotecan as a radiosensitizer for brainstem glioma of childhood: first report of the Children's Cancer Group-0952. *Neuro Oncol*. 2003;5:8–13.

Saran FH, Baumert BG, Khoo VS, et al. Stereotactically guided conformal radiotherapy for progressive low-grade gliomas of childhood. *Int J Radiat Oncol Biol Phys*. 2002;53:43–51.

Schmandt SM, Packer RJ, Vezina LG, et al. Spontaneous regression of low-grade astrocytomas in childhood. *Pediatr Neurosurg*. 2000;32:132–136.

Sposto R, Ertel IH, Jenkin RD, et al. The effectiveness of chemotherapy for treatment of high grade astrocytoma in children: results of a randomized trial. A report from the Children's Cancer Study Group. *J Neurooncol*. 1989;7:165–177.

Tao ML, Barnes PD, Billett AL, et al. Childhood optic chiasm gliomas: radiographic response following radiotherapy and long-term clinical outcome. *Int J Radiat Oncol Biol Phys*. 1997;39:579–587.

Thorarinsdottir HK, Santi M, McCarter R, et al. Protein expression of platelet-derived growth factor receptor correlates with malignant histology and PTEN with survival in childhood gliomas. *Clin Cancer Res*. 2008;14:3386–3394.

Warren KE, Goldman S, Pollack IF, et al. Phase I trial of lenalidomide in pediatric patients with recurrent, refractory, or progressive primary CNS tumors: Pediatric Brain Tumor Consortium study PBTC-018. *J Clin Oncol*. 2011;29:324–329.

Wisoff JH, Boyett JM, Berger MS, et al. Current neurosurgical management and the impact of the extent of resection in the treatment of malignant gliomas of childhood: a report of the Children's Cancer Group Trial No. CCG-945. *J Neurosurg*. 1998;89:52–59.

Wisoff JH, Sanford RA, Heier LA, et al. Primary neurosurgery for pediatric low-grade gliomas: a prospective multi-institutional study from the Children's Oncology Group. *Neurosurgery*. 2011;68:1548–1555.

Wolff JE, Driever PH, Erdlenbruch B, et al. Intensive chemotherapy improves survival in pediatric high-grade glioma after gross total resection: results of the HIT-GBM-C protocol. *Cancer*. 2010;116:705–712.

Wolff JE, Gnekow AK, Kortmann RD, et al. Preradiation chemotherapy for pediatric patients with high-grade glioma. *Cancer*. 2002;94:264–271.

Embryonal Tumors: Medulloblastomas, Primitive Neuroectodermal Tumors, and Atypical Teratoid/Rhabdoid Tumors

Aldosari N, Bigner SH, Burger PC, et al. MYCC and MYCN oncogene amplification in medulloblastoma. A fluorescence in situ hybridization study on paraffin sections from the Children's Oncology Group. *Arch Pathol Lab Med*. 2002;126:540–544.

Bergthold G, El Kababri M, Varlet P, et al. High-dose busulfan-thiotepa with autologous stem cell transplantation followed by posterior fossa irradiation in young children with classical or incompletely resected medulloblastoma. *Pediatr Blood Cancer*. 2014;61:907–912.

Biegel JA, Janss AJ, Raffel C, et al. Prognostic significance of chromosome 17p deletions in childhood primitive neuroectodermal tumors (medulloblastomas) of the central nervous system. *Clin Cancer Res*. 1997;3:473–478.

Biegel JA, Kalpana G, Knudsen ES, et al. The role of INI1 and the SWI/SNF complex in the development of rhabdoid tumors: meeting summary from the workshop on childhood atypical teratoid/rhabdoid tumors. *Cancer Res*. 2002;62:323–328.

Burger PC, Yu IT, Tihan T, et al. Atypical teratoid/rhabdoid tumor of the central nervous system: a highly malignant tumor of infancy and childhood frequently mistaken for medulloblastoma. A Pediatric Oncology Group study. *Am J Surg Pathol*. 1998;22:1083–1092.

Butturini AM, Jacob M, Aquajo J, et al. High-dose chemotherapy and autologous hematopoietic progenitor cell rescue in children with recurrent medulloblastoma and supratentorial primitive neuroectodermal tumors. *Cancer*. 2009;115(13):2956–2963.

Chi SN, Gardner SL, Levy AS, et al. Feasibility and response to induction chemotherapy intensified with high-dose methotrexate for young children with newly diagnosed high-risk disseminated medulloblastoma. *J Clin Oncol*. 2004;22:4881–4887.

Chi SN, Zimmerman MA, Yao X, et al. Intensive multimodality treatment for children with newly diagnosed CNS atypical teratoid rhabdoid tumor. *J Clin Oncol*. 2009;27:385–389.

Cogen PH, Daneshvar L, Metzger AK, et al. Deletion mapping of the medulloblastoma locus on chromosome 17p. *Genomics*. 1990;8:279–285.

Cohen BH, Zeltzer PM, Boyett JM, et al. Prognostic factors and treatment results for supratentorial primitive neuroectodermal tumors in children using radiation and chemotherapy: a Children's Cancer Group randomized trial. *J Clin Oncol*. 1995;13:1687–1696.

Dufour C, Kieffer V, Varlet P, et al. Tandem high-dose chemotherapy and autologous stem cell rescue in children with newly diagnosed high-risk medulloblastoma or supratentorial primitive neuro-ectodermic tumors. *Pediatr Blood Cancer*. 2014;61(8):1398–1402.

Dunkel IJ, Gardner SL, Garvin JH Jr, et al. High-dose carboplatin, thiotepa, and etoposide with autologous stem cell rescue for patients with previously irradiated recurrent medulloblastoma. *Neuro Oncol*. 2010;12:297–303.

Eberhart CG, Kepner JL, Goldthwaite PT, et al. Histopathologic grading of medulloblastomas: a Pediatric Oncology Group study. *Cancer*. 2002;94: 552–560.

Ellison DW, Dalton J, Kocak M, et al. Medulloblastoma: clinicopathological correlates of SHH, WNT, and non-SHH/WNT molecular subgroups. *Acta Neuropathol*. 2011;121:381–396.

Evans AE, Jenkin RDT, Sposto R, et al. The treatment of medulloblastoma. Results of a prospective randomized trial of radiation therapy with and without CCNU, vincristine, and prednisone. *J Neurosurg*. 1990;72:572–582.

Fangusaro J, Finlay J, Sposto R, et al. Intensive chemotherapy followed by consolidative myeloablative chemotherapy with autologous hematopoietic cell rescue (AuHCR) in young children with newly diagnosed supratentorial primitive neuroectodermal tumors (sPNETs): report of the Head Start I and II experience. *Pediatr Blood Cancer*. 2008;50:312–318.

Gajjar A, Chintagumpala M, Ashley D, et al. Risk-adapted craniospinal radiation therapy followed by high-dose chemotherapy and stem-cell rescue in children with newly diagnosed medulloblastoma (St Jude Medulloblastoma-96): long-term results from a prospective, multicentre trial. *Lancet Oncol*. 2006;7:813–820.

Gajjar A, Hernan R, Kocak M, et al. Clinical, histopathologic, and molecular markers of prognosis: toward a new disease risk stratification system for medulloblastoma. *J Clin Oncol*. 2004;22:984–993.

Gajjar A, Stewart CF, Ellison DW, et al. Phase I study of vismodegib in children with recurrent or refractory medulloblastoma: a pediatric brain tumor consortium study. *Clin Cancer Res*. 2013;19:6305–6312.

Gerber NU, von Hoff K, Resch A, et al. Treatment of children with central nervous system primitive neuroectodermal tumors/pinealoblastomas in the prospective multicentric trial HIP 2000 using hyperfractionated radiation therapy followed by maintenance chemotherapy. *Int J Radiat Oncol Biol Phys*. 2014;89:863–871.

Gerber NU, von Hoff K, von Bueren AO, et al. Outcome of 11 children with ependymoblastoma treated within the prospective HIT-trials between 1991 and 2006. *J Neurooncol*. 2011;102:459–469.

Geyer JR, Sposto R, Jennings M, et al. Multiagent chemotherapy and deferred radiotherapy in infants with malignant brain tumors: a report from the Children's Cancer Group. *J Clin Oncol*. 2005;23:7621–7631.

Gibson P, Tong Y, Robinson G, et al. Subtypes of medulloblastoma have distinct developmental origins. *Nature*. 2010;468:1095–1099.

Gilheeney SW, Saad A, Chi S, et al. Outcome of pediatric pineoblastoma after surgery, radiation and chemotherapy. *J Neurooncol*. 2008;89:89–95.

Goldwein JW, Radcliffe J, Packer RJ, et al. Results of a pilot study of low-dose craniospinal radiation therapy plus chemotherapy for children younger than 5 years with primitive neuroectodermal tumors. *Cancer*. 1993;71:2647–2652.

Grill J, Lellouch-Tubiana A, Elouahdani S, et al. Preoperative chemotherapy in children with high-risk medulloblastomas: a feasibility study. *J Neurosurg*. 2005;103:312–318.

Grill J, Sainte-Rose C, Jouver A, et al. Treatment of medulloblastoma with post-operative chemotherapy alone: an SFOP prospective trial in young children. *Lancet Oncol.* 2005;6:573–580.

Grotzer MA, Hogarty MD, Janss AJ, et al. MYC messenger RNA expression predicts survival outcome in childhood primitive neuroectodermal tumor/medulloblastoma. *Clin Cancer Res.* 2001;7:2425–2433.

Grotzer MA, Janss AJ, Phillips PC, et al. Neurotrophin receptor Trk C predicts good clinical outcome in medulloblastoma and other primitive neuroectodermal brain tumors. *Klin Padiatr.* 2000;212:196–199.

Hilden JM, Meerbaum S, Burger P, et al. Central nervous system atypical teratoid/rhabdoid tumor: results of therapy in children enrolled in a registry. *J Clin Oncol.* 2004;22:2877–2884.

Horvestadt V, Jones DT, Picelli S, et al. Decoding the regulatory landscape of medulloblastoma using DNA methylation sequencing. *Nature.* 2014;510:537–541.

Jakacki RI, Zeltzer PM, Boyett JM, et al. Survival and prognostic factors following radiation and/or chemotherapy for primitive neuroectodermal tumors of the pineal region in infants and children: a report of the Children's Cancer Group. *J Clin Oncol.* 1995;13:1377–1383.

Jones DT, Jager N, Kool M, et al. Dissecting the genomic complexity underlying medulloblastoma. *Nature.* 2012;488:100–105.

Komori T, Scheithauer BW, Anthony DC, et al. Papillary glioneuronal tumor: a new variant of mixed neuronal-glial neoplasm. *Am J Surg Pathol.* 1998;22:1171–1183.

Korshunov A, Sturn D, Ryzhova M, et al. Embryonal tumor with abundant neuropil and true rosettes (ETANTR), ependymoblastoma, and medulloepithelioma share molecular similarity and comprise a single clinicopathological entity. *Acta Neuropathol.* 2014;128(2):279–289.

Kortmann RD, Kuhl J, Timmermann B, et al. Postoperative neoadjuvant chemotherapy before radiotherapy as compared to immediate radiotherapy followed by maintenance chemotherapy in the treatment of medulloblastoma in childhood: results of the German prospective randomized trial HIT 91. *Int J Radiat Oncol Biol Phys.* 2000;46:269–279.

Li M, Lee KE, Lu Y, et al. Frequent amplification of a chr19q13.41 microRNA polycistron in aggressive primitive neuroectodermal brain tumors. *Cancer Cell.* 2009;16:533–546.

Lusher ME, Lindsey JC, Latif F, et al. Biallelic epigenetic inactivation of the RASSF1A tumor suppressor gene in medulloblastoma development. *Cancer Res.* 2002;62:5906–5911.

McNeil DE, Cote TR, Clegg L, et al. Incidence trends in pediatric malignancies medulloblastoma/primitive neuroectodermal tumor: a SEER update. Surveillance Epidemiology and End Results. *Med Pediatr Oncol.* 2002;39:190–194.

Michaels EM, Weiss MM, Hoovers JM, et al. Genetic alterations in childhood medulloblastoma analyzed by comparative genomic hybridization. *J Pediatr Hematol Oncol.* 2002;24:205–210.

Miller S, Rogers HA, Lyon P, et al. Genome-wide molecular characterization of central nervous system primitive neuroectodermal tumor and pineoblastoma. *Neuro Oncol.* 2011;13:866–879.

Morfouace M, Shelat A, Jacus M, et al. Pemetrexed and gemcitabine as combination therapy for the treatment of group 3 medulloblastoma. *Cancer Cell.* 2014;25:1–14.

Needle MN, Molloy PT, Geyer JR, et al. Phase II study of daily oral etoposide in children with recurrent brain tumors and other solid tumors. *Med Pediatr Oncol.* 1997;29:28–32.

Nicholson HS, Kretschmar CS, Krailo M, et al. Phase 2 study of temozolomide in children and adolescents with recurrent central nervous system tumors: a report from the Children's Oncology Group. *Cancer.* 2007;110:1542–1550.

Northcott PA, Lee C, Zichner T, et al. Enhancer hijacking activates GFI1 family oncogenes in medulloblastoma. *Nature.* 2014;511:428–434.

Northcott PA, Shih DJ, Peacock J, et al. Subgroup-specific structural variation across 1,000 medulloblastoma genomes. *Nature.* 2012;488:49–56.

Northcott PA, Shih DJ, Remke M, et al. Rapid, reliable, and reproducible molecular sub-grouping of clinical medulloblastoma samples. *Acta Neuropathol.* 2012;123:615–626.

Oyharcabal-Bourden V, Kalifa C, Gentet JC, et al. Standard-risk medulloblastoma treated by adjuvant chemotherapy followed by reduced-dose craniospinal radiation therapy: a French Society of Pediatric Oncology Study. *J Clin Oncol.* 2005;23:4726–4734.

Packer RJ, Biegel JA, Blaney S, et al. Atypical teratoid/rhabdoid tumor of the central nervous system: report on workshop. *J Pediatr Hematol Oncol.* 2002;24:337–342.

Packer RJ, Gajjar A, Vezina G, et al. Phase III study of craniospinal radiation therapy followed by adjuvant chemotherapy for newly diagnosed average-risk medulloblastoma. *J Clin Oncol.* 2006;24:4202–4208.

Packer RJ, Goldwein J, Nicholson HS, et al. Treatment of children with medulloblastomas with reduced-dose craniospinal radiation therapy and adjuvant chemotherapy: a Children's Cancer Group Study. *J Clin Oncol.* 1999;17:2127–2136.

Packer RJ, Sutton LN, Elterman R, et al. Outcome for children with medulloblastoma treated with radiation and cisplatin, CCNU, and vincristine chemotherapy. *J Neurosurg.* 1994;81:690–698.

Picard D, Miller S, Hawkins CE, et al. Markers of survival and metastatic potential in childhood CNS primitive neuro-ectodermal brain tumours: an integrative genomic analysis. *Lancet Oncol.* 2012;13:836–848.

Pigott TJ, Punt JA, Lowe JS, et al. The clinical, radiological and histopathological features of cerebral primitive neuroectodermal tumours. *Br J Neurosurg.* 1990;4:287–297.

Pomeroy SL, Tamayo P, Gaasenbeek M, et al. Prediction of central nervous system embryonal tumour outcome based on gene expression. *Nature.* 2002;415:436–442.

Pugh TJ, Weeraratne SD, Archer TC, et al. Medulloblastoma exome sequencing uncovers subtype-specific somatic mutations. *Nature.* 2012;488:106–110.

Ramaswamy V, Remke M, Bouffet E, et al. Recurrence patterns across medulloblastoma subgroups: an integrated clinical and molecular analysis. *Lancet Oncol.* 2013;14:1200–1027.

Reddy AT, Janss AJ, Phillips PC, et al. Outcome for children with supratentorial primitive neuroectodermal tumors treated with surgery, radiation, and chemotherapy. *Cancer.* 2000;88:2189–2193.

Rickert CH, Paulus W. Chromosomal imbalances detected by comparative genomic hybridization in atypical teratoid/rhabdoid tumours. *Childs Nerv Syst.* 2004;20:221–224.

Rudin CM, Hann CL, Laterra J, et al. Treatment of medulloblastoma with hedgehog pathway inhibitor GDC-0449. *New Engl J Med.* 2009;361:1173–1178.

Rutkowski S, Bode U, Deinlein F, et al. Treatment of early childhood medulloblastoma by postoperative chemotherapy alone. *N Engl J Med.* 2005;352:978–986.

Rutkowski S, von Hoff K, Emser A, et al. Survival and prognostic factors of early childhood medulloblastoma: an international meta-analysis. *J Clin Oncol.* 2010;28:4961–4968.

Schabet M, Martos J, Buchholz R, et al. Animal model of human medulloblastoma: clinical, magnetic resonance imaging, and histopathological findings after intra-cisternal injection of MHH-MED-1 cells into nude rats. *Med Pediatr Oncol.* 1997;29:92–97.

Shih DJ, Northcott PA, Remke M, et al. Cytogenetic prognostication within medulloblastoma subgroups. *J Clin Oncol.* 2014;32:886–896.

Sutton LN, Phillips PC, Molloy PT. Surgical management of medulloblastoma. *J Neuro Oncol.* 1996;29:9–21.

Tait DM, Thornton-Jones H, Bloom HJ, et al. Adjuvant chemotherapy for medulloblastoma: the first multi-centre control trial of the International Society of Pediatric Oncology (SIOP I). *Eur J Cancer.* 1990;26:464–469.

Taylor MD, Northcott PA, Korshunov A, et al. Molecular subgroups of medulloblastoma: the current consensus. *Acta Neuropathol.* 2012;123:465–472.

Thomas PR, Deutsch M, Kepner JL, et al. Low-stage medulloblastoma: final analysis of trial comparing standard-dose with reduced-dose neuraxis irradiation. *J Clin Oncol.* 2000;18:3004–3011.

Timmermann B, Kortmann RD, Kuhl J, et al. Role of radiotherapy in the treatment of supratentorial primitive neuroectodermal tumors in childhood: results of the prospective German brain tumor trials HIT 88/89 and 91. *J Clin Oncol.* 2002;20:842–849.

Vincent S, Dhellemmes P, Maurage CA, et al. Intracerebral medulloepithelioma with a long survival. *Clin Neuropathol.* 2002;21:197–205.

Von Bueren AO, von Hoff K, Pietsch T, et al. Treatment of young children with localized medulloblastoma by chemotherapy alone: results of the prospective, multicenter trial HIT 2000 confirming the prognostic impact of histology. *Neuro Oncol.* 2011;13:669–679.

Weil MD, Lamborn K, Edwards MS, et al. Influence of a child's sex on medulloblastoma outcome. *JAMA.* 1998;279:1474–1476.

Weiner HL, Bakst R, Hurlbert MS, et al. Induction of medulloblastomas in mice by sonic hedgehog, independent of Gli1. *Cancer Res.* 2002;62:6385–6389.

Zaky W, Dhall G, Ji L, et al. Intensive induction chemotherapy followed by myeloablative chemotherapy with autologous hematopoietic progenitor cell rescue for young children newly-diagnosed with central nervous system atypical teratoid/rhabdoid tumors: the Head Start III experience. *Pediatr Blood Cancer.* 2014;61:95–101.

Ependymomas

Atkinson JM, Shelat AA, Carcaboso AM, et al. An integrated in vitro and in vivo high-throughput screen identifies treatment leads for ependymoma. *Cancer Cell.* 2011;20:384–399.

Duffner PK, Horowitz ME, Krischer JP, et al. Postoperative chemotherapy and delayed radiation in children less than three years of age with malignant brain tumors. *N Engl J Med.* 1993;328:1725–1731.

Garvin JH Jr, Selch MT, Holmes E, et al. Phase II study of pre-irradiation chemotherapy for childhood intracranial ependymoma. Children's Cancer Group protocol 9942: a report from the Children's Oncology Group. *Pediatr Blood Cancer.* 2012;59:1183–1189.

Gilbertson RJ, Bentley L, Hernan R, et al. ERBB receptor signaling promotes ependymoma cell proliferation and represents a potential novel therapeutic target for this disease. *Clin Cancer Res.* 2002;8:3054–3064.

Good CD, Wade AM, Hayward RD, et al. Surveillance neuroimaging in childhood intracranial ependymomas: how effective, how often, and for how long? *J Neurosurg.* 2001;94:27–32.

Granzow M, Popp S, Weber S, et al. Isochromosome 1q as an early genetic event in a child with intracranial ependymoma characterized by molecular cytogenetics. *Cancer Genet Cytogenet.* 2001;130:79–83.

Grundy RG, Wilne SA, Weston CL, et al. Primary postoperative chemotherapy without radiotherapy for intracranial ependymoma in children: the UKCCSG/SIOP prospective study. *Lancet Oncol.* 2007;8:696–705.

Horn B, Heideman R, Geyer R, et al. A multi-institutional retrospective study of intracranial ependymoma in children: identification of risk factors. *J Pediatr Hematol Oncol.* 1999;21:203–211.

Johnson RA, Wright KD, Poppleton H, et al. Cross-species genomics matches driver mutations and cell compartments to model ependymoma. *Nature.* 2010;466:632–636.

Korshunov A, Golanov A, Sycheva R, et al. The histologic grade is a main prognostic factor for patients with intracranial ependymomas treated in the microneurosurgical era: an analysis of 258 patients. *Cancer.* 2004;100:1230–1237.

Kramer DL, Parmiter AH, Rorke LB, et al. Molecular cytogenetic studies of pediatric ependymomas. *J Neurooncol.* 1998;37:25–33.

Merchant TE, Mulhern RK, Krasin MJ, et al. Preliminary results from a phase II trial of conformal radiation therapy and evaluation of radiation-related CNS effects for pediatric patients with localized ependymoma. *J Clin Oncol.* 2004;22:3156–3162.

Modena P, Buttarelli FR, Miceli R, et al. Predictors of outcome in an AIEOP series of childhood ependymomas: a multifactorial analysis. *Neuro Oncol.* 2012;14:1346–1356.

Needle MN, Goldwein JW, Grass J, et al. Adjuvant chemotherapy for the treatment of intracranial ependymoma of childhood. *Cancer.* 1997;80:341–347.

Strother DR, Lafay-Cousin L, Boyett JM, et al. Benefit from prolonged dose-intensive chemotherapy for infants with malignant brain tumors is restricted to patients with ependymoma: a report of the Pediatric Oncology Group randomized controlled trial 9233/34. *Neuro Oncol.* 2013;16(3):457–465.

Sutton LN, Goldwein J, Perilongo G, et al. Prognostic factors in childhood ependymomas. *Pediatr Neurosurg.* 1990;16:57–65.

Tabori U, Ma J, Carter M, et al. Human telomere reverse transcriptase expression predicts progression and survival in pediatric intracranial ependymoma. *J Clin Oncol.* 2006;24:1522–1528.

Taylor MD, Poppleton H, Fuller C, et al. Radial glia cells are candidate stem cells of ependymoma. *Cancer Cell.* 2005;8:323–335.

Timmermann B, Kortmann RD, Kuhl J, et al. Combined postoperative irradiation and chemotherapy for anaplastic ependymomas in childhood: results of the German prospective trials HIT 88/89 and HIT 91. *Int J Radiat Oncol Biol Phys.* 2000;46:287–295.

Van Veelen-Vincent ML, Pierre-Kahn A, Kalifa C, et al. Ependymoma in childhood: prognostic factors, extent of surgery, and adjuvant therapy. *J Neurosurg.* 2002;97:827–835.

Witt H, Mack SC, Ryzhova M, et al. Delineation of two clinically and molecularly distinct subgroups of posterior fossa ependymoma. *Cancer Cell.* 2011;20:143–157.

Zacharoulis S, Ashley S, Moreno L, et al. Treatment and outcome of children with relapsed ependymoma: a multi-institutional retrospective analysis. *Childs Nerv Syst.* 2010;26:905–911.

Germ Cell Tumors

Benesch M, Lackner H, Schagerl S, et al. Tumor- and treatment-related side effects after multimodal therapy of childhood intracranial germ cell tumors. *Acta Paediatr.* 2001;90:264–270.

Caliminus G, Kortmann R, Worch J, et al. SIOP CNS GCT 96: final report of outcome of a prospective, multinational nonrandomized trial for children and adults with intracranial germinoma, comparing craniospinal irradiation alone with chemotherapy followed by focal primary site irradiation for patients with localized disease. *Neuro Oncol.* 2013;15:788–796.

Drummond KJ, Rosenfeld JV. Pineal region tumours in childhood. A 30-year experience. *Childs Nerv Syst.* 1999;15:119–126.

Echevarria ME, Fangusaro J, Goldman S. Pediatric central nervous system germ cell tumors: a review. *Oncologist.* 2008;13:690–699.

Kellie SJ, Boyce H, Dunkel IJ, et al. Primary chemotherapy for intracranial non-germinomatous germ cell tumors: results of the second international CNS germ cell study group protocol. *J Clin Oncol.* 2004;22:846–853.

Kretschmar C, Kleinberg L, Greenberg M, et al. Pre-radiation chemotherapy with response-based radiation therapy in children with central nervous system germ cell tumors: a report from the Children's Oncology Group. *Pediatr Blood Cancer.* 2007;48:285–291.

Modak S, Gardner S, Dunkel IJ, et al. Thiotepa-based high-dose chemotherapy with autologous stem-cell rescue in patients with recurrent or progressive CNS germ cell tumors. *J Clin Oncol.* 2004;22:1934–1943.

Roberge D, Kun LE, Freeman CR. Intracranial germinoma: on whole ventricular irradiation. *Pediatr Blood Cancer.* 2005;44:358–362.

Schneder DT, Zahn S, Sievers S, et al. Molecular genetic analysis of central nervous system germ cell tumors with comparative genomic hybridization. *Mol Pathol.* 2006;19:864–873.

Lymphomas

Abla O, Sandlund JT, Sung L, et al. A case series of pediatric primary central nervous system lymphoma: favorable outcome without cranial irradiation. *Pediatr Blood Cancer.* 2006;47:880–885.

Cheng AL, Yeh KH, Uen WC, et al. Systemic chemotherapy alone for patients with non-acquired immunodeficiency syndrome-related central nervous system lymphoma. A pilot study of the BOMES protocol. *Cancer.* 1998;82:1946–1951.

DeAngelis LM. Primary central nervous system lymphomas. *Curr Treat Options Oncol.* 2001;2:309–318.

DeAngelis LM, Seiferheld W, Schold SC, et al. Combination chemotherapy and radiotherapy for primary central nervous system lymphoma: Radiation Therapy Oncology Group Study 93-10. *J Clin Oncol.* 2002;20:4643–4648.

DeAngelis LM, Yahalom J, Thaler HT, et al. Combined modality therapy for primary CNS lymphoma. *J Clin Oncol.* 1992;10:635–643.

Mohile NA, DeAngelis LM, Abrey LE. The utility of body FDG PET in staging primary central nervous system lymphoma. *Neuro Oncol.* 2008;10:223–228.

Silfen ME, Garvin JH Jr, Hays AP, et al. Primary central nervous system lymphoma in childhood presenting as progressive panhypopituitarism. *J Pediatr Hematol Oncol.* 2001;23:130–133.

Meningiomas and Mesenchymal Tumors

Amirjamshidi A, Mehrazin M, Abbassioun K. Meningiomas of the central nervous system occurring below the age of 17: report of 24 cases not associated with neurofibromatosis and review of the literature. *Childs Nerv Syst.* 2000;16:406–416.

Erdincler P, Lena G, Sarioglu AC, et al. Intracranial meningiomas in children: review of 29 cases. *Surg Neurol.* 1998;49:136–140.

Greenberg SB, Schneck MJ, Faerber EN, et al. Malignant meningioma in a child: CT and MR findings. *Am J Radiol.* 1993;160:1111–1112.

Liu Y, Li F, Zhu S, et al. Clinical features and treatment of meningiomas in children: report of 12 cases and literature review. *Pediatr Neurosurg.* 2008;44:112–117.

Pedersen M, Küsters-Vandevelde HV, Viros A, et al. Primary melanoma of the CNS in children is driven by congenital expression of oncogenic NRAS in melanocytes. *Cancer Discov.* 2013;3:458–459.

Perry A, Giannini C, Raghavan R, et al. Aggressive phenotypic and genotypic features in pediatric and NF2-associated meningiomas: a clinicopathologic study of 53 cases. *J Neuropathol Exp Neurol.* 2001;60:994–1003.

Schiariti M, Goetz P, El-Maghraby H, et al. Hemangiopericytoma: long-term outcome revisited. Clinical article. *J Neurosurg.* 2011;114:747–755.

Somers KE, Almast J, Biemiller RA, et al. Diagnosis of primary CNS melanoma with neuroimaging. *J Clin Oncol.* 2013;e9–e11.

Late Effects of Treatment and Quality of Life

Andersen PB, Krabbe K, Leffers AM, et al. Cerebral glucose metabolism in long-term survivors of childhood primary brain tumors treated with surgery and radiotherapy. *J Neurooncol.* 2003;62:305–313.

Bandopadhayay P, Bergthold G, London WB, et al. Long-term outcome of 4,040 children diagnosed with pediatric low-grade gliomas: an analysis of the Surveillance Epidemiology and End Results (SEER) database. *Pediatr Blood Cancer.* 2014;61:1173–1179.

Barr RD, Simpson T, Webber CE, et al. Osteopenia in children surviving brain tumors. *Eur J Cancer.* 1998;34:873–877.

Barr RD, Simpson T, Whitton A, et al. Health-related quality of life in survivors of tumours of the central nervous system in childhood—a preference-based approach to measurement in a cross-sectional study. *Eur J Cancer.* 1999;35:248–255.

Bell J, Parker KL, Swinford RD, et al. Long-term safety of recombinant human growth hormone in children. *J Clin Endocrinol Metab.* 2010;95:167–177.

Bhat SR, Goodwin TL, Burwinkle TM, et al. Profile of daily life in children with brain tumors: an assessment of health-related quality of life. *J Clin Oncol.* 2005;23:5493–5500.

Brière ME, Scott JG, McNall-Knapp RY, et al. Cognitive outcome in pediatric tumor survivors: delayed attention deficit at long-term follow-up. *Pediatr Blood Cancer.* 2007;49:298–305.

Cardarelli C, Cereda C, Masiero L, et al. Evaluation of health status and health-related quality of life in a cohort of Italian children following treatment for a primary brain tumor. *Pediatr Blood Cancer.* 2006;46:647–644.

Carlson-Green B, Morris RD, Krawiecki N. Family and illness predictors of outcome in pediatric brain tumors. *J Pediatr Psychol.* 1995;20:769–784.

Constine LS, Woolf PD, Cann D, et al. Hypothalamic-pituitary dysfunction after radiation for brain tumors. *N Engl J Med.* 1993;328:87–94.

Foreman NK, Faestel PM, Pearson J, et al. Health status in 52 long-term survivors of pediatric brain tumors. *J Neurooncol.* 1999;41:47–53.

Gleeson HK, Stoeter R, Ogilvy-Stuart AL, et al. Improvements in final height over 25 years in growth hormone (GH)-deficient childhood survivors of brain tumors receiving GH replacement. *J Clin Endocrinol Metab.* 2003;88:3682–3689.

Grill J, Kieffer V, Kalifa C. Measuring the neuro-cognitive side-effects of irradiation in children with brain tumors. *Pediatr Blood Cancer.* 2003;42:452–456.

Gurney JG, Kadan-Lottick NS, Packer RJ, et al. Endocrine and cardiovascular late effects among adult survivors of childhood brain tumors: childhood cancer survivor study. *Cancer.* 2003;97:663–673.

Gurney JG, Ness KK, Stovall M, et al. Final height and body mass index among adult survivors of childhood brain cancer: childhood cancer survivor study. *J Clin Endocrinol Metab.* 2003;88:4731–4739.

Heikens J, Ubbink MC, van der Pal HP, et al. Long term survivors of childhood brain cancer have an increased risk for cardiovascular disease. *Cancer.* 2000;88:2116–2121.

Jakacki RI, Goldwein JW, Larsen RL, et al. Cardiac dysfunction following spinal irradiation during childhood. *J Clin Oncol.* 1993;11:1033–1038.

Jakacki RI, Schramm CM, Donahue BR, et al. Restrictive lung disease following treatment for malignant brain tumors: a potential late effect of craniospinal irradiation. *J Clin Oncol.* 1995;13:1478–1485.

Kennedy C, Bull K, Chevignard M, et al. Quality of survival and growth in children and young adults in the PNET4 European controlled trial of hyper-fractionated versus conventional radiation therapy for standard-risk medulloblastoma. *Int J Radiat Oncol Biol Phys.* 2014;88:292–300.

Khan RB, Marshman KC, Mulhern RK. Atonic seizures in survivors of childhood cancer. *J Child Neurol.* 2003;18:397–400.

Laughton SJ, Merchant TE, Sklar CA, et al. Endocrine outcomes for children with embryonal brain tumors after risk-adapted craniospinal and conformal primary-site irradiation and high-dose chemotherapy with stem-cell rescue on the SJMB-96 trial. *J Clin Oncol.* 2008;26:1112–1118.

Lustig RH, Post SR, Srivannaboon K, et al. Risk factors for the development of obesity in children surviving brain tumors. *J Clin Endocrinol Metab.* 2003;88:611–616.

Macedoni-Luksic M, Jereb B, Todorovski L. Long-term sequelae in children treated for brain tumors: impairments, disability, and handicap. *Pediatr Hematol Oncol.* 2003;20:89–101.

Maule M, Scélo G, Pastore G, et al. Risk of second malignant neoplasms after childhood central nervous system malignant tumours: an international study. *Eur J Cancer.* 2008;44:830–839.

Micklewright JL, King TZ, Morris RD, et al. Quantifying pediatric neuro-oncology risk factors: development of the neurological predictor scale. *J Child Neurol.* 2008;23:455–458.

Morris EB, Gajjar A, Okuma JO, et al. Survival and late mortality in long-term survivors of pediatric CNS tumors. *J Clin Oncol.* 2007;25:1532–1538.

Mulhern RK, Palmer SL, Merchant TE, et al. Neurocognitive consequences of risk-adapted therapy for childhood medulloblastoma. *J Clin Oncol.* 2005;23:5511–5519.

Mulhern RK, Reddick WE, Palmer SL, et al. Neurocognitive deficits in medulloblastoma survivors and white matter loss. *Ann Neurol.* 1999;46:834–841.

Nathan PC, Patel SK, Dilley K, et al. Guidelines for identification of, advocacy for, and intervention in neurocognitive problems in survivors of childhood cancer: a report from the Children's Oncology Group. *Arch Pediatr Adolesc Med.* 2007;161:798–806.

Oberfield SE, Chin D, Uli N, et al. Endocrine late effects of childhood cancers. *J Pediatr.* 1997;131(pt 2):S37–S41.

Odame I, Duckworth J, Talsma D, et al. Osteopenia, physical activity and health-related quality of life in survivors of brain tumors treated in childhood. *Pediatr Blood Cancer.* 2005;46:357–362.

Olshan JS, Gubernick J, Packer RJ, et al. The effects of adjuvant chemotherapy on growth in children with medulloblastoma. *Cancer.* 1992;70:2013–2017.

Packer RJ, Boyett JM, Janss AJ, et al. Growth hormone replacement therapy in children with medulloblastomas: use and effect on tumor control. *J Clin Oncol.* 2001;19:480–487.

Packer RJ, Gurney JG, Punyko JA, et al. Long-term neurologic and neurosensory sequelae in adult survivors of a childhood brain tumor: childhood cancer survivor study. *J Clin Oncol.* 2003;21:3255–3261.

Pietilä S, Ala-Houhala M, Lenko HL, et al. Renal impairment and hypertension in brain tumor patients treated in childhood are mainly associated with cisplatin treatment. *Pediatr Blood Cancer.* 2005;44:363–369.

Reimers TS, Ehrenfels S, Mortensen EL, et al. Cognitive deficits in long-term survivors of childhood brain tumors: identification of predictive factors. *Med Pediatr Oncol.* 2003;40:26–34.

Ross L, Johansen C, Dalton SO, et al. Psychiatric hospitalizations among survivors of cancer in childhood or adolescence. *N Engl J Med.* 2003;349:650–657.

Silber JH, Radcliffe J, Peckham V, et al. Whole-brain irradiation and decline in intelligence: the influence of dose and age on IQ score. *J Clin Oncol.* 1992;10:1390–1396.

Sklar CA, Mertens AC, Mitby P, et al. Risk of disease recurrence and second neoplasms in survivors of childhood cancer treated with growth hormone: a report from the childhood cancer survivor study. *J Clin Endocrinol Metab.* 2002;87:3136–3141.

Sonderkaer S, Schmiegelow M, Carstensen H, et al. Long-term neurological outcome of childhood brain tumors treated by surgery only. *J Clin Oncol.* 2003;21:1347–1351.

Spoudreas HA, Charmandari E, Brook CG. Hypothalamo-pituitary-adrenal axis integrity after cranial irradiation for childhood posterior fossa tumours. *Med Pediatr Oncol.* 2003;40:224–229.

Swerdlow AJ, Reddingius RE, Higgins CD, et al. Growth hormone treatment of children with brain tumors and risk of tumor recurrence. *J Clin Endocrinol Metab.* 2000;85:4444–4449.

Zebrack BJ, Gurney JG, Oeffinger K, et al. Psychological outcomes in long-term survivors of childhood brain cancer: a report from the childhood cancer survivor study. *J Clin Oncol.* 2004;22:999–1006.

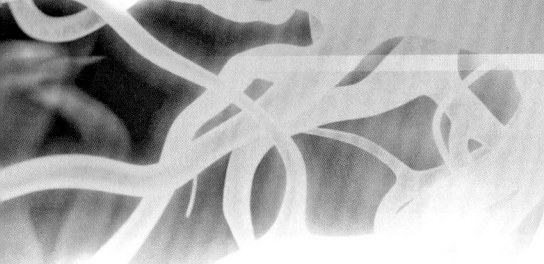

Pediatric Brain Injury and Shaken Baby Syndrome 146

Joshua Cappell and Steven G. Kernie

INTRODUCTION

The still-developing nervous system holds the potential for greater recovery from traumatic brain injury while also carrying the risk of disordered development, dysplasia, and other adverse sequelae. At the same time, mechanical factors may differentiate pediatric from adult injury such as the unfused or less mineralized calvarium and the narrower subarachnoid and sulcal spaces. Pediatric head trauma also differs not only from adult but also within the childhood age spectrum. The mechanisms, including not only the velocity but also the *intentionality*—whether the injury was accidental—strongly affect the severity distribution. Greater impact force, as seen in vehicular (especially unrestrained)-induced injury or nonaccidental injury, skews the distribution toward more severe presentation and worse outcomes.

EPIDEMIOLOGY

Trauma is the major cause of morbidity and mortality in childhood and nervous system involvement is the biggest determinant of severity. Children account for about one-half million incidents of traumatic brain injury (TBI) per year in the United States, a rate disproportionately high for their part of the overall population. Although the mechanisms and circumstances vary across the pediatric age range—with child abuse dominant in infancy and self or mutual violence, vehicular, firearm use, and other high-risk behaviors prevalent in adolescence—it remains true across the pediatric age range that the causes are to a great extent socially influenced rather than purely sporadic and therefore often at least potentially preventable. As such, the reduction of the immense toll of brain injury relies on two distinct approaches: prevention of primary injury and of secondary injury.

The former is an educational and legal as much as medical task. Initiatives such as infant car seats, bike helmets, and statewide abuse recognition and reporting systems are critical components. Although recent public attention to cumulative and late effects of concussion was largely generated by cases of prominent adult athletes, much of the response has been to change practice from middle school through college, the duration of the athletic careers of most of the public.

PATHOGENESIS

The pathophysiology of primary and secondary brain injury is distinct. The primary injury depends on linear and angular velocity, mechanism (penetrating or closed), biomechanical factors (contrecoup injury), trajectory, and compartment. The consequences can be considered based on the tissue impacted. Epidural and subdural bleeds contribute to injury largely due to the pressure they cause by stealing intracranial space. Gray matter architecture can be disrupted in concussion, contusion, or abrasion. Cortical projections and corticocortical connections can be interrupted by penetrating foreign bodies or bone fragments. Less obvious on initial computed tomography imaging but highly influential on outcome is the diffuse axonal injury, the shearing of fiber tracts from torsional forces. Cerebral ischemia due to vascular dissection, occlusion, and thrombosis can be as injurious as force to the parenchyma directly. In intentionally inflicted trauma, multiple mechanisms may have contributed. The injuries of the "shaken baby" can be compounded by impact, partial strangulation, or carotid compression.

Secondary injury encompasses all subsequent deleterious processes at various levels of organization (Table 146.1). On a macroscopic scale, the pediatric brain is at high risk from loss of volume. As brain growth drives skull growth in childhood and the atrophy of adulthood is not yet present, accommodation of hematoma and cerebral edema (which evolves largely over the first 3 days post injury) is poor. Although the dura and unfused calvarium of the neonate and infant flexibly allows reshaping (as required during parturition), it maintains intracranial volume nearly constant as it is inelastic to outward stretch. Consequently, babies too are subject to severe restriction of the intracranial vault. Pressure can cause herniation, compromise cerebral perfusion pressure globally, or compress adjacent cerebral vessels exacerbating tissue compromise.

TABLE 146.1	Example Mechanisms of Secondary Brain Injury after Trauma

Systemic

Hypoperfusion due to the following:

- Respiratory cause: hypoventilation, airway obstruction, lung injury
- Cardiac causes: commotio cordis, stunned myocardium, arrhythmia
- Vascular cause: hypotension due to hemorrhagic hypovolemia, spinal shock, adrenal injury or insufficiency, dysautonomia, especially associated with delirium
- Electrolyte abnormalities of central cause but with systemic effect (salt wasting, diabetes insipidus [DI], syndrome of inappropriate antidiuretic hormone secretion [SIADH])

Intracranial

- Hypoperfusion due to expanding mass
- Subdural, epidural, parenchymal hematoma (which can be due to loss of clotting factors to systemic injury), hydrocephalus, or swelling of diffuse axonal injury
- Excitotoxicity and energy exhaustion due to seizures

Injury to Intervening and Adjacent Structures

- Carotid occlusion or dissection, poor jugular drainage
- Infection due to penetrating injury, of particular concern with injury to the sinuses

Multiple factors threaten the already wounded cortical tissue. Cerebral autoregulation is less robust after injury, increasing the risk that cerebral perfusion pressure will fall beneath the compensated range. Injury to the normally well-sealed and precisely regulated blood–brain barrier implies loss of control of the neuronal microenvironment.

At the cellular level, excitotoxicity due to excessive glutamate release, calcium entry, and hyperactivated intrinsic membrane conductances place increased metabolic demands and interfere with cell volume regulation. At the same time, mitochondrial dysfunction and impaired perfusion make the cells less able to meet these increased demands, leading to cell death.

Although overlapping with mechanisms of secondary injury in the adult, the distribution of injury may differ in the child because of incomplete myelination and selective expression of transmitter and voltage-dependent conductances in specific developmental windows.

CLINICAL ASSESSMENT AND TREATMENT

Medical management is directed toward secondary prevention, providing, through optimized care, the best possible outcome obtainable given that an injury has already occurred. This is the medical challenge commonly faced by practitioners in a chain from the first responder to the emergency room and the pediatric intensive care unit (ICU). To date, few modalities are available to promote reversal of injury, and neuroprotection in the strictest sense, of physiologically isolating the brain from systemic changes, remains largely experimental. Consequently, the focus of management in the acute period is on preventing additional injury so that the body may gradually heal itself to the maximum extent to which it is intrinsically capable rather than extrinsically promoting healing.

The mechanisms of potential secondary injury to be intercepted are several: Head trauma is often accompanied by systemic trauma. This in turn can cause brain hypoperfusion at the very moment that the brain is most susceptible to hypoperfusion due to impairment of the usual protective reflexes that ordinarily prioritize the maintenance of cerebral blood flow. Consequently, the highest priority in the acute management of pediatric brain injury is on stabilizing perfusion: providing adequate oxygenation, ventilation, and blood pressure. Hypotension in particular is common due to many mechanisms (see Table 146.1) and has been shown to be quite deleterious, independent of other factors. It should be combatted aggressively by fluid resuscitation and, as needed, by pressor support and transfusion.

Differences between pediatric and adult TBI are emphasized by improved outcomes when children are treated at pediatric-experienced centers. Direct admission to such a center is superior to secondary transfer.

Although the perception of some practitioners may be that highly specialized elective procedures or workups mandate tertiary care, whereas trauma is the "bread and butter" of community hospitals, studies show to the contrary that not only is trauma experience important but also pediatric-specific experience in particular matters in childhood injury.

As in all cases of pediatric trauma, clinicians must always consider whether the child presenting with TBI has injuries consistent—in both severity and wound age—with the reported mechanism. Infants are most vulnerable both because they are affected at higher rates and because they are unable to recount events. Difficult legal and ethical questions arise often, as many traumas result from poor

TABLE 146.2	**Considerations in Evaluation of Possible or Suspected Nonaccidental Trauma**

- Establish age of injury or injuries and determination of consistency with reported history.
- Social work screen, discuss with child protective services, police, or district attorney's office
- Ophthalmology consult with dilated examination
- Skeletal survey and/or radionucleotide study for reactive changes of older, healing bone injury
- Exclude (by clinical findings or lab test) other causes such as coagulopathy, osteogenesis imperfecta, or glutaric aciduria.

supervision, raising concern for negligence even when there was no intent to harm. In inadequately explained trama, a social or home safety screening, involvement of child protection specialist, and discussion with the jurisdictional agency is imperative. Screenings are mandated whenever even a concern has been raised by a presentation not only when there is a high suspicion or certainty. As such, it is most constructive for parents to regard reporting as a chance to assess and mitigate risks rather than an accusation, much less a determination, of criminality. Factors to be considered are shown in Table 146.2.

SEVERITY GRADATION AND MINOR TRAUMATIC BRAIN INJURY

Patients presenting with a Glasgow Coma Scale (GCS) score of 8 or less (see Table 46.3) are defined by most studies as having severe head trauma. Patients with a GCS of 14 or 15 are generally regarded as having minor head trauma. This category often overlaps with concussion, defined as a head injury causing transient loss or alteration of consciousness or loss of memory. Increasing evidence that lasting encephalopathy can result from the cumulative effects of even minor head trauma in professional sports has made this a source of greater societal and parental concern. American Academy of Neurology (AAN) guidelines recommend refraining from activities with recurrent injury risk (practice or play) until resolution of concussion and associated symptoms such as headache. American Academy of Pediatrics (AAP) guidelines also recommend "cognitive rest" including reducing academic activities to prevent exacerbation of symptoms However, there is no evidence supporting this as either necessary or beneficial for recovery.

INDICATIONS FOR HEAD COMPUTED TOMOGRAPHY IMAGING

Several studies have established criteria mandating a head computed tomograph (CT) in infants and children presenting with injury, aiming to eliminate unnecessary scans while assuring that no potentially actionable findings are missed by not scanning. The Canadian Assessment of Tomography in Childhood Head Injury or "CATCH" rule is to scan any child with any of the following: GCS less than 14, suspected open or depressed skull fracture, worsening headaches, or irritability on exam. Application of this rule identified 98% of patients with CT findings of injury and all patients requiring surgical intervention among the 2,043 CTs performed.

The Pediatric Emergency Care Applied Research Network (PECARN) conducted a large study across 25 centers to identify and validate a decision rule to determine necessity of head CT for children (younger than 18 years) presenting with a GCS of 14 or 15 [**Level 1**].[1] Among children younger than 2 years of age, criteria with predictive value were alteration of mental status per examiner *or* not at baseline per parent, presence of nonfrontal scalp hematoma, loss of consciousness longer than 5 seconds, severe mechanism (vehicular, hit by high-velocity object or >3 feet fall), or palpable fracture. Absence of these elements had a predictive value approaching 100% for excluding clinically important injury warranting CT scanning. In the children 2 years or older, validated criteria were any alteration of mental status, *any* loss of consciousness (even <5 seconds), emesis, severe injury (in these meaning vehicular, high-velocity object or >5 feet fall), signs of basilar skull fracture (Battle's or "raccoon" sign, hematotympanum, or cerebrospinal fluid oto- or rhinorrhea), and severe headache. Absence of these factors was greater than 99% predictive for the absence of a clinically significant injury to be found on imaging, providing a level I evidence basis for decision making.

SEVERE TRAUMATIC BRAIN INJURY

In an effort to improve and standardize the management of severe pediatric TBI, a collaborative literature review was undertaken to assemble evidence-based guidelines. These have recently been updated and are the basis of Table 146.3. Regarding some interventions, large, well-designed trials have been performed, for example, showing that cooling did not show a demonstrable neuroprotective benefit in children, nor did steroids in a large adult trial. In Table 146.4, the order in which interventions are implemented is presented with higher "tiers" offering more aggressive measures for the circumstance that the prior, less invasive tier has failed to adequately control intracranial pressure (ICP). Particular management considerations and evidence are described in the following text.

INTRACRANIAL PRESSURE IN CHILDREN

Normal ICP in children ranges up to 28 cm H_2O corresponding to 20 mm Hg. Elevations of ICP after trauma have been associated with higher mortality in observational studies, especially if elevated ICP has been unresponsive to interventions. Although ICP monitors have not been directly demonstrated to improve outcomes, they do allow the titration of therapies that reduce ICP. Lower ICP, even when achieved by intervention, correlates with better outcome. Consequently, the latest pediatric TBI guidelines include a level III recommendation for the consideration of ICP monitoring in severe TBI. A recent trial in Bolivia and Ecuador directly comparing management with and without the use of ICP monitoring included some adolescents (age older than 13 years). However, the study was not powered to analyze teenagers separately. No corresponding study yet exists for younger children.

Hypothermia as a treatment modality after TBI was carefully evaluated by the Canadian Critical Care Trials Group in the Hypothermia Pediatric Head Injury Trial [**Level 1**].[2] Two hundred twenty-five children were randomly assigned to either hypothermic therapy 90.5°F, initiated within 8 hours of the injury and maintained for 24 hours or normothermia. No advantage was found for hypothermia, a level I evidence finding (this and other level I designations in the present chapter are based on criteria comparable to the original version of the pediatric severe TBI guidelines, generally corresponding to level II in the second edition). In fact, more hypotension was seen in the hypothermia group with a possible trend toward greater mortality. Whether there exist individual subgroups, such as refractory elevated ICP awaiting decompression,

TABLE 146.3	**Best Evidence Management for Severe Traumatic Brain Injury**

Invasive pressure monitoring

Use of ICP monitoring may be considered in infants with severe TBI (level III).

Intracranial pressure

Treatment of ICP may be considered at a threshold of 20 mm Hg (level III).

Cerebral perfusion pressure

A CPP threshold of 40–50 mm Hg may be considered. There may be age-specific thresholds with infants at the lower end and adolescents at the higher end of this range (level III).

Advanced neuromonitoring

IF brain oxygenation monitoring is used, maintenance of a partial pressure of brain tissue oxygen >10 mm Hg may be considered (level III).

Hypothermia

Moderate hypothermia (89.6°F to 91.4°F) beginning early after severe TBI and continuing for only 24 h should be avoided (level II). Moderate hypothermia (89.6°F to 91.4°F) beginning early after severe TBI and continuing for 48 h may be considered (level III).

Hyperventilation

Avoidance of severe hypoventilation (<30 mm Hg) may be considered in the 48 h after severe TBI (level II).

Anticonvulsant therapy

Prophylactic treatment with phenytoin may be considered to reduce the risk of early posttraumatic seizures in pediatric patients with severe TBI (level III).

Use of steroids

The use of steroids is NOT recommended to improve outcome or reduce ICP for children with severe TBI (level II).

Sedatives

Etomidate and thiopental may be considered to reduce refractory ICP. For etomidate, risks of adrenal suppression must be considered (level II).

Reimaging

In the absence of neurologic deterioration or increase in ICP, obtaining a routine repeat CT scan >24 h after admission and initial follow-up study may not be indicated for the decisions about neurosurgical intervention (level III).

Hyperosmolar therapy

Hypertonic saline (3%) should be considered for the acute management of severe pediatric TBI associated with intracranial hypertension. The effective dose for acute therapy ranges 6.5–10 mL/kg (level II).

As a continuous infusion the effective dose range is 0.1–1 mL/kg per hour. The minimum dose needed to maintain ICP <20 mm Hg should be used; serum osmolarity should be maintained <360 mOsm/L.

ICP, intracranial pressure; TBI, traumatic brain injury; CPP, cerebral perfusion pressure; CT, computed tomography.

Based on Kochanek P, Carney N, Adelson PD, Wong H, et al. Guidelines for the acute medical management of severe traumatic brain injury in infants, children, and adolescents. 2nd ed. *Pediatr Crit Care Med.* 2012;13:S1–S82.

Levels shown here are their designations.

TABLE 146.4	Stepwise Approach to Management of Elevated Intracranial Pressure
Tier 1	
• Head of bed elevation	
• Sedation and neuromuscular blockade	
• Mechanical ventilation to normal arterial carbon dioxide pressure	
• Active normothermia	
• Hyperosmolar therapy	
• External ventricular drainage	
Tier 2	
• Moderate hyperventilation	
• Mild hypothermia (to 35°C)	
• Thiopental infusion	
Tier 3	
• Decompressive craniectomy	

who may benefit, remains uncertain. Meanwhile, routine use of hypothermia cannot be recommended for pediatric TBI.

SEIZURE PROPHYLAXIS

The original Temkin study in 1990 established a benefit to the short-term use of phenytoin in patients older than 16 years of age to reduce seizures in the week after injury. Indications for prophylaxis were the presence of intracranial blood and/or a depressed skull fracture [**Level 1**].[3] In a retrospective analysis of pediatric cases, low GCS scores were most predictive of early seizures, and treatment with phenytoin was associated with a lower seizure rate. In one prospective trial, no benefit for rate of seizures within 48 hours was seen in children receiving phenytoin within 1-hour of arrival [**Level 1**].[4] However, benzodiazepines given for elevated ICP or intubation may have masked the effect. The current pediatric TBI guidelines include a level II recommendation for consideration of phenytoin prophylaxis. Since the introduction of intravenous levetiracetam, this is an increasingly chosen option because of a perceived high degree of efficacy and a favorable side effect profile. The feasibility of this was demonstrated by a phase II trial in 2013 in which levetiracetam 55 mg/kg/day, divided twice a day (b.i.d.), was administered to children ages 6 to 17 years for 30 days. A prospective trial will be needed to confirm benefit.

REPEAT IMAGING

Criteria for repetition of imaging in pediatric TBI are not well established. In one analysis, worsening was found in 13% of follow-up scans. However, among these, all requiring surgical intervention had clinical indications of worsening neurologic status. Consequently, the pediatric TBI guidelines include a level II recommendation suggesting that repeat imaging may not be warranted in the absence of clinical change or increasing ICP. On the other hand, in a separate large retrospective case series, 27% of patients showed worsening, of whom less than a fifth had accompanying clinical signs. Furthermore, among those whose CTs led to surgical intervention, two-thirds did not have clinical signs. This would suggest that high clinical concern based on initial findings or clinical picture in addition to worsening or rising ICP is sufficient justification for repeat CT.

The recent DEcompressive CRAniectomy (DECRA) trial which did not show a survival benefit to decompressive craniectomy as a rescue therapy did not include children. A prospective but small early pediatric trial found a trend toward benefit of decompressive bitemporal craniectomy in patients with medically refractory ICP. However, the decompression in this study was performed without duraplasty, different from the techniques more commonly employed. A larger study in children including duraplasty has yet to be done, and the use of decompressive craniectomy including duraplasty is regarded as a level III option in the pediatric TBI guidelines.

OUTCOME

Except in the most severe of cases, the degree of injury, whether by clinical criteria or imaging, incompletely predicts ultimate outcome. Consequently, prognostic prediction during the acute treatment should be cautious. In children, recovery may continue long after the injury. Diffusion tensor imaging (DTI) is emerging as the best predictor, especially for the extent of white matter damage in diffuse axonal injury. There is less clinical experience with the use of serum markers for gradation in trauma.

Patients with moderate and severe injuries typically will require inpatient rehabilitation after their stabilization. Impairments of gross and fine motor skills are easily identified and readily justify the need for physical and occupational therapy. However, parents should be forewarned of the possibility of more subtle deficits that may even be unapparent on screening neurologic exam but can impose large burdens as the patient attempts to resume activities of daily living and education. Posttraumatic changes in memory, attention, motivation, as well as migraine or tension-like headaches can all interfere with return to school. Neuropsychological testing can be helpful in identifying cognitive disabilities. Schools can be asked to structure an individualized education plan or supplemental services and accommodation (commonly known as a *504 plan*, referring to Section 504 of Federal Disability Law) to smooth the transition.

Neurologic follow-up may be warranted to treat sequela such as headaches or chronic posttraumatic seizures. Also, in infants, screening may be needed to identify failure of proper skull healing. The incompletely fused or partially mineralized pediatric skull can undergo aberrant healing. Pressure on a fracture or diastasis of an existing suture can lead to a "growing fracture." Over a period of weeks to months, this can allow formation of so-called leptomeningeal cysts, a misnomer used to describe what is actually a dural herniation through the skull defect. This entity, extremely rare in adults, can be ruled out in young children with severe TBI by a follow-up skull film 6 weeks to 3 months after injury.

LEVEL 1 EVIDENCE

1. Kuppermann N, Holmes JF, Dayan P, et al. Identification of children at very low risk of clinically-important brain injuries after head trauma. A prospective cohort study. *Lancet.* 2009;374:1160–1170.
2. Hutchison JS, Ward RE, Lacroix J, et al. Hypothermia therapy after traumatic brain injury in children. *N Engl J Med.* 2008;358:2447–2456.
3. Temkin NR, Dikmen SS, Wilensky AJ, et al. A randomized, double-blind study of phenytoin for the prevention of posttraumatic seizures. *N Engl J Med.* 1990;323:497–502.

4. Young KD, Okada PJ, Sokolove PE, et al. A randomized, double-blinded, placebo-controlled trial of phenytoin for the prevention of early posttraumatic seizures in children with moderate to severe blunt head injury. *Ann Emerg Med.* 2004;43(4): 435–446.

SUGGESTED READINGS

Chesnut RM, Temkin N, Carney N, et al; Global Neurotrauma Research Group. A trial of intracranial-pressure monitoring in traumatic brain injury. *N Engl J Med.* 2012;367:2471–2481.

Cooper DJ, Rosenfeld JV, Murray L, et al; DECRA Trial Investigators and the Australian and New Zealand Intensive Care Society Clinical Trials Group. Decompressive craniectomy in diffuse traumatic brain injury. *N Engl J Med.* 2011;364:1493–1502.

Duhaime AC, Christian CW, Rorke LB, et al. Nonaccidental head injury in infants—the "shaken-baby syndrome." *N Engl J Med.* 1998;338:1822–1829.

Figg RE, Stouffer CW, Vander Kolk WE, et al. Clinical efficacy of serial computed tomographic scanning in pediatric severe traumatic brain injury. *Pediatr Surg Intern.* 2006;22(3):215–218.

Giza CC, Kutcher JS, Zafonte R, et al. Summary of evidence-based guideline update: evaluation and management of concussion in sports. *Neurology.* 2013;80(24):2250–2257. http://www.neurology.org/content/80/24/2250.full. Accessed June 1, 2015.

Halstead ME, Walter KD; Council on Sports Medicine and Fitness. Sport-related concussion in children and adolescents. *Pediatrics.* 2010;126(3):597–615. http://pediatrics.aappublications.org/content/126/3/597.full. Accessed June 1, 2015.

Hollingworth W, Vavilala MS, Jarvik JG, et al. The use of repeated head computed tomography in pediatric blunt head trauma: factors predicting new and worsening brain injury. *Pediatr Crit Care Med.* 2007;8(4):348–356.

Kochanek P, Carney N, Wong H, et al. Guidelines for the acute medical management of severe traumatic brain injury in infants, children, and adolescents. 2nd ed. *Pediatr Crit Care Med.* 2012;13:S1–S82. http://www.braintrauma.org/pdf/guidelines_pediatric2.pdf. Accessed June 1, 2015.

Lewis RJ, Yee L, Inkelis SH, et al. Clinical predictors of post-traumatic seizures in children with head trauma. *Ann Emerg Med.* 1993;22:1114–1118.

Pearl PL, McCarter R, McGavin CL, et al. Results of phase II levetiracetam trial following acute head injury in children at risk for posttraumatic epilepsy. *Epilepsia.* 2013;54(9):e135–e137.

Pinto PS, Poretti A, Meoded A, et al. The unique features of traumatic brain injury in children. Review of the characteristics of the pediatric skull and brain, mechanisms of trauma, patterns of injury, complications and their imaging findings—part 1. *J Neuroimaging.* 2012;22(2):e1–e17.

Pinto PS, Meoded A, Poretti A, et al. The unique features of traumatic brain injury in children. Review of the characteristics of the pediatric skull and brain, mechanisms of trauma, patterns of injury, complications and their imaging findings—part 2. *J Neuroimaging.* 2012;22(2):e18–e41.

Taylor A, Butt W, Rosenfeld J, et al. A randomized trial of very early decompressive craniectomy in children with traumatic brain injury and sustained intracranial hypertension. *Childs Nerv Syst.* 2001;17:154–162.

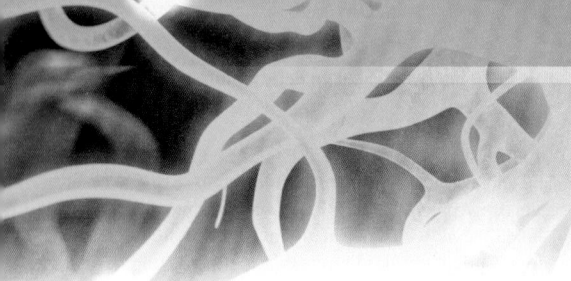

Claudia A. Chiriboga

PEDIATRIC AIDS AND HIV INFECTION

Most children with AIDS in the United States are infected perinatally. Intravenous (IV) drug abuse and sexual contact with HIV-infected partners are the maternal risk factors in nearly all perinatal cases. Mother-to-child HIV transmission rates have dropped below 2% with the use of highly active antiretroviral drugs treatment (HAART) during pregnancy from a rate of 25% without prophylaxis. In the United States, 166 children younger than the age of 13 years were diagnosed with HIV in 2009, 13 of whom were diagnosed with AIDS. In contrast, among older children (older than age 13 years), the incidence of HIV infection continues to rise mostly in boys as a result of male-to-male sexual transmission. Racial and ethnic minority children are disproportionately affected by perinatal HIV infection accounting in 2009 for 90% of HIV infections. Most infections occur in the last trimester of pregnancy and at the time of delivery. Risk factors for vertical transmission are recent maternal HIV seroconversion, high viral burden, and maternal AIDS. Premature infants are also at increased risk of infection. Infection may result from exposure to blood and other body fluids at delivery. Breastfeeding is, thus, not recommended in the United States; cesarean section is not routinely recommended unless maternal viral burden is high.

Determining transmission of HIV infection to offspring based on detection of HIV antibody has been replaced by infant HIV polymerase chain reaction (PCR). Further, maternal HIV infection status is no longer required to determine infant HIV infection status. The Centers for Disease Control and Prevention (CDC) surveillance definition states a child is considered definitively infected if he or she has positive virologic results on two separate specimens or is aged older than 18 months and has either a positive virologic test or a positive confirmed HIV antibody test. HIV-seropositive children who do not meet these criteria are considered perinatally exposed and later seroreverters when antibodies turn negative. The 1994 clinical classification system for confirmed cases of HIV infection in children has been replaced by a five staging system that applies to both adults and children: 0, 1, 2, 3, or unknown. Stage 0 corresponds to early infection as noted by a negative HIV test within 6 months of HIV diagnosis. Stages 1 to 3 are classified immunologically (absolute CD4 count or percent CD4 count) depending on the child's age (younger than 12 months, 1 to 5 years, and older than 6 years): stage 1, no evidence of immune suppression; stage 2, moderate immune suppression; and stage 3, severe immune suppression (either a low CD4 count or whether an opportunistic illness was diagnosed) (Table 147.1). T-cell counts in infants and toddlers are higher for a specific immune category and reach adult levels after age 6 years.

DIAGNOSTIC TESTS

Because of early testing, most HIV-positive children are identified soon after birth, especially in States with universal perinatal screening. HIV DNA PCR is the preferred diagnostic method, whereas quantitative HIV RNA PCR is more sensitive in determining plasma concentration (copies/mL) of HIV RNA, commonly referred to as *plasma viral load*. By age 6 months, 100% of HIV-infected children are identified by a positive PCR. In newborns, a negative PCR test for HIV does not exclude infection but decreases the risk of HIV infection to 3%. Viral load runs higher in asymptomatic children than in asymptomatic adults. Sustained high viral load and low CD4 count predict progression to AIDS. High viral loads in early infancy predict early onset of symptomatic HIV disease. In the post-HAART era, most progression to AIDS is related to nonadherence to HAART of any cause (i.e., medical or social), which in turn facilitates development of drug resistance. HIV-1 syncytial-inducing phenotypes are linked to aggressive early symptomatic disease.

CLINICAL MANIFESTATIONS

Mild HIV infection includes diarrhea, unexplained persistent fever, lymphadenopathy, and parotitis. Lymphoid interstitial pneumonitis and recurrent bacterial infections are seen in HIV-infected children but not in infected adults. Prior to the advent of antiretroviral therapy, severe manifestations in early infancy, such as progressive encephalopathy or opportunistic infections (e.g., *Pneumocystis carinii*), carried a poor prognosis for survival but with effective antiretroviral therapy, these disorders are compatible with survival to adulthood.

TABLE 147.1	Infection Stage Based on Age-Specific CD4+ T-lymphocytes Count or Age-Specific CD4+ T-lymphocyte Percentage of Total Lymphocytes						
		<12 mo		1–5 yr		>6 yr	
Stage	Immunologic Category	Cells/μL	(%)	Cells/μL	(%)	Cells/μL	(%)
1	No evidence of suppression	≥1,500	(≥34)	≥1,000	(≥30)	≥500	(>26)
2	Moderate suppression	750–1,499	(26–33)	500–999	(22–29)	200–499	(14–25)
3	Severe suppression	<750	(<26)	<500	(<22)	<200	(<14)

Adapted from Selik RM, Mokotoff, ED, Branson B, et al. Revised surveillance case definition for HIV infection—United States, 2014. *MMWR Morb Mortal Wkly Rep*. 2014;63:1–10.

MECHANISM OF ACTION

HIV infection is maintained by viral persistence in helper T lymphocytes and macrophages. HIV strains with tropism for monocyte-derived macrophages have a predilection to infect cerebral vascular endothelium and the central nervous system (CNS). Infected macrophages traverse the blood–brain barrier and infect microglial cells; astrocytes are infected nonproductively, whereas neurons are spared from direct infestation. Neuronal dropout is seen as the disease advances, but it is not known how HIV induces neural damage. Postulated mechanisms include release of soluble neurotoxins by HIV-infected macrophages and lymphocytes (e.g., cytokines, quinolinic acid, viral antigens, or undefined viral products), neurotoxin amplification by astrocyte–macrophage interaction, and impaired blood–brain barrier function secondary to HIV-related endothelial damage. Nonproductive infection of a portion of astrocytes is reported to amplify bystander neurotoxicity. These neurotoxins are thought to produce a reversible metabolic encephalopathy that may disappear with effective antiretroviral treatment.

PATHOLOGY

Glial nodules and endothelial hyperplasia with calcification, dystrophic calcification, and perivascular mononuclear inflammation are common pathologic findings of subacute encephalitis in HIV-infected brains. The glial nodule comprises a cluster of chronic inflammatory cells in the neuropil and is often associated with multinucleated giant cells that are presumed to arise from coalescent microglia.

HIV ENCEPHALOPATHY

Two types of encephalopathy are seen in children: progressive and static. The evolution of the progressive encephalopathy may be fulminant, inexorably progressive, or stepwise. Progressive encephalopathy is characterized by loss of developmental milestones, progressive pyramidal tract dysfunction, and acquired microcephaly or impaired brain growth. The static encephalopathy is less well defined and may not be related to direct HIV CNS disease.

The neurologic abnormalities commonly include abnormalities of muscle tone, hyperreflexia, clonus, and impaired head growth. Hypotonia with corticospinal tract dysfunction may be seen in infants early in the course of the encephalopathy and evolves into a spastic diparesis; with newer antiretroviral treatments, progression to a spastic tetraparesis, with or without pseudobulbar palsy, is seldom seen. Ataxia and rigidity are uncommon. Prior to HAART, progressive neurologic dysfunction was the first evidence of progression to AIDS in 10% of infected children. In young children, early presentation may mimic a leukodystrophy. At the time of onset of neurologic symptoms, there is always evidence of underlying HIV infection, such as immunologic compromise (low CD4 counts) or high viral load. Many infected children exhibit global developmental delay, regardless of neurologic findings.

The rate of neurologic abnormalities reported in HIV-infected cohorts before the advent of antiretroviral treatments was 15% to 30%. The incidence of progressive HIV encephalopathy in 2000 was less than 2% in the cohort followed. Children most at risk are those who have recovered from HIV encephalopathy. Older HIV-infected children may show problems in visual–spatial processing functions and expressive language and may develop AIDS dementia complex indistinguishable from that described in adults. Children with HIV encephalopathy who respond to antiretroviral therapy may show reversal of microcephaly and cognitive impairments. The most frequent sequelae of "arrested" HIV encephalopathy are learning difficulty and nonprogressive mild spastic diparesis.

HIV-associated myelopathy, polyneuropathy, and myopathy are rare in children. Spinal cord pathology may show demyelinating changes of the corticospinal tracts, vacuolar changes, or myelitis attributable to HIV or other virus. Acute inflammatory demyelinating polyneuropathy is a rare complication in pediatric HIV.

FOCAL MANIFESTATIONS

HIV brain infection is nonfocal and subcortical. Seizures are not common. Focal signs or seizures raise the possibility of neoplasm, strokes, or, less likely, opportunistic infections.

Primary Central Nervous System Lymphoma

Rates of CNS lymphoma have decreased since the advent of HAART from an incidence ratio (IR; HIV-infected children/uninfected children) of 1,994 down to an IR of 1,088. CNS lymphoma is still the most common cause of focal cerebral signs in HIV-infected children (see also Chapter 99). It is often multifocal, and seizures are reported in about 33% of patients. It may be difficult to differentiate this tumor from a toxoplasmic brain abscess by neuroimaging, but a positive PCR for Epstein–Barr virus (EBV) in cerebrospinal fluid (CSF) is highly suggestive of CNS lymphoma. Thallium single-photon emission computed tomography (SPECT) and magnetic resonance (MR) spectroscopy may prove helpful in distinguishing CNS toxoplasmosis from lymphoma (Table 147.2). Diagnostic confirmation may require brain biopsy.

Stroke

Untreated HIV infection produces inflammation of cerebral vessels, increasing the risk of stroke, which occurred at a rate of 1.3% a year in symptomatic HIV-infected children. More than 50% of strokes were hemorrhagic and occurred with thrombocytopenia (especially immune thrombocytopenic purpura) or CNS neoplasia. Nonhemorrhagic stroke and subarachnoid hemorrhage are attributed to an arteriopathy of large vessels in the circle of Willis (fusiform aneurysms) or meninges (Fig. 147.1). HIV-related strokes may be clinically silent, so the true incidence is probably higher. In cases of stroke, varicella-zoster virus (VZV) should be excluded as the etiologic agent by CSF PCR, especially when small intracranial vessels are involved. Ocular involvement should be excluded by pupillary dilatation for ophthalmologic assessment. Any vasculopathy in an HIV-infected patient is presumed to be infectious (from either HIV

TABLE 147.2	Distinguishing Features between Central Nervous System Lymphoma and Toxoplasmosis Abscess	
	Lymphoma	**Toxoplasmosis**
Distribution of lesion	Often solitary, subependymal spread	Typically multifocal, basal ganglia or corticomedullary junction
Enhancement	Typically homogenous	Often ring or nodular
MR perfusion	Increased rCBV	Decreased rCBV
SPECT	Increased uptake	Decreased uptake
MRS	Increased choline peak	Decreased choline peak

MR, magnetic resonance; rCBV, relative cerebral blood volume; SPECT, single-photon emission computed tomography (thallium); MRS, magnetic resonance spectroscopy.

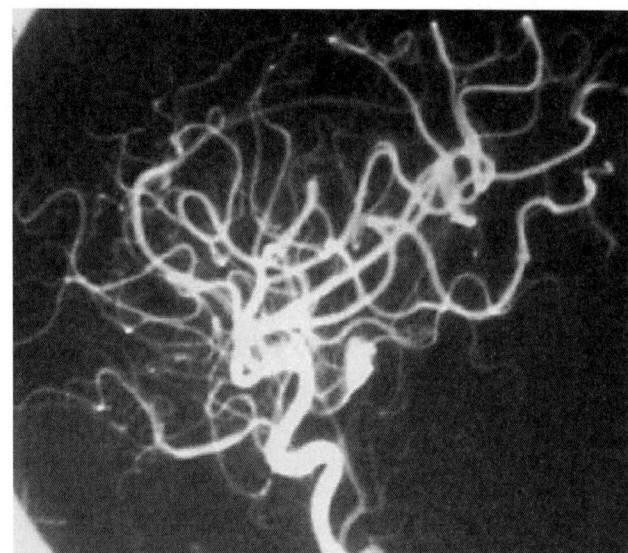

FIGURE 147.1 Fusiform aneurysm in a child with advanced HIV encephalopathy presenting with intraventricular hemorrhage and stroke.

or VZV) and should be treated with appropriate antiretroviral and antiviral medication.

Opportunistic Central Nervous System Infection

As opposed to adults, opportunistic infections (OIs) in children involve primary infections rather than reactivation. Exposure rates to OI pathogens are cumulative and approximate adult rates by adolescence. Hence, rates of CNS OI occur less frequently in HIV-infected young children. Presentation and treatment of OIs are akin to what is described among HIV-infected adults (see Chapter 67). Survival of children with progressive multifocal leukoencephalopathy (PML) has increased with antiretroviral treatment (e.g., cidofovir) and effective antiretroviral combination therapy.

IMAGING

In children with HIV encephalopathy, brain atrophy (cortical and subcortical) is the most common imaging abnormality (Fig. 147.2). Periventricular or parietooccipital demyelination can be observed on magnetic resonance imaging (MRI) (Fig. 147.3). Frontal lobe or basal ganglia enhancement and calcifications are late manifestations of HIV encephalopathy, best seen on computed tomography (CT), and occur primarily in symptomatic infants (see Fig. 147.2). Imaging findings may be indistinguishable from Aicardi–Goutières syndrome. HIV myelopathy may show a high signal on spinal MRI but is usually normal. Bilateral cerebral lesions may mimic myelopathy and must be excluded with MRI or CT. Lesions of PML are commonly located in the parietooccipital or frontal regions, affecting both periventricular and subcortical white matter. These lesions may be difficult to distinguish from HIV demyelination.

CEREBROSPINAL FLUID

CSF findings are commonly normal in children with HIV infection. In the absence of OI, CSF analysis in children with progressive encephalopathy may show nonspecific changes of lymphocytic pleocytosis and elevated protein content. Intra–blood–brain barrier synthesis of HIV-specific antibody or antigen detection in CSF has not been useful in predicting encephalopathy. CSF viral load,

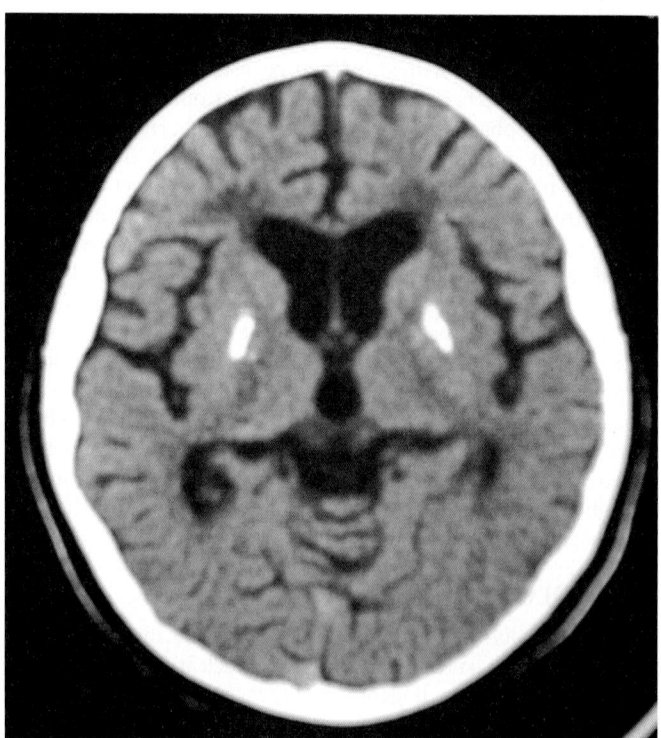

FIGURE 147.2 CT scan of an infant with HIV encephalopathy showing cortical and subcortical atrophy, basal ganglia, and frontal lobe calcifications. (Courtesy of Dr. Ram Kairam.)

although not routinely available, may prove useful in determining HIV encephalopathy in children, especially in cases of compartmentalization (i.e., a sequestered HIV reservoir in the CNS), in which systemic measures of viral load do not parallel the CNS level of viral replication.

ANTIRETROVIRAL THERAPY

HAART, consisting of a protease inhibitor (PI) or a nonnucleoside reverse transcriptase inhibitor (NNRTI) administered in combination with nucleoside reverse transcriptase inhibitors (NRTIs), have been reported to suppress viral replication, improve immune function, and decrease AIDS-related death as well as diminish rates of HIV encephalopathy. High systemic viral load tends to predict the development of HIV encephalopathy, whereas CD4 counts tend to predict HIV disease progression primarily from OIs. Children younger than 1 year tend to be at greatest risk for progression and should be treated regardless of symptomatology. After 12 months, treatment is not indicated if child is asymptomatic or minimally symptomatic.

ANTIRETROVIRAL THERAPY SIDE EFFECTS

Treatment with nucleoside inhibitors of viral reverse transcriptase can alter mitochondrial (mt) function by inhibiting mtDNA polymerase-γ, which is responsible for the replication of mtDNA. Inhibition of mtDNA results in diminished synthesis of respiratory chain enzymes, causing the syndrome of mt depletion. Antiretroviral-induced mt dysfunction in turn is responsible for diverse adverse effects frequently observed in HIV-infected patients. Nonneurologic side effects include hepatic steatosis, lactic acidemia (>2 mmol/L), and lipodystrophy, a disorder characterized by the accumulation of visceral fat, breast adiposity, cervical fat pads, hyperlipidemia,

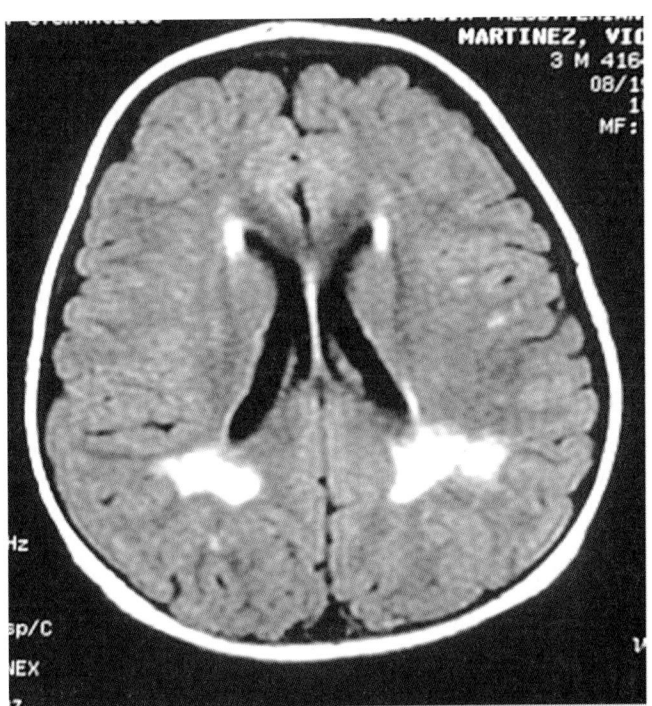
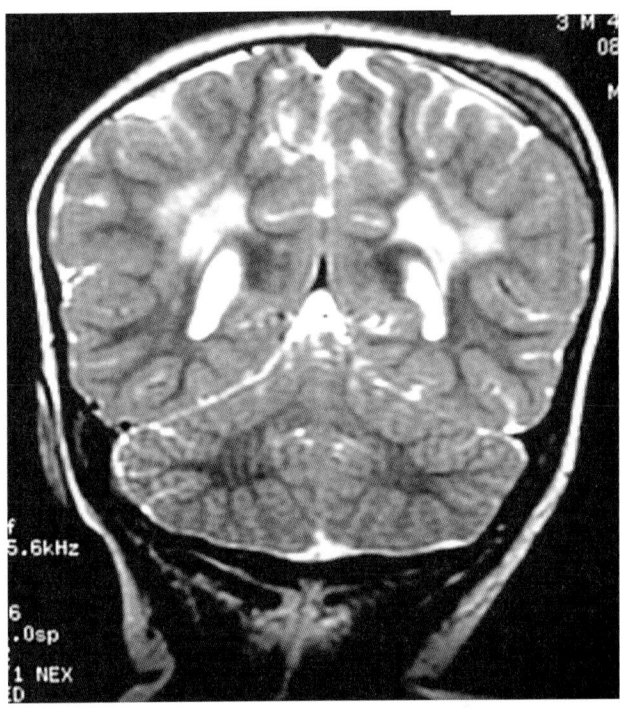

FIGURE 147.3 Parietal occipital demyelination on **(A)** axial fluid-attenuated inversion recovery (FLAIR) and **(B)** coronal T2 images in a child with advanced HIV encephalopathy and high viral load (RNA HIV = 1.5 million copies per milliliter).

insulin resistance, and fat wasting in face and limbs. Neurologic side effects include myopathy, peripheral neuropathy, and parkinsonism. Mt depletion myopathy can be seen in children treated with combination therapy, especially with NRTI that have a high affinity to mt polymerase-γ. Low-dose treatment with didanosine (ddI) causes a painful sensory neuropathy in less than 10% of patients treated. The neuropathy is dose related and usually clears with cessation of treatment. ddI, stavudine, and zalcitabine have a high affinity for binding polymerase-γ, whereas zidovudine, abacavir, tenofovir, and lamivudine have a lower affinity for that enzyme. Changing antiretroviral agents usually relieves the symptoms.

In the immune reconstitution syndrome (IRS), worsening or de novo manifestations of OI (clinically or radiographically) are seen after introduction of HAART. The syndrome coincides with improving CD4 count and is not caused by treatment failure or a new infection. In a Johns Hopkins cohort, the independent predictors of IRS in adults were boosted (with ritonavir) PI and rapid decline of viral load (>2.5 log). The infection most commonly reported in adult IRS is cryptococcal meningitis, but PML and HIV dementia have also been reported. Among immune-suppressed (i.e., CD4 <15%) Thai children, the incidence of IRS following HAART was 19%, the median time of onset was 4 weeks, and the primary pathogens involved were VZV and tuberculosis. Most cases of IRS occur within the first 3 months of treatment, although delayed cases are reported.

FETAL ALCOHOL SYNDROME

Fetal alcohol syndrome (FAS) affects children of chronic alcoholic women but also occurs with binge drinking, as defined by five drinks or more on one occasion. Fetal susceptibility to the effects of alcohol is greatest during the first trimester of pregnancy. FAS is characterized by abnormalities of growth, CNS, and facial features;

birth defects are common (Table 147.3). The severity of the facial dysmorphology correlates with neurodevelopmental impairment. FAS rates in the United States range from 0.3 to 1.5 cases per 1,000 live births. Rates of FAS are highest among Alaska Native and Native American populations. FAS is confined to infants of alcohol-abusing women and occurs in about 2% to 4% of their offspring. Risk factors for FAS include poverty, poor maternal nutrition, and advanced maternal age. Risk of FAS is modulated by genetic factors: Certain enzyme polymorphisms confer protection (e.g., alcohol dehydrogenase [ADH] enzyme and cytochrome P4502E1), whereas others increase risk (absence of ADH2).

TABLE 147.3 Fetal Alcohol Syndrome

Growth Impairment

- Prenatal and postnatal growth impairment (weight or length <10th percentile)

CNS abnormalities

- Structural: head circumference <10th percentile or abnormal brain structure on neuroimaging

- Neurodevelopmental (neurological, cognitive or developmental impairments)

Dysmorphic Features

- Microphthalmia, short palpebral fissures, or both

- Poorly developed philtrum

- Thin upper lip

- Flattening of the maxillary area

Most children with FAS are mildly or moderately retarded, with mean IQ scores of 65 to 70, but intellectual ability varies widely. In families with several affected siblings, the youngest child is usually the most cognitively impaired. Learning disabilities—in particular, difficulty with arithmetic, speech delay, and hyperactivity—are commonly observed.

Less severe alcohol-related effects, termed *fetal alcohol effects*, are associated with different patterns of drinking and lack the typical facial dysmorphology seen with FAS. Fetal alcohol effects are probably a low point on the continuum of alcohol effects on the fetus. Maternal alcohol abuse increases the risk of spontaneous abortions, infant mortality, intrauterine growth retardation, and prematurity. Birth defects are common; congenital anomalies occur in about a third of infants born to heavy drinkers, compared with 9% of minor anomalies in infants of women who abstain from alcohol. Decreasing alcohol intake during pregnancy is beneficial to offspring, reducing the frequency of growth retardation and dysmorphic features. Heavy alcohol exposure prenatally, but not mild or moderate exposure, has been linked to lower IQ scores, hyperactive behavior, attention problems, learning difficulty, and speech disorders. Neuroimaging abnormalities are common among alcohol-exposed infants and commonly include volume loss/microcephaly and developmental anomalies of cerebellum or corpus callosum (agenesis, hypoplasia). Neuroimaging abnormalities correlate with neurocognitive impairments.

POSTNATAL ALCOHOL EXPOSURE

Alcohol transferred through breast milk impairs motor development but not mental development at age 1 year. Ingestion of alcohol by children may lead to hypoglycemic seizures.

WITHDRAWAL SYNDROME

Infants born to women who drink large amounts of alcohol during pregnancy may rarely exhibit signs of withdrawal. Restlessness, agitation, tremulousness, opisthotonus, and seizures are seen shortly after birth and disappear within a few days.

PRENATAL COCAINE EXPOSURE

Although the cocaine epidemic has abated, cocaine is still one of the most frequent hard drugs of abuse in urban centers, whereas methamphetamine is the preferred substance of abuse in rural settings (with effects similar to those of cocaine).

Cocaine use during pregnancy has been linked to spontaneous abortion, abruptio placentae, stillbirth, and premature delivery. These events may immediately follow a large intake of cocaine and are attributed to drug-induced vasoconstriction of intrauterine vessels. Women who use cocaine tend to resort to prostitution, increasing risks for syphilis and HIV. They also tend to lack prenatal care, adding to the risks of infant death, low birth weight, and prematurity.

Low birth weight and intrauterine growth retardation are common among cocaine-exposed infants. Fetal brain growth is impaired independently of birth weight or gestational age. Sudden infant death syndrome (SIDS) has also been linked to cocaine exposure in utero. In addition to any specific cocaine-related effects, offspring are at increased risk because of polydrug exposure, as cocaine is rarely the only drug used.

NEUROBEHAVIOR

State regulation difficulties are well described among cocaine-exposed newborns. Findings vary from irritability and excitability to decreased organizational response and interactive behavior, even if the exposure to cocaine was limited to the first trimester of pregnancy. Modulation of attention is impaired among cocaine-exposed infants who, unlike unexposed infants, prefer higher rates of stimuli when in a high level of arousal. Infant processing abilities, as reflected by looking time at novel stimuli, are also affected by prenatal cocaine exposure. Exposed infants show motor and movement abnormalities, including excessive tremor and hypertonia. Dose–response effects of cocaine on state regulation and neurologic findings that tend to be transient are reported in newborns and infants. Some studies show no neurobehavioral effects, however.

STROKES

Experimentally, cocaine and its main metabolite, benzoylecgonine, cause vasoconstriction of fetal cerebral vessels. Neonatal stroke and porencephaly have been associated with prenatal cocaine exposure. Some cases may be related to other neonatal stroke risk factors that accompany fetal cocaine exposure, such as abruptio placentae or birth asphyxia. Intraventricular hemorrhage is observed among infants more heavily exposed to cocaine.

SEIZURES

Focal seizures may occur in cocaine-exposed newborns with strokes. EEGs in cocaine-exposed infants show bursts of sharp waves and spikes that are often multifocal. These findings do not correlate with clinical seizures or neurologic abnormalities and may disappear in 3 to 12 months. Cocaine-exposed premature infants are at increased risk of neonatal seizures. Seizures are rare if there is no stroke.

MALFORMATIONS

Prenatal cocaine exposure has been linked with urogenital malformations, limb reduction deformities, and intestinal atresia and infarction. Agenesis of the corpus callosum and septo-optic dysplasia has also been noted. These teratogenic effects may result from cocaine-induced vasoconstriction and fetal vascular disruption in early organogenesis.

NEURODEVELOPMENTAL IMPACT

In experiment models, prenatal cocaine has been reported to affect serotonin, norepinephrine, dopaminergic, and GABA systems. Lower CSF levels of homovanillic acid found in human newborns exposed to cocaine suggest dopaminergic involvement. In infancy, there may be a high incidence of global hypertonia that resolves prior to age 24 months (Table 147.4). Many studies in toddlers and school-aged children have failed to show that prenatal cocaine exposure adversely affects cognition, except as mediated through cocaine effects on brain growth. Cocaine-exposed children seem to suffer from language delays and an excess of neurobehavioral abnormalities, including irritability, impaired attention, inhibitory control, impulsivity, and aggressive behavior. Early neurobehavior involving orientation and irritability tend to improve over the first 2 years of life. Heavy prenatal cocaine exposure has been associated with delinquent behavior in both genders at older ages.

COCAINE EXPOSURE IN CHILDHOOD

Passive intoxication with cocaine may be caused by breastfeeding or passive inhalation of free-base cocaine (crack). Seizures are the chief manifestation of symptomatic intoxication, but intoxication may be unsuspected. Urine toxicology screening is used to detect

TABLE 147.4	Neurologic Fetal Cocaine Effects and Associations

Neonatal Period

Microcephaly

Vascular abnormalities

Stroke

Porencephaly

Intraventricular hemorrhage

Seizures

Symptomatic (secondary to vascular complications)

Primary (owing to cocaine or its metabolites)

Brain malformations

Agenesis of corpus callosum

Septo-optic dysplasia

Skull defects

Encephalocele

Abnormal neurobehavior

Impaired organizational state

Depressed sensorium

Hypertonia

Coarse tremor

Irritability/excitable state

Infancy and Childhood

Neurologic

Hypertonia in infancy

Developmental

Language delays

Semantic delays

Behavioral

Inattentiveness

Temperamental differences

Impulsivity

Aggressive or delinquent behavior

illicit substances in evaluating seizures in infants and children, regardless of socioeconomic status.

WITHDRAWAL SYMPTOMS

There is no evidence of a cocaine-induced withdrawal syndrome. Even with remote prenatal cocaine exposure, cocaine-exposed infants may show hypertonicity and tremor, which are probably manifestations of a transient embryopathy resulting from cocaine-related perturbations.

PRENATAL OPIATE EXPOSURE

Cheap and abundant supplies of heroin are fueling a nationwide epidemic of late, especially in urban centers. Prospective studies, however, on the developmental impact of prenatal heroin exposure are sparse. Methadone, on account of its controlled administration,

has been more extensively studied. The main risk factor linked to developmental effects and lower IQ scores is the presence of neonatal withdrawal syndrome.

WITHDRAWAL SYMPTOMS

A neonatal withdrawal syndrome is well described in infants born to opiate-dependent mothers (Table 147.5). It is characterized by signs and symptoms of central nervous system hyperirritability, gastrointestinal dysfunction, respiratory distress, and autonomic disturbances. CNS signs and symptoms consist of hypertonicity, tremor, hyperreflexia, irritability, sleep disturbances, feeding difficulties, and occasionally seizures. Onset of neonatal withdrawal from heroin usually begins within 24 hours of birth, withdrawal from methadone usually starts around 24 to 72 hours of age, and withdrawal to buprenorphine starts at around 40 hours and peaks in severity at 70 hours of age. The neonatal withdrawal syndrome associated with methadone is more severe and occurs more often (84%) than that described with buprenorphine (60%). For both opioids, signs of withdrawal may be delayed in onset until 5 to 7 days of age or later. Among neonates acutely withdrawing from opioids, seizures are observed in 2% to 11% and EEG abnormalities without evidence of seizures in over 30%. Mild withdrawal does not require treatment, other than swaddling and a quiet room, but symptomatic infants are likely to require pharmacologic intervention. The two most popular agents used to treat withdrawal are paregoric (camphorated tincture of opium) and phenobarbital. Of the two, paregoric is more physiologic because it substitutes for the substance causing withdrawal but is only effective for opiate withdrawal. Other opiates studied include morphine and buprenorphine. For suspected polydrug exposure, phenobarbital may be preferable.

The most widespread scale in use to assess the severity of withdrawal syndrome is that developed by Finnegan: It assesses 21 signs in three domains: CNS, gastrointestinal, and autonomic/sleep/respiratory. Assessments are recommended every 2 to 4 hours after birth, and treatment is suggested for withdrawal scores 8 or higher.

TABLE 147.5	Opiate Withdrawal Syndrome

Central Nervous System

- Jitteriness/tremors
- Irritability
- Hypertonia
- High-pitch cry
- Generalized convulsions

Autonomic

- Fever
- Nasal stuffiness
- Mottling of skin
- Sweating
- Tachypnea

Gastrointestinal

- Vomiting
- Diarrhea
- Poor feeding

Paregoric or phenobarbital is then titrated according to the severity of withdrawal score. There is no agreed upon standard treatment protocol to manage neonatal abstinence. When using phenobarbital, one can choose to load (15 mg/kg) prior to titrating maintenance (5 to 8 mg/kg) dose. Paregoric doses may start at 0.2 mL q3h and titrate by 0.05 mL according to withdrawal score. Tapering of the dose may commence by the end of the second week as tolerated.

SUGGESTED READINGS

Behnke M, Smith VC; Committee on Substance Abuse. Prenatal substance abuse: short- and long-term effects on the exposed fetus. *Pediatrics.* 2013;131:e1009.

Centers for Disease Control and Prevention. Achievements in public health: reduction in perinatal transmission of HIV infection—United States, 1985–2005. *MMWR Morb Mortal Wkly Rep.* 2006;55:592–597.

Chiriboga CA, Fleishman S, Champion S, et al. Incidence and prevalence of HIV encephalopathy in children with HIV infection receiving highly active anti-retroviral treatment (HAART). *J Pediatr.* 2005;146(3):402–407.

Ernst TM, Chang L, Witt MD, et al. Cerebral toxoplasmosis and lymphoma in AIDS: perfusion MR imaging experience in 13 patients. *Radiology.* 1998;208(3):663–669.

George R, Andronikou S, du Plessis J, et al. Central nervous system manifestations of HIV infection in children. *Pediatr Radiol.* 2009;39(6):575–585.

Hudak ML, Tan RC; Committee on Drugs and the Committee on the Fetus and Newborn. Neonatal drug withdrawal. *Pediatrics.* 2012;129:e540–e560.

Ismail S, Buckley S, Budacki R, et al. Screening, diagnosing and prevention of fetal alcohol syndrome: is this syndrome treatable? *Dev Neurosci.* 2010;32(2):91–100.

Lebel C, Roussotte F, Sowell ER. Imaging the impact of prenatal alcohol exposure on the structure of the developing human brain. *Neuropsychol Rev.* 2011;(2):102–118.

Manabe YC, Campbell JD, Sydnor E, et al. Immune reconstitution inflammatory syndrome: risk factors and treatment implications. *J Acquir Immune Defic Syndr.* 2007;46(4):456–462.

Mazzoni, P, Chiriboga CA, Millar WS, et al. Intracerebral aneurysms in human immunodeficiency virus infection: case report and literature review. *Pediatr Neurol.* 2000;23:252–255.

Panel on Treatment of HIV-Infected Pregnant Women and Prevention of Perinatal Transmission. Recommendations for use of antiretroviral drugs in pregnant HIV-1 infected women for maternal health and interventions to reduce perinatal HIV transmission in the United States. Available at http://aidsinfo .nih.gov/contentfiles/lvguidelineslvguidelines/PerinatalGL.pdf. Accessed May 30, 2015.

Selik RM, Mokotoff, ED, Branson B, et al. Revised surveillance case definition for HIV infection—United States, 2014. *MMWR Morb Mortal Wkly Rep.* 2014;63:1–10.

Siberry GK, Abzug MJ, Nachman S, et al. Guidelines for the prevention and treatment of opportunistic infections in HIV-exposed and HIV-infected children: recommendations from the National Institutes of Health, Centers for Disease Control and Prevention, the HIV Medicine Association of the Infectious Diseases Society of America, the Pediatric Infectious Diseases Society, and the American Academy of Pediatrics. *Pediatr Infect Dis J.* 2013;32(suppl 2):i–KK4.

Psychosis 148

Jacob S. Ballon and T. Scott Stroup

INTRODUCTION

Psychosis is characterized as a detachment from reality, often including hallucinations or delusions. Psychotic symptoms are a core feature of schizophrenia but may also be seen in other serious psychiatric disorders including bipolar disorder, major depressive disorder, and posttraumatic stress disorder (PTSD). Importantly, psychosis may also be a prominent symptom in many neurologic disorders, other medical conditions, substance intoxications, and withdrawal syndromes. New-onset psychosis should prompt a thorough workup to determine the etiology of such symptoms.

Psychotic experiences can be characterized as phenomena in which sensory experiences are generated by aberrant brain stimuli rather than external inputs. Hallucinations can be auditory (e.g., hearing voices), visual (seeing objects that are not there), or can occur in other sensory domains, although olfactory, tactile, and gustatory hallucinations are less typical of psychiatric illness. Hallucinations can be differentiated from illusions by having no basis in reality, whereas illusions are misperceptions of natural sensations. Delusions are fixed, false beliefs that persist in spite of contradictory evidence. Often, delusions are paranoid (e.g., a feeling of being watched or followed) or grandiose (e.g., possessing special powers or relationships with powerful people). Hallucinations and delusions must be considered within the relevant cultural context.

The lifetime prevalence of psychosis is between 3% and 5% in the general population. Most cases of psychosis are due to causes other than schizophrenia. The majority of nonschizophrenia psychosis is seen in drug-induced psychosis, mood disorders, and general medical causes.

SCHIZOPHRENIA AND OTHER PSYCHOTIC DISORDERS

EPIDEMIOLOGY

Globally, estimates suggest that almost 1% of the population will develop schizophrenia in their lifetime. The typical age of onset of schizophrenia is the late teens or early 20s, with men diagnosed on average a few years younger than women. Most people who develop schizophrenia have a prodromal period of illness before they meet the threshold for diagnosis characterized by subthreshold psychotic symptoms in conjunction with declines in social and occupational functioning. Schizophrenia typically follows a relapsing and remitting course characterized by periods of stability with episodic exacerbations of symptoms. Although antipsychotic medications are efficacious in reducing psychotic symptoms, many individuals may still have symptoms despite usual treatment.

NEUROBIOLOGY

Scientists debate whether schizophrenia is a degenerative brain disease, neurodevelopmental disease, or a combination of both. Several studies have shown that there are neuroanatomic differences in ventricle size, cortical thickness, gray and white matter, and overall brain volume in people with schizophrenia. Supporting neurodevelopmental hypotheses, neuroanatomic differences are seen before the onset of psychosis. However, favoring degenerative hypotheses, these differences increase over the course of illness. Further, although many studies have shown that cognitive decline predates the onset of psychosis, there is some evidence that cognitive deficits worsen over time. It is difficult to isolate a specific degenerative impact of schizophrenia itself apart from other environmental factors such as chronic exposure to antipsychotic drugs.

Much work has been done to isolate the specific neurotransmitter systems responsible for psychosis and schizophrenia. Although no single system is responsible for the overall psychotic phenotype, several have been shown to contribute to the development of symptoms. Dopamine is often most closely associated with psychosis and all currently marketed antipsychotic drugs are dopamine D2 antagonists but those drugs do not address all facets of the illness. Other neurotransmitters implicated include serotonin, glutamate, and acetylcholine.

CLINICAL FEATURES AND DIFFERENTIAL DIAGNOSIS

Schizophrenia is a serious mental illness responsible for significant morbidity, diminished quality of life, loss of productivity, and premature mortality. There is a 5% to 10% risk of suicide, and schizophrenia is a leading cause of disability throughout the world. Symptoms of schizophrenia can be categorized into positive, negative, and cognitive domains. Positive symptoms refer to delusions, hallucinations, and disorganized speech or behavior. Negative symptoms include apathy and avolition and generally refer to deficits in functioning. Cognitive symptoms affect multiple domains including primarily executive functioning, verbal learning, and working memory.

Although schizophrenia cannot be diagnosed until psychosis has been present for at least 1 month, nonspecific symptoms have been seen from early childhood in people who later develop schizophrenia. For example, young children who go on to develop schizophrenia have increased incidence of deficits in motor skills compared to children who do not develop schizophrenia or other psychiatric disorders.

The *Diagnostic and Statistical Manual of Mental Disorders*, 5th edition (*DSM-5*), which was released in 2013, modified the criteria for psychotic disorders (Fig. 148.1). A schizophrenia diagnosis requires at least two out of five symptoms including hallucinations,

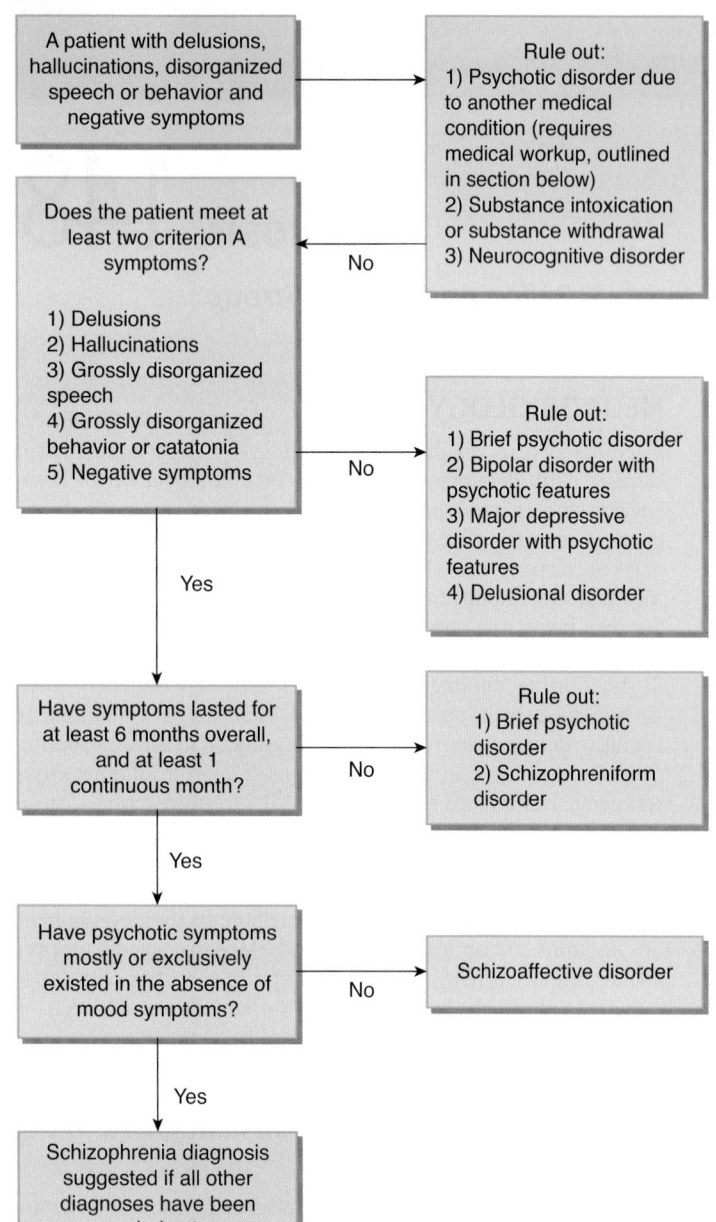

FIGURE 148.1 Diagnostic algorithm for a patient with psychotic symptoms. (Based on American Psychiatric Association. *Diagnostic and Statistical Manual of Mental Disorders.* 5th ed. Washington, DC: American Psychiatric Association; 2013.)

delusions, disorganized speech, disorganized behavior, or negative symptoms for at least 1 month and with an overall duration of illness of at least 6 months. New in *DSM-5* is a requirement for hallucinations, delusions, or disorganized speech; only having disorganized behavior and negative symptoms does not meet the new criteria. If mood symptoms are present, a timeline is essential to determining the correct diagnosis. If there are concurrent mood symptoms along with the hallucinations or delusions, the criteria for schizoaffective disorder are met if the psychotic symptoms persist for at least 2 weeks in the absence of mood symptoms and if the mood symptoms are present for the majority of the entire illness. If the psychotic symptoms occur only in the context of a mood disorder (bipolar disorder or major depressive disorder), then the diagnosis is bipolar disorder or major depressive disorder with psychotic features. If the only psychotic symptom is a delusion, then the diagnosis may be delusional disorder, particularly if there is limited functional impairment. Catatonia is a constellation of

psychomotor features that may include stupor, posturing, mutism, stereotypy, and other odd mannerisms. Catatonia is often associated with schizophrenia but can be present in most other serious mental illnesses. Catatonia is included in the *DSM-5* as a specifier for several mental disorders and is seen in approximately 10% of patients hospitalized with schizophrenia.

Psychotic symptoms frequently occur in other psychiatric disorders. Up to 60% of people with bipolar disorder have a history of at least one psychotic symptom, and psychosis is seen in up to 50% of manic episodes. Psychosis may also be present in depression, especially when it is severe. Overall, people with depression are three times more likely to have hallucinations and nine times more likely to have delusions compared to those without depression. Up to 15% of people with schizophrenia have comorbid obsessive–compulsive symptoms. People with social phobia and general anxiety also have an increased incidence of psychosis. Data from the National Comorbidity Survey suggests that psychosis should lead to a separate subtype categorization of PTSD and a subtype of "with dissociative symptoms" was added to *DSM-5*. Substance abuse and schizophrenia frequently co-occur, with rates of substance use disorders as high as 70% in people with schizophrenia. In a large European study of first-episode schizophrenia, already 31.1% of patients reported a comorbid substance use disorder, including 22.2% who used marijuana. Comorbid substance use is associated with poorer medication adherence, more hospitalizations, and overall worse functional outcomes, with the worst effects seen in heavy substance users.

SCHIZOPHRENIA-SPECTRUM CASE

A 21-year-old male collegian is brought to the student health service by his resident advisor (RA). The RA notes that over the past several months, the student has withdrawn from fellow students and stopped participating in dormitory activities. His grades have suffered, and he was caught smoking marijuana in his room. He recently began putting tape over the cameras in the computer lab and foil over the windows of his room. When asked about these behaviors, the student said that the Central Intelligence Agency (CIA) was tracking his movements through a vast network of computers. He spent several nights sleeping in the library or in a local 24-hour coffee shop to avoid detection. He believed that the CIA considered him to have special knowledge of operations within the government. The student believed that everyone knew about him because the CIA had put up a website about him. He said that he could hear agents and other people talking to him through the walls of his room, commenting on his behaviors, and telling him that he was stupid. His sleep was poor and he was using marijuana to help sleep and to manage his anxiety.

TREATMENT/OUTCOME

Antipsychotic Medication

The mainstay of treatment for schizophrenia and other psychotic disorders is antipsychotic medication. Antipsychotics reduce psychotic symptoms and reduce relapse rates [**Level 1**].[1] All currently available antipsychotic medications antagonize dopamine D2 receptors in the brain, which is thought to be their primary mechanism of action. Historically, antipsychotic medications have been categorized based on their potency at the D2 receptor into high-potency and low-potency categories. Antipsychotics also affect other neurotransmitters including serotonergic, histaminergic, and adrenergic receptors. Effects on the various neurotransmitters determine therapeutic and adverse effects.

All antipsychotic drugs are capable of inducing neurologic side effects including abnormal involuntary movements known as *tardive dyskinesia* (TD), *akathisia* (restlessness), *dystonia*, and *pseudoparkinsonism* (tremor, rigidity, and bradykinesia) (Table 148.1). By definition, TD is associated with prolonged (at least 3 months) exposure to an antipsychotic agent. Increased age, female gender, and duration of exposure are the greatest risk factors for TD. Newer (or second-generation) antipsychotics tend to have lower risk of TD but risk varies according to individual drug characteristics, as well as dose and duration of exposure. Drugs with lower potency at the D2 receptor tend to be associated with more adverse metabolic side effects (weight gain, diabetes, dyslipidemia), whereas those with higher potency are more likely to cause neurologic side effects. Severe dystonias, especially those involving laryngeal or extraocular muscles, require emergency treatment with intramuscular diphenhydramine (50 mg) or benztropine (2 mg). Oral benztropine (1 to 4 mg daily) is effective for treatment

of antipsychotic-induced tremors, and propranolol (30 to 90 mg daily) is often used for treatment of akathisia.

Metabolic side effects are closely associated with many antipsychotic treatments, in particular clozapine, olanzapine, quetiapine, and risperidone. The mechanism by which antipsychotics cause these effects is not conclusively known. Schizophrenia has long been associated, even before the introduction of antipsychotic medications, with increased rates of diabetes and obesity compared the general population. Clozapine, olanzapine, and quetiapine are potent antihistaminergic agents and thus are associated with drowsiness and central histamine H1 receptor activity, which may contribute to their risk of weight gain. Other theories regarding the metabolic effects focus on shared signaling pathways between insulin regulation and psychosis involving the kinase *AKT1* in the brain, pancreas, and liver. Peripheral response to antipsychotic drugs may feedback to the brain in a way that alters insulin secretion, which may have effects on weight. Although diabetes may often result from the central adiposity associated with antipsychotics, there are likely multiple pathways responsible for these metabolic effects, as people may develop insulin resistance and diabetes in the absence of weight gain and vice versa.

A dangerous but rare side effect of antipsychotic drugs is neuroleptic malignant syndrome (NMS). NMS is characterized by tremors, muscle rigidity and myalgias, extreme fever, other autonomic instability, and altered mental status. The muscle rigidity ultimately leads to rhabdomyolysis, with increased creatine kinase (CK) and white blood cell counts. The resultant muscle breakdown products can lead to acute renal failure. Without rapid and intensive intervention, NMS can be fatal and is in nearly 10% of cases. Treatment of NMS focuses on stopping the antipsychotic immediately, cooling the hyperthermia rapidly, and protecting the kidneys from myoglobinemia through aggressive hydration.

Antipsychotics differ mainly in side effects, but some small to moderate differences in efficacy have also been detected. All three of the medicines with better efficacy that are available in the United States (clozapine, olanzapine, and risperidone) are associated with adverse metabolic effects. This finding leads to a clinical dilemma in which clinicians and patients must balance the opportunity for maximum symptom improvement with significant metabolic risk.

Clozapine has a special role because it is more efficacious than other antipsychotics in patients with treatment-resistant schizophrenia and has been shown to decrease suicidality and to cause the fewest abnormal involuntary movements. However, in addition to weight gain and significant metabolic side effects, clozapine is also associated with agranulocytosis and subsequent risk of death due to infection. Therefore, patients taking clozapine must be enrolled in a clozapine registry and monitored carefully for decreases in granulocyte counts. Other risks of clozapine include myocarditis and seizures. However, with close clinical monitoring, clozapine can be highly effective for many patients.

Nonpharmacologic Treatment

Nonpharmacologic treatments for schizophrenia that are supported by some evidence include repetitive transcranial magnetic stimulation (rTMS) for auditory hallucinations that do not respond to antipsychotic medications [**Level 1**].[1] Several psychosocial treatments are effective for specific problems associated with persistent psychotic illnesses. For example, multidisciplinary teams known as *Assertive Community Treatment* (ACT) teams provide outreach and comprehensive care, which reduces rates of hospitalization [**Level 1**].[2] Supported employment programs are effective in helping people with schizophrenia obtain jobs [**Level 1**].[2]

TABLE 148.1 Selected Information on Commonly Used Antipsychotics

Antipsychotic Medication	Haloperidol	Aripiprazole	Clozapine	Olanzapine	Paliperidone	Quetiapine	Risperidone	Ziprasidone	Lurasidone
Typical dose range for maintenance treatment of schizophrenia	Oral: 2–12 mg	Oral: 10–30 mg	Oral: 150–600 mg	Oral: 10–30 mg	Oral: 6–12 mg	Oral: 300–800 mg	Oral: 2–8 mg	Oral: 80–160 mg	Oral: 40–80 mg
Side Effect Risk									
Akathisia/parkinsonism	+++	+	0/+	+	++	0/+	++	+	++
QT prolongation on ECG	+	+	+	+	+	+	+	++	0
Glucose abnormalities	+	+	+++	+++	+	++	+	0/+	+
Lipid abnormalities	+	+	+++	+++	++	++	++	0/+	+
Orthostatic hypotension	0/+	0/+	+++	++	++	++	++	+	0
Weight gain	0/+	+	+++	+++	++	++	++	0/+	0/+
Serum prolactin elevation	++	0	0	+	+++	0/+	+++	+	+
Sedation	+	+	+++	++	+	++	+	+	+

0, no or minimal risk; +, low risk/mild effects; ++, medium risk/moderate effects; +++, high risk/severe effects; ECG, electrocardiogram.

Data from Stroup TS, Lawrence R, Abbas AI, et al. Schizophrenia spectrum and other psychotic disorders. In: Hales RE, Yudofsky SC, Roberts LW, eds. *The American Psychiatric Publishing Textbook of Psychiatry*. 6th ed. Washington, DC: American Psychiatric Publishing; 2014:173–206; and Buchanan RW, Kreyenbuhl J, Kelly DL, et al. The 2009 schizophrenia PORT psychopharmacological treatment recommendations and summary statements. *Schizophr Bull*. 2010;36(1):71–93.

OTHER CAUSES OF PSYCHOSIS

When a patient presents with psychosis for the first time, it is important to remember that psychotic symptoms are associated with numerous brain conditions and the cause may not always be identifiable. A thorough workup should be conducted to make sure that potentially reversible causes of psychosis are ruled out (Table 148.2).

The workup for reversible causes of psychosis should start broadly and then focus more narrowly according to the specific presentation. Laboratory tests are used to investigate possible metabolic or nutritional abnormalities, signs of infection/inflammation, and autoimmune processes. Neuroimaging may be indicated, particularly if there are focal neurologic deficits or an acute personality change. Lumbar puncture (LP) and electroencephalogram may also be part of a workup when associated symptoms suggest the possibility of infection.

Delirium is a common cause of psychosis and should be suspected in any patient with acute psychosis, particularly those who are older than typical first-episode psychosis patients (Table 148.3). Although the definitive intervention for delirium is treatment of the underlying medical condition, there are important steps to take while the underlying cause is sought and treated. The first step is to ensure the patient's physical safety. Efforts to normalize the sleep–wake cycle should be a priority. Frequent reminders of location, time, and situation are helpful to reorient patients to their surroundings. Medications that cause or exacerbate delirium,

TABLE 148.2	**Suggested Medical Workup for Psychosis**

In all patients:

- Complete blood count (CBC)
- Glucose, chemistries, liver function tests
- Thyroid-stimulating hormone (TSH)
- Vitamin B_{12} and folate
- Urinalysis
- Urine drug screen
- HIV test

Secondary testing to be done as clinically indicated:

- Brain imaging with CT or MRI
- Electroencephalogram
- Lumbar puncture
- Chest radiography
- Blood and urine cultures
- Arterial blood gases
- Serum cortisol levels
- Antinuclear antibodies (to test for autoimmune disorders such as systemic lupus erythematosus)
- Ceruloplasmin (to test for Wilson disease)
- Rapid plasma reagin (to test for syphilis)
- Toxin search/drug levels

CT, computed tomography; MRI, magnetic resonance imaging.
Based on Freudenreich O, Schulz SC, Goff DC. Initial medical work-up of first-episode psychosis: a conceptual review. *Early Interv Psychiatry*. 2009;3(1):10–18.

TABLE 148.3	**Medical Conditions that Can Present with Psychosis**

Delirium
Dementia/neurodegenerative disorders
Neoplasms
Seizures
Intoxications/medications
HIV/AIDS/other infections
Autoimmune/limbic encephalitis
Systemic lupus erythematosus
Neurovascular events
Leukodystrophies
Endocrine disorders
Mitochondrial disorders

including anticholinergic agents, should be avoided as much as possible. Benzodiazepines should also be avoided in nonalcoholic delirium. Antipsychotic medications can be useful in symptomatic treatment of delirium and associated psychosis. Antipsychotics have been shown to shorten the duration of delirium episodes with similar efficacy seen across multiple agents.

Psychosis is associated with drug intoxication and withdrawal states. In severe alcohol and benzodiazepine withdrawal, patients may experience delirium tremens (DTs), which is fatal in approximately 1% of cases. This is characterized by autonomic instability, hallucinations, and agitation. Benzodiazepines (e.g., lorazepam 2 mg every 2 hours as needed) are the mainstay of treatment for significant alcohol withdrawal and DTs [**Level 1**].[3] Many drug intoxications can yield psychotic symptoms. Cannabis, particularly as it has become more potent in recent years, often causes a transient psychotic state characterized mostly by paranoia. Sympathomimetic drugs, such as amphetamine or methamphetamine, can cause paranoia and hallucinations with acute and chronic use. N-methyl-D-aspartate (NMDA) antagonists such as PCP and ketamine are also associated with auditory hallucinations, paranoia, and negative symptoms. These drugs, as well as amphetamines, are often used in animal models of schizophrenia because of the similarity in presentation to schizophrenia. Tactile hallucinations are often seen with amphetamines and cocaine.

Psychosis is also common in major neurocognitive disorders such as dementias. Patients with dementia often report paranoid delusions or feelings that people are stealing from them. In dementia with Lewy bodies (DLB), many patients report delusions and visual hallucinations (including "lilliputian hallucinations" of little people/animals) and develop pseudoparkinsonism even with low doses of antipsychotics. Antipsychotics can be helpful in treating these psychotic symptoms and can help reduce dementia-related agitation but should be used with caution and in low dosages. In many circumstances, cholinesterase inhibitors are effective and should be considered first in DLB. If using antipsychotics in treating patients with DLB, quetiapine, at low doses (e.g., 25 to 50 mg daily), is a good first choice. Clozapine (e.g., 25 to 50 mg daily) is a second choice if quetiapine is not effective. Dementia is not an U.S. Food and Drug Administration (FDA)–approved indication for antipsychotics, and all antipsychotics carry a black box warning for this use because of an increased risk of mortality for elderly dementia patients. The possible benefits of antipsychotics in reducing psychosis or agitation must be weighed against the small but significant risk of increased mortality as well as the other adverse effects of antipsychotics. Importantly, if an antipsychotic is used for a patient with dementia, it should be discontinued unless there are clear benefits.

Because brain tumors can have many psychiatric manifestations, including psychosis, the workup for new-onset psychotic symptoms should include neuroimaging. Although rare, the presence of other focal neurologic findings should raise the index of suspicion for psychosis secondary to a brain lesion. Peripheral tumors including small cell lung cancer (and resultant paraneoplastic syndrome), steroid-producing hormones such as adrenal tumors (Cushing disease), and pheochromocytoma may also cause psychosis. Another rare cause of psychosis is autoantibodies to the NMDA receptor. These antibodies, most often seen in young women, often derive from ovarian teratomas or other tumors; surgical removal of the tumors may resolve the symptoms. Immunotherapy (e.g., steroids, intravenous immunoglobulins, and plasmapheresis) can also be used to treat the psychosis and associated symptoms with good effect.

Seizures may also cause psychotic symptoms, and the presence of other seizure sequelae, such as auras or postictal periods, should prompt testing in that domain including electroencephalogram. Psychosis may occur intraictally or postictally. Temporal lobe epilepsy is classically associated with psychotic symptoms including déjà vu (a sense of reexperiencing something that is novel), fear without identifiable cause, or olfactory hallucinations. Treatment of epileptic-related psychosis can be complicated because antipsychotic medications can lower the seizure threshold. However, this effect is generally not clinically significant except in the case of clozapine (e.g., at doses $\geq$600 mg daily or when blood levels rise rapidly). Some antiepileptic drugs (AEDs) including levetiracetam, vigabatrin, and topiramate can worsen psychosis. In addition, carbamazepine induces antipsychotic drug metabolism and may lead to decreased blood levels, resulting in the emergence of psychotic symptoms. On the other hand, valproic acid (e.g., 500 to 1,500 mg daily) is commonly used off-label as adjunctive agent to potentiate the initial efficacy of antipsychotic drugs in the treatment of schizophrenia, although the efficacy of this strategy is uncertain. Ultimately, if antipsychotics are indicated in someone with a seizure disorder, then the choice of drug depends largely on tolerance for side effects and drug–drug interactions.

Several infections can cause psychotic symptoms. Infections that yield brain lesions, such as neurocysticercosis or other fungal infections, seen as ring-enhancing lesions on magnetic resonance imaging (MRI), can cause both seizure activity and associated psychosis. Up to 15% of HIV patients may experience psychotic symptoms generally through opportunistic infections, HIV-associated neoplasms, or HIV-associated delirium/dementia. More commonly, HIV is associated with psychotic symptoms, both through progression of the illness or through drug interactions with antiretroviral therapy or from highly active antiretroviral therapy (HAART) medications themselves. Other infections sometimes associated with psychosis include Lyme disease, herpes, and neurosyphilis. Herpes encephalitis, the most common sporadic viral encephalitis in the United States, requires immediate attention because there is a high risk of mortality if not treated promptly. Acyclovir (30 mg/kg/day) should be started while waiting for the results of LP and imaging studies.

Many medications are associated with psychosis. Steroids are most commonly implicated in causing psychotic symptoms and can also cause other significant emotional side effects including depression and anxiety. Treatment of Parkinson disease is often complicated by psychosis when using prodopaminergic agents. Low doses of quetiapine (25 to 50 mg daily) or clozapine (25 to 50 mg daily), which have a relatively low risk of pseudoparkinsonism, are recommended for treating psychotic symptoms in patients with Parkinson disease. Psychoactive medications including sympathomimetic agents, opioids, and benzodiazepines can cause psychosis, particularly in high dosages. Psychosis has also been reported to be associated with antibiotics, antimalarials (particularly mefloquine), antituberculous drugs, and muscle relaxants.

DELIRIUM WITH PSYCHOSIS CASE

A 73-year-old man is admitted to orthopedic surgery for surgical repair of his left hip. On postoperative day 2, nurses report that he is agitated and complaining that he sees a "crippled equestrian" near the air conditioning vent. Nurses also report that he was awake much of the night and sleeping during the day. He was given lorazepam last night to help him sleep, but the report from nursing staff is that it made him agitated, and he needed to be placed on 1:1 observation because he did not sleep and tried to get out of bed unsafely. He's been picking at his bed sheets and nearly pulled out his intravenous (IV) line. When you see him at the bedside, he says that the year is 1968 and he is at a racetrack. His vital signs show a low-grade fever and tachycardia, and his complete blood count (CBC) shows a mildly elevated white count.

CONCLUSION

Psychosis presents in many psychiatric and other medical conditions and is generally a sign of a severe underlying problem. Not all cases of psychosis are due to a primary psychotic disorder such as schizophrenia, and many represent urgent medical problems. This is particularly important in older patients and in cases that do not otherwise fit the typical pattern of schizophrenia onset. A broad differential should be considered to identify reversible and potentially progressive causes of psychosis. Prompt, appropriate treatment will lead to improved outcomes.

LEVEL 1 EVIDENCE

1. Buchanan RW, Kreyenbuhl J, Kelly DL, et al. The 2009 schizophrenia PORT psychopharmacological treatment recommendations and summary statements. *Schizophr Bull.* 2010;36(1):71–93.
2. Dixon LB, Dickerson F, Bellack AS, et al. The 2009 schizophrenia PORT psychosocial treatment recommendations and summary statements. *Schizophr Bull.* 2010;36(1):48–70.
3. Awissi DK, Lebrun G, Coursin DB, et al. Alcohol withdrawal and delirium tremens in the critically ill: a systematic review and commentary. *Intensive Care Med.* 2013;39(1):16–30.

SUGGESTED READINGS

Achim AM, Maziade M, Raymond E, et al. How prevalent are anxiety disorders in schizophrenia? A meta-analysis and critical review on a significant association. *Schizophr Bull.* 2011;37(4):811–821.

Adachi N, Kanemoto K, Toffol B, et al. Basic treatment principles for psychotic disorders in patients with epilepsy. *Epilepsia.* 2013;54(suppl 1):19–33.

Addington J, Heinssen R. Prediction and prevention of psychosis in youth at clinical high risk. *Annu Rev Clin Psychol.* 2012;8(1):269–289.

Allison DB, Mentore JL, Heo M, et al. Antipsychotic-induced weight gain: a comprehensive research synthesis. *Am J Psychiatry.* 1999;156(11):1686–1696.

American Psychiatric Association. *Diagnostic and Statistical Manual of Mental Disorders.* 5th ed. Washington, DC: American Psychiatric Association; 2013.

American Psychiatric Association. Practice guideline for the treatment of patients with HIV/AIDS. Work Group on HIV/AIDS. *Am J Psychiatry.* 2000;157(11)(suppl):1–62.

Ballard C, Aarsland D, Francis P, et al. Neuropsychiatric symptoms in patients with dementias associated with cortical Lewy bodies: pathophysiology, clinical features, and pharmacological management. *Drugs Aging.* 2013; 30(8):603–611.

Ballon J, Stroup TS. Polypharmacy for schizophrenia. *Curr Opin Psychiatry.* 2013;26(2):208–213.

Bartolommei N, Lattanzi L, Callari A, et al. Catatonia: a critical review and therapeutic recommendations. *J Psychopathol.* 2012;18:234–246.

Bleakley S. Identifying and reducing the risk of antipsychotic drug interactions. *Prog Neurol Psychiatry.* 2012;16(2):20–24.

Bousman CA, Glatt SJ, Everall IP, et al. Methamphetamine-associated psychosis: a model for biomarker discovery in schizophrenia. In: Ritsner MS, ed. *Handbook of Schizophrenia Spectrum Disorders.* Vol 1. Dordrecht, The Netherlands: Springer Science and Business Media BV; 2011:327–343.

Clegg A, Young JB. Which medications to avoid in people at risk of delirium: a systematic review. *Age Ageing.* 2011;40(1):23–29.

Dixon L. Dual diagnosis of substance abuse in schizophrenia: prevalence and impact on outcomes. *Schizophr Res.* 1999;35(suppl):S93–S100.

Fallon BA, Levin ES, Schweitzer PJ, et al. Inflammation and central nervous system Lyme disease. *Neurobiol Dis.* 2010;37(3):534–541.

Foster R, Olajide D, Everall IP. Antiretroviral therapy-induced psychosis: case report and brief review of the literature. *HIV Med.* 2003;4(2):139–144.

Freudenreich O, Schulz SC, Goff DC. Initial medical work-up of first-episode psychosis: a conceptual review. *Early Interv Psychiatry.* 2009;3(1):10–18.

Gutierrez B, Heiber G, Torres-Gonzalez F, et al. The role of microbial agents in the etiology of schizophrenia: an infectious hypothesis for psychosis? *Curr Immunol Rev.* 2011;7(1):57–63.

Hor K, Taylor M. Suicide and schizophrenia: a systematic review of rates and risk factors. *J Psychopharmacol.* 2010;24(4)(suppl):81–90.

Kahn RS, Keefe RE. Schizophrenia is a cognitive illness: time for a change in focus. *JAMA Psychiatry.* 2013;70(10):1107–1112.

Karam CS, Ballon JS, Bivens NM, et al. Signaling pathways in schizophrenia: emerging targets and therapeutic strategies. *Trends Pharmacol Sci.* 2010;31(8):381–390.

Keck PE Jr, McElroy SL, Havens JR, et al. Psychosis in bipolar disorder: phenomenology and impact on morbidity and course of illness. *Compr Psychiatry.* 2003;44(4):263–269.

Kerfoot KE, Rosenheck RA, Petrakis IL, et al. Substance use and schizophrenia: adverse correlates in the CATIE study sample. *Schizophr Res.* 2011;132 (2–3):177–182.

Kessler RC, Birnbaum H, Demler O, et al. The prevalence and correlates of nonaffective psychosis in the National Comorbidity Survey Replication (NCS-R). *Biol Psychiatry.* 2005;58(8):668–676.

Kohen D. Diabetes mellitus and schizophrenia: historical perspective. *Br J Psychiatry Suppl.* 2004;184(47):s64–s66.

Kroeze WK, Hufeisen SJ, Popadak BA, et al. H1-histamine receptor affinity predicts short-term weight gain for typical and atypical antipsychotic drugs. *Neuropsychopharmacology.* 2003;28(3):519–526.

Krystal JH, Karper LP, Seibyl JP, et al. Subanesthetic effects of the noncompetitive NMDA antagonist, ketamine, in humans: psychotomimetic, perceptual, cognitive, and neuroendocrine responses. *Arch Gen Psychiatry.* 1994;51(3):199–214.

Kuepper R, van Os J, Lieb R, et al. Continued cannabis use and risk of incidence and persistence of psychotic symptoms: 10 year follow-up cohort study. *BMJ.* 2011;342:d738.

Lee KC, Ladzinski B. Mucocutaneous manifestations of illicit drug use. *Int J Dermatol.* 2014;53(8):1048–1051.

Leucht S, Cipriani A, Spineli L, et al. Comparative efficacy and tolerability of 15 antipsychotic drugs in schizophrenia: a multiple-treatments meta-analysis. *Lancet.* 2013;382(9896):951–962.

Lonergan E, Britton AM, Luxenberg J, et al. Antipsychotics for delirium. *Cochrane Database Syst Rev.* 2007;2:CD005594.

Mahajan SK, Machhan PC, Sood BR, et al. Neurocysticercosis presenting with psychosis. *J Assoc Physician India.* 2004;52:663–665.

Meltzer HY, Alphs L, Green AI, et al. Clozapine treatment for suicidality in schizophrenia: International Suicide Prevention Trial (InterSePT). *Arch Gen Psychiatry.* 2003;60(1):82–91.

Murray CJ, Vos T, Lozano R, et al. Disability-adjusted life years (DALYs) for 291 diseases and injuries in 21 regions, 1990–2010: a systematic analysis for the Global Burden of Disease Study 2010. *Lancet.* 2012;380(9859):2197–2223.

Ohayon MM, Schatzberg AF. Prevalence of depressive episodes with psychotic features in the general population. *Am J Psychiatry.* 2002;159(11): 1855–1861.

Olabi B, Ellison-Wright I, McIntosh AM, et al. Are there progressive brain changes in schizophrenia? A meta-analysis of structural magnetic resonance imaging studies. *Biol Psychiatry.* 2011;70(1):88–96.

Ondo WG, Tintner R, Voung KD, et al. Double-blind, placebo-controlled, unforced titration parallel trial of quetiapine for dopaminergic-induced hallucinations in Parkinson's disease. *Mov Disord.* 2005;20(8):958–963.

Perälä J, Suvisaari J, Saarni SI, et al. Lifetime prevalence of psychotic and bipolar I disorders in a general population. *Arch Gen Psychiatry.* 2007;64(1):19–28.

Rolinski M, Fox C, Maidment I, et al. Cholinesterase inhibitors for dementia with Lewy bodies, Parkinson's disease dementia and cognitive impairment in Parkinson's disease. *Cochrane Database Syst Rev.* 2012;3:CD006504.

Saha S, Chant D, Welham J, et al. A systematic review of the prevalence of schizophrenia. *PLoS Med.* 2005;2(5):e141.

Schmitz B. Effects of antiepileptic drugs on mood and behavior. *Epilepsia.* 2006;47:28–33.

Schneider LS, Tariot PN, Dagerman KS, et al. Effectiveness of atypical antipsychotic drugs in patients with Alzheimer's disease. *N Engl J Med.* 2006;355(15):1525–1538.

Schwarz C, Volz A, Li C, et al. Valproate for schizophrenia. *Cochrane Database Syst Rev.* 2008;3:CD004028.

Sellner J, Trinka E. Seizures and epilepsy in herpes simplex virus encephalitis: current concepts and future directions of pathogenesis and management. *J Neurol.* 2012;259(10):2019–2030.

Shevlin M, Armour C, Murphy J, et al. Evidence for a psychotic posttraumatic stress disorder subtype based on the National Comorbidity Survey. *Soc Psychiatry Psychiatr Epidemiol.* 2011;46(11):1069–1078.

Smith MJ, Thirthalli J, Abdallah AB, et al. Prevalence of psychotic symptoms in substance users: a comparison across substances. *Compr Psychiatry.* 2009;50(3):245–250.

Stevens JR, Jarrahzadeh T, Brendel RW, et al. Strategies for the prescription of psychotropic drugs with black box warnings. *Psychosomatics.* 2014;55(2):123–133.

Strawn JR, Keck PE Jr, Caroff SN. Neuroleptic malignant syndrome. *Am J Psychiatry.* 2007;164(6):870–876.

Stroup TS, Lawrence R, Abbas AI, et al. Schizophrenia spectrum and other psychotic disorders. In: Hales RE, Yudofsky SC, Roberts LW, eds. *The American Psychiatric Publishing Textbook of Psychiatry.* 6th ed. Washington, DC: American Psychiatric Publishing; 2014:173–206.

Titulaer MJ, McCracken L, Gabilondo I, et al. Treatment and prognostic factors for long-term outcome in patients with anti-NMDA receptor encephalitis: an observational cohort study. *Lancet Neurol.* 2013;12(2):157–165.

Wahab S, Md Rani SA, Sharis Othman S. Neurosyphilis and psychosis. *Asia Pac Psychiatry.* 2013;5(suppl 1):90–94.

Walker EF, Savoie T, Davis D. Neuromotor precursors of schizophrenia. *Schizophr Bull.* 1994;20(3):441–451.

Wobrock T, Falkai P, Schneider-Axmann T, et al. Comorbid substance abuse in first-episode schizophrenia: effects on cognition and psychopathology in the EUFEST study. *Schizophr Res.* 2013;147(1):132–139.

Zipursky RB, Reilly TJ, Murray RM. The myth of schizophrenia as a progressive brain disease. *Schizophr Bull.* 2013;39(6):1363–1372.

Mood Disorders 149

Licínia Ganança, Alejandro S. Cazzulino, and
Maria A. Oquendo

INTRODUCTION

Mood disorders are defined by the presence of a distinct period of persistently altered disposition, specifically, depressed, manic, or hypomanic states. These states are categorized as depressive or bipolar disorders depending on the presenting symptoms and the longitudinal course of the illness. Comorbidity between mood and neurologic disorders occurs frequently. Furthermore, not only may mood, especially depressive, symptoms be part or precede the clinical presentation of some neurologic disorders (e.g., Huntington disease [HD]) but they may also increase the risk for cerebrovascular disorders, and possibly some dementias, and therefore have a considerable impact in the prognosis and quality of life of primary neurologic disorders.

EPIDEMIOLOGY

Major depression is one of the leading causes of disability in the United States and worldwide. It ranked 11th in terms of disability-adjusted life years (DALYs) in a study of 291 diseases and injuries conducted in 21 regions. Moreover, according to the National Mental Health Association, depression affects 1 in every 33 children and 1 in every 8 adolescents. In any given year, about 21 million people in the United States will suffer from major depression (http://www.nimh.nih.gov/health/publications/the-numbers-count-mental-disorders-in-america/index.shtml#MajorDepressive).

The incidence of depression is nearly twice as high in women as it is in men, and suicide attempts are more numerous in women. However, death from suicide is far more common in men. Additionally, postpartum depression occurs after as many as 10% of all deliveries. The 12-month prevalence of depression in the U.S. population is estimated to be around 8.1% for women and 4.6% for men.

Bipolar disorder has a lifetime risk of 0.3% to 1.5%, with equal prevalence among men and women. It is estimated that around 10% of depressed patients may in fact be bipolar but have yet to be diagnosed.

PATHOPHYSIOLOGY

Although the underlying biology of depression has not been fully elucidated, it is clear that several key systems are involved. These include the serotonergic, glutamatergic, noradrenergic, and dopaminergic systems. Other putative pathophysiologic processes include neuroinflammation, hypothalamic–pituitary–adrenal axis dysfunction, and neuroplasticity.

Genetic factors are thought to be relevant due to the high heritability of mood disorders, estimated at about 30% to 40%. The data from twin studies indicates that environmental factors also play an important role in the expression of mood disorders. Nonetheless, the risk of becoming ill increases two- to threefold for first-degree family members of patients with mood disorders. Of note, despite early suggestions that bipolar disorder is more heritable than depressive disorders, the evidence that genetic vulnerability or heritability of mood disorders differs between bipolar and unipolar conditions is mixed and far from definitive.

The serotonergic system plays a key role in depression, with studies demonstrating an overall decrease in serotonin (5-HT) function. Brain imaging studies demonstrate increased 5-HT1A-receptor binding and fewer brain 5-HT reuptake sites. Tryptophan (serotonin's precursor) depletion has been shown to produce rapid depressive relapses in patients with a history of depression but no change in subjects with no personal or familial history of mood disorders. This suggests that low levels of 5-HT in the brain are not sufficient to cause depression but may act in concert with other factors in vulnerable individuals to cause symptoms. Indeed, many antidepressants exert their action through modulation of serotonin transmission.

Other neurotransmitter systems have been implicated in depression as well. For example, norepinephrine is linked to the pathophysiology of severe depression, as is dopamine, a neurotransmitter involved in incentive behavior and reward. Low cerebrospinal fluid levels of the dopamine metabolite, homovanillic acid, have been documented in depressed patients and exposure to dopamine-depleting drugs such as reserpine is known to precipitate depression. Changes in other neurotransmitters such as glutamate have also been identified. Glutamate, the main excitatory neurotransmitter appears to be increased in major limbic and cortical systems, possibly in response to stress, and may exert pathogenic effects either by limiting neurogenesis or dendritic remodeling directly or in concert with other factors that have similar effects on neuroplasticity.

Stress is implicated in the pathophysiology of depression, not only as mediated through glutamatergic changes in response but also as exemplified by prominent changes to the neuroendocrine system, especially in the hypothalamic–pituitary axis (HPA). Under normal conditions, stress prompts the HPA axis to secrete serum cortisol. In mood disorders, the HPA axis may become unresponsive to normal negative feedback loop, leading to a failure to restore cortisol to normal levels once the stressor is removed. These changes may be accompanied by the loss of normal diurnal variation in cortisol levels. Whether these changes are linked to early life experiences, leading to enduring changes in the HPA axis thereby increasing the probability of developing a mood disorder later in life, is not known.

Another hypothesis about the pathophysiology of depression posits that depression is a neuroinflammatory process, a concept bolstered by the observation that depressive symptoms (fatigue, anhedonia, anorexia, etc.) could be viewed as "sickness behaviors." Indeed, changes in inflammatory markers, such as increased interleukin (IL)-6 and tumor necrosis factor (TNF)-α levels have been consistently found in patients with depression. Furthermore, administration of therapeutic cytokines has been shown to cause significant depressive symptoms in 50% of exposed individuals, providing further evidence for the role of neuroinflammation.

As noted earlier, neuroplastic changes in the hippocampus have been linked to depression. Chronic stress is associated with decreased hippocampal neurogenesis, a phenomenon often observed in animal models of depression and postmortem tissue. Treatments with antidepressants seem to reverse these hippocampal deficits in neurogenesis. Both stress and antidepressants have been shown to affect levels of brain-derived neurotrophic factor (BDNF), which is normally highly expressed in hippocampus and prefrontal cortex and plays a major role in neuronal growth, survival, and maturation. BDNF also seems to have antidepressant-like actions and can induce molecular transcription in several key pathways.

Most psychosocial models focus on loss as the cause of depression in vulnerable, or less resilient, individuals. Exogenous factors may include social rejection or loss (interpersonal, financial, or health-related). Certainly, loss of income, job, social status, or the failure to achieve a life goal may produce profound mourning. Regardless, clinical manifestations in response to these stressors are ultimately mediated through brain circuitry and neurochemistry.

The pathophysiology of bipolar disorder is still being clarified, but studies have shown both structural and functional changes in those with the condition. Structural evidence from brain imaging studies shows a reduction of neurons and glial cells in areas such as the prefrontal cortex, amygdala and striatal regions, as well as white matter hyperintensities. Positron emission tomography (PET) studies suggest serotonergic abnormalities reflected in fewer serotonin transporters and more serotonin 1a receptors. Other relevant neurotransmitters include dopamine and glutamate. For instance, drugs that increase dopamine release, such as amphetamines, can induce manic-like symptoms. Similarly, decreased dopamine reuptake and reductions in dopamine transporter availability are linked to bipolar disorder. In addition, increased cortical glutamate levels and vesicular glutamate transporter gene expression are also implicated in the neurobiology of bipolar disorder.

As with depression, bipolar disorder can be viewed as a disorder related to synaptic plasticity involving dysfunction of neuroprotective pathways and impaired neuronal resilience. Multiple pathways related to plasticity are implicated including impaired regulation of calcium signaling cascades, associated with oxidative stress, and mitochondrial and endoplasmic reticulum stress response dysfunction.

Several intracellular molecular pathways affected by lithium and pertinent to neuroplasticity have been investigated as potential pathophysiologic contributors. The phosphoinositol pathway, involved in protein kinase C activation, regulates expression of several genes including BDNF. In fact, altered levels of BDNF are posited to contribute to the polarity switch process. Another lithium target, glycogen synthase kinase-3 (GSK3) is a key component of Wnt signaling and has effects on neurotransmission, neuroplasticity, neuronal growth, and metabolism.

CLINICAL FEATURES

DEPRESSIVE DISORDERS

A depressive episode is distinct from the normal emotional feelings of sadness or loss or a passing state of these emotions. Functional impairment and significant distress are key criteria and indeed, depression encompasses dysfunction in affective, cognitive, behavioral, and psychomotor domains.

In order to make the diagnosis, at least one of two gateway symptoms must be present for a minimum of 2 weeks: depressed mood and/or substantial decrease in interest or pleasure. Interestingly, depressed mood can manifest in a variety of ways and patients may report feeling down, sad, depressed, anxious, angry, or irritable. Of note, males may be more likely to present with irritability or anger, sometimes making the diagnosis more challenging to identify. Women more often present with "classic" sadness or depression. Anhedonia, or inability to feel pleasure, manifests as a reduction or loss of interest in things, people, or activities. As "gateway symptoms," the diagnosis of depression cannot be made in the absence of at least one of them.

Cognitively, patients may experience difficulty concentrating or making decisions, a decrease in productivity, forgetfulness, and slowed thoughts. In addition, patients often report distorted thoughts that are negative and pessimistic, including feelings of worthlessness, loss of self-esteem, and unreasonable self-blame or guilt. The future is regarded with a sense of doom or dread and hopelessness. Moreover, negative memories from the past may be preferentially recalled. At times, such cognitive distortions may be of delusional intensity. For example, patients may become convinced they are gravely ill or impoverished and unable to process or "believe" results from medical tests or bank reports. Other delusions typical of depression with psychotic features focus on pessimism or deserved punishment. Auditory hallucinations that are usually simple and mood congruent may be present as well.

The behavioral symptoms of depression include changes in appetite and weight and disruptions of sleep patterns. Sleep disturbances include difficulty falling asleep (early insomnia), waking up in the middle of the night (middle insomnia), and waking up earlier than usual (terminal insomnia). Middle and terminal insomnias are more specific to depression than early insomnia, which is more common in the absence of a mood disorder. However, some patients experience hypersomnia rather than insomnia. Similarly, patients often report poor appetite and weight loss, although increased appetite and weight are sometimes observed, too. Other behavioral symptoms include loss of libido.

Psychomotor activity is usually diminished in depression and low energy and physical fatigue are often present. Patients may experience difficulty completing day-to-day activities and self-care or find that these activities require greater effort. In extreme cases, patients may become virtually immobile and mute, and this condition combined with loss of appetite and overall self-neglect can result in a medical emergency due to dehydration or poor nutrition. In contrast, some patients exhibit psychomotor agitation, which is often accompanied by intense anxiety. Agitation can often be seen in depressed patients but may also result from the side effects of antidepressant medications.

Perhaps, the most worrisome symptom of depression is suicidal thinking or behavior. Suicidal ideation may range from passing thoughts that life is not worth living to well-defined plans with intent to kill oneself. About 15% of patients with depression acknowledge a suicide attempt at some point in their lives and between 2% and 12% of patients with depression commit suicide. This is another way in which depression can lead to morbidity and mortality.

On examination, depressed patients characteristically exhibit a dejected posture, with bent shoulders, frowning, and a downcast gaze. Gestural movements and facial expressions are reduced, and grooming may be neglected. Patients usually take more time to start answering questions and speak slowly and softly.

BIPOLAR DISORDERS

The distinguishing feature of bipolar disorder is the presence of a manic or hypomanic state that lasts a week or longer (can be less for hypomania). As with depressive disorders, there are impairments in affective, cognitive, psychomotor, and behavioral domains.

Mania, lasting a minimum of 1 week, is characterized by abnormally elevated or euphoric feelings. As with depression, there can be significant irritability and anger, especially when the patient is frustrated. Patients often appear exaggeratedly cheerful and happy.

Cognitive abnormalities include rapid or even racing thoughts, which may translate into rapid, pressured speech that can, as the severity of mania progresses, become increasingly disorganized. As thoughts become disorganized, speech can exhibit flight of ideas or loosening of associations. In addition, patients are easily distracted and have difficulty focusing on tasks that require concentration. Patients also frequently exhibit impaired judgment and engage in activities they would normally eschew if well. Patients may go on spending sprees, engage in promiscuous sexual behaviors, or make risky business decisions. Cognitive distortions in mania often include inflated self-esteem and grandiose ideas such as a sense of being special, capable of anything, or possessing special powers. As in depression, the cognitive distortions can cross the line into delusional or psychotic thinking. Grandiose delusions are a common psychotic feature in mania.

Behaviorally, manic patients are usually overactive with increased energy levels and engage in multiple activities. Typically, the number of hours of sleep is reduced, without the sensation of fatigue or sleepiness. In fact, insomnia is often the first recognizable symptom of a manic episode. Appetite is usually reduced and combined with increased activity can lead to significant weight loss. Manic patients classically dress with bright colors, use excess make up, or wear extravagant clothing. Movements are exaggerated or theatrical, and patients may express excessive familiarity toward strangers.

From a psychomotor vantage, manic patients frequently have increased psychomotor activity. They may engage in both goal-oriented activities at an accelerated pace or be overactive in a general way, with pacing or fidgeting.

Interviewing can be very difficult, as manic psychopathology tends to block communication. It is usually counterproductive for the physician to spend time arguing with or countering the illogical thinking of the patient. Insight is absent in virtually all cases and, therefore, patients typically object to treatment.

Hypomania has a similar clinical presentation but may be briefer, cause less functional impairment, and has no psychotic symptoms.

Although the presence of manic or hypomanic episodes differentiates bipolar from depressive disorders, depression is prominent in bipolar disorder. In fact, over the course of the disorder, most bipolar patients spend significantly more time depressed than manic or hypomanic. Bipolar depression usually has an earlier onset, greater risk of suicidal behavior, likely linked to the greater time spent depressed, and more episodes of illness.

DIAGNOSIS

There is no pathognomonic sign or symptom and, as of yet, no biologic or neuroimaging markers that can establish the diagnosis of a mood disorder. Therefore, mood disorder diagnoses are established according to their clinical features. Each category has specific criteria, which are defined by consensus and described in manuals such as the *Diagnostic and Statistical Manual of Mental Disorders*, 5th edition (*DSM-5*). It is likely that these diagnoses will ultimately be understood as a grouping of multiple distinct disorders and more specific entities within the current disorders will be defined using genetics, epigenetics, brain imaging, and other methods.

Major depressive disorder (MDD) is diagnosed by the presence of at least one major depressive episode. Episodes can occur a single time but, more often, they are recurrent.

Persistent depressive disorder is a form of depression that has less than 5 symptoms, as required in MDD, but lasting for at least 2 years, with little or no remission during that time. Typical symptoms include low mood, lack of energy and interest, low self-esteem, and irritability. Chronic forms of depressive disorders are associated with poorer response to treatment, slower rate of improvement over time, younger age of onset, longer episodes, greater disease burden, higher rates of medical and psychiatric co-morbidity, and higher rates of suicidal ideation.

Mood and associated physical symptoms may occur in relation to the menstrual cycle. **Premenstrual dysphoric disorder** is diagnosed if symptoms are present during the last week of the luteal phase, remit within a few days of the follicular phase, and are absent in the week following menses. A prospectively documented cyclical pattern over at least 2 consecutive months must be present to confirm the diagnosis.

Mood disorders in children and adolescents bring specific diagnostic challenges. Behavioral problems are common and include withdrawal, sullenness, truancy, poor grades, and tantrums. Children and adolescents showing persistent irritability, which manifests as frequent temper outbursts and angry, irritable mood in between outbursts, may be eligible for the diagnosis of **disruptive mood dysregulation disorder** (DMDD).

The presence of at least one manic episode is required to diagnose a **bipolar I disorder**. In contrast, a **bipolar II disorder** diagnosis requires a history of both depressive and hypomanic episodes. Recurrence of episodes, interspersed with periods of normal mood (euthymia), is the norm, although single episodes are possible. In some cases, patients never fully recover and continue on a chronic course.

Patients with **cyclothymia** alternate between mild, short-lived depressions and hypomania. The cycles may be continuous and last for several weeks to several months. Rarely do these patients complain specifically about the highs and lows they experience. More commonly, patients will complain only of being depressed at times, not realizing that they have been hypomanic at other times. Cyclothymia is sometimes a precursor to the more classic form of bipolar disorder.

Substance/medication-induced bipolar or depressive disorders can occur when mood episodes develop during or soon after substance intoxication or withdrawal or alternatively after exposure to a medication. Note that in cases where mania or hypomania ensues after treatment with an antidepressant, the diagnosis of bipolar disorder is warranted if the manic/hypomanic symptoms do not remit upon withdrawal of the antidepressant (considering the time needed for metabolic elimination of the compound). Similarly, **bipolar or depressive disorders due to another medical condition** occur when there is evidence from the history, medical examination, or laboratory findings that the mood episode is a direct pathophysiologic consequence of another medical condition. See Table 149.1 for a list of common neurologic disorders associated with mood symptoms.

When patients present with the characteristic symptoms of a depressive or bipolar disorders but do not meet all the full criteria, a diagnosis of **other specified bipolar or depressive disorders** can be established if the condition causes clinically significant distress or impairment.

DIFFERENTIAL DIAGNOSIS

Sadness is a normal reaction to life adversity and is characterized by an adequate response in proportion to the provoking stimulus,

TABLE 149.1	Neurologic Disorders Commonly Associated with Mood Symptoms	
Depressive Symptoms	**Manic Symptoms**
• Stroke (depression as both risk factor and sequelae)	• Focal strokes in right baso-temporal and inferofrontal region
• Parkinson disease	• Stroke/tumor in perihypo-thalamic region
• Huntington disease	• Huntington disease
• Essential tremor	• Multiple sclerosis
• Multiple sclerosis	• Head trauma
• Epilepsy	• Neurosyphilis
• Dementia	• Creutzfeldt–Jakob disease
	• Frontotemporal dementia

relatively brief duration, and lack of a major impact on psychosocial functioning. In normal bereavement and adjustment disorders, there is typically a reduction in depressive symptoms after the removal of provoking stressors.

Some medical conditions cause prominent mood symptoms. In addition to the history and physical examination, laboratory testing should include hepatic and thyroid function, studies of electrolytes, calcium, blood urea nitrogen, creatinine, a complete blood count, and a urinalysis (for drug abuse screening).

DIFFERENTIAL DIAGNOSIS WITH NEUROLOGIC DISORDERS

Twenty-five percent to 40% of patients with neurologic conditions, including Parkinson disease (PD) and HD, as well as Alzheimer dementia, develop a marked depressive syndrome at some point over the course of the illness. Evidence shows that mood symptoms may even precede neurologic manifestations in the cases of PD, HD, and essential tremor (ET). Critically, PD shares some symptoms with major depression, such as bradykinesia, decreased or even expressionless faces, bradyphrenia, stooped posture, loss of interest and concentration, and reduced libido. Comorbidity between the two disorders is highly prevalent, around 40%. Bromocriptine treatment is also associated with depressive symptoms. Features that facilitate the diagnosis of depression in these patients include the presence of a pervasive low mood (sometimes with diurnal variation), early morning awakening, pessimism (not proportional to the level of neurologic disability), and suicidal ideation. Of note, some psychiatric drugs directly affect dopaminergic transmission, such as first- and second-generation antipsychotics or some specific selective serotonin reuptake inhibitors (SSRIs) in high doses, and can cause or worsen parkinsonian symptoms or cause tardive dyskinesias.

Depressive symptoms can occur in patients with ET with prevalences as high as 49%. Not only do these symptoms result from the functional impairment associated with a disabling tremor but also may be a part of the pathophysiologic process and in some cases even precede the onset of motor symptoms. A recent study revealed lower scores on items such as "reported sadness," "inability to feel," and "pessimistic thoughts" in depressed patients with ET.

Euphoria can also be seen in organic states. Frontal lobe lesions can manifest with euphoria, often in the form of silliness and lack of foresight. Extreme social disinhibition, in the absence of other features of mania, strongly suggests frontal lobe pathology.

Patients suffering from dementia may present with manic-like agitation or depression. Cognitive and behavioral changes mimicking depression, such as apathy and loss of concentration, are more common than those that mimic mania, such as restlessness and combativeness. The medical evaluation is most important in elderly patients because they are at the greatest risk of having another illness comorbid with depression. They may also have a different medical condition presenting as depression. Although "pseudodementia" may be a sign of depression in the elderly, this assumption should be regarded as a diagnosis of exclusion. The appearance of a late-life affective disorder, especially in patients with no family history of such a condition, suggests a medical etiology.

Psychiatric symptoms, such as irritability, impulsivity, anxiety, and depressed mood, are almost ubiquitous in HD, which may initially present as a depressive illness. Depression may predate the neurologic diagnosis by 4 to 10 years. Apathy is a symptom that typically worsens as the disease progresses and may be related to the disorder itself. Suicide and suicide attempts are common. Manic symptoms can occur but are not as common. Family history is indicative of HD, and the definitive diagnosis is made through genetic testing.

Mood disorders are very common in epilepsy, 55% of epileptics report depression, and they tend to have a pleomorphic presentation, sometimes not meeting full *DSM-5* criteria. Depressed mood, irritability, and anxiety are common. Mood disorders are classified according to their temporal relation to the occurrence of seizures as ictal, interictal, or postictal.

In some situations, as in the so-called masked depression, patients fail to report feeling sad or depressed and can present with pain, fatigue, and other vague medical complaints. The presence of at least five of the necessary symptoms establishes the correct diagnosis. The differential diagnosis is especially important in neurology, as these patients often complain of headaches or backaches that are not amenable to conventional treatments with pain medication.

Sleep apnea can cause fatigue, diminished concentration, and other symptoms similar to those of depression. A polysomnographic study may be warranted, especially in obese patients presenting with depressive symptoms.

DIFFERENTIAL DIAGNOSIS WITH OTHER PSYCHIATRIC DISORDERS

The distinction between mood disorders and other psychiatric disorders can be difficult and further complicated by the fact that comorbidity is very common. The negative symptoms of schizophrenia, such as apathy, anhedonia, decreased motor activity, social withdrawal, and cognitive decline can resemble depression. On the other hand, patients with schizophrenia can present with grandiose delusions and florid agitation similar to mania. In mood disorders, delusional themes tend to be congruent with the main presenting mood. A history of periodic psychotic illnesses with a return to proper functioning between episodes is more suggestive of an affective disorder, whereas a history of chronic or deteriorating functioning is more suggestive of schizophrenia. A diagnosis based on a longitudinal evaluation is the most reliable. In the case of schizoaffective disorder, in which psychotic and mood symptoms coexist, the persistence of psychotic symptoms after resolution of mood symptoms validates the diagnosis.

Comorbidity with substance abuse disorders is prominent. In community samples, over 50% of individuals with mood disorders meet criteria for alcohol and/or substance abuse disorders. Patients may view substance abuse as a form of "self-medication" but often, symptoms are in fact caused or exacerbated by the substance. Such changes may be limited to the period of intoxication or occur after intoxication. If intoxication occurs frequently, it may produce diagnostic uncertainty, and prolonged abstinence may be necessary to make an accurate diagnosis. Patients with mood disorders who abuse both alcohol and drugs are more difficult to treat and have a higher rate of suicide attempts and suicide. Alcohol is often used in suicide attempts and may be the factor that triggers impulsive, self-destructive behavior or that intensifies the effects of an overdose.

Depressed patients often have severe anxiety and sometimes experience panic attacks as part of their illness. Predominance of either anxiety or depressive symptoms usually helps to establish the correct diagnosis. Nevertheless, there is a high rate of comorbidity with depression and all forms of anxiety disorders.

In the case of personality disorders, especially borderline personality disorder, the differential diagnosis is made if characteristic personality features, such as feelings of emptiness, extreme rejection sensitivity, and frantic efforts to avoid perceived abandonment, exist outside mood episodes.

TREATMENT

TREATMENT OF DEPRESSIVE DISORDERS

Depression can be treated with either pharmacotherapy or manualized therapies such as cognitive behavioral therapy or interpersonal therapy. More severe depression may require both medication and psychotherapy as opposed to one treatment approach alone. Hospitalization may be necessary, especially for actively suicidal patients or for those whose personal care is so impaired that around the clock nursing is essential.

A family history of effective drug response or previous response to a medication may be used to inform treatment selection. It is best with most medications to start with a low dose and increase slowly. Full benefit may take up to 4 to 6 weeks. After an initial episode, treatment should continue for 6 to 9 months at full dosage after the acute phase in order to prevent relapse.

Symptomatic relief with treatment may not result in immediate improvement of psychosocial function, which may be delayed. Relapses occur in up to 20% of patients in 6 months and over 30% in 1 year according to Keller. The risk of recurrence increases by 16% with each recurrent episode. The high rates of relapse have led to recommendations of maintenance treatment with drug therapy and prophylactic psychotherapy for patients with at least two episodes of depression.

Fifty percent to 60% of patients respond (50% improvement or better) to an initial course of antidepressant, whereas only 10% to 20% of severely depressed patients improve when given placebo. However, remission (return to baseline or near baseline) is harder to attain and only about a third of patients remit after a first antidepressant treatment, requiring use of a different medication or augmentation strategies (see in the following text).

Antidepressant medications are classified by molecular structure or by effects on neurotransmitters.

SSRIs and other new-generation antidepressants (mirtazapine, bupropion) are the drugs of choice for the treatment of depression. Common side effects include gastrointestinal disturbance, agitation (especially early in treatment), and sexual dysfunction. Note that patients with psychotic depression rarely respond to antidepressants alone and require either the addition of an antipsychotic drug or a course of electroconvulsive therapy (ECT) (see the following text).

Although in general, SSRIs are as effective as tricyclic antidepressants (TCAs) and monoamine oxidase inhibitors (MAOIs) in mild to moderate depression, TCAs and MAOIs introduced in the 1960s are often still used for patients who do not respond to one or more of the newer medications. The relative reluctance to use TCAs and MAOIs is due to issues of tolerability and/or serious side effects, as well as the fact that they may be lethal if used in a suicide attempt. The most common adverse reactions when using TCAs are mainly due to their cardiovascular and anticholinergic effects.

As with any medication, drug interactions may occur and cross checking for these is key. MAOIs have important, life-threatening interactions with several drugs as well as interactions with food and, therefore, dietary precautions are essential.

Depression is often resistant to treatment. Several strategies have been developed to overcome this issue, such as combining antidepressants or augmenting antidepressant efficacy by adding other drugs such as lithium, stimulants (e.g., dextroamphetamine or methylphenidate), antipsychotics, buspirone, or thyroid hormone. Empirical data driving decision making around intervention selection for treatment-resistant depression is still lacking. Studies comparing outcomes have not shown an advantage for any of the augmentation or second-tier strategies described thus far.

Electroconvulsive treatment is indicated for patients with the following characteristics:

1. Failure to respond to adequate antidepressant pharmacotherapy trials
2. Depression with psychotic or catatonic features
3. Actively suicidal patients or manic patients so severely agitated that they must be rapidly controlled
4. Intolerance of side effects, as can happen in patients with PD, or allergies to multiple antidepressants
5. Inability to participate in pharmacotherapy or psychotherapy due to refusal to eat or drink or markedly slowed speech and cognition

ECT is a safe treatment and generally well tolerated. The most common side effect is mild, temporary memory loss. Because it is administered under general anesthesia, risks associated with anesthesia are also present. With proper medical preparation and screening, treatments may be administered even in the presence of neurologic or cardiovascular conditions. At the end of the course of treatment, a maintenance regimen must be instituted to prevent relapse. This can take the form of antidepressant medications, usually in combination, or "maintenance" ECT, generally administered monthly.

TREATMENT OF BIPOLAR DISORDERS

Mood stabilization treatment is the gold standard for bipolar disorders. It serves to both control acute phases of the disease and prevent future episodes. Lithium is a potent antimanic. Remission is achieved in about 60% to 70% of cases, especially for patients with euphoric mania and infrequent episodes, although it takes several weeks for it to fully exert its therapeutic benefits. Lithium therapy requires regular blood level monitoring to prevent toxicity, which manifests at higher levels and can be life threatening. Agitated and medically ill patients are at increased risk for toxicity. Lithium can cause hypothyroidism in 10% to 20% of patients and is relatively contraindicated in renal disease. Tremor is a common side effect.

Anticonvulsants such as valproate or carbamazepine can be used with good results in dysphoric mania or rapid cycling. They are often combined with lithium. Mood stabilization with second-generation antipsychotics (olanzapine, quetiapine, risperidone, or lurasidone) is usually quicker and may also be more effective when psychotic symptoms are present. Sedating agents can also be used as adjunctive therapy for rapid control of agitated patients. The anticonvulsant lamotrigine has been shown to prevent recurrence of depression, but the data on its ability to control manic or hypomanic phases is weak.

In the case of bipolar depression, treating a depressive episode with antidepressants alone carries the risk of switching to mania or hypomania. Nonetheless, aggressive treatment of depression is essential in bipolar disorder because it is in this phase that suicidal behavior occurs. Thus, although less dramatic than mania, it is certainly just as dangerous, if not more. Using mood stabilizers alone is only effective in a few cases. Most commonly, bipolar depression is treated with a combination of antidepressants and mood stabilizers. Quetiapine and lurasidone both have antidepressant effects and are U.S. Food and Drug Administration (FDA) approved for monotherapy in bipolar depression.

Manic relapse may be spontaneous, induced by therapeutic drugs, or induced by substances. With continued use of a mood stabilizer, the risk of antidepressant-induced mania is about 10%. Data suggest that newer antidepressants are less likely than tricyclics to precipitate manic "switches."

After the second bipolar episode, regardless of polarity, patients should be treated indefinitely because relapse is almost certain. The treatment goal is to maintain euthymia and prevent either depression or manic episodes. Lithium has been the prophylactic drug of choice for decades, but the antipsychotic mood stabilizers are also approved for long-term prophylaxis. Consideration of side effect profiles as well as therapeutic benefits is essential when considering treatment selection.

TREATMENT OF MOOD DISORDERS COMORBID WITH NEUROLOGIC DISORDERS

Patients with dementia frequently develop psychiatric symptoms, including depression; elation; delusions; hallucinations; and periods of extreme irritability, agitation, or disinhibition, and dementia may be accompanied by full-blown psychiatric syndromes. These episodes are often brief. Nevertheless, modest doses of antidepressants may be of use. Side effects may be minimal with low doses. Antipsychotic medications must be used with extreme care but may be useful to treat agitation. They may induce extrapyramidal symptoms, especially the conventional ones. Depression and depression with dementia occur in almost 25% of patients with PD. The depressive symptoms respond well to low doses of antidepressants including the SSRIs. Occasionally, SSRI therapy increases the parkinsonism, especially sertraline at higher doses, wherein the drug's selective affinity for serotonin transporters is obviated. ECT is safe and effective and may improve both the depression and the motor symptoms of PD. In the case of HD, manic symptoms should be treated with the usual medications but often require smaller (one-third to one-half) doses. At times, ECT may be lifesaving. Treatment of mood disorders associated with epilepsy depends on whether the episode in question is ictal or peri-ictal. The latter is treated as usual with pharmacotherapy and/or psychotherapy, whereas in the case of ictal episodes, complete resolution of the seizure episode is needed to achieve mood remission. Drugs used to treat mood disorders, including for example, lithium or valproic acid may cause or exacerbate tremor. See Table 149.2 for a list of neurologic adverse effects of common drugs used to treat mood disorders.

TABLE 149.2	Neurologic Side Effects Associated with Drugs Used for Mood Disorders Treatment
Side Effect	**Drug**
Seizures	(All antidepressants and antipsychotics can potentially induce seizures.) Bupropion Maprotiline Amoxapine Imipramine Escitalopram Clozapine Selegiline
Tremor	Bupropion Lamotrigine SSRIs Antipsychotics (especially conventional) Phenelzine Trazodone Lithium Valproic acid
Akathisia	Aripiprazole and other antipsychotics SSRIs
Dyskinesia	Selegiline
Tardive dyskinesia	Conventional antipsychotics (theoretical risk for new-generation antipsychotics)
Cerebrovascular events	Increased risk with atypical antipsychotics in elderly
Headaches	Trazodone Venlafaxine
Ataxia	Lamotrigine Nefazodone
Aseptic meningitis	Lamotrigine (rare)

SSRIs, selective serotonin reuptake inhibitors.

OUTCOME

Mood disorders are a major cause of disability and are highly associated with poor psychosocial functioning, mainly due to depressive episodes, which are much more common and longer lasting.

First-onset MDD typically peaks from ages 14 to 19 years, although first depressive episodes can appear at any age. If untreated, an episode lasts on average 6 to 9 months. Fifty percent to 70% of patients with major depression have recurrent episodes in their lifetimes. Young age, presence of a severe preceding episode, persistence of even mild depressive symptoms, and a history of multiple episodes increase the likelihood of recurrence. Symptom profiles can often change from one episode to another. Around 12% to 20% of patients will present a chronic course. Risk factors for chronicity include a strong family history of depression, older age, longer duration of illness before treatment is sought, alcoholism, medical illness, disability of spouse, or multiple recent deaths of family members.

Bipolar disorder usually has an earlier age of onset than major depression. The first episode is more frequently depressive, with a peak incidence at age 17 years. Late-onset bipolar disorder is rare and is usually associated with organic disease. Mania typically ensues within 5 years of the first depressive episode.

In terms of the polarity of episodes, very few patients present only recurrent manic episodes with little or no depression. Rather, depressive episodes and symptoms tend to dominate the longitudinal course of bipolar disorder. Bipolar disorder can also vary in terms of the frequency of episodes. Almost all patients with bipolar disorder have recurrent episodes and episodes are more frequent and numerous than in depressive disorders. In some cases, patients may experience four or more mood episodes in a year, termed *rapid cycling*. Once thought to be a characteristic of the patient, rapid cycling can occur and later resolve itself with a return to less frequent episodes.

Bipolar patients usually function well when medicated. Nevertheless, although many patients are able to resume normal activities within several weeks to months after recovery, approximately 40% of patients have significant social dysfunction for up to 2 years after an episode. Persistent cognitive deficits are documented as well. Neurobiologic deterioration from repeated episodes may play a role in this phenomenon.

Suicide is the most dreaded outcome of mood disorders. The suicide rate in bipolar illness is higher than in any other psychiatric illness, responsible for the death of 8% to 15% of patients, and patients with bipolar disorder carry a 15-fold greater risk of suicide than in the general population. Risk is even greater in the case of comorbidity with substance abuse disorders.

SUGGESTED READINGS

Andreazza AC, Young LT. The neurobiology of bipolar disorder: identifying targets for specific agents and synergies for combination treatment. *Int J Neuropsychopharmacol.* 2014;17(7):1039–1052. doi:10.1017/S1461145713000096.

Aprahamian I, Nunes PV, Forlenza OV. Cognitive impairment and dementia in late-life bipolar disorder. *Curr Opin Psychiatry.* 2013;26(1):120–123.

Bauer M, Adli M, Ricken R, et al. Role of lithium augmentation in the management of major depressive disorder. *CNS Drugs.* 2014;28(4):331–342.

Berent D, Zboralski K, Orzechowska A, et al. Thyroid hormones association with depression severity and clinical outcome in patients with major depressive disorder. *Mol Biol Rep.* 2014;41(4):2419–2425.

Cardamone L, Salzberg MR, O'Brien TJ, et al. Antidepressant therapy in epilepsy: can treating the comorbidities affect the underlying disorder? *Br J Pharmacol.* 2013;168(7):1531–1554.

Cipriani A, Hawton K, Stockton S, et al. Lithium in the prevention of suicide in mood disorders: updated systematic review and meta-analysis. *BMJ.* 2013;346:f3646.

Cipriani A, Reid K, Young AH, et al. Valproic acid, valproate and divalproex in the maintenance treatment of bipolar disorder. *Cochrane Database Syst Rev.* 2013;10:CD003196.

Coplan J, Gugger JJ, Tasleem H. Tardive dyskinesia from atypical antipsychotic agents in patients with mood disorders in a clinical setting. *J Affect Disord.* 2013;150(3):868–871.

Heim C, Binder EB. Current research trends in early life stress and depression: review of human studies on sensitive periods, gene-environment interactions, and epigenetics. *Exp Neurol.* 2012;233(1):102–111.

Hellmann-Regen J, Piber D, Hinkelmann K, et al. Depressive syndromes in neurological disorders. *Eur Arch Psychiatry Clin Neurosci.* 2013;263 (suppl 2):S123–S136.

Kessler RC, Petukhova M, Sampson NA, et al. Twelve-month and lifetime prevalence and lifetime morbid risk of anxiety and mood disorders in the United States. *Int J Methods Psychiatr Res.* 2012;21(3):169–184.

Kudlow PA, Cha DS, Lam RW, et al. Sleep architecture variation: a mediator of metabolic disturbance in individuals with major depressive disorder. *Sleep Med.* 2013;14(10):943–949.

Kupfer DJ, Frank E, Phillips ML. Major depressive disorder: new clinical, neurobiological, and treatment perspectives. *Lancet.* 2012;379(9820):1045–1055.

Mann JJ. The serotonergic system in mood disorders and suicidal behaviour. *Philos Trans R Soc Lond B Biol Sci.* 2013;368(1615):20120537.

McGrath CL, Kelley ME, Holtzheimer PE, et al. Toward a neuroimaging treatment selection biomarker for major depressive disorder. *JAMA Psychiatry.* 2013;70(8):821–829.

Miller JM, Hesselgrave N, Ogden RT, et al. Brain serotonin 1A receptor binding as a predictor of treatment outcome in major depressive disorder. *Biol Psychiatry.* 2013;74(10):760–767.

Oquendo MA, Ellis SP, Chesin MS, et al. Familial transmission of parental mood disorders: unipolar and bipolar disorders in offspring. *Bipolar Disord.* 2013;15(7):764–773.

Perera TD, Thirumangalakudi L, Glennon E, et al. Role of hippocampal neurogenesis in mnemonic segregation: implications for human mood disorders. *World J Biol Psychiatry.* 2013;14(8):602–610.

Proudfoot J, Whitton A, Parker G, et al. Triggers of mania and depression in young adults with bipolar disorder. *J Affect Disord.* 2012;143(1–3): 196–202.

Rist PM, Schürks M, Buring JE, et al. Migraine, headache, and the risk of depression: prospective cohort study. *Cephalalgia.* 2013;33(12):1017–1025.

Robillard R, Naismith SL, Hickie IB. Recent advances in sleep-wake cycle and biological rhythms in bipolar disorder. *Curr Psychiatry Rep.* 2013;15(10):402.

Rosenblat JD, Cha DS, Mansur RB, et al. Inflamed moods: a review of the interactions between inflammation and mood disorders. *Prog Neuropsychopharmacol Biol Psychiatry.* 2014;53C:23–34.

Salvadore G, Quiroz JA, Machado-Vieira R, et al. The neurobiology of the switch process in bipolar disorder: a review. *J Clin Psychiatry.* 2010;71(11):1488–1501.

Sanacora G, Banasr M. From pathophysiology to novel antidepressant drugs: glial contributions to the pathology and treatment of mood disorders. *Biol Psychiatry.* 2013;73(12):1172–1179.

Sanacora G, Treccani G, Popoli M. Towards a glutamate hypothesis of depression: an emerging frontier of neuropsychopharmacology for mood disorders. *Neuropharmacology.* 2012;62(1):63–77.

Vázquez GH, Tondo L, Undurraga J, et al. Overview of antidepressant treatment of bipolar depression. *Int J Neuropsychopharmacol.* 2013;16(7):1673–1685.

Verdelho A, Madureira S, Moleiro C, et al; LADIS Study. Depressive symptoms predict cognitive decline and dementia in older people independently of cerebral white matter changes: the LADIS study. *J Neurol Neurosurg Psychiatry.* 2013;84(11):1250–1254.

Vieta E, Popovic D, Rosa AR, et al. The clinical implications of cognitive impairment and allostatic load in bipolar disorder. *Eur Psychiatry.* 2013;28(1):21–29.

Vilalta-Franch J, López-Pousa S, Llinàs-Reglà J, et al. Depression subtypes and 5-year risk of dementia and Alzheimer disease in patients aged 70 years. *Int J Geriatr Psychiatry.* 2013;28(4):341–350.

Wu KY, Chang CM, Liang HY, et al. Increased risk of developing dementia in patients with bipolar disorder: a nested matched case-control study. *Bipolar Disord.* 2013;15(7):787–794.

Zahodne LB, Marsiske M, Okun MS, et al. Components of depression in Parkinson disease. *J Geriatr Psychiatry Neurol.* 2012;25(3):131–137.

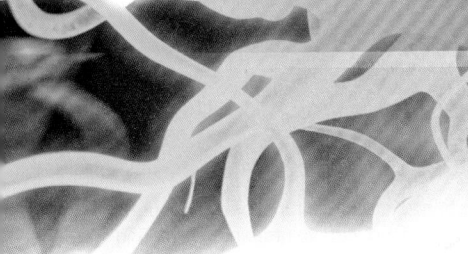

Anxiety Disorders, Posttraumatic Stress Disorder, and Obsessive–Compulsive Disorder

Franklin R. Schneier

INTRODUCTION

Anxiety is an adaptive emotional state related to anticipation of threat; it can encompass fearful thoughts, symptoms of physiologic arousal, and preparation for fight or flight. *Anxiety disorders* are characteristic syndromes of maladaptation to various types of anticipated threat. Examples include dangers from predators, interpersonal conflicts, germs, and other hazards. Anxiety disorders are distinguished from mild episodes of anxiety by their persistence and intensity and also by the diagnostic requirement that they cause marked distress or impairment in functioning.

Anxiety disorders have historically included panic disorder, agoraphobia, specific phobias, social anxiety disorder, generalized anxiety disorder, obsessive–compulsive disorder (OCD), acute stress disorder, and posttraumatic stress disorder (PTSD). The recent revision of the *Diagnostic and Statistical Manual of Mental Disorders,* 5th edition (*DSM-5*), places OCD in a separate category of obsessive–compulsive and related disorders and PTSD in a separate category of trauma- and stressor-related disorders, in recognition of their unique features. Two disorders previously categorized as childhood disorders, separation anxiety disorder and selective mutism, are now also recognized as anxiety disorders that can persist into adulthood.

Anxiety and anxiety disorders may co-occur with neurologic disease through a variety of mechanisms. Neurologic disease processes may cause anxiety symptoms directly by dysregulating function of brain circuits that subserve anxiety. Alternatively, primary neurologic illnesses may lead to anxiety via psychological mechanisms as when visible signs of a movement disorder lead to embarrassment and social anxiety or when an uncertain or poor prognosis leads to anticipatory anxiety. A primary anxiety disorder or its treatment may generate neurologic manifestations, such as syncope secondary to hyperventilation in panic disorder, or a seizure due to abrupt discontinuation of a benzodiazepine. Neurologic and psychiatric conditions may also co-occur secondary to another causal agent as when combat trauma leads to both traumatic brain injury (TBI) and PTSD.

EPIDEMIOLOGY

The historical category of anxiety disorders constitutes the most common type of psychiatric disorder with a lifetime prevalence of over 25%. Anxiety disorders are more common in women by a 2:1 ratio, have an age of onset before 30 years in most cases, and tend to be chronic. Community prevalence rates for individual anxiety disorders range from 5% to 12% for social anxiety disorder and specific phobias to 1% to 2% for panic disorder and OCD with intermediate rates for PTSD and generalized anxiety disorder.

PATHOBIOLOGY

The neural circuits, neurochemistry, and behaviors mediating human anxiety share features with neural systems that mediate withdrawal responses to aversive stimuli across species. In humans, these responses incorporate higher cortical functions such as anxious anticipation and adaptations based on life experiences and culture. Twin studies show heritability of specific anxiety disorders in the range of 10% to 60%, but findings for individual genes explain only very small proportions of the overall risk. Environmental risk factors for anxiety disorders include early childhood trauma and acute stressors, such as interpersonal loss.

Studies in rodents and humans have implicated central nervous system (CNS) fear circuitry, including the amygdala, hippocampus, and prefrontal cortex, in the development and maintenance of conditioned fear; this circuitry is activated when persons with social anxiety disorder, specific phobias, or PTSD are exposed to fear-inducing stimuli (Fig. 150.1). Anxiety disorders also have been shown to be associated with dysfunction of several neurotransmitter systems, including serotonin, norepinephrine, γ-aminobutyric acid (GABA), and glutamate. Dopamine dysfunction has also been reported, and elevated rates of panic disorder, generalized anxiety disorder, and social anxiety disorder have been reported in Parkinson disease. Sympathetic nervous system and hypothalamic–pituitary axis abnormalities have been found across anxiety disorders. Panic disorder has been associated with hyperventilation, hypocapnia, and disordered CO_2 regulation.

The pathobiology of OCD shows some differences from other anxiety disorders. Anatomic and brain imaging evidence suggest hyperactivity in a circuit involving the orbitofrontal cortex, basal ganglia, and thalamus. Acquired lesions in the corticostriato-thalamic circuit, parietal and temporal cortex, cerebellum, and brain stem have been reported to induce compulsivity. OCD has been associated with other neurologic conditions involving the basal ganglia, such as Tourette syndrome, Huntington disease, and Sydenham chorea.

CLINICAL FEATURES

Anxiety disorder patients may present with anxiety, avoidance, physical symptoms, secondary depression, or substance abuse. Complaints of anxiety should be assessed with respect to symptoms and cognitions, frequency and intensity, environmental precipitants, avoidance, and interference with functioning. Some anxiety disorder features can occur across these disorders. *Anticipatory anxiety* refers to apprehension in anticipation of a feared situation and may include worry, difficulty concentrating, or physical symptoms. Anxiety disorders are often marked by a failure of the habituation that normally occurs during continuing exposure to a feared situation. A *panic attack* is defined by intense fear that reaches a peak in minutes and includes a group of physical anxiety symptoms, often with feelings of unreality, dizziness, paresthesias, dyspnea, and fear of dying. *Phobic avoidance* involves excessive avoidance of circumscribed feared situations, and it is often the most directly disabling of anxiety disorder features.

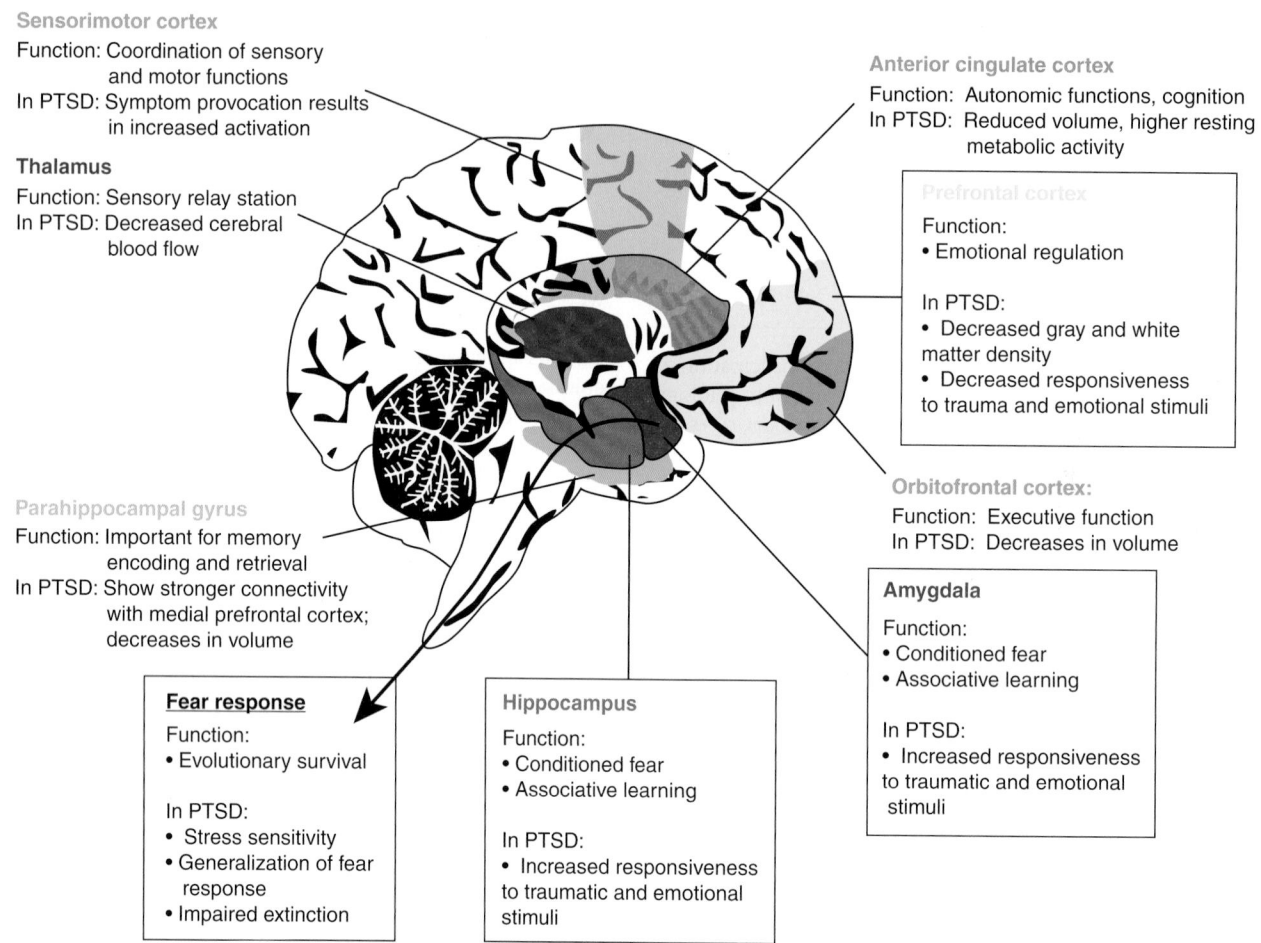

Sensorimotor cortex
Function: Coordination of sensory and motor functions
In PTSD: Symptom provocation results in increased activation

Thalamus
Function: Sensory relay station
In PTSD: Decreased cerebral blood flow

Anterior cingulate cortex
Function: Autonomic functions, cognition
In PTSD: Reduced volume, higher resting metabolic activity

Prefrontal cortex
Function:
• Emotional regulation
In PTSD:
• Decreased gray and white matter density
• Decreased responsiveness to trauma and emotional stimuli

Orbitofrontal cortex:
Function: Executive function
In PTSD: Decreases in volume

Parahippocampal gyrus
Function: Important for memory encoding and retrieval
In PTSD: Show stronger connectivity with medial prefrontal cortex; decreases in volume

Amygdala
Function:
• Conditioned fear
• Associative learning
In PTSD:
• Increased responsiveness to traumatic and emotional stimuli

Fear response
Function:
• Evolutionary survival
In PTSD:
• Stress sensitivity
• Generalization of fear response
• Impaired extinction

Hippocampus
Function:
• Conditioned fear
• Associative learning
In PTSD:
• Increased responsiveness to traumatic and emotional stimuli

FIGURE 150.1 Brain regions associated with PTSD. PTSD, posttraumatic stress disorder. (From Mahan AL, Ressler KJ. Fear conditioning, synaptic plasticity and the amygdala: implications for posttraumatic stress disorder. *Trends Neurosci.* 2012;35[1]:24–35.)

Anxiety often leads to symptoms of depression, so anxious patients should be evaluated for depressed mood, loss of pleasure, change in weight, sleep disturbance, fatigue, poor concentration, and suicidal ideation. Substance abuse is also common in anxiety disorder patients and may be either a precipitant of anxiety or a response to it. People with anxiety disorders are usually aware that the symptoms are related to an excessive or unrealistic reaction on their part, and in this way, they differ from patients with psychotic disorders with delusional fears.

Anxiety disorders may interact with other medical conditions so that patients with asthma may also experience dyspnea related to panic attacks, and individuals with disorders that attract unwanted attention (e.g., essential tremor) may be impaired by excessive fear of embarrassment as in social anxiety disorder. Medical conditions that can directly mimic anxiety symptoms include hyperthyroidism; hyperparathyroidism; cardiac arrhythmias; reactions to caffeine, cocaine, or marijuana; pheochromocytoma; and vestibular dysfunction.

DIAGNOSIS

See Table 150.1 for key diagnostic features.

PANIC DISORDER AND AGORAPHOBIA

The essential feature of panic disorder, as described in *DSM-5*, is recurrent unexpected panic attacks followed by persistent concerns or significant changes in behavior related to fear of another attack. Patients with panic disorder are often first seen medically because of fears that they are having a heart attack or stroke. Panic attacks may become cued by specific situations most commonly involving situations in which the person anticipates difficulty escaping or getting help in the event of an attack, such as traveling away from home, being in a crowd, or being alone. When people fear and avoid such situations, the diagnosis of agoraphobia is made.

Case Example of Panic Disorder

A 23-year-old woman presented to the emergency department complaining of 1-hour duration of light-headedness, weak legs, difficulty breathing, tingling sensations in her hands, and fear that she was having a stroke. Symptoms came on suddenly with no specific trigger, although she was feeling stressed after having had an argument with her boyfriend yesterday. Medical and neurologic evaluation was unremarkable. The patient was told that her symptoms were due to anxiety, and they subsequently resolved over a couple of hours. However, the patient developed daily recurrences of attacks over the next week, with fear that the symptoms would be persistent and disabling, even if they were not life-threatening. She called in sick to work and asked a family member to stay with her. Following 8 weeks of treatment with a selective serotonin reuptake inhibitor (SSRI) medication and cognitive behavioral therapy (CBT), her panic attacks remitted, although she continued to experience occasional brief surges of mild anxiety.

TABLE 150.1	**Key Diagnostic Features of Anxiety Disorders**
Diagnosis	**Key Diagnostic Features**
Panic disorder	Recurrent unexpected panic attacks
Agoraphobia	Avoidance of situations where escape might be difficult in the event of experiencing panic-like symptoms
Social anxiety disorder	Persistent and excessive fears of negative evaluation in social or performance situations
PTSD and acute stress disorder	After a traumatic event, persistent intrusive thoughts, avoidance of reminders, dysphoria, and hyperarousal
Obsessive–compulsive disorder	Obsessive thoughts and repetitive compulsive behaviors
Generalized anxiety disorder	Excessive anxiety and worry about multiple issues
Specific phobia	Persistent and excessive fear of a specific object or situation
Separation anxiety disorder	Persistent and excessive fear of separation from an attachment figure
Selective mutism	Persistent failure to speak in specific social situations (e.g., school); usually seen in young children

PTSD, posttraumatic stress disorder.

SOCIAL ANXIETY DISORDER (SOCIAL PHOBIA)

Social anxiety disorder, also known as *social phobia*, is characterized by an excessive fear of social situations due to fears of negative evaluation. The person may avoid social or performance situations or endure them with great distress. Physical symptoms, such as sweating, tremor, and blushing, may be present, but they are not necessary for the diagnosis as per *DSM-5*. The scope of feared situations may encompass most situations and appear similar to extreme shyness or may be limited to performance situations, such as public speaking. Social anxiety disorder is distinguished from normal shyness by its greater persistence and severity and its associated distress or impairment. Persons with social anxiety disorder often have difficulty participating in classroom settings or work meetings, dating, or engaging in social gatherings.

POSTTRAUMATIC STRESS DISORDER AND ACUTE STRESS DISORDER

Stress disorders occur in persons exposed to a traumatic event in which the person experienced, witnessed, or was confronted with actual or threatened death, serious injury, or sexual violence to self or others. PTSD features according to *DSM-5* include more than 1 month of (1) intrusive memories, dreams, or flashbacks or intense psychological and physiologic distress at exposure to reminders of the trauma; (2) avoidance of stimuli associated with the trauma; (3) alterations in cognition or mood, such as self-blame or inability to experience positive emotions; and (4) symptoms of increased arousal, such as hypervigilance, insomnia, poor concentration, irritability, or reckless behavior. Acute stress disorder is diagnosed when a similar syndrome is present in the month after

trauma exposure, and it may progress to PTSD. When a TBI co-occurs, PTSD symptoms may overlap TBI-related neurocognitive symptoms.

OBSESSIVE–COMPULSIVE DISORDER

OCD is defined in *DSM-5* by recurrent obsessions or compulsions that are time-consuming (more than 1 h/day) or cause significant distress and impairment. Obsessions are recurrent and persistent thoughts, urges, or images that are experienced as intrusive and unwanted and cause marked anxiety or distress. The individual attempts to ignore or suppress the obsessions or to neutralize them with some other thought or action. Insight into the truth of obsessive beliefs may vary. Compulsions are repetitive behaviors, such as washing or checking, or mental acts, such as counting, that an individual feels driven to perform in response to an obsession or according to rigid rules. The individual may have ideas that the behaviors prevent distress or that they somehow prevent a dreaded event (e.g., death of a loved one). However, these behaviors are not realistically connected with what they are intended to prevent, or they are clearly excessive. Up to 30% of individuals with OCD have a lifetime tic disorder, and in such cases, the diagnosis should be specified as *tic-related*.

GENERALIZED ANXIETY DISORDER

Generalized anxiety disorder is characterized, according to *DSM-5*, by excessive anxiety and worry about a number of events or activities occurring more days than not for at least 6 months. The individual finds it difficult to control the worry, which is associated with three or more of (1) restlessness or feeling keyed up, (2) fatigue, (3) difficulty concentrating, (4) irritability, (5) muscle tension, and (6) sleep disturbance. Generalized anxiety disorder is highly comorbid with depression.

SPECIFIC PHOBIAS

Persons with a specific phobia exhibit persistent fear of a specific object or situation, exposure to which evokes a fear response out of proportion to the actual danger. As specified in *DSM-5*, common types are the following: animal (e.g., spiders or dogs), natural environment (e.g., storms, heights), situational (e.g., airplanes, enclosed places), and blood–injection–injury (e.g., needles, dentist). A vasovagal response has been specifically associated with blood–injection–injury phobia.

SEPARATION ANXIETY DISORDER

Separation anxiety disorder is characterized in *DSM-5* by an excessive fear of separation from an attachment figure as evidenced by at least three of the following: excessive distress related to separation, excessive worry about harm to an attachment figure, excessive worry about an untoward event that results in separation, reluctance to go out (e.g., to work), reluctance to be alone, reluctance to sleep away from an attachment figure, nightmares about separation, and physical symptoms when separated. Adults often worry about a significant other or a child.

SELECTIVE MUTISM

Selective mutism is generally diagnosed in young children but may persist into adulthood. As described in *DSM-5*, the diagnosis is based on observation that an individual manifests a persistent failure to speak in specific social situations (e.g., school) despite speaking in other situations. The behavior interferes with functioning and is not due to a lack of knowledge of the spoken language or a communication disorder (e.g., childhood-onset fluency disorder). A child with selective mutism may be unable to offer an explanation for his or her silence, although high levels of social anxiety often appear to be associated with this reticent behavior.

ANXIETY AND NEUROLOGIC DISEASE: COMORBIDITY AND DIFFERENTIAL DIAGNOSIS

Anxiety disorder symptoms can overlap greatly with symptoms of a variety of neurologic disorders, including movement disorders, epilepsy, or cerebrovascular disease. For example, tremor is a common manifestation of anxiety, and it is particularly common in performance situations for individuals with social anxiety disorder. Light-headedness, occasionally even leading to syncope, is common during panic attacks. Panic-related light-headedness is usually of short duration and accompanied by dyspnea, hyperventilation, and intense fear. Paresthesias, tinnitus, vertigo, impaired concentration, derealization, and depersonalization may also occur during panic attacks or other periods of high anxiety. Importantly, the presence of psychopathology does not rule out the presence of concurrent neurologic disorder, and symptoms of a primary neurologic disorder, such as tremor or vertigo, may be exacerbated by situational anxiety. When a comorbid anxiety disorder complicates a neurologic disorder, treatments targeted at each condition may be necessary.

Obsessive–compulsive symptoms have been specifically associated with several neurologic disorders sharing dysfunction of frontostriatal circuitry, including Huntington disease and Gilles de la Tourette syndrome. In patients with Huntington disease, obsessive–compulsive symptoms, particularly obsessive checking, pathologic impulses, and compulsive rituals, have been reported in 15% to 50% of cases. OCD symptoms are also elevated in persons with the genetic mutation for Huntington but who have not yet met criteria for the diagnosis.

Tics have a compulsive quality, and like compulsions, if resisted, they result in internal tension that is relieved by performance of the behavior. The compulsions of OCD, however, are often accompanied by a complex thought process (e.g., need to relieve a sense of contamination) that seems to motivate the compulsive behavior. Compulsions that are present in patients with Tourette syndrome tend to be related to symmetry, counting, or "just right" thoughts and less likely to relate to fears of contamination or harm to others. Pediatric autoimmune neuropsychiatric disorders associated with streptococcal infections (PANDAS) is a controversial variant of Gilles de la Tourette syndrome and childhood-onset OCD in which both conditions may be associated with the development of an immune response against group A β-hemolytic *Streptococcus*.

In epilepsy, there is an increased rate of anxiety disorders, and panic disorder symptoms are the anxiety symptoms most likely to be generated directly by a seizure. Patients with primary panic attacks are less likely than seizure patients to experience automatisms, impaired consciousness, or déjà vu experiences and more likely to have accompanying phobias, depression, and anticipatory anxiety.

Dementia is accompanied by elevated rates of anxiety, often in the form of generalized anxiety disorder symptoms. Rates of anxiety symptoms may be particularly greater in vascular dementia and frontotemporal dementia. The presence of anxiety in dementia is associated with a variety of worse outcomes, including more impairment in quality of life, activities of daily living, nighttime awakenings, and neuropsychological performance.

Males with the genetic syndrome fragile X commonly experience symptoms of multiple anxiety disorders, particularly social anxiety symptoms of poor eye contact and excessive shyness. They also have elevated rates of separation anxiety, panic attacks, and agoraphobia. Compulsive behaviors are present in most patients, but these often involve pleasurable activities rather than the unwanted compulsions characteristic of OCD.

In patients with multiple sclerosis, anxiety disorders occur at three times the rate of the general population. Generalized anxiety disorder, OCD, panic disorder, and social anxiety disorder have been found to be elevated in some studies. Anxiety is associated with confirmed exacerbations and pseudoexacerbations of multiple sclerosis and with greater impairment, although it has not been specifically linked to progression of brain lesions.

TREATMENT

GENERAL APPROACHES TO ANXIETY DISORDERS

Psychological and pharmacologic treatments (Table 150.2) have well-established efficacy for anxiety disorders. The two best established first-line treatments for most of the anxiety disorders are CBT and SSRI medications, based on dozens of controlled trials in specific anxiety disorders. Other psychotherapies, such as short-term psychodynamic therapies, and other medications, such as benzodiazepines, have been demonstrated efficacious in certain anxiety disorders. This section will describe the general features of CBT and classes of medication used for anxiety disorders, as well as their unique adaptations for specific anxiety disorders.

CBTs for anxiety disorders are short-term psychotherapies based on the observation that patients manifest cognitive distortions (irrational negative thoughts) that maintain anxiety and avoidance behaviors, and that deny them opportunities to disprove those fears or to experience habituation of anxiety symptoms. Components of this therapy may include cognitive restructuring, exposure, and relaxation techniques. Typically, an active therapist helps the patient identify his or her cognitive distortions and avoidance behaviors and introduces alternative approaches for coping with feared situations. Therapist and patient collaborate to conduct exposures to the feared situations in the presence of the therapist and through homework assignments. As the patient uses new coping skills to manage the anxiety induced by the exposure without resorting to avoidance or rituals, new learning takes place and the habitual cycle of fear and avoidance recedes. A far smaller body of evidence exists for efficacy of other psychotherapy approaches to anxiety, including psychodynamic therapy. Disorder-specific features of CBT and other psychotherapies are discussed below under specific disorder sections.

SSRIs and serotonin–norepinephrine inhibitors (SNRIs) have emerged as first-line treatments for each of the anxiety disorders (with the exception of specific phobias) based on efficacy and acceptability. No single SSRI has been shown to be superior to others, although individuals often have different responses to different agents. Dosages are similar to those recommended for treatment of depression. Responses typically become apparent after 2 to 4 weeks of treatment, but an adequate acute trial may require 8 to 12 weeks of treatment, and nonresponders should have the dosage gradually increased to the maximum as tolerated. Common side effects include nausea, insomnia, fatigue, weight gain, and sexual dysfunction. Treatment guidelines tend to recommend that responders to an acute trial of medication be maintained on the effective dose for

TABLE 150.2	**Medications Used in the Treatment of Anxiety Disorders**		
Medication	**Initial Dose (mg/day)**	**Target Dose (mg/day)**	**Indication (Level 1 Evidence)**
Selective Serotonin Reuptake Inhibitors			
Sertraline	50[a]	50–200	OCD,[9] PD,[2] SAD,[6] PTSD,[7] GAD[12]
Paroxetine	10[a]	10–60	OCD,[9] PD,[2] SAD,[6] PTSD,[7] GAD[12]
Paroxetine CR	12.5[a]	12.5–75	SAD[6]
Citalopram	10[a]	20–40	PD,[2] OCD[9]
Escitalopram	5[a]	5–20	GAD[12]
Fluvoxamine	50[a]	50–300	OCD,[9] PD[2]SAD[6]
Fluoxetine	20	20–80	OCD,[9] SAD,[6] PTSD[7]
Serotonin–Norepinephrine Reuptake Inhibitors			
Venlafaxine XR	75[a]	75–375	SAD,[6] PD,[2] PTSD,[7] GAD[12]
Duloxetine	30[a]	30–60	GAD[12]
Other Antidepressants			
Nefazodone	200	200–600	PTSD[7]
Mirtazapine	15	30–60	SAD,[6] PD[2]
Clomipramine	25	50–250	OCD,[10] PD[5]
Imipramine	25	50–300	PD[4]
Phenelzine	15	30–90	SAD[6]
Benzodiazepines			
Clonazepam	0.25	.5–4	SAD,[6] PD[3]
Alprazolam	.25	.5–6	PD,[3] GAD[15]
Lorazepam	.5	1–2	GAD[15]
Diazepam	5	20	GAD[15]
Other Classes			
Buspirone	10	30–60	GAD[13]
Hydroxyzine	25	50	GAD[14]
Gabapentin	600	900–3,600	SAD[6]
Pregabalin	300	600	SAD,[6] GAD[12]
Prazosin	1	2–6	PTSD[8]
Risperidone	0.5	0.5–6	PTSD[7]
Quetiapine ER	50	50–300	GAD[16]

[a]For PD, antidepressants are commonly initiated at half the usual initial dose.

PTSD, posttraumatic stress disorder; PD, panic disorder; SAD, social anxiety disorder; OCD, obsessive–compulsive disorder; GAD, generalized anxiety disorder.

6 to 12 months, and when medication is discontinued, it should be tapered to minimize risk of withdrawal symptoms and relapse.

Medication is commonly combined with CBT, although evidence for additive efficacy is limited. Other medications, including some classified as benzodiazepines, tricyclic antidepressants, monoamine oxidase inhibitors, anticonvulsants, and antipsychotics, have also been shown to be effective for some of the anxiety disorders. These are discussed where relevant in the following text under specific anxiety disorders.

PANIC DISORDER AND AGORAPHOBIA

CBT for panic and agoraphobia has been shown efficacious in multiple randomized controlled trials (RCTs) [Level 1].[1] It helps patients decatastrophize their beliefs about physical symptoms through cognitive restructuring and interoceptive exposure, which involves purposefully inducing feared physical symptoms (e.g., by exercise or hyperventilation). Patients with agoraphobia purposefully approach their feared situations. Among pharmacologic treatments for panic disorder, SSRIs [Level 1][2] and SNRIs [Level 1][2] are first-line treatments. Benzodiazepines [Level 1],[3] the antidepressant mirtazapine [Level 1],[2] and the older class of tricyclics (e.g., imipramine) [Level 1][4] and clomipramine [Level 1][5] have also been shown to be efficacious. Antidepressants are typically started at half of the usual starting dose, as some panic disorder patients will report excessive stimulation with initial dosing. Benzodiazepines are often prescribed on an as-needed basis for intermittent anxiety, but for panic disorder and social anxiety disorder (see the following section), they are most effectively used with standing doses. Alprazolam and clonazepam are the benzodiazepines that have been best studied in panic disorder. Benzodiazepines have rapid onset of effect and a relatively low rate of side effects other than sedation. They are sometimes used in combination with SSRIs. Disadvantages include potential for abuse, cognitive and motor impairment, risk of severe withdrawal symptoms if discontinued abruptly, and lack of efficacy for comorbid depressive symptoms.

SOCIAL ANXIETY DISORDER

CBT [Level 1][1] is effective in either individual or group formats, incorporating role-playing techniques to practice exposure to feared social scenarios. SSRIs and the SNRI venlafaxine are first-line treatments based on numerous RCTs [Level 1].[6] A smaller number of RCTs support use of the benzodiazepine clonazepam; the antidepressant mirtazapine, gabapentin, and pregabalin, which act at calcium channels; and the older antidepressant class of monoamine oxidase inhibitors (e.g., phenelzine) [Level 1].[6] β-Adrenergic blockers (e.g., propranolol), taken on an as-needed basis, are commonly used for anxiety that is limited to predictable performance situations.

POSTTRAUMATIC STRESS DISORDER AND ACUTE STRESS DISORDER

Efficacy of CBT for acute stress disorder and PTSD has been established by more than two-dozen controlled trials [Level 1].[1] Goals of psychotherapy for acute stress disorder are to reestablish a sense of safety, build a therapeutic alliance, provide information, and allow ventilation of emotion only after the perceived threat ends. Treatment of PTSD involves education about the normal course of stress response, relaxation techniques, cognitive therapy to address pathogenic beliefs, and exposure to trauma-related stimuli through imaginal techniques, such as reviewing a script of the trauma, and through in vivo exposure.

Pharmacologic treatments for PTSD are used primarily as an adjunct to psychotherapy. The SSRIs paroxetine, fluoxetine, and sertraline and the SNRI venlafaxine each have a few RCTs supporting efficacy [Level 1].[7] Benzodiazepines, however, have not been shown to be effective. Single controlled trials have supported efficacy for the serotonergic antidepressant nefazodone [Level 1][7] and the α1 antagonist prazosin [**Level 1**],[8] and two very small RCTs have suggested efficacy for the atypical antipsychotic risperidone [**Level 1**].[7]

OBSESSIVE–COMPULSIVE DISORDER

Exposure and response prevention is the most effective treatment of OCD based on many controlled trials including comparisons to medication treatment [**Level 1**].[1] This CBT involves systematically exposing a patient to feared situations and preventing ritualizing (e.g., touching dirt without washing, leaving home without checking the lock). Clinical trials report high response rates in patients who participate in this therapy.

SSRIs [**Level 1**][9] and the serotonergic tricyclic antidepressant clomipramine [**Level 1**][10] are the only established pharmacologic monotherapies for OCD. Patients may require maximal dosage and a 12-week trial to assess efficacy, and most patients achieve only partial benefit from these medications. The only pharmacologic augmentation strategy shown to be effective for partial responders to SSRIs, on the basis of several small RCTs, is the use of antipsychotic agents, such as haloperidol or risperidone [**Level 1**].[11] Refractory OCD has occasionally been treated neurosurgically by anterior cingulotomy, subcaudate tractotomy, or anterior capsulotomy. Deep brain stimulation has been studied in over 100 patients to date with some reports of at least short-term benefit.

SPECIFIC PHOBIAS

Desensitization by exposure is the preferred treatment for specific phobias, and it is highly effective. Medications have received little study, but benzodiazepines, taken as needed, are useful for feared situations that are encountered only occasionally.

GENERALIZED ANXIETY DISORDER

CBT for generalized anxiety disorder has established efficacy [**Level 1**][1] and often incorporates self-monitoring of symptoms and their triggers, and relaxation techniques. In addition to SSRIs and SNRIs, which have established efficacy in multiple RCTs [**Level 1**],[12] other drugs with evidence for efficacy from RCTs include pregabalin [**Level 1**],[12] the serotonin 1a receptor agonist–antagonist buspirone [**Level 1**],[13] and antihistamines (e.g., hydroxyzine) [**Level 1**].[14] Although benzodiazepines were once a mainstay for generalized anxiety, recent studies have questioned the quality of the early trials in generalized anxiety disorder that established efficacy of these medications [**Level 1**].[15] The antipsychotic quetiapine has appeared efficacious in several controlled trials but carries a risk of serious adverse effects, such as tardive dyskinesia [**Level 1**].[16]

SEPARATION ANXIETY DISORDER AND SELECTIVE MUTISM

There have been no studies of treatment of either of these disorders in adults. Controlled trials in children suggest that both SSRIs and CBT are beneficial for separation anxiety disorder. Studies of selective mutism similarly suggest a role for SSRIs and CBT.

TREATMENT OF ANXIETY DISORDERS COMORBID WITH NEUROLOGIC DISORDERS

Although there is little data to guide approaches to these patients, existing studies suggest that standard treatments for the comorbid anxiety disorder can be effective in reducing anxiety symptoms and impairment. For example, CBT has been shown to reduce anxiety symptoms and social adjustment in epilepsy patients with mixed psychiatric problems even in the absence of reduction in seizure frequency. GABAergic anticonvulsants such as benzodiazepines and pregabalin often benefit comorbid anxiety, and SSRIs can be used with only small effects on seizure threshold. In dementia, psychosocial interventions are preferred for anxiety, as benzodiazepines and antipsychotics carry increased risks for the elderly and cognitively impaired. In Tourette syndrome, CBT and SSRIs should be considered for patients with comorbid OCD. Open trials for poststroke anxiety have suggested possible benefit for buspirone and for SSRIs plus psychotherapy.

OUTCOME

Efficacious psychological and pharmacologic treatments have been well established for most of the anxiety disorders. CBTs have yielded response rates upwards of 80% in some studies for those patients able to complete a course of treatment. Response rates to an initial trial of SSRI medication typically range from 50% to 70%, but less than half of these responders attain remission. These same approaches appear to be useful for anxiety disorders that are comorbid with neurologic disorders. Research is ongoing into exploring anxiety disorder treatments with novel mechanisms, improving treatment selection through personalized medicine, and developing alternative strategies for patients who do not respond fully to first-line treatments.

LEVEL 1 EVIDENCE

1. Hofmann SG, Smits JA. Cognitive-behavioral therapy for adult anxiety disorders: a meta-analysis of randomized placebo-controlled trials. *J Clin Psychiatry.* 2008;69:621–632.

2. Andrisano C, Chiesa A, Serretti A. Newer antidepressants and panic disorder: a meta-analysis. *Int Clin Psychopharmacol.* 2013;28:33–45.

3. Stein M, Steckler T, Lightfoot JD, et al. Pharmacologic treatment of panic disorder. *Curr Top Behav Neurosci.* 2010;2: 469–485.

4. Barlow DH, Gorman JM, Shear MK, et al. Cognitive-behavioral therapy, imipramine, or their combination for panic disorder: a randomized controlled trial. *JAMA.* 2000;283:2529–2536.

5. Bakker A, van Dyck R, Spinhoven P, et al. Paroxetine, clomipramine, and cognitive therapy in the treatment of panic disorder. *J Clin Psychiatry.* 1999;60:831–838.

6. Schneier FR. Pharmacotherapy of social anxiety disorder. *Expert Opin Pharmacother.* 2011;12:615–625.

7. Ipser JC, Stein DJ. Evidence-based pharmacotherapy of posttraumatic stress disorder (PTSD). *Int J Neuropsychopharmacol.* 2012;15:825–840.

8. Raskind MA, Peterson K, Williams T, et al. A trial of prazosin for combat trauma PTSD with nightmares in active-duty soldiers returned from Iraq and Afghanistan. *Am J Psychiatry.* 2013;170:1003–1010.

9. Soomro GM, Altman D, Rajagopal S, et al. Selective serotonin re-uptake inhibitors (SSRIs) versus placebo for obsessive compulsive disorder (OCD). *Cochrane Database Syst Rev.* 2008;23:CD001765.

10. Foa EB, Liebowitz MR, Kozak MJ, et al. Randomized, placebo-controlled trial of exposure and ritual prevention, clomipramine, and their combination in the treatment of obsessive-compulsive disorder. *Am J Psychiatry.* 2005;162: 151–161.

11. Fineberg NA, Reghunandanan S, Brown A, et al. Pharmacotherapy of obsessive-compulsive disorder: evidence-based treatment and beyond. *Aust N Z J Psychiatry*. 2013;47: 121–141.

12. Baldwin DS, Waldman S, Allgulander C. Evidence-based pharmacological treatment of generalized anxiety disorder. *Int J Neuropsychopharmacol*. 2011;14:697–710.

13. Chessick CA, Allen MH, Thase M, et al. Azapirones for generalized anxiety disorder. *Cochrane Database Syst Rev*. 2006;(3):CD006115.

14. Guaiana G, Barbui C, Cipriani A. Hydroxyzine for generalised anxiety disorder. *Cochrane Database Syst Rev*. 2010;(12):CD006815.

15. Martin JL, Sainz-Pardo M, Furukawa TA, et al. Benzodiazepines in generalized anxiety disorder: heterogeneity of outcomes based on a systematic review and meta-analysis of clinical trials. *J Psychopharmacol*. 2007;21:774–782.

16. Maher AR, Maglione M, Bagley S, et al. Efficacy and comparative effectiveness of atypical antipsychotic medications for off-label uses in adults: a systematic review and meta-analysis. *JAMA*. 2011;306:1359–1369.

SUGGESTED READINGS

American Psychiatric Association. *Diagnostic and Statistical Manual of Mental Disorders*. 5th ed. Washington, DC: American Psychiatric Association; 2013.

Dissanayaka NN, Sellbach A, Matheson S, et al. Anxiety disorders in Parkinson's disease: prevalence and risk factors. *Mov Disord*. 2010;25:838–845.

Etkin A, Wager TD. Functional neuroimaging of anxiety: a meta-analysis of emotional processing in PTSD, social anxiety disorder, and specific phobia. *Am J Psychiatry*. 2007;164:1476–1488.

Fibbe LA, Cath DC, van den Heuvel OA, et al. Relationship between movement disorders and obsessive-compulsive disorder: beyond the obsessive-compulsive-tic phenotype. A systematic review. *J Neurol Neurosurg Psychiatry*. 2012;83:646–654.

Figee M, Wielaard I, Mazaheri A, et al. Neurosurgical targets for compulsivity: what can we learn from acquired brain lesions? *Neurosci Biobehav Rev*. 2013;37:328–339.

Goodman WK, Alterman RL. Deep brain stimulation for intractable psychiatric disorders. *Annu Rev Med*. 2012;63:511–524.

Jenike MA. Clinical practice. Obsessive–compulsive disorder. *N Engl J Med*. 2004;350:259–265.

Leahy RL, Holland SJF, McGinn LK. *Treatment Plans and Interventions for Depression and Anxiety Disorders*. 2nd ed. New York: Guilford Press; 2012.

Leonardo E, Hen R. Anxiety as a developmental disorder. *Neuropsychopharmacology*. 208;33:134–140.

Liberzon I, Sripada CS. The functional neuroanatomy of PTSD: a critical review. *Prog Brain Res*. 2008;167:151–169.

Martino D, Defazio G, Giovannoni G. The PANDAS subgroup of tic disorders and childhood-onset obsessive-compulsive disorder. *J Psychosom Res*. 2009;67:547–557.

Perugi G, Frare F, Toni C. Diagnosis and treatment of agoraphobia with panic disorder. *CNS Drugs*. 2007;21:741–764.

Schneier FR. Clinical practice: social anxiety disorder. *N Engl J Med*. 2006;355:1029–1036.

Simpson HB, Neria Y, Lewis-Fernandez R, et al, eds. *Anxiety Disorders: Theory, Research and Clinical Perspectives*. Cambridge, United Kingdom: Cambridge University Press; 2010.

Stein DJ, Hollander E, Rothbaum BO, eds. *Textbook of Anxiety Disorders*. 2nd ed. Washington, DC: American Psychiatric Publishing; 2010.

Anna Lopatin Dickerman and Philip R. Muskin

INTRODUCTION

Somatic symptom disorders are a group of psychiatric illnesses in which patients experience bodily symptoms along with associated abnormal thoughts, feelings, and behaviors that cause clinically significant distress and functional impairment. Patients with somatic symptom disorders tend to initially present in medical or neurologic settings. The disorders account for medical and psychiatric morbidity among patients, as well as increased costs due to greater chronicity of symptoms, health care use, and higher rates of disability. Patients with somatic symptom disorders can be among the most challenging for both psychiatric and nonpsychiatric clinicians alike, as their presentation initially appears "real." Evidence-based treatments exist for these illnesses, and timely recognition and appropriate referral may significantly improve outcomes. Therefore, it behooves all clinicians—and in particular neurologists, who often encounter these patients before psychiatrists—to be familiar with these complex conditions. Patients with somatic symptom disorders can present with almost any neurologic complaint, including (but not limited to) headache, sensorimotor loss, problems with gait, tremor and other movement disturbances, cognitive complaints, ocular symptoms, and urogenital symptoms. This chapter provides an overview of the different types of somatic symptom disorders, their epidemiology and pathophysiology, and treatment strategies.

SOMATIC SYMPTOM DISORDERS IN *DIAGNOSTIC AND STATISTICAL MANUAL OF MENTAL DISORDERS*, 5TH EDITION

The somatic symptom disorders have undergone significant diagnostic criteria revision in *Diagnostic and Statistical Manual of Mental Disorders*, 5th edition (*DSM-5*) (Table 151.1).

There were several problematic issues with the *Diagnostic and Statistical Manual of Mental Disorders*, 4th edition (*DSM-IV*), criteria for somatic symptom disorders (formerly referred to as *somatoform disorders*). Clinicians underdiagnosed these illnesses because of confusion about terminology. The *DSM-IV* diagnostic criteria were particularly challenging for nonpsychiatric clinicians, who are often the first to encounter these patients. Furthermore, the hallmark of somatoform disorders in *DSM-IV* was the absence of a medical explanation for the somatic symptoms. This resulted in a problematic mind–body dualism that does not conform well to actual clinical experience. Conditions that are medically "unexplained" are not necessarily psychogenic in origin, that is, fibromyalgia and chronic fatigue syndrome are not considered psychiatric illnesses. Having a medically unexplained symptom is insufficient to make a psychiatric diagnosis; conversely, it is possible to have a documented medical condition and still have an abnormal psychological response to the physical symptoms. Patients with somatic symptom disorders *may or may not have a comorbid diagnosed medical condition*. The distinctive characteristic of these disorders has been shifted away from the somatic symptoms or their underlying etiology per se and focused on the maladaptive way in which the patient presents and interprets symptoms.

The terminology of somatic symptom disorders in *DSM-5* reduces the number of disorders and subcategories to minimize problematic overlap and diagnostic confusion. Somatic symptom disorders are defined on the basis of *positive* psychiatric symptoms rather than the *absence* of medical explanation for symptoms. Diagnosis no longer requires an exhaustive workup necessitating that the clinician rule out any physiologically based medical condition. The notable exceptions to this new rule are conversion disorder (functional neurologic symptom disorder) and pseudocyesis. *DSM-5* also eliminates the use of arbitrarily high symptom requirements that existed in *DSM-IV* diagnostic criteria for somatoform disorders. A large body of research has shown that the relationship between somatic symptoms and psychopathology exists along a spectrum that was not adequately reflected by these symptom count prerequisites.

The *DSM-IV* diagnosis of body dysmorphic disorder has been moved to the chapter on obsessive–compulsive disorder and related illnesses in *DSM-5*, as there is a large body of research establishing pathophysiologic connections between obsessive–compulsive illness and body dysmorphia. Body dysmorphic disorder is thus no longer considered a somatic symptom disorder. This research has considerable treatment implications. Somatization disorder, hypochondriasis, pain disorder, and undifferentiated somatoform disorder (all diagnoses in *DSM-IV*) have been removed and incorporated into two central diagnoses in *DSM-5*: somatic symptom disorder

TABLE 151.1	*DSM-IV* Somatoform Disorders and New *DSM-5* Somatic Symptom Disorders	
***DSM-IV* Somatoform Disorders**	***DSM-5* Somatic Symptom Disorders**
Somatization disorder	Somatic symptom disorder
Hypochondriasis	Illness anxiety disorder
Conversion disorder	Conversion disorder (functional neurologic symptom disorder)
Pain disorder	Factitious disorder
Body dysmorphic disorder	Psychological factors affecting other medical conditions
Undifferentiated somatoform disorder	Other specified somatic symptom and related disorder
Somatoform disorder NOS	Unspecified somatic symptom and related disorder

DSM-IV, Diagnostic and Statistical Manual of Mental Disorders, 4th edition; *DSM-5, Diagnostic and Statistical Manual of Mental Disorders*, 5th edition; NOS, not otherwise specified.

TABLE 151.2   Clinical Characteristics of *DSM-5* Somatic Symptom Disorders

Somatic symptom disorder	• One or more distressing somatic symptoms (including pain) • Maladaptive thoughts/feelings/behaviors related to the symptom(s) • Lasts at least 6 mo
Illness anxiety disorder	• Preoccupation with having or acquiring a serious illness • Somatic symptoms *mild or absent* • High level of health anxiety disproportionate to actual physical illness or risk of illness • Lasts at least 6 mo
Psychological factors affecting other medical conditions	• Psychological or behavioral symptoms that adversely impact an underlying medical or neurologic condition (either by interference with treatment, by constituting additional health risks, or by adversely impacting underlying pathophysiology)
Conversion disorder (functional neurologic symptom disorder)	• One or more symptoms of altered voluntary motor or sensory functions that cause significant distress or impairment • Symptom(s) incompatible with recognized neurologic or medical condition
Factitious disorder	• Falsified physical or psychological signs/symptoms via *identified deception* • Patient presents himself or herself (or his or her relative) as ill, impaired, or injured. • Deceptive behavior in the *absence of obvious external reward*

and illness anxiety disorder. Factitious disorder is now considered a somatic symptom disorder in *DSM-5*, as these patients often present with somatic symptoms in general medical settings. Psychological factors affecting other medical conditions is now a psychiatric diagnosis in *DSM-5*. The diagnosis is quite prevalent in medical and surgical patients. The revised *DSM-5* criteria should result in a reduction of the stigmatization of patients and to an improvement of diagnostic accuracy across various medical disciplines.

Table 151.2 summarizes the hallmark features of the *DSM-5* somatic symptom disorders.

SOMATIC SYMPTOM DISORDER

Somatic symptom disorder (somatization disorder in *DSM-IV*) is defined as an illness in which patients experience at least 6 months of one or more distressing somatic symptoms in addition to maladaptive thoughts, feelings, and behaviors related to these symptoms. This may include disproportionate or persistent thoughts about symptoms, an abnormally high level of anxiety about symptoms, and/or excessive time and energy devoted to the symptoms.

SAMPLE CASE

A 50-year-old woman complains of constant back pain. She is reluctant to take any narcotic analgesics for fear of addiction. Magnetic resonance imaging (MRI) of her back is not diagnostic. She continues to go to work daily but finds herself so exhausted at the end of the day from her pain that she goes to bed immediately when she returns home, unable to participate in any of the family's activities. Each time she improves and the neurologist recommends she return in 6 months, her pain increases and she seeks out a new physician.

EPIDEMIOLOGY

The prevalence of somatic symptom disorder is approximately 5% to 7% in the general adult population. Females report distressing somatic symptoms more frequently than males. Initial symptoms can begin at any age and usually appear by early adulthood.

Certain demographic factors are associated with a more severe clinical course, including female gender and older age. In elderly

individuals, somatic symptom disorder is more likely to go unrecognized because of comorbid medical illness. The physical complaints of older patients may also be misattributed to "normal aging" or "understandable" concern.

Somatic symptom disorder occurs more frequently in individuals with lower educational/socioeconomic status. They have more severe illness and worse outcomes. Demographic factors that adversely affect clinical course include unemployment, history of childhood physical or sexual abuse or other adversity, medical and psychiatric comorbidity, and external factors that reinforce the illness (e.g., disability payments).

PATHOPHYSIOLOGY AND ETIOLOGY

As is the case for most psychiatric illnesses, there are biologic, psychological, and social factors that contribute to the development of somatic symptom disorder. Biologic risk factors include genetic vulnerability to increased sensitivity to pain and other physical sensations. There is also an emerging literature to suggest a potential role for psychoneuroimmune mechanisms of somatic symptom amplification. Proinflammatory cytokines are known to be involved in the production of illness behavior; chronic activation or sensitization of this system may result in nonspecific somatic symptoms and chronic pain. Some have hypothesized that immunologic mechanisms in the setting of infectious triggers may contribute to the development of somatic symptom disorders. Functional neuroimaging studies have demonstrated aberrant cortical and limbic activity that may impact conscious processing of mild or chronically painful stimuli.

Psychosocial risk factors for somatic symptom disorder include early childhood trauma such as physical, sexual, or emotional abuse and/or neglect. Social learning mechanisms such as the attention gained from physical illness or lack of reinforcement of nonsomatic (emotional) expressions of distress may also contribute to the occurrence of somatic symptom disorder. Intrinsic temperamental factors may correlate with a higher risk of developing somatic symptom disorder, including alexithymia (difficulty identifying inner emotional states) and neuroticism (high levels of negative affect). Difficulties in communication—from intellectual, emotional, or social limitations—can predispose to bodily expression of distress.

DIFFERENTIAL DIAGNOSIS AND COMORBIDITY

Patients with psychiatric illness often present with somatic symptoms. Patients with major depressive disorder may experience prominent fatigue, whereas patients with anxiety disorders may experience tachycardia or abdominal pain. Usually the cardinal feature of these other illnesses is a pronounced mood disturbance accompanied by numerous other physical and mental symptoms, whereas the distress in somatic symptom disorders emanates predominantly from the physical symptoms themselves. Mood and anxiety disorders frequently co-occur with somatic symptom disorders. Depressive disorders are common in patients with somatic symptom disorder, particularly in the elderly. Patients with somatic symptom disorder are at risk to develop secondary substance use disorders.

Medical comorbidity is common among patients with somatic symptom disorder, which may further complicate the diagnosis. Iatrogenic creation of symptoms may be subsequently mislabeled as psychogenic. Common complications of somatic symptom disorder include iatrogenic harm from invasive procedures or dependence on habit-forming substances such as opiates. Greater medical and psychiatric comorbidity is typically associated with greater severity of illness, degree of distress, and functional impairment.

Cultural factors are crucial when considering the diagnosis of somatic symptom disorder; many culture-bound syndromes present with prominent physical symptoms. Differences in medical care across cultures can also affect the presentation and course of somatic symptom disorders. The ways in which individuals recognize and respond to bodily sensations is influenced by numerous interacting factors that occur within a given social and cultural context, which affects the way in which the patient perceives illness and seeks medical attention.

TREATMENT

Somatic symptom disorder is difficult to treat, and the literature does not suggest a single superior treatment approach. It is recommended that the patient form a stable relationship with a primary care physician who regularly and reliably follows up on a predetermined scheduled basis. When talking to the patient with suspected somatic symptom disorder, a thorough/empathic approach will put the patient at ease and facilitate successful psychiatric referral and follow-up. Objectively corroborated problems should be judiciously investigated; however, unnecessary exhaustive diagnostic testing should be avoided, as this may inadvertently reinforce the development of new somatic symptoms or even cause iatrogenic harm. The therapeutic focus shifts from "cure" toward symptom management. In the case of somatic symptom disorder with predominant pain, use of addictive substances should be avoided.

Early psychiatric intervention is likely to improve outcomes for patients with somatic symptom disorder; greater chronicity of undiagnosed somatization is correlated with worse outcomes and makes subsequent mental health treatment more challenging. An interdisciplinary "team" approach to the patient is crucial; close collaboration between the mental health practitioner and the medical care provider can help minimize errors of diagnostic omission in either domain. Frequent communication between treatment disciplines helps maximize consistency and reduce the likelihood of the patient feeling dismissed or abandoned.

When discussing a suspected diagnosis of somatic symptom disorder with a patient, the clinician may emphasize that stress can generate physical symptoms without the patient's awareness.

Providing education about the illness and giving patients a list of psychiatric diagnostic criteria is helpful in legitimizing and validating their complaints by giving them a "genuine" diagnosis. Developing a relationship with the patient's family may also be helpful for understanding and managing the greater social context in which somatic symptoms tend to occur.

Various treatments are successful for somatic symptom disorders. Psychotherapy is the mainstay of treatment for somatizing patients; such approaches include cognitive behavioral therapy [**Level 1**][1,2] and psychodynamic psychotherapy [**Level 1**].[3]

Data suggests that pharmacotherapy can be helpful in the management of somatic symptom disorder. Serotonergic antidepressants are moderately effective in reducing intensity of functional somatic symptoms. Medications are helpful in treating the comorbid depressive and anxiety disorders. Agents commonly used for neuropathic pain such as mixed noradrenergic/serotonergic antidepressants, tricyclic antidepressants, and certain anticonvulsants may be helpful. The mechanism of action for these agents remains to be fully elucidated, but recent research findings suggest potential modulation of the psychoneuroimmune pathophysiology described earlier.

When treating patients with somatic symptom disorder, consider the reinforcing role of secondary gain in maintaining symptoms. Although patients with somatic symptom clearly suffer, they may also obtain relief from certain societal, personal, and professional responsibilities as a result of their illness. Any successful treatment of somatic symptom disorder will seek as much as possible to eradicate these reinforcing agents and help reduce the possibility of further iatrogenic harm.

ILLNESS ANXIETY DISORDER

Illness anxiety disorder, formerly termed *hypochondriasis*, is characterized by a preoccupation with having or acquiring a serious medical illness that leads to clinically significant distress and dysfunction in social and/or occupational function. In this condition, bodily complaints and symptoms are often absent or mild. The hallmark of illness anxiety disorder is distress and preoccupation related to the individual's *anxiety about the meaning or significance* of the somatic complaint rather than the actual symptoms. Patients with illness anxiety disorder have a high level of health anxiety, disproportionate to their actual physical illness or risk of illness. They may engage in excessive health-related behaviors, including frequently checking their body or researching diseases on the Internet. Medical reassurance or negative diagnostic tests are unlikely to alleviate these patients' excessive concerns.

SAMPLE CASE

A 35-year-old woman finds what she thinks is a lump in her breast. She has a strong family history of breast cancer. She requests an "emergency appointment" with a surgeon who tells her that she does not feel a mass. Imaging of the woman's breast shows no pathology. The woman continues to fear she has breast cancer, examining her breast repeatedly and calling her gynecologist's office weekly regarding her concerns that she might have breast cancer.

EPIDEMIOLOGY

Estimates of the prevalence of illness anxiety disorder are based on epidemiologic studies on the *DSM-IV* diagnosis of hypochondriasis. These community surveys and population-based samples demonstrate a 1- to 2-year prevalence of health anxiety and/or disease conviction ranging from 1.3% to 10%. In ambulatory medical populations, the 6-month/1-year prevalence rates are between 3% and 8%. Illness anxiety is equally prevalent in males and females.

Illness anxiety disorder is a chronic/relapsing condition that begins in early to middle adulthood. In the general population, health-related anxiety increases with age, often focusing on cognitive deficits. In medical settings, no significant age differences have been found between those with low and those with high levels of illness anxiety.

PATHOPHYSIOLOGY AND ETIOLOGY

There are biologic and psychosocial components to the development of illness anxiety disorder. A history of childhood abuse/neglect or serious childhood illness is a risk factor for the development of illness anxiety disorder in adulthood. Major life stressors or illnesses are factors that may trigger the development of illness anxiety disorder.

DIFFERENTIAL DIAGNOSIS AND COMORBIDITY

It is important to consider the presence of underlying medical or neurologic disease. Anxiety related to health and feeling well is a normal response to being diagnosed with a major medical illness. In order to make a diagnosis of illness anxiety disorder, symptoms must be *disproportionate* to the underlying physical disease; the patient must have severe and continuous anxiety that causes significant distress for a minimum 6 months.

Major mood and anxiety disorders are other differential diagnostic considerations. Depressed patients can become preoccupied with concerns about their body and health. What distinguishes illness anxiety disorder from depressive and anxiety disorders is the patient's narrowed and persistent focus on health-related anxiety. Patients who are psychotic and have somatic delusions typically have other symptoms of psychosis. Patients with illness anxiety disorder may develop depression; this may make it difficult to tease apart which of the two is the primary psychiatric diagnosis. Patients with mood disorders and psychotic disorders may develop somatic delusions. Delusions are fixed, false beliefs that are held with a degree of conviction and intensity that is not typically seen in illness anxiety disorder. Patients with delusions are not able to reality-test, whereas patients with illness anxiety disorder are usually able to accept the possibility that they may not be as sick as they fear. Somatic delusions are often more bizarre or striking than the fears associated with illness anxiety disorder (e.g., delusions of complete bodily decay).

Illness anxiety disorder is a new diagnosis, therefore exact rates of comorbidities are not yet known. Prior research on hypochondriasis suggests that comorbidity is high in these patients. As many as two-thirds of illness anxiety disorder patients are likely to have at least one other major mental illness. Patients with significant illness anxiety are particularly likely to have comorbid depressive and anxiety disorders. Other common comorbid syndromes include somatic symptom disorder and personality disorders.

TREATMENT

The treatment of illness anxiety disorder has not been thoroughly researched. Patients referred early for psychiatric evaluation tend to have a better prognosis compared to those who receive only medical assessment and treatment. Psychiatric referral should be presented as a supplement, rather than an alternative or replacement for ongoing medical care and evaluation. Regularly scheduled, supportive treatment visits with a consistent primary care physician are helpful.

Evidence suggests that serotonergic antidepressants may be effective for somatic symptom disorders characterized by predominant illness anxiety [Level 1].[4,5] Therapeutic dosages may be higher than those for depressive and anxiety disorders. Cognitive behavioral therapy may be a particularly effective form of psychotherapy [Level 1],[5,6] with response rates at 12 months as high as 57%.

CONVERSION DISORDER (FUNCTIONAL NEUROLOGIC SYMPTOM DISORDER)

Patients with conversion disorder exhibit one or more symptoms of altered voluntary motor or sensory functions that cause significant distress or functional impairment. *DSM-5* specifies that *conversion disorder symptoms must be incompatible with recognized medical or neurologic conditions*. The diagnosis should not be made simply because diagnostic tests are normal or because the symptom is "bizarre." Functional neurologic symptoms may be acute or chronic and may affect various sensory or motor modalities. The diagnosis of conversion disorder in *DSM-5* does *not* require that a psychological stressor precede the development of symptoms. This decision was made by experts in the field in recognition of the fact that it is not always possible to immediately identify an antecedent stressor in conversion disorder. Nevertheless, it is important to make the diagnosis as quickly as possible in order to minimize morbidity or iatrogenic complications. The change in the diagnostic criteria is not meant to imply that psychological factors are not present or important for the patient and the symptoms.

The conventional psychodynamic model of conversion is that patients with conversion disorder unconsciously transmute their psychic distress into physical symptoms. It can be difficult to definitively eliminate the possibility of conscious feigning when initially encountering a patient with conversion disorder. Therefore, the assessment of conscious versus unconscious production of symptoms is unreliable. Thus, the new diagnostic criteria for conversion disorder no longer require a definitive judgment that the symptoms are unconsciously produced.

SAMPLE CASE

A 33-year-old woman is admitted to after sudden loss of function of her right arm. She smokes one pack per day, is overweight, and is on oral contraceptives. The loss of function in her arm occurred during an argument with her ex-husband when she admits she felt like "bopping him." When hypnotized by the psychiatric consultant, she is able to lift her right arm while in the trance; however, the arm becomes limp when she is out of the trance state.

PRESENTATION AND EPIDEMIOLOGY

Methodologic differences in epidemiologic studies of conversion disorder have led to great variability in the reported rates of prevalence. Lifetime prevalence rates in the general population range from 11 in 100,000 to 500 in 100,000. In the general hospital setting and the outpatient neurologic setting, lifetime prevalence rates are 4% to 15%.

Conversion disorder usually presents in early adult life, and is approximately two to three times more likely to occur in females. Conversion disorder is also more frequently seen in those belonging to groups of lower socioeconomic status and those with relatively less education. As with the other somatic symptom disorders, psychiatric comorbidity is high, for example, depressive and anxiety disorders and posttraumatic stress disorder as well as personality disorders and impairment of psychosocial functioning. Although conversion symptoms can be short-lived, it is not unusual for symptoms to recur in the same individual; 1-year relapse rates can be as high as 20% to 25%.

There is great variation in the degree of symptom severity among patients with conversion disorder. Good prognostic factors include acute onset and short duration of symptoms, presence of an identifiable stressor at the onset of illness, short interval between onset and referral to treatment, higher intelligence, and willingness to accept a psychological component to the illness. Underlying personality disorder is a poor prognostic indicator, as is comorbid somatic symptom disorder. The more long-standing the conversion symptoms, the more difficult it becomes to treat the disorder. This may be because of the accumulation of associated benefits over time (e.g., secondary gain). Comorbid psychiatric and medical illness is also associated with worse outcome.

PATHOPHYSIOLOGY AND ETIOLOGY

An underlying personal or family history of organic neurologic disease is a risk factor for the development of conversion symptoms. For example, patients with epilepsy are more likely to develop psychogenic nonepileptic seizures (PNES) than the general population; the estimated comorbidity of PNES in epilepsy patients is approximately 10%. Maladaptive coping style and personality traits as well as difficulty identifying and expressing emotion (alexithymia) may predispose an individual to development of conversion symptoms.

Patients with PNES have been found to have higher basal cortisol levels compared with healthy volunteers, a marker of overall greater stress level that is unrelated to seizure frequency, physical activity, or acute psychological stress. Statistically significant pre-ictal heart rate increases and postictal heart rate reductions normalized to baseline have also been identified in those with PNES compared to patients with complex partial seizures.

Environmental factors such as childhood abuse/neglect and other stressful or traumatic life events are also associated with the development of conversion disorder. Dissociation, a commonly seen psychological response to trauma, has also been described in patients with conversion disorder, particularly those with PNES. Researchers have hypothesized similar psychological processes underlying conversion and dissociative disorders despite the descriptive differences between the two conditions. Any clinician treating patients with conversion disorder should be aware of the potential role of past trauma in this illness and should be sensitive to therapeutic implications in the management of a traumatized patient (particularly as it relates to forming a stable treatment alliance).

Neuroimaging studies in patients with conversion disorder show different patterns of brain activation and deactivation compared to patients who consciously feign symptoms. Although there is no commonly accepted theory about the functional neuroanatomy of conversion disorder, available evidence suggests that the illness may represent a "functional unawareness syndrome" involving networks involved in the processing of emotion and affect. Several authors have established the presence of abnormal limbic–motor connectivity in conversion disorder.

DIFFERENTIAL DIAGNOSIS AND COMORBIDITY

A diagnosis of conversion disorder should only be made following a thorough neurologic assessment, including detailed history and examination and relevant imaging or other studies. Conversion disorder can be differentiated from organic illness by its incompatibility with known features of neurologic disease; however, as with the other somatic symptom disorders, actual physical illness and conversion disorder (or other apparent functional overlay) are not mutually exclusive. Overt evidence of deliberate feigning or exaggeration of symptoms should guide one away from a diagnosis of conversion disorder and more toward factitious disorder or malingering.

TREATMENT

Effective treatment of conversion disorder begins with empathic and positive communication of the diagnosis. It is generally best to avoid any comments that suggest to the patient that there is nothing "biologically" wrong with him or her in order to prevent embarrassment. It is helpful to inform the patient that he or she is clearly suffering from real symptoms that are concerning and disruptive but the expectation is that he or she will ultimately recover. The patient should be told that there is no need to be exposed to unnecessary medication or studies but that treatment focusing on managing the emotional issues and distress associated with the symptoms is very important for ultimate improvement. This type of phrasing can help engage the patient in a dialogue about any stress associated with the symptoms. Although the psychological conflict producing the symptoms may seem obvious to the physician, delicacy is required in presenting an interpretation of the proposed etiology to the patient. The most common "precipitants" are aggressive and sexual thoughts that are unacceptable to the patient; however, if the patient could easily cope with such thoughts, then the symptoms would not be manifested.

Despite the illness burden of conversion disorder and the therapeutic challenges inherent in its management, there is a lack of empirical data on effective treatment strategies. The majority of evidence for the treatment of conversion disorder is in the form of uncontrolled case series and reports. In general, the cornerstone of management for conversion disorder has been psychotherapy of various sorts. There is little clinical evidence to support the use of pharmacotherapy in the absence of other comorbid psychiatric conditions such as depressive or anxiety disorders. Some success has been reported with antidepressants and antipsychotics. Treatment with the antipsychotics is problematic given the potential for neuroleptic-induced movement disorder in patients who may already have psychogenic movement disorders.

Psychotherapy of patients with conversion disorder should be geared to helping the individual develop more adaptive coping strategies to deal with emotional conflicts and more effective ways of communicating distress. Cognitive behavioral therapy is one such therapeutic modality [**Level 1**].[7] Psychoanalytic and psychodynamic approaches to conversion can also be quite effective [**Level 1**].[8]

In addition to psychotherapy, there are studies of small sample sizes with preliminary findings suggesting possible efficacy for hypnosis [**Level 1**],[9,10] behavioral therapy and rehabilitation, physical therapy, and paradoxical intention. These treatments can be potentially "face-saving" for the patient, as they are based on a physical model of recovery, and may be particularly helpful for patients who have difficulty engaging in psychotherapy.

FACTITIOUS DISORDER

Unlike the other somatic symptom disorders, factitious disorder involves *intentional falsification* of physical and/or psychological symptoms or induction of injury or disease. The individual is aware of the deception and presents himself or herself as ill, injured, or impaired. A subtype of factitious disorder involves the presentation of someone else close to the patient as ill, injured, or impaired. This was previously called *factitious disorder by proxy* in *DSM-IV* and is now referred to in *DSM-5* as *factitious disorder imposed on another*. Patients with factitious disorder may present with single or recurrent episodes. Munchhausen syndrome is a particularly chronic and intractable form of factitious disorder.

Unlike the malingering patient, those with factitious disorder exhibit deceptive behavior *in the absence of any obvious external reward*. The traditional model of this illness rests on the idea that patients seek secondary gain via assumption of the sick role; however, *DSM-5* does not specifically list this as a diagnostic criterion because it is often not possible to reliably infer this early on in the disease course.

Common clinical characteristics often include a history of numerous prior medical evaluations and treatments, particularly hospitalizations, surgeries, and other invasive procedures. Other features that suggest the diagnosis include a dramatic or inconsistent history that is vague or variable in its detail, inexplicable laboratory results, inconsistent physical examination findings, use of highly medicalized jargon, minimization of the presence of scars from prior invasive procedures, or confabulation of details when attempts are made to corroborate history. Patients may also demonstrate remission of neurologic deficits when they believe no one is observing. The classic example of a patient with factitious disorder is someone who migrates to different treatment settings in order to avoid discovery of the psychopathology.

SAMPLE CASE

A 48-year-old woman is admitted for evaluation of an inoperable brain tumor. She has extensive records from prior hospitalizations. Neuroimaging reveals no pathology. When confronted, the patient reveals that she falsified the records for her "brain tumor." She reports that she planned to commit suicide and wanted her family to think she had an incurable cancer and would not be upset when she took her life.

EPIDEMIOLOGY

Because of the level of deception in patients with factitious disorder, exact estimates of prevalence are unknown. In the general hospital setting, approximately 1% of individuals meet criteria for the disorder, but rates may be higher in specialized treatment settings. The typical course of factitious disorder is recurrent, intermittent episodes that last over the course of the life span. Patients usually present during adulthood. Factitious disorder is more common in women, but its course is often more severe and refractory in men.

PATHOPHYSIOLOGY AND ETIOLOGY

Factitious disorder often presents following a hospitalization for a medical condition or mental disorder. In factitious disorder imposed on another, it is following the child or dependent party's hospitalization. Risk factors include a history of childhood abuse, disturbed parental relationships/emotional deprivation, early life illness or extended hospitalizations, and exposure to or employment in the medical setting.

There are several psychodynamic and cognitive, social learning, and behavioral theories that have been posited for the development of factitious disorder. Neurobiologic findings of functional imaging studies have been inconsistent.

DIFFERENTIAL DIAGNOSIS AND COMORBIDITY

The major differential diagnostic consideration in factitious disorder is malingering. Patients may have features or elements of both conditions, that is, a patient who may be subconsciously motivated complain of pain while enjoying access to opiates.

Many clinicians have difficulty differentiating between the somatic symptoms of factitious disorder and those of conversion disorder. The hallmark of factitious disorder is deliberate deception or fabrication of symptoms. In conversion disorder, patients do not intentionally produce symptoms.

Patients with factitious disorder who injure themselves do so specifically in order to assume the sick role. They are not attempting to kill themselves or to obtain affective or emotional release from the self-injury. This distinguishes their self-harming behavior from those of patients with mood or personality disorders. Patients with factitious disorder may have comorbid personality disorders and have frequent comorbid substance use disorders.

TREATMENT

Factitious disorder is one of the most difficult psychiatric illnesses to treat. Not surprisingly, clinicians often have strong negative emotional reactions to patients who falsify symptoms. Care providers may feel exploited, humiliated, or angered. It is important to remember when treating the patient with factitious disorder that he or she is in fact quite ill but not in the way he or she presents. These patients are at significant risk of self-inflicted injury or death. If a diagnosis of factitious disorder is suspected, it is often helpful to confer with hospital administrative and legal services.

An additional therapeutic challenge is the fact that patients often abruptly flee from care once they are confronted about the false nature of their symptoms; other responses include denial or threats of litigation. There is a dearth of comparative literature examining the efficacy of various treatment approaches. In general, it is recommended that treatment be collaborative, involving interdisciplinary team meetings and communication among providers to coordinate efforts and manage negative emotions. Psychodynamic and behavioral approaches have been used to treat the disorder. Pharmacotherapy has a role in treating specific comorbid symptoms, such as mood or psychotic disorders, if present.

PSYCHOLOGICAL FACTORS AFFECTING OTHER MEDICAL CONDITIONS

Psychological or behavioral factors that adversely affect other medical conditions (PFAOMC) are very common. This diagnosis is included in the group of somatic symptom disorders because of its usual appearance in primary care and other medical settings. Psychological or behavioral symptoms may include psychological distress, patterns of interpersonal interaction, coping styles, and maladaptive coping strategies such as denial or poor adherence. These thoughts, feelings, and behaviors can adversely affect known medical conditions in a variety of ways. A common example of this is denial of the significance of physical symptoms, which may in turn lead to delayed medical intervention.

There may be a temporal relationship between psychological factors and development or exacerbation of a medical condition, as in the example of a depressed patient with diabetes mellitus who begins to neglect glucose control. Psychological factors may also interfere with treatment of a medical condition. Patients with a history of trauma may be particularly sensitive to certain invasive procedures and become resistant to medical workups. Psychological factors can constitute additional health risks or adversely influence underlying pathophysiology. A hypoxic patient with pulmonary disease who subsequently develops anxiety will experience vasoconstriction secondary to release of catecholamines, resulting in further reduction of oxygen delivery to tissues and a positive feedback loop contributing to exacerbation of both hypoxia and anxiety.

SAMPLE CASE

A patient with documented epilepsy is admitted in status epilepticus. When he recovers, he states that he has taken all of his medications regularly; however, his serum levels of the anticonvulsants are zero. When confronted with this information, he admits that it is not "strong" to take medication and he stopped his medication.

EPIDEMIOLOGY

The exact prevalence of PFAOMC is unknown; however, private insurance billing data from the United States indicates that this diagnosis is made more commonly than somatic symptom disorder. Psychological factors may affect a medical illness at any point during the life cycle. Denial of medical illness is not currently a diagnosable disorder in *DSM-5* but is commonly seen in clinical settings.

DIFFERENTIAL DIAGNOSIS AND COMORBIDITY

By definition, the diagnosis of PFAOMC necessitates the presence of a comorbid medical illness along with a psychological symptom or behavior. The hallmark of PFAOMC is the directionality of psychological factors adversely affecting underlying medical or neurologic disease. Conversely, when psychiatric symptoms develop predominantly in response to the stressor of medical illness, a diagnosis of adjustment disorder is more appropriate. In actual clinical practice, psychological syndromes often co-occur with medical illness in a mutually exacerbating fashion, making it difficult to determine the exact direction of causality. If the symptoms leading to aggravation of medical illness are best explained by another major mental illness such as major depressive disorder, then it is this condition that should be noted rather than PFAOMC.

CONCLUSIONS

Somatic symptom disorders are a costly group of psychiatric illnesses that cause much suffering on the part of the patient and frequent frustration on the part of the clinician. This chapter has reviewed major recent findings on epidemiology and pathophysiology specific to each of the somatic symptom disorders. Fortunately, a variety of evidence-based therapeutic modalities are available for some of these disabling disorders. Treatment should be focused on understanding and treating dysfunctional thoughts, feelings, and behaviors related to the somatic symptoms, as opposed to attempting to completely eliminate the symptoms themselves. Invasive workups should be initiated with caution. Early recognition and appropriate referral by general and medical neurologic practitioners remains the initial crucial step in facilitating treatment and may significantly improve outcomes. Neurologic follow-up is important to prevent feelings of abandonment and ensure that relevant medical or neurologic illness has not been missed.

LEVEL 1 EVIDENCE

1. Allen L, Woolfolk R. Cognitive behavioral therapy for somatoform disorders. *Psychiatr Clin North Am.* 2010;33:579–593.
2. Kroenke K. Efficacy of treatment for somatoform disorders: a review of randomized controlled trials. *Psychosom Med.* 2007;69:881–888.
3. Abbass A, Kisely S, Kroenke K. Short-term dynamic psychotherapy for somatic disorders: systematic review and meta-analysis. *Psychother Psychosom.* 2009;78(5):265–274.
4. Fallon BA, Petkova E, Skritskaya N, et al. A double-masked, placebo-controlled study of fluoxetine for hypochondriasis. *J Clin Psychopharmacol.* 2008;28:638–645.
5. Greeven A, van Balkom AJLM, Visser S, et al. Cognitive behavior therapy and paroxetine in the treatment of hypochondriasis: a randomized controlled trial. *Am J Psychiatry.* 2007;164:91–99.
6. Barsky AJ, Ahern DK. Cognitive behavior therapy for hypochondriasis. *JAMA.* 2004;291:1464–1470.
7. Speckens AE, van Hemert AM, Spinhoven P, et al. Cognitive behavioral therapy for medically unexplained physical symptoms: a randomized controlled trial. *BMJ.* 1995;311:1328–1332.
8. Hinson VK, Weinstein S, Bernard B, et al. Single-blind clinical trial of psychotherapy for treatment of psychogenic movement disorders. *Parkinsonism Relat Disord.* 2006;12:177–180.
9. Moene FC, Spindhoven P, Hoogduin KA, et al. A randomized controlled clinical trial on the additional effect of hypnosis in a comprehensive treatment program for in-patients with conversion disorder of the motor type. *Psychother Psychosom.* 2002;71:66–76.
10. Moene FC, Spindhoven P, Hoogduin KA, et al. A randomized controlled clinical trial of a hypnosis based treatment for patients with conversion disorder, motor type. *Int J Clin Exp Hypn.* 2003;51:29–50.

SUGGESTED READINGS

Allin M, Streeruwitz A, Curtis V. Progress in understanding conversion disorder. *Neuropsychiatr Dis Treat.* 2005;1(3):205–209.

American Psychiatric Association. *Diagnostic and Statistical Manual of Mental Disorders.* 5th ed. Washington, DC: American Psychiatric Publishing; 2013.

Andrade C, Bhakta SG, Singh NM. Systematic enhancement of functioning as a therapeutic technique in conversion disorder. *Indian J Psychiatry.* 2009;51(2):134–136.

Ataoglu A, Ozcetin A, Icmeli C, et al. Paradoxical therapy in conversion reaction. *J Korean Med Sci.* 2003;18:581–584.

Bakvis P, Spinhoven PH, Giltav EJ, et al. Basal hypercortisolism and trauma in patients with psychogenic non-epileptic seizures. *Epilepsia.* 2010;51(5):752–759.

Bakvis P, Spinhoven P, Roelofs K. Basal cortisol is positively correlated to threat vigilance in patients with psychogenic nonepileptic seizures. *Epilepsy Behav.* 2009;16:558–560.

Ballmeier M, Schmidt R. Conversion disorder revisited. *Functional Neurol.* 2005;20(3):105–113.

Barsky AJ, Orav EJ, Bates DW. Somatization increases medical utilization and costs independent of psychiatric and medical comorbidity. *Arch Gen Psychiatry.* 2005;62:903–910.

Binzer M, Andersen PM, Kullgren G. Clinical characteristics of patients with motor disability due to conversion disorder: a prospective control group study. *J Neurol Neurosurg Psychiatry.* 1997;63(1):83–88.

Bodde NM, Brooks JL, Baker GA, et al. Psychogenic non-epileptic seizures—diagnostic issues: a critical review. *Clin Neurol Neurosurg.* 2009;111:1–9.

Bourgeois JA, Chang CH, Hilty DM, et al. Clinical manifestations and management of conversion disorders. *Curr Treat Options Neurol.* 2002;4: 487–497.

Bowman ES. Why conversion seizures should be classified as a dissociative disorder. *Psychiatr Clin North Am.* 2006;29:185–211.

Brown RJ, Cardena E, Nijenhuis E, et al. Should conversion disorder be reclassified as a dissociative disorder in DSM V? *Psychosomatics.* 2007;48: 369–378.

Carson AJ, Ringbauer B, Stone J, et al. Do medically unexplained symptoms matter? A prospective cohort study of 300 new referrals to neurology outpatient clinics. *J Neurol Neurosurg Psychiatry.* 2000;68:207–201.

Cloninger CR. Somatoform and dissociative disorders. In: Winokur G, Clayton P, eds. *The Medical Basis of Psychiatry.* 2nd ed. Philadelphia: WB Saunders; 1994:169–192.

Creed FH, Davies I, Jackson I, et al. The epidemiology of multiple somatic symptoms. *J Psychosomatic Res.* 2012;72:311–317.

Deka K, Chaudhury PK, Bora K, et al. A study of clinical correlates and socio-demographic profile in conversion disorder. *Indian J Psychiatry.* 2007;49(3):205–207.

Dickinson P, Looper KJ. Psychogenic nonepileptic seizures: a current overview. *Epilepsia.* 2012;53:1679–1689.

Dikel TN, Fennel EB, Gilmore RL. Posttraumatic stress disorder, dissociation, and sexual abuse history in epileptic and nonepileptic seizure patients. *Epilepsy Behav.* 2003;4:644–650.

Eisendrath SJ, Feder A. Management of factitious disorders. In: Feldman MD, Eisendrath SJ, eds. *The Spectrum of Factitious Disorders.* Washington, DC: American Psychiatric Press; 1996:63–78.

Eisendrath S, McNiel D. Factitious physical disorders, litigation, and mortality. *Psychosomatics.* 2004;45:350–353.

Evren C, Can S. Clinical correlates of dissociative tendencies in male soldiers with conversion disorder. *Isr J Psychiatry Relat Sci.* 2007;44(1):33–39.

Feinstein A. Conversion disorder: advances in our understanding. *CMAJ.* 2011;183(8):915–920.

Feldman M, Feldman J. Tangled in the web: countertransference in the therapy of factitious disorders. *Int J Psychiatry Med.* 1995;25:389–399.

Feldman MD, Hamilton JC, Deemer HN. Factitious disorders. In: Phillips K, ed. *Somatoform and Factitious Disorders.* Washington, DC: American Psychiatric Publishing; 2001:129–166.

Ford CV. *Lies! Lies!! Lies!!! The Psychology of Deceit.* Washington, DC: American Psychiatric Press; 1996.

Ford CV, Folks DG. Conversion disorders: an overview. *Psychosomatics.* 1985;26:371–383.

Garcia-Campayo J, Fayed N, Serrano-Blanco A, et al. Brain dysfunction behind functional symptoms: neuroimaging and somatoform, conversive, and dissociative disorders. *Curr Opin Psychiatry.* 2009;22:224–231.

Goldstein LH, Deale AC, Michell-O'Malley SJ, et al. An evaluation of cognitive behavior therapy as a treatment for dissociative seizures: a pilot study. *Cogn Behav Neurol.* 2004;7:41–49.

Goldstein LH, Drew C, Mellers J, et al. Dissociation, hypnotizability, coping styles and health locus of control: characteristics of pseudoseizure patients. *Seizure.* 2000;9:314–322.

Goldstein LH, Mellers JDC. Ictal symptoms of anxiety, avoidance behavior, and dissociation in patients with dissociative seizures. *J Neurol Neurosurg Psychiatry.* 2006;77:616–621.

Harden CL. Pseudoseizures and dissociative disorders: a common mechanism involving traumatic experiences. *Seizures.* 1997;6:151–155.

Hirsch M. The body as a transitional object. *Psychother Psychosom.* 1994;62: 78–81.

Hurtwitz TA. Somatization and conversion disorder. *Can J Psychiatry.* 2004;49:172–178.

Kanaan RAA, Craig TKJ, Wessely SC, et al. Imaging repressed memories in motor conversion disorder. *Psychosom Med.* 2007;69:202–205.

Krahn L, Li H, O'Connor M. Patients who strive to be ill: factitious disorder with physical symptoms. *Am J Psychiatry.* 2003;160:1163–1168.

Kranick S, Gorrindo T, Hallett M. Psychogenic movement disorders and motor conversion: a roadmap for collaboration between neurology and psychiatry. *Psychosomatics.* 2011;52(2):109–116.

Lacourt TE, Houtveen JH, Smeets HM, et al. Infection load as a predisposing factor for somatoform disorder: evidence from a Dutch general practice registry. *Psychosom Med.* 2013;75(8):759–764.

Leary PM. Conversion disorder in childhood: diagnosed too late, investigated too much? *J Royal Soc Med.* 2003;96:436–438.

Mace CJ, Trimble MR. Ten-year prognosis of conversion disorder. *Br J Psychiatry.* 1996;169:282–288.

Masuda D, Hayashi Y. A case of dissociative (conversion) disorder treated effectively with haloperidol: an adolescent boy who stopped talking *Seishin Igaku (Clinical Psychiatry).* 2003;45:663–665.

Milrod B. A 9-year-old with conversion disorder, successfully treated with psychoanalysis. *Int J Psychoanal.* 2002;83:623–631.

Muskin PR, Feldhammer T, Gelfand JL, et al. Maladaptive denial of physical illness: a useful new "diagnosis." *Int J Psychiatry Med.* 1998;28:503–517.

Nash SS, Kent LK, Muskin PR. Psychodynamics in medically ill patients. *Harv Rev Psychiatry.* 2009;17(6):389–397.

Ness D. Physical therapy management for conversion disorder: case series. *J Neurol Phys Ther.* 2007;31:30–39.

Noyes R, Carney CP, Hillis SL, et al. Prevalence and correlates of illness worry in the general population. *Psychosomatics.* 2005;46:529–539.

Perez DP, Barsky A, Daffner K, et al. Motor and somatosensory conversion disorder: a functional unawareness syndrome? *J Neuropsychiatry Clin Neurosci.* 2012;24:141–151.

Plassman R. Inpatient and outpatient long-term psychotherapy of patients suffering from factitious diseases. *Psychother Psychosom.* 1994;62:96–107.

Plassman R. Muchausen syndromes and factitious diseases. *Psychother Psychosom.* 1994;62:7–26.

Plassman R. Structural disturbances in the body self. *Psychother Psychosom.* 1994;62:91–95.

Reinsberger C, Perez DL, Murphy MM, et al. Pre- and postictal, not ictal, heart rate distinguishes complex partial and psychogenic nonepileptic seizures. *Epilepsy Behav.* 2012;23(1):68–70.

Rolfs K, Kaisers GP, Hoogduin KA, et al. Child abuse in patients with conversion disorder. *Am J Psychiatry.* 2002;159:1908–1913.

Rosebush PI, Mazurek MF. Treatment of conversion disorder in the 21st century: have we moved beyond the couch? *Curr Treat Options Neurol.* 2011;13(3):255–266.

Scher LM, Knudsen P, Leamon M. Somatic symptom and related disorders. In: Hales RE, Yudofsky SC, Roberts LW, eds. *The American Psychiatric Publishing Textbook of Psychiatry.* 6th ed. Washington, DC: American Psychiatric Publishing; 2014:531–556.

Schweitzer J, Zafar U, Pavlicova M, et al. Long-term follow-up of hypochondriasis after selective serotonin reuptake inhibitor treatment. *J Clin Psychopharmacol.* 2011;31:365–368.

Shapiro AP, Teasell RW. Behavioral interventions in the rehabilitation of acute v. chronic non-organic (conversion/factitious) motor disorders. *Br J Psychiatry.* 2004;185:140–146.

Spence SA, Crimlisk HL, Cope H, et al. Discrete neurophysiological correlates in prefrontal cortex during hysterical and feigned disorder of movement [letter]. *Lancet.* 2000;355:1243–1244.

Spitzer C, Barnow S, Gau K. et al. Childhood maltreatment in patients with somatization disorder. *Aust N Z J Psychiatry.* 2008;42:335–341.

Steinhausen HC, von Aster M, Pfeiffer E, et al. Comparative studies of conversion disorders in childhood and adolescence. *J Child Psychol Psychiatry.* 1989;30:615–621.

Stone J, Warlow C, Sharpe M. The symptom of functional weakness: a controlled study of 107 patients. *Brain.* 2010;133:1537–1551.

Stone J, Zeman A, Simonotto E, et al. FMRI in patients with motor conversion symptoms and controls with simulated weakness. *Psychosom Med.* 2007;69(9):961–969.

Strauss DH, Spitzer RL, Muskin PR. Maladaptive denial of physical illness: a proposal for DSM-IV. *Am J Psychiatry.* 1990;147:1168–1172.

Sutherland A, Rodin G. Factitious disorders in a general hospital setting: clinical features and a review of the literature. *Psychosomatics.* 1990;31:392–399.

Teasell RW, Shapiro AP. Strategic-behavioral intervention in the treatment of chronic nonorganic motor disorders. *Am J Phys Med Rehabil.* 1994;73: 44–50.

van Beilen M, de Jon BM, Gieteling EW, et al. Abnormal parietal function in conversion paresis. *PLoS One*. 2011;6(10):e25918. doi:10.1371/journal .pone.0025918.

Viederman M. Metaphor and meaning in conversion disorder: a brief active therapy. *Psychosom Med*. 1995;57:403–409.

Voon V, Lang AE. Antidepressant treatment outcomes of psychogenic movement disorders. *J Clin Psychiatry*. 2005;66:1529–1534.

Vuilleumier P. Chicherio C, Assal F, et al. Functional neuroanatomical correlates of hysterical sensorimotor loss. *Brain*. 2001;124:1077–1090.

Ward NS, Oakley DA, Frackowiak RS, et al. Differential brain activations during intentionally simulated and subjectively experienced paralysis. *Cogn Neuropsychiatry*. 2003;8:295–312.

Williams DT, Harding KJ, Fallon BA. Somatoform disorders. In: Rowland LP, Pedley TA, eds. *Merrit's Neurology*. 12th ed. Philadelphia: Lippincott Williams and Wilkins; 2010:1069–1075.

Wise MG, Rundell JR. *Clinical Manual of Psychosomatic Medicine: A Guide to Consultation-Liaison Psychiatry*. Washington, DC: American Psychiatric Publishing; 2005.

Neurologic Rehabilitation 152

Heidi Schambra and Laura Lennihan

INTRODUCTION

Neurologic disorders commonly cause impairments that impede intellectual and physical activities. Neurologists play an important role in prescribing and monitoring rehabilitation therapies to maximize functional recovery and in optimizing patient health for maximal engagement in these therapies. The selection and timing of these therapies substantially contribute to the optimal quality of life for patient and family. There is significant variability in access to rehabilitation services, and many people with acute and chronic neurologic conditions do not receive adequate rehabilitation therapy. When given proper training and equipment, these patients may improve in independence, access to the community, and ease with which caregivers assist them. The medical and neurologic management of patients with neurologic injury begins in the acute setting and continues throughout the course of their care, through varied institutional and home settings. Experience with neurorehabilitation is essential in the management continuum of acute to chronic neurologic disorders.

The World Health Organization's (WHO) *International Classification of Functioning, Disability and Health* (ICF) defines limitations caused by disease in three broad categories: bodily functions, personal activities, and societal participation. These definitions provide a structure for understanding the impact of disease on personal independence and integration into society and can help to identify patients who may benefit from rehabilitation. The planning and prescription of a rehabilitation program for a neurologically impaired individual requires characterization of the neurologic disorder in terms of natural history, localization, and extent of nervous system involvement; determination of functional disabilities caused by cognitive and physical impairments; and definition of these disabilities in the context of the patient's physical and social environment. Combining this information with knowledge of available resources for postacute care, the type and intensity of rehabilitation therapies can be planned.

Impairments caused by neurologic disease or injury frequently affect an individual's ability to perform functions, such as activities of daily living (ADLs) and instrumental activities of daily living (IADLs). ADLs include the basic activities an individual performs daily, including feeding, grooming, dressing, toileting, bathing, and mobility. IADLs are activities beyond basic self-care that allow a patient to participate in the home and community, such as meal preparation, housekeeping, laundry, shopping, using a telephone/technology, driving a car/using transportation, and money management. The most commonly used ADL measurement tool in an acute rehabilitation population is the functional independence measure (FIM). The FIM is a seven-point ordinal scale of function, addressing self-care, bladder and bowel continence, mobility, and social cognition. The minimum score is 18 and the maximum is 126, and scores grossly indicate levels of patient dependency and burden of care. A typical trajectory of improvement in the FIM score following an acute stroke in a patient receiving daily intensive comprehensive rehabilitation is about one point per day. Of note, because the FIM evaluates ADLs at the level of task completion, it does not distinguish between gains made from reduced neurologic impairment and gains made using compensatory strategies.

COMPENSATION AND RECOVERY

Two principal approaches are used in neurorehabilitation programs: compensating for impairment and training to reduce impairment. *Compensation* teaches adaptive techniques using preserved neurologic function to circumvent neurologic impairment. For example, a person with a paralyzed arm can be trained in one-handed techniques using the normal arm, a patient unable to walk can learn to use a wheelchair, or a patient with expressive aphasia can communicate with a picture board. Although this approach yields faster results and improves functional independence by reducing disability at task level, it does little to diminish the original neurologic impairment. Troublingly, rodent models suggest that training compensation after stroke (e.g., using the nonparetic limb to grasp a food pellet) impedes the beneficial effects of training to reduce impairment in the paretic limb.

Training to reduce impairment augments spontaneous neurologic recovery and facilitates the return of neurologic function. For example, a patient practices reaching and grasping with a paretic arm to improve motor control, a patient with gait dysfunction practices locomotion, or a patient with visual neglect practices shifting visual attention to the neglected space. This approach requires intensive training for weeks to months and is superior for the biologic restoration of function. However, in patients who are unable to engage in training due to the severity of their impairment, it may not be a suitable main approach.

Some combination of both strategies is commonly applied in neurorehabilitation programs. However, given ever diminishing lengths of stay and the cost–benefit considerations of compensatory and impairment training, a personalized selection of rehabilitation approaches is warranted. Tailoring the rehabilitative approach based on recovery potential is an area of current clinical research. Knowing a patient's potential would enable clinicians to set sensible rehabilitation goals and could guide the team toward the most appropriate therapeutic approach. A clinical trial is currently underway validating an algorithm for predicting motor recovery potential, which takes into account a patient's motor function and corticospinal tract integrity.

In addition to task-oriented training to reduce motor impairments in patients with motor dysfunction, exercises to increase the strength of muscle groups are also commonly used. However, cortical map reorganization in animal models does not result from resistance training, and there is insufficient evidence from clinical trials to support the use of resistance training to aid in recovery [**Level 1**].[1]

Most patients who have marked neurologic injury, particularly those with stroke, are deconditioned and have limited exercise capacity and aerobic reserve. Rehabilitation therapy with mobilization and exercise helps to increase general conditioning and tolerance for exercise. In animal models, cardiovascular exercise increases production of brain-derived neurotrophic factor (BDNF), which supports synaptogenesis and synapse stabilization. A recent meta-analysis of human stroke rehabilitation trials showed improvement in disability with cardiorespiratory training, largely attributed to improved gait and balance metrics [**Level 1**].[1]

NEUROPLASTICITY AND RECOVERY

Following focal injury, the central nervous system (CNS) undergoes long-lasting structural and functional changes. Neuroplasticity is heightened by the injury itself, which can be leveraged for enhancing activity-dependent gains made through rehabilitative training. Injury-induced plasticity after CNS injury and activity-dependent plasticity share many common mechanisms and substrates. Importantly, it is the combination of both that produces maximal recovery gains.

INJURY-INDUCED PLASTICITY

Injury to the CNS activates neurobiologic recovery processes. Elucidating the underlying neurobiology of spontaneous recovery, particularly after focal CNS lesions, is a rapidly evolving field. Animal models of CNS injury have helped build our understanding of the complex molecular and cellular aspects of recovery in the brain and spinal cord. Rapid, significant changes in gene expression and protein production which occur after injury, help or hinder plasticity in perilesional and remote brain and spinal cord areas.

At the cellular level, processes that promote plasticity include neuronogenesis and angiogenesis, axonal sprouting, dendritic arborization, synaptogenesis and silent synapse unmasking, changes in synaptic strength, and changes in glutamatergic and GABAergic tone. Processes that limit plasticity include excitotoxicity, free radical formation, delayed neuronal death, edema, inflammation, expression of growth inhibitors, and glial scar formation. Importantly, these processes peak and wane within the first weeks to early months after injury, underscoring the limited time window for optimized combination with rehabilitation training.

Research in targeting these plasticity modifiers, either by upregulating or downregulating their effects, is actively underway. For example, in animal models, selective serotonin reuptake inhibitors (SSRIs) increase expression of BDNF and synaptogenesis. A recent multicenter, double-blinded, randomized controlled trial compared 3 months of fluoxetine versus placebo in severely impaired stroke patients, started within 5 to 10 days after stroke. Both groups received conventional rehabilitation. At 3 months, patients who received fluoxetine had significantly improved motor impairment and disability scores than those who received placebo [**Level 1**].[2] There appears to be a modest class-wide effect on recovery [**Level 1**].[3]

ACTIVITY-DEPENDENT PLASTICITY

Using training to capitalize on neuroplasticity after brain injury is the objective of neurorehabilitation. The optimal type, timing, and dose of training required to maximize activity-dependent plasticity

after CNS injury is an area of active basic and clinical research. Some direction about best practices can be gained from animal stroke studies in the motor system. One clear principle that has emerged from animal models is that injury-induced plasticity requires adjunctive paretic limb training in order to promote recovery. In animal studies, intracortical microstimulation techniques may be used to track in vivo neuroplastic cortical map changes. In healthy animals, skilled training results in the expansion of cortical representations of the training effectors, whereas rote, unskilled movements lead to no change. These cortical map changes are associated with increased synaptogenesis and dendritic arborization. In a nonhuman primate model of motor stroke recovery, lost cortical motor representations do not spontaneously reappear if the paretic arm is not trained and the nonparetic arm is used to compensate. In animals trained to reach and grasp with their paretic arm, perilesional distal forearm representations expand into areas that previously subserved the proximal arm. These results suggest that training directed at reducing impairment promotes neuroplasticity.

How early to begin therapy is a point of debate, given concerns about glutamate excitotoxicity after CNS injury. In rodent models of stroke, paretic limb training started 5 days after stroke results in greater functional gains than the same amount of training started 30 days after stroke. In a recent phase II randomized controlled trial, a faster return to unassisted ambulation was found in patients who were mobilized earlier (<24 hour after stroke) and who received more intensive gait training compared to those receiving standard of care; a large phase III clinical trial testing this early intervention is currently underway.

The dose of therapy is also an issue of exploration. From animal and human motor learning studies, it is clear that high doses of repetitive, goal-directed practice are required for long-term skill gains. A recent observational study of inpatient and outpatient rehabilitation sessions found the number of functional repetitions to be an order of magnitude less than would be needed for conventional skill gains. Meta-analyses of dose response to training modestly support improved motor outcomes at higher doses of exercise-based therapy.

However, it is possible that too much therapy, particularly initiated early after injury, may be suboptimal. For example, a recent randomized, single-blind phase II trial investigated the long-term motor benefits of different doses of constraint-induced movement therapy (CIMT) initiated within 2 weeks post stroke. CIMT forces the use of the paretic arm through restraint of the unaffected arm. CIMT performed equally well to dose-matched traditional therapy. However, high-dose CIMT, which restrained the nonparetic arm for 90% of waking hours, resulted in less motor improvement. From these results, it appears that moderately intensive therapy delivered early after an acute CNS insult may be optimal for impairment reduction.

LEVELS OF CARE

Rehabilitation services are provided in a variety of settings and at varied levels of intensity and duration. Postacute care can occur in inpatient rehabilitation facilities (IRFs), in skilled nursing facilities (SNFs), from home health agencies (HHAs), or at outpatient facilities. At IRFs, patients receive 3 hours of therapy 5 to 7 days per week for usually less than 1 month. There is daily physiatrist or neurologist oversight. At SNFs, patients receive 0.5 to 2 hours of therapy 5 to 6 days per week for usually less than 2 months. There is weekly to monthly physician oversight, usually by a general practitioner, internist, or geriatrician. In outpatient therapy, be it in-home or at a facility, patients receive 0.5 to 1 hour of therapy 2 to 3 times per week, durations average 1 month, and there is no physician oversight.

In an IRF, the most common neurologic diagnoses are stroke, traumatic brain injury, and spinal cord injury; also seen are multiple sclerosis (MS), Parkinson's disease, and peripheral neuropathies (particularly critical illness neuromyopathy and acute inflammatory polyneuropathy). For patients hospitalized with acute neurologic injury, functional outcome is improved by an experienced, coordinated interdisciplinary team providing a comprehensive rehabilitation program. Stroke patients who receive rehabilitation therapies on a stroke rehabilitation unit have better functional outcomes and shorter hospital stays than those treated on a general neurology ward, and benefits persist over time. Similarly, stroke patients admitted to hospital-based intensive rehabilitation programs have better functional recovery and are more likely to return home than those treated in a low-intensity rehabilitation program at an SNF.

Multiple considerations go into determining the best placement for the medically stable neurologic patient. For admission to an IRF, the patient must have impairments that necessitate at least two therapy types (see the following text), must tolerate at least 3 hours of therapy daily, and must have 24-hour medical and nursing needs. Placement at an SNF typically occurs when the patient is unable to tolerate a high intensity of rehabilitation or has low capacity for functional improvement and has reduced medical and nursing needs. Outpatient therapy is appropriate for patients with mild and limited deficits or follows a course of inpatient rehabilitation to extend functional training at home or in the community. Interestingly, availability of postacute care is a more powerful predictor of its use than the clinical characteristics of the patients. Nonclinical factors that strongly influence placement include availability, convenience, distance to provider, demographic factors (age, race, and marital status), insurance status, local practice patterns, and characteristics of the discharging hospital (size, ownership, status as a teaching hospital, etc.).

THE DISCIPLINES

A comprehensive inpatient neurorehabilitation program requires an interdisciplinary team composed of the physician, physical therapist, rehabilitation nurse, occupational therapist, speech language pathologist, neuropsychologist, social worker, and recreational therapist. All team members participate in formulating a treatment and discharge plan, working together to attain collective goals of reducing patient disability, and in educating and training the patient and family in preparation for return home. Importantly, patients must also shift from being passive recipients of medical treatment in the acute setting to being active participants in their own therapy to maximize their neurologic recovery.

PHYSICIAN

The physician, as team leader, defines the type and prognosis of the neurologic disorder, sets realistic treatment goals, and coordinates the rehabilitation services. The major role of the physician is to optimize patient engagement in therapy through management of medical issues (e.g., orthostatic hypotension, depression, pain, constipation or incontinence, infection, nutrition and hydration, etc.). With the team, the physician reviews progress toward attaining functional goals that allow the patient to return home.

Roadblocks, alternative strategies, and discharge dispositions are discussed at weekly team rounds. Postdischarge plans for home care and outpatient therapy are coordinated with the patient and family.

REHABILITATION NURSING

Rehabilitation nurses provide general medical and more targeted nursing for patients with neurologic dysfunction. A major nursing focus for the neurologically impaired patient is prevention of pressure ulcers due to immobility and management of bowel and bladder incontinence (see the following section). In the inpatient setting, the nurse helps incorporate skills learned in therapy into the patient's daily routines. The nurse also educates the patient and family in medication administration, self-catheterization, and skin care.

PHYSICAL THERAPY

Physical therapy (PT) focuses on bed mobility, transferring to chair or toilet, ambulating, and stair climbing. Techniques and orthotics are chosen to maximize safe and independent mobility; to optimize energy efficiency; to prevent decubitus skin ulcers, tendon contractures, and falls; and to enhance motor recovery. Limitations in mobility and sensorimotor function are addressed by strengthening exercises, gait and balance training, and stretching. PTs also concentrate on musculoskeletal and orthopedic injuries. Typical problems associated with neurologic injury include musculoskeletal pain, muscle spasm, joint pain, heterotopic ossification, and contractures.

Leg and trunk weakness, impaired postural reflexes, ataxia, proprioceptive loss, and hemineglect may all interfere with ambulation and are actively managed. Bracing, assistive devices (e.g., cane, walker), or a wheelchair are used as compensatory strategies for safe completion of ADLs. Although a person may not be able to walk immediately after neurologic injury, ambulation usually becomes possible with the use of a walker or cane and a combination of bracing at the ankle and sometimes the knee. When ambulation is not possible, mobility is attained through training in the use of a wheelchair of the correct size and height, occasionally employing a special seat to prevent skin breakdown or cushions for trunk support.

OCCUPATIONAL THERAPY

Occupational therapy (OT) focuses on functional loss in ADLs and limitations in the patient's occupational and social role caused by neurologic injury. OTs treat patients with the goal of enabling patients to return to home, community, and work (which was traditionally its focus, hence its name). Typically, OTs concentrate on impairments affecting the use of the arms and hands, such as weakness, sensory loss, ataxia, and abnormal tone. Improving motor skills is only one of the important components in enhancing performance of ADLs. OTs thus also address impaired attention, judgment, cognition, and memory; visuospatial neglect; and apraxia. Training focuses on restoring upper extremity functional skills that are important for self-care at home and autonomy in the community. If necessary, adaptive aids are used to increase the use of the impaired arm and hand, such as hand and wrist orthoses, reachers, Velcro closures, and built-up utensils. When the impairment is unilateral and severe, an occupational therapist may select adaptive equipment and train the patient and family to compensate. Advanced programs may include learning special one-sided techniques, such as driving with the left hand and foot.

OTs additionally manage paretic shoulder subluxation to forestall shoulder–hand syndrome and select orthotics such as wrist and hand splints to prevent contractures. They also optimize safety and functionality in the home environment by training the patient and the family in use of adaptive equipment (e.g., tub benches, elevated toilet seats, ramps, grab bars, safety rails).

SPEECH, LANGUAGE, AND COGNITIVE THERAPY

The speech–language pathologist (SLP) focuses on dysphagia (see the following section), dysarthria, aphasia, and cognitive dysfunction in the neurologically impaired patient.

Treatment of dysarthria aims to improve intelligibility and includes methods such as slowing and exaggerating articulation, increasing breath support, and pacing speech rate. For aphasia, the SLP identifies areas of strength and weakness in receptive and expressive language. Areas of strength may then be used for compensatory purposes, such as using better preserved written expression in lieu of verbal expression. Therapeutic approaches vary widely but can employ visual and verbal cueing, melodic intonation, and constraint-induced language therapy. For example, use of visual imagery as an internal cue may help to overcome the word blocking of expressive aphasia.

For cognitive rehabilitation, speech and occupational therapists collaborate on program development and implementation, and all members of the rehabilitation team contribute. Neurobehavioral impairments and how they interfere with function are first identified. Diffuse brain injury may affect several cognitive domains, and the therapeutic approach is tailored to the nature and complexity of the symptoms. For example, inattention and distractibility may preclude participation in group activities such as business meetings, or memory impairment may lead to failure at school. In diffuse or multifocal brain injury that impairs attention, behavior, cognition, and language, it is necessary to provide a structured program that minimizes distractions by controlling the noise and activity in the environment. Strategies are used to help compensate for impairments across multiple cognitive domains. For example, memory cues help to improve retention of techniques learned in PT or OT; breaking a task into individual steps and then teaching one step at a time helps to overcome attentional and constructional problems. Finally, the SLP educates the patient and family about aphasia and other cognitive problems. This is essential to reduce frustration with impaired communication, memory, and abnormal behavior.

NEUROPSYCHOLOGY

Neuropsychologists concentrate on the mood, behavioral, and cognitive problems that occur after injury to the brain. They perform detailed neuropsychological testing of the patient to identify cognitive and affective disorders and make therapeutic recommendations to the team. Neuropsychologists may also counsel the patient and family in the management of their disorders.

SOCIAL WORK

Social workers identify concrete resources that will enable the patient to succeed at home, such as finances, availability of caregivers, and community services. They provide counseling, support, and education to the family, who often take on a caregiving role for the patient. Social workers or case managers may directly interact with the patient's insurance provider, supplying medical updates and obtaining authorizations. They also coordinate home services and delivery of adaptive equipment and facilitate discharge planning.

RECREATIONAL THERAPY

Recreational therapy focuses on the patient's social and emotional health through use of enjoyable recreation, with a goal of reintegration into the community. Group activities such as games, karaoke, gardening, and arts and crafts encourage socialization and engage patients physically and cognitively.

SPECIALIZED NEUROLOGIC AND MEDICAL MANAGEMENT

DYSPHAGIA

Swallowing is a complex act involving voluntary and involuntary pairs of muscles including facial, lingual, masticatory, pharyngeal, esophageal, and respiratory muscles. Neurologic disorders that disturb coordinated contraction and interaction of these muscles can cause dysphagia and, secondarily, dehydration, malnutrition, aspiration pneumonia, and airway obstruction. Dysphagia evaluation is indicated for patients who have any of these complications; who report coughing, choking, or nasal regurgitation while eating; who are dysarthric; or who have a disease commonly associated with dysphagia, such as motor neuron disease, myasthenia gravis, or brain stem stroke. Dysphagia is identified with bedside testing and with video fluoroscopic or fiberoptic endoscopic evaluations of swallowing. Therapeutic approaches include altering the consistency of foods and thickening liquids, using head repositioning strategies such as a chin-tuck technique, and reducing the rate and amount of intake.

BLADDER AND BOWEL DYSFUNCTION

Loss of control of bladder or bowel emptying is a devastating condition and should be addressed by any comprehensive neurorehabilitation programs. The cause of impaired bladder emptying or sphincter incompetence, and therefore the treatment, depends on the site of the neural injury. Evaluation includes clinical observations about incontinence and retention; search for nonneurologic factors, such as infection or mechanical problems, particularly urethral obstruction by prostatic enlargement; and cystometrographic measurements of bladder and sphincter functions. The neurorehabilitation nurse plays a crucial role in the treatment of bladder and bowel disorders, including implementation of voiding programs and training patient and family to use urethral catheters.

The goal of bladder rehabilitation is to allow the bladder to fill under low pressure to a volume of 250 to 500 mL, then empty, whether volitionally or mechanically and without incontinence between emptying. Incontinence characterized by bladder hyperreflexia, in which the bladder contracts at low urine volumes and voluntary inhibition of bladder contraction and sphincter relaxation fails, commonly complicates cerebral, particularly frontal lobe, injury. Lack of awareness or indifference may impede achievement of continence, but neurologic recovery usually reduces incontinence. Prompted voiding at 2-hour intervals contributes to regaining continence. Detrusor-sphincter dyssynergia, in which dissociated bladder contraction and sphincter relaxation results in the bladder contracting against a closed sphincter, is usually a consequence of lower brain stem or spinal cord lesions. Bladder emptying, if it occurs at all, is incomplete and occurs at high vesicular pressure. Treatment includes bladder antispasmodic drugs and intermittent catheterization at 4- to 6-hour intervals. Hydronephrosis, renal failure, and bladder wall hypertrophy with consequent volume loss are potential complications of a chronically high-pressure bladder.

TABLE 152.1   Morbidity in Rehabilitation

Preventable Morbidities	Common Preexisting Comorbidities Requiring Regulation	Secondary Effects
• Deep vein thrombosis	• Hypertension	• Partial or generalized seizures
• Recurrent or progression of stroke	• Diabetes	• Depression
• Aspiration pneumonia	• Osteoarthritis	• Cognitive impairment
• Urinary tract infections	• Coronary artery disease	• Intracerebral bleeding
• Fecal impaction	• COPD	• Hydrocephalus
• Pressure ulcers	• Peripheral vascular disease	• CSF leakage
• Falls	• Substance abuse	• Autonomic dysreflexia
• Dehydration	• Impairments of hearing and vision	• Heterotopic ossification
• Malnutrition	• Poor dentition	• Surgical site complications
• Influenza or pneumococcus infection	• Sleep apnea	• Infection
• Accelerated osteoporosis		• Fever
		• Pain
		• Musculoskeletal injury

COPD, chronic obstructive pulmonary disease; CSF, cerebrospinal fluid.

Conversely, peripheral nerve diseases involving the nerves innervating the bladder may cause bladder flaccidity. Bladder emptying, at low pressures, is incomplete, and incontinence occurs between voluntary voiding. Cholinergic agents may improve emptying, but intermittent catheterization is often necessary.

Neurologic disorders leading to immobility, decreased fluid access and intake, and loss of cortical control over rectal sphincters may cause severe constipation or impaction. Prevention combines a high-fiber diet, adequate hydration, stool softeners, and regularly scheduled evacuation using suppositories, enemas, and/or digital rectal stimulation. Bowel incontinence can also be lessened by scheduled toileting, providing regular clearance of the rectal vault.

MEDICAL CARE

An important component of rehabilitation neurology is the prevention of secondary complications, the optimized management of existing comorbidities, and the early recognition and treatment of known complications or effects of injury (Table 152.1). Comorbidities are extremely common and are often dysregulated or exacerbated by the changes in activity, diet, and medications that occur after sudden neurologic injury. For example, poststroke rehabilitation has goals of gradual reduction in blood pressure (BP) to achieve Joint National Committee (JNC) 7 guidelines, proper control of diabetes, dyslipidemia management, appropriate administration of anticoagulation or antiplatelet agents, and counseling on lifestyle changes (e.g., cessation or reduction of alcohol and tobacco use, increase in exercise) [**Level 1**].[4] Low molecular weight heparins are used to prevent deep vein thrombosis; appropriate oral consistencies are chosen to minimize the risk of aspiration and to maximize nutrition and hydration; and preventative measures are put in place to minimize the risk of falls. A patient may also be given fluoxetine for the potentiation of motor recovery and for the treatment of poststroke depression.

The goal of the physician is to optimize the medical management and lifestyle changes that will reduce comorbities and secondary effects of brain injury and to coordinate with the patient's primary physician for continuation of optimum outpatient care.

LEVEL 1 EVIDENCE

1. Saunders DH, Sanderson M, Brazzelli M, et al. Physical fitness training for stroke patients. *Cochrane Database Syst Rev.* 2013;10:CD003316.
2. Chollet F, Tardy J, Albucher JF, et al. Fluoxetine for motor recovery after acute ischaemic stroke (FLAME): a randomised placebo-controlled trial. *Lancet Neurol.* 2011;10(2):123–130.
3. Mead GE, Hsieh CF, Lee R, et al. Selective serotonin reuptake inhibitors (SSRIs) for stroke recovery. *Cochrane Database Syst Rev.* 2012;11:CD009286.
4. Kernan WN, Ovbiagele B, Black HR, et al. Guidelines for the prevention of stroke in patients with stroke and transient ischemic attack: a guideline for healthcare professionals from the American Heart Association/American Stroke Association. *Stroke.* 2014;45(7):2160–2236.

SUGGESTED READINGS

Allred RP, Maldonado MA, Hsu And JE, et al. Training the "less-affected" forelimb after unilateral cortical infarcts interferes with functional recovery of the impaired forelimb in rats. *Restor Neurol Neurosci.* 2005;23(5–6):297–302.

Buntin MB, Garten AD, Paddock S, et al. How much is postacute care use affected by its availability? *Health Serv Res.* 2005;40(2):413–434.

Cooke EV, Mares K, Clark A, et al. The effects of increased dose of exercise-based therapies to enhance motor recovery after stroke: a systematic review and meta-analysis. *BMC Med.* 2010;8:60.

Cramer SC. Repairing the human brain after stroke: I. Mechanisms of spontaneous recovery. *Ann Neurol.* 2008;63(3):272–287.

Cramer SC. Repairing the human brain after stroke. II. Restorative therapies. *Ann Neurol*. 2008;63(5):549–560.

Cumming TB, Thrift AG, Collier JM, et al. Very early mobilization after stroke fast-tracks return to walking: further results from the phase II AVERT randomized controlled trial. *Stroke*. 2011;42(1):153–158.

Deutsch A, Granger CV, Heinemann AW, et al. Poststroke rehabilitation: outcomes and reimbursement of inpatient rehabilitation facilities and subacute rehabilitation programs. *Stroke*. 2006;37(6):1477–1482.

Dobkin BH. *The Clinical Science of Neurologic Rehabilitation*. 2nd ed. New York: Oxford University Press; 2003.

Dromerick AW, Lang CE, Birkenmeier RL, et al. Very Early Constraint-Induced Movement during Stroke Rehabilitation (VECTORS): a single-center RCT. *Neurology*. 2009;73(3):195–201.

Foley N, Teasell R, Salter K, et al. Dysphagia treatment post stroke: a systematic review of randomised controlled trials. *Age Ageing*. 2008;37(3):258–264.

Good DC, Couch JR, eds. *Handbook of Neurorehabilitation*. New York: Marcel Dekker; 1994.

Kwakkel G, van Peppen R, Wagenaar RC, et al. Effects of augmented exercise therapy time after stroke: a meta-analysis. *Stroke*. 2004;35(11):2529–2539.

Lang CE, Macdonald JR, Reisman DS, et al. Observation of amounts of movement practice provided during stroke rehabilitation. *Arch Phys Med Rehabil*. 2009;90(10):1692–1698.

Miller EL, Murray L, Richards L, et al. Comprehensive overview of nursing and interdisciplinary rehabilitation care of the stroke patient: a scientific statement from the American Heart Association. *Stroke*. 2010;41(10):2402–2448.

Nudo RJ. Recovery after brain injury: mechanisms and principles. *Front Hum Neurosci*. 2013;7:887.

Overman JJ, Carmichael ST. Plasticity in the injured brain: more than molecules matter. *Neuroscientist*. 2014;20(1):15–28.

Stinear CM, Barber PA, Petoe M, et al. The PREP algorithm predicts potential for upper limb recovery after stroke. *Brain*. 2012;135(pt 8):2527–2535.

Stroke Unit Trialists' Collaboration. Organised inpatient (stroke unit) care for stroke. *Cochrane Database Syst Rev*. 2013;9:CD000197.

World Health Organization. *International Classification of Functioning, Disability and Health*. Geneva, Switzerland: World Health Organization; 2001. http://www.who.int/classifications/icf/en/. Accessed April 25, 2015.

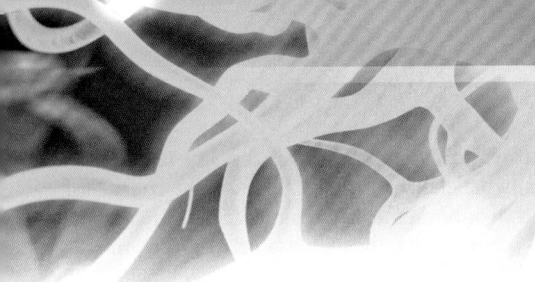

Ethical and End-of-Life Issues in Neurology 153

Fred Rincon, Lewis P. Rowland, and
Stephan A. Mayer

INFORMED CONSENT

The concept of informed consent originates from the notion that individuals are autonomous. Rational individuals with decisional capacity, or competency in legal terms, are uniquely qualified to decide what is best for them. It also means that people should be allowed to do what they want, even if doing so involves considerable risk or would be considered foolish by others. This of course is supported only if the individual's decision does not infringe on the autonomy or welfare of another individual (Table 153.1).

When a patient is found not to have decision-making capacity, the health care provider must seek an alternate way to obtain consent. The options in these cases are as follows: (1) to seek a written advance directive such as a living will or durable power of attorney (for health care) or (2) in the absence of an advance directive, the physician must seek the substituted judgment of a proxy or surrogate authorized by the jurisdictional law.

ADVANCE DIRECTIVES

Advance directives are legal documents that can be used to direct care in the event of incapacity and are most often helpful in situations related to terminal conditions. These documents are able to specify the individual's preferences in regard to end-of-life treatments under specific circumstances and may also appoint surrogate decision makers if the individual is not competent to make decisions at some future time. Shortcomings of these documents are as follows: (1) that the health care provider may not find instructions that clearly guide certain treatment decisions and (2) the ethical argument that a person may not be able to predict his own reaction if faced with a disability. Studies have demonstrated

a tendency among the nondisabled to view disability as equivalent to death and historically, investigators frequently equate death with the severe disability. In this sense, advance directives or living wills, even if legally valid, are suboptimal to find treatment directions in certain terminal illness particularly when goals of self-determination and perceptions that guide one's chosen moral course may change.

SUBSTITUTED JUDGMENT STANDARD

Obtaining informed consent by an authorized surrogate decision maker is an alternative to direct informed consent. Appointees by advance directive, or living will, or durable power of attorney (for health care decisions), or a family member identified by jurisdictional law are expected to make the same decisions as the patient would if the patient's capacity were intact and usually based on knowledge of the patient's general values and preferences. Shortcomings of this mechanism are related to the poor accuracy of the proxy's ability to predict the patient's wishes, which some studies have found to be no better than random chance. The inherent difficulty of making decisions for other persons may also make proxies reluctant to participate in the consent process on any level. This can lead to increased reliance on the physician's expertise without fully considering the risks and benefits associated with an intervention.

BEST INTEREST STANDARD

When other sources for consent are lacking, a legal exception may be invoked in emergency situations, in which case the consent of a reasonable person to appropriate treatment is implied, so the *best interest standard* may be applied in these circumstances.

TABLE 153.1	The Informed Consent Process
Components	**Example**
Verifying that the patient has decision-making capacity	This component verifies that the patient has insight into the proposed procedure or research. A bedside evaluation assessing if the patient can (1) understand the information; (2) understand the current situation and its consequences; (3) rationally consider information in light of one individual's values; and (4) retain the information given, analyze it, and make an informed decision.
Full disclosure	This component is designed to explain the risks and benefits, ratio, complications, and alternatives of the procedure or research. Without disclosure, voluntary choice and competence cannot be properly exercised.
Understanding	In this component, the agent verifies that the patient understands fully the risks and benefits, specifically if the ratio (risk/benefit) is in favor or not.
Voluntary choice	In this component, the agent verifies that there is deliberate informed consent. The informed consent process should be guided by the freedom to act voluntarily without coercive forces or due influence.
Formal authorization	In some jurisdictions, a written document is necessary to fully execute the procedure or research for which the subject has been asked to consent. This should include a statement of risk/benefit and potential complications and alternatives and the signatures of the health care provider, patient or surrogate, and in some instances, a witness.

The emergency doctrine of "implied consent" allows providers to deliver certain interventions that if not performed in a timely basis could potentially lead to increase morbidity and mortality. The requirements to meet the best interest standard for emergency situations are as follows: (1) The treatment in question represents the usual and customary standard of care for the condition being treated; (2) it would be clearly harmful to the patient to delay treatment awaiting explicit consent; and (3) patients ordinarily would be expected to consent for the treatment in question if they had the capacity to do so. This principle is also applicable in those cases when the burden of a therapy outweighs the benefits and the pain of interventions which would make them inhumane. Despite widely held beliefs to the contrary, it is not necessary to obtain legal counsel before withdrawing life-sustaining therapy. One of the shortcomings of using the *best interest standard* is the possibility of the health care provider being judge as paternalistic based on their inherent role to prevent evil or harm by promoting good and welfare for others.

In some jurisdictions of the United States and the world, the principle of "clear and convincing evidence" may be used in lieu of the *substituted judgment standard*. This is one of the legal principles used in the United States legal system (the other two being beyond the reasonable doubt and preponderance of evidence). This principle can be used by physicians in certain jurisdictions of the United States (Missouri, New York, Florida) to withdraw life support or any other intervention when there is *clear and convincing evidence* of previous patient's statements and in the absence of a "declaration" such as a living will, advance directive, or durable power of attorney. This principle is valid in many places of the world. However, the logistics and, whether or not the court system needs to be involved are rather jurisdiction specific.

END-OF-LIFE CARE

Neurologic diseases have been at the center of discussions on issues at the end of life. To this end, end-of-life conversations are routine between health care providers and patients suffering certain neurologic diseases. The American Academy of Neurology (AAN) has set standards for the determination of death based on neurologic criteria, prediction of outcome in comatose survivors of cardiac arrest, and for the persistent vegetative state (PVS). Additional diseases such as amyotrophic lateral sclerosis (ALS) and Alzheimer disease have been the focus of debates about physician-assisted suicide. Health care providers practicing in neuro–intensive care units (ICUs) also face end-of-life discussions when withholding or withdrawing life-sustaining therapies. Finally, presymptomatic diagnosis is available for incurable conditions like Huntington disease, creating additional ethical challenge.

INEFFECTIVE, INAPPROPRIATE, AND FUTILE THERAPIES

Health care providers may often encounter clinical situations in which therapies may found to be ineffective at achieving certain goals. Health care providers don't know whether a therapy, in a particular neurologic condition, will be effective unless the therapy is trialed. In this case, it is always better to attempt a "trial of intervention" by setting up reasonable goals of care, determining whether those goals can be achieved by ongoing reassessment, and allowing the health care provider to find if the therapy is ineffective while maintaining good communication with patient's families, friends, and surrogates. This approach would allow the health care team to withdraw an ineffective therapy rather than withhold a potentially beneficial treatment, limiting the chance for undertreatment and avoiding ethical dilemmas. Some treatments may be considered inappropriate or inadvisable. Such treatments are characterized by extremely low likelihood of achieving the intended goal, minimally or potentially beneficial but extremely expensive, and of uncertain or controversial benefit. Finally, some other treatments may be labeled as futile. There is still controversy about the medical definition of futility, but in general, futile medical interventions serve no meaningful purpose no matter how often they are repeated. Therefore, a futile medical intervention is that for which there is *de facto* knowledge that it will not accomplish its intended goal. Characteristics of a futile therapy are that the intervention has no pathophysiologic rationale, that the intervention has already failed in the patient, and that the unintended effect occurs despite maximal treatment. Futile, inappropriate, or inadvisable cases are fortunately rare but very complicated from the ethical perspective, as they bring the values of the patient, surrogates, health care providers, and the society at odds. For this reason, resolution of these conflicts requires conscientious ethical analysis and a fair process that usually involves a multidisciplinary team, and a bilateral or shared conflict resolution.

WITHHOLDING AND WITHDRAWING

When facing withholding or withdrawal of medical interventions, ethical questions can not be addressed successfully unless the probability of outcomes is entertained. To attain a balanced view of the impact of therapeutic decisions and the expected disability to the patient, the effort requires understanding of disease in question and a multidisciplinary team approach. Morally, there may be no difference between withholding and withdrawing life-sustaining therapies. However, patients, families, and health care providers have strong and divergent views. Some may feel comfortable with both situations, some may feel comfortable only when deciding not to start a therapy, but some may feel uncomfortable deciding when to stop that therapy. According to Miller and Truog, "what distinguishes withdrawing from withholding, is that in the former, the agent initiates the fatal consequence, as distinct from merely permitting it to continue without intervention to stop it." The distinction between withdrawing and withholding may cause feelings of reluctance but is morally irrelevant and can be dangerous. From the legal standpoint, the courts in the United States have upheld the concept that there is no difference between withdrawing and withholding. Both are medical decisions that entail a duty to inform the patient and his or her representative.

DEATH, DYING, AND PALLIATIVE CARE

According to the World Health Organization (WHO), health in its broader sense is defined as "a state of complete physical, mental, and social well-being and not merely the absence of disease or infirmity." Because this "state" is sometimes hard to achieve at the end of life, patients suffering terminal neurologic diseases should also have access to therapies that carry different goal in mind: the relief of pain and suffering.

Palliative care is defined by the WHO as "the active total care of patients whose disease is not responsive to curative treatment, where the control of pain, of other symptoms and of psychological, social, and spiritual problems is paramount, and where the goal is the achievement of the best quality of life for patients and their families."

In the case of Karen A. Quinlan (*in the matter of Quinlan, an alleged incompetent, 70 NJ 10, 1976*), the Supreme Court of New Jersey established the concepts that provided the framework for the development of a more patient-centered than physician-centered medical decision-making paradigm and nurtured the palliative care movement in the United States. Ms. Quinlan was a young patient that lapsed into a PVS after suffering hypoxic brain injury. A legal battle ensued between the county's prosecutor, the hospital, and the health care providers that argued that Ms. Quinlan should be kept on life support and never be allowed to die (as there was no advanced directive to guide care) and the family members (devout Catholics) that argued that Ms. Quinlan should be allowed to die with dignity based on known wishes that established that she would have never wanted to live that way. After many years of litigation, the Court finally granted the family's wishes and determined that (1) a guardian *ad litem* (appointed by court order) was not necessary to represent a patient independently in a particular case and (2) allowed family members to make decisions on the patient's behalf. The ruling was rooted on the United States Constitution's individual right to privacy, preventing the Government to prohibit treatments or the refusal of them (under certain circumstances) under the sole argument of Government's interest on preserving life. The Court granted the ability to family members to make assertions on behalf of patients using their own best judgment (see "Substituted Judgment Standard"). The Court's decision included legal immunity for the physicians and the suggestion to involve ethics committees.

A *hospice program* is often the venue for palliative care. This is sometimes carried out in a hospital or separate physical facility but is increasingly a home care program. Although most Americans express their desire to die at home, relatively few actually die there and die in hospitals or nursing homes. In a study of terminally ill patients, Pritchard et al. shown that terminally-ill patients died at teaching hospitals (56%) more often than home (25%), nursing home (9%), hospice (9%), and en route to the hospital (1%). Many factors affect how individuals die and where they die.

Nationwide, hospice care is used by only 17% of people who are dying. Reasons for the relatively low rate of hospice care include the following: (1) Physicians are uncomfortable about talking with patients about terminal events long enough in advance; (2) it may be difficult to determine precisely the expected time of death; (3) hospices emphasize home care, and family members may not be able to commit the time required or there may be no family members; and (4) financial issues. Although in the United States, a Medicare disease-related group (DRG) provides reimbursement for the care of patients who are not expected to survive for more than 6 months, many Americans, based on the lack of coverage, may still have to pay out of pocket for some of the palliative care expenses. Another drawback to the use of home or hospice care is the insensitivity of United States physicians to the advance directives of their patients, as detected by the 1995 to 2000 Study to Understand Prognoses and Preferences for Outcomes and Risks of Treatment (SUPPORT), which analyzed end-of-life care in over 3,000 hospitalized patients who died. Fifty percent of the physicians polled did not respect or did not know their patient's advance directives; most do-not-resuscitate (DNR) orders were not written until 24 hours before death; and 40% of the patients had severe pain for several days before death. In a follow-up study, an intervention to improve communication resulted in reduction in total ICU days prior to death and no increase in the proportion of patients with a DNR order, which were not written in 50% of the patients surveyed.

PRINCIPLE OF DOUBLE EFFECT

At least 43% of Americans will be admitted to nursing homes prior to death, and more than 1.5 million are currently being cared for in these establishments. According to Teno et al., nearly 15% of these patients are in pain at the time of the initial assessment and approximately 41% are in severe pain later on. Pain management is therefore an important aspect of palliation. Some actions during palliative care aimed at controlling pain are morally and ethically acceptable and may have foreseeable but unintended and undesirable outcomes; the morality of the action depends on the morality of the intended outcome, not the unintended one. Several conditions must be met: (1) The action to be carried out must be morally or ethically acceptable or at least neutral, (2) the good effect must not depend on the undesired or bad effect, and (3) the good effect must be sufficient to justify the risk of the unintended outcome. In practice, this principle makes it possible to administer sufficient analgesic and sedative medication to keep a patient comfortable even though the treatment will not prolong life. The principle of *double effect* is the basis of the hospice program (Table 153.2).

PALLIATIVE SEDATION

In certain circumstances, the burden of a neurologic disease at the end of life may be higher than expected. Certain patients may not achieve adequate relief of symptoms even with palliative care measures that usually include the titration of opioids. As defined by Broeckaert and Nunez-Olarte, "palliative sedation is the intentional administration of sedative drugs in dosages and in combinations required to reduce the consciousness of a terminal patient as much as necessary to adequately relieve one or more refractory symptoms." This is usually achieved by the use of benzodiazepines, propofol, and barbiturates. It's intended to achieve the relief of overwhelming symptoms when other conventional palliative care strategies have failed. The AMA Council on Ethical and Judicial Affairs has provided support for the use of palliative sedation at the end of life when (1) patients are in the final stages of their disease and are expected to die shortly, (2) conventional treatments have failed to control the symptoms, (3) consent has been obtained from the patient or surrogates, (4) a multidisciplinary team of experts have already assessed the patients symptoms, (5) palliative sedation will not be used to solely relief existential experiences (anxiety, depression, feelings of isolation, etc.), and (6) it will not be used to intentionally cause a patient's death.

Palliative sedation is usually reserved for the ICU environment or for units designed to fulfill that purpose. Some ethicists have argued about the difference between palliative sedation and euthanasia. The difference lies in the concept of intent and the timing of the procedure. Palliative sedation is used to achieve a control of symptoms during the process of death (last resort), when other measures have failed, and exclusively in actively dying patients.

REFUSAL OF THERAPY, PHYSICIAN-ASSISTED SUICIDE, AND EUTHANASIA

A competent patient's refusal of therapy should not be interpreted as suicidal. In 1983, the President's Commission for the Study of Ethical Problems in Medicine and Biomedical and Behavioral Research published its report entitled *Deciding to Forego Life-Sustaining Treatment*. The conclusion from the President's Commission was that decisions regarding health care, including the refusal or withdrawal of life-sustaining treatment, rest ultimately with the competent patient and exercised through the country's long tradition of procedures for informed consent. On the other hand, refusal or

TABLE 153.2 Palliative Care Protocol during Withdrawal of Life Support

Steps	Procedures
Prewithdrawal of LST	• Meet with surrogates and family to discuss withdrawal of LSTs.
	• If patient is conscious, involve him or her in the discussion.
	• Prepare to discuss other issues such as organ donation.
	• Establish a time frame and additional needs: pastoral care, etc.
	• Document plan and discussion in the chart.
	• Discuss with clinical team.
	• Review LSTs to be withdrawn (ventilator, medications[a], IV or enteral fluids, parenteral or enteral nutrition, pacemakers, IABPs, RRT, blood draws, etc).
Sedayion/analgesia	
• Lorazepam	• If any, continue current infusion if patient is comfortable, then bolus same as hourly dose. May increase by 25%–50%.
	OR
	• Begin with a bolus of 2.5–10 mg IV. May repeat boluses every 15 min as needed.
	OR
	• Begin continuous infusion at 2.5–5.0 mg/h.
• Morphine	• If any, continue current infusion if patient is comfortable, then bolus same as hourly dose for signs of distress. May increase by 25%.
	OR
	• Begin with a bolus of 10 mg IV and begin infusion at 5–7 mg/h. If discomfort, repeat boluses equal to hourly infusion dose and increase rate by 25%–50%.
• Fentanyl	• If any, continue current infusion if patient is comfortable, then bolus 25%–50% of the hourly dose and increase by 25%.
	OR
	• Begin with a bolus of 25–100 μg IV and begin infusion at 25–100 μg/h. If discomfort, repeat boluses 50% of hourly infusion dose and increase rate by 25%–50%.
Withdrawal of LST	• Adjust analgosedation to achieve no distress before withdrawal of LST (see above).
	• Reduce or eliminate alarm settings and monitors.
	• Disconnect cardiac monitors.
	• Disconnect other monitoring devices (arterial lines, ICP lines, etc.).
	• Disconnect supplemental oxygen.
	• Remove lines and enteric feeding tubes, if any.
	• Suction and control secretions if needed.
After death	• Inform family and surrogates about official time of death.
	• Allow family and staff to surround the patient.
	• Allow family to visit patient postmortem if they choose to.
	• Assist with postmortem decisions and fill-in pertinent paperwork.
	• Document a death note in the chart.

[a]Medications that can be continued to provide comfort are, for example, antiepileptics (seizures), antiemetics (rare), and skin or local oral care (glycerine creams, etc.).
LST, life-sustaining therapy; IV, intravenous; IABP, intra-aortic balloon pump; RRT, renal replacement therapy; ICP, intracranial pressure.

withdrawal of therapies by surrogates on behalf of incompetent patients that remain conscious are ethically and legally permissible as long as there are written statements or in accordance with the patient's "wishes to the extent known." In the absence of these, the decision-making process is based on the patient's best interest.

In 1994, Oregon became the only state to legalize physician-assisted suicide (PAS) when voters, through a citizen's initiative election, enacted the Oregon Death with Dignity Act (DWDA) through a 51% approval. In order to qualify for PAS in Oregon, the individual must reside in that state, be at least 18 years of age, have the ability to communicate regarding health care issues, and be diagnosed with a terminal disease with 6 months of less of life expectancy (confirmed by two independent physicians). As specified by law in the state of Oregon, it is permissible for a physician to prescribe medication to be used by a patient for the purpose of suicide. However, the physician may not actually administer the drug. Additional states that legalized PAS are Washington,

Vermont (via court ruling), and New Mexico. PAS is currently under debate in New Jersey. Although PAS is legal in these states, the United States Supreme Court has upheld criminal statutes that prohibited PAS in New York and Washington negating the constitutionality of the individual's right to PAS. However, it also negates the constitutionality of prohibiting PAS at the state level.

Neurologic diseases generate problems for PAS. Patients may be incompetent and unable to give consent. Other patients may lose the use of their hands from motor neuron diseases such as ALS. Under these circumstances, the patients themselves cannot fill the prescription and take the drug; someone else must assist them physically, which would be euthanasia and specifically banned by the Oregon and others laws. Many authorities have debated the desirability of PAS. Medical and nursing organizations have uniformly opposed legalization.

If in compliance with a patient's request a physician administers a lethal drug by injection or other means, the act is euthanasia, which is illegal in the United States. In euthanasia, the health care provider intends the death of the patient. In doing so, the health care provider selects the type of drugs and doses that are lethal by all objective measures. In the process, the health care provider administers the drug and causes unconsciousness and cardiac arrest. Only if the outcome is achieved, the health care provider can conclude that the intervention was successful. These contrast with the objective of palliative sedation and palliative care, where the intent is to relieve otherwise unmanageable symptoms (see "Principle of Double Effect").

The public, physicians, and courts have had difficulty separating refusal or discontinuation of therapy, which are legal, from assisted suicide and euthanasia, which are not. The distinction between PAS and euthanasia is the most controversial of all. The Supreme Court concluded that palliative care and palliative sedation are permissible but referred the question of PAS back to legislation by the states.

This issue was highlighted in 2002 when Veldink et al. reported experience in the Netherlands, where euthanasia is legal. Among 279 patients who died of ALS, 17% chose euthanasia and 3% died as a result of PAS. Another 24% received palliative care, "which probably shortened their lives." In an accompanying editorial and correspondence, Ganzini and Block attributed the high rates of assisted death to inadequate palliative care. However, this has been recently contended by the authors.

CONCLUSION

The issues discussed here are among the most controversial in modern life. Consensus is not easy to achieve, but views are changing and current practices are likely to change as well. Already, pain control and palliative care have come to the fore and provide effective alternatives to assisted suicide. Documenting the preventive value of palliative care is a challenge for all concerned. Legal changes may be anticipated but do not seem imminent.

SUGGESTED READINGS

Beauchamp TL, Childress JF. *Principles of Biomedical Ethics*. New York: Oxford University Press; 2009.

Bernat JL. *Ethical Practice. Ethical Issues in Neurology*. 3rd. ed. Philadelphia: Lippincott Williams & Wilkins; 2008:24–48.

Billings JA, Block SD. Slow euthanasia. *J Palliat Care*. 1996;12:21–30.

Broeckaert B. Palliative sedation, physician-assisted suicide, and euthanasia: "same, same but different"? *Am J Bioeth*. 2011;11:62–64.

Enck RE. Drug-induced terminal sedation for symptom control. *Am J Hosp Palliat Care*. 1991;8:3–5.

Enck RE. Terminal sedation. *Am J Hosp Palliat Care*. 2000;17:148–149.

Fleck LM, Hayes OW. Ethics and consent to treat issues in acute stroke therapy. *Emerg Med Clin North Am*. 2002;20:703–715, vii–viii.

Ganzini L, Block S. Physician-assisted death—a last resort? *N Engl J Med*. 2002;346:1663–1665.

Gostin LO. Deciding life and death in the courtroom. From Quinlan to Cruzan, Glucksberg, and Vacco—a brief history and analysis of constitutional protection of the "right to die". *JAMA*. 1997;278:1523–1528.

Howland J. Questions about palliative sedation: an act of mercy or mercy killing? *Ethics Medics*. 2005;30:1–2.

Kottow M. The battering of informed consent. *J Med Ethics*. 2004;30:565–569.

Kummer HB, Thompson DR. *Critical Care Ethics*. Mount Prospect, IL: Society of Critical Care Medicine; 2009.

Louw SJ, Keeble JA. Stroke medicine-ethical and legal considerations. *Age Ageing*. 2002;31(suppl 3):31–35.

Miller FG, Truog RD. Withdrawing life-sustaining therapy: allowing to die or causing death? In: Miller FG, Truog RD, eds. *Death, Dying, and Organ Transplantation*. New York: Oxford Press; 2012:1–25.

President's Commission for the Study of Ethical Problems in Medicine and Biomedical and Behavioral Research. *Deciding to Forego Life-Sustaining Treatment*. Washington, DC: Government Printing Office; 1983.

Pritchard RS, Fisher ES, Teno JM, et al. Influence of patient preferences and local health system characteristics on the place of death. SUPPORT Investigators. Study to understand prognoses and preferences for risks and outcomes of treatment. *J Am Geriatr Soc*. 1998;46:1242–1250.

Stein J. The ethics of advance directives: a rehabilitation perspective. *Am J Phys Med Rehabil*. 2003;82:152–157.

ten Have H, Welie JV. Palliative sedation versus euthanasia: an ethical assessment. *J Pain Symptom Manage*. 2014;47:123–136.

The Belmont Report: ethical principles and guidelines for the protection of human subjects of research. http://www.hhs.gov/ohrp/humansubjects/guidance/belmont.html. Accessed July 20, 2011.

Veldink JH, Wokke JH, van der Wal G, et al. Euthanasia and physician-assisted suicide among patients with amyotrophic lateral sclerosis in the Netherlands. *N Engl J Med*. 2002;346:1638–1644.

World Health Organization. *Constitution of the World Health Organization. Basic Documents*. 45th ed. Geneva, Switzerland: World Health Organization; 2006.

Index

Note: Page numbers followed by *f* indicate figure; those followed by *t* indicate table.

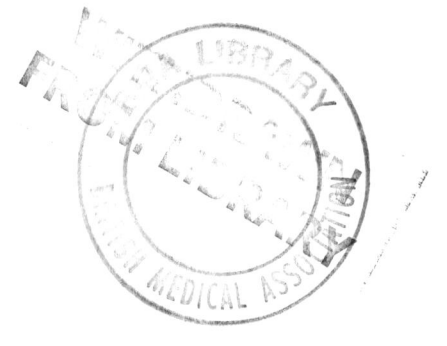